Continued

PRIMARY CARE

A COLLABORATIVE PRACTICE

PRIMARY CARE

A COLLABORATIVE PRACTICE

THIRD EDITION

TERRY MAHAN BUTTARO, MS, APRN, BC, ANP, GNP, CEN, CCRN
Clinical Assistant Professor
Simmons College, Boston, Massachusetts;
Lahey Amesbury, Amesbury, Massachusetts;
Coastal Medical Associates, Salisbury, Massachusetts;
Beth Israel Deaconess Medical Center North, Chelsea, Massachusetts

JOANN TRYBULSKI, PhD, APRN, BC, ARNP
Associate Dean for Master's Programs
University of Miami School of Nursing and Health Studies, Miami, Florida

PATRICIA POLGAR BAILEY, MS, MPH, APRN, BC, FNP, BC-ADM, CDE
Family Nurse Practitioner
The Queen's Medical Center, Honolulu, Hawaii

JOANNE SANDBERG-COOK, MS, APRN, BC ANP, GNP, BC-PCM
Adult/Gerontologic Nurse Practitioner
Dartmouth-Hitchcock Medical Center, Lebanon, New Hampshire;
Instructor in Medicine
Dartmouth Medical School, Hanover, New Hampshire

MOSBY

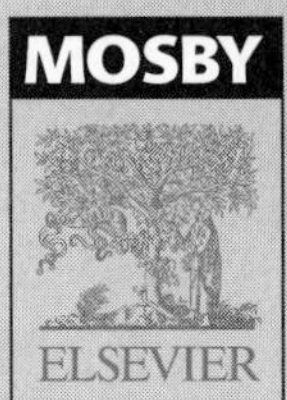

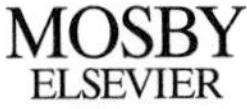

11830 Westline Industrial Drive
St. Louis, Missouri 63146

PRIMARY CARE: A COLLABORATIVE PRACTICE, ed 3 ISBN: 978-0-323-04742-5

Notice

Knowledge and best practice in this field are constantly changing. As new research and experience broaden our knowledge, changes in practice, treatment, and drug therapy may become necessary or appropriate. Readers are advised to check the most current information provided (i) on procedures featured or (ii) by the manufacturer of each product to be administered, to verify the recommended dose or formula, the method and duration of administration, and contraindications. It is the responsibility of the practitioner, relying on their own experience and knowledge of the patient, to make diagnoses, to determine dosages and the best treatment for each individual patient, and to take all appropriate safety precautions. To the fullest extent of the law, neither the Publisher nor the Editors assume any liability for any injury and/or damage to persons or property arising out or related to any use of the material contained in this book.

The Publisher

Library of Congress Control Number: 2007927357

Senior Acquisitions Editor: Sandra Clark Brown
Senior Developmental Editor: Cindi Anderson
Publishing Services Manager: Deborah L. Vogel
Senior Project Manager: Deon Lee
Senior Designer: Teresa McBryan

Printed in the United States of America

Last digit is the print number: 9 8 7 6 5 4 3 2

We would like to dedicate this book to the people most directly impacted by our involvement in this project. We are most grateful to our husbands and children, who have been endlessly patient and supportive. We would also like to thank our professional colleagues, without whose close collaboration we would not have been able to sustain the energy needed for a project of this size and scope.

CONTRIBUTORS

Marie A. Bakitas, DNSc, ARNP, FAAN
Post Doctoral Fellow
Yale University School of Nursing
New Haven, Connecticut;
Adult Nurse Practitioner, Palliative Care
Section of Palliative Medicine
Dartmouth-Hitchcock Medical Center
Lebanon, New Hampshire
Chapter 15: Palliative and End-of-Life Care

Claire Barrett, RN, MS
Program Director
Senior Living on Bellingham Hill
Chelsea, Massachusetts
Chapter 260: Bipolar Disorder

Cynthia Erskine Bashaw, APRN-BC, FNP
Assistant Professor
Regis College
Weston, Massachusetts
Chapter 20: Screening for Cancer

Jena Beach, NP, MSN
Nurse Practitioner
Merrimack Valley Nephrology
Pentucket Medical Associates
Methuen, Massachusetts
Chapter 96: Rhinitis; Chapter 97: Sinusitis

Katherine E. Beben, BA, BS, MSIII
Medical Student, Third Year
University of Connecticut School of Medicine
Farmington, Connecticut
Chapter 50: Animal and Human Bites; Chapter 209: Infections of the Central Nervous System

Kathleen M. Benedetti, MSN, RN
Clinical Assistant Professor
Department of Nursing
School for Health Studies
Simmons College
Boston, Massachusetts
Chapter 41: Syncope

Martin Jan Bergman, MD, FACR, FACP
Clinical Assistant Professor of Medicine
Drexel University College of Medicine
Media, Pennsylvania
Chapter 250: Lyme Disease

Cathy Cramer Bertram, PhD, APRN
Women's Health Nurse Practitioner
The Queen's Medical Center
Honolulu, Hawaii
Chapter 176: Pap Smear Abnormalities

Wendy L. Biddle, PhD, CFNP
Nurse Practitioner
Digestive and Liver Disease Specialists
Norfolk, Virginia
Chapter 144: Hepatitis; Chapter 145: Inflammatory Bowel Disease

Rosemary Bill-Fleury, MSN, ANP, CDE
Nurse Practitioner
Department of Internal Medicine and Cardiology
North Suburban Cardiology
Stoneham, Massachusetts
Chapter 218: Diabetes Mellitus

Margaret Firer Bishop, MS, ARNP
Adult Nurse Practitioner, Palliative Care
Section of Palliative Medicine
Dartmouth-Hitchcock Medical Center
Lebanon, New Hampshire
Chapter 15: Palliative and End-of-Life Care

Maureen B. Boardman, MSN, FNP, BC
Little Rivers Health Care
Bradford, Vermont
Department of Community and Family Medicine
Dartmouth College
Hanover, New Hampshire
Chapter 111: Chronic Obstructive Pulmonary Disease

Alice Bolton, ARNP, MS, CS, BC
Private Practice
Psych-Mental Health
Sarasota, Florida
Chapter 263: Grief; Chapter 266: Somatization Disorder

Nancy D. Bolton, RN, MSN, ANP, CCRC
Director of Clinical Research
Charlottesville Medical Research
Charlottesville, Virginia
Chapter 142: Gastroesophageal Reflux Disease

Christine A. Boodley, RN, PhD, FNP, FAANP
Associate Professor
Master's Program; School of Nursing
University of Texas Medical Branch School of Nursing
Galveston, Texas
Chapter 89: Inner Ear Disturbances; Chapter 90: Otitis Externa; Chapter 91: Otitis Media

Karen Borden, NP
Nurse Practitioner
Gillette Center for Gynecologic Oncology
Massachusetts General Hospital Cancer Center
Boston, Massachusetts
Chapter 253: Basic Principles of Oncology Treatment

Marie Elena Botte, APRN-BC, CDE
Family Nurse Practitioner
Certified Diabetes Educator
The Lowell Diabetes & Endocrine Center
Lowell, Massachusetts
Chapter 165: Amenorrhea; Chapter 166: Bartholin's Gland Cysts and Abscesses; Chapter 170: Dyspareunia; Chapter 171: Ectopic Pregnancy; Chapter 174: Infertility

Sharon M. Bouvier, RN, MS
Nursing Director, Vascular Surgery
Massachusetts General Hospital
Boston, Massachusetts
Chapter 125: Carotid Artery Disease

Jennifer C. Braimon, MD
Staff Endocrinologist
Department of Endocrinology and Metabolism
Lahey Clinic
Peabody, Massachusetts
Chapter 225: Thyroid Disorders

Christell O. Bray, RN, FNP, PhD, FAANP
Associate Professor
Texas A&M University—Corpus Christi
Corpus Christi, Texas
Chapter 85: Auricular Disorders; Chapter 86: Cerumen Impaction; Chapter 87: Cholesteatoma

Lin A. J. Brown, MD
Associate Professor of Medicine
Dartmouth Medical School Program Director
Rheumatology Fellowship Program and Staff Rheumatologist
Dartmouth-Hitchcock Medical Center
Lebanon, New Hampshire
Chapter 186: Fibromyalgia and Myofascial Pain Syndrome; Chapter 234: Raynaud's Phenomenon

Ann S. Bruner-Welch, PA-C
Physician Assistant, Surgical 1st Assistant
Department of Orthopedics
Kaiser Permanente
Santa Rosa, California
Chapter 189: Hip Pain; Chapter 194: Osteoarthritis

Terry Mahan Buttaro, MS, APRN, BC, ANP, GNP, CEN, CCRN
Clinical Assistant Professor
Simmons College
Boston, Massachusetts;
Lahey Amesbury
Amesbury, Massachusetts;
Coastal Medical Associates
Salisbury, Massachusetts;
Beth Israel Deaconess Medical Center North
Chelsea, Massachusetts
Chapter 1: Collaborative Practice; Chapter 4: The Provider-Patient Relationship; Chapter 28: Preparticipation Sports Physical; Chapter 31: Anaphylaxis; Chapter 32: Bites and Stings; Chapter 33: Bradycardia; Chapter 34: Cardiac Arrest; Chapter 36: Electrical Injuries; Chapter 37: Head Trauma; Chapter 39: Poisoning; Chapter 42: Tachycardia; Chapter 134: Valvular Heart Disease and Cardiac Murmurs; Chapter 135: Abdominal Pain and Infections; Chapter 136: Anorectal Complaints; Chapter 138: Cirrhosis; Chapter 139: Constipation; Chapter 221: Hypernatremia and Hyponatremia

Cindy Campbell, ANP, ND, BC
Advanced Nurse Practitioner
Behavioural Health
Alaska Native Primary Care Center
Anchorage, Alaska
Chapter 265: Psychotic Disorders; Chapter 266: Somatization Disorder

David R. Campbell, MD
Associate Clinical Professor, Surgery
Harvard Medical School
Department of Vascular Surgery
Beth Israel Deaconess Medical Center
Boston, Massachusetts
Chapter 131: Peripheral Arterial Insufficiency; Chapter 133: Peripheral Venous Insufficiency

Virginia Capasso, PhD, APRN, BC
Co-Director, Nurse Practitioner, Wound Care Center
Nurse Scientist
Munn Center for Nursing Research
Massachusetts General Hospital
Boston, Massachusetts
Chapter 125: Carotid Artery Disease

Catherine E. Carter, RN, MSN, FNP-C
Family Nurse Practitioner
PhyAmerica, Government Services, Inc.
Oak Harbor, Washington
Chapter 57: Dry Skin; Chapter 67: Psoriasis

Joanne N. Casaletto, MSN, MSPH, APRN, WHNP, COHN
Nurse Practitioner
Harvard University Health Service
Cambridge, Massachusetts
Chapter 193: Neck Pain

Emily Chandler, PhD, MDiv, APRN, BC
Consultant
Private Practice
Rockport, Massachusetts
Chapter 14: Psychosociospiritual Issues

Debra Connolly, NP
Nurse Practitioner
Gillette Center for Gynecologic Oncology
Massachusetts General Hospital Cancer Center
Boston, Massachusetts
Chapter 253: Basic Principles of Oncology Treatment

Margaret Costello, RNCS, MHA, MSN
Instructor
Simmons College
Boston, Massachusetts
Chapter 143: Gastrointestinal Hemorrhage; Chapter 150: Pancreatitis

Erin Cox, MS, APRN-BC, CCRN
Clinical Nurse Specialist, Vascular Surgery
Massachusetts General Hospital
Boston, Massachusetts
Chapter 125: Carotid Artery Disease

Kathleen M. Craig, RNc, BSN, IBCLC
Staff Nurse, Lactation Consultant
Birthing Pavilion
Dartmouth-Hitchcock Medical Center
Lebanon, New Hampshire
Chapter 12: Lactation

Constance Dahlin, MSN, APRN, BC, PCM
Nurse Practitioner; Clinical Nurse Specialist
Palliative Care Service
Massachusetts General Hospital
Boston, Massachusetts
Chapter 15: Palliative and End-of-Life Care; Chapter 16: Chronic Pain

Terry Davies, MSN, RNAP-BC
Associate Clinical Faculty
Simmons College
Advanced Practice Nurse
Urgent Care/Emergency Department
Boston Medical Center
Boston, Massachusetts
Chapter 140: Diarrhea, Noninfectious; Chapter 148: Nausea and Vomiting; Chapter 249: Infectious Diarrhea

Henry DeGroot III, MD
Private Practice
Orthopedic Surgery
Newton, Massachusetts
Chapter 183: Bone Tumors

Eileen M. Deignan, MD
Concord, Massachusetts
Chapter 45: Surgical Office Procedures; Chapter 48: Acne Vulgaris; Chapter 49: Alopecia; Chapter 51: Burns (Minor); Chapter 52: Cellulitis; Chapter 53: Contact Dermatitis; Chapter 58: Eczematous Dermatitis (Atopic Dermatitis); Chapter 59: Fungal Infections (Superficial); Chapter 60: Herpes Zoster (Shingles); Chapter 69: Scabies; Chapter 70: Seborrheic Dermatitis; Chapter 73: Warts

Karen Dick, PhD, APRN-BC, FAANP
Graduate Program Director and Coordinator
Adult/Gerontologic Nurse Practitioner Program
University of Massachusetts Boston
Boston, Massachusetts
Chapter 204: Delirium; Chapter 205: Dementia

Karin C. Dieselman, MS, RNCS, ANP
Adult Nurse Practitioner
Department of Occupational Health
Anna Jaques Hospital
Newburyport, Massachusetts
Chapter 30: Altitude Illness; Chapter 188: Hand and Wrist Pain

Susan DiMattia, RN, NP
Cardiology Nurse Practitioner
Massachusetts General Hospital
Boston, Massachusetts
Chapter 124: Cardiac Arrhythmias

Wendye DiSalvo, MSN, ARNP, AOCN®
Advanced Registered Nurse Practitioner
Department of Thoracic Oncology
Norris Cotton Cancer Center
Dartmouth-Hitchcock Medical Center
Lebanon, New Hampshire
Chapter 114: Lung Cancer

Zita Dubauskas, PA-C
Physician Assistant
Department of Genitourinary Medical Oncology
The University of Texas MD Anderson Cancer Center
Houston, Texas
Chapter 257: Oncology Complications and Paraneoplastic Syndromes

Heather Elias, MD
Medical Resident
Department of Internal Medicine
Lahey Clinic
Burlington, Massachusetts
Chapter 225: Thyroid Disorders

Walter Elias, III, MD
Head, Clinical/Business Operations
Naval Healthcare Support Office San Diego
San Diego, California
Chapter 35: Chemical Exposure; Chapter 47: Screening for Skin Cancer

Nancy Evans, BS, PT
Director of Rehabilitation
Kendal at Hanover
Hanover, New Hampshire
Chapter 200: Stretch Exercises

Kathy J. Fabiszewski, PhD, RN, CS
Nurse Practitioner
Harvard Vanguard Medical Associates
Peabody, Massachusetts;
Assistant Professor
College of Nursing
Division of Corporate, Continuing, and Distance Education
University of Massachusetts Boston
Boston, Massachusetts
Chapter 198: Shoulder Pain

Julie P. Fago, MD
Associate Professor of Medicine and Community and Family Medicine
Department of Internal Medicine
Dartmouth-Hitchcock Medical Center
Lebanon, New Hampshire
Chapter 197: Paget's Disease of the Bone

Mary E. Farrell, RN, PhD, CCRN
Professor and Chairperson
School of Nursing
Salem State College
Salem, Massachusetts
Chapter 199: Sprains, Strains, and Fractures

Patricia Fergus, RN, RRT
Department of Pulmonary Rehabilitation/Respiratory Care
St. John's Mercy Medical Center
St. Louis, Missouri
Chapter 24: Lifestyle Assessment

Michele DuBois Finnell, MSN
Nurse Practitioner
Department of Rheumatology
Beth Israel Deaconess Medical Center
Boston, Massachusetts
Chapter 192: Low Back Pain

Jane Flanagan, PhD, APRN, BC
Assistant Professor
Connell School of Nursing
Boston College
Chestnut Hill, Massachusetts
Chapter 27: Presurgical Clearance

Laurie L. Flanagan, MSN, RN
Doctoral Student
William F. Connell School of Nursing
Boston College
Chestnut Hill, Massachusetts
Chapter 262: Eating Disorders

Debra Fournier, MSN, ARNP, BC
Adult Nurse Practitioner and Psychiatric Nurse Practitioner
Department of Physical Medicine and Rehabilitation
Dartmouth-Hitchcock Medical Center
Lebanon, New Hampshire
Chapter 261: Depressive Disorders; Chapter 264: Posttraumatic Stress Disorder

Michelle Freshman, MPH, MSN, APRN, BC, MSCN
Nurse Practitioner
Department of Medicine
Newton-Wellesley Hospital
Newton, Massachusetts
Chapter 219: Hirsutism; Chapter 239: Fatigue; Chapter 241: Lymphadenopathy; Chapter 242: Weight Loss

Elizabeth Friedlander, PhD, APRN, BC
Division of Gastroenterology
Beth Israel Deaconess Medical Center
Boston, Massachusetts
Chapter 146: Irritable Bowel Syndrome

Denise DeJoseph Gauthier, MS, RN, CS
Acute Care Nurse Practitioner
Cardiology Division
Massachusetts General Hospital
Boston, Massachusetts
Chapter 127: Infective Endocarditis

Kelli Gershon, APRN, PCM-BC
Advanced Practice Nurse
Department of Palliative Care
The University of Texas MD Anderson Cancer Center
Houston, Texas
Chapter 256: Management of Cancer Pain

Maryjane Giacalone, MS, ANP, ACNP-CS
Department of Cardiology
Massachusetts General Hospital
Boston, Massachusetts
Chapter 129: Hypertension

Karen Gilbert, MS, ARNP, CNRN
Nurse Practitioner/Coordinator
Dartmouth Epilepsy Program
Dartmouth-Hitchcock Medical Center
Lebanon, New Hampshire
Chapter 213: Seizure Disorder

Patricia Gillett, RN, MSN, FNP-BC, ACNP-BC
Acute Care Nurse Practitioner Concentration Coordinator
College of Nursing
University of New Mexico
Albuquerque, New Mexico
Chapter 75: Evaluation of the Eyes; Chapter 76: Cataracts; Chapter 77: Chalazion, Hordeolum, and Blepharitis; Chapter 78: Conjunctivitis; Chapter 79: Corneal Surface Defects and Ocular Surface Foreign Bodies; Chapter 80: Dry Eye Syndrome; Chapter 81: Nasolacrimal Duct Obstruction and Dacryocystitis; Chapter 82: Orbital and Periorbital Cellulitis; Chapter 83: Pingueculum and Pterygium; Chapter 84: Traumatic Ocular Disorders

Donna M. Glynn, MS, APRN, BC
Adult Nurse Practitioner
Compass Medical
Brockton, Massachusetts
Chapter 152: Ulcer Disease

Kate Goldblum, MSN, NP, CRNO
Nurse Practitioner
Goldblum Family Eye Care
Albuquerque, New Mexico
Chapter 75: Evaluation of the Eyes; Chapter 76: Cataracts; Chapter 77: Chalazion, Hordeolum, and Blepharitis; Chapter 78: Conjunctivitis; Chapter 79: Corneal Surface Defects and Ocular Surface Foreign Bodies; Chapter 80: Dry Eye Syndrome; Chapter 81: Nasolacrimal Duct Obstruction and Dacryocystitis; Chapter 82: Orbital and Periorbital Cellulitis; Chapter 83: Pingueculum and Pterygium; Chapter 84: Traumatic Ocular Disorders

Deanna Gordon, RN, PhD, MPH
Professor and Director
Traditional Undergraduate Program
School of Nursing
Capital University
Columbus, Ohio
Chapter 24: Lifestyle Assessment

John Joseph Graykoski, PA-C, MPAS
Physician Assistant, Emergency Department
Luther Middlefort, Northland, Mayo Health Systems
Barron, Wisconsin
Chapter 203: Cerebrovascular Events; Chapter 229: Lymphomas

Marilyn Bleiler Green, MS, APRN, BC, AE-C
Adult Nurse Practitioner
Granite Medical
Quincy, Massachusetts
Chapter 21: Screening for Sexually Transmitted Diseases; Chapter 156: Infectious Processes: Urinary Tract Infections and Sexually Transmitted Diseases

Glen P. Greenough, MD
Assistant Professor of Medicine (Neurology) and Psychiatry (Sleep Medicine)
Director, Fellowship in Sleep Medicine
Dartmouth-Hitchcock Medical Center
Lebanon, New Hampshire
Chapter 19: Sleep Disorders

Brenda Hage, PhD(c), CRNP, APRN, BC
Assistant Professor, Nursing
Coordinator, Health Care Informatics Program
College Misericordia
Dallas, Pennsylvania
Chapter 9: Health Literacy; Chapter 18: Rehabilitation

Rosemary F. Hall, PhD, RN
Associate Professor of Nursing
University of Miami School of Nursing and Health Studies
Coral Gables, Florida
Chapter 6: Population-Based Health Care and the Role of the Advanced Practice Nurse; Chapter 7: Chronic Disease Management Teams

Tara Jayne Hamilton, MD
Fellow, Endocrinology, Diabetes, and Metabolism
Boston Medical Center
Boston, Massachusetts
Chapter 224: Parathyroid Gland Disorders

Simon M. Helfgott, MD
Associate Professor of Medicine
Harvard Medical School
Boston, Massachusetts
Chapter 237: Vasculitis

Debra Hobbins, MSN, APRN, NP
Nurse Practitioner
Discovery House/Intermountain Healthcare
Salt Lake City, Utah
Chapter 11: Pregnancy; Chapter 132: Peripheral Edema; Chapter 178: Preconception Care

Susan Hoch, MD
Chief
Division of Rheumatology
Crozer-Chester Medical Center
Drexel University College of Medicine
Upland, Pennsylvania
Chapter 232: Ankylosing Spondylitis and Related Disorders; Chapter 233: Polymyalgia Rheumatica and Temporal Arteritis

Todd Douglas Hultman, PhD, APRN, ACHPN
Assistant Professor of Nursing
University of Massachusetts Lowell
Lowell, Massachusetts
Chapter 14: Psychosociospiritual Issues

Eric M. Isselbacher, MD
Associate Professor of Medicine
Harvard Medical School
Associate Director
Massachusetts General Hospital Heart Center
Boston, Massachusetts
Chapter 127: Infective Endocarditis

Dorothy Johnson, DNSc
Nurse Practitioner
Department of Internal Medicine, Rheumatology
Los Angeles County and University of Southern California, Los Angeles, Medical Center
Los Angeles, California
Chapter 235: Rheumatoid Arthritis; Chapter 236: Systemic Lupus Erythematosus

Brenda L. Jordan, MS
Nurse Practitioner and Clinical Instructor
Dartmouth-Hitchcock-Kendal
Dartmouth Medical School
Dartmouth-Hitchcock Medical Center
Lebanon, New Hampshire
Chapter 212: Parkinson's Disease

Brooke G. Judd, MD
Assistant Professor of Psychiatry and Medicine
Dartmouth Medical School
Lebanon, New Hampshire
Chapter 19. Sleep Disorders

Alexander J. Kallen, MD, MPH
Staff Physician
Department of Internal Medicine
VA Medical Center
White River Junction, Vermont;
Instructor, Internal Medicine
Dartmouth Medical School
Lebanon, New Hampshire
Chapter 195: Osteomyelitis

Kevin D. Kerin, MD
Section of Rheumatology
VA Medical Center
White River Junction, Vermont
Chapter 190: Infectious Arthritis

Nancy W. Knee, MS, ARNP
Family Nurse Practitioner
Concord Family Medicine
Concord, New Hampshire;
Dartmouth-Hitchcock Medical Center
Lebanon, New Hampshire
Chapter 56: Dermatitis Medicamentosa; Chapter 63: Intertrigo; Chapter 64: Nail Disorders; Chapter 71: Stasis Dermatitis

Janelle Koo, MPA, DCSW, LCSW, CSAC
Service Area Administrator
Department of Health
Adult Mental Health Division
Kauai, Hawaii
Chapter 24: Lifestyle Assessment; Chapter 40: Sexual Assault

Patricia A. Lamb, RN, MN, CNS, CRNO
President/Owner
Opthalmic Nursing Care of Arizona, Inc.
Phoenix, Arizona
Chapter 75: Evaluation of the Eyes

Cheryl A. Cahill Lawrence, PhD, RN
Amelia Peabody Professor of Nursing
Massachusetts General Hospital Institute of Health Professions
Boston, Massachusetts
Chapter 2: Collaboration in Research: The Partnership Between Clinicians and Academic Clinical Researchers; Chapter 3: Weighing the Evidence for Clinical Practice

Nancy McQueen Le, RNC, MS, GNP, CNRN
Nurse Practitioner, Neurology
Department of Neurology
Boston University
Boston, Massachusetts;
Braintree Rehabilitation Hospital
Braintree, Massachusetts
Chapter 206: Dizziness and Vertigo; Chapter 210: Movement Disorders and Essential Tremor; Chapter 211: Multiple Sclerosis

Noreen M. Leahy, MS, RN
Nurse Practitioner
Department of Patient Care Services
Massachusetts General Hospital
Boston, Massachusetts
Chapter 201: Amyotrophic Lateral Sclerosis; Chapter 202: Bell's Palsy; Chapter 214: Trigeminal Neuralgia

Kelley Hamill Lemay, MSN, ARNP
Urology Nurse Practitioner
Female Urology and Voiding Dysfunction
Section of Urology, Department of Surgery
Dartmouth-Hitchcock Medical Center
Lebanon, New Hampshire
Chapter 155: Incontinence; Chapter 157: Obstructive Uropathy

Renato Lenzi, MD
Clinical Associate Professor
Gastrointestinal Medical Oncology
The University of Texas MD Anderson Cancer Center
Houston, Texas
Chapter 254: Unknown Primary Carcinoma

V. Ted Leon, MD, MPH
Travel Clinic
The Queen's Medical Center
Honolulu, Hawaii
Chapter 26: Health Care of the International Traveler

Jane Leonard, RN, MSN, FNP
Assistant Professor
School of Nursing
University of Texas Medical Branch
Galveston, Texas
Chapter 88: Impaired Hearing; Chapter 92: Tympanic Membrane Perforation

Katherine Griffis Low, RN, MS, ARNP, AOCN®
Nurse Practitioner
Malignant Hematology Program
H. Lee Moffitt Cancer Center and Research Institute
University of South Florida
Tampa, Florida
Chapter 226: Anemia

Alan Ona Malabanan, MD
Physician
Beth Israel Deaconess Medical Center
Boston, Massachusetts
Chapter 196: Osteoporosis; Chapter 216: Acromegaly; Chapter 220: Hypercalcemia and Hypocalcemia; Chapter 224: Parathyroid Gland Disorders

Maura Malone, MSN, RN
Clinical Nurse Specialist, Hemophilia and Thrombophilia
Dartmouth-Hitchcock Medical Center
Lebanon, New Hampshire
Chapter 227: Blood Coagulation Disorders

Bryan J. Marsh, MD
Associate Professor of Medicine
Acting Chief, Section of Infectious Disease and International Health
Dartmouth-Hitchcock Medical Center
Lebanon, New Hampshire
Chapter 246: HIV Infection

Margaret McAllister, PhD, FNP-C, FAANP
Director
Post-Master's Certificate Program
College of Nursing and Health Sciences
University of Massachusetts, Boston
Boston, Massachusetts
Chapter 44: Examination of the Skin and Approach to Diagnosing Skin Disorders; Chapter 54: Corns and Calluses; Chapter 61: Hidradenitis Suppurativa (Acne Inversa); Chapter 62: Hyperhidrosis; Chapter 65: Pigmentation Changes (Vitiligo)

Kathleen Golden McAndrew, MSN, APRN, BC, ANP, COHN-S, CCM, FAAOHN, FAANP
Assistant Vice Chancellor, Student Affairs
Executive Director, University Health Services
University of Massachusetts, Boston
Boston, Massachusetts
Chapter 22: Principles of Occupational and Environmental Health in Primary Care

Talli McCormick, MSN, GNP
Clinical Assistant Professor
Graduate Program in Nursing
Massachusetts General Hospital Institute of Health Professions
Boston, Massachusetts
Chapter 149: Oropharyngeal Dysphagia

Dennis M. McCullough, MD
Associate Professor
Department of Community and Family Medicine
Dartmouth Medical Center
Hanover, New Hampshire
Chapter 217: Adrenal Gland Disorders

Matthew Stiles McDonald, MD
Clinical Fellow
Section of Allergy and Clinical Immunology
Yale University School of Medicine
New Haven, Connecticut
Chapter 240: Immunodeficiency

Eran D. Metzger, MD
Associate Director of Psychiatry
Hebrew Senior Life
Boston, Massachusetts
Chapter 262: Eating Disorders

Louise P. Meyer, MS, ARNP, AOCN®
Nurse Practitioner
Department of Hematology/Oncology
Dartmouth-Hitchcock Medical Center
Lebanon, New Hampshire
Chapter 141: Diverticular Disease; Chapter 147: Jaundice; Chapter 151: Tumors of the Gastrointestinal Tract

Cheryl A. Miller, MSN, APRN, GNP
Gerontologic Nurse Practitioner
Long Term Care of Virginia
Norfolk, Virginia
Chapter 25: Immunizations

Catharine Moffett, RN, MSN, APRN, FNP
Director, Student Health Services
Connecticut College
New London, Connecticut
Chapter 23: College Health

H. A. Morcos, MD, PhD
Chair of Pharmacology
American University of Antigua
College of Medicine
St. John's, Antigua, West Indies
Chapter 130: Myocarditis

Debra S. Munsell, MPAS, PA-C
Assistant Professor, Clinical Specialist
Physician Assistant Studies
Department of Otolaryngology
University of Texas Medical Branch—Galveston
Galveston, Texas
Chapter 100: Dental Abscess; Chapter 101: Diseases of the Salivary Glands; Chapter 102: Epiglottitis; Chapter 103: Oral Infections; Chapter 104: Parotitis; Chapter 105: Peritonsillar Abscess; Chapter 106: Pharyngitis and Tonsillitis

David Patrick Murphy, MD, FCCP
Director of Medical Services
Head, Pulmonary/Critical Care Medicine
US Naval Hospital
Okinawa, Japan
Chapter 112: Dyspnea

Jennifer A. Neves, APRN, BC
Nurse Practitioner
Preadmission Clinic
Massachusetts General Hospital
Boston, Massachusetts
Chapter 27: Presurgical Clearance

Patrice K. Nicholas, DNSc, MPH, APRN-BC
Director of Global Health and Academic Partnerships
Brigham and Women's Hospital
Professor, Graduate Program in Nursing
Massachusetts General Hospital Institute of Health Professions
Boston, Massachusetts
Chapter 93: Chronic Nasal Congestion and Discharge; Chapter 94: Epistaxis; Chapter 95: Nasal Trauma; Chapter 98: Smell and Taste Disturbances; Chapter 99: Tumors and Polyps of the Nose

Janice D. Nunnelee, PhD, RN, ANP-BC, CVN
Professor
Chamberlain College of Nursing
St. Louis, Missouri
Chapter 123: Abdominal Aortic Aneurysm

Karen Koozer Olson, RN, FNP, PhD, FAANP
Professor of Nursing
College of Nursing and Health Professions
Texas A & M University—Corpus Christi
Corpus Christi, Texas
Chapter 85: Auricular Disorders; Chapter 86: Cerumen Impaction; Chapter 90: Otitis Externa; Chapter 91: Otitis Media

Daniel W. O'Neill, MD
Associate Professor of Family Medicine
University of Connecticut
Farmington, Connecticut
St. Luke's Family Practice
Putnam, Connecticut
Chapter 50: Animal and Human Bites; Chapter 66: Pruritus; Chapter 209: Infections of the Central Nervous System

Marie-Eileen Onieal, PhD, MMHS, RN, CPNP, FAANP
Revere, Massachusetts
Chapter 182: Ankle and Foot Pain; Chapter 191: Knee Pain

Angela Patterson, MS, APRN, BC
Co-owner and Clinical Director
Atreva Health Care
Adjunct Instructor
School for Health Studies
Simmons College
Boston, Massachusetts
Chapter 8: Reimbursement for Nurse Practitioner Services

Donna Jenell Pease, MSN, ANP/GNP, CDE, BC-ADM
Diabetes Nurse Practitioner
Adult Medicine Clinic
Tripler Army Medical Center
Honolulu, Hawaii
Chapter 223: Metabolic Syndrome

Joanne Marie Petrelli, RN, MSN, CRNP-Adult, LCDR, NC, USN
Department of Internal Medicine
Naval Medical Center San Diego
San Diego, California
Chapter 55: Cutaneous Herpes

Timothy J. Phillips, MD
Senior Medical Officer
Branch Medical Clinic
Marine Corps Air Station (MCAS) Yuma
Yuma, Arizona
Chapter 43: Thermal Injuries

Patricia Polgar Bailey, MS, MPH, APRN, BC, FNP, BC-ADM, CDE
Family Nurse Practitioner
The Queen's Medical Center
Honolulu, Hawaii
Chapter 107: Acute Bronchitis; Chapter 108: Asthma; Chapter 109: Chest Pain (Noncardiac); Chapter 110: Chronic Cough; Chapter 113: Hemoptysis; Chapter 115: Occupational Respiratory Disease; Chapter 116: Pleural Effusions; Chapter 117: Pleurisy; Chapter 153: Male Sexual Dysfunction; Chapter 156: Infectious Processes: Urinary Tract Infections and Sexually Transmitted Diseases; Chapter 158: Renal Disease and Pregnancy; Chapter 162: Testicular Disorders; Chapter 167: Breast Disorders; Chapter 169: Dysmenorrhea; Chapter 172: Fertility Control; Chapter 173: Genital Tract Cancers; Chapter 177: Pelvic Inflammatory Disease; Chapter 179: Sexual Dysfunction, Female; Chapter 180: Unplanned Pregnancy; Chapter 181: Vulvar and Vaginal Disorders; Chapter 245: Tuberculosis; Chapter 248: Infectious Mononucleosis

JoNell Efantis Potter, PhD, RN, ARNP
Associate Professor of Clinical Obstetrics and Gynecology
Director of Division of Research and Special Projects
Department of Obstetrics and Gynecology
University of Miami Miller School of Medicine
Miami, Florida
Chapter 175: Menopause

Joyce Powers, RN, MSN, ACNP, FNP
Nurse Practitioner
Department of Cardiology
Veterans Administration
Albuquerque, New Mexico
Chapter 75: Evaluation of the Eyes; Chapter 76: Cataracts; Chapter 77: Chalazion, Hordeolum, and Blepharitis; Chapter 78: Conjunctivitis; Chapter 79: Corneal Surface Defects and Ocular Surface Foreign Bodies; Chapter 80: Dry Eye Syndrome; Chapter 81: Nasolacrimal Duct Obstruction and Dacryocystitis; Chapter 82: Orbital and Periorbital Cellulitis; Chapter 83: Pingueculum and Pterygium; Chapter 84: Traumatic Ocular Disorders

William R. Prebola, Jr., MD
Northeastern Rehabilitation Associates
John Heinz Institute of Rehabilitation
Wilkes-Barre, Pennsylvania
Chapter 18: Rehabilitation

Judy Ptak, RN, MSN
Infection Prevention Practitioner
Collaborative Healthcare-Associated Infection Prevention Program
Dartmouth-Hitchcock Medical Center
Lebanon, New Hampshire
Chapter 247: Influenza

Francisco P. Quismorio, Jr., MD, MACP, FACP
Professor of Medicine and Pathology
Vice Chief, Division of Rheumatology and Clinical Immunology
Keck School of Medicine
University of Southern California
Los Angeles, California
Chapter 235: Rheumatoid Arthritis; Chapter 236: Systemic Lupus Erythematosus

Joseph Rampulla, MS, APRN
Nurse Practitioner
Boston Health Care for the Homeless Program
Medical Walk-in Unit
Massachusetts General Hospital
Boston, Massachusetts
Chapter 258: Alcohol Abuse; Chapter 267: Substance Abuse

Roberta N. Regan, APRN, BC
Adult Nurse Practitioner
Evercare, Nova Psychiatric Services
Waltham, Massachusetts
Chapter 128: Heart Failure

Elvi N. Rigby, MS, RN
Nurse Administrator
Patient Care Services
Brigham and Women's Hospital
Boston, Massachusetts
Chapter 93: Chronic Nasal Congestion and Discharge; Chapter 94: Epistaxis; Chapter 95: Nasal Trauma; Chapter 98: Smell and Taste Disturbances; Chapter 99: Tumors and Polyps of the Nose

Joanne Sandberg-Cook, MS, APRN, BC ANP, GNP, BC-PCM
Adult/Gerontologic Nurse Practitioner
Dartmouth-Hitchcock Medical Center
Lebanon, New Hampshire;
Instructor in Medicine
Dartmouth Medical School
Hanover, New Hampshire
Chapter 13: Aging and Common Geriatric Syndromes; Chapter 68: Purpura; Chapter 121: Sarcoidosis; Chapter 200: Stretch Exercises; Chapter 207: Guillain-Barré; Chapter 215: Tumors of the Brain; Chapter 238: Barotrauma and Other Diving Injuries; Chapter 249: Infectious Diarrhea

Michael J. Sateia, MD
Professor of Psychiatry
Chief, Section of Sleep Medicine
Dartmouth Medical School
Lebanon, New Hampshire
Chapter 19: Sleep Disorders

Anna D. Schaal, RN, BSN, MS
Advanced Practice Nurse, Nurse Practitioner
Department of Hematology/Oncology
Norris Cotton Cancer Center at Dartmouth-Hitchcock Medical Center
Lebanon, New Hampshire
Chapter 230: Myelodysplastic Syndromes

Naomi Schlesinger, MD
Associate Professor of Medicine
Director, Clinical Rheumatology
Robert Wood Johnson Medical School
University of Medicine and Dentistry of New Jersey
New Brunswick, New Jersey
Chapter 187: Gout

Willadene "Billie" Walker Schmucker, ARNP, CS, BC, MS, MAEd, PhD
Owner, Nurse Practitioner
The Alternative
Faculty
University of Phoenix
Sarasota, Florida
Chapter 259: Anxiety Disorders; Chapter 266: Somatization Disorder

Elizabeth C. Sensenig, MSN, ARNP
Nurse Practitioner, Clinical Instructor
Obstetrics and Gynecology
Department of Reproductive Endocrinology and Infertility
Dartmouth-Hitchcock Medical Center
Lebanon, New Hampshire
Chapter 168: Chronic Pelvic Pain

Scott W. Shiffer, MSN, FNP-C
Department of Family Practice
Naval Branch Health Clinic
Milton, Florida
Chapter 137: Cholelithiasis and Cholecystitis; Chapter 184: Bursitis

Robert H. Shmerling, MD
Associate Physician, Department of Medicine
Clinical Chief, Division of Rheumatology
Beth Israel Deaconess Medical Center
Associate Professor of Medicine
Harvard Medical School
Boston, Massachusetts
Chapter 231: Common Diagnostics in Rheumatologic Disorders

Jeanne H. Siegel, PhD(c), ARNP, BC
Research Project Director
Nursing School
University of Miami
Coral Gables, Florida
Chapter 17: Obesity

Joanna D. Sikkema, MSN, APRN-BC, FAHA
Clinical Faculty
University of Miami
Miami, Florida
Chapter 122: Cardiac Diagnostic Testing: Noninvasive Assessment of Coronary Artery Disease; Chapter 126: Chest Pain and Coronary Artery Disease

Trudi Simon, MSN, ARNP
Women's Health Nurse Practitioner
Department of Obstetrics and Gynecology
University of Miami
Miami, Florida
Chapter 175: Menopause

Cathy J. Sizer, MS, RN, CPNP
Certified Pediatric Nurse Practitioner
Salerno Pediatric Care
Hilton Head Island, South Carolina
Chapter 10: Adolescent Issues

Laura Stempkowski, MS, CUNP, AOCN®
Nurse Practitioner, Genitourinary Oncology
Department of Urology
Dartmouth-Hitchcock Medical Center
Lebanon, New Hampshire
Chapter 153: Male Sexual Dysfunction; Chapter 163: Tumors of the Genitourinary Tract (Kidneys, Ureters, Bladder)

Robbyn K. Takeuchi, MSW
Case Management and Support Services Director
Adult Mental Health Division
State of Hawaii, Department of Health
Honolulu, Hawaii
Chapter 24: Lifestyle Assessment; Chapter 40: Sexual Assault

Elizabeth A. Talbot, MD
Assistant Professor of Medicine
Infectious Disease and International Health Section
Dartmouth Medical School
Dartmouth-Hitchcock Medical Center
Lebanon, New Hampshire
Chapter 244: Fever

Thomas H. Taylor, MD
Chief, Infectious Diseases and Rheumatology
Department of Medicine
White River Junction VA Hospital
White River Junction, Vermont
Chapter 195: Osteomyelitis; Chapter 243: Emerging and Reemerging Infectious Diseases; Chapter 249: Infectious Diarrhea; Chapter 251: West Nile Virus

Sara Tinsley, MS, ARNP, AOCN®
Nurse Practitioner
Department of Malignant Hematology
H. Lee Moffitt Cancer Center
Tampa, Florida
Chapter 228: Leukemias

Derrick J. Todd, MD, PhD
Rheumatology Fellow
Orthopedic and Arthritis Center
Brigham and Women's Hospital
Boston, Massachusetts
Chapter 237: Vasculitis

JoAnn Trybulski, PhD, APRN, BC, ARNP
Associate Dean for Master's Programs
University of Miami School of Nursing and Health Studies
Miami, Florida
Chapter 1: Collaborative Practice; Chapter 4: The Provider-Patient Relationship; Chapter 29: Acute Bronchospasm; Chapter 38: Hypotension; Chapter 130: Myocarditis; Chapter 134: Valvular Heart Disease and Cardiac Murmurs

Susan R. Tussey, CRNP, MSN, CDR, NC, USN
Family Nurse Practitioner
Family Practice Clinic
Naval Health Clinic Hawaii
Pearl Harbor, Hawaii
Chapter 72: Urticaria

Gretchen Van Buren, MSN, ARNP
Adult Nurse Practitioner
Department of Orthopedics—Inpatient
Dartmouth-Hitchcock Medical Center
Lebanon, New Hampshire
Chapter 208: Headache

Denise A. Vanacore, PhD, CRNP, APRN, BC, ANP, PsyNP
Coordinator, Nurse Practitioner Program
Director, Primary Care Services
Gwynedd Mercy College
Gwynedd Valley, Pennsylvania
Chapter 37: Head Trauma; Chapter 39: Poisoning; Chapter 46: Principles of Dermatologic Therapy; Chapter 47: Screening for Skin Cancer; Chapter 185: Elbow Pain

Carol A. Whelan, APRN
Primary Care Division
Yale University School of Nursing
New Haven, Connecticut
Department of Medicine
Rocky Hill Veteran's Home and Hospital
Rocky Hill, Connecticut
Chapter 118: Pneumonia; Chapter 119: Pneumothorax; Chapter 120: Pulmonary Hypertension; Chapter 154: Hypokalemia and Hyperkalemia; Chapter 159: Prostate Disorders; Chapter 160: Proteinuria and Hematuria; Chapter 161: Renal Failure; Chapter 164: Urinary Calculi

Patricia A. White, PhD, APRN, BC
Assistant Professor, Nursing Programs
School for Health Studies
Simmons College
Boston, Massachusetts
Chapter 5: Ethical Analysis and Decision Making in Primary Care

Jane Williams, MSN, RN, FNP, BC
Family Nurse Practitioner and Manager
Department of Genitourinary Medical Oncology
The University of Texas MD Anderson Cancer Center
Houston, Texas
Chapter 252: Collaborative Management of the Oncology Patient;
Chapter 255: Gastrointestinal Symptoms in the Oncology Patient;
Chapter 257: Oncology Complications and Paraneoplastic Syndromes

Christine Wilson, PhD, ARNP, BC
Family Nurse Practitioner
Tampa, Florida
Chapter 199: Sprains, Strains, and Fractures

Barbara E. Wolfe, PhD, APRN, FAAN
Professor
Psychiatric-Mental Health Nursing
Boston College, William F. Connell School of Nursing
Chestnut Hill, Massachusetts
Chapter 262: Eating Disorders

Mary Young, MSN, ARNP, BC
Nurse Practitioner
Department of Cardiology
Dartmouth-Hitchcock Medical Center
Lebanon, New Hampshire
Chapter 74: Wound Management; Chapter 222: Lipid Disorders

Randall M. Zusman, MD
Associate Professor of Medicine
Harvard Medical School
Director, Hypertension Section, Cardiology Division
Massachusetts General Hospital, Boston
Boston, Massachusetts;
Consultant (Cardiology)
Medical Department
Massachusetts Institute of Technology
Cambridge, Massachusetts
Chapter 129: Hypertension

CONTRIBUTORS TO PREVIOUS EDITIONS

James L. Abbruzzese, MD; Saralynn H. Allaire, ScD, RN; Murat Anamur, MD; Joseph C. Aquilina, MD; Mary Attardo, MSN, RN,C, ANP; Sheryl M. Barkan, MSN, RN, CS, ANP; Rita Beckman-Williams, RNC, MSN; Heather E. T. Bell, MPH, RD, LDN, CHES; Bonnie L. Bermas, MD; Joyce S. Billue, EdD, RN, CS, RNP; Kathryn Blum, RN, BS, MSN, ANP; David A. Bradshaw, MD, CDR, MC, USN; Susan Browne, MD, FAAP, IBCLC; Han Q. Bui, MD; Leslie Burton, RN, MSN, CNN, ANP; Denise T. Bynum, RN, MSN, FNP; Diane L. Carroll, PhD, RN; Gretchen Carrougher, MN, RN; Jackie Cassidy, MS, CCC-SP; Tamera D. Cauthorne-Burnette, RN, MSN, FNP; Sharon G. Childs, MS, APRN-BC, CS, CEN, ONC; Alison B. Christopher, LCSW; Dorothy S. Cluff, RN, MSN, CFNP; Leslie J. Collins, RN; Noreen Connolly, RN, CS, MSN; Inge B. Corless, PhD, RN, FAAN; Cornelius J. Cornell, MD; Sandra L. Creamer, RN, CS, PhD, OCN®; Susan Cross-Skinner, MSN, RNCS; Stephen T. Cruz, MD; Maureen Cullen, RN, MS, CCRN, CEN, EMT; William L. Daley, MD, MPH; Jeffrey B. Dattilo, MD; Denise A. DeJoseph, RNCS, ANP; Sallustio Del Re, MD, FCCP; Thomas G. DiSalvo, MD, MPH; Susan Waldrop Donckers, RN, EdD, CS, FNP; Linda M. Douville, MS, ARNP; Richard J. Dowling, MD; Claire Ford Dunbar, ANP-C, MS; Annabel D. Edwards, RN, MSN, ANP; Richard W. Emerine, MD, NPH, FAAFP; Jackie S. Fantes, MD; Diana G. French, PhD, RN, FNP, GNP; Cynthia J. Gantt, RN, PhD, CFNP; Annette Gary, RNC, PhD, CNAA, FNP; Denise Ladd Goksel, RN, MSN, MSc, FNP; Susan Harvey, MSN, RN-CS, FNP; Barbara Kingsley Hathaway, C-RNP, ANP, MIH; Judith M. Haywood, ARNP, EdD; Bonnie Hooper, RN, ANP, MSN, DNC; Elizabeth Hossan, MD; Susan Crocker Houde, PhD, RN; Lorraine K. Jacobsohn, RN, MS, CS; Thomas W. Jenkins, MS, PA-C; David C. Jimerson, MD; Vicki Y. Johnson, RN, PhD, CURN; Patricia A. Joyce, RN, MSN, ANP, CS; E. Lynne Kelley, MD; Marianne Kelly, RN, BS; Phillip E. Knapp, MD; Nancy Kotzuba, RN, MSN, CS, PNP; Frances J. Lagana, DPM; Margaret LaGrange, MSN, RN, CS, ANP; Laurie Landry, MS, RN, CS; Diane Panton Lapsley, MS, RN, CS; Eric Larsen, MD; Dara K. Lee, MD; Pamela V. Lehmberg, MSN, RN, CS; Anne LeMaitre, PT; Ann H. Lewis, PhD; Naaznin Lokhandwala, MD; Patricia Lowry, MS, ARNP; Jane Maffie-Lee, MSN, RN, CS, FNP; Nancy S. Mahan, MS; Elyse Mandell, MSN, RNCS; Sheryl A. Martz, MSN, RN, CS, NP-C; Karlwin J. Matthews, MD; Timothy E. McAlindon, MD, MPM; Claire McGowan, MS, RN, CCRN; Laurel McKernan, MSN, RN; Steven T. Meister, MD; Ruth M. Messer, RN, BSN, OCN®; Patricia J. Mian, RN, MS, CS; Virginia Pender Michel, RN, MSN, ANP; Sally-Ann Milne, CRNI, OCN®, CEN; Virginia McNally Minchiello, MS, APRN-BC; Katherine B. Mishaw, BSN, MS; Diane Mitchell, RN, MSN, ANP; Catherine Morency, MS, RNC; Brian S. Morris, MD; Denise J. Mullaney, MSN, RNCS, ANP, ACNP; Kathleen L. Neill, RN, CS-ANP, MSN, MA; Laura K. Neilley, RN-C, MSN, ANP, GNP; Cynthia H. Nichols, FNP, RN; Nancy H. Nicholson, RN, MSN, NP; Noreen Heer Nicol, MS, RN, FNP; Kathlyn Nowak, RNC, MS; Cheryl A. Ostrowski, MD; Maureen O'Hara Padden, MD, MPH; Julie A. Patterson, MD; Marcia L. Patterson, MSN, RN, NP-Cf; Alexandra Paul-Simon, PhD, RN; Samara Peña, MD; Lisa Presutto-Curley, RPT; Richard D. Quattrone, DO, LT, MC, USN; Joseph N. Ragan, MD; Jennifer A. Ramin, MSN, RN, CS; Martha G. Regan-Smith, MD, EdD; Jacqueline Rhoads, PhD; Catherine Rhuda, RN, MSN, CS; Suzanne Mary Rieke, MD; Robert J. Riggen, MD, MS; Barbara Jean Roberge, PhD, RN, CS; Thomas P. Rocco, MD; G.V.R.K. Sharma, MD; Sharon R. Smart, MS, RN, CS, FNP; LT Clayton M. Smiley, MD; Chad J. Smith, DO; Daniel H. Solomon, MD; Jean E. Steel, PhD, FAAN; Laura M. Sterling, MD; William S. Strauss, MD; Tim Stryker, MD; Paul S. Sullivan, DO; Stacey A. Swaika, MD; Viva Jane Tapper, MSN, ARNP; Janet E. Tatman, PhD, PA-C; Kathleen Thaney, MS, CRNP-A; Elizabeth Renee Thomas, JD, RN, MSN; Deborah M. Thorpe, PhD, RN, CS; Debra Toran, MSN, RN, CS; Cheryle M. Totte, MS, RNC; Catherine E. Turner, MSN, FNP-C; Eugene G. Tutko, MD; Peter J. Ungvarski, MS, RN, FAAN, ACRN; Lynn Valentine, DNSc, FNP, RN; Janet H. Van Cleave, RN, ACNP-CS, AOCN®; Peggy Vernon, RN, MA, C-PNP; Monika Walzak, MD; Vera L. N. Wekullo, MD; Joan Domigan Wentz, MSN, RN, CS, ANP; Karen G. Wiberg, MSN, RNC; Cynthia M. Williams, DO, MAEd, CAPT, MC, USN; Leila S. L. Williams, DO, LT, USN, MC; Barbara Willson, PhD, MSN; Gerri Wittrock-Walton, MS, RN, CS; Nancy M. Youngblood, PhD, CRNP, FNP; Leo Zacharski, MD

REVIEWERS

Maureen Dever-Bumba, DrPH, MSN, CFNP, PNP-C
Assistant Professor and Coordinator, NP Programs
School of Nursing
Medical College of Georgia
Augusta, Georgia

Jane F. Kapustin, PhD, RN, MS, CRNP
Assistant Professor of Nursing
School of Nursing
University of Maryland, Baltimore
Baltimore, Maryland

PREFACE

In the first edition of *Primary Care: A Collaborative Practice,* we recognized that collaboration would be the hallmark for health care delivery in the new millennium. In our second edition we were challenged to articulate the evidence base for care. Building the evidence base for practice requires collaboration among researchers and clinicians of multiple disciplines to identify "best practices" and evaluate support for previously unchallenged therapeutic interventions.

In this, the third edition, two new chapters titled "Collaboration in Research: the Partnership Between Clinicians and Academic Clinical Researchers" and "Weighing the Evidence for Clinical Practice" represent the essence of our philosophy: primary care practice is collaborative and changes in practice are based on knowledge shaped by research. In today's health care environment, practitioners must be astute research consumers in order to provide the highest quality patient care. In this third edition we continue to present the research necessary for evidence-based practice while acknowledging that the evidence is constantly evolving and that there are challenges to providing comprehensive care in the face of declining human and financial resources.

This edition addresses the evolution of thought inherent in any practice discipline. New chapters have been added, and previous chapters have been evaluated and updated with the latest information from an evidence-based perspective. We are pleased with the addition of a new infectious disease section because there is considerable concern about emerging infectious diseases and the resurgence of diseases once thought to have been eradicated.

The response to the previous editions validated our efforts to provide a multidisciplinary resource for learning and practice. We welcomed comments from practicing clinicians, students, and faculty and tried, in this edition, to preserve the balance between a comprehensive and a concise approach to each disorder.

FORMAT

The third edition of *Primary Care: A Collaborative Practice* continues to recognize the increasing complexity of primary care and its inherent challenge for the primary care provider. Increasingly health care providers are providing comprehensive care to patients, either a specific population (e.g., geriatric patients or women) or to a diverse cohort with the same illness (e.g., blood coagulation disorders or HIV). The scope of primary care practice is immense, multifaceted, and in a constant state of change. Issues commonly encountered in the delivery of primary care are presented in this text within a framework that encourages comprehensive and cost-effective care. The format of each chapter remains consistent. A health promotion section has been incorporated in many sections to highlight the importance of health teaching and health promotion in the care of patients.

EMERGENCY AND PHYSICIAN REFERRAL ICONS

This text takes a unique approach by recognizing that collaboration among interdisciplinary team members is enhanced when communication is encouraged and the scope of practice of each provider is well defined and understood. This text has clear guidelines for referrals, and icons highlight conditions that require immediate consultation. Because experience and skills vary among primary care providers, these icons are organized into the following levels:

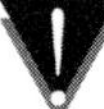

The emergency icon represents circumstances concerning specific emergent conditions. Any patient experiencing these signs and symptoms requires immediate emergency department and/or physician referral.

The physician referral icon represents the need for physician consultation for diagnosis or management. The phrase "Physician consultation is indicated" is used for situations in which a physician's consultation is necessary. The phrase "Physician consultation is recommended" is used for situations in which physician consultation may depend on the primary care provider's level of experience.

The reader should be aware that more comprehensive referral or consultation criteria are contained in the text of the chapters that have these special icons. The reader should also realize that the emergency icons might not include all the conditions requiring emergency referral. The Editors are also aware that experienced providers may not require consultation for all the specified circumstances. In addition, state practice regulations may mandate referral under certain circumstances; these regulations supersede any reference to consultation points detailed in this text.

DIAGNOSTICS AND DIFFERENTIAL DIAGNOSIS BOXES

In any patient encounter, critical thinking skills are necessary to create an appropriate management plan. This text is constructed to assist providers in determining the correct diagnostics and differential diagnoses. Diagnostics boxes list appropriate tests, and Differential Diagnosis boxes list possible differentials. Diagnostics boxes can include up to four categories of testing: (1) initial tests (tests that may be performed in the office setting, such as peak flow measurement or pulse oximetry), (2) laboratory tests (diagnostic tests performed in a medical laboratory, such as blood hematologies or chemistries), (3) imaging tests (radiographic, ultrasound, and nuclear or magnetic resonance studies), and (4) other tests (miscellaneous studies that may be necessary in the evaluation of the disorder, such as EEGs or biopsies). Because the clinical presentation differs with each patient, not all diagnostic tests listed may be necessary in each circumstance. An asterisk is placed beside those tests that may be indicated by clinical presentation and physical examination findings. For more detailed information, the reader should refer to the Diagnostics and Differential Diagnosis sections included with each disorder.

MANAGEMENT

The management sections make every attempt to incorporate the research contributions that create evidence base for practice. Specialty organization guideline recommendations for management, as well as current, ongoing research findings, are presented when they exist. As with any evolving science, recommendations can be in a state of flux. Management recommendations may change, and new recommendations for practice supersede the management recommendations presented in this text. In addition, the reader is directed to check drug indications and dosages in medication product information before administering any medication.

ACKNOWLEDGMENTS

This text represents a collaborative effort. We remain indebted to our contributors, who generously provided their expertise to make this text the resource it is. Their efforts model collaboration, and we are grateful for their patience with questions and revisions. We must also acknowledge the contributions made by our patients, students, and colleagues. We continue to try to incorporate your suggestions to make this text a useful one for practicing clinicians and students alike.

The support of everyone at Elsevier is greatly appreciated. Still, we are particularly appreciative of Cindi Anderson and Deon Lee, who patiently guided the editing and production process, and for Sandra Clark Brown, who encouraged us through this third edition. Finally, our spouses, children, and friends deserve eternal thanks. They continue to sustain and support us, even when this project has competed with them for our attention.

Terry Mahan Buttaro
JoAnn Trybulski
Patricia Polgar Bailey
Joanne Sandberg-Cook

CONTENTS

PART 1

Introduction

JOANN TRYBULSKI, *Section Editor*

CHAPTER 1

Collaborative Practice

Jean E. Steel
Updated by Terry Mahan Buttaro and
JoAnn Trybulski

During the twentieth century a major explosion of scientific knowledge significantly affected health care. New technologies and treatments proliferated. In response to this influx of knowledge and technology, professional education, standards, and domains of practice expanded, and the concept of interdisciplinary teams of health care professionals was introduced.

In today's health care environment, patient care concerns are complex. Meeting these concerns requires that a professional team work together to design, implement, and evaluate patient care. Dialogue among collaborating disciplines is essential to building and maintaining trust during every facet of managing care. The essence of collaborative practice is a collective or a network of professionals that jointly designs, delivers, and evaluates outcomes of care. Patients benefit when the interdisciplinary team focuses attention on planning and managing health care concerns.

A HISTORICAL PERSPECTIVE

In the 1960s the U.S. government began to encourage team training for health care professionals. In 1972 the American Medical Association and the American Nurses Association formed the National Joint Practice Commission (NJPC). The purpose of the NJPC was to describe, research, and refine the value of collaborative practice for nurses and physicians. The NJPC published descriptions of collaborative practices and guidelines for establishing a collaborative practice.[1,2] The NJPC also concluded that joint practice results in improved quality of care, increased patient and provider satisfaction, decreased morbidity and mortality, and decreased hospital length of stay.[1]

Numerous articles and studies have described collaborative practice and have shown multidisciplinary collaboration to be an effective and efficient model of health care delivery.[3-10] Most collaborative practice research has occurred in specialty areas and has linked improved patient outcomes to interdisciplinary collaboration.[11-21] Collaborative practice has provided high-quality health care services in many settings, but at times it has failed to fulfill its potential.

The unfulfilled promise of interdisciplinary practice, its impact on patient care, and the resultant financial burden on the health care system are well described in the first and second reports of the Committee on the Quality of Health Care in America.[22,23] The committee recognized that, despite rapid advances in medicine and technology, the health care system has not been able to offer reliable, high-quality, cost-efficient care to patients in this country.[23] The failure of our health care system is multifactorial. However, one significant recommendation of the Institute of Medicine is the need for "cooperation among clinicians"[23] to ensure coordinated care. Further suggestions include the importance of developing multidisciplinary teams to ensure close patient monitoring and follow-up, as well as improved patient information and education.[23] Perhaps one of the most important concepts addressed by the Institute of Medicine is the recognition that collaborative practice includes the patient in shared decision making.[23]

ELEMENTS OF COLLABORATIVE PRACTICE

Recognition of Patient Needs

The patient is the focus and shapes the elements of collaborative practice. Patient concerns determine the discipline that leads the collaborative care effort. Sometimes medicine or nursing directs the health care team; at other times social services or physical therapy coordinates patient care. The focus of care and attention must be the patient and his or her significant others; therefore leadership of the health care team varies as the patient's needs change.

Trust

Collaborative practice requires respect for each other's knowledge, skill, and clinical decisions. To achieve trust, team members must have a broad understanding of the strength and contributions of each health care discipline to patient care. Each health care professional involved in collaboration should understand the others' assessments of the patient and value the decisions made for this patient.

Recognition of Each Discipline's Contribution

Although state practice laws and professional associations describe responsibility and accountability for practice, these laws, standards, and scopes of practice descriptions may permit several disciplines to provide the same service, thereby increasing access to care. Clearly, health care knowledge and skills are not segregated in a single discipline. Rather, multiple health care disciplines possess common knowledge; in many areas, however, the depth and focus of that knowledge differs. Thus each discipline potentially offers a unique perspective.

Knowledge and understanding of each collaborator's education and experience are vital to the success of collaboration. Educational standards for professional disciplines may appear to be similar, but each has a different emphasis. For example, nurse practitioners value and include health education for patients. Thus the nurse practitioner curriculum has a strong emphasis on illness prevention and health promotion. The physical therapist examines movement dysfunction and develops and implements exercise interventions to enhance functional outcomes. Both the nurse and the physical therapist are concerned about prevention, health promotion, and functional outcomes; however, the physical therapist has more education and experience with musculoskeletal functions.

Another feature of collaborative practice is the delegation of tasks and responsibilities to other caretakers. Accountability with delegation may vary from situation to situation. State laws also guide accountability in the case of delegation. It is always wise for the professional to determine the line of authority and responsibility when delegating tasks to another professional or lay individual.

Time

Another aspect of collaborative practice centers on the provision of time. Time for discussion and planning of care is essential to ensure that the patient focus remains and that the most appropriate member of the collaborating team directs the effort. Additionally, each professional must believe in the value of collaboration for the patient. By attending patient care planning meetings, each member of the interdisciplinary team is able to contribute his or her unique perspective and expertise. Administrative personnel also need to recognize and support the need for time dedicated to this activity.

CHALLENGES INHERENT IN COLLABORATIVE PRACTICE

In some cases, legal regulations, longstanding traditions, and territorial concerns have hindered the development of collaborative practice among different professions. However, as professional domains of practice have changed in the past few years, there is more evidence of shared activities among professional disciplines. Today advanced practice nurses are willing and able to initiate care based on professional standards, education, and scope of practice and experience. In collaborative practice, each discipline is expected to practice according to its own standards and laws in meeting patient needs. Interdisciplinary teams recognize the value of collaboration and the need to value and acknowledge each other's expertise. However, health care providers also must recognize the inherent difficulties in collaborative relationships, identify each others' strengths and weaknesses, and construct a collaborative framework to ensure professional unity.[24]

VALUE OF COLLABORATIVE PRACTICE

The professional literature has reported the benefits of collaborative practice. From the NJPC descriptions of reduced morbidity and mortality, patient and provider satisfaction, and shortened lengths of stay to many of the current reviews, evidence is increasing that collaborative practice improves patient care. Ongoing outcomes research is providing additional information about the value of collaborative practice and is examining the effect of collaborative practice on cost containment and the economics of health care.

The value of outcomes research on collaboration can be seen in gerontology nursing practice. Studies in gerontology practice uncovered a need for significant improvement in care as demonstrated by reduced hospitalizations. Consequently, many evaluation and chronic disease management clinics for patients and their families have been developed using collaborative staffing. Subsequent investigations point to a significant reduction in hospitalizations. Other studies have indicated that, through collaborative practice, patients have greater comprehension of their condition and its management, fewer broken appointments, fewer hospitalizations, and more efficient use of physician time.[25,26]

BUILDING COLLABORATIVE PRACTICE

Practitioners in a discipline share common education, language, and paradigm (world view). The language and paradigm of practitioners of one discipline may be foreign to practitioners of another discipline. This situation can contribute to practitioners of different disciplines working in "silos," without effective interactions across disciplines. For effective collaboration to occur, health care providers must have knowledge of the elements of successful cooperation and seek opportunities to collaborate with other disciplines.

Working together on issues that affect two or more disciplines can create opportunities for collaboration. Interdisciplinary research teams not only represent an occasion for collaboration in patient care, but also have become a crucial aspect of qualifying for research funding from the National Institutes of Health (see Chapter 2). In clinical practice a problem with access to care or the implementation of a new treatment standard may be the impetus for a collaborative venture.

When initiating a collaborative venture, the participants must be aware of personal, institutional, or administrative factors that can be barriers to collaboration. If barriers are identified, participants must devise strategies to reduce them or risk failure of the collaborative venture. Many times what appears to be a barrier is merely distrust or inaccurate knowledge concerning the intent or ability of one discipline. This barrier can be overcome by providing specific information concerning the purpose of the proposed collaboration and the benefits to each of the collaborating disciplines, in conjunction with information about the education and role of each of the collaborating disciplines.

CONCLUSION

One of the most significant values of collaboration is the enhancement and expansion of efforts and results. Collaborative research is exponentially productive as it combines resources, expertise, and thinking in the creation of knowledge for practice. Collaborative leadership allows more individuals to participate, and the outcome derives from a collective of minds. Collaboration in clinical practice offers improved quality of care for patients and significant others as professionals share expertise.

The ingredients for successful collaborative practice include a significant and constant degree of trust among members of the team. An understanding of each member's education, expertise, challenges, and scope of practice is essential for successful implementation of collaborative practice. Protected time for planning and evaluating must be allotted within the settings, or the delivery of services may be compromised. Continuing research needs to focus on patient care outcomes.

Collaborative practice represents the best response that a group of interdisciplinary medical expert clinicians can offer patients and their families. Collaborative practice efforts are indicators of high-quality primary care and should be the goal of every health care provider.

REFERENCES

1. National Joint Practice Commission: *Guidelines for establishing joint or collaborative practice in hospitals*, Chicago, 1981, The Commission.
2. Roueche B: *Together: a casebook of joint practices in primary care*, Chicago, 1977, National Joint Practice Commission.
3. Baggs JG, Schmitt MH: Collaboration between nurses and physicians, *Image J Nurs Sch* 20:145-149, 1988.
4. Devereux PM: Does joint practice work? *J Nurs Admin* 11:39-43, 1981.
5. Styles MM: Reflections on collaboration and unification, *Image J Nurs Sch* 16:21-23, 1984.

6. Steel JE: *Issues in collaborative practice*, Orlando, 1986, Grune & Stratton.
7. Prescott PA, Bowen SA: Physician-nurse relationships, *Ann Intern Med* 103:127-133, 1985.
8. Baggs JG, Schmitt MH: Collaboration between nurses and physicians, *Image J Nurs Sch* 20:145-149, 1988.
9. Safriet BJ: Health care dollars and regulatory sense: the role of advanced practice nursing, *Yale J Regul* 9(2):417-488, 1992.
10. Fagin CMN: Collaboration between nurses and physicians: no longer a choice, *Acad Med* 67:295-303, 1992.
11. Thorne S, Paterson B: Shifting images of chronic illness, *Image J Nurs Sch* 30(2):173-177, 1998.
12. Schaffer J, Wexler LF: Reducing low-density lipoprotein cholesterol levels in an ambulatory care system: results of a multidisciplinary collaborative practice lipid clinic compared with physician-based care, *Arch Intern Med* 155(21):2330-2335, 1995.
13. Grindel CG, Peterson K, Kinneman M, and others: The Practice Environment Project: a process for outcome evaluation, *J Nurs Admin* 26(5):43-51, 1996.
14. Schmitt MH, Watson N, Feiger SM, and others: Conceptualizing and measuring of outcomes of interdisciplinary team care for a group of long-term, chronically ill, institutionalized patient. In Bachman JE, editor: *Interdisciplinary health care: proceedings of the Third Annual Conference on Interdisciplinary Team Care*, Kalamazoo, Mich, 1981, Center for Human Services, Western Michigan University.
15. Michelson EL: The challenge of nurse-physician collaborative practices: improved patient care provision and outcomes, *Heart Lung* 17:390-391, 1988.
16. Daly BJ, Phelps C, Rudy EB: A nurse-managed special care unit, *J Nurs Admin* 21(7/8):31-38, 1991.
17. Anvaripour PL, Jacobson L, Schweiger J, and others: Physician-nurse collegiality in the medical school curriculum, *Mt Sinai J Med* 58(1):91-94, 1991.
18. Baggs JG, Ryan SA: Intensive care unit nurse-physician collaboration and sure satisfaction, *Nurs Econ* 8:386-392, 1990.
19. Evans SA, Carlson R: Nurse/physician collaboration: solving the nursing shortage crisis, *Am J Crit Care* 1(1):25-32, 1992.
20. King ML, Lee JL, Henneman E: A collaborative practice model for critical care, *Am J Crit Care* 2:444-449, 1993.
21. Institute of Medicine: *Primary care: America's health in a new era*, Washington, DC, 1996, National Academy Press.
22. Institute of Medicine: *To err is human: building a safer healthcare system*, Washington, DC, 1999, National Academy Press.
23. Institute of Medicine: *Crossing the quality chasm: a new health care system for the 21st century*, Washington, DC, 2001, National Academy Press.
24. Hornby S, Atkins J, Beale H, and others: *Collaborative care: interprofessional, interagency, and interpersonal*, Boston, Mass, 2001, Blackwell.
25. Hankins GD, Shaw SB, Cruess DF, and others: Patient satisfaction with collaborative practice, *Obstet Gynecol* 88(6):1011-1015, 1996.
26. Henneman EA, Lee JL, Cohen JI: Collaboration: a concept analysis, *Adv Nurs* 21:103-109, 1995.

CHAPTER 2

Collaboration in Research: The Partnership Between Clinicians and Academic Clinical Researchers

Cheryl A. Cahill Lawrence

Collaborative practice models among clinicians have succeeded because they develop the synergy among each medical professional's unique skills. Similarly, collaborations between clinicians and academic researchers maximize the expertise of each partner to yield timely and effective clinical research. Since clinicians and academics often work in orbits that seldom intersect, such collaborations have been rare; however, the climate is changing. The purpose of this chapter is to discuss some strategies that may be useful in forging such collaborations.

THE NATIONAL INSITUTES OF HEALTH ROADMAP

The National Institutes of Health (NIH) Roadmap has been proposed as a way to accelerate translation of basic science discoveries into clinical treatments and to generate innovative approaches to disease management and health-promoting interventions. Implementation of the Roadmap calls for greater cooperation between scientists and clinicians. Several new initiatives have been inaugurated to support the "re-engineering of the clinical research enterprise."[1]

The new initiatives include five general approaches:

1. Clinical Research Networks and National Electronics Clinical Trials and Research (NECTAR)
2. Clinical Outcomes Assessment
3. Clinical Research Training
4. Clinical Research Policy Analysis and Coordination
5. Translational Research

Each new initiative has been designed to overcome historical barriers to collaborations between academic researchers and clinicians.

Clinical Research Networks and National Electronics Clinical Trials and Research Program

The NECTAR program aims to enhance interactions among existing networks of clinical investigators by supporting infrastructure enhancements to foster data and sample sharing, thus reducing duplications in clinical trials research. Funds for feasibility studies will be provided through "a Broad Agency Announcement." Among the activities included under this initiative is enhancement of informatics to support clinical research collaborations, and several projects have been funded. Capturing characteristics of clinical collaborations across clinical research networks will assist in the identification of barriers and incentives to collaborative work. Clinical Research Network initiatives are intended to generate the formation of collaborative groups that can rapidly conduct high-quality clinical studies in a variety of specialty areas. A searchable database of existing clinical research networks is available at https://clinicalresearchnetworks.org/default.asp.[2] Clinicians and investigators interested in participating in a clinical research network will find this database informative and helpful in finding possible collaborators.

Clinical Outcomes Assessment

Clinical Outcomes Assessment is focused on development of new methods to evaluate clinical outcomes. Of particular interest in this initiative are new methods to assess symptoms, the reported consequences of disease. Often symptom change is difficult to measure because current methods rely on self-reports. Self-reported symptom severity appears to depend on several unknown factors that are unique to individual subjects. If change in symptom severity is to be used as a major outcome of an intervention, the unknown nature of individual variation usually requires a large sample size to achieve sufficient power to draw conclusions. The Patient-Reported Outcomes Measurement Information System (PROMIS)[3] will receive $6 million in federal funding to support the development of a publicly available computerized system to assess patient self-reported disease variables. Data will be collected from diverse populations of individuals with a variety of clinical diagnoses. Standardized valid and reliable measures of self-reported clinical symptoms will contribute to more effective and efficient clinical outcomes research. Interested scientists will be invited to a variety of public forums to capture a wide range of perspectives during the development and refinement of PROMIS. The forums will be announced on the website http://www.nihpromis.org.[3]

Clinical Research Training

Clinical Research Training initiatives will build on and expand the current capacities in clinical research. The new and expanded workforce will be trained in a variety of disciplines, including epidemiology, behavioral medicine, and patient-oriented research. Special emphasis will be placed on the capacity of investigators and team members who can rapidly and effectively devise and conduct research into complex health problems. To achieve these goals, several new initiatives are envisioned that will require greater cooperation among the various institutes at and programs currently housed within the NIH. The Multidisciplinary Clinical Research Career Development Program will provide funds for the training of a diverse mix of health care professionals, including nurses, physicians, and dentists, in ways to best manage large, complex multidisciplinary programs of research.[4]

National Clinical Research Associates Program. The NIH Roadmap is an ambitious reordering of how human health sciences research is conducted. To achieve the vision as it has been set out, it will be necessary to rapidly expand the number and the expertise of those engaged in the enterprise. Given the fiscal restraints imposed on federal programs, one way to rapidly expand is to engage professionals who are not usually participants in NIH projects. The National Clinical Research Associates program is intended to engage health care providers working in community-based clinical settings by encouraging them to refer their patients to research protocols and to continue to follow and assess them while they are serving as research subjects.[5]

Predoctoral Clinical Research Training Program. The Predoctoral Clinical Research Training program has been established to sustain the availability of clinical research investigators. This predoctoral training program will prepare the investigators of the future. Programs established under this program must include a specific didactic core and short-term research experiences that will prepare students for the re-envisioned research agenda.[6] To date, funds have been awarded to 10 universities to establish programs to promote clinical investigation training at the predoctoral level.

The NIH Clinical Research Training Center has been operating on the NIH campus since 1997 and will continue under the new initiatives. Medical and dental students who attend this program are trained in the conduct of clinical research. An annual scientific meeting is supported by this program. Over the next several years the program will expand to include more students.

Clinical Research Policy Analysis and Coordination

The Clinical Research Policy Analysis and Coordination initiative will examine the various regulations that investigators must satisfy to conduct research with human beings. Policies that are currently in place are at times redundant and draw investigators' attention and talent away from the research enterprise. The purpose of this initiative is to explore ways to streamline processes and especially reporting procedures without compromising the safety of the clinical research establishment. Management of this program will reside in the office of the director of NIH.[7]

Translational Research

Translational research is defined as an effort to make new scientific discoveries useful in the clinical care of Americans. Initially this term referred to the "translation" of scientific discoveries from the "bench to the bedside." However, over time the importance of clinical observations in seeding bench questions has been recognized. In the past, translational research has been impeded by difficulties associated with human-based research. Other initiatives to reorder the clinical research infrastructure may alleviate some of these difficulties, but if the Roadmap is to be fully realized, greater emphasis must be placed on translational research. To that end, several programs have been proposed.[8]

Initiatives to Facilitate Translation of Research Findings: CTSA Program. The institutional Clinical and Translational Science Awards (CTSA) program was established to "assist institutions to forge a uniquely transformative, novel, and integrative academic home for Clinical and Translational Science that has the consolidated resources to: (1) captivate, advance, and nurture a cadre of well-trained multi- and inter-disciplinary investigators and research teams; (2) create an incubator for innovative research tools and information technologies; and (3) synergize multi-disciplinary and interdisciplinary clinical and translational research and researchers to catalyze the application of new knowledge and techniques to clinical practice at the front lines of patient care."[9]

The CTSA program will be managed by the National Center for Research Resources, which has been responsible for administering the General Clinical Research Center (GCRC) program. The GCRC program will be phased out. Institutions have been encouraged to transform existing GCRC activities into a CTSA. This proposal has many controversial elements, and a discussion of them is far beyond the scope of this chapter. However, in the past, GCRCs have been a rich resource for new clinical investigators. It remains to be seen whether the CTSA will meet that need. Surely, the emphasis on multidisciplinary research teams and especially the explicit mention of nonphysician clinical experts (nurses and dentists) are encouraging.

Initiatives to Facilitate Translation of Research Findings: RAID Pilot. The last program proposed under the translational research domain is the establishment of translational research core services at the NIH. The first initiative will be the establishment of the NIH Rapid Access to Interventional Development (RAID) Pilot. Under this program essential resources will be made available to develop small-molecule therapeutic agents.[10]

The NIH Roadmap establishes a context and in some cases opportunities for partnerships between clinicians and academic researchers, as well as partnerships among academic investigators from diverse disciplines in the clinical research arena. The remainder of this chapter discusses several factors that will assist each in the process of partnering.

FORMING RESEARCH PARTNERSHIPS

Research partnerships form for a variety of reasons. In general, each member of the partnership brings a unique research perspective or skill to the research question. Collaborations of this nature are common and may often be limited to a specific experiment or set of experiments. Team approaches to investigations of health care will likely be long-lasting partnerships, perhaps lasting for the researchers' entire careers. This section offers some general observations about the nature of the processes governing interdisciplinary teams. These observations are based on the author's experiences in a variety of major academic health centers and her efforts to conduct interdisciplinary research.

Initiating Collaboration

Initial contacts among investigators often begin in a social setting. Once individuals determine that they have sufficient comfort with communication styles, they begin efforts to determine the scientific skill and intellectual characteristics of potential collaborators. This stage of exploration can be stimulating and interesting but also challenging, depending on the styles of the participants. The critical outcome of this exploration is the determination of the strengths and weaknesses of team members. Optimally, the strengths of the whole balance the weaknesses of individual potential team members.

Another important outcome of these early formative interactions is a new articulation of the theoretical focus of the research collaboration. Investigators come together initially because of some common interest. In the case of the NIH Roadmap, the common interest may be a particular disease or patient population. Each investigator may represent a particular discipline (e.g., medicine, nursing, molecular biology). Each potential collaborator may be an expert investigator within his or her discipline, but most likely each approaches the research question in a different way and perhaps conceptualizes the question differently. If the team is to investigate the problem from a truly interdisciplinary perspective, the question must be reframed to incorporate the unique points of view of each discipline represented. This new conceptualization is the innovation at the crux of the reform envisioned in the Roadmap.

Clinicians and Researchers: Merging Perspectives

Inclusion of expert clinicians is envisioned in the Roadmap proposal. The expectation is that active clinicians will bring an orientation to the research enterprise that reflects the "real world" of health care. Targeting the most relevant aspects of the clinical research conundrum under study will likely result in findings more immediately applicable to clinical solutions. Investigators may experience some angst in accommodating the clinical perspective because it may mean leaving some pertinent but perhaps less germane questions unanswered. In some cases, for example, a clinician may be more interested in finding a solution that works and be less interested in why it does. This pragmatic approach to scientific development is not the norm and may not be the most interesting to investigators motivated by the search for knowledge. However, both perspectives must be incorporated because the how and the why—the mechanisms of the intervention—are essential building blocks of clinical diagnosis and treatment. Treatment outcome variables are, in fact, measures of the mechanistic elements of disease or healthy life processes. The merger of the two perspectives will achieve an efficient research enterprise related to human health and illness.

During the formative period, several other logistical issues must be determined. Who will be the lead investigator? How will day-to-day operations be managed? Who will control and be accountable for the budget? How will authorship of findings be parsed? Many of these issues have been written about elsewhere. Leadership issues are generally decided pragmatically. Who has the track record, the degree, or the leadership position? Answers to these questions are governed by many factors, including grantsmanship strategies.

Strategies to Increase Grant Success (Grantsmanship)

Grantsmanship strategies include the cogent formulation of the research enterprise to accentuate and optimize those characteristics of a team, the proposed study, and the expected results that increase the likelihood an application will succeed. Analyses of the factors that predict funding of an application at NIH suggest that having received funding in the past from NIH significantly increases the chance of new awards. Thus, if one team member has a stellar résumé of grants funding and publication record, he or she may be the strongest candidate to serve as project director. There must also be congruence between the focus of the new proposal and the past record of research. Past experience in management of a team of investigators may also be a consideration; however, simply holding an administrative position within an organization is probably not sufficient reason to elect an individual to the project director's position.

Importance of Team Composition and Roles. Composition of the research team will be influenced by grantsmanship strategies. Scientists from nursing, dentistry, and other disciplines not well represented in the current NIH portfolio are targeted for inclusion in Roadmap initiatives. If the team member from an underrepresented clinical discipline is selected because of her or his clinical expertise or access to clinical populations, the specific contributions must be carefully delineated and the clinical usefulness of the results strongly evident in the application. There must be a clear description of the ways the clinician will participate in the scientific development of the proposal and implementation of the protocol. The clinician's role in this case will not be trivial. It will not be sufficient to simply charge the clinician with the recruitment of subjects.

Inclusion of scientists from underrepresented disciplines on the research team may also be a grantsmanship strategy. Because there are fewer seasoned investigators in these disciplines, an inexperienced but interested, credentialed individual may be recruited. For example, senior investigators seeking to add a novice nurse-scientist to the team may actually be assuming a mentorship role. It may be necessary to specify in the grant application what this support will include. At the very least, the responsibilities of each investigator must be clarified and the responsibilities must be consistent with the percentage of effort funded by the project and the expertise of the individual.

Critical Grantsmanship Strategies. Other grantsmanship factors are obvious but are mentioned here for the sake of completeness. They include responding to specific requests for applications or other program announcements and selecting research focuses that are consistent with the expertise of the team members and that affect a sufficient percentage of the American public. Communication with the program managers of the targeted institute at NIH is a good way to determine the appropriateness of the research question. The investigators should determine their main competitors and become familiar with their research program and in particular their interpretation of the data to date. Since all new applications are reviewed by accomplished researchers, it is likely that the investigators' main competitor will be represented in some way in the review. The team can deter criticism by explaining where and why their perspective may diverge from that of other scientists (Box 2-1).

TEAMING UP

Volumes have been written about team building within organizations. Most seem to emphasize the need for clear and accurate communication regarding roles and responsibilities. As stated earlier, many decisions regarding the leadership of the research team and allocation of responsibilities will be driven by grantsmanship issues, but allocation of resources to support those activities and communication processes must be explicitly negotiated and codified from the beginning.

BOX 2-1

CRITICAL GRANTSMANSHIP STRATEGIES

- Respond to requests for application or program announcements.
- Select timely research focus.
- Assemble an interdisciplinary team.
- Communicate with the National Institutes of Health institute program manager before grant submission.
- Identify and assess the status of any grant competitors.
- Anticipate and address potential criticism in the grant.

Application Process: Development of the Research Question, Proposal, and Research Protocol

During the application process, the focus is on formulation of the research question and the generation of a strong proposal. Considerable discussion of the protocol will be used to generate data and assignment of responsibility for implementation of the protocol. In large projects, advisory responsibilities may be assigned.

The time between submission of the application and the award of a grant may be as long as 1 year. During that time it is useful for the team to continue to meet and work on the project. If the generation of pilot data was part of the preparation process, these meetings could focus on data analysis and interpretation. Such discussions will help solidify the intellectual connections among team members. Furthermore, the contributions of each team member will be clearly identified. Failure to maintain the team and to use the exuberance of the application process will mean that team building will coincide with implementation of the protocol. Furthermore, over time, individuals will move on. Perhaps they will accept other responsibilities and be unavailable to participate. If leaders forget to include newer team members in grant preparation deliberations, this may gravely affect team dynamics.

Role of the Team Leader

Team building is a crucial step in collaborative research whether the collaboration is between scientists and clinicians or diverse group of scientists. It is essential that all team members feel they are integral to the project's success. The team leader must be extremely attentive to communication among team members. Open communication is essential. No coinvestigator should be excluded from administrative meetings by design or by accident. Leaders should not assume that a named investigator is "not interested" in any element of the implementation of the project. Leaders should provide feedback as to the effectiveness of each member and seek feedback about leadership style and communication. They also must make time to find out about the progress of each investigator's activities. Team leaders have the responsibility to assess availability of and plan for allocation of resources.

Resource Issues

Attached to all NIH grants is subsidy funding for administrative costs associated with managing grant funds. These indirect costs are allocated in various ways within institutions, but often some portion is passed to the department of the principal investigator. In the case of team research, this arrangement could be a barrier to interdepartmental cooperation. In rare instances it could lead to in-fighting about who the lead investigator should be when grantsmanship considerations should take precedence. Administrators must address solutions to abate this potential issue of contention. Investigators invited to join research teams should consult with department leaders early in the process.

Another area of communication that can cause some difficulties in team research is related to resource allocation and utilization. Many of these issues are negotiated during the application process. However, departmental or organizational resources differ across disciplines and clinical settings. Generally, departmental resources are greater in departments with several successful investigators. It may be necessary to provide similar support services to all investigators. If it is important for the research team to participate in professional meetings, it may be necessary to provide funds through direct grant funding. Access to research support from statisticians, research coordinators, and editors may be available within some departments and not others. Team leaders need to assess the needs of each investigator and secure access to needed resources if the entire team is to be successful. Over time, support for interdisciplinary team research by academic health centers and universities will be allocated. The playing field will be level regardless of discipline, and some of these concerns will abate.

Enhancing the Research Infrastructure: Interdisciplinary Team Building

Reformation of the research enterprise supported by NIH will affect and perhaps reform the research enterprises of academic health centers and universities. Many such institutions are organized around disciplinary lines. Thus it may be difficult to meet or become acquainted with scientists and clinicians affiliated with other organizational units. There may be barriers to cross-departmental collaboration as well. Consequently, research administrators may need to formulate strategies to encourage and support interdisciplinary research activities.

Administrators may need to be proactive in encouraging interdisciplinary team building, since such collaborations are rare. Many academic organizations are structured in disciplinary silos. For example, it is rare for the faculty of medical schools and nursing schools to co-teach classes or to share research space. Both would be natural venues for each specialist to become familiar with the other's work. Seminars may be organized that bring together investigators from throughout the organization. They may focus on an area of research or on process elements of collaborative research. Searchable databases of researcher interests and expertise may be useful tools for those seeking research partnerships. Incentives such as seed funding for new research partnerships may provide the impetus to forge partnerships and may actually be required to generate preliminary data to support applications to NIH. Over time, if the goals of the Roadmap are achieved, permanent restructuring of academic settings may occur.

Career Development Issues with Research Collaboration

Academic health centers and universities have established criteria to measure career development and scholarly achievement. Progression to professor status generally requires national or international recognition as a leader in a particular field of research. If team research is to become a norm, how will career development and achievement be judged? It is beyond the scope of this chapter to propose those norms, but it is important that the question be framed.

In institutions with tenure, faculty members are on a timeline to achieve promotion criteria. If the criteria require that the individual be the principal recipient of a research grant, participation in team research may jeopardize his or her career. On the other hand, the ability to join an accomplished investigator who is willing to serve as a mentor may result in rapid development of research experience and selection as the lead investigator in subsequent team research. As the reformed variety of the clinical research enterprise at NIH becomes the norm, criteria are likely to change to recognize the importance of the team. In the meantime, it behooves investigators to discuss implications of collaborative research with the leadership of the department and the chairperson of the committee charged with recommending promotion and tenure.

Collaborative Research as a Strategy for Career Development

Although the proposed new NIH Roadmap serves as a unique impetus for formation of research teams, collaborative research is not new. In fact, it has been successfully used to launch research careers in resource-limited organizations. Rarely is an investigator successful in obtaining grant funding without providing some evidence that he or she can generate the data proposed. Presentation of pilot or feasibility data is the usual way this is done. Ordinarily these data cannot be generated without cost. So a new investigator may negotiate with a senior investigator to assist with the latter's research in exchange for amending the protocol to include needed pilot data.

In negotiating this relationship, the researchers must explore similar concerns related to the nature of the relationship, communication, access to resources, and data ownership. In the case of time-limited collaborations, these concerns assume new meaning. The negotiation period is likely to be shorter and more targeted. The novice investigator will have to make it clear to the senior investigator what the advantages of the ongoing research program will be. The novice must recognize that his or her work will be of secondary importance. Some new investigators will not enjoy the subordinate role that may be available. Since it would likely adversely affect the ongoing program, it would be difficult to withdraw without completing the project. Thus it will be important to evaluate the management style of the senior investigator. Speaking with current and past employees can help a researcher discern the compatibility of the style with his or her own.

Benefits of Having a Mentor

In academic centers and universities, senior investigators usually hold teaching or mentoring roles. Most embrace them and see them as essential to the satisfaction they feel in their jobs. Ordinarily they do not differentiate mentoring a colleague from mentoring a student. So a successful collaboration begun as a way of launching an academic career may have long-term benefit. A senior investigator within an organization has knowledge of the bureaucracy associated with the research enterprise. Navigating that bureaucracy is rarely simple. Having someone to "show you the ropes" can be invaluable. Senior investigators will also know how to access support services that may not be readily evident. Usually these resources are oversubscribed, so having someone experienced in accessing the service is important.

Seasoned investigators have knowledge of the personal characteristics required to succeed as a scientist. If the selected mentor is willing and the protégé is amenable, the novice will be able to progress rapidly and develop the skills required to be a successful investigator and professor. A successful collaborative research experience is a win-win situation for all concerned—especially the organization.

INTERNATIONAL COLLABORATION AMONG CLINICIANS AND ACADEMIC RESEARCHERS

Concerns about bird flu and the recent tuberculosis and HIV pandemics have increased opportunities to collaborate with investigators in other countries. The characteristics of international collaborations are not unlike those discussed thus far. However, distance and cultural differences may raise additional issues.

Work Expectations in American Academia

The work ethic of American academics is extraordinary. Contrary to recent arguments that university professors teach only a few hours per week, the majority of academics work far more than 40 hours per week. Most university professors conduct research and provide service to their profession and university in addition to teaching. Most feel privileged to have the opportunity to discover new information, promote student learning, and participate in world-class educational institutions. Academics all over the world share these sentiments, but the work patterns may differ.

The energy exhibited by Americans in completing research-related tasks is not always matched by international collaborators, who have different demands placed on their time. It is easy to become frustrated with delays in communication and task completion. When investigators depend on international collaborators to conduct studies in their countries with their populations, Americans have no choice but to be patient. However, some strategies may help move the process forward.

Communication Issues in International Collaborations

Communication among team members is essential if the goals of the collaboration are to be achieved. Communication across campus can be difficult; across the world it can be enormously complicated. Time changes alone affect scheduling of meetings. An e-mail sent at the end of the day in the United States reaches European collaborators long after the end of the workday. In resource-poor countries, international collaborators may have limited access to e-mail, facsimile transmissions, and telephones. During the development of international collaborations it is important to establish communication patterns that are acceptable to both parties. Telephoning is useful but usually requires scheduled meetings. Internet-based meeting software is becoming more widely useful, but if the international collaborator does not have the technical support to make it work, it will be more stressful than helpful. Face-to-face meetings require long trips at some expense. Most of these complications can be overcome with patience and in some cases adequate funding. Recognizing cultural differences and accommodating them can be most difficult.

Issues with Funding

Often the international collaborator is interested in collaborative research because of promised funding for the project. It is extremely important to be clear that funds may not be used to supplement usual income. Confirmation with the targeted funding agency is recommended to clarify this issue. If seed funding from the United States is available to pay for collaborative participation in project developments, some of the issues related to timely achievement of tasks may be eliminated. During the planning process it must be made clear to collaborators that, if funded, they will be required to perform the designated tasks on the time line outlined. Clarity will prevent future problems and enable collaborators to perform as expected.

SUMMARY

The time required to form international partnerships varies, but usually it will take longer than similar collaborations in the United States. U.S. investigators must spend time in the other country so they can understand the culture of the academic enterprise there. Recognizing and embracing cultural differences will enhance the collaboration and relieve the stress of long-distance relationships. Frequent visits will accelerate the process of collaboration because familiarity and personal relationships are essential to successful international collaborations.

Although the newly proposed NIH Roadmap will generate new teams of researchers, collaborative research is not a new phenomenon. Teams of investigators coalesce around common research interests. Each member of the team brings unique skills to the research process and is integral to the project's success. International research projects are proliferating. Successful collaborative national and international research teams are based on clear and accurate communication of the roles and responsibilities of each member and respect for the perspective each discipline brings to the collaboration.

REFERENCES

1. National Institutes of Health: *The National Institutes of Health (NIH) roadmap for biomedical research*, 2006, retrieved from http://nihroadmap.nih.gov/clinicalresearch.
2. National Institutes of Health: The Clinical Research Networks and National Electronics Clinical Trials and Research (NECTAR). In *The National Institutes of Health (NIH) roadmap for biomedical research*, 2006, retrieved from https://clinicalresearchnetworks.org/default.asp.
3. National Institutes of Health: Patient-Reported Outcomes Measurement Information System (PROMIS). In *The National Institutes of Health (NIH) roadmap for biomedical research*, 2006, retrieved from

http://www.nihpromis.org.
4. National Institutes of Health: Clinical research training. In *The National Institutes of Health (NIH) roadmap for biomedical research,* 2006, retrieved from http://nihroadmap.nih.gov/clinicalresearch/overview-training.asp.
5. National Institutes of Health: National clinical research associates. In *The National Institutes of Health (NIH) roadmap for biomedical research,* 2006, retrieved from http://nihroadmap.nih.gov/clinicalresearch/overview-training.asp.
6. National Institutes of Health: Predoctoral clinical research training. In *The National Institutes of Health (NIH) roadmap for biomedical research,* 2006, retrieved from http://nihroadmap.nih.gov/clinicalresearch/clinicaltraining/predoc_factsheet.asp.
7. National Institutes of Health: Clinical research policy analysis and coordination. In *The National Institutes of Health (NIH) roadmap for biomedical research,* 2006, retrieved from http://nihroadmap.nih.gov/clinicalresearch/overview-policy.asp.
8. National Institutes of Health: Translational research. In *The National Institutes of Health (NIH) roadmap for biomedical research,* 2006, retrieved from http://nihroadmap.nih.gov/clinicalresearch/overview-policy.asp.
9. National Institutes of Health: Institutional Clinical and Translational Science Awards. In *The National Institutes of Health (NIH) roadmap for biomedical research,* 2006, retrieved from http://nihroadmap.nih.gov/clinicalresearch/overview-translational.asp.
10. National Institutes of Health: NIH Rapid Access to Interventional Development (NIH-RAID Pilot). In *The National Institutes of Health (NIH) roadmap for biomedical research,* 2006, retrieved from http://nihroadmap.nih.gov/raid/.

CHAPTER 3

Weighing the Evidence for Clinical Practice

Cheryl A. Cahill Lawrence

The translation of research findings into clinical practice is an essential element of the clinician's responsibility. However, decisions regarding the sufficiency of evidence to alter usual practices may be difficult to make. This chapter provides clinicians with some guidelines that may be useful in making decisions about evidence-generated changes in care.

Rarely are the results of a single research study sufficient for clinicians to change the usual practice guidelines and standards. Careful evaluation of individual studies to ensure that the study or research question, design, analysis, and conclusions are appropriate is the essential first step. Consistent results from multiple studies are necessary to support changes in practice standards. Because the ultimate purpose of health-related research is to develop and test treatments that prevent illness or restore health, the requisite body of evidence is a clear demonstration of cause-and-effect mechanisms governing the phenomenon of interest. Without an understanding of the mechanisms that regulate the phenomenon of interest, prescriptions and interventions with predictable and consistent outcomes are limited. A systematic investigation is carried out to develop a sufficient understanding of regulatory mechanisms. This investigation begins with identifying the characteristics of the phenomenon and leads to demonstrations of cause-and-effect relationships among variables.

Once cause-and-effect relationships are determined, clinical investigators postulate and test interventions with predictable outcomes. By identifying the level of the question addressed in a single research project, the clinician may determine what is known about the phenomenon of interest and apply that knowledge to clinical practice. This hierarchical view of evidence provides the clinician with a context for evaluating study results for clinical applicability.

LEVEL I RESEARCH QUESTIONS: DESCRIPTION OF CHARACTERISTICS

The progression from description to intervention may be conceptualized as passing through four levels. Determining the level of the question within this hierarchy is the first step in evaluating the clinical utility of a particular study. The purpose of a level I question is to describe the pertinent characteristics of the phenomenon of interest.[1] The question usually includes the stem "What is...?"; for example, "What is the experience of individuals diagnosed with HIV?"

To answer this question, investigators apply qualitative methods such as structured interviews. Qualitative data may be analyzed with a variety of techniques that guide the investigators to identify ranges of typical responses. Alternatively, investigators may use quantitative methods such as a survey.

Analysis of the quantitative data generated in level I studies includes nonparametric statistics, which generate measures of central tendency and dispersion. These measures indicate typical responses by determining the average response (mean, mode, median) and variability of responses (range of responses, standard deviation, other measures of dispersion). The results from this type of study may be used by clinicians to expand the usual assessment parameters but generally do not guide the selection of an intervention or a treatment.

LEVEL II RESEARCH QUESTIONS: RELATIONSHIPS AMONG OR BETWEEN VARIABLES

The results of level I questions provide the basis for level II questions. Once the fundamental characteristics of a phenomenon have been described, the next logical step is to describe the relationships between and among characteristics or variables. The purpose of level II questions is to establish associations or differences between variables. Level II questions include the stem "What is the relationship...?" or "What are the differences between...?"; for example, "What is the association between a history of cigarette smoking and the incidence of heart disease in women over 40 years of age?"

Several approaches to this type of question are applicable. For example, investigators may carry out epidemiologic studies in large data sets. This approach has been used to identify the risk factors commonly used to assess patients, to gather specific diagnostic data, and to counsel persons to change behavior. Other studies may be designed to compare the differences in variables between two or more groups. For example, an investigator may measure selected variables in a group of persons with HIV and a group of matched persons without HIV to determine associations between CD4 counts and fatigue levels. The results of these studies simply describe the associations and differences between the groups and suggest that the differences may be associated with group membership.

The data analysis techniques used in level II studies are measures of association (e.g., correlation coefficients) and differences between and among the research study groups (e.g., *t*-tests and analysis of variance).[1,2] The evidence generated with this question level is probably insufficient to demonstrate a mechanistic cause-and-effect relationship between the variables. Demonstrating such a relationship requires more rigorous control of extraneous variables and active manipulation of the independent variable (the variable thought to be the causal variable). The clinician may suggest a change in behavior because of the results of a level II question, but the results do not guide methods to change those behaviors, nor do they explain how the behavioral change will be effective.

LEVEL III RESEARCH QUESTIONS: CAUSE AND EFFECT

Armed with the results of level II studies, investigators can design level III studies. The purpose of level III studies is to identify the mechanistic relationships among characteristic variables associated with the phenomenon of interest.[1] Level III research questions are more complicated because the investigator has a hypothesis about the nature of the relationships among variables (i.e., which is the causal variable and which is the effect variable). Rather than a research question, the putative relationship tested in the study is often stated as a hypothesis. The format of a hypothesis is a declarative sentence that asserts the relationship: changes in A (the independent variable) cause changes in B (dependent variables). Depending on the amount of preliminary evidence or on the theoretical model proposed by the investigator, the investigator might suggest a directional relationship (e.g., as A increases, B decreases). The design applied to this level of question is either experimental or quasi-experimental.

True Experimental Design

To demonstrate a causal relationship, the investigator must exercise maximum control over the study. A true experiment provides this level of maximum control. A true experiment is characterized by random selection of participants and manipulation of the independent or causal variable. The random selection of subjects ensures that the sample is representative of a population. Several strategies may be used to ensure a representative sample, with each strategy engineered such that each eligible member of the population has an equal chance of being included in the study.[1]

If human subjects are used in a level III study, considerable care must be taken to control extraneous variables. Extraneous variables are those characteristics of the subject or setting that may influence the behavior of the dependent variable. In addition to random selection of participants, random assignment to the treatment group or the control group provides further control of extraneous variables. For example, if the study's purpose is to demonstrate that slow and rhythmic breathing by persons with essential hypertension results in lower systolic blood pressure, investigators may send a letter asking for volunteers to all persons being treated at a particular clinic. Because participation in a research study must be voluntary, it is safe to assume that participants "self-select" the study. Willingness to participate in a study may differentiate study participants from the overall population. Therefore random assignment to either the control group or the experimental group helps ensure that the sampling methods did not contribute to errors.

Similarly, the investigator may consider other inclusion and exclusion criteria to guide subject recruitment. For example, the investigator may specify that subjects must be following a particular pharmacologic treatment regimen. Because these types of controls increase the complexity of recruitment, the investigator may select persons who are newly diagnosed with hypertension and test them before they begin rhythmic breathing treatments and again after a specified period of treatment. The study may include a control group of newly diagnosed persons who are monitored in exactly the same way as the experimental group but do not change their respiratory pattern. One way to ensure that environmental stimulation is the same for all subjects is to conduct the experimental sessions in the same laboratory setting. Subjects return at the same time after the initiation of treatment. By contrasting the blood pressure measures of the experimental group with those of the control group, the investigator is able to differentiate the effects of changes in breathing patterns alone from the effects of pharmacologic treatment alone and from the effects of both changes in breathing patterns and pharmacologic treatment (Table 3-1).

TABLE 3-1 True Experimental Design

Group	Baseline	Treatment
Control	No treatment	Pharmacologic treatment
Experimental	Rhythmic breathing treatment	Rhythmic breathing treatment *and* pharmacologic treatment

The purpose of this study is to evaluate the effectiveness of intermittent rhythmic breathing exercises to control hypertension in newly diagnosed persons. During the baseline period, the control group receives no treatment, whereas the experimental group practices the rhythmic breathing treatment. During the treatment period, the control group receives the usual treatment—pharmacologic treatment. The experimental group also receives the usual pharmacologic treatment, since it would be unethical to withhold treatment given the complications of untreated hypertension. A comparison of data from each cell reveals the effects of no treatment, pharmacologic treatment alone, rhythmic breathing treatment alone, and rhythmic breathing with pharmacologic intervention.

Quasi-Experimental Design

In many cases it is not possible to randomly select participants or to randomly assign them to treatment and control groups. For example, if an investigator is interested in the effects of a disease, it would not be possible to assign some subjects to have the disease and others to be free of a disease. In such cases the disease would be the treatment variable. For example, suppose that an investigator is interested in understanding the pathology of HIV in the immune system. Clearly it would be unethical to randomly assign persons to an experimental group to be infected with HIV. Instead, the investigator monitors persons diagnosed with HIV at baseline and at regular intervals thereafter.

The comparison of baseline data to subsequent observations allows the investigator to characterize the causal relationship between HIV infection and changes in immune parameters. This type of design is referred to as *quasi-experimental* because there is no random assignment to the experimental condition. Sometimes this type of design is called a *repeated measures design*, and it is argued that the subject serves as his or her own control.[2] In some ways this type of design ensures better control of extraneous variables associated with the constitution of individual subjects. However, the investigator should demonstrate with some assurance that every subject is representative of the general population. For example, if the sample lacks diversity of gender, age, and ethnicity, one would wonder to what degree the sample represents the overall population. The results can be applied only to those individuals represented in the sample. In other words, if the sample is not representative of the target population, then the results may not be extrapolated to the population.

Analysis of level III data tests hypothesized relationships between independent and dependent variables. For example, regression techniques generate a mathematical model to predict the change in dependent variables in response to changes in the independent variable. The value of level III studies to clinicians is that they may provide a degree of confidence in their prediction of outcomes. Clinicians who attempt to anticipate the clinical course of a disease state may use the results of level III studies.

LEVEL IV RESEARCH QUESTIONS: RANDOMIZED CLINICAL TRIALS

Level IV studies demonstrate the effectiveness of an intervention or treatment. The mechanistic relationships among variables identified by level III studies support the proposition of the interventions and treatments tested in level IV questions. The randomized, placebo-controlled, double-blind clinical trial is the definitive way of conducting this type of study because it provides the investigator maximum control of the sources of error inherent in human clinical investigations.

Random Selection and Random Assignment

The random selection of participants for a study is one way to achieve a study sample that is representative of the targeted population.[1] Investigators in level IV studies use several methods to ensure that all eligible subjects have an equal chance of being included in the study. When the availability of subjects is limited, investigators may conduct the study at a variety of sites. Within each site, all potential subjects are informed of the study and are offered the opportunity to participate. By casting the widest possible net, investigators are ensured of a representative sample.

Random assignment to a treatment group helps ensure that the groups are comparable. If random assignment is not made, individuals who are significantly better or worse may end up being assigned to a specific group. For example, if an investigator were free to assign the treatment group, he or she might inadvertently assign those most likely to respond to the new treatment to that group. There might also be a bias toward one treatment over another. A surgeon participating in a randomized clinical trial testing the effectiveness of a lumpectomy in comparison to the usual treatment of mastectomy may prefer to assign young women to the lumpectomy group because of the disfigurement associated with mastectomy.

Placebos

Placebos, or sham interventions or treatments, exclude the possibility that changes in patient behavior are due to a desire to please a researcher. The Hawthorne effect must also be acknowledged in any research. The Hawthorne effect produces improvements in performance because subjects are aware they are being observed. Observation of the placebo control group permits investigators to demonstrate effects such as accelerated resolution of symptoms or palliative effects rather than curative effects. For conditions in which an effective treatment exists for the targeted population, those in the placebo group receive the usual treatment rather than a placebo, since in most cases it would be unethical to withhold treatment.

Blinding the Subject and Researcher

Blinding the subject and the researchers and caregivers as to group membership (control group or experimental group) prevents the contamination of results by personal biases. Investigators who are invested in obtaining positive results may be biased in their observations. In the case of pharmaceuticals, only the pharmacist may know which patient is receiving the investigational treatment. Patients who enroll in studies may do so simply because there is no alternate therapy. Hope for a positive effect could bias their reports of effects.

Data Analysis Methods

The aim of data analysis is to demonstrate groupwise differences in treatment effects. Analysis of variance methods or *t*-tests are most often used, but regression analysis may also be done. The quandary investigators face is how to treat the numbers relative to subjects who do not complete a study. Obviously, it is important to know if significantly more subjects died in the treatment group, but what about subjects who withdraw from the study?

One of the important aspects to evaluate in any new treatment is patient preference and a tolerance for side effects. Some have argued that an "intent-to-treat" approach to these data ought to be used. In this approach, subjects who withdraw or die are counted as treatment failures, thus raising the standard for significant results. Consider a case in which 100 subjects are recruited for a study (Table 3-2). Fifty subjects are randomly assigned to the usual treatment, and 50 are assigned to the new treatment. At the end of the study, 10 in each group have died. No subjects withdrew from the usual treatment, but 10 withdrew from the new treatment group. At the end of the study, 20 subjects "got better" with the usual treatment and 20 subjects showed improvement with the new treatment. When investigators calculate success rates, if the number of persons *completing* the study is used as the denominator, the success rate for the usual treatment group is 20 out of 40 (50%) compared with 20 out of 30 (66%) for the new treatment or experimental group. The experimental treatment would appear to be superior. However, if instead the number who *began* the study is used as the denominator, the success rate in the usual treatment group is 20 out of 50 (40%) compared with 20 out of 50 (40%) in the new treatment group, which suggests no difference between the groups. Thus, with the intent-to-treat approach, one would conclude no difference in success rate between the two treatments and a twofold increase in the failure rate for the new treatment.

ADDITIONAL STUDY PARAMETERS NEEDING EVALUATION

Identification of the level of the question simply informs the clinician of the possible usefulness of the results. The decision to actually modify clinical practices because of the study results must also include some evaluation of the design, subject selection, methods, data analysis scheme, and resultant conclusions. Table 3-3 summarizes some of these elements as they relate to the level of the question. Inherent in the progression from description of the phenomenon to clinical trials is an increasing amount of control that the investigator can exert over the study's conduct. The purpose of the increase in control is to control error. Error is that portion of the measurement that cannot be explained. A simplistic way of describing a statistic is the ratio between the effect of the experiment and the error.

STATISTICAL ANALYSIS PRINCIPLES

Although it is beyond the scope of this chapter to fully explore statistical methods, it may be helpful to review some basic principles of statistics. The purpose of any statistic is to provide a mathematic measure of the effects of study variables while accounting for error. At the core of statistical analysis is the assumption that variance is normally distributed within a given population. A *population* is defined as all units targeted by the study. A *sample* is defined as that portion of units selected for study that represent the population.

Type I and Type II Errors

One significant source of error in any study is an investigator's failure to include units that represent all characteristics of the population. As discussed previously, one way to avoid this error is to select study participants carefully. A basic element of these strategies is the accrual of a sufficient sample size to ensure that all characteristic elements of the population are included. If a sample is insufficiently representative of a population, the investigator may report false results and may erroneously conclude that the research hypothesis is supported—that is, that the effect of the study may be sufficiently robust to conclude that differences or associations exist between baseline and outcome or between the experimental groups and control groups when in fact there is no difference. This type of error is a type I error. The investigator also risks what is known as a type II error, or the failure to detect significant associations or differences when they are present. During the design of a study the investigator may protect the study from these errors by conducting a power analysis.[1]

TABLE 3-2 Intent-to-Treat Table

Participants	Usual Treatment			Experimental Treatment		
	N	Total Intent-to-Treat (%)	Complete (%)	N	Total Intent-to-Treat (%)	Complete (%)
Admitted	50	100	80	50	100	60
Died	10	20	NA	10	20	NA
Withdrew	0	0	NA	10	20	NA
Completed, improved	20	40	50	20	40	66
Completed, did not improve	20	40	50	10	20	33
Total completing	40	80	100	30	60	100

The analysis of data from a clinical trial may be carried out in several ways. Of main concern is how investigators handle participant attrition. The inclusion of participants who begin a study but fail to complete it is referred to as the intent-to-treat approach. This table illustrates the difference of results with an intent-to-treat scheme versus an approach that disregards attrition.

TABLE 3-3 Summary of Study Parameters

Level of Question	Purpose	Methods	Analysis	Application
I. What is it?	To describe or define a phenomenon of interest To identify pertinent variables or characteristics	Qualitative methods Structured interviews Questionnaires Surveys	Content analysis Ethnography Nonparametric statistics Measures of central tendency	May suggest assessment parameters (Do you experience . . . ?)
II. What is happening here?	To identify relationships between variables—associations and differences	Epidemiologic studies Cross-section studies Correlational studies Studies of groupwise differences	Correlations among variables Differences between variables or groups Mann-Whitney *U*; analysis of variance; *t*-test	Suggests avenues of further assessment (If you observe *x*, what is likelihood that *y* will occur?)
III. What is the nature of the relationship among variables (cause-and-effect relationship)?	To determine cause-and-effect relationships among variables To explicate mechanisms mediating the phenomenon of interest	Experimental designs Quasi-experimental designs	Analysis of variance Regression analysis	Suggests underlying pathologic conditions that may be treated
IV. What is the therapeutic effect of a proposed intervention? What is the proper dose of a treatment to achieve a predictable outcome?	To determine predictability of hypothesized outcome at specific dose in selected population	Randomized clinical trial	Intent-to-treat analysis Analysis of variance Regression analysis	Demonstrates usefulness of particular treatment for patient population; with sufficient replication, clinician may be reasonably sure that treatment will be effective

Power Analysis

Simply defined, *power* is an estimate of the probability of detecting significant effects at a given probability of a type II error.[1] In other words, power is an indication of the confidence one may have that the results are true. In general, research reports discuss power analysis as a way of calculating the sample size needed to adequately represent the target population. In general, the proportional risk of a type II error is set at 0.80; that is, the investigator estimates that the risk of failure to detect significant results is 2 in 10. If a power analysis has been done, clinicians should be assured that care was taken to ensure that the sample is representative of the target population.

Analysis of Research Study Results

Description of Data and Measures of Central Tendency. A description of the sample and general findings is usually the first step in analyzing the results of a study. Descriptive statistics summarize data. They include measures of central tendency, dispersion, and association. The simplest descriptive statistic may be a graphic representation of the data. A pie chart, bar graph, or line graph is a pictorial representation of the distribution of the data.

Measures of central tendency indicate the "typicalness" of the data set. The appropriate measure of central tendency is determined by the way the variable of interest is scaled. The typical representation of gender is categorized as male or female in a sample by the actual number of participants in each level of the variable or by the value as a proportion of the total.

In a case in which the variable of interest may have three or more possible responses, the appropriate measure of central tendency is the mode.[2] The *mode* is the category most frequently selected. For example, suppose the variable of interest was an evaluation of the effectiveness of an educational program for newly diagnosed diabetic patients. The evaluation tool consists of a list of statements attached to a scale with five possible responses: 1 represents strongly agree; 2, agree; 3, neutral; 4, disagree; and 5, strongly disagree. These responses represent categories with unknown relationships. Therefore the appropriate measure of central tendency for these questions is the mode, or the category with the most responses.

The *median* is an appropriate measure of central tendency for rank order data such as income of participants in a study.[2] Participants are often asked to indicate their annual income by selecting from a range of annual incomes. The median is the point on the scale with 50% of the responses below and 50% above. For example, census data generally report the median income in a community or the median price of a home.

The appropriate measure of central tendency for discrete data is the *mean*, which is simply the arithmetic mean.[2] For example, a study of the effects of stress on systolic blood pressure might indicate the mean, or average baseline, systolic blood pressure for the sample.

Standard Deviation. Dispersion is a measure of the variability of the data, or the degree to which data deviate from each other. The range is the difference between the highest score and the lowest score. Standard deviation is a measure of dispersion commonly reported for discrete data. The standard deviation is a summary of the average amount of difference among the data points.[2] A complete description of discrete data would include the mean plus or minus the standard deviation. Assuming that the study group is truly representative of the population, the mean, plus and minus the standard deviation, may represent the "normal" range of responses the clinician may expect to see.

Normal Distribution and Error. If the responses from everyone in a population across the range of possible responses are counted and graphed, the majority of responses fall in the middle, with the rest evenly distributed above and below the middle (Figure 3-1). This sort of distribution is referred to as *normal distribution*. Underlying the parametric statistics is the assumption that all responses to an experimental condition are normally distributed.[1] If participants have been truly selected at random from the same population, then the sum of responses should be normally distributed. Individual responses are therefore a result of chance. By randomly sampling from a population, the investigator assumes that the sample is representative of the overall population. The distribution of responses of the sample should therefore mirror the distribution of responses of the population. Deviation from a normal distribution model is assumed to be due to error. A well-designed study is engineered to reduce error, and instruments with demonstrated validity and reliability are used. Subject selection is based on clear and reasoned inclusion and exclusion criteria so that only members of the targeted population are included. Data collection protocols are rigorously followed. Despite these best practice methods, however, some error is inevitable.

Statistical Significance (Alpha Values). The purpose of statistical analysis is to estimate the amount of error. Because error is inevitable, the investigator decides before data are collected how much error can be tolerated and still demonstrate significant effects. The amount of tolerable error is defined as the *alpha* (α) *value*. The α value is expressed as a decimal representation of the proportional risk for error. An α of 0.05 is interpreted as 5 chances in 100 that an error may occur. Similarly, 0.01 is interpreted as 1 chance in 100. The maximum risk for error is generally set at 0.05.[1]

More rigorous or lower α values are specified to prevent a wrong conclusion that the research has demonstrated positive or significant results. For example, an investigator evaluating a new therapy might decide that the risk of the therapy being ineffective 5 out of 100 times is too high. The α could be set at 0.01, or 1 chance in 100. If that is done, then the results are reported as not significant if statistical analysis demonstrates a p value (the actual proportion of error) of 0.05 at the completion of the study. The clinician may use the strength of the statistical significance to determine the robustness of the effect of the intervention when deciding to change a therapeutic routine. Suppose a study is conducted to compare the usual treatment (drug A) to a new treatment (drug B). The α has been set a priori (beforehand) at 0.05. The reported p values at the end of the study are 0.05, which suggest that the new treatment is better than the old. The clinician must decide whether the 5% risk that this conclusion is not true is sufficiently low to change the usual prescription.

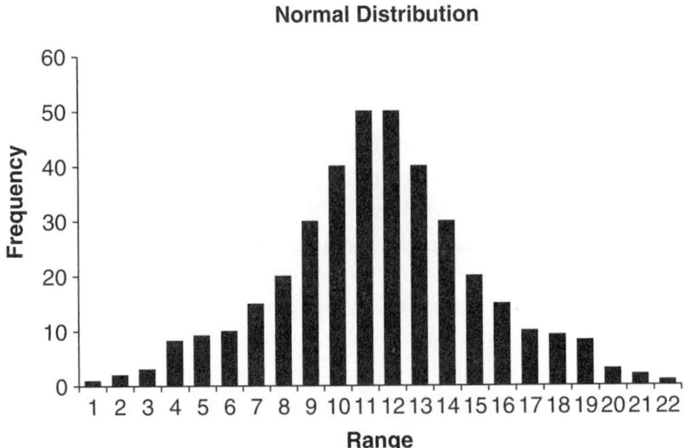

Figure 3-1

A graph of a theoretical normal distribution. The x axis represents all possible responses, and the y axis is simply the number of responses. This graph demonstrates that the majority of responses cluster in the middle range of possible responses and that the rest are evenly distributed above and below the middle.

Statistics of Differences and Associations. Statistics measure associations among variables or differences between variables. During the design of a study the investigator plans to demonstrate that participants behave in similar or different ways. Association statistics evaluate the similarities among the data. Association statistics compare the distribution of the variables of interest and evaluate whether they are consistently similar enough to conclude that they are related. The appropriate association statistic depends on the way the variables are scaled. For example, associations between two categorical variables (the values of the variables are not on a numeric continuum) are evaluated using a goodness-of-fit-statistic, whereas an association between two ranked variables (the values of these variables are in hierarchical order) are evaluated using a rank order correlation statistic. Associations among continuous data are determined by calculating correlation coefficients.[2] Strong correlations among variables may indicate to clinicians that if one symptom is observed, a second may also be present.

Many times an investigator is interested in discerning the differences among variables or groups. For example, if the study's purpose is to evaluate the effects of a treatment, the investigator would be interested in demonstrating that a significant difference has occurred. Therefore difference statistics compare the distribution of variables to determine if they are sufficiently different. Because an assumption that all data are normally distributed is central to statistics, difference statistics evaluate the difference between the appropriate measure of central tendency and dispersion to ensure that the distributions are actually independent. In the case of categorical data, differences are determined by the chi-square (χ^2) statistic.[2] For continuous data, a comparison between two variables is evaluated by a t-test. More than two discrete variables are evaluated with some type of analysis of variance (ANOVA).[2]

The appropriateness of analytic methods is an essential element that the clinician needs to consider when using specific research findings. In general, if the results are consistent across several studies and the analytic methods are similar, the clinician may feel comfortable that the conclusions are correct.

Clinical Significance Versus Statistical Significance. The definitive method for determining the correctness of a research finding is whether the statistical analysis yields significant results. However, occasionally an investigator will report the results to be clinically significant despite no statistically significant result. Such an assertion is usually made when the level of significance has approached the 0.05 level. If it is kept in mind that the α is the minimally acceptable risk that a false report is made, then this argument is for increasing that risk. A slightly lower significance is usually the result of small sample sizes. Pragmatically speaking, the time, energy, and resources needed to gather some clinical data may preclude increases in sample sizes. Therefore the clinician must be cautious when considering the usefulness of such data. In these cases clinicians may be advised to wait for additional studies to be reported before changing their usual practices.

SUMMARY

Clinicians require accurate and precise information to deliver safe and effective care. However, the demands of day-to-day practice environments make it difficult to keep up. This chapter identifies general guidelines useful in evaluating individual studies. The progression of knowledge from description of a phenomenon, disease, or syndrome to effective clinical management requires systematic investigation. Descriptive studies (level I) characterize the phenomenon of interest and may be used by clinicians to hone their assessment skills. Level II studies aim to detail the essential characteristics of a phenomenon and to demonstrate the relationships among those elements. Clinicians may use these results to guide the diagnosis or recognition of a condition. Level III studies are designed to demonstrate cause-and-effect relationships among variables or elements. Clinicians may use proof of causation to treat. Level IV studies test treatments or interventions. Clinicians use the results of these studies to predict the effectiveness of a particular treatment for an individual. This hierarchical conceptualization of scientific progression is an important aspect of evidence-based practice.

REFERENCES

1. Burns N, Grove SK: *The practice of nursing research,* ed 5, St Louis, 2005, Elsevier.
2. Munro BH: *Statistical methods for health care research,* ed 5, Philadelphia, 2006, Lippincott, Williams & Wilkins.

CHAPTER 4

The Provider-Patient Relationship

Terry Mahan Buttaro and JoAnn Trybulski

The purpose of primary care is to encourage wellness, prevent illness, treat chronic disease, and provide palliative care. The majority of primary care visits provide treatment for minor problems or continuing care for chronic diseases. Often, however, the chief complaint is not the real problem. Careful listening in a supportive environment can help identify the unique health care needs of each individual patient. Since many of our patients are from diverse cultural and ethnic backgrounds, it is also necessary for primary health care providers to work collaboratively with medical interpreters to deliver culturally sensitive, holistic care.

Textbooks detail the common symptoms of illness and assemble epidemiologic and diagnostic data to permit swift diagnosis and expeditious treatment. However, health care is not a commodity—it is a relationship between the patient and the provider. Historically this has been an intimate partnership based on caring, respect, and trust, but the changing health care environment has wrought widespread changes. A sizable number of health care providers are employees of large corporations. They are now managers responsible for coordinating care and monitoring referrals and prescriptive practices.

HOLISTIC CARE

Caring, sensitive providers understand that patients are more than the sum of their physiologic systems. This belief underlies the concept of holism. The holistic approach to a patient recognizes and incorporates the complex interactions among the biologic, psychologic, sociologic, and spiritual dimensions in every encounter. The holistic approach also considers the patient to be part of a larger entity, a family and a community. Holistic providers value each individual's reality of health, health beliefs, health practices, and values.[1]

THE HEALTH CARE PROVIDER

In the current health care milieu there is an urgent need for health care providers to do what they have done so capably for hundreds of years: care for the sick, support their families and friends, and provide education about health. Patients need to feel connected to their provider and know that each infirmity and each anxiety is heard with compassion. Providers must advocate for their patients, ensure high-quality care, and assist patients in the negotiation of a confusing health care network. All health care disciplines must collaborate to develop plans for care and programs that promote well-being and acknowledge each individual's worth.

All these functions are components of the provider-patient relationship. In addition, certain provider attributes are important. The first is attentiveness, or the ability to thoughtfully listen and observe. The second is respect for the patient as an individual and for his or her belief system. The third is humility, or that quality of recognizing one's strengths and limitations. The final quality is fortitude, or enduring courage in the face of opposition.

Provider-patient relationships that incorporate the characteristics of respect, trust, and caring will be therapeutic and fruitful. Providers who approach relationships with patients from this perspective will increase their effectiveness as health care providers and enhance the quality of their patient interactions.

THE PATIENT ENCOUNTER

Time management has become an essential requirement in medical practice today. The key to efficiency is focus. Distractions must be kept to a minimum; the provider's focus is the patient. A quiet room is crucial to encourage patients to relate their concerns and anxieties. An accurate clinical picture is imperative and is achieved by obtaining a complete history and understanding the patient's family role, work environment, spirituality, social supports, and psychologic profile.

The history is usually obtained first. The physical examination is based on the patient's complaint, and the history can be obtained after the examination. The history should be reviewed with the patient for clarification. Providers must assess a patient's eating, sleeping, and elimination habits, as well as any personal life or work stress for the effect these may have on a patient's situation. Experience demonstrates that patients return for care until they are satisfied with their management options or until their problem is resolved. If patients are comfortable that their concerns have been addressed, corporate cost-containment and time-efficiency goals may be achieved by eliminating unnecessary tests and visits.

ENCOUNTERS WITH MEDICAL INTERPRETATION

Increasingly, providers and patients may not share English as their primary language. Health care providers should assess each patient for English proficiency. When a patient has limited English proficiency, providers need to collaborate with an interpreter. Ideally, trained medical interpreters should be used. However, these may not be available or patients may prefer to have only a trusted family member present during their interaction with their health care provider. When trained medical interpreters are not available, options include telephone interpreting services, interpreters who may be shared with other providers or clinics, community-based resources, or volunteers with language fluency from local universities.[2] Bilingual employees can be used; the provider should consult state health laws concerning who may act as a medical interpreter.[3] See Box 4-1 for tips on working successfully with bilingual staff members as interpreters.

Before discharge, providers should have the patient or his or her family members restate any care instructions, follow-up times, and signs and symptoms that necessitate a call or return to the clinic or office. This is to ensure that the discharge instructions are clearly understood. When medications are prescribed, providers should give written information in the patient's preferred language and ask the patient or family member to state the name, dose, frequency, route, and length of time to use the medicine. The ability of the patient or family to describe potential adverse signs or symptoms and the appropriate action to take is also essential.[2]

BOX 4-1

WORKING WITH BILINGUAL STAFF MEMBERS AS INTERPRETERS

- Check state laws to ensure that staff members can provide interpretation services.
- Preview what the general topics will be with the interpreter before entering the patient's room.
- Introduce the interpreter; make certain the patient is comfortable with the interpreter.
- Face the patient, and address questions to the patient, not the staff member.
- Make certain the staff member uses a universal form of the language, not a dialect.
- Monitor the interaction to ensure information is not being filtered by the interpreter.
- Do not interrupt the patient.
- Tell the interpreter to translate everything that is said; redirect the interpreter if you detect extra conversation.

Adapted from Sevilla Matir JF, Willis DR: Using bilingual staff members as interpreters, *Fam Pract Manage* 11(7):34-36, 2004, retrieved from http://www.aafp.org/fpm/20040700/34usin.pdf.

SUMMARY

The provider-patient relationship is a privileged one. The bond between provider and patient is a confidential, intimate relationship rooted in caring and trust and based on mutual respect. Each encounter should inspire confidence. There may be little control over disease progression, but hope and dignity should be sustained. Box 4-2 provides strategies to facilitate interactions between the provider and the patient. Box 4-3 shows online resources.

BOX 4-2

STRATEGIES TO ENHANCE PROVIDER-PATIENT INTERACTIONS

- Always introduce yourself and shake hands.
- Allow the patient to remain in street clothes during the initial contact; this may make him or her feel more comfortable.
- Sit at eye level with the patient to facilitate eye contact.
- Begin the encounter by inquiring how you may help the patient.
- Be focused. Keep distractions to a minimum.
- Be committed to the patient by listening.
- Do not allow provider prejudices to affect the relationship.
- Allow patient participation in planning therapeutic interventions; this is critical.
- Provide an opportunity for follow-up.
- Close the encounter by asking if the patient has any other concerns.

BOX 4-3

ONLINE RESOURCES

Language Line Services: http://www.languageline.com
National Council on Interpreting in Health Care: http://www.ncihc.org

REFERENCES

1. Frisch NC: Standards for holistic nursing practice: a way to think about our care that includes complementary and alternative modalities, *Online J Issues Nurs* 6(2), 2001, retrieved from http://www.nursingworld.org/ojin/topic15/tpc15_4.htm.
2. Flores G: Language barrier, *Morbid Mortal Rounds Web,* retrieved May 2006 from http://www.webmm.ahrq.gov/printview.aspx?caseID=123.
3. Sevilla Matir JF, Willis DR: Using bilingual staff members as interpreters, *Fam Pract Manage* 11(7):34-36, 2004, retrieved 12/2/06 from http://www.aafp.org/fpm/20040700/34usin.pdf.

CHAPTER 5

Ethical Analysis and Decision Making in Primary Care

Patricia A. White

Health care providers in today's health care system continue to find themselves in clinical situations that involve ethical conflict. Increasing role responsibilities for advanced practice nurses have generated a need for leadership in identifying and managing clinical situations that involve ethical issues and conflicts. Changes in the health care delivery system have created an environment in which ethical dilemmas are more likely to occur, posing difficult choices for patients and providers. Managed care and the availability of technologic interventions add to the complexity of these dilemmas. To advocate for patients in this health care environment, health care providers need to be well informed about ethical principles and analysis.

This chapter presents a brief overview of the types of ethical dilemmas faced by health care providers and the ethical principles involved. Contemporary ethical theories that predominate in the health care delivery environment are also outlined. An approach to analyzing situations that involve ethical dilemmas is provided along with a discussion of ethical principles and how they are used in such analyses. Finally, the role of health care providers as ethical decision makers is reinforced, with suggestions for an advanced role in the practice arena and in the larger health care delivery system.

ETHICAL PRINCIPLES

Ethical dilemmas in clinical situations occur when the perspectives of patients and providers differ regarding the approach to complicated clinical scenarios. Patients and providers often have varied perspectives of the same clinical situation. Patients' values and priorities often differ from those of providers as they view the dilemmas from the perspective of their own life histories and current health status. Patients and providers also differ in their adherence to various ethical principles.

Essential Principles

The major ethical principles to consider when ethical dilemmas arise are autonomy, beneficence, nonmaleficence, fidelity, justice, and veracity.[1]

Autonomy is considered an essential ethical principle because it refers to an individual's right to make health care decisions. Federal and state laws and regulations protect the right of all citizens to exert autonomy unless an individual is deemed incompetent by the legal system. Many ethical dilemmas arise in relation to this principle, since a patient's right to decide often conflicts with a family member's or health care provider's wishes to protect the patient from harm or to prolong his or her life through medical means. Family members often struggle with a loved one's decision to forgo what might be lifesaving treatment.

Justice, fidelity, and veracity are ethical principles that health care providers use to guide their professional interactions. When health care providers treat all with respect and address their patient's health care needs, they are following the principle of justice. Adherence to the principle of fidelity mandates that health care providers honor their commitments, while adherence to veracity compels health care providers to tell the truth and not be deceptive.[1]

Providers also remain faithful to the ethical principles of beneficence and nonmaleficence when they act on behalf of patients' wishes and try to protect patients from harm. Adherence to these principles is commendable but is sometimes seen as paternalistic. Concerns also arise in adherence to these principles when a patient makes a decision that may affect his or her safety. Careful identification of the principles involved allows everyone a voice and an opportunity to identify sometimes worthy but competing principles.

Patient and Provider Perspectives

Researchers have examined the perspectives of patients regarding ethical dilemmas. Pinch and Parsons[2] studied the older population's views about dilemmas regarding end-of-life decisions. They discovered that patients rely heavily on provider input when making health care decisions. Spielman[3] identified the ethical dilemmas that arise when caring for older adults with dementia, who often are unable to express their wishes yet need to be respected as individuals. This research is critical for clarifying patients' perspectives, which often are not considered when decisions are made. Patients' reliance on provider input, as illustrated in this research, highlights the care and responsibility inherent in providers' roles as advocates for clients. Vulnerable populations are particularly at risk of not having their views well represented when difficult and life-changing decisions are made.

Providers have varied personal views and professional experience, including adherence to their professional codes of ethics. The code of ethics of the American Nurses Association (ANA) requires nurses to consider the consequences of their ethical decisions and ethical principles.[4] Nurses are obligated to demonstrate respect for human dignity and the uniqueness of the individual. The 2001 ANA code of ethics provides additional perspectives for adherence to principles grounded in nursing's long tradition and commitment to ethical practice. This updated code of ethics builds on the old code by reiterating the nurse's obligation to uphold the patient's dignity, worth, and uniqueness. The 2001 code highlights the need to extend this respect to colleagues, employees, and students, and it emphasizes respect for dignity as a fundamental principle.

Another fundamental value identified in the code of ethics is protection of patients, particularly concerning their right to privacy. The code also delineates the nurse's responsibility to protect patients from the negligent practice of colleagues that is deemed illegal, incompetent, or unethical. Furthermore, this revised code underscores nurses' obligation to maintain professional competency and contribute to knowledge development through research. The code also addresses workplace conditions, with an emphasis on identifying a work environment that is conducive to safe practice as an important right of the profession. In addition, the code accentuates the nurse's responsibility to maintain the integrity of the profession by advocating for the protection of the public from deceptive advertising and false claims from any source. Finally, the code advocates health promotion through nurses' support of public health initiatives and support of policy that positively affects access to care and social change.

ETHICAL DILEMMAS

Providers and patients often differ in their approach to health care decisions because they highlight certain ethical principles over others. Specific examples of ethical dilemmas include providers' concerns about patient safety conflicting with patients' perspectives regarding their right to autonomy in decision making about health-related issues. Ethical conflicts also arise when patients and family members disagree about what ought to be done in a particular health care situation.

Providers often experience conflict when environmental constraints such as insurance regulations or practice policies dictate an approach that conflicts with adherence to specific ethical principles. The ethical principle of justice, which emphasizes doing the most good for the most people, often conflicts with the desire to assist individuals in their access to certain types of care. Managed care regulations often dictate which treatment a patient should receive based on data suggesting that monies might be better spent on providing a preventive approach to more patients. Concerns arise in settings when capitation practices allow only a certain number of visits to specialists but a patient or provider believes that additional services are warranted.

Clarifying the principles that both the provider and patient consider significant is important when analyzing scenarios that involve ethical dilemmas. The following section identifies the two major traditions in ethical theory in which consideration of ethical principles takes place.

Ethical Theories

Current tension in the field of ethics stems from a belief in persons as rational and individualistic, in contrast to a belief that persons exist in relation to others. Waithe[5] describes the historical view of the justice- and virtue-based traditions that underpin the current tension between the person-centered view and the worldview of individuals as principled and independent. The justice-based, or principle-based, tradition emphasizes adherence to principles as primary in the analysis of ethical dilemmas. The virtue-based, or care-based, tradition not only emphasizes care and concern for others but also considers the particulars of a clinical situation as primary in the analysis of a case.[6]

The polarization of these two traditions has continued to dominate current ethical theory. Fry, Killen, and Robinson[7] speak of the importance of discovering ways to reconcile these two traditions; the goal is the consideration of ethical principles in relation to the patient's situation. The consideration of ethical principles in a clinical situation with ethical dilemmas most often needs to take into account the contextual features of the patient care situation. Considering the ethical principles involved with this contextual approach can bring the best of both traditions to discussions of compelling and difficult dilemmas.

ANALYSIS OF ETHICAL DILEMMAS

The analysis of ethical dilemmas requires a thoughtful approach to each case presentation. Veatch and Fry[8] pose four questions that can be used as a guide to analysis. The first question involves distinguishing between moral and nonmoral evaluations and determining who ought to decide the outcome of a clinical scenario. The second question concerns what types of acts are right and requires consideration of the principles involved in the dilemma and how to balance the principles of the parties involved. The third question involves how the rules or principles apply to the specific situation. The application of the principles is a central feature of ethical conflict, since the principles themselves are often competing. How people interpret and view principles is often a concern, since some view principles as guides to behavior without regard to context. The fourth question involves what should be done in a particular situation. This stage is the culmination of ethical analysis and should be entered only after careful conideration of all perspectives. These four questions can be used as a guide to decide if ethical dilemmas and conflict do exist.

RESEARCH IN NURSING ETHICS

Although the understanding and practice of ethics have derived mostly from the previously reviewed ethical theories and principles, research in nursing suggests we need to be more mindful of ethical practice as embodied in the everyday experiences of nurses, patients, and other health care providers. A number of studies have yielded important information in deciphering the nature of ethical dilemmas that arise in the "everydayness" of practice. Varcoe, Doane, Pauly, and colleagues[9] studied the ethical experiences of nurses working in a variety of settings. Through focus groups, the researchers found that nurses act as moral agents on behalf of patients in very contextual ways. In addition to working with patients and families when ethical issues and dilemmas arise, nurses also reported the tension involved in working in environments where their values were not always supported. Resource constraints, the dominance of physicians in health care setting, the deference paid to physicians, and the lack of leadership for guidance in ethically difficult circumstances were all cited as issues that often compromised their ability to act as moral agents. Further research is suggested that addresses the shifting environment in which nurses practice and the effect it has on their ability to practice as moral agents.

Enes and de Vries[10] studied ethical issues faced by 135 registered nurses caring for terminally ill older adults in nursing homes and community hospital settings in the United Kingdom. Results from this study demonstrated that the ethical issues of most concern involved preparation for death and the need for patients and families to maintain bonds through illness and the end of life. The areas of ethical conflict or difficulty identified by the nurses surveyed centered on the quality of the elderly patients' death. The nurses identified decisions about treatment and who should make these decisions as areas where conflicts frequently arose. It is interesting to note that nurses identified ethical dilemmas and classified them as either issues or conflicts. Nurses expect issues to arise. However, when identifying conflicts and dilemmas, nurses seem to believe that more education and support regarding end-of-life and palliative care for patients, families, and physicians would assist in making these ethical issues less conflictual. Ongoing concern on the part of nurses in this study in terms of conflicts with physicians is consistent with research in the United States. The need for more efforts to professionalize the relationships between physicians and nurses is paramount, as this tension and conflict add to the environmental stressors nurses cite as creating environments not conducive to ethical practice.

Smith[11] identified ethical issues most often cited by older adults. The most interesting finding is that older adults identify attentiveness to their needs and respect for their persons in everyday interactions as their major ethical concerns. Although major ethical issues dominate much writing and discussion about ethics and health care, patients identify issues that are less dramatic yet highlight their needs and concerns relative to preserving their dignity as they age. Although the study was a small pilot study, it provides important perspectives about patients' identification and definition of ethical concerns.

HEALTH CARE PROVIDERS AS ETHICAL DECISION MAKERS

Health care providers have many leadership opportunities as thoughtful decision makers about the ethical dilemmas that arise in their settings. Using knowledge of the nature of ethical dilemmas and analyzing situations as outlined in this chapter will provide guidelines for this process. Future research needs to consider more carefully the experience of patients involved in ethical dilemmas. There must also be a careful analysis of the types of conflicts and dilemmas as seen from this most important perspective. Research needs to outline the providers' perspective in ethical dilemmas and should determine how environmental factors affect decision making. Particular attention needs to be given to vulnerable populations, whose voice is often not heard when ethical dilemmas arise. Involving patients in decision making and providing a voice for the vulnerable should be at the heart of providers' concerns when ethical dilemmas arise.

As additional research highlights ongoing ethical dilemmas and approaches, advanced practice nurses can continue to bring to their role important reflections regarding ethics. Ethics advisory boards are one way to ensure that a forum exists for providers to discuss and deliberate ethical dilemmas. An interdisciplinary group with community representation can provide an important mechanism to discuss and consider these issues. Clarification of important ethical issues can be a useful outcome of case presentations to advisory boards. Ensuring that a patient has a health care proxy is another way to address patient perspectives and wishes if his or her decision-making capacity becomes impaired.

Patients and health care providers will benefit from thoughtful ethical analysis and decision making. Clarification of the principles involved for both can contribute to patient well-being and professional satisfaction. Future research will assist in the use of principles within the context of compelling clinical situations. Continued clarification of the perspectives of both providers and patients will also assist health care providers in their roles as ethical decision makers.

ETHICAL ISSUES IN HUMAN EXPERIMENTATION AND RESEARCH

The history of medical progress is, to a large extent, the history of medical experimentation. Human experimentation and research are based on the philosophy that no patient is ever under any obligation to participate in research.[12] The process of research and human experimentation occurs when the health care provider departs from standard medical practice to obtain new, generalizable knowledge or to test a hypothesis using the scientific method.[12,13]

The ethics of human experimentation and the research process are based on the tenets of the Nuremberg Code, written in 1947 after the trial of Nazi physicians for crimes against humanity. The Nuremberg Code addresses the boundaries of human experimentation on the basis of 10 principles. The first principle states that "the voluntary consent of the human subject is absolutely essential." Implicit in voluntary consent is the requirement that the individual not only have the legal capacity to provide consent but also have sufficient knowledge and comprehension of the choices available in the health care process.

The nine other principles of the Nuremberg Code address facets of the research process, including the benefits of research to society; the study design and its basis in the natural history of a disease; and the avoidance of physical injury and harm, death, or disability during the experimental process. These principles also state that the degree of experimental risk should not exceed the humanitarian importance of the problem, that scientifically qualified persons must conduct the experiment, that the patient may choose to end participation at any time in the research process, and that the researcher must terminate the research process if untoward effects related to the experiment occur.

Within any health care organization, the institutional review board (IRB) is responsible for the review and oversight of proposed research. The role of the IRB is to review research protocols and protect human subjects. Review of informed consent related to any research study is a major function of the IRB. Specific requirements addressed by the IRB in the review relate to minimization of risks, the balance of risks with the anticipated benefits of the research, careful consideration of the selection of human subjects in the study design, and the requirement for obtaining informed consent.

REFERENCES

1. Beauchamp TL, Childress JF: *Principles of biomedical ethics,* ed 4, New York, 1994, Oxford University Press.
2. Pinch WJ, Parsons ME: The ethics of treatment decision making: the elderly patient's perspective, *Geriatr Nurs* 14(6):289-293, 1993.
3. Spielman K: Demented residents' right to refuse treatment, *Clin Excell Nurse Pract* 1(6):376-381, 1997.
4. American Nurses Association: *Code of ethics with interpretative statements,* Silver Spring, Md, 2001, The Association.
5. Waithe ME: Twenty three hundred years of women philosophers: toward a gender undifferentiated moral theory. In Brabeck MM, editor: *Who cares? Theory, research and educational implications of the ethic of care,* Westport, Conn, 1989, Praeger.
6. Cooper MC: Principle-oriented ethics and the ethic of care: a creative tension, *Adv Nurs Sci* 14(2):22-31, 1991.
7. Fry ST, Killen AR, Robinson EM: Care based reasoning, caring and the ethic of care: a need for clarity, *J Clin Ethics* 7(1):41-47, 1996.
8. Veatch RM, Fry ST: Four questions of ethics. In Veatch RM, Fry ST, editors: *Case studies in nursing ethics,* Boston, 1995, Jones & Bartlett.
9. Varcoe C, Doane G, Pauly B, and others. Ethical practice in nursing: working the in-betweens, *J Adv Nurs* 45(3):316-325, 2004.
10. Enes P, de Vries K: A survey of ethical issues experienced by nurses caring for terminally ill people, *Nurs Ethics* 11(2):150-164, 2004.
11. Smith KV: Ethical issues related to health care: the older adult's perspective, *J Gerontol Nurs* 31(2):32-39, 2005.
12. Annas GJ: *The rights of patients,* ed 2, Carbondale, Ill, 1989, Southern Illinois University Press.
13. Munson R: *Intervention and reflection: basic issues in medical ethics,* ed 5, New York, 1996, Wadsworth.

CHAPTER 6

Population-Based Health Care and the Role of the Advanced Practice Nurse

Rosemary F. Hall

Population-based nursing and the role of the advanced nurse practitioner are integral components of health promotion and disease prevention. Primary care practice emphasizes risk assessment, health maintenance, health promotion, and disease prevention through health education, behavioral change, and preventive treatment for individuals, whereas the focus of population-based nursing care is to target groups and improve the health of the whole community.[1] In population-based health care, the advanced nurse practitioner must take an active role at the primary or secondary level of intervention to focus on community health by addressing populations, health care systems, and geographic areas as a target of practice. The focus of practice is not removed from the individual but is directed to health promotion and disease prevention in populations to prevent illness and/or reduce its devastating effects.[2] The importance of population-based care is bolstered by changing demographics, escalating health care costs, health insurance inadequacies, new and re-emerging communicable diseases, the increasing incidence and prevalence of chronic diseases, health disparities, environmental concerns, and lifestyle behaviors.

The impetus for population-based care is in part related to the mandate of *Healthy People 2010*[3] to engage health care providers, health care systems, and communities to promote health and enhance quality of life. However, the fact that 97% of health care dollars are spent on secondary and tertiary prevention also suggests that curative care is not the answer.[2] To control health care costs and improve the nation's health, care needs to be directed to populations with an emphasis on primary prevention.

POPULATION-BASED HEALTH CARE

The population-based approach to health care refers to care provided to groups of human beings, who may be well or sick, indigent or nonindigent. It may be limited to a defined geographic location, a defined population (or entire populations in a geographic location), an organization, or a group of individuals or aggregate of people with at least one defining common characteristic (e.g., a group of pregnant adolescents). The focus of the population-based approach encompasses health promotion, disease prevention, primary care, public health, and the overall, overarching state of health. The interventions in population-based health care are group specific, reflecting the culture and health needs of the individuals in the population group.

The population-based health care approach starts with primary prevention then proceeds to secondary and tertiary prevention. It encompasses case finding, collection of health status data, analysis of data, and development of efficient primary interventions at the population level. In essence, the population-based approach to care is an organizational framework that focuses on illness prevention and health promotion specific to disease dissemination and health determinants.[2,4,5] Box 6-1 contains questions to help determine what the health care needs may be in a population.

BOX 6-1

QUESTIONS TO DETERMINE HEALTH CARE ISSUES IN A POPULATION

- What major health problems or potential health issues are present?
- What populations are at the greatest risk?
- Are health care risks or people with a specific health care risk geographically distributed?
- What services are available to address the health care issues?
- If the services are available, what is the level of quality?
- How do community organizations or citizens view the health needs of the community?
- What is the history of the community's collaborative process to work together to address the health issues?

COMMUNITY-BASED NURSING CARE

The community-based approach to nursing is often confused with the population-based approach, yet there is a distinct difference between the two. Community-based nursing refers to a philosophy of care given to individuals and families wherever they are.[6] The care may be where they live, play, or go to school; however, the focus of care is family centered. In community-based nursing the nurse provides care to help individuals and their families achieve common goals in managing acute or chronic conditions to promote health.[6] The nurse may be the direct caregiver, assessing and prioritizing needs, acting as an educator and counselor, and assisting with referrals and follow-up care.

With population- and community-based nursing care, the roles do overlap. The difference is that population-based care focuses on aggregate groups and community-based care focuses primarily on individuals and families in communities. Population-based care emphasizes health promotion and primary prevention, whereas community-based care generally focuses on tertiary care issues such as access and curative care services.

PRINCIPLES OF POPULATION-BASED CARE

The principles of population-based care are derived from the principles of public health and community health nursing. Public health practice is at the forefront of population-based health care. In the 1988 report *The Future of Public Health Practice,* the Institute of Medicine stated, "Public health in combination with nursing practice is a unique field created to focus on the health of population groups."[7] This report defined the core functions of public health as assessment, policy development, and assurance (links within the community to health services, assurance that health care providers are competent, and evaluation of the health services for access, effectiveness, and quality of policy compliance). In addition, the Quad Council consisting of four organizations—the American Nurses Association (ANA), the Association of Community Health Nursing Educators, the American Public Health Association, and the Association of State and Territorial Directors of Nursing—endorses these functions within nursing and the standard and scope of public health.[4]

ROLE OF THE ADVANCED PRACTICE NURSE IN POPULATION-BASED CARE

Advanced practice nurses are in a primary position to institute a population-based approach to improve health care for the groups they serve. The following three attributes of advanced practice nurses contribute to their important role in population-based health care:

1. Educational preparation that includes knowledge of epidemiology, public health, cultural competence, health determinants, and health disparities
2. The integration of nursing process into the public health core functions of assessment, development of health policy, and assurance
3. The ANA's Standards of Care for Advanced Practice, which include the obligation to perform a holistic assessment of mind and body focusing on the social, psychologic, physical, and environmental entities that contribute to health promotion and illness prevention

The advanced practice nurse practicing in a primary care setting is in a unique position to understand the populations being served, including the demographics of those seeking care and the major reasons for seeking care. The advanced practice nurse also has the ability to case find, conduct disease prevalence assessment, and monitor the trajectory of diseases and other health-related conditions. He or she is aware of the available community resources, the appropriate community contacts, and the critical community stakeholders and their willingness to participate in health ventures to promote health and prevent illness. Therefore the advanced practice nurse is in a pivotal position to promote population-based health through the following:

- Conduct surveys to determine what patients seeking care would like addressed for health promotion and prevention.
- Collaborate with health care professionals in the primary setting to assess the needs of the population served.
- Work with administrators to provide time for community outreach in park or recreational settings and housing developments, using the health survey previously mentioned.
- Use an interdisciplinary approach to address population needs.[8]
- Attend community meetings to establish a partnership with community members to assist with population-based health promotion.
- Design community-level interventions to address the health needs of the community.

DISEASE PREVENTION, HEALTH PROMOTION, AND PREVENTION LEVEL–SPECIFIC INTERVENTIONS

Disease prevention and health promotion are fundamental concepts in population-based care, yet these are two distinct concepts. Disease prevention is the step or interventions designed to prevent the development of disease or its related consequences.[9] Health promotion activities are related to lifestyle behaviors and are concerned with promoting or improving health. Pender further relates that health promotion constitutes "behaviors directed toward increasing the level of well-being and actualizing the health potential of individuals, families, communities, and society."[10] Disease prevention and health promotion are strategies designed to increase physical, social, and emotional health and well-being of individuals, families, and communities.[2]

Intertwined within disease prevention and health promotion are interventions developed for primary, secondary, and tertiary prevention at the individual, family, and community level. Some activities or strategies for primary prevention are health education and counseling, immunizations, and occupational injury prevention programs. Actions specific to secondary prevention, or the early diagnosis and treatment of disease, include health screenings, community assessment, and health care for early treatment of disease. Tertiary prevention, or interventions designed to prevent complications of a disease, may include public availability of treatment programs such as physical therapy or mental health therapy. These combined levels of intervention are used by community members, leaders, and stakeholders working collaboratively to promote a community's well-being.

MODELS OF POPULATION-BASED CARE

The concept of population-based health care is not new. Health care providers have long explored effective strategies to deliver population-based care. Successful models for population-based care include the public health nursing practice model, the community-oriented primary care model, and the community as partner model.

Public Health Nursing Practice Model

The public health nursing practice model of primary health care is specific to health promotion and disease prevention for population health. This model encompasses six steps to guide population-based care and provide evidence of the quality of services provided.[11] The standards follow the practice delineated by the Quad Council and encompass the core functions of public health. The six specific steps in the public health nursing practice model are assessment, diagnosis, outcome identification, planning, assurance, and evaluation (Box 6-2).[12]

Community-Oriented Primary Care Model

The model of community-oriented primary care (COPC) was developed in rural South Africa by two African physicians, Sidney and Emily Kark.[13] These two physicians were challenged to establish a system of health care to treat illness and to work with tribal leaders of South Africa. They brought tribal leaders together to develop strategies that would engage community outreach workers in population assessment and design of effective health promotion and primary prevention activities.

Following their work in South Africa, the Karks joined the Hebrew University in Israel and began teaching clinicians, public health workers, and epidemiologists, blending the

BOX 6-2

STEPS IN THE PUBLIC HEALTH NURSING PRACTICE MODEL

1. **Assessment:** The assessment step involves careful analysis of existing data about population health, knowledge of and analysis of health resources in the community or outlying community, identification of potential or actual health problems needing immediate attention, and identification of barriers to ensure that health services are available.
2. **Diagnosis:** After the assessment step, a community diagnosis can be developed. This mechanism provides the basis for establishing a surveillance system to monitor the health risks or hazards of early identification or actual problem present.
3. **Outcome identification:** With other community partners, outcome objectives are established to develop strategies to address the identified problem.
4. **Planning:** The primary purpose of this step is the continuous assessment of the programs, services, and policies present. Planning provides the visual picture of what is available and what is still needed to ensure that interventions are present to address actual or potential health problems.
5. **Assurance:** This is the ongoing process of having a network of competent community providers available to link aggregate populations with the services needed outside the primary community setting.
6. **Evaluation:** This involves the careful assessment of the health status of populations, addressing morbidity, mortality, health risks, and improvement of health conditions.

Adapted from Quad Council of Public Health Nursing Organizations: *Scope and standards of public health nursing practice.* Washington, DC, 1999, American Nurse Publishing.

BOX 6-3

EXAMPLE OF COMMUNITY-ORIENTED PRIMARY CARE MODEL INTERVENTION FOR DIABETIC PATIENTS IN A PRIMARY CARE PRACTICE

1. Identify all individuals in the practice with diabetes, and collect demographic data and geographic mapping of the patients.
2. Hold a meeting with this diabetic patient group, and ask the group what they believe their needs are.
3. Use the information from the diabetic group meeting to assess the effectiveness of current services. Develop programs the group expressed an interest in, such as exercise and self-monitoring of blood glucose classes.
4. To reach out to the community, the clinicians in the community-oriented primary care intervention model practice should reach out to the network of health care practitioners from other primary settings and encourage meetings with other groups of diabetic patients in the community to establish useful programs.

principles of primary care and public health. Over the half century since then, their philosophy of care has spread into England, Israel, Spain, the U.S. Indian Health Service, and other parts of the United States. HMOs, major universities, physicians, nurses, social workers, and community leaders have embraced this philosophy and model of care.

This innovative blending of public health and primary care delivery fulfills the concept of population-based care as it focuses on health determinants of populations, as well as primary prevention and health promotion approaches for disease prevention for the systematic improvement in quality of care.[14-16] In essence, COPC is a mechanism that engages the community as active partners in making decisions that improve the health of the entire community. COPC is an interactive framework that defines and characterizes the community, identifies community health problems, develops interventions, and monitors the impact of the interventions.[17]

The role of the health care provider in the COPC model is to redirect thinking from the focus of the individual unit of care to the community approach and to envision patients as members of a population.[18] The first stage in this process is to look at active users and nonusers within the setting, using epidemiology to identify those at risk and to monitor incidence and prevalence of disease morbidity and mortality. The second step is to assess the health risks and actual patterns of disease within the community. The final phase is to engage multiple community and health professional participants with a wide range of skills to provide community outreach through the development of intervention programs (see Box 6-3 for an example of a COPC intervention in practice). For success, it is important to engage community leaders, health care providers, and patient groups in the community.

Community as Partner Model of Care

Community assessment is a framework to guide the health care provider in assessment, analysis, planning, implementation, and evaluation of communities or populations. In this model, assessment involves a critical evaluation of the strengths, resources, and level of functioning of community members to identify gaps, barriers, and forthcoming needs. There are many models for assessment; however, the community as partner (CAP) model[19] uses the nursing process, thus providing explicit direction for advanced practice nurses to determine the uniqueness and intricacies of populations in communities they are serving.

The CAP model (Box 6-4) essentially uses the steps of nursing process that emphasize primary prevention, community participation, and partnership building. The model is composed of the eight subsystems of a community in conjunction with the community core, or the sense of the community as a whole. The eight subsystems of the CAP model are physical environment, education, safety and transportation, politics and government, health and social services, communication, economics, and recreation. When performing a community assessment, health care providers ascertain the status of each of these subsystems.[19]

The community core is composed of those dimensions of the community which are "essential, basic, and enduring."[19] Critical community dimensions—structure, status, and process—are aspects of this community core and form the characteristic picture of the overall health of the people of the community.

The structure dimension is the availability and adequacy of services and resources specific to demographic statistics of a community. The dimension of community status has physical, emotional, and social components. Examples of the physical components are morbidity and mortality statistics, life-expectancy indexes, and risk profiles. The process dimension

BOX 6-4

COMMUNITY AS PARTNER MODEL FOR POPULATION-BASED CARE INTERVENTIONS

STEP 1: ASSESSMENT

Collect community data.

- Identify the community and assess the community core.
- Assess subsystems: physical environment, education, safety and transportation, politics and government, health and social services, communication, economics, and recreation.
- Assess residents' perceptions and the health care provider's perceptions. Perception data include identification of feelings in the community with a focus on strengths and weaknesses.
- Form partnerships with community groups.

STEP 2: DATA ANALYSIS

Categorize data according to the subsystems. Analyze each for its effect on the population or core.

STEP 3: PRIORITIZATION OF PROBLEMS

Present problem(s) to the community partnership for prioritization.

Questions to assist with prioritization of problems include:

- How aware is the community of the problem?
- Is the community motivated to resolve or better manage the problem?
- Is the provider able to influence the problem situation?
- Are experts available to solve the problem?
- How severe is the outcome if the problem is not addressed?
- How quickly can the problem be addressed?[21]

STEP 4: PLANNING

Develop a community-focused plan that delineates the long-term goal, short-term goals, objectives, and actions (interventions) with projected completion dates.

STEP 5: IMPLEMENTATION

Align intervention activities directly to the goals and objectives according to priority of need. For success, the plan should delineate precise activities and how each activity will be done.

STEP 6: EVALUATION

Critically evaluate the data for effects of the interventions and/or program. Ongoing evaluation allows the partners to diagnose and troubleshoot problems before the program ends and the objectives are not reached.

is the ability of community leaders and organizations (e.g., government, police) to function collaboratively and effectively, intervening with problem-solving mechanisms when presented with actual or potential problems. The ability of the community members, leaders, and stakeholders to collaboratively analyze the dimensions and work together in a flexible, negotiable, and informed manner affects these dimensions. Thus the inclusion of community members in the partnership is critical to achieve the goal of improving the community's health.

PLANNING MODELS FOR PRIMARY PREVENTION INTERVENTIONS

Since primary prevention is the key to improving the health of a population and meeting *Healthy People 2010* goals, models for primary prevention interventions are critical to population-based care. Several frameworks have been found to be useful: the planned approach to community health (PATCH), the PRECEDE-PROCEED model, and the population-based public health nursing interventions wheel.[4,5,20]

PATCH

The PATCH model of care, developed by Centers for Disease Control and Prevention in 1985, provides direction for public health agencies to focus on assessment data of communities and addresses five key aspects specific to program planning.[4] This model can be a guide for the health care provider when addressing problems of an aggregate or population. The model stresses active participation of community members, use of data to determine health priorities, program development based on health priority and resource assessment, evaluation with an emphasis on quality improvement, and education of community members to improve health. In this model, a health care provider can enhance the work of the local health department by working as a partner to provide assessment data (incidence and prevalence of disease and specific needs of the population he or she cares for) and can incorporate designed interventions of the local health department into the primary care setting.

PRECEDE-PROCEED Model

The PRECEDE-PROCEED model is primarily an education model that "is oriented toward outcomes and asks 'Why' before it asks 'How.'"[21] This model is especially useful for the health care provider when designing educational programs for primary prevention. It focuses on the varied factors needed for an effective program. The *PRECEDE* acronym focuses on Predisposing, Reinforcing, Enabling, Causes in, Educational, Diagnosis, and Evaluation. The *PROCEED* acronym focuses on Policy, Regulatory, Organizational, Constructs in, Educational, Environmental, and Development. The emphasis is directed toward designing programs that focus on the uniqueness of the populations as revealed in assessment data; for example, What are the needs of the learner? Using assessment data and unique characteristics of the population, the provider tailors the educational plan to the learner. An especially important piece of the model is asking populations what they see as the need, assessing the environment in which the group lives, working with groups to problem solve to reach ways to adapt health behaviors, and finally, determining whether the needs were met and the behaviors sustained.

Public Health Nursing Intervention Wheel

The public health nursing intervention framework was developed by public health nurses in the Minnesota Department of Health. It began as a search to define what public health nurses do and explain the population-based approach to interventions that contribute to improving health outcomes. The model integrates three levels of care focusing on the individual, community, and health care system.[5,20]

From the seminal work that began in 1994, 17 nursing interventions have been researched and validated as evidence based. The interventions address the core functions of public health and focus on determination of health status of communities. The model addresses intervention at the individual, community, and systems level, an approach that in turn promotes health of populations in their entirety.

The 17 interventions are advocacy, case management, coalition building, collaboration, community organizing, consultation, counseling, delegated medical treatment and observations, disease investigation, health teaching, outreach or case findings, policy development, provider education, referral and follow-up, screening, social marketing, and surveillance. Most of the interventions are familiar to nurses; however, some interventions, such as coalition building, community organizing, social marketing, and policy development, are often not thought about for promoting the health of communities.[20]

SUMMARY

Building healthy communities is the key to population-based health. The advanced practice nurse is an essential collaborator in the formation of healthy communities, focused on the reduction of health disparities and the promotion of the *Healthy People 2010* goals. The advanced practice nurse can promote healthy communities by assuming a leadership role to convene group members, collect data to validate community needs or problems, conduct focus groups, use effective strategies to prevent or reduce conflicts among group members, rank and prioritize problems, address cultural-specific issues, engage others to locate hidden and current community resources, and ascertain the strengths and weaknesses of the community resources. This leadership role is necessary to develop a well-articulated plan with goals, objectives, assigned tasks, and a time line for achievement.

Population-based care extends beyond the individual to address the needs of population groups. Performing population-based care in primary care settings is mandated in today's world of managed care, escalating health care costs, increasing complexity of chronic illnesses and communicable diseases, and emergence of old and new diseases. Population-based care is differentiated from community-based care in that its primary goal is to promote health with primary prevention to groups of people.

REFERENCES

1. Drevdahl D, Dorcy KS, Grevadstad L: Integrating principles of community-centered practice in a community health nursing practicum, *Nurs Educ* 26(5):234-239, 2001.
2. Stanhope M, Lancaster J: *Foundations of community health nursing,* St Louis, 2002, Mosby.
3. US Government Printing Office: *Healthy people 2010,* retrieved Dec 2, 2006, from http://www.healthypeople.gov/Document/.
4. Porsche DJ: *Public and community health nursing practice,* Thousand Oaks, Calif, 2004, Sage Publications.
5. Keller LO, Strohschein MS, Lia-Hoagberg B, and others: Population-based public health interventions: practice based and evidence supported, part 1, *Pub Health Nurs* 21(5):453-468, 2004.
6. Zotti ME, Brown P, Stotts RC: Community-based nursing versus community-health nursing: what does it mean? *Nurs Outlook* 9(10):211-217, 1996.
7. Institute of Medicine: *The future of public health,* Washington, DC, 1988, National Academy Press.
8. Gerrish K: Teamwork in primary care: an evaluation of the contribution of integrated nursing teams, *Health Soc Care Commun* 7(5):367-375, 1999.
9. Thomas S: Caring in community-health nursing. In Hitchcock J, Schubert P, Thomas S, editors: *Community health nursing: caring in action,* Boston, 1999, Delmar.
10. Pender NJ: *Health promotion in nursing practice,* ed 3, Stamford, Conn, 1996, Appleton & Lange.
11. Mondy C, Cardena D, Avila M: The role of the advanced practice public health nurse in bioterrorism preparedness, *Pub Health Nurs* 20(6):422-436, 2003.
12. Quad Council of Public Health Nursing Organizations: *Scope and standards of public health nursing practice,* Washington, DC, 1999, American Nurse Publishing.
13. Mullan F, Epstein L: Community-oriented primary care: new relevance in a changing world, *Am J Pub Health* 92(11):1748-1755, 2002.
14. Nutting PA, Strotz C, Shorr GI: Reduction of gastroenteritis morbidity in high-risk infants [abstract], *Pediatrics* 55:354-358, 1975.
15. Nutting PA, Barrick JE, Logue SC: The impact of a maternal and child health program in the quality of pre-natal care: an analysis by risk group, *J Commun Health* 4:267-279, 1979.
16. Shorr GI, Nutting PA: A population-based assessment of the continuity of ambulatory care, *Med Care* 15:455-464, 1977.
17. Rhyme R, Bogue R, Kukulka G, and others: *Community-oriented primary care: health care for the 21st century,* Washington, DC, 2005, American Public Health Association.
18. Overall NA, Williamson J: *Community-oriented primary care in action: a practice manual for primary care settings,* Berkeley, Calif, 1984, University of California at Berkeley.
19. Anderson ET, McFarlane J: *Community as partner: theory and practice in nursing,* ed 3, Philadelphia, 2004, Lippincott, Williams & Wilkins.
20. Keller LO, Strohschein S, Lia-Hoagberg B, and others: Population-based public health nursing interventions: a model from practice, *Pub Health Nurs* 15(30):207-215, 1998.
21. Stanhope M, Lancaster J: *Foundations of nursing in the community*, St Louis, 2006, Mosby.

CHAPTER 7

Chronic Disease Management Teams

Rosemary F. Hall

Despite sophisticated medical technology, the incidence of chronic disease continues to rise, especially in people 65 years and older. Living with a condition for longer than 6 months that is not curable causes ongoing physical, psychosocial, and financial hardships for individuals, families, and populations. Health care systems also experience the burden of chronic illnesses, as these disorders contribute to rising health care costs. Studies show that prevention of emergency department visits and rehospitalization for chronic and acute illness is necessary to reduce these escalating costs, which account for about 70% of overall health spending.[1] However, any initiatives to reduce health care costs must also incorporate measures to reduce the longitudinal effects of chronic disease and its associated burdens.

Escalating costs of chronic illness, specifically arthritis, cardiovascular disease, diabetes, asthma, and mental illness, have forced public and private health care systems (managed care companies, employers, Medicaid, and Medicare) to embrace the concept of chronic disease management. Chronic disease management involves sometimes complex health interventions to treat chronic disease exacerbations; reduce severity of illness; prolong symptom-free periods; and promote quality of life for the individual, family, and community.

Chronic disease management teams are organizations of health care providers (physicians, nurses, social workers, educators, pharmacists, and trained community workers) who collaborate effectively to execute evidence-based treatment guidelines for populations. The goal of chronic disease teams is to institute a holistic approach to care and achieve better chronic disease outcomes. In a chronic disease management team, health care providers, trained community health workers, and the individual patient and his or her family collaborate to reduce the devastation and long-term effects of chronic disease. The chronic disease management team members collaborate to ensure that interventions are evidence based and effective in achieving the goals of disease self-management, health maintenance, health promotion, and disease prevention.

The interdisciplinary team selects a disease manager or leader with expert clinical skills and leadership. This leader, often an advanced practice nurse, is the catalyst within the disease management team. The team provides more than case management; team members deliver health care for individuals with chronic illness to diminish the symptoms associated with the illness, enhance activity, and increase independence to promote health and quality of life.

CASE MANAGEMENT, CARE MANAGEMENT, AND DISEASE MANAGEMENT

Case management, care management, and *disease management* (DM) are terms that often overlap or are not understood. To enhance understanding and eliminate confusion, a brief overview of the three approaches is provided. Fundamental to understanding each term is the role of nursing and the importance of educational preparation for these roles.[1]

Case Management

Case management and *care management* are terms used interchangeably to describe patient care management on discharge from an acute setting to a rehabilitation setting to home. The Case Management Society of America and the National Case Management Task Force[2] definition of case management is "a process of care that engages a case manager, who participates in a collaboration process, which assesses, plans, implements, coordinates, monitors, and evaluates the options and services required to meet an individual's health needs using communication and available resources to promote quality, cost-effective outcomes."[2,3] Stanhope and Lancaster address the process similarly but describe it as a nursing function of advocacy and case management to provide uninterrupted access to health care delivery that responds to an individual's health care needs.[4]

Care Management

Care management is a part of case management, but the focus of care is shifted. Providers who perform care management monitor the health status, resources, and outcomes of an "aggregate," or "a targeted segment of a population or a group of human beings with at least one common characteristic."[4]

Comparison: Case Management vs. Care Management

From assessment to evaluation, nursing process is the integral component of case management. The focus is on the patient as the center of care. The case manager incorporates nursing process in many roles (broker, consultant, coordinator, educator, etc.) and must have clinical experience and an understanding of financial management systems and care resources. The case manager works closely with insurance providers, monitoring costs to ensure the provision of high-quality care in an efficient manner. An example of case management, as outlined by Aubert, Herman, Waters, and colleagues, addresses the role of the advanced practice nurse working *individually* with patients on lifestyle and medication changes in the management of diabetes.[5]

Case management is traditionally directed to the individual, whereas care management commonly occurs in a community setting. A notable example is the model of care for the aggregate of elders enrolled in Medicare and HMOs at St. Mary's Hospital in Tucson, Arizona. In this model the care manager directs health care services provided to individuals in a home setting, embracing assessment, counseling, education, individual health care planning, and linkage to community resources, in addition to facilitating communication between family members and monitoring services for outcomes. This model was successful in cutting health care costs by reducing lengths of stay in the acute setting.[4,6]

Disease Management

Background. Disease management (DM) is a relatively new concept of care being adopted by DM companies, employers, and insurance companies. It espouses the concept of population-based care and focuses on a delivery system design identified as a DM team. This interdisciplinary team can include physicians, nurses, social workers, dietitians, health educators, pharmacists, and community lay workers. DM is defined by the Disease Management Association of America as "a system of coordinated healthcare interventions and communication with populations with conditions in which patient self-care efforts are significant."[3] In the center of the coordinated team of care is the disease manager, who works closely with members of the DM team. The goal of DM is ultimately to improve care, improve health outcomes, reduce inpatient hospitalization days, and reduce emergency department visits to lower the total cost of care.[7]

The concept of DM began in the 1990s with DM companies to reduce hospital lengths of stay and ultimately reduce the cost of chronic disease care. The process focused on the specialization of services for groups of populations with one or two diseases. Specialization of services began with management of diabetes and asthma, since there was evidence that DM teams could follow treatment protocols to reduce hospitalizations or lengths of stay and health care costs for patients with diabetes and asthma. These guidelines reconfirmed the importance of a systematic plan of collaborative care that included team members with individual expertise. The team members were able to provide seamless interventions for diabetes and asthma patients that affected DM outcomes. Since then, DM teams have been used in hospitals, outpatient clinics, specialty clinics, health plan environments, DM companies, and pharmacies.[2]

Role of the Disease Management Team. The DM teamwork approach of longitudinal, chronic DM engages diverse health care providers with a wide range of skills. It brings together a team that is goal directed to reach defined populations with defined interventions of assessments and treatment. The treatment plan has defined protocols, specified interventions, and delegated assignments for each team member.[8] The team collaborates in an interdisciplinary approach, meets regularly to discuss the care of a defined population group, follows the care plan, and evaluates the outcomes.[8,9]

The goal of the DM team is to promote population-based health by empowering populations (groups of people with defined chronic disease) to become self-motivated and proactive to gain knowledge concerning disease symptom management, treatment regimens, healthy lifestyle behavior, peer communication, supportive care for specialty care referral, financial assistance, psychosocial needs, and mobility needs. In essence, DM teams target populations with chronic disease to achieve the goal of creating well-informed health care providers and consumers.[7]

THE DISEASE MANAGEMENT TEAM

Team Composition

The team can consist of two professionals (physician and nurse) or multiple health care providers, including pharmacists, who follow defined guidelines and tasks. The team members practice according to guidelines, and their collaboration results in successful DM.

Wagner[8] addresses specific team roles. Typically, teams may be composed of the disease or case manager, medical specialists, the clinical pharmacist, the social worker, and a lay health worker.

The disease manager is usually an advanced practice nurse but may be a professional nurse with additional experience in the clinical and behavioral treatment of chronic disease. The nurse is skilled in population-based care, leadership, and holistic care and assumes the role of provider, manager, initiator, and evaluator. The nurse disease manager's role includes clinical care organization, planning, and direction.

The complexity of chronic disease care mandates care by medical specialists (in kidney disease, diabetes, internal medicine, education, etc.). These specialists generally rotate between sites and see patients by referrals initiated by the other members of the team. Patients in DM have comorbidities and may have multiple specialists involved in their care.

The clinical pharmacist is a pivotal DM team member. Studies demonstrate that clinical pharmacists have positive effects on the patient care outcomes. These effects include optimizing drug-prescribing behavior and monitoring drug regimens to reduce adverse drug effects and use of health services.[10-12]

The social worker has long been involved with health care both as a clinician and as a resource for patients, families, and other health care team members. The social worker's expertise is considered essential as part of the DM team to facilitate the use of community services.

The lay health care worker may be a less familiar addition to the DM team. These lay workers help bridge any gaps in accessing or adherence to care, especially in low-income communities. These lay team members help with the integration of care and education, thus preventing cultural misunderstanding or confusion.

Essential Characteristics of Care by Disease Management Teams

The characteristics of DM by teams are "treatment planning, evidence-based clinical management, self-management support, effective consultation, and sustained follow-up."[8,13] When teams of health care providers manage diseases, the plans for the treatment they manage are specific to both the disease process and the population of patients.[8,13] To provide competent clinical care, these DM team members utilize protocols and evidence-based guidelines; this is essential, given patients' multiple comorbidities coupled with their increasingly complex medication and treatment regimens.[8,13]

A goal for patients managed by a DM team is the ability for patients to self-manage treatment and symptoms. Self-management support by the DM team can help patients change unhealthy behaviors and improve patient outcomes in many chronic illnesses.[14,15] There are distinct advantages for the patients as well as for the DM team when a nurse or other professional trained in behavioral counseling can assist in promoting changes in self-efficacy.[10-12]

DM teams are characterized by effective consultation practices; patients with the same diagnosis are managed in one clinic, and several patients may be seen at once, as a group. Beck, Scott, Williams, and colleagues[16] report that group consultations with several patients at once result in improved patient satisfaction, more current preventive care, and less frequent use of health services.

Finally, any DM team must have effective systems for sustained follow-up. These include computerized tracking systems or other designed systems (such as tickler computer systems) that allow close follow-up (including telephone management). These systems are essential for early detection of adverse effects, problems in compliance, failure to respond to treatment, and recurrence of symptoms.[8]

CONCLUSION

Chronic DM teams are an effective strategy for management of chronic disease(s) with populations. Chronic DM teams have been integrated into hospitals, outpatient settings, DM companies, and federal programs. Defined roles for the members of the interdisciplinary team and their collaboration with each other are essential components to empower populations to engage in health-promoting DM regimens.

REFERENCES

1. Short A, Mays G, Mittler J: Disease management: a leap of faith to lower-cost, higher-quality health care, *Issue Brief Cent Stud Health Syst Change* 69:1-4, 2003.
2. Mullahy CM: *The case manager handbook*, ed 2, Gaithersburg, Md, 1998, Aspen.
3. Howe R: Disease manager: an emerging profession? *Case Manage* 10(7):1-4, 2003.
4. Stanhope M, Lancaster J: *Foundations of nursing in the community*, St Louis, 1998, Mosby.
5. Aubert RE, Herman WH, Waters J, and others: Nurse case management to improve glycemic control in diabetic patients in a health maintenance organization: a randomized control trial, *Ann Intern Med* 129:605-612, 1998.
6. Zander K, Etheredge ML, Bower KA: *Nursing case management: blueprint for transformation*, Waban, Mass, 1987, Winslow.
7. Weingarten SC, Henning JM, Badamgarav E, and others: Interventions used in disease management programmes for patients with chronic illness—which ones work? Meta-analysis of published reports, *BMJ* 325:925-950, 2002.
8. Wagner EH: The role of patient care teams in chronic disease management, *BMJ* 320:569-572, 2000.
9. Starfield B: *Primary care: concept, evaluation, and policy*, New York, 1992, Oxford University Press.
10. Bero LA, Mays NB, Barjesteh K, and others: Abstract of review: expanding outpatient pharmacists' roles and health services utilisation, costs and patient outcomes, *Cochrane Library*, issue 1, Oxford, 2000, Update Software.
11. Hanlon JT, Weinberger M, Samsa GP, and others: A randomized, controlled trial of a clinical pharmacist intervention to improve inappropriate prescribing in elderly outpatients with polypharmacy, *Am J Med* 110:428-437, 1996.
12. Leape LL, Cullen DJ, Clapp MD, and others: Pharmacist participation on physician rounds and adverse drug effects in the intensive care unit, *JAMA* 21:267-270, 1999.
13. Wagner EH: Population-based management of diabetes care, *Patient Educ Couns* 26:225-230, 1995.
14. Von Korff M, Gruman J, Schaefer J, and others: Collaborative management of chronic illness: essential elements, *Ann Intern Med* 127:1097-1102, 1997.
15. Lorig KR, Mazonson PD, Holman HR: Evidence suggesting that health education for self-management in patients with chronic arthritis has sustained health benefits while reducing health care costs, *Arthritis Rheum* 36:439-446, 1993.
16. Beck A, Scott J, Williams P, and others: A randomized trial of group outpatient visits for chronically ill older HMO members: the Cooperative Health Care Clinic, *J Am Geriatr Soc* 45:543-549, 1997.

CHAPTER 8

Reimbursement for Nurse Practitioner Services

Angela Patterson

In recent years, health care practices, facilities, and agencies have recognized the contribution of nurse practitioner (NP) services in ensuring the provision of high-quality and cost-effective care. However, the problem of deciphering how federal and state law, often written in general terms, applies to a specific practice situation can deter health care organizations from using NPs to their full potential. Furthermore, wide variances in states' laws and significant differences in the policies of third-party payers regarding reimbursement for NP services make the quest for payment a challenging task.

The integration of the NP role into the health care economy has lagged behind acceptance of its clinical contributions and responsibilities. Confusion remains about NP reimbursement and what differentiates NPs from physicians (medical doctors) and physician assistants. This stems in part from the peculiarities of our federal health care insurance and regulatory system. Medicare sets the standard and tone for Medicaid, all health maintenance organizations (HMOs), and other insurers in the United States. Medicare supports NPs as cost-effective, high-quality providers who can act independently, but defers to states in terms of regulatory guidelines that govern the NP's scope of practice. Each of the 50 states' legal language and process are influenced by their own legislators, governors, lobbyists, medical associations, and nursing associations. The result is Medicare's variable support of NPs across the states, allowing NP roles to evolve at different rates.

The wide array of patient needs, providers, and third-party payers in the U.S. health care industry creates continually evolving delivery systems and practice arrangements. Providers find that specific situations are not addressed in the rules and frequently call on the government to issue new regulations to address questions that arise. As a result, rules often proliferate among the states. In addition, much of federal law was enacted when NPs were not as prevalent or accepted as they are today. The development of new language or rules and regulations requires changes in the law. Enacting these changes takes time and depends on a proponent for change who is more effectual than any opposing group or agency.

NPs have the right to work independently, in some states absent collaboration with physicians, and, like physicians, are authorized to bill Medicare directly for their services when furnished in any area or setting. In certain states and settings NPs legally act and are paid for services as independent primary care providers (PCPs) and as attending physicians.[1] NPs are covered by Medicare for many of the types of services that are reimbursable under federal law if they are provided by a physician, thus allowing NPs to "furnish services billed under all levels of evaluation and management codes and diagnostic tests."[2] Medicare requires NPs to have a *collaborative*, not supervisory, arrangement with a physician.[2] This consultative arrangement implies greater responsibility, autonomy, and liability than a supervisory arrangement. A physician does not need to be present with the NP when services are furnished and is not required to make an independent evaluation of each patient who is seen by the NP.

REIMBURSEMENT ENTITIES: THIRD-PARTY PAYERS

Except for a small minority of patients who pay out of pocket for their own medical expenses, every billable patient encounter is composed of three participants: the patient, the provider, and a third-party payer. The categories of third-party payers who may reimburse for NP services include Medicare, Medicaid, commercial indemnity insurers, commercial managed care organizations (MCOs) or HMOs, and businesses or schools wanting health services for employees or students.

Medicare and Medicaid strongly influence other third-party payers through their policies, rules, and regulations. However, each type of third-party payer has its own reimbursement policies and fee schedules, and each operates under a separate body of law. It is crucial that NPs fully understand Medicare and Medicaid as well as the structure, reimbursement rules, and regulations of third-party payers in order to negotiate for direct reimbursement.

Medicare

Medicare is a federal program, administered nationally by the Centers for Medicaid and Medicare Services and locally by Medicare carrier agencies. Medicare provides health care coverage to (1) persons 65 years of age and older who have enrolled in the program and pay premiums and (2) disabled individuals who qualify for Social Security disability payments and benefits.[3]

Medicare is subdivided into two parts. Medicare Part A, or "hospital insurance," covers inpatient hospital services, some posthospital nursing care, and some home health care. Part A is paid for through federal payroll taxes. NPs cannot bill independently for their inpatient care under Medicare Part A but must bill under their collaborative physician.[3] Hospitals providing care to Medicare patients require NPs to provide services only under the delegation from a physician. This is considered a significant limitation for NPs who currently maintain hospital admitting privileges.

Medicare Part B, also known as Supplemental Medical Insurance, covers outpatient services of physicians and other selected providers, home health visits, and rural health clinic services. Part B is paid for from general tax funds and patient premiums. NPs can be reimbursed directly for services provided under Medicare Part B, provided that they are "physician services" (i.e., diagnosis, therapy, surgery, consultation, and care plan management). Medicare will not reimburse NPs for services considered to be exclusive to nursing.

Medicaid

Medicaid is a federal program administered by each state that provides health care coverage to low-income families, women and children who qualify on the basis of poverty, the aged, and those with short-term disabilities. Each state establishes its own Medicaid rules regarding eligibility and services under federal guidelines.

Federal law provides that Medicaid will cover the services of pediatric NPs and family NPs, whether or not the NP is employed or supervised by a physician. It does not, however, mention adult NPs, geriatric NPs, or NPs trained in other specialties. States may elect to enhance federal law and reimburse NPs trained in specialties other than pediatrics or family medicine. Variations of this option are noted state to state.

Commercial Indemnity Insurers

An indemnity insurer is an insurance company that pays for the medical care of its insured members, but does not deliver health care. Indemnity insurers typically allow patients to choose their own providers and often apply deductibles and co-insurance payments. Health care providers are paid on a per-visit, per-procedure basis known as *fee-for-service.* To obtain reimbursement for service, the NP submits a billing form to the insurance company. Indemnity insurers have fee schedules based on *usual and customary charges*, an insurance industry term for a charge that is (1) usual and customary when compared with the charges made for similar services and supplies, and (2) made to persons having similar medical conditions in the county of the policyholder or such larger area than a county as is needed to secure a representative cross section of fees. "Usual and customary" varies from insurer to insurer; thus some indemnity insurers may reimburse at higher rates than others for the same services.

Managed Care Organizations

An MCO is an insurer that provides both health care services and payment for the services. *MCO* is considered an umbrella term that may include HMOs, provider-sponsored organizations, or physician-hospital organizations.

Over recent years, NPs are increasingly being credentialed by MCOs and achieving admittance to MCO provider panels. Once a panel member, the NP attains the designation of PCP. PCP status implies a contract between the NP and the MCO for the provision of care, credentialing, directory listing, and reimbursement. An NP with PCP status assumes full responsibility for a patient's primary care, including (1) complying with the MCO's quality, utilization, and patient satisfaction standards; (2) coordinating care with specialists, hospitals, or long-term care facilities; (3) approving or disapproving referrals for specialty care; (4) practicing cost-containment care while maintaining quality; and (5) providing a system for 24-hour access to care.

MCOs reimburse PCPs on a fee-for-service basis (reimbursed for each covered service provided), a capitated basis (set payment per-member per-month from the third-party payer to the provider or provider network), or a combination of fee-for-service and capitation. Each MCO negotiates a payment arrangement with each health care facility, practice, or provider on its panel. Contractual relationships with MCOs cover not only compensation, but many other issues concerning practice. NPs seeking to contract with an MCO are encouraged to seek the counsel of an attorney experienced in negotiating contracts with MCOs, since there are distinct challenges regarding NP reimbursement in these organizations.[1]

Direct Contracts for Health Care

Currently no rules or regulations limit an NP's ability to directly contract with businesses or agencies for reimbursement of furnished health care services. Examples of this ability to directly contract for reimbursement of health care services include NPs who contract with government agencies to provide school-based health services, colleges to provide college health services, and businesses to provide occupational health services.

REGULATIONS SURROUNDING NURSE PRACTITIONER REIMBURSEMENT

General Information

According to the Centers for Medicare and Medicaid Services, the professional services of an NP may be covered if she or he meets the qualifications and is legally authorized to furnish services in the state where the services are being rendered. Payments are permitted for assistance in surgical services and services furnished in all areas and settings permitted under applicable state licensure laws. NPs are also authorized to bill the Medicare program directly for their services when furnished in any area or setting. Medicare will not make a separate payment when a facility or another provider, such as a physician, charges or is paid any amount for delivering the same professional services as identified in the NP's reimbursement claim. A facility or other provider includes a hospital, skilled nursing facility, nursing facility, comprehensive outpatient rehabilitation facility, ambulatory surgical center, community mental health center, rural health center, or federally qualified health center.[2]

Health care services must be deemed "medically necessary" to be covered for reimbursement. Specifically, the services must be ordered by an NP or physician, required for symptom management, and provided in accordance with approved and generally accepted medical-surgical practice.[4]

Types of Nurse Practitioner Services That May Be Covered

In determining the types of NP services eligible for reimbursement, the state's laws or regulations that govern an NP's scope of practice in the state in which the services are rendered apply. Also, if authorized under the scope of their state license, NPs may be reimbursed for services billed under all levels of the Evaluation and Management Codes and Diagnostic Tests if furnished in collaboration with a physician.

Nurse Practitioner Services Not Covered

Under Medicare regulations, the following NP services are not eligible for reimbursement:

- Services to patients enrolled in hospice where the beneficiary has not selected an NP as attending physician
- Admission evaluation for patients in skilled nursing facility services
- The monthly *comprehensive* evaluation of patients in skilled nursing facilities (Other monthly billing levels are covered.)

- Certification and recertification of patients for home care

Collaboration

Collaboration is defined in federal law as a process in which an NP works in association with one or more physicians for the purpose of delivering health care services with medical direction and appropriate supervision, as required by the law of the state in which the services are rendered. In those states in which the laws do not specifically address collaboration, NPs are required to provide evidence of the existence of collaboration by specifically documenting their scope of practice and outlining in writing the process by which consultation with a physician is carried out when dealing with issues outside of the defined NP scope of practice. The collaborating physician does not need to be physically present when the NP renders services or to make an independent evaluation of each patient who is seen by the NP.[2]

"Incident To"

Services provided by NPs, if certain conditions are met, may be reimbursed by billing "incident to" a physician services, that is, as if the physician had provided the service directly. This method of billing allows for slightly higher reimbursement of the service provided, 100% of the physician fee scale, when compared with direct billing, which is paid out at 85% of the physician fee scale; however, "incident to" billing identifies the physician as the servicing provider and not the NP.[3]

Nursing Facilities

Medicare defines the term *skilled nursing facility* as "an institution which is primarily engaged in providing skilled nursing care and related services for residents who require medical or nursing care or rehabilitation services for the rehabilitation of injured, disabled, or sick persons and is not primarily for the care and treatment of mental diseases." Medicaid uses the term *nursing facility* and defines it as "an institution which is primarily engaged in providing to residents, skilled nursing care and related services for residents who require medical or nursing care rehabilitation services for the rehabilitation of injured, disabled, or sick persons, or, on a regular basis, health-related care and services to individuals who because of their mental or physical condition require care and services which can be made available to them only through institutional facilities, and is not primarily for the care and treatment of mental diseases."[5] Appreciating the distinction between skilled nursing facilities and nursing facilities is essential because federal rules and regulations regarding NP services differ depending on whether the patient is in a skilled nursing or nursing facility.

Hospital Visits and Procedures

Hospitals and physicians are increasingly hiring acute care NPs to provide services to their hospitalized patients. NP services furnished to hospitalized patients are eligible for third-party payer reimbursement provided those services are within the scope of practice of an NP according to state law. Under common state law, assessment and management of acute and chronic illnesses are within an NP's scope of practice. Many states also authorize NPs to perform diagnostic and therapeutic procedures. In those states with vague or obscure law, the NP may perform procedures when specifically delegated by a physician. In any state, NPs are not permitted to independently assume full responsibility for the care of a hospitalized patient. Federal law governing hospitals clearly states that, in a hospital setting, each and every patient must be under the care of a physician provider.[5]

Hospice

Hospice is defined as a provider entity and is subject to the regulatory requirements as outlined in federal law. The election of hospice coverage is available to those patients who have been determined to have a life expectancy of 6 months or less should their illness follow its usual course. When a patient selects hospice coverage, all rights to Medicare Part B benefits are waived.[2]

Home Visits

Under Medicare Part B, medically necessary physician services provided in a patient's home by either a physician or NP are eligible for reimbursement. A physician's order or referral is not required to furnish these services, and the patient does not need to be confined to the home. However, it is critical that NPs understand the difference between what is defined as *physician services* vs. *nursing services* to appropriately bill for home visits.

Physician services are defined as those services which are considered typical of a physician's work and would be reimbursed if a physician had directly performed the service, such as assessment and management of a patient's congestive heart failure. *Nursing services* are defined as those services which are unique to the nursing profession, such as the parenteral administration of medications or wound dressing changes. When an NP provides services to the home-bound patient and seeks reimbursement from Medicare Part B, only physician services are reimbursable—nursing services are *not* eligible for reimbursement.[2]

When medically necessary services are provided in the home, physician services are reimbursed under Medicare Part B and may be furnished by an NP or physician. The appropriate procedure (CPT) and diagnosis (ICD-9) codes are submitted together with the provider's name and Medicare number. "Incident to" is not an option in this setting. When nursing services are provided in the home, several conditions must be met to receive reimbursement, including (1) the services are performed by a nurse or NP who is employed by a home care agency, (2) the services are provided under the direction of a physician's order, (3) the patient has been certified for home care by a physician, (4) the patient meets Medicare's definition of "home bound," and (5) the home care agency is enrolled as a provider with Medicare and is compliant with state regulations. In this situation, the provision of nursing services is reimbursed under Medicare Part A.[5]

With regards to non-Medicare payers, both NP and physician reimbursement eligibility for physician services provided to home-bound patients is variable. Providers wishing to bill non-Medicare payers for physician services provided in the patient's home are required to contact the insurer for information regarding its policies and procedures.

HOW TO APPLY FOR PROVIDER STATUS

As of May 23, 2007, all practitioners have been issued a National Provider Identifier (NPI). The NPI replaces all existing billing provider numbers and is the practitioner's sole billing ID for the entire time he or she practices.

Medicare

Nurse practitioners apply for a Medicare provider number by appropriately completing and submitting a CMS-855I form. Contact information is available online at http://www. medicare.gov/Contacts/Home.asp. The CMS-855I form can be obtained at: http://cms.hhs.gov/providers/enrollment/forms.

Once a Medicare provider number is obtained, reimbursement for NP services to Medicare patients can be attained by appropriately completing and submitting a claim form referred to as the HCFA-1500. Information required to complete the HCFA-1500 includes the patient's full name and identifying information, the diagnosis code (ICD-9), the procedure code (CPT), the charge, and the NP's provider number.

Medicaid

NPs apply for a Medicaid provider number by contacting the state agency that administers the plan, asking for the provider relations department, and requesting an NP provider application. A list of state agencies and contact information can be obtained at http://www.cms.hhs.gov.

Once a Medicaid provider number is obtained, reimbursement for NP services to Medicaid patients can be obtained by appropriately completing and submitting a HCFA-1500 claim form. Information necessary on the HCFA-1500 includes the patient's name and identifying information; the ICD-9 code; the CPT code; the charge; and the NP's name, Medicaid provider number, and location.

Managed Care Organizations

Each MCO has individually developed rules and regulations regarding which provider types are eligible for credentialing and the credentialing and reimbursement process as a whole. This requires that NPs who seek credentialing for reimbursement of services contact the provider relations department of each MCO for which provider status is sought. This allows the NP to determine the MCO's policies and how to proceed with credentialing so that it is consistent with the organization's process.

Should a specific MCO deny NP admission to its provider panel, the NP should (1) note the reason for the rejection, (2) ask the provider relations department to forward in writing the rejection and the reasons for the rejection, and (3) contact state agency in charge of insurance law.[1] In some states an HMO is prohibited from discriminating against providers on the basis of license class. In other states HMOs can accept or reject provider types at will. If the latter is the case, seek an opportunity with the MCO to present a case for NP admittance to provider panels. MCO credentialing can be pursued through meetings, presentations, letters, telephone calls, and enlisting the assistance of colleagues, politicians, and patients in this endeavor.

Commercial Indemnity Insurers

Like MCOs, each commercial indemnity insurer has individually developed and executed rules regarding provider credentialing and reimbursement. If the payer prohibits the NP from receiving credentialing and reimbursement, proceed with the steps outlined under Managed Care Organizations.

If the payer does not require a provider number, submit a HCFA-1500 claim form for the NP services provided. Complete the form in its entirety. If the indemnity insurer rejects the claim, it will return the claim form with a written statement explaining the rejection. In this case, address the rejection by forwarding the company a letter of protest. If an error was cited, fully explain and correct the error or supply any further information required. In these situations repeated correspondence with the company may be needed before the claim is paid. On rare occasions, submission of a legal letter by the NP's practice attorney is required. Should the indemnity insurer continue to reject the claim, the patient is then held liable for the reimbursement charge.

BILLING THIRD-PARTY PAYERS

Billable NP services are those which involve a face-to-face visit between the patient and the NP. The encounter may occur in the provider's office, an inpatient facility, or the patient's home. Each billable visit must be assigned a procedural code according to CPT guidelines and be identified as a diagnostic visit with an appropriate ICD-9 code.

Billing third-party payers for the purpose of reimbursement of NP services requires the completion and filing of standard billing forms, which include appropriate identification of procedural and diagnostic codes. The standard billing form to be used is the HCFA-1500. Electronic versions of the HCFA-1500 are available at http://www.osmre.gov/pdf/form1500-90.pdf.

Coding

Coding systems were established to identify and specifically communicate to third-party payers the services and rationale for services that have been furnished to patients. Current Procedural Technology (CPT) codes describe medical or psychiatric procedures performed by physicians and other health care providers. The International Classification of Diseases (ICD-9) is a system developed by the National Center for Health Statistics that identifies particular illnesses and diseases. It is used by the World Health Organization and the National Center for Health Statistics to track morbidity and mortality rates. For the purposes of billing and coding, ICD-9 codes are used to communicate a patient's disease or medical condition to third-party payers.[6]

CPT codes were developed by the Centers for Medicaid and Medicare Services to assist in the assignment of reimbursement amounts to providers by Medicare carriers. Over the years, growing numbers of managed care and other third-party payers have adopted the CPT codes and reimbursement values established by the centers.[7]

Documentation

Each billable visit requires documentation in the patient's medical record to support the level of care billed. Third-party payer examiners investigate fraud and abuse in billing by inspecting documentation of medical services in patient charts. Overcoding or underdocumentation can lead to charges of fraudulent billing, which may result in fines, criminal prosecution, loss of provider status, or loss of professional licensure.[4]

Generally accepted principles of documentation for Evaluation and Management Services applicable to NP services furnished in all settings include:

- The medical record should be complete and legible.
- The documentation of each patient encounter should include reason for the encounter and relevant history; physical examination findings and prior diagnostic tests; assessment, clinical impression, or diagnosis; care plan; and date and legible identity of the examiner.
- If not documented, the rationale for ordering diagnostic and other ancillary services should be easily inferred.
- Past and present diagnoses should be accessible to the treating and/or consulting health care provider.
- Appropriate health risk factors should be identified.
- The patient's progress, response to and changes in treatment, and revision of diagnosis should be documented.
- The CPT and ICD-9 codes reported on the health insurance claim form should be supported by the documentation in the patient's medical record.[8]

REFERENCES

1. Buppert C: *Nurse practitioner's business practice and legal guide,* Sudbury, Mass, 2003, Jones & Bartlett.
2. *Medicare Part B: physician assistant, nurse practitioner, and clinical nurse specialist billing guide,* Sept 2004, National Heritage Insurance and Centers for Medicare and Medicaid Services, REF-EDO-0020, Version 3.0, retrieved Nov 26, 2006, from http://www.acnpweb.org/files/public/Medicare_PartB_PA_NP_CNS_Billing_Guide_Sept04.pdf.
3. Lindeke L: *Reimbursement realities for advanced practice nurses,* Minneapolis, Minn, 2000, Collaborative Rural Nurse Practitioner Project, retrieved March 1, 2006, from http://www.nursing.umn.edu/professional/reimbursement.
4. Buppert C: Billing for nurse practitioner services—update 2005: guidelines for NPs, physicians, employers, and insurers, *Medscape,* 2005, retrieved March 22, 2006, from http://www.medscape.com/viewprogram/4321.
5. Buppert C: *Billing physician services provided by nurse practitioners,* Annapolis, Md, 2004, Law office of Carolyn Buppert.
6. Mills C, Moroney S, Kochman C, and others: *Guide to nurse practitioner practice in Massachusetts,* Littleton, Mass, 2003, Massachusetts Coalition of Nurse Practitioners.
7. Abood S, Keepnews D: *Understanding payment for advanced practice nursing services,* vol 1, Medicare reimbursement, Washington, DC, 2000, American Nurses Association.
8. Health Care Financing Administration: *1997 Documentation guidelines for evaluation and management services,* Centers for Medicare and Medicaid Services, retrieved Nov 17, 2005, from http://www.cms.hhs.gov/MLNProducts/Downloads/MASTER1.pdf.

OTHER RESOURCES

2005 ACNP public policy agenda, Washington, DC, 2005, American College of Nurse Practitioners.

American Medical Association: *Physicians Current Procedural Terminology (CPT),* Chicago, 2006, The Association.

Bodenheimer TS, Grumback K: *Understanding health policy: a clinical approach,* ed 4, New York, 2002, McGraw-Hill.

Centers for Medicare and Medicaid Services: "Incident to" services, *MLN Matters,* no SE0441, retrieved March 1, 2006, from http://www.cms.hhs.gov/MLNMattersArticles.

Centers for Medicare and Medicaid Services: *Medicare carriers manual,* part 3, chapter II, section 2050, retrieved from http://www.cms.hhs.gov.

Centers for Medicare and Medicaid Services: Nurse practitioners as attending physicians in the Medicare hospice benefit, *MLN Matters,* no MM3226, retrieved Feb 26, 2006, from http://www.cms.hhs.gov/MLNMattersArticles.

CPT Code Training Module, 2005, American Academy of Child and Adolescent Psychiatry, retrieved Dec 15, 2005, from http://www.aacap.org/clinical/cptcode.htm.

Druss B, Marcus S, Olfson M, and others: Trends in care by nonphysician clinicians in the United States, *N Engl J Med* 348(3):130-136, 2003.

Greenberg SA: *Nurse practitioners: evolution of advanced practice,* ed 4, New York, 2003, Springer.

Hickey JV, Ouimette RM, Venegoni SL: *Advanced practice nurses: changing roles and clinical applications,* ed 2, Philadelphia, 2000, Lippincott.

ICD-9-CM 2006: International classification of diseases, Chicago, 2006, American Medical Association.

Jones DC: *Professional and legislative issues related to pediatric nurse practitioner practice,* 2003, retrieved Feb 28, 2006, from http://www.medscape.com/viewarticle/45583.

LeClaire J: Nurse practitioners fill gap left by shortage of doctors, *Sacramento Bus J,* April 8, 2005.

Making sense of the new reimbursement laws: Q & A, *Nurs World,* retrieved April 18, 2006, from http://www.nursingworld.org/gova/medreqa.htm.

Moore K: Billing for NP services: what you need to know, *Medicare Update,* 1998, retrieved Feb 26, 2006, from http://www.aafp.org/fpm/980500fm/billing.html.

Moore PL: Discover the power of positive coding: five ways to code better and stay in control, *Phys Practice Digest,* March/April:16-30, 2002.

Moore PL: Why billing low can bring you down—and how to get back up, *Phys Practice Digest,* March/April:12-62, 2001.

Mundinger M, Kane R, Lenz E, and others: Primary care outcomes in patients treated by nurse practitioners or physicians, *JAMA* 283(1):59-68, 2000.

Nagelkerk J: *Starting your practice: a survival guide for nurse practitioners,* St Louis, 2006, Mosby.

Newton DA, Grayson MS: Trends in career choice by U.S. medical school graduates, *JAMA* 290(9):1179-1182, 2003.

Nurse Practitioner Association New York: *The nurse practitioner resource guide,* ed 3, 2003, The Association, retrieved April 22, 2006, from http://www.thenpa.org/associations/1031/files/NPResourceGuide10-03.pdf.

Pearson LJ: The Pearson report: a national overview of nurse practitioner legislation and healthcare issues, *Am J Nurse Pract* 10(1):15-84, 2006.

Reel S, Abraham I: *Business and legal essentials for nurse practitioners: from negotiating your first job through owning a practice,* St Louis, 2007, Mosby.

Vanderbilt M: HCFA issues: instructions implementing NP/CNS reimbursement, *Nurs World,* retrieved March 21, 2006, from http://www.nursingworld.org/gova/hcfamem.htm.

CHAPTER 9

Health Literacy

Brenda Hage

SCOPE OF THE PROBLEM

Many factors have been attributed to the rapidly escalating health care costs in today's society. Some of these factors include the ever-increasing use of technology, an aging population, and an increasing incidence of chronic disease. One of the most important and least considered factors in the cost of health care is health literacy. Sources estimate that inadequate health literacy costs the U.S. health care system between $29 billion and $73 billion dollars annually.[1,2] The National Adult Literacy Survey (NALS) represents the largest household-based literacy assessment conducted in the United States. The NALS survey found that between 40 million and 44 million adults in this country have significantly limited reading skills, leaving them unable to read a food label or complete an application form. An additional 40 million to 50 million adults were found to have a slightly higher level of literacy, still limiting their ability to synthesize complex information or to complete sequential numeric operations.[3]

Health literacy has been defined as the ability of individuals to obtain, process, and understand basic information and services needed to make appropriate health decisions. According to the Institute of Medicine's report, *Health Literacy: A Prescription to End the Confusion,* approximately 90 million people—or close to half of all adults in the United States—have inadequate health literacy.[4] *Healthy People 2010* has a major goal focused on improving health communication, which addresses the need to improve health literacy for "persons with inadequate or marginal literacy skills."[5] A large-scale study examining the reading and health literacy levels of 3260 Medicare enrollees ages 65 and above found that 34% of English-speaking and 54% of Spanish-speaking patients had inadequate or marginal health literacy. Variables associated with low health literacy included having a poor education, having a blue collar occupation, being older, living in rural areas, belonging to a racial or ethnic minority group, or being an immigrant.[6,7]

HEALTH OUTCOMES AND HEALTH LITERACY

Patients with inadequate health literacy are at increased risk for medication errors, missed appointments, and misunderstood consent forms[8] (Box 9-1). Affected individuals are also less likely to use preventive health services such as mammography, cervical cancer screening, and immunizations.[9] Studies found patients with inadequate health literacy had less knowledge about their health conditions, fewer self-management skills, poorer physical functioning and mental health, higher rates of hospitalization, and greater difficulties with instrumental activities of daily living.[9-11]

BOX 9-1

RISKS ASSOCIATED WITH INADEQUATE HEALTH LITERACY MEDICATION ERRORS

- Misunderstood consent forms
- Missed appointments
- Poor use of preventive health measures, including recommended health screenings
- Inadequate knowledge about personal health conditions
- Higher hospitalization rates
- Decreased self-management skills

IDENTIFYING AND MANAGING INADEQUATE HEALTH LITERACY

Level of education completed cannot be used to determine health literacy, since many individuals may read well below grade level attained. Several validated tests exist for health literacy; however, many are lengthy and may be potentially embarrassing to patients.[12] Two examples of literacy assessments include the Rapid Estimate of Adult Literacy in Medicine (REALM)[13] and the Test of Functional Health Literacy in Adults (TOFHLA),[14] which also has a short form, the S-TOFHLA.

The REALM test is a 66-item word pronunciation test requiring patients to correctly read and pronounce medical words. It takes 2 to 3 minutes to administer and score. The REALM has been validated by multiple studies, but some studies have shown discordance in results between Caucasians and African-Americans,[15] and the REALM does not assess numeric literacy.

The TOFHLA is specifically focused on identifying functional health literacy and evaluates both reading comprehension and numeracy. Reading comprehension of health information is evaluated by a 50-item test using the modified cloze procedure, where every fifth or seventh word is omitted and the reader must select the correct choice to fill in the missing information. Numeracy is assessed using actual medication prescription labels and hospital forms to test the individual's ability to understand directions for taking medications, keeping appointments, and obtaining financial assistance. The S-TOFHLA assesses reading and comprehension through a 36-item reading assessment, which takes about 7 minutes to administer. The TOFHLA and the S-TOFHLA score levels of health literacy as adequate, inadequate, or marginal.[14] A recent study identified three questions from the S-TOFHLA that were highly associated with inadequate health literacy: "How often do you have someone help you read hospital materials?" "How confident are you filling out medical forms by yourself?" and "How often do you have problems learning about your medical conditions because of difficulty understanding written information?" The researchers found that the three questions were weaker in identifying marginal health literacy; however, the questions may be helpful as a quick preliminary screening for inadequate health literacy; more extensive testing could follow if needed[12] (Box 9-2).

It is important to remember that health literacy can change due to illness, decreased cognition, or increased stress.

BOX 9-2

PRELIMINARY SCREENING QUESTIONS TO ASSESS HEALTH LITERACY

- How often do you have someone help you read medical pamphlets or instruction sheets?
- How confident are you filling out medical forms by yourself?
- How often do you have problems learning about your medical conditions because of difficulty understanding written information?

Adapted from Chew L, Bradley KA, Boyko EJ: Brief questions to identify patients with inadequate health literacy, *Fam Med* 36(8):588-594, 2004.

BOX 9-3

MEASURES TO REDUCE BARRIERS TO HEALTH LITERACY

1. Screen patients for health literacy.
2. Provide written patient education materials at reading level appropriate for every patient.
3. Use pictographs and symbols to convey information in patient education materials.
4. Use the talk-back method to assess patient's understanding of instructions and explanations.
5. Always address the following with all patients:
   - Their main problem
   - What they need to do
   - Why this is important for them to do

BOX 9-4

HEALTH LITERACY RESOURCES

AMA Foundation on Health Literacy has a health literacy toolkit and streaming video presentations on the problems of health literacy for patients and providers; available at http://www.ama-assn.org/ama/pub/category/8115.html.

AskMe3 offers helpful information about improving health communication and has education materials for patients and providers about low health literacy; available at http://www.askme3.org.

Institute of Medicine Report, "Health Literacy: A Prescription to End Confusion," 2004, is available at http://www.iom.edu/CMS/3775/3827/19723.aspx.

Pfizer Principles for Clear Health Communication, ed 2, 2004, offers valuable information for creating appropriate patient education materials incorporating health literacy principles; available at http://www.pfizerhealthliteracy.com/pdfs/Pfizers_Principles_for_Clear_Health_Communication.pdf.

Adequate health literacy does not guarantee that patients' behavior will change in a desired way.[16]

Multiple studies examining the reading grade level of health-related printed materials have found that the reading abilities of average adults are much lower than are required to read and comprehend health-related print materials such as consent forms, educational handouts, and patient instructions.[5] The American Academy of Family Physicians (AAFP) conducted an analysis of a random sample of AAFP patient education materials available on the Internet.[17] Using the Simplified Measure of Gobbledygook (SMOG) readability formula,[18] the study found the mean reading level for the patient education materials was at approximately the ninth-grade level, much higher than the reading level of the average U.S. adult.[14] The use of pictures and symbols may also be useful in conveying information in patient instructions and education materials.[19] Health care providers should carefully assess the appropriateness of the reading level of the education materials used with their patient populations.

An important new resource for those with inadequate health literacy has been developed by the Partnership for Clear Health Communication, a consortium of health professional organizations, including the American Nurses Association and American Medical Association. This resource, AskMe3, uses three main questions that patients are encouraged to ask their health care provider to enhance patient-provider communication. These questions are: "What is my main problem?" "What do I need to do?" and "Why is it important for me to do this?" This simple yet effective framework helps patients and caregivers initiate communication with their health care provider about their health concerns.

When providing patient instructions, health care providers are encouraged to use the "talk-back" method, which asks patients to verbalize their understanding of the information presented to help ensure comprehension. The AskMe3 website (http://www.askme3.org/PFCHC) offers helpful resources for providers, including bilingual training materials in English and Spanish and ideas for making office practices more user-friendly for patients with inadequate health literacy. Some of these ideas include examining processes for making appointments, obtaining consent forms, and completing insurance applications. Signage and facility maps should also be evaluated.

To effectively meet the needs of patients with low health literacy, providers must develop the necessary awareness, knowledge, and skills required to address this complex issue. Screening should be offered to patients at risk for this problem. Patient education materials should be developed at a reading level appropriate for each individual patient's needs. The talk-back method should be used to assess patient understanding of health information and instructions. Office processes for patient procedures should also be evaluated (Box 9-3). With a concerted effort, providers can play a significant role in removing barriers for those with inadequate health literacy.

Box 9-4 provides a sampling of health literacy resources.

REFERENCES

1. Smoak RD: AMA Foundation to improve health literacy, *Am Med Assoc News* 40(13):20, 2000.
2. The health literacy initiative: enhancing communications for better outcomes, *Clin News* 9(4):1, 10-11, 2005.
3. Artinian NT, Lange MP, Templin TN, and others: Functional health literacy in an urban primary care clinic, *Internet J Adv Nurs Pract* 5(2):8, 2003.
4. Institute of Medicine: *Health literacy: a prescription to end the confusion,* Washington, DC, 2004, U.S. Department of Health and Human Services.

5. U.S. Department of Health and Human Services, O.D.P.H.P.: Health communication objective. In *Healthy people 2010,* vol 1, section 11, Washington, DC, 2000, The Department.
6. Gazmararian JA, Baker DW, Williams MV, and others: Health literacy among Medicare enrollees in a managed care organization, *JAMA* 281(6):545-551, 1999.
7. Davis TC, Wolf MS: Health literacy: implications for family medicine, *Fam Med* 36(8):595-598, 2004.
8. Scott T, Gazmararian JA, Williams MV, and others: Health literacy and preventative health care use among Medicare enrollees in a managed care organization, *Med Care* 40(5):395-404, 2002.
9. Williams MV, Baker DW, Parker RM, and others: Relationship of functional health literacy to patients' knowledge of their chronic disease, *Arch Intern Med* 158:166-172, 1998.
10. Williams MV, Baker DW, Homig EG, and others: Inadequate literacy is a barrier to asthma knowledge and self-care, *Chest* 114:1008-1015, 1998.
11. Wolf MS, Gazmararian JA, Baker DW: Health literacy and functional status among older adults, *Arch Intern Med* 165:1946-1952, 2005.
12. Chew L, Bradley KA, Boyko EJ: Brief questions to identify patients with inadequate health literacy, *Fam Med* 36(8):588-594, 2004.
13. Davis TC, Long SW, Jackson RH, and others: Rapid Estimate of Adult Literacy in Medicine: a shortened screening instrument, *Fam Med* 25(6):391-395, 1993.
14. Parker RM, Baker DW, Williams MV, and others: The test of functional health literacy in adults: a new instrument for measuring patients' literacy skills, *J Gen Intern Med* 10:537-541, 1995.
15. Shea JA, Beers BB, McDonald VJ, and others: Assessing health literacy in African American and Caucasian adults: disparities in Rapid Estimate of Adult Literacy in Medicine (REALM) scores, *Fam Med* 36(8):575-581, 2004.
16. Rudd RE, Moeykens BA, Colton TC: Health and literacy: a review of medical and public health literature. In Comings JP, Garner B, Smith C, editors: *The annual review of adult learning and literacy,* San Francisco, 2000, Jossey-Bass.
17. Silver Wallace L, Lennon ES: American Academy of Family Physicians patient education materials: can patients read them? *Fam Med* 36(8):571-574, 2004.
18. McLaughlin GH: SMOG grading: a new readability formula, *J Reading* 12:639-646, 1969.
19. Schillinger D, Machtinger EL, Wang F, and others: Language, literacy, and communication regarding medication in an anticoagulation clinic: are pictures better than words? *Adv Patient Safety* 2:199-210, 2005.

PART 2

Primary Care: Adolescence Through Adulthood

JOANN TRYBULSKI, *Section Editor*

CHAPTER 10

Adolescent Issues

Cathy J. Sizer

Adolescence is the interval in physical, cognitive, emotional, and psychosocial development that occurs between 10 and 21 years of age. Often it is described as a time of intense upheaval for the adolescent and anxiety for the parents. However, these normal developmental changes usually occur without major difficulties.

Successful metamorphosis from adolescence to adulthood involves the attainment of economic and emotional independence from parents, the cultivation of a workable value system, the evolution of a sexual identity, and the development of new and meaningful relationships.[1] Adolescence is also a time when individuals may engage in intentional or unintentional risky behaviors that can lead to significant consequences and complicate their future care.[2] Each year 15,000 to 18,000 adolescents die in accidents.[3] Another 6000 adolescents are homicide victims each year, and approximately 24% of ninth to twelfth graders attempt suicide.[3] These facts mandate increased health promotion, safety awareness, and risk prevention for these young adults. Specific interventions and guidance should be tailored to each adolescent's individual period of development.

Three distinct periods of adolescence characterize the transformation that occurs within this decade of life. Early adolescents (those ages 10 to 14) challenge authority, experience wide mood swings, reject the activities and ideation of childhood, can be argumentative or disobedient, and desire more privacy. There is an intense preoccupation with normal body changes. Anxieties regarding menses or nocturnal emissions ("wet dreams") and differences in the size of sexual body parts may or may not be expressed. An imaginary judgmental audience may influence behavior and increase insecurities. Peer groups, manifested by close friendships with the same sex along with contact with the opposite sex in groups, may become more important than parental influence. These adolescents may express future plans and an emerging value system; although these ideations are initially idealistic, they may change frequently.[4] During this stage, health promotion should focus on the immediate impact of behaviors. Goals include the prevention of cigarette smoking, street drug use, alcohol use, and sexual activity.[5]

Middle adolescents (those ages 15 to 17) are strongly influenced, positively or negatively, by peer groups. Despite this powerful support system, this period is often a lonely one. Family conflict occurs and may escalate as the adolescent strives for independence. Concern about body image decreases, whereas anxiety about attractiveness increases. In addition, the "tired teenager" surfaces, sexual drive heightens, and fad behavior predominates. This is the age of experimentation with sex, drugs, different types of friends, and risk-taking behaviors. However, future goals seem more realistic as the adolescent gains awareness of his or her strengths and limitations. Finally, the adolescent has an increased intellectual ability that includes emerging abstract thought, creativity, and contemplation of the future.[4] Health promotion goals continue to include prevention of cigarette smoking, street drug use, alcohol use, and sexual activity, with additional counseling for those engaging in alcohol use or abuse or sexual activity, especially unprotected sexual activity.[5]

As they become emancipated from the nuclear family, late adolescents (those ages 18 to 21) begin to assimilate adult roles. At this age adolescents are usually comfortable with their body image, and abstract thinking matures. Peer influence diminishes, and decisions relate more to the individual or to his or her partner. At this age successful adolescents pursue realistic goals, understand the consequences of their behavior, and relate to the family as adults. They realize their own limitations and mortality and have established a sexual identity and an ethical and moral value system.[4] The long-term negative health effects of alcohol abuse, unsafe sex, use or abuse of street drugs, and cigarette smoking should be stressed.[5]

PHYSICAL DEVELOPMENT

Although growth occurs over a continuum, adolescence is marked by a 15% to 18% growth spurt, during which time about 95% of the adult size is reached.[1] Before that growth spurt occurs, other specific pubertal physical changes take place. These changes are regulated by the endocrine feedback systems, including the somatotropic, the adrenal, and the hypothalamic pituitary gonadal axes, as well as by interplay with the thyroid axis. For girls, physical changes usually begin with breast development or breast buds around age 10 years. For boys, testicular enlargement at an average age of 11.5 years marks the initiation of puberty.

The average age for menarche, which follows a growth spurt, is 12.5 years; African-American girls may experience an earlier menarche. Dysmenorrhea is rare, since the first few periods are usually anovulatory. Girls acquire fat during puberty, since a body fat composition of nearly 22% is necessary to maintain regular ovulatory cycles.[6] Girls may have asymmetric breast development in the early stages, as well as extra nipples. Physiologic leukorrhea, which begins several months before menarche, may continue for several years. Puberty for female adolescents is completed with the sculpting of the body that results in the familiar adult shape.

For male adolescents, nocturnal emissions begin after testicular and penile growth is underway because dreams become more sexual in nature under the influence of hormones. Male adolescents may have tender or nontender gynecomastia or unilateral breast buds, which may be present for about 1 year. Testicular asymmetry is also common. These adolescents may need reassurance that the size of the penis is not an indication of sexual functioning, and they should be made aware that impregnation is a possibility because the testicles are probably capable of producing a few sperm at ejaculation. The remaining male physical developmental changes include voice deepening, axillary hair, and facial hair.

Pubertal changes occur in the same sequence for all adolescents. These changes should be tracked with each physical examination using the Sexual Maturation Scale or Tanner stages. Often the family history will dictate the timing of puberty, but it is worrisome for boys when testicular enlargement occurs before ages 9.5 to 10 years (precocious) or when no changes have occurred by age 13.5 years (delayed). It is equally worrisome for girls when breast buds appear before ages 8 to 8.5 years (precocious) or when no breast buds have appeared by age 13 years (delayed). An easy and inexpensive intervention to evaluate these variations is the bone age radiograph. If the bone age (wrist) is less than the chronologic age but is still appropriate for height, no further diagnostic testing is necessary.

COGNITIVE DEVELOPMENT

Piaget first recognized what is now thought to be the distinguishing feature of adolescent thought: abstract reasoning. By late adolescence, many adolescents can understand and create general principles or formal rules to explain many aspects of human experience. Piaget called this last stage of cognitive development, which is ideally attained by approximately age 15 years, formal operational thought. However, many adolescents arrive at this cognitive stage later than age 15 years, and some adults never achieve this level of cognition.[7] One of the qualities of adolescence that is most exasperating to parents is the adolescents' ability to reason well in academic subjects but at the same time exhibit illogical thinking about their own lives.[7]

With increasing sophistication and mental agility, an egocentric attitude emerges and peaks at about age 13 years. The belief that they can handle anything and that adults do not understand them can lead adolescents to engage in risk-taking behaviors such as drug use and unprotected sex. As part of this egocentrism, adolescents create the aforementioned judgmental imaginary audience. This same egocentrism sometimes causes adolescents to seek public attention in any way possible.[7] Other aspects of this egocentrism include the "personal fable," or the belief of adolescents that they are special and that the usual laws of nature do not apply to them; "overthinking," or the tendency to make daily circumstances more complicated than necessary; and "apparent hypocrisy," or the belief that rules apply differently to them than to others.[6] An understanding of this as normal development may make communication less difficult and frustrating.

EMOTIONAL DEVELOPMENT

The quest for identity, a major task of adolescence, is accomplished by the development of new goals and the abandonment of childhood aspirations. This ideation is usually positive but can be negative, and it helps explain the apathy, insecurity, or socially unacceptable attributes and behaviors that may occur, such as outrageous hairstyles, hair colors, or clothing; drug use; or pregnancy.[7]

Given the ongoing turmoil, conflict, and change that an adolescent experiences, it is no wonder that self-esteem suffers. This can be manifested by depression or suicide. Beginning in seventh grade (a time of overwhelming transition) through the middle to late adolescence periods, many factors contribute to the increasing risk of suicide. Poverty, racial minority status, parental depression, confused sexual identity, rejection by one's peer group, anger, chronic illness, drug use, adolescent impulsivity, a history of corporal punishment, and divorce are considered potential precipitating factors.[8]

SOCIAL DEVELOPMENT

Successful identity formation in society depends on the support of family and friends. Peer groups buffer the transition between childhood dependency and adult independence and must be respected.[7] These groups identify and define the adolescent. Peer group pressure is positive if it eases the transition to adulthood by decreasing dependence on parents. However, it may also be negative and can lead to experimentation and destructive behaviors.

Given the developmental tasks of adolescence, some parental conflict is inevitable. A consistent and fair parenting style can help alleviate the ongoing conflict. Parents can be influential, especially if family members respect one another and engage in rational discussion. If parents recognize and become more comfortable with the growing autonomy of their adolescent, the difficulties will usually diminish with time.

Community and school are also important influences on development. "Rites of passage" such as bar mitzvahs or bas mitzvahs, achievement awards, "sweet sixteen" parties, driver's licenses, voter registration, and graduation from high school or college foster, focus, celebrate, and further the attainment of adult identity.[7]

DEVELOPMENTAL HISTORY

The Guidelines for Adolescent Preventive Services (GAPS) have been developed by the American Medical Association and provide a framework for a complete screening history, physical assessment, appropriate testing, and immunization update.[9] Anticipatory guidance for health promotion, safety, and risk issues is also addressed. The focus of these guidelines varies with each stage of adolescence. Therefore modifications based on variations of patient populations are recommended.

THE ADOLESCENT HEALTH VISIT

The initial comprehensive adolescent health visit, with the parent present, begins with an interview to assess the family medical history. Family practices such as household smoking, smoke detector use, and firearm storage are discussed in addition to routine health screening questions.

The parent's presence at the beginning of the adolescent interview affords the opportunity to observe the relationship between the adolescent and the parent. The adolescent should remain dressed at this stage of the visit. Careful explanation of the changing provider-patient relationship for adolescents and the safeguarding of their privacy are stressed. At this time, parents should be asked about their current concerns or stressors.[10]

The interview continues in private with the adolescent. The format of the visit should be explained. Assuring the adolescent of confidentiality, and what the limits of the confidentiality are, is essential. The health history can be organized around the mnemonic *HEADSS FIRST.* In this assessment, adolescents are asked about *H*ome, *E*ducation, *A*ctivities, *D*rugs, *S*exual activity, *S*uicide/depression, *F*riends, *I*mage, *R*ecreation, *S*afety issues, and *T*hreats.[2]

Affirmative answers to questions concerning the use of street drugs or alcohol can be further explored with two other useful mnemonics: *CAGE* and *RAFTT*. The *CAGE* mnemonic stands for the following questions: "Have you ever felt the need to Cut down on your use of alcohol or drugs?" "Have you gotten Annoyed by someone's criticism of your drug or alcohol use?" "Do you ever feel Guilty about your alcohol or drug use?" and "Do you Ever need a drink or drugs in the morning before school?" A positive screen result consists of two or more "yes" answers.[11] The *RAFFT* mnemonic refers to the following questions: "Do you use alcohol or drugs to Relax, feel better about yourself, or fit in?" "Do you ever drink or use drugs when you are Alone?" "Do any of your close Friends drink or use drugs?" "Do any close Family members have a problem with alcohol or drugs?" and "Have you ever gotten in Trouble from drinking or taking drugs?" A positive screen result consists of two or three "yes" answers.[11]

An increased risk for drug use is associated with a family history of alcoholism, parental use of alcohol or drugs, overly permissive or controlling parents, the availability of alcohol or drugs, alcohol- or drug-using friends, school problems, attention deficit hyperactivity disorder with impulsivity, past physical or sexual abuse, depression or other psychiatric problems, low self-esteem, low religiosity, and the need for peer acceptance.[11]

Mental health problems afflict a sizable proportion of adolescents.[12] Unlike adult depression, adolescent depression is not associated with powerlessness or pessimism about the future. Instead, it is directly affected by negative beliefs about self and low parental support. Adolescents tend to mask their depression and exhibit behavioral symptoms such as anger and self-destructive activities. These behaviors are used as a defense mechanism to protect the adolescent from feeling or appearing vulnerable or dependent.[13,14] A referral for immediate psychiatric assessment is indicated if the adolescent has made a suicide plan or has actually attempted suicide. Suicide risk factors are listed in Box 10-1.[15]

The prevalence of violence in society necessitates a violence risk screening (Box 10-2).[14] Affirmative answers to any of the questions in Box 10-2 suggest the need for further intervention. A referral to appropriate professionals for conflict resolution, anger management, or assertiveness training should be considered. A suspicion of abuse mandates reporting according to the laws in each state.

BOX 10-1

SUICIDE RISK FACTORS

- Recent loss of a family member
- Social isolation
- Family history of affective disorders
- Interpersonal problems with peers
- Sexual identity concerns
- Abuse or neglect
- Exposure to suicide
- Prior attempts
- Suicidal ideation
- Physical illness or injury
- Intense life stresses
- Poor coping skills

BOX 10-2

VIOLENCE SCREENING QUESTIONS

- How many fights have you been in during the past year?
- How many of those fights were serious?
- How do you get out of a fight?
- Have you ever been threatened with a weapon?
- Have you ever carried a weapon?
- Does anyone in your family carry a weapon?
- Do your parents physically fight in front of you?
- What is your favorite television show or movie?

Sexually active adolescents need counseling concerning the risks of sexual activity and the benefits of delaying future sexual encounters. Particularly, the risks of sexually transmitted diseases (STDs) and HIV infection, as well as the necessity of screening, are discussed. The use and limitations of condoms should be explained. Contraception options are also addressed during this discussion.

The Advisory Committee on Immunization Practice (ACIP) and GAPS recommend a routine comprehensive adolescent visit at age 11 years to lay the groundwork for future annual visits. Immunizations should be reviewed and updated at these annual visits. By 15 years of age, all adolescents should have received three hepatitis B vaccine doses (some states allow a two-dose schedule, with 10 mcg given at each dose and 4 to 6 months between doses); two measles-mumps-rubella (MMR) vaccine doses; four polio vaccine doses; one booster dose of tetanus vaccine using one of two new Tdap (tetanus-diphtheria vaccine booster with the addition of pertussis) vaccines (Boostrix [manufactured by Glaxo Smith Kline and licensed for children 10 to 18 years of age] or ADACEL [manufactured by Sanofi Pasteur and licensed for persons 11 to 64 years of age], if at least 5 years have passed since the last dose of diphtheria, tetanus, and pertussis vaccine). At this time, Tdap is only approved for a single dose. It should not be used for all the doses of Td in a previously unvaccinated person 7 years or older.[16] Varicella vaccine (Varivax) should be administered if there is no reliable history of chickenpox or evidence of varicella immunity.[16] Two doses of Varivax separated by 4 to 8 weeks are required for adolescents ages 13 years or older. Routine meningococcal vaccination is now recommended for all adolescents due to the disproportionate increase of meningococcal disease in this age group. Meningococcal conjugate vaccine (MCV4), Menactra, is now recommended for all children 11 to 12 years of age, as well as unvaccinated adolescents at high school entry. The previously licensed meningococcal polysaccharide vaccine (MPSV4), Menomune, is no longer recommended for routine vaccination because of its relative ineffectiveness in certain age groups and its relatively short duration of protection.[16] MCV4 is expected to provide longer protection than MPSV4 however, additional studies are necessary to confirm this assumption. At this time, routine revaccination is not recommended after receipt of MCV4. Antibody levels of MPSV4 decline rapidly in the first 2 to 3 years after vaccination, and revaccination with MCV4 is recommended for persons 11 to 55 years of age who received MPSV4, if indications still exist for vaccination.[16] MPSV4 is still used in children aged 2 to 10 years and adults older than 55 years who are at risk for meningococcal disease.[17] Gardasil, a vaccine to prevent cervical cancer, is recommended for females 9 to 26 years of age.[18]

Routine tuberculosis (TB) screening (using purified protein derivative, or PPD) is not usually performed unless the patient has risk factors for TB or the test is required for college admission. High-risk groups include close contacts of a person with infectious disease, foreign-born persons from areas where TB is common, and persons from medically underserved and low-income populations, including certain racial and ethnic groups (see Chapter 245).

A complete gynecologic examination is necessary for female adolescents once they become sexually active. This examination should include screening for STDs annually or more frequently depending on risk, and a Papanicolaou smear screening should be initiated within 3 years after the first episode of intercourse or by age 21 years and annually thereafter.

Annual adolescent preventive visits continue to age 21 years and include appropriate anticipatory guidance and a complete physical examination.[15] Height, weight, and body mass index should be plotted on growth charts at each well visit. When the health visit is for an evaluation for a sports physical, it should be sport-specific; at a minimum, the evaluation includes height, weight, blood pressure, visual acuity, cardiovascular assessment, abdominal palpation, testicular and inguinal examination for male adolescents, and a screening orthopedic examination.[19]

Precollege visits are an opportune time to update the adolescent's records, including immunization status, and to offer anticipatory guidance regarding sexuality (e.g., contraception, risks and prevention of STDs and HIV, responsible sexual behavior, prevention of sexual assault), cardiovascular health (e.g., nutrition, exercise, smoking), injury prevention (e.g., automobile and campus safety), obesity prevention, and mental health (e.g., stress, substance abuse, eating disorders). Patient education should occur at each visit. Box 10-3 lists some available resources.

Good health maintenance habits such as self-examination of the breast or testicles can be discussed during the physical examination. The presence of any abnormal medical conditions should be noted and the adolescent referred to other health professionals as needed. Screenings for preventable or treatable conditions (e.g., CBC, urinalysis, lipid profile) should be included with each health visit.[8,15] Consent for interventions may depend on the individual state regulations regarding emancipation of minors.

Caring for adolescents is challenging. However, the rewards are incalculable because the health care provider is a privileged witness to the formation of an adult. The potential for the health care provider to be a positive influence for the emerging adult is immeasurable.

BOX 10-3

RESOURCES FOR CARING FOR ADOLESCENTS

AMERICAN ACADEMY OF CHILD AND ADOLESCENT PSYCHIATRY
3615 Wisconsin Ave., NW
Washington, DC 20016-3007
(800) 333-7636
http://www.aacap.org

AMERICAN ACADEMY OF PEDIATRICS
141 Northwest Point Blvd.
Elk Grove Village, IL 60007
(847) 434-4000
http://www.aap.org

CENTER FOR YOUNG WOMEN'S HEALTH, CHILDREN'S HOSPITAL BOSTON
333 Longwood Ave., 5th floor
Boston, MA 02115
(617) 355-2994
http://www.youngwomenshealth.org

CHILDREN NOW
1212 Broadway, 5th floor
Oakland, CA 94612
(510) 763-2444
http://www.childrennow.org

DEPARTMENT OF CHILD AND ADOLESCENT HEALTH AND DEVELOPMENT, WORLD HEALTH ORGANIZATION
Avenue Appia 20, CH-1211
Geneva 27, Switzerland
(+00 41 22) 791 21 11
http://www.who.int/child-adolescent-health

KEEP KIDS HEALTHY
http://www.keepkidshealthy.com/adolescent/adolescent.html

PFLAG—PARENTS, FAMILIES, AND FRIENDS OF LESBIANS AND GAYS
1726 M St., NW, Suite 400
Washington, DC 20036
(202) 467-8180
http://www.pflag.org

SUICIDE PREVENTION HOTLINE
(800) 621-4000

REFERENCES

1. Robinson P: Puberty—am I normal? *Pediatr Ann* 26(2 suppl):S133-S136, 1997.
2. Cavanaugh R: Anticipatory guidance for the adolescent: has it come of age? *Pediatr Rev* 15(12):485-489, 1994.
3. Update: cardiovascular screening for athletes, *Contemp Pediatr* 13(10):16, 1996.
4. Boschere S: Tailor the message to age group, *Pediatr News* 31(7):32, 1997.
5. Burns CE, Dunn AM, Brady MA, and others: *Pediatric primary care*, Philadelphia, 2004, Saunders.
6. Greydanus D, editor: *Caring for your adolescent*, New York, 1991, Bantam Books.
7. Nelms B: Suicide—can we help prevent it? *J Pediatr Health Care* 10(3):97-98, 1996.
8. Morris G: Tasks of the times, *Contemp Pediatr* 13(6):94-104, 1996.
9. Elster AB, Kuntz NJ, editors: *AMA guidelines for adolescent preventive services (GAPS)*, Baltimore, 1994, Williams & Wilkins.

10. Knight J: Adolescent substance use: screening, assessment, and intervention, *Contemp Pediatr* 14(4):45-72, 1997.
11. Jenkins R, Saxena S: Keeping adolescents healthy, *Contemp Pediatr* 12(6):76-89, 1995.
12. Brown-Jones L, Orr D: Enlisting parents as allies against depression, *Contemp Pediatr* 13(11):67-86, 1996.
13. Morgan IS: Recognizing depression in the adolescent, *MCN* 19:148-155, 1994.
14. Maurer K: Guidelines offer questions to screen for violence, *Pediatr News* 31(2), 1997.
15. Jones CP: ACIP recommends early adolescent health check, *Infect Dis Child*, Jan 1995, pp 1-17.
16. Centers for Disease Control and Prevention, Atkinson W, Hamborsky J, McIntyre L, and others, editors: *Epidemiology and prevention of vaccine-preventable diseases*, ed 9, Washington, DC, 2006, Public Health Foundation.
17. Centers for Disease Control and Prevention: Meningococcal vaccines, what you need to know. Retrieved Dec 16, 2006, from http://www.cdc.gov/nip/publications/VIS/vis-mening.pdf.
18. Merck & Co.: *Gardasil—the only cervical cancer vaccine*, retrieved March 25, 2007, from http://www.gardasil.com.
19. Andrews JS: Making the most of the sports physical, *Contemp Pediatr* 14(3):183-205, 1997.

CHAPTER 11

Pregnancy

Debra Hobbins

Adequate, effective prenatal care has been associated with improved birth outcomes.[1-3] There are insufficient data to explain this relationship, however, in part because many studies have evaluated the adequacy of prenatal care by the quantity and early initiation of visits rather than by the specific content of the prenatal care visit.[3-5] The current prenatal care framework of first visit by 16 weeks, with subsequent monthly visits until 28 weeks, every 2 weeks after 28 weeks, and every week beginning at 36 weeks, has been the standard for nearly a century, without an evidence base. This care framework is based on number of visits and specific scheduling.[6] A tragic fact is that, even though the United States has more prenatal visits than any other country, in 2002 we ranked 28th out of 37 countries in infant mortality.[7]

In 1989 the U.S. Public Health Service[8] published specific guidelines for effective routine prenatal care, recommending that low-risk women receive eight visits instead of the usual 14 to 16 visits. Three basic components of prenatal care were identified: (1) early and continuing risk assessment, (2) health promotion, and (3) medical and psychosocial interventions and follow-up. The U.S. Public Health Service document[8] describes the critical components of each prenatal care visit, including laboratory tests, examinations, and health promotion activities, based on the gestational age of the pregnancy. In 1994, in an effort to define and strengthen prenatal care globally, the World Health Organization[9] convened a working group to formulate recommendations for prenatal care at the health center level. Seven essential areas of health behavior advice are recommended for all pregnant women: (1) breastfeeding; (2) reducing or eliminating alcohol; (3) reducing or eliminating smoking; (4) not using illegal drugs; (5) eating the proper foods; (6) taking vitamin and mineral supplementation, including folic acid; and (7) gaining appropriate weight during pregnancy. Unfortunately, prenatal care is primarily capable of providing secondary prevention. Primary prevention lies within the purview of integrated health care for women, a critical component of which is preconceptional health promotion.[10]

The group model of providing complete prenatal care is the most ambitious and revolutionary approach to prenatal care in almost a century. This innovative and promising approach is known as Centering Pregnancy and has been used in the United States since the mid-1990s.[6,11,12] Centering Pregnancy underscores the fact that pregnancy is a normal physiologic process involving psychosocial and physical adaptations and preparation for labor and parenting. Inherent in this model is recognition of the value of supportive relationships among patients and among patients and their support system. Centering Pregnancy is relationship oriented and promotes new ways of nonhierarchic interaction between women and their providers.[13]

Although this chapter may seem to concentrate heavily on the medical or technical aspects of a woman's prenatal care, the impact of the psychosocial aspects of a woman's life and her pregnancy on her emotional well-being and relationship with her infant cannot be overemphasized. The implications of childbirth on families and society are acknowledged and briefly addressed. There is an association between a woman's social situation, her health, and her use of health services.[14]

Waldenstrom[15] encourages health care providers to consider different perspectives of childbirth when providing care for childbearing women. From a psychologic viewpoint, childbirth has implications for a woman's identity as a woman, her maturation into motherhood, and her relationship with her infant. From a psychosocial perspective, childbirth has ramifications for a woman's relationships with other people, particularly her partner and parents. From a social point of view, the role of motherhood has implications for all other roles, including professional roles. Childbirth also has economic consequences for the family and society. The birth itself and procedures surrounding the event are colored by the cultural, ethical, and religious beliefs held by the woman and her family. Therefore, social and psychologic support are integral elements of all care provided to pregnant women.[14]

Physician consultation is indicated for many disorders associated with pregnancy. Some patients require emergent evaluation, whereas others require consultation with the appropriate specialist, obstetrician, or health care provider. Pregnant women with severe hypertension, preeclampsia, or eclampsia; gestational, type 1, or type 2 diabetes; new-onset hyperthyroidism; vaginal bleeding; pyelonephritis; congenital or suspected heart disease; ectopic pregnancy; or asthma exacerbation may require both physician consultation and hospitalization.

GOALS OF PRENATAL CARE

Ideally, prenatal care includes individualized health education, screening, diagnosis, risk assessment, treatment, referral, skills building, and support.[9,13] The traditional goal of prenatal care has been to reduce maternal and fetal morbidity and mortality. The current goals of prenatal care have been broadened to include health promotion for the mother, fetus, and family and have been extended longitudinally through the first year to encompass family development and parenting skills; reduction of family violence and neglect, injuries, and accidents; prevention of acute illness; treatment and stabilization of chronic illnesses; and family planning.[8,16]

BARRIERS TO PRENATAL CARE

Some effort has been made to reduce the traditional barriers to prenatal care in areas such as affordability, transportation, child care, and availability of health care providers. Nonstructural barriers to prenatal care in relation to areas such as attitudes, beliefs, social setting, and culture also exist and may significantly influence a woman's decision about obtaining care, particularly during the first trimester.[17,18] Three cognitive factors are significantly correlated with earlier presentation for prenatal care: (1) the desire for pregnancy, (2) a wish for early confirmation of pregnancy, and (3) an experience of early pregnancy symptoms. The decision to use prenatal care is made within a social, cultural, and historical context that depends on social interpretations.[17]

AMBULATORY PRENATAL CARE

Prenatal care can be effectively and efficiently provided by defining the capabilities and expertise of health care providers and by ensuring that pregnant women receive risk-appropriate care. All providers must be able to identify a full range of medical and psychosocial risks and refer patients for appropriate care throughout their pregnancy.[19]

Basic prenatal care includes the prenatal care record, physical examination and interpretation of findings, routine laboratory tests, assessment of gestational age and normal progression of pregnancy, ongoing risk identification with consultation and referral mechanisms, psychosocial support, childbirth education, and care coordination. This level of care is safely and appropriately provided by certified nurse midwives, nurse practitioners, and physician assistants with experience, training, and demonstrated competence.[19] Considering the shortcomings of prenatal care in the United States, Strong[20] stoutly recommended that nurse-midwives become the providers of choice for all low-risk women in America. Indeed, based on the evidence in reviews of randomized controlled trials in the Cochrane Pregnancy and Childbirth Database, routinely involving physicians and obstetricians in the care of all women during pregnancy and childbirth is not uniformly beneficial.[14,21]

Specialty care, which includes additional fetal diagnostic testing and expertise in managing medical and obstetric complications, is generally provided by obstetricians/gynecologists (OB/Gyns). Subspecialty care consisting of advanced fetal diagnoses; medical, surgical, neonatal, and genetic consultation; and management of severe maternal complications is provided by maternal-fetal medicine (MFM) specialists and reproductive geneticists.[22] Consultation and referral among providers of basic, specialty, and subspecialty levels of prenatal care are instituted on the basis of the patient's circumstances and the expertise of the individual provider. Conditions requiring consultation may be present before conception or may become apparent, arise, or be exacerbated during the pregnancy (Tables 11-1 and 11-2). Follow-up care is determined jointly at the time of consultation, resulting in continued care by collaboration or transfer of care.[19]

CONTENT OF PRENATAL CARE

Although more women are receiving prenatal care, the staggering incidence of low-birth-weight infants and preterm labor is increasing, suggesting the need for critical evaluation of levels of care and the clinical significance of that care.[23] It has been suggested that the quality of prenatal care, particularly in terms of the patient's receiving all of the recommended health behavior advice, is independent of the quantity of care (number of visits) in predicting improved birth outcomes.[8] It has also been suggested that women who are at greater risk of adverse birth outcomes benefit most from educational health care messages.[3,5] It may simply be that educating women and their significant others is of more value in positive perinatal outcomes than measuring the fundus, listening to heart tones, and dipping urine.

TABLE 11-1 Early Pregnancy Indications for Consultation

Indication	Consultant
HEALTH HISTORY AND CONDITIONS	
Asthma	
Symptomatic (on medication)	Ob/Gyn
Severe (multiple hospitalizations)	MFM
Autoimmune disease (systemic lupus erythematosus, rheumatoid arthritis, scleroderma, ankylosing spondylitis, Sjögren's syndrome, polymyositis or dermatomyositis)	Ob/Gyn
Cardiac disease	
Congenital heart disease	MFM
Cyanosis, prior myocardial infarction, aortic stenosis, primary pulmonary hypertension, prosthetic valve, American Hospital Association class II or greater	MFM
Other	Ob/Gyn
Diabetes mellitus	
Class A-C	Ob/Gyn
Class D or greater	MFM
Drug or alcohol use	Ob/Gyn
Epilepsy (on medication)	Ob/Gyn
Family history of genetic problems (Down's syndrome, Tay-Sachs disease, cystic fibrosis, Duchenne's muscular dystrophy)	MFM
Hemoglobinopathy (SS-, SC-, S-thalassemia)	MFM
Hypertension	
Chronic with renal or heart disease	MFM
Chronic without renal or heart disease	Ob/Gyn
Phenylketonuria	MFM
Prior pulmonary embolus or deep venous thrombosis	Ob/Gyn
Psychiatric illness	Ob/Gyn
Pulmonary disease	
Severe obstructive or restrictive	MFM
Moderate	Ob/Gyn
Renal disease	
Chronic, creatinine ≥3 mg/dl, with or without hypertension	MFM
Chronic, other	Ob/Gyn
Requirement for prolonged anticoagulation	MFM
Severe systemic disease	MFM
OBSTETRIC HISTORY AND CONDITIONS	
Age ≥35 yr at estimated date of birth	Ob/Gyn
Cesarean birth, prior classic or vertical incision	Ob/Gyn
Incompetent cervix	Ob/Gyn
Prior fetal structural or chromosomal abnormality	MFM
Prior neonatal death	Ob/Gyn
Prior fetal death	Ob/Gyn
Prior preterm birth or preterm premature rupture of membranes	Ob/Gyn
Prior low birth weight (<2500 g)	Ob/Gyn
Second-trimester pregnancy loss	Ob/Gyn
Uterine leiomyomas or malformation	Ob/Gyn
INITIAL LABORATORY TESTS	
HIV	Ob/Gyn
Symptomatic or low CD4 count	MFM
Other	Ob/Gyn
CDE (Rh) or other blood group isoimmunization (excluding ABO, Lewis)	MFM
INITIAL EXAMINATION	
Condylomas (extensive, covering vulva and vaginal opening)	Ob/Gyn

Modified from American Academy of Pediatrics, American College of Obstetricians and Gynecologists: *Guidelines for perinatal care,* ed 4, Washington, DC, 1997, The College.
MFM, Maternal-fetal medicine specialist; *Ob/Gyn,* obstetrician/gynecologist.

Diagnosis of Pregnancy

A diagnosis of pregnancy is usually based on a patient's history of missed menses and a positive urine pregnancy test. A home pregnancy test should be confirmed by an office test for urinary human chorionic gonadotropin (HCG) to rule out false-positive or false-negative results.[16]

Estimated Date of Birth

The age of the pregnancy or a clinical estimated date of birth (EDB), date of delivery, or time of arrival should be determined by 20 weeks' gestation, since dating becomes increasingly inaccurate after that time. Accurate dating is important for the management of some pregnancy problems and for the application and interpretation of certain laboratory tests, such as maternal serum alpha-fetoprotein (MSAFP).[19]

Nägele's rule is commonly used to determine the EDB by counting back 3 months from the first day of the last normal menstrual period (LMP) and adding 7 days. For example, if the LMP was April 5, the EDB would be January 12.[24] The duration of a pregnancy is 40 weeks ± 2 weeks. The incidence of pregnancies continuing beyond 42 weeks is 3% to 12%.[25] If a size-date discrepancy exists or menstrual dates are uncertain, ultrasound imaging for dating should be performed; this is most accurate before 20 weeks' gestation. An ultrasound evaluation is considered consistent with menstrual dates if there is gestational age agreement to within 7 days when the imaging is done at 6 to 11 weeks' gestation, or within 10 days when the imaging is done at 12 to 20 weeks' gestation.[19] The use of routine early ultrasound reduces the incidence of postterm pregnancy, and routine induction of labor at 41 weeks' gestation reduces perinatal mortality with no effect on cesarean birth.[26]

Timing of Visits

Traditionally, prenatal visits have been scheduled every 4 weeks from 8 to 28 weeks' gestation, every 2 weeks until 36 weeks' gestation, and weekly thereafter, for a total of 14 visits.[27] A schedule of fewer visits for healthy low-risk women, with visits limited to specific purposes during the first 6

TABLE 11-2 Ongoing Pregnancy Indications for Consultation

Indication	Consultant	Indication	Consultant
HEALTH HISTORY AND CONDITIONS		Hyperemesis persisting beyond first trimester	Ob/Gyn
Proteinuria (≥2+ detected by catheter sample, unexplained by urinary tract infection)	Ob/Gyn	Multiple gestation	Ob/Gyn
Pyelonephritis	Ob/Gyn	Oligohydramnios suspected by ultrasound	Ob/Gyn
Severe systemic disease affecting pregnancy	MFM	Preterm labor, threatened at <37 weeks	Ob/Gyn
Substance abuse	Ob/Gyn	Premature rupture of membranes	Ob/Gyn
OBSTETRIC HISTORY AND CONDITIONS		Vaginal bleeding ≥14 weeks	Ob/Gyn
Blood pressure elevation (diastolic ≥90 mm Hg), no proteinuria	Ob/Gyn	**LABORATORY AND EXAMINATION FINDINGS**	
Fetal abnormality suspected by ultrasound	Ob/Gyn	Abnormal MSAFP (low or high)	Ob/Gyn
Anencephaly	MFM	Abnormal Pap test	Ob/Gyn
Other	Ob/Gyn	Anemia (hematocrit <28%, unresponsive to iron therapy)	Ob/Gyn
Fetal death	Ob/Gyn	CDE (Rh) or other blood group isoimmunization (excluding ABO, Lewis)	MFM
Fetal growth restriction suspected	Ob/Gyn	Condylomas (extensive, covering labia and vaginal opening)	Ob/Gyn
Gestational age 41 weeks (seen by 42 weeks)	Ob/Gyn	HIV	
Gestational diabetes mellitus	Ob/Gyn	Symptomatic or low CD4 count	MFM
Herpes, active lesions at 36 weeks	Ob/Gyn	Other	Ob/Gyn
Hydramnios suspected by ultrasound	Ob/Gyn		

Modified from American Academy of Pediatrics, American College of Obstetricians and Gynecologists: *Guidelines for perinatal care*, ed 4, 1997, Washington, DC, The College.
MFM, Maternal-fetal medicine specialist; *MSAFP*, maternal serum alpha-fetoprotein; *Ob/Gyn*, obstetrician/gynecologist.

months, has been recommended.[24] The revised schedule consists of visits at 6 to 8, 14 to 16, 24 to 28, 32, 36, 38, 39, and 40 weeks' gestation, for a total of eight visits. In low-risk women, this schedule has produced no increases in adverse maternal or perinatal outcomes.[20,27-29] Whatever the visit schedule, the most important element of care is the ongoing risk assessment of the woman. Visits must be tailored to her specific needs, avoiding a "cookie cutter approach" to providing prenatal care.[6]

Prenatal Visits

A comprehensive summary of recommendations on the diagnostic and educational content of visits is presented in Box 11-1.[30] A version of this summary can be used in clinical practice with dates placed by each item as discussed, ordered, or evaluated. It should be noted that the routine early use of ultrasound has been shown to have a trade-off between beneficial and adverse effects.[14]

During pregnancy, only anemia is more common than violence against women. Because of the prevalence of violence against women; the increase in violence associated with pregnancy; and the association of pregnancy complications, perinatal morbidity and mortality, and substance abuse with domestic violence, the "abuse screen" item in Box 11-1 is mandatory. The abuse screen consists of the questions and interventions provided in Boxes 11-2 and 11-3.[19,31]

Although prospective studies have not confirmed an association between hyperthermia and birth defects, animal studies and some human data suggest an association with neural tube defects and impaired brain development. It is recommended that pregnant women not use a hot tub or sauna with a temperature greater than 38.9° C (102° F), and that exposure be limited to 10 minutes.[25,32]

COMPLICATIONS OF PREGNANCY

Nausea and Vomiting

Nausea and vomiting are the most common symptoms experienced in early pregnancy: 70% to 85% of women experience nausea, and 50% experience vomiting. A review of randomized controlled trials reveals that vitamin B_6 (pyridoxine) is effective in reducing the severity of nausea; ginger may be of benefit although the evidence is weak. Antiemetics reduce the frequency of nausea, but little information is available on the effects on fetal outcomes.[33] A sea-sick wrist band has been helpful to some women with nausea and vomiting.

Constipation

Constipation is a common problem during pregnancy and is possibly caused by increased levels of circulating progesterone. Bran or wheat fiber increases the frequency of defecation. Stimulant laxatives (bisacodyl, senna) are more effective than bulk-forming laxatives (psyllium, calcium polycarbophil), but they may cause more side effects.[34]

First-Trimester Bleeding

Approximately 20% to 25% of women experience vaginal spotting or heavier bleeding during the first half of pregnancy; of these women, half will abort. Bleeding may be physiologic and occur around the time of the expected menses. It may be caused by cervical lesions or erosion (especially after intercourse) or by cervical polyps.[24] Most women who are threatening to abort will do so no matter what interventions are instituted. Bleeding accompanied by pelvic or back pain requires a cervical and bimanual examination; the prognosis for the pregnancy is poor. Viability may be assessed with transvaginal ultrasound and/or serial quantitative HCG levels, which should increase by at least 65% every 48 hours.[24]

BOX 11-1

PRENATAL CARE PROTOCOL: RECOMMENDED DIAGNOSTIC AND EDUCATIONAL COMPONENTS OF VISITS

INITIAL COMPREHENSIVE EVALUATION

History
- Social
- Obstetric
- Medication
- Menstrual
- Health
- Family

Abuse screen

Physical examination (including blood pressure, teeth [periodontal disease], height, weight, and pelvic examination)

Laboratory tests
- Cervical cytology
- *Chlamydia trachomatis*
- *Neisseria gonorrhoeae*
- Wet mount (bacterial vaginosis)
- Prenatal labs (CBC, HIV, blood type/Rh, antibody screen, serology, hepatitis B antigen, rubella titer, hepatitis C antigen as indicated)
- Urine for quantitative culture and protein

Fundal height (FH)

Fetal heart tones (FHTs)

Education
- Office care and timing of visits
- Danger signs and who to call (vaginal bleeding, swelling of face or fingers, severe or continuous headache, dimness or blurring of vision, abdominal pain, persistent vomiting, chills, or fever ≥38.3° C [101° F], dysuria, escape of fluid from vagina, marked change in frequency or intensity of fetal movements)
- Medication counseling (consider alternative needs for chronic conditions; no ibuprofen, aspirin, loratadine)
- Alcohol, smoking, illegal drug cessation
- Eating proper foods
- Taking vitamins, minerals, and folic acid
- Weight gain
- Breastfeeding infant
- Schedule breastfeeding class
- Toxoplasmosis awareness (not handling kitty litter, eating well-cooked meat, wearing gloves in garden)
- Listeriosis awareness (not drinking or eating foods made with unpasteurized milk, avoiding ready-to-eat meats [deli])
- Parvovirus B19 (fifth disease, slapped cheek syndrome) and cytomegalovirus awareness (young children at home, working with young children)
- Tuberculosis (TB) (HIV positive; abnormal chest radiography; recent contact with active case of TB; foreign born; IV drug users who are HIV negative, are low income, or have a medical condition that increases the risk for TB)
- Morning sickness measures
- Daily fluid intake of 2 quart minimum
- Health maintenance practices (e.g., rest, seat belt)

ALL FOLLOW-UP PRENATAL VISITS

Blood pressure, weight, FHTs, FH, urine glucose and protein, fetal movement

8-18 WEEKS

Screening and dating ultrasound

Chorionic villus sampling

Amniocentesis

Education
- Review laboratory results
- Review Pap test results
- Exercise and activity
- Travel
- Discomforts of pregnancy
- Sexuality

16-18 WEEKS

Maternal serum alpha-fetoprotein (MSAFP)

Education
- Prenatal vitamin follow-up
- Financial assistance

26-28 WEEKS

1-hour glucose tolerance (as indicated)

Repeat hemoglobin (Hgb) or hematocrit (Hct)

Repeat antibody test and prophylactic administration of RhoGam for unsensitized Rh-negative women

Repeat HIV testing

Education
- Fetal movement counts
- Preterm labor signs and symptoms
- Contraception postpartum
- Sign up for classes
- Labor companion(s)
- Alcohol, smoking, illegal drug cessation

Abuse screen

32-36 WEEKS

Testing for sexually transmitted diseases as indicated

Repeat Hgb or Hct

Presenting part

Education
- Preeclampsia signs and symptoms
- Confirm class attendance
- Left side-lying position
- Push fluids, protein
- Require car seat for infant

36-40 WEEKS

Presenting part or station

Group B streptococci culture (35-37 weeks)

Education
- Labor signs and symptoms, when to call
- Labor and delivery procedures
- Labor and birth preferences
- Early labor
- Anesthesia
- Circumcision
- Contraception postpartum
- Breastfeeding or bottle feeding
- Discharge planning
- Parenting and child care

Blood type and Rh should be determined in cases of threatened, spontaneous, or induced abortion; ectopic gestation; any procedure associated with possible fetal-to-maternal bleeding (e.g., chorionic villus sampling and amniocentesis); and conditions associated with fetal-maternal hemorrhage (e.g., abdominal trauma or abruptio placentae). Women who are unsensitized Rh (D) negative should receive RhoGam within 72 hours. Administration of 300 mcg of RhoGam will provide protection in the presence of a fetal-to-maternal bleed of 30 ml. A Kleihauer-Betke test may be used to detect a fetal-

BOX 11-2

ABUSE SCREEN

These questions may be asked verbally or on a written form. Complete privacy, with only the patient and health care provider present, is necessary.

1. Have you ever been emotionally or physically abused by your partner or someone important to you?
2. In the year before you were pregnant, were you pushed, shoved, slapped, hit, kicked, or otherwise physically hurt by someone?
3. Since the pregnancy began, have you been pushed, shoved, slapped, hit, kicked, or otherwise physically hurt by someone?
4. In the year before you were pregnant, did anyone force you to have sexual activities?
5. Since the pregnancy began, has anyone forced you to have sexual activities?
6. Are you afraid of your partner or anyone you listed above?

Modified from McFarlane J, Parker B, Soeken K, and others: Safety behaviors of abused women after an intervention during pregnancy, *JOGNN* 27(1):64-69, 1998.

BOX 11-3

SAFETY PLAN

Try to do the following:

- Hide money.
- Hide an extra set of house and car keys.
- Establish a code with family and friends.
- Ask a neighbor to call police if violence begins.
- Remove weapons.

Have available:

- Social Security numbers (his, yours, children's)
- Rent and utility receipts
- Birth certificates (yours and children's)
- Drivers license (yours and children's)
- Bank account numbers
- Insurance policies and numbers
- Marriage license
- Valuable jewelry
- Important phone numbers

Hide a bag with extra clothing.

Modified from McFarlane J, Parker B, Soeken K, and others: Safety behaviors of abused women after an intervention during pregnancy, *JOGNN* 27(1):64-69, 1998.

maternal hemorrhage greater than 30 ml that would require additional RhoGam.[19]

Second- and Third-Trimester Bleeding

The incidence of second-trimester bleeding is higher than that of third-trimester bleeding and is associated with a perinatal mortality rate of 23% to 32%. Placenta previa, premature placental separation (abruption), molar gestation, and cervical or vaginal lesions are the most common causes of second- and third-trimester bleeding.[25]

The incidence of placenta previa is 1 out of 200 births, occurring in 1 out of 20 births for grand multiparas, and is associated with an increased risk of congenital abnormalities and intrauterine growth restriction (IUGR). Presentation is typically painless vaginal bleeding at a mean of 32.5 weeks' gestation, with blood loss from the first bleed rarely fatal. Ultrasound imaging is the diagnostic technique of choice; vaginal and rectal examinations are not performed. An immediate hospital referral is required.[25,35]

The most common cause of third-trimester bleeding (>80%) is abruptio placentae, which complicates 1 out of 120 pregnancies. The most common clinical correlate of moderate to severe abruption is chronic or pregnancy-related hypertension. Other risk factors are cigarette smoking, cocaine use, and trauma. Abruption is commonly accompanied by uterine pain and tenderness; back pain; and frequent, low-amplitude contractions. Immediate hospital referral is required.[25,35]

Gestational Diabetes

Gestational diabetes is a form of type 2 diabetes. Women with a history of gestational diabetes have a 30% to 70% risk of developing type 2 diabetes, the highest risk being for women who had early diagnosis, severe disease, a need for insulin, and impaired glucose tolerance during the postpartum period. Diet therapy is the initial intervention; oral or insulin therapy is added after the diet has failed to control glucose levels.[36]

Pregnancy-Related Hypertension

Pregnancy-related hypertension is hypertension that develops as a consequence of pregnancy and regresses postpartum. The archaic terminology *toxemia of pregnancy* has been abandoned. Risk factors include nulliparity, age, race, a family history of preeclampsia or eclampsia, preexisting hypertensive vascular and autoimmune disease, diabetes, obesity, multiple gestations, trisomy 13, hydatidiform mole (earlier than 20 weeks' gestation), and nonimmune or alloimmune fetal hydrops.[24,25,37]

There are four categories of pregnancy-related hypertension: (1) chronic hypertension, (2) preeclampsia and eclampsia, (3) preeclampsia superimposed on chronic hypertension, and (4) gestational hypertension.[37,38] Chronic hypertension is hypertension that is present and observable before pregnancy or is diagnosed before the 20th week of gestation when blood pressure is 140/90 mm Hg. Preeclampsia is increased blood pressure, greater than 140/90 mm Hg, accompanied by proteinuria (+1 dipstick). Diastolic blood pressure is determined by the disappearance of Korotkoff's V sounds. Preeclampsia is a spectrum, arbitrarily divided into mild and severe forms. Severe preeclampsia is diagnosed when the following are present: (1) blood pressure over 160/110 mm Hg; (2) more than 2 g proteinuria in 24 hours; (3) serum creatinine greater than 1.2 mg/dl, unless previously elevated; (4) persistent headache or cerebral or visual disturbances; (5) persistent epigastric pain; and (6) platelets less than 100,000/mm^3 and/or evidence of microangiopathic hemolytic anemia. Eclampsia is the occurrence of seizures in a preeclamptic woman that are not attributable to other causes. Edema is no longer a marker for preeclampsia.[37]

Superimposed preeclampsia is probable with the following conditions: (1) new-onset proteinuria in a woman with hypertension and no proteinuria before 20 weeks' gestation; and (2) in a woman with hypertension and proteinuria before 20 weeks' gestation: (a) sudden increase in proteinuria, 2 dipsticks of 2+, 4 hours apart, without evidence of urinary tract infection; (b) sudden increase in blood pressure in a woman whose blood pressure had been normal; (c) thrombocytopenia of less than 100,000/mm^3; and (d) an increase in alanine aminotransferase (ALT) or aspartate aminotransferase (AST) to abnormal levels. Gestational hypertension is blood pressure elevation detected for the first time during pregnancy, without proteinuria. If preeclampsia does not develop and blood pressure returns to normal by 12 weeks postpartum, the diagnosis is transient hypertension of pregnancy. If blood pressure elevation persists, the diagnosis is chronic hypertension.[37]

Gallbladder Disease

The most common type of gallbladder disease, cholelithiasis, is four times more common in women than in men and occurs in approximately 3% to 4% of pregnant women. The majority of these women are asymptomatic. Pregnancy increases the risk of gallstones primarily as a result of incomplete emptying of the gallbladder and the formation of biliary sludge.[24] Rarely, a stone enters the cystic duct, and one of three disorders may occur: biliary colic, acute cholecystitis (accompanied by bacterial infection in 50% to 85% of cases), or obstructive jaundice and pancreatitis. The diagnosis of cholelithiasis is made by ultrasound evaluation of the gallbladder, cystic duct, common bile duct, and liver.[25,39]

Depending on the severity of the disease, patients can usually be managed medically and may require hospitalization for bed rest, nasogastric suctioning, IV hydration, analgesic administration, and broad-spectrum antiinfective coverage. Laboratory tests include a CBC, liver function tests, urinalysis, urine culture, serum amylase to exclude pancreatitis, blood cultures in febrile patients, and evaluation of stool color. Surgery for acute gallbladder disease is not common in pregnancy and should be postponed until the postpartum period to avoid the 5% pregnancy loss associated with its performance in the second and third trimesters. More aggressive surgical management is indicated with concomitant biliary pancreatitis. Laparoscopic cholecystectomy has become the treatment of choice.[25,26,39]

MANAGEMENT OF CHRONIC CONDITIONS

Asthma

The effect of pregnancy on asthma is unpredictable—one third of patients improve, one third become worse, and one third remain the same. The course of asthma is often similar in subsequent pregnancies. Maternal asthma is associated with diabetes, fertility treatments, IUGR, hypertensive disorders, premature rupture of membranes, and higher rates of cesarean births.[40] In addition, chronically poor asthma control during pregnancy is associated with uterine hemorrhage, preterm birth, low birth weight, and congenital malformations.[41]

Women with moderate to severe asthma need to measure and record their daily peak expiratory flow rates (PEFRs) with a portable peak flow meter at home on rising and 12 hours later. Changes in PEFR values signifying early signs of deterioration often appear before symptoms. PEFR values range from 380 to 550 L/min, with each woman having her own baseline. Adjustments in therapy are made using these measurements. Patients can be symptomatic if they have PEFR variations of 20% or more.

Maintenance therapy for chronic asthma with mild, infrequent symptoms consists of inhaled β-adrenergic agonists (metaproterenol, albuterol, terbutaline, isoproterenol) as needed, theophylline, inhaled cromolyn sodium 2 puffs q.i.d., and inhaled corticosteroids (beclomethasone 42 mcg, 4 puffs b.i.d.) for individuals uncontrolled with bronchodilators. Asthma-associated medications to avoid in pregnancy are α-adrenergic compounds other than pseudoephedrine, epinephrine, iodides, sulfonamides (late in pregnancy), tetracyclines, and quinolones.[40-43]

Diabetes

During the first trimester, maternal hyperglycemia and derangements in maternal metabolism may lead to rates of major fetal malformation that are 10% or higher. Maternal glycosylated hemoglobin levels should be checked in the first trimester to assess control during the prior 4 to 6 weeks. MSAFP determinations should be performed at 16 weeks' gestation, comprehensive ultrasound evaluation at 16 to 18 weeks' gestation, and fetal echocardiography at 20 weeks' gestation.[44]

Antepartum care consists of glucose monitoring, oral or insulin therapy, and diet. Capillary glucose should be monitored and recorded: morning fasting values, 1 to 2 hours after breakfast, before and after lunch, before dinner, and at bedtime. Ideal whole blood glucose values are fasting, less than 95 mg/dl; 1-hour postprandial, less than 130 to 140 mg/dl; and 2-hour postprandial, less than 120 mg/dl. It has been suggested that peak postprandial glucose levels taken 1 hour after beginning a meal are the best predicators of fetal macrosomia.[36] Glycosylated hemoglobin levels should be measured every 4 to 6 weeks during pregnancy to provide feedback to the woman on her success at keeping her blood glucose within a narrow range. Oral and insulin therapy is beyond the scope of this chapter and quite involved. Oral agents now used to augment glucose control are sulfonylurea with insulin, metformin and troglitazone for insulin resistance, and acarbose for postprandial hyperglycemia. Medical nutritional therapy should be supervised by a registered dietitian. Dietary intake consists of three meals and three snacks with nonglycemic foods, no more than 50% carbohydrates, with 25% protein and 25% fats.[36,45,46]

Fetal evaluation to prevent demise consists of ongoing maternal assessment of fetal activity beginning at 28 weeks' gestation; nonstress tests twice weekly and contraction stress tests weekly at 28 to 34 weeks' gestation in an insulin-dependent woman, and at 36 weeks in a woman with diet-controlled gestational diabetes; and ultrasound biophysical profile weekly.[36,37,45]

Thyroid Disease

During pregnancy the thyroid gland is moderately enlarged, with increased uptake of radioiodine. Total serum thyroxine (T_4) and triiodothyronine (T_3) concentrations rise sharply as early as the second month. Daily T_4 secretion is probably increased, with substantial amounts transferred from the mother to the fetus. Thyroid-binding globulin is increased considerably, and thyroid-releasing hormone and thyroid-stimulating hormone (TSH), or thyrotropin, concentrations are unchanged. Transient lowering of serum TSH is associated with direct stimulation of the maternal thyroid gland by elevated levels of HCG.[47]

Hypothyroidism

Women with untreated hypothyroidism who do become pregnant have a high incidence of preeclampsia and placental abruption, with a correspondingly high number of low-birth-weight and stillborn infants, an increased incidence of fetal distress, and an increased frequency of heart failure. Correction of hypothyroidism can prevent these problems. The drug of choice in the treatment of hypothyroidism is levothyroxine. The optimum dose of thyroid hormone is unclear, but the dose should be adjusted so that serum TSH levels are within the normal range. More than 50% of women with hypothyroidism need an increase in thyroid dosage during pregnancy.[24,48]

Hyperthyroidism

Most cases of hyperthyroidism are due to Graves' disease (85%), although nodular goiter and Hashimoto's thyroiditis are occasionally responsible. Early in pregnancy, hydatidiform mole may manifest with symptoms consistent with thyrotoxicosis. The diagnosis of hyperthyroidism is confirmed by the presence of increased free thyroxine (FT_4) or free thyroxine index (FT_4I); decreased TSH; and, in Graves' disease, TSH receptor antibody (TRAb). When the diagnosis is suspected, an endocrinologist should be consulted to assist with diagnosis and management.

Methimazole (10 to 20 mg b.i.d.) or propylthiouracil (100 to 150 mg t.i.d.) are both category D (positive evidence of risk, investigational or postmarketing data show risk to the fetus, potential benefits may outweigh the potential risk) in pregnancy. However, propylthiouracil is usually the preferred treatment because methimazole may be associated with more serious congenital defects. Propylthiouracil should be titrated to the lowest effective dose to minimize the risk for hypothyroidism or goiter in the fetus. Most patients respond to therapy, with an improvement in symptoms and thyroid values within 2 to 4 weeks. When the FT_4I improves, the drug dosage is reduced by one half. When the patient is euthyroid, the dosage is further reduced until the total dose is 15 mg of methimazole or 50 mg of propylthiouracil daily. A high titer of TRAb (>50%) in the mother at the end of pregnancy is predictive of neonatal hyperthyroidism.[48]

Heart Disease

Pregnancy causes marked changes in the heart. The resting pulse rate increases 10 to 15 beats per minute, and the heart is displaced to the left and upward and is rotated partially on its long axis so the apex is displaced laterally. There is an increase in the cardiac silhouette, and normal pregnant women have some degree of benign pericardial effusion. Heart sounds may also be altered during pregnancy. There may be an exaggerated splitting of the first heart sound with increased loudness of both components; a loud, easily heard third sound; a systolic murmur in 90% of pregnant women (intensified in either inspiration or expiration); a soft diastolic murmur in 20%; and continuous murmurs arising in the breast vasculature in 10%. Pregnancy produces no changes in the ECG other than slight deviation of the electrical axis to the left.[24]

Cardiac disease should be suspected in women with complaints of dyspnea, chest pain, palpitations or arrhythmia, and cyanosis. Increased attention should be given to women with a history of exercise intolerance, heart murmurs before pregnancy, or rheumatic fever. A general evaluation of heart disease in pregnancy includes a thorough history and physical examination, chest radiographs, ECG, arterial blood gases, and an echocardiogram. If this evaluation suggests cardiac disease, a prompt referral is indicated to classify the type of disorder and evaluate the functional status and reserve in order to counsel the woman regarding the risks to and prognosis for her and her fetus.[24]

Women with congenital heart disease should be referred immediately on discovery of pregnancy to an MFM specialist.

ACUTE EPISODIC ILLNESS

The incidence of asymptomatic bacteriuria varies from 2% to 7% depending on parity, race, and socioeconomic status. It is typically present at the first prenatal visit and is diagnosed by the presence of more than 100,000 organisms of a single uropathogen per milliliter in a clean-voided specimen. After an initial negative urine culture, less than 1% of women develop a urinary tract infection during pregnancy. If asymptomatic bacteriuria is not treated, 25% of women will develop an acute symptomatic infection. Renal bacteriuria is present in approximately 50% of cases. Treatment regimens include nitrofurantoin macrocrystals, 100 mg/day for 10 days; or ampicillin, amoxicillin, a cephalosporin, nitrofurantoin, or a sulfonamide for a minimum of 3 days. Prophylactic therapy with 100 mg of nitrofurantoin at bedtime for the duration of the pregnancy is indicated for women with persistent or frequent recurrences of bacteriuria.[24]

Symptoms of cystitis include dysuria, urgency, and frequency, with pyuria, bacteriuria, and hematuria microscopically. More than 90% of infections are limited to the bladder, as opposed to asymptomatic bacteriuria with renal involvement. Treatment is the same as for asymptomatic bacteriuria, with the exception that ampicillin, a sulfonamide (cannot be used in the third trimester), nitrofurantoin, or a cephalosporin is given for 10 days.[24]

Upper respiratory tract infections are treated conservatively with rest, hydration, humidification, and medication for the relief of symptoms. Medications include decongestants (pseudoephedrine, 60 mg up to q.i.d., 120-mg sustained-release capsules or tablets b.i.d., or saline nasal spray or drops up to 5 days), antihistamines (chlorpheniramine, 4 mg up to q.i.d. or 8- to 12-mg sustained-release capsules or tablets b.i.d.; or tripelennamine, 25 to 50 mg up to q.i.d. or 100-mg sustained-release capsules or tablets b.i.d.), and cough suppressants (guaifenesin or dextromethorphan, 2 teaspoons q.i.d.). Sinusitis is treated with amoxicillin for 3 weeks (if the patient is not allergic to penicillin).[42]

In general, penicillins are safe and lack toxicity for the woman and her fetus; however, there is little experience in pregnancy with the newer penicillins (piperacillin, mezlocillin, and azlocillin), and these should be used only when another, better-studied antibiotic is not effective. There is no evidence of teratogenicity of cephalosporins; the third-generation agents have had limited use in pregnancy. Sulfonamides are not teratogenic but should not be used in a woman with glucose-6-phosphate dehydrogenase deficiency or during the third trimester because of an increased risk of hyperbilirubinemia in the neonate. During the second and third trimesters, tetracyclines can cause a brown discoloration of the teeth, hypoplasia of the enamel, inhibition of bone growth, and other skeletal abnormalities. First-trimester exposure has not been associated with a teratogenic risk. However, tetracycline is considered category D in pregnancy. As an alternate to penicillin, erythromycin is the drug of choice for many diseases in pregnancy. Erythromycin estolate has been associated with reversible hepatotoxicity during pregnancy, but all other forms are recommended. Metronidazole has not been found to increase the incidence of congenital defects or other adverse outcomes of pregnancy for mothers or infants. Because there is some controversy surrounding this drug, deferring therapy until after the first trimester is wise.[49]

INTEGRATED HEALTH CARE FOR WOMEN

As primary prevention continues to gain momentum in the United States, it is likely that the potential for prenatal care visits to provide a venue for intervention will increasingly be recognized. Prenatal care continues to improve some outcomes of pregnancy, whereas other outcomes are seemingly unaffected by prenatal care. Preconceptional health promotion, a critical component of integrated health care for women, addresses many of the outcomes not affected by prenatal care. It is clear that additional research is needed.

Peoples-Sheps[4] asserts that, in the years to come, prenatal care will be characterized by (1) increasing recognition and use of components of care that have been shown to be effective; (2) research on psychosocial interventions, preconception care, and the timing of visits; (3) emphasis on balancing the medical and obstetric components of care with psychosocial components to meet the needs of individual patients; (4) interventions to eliminate smoking during pregnancy; and (5) development and evaluation of more effective ways of delivering services to the poor and to people of color.

Integrated health care for women and Centering Pregnancy are characterized by precisely those elements described. What has been heretofore referred to as *enhanced services*—such as Women, Infants, and Children (WIC) services, nutrition counseling, social work services, health education, childbirth and parenting education, social support, and violence intervention—are actually the basic services, with measuring fundal height and fetal heart tones the "enhanced" or even unnecessary services.[13,50]

REFERENCES

1. Enkin MW: Effective care in pregnancy and childbirth: the Cochrane Pregnancy and Childbirth Database, *J Perinat Educ* 4(4):23-35, 1995.
2. Haas JS, Berman S, Goldberg AB, and others: Prenatal hospitalization and compliance with guidelines for prenatal care, *Am J Pub Health* 86(6):815-819, 1996.
3. Sable MR, Herman AA: The relationship between prenatal health behavior advice and low birth weight, *Pub Health Rep* 112(4):332-339, 1997.
4. Peoples-Sheps MD: Prenatal care: will the past predict the future? *Women's Health Issues* 6(4):235-236, 1996.
5. Kogan MD, Alexander GR, Kotelchuck M, and others: Relation of the content of prenatal care to the risk of low birth weight: maternal reports of health behavior advice and initial prenatal care procedures, *JAMA* 271(17):1340-1345, 1994.
6. Moos MK: Prenatal care: limitations and opportunities, *JOGNN* 35(2):278-285, 2006.
7. Maternal and Child Health Bureau: *Comparisons of national infant mortality rates*, retrieved April 30, 2006, from http://mchb.hrsa.gov/chusa02/main_pages/page_22.htm.
8. US Public Health Service: *Caring for our future: the content of prenatal care,* Washington, DC, 1989, US Government Printing Office.
9. Berg CJ: Prenatal care in developing countries: the World Health Organization Technical Working Group on antenatal care, *JAMA* 50(5):182-186, 1995.
10. Hobbins D: Every woman, every time: state-of-the-science, state-of-the-art, *J Pernat Neonat Nurs* 20:43-45, 2006.
11. Rising SS: Centering Pregnancy: an interdisciplinary model of empowerment, *J Nurse Midwifery* 43:46-54, 1998.
12. Rising SS, Kennedy HP, Klima CS: Redesigning prenatal care through Centering Pregnancy, *J Midwifery Women's Health* 49:398-404, 2004.
13. Massey Z, Rising SS, Ickovics J: Centering Pregnancy group prenatal care: promoting relationship-centered care, *JOGNN* 35(2):286-294, 2006.
14. Enkin MW, Keirse MJNC, Renfrew M, and others: *A guide to effective care in pregnancy and childbirth,* ed 2, Oxford, 1995, Oxford University Press.
15. Waldenstrom U: Modern maternity care: does safety have to take the meaning out of birth? *Midwifery* 12:165-173, 1996.
16. Byrd J: Content of prenatal care. In Ratcliffe SD, Byrd JE, Sakornbut EL, editors: *Handbook of pregnancy and perinatal care in family practice: science and practice,* Philadelphia, 1996, Hanley & Belfus.
17. Campbell JD, Stanford JB, Ewigman B: The social pregnancy interaction model: conceptualizing cognitive, social, and cultural barriers to prenatal care, *Appl Behav Sci Rev* 4(1):81-97, 1996.
18. Brown SS, editor: *Prenatal care: reaching mothers, reaching infants,* Washington, DC, 1998, National Academy Press.
19. American Association of Pediatrics, American College of Obstetricians and Gynecologists: *Guidelines for perinatal care,* ed 4, Washington, DC, 1997, The College.
20. Strong TH: *Expecting trouble: what expectant parents should know about prenatal care in America,* New York, 2000, University Press.
21. Villar J, and others: Patterns of routine antenatal care for low-risk pregnancy (Cochrane Review). In *The Cochrane Library,* No 4, Oxford, 2001, Update Software.
22. Lockwood CJ: Autoimmune disease. In Queenan JT, Hobbins JC, editors: *Protocols for high-risk pregnancies,* ed 3, Cambridge, Mass, 1996, Blackwell Science.
23. Kogan MD, Martin JA, Alexander GR, and others: The changing pattern of prenatal care utilization in the United States, 1981-1995, using different prenatal care indices, *JAMA* 279:1623-1628, 1998.
24. Cunningham FG, Gilstrap LC, Leveno KJ, and others: *Williams obstetrics,* ed 22, Stamford, Conn, 2005, Appleton & Lange.
25. Scott JR, Hammond C, Spellacy WN, and others: *Danforth's handbook of obstetrics and gynecology,* Philadelphia, 1996, Lippincott-Raven.
26. Crowley P: Interventions for preventing or improving the outcome of delivery at or beyond term (Cochrane Review). In *The Cochrane Library,* No 4, Oxford, 2001, Update Software.
27. McDuffie RS, Beck A, Bischoff K, and others: Effect of frequency of prenatal care visits on perinatal outcome among low-risk women: a randomized controlled trial, *JAMA* 275(11):847-851, 1996.
28. Binstock MA, Wolde-Tsadik G: Alternative prenatal care: impact of reduced visit frequency, focused visits and continuity of care, *J Reprod Med* 39:1-6, 1994.
29. Partridge CA, Holman JR: Effects of a reduced-visit prenatal care clinical practice guideline, *J Am Board Fam Pract* 18(6):555-560, 2005.
30. Farrington PF, McElligott K, Hobbins-Garbett D: *Prenatal protocol,* unpublished document, Salt Lake City, 1997, Teen Mother and Child Program, University of Utah.
31. McFarlane J, Parker B, Soeken K, and others: Safety behaviors of abused women after an intervention during pregnancy, *JOGNN* 27(1):64-69, 1998.

32. Speroff L: Exercise. In Queenan JT, Hobbins JC, editors: *Protocols for high-risk pregnancies*, ed 3, Cambridge, Mass, 1996, Blackwell Science.
33. Jewell D, Young G: Interventions for nausea and vomiting in early pregnancy (Cochrane Review). In *The Cochrane Library*, No 4, Oxford, 2001, Update Software.
34. Jewell DJ, Young G: Interventions for treating constipation in pregnancy (Cochrane Review). In *The Cochrane Library*, No 4, Oxford, 2001, Update Software.
35. Lockwood CJ: Third trimester bleeding. In Queenan JT, Hobbins JC, editors: *Protocols for high-risk pregnancies*, ed 3, Cambridge, Mass, 1996, Blackwell Science.
36. Jovanovic L: *Diabetes and pregnancy: glucose-mediated macrosomia and the fetus*, 61st Scientific Sessions of the American Diabetes Association, Philadelphia, 2001.
37. Roberts JM: Pregnancy-related hypertension, In Creasy RK, Resnik R, editors: *Maternal-fetal medicine: principles and practice*, ed 5, Philadelphia, 2004, Saunders.
38. Gifford R, and others: *Report of the National High Blood Pressure Education Program Working Group on High Blood Pressure in Pregnancy*, Bethesda, Md, 2000, National Institutes of Health and National Heart, Lung, and Blood Institute.
39. Collea JV: Gallbladder. In Queenan JT, Hobbins JC, editors: *Protocols for high-risk pregnancies*, ed 3, Cambridge, Mass, 1996, Blackwell Science.
40. Sheiner E, Mazor M, Levy A, and others: Pregnancy outcome of asthmatic patients: a population-based study, *J Matern Fetal Neonat Med* 18(4):237-240, 2005.
41. Tan KS, Thomson NC: Asthma in pregnancy, *Am J Med* 109(9):727-733, 2000.
42. Working Group on Asthma and Pregnancy: *Executive summary: management of asthma during pregnancy*, NIH Pub No 93-3279A, Washington, DC, 1993, National Institutes of Health.
43. Whittey JE, Dombrowski MP: Respiratory diseases in pregnancy. In Creasy RK, Resnik R, editors: *Maternal-fetal medicine: principles and practice*, ed 5, Philadelphia, 2004, Saunders.
44. Kochenour NK: Asthma. In Queenan JT, Hobbins JC, editors: *Protocols for high-risk pregnancies*, ed 3, Cambridge, Mass, 1996, Blackwell Science.
45. Gabbe SG: Diabetes mellitus. In Queenan JT, Hobbins JC, editors: *Protocols for high-risk pregnancies*, ed 3, Cambridge, Mass, 1996, Blackwell Science.
46. Moore TR: Diabetes in pregnancy. In Creasy RK, Resnik R, editors: *Maternal-fetal medicine: principles and practice*, ed 5, Philadelphia, 2004, Saunders.
47. Glinoer D: What happens to the normal thyroid during pregnancy? *Thyroid* 9(7):631-635, 1999.
48. Mestman JH: Hypothyroidism. In Queenan JT, Hobbins JC, editors: *Protocols for high-risk pregnancies*, ed 3, Cambridge, Mass, 1996, Blackwell Science.
49. Reece EA, Petrie RH, Hobbins JC, and others: *Handbook of medicine of the fetus and mother*, Philadelphia, 1995, Lippincott.
50. Mahan CS: Prenatal care indices: how useful? *Pub Health Rep* 111:419, 1996.

CHAPTER 12

Lactation

Kathleen M. Craig

Lactation counseling begins during pregnancy with verbal and written health education regarding what to expect in the immediate postpartum period. Expectant mothers should be informed about the benefits of breastfeeding and about recommendations from the American Academy of Pediatrics (AAP) that infants be breastfed for the first year of life (or longer if the infant and mother desire).[1] Mothers should also know that they can breastfeed even if they are returning to work.[2]

Mothers should expect to keep their infant close to them in the first 2 weeks as the infant learns to nurse[3] and to plan to sleep when the infant sleeps. The AAP Task Force on SIDS has issued a policy statement recommending that infants sleep on their backs on firm mattresses in separate beds or bassinets in the mother's room. Soft objects and loose bedding should be kept out of the crib. Important teaching topics for prospective nursing mothers include good attachment principles that minimize breast engorgement and sore nipples and avoidance of bottles and supplements during the initial period of lactation, unless medically indicated.[4] Pacifier use, also included in the SIDS reduction recommendations, should be delayed until 1 month of age to ensure that breastfeeding is firmly established.[5]

After the infant is born, mothers are instructed in how to help the baby latch on correctly and how to assess colostrum transfer and milk production. Mothers are taught that the infant feeds frequently in the first 2 weeks and, in general, will begin to space out the feedings thereafter.[6] Mothers are encouraged to feed the baby on demand and to wake a sleepy baby to feed. Health care providers can support mothers in working with the baby to establish effective breastfeeding by teaching them that mother-infant dyads that make it through the first 2 weeks of breastfeeding generally go on to meet the mother's breastfeeding goals.[7] The mother should be provided with a list of community-based lactation resources. Problems that threaten continued lactation should be referred to lactation consultants.[8]

DISCHARGE INSTRUCTIONS

Discharge instructions should be in writing and reviewed with the mothers to assess their understanding.[9] Mothers need to monitor their infants for signs of adequate milk intake. Feeding requirements for breastfed infants depend on many factors, such as gestational age, size for gestational age, birth history, and early adaptation to extrauterine life. Premature infants have fewer reserves and are vulnerable to complications such as low blood glucose and low weight gain. Infants who are large for gestational age or small for gestational age require careful observation of feeding behaviors as well.[10]

It is preferable to teach mothers the expected goals and to teach them to report concerns, rather than teach them the "danger" signs, since once these signs appear, the infant's condition may be serious. Mothers need to recognize and report whether their infant is not meeting the standard for a "good" intake, since early intervention is critical. For example, newborns are vulnerable to hypernatremic dehydration starvation syndrome and will continue to produce some urine even when the situation is life threatening.[11]

Discharge instructions include a description of the normal progression of the stool and the optimum feeding and voiding patterns. Newborns should feed at least 8 to 12 times per day. The stool initially will be meconium, dark and tarry. Transitional stool is brown, and after the milk comes in, usually by day 3 or 4, the stools will become yellow with milk curds. For the first week of life, the number of stools and the number of voids should match the age in days. After this, the infant will develop a personal pattern of elimination that may change again at 1 month of age. Any changes in an infant's established pattern should be evaluated. With an optimum feeding pattern, the infant should latch on securely to the breast and suck and swallow rhythmically and vigorously for at least 10 minutes on each breast. Suckling time at the breast should not be limited, since some babies are less efficient than others. Mothers should assess for milk transfer.[12]

Mothers should keep a feeding log for the first week. The feeding log tracks the number and quality of feeds and the number of stools and voids. A feeding log helps the parents determine whether the infant is feeding well. The breasts should soften after feeding, and the infant should be satisfied and may fall asleep after suckling at the second breast.[13]

Mothers are instructed to call the provider if the infant develops jaundice or has difficulty feeding. Infants should be evaluated 1 to 3 days after discharge for hyperbilirubinemia and to assess weight.[14] Infants may lose up to 10% of their birth weight during the first week of life. A supplemental feeding plan should be initiated for infants who lose greater than 10% of their birth weight (Box 12-1).[15]

BOX 12-1

COMPONENTS OF A PLAN TO IMPROVE BREAST MILK INTAKE

1. Evaluate the breastfeeding and correct any problems with attachment technique or positioning.
2. Suggest the appropriate feeding frequency and duration based on individual assessment.
3. Use a hospital-grade breast pump with a double-pump setup (pumping both sides at once) to increase breast emptying and stimulation. Use the pumped milk to supplement breastfeeding.
4. Assess adequacy of feeding by closely following weight gain. If the maternal supply is adequate, weight gain should be about 1 ounce a day. If the supply is less than required, supplemental feedings of formula or banked human milk may be required temporarily. Taper them as soon as the supply is increased and weight gain is improved.
5. Slowly taper the pumping sessions after the infant has gained the appropriate weight and is breastfeeding without supplement.
6. If the breastfeeding problem is not improved by improving technique and supply, contact the referral network for expert help. Continue to maintain contact with the mother and specialists.

MANAGEMENT OF BREASTFEEDING PROBLEMS

Breast Engorgement

Breast engorgement may occur on the third or fourth postpartum day. It can usually be minimized by feeding the infant 8 to 12 times each day in the days leading up to the milk coming in. This may mean waking the infant to nurse. Mothers should keep a feeding log. Mothers should be taught to evaluate the difference between sustained and intermittent suckling. Some women with engorgement may need to express some milk manually or with a pump to soften the areola enough to allow the infant to latch on. When an engorged breast is not well emptied, the resulting back pressure on the milk glands can result in decreased milk production.[16] If a mother develops sore nipples, the primary care provider or a lactation consultant should be notified.

Infants need to be latched deeply onto engorged breasts to extract the milk. Mothers with engorgement may need to compress their breasts manually to form it for the infant's mouth. Deep asymmetric latch-on will resolve most nipple problems and engorgement. If the engorgement is serious, ice packs or cabbage leaves can be applied to the breasts between feedings, and hot packs can be applied before feedings.[17] If the mother cannot get her infant to latch on, direct observation of feeding is required. The mother should have a breastfeeding support plan at discharge. This may include visiting nurses, a lactation nurse, or other health care providers. Obstetric nurses can provide 24-hour phone support to triage concerns and to address early breastfeeding initiation problems.[18]

Latch-On Problems

An infant's inability to suckle effectively is often caused by inappropriate positioning or attachment. Mothers are taught to evaluate the latch-on and how to present the breast to the infant. Sucking on the nipple tip causes pain and poor let-down.

The ideal breastfeeding position for the mother is comfortably upright with pillows for support. It is important that she not be in a semireclining position, since this causes breast tissue to fall back to her chest wall. A cross-legged position with pillows for back and thigh support is comfortable for most women, even those who have had a cesarean section. The infant should be "unfolded" from the prenatal position so that the upper body is slightly extended. The infant's head should not be cradled in the crook of her arm or cupped in the mother's hand. Instead the infant is held in the cradle position with the head allowed to fall over mother's arm so that the baby is looking up to the breast.

The cross-cradle position provides more control of the baby's head. In the cross-cradle position the mother holds the baby in the arm opposite the breast by grasping the baby's shoulders and upper back and tucking the baby closely under both breasts; this allows the head to fall through the web space in her hand. The baby's head will tip back, creating plenty of room between the chin and chest so that the mouth can open wide. The baby will be able to open the mouth widely if the mother entices him or her by moving the baby, not the breast. The mother's hand should grasp the breast well behind the areola, compressing and projecting the breast forward so that when the infant latches on with flanged lips, he or she connects deeply with the tissue behind the areola to extract colostrum or milk. The infant should be attached asymmetrically, with more of the underside of the breast laid on the baby's gaping lower jaw and the nipple tucked into the baby's mouth last, disappearing just under the upper gum line. The baby needs to be drawn into the mother's body deeply. Latching asymmetrically allows the baby to strip the breast effectively, minimizing nipple trauma and maximizing colostrum or milk transfer.[19] A parent handout with diagrams of asymmetric latch developed by Ann Barnes, titled "When Latching," is available at http://www.breastfeedingonline.com/newman.shtml.

Every mother-infant pair should have frequent assessment of latch-on during the early postpartum period. This is an opportunity to teach the parents about their infant's unique characteristics and to practice good attachment techniques. An infant who is consistently dissatisfied after feeding for long periods is probably not getting enough to eat at the breast and may not be latched on correctly. If the mother reports poor feeding after the infant has been discharged, the infant should be brought to the clinic for evaluation. If the mother is still hospitalized, skilled personnel should work with the mother and infant to improve latch-on and assess colostrum or milk transfer. Sustained suckling with deep attachment promotes effective colostrum and milk extraction. Babies who are suckling intermittently should be assessed for deep latch. After attaining deep latch, the baby may improve his or her feeding behavior with facilitated feeding techniques such as using breast compression to encourage swallowing. Mother may massage baby as well to encourage active feeding and to keep baby from falling asleep. After milk production has been established, the breasts should soften after feeding and the infant's stooling pattern will increase. The mother will not need to provide as much structure and guidance for the baby after breastfeeding is established.[20]

Let-Down (Milk Ejection) Problems

Let-down, or milk ejection, results from smooth muscle contraction of the myoepithelial cells surrounding the secretory alveoli (glands) of the breast. Oxytocin produced in response to the infant's suckling, as well as to the sight, sound, and smell of the infant, causes this contraction and the resultant milk flow. Uterine cramping signals early oxytocin production, and the presence of these cramps is a good predictor of ultimate breastfeeding success. The cramping is usually worse with second and subsequent infants. Mothers may need analgesics in the early postpartum period to manage the "afterpains."

After a few weeks the let-down response can be sensed as a tingling sensation throughout the breasts followed by milk leaking from the nipple. Let-down is inhibited by stress, pain, and alcohol. The let-down response is enhanced through breast massage, thoughts of the infant, and relaxation. It is important for mothers to condition their let-down response if they need to pump milk from their breasts, such as providing milk for feeding their premature infants or for feeding their infants while they are at work.[21,22]

Inadequate Milk Production

Inadequate milk production usually results from inadequate suckling and breast emptying. It may also result from inadequate prolactin or from inadequate mammary glandular tissue. Prolactin levels in the mother measured before and after breastfeeding should show a threefold increase after suckling. A similar increase in prolactin levels occurs after the mother pumps her breasts. If the problem is the infant, infant suckling produces less milk and lower prolactin levels after breastfeeding than after the mother pumps. If the prolactin levels are uniformly low, it suggests an endocrine basis for the low milk supply. In the case of inadequate glandular tissue, the amount of milk production is decreased, while prolactin levels demonstrate the expected increase after stimulation in conjunction with a normal let-down response.[23] Assessing breast glandular tissue to determine if an adequate amount exits is part of prenatal maternal assessment.[24] If an inadequate amount of breast tissue is detected, the health care provider should develop a feeding plan for the infant, including close follow-up and early supplementation. Supporting the infant with supplemental feedings while increasing breast stimulation with a breast pump may improve milk production in cases of inadequate amounts of breast tissue.

In some cases, milk production (galactagogue) stimulators, including metoclopramide (10 mg t.i.d. for 1 week and then tapered over 4 days), are prescribed. Metoclopramide has been demonstrated to increase prolactin levels,[25] but not all mothers with low supply will respond.[26] Lactogenesis is a complex and not completely understood biochemical and psychosocial process.[27] Mothers who are suboptimally producing milk must be assessed for physiologic, psychologic, and social support variables that may be influencing supply. The mother can use herbal galactagogues such as fenugreek, but these galactagogues are not consistently reliable.[28] Double pumping in addition to nursing produces the best results for increasing supply.

Low Infant Weight Gain

Low infant weight gain in the first few weeks after birth is a problem that is usually caused by inappropriate breastfeeding management in the hospital and during the immediate postdischarge period. Infants who have lost 8% or more of their birth weight must be monitored to prevent significant problems. Infants who are feeding well should have four or more milk curd stools per day by the fourth day and at least six wet diapers per day. They should be easily arousable and feeding at least eight times per day for a minimum of 10 minutes of audible sucking and swallowing.

When assessing an infant with low weight gain, providers must observe a breastfeeding session. Strategies to increase success include infant arousal techniques, increased feeding frequency, and breast pumping to increase the milk supply. Techniques to arouse sleepy infants include stroking the infant's back, talking softly to the infant, stroking the feet, changing the diaper, or placing the infant on the mother (skin-to-skin contact). Sometimes it is necessary to offer the infant supplemental pumped milk or formula. Ideally, this is done while the infant is feeding at the breast using a supplemental nursing system. Significant infant weight loss or difficult management problems require careful evaluation and follow-up. Consultation with lactation consultants or physicians experienced with breastfeeding management and care of infants with failure to thrive may be necessary.[29]

Cracked Nipples

Cracked nipples are usually caused by attachment or latch-on problems. When the infant latches on to only the tip of the nipple instead of the underside of the breast followed by the nipple, the nipple becomes abraded. Therefore mothers should be taught the asymmetric latch-on technique. Treatment includes correcting the attachment and supporting milk extraction. Some mothers require 24 hours of nipple rest and pumping to allow for some healing of the irritated nipples to resume breastfeeding. Close interval assessment of the mother-infant dyad breastfeeding sessions will limit the need for nipple rest, since nipples can heal while the baby is breastfeeding if the attachment is corrected. The mother should be taught to listen for audible swallowing to determine when the infant is actively feeding. She can remove the infant from the breast after the nursing rhythm changes from active deep suckling that removes milk (active feeding) to leisurely comfort sucking.[30] The mother should be taught to use her finger to detach the baby by sliding her finger over the baby's lips, over the gum line, all the way back to the hinge of the baby's jaw. This will protect the nipple from further damage.

Medical-grade lanolin may improve breastfeeding comfort if the nipples are dry and cracked. For severely damaged nipples, hydrogel dressings are useful to maintain a moist wound healing environment. In addition, mothers must avoid overdrying their nipples and should apply warm, moist compresses after feedings to soothe and promote healing. Sometimes the pain of breastfeeding is so severe that pumping or hand expression is required to maintain the supply and prevent engorgement while healing begins. Nipple soreness generally improves after a rest from breastfeeding for 24 hours and institution of the correct attachment position. Mothers will need to pump every 3 hours while not breastfeeding. It generally takes 10 days for sore nipples to heal completely. If there is no improvement, the health care provider must reevaluate the breastfeeding technique and treatment plan; a referral to a lactation specialist may be indicated.[31]

Mastitis

Mastitis, or cellulitis of the interlobular connective tissue of the breast, is often a marker for breastfeeding problems. Mastitis usually manifests with fever, generalized malaise, flulike symptoms, local erythema, and breast warmth and tenderness. A combination of unrelieved breast engorgement with cracked or abraded nipples is often the reason why bacteria gains entry to breast tissue.

Treatment for mastitis includes the application of warm packs to the breast and frequent breastfeeding or pumping. In addition to these nonpharmacologic interventions, the infection is treated with antibiotics such as amoxicillin and clavulanate, dicloxacillin, or a broad-spectrum cephalosporin to cover a probable staphylococcal or streptococcal infection. The infant's sucking technique and the mother's breastfeeding pattern and support system should also be evaluated. Mastitis can progress to abscess if early intervention is not instituted. Therefore any occurrence of flulike symptoms in a breastfeeding mother requires an evaluation for mastitis.[32]

Infant Jaundice

Most newborns become mildly jaundiced between the third and fifth days of life. Excessive jaundice in a full-term newborn may be a sign of inadequate fluid intake. Newborns should be assessed for risk of developing hyperbilirubinemia before discharge. Risk factors include jaundice that develops in the first 24 hours, blood group incompatibility, gestational age less than 37 weeks, cephalhematoma, significant bruising, excessive weight loss, difficulty establishing breastfeeding, East Asian race, and a previous sibling requiring phototherapy. Babies with a high direct or conjugated bilirubin level need to be evaluated for biliary obstruction or hepatitis.

The most common cause of indirect or unconjugated hyperbilirubinemia in the first 5 to 10 days of life is infrequent feeding and low milk intake, resulting in an exaggerated physiologic jaundice. Frequent feedings generally result in frequent stools, and bowel movements are the primary excretion route for bilirubin. When feedings and associated stools are infrequent, the bilirubin in the meconium stool is reabsorbed into the bloodstream, which raises the serum bilirubin level and results in clinical jaundice. This is commonly referred to as *no breast milk* jaundice and is generally associated with less than optimum breastfeeding. It responds to increased breastfeeding, which may require the use of a breast pump to increase the mother's supply. Supplementing with water and sugar water are not recommended. Frequent breastfeeding, once the mother's milk is in, will usually improve the jaundice. Formula supplementation may be required in cases of low milk supply. If the baby is lethargic, the mother may extract the milk with a breast pump and feed it to the baby with a bottle or cup until the baby regains the vigor to extract milk directly from the breast.

The AAP has developed phototherapy guidelines specific to the rate of rise of the bilirubin levels plotted against the baby's age in hours. Newborn care providers must familiarize themselves with the guidelines and develop follow-up plans to assess the baby during the most vulnerable period, 3 to 5 days of age.[14]

True breast milk jaundice usually occurs after 1 to 2 weeks of age, after breastfeeding is well established, and occurs in the setting of appropriate weight gain. True breast milk jaundice may be caused by an inheritable enzymatic defect that inhibits glucuronyl transferase and prevents the conjugation of bilirubin. It results in late-onset, prolonged, unconjugated hyperbilirubinemia. The infant with true breast milk jaundice is typically thriving, gaining weight, and producing four or more milk curd stools per day. A temporary cessation of breastfeeding for 12 to 24 hours can be tried in cases when the bilirubin level exceeds 20 mg/dl. The mother's milk supply should be maintained by pumping while breastfeeding is interrupted. Once the bilirubin level has dropped, breastfeeding can be resumed. The bilirubin level may rise slightly, but not usually to clinically significant levels.[14]

Weaning

Weaning is a natural process. It is physically and emotionally less painful when it is done gradually and the infant leads the process. As the infant grows, other activities and other foods often replace the need to breastfeed. Weaning can happen as early as 6 to 7 months of age, when solids are introduced, or as late as 2 or 3 years of age. Some mothers and infants choose to breastfeed into the toddler years, and there is no reason to oppose a continuation of this bond. The ethnographic literature suggests that, before the widespread use of artificial infant formulas, children were traditionally nursed for 3 to 4 years.[33]

When mothers desire weaning, feedings should be replaced by supplemental milk or formula (depending on the infant's age), one feeding at a time over a period of a few weeks until all feedings have been replaced. Infants who are less than 1 year of age should receive breast milk or formula. Cow's milk should be withheld until infants are older than 1 year of age. When weaning toddlers, mothers may replace some feedings with activities instead of food.

CO-MANAGEMENT ISSUES

Expectant and new mothers may be referred to breastfeeding support groups such as La Leche League International; Nursing Mothers' Council; and Women, Infants, and Children (WIC) services. Patients who need additional assistance or specialized help should be referred to breastfeeding or lactation specialists. The Academy of Breastfeeding Medicine, La Leche League International Medical Associates, and the International Board of Lactation Consultant Examiners can provide referrals to lactation consultants.

SPECIAL PROBLEMS IN BREASTFEEDING MANAGEMENT

Working Mothers

Mothers who must return to work or school or be separated from their infants for regular periods can usually continue breastfeeding. The milk supply will adjust to the demands. Depending on the mother and the child's age, the mother may need to pump the breasts two or three times per day to maintain the milk supply and collect it to give to the caregiver for the infant's bottle feedings.

Multiple Births

Mothers of twins or triplets can breastfeed successfully. With proper support and encouragement they can expect to have a sufficient supply. Initially, twins may need to be breastfed separately until they learn how to nurse. After the infants learn how to nurse, they can be breastfed simultaneously. The need for supplemental feedings depends on both the mother's milk supply and the infants' needs.

Breast Pumps

Breast milk can be expressed by hand or by using a breast pump. Hand expression is a learned skill that can be taught easily. Many different types of manual and electric pumps are available. Mothers should choose one designed for their needs. Department store breast pumps are usually not well designed and may compromise supply. Hospital-grade electric pumps are available for rent, and effective single user pumps can be purchased from vendors specializing in breastfeeding support. Mothers should be provided with written instructions about milk storage and handling.[34]

REFERENCES

1. American Academy of Pediatrics Work Group on Breastfeeding: Breastfeeding and the use of human milk, *Pediatrics* 100:1035-1039, 1997.
2. Neilsen J: Return to work: practical management of breastfeeding, *Clin Obstet Gynecol* 47(3):656-675, 2004.
3. Lindenberg CS, Cabrera Artola R, Jimenez V: The effect of early postpartum mother-infant contact and breastfeeding promotion on the incidence and continuation of breastfeeding, *Int J Nurs Stud* 27(3):170-186, 1990.
4. Saadeh R, Akre J: Ten steps to successful breastfeeding: a summary of the rationale and scientific evidence, *Birth* 23(3):154-160, 1996.
5. American Academy of Pediatrics Task Force on Sudden Infant Death Syndrome: The changing concept of sudden infant death syndrome: diagnostic coding shifts, controversies regarding the sleeping environment, and new variables to consider in reducing risk, *Pediatrics* 116(5):1245-1255, 2005.
6. Neifert M: Early assessment of the breastfeeding infant, *Contemp Pediatr* 13:142-166, 1996.
7. Cernadas JM, Noceda C, Barrera L, and others: Maternal and perinatal factors influencing the duration of exclusive breastfeeding during the first 6 months of life, *J Hum Lact* 19(2):125-130, 2003.
8. Fairbank L, O'Meara S, Renfrew MJ, and others: A systematic review to evaluate the effectiveness of interventions to promote the initiation of breastfeeding, *Health Technol Assess* 4(25):1-17, 2000.
9. Bertini G, Perugi S, Dani C, and others: Maternal education and the incidence and duration of breastfeeding: a prospective study, *J Pediatr Gastroenterol Nutr* 37(4):447-452, 2003.
10. Spatz DL: Ten steps for promoting and protecting breastfeeding for vulnerable infants, *J Perinat Neonat Nurs* 18(4):385-396, 2004.
11. Yaseen H, Salem M, Darwich M: Clinical presentation of hypernatremic dehydration in exclusively breastfed neonates, *Indian J Pediatr* 71(12):1059-1062, 2004.
12. Shrago L: The relationship between bowel output and adequacy of breastmilk intake in neonates' first weeks of life. In Anaheim, Calif, 1996, Association of Women's Health, Obstetric and Neonatal Nurses.
13. Academy of Breastfeeding Medicine Protocol Committee: *Clinical protocol #5: peripartum breastfeeding management for the healthy mother and infant at term,* 2003, retrieved Dec 4, 2006, from http://www.bfmed.org/ace-files/protocol/supplementation.pdf.
14. American Academy of Pediatrics Subcommittee on Hyperbilirubinemia: Management of hyperbilirubinemia in the newborn infant 35 or more weeks of gestation, *Pediatrics* 114:297-316, 2004.
15. Academy of Breastfeeding Medicine Protocol Committee: *Clinical protocol #3: hospital guidelines for the use of supplemental feedings in the healthy term breastfed neonate,* 2003, retrieved Dec 4, 2006, from http://www.bfmed.org/ace-files/protocol/supplementation.pdf.
16. Neville MC, Morton J: Physiology and endocrine changes underlying human lactogenesis II, *J Nutr* 131:3005S-3008S, 2001.
17. Nikodem VC, Danziger D, Gebka N, and others: Do cabbage leaves prevent breast engorgement? A randomized controlled study, *Birth* 20(2):61-64, 1993.
18. Humenick S, Hill P, Spiegelberg P: Breastfeeding and health professional encouragement, *J Hum Lact* 14(4):305-310, 1998.
19. Ingram J, Johnson D, Greenwood R: Breastfeeding in Bristol: teaching good positioning, and support from fathers and families, *Midwifery* 18(2):87-101, 2002.
20. Ramsay DT, Hartmann PE: Milk removal from the breast, *Breastfeeding Rev* 13(1):5-7, 2005.
21. Matthisen AS, Ransjo-Arvidson AB, Nissen E, and others: Postpartum maternal oxytocin release by newborns: effects of infant hand massage and sucking, *Birth* 28(1):13-19, 2001.
22. Dewey KG: Maternal and fetal stress are associated with impaired lactogenesis in humans, *J Nutr* 131:3012S-3015S, 2001.
23. Ingram JC, Woolridge MW, Greenwood RJ, and others: Maternal predictors of early breast milk output, *Acta Paediatr* 88(5):493-499, 1999.

24. Neifert M, DeMarzo S, Seacat J, and others: The influence of breast surgery, breast appearance, and pregnancy-induced breast changes on lactation insufficiency as measured by infant weight gain, *Birth* 17:31-38, 1999.
25. Kaupila A, Kivinen S, Ylikorkala O: A dose response relation between improved lactation and metoclopramide, *Lancet* 1(8231):1175-1177, 1981.
26. Hansen W, McAndrew S, Harris K, and others: Metoclopramide effect on breastfeeding the preterm infant: a randomized trial, *Obstet Gynecol* 105:383-389, 2005.
27. Hill P, Aldag J, Chatterton R, and others: Primary and secondary mediators' influence on milk output in lactating mothers of preterm and term infants, *J Hum Lact* 21(2):138-150, 2005.
28. Betzold C: Galactogogues, *J Midwifery Women's Health* 49(2):151-154, 2004.
29. Dewey KG, Nommsen-Rivers LA, Heinig MJ, and others: Risk factors for suboptimal infant breastfeeding behavior, delayed onset of lactation, and excess neonatal weight loss, *Pediatrics* 112:607-619, 2003.
30. Neifert M: Breastmilk transfer: positioning, latch-on, and screening for problems in milk transfer, *Clin Obstet Gynecol* 47(3):656-675, 2004.
31. Centuori S, Burmaz T, Ronfani L, and others: Nipple care, sore nipples, and breastfeeding: a randomized trial, *J Hum Lact* 15(2):125-130, 1999.
32. Foxman B, D'Arcy H, Gillespie B, and others: Lactation mastitis: occurrence and medical management among 946 breastfeeding women in the United States, *Am J Epidemiol* 155(2):103-114, 2002.
33. Stuart-Macadam P, Dettwyler K, editors: *Breastfeeding: biocultural perspectives*, New York, 1995, Walter de Gruyter.
34. Hands A: Safe storage of expressed breast milk in the home, *MIDIRS Midwifery Digest* 13:378-385, 2003.

CHAPTER 13

Aging and Common Geriatric Syndromes

Joanne Sandberg-Cook

Demographic predictions for society are for both greater numbers of older adults and increased longevity of the population. By 2020, 1 in 6 Americans will be elderly, and by 2050, 1 in 5. The fastest-growing cohort in the late twentieth century was the group identified as "old old" (over age 85 years), and the number of centenarians increased the fastest.[1]

Because of this anticipated increase in elderly persons, as well as their ethnic diversity, this age-group will have an unprecedented need for services and goods. Heart disease, cancer, and cerebrovascular disease continue to be the chief causes of death and disability among older adults. The most common chronic conditions include arthritis, heart disease, hypertension, diabetes, and hearing and vision impairment.[2]

CHALLENGES IN PRIMARY CARE

The goal of geriatric primary care is to maximize independence and functional status and shorten the morbidity period in the life of each older adult. The challenges in achieving this goal include ageism, a lack of geriatric education in the nation's health professional schools, the complexity of illness in older adults, the increasing dependence of older adults, and cost.

Robert Butler coined the term *ageism* in 1965 to describe the culturally rooted discomfort with growing older. He observed not only revulsion on the part of young people but also fear of losses associated with aging.[3] Neither older adults nor health care providers are immune to ageism. Older adults themselves determine when to seek screening or treatment and are known to assume that many symptoms of disease are a result of advanced age and therefore have no effective treatment available.

Health care providers continue to receive minimum education in gerontology and geriatrics.[4] This is in spite of the fact that greater than 50% of hospitalized patients are over age 65, and a much higher proportion of the office practice is elderly. Research demonstrates that the presentation of disease is often atypical in an aging patient. Treatment must be based on an understanding of the body's ability to adapt to aging and the effect of aging on pharmacokinetics. Although the human body demonstrates remarkable compensation for aging, stress disrupts this adaptation.

An individual experiencing the usual aging pattern is increasingly vulnerable to multiple health problems and experiences losses that affect stamina, motivation for self-care, and the ability to function effectively. Functional problems affecting the older adult's mental and physical status and care are aggravated by many factors, including a lack of exercise, constipation, sleep disturbances, failing cognition, social isolation, and depression. Nonprescription drugs and prescriptions from multiple medical specialists can result in a dangerous mix of medications, which must be identified to avoid interactions. Reduction of memory and sensory input further complicates the diagnosis and treatment plans. Additional challenges arise from the use of alcohol and tobacco and from poor nutrition.[5]

MENTAL STATUS AND FUNCTIONAL ASSESSMENTS

Geriatric specialists have multiple functional assessment tools, such as the Folstein Mini-Mental State Examination, the Short Portable Mental Status Questionnaire, and the Geriatric Evaluation of Mental Status, to differentiate short-term memory loss from dementia and to observe the progression of cognitive impairment. A detailed history of cognitive change and of lifelong habits is a vital element in the differential diagnosis of dementia and often necessitates an interview with an observant family member or friend. Maintaining a record of the patient's baseline mental status and the results of subsequent mental status testing is essential for accurate diagnosis and management.

Tools for the assessment of functional status, including the Barthel Index, the Physical Self-Maintenance Scale, and the Katz Index, are also well developed, validated, and easily administered. Function is addressed on two levels: (1) basic activities of daily living, including feeding, bathing, dressing, ambulation, and toileting; and (2) the more complex, instrumental activities of daily living, including cooking, shopping, using the telephone, reading, writing, and managing money. Poor performance on functional or mental status testing might explain a failure to respond to medications, noncompliance with exercise or diet recommendations, falls and injuries, or the occurrence of depression or anxiety.

ISSUES WITH HEALTH SCREENING

Routine screening of older adults for disease remains controversial simply because little outcomes data exist for elderly patients. Screening should be individualized based on the patient's general health and personal and family history. It is reasonable to assess an older person's anticipated life expectancy, considering all co-morbidities and his or her personal preferences, before embarking on routine screening. Many older patients refuse invasive screening or treatment programs, choosing comfort and quality of life over longevity. Annual examinations should be comprehensive, are necessarily time-consuming, and should include responsible family members.

COUNSELING ELDERLY DRIVERS

Providing useful assessment and counseling to the elderly driver often falls to health care providers. The incidence of crashes, especially fatal ones, is high among elderly drivers.[6] Assessment of cardiovascular status, mental status, vision, balance, and gait and range of motion of hips and knees can provide information regarding the elderly person's ability to drive. Those drivers judged at risk should be referred for a road test by the registry of motor vehicles or to a private rehabilitation facility. Frank discussions with patients and families that elaborate the risks of driving can be difficult but are essential to protect the safety of the elderly driver and the public at large. Mandatory reporting of unsafe drivers is the law in many states.

IMPORTANCE OF ADVANCE DIRECTIVES

The primary care of older adults includes a discussion of advance directives and the identification of a health care proxy or durable power of attorney for health care. A living will or similar document, which describes in detail the patient's wishes in regard to resuscitation, hospitalization, treatment, and a health care proxy, should be part of each patient's health care record.

The challenge for the health care provider who treats older adults is to recognize the individual aging process of each older adult, promote optimum health and functioning, provide care and comfort during illness, and minimize the length and severity of the premorbid illness and disability period, thus helping both patient and his or her family with the final life transition.

COMMON GERIATRIC SYNDROMES

Primary care, including health promotion and disease prevention, as well as the prevention of disease exacerbation, complications, or disability, must continue in all settings in which older adults live and must be provided by a coordinated team of health care professionals. Geriatric syndromes are complex, multicausal entities that test the diagnostic powers of the health care provider. Chaos may reign, but therein lies the challenge in meeting the primary care needs of older patients. This chapter discusses six common syndromes seen in older adults: polypharmacy, cognitive impairment, dehydration, falls, failure to thrive, and elder abuse.

POLYPHARMACY

Definition and Etiology

Polypharmacy is the use or misuse of multiple drugs, both prescription and nonprescription, and their interaction with one another. It is a common cause of iatrogenic illness in older adults, who account for 14% of the population but consume 30% of all prescription drugs. Polypharmacy has multiple "causes," including multiple prescribers for the same patient, fear of accusation of ageism or cultural bias, and good intentions to treat side effects of one medication with another.[7]

Pathophysiology

Drug distribution and clearance are affected by normal aging changes, including a reduction in lean body mass and blood flow to the kidney and liver and an increase in body fat. These issues are compounded in frail older adults because, in addition to normal aging changes, disease alters the function of specific organ systems and affects pharmacokinetics. Abnormalities in the cardiac conduction system, decreased gastric acid production, decreased total body water, and increased total body fat all affect drug absorption and metabolism. Age-related renal changes lead to increased drug levels and potentially toxic effects of renally excreted drugs.[8]

Clinical Presentation

The clinical presentation varies, covering a wide range of signs and symptoms. A drug-related side effect should be considered for any presenting symptom until proven otherwise. The number of possible adverse reactions and drug interactions is staggering, since the addition of just one drug may precipitate a toxic effect.

Management

To avoid the negative consequences of polypharmacy, it is important to review all medications at each patient contact and to maintain good communication with consultants. Patients should be encouraged to carry an up-to-date list of their medications and have one readily available to give emergency medical providers in the event of an emergency. Patients should be encouraged to order drugs from a pharmacy with computerized drug data whenever possible. As an educator for both the patient and the health care provider, the pharmacist plays an important role in preventing poor outcomes from polypharmacy.

The drug risk/benefit ratio should be determined when considering the use of any new drug. The general principles of drug therapy in geriatrics are first considered, such as the pharmacodynamics of the drug class and common adverse effects experienced by older adults (Box 13-1). For example, older adults are more susceptible than younger adults to the anticholinergic effects of drugs. Second, the specific side effect profiles of a drug class and a patient's history of previous adverse effects, morbidity, and general nutritional state are considered. The known or suspected risk is weighed against the presumed benefit of administering the drug. "Start low and go slow" is common advice when prescribing for older adults. Based on a literature review and expert panel recommendations, Knight and Avorn developed 12 quality indicators for appropriate medication use.[9] These indicators are presented in Table 13-1 along with the level of supporting evidence.

BOX 13-1

MEDICATION ANALYSIS: GENERAL CONSIDERATIONS

DRUG ISSUES RELATED TO DRUG CLASS

1. Pharmacokinetic properties of class (e.g., ACE inhibitors affect renal excretion)
2. Common side effects (e.g., ACE = hyperkalemia)

PATIENT ISSUES

1. Common adverse effects in older adults:
   - Anticholinergic effects
   - Constipation or diarrhea
   - Indigestion
   - Delirium
   - Dizziness
   - Depression
   - Dermatologic effects
2. Specific prior problems in older adults that affect medication risks:
   - Renal failure
   - Dehydration
   - Malnutrition
   - Poor compliance
   - Drug cost

ACE, Angiotensin-converting enzyme.

COGNITIVE IMPAIRMENT

Definition and Etiology

The most common and feared cause of a decline in cognition is dementia, and the most prevalent form of dementia is Alzheimer's disease (AD) (see Chapter 205). The cost of treating AD approaches $100 billion annually in the United States. The incidence of AD doubles every 5 years after age 65 and approaches 50% by age 85.[10]

Clinical Presentation

AD is a chronic, irreversible illness with a gradual onset and a steady decline in cognition. Short-term memory loss is the primary symptom in AD, along with one or more of the following: disorientation; disturbance in executive functioning (planning, organizing, and abstract thinking); problems with activities of daily living; and one of three common neurologic disorders: aphasia, apraxia, or agnosia. Day-night sleep cycles are often reversed; consciousness and psychomotor changes are not evident until late in the disease. Irritability, withdrawal, and apathy may be exhibited in the early stages of the disease. Psychotic symptoms such as paranoia and agitation can be seen later in the disease.

Delirium, a common cause of cognitive change in the sick or hospitalized elderly, is a transient waxing and waning level of consciousness. It is characterized by acute onset and fluctuations in orientation and attention. The incidence in hospitalized elders is high and associated with longer lengths of stay and increased rates of admission to nursing homes (see Chapter 204).

DEHYDRATION

Definition and Etiology

Dehydration is more prevalent in older adults and has a greater likelihood of a negative outcome than in younger adults. It is defined as a state of fluid intake deprivation and/or excess fluid loss. Accompanying electrolyte imbalances may ensue (see Chapter 221). The most significant electrolyte abnormality is sodium imbalance. Because of this, dehydration is further categorized by the associated relationship between free water and sodium[11]:

Isotonic dehydration occurs with a balanced loss of water and sodium. An example of this is vomiting and diarrhea, with equal losses of water and electrolytes.

Hypertonic dehydration, also called *hypernatremic dehydration,* occurs when water loss is greater than sodium loss. Febrile illnesses and poor fluid intake result in hypertonic dehydration.

Hypotonic dehydration occurs when sodium loss is greater than water loss, resulting in hyponatremia. The inappropriate use of diuretics can cause this type of dehydration.

In older adults, dehydration is often multicausal (Box 13-2). Environmental issues, polypharmacy, and diseases prevalent in older adults predispose this group to dehydration, as do age-related changes in plasma osmolality and thirst response.

Pathophysiology

Three principal changes in the homeostatic mechanism that controls the volume and osmolality of extracellular fluids occur in older adults. These normal changes result in a

TABLE 13-1 Quality Indicators: Appropriate Medication Use in Vulnerable Older Adults

Quality Indicator for Vulnerable Older Adults	Supporting Evidence
All drugs should have a clearly defined indication documented to avoid indefinite continuation of unnecessary drugs.	No clinical trials, expert panel
Drug education may improve adherence and outcomes and alert patient to the side effects.	Meta-analysis review and randomized control trial (RCT)
All patient records should contain an up-to-date medication list to eliminate inappropriate duplication and avoid drug interactions.	Cohort study
For chronic diseases, document the drug response at a minimum within 6 months of prescribing to provide a basis for continuation.	Expert panel
Review the patient's drug regimen at least annually to provide an opportunity for discontinuation and to include new prevention regimens.	Criteria-based literature; 1 RCT; outcomes studies on computer-based retrospective drug-use review, which found no change in status, mortality, or morbidity
International normalized ratio should be performed within 4 days of initiating warfarin and at least every 6 weeks. The risk of adverse events is greatest in vulnerable older adults.	Expert panel
Electrolytes should be measured within 1 week of initiating thiazide or a loop diuretic and then a minimum of every year.	No studies of monitoring electrolytes on outcomes; RCT demonstrated the association of hypokalemia with these diuretics; twofold increased risk of ventricular arrhythmias with potassium <3.0 mEq/L
Avoid the use of chlorpropamide (Diabinese) because of its prolonged half-life.	473 case-based review plus expert panel
Avoid drugs with strong anticholinergic properties, which have the potential for adverse effects.	RCTs
Barbiturates should not be used if seizure control is not needed because of the potent CNS depressant and addictive properties, the high incidence of drug interactions, and an increased fall risk.	Epidemiologic study of fall rate and barbiturate use
Avoid the use of meperidine (Demerol) in vulnerable older adults because of the high risk of delirium.	Case-based study plus RCT comparing meperidine; found to be no more effective than NSAIDs for acute pain
Check electrolytes within 1 week of initiating therapy with ACE inhibitors because they may cause renal insufficiency and hyperkalemia.	Epidemiologic study plus case-based study; greater risk for developing renal dysfunction immediately after initiating drug, but risk persists for duration of therapy

Modified from Knight EL, Avorn J: Quality indicators for appropriate medication use in vulnerable elders, *Ann Intern Med* 135(8 pt 2):703-710, 2001.
ACE, Angiotensin-converting enzyme.

reduced adaptability and reserve to deal with system stressors. First, the thirst response, which is stimulated by dehydration, is diminished and results in an increased solute/water ratio. Second, decreased renal plasma flow may be responsible for a decline in the body's ability to concentrate urine. The inability to concentrate urine prevents the body from retaining enough fluid to avert dehydration. Finally, vasopressin release stimulated by low fluid volume is diminished. Therefore the inherent homeostatic mechanism that prevents the sequela of hypovolemia is blunted.[11]

Clinical Presentation

The presenting symptoms of dehydration are often vague and nonspecific. These include confusion, lethargy, rapid weight loss, and functional decline. Dehydration is often a feature of failure to thrive. The history should include an assessment of fluid intake, functional status, weight, and cognition. The presence of constipation may indicate a lack of water intake (see Box 13-2).

Physical Examination

The physical examination includes a cardiovascular assessment and may reveal an orthostatic drop in blood pressure and a rise in pulse, indicating volume depletion. Temperature may be elevated as a result of dehydration or an inflammatory process. Mucous membranes are often not noticeably dry until severe dehydration is present. Because of changes in skin collagen, poor skin turgor, often used as a sign of dehydration in younger individuals, is unreliable in older adults. The tongue may be swollen and furrowed.

Diagnostics

Laboratory data include a review of serum electrolytes, BUN/creatinine ratio, osmolality, hematocrit and hemoglobin, and glucose. A BUN/creatinine ratio of 25:1 or more suggests dehydration. Dehydration is present when the sodium level is greater than 148 mEq/L. However, with isotonic or hypotonic dehydration, serum sodium is normal or low, respectively. Hematocrit is elevated compared with the level of hematocrit when the patient is well hydrated. Respiratory and genitourinary infections are common, and a urinalysis and chest x-ray studies may be appropriate.

Differential Diagnosis

Fever, poor fluid intake, iatrogenic drug use, and gastrointestinal fluid losses are the most common causes of

BOX 13-2

COMMON CAUSES OF DEHYDRATION

INTAKE (FLUID DEPRIVATION)

Environmental Factors
- Restricted ambulation
- Decreased hearing or vision

Increased Metabolic Demands
- Infections (resulting in malaise, reduced appetite, and poor intake)

Dehydration
- Poorly fitting dentures
- Esophageal lesions
- Neurologic disease

Pharmacologic Factors
- Narcotics
- Sedatives
- Neuroleptics
- Anticholinergics

Normal Aging Changes
- Ineffective water conservation
- Decreased thirst drive

Poor Appetite
- Fatigue
- Constipation
- Depression

Fluid Limitations
- Before a procedure or operation
- Prevention of urinary incontinence
- Management of heart failure
- Management of hyponatremia

OUTPUT (FLUID EXCESS)

Environmental Factors
- Hot weather
- Alcohol intake

Increased Metabolic Demands
- Infections (resulting in tachypnea and sweating)
- Diarrhea
- Vomiting
- Sweating

Endocrine Disorders
- Diabetes insipidus
- Hyperglycemia or glycosuria

Pharmacologic Factors
- Diuretics
- Laxatives

Normal Aging Changes
- Ineffective salt conservation

dehydration in older adults. Other causes of dehydration should be pursued if electrolyte imbalances persist after treatment, with a focus on the endocrine system. However, older adults respond slowly to the treatment of severe electrolyte abnormalities.

Hyponatremia, a common and often misdiagnosed clinical finding in older adults, results from an inability to excrete free water. This is due to increased vasopressin release, which causes the kidneys to conserve water and thus increases the ratio of free water to sodium solute. This syndrome is termed the *syndrome of inappropriate antidiuretic hormone (SIADH)*. In SIADH, urine osmolality is greater than 300 mOsm/kg with a low serum sodium level. This high urine osmolality differentiates SIADH from low sodium dehydration. The treatment is limitation of free water, which may then result in dehydration if the patient is not monitored closely.[11]

Management

As described in Table 13-2, management of dehydration is driven by the severity of electrolyte imbalance, the treatment setting, and goals. This distinction is important because all three must be carefully defined before treatment is planned.

Guidelines for oral rehydration have been proposed.[12] An oral fluid prescription for a patient should be written with the patient's family and caregivers in mind; it is important to inform the staff and the family that it is difficult to overhydrate a dehydrated patient with fluids by mouth. Rehydration prescriptions for the first 24 hours include replacement of one half of the fluid deficit plus ongoing loss and maintenance fluid of at least 1500 ml/day. Over the next 2 or 3 days the remainder of the fluid deficit is replaced, and maintenance fluids are given. A simple formula for estimating fluid loss or deficit (based on the fact that 1 L of water weighs 1 kg) has been devised[11]:

$$\text{Preillness weight (kg)} - \text{Current weight (kg)} = \text{Fluid deficit (L)}$$

Because the primary care of older adults occurs in multiple settings, health care providers may be involved in hypodermoclysis (clysis), the infusion of fluids subcutaneously, or IV fluid administration. A survey of the geriatric literature suggests that clysis is gaining in popularity. During this treatment it is best to avoid electrolyte-free or hypertonic solutions because they are poorly absorbed and may precipitate circulatory collapse and death.[13] It should be noted that these recommendations are from poorly designed, older studies using hypertonic solutions (10% to 25% glucose) that are rarely used today.[13]

The choice of subcutaneous or IV fluids depends on the serum sodium level and the degree of hypovolemia. If the serum sodium level is normal or low, isotonic saline (0.9%) is infused. If the serum sodium level is high, then 5% dextrose in half normal (0.45%) saline is appropriate after hemodynamic stabilization. If hypotension, orthostasis, and decreased urinary output are present (signaling hemodynamic collapse), the initial IV therapy is rapid infusion of isotonic saline to stabilize these parameters. Hospitalization may be appropriate depending on the treatment goals. After hydration is treated, a return to the premorbid mental status and functional level may take weeks.

Hemodynamic collapse will occur if dehydration is severe and manifests as hypotension, orthostasis, and decreased urinary output. Overzealous rehydration, or an attempt to replace total water loss within 24 hours, may result in death from cerebral edema.

Education focuses on the prevention of dehydration (Box 13-3). When it occurs, the amounts and types of fluids to ingest are included in the educational plan. Fluids high in sodium (e.g., tomato juice, bouillon, or sports drinks) are

TABLE 13-2 Dehydration Management

	Low Risk*		High Risk*	
Setting	**Treatment**	**Comfort**	**Treatment**	**Comfort**
Office practice	OR†	OR	NA	OR
Home	OR/clysis	OR	NA	OR
Nursing home	OR/clysis	OR	Clysis/IV	OR
Hospital	OR	OR	IV	OR

OR, Oral rehydration; *NA,* not applicable.
*Risk is defined by clinical parameters and may include severity of electrolyte imbalance. High risk may be defined as a serum sodium ≥150 mEq/L, an inability to take sufficient fluids by mouth, or co-morbid conditions that increase the risk of complications from rehydration (e.g., congestive heart failure). This definition of risk is not research based.
†OR is used while fluids by mouth are possible.

BOX 13-3

DEHYDRATION PREVENTION

- Drink six to eight 8-ounce glasses of water or juice daily.
- Take a full glass of water or juice with medications.
- Drink more than usual in hot weather or when you have a fever.
- Keep a fluid intake record for 2 days.
- Poor dental hygiene, missing teeth, or poorly fitting dentures will interfere with food and fluid intake.
- People with memory problems need fluid monitoring.

appropriate for those with low sodium levels, whereas water is appropriate for those with high sodium levels. Caffeinated beverages have a mild diuretic effect and should be avoided.

FALLS

Definition and Etiology

Falling is an unintentional loss of balance that results in a position change and contact with the ground. The most feared sequela of a fall is a fracture. Quality of life may be severely affected by a "fear of falling," with self-imposed isolation and immobility causing a vicious cycle of risk. Fall assessment focuses on known risk factors, including sensory abnormalities and abnormalities of the central and peripheral nervous system, musculoskeletal system, and cognition.[14]

In a community sample, one third to one half of older adults fell each year. The probability of falling increases with age. In long-term care the annual fall incidence per resident is greater than 50%. Approximately 40% of falls result in minor injuries, and 3% to 5% of falls result in fractures. Falls contribute to 40% of nursing home admissions.[15]

Pathophysiology

Falls are multifactorial in origin. The majority occur during walking, stepping, or position changes and not during more hazardous activities. Contributing factors are lower extremity weakness, poor balance, orthostatic hypotension, central nervous system disease, cognition and sensory abnormalities, and unsafe environments. The role of lower extremity weakness as a marker of preclinical disability has been well demonstrated.

Sensory input from vision, hearing, vestibular function, and proprioception is important in preventing falls. Visual impairment increases as a result of normal age-related changes and the increased prevalence of ocular diseases. Normal age-related changes cause glare intolerance and slower adaptation to the dark than in younger adults.

Balance depends on sensory cues and vestibular function, both peripheral and central. Disequilibrium and unsteadiness are common in older adults and are related to aging changes and disease in the inner ear, as well as to changes in the transmission of signals from the periphery. Acute and chronic changes in mental status and depression contribute to falls, but the mechanism of action is unclear. Drugs causing sedation, postural hypotension, and electrolyte imbalance have been implicated in the risk for falls. The use of four or more medications increases the risk for falls, regardless of the type of medication.[14]

Normal aging changes in the cardiovascular system blunt the homeostatic mechanisms that maintain adequate organ perfusion and blood pressure control, causing hypotension, threatening the ability to maintain balance. Musculoskeletal and joint diseases affect balance and gait, as do environmental factors, such as loose rugs, cords, and clutter in the home. A fall erodes the self-confidence of older adults and intensifies their fear of dependence and loss of control over their lives. The fear of falling is an independent risk factor for further falls.

Clinical Presentation

The clinical presentation of falling is varied. The health history should focus on previous falls and events surrounding a fall, including episodes of syncope, unsteadiness, and dizziness. The mnemonic *DDROPP* (Diseases, Drugs, Recovery, Onset, Prodrome, and Precipitants) helps ensure a complete postfall assessment. The assessment should also focus on any history of coronary artery disease or arrhythmias, vision and hearing problems, neurologic dysfunction, fractures, cognitive changes, and medications.

Self-reported functional scales quickly supplement the history with information on mobility, self-care abilities, mood, hospitalizations, and nutrition. It is important to ask questions in reference to current activities. The reply to "How did you get to this appointment?" is immensely informative, as is simply watching how a patient enters the examination room and with whom.

Physical Examination

A complete physical examination with a focus on postural vital signs is necessary and should include a cardiovascular and neurologic examination, including Romberg's test with a sternal nudge and a check for nystagmus. Mobility (including gait and balance), upper extremity function and strength, cognition, vision, and hearing are also examined. Quick and easy mobility and gait tests are now available and correlate positively with the risk for falls and a decline in self-care ability. With the "get up & go" test, the patient is asked to get up from a chair with his or her arms folded across the chest, walk 10 feet, return to the chair, and sit down using regular footwear and any regular walking aid.[16] The ease of gait, balance, position change, and turning are evaluated. Completion of the task in 20 seconds or less correlates with functional independence; those taking 30 seconds or more are considered functionally dependent.

Lower extremity balance is tested by evaluating the patient standing with the feet side by side, semitandem and tandem, and balancing for 10 seconds. The functional reach test for balance is completed by asking the individual to reach forward in a parallel plane without taking a step.[17] Patients with a reach of less than 17.8 cm (7 inches) are considered very frail and at higher risk of falling. Patients should be closely monitored by a member of the clinical team while performing any activity that may be associated with falling.

Diagnostics

The initial evaluation should include a CBC (to rule out anemia and infections), electrolytes, BUN, creatinine (to look for dehydration and electrolyte imbalance), serum glucose, and a stool occult blood test. An ECG can help rule out rhythm disturbances. If syncope and ECG abnormalities are present, a myocardial infarct must be excluded, and a careful examination and diagnostic workup for ischemic disease are indicated. If the neurologic examination is positive, an MRI will rule out brain or spinal cord lesions or other abnormalities. The patient with true vertigo is most likely to suffer from inner ear disease. Benign positional vertigo (BPV) is common in older adults. The vertigo of BPV is episodic and is provoked by position changes.

Management

The goal of treatment and education is to alter modifiable risk factors (Box 13-4). Experts have proposed guidelines for fall prevention.[18,19] If lower extremity weakness is present, a referral to a physical therapist for strength training is recommended. Resistance training benefits even those of advanced age and frailty.[20] If balance is altered, balance training consists of having the patient stand on one foot for 10 seconds and gradually increase the time and frequency. Low-intensity Tai Chi has been demonstrated to improve balance.[21] Balance may also be improved by proper footwear and the use of assistive devices. Drug reduction and the avoidance of alcohol are important if hypotension is present. A home safety evaluation or checklist is indicated if trips and falls are prevalent.

Serious complications of falls (e.g., subdural hematoma, hip fracture, or cervical fracture) occur 3% to 5% of the time. Because of the high incidence of osteoporosis in older adults, fractures requiring surgical intervention occur with falls. The most feared fractures are of the hip, but wrist and humerus fractures are common and disabling. Soft tissue injury is a more common outcome. Consultation should be considered if complications are suspected, particularly if fracture, syncope, true vertigo, or abnormal cardiovascular or neurologic findings are present.

Fall prevention is an excellent example of success through the collaborative effort of a multidisciplinary team. Physical and occupational therapists provide appropriate exercise, balance, and gait-training programs and teach patients about environmental hazards. Physicians, nurse practitioners, and physician assistants assess medication usage and monitor the treatment of orthostatic hypotension, peripheral vascular disease, and incontinence (a few of the immediate causes of falls). Nutritionists prevent dehydration and anemia through teaching sessions. When falls are prevented, pain, disability, hospitalization, and possibly iatrogenic disaster are also prevented.

BOX 13-4

FALL PREVENTION

- Evaluate the home to eliminate loose cords, clutter, and slippery surfaces.
- Install and use bathroom and stair rails.
- Change position slowly.
- Treat foot problems and wear well-fitting, low-heeled footwear.
- Light the environment well.
- Exercise to maintain lower leg strength.
- Join a Tai Chi class for balance training.
- Bring all medications, including nonprescriptions, to your health care provider at each visit.
- Have regular hearing and vision testing.

FAILURE TO THRIVE (FRAILTY)

Definition and Etiology

Failure to thrive (FTT) is a syndrome described as a progressive loss of function and general deterioration. A physiologic vulnerability results from reduced reserve and capacity to withstand stress. Patients exhibit signs of anorexia, weight loss, skeletal muscle loss (sarcopenia), and functional decline. The result of these signs can be osteopenia, balance and gait disorders, undernutrition, deconditioning, and slow gait speed.[20]

The diagnostic evaluation of FTT seeks to differentiate reversible from irreversible causes. Because of inconsistent definitions of the syndrome, its incidence is unknown. Approximately 15% of hospitalized older adults with FTT die during hospitalization, and 30% of the survivors are discharged to nursing homes.[22]

Pathophysiology

FTT, also known as frailty, is strongly associated with age and not specific disease. Weight loss and sarcopenia are strongly associated with age and undernutrition. This results in decreased strength and endurance, weakness, and fatigue. Loss of muscle mass may result in decreased bone density and slowing of metabolic rate, thereby disrupting thermoregulation and leading to heat and cold intolerance. Age-related changes in lean body mass are partially due to changes in growth hormone, estrogen, and androgen secretion. Administering these hormones increases lean body mass but does not necessarily improve functional capacity and strength. The immune system changes with age, including an overall decline in T cells and decreased effectiveness of T memory cells. This decline may explain the shorter duration of effectiveness of immunizations in older individuals and their increased vulnerability to infections.[20] End-stage chronic diseases (e.g., heart failure, pulmonary disease) and malignancy cause weight loss, general weakness, and debility.

Clinical Presentation

Patients with FTT may be seen by their health care provider with any of the following symptoms: weakness, inability to care for self, dizziness, weight and memory loss, and depression. Weight loss in FTT is often gradual. The health history focuses on chronic diseases with signs of organ failure, the presence of gastrointestinal malabsorption, cancer risk factors, infection, thyroid abnormalities, depression, and changes in memory. Nutritional intake and the progression of weight loss are calculated. Adverse reactions to medications, including confusion or anorexia, may be partially responsible for FTT. A history of smoking and alcohol use may be helpful in discovering cause. Reversible causes of FTT are sought (Box 13-5).[20]

Physical Examination and Diagnostics

An unplanned loss of 10% or more of body weight in less than a year requires a search for a reversible cause. A complete physical examination should focus on symptoms, organ failure, infections, and malignancy. A skin, mucous membrane, and eye examination may reveal muscle wasting; ulcerative lesions; and signs of vitamin deficiency, anemia, and dehydration. A complete oral examination, including an evaluation of the dentition and denture fit, is necessary. Tests of swallowing ability and the gag reflex are included in the neurologic examination. A thorough breast examination, a Papanicolaou test, and a rectal examination for occult blood loss will evaluate for malignancy. Many older women have not had a vaginal or breast examination for years, if ever; thus it is important to explain the purpose and importance of these examinations. Because of the heterogeneity of older adults, biologic age should not be the only deciding factor in omitting breast and pelvic examinations.

Screening tests should include a CBC, electrolytes, kidney and thyroid studies, fasting blood glucose, liver function tests, calcium levels, urinalysis, and a chest x-ray examination. Additional diagnostics may be indicated, depending on initial testing, examination, and patient preference.

Any irreversible cause of FTT, such as malignancy or end-stage organ disease, should be evaluated. The patient, family, or both need to be involved in all decisions to perform diagnostic testing. The patient or proxy does not always desire treatment of potentially life-threatening conditions, making expensive and invasive diagnostic testing moot. End-of-life support and comfort may be a reasonable approach after discussion and preliminary evaluation.

A lifelong history of anorexia because of body image concerns has been reported in the literature. Older adults may have lifelong patterns of dieting and anorexia nervosa–like symptoms, which can be overlooked as a cause of weight loss in this population.[23]

BOX 13-5

FAILURE-TO-THRIVE CAUSES

DISEASE

- Organ failure
- Metastases
- Infection
- Stroke
- Thyroid disease
- Fractures

MEDICATION

- Cognitive changes
- Anorexia
- Dehydration

ENVIRONMENTAL CAUSES

- Isolation
- Neglect
- Poverty

PSYCHIATRIC CAUSES

- Depression
- Dementia
- Psychosis
- Delirium

GASTROINTESTINAL CAUSES

- Malabsorption
- Dysphagia
- Dental problems
- Diarrhea
- Vitamin deficiency

Management

Adequate protein and caloric intake is mandatory. Meals on Wheels and other community support organizations may be necessary if isolation or functional decline is present. High-calorie and high-protein supplements are beneficial. A daily multivitamin supplement and 800 IU of vitamin D are beneficial. Appetite stimulants are not recommended. Depression is treated with an antidepressant.

Regular exercise is possible and helpful in building strength in even the very old, deconditioned nursing home patient. In one study weight training coupled with nutritional supplements over a 10-week period in nursing home patients ages 85 and older improved muscle strength by more than 125% compared with 3% in the control group.[24]

Creative solutions and their dissemination to prevent malnutrition in nursing home residents have been proposed and include small group dining for dementia patients, the use of volunteers to assist at dinner time, and ethnically appropriate foods.[25] Families need to be included in education and support measures. Often they are the ones to urge patients to seek health care when the patients themselves are reluctant to do so. Patient autonomy must be preserved as long as dementia and depression have been excluded. If irreversible causes of FTT are not found, it may be the natural course of life's end.

ELDER ABUSE

Definition

Elder abuse is defined as the maltreatment of an elderly person living at home, in the home of a caregiver, or in an institution. *Self-neglect* refers to the behavior of an elderly person living alone that threatens his health or safety. There are seven kinds of elder abuse: physical, sexual, psychologic, financial, neglect, abandonment, and self-neglect.[26] It is difficult to get accurate information on the incidence and prevalence of elder abuse, but the best estimate is that between 1 million and 2 million elderly people are reported abused each year in the United States.[27] Shame, guilt, and poor reporting all contribute to lack of hard data. The incidence is likely much higher.

Clinical Presentation

Older adults who come into the health care provider's office or hospital with bruises, pressure or rope marks, broken bones, or burns may be suffering physical abuse. Bruising of the breasts or genital area may indicate sexual abuse. Sudden withdrawal from usual activities or a change in behavior or alertness may indicate psychologic abuse. A change in financial situation or checks signed by unauthorized persons raises suspicions of financial exploitation. Bedsores, unattended medical needs, poor hygiene or nutritional status, hoarding, or inappropriate clothing for the weather can be signs of neglect or self-neglect. The suffering is often in silence, but an alert health care provider will notice subtle changes and start to question causes.[27]

Management

Any suspicion of abuse is reported to the state adult protective services, the long-term care ombudsman, or, if the risk is immediate, the police. Older adults can reduce the risk of abuse by seeking professional help for medical, psychologic, and substance abuse problems; choosing a trusted person to hold durable power of attorney or be a guardian; and knowing their rights as patients, residents of long-term care facilities, and individuals.

INDICATIONS FOR REFERRAL AND CONSULTATIONS

Comprehensive geriatric assessment by an interdisciplinary team may be the preferred approach to problems that clearly involve medical, mental, and social disability. Specialized geriatric assessment focuses on prioritizing problems and approaches, improving functional capacity, and minimizing invasive and expensive medical care.

REFERENCES

1. Goldstein A, Damon B: *We the elderly,* US Department of Commerce, Bureau of Census, retrieved Dec 12, 2003, from http://www.census.gov/apsd/wepeople/we-9.pdf.
2. National Center for Health Statistics: *Death rates for 72 selected causes by 10-year age groups, race and sex,* Washington, DC, 1995, US Department of Health and Human Services.
3. Butler R: Ageism: another form of bigotry, *Gerontologist* 9(4):243-246, 1969.
4. American Geriatrics Society: A statement of principles: toward improved care of older patients in surgical and medical specialties, *J Am Geriatr Soc* 49:782-787, 2000.
5. Rowe J, Kahn T: Successful aging, *Gerontologist* 37(4):443-440, 1997.
6. National Center for Statistics and Analysis: *Traffic safety facts 2005: older population,* retrieved Dec. 4, 2006, from http://www-nrd.nhtsa.dot.gov/pdf/nrd-30/NCSA/TSF2005/ OlderPopulationTSF05.pdf.
7. Jackson SHD, Mangoni AA, Batty GM: Optimization of drug prescribing, *Br J Clin Pharmacol* 57(3):231-236, 2003.
8. Day H, Weinryb J, Lavizzo-Mourey R: Clinical problems in geriatrics. In Branch WT, editor: *Office practice of medicine,* Philadelphia, 2003, Saunders.
9. Knight EL, Avorn J: Quality indicators for appropriate medication use in vulnerable elders, *Ann Intern Med* 134(8 pt 2):703-710, 2001.
10. Morris J: Is Alzheimer's disease inevitable with aging? *J Clin Invest* 104(9):1171-1173, 1999.
11. Warren JL, Bacon WE, Harris T, and others: The burden and outcomes associated with dehydration among US elderly, *Am J Pub Health* 84(8):1265-1269, 1994.
12. Hebrew Rehabilitation for the Aged: *Quality care in the nursing home,* St Louis, 1997, Mosby.
13. Rochon P, Gill SS, Litner J, and others: A systematic review of the evidence for hypodermoclysis to treat dehydration in older people, *J Gerontol* 52A(3):M169-M175, 1997.
14. Tinetti M, Speechley M, Ginter S: Risk factors for falling among elderly persons living in the community, *N Engl J Med* 319:1701-1707, 1988.
15. Edelberg E: *Falls in the elderly* (geriatric medicine course), Boston, 1998, Harvard Medical School Division on Aging
16. Podsiadlo D, Richardson S: The timed "up & go": a test of basic functional mobility for frail elderly persons, *J Am Geriatr Soc* 39(2):142-148, 1991.
17. Weiner DK, Duncan PW, Chandler J, and others: Functional reach: a marker of physical frailty, *J Am Geriatr Soc* 40:203-207, 1992.
18. Tinetti M: Preventing falls in elderly persons, *N Engl J Med* 348(1):42-49, 2003.
19. Panel on Fall Prevention: Guidelines for the prevention of falls in older persons, *J Am Geriatr Soc* 49:664-672, 2001.
20. Sandberg-Cook J: Frailty. In Paulman P, Susman J, Harrison J, and others, editors: *A family medicine clerkship guide,* St Louis, 2005, Mosby.
21. Wolfson L, Whippler R, Derby C, and others: Balance and strength training in older adults: intervention gains and Tai Chi maintenance, *J Am Geriatr Soc* 44:498-506, 1996.
22. Sarkisian C, Lachs M: Failure to thrive in older adults, *Ann Intern Med* 124:1072-1078, 1996.
23. Miller DK, Morley JE, Rubenstein LZ, and others: Abnormal eating attitudes and body image in older undernourished individuals, *J Am Geriatr Soc* 39:462-466, 1991.
24. Fiatarone MA, O'Neill EF, Ryan ND, and others: Exercise training and nutritional supplements for physical frailty in very old people, *N Engl J Med* 330:1769-1775, 1994.
25. Burger SG, Kayser-Jones J, Bell JP: *Malnutrition and dehydration in nursing homes: key issues in prevention and treatment,* Pub No 386, Boston, June 2000, Commonwealth Fund.
26. National Center on Elder Abuse: *Frequently asked questions,* retrieved Nov 27, 2005, from http://www.elderabusecenter.org/default.cfm?p=faqs.cfm.
27. National Center on Elder Abuse: *Elder abuse prevalence and incidence,* retrieved Nov 27, 2005, from http://ncea@nasua.org.

CHAPTER 14

Psychosociospiritual Issues

Todd Douglas Hultman and Emily Chandler

It is now axiomatic that nursing involves care of the whole person in body, mind, and spirit. From the beginning to the end of life, there are moments and events that lead to not only disease of the body, but also "dis-ease" of the mind and spirit. This "dis-ease" of the mind and spirit is often called *suffering*. And although suffering may occur at any time in the human life span, it is frequently recognized in the context of life-threatening illnesses, traumatic injuries, psychologic traumas, and end-of-life experiences.

END OF LIFE

Recent discussions surrounding end-of-life issues are often grounded in apprehension of pain, loss of control, and diminished quality of life. These problems are far more complex than either legalistic solutions or physical symptom management would allow.[1] The mystery of death is at the root of concern for patients and their families. A 1997 Gallup Poll offered revealing answers to the question of what dying patients want. Most reported that they wanted to die at home, be with someone close to them, and have someone pray with them.[2] But the end of life is fraught with potential crises: physical, psychologic, social, and spiritual. With meaningful support, dying can be healing, peaceful, and even fulfilling for patients and those closest to them.

The physical aspects of dying are usually more familiar to the health care provider than the more elusive psychologic and spiritual elements of the process. An appreciation for the psychosociospiritual needs that accompany the journey of the dying is essential to reducing suffering and promoting a peaceful death. Health care providers are ethically obligated to develop a repertoire of skills for attending to all aspects of the patient as an individual.[3]

IMPACT OF CRISES

The journey with a patient and family through a terminal illness to the end of life is not without its emotional risks. This course brings the health care provider face to face with his or her own experiences of loss. Losses that are unresolved can creep up and surprise with their tenacity whenever witnessing another's suffering. When contemplating the unknown, everyone is confronted with feelings of hopelessness and hope, sadness and peace, fear and trust. A poignant balance is often maintained between these polarized feelings and between the players who, at various points in the process, become the custodians of the feelings. Central to the experience is sorting out which feelings belong to whom.

The health care provider's own unresolved issues need to be confronted so that any work with patients and families is not blunted by a need to protect the self from being overwhelmed. This is particularly important in the face of compound crises with the pressure of a caseload filled with too many patients—each of whom needs the best the provider can give. Embracing loss and suffering is the starting point for compassionate and trustworthy care that allows others their feelings and experiences without losing hold of the self.

Everyone who deals with crises on a daily basis is at risk for posttraumatic stress disorder (PTSD). Mirroring the fear of patients and the sadness and grief of family members, providers who are exposed to stress without adequate coping strategies can become distant and walled off from their feelings. Being overwhelmed by cumulative crises can precipitate the classic symptoms of PTSD: negativism, withdrawal, irritability, blaming, depression, physical complaints, impoverished interpersonal relationships, and, the hallmark of PTSD, psychic numbing. When the system cannot bear any more pain, it simply shuts down.

Health care providers who care for terminally ill patients and their families in the context of other professional demands are at risk for avoiding the patient's and family's sadness in an attempt to prevent the stress from becoming too much. An unconscious triage is always a possibility: focusing care on those patients who are most likely to improve. What is needed to meet patients' needs is a basic knowledge of crisis intervention, a family systems orientation, and familiarity with spiritual care—in short, psychosociospiritual care.

CRISIS INTERVENTION

Death and loss represent a normal, anticipated, developmental crisis in the course of the human life span. The circumstances surrounding the illness and death may compound the crisis. Sudden death, violent death, and the death of a child deepen the suffering. Other developmental crises, such as marriage or birth of a child, and situational stressors, such as unemployment or relocation, often occur simultaneously within families. The human response to stress, particularly in regard to universal experiences, often has recurring patterns. Guidelines for responding to those patterns are the crux of well-known crisis intervention strategies.[4] Crisis intervention is no longer the prerogative of mental health practitioners alone. Although it may not be specifically named as such, it is continually practiced in primary care.

Model for Crisis Phase Assessment and Intervention

Increasingly, health care providers may find themselves as the primary providers of care. With this reality in mind, a model for identifying phases of crises at the end of life and the interventions specific to those phases can aid in the assessment of patients and their families (Table 14-1). The model as proposed is offered as a way of quickly assessing patients' responses to the specific crisis of dying, but it also can prove useful in other contexts.

During the impact phase, which begins with the diagnosis of a terminal illness or the news of the sudden death of a loved one, denial and anger can be most apparent. The patient or family member may be in shock and disbelief, unable to incorporate either information or an emotional response. A steady,

TABLE 14-1 Phases of Crises Related to Dying, Death, and Bereavement

Phase	Duration	Intervention
Impact	Minutes to hours	Being present
Recoil	Hours to week 2	Initiating overtures
Disorganization	Week 3	Actively intervening
Reorganization	Weeks 4-6	Gradually withdrawing
Reemergence	Weeks 6+	Terminating

caring presence is critical at this juncture. Being present means staying with the patient, witnessing the grief, listening to the rage, and feeling the stunned reaction that accompanies the news. There is nothing to say. False reassurance is seen as untrustworthy, and an important connection is lost. Small, symbolic gestures say what words cannot; offering tissues and taking them back to discard them is a way of participating in the grief and giving permission to weep. Even offering a glass of water or cup of coffee is a way of attending to the arid reality of the impact phase. Remaining with patients and their families during this aspect of care requires a well-rooted certainty of hope and healing that will come in its own time. The capacity to be fully present with someone in pain, no matter how briefly, sets the stage for future interventions that can be extremely effective as the crisis evolves.

The recoil phase typically lasts somewhat longer—hours to days—and is characterized by a need to withdraw from the reality of the event. Patients may avoid scheduled appointments or decide that treatment is unwarranted. They may look to other providers in their search for answers. They may become rejecting, bitter, and angry. It becomes extremely important to initiate overtures at this point, even if one expects to be rebuffed. Patients and families often remember the overture as helpful long after the event, even though they seemed indifferent at the time. The recoil phase is one of lonely reality testing as the person tries to come to grips with the enormity of what is happening. The growing awareness of dying with anticipatory bereavement, as well as the attempt to escape its reality, overshadows everything else.

As the inevitability of the circumstance settles on the family, both the patient and family may undergo profound disorganization. This experience may be prolonged, especially if the dying process is slow. Attending to simple activities of daily living, shopping, preparing meals, and caring for children become insurmountable chores. Anxiety, insomnia, and depression aggravate the loss of routine even further. Providing direct, active intervention at this point helps the family carry on in spite of the confusion and exhaustion. Marshaling the forces that have proffered comfort and support may be the most important function for the health care provider. Most family members are too upset during this phase to organize assistance for themselves. Brief home visits are particularly appropriate at this point. They give the provider a wealth of information and give the patient and family an occasion to feel empowered. The opportunity to be part of a community of care becomes as much a privilege as a responsibility for the health care provider at this time.

The reorganization phase is one of gradual withdrawal for both the patient and the caregivers. In some instances the term *acceptance* is perhaps too strong, but resolve occurs. The patient who is dying and the family or loved one who is grieving come to terms with the reality of what is happening or will happen. It is important to recognize this turn of events and respect the distance that may now be required. Supporting the patient and family indirectly with psychic and spiritual energy becomes indicated. Shorter visits, brief telephone calls, and a short note may be helpful. The amount and timing of contact are determined by clinical judgment that considers the dying patient's physical condition and the family's need for support. Premature withdrawal should be avoided; the temptation to retreat before the end can be overwhelming. Being aware of one's own ambivalence about death is critical.

On the other hand, staying too involved to fulfill some unmet personal need betrays the trust the patient has placed in the health care provider. Patients and families depend on providers to meet their needs as they are able; patients cannot be expected to meet the needs of providers. The intensity needed to connect with a dying patient and his or her family can draw the provider into more intimacy than may be healthy. Discussing cases at staff meetings or with peers safeguards against the tendency to care too much.

Terminating contact during the reemergence phase of the process is as necessary for the provider as it is for the family. When such intimate moments as death are shared with families, there is often a pull to stay involved, particularly with loved ones who seem especially alone. Such involvement is not helpful, and it usually promises more than can be given. Saying good-bye is a lesson that the caregiver and the cared for must both learn.

FAMILY SYSTEMS AND CRISIS SITUATIONS

Every patient comes from a family of origin and from a functional family context, both of which profoundly affect the patient's experience of a health crisis.[5] One of the most useful concepts from family systems theory is the notion of *interface*, or the overlapping connection points between and among family members. Applying that concept to families in crisis directs the health care provider toward the relationships that are the most involved and those with the strongest interfaces. Those closest to the patient will become either allies or antagonists in the patient's care, depending on how they are approached. A little consideration will prove to be a wise investment of time and energy.

A crisis for one member of a family can lead to threatening change for all the members within the family system.[6] Even family members who have had marginal contact appear drawn into the crisis of illness—especially terminal illness. The intensity of the reactions of family members and significant others is directly related to grief and unresolved relationship issues. Fears, guilt, and grief all come into play and masquerade as anger, rage, and demanding behavior.

These reactions can be enormously frustrating—not to mention provoking—for the provider, whose goal is the patient's care and well-being. A measured response is critical. A referral to a social worker, a mental health clinician, or pastoral care may be appropriate. At the very least, simply acknowledging the existence of those complex emotions and responding with warmth and empathy will lower the anxiety level in the patient's immediate circle.

THE ROLE OF SPIRITUAL CARE

Spiritual care has historically been a central component of nursing care. Nightingale recognized that caring for the spiritual aspect of the patient was part of the nursing ideal.[7] Confusion, distortion, and numerous interpretations of what spirituality actually is have hampered our understanding and compromised our care.[8] As clearer definitions have emerged, research from a variety of fields has focused on the significance of spiritual care to the patient.[9,10] At this point it is commonly assumed that the importance of spirituality in nursing theory and practice continues to grow, that spirituality is part of the patient, and that supporting the spiritual aspect of a patient can mitigate the experience of loss and suffering.[11]

When under the strain of life-threatening illness, patients can develop spiritual distress. This distress is heard in questions such as "Why me?" or "What did I do to deserve this?" Such questions reflect a search for meaning in the experience, an effort to make sense out of the incomprehensible. Patients may begin to question their sense of connectedness to a higher power or whatever relationships they experience as sacred. At this time the role of the health care provider is not that of a theologian, but of an intuitive listener who remains present with the patient.[12] The healing occurs in the telling of the story.

Giving the spiritual domain its due can present a challenge for those who would not claim to be particularly conversant with the language of the spirit. Although it may be more comfortable for those who are intentional about their own faith journey, spiritual care does not depend on the caregiver's own experience of the spiritual, faith, or religion. In fact, projecting one's own belief systems onto the patient would be inappropriate. What spiritual care does require is an appreciation of mystery and a willingness to be open to the patient's experience.

One clear opportunity to appreciate mystery is *nearing death awareness*.[13] This term has been suggested for what happens with many patients as death is imminent; it is the sense of setting out on a journey and seeing or speaking to loved ones long dead. One might name their experience *confusion* or *disorientation* or diagnose it as hypoxia, and search for explanations. One might also simply accept that there are phenomena that cannot be explained but simply described. Because the experience of dying is so difficult to articulate, the language used is often symbolic. Listening intently and being attuned to the possible use of metaphor, story, and symbol, the provider not only stays in communication with patients but also becomes aware of their peaceful, even joyful experiences.

PSYCHOSOCIOSPIRITUAL CARE: ACTIVATING HOPE IN THE HOPELESS

The question then becomes, "What exactly are we to do for patients when it appears there is nothing to be done?" This is the place for presence and for a transition to being. This is the time for psychosociospiritual interventions. Most nurses instinctively know that their most meaningful interventions involve the simplest gestures: the touch of a hand, a nod of affirmation, and a look of full and complete attention that exudes presence.

As a sense of hopelessness emerges in the patient, it is incumbent on the health care provider to determine meaningful, empowering interventions. Assessing prior coping strategies provides a basis for intervening. Such assessment must include examining the social support for the patient. Connections with others often allow the patient to recognize a connection to a higher power, if the patient is a believer.

For patients who have relied more on cognitive coping strategies, often providing information or anticipatory guidance, using the patient's language, is useful. Patients may wish to know what to expect as they approach the end of life and to have their beliefs regarding end-of-life experiences validated. Caregivers may also benefit from such intervention as their beliefs about the patient making a transition to a more positive spiritual experience are supported. Statements made by patients and caregivers such as "joining [a dead loved one]" or "going to rest" serve as empowering affirmations in the midst of hopelessness that are strengthened from confirmation by the provider.

But as intellectual faculties fade or are overwhelmed, nothing is more powerful or more spiritual than touching another soul with one's own. Strategies for intervention that intentionally include spiritual care encourage the patient's own search for meaning and experience of the sacred. Allowing for a spiritual experience that involves the senses—sensory spirituality—is a natural access point for nursing.[14]

As body, mind, and spirit are bound together, spiritual care can take the form of relaxation, allowing the patient to exercise some control over his or her body and its sensory experiences. Tired bodies and discouraged spirits respond to complementary modalities as a spiritual experience.[15] Relaxation and comfort can quickly be attained through interventions intended to heal the spirit. Therapies such as acupuncture, therapeutic touch, biofeedback, Reiki, reflexology, aromatherapy, chiropractic therapy, and massage serve as physical forms of care for the whole patient. Guided imagery can draw on music, voices, images, and color to induce a period of helpful relaxation and meditation. Using the arts with patients suffering from chronic pain, or particularly when they are dying, promotes a peaceful environment, can reduce anxiety and fear, and, most important, can facilitate their own sense of the spiritual. Music therapy, such as that promoted by music thanatologists at the Chalice of Repose Project in Mount Angel, Oregon, can be used to create deeply sacred moments that are soothing to both patient and caregiver.[16]

This approach is as nourishing to the provider as it is to the patient. When one tries to preserve empathy and the capacity to cope simultaneously, recognizing the images, symbols, metaphors, and rituals that activate hope protects one's own reservoir of compassion. What is good for patients is good for us.

RESOURCES FOR PSYCHOSOCIOSPIRITUAL CARE

Multiple collaborative resources are available to the health care provider, ranging from mental health providers to chaplains or spiritual counselors. Nurses engaged in health ministries and the emerging field of parish nursing can play a critical role in psychosociospiritual care and are an important source of information on resources for spiritual care with patients and families. Nurse specialists involved in hospice care and mental health are important resources and have developed tools for assessing and intervening with the whole patient. In addition, holistic health care practitioners can contribute to psychosociospiritual care and enjoy increasing support from the general public.

Models of spiritual assessment, especially those tailored for brief intervention, are useful and easily adapted to multiple settings.[17,18] Exploring ways to integrate psychosociospiritual interventions into primary care with patients at the end of life can undoubtedly demonstrate the effectiveness of such a model in the care of all patients in crisis. Staring death in the face puts life in perspective. Nothing is ever the same again. The world is viewed with a type of "wiseheartedness" that only the journey into the valley of the darkness can provide. Every decision, every priority, every relationship, every wish, and every hope is transformed from that time forward. The provider, too, has become a little more healed and a little more whole in body, mind, and spirit.

REFERENCES

1. Agrawal M, Emanuel EJ: Attending to psychological symptoms and palliative care, *J Clin Oncol* 20(3):624-626, 2002.
2. Gallup G: *Spiritual beliefs and the dying process,* Princeton, 1997, George H Gallup International Institute.
3. American Nurses Association: *Code of ethics for nurses with interpretive statements*, 2001, retrieved Jan 2, 2006, from http://www.nursingworld.org/ethics/code/protected_nwcoe303.htm#1.1.
4. Augliera DC: *Crisis intervention: theory and methodology,* ed 8, St Louis, 1998, Mosby.
5. Van Horn E, Fleury J, Moore S: Family interventions during the trajectory of recovery from cardiac event: an integrative literature review, *Heart Lung* 31(3):186-198, 2002.
6. Wright LM, Leahey M: *Nurses and families: a guide to family assessment and intervention,* ed 3, Philadelphia, 2000, Davis.
7. Delgado C: A discussion of the concept of spirituality, *Nurs Sci Q* 18(2):157-162, 2005.
8. Lemmer CM: Recognizing and caring for spiritual needs of clients, *J Holis Nurs* 23(3):310-332, 2005.
9. Baldacchino D, Draper P: Spiritual coping strategies: a review of the nursing research literature, *J Adv Nurs* 34(6):833-841, 2001.
10. Mueller P, Plevak DJ, Rummans TA: Religious involvement, spirituality, and medicine: implications for clinical practice, *Mayo Clin Proc* 76(12):1225-1235, 2001.
11. Henery N: Constructions of spirituality in contemporary nursing theory, *J Adv Nurs* 46(6):550-557, 2003.
12. Sawatzky R, Pesut B: Attributes of spiritual care in nursing practice, *J Holis Nurs* 23(1):19-33, 2005.
13. Callanan M, Kelley P: *Final gifts: understanding the special awareness, needs, and communications of the dying,* New York, 1993, Bantam.
14. Chandler E: Spirituality, *Hosp J* 14(3-4):63-74, 1999.
15. Brown-Saltzman K: Replenishing the spirit by meditative prayer and guided imagery, *Semin Oncol Nurs* 13(4):255-259, 1997.
16. Schroeder-Sheker T: Music for the dying: a personal account of the new field of music thanatology: history, theories, and clinical narratives, *J Holis Nurs* 12(1):83-99, 1994.
17. Larson K: The importance of spiritual assessment: one clinician's journey, *Geriatr Nurs* 24(6):370-371, 2003.
18. Maddox M: Spiritual assessments in primary care, *NP* 27(2):12, 14, 2002.

CHAPTER 15

Palliative and End-of-Life Care

Marie A. Bakitas, Constance Dahlin, and Margaret Firer Bishop

Almost every health care provider at some point interacts with patients who are dying. With dramatic advances in biomedical research and the ability to treat disease and prolong life, however, modern medicine—until recently—has neglected its traditional role of comforting patients and their families when "end of life is near."[1]

Entire texts are devoted to birth and obstetric care, yet most medical references barely mention care of the dying patient.[2,3] Unlike the unmistakable signals of impending birth, the objective signs of dying and death are more elusive, depending on a patient's diagnosis. Accurately predicting the prognosis is a poorly developed skill in most providers. A challenge in health care is to determine who is dying. A large study of seriously ill patients attempted to answer this question and found that, although patients with incurable cancer follow a linear downward path, those dying of chronic cardiopulmonary illness follow a less predictable course.[4] Rather than attempting to determine which patient is "actively" dying, the "surprise" question may be more helpful: "Would you be surprised if this patient died in the next 6 months to a year?"[5] Considering the population in this way can ease transitions and lead to an earlier integration of a palliative approach to care.

The key concept is to replace a dichotomous model of cure versus palliation with one that focuses on palliation in increasing degrees from the time of diagnosis with the life-threatening illness[6] (Figure 15-1). It is appropriate to begin to use a palliative philosophy long before death is imminent but when life-prolonging therapy options have become less effective.[7,8] Health care providers focused on continuity of care are in a unique position to help patients and families understand the concept of palliative care. Some basic strategies for providers may improve care for patients with incurable illnesses and their families. This chapter describes selected principles of palliative and end-of-life care and symptom management that are appropriate for adults with life-threatening illnesses.

PALLIATIVE CARE

Definition and Epidemiology

According to the World Health Organization, palliative care is "an approach which improves the quality of life of patients and their families facing life-threatening illness, through the prevention, assessment and treatment of pain and other physical, psychosocial and spiritual problems."[8] The goals of palliative care are listed in Box 15-1.

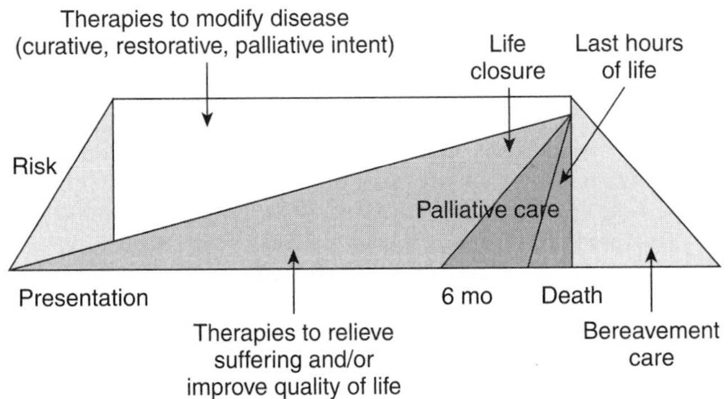

FIGURE 15-1

World Health Organization palliative care model. (As modified by Ferris FD: *Establishing a palliative care program: rationale*, Center for the Advancement of Palliative Care Management Training Seminar, Oakland, Calif, July 2001, retrieved Dec 2001 from http://www.capc.org.)

BOX 15-1

GOALS OF PALLIATIVE CARE

Palliative care:

- Provides relief from pain and other distressing symptoms
- Affirms life and regards dying as a normal process
- Intends neither to hasten nor postpone death
- Integrates the psychological and spiritual aspects of patient care
- Offers a support system to help patients live as actively as possible until death
- Offers a support system to help the family cope during the patient's illness and in their own bereavement
- Uses a team approach to address the needs of patients and their families, including bereavement counseling, if indicated
- Will enhance quality of life, and may also positively influence the course of illness
- Is applicable early in the course of illness, in conjunction with other therapies that are intended to prolong life, such as chemotherapy or radiation therapy, and includes those investigations needed to better understand and manage distressing clinical complications

From World Health Organization: *Palliative care,* 2003, retrieved April 2003 from http://www.who.int/hiv/topics/palliative/care/en.

Access to Care

The Clinical Practice Guidelines for Quality Palliative Care, developed by the National Consensus Project, emphasize that palliative care is a critical dimension of health care. All persons should have access to health care providers who have basic knowledge and skills in palliative care practices.[9] Furthermore, appropriate interdisciplinary palliative care should be accessible to all patients regardless of care setting or disease.[9] Health care providers can provide palliative care support and expertise to their panel of patients; at times, however, consultation with a specialty palliative care or hospice interdisciplinary team or service may be desirable. Palliative care consultation services and interdisciplinary teams have become widely available in hospitals or as an expansion of community hospice services.[10] Some also provide this focus within skilled or extended-care and assisted-living facilities. Resources for learning about palliative care approaches and specialists are listed in Box 15-2.

Most Americans express a wish to spend their final days in their own home, surrounded by loved ones. The reality of dying in the United States in the twenty-first century is very different. Up to 50% of people will die in the hospital, and another 25% will die in nursing homes. Only 30% of those dying will receive hospice services.[11] The 1997 Institute of Medicine report titled *Approaching Death*[7] proposed a model of a "good death" as a target for improvements in the health care system. It stated the following:

> People should be able to expect and achieve a decent and good death—one that is free from avoidable distress and suffering for patients, families and caregivers; in general accord with the patient's and family's wishes; and reasonably consistent with clinical, cultural, and ethical standards.

In truth, palliative care is simply "good" medical care—care that can be provided by any skilled health care provider in the patient's home or community or, when necessary, in a hospital or extended-care facility.

ADVANCE CARE PLANNING

In a primary care practice the first step is to understand the patient's preferences and help identify goals of care that may change as the disease progresses. The health care provider should initiate such discussions as a component of the initial history of all adult patients, regardless of age or health status, as an important aspect of preventive care. It is an ongoing process that needs to be revisited whenever a patient's health status or life goals change. Advance care planning includes discussion and documentation of the patient's values and care preferences through the completion of advance directives (see Chapter 13). To be complete, it should include the type of care the patient does or does not wish at the end of life, and name the proxy decision maker if the patient lacks the capacity to express his or her preferences.

Most standardized advance directive forms are written in a defensive tone, indicating the type of care a patient does *not* want. Another, more comprehensive approach to this type of documentation, called "Five Wishes," addresses the type of care a patient *does* want as disease progresses (Box 15-3). For example, patients can describe their wish to shift the focus of medical interventions to "comfort care" when they are very near death. This type of care involves minimizing procedures that do not contribute to comfort. Some common medical procedures may be "invisible" to the provider but uncomfortable for the patient (e.g., daily weights, laboratory tests, vital signs) and hence not appropriate at the very end of life.[12]

Health care providers should ensure that patients' wishes are carried out even when they are not able to speak for themselves. For example, for patients wishing to die at home, it is critical that the proxy decision maker (usually a family member) is prepared to anticipate symptom crises or the moment of natural death. Unprepared family members may panic in such circumstance and call 911. Most do not realize that, when the 911 system is activated, emergency medical personnel are obligated by law to perform life-sustaining measures, including CPR and intubation, unless a do-not-resuscitate (DNR) order is written for the home. Many states

BOX 15-2

PALLIATIVE CARE WEB RESOURCES

American Academy of Hospice and Palliative Medicine (http://www.AAHPM.org) is a national professional organization dedicated to promoting palliative medicine. Features include publications, education, competencies, and certification.

Americans for Better Care of the Dying (http://www.abcd-caring.org) is dedicated to social, professional, and policy reform aimed at improving the care system for patients with serious illness and for their families.

Center to Advance Palliative Care (CAPC) (http://www.capc.org) provides technical assistance needed to establish palliative care programs, as well as opportunities to network with colleagues in the palliative care community. Features include CAPC publications, education calendar, and information about advocacy activities.

Dying Well (http://www.dyingwell.org) offers resources and referrals to organizations, websites, and books to empower persons with life-threatening illnesses and their families to live as fully as possible during the dying process. It provides a link to the Missoula Demonstration Project, which demonstrates a community-based approach to end-of-life care.

Education for Palliative and End-of-Life Care (EPEC) (http://www.epec.net) educates physicians, through its core curriculum, on essential clinical competencies required to provide quality end-of-life care.

End-of-Life Nursing Education Consortium (ELNEC) (http://www.aacn.nche.edu/ELNEC/about.htm) project is a national education initiative to improve end-of-life care in the United States. The project provides training for undergraduate and graduate nursing faculty, continuing education providers, staff development educators, pediatric and oncology specialty nurses, and other nurses in end-of-life care so they can teach this essential information to nursing students and practicing nurses.

End of Life/Palliative Education Resource Center (EPERC) (http://www.eperc.mcw.edu) assists physician educators and others in locating high-quality, peer-reviewed training materials. Visitors to the website can search for educational materials indexed by end-of-life care topic areas and educational formats.

Growth House (http://www.growthhouse.org) is a search engine that offers access to the Internet's most comprehensive collection of reviewed resources for end-of-life care.

Hospice and Palliative Nurses Association (HPNA) (http://www.hpna.org) exchanges information, experiences, and ideas; promotes understanding of the specialties of hospice and palliative nursing; and studies and promotes hospice and palliative nursing research. A listserv is available for advance practice nurses.

Hospice Foundation of America (http://www.hospicefoundation.org) provides education and information about death and dying in America.

Innovations in End-of-Life Care (http://www.edc.org/lastacts) is an online journal featuring peer-reviewed examples of promising practices in end-of-life care. Each bimonthly issue focuses on a different theme.

National Board for Certification of Hospice & Palliative Nurses (http://www.nbchpn.org) promotes a certification process that advances quality in the provision of end-of-life care. The advanced practice examination results in the following credential: APRN, BC-PCM (advanced practice registered nurse, Board Certified–Palliative Care Management).

National Consensus Project for Quality Palliative Care (http://www.nationalconsensusproject.org) promotes the implementation of clinical practice guidelines that ensure care of consistent and high quality, and that guide the development and structure of new and existing palliative care services.

National Hospice and Palliative Care Organization (http://www.nhpco.org) is the industry's largest association and leading resource for professionals and volunteers committed to and providing service to patients and their families during end of life.

On Our Own Terms: Moyers on Dying (http://www.thirteen.org/onourownterms) supports the On Our Own Terms outreach campaign with various tools, articles, personal stories, audio and video clips, and interactive opportunities.

BOX 15-3

FIVE WISHES

- The person I want to make care decisions for me when I can't
- The kind of medical treatment I want or don't want
- How comfortable I want to be
- How I want people to treat me
- What I want my loved ones to know

From *Five wishes: an advanced directives document*, available from Aging with Dignity, (888) 594-7437 or http://www.agingwithdignity.org.

have provisions for "No Code" or DNR orders for patients at home; such provisions allow emergency personnel to provide "comfort care" rather than CPR if they are called to the home by family members or if patients are brought to an emergency department with a need for symptom control.[13] Because DNR orders are generally nonportable, provisions should be made to avoid unwanted care when the dying patient is at home or in a nursing home.

SYMPTOM MANAGEMENT IN PALLIATIVE CARE

Holistic symptom care of the patient at the very end of life addresses physical, psychologic, social, and spiritual distress of the patient and the family (Figure 15-2). This section describes common symptoms and palliative care management strategies that can be applied by health care providers who care for patients with life-limiting illnesses.[14]

ANOREXIA AND CACHEXIA

Definition

Anorexia is the reduced desire to eat. Because food is the essence of life and often represents love, a loss of interest in food can be upsetting to the family. Anorexia is characterized by a loss of appetite and a loss of interest in food. Food is not appealing, and the patient may be too tired or may lose the desire to eat. Cachexia is a state of general malnutrition marked by weight loss, malnutrition, weakness, and emaciation. It is usually induced by anorexia and is marked by an equal loss of fat, muscle, and bone mineral content. There is often no improvement with nutritional supplements or increased intake.[15,16]

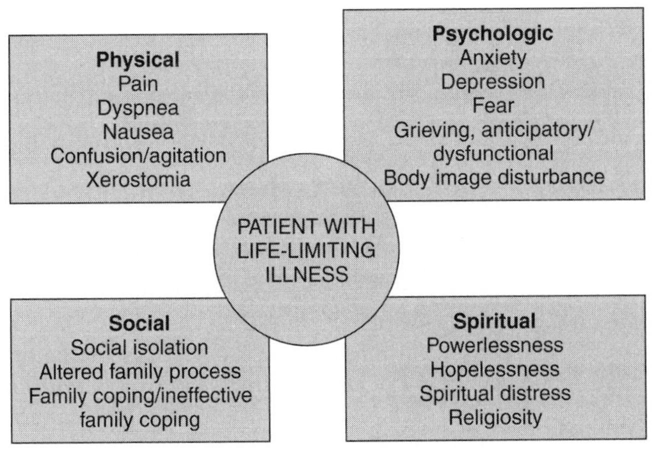

FIGURE 15-2

Symptom model for palliative care patients.

Pathophysiology

Anorexia is common in patients with HIV infection and is the second most common symptom in patients with cancer. Causes include impaired situational coping, unrelated illnesses, treatment side effects, anxiety, and depression.[17] Physiologic causes include impaired gastric emptying, constipation, pain, medications, oral infections, intracranial disease, and tumor-produced peptides.[17] Progressive anorexia occurs as the patient nears death and is a natural part of the dying process.

Clinical Presentation and Physical Examination

Comprehensive assessment of anorexia is important. The assessment includes preferred foods, problems with taste or smell, dry mouth, chewing difficulties, bowel assessment, and a social history (including the enjoyment of alcoholic drinks).[17] The physical examination includes an observation of cognition, an oral examination that looks for dryness or lesions, an observation of skin turgor and muscle strength, and an abdominal examination (including a rectal examination). Blood studies may sometimes be appropriate, with particular attention given to nutritional markers, including total lymphocytes, hemoglobin, albumin, and iron.

Management

Education is the cornerstone to care. A loss of appetite is common in dying patients because they cannot tolerate premorbid calorie intake, nor do they want to eat. Anorexia usually generates many issues because food as seen as the sustenance and essence of life. Family and friends may not understand the patient's inability to eat and should be counseled about the pros and cons of artificial nutrition and hydration.[18] When discussing artificial nutrition and hydration, it is important to avoid using the terms *food and water.* Rather, discussing *medically provided* or *artificial* nutrition and hydration helps define these as medical interventions, different from the natural impulses of eating and drinking. Friends and family members also worry their loved one will experience thirst or hunger. The sensation of thirst is best relieved by keeping the mouth moist (see Dry Mouth [Xerostomia]) rather than administering IV fluids. As nutritional intake declines, ketones are released that promote a sense of well-being.

In particular, family members must be informed that anorexia and cachexia are a natural part of death. Although IV fluids or feedings by means of total parenteral nutrition or a nasogastric or gastrostomy tube can prolong life, they may also cause discomfort. The dying patient may experience fluid overload from such strategies because the body is unable to metabolize fluids and proteins in the same way as a "normal, healthy" person. This can result in edema in the arms, legs, and abdomen; incontinence and skin breakdown; and pulmonary congestion and ascites causing dyspnea as the abdomen pushes up on the diaphragm.

Realistic goals of nutritional intake (e.g., relief of hunger or thirst, socialization at mealtimes) should be encouraged. The focus should be on giving patients preferred foods that improve their quality of life, offering welcome relief from lifelong dietary restrictions (e.g., diabetic, low-salt, or low-cholesterol diets). Eliminating blood glucose monitoring and evaluating the need for other diet-related medications (e.g., cholesterol-lowering agents) reduces the burden of treatment at this time. An appetite stimulant may be offered if the patient wishes. A progesterone steroid such as megestrol (Megace) 200 to 800 mg/day or dronabinol (Marino) 2.5 mg b.i.d. may be helpful. Other short-term symptom relief medications for depression (e.g., methylphenidate [Ritalin]) or for pain (e.g., dexamethasone [Decadron]) may have the added benefit of helping to increase appetite.[15] A glass of beer, sherry, or wine may stimulate the appetite, particularly if this has been a part of the patient's established routine.

ANXIETY AND FEAR

Definition

Anxiety is a sense of deep unease. It is related to fear and is characterized by a constellation of signs and symptoms, including insomnia, headache, shortness of breath, weakness, chest pain, palpitations, a sensation of butterflies in the stomach, urinary frequency, pallor, restlessness, tremor, and sweating. The difference between fear and anxiety is that *fear* has a definable quality or cause.

Pathophysiology

Causes of anxiety at the end of life include situational issues (e.g., financial or family worries, unfinished business, fears, and adjustment to disease) and organic causes (e.g., uncontrolled pain or dyspnea, psychiatric causes, medications, existential distress, altered physiologic status, and a lack of control).[19] (See Chapter 259 for a more detailed discussion of the pathophysiology of anxiety.)

Clinical Presentation and Physical Examination

Assessment of anxiety begins with understanding the patient's knowledge of his or her disease, specifically if there are any fears about dying or death.[20] The patient should be asked about troubling symptoms, previous stressful incidents, and his or her previous coping style with stress and illness. Complaints of tremors, weakness, agitation, limb numbness, or shortness of breath should be noted. The patient may also complain of gastrointestinal upset, palpitations, muscle aches, and sleep disorders.

The physical assessment includes vital signs, noting rapid pulse, high blood pressure, or hyperventilation. Generalized signs, including flushing, wheezing, sweating, or tremor, may be found on examination. Muscle tightness, nausea, or vomiting can also occur.

Management

Treatment focuses on pharmacologic interventions and, if possible, alleviation of the specific problem, particularly if the problem is behavioral. This includes the provision of factual information accompanied by the use of psychosocial or spiritual therapists. Pharmacologic interventions include the use of anxiolytics (e.g., benzodiazepines such as lorazepam 0.5 to 2 mg PO/IV/sublingually q 3-6 hr, or diazepam 2.5 to 10 mg q 3-6 hr). Because of expense, the lack of an oral form, and short-term effects, midazolam administered as a continuous infusion should be reserved for those patients who are unable to swallow and have intractable anxiety.

Alleviation of anxiety may also require relief of a symptom cluster, such as the cycle of pain, dyspnea, and anxiety. In such cases it may be impossible to separate and treat the "initiating event." The selection of agents that treat multiple symptoms (e.g., morphine, which can relieve pain and dyspnea and provide a calming effect) is often the best approach.

DELIRIUM

Definition

Delirium is defined as a reversible, sudden, and acute confusional state. It is characterized by sudden changes in mental status, a mental status that waxes and wanes, a reduced attention span, and hyperactivity or hypoactivity.[21]

Pathophysiology

Delirium is common in patients with advanced disease. It may be caused by tumor pressure in the brain; medication side effects, withdrawal, or overdose; uncontrolled pain; metabolic changes; liver or kidney dysfunction; infections; or nutritional deficiencies. More than half of all dying patients experience delirium as they approach death.[21,22] This may be attributed to the actual dying process or to one of the previously listed causes.

Clinical Presentation and Physical Examination

Delirium often occurs suddenly and may fluctuate during the course of the day. It often worsens in the late afternoon or at night, disturbing the patient's sleep-wake cycle. Speech may be incoherent or inappropriate to the situation. The patient may have altered perceptions that manifest as hallucinations or delusions. Disorientation to person, place, date, and time, as well as agitation, restlessness, aggressiveness, and paranoia, is also possible (see Chapter 204).

A Mini-Mental Status Examination is a simple and reliable initial assessment of cognitive function. This test includes orientation to person, place, date, and residence; memory and recall of three objects; attention and calculation; language; response to commands; and ability to copy a design. This assessment can begin to define the degree of disturbance and is best used when a baseline examination is done. A thorough neurologic examination may provide further clues to the etiology.

Diagnostics

Diagnostic studies should be undertaken only if the results are likely to change patient management. For example, correcting dehydration, metabolic abnormalities, or hypercalcemia can sometimes reverse delirium, especially if death is not imminent. Other simple blood studies may reveal easily reversible causes of delirium such as glucose levels, kidney function, liver function, and oxygen saturation levels.

Management

First and foremost, educating the family about delirium, its causes (if known or suspected), and its prognosis is critical. If otherwise beneficial medications are the cause, the family needs to assist in identifying the patient's priorities for comfort. Older adults are particularly sensitive to medications for pain and symptom control and hence are at high risk for delirium.

Treatment of delirium in a patient whose death is not imminent includes identifying and treating the reversible causes while keeping the patient in a safe and comfortable environment. The environment should be modified immediately to reduce stimuli, the patient should be reoriented (if possible), and neuroleptics should be administered.[23] If the delirium is a result of opioid or benzodiazepine withdrawal, slowing the tapering process can help. Long-term, high-dose opioids may cause delirium due to the accumulation of metabolites.[24] This is especially common in patients who were previously stable on a particular dose and experience acute dehydration or renal insufficiency. It is usually unrealistic to discontinue opioids in a dying patient. If the current opioid regimen is believed to be the cause of delirium, however, a different opioid in an equianalgesic dose may provide pain relief without delirium. For example, methadone, hydromorphone, and oxycodone may be less deliriogenic than morphine or meperidine. The former agents lack the metabolites that can accumulate and cause delirium.

For the patient who is close to death, the family needs to be counseled that delirium may signal impending death. This subtlety is often missed, resulting in missed opportunity for closure. Neuroleptic medications such as haloperidol are the drugs of choice for patients who are delirious in the last few days of life (Table 15-1).[22,23] These medications may be given to help calm the patient and to ease fear and panic. IV dosing is recommended to initially provide rapid relief and to minimize the extrapyramidal symptoms. Once a dose is established, converting to an equivalent oral dosing regimen (whenever possible) on a scheduled basis can maintain a calm state. Treatment of delirium using a benzodiazepine alone can result in paradoxical effects and actually worsen the delirium. Hence this often prescribed approach to calm or quiet a delirious patient is discouraged in the dying patient.[23] However, for some cases of intractable delirium, palliative sedation (described later) may be necessary.

TABLE 15-1 Medications Used for Terminal Delirium/Sedation at End of Life

Generic Name	Approximate Daily Dosage	Route
NEUROLEPTICS		
Haloperidol	0.5-5 mg q 2-12 hr	PO, IV, SC, IM
Chlorpromazine	12.5-50 mg q 4-12 hr	PO, IV, IM
Droperidol	0.5-5 mg q 12 hr	PO
BENZODIAZEPINES		
Lorazepam	0.5-2.0 mg q 1-4 hr	PO, IV, 1M
Midazolam	30-100 mg/24 hr	IV, SC

SC, Subcutaneous; *IM*, intramuscular.

DEPRESSION

Definition

Depressive disorders are illnesses that affect mood and result in a variety of symptoms, including anhedonia, helplessness, hopelessness, worthlessness, and guilt. Feelings of personal failure are strong.

Diagnosis of depression in a terminally ill patient can be a challenge because the neurovegetative signs that are typically part of the diagnostic criteria of depression are often normally present in patients with advanced terminal disease, particularly cancer. Observing the patient for psychologic and cognitive symptoms of worthlessness, hopelessness, excessive guilt, and suicidal ideation may be more diagnostic.[21] Box 15-4 provides a helpful acronym for diagnosis.

Depression with serious or terminal illness should not be considered normal, or "the norm." Although sadness and grief may be anticipated in terminally ill patients, a mood of total despair can lead to suicide, a request for assisted suicide, or other attempts at a "hastened death." The desire for a hastened death is highly linked to depression and unmanaged symptoms.[20] Conversely, treating depression in terminally ill patients can allow them to experience pleasure in life, finish the emotional work of saying good-bye, make meaning of their lives, and perform other important activities of life closure.[20]

Clinical Presentation and Physical Examination

The assessment of depression in the terminally ill patient is multifaceted with particular sensitivity to culture and religion. The patient's appearance, including dress and grooming, is important. Affect, speech, and orientation are all factors in the examination. Obtaining a history with attention to substance abuse and previous depressive or bipolar episodes is critical.

Assessment also includes mood and lifestyle changes. A history of sleep disturbances, weight loss, impaired concentration, psychomotor changes, loss of interest in life, feelings of guilt, loss of energy, fatigue, and suicidal thoughts should be noted. Patients must be asked directly about whether they feel depressed, whether they have contemplated taking their own lives, and if they have a plan for doing so (see Chapter 261).

BOX 15-4

SIGECAPS MNEMONIC TO ASSESS DEPRESSION

- **S** *S*leep changes (increased or decreased)
- **I** *I*nterest changes (increased or decreased)
- **G** *G*uilt
- **E** *E*nergy changes (fatigue or loss of energy)
- **C** *C*oncentration changes (inability to focus)
- **A** *A*ppetite (decreased or increased)
- **P** *P*sychomotor agitation
- **S** *S*uicidal thoughts

Diagnostics

Diagnostic testing is indicated to exclude other causes of mood disorders and includes CBC, serum electrolytes, calcium, BUN, creatinine, and thyroid-stimulating hormone.

Management

Treatment includes pharmacologic and psychotherapeutic modalities. Pharmacologic treatment depends on the prognosis. A psychostimulant or steroid may be the drug of choice if death is likely within 1 month.[25] Methylphenidate is rapid acting and may reduce pain. It can be started at 2.5 to 5 mg/day and increased to 10 to 20 mg/day. This medication is given early in the morning, with the same dose repeated at noon to allow the peak effect to wear off by bedtime. Dosing later in the day may cause insomnia, although some patients may do better with more frequent dosing. Both psychostimulants and steroids may help improve multiple common end-of-life symptoms, including depression, loss of appetite, and sedation.

A trial of tricyclic antidepressants (TCAs) or selective serotonin reuptake inhibitors (SSRIs) is appropriate if death is not likely within 1 month. TCAs can help with neuropathic pain, depression, and insomnia. They are inexpensive, but the sedating and autonomic properties may cause more side effects. The starting dosage for amitriptyline, imipramine, desipramine, or nortriptyline is 10 to 25 mg/day. The dosage can be increased to 25 to 100 mg/day. TCAs should be taken at bedtime because they cause sedation. SSRIs are often considered as a first-line choice because of an improved side effect profile over TCAs.[26] Sertraline is initiated at 12.5 to 25 mg/day with a range up to 50 to 100 mg/day. Fluoxetine is started at 10 mg/day and increased to 20 to 40 mg/day. Paroxetine is started at 10 mg/day. Psychostimulants can be used over the short term while initiating an SSRI, then weaned as the TCA or SSRI becomes effective.[21]

Some patients benefit from St. John's wort or other herbal remedies. It is important that patients and families understand that herbal remedies are also pharmacologic agents with side effects and adverse effects. Consultation with an herbalist or naturopath may be indicated.

Indications for Referral or Hospitalization

Substantial literature documents that the best treatment for depression includes both pharmacologic interventions and counseling. Referrals for the patient and family members to a psychiatrist, psychologist, social worker, pastoral counselor, or hospice worker can help in the understanding and management of depression at the end of life. Psychotherapeutic approaches can encourage the patient to talk about past and present experiences, as well as the dying experience.

Behavioral interventions and cognitive restructuring may also be helpful. A formal psychiatric evaluation may be used to determine the appropriateness of antidepressant medications for patients with co-morbid conditions and for stoic patients who may not be willing to admit depression to their family or health care provider for fear of causing disappointment or appearing weak.

A multidisciplinary approach may be helpful in engaging the patient and acknowledging his or her feelings. Reiteration of the goals of pain and symptom management may provide reassurance and promote feelings of support.

DYSPNEA

Definition and Pathophysiology

Dyspnea is a subjective sense of shortness of breath, difficulty breathing, or an uncomfortable awareness of breathing. The patient may feel as if he or she is suffocating or choking. This shortness of breath may be accompanied by fear, anxiety, or panic.[27] Dyspnea is common in patients with lung cancer, lung disease, and cardiac disease. Causes include the effects of tumors, the effects of cancer treatment, lung disease, heart disease, infection, muscle weakness, and anxiety.

Clinical Presentation and Physical Examination

A patient's self-report of dyspnea is the most important assessment criterion.[28] The patient may appear short of breath but may deny shortness of breath, or may report being short of breath without appearing so. The use of a scale similar to that indicating pain may be helpful. A 0 to 10 scale can be used, with 0 being no problem and 10 being the worst trouble breathing the patient can imagine. A history of shortness of breath, including onset, frequency, and contributing factors, should be obtained.

In addition to subjective reporting, objective examination includes chest auscultation, observations of the patient's breathing, and oxygen saturation. Pulse oximetry should be obtained with the patient at rest, during activity, and in different positions. Radiologic procedures, including chest x-ray films for possible pneumonia, pleural effusions, and disease progression, or a spiral CT scan for possible pulmonary embolism, can be helpful. However, these examinations should be performed only if the data would change treatment and the patient is not actively dying, since they are exhausting for the patient and expensive.

Management

In treating dyspnea, it is important to consider the prognosis and the patient's values and preferences regarding the treatment of any underlying disease such as infection or progressive cancer. The risks and benefits of the treatment and the potential improvement of the patient's symptoms should be considered.[27] If comfort is the goal and the patient is close to death, some simple maneuvers can be helpful. Merely repositioning the patient in an upright sitting position may help. Oxygen administration via nasal cannula (and humidification) rather than a face mask is usually more comfortable and may also be beneficial. A fan blowing gently on the face reduces the perception of breathlessness by stimulating the receptors in the buccal mucosa.[29]

Opioids and benzodiazepines may also relieve dyspnea. Since opioids are the mainstay of therapy, morphine is the drug of choice, with a starting dosage of 5 to 10 mg PO q 3-4 hr in the opioid-naive patient. Dosages for older adults can be smaller, starting at 2 to 5 mg PO or subcutaneously q 3-4 hr. Oxycodone 5 to 10 mg q 3-4 hr may be substituted for older adults or morphine-sensitive patients. Antianxiety agents include lorazepam, 0.5 to 2 mg PO q 4-6 hr, or diazepam, 2.5 to 10 mg q 4-6 hr. Lorazepam is usually shorter acting than diazepam. The use of nebulized opioids or other nebulized medications (e.g., bronchodilators, steroids for relief of specific symptoms) should be matched to the clinical situation. Many of these interventions lack an evidence base in improving symptoms at the end of life but are perceived by providers and patients as beneficial.[28]

At the very end of life, a patient may experience upper airway congestion or a "death rattle," caused by the relaxation of throat muscles with saliva pooling on the vocal cords. This is usually more distressing to the family than to the patient. Reducing fluid intake, especially IV fluids, can help. This must be done sensitively, with consideration for the patient's and family's culture and religion. If complete discontinuation of an IV is not appropriate, decreasing fluids to a minimum can provide significant relief. Anticholinergic agents may provide some additional relief from this distressing end-stage symptom. These agents include 1.5-mg scopolamine patches (Transderm Scōp, 1 to 4 patches q 72 hr), which take 3 to 4 hours to reach peak onset; hyoscyamine (Levsin) in drops or pills (0.125 to 0.25 mg q 4-6 hr); or glycopyrrolate (Robinul) in either an oral (1 to 2 mg q 6 hr), IV, or nebulized form, which has more immediate effect. Atropine 1% ophthalmic drops used sublingually (2 drops q 4 hr p.r.n) has also been useful in patients who are nonresponsive. Oral cavity suctioning may help, but secretions will reaccumulate. Deep suctioning is rarely effective and may cause more distress than benefit in the dying person.

DRY MOUTH (XEROSTOMIA)

Definition

Dry mouth, or xerostomia, is the sensation of oral dryness. It is accompanied by decreased salivary secretions and is commonly experienced by patients with advanced progressive disease.[30] It may be difficult to identify the exact underlying cause and contributing factors. However, treatment offers much comfort and relief to patients.

Pathophysiology

Half of all palliative care patients report serious distress from dry mouth, but providers may not recognize it as a priority. Common causes of dry mouth in terminally ill patients include medication side effects; mouth breathing; side effects of oxygen administration; infection; ulcers; and treatments such as surgery, chemotherapy, or radiotherapy.

Clinical Presentation and Physical Examination

Assessment begins with a thorough oral examination that includes inspection for mucosal and buccal dryness; pallor; a dry, fissured tongue or cracked lips; absence of salivary pooling; and oral ulcerations, gingivitis, or candidiasis.

Two quick bedside tests are the cracker biscuit test and the tongue blade test. The cracker biscuit test involves giving the patient a dry cracker or biscuit. If the patient cannot eat it, xerostomia is present. The tongue blade text is an extension of the mouth examination. After inspection is complete, the tongue blade is placed on the tongue. If it sticks, xerostomia is present.[30]

Management

Treatment of xerostomia includes:

1. Treatment of any underlying infection or disease, such as yeast or mucositis
2. Review, and if necessary, alteration of current medications, such as antihistamines or anticholinergics
3. Stimulation of salivary flow, using both nonpharmacologic (peppermint water, vitamin C, chewing gum, and mints) and pharmacologic interventions

Pharmacologic interventions can include pilocarpine 2.5 mg PO t.i.d., slowly titrated up to 10 mg PO t.i.d. Saliva production is greatest after a dose, and the response lasts for approximately 4 hours and varies with severity of xerostomia. Lost secretions are replaced with water and artificial saliva if necessary. An inexpensive spritzer filled with nine parts water and one part fine oil (e.g., grapeseed oil) can be helpful. The teeth should be protected with frequent oral hygiene, and the lips should be lubricated with lip balm. Topical rehydration with water or ice chips is a more subjectively effective remedy to dry mouth and thirst than is IV hydration.[17] Dietary modifications such as the avoidance of spicy or salty foods may help.

NAUSEA AND VOMITING

Definition

Vomiting is the expulsion of the contents of the stomach, duodenum, or jejunum through the mouth. Nausea is a feeling of queasiness or a desire to vomit. Nausea manifests itself in a wavelike sensation and can be accompanied by a cold sweat, fast heart rate, or diarrhea.

Pathophysiology

Nausea and vomiting are common at some time during the terminal stage of illness. Causes include delayed stomach emptying, constipation, bowel obstruction, infection, radiotherapy, medications, metabolic disturbances, and increased intracranial pressure.

Clinical Presentation and Physical Examination

Understanding the etiology of nausea and vomiting is critical to facilitate treatment, and therefore a good history is crucial. History of nausea should review onset, related factors, and pattern, along with presence of peptic ulcer disease, constipation, intracranial pressure, and nausea-inducing medications. Other important considerations include epigastric pain, pain on swallowing, thirst, hiccups, heartburn, and last bowel movement.

Physical assessment includes an oral examination, an abdominal examination (with particular emphasis on bowel sounds), a rectal examination, and a neurologic assessment. Studies may include an abdominal x-ray study and, if there is a concern about bowel obstruction, a gastroenterology consultation.

Management

Treatment of nausea and vomiting depends on the cause. First, the underlying cause is treated if possible. Different classes of antiemetics, alone or in combination, can be administered orally, subcutaneously, intravenously, or via a suppository for symptomatic relief.[31] Phenothiazines (prochlorperazine, chlorpromazine), butyrophenones (haloperidol), serotonin receptor antagonists (ondansetron, dolasetron), steroids, peristaltic agents (metoclopramide), benzodiazepines (lorazepam), or cannabinoids provide a vast array of choices, combinations, and expense.

Nonpharmacologic therapy includes relaxation, distraction, imagery, acupressure, cold therapy, aromatherapy, and music therapy. Diet modifications include eating dry crackers on awakening and eating fewer spicy and greasy foods. Holding or slowing down tube feedings may eliminate nausea induced by bloating. If nausea and vomiting are caused by an obstruction that cannot be relieved, placement of a venting gastrostomy rather than a nasogastric tube may decrease these symptoms, allow the patient the pleasure of eating, and increase the patient's overall quality of life.

CONSTIPATION

Definition

Constipation is infrequent rectal emptying (usually defined as less than every 3 days) or physical difficulty in emptying the rectum. This may vary according to patient's usual elimination pattern. Constipation is also characterized by hard or infrequent stools.[32]

Pathophysiology

Constipation is a common problem in terminal care resulting from narcotic therapy, immobility, and decreased fluid and food intake. However, constipation may also be age related, neurologically induced, or associated with colorectal tumors or lesions such as fissures or hemorrhoids.[17,32]

Clinical Presentation and Physical Examination

A bowel history is essential in assessing constipation and includes the patient's usual pattern, day of last bowel movement, use of laxatives or other interventions in an effort to move the bowels, and current drug regimen with special attention to the use of opioids. Physical assessment includes bowel sounds, inspection and palpation of the abdomen, and a rectal examination to check for stool.

Management

If possible and appropriate, the patient's fluid intake should be increased and a bowel regimen initiated (e.g., senna with stool softener, 1 to 4 tablets once or twice daily). An aggressive prophylactic bowel regimen needs to be prescribed concomitantly when opioids are initiated or increased. Lactulose 15 to 30 ml one to three times daily, milk of magnesia 15 to 30 ml b.i.d., and citrate of magnesia are alternative stimulants if senna and softener are not adequate. A senna-based tea such as Smooth Move tea each day is also beneficial. An enema or disimpaction may be necessary if there is no stool for several days.[17,32] Relief of constipation remains a major comfort measure even toward the very end of life because of its adverse effects on lower abdominal pain, nausea, and restlessness.

BOWEL OBSTRUCTION

Definition

Bowel obstruction is the total or partial occlusion of the bowel lumen and/or the alteration of normal peristaltic motion.[32,33] It is most likely to occur with advanced abdominal or pelvic cancers, such as ovarian, colorectal, and pancreatic cancer. Symptoms can be mild to severe and intermittent or continuous and include distention, intractable nausea and vomiting, and a colicky pain.

Clinical Presentation and Physical Examination

Assessment includes an abdominal examination. Bowel sounds may be normal to absent and hyperactive or hypoactive depending on the location, etiology, and degree of obstruction. Distention will be noted. An abdominal x-ray study and a CT scan will reveal the obstruction.

Management

Treatment depends in part on the patient's prognosis. Acute management is aimed at the immediate relief of symptoms and includes stopping oral intake and inserting a nasogastric tube to alleviate gastric distention. This is the treatment of choice for patients who have a longer prognosis and are able to withstand surgery. Occasionally, endoscopically placed stents can provide relief. Finally, a venting gastrostomy can provide decompression of gas and fluids.[32,33]

A conservative approach to providing comfort for very ill patients can be accomplished through the use of subcutaneously or intravenously administered agents. Analgesics reduce the pain of abdominal distention. Morphine starting at 1 mg/hr and titrating to the appropriate level to treat the pain is effective. Antiemetics such as prochlorperazine PO or per rectum (PR) or haloperidol 0.5 to 1.5 mg/24 hr can help. Prokinetic agents such as metoclopramide can help in partial obstructions by increasing peristalsis but should be avoided if complete obstruction is suspected. Antiinflammatories (e.g., corticosteroids) help reduce the inflammatory response and may partially alleviate the obstruction. Dexamethasone 8 to 20 mg/24 hr can reduce inflammatory edema and also help decrease nausea. Somatostatin analogues such as octreotide, 300 to 600 mcg/24 hr, are thought to inhibit the cascade effect of the glandular secretions and inhibit peristalsis and blood flow to the splanchnic area.

PAIN

Definition

Pain at the end of life is the most feared symptom. It most often occurs when the underlying diagnosis is cancer. However, discomfort at the end of life can stem from many other conditions, including arthritis, low back pain, pathologic or compression fractures, pressure sores, and cardiac or other ischemic pain. Patients who continue to follow normal routines and receive unnecessary procedures such as daily weights, laboratory tests, vital signs, and prescribed position changes may also experience unnecessary discomfort. Providing comfort to family members and asking their assessment of patient comfort when the patient cannot communicate is essential to good pain assessment. The following section briefly addresses pain issues specific to end-of-life. (Chapter 16 provides a comprehensive review of many similar principles of chronic pain management.)

Management

Unrelieved pain at the end of life is unnecessary and with few exceptions treatable. Practical issues can be the most challenging, including the loss of oral route for medication administration, a wish to die at home, non-opioid–responsive "total pain" or suffering, and a fear that the pain may indicate a hastening death.[20] With the skill and expertise of hospice or home care support, all of the previously mentioned strategies for expert pain relief are available at home or in long-term care settings. Alternatives to oral opioid administration include equianalgesic dosing, rectally (including enteric-coated tablets or suppositories), transdermally, sublingually (via high-concentrate solutions administered to the oral cavity), or subcutaneously (continuously, intermittently, or via a patient-controlled pump).[34] Given these options, there rarely is a need for IV catheters, which can be painful to insert and provide interrupted analgesia when infiltrated. There is no ceiling dose of opioids, and therefore carefully increased dosing in response to pain provides an acceptable ethical and clinical approach even if adequate analgesia comes only with sedation.[35,36]

There is great fear that administering escalating doses of opioids will hasten death. This fear is controversial and difficult to evaluate. Patients who are dying of a terminal illness should continue to receive opioids for pain relief or dyspnea until the time of death. It is important to remember that respirations will ultimately cease from the dying process itself, not the opioids. Respiratory depression from opioids is known to occur most often in the opioid-naive person. Careful upward titration in response to pain rarely causes respiratory depression, since pain is a natural stimulant to the respiratory center. Patients, families, and nursing staff should be educated about the appropriate use of pain medications for symptom control.[37]

SEDATION FOR MANAGEMENT OF INTRACTABLE SYMPTOMS IN PATIENTS NEAR DEATH

The term *terminal sedation* was first applied to the practice of using sedating medications to induce a state of unconsciousness and hence allow a patient to escape physical suffering at the end of life. This language has been changed to eliminate any misunderstanding that the purpose of the sedation is to end the patient's life. More recent terms are *palliative sedation* or *sedation at the end of life*.

Palliative sedation is an appropriate "treatment of last resort" in the rare instances in which death is imminent and symptoms such as pain, delirium, dyspnea, and anxiety have become totally refractory to treatment or management. The goal of sedation is to alleviate the suffering caused by the unrelieved symptom. An evaluation of the values and beliefs of the patient, family, and providers concerning the acceptability of this approach and the development of a consensus is critical to ensure the success of this strategy. All those involved in caring for the patient should participate in the discussion and have their questions answered regarding the proposed treatment modalities and their intended effects. A patient and family educational guide is available to help clinicians discuss this sensitive topic.[35,36]

REFERENCES

1. Cassel C, Foley K: *Principles for care of patients at the end of life: an emerging consensus among the specialties of medicine*, New York, 1999, Milbank Memorial Fund.
2. Ferrell BR, Virani R, Grant M: Analysis of end of life content in nursing textbooks, *Oncol Nurs Forum* 26(5):869-876, 1999.
3. Carron AT, Lynn J, Keaney P: End-of-life care in medical textbooks, *Ann Intern Med* 130:82-86, 1999.
4. SUPPORT Principal Investigators: A controlled trial to improve care for seriously ill hospitalized patients, *JAMA* 274(20):1591-1598, 1995.
5. Lynn J, Schuster JL: *Improving care for the end of life: a sourcebook for health care managers and clinicians,* New York, 2000, Oxford University Press.
6. Ferris F: *Establishing a palliative care program: rationale*, Dec 2005, Center for the Advancement of Palliative Care, retrieved from http://www.capc.org.
7. Field MJ, Cassel CK: *Approaching death: improving care at the end of life*, Washington, DC, 1997, National Academy Press.
8. World Health Organization: *Palliative care,* 2003, retrieved April 2003 from http://www.who.int/hiv/topics/palliative/care/en.
9. National Consensus Project: *Clinical practice guidelines for quality palliative care,* Brooklyn, NY, 2004, National Consensus Project for Quality Palliative Care, retrieved Dec 5, 2006, from http://www.nationalconsensusproject.org/Guidelines_Download.asp.
10. National Hospice and Palliative Care Organization: *Facts and figures on hospice care in America,* Alexandria, Va, 2003, National Hospice and Palliative Care Organization, retrieved Dec 5, 2006, from http://www.nhpco.org/templates/1/homepage.cfm.
11 Wennberg J, Fisher ES, Stukel TA, and others: Use of hospitals, physician visits, and hospice care during last 6 months of life among cohorts loyal to highly respected hospitals in the United States, *BMJ* 328:1-5, 2004.
12. Bakitas M, Daretany K: Hospital-based palliative care. In Ferrell BR, Coyle N, editors: *Textbook of palliative care*, Oxford, 2005, Oxford University Press.
13. Sabatino CP: *Survey of state EMS-DNR laws and protocols: Commission of Legal Problems of the Elderly*, Washington, DC, 1999, American Bar Association.
14. Walsh D, Doona M, Molnar M, and others: Symptom control in advanced cancer: important drugs and routes of administration, *Semin Oncol* 27(1):69-83, 2000.
15. Von Roenn J, Paice J: Control of common, non-pain cancer symptoms, *Semin Oncol* 32:200-210, 2005.
16. McCarthy DO: Rethinking nutritional support for persons with cancer cachexia, *Biol Res Nurs* 5(1):3-17, 2003.
17. Waller A, Caroline N: *Handbook of palliative care in cancer*, ed 2, Boston, 2002, Butterworth-Heinemann.
18. Mayo T: Foregoing artificial nutrition and hydration: legal and ethical considerations, *Nutr Clin Pract* 11(6):254-264, 1996.
19. Passik SD, Kirsh KL: *Diagnosis of psychiatric and psychologic disorders in patients with cancer*, Feb 2005, retrieved from http://www.uptodate.com.
20. Brietbart W, Rosenfeld B, Pessin H, and others: Depression, hopelessness, and desire for hastened death in terminally ill patients with cancer, *JAMA* 284(22):2907-2911, 2000.
21 Block S: Assessing and managing depression in the terminally ill patient, *Ann Intern Med* 132(3):209-218, 2000.
22. Lawlor P, Bruera E: Delirium in patients with advanced cancer, *Hematol Oncol Clin North Am* 16:701-714, 2002.
23. Brietbart W, Marotta R, Platt MM, and others: A double blind trial of haloperidol, chlorpromazine and lorazepam in the treatment of delirium in hospitalized AIDS patients, *Am J Psychiatry* 153:231-237, 1996.
24. Andersen G, Christrup L, Sjogren P: Relationships among morphine metabolism, pain, and side effects during long-term treatment: an update, *J Pain Symptom Manage* 25(1):74-91, 2003.
25. Rozans M, Dreisbach A, Lertora JJ, and others: Palliative uses of methylphenidate in patients with cancer: a review, *J Clin Oncol* 20:335-339, 2002.
26. Paulsen R, Katon W, Ciechanowski P: *Treatment of depression,* March 2005, retrieved from http://www.uptodate.com.
27. Jacobs L: Managing respiratory symptoms at the end of life, *Clin Geriatr Med* 19:225-239, 2003.
28. Dudgeon D: Dyspnea, death rattle, and cough. In Ferrell BR, Coyle N, editors: *Textbook of palliative nursing,* Oxford, 2006, Oxford University Press.
29. Schwartzstein R, Lahive K, Pope A: Cold facial stimulation reduces breathlessness induced in normal subjects, *Am Rev Respir Dis* 136:58-61, 1987.
30. Dahlin C, Goldsmith T: Dysphagia, xerostomia, and hiccups. In Ferrell BR, Coyle N, editors: *Textbook of palliative nursing*, Oxford, 2006, Oxford University Press.
31. King C: Nausea and vomiting. In Ferrell BR, Coyle N, editors: *Textbook of palliative nursing*, Oxford, 2006, Oxford University Press.
32. Economou D: Bowel management: constipation, diarrhea, obstruction, ascites. In Ferrell BR, Coyle N, editors: *Textbook of palliative nursing*, Oxford, 2006, Oxford University Press.
33. Ripamonti C, Fagnoni E, Magnj A: Management of symptoms due to inoperable bowel obstruction, *Tumori* 91:233-236, 2005.
34. Anderson S, Shreve S: Continuous subcutaneous infusion of opiates at end-of-life, *Ann Pharmacother* 38:1015-1023, 2004.
35. Brender E, Burke A, Glass RM: Palliative sedation, *JAMA* 294(14): 1850, 2005.
36. Lo B, Rubenfeld G: Palliative sedation in dying patients: "we turn to it when everything else hasn't worked," *JAMA* 294(14):1810-1816, 2005.
37. Morita T, Tsunoda J, Inoue S, and others: Effects of high dose opioids and sedatives on survival in terminally ill cancer patients, *J Pain Symptom Manage* 21(4):282-289, 2001.

CHAPTER 16

Chronic Pain

Constance Dahlin

DEFINITION AND EPIDEMIOLOGY

Although pain is a normal physiologic response that serves as a mechanism of protection against harmful stimulation, chronic pain contributes to morbidity and mortality.[1] It is a poorly understood condition and is therefore undertreated in primary care.[2] Chronic pain, defined as pain that lasts longer than 6 months or persists beyond the expected time of healing, usually encompasses a mechanism separate from that of the original insult.[3] Thus the focus of chronic pain control turns away from repairing damage that may be causing the pain and toward rehabilitation. Rehabilitation focuses on promoting optimum functioning, coping, and quality of life.

Chronic pain can include conditions such as headaches, low back pain, neck pain, musculoskeletal injury or soft tissue disease, degenerative joint pain, peripheral neuropathy, or neuralgia.[1,3] Chronic pain is not merely a symptom of disease; it also describes a syndrome that includes both physical and psychologic distress. Specifically, the patient may experience depression, along with alterations in daily activities, function, and personality.[1,3] The side effects of pain in the older adult can be deleterious, since unrelieved pain inhibits respiration, decreases mobility, and impairs functional status, with consequent pneumonia, constipation, and deep venous thrombosis.[4]

Chronic pain is a complex, highly subjective health problem that affects more than 50 million people in the United States.[1,3] Unlike acute pain, chronic pain serves no protective function. The causes are often multifactorial, and patients' responses are equally varied and individualistic. These patients generally seek a health care provider at initial presentation for headaches, abdominal pain, musculoskeletal discomfort, or neurologic pain. Such pains often are the result of work-related stresses or injuries. Low back pain usually is the result of work or automobile accidents and trauma.[1] However, pain can also be secondary to other organic disorders, including diabetes, end-stage renal disease, alcoholism, or postherpetic syndromes.[1,5]

PATHOPHYSIOLOGY

According to Bonica, "Chronic pain is caused by a chronic pathologic process in somatic structures or viscera, or by prolonged and sometimes permanent dysfunction of the peripheral and central nervous system or both." Moreover, states Bonica, "The physiologic, affective, and behavioral responses to chronic pain are quite different from those in acute pain."[3]

Pain is a subjective impression that is unique to each patient. Pain is categorized pathophysiologically as either organic or idiopathic (previously referred to as *psychogenic pain*). Organic pain is further delineated as nociceptive or neuropathic.

Nociceptive pain is caused by either direct or threatened injury to tissue and results from the activation of nociceptors, which are peripheral afferent nerve endings that are both sensitive to and transmitters of painful stimuli. Bradykinins, prostaglandins, and other chemical mediators of inflammation found in injured tissue contribute to the pathogenesis of nociceptive pain.[1] Nociceptive pain can manifest as either somatic or visceral pain.

Somatic pain is caused by the activation of nociceptors in the peripheral tissues. Somatic pain is usually described as well localized and is characterized as stabbing, aching, or throbbing. In contrast, visceral pain is usually poorly localized; often is not attributable to the involved organ (i.e., referred pain); and may be described as dull, crampy, or deep. Visceral nociceptive pain can be referred in a dermatomal distribution.

Organic neuropathic pain occurs because of injury to or disease of the nervous system. Neuropathic pain is most often described as burning, shooting, or tingling, and it can follow a dermatomal distribution. Although neuropathic pain may occur spontaneously, evoked pain is the hallmark of neuropathic pain and can be experienced as dysesthesia (altered or abnormal sensations), paresthesia (sensation of electrical shock), hyperalgesia (increased sensitivity to painful stimulation), or allodynia (pain resulting from ordinarily nonpainful causes, such as cool air or light touch).[1]

Idiopathic pain may not demonstrate any clinical evidence of an associated organic cause but might include additional psychologic elements at the time of clinical presentation. Because the experience of pain is subjective, the reality of patients' idiopathic pain is comparable to that of organic pain, and it must be treated.

CLINICAL PRESENTATION

The clinical picture of chronic pain is nonspecific and may be noted only in terms of a retrospective review of patient care. Both physical and psychologic perspectives must be considered in a patient with chronic pain. Certain patterns may emerge. First, chronic pain continues for a prolonged period and beyond a "reasonable" healing time for a specific injury.

Second, as the autonomic nervous system adapts to the chronicity of the pain, there can be disparity between objective and functional findings because of the lack of signs of heightened sympathetic activity. Therefore the objective physical examination and diagnostic testing may not reveal or provoke a pain response consistent with the patient's subjective description of the pain. However, the patient is adamant that pain exists.

Third, a patient complaining of pain may also have depression or other psychiatric conditions. The pain as described by the patient may have emotional labels resulting in sadness, anxiety, and irritability.[6] A diagnosis of chronic pain syndrome may be considered in patients whose continued chronic pain is compounded by psychologic and behavioral changes that lead to functional impairment and emotional distress.[1] Patients with chronic pain may manifest their distress through relationship difficulties, decreased coping abilities, or an inability to work.

Fourth, a pattern of excessive use of the health care system may become apparent as the patient continues to seek various treatment options or additional consultations because of existing pain.[1]

Fifth, the patient may have a history of prolonged or excessive use of opiates, benzodiazepines, or alcohol.[1] Initially the patient may take these substances to promote relaxation and rest, but their excessive use may have become counterproductive to healing. At the same time, the patient may have developed a tolerance to these medications, possibly leading to substance abuse.

PHYSICAL EXAMINATION

Pain is often managed inadequately because of poor clinical assessment. Therefore it is critical that pain assessment be integrated into the patient's detailed history and physical assessment, with reassessment at each visit. A review of previous diagnostic studies and medical interventions, as well as an assessment of co-existing conditions, is also necessary.[1,6]

Pain assessment can be aided by the mnemonic device *PQRST*: *P*rovocative-palliative factors, *Q*uality, *R*egion, *S*everity, *T*emporal (i.e., time of day or season in which the pain is more constant or the duration longer). The use of simple pain intensity scales (e.g., 1 = no pain, 5 = moderate pain, 10 = worst possible pain) describes and documents the patient's chronicity and severity of pain; individual pain diaries can also be valuable.[6] A psychiatric assessment, including a history of alcohol or other substance use or abuse for pain management, should be performed.[1] Signs and symptoms of depression such as fatigue, insomnia, decreased appetite, and decreased activities should be elicited, and the patient's activities of daily living and usual patterns of coping under duress should be reviewed. Finally, it is important to determine how the easing or absence of pain would improve the patient's quality of life.[1]

In addition, it is beneficial to focus not only on the patient's functional disability but also on possible psychologic distress. What is the meaning of the pain to the patient? What are the past experiences of pain? What are the meaning and expression of pain within the patient's culture?

DIAGNOSTICS

No specific diagnostics are indicated, but ECGs; x-ray studies; and laboratory tests such as CBC, SMA 20 (sequential multiple analysis of 20 chemical constituents), and a urinalysis should be ordered when appropriate.[1] An electromyogram may also be necessary to localize neurologic pain.

DIFFERENTIAL DIAGNOSES

Multiple disorders are associated with chronic pain syndromes. Causes of chronic pain syndromes include trauma to the cervical and lumbar spine; cervical and lumbar disc disease; vascular headaches; arthritis; connective tissue disorders; fibromyalgia; complications from surgical diseases; and neuropathies caused by various viruses, toxins, and diseases.[1]

MANAGEMENT

Many issues may affect the experience of chronic pain, including personal implications of injury, developmental history and past experience of coping, ethnocultural influences, premorbid psychologic health, secondary gain from injury, and environmental factors.[1] Therefore each patient reacts uniquely to pain. It is essential to believe the patient's report of pain.[7] In addition, it is critical to set realistic goals concerning pain control. Except in rare circumstances, a patient with a chronic pain syndrome will not be pain free. Thus the most realistic goal is to make the person as comfortable as possible and to encourage the maintenance of optimum mobility and daily functioning.[2] To accomplish this goal, the health care provider must enter into a partnership with the patient to work together to decrease, rather than eliminate, the pain and optimize the quality of life.

An individual treatment plan that focuses on both the psychologic and physical components is necessary. Evaluating strategies that have been beneficial in the past may be helpful in developing a manageable care plan for chronic pain. The goal of chronic pain management is not analgesia but rather preserving and maximizing function and enhancing coping skills. In particular, the patient is offered alternative approaches to dealing with the pain, which increases self-promoting behaviors to decrease the pain's negative impact on the quality of life.

Pharmacologic Interventions

Pharmacologic interventions follow the guidelines of the three-step analgesic ladder for pain control developed by the World Health Organization (WHO) and endorsed by the American Pain Society.[8] However, cost may also be a consideration, since insurance coverage for some medications is changing with new Medicare regulations from the Medicare Modernizations Act of 2003. Step 1 begins with the use of nonopioids and adjuvants, including NSAIDs, tricyclic antidepressants (TCAs), selective serotonin reuptake inhibitors (SSRIs), anticonvulsants, or antiarrhythmics.

Although NSAIDs have not been proven to be efficacious in chronic pain, their effectiveness in acute pain is well documented. Thus it is worthwhile to use ibuprofen or naproxen in cases of chronic pain. The new cylcooxygenase-2 (COX-2) class of NSAIDs may relieve pain, with fewer side effects. However, the cardiac side effect profile should be individually evaluated against the patient's cardiac history. Rofecoxib (Vioxx) was taken off the market, but celecoxib (Celebrex) currently remains available.[1]

TCAs are the initial drugs of choice because they can simultaneously treat the depressive aspects of chronic pain and the physiologic nerve pain. Pharmacologic agents include amitriptyline, nortriptyline, imipramine, or desipramine, effective at a starting dose of 25 mg PO at bedtime. This may also enhance sleep, since TCAs are sedating. Further consideration must be given to older adults, whose starting dose would be lower. Failure of one medication in this class does not necessarily indicate complete failure of TCAs, so it may be worthwhile to at least try two agents in this class. Common side effects include dry mouth, constipation, and a feeling of being "hung over." Monitoring blood levels when possible can prevent or lessen these side effects.[8]

Second-line medications are anticonvulsants, including phenytoin, carbamazepine, and valproic acid. The anticonvulsants are especially helpful in cases of neuralgia and paresthesia. Initial dosing should be low, such as 50 mg at bedtime for an older adult or 100 mg for a younger patient. Again bedtime doses are important due to the sedating side effect. Blood levels must be monitored and are kept in the same range as for treating seizures.[8]

The SSRIs, which include fluoxetine, sertraline, and paroxetine, are particularly appropriate for patients who are unresponsive to or have suffered side effects from TCAs. Side effects of the SSRIs can include rash, urticaria, dizziness, and drowsiness.

Step 2 of the WHO three-step analgesic ladder includes mild opiates such as oxycodone and acetaminophen (Percocet), codeine, and acetaminophen and codeine phosphate (Tylenol No. 3), along with adjuvant medications. Side effects include drowsiness and constipation. Tramadol (Ultram) may initiate addiction. This is a concern because tramadol is a synthetic opioid. Patients may not be aware of the potential for the reinitiation of abuse. The newer drug Ultracet (tramadol with acetaminophen) has a similar potential.

Step 3 medication interventions involve opiates.[8,9] Opiates should be considered only after all other reasonable attempts at analgesia have failed. They have traditionally been underused because of concerns regarding addiction, tolerance, and side effects such as diversion.[1] Step 3 medications include morphine, fentanyl patches, oxycodone, and hydromorphone. Meperidine (Demerol) should not be used for chronic pain because the long-acting metabolites can cause central nervous system toxicity, and repetitive injections can cause skin problems. Adjuvant medications such as NSAIDs, tricyclics, SSRIs, anticonvulsants, or antiarrhythmics may be used in combination with opiates.[8,9]

Nonpharmacologic Interventions

Patients often use both traditional medicine and alternative therapy. This tandem effect can be effective, particularly if the traditional and alternative practitioners collaborate. For patients not exposed to alternative therapy, it is important to provide information regarding how such therapies can enhance pain management. Nonpharmacologic interventions include[1,10]:

Cognitive behavior interventions: Relaxation, biofeedback, distraction, hypnosis, and support groups. Pain often drains a person's focus and energy. Cognitive behavior interventions can temporarily raise the pain threshold, thereby allowing the patient's attention to be directed toward something other than the pain.

Exercise: Physical therapy, occupational therapy, and exercise programs, including hydrotherapy. Exercise can improve general conditioning, thereby improving stamina and endurance. In addition, exercise can promote the production of endorphins, which are the body's natural pain relievers. Stress reduction is a secondary benefit of an exercise program and can assist in overall coping behaviors.

Alternative therapies: Chiropractic treatment, acupuncture, massage therapy, herbal therapies, and homeopathy.

Transcutaneous electrical nerve stimulation: A process in which a low-voltage electrical pulse is directed through the skin. It is believed to stimulate nerve fibers and interfere with the conduction of painful stimuli.

Nerve blocks: Anesthetic given within a nerve to stop painful conduction.

Heat or cold therapy: Act as counterirritants or reduce muscle spasm.

Co-Management with Specialists

Because chronic pain encompasses both physical and psychologic components, pain control is more effective and successful when using a multidisciplinary team approach.[1,3] However, it is crucial for one provider to take responsibility for all prescriptions, which allows for a systematic approach to pain medications, permits an adequate trial of medications before change, and prevents polypharmacy.

LIFE SPAN CONSIDERATIONS

Chronic pain is rare in a child unless he or she has undergone a surgical procedure that initiates a response. Usually, a chronic pain syndrome begins in young adulthood, precipitated by an accident, incident, or soft tissue injury. It then progresses in middle-aged and older adults where age-related factors may exacerbate the problem. When onset begins in older adults, it is usually caused by degenerative joint pain.

COMPLICATIONS

Complications can arise with medication misuse or abuse. It is important to monitor a patient's use of NSAIDs for toxic effects and the use of opiates because of their potential for abuse. As stated previously, it is important to treat not only the pain, but also the psychologic issues that accompany the pain.

INDICATIONS FOR REFERRAL OR HOSPITALIZATION

Chronic pain is difficult to manage within one discipline. It may be helpful to initiate consultations with social work, psychology, and psychiatry to assist in identification of ineffective coping mechanisms, introduction of more effective mechanisms, and treatment of other mental health issues such as depression. If there is a history of substance abuse, a referral to or consultation with a substance abuse counselor may be helpful.[1] If pain is localized to a specific area, a specialist consultation may be indicated. For example, chronic abdominal pain may require a gastroenterology consultation. Referral to an outpatient pain clinic or pain specialist may also be considered.[1] Some patients may require pain management within a specialist program setting, which is appropriate if other pain management interventions have failed. Both inpatient and outpatient pain clinic and rehabilitation programs may be used. Consideration of insurance coverage of these programs and the availability of a program within a reasonable geographic proximity are important.

PATIENT AND FAMILY EDUCATION

Education is the critical core of pain management. Included in patient education are the explanation of the physiology of the affected body system, the pain cycle, and the purpose and side effects of the medications.[1] Education engenders self-assertion and empowers the patient in decisions regarding chronic conditions, possibly ameliorating the lethargy or depression that may be part of the chronic pain syndrome. Education also may provide realistic hope about the pain—that the pain may not be totally eliminated but rather that the quality of life can be improved.

HEALTH PROMOTION

Health promotion activities include good education surrounding activities of daily living. This includes continued participation, distraction, positive behaviors to avoid dependency on medications, and the use of various methods in coping with pain.

REFERENCES

1. Hainline B: Chronic pain: physiological, diagnostic, and management considerations, *Psychiatr Clin North Am* 28(3):713-735, 2005.
2. Chelminski PR, Ives TJ, Felix KM, and others: A primary care, multidisciplinary disease management program for opioid-treated patients with chronic non-cancer pain and a high burden of psychiatric comorbidity, *BioMed Central*, retrieved Dec 5, 2006, from http://www.biomedcentral.com/1472-6963/5/3.
3. Bonica J: General considerations of chronic pain. In Bonica J, editor: *Management of chronic pain*, Philadelphia, 2001, Lea & Febiger.
4. Barkin RL, Barkin SJ, Barkin DS: Perception, assessment, and treatment of pain in the elderly, *Clin Geriatr Med* 21(3):465-490, 2005.
5. Davison S: Chronic pain in end-stage renal disease, *Adv Chronic Kidney Dis* 12(3):326-334, 2005.
6. Hitchcock LS, Ferrell BR, McCaffrey M: The experience of chronic nonmalignant pain, *J Pain Symptom Manage* 9(5):312-318, 1994.
7. Fishman S: The mysteries of chronic pain. In Fishman S, Berger L, editors: *The war on pain*, New York, 2002, Harper Collins.
8. American Pain Society: *Principles of analgesic use in the treatment of acute pain and cancer pain*, ed 4, Skokie, Ill, 2004, The Society.
9. Gardner-Nix J: Principles of opioid use in chronic noncancer pain, *CMAJ* 169(1):38-43, 2003.
10. Loder E, Herbert P, McAlary P: Chronic pain rehabilitation. In Ballantyne J, Fishman S, Abdi S, editors: *The Massachusetts General Hospital handbook of pain management*, ed 2, Philadelphia, 2002, Lippincott Williams & Wilkins.

CHAPTER 17

Obesity

Jeanne H. Siegel

Obesity has reached epidemic proportions in the United States and around the globe. The Centers for Disease Control and Prevention (CDC) estimate that 65% of Americans are overweight, of which 23% are considered obese.[1] This predisposes more than 97 million Americans to obesity-related chronic diseases and conditions. In the United States alone approximately 112,000 deaths a year are associated with obesity.[2,3]

Worldwide incidence of obesity is also increasing, as reflected in the term *globesity*. The World Health Organization (WHO) published a report titled "Obesity: Preventing and Managing the Global Epidemic," which classified obesity as a growing epidemic.[4] The International Obesity Taskforce, a collaborative program of the International Association for the Study of Obesity and the WHO, estimated that worldwide 1.7 billion individuals are overweight.[5]

DEFINITION AND EPIDEMIOLOGY

Obesity is a chronic condition in which the body's natural energy stores, stored in the fatty tissues, increase to a point where significant risk for health consequences exists. Body mass index (BMI) is the most widely used calculation of body fat in human beings. An individual's BMI is calculated by dividing his or her weight in kilograms by the height in meters squared. Different formulas are used for metric versus American standard measurement systems (Box 17-1). Other methods of determining body fat include skin fold measurement, waist/hip ratio, underwater weighing, bioelectrical impedance analysis, and ultrasound measurement of abdominal fat.[6] Alternative methods are rarely used due to concerns with reliability, availability, and cost.

The CDC and WHO both use BMI for classifying body fat but differ slightly in their definitions. The WHO published guidelines in 1997 classifying individuals with BMIs greater than 25 as overweight. Individuals with BMIs greater than 30 were classified as obese (obese class I) or moderately obese, and those with BMIs greater than 35 are severely obese (class II). Individuals considered morbidly obese, with BMIs of 40 or greater (class III), are considered at a higher risk of morbidity and mortality because of their excess weight.[4]

BOX 17-1

CALCULATING BMI

METRIC

Weight in kilograms/(Height in meters)^2

AMERICAN STANDARD

Weight in pounds/(Height in inches)^2 × 703

The CDC uses BMI to indicate levels of body fat that have been shown to increase the chance of certain diseases and other health problems. BMIs less than 18.5 are considered underweight, and 18.5 to 24.9 are normal weight. Individuals with BMIs of 25 or greater are considered overweight, with those higher than 30 considered obese.[2]

There are some concerns with using BMI as the standard for determining body fat. The BMI was designed to be used for individuals with sedentary lifestyles. BMI cannot distinguish between body fat, muscle mass, and bone mass. Interpretation of BMI becomes challenging in athletes, children, and older adults. Because muscle weighs more than fat, it is not unusual for professional athletes to have BMIs high enough to classify them as obese. In children, it is best to use the BMI-for-age calculation to improve interpretation.[2]

PATHOPHYSIOLOGY

The actual cause of obesity appears quite simple: increasing energy consumption, decreasing energy expenditure, or a combination of both results in a positive energy balance.[7] A positive energy balance leads to a gain in weight over time. As little as an extra 100 kcal/day can result in the gain of 4.5 kg (10 pounds) per year.

The difficulty in explaining the etiology of obesity begins with the plethora of factors that can affect the way we consume food and burn energy. Most providers agree that the cause of obesity is multifactorial. This interaction of multiple factors contributes to the difficulty in developing successful interventions. The factors that contribute to the development of obesity are resting metabolic rate (RMR); excessive caloric intake; insufficient exercise or sedentary lifestyle; genetics; parental influences; and, to a lesser degree, medical conditions, including metabolic and eating disorders. Several environmental factors have emerged in the research on obesity that may shed light on the dramatic rise of obesity in the past 30 years. The increase in stress and decrease in sleeping time (also called short sleep duration) cause some physiologic changes that may lead to increased weight.

Resting Metabolic Rate

An individual's weight status can be affected by the RMR, which is the minimum number of calories the body needs to support its basic physiologic functions, including breathing, circulating blood, and all of the numerous biochemical reactions required to keep an individual alive. An individual's RMR is generally 60% to 75% of the total daily caloric expenditure. The RMR also affects energy expended and varies widely, influenced by lean muscle mass, age, gender, activity, and heredity (genetic characteristics).

Excessive Calorie Intake

Lifestyle changes related to how and what we eat have contributed to an increase in calorie and fat consumption. Consumer food choices are more motivated by taste, cost, and convenience than by health and variety.[8] Dietary changes over the past 3 decades, including increased availability of fast foods, pressures on families to decrease food costs, decreased preparation time, and changes in the composition of our diets, may also contribute to the obesity problem.[9] Families are consuming fewer fruits and vegetables because of cost and availability.

Portion size is a likely contributor to the obesity epidemic.[10] This environmental factor, consisting of large portions of energy-dense foods that are excessive for an individual's caloric needs, leads to weight gain. Individuals over the age of 5 years demonstrate a tendency to eat in portions, and larger portions mean increased calories. There is evidence that portion size and the obesity epidemic have increased in parallel, supporting the need for further investigation.[10]

Insufficient Physical Activity

As individuals consume more calories, they are not compensating by increasing their activity levels. Despite the apparent benefits, less than half of American adults engage in moderate activity 30 minutes a day as recommended by the surgeon general; nearly 26% percent report no physical activity at all.[11] A variety of factors affect the exercise habits of individuals. These include the increased use of automobiles, unsafe neighborhoods, decreased school physical education and after-school programs, increased demands on free time, and cost of programs and equipment.

Genetics

Several studies support the theory that an interaction of multiple genes may contribute to the development of obesity. As many as 340 genes have been reported to have an influence on weight control. Most of these genes appear to increase the likelihood of weight gain, but a number are protective against excessive gain. A well-known study of twins in 1976 in Scandinavia estimated that obesity could be 88% inherited.[12]

The presence of a genetic tendency in combination with exposure to a variety of risk factors may explain why some individuals gain weight more easily than others. The prevalence of obesity has doubled in adults and tripled in children over the past 20 years.[2] Genetics may be one factor contributing to this excess weight gain, but it is not an explanation for the recent epidemic of obesity.[9] The genetic characteristics of populations have not changed over the past 2 decades, which suggests that behavioral and environmental factors, rather than genetic factors, are to blame.[7]

Parental Influence

Researchers have observed a relationship between parental obesity and obesity in their children. This relationship is hard to define because the relationship could be genetic, environmental, or a pattern of learned behavior. In a study of the incidence of parental obesity in overweight individuals, Noble[13] found a relationship that appeared to be stronger when the mother was the obese parent. There was a far greater prevalence of obese mothers than fathers. Noble also found a higher incidence of obese grandmothers than grandfathers when the weight status of the grandparents was explored.[13] Having obese parents more than doubles a child's risk of being overweight. Mother-only obesity occurred almost three times more often than father-only obesity. This study suggests that mothers are more likely to be the determining influence in a child's eating habits. It is not surprising that family environment is a factor in obesity.[13]

Environmental Factors

Inadequate sleep and insomnia have become frequent complaints from primary care patients. Several studies have reported an association between short sleep duration and increased body fat. Over the past 4 decades sleep duration in the United States has declined by 1 to 2 hours a night, and the proportion of young adults reporting less than 7 hours of sleep a night has more than doubled.[14] In a recent study, short sleep duration was found to be associated with decreased leptin levels, increased ghrelin levels, and increased hunger and appetite.[15] Leptin, a hormone, and ghrelin, a prehormone, contribute to the central regulation of food intake.[15] Leptin, which is produced primarily in the white adipose tissues, is active in energy expenditure and appetite regulation (decreasing hunger and food consumption). Ghrelin, which is produced primarily in the stomach, stimulates appetite and promotes food intake.[6] Ghrelin also stimulates growth hormone secretion. If leptin levels are decreased, increased food consumption and decreased activity are likely to occur. If this is combined with increased ghrelin, which stimulates appetite, overeating and sedentary activity may result.

Stress

Stress and its associated physical symptoms have become common problems in today's fast-paced societies. Obesity secondary to the physiologic changes created by stress reactions is the subject of study. *Stress reactions* are defined as circumstances followed by activation of the hypothalamic-pituitary-adrenal axis and the sympathetic nervous system.[16] When individuals are exposed to prolonged stress, the hypothalamus is activated, leading to a hormonal cascade that results in the release of cortisol from the adrenal cortex.[17] Clinical experience has repeatedly demonstrated that patients treated with corticosteroids have insatiable appetites that frequently lead to excessive weight gain.[16] These clinical observations suggest that cortisol and other glucocorticords may be involved in increased caloric intake, desire for high-caloric fatty and sugar-laden foods, relocation of fat deposits to the abdominal area, and the eventual development of obesity.[17]

CLINICAL PRESENTATION

Patients who are obese generally have no outward distinguishing characteristic other than excessive weight.[18] Obese individuals generally come to a primary care setting with a large number of complaints. The complaints are often associated with the effects of obesity on the body. They may complain of weight gain, garments that are too tight, and inability to diet or lose weight.[18] Common complaints expressed by overweight and obese individuals also include exercise intolerance, dyspnea on exertion, skin ailments, and joint pain.

The existence of co-morbid conditions is significant and suggests further testing. A complete list of medications, including over-the-counter and herbal preparations, may provide useful information. Determining what interventions have already been attempted will assist the provider in determining an effective plan of action and discovering a pattern of chronic dieting associated with weight loss and regain.

It is important to rule out weight gain from fluid retention, as seen in patients with kidney disease or heart failure. Severe hypothyroidism can lead to a decreased metabolic need and to weight gain.[18] Some commonly prescribed drugs can lead to weight gain by causing fluid retention or stimulating appetite.

PHYSICAL EXAMINATION AND DIAGNOSTICS

The goal of treatment in the overweight patient is to reduce the patient's weight and control any existing co-morbid conditions caused or affected by the excess weight. A complete patient history, including a family history, is a necessary starting point for the treatment of obesity. The age onset of any weight gain in family members is helpful. To evaluate for co-morbid conditions, a complete physical assessment is needed, including accurate measurement of height, weight, and abdominal circumference. Self-reports of height and weight are frequently inaccurate in overweight patients.

The effect of obesity on imaging examinations is important to practitioners ordering diagnostic tests. In the past 15 years there has been a small but significant increase in the number of poor-quality radiology reports labeled "limited by body habitus."[19] These poor-quality radiology readings occurred despite advances in imaging technology and affect the diagnostic ability of the examinations. The diagnostic tests most affected by obesity were abdominal ultrasound, followed by chest radiography, abdominal radiography, abdominal CT, chest CT, and MRI (for all anatomic regions). Diagnostic equipment may also be affected by the girth or the weight of the patient. Standard CT tables can manage patients weighing up to 204 kg (450 pounds), whereas MRI machines typically handle patients weighing 158.8 kg (350 pounds). Many of the newer machines are being designed to accommodate individuals as heavy as 249.5 kg (550 pounds).

DIFFERENTIAL DIAGNOSIS

Physiologic factors, excessive caloric intake, drugs, edema syndromes, and metabolic causes are significant considerations in the differential diagnosis of weight gain[18] (Box 17-2). Physiologic factors that can explain weight gain include pregnancy and premenstrual fluid retention. Excessive caloric intake leading to increased adipose tissue storage, the most common cause of weight gain, is often subtle and unnoticed by the patient until a significant amount of weight has been gained. The root cause of overeating may be an emotional factor such as anxiety, guilt, or depression.[20] Drugs that are often associated with weight gain include steroids, NSAIDs, lithium, antipsychotics, antidepressants, propranolol, and oral contraceptives.

MANAGEMENT

Lifestyle modifications are a good starting point in the management of obesity and should include improving diet, decreasing sedentary activity, reducing stress, and improving sleeping habits. Patients will achieve greater success if these lifestyle modifications are structured. Structured lifestyle modifications include detailed instructions for the patient,

BOX 17-2

IDENTIFICATION OF PATIENTS AT HIGH AND VERY HIGH ABSOLUTE RISK FOR CHD

CONDITIONS DENOTING HIGH ABSOLUTE RISK*

- Cigarette smoking
- Hypertension
- High-risk LDL cholesterol
- Low HDL cholesterol
- Impaired fasting glucose
- Family history of premature CHD
- Male ≥45 years, female ≥55 years (or postmenopausal)

CONDITIONS DENOTING VERY HIGH ABSOLUTE RISK

- Established CAD
- History of myocardial infarction
- History of angina pectoris (stable or unstable)
- History of coronary artery surgery
- History of coronary artery procedures (angioplasty)
- Presence of other atherosclerotic diseases
- Peripheral arterial disease
- Abdominal aortic aneurysm
- Symptomatic CAD
- Type 2 diabetes
- Sleep apnea

From National Institutes of Health and National Heart, Lung, and Blood Institute: *Clinical guidelines on the identification, evaluation, and treatment of overweight and obesity in adults: the evidence report*, Washington, DC, 1998, The Institute.

CAD, Coronary artery disease; *CHD*, coronary heart disease; *HDL*, high-density lipoprotein; *LDL*, low-density lipoprotein.

*Patients must have 3 or more of these risk factors to meet the criteria for high absolute risk.

including time frames and goals. Practitioners who provide the overweight patient with written information on the benefits of recommended modifications and the tools necessary to achieve them will increase the probability of success. Writing a prescription for the lifestyle modification reinforces the desired activity.

The management of diet includes reducing calories, limiting fats and carbohydrates, eating foods only from certain food groups, and following a number of commercial diet programs. One randomized trial comparing the Atkins, Ornish, Weight Watchers, and Zone diets found that each popular diet resulted in modest reductions in body weight and several cardiac risk factors.[21]

The CDC and the American College of Sports Medicine recommend that all adults achieve moderate-intensity physical activity for at least 30 minutes on most, preferably all, days of the week to improve their cardiovascular fitness.[2] Diet modifications should include a plan for changing a patient's eating habits for the long term. Diets are generally unsuccessful because of a tendency to return to previous eating habits, leading to "yo-yo dieting," or the regaining of lost weight as soon as old habits resume.

Providers need to implement multicomponent, individually tailored care plans that combine counseling with behavior modification, including written prescriptions, goal setting, follow-up communications, and specific lifestyle modifications that address weight loss.[22] Lifestyle modifications do not need to be drastic to be successful. Reducing daily caloric intake by 100 to 200 kcal and walking 2000 additional steps a day (approximately 1.6 km [1 mile]) can have a healthy effect over time without complaints of hunger and sore muscles. Many programs now recommend a pedometer to reinforce their walking programs and give participants a tangible measurement of success.

Recent studies have demonstrated that overweight adults are not consistently counseled on the importance of maintaining a healthy weight. Only 42% of obese adults had been counseled by a health care provider to lose weight during the previous year.[23] Other studies suggest that the rates may be significantly lower.[24,25] Diet counseling rates were found to be 45% or less and physical activity counseling 30% or less in adult patients with hyperlipidemia, hypertension, obesity, or diabetes in an analysis of the National Ambulatory Medical Care Survey and the National Hospital Ambulatory Medical Care Survey.[26]

Drugs and surgery cannot replace decreased calorie intake, exercise, and lifestyle modifications in the treat of obesity. However, in patients who are unsuccessful with structured lifestyle modifications, the use of medications and surgical interventions may be indicated. Research is currently underway to develop pharmacologic interventions to combat obesity. The only medications that are approved for long-term treatment of diet- and exercise-resistant obesity include orlistat (Xenical) and sibutramine (Meridia).[27] Orlistat is an inhibitor of pancreatic lipase, which reduces intestinal fat absorption. Sibutramine is an anorectic, or appetite suppressant. Noradrenergic medications, including diethylpropion (Tenuate), mazindol (Sanorex), phendimetrazine (Plegine), and phentermine (Fastin), are also used as short-term appetite suppressants that act through a centrally mediated pathway in the hypothalamus and result in anorexia.[27]

Rimonabant (Acomplia), a cannabinoid-1 (CB_1) receptor blocker, is currently in the Food and Drug Administration (FDA) drug approval process. The central CB_1 receptors are believed to play a role in controlling food consumption. Selective CB_1 receptor blockade with rimonabant significantly reduces body weight and abdominal obesity, improving the profile of several metabolic risk factors in high-risk patients who are overweight or obese. When used with lifestyle and behavior modification, it has demonstrated effectiveness in treating multiple cardiometabolic risk factors, including abdominal obesity and smoking.[28]

Numerous over-the-counter dietary supplements for weight loss are available. Caution should be used in recommending these substances because, of the 50 different dietary supplements and the more than 125 commercially available combinations of these substances, no current weight loss supplements meet the criteria for recommended use.[29] Evidence of moderate weight loss secondary to ephedra-caffeine products exists, but the FDA has banned the sale secondary to potentially serious adverse effects.[29]

Weight loss intervention can be frustrating for both patient and provider. Despite the difficulty encountered in weight loss efforts, even small or modest weight loss can result in significant improvements in health. One study found that intentional weight loss can improve or prevent some of the obesity-related risk factors for coronary heart disease (CHD), including insulin resistance, type 2 diabetes, dyslipidemia, hypertension, and inflammation.[30]

LIFE SPAN CONSIDERATIONS

Obesity is at epidemic proportions across the life span. As previously discussed, rates of obesity in adolescents have tripled in the past 20 years. Unfortunately, recent studies have shown that the majority of obese children will remain obese into adulthood. This increase in childhood obesity will lead to earlier onset of the co-morbid conditions associated with obesity and increased prevalence of obesity in adulthood.

COMPLICATIONS

The consequences of obesity include an increased risk of type 2 diabetes, heart disease, dyslipidemia, metabolic syndrome, sleep apnea, gallbladder disease, and certain cancers. Obese individuals are prone to develop a variety of orthopedic conditions, including arthritis. The burden of the weight on organs and joints, impairment of the immune system, and excess release of endogenous hormones and proinflammatory cytokines all appear to contribute to the development of these conditions (Table 17-1).

Co-morbid conditions are common among obese individuals. In a sample derived from the original Framingham Study cohort, researchers found that 62% of obese women and 56% of obese men had two or more coronary risk factors.[31] In addition, this study found that only 9% of obese women and 12.8% of obese men had no coronary risk factors. In the Framingham Study, excess weight accounted for 40% to 70% of the hypertension observed.[32]

One constellation of co-morbid conditions, termed *metabolic syndrome,* includes central obesity (excess waist circumference), elevated triglycerides, reduced high-density lipoprotein, elevated blood pressure, and impaired fasting glucose. The definition of metabolic syndrome remains controversial, but the effects of individual and combined co-morbid conditions are not. The evidence is mounting that the presence of any of the components of metabolic syndrome can increase an individual's chance of heart disease. One study determined that three or more of the components of metabolic syndrome increase the risk of CHD 2.39 times in men and 5.9 times in women.[33]

Obesity is associated with a significant decrease in life expectancy and an increase in early mortality, according to a prospective study follow-up of the Framingham Study.[34] In a study of individuals with severe obesity, it was estimated that excess weight contributed to a decreased life expectancy of 5 to 20 years.[35] Additionally, obesity has been associated with increasing death rates from a variety of causes, including cardiovascular disease, diabetes, and accidents.[36]

According to the National Cancer Institute, obesity increases the risk of breast cancer in postmenopausal women and of the uterus (endometrium), colon, kidney, and esophagus.[37] Additionally, excess weight can make it difficult to

TABLE 17-1 Differential Diagnoses to Consider in Obese Patients

Disorder	Clinical Presentation	Diagnostics
Hyperinsulinemia	Use of exogenous insulin Hyperglycemia Use of exogenous steroids, signs of Cushing's disease Polycystic ovary disease	Glucose Insulin levels
Cushing's disease	Moonface Buffalo hump Electrolyte abnormalities Hypertension resistant to medication Tachycardia	Cortisol challenge test Electrolytes Glucose
Polycystic ovary disease	Hirsutism History of oligomenorrhea Infertility	Follicle-stimulating hormone Luteinizing hormone
Hypothyroidism	Mild obesity Hyporeflexivity Cold intolerance Hair loss Dry skin Amenorrhea Decreased libido	Thyroid-stimulating hormone Free T_4 (thyroxine)
Hypothalamic state (craniopharyngioma)	Delayed sexual development Headache Papilledema Mental deterioration Hypogonadism	CT scan
Growth hormone deficiency (rare)	History of pituitary resection or dysfunction Dwarfism	Growth hormone

diagnose tumors early, catch recurrences, determine optimum chemotherapy doses, and administer radiotherapy. In a prospective study of 900,000 U.S. adults from the Cancer Prevention Study II, an estimated 90,000 deaths each year were related to excess body weight.[38]

INDICATIONS FOR REFERRAL OR HOSPITALIZATION

For patients with significant obesity or co-morbid conditions, referral to a nutritionist and exercise program is advisable. Complaints of overweight or obesity, chronic fatigue, loud snoring, nocturnal breathing pauses, choking, gasping, excessive daytime sleepiness, restless sleep, or frequent episode of waking each night require an immediate referral for a sleep study to rule out sleep apnea and associated sleep disorders.[39] Significant others are frequently a good source of information on a patient's sleep patterns. Many patients are reluctant to carry out this test because they must sleep at a testing center. Provider encouragement and follow-up may be required to ensure completion of this examination.

For patients with a BMI greater than 40 who fail to achieve weight loss goals, or those who have a BMI greater than 35 with related complications, a referral for bariatric surgery may be indicated. Before bariatric surgery the patient undergoes a series of evaluations, including medical, surgical, psychologic, and nutritional examinations. Bariatric surgery should be offered to candidates who meet the criteria, but only after they have completed a multidisciplinary evaluation.[40]

Bariatric surgery results in a decreased stomach capacity, which reduces the amount of food that can be consumed. This decreased calorie consumption leads to weight loss over time. The patient needs to be apprised of the complications and the lifelong physical alterations that result from the surgery. The adjustable gastric band—a silicone ring placed around the top of the stomach, restricting the amount of food that can be eaten—was approved by the FDA in 2001, is considered one of the safest surgical interventions, and is completely reversible.[40]

Other methods of gastric bypass result in permanent alteration of the digestive system. The Roux-en-Y gastric bypass has become the most common procedure for patients undergoing bariatric surgery.[40] This procedure carries a 1% risk for mortality and 10% risk for serious complications.[40] Pulmonary emboli, anastomotic leaks, and respiratory failure account for 80% of all deaths that occur within 30 days of bariatric surgery.[40]

Weight loss surgeries should not be considered lightly, and the risks of the surgery should be balanced with the risks of being obese. Surgery is not a magical solution to obesity. It can help patients eat less but cannot choose what they eat. A long-term commitment to eat properly is required for success.

PATIENT AND FAMILY EDUCATION

Many providers attempt to involve the entire family in efforts to reduce caloric intake and increase physical activity. This requires careful evaluation of the family structure and education of the family members responsible for shopping and preparing meals in the home. This is very time-consuming and impractical in most practices.

Several programs exist to assist the provider in discussing overweight and obesity. The Aim for a Healthy Weight Education Kit provides information on weight gain and interactive tools based on established clinical guidelines.[41] Tools include a BMI calculator, a menu planner, portion distortion quiz, and information that encourages healthy eating and increased physical activity.[41]

HEALTH PROMOTION

Prevention is the key to ending the obesity epidemic. Obesity by its nature is difficult to treat and presents a lifelong struggle for many adults. Early diagnosis and aggressive treatment are essential. Recognizing the need for a nationwide comprehensive effort to prevent obesity, several government organization have developed activity and education programs to assist communities and practitioners in preventing and treating obesity (Table 17-2). These communication programs are designed to get the message to communities that obesity is preventable if changes in the way we eat and exercise are implemented. Programs like Hearts N' Parks are designed

TABLE 17-2 Motivational Stages and Processes of Change

Stage of Change	Characteristics	Processes and Techniques
Precontemplation	Patient does not acknowledge a problem; is not considering change within the next 6 months.	Establish rapport: validate patient's lack of readiness, acknowledge that the decision belongs to *patient.* Raise patient consciousness of personal risks to health and happiness. Ask about the impact of the problem on significant others.
Contemplation	Patient is ambivalent about change; not considering change within the next month.	Establish rapport: validate lack of readiness, acknowledge that the decision belongs to *patient.* Encourage evaluation of the pros and cons of behavior change. Identify and promote new, positive outcome expectations.
Preparation	Patient is intending to take action within the month, and small steps toward change may have already occurred.	Praise the decision to change. Verify that the patient has the necessary skills for successful change. Identify and assist in problem solving with regard to obstacles. Assist patient in identifying social supports. Encourage small, reasonable "practice" steps.

Data from *Motivating health behavior change: powerful conversations in the exam room,* courtesy of Steve Taylor, DHSc, St. Anthony Family Medicine Residency Program, Denver; and Greene GW, Rossi SR, Rossi JS, and others: Dietary applications of the stages of change model, *J Am Diet Assoc* 99:673-678, 1999.

for all members of the family to learn about eating healthy and increasing daily physical activity.

To aid in the prevention of obesity, practitioners should include in their routine screening questions on dietary habits and physical activity. The key to primary prevention is to openly discuss this potential problem and have resources readily available to reinforce education. Health care providers have a pivotal role in reversing the obesity epidemic.

REFERENCES

1. Centers for Disease Control and Prevention: *Health, United States 2005*, retrieved July 23, 2006, from http://www.cdc.gov/nchs/hus.htm.
2. Centers for Disease Control and Prevention: *Frequently asked questions about calculating obesity related risk*, retrieved July 26, 2006, from http://www.cdc.gov/doc.do/id/0900f3ec803207fd
3. Flegal KM, Graubard BI, Williamson DF: Methods of calculating deaths attributed to obesity, *Am J Epidemiol* 160(4):331-338, 2004.
4. World Health Organization: *Obesity: preventing and managing the global epidemic*, Geneva, 2000, WHO Technical Report Series, No 894, retrieved July 29, 2006, from http://www.who.int/nutrition/publications/obesity/en/index.html.
5. International Obesity Taskforce: *Call for obesity review as overweight numbers reach 1.7 billion*, March 17, 2003, retrieved Aug 2, 2006, from http://www.iotf.org/media.
6. Daniels J: Obesity: America's epidemic, *AJN* 106(1):40-49, 2006.
7. Stein CJ, Colditz GA: The epidemic of obesity, *J Clin Endocrinol Metab* 89(6):2522-2525, 2004.
8. Glanz K, Basil M, Maibach E, and others: Why Americans eat what they do: taste, nutrition, cost, convenience, and weight control as influences on food consumption, *J Am Diet Assoc* 98:1118-1126, 1998.
9. Institute of Medicine: *Preventing childhood obesity: health in the balance,* Washington, DC, 2005, National Academies Press.
10. Rolls BJ: The supersizing of America: portion size and the obesity epidemic, *Nutr Today* 28(2):42-53, 2003.
11. Centers for Disease Control and Prevention: Prevalence of physical activity, including lifestyle activities among adults—United States, 2000-2001, *MMWR* 52(32):764-769, 2003.
12. Borjeson M: The aetiology of obesity in children: a study of 101 twin pairs, *Acta Paediatr Scand* 65(3):279-287, 1976.
13. Noble RE: The incidence of parental obesity in overweight individuals, *Int J Eating Disord* 22(3):265-271, 1997.
14. Lauderdale DS, Kntson KL, Yan LL: Objectively measured sleep characteristics among early middle aged adults: the Cardia Study, *Am J Epidemiol* 164:5-16, 2006.
15. Spiegel K, Tasali E, Penev P, and others: Brief communication: sleep curtailment in healthy young men is associated with decreased leptin levels, elevated ghrelin levels, and increased hunger and appetite, *Ann Intern Med* 141:846-850, 2004.
16. Bjorntorp B: Do stress reactions cause abdominal obesity and comorbidities? *Obes Rev* 2(2):73-86, 2001.
17. Maglione-Garves CA, Kravitz L, Schneider S: Cortisol connection: tips on managing stress and weight, *ACSM's Health Fitness J* 9(5):20-23, 2005.
18. Seller RH: *Differential diagnosis of common complaints,* ed 4, Philadelphia, 2000, Saunders.
19. Uppot RH, Sahani DV, Hahn PF, and others: Effect of obesity on image quality, *Radiology* 240(2):435-439, 2006.
20. Springhouse Publishing, editor: *Rapid differential diagnosis,* Philadelphia, 2002, Lippincott Williams & Wilkins.
21. Dansinger ML, Augustin GJ, Griffith JL, and others: Comparison of the Atkins, Ornish, Weight Watchers, and Zone diets for weight loss and heart disease risk reduction: a randomized trial, *JAMA* 293(1):43-53, 2005.
22. Calfas KJ, Sallis JF, Zabinski MF, and others: Preliminary evaluation of a multicomponent program for nutrition and physical change in primary care: PACE + for adults, *Prev Med* 34:153-161, 2002.
23. Galuska DA, Will JC, Serdula MK, and others: Are health care professionals advising obese patients to lose weight? *JAMA* 282:1576-1578, 1999.
24. Wee CC, McCarthy EP, Davis RB, and others: Physician counseling about exercise, *JAMA* 282:1583-1588, 1999.
25. Stafford RS, Farhat JH, Misra B, and others: National patterns of physician activities related to obesity management, *Arch Fam Med* 9:631-638, 2000.
26. Ma J, Urizar GG, Alegn T, and others: Diet and physical activity counseling during ambulatory care visits in the United States, *Prev Med* 39:815-822, 2004.
27. Kroner J, Aronne LJ: Pharmacological approaches to weight reduction: therapeutic targets, *J Clin Endocrinol Metab* 89(6):2616-2621, 2004.
28. Gelfand EV, Cannon CP: Rimonabant: a cannabinoid receptor type 1 blocker for management of multiple cardiometabolic risk factors, *J Am Coll Cardiol* 47(10):1919-1926, 2006.
29. Saper RB, Eisenberg DM, Phillips RS: Common dietary supplements for weight loss, *Am Fam Phys* 70(9):1731-1738, 2004.
30. Klein S, Burke LE, Bray GA, and others: Clinical implications of obesity with specific focus on cardiovascular disease: a statement for professionals from the American Heart Association Council on Nutrition, Physical Activity, and Metabolism, *Circulation* 110:2952-2967, 2004.
31. Kannel WB, Wilson WF, Nam B, and others: Risk stratification of obesity as a coronary risk factor, *Am J Cardiol* 90(7):697-701, 2002.
32. Garrison RJ, Kannel WB, Stokes J, and others: Incidence and precursors of hypertension in young adults: the Framingham Study, *Prev Med* 16:235-251, 1987.
33. Vega GL: Obesity, the metabolic syndrome, and cardiovascular disease, *Am Heart J* 142(6):1108-1116, 2001.
34. Peeters A, Barendregt JJ, Willekens F, and others: Obesity in adulthood and its consequences for life expectancy, *Ann Intern Med* 138:24-32, 2003.
35. Olshansky SJ, Passaro DJ, Hershow RC, and others: A potential decline in life expectancy in the United States in the 21st century, *N Engl J Med* 352(11):1138-1146, 2005.
36. Tsai SP, Donnelly RP, Wendt JK: Obesity and mortality in a prospective study of middle aged industrial population, *J Occup Environ Med* 48:22-27, 2006.
37. National Cancer Institute: *Obesity and cancer: fact sheet*, retrieved Aug 14, 2006, from http://www.cancer.gov/newscenter/obesity1.
38. Calle EE, Rodriguez C, Walker-Thurmond K, and others: Overweight, obesity, and mortality from cancer in a prospectively studied cohort of US adults, *N Engl J Med* 348(17):1625-1638, 2003.
39. Young T, Skatrud J, Peppard PE: Risk factors for obstructive sleep apnea in adults, *JAMA* 291(16):2013-2016, 2004.
40. Virji A, Murr MM: Caring for patients after bariatric surgery, *Am Fam Phys* 73(8):1403-1408, 2006.
41. Donato KA: National health education programs to promote healthy eating and physical activity, *Nutr Rev* 64(2):S65-S70, 2006.

CHAPTER 18

Rehabilitation

Brenda Hage and William R. Prebola, Jr.

Approximately 54 million people in the United States—almost 1 in 5 Americans—have some type of developmental, physical, or medical disability.[1] The prevalence of disabilities is disproportionately higher among minority populations, rural populations, and those with lower socioeconomic status. These disabling conditions include physical impairments (affecting mobility, vision, speech, or swallowing) or emotional or mental impairments and can limit one or more of the affected individual's activities of daily living (ADLs).[1] Significant efforts must be directed toward increasing the functional status of the disabled. Rehabilitation seeks to assist individuals with restoration of function and maintenance of health and has been described as aiding the individual in reaching maximum physical, psychosocial, educational, vocational, and avocational potential consistent with the patient's abilities and limitations.[2]

Rehabilitation uses an interdisciplinary team approach, with a patient- and family-centered care plan and mutual goal setting in which the patient is an active participant. Several disciplines are involved in the rehabilitative process. A *physiatrist,* also known as a physical and rehabilitation medicine specialist, is a physician trained in the care of patients with loss of function and usually serves as the leader of the rehabilitation team. Rehabilitation nurses are skilled in caring for patients with disabilities and altered functional ability and in providing patient and family education. Advanced practice nurses such as nurse practitioners and clinical nurse specialists provide clinical follow-up care, coordination of care, and staff consultation. Physical therapists focus on gait and mobility issues, and occupational therapists promote self-care abilities used in ADLs and activities related to vocational and avocational functioning. Speech and language therapists assist patients with dysphagia, cognition, and language problems. Dietitians offer consultation regarding nutritional needs. Psychologists provide supportive counseling and diagnostic testing for cognitive problems. Recreational therapists offer patients opportunities to develop and participate in leisure interests. Social workers and case managers coordinate discharge planning. Other health care professionals, such as cognitive therapists, may offer additional services.

The rehabilitation team works together to assist the patient and family. Rehabilitation services may be provided in a variety of settings, such as the home, outpatient programs, inpatient rehabilitation units or centers, acute care hospitals, and skilled nursing facilities. The setting is selected on the basis of the patient's underlying function, potential abilities, and individual problems. It is often necessary to use several different settings as the patient moves through the continuum of rehabilitation care.

ASSESSMENT

A comprehensive functional history and assessment are essential to developing the patient's care plan and measuring patient progress. The key elements of the functional history include the patient's ability to complete ADLs (both currently and before the present illness) and the degree of assistance required. Information regarding the use of wheelchairs, walkers, canes, prosthetics (artificial limbs), orthotics (splints, braces), and any other adaptive equipment, as well as accessibility within the patient's home, is also important. The level of family and social support available and the use community support services such as the city or county department providing elder services or Meals on Wheels should also be assessed.

Indexes of functional assessment include the ability to perform self-care activities (e.g., dressing, bathing, toileting, grooming, hygiene, eating) and mobility (e.g., ambulation, transfers, bed and wheelchair mobility). Social and cognitive functions are also assessed. Some of the many instruments available include the Katz Index of ADL, the Barthel Index, the Kenney Self-Care Evaluation, and the Functional Independence Measure (FIM). The FIM scoring system is the most widely used and consists of 18 functional categories that are further subdivided into mobility, locomotion, self-care, sphincter control, communication, and social cognition.[3] Although sometimes complex and time intensive, the use of FIM scoring or other assessment tools is a valuable means of establishing the patient's baseline functional abilities, measuring treatment outcomes, and facilitating communication with the rehabilitation team. These tools are used at rehabilitation staffing meetings to assist in coordinating the patient's individualized care plan and in discharge planning. FIM scoring and other assessment measures are also important in fulfilling the documentation requirements of third-party payers, which often require updates showing patients' progress for continued rehabilitation eligibility.

PAIN MANAGEMENT

Pharmacologic pain management in rehabilitation is based on many factors, including the patient's age, co-morbid medical problems, medication side effect profile, ease of use, and cost. NSAIDs and acetaminophen are helpful for mild to moderate pain. NSAIDs used concomitantly with opioid analgesics allow for lower medication dosages and decrease the incidence of adverse side effects.[4] Chronic, painful conditions such as peripheral neuropathy, lumbar radiculopathy, and fibromyalgia respond well to the analgesic effect of tricyclic antidepressants such as amitriptyline (Elavil) and to selective serotonin reuptake inhibitors (SSRIs) such as sertraline (Zoloft), duloxetine (Cymbalta), or citalopram (Celexa). Anticonvulsants such as valproic acid (Depakene), divalproex sodium (Depakote), levetiracetam (Keppra), pregabalin (Lyrica), gabapentin (Neurontin), and carbamazepine (Tegretol) may also be beneficial in relieving pain associated with neuropathic pain syndromes.[5] Metaxalone (Skelaxin), cyclobenzaprine (Flexeril), or other antispasmodic agents can be prescribed for short-term use to treat pain related to myofascial spasm. Topical agents, including lidocaine (Lidoderm) patches and capsaicin cream, are also helpful adjuncts in pain relief.[6]

Chronic, persistent pain associated with reflex sympathetic dystrophy and postherpetic neuralgia may respond well to sympathetic anesthetic blocks, such as a stellate ganglion block.[5] Injections of corticosteroids into joints, the spinal canal (epidural), and the soft tissues are useful in reducing pain and inflammation and may be used in conjunction with other conservative methods.[7] Biofeedback, relaxation techniques, behavioral-cognitive therapy, and other nonpharmacologic measures of pain relief are also useful adjuncts to pain management.[8]

The use of alternative and complementary health modalities is on the rise. It has been estimated that approximately 15 million adults use herbal products and megavitamins concurrently with prescription medications. Patients often do not disclose the use of these products to their health care provider, thus placing them at risk for untoward adverse drug reactions.[9] The health care provider should assess the use of herbal and vitamin therapies each time a medication history is obtained. It is imperative that providers maintain an open line of communication with patients regarding self-care practices and health beliefs to develop an efficacious, acceptable, and safe care plan.

Some sources suggest that the use of vitamin and herbal therapies may be helpful in the management of chronic pain. Before recommending such therapies, providers should carefully research the empirical data regarding the use of these alternative and complementary therapies and evaluate their validity, reliability, and potential for interactions with any prescription medications taken by the patient. As with all therapeutic treatment options, the risk/benefit ratio must be considered. Ginger and turmeric are two culinary herbs that appear to offer some antiinflammatory properties. The recommended dose of ginger is 1 g/day (in 2 capsules) taken with food to avoid irritating the stomach. Exact dosing for turmeric is less clear, but it can be used as a spice for cooking foods such as curries. Whole herbal products of turmeric are not yet readily available, and extracts of partial ingredients do not appear to be as effective as the whole herb.[10] The food supplement glucosamine has been widely studied with conflicting results regarding its efficacy. A major multicenter clinical trial by the National Institutes of Health, Glucosamine/Chondroitin Arthritis Intervention Trial, has been conducted to assess the separate and combined effects of the dietary supplements glucosamine and chondroitin on the cessation or reduction of the progression of knee osteoarthritis. The results indicated that the only subgroup that showed significant pain relief were patients with moderate to severe osteoarthritis; the study is still ongoing to assess any effect on arthritis progression.[11]

PHYSICAL MODALITIES

Cryotherapy (cold) can be used to control postoperative pain and, initially, to control pain after musculoskeletal and soft tissue injuries. Chronic problems such as muscle spasm, trigger points, bursitis, and tendonitis also respond well to cold. Hydrotherapy, hot packs, paraffin baths, and ultrasound are all types of therapeutic heat that are useful in pain relief.[8] Transcutaneous electrical nerve stimulation units may benefit patients with postoperative pain and acute pain syndromes. Acupuncture and therapeutic massage have also been shown to be effective in providing pain relief. Interested patients should be referred to a qualified acupuncturist or massage therapist.[12] Prescribing providers should be knowledgeable about the various contraindications associated with physical modalities.

THERAPEUTIC EXERCISE

The main goal of therapeutic exercise is mobilization of the patient. The benefits of exercise include preventing or minimizing complications of immobility such as skin breakdown, pneumonia, atrophy, contractures, and deconditioning. Therapeutic exercise should begin when the patient is medically stable. Initially patients are encouraged to remain out of bed for short periods. Gradually these periods are increased in length and frequency. A reconditioning program should then be instituted. Isometric and isotonic exercises can be used in conjunction with a gentle strengthening regimen. As the patient's endurance increases, ambulation and transfer training should begin with functional transfers to the wheelchair and commode. With improvement in stamina and mobility, stair training can usually be initiated. The use of exercise bikes and treadmills also aids in improving conditioning and endurance. Later, outdoor ambulation and higher-level transfers with a cane, walker, or other assistive device may be tried.

HOME CARE

Home evaluations by occupational therapists, physical therapists, and home health nurses are useful in identifying equipment needs, environmental and architectural barriers, or other safety hazards within the patient's home. These evaluations, in conjunction with family training sessions, offer additional insights into caregivers' abilities to assist the patient. Patient and family expectations for discharge from the inpatient setting can sometimes be unrealistic; therefore observing the patient's function in the home setting may provide a more realistic picture of both the patient's and caregiver's abilities.

INDICATIONS FOR REFERRAL OR HOSPITALIZATION

A referral to the physiatrist should be considered after any major medical illness or injury that results in severe impairment and disability with profound limitation of function. Patients with multiple concomitant medical problems and chronic pain syndromes with significant limitations should also be referred. Physiatrists are also skilled in electrodiagnostic testing such as electromyography. Patients who require expensive orthotic or prosthetic devices for foot drop or amputation also benefit from physiatric evaluation. The physiatrist can aid in cost containment by determining whether patients require standardized, "off-the-shelf" equipment vs. customized prescriptions for complex bracing, wheelchair and seating systems, or other appropriate adaptive equipment, thus avoiding unnecessary or inappropriate expenditures.

Early rehabilitation is essential to maximize and maintain the functional abilities of the disabled patient. Individuals with disabilities can enjoy a higher quality of life with an appropriate rehabilitation program.

REFERENCES

1. US Department of Health and Human Services: *HHS programs serve Americans with disabilities* (fact sheet), retrieved Dec 29, 2001, from http://www.hhs.gov/news/press/2001pres/01fsdisabilities.html.
2. Stein SA, O'Young B, Young MA: The person, disablement, and the process of rehabilitation. In O'Young B, Young MA, Stein SA, editors: *Physical medicine and rehabilitation secrets,* St Louis, 1996, Mosby.
3. Ottenbacher KJ, Hsu Y, Granger CV, and others: The reliability of the Functional Independence Measure: a quantitative review, *Arch Phys Rehabil Med* 77(12):1226-1232, 1996.
4. Goddard MJ, Dean BZ, King JC: Basic science, acute pain, and neuropathic pain, *Arch Phys Rehabil Med* 75(5 Spec No):S4-S8, 1994.
5. Dean BZ, Williams FH, King RC, and others: Therapeutic options in pain management, *Arch Phys Rehabil Med* 75(5 Spec No):S21-S30, 1994.
6. McCaffery M, Pasero C: *Pain: clinical manual,* St Louis, 1999, Mosby.
7. Tan JC: *Practical manual of physical medicine and rehabilitation,* St Louis, 1998, Mosby.
8. Williams FH, Maly BJ: Cancer pain, pelvic pain, and age-related considerations, *Arch Phys Rehabil Med* 75(5 Spec No):S15-S20, 1994.
9. Eisenberg DM: Advising patients who seek alternative medical therapies, *Ann Intern Med* 121:61-69, 1997.
10. Weil A: *Healthy aging: a lifelong guide to your physical and spiritual well-being,* New York, 2005, Knopf.
11. Clegg DO, Reda DJ, Harris CL, and others: Glucosamine, chondroitin sulfate, and the two in combination for painful knee osteoarthritis. *N Engl J Med* 354(8):795-808, 2006.
12. Giusto J, Helms JM: Acupuncture. In O'Young B, Young MA, Steins SA, editors: *Physical medicine and rehabilitation secrets,* St Louis, 1996, Mosby.

CHAPTER 19

Sleep Disorders

Michael J. Sateia, Glen P. Greenough, and Brooke G. Judd

Sleep disorders are associated with major functional impairments, including loss of productivity, work-related and vehicular accidents, social impairment, and cognitive and mood disturbances, as well as morbidity and mortality related to cardiovascular, endocrine, and immune disturbances. Given the significance and lack of recognition of these disorders, health care providers are increasingly obligated to recognize the symptoms of sleep disorders, make accurate diagnoses, initiate sound referrals, and develop successful treatment plans in collaboration with sleep disorders specialists.

This chapter presents an overview of normal sleep and describes the most common disorders of sleep. The most recent edition of the *International Classification of Sleep Disorders*[1] (ICSD) organizes the conditions into eight major categories: insomnias, sleep-related breathing disorders, central nervous system (CNS) hypersomnias (excessive sleepiness not related to other sleep disorders), circadian rhythm disorders, movement disorders, parasomnias (abnormal behaviors or events arising from sleep), isolated sleep-related symptoms (e.g., sleep starts), and other sleep disorders. These categories, which are largely symptom based (e.g., insomnia or hypersomnias), serve as a guide to obtaining a detailed history and initiating essential diagnostic procedures.

From a practical standpoint, fundamental assessment of sleep, which should be part of any complete patient history, can begin with three basic questions: How are you sleeping at night? Are you excessively sleepy during the daytime? Are there any unusual events or problems with your sleep, especially heavy snoring? More detailed aspects of assessment are included in individual sections within this chapter.

NORMAL SLEEP

DEFINITION AND PHYSIOLOGY

Sleep is an active, dynamic physiologic process. Normal human sleep consists of two major states of consciousness: non–rapid eye movement (NREM) and rapid eye movement (REM) sleep. NREM sleep is further divided into four stages from lightest (stage 1) to deepest (stages 3 or 4, also referred to as slow wave or delta) sleep. These stages unfold in a predictable, repeated cycle, as illustrated in Figure 19-1. In young adults NREM sleep occupies about 75% of the night and REM the remaining 25%. Delta sleep is most prominent in young children and gradually diminishes through the life cycle. REM sleep (or its ontogenetic precursor) is seen in high percentages in neonates and infants but diminishes rapidly in the first years of life and remains fixed at about 25% thereafter.

Normal total sleep time varies considerably with age.[2] Although young children require longer sleep times, total sleep

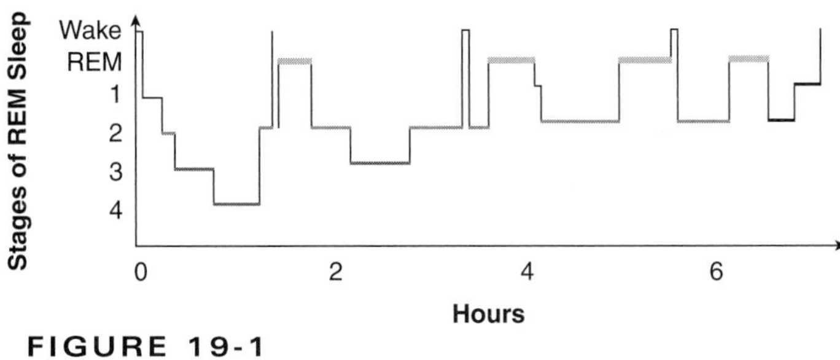

FIGURE 19-1

Sleep histogram. *REM*, Rapid eye movement.

time begins to decline by the second decade, remains relatively stable from the third decade through the fifth decade, and falls off more dramatically after age 70. It remains unclear to what extent the decline in nocturnal sleep in older individuals is a function of diminished sleep need as opposed to decreased ability to sleep. Time to fall asleep (sleep latency) and wake time after sleep onset are increased in the elderly, as is daytime napping.

NREM sleep is associated with a decline in respirations, heart rate and blood pressure, muscle relaxation, and cognitive activity. Sleep starts (sudden muscle contractions involving part or all of the body) may occur during wake-sleep transitions. REM sleep is marked by pronounced changes in physiology, including skeletal muscle atonia; increased variability in heart rate, blood pressure, respiration, and autonomic function; REM; and heightened cognitive activity associated with dreaming. Ventilatory drive to hypoxia and hypercapnia is decreased during NREM sleep and reaches its lowest point in REM sleep.

Current theories of sleep regulation focus on the two-process model.[3] This model suggests that sleep is regulated by two factors: homeostatic drive, which increases progressively during wake time, and circadian drive, which is based on the oscillating 24-hour rhythm of the major circadian clock, located in the suprachiasmatic nucleus of the hypothalamus. Thus the timing and amount of sleep are influenced by complex interactions between the biologic rhythms and the length of time since the last sleep period. Average human circadian cycles naturally run slightly longer than 24 hours (about 24.2 hours) but are reset daily (entrained) to a 24-hour rhythm by a variety of environmental cues, the most important of which is exposure to light. Sleep-wake rhythms are normally synchronized with myriad other clock-regulated physiologic functions, including endocrine-metabolic, immune, and cardiovascular.

INSOMNIA AND NONRESTORATIVE SLEEP

DEFINITION AND EPIDEMIOLOGY

Current epidemiologic data indicate that about 30% to 35% of individuals in Western society report at least occasional insomnia.[4] Multiple studies place the prevalence of chronic insomnia around 10%. Insomnia is a complex condition that may represent a final common pathway with numerous contributing factors. Acute or transient insomnia (days to a few weeks) is an almost universal problem that is typically related to acute stress or a time-zone shift (i.e., jet lag) and is generally self-resolving. Good sleep hygiene and, for some patients, short-term sleep medication are usually adequate. The major concern regarding short-term insomnia problems is that some patients begin to exhibit cognitions and behaviors that establish a foundation for development of a chronic insomnia problem.

PATHOPHYSIOLOGY

A widely accepted model of chronic insomnia suggests that it is a function of predisposing, precipitating, and perpetuating factors.[5] Little is known about predisposing biologic or psychologic factors, although it does seem clear that certain persons are at greater risk for the development of a chronic insomnia problem than others. Precipitating factors (which are sometimes referred to as "causes" of chronic insomnia) are identified in Box 19-1 and are discussed in greater detail below.

A unifying concept in the pathophysiology of chronic insomnia is that of *hyperarousal*.[6] Data indicate that patients with this condition exhibit evidence of both physiologic and cognitive hyperarousal, in the form of increased 24-hour metabolic rate, increased temperature, muscle tension, sleep EEG frequency, overactivity of the hypothalamic-pituitary-adrenal axis, and cognitive activity. It remains unclear how this hyperarousal develops, although preliminary data suggest that it is, at least in part, acquired and is amenable to change with therapeutic interventions such as cognitive-behavioral treatment.

CLINICAL PRESENTATION

Psychiatric disorders, especially major depression, are the most common precipitating factors. Generalized anxiety, panic, and posttraumatic stress disorders are also associated with elevated rates of insomnia. Substance abuse or dependence, including alcohol, sedative-hypnotics, stimulants, and opiates, frequently manifests with insomnia, which may persist even after discontinuation of the substance. Excessive use of caffeine, or even moderate use later in the day, may also be problematic.

Circadian disorders, especially shift work and delayed sleep phase disorders, are commonly associated with sleep complaints. High percentages of night shift workers experience abnormal sleep, with reduced total sleep times and poor-quality sleep. This pattern does not tend to improve over long periods of night work for most shift workers. As a result of these disturbances, shift workers are at increased risk for accidents. Delayed sleep phase disorder occurs most commonly in adolescents and younger adults and is characterized by an inability to sleep at normal clock times, with normal sleep onset occurring late (e.g., 4 AM) and subsequent inability to arise at conventional times (e.g., noon awakening). Sleep is otherwise restorative and normal, but the schedule is clearly inconsistent with normal school or work times. Advanced sleep phase disorder is a less common circadian rhythm disorder, with normal sleep quantity and quality occurring early in the 24-hour day (e.g., 6 PM to 2 AM). It appears to be most common in older adults.

BOX 19-1

SOME KEY PRECIPITANTS OF CHRONIC INSOMNIA

PSYCHIATRIC DISORDERS

Adjustment disorders
Mood disorders
- Major depressive disorder
- Bipolar disorder
- Dysthymic disorder

Anxiety disorders
- Generalized anxiety disorder
- Posttraumatic stress disorder
- Panic disorder

Psychotic disorders
Personality disorders

SUBSTANCES AND MEDICATIONS

Alcohol
Stimulants
- Amphetamines, methylphenidate, modafinil, cocaine, Ecstasy (MDMA, or 3,4-methylenedioxymethamphetamine), or caffeine
- Steroids
- Bronchodilators
- Some anithypertensives

Some antidepressants
Cholesterol-lowering agents

MEDICAL AND NEUROLOGIC DISORDERS

Degenerative neurologic diseases
Stroke
Recurrent nocturnal headache
Traumatic brain injury
Chronic obstructive pulmonary disease, nocturnal dyspnea, cough
Nocturnal angina
Gastroesophageal reflux disease, other nocturnal gastrointestinal disturbance
Pain from any source
Nocturia
Endocrine disorders

OTHER SLEEP DISORDERS

Obstructive or central sleep apnea
Restless legs syndrome, periodic limb movements
Nightmare disorder
Circadian rhythm disorders

Medical conditions and medications may contribute to sleep disturbance. Among the most common are those associated with nocturnal pain, chronic lung disease, end-stage organ failure, endocrine disorders and other metabolic conditions, and especially neurodegenerative diseases. Likewise, many medications may aggravate sleep, most notably, steroids, methylxanthines, some antihypertensives, stimulants, and certain antidepressant medications.

Other physiologic sleep disorders may result in an insomnia problem. The patient with restless legs syndrome (RLS) complains of annoying, "creepy-crawly" sensations in the legs or, less commonly, the arms. The sensation is associated with an irresistible urge to move the extremities. The sensations may interfere with sleep onset. RLS is often associated with periodic limb movement in sleep (PLM), which is characterized by repetitive, periodic (every 20 to 40 seconds) limb movements, often resulting in arousals that the sleeper is unaware of (much as in obstructive sleep apnea [OSA]). These disorders are discussed in greater detail in the Sleep-Related Movement Disorders section.

Although OSA is most often associated with complaints of daytime sleepiness, rather than insomnia, these patients may be seen with clinically significant complaints of insomnia. Therefore OSA must also be considered in the differential diagnosis, particularly in obese patients or those with heavy snoring.

The essential features of psychophysiologic (primary) insomnia (PPI) are conditioned arousal in response to efforts to sleep and negative expectations regarding the ability to sleep. Individuals with PPI may be able to sleep better when not trying to fall asleep or in settings other than their own bedroom. Symptoms may include difficulty getting to sleep and trouble returning to sleep following awakening. This type of insomnia exists commonly as a disorder in its own right. However, the hyperarousal and negative conditioning that occur in this disorder are frequent complicating factors in insomnia that is associated with the numerous precipitating factors described above. Often, when an initial precipitating factor (e.g., major depression, acute stress, or medical illness) resolves, these conditioned psychophysiologic elements serve as the perpetuating factors noted earlier in this chapter.

DIAGNOSTICS

The essential element in the evaluation of an insomnia complaint is the history. The nature of the onset, course, complications, and treatments of the condition must be elicited in detail. Sleep-wake schedule, including napping, is critical to assessment. Sleep logs, usually conducted for 1 to 2 weeks, can be a helpful adjunct to history. The log should contain the following information for each night: time of getting into bed, time lights are actually turned out (e.g., after television, reading), estimate of sleep latency (time to fall asleep after lights out), estimate of the number of awakenings and total awake time across the night, time of final awakening, and time of actual arising. Evidence of other sleep-related symptoms (e.g., snoring or observed pauses in breathing, limb movement or restless legs, nightmares, behavioral disturbances, headaches, pain, gastroesophageal reflux disorder, and the like) must be sought from the patient and, whenever possible, the bed partner. Daytime consequences, particularly evidence of significant sleepiness, should be assessed. Medical, neurologic, and psychiatric evaluations are essential, as are pertinent physical examination and appropriate laboratory procedures.

Polysomnography (PSG) (overnight sleep recording) contributes little to the diagnosis of most insomnia patients and is usually reserved for those cases in which demonstrable physiologic disturbances are suspected, typically breathing disorders, hypersomnias, and some parasomnias. Patients with treatment-refractory insomnia may also be appropriate for PSG.

MANAGEMENT

The management of insomnia begins with careful identification of the contributing factors. Treatment is tailored based on those factors. When clear precipitating causes are present (e.g., major depression or PLM), specific therapies appropriate to those factors must be instituted (e.g., antidepressant medication or dopamine agonists for PLM). Attention must also be directed to substances or medications that may be disturbing sleep. Sleep hygiene education is an essential component for management of any insomnia problem, but is typically not sufficient treatment in its own right.

Treatment of circadian rhythm sleep disorders is often complex and is best administered by sleep medicine specialists. Bright light therapy and melatonin have demonstrated therapeutic benefit in certain patients with sleep-wake schedule disorders. Chronotherapy (planned behavioral adjustments of schedule) involving progressive phase delay has also been used for patients with delayed sleep phase disorder.

Dopaminergic agents (e.g., ropinirole or pramipexole) are the first-line treatment for the patient with RLS or periodic limb movement disorder (PLMD). Treatment of breathing disorders is discussed in a later section.

Once precipitating factors have been evaluated and treated, additional therapeutic approaches lie largely in the pharmacologic and behavioral realm. The most commonly employed hypnotic medications are nonbenzodiazepines, so titled because they act selectively at the benzodiazepine receptor but are chemically distinct from the benzodiazepine class of sleeping pills. The major agents in this class are zolpidem (Ambien), zaleplon (Sonata), and eszopiclone (Lunesta).

These agents have comparable efficacy and, like the benzodiazepines themselves, differ primarily with respect to the clinical duration of action. Although hypnotic medications have been indicated only for short-term use until recently, emerging data suggest that long-term use of nonbenzodiazepines is safe and effective, without dosage escalation or evidence of dependency.[7] However, a clear algorithm for long-term use of pharmacologic therapies, and the interaction of these therapies with nonpharmacologic approaches, has yet to be elucidated.

Cognitive-behavioral therapies for chronic insomnia, particularly PPI, are brief and produce sustained benefit.[8] Compared to short-term courses of medication, cognitive-behavioral therapies produce durable improvement, whereas improvements seen with time-limited courses of hypnotics tend to dissipate rapidly after drug discontinuation. Behavioral therapies include sleep restriction therapy, stimulus control, and relaxation training. These therapies are often combined on a case-by-case basis. The common component of the most successful therapeutic approaches is marked reduction of the time spent in bed awake. In addition to the behavioral components, successful regimens also include cognitive restructuring to identify and alter the distorted cognitions that are often part of the fabric of insomnia.

DIFFERENTIAL DIAGNOSIS

Chronic Insomnia

- Insomnia secondary to mental disorder
- Insomnia secondary to medication or substances
- Circadian rhythm disorders
- Shift work
- Delayed or advanced sleep phase
- Insomnia secondary to medical or neurologic condition
- Other primary sleep disorder
- Restless legs syndrome or periodic limb movement in sleep
- Sleep-related breathing disorder
- Primary insomnia
- Psychophysiologic insomnia

Access to cognitive-behavioral therapies for insomnia by skilled and experienced clinicians can be problematic, particularly in primary care settings outside of larger centers. Training in behavioral therapy for insomnia is available to health care providers in brief continuing education courses, and a referral to a psychologist familiar with the use of these therapies should be readily available in most urban communities.

SLEEP-RELATED BREATHING DISORDERS

DEFINITION AND EPIDEMIOLOGY

The sleep-related breathing disorders encompass a number of disorders, including OSA, upper airway resistance syndrome (UARS), and central sleep apnea (CSA). OSA is the most common sleep-related breathing disorder. Clinically significant OSA occurs in at least 2% to 4% of women and 4% to 10% of men in North America.[9] The predominant physiologic derangement in OSA is repetitive upper airway narrowing or closure, which occurs during sleep, leading to increased efforts to breathe, finally ending with a brief CNS arousal to reestablish patency of the upper airway. The closures (or near closures) can occur many times a night, leading to significant sleep fragmentation and poor-quality sleep. More recently, UARS has been recognized as a disorder.[10] In UARS, there is increased resistance due to narrowing in the upper airway, which causes the individual to increase respiratory efforts to maintain airflow. While airflow (tidal volume) remains at essentially normal levels, the increasing respiratory efforts still may lead to brief CNS arousals and thus have many of the same consequences as the more overt OSA.

CSA is significantly less common than OSA. The primary derangement in CSA is altered CNS respiratory drive, such that the patient does not receive the usual metabolic feedback to the CNS during sleep to drive the breathing. This leads to repetitive cycles characterized by cessation of airflow because of lack of respiratory effort, which terminates once the metabolic trigger to breathe (usually blood carbon dioxide levels) increases sufficiently to drive respiratory output from the CNS. As with OSA, there are often brief CNS arousals associated with these events, leading to fragmented sleep.

CLINICAL PRESENTATION

A history of OSA and UARS is most often suggested by loud, disruptive snoring, with or without witnessed apneas, nocturnal gasping, or choking. Patients may complain of frank excessive daytime sleepiness (EDS), daytime fatigue and tiredness without unintentional sleep, or even vague depressive symptoms. They are often not aware of fragmented sleep, since the respiratory-related arousals are often too brief to be consciously registered during the night. In fact, patients not uncommonly report that they sleep well through the night and are puzzled by their daytime sleepiness. Nocturia is a frequent complication of the disorder.

The most common risk factor for OSA is obesity, and patients may be able to relate the onset of their symptoms to weight gain. The disorder is more common in men, although the prevalence rate in postmenopausal women approaches the same level as in men. A substance history is helpful in that particular substances may alter airway muscle tone and further increase risk for obstructive respiratory events. This includes the use of alcohol, opiates, or muscle relaxant medication such as the benzodiazepines in the evening. It is also helpful to elicit other medical history, such as heart disease, hypertension, or stroke, since these disorders may be seen with OSA. On physical examination, the presence of obesity and a crowded oropharynx may be suggestive of OSA in a patient with symptoms associated with the disease.

In addition to leading to EDS and impairment of daytime functioning, untreated OSA has more recently been found to have associations with a variety of more long-term health consequences. There is substantial convincing evidence that untreated OSA is an independent cause of systemic hypertension.[11] Multiple studies also demonstrate an association between untreated OSA and cardiac disease and stroke.[12]

Individuals with CSA may be noted by their bed partner to have pauses in their breathing, which may or may not be followed by a period of more rapid breathing. They typically will not, however, have a history of snoring. These patients may also have complaints of EDS or daytime fatigue, since the central apneic events disrupt sleep in a way similar to OSA events. Risk factors for CSA include decompensated congestive heart failure or the use of opioid medications, especially methadone.

DIAGNOSTICS

Overnight PSG is the standard test to establish the diagnosis of OSA, UARS, and the other sleep-related breathing disorders. Unattended home PSG is employed in some settings, but current clinical standards do not support its reliability in the routine diagnosis of OSA.[13] Overnight pulse oximetry is not sufficiently sensitive to be a reliable screening test for sleep apnea.

MANAGEMENT

OSA and UARS are most commonly treated with nasal continuous positive airway pressure (nCPAP). This is the most effective treatment, with efficacy rates of 95%, and is essentially free of dangerous side effects. The major impediments to successful nCPAP therapy are comfort and acceptance. Careful counseling and initial attention to equipment fit can go a long way toward ensuring patient adherence to the device. Weight loss may also be helpful in the overall management strategy, although this should not be used as the sole treatment modality in patients with anything more than mild OSA. Other potential treatment options include custom-fit dental appliances designed to increase posterior airway dimensions and upper airway surgical procedures designed to remove upper airway excessive tissue. These modalities, however, are less effective than nCPAP, and success cannot be predicted before treatment. Less commonly, appropriate treatment choices may include tracheotomy or, in patients who have undergone a careful preoperative evaluation and failed less invasive therapies, more extensive maxillofacial surgery.

CENTRAL NERVOUS SYSTEM HYPERSOMNIAS

DEFINITION AND EPIDEMIOLOGY

The primary disorders of hypersomnolence are characterized by an intrinsic CNS deficit that results in a sleep-wake system that is inadequate for maintaining wakefulness and/or overactive in promoting sleep. The predominant clinical characteristic of these syndromes is EDS not caused by disturbed nocturnal sleep or misaligned circadian rhythms.

The primary hypersomnias include narcolepsy, idiopathic hypersomnia, and posttraumatic hypersomnia. Narcolepsy, the best defined of the primary hypersomnias, is characterized by EDS and inappropriate manifestations of REM sleep. These include such phenomena as cataplexy (sudden onset of REM-related muscle atonia precipitated by emotion during wakefulness) and hallucinations and paralysis occurring at sleep onset (hypnagogic) or offset (hypnopompic) related to inappropriately timed REM. The EDS and the REM-related symptoms can be extremely disabling and potentially dangerous, depending on when they occur.

Idiopathic CNS hypersomnia also involves CNS sleep system dysfunction, which results in profound EDS. However, with idiopathic CNS hypersomnia, there is no known disease of the REM system, and other symptoms present in narcolepsy are absent. Posttraumatic hypersomnia is not readily distinguishable from idiopathic hypersomnia, other than that the symptoms follow head injury or another CNS insult such as an infection.

CLINICAL PRESENTATION

Assessment of the patient with EDS usually begins with either the patient or a family member complaining of sleepiness or unintentional sleep in undesired situations. This may include falling asleep unintentionally while watching television or reading, in noisy gatherings, at work, in conversation, or even while driving. Information obtained from a family member can be essential to accurate diagnosis, since patients with EDS may not recognize or may minimize the severity of their symptoms. It is important to obtain a full sleep history, including 24-hour sleep-wake schedules, time and duration of naps, and associated symptoms that may point to the underlying cause of the EDS symptoms.

The key clinical feature of narcolepsy is EDS. Cataplexy; hypnagogic or hypnopompic hallucinations; sleep paralysis; and fragmented, disturbed nocturnal sleep may be present but are not all required for the diagnosis. Cataplexy is seen almost exclusively in narcolepsy and is characterized by sudden episodes of muscle atonia during wakefulness. Cataplexy is often brought on when the patient is experiencing a strong emotion, particularly laughter. Such episodes may pose potential danger, depending on when and where they occur. They are often only seconds in duration but can last for minutes or longer in some cases. The sleep paralysis involves REM-related atonia (excluding the ocular muscles and diaphragm) and is often described as terrifying by patients. The hypnagogic or hypnopompic hallucinations are dreamlike and often frightening fragments that occur near sleep onset or offset and typically involve patient confusion about whether he or she is awake or asleep. The typical onset of narcolepsy symptoms is in the second or third decade, although it can occur earlier or later in life. There is no gender predominance. There are no features on physical examination that are particularly helpful in identifying narcolepsy.

The diagnosis of idiopathic CNS hypersomnia is most often a diagnosis of exclusion. Patients typically have complaints of EDS despite adequate or prolonged total sleep time, and they do not have the symptoms that otherwise characterize narcolepsy. A careful history should be obtained regarding possible CNS insult from infection or trauma.

In addition to using the history to identify the above disorders, the health care provider should also question the patient for symptoms suggestive of RLS or PLM (discussed in further detail later in this chapter). The patient's sleep-wake schedule should also be evaluated to make certain that insufficient sleep is not playing a role, and a complete medication and substance history should be obtained, since many medications and drugs may cause sleepiness as a side effect.

DIFFERENTIAL DIAGNOSIS

Excessive Daytime Somnolence

- Insufficient sleep
- Sleep-wake system deficit
- Narcolepsy
- Idiopathic CNS hypersomnia
- Posttraumatic hypersomnia
- Sleep fragmentation
- Obstructive or central sleep apnea
- Periodic limb movement disorder
- Circadian rhythm disorder
- Substances, medication, or primary medical or neurologic disorder

DIAGNOSTICS

Overnight PSG is generally employed when assessing the primary hypersomnias. The purpose is to exclude other underlying causes of the patient's sleepiness symptoms, such as an occult sleep-related breathing disorder. If no cause of EDS is identified on the overnight PSG, the next step is to perform a multiple sleep latency test (MSLT).[14] The MSLT is used to determine one's propensity for daytime sleep. The subject is given multiple opportunities to nap under standardized conditions, and a mean sleep onset latency (i.e., time to fall asleep) is determined and compared with normative values. This is the most objective means of determining EDS. The presence of sleep-onset REM episodes on the MSLT is a required diagnostic finding for narcolepsy.

MANAGEMENT

EDS as a result of CNS-based disorders has historically been treated with psychostimulants (e.g., dextroamphetamine or methylphenidate). The non–habit-forming stimulant modafinil is increasingly used. Cataplexy is treated by using REM-suppressing medications. Most commonly these have included the tricyclic antidepressants and the SSRI-type antidepressants. More recently, g-hydroxybutyrate has become available as a therapy to treat cataplexy.

SLEEP-RELATED MOVEMENT DISORDERS

DEFINITION AND EPIDEMIOLOGY

Sleep-related movement disorders are conditions in which patients have stereotyped movements or other sleep-related monophasic movements that may disturb sleep. Sleep-related leg cramps, sleep-related rhythmic movement disorder, PLMD, and sleep-related bruxism are disorders that fall into this category. RLS, because of its association with PLMs, is included in this category. Because RLS is so common (5% to 10% in populations derived from Western Europe),[1] this will be the focus of this section. The prevalence of this disorder increases with age, but symptoms may start in childhood. RLS is seen more commonly in women. RLS is an uncomfortable sensation, usually in the legs, associated with a strong desire to move the legs. Because this discomfort occurs primarily in the evening, it may lead to sleep difficulties.

The pathophysiology of RLS is unclear. RLS may occur in association with a wide variety of conditions. Pregnancy, renal failure, and ferritin levels less than 50 mcg/L have the most well-established associations. Peripheral neuropathy and Parkinson's disease may also be associated with RLS. A number of widely used medications, including most antidepressants, sedating antihistamines, and dopamine antagonists, may cause or exacerbate RLS.[1] RLS, however, is often idiopathic. Given the efficacy of dopaminergic agents in treating RLS, a CNS dysfunction in a dopaminergic system has been postulated as an etiology for this syndrome.

CLINICAL PRESENTATION AND DIAGNOSTICS

Patients suffering from RLS may come to see their health care provider because they find the discomfort bothersome or possibly because of the sleep onset problems caused by the discomfort. RLS has four principal diagnostic criteria. The first is an urge to move the legs, usually accompanied or caused by an uncomfortable sensation in the legs. The second and third criteria are that this urge begins or worsens during inactivity or rest and is at least partially ameliorated by activity or movement such as stretching or walking. The final criterion is that the urge or sensations are worsened or occur exclusively in the evening or at night. A family history is supportive of the diagnosis. A therapeutic response to levodopa or a dopamine agonist would also be supportive of the diagnosis of RLS.

The physical examination is normal unless it occurs in the setting of an associated medical condition (e.g., peripheral neuropathy). PLMs are triple flexion (hip, knee, ankle) responses of the legs that occur every 10 to 60 seconds during sleep. PLMs are present on PSG in up to 90% of people with RLS. The presence of PLMs would then be supportive of the diagnosis of RLS. PLMs, however, can occur in association with other sleep disorders such as sleep-disordered breathing, narcolepsy, and REM sleep behavior disorder. PLMs can also be seen in patients without sleep disorders and are not labeled as a disorder (PLMD) unless they lead to disturbed sleep. PLMD is probably rare. PSG is useful in assessing for the presence of PLMs but is not necessary for the diagnosis of RLS, which is typically a clinical diagnosis.

RLS must be distinguished from other forms of lower extremity discomfort such as arthritis, neuropathy, and vascular disease. The response of RLS to dopaminergic agents and the irresistible urge to move the legs in RLS can help distinguish it from these other disorders. Leg cramps can be distinguished from RLS in that typical leg cramps involve a specific muscle, which often visibly hardens. Stretching of the specific muscle improves the condition. In patients with suspected RLS, screening for the associated conditions listed previously (e.g., ferritin level, renal function) is prudent.

MANAGEMENT

Mild forms of RLS can potentially be addressed with good sleep hygiene, massage, hot baths, or exercise. If medication is desired, the dopaminergic agents are the best studied and most successful agents.[15] Carbidopa-levodopa was commonly used for this disorder in the past but, because of rebound symptoms and augmentation (appearance of symptoms earlier in the day), it has been largely replaced by the dopamine agonists. In particular the agents pramipexole and ropinirole have been shown to be effective. Alternate therapies include anticonvulsants (gabapentin), opiates, or benzodiazepines (clonazepam). Patients with ferritin levels less than 50 mcg/L may respond to iron replacement. Reduction in the dose or discontinuation of a medication known to cause RLS may also offer relief. PLMs as part of RLS or PLMD are often treated with the same medications as RLS alone.

PARASOMNIAS

DEFINITION AND EPIDEMIOLOGY

Parasomnias, as defined by the ICSD, are undesirable physical events or experiences that occur during entry into sleep, within sleep, or during arousals from sleep.[1] The pathophysiology of this heterogeneous group of disorders is variable and depends in part on which stage of sleep they arise from. In the case of disorders of arousal from NREM sleep (e.g., sleepwalking, sleep terrors, confusional arousals), the mechanism is an abrupt and abnormal arousal from delta (stage 3/4) sleep. Any factor that increases delta sleep or leads to fragmentation of delta sleep could predispose the person to this group of disorders, although genetic predisposition may be an important factor for many affected individuals.

This group of disorders most often occurs in children but can occur in adults. In contrast, one REM-sleep parasomnia (REM sleep behavior disorder [RBD]) results from the loss of normal REM muscle atonia, typically in men over the age of 50. In this disorder the patient enacts dreams, often in a potentially dangerous fashion. Nightmares are terrifying dreams that are common on an occasional basis among adults and children. When such dreams are frequent and disturbing, nightmare disorder, another REM-sleep parasomnia, should be considered. Nightmare disorder may result from psychologic factors, inherited factors, prior sleep deprivation, or the use or withdrawal of certain medications. Specifically the cessation of most types of antidepressant medications will predispose the patient to a transient increase in nightmares. Nightmares are especially common in posttraumatic stress disorder patients.

CLINICAL PRESENTATION AND DIAGNOSTICS

Patients may be initially seen with a chief complaint of disturbing behaviors during sleep. A careful history is helpful in distinguishing NREM from REM parasomnias. The disorders of arousal from NREM sleep (confusional arousals, sleep walking, sleep terrors) arise from slow wave sleep, which occurs primarily in the first third of night. The patient usually is amnestic for the event, so a description of the events from an observer is helpful. Confusional arousals consist of mental confusion or confusional behavior precipitated by an arousal from sleep. In adults this disorder may occur in association with a disorder that increases sleep drive while simultaneously promoting repetitive arousal (e.g., sleep apnea).

Sleep terrors consist of episodes in which the patient sits up and screams with a terrified expression. There are accompanying signs of autonomic arousal (mydriasis, tachypnea, tachycaradia). Patients will be amnestic or recall an image but not a complex dream as would be the case with a nightmare. The episodes last 30 seconds to 3 minutes. There may be associated psychopathology in adults with this disorder.

Sleepwalking (somnambulism) consists of walking and automatic behaviors without awakening, usually for less than 5 minutes. Complex behaviors such as eating or driving may occur. The subject may be violent, particularly if an attempt is made to awaken him or her. A family history of sleepwalking is common.

Disorders of arousal from NREM sleep are typically diagnosed by history. PSG can be helpful in detecting precipitating or associated disorders such as OSA and may also reveal an increase in slow wave sleep percentage. The physical examination is generally unremarkable in these conditions.

In RBD enactment of an often violent dream occurs. The patient and bed partner are at risk for injury during these events. Unlike the disorders of arousal in NREM sleep, there is typically an associated dream with a coherent story line. During PSG confirmation of this disorder, the muscle tone in REM sleep may be elevated and PLMs may be observed. Although RBD is most often idiopathic, it may be associated with other neurologic disorders, making further neurologic assessment in newly diagnosed RBD patients a necessity. The strongest association is with the α-synucleinopathies (Parkinson's disease, dementia with Lewy bodies, and multiple-system atrophy). There may be a latency of years from the development of RBD until the onset of the parkinsonism.

Nightmare disorder is characterized by awakenings from sleep associated with recall of a disturbing dream. Generally the patient is fully alert on awakening with clear recall of the dream. The patient may be so distressed as to have a delay in the return to sleep. Events typically occur in the second half of the night when REM sleep is most common. As one would expect, physical examination is typically normal.

TABLE 19-1 Distinguishing Seizures in NFLE from NREM Parasomnias

	NREM Parasomnia	Seizure in NFLE
Episodes per month	<1 or a few	Usually >10
Episodes per night	1	>1
Type of episode	Nonstereotyped	Stereotyped
Episode duration	Minutes	Seconds

Adapted from Malow BA, Plazzi G: Nocturnal seizures. In Chokroverty S, Hening WA, Walters AS, editors: *Sleep and movement disorders,* Philadelphia, 2003, Butterworth Heinemann.
NFLE, Nocturnal frontal lobe epilepsy; *NREM,* non–rapid eye movement.

Some disorders present during waking hours may also occur during sleep. Up to 50% of patients with panic disorder experience panic attacks at some point in their lifetime that arise out of sleep, typically NREM.[16] Some patients have only sleep-related attacks and never experience daytime panic attacks. Nocturnal seizures are another group of disorders that may arise from sleep. Certain types of nocturnal seizures, especially nocturnal frontal lobe epilepsy (NFLE), may arise exclusively from sleep. The sometimes bizarre nature of seizures in NFLE may make diagnosis a challenge. Clinical features can help distinguish NFLE from NREM parasomnias (Table 19-1), although overnight PSG or video-EEG monitoring is often required.

MANAGEMENT

Many disorders of arousal from NREM sleep do not require pharmacologic treatment. Reassurance of the patient or parents, coupled with attention to safety issues, may be sufficient. Addressing predisposing factors such as sleep deprivation, medications, or stress may be helpful. Benzodiazepines and tricyclic antidepressants have been successfully used in sleepwalking and night terrors. Sedating medications, however, may also precipitate confusional arousals, making it more difficult for the patient to awaken. RBD responds to clonazepam in 90% of cases.[17] Dosing is begun at 0.5 mg at bedtime and is titrated upward as needed, generally to a maximum dose of 2 mg at bedtime. Alternatives to clonazepam include melatonin (3 to 12 mg at bedtime), pramipexole, and levodopa. Nightmare disorder may respond to cognitive behavioral therapies such as systematic desensitization, relaxation techniques, imagery rehearsal, and hypnosis among others.[18]

DIFFERENTIAL DIAGNOSIS

Parasomnias

Arousals secondary to sleep fragmentation from sleep apnea, gastroesophageal reflux disease, or other factors
- Confusional arousals
- Sleepwalking
- Sleep terrors
- Posttraumatic stress disorder
- Nightmares
- Rapid eye movement sleep behavior disorder
- Dissociative disorder
- Nocturnal panic attacks
- Nocturnal seizures
- Other

REFERENCES

1. American Academy of Sleep Medicine: *International classification of sleep disorders,* ed 2, Westchester, Ill, 2005, The Academy.
2. Sheldon S: *Pediatric sleep medicine,* Philadelphia, 1992, Saunders.
3. Borbely AA: A two-process model of sleep regulation, *Hum Neurobiol* 1:195-204, 1982.
4. Sateia MJ: Epidemiology, consequences and evaluation of insomnia. In Lee-Chiong TL, Sateia MJ, Carskadon MA, editors: *Sleep medicine,* Philadelphia, 2002, Hanley & Belfus.
5. Spielman AJ, Caruso LS, Glovinsky PB: A behavioral perspective on insomnia treatment, *Psychiatr Clin North Am* 10(4):541-553, 1987.
6. Sateia MJ, Nowell PN: Insomnia, *Lancet* 364:1959-1973, 2004.
7. Krystal A, Walsh J, Laska E, and others: Sustained efficacy of eszopiclone over 6 months of nightly treatment: results of a randomized, double-blind, placebo-controlled study in adults with chronic insomnia, *Sleep* 26(7):793-799, 2003.
8. Morin CM, Hauri PJ, Espie CA, and others: Nonpharmacologic treatment of chronic insomnia: an American Academy of Sleep Medicine review, *Sleep* 22(8):1134-1156, 1999.
9. Young T, Peppard PE, Gottlieb DJ: Epidemiology of obstructive sleep apnea: a population health perspective, *Am J Respir Crit Care Med* 165(9):1217-1239, 2002.
10. Guilleminault C, Stoohs R, Clerk K, and others: A cause of excessive daytime sleepiness: the upper airway resistance syndrome, *Chest* 104:781-787, 1993.
11. Narkiewicz K, Wolf J, Lopez-Jimenez F, and others: Obstructive sleep apnea and hypertension, *Curr Cardiol Rep* 7(6):435-440, 2005.
12. Thorpy MJ: Obstructive sleep apnea syndrome is a risk factor for stroke, *Curr Neurol Neurosci Rep* 6(2):147-148, 2006.
13. Chesson AL, Berry RB, Pack A: Practice parameters for the use of portable monitoring devices in the investigation of suspected obstructive sleep apnea in adults, *Sleep* 26(7):907-913, 2003.
14. Arand D, Bonnet M, Hurwitz T, and others: The clinical use of the MSLT and MWT, *Sleep* 28(1):123-144, 2005.
15. Montplaisir J, Allen R, Walters A, and others: Restless legs syndrome and periodic limb movement disorder. In Kryger MH, Roth T, Dement WC, editors: *Principles and practice of sleep medicine,* ed 4, Philadelphia, 2005, Saunders.
16. Stein MB, Mellman TA: Anxiety disorders. In Kryger MH, Roth T, Dement WC, editors: *Principles and practice of sleep medicine,* ed 4, Philadelphia, 2005, Saunders.
17. Mahowald MW, Schenck CH: REM sleep parasomnias. In Kryger MH, Roth T, Dement WC, editors: *Principles and practice of sleep medicine,* ed 4, Philadelphia, 2005, Saunders.
18. Krakow B, Kellner R, Pathak D, and others: Imagery rehearsal treatment for chronic nightmares, *Behav Res Ther* 7:837-843, 1995.

PART 3

Health Maintenance

JOANN TRYBULSKI, *Section Editor*

CHAPTER 20

Screening for Cancer

Cynthia Erskine Bashaw

DEFINITION AND EPIDEMIOLOGY

Cancer is the second most common cause of death in the United States, accounting for 1 in every 4 deaths.[1] Regular screening can result in the detection of certain precancerous tissue changes and certain cancers at earlier stages, when treatment is more likely to be successful. Screening has been shown to reduce mortality for cancers of the breast, cervix, colon, and rectum.[2] Although the evidence is less certain, there are other cancers, most notably cancer of the prostate, for which screening may be associated with lower mortality rates.[2]

A cancer-related check-up is ideally incorporated into the periodic health visit; however, since many individuals do not schedule routine examinations, it is incumbent on the health care provider to address cancer-related screening issues during visits for other reasons. A thorough cancer-related check-up includes a complete history to screen for risk factors and early symptoms of disease and a thorough physical examination. Inspection of the skin, oral cavity, breasts, external genitals, and cervix is generally recommended, as is palpation of the breasts, oral cavity, thyroid, rectum, prostate, testes, ovaries, uterus, and lymph nodes. Health counseling regarding tobacco, sun exposure, diet and nutrition, risk factors, sexual practices, and environmental and occupational exposures should be incorporated into this visit.[2,3]

Specific screening guidelines exist for several cancers. *Screening* is defined as a means of accomplishing early detection of disease in asymptomatic people. Screening tests and procedures are usually not diagnostic but serve to sort out persons who are under suspicion for the presence of cancer from those who are not. Screening guidelines are developed in accordance with two requirements: (1) evidence that a test or procedure will detect cancer earlier than if the cancer were detected as a result of the development of symptoms, and (2) evidence that treatment at an earlier stage of the disease will result in an improved outcome.[4] See Table 20-1 for screening guidelines from the American Cancer Society (ACS).

The following review of current cancer screening recommendations includes a discussion of risk factors for each disorder. Individuals at high risk for a particular disease may require a more aggressive screening approach than is recommended by the existing guidelines that have been developed for the general population.

BREAST CANCER

Breast cancer is the most commonly diagnosed noncutaneous cancer in women and is second only to lung cancer as a cause of cancer deaths in women.[1,5] It is one of the few cancers for which the benefits of screening (namely, mammography) have been unequivocally demonstrated. Tumors of the breast typically metastasize late in the preclinical course or before reaching clinically detectable size. Early detection in the preclinical phase (before metastasis) is possible with mammography, which can detect tumors as small as 1 mm.[6] Numerous large-scale randomized clinical trials have shown reductions in breast cancer mortality with regular mammography, and its value as a screening tool is widely accepted.[5,7-10] Overall, screening mammography detects 80% to 90% of breast cancers.[5]

Specific recommendations for breast cancer screening vary somewhat from organization to organization; however, all advocate for some form of regular screening inclusive of mammography. The ACS has been steadfast since 1997 in its recommendation for annual screening mammography for all women beginning at age 40.[11] The U.S. Preventive Services Task Force (USPSTF) notes strong support in the research for its recommendation for screening mammography every 1 to 2 years for women over age 40. The rationale for this recommendation notes that the strongest evidence for reduction in mortality occurs in the 50- to 69-year age range, with a smaller absolute benefit being seen in the 40- to 49-year age range because of the lower incidence of the disease in this group.[9] Neither the ACS nor the USPSTF specifies an age for cessation of screening in women whose life expectancy is not compromised by co-morbid disease.[5,9] Although the benefit of screening mammography is less clear and less well studied in women over 70 years, it must be remembered that the annual risk of a 70-year-old being diagnosed with breast cancer is three times that of a 40-year-old and that she has a five times greater annual risk of dying from breast cancer.[8-10]

In addition to screening mammography, the ACS recommends that clinical breast examinations (CBEs) be included as part of the periodic health examination every 3 years for women in their twenties to thirties and annually for women 40 or older. CBE is recommended as a complement to mammography that may contribute to earlier detection for the small percentage of breast cancers that are not detected by mammography. It is recommended that the CBE occur shortly before the mammogram.[5] The USPSTF found insufficient evidence in the research to recommend for or against the use of CBE and simply recommends a mammogram every 1 to 2 years either with or without CBE beginning at age 40.[9]

Neither the ACS nor the USPSTF recommends breast self-examination (BSE) as part of breast cancer screening. The ACS dropped its recommendation for monthly BSE, leaving it as an option, but noting that the research has determined "self-awareness" is more effective than a structured examination. The ACS notes that most women who find lumps do so while going about daily activities such as dressing or showering. An awareness of the appearance and feel of the breasts is encouraged, as is prompt reporting of any changes or concerns.[5] The USPSTF did not find sufficient evidence to recommend for or against teaching BSE, noting poor evidence that it influences mortality from breast cancer and in fact finding fair evidence that it was associated an increased risk of false-positive results and unnecessary biopsies.[9]

Modalities are emerging that hold promise in the early detection of breast cancer. Mammography is being improved by the use of computer-assisted diagnosis from digital images in addition to human interpretation of x-ray films.[5] A recent National Cancer Institute trial comparing digital to film

TABLE 20-1 Screening Guidelines for the Early Detection of Cancer in Asymptomatic People

Site	Recommendation
Breast	Yearly mammograms are recommended starting at age 40. The age at which screening should be stopped should be individualized by considering the potential risks and benefits of screening in the context of the overall health status and longevity. Clinical breast examination should be part of a periodic health examination, about every 3 years for women in their 20s and 30s and every year for women 40 and over. Women should know how their breasts normally feel and report any breast change promptly to their health care providers. Breast self-examination is an option for women starting in their 20s. Women at increased risk (e.g., family history, genetic tendency, past breast cancer) should talk with their doctors about the benefits and limitations of starting mammography screening earlier, having additional tests (i.e., breast ultrasound or MRI), or having more frequent examinations.
Colon and rectum	Beginning at age 50, men and women should begin screening with one of the examination schedules below: • A fecal occult blood test (FOBT) or fecal immunochemical test (FIT) every year • A flexible sigmoidoscopy (FSIG) every 5 years • Annual FOBT or FIT and flexible sigmoidoscopy every 5 years* • A double-contrast barium enema every 5 years • A colonoscopy every 10 years
Prostate	The prostate-specific antigen (PSA) test and the digital rectal examination should be offered annually, beginning at age 50, to men who have a life expectancy of at least 10 years. Men at high risk (African American men and men with a strong family history of one or more first-degree relatives diagnosed with prostate cancer at an early age) should begin testing at age 45. For both men of average risk and men at high risk, information should be provided about what is known and what is uncertain about the benefits and limitations of early detection and treatment of prostate cancer so that they can make an informed decision about testing.
Uterus	**Cervix:** Screening should begin approximately 3 years after a woman begins having vaginal intercourse, but no later than 21 years of age. Screening should be done every year with regular Pap tests or every 2 years using liquid-based tests. At or after age 30, women who have had three normal Pap test results in a row may get screened every 2 to 3 years. Alternatively, cervical cancer screening with human papillomavirus DNA testing and conventional or liquid-based cytology could be performed every 3 years. However, doctors may suggest a woman get screened more often if she has certain risk factors, such as HIV infection or a weak immune system. Women 70 years and older who have had 3 or more consecutive normal Pap tests in the last 10 years may choose to stop having cervical cancer screening. Screening after total hysterectomy (with removal of the cervix) is not necessary unless the surgery was done as a treatment for cervical cancer. **Endometrium:** The American Cancer Society recommends that at the time of menopause, all women should be informed about the risks and symptoms of endometrial cancer and strongly encouraged to report any unexpected bleeding or spotting to their physicians. Annual screening for endometrial cancer with endometrial biopsy beginning at age 35 should be offered to women with or at risk for hereditary nonpolyposis colon cancer (HNPCC).
Cancer-related check-up	For individuals undergoing periodic health examinations, a cancer-related check-up should include health counseling and, depending on a person's age and gender, might include examinations for cancers of the thyroid, oral cavity, skin, lymph nodes, testes, and ovaries, as well as for some nonmalignant diseases.

American Cancer Society guidelines for early cancer detection are assessed annually in order to identify whether there is new scientific evidence sufficient to warrant a reevaluation of current recommendations. If evidence is sufficiently compelling to consider a change or clarification in a current guideline or the development of a new guideline, a formal procedure is initiated. Guidelines are formally evaluated every 5 years regardless of whether new evidence suggests a change in the existing recommendations. There are 9 steps in this procedure, and these "guidelines for guideline development" were formally established to provide a specific methodology for science and expert judgment to form the underpinnings of specific statements and recommendations from the Society. These procedures also constitute a deliberate process to ensure that all Society recommendations have the same methodological and evidence-based process at their core. This process also employs a system for rating strength and consistency of evidence that is similar to that employed by the Agency for Healthcare Research and Quality (AHRQ) and the U.S. Preventive Services Task Force (USPSTF).

From American Cancer Society: *Cancer prevention and early detection facts and figures 2005,* Atlanta, 2005, The Society, p 36, retrieved from http://www.cancer.org/downloads/STT/CPED2005v5PWSecured.pdf.

*Combined testing is preferred over either annual FOBT or FIT, or FSIG every 5 years, alone. People who are at moderate or high risk for colorectal cancer should talk with a doctor about a different testing schedule.

mammography demonstrated no difference in the general population, but suggested benefits of digital over film for women under the age of 50, premenopausal and perimenopausal women, and women with radiographically dense breasts.[12] Ultrasound is also being used increasingly as an adjunct to mammography to find tumors in women with dense breast tissue. Also, MRI screening is being used increasingly for women at high risk for developing breast cancer (those with genetic predisposition), since it has been shown to find more cancers than standard mammograms. Whether this difference is great enough to save additional lives has yet to be demonstrated.[5]

In assessing risk factors for breast cancer, it is important to recognize that approximately 75% of breast cancers occur in women without known risk factors aside from age and gender.[10] The risk is known to be higher for women who have a personal or family history of breast cancer, biopsy-confirmed atypical hyperplasia, early menarche and/or late menopause, nulliparity or history of first child after age 30, obesity after menopause, postmenopausal hormone replacement, or excessive alcohol consumption.[5] Possible links to breast density and physical inactivity are under study. Research regarding *BRCA1* and *BRCA2* susceptibility genes is ongoing. General screening of the population for these genes is not recommended.[5] Only 5% of breast cancers are related to these genes.[13] Those at high risk, particularly those with a strong multigenerational family history of breast cancer, may warrant an individualized plan of screening and follow-up monitoring.

COLORECTAL CANCER

Colorectal cancer is the third most commonly diagnosed cancer and the second leading cause of cancer death in the United States.[14] When cancer of this type is confined to the colon-rectum, the 5-year survival rate is 90%. The 5-year survival rate falls to 65% when the cancer spreads to surrounding tissue and to 10% with distant spread.[14] The tragedy of these figures is that only 39% of colorectal cancers are diagnosed in the localized stage. This is due in large part to the fact that screening rates remain low. Despite nearly universal agreement that persons 50 years of age and older should be screened for colon cancer, the ACS reports that fewer than 50% of those ages 50 and older have had a recent test.[14] Beyond the benefits of early detection, screening actually results in the prevention of many cases of colorectal cancer in that it detects adenomatous polyps, benign growths from which the majority of colon cancers arise. These polyps are usually present for several years before their evolution to cancer. With proper screening they are often detected and can be removed before becoming cancerous.[14]

ACS screening guidelines recommend that all men and women of average risk have one of the following beginning at age 50 years: (1) annual fecal occult blood test (FOBT) or fecal immunochemical test (FIT) every year, (2) flexible sigmoidoscopy every 5 years, (3) FOBT or FIT every year and flexible sigmoidoscopy every 5 years, (4) double-contrast barium enema (DCBE) every 5 years, or (5) colonoscopy every 10 years.[14] The digital rectal examination (DRE) and office-based single-specimen testing for fecal occult blood is not a recommended option for colon cancer screening.[14,15] The USPSTF also strongly recommends that providers screen patients for colorectal cancer starting at age 50 years. The recommendation reviews the various screening options and recommends screening intervals for the various methods similar to those of the ACS.[15]

The choice among the recommended options is made on an individual basis with an eye toward enhancing compliance. Each method has its benefits and drawbacks. Generally the choice is made jointly between the provider and the patient with individual variables, such as patient preference, taken into consideration. As the discussion continues and research continues to emerge regarding which screening method is optimum, it is important for the provider to recognize that getting the patient screened is more important than which method is used.

FOBT is accomplished via the collection and testing of six samples from three consecutive stools and has been shown to decrease the risk of death from colon cancer by 15% to 33%.[14] FOBT is low cost, can be done at home, involves no bowel preparation, and does not carry the risk of bowel tears or infections. However, it requires annual commitment and the inconvenience of eliminating aspirin and NSAIDs, red meat, vitamin C, and citrus juices several days before the test, making compliance issues a consideration. Additionally, with the exception of large bleeding polyps, it has limited value in the detection of adenomatous polyps. A positive test should be followed up with a colonoscopy.[14-16]

Flexible sigmoidoscopy, when performed every 5 years, also shows a significant reduction in mortality. Although it allows for visualization of only the distal third of the colon, it identifies 70% to 80% of people who have significant neoplasms in the colon when positive findings are followed up with a colonoscopy.[14,15] The procedure can be done in the office without sedation, involves minimum bowel preparation, typically causes only mild abdominal discomfort, and can be completed in 10 to 15 minutes. The main drawback is that positive findings must be followed up by colonoscopy. The procedure also carries a small risk of bowel tears or bleeding.[14-16] It is more costly than FOBT but less so than DCBE or colonoscopy.[14]

The ACS prefers the combination of the annual FOBT and the every-5-year sigmoidoscopy over either FOBT or sigmoidoscopy alone. Combined testing is better than one or the other alone. FOBT potentially detects blood from lesions anywhere in the colon, including areas that are beyond the reach of the sigmoidoscope, whereas sigmoidoscopy is superior for detecting lesions in the distal colon and for detecting nonbleeding lesions.[2,14]

Colonoscopy is considered the definitive test for colon cancer screening, since it is the most sensitive and specific in the detection of both colon cancer and adenomatous polyps.[14,16] It is estimated that periodic colonoscopy could prevent 76% to 90% of colon cancers.[14] It allows for direct visualization of the entire colon and for screening, diagnosis, and polyp removal in a single visit. Provided there are no positive findings, the interval for screening by colonoscopy for those at average risk is every 10 years. Drawbacks include the need for a full bowel preparation, the necessity of sedation and all its inherent risks, often a lost day of work, and the potential for bowel tears and infections. It is also expensive and requires a skilled examiner.[14-16]

The DCBE is an alternative method of examining the entire colon. It is less costly than colonoscopy, but still expensive. Like colonoscopy it requires a full bowel preparation; however, it does not require sedation. It is less effective in detecting polyps and cancers than the colonoscopy; hence the recommendation of the shorter 5-year interval for screening. Another drawback is that, unlike colonoscopy, it does not allow for excision of suspicious areas during the same procedure. Positive findings must be followed up with a colonoscopy.[14-16]

CT-assisted colonography (virtual colonoscopy) and molecular screening of stool DNA are methods being evaluated as potential screening tools. CT-assisted colonography involves a full bowel preparation and the insufflation of the colon with air. The colon is then scanned as the patient assumes different positions. Positive findings need to be followed up with colonoscopy. Molecular screening of stool DNA is a new noninvasive method of extracting colorectal epithelial DNA from stool samples to detect neoplasia. These methods hold promise for the future; however, currently there are insufficient studies to evaluate their effectiveness in reducing colorectal cancer mortality.[14-16]

Special attention needs to be given to individuals who are at higher than average risk for developing colon cancer, since different screening recommendations apply. Individuals are classified as having an elevated risk of developing colorectal cancer if they have a history of one or more first-degree relatives (sibling, parent, child) with colon cancer or adenomatous polyps, particularly before the age of 60; a personal history of adenomatous polyps or colon cancer; a history of inflammatory bowel disease; or a family history of a hereditary colorectal cancer syndrome.[14,16] People in this category of risk should consult with a gastroenterologist and begin screening earlier or undergo screening more often; also, for persons with this degree of risk, colonoscopy is typically the preferred screening modality. Other risk factors include age (90% are more than 50 years of age); high-fat, low-fiber diet; and physical inactivity.[14] It is important to recognize, however, that 80% to 85% of all colorectal cancers occur among people with no increased risk except for age.[14,16]

CERVICAL CANCER

The 2006 estimates for cervical cancer predicted that 9710 new cases of invasive cervical cancer would be diagnosed and that approximately 3500 women would die of the disease.[1,17] Between 1955 and 1992 the number of cervical cancer deaths in the United States dropped by 74%, primarily because of the increased use of the Papanicolaou (Pap) test, which detects precancerous lesions and early cervical cancers at a treatable stage. The death rate from cervical cancer continues to fall by nearly 4% per year.[17] The 5-year survival rate nears 100% for those with preinvasive lesions and 92% for those with early invasive cervical cancer.[17,18] In addition, cervical cancer has a long lead time and progresses through a series of identifiable, premalignant stages before becoming invasive. Detection of these precancerous changes allows for a variety of treatment options when the disorder is almost certainly curable, thereby decreasing not only mortality from cervical cancer but also its incidence.[18]

Major revisions to cervical cancer screening recommendations were issued in 2002 and 2003. Recommendations by the ACS, the USPSTF, and the American College of Obstetricians and Gynecologists (ACOG) have all been changed to reflect an improved understanding of the role of the human papillomavirus (HPV) relative to cervical cancer causation, and to incorporate new technologies such as the liquid-based Pap test and HPV testing. Each of the previously mentioned organizations now recommends that screening with a Pap test begin approximately 3 years after first sexual intercourse or by age 21, whichever comes first.[18-20] The basis of this recommendation for later initiation of screening is the acknowledgment that cervical cancers and the high-grade squamous intraepithelial lesions that precede them are related almost entirely to certain high-risk types of HPV that are acquired during vaginal intercourse; lesions do not occur until 3 to 5 years after exposure.[18-20]

Recommendations for the intervals at which Pap testing should occur vary somewhat and incorporate issues related to the prevalence of HPV in different age-groups and also those related to liquid-based cytology and HPV testing. Women under 30 years of age have a higher likelihood than older women of acquiring high-risk types of HPV that cause premalignant cervical changes and cervical cancer.[18,20] The ACS and ACOG acknowledge this fact by recommending more frequent Pap testing for those under age 30 than for those ages 30 and over. Changes also reflect the newly available testing. Liquid-based cytology may be more sensitive than the conventional Pap test, and the ACS allows for lengthening the screening interval when this type of test is used.[18] Additionally, it is now possible to test directly for HPV DNA at the time of the Pap test. Both the ACS and ACOG support the option of lengthening the screening interval when both the Pap test and the HPV test are negative.[18,20]

It must be noted, however, that HPV testing is approved only for those over the age of 30. HPV infection is common under the age of 30 and frequently clears on its own, making its significance difficult to interpret.[18,20] Based on this information, the ACS recommends that screening be done annually with regular Pap tests or every 2 years with liquid-based tests until the age of 30. At or after the age of 30, if a woman has had three consecutive negative test results, the interval may be lengthened to every 2 to 3 years. Alternatively, for women over 30, cervical cancer screening with both HPV DNA testing and a Pap test (liquid-based or conventional) may be used at an interval of every 3 years provided both test results are negative. Note that these longer intervals are not appropriate for women with other risk factors such as diethylstilbestrol (DES) exposure, HIV, or other forms of immunocompromise.[18] The ACOG guideline differs only slightly in that it does not recommend lengthening the screening interval from 1 to 2 years when the liquid-based test is used, finding insufficient evidence to support such a change.[20] The USPSTF found insufficient evidence to recommend either for or against the liquid-based test or HPV testing, and simply recommends a Pap test at least every 3 years.[19]

An upper age limit when cervical cancer screening ceases to be effective is not known.[18-20] Currently the ACS suggests that women ages 70 and older who have had three or more consecutive normal Pap tests and who have had no abnormal Pap tests within the previous 10 years may discontinue screening. Note that the incidence of cervical cancer in older women is almost entirely confined to the unscreened and the underscreened; if an older woman has never or not recently been screened, there is clear indication for doing so.[18] The USPSTF likewise notes the low yield of cervical cancer screening in previously screened older women and recommends discontinuing screening after age 65.[19] ACOG does not establish an upper age limit, preferring that the decision to discontinue screening be made individually considering a woman's medical history and risk factors.[20]

Finally, if a woman has had a total hysterectomy for benign reasons and has no history of high-grade lesions, screening with a Pap test is not necessary or recommended.[18-20]

UTERINE CORPUS (ENDOMETRIAL) CANCER

The ACS recommends that at the time of menopause all women should be informed about the risks and symptoms of endometrial cancer and strongly encouraged to report any unexpected bleeding or spotting. Additionally, beginning at age 35, annual screening for endometrial cancer with endometrial biopsy should be offered to women with or at risk for hereditary nonpolyposis colon cancer (HNPCC), a form of colon cancer related to genetic mutation.[2]

Uterine cancer is the most common gynecologic cancer in women in the United States. It was expected that 40,880 cases would be diagnosed in 2005 and that 7310 cases would be fatal.[1] Fortunately, most (77%) of cases are diagnosed early when the disease is highly treatable; the 5-year survival rate for localized disease is 96%.[21] Early diagnosis is typically accomplished based on signs and symptoms, namely, abnormal or postmenopausal uterine bleeding or frequent spotting.[21]

Uterine cancer is uncommon before the age of 40, with a peak incidence between 75 and 79.[21] Other than advancing age, risk factors include unopposed estrogen therapy, obesity, tamoxifen therapy, early menarche, late menopause, late primiparity, polycystic ovarian disease, infertility, and diabetes. A final risk factor, HNPCC or being at risk for this disease, confers special risk.[1,21]

Previously the ACS recommended that all women at increased risk for endometrial cancer be considered for periodic screening with endometrial biopsy beginning at menopause. However, in a change from that recommendation, with the exception of those with or at risk for HNPCC, the ACS no longer recommends screening women at increased risk. As with women at average risk, women at increased risk should be educated about the signs and symptoms of endometrial cancer and encouraged to report them to their health care provider promptly. The rationale is the high percentage of cases that are diagnosed because of an alerting symptom, namely, abnormal uterine bleeding. Women with or at risk for HNPCC based on family history, however, should be offered annual screening with endometrial biopsy beginning at age 35, since they have a 22% to 50% lifetime risk of developing uterine cancer and of having it develop at younger ages.[21]

PROSTATE CANCER

Prostate cancer is the most commonly diagnosed cancer in men; 234,460 new cases were expected in 2006.[1] The only known risk factors are age, family history of the disease, and ethnicity. It is a disease of aging, with more than 70% of cases being diagnosed in men older than 65 years. It is estimated that strong familial predisposition may be responsible for 5% to 10% of prostate cancers. African American men and Jamaican men of African descent have the highest rates of prostate cancer in the world.[1] There is also a possible association of prostate cancer with diets high in fat and with obesity.[1]

Over the past 20 years the 5-year survival rate for all stages combined has increased from 67% to 99%. This dramatic improvement is partly due to improved early diagnosis but also a result of improvements in treatment.[1] However, considerable controversy exists with regard to screening. Both the USPSTF and the ACS find insufficient evidence to recommend for or against screening for prostate cancer using the prostate-specific antigen (PSA) blood test or DRE.[1,22] The ACS, however, notes that evidence supporting screening is stronger now than it has been at any time in the past and incorporates in its recommendation that men in the appropriate age range be offered prostate cancer screening along with information about the benefits and limitations of early detection.[21]

Data on screening are limited and conflicting. Despite good evidence that DRE and the PSA blood test have value for early detection, it is not clear that early detection improves health outcomes.[21,22] Additionally, screening is associated with significant harms. PSA testing is prostate-tissue specific, not prostate-*cancer* specific. Therefore there is no absolute value that is applicable to all men. Elevations may occur in response to other conditions such as benign prostatic hypertrophy or prostatitis. These men may be subjected to further invasive testing unnecessarily.[21] False-positive results may also cause unnecessary anxiety. Furthermore, screening may result in treatment complications for some PSA-detected cancers that are latent or indolent and would have been unlikely to affect survival.[21] Some men, particularly older men, may well have died of other causes before the disease was able to manifest itself.[21]

The normal range of the PSA is also under discussion. Conventionally, "normal" PSA has been considered to be between 0 and 4 ng/dl. Emerging evidence suggests that an upper cutoff of 2.5 ng/dl would improve early detection of organ-confined cancers but would also increase the number of men without disease undergoing biopsy.[21]

In acknowledgment of these issues, the ACS specifies in its guidelines that men should be given information about the benefits and limitations of early detection and screening methods so that an informed choice can be made. The guidelines state that, beginning at age 50 years, men with a life expectancy of at least 10 years should be offered both PSA testing and DRE annually. Men at high risk (African American men and men with a first-degree relative who developed prostate cancer at a young age) should begin testing at age 45.[2] Men who are at even higher risk (multiple first-degree relatives affected at an early age) could begin testing at age 40 and, depending on the results of this initial test (i.e., PSA <1.0 ng/dl), may need no further testing until age 45.[21,23] The ACS further specifies that men who ask their health care provider to make the decision regarding screening on their behalf should be tested. Discouraging testing is not appropriate, nor is not offering testing.[21,23]

On a final note, the PSA test is superior to DRE in the detection of prostate cancer. Nevertheless, DRE should be included in testing whenever appropriate. If DRE is an obstacle to testing, PSA testing alone is an acceptable alternative.[21]

OTHER CANCERS

For persons undergoing periodic heath examinations, the ACS suggests that a cancer-related check-up should include health counseling and, depending on age and gender, might include examinations for cancers of the thyroid, oral cavity, skin, lymph nodes, testes, and ovaries.[2] There are no specific screening recommendations for these cancers.

SUMMARY

Cancer screening is a vital part of ongoing efforts to decrease cancer mortality. Its success depends on awareness and the use of available screening tools by both patients and health care providers. When integrated into a total approach focusing on healthy lifestyles and disease prevention, it has the potential to increase longevity and enhance quality of life.

REFERENCES

1. American Cancer Society: *Cancer facts and figures 2006*, retrieved Dec 11, 2006, from http://www.cancer.org/downloads/STT/CAFF2006PWSecured.pdf.
2. American Cancer Society: *Cancer prevention and early detection, facts and figures 2005*, retrieved Jan 2006 from http://www.cancer.org/docroot/STT/stt_0_2005.asp?sitearea=STT&level=1.
3. American Cancer Society: *Cancer detection guidelines*, retrieved Jan 2006 from http://www.cancer.org/docroot/STT/stt_0_2005.asp?sitearea=STT&level=1.
4. National Cancer Institute: *Cancer screening overview*, retrieved Jan 2006 from http://www.cancer.gov/cancertopics/pdq/screening/overview/healthprofessional.
5. American Cancer Society: *Breast cancer facts and figures 2005-2006*, retrieved Jan 2006 from http://www.cancer.org/docroot/STT/stt_0_2005.asp?sitearea=STT&level=1.
6. Crane R: Breast cancers. In Otto S: *Oncology nursing*, St Louis, 1997, Mosby.
7. Smart CR, Bryne C, Smith RA, and others: Twenty-year follow-up of the breast cancers diagnosed during the breast cancer detection demonstration project, *CA Cancer J Clin* 47(3):134-149, 1997.
8. National Cancer Institute: *Breast cancer: screening and testing*, retrieved Jan 2006 from http://www.cancer.gov/cancertopics/pdq/screening/breast/healthprofessional.
9. US Preventive Services Task Force: *Screening for breast cancer*, retrieved Jan 2006 from http://www.ahrq.gov/clinic/3rduspstf/breastcancer/brcanrr.htm.
10. Lippman ME: Breast cancer. In Braunwald E, Fauci AS, Kasper DL, and others: *Harrison's principles of internal medicine*, ed 15, New York, 2001, McGraw-Hill.
11. American Cancer Society: *Chronological history of ACS recommendations on early detection of cancer*, retrieved Jan 2006 from http://www.cancer.org/docroot/PED/content/PED_2_3X_Chronological_History_of_ACS_Recommendations_on_Early_Detection_of_Cancer.asp?sitearea=PED.
12. National Cancer Institute: *Digital mammography trial results announced: women with dense breasts, women younger than 50, and those who are perimenopausal may benefit from digital mammograms*, retrieved Jan 2006 from http://www.cancer.gov/newscenter/pressreleases/DMISTrelease.
13. National Cancer Institute: *Genetics of breast and ovarian cancer*, retrieved Jan 2006 from http://www.cancer.gov/cancertopics/pdq/genetics/breast-and-ovarian/healthprofessional.
14. American Cancer Society: *Colorectal cancer facts and figures: special edition 2005*, retrieved Jan 2006 from http://www.cancer.org/docroot/STT/stt_0_2005.asp?sitearea=STT&level=1.
15. US Preventive Services Task Force: *Screening for colon cancer*, retrieved Jan 2006 from http://www.ahrq.gov/clinic/3rduspstf/colorectal/colorr.htm.
16. Cahill BA: Colorectal cancer: which test is best? *Adv Nurse Pract* 13(1):71-74, 2005.
17. American Cancer Society: *What are the key statistics about cervical cancer?* retrieved Jan 20006 from http://www.cancer.org/docroot/CRI/content/CRI_2_4_1X_What_are_the_key_statistics_for_cervical_cancer_8.asp?sitearea=.
18. Saslow D, Runowicz CD, Solomon D, and others: American Cancer Society guideline for the early detection of cervical neoplasia and cancer, *CA Cancer J Clin* 52:342, 2002; retrieved Jan 2006 from http://caonline.amcancersoc.org/cgi/content/full/52/6/342?maxtoshow=&HITS=10&hits=10&RESULTFORMAT=&fulltext=saslow&searchid=1&FIRSTINDEX=0&resourcetype=HWCIT.
19. US Preventive Services Task Force: *Screening for cervical cancer*, retrieved Jan 2006 from http://www.ahrq.gov/clinic/3rduspstf/cervcan/cervcanrr.htm.
20. American College of Obstetricians and Gynecologists: *Cervical cancer screening: testing can start later and occur less often under new ACOG recommendations*, retrieved Jan 2006 from http://www.acog.org/from_home/publications/press_releases/nr07-31-03-1.cfm.
21. Smith RA, von Eschenbach AC, Wender R, and others: American Cancer Society Guidelines for the early detection of cancer: update of early detection guidelines for prostate, colorectal, and endometrial cancers, *CA Cancer J Clin* 51:38-75, 2001; retrieved Jan 2006 from http://caonline.amcancersoc.org/cgi/content/full/51/1/38?maxtoshow=&HITS=10&hits=10&RESULTFORMAT=&fulltext=smith%2C+RA&searchid=1&FIRSTINDEX=0&resourcetype=HWCIT.
22. US Preventive Services Task Force: *Screening for prostate cancer*, retrieved Jan 2006 from http://www.ahrq.gov/clinic/3rduspstf/prostatescr/prostaterr.htm#clinical.
23. American Cancer Society: *ACS cancer detection guidelines*, retrieved Jan 2006 from http://www.cancer.org/docroot/PED/content/PED_2_3X_ACS_Cancer_Detection_Guidelines_36.asp?sitearea=PED.

CHAPTER 21

Screening for Sexually Transmitted Diseases

Marilyn Bleiler Green

DEFINITION AND EPIDEMIOLOGY

The term *sexually transmitted disease* (STD) includes the more than 25 diseases that are spread through sexual contact. In the United States the most common STDs include chlamydia, gonorrhea, syphilis, genital herpes, human papillomavirus (HPV), and hepatitis B.

Despite efforts to promote safer sex practices, STDs—often referred to as the "hidden epidemic"[1]—continue to afflict a large number of people in the United States and remain a public health challenge. The Centers for Disease Control and Prevention (CDC) estimate that more than 65 million people in the United States are currently living with an incurable STD. An additional 19 million people will become infected each year, and of these about half will develop a lifelong infection. Almost half of these infections occur in people ages 15 to 24.[2]

Efforts to curb and prevent the acquisition and spread of STDs include screening certain higher-risk populations. A group is classified as high risk based on age, gender, sexual practices, locale, and other social behaviors or practices that place them at risk for acquiring an STD. This chapter reviews the screening recommendations for selected, commonly screened STDs based on recommendations from the CDC and the third report of the U.S. Preventive Services Task Force (USPSTF).[3,4]

The goal of screening for disease is early detection of a condition to reduce morbidity and mortality. The value of screening asymptomatic persons must take into consideration the benefits, risks, costs, and effectiveness of screening practices. Effectiveness is determined in part by the characteristics of the screening test; the ease and skill required to perform the test or collect the specimen; and the characteristics of the target population, including age and gender. The USPSTF has developed evidence-based recommendations for a number of diseases. The CDC is continually revising its recommendation for the prevention, detection, and treatment of STDs. The guidelines in this chapter are based on the recommendations of both groups.

CHLAMYDIA

Chlamydia is an STD caused by an intracellular, parasitic organism, *Chlamydia trachomatis*. Currently *C. trachomatis* has at least 15 recognized serotypes. Clinical syndromes associated with certain *C. trachomatis* serotypes include nongonococcal urethritis (NGU), mucopurulent cervicitis, pelvic inflammatory disease (PID), lymphogranuloma venereum, acute urethral syndrome in female patients, ocular infections, proctocolitis, epididymitis, and Reiter's syndrome in adults. *C. trachomatis* may be acquired by infants through an infected birth canal, causing pneumonia and conjunctivitis in newborns.[5]

Chlamydia is the most commonly reported infectious disease in the United States. Each year, an estimated 3 million new cases of genital infection caused by *C. trachomatis* occur in the United States at a cost of $2.4 billion.[1,3] Chlamydial infection is especially prevalent among adolescents, especially girls. In the past 2 decades, genital chlamydial infection has been identified as a major public health problem because of its association with several disease syndromes, including NGU, mucopurulent cervicitis, and PID.[5,6] Up to 40% of women with untreated chlamydia will develop PID, infertility, and tubal pregnancy. Although the disease may be asymptomatic in women, chlamydia causes a painful genital infection in men. Moreover, chlamydia increases the risk for HIV infection in both men and women. In addition, infants born to women with chlamydia can develop eye infections and pneumonia. From 2003 to 2004 there was a 5.9% increase in the number of reported cases of chlamydia. This may be due in part to increased screening and the advances in diagnostic tests that allow for coupling the liquid-based Papanicolaou (Pap) test with a test for chlamydia and the availability of urine tests for chlamydia.[3]

The third USPSTF report recommends routine screening for chlamydia in all sexually active women ages 25 years and younger and in all women who may be otherwise at risk, whether or not they are pregnant.[3] Evidence suggests that the cost of screening women who are at risk for chlamydia may be less than the cost of treating chlamydia and its complications. Screening patients at greatest risk is more cost-effective than screening all patients. There is no recommendation for or against screening for asymptomatic women ages 26 years and older who are at low risk for infection. There is some evidence that routine screening may be beneficial for all asymptomatic pregnant women ages 25 years or younger and other pregnant women at increased risk for infection. If screened, pregnant women should be screened for chlamydia during their third trimester. There is unclear or insufficient evidence for or against routine screening of asymptomatic men.[3,4]

An age of 25 years or younger is the strongest risk factor for chlamydial infection.[4] Other risk factors include having more than one sexual partner, history of a prior STD, and inconsistent or incorrect condom use. The greatest risk for women is not knowing that chlamydial infection is present. Chlamydia may be asymptomatic, but the infection still produces damage.[4]

GONORRHEA

Gonorrhea is the second most commonly reported infectious disease in the United States.[7] It primarily involves mucocutaneous surfaces of the genitourinary tract, pharynx, conjunctiva, and anus. In men it is often characterized by a purulent urethral discharge, whereas in up to 80% of women it is asymptomatic. Gonorrhea rates fell to 113.5 per 100,000 in 2004, representing a 76% decline since reporting began in 1946.[2] Like chlamydia, gonorrhea is often undiagnosed and underreported. Populations at risk for gonorrhea include young, sexually active individuals and other individuals who engage in high-risk behaviors such as illegal drug use or prostitution. African American men remain the group most affected. Recently, researchers have seen indications that gonorrhea may be on the increase among gay and bisexual men. Up to 50% of persons with gonorrhea have a coexistent chlamydial infection.[2,7]

Testing for gonorrhea includes the nucleic acid amplification test on endocervical swab and urine, as well as culture. Gonorrhea, like chlamydia that is present in the cervix or urethra, can be tested with a urine specimen.[8] Testing is also possible by coupling the test for gonorrhea (and chlamydia) with liquid-based cervical cytology.

There is unclear or insufficient evidence to recommend for or against routine screening of asymptomatic high-risk men; however, testing may be indicated on other grounds.

There is fair evidence to recommend routine screening for gonorrhea for high-risk, asymptomatic women and pregnant women. A test for gonorrhea should be performed during the first prenatal visit for women who are at risk or are living in an area in which the prevalence of gonorrhea is high. After delivery, there is clear evidence to recommend routine ophthalmic antibiotic in newborns.[3]

SYPHILIS

Syphilis is a complex systemic STD caused by *Treponema pallidum*. Syphilis has been classified by the CDC into several stages depending on the length of infection. Patients may be seen with signs and symptoms of primary infection (ulcer or chancre at the infection site; see Color Plate 6), secondary infection (rash, mucocutaneous lesions, and adenopathy), or tertiary infection (cardiac, neurologic, ophthalmic, auditory, or gummatous lesions).[9]

The signs of primary and secondary syphilis may resolve spontaneously even without treatment. The patient then enters the latent stage of the disease, in which there are generally no clinical signs or symptoms of infection and diagnosis is made on the basis of serology. Tertiary syphilis is manifested after a variable period of latency in approximately one third of patients who fail to receive treatment. Late-stage syphilis may occur 10 to 20 years after initial infection. It may present as gummatous disease (rubbery lumps or lesions found in subcutaneous tissue), cardiovascular disease, or, in one third of untreated patients, neurosyphilis. However, neurosyphilis can occur in all stages of syphilis. The diagnosis of neurosyphilis is based on clinical findings and examination of the serum and cerebrospinal fluid.[9]

The latent stage of syphilis is dangerous for pregnant women. Even though she may not have symptoms, a pregnant woman with latent disease can infect her fetus.[10]

Dark-field examinations and direct fluorescent antibody tests of lesion exudate or tissue are the definitive methods for diagnosing early syphilis. Serologic nontreponemal tests (e.g., Venereal Disease Research Laboratory [VDRL] or rapid plasma reagin [RPR]) and treponemal tests (e.g., fluorescent treponemal antibody absorbed [FTA-ABS] or microhemagglutination assay for antibody to *T. pallidum* [MHA-TP]) are tests performed to establish a diagnosis. The use of one test alone is not sufficient. A nontreponemal test may be used as the initial screening test. These tests correlate with disease activity and are reported quantitatively. However, false-positive nontreponemal test results are associated with hepatitis, viral pneumonia, pregnancy, infectious mononucleosis, and other viral infections.[9] In addition, chronic false-positive findings are associated with connective tissue diseases such as systemic lupus erythematosus.[10] A treponemal test is used to confirm the diagnosis.[9,11] Treponemal tests are not used for screening because they remain reactive after the infection is treated.

Both treponemal and nontreponemal tests are used to screen patients with past suspected syphilis infection. Patients treated for early syphilis whose nontreponemal test either shows an increase or fails to show a fourfold decline in *T. pallidum* within 6 months should be retreated. Treponemal tests are used to screen patients for late syphilis when the nontreponemal tests are negative, yet late syphilis is suspected. In later stages of syphilis, antibody titers decline and may be undetectable. All patients who have syphilis should be offered testing for HIV infection.[9]

Clear evidence exists to recommend routine screening for syphilis for all pregnant women and all persons at increased risk of infection (commercial sex workers; persons who exchange sex for drugs; those with other STDs, including HIV; and contacts of persons with active syphilis).[3] A serologic test for syphilis should be performed on all pregnant women at the first prenatal visit. For those women at high risk, screening should be repeated in the third trimester and again at delivery. Any woman who delivers a stillborn infant should be tested for syphilis.[9]

GENITAL HERPES

Herpes simplex virus (HSV) infection is a condition characterized by a primary infection with visible, painful, genital or anal lesions or grouped vesicles at the site of inoculation and regional lymphadenopathy. Recurrent HSV infection is characterized by a normal course of recurring outbreaks of vesicles at the same site.[12]

It is estimated that approximately 1 in 5 of the U.S. adult population is HSV-2 seropositive.[3,13] In 1999 the estimated prevalence was 19% among the general population between 14 and 49 years old. As many as 1.6 million people in the United States become infected each year.[1] This does not include the contribution of sexually acquired HSV-1.

Spread of genital herpes is by direct contact because secretions can transmit the virus. Transmissibility is higher with active lesions, but asymptomatic shedding of virus with transmission is also possible. Asymptomatic shedding occurs more often during the first 3 months after primary infection.[13] About 75% of patients with primary infection are asymptomatic. Antibody response occurs 2 to 12 weeks after infection and is lifelong.[14]

About 75% of patients with primary infection are asymptomatic. Diagnosis of HSV is often a clinical decision based on the patient's history and the morphology of the lesions. The diagnosis is confirmed with a culture or polymerase chain reaction (PCR) swab test on tissue taken from the base of a lesion or unroofed vesicle.[12,13,15] Lesions in the process of healing may affect the sensitivity of virologic testing, giving false-negative results.

Routine screening for genital HSV infection is not recommended for asymptomatic persons, including asymptomatic pregnant women. The USPSTF recommends against routine serologic screening for HSV in asymptomatic adolescents and adults. There is unclear or insufficient evidence available at present to recommend for or against the examination of pregnant women in labor for signs of active genital HSV lesions, although recommendations to do so may be made on other grounds.[3,14] Experts have recommended that any serologic testing for HSV use type-specific assays.[16]

HUMAN PAPILLOMAVIRUS

HPV is a virus associated with a group of viruses that infect the epithelium of the skin and mucous membranes. HPV has a number of distinct serotypes. The infections they cause may be asymptomatic, produce warty lesions, or be associated with a variety of benign or malignant neoplasias. More than 70 types of HPV are recognized, and distinct types are associated with specific clinical manifestations. Of the 70 types, 30 can infect the genital area. Some cause genital warts, or condyloma acuminata. Others may cause subclinical infections that cannot be seen initially. These subclinical infections are more common and can lead to cervical, penile, or anal cancer. On the other hand, genital warts can be treated and cured.[15,17]

It is estimated that 6.2 million people in the United States become infected with HPV each year. Currently, 20 million people in the United States are infected. Women seem to be at higher risk, since persistent cervical infection in women is the single most important risk factor for cervical cancer.[2] Of the oncogenic types of HPV, type 16 accounts for 50% of cervical cancers and high-grade dysplasias. Type 16 (along with types 18, 31, and 45) accounts for 80% of cervical cancers.[2] According to the CDC, levels of infection with HPV appear to be similar among both men and women.[18] Research indicates that approximately 1% of sexually active adults in the United States have genital warts.[2]

High-risk types (HPV 16, 18, 31, 33, 35, 39, 45, 51, 52) are associated with low- and high-grade squamous intraepithelial lesions (LSIL and HSIL) and invasive cancer; low-risk types (HPV 6, 11, 42, 43, 44) are primarily associated with genital warts and LSIL. Women with persistent HPV infection, especially high-risk types, are at a greatest risk for developing cervical intraepithelial neoplasia (CIN) and CIN lesions that progress rather than regress. Studies indicate that infection with high-risk and multiple types of HPV and older age are associated with persistent infection.[18]

Genital warts are diagnosed by inspection. They appear as soft, moist, pink or red swellings. They can be flat, single or multiple, and small or large. Some cluster, forming a cauliflower shape. They can appear on the vulva or in or around the anus or vagina, penis, scrotum, groin, or thigh. Incubation varies from weeks (4 to 8) to months.[7,16] Subclinical lesions may be detected with Pap testing, colposcopy, or biopsy or by the application of acetic acid to lesions with light and magnification.

A definitive diagnosis of HPV depends on the detection of viral nucleic acid (DNA or RNA) or capsid protein. Pap smear diagnosis of HPV does not always correlate with the detection of HPV DNA in cervical cells. As with mild dysplasia, cell changes attributed to HPV often regress without treatment. Screening for HPV using HPV and RNA tests or acetic acid is not recommended.[9] Recent advance in liquid-based technology has changed the concept of a traditional Pap test. HPV DNA testing was recently approved by the U.S. Food and Drug Administration (FDA) for use as an adjunct routine cervical cancer screening based on use of the liquid-based cytology. Because of limited data, there are conflicting recommendations regarding use of HPV testing with cervical cancer screening. The American Cancer Society concludes that it would be reasonable to consider in women over 30 years of age. The American College of Obstetricians and Gynecologists has developed interim guidelines for the use of HPV DNA testing as an adjunct to cervical cytology screening that are based on a consensus workshop convened in 2003. The consensus was reached based on literature review, expert opinion, and unpublished results from large screening studies. One conclusion was that HPV DNA testing may be added to cervical cytology for screening in women ages 30 years or over. An algorithm is provided to assist clinicians. It must be noted that at the time of this writing that this is a consensus opinion.[3,7]

The USPSTF concluded that there is insufficient evidence to recommend for or against routine use of the HPV testing as a primary screen for cervical cancer.[3]

HUMAN IMMUNODEFICIENCY VIRUS

HIV was first clinically recognized in 1981 when the CDC noticed increased cases of *Pneumocystis carinii* pneumonia in previously healthy young men.[19,20] The disease soon became recognized in male and female injection drug users. At the same time similar occurrences were being reported in Africans attending European centers for treatment. In 1983 HIV was isolated from a patient and shown to be the causative agent of acquired immunodeficiency syndrome (AIDS).

Over the years the case definition of AIDS has undergone several revisions. The etiologic agent of AIDS is HIV, a member of a family of retroviruses and the subfamily of *Lentivirinae*. Infection with HIV produces a spectrum of diseases that progress from a clinical latent state or asymptomatic state to AIDS as a late manifestation. The rate of progression is variable. Viral replication is active during all states and increases as the immune system deteriorates. HIV is an RNA virus whose hallmark is the reverse transcription of its RNA to DNA by the enzyme reverse transcriptase. HIV is transmitted by both heterosexual and homosexual contact; by blood and blood products; and by infected mothers to infants either intrapartum, perinatally, or by breast milk.[19,21] HIV is predominantly an STD. It is characterized by a gradual deterioration of immune functions. During the course of infection, crucial immune cells (CD4 T cells) are disabled and killed and their numbers progressively decline. After a variable period the CD4 T cell count falls below a critical level, and the patient becomes highly susceptible to opportunistic disease.[19,21]

The most common cause of HIV disease throughout the world and in the United States is HIV-1.[9] The prevalence of HIV-2 in the United States is extremely low.[9] Approximately 800,000 to 900,000 persons in the United States are infected with HIV, and approximately 275,000 of these persons might not know they are infected.[21] Early detection of HIV infection is now recognized as a critical component in controlling the spread of HIV infection.[21,22]

Only HIV tests approved by the FDA should be used for diagnostic purposes. Several HIV test technologies have been approved by the FDA for diagnostic use in the United States. These tests enable testing of different fluids (i.e., whole blood, serum, plasma, oral fluid, and urine). Informed consent must be obtained before an HIV test is performed.[9] HIV-1 testing consists of initial screening with an electroimmunoassay (EIA) to detect antibodies to HIV-1. Specimens with a nonreactive result from the initial EIA are considered HIV negative unless new exposure to an infected partner or partner of unknown HIV status has occurred. Specimens with a reactive EIA result are retested in duplicate. If the result of either duplicate test is reactive, the specimen is reported as repeatedly reactive and undergoes confirmatory testing with a more specific supplemental test (e.g., Western blot or, less commonly, an immunofluorescence assay). An HIV test result should be considered positive only after screening and confirmatory tests are reactive.[21]

A Western blot test may be reported as indeterminate. This may represent the evolving antibody response of a recent infection or may be produced by the presence of nonspecific antibodies. If the indeterminate result was found in a patient who was seronegative for HIV on previous tests, there is concern that this indeterminate result is caused by a new HIV infection. If the result remains indeterminate for 6 months, this probably represents a nonspecific antibody response.

Most infected persons develop a detectable HIV antibody within 3 months of exposure. If the initial negative HIV test was conducted within the first 3 months after exposure, repeat testing should be considered 3 months or longer after the exposure occurred to account for the possibility of a false-negative result. If the follow-up test is nonreactive, it is unlikely that the patient is HIV positive. However, if the patient was exposed to a known HIV-infected person or if provider or patient concern remains, a second repeat test might be considered 6 months or more from the exposure.[21]

Providers are encouraged to perform HIV testing in all patients. Individual risk can be ascertained through risk screening. Under certain circumstances of perinatal transmission, acute occupational exposure, and acute nonoccupational exposure (e.g., high-risk sex or needle sharing), providers should recommend HIV CTR regardless of setting prevalence or behavioral or clinical risk.[21]

At the end of 2003 an estimated 1,039,000 to 1,185,000 persons in the United States were living with HIV/AIDS, with 24% to 27% undiagnosed and unaware of their infection. By April 2004, all states had adopted some type of system for reporting HIV diagnoses to the CDC. A major advance in surveillance is the development of the serologic testing algorithm for recent HIV seroconversion.[23]

It is estimated that 120,000 to 160,000 infected women live in the United States. Of these women, 80% are of childbearing age. Approximately 25% of HIV-infected pregnant women who are not treated during pregnancy can transmit HIV to their infants during pregnancy, labor and delivery, or breastfeeding. Effective interventions for HIV-infected pregnant women can protect their infants from acquiring HIV and can prolong the survival and improve the health of these mothers and their children. For these reasons, HIV testing is recommended for all pregnant women. All health care providers should recommend HIV testing to all of their pregnant patients, pointing out the substantial benefit of knowledge of HIV status for the health of women and their infants. HIV screening should be a routine part of prenatal care for all women.[22] Regulations, laws, and policies regarding HIV screening of pregnant women and infants are not standardized throughout all states. Health care providers should be aware of and adhere to the laws and regulations governing their areas of practice related to HIV screening.[22]

Because of recent advances in both antiretroviral and obstetric interventions, pregnant women infected with HIV who know their status prenatally can reduce their risk for transmitting HIV to their infants to 2% or less. Finally, all HIV testing should include counseling, both pretest and posttest.

The USPSTF strongly recommends that providers screen for HIV all adolescents and adults at increased risk for HIV infection. The USPSTF makes no recommendation for or against routinely screening for HIV adolescents and adults who are not at risk for HIV infection.[24]

REFERENCES

1. Institute of Medicine, Committee on Prevention and Control of Sexually Transmitted Diseases: *The hidden epidemic: confronting sexually transmitted diseases,* Washington, DC, 1997, National Academy Press.
2. Centers for Disease Control and Prevention: *STD surveillance 2004: trends in reportable STDs in the United States,* 2004, retrieved Dec 2006 from http://www.cdc.gov/nchstp/dstd/Stats_Trends/Stats_and_Trends.htm.
3. US Preventive Services Task Force: *Guide to clinical preventive services: periodic updates,* ed 3, Washington, DC, 2003, US Department of Health and Human Services.
4. *Screening for chlamydia infection: what's new from the third USPSTF,* Rockville, Md, March 2001, AHRQ Pub No APPIP01-0010, Agency for Healthcare Research and Quality, retrieved Dec 2001 from http://www.ahrq.gov/clinic/prev/chlamwh.htm.
5. Peeling RW, Brunham RC: Chlamydia as pathogens: new species and new issues, *Emerg Infect Dis* 2(4):307-319, 1996.
6. Centers for Disease Control and Prevention: Screening test to detect *Chlamydia trachomatis* and *Neisseria gonorrhoeae* infections—2002, *MMWR* 51(No RR-15):1-80, 2002.
7. Wright WC, Schiffman M, Solomon D, and others: Interim guidance for the use of human papillomavirus DNA testing as an adjunct to cervical cytology screening, *Obstet Gynecol* 103(2):304-309, 2004.
8. Sexually transmitted diseases and HIV infection. In US Department of Health and Human Services: *Clinicians' handbook of preventive services: put prevention into practice,* Washington, DC, 1994, US Government Printing Office.
9. Centers for Disease Control and Prevention: Sexually transmitted diseases treatment guidelines 2002, *MMWR* 51(No. RR-6):1-80, 2002.
10. Larson S, Steiner B, Rudolph A: Laboratory diagnosis and interpretation of tests for syphilis, *Clin Microbiol Rev* 8(1):1-19, 1995.
11. Borgatta L, and others: A contemporary approach to curbing STDs, *Patient Care* 30(20):30-42, 1996.
12. Fitzpatrick TB, Johnson RA, Wolff K, and others: *Color atlas and synopsis of clinical dermatology,* ed 3, New York, 1997, McGraw-Hill.
13. Dorsky D: Herpes simplex virus infections. In STD/HIV Prevention Training Center of New England: *Home study module* (3-day intensive course), Boston, 1997, Boston University School of Medicine
14. US Preventive Services Task Force: *Screening for genital herpes simplex: brief update,* March 2005, retrieved March 31, 2006, from http://ahrq.gov/clinic/uspstf05/herpes/herpesup2.htm.
15. Warren T: Serologic testing to diagnose herpes simplex virus infections, *J Nurse Practitioners* 1(2):84-90, 2005.
16. Centers for Disease Control and Prevention, US Department of Health and Human Services: *Proposed approaches for herpes prevention: report*

of the Genital Herpes Prevention Consultants Meeting, May 5-6, 1998, retrieved Dec 8, 2006, from http://www.cdc.gov/nchstp/dstd/Reports_Publications/herpes-98/Herpes_Prevention.htm.
17. Centers for Disease Control and Prevention: *CDC issues major new report on STD epidemics*, Dec 5, 2000, retrieved Dec 2001, from http://www.cdc.gov/nchstp/dstd/Press_Releases/STDEpidemics2000.htm.
18. US Department of Health and Human Services, Division of STD Prevention: *Prevention of genital HPV infection and sequelae: report of an external consultants meeting*, Atlanta, 1999, Centers for Disease Control and Prevention.
19. Fauci AS, Lane HC: Human immunodeficiency virus. In Fauci A, and others, editors: *Harrison's principles of internal medicine*, New York, 1998, McGraw-Hill.
20. Wisdom A, Hawkins, DA: *Diagnosis in color: sexually transmitted diseases*, ed 2, London, 1997, Mosby-Wolfe.
21. Centers for Disease Control and Prevention: Revised guidelines for HIV counseling, testing and referral, *MMWR* 50(RR19):1-58, 2001.
22. Centers for Disease Control and Prevention: Revised recommendation for HIV screening of pregnant women, perinatal counseling and guideline consultation, *MMWR* 50(RR19):59-68, 2001.
23. US Department of Health and Human Services, Centers for Disease Control and Prevention: *HIV/AIDS surveillance report, 2004*, vol 16, Atlanta, 2005, The Centers.
24. US Preventive Services Task Force: *Screening for HIV: recommendation statement*, AHRQ Pub No 05-0580-A, July 2005, Rockville, Md, 2005, Agency for Healthcare Research and Quality, retrieved Oct 19, 2006, from http://ahrq.gov/clinic/uspstf05/hiv/hivrs.htm.

CHAPTER 22

Principles of Occupational and Environmental Health in Primary Care

Kathleen Golden McAndrew

Occupational and environmental health care is the specialty focused on prevention and management of environmental and occupational injuries, illness, and disability. Occupational and environmental health care also includes the promotion of health and productivity in workers, their families, and their communities.[1]

Health care providers may offer occupational health care as part of their practices. The provider's role in delivering occupational health-related services may vary. Involvement depends on the defined scope of service of the practice setting, its proximity to an occupational medicine health care provider or program, and the knowledge base and interest of the health care provider.

Primary health care providers evaluate and treat workers' compensation injuries, identify workplace hazards, provide standard medical evaluations and health screenings, and treat employees' illnesses. They may assist occupational and environmental health professionals with evaluating employees for fitness-for-duty or return-to-work issues.

Regardless of the role the health care provider plays in providing occupational and environmental health services, including an occupational and environmental health history as part of the medical history and understanding the risks associated with each patient's job will assist in monitoring and maintaining the health of the working population. An occupational and environmental health history should include at least the following[2,3]:

- Current and past positions held
- Previous employers, years employed, type of industry or employer, and products manufactured or developed
- A brief description of job duty requirements
- Known health hazards in the workplace
- Any current or past exposure to chemicals or other hazardous substances, noise, radiation, heat, vibration, or repetitive motion
- Use of personal protective equipment
- Time off work for a health problem or injury
- Changed residence because of health problems
- Spousal contact with dust or chemicals at work
- Use of pesticides in gardens or around the home

HEALTH PROMOTION

Health promotion and education are important in maintaining a healthy, productive, creative, and engaged workforce.[4] A healthy workforce results in reduced risk of work-related injuries, less sick time usage, and improved employee morale. To assist with improving the health and well-being of their employees, many companies offer health promotion programs at the worksite. These offerings may include on-site exercise programs; health screening for high-risk health indicators; and health education programs on topics such as smoking cessation, nutrition, exercise, stress reduction, and personal safety. Medical clearance from health care providers is sometimes requested before employees may participate in programs that involve strenuous physical activity.

Companies offering health screening programs at the worksite may screen for risk factors such as measurement of blood pressure, weight, blood glucose, cholesterol, and body mass index. Results from the screenings are used to educate employees on risk reduction through lifestyle changes, and also serve as a basis for establishing future health promotion programs that target employees' needs. Results that require evaluation or monitoring are referred to the employee's health care provider for further evaluation and, as indicated, treatment.

PREPLACEMENT HEALTH EVALUATION

Most employers require some form of preplacement screening or a physical examination before an employee may begin work. Health care providers who offer preplacement evaluations as part of their practice must understand the purpose and focus of these examinations.

The provider's focus in a preplacement evaluation is to ensure that the employee is free from any medical condition that may preclude him or from performing the job, become aggravated during performance of job duties, or affect the health and safety of others.[5,6] During the evaluation the health care provider establishes a baseline health status for comparison when work-related injuries, illnesses, or exposures occur. The provider also gathers information for recommendations for health promotion and wellness programs. Employees in certain occupations, such as truck drivers or airline pilots, must have specific tests that are required by federal law as part of their preemployment evaluation.[5] Therefore it is essential that the health care provider be provided with and understand the job duty requirements and the work environment associated with the job, as well as any mandated testing or evaluation components.

Components of the preplacement evaluation should include a job-specific physical examination and appropriate ancillary testing.[5] Job-specific ancillary testing may include spirometry, audiometry, vision screening, a baseline chest x-ray study, various blood studies, and urinalysis. Drug testing or regulatory agency–required testing for certain licenses or certificates may be necessary.

The health care provider may uncover significant health findings that are incidental to the patient's job performance. Although these findings need to be addressed and plans for follow-up discussed, they should not be addressed as part of the preplacement evaluation or included in the clearance or report to the employer, unless the findings directly affect the employee's ability to perform his or her job.

After completion of the evaluation, any recommendations, restrictions, abnormal findings, identified special protective measures, or other issues should be discussed with the employee. Recommendations for periodic screening should also be brought to the employee's attention. In addition, the provider should emphasize the need to use appropriate protective equipment and review proper body mechanics as they relate to the employee's job duties.

A written recommendation on work fitness should be provided to the employer. The recommendation should be limited to whether the employee is cleared for full work duty or whether any restrictions are recommended. Documentation of restrictions should be specific and described by function. In addition, restrictions should be listed without including the underlying medical reason, since medical information should not be provided to the employer without the employee's written consent.

MEDICAL SURVEILLANCE

When performing occupational health medical surveillance, health care providers collect, analyze, and disseminate data on groups of workers and workplaces to prevent illness and injury.[6] These surveillances are conducted according to government requirements. In them, health care providers survey the workplace environment for potential hazards, monitor the health status of employees for exposure to harmful substances, and assess the employee's ability to perform his or her job duties.[2]

Potential workplace hazards can be biologic, chemical, physical, or ergonomic. The personnel responsible for OSHA compliance at the worksite performs a needs assessment to determine whether a surveillance program is necessary. Health care providers are often requested to provide some of the components of the surveillance program, such as medical examinations, biologic tests, or other health screenings that are used as part of the overall program monitoring.

Both the nature and frequency of medical surveillance are determined by national or state Occupational Safety and Health Administration (OSHA) requirements and by individual employers. Standards are available for each hazard (e.g., lead, asbestos, noise) to which workers are exposed. These standards detail the specifics of both routine medical surveillance (e.g., for workers requiring respiratory protection such as firefighters) and surveillance after exposure (e.g., exposure to noise or blood-borne pathogens). Specific requirements are listed in each code and should be referenced before performing evaluations.

DRUG AND ALCOHOL TESTING

Drug and alcohol testing is required of employees who work for companies covered by agencies of the Department of Transportation (DOT) and whose jobs are identified as safety sensitive. In addition, companies or contractors whose federal grants exceed $25,000 are required to establish a drug-free workplace policy that includes drug screening. Individual companies also may choose to implement their own drug-free workplace requirements.[7]

Drug and alcohol testing may be performed at the time of preplacement screening, at random intervals, after accidents, and when there is suspicion of impairment from substances (or "for cause"). The most common drugs tested include the panel required by the DOT and other federal agencies. This panel includes marijuana (tetrahydrocannabinol [THC] metabolite), cocaine, amphetamines, opiates, and phencyclidine (PCP). Private companies may screen for other drugs, such as barbiturates, hallucinogens, inhalants, or designer drugs.[7,8] Special panels are sometimes used that include multiple drugs with potential for abuse among those with specific occupations. Most drug-testing programs adopt federal regulations, including their cutoff levels and chain-of-custody procedures required during specimen collection.

Drug screens are normally performed on urine and must be collected by staff who are knowledgeable of federal guidelines. Ethanol (alcohol) testing is done using a breathalyzer test performed by certified breath alcohol technicians or screening test technicians. Specimens are analyzed by laboratories certified to perform these tests by the Substance Abuse and Mental Health Services Administration. Results of the substance testing are sent to a designated medical review officer, whose role is to interpret drug screen results and determine whether there is a medical or other explanation for positive results before contacting the employer.

Guidelines must be strictly followed with every specimen collection, and facilities must be set up to meet the specifications for collection (e.g., dry bathrooms). Therefore most primary care practices defer drug and alcohol testing to occupational medicine programs or to private laboratories that offer drug collection as part of their services.

TREATMENT OF WORK-RELATED INJURIES, ILLNESSES, AND EXPOSURES

Workers' compensation is a system that provides medical care, wage replacement benefits, and, when necessary, rehabilitation for workers who incur injuries or illnesses as a result of workplace exposure or activity. With few exceptions for federally administered programs, most are regulated by the individual states.

Many potential hazards in the workplace can cause a work-related injury, illness, or exposure. Some of these injuries may be similar to others or already encountered within a primary care practice. Such hazards include physical hazards of the work environment that may cause injuries (e.g., from objects, falls, noise, heat, or cold). Poor ergonomics is the cause of a large number of work-related injuries, including back injuries and injuries caused by repetitive motion or cumulative trauma. It is imperative that the work setting be evaluated and altered to lessen the chance of recurrence in these situations.

Exposures may occur when employees work around potentially toxic chemicals or biologic agents. Chemical-related injury, illness, or exposure may occur as a result of normal working conditions or through accidents. These episodes require the primary care provider to have a basic understanding of toxicology. Familiarization with material safety data sheets or access to computerized databases or poison control centers can assist in determining actual exposure and necessary treatment. For biologic exposures the epidemiology, including mode of transmission, incubation, employee's immunity status, and appropriate or required follow-up testing, must be known for each exposure. Workers such as health care facility employees, emergency responders, and employees in laboratory and research facilities may encounter biologic hazards.

Workers' Compensation

Numerous professionals are usually involved in workers' compensation cases. The number of professionals and their titles may vary depending on the manner in which each employer is insured. Required forms and regular reports that reflect the employee's status must be completed within defined time frames. The health care provider usually must obtain preauthorization before referring the patient to specialty or adjunct treatment modalities or before ordering diagnostic tests.

Requirements governing workers' compensation certification vary by employer and state. Health care providers who are interested in providing workers' compensation as part of their practice should ensure that they and their support staff have a basic understanding of what is required for each patient situation. They should review state regulations and employer requirements for compliance with each case. Attending conferences in the area of workers' compensation is also helpful.

Principles of medical confidentiality regarding work-related injuries and illness must be followed. These principles limit the information employers receive regarding the exact nature of the occupational illness or injury, specifics about treatment, reasons for restrictions and limitations, and details of the plan for continual care.[6,9] After each workers' compensation visit the treating health care provider notifies the case manager or representative of the plan concerning further medical treatment and designated work restrictions.[6]

In many situations the injured employee may not be able to perform his or her complete duties while recovering but may be able to perform parts of the job or other tasks. In these cases the health care provider works with the employer to identify how temporary accommodation of these employees can be provided through modified or light duty.[7] Many companies are mandated or volunteer to develop modified-duty programs. To recommend modified duty, the health care provider must understand the job requirements of each injured employee. It is important that the employer provide information concerning physical job demands. The provider should describe limitation or restrictions by function and qualify and quantify restrictions in as much detail as possible to avoid confusion and to assist the employer in accommodating these restrictions.

REGULATORY AGENCY REQUIREMENTS

In addition to understanding the basics of workers' compensation, health care providers who choose to address occupational health–related medical issues need to be familiar with other regulations that apply to treatment and screening of employees. Copies of these regulations can be obtained through the respective agency responsible for the regulation, or they can be found on the Internet.

Occupational Safety and Health Administration

Created by Congress in 1970, OSHA requires each employer to provide "a place of employment, which is free from recognized hazards that are causing or are likely to cause death or serious physical harm to employees."[10] OSHA functions under the Department of Labor. It has the authority to fine or imprison employers who are found to be in violation of its regulations. Although most of OSHA's regulations deal with safety-related concerns, this organization has also issued a number of standards that specify medical evaluations and the testing of employees who may be exposed to certain workplace hazards. Testing is required when exposures meet or exceed a certain level. Other standards require that employees receive medical clearance before using the required protective equipment.

National Institute for Occupational Safety and Health

The National Institute for Occupational Safety and Health (NIOSH) was established under the Occupational Safety and Health Act of 1970 and is part of the U.S. Department of Health and Human Services. Its function is to conduct research and to advise OSHA on issues regarding hazards in the workplace. NIOSH provides educational information to health care providers, employers, and employees.

Americans with Disabilities Act

Congress enacted the Americans with Disabilities Act (ADA) in 1990 to protect disabled workers from discrimination in the workplace. This act must be considered when offering many occupational health–related evaluations. The ADA requires that an employer make reasonable accommodations so the disabled employee is able to perform those job functions considered essential to the position.[11] In addition, it is necessary to determine whether disabled employees can perform the job without posing a "direct threat" to the health and safety of themselves or others.[11]

Professional Organizations

Professional organizations such as the American College of Occupational and Environmental Medicine, the American Association of Occupational Health Nurses, and the American Conference of Governmental Industrial Hygienists offer texts, guidelines, and other information that can assist the health care provider with occupational health–related issues.

REFERENCES

1. American College of Occupational and Environmental Medicine: *Mission statement*, 2005, retrieved Dec 8, 2006, from http://www.acoem.org/general/vision.asp.
2. Burgel B: Direct care in the occupational setting. In Salazar MK, editor: *AAOHN core curriculum for occupational and environmental health nursing,* ed 3, Philadelphia, 2006, Saunders.
3. Wright WE: Case report: discovery of occupational disease. In McCunney RJ, editor: *A practical approach to occupational and environmental medicine,* ed 3, Philadelphia, 2003, Lippincott Williams & Wilkins.
4. Campbell K: Health promotion and adult education. In Salazar MK, editor: *AAOHN core curriculum for occupational and environmental health nursing,* ed 3, Philadelphia, 2006, Saunders.
5. McCunney RJ: Occupational medical services. In McCunney RJ, editor: *A practical approach to occupational and environmental medicine,* ed 3, Philadelphia, 2003, Lippincott Williams & Wilkins.
6. Harber P, Colon C, McCunney RJ: Occupational medical surveillance. In McCunney RJ, editor: *A practical approach to occupational and environmental medicine,* ed 3, Philadelphia, 2003, Lippincott Williams & Wilkins.
7. Golden McAndrew K, McAndrew S: Workplace substance abuse impairment, *AAOHN J* 48(1):32-45, 2000.
8. Gochnour MK, Bruck A, Souza D: Examples of occupational health and safety programs. In Salazar MK, editor: *AAOHN core curriculum for occupational and environmental health nursing,* ed 3, Philadelphia, 2006, Saunders.
9. Golden McAndrew K: AAOHN advisory: nurse practitioners in occupational and environmental health, *AAOHN J* 47(1 suppl 1-2), 1999, updated 2004.
10. US Department of Labor, Occupational Safety and Health Administration: *General industry OSHA safety and health standards,* 29 CFR 1910, OSHA 2206,Washington, DC, 2004, US Government Printing Office.
11. Peterson KW, Rischitelli DG: The Americans with Disabilities Act. In McCunney RJ, editor: *A practical approach to occupational and environmental medicine,* ed 3, Philadelphia, 2003, Lippincott Williams & Wilkins.

CHAPTER 23

College Health

Catharine Moffett

College or university health services often reflect campus culture and are varied in composition and services. A large university with a medical center can offer a wider variety of providers and specialists than can a small rural college health center. However, one nurse working collaboratively with a local physician at a smaller college might be acquainted with every student.

The mission of a college or university health services is to provide primary care for the student, to promote the well-being of the institution's citizens through health education and illness prevention programs, and to contribute ultimately to the academic success of its patients (students).[1] Student health services may also position itself as the student's "interim" health care provider, with the understanding that communication with the student's provider at home will be ongoing.

Student health services may also be in the position to advise or create the institution's emergency preparedness plan or health policy, particularly concerning infectious disease issues such as avian flu pandemic or bioterrorism.

ROLES OF UNIVERSITY HEALTH CARE PROVIDERS

In college or university health services, the health care provider has an ideal opportunity to affect the young adult at a critical time of development. The college years are a transitional stage between the end of adolescence and the beginning of adulthood. A college health care provider can assist in that transition by explaining issues of confidentiality (often a new concept to the student), modeling the practice of partnership between provider and patient in treatment or care decisions, and instructing a student in the often confusing world of health insurance. In such encounters, a college health care provider can positively influence the student's developmental stage from dependent living at home to independent living, and from pediatric to adult health care.

Health education plays a critical role in the services offered to students. Some institutions have wellness programs at designated "wellness centers." Ideally, health education programs are a collaboration among the college health services, counseling services, health educator, peer educators, and residential life staff. With these various talents and teaching skills, programs can target the current trends on campus, including risk-taking behavior and drug use, and tailor programs to specific issues and audiences.

TOPICS IN COLLEGE HEALTH

Confidentiality

For some students, the college setting marks the first time they receive health care without a parent present. If the student is more than 18 years old, he or she is legally able to make a health care decision without parental involvement. Clearly explaining to the student the right to confidentiality can foster more open communication with the provider. Obtaining a student's written permission to discuss a specific illness episode with a parent, professor, or administrator confirms the legal nature of the information in the student's medical chart. On the other hand, parents often need the reassurance that, although their over-18-year-old child may desire privacy regarding visits to the college health center, serious or life-threatening illnesses can and will be made known to parents at the discretion of the professional staff.

If a student is covered by a parent's medical insurance plan, confidential information may be inadvertently revealed to the policyholder (parent) as a result of routine billing procedures and documents. When students have the privacy of their own policy, they may be less hesitant in seeking gynecologic care, contraception, or treatment for sexually transmitted diseases (STD). Costs of these services should never be a barrier.

Health Care Issues: Female College Students

For some young women, being away from home provides an opportunity for more intimate sexual relationships and the concomitant responsibilities. A first gynecologic visit to the student health services should include enough time for a first pelvic examination (for some), a thorough sexual history, STD education, and contraceptive counseling. Some institutions schedule this as a two-part visit.

Appointments requested specifically for STD screening or emergency contraception create opportunities for the provider to explore the college woman's sense of control in a sexual situation, the impact of drug or alcohol use on her decisions, and any sense of guilt or regret connected to her sexual experience. Although sexual assault is covered elsewhere (Chapter 40), it must be noted here that research suggests that college women are at greater risk for sexual assault than are women of a comparable age in the general population.[2] In a survey conducted by the American College Health Association, 6% of college women reported an attempted or completed rape in 2005.[3] Other studies put the annual (9-month) incidence at 3%.[2] Discrepancies in numbers may be based on underreporting due to certain barriers such as fears about confidentiality; fear of sanction and guilt over alcohol use; differences in definitions of dating violence, sexual assault, or rape; or institutional misunderstanding or ignorance about the guidelines for reporting the data. Several legislative acts (1990-1998), including the Clery Act, have mandated that colleges and universities make available campus crime statistics, including sexual assault, and that schools have policies to address sexual assault.[4] The student health services are an active participant in reporting such crimes and in preventive programs related to sexual assault. As a supportive member of the community, student health services should have a thorough understanding of the institution's policies and procedures for reporting rape, sexual misconduct, and sexual harassment.

Understanding the student's level of risk-taking behavior enables the provider to guide the student in contraceptive care, provide a referral to student counseling services or alcohol or drug programs, or schedule a follow-up appointment at student health services to continue in the educational and supportive aspect of her care. Unplanned pregnancies can require the collaboration of student health services, student counseling services, and other appropriate community services.

All students, particularly women, who visit student health services should be observed for evidence of an eating disorder. Diagnosis and management of anorexia nervosa or bulimia are addressed elsewhere in this text; however, diagnosis and treatment in the college setting have some unique aspects. Female students are acutely aware of the myth of the "freshman 15," which purports that freshmen women will gain 15 pounds during their first year on campus.[5] Students with an eating disorder in remission who find college life stressful are prone to regression. Women pressured to compete socially or athletically may respond with disordered eating at college, which can progress to a full eating disorder.

Students living in dorms or sororities and students participating in activities such as athletic teams, dance, or theater groups may notice fellow students exhibiting behavior indicative of an eating disorder. These students, as well as coaches, professors, or student leaders, should be encouraged to approach student health services to seek advice concerning treatment for a friend or classmate. Whether working alone or in concert with student counseling services, the student health services staff must proceed carefully to protect the individual, while also reassuring the group concerned about their friend or classmate. Depending on the clinical situation, remaining in treatment and meeting established goals to remain in college can serve as strong motivating factors for the student with an eating disorder. Unfortunately, the health services are powerless if the student never seeks treatment on her own. Mandated visits have limited value beyond possible diagnosis and can sabotage future treatment.

Health Care Issues: Male College Students

Males 16 to 20 years of age have far fewer health care visits than younger males (11 to 15 years old) or their female contemporaries.[6] Male college students visit the health center episodically for sick visits or injuries. Therefore there are fewer opportunities for health education or risk-reduction counseling than for college-age women. Efforts to reach this population through outreach programs in dormitories, fraternities, or athletic teams can help bridge this gap.

Young men also come to the health center for STD screening. This occasion provides the opportunity to screen for high-risk behaviors, including drug and alcohol use, violence, nonrelational sexual activity, and condom use. The STD screening visit is an excellent opportunity for one-on-one teaching of college men. Because testicular cancer is more prevalent in this age-group, education about testicular cancer and self-examination should be offered to the individual and promoted in wellness efforts. The proper use of condoms can also be taught at an STD screening visit.

Injuries related to violence as a result of male clubs, organizations, or initiation rites are cause for concern and must be discussed with the student. However, the student may be conflicted about giving information, particularly if the student took an oath of confidentiality. Understanding the institution's policies about these activities will help guide the provider's response. All forms of campus violence—whether sexual, psychologic, physical, or verbal—impede the educational mission of the college campus. Providers in college health have a critical role in prevention, reporting, and care for the victims of violence.

Gay, Lesbian, Bisexual, and Transgender Students

Gay, lesbian, bisexual, and transgender students face multiple challenges on college campuses. Student health services must initiate outreach to the gay, lesbian, bisexual, and transgender student communities, since these students may be reluctant to have contact with student health services. Student health services can be visible to these communities and understand their special needs by speaking with student gay, lesbian, bisexual, and transgender organizations and requesting feedback on the health services and programs.

Mental Health Issues

As a result of advancements in pharmacologic treatment, increasing numbers of college students have complex psychiatric diagnoses and need various types of on-campus support.[7] Student health services can be involved in medical maintenance, treatment, referral, or co-management of students with mental health needs. The relationship of student health services with student counseling services can range from a merged, fully integrated center to separate services with shared administration, to completely independent services. Regardless of the structure, health services and counseling services must collaborate when necessary for optimum care for the student while maintaining confidentiality.

Transfer or coordination of mental health care from home to the college setting can cause various concerns. As with any chronic illness, students may have established a therapeutic relationship with their mental health provider and may be reluctant to establish a new relationship with an unfamiliar therapist. Outreach to students who may benefit from on-site counseling services is crucial. Students with mental health needs may be identified via information on their health form, which should record chronic psychiatric medications. Student health services can serve as a conduit to campus counseling services when the health services are asked by the athletic or dance department to evaluate a student with a potential eating disorder. The academic or student life department may also refer a student with a potential mood, thought, or adjustment disorder. Health care providers must be sensitive to the fact that, for some, the stigma of seeking mental health services can be a barrier to care, and that access through a medical service or for a medically related complaint can be more acceptable. Students should be encouraged to sign a release when the referral is made to allow for a collaborative approach to treatment.

The college years are acutely stressful and accompanied by periods of hopelessness for some students. It is essential that college and university health providers and counselors maintain a high level of vigilance for suicide risk when assessing all students.

Sleep

Whether a result of academic, social, athletic, work schedules, psychologic, or pharmacologic reasons, college students are notorious for not getting adequate sleep. A recent survey showed that only 11% of the students studied got an adequate amount of sleep.[8] Sleeping problems can be a symptom of depression or a precipitant of depression. By resetting their biologic clocks, sleep-deprived students can develop concentration difficulties, impaired immune systems, anxiety, irritability, and possibly increased drug or alcohol abuse.[9] Consideration of sleep habits and sleep disorders must be included in a clinical visit for fatigue, illness, or depression.

Tobacco and Alcohol

Alcohol use in the college population continues to be a problem despite institutional efforts to curb its use.[10] Secondary effects of binge drinking include academic failure, sexual assault, violence, property damage, motor vehicle accidents, and death. Among the strategies most often used to curb alcohol consumption are alternative late-night alcohol-free events, increased sanctions, student involvement in campus policies and adjudication, and peer education. Student health services treat both the acute and secondary effects of alcohol intoxication. This encounter affords the opportunity to educate the student on issues connected with alcohol use. In addition, referrals to counseling services, on-campus alcohol education programs, or community alcohol treatment programs may be appropriate.

Tobacco use on the college campus has increased in the past decade; 28% of college smokers begin to smoke regularly at or after age 19 years (when most are already in college).[11] Although most public buildings and most college buildings prohibit smoking, only 27% of the campuses surveyed prohibit smoking in student dormitories.[12]

College or university health care providers have a role both in advocating for policies that restrict smoking and in promoting smoking cessation. Tobacco use should be the "fifth vital sign" in student sick visit encounters, to initiate the opportunity to discuss smoking cessation. Even when there is little student demand for formal cessation programs, these programs must remain part of the wellness armamentarium for the student health center.

SCREENINGS AND IMMUNIZATIONS

Evidence of immunity or current immunization to measles and rubella is usually required for college enrollment. Immunizations or evidence of immunity to hepatitis B, chickenpox, and tetanus are recommended. Prematriculation immunizations are mandated by colleges and universities and by state law. Student health services are responsible for ensuring student compliance with these mandates, including documentation of students who are not immunized because of religious beliefs. The most recent recommendations by the Centers for Disease Control and Prevention Advisory Committee on Immunization Practices, as well as by the American College Health Association, advise students and parents to be educated about the risks of meningococcal disease in the college population and encourage vaccination.[13] Students arriving from tuberculosis (TB)-endemic countries within the past 5 years must typically receive tuberculin skin testing before enrollment.[1] Students studying abroad during college need advice on travel immunizations and information on infectious disease prevention. After returning from a TB-endemic country, students should be rescreened.

CULTURAL ISSUES

Cultural competency is crucial to the student health services' success in caring for a diverse student population. Cultural competency is more than cultural awareness (knowledge) and cultural sensitivity (knowledge plus some experience with the culture). Cultural competency encompasses the ability to think about power differentials in relationships and respond with varied skills to establish rapport with diverse individuals.[14] Student health care providers must be sensitive to voice, body language, and gestures as they communicate with patients. There may be culture-specific meanings for aspects of health care such as pain and reproductive issues in patient populations. University or college providers can expect to experience multiple cultures on their campus and must be leaders in modeling and fostering cultural competency.

RESOURCES

The American College Health Association, with membership representing more than 2500 health care providers and 920 institutions of higher education, provides useful standards and guidelines for college health programs and services. Its website can be accessed at http://www.acha.org.

REFERENCES

1. American College Health Association: *General statement of ethical principles and guidelines,* retrieved Dec 2006 from http://www.acha.org./info_resources/ethics_stmnt.pdf.
2. Fisher BS, Cullen FT, Turner MG: *The sexual victimization of college women* (NCJRS Pub No 182369), Washington, DC, 2000, US Department of Justice, National Criminal Justice Reference Service.
3. American College Health Association: *ACHA—National College Health Assessment: selected data highlights,* Fall 2005, retrieved Dec 2006 from http://www.acha.org/projects_programs/ncha_sampledata.cfm.
4. Security on Campus: *Clery Act,* retrieved Dec 2006 from http://www.securityoncampus.org./schools/cleryact/cleryact.html.
5. Graham MP, Jones AL: Freshman 15: valid theory or harmful myth? *J Am Coll Health* 50(4):171-173, 2002.
6. Marcell AV, Klein JD, Fischer I, and others: Male adolescent use of health care services: where are the boys? *J Adolesc Health* 30:35-43, 2002.
7. Gallagher RP, Zhang B, Taylor R: *National survey of counseling center directors, 2003,* Alexandria, Va, 2003, International Association of Counseling Services, retrieved Dec 2006 from http://www.education.pitt.edu/survey/nsccd/archive/2003/toc.pdf.
8. Buboltz WC Jr, Brown F, Soper B: Sleep habits and patterns of college students, *J Am Coll Health* 50(3):131-135, 2001.
9. Kadison R, DiGeronimo T: *College of the overwhelmed,* San Francisco, 2004, Jossey-Bass.
10. Wechsler H, Lee JE, Kuo M, and others: Trends in college binge drinking during a period of increased prevention efforts, *J Am Coll Health* 50(5):203-217, 2002.
11. Wechsler H, Rigotti NA, Gledhill-Hoyt J, and others: Increased level of cigarette use among college students, *JAMA* 280(19):1673-1678, 1998.
12. Wechsler H, Kelley K, Seibring M, and others: College smoking policies and smoking cessation programs: results of a survey of college health center directors, *J Am Coll Health* 49(4):1-8, 2001.
13. Meningococcal disease in college students. Recommendations of the Advisory Committee on Immunization Practices (ACIP), *MMWR* 49(RR-7):13-20, 2000.
14. American College Health Association: *Cultural competency statement,* retrieved Dec 9, 2006, from http://www.acha.org./info_resources/cult_comp_stmnt.pdf.

CHAPTER 24

Lifestyle Assessment

Deanna Gordon, Patricia Fergus,
Janelle Koo, and Robbyn K. Takeuchi

LIFESTYLE MANAGEMENT

Diseases of contemporary society are often caused by nutritive deficiencies or excesses, inactivity, and ineffective stress management. Nutrition, physical activity, and stress are the dominant lifestyle features that contribute to the three main causes of death in the United States. Heart disease is the major cause of death, followed by cancer and stroke. In 2003, there were 2,443,930 deaths in the United States, or a rate of 840 deaths per 100,000, as reported in the National Vital Statistics Reports. The age-adjusted death rate was 235 per 100,000 for heart disease, 191 per 100,000 for cancer, and 54 per 100,000 for stroke.[1]

Healthy People 2010 has incorporated morbidity and mortality data in setting objectives for the nation's health. The document offers a plan to enhance health through health promotion and disease prevention efforts. It has two major goals. The first is to increase life expectancy and quality of life for all, and the second is to eradicate health disparities among the various subgroups of the population. As reported, environmental influences and individual behaviors account for 70% of premature deaths. Two of the major focus areas for healthy lifestyle goals are (1) nutrition and weight management and (2) physical activity and fitness.[2]

In addition to adverse clinical outcomes, profound financial consequences are associated with lifestyle choices. Health problems caused by overweight or obesity accounted for 9.1% of expenditures for medical care in 1998, or as much as $78.5 billion, half of which was paid through Medicare and Medicaid reimbursement.[3] Further, consumers spend an estimated $33 billion annually on weight loss programs and products.[4]

INTERCONNECTION AMONG LIFESTYLE COMPONENTS

Lifestyle influences are not mutually exclusive but are interconnected in ways that affect health and well-being. The epidemiology of chronic disease refers to this interconnection as a "web of causation," or multifactorial causation. Nutrition and stress are interrelated in that poor nutritional status may be a stressor. For example, a diet lacking in calcium will likely lead to osteoporosis. Conversely, states of stress may influence eating behaviors. Some individuals consume greater quantities of food when they are under stress, whereas others lose their appetites. Food intake and exercise are linked through metabolic processes. Exercise enhances the effectiveness of metabolic processes, and food is the necessary fuel. Exercise and levels of stress are connected. On one hand, exercise is an effective means to diffuse the tension associated with stress. Conversely, humans need some stress to perform at peak levels, and exercise affords an opportunity to experience positive stress through the exhilaration of engaging in physical activity.

Overweight and obesity are linked to cardiovascular problems and some forms of cancer. An imbalance in lifestyle influences is associated with a multitude of medical conditions, including type 2 diabetes, sleep apnea, gallbladder disease, hypertension, musculoskeletal injuries, and psychiatric illnesses.

Obesity

The Centers for Disease Control and Prevention reported that in 2000, approximately 19% of the population was obese.[5] By 2005, according to data from the National Health Interview Survey (NHIS), the percentage increased to 25.4%. In the 20- to 39-year age range, the rate is 22%; for those 40 to 59 years, the rate is 29%; and in those over 60 years of age, 25% are obese.[6] In the younger age-groups, more men than women are obese, whereas after age 60, more women are affected.[6] In the Hispanic population, the prevalence is 33% for women and 25% for men. For African Americans, the percentages are 29% for men and 37% for women. In the Caucasian population, 25% of men and 22% of women are obese.[6] Hence, an obesity epidemic exists in the United States.[6] Associated with the epidemiologic characteristics of age, gender, and ethnicity, the level of education is significant. Among those with less than a high school education, more than one fourth are obese, compared with one fifth of high school graduates. Obesity in college graduates is the lowest, at 15%.[7]

Regrettably, more than half of all Americans are considered overweight.[8] An evidence-based report prepared by a consortium of the National Heart, Lung, and Blood Institute (NHLBI) reported that approximately 97 million adults are overweight or obese. The expert panel has defined overweight as a body mass index (BMI) from 25 to 29.9 kg/m^2. Obesity is identified as a BMI of 30 kg/m^2 or more.[9]

Sedentary Lifestyle

Exacerbating the problem of overweight is the sedentary lifestyle of the majority of Americans. Data collected in the NHIS indicate that, adjusted for age, 31% of individuals participate in regular physical activity during leisure time. Men are more likely to be physically active than women. Among Caucasians, 35% are physically active. For African Americans, the percentage drops to 22%, and it is even less for Hispanics, with 20% being physically active.[10] See Chapter 17 for more information regarding obesity and primary care.

Stress

The American Institute of Stress, a nonprofit organization, is a clearinghouse for all information related to stress. The institute emphasizes that stress is the number one health problem in the United States. Research conducted during the past 20 years reveals the impact of stress on health. Health conditions caused by stress affect 43% of adults, and stress-related conditions account for 75% to 95% of visits to health care providers.[11] Job-related stress is gaining recognition along with the increased incidence of violence in the workplace. Unmanaged stress is linked to hypertension, heart disease, some forms of cancer, gastrointestinal problems, and some emotional health disorders.

LIFESTYLE CHOICES

The effects of lifestyle choices are often readily apparent to the experienced provider when the patient comes in for a physical examination. Clues can be gleaned by observing body size, movement, and affect. The negative effects of poor lifestyle choices are cumulative and usually require a long incubation period before manifestation. Family history may include health conditions that tend to run in the family, such as hypertension and diabetes.

Nutrition

The patient history will provide important clues to lifestyle, including those related to cultural and religious practices that influence food preparation and consumption. Eating habits related to frequency of eating and types of food consumed should be identified. For an individual with weight management problems, the provider should evaluate dietary intake of sugar and fats, inclusion of foods high in fiber content, amount of fruits and vegetables, and amount of food consumed. The consumption of stimulants such as caffeine is important because caffeine may be associated with a pleasant and uplifting feeling for some but may cause irritability and jitteriness in others.

The National Cholesterol Education Program (NCEP), under the auspices of the NHBLI of the National Institutes of Health, has established a dietary questionnaire based on the mnemonic *CAGE* for providers to use in assessing the fat and cholesterol consumption of patients[12] (Box 24-1). This measure enables the diagnostician to quickly identify potentially detrimental fat consumption.

Exercise

Physical activity must also be considered as a part of the lifestyle assessment. An insufficient amount has harmful consequences, not only for cardiovascular health and flexibility but also for psychologic well-being. Sedentary patients are unlikely to describe themselves as "energetic"; indeed, patients may report becoming easily fatigued. The history should include information about the type and frequency of physical activity. Consequences of the activity, as well as any adverse events, are important considerations for lifestyle influences on health.

BOX 24-1

DIETARY CAGE QUESTIONS FOR ASSESSMENT OF INTAKE OF SATURATED FAT AND CHOLESTEROL

C Cheese (and other sources of dairy fats—whole milk, 2% milk, ice cream, cream, whole-fat yogurt)
A Animal fats (hamburger, ground meat, frankfurters, bologna, salami, sausage, fried foods, fatty cuts of meat)
G Got it away from home (high-fat meals either purchased and brought home or eaten in restaurants)
E Eat (extra) high-fat commercial products: candy, pastries, pies, doughnuts, cookies

Courtesy US Department of Health and Human Services: *Third report of the National Cholesterol Education Program on Detection, Evaluation, and Treatment of High Blood Cholesterol in Adults,* Washington, DC, 2001, US Government Printing Office.

Stress

Stress is a subjective experience with the potential for detrimental effects on cardiovascular health. To evaluate the impact of a stressor on a patient and to plan effective interventions, an understanding of the nature of the stressor is important. The provider should explore attributes of stress with the patient. What is the source of the stress? Is there a single stressor, or are there multiple stressors? What is the acuity level of the stress? Some stressors are chosen, whereas others present themselves. Is the stress longstanding or newly acquired? Does the patient have prior experience in coping with the particular stressor? How effective are the patient's usual means of managing stress?

Schafer has identified and described behavioral and physical distress symptoms, direct behavioral distress symptoms, and indirect symptoms of stress.

Behavioral signs are manifested physically by rigidity and tightness of the body, such as folded or crossed arms or legs. Fists may be clenched to indicate anxiety, or the forehead may be furrowed to signify worry. Direct behavioral distress symptoms reflect internal states and include teeth grinding, irritability, compulsiveness, rapid speech, stuttering, verbal aggression, a withdrawn demeanor, and crying spells. Indirect symptoms encompass addictive and escape behaviors. An elevated level of stress can increase the frequency of unhealthy behaviors. Addictions may be observed in increased smoking, alcohol consumption, the use of drugs to mitigate tension or induce sleep, and excessive consumption of caffeinated products. Common escape modalities are sleeping and television viewing.[13]

Signs of stress may be apparent in the patient's self-report or in distracting mannerisms such as agitation. When questioned about stress in their lives, patients are often forthcoming with evidence and usually can identify their most significant stressors. Stress related to overload is common and is characterized by an urgency about time. Other common sources of stress are interpersonal relationships, relationships within social or work domains, financial worries, and major life changes.

In general, stress is associated with distress. However, happy events and occasions can create a type of stress known as *eustress*. These events may include a wedding, the birth of a baby, or winning the lottery. The stress accompanies the modifications in behavior required to adapt and adjust to the change. However, the stress associated with the changes accompanying these pleasant events is often not acknowledged.

PHYSICAL EXAMINATION

Assessment of the patient's overall appearance when he or she is first seen is an important preliminary diagnostic activity. Measurement of vital signs should be taken into account, as well as height and weight. The patient who is well nourished is alert, has good color and smooth skin, stands erect, and is of normal weight for body build and age.[14] A poorly nourished patient is languid with pale, dry skin and poor posture; weighs more or less than normal for body build; and may appear to be high strung.[14] Ease of movement can be observed to give some indication of body flexibility. Conversely, limited movement may be apparent. A patient under great stress may have signs such as agitation, excessive perspiration, impatience, anxiety, and perhaps even mental dullness.

Established guidelines from the Obesity Education Initiative (OEI) of the NHLBI recommend the use of surrogate measures to assess body fat.[9] Although technologically sophisticated measures exist, they are expensive and unavailable to many providers; therefore BMI and waist circumference should be used. The BMI may be calculated by using one of the following equations:

$$\text{BMI} = \text{Weight (kg)} \times \text{Height (m) squared}$$

$$\text{BMI} = \text{Weight (lb)} \times 703 \div \text{height (in) squared}$$

The expert panel has defined overweight as BMI ranging from 25 to 29.9 kg/m^2 and obesity as a BMI of more than 30 kg/m^2.

In addition, the OEI recommends using waist circumference to measure abdominal fat. A measuring tape is placed on the upper hip bone and at the top of the right iliac crest so it is horizontal and parallel with the floor. The tape measure is extended around the waist in a snug manner but not so as to compress the skin. The measure is made at the end of a normal expiration. For men, a high-risk value is 102 cm or more (≥40 inches). A measure of more than 89 cm (>35 inches) is considered high risk for women.

The physical examination should include evaluation of cardiovascular fitness, musculature, and flexibility. The heart rate is one indicator of cardiovascular fitness. A fit person will have a lower heart rate with greater muscle strength and endurance, plus full range of motion. Patients who are not fit may have dyspnea or chest pain with exertion, be unable to participate in activities for extended periods, have less muscle tone and mass, and have limited range of motion.

DIAGNOSTICS

Identification of individuals at risk for health problems is key. Evaluation of blood glucose concentrations will identify those with type 2 diabetes. Lipid profile testing is important to detect individuals at risk for coronary artery disease. Lipoprotein analysis includes the measurement of concentrations of triglycerides, total cholesterol, α-lipoproteins (high-density lipoproteins [HDLs]), β-lipoproteins (low-density lipoproteins [LDLs]), and pre–β-lipoproteins (very low–density lipoproteins [VLDLs]). Epidemiologic investigations suggest that HDL cholesterol is inversely related to coronary disease, with high levels offering protection and lower levels increasing risk.[15] High cholesterol levels may be caused by some drugs, such as corticosteroids, and by diseases such as hypothyroidism, biliary obstruction, and pancreatic dysfunction.

An at-risk individual over 35 years of age who plans to begin an exercise program should undergo a stress ECG test as a precautionary measure. Younger patients with blood chemistry values and blood pressure readings indicating risk for metabolic or cardiopulmonary disease also need a complete physical examination and stress ECG test.[16] Bone density studies should be conducted on postmenopausal women to ascertain their risk for fracture and to diagnose osteopenia and osteoporosis.

LIFESTYLE-RELATED MEDICAL PROBLEMS

Hypertension

Guidelines from the American Heart Association state that a diagnosis of hypertension is based on an average of at least two blood pressure readings taken during two or more office visits after the initial measurement.[17] An optimum reading is less than 120 mm Hg for systolic blood pressure and less than 80 mm Hg for diastolic blood pressure. Prehypertension is systolic blood pressure in the 130 to 139 mm Hg range and diastolic blood pressure in the 80 to 89 mm Hg range. These patients should monitor their blood pressure on a regular basis. For more in-depth information on hypertension, see Chapter 129.

Hyperlipidemia

Cholesterol is a sterol that is synthesized in the liver from fats consumed in the diet and endogenously within body cells.[18] Cholesterol is essential for the production of bile acids, steroids, cell membranes, and sex hormones. Cholesterol enters the bloodstream via lipoproteins, with almost 75% being bound to LDLs.[15] Normally, a value of less than 200 mg/dl is considered an acceptable cholesterol level. Table 24-1 presents the normal ranges of total cholesterol, HDL, and LDL for men and women, allowing for a 10% higher range for African Americans. The blood triglyceride levels for men and women are presented in Table 24-2.

Diabetes

The concentration of blood glucose varies depending on the time since and contents of the last meal. In general, acceptable glucose levels for whole blood range from 60 to 89 mg/dl for adults under 60 years of age and from 68 to 98 mg/dl for individuals over 60 years of age. The acceptable range for blood serum levels is 70 to 105 mg/dl for adults under 60 years of age and 80 to 115 mg/dl for those over 60 years of age.[18]

Metabolic Syndrome

A cluster of risk factors significantly increases the risk for coronary artery disease. In combination the factors increase the risk for coronary heart disease with any level of LDL, according to the NCEP, and the presence of three or more of the risks is sufficient to support a diagnosis of metabolic syndrome[12] (Table 24-3).

LIFE SPAN ISSUES

Adverse health consequences from lifestyle influences have long incubation periods, ranging up to several decades. It follows that interventions in risk factors at an early age will produce better health outcomes later in life. Risk factors that can be modified are dietary habits, physical activity, and stress management. In addition, methods to intervene in addictions, such as smoking and alcohol consumption, will result in a longer life with more healthy years.

In general, it is not until the middle years of life that problems rooted in earlier patterns of health behaviors begin to arise; these problems include hyperlipidemia and type 2 diabetes, which are currently seen at increasingly early ages. Men are more likely to have coronary problems than are

TABLE 24-1 Blood Cholesterol*

Age	Male		Female	
	mg/dl	SI Units (mmol/L)	mg/dl	SI Units (mmol/L)
TOTAL CHOLESTEROL				
Adults (10% Higher Levels for African Americans)				
20-24 years	124-218	3.21-5.64	122-216	3.16-5.59
25-29 years	133-244	3.44-6.32	128-222	3.32-5.75
30-34 years	138-254	3.57-6.58	130-230	3.37-5.96
35-39 years	146-270	3.78-6.99	140-242	3.63-6.27
40-44 years	151-268	3.91-6.94	147-252	3.81-6.53
45-49 years	158-276	4.09-7.15	152-265	3.94-6.86
50-54 years	158-277	4.09-7.17	162-285	4.20-7.38
55-59 years	156-276	4.04-7.15	172-300	4.45-7.77
60-64 years	159-276	4.12-7.15	172-297	4.45-7.69
65-69 years	158-274	4.09-7.10	171-303	4.43-7.85
≥70 years	144-265	3.73-6.86	173-280	4.48-7.25
HIGH-DENSITY LIPOPROTEIN CHOLESTEROL (HDL)				
Adult (African-American Levels Approximately 10 mg/dl Higher)				
20-24 years	30-63	0.78-1.63	33-79	0.85-2.04
25-29 years	31-63	0.80-1.63	37-83	0.96-2.15
30-34 years	28-63	0.72-1.63	36-77	0.93-1.99
35-39 years	29-62	0.75-1.60	34-82	0.88-2.12
40-44 years	27-67	0.70-1.73	34-88	0.88-2.28
45-49 years	30-64	0.78-1.66	34-87	0.88-2.25
50-54 years	28-63	0.72-1.63	37-92	0.96-2.38
55-59 years	28-71	0.72-1.84	37-91	0.96-2.35
60-64 years	30-74	0.78-1.91	38-92	0.98-2.38
65-69 years	30-75	0.78-1.94	35-96	0.91-2.48
≥70 years	31-75	0.80-1.94	33-92	0.85-2.38
LOW-DENSITY LIPOPROTEIN CHOLESTEROL (LDL)				
Adult				
20-24 years	66-147	1.71-3.81	57-159	1.48-4.12
25-29 years	70-165	1.81-4.27	71-164	1.84-4.25
30-34 years	78-185	2.02-4.79	70-156	1.81-4.04
35-39 years	81-189	2.10-4.90	75-172	1.94-4.45
40-44 years	87-186	2.25-4.82	74-174	1.92-4.51
45-49 years	97-202	2.51-5.23	79-186	2.05-4.82
50-54 years	89-197	2.31-5.10	88-201	2.28-5.21
55-59 years	88-203	2.28-5.26	89-210	2.31-5.44
60-64 years	83-210	2.15-5.44	100-224	2.59-5.80
65-69 years	98-210	2.54-5.44	92-221	2.38-5.72
≥70 years	88-186	2.28-4.82	96-206	2.49-5.34

Modified from Chernecky C, Berger B, editors: *Laboratory tests and diagnostics procedures*, ed 3, Philadelphia, 2001, Saunders.
***Norm:** There is variation in recommended norms in the literature. (NOTE: Range given applies to a healthy population consuming a typical North American diet.)

women, although postmenopausal women have risks similar to those of men. The incidence of lung cancer has increased among women, who are more likely to begin smoking at younger ages. Postmenopausal women are at risk for calcium deficiency, which contributes to osteopenia or osteoporosis.

Older persons are particularly susceptible to malnutrition because of decreased physiologic functioning and changes associated with social factors, such as living alone. Suboptimum nutrition is often manifested by osteoporosis, iron deficiency anemia, weight management issues, and constipation.[19] Because malnutrition in the older patient is difficult to remedy, early detection is imperative.[20]

Older persons often erroneously believe that they have less need for physical activity. In reality, however, moderate to high levels of exercise boost their physiologic functioning, thereby optimizing functional status. In one study, exercise was shown to improve muscle strength, reaction time, and even control over body sway.[21]

COMPONENTS OF A HEALTHY LIFESTYLE

Lifestyle change is difficult, and the course is usually not smooth. There will be setbacks, but it is imperative that the patient begin anew and not be deterred. The therapeutic plan should be as simple as possible because one that is perceived

TABLE 24-2 Triglycerides

	Serum Values	
	mg/dl	SI Units (mmol/L)
ADULT WOMEN		
20-29 years	10-100	0.11-1.13
30-39 years	10-110	0.11-1.24
40-49 years	10-122	0.11-1.38
50-59 years	10-134	0.11-1.51
>59 years	10-147	0.11-1.66
ADULT MEN		
20-29 years	10-157	0.11-1.77
30-39 years	10-182	0.11-2.05
40-49 years	10-193	0.11-2.18
50-59 years	10-197	0.11-2.22
>59 years	10-199	0.11-2.24
CLASSIFICATION OF TRIGLYCERIDE LEVELS		
Borderline high	200-400	2.3
High	400-1000	4.5-11.3
Very high	>1000	>11.3

Modified from Chernecky C, Berger B, editors: *Laboratory tests and diagnostics procedures*, ed 3, Philadelphia, 2001, Saunders.

TABLE 24-3 Clinical Identification of Metabolic Syndrome

Risk Factor	Defining Level
Abdominal obesity*	Waist circumference†
Men	>102 cm (>40 in)
Women	>88 cm (>35 in)
Triglycerides	≥150 mg/dl
HDL cholesterol	
Men	<40 mg/dl
Women	<50 mg/dl
Blood pressure	≥130/85 mm Hg
Fasting glucose	≥110 mg/dl

Courtesy US Department of Health and Human Services: *Third report of the National Cholesterol Education Program on Detection, Evaluation, and Treatment of High Blood Cholesterol in Adults*, Washington, DC, 2001, US Government Printing Office.

*Overweight and obesity are associated with insulin resistance and metabolic syndrome. However, abdominal obesity is more highly correlated with metabolic risk factors than is an elevated body mass index (BMI). Therefore the simple measure of waist circumference is recommended to identify the body weight component of the metabolic syndrome.

†Some male patients can develop multiple metabolic risk factors when the waist circumference is only marginally increased (e.g., 94-102 cm [37-39 in]). Such patients may have a strong genetic contribution to insulin resistance. They should benefit from changes in life habits, similarly to men with categorical increases in waist circumference.

as too complicated will become a disincentive. According to the NHIS, 66% of individuals report that they have either excellent or very good health. There is a discrepancy based on race, with 57% of Hispanics and African Americans rating their health as excellent or good and 70% of Caucasians using these descriptors.[6]

Lifestyle counseling is essential to primary prevention of disease and disability and will have a positive effect on modifiable risk factors such as hypertension and hyperlipidemia. At the level of primary prevention, health education and counseling regarding nutrition, physical activity, and stress management will produce positive results for the patient.

Nutrition

The American diet has changed substantially during the past few decades. More meals are consumed on the run, away from home and family. Much of the food consumed is fast food, which is usually high in fat, calories, and salt. Over time, there is a cumulative effect on the body, with an increase in girth. Early on, the patient needs encouragement to make better food selections. The U.S. Department of Agriculture revised the Food Pyramid to allow for a more personalized approach to nutrition (Figure 24-1). The website http://www.mypyramid.gov allows users to customize a food plan based on their needs and preferences.

Eating well has several benefits, including providing a sense of vitality, maintaining a better weight, and giving a better overall appearance. Identifying factors that influence food consumption behaviors will enable the health care provider to adapt health counseling to the patient's circumstances. Motives that influence food selection and consumption may relate to culture, habit, or convenience. Cultural practices must be acknowledged and accommodated in health counseling. Habits related to food intake probably require a program of behavioral change. Food consumption behaviors born out of convenience, such as reaching for chips when hunger is felt, may be amendable through health education.

Adequacy of nutritional intake should be ensured. Sufficient intake of daily dietary fiber is often neglected. Fiber in the form of whole-grain foods, fruits, and vegetables is essential to good health and aids in reducing heart disease and cancer. Fiber-rich foods are often neglected because they often require cleaning and preparation. These nutrients are often replaced with prepackaged snack foods. One technique that can be used to avoid convenience foods is to have clean fruits and vegetables prepared in advance and stored so they are ready to eat when a quick snack is desired.

Middle-aged women may be at risk for hypocalcemia resulting from a diet that lacks calcium-rich foods. The ingestion of calcium-enriched orange juice, almonds, spinach, broccoli, kale, turnip greens, milk, cheese, and yogurt should be encouraged. However, caution is advised because overconsumption of calcium may result in hypercalcemia, which is related to the formation of renal calculi.

Caffeine has been classified as a drug because of its effects on the body. Caffeine is used for its stimulating effect, which increases alertness. Excess caffeine, however, can induce caffeinism, which is characterized by headaches, irritability, anxiety, insomnia, and heart palpitations. Recent studies suggest that moderate intake of caffeine may not have the detrimental consequences once associated with its use. Moderate use is generally considered to be less than 250 mg/day, or the equivalent of two or three 5-ounce cups of coffee; percolated coffee has 64 to 124 mg of caffeine per 5 ounces, whereas drip-brewed coffee has 110 to 150 mg of caffeine per 5 ounces.[22] Coca-Cola has 46 mg of caffeine in a 12-ounce can, and Mountain Dew has 54 mg.[23]

Anatomy of MyPyramid

One size doesn't fit all

USDA's new MyPyramid symbolizes a personalized approach to healthy eating and physical activity. The symbol has been designed to be simple. It has been developed to remind consumers to make healthy food choices and to be active every day. The different parts of the symbol are described below.

Activity
Activity is represented by the steps and the person climbing them, as a reminder of the importance of daily physical activity.

Moderation
Moderation is represented by the narrowing of each food group from bottom to top. The wider base stands for foods with little or no solid fats or added sugars. These should be selected more often. The narrower top area stands for foods containing more added sugars and solid fats. The more active you are, the more of these foods can fit into your diet.

Personalization
Personalization is shown by the person on the steps, the slogan, and the URL. Find the kinds and amounts of food to eat each day at MyPyramid.gov.

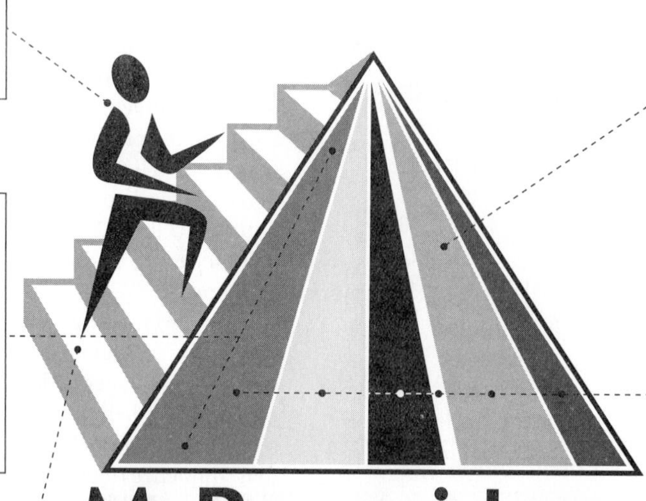

Proportionality
Proportionality is shown by the different widths of the food group bands. The widths suggest how much food a person should choose from each group. The widths are just a general guide, not exact proportions. Check the Web site for how much is right for you.

Variety
Variety is symbolized by the 6 color bands representing the 5 food groups of the Pyramid and oils. This illustrates that foods from all groups are needed each day for good health.

Gradual Improvement
Gradual improvement is encouraged by the slogan. It suggests that individuals can benefit from taking small steps to improve their diet and lifestyle each day.

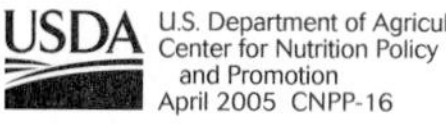

U.S. Department of Agriculture
Center for Nutrition Policy and Promotion
April 2005 CNPP-16

USDA is an equal opportunity provider and employer.

GRAINS | VEGETABLES | FRUITS | OILS | MILK | MEAT & BEANS

FIGURE 24-1

The Food Guide Pyramid. (Courtesy U.S. Department of Agriculture and U.S. Department of Health and Human Services.)

The Vegetarian Diet. Many individuals have chosen to become vegetarians. Reasons for this include personal life philosophy, concern about excess consumption of saturated fat in beef products, concern about food-borne illnesses associated with meat consumption, and a desire for a healthier lifestyle. Vegetarians should follow the principle of complementation when selecting foods. To ensure that the required amino acids are supplied, complementation combines a grain with legumes or a dairy product (for lactovegetarians). Possible combinations include a peanut butter and jelly sandwich, beans and corn, brown bread and baked beans, a flour tortilla and beans, macaroni and cheese, and rice and milk. A major health concern is the adequacy of vitamin B intake, since meats are the major source of this nutrient. Because vegetarians may not deliberately plan their meals to incorporate essential nutrients, they should be advised to take a daily multivitamin.

Weight Management. The practice guidelines released by the OEI of the NHLBI advise that management of overweight and obesity has many components, including behavioral, dietary, physical, and pharmacologic.[9] The expert panel offers several suggestions from a behavioral perspective. The provider must communicate with the patient in a nonjudgmental manner. Some individuals are exceptionally sensitive about weight and likely to have a long history of frustration and trouble with weight control. In addition, providers need to examine their own attitudes toward the condition.

Experts liken obesity to a chronic disease, such as diabetes. Behavioral change is required, and compliance with a long-term regimen of behavioral change is generally poor. Providers are advised to build a partnership with the patient, taking into account the patient's weight management goals. Goal setting should be specific yet achievable. A reasonable goal for weight loss can be a reduction of 10% of body weight over a 6-month period. Weight control is not a destination but rather a journey; therefore frequent contact with the health care provider is beneficial to the patient. This can be achieved through frequent monitoring of weight, which has the advantage of being an effective motivator.

Dietary Considerations. According to the OEI practice guidelines, the patient's motivation or inclination toward weight loss is of primary concern.[9] Diet is the cornerstone of a weight management program. According to the recommendations, there are many topics to cover in a patient education program. The patient needs basic instructions on the composition of foods, including information on calorie content, how to read food labels, and what constitutes a serving size. In addition, the patient may need coaching on how to make wise food purchases and techniques for low-calorie food preparation. The patient should understand the value of adequate water intake and the importance of limiting alcohol consumption. Suggested food plans for 1200- and 1600-calorie diets are presented in Tables 24-4 and 24-5. A guide to food exchanges is presented in Box 24-2.

TABLE 24-4 1200-Calorie Diet

	Calories	Fat (g)	Fat (%)	Exchange For:
BREAKFAST				
Whole wheat bread, 1 medium slice	70	1.2	15	1 bread/starch
Jelly, regular, 2 tsp	30	0	0	1/2 fruit
Cereal, shredded wheat, 1/2 cup	104	1	4	1 bread/starch
Milk, 1%, 1 cup	102	3	23	1 milk
Orange juice, 3/4 cup	78	0	0	1 1/2 fruit
Coffee, regular, 1 cup	5	0	0	Free
Breakfast total	**389**	**5.2**	**10**	
LUNCH				
Roast beef sandwich:				
Whole wheat bread, 2 medium slices	139	2.4	15	2 bread/starch
Lean roast beef, unseasoned, 2 oz	60	1.5	23	2 lean protein
Lettuce, 1 leaf	1	0	0	—
Tomato, 3 medium slices	10	0	0	1 vegetable
Mayonnaise, low calorie, 1 tsp	15	1.7	96	1/3 fat
Apple, 1 medium	80	0	0	1 fruit
Water, 1 cup	0	0	0	Free
Lunch total	**305**	**5.6**	**16**	
DINNER				
Salmon, 2 oz edible	103	5	44	2 lean protein
Vegetable oil, 1 1/2 tsp	60	7	100	1 1/2 fat
Baked potato, 3/4 medium	100	0	0	1 bread/starch
Margarine, 1 tsp	34	4	100	1 fat
Green beans, seasoned, with margarine, 1/2 cup	52	2	4	1 vegetable, 1/2 fat
Carrots, seasoned	35	0	0	1 vegetable
White dinner roll, 1 small	70	2	28	1 bread/starch
Iced tea, unsweetened, 1 cup	0	0	0	Free
Water, 2 cups	0	0	0	Free
Dinner total	**454**	**20**	**39**	
SNACK				
Popcorn, 2 1/2 cups	69	0	0	1 bread/starch
Margarine, 3/4 tsp	30	3	100	3/4 fat
Total	**1247**	**34-36**	**24-26**	

Modified from National Heart, Lung, and Blood Institute: *The practical guide to the identification, evaluation, and treatment of overweight and obesity in adults,* Bethesda, Md, 2000, NHLBI Information Center.

Traditional American Cuisine—1200 calories

You can use the exchange list in Box 24-2 to give yourself more choices.

Calories	1247	Saturated fat, % kcals	7
Total carbohydrate, % kcals	58	Cholesterol, mg	96
Total fat, % kcals	26	Protein, % kcals	19
*Sodium, mg	043		

NOTE: Calories have been rounded.

1200: 100% RDA met for all nutrients except vitamin E 80%, vitamin B_2 96%, vitamin B_6 94%, calcium 68%, iron 63%, and zinc 73%.

*No salt added in recipe preparation or as seasoning. Consume at least 32 oz of water.

TABLE 24-5 1600-Calorie Diet

	Calories	Fat (g)	Fat (%)	Exchange For:
BREAKFAST				
Whole wheat bread, 1 medium slice	70	1.2	15.4	1 bread/starch
Jelly, regular, 2 tsp	30	0	0	1/2 fruit
Cereal, shredded wheat, 1/2 cup	207	2	8	2 bread/starch
Milk, 1%, 1 cup	102	3	23	1 milk
Orange juice, 3/4 cup	78	0	0	1 1/2 fruit
Coffee, regular, 1 cup	5	0	0	Free
Milk, 1%, 1 oz	10	0.3	27	1/8 milk
Breakfast total	**502**	**6.5**	**10**	
LUNCH				
Roast beef sandwich:				
Whole wheat bread, 2 medium slices	139	2.4	15	2 bread/starch
Lean roast beef, unseasoned, 2 oz	60	1.5	23	2 lean protein
American cheese, low fat and low sodium, 1 slice, 3/4 oz	46	1.8	36	1 lean protein
Lettuce, 1 leaf	1	0	0	—
Tomato, 3 medium slices	10	0	0	1 vegetable
Mayonnaise, low calorie, 2 tsp	30	3.3	99	2/3 fat
Apple, 1 medium	80	0	0	1 fruit
Water, 1 cup	0	0	0	Free
Lunch total	**366**	**9**	**22**	
DINNER				
Salmon, 2 oz edible	155	7	40	3 lean protein
Vegetable oil, 1 1/2 tsp	60	7	100	1 1/2 fat
Baked potato, 3/4 medium	100	0	0	1 bread/starch
Margarine, 1 tsp	34	4	100	1 fat
Green beans, seasoned, with margarine, 1/2 cup	52	2	4	1 vegetable, 1/2 fat
Carrots, seasoned, with margarine, 1/2 cup	52	2	4	1 vegetable, 1/2 fat
White dinner roll, 1 small	80	3	33	1 bread/starch
Ice milk, 1/2 cup	92	3	28	1 bread/starch, 1/2 fat
Iced tea, unsweetened, 1 cup	0	0	0	Free
Water, 3 cups	0	0	0	Free
Dinner total	**625**	**28**	**38**	
SNACK				
Popcorn, 2 1/2 cups	69	0	0	1 bread/starch
Margarine, 3/4 tsp	58	6.5	100	1 1/2 fat
Total	**1620**	**50**	**28**	

Modified from National Heart, Lung, and Blood Institute: *The practical guide to the identification, evaluation, and treatment of overweight and obesity in adults,* Bethesda, Md, 2000, NHLBI Information Center.

Traditional American Cuisine—1600 calories

You can use the exchange list in Box 24-2 to give yourself more choices.

Calories	1613	Saturated fat, % kcals	8
Total carbohydrate, % kcals	55	Cholesterol, mg	142
Total fat, % kcals	29	Protein, % kcals	19
*Sodium, mg	1341		

NOTE: Calories have been rounded.

1600: 100% RDA met for all nutrients except vitamin E 99%, iron 73%, and zinc 91%.

*No salt added in recipe preparation or as seasoning. Consume at least 32 oz of water.

Dietary Influences on Heart Health

Brunner, Thorogood, Rees, and colleagues reviewed the scientific literature on the effects of dietary advice given to healthy adults to assess the consequences of diet on cardiovascular health.[22] Dietary teaching included decreasing salt and fat intake and increasing vegetables, fruit, and fiber. They concluded that there were modest benefits with a modified diet and that the most change was in women, who were more likely to decrease fat intake.

The American Heart Association published a scientific paper by Appel, Brands, Daniels, and colleagues on the dietary factors associated with hypertension treatment and control: less dietary salt; alcohol use in moderation; weight loss; increased potassium; and adherence to a food plan based on

BOX 24-2

FOOD EXCHANGE LIST

Within each group, these foods can be exchanged for each other. You can use this list to give yourself more choices.

VEGETABLES

Contain 25 calories and 5 g of carbohydrate. One serving equals:

- 1/2 cup cooked vegetables (e.g., carrots, broccoli, zucchini, cabbage)
- 1 cup raw vegetables or salad greens
- 1/2 cup vegetable juice

If you're hungry, eat more fresh or steamed vegetables.

FAT-FREE AND VERY-LOW-FAT MILK

Contains 90 calories and 12 g of carbohydrate per serving. One serving equals:

- 8 oz milk, fat free or 1% fat
- 3/4 cup yogurt, plain nonfat or low fat
- 1 cup yogurt, artificially sweetened

VERY LEAN PROTEIN

Choices have 35 calories and 1 g of fat per serving. One serving equals:

- 1 oz turkey breast or chicken breast, skin removed
- 1 oz fish fillet (flounder, sole, scrod, cod, haddock, halibut)
- 1 oz canned tuna in water
- 1 oz shellfish (clams, lobster, scallop, shrimp)
- 3/4 cup cottage cheese, nonfat or low fat
- 2 egg whites
- 1/4 cup egg substitute
- 1 oz fat-free cheese
- 1/2 cup beans—cooked (black beans, kidney, chickpeas, or lentils); count as 1 starch/bread and 1 very lean protein

FRUITS

Contain 15 g of carbohydrates and 60 calories. One serving equals:

- 1 small apple, banana, orange, nectarine
- 1 medium fresh peach
- 1 kiwi
- 1/2 grapefruit
- 1/ mango
- 1 cup fresh berries (strawberries, raspberries, or blueberries)
- 1 cup fresh melon cubes
- 1/8 honeydew melon
- 4 oz unsweetened juice
- 4 tsp jelly or jam

LEAN PROTEIN

Choices have 55 calories and 2 to 3 g of fat per serving. One serving equals:

- 1 oz chicken—dark meat, skin removed
- 1 oz turkey—dark meat, skin removed
- 1 oz salmon, swordfish, herring, catfish, trout
- 1 oz lean beef (flank steak, London broil, tenderloin, roast beef)*
- 1 oz veal, roast or lean chop*
- 1 oz lamb, roast or lean chop*
- 1 oz pork, tenderloin or fresh ham*
- 1 oz low-fat cheese (3 g or less of fat per ounce)
- 1 oz low-fat luncheon meats (with 3 g or less of fat per ounce)
- 1/4 cup 4.5% cottage cheese
- 2 medium sardines

MEDIUM-FAT PROTEINS

Have 75 calories and 5 g of fat per serving. One serving equals:

- 1 oz beef (any prime cut), corned beef, ground beef
- 1 oz pork chop
- 1 oz whole egg (medium)
- 1 oz mozzarella cheese
- 1/4 cup ricotta cheese
- 4 oz tofu (a heart-healthy choice)

STARCHES

Contain 15 g of carbohydrate and 80 calories per serving. One serving equals:

- 1 slice bread (white, pumpernickel, whole wheat, rye)
- 2 slices reduced-calorie or "lite" bread
- 1/4 (1 oz) bagel (varies)
- 1/2 English muffin
- 1/2 hamburger bun
- 3/4 cup cold cereal
- 1/3 cup rice, brown or white—cooked
- 1/3 cup barley or couscous—cooked
- 1/3 cup legumes (dried beans, peas, or lentils)—cooked
- 1/2 cup pasta—cooked
- 1/2 cup bulgur—cooked
- 1/2 cup corn, sweet potato, or green peas
- 3 oz baked sweet or white potato
- 3/4 oz pretzels
- 3 cups popcorn, hot-air popped or microwave (80% light)

FATS

Contain 45 calories and 5 g of fat per serving. One serving equals:

- 1 tsp oil (vegetable, corn, canola, olive, etc.)
- 1 tsp butter
- 1 tsp stick margarine
- 1 tsp mayonnaise
- 1 Tbsp reduced-fat margarine or mayonnaise
- 1 Tbsp salad dressing
- 1 Tbsp cream cheese
- 2 Tbsp light cream cheese
- 1/8 avocado
- 8 large black olives
- 10 large stuffed green olives
- 1 slice bacon

Modified from National Heart, Lung, and Blood Institute: *The practical guide to the identification, evaluation, and treatment of overweight and obesity in adults,* Bethesda, Md, 2000, NHLBI Information Center. Based on the American Dietetic Association Exchange List.
*Limit to 1 or 2 times per week.

the Dietary Approaches to Stop Hypertension eating plan, also know as the DASH diet.[24] The authors concluded that, in particular, African Americans and the elderly benefit from the diet. The DASH diet presented in Table 24-6 is from the National Institutes of Health.[25]

Exercise

Patients who do not participate in any type of physical activity may have a plethora of excuses. Among the most familiar are lacking time, feeling tired, being too busy, and disliking exercise. Older adults may use their age to justify a lack of physical activity. However, physical activity has been called a "magic bullet" that can ward off heart disease and should be encouraged.

Before encouraging any type of exercise program, the health care provider must be aware of the patient's existing level of fitness. A patient in mid-life or one who is sedentary and significantly overweight may need medical clearance to begin

TABLE 24-6 The DASH Diet*

Food Group	Daily Servings	Serving Sizes	Examples and Notes	Significance of Each Food Group to DASH Diet Pattern
Grains and grain products	7-8	1 slice bread 1/2 cup dry cereal 1/2 cup cooked rice, pasta, or cereal	Whole wheat bread, English muffin, pita bread, bagel, cereals, grits, oatmeal	Major sources of energy and fiber
Vegetables	4-5	1 cup raw leafy vegetable 1/2 cup cooked vegetable 6 oz vegetable juice	Tomatoes, potatoes, carrots, peas, squash, broccoli, turnip greens, collards, kale, spinach, artichokes, sweet potatoes, beans	Rich sources of potassium, magnesium, and fiber
Fruits	4-5	6 oz fruit juice 1 medium fruit 1/4 cup dried fruit 1/2 cup fresh, frozen, or canned fruit	Apricots, bananas, dates, oranges, orange juice, grapefruit, grapefruit juice, mangoes, melons, peaches, pineapples, prunes, raisins, strawberries, tangerines	Important sources of potassium, magnesium, and fiber
Low-fat or nonfat dairy foods	2-3	8 oz milk 1 cup yogurt 1.5 oz cheese	Skim or 1% milk, skim or low-fat buttermilk, nonfat or low-fat yogurt, part skim mozzarella cheese, nonfat cheese	Major sources of calcium and protein
Meats, poultry, and fish	2 or less	3 oz cooked meats, poultry, or fish	Select only lean; trim away visible fats; broil, roast, or boil, instead of frying; remove skin from poultry	Rich sources of protein and magnesium
Nuts, seeds, and legumes	4-5 per week	1.5 oz or 1/3 cup nuts 1/2 oz or 2 Tbsp seeds 1/2 cup cooked legumes	Almonds, filberts, mixed nuts, peanuts, walnuts, sunflower seeds, kidney beans, lentils	Rich sources of energy, magnesium, potassium, protein, and fiber

THE DASH DIET SAMPLE MENU†

Food	Amount	Servings Provided
Breakfast		
Orange juice	6 oz	1 fruit
1% low-fat milk	8 oz (1 cup)	1 dairy
Corn flakes (with 1 tsp sugar)	1 cup	2 grains
Banana	1 medium	1 fruit
Whole wheat bread (with 1 Tbsp jelly)	1 slice	1 grain
Soft margarine	1 tsp	1 fat
Lunch		
Chicken salad	3/4 cup	1 poultry
Pita bread	1/2, large	1 grain
Raw vegetable medley:		1 vegetable
Carrot and celery sticks	3-4 sticks each	
Radishes	2	
Loose-leaf lettuce	2 leaves	
Part-skim mozzarella cheese	1.5 slice (1.5 oz)	1 dairy
1% low-fat milk	8 oz (1 cup)	1 dairy
Fruit cocktail in light syrup	1/2 cup	1 fruit
Dinner		
Herbed baked cod	3 oz	1 fish
Scallion rice	1 cup	2 grains
Steamed broccoli	1/2 cup	1 vegetable
Stewed tomatoes	1/2 cup	1 vegetable
Spinach salad:	1/2 cup	1 vegetable
Raw spinach	1/2 cup	
Cherry tomatoes	2	
Cucumber	2 slices	

*Available at http://www.nhlbi.nih.gov/health/public/heart/hbp/dash/new_dash.pdf.
†Based on 2100 calories/day.

TABLE 24-6 The DASH Diet*—cont'd

THE DASH DIET SAMPLE MENU† —CONT'D

Food	Amount	Servings Provided
Dinner—cont'd		
Light Italian salad dressing	1 Tbsp	1/2 fat
Whole wheat dinner roll	1 small	1 grain
Soft margarine	1 tsp	1 fat
Melon balls	1/2 cup	1 fruit
Snacks		
Dried apricots	1 oz (1/4 cup)	1 fruit
Mini-pretzels	1 oz (3/4 cup)	1 grain
Mixed nuts	1.5 oz (1/3 cup)	1 nuts
Diet ginger ale	12 oz	—

TOTAL NUMBER OF SERVINGS IN 2100 CALORIES/DAY MENU

Food Group	Servings
Grains	6-8
Vegetables	4 -5
Fruits	4-5
Dairy foods	2-3
Meats, poultry, and fish	6 oz
Nuts, seeds, and legumes	4-5/week
Fats and oils	2-3

TIPS ON EATING THE DASH WAY

- Start small. Make gradual changes in your eating habits.
- Center your meal around carbohydrates, such as pasta, rice, beans, or vegetables.
- Treat meat as one part of the whole meal, instead of the focus.
- Use fruits or low-fat, low-calorie foods such as sugar-free gelatin for desserts and snacks.

REMEMBER!

If you use the DASH diet to help prevent or control high blood pressure, make it part of a lifestyle that includes choosing foods lower in salt and sodium, keeping a healthy weight, being physically active, and, if you drink alcohol, doing so in moderation.

exercising based on clinical findings in the history and physical examination.

For the sedentary patient, it is extremely important to begin a physical fitness program slowly so that the body can acclimate to the new demands imposed on it. Moreover, a slow start safeguards against injury. An overzealous exercise program is likely to have a negative impact on motivation (i.e., the exercise prescription may serve as a deterrent if it is too rigorous early on). The patient must be committed to carrying out the program. Most individuals are aware of the value of incorporating exercise into their daily schedules, yet many do not follow through. Because exercise requires a personal commitment, individuals need to be deliberate about making time for exercise in their daily lives. Wilbur, Chandler, and Miller investigated women's adherence to a home-based walking program.[26] Frequency of participation proved to be most problematic; however, once the 24 women began walking, they walked for the prescribed length of time and at the appropriate intensity. Thus patients may need suggestions for scheduling physical activities into their daily routines to ensure frequency of participation in physical activity.

The OEI recommends 30 to 40 minutes of moderate activity 3 to 5 days a week. Good results can be achieved through a program of walking.[9] Table 24-7 provides a suggested plan from the OEI expert panel.

Aerobic activity is particularly recommended for cardiac health because it strengthens the heart muscle. Aerobic endurance training consists of three phases: the warm-up, aerobics, and the cool down. Warming up for the intensity of aerobic training begins to raise the pulse rate and prepares the muscles and joints. This generally takes 3 to 5 minutes but may take longer in lower temperatures. Often, the warm-up activity is a gentler motion of the same type of physical activity that is part of the aerobic exercise and may involve stretching. The aerobic portion encompasses the dimensions of frequency, intensity, and time (known by the acronym *FIT*). The recommended frequency is three to five times per week, with a day off between workouts being desirable.

TABLE 24-7 Sample Walking Program

	Warmup	Exercising	Cool Down	Total Time
Week 1				
Session A	Walk 5 minutes.	Then walk briskly 5 minutes.	Then walk more slowly 5 minutes.	15 minutes
Session B	Repeat above pattern.			
Session C	Repeat above pattern.			
Continue with at least 3 exercise sessions during each week of the program.				
Week 2	Walk 5 minutes.	Walk briskly 7 minutes.	Walk 5 minutes.	17 minutes
Week 3	Walk 5 minutes.	Walk briskly 9 minutes.	Walk 5 minutes.	19 minutes
Week 4	Walk 5 minutes.	Walk briskly 11 minutes.	Walk 5 minutes.	21 minutes
Week 5	Walk 5 minutes.	Walk briskly 13 minutes.	Walk 5 minutes.	23 minutes
Week 6	Walk 5 minutes.	Walk briskly 15 minutes.	Walk 5 minutes.	25 minutes
Week 7	Walk 5 minutes.	Walk briskly 18 minutes.	Walk 5 minutes.	28 minutes
Week 8	Walk 5 minutes.	Walk briskly 20 minutes.	Walk 5 minutes.	30 minutes
Week 9	Walk 5 minutes.	Walk briskly 23 minutes.	Walk 5 minutes.	33 minutes
Week 10	Walk 5 minutes.	Walk briskly 26 minutes.	Walk 5 minutes.	36 minutes
Week 11	Walk 5 minutes.	Walk briskly 28 minutes.	Walk 5 minutes.	38 minutes
Week 12	Walk 5 minutes.	Walk briskly 30 minutes.	Walk 5 minutes.	40 minutes
Week 13 on	Gradually increase your brisk walking time to 30 to 60 minutes, 3 or 4 times a week. Remember that your goal is to get the benefits you are seeking and enjoy your activity.			

From National Heart, Lung, and Blood Institute: *The practical guide to the identification, evaluation, and treatment of overweight and obesity in adults,* Bethesda, Md, 2000, NHLBI Information Center.

Heart rate is a measure of intensity. The maximum heart rate, calculated by subtracting one's age from 220, represents the heart rate that should not be exceeded during exercise. For example, an individual who is 55 years of age should not have a pulse rate in excess of 165 beats per minute during training. The target heart rate is recommended for maximum effectiveness of aerobic activity and is represented by a range of values between 60% and 80% of the maximum heart rate. Thus the 55-year-old individual is well advised to keep the pulse rate between 99 beats per minute (165 maximum heart rate × 60% = 99) and 132 beats per minute (165 × 80% = 132). The aerobic portion of activity should be at least 20 minutes long, with the heart beating within the range of the target heart rate. Conditioned individuals may extend their workouts to up to 1 hour.

Any activity that requires rhythmic, continuous movement and the use of the large muscles of the arms and legs may be selected. Bicycling, cross-country skiing, and some forms of dancing are examples of aerobic activities. The final component of the workout is the cool down, during which the heart rate gradually returns to normal. Because the muscles are warm, stretching exercises may be incorporated to enhance flexibility.

Resistance training for muscle strength and endurance may be performed before an aerobic activity training or on opposite days. Some individuals lift weights as part of the warm-up. Musculoskeletal training may be achieved through the use of weights or through calisthenics.

The American Heart Association advises that individuals be aware of any sensation of pressure or pain in the middle or left chest area and of pallor, cold sweat, sudden lightheadedness, or fainting during a workout.[27] The patient should be advised that, if any of these events occur, he or she needs to stop exercising and call the health care provider.

Physical Activity and Chronic Illness

Evidence strongly suggests that physical activity has a significant positive effect on patients with chronic diseases. Sally Fitts, PhD, of the Department of Rehabilitation Medicine at the University of Washington, discovered that stationary bicycling during hemodialysis is beneficial for patients with chronic renal failure and end-stage renal disease.[28] The exercise not only is safe but also increases the efficiency of fluid removal and decreases common problems that accompany dialysis, such as chills, fatigue, and muscle cramping. Fitts cautions that the target heart rate is not a useful measure for patients with end-stage renal disease and instead recommends that the patient's report of perceived exertion be used to determine fitness and intensity.

Patricia Deuster, PhD, MPH, of the Department of Military and Emergency Medicine of the Uniformed Services University of the Health Sciences, affirms that physically active women have a reduced breast cancer risk and that those with osteoporosis, fibromyalgia, or rheumatoid arthritis also benefit from exercise.[29] Osteoporosis, a disease that affects not only postmenopausal women but also female athletes who are amenorrheic, is linked to a low bone mineral density. The condition is averted through impact and weight-bearing exercises. For those with fibromyalgia, cardiovascular conditioning enhances fitness and elevates the pain threshold. Arthritic patients benefit both physically and psychologically. Muscle strength and joint flexibility are improved, and morning stiffness is decreased; psychologically, anxiety and depression are decreased. Exercise regimens that are particularly effective with arthritic patients are water-based exercises and modified dance exercises. Although these preliminary observations hold promise, definitive guidelines must be deferred until the appropriate frequency, intensity, and duration of exercise have been determined.[29]

Stress Management

Behaviors that are beneficial to physiologic wellness, such as engaging in physical activity and a healthy diet, also afford protection against the adverse effects of stress. Excessive stress is harmful because it interferes with the function of the immune system, and high levels of stress can impede disease protection.[30] Fortunately, there are many ways to minimize the detrimental consequences, including adequate amounts of sleep, cultivation of interpersonal relationships, relaxation techniques, good time management skills, prayer, a perspective on life, and a sense of humor.

Sleep. Impairment secondary to insufficient sleep is in itself a common health problem that increases the risk for errors in performance and problem solving. Originally, it was believed that sleep was essential to rejuvenate the body physically. Current interest in sleep research centers on the effect of sleep on the prefrontal cerebral cortex, the part of the brain associated with higher-level thinking abilities. For many, sleep is a low priority and is often sacrificed to make time for other activities. Sleep-deprived individuals are more at risk for automobile accidents, anxiety, and depression; are less productive; and are poorer at problem solving. To operate at peak performance, most individuals require 7 to 8 hours of sleep each day. Some individuals can manage with fewer than 5 hours of sleep, but they represent the exception.

To guarantee adequate time for sleep, patients can use time management techniques to deliberately block out the time needed for adequate rest. The sleep schedule should be regular, which means arising at the same time daily. Caffeinated products should be avoided for a minimum of 6 and up to 11 hours before retiring. Sleeping pills and alcohol should be avoided as aids to sleep. A glass of warm milk or a slice of turkey may be helpful because these foods contain the amino acid tryptophan, which is a natural sedative. Daily exercise is also an effective sleep inducer, although it should be avoided before bedtime, when it may have a stimulating effect. Cares and worries should not preoccupy the patient during the time before dozing off. Instead, noting concerns and planning courses of action before going to bed may be helpful. Bedtime rituals are also effective for sleep preparation. These may include reading, praying, preparing for the next day, and bathing.

Interpersonal Relationships. Healthy and satisfying personal relationships are not only rewarding but also buffer some of the stressors in life. Encouraging patients to nurture, maintain, and cherish relationships with family and friends is beneficial. In addition, patients need to have realistic expectations of what to expect from their relationships with others. The quality of relationships takes precedence over quantity; therefore a few good friends confer greater resistance to stress than do many superficial ones.

Relaxation. The relaxation response is an antidote to the physiologic alterations triggered by exposure to a stressor. Blood glucose levels decrease with relaxation, as do the heart rate, respiration rate, and blood pressure. Muscles relax as well. Psychologic advantages may include decreased anxiety and an enhanced ability to cope with fearful situations.

Napping, walking, stroking a pet, participating in a hobby, listening to soothing music, and other activities can elicit the relaxation response. Breathing techniques are also effective for decreasing stress. Deep breathing involves two steps: (1) inhaling through the nose with the intention of inflating the lungs, and (2) exhaling through the mouth at a slower rate than inhaling. This is the "cleansing breath" many individuals learn in Lamaze classes. Another technique involves diaphragmatic breathing (i.e., using the diaphragm to regulate respiration). This is sometimes called "belly breathing," which can be observed in the way an infant breathes. The belly is thrust outward as a long, deep breath is taken. Because the relaxation occurs on exhalation, the exhalation should be long and slow.

Time Management. Time is a precious commodity and must be managed wisely. Americans are overextended by the sheer volume of tasks they hope to complete daily. Even youths are beginning to complain of not having enough time in the day—a phenomenon previously reserved for adulthood and its concomitant responsibilities. A common time management technique is to apply an *A, B, C* format to the list of tasks that need to be achieved on a given day. *A* represents what must be achieved during the day, *B* signifies an important task, and *C* means that the activity can wait for another day. The goal is to achieve tasks assigned to the *A* group, make progress on those in the *B* group, and possibly begin the tasks in the *C* group. To ensure successful completion of required and important tasks, individuals should schedule themselves at 75% capacity. Inevitably, tasks, projects, and assignments consume more time than originally allocated. "Underscheduling" will probably convert to a full, rather than overloaded, slate of activities. As the day progresses, it is helpful to ask the question, "What is the best use of my time right now?" Breaks are important and can be used during transition times between activities. A break may be filled by having a meal, engaging in a physical activity (e.g., walking around the block, jumping rope), or calling a friend on the telephone. In the long run, continuously working without a break will diminish productivity and may lead to psychologic burnout.

Prayer. In the aftermath of the events of September 11, 2001, many Americans felt that their basic sense of psychologic security had been violated. Some experienced depression, requiring medication for symptom relief. Others responded by becoming more spiritual and turning to a higher power for assistance in the face of adversity. Overall, those with an active prayer life tend to be more optimistic in their outlook.

Certainly the spiritual domain of health must be acknowledged and faith practices encouraged.

Perspective on Life. Optimists seem to fare better than do pessimists. Patients can be encouraged and supported in their attempts to keep a positive perspective. Care needs to be taken with unduly upset patients or with those who are experiencing a significant personal loss. To coach these individuals in optimism would be to trivialize their needs. These patients could be better served by identifying a source of hope for them.

Humor. A sense of humor serves many purposes. Certainly, it enables one to laugh rather than cry about a situation. Not only does laughter diffuse stress in an individual, but, when used appropriately, humor may subdue interpersonal tension in social situations.

Safety

Home Safety. Many regard home as a "safe" haven, yet it is the scene for most accidents and injuries. Falls result from navigating cluttered rooms and steps. Kitchen fires can arise from cooking fats and improperly using small appliances. Poisonings occur from chemicals commonly found in household cleaning solutions. In addition, toxic fumes in the form of carbon monoxide or radon may be emitted within homes. Larger appliances, power tools, and electrical cords also pose potential dangers. The use of goggles or safety glasses and ear plugs may be warranted with some types of tools.

Safety at home requires knowledge of potential sources of trauma and injury. Smoke detectors are recommended for each level of the house. If the smoke detectors are battery powered, batteries should be checked twice a year and replaced as necessary. The schedule should coincide with an event, such as resetting the clock for daylight savings time in spring and for standard time in fall. Carbon monoxide detectors may be useful for detecting carbon monoxide leaks. Radon, another poisonous gas, can also be detected with a home testing kit. Ventilation systems also need to be checked.

Lighting needs to be assessed for adequacy. In dark homes and in homes with small children or older adults, nightlights may prevent injury from tripping or falling. Floor rugs need to be anchored securely to prevent falls, and stairs should be free of clutter. Slippery floors may also cause household accidents. Electrical cords should not be frayed and should be out of the path of normal daily activity.

Hazardous cleaning supplies need to be stored safely and toxic supplies disposed of properly. Medications should be labeled and kept out of the reach of children. If firearms are kept in the home, extra care needs to be exercised to reduce the risk of injury. Guns should be stored unloaded and be secured under lock and key. Ammunition should be stored away from the firearm, preferably in a locked compartment or container.

Personal Preparedness. The incidence of natural disasters, such as flooding, has increased. Thus it is important for families to have mapped out emergency plans. Important papers and documents, such as birth certificates and Social Security cards for all family members, should be kept in a central place so they are available in case household members need to evacuate quickly. Moreover, a supply of any necessary medications should be on hand. A central meeting place should be designated, or an extended family member or representative away from the residence should be identified as a communication link should household members become separated in an emergency.

Biologic Threats and Epidemics. There is an ever-present danger related to biologic threats to health, most recently taking the form of the H5N1 virus, which causes avian flu. The threat of a virulent, infectious disease with the potential for high mortality rates and widespread social disruption has prompted the federal government to develop guidelines for the general population. The government is advocating that households keep a supply of food and water, in case people are confined to their homes.[31] More information is available at http://www.pandemicflu.gov.

Sports and Vehicular Safety. Seat belts should always be worn in vehicles. Although some may argue that seat belt use may be responsible for some injuries or deaths by trapping individuals in the vehicle, this is the rare exception. In the vast majority of cases, seat belts save lives. Drivers need to be alert to the possibility of "road rage" or aggression by other drivers on the road. When encountering an enraged individual, one should avoid eye contact and be alert for opportunities for safety, such as escape routes.

Eye protection should be worn to prevent unintentional injuries to the eyes during sporting activities. Mouth guards are advised when participating in upper body contact sports, such as soccer, basketball, and football. If there is any possibility of being forcefully thrown in a sport, such as horseback riding or bicycling, a helmet should be worn. Patients should be advised that additional protective devices such as wrist guards and elbow and knee protectors prevent traumatic injuries during in-line skating.

SMOKING CESSATION

Cigarette smoking is the single most preventable cause of premature death in the United States. Each year, more than 400,000 Americans die from cigarette smoking. In fact, 1 in every 5 deaths in the United States is smoking related. From 1997 to 2001, smoking was the cause of death in 259,494 men and 178,408 women.[32]

The causes of smoking are varied; the appeal is different for each smoker. Smoking is pleasurable for some and a habit for others. Tobacco has more than 4000 components, many of which have biologic activity. Nicotine, a vasoconstrictor, is the most widely known constituent of cigarette smoke. With inhalation of cigarette smoke, nicotine is distributed throughout the body within 10 seconds.[33] At high exposure levels, nicotine is a potentially lethal poison that may cause intoxication in young children who ingest cigarettes. Long-term nicotine exposure affects many organ systems and has been associated with cancer, hypertension, cardiovascular disease, and gastrointestinal and reproductive disorders.

EFFECTS OF NICOTINE

Most smokers use tobacco products regularly because they are addicted to nicotine. Addiction is defined as "compulsive drug seeking and use, even in the face of negative health consequences."[33] Health care providers should remember that approximately 35 million smokers attempt to quit annually but fewer than 7% of them are able to achieve 1 year of abstinence without help.[33] Cigarettes are very efficient and highly engineered drug delivery systems. Because a typical smoker inhales an average of 10 puffs per cigarette, if that person smokes one pack a day, there will be on average 200 hits a day, which strongly reinforces the habit.[33]

Neurochemical Effects of Nicotine

Nicotine affects how a person feels and thinks by activating nicotine receptor sites in the brain. These receptors affect both the mesolimbic dopaminergic pathway and the locus ceruleus. Dopamine causes cognitive arousal, which leads to feeling alert and vigorous, as well as the perception of pleasure. Activation of the locus ceruleus causes the smoker to feel more alert and cognitively aroused, which leads to memory formation, storage, retention, and recall. Analytical thinking, arithmetic, and verbal skills are enhanced.[34] The number of nicotine receptor sites is increased by two or three times in as little as 3 to 6 weeks of regular cigarette smoking. Unfortunately, this is not reversible.

Nicotine Withdrawal

When a smoker stops "cold turkey," he or she may experience one or more withdrawal symptoms from the sudden removal of nicotine from the receptor sites. The most common are dysphoria and difficulty thinking. This usually occurs 1 or 2 days after stopping smoking. These symptoms can be ameliorated by the use of nicotine replacement therapy (NRT).

Genetics of Nicotine Addiction

Central nervous system sensitivity and response to nicotine are genetically determined. If a smoker does not have the proper genetic substrate, he or she cannot become addicted to nicotine.[34] About 10% of smokers lack the genes for nicotine dependence and can smoke rarely without having withdrawal symptoms. These individuals are social smokers and are able to control when and where they smoke. These "chippers" can readily stop without assistance.

However, the majority of smokers are addicted to nicotine and will benefit from treatment that addresses the real symptoms they experience when withdrawing from nicotine. The effects of smoking are potentially reversible; smoking represents a treatable condition. Most smokers are aware of the dangers and want to stop but find this difficult to do. Despite this knowledge, health care providers may not consistently inquire about a patient's smoking history or counsel patients to stop smoking. One study looked at primary care physicians and found that fewer than half of smokers reported that they even had been advised to quit.[35] Another study found that tobacco was discussed during 633 out of 2963 encounters (21%).[36] Yet the Agency for Healthcare Research and Policy Smoking Cessation Guideline found that just a few minutes of counseling can be an effective mechanism to aid patients in smoking cessation.[37]

STRATEGIES TO HELP PATIENTS QUIT SMOKING

In the early 1980s psychologists James Prochaska and Carlo DiClimente sought to understand how people can change behavior, with or without professional intervention. They theorized that patients' willingness to change addictive behavior depended on their state of readiness. There are six distinct phases of change that patients must experience to stop smoking[38] (Table 24-8).

The first stage is *precontemplation,* in which the patient is not considering change. If a patient is not considering change, the health care provider must be careful not to argue or defend a position on smoking. Arguments are counterproductive, and resistance is a signal to change strategies. Patients should be asked if they smoke and are thinking of quitting. If they say that they smoke and are not thinking of quitting, they should be advised to quit and given some literature to read "in case they change their mind." The subject is not pursued at this visit.

Patients may be in denial. Patients who are in denial will disagree with the provider, will express no need for help, and will not accept help if it is offered.[38] Patients who are in denial may perceive further advice as nagging, which may trigger a

TABLE 24-8 Six Processes of Change

Process of Change	Description	Intervention Strategies
Precontemplation	Patient is not considering change.	Raise doubts; increase perception of risks.
Contemplation	Patient shows awareness of a problem.	Evoke reasons to change; list risks of not changing.
Determination	Patient says, "I've got to do something."	Help patient determine steps to take (if no intervention in this stage, patient may slip back to precontemplation stage).
Action	Patient stops smoking.	Help patient take steps toward change.
Maintenance	Patient sustains change.	Help patient identify strategies to prevent relapse (self-efficacy is important).
Relapse	"Slips" occur.	Help patient avoid demoralization and discouragement (sends him or her back to contemplation).

Data from DiClimente CC, Prochaska JO, Fairhurst SK, and others: The process of smoking cessation: an analysis of precontemplation and preparation stages of change, *J Consult Clin Psychol* 59:295-304, 1991.

paradoxical response. If their anxiety levels are increased and they perceive that their freedom is being threatened, they may respond to this threat by increasing smoking.[38]

This does not mean that the provider never brings up the subject again. Patients should be questioned about smoking and offered help at each visit, but the provider's response should be determined by the patient's response. The provider can look for a "teaching moment," raise doubts about smoking, and help the patient increase his or her understanding of the risks of smoking. The provider can point out links between smoking and specific health concerns of the patient (e.g., the number of colds this year).

Awareness of a problem is the next step toward changing behavior. Once a patient admits there is a problem, he or she is in the *contemplation* stage of change. The provider must "tip the balance" at this point by evoking reasons to change and pointing out the risks of not changing behavior.

When a patient makes statements such as "I've got to do something," he or she has entered the *determination* stage. The best course of action should be planned together with the patient. This is the crucial point in the stages of change model. If there is no intervention at this stage, the patient will return to the precontemplation stage. Any barriers to treatment should be explored and removed if possible. Self-efficacy is an important tool for patients to become successful in their goal. The provider should give the patient information and determine the patient's reaction. Patients should be asked to list the rewards and problems of smoking and identify any past unsuccessful attempts; they should be asked why they thought they did not succeed and what they would do differently this time.

Patients have reached the *action* phase of the model when they have smoked their last cigarette. The patient must have a specific plan by this stage and should have a follow-up visit scheduled so that there is something invested in the smoking cessation attempt.

Maintenance is the phase in which patients must sustain change. The patient needs help identifying strategies to make this a success. The patient needs to be encouraged to find other ways to deal with the urge to smoke, such as taking a walk or doodling, and should be warned of the inherent dangers in thinking of smoking and the importance of substituting alternate behaviors at those times.

Unfortunately, many patients *relapse*. DiClimente, Prochaska, Fairhurst, and colleagues found that smokers ordinarily went around the wheel of change three or four times before a stable change was effected.[38] If the patient relapses, the provider should point out that a coping behavior is learned on each attempt. This can lessen the feeling of failure.

Patients should be continually moved toward their goal and counseled to quit on every visit. This does not need to be a formal counseling session; a brief talk should suffice. The American Cancer Society advises health care providers to cover the "four *A*'s"[39]:

- Ask about smoking at every visit.
- Advise patients of the health benefits of quitting smoking (e.g., "As your health care provider, I must advise you to stop smoking now").
- Assist the patient in stopping. Identify and remove any barriers to treatment.
- Arrange a follow-up visit.

When patients discover what drives them to smoke, interventions can be designed to help meet those needs. By interviewing the patient to determine specific motivators for smoking, the health care provider can assist patients in designing a program that is tailored to them (Table 24-9).

Recently, Prochaska, Velicer, Fava, and colleagues conducted a study to determine whether the use of a computer-generated "expert system" would improve outcome rates.[40] Individualized and interactive computer reports were given to patients at 0, 3, and 6 months after randomization. At 24 months, the expert system resulted in 12% sustained abstinence, demonstrating a measurable difference when the message is individualized.

It is important to keep in mind that what the provider says and how he or she says it influence how the patient receives the message. Researchers have studied counseling styles, comparing autonomy-supportive and controlling interpersonal styles in brief counseling of smokers. Autonomy-supporting styles, although not directly affecting smoking cessation rates, resulted in an increase in patients' active involvement in the counseling session. Active involvement in turn increases continuous abstinence rates over 30 months.[41]

Modifying the Approach

Patients have different smoking issues that vary by age and gender.[42] The message that the patient is given has greater impact if it is directed toward his or her needs and drives. Women often worry about weight gain after quitting. They should be encouraged to have low-calorie snacks on hand (e.g., carrot sticks) to substitute for handling a cigarette. If it is medically appropriate, women should also incorporate an exercise program into their quitting plan to increase their metabolic rate and make up for the lowered metabolism that results from the drop in nicotine levels.

TABLE 24-9 Smoking Motivation and Strategies for Cessation

Motivations for Smoking	Strategies for Cessation
To keep from slowing down; to perk up; to get a lift	Change activity with urge to smoke; stimulate mouth with mouthwash or brush teeth; avoid fatigue.
Enjoys handling cigarettes; enjoys steps in lighting up; enjoys watching exhaled smoke	Doodle; do crosswords; handle a small object.
Because smoking is pleasant, relaxing; because smoking is pleasurable; to relax	List pleasures of not smoking; contemplate harmful effect of smoking; go to a movie or read to substitute.
When upset; when uncomfortable; when "blue"	Identify what is needed when upset; do deep breathing or relaxation exercises; take up hobby or sport.

Moreover, women who are at different stages of their life need different approaches. A young mother should be warned of the dangers to her born and unborn children. England, Kendrick, Wilson, and colleagues studied the effect of tobacco exposure during pregnancy on the birth weight of term infants.[43] They found that "as third trimester cigarette use increased, birth weight declined sharply but leveled off at more than 8 cigarettes per day. Women who smoke during pregnancy may need to reduce to low levels of exposure (<8 cigarettes/day) to improve infant birth weight."

Health care providers have an obligation to inform patients that any maternal smoking also increases the danger of fetal death and congenital heart anomalies. Nicotine is contained in breast milk, and infants who breathe environmental tobacco smoke are more prone to otitis media and upper respiratory tract infections. Parents of asthmatic children should be advised to never allow them to be in an environment with tobacco smoke. Infants are at greater risk than older children because their systems are more immature and they are less able to independently escape a smoky environment.

On the other hand, young men may be more interested in the image they convey by smoking. Professional athletes are often shown using smokeless tobacco. Young men should be encouraged to make their own decisions about nicotine use in any form and to not rely on marketing information to make this important health decision.

In addition, adolescents are not convinced of their own mortality; therefore health concerns associated with smoking have a lesser impact on their smoking decisions. Instead, counseling highlights nicotine's effect on appearance (e.g., yellow teeth and fingers, hair and clothes that smell like smoke, bad breath). Factors associated with the initiation of adolescent smoking include poor academic performance in middle or high school and prior smoking behavior. Other predictors are a younger age than grade cohorts, an intention to smoke in the following 6 months, and underage drinking. Adolescents who did not start smoking until age 18 and had few friends who smoked were more likely to quit by age 23. The results of this study underscore the importance of early smoking prevention courses and the continuation of these throughout the high school level.[44]

Adults are more receptive to the messages about health concerns with smoking. Counseling should include the effects on blood pressure, the cardiovascular system, and the lungs. The encouragement to stop or refrain from smoking can be individualized according to the patient's personal and family medical history. Patients with high cardiovascular risk factors can be informed of the results of a clinical trial which found that only 8 weeks of smoking reduction resulted in an improvement in fibrinogen levels, WBC counts, and HDL/LDL ratios.[45]

Other health implications of smoking are its effect on mood and affect. Smoking has been found to have palliative effects on sadness in men, as well as palliative effects on anger in both men and women.[46] Therefore patients with depression or anxiety disorders are at particular risk for nicotine addiction. With these patients it may be helpful to augment therapy with an antidepressant, such as bupropion (Wellbutrin). If the patient has a personal or family history of a psychiatric disorder, nicotine withdrawal may exacerbate symptoms of depression or anxiety. Many of these patients require more extensive psychiatric treatment, behavioral therapy, and support.[47]

Pharmacologic Interventions

Health care providers should remember that pharmacologic adjuncts are most successful when combined with behavior modification strategies or a formalized smoking cessation class. Classes are usually offered at area hospitals or through the American Cancer Society or American Lung Association.

There are basically two types of pharmacologic interventions: one aimed at nicotine replacement and the other aimed at neurochemical mechanisms of the brain pathways. Currently, four medications are available for NRT: gum, patches, inhalers, and nasal spray. Nicotine gum is available in 2- or 4-mg doses. The patient must refrain from smoking while using NRT. With cardiovascular disease patients, nicotine gum should be used only after considering the risk/benefit ratio because nicotine is a potent vasoconstrictor and can precipitate arrhythmias. Other adverse effects include mouth soreness, hiccups, dyspepsia, and jaw ache; these are usually mild and transient.

Generally, when commencing NRT, the patient initially uses the 2-mg dose. Patients using the 2-mg dose should have a maximum of 24 pieces per day, and patients using the 4-mg dose should have a maximum of 20 pieces per day.[48] The gum is chewed until a peppery taste emerges and then is held between the cheek and gum. The patient is instructed to chew and hold intermittently for 30 minutes and to avoid eating or drinking anything but water for 15 minutes beforehand; this prevents any interference with buccal absorption.

Nicotine patches are available in varying doses depending on the manufacturer. Most manufacturers recommend using the higher dose for the first 4 weeks and then switching to lower doses at 2-week intervals. An interval of 8 weeks has been found to be the most effective length of treatment.[49] Light smokers may experience more side effects and may need to begin at a lower dose. The patient must refrain from smoking while using the patch. The same precautions as with the gum apply to patients with cardiovascular disease.

The patch is placed on a relatively hairless location between the neck and waist. Patients should be advised to place the patch on awakening on their quit day. The location should be changed daily. Up to 50% of patients may experience a localized skin reaction, which is usually mild and self-limiting.[48] The reaction can be treated locally with 5% hydrocortisone cream or 0.5% triamcinolone cream if necessary. Rotating patch sites will decrease the likelihood of a skin rash.

Dosing for a nicotine nasal spray begins at 2 to 4 sprays per hour, which may be increased to a maximum of 40 sprays daily. Treatment is recommended for 8 weeks, followed by gradual tapering over 4 to 6 weeks. Proper technique for dosing with nicotine nasal spray begins by gently blowing the nose, then tilting back the head slightly and spraying the nares. The spray should be aimed toward the center of the nasal opening while avoiding direct spraying of the nasal septum. Sniffing, swallowing, or inhaling the spray should be avoided. Side effects include nasal irritation, blisters or tingling, watery eyes, sneezing, coughing, and change in taste or smell. Additional rarely reported side effects are chest pain, muscle weakness, speech problems, dyspnea, and rash.

The dosage for nicotine inhalers is 6 to 16 cartridges daily. This dosage is maintained for 3 months and gradually tapered over the next 3 months. Maximum treatment duration is 6 months. Side effects include headache; mouth, tooth, or throat irritation; cough; nasal congestion; change in taste; dyspepsia; and diarrhea. Rarely reported side effects are tachycardia and chest pain.

NRT alone has been proved to double the quit rate of smokers. However, even with this increase, only 10% to 30% of smokers remain continuously abstinent for 1 year.[50] There are two hypotheses for low success rates. The first is that "no current formulation mimics the extremely rapid, rewarding high arterial nicotine concentrations from inhaled tobacco smoke."[51] The second possible explanation is underdosing of NRT by the user. All standard NRT therapies average half the plasma nicotine concentrations of a heavy smoker. Underdosing is thought to result either from incorrect technique or from the user finding the side effects unpleasant.

Bupropion has been found to be an aid in smoking cessation. Initially marketed and formulated as an antidepressant, bupropion has the unexpected result of enabling patients to quit smoking. The drug has been remarketed under the name Zyban. The efficacy of bupropion may be explained in part by its effect on the neural uptake of dopamine, prolonging the action of this neurotransmitter. Nicotine, like all addictive drugs, is believed to stimulate increases in the neurotransmitter dopamine. Bupropion should not be prescribed for patients with a seizure disorder, patients with an eating disorder, or patients who are concurrently taking Wellbutrin or any other medication containing bupropion. The dosage may need to be reduced for patients with liver or renal dysfunction. The most common side effect is insomnia. The usual dosage is 150 mg b.i.d. Therapy should begin at 150 mg q day for the first 3 days and then be increased to 150 mg b.i.d. Patients may smoke while taking bupropion, and it is recommended that the patient start bupropion 1 to 2 weeks before the intended quit date to allow for stabilization of blood levels.

U.S. Food and Drug Administration approval was recently granted for varenicline (Chantix), manufactured by Pfizer. The mechanism of action is similar to that of NRT (i.e., nicotine receptors are bound and thus deactivated). Varenicline is designed to bind potently with the nicotine receptors that stimulate the mesolimbic dopamine system, which is believed to be the neuronal mechanism underlying reinforcement and reward experienced on smoking.

Treatment length in the six reported phase 2 clinical trials varied from 9 to 52 weeks. By weeks 9 through 12, 45% had carbon monoxide (CO)–confirmed abstinence in the group randomized to Chantix vs. 12% in the placebo group. The numbers of subjects who remained abstinent with Chantix by week 40 dropped to 29%, vs. 9% of the placebo subjects. By 52 weeks, 23% of subjects taking Chantix had CO-confirmed abstinence, vs. 8% of subjects taking placebo and 16% of subjects taking bupropion SR. Additionally, based on responses to the Brief Questionnaire of Smoking Urges and the Minnesota Nicotine Withdrawal scale "Urge to Smoke" item, patients treated with Chantix had a reduced urge to smoke compared with patients taking placebos in all studies.[52]

Dosing for Chantix should be initiated 1 week before the target quit date, beginning at one 0.5-mg tablet daily for the first 3 days, then b.i.d. dosing for the next 4 days. On day 8, dosage is increased to 1 mg b.i.d. Nausea was the most commonly reported adverse event. Pfizer reported that most of the nausea was described as mild or moderate and was often transient. The incidence was dose dependent: 30% reported nausea in the group treated with the 1-mg dose and 16% in the group treated with the 0.5-mg dose.

A vaccine, NicVAX, is under investigation. The vaccine facilitates nicotine antibody development. The antibody binds to nicotine in the blood and prevents nicotine from reaching the brain, thus reducing nicotine's pleasurable sensation. Large-scale trials are in progress.

Individualizing Therapeutic Regimens

Deciding on the most efficacious therapeutic regimen can increase the chances of the successful transition from smoker to ex-smoker. Using one NRT product alone has only a 20% success rate; combining NRT products is another avenue to pursue. Using the patch to keep steady plasma levels (especially overnight) with the addition of faster-acting preparations for breakthrough cravings and withdrawal symptoms has been demonstrated to improve quit rates. However, data are not robust and further studies seem warranted.[53]

Studies conducted in the United Kingdom have recommended a four-tiered approach[54]:

Recommendation 1 (for all patients): Systematically record smoking status. This prompts primary caregivers to discuss smoking with all patients.

Recommendation 2 (for motivated light smokers [<10 cigarettes per day]): Give brief advice and refer to formalized smoking cessation program as indicated.

Recommendation 3 (for motivated heavy smokers [average >10 cigarettes per day]): Provide NRT and behavioral support (either in-house or local smoking cessation classes).

Recommendation 4 (for motivated heavy smokers [>15 cigarettes per day]): Provide NRT and behavioral support. If unsuccessful, consider adding bupropion and more interventional behavioral support.

Smokers in the relapse phase have been shown to experience a lower incidence of relapse if they remain on bupropion for more than 7 weeks. A clinical trial was performed that included smokers who were prescribed bupropion for 7 weeks. Participants were randomly divided into one group that received bupropion for 45 additional weeks and another that received a placebo for 45 weeks. Of the participants who received bupropion after 7 weeks, 55.1% remained smoke free at week 52 compared with 42.3% of participants in the placebo group. By week 78, the numbers had decreased to 47.7% in the bupropion group and 37.7% in the placebo group. However, by week 104, these numbers had leveled off to 41.6% (bupropion) and 40.0% (placebo). This could either reflect a lack of bupropion for 52 weeks or the lack of efficacy of bupropion in long-term smoking abstinence. Interestingly, bupropion was also shown to increase median time to relapse in those smokers who relapsed. Relapse time for smoking was 156 days in the bupropion group vs. 65 days in the placebo group.[55]

Incorporating Smoking Cessation with Primary Care Strategies

Health care providers should remember that it is possible to incorporate basic, brief primary care interventions into a busy practice setting. The five elements of smoking cessation intervention are a strong message to quit smoking, self-help motivational quitting and relapse materials, brief counseling that includes a quit date, use of pharmacologic interventions when indicated, and follow-up support.[56]

Patients may report that they have cut down on the number of packs they smoke per day; while commending their effort, providers should remind these patients that as long as they continue to smoke, carbon monoxide levels will be elevated and mucociliary clearance affected. Providers should stress that "cold turkey" quitters have the best overall success rates and that withdrawal symptoms are short lived and can be ameliorated by the use of pharmacologic adjuncts. Gradual withdrawal usually makes for more miserable smokers who quickly revert to their previous smoking rate.

A good resource to develop a more structured program can be found in the pamphlet *How to Help Your Patients Stop Smoking,* which is available from the National Institutes of Health in conjunction with the American Cancer Society.[39] Another resource is available at http://www.surgeongeneral.gov/tobacco/default.htm through the office of the surgeon general. It offers a 5-day plan for quitting smoking and tips for the first week. Other organizations with materials for smoking cessation include:

American Cancer Society: (800) ACS-2345; http://www.cancer.org

American Lung Association: (800) LUNG USA; http://www.lungusa.org

Office of Cancer Communications, National Cancer Institute: (800) 4-CANCER; http://www.cancer.gov/aboutnci/office-of-communications/page1

Tobacco Information and Prevention Source, National Center for Chronic Disease Prevention and Health Promotion, Centers for Disease Control and Prevention: (800) CDC-INFO; http://www.cdc.gov/tobacco/question.htm

DOMESTIC VIOLENCE

DEFINITION AND EPIDEMIOLOGY

Domestic violence is a significant health care problem with widespread and devastating effects for patients and their children, families, and communities. Approximately 4.8 million intimate partner rapes and physical assaults are perpetrated against women in the United States each year.[57] Domestic violence is the cause of more than 1300 deaths and more than 2 million injuries annually.[58] In the past, domestic violence was thought to be a social and judicial concern rather than a health care issue. However, recent research has consistently demonstrated that women seek help in various health care settings and that their health is seriously affected by ongoing abuse. Men can be victims of domestic violence as well, although the incidence in men is less than the incidence in women. About 1 million women and 371,000 men are stalked by intimate partners yearly.[59]

The overall cost of domestic violence is staggering. The annual cost has been calculated at more than $5.8 billion, with $4.1 billion for direct medical and mental health expenditures.[58]

Intimate murder accounts for about 9% of all murders nationwide and 30% of female murders; intimate partner violence made up 20% of all nonfatal violent crimes experienced by women in 2001.[60] One Midwestern family practice clinic reported that 23% of female patients were assaulted within the past year; 39% had been assaulted at some time during their life.[61] In one primary care setting, 1 in 7 women reported domestic abuse.[62]

Domestic violence is defined as a pattern of coercive and controlling behavior exercised by one partner over the other. Behaviors can range from economic control, social isolation, and emotional abuse, to sexual assault and threats of or actual physical violence. Abusive behavior by the batterer may be sporadic but generally is cyclic and usually escalates in terms of frequency and severity. The majority of victims of domestic violence appear to be women; however, domestic violence occurs in all age, racial, socioeconomic, and sexual orientation groups. Because of the disproportionate representation of women as victims, and for the ease of writing, this chapter may generalize and refer to victims of domestic violence as women.

The myth that domestic violence occurs in certain populations can result in the error of screening only those believed to be at risk. Despite the prevalence of domestic violence and its significant ramifications for individuals and communities, a variety of barriers to identification and treatment remain. This chapter explores these barriers and the basic principles of domestic violence and identifies specific techniques for assessment and intervention for the health care provider.

Barriers to Treatment

Power and Control. The relationship dynamics inherent in domestic violence are significant to understanding the barriers patients encounter in obtaining treatment. All abusive relationships are based on an imbalance of power and control and incorporate the use of specific tactics to maintain this imbalance. The perpetrator's desire for increased control over the partner generates a sense of power over the victim and an imbalance of power in the overall relationship.

Abusive control and controlling behavior can be exercised in many different ways. Fear is often a powerful deterrent to women seeking appropriate treatment. This includes the use of coercion and threats of physical, psychologic, or economic harm; intimidation; and physical or sexual violence. Abusive partners attempt to further exert psychologic, emotional, and financial control over their partners through verbal degradation, isolation, and economic abuse. The perpetrator often minimizes or denies the abuse and may blame the victim for the abuse, shifting the responsibility for the abusive behavior. If children are present, the abuser may use them to create guilt or manipulate the victim, or make threats to have them taken away or harmed in a further attempt to control the victim's emotions and reactions. For female victims, the perpetrator commonly claims male privilege, defining and devaluing the woman's role in the household.

Clearly, a perpetrator can use countless tactics to exert emotional, physical, and social control over the victim. The more control one partner exercises over the other, the greater the sense of power he feels. Likewise, the less control the victim feels she has in the relationship and in her life as a whole, the less power she perceives she has. The more powerless the victim feels, the less likely and able she is to leave the abusive relationship or seek treatment and help.

Cycle of Abuse. Along with the interpersonal dynamics between the abuser and the victim, the evolving dynamics of the relationship itself are important factors to consider while exploring barriers to treatment. The dynamics of abusive relationships are often a part of a systematic pattern of dominance and control characterized as a cycle; each turn of the cycle perpetuates the dynamics of the ongoing violence and controlling behavior. The first stage of the cycle often represents the baseline of the relationship without any acute issues at hand. Slowly, the relationship may enter a tension-building phase in which stress level and tension are raised, ultimately leading to an explosive event. This may be characterized by a verbal argument or may also result in physical or sexual abuse. After this explosion the tension and stress that had been building are expelled, and a false sense of calm returns to the relationship. Often after an explosive event the relationship goes through a phase commonly referred to as the "honeymoon period." During this time the abuser often appears more loving and sensitive toward the partner, perhaps in some respect atoning for the recent abusive episode. The relationship at this time may even appear to have improved, which often persuades the victim that the partner is changing and the abuse will end. Unfortunately, over time, the cycle repeats itself with some modifications. As the cycle of abuse self-perpetuates over time, it appears that the length of the honeymoon period shortens with each turn of the cycle, thereby increasing the frequency and severity of abusive episodes.

Barriers to Identification

Despite the prevalence of domestic violence, abuse is often not identified, and an opportunity to intervene and offer resources and follow-up support is missed. The reason for this is twofold and can be attributed to the patient's reluctance to disclose this information and barriers posed by the health care provider.

Patient Barriers. Aside from the interpersonal and relationship dynamics that often hinder access to treatment, other factors also contribute to the difficulty in identifying abuse. Patients may be reluctant to disclose information because of shame, embarrassment, or a cultural belief that it is inappropriate to discuss their intimate relationships with others. Sometimes, after negative or unhelpful experiences with past disclosure of abuse, patients are reluctant to repeat this experience. This negative experience may include not being asked by the provider despite the patient's attempts to raise the issue herself, or not being asked in a caring or empathic manner. The victim's impaired insight or awareness concerning her abusive situation may also present a barrier to identification; these ongoing patterns of abusive power and control may seem normal to victims, thereby hindering their ability to recognize the lethality of their situations.

Often patients who may be willing to seek assistance face another challenge imposed by the medical system itself. Treatment and intervention may be prohibited because of lack of insurance or resources to pay for out-of-pocket medical expenses. Further, patients who are reluctant to use insurance in an attempt to seek help because it might alert their abusive partners may encounter difficulty in accessing care or place themselves at greater risk for harm by attempting to obtain assistance.

Provider Barriers. Health care providers unfortunately create their own barriers to identification as well. The greatest barrier to the identification of abuse is often providers simply not asking about abuse. Health care providers may be unaware of the prevalence of abuse or have inadequate understanding about domestic violence, including misconceptions about abuse risks, settings, and lethality. Thus they miss opportunities for screening. These false stereotypes may also result in practitioners thinking that abuse does not occur within the population they serve, and they may be concerned about offending their patients by asking.

Providers may also feel powerless to address the problem and therefore ill equipped to deal with the situation and provide adequate intervention. However, one study clearly indicated that health care providers can be effective in helping victims of domestic violence, and they were rated almost as highly as counselors and support groups.[63] The magnitude of the problem may also overwhelm providers, who believe they lack the time or resources to address the situation. However, findings suggest that providers can improve their ability to respond to these situations by educating themselves and their patients about domestic violence and familiarizing themselves with local resources available to provide support for these patients.[63]

CLINICAL PRESENTATION

Domestic violence is the number one reason for admission into emergency departments for women in the United States.[63] Therefore a history of recent visits to the emergency department for repeated physical injuries may indicate that the patient is in a violent domestic situation. Likewise, repeated office visits for either physical injuries or complaints may suggest that abuse may be occurring. The National Violence Against Women Survey found that physical or sexual violence resulted in more than 320,000 outpatient visits annually.[57] A patient who has been battered may show obvious signs of abuse, or the symptoms may be more obscure. In general, clinical indicators of domestic violence may be categorized into physical complaints, psychosocial indicators, or a combination of the two.

Physical Complaints

Injuries to the head and neck are the most common injuries in domestic abuse situations, followed by upper extremity, breast, back, and buttock injury.[64] In a large domestic violence study done in a primary care setting, researchers found that frequent or serious bruises or cuts, sprains, broken bones, and various pains (e.g., chest, stomach, pelvic, and genital) were associated with high levels of abuse.[65] Some of the less obvious signs and symptoms include loss of appetite, eating binges and self-induced vomiting, vaginal discharge, diarrhea or constipation, fainting, difficulty passing urine, hyperventilation, and headaches. Other indicators of domestic violence include injuries in various stages of healing, repeated office visits, delayed treatment for an injury, reluctance to talk about an injury, or explanations that are inconsistent with the type of injury.[66]

Sexual assault can occur with the physical or emotional abuse, or it can be the only form of abuse in the relationship. Intimate partner sexual assault includes any forced sex acts that occur within the context of any intimate relationship, and it may include the use of objects, rape, or uncomfortable or embarrassing sexual experiences.[67] Studies in San Francisco and Boston revealed that 8% to 10% of participants were victims of intimate partner rape.[57] Men who sexually abuse their partners are particularly dangerous, which means that women are at greater risk of death.[68] Although approximately one third of women injured in their most recent incident of intimate partner rape seek medical treatment, only one fifth of these cases are reported to the police.[57] This disparity supports the critical role of health care providers in identifying domestic violence and offering support and resources to their patients. Evidence of sexual assault should automatically prompt further exploration by providers. This form of violence can result in problems such as pelvic inflammatory disease, sexually transmitted diseases (STDs), HIV/AIDS, vaginal or anal tearing, urinary tract infections, dysmenorrhea, unexplained vaginal bleeding, or pelvic pain.[64] The male partner may exert control over his partner by not using a condom, thereby increasing her risk for STDs and an unintended pregnancy.

Physical abuse during pregnancy poses a significant health risk for mother and fetus; therefore assessment for abuse during pregnancy should be part of routine prenatal care.[65] For some relationships, domestic violence may begin when a woman becomes pregnant; if domestic violence is already occurring, it may escalate during pregnancy. Research indicates that 1 in 6 women is battered during pregnancy.[69] Possible complications of domestic violence during pregnancy include low birth weight and miscarriage. Both of these symptoms could result from abdominal trauma, inadequate prenatal care, suboptimal weight gain, an unhealthy diet, or severe stress.[70] The stress from abuse may increase the likelihood that the pregnant woman would smoke or abuse substances, which would be another cause for low birth weight.[71] Since pregnancy may be the only time healthy women come in frequent contact with health care providers, this is an opportune time to ask about domestic violence.[66]

Psychosocial Indicators

In addition to physical injuries and complaints, patients may experience a variety of psychosocial problems. A recent study supports the need for better understanding of the effects of nonphysical forms of abuse. Women may be treated for symptoms of depression or anxiety without assessment for domestic violence; if these symptoms are taken out of context of the abuse, treatment may be ineffective.[63] Psychologically, the patient can experience a complex traumatic stress response, which includes the symptoms of posttraumatic stress disorder (i.e., intrusive thoughts, nightmares, disassociated flashbacks, psychic numbness, hypervigilance, and exaggerated startle response).[71] Victims commonly experience depression; anxiety; and their related symptoms, including anhedonia, difficulty concentrating, changes in sleep and eating patterns, depressed mood, somatization, decreased self-esteem, and suicidal ideations. There may be an alteration in affect (predominantly depressed or restricted), alteration in perceptions of the perpetrator (seeing the abuser as omnipotent), and an alteration in the sense of self (disappearance of self and increased feelings of self-blame).[70] This complex traumatic response can be immobilizing and prevent the victim from escaping the abusive relationship or seeking help.

PHYSICAL EXAMINATION

It is important to address patients' health care needs at the time of the visit, urgent and nonurgent, time permitting. Some victims of domestic violence may have difficulty returning to the health care provider's office for follow-up. Patients who report domestic violence and who are not ready to leave the abusive relationship may benefit from education and services targeting the prevention of unintended pregnancy. When treating the patient's illness or injuries, the provider must take care to not prescribe any medication that could impair the patient's judgment or ability to respond, since this would place her at increased risk for further harm. If necessary, the patient can be referred to a specialist for additional health care needs.

The documentation of the patient's visit is important and may be needed for legal proceedings. The patient's account of domestic violence should be documented in the medical record using the patient's own words, when possible. It is advisable to avoid using the term *alleges*. An appropriate substitute is "patient reports" or "patient states." Caution should be used when documenting the patient's demeanor. Since the patient's medical record may be used in legal proceedings, accuracy is important. Documentation should also indicate the patient's report on when and how the patient sustained the injuries. It should include the identity of the person who caused the injury. It is important that the health care provider stick to his or her area of expertise. Documented inferences that are out of the provider's area of expertise may create legal difficulties for a patient who pursues legal action against the abuser.[72] Documentation should include a detailed description of the injuries and a body map to identify the location of injuries. Care should be taken to not attempt to place a date on when injuries occurred based on the appearance of the injuries; rather the provider should document objective data, such as color and size of bruises. Dating injuries can create complications with legal proceedings.

If possible, the provider should offer to photograph the patient's injuries. The patient's written consent is required before pictures are taken, and all pictures must be labeled with the patient's name and medical record number. When appropriate, an object of standard size (e.g., a tape measure or coin) can be placed in the picture, near the injury, to illustrate size. This will aid in providing an accurate perspective of the injuries should the patient need the photographs as evidence of the assault for legal purposes. Care should be taken to preserve the patient's dignity during photographing, and the patient should not be asked to remove more clothing than is necessary. Some of the photographs of the injuries should include the patient's face, when possible, to protect against a possible dispute over the identity of the person photographed.[72]

If a patient was recently sexually assaulted, before beginning the physical examination, the provider should consider referring the patient to an emergency department that has a program to assist victims of sexual assault. Personnel there can assist in securing evidence that may be lost during a regular physical examination. This referral should be encouraged even if the patient is not considering notifying law enforcement at the time of disclosure of sexual assault. There are time restrictions on these types of services; therefore providers should check with the local hospital for service guidelines.

MANAGEMENT

Clinical Intervention

The health care provider can assist the patient who admits to being a victim of domestic violence by assessing and treating medical problems, educating about the dynamics of domestic violence, discussing safety issues, and providing referrals.

Universal Screening. All patients seen in primary care settings should be routinely screened for domestic violence. Because many patients are reluctant to disclose that they are being abused the first time that the subject is raised, they may be more likely to disclose information after they have developed some level of trust with the provider. Therefore screening should not be limited to the first visit; providers should continue to screen at subsequent visits. Research with survivors of domestic violence revealed that, with or without direct disclosure and identification, compassionate asking from health care professionals provided validation and helped victims change their situations and move toward safety.[73]

Framing the Question. When screening or interviewing a patient about domestic violence, the provider must remember that privacy and confidentiality are essential. The patient's partner or a third party should never be informed that the patient is being screened for domestic violence, since this may place the patient and provider at risk for retaliation. Providers should use their own style of communication to introduce the subject and convey the need for screening because of the seriousness and prevalence of domestic violence. It may be helpful to normalize the process for patients by using statements such as "Since domestic violence is so prevalent, I have started screening all my patients." It is usually most beneficial to ask direct questions when screening,[74] such as:

- Have you ever been hit, slapped, kicked, or otherwise physically hurt by someone? If yes, by whom?
- Have you ever been threatened, controlled, or forced to do things you did not want to do? If yes, by whom?
- Are you afraid of your partner or anyone else?

The provider's demeanor when screening a patient can negatively influence the patient's willingness to disclose her victimization. If the provider is not comfortable with the subject matter and the screening process, it is advisable to have an appropriate staff member screen patients. It is essential that the provider be aware of not only how to appropriately interview patients to screen for domestic violence but also how to respond to them when the screening has been completed. It is recommended that the provider compile a list of resources and related brochures and have them available to aid in the education of the patient regarding domestic violence.

Patient Denial of Abuse. If the patient denies abuse, the provider should document in the patient's chart that the screening was completed. If the patient has injuries that are inconsistent with the explanation as to how they occurred and denies abuse, the provider documents in the patient's chart that the "injury is inconsistent with explanation." There is generally no therapeutic benefit in challenging the patient's explanation. Consider the need to report to appropriate authorities if the patient is a minor or a dependent adult. Providers should acquaint themselves with the mandatory reporting laws in the state in which they practice, since the laws vary greatly from state to state. Even when a patient denies abuse and is well known to the provider, the patient should be rescreened at subsequent visits. Providers should continue to convey to the patient that they are available to assist, if needed.

Patient Disclosure of Abuse. When a patient discloses that she is being abused, the provider can use the opportunity to convey concern, educate, and provide information on available resources. The patient should be assured that she is not at fault for the battering, regardless of what she may or may not have done. The provider should not try to verify the patient's report with her partner or other family members. The primary focus should be on the patient's safety and the provision of appropriate referrals. It is important to remember that victims of domestic violence will react in many different ways. If the victim does not cry or appear distraught when disclosing incidences of abuse or violence, it does not mean that she has not been victimized.

Psychosocial Intervention

Repeated abuse can have a monumental psychologic impact on the victim. Care should be taken to discuss the patient's psychologic well-being. Patients may experience feelings of intense fear and helplessness. Some victims may develop posttraumatic stress disorder.[75] Victims of chronic abuse should be screened for suicidal and homicidal ideations, since they may feel that there is no way out of the abusive relationship other than death. If appropriate, the patient should be referred for crisis intervention. Referrals to individual counseling and support groups specific to domestic violence are also appropriate. However, couples counseling is highly discouraged because of the potential for further harm to the patient. The provider should inform the patient about how to access emergency shelters and financial and legal assistance.

Children who are exposed to family violence should be referred to age-appropriate counseling. Many organizations that provide services to adult victims of domestic violence also have services for children. Victims should be encouraged to have a pediatrician examine their children to assess their well-being, physically and psychologically. Many people mistakenly think that if a child was not physically assaulted, he or she is not in need of services. Children who are exposed to violence are at significant risk for using violence themselves, becoming delinquent, experiencing school and behavioral problems, and having serious and possibly life-long mental health problems.[76]

Safety Assessment and Planning. On identification and discussion of a domestic violence situation, the health care provider should do a thorough assessment and discuss a safety plan. The provider should obtain information on the history of the violence, including when the violence first occurred, types of incidents, whether weapons were used, and frequency of assaults. This will assist in determining whether the violence is escalating and in raising the victim's awareness of the progression of violence. The presence of weapons in the home increases the potential lethality of the situation. Patients need to make their own decisions about their safety and whether they should leave the abusive relationship. Violence often escalates when the victim attempts to leave; as a result, patients should be advised to take extra precautions to protect their safety when leaving a relationship.

If the patient is in immediate danger while in the clinical setting, immediately contact the appropriate security services. The health care provider should not attempt to mediate between the victim and her partner.

The safety plan should consider various scenarios that the patient may find herself in and need to escape from. It may include having the patient develop a code with someone she trusts who lives in the home, or next door, that would indicate the patient needs help and that the police should be notified. Details should be discussed regarding where the patient would go if the home is not safe. Patients should be encouraged to use domestic violence shelters to protect their safety, rather than going to family or friends' homes where the abuser may be able to locate them. Providers should encourage patients to compile important documents such as birth certificates and photo identification, an address book, checkbook, bank cards, medical cards, Social Security cards, chronic medication, and clothing. The patient's safety is of the utmost importance, so if compiling documents places her at greater risk, she should be advised not to do so. Providers should help the patient identify people and agencies that are able to assist. A follow-up appointment, as appropriate, should be scheduled before the patient leaves. Further, the health care provider should inquire about whether the patient can be contacted through the mail or on the phone. The provider's good intention of calling the patient later to inquire about her well-being may actually further jeopardize her safety.

A determination of the success of an intervention should not hinge on whether the patient leaves the abusive relationship. A successful intervention is one in which the provider has acknowledged and validated the situation and offered appropriate referrals. The patient may decide at a later date to seek services based on the groundwork that was laid at a previous visit.

LIFE SPAN CONSIDERATIONS

Domestic violence occurs across the life span, and therefore health care practitioners must maintain the same standards of screening and identification of all patients. Studies have indicated that women ages 35 to 49 were the most vulnerable to intimate murder, whereas females ages 16 to 24 were the most vulnerable to nonfatal violence.[60] However, from 1993 to 1999, of all female murder victims ages 20 to 24, 45% of them were killed by a current or former intimate partner.[60] Additional statistics have been gathered regarding the marital status of domestic violence victims, and it was determined that women separated from their husbands were victimized by an intimate at rates higher than married, divorced, widowed, or never married women.[60] This underscores the significance of developing safety plans with patients who are still in the process of leaving an abusive relationship.

A further consideration regarding life span issues is the impact of domestic violence on children. Findings indicate that more than half of the female victims live in households with children under 12 years of age.[60] The psychologic and emotional impact on these children often continues throughout their lives, extending the effects of domestic violence across the life span.

PATIENT AND FAMILY EDUCATION

Patients and their families are often unaware of the prevalence of this issue. The isolative nature of domestic violence results in a lack of awareness of this problem among patients and their families. Individuals are frequently unaware that they are not dealing with these issues alone and can gain support from others who have survived similar experiences. Educating patients and their families regarding controlling behaviors that often escalate into violence may prompt change before the violence occurs. Health care providers should offer additional education regarding community programs and resources to further support victims of domestic violence. Finally, because most victimizations are perpetrated against women by current and former intimates and because women are more likely to be injured if their assailant is a current or former intimate, violence prevention strategies for women that focus on how they can protect themselves from intimate partners are needed.[57]

HEALTH PROMOTION

Studies show that only about half of female victims of nonlethal intimate violence reported the incident to law enforcement.[60] Of that total, 1 in 3 (and 1 in 6 of all female victims of intimate violence) said that they had considered the victimization a "private or personal matter"; the second most common reason for nonreporting was fear of offender retaliation.[60] These results indicate that many more episodes of intimate partner violence occur than are reported, and women frequently feel ashamed of raising the issue with others. As a result, health care providers who act as on the "front line" with these women can help tremendously with the identification of and interventions for domestic violence by initiating simple screening mechanisms in their practice. A study piloted for a self-administered questionnaire developed for the early detection of intimate partner violence risk factors during routine health care visits in an urban primary care clinic revealed surprisingly high rates of multiple risk markers that might not ordinarily raise provider suspicion.[77] These findings confirmed the value of early identification and intervention. The addition of a single question pertaining to domestic violence in routine health screening can increase identification of domestic violence by as much as 11%.[78]

Although patient disclosure and secondary prevention are the ideal practitioners aim for, the value of simply beginning the discussion regarding domestic violence cannot be overemphasized. Data from a national study on violence against women highlight the need to focus identification efforts on building a respectful patient-provider relationship and creating openings for future disclosure, rather than on "fixing the problem" or controlling the outcome.[73]

REFERENCES

1. National Vital Statistics Reports: *Deaths: preliminary data for 2003,* retrieved Dec 9, 2006, from http://www.cdc.gov/nchs/data/hestat/finaldeaths03_tables.pdf.
2. US Department of Health and Human Services: *Healthy people 2010,* ed 2, Washington, DC, 2000, US Government Printing Office.
3. Centers for Disease Control and Prevention: *Overweight and obesity: economic consequences,* retrieved May 4, 2006, from http://www.cdc.gov/nccdphp/dnpa/obesity/economic_consequences.htm.
4. MedHelp International: *Statistics related to overweight and obesity,* retrieved May 3, 2006, from http://www.medhelp.org/NIHlib/GF-367.html#research.
5. Mokdad AH, Bowman BA, Ford ES, and others: Obesity trends among US adults, *JAMA* 286(10):1195-1200, 2001.
6. Centers for Disease Control and Prevention, National Center for Health Statistics: *Early release of selected estimates based on data from the January-September 2005 National Health Interview Survey,* retrieved May 3, 2006, from http://www.cdc.gov/nchs/about/Major/nhis/released200603.htm.
7. Centers for Disease Control and Prevention, National Center for Chronic Disease Prevention and Health Promotion: *Nutrition and physical activity obesity trends: prevalence of obesity among U.S. adults, by characteristics: Behavioral Risk Factor Surveillance System (1991-2000); self-reported data,* retrieved Aug 12, 2002, from http://www.cdc.gov/nccdphp/dnpa/obesity/trend/prev_char.htm.
8. National Center for Chronic Disease Prevention and Health Promotion: *Nutrition and physical activity. Centers for Disease Control and Prevention: Obesity trends: U.S. obesity trends 1985-2000,* retrieved Dec 9, 2006, from http://www.cdc.gov/nccdphp/dnpa/obesity/trend/index.htm.
9. National Heart, Lung, and Blood Institute: *The practical guide to the identification, evaluation, and treatment of overweight and obesity in adults,* Bethesda, Md, 2000, NHLBI Information Center.
10. Centers for Disease Control and Prevention, National Center for Chronic Disease Prevention and Health Promotion: *Physical activity and health: a report of the surgeon general—adults,* retrieved Aug 12, 2002, from http://www.cdc.gov/nccdphp/sgr/adults.htm.
11. American Institute of Stress: *America's #1 health problem: why is there more stress today?* retrieved Aug 12, 2002, from http://www.stress.org/problem.htm.
12. US Department of Health and Human Services: *Third report of the National Cholesterol Education Program on Detection, Evaluation, and Treatment of High Blood Cholesterol in Adults,* Washington, DC, 2001, US Government Printing Office.
13. Schafer W: *Stress management for wellness,* Austin, Tex, 1996, Holt, Rinehart & Winston.
14. Stanhope M, Knollmueler RN: *Public and community health nurse's consultant: a health promotion guide,* St Louis, 1997, Mosby.
15. Pagana K, Pagana T: *Mosby's diagnostic and laboratory test reference,* ed 5, St Louis, 1999, Mosby.
16. Maud PJ, Foster C: *Physiological assessment of human fitness,* Champaign, Ill, 1995, Human Kinetics.
17. American Heart Association: *Blood pressure levels,* retrieved Aug 12, 2002, from http://216.185.112.5/presenter.jhtml?identifier=4450.
18. Chernecky C, Berger B, editors: *Laboratory tests and diagnostic procedures,* ed 3, Philadelphia, 2001, Saunders.
19. Fisher C: Nutrition and quality of life, *Can Nurs Home* 4(1).
20. Guigoz Y, Vellas B, Garry PJ: Assessing the nutritional status of the elderly: the mini nutritional assessment as part of the geriatric evaluation, *Nutr Rev* 54(1 Pt 2):559-565, 1996.
21. Lord S, Castell S: Effect of exercise on balance, strength and reaction time in older people, *Arch Phys Med Rehabil* 75(6):648-652, 1994.
22. Brunner EJ, Thorogood M, Rees K, and others: Dietary advice for reducing cardiovascular risk, *Cochrane Database Syst Rev* (4): CD002128.DOI:10.1002/14651858.pub2, 2005.
23. Payne WA, Hahn DB: *Understanding your health,* ed 4, St Louis, 1995, Mosby.
24. Appel LJ, Brands MW, Daniels SR, and others: Dietary approaches to prevent and treat hypertension, *Hypertension,* retrieved May 4, 2006, from http://hyper.ahajournals.org/cgi/content/full/47/2/296.
25. National Institutes of Health: *The DASH diet,* retrieved May 4, 2006, from http://www.nih.gov/news/pr/apr97/Dash.htm.
26. Wilbur J, Chandler P, Miller A: Measuring adherence to a women's walking program, *West J Nurs Res* 23(1):8-32, 2001.
27. American Heart Association: *Exercise and your heart: a guide to physical activity,* Dallas, 1993, The Association.
28. Fitts SS: Physical benefits and challenges of exercise for people with chronic renal disease, *J Renal Nutr* 7(3):123-128, 1997.
29. Deuster PA: Exercise in the prevention and treatment of chronic disorders, *Women's Health Issues* 6(6):320-331, 1996.
30. Lego S: Women and stress, *Imprint* 43(2):57-60, 1996.
31. Centers for Disease Control and Prevention: *Individuals and families planning,* retrieved Dec 9, 2006, from http://www.pandemicflu.gov/plan/tab3.html.
32. Centers for Disease Control and Prevention: Smoking-attributable mortality and years of potential life lost—United States, 2005, *MMWR* 54(25):625-628, 2005.
33. National Institute on Drug Abuse: *NIDH research report series: nicotine addiction,* NIH Pub No 01-4342 (revised 2006), Rockville, Md, 2006, National Institutes of Health.
34. Hodgkin JE, Celli BR, Connors GL: *Pulmonary rehabilitation; guidelines to success,* ed 3, Philadelphia, 2000, Lippincott Williams & Wilkins.
35. Park E, Eaton CA, Goldstein MG, and others: The development of a decisional balance measure of physician smoking cessation interventions, *Prev Med* 33(4):261-267, 2001.
36. Ellerbeck EF, Ahluwalia JS, Jolicoeur DG, and others: Direct

observation of smoking cessation activities in primary care practice, *J Fam Pract* 50(8):688-693, 2001.
37. Amar S, Tiben N, Karkabi K, and others: The efficacy of a doctor-patient appointment in a primary care setting dedicated to preventative medicine, *Harefuah* 140(8):689-693, 2001 (in Hebrew).
38. DiClimente CC, Prochaska JO, Fairhurst SK, and others: The process of smoking cessation: an analysis of precontemplation and preparation stages of change, *J Consult Clin Psychol* 59:295-304, 1991.
39. Glynn TJ, Manley M: *How to help your patients stop smoking: a National Cancer Center Institute manual for physicians,* NIH Pub No 95-3064, Washington, DC, 1995, National Cancer Institute.
40. Prochaska JO, Velicer WF, Fava JL, and others: Evaluating a population-based recruitment approach and a stage-based expert system intervention for smoking cessation, *Addict Behav* 26(4):583-602, 2001.
41. Williams GC, Deci EL: Activating patients for smoking cessation through physician autonomy support, *Med Care* 39(8):813-823, 2001.
42. Goring S, Arnold J: *Health promotion handbook,* St Louis, 1998, Mosby.
43. England LJ, Kendrick JS, Wilson HG, and others: Effects of smoking reduction during pregnancy on the birth weight of term infants, *Am J Epidemiol* 154(8):694-701, 2001.
44. Ellickson PL, McGuigan KA, Klein DJ: Predictors of late-onset smoking and cessation over 10 years, *J Adolesc Health* 29(2):101-108, 2001.
45. Eliasson B, Hjalmarson A, Kruse E, and others: Effects of smoking reduction and cessation on cardiovascular risk factors, *Nicotine Tob Res* 3(3):249-255, 2001.
46. Delfino RJ, Jamner LD, Whalen CK: Temporal analysis of the relationship of smoking behavior and urges to mood states in men versus women, *Nicotine Tob Res* 3(3):245-248, 2001.
47. Ziedonis D, Brady K: Dual diagnosis in primary care: detecting and treating both the addiction and mental illness, *Med Clin North Am* 81:1017-1036, 1997.
48. Hodgson BB, Kizior RJ: *Nursing drug handbook,* Philadelphia, 2002, Saunders.
49. Silagy C, Mant D, Fowler G, and others: Nicotine replacement therapy for smoking cessation, *Cochrane Database Syst Rev* (3):CD000146, 2000.
50. Wagena EJ, Huibers MJ, van Schaych CP: Therapies for smoking cessation (antidepressants, nicotine replacement and counseling) and implications for the treatment of patients with chronic obstructive pulmonary disease, *Ned Tijdsch Geneach* 145(31):1492-1496, 2001.
51. Stapleton J: Commentary: progress on nicotine replacement therapy for smokers, *BMJ* 318(7179):289, 1999.
52. Pfizer: *Chantix: A different way to help you quit smoking,* retrieved Jan 23, 2007, from http://www.chantix.com/content/Chantix_Branded_Homepage.jsp?setShowOn=../content/Chantix_Branded_Homepage.jsp&setShowHighlightOn=../content/Chantix_Branded_Homepage.jsp.
53. Sweeney CT, Fant RV, Fagerstrom KO, and others: Combination nicotine replacement therapy for smoking cessation: rationale, efficacy, and tolerability, *CNS Drugs* 15(6):453-467, 2001.
54. Coleman T: Smoking cessation: integrating recent advances into clinical practice, *Thorax* 56:579-582, 2001.
55. Hays JT, Hurt RD, Rigotti NA, and others: Sustained-release bupropion for pharmacological relapse prevention after smoking cessation: a randomized, controlled trial, *Ann Intern Med* 135(6):423-433, 2001.
56. Goring S, Arnold J: *Health promotion handbook,* St Louis, 1998, Mosby.
57. National Institute of Justice and the Centers for Disease Control and Prevention: *Findings from the national violence against women survey,* US Department of Justice, 2000, Washington, DC.
58. Centers for Disease Control and Prevention: *Costs of intimate partner violence against women in the United States,* Atlanta, 2003, National Center for Injury Prevention and Control, retrieved Dec 2006, from http://www.cdc.gov/ncipc/pub-res/ipv_cost/ipv.htm.
59. Tjaden P, Thoennes N: Extent, nature, and consequences of intimate partner violence: findings from the National Violence Against Women Survey, Washington, DC, 2000, Department of Justice, Publication No NCJ 181867.
60. US Department of Justice: *Intimate partner violence,* Washington, DC, 2003, US Department of Justice Bureau of Justice Statistics.
61. Hamburger K, Saunders DG, Hovey M: Prevalence of domestic violence in community practice and rate of physician inquiry, *Fam Med* 24:283-287, 1992.
62. Freund K, Blackhall L: Detection of domestic violence in a primary care setting, *Clin Res* 38:736A-738A, 1990.
63. Gordon J: *Helping survivors of domestic violence,* New York, 1998, Garland.
64. Eisenstat SA: Domestic violence. In Carlson K, Eisenstat SA, editors: *Primary care of women,* St Louis, 1995, Mosby.
65. McCauly J, Kern DE, Kolodner K, and others: The "battering syndrome": prevalence and clinical characteristics of domestic violence in primary care internal medicine, *Ann Intern Med* 123(10):737-746, 1995.
66. Alpert EJ: Violence in intimate relationships and the practicing internist: new "disease" or new agenda? *Ann Intern Med* 123(10):774-781, 1995.
67. Campbell JC, Alford P: The dark consequences of marital rape, *Am J Nurs* 89(7):946-949, 1989.
68. Council of Scientific Affairs, American Medical Association: Violence against women: relevance for medical practitioners, *JAMA* 267(23):3184-3189, 1992.
69. McFarlane J, Parker B, Soeken K, and others: Assessing for abuse during pregnancy: severity and frequency of injuries and associated entry into prenatal care, *JAMA* 267(33):3176-3178, 1992.
70. Campbell JC, Lewandowski LA: Mental and physical health effects of intimate partner violence on women and children, *Psychiatr Clin North Am* 20(2):353-374, 1997.
71. Herman J: *Trauma and recovery,* New York, 1994, Basic Books.
72. Schornstein S: *Domestic violence and health care: what every professional needs to know,* Thousand Oaks, Calif, 1997, Sage.
73. Gerbert B, Caspers N, Bronstone A, and others: A qualitative analysis of how physicians with expertise in domestic violence approach the identification of victims, *Ann Intern Med* 131(8):578-584, 1999.
74. Feldhaus KM, Koziol-McLain J, Amsbury HL, and others: Accuracy of three brief screening questions for detecting violence in the emergency department, *JAMA* 277(17):1357-1361, 1997.
75. Kubany E, McKenzie W, Owens J, and others: PTSD among women survivors of domestic violence in Hawaii, *Hawaii Med J* 55:164-165, 1996.
76. Walker L: *The battered woman syndrome,* New York, 2000, Springer.
77. Ross J, Walther V, Epstein I: Screening risks for intimate partner violence and primary care settings: implications for future abuse, *Soc Work Health Care* 38(4):1-23, 2004.
78. Freund KM, Bak SM, Blackhall L: Identifying domestic violence in primary care practice, *J Gen Intern Med* 11(1):44-46, 1996.

CHAPTER 25

Immunizations

Cheryl A. Miller

Vaccine-preventable infectious diseases, such as influenza and pneumococcal pneumonia, continue to be leading causes of significant medical costs, morbidity, and mortality.[1] According to *Healthy People 2010,* pneumonia and influenza combined are the sixth leading cause of death in this country. Increased mortality results not only from the diseases themselves but from cardiopulmonary and other chronic diseases that can be exacerbated by influenza. Significant progress has been made in improving adult immunization rates in certain population groups. For example, in 2003, 66% of persons aged 65 years and older received influenza vaccine in the previous year.[2] In addition, many vaccine-preventable diseases, such as measles and smallpox, are under control or essentially have been eradicated.

As a result of successful immunization practices geared toward infants and children in the United States, the incidence of childhood vaccine-preventable disease has also declined dramatically. However, both young and older adults are often unaware of the need for adult immunizations, and as a result, most of the vaccine-preventable diseases in the United States occur in these populations.[2] Many adolescents also do not receive the recommended immunizations.[1] Although immunization rates have improved in some populations, poor access to health care and inadequate public education continue to result in lower immunization rates among minority populations.[2]

One of the goals of *Healthy People 2010* is to prevent disease, disability, and death from vaccine-preventable illnesses. Vaccine schedules have been clarified and combination vaccines are helpful in decreasing the number of vaccines required. There is no contraindication to the *simultaneous* administration of any vaccine, and only live parenteral (injected) vaccines (e.g., MMR, varicella and yellow fever, live attenuated influenza vaccine) need to be separated by at least 4 weeks if not administered simultaneously.[2]

Health care providers in all settings, including schools, colleges, outpatient clinics, workplaces, and emergency departments, should take advantage of the opportunities to discuss immunization history, including past and present illnesses, age, employment, family history, and risk factors. This history should also include allergies and prior allergic or untoward reactions. Women of childbearing age should be questioned about the possibility of pregnancy, because certain vaccines are contraindicated during pregnancy (e.g., varicella [Varivax], MMR). Adolescents should have their immunization history updated at age 11 or 12 years.[3,4] Patients must be educated about the potential side effects of each vaccine and should be encouraged to keep a record of their vaccination history. Vaccine doses should not be administered at intervals less than the recommended intervals or earlier than the minimal ages.[2] As with any injected medication, observation for a minimum of 30 minutes is recommended because of the danger of anaphylaxis. Immunosuppressed patients (e.g., patients with HIV infection or leukemia, or patients receiving chemotherapy or steroids) should not be given live vaccines because this may lead to vaccine-induced illness or disseminated disease.

Table 25-1 provides information, including dosages and side effects, on the currently recommended vaccines.[2,6,7] Figures 25-1 and 25-2 include the recommended childhood/adolescent and adult immunization schedules, respectively. Other information regarding immunizations can be obtained by calling the Centers for Disease Control and Prevention Hotline (800-232-4636) or sending immunization and vaccine-preventable disease questions to the CDC at nipinfo@cdc.gov. nipinfo@cdc.gov. Other resources include the Immunization Action Coalition (www.immunize.org) and state immunization programs.

Text continued on p. 158.

TABLE 25-1 Quick Reference for Routine Immunizations

Vaccine Antigen Dose and Route	Routine Administration Schedule*	Precautions and Contraindications†‡	Adverse Reactions	Serious Adverse Reactions	Education Indications
DTP					
Diphtheria-tetanus-pertussis§ Child: 0.5 ml IM Adult: see Td D—Toxoid T—Toxoid P—Bacteria	2, 4, 6, 12-15 months Booster: 4-6 years (contains aluminum) Administer deep IM; avoid compressing plunger when withdrawing needle to prevent leakage into subcutaneous fat 6 months should elapse between 3rd and 4th doses	Neurologic disorder with progressive developmental delay or changed neurologic findings Neurologic condition predisposing to seizures or neurologic deterioration ≥7 yr Serious adverse reactions to previous immunization, including anaphylaxis, shock, fever (>40.5° C [>104.9° F]) of unknown origin within 2 days after vaccine administration, encephalopathy within 7 days of previous vaccination, or seizure related to previous DtaP[8]	Local pain, erythema Fussiness Fever <40.5° C (<104.9° F) Sleepiness Painless lump at injection site that may last several weeks	Once for every 100-1000 doses: Fever >40.5° C (>104.9° F) within 48 hours of dose Persistent, inconsolable cry for >3 hours or high-pitched cephalic cry within 48 hours of dose Once for every 1750 doses: Convulsions, facial neurologic signs, alteration in consciousness Collapse or shocklike state Very rarely: Anaphylaxis Coma	Apply a warm compress to injection site if red, swollen. Report serious adverse reactions to health care provider. Give acetaminophen for fever. Adverse effects may last 12-24 hours.
Tdap (tetanus, diphtheria, acellular pertussis) 0.5 ml IM	Indicated for active booster immunization for the prevention of tetanus, diphtheria, and pertussis as a single dose in persons 11-64 years old (replaces Td in this age group)	Life-threatening allergic reaction to DTP, DTap, DT, or Td Severe allergy to any component of vaccine Patients with epilepsy or an unstable neurologic condition should consult a physician.	Pain and swelling at the injection site	Hives Shortness of breath Wheezing Angioedema	Minimum recommended interval between Td and Tdap is 2 years
DTaP	Consider 4th and 5th doses only for children ≥15 months old				

Adapted from Centers for Disease Control and Prevention; Atkinson W, Hamborsky J, McIntyre L, and others, editors: *Epidemiology and prevention of vaccine-preventable diseases,* ed 9, Washington, DC, 2006, Public Health Foundation.

*Recommended schedules differ for infants and children who do not begin immunizations at usual time or who are behind schedule. See specific guidelines from AAP or ACIP, USDHHS/CDC.

†No immunization should be given to a client who is moderately or severely ill.

‡Pregnancy is a precaution with any immunization. Special cases must be considered on an individual basis.

§DTP/Hib combination vaccines are available. See specific guidelines from Advisory Committee on Immunization Practices, USDHHS/CDC, and American Academy of Pediatrics.

Continued

TABLE 25-1 Quick Reference for Routine Immunizations—cont'd

Vaccine Antigen Dose and Route	Routine Administration Schedule*	Precautions and Contraindications†‡	Adverse Reactions	Serious Adverse Reactions	Education Indications
DT					
Diphtheria-tetanus (pediatric) 0.5 ml IM	Only used if child had serious reaction to DTP; "D" (larger dose of diphtheria) is not given to children ≥7 years old.		Local pain at injection site		
TD					
(Tetanus diphtheria) 0.5 ml IM	Unvaccinated children ≥7 years old All adults (18-65) who did not complete a primary series in childhood Dose 1 Dose 2: at least 6 weeks later Dose 3: 6-12 months after 2nd dose	History of neurologic reaction or severe hypersensitivity (anaphylaxis or generalized urticaria)	Local reactions (induration and erythema) Arthus-type hypersensitivity—severe local reaction, fever, and malaise—may occur if tetanus boosters given too often.	Very rarely: Serious allergic reaction Deep, aching pain and muscle wasting in upper arm 2 days to 4 weeks after the injection; may last months	Td is recommended for persons seeking medical attention for clean, minor wounds if more than 10 years since last dose. Td is recommended for deep puncture wounds if more than 5 years since last dose.
POLIOMYELITIS					
IPV killed virus 0.5 ml SQ (OPV no longer recommended in U.S.)	2, 4, 6 months (dosage may be given through 18 months) Booster: 4-6 years Can be substituted for some or all doses of OPV	Altered immunity in recipient or household HIV positive Larger dose corticosteroid ≥18 years Allergic reaction to neomycin or streptomycin	Local pain at injection site	1 case for every 1.5 million after 1st dose 1 case for every 30 million later doses Paralytic polio in recipient or close contact (more common in adults) Anaphylaxis	Virus can be shed in stool for 4-6 weeks—need for good handwashing and proper disposal of diapers. IPV is recommended for previously unvaccinated adults—travelers to areas where wild poliovirus is endemic and epidemic
MMR					
Measles, mumps, rubella Live virus Mix with diluent and give contents of single-dose vial SQ. Measles, mumps, and rubella vaccines may be administered separately (see insert recommendations).	12-15 months Booster: either at 4-6 or 11-12 years Adults: 1 dose MMR, unless contraindicated, if not immunized as a child (ACIP recommends a 2nd dose of MMR for certain high-risk individuals: those entering post–high school educational settings, persons in health care settings with direct patient care contact, travelers to areas with endemic measles)	Severe allergy to eggs, neomycin, or gelatin[8] Serum immune globulin, whole blood, or blood products within past 3 months Altered immunity in recipient Large-dose corticosteroid Pregnancy contraindicated for 3 months after rubella immunization (use contraception)	Mild burning sensation at injection site Measles: Fever starting 5-12 days after vaccination Rash Mumps: Swelling of salivary glands Fever Rubella: Joint pain, swelling 1-3 weeks after immunization, lasting 1 day to 3 weeks; more common among older, not previously immunized patients	Very rarely: Serious allergic reaction Anaphylaxis Postvaccination encephalitis Coma Residual seizure disorder Thrombocytopenia—usually temporary	All adults born in 1957 or later should receive 1 dose of measles-mumps vaccine unless there is laboratory evidence of immunity. Rubella vaccine is recommended for adults (especially women) without proof of vaccination or laboratory immunity. There is no evidence that revaccination with MMR in persons with natural or acquired immunity, to any or all three diseases, causes increased risk. Measles vaccine may suppress tuberculin activity for 4-6 weeks.

TABLE 25-1 Quick Reference for Routine Immunizations—cont'd

Vaccine Antigen Dose and Route	Routine Administration Schedule*	Precautions and Contraindications†‡	Adverse Reactions	Serious Adverse Reactions	Education Indications
HIB					
0.5 ml IM DTP/Hib combination vaccines are available. See specific guidelines from AAP and ACIP and review package insert information. After the primary infant Hib conjugate vaccine series is completed, any other licensed Hib conjugate vaccines may be used for 12-15 month booster dose.	2, 4, 6 months (Children who received PRP-OMP at 2 and 4 months do not require a dose at 6 months.) Booster: 12-15 months	≥5 years of age (unimmunized children ≥5 years with chronic disease that is associated with *Haemophilus influenzae* should receive 1 dose) Previous anaphylactic reaction to diphtheria toxoid if using HbOC (HibTITER) or PRP-D (ProHIBIT); these vaccines contain small amounts of diphtheria toxoid	Local pain at injection site Mild fever		Hib protects child against some illnesses caused by *H. influenzae* (e.g., *H. influenzae* meningitis, pneumonia).
HEPATITIS B					
Recombinant antigen Infants: 0.25 ml IM (The dose for infants born to HBsAg-positive mothers is 0.5 ml IM. These infants are also given hepatitis B immune globulin [HBIG] at birth.) Child <11 years 0.25 ml IM Child 11-19 years: 0.5 ml IM Adult ≥20 years: 1 ml IM Recombivax HB dialysis formulation is recommended for adult predialysis and dialysis patients (see package insert).	Infants: series of 3 doses Option 1: at birth, 1-2 months, 6-18 months Option 2: 1-2, 4, and 6-18 months Infants born to HBsAg-positive mothers should receive hepatitis B immunoprophylaxis before hospital discharge. 7 years–adult: series of 3 doses—at 1st visit, then 2 months later, then 6 months after 2nd dose	Hypersensitivity to yeast or previous anaphylaxis related to Hep B vaccine[8] If symptoms of sensitivity occur after an injection, do not give additional immunizations.	Local pain, erythema, swelling Fatigue, weakness, headache Fever (≥37.8° C [≥100° F]), malaise	Anaphylaxis	3-dose regimen provides a protective level against hepatitis B viral infection. Hepatitis B can cause cirrhosis and cancer of the liver. Duration of protection is generally 7 years. Vaccination is recommended for following at-risk groups: 1. Health care and public safety personnel 2. Employees of chronic care facilities 3. Subpopulations with a known high incidence of disease—Alaskan Eskimos, Indochinese, Haitians, and sub-Saharan refugees 4. Illicit injectable drug users 5. Prisoners 6. Morticians 7. Persons who have heterosexual activity with multiple partners, persons who repeatedly contract STDs, homosexually active males, prostitutes

Continued

TABLE 25-1 Quick Reference for Routine Immunizations—cont'd

Vaccine Antigen Dose and Route	Routine Administration Schedule*	Precautions and Contraindications†‡	Adverse Reactions	Serious Adverse Reactions	Education Indications
HEPATITIS B—CONT'D					
					8. Patients who frequently require blood transfusions or clotting factor concentrates 9. Household contacts of HBV carriers 10. Military personnel and travelers to areas with high endemic levels
HEPATITIS A					
Recommended for all children at 12-23 months of age Also recommended for persons at increased risk of hepatitis A infection or who are at increased risk for complications of hepatitis A infection	Children 2-18 years of age: 0.5 ml IM of the pediatric formulation, followed by a booster dose 6 months after the first dose Adults: 0.5 ml IM of the adult formulation, followed by a booster dose 6-18 months after the first dose Combination hepatitis A and hepatitis B vaccine (Twinrix) approved for persons ≥18 years. Schedule 0, 1, 6 months	History of severe allergic reaction to a vaccine component or following a prior dose of hepatitis A vaccine, hypersensitivity to alum, or in the case of HAVRIX, hypersensitivity to the preservative 2-phenoxyethanol Vaccinations of persons with moderate or severe acute illness should be deferred. Safety in pregnancy has not been determined; however, because it is an inactivated vaccine, the theoretical risk to the fetus is low.	Local reactions at the injection site (pain, erythema, or swelling), which tend to be mild or self-limited		Hepatitis A infection produces lifelong immunity to hepatitis A, so there is no benefit to vaccinating someone with serologic evidence of past hepatitis A infection. Routine serologic testing is not indicated except for persons who were born or have lived for extended periods in geographic areas that have a high endemicity of hepatitis A infection.
INFLUENZA					
Trivalent inactivated influenza vaccine (TIV) (only subviron or split virus available in the U.S.) Children: 1 or 2 doses (children <9 years who are receiving influenza vaccine for the 1st time should be given 2 doses, at least 1 month apart.)	Annually in the fall Administered IM	History of allergy to eggs or previous serious reaction to influenza vaccine Pregnancy—postpone immunization to 2nd or 3rd trimester. Defer influenza vaccine in patients with fever and acute illness.	Soreness at the injection site Myalgia, fever, flulike symptoms		CDC targets the following high-risk groups: 1. Persons >65 years old 2. Residents of nursing homes or other chronic care facilities 3. Adults and children with chronic disorders of pulmonary or cardiovascular system (e.g., asthma, bronchopulmonary dysplasia)

TABLE 25-1 Quick Reference for Routine Immunizations—cont'd

Vaccine Antigen Dose and Route	Routine Administration Schedule*	Precautions and Contraindications†‡	Adverse Reactions	Serious Adverse Reactions	Education Indications
INFLUENZA—CONT'D					
6-35 months: 0.25 ml IM of split virus at least 1 month apart in anterolateral thigh 3-9 years: 1 or 2 doses of 0.5 ml IM of split virus in anterolateral thigh or deltoid ≥9 years: 1 dose of 0.5 ml IM in deltoid Adult: 0.5 ml IM in deltoid					4. Persons who required regular medical follow-up or hospitalization during previous year because of chronic metabolic diseases (e.g., diabetes, renal dysfunction), hemoglobinopathies, or immunosuppressants (e.g., HIV, AIDS, or immunosuppression because of medications) 5. Family members, health care providers, and employees and volunteers who are potentially capable of transmitting influenza to high-risk patients
Live attenuated influenza vaccine (LAIV) approved only for use among healthy persons ages 5-49 yr	Administered intranasally	Close contacts of persons at high risk for influenza infection should not receive LAIV.	Significantly increased risk of asthma or reactive airway disease in children 12-59 months of age Significantly increased risk of cough, runny nose, nasal congestion, sore throat, and chills reported in adults	No serious adverse reactions identified.	Persons with chronic medical conditions including asthma, reactive airway disease, or other chronic pulmonary or cardiovascular conditions; metabolic diseases such as diabetes or renal disease; or hemoglobinopathies such as sickle cell disease should not receive LAIV. Children and adolescents receiving long-term therapy with aspirin or other salicylates should not receive LAIV because of the association with Reye syndrome.

Continued

TABLE 25-1 Quick Reference for Routine Immunizations—cont'd

Vaccine Antigen Dose and Route	Routine Administration Schedule*	Precautions and Contraindications†‡	Adverse Reactions	Serious Adverse Reactions	Education Indications
PNEUMOCOCCAL					
Pneumococcal polysaccharide vaccine (23 valent) Inactivated antigen Child: 0.5 ml IM or SQ Adults: 0.5 ml IM or SQ (Persons who received the 14-valent vaccine should not be reimmunized unless they are very high risk.)	Adults ≥65 years: 1 dose; revaccination recommended only for those at highest risk ≥6 years after 1st dose Persons ≥2 years with chronic illness, anatomic or functional asplenia, immunocompromised, HIV infection, and environments or settings with increased risk Not effective in children <2 years.	For both the polysaccharide and conjugate vaccines, severe allergic reaction to a vaccine component or following a prior dose of the vaccine Moderate or severe acute illness Safety in pregnancy has not been evaluated, although no adverse consequences have been reported among newborns whose mothers were inadvertently vaccinated during pregnancy.	Localized pain and erythema at the injection site Low-grade fever for 24 hours		CDC targets the following high-risk groups: 1. Adults ≥65 years old 2. Children or adults with chronic cardiac or respiratory illnesses or at risk for respiratory illness 3. Immunocompromised children or adults (e.g., splenic dysfunction, HIV, AIDS, sickle cell disease) 4. Revaccination considered ≥6 years after the 1st dose for those at highest risk of fatal pneumococcal disease or rapid decline in antibody levels
Pneumococcal conjugate vaccine (7 serotypes)	Routine vaccination of children age <24 months and children 24-59 months with a high-risk medical condition Children: 1 dose at ages 2, 4, and 6 months, with a booster dose at 12-15 months Age ≥24 months: give 1 or 2 doses at least 6-8 weeks apart		Local reactions and fever and myalgias	Rare	

TABLE 25-1 Quick Reference for Routine Immunizations—cont'd

Vaccine Antigen Dose and Route	Routine Administration Schedule*	Precautions and Contraindications†‡	Adverse Reactions	Serious Adverse Reactions	Education Indications
MENINGOCOCCAL					
MCV (meningococcal conjugate vaccine)	Recommended for all children at routine preadolescent visit (11-12 years) and for others at increased risk of meningococcal disease. MCV is the preferred vaccine for routine vaccination of persons 11-55 years of age who are at increased risk of meningococcal disease. Single dose 0.5 ml IM	Allergic reaction to previous dose or prior history of Guillain-Barré syndrome Allergy to any vaccine component Anyone moderately or severely ill should wait until recovery.	Local reactions at the injection site Headache and malaise (within 7 days of vaccination)	Anaphylaxis	Family members and close contacts of infected persons are at increased risk for meningococcal disease and should be vaccinated. Risk factors for the development of meningococcal disease include deficiencies in the terminal common complement pathway, functional or anatomic asplenia, HIV, and certain genetic factors (e.g., tumor necrosis factor).
MPSV (meningococcal polysaccharide vaccine)	Approved for children ≥2 years of age Not recommended for routine immunization of civilians Should be used only for persons at increased risk of *Neisseria meningitidis* infection who are 2-10 or >55 years of age, or if MCV is not available Single 0.5 ml dose SQ Revaccination may be indicated for persons previously vaccinated with MPSV who remain at increased risk if 5 years have elapsed since vaccination with MPSV.	Same as for MCV	Same as for MCV	Same as for MCV	

Continued

TABLE 25-1 Quick Reference for Routine Immunizations—cont'd

Vaccine Antigen Dose and Route	Routine Administration Schedule*	Precautions and Contraindications†‡	Adverse Reactions	Serious Adverse Reactions	Education Indications
VARICELLA					
Recommended for all children without contraindications at 12-18 months of age Also recommended for all persons ≥13 years of age without evidence of varicella immunity	12 months–12 years: 0.5 ml SQ >12 years: 1st dose of 0.5 ml SQ, then a repeat dose in 4-8 weeks (same for adults who have never received this immunization)	Anaphylactic allergy to gelatin or neomycin Pregnancy Immunocompromised patients (e.g., HIV, leukemia, lymphoma) should not be vaccinated[8] Acute febrile illness Blood dyscrasias, leukemia, lymphoma Active, untreated TB Defer vaccination for 5 months after blood transfusions or administration of immune globulin or VZIG. Avoid use of salicylates for 6 weeks after vaccination.	Mild local pain at injection site Rare: mild varicella-like illness with a few fever vesicles	Anaphylaxis	Offer to high-risk groups with no history of varicella illness: teachers of young children, day care workers, health care workers. Children who receive varicella vaccine should not receive aspirin or aspirin-related products for at least 6 weeks.[8]
HERPES ZOSTER					
(Shingles) Zostavax Recommended for persons >60 years of age	Single dose of 0.65 ml administered SQ	Allergic reactions or hypersensitivity to any of its ingredients, including allergies to gelatin or neomycin Disease or condition resulting in a compromised immune system such as leukemia, lymphoma, HIV/AIDS or high doses of oral steroids Active TB that is not being treated Pregnancy or the possibility of pregnancy	Local reactions (redness, pain, swelling, itching, warmth) at the injection site, as well as headache		Persons >60 without a known history of varicella are presumed to have had varicella exposure and do not need to have varicella antibody titers done prior to vaccination.
HUMAN PAPILLOMA VIRUS					
(HPV) Approved for girls and women 9-26 years of age	Series of 3 IM injections administered at 0, 2, 6 months	Allergic reactions or hypersensitivity to any of its ingredients or after getting a dose of the vaccine	Local reactions (pain, swelling, itching or redness) at the injection site, as well as fever		An estimated 50% of sexually active people acquire HPV during their lifetime. Persons of any age taking part in any kind of sexual activity involving genital contact are at risk.

Department of Health and Human Services • Centers for Disease Control and Prevention

Recommended Childhood and Adolescent Immunization Schedule UNITED STATES • 2006

Vaccine ▼ / Age ▶	Birth	1 month	2 months	4 months	6 months	12 months	15 months	18 months	24 months	4–6 years	11–12 years	13–14 years	15 years	16–18 years
Hepatitis B[1]	HepB	HepB		*HepB[1]*		HepB					HepB Series			
Diphtheria, Tetanus, Pertussis[2]			DTaP	DTaP	DTaP		DTaP			DTaP	Tdap		Tdap	
Haemophilus influenzae type b[3]			Hib	Hib	*Hib[3]*	Hib								
Inactivated Poliovirus			IPV	IPV		IPV				IPV				
Measles, Mumps, Rubella[4]						MMR				MMR		MMR		
Varicella[5]							Varicella				Varicella			
Meningococcal[6]							Vaccines within broken line are for selected populations		MPSV4		MCV4	MCV4	MCV4	
Pneumococcal[7]			PCV	PCV	PCV	PCV			PCV		PPV			
Influenza[8]						Influenza (Yearly)					Influenza (Yearly)			
Hepatitis A[9]									HepA Series					

This schedule indicates the recommended ages for routine administration of currently licensed childhood vaccines, as of December 1, 2005, for children through age 18 years. Any dose not administered at the recommended age should be administered at any subsequent visit when indicated and feasible. ■ Indicates age groups that warrant special effort to administer those vaccines not previously administered. Additional vaccines may be licensed and recommended during the year. Licensed combination vaccines may be used whenever any components of the combination are indicated and other components of the vaccine are not contraindicated and if approved by the Food and Drug Administration for that dose of the series. Providers should consult the respective ACIP statement for detailed recommendations. Clinically significant adverse events that follow immunization should be reported to the Vaccine Adverse Event Reporting System (VAERS). Guidance about how to obtain and complete a VAERS form is available at **www.vaers.hhs.gov** or by telephone, **800-822-7967.**

Range of recommended ages | **Catch-up immunization** | **11–12 year old assessment**

1. **Hepatitis B vaccine (HepB).** ***AT BIRTH:*** **All newborns** should receive monovalent HepB soon after birth and before hospital discharge. **Infants born to mothers who are HBsAg-positive** should receive HepB and 0.5 mL of hepatitis B immune globulin (HBIG) within 12 hours of birth. **Infants born to mothers whose HBsAg status is unknown** should receive HepB within 12 hours of birth. The mother should have blood drawn as soon as possible to determine her HBsAg status; if HBsAg-positive, the infant should receive HBIG as soon as possible (no later than age 1 week). **For infants born to HBsAg-negative mothers,** the birth dose can be delayed in rare circumstances but only if a physician's order to withhold the vaccine and a copy of the mother's original HBsAg-negative laboratory report are documented in the infant's medical record. ***FOLLOWING THE BIRTHDOSE:*** The HepB series should be completed with either monovalent HepB or a combination vaccine containing HepB. The second dose should be administered at age 1–2 months. The final dose should be administered at age ≥24 weeks. It is permissible to administer 4 doses of HepB (e.g., when combination vaccines are given after the birth dose); however, if monovalent HepB is used, a dose at age 4 months is not needed. **Infants born to HBsAg-positive mothers** should be tested for HBsAg and antibody to HBsAg after completion of the HepB series, at age 9–18 months (generally at the next well-child visit after completion of the vaccine series).
2. **Diphtheria and tetanus toxoids and acellular pertussis vaccine (DTaP).** The fourth dose of DTaP may be administered as early as age 12 months, provided 6 months have elapsed since the third dose and the child is unlikely to return at age 15–18 months. The final dose in the series should be given at age ≥4 years.
   Tetanus and diphtheria toxoids and acellular pertussis vaccine (Tdap – adolescent preparation) is recommended at age 11–12 years for those who have completed the recommended childhood DTP/DTaP vaccination series and have not received a Td booster dose. Adolescents 13–18 years who missed the 11–12-year Td/Tdap booster dose should also receive a single dose of Tdap if they have completed the recommended childhood DTP/DTaP vaccination series. Subsequent **tetanus and diphtheria toxoids (Td)** are recommended every 10 years.
3. ***Haemophilus influenzae*** **type b conjugate vaccine (Hib).** Three Hib conjugate vaccines are licensed for infant use. If PRP-OMP (PedvaxHIB® or ComVax® [Merck]) is administered at ages 2 and 4 months, a dose at age 6 months is not required. DTaP/Hib combination products should not be used for primary immunization in infants at ages 2, 4 or 6 months but can be used as boosters after any Hib vaccine. The final dose in the series should be administered at age ≥12 months.
4. **Measles, mumps, and rubella vaccine (MMR).** The second dose of MMR is recommended routinely at age 4–6 years but may be administered during any visit, provided at least 4 weeks have elapsed since the first dose and both doses are administered beginning at or after age 12 months. Those who have not previously received the second dose should complete the schedule by age 11–12 years.
5. **Varicella vaccine.** Varicella vaccine is recommended at any visit at or after age 12 months for susceptible children (i.e., those who lack a reliable history of chickenpox). Susceptible persons aged ≥13 years should receive 2 doses administered at least 4 weeks apart.
6. **Meningococcal vaccine (MCV4).** Meningococcal conjugate vaccine (MCV4) should be given to all children at the 11–12 year old visit as well as to unvaccinated adolescents at high school entry (15 years of age). Other adolescents who wish to decrease their risk for meningococcal disease may also be vaccinated. All college freshmen living in dormitories should also be vaccinated, preferably with MCV4, although **meningococcal polysaccharide vaccine (MPSV4)** is an acceptable alternative. Vaccination against invasive meningococcal disease is recommended for children and adolescents aged ≥2 years with terminal complement deficiencies or anatomic or functional asplenia and certain other high risk groups (see *MMWR* 2005;54 [RR-7]:1-21); use MPSV4 for children aged 2–10 years and MCV4 for older children, although MPSV4 is an acceptable alternative.
7. **Pneumococcal vaccine.** The heptavalent **pneumococcal conjugate vaccine (PCV)** is recommended for all children aged 2–23 months and for certain children aged 24–59 months. The final dose in the series should be given at age ≥12 months. **Pneumococcal polysaccharide vaccine (PPV)** is recommended in addition to PCV for certain high-risk groups. See *MMWR* 2000; 49(RR-9):1-35.
8. **Influenza vaccine.** Influenza vaccine is recommended annually for children aged ≥6 months with certain risk factors (including, but not limited to, asthma, cardiac disease, sickle cell disease, human immunodeficiency virus [HIV], diabetes, and conditions that can compromise respiratory function or handling of respiratory secretions or that can increase the risk for aspiration), healthcare workers, and other persons (including household members) in close contact with persons in groups at high risk (see *MMWR* 2005;54[RR-8]:1-55). In addition, healthy children aged 6–23 months and close contacts of healthy children aged 0–5 months are recommended to receive influenza vaccine because children in this age group are at substantially increased risk for influenza-related hospitalizations. For healthy persons aged 5–49 years, the intranasally administered, live, attenuated influenza vaccine (LAIV) is an acceptable alternative to the intramuscular trivalent inactivated influenza vaccine (TIV). See *MMWR* 2005;54(RR-8):1-55. Children receiving TIV should be administered a dosage appropriate for their age (0.25 mL if aged 6–35 months or 0.5 mL if aged ≥3 years). Children aged ≤8 years who are receiving influenza vaccine for the first time should receive 2 doses (separated by at least 4 weeks for TIV and at least 6 weeks for LAIV).
9. **Hepatitis A vaccine (HepA).** HepA is recommended for all children at 1 year of age (i.e., 12–23 months). The 2 doses in the series should be administered at least 6 months apart. States, counties, and communities with existing HepA vaccination programs for children 2–18 years of age are encouraged to maintain these programs. In these areas, new efforts focused on routine vaccination of 1-year-old children should enhance, not replace, ongoing programs directed at a broader population of children. HepA is also recommended for certain high risk groups (see *MMWR* 1999; 48[RR-12]1-37).

The Childhood and Adolescent Immunization Schedule is approved by:
Advisory Committee on Immunization Practices www.cdc.gov/nip/acip • American Academy of Pediatrics www.aap.org • American Academy of Family Physicians www.aafp.org

Continued

Figure 25-1

Recommended childhood and adolescent immunization schedules. (From Department of Health and Human Services, Atlanta, 2006, Centers for Disease Control and Prevention.)

Recommended Immunization Schedule for Children and Adolescents Who Start Late or Who Are More Than 1 Month Behind

UNITED STATES • 2006

The tables below give catch-up schedules and minimum intervals between doses for children who have delayed immunizations. There is no need to restart a vaccine series regardless of the time that has elapsed between doses. Use the chart appropriate for the child's age.

CATCH-UP SCHEDULE FOR CHILDREN AGED 4 MONTHS THROUGH 6 YEARS

Vaccine	Minimum Age for Dose 1	Minimum Interval Between Doses			
		Dose 1 to Dose 2	Dose 2 to Dose 3	Dose 3 to Dose 4	Dose 4 to Dose 5
Diphtheria, Tetanus, Pertussis	6 wks	4 weeks	4 weeks	6 months	6 months[1]
Inactivated Poliovirus	6 wks	4 weeks	4 weeks	4 weeks[2]	
Hepatitis B[3]	Birth	4 weeks	8 weeks (and 16 weeks after first dose)		
Measles, Mumps, Rubella	12 mo	4 weeks[4]			
Varicella	12 mo				
Haemophilus influenzae type b[5]	6 wks	**4 weeks** if first dose given at age <12 months **8 weeks (as final dose)** if first dose given at age 12-14 months **No further doses needed** if first dose given at age ≥15 months	**4 weeks[6]** if current age <12 months **8 weeks (as final dose)[6]** if current age ≥12 months and second dose given at age <15 months **No further doses needed** if previous dose given at age ≥15 mo	**8 weeks (as final dose)** This dose only necessary for children aged 12 months–5 years who received 3 doses before age 12 months	
Pneumococcal[7]	6 wks	**4 weeks** if first dose given at age <12 months and current age <24 months **8 weeks (as final dose)** if first dose given at age ≥12 months or current age 24–59 months **No further doses needed** for healthy children if first dose given at age ≥ 24 months	**4 weeks** if current age <12 months **8 weeks (as final dose)** if current age ≥12 months **No further doses needed** for healthy children if previous dose given at age ≥24 months	**8 weeks (as final dose)** This dose only necessary for children aged 12 months–5 years who received 3 doses before age 12 months	

CDC SAFER • HEALTHIER • PEOPLE™

CATCH-UP SCHEDULE FOR CHILDREN AGED 7 YEARS THROUGH 18 YEARS

Vaccine	Minimum Interval Between Doses		
	Dose 1 to Dose 2	Dose 2 to Dose 3	Dose 3 to Booster Dose
Tetanus, Diphtheria[8]	4 weeks	6 months	**6 months** if first dose given at age <12 months and current age <11 years; otherwise **5 years**
Inactivated Poliovirus[9]	4 weeks	4 weeks	IPV[2,9]
Hepatitis B	4 weeks	8 weeks (and 16 weeks after first dose)	
Measles, Mumps, Rubella	4 weeks		
Varicella[10]	4 weeks		

1. **DTaP.** The fifth dose is not necessary if the fourth dose was administered after the fourth birthday.
2. **IPV.** For children who received an all-IPV or all-oral poliovirus (OPV) series, a fourth dose is not necessary if third dose was administered at age ≥4 years. If both OPV and IPV were administered as part of a series, a total of 4 doses should be given, regardless of the child's current age.
3. **HepB.** Administer the 3-dose series to all children and adolescents<19 years of age if they were not previously vaccinated.
4. **MMR.** The second dose of MMR is recommended routinely at age 4–6 years but may be administered earlier if desired.
5. **Hib.** Vaccine is not generally recommended for children aged ≥5 years.
6. **Hib.** If current age <12 months and the first 2 doses were PRP-OMP (PedvaxHIB® or ComVax® [Merck]), the third (and final) dose should be administered at age 12–15 months and at least 8 weeks after the second dose.
7. **PCV.** Vaccine is not generally recommended for children aged ≥5 years.
8. **Td.** Adolescent tetanus, diphtheria, and pertussis vaccine (Tdap) may be substituted for any dose in a primary catch-up series or as a booster if age appropriate for Tdap. A five-year interval from the last Td dose is encouraged when Tdap is used as a booster dose. See ACIP recommendations for further information.
9. **IPV.** Vaccine is not generally recommended for persons aged ≥18 years.
10. **Varicella.** Administer the 2-dose series to all susceptible adolescents aged ≥13 years.

Report adverse reactions to vaccines through the federal Vaccine Adverse Event Reporting System. For information on reporting reactions following immunization, please visit www.vaers.hhs.gov or call the 24-hour national toll-free information line 800-822-7967. Report suspected cases of vaccine-preventable diseases to your state or local health department.

For additional information about vaccines, including precautions and contraindications for immunization and vaccine shortages, please visit the National Immunization Program Website at www.cdc.gov/nip or contact 800-CDC-INFO (800-232-4636) (In English, En Español — 24/7)

Figure 25-1—cont'd

Recommended Adult Immunization Schedule
United States, October 2006–September 2007

Recommended adult immunization schedule, by vaccine and age group

<table>
<tr><th>Age group (yrs) ▶
Vaccine ▼</th><th>19–49 years</th><th>50–64 years</th><th>≥65 years</th></tr>
<tr><td rowspan="2">Tetanus, diphtheria, pertussis (Td/Tdap)[1]*</td><td colspan="3">1-dose Td booster every 10 yrs</td></tr>
<tr><td colspan="2">Substitute 1 dose of Tdap for Td</td><td></td></tr>
<tr><td>Human papillomavirus (HPV)[2]*</td><td>3 doses (females)</td><td></td><td></td></tr>
<tr><td>Measles, mumps, rubella (MMR)[3]*</td><td>1 or 2 doses</td><td colspan="2">1 dose</td></tr>
<tr><td>Varicella[4]*</td><td>2 doses (0, 4–8 wks)</td><td>2 doses (0, 4–8 wks)</td><td></td></tr>
<tr><td>Influenza[5]*</td><td>1 dose annually</td><td colspan="2">1 dose annually</td></tr>
<tr><td>Pneumococcal (polysaccharide)[6,7]</td><td colspan="2">1–2 doses</td><td>1 dose</td></tr>
<tr><td>Hepatitis A[8]*</td><td colspan="3">2 doses (0, 6–12 mos, or 0, 6–18 mos)</td></tr>
<tr><td>Hepatitis B[9]*</td><td colspan="3">3 doses (0, 1–2, 4–6 mos)</td></tr>
<tr><td>Meningococcal[10]</td><td colspan="3">1 or more doses</td></tr>
</table>

Recommended adult immunization schedule, by vaccine and medical and other indications

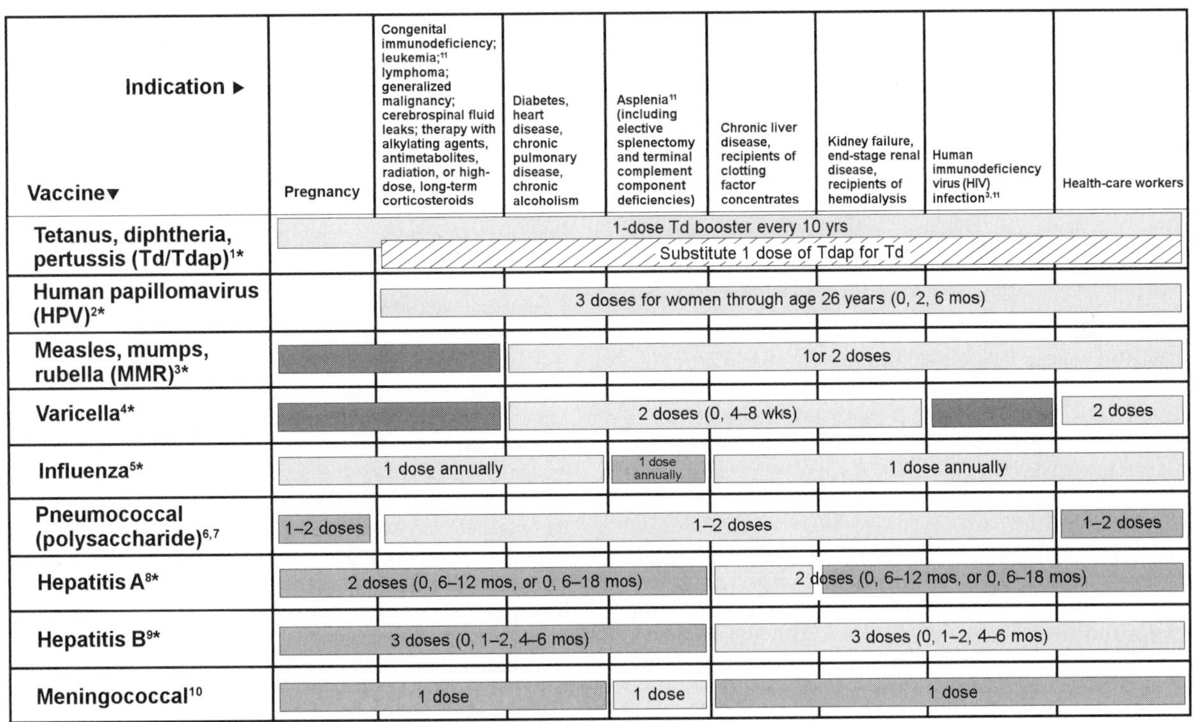

<table>
<tr><th>Indication ▶
Vaccine ▼</th><th>Pregnancy</th><th>Congenital immunodeficiency; leukemia;[11] lymphoma; generalized malignancy; cerebrospinal fluid leaks; therapy with alkylating agents, antimetabolites, radiation, or high-dose, long-term corticosteroids</th><th>Diabetes, heart disease, chronic pulmonary disease, chronic alcoholism</th><th>Asplenia[11] (including elective splenectomy and terminal complement component deficiencies)</th><th>Chronic liver disease, recipients of clotting factor concentrates</th><th>Kidney failure, end-stage renal disease, recipients of hemodialysis</th><th>Human immunodeficiency virus (HIV) infection[3,11]</th><th>Health-care workers</th></tr>
<tr><td rowspan="2">Tetanus, diphtheria, pertussis (Td/Tdap)[1]*</td><td colspan="8">1-dose Td booster every 10 yrs</td></tr>
<tr><td></td><td colspan="7">Substitute 1 dose of Tdap for Td</td></tr>
<tr><td>Human papillomavirus (HPV)[2]*</td><td></td><td colspan="7">3 doses for women through age 26 years (0, 2, 6 mos)</td></tr>
<tr><td>Measles, mumps, rubella (MMR)[3]*</td><td colspan="2"></td><td colspan="6">1or 2 doses</td></tr>
<tr><td>Varicella[4]*</td><td colspan="2"></td><td colspan="4">2 doses (0, 4–8 wks)</td><td></td><td>2 doses</td></tr>
<tr><td>Influenza[5]*</td><td colspan="3">1 dose annually</td><td>1 dose annually</td><td colspan="4">1 dose annually</td></tr>
<tr><td>Pneumococcal (polysaccharide)[6,7]</td><td>1–2 doses</td><td colspan="6">1–2 doses</td><td>1–2 doses</td></tr>
<tr><td>Hepatitis A[8]*</td><td colspan="4">2 doses (0, 6–12 mos, or 0, 6–18 mos)</td><td colspan="4">2 doses (0, 6–12 mos, or 0, 6–18 mos)</td></tr>
<tr><td>Hepatitis B[9]*</td><td colspan="4">3 doses (0, 1–2, 4–6 mos)</td><td colspan="4">3 doses (0, 1–2, 4–6 mos)</td></tr>
<tr><td>Meningococcal[10]</td><td colspan="3">1 dose</td><td>1 dose</td><td colspan="4">1 dose</td></tr>
</table>

* Covered by the Vaccine Injury Compensation Program

These recommendations must be read along with the footnotes, which can be found on the next 2 pages of this schedule.

- (light) For all persons in this category who meet the age requirements and who lack evidence of immunity (e.g., lack documentation of vaccination or have no evidence of prior infection)
- (medium) Recommended if some other risk factor is present (e.g., on the basis of medical, occupational, lifestyle, or other indications)
- (dark) Contraindicated

Continued

Figure 25-2

Recommended adult immunization schedule. (From Department of Health and Human Services, Atlanta, 2006, Centers for Disease Control and Prevention.)

Footnotes

1. Tetanus, diphtheria, and acellular pertussis (Td/Tdap) vaccination. Adults with uncertain histories of a complete primary vaccination series with diphtheria and tetanus toxoid–containing vaccines should begin or complete a primary vaccination series. A primary series for adults is 3 doses; administer the first 2 doses at least 4 weeks apart and the third dose 6–12 months after the second. Administer a booster dose to adults who have completed a primary series and if the last vaccination was received ≥10 years previously. Tdap or tetanus and diphtheria (Td) vaccine may be used; Tdap should replace a single dose of Td for adults aged <65 years who have not previously received a dose of Tdap (either in the primary series, as a booster, or for wound management). Only one of two Tdap products (Adacel® [sanofi pasteur, Swiftwater, Pennsylvania]) is licensed for use in adults. If the person is pregnant and received the last Td vaccination >10 years previously, administer Td during the second or third trimester; if the person received the last Td vaccination in <10 years, administer Tdap during the immediate postpartum period. A one-time administration of 1-dose of Tdap with an interval as short as 2 years from a previous Td vaccination is recommended for postpartum women, close contacts of infants aged <12 months, and all health-care workers with direct patient contact. In certain situations, Td can be deferred during pregnancy and Tdap substituted in the immediate postpartum period, or Tdap can be given instead of Td to a pregnant woman after an informed discussion with the woman (see http://www.cdc.gov/nip/publications/acip-list.htm). Consult the ACIP statement for recommendations for administering Td as prophylaxis in wound management (http://www.cdc.gov/mmwr/preview/mmwrhtml/00041645.htm).

2. Human Papillomavirus (HPV) vaccination. HPV vaccination is recommended for all women aged <26 years who have not completed the vaccine series. Ideally, vaccine should be administered before potential exposure to HPV through sexual activity; however, women who are sexually active should still be vaccinated. Sexually active women who have not been infected with any of the HPV vaccine types receive the full benefit of the vaccination. Vaccination is less beneficial for women who have already been infected with one or more of the four HPV vaccine types. A complete series consists of 3 doses. The second dose should be administered 2 months after the first dose; the third dose should be administered 6 months after the first dose. Vaccination is not recommended during pregnancy. If a woman is found to be pregnant after initiating the vaccination series, the remainder of the 3-dose regimen should be delayed until after completion of the pregnancy.

3. Measles, Mumps, Rubella (MMR) vaccination. *Measles component:* adults born before 1957 can be considered immune to measles. Adults born during or after 1957 should receive ≥1 dose of MMR unless they have a medical contraindication, documentation of ≥1 dose, history of measles based on health-care provider diagnosis, or laboratory evidence of immunity. A second dose of MMR is recommended for adults who 1) have been recently exposed to measles or in an outbreak setting; 2) were previously vaccinated with killed measles vaccine; 3) have been vaccinated with an unknown type of measles vaccine during 1963–1967; 4) are students in postsecondary educational institutions; 5) work in a health-care facility, or 6) plan to travel internationally. Withhold MMR or other measles-containing vaccines from HIV-infected persons with severe immunosuppression. *Mumps component:* adults born before 1957 can generally be considered immune to mumps. Adults born during or after 1957 should receive 1 dose of MMR unless they have a medical contraindication, history of mumps based on health-care provider diagnosis, or laboratory evidence of immunity. A second dose of MMR is recommended for adults who 1) are in an age group that is affected during a mumps outbreak; 2) are students in postsecondary educational institutions; 3) work in a health-care facility; or 4) plan to travel internationally. For unvaccinated health-care workers born before 1957 who do not have other evidence of mumps immunity, consider giving 1 dose on a routine basis and strongly consider giving a second dose during an outbreak. *Rubella component:* administer 1 dose of MMR vaccine to women whose rubella vaccination history is unreliable or who lack laboratory evidence of immunity. For women of childbearing age, regardless of birth year, routinely determine rubella immunity and counsel women regarding congenital rubella syndrome. Do not vaccinate women who are pregnant or who might become pregnant within 4 weeks of receiving vaccine. Women who do not have evidence of immunity should receive MMR vaccine upon completion or termination of pregnancy and before discharge from the health-care facility.

4. Varicella vaccination. All adults without evidence of immunity to varicella should receive 2 doses of varicella vaccine. Special consideration should be given to those who 1) have close contact with persons at high risk for severe disease (e.g., health-care workers and family contacts of immunocompromised persons) or 2) are at high risk for exposure or transmission (e.g., teachers of young children; child care employees; residents and staff members of institutional settings, including correctional institutions; college students; military personnel; adolescents and adults living in households with children; non-pregnant women of childbearing age; and international travelers). Evidence of immunity to varicella in adults includes any of the following: 1) documentation of 2 doses of varicella vaccine at least 4 weeks apart; 2) U.S.–born before 1980 (although for health-care workers and pregnant women, birth before 1980 should not be considered evidence of immunity); 3) history of varicella based on diagnosis or verification of varicella by a health-care provider (for a patient reporting a history of or presenting with an atypical case, a mild case, or both, health-care providers should seek either an epidemiologic link with a typical varicella case or evidence of laboratory confirmation, if it was performed at the time of acute disease); 4) history of herpes zoster based on health-care provider diagnosis; or 5) laboratory evidence of immunity or laboratory confirmation of disease. Do not vaccinate women who are pregnant or might become pregnant within 4 weeks of receiving the vaccine. Assess pregnant women for evidence of varicella immunity. Women who do not have evidence of immunity should receive dose 1 of varicella vaccine upon completion or termination of pregnancy and before discharge from the health-care facility. Dose 2 should be administered 4–8 weeks after dose 1.

5. Influenza vaccination: *Medical indications:* chronic disorders of the cardiovascular or pulmonary systems, including asthma; chronic metabolic diseases, including diabetes mellitus, renal dysfunction, hemoglobinopathies, or immunosuppression (including immunosuppression caused by medications or HIV); any condition that compromises respiratory function or the handling of respiratory secretions or that can increase the risk of aspiration (e.g., cognitive dysfunction, spinal cord injury, or seizure disorder or other neuromuscular disorder); and pregnancy during the influenza season. No data exist on the risk for severe or complicated influenza disease among persons with asplenia; however, influenza is a risk factor for secondary bacterial infections that can cause severe disease among persons with asplenia. *Occupational indications:* health-care workers and employees of long-term–care and assisted living facilities. *Other indications:* residents of nursing homes and other long-term–care and assisted living facilities; persons likely to transmit influenza to persons at high risk (i.e., in-home household contacts and caregivers of children aged 0–59 months, or persons of all ages with high-risk conditions); and anyone who would like to be vaccinated. Healthy, nonpregnant persons aged 5–49 years without high-risk medical conditions who are not contacts of severely immunocompromised persons in special care units can receive either intranasally administered influenza vaccine (FluMist®) or inactivated vaccine. Other persons should receive the inactivated vaccine.

Figure 25-2—cont'd

Footnotes

6. Pneumococcal polysaccharide vaccination. *Medical indications:* chronic disorders of the pulmonary system (excluding asthma); cardiovascular diseases; diabetes mellitus; chronic liver diseases, including liver disease as a result of alcohol abuse (e.g.,cirrhosis); chronic renal failure or nephrotic syndrome; functional or anatomic asplenia (e.g., sickle cell disease or splenectomy [if elective splenectomy is planned, vaccinate at least 2 weeks before surgery]); immunosuppressive conditions (e.g., congenital immunodeficiency, HIV infection [vaccinate as close to diagnosis as possible when CD4 cell counts are highest], leukemia, lymphoma, multiple myeloma, Hodgkin disease, generalized malignancy, organ or bone marrow transplantation); chemotherapy with alkylating agents, antimetabolites, or high-dose, long-term corticosteroids; and cochlear implants. *Other indications:* Alaska Natives and certain American Indian populations and residents of nursing homes or other long-term–care facilities.

7. Revaccination with pneumococcal polysaccharide vaccine. One-time revaccination after 5 years for persons with chronic renal failure or nephrotic syndrome; functional or anatomic asplenia (e.g., sickle cell disease or splenectomy); immunosuppressive conditions (e.g., congenital immunodeficiency, HIV infection, leukemia, lymphoma, multiple myeloma, Hodgkin disease, generalized malignancy, or organ or bone marrow transplantation); or chemotherapy with alkylating agents, antimetabolites, or high-dose, long-term corticosteroids. For persons aged ≥65 years, one-time revaccination if they were vaccinated ≥5 years previously and were aged <65 years at the time of primary vaccination.

8. Hepatitis A vaccination. *Medical indications:* persons with chronic liver disease and persons who receive clotting factor concentrates. *Behavioral indications:* men who have sex with men and persons who use illegal drugs. *Occupational indications:* persons working with hepatitis A virus (HAV)–infected primates or with HAV in a research laboratory setting. *Other indications:* persons traveling to or working in countries that have high or intermediate endemicity of hepatitis A (a list of countries is available at http://www.cdc.gov/travel/diseases.htm) and any person who would like to obtain immunity. Current vaccines should be administered in a 2-dose schedule at either 0 and 6–12 months, or 0 and 6–18 months. If the combined hepatitis A and hepatitis B vaccine is used, administer 3 doses at 0, 1, and 6 months .

9. Hepatitis B vaccination. *Medical indications:* Persons with end-stage renal disease, including patients receiving hemodialysis; persons seeking evaluation or treatment for a sexually transmitted disease (STD); persons with HIV infection; persons with chronic liver disease; and persons who receive clotting factor concentrates. *Occupational indications:* health-care workers and public-safety workers who are exposed to blood or other potentially infectious body fluids. *Behavioral indications:* sexually active persons who are not in a long-term, mutually monogamous relationship (i.e., persons with >1 sex partner during the previous 6 months); current or recent injection-drug users; and men who have sex with men. *Other indications:* household contacts and sex partners of persons with chronic hepatitis B virus (HBV) infection; clients and staff members of institutions for persons with developmental disabilities; all clients of STD clinics; international travelers to countries with high or intermediate prevalence of chronic HBV infection (a list of countries is available at http://www.cdc.gov/travel/diseases.htm); and any adult seeking protection from HBV infection. Settings where hepatitis B vaccination is recommended for all adults: STD treatment facilities; HIV testing and treatment facilities; facilities providing drug-abuse treatment and prevention services; health-care settings providing services for injection-drug users or men who have sex with men; correctional facilities; end-stage renal disease programs and facilities for chronic hemodialysis patients; and institutions and nonresidential daycare facilities for persons with developmental disabilities. *Special formulation indications:* for adult patients receiving hemodialysis and other immunocompromised adults, 1 dose of 40 μg/mL (Recombivax HB®) or 2 doses of 20 μg/mL (Engerix-B®).

10. Meningococcal vaccination. *Medical indications:* adults with anatomic or functional asplenia, or terminal complement component deficiencies. *Other indications:* first-year college students living in dormitories; microbiologists who are routinely exposed to isolates of *Neisseria meningitidis*; military recruits; and persons who travel to or live in countries in which meningococcal disease is hyperendemic or epidemic (e.g., the "meningitis belt" of Sub-Saharan Africa during the dry season [December–June]), particularly if contact with local populations will be prolonged. Vaccination is required by the government of Saudi Arabia for all travelers to Mecca during the annual Hajj. Meningococcal conjugate vaccine is preferred for adults with any of the preceeding indications who are aged ≤55 years, although meningococcal polysaccharide vaccine (MPSV4) is an acceptable alternative. Revaccination after 5 years might be indicated for adults previously vaccinated with MPSV4 who remain at high risk for infection (e.g., persons residing in areas in which disease is epidemic).

11. Selected conditions for which *Haemophilus influenzae* type b (Hib) vaccination may be used. Hib conjugate vaccines are licensed for children aged 6 weeks–71 months. No efficacy data are available on which to base a recommendation concerning use of Hib vaccine for older children and adults with the chronic conditions associated with an increased risk for Hib disease. However, studies suggest good immunogenicity in patients who have sickle cell disease, leukemia, or HIV infection or have had splenectomies; administering vaccine to these patients is not contraindicated.

This schedule indicates the recommended age groups and medical indications for routine administration of currently licensed vaccines for persons aged ≥19 years, as of October 1, 2006. Licensed combination vaccines may be used whenever any components of the combination are indicated and when the vaccine's other components are not contraindicated. For detailed recommendations on all vaccines, including those used primarily for travelers or that are issued during the year, consult the manufacturers' package inserts and the complete statements from the Advisory Committee on Immunization Practices (http://www.cdc.gov/nip/publications/acip-list.htm).

Report all clinically significant postvaccination reactions to the Vaccine Adverse Event Reporting System (VAERS). Reporting forms and instructions on filing a VAERS report are available at http://www.vaers.hhs.gov or by telephone, 800-822-7967.

Information on how to file a Vaccine Injury Compensation Program claim is available at http://www.hrsa.gov/vaccinecompensation or by telephone, 800-338-2382.To file a claim for vaccine injury, contact the U.S. Court of Federal Claims, 717 Madison Place, N.W., Washington, D.C. 20005; telephone, 202-357-6400.

Additional information about the vaccines in this schedule and contraindications for vaccination is also available at http://www.cdc.gov/nip or from the CDC-INFO Contact Center at 800-CDC-INFO (800-232-4636) in English and Spanish, 24 hours a day, 7 days a week.

Approved by the Advisory Committee on Immunization Practices, the American College of Obstetricians and Gynecologists, and the American Academy of Family Physicians

Figure 25-2—cont'd

REFERENCES

1. US Department of Health and Human Services: *Healthy people 2010,* ed 2, Washington, DC, 2000, US Government Printing Office.
2. Centers for Disease Control and Prevention; Atkinson W, Hamborsky J, McIntyre L, and others, editors: *Epidemiology and prevention of vaccine-preventable diseases,* ed 9, Washington, DC, 2006, Public Health Foundation.
3. LoBuono C: Steps to improve immunization rates, *Patient Care* 34(9):93-111, 2000.
4. Schaffer S, Humiston SG, Shone LP, and others: Adolescent immunization practices: a national survey of US physicians, *Arch Pediatr Adolesc Med* 155(5):566-571, 2001.
5. Reid K, Grizzard T, Poland G: Adult immunizations: recommendations for practice, *Mayo Clin Proc* 74(4):377-384, 1999.
6. Waldrop J: Childhood vaccination update: a new weapon against pneumococcal bacteria, *Adv Nurse Pract* 9(2):34-40, 2001.
7. CDC Office of Communication Press Release: *Advisory Committee on Immunization Practice recommends adult vaccination with new tetanus, diphtheria and pertussis vaccine (Tdap),* retrieved Nov 9, 2005, from http://www.cdc.gov/od/oc/media/pressrel/r051109.htm.
8. Lehna RA: *Pharmacology for nursing care,* ed 6, St Louis, 2007, Mosby.

CHAPTER 26

Health Care of the International Traveler

V. Ted Leon

According to the World Tourism Organization, the number of international travelers worldwide has increased from 690 million persons crossing an international border in 2003, to an all-time high of 763 million persons crossing an international border in 2004. About 50 million of these travelers were residents of wealthy developed countries, traveling for business or pleasure to an undeveloped or developing country.[1] The total number of Americans who traveled internationally in 2004 is estimated at 40 million, with most traveling to Europe and Canada, where the risk of infection is low. However, nearly 4 million U.S. residents traveled to Mexico, 3.5 million traveled to Asia, 3 million traveled to Central or South America, and 200,000 traveled to Africa.[2] Thus as many as 10 million of the 40 million international trips taken by U.S. residents in 2004 were to countries or regions that could be considered at higher risk for infectious diseases, and also as less capable of providing adequate hospital services for major injuries or illnesses. Even among the American travelers in Europe, the idea of hospitalization in a foreign country is a discomforting thought.

It is estimated that approximately 1300 Americans die while traveling abroad each year. Many people are surprised to learn that the leading causes of death for the traveler are not rare and exotic infectious diseases, but rather natural causes.[3,4] About 50% of deaths are due to cardiovascular events, mostly in elderly travelers, who presumably might have had the same problems at home. Another 25% of the deaths are due to motor vehicle accidents, and 15% are due to other accidents, including falls and drownings. The remaining 10% of deaths are due to infectious causes, but even these may often be ordinary pathogens such as the influenza virus or the *Pneumococcus* bacteria, which are prevalent throughout the world. It is thought that only 1% to 4% died from a uniquely tropical infectious disease.[5,6] Nevertheless, the World Health Organization[7] estimates that in 2004 there were 300 million new cases of malaria, 200 million individuals infected with schistosomiasis, 50 million new cases of dengue fever, and 200,000 new cases of yellow fever, to highlight just a few of the major tropical pathogens. Travelers to regions where these and other diseases are endemic need to take appropriate precautions and preventive measures.

Despite recent trends toward more international travel, more adventure travel, more travel to Third World countries, and more travel by elderly persons with significant underlying chronic illness, some recent studies have shown that many European and American travelers are not seeking out pretravel advice, nor are they carrying antimalarials or getting vaccinated appropriately. A 2003 European study looked at 5465 travelers about to depart from nine major European airports to areas known to be high risk for hepatitis A or malaria.[8] Only 52% had sought any pretravel health advice, and just 42% had been vaccinated against hepatitis A and 31% against hepatitis B. Although 84% of travelers to *high*-risk malaria zones were carrying antimalarial medications, just 22% of travelers to areas with at least *some* malaria risk carried antimalarials. To further demonstrate the disconnect between perceived and actual risk, about 13% of the travelers to countries with *no* malaria risk were planning to take malaria prophylaxis.

A similar American study of 404 travelers from JFK Airport in New York to high-risk areas for hepatitis A and malaria found that only 36% had sought pretravel health advice of any kind.[9] Only 14% had been vaccinated against hepatitis A, only 13% had been vaccinated against hepatitis B, and just 11% of adults had received a tetanus booster in the past 10 years as routinely recommended. Moreover, only 46% of U.S. travelers to malarial regions were carrying antimalarial prophylaxis, and of the travelers to sub-Saharan Africa, where chloroquine is not recommended because of widespread drug resistance, 42% were carrying only chloroquine—the wrong medication. Since 57% of the Europeans and 60% of the Americans who sought pretravel advice stated that they got their information from their primary care physician, it is evident that primary care providers have an important role in education and provision of services.

Patients who need pretravel advice, vaccines, or medications have a choice of both location and providers, primary care providers, employee health, student health, urgent care clinic; and a specialized travel medicine clinic. In a primary care office, it can be difficult to offer a full range of services because of the logistics of maintaining a complete stock of all the recommended travel vaccines. In addition, some health care providers understandably do not feel comfortable prescribing medications or giving advice for diseases they have never had to treat. In an employee health, student health, or urgent care clinic, there is a greater economy of scale in terms of vaccine supply, and the provision of vaccines is often more efficient than in a private office, but the level of interest and knowledge of travel medicine among the providers are variable. In a travel clinic, on the other hand, the vaccines are readily available and the providers are more likely to be interested, knowledgeable, and experienced with some of the travel-related health problems and country-specific diseases that are likely to arise on an international trip (Box 26-1).

Unfortunately, often the patient who comes for travel medicine services is not already well known to the provider. In these instances, it is important to quickly assess the patient's expectations and to discover whether he or she is coming primarily to receive "pills and shots," or also for travel health education, advice, and consultation. An intake form (Figure 26-1) can help clarify these expectations. Unless patients are coming strictly for a particular vaccine that their health care provider recommended but was unable to provide, it is helpful to learn more about the travelers and their upcoming trip. In addition to the usual questions about itinerary and duration of stay, it is important to know if the travelers are experienced or have traveled on this particular itinerary before. Will they be traveling alone, with family and friends, or on an organized tour? Do they have any chronic medical conditions that could worsen on this trip? Do they already have a caring and established relationship with a health care provider? What is their work status and marital status? Although privacy may be a concern for some, most patients will welcome the provider's interest in these aspects of their life.

BOX 26-1

PROVIDERS OF TRAVEL MEDICINE SERVICES

Travel medicine services are usually provided by nurse practitioners or by physicians trained in family medicine or internal medicine. Some physicians who practice travel medicine are also board certified in preventive medicine, occupational medicine, or infectious disease. Although there is no board certification in either travel medicine or tropical medicine, some providers receive a Certificate of Knowledge in Travel Health from the International Society of Travel Medicine (http://www.istm.org), and some physicians who have international experience take an 8- to 12-week course in tropical medicine, pass a written examination, and receive a Certificate of Knowledge in Clinical Tropical Medicine and Traveler's Health from the American Society of Tropical Medicine and Hygiene (http://www.astmh.org).

Although a detailed travel medicine initial consultation is ideal, occasionally these are not covered by insurance, or the patient may express a strong preference to come in just for a vaccination without incurring the cost of an office visit. For a seasoned traveler going to a low-risk country, who either has no medical problems or has these problems well controlled by a health care provider, it seems reasonable to administer an immunization without a formal travel medicine consultation. But for most travelers who have questions and concerns; have underlying health problems; or are traveling anywhere in the developing regions of Asia, Africa, or South America, a full travel consultation is more appropriate.

As the purpose and details of the trip are described, it is the health care provider's duty to anticipate the various problems that are likely to arise. This includes accident prevention; secondary prevention of any worsening of the underlying health problems; and reduction of physical hazards and chemical or infectious exposures through the judicious use of personal protective devices, behavior change, or medications and vaccines. Most noxious chemicals enter the human body via the respiratory or gastrointestinal tract or via the skin and mucous membranes. Infectious pathogens, spread from human to human, also tend to enter via the respiratory or gastrointestinal tract, but it is important to also consider the special categories of sexually transmitted diseases; all the diseases transmitted by insect vectors; and all the zoonotic diseases such as rabies, avian influenza, or leptospirosis, which can inadvertently cause disease in humans because of proximity to diseased animal or their secretions.

Travelers should be given the relevant patient education brochures and be directed toward relevant resources in print or on the Internet (Box 26-2). Above all, they should be given ample time to get all their travel health questions answered.

PRETRAVEL PREPARATION AND PATIENT EDUCATION

Some health insurance plans do not provide coverage for travelers outside the United States. Medicare, for example, will

Initial Travel Medicine Consultation

Name: ______________________ Age: __________ Male/Female *(circle one)*

Height: __________ Weight: __________

Today's date: __________ Departure date: __________ Trip duration: __________

• Do you need pretravel vaccines?	Yes	No	Not sure
• Do you need pretravel medications?	Yes	No	Not sure
• Do you need any travel-related medical advice?	Yes	No	Not sure
• Do you have any travel-related health questions?	Yes	No	

Itinerary: City/province/country → Duration (days/weeks)

1. ______________________
2. ______________________
3. ______________________
4. ______________________

• Have you ever traveled to these countries on this itinerary before? Yes No

We are eager to help you have a safe trip and to avoid any health problems along the way. Please take a moment to answer the following questions regarding your upcoming trip and your general health history so that we may give you all the necessary vaccines, medications, and relevant health information. Please circle all that apply; you may leave a question blank if privacy is a concern.

Type of trip

1. Business
2. Visiting family/friends
3. Studying, teaching, or missions
4. Vacation, cruise, or relaxation
5. Adventure travel: trek, raft, or bike
6. Safari

How are you traveling?

1. Alone
2. With spouse or partner
3. With children
4. With friends
5. With work colleagues
6. With an organized group tour

Mode of transport

Airplane Ship or ferry Rail Bus Taxi Car Motorbike

Lodging

Tent Local hotel Western-style hotel Ship cabin Private home

Travel health risks: Will you be...

Climbing about 8000 feet/2500 meters?	Yes	No
Exposed to insects or other pests?	Yes	No
Swimming in freshwater lakes?	Yes	No
Eating at local restaurants and from street vendors?	Yes	No

FIGURE 26-1

Form for initial travel medicine consultation.

not provide coverage for illness or accidents occurring outside the United States, including Canada.[5] Thus all travelers should be encouraged to closely examine their health care policies. If provisions for foreign travel are not included, the traveler should obtain a short-term policy to cover episodic medical needs that could occur while traveling. Travelers with serious preexisting medical conditions that might require hospitalization should also purchase air evacuation insurance, unless they are comfortable with the quality of hospital services in the countries they plan to visit.[10]

Travelers with chronic health conditions should carry a written summary of their health problems, a list of current medications and allergies, and a copy of a recent ECG if they have any cardiac history. A complete list of suggested travel documents is shown in Box 26-3. Travelers who use inhalers (which may arouse suspicion), require needles or syringes (e.g., for insulin administration), or use controlled substances may find it worthwhile to carry a letter from their physician certifying their diagnosis and need for treatment, in case of customs or security questions.

Travelers should bring an adequate supply of their routine medications and keep them in clearly labeled bottles. They may want to wear identification bracelets listing major allergies or illnesses and carry a backup pair of eyeglasses.

BOX 26-2

RESOURCES FOR TRAVEL HEALTH

INTERNET SITES

International Society of Travel Medicine (ISTM) (http://www.istm.org) lists courses, conferences, and travel medicine providers around the world. ISTM has an excellent link to news from the World Health Organization and Centers for Disease Control and Prevention, which is updated monthly, and publishes the *Journal of Travel Medicine.*

American Society of Tropical Medicine and Hygiene (http://www.astmh.org) is similar to the ISTM website, with several publications and a travel clinic directory, but focused on infectious and communicable diseases commonly seen in the tropics.

Centers for Disease Control and Prevention (CDC) (http://www.cdc.gov) has a wide range of information available by clicking on "Travelers' health."

World Health Organization (http://www.who.int) has an excellent on-line publication, *International Travel and Health,* updated in 2006. Click on "Countries" or on "Health topics, then "Travel."

PRINT RESOURCES

The CDC's *Health Information for International Travel:* known as the Yellow Book, this valuable resource is updated biannually

The Travel and Tropical Medicine Manual, ed 3: a popular and concise textbook by Elaine Jong and Russel McMullen (Saunders, 2003)

HOTLINES

CDC public inquiries: (404) 639-3534 or (800) 311-3435

CDC Traveler's Hotline: (888) 232-3299 (for faxed information)

Malaria Hotline: (404) 488-7788 (during business hours) and (770) 488-7100 (after hours and on weekends)

TRAVEL EVACUATION INSURANCE

International SOS Assistance: (800) 523-8930 or (215) 942-8000; http://www.internationalsos.com

Medex Assistance Corporation: (800) 732-5309 or (410) 453-6300; http://www.medexassist.com

Medic Alert Foundation: (800) 863-3427; http://www.medicalert.org

MedjetAssist: (800) 963-3538; http://www.medjetassistance.com

Travelex: (800) 228-9792; http://www.travelex.com

Travel Guard: (800) 826-4919; http://www.travelguard.com

International Medical Group (IMG): (800) 628-4664 or (309) 296-0600; http://www.imglobal.com

BOX 26-3

TRAVEL DOCUMENTATION

- Passport and visa information
- International driver's permit and photo identification
- Emergency contact information for family, health care provider, and any other specialists you may need to contact from overseas
- List of physicians and hospitals in the host countries where you intend to travel
- Evidence of yellow fever vaccination, if traveling to countries where yellow fever is present or that require evidence of vaccination, recorded on the Traveler's International Certificate of Vaccination (yellow passport insert)
- Complete and up-to-date list of all routine and travel immunizations, including recent PPD (purified protein derivative [tuberculin]) results, recorded on the yellow passport insert
- Copy of recent HIV test results (may be needed for entry to some countries)
- Copy of current ECG if any relevant cardiac history
- Physician's letter listing traveler's specific health needs, including all prescription medications, syringes, and exemption from vaccines with reason for exemption

IMMUNIZATIONS

The pretravel visit is an ideal time to update all routine immunizations and to provide all the required and recommended immunizations (Table 26-1). Currently the only vaccines that are "required" and would block the traveler's entry to certain countries if documentation were absent are yellow fever and meningococcal vaccines, but many more vaccines are frequently "recommended" to protect the traveler. These may include hepatitis A and B, typhoid fever, polio, Japanese encephalitis, and rabies. The traveler's decision to be vaccinated should be an informed choice based on the destination, length of stay, current disease outbreaks, prior destinations, and other factors. Immunization requirements should be reviewed at least 6-8 weeks before travel commences to ensure adequate time for antibody response, as well as sufficient time to complete certain vaccines that need to be administered as a two- or three-dose series. Country-specific guidelines for recommended and required immunizations are found in the CDC documents (see Box 26-2).

MEDICATIONS AND PRESCRIPTIONS

Malaria

Malaria is the most deadly parasite in the world and the fifth leading infectious cause of death overall, trailing only lower respiratory tract infections, AIDS, diarrheal diseases, and complications of tuberculosis (Table 26-2). The malaria parasite is considered one of the "big three" pathogens in terms of global importance, along with HIV and the tuberculosis bacillus.

Malaria is transmitted from human to human, primarily through the bite of an infected female *Anopheles* mosquito. Currently malaria is present in more than 100 countries, including almost all countries in the tropics. An estimated 300 million cases and 1.1 million deaths occur annually because of the malaria parasite. Unfortunately, as of 2006, there is no commercially available malaria vaccine and little hope for eradication of the parasite. It will remain a scourge, especially for Africa, for years to come.

For the traveler, however, most cases of malaria can be prevented by avoiding mosquito bites with protective clothing, mosquito netting, and DEET-containing insect repellants, and by taking a prophylactic medication before, during, and after travel to the malaria-endemic region. Medication options include chloroquine, mefloquine, atovaquone and proguanil (Malarone), and doxycycline. Chloroquine is still a useful medication in a few areas (e.g., Central America, Haiti, Dominican Republic, Iraq, Egypt, Turkey, northern Argentina, and Paraguay). However, for most malarial regions, travelers are advised to take one of the other three medications as prophylaxis. Mefloquine has the advantage of weekly dosing, but its utility has been limited by severe neuropsychiatric side effects in some patients. Malarone appears to have fewer side effects, but it is expensive and must be taken daily. Doxycyline is an inexpensive and effective alternative, and in fact is the first-line drug in the Thai-Cambodia border areas where mefloquine resistance has emerged. However, it too must be taken daily, and it cannot be taken by pregnant women or children. It can also cause some photosensitivity and gastrointestinal upset. Regardless of which antimalarial is used, the traveler needs to be educated about fever and other symptoms

TABLE 26-1 Vaccine Information

Vaccine	Dosing
ROUTINE IMMUNIZATIONS	
Tetanus-diphtheria-pertussis (Tdap) or Td	Booster every 10 years
Measles-mumps-rubella (MMR)	1 dose for adults born after 1957 if not immune
Chickenpox (varicella)	2 doses to all >13 years old if no history of varicella or evidence of immunity
Flu shot (influenza)	Annually for all >50 years old or earlier if h/o chronic disease
Pneumococcal	Once at age 65 years or earlier if h/o chronic disease
Hepatitis B	0-1-4 month series
TRAVEL VACCINES AND BOOSTERS	
Polio (IPV)	One booster if primary series >10-15 years ago
Hepatitis A	2 doses 0, 6-12
Hepatitis B	3 doses 0, 1, 6 months
Hepatitis A and B (inactivated; Twinrix)	3 doses 0, 1, 6-12 month (booster after 10 years?)
Typhoid Ty21a (oral live attenuated)	1 capsule on day 0, 2, 4, 6; booster every 5 years
Typhoid Vi (capsular polysaccharide)	1 doses IM booster every 2 years
Rabies	3 doses 0, 7, 21-28 days
Japanese encephalitis	3 doses 0, 7, 30 days; booster every 2 years
Meningococcal conjugate	1 dose IM
Yellow fever	1 dose SQ, booster every 10 years

Adapted from Centers for Disease Control and Prevention: Health information for international travel 2005-2006, Atlanta, 2005, US Department of Health and Human Services, Public Health Service.

ID, Intradermal; *IPV,* inactivated polio vaccine; *HDCV,* human diploid cell rabies vaccine; *RVA,* rabies vaccine adsorbed.

of malaria and be encouraged to seek medical treatment promptly should such symptoms occur.

Any fever in a *returned* traveler from a malaria-endemic region must be considered as suspicious for malaria until proven otherwise. Thin and thick blood smears should be taken to look for evidence of the parasite. In a recent European study of 147 consecutive febrile hospitalized patients who had a history of travel to the tropics in the previous 6 months, malaria was the most common diagnosis.[11] It was reported that 70 of the 147 admissions (47.6%) were cause by malaria. The other most common causes of fever in that study included 13 admissions for viral hepatitis (8.8%), 7 cases of gastroenteritis (4.8%), 7 cases of schistosomiasis (4.8%), 6 cases of typhoid fever (4.1%), and 5 cases of dengue fever (3.4%).

TABLE 26-2 Death from Infectious Diseases (Worldwide)

Cause of Death	Number of Deaths (millions)
Lower respiratory tract infection	3.9
HIV/AIDS	2.9
Diarrheal diseases	2.0
Tuberculosis	1.6
Malaria	1.1
Measles	0.7

From World Health Organization, 2002.

Food and Water Precautions and Traveler's Diarrhea

Diarrhea is the most common health problem among travelers to underdeveloped and tropical countries. Although it is rarely life threatening if properly treated, traveler's diarrhea is notorious for causing many work and vacation days to be lost to illness.

Diarrhea is spread through contaminated food and water, which carry pathogenic bacteria, parasites, and viruses. The most common cause of traveler's diarrhea is the bacterium *Escherichia coli.* Other common bacterial causes include *Salmonella, Shigella,* and *Campylobacter* organisms.

It is important for the traveler to note if the diarrhea is watery, contains any blood or pus, and is associated with fever or abdominal pain. Watery diarrhea is often caused by intestinal viruses such as the rotavirus or Norwalk virus and responds primarily to oral rehydration solution or IV fluids. Bloody diarrhea, on the other hand, is more commonly caused by bacteria or parasites. Simple dysentery without fever is often due to the parasite *Entamoeba histolytica* (amebas), which is treatable with metronidazole, but dysentery can also be caused by other parasites, including *Cryptosporidium, Schistosoma,* and *Cyclospora* organisms. Bloody diarrhea *with* fever or abdominal pain is usually bacterial and requires immediate medical attention.

A small number of travelers develop a chronic diarrhea, which is usually caused by the *Giardia lamblia* parasite. The *Giardia* parasite often causes bloating and belching or flatulence with a characteristic "rotten egg" or sulfur smell. It is usually treated with metronidazole. Among expatriates and long-term travelers, chronic diarrhea can also be caused by a condition called *tropical sprue.*

Because most cases of traveler's diarrhea are caused by bacteria, antibiotics are often indicated. For a mild case of traveler's diarrhea caused by *E. coli,* one or two doses of a quinolone such as ciprofloxacin or levofloxacin are sufficient. For the sicker traveler with salmonella or shigella, a 5-day course of ciprofloxacin, 500 mg b.i.d., may be necessary. For children, pregnant women, or patients thought to have *Campylobacter* infection, the macrolide azithromycin should be used, 500 mg/day for 3 days. Because of increasing resistance to trimethoprim-sulfamethoxazole, sulfa drugs such as Bactrim are no longer the drug of choice.

In addition to antibiotics, travelers may use bismuth subsalicylate (Pepto-Bismol) or antimotility drugs such as loperamide (Imodium) to treat diarrhea. Both these medications reduce the number of unformed stools and usually make the patient feel better. Some providers believe that loperamide and other antimotility drugs may actually prolong the duration of illness, but this has not been observed in most cases of travel-related watery diarrhea. However, antimotility drugs are contraindicated if the patient has a fever or blood in the stool.

Education about proper food and water precautions is imperative. The adage "boil it, cook it, peel it, or forget it" is helpful to pass on to travelers: eat well-cooked foods served hot, or peeled fruits and vegetables, and drink only bottled beverages or hot tea and coffee that were made with boiled water. Travelers should avoid milk and milk products that have not been pasteurized, ice, and uncapped or locally bottled water. Even clear wilderness stream and lake water can be contaminated with *Giardia* or *Campylobacter* organisms. Finally, travelers should try to avoid eating food from street vendors or in establishments where the kitchen or restrooms are unclean.

AIR TRAVEL RISKS

Air travel of more than 6 hours' duration increases the risk of deep venous thrombosis and peripheral edema. To minimize this risk, travelers should be encouraged to get out of their seats and walk around every 1 to 2 hours. On most flights cabin pressure is maintained at a level equivalent to that of altitudes of 8000 feet or lower, which does result in some reduction in available oxygen. As a result, travelers with chronic pulmonary or cardiac disease may require supplemental oxygen. Travelers should wait at least 3 weeks after a myocardial infarction to fly and should be aware that supplemental oxygen may be needed for up to 4 months after the event.[12] Air travel during pregnancy is generally considered safe up until about 36 weeks' gestation.

Travelers with diabetes must monitor their serum glucose levels more closely, since changes in time zone, diet, and exercise routines can cause significant changes even in those with good control. Travelers with recently diagnosed and unstable diabetes should be advised to wait until glycemic control is stabilized before traveling. Stuart Rose's *International Travel Health Guide* includes protocols for adjusting insulin dosages across multiple time zones based on the direction and duration of travel.[5]

TRAVEL SAFETY

All travelers should be aware of safety risks while traveling and take appropriate measures to mitigate those risks. Crime is a problem in most parts of the world, and travelers should take precautions to avoid being robbed. Travelers should keep valuables in a hotel safe if available, refrain from wearing expensive jewelry, minimize the amount of cash carried, use travelers' checks wherever possible, and dress modestly and inconspicuously.

The most common cause of death while overseas for most healthy travelers is a motor vehicle accident. Motor vehicle accidents rank above all other accidents, including falls and drowning, burns, gunshot wounds, and plane and boating accidents. Only heart attacks kill more travelers, and these are typically among the subset of elderly travelers with known coronary artery disease. Every year approximately 1.2 million people are killed and 20 million to 50 million badly injured or disabled in a motor vehicle accident. This represents about 2.1% of total global mortality.[13] Despite many fewer average road miles per person per year in the developing world, about 85% of the global motor vehicle deaths occur in low- and middle-income countries, mostly because roads and vehicles are less safe. Compared with road travel in the United States, seat belts are rarely used or available, and traffic is less regulated. Moreover, when a major accident does occur, the hospital and trauma services are often lacking, and there may be insufficient time to evacuate the traveler to a major trauma center. As a result, the relative risk of actually dying in a motor vehicle accident is higher when driving overseas than it is in the United States. The magnitude of that increased risk varies between 2.5 to 1 and 40 to 1, depending on the country studied. Even in Europe as a whole, the risk is greater than in the United States, at an estimated 5.4 to 1.

Travelers should be advised that air travel is still the safest mode of transport, followed by rail, ship, and finally road travel. Seat belts should be worn at all times, and all travelers in the developing world should avoid traveling by road at night if possible. Depending on the length of stay and the countries visited, and whether a major trauma center exists with a safe blood supply, even young healthy travelers to urban areas should consider obtaining medical evacuation insurance, known as "SOS insurance," mostly because of this risk of death or serious injury in a major motor vehicle accident. For older travelers or travelers to rural areas with more infectious disease, the argument for SOS insurance is even more compelling. Several companies are listed in Box 26-2.

SUMMARY

As international travel becomes more common, health care providers will need to become more knowledgeable about travel medicine and the relevant health care issues for international travel. At the very least, providers should have fully explored the health care options around them and be prepared to make referrals for travelers requiring additional services. Travelers with any underlying or chronic illness should be well prepared to manage the common minor complications or manifestations of their illness for themselves, and know which signs and symptoms should prompt them to seek professional medical care. All travelers should attend to their routine health care maintenance needs before travel and be educated about how to improve their personal safety and reduce their risk from injury in a motor vehicle accident. All travelers should be encouraged to receive the vaccines that are required (e.g., yellow fever) or recommended (e.g., hepatitis A and B, typhoid fever) for their particular itinerary, and be given malaria prophylaxis if appropriate. In addition, travelers should clearly understand basic food and water precautions and how to manage traveler's diarrhea. They should also know how to protect themselves against the myriad pathogens spread person to person via the respiratory tract.

An example of a travel medicine "toolbox" is shown in Box 26-4. It lists commonly used medications, vaccines, and patient education brochures or handouts. Many of the vaccines and medications have already been discussed. However, it is equally important to create or collect good patient education materials. General and country-specific travel education should include handouts about jet lag, motion and altitude sickness, traveler's diarrhea, and protection against diseases spread by insect vectors (e.g., malaria, dengue fever, yellow fever). Travelers should know how to protect themselves against sexually transmitted diseases and HIV, through

BOX 26-4

PROVIDER TOOLBOX FOR TRAVELERS: BROCHURES, VACCINES, AND MEDICATIONS

BROCHURES
- Vaccine safety and indications
- Malaria prevention
- Traveler's diarrhea
- Food and water safety
- Insect and sun avoidance
- First aid kit
- Personal and transport safety
- Evacuation insurance
- Sexually transmitted disease and HIV prevention
- Animals and rabies risk
- Fresh water and schistosomiasis risk
- High-altitude sickness
- Jet lag and motion sickness
- Exercise and travel

VACCINES
- Tdap (tetanus-diphtheria-pertussis) or Td (tetanus-diphtheria)
- MMR (measles-mumps-rubella)
- Varicella
- Influenza
- Pneumococcal
- Hepatitis A
- Hepatitis B
- Typhoid
- Polio
- Rabies
- Japanese encephalitis
- Yellow fever
- PPD (purified protein derivative [tuberculin]) testing

MEDICATIONS (USES)
- Chloroquine (malaria)
- Doxycycline (malaria)
- Mefloquine (malaria)
- Atovaquone and proguanil (Malarone) (malaria)
- Primaquine (malaria)
- Bismuth subsalicylate (traveler's diarrhea, gastrointestinal upset)
- Loperamide (traveler's diarrhea)
- Ciprofloxacin (traveler's diarrhea)
- Azithromycin (*Campylobacter* infection)
- Metronidazole *(Entamoeba histolytica)*
- Meclizine (motion sickness)
- Scopolamine (motion sickness)
- Acetaminophen (pain or fever)
- Ibuprofen (pain or fever)

abstinence or the proper use of condoms, and receive patient education handouts as needed. They should know how to protect themselves against zoonotic diseases (rabies, avian influenza, leptospirosis, etc.) by avoiding potentially diseased animals and by receiving a vaccine or taking prophylactic medications if close contact is unavoidable or unpredictable. Finally, travelers should be advised to research the best sources of medical care in the countries they will be visiting and make an informed decision about whether they will obtain medical evacuation insurance.

REFERENCES

1. Castelli F: Human mobility and disease: a global challenge, *J Travel Med* 11(1):1-2, 2004.
2. Virk A: Travel: risks and prevention. In Lang RS, Hensrud DD, editors: *Clinical preventive medicine,* ed 2, Chicago, 2004, American Medical Association.
3. MacPherson D: Death and dying abroad: the Canadian experience, *J Travel Med* 7:227-234, 2000.
4. Jong E, McMullen R: *Travel and tropical medicine manual,* ed 3, Philadelphia, 2003, Saunders.
5. Rose SR: *International travel health guide,* Northampton, Mass, 1999, Travel Medicine.
6. Hargarten SW, Baker TD, Guptil K: Overseas fatalities of United States citizen travelers: an analysis of deaths related to international travelers, *Ann Emerg Med* 20:622-626, 1991.
7. World Health Organization: http://www.who.int/en/.
8. Van Herck K, Van Damme P, Castelli F, and others: Knowledge, attitudes and practices in travel-related infectious disease: the European Airport Survey, *J Travel Med* 11(1):3-8, 2004.
9. Hamer D, Connor B: Travel health knowledge, attitudes and practices among United States travelers, *J Travel Med* 11(1):23-26, 2004.
10. Bratton RL: Advising patients about international travel: what they can do to protect their health and safety, *Postgrad Med* 106(1):57-64, 1999.
11. Antinori S, Galimberti L, Gianelle E, and others: Prospective observational study of fever in hospitalized returning travelers and migrants from tropical areas, 1997-2001, *J Travel Med* 11(3):135-142, 2004.
12. Aerospace Medical Association, Air Transport Medicine Committee: Medical guidelines for air travel, *Aviat Space Environ Med* 667(10 suppl):B1-B16, 1996.
13. Peden M: *The World Report on Road Traffic Injury Prevention*, Symposia No SY02.01, International Society of Travel Medicine conference, Lisbon, May 2005.

CHAPTER 27

Presurgical Clearance

Jane Flanagan and Jennifer A. Neves

DEFINITION AND EPIDEMIOLOGY

Before the late 1980s, patients were hospitalized at least 1 day before surgery for presurgical clearance. During that time they were assessed by a surgical team that included anesthesiologists, surgeons, and nurses. In addition, they had presurgical preparation and tests completed. As surgical and anesthesia techniques improved, the need for extensive testing and preparation declined. Concurrently, patients expressed a desire to be home with family or loved ones the night before surgery. There was also an increasing demand to implement cost-containment measures by health care organizations.[1,2]

By the late 1980s, presurgical clinics were created in hospitals throughout the United States in an effort to provide patients and their families with the same level of surgical preparation that they had received previously.[2] Initially, these clinics were established to prepare patients undergoing minor surgeries. However, continued concerns about cost containment combined with improvements in surgical technologies provided the impetus to prepare a diverse and a more acute population of patients for surgery. Presurgical clinics are one reason that the patient length of stay for surgical procedures has decreased nationwide. For example, in the 1980s, the average length of stay for major joint repair was 4 weeks. This hospitalization often would have included 1 or 2 preoperative days. Yet, by 1995 to 1997, the average length of stay for a major joint repair had decreased to 4 days.[3]

More recently the number of surgical procedures performed has increased. In one Massachusetts hospital the number of people having surgery requiring a hospital stay increased from 21,000 to 22,000 between 1999 and 2000. Ninety percent of these surgical patients were admitted on the same day of surgery.[4]

PATHOPHYSIOLOGY

The types of adult patients entering a presurgical clinic vary greatly by age, medical condition, and diagnosis. Patients can be young and healthy or older with varied co-morbid conditions. The one common characteristic of all these surgical patients is that their surgeries and hospitalizations are considered elective, nonemergent admissions. It is this characteristic which serves as a basis for classifying these patients from an anesthesia risk perspective.

CLINICAL PRESENTATION

All patients who are admitted to a presurgical clinic are considered outpatients. They can come from home, rehabilitation centers, nursing facilities, or other extended-care environments. The intent is that these patients will return to these environments after clearance. Presurgical clearance can occur 1 to 30 days before surgery and ideally occurs far enough in advance of the surgical procedure to allow necessary consultations and evaluations by the appropriate health care providers. For example, if a patient scheduled for an open, elective abdominal aortic aneurysm repair develops new-onset angina, there should, if possible, be enough time to schedule cardiac stress testing and review the results with the anesthesia team. The anesthesiologists will then determine the appropriate anesthetic plan for this patient based on the cardiac stress test results.

A general review of systems plus smoking history; drug and alcohol use or abuse; intake of herbal remedies, vitamins, or other over-the-counter medications (especially aspirin or NSAIDs, which could cause bleeding perioperatively); latex or medication allergies; recent blood transfusions; pregnancy (term or incomplete); recent history of chemotherapy or radiation; and family history of problems with anesthesia should be obtained. In-depth information about medical conditions such as cardiac disease, respiratory disease, diabetes, gastrointestinal problems, psychiatric issues, or bleeding problems is also necessary. Additionally, patients should be specifically queried about exercise capacity, since an inability to walk four blocks or climb two flights of stairs has been associated with increased postoperative complications.[5]

PHYSICAL EXAMINATION

The physical examination focuses around the presenting surgical problem and expected type of anesthesia. The general examination should include generalized appearance, height, weight, and baseline vital signs, including oxygen saturation. Evaluation of the airway, dentition, and range of motion of head and neck is necessary. Abnormalities should be noted in the appearance of neck veins; presence of bruits; and auscultation of the heart, lungs, and abdomen. Further evaluation for abdominal masses, genitourinary or rectal problems, peripheral pulses, and cranial nerve deficits could also be warranted, depending on the reason for presentation, the medical history, and the anesthetic plan. For example, the physical examination of a 32-year-old healthy man with a herniated lumbar disc should include all of the above, since this patient may manifest neurologic or peripheral vascular changes or these changes could occur postoperatively. Additionally, sexual, urinary, and bowel function could be a presenting symptom associated with his back problem or may develop postoperatively as an untoward result of the surgery.

DIAGNOSTICS

Diagnostic testing for presurgical clearance is variable and depends on several factors: (1) the presenting diagnosis, (2) the patient's age, (3) the patient's co-morbidities, and (4) the type of anesthetic agent planned. Much of what was considered necessary preoperative testing in the past has been reviewed by collaborating staff, and in many presurgical clinics guidelines have been developed that are consistent with research in this area.[6] Guidelines used in one presurgical clinic are outlined in Table 27-1.

DIFFERENTIAL DIAGNOSIS

Patients who come into a presurgical clinic have a known diagnosis requiring surgery. Most patients are referred by their health care provider to a surgical specialist who performs

TABLE 27-1 Tests for Presurgical Clearance

Test	Indications for Performing Test
Chest x-ray	Patient over age 60; smoking history of >20 pack years; history of cardiovascular or pulmonary diseases, having thoracic procedure, or presence of malignant disease
ECG	Men >45 years of age, women >55 years of age; history or symptoms of cardiac disease, diabetes, morbid obesity, significant pulmonary disease, or cocaine abuse
Pulmonary function testing	All patients undergoing major thoracic surgery; history of severe chronic obstructive pulmonary disease
CBC	Patient over age 60; history of pulmonary, cardiovascular or renal disease; smoking history of >20 pack years; history of radiation, chemotherapy, or bleeding disorder; symptoms of infectious process (increased temperature and cough)
Coagulation studies	Patient currently on coagulation therapy; history of alcohol abuse, hepatic disease, easy bruising (family or personal history), bleeding disorders, or malignant disease; undergoing procedures with associated blood loss or postoperative coagulation therapy
Pregnancy test	All women who are of childbearing age except those who have had oophorectomy
Electrolytes	Patient on dialysis; diabetes; hypertension or heart disease; potential for alterations in electrolytes because of other disease processes or medications
Liver function tests	Patient with history of alcohol abuse, hepatitis, or known hepatic disease
Urinalysis or urine culture and sensitivity	Patient undergoing urologic procedure who has a history of frequent urinary tract infections or is receiving a graft, prosthetic, and/or implantable device
Albumin	Patient who is malnourished or has a history of alcohol abuse or hepatic or malignant disease

appropriate and specific diagnostic testing before determining the exact diagnosis and referring them to the presurgical clinic. Therefore there are few, if any, instances when a differential diagnosis is necessary.

MANAGEMENT

Ideally, patients who come into a presurgical clinic will have had good primary care and will have underlying medical conditions well managed on presentation. In two instances the health care provider must provide management of co-morbid disease processes: (1) when a patient does not have appropriate primary care, and (2) when a patient does have good primary care, but needs further testing because of the anesthesia plan and co-morbid diseases.

When the patient does not have a primary care provider (PCP), it is important that the person performing the presurgical clearance determine the need for a preoperative evaluation by a primary care healthcare provider. If a primary care evaluation is not indicated before the surgical procedure, the patient progresses through presurgical clearance. However, the patient is educated about the importance of primary care. If the patient needs evaluation by a PCP before surgery, the surgeon is contacted by the person performing the presurgical clearance, and the patient is referred to a PCP before surgery.

At other times a patient has been well managed by a PCP, but the PCP is uncertain about appropriate diagnostic testing for surgery. In these instances, the health care provider in the presurgical clinic makes recommendations for the appropriate diagnostic testing and refers the patient to the PCP. For example, a patient scheduled for general anesthesia for a total hip replacement who has a history of well-managed angina but has not had a recent stress test will need a stress test before surgery. This may be arranged in collaboration with the PCP, or the patient may be referred back to the PCP, who will order the test and send the results to the presurgical clinic. Other diagnostic tests that may be required because of the anesthesia plan include echocardiograms in patients with known valvular disease or pulmonary function tests in patients with severe chronic obstructive pulmonary disease (COPD).

Medication and fasting requirements are other management issues addressed in the presurgical clinic. Herbal medications and vitamin E should be stopped 2 weeks before surgery. Medications used to control medical conditions such as hypertension, heart disease, eye problems, anxiety, pain, and COPD should be continued and taken on the morning of surgery.

Oral diabetic agents should not be taken the morning of surgery except for metformin (Glucophage), which should be stopped for 24 hours before surgery. Patients who are taking insulin are generally instructed to take half their usual dose of the longer-acting agent and to withhold the shorter-acting insulin. Consultation with the endocrinologist for confirmation or more tailored management is also recommended.[7]

Fasting guidelines vary among hospitals. However, it is generally acknowledged that patients can have clear fluids up until 5 hours before surgery, unless the patient has gastroesophageal reflux disease (GERD) or is scheduled to have surgery requiring a prone position. These patients need to fast from both food and fluids for 8 hours before surgery. Since the presence of upper gastrointestinal disease (including GERD) can predispose a patient to aspiration of stomach contents during intubation, these patients should take an H_2-receptor antagonist on the night before and the morning of surgery to diminish the risk of aspiration.[8]

LIFE SPAN CONSIDERATIONS

Patients coming to the hospital for surgery are unique, and the ways in which they cope cannot be predicted or assumed. Although providers might expect that an older, more medically complex patient undergoing a life-threatening surgery could be anxious and that a younger healthy patient undergoing a minor surgery would be calm, the opposite may in fact be the case. Anxiety level and coping style are not predictable in this setting and are often more related to current life stresses, perceived level of support, and psychosocial development issues than the age or illness. Therefore a careful assessment of these factors is necessary to accurately evaluate and plan for each individual's care.

COMPLICATIONS

Complications related to anesthesia are multiple and range from major life threatening (rare) to the more benign and easily resolved (more common). Complications vary by anesthetic type, but co-morbid conditions can increase risk. For general anesthesia, complications include nausea, vomiting, sore throat, fatigue, stroke, myocardial infarction, allergic reaction, and death. For spinal or other regional anesthesia, complications can include headache, nerve damage, infection, and limb loss. All potential complications are considered in the presurgical clinic to stratify risk and minimize perioperative morbidity and mortality. The potential risks and complications are readdressed by the anesthesiologist or anesthetist providing care on the day of surgery before obtaining consent.

INDICATIONS FOR REFERRAL

The health care provider in the presurgical clinic collaborates with the PCP, the surgeon, and the anesthesiologist who will be providing anesthesia to establish the appropriate care plan for the patient. In conjunction with the PCP and surgeon, referrals to cardiologists and other specialists are provided as needed to determine the safest anesthesia plan. The presurgical clinic health care provider and anesthesiologist will review the results of any diagnostic tests and discuss with the surgeon the proposed anesthesia plan. The proposed plan is then communicated to the PCP.

Patients in presurgical clinics should have their general health managed in the primary care setting, but in some instances this is not being done. If this is the case, the trip to the presurgical clinic is an excellent opportunity to review the importance of good primary care and refer the patient to a PCP in a convenient location.

The American College of Cardiology and the American Heart Association have established clinical predicators of increased perioperative cardiac risk.[9,10] The clinical predictors are divided among three categories: major, intermediate, and minor predictors (Table 27-2). Consideration of five other factors in addition to these clinical predictors helps determine whether preoperative cardiac evaluation is required. A decision tree related to these five factors is shown in Table 27-3.

TABLE 27-2 Clinical Predictors of Increased Perioperative Cardiac Risk

Type of Clinical Predictors	Specific Predictors That Increase Risk
Major	Myocardial infarction within past 30 days Unstable angina Decompensated heart failure High-grade atrioventricular block Symptomatic ventricular arrhythmia Supraventricular arrhythmias with uncontrolled ventricular rate Severe valvular disease
Intermediate	Mild angina Previous myocardial infarction by history or pathologic Q waves, compensated or previous heart failure Diabetes (especially type 1) Renal insufficiency
Minor	Advanced age Abnormal ECG Rhythm other than sinus Low functional capacity History of stroke Uncontrolled hypertension

PATIENT AND FAMILY EDUCATION

Patient and family education in the presurgical clinic is related to the surgical and anesthesia care plan. After the patient has been assessed individually, the family should be brought into the setting to discuss preoperative and postoperative teaching and expectations about the patient's care on discharge either to home or another facility. Teaching about the anesthesia care plan is also completed by the nurse practitioner or other

TABLE 27-3 Factors to Consider for Preoperative Cardiac Evaluation

Question	If "Yes"	If "No"
Is surgery emergent?	Proceed to surgery.	Obtain cardiac evaluation.
Has the patient undergone coronary revascularization in the past 5 years and currently is without cardiac-related symptoms?	Proceed to surgery.	Obtain cardiac evaluation.
Has the patient had a recent favorable cardiac evaluation?	Proceed to surgery.	Obtain cardiac evaluation.
Can the patient climb 2 flights of stairs (as one measure of functional capacity)?	Proceed to surgery.	Obtain cardiac evaluation.
Is the level of risk for the surgery low?	Proceed to surgery.	If no, as in surgeries such as abdominal aortic aneurysm repair, obtain cardiac evaluation.
Are any of the clinical predictors listed in Table 27-2 present?	If intermediate or major, obtain cardiac evaluation; if low, proceed to surgery.	Proceed to surgery.

health care provider in this setting and includes possible complications and effects of anesthesia and pain management concerns during and after surgery.

HEALTH PROMOTION

Lifestyle issues can promote or exacerbate disease processes. The presurgical clinic setting provides the health care provider an opportunity to encourage lifestyle changes and appropriately refer the patient to programs that address alcohol or drug abuse, smoking cessation, stress management, nutritional counseling, exercise, home safety, or domestic violence.

REFERENCES

1. Jones D, Coakley A, Flanagan J: Nursing diagnosis at 24 and 72 hours following same day surgery with general anesthesia. In Rantz M, LeMore P, editors: *Proceedings of the 13th North American Nursing Diagnosis,* Glendale, Calif, 1999, CINAHL Information Systems.
2. Flanagan J: Creating a healing environment for staff and patients in a presurgery clinic. In Picard C, Jones D, editors: *Giving voice to what we know: Margaret Newman's theory of health as expanding consciousness in nursing practice, research and education,* Sudbury, Mass, 2004, Jones & Bartlett.
3. Lagoe R, Arnold K, Noetscher C: Benchmarking hospital lengths of stay using histograms, *Nurs Econ* 17:75-92, 1999.
4. Kowalczyk L: Elective surgeries soar, *Boston Globe* 258:A1, B4, 2000.
5. Reilly DF, McNeeley MJ, Doerner D, and others: Self-reported exercise tolerance and the risk of serious perioperative complications, *Arch Intern Med* 159:2185, 1999.
6. Everett L, Kallar S: *Pre-surgical evaluation and laboratory testing.* In Twersky R, editor: *The ambulatory anesthesia handbook,* St Louis, 2005, Mosby.
7. Cygan R, Waitzkin H, Hsaio R: When to stop and restart medications in the perioperative period, *Intern Med* 11:29, 1993.
8. Moyers JR, Vincent CM: Preoperative medication. In Barash PG, Cullen BF, Stoelting RK, editors: *Clinical anesthesia,* Philadelphia, 2001, Lippincott Williams & Wilkins.
9. American College of Cardiology Foundation: *ACC/AHA guideline update for perioperative cardiovascular evaluation for noncardiac surgery,* 2002, retrieved Dec 6, 2006, from httpp://www.acc.org/clinical/guidelines/perio/update/periupdate_index.htm.
10. Holman J: Preoperative evaluation: priorities and pointers, part 1, Cardiac assessment, *Consultant* 45(12):1296-1301, 2005.

CHAPTER 28

Preparticipation Sports Physical

Terry Mahan Buttaro

Health care providers are often asked to do preparticipation examinations (PPEs) for student athletes. Most states require these examinations for both middle and high school athletes. Physicians experienced in sports medicine recommend that student athletes have a preparticipation physical for middle school, junior high school, high school, and college athletics.[1] The American Heart Association recommends cardiovascular preparticipation screening and a history and physical examination for all athletes participating in high school and college sports and prefers that a physician perform the examination.[2] Some states allow nurse practitioners and physician assistants to perform sports physicals, and others do not.[2]

Historically, the primary goal for these examinations has been to identify adolescent athletes at risk for a cardiovascular event. It is also necessary that other medical problems be identified and treated before the student is cleared to participate in any athletics. Determining the athlete's overall health, providing counseling, and strengthening the provider-patient relationship are other objectives. The preparticipation sports physical is an excellent opportunity to educate the student on healthy behaviors and injury prevention, in addition to identifying risk factors that affect adolescent well-being. Still, the importance of the sports participation PPE cannot be overstated. The examiner must be skilled and have sufficient experience in performing both the cardiovascular and musculoskeletal examination to identify any condition that would prohibit participation in the chosen sport.

Although some PPEs have been performed in the school in the past, it is preferable to perform the examination in the office so that adequate time can be spent ascertaining the student's and family's health history and performing the examination. If possible, the examination should be performed at least 6 weeks before the beginning of the sports season. It is also important that a parent accompany the student to the examination to fully establish the family history and cardiovascular risk factors. It is often helpful to have the student and parent complete and sign a preparticipation health history form before the examination. *It is essential that the provider review the form with the student and parent and specifically question the parent and student about each item on the health history form.*

Physician consultation is recommended for preparticipation sports physical.

HISTORY

Allergies, current and past medications, and the personal and family history should be carefully assessed. Answers to the following questions should be determined before the examination commences.

1. Medical history, including:
   - Allergic or untoward reactions to exercise, medications, pollens, foods, and stinging insects (including the specific nature of the reaction)
   - Current medications, including vitamins or herbal supplements, prescribed or over-the-counter medications, and nutritional supplements
   - Habits such as smoking, caffeine, and alcohol or drug use
   - Immunization history: tetanus, hepatitis, chickenpox, and MMR (measles, mumps, rubella)
   - Previous surgeries (particularly orthopedic, genital, kidney, or eye surgeries)
   - Previous hospitalizations
   - Loss of an organ such as eye, kidney, or testicle
2. Present or past illness, including:
   - Recent viral illness such as mononucleosis or myocarditis
   - Recent weight loss or gain
   - Previous sports restriction
   - History of heat-related illness
   - Skin reactions (hives, rashes, infections)
   - Head injury, neck injury, loss of consciousness, fainting, concussion, headaches, seizures
   - Visual problems such as blurred vision or a history of detached retina; whether the patient wear glasses or contacts
   - History of heart surgery, hypertrophic cardiomyopathy, myocarditis, mitral valve prolapse, prior embolic event, commotio cordis, or coronary artery abnormalities; history of chest pain, dizziness, fatigue or weakness, syncope, or palpitations (heart racing or skipped heart beats) with or after exercise; history of hypertension; history of murmur or syncope[1]
   - Breathing problems such as wheezing, coughing, or trouble breathing with or after exercise; history of asthma
   - History of musculoskeletal injury such as fracture or dislocation; injury or pain in neck, shoulder, back, elbow, hand, finger, knee, ankle, foot, or toe
   - History of use of special equipment for sports-related activities
   - History of numbness or tingling in the upper or lower extremities
   - History of eating disorder, excessive fatigability, diabetes, bleeding problems, anemia, hepatitis, mononucleosis
   - History of stress, anxiety, or depression
   - Menstrual history: menarche, last menstrual period, frequency of menses (number of menstrual periods in the past year), history of amenorrhea or other menstrual dysfunction
   - History of anemia or sickle cell disease
3. Family history, including:
   - History of premature or sudden death, short QT syndrome,* long QT syndrome, Wolfe-Parkinson-White syndrome, arrhythmias, hypertrophic or dilated cardiomyopathy, Marfan's syndrome, or Brugada's syndrome†
   - Family history of coronary artery disease

*Sudden death in individuals with structurally normal hearts associated with short QT interval.[3]

PHYSICAL EXAMINATION

The physical examination should be focused and thorough to determine the presence of an acute infection or any impairment that would prohibit participation in the selected sport. General appearance, posture, overall health, height, weight, and percentage of body fat should be determined. It is vital to note congenital deformities such as arachnodactyly or other signs of Marfan's syndrome. Additional components of the physical examination should include:

1. Visual acuity with Snellen chart (Corrected visual acuity should be 20/40 or better.)
2. Vital signs
3. Blood pressure and heart rate at rest, 3 minutes after exercise, and again 6 minutes after exercise
4. Skin evaluation for signs of fungal, candidal, or other infection
5. Head, eyes, ears, nose, and throat (HEENT) evaluation to determine infectious processes and evaluate any lymphadenopathy
6. Cardiovascular examination
   - Note any pectus deformity of the anterior chest, since this could indicate Marfan's syndrome.[1]
   - Assess the heart sounds with the patient in the supine, standing, and squatting positions. Special emphasis is necessary to determine the presence of any murmurs or arrhythmias. Arrhythmias, extra heart sounds (S_3, S_4), a new murmur, a diastolic murmur, a systolic murmur grade 3/6 or higher, a systolic murmur that increases in intensity with Valsalva's maneuver, or a mitral valve click accompanied by a murmur requires further evaluation before clearance for sports participation can be given.
   - Radial and femoral pulses should be symmetric to exclude coarctation of the aorta.
   - Blood pressure must be compared with age-adjusted tables. Elevated blood pressure requires treatment, and it must be within the accepted range before medical clearance is given. The use of beta blockers and/or diuretics may preclude athletic participation in some states.[1]
7. Pulmonary examination; an assessment of lung sounds anteriorly and posteriorly
8. Abdominal examination; further evaluation if organomegaly is detected‡
9. Genitourinary examination
   - The testes must be descended.
   - The presence of inguinal hernias must be determined.
10. Musculoskeletal examination
    - Is there neck pain on examination or with range of motion (ROM)?‡

†Sudden death in individuals with normal hearts associated with ST-segment elevation in right precordial leads.[4]

‡Any pain or deficit requires further evaluation before medical clearance is given for sports participation.

- With the patient standing, the back should be evaluated for scoliosis, flexibility, and pain with ROM.*
- All extremities, muscles, and joints, including the shoulders/arms, elbow/forearm, wrist/hand, hip/thigh, knee, leg/ankle, foot, and acromioclavicular joint, must be evaluated for muscle atrophy, flexibility, symmetry, tenderness, and ROM. Resisted shoulder shrug and resisted flexion and extension must be determined.* Asymmetry or pain with ROM requires further evaluation.
- The physical signs of Marfan's syndrome should be excluded.
- Can the patient "duck walk" at least four steps?
- Can the patient hop on each foot several times?

11. Neuromuscular examination
    - Cranial and sensory nerves
    - Deep tendon reflexes
    - Cerebellar function

DIAGNOSTICS

Diagnostics are not usually necessary, although some states require urinalysis to determine the presence of protein or glucose in the urine. Other diagnostics such as ECG, exercise stress test, or echocardiogram are necessary if the history and physical examination suggest any cardiac abnormalities. Hemoglobin and hematocrit should be determined as necessary in female athletes.

MEDICAL CLEARANCE

Physician consultation or referral is indicated and medical clearance deferred if there is a history of detached retina; posttraumatic convulsive disorder; or the absence of an eye, kidney, or testicle (these conditions usually prohibit participation in any contact sport). Appropriate consultation or referral is also indicated if the student is unable to perform duck walk maneuvers or has evidence of diminished visual acuity, hypertension, an acute systemic infection, cardiac abnormalities, neurologic deficit, neck pain or history of cervical stenosis, shoulder asymmetry, joint tenderness, or pain with ROM. Medical clearance is deferred pending specialist evaluation. Patients with significant lymphadenopathy, abdominal organomegaly, uncontrolled diabetes or asthma, obesity, and eating disorders also require further evaluation before medical clearance can be provided. Students with controlled asthma, diabetes, or other chronic illness can participate in sports but must have careful medical management.[5]

PATIENT AND FAMILY EDUCATION

Students, parents, and coaches can exert considerable pressure on the health care provider to provide medical clearance for the athlete. However, the health care provider's fundamental responsibility is to protect the student from harm. Any concerns elicited during the history or physical examination must be carefully explained to both the parent and student. It is important that both the parent and student understand that medical clearance cannot be given until the results of diagnostic testing and specialist evaluation are known. The parent and student should also understand that a preparticipation sports physical examination has limitations and cannot completely eliminate the risks inherent in any athletic activity.

REFERENCES

1. Hergenroeder AC: *The preparticipation sports physical in children and adolescents,* retrieved Dec 29, 2005, from http://www.uptodate.com.
2. Lyznicki JM, Nielsen NH, Schneider JF: Cardiovascular screening of student athletes, *Am Fam Phys* 62(4):765-774, 2000.
3. Gaita F, Giustetto C, Bianchi F, and others: Short QT syndrome: a familial cause of sudden death, *Circulation* 108(8):965-970, 2003.
4. Antzelevitch C, Brugada P, Brugada J, and others: Brugada syndrome: 1992-2002: a historical perspective, *J Am Coll Cardiol* 41(10):1665-1671, 2003.
5. American Academy of Pediatrics: Medical conditions affecting sports participation, *Pediatrics* 107(5):1205-1209, 2001; retrieved Dec 5, 2006, from http://aappolicy.aappublications.org/cgi/content/full/pediatrics;107/5/1205#T3.

*Any pain or deficit requires further evaluation before medical clearance is given for sports participation.

PART 4

Office Emergencies

TERRY MAHAN BUTTARO, *Section Editor*

CHAPTER 29

Acute Bronchospasm

JoAnn Trybulski

DEFINITION AND EPIDEMIOLOGY

Bronchospasm, or constriction of the bronchioles, occurs in conjunction with multiple entities. Bronchospasm may develop in a patient as a reaction to medication administered in the office, or the patient may already have bronchospasm when he or she comes to the office for an examination.

Clinical conditions that are associated with bronchospasm include anaphylactic reactions to medications or other allergens, congestive heart failure, pulmonary embolism, asthma, chronic obstructive pulmonary disease, lower respiratory tract infection, mechanical airway obstruction by anatomic changes or tumor, and vocal cord dysfunction.[1] The actual incidence of bronchospasm is difficult to determine because many cases are intermittent and the conditions that cause bronchospasm are multiple.

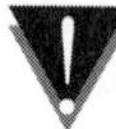

Immediate emergency department referral or physician consultation is indicated for patients in acute respiratory distress.

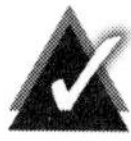

Physician consultation is indicated for patients with an Sao_2 of less than 92% on room air and failure to improve with nebulizer treatment given three times or epinephrine injection administered three times or to a peak flow of greater than 80% of predicted.

PATHOPHYSIOLOGY

Bronchospasm results when hyperreactivity of the airways, caused by inflammatory substances, produces airway bronchoconstriction, edema, and obstruction. The bronchospasm may be intermittent and resolve without treatment, or the obstruction may progress to respiratory arrest, with its potential for death.

CLINICAL PRESENTATION

Patient presentations can vary from mild anxiety to acute respiratory distress. Most often, wheezing, coughing, and dyspnea are present. A repetitive, spasmodic cough may be the only sign of bronchospasm. The patient's inability to speak a full sentence without pausing to breathe indicates severe bronchospasm. Patients' psychologic states vary according to their previous experience with this condition and the severity of symptoms. Patients with a history of asthma may have experienced bronchospasm frequently and may have even come to accept this as a usual daily pattern, whereas patients who experience their first episode or a severe episode may understandably be anxious.

PHYSICAL EXAMINATION

Vital signs may show tachypnea, tachycardia, and a normal or slightly elevated blood pressure. Hypotension occurs in an allergic reaction with anaphylaxis. The presence of pulsus paradoxus of greater than 25 mm Hg is a uniform indicator of severe respiratory compromise.[2]

Skin color may be normal, flushed, or pale. The presence of pruritus or a rash is a diagnostic aid with an allergic etiology.

The use of accessory muscles is noted as a sign of more severe bronchospasm. Wheezing may be audible or detected during auscultation on inspiration or expiration. The finding of a silent chest indicates severe spasm and is an ominous sign. With audible wheezing, the trachea should be auscultated to discern whether these sounds are indicative of laryngospasm or partial airway obstruction with a foreign body.

DIAGNOSTICS

Peak flow measurements will be reduced from the patient's normal or from what is considered normal for age and height. Pulse oximetry values below 90% in adults indicate more severe bronchospasm. Arterial blood gas (ABG) analysis is best performed in an emergency department.

Chest radiographs may delineate the cause of bronchospasm. With asthma or allergy, the chest radiograph can be normal or show hyperinflation.

DIFFERENTIAL DIAGNOSIS

Potentially fatal conditions require immediate exclusion. The presence of an urticarial rash with decreasing blood pressure is a sign of anaphylaxis, necessitating immediate treatment with supplemental oxygen via nasal cannula or mask and diphenhydramine (Benadryl) 25 or 50 mg IV or IM, or epinephrine 0.3 mg SQ or IM, depending on the patient's condition and cardiac status.

Cardiac failure may manifest as bronchospasm in the setting of known cardiac disease. Clinical presentation with paroxysmal nocturnal dyspnea, distended neck veins, or pedal edema confirms the diagnosis. Vascular redistribution or pleural effusion may be seen on chest radiographs. Obtaining chest radiographic studies should not delay treatment for cardiac failure.

Bronchospasm with acute dyspnea may herald impending respiratory failure in patients with chronic lung disease. Other causes of respiratory failure include depressed respiratory drive, pneumonia, atelectasis, asthma, airway obstruction, pulmonary edema, pulmonary hemorrhage, pulmonary contusion, and acute respiratory distress syndrome. The history and clinical presentation indicate the origin of the respiratory failure.

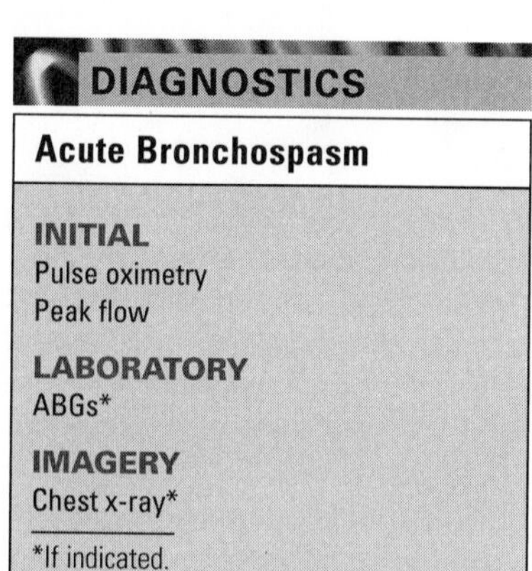

DIAGNOSTICS

Acute Bronchospasm

INITIAL
Pulse oximetry
Peak flow

LABORATORY
ABGs*

IMAGERY
Chest x-ray*

*If indicated.

Pulmonary embolization should be suspected when bronchospasm occurs in a patient at risk for a pulmonary embolus. These patients include those who smoke and those with signs of vascular thrombosis, a history of atrial fibrillation, or a history of oral contraceptive use.

Recurrent bronchospasm or a poor response

to bronchodilation medication indicates the need for reassessment and thorough evaluation for mechanical airway obstruction caused by anatomic changes or tumor, as well as vocal cord dysfunction, a missed case of heart failure, or pulmonary embolus.

INITIAL STABILIZATION AND MANAGEMENT

Acute bronchospasm occurring in the setting of lower respiratory tract infection, asthma, or chronic obstructive pulmonary disease is initially managed by supplemental oxygen via nasal cannula or mask and inhalation of a beta agonist via a metered-dose inhaler (MDI) or nebulizer. Treatment via an MDI (90 mcg/puff) consists of 4 to 8 puffs of albuterol every 20 minutes; up to 4 hours may be given to reverse bronchospasm as long as tachycardia does not increase or palpitations are not precipitated by the treatments.[3] As an alternative, nebulizer treatment with 2.5 to 5 mg albuterol is given every 20 minutes for up to three treatments, then 2.5 to 10 mg every 1 to 4 hours as needed.[3] Alternatively, continuous nebulizer treatment with albuterol at a rate of 10 to 15 mg/hr can be used.[3] For best results, the albuterol should be diluted with saline to a volume of at least 3 ml and delivered at an oxygen flow of 6 to 8 L/min.[3] Ipratropium bromide 0.5 mg may be added to the nebulizer solution with saline for dosing every 30 minutes for three doses, then given every 2 to 4 hours as needed to augment and prolong bronchodilation.[3]

Recent investigations have centered on alternative routes and procedures for albuterol administration. Endotracheal administration of albuterol has been used successfully in two case reports involving children.[4] Use of resuscitator bag device as a spacer device for albuterol has been reported.[5] A continuous nebulizer treatment using albuterol at a rate of 7.5 mg/hr was found to be as effective as a rate of 15 mg/hr in cases of moderate to severe bronchospasm in one study.[6]

DIFFERENTIAL DIAGNOSIS

Acute Bronchospasm

- Anaphylaxis
- Congestive heart failure
- Respiratory failure
- Pulmonary embolism
- Tremor
- Vocal cord dysfunction

Worsening respiratory status, increased respiratory difficulty, decreasing pulse oximetry values, and failure to respond to beta agonist therapy indicate impending respiratory failure. The health care provider should be prepared to support respiration via intubation and mechanical ventilation while transferring the patient to the nearest emergency facility for other therapeutic modalities. Once acute bronchospasm is resolved, oral prednisone (starting at 120 to 180 mg/day in three or four divided doses for the first 48 hours, followed by 60 to 80 mg/day until peak expiratory flow reaches 70% of predicted or personal best, then tapered) is generally prescribed to reduce inflammation.[3] No advantage has been found for IV steroid administration over oral, provided that gastrointestinal transit time is not increased or absorption is not impaired.[3] Recent studies point to the efficacy of using magnesium sulfate IV as an adjunct to treat acute bronchospasm.[7] Doses for magnesium sulfate IV reported in a meta-analysis ranged from 10 to 25 mg/kg with infusion over 20 minutes.[7]

DISPOSITION AND REFERRAL

The health care provider should be acquainted with the capabilities of the local emergency medical services (EMS) system and have a plan for the emergency transport of patients. Patients who fail to respond to treatment or who do not improve with initial therapy should be transported to an emergency treatment facility.

PREVENTION AND PATIENT EDUCATION

The health care provider needs to be prepared to manage acute bronchospasm in the office setting and must have a plan for EMS support. Equipment and supplies needed in initial patient management include, at a minimum, oxygen, peak flow meters (disposable or capable of being decontaminated), beta-agonist inhalers (albuterol), and epinephrine. If an emergency department is not readily available, additional recommended supplies include IV access capability, parenteral steroids, anticholinergic medication (ipratropium), intubation equipment, and a hand-held nebulizer. Increasingly, medical offices have access to pulmonary function testing machines and pulse oximetry. Office personnel who triage telephone calls and make appointments should receive guidelines for which patients to reroute to the emergency department via ambulance.

Patients with known asthma need to have a management plan devised that includes parameters for seeking medical evaluation. These patients also require extensive education regarding their medication regimens, care and use of inhalers, and use of peak flow measurements.

REFERENCES

1. Richmond E: Asthma diagnosis and management, *Clin Rev* 7(8):76-112, 1997.
2. Abou-Shala N, MacIntyre N: Emergent management of acute asthma, *Med Clin North Am* 80(4):677-699, 1996.
3. Expert Panel Report: *Guidelines for the diagnosis and management of asthma,* NIH Pub No 02-5074, Bethesda, 2003, National Institutes of Health, retrieved Dec 5, 2006, from http://www.nhlbi.nih.gov/guidelines/asthma/index.htm.
4. Carroll CL: Endotracheal albuterol treatment of acute bronchospasm (letter to the editor), *Am J Emerg Med* 22(6):506, 2004.
5. Schleufe P, Domurath H, Piepenbrock S: Beta$_2$-agonist delivery via a resuscitator bag (Ambu MediBag): a comparison with a metered dose inhaler using the Volumatic-Spacer, *Resuscitation* 61(3):327-331, 2004.
6. Stein J, Levitt MA: A randomized, controlled double-blind trial of usual-dose versus high-dose albuterol via continuous nebulization in patients with acute bronchospasm, *Acad Emerg Med* 10(1):31-36, 2003.
7. Alter HJ, Koepsell TD, Hilty WM: Intravenous magnesium as an adjuvant in acute bronchospasm: a meta-analysis, *Ann Emerg Med* 36(3):191-197, 2000.

CHAPTER 30

Altitude Illness

Karin C. Dieselman

DEFINITION AND EPIDEMIOLOGY

Altitude illness is a syndrome complex of mild to severe symptoms that results from rapid ascent into a hypoxic environment, especially in nonacclimatized people. This syndrome complex is manifested as acute mountain sickness (AMS), high-altitude periodic breathing of sleep, high-altitude pulmonary edema (HAPE), high-altitude retinal hemorrhage, and high-altitude cerebral edema (HACE). AMS, HAPE, and HACE are separate clinical syndromes with a continuum of mild to severe symptoms.[1] This complex of symptoms can cause coagulation abnormalities, focal neurologic deficits, syncope, peripheral edema, retinopathy, pharyngitis, bronchitis, immunosuppression, and flatus expulsion. High-altitude periodic breathing of sleep is thought to be a subset of AMS and the cause of the sleeplessness that can occur at high altitudes.[2]

More than 300 million people worldwide inhabit high-altitude regions, with 50% living above 2438 m (8000 feet).[3] In the United States more than 40 million people travel above 2438 m annually.[4,5]

AMS occurs within the first 24 hours of a rapid ascent to 2011 m (6600 feet) or higher and is seen in 33% of climbers.[4] This syndrome develops in nearly 3 out of 4 climbers to 4572 m (15,000 feet). The incidence at 2195 m (7200 feet) and 2743 m (9000 feet) is 17% and 40%, respectively. AMS occurs in 40% of trekkers in Nepal on the path to Mount Everest; this number increases to 70% during ascent to the top.[6] Two thirds of the climbers of Mount Rainier and 25% of travelers to Colorado ski resorts experience AMS.[3]

Men and women are equally susceptible to AMS; children and individuals with preexisting diseases (e.g., arteriosclerotic cardiovascular disease [ASCVD], chronic obstructive pulmonary disease [COPD], congestive heart failure, sickle cell anemia) are more susceptible. HAPE is less common, occurring in 1% to 2% of those who rapidly ascend to 3048 m (10,000 feet).[4] HAPE is more common in climbers and skiers who have not acclimatized. With HAPE, 20 deaths worldwide are reported annually, with men having a preponderance of 87% over women.[5]

Risk factors for these disorders include previous history of high-altitude disease, rapid ascent to a high altitude, and marked physical effort. Other possible causes include age less than 50 years, primary residence at an altitude less than 914 m (3000 feet), and obesity.

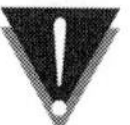

Immediate emergency department referral or physician consultation is indicated for patients with altitude illness.

PATHOPHYSIOLOGY

AMS results in a decrease of oxygen delivery to the tissues at the alveolar level. At 1524 m (5000 feet), Pa_{O_2}, as measured with arterial blood gas (ABG) sampling, is 80 mm Hg; at 2286 m (7500 feet), 70 mm Hg; and at 4572 m (15,000 feet), 50 mm Hg. Hypoxia ensues, which stimulates changes in the lungs, heart, brain, and kidneys.

The pulmonary effects of AMS include hyperventilation and increased tidal volume, which lead to a decrease in P_{CO_2} or respiratory alkalosis. Pulmonary circulation constricts, resulting in increased pressure that leads to pulmonary edema. Hypoxia stimulates the hypoxic ventilatory response of the peripheral chemoreceptors in the carotid bodies. The inhibition of central chemoreceptors results in a decrease in minute ventilation. This interaction controls respiratory rate and heart rate and is indirectly responsible for the renal control of bicarbonate. In AMS the hypobaric hypoxia is the underlying cause. Although the exact sequence of events is unclear, an increase in aldosterone and antidiuretic hormone levels and renin-angiotensin secretion interaction results in fluid overload, which leads to cerebral and pulmonary edema.

In HAPE, pulmonary hypertension is present as a result of the hypoxia. Pulmonary wedge pressures and left ventricular function are not affected. Theories include overperfusion (fluid leakage into alveoli), pulmonary venous obstruction, and capillary permeability.[5] With HACE, there is alteration in the blood-brain barrier and increased cerebral blood flow, which lead to cerebral edema.

CLINICAL PRESENTATION

AMS, HAPE, and HACE are separate clinical syndromes that fall on a continuum of mild to increasingly severe symptoms (Table 30-1). AMS manifests within 6 hours of arrival or even after 1 day or longer and is similar to an alcoholic hangover. The headache is bifrontal and worsens when bending over or performing Valsalva's maneuver. The gastrointestinal and constitutional symptoms are outlined in Table 30-2. There is

TABLE 30-1 Altitude-Related Findings

	High Altitude	Very High Altitude	Extreme Altitude
Elevation (in meters)	1500-3500	3500-5500	>5500
Elevation (in feet)	~4900-11,500	11,500-18,000	>18,000
Pa_{O_2}	>90%	<90%	<70%-90%
Impairment of oxygen transport	No	Yes	Yes
Severity	Mild	Moderate to severe	Severe and life threatening
Findings	↓ Exercise performance ↑ Respiratory rate	Mild to moderate hypoxemia	Severe hypoxemia Death without oxygen

TABLE 30-2 Altitude Illness

Onset	Symptoms	Physical Examination	Management	Prevention
ACUTE MOUNTAIN SICKNESS (AMS)				
1-6 hours to several days Rapid	Headache Anorexia Cough Nausea Emesis Weakness Insomnia	Increased heart rate, decreased blood pressure, fluid retention	Descend ≥500 m, or stop, rest, acclimatize Acetazolamide 125-250 mg PO, emetics, and analgesics	Ascend slowly. Avoid strenuous exertion and rapid ascent >2743 m (9000 feet). Consider acetazolamide 1 day before and 2 days after ascent to high altitude. Spend night at intermediate altitude.
Moderately Severe AMS				
			Oxygen 1-2 L/min Dexamethasone 4 mg PO or IM q 6 hr until symptoms resolve	
HIGH-ALTITUDE PULMONARY EDEMA				
6 hours to 4 days	Fatigue Irritability Shortness of breath Cough Confusion Hemoptysis Nocturnal illness	Increased heart and respiratory rates Decreased blood pressure Cyanosis Frothy sputum Oliguria Mental status changes Rales Ataxia	Immediate descent Portable hyperbaric chamber or oxygen 4-6 L/min, then 2-4 L/min Nifedipine 10 mg × 1, then 30 mg extended release q 12 hr initially, then 4 mg q 6 hr Dexamethasone if neurodeterioration	Ascend slowly. Avoid overexertion. Consider nifedipine ER 20 mg PO q 8 hr in persons with prior episode.
HIGH-ALTITUDE CEREBRAL EDEMA				
Hours to days	Nausea Emesis Irritability Severe headache Insomnia Ataxia Irrationality Hemiplegia Seizures Coma	Decreased loss of consciousness Cranial nerve palsies Seizures Coma Rales	Oxygen 2-4 L/min Descend as soon as possible Hyperbaric chamber Dexamethasone 8 mg PO, IM, or IV initially, then 4 mg PO q 6 hr Acetazolamide if descent delayed	Ascend slowly at graded rate. Avoid overexertion. Consider acetazolamide 125- 250 mg 1 day before and 2 days after being at high altitude.*

Modified from Hackett PH, Roach RC: High altitude illness, *N Engl J Med* 345(2):107-113, 2001.
*For persons with repeated episodes.

irritability, a worsening headache, emesis, and dyspnea. In its most severe form, AMS can lead to HAPE, HACE, and coma within 12 hours.

HAPE manifests between 6 hours and 4 days after arrival in a high-altitude environment (see Table 30-2). Many of the symptoms appear nocturnally as a result of arterial desaturation during sleep. The onset can be gradual or acute, and symptoms can be mild (dyspnea on exertion, dry cough), moderate (weakness, fatigue with walking, raspy cough, headache), or severe (dyspnea at rest, productive cough, orthopnea, stupor, or coma). The progression of the cough from dry to wet and mental status changes indicate a worsening condition. Coma and death occur quickly if HAPE is left untreated.

HACE, the advanced stage of AMS, is characterized by a worsening of the AMS symptoms listed in Table 30-2. As with HAPE, the onset can be gradual or acute. Initial symptoms include a headache or confusion. Additional signs and symptoms include visual problems, papilledema, paralysis, progressive neurologic involvement, coma, and rarely seizures.[4]

PHYSICAL EXAMINATION

The physical findings for altitude illness vary and depend on the severity of the condition; see Table 30-2 for a comparison. With mild AMS the findings are nonspecific. Fluid retention is the hallmark.

In HAPE the physical findings vary with the severity of the illness. Hackett and Rabold classify this severity as follows: mild HAPE reveals a normal heart rate, a normal respiratory rate, dusky nail beds, and, possibly, pulmonary rales. Moderate HAPE reveals a normal heart rate, a respiratory rate of 16 to 30 breaths per minute, cyanotic nail beds, rales, and ataxia. Severe HAPE includes tachycardia (>110 beats per minute), a respiratory rate of greater than 30 breaths per minute, facial and nail bed cyanosis, and ataxia.[5,6]

The progressive neurologic signs of HACE are listed in Table 30-2. Focal neurologic findings are a result of increased intracranial pressure and include the third and sixth cranial nerve palsies, papilledema, and pulmonary rales.

DIAGNOSTICS

The clinical presentation and physical findings indicate the diagnosis. Pulse oximetry, ABG analysis, and chest x-ray studies confirm the severity of the presentation of AMS. Pulse oximetry values vary depending on the severity of AMS. Normal values are greater than 90% in adults and greater than 94% in infants and children. The chest x-ray study will be normal in patients with AMS, but with HAPE or HACE there is a patchy bilateral interstitial edema.

DIFFERENTIAL DIAGNOSIS

Unlike with a viral illness, a patient with uncomplicated AMS does not manifest a fever or myalgia. Hangover, exhaustion, and dehydration may be difficult to differentiate. A history of alcohol intake, recent vigorous activity, and other reasons for lack of water intake may assist the provider. Hypothermia and the use of sedatives may slow the mental processes and cause ataxia.[3] With HAPE, patients with preexisting cardiac (ASCVD), hematologic (sickle cell anemia), and pulmonary (COPD) diseases need to be differentiated through the history, physical examination, chest x-ray study, and ECG. HACE may mimic transient ischemic attacks or cerebrovascular accidents. Brain tumors have similar manifestations.

INITIAL STABILIZATION AND MANAGEMENT

Preventive measures and early recognition by the patients and timely intervention by the provider result in timely and effective management (Box 30-1). In all cases, the ascent should be stopped and a descent initiated. General measures on presentation include a complete medical history, physical examination, and pulse oximetry.

AMS, the most common of the syndromes, rapidly improves over 24 to 48 hours as acclimatization occurs. Simple measures, such as rest and adequate fluid intake, ameliorate the symptoms; a descent of 152 to 305 m (500 to 1000 feet) will help for associated sleep disturbances. Continued ascent is not recommended. More severe symptoms require acetazolamide 250 mg b.i.d. (5 mg/kg/day in divided doses), supplemental oxygen 1 to 2 L/min, prochlorperazine (Compazine) 5 to 10 mg IM t.i.d. p.r.n. for nausea, dexamethasone 4 mg q 6 hr, and/or diuretics (furosemide [Lasix] 20 to 40 mg q 12 hr). Hyperbaric bags reduce altitude sickness and diminish symptoms in 1 to 2 hours.[3,5,6]

HAPE usually resolves with an immediate descent of 305 m (1000 feet). Severe cases should initially be managed as AMS is managed. Although no definitive studies exist, urgent management should also include immediate treatment with nifedipine 10 mg PO. Nifedipine ER 30 mg PO should be continued q 12-24 hr.[4,7,8] Oxygen 4 to 6 L/min is also indicated until improvement is noted; the flow rate can then be decreased to 2 to 4 L/min to conserve the supply. The use of diuretics has had mixed results and may in fact worsen symptoms.[4,5] Despite therapy, the overall mortality rate is 11% for those who descended and 44% for those who did not.[4]

HACE requires emergent evacuation. Treatment may include oxygen 2 to 4 L/min and dexamethasone 8 mg PO, IM, or IV followed by 4 mg q 6 hr.[7] Acetazolamide can be administered if descent is delayed. Supportive measures may include basic cardiac life support, advanced cardiac life support, and seizure control. Hyperventilation in patients who are intubated may decrease intracerebral pressure.

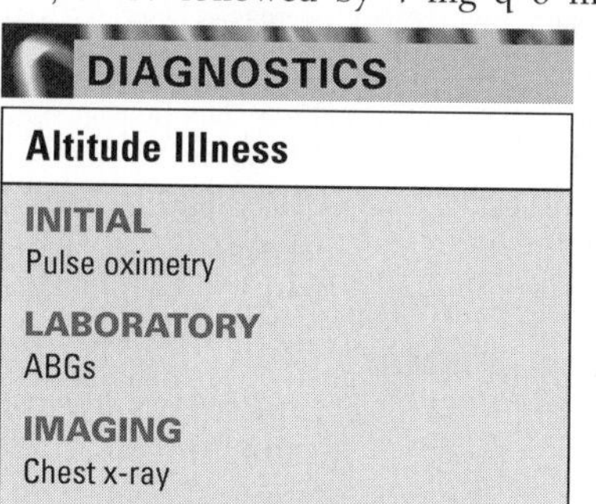
DIAGNOSTICS

Altitude Illness

INITIAL
Pulse oximetry

LABORATORY
ABGs

IMAGING
Chest x-ray

DISPOSITION AND REFERRAL

Patients with AMS that does not improve should be evacuated; hospital admission for more intensive treatment monitoring is essential. HAPE and HACE require immediate descent and urgent treatment.

PREVENTION AND PATIENT EDUCATION

AMS is best prevented with acclimatization with a slow ascent of 305 m (1000 feet) per day. Adequate hydration and the avoidance of alcohol, strenuous activity, or abrupt ascents are additionally recommnded.[4,6,7,9] Acetazolamide 125 to 250 mg b.i.d. for 24 to 48 hours before ascent is helpful, especially for those with a history of AMS or for abrupt ascent without acclimatization. This treatment is continued for 2 days and stopped unless symptoms recur.[6,7] Nifedipine 20 mg t.i.d. 24 hours before ascent may help prevent HAPE. Spending 1 night at 1524 to 2012 m (5000 to 6600 feet) before ascent and sleeping at altitudes below 2500 m (8200 feet) will be beneficial. Gradually ascending 305 m (1000 feet) per day, avoiding abrupt ascents to more than 3048 m (10,000 feet), and allowing 2 nights for each 800- to 1000-m (2624- to 3280-foot) altitude gain may prevent AMS. For altitude climbing, Zafren and Honigman recommend the maintenance rule, "climb high, sleep low."[3] Patients who have experienced HAPE have a recurrence rate of 66%.[8]

BOX 30-1

TREATMENT OF ALTITUDE ILLNESS

ACUTE MOUNTAIN SICKNESS
- Analgesics, descent, avoidance of alcohol, benzodiazepines
- Use of acetazolamide, prochlorperazine (Compazine), oxygen, dexamethasone, hyperbaric bag, diuretics (if indicated)

HIGH-ALTITUDE PULMONARY EDEMA
- Immediate descent, rest, evacuation (if not improved)
- Nifedipine, oxygen, hyperbaric bag

HIGH-ALTITUDE CEREBRAL EDEMA
- Immediate descent and evacuation
- Dexamethasone, hyperbaric bag, basic cardiac life support, advanced cardiac life support, seizure control (if indicated)

DIFFERENTIAL DIAGNOSIS

Altitude Illness

ACUTE MOUNTAIN SICKNESS (AMS)
- Viral illness or bacterial infection
- Hangover
- Dehydration
- Exhaustion
- Hypoglycemia
- Hyponatremia
- Hypothermia
- Sedatives, alcohol, or other medications
- Transient ischemic attack or cerebrovascular accident
- Psychosis
- Brain tumor
- Carbon monoxide poisoning
- Seizure
- Migraine

HIGH-ALTITUDE PULMONARY EDEMA (HAPE)
- Transient ischemic attack or cerebrovascular accident
- Brain tumor
- Sickle cell anemia
- Chronic obstructive pulmonary disease
- Cardiac disease or congestive heart failure
- Brain tumors
- Asthma
- Bronchitis
- Pneumonia
- Pulmonary edema
- Pulmonary embolus

HIGH-ALTITUDE CEREBRAL EDEMA (HACE)
- Transient ischemic attack or cerebrovascular accident
- Brain tumor

REFERENCES

1. West JB: The physiologic basis of high-altitude diseases, *Ann Intern Med* 141:789-800, 2004.
2. Eichenberger U, Weiss E, Reimann D, and others: Nocturnal periodic breathing and the development of acute high altitude illness, *Am J Respir Crit Care Med* 154(6):1748-1754, 1996.
3. Zafren K, Honigman B: High-altitude medicine, *Emerg Med Clin North Am* 15(1):191-222, 1997.
4. Braun R, Krishel S: Environmental emergencies, *Emerg Med Clin North Am* 15(2):451-476, 1997.
5. Hultgren HN: High-altitude pulmonary edema: current concepts, *Ann Rev Med* 47:267-284, 1996.
6. Hackett PH, Rabold M: High altitude medical problems. In Tintinalli JE, Ruiz E, Krome RL, editors: *Emergency medicine: a comprehensive study guide*, New York, 1996, McGraw-Hill.
7. Hackett PH, Roach RC: High altitude illness, *N Engl J Med* 345(2):107-113, 2001.
8. Harris MD, Terrio J, Miser WF, and others: High-altitude medicine, *Am Fam Phys* 57(8):1907-1914, 1998.
9. Dumont L, Mardirosoff C, Tramer MR: Efficacy and harm of pharmacologic prevention of acute mountain sickness: quantitative systematic review, *BMJ* 321(29):267-272, 2000.

CHAPTER 31

Anaphylaxis

Terry Mahan Buttaro

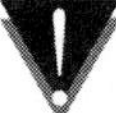

Immediate emergency department referral or physician consultation is indicated for patients with angioedema, respiratory distress, and vascular collapse.

DEFINITION AND EPIDEMIOLOGY

Anaphylaxis is a systemic, life-threatening allergic reaction characterized by urticaria, pruritus, angioedema (Color Plate 8), gastrointestinal symptoms, respiratory distress, and cardiovascular collapse. Anaphylactic reactions are commonly underreported, and the exact number of individuals affected by this disorder is uncertain. However, it is estimated that more than 40 million people are at risk for anaphylaxis and that this disorder causes approximately 500 to 1000 deaths in the United States each year.[1] Although individuals may respond differently, anaphylactic reactions usually occur within seconds to minutes after sensitization to a specific antigen. The response is typically immediate, but reactions can occur several hours after the exposure. To prevent death, prompt recognition and treatment are essential. Antibiotics are commonly associated with anaphylaxis, but food reactions are actually the most common cause of anaphylaxis and account for 150 to 200 deaths each year.[2] Latex, other medications, food additives, hymenoptera stings, venoms, chemicals, exercise, cold urticaria, and even glucocorticoids can also cause anaphylaxis, but often the cause is idiopathic[3] (Box 31-1).

PATHOPHYSIOLOGY

An immunoglobulin E (IgE)–mediated response, anaphylaxis is a profound, immediate allergic reaction with life-threatening bronchospasm, hypoxemia, and hypotension. A similar presentation occurs in an anaphylactoid reaction, a non–antigen-, non–antibody-mediated response.[4] Both reactions are caused by mediators from basophils and mast cells, which precipitate the release of histamines, causing increased capillary permeability, vasodilation, and bronchospasms. Urticaria and pruritus are a result of mild allergic reactions, whereas facial angioedema (well-defined subcutaneous edema), respiratory distress, and vascular collapse indicate a severe reaction.

CLINICAL PRESENTATION

Within seconds of exposure to the offending agent, the individual can experience a variety of symptoms, including weakness, pruritus, urticaria, nausea, vomiting, abdominal cramping, diarrhea, incontinence, throat tightness, stridor, a "lump" in the throat, hoarseness, wheezing, angioedema, or chest tightness. Most reactions are uniphasic. These reactions are fairly immediate, occurring 1 to 45 minutes after exposure to the allergen. Some patients have a biphasic reaction, with a second phase of anaphylaxis occurring several hours after an

BOX 31-1

COMMON ALLERGENS ASSOCIATED WITH ANAPHYLAXIS

Allergen extracts: pollen and nonpollen extracts
Antiserums
Blood products
Dyes (fluorescein, radiographic contrast media)
Environmental allergens (dust, mold, grasses, trees, animals)
Enzymes
Exercise
Foods
- Additives such as monosodium glutamate (MSG)
- Beans (including soybeans)
- Chocolate
- Cottonseed oil
- Eggs
- Grains
- Mango
- Milk
- Nuts (especially peanuts and tree nuts)
- Seafood (particularly shellfish)
- Sesame and sunflower seeds
- Spices: mustard
- Strawberries
- Wheat, buckwheat

Hormones (insulin, progesterone, vasopressin)
Hymenoptera stings (bees, wasps, yellow jackets, hornets, imported fire ants)
Idiopathic
Intravenous colloids: dextran
Medications
- Anesthetics
- Angiotensin-converting enzyme inhibitors
- Antibiotics, particularly penicillins, cephalosporins
- Antineoplastic compounds
- Aspirin
- Corticosteroids
- Insulin
- Iron dextran
- Lidocaine
- Muscle relaxants
- Nitrofurantoin
- NSAIDs
- Opiates
- Procaine
- Vaccines
- Vitamins: thiamine, folic acid

Mite-contaminated foods
Occupational chemicals and proteins
- Ethylene oxide
- Latex
- Rubber products

Venom

asymptomatic interval of up to 8 hours.[5] A careful history is important to elicit information about previous exposure to offending agents, onset of symptoms, other illnesses, medications, and allergies.

PHYSICAL EXAMINATION

Physical examination reveals characteristic pruritic, urticarial eruptions. Facial angioedema may be significant and associated with vocal changes, stridor, or wheezing, indicating the need for intubation and immediate transfer to the nearest emergency facility. Tearing, rhinorrhea, pallor, cyanosis, confusion, restlessness, anxiety, tachycardia, bronchospasm, arrhythmias, hypoxia, accessory muscle use, distant heart and lung sounds, and hypotension are other common physical findings. Airway obstruction and cardiopulmonary arrest can occur within minutes to hours after allergen exposure.

DIAGNOSTICS

The ECG may reveal ST-segment elevation, hyperacute or inverted T waves, arrhythmias, or asystole. Arterial blood gas analysis, if available, is indicated. A chest x-ray examination also may be appropriate.

DIFFERENTIAL DIAGNOSIS

The presentation and history are usually sufficient to accurately diagnose an anaphylactic reaction, although acute bronchospasm, upper airway obstruction, and pulmonary edema should be considered in the differential diagnosis. However, these disorders do not cause urticaria or angioedema and are not usually associated with gastrointestinal symptoms. Identification of the offending antigen, if possible, will aid in the prevention of future reactions.

INITIAL STABILIZATION AND MANAGEMENT

High-flow oxygen; continuous monitoring of airway, breathing, and circulation (ABCs); and immediate transport to an emergency facility are indicated, since endotracheal intubation, tracheostomy, or even cricothyroidotomy may be necessary. Immediate epinephrine is recommended to stimulate vasoconstriction and bronchial smooth muscle relaxation and reduce capillary permeability. For mild or moderate reactions, immediate intramuscular epinephrine (0.3 to 0.5 ml of a 1:1000 solution for adults; 0.01 mg/kg for children) injected into the vastus lateralis muscle (lateral thigh) results in better absorption of the epinephrine.[6-9] For adults, the dose can be repeated at 10- to 15-minute intervals, if necessary. Patients with severe bronchospasm, angioedema, or hypotension have critical anaphylaxis and require IV epinephrine (0.5 to 1 ml of a 1:10,000 solution slow IV push at 5- to 10-minute intervals) or a continuous epinephrine infusion (1 to 10 mcg/min) and aggressive isotonic (0.9% normal saline) fluid resuscitation through a large-bore (14 or 16 gauge) IV catheter. Physician consultation and hospitalization are indicated because epinephrine can cause myocardial ischemia, arrhythmias, seizures, and severe systolic hypertension.[10] Sublingual or endotracheal epinephrine can be given in life-threatening situations if IV access is unobtainable. Physician consultation is also indicated for patients receiving beta-blocker therapy. These patients can be resistant to epinephrine and require glucagon 1 mg IV.[4]

H_1 and H_2 blockers are indicated in mild, moderate, or severe reactions. Diphenhydramine, 50 to 100 mg PO with mild symptoms, or 25 to 50 mg IM or IV q 4-6 hr with more severe symptoms, will help alleviate urticaria and angioedema. Ranitidine, 50 mg IV, or cimetidine, 300 mg IV, are given at the same time as the H_1 blocker and continued every 8 hours until the anaphylaxis resolves.[11] Although not effective immediately, hydrocortisone 100 mg IV q 6 hr should be discussed with the physician to prevent recurrent anaphylaxis.

DIAGNOSTICS

Anaphylaxis

INITIAL
Pulse oximetry
ECG

LABORATORY
ABGs
24-hour urine for N-methyl histamine*
Plasma histamine*: to confirm anaphylaxis
Serum or urinary tryptase*: to confirm anaphylaxis

IMAGERY
Chest x-ray

*If indicated.

Bronchodilator therapy with an inhaled β_2 agonist can be beneficial for patients with bronchospasms. Recent evidence also suggests that placing the patient in a supine or Trendelenburg's position can decrease mortality, though a recumbent position could be uncomfortable for a patient experiencing respiratory distress.[10]

If the reaction has occurred in response to an insect bite, the area should be carefully examined and the stinger, if present, removed (see Chapter 32). The area should be carefully cleaned and cool packs applied to the area.

DIFFERENTIAL DIAGNOSIS

Anaphylaxis

- Bronchospasm
- Upper airway obstruction
- Pulmonary edema
- Panic attack

DISPOSITION AND REFERRAL

The patient should be immediately transferred to an emergency facility even if initial stabilization and treatment are effective. All patients require continued observation in the emergency department or hospital for 24 hours because, in 20% of patients, the anaphylactic reaction can be biphasic, with the second phase occurring 8 to 24 hours after the initial phase.[5]

PREVENTION

The prevention of future anaphylactic reactions is the primary goal. Patients identified as being allergic to aspirin should understand the importance of avoiding all aspirin- and NSAID-containing products. Any allergens must be forever avoided, and consultation with an allergist is recommended. Radioallergosorbent (RAST) and skin testing may be recommended to determine the cause of the reaction, although skin testing should not be conducted within 6 weeks of any anaphylactic event. With all allergy testing, there is the potential risk of precipitating a fatal anaphylactic reaction.

For reactions associated with venom stings, a referral for desensitization is strongly recommended. The importance of wearing shoes outdoors and avoiding perfumes and bright clothing should be stressed. Beta blocker therapy may be contraindicated for patients with a history of hymenoptera stings.

Patients with a food allergy must be particularly attentive, since fatal reactions in this population are not uncommon.[12] The importance of reading labels carefully and always carrying an epinephrine pen should be frequently reiterated. Recent studies suggest that anti-IgE therapy may be helpful in preventing food-related anaphylaxis.[13]

PATIENT AND FAMILY EDUCATION

Individuals who have experienced an anaphylactic reaction should wear a medical alert bracelet. Patients, families, and co-workers should be instructed in the use of a home epinephrine kit, which should contain a premeasured, disposable syringe of 1:1000 epinephrine and an antihistamine tablet. The importance of having immediate access to the kit at all times; of urgently administering epinephrine and antihistamine; and of calling 911 immediately if wheezing, breathing difficulties, or facial, lip, or tongue swelling occurs should be emphasized and understood by the individual and family members. Patients should be reminded to replace the medication in the home epinephrine kit yearly.

In addition, a trained health care provider should teach patients, teachers, and caregivers how to use the epinephrine autoinjector pen.[14] It is also important to explain (and demonstrate) that the epinephrine should be given intramuscularly in the lateral aspect of the patient's thigh to facilitate the most rapid absorption.[6]

REFERENCES

1. Neugut AI, Ghotek AT, Miller RL: Anaphylaxis in the United States: an investigation into its epidemiology, *Arch Intern Med* 161(1):15-21, 2001.
2. Clark S, Camargo CA: Emergency management of food allergy: systems perspective, *Curr Opin Allergy Clin Immunol* 5(3):293-298, 2005.
3. Erdmann SM, Abuzahra F, Merk HF, and others: Anaphylaxis induced by glucocorticoids, *J Am Board Fam Pract* 18(2):143-146, 2005.
4. O'Dowd L, Zweiman B: *Anaphylaxis*, retrieved May 23, 2005, from http://www.uptodate.
5. Ellis AK, Day JH: Diagnosis and management of anaphylaxis, *CMAJ* 169(4):307-311, 2003.
6. Simons FE: First-aid treatment of anaphylaxis to food: focus on epinephrine, *J Allergy Clin Immunol* 113(5):837-844, 2004.
7. Simons FE, Gu X, Simons KJ: Epinephrine absorption in adults: intramuscular versus subcutaneous injection, *J Allergy Clin Immunol* 108(5):871-873, 2001.
8. Sicherer SHL: Advances in anaphylaxis and hypersensitivity reactions to foods, drugs, and insect venom, *J Allergy Clin Immunol* 111(3 suppl):S829-S834, 2003.
9. Ellis AK, Day JH: The role of epinephrine in the treatment of anaphylaxis, *Curr Allergy Asthma Rep* 3(1):11-14, 2003.
10. Brown SG: Cardiovascular aspects of anaphylaxis: implications for treatment and diagnosis, *Curr Opin Allergy Clin Immunol* 5(4):359-364, 2005.
11. O'Dowd LC, Zweiman B: *Anaphylaxis in adults*, retrieved Dec 27, 2005, from http://www.uptodate.com.
12. Bock SA, Munoz-Furlong A, Sampson HA: Fatalities due to anaphylactic reactions to foods, *J Allergy Clin Immunol* 107(1):191-193, 2001.
13. Leung DY, Shanahan WR, Li XM, and others: New approaches in the treatment of anaphylaxis, *Novartis Found Symp* 257:248-285, 2004.
14. Grouhi M, Alshehri M, Hummel D: Anaphylaxis and epinephrine auto-injector training: who will teach the teachers? *J Allergy Clin Immunol* 104(1):190-193, 1999.

CHAPTER 32

Bites and Stings

Jackie S. Fantes
Updated by Terry Mahan Buttaro

INSECT BITES AND STINGS

DEFINITION AND EPIDEMIOLOGY

More species of insects are in existence than any other form of multicellular life. Insects that bite and infest include mosquitoes, flies, bedbugs, kissing bugs, fleas, lice, blister beetles, centipedes, millipedes, scabies, chiggers, and ticks. Stinging insects include vespids, bees, and ants. The medical importance of insects is that they bite, sting, and envenomate; are vectors for infectious pathogens; and cause hypersensitivity reactions. Insect bites and stings can cause toxic reactions that range from local and mild to life threatening.[1]

Immediate emergency department referral or physician consultation is indicated for anaphylaxis and suspected black widow or brown recluse spider bites.

PATHOPHYSIOLOGY AND CLINICAL PRESENTATION

Although many insect bites and stings are simply a nuisance, some patients can have severe skin or systemic reactions. Vespids (yellow jackets, hornets, and wasps), bees (honeybees and bumblebees), and ants inject venom with a stinger. The sting results in immunoglobulin E (IgE)–mediated systemic reactions that cause the release of mediators (histamines, the slow-reacting substance of anaphylaxis, and eosinophil chemotactic factors of anaphylaxis)[2] from mast cells, culminating in local inflammation involving many cell types and numerous mechanisms.[3]

These stings induce local, toxic, systemic, and delayed reactions. A local reaction consists of erythema, edema, and pruritus at the sting site. A toxic reaction is initially seen as gastrointestinal distress, light-headedness, syncope, headache, fever, drowsiness, muscle spasms, edema, and occasionally seizures. A systemic reaction is anaphylaxis, which initially manifests as itchy eyes, facial flushing, generalized urticaria, and dry cough. Anaphylaxis can quickly intensify to respiratory distress, and it may deteriorate to respiratory or cardiovascular failure. A delayed reaction can occur 10 to 14 days after the sting and cause fever, malaise, headache, urticaria, lymphadenopathy, polyarthritis, or more systemic autoimmune illnesses (i.e., leukocytoclastic vasculitis or Henoch-Schönlein purpura).[2,4] Table 32-1 describes the pathophysiology and clinical presentation of other insect bites and stings.[1]

PHYSICAL EXAMINATION

The initial assessment of bites and stings should determine any compromise in airway, breathing, and circulation (i.e., evidence of anaphylaxis). A thorough examination of the bite or sting and surrounding area should be made to determine the extent of envenomation and any associated infection.

DIAGNOSTICS

Adults with systemic allergic reactions should be considered for venom immunotherapy, which is successful in virtually all patients. The diagnosis of insect sting allergy can be made on the basis of a history of anaphylaxis with a sting, positive

TABLE 32-1 Summary of Insect Bites and Stings

Insect	Clinical Presentation	Pathophysiology
Wasps, bees, ants, hornets, yellow jackets	Local reaction Toxic reaction Systemic reaction Delayed reaction	Inject venom with stinger
Fire ants	Papule progressing to sterile pustule in 6-24 hours	Inject venom with stinger
Mosquitoes, flies	Pruritic, painful papule Secondary infection common	Inject salivary material
Bedbugs, kissing bugs	Clustered, erythematous, pruritic nodules	Painlessly suck blood
Fleas	Pruritic grouped welts, papules, vesicles Secondary infection common	Deposit saliva in bite
Lice	Pruritus Nits in scalp, body, or pubic hair	Deposit saliva in bite
Blister beetles	Large blisters	Release hemolymph
Centipedes	Pain and itching with local necrosis	Inject venom with fangs
Millipedes	Brown-stained area with blistering	Excrete toxic chemicals
Scabies	Burrow lesion with pruritus Secondary infection common	Burrow in epidermis
Chiggers	Pruritic papules or vesicles Secondary infection common	Release digestive substances in bite
Ticks	Pruritic papule with tick present Secondary infection common	Attach to victim with painless bite

skin tests, or radioallergosorbent tests (RASTs).[3] Otherwise, no specific laboratory evaluation is required unless indicated by the clinical course.

DIFFERENTIAL DIAGNOSIS

The diagnosis of all insect bites and stings is made by obtaining a careful history. It is helpful if the patient brings in the insect. Insect bites are commonly confused with contact dermatitis and viral exanthemas. Flea bites may resemble varicella. Reactions to blister beetles may resemble bullous impetigo and burns. Because of such similarities, a history of exposure may be the only diagnostic clue.[5]

INITIAL STABILIZATION AND MANAGEMENT

The management of all insect bites and stings begins with local wound care, including removal of the stinger and the use of ice packs, antihistamines (H_1- and H_2-blockers) for itching, topical steroids for inflammation, topical or systemic antibiotics for secondary infection, and NSAIDs to relieve discomfort.[5] Any evidence of a systemic reaction must be treated as anaphylaxis.

Management also includes eradication of the insect. For flea infestation it is necessary to vacuum thoroughly; wash the rugs, pets, and beds; and use an insecticide. Lice and scabies are eradicated by applying 1% lindane lotion or shampoo (Kwell, Scabene) on two consecutive nights. Permethrin (NIX, Elimite) is another effective scabies treatment.

According to Gammons and Salam, ticks are effectively removed with blunt, angled, medium-tipped forceps. The tick should be removed as soon as possible by grasping it close to the mouth, flipping the tick so the backside is closest to skin, and pulling.[6] An alternative method is to suffocate the tick with mineral oil, nail polish, petrolatum, or chloroform. After removing the tick, the health care provider must explore the bite area for retained mouth parts, then carefully clean it with an antiseptic.[4,6] Antibiotic prophylaxis is indicated wherever Lyme's disease is endemic (see Chapter 250).

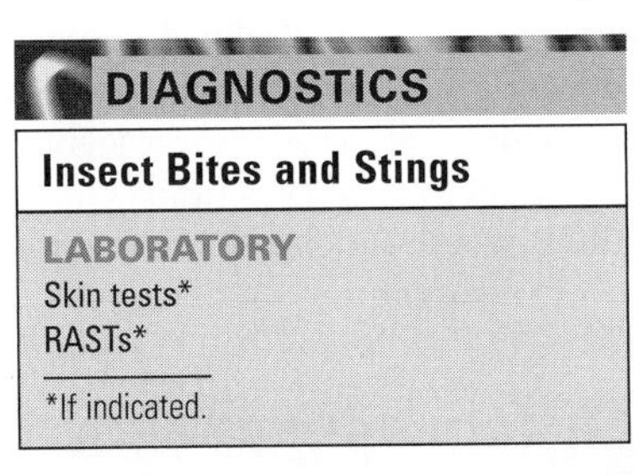
DIAGNOSTICS

Insect Bites and Stings

LABORATORY
Skin tests*
RASTs*

*If indicated.

DIFFERENTIAL DIAGNOSIS

Insect Bites and Stings

- Contact dermatitis
- Varicella
- Viral exanthemas
- Bullous impetigo
- Burns

DISPOSITION AND REFERRAL

Systemic reactions to bites and stings may be life threatening. Thus any systemic or anaphylactic reaction requires a referral to the emergency department for definitive management and possible hospitalization.

PREVENTION AND PATIENT EDUCATION

Preventive management against bites and stings includes avoidance and protective clothing. Repellents can be used, including diethyltoluamide (DEET), dimethyl phthalate, dimethyl carbate, ethyl hexanediol, butopyronoxyl (Indalone), and benzyl benzoate.[7] Any person with a history of anaphylaxis from wasp or bee stings should be given medical warning tags, epinephrine injector kits, and a referral for venom immunotherapy.[2,8,9]

SPIDER BITES

DEFINITION AND EPIDEMIOLOGY

More than 30,000 species of spiders, 50 of which are medically important to humans, are found worldwide.[2] In the United States problems are caused by the bites of only two spiders: brown recluse spiders and black widow spiders.[10] However, the hairs of other spiders (e.g., the tarantula) are associated with anaphylaxis.[11]

The brown recluse spider is a six-eyed nocturnal spider that avoids people. It is yellow, brown, or black with thin legs that are five times the body length; the entire spider is approximately the size of a quarter. It has a violin-shaped marking on its back. The brown recluse spider is found in warm, dry areas such as abandoned buildings, woodpiles, and cellars.[2]

The female black widow spider is the most venomous of all spiders and has a body size of approximately 1.5 cm (0.6 inch) and a leg span of 4 to 5 cm (1.6 to 2 inches).[2] Despite the name *black* widow, these spiders may be black, brown, tan, or variegated.[10] The classic orange-red, hourglass-shaped marking is actually found on only one species (*Latrodectus mactans*) and may be merely an indistinct yellow or orange spot. The male spider is only one third the size of the female; its bite cannot penetrate human skin. Black widow spiders are aggressive and tend to live in basements, woodpiles, and garages.[2]

PATHOPHYSIOLOGY AND CLINICAL PRESENTATION

The venom of the brown recluse spider is chemotactic, which results in endothelial injury and subsequent thrombosis.[10] It is a neurotoxin that causes the release of acetylcholine and norepinephrine at the neurosynaptic junction.[2] The bite of the brown recluse spider is almost painless and most commonly manifests as a mild, erythematous lesion that may become firm and then heal over several days to weeks. The bite can also be more severe, causing erythema, blistering, and a bluish discoloration within 24 hours and possibly becoming necrotic within 3 to 4 days. The lesions can vary in size from 1 to 30 cm (0.4 to 11.8 inches) and take 6 weeks to 4 months to heal. The victim may have a systemic response and experience fevers, chills, nausea, vomiting, myalgia, arthralgia, petechiae, hemolysis, or seizures within 24 to 48 hours of the bite. Severe systemic manifestations can lead to hemoglobinuria, renal failure, disseminated intravascular coagulation, and death.[2]

The bite of the black widow spider is mildly to moderately painful, with erythema, swelling, and muscle cramps beginning at the site within 30 minutes to 12 hours. The muscle cramping progresses to large muscle groups and the abdomen and can mimic peritonitis. The muscle pain can subside over a few hours but can flare over 2 to 3 days, with muscle weakness and intermittent spasms persisting for weeks to months.

Hypertension can be a serious complication. Anxiety or confusion can also occur. Severe envenomation may lead to shock, coma, or respiratory failure secondary to muscle paralysis.[10]

HISTORY AND PHYSICAL EXAMINATION

The history and physical examination of the patient should be thorough. The history is important to elicit associated symptoms such as fever, nausea, or pain in addition to information on when and where the suspected bite occurred. In areas where spider bites are not endemic, a recent history of travel should be determined if a spider bite is suspected.

The primary survey should determine any compromise of the airway, breathing, or circulation (i.e., evidence of anaphylaxis). Vital signs and a thorough examination, including a careful evaluation of the bite and surrounding area, is then necessary to determine the extent of envenomation and any associated infection.

DIAGNOSTICS

If a brown recluse spider bite is suspected, CBC, BUN, electrolytes, blood glucose, creatinine, coagulation profile, and urinalysis (for hemoglobinuria) tests should be ordered. No specific laboratory tests are indicated for a suspected black widow spider bite.[2] However, CBC, urinalysis, BUN, creatinine, glucose, electrolytes, and an acute abdominal series may be indicated, since the presentation may mimic an acute abdomen.

DIFFERENTIAL DIAGNOSIS

Brown recluse and black widow spider bites should be included in the differential diagnosis of any spider bite. However, the diagnosis of either of these spider bites can be difficult, especially in the absence of the actual spider. The unusual presentation of acute abdominal pain requires that all causes of acute abdomen be considered in the differential diagnosis.

INITIAL STABILIZATION AND MANAGEMENT

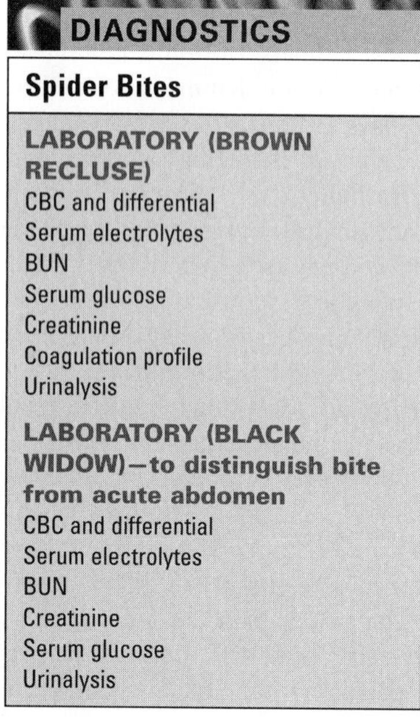
DIAGNOSTICS

Spider Bites

LABORATORY (BROWN RECLUSE)
CBC and differential
Serum electrolytes
BUN
Serum glucose
Creatinine
Coagulation profile
Urinalysis

LABORATORY (BLACK WIDOW)—to distinguish bite from acute abdomen
CBC and differential
Serum electrolytes
BUN
Creatinine
Serum glucose
Urinalysis

The bite of the brown recluse spider requires no medications, and currently no antivenom is available. Tetanus prophylaxis and supportive measures should be provided. Antibiotics are indicated only if infection is suspected. Pain relief may be required in some cases. Daily wound care is important for necrotic lesions, and surgery may be required for necrotic lesions larger than 2 cm (0.8 inch).[2]

The initial therapy for black widow spider bites is basic supportive care—airway, breathing, and circulation. Local wound care and tetanus prophylaxis should always be provided. Narcotic analgesics, benzodiazepines, and calcium gluconate are all effective means of pain relief and muscle relaxation. Antivenom is indicated only for a severe bite because of the risk of anaphylaxis and serum sickness and can be given only to patients who have not previously had exposure to horse serum.[10]

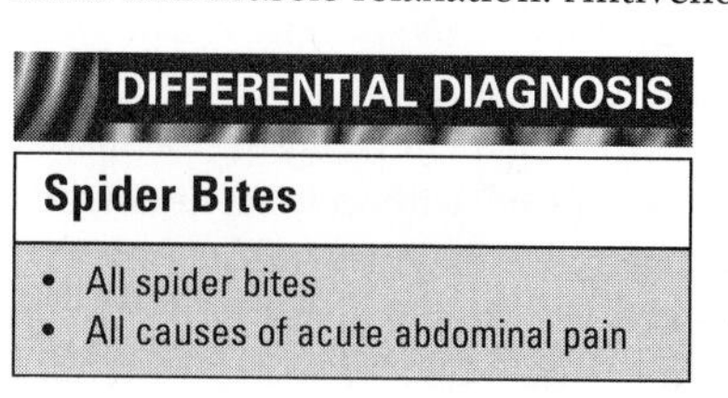
DIFFERENTIAL DIAGNOSIS

Spider Bites

- All spider bites
- All causes of acute abdominal pain

The wolf spiders, of which the tarantula is the most common, cause bites the equivalent of a wasp sting without necrosis. These bites usually require only supportive care.[5]

DISPOSITION AND REFERRAL

Adults and children with evidence of significant systemic reactions should be referred for hospitalization and close observation. Patients with black widow spider bites that require antivenom should always be referred to the emergency department and/or for hospital admission.

PREVENTION AND PATIENT EDUCATION

Everyone in endemic areas should be taught to recognize the brown recluse spider and avoid its habitats. Clothing, bed linens, attics, closets, and woodpiles should be examined closely in endemic areas because the spider is aggressive only if forced into contact with the substrate.[12]

Black widow spiders are more commonly found in their webs at night. Therefore the webs should be cleaned cautiously at night and the spider mechanically destroyed. Professional exterminators are indicated for heavy infestations. Everyone in endemic areas should be taught to recognize the black widow spider. Protective sleeves and gloves are recommended in handling wood and brush in infested areas.[12]

REPTILE BITES AND SCORPION STINGS

DEFINITION AND EPIDEMIOLOGY

In the United States the venomous snakes include the pit vipers and coral snakes. Pit vipers include rattlesnakes, copperheads, cottonmouths (water moccasins), and bushmasters. Worldwide 100,000 to 125,000 deaths occur each year from snake bites, but in the United States 5000 snakebites are reported annually.[13,14] Only one third to one half of these are caused by venomous snakes. The most severe envenomations tend to occur with rattlesnakes, but copperheads, coral snakes, and snakes imported from other countries are other causes of snakebites. Of the venomous snakebites, 20% result in no envenomation and 40% result in only mild envenomation.[15]

Other reptiles to consider are Gila monsters, which are slow-moving lizards in the deserts of the southwestern United States. Medically significant scorpion stings also occur in the southwestern United States from the bark scorpion[10] (so named because it often lives under the bark of trees).[16]

PATHOPHYSIOLOGY

The venom of the pit viper is a complex mixture of cytotoxic, hemotoxic, and neurotoxic enzymes that cause local tissue injury, systemic vascular damage, hemolysis, fibrinolysis, and neuromuscular dysfunction.[2] Coral snake venom is neurotoxic.[2] Gila monster venom is as toxic as rattlesnake venom, but Gila monsters lack the apparatus to effectively inject it; they have short, grooved teeth and therefore require a prolonged bite for envenomation.[2] Scorpion venom is primarily neurotoxic and is composed of proteins and polypeptides that activate sodium channels to produce a hyperadrenergic state.[16]

CLINICAL PRESENTATION

The history is particularly important in identifying the type of bite. An attempt should be made to determine whether the bite is venomous. Venomous rattlesnakes have fangs, whereas nonvenomous rattlesnakes do not have fangs.[13,14] Poisonous coral snakes also have fangs and, according to Cheng, are easily identified by their red and yellow bands.[13] Associated symptoms such as pain, dizziness, nausea, vomiting, or paresthesias are important to elicit.[13]

For the bites in which there is no envenomation, the only clinical finding is the puncture wound. The clinical picture of patients who are envenomated depends on several factors: amount of venom introduced; anatomic location of the bite; and the patient's size, age, and overall health. The bites are classified by the degree of envenomation: none, minimum, moderate, or severe. The presentation of no envenomation is minimum pain and no significant swelling. Minimum envenomation manifests as local swelling of less than 15 cm (6 inches) from the bite wound and no systemic manifestations. Moderate envenomation has local swelling of 15 to 30 cm (6 to 12 inches) with systemic signs and symptoms. Severe envenomation has local swelling of more than 30 cm with severe systemic signs and symptoms, including coagulation abnormalities.[15]

Coral snake bites resemble scratch marks and are somewhat painful. Patients are initially seen with neurologic symptoms such as tremors, salivation, dysarthria, diplopia, dysphagia, dyspnea, and seizures. These symptoms, which are usually delayed 1 to 6 hours or even up to 12 hours, may progress to respiratory muscle paralysis and death.[15] In most cases the bite of the Gila monster causes only local pain and swelling that worsens over several hours and then subsides over the next several hours. Only occasionally will a systemic reaction occur, with weakness, light-headedness, paresthesias, diaphoresis, or hypertension.[2] Scorpion stings may manifest mild symptoms with only local pain and/or paresthesias, or they may progress to somatic or cranial nerve dysfunction. Motor nerve effects include roving eye movements, fasciculations, dysphagia, and the autonomic effects of tachycardia and excessive secretions.[16]

PHYSICAL EXAMINATION

The physical examination of the patient should be thorough. First, any compromise of the airway, breathing, or circulation (i.e., anaphylaxis) should be determined. This is followed by assessing vital signs; evaluating the patient for bleeding; and thoroughly examining the bite and surrounding area to determine the extent of envenomation, tissue damage, and associated lymphadenopathy. A careful neurologic examination and documentation are necessary initially and should be routinely repeated to assess for neurologic involvement.

DIAGNOSTICS

Reptile Bites and Scorpion Stings

LABORATORY
CBC and differential
Coagulation studies: PT/PTT, clotting time
Fibrinogen
Serum electrolytes
BUN
Creatine kinase
Creatinine
Urinalysis

DIAGNOSTICS

Several corroborating laboratory studies are needed, including CBC, coagulation studies, fibrinogen, electrolytes, BUN, creatinine, and urinalysis. A type and crossmatch for blood, an arterial blood gas analysis, and an ECG are needed if the envenomation is severe.[15]

DIFFERENTIAL DIAGNOSIS

The diagnosis is made on the basis of a history of a snakebite or scorpion bite, with a clinical presentation consistent with envenomation. It is helpful if the victim can identify the snake or scorpion with use of a picture.

INITIAL STABILIZATION AND MANAGEMENT

First aid measures must be instituted first, but all patients bitten by venomous snakes or scorpions must be taken to a health care facility. First aid measures include retreating beyond striking range, remaining calm, immobilizing the extremity involved, minimizing physical activity, wiping the bite site, identifying the snake if it can be done safely, and closely observing the patient's respiratory status. Incision of the wound, suction of the wound, and tourniquets are not recommended.[17] In the prehospital or office setting, management includes providing advanced cardiac life support as appropriate, immobilizing the limb, establishing IV access, and administering oxygen. The wound should be cleaned and tetanus prophylaxis administered.[16]

The major determinant of the required therapy is the degree of envenomation, with the mainstay of therapy for moderate to severe venomous snakebites being antivenom.[15] For Gila monsters, local wound care is probably sufficient and must include the removal of any teeth in the wound; no antivenom is available.[2] For scorpion bites, management is supportive with analgesics and wound care; there is antivenom for severe bites, but it is available only in Arizona and is rarely used.[16]

DISPOSITION AND REFERRAL

Because the clinical symptoms can be delayed, all bites by venomous snakes and scorpions need to be observed for a minimum of 12 hours. The patient must be in an emergency department or hospital setting in which antivenom is available. For snakebites, consultation with a physician or poison control center familiar with envenomation is always recommended.[15]

PREVENTION AND PATIENT EDUCATION

Knowledge of reptile habits and habitats can help prevent envenomation. Anyone who may come in contact with these reptiles should be educated on their habits.

REFERENCES

1. Schlossberg D: Arthropods and leeches. In Cecil RL, Goldman L, Bennett JC, editors: *Cecil textbook of medicine,* Philadelphia, 2000, Saunders.
2. Salluzzo RI: Insect and spider bites. In Tintinalli JE, editor: *Emergency medicine: a comprehensive study guide,* New York, 1996, McGraw-Hill.
3. Lichtenstein L: Insect sting allergy. In Cecil RL, Goldman L, Bennett JC, editors: *Cecil textbook of medicine,* Philadelphia, 2000, Saunders.
4. Fernández M, Arredondo N: *Bites, stings,* retrieved May 23, 2006, from http://www.emedicine.com/EMERG/topic62.htm.
5. Nichols CG: Insect bites and infestations. In Harwood-Nuss AL, editor: *The clinical practice of emergency medicine,* Philadelphia, 1996, Lippincott-Raven.
6. Gammons M, Salam G: Tick removal, *Am Fam Physician* 66(4):643-645, 2002.
7. Elston DM: Bugs and bites, *Dela Med J* 68(9):445-450, 1996.
8. Ditto AM: Hymenoptera sensitivity: diagnosis and treatment, *Allergy Asthma Proc* 23(6):381-384, 2002.
9. Golden DB: Stinging insect, allergy, *Am Fam Phys* 67(12):2541-2546, 2003.
10. Gateley A, McKinney P: Arthropod envenomation. In Noble J, editor: *Textbook of primary care medicine,* ed 3, St Louis, 2001, Mosby.
11. Castells MC: *Spider bites,* retrieved May 24, 2006, from http://www.uptodate.com.
12. Allen C: Arachnid envenomations, *Emerg Med Clin North Am* 10(2):269-298, 1992.
13. Cheng AC: *Snake bite management in the United States (2005),* retrieved May 24, 2006, from http://www.uptodate.com.
14. White J: Snake venoms and coagulopathy, *Toxicon* 45(8):951, 2005.
15. Adam R, Sullivan J: Venomous snake bites. In Cecil RL, Goldman L, Bennett JC, editors: *Cecil textbook of medicine,* Philadelphia, 2000, Saunders.
16. Walter F, Bilden E, Gibly R: Environmental emergencies, *Crit Care Clin* 15(2):353-386, 1999.
17. Alberts MB, Shalit M, LoGalbo F: Suction for venomous snakebite: a study of "mock venom" extraction in a human model, *Ann Emerg Med* 43:181-186, 2004.

CHAPTER 33

Bradycardia

Terry Mahan Buttaro

DEFINITION AND EPIDEMIOLOGY

Absolute bradycardia is defined as a heart rate of less than 60 beats per minute. Athletes, older adults, and other individuals may have normally slow heart rates, and bradycardia may not be pathologic during sleep or after Valsalva's maneuver or other vagal stimulation. Relative bradycardia occurs when the heart is unable to respond as expected to traumatic or hypovolemic hypotension.[1] Although the heart rate in relative bradycardia can be greater than 60 beats per minute, medications or sinoatrial node dysfunction can repress the heart rate.

Medications, cardiac disease, hypothyroidism, electrolyte abnormalities, sleep apnea, infections, increased intracranial pressure, hypothermia, hypoxemia, acidemia, and other disease states can also produce bradycardia.[2] Asymptomatic bradycardia does not require urgent intervention. However, careful monitoring and therapy are indicated if the bradycardia causes symptoms or is related to type II second-degree (Mobitz type II) or third-degree atrioventricular (AV) block.

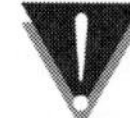

Immediate emergency department referral or physician consultation is indicated for patients with symptomatic bradycardia or Mobitz type II or third-degree heart block.

PATHOPHYSIOLOGY

Bradycardia may result from sinus node dysfunction or AV block. Sinus node dysfunction can be a result of increased vagal tone, as seen in athletes or conditioned young people or in older adults as the result of underlying disease processes, medications, or toxicity. AV block is also associated with various disease processes, including myocardial infarction, coronary artery spasm, digitalis toxicity, cardiac mesotheliomas, and infectious processes. Medications, particularly beta blockers and calcium channel blockers, may induce either sinus node or AV dysfunction.

CLINICAL PRESENTATION

Some symptoms may be nonspecific, but dizziness, fatigue, and syncope are complaints commonly identified with bradycardia. Nausea, vomiting, and confusion have also been correlated with bradycardia. Any bradyarrhythmia associated with chest pain, shortness of breath, exercise intolerance, decreased level of consciousness, hypotension, seizure, congestive heart failure, or myocardial infarction is considered a prearrest condition. A careful symptom analysis and review of the patient's medical history, including allergies and medications, is necessary to discern the cause of the bradycardia so that appropriate treatment can be initiated.

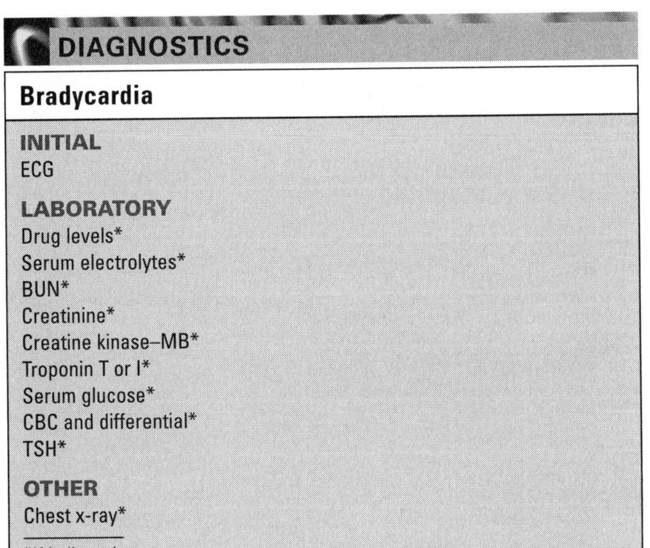

DIAGNOSTICS

Bradycardia

INITIAL
ECG

LABORATORY
Drug levels*
Serum electrolytes*
BUN*
Creatinine*
Creatine kinase–MB*
Troponin T or I*
Serum glucose*
CBC and differential*
TSH*

OTHER
Chest x-ray*

*If indicated.

PHYSICAL EXAMINATION

Although associated symptoms will often guide the physical examination, a focused history and physical examination are necessary. The patient's level of responsiveness and vital signs (including temperature, blood pressure, pulse, respiratory rate, and oxygen saturation) are significant and should be continually reassessed. Hypotension, ventricular arrhythmias, and pulmonary congestion are serious signs indicating the need to identify the cardiac rhythm and institute rapid, appropriate treatment.

DIAGNOSTICS

An ECG is necessary for rhythm analysis and appropriate management. Further diagnostics are guided by the history and physical examination but can include drug levels, electrolytes, glucose, BUN, creatinine, CBC, creatine kinase muscle-brain (MB) fraction, troponin T or I, thyroid studies, and chest x-ray studies.

DIFFERENTIAL DIAGNOSIS

DIFFERENTIAL DIAGNOSIS

Bradycardia

- Medication induced
- Infection
- Vasovagal syncope
- Myocardial infarction
- Digitalis toxicity
- Sick sinus syndrome
- Hypothyroidism
- Bradycardia-tachycardia syndrome

Determination of the bradyarrhythmia and associated pathology is essential for treatment (see Chapter 124). Common causes include medications, infections, vasovagal syncope, myocardial infarction, digitalis toxicity, sick sinus syndrome, bradycardia-tachycardia syndrome, hypothyroidism, and other disease states.

INITIAL STABILIZATION AND MANAGEMENT

The American Heart Association recommends supplementary oxygen, cardiac monitoring, IV access, and continuous assessment of the patient (including vital signs and oxygen saturation).[3] It is crucial to differentiate the symptoms caused by the bradycardia from those not related to the slow rate. No intervention is necessary if the patient is stable and asymptomatic, but continued monitoring is indicated to ensure patient well-being.

To correctly identify the cardiac rhythm, a 12-lead ECG is necessary. Patients with suspected myocardial infarction (Figure 33-1) should be treated for acute coronary syndrome according to the 2005 American Heart Association guidelines (with oxygen, aspirin [160 to 325 mg chewed, if not aspirin allergic], nitroglycerin, morphine, and, if appropriate, reperfusion therapy).[3]

Symptomatic patients with worsening clinical symptoms or prearrest conditions related to the bradycardia may require urgent intervention before a definitive underlying condition is identified (Figure 33-2). The American Heart Association recommends transcutaneous pacing (class I intervention) for patients with symptomatic bradycardia, especially if the bradycardia is associated with Mobitz type II second-degree heart block or third-degree heart block.[3] If a pacer is unavailable, atropine 0.5 mg IV push q 3-5 min (total dose 3 mg) may be indicated.[3] However, atropine, a class IIa intervention, can induce cardiac ischemia, precipitate ventricular tachycardia or fibrillation, and be deleterious for patients with a history of cardiac transplantation.[3] In the presence of Mobitz type II second-degree heart block or third-degree heart block associated with wide-complex ventricular escape beats, atropine should be avoided and a transcutaneous pacer applied as soon as possible.[3] Although often not available, these pacers are currently obtainable with some defibrillator monitors.

For patients unresponsive to atropine or pacing, IV epinephrine (a class IIb intervention) of 2 to 10 mcg/min can be used to treat critical bradycardia.[3] A dopamine infusion of 2 to 10 mcg/kg/min can also improve cardiac output and increase blood pressure and may be used alone or in conjunction with an epinephrine infusion.[3]

For patients with a drug-induced bradycardia related to beta blockers or calcium channel blockers, IV glucagon 3 mg may be helpful.[3] The initial glucagon bolus can be followed by a glucagon infusion to run at 3 mg/hr.[3]

DISPOSITION AND REFERRAL

Patients experiencing signs and symptoms related to bradyarrhythmias require constant reassessment and definitive management in an emergency department. Immediate transfer to an emergency center is required.

PREVENTION

Prevention, when possible, may avert complications or serious injury. Patients who complain of syncope, fatigue, or other symptoms that may be related to bradycardia require diagnostic assessment. A permanent pacemaker may be indicated for bradycardia associated with sinus node dysfunction and certain heart blocks (e.g., fascicular block or acquired AV block).[4]

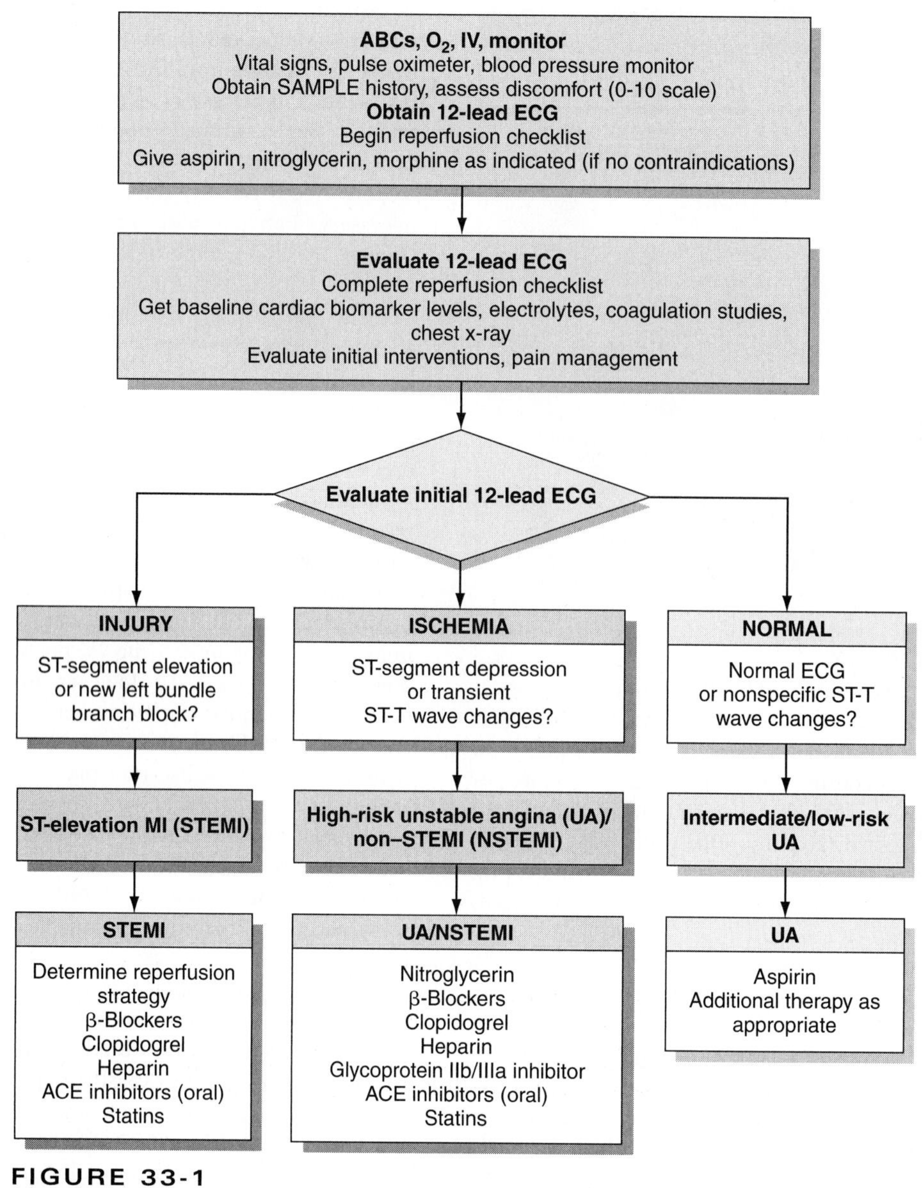

FIGURE 33-1

Ischemic chest pain/discomfort algorithm. *ACE,* Angiotensin-converting enzyme; *MI,* myocardial infarction; *SAMPLE,* signs/symptoms, allergies, medications, past medical history, last oral intake, events leading up to illness/injury; *STEMI,* ST-elevation myocardial infarction; *UA,* unstable angina. (From Aehlert B: *ACLS study guide,* ed 3, St Louis, 2007, Mosby.)

PATIENT AND FAMILY EDUCATION

Patients should understand the importance of calling their health care provider if they experience syncope, lightheadedness, or a slow heart rate that hinders activities. In addition, patients and caregivers should know how to activate the emergency medical system (911) if these symptoms occur with chest discomfort or shortness of breath.

Careful explanation and supportive therapy will enhance patient and family understanding. These measures will also help allay the anxiety inherent in an emergent situation. Medication regimens, if associated with the bradyarrhythmias, should be reviewed to prevent misinterpretation.

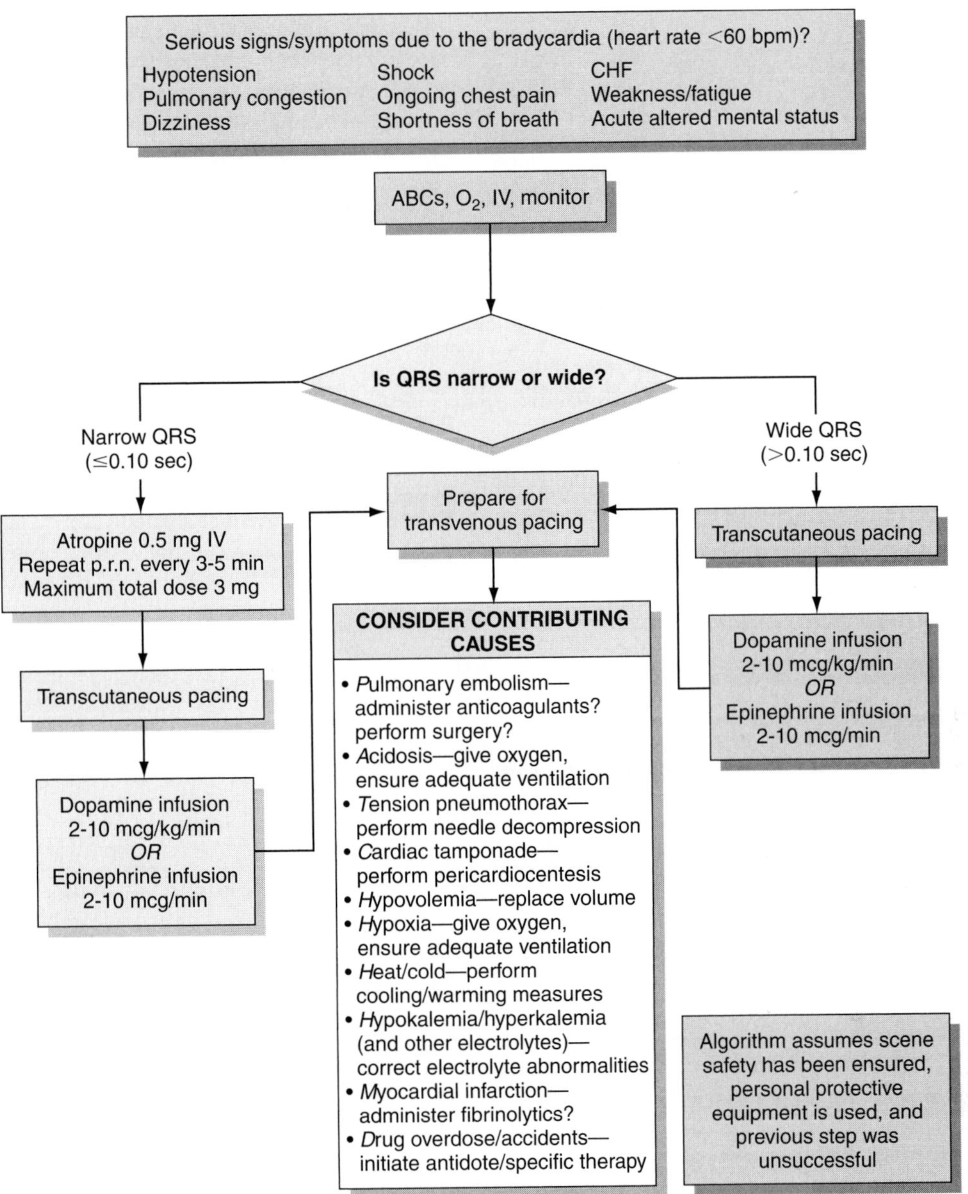

FIGURE 33-2

Symptomatic bradycardia. *ABCs,* Airway, breathing, circulation; *CHF,* congestive heart failure. (From Aehlert B: *ACLS study guide,* ed 3, St Louis, 2007, Mosby.)

REFERENCES

1. Demetriades D, Chan LS, Bhasin P, and others: Relative bradycardia in patients with traumatic hypotension, *J Trauma* 45(3):534-539, 1998.
2. Livingston M, Overton D: *Sinus bradycardia,* retrieved March 9, 2006, from http://www.emedicine.com/emerg/topic534.htm.
3. American Heart Association: 2005 American Heart Association guidelines for cardiopulmonary resuscitation and emergency cardiovascular care, *Circulation* 112(24):IV 67-77, 2005.
4. Gregoratos G: Indications and recommendations for pacemaker therapy, *Am Fam Phys* 71(8):1563-1570, 2005.

CHAPTER 34

Cardiac Arrest

Terry Mahan Buttaro

DEFINITION AND EPIDEMIOLOGY

According to the American Heart Association (AHA), 1 in 3 Americans has some form of cardiovascular disease, and more than 163,000 out-of-hospital cardiac arrests occur in this country each year.[1,2] Nearly one third of the victims die, usually within the first hour, the result of the abrupt cessation of normal heart rhythm. Most often the result of malignant ventricular arrhythmias or ventricular fibrillation (VF), cardiac arrest can also be caused by asystole or pulseless electrical activity.[2,3]

Unfortunately, some patients are first seen by their health care provider with prearrest conditions. If cardiac arrest does occur, resuscitative efforts should be initiated immediately.[2] Trained personnel should begin basic life support (BLS) to maintain airway, breathing, and circulation (ABCs) until advanced life support (ALS) is available[1,2] (Figure 34-1). Preplanning requires that each member of the office team have a specified role if a cardiac arrest occurs and that providers be trained in BLS and ALS.

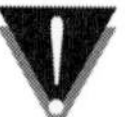

Immediate emergency department referral or physician consultation is indicated for cardiac arrest.

PATHOPHYSIOLOGY

Cardiac arrest may result from either cardiac causes or extraneous circumstances. The net effect is the cessation of cardiac rhythm and the resultant tissue hypoxia and acidosis. Biologic death will occur if resuscitative measures are not instituted immediately.

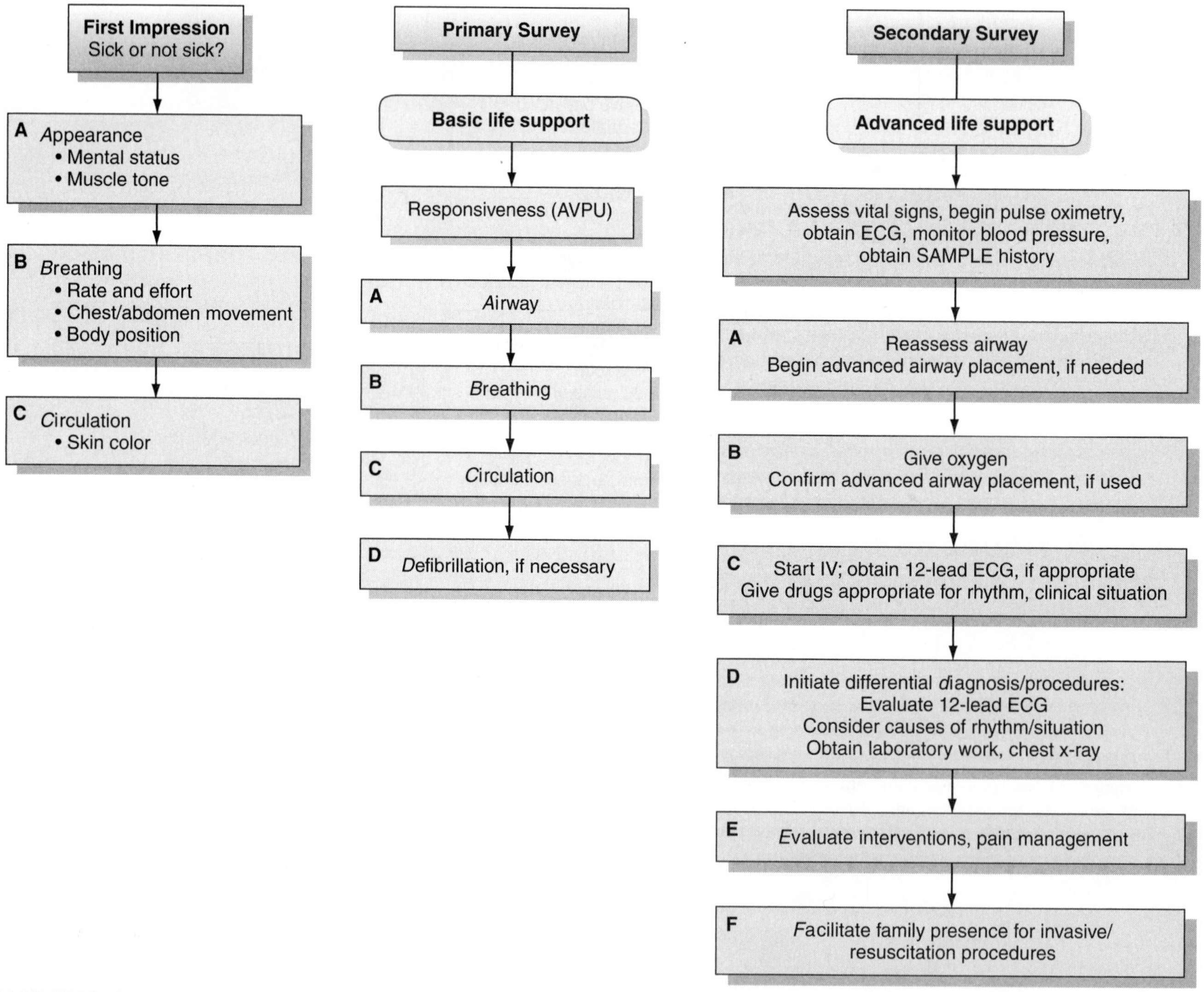

First Impression
Sick or not sick?

A *Appearance*
- Mental status
- Muscle tone

B *Breathing*
- Rate and effort
- Chest/abdomen movement
- Body position

C *Circulation*
- Skin color

Primary Survey

Basic life support

Responsiveness (AVPU)

A *Airway*

B *Breathing*

C *Circulation*

D *Defibrillation, if necessary*

Secondary Survey

Advanced life support

Assess vital signs, begin pulse oximetry, obtain ECG, monitor blood pressure, obtain SAMPLE history

A Reassess airway
Begin advanced airway placement, if needed

B Give oxygen
Confirm advanced airway placement, if used

C Start IV; obtain 12-lead ECG, if appropriate
Give drugs appropriate for rhythm, clinical situation

D Initiate differential *d*iagnosis/procedures:
Evaluate 12-lead ECG
Consider causes of rhythm/situation
Obtain laboratory work, chest x-ray

E *E*valuate interventions, pain management

F *F*acilitate family presence for invasive/resuscitation procedures

FIGURE 34-1

Patient assessment: secondary survey. *AVPU,* Alert, verbal, painful, unresponsive; *SAMPLE,* signs/symptoms, allergies, medications, past medical history, last oral intake, events leading up to illness/injury. (From Aehlert B: *ACLS study guide,* ed 3, St Louis, 2007, Mosby.)

CLINICAL PRESENTATION

There may be no warning that an acute event is about to occur. Presentation can include the classic midsternal, crushing, "viselike" chest pressure with radiation to the arm, neck, or jaw and accompanying diaphoresis, or it may consist of vague, nonspecific symptoms that include chest tightness, discomfort, nausea, shortness of breath, palpitations, lightheadedness, or syncope. A recent history of angina, fatigue, and other nonspecific complaints is also reported. A medical history of smoking, hypertension, elevated cholesterol level, diabetes, and a sedentary lifestyle and family history of coronary artery disease (CAD) are significant risk factors for cardiac arrest; therefore obtaining this information is beneficial. If information cannot be elicited from the patient, family members or others should be questioned to determine the patient's medical history and details of the circumstances surrounding the event.

PHYSICAL EXAMINATION

Assessing unresponsiveness in a calm but efficient manner is critical in the initial management of cardiac arrest. The AHA recommends tapping the victim on the shoulder and asking, "Are you okay?" [2] If unresponsiveness is confirmed in an adult patient, it is necessary to immediately call 911 to activate the emergency medical services (EMS) system to enable rapid procurement of an automated external defibrillator (AED) or a conventional defibrillator.[1,2]

If a second person is available to activate the EMS system, the provider should place the victim in a supine position on a hard, firm surface. With the provider kneeling beside the victim's thorax, the primary survey consists of opening and inspecting the airway with the head tilt–chin lift maneuver (if there is evidence of a head or neck injury, the jaw thrust maneuver [without neck extension] is recommended), then assessing breathlessness by looking, listening, and feeling for breathing. If the victim is not breathing effectively, two regular breaths (1 second per breath) should be given with enough volume to make the chest rise. The carotid pulse can then be checked. If there is no pulse in 10 seconds, chest compressions according to the standards established by the AHA should be initiated (100 compressions per minute with a compression depth of 3.8 to 5 cm [1½ to 2 inches]; 30 compressions to two breaths). The chest should be allowed to recoil completely after each compression. The AHA recommends that interruptions to CPR be limited and that victims of a witnessed arrest be defibrillated as soon as possible (preferably within 3 to 5 minutes).[1,2] There is *limited evidence* suggesting the benefit of a precordial thump in the witnessed arrest of a pulseless patient when an AED or conventional defibrillator is unavailable. However, the AHA considers the precordial thump to be an acceptable intervention for health care providers if a defibrillator or AED is not available.[2] As soon as an AED or conventional defibrillator is available, the leads should be attached to the victim, the rhythm assessed, and, if appropriate, the victim defibrillated according to AHA standards[2] (see Figure 34-1).

Assessment of ABCs and the need for defibrillation (ABCD) is ongoing. At frequent intervals the provider should reassess heart rate; blood pressure; oxygen saturation; and the effectiveness of intubation, CPR, and defibrillation.

DIAGNOSTICS

DIAGNOSTICS

Cardiac Arrest

INITIAL
Pulse oximetry
ECG

LABORATORY
Serum electrolytes
Drug levels*
Cardiac enzymes
ABGs

*If indicated

An ECG, defibrillator monitor, or AED is needed to determine cardiac rhythm, which indicates the necessity of defibrillation and appropriate ALS intervention. Serum electrolytes, drug levels, and cardiac enzymes are required for more definitive diagnosis but are deferred to emergency department management.

DIFFERENTIAL DIAGNOSIS

DIFFERENTIAL DIAGNOSIS

Cardiac Arrest

- Arrhythmias
- Cardiac tamponade
- Electric shock
- Hypotension
- Shock
- Pulmonary edema
- Pulmonary embolus
- Tension pneumothorax
- Toxicologic cardiac emergencies
- Metabolic abnormality
- Near-drowning
- Hypothermia
- Lightning strike

Sudden cardiac death is often associated with VF. Other emergency situations associated with cardiac arrest include significant but nonlethal arrhythmias, hypotension, shock, pulmonary edema, pulmonary embolus, toxicologic cardiac emergencies, metabolic imbalance, near-drowning, hypothermia, cardiac tamponade, tension pneumothorax, electric shock, and lightning strike. It is important to consider, determine, and treat reversible causes of the arrest.

INITIAL STABILIZATION AND MANAGEMENT

Management should follow the guidelines of the AHA[2] (see Figure 34-1). If the patient's collapse may have caused trauma, the head, neck, and spine must be maintained in a straight line to stabilize the cervical spine. After activation of the EMS system, the patient should be positioned on a flat, firm surface, and BLS should be initiated. The cause of the cardiac arrest should be considered throughout the resuscitative effort to facilitate appropriate interventions and promote successful resuscitation.

Because most victims of cardiac arrest are in VF, the AHA still considers early defibrillation the most effective treatment for adult victims of cardiac arrest[2] (Figure 34-2). There is evidence suggesting the benefit of early CPR and defibrillation; approximately 85% to 90% of cardiac arrest victims respond to early CPR and defibrillation. Therefore defibrillation with a biphasic defibrillator, a conventional defibrillator, or an AED should occur as soon as the defibrillator is available. Defibrillation now consists of one shock, rather than a series of stacked shocks.[1,2] Chest compressions should be restarted immediately after defibrillation. After five cycles (or 2 minutes) of CPR, the cardiac rhythm should be reanalyzed. If a shockable rhythm is present, the victim should be defibrillated

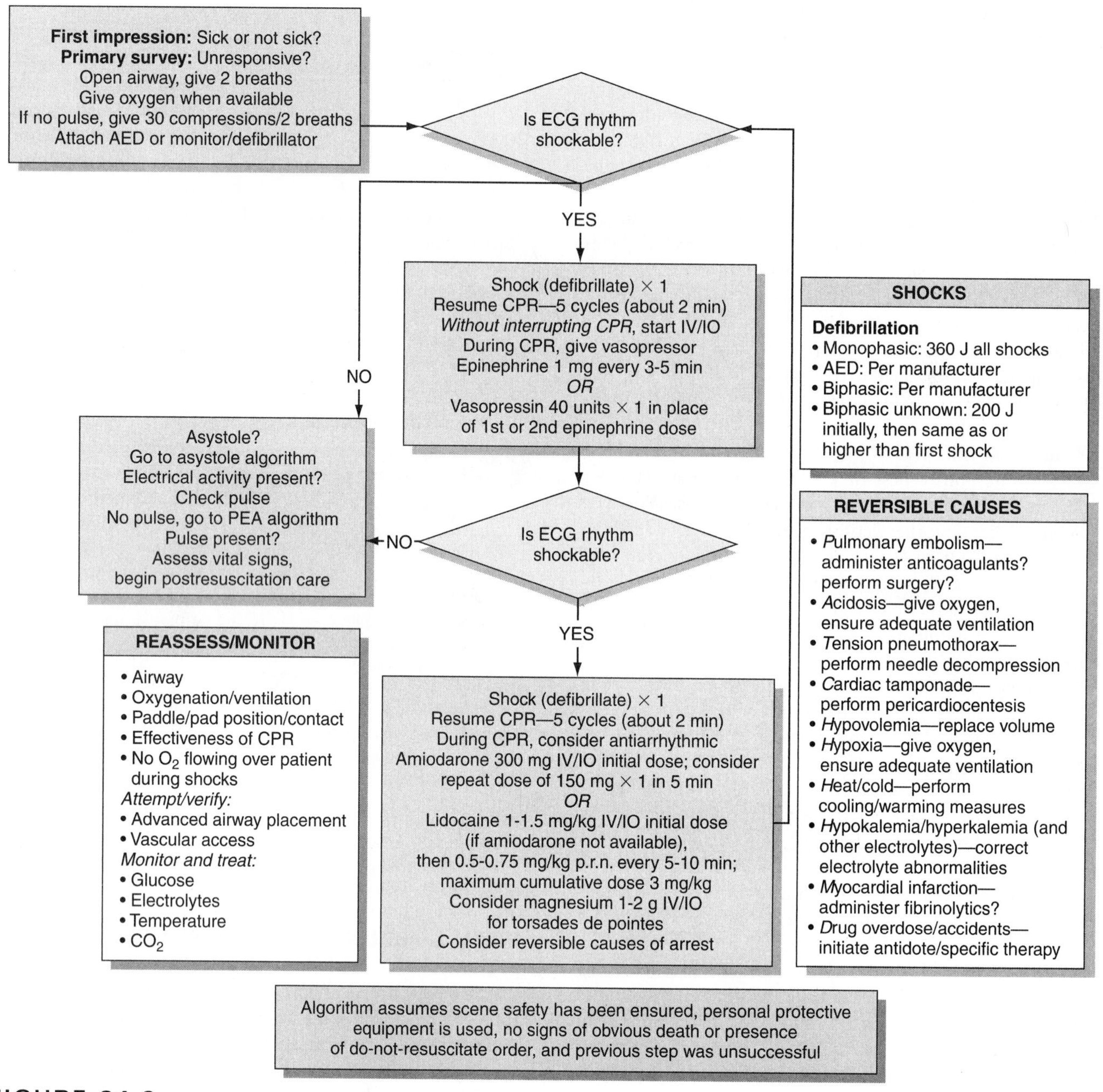

FIGURE 34-2

Pulseless ventricular tachycardia–ventricular fibrillation algorithm. *AED,* Automated external defibrillator; *IO,* intraosseous; *PEA,* pulseless electrical activity. (From Aehlert B: *ACLS study guide,* ed 3, St Louis, 2007, Mosby.)

again and CPR immediately restarted after the defibrillation. Interruptions to CPR should be kept at a minimum to ensure oxygenation to the myocardium. As soon as possible, the patient should be transported to the nearest emergency facility by trained EMS personnel.

COMPLICATIONS

Death will ensue rapidly if CPR, defibrillation, and treatment are not immediately initiated; few victims will survive if CPR is not started within 4 minutes. Those who do survive cardiac arrest may sustain central nervous system injury, hemodynamic instability, and arrhythmias.

DISPOSITION AND REFERRAL

Circulation has been restored if a pulse is present. ABCs should be supported and the patient transported to the nearest emergency department. Emergency department personnel should be advised of pertinent medical information.

PREVENTION

Primary prevention of cardiac arrest is the ultimate goal. Patients with dyspnea, light-headedness, angina, palpitations, or fatigue should be evaluated for underlying CAD. The identification of risk factors for CAD and the appropriate interventions are indicated to decrease the number of sudden cardiac deaths. In addition, community programs enhance the understanding of coronary disease, reinforce early management of chest pain, and promote early access to the EMS system.

Training in CPR and emergency cardiac care is essential for any health care provider. Caregivers of patients with CAD should also be trained in BLS and understand the warning signs associated with sudden cardiac death.

If the cardiac arrest was the result of sustained ventricular tachycardia, the victim will need therapy to reduce the chance of future events. An automated implantable cardioverter-defibrillator (ICD) or cardiac surgery may be the most appropriate intervention.[4] Antiarrhythmic pharmacologic therapy may not be useful for the prevention of ventricular arrhythmias and in fact may be proarrhythmic. According to Trappe, Brandts, and Weismueller, amiodarone and ibutilide have been used successfully to treat arrhythmias in the acute care setting.[5] However, recent evidence suggests there is increased long-term survival with the ICD.[4,6]

PATIENT AND FAMILY EDUCATION

Patients and caregivers should be aware that chest discomfort that increases in intensity or is associated with sweating; palpitations; irregular heartbeat; shortness of breath; lightheadedness; nausea or vomiting; loss of consciousness; or discomfort that radiates to the jaw, neck, or arm necessitates calling 911 or other emergency service immediately. It is important to explain that presentation can be atypical, particularly in women, diabetic persons, or older adults. Everyone should be encouraged to learn BLS, but families who have loved ones with CAD should know how to perform CPR. In addition, patients with risk factors for CAD should be constantly encouraged to make lifestyle changes to reduce the risk of cardiac arrest.

REFERENCES

1. American Heart Association: *Heart disease and stroke statistics—2006 update*, retrieved Jan 9, 2006, from http://www.americanheart.org/downloadable/heart/1136308648540statupdate2006.pdf.
2. American Heart Association: Highlights of the 2005 American Heart Association guidelines for cardiopulmonary resuscitation and emergency cardiovascular care, *Curr Cardiovasc Care* 16(4):2005-2006.
3. Thel MC, O'Connor CM: Cardiopulmonary resuscitation: historical perspective to recent investigations, *Am Heart J* 137(1):39-48, 1999.
4. Stevenson WG, Ellison KE, Sweeney MD, and others: Management of arrhythmias in heart failure, *Cardiol Rev* 10(1):8-14, 2002.
5. Trappe HJ, Brandts B, Weismueller P: Arrhythmias in the intensive care patient, *Curr Opin Crit Care* 9(5):345-355, 2003.
6. Arya A, Haghjoo M, Sadr-Ameli MA: Can amiodarone prevent sudden cardiac death in patients with hemodynamically tolerated sustained ventricular tachycardia and coronary artery disease? *Cardiovasc Drug Ther* 19(3):219-226, 2005.

CHAPTER 35

Chemical Exposure

Walter Elias, III

DEFINITION AND EPIDEMIOLOGY

Harmful chemicals are found in every aspect of life, particularly the home and workplace. Chemical exposures can occur by inhalation, ingestion, injection, or absorption through the skin and mucous membranes. Any suspected chemical exposure requires evaluation in the nearest emergency department to initiate immediate treatment.

Common household chemicals that are dangerous include shoe polishes, cosmetics, over-the-counter and prescription medications, alcohols (isopropyl alcohol, methanol, and ethanol), detergents, cleaning products (especially chlorine, ammonia, or lye-containing cleaners), rodent and insect poisons, common yard chemicals, and paints and paint products. Household chemicals are often associated with poisonings in children, but chemical exposures in the home affect people of all ages.

Chemicals abound in the workplace, and many of these cause irritation or toxicity if exposed to the human body. The Occupational Safety and Health Administration (OSHA) requires that all employers and employees be advised of chemical hazards by means of a hazards communication program, which includes having a material safety data sheet (MSDS) for each chemical used in the workplace. The employer must ensure that MSDSs are readily accessible to employees during each work shift when they are in the work area.[1] MSDSs are fact sheets provided by chemical manufacturers that list chemical, physical, and health hazard data for a particular substance. Health hazard data include routes of entry, acute and chronic effects, signs and symptoms of exposure, and emergency and first aid procedures.[2] For safety reasons and because federal law requires accurate labeling on chemical containers, it is wise to avoid the unnecessary transfer of potentially dangerous chemicals into any other containers. If transfer to another container is necessary, OSHA labeling requirements must be followed.[1]

In 2003 poisoning was the third leading cause of unintentional injury or death in the United States, resulting in 13,000 deaths.[3] These statistics demonstrate the importance of taking preventive measures against accidental chemical exposures. Prevention is best achieved by keeping medications and cleaners out of the sight and reach of children[3] and by keeping the materials clearly labeled.[1] Essential first aid materials for poisoning and the telephone number of the poison control center should also be readily available.

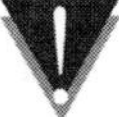

Immediate emergency department referral, physician consultation, and contact with a poison control center are indicated for chemical exposure.

PATHOPHYSIOLOGY

The pathophysiologic and systemic effects of a chemical exposure depend on the characteristics and effects of the substance, the degree and route of exposure, and patient co-morbidities.

CLINICAL PRESENTATION

For poisoning, the history should address the "Five W's": *who*—the patient's age, weight, sex, and relationship to others present; *what*—the name and dosage of the substance, co-ingestants, and amount ingested; *when*—the time and date of ingestion; *where*—both the route of poisoning and the geographic location in which the poisoning occurred, and *why*—whether the ingestion was intentional or unintentional, plus associated details. A detailed medical history should be obtained, including previous poisonings, medical conditions, and concurrent medications that might affect the patient's response to and the metabolism or elimination of ingestants; psychiatric history; and history of substance abuse. Particular attention should be given to eliciting a history of alcoholism and renal or hepatic disease.[4]

The patient who has had a toxic exposure may be affected in many different ways. The presentation of chemical exposures can range from a viral, respiratory-like syndrome to severe burns or coma.[5] With children, there often is physical evidence (e.g., a smell of cleaning products, pill or plant fragments, nonfood stains, open bottles or containers), which can be more suggestive than the symptoms themselves.[6] Adults commonly know the type of exposure unless they are incapacitated by it, in which case witnesses can usually identify the exposure. If the exposure is occupational, the chemical may be readily identifiable. Reviewing MSDSs for pertinent information after an occupational exposure may be helpful.

The following paragraphs describe a few common presentations of chemical exposure related to specific classes of chemicals. *Anticholinergics* include prescription medications such as dimenhydrinate, diphenhydramine, astemizole, loratadine, meclizine, promethazine, and tricyclic antidepressants; and household and wild plants such as mandrake, jimsonweed ("loco weed"), and nightshade. Anticholinergics cause a syndrome that is best remembered by the mnemonic "hot as Hades, blind as a bat, red as a beet, dry as a bone, mad as a hatter," which describes the syndrome of hyperthermia; mydriasis; flushed skin; dry mucous membranes, urinary retention, and decreased bowel motility; and hallucinations or frank psychosis, respectively.[7]

Alkalis are found in numerous household cleaning products, batteries, and other substances and cause irritation to the oral mucosa, esophagus, and stomach. This irritation ranges from mild to extremely severe. Both acids and alkalis cause extensive tissue damage to mucous membranes and the gastric system. The alkalis, however, are associated with a much more serious prognosis because they tend to penetrate tissues more deeply and rapidly than do the acids, particularly if the eye is involved.[7]

Hydrocarbons are the basis of many chemicals commonly used in industry and are found in garages and sheds. These substances cause a host of reactions, including coughing, vomiting, a chemical odor to the breath, and, in severe exposure, unconsciousness and coma.

PHYSICAL EXAMINATION

The initial physical examination for chemical exposure must be rapid and focused. Airway, breathing, and circulation (ABCs) must be supported and cardiac function monitored. Vital signs and cardiac function should be frequently reassessed, and a possible deterioration in the patient's status should be anticipated. The examination must focus on systems (e.g., pupils, skin, mucous membranes) to help determine clues to the chemical exposure and on adjuvant diagnostic laboratory studies.

DIAGNOSTICS AND DIFFERENTIAL DIAGNOSIS

Useful diagnostic studies in the evaluation of a chemical exposure include CBC, an electrolyte panel to calculate the anion gap, and liver function tests. If an inhalation injury is suspected, arterial blood gas studies are indicated to assess ventilation or perfusion problems related to the possible exposure. Other diagnostics should be ordered as the history warrants; examples include methemoglobin level for possible carbon monoxide toxicity or blood serum measurements of specific chemicals such as lead, arsenic, or mercury.

The differential diagnosis depends on the type, length, and route of exposure as well as on the patient's presenting signs and symptoms. Etiologies not related to the exposure (e.g., head trauma in a patient with altered mental status) and co-morbid conditions should be considered in the differential diagnosis. The poison control center and appropriate texts should be consulted for specific recommendations.

INITIAL STABILIZATION AND MANAGEMENT

The initial objective in the treatment of any chemical exposure or poisoning is to first protect or establish an airway and breathing and to ensure adequate circulation. Intubation is recommended for obtunded or comatose patients if gastric lavage is considered.[8] Once the ABCs have been established, it is important to consult the nearest poison control center and carefully examine the patient. Poison control center personnel are able to help identify the chemical and guide appropriate treatment. The main poison control telephone number ([800] 222-1222) will lead callers to their specific regional centers, and *all health care providers should be aware of the location of the main telephone number or the number to their regional poison control center.*

Physical examination findings may indicate the type of toxicologic emergency. Vital signs are particularly important, since poisonings may cause significant hypertension, hemodynamic instability, cardiac arrhythmias, conduction defects, respiratory depression, or coronary ischemia.[8] State of consciousness and presence of agitation, ocular or facial burns, and cardiopulmonary status are essential to determine.

For ingestions, therapy depends on the material ingested. It is essential to check toxicologic clinical guidelines for specific recommendations based on the substance. Possible therapeutic modalities can include gastrointestinal decontamination via gastric lavage or with activated charcoal. Gastric lavage is accomplished by inserting an orogastric tube through the mouth to the stomach and then instilling and withdrawing warmed water or normal saline solution using a syringe. Gastric lavage is acceptable for some ingestions, such as for a patient who has ingested a potentially life-threatening amount of poison, and the procedure can be undertaken within 60 minutes of ingestion.[8,9] Because the act of lavage often initiates vomiting in the victim, adequate airway protection must always be ensured. Ipecac should not be administered routinely in the management of poisoned patients.[9] It should

DIAGNOSTICS

Chemical Exposure

INITIAL

Pulse oximetry, if inhalation exposure

LABORATORY

CBC and differential
Serum electrolytes
BUN
Creatinine
Serum glucose
Anion gap
LFTs
ABGs, if inhalation exposure
Methemoglobin for carbon monoxide
Serum lead, arsenic, mercury, or other specific chemical tests*
Alcohol and drug levels*

IMAGERY

Chest x-ray for inhalation exposure*

*If indicated.

not be administered to a patient who has a decreased level or impending loss of consciousness or who has ingested a corrosive substance or hydrocarbon with high aspiration potential.[9] However, it may be useful for the telephone management of childhood ingestion in non–high-risk patients when the patient cannot reach medical care within 1 hour.[4]

Activated charcoal 1 to 2 g/kg is the mainstay of gastrointestinal decontamination. The charcoal absorbs ingested substances because of its higher exposed surface area, thereby reducing absorption by the gastrointestinal tract. However, it is not helpful for caustic acids and alkalis, alcohols, lithium, or heavy metals.[4] Activated charcoal may be given with any diluent (e.g., water, magnesium citrate, sorbitol) mixed at 240 ml/30 g of charcoal. Magnesium citrate and sorbitol can enhance gastric motility and reduce the body's absorption of the toxin.[4] Cathartics should not be administered to children younger than 1 year of age.[10]

Specific toxins have specific antidotes. The poison control center is the single best source to quickly determine these antidotes. Table 35-1 can be used as a supplementary guide until the poison control center can be reached.

TABLE 35-1 Common Chemical Exposures and Initial Management

Toxin	Symptoms and Physical Examination	Initial Stabilization	Management
Acids (toilet cleaner, drain cleaner, hydrochloric acid, sulfuric acid, battery acid)	Burns of oral mucosa, drooling, odynophagia, abdominal pain	Airway maintenance, circulatory support; sucralfate 1 g PO (may decrease symptoms but not complications)	Copiously wash mouth with cold water. Do not induce vomiting, perform lavage, or administer charcoal.
Alkalis	Caustic—burns	Dilution with water	Do not induce vomiting or perform lavage. Ingest only large amounts of water or milk. Avoid causing emesis.
Anticholinergics	Flushing of skin, blurred vision or mydriasis, tacky mucous membranes, hypoactive bowel sounds	Physostigmine	Provide 0.5-2.0 mg IV or IM over 2 minutes, q 30-60 min p.r.n.
Carbon monoxide	Headache, cherry red lips, altered consciousness, coma	Oxygen	Provide 100% hyperbaric oxygen if available.
Ethylene glycol	Cough, dizziness, headache, abdominal pain, dullness, nausea, unconsciousness, vomiting	Ethanol	Provide 10 ml/kg of a 10% ethanol solution in D5W over 30 minutes followed by 1.5 ml/kg/hr of a 10% ethanol solution to maintain blood alcohol level of 100-150 mg/dl. *OR* Provide IV fomepizole.
Isopropyl alcohol	Ethyl alcohol–like (ETOH-like) effects (altered consciousness, stupor, slurred speech)	Lavage with charcoal	Do not induce emesis; lavage is indicated if performed within 30 minutes of ingestion.
	Dizziness, gastroenteritis, stupor to coma, incoordination	Emesis, gastric lavage, correction of electrolyte alterations	Perform nasogastric or orogastric intubation with lavage; may require dialysis.
Methanol	Cough, dizziness, headache, nausea, dry skin, redness	Ethanol	See *Ethylene glycol.*
Petroleum products	Vomiting, chest or abdominal pain, cough, dyspnea, fever, arrhythmias, seizures, altered level of consciousness	Prompt gastric lavage, oxygen, respiratory support, and airway management	Initiate gastric emptying by ipecac in the alert patient (1 time only); use intubation and lavage in the unconscious or stuporous patient. Activated charcoal is controversial. Support respiration and metabolic parameters.

Most skin exposure to chemicals must be treated immediately with copious irrigation with water (i.e., "dilution is the solution to pollution"). Removal of saturated clothing and vigorous showering off of the chemical with large quantities of water are essential to prevent further damage to the patient. Exposed areas should be irrigated for at least 15 to 30 minutes. This minimizes the time the offending agent is in direct contact with the skin, thus limiting the damage caused by the chemical agent. Health care providers should be cautious during the decontamination process to avoid contaminating themselves.[11]

DISPOSITION AND REFERRAL

Once a patient's condition has been initially stabilized, he or she should be referred for definitive care. If the exposure has been minimal, follow-up with the health care provider may be all that is necessary. Severe intoxication may warrant admission to the ICU. Hospital admission should be considered if the extent of exposure is unknown or significant; this is especially true for older adults and the very young.

PREVENTION AND PATIENT EDUCATION

Toxic and chemical exposure can be easily prevented by correctly labeling, storing, and locking up potentially harmful agents and by using appropriate protective measures such as wearing appropriate personal protective equipment. Patients should be reminded to handle and dispose of hazardous chemicals appropriately, plus they should be able to recognize the signs and symptoms of chemical exposure: dizziness, headache, blurred vision, unsteady gait, clumsiness, poor coordination, difficulty breathing, nausea, abdominal cramping, skin discoloration or irritation, and eye or mucous membrane irritation. MSDSs are available online at http://www.ilpi.com/msds. The telephone number for the local poison control center should be posted on every home and business telephone for ready access if required. The U.S. national poison control hotline is (800) 222-1222.

REFERENCES

1. Occupational Safety and Health Administration: *OSHA regulations: standards—29 CFR, Hazards communication in the 21st century workplace—2004,* retrieved Dec 2, 2006, from http://www.osha.gov/SLTC/hazardcommunications/index.html.
2. Occupational Safety and Health Administration: *Appendix III material safety data sheet,* retrieved Dec 2, 2006, from http://www.oshttp://www.osha.gov/pls/oshaweb/searchresults.category?p_text=Appendix%20III%20MSDS&p_title=&p_status=CURRENT.
3. National Safety Council: *Report on injuries in America,* 2004, retrieved June 27, 2006, from http://www.nsc.org/library/report_injury_ usa.htm.
4. Larsen LC, Cummings DM: Oral poisonings: guidelines for initial evaluation and treatment, *Am Fam Phys* 57(1):85-92, 1998.
5. Verdon ME: Common clinical presentations of occupational respiratory disorders, *Am Fam Phys* 52(3):939-946, 1995.
6. Rakel RE: *Saunder's manual of medical practice,* Philadelphia, 1996, Saunders.
7. Tintinalli JE, Ruiz E, Krome RL: *Emergency medicine: a comprehensive study guide,* ed 4, New York, 1996, McGraw-Hill.
8. American Heart Association: Toxicology in emergency cardiovascular care, *Circulation* 112(24):IV 126-132, 2005.
9. Krenzelok EP, McGuigan M, Lheur P: Position statement: ipecac syrup: American Academy of Clinical Toxicology; European Association of Poisons Centres and Clinical Toxicologists, *J Toxicol Clin Toxicol* 35(7):699-709, 1997.
10. Hay WW, Hay W, Groothuis J, and others: *Current pediatric diagnosis and treatment,* ed 13, Stanford, Calif, 1997, Appleton & Lange.
11. Simpson WM Jr, Schuman SH: Recognition and management of acute pesticide poisoning, *Am Fam Phys* 65(8):1599-1604, 2002.

CHAPTER 36

Electrical Injuries

Updated by Terry Mahan Buttaro

DEFINITION AND EPIDEMIOLOGY

Injuries from an electrical accident can be minor or can cause severe damage, electrocution, or death from cardiopulmonary arrest. In the United States approximately 50,000 people are hospitalized yearly for electrical injuries.[1] One thousand are killed each year in electrical accidents.[2] Although the actual number of accidental and environmental electrical injuries is uncertain, the second leading cause of death in the workplace is electrical injury.[3] Lightning is the most common lethal natural phenomenon, causing approximately 300 to 600 deaths yearly.[1] From 20% to 30% of persons struck by lightning die; 70% of the survivors have permanent sequelae. Electrical injuries caused by low-voltage current account for 60% to 70% of reported electrical injury and are responsible for nearly half of deaths from electrical shock and 1% of accidental deaths in the home.[4] The majority of household electrocutions involve 110- or 220-V current and are usually due to failure to ground tools or appliances or the use of hair dryers or other electrical devices near water. Contact with low- and high-voltage electrical current is responsible for a significant number of injuries in children.[5] The most common cause of electrical injury in children under age 6 years is oral contact with electrical cords or wall sockets and the placement of conductive bodies in wall sockets. Adolescent boys 11 to 18 years of age often sustain high-voltage injuries.[5]

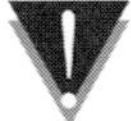

Immediate emergency department referral or physician consultation is indicated for patients with electrical injuries.

PATHOPHYSIOLOGY

Electrical injuries result from the direct effects of current and from the conversion of electrical energy into thermal energy as current passes through body tissues. Factors that determine the severity and distribution of injury include the type of current, voltage, amperage, tissue resistance, surface contacted, pathway of current, duration of contact, and other associated trauma.[6] Alternating current (AC), the more common cause of electrical injuries, is more dangerous than direct current (DC) because it can produce tetanic skeletal muscle contractions and prevent the victim from letting go of the energized source, thus increasing current delivery to the victim. AC voltage at 25 to 300 Hz and 25 to 220 V, the common household current level, can easily cause ventricular fibrillation if the pathway of the current includes the heart. Low-voltage contact, although potentially lethal, does not result in the magnitude of tissue necrosis seen with high-voltage injury. The voltage in a lightning strike is in the range of 10 million to 2 billion V, but the duration of a lightning strike is short.

Heat generation is responsible for most burns seen with electrical injuries. Heat damage is proportional to tissue resistance. Tissues with high fluid and electrolyte content conduct electrical current better than others. Listed in decreasing order of magnitude of tissue necrosis are nerves, blood vessels, muscle, skin, tendon, fat, and bone. Nerve tissue has the least resistance to direct flow and therefore is most easily damaged.[7] Electrical current passing through the head or crossing the thorax is more likely to cause respiratory arrest or ventricular fibrillation than current passing through the leg. Skin, the initial barrier to current flow, is an effective insulator to deeper tissues. As current flows from the contact point, tissue with the least electrical resistance sustains the greatest current density and destructive injury. The most severe cutaneous and deep injuries are adjacent to contact sites, and the damage decreases with increasing distance from damage points.

CLINICAL PRESENTATION

The spectrum of electrical injury ranges from a transient unpleasant sensation to instantaneous death. Cardiopulmonary arrest is the primary cause of immediate fatalities from electrical injury and is common in patients with high-voltage electrical and lightning injury. In lightning injuries cardiac activity can spontaneously return, but the associated respiratory arrest often continues, causing death.[6] Common sequelae are hypertension; tachycardia; cardiac muscle necrosis; respiratory paralysis; burns; fractures; ruptured tympanic membrane; hyphema; vitreous hemorrhage; and injuries to the spinal cord, peripheral nervous system, and vascular systems.[3,8] Oliguria or anuria from deep tissue damage and rhabdomyolysis can cause acute renal failure.[8] Visible myoglobinuria indicates massive acute muscle necrosis and impending renal failure. Disseminated intravascular coagulation can result from massive trauma.[8] Neurologic deficits are sometimes evident immediately after the current exposure. However, complications such as reflex sympathetic dystrophy and motor neuron disease may not become apparent for days to months after the electrical trauma.[8,9] Long bone fracture often occurs with falls, and fractures (particularly of the vertebral column) can result from tetanic muscle contraction at the time of electrocution.[10] Cataracts can form up to 2 years after such injury. Direct injury to internal organs is uncommon.

PHYSICAL EXAMINATION

When evaluating a victim with an electrical injury, the health care provider should always completely undress the patient to determine entry and exit wounds and associated injuries. Patients should be assessed for associated cranial, spinal, or other trauma, and the neck should initially be treated as being unstable, particularly with DC injuries. Arrhythmic conduction disturbances and infarct patterns can be present on the ECG. Cardiopulmonary presentations vary, and most patients lack the characteristic chest discomfort indicative of myocardial ischemia. Transient, mild paresthesias and complete and irreversible impairment of sensory or motor function, or both, can be present in patients with electrical injuries. Absent pulses, decreased peripheral perfusion, and impaired neurologic function are also seen in patients with acute vascular complications from electrical trauma.

Injuries consistent with findings of blunt trauma to the head, spinal cord, musculoskeletal, intrathoracic, and intraabdominal areas can be present in patients who were thrown from the energized current source, had forceful tetanic muscle contractions associated with AC injuries, or fell after losing consciousness and muscle control. Skin wounds are typically leathery or charred areas of full-thickness skin loss. The patient with lightning injury may have linear, punctate, feathery burns that often are referred to as Lichtenberg's flowers. The entry and exit sites are usually depressed, giving the appearance that current exploded the tissue. Underlying injury to a major muscle compartment is accompanied by edema formation. Circulatory integrity is best judged with Doppler ultrasound of distal pulses.

DIAGNOSTICS

Initial studies include CBC, electrolytes, glucose, BUN, creatinine, coagulation profile, arterial blood gas analysis, creatinine phosphokinase level, creatine kinase muscle-brain (MB) fraction, and myoglobin level.[11] A 12-lead ECG and continuous cardiac monitoring are necessary for all patients with electrical injury. Fetal monitoring is necessary if the victim is pregnant.[12] Patients with suspected spinal injuries should undergo cervical spine radiographs. Other x-ray studies are indicated to exclude fracture if localized edema and pain are present.[10] Consideration of other diagnostic studies should be coordinated with the consulting specialists.

DIAGNOSTICS

Electrical Injuries

INITIAL
ECG

LABORATORY
CBC and differential
Serum electrolytes
BUN
Creatinine
Serum glucose
Coagulation studies
ABGs
Creatinine phosphokinase level
Creatine kinase muscle-brain (MB) fraction
Myoglobin

DIFFERENTIAL DIAGNOSIS

The diagnosis of electrical injury may be unclear, particularly in unwitnessed cases in which the victim is confused, amnestic, or unconscious or in instances in which external signs of injury are absent. In these cases, several conditions should be considered as part of the differential diagnosis: cardiopulmonary arrest, arrhythmias, peripheral neuropathies, seizures, and nonelectrical trauma. Circumstances surrounding the electrical injuries should also be sought to determine the possible mechanism of the injury. Precipitating factors such as intoxication, suicidal intention, or foul play should be considered.

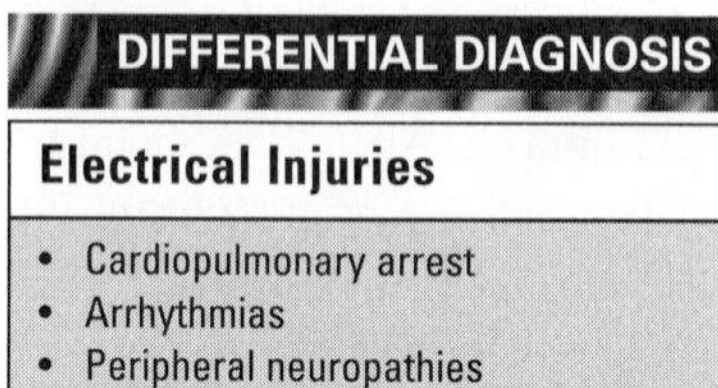
DIFFERENTIAL DIAGNOSIS

Electrical Injuries

- Cardiopulmonary arrest
- Arrhythmias
- Peripheral neuropathies
- Seizures
- Nonelectrical trauma

INITIAL STABILIZATION AND MANAGEMENT

Immediate priorities for patients include the airway, breathing, and circulation (ABCs) taught in basic life support and advanced cardiac life support classes. The cervical spine should be immobilized and the airway secured while supporting respiration, with adequate oxygenation and stabilization of circulation if required. CPR must be initiated, and the emergency medical services system should be activated if necessary. Defibrillation is indicated for ventricular tachycardia or ventricular fibrillation, and early intubation is recommended for patients with facial or neck burns.[6] Continued thermal damage can be limited by removing affected clothing.[6] Intravascular volume is replenished with lactated Ringer's or normal saline solution with a bolus of 10 to 20 ml/kg to maintain urinary output at approximately 1 ml/kg/hr. Myoglobinuria is treated by alkalinizing the urine by adding sodium bicarbonate to the IV fluids (i.e., 44 to 50 mEq of bicarbonate to 1 L of lactated Ringer's or normal saline solution).[13]

Wound care involves treating both cutaneous and deep soft tissue injuries with a saline dressing. Consultation with a surgeon should be considered to evaluate the need for formal wound exploration and debridement. Tetanus prophylaxis should be updated. Prophylactic antibiotics have not been shown to decrease episodes of infection and usually are not indicated. Management of other complications resulting from electrical trauma generally follows standard emergency therapy.

DISPOSITION AND REFERRAL

Prompt specialty consultation is required in addition to the liberal involvement of surgical specialists. All patients who have lost consciousness or sustained cardiac or respiratory arrest, as well as those with ischemic chest pain, myoglobinuria, or significant burn wounds, should be hospitalized. Referral to a burn center is often necessary for electrical burns because considerable injury to deeper neurovascular and musculoskeletal structures may not be obvious until several days after the injury.

PREVENTION AND PATIENT AND FAMILY EDUCATION

All discharged patients should have reliable home support. Patients should be advised to return immediately to their health care provider if any symptoms occur. A specific follow-up visit should be arranged with a health care provider familiar with electrical injuries, and patients should receive careful explanation of the injury and recuperative process.

Open sockets and outlets must be covered with "child-proof" devices, and children must be watched carefully. Plug-in electrical appliances should be kept away from the bathtub. Community education programs, particularly at school and at work, are necessary to help prevent accidents. Safety standards in industry and in the community must be constantly updated and enforced.[14]

REFERENCES

1. American Burn Association: *Look up and live: prevention for electrical injuries*, 2005, retrieved June 26, 2006, from http://www.ameriburn.org/Preven/2005Prevention/ABA2005PreventionCampaign.pdf.
2. Martinez JA, Nguyen T: Electrical injuries, *South Med J* 12:1165-1167, 2000, retrieved June 26, 2006, from http://www.medscape.com/viewarticle/410681_3.
3. Pinto DS, Clardy P: *Environmental electrical injuries*, retrieved June 26, 2006, from http://www.uptodate.com.
4. Rakel R: *Textbook of family practice,* ed 5, Philadelphia, 1995, Saunders.

5. Rai J, Jeschke MG, Barrow RE, and others: Electrical injuries: a 30-year review, *J Trauma* 46(5):933-936, 1999.
6. American Heart Association: Electric shock and lightning strikes, *Circulation* 112(24):IV 154-155, 2005.
7. Tintinalli J, Ruiz E, Krone R: *Emergency medicine,* New York, 1996, McGraw-Hill.
8. Fish RM: Electrical injuries, part 2, Specific injuries, *J Emerg Med* 18(1):27-34, 2000.
9. Jafari H, Couratier P, Camu W: Motor neuron disease is a potential complication of lightning or electrical shock, *J Neurol Neurosurg Psychiatr* 71(2):265-267, 2001.
10. Hostetler MA, Davis CO: Galeazzi fracture resulting from electrical shock, *Pediatr Emerg Care* 16(4):258-259, 2000.
11. Schwartz GR: *Principles and practice of emergency medicine,* Philadelphia, 1992, Lea & Febiger.
12. Fish RM: Electrical injuries, part 3, Cardiac monitoring indications, the pregnant patient, and lightning, *J Emerg Med* 18(2):181-187, 2000.
13. Bennett J, Plum F: *Cecil textbook of medicine,* ed 21, Philadelphia, 1996, Saunders.
14. Marx JA, Hockberg RS, Walls RM, and others: *Rosen's emergency medicine: concepts and clinical practice,* ed 6, Philadelphia, 2006, Mosby.

CHAPTER 37

Head Trauma

Denise A. Vanacore and
Terry Mahan Buttaro

DEFINITION AND EPIDEMIOLOGY

Traumatic brain injury (TBI) is a significant cause of morbidity and mortality in this country. Each year more than 50,000 people die from TBI, and an additional 235,000 people are hospitalized.[1] Most of these deaths are related to motor vehicle accidents, violence, or falls. Other causes include sports injuries and bicycle accidents. Among children, bicycle accidents account for an estimated 140,000 head injuries each year.[1] Head injuries from falls occur most often in children younger than 2 years of age and in persons older than 65 years of age, whereas motor vehicle accidents are the leading cause of brain injury in persons ages 5 to 64 years.[1,2] Approximately 11% of fall-related TBIs are fatal.[1] Older patients are particularly vulnerable and can sustain a subdural hematoma even when the head injury is not associated with loss of consciousness.[3]

The National Center for Injury Prevention and Control reports that 5.3 million Americans have a TBI-related disability.[1] Brain injury can be mild or severe enough to dramatically affect a patient's intellectual and physical capacity, as well as his or her psychologic, social, and economic well-being. Loss of consciousness is one of the most significant indicators of brain injury.

The severity of damage can be described by an injury-rating system such as the Glasgow Coma Scale (GCS) score (Table 37-1). The GCS assesses eye opening responses, motor

TABLE 37-1 Glasgow Coma Scale

Sign	Score
EYE OPENING	
Spontaneous	4
To verbal command	3
To pain	2
No response	1
BEST MOTOR RESPONSE	
Obeys verbal commands	6
Localizes pain	5
Movement or withdrawal to pain	4
Flexion response to pain (decorticate)	3
Extension response to pain (decerebrate)	2
No response	1
BEST VERBAL RESPONSE	
Alert and oriented	5
Converses but confused/disoriented	4
Nonsensical/inappropriate words	3
Nonspecific sounds	2
No response	1

responses, and verbal responses. Numbers are assigned for the level of function attained in each category and then totaled. A normal patient has a score of 15, whereas a patient who is brain dead has a score of 3. Minor head trauma is defined as an initial GCS of 13 to 15 and a period of unconsciousness of less than 20 minutes. Moderate head injury refers to an initial GCS score of 9 to 12 with or without loss of consciousness. Severe head trauma is defined as an initial GCS of less than 8 or a comatose state for 6 hours or more.[4]

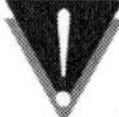

Immediate emergency department referral or physician consultation is indicated for head trauma with alteration in level of consciousness, paralysis, paresthesia, rhinorrhea, raccoon's sign (ecchymosis beneath both eyes), Battle's sign, otorrhea, and hemotympanum.

PATHOPHYSIOLOGY

Head trauma can consist of soft tissue injury, skull fracture, or both. Brain injury from trauma can occur in two stages: primary and secondary. Primary injury is sustained as a direct result of the initial insult and may result from blunt trauma, penetrating injury, coup-contrecoup lacerations or contusions of the brain, or direct disruption of brain tissue by the shearing of axons. Secondary injury may occur as a result of increased intracranial pressure (ICP), cerebral hypoxia, systemic hypotension, or decreased cerebral blood flow. This may cause further neuronal damage, which can compromise an already injured brain. The cranial vault is a fixed space that contains the brain, cerebrospinal fluid (CSF), and blood. Because the skull limits intracranial volume, neurologic damage after head injury can be directly related to cerebral edema that causes increased ICP, which in turn decreases cerebral blood flow and causes cerebral ischemia.

CLINICAL PRESENTATION

It is important to establish the mechanism of the trauma, the stability or progression of the patient's symptoms, the patient's prior condition, and the patient's significant medical history. The cause of the injury should be determined: Was it accidental or intentional?[2] Changes in mentation and level of consciousness should be noted and elicited from witnesses. A history of amnesia concerning the traumatic event often indicates altered consciousness. It is also necessary to ascertain consciousness before the head injury to identify other pathologic conditions such as stroke, myocardial infarction, or respiratory distress. Additional causes of altered mental status, such as hypoglycemia, drug overdose, hyperthermia, or arrhythmias, must also be investigated. Alcohol intoxication can mask the signs and symptoms of a head injury; therefore it is important to determine if alcohol was involved. The history should also elicit complaints of headache, nausea, vomiting, unsteady gait, visual changes, tinnitus, difficulty concentrating, and emotional lability.

PHYSICAL EXAMINATION

The patient with head trauma can fluctuate from being awake and alert to being comatose and in respiratory distress. The initial evaluation should follow the standard protocol developed for all trauma patients. The patient's airway, breathing, and circulation (ABCs) and cervical spine must be evaluated and stabilized. The initial observation should focus on the patient's level of consciousness, vital signs, and determination of GCS score. A quick but thorough neurologic examination is necessary to assess brain injury, focal deficits, and patient stability. The neurologic examination should include pupillary response, extraocular motion, Romberg's test, gait, finger to nose test, memory, and concentration. The skull must also be examined for fractures, penetrating injuries, lacerations, or CSF drainage. Clinical signs of skull fracture include raccoon's sign (bruising around the orbit), Battle's sign, and blood in the external auditory canal. It is also important to perform repeated neurologic examinations to determine whether the patient's condition is stable, improving, or deteriorating. However, a normal neurologic examination does not eliminate the possibility of brain injury. The severity of injury and prognosis are indicated by the amount of retrograde or posttraumatic amnesia.

DIAGNOSTICS

Because patients with head injury can have an associated cervical spine fracture, an x-ray examination of the cervical spine is necessary. A nonenhanced CT scan or x-ray is indicated for patients with a depressed or deteriorating level of consciousness, skull fracture, neurologic deficit, open head wound, penetrating head injury, amnesia, or high risk of intracranial injury. Repeat CT scans may be necessary if neurologic deficits develop.[5] Although an MRI has a limited role in head injury, it does reveal anatomic detail and can identify diffuse axonal injury. Laboratory studies should include CBC, electrolytes, serum glucose, urinalysis, arterial blood gases (ABGs), coagulation panel, blood alcohol level, and, if indicated, a drug/ alcohol screen. Blood should be sent immediately for type and crossmatch. Further examinations may be indicated in cases of severe trauma.

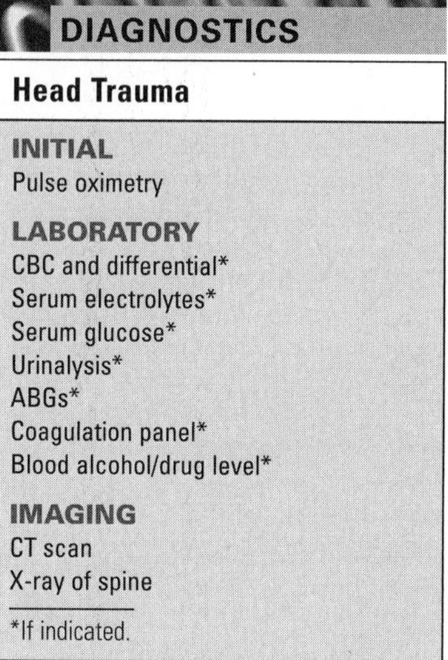

DIAGNOSTICS

Head Trauma

INITIAL
Pulse oximetry

LABORATORY
CBC and differential*
Serum electrolytes*
Serum glucose*
Urinalysis*
ABGs*
Coagulation panel*
Blood alcohol/drug level*

IMAGING
CT scan
X-ray of spine

*If indicated.

DIFFERENTIAL DIAGNOSIS

The differential diagnosis must include skull fracture, concussion, cerebral contusion, epidural hematoma, subdural hematoma, subarachnoid bleeding, cerebral edema, and penetrating injuries. *Cerebral concussion* is defined as the loss of consciousness without significant anatomic damage to the brain. The severity of the injury is quantified

DIFFERENTIAL DIAGNOSIS

Head Trauma

- Skull fracture, concussion, or contusion
- Epidural or subdural hematoma
- Subarachnoid bleed
- Cerebral edema
- Penetrating injuries

by the duration of amnesia—the length of amnesia concerning the time before impact (antegrade amnesia) plus the length of amnesia after impact (retrograde amnesia). It is usually helpful to determine the time interval between the first thing and the last thing remembered. Cerebral contusions usually occur on the undersurface of the poles of the frontal lobes or on the poles of the temporal lobes. The patient is typically awake and alert after the initial injury, but increasing ICP, decreased level of consciousness, and focal neurologic deficits may develop as the contusion mass increases in size.

INITIAL STABILIZATION AND MANAGEMENT

The main priority in the patient with head injury is the same as that for all trauma patients—management of the ABCs and cervical spine. Once that is achieved, the principal goal is to assess the primary injury and to rapidly recognize a surgically correctable lesion. CT scans are not indicated for patients with minor head trauma or a GCS score of 15 or more. Patients without loss of consciousness, amnesia, focal neurologic deficits, or depressed skull fracture do not require a CT scan. These patients may be discharged home if observation is available and instructions are given on proper patient evaluation. Minor head injuries (loss of consciousness for less than 5 minutes, amnesia, a GCS score of 12 to 14, impaired alertness, or depressed skull fracture) require a diagnostic CT scan.[5]

Health care providers must always be aware of the "talk and deteriorate" syndrome. Patients with this syndrome utter recognizable words after the head injury and then deteriorate to a severe, brain-injured condition within 48 hours. The most common neurologic findings are altered mental status and focal hemispheric deficits. Early and appropriate use of CT scanning is helpful in detecting significant intracranial lesions before clinical neurologic deterioration occurs.

DISPOSITION AND REFERRAL

The patient may be discharged home with proper instructions if the CT scan is normal and if a family member or friend can provide close observation for 24 hours. If no one is available to monitor the patient or if there is evidence of a pathologic condition, the patient should be admitted to the hospital for observation. A patient who has had more than 5 minutes of unconsciousness, posttraumatic seizures, a GCS score of 12 to 14, focal neurologic deficits, a lesion on the CT scan, or a moderate head injury (a GCS score of 9 to 12) should be hospitalized, stabilized, and closely observed for any neurologic deterioration; a neurosurgical evaluation is also indicated. Patients with severe head trauma (a GCS score of 8 or less, penetrating skull injuries, or compound skull fractures) should be evaluated at the nearest hospital and have a neurosurgical evaluation.

PATIENT AND FAMILY EDUCATION

Specific instructions must be provided to those who will be observing the patient who is discharged home. The patient should remain in the care of a competent caregiver and rest in a quiet environment for the first 24 hours after discharge. The first 24 hours after the injury are the most important. The patient should return for treatment if any of the following develop: drowsiness or difficulty awakening (the patient should be awakened every 2 hours during sleep), continuous nausea, vomiting more than twice, seizures or convulsions, visual disturbances or pupillary changes, new-onset weakness or an inability to move body parts, severe headache, confusion, personality changes, unusual restlessness, difficulty breathing, dizziness, or difficulty walking.[4] Aspirin (and medications that contain aspirin), alcohol, and narcotics should not be taken for 1 week after the injury.

Patients should also be informed about the posttraumatic or postconcussion syndrome, which is not life threatening but may disable a patient for weeks to months. Symptoms may include headache, tinnitus, memory loss, dizziness, giddiness, poor concentration, emotional lability, irritability, nervousness, disturbed sleep, fatigue, and decreased libido. Symptoms last for 2 to 6 weeks in most cases but can be present for 1 to 2 years. Treatment consists of rest, reassurance, and analgesics. It is also extremely important that patients return to work as soon as possible, even if a reduced workload is necessary.

Patients must be educated regarding safety issues such as the proper use of bicycle helmets, seat belts, and car seats for infants and children. Safety issues in the home should also be reviewed (e.g., staircases, gates, throw rugs, and lighting) in an attempt to reduce falls in children and older adults.

REFERENCES

1. National Center for Injury Prevention and Control: retrieved May 9, 2006, from http://www.cdc.gov/ncipc/didop/StateInjuryIndicatorsTBI.htm.
2. Caviness AC: *Skull fractures in children*, retrieved May 30, 2002, from http://www.uptodate.com.
3. Evans RW: Geriatric headache, *Ann Long-Term Care* 10(5):28-35, 2002.
4. Logan P: *Principles of practice for the acute care nurse practitioner*, Stamford, Conn, 1999, Appleton & Lange.
5. Odishoo TA: CT imaging for minor head injury, *Nurse Pract* 31(9):49-56, 2005.

CHAPTER 38

Hypotension

JoAnn Trybulski

DEFINITION AND EPIDEMIOLOGY

Hypotension, or low blood pressure, is a relative term, and its evaluation in the office setting presents a challenge. Whatever the absolute blood pressure measurement or cause, health care providers must be prepared to manage hypotension in the ambulatory setting.

In those patients accustomed to elevated pressures, a sudden decrease to 110 mm Hg systolic may cause symptoms. On the other hand, some patients may routinely have a systolic blood pressure in the 90s and be asymptomatic. Clinical conditions may also produce symptomatic low blood pressure. Postural (orthostatic) hypotension is low blood pressure that results from assumption of the upright position and has been found in epidemiologic surveys to affect from 5% to 20% of patients over 65 years of age.[1] Another form of hypotension, postprandial hypotension, occurs after meals. The causes of symptomatic hypotension are multiple, and the morbidity ranges from the transient symptoms of vasovagal episodes to life-threatening conditions such as hemorrhage, pulmonary embolus, myocardial failure, myocardial infarction, or arrhythmia.

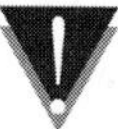

Immediate emergency department referral and physician consultation are indicated for unstable, hemodynamically compromised patients.

PATHOPHYSIOLOGY

When blood pressure is decreased, there is an alteration in one of the three basic components necessary for the maintenance of blood pressure. The first component is the state of contraction of the muscles in the vessel walls themselves. Some physiologic endocrine states or autonomic nervous system dysfunction may cause abnormal relaxation of the muscles in the vessel walls, sequestering blood and causing a decrease in blood pressure. The second component is the intravascular volume. When fluid is depleted through bleeding, vomiting, or diarrhea, this decrease in intravascular volume produces low blood pressure. The final component is the state of the cardiac muscle. Any failure in critical pumping function of the heart produces decreased pressure in the vascular system.

The pathophysiologic mechanisms for postural hypotension involve autonomic failure or volume depletion. Autonomic failure represents a dysfunction of the postganglionic sympathetic nerves in which these neurons fail to release appropriate amounts of norepinephrine, producing impaired vasoconstriction, thus reducing intravascular volume and producing hypotension.[1] Autonomic failure is produced by some medications (e.g., antihypertensives, vasodilators, nitrates, calcium channel blockers, antidepressants, opiates, alcohol) or as a result of neurologic conditions such as reflex syncope (e.g., carotid sinus hypersensitivity, micturition syncope, defecation syncope), postural orthostatic tachycardia syndrome, degenerative neurologic diseases, and some peripheral neuropathy syndromes.[1] Decreased baroreceptor sensitivity is the pathophysiologic mechanism for the often observed, milder form of postural hypotension seen in older persons.[1]

The mechanism of postprandial hypotension is poorly understood. Normally, there is meal-induced pooling of blood in the splanchnic circulation, with resulting sympathetic nervous system activation as compensatory mechanism. A default in this sympathetic compensation produces a decrease in cardiac output and systemic vascular resistance, resulting in hypotension.[1] Other factors implicated include vasodilation produced by postprandial insulin release or gastrointestinal peptides that have vasoactive effects.[1]

Symptomatic hypotension produces low perfusion of all body tissues. Vital organs such as the kidneys, brain, and heart are particularly at risk in hypoperfusion states. Hypoperfusion of the kidneys precipitates failure. With inadequate oxygen supplied to the brain, function and consciousness are impaired. Moreover, hypoperfusion of cardiac muscle carries the risk of myocardial ischemia.[2]

CLINICAL PRESENTATION

Most patients with hypotension complain of being dizzy or light-headed. Some may relate that their symptoms occur only when they sit or stand. Patients exhibiting a vasovagal response also describe a sensation of impending syncope. Tachycardia is produced as a compensatory attempt to maintain blood pressure. The existence of associated signs and symptoms, such as vomiting, chest pain, diaphoresis, urticaria, dyspnea, hematochezia, or palpitations, provides important clues concerning the etiology of the hypotension.

PHYSICAL EXAMINATION

Pulse and blood pressure are measured with the patient in the lying, sitting, and standing positions (if patient response allows it). A low blood pressure, absolute or in comparison with the patient's normal pressure, when the patient is lying down confirms the diagnosis, particularly if the decrease is associated with dizziness, light-headedness, or tachycardia.

DIAGNOSTICS

A 20 mm Hg decrease in systolic blood pressure, a 10 mm Hg decrease in diastolic blood pressure, or symptoms of dizziness or light-headedness when the patient changes position from lying to standing confirm the diagnosis of postural or orthostatic hypotension.[3] Failure to increase the pulse with the decrease in blood pressure is indicative of cardiac disorder or autonomic dysfunction.[3] However, young patients may maintain their systolic blood pressure and exhibit an increased pulse with a position change in conjunction with symptoms of cerebral hypoperfusion (fatigue, light-headedness, exercise intolerance, or cognitive impairment); this represents the syndrome of postural autonomic tachycardia.[1]

Additional physical examination and diagnostic tests, including an ECG, electrolytes, glucose, BUN, creatinine, chest x-ray examination, tilt-table test, CT or lung scan, and endocrine studies, are obtained to confirm or eliminate conditions as the cause of hypotension, based on the patient's presentation. In addition, a thorough medication history is

DIAGNOSTICS

Hypotension

INITIAL
ECG*

LABORATORY
Serum electrolytes
BUN
Creatinine
Serum glucose
CBC and differential
Urinalysis
Endocrine studies*

IMAGERY
Chest x-ray*
CT scan

OTHER
Tilt-table test*

*If indicated.

obtained and a side effect profile for each drug is reviewed, since many hypertension medications, psychotropics, or muscle relaxants have hypotension as a potential side effect.

DIFFERENTIAL DIAGNOSIS

See the Differential Diagnosis box for possible causes of hypotension.

INITIAL STABILIZATION AND MANAGEMENT

The patient with hypotension initially should be placed in a recumbent position. Supplemental oxygen is essential for those patients in whom bleeding, myocardial infarction or failure, arrhythmia, or pulmonary embolus is suspected or for any patient with breathing difficulty. If hypovolemia is suspected, a fluid challenge of 250 to 500 ml of normal saline solution is administered intravenously, and its effect on the blood pressure is assessed.[4]

DIFFERENTIAL DIAGNOSIS

Hypotension

- Hypovolemia
- Vasovagal response
- Myocardial disease
- Heart failure
- Active bleeding
- Pulmonary embolus
- Arrhythmia
- Diabetic neuropathy
- Malnutrition
- Adrenal insufficiency
- Drug-induced condition
- Organic dementia
- Anaphylaxis
- Heat exhaustion
- Autonomic dysfunction

The suspected cause of the hypotension guides further diagnostic evaluation and management. Nonpharmacologic interventions for postural (orthostatic) hypotension include arising slowly; avoiding coughing, straining, or walking in hot weather; raising the head of the bed 10 to 20 degrees for sleep; using custom-fitted elastic stockings (although these may not be tolerated by patients with motor dysfunction or neuropathies); exercising; increasing water intake; and crossing the legs to stand.[5] Additional interventions for orthostatic hypotension are dorsiflexing the feet several times before arising; eating small, frequent meals; increasing fluid and salt intake; elevating the head of the bed 5 to 20 degrees; wearing compression stockings; and reserving vigorous activities until later in the day.[6] Postprandial hypotension treatment recommendations include reducing carbohydrate intake, avoiding large meals, limiting alcohol ingestion, and reducing activity immediately after eating.[5]

Pharmacologic therapy is instituted in conjunction with physician consultation. Medications used include fludrocortisone as a first-line agent for orthostatic hypotension; second-line agents are sympathomimetics such as midodrine.[5] Supplementary agents such as NSAIDs and caffeine are used in conjunction with first- or second-line medications.[5] In cases of autonomic failure associated with anemia or decreased red cell mass, erythropoietin is used.[6] There are a variety of third-line agents and investigational medications.

DISPOSITION AND REFERRAL

Patients with hypotension as a result of dehydration may be hydrated on an outpatient basis. Patients with poor response to a fluid challenge may need rapid transport to an emergency facility for further diagnosis, consultation, and treatment.

PREVENTION AND PATIENT EDUCATION

Patients taking medications that have orthostatic hypotension as a side effect are taught to change position or to arise from sitting slowly. Maintaining adequate fluid intake while in a hot environment, and when vomiting or diarrhea occurs, is essential to avoid hypovolemia from dehydration. Patients at risk for dehydration (or their caregivers) are instructed to report any signs of dehydration (e.g., dry mucous membranes, light-headedness, altered mentation, or diminished urinary output) to the health care provider.

REFERENCES

1. Kaufman H, Kaplan NM, Freeman R: *Mechanisms and causes of orthostatic and postprandial hypotension,* retrieved Jan 18, 2001, from http://www.uptodate.com.
2. Beique F, Ramsey V: Cardiopulmonary circulation in the critically ill. In Garrard C, Foex P, Westaby S, editors: *Principles and practices of critical care,* New York, 1997, Oxford University Press.
3. Reilly BM, editor: *Practice strategies in outpatient medicine,* ed 2, Philadelphia, 1991, Saunders.
4. Iseke RJ: Heat related illnesses. In Noble J, editor: *Textbook of primary care medicine,* ed 3, St Louis, 1996, Mosby.
5. Kaufman H, Freeman R, Kaplan NM: *Treatment of orthostatic and postprandial hypotension,* retrieved May 6, 2006, from http://www.uptodate.com.
6. Bradley JG, Davis KA: Orthostatic hypotension, *Am Fam Phys* 68:2393-2398, 2003.

CHAPTER 39

Poisoning

Denise A. Vanacore
Updated by Terry Mahan Buttaro

DEFINITION AND EPIDEMIOLOGY

Although poisonings are most commonly associated with ingestion, toxic effects can also be caused by injection, inhalation, or absorption through skin or mucous membranes. The effects of the poisoning are not always initially obvious, but the toxic substances can subsequently affect various organ systems. The American Association of Poison Control Centers (AAPCC) reports more than 2 million poisonings annually, although accidental and intentional ingestions of toxic substances are not always reported. In 2000, 2.2 million poison exposures were reported in the United States; 920 deaths occurred as a result of these exposures.[1] Poisoning remains one of the leading causes of death in the United States and in 2000 was the primary cause of death in the home.[2] More than 50% of poisonings occur in children less than 6 years of age.[1] Fortunately, the AAPCC is available 24 hours a day ([800] 222-1222) to provide treatment information regarding toxicologic substances.[3]

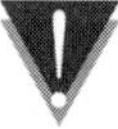

Immediate emergency department referral or physician consultation is indicated for victims of poisoning. The goal is to treat the patient as soon as possible after the event.

PATHOPHYSIOLOGY

Pathophysiology depends on the poisonous substance and on the route, duration, and amount of exposure. The patient's underlying physical condition and initial first aid measures will also affect the impact of the toxin.

CLINICAL PRESENTATION

Specific signs and symptoms sometimes enable medical personnel to identify the type of poisoning. A thorough history and physical examination also can aid in identifying the substance. Often, however, these details are not readily available because of the patient's mental status and physical condition. The toxin, time and amount of exposure, and cause (accidental vs. intentional) are important details that sometimes can be elicited from family, friends, or witnesses, or can be determined by examination of the patient's clothes or valuables or objects noted at the scene of the exposure. In addition, some toxins cause a characteristic group of symptoms called *toxidromes* (a constellation of signs and symptoms related to a particular toxic substance), which can alert the provider to the presence of a particular substance (Table 39-1). Acetaminophen and other over-the-counter pain medications should be considered with patients with a past medical history of chronic pain syndrome.[4]

PHYSICAL EXAMINATION

The physical examination should assess mental status and vital signs and determine the presence of any toxidromes. A focused but complete examination of the cardiovascular, respiratory, and neurologic systems is essential. The toxicologic substance and type of poisoning will dictate the need for additional evaluation (e.g., skin, gastrointestinal [GI] tract).

TABLE 39-1 Symptoms and Substances

Symptom	Toxic Substances
Hallucinations	Atropine, cocaine, PCP, LSD
Seizures	Strychnine, anticholinergics, isoniazid, theophylline, nortriptyline
Increased vital signs	Sympathomimetics, anticholinergics
Mydriasis	Anticholinergics, sympathomimetics
Miosis	Organophosphates, narcotics, bromide, acetone, clonidine, heroin
Nonreactive pupils	Anticholinergics
Horizontal nystagmus	Alcohol, lithium, carbamazepine, solvents, memprobamate, quinine, primidone
Decreased respirations	Opiates, organophosphates, barbiturates, beta blockers, benzodiazepines, alcohol, clonidine
Bradycardia	Opiates, organophosphates, barbiturates, beta blockers, benzodiazepines, alcohol, clonidine
Decreased temperature	Opiates, organophosphates, barbiturates, beta blockers, benzodiazepines, alcohol, clonidine
Periorbital edema	Fish poisoning
Abdominal cramps, nausea or vomiting, diarrhea	Fish poisoning, corrosive materials (lye, iodine), cocaine
Tachycardia	Cyclic antidepressants, strychnine, cocaine

LSD, Lysergic acid diethylamide, *PCP*, phencyclidines.

Many substances can cause changes in mental status, ranging from agitation or delirium to coma. Some characteristic signs and symptoms may suggest a particular substance. Atropine, cocaine, phencyclidine (PCP), and lysergic acid diethylamide (LSD) may cause hallucinations. Strychnine can cause seizures in an otherwise alert patient. Other drugs that are known to cause seizures include anticholinergics, isoniazid, and theophylline. Sympathomimetics and anticholinergics cause increased vital sign values. A below-normal temperature, respiratory rate, and heart rate may be a result of opiates, organophosphates, barbiturates, beta blockers, benzodiazepines, alcohol, or clonidine. Anticholinergic and sympathomimetic substances can cause mydriasis, whereas organophosphates, narcotics, bromide, acetone, clonidine, and nicotine may cause miosis. Cocaine does not interfere with reactivity of the pupils, but anticholinergics cause nonreactive pupils. Nystagmus can be caused by a variety of substances. Alcohol, lithium, carbamazepine (Tegretol), solvents, meprobamate, quinine, and primidone may cause horizontal nystagmus. Sometimes characteristic odors emanate from patients and may aid in identification.

DIAGNOSTICS

In addition to vital signs and physical findings, laboratory values can be an important aspect of the diagnostic evaluation and aid in management. Diagnostic tests should be dictated by the toxicologic exposure. Some substances, including alcohol,

DIAGNOSTICS

Poisoning

INITIAL
Pulse oximetry
ECG

LABORATORY
Urine drug screen
CBC and differential
Serum electrolytes
BUN
Serum glucose
Creatinine
LFTs
Drug and alcohol screen
Serum human chorionic gonadotropin*
Anion gap
ABGs*
Carboxyhemoglobin*
Serum, gastric, and suspected substance analysis*

*If indicated.

aspirin, acetaminophen, illicit drugs, iron, lead, mercury, carboxyhemoglobin, and ethylene glycol, can be measured directly. In addition, many psychopharmacologic substances, including lithium hydroxide, divalproex sodium (Depakote), carbamazepine, oxcarbazepine (Trileptal), gabapentin (Neurontin), and nortriptyline (Pamelor), can be calculated. Assessment of arterial blood gases, the anion gap, the osmolar gap, and the oxygen saturation gap may provide additional information.

Other laboratory studies are helpful in assessing end-organ involvement and should include electrolytes, glucose, BUN, creatinine, and liver function tests. Urine screens may be indicated if cocaine, opiates, or marijuana is suspected. A pregnancy test should be obtained, if indicated. An ECG is necessary with specific poisons and in some instances will need repeated assessment.[5] Further evaluation is indicated if abnormalities such as acidosis or hypoxia are discovered.

DIFFERENTIAL DIAGNOSIS

Poisoning

- Trauma
- Metabolic abnormality
- Neurologic injury
- Alcohol
- Medications
- Illicit substances
- Iron
- Plants
- Food
- Insecticides
- Carbon monoxide
- Heavy metals
- Cyanide
- Inhalation
- Petroleum distillates
- Transient ischemic attack
- Gastrointestinal disorders

DIFFERENTIAL DIAGNOSIS

Initial diagnostic determination and treatment are usually based on the history and physical examination. If the patient is confused or comatose, all potential causes for the change in mental status should be considered. Laboratory analysis and the patient's response to therapeutic intervention provide additional diagnostic information. The differential diagnosis should include trauma; metabolic abnormality; neurologic injury; and poisoning from alcohol, medications, illicit substances, cleaning agents, plants, insecticides, food, carbon monoxide, heavy metals, cyanide, inhalation, and petroleum distillates. If GI symptoms are present, the differential diagnosis should include any possible GI disorders.

INITIAL STABILIZATION AND MANAGEMENT

Regardless of the poison, the initial assessment and frequent reassessment of the poisoned patient require attention to airway, breathing, and circulation. Oxygen and continuous airway maintenance are critical. IV access is also necessary. If the patient is comatose, a standard cocktail of glucose 25 to 50 g IV, thiamine 100 mg IV, and naloxone 2 mg IV, IM, or SQ has been recommended in the past, and the benefits of this regimen seem to outweigh the potential risks.[6,7] In opiate poisoning, repeat doses of naloxone can be necessary every 3 to 5 minutes.[8] *Ambulance transport to the nearest emergency department and contact with the regional poison control center are vital.* When the specific substance is known, the local poison control center can provide specific management and treatment recommendations.[8] Further management should be directed to reverse the known side effects. Gastric lavage is most useful in severe, potentially fatal poisonings and is now recommended only within the first hour after ingestion.[9] Ipecac, at one time used frequently, is no longer routinely recommended and should be used only after consultation with the poison control center.

Considering the large number of substances that could potentially act as toxins, a relatively small number of antidotes are available. Some commonly used antidotes include *N*-acetylcysteine, flumazenil, and naloxone. *N*-acetylcysteine is administered at an initial dose of 140 mg/kg by a standard protocol based on a nomogram to determine the necessity of treatment for acetaminophen overdoses. Flumazenil administered intravenously in 0.2-mg doses every minute to a maximum of 1 to 3 mg reverses the effects of benzodiazepines but could be detrimental if given to patients with benzodiazepine dependence, mixed substance overdose, alcohol overdose, or seizure history.[7,8] Naloxone is an opiate antagonist and is given in doses of 0.4 to 0.8 mg IV for adults to a maximum of 8 to 22 mg and in doses of 0.01 mg/kg IV for children.[5,10] More detailed listings that include antidotes for other substances are available at http://www.aapcc.org/FinalizedPMGdlns/finalizedPMGuidelines.htm.[3,5,7,8]

DISPOSITION AND REFERRAL

Immediate transfer or referral to an emergency department is recommended. Most patients who are treated for poisoning require a minimum observation period, if not hospitalization.

PREVENTION AND PATIENT EDUCATION

Education about the prevention of accidents and injuries is of utmost importance. To prevent exposures to potentially harmful substances, patients must understand the risks of inappropriate contact with medications and other household or work-related items. Information regarding the toxic effects of specific substances and the safe usage, storage, and handling of potential toxins at home and in the workplace is always useful and is an important reminder for us all. For patients with children, reminders about child proofing the home (particularly the importance of locking medications and cleaning agents in a child-proof cabinet) can potentially prevent accidental exposures.

REFERENCES

1. Centers for Disease Control and Prevention, National Center for Injury Prevention and Control: *Poisonings: fact sheet*, Atlanta, 2006, The Centers, retrieved May 12, 2006, from http://www.cdc.gov/ncipc/factsheets/poisoning.htm.
2. National Safety Council: *Injury facts*, retrieved May 12, 2006, from http://www.nsc.org.
3. American Association of Poison Control Centers: *Poison Control and Prevention Center directory*, retrieved May 12, 2006, from http://www.aapcc.org/findyourcenter.htm.
4. Bramson R: OTC and Rx drugs require rapid screen in overdose, *Med Lab Observer* Nov 2005.
5. Bone R: Approach to the poisoned patient, *Dis Mon* 42(9):511-607, 1996.
6. Kirk M, Pace S: Pearls, pitfalls, and updates in toxicology, *Emerg Med Clin North Am* 15(2):427-429, 1997.
7. Tintinalli JE, Ruiz E, Krome RL: *Emergency medicine*, ed 4, San Francisco, 1996, McGraw-Hill.
8. American Heart Association: Toxicology in emergency cardiovascular care, *Circulation* 112(Suppl I):IV-126–IV-132, 2005.
9. Chyka PA, Seger D, Krenzelok EP, and others: Position paper: single dose activated charcoal, *Clin Toxicol (Phila)* 43(2):61-87, 2005.
10. Hodgson BB, Kizior RJ: *Saunders nursing drug handbook*, Philadelphia, 2002, Saunders.

CHAPTER 40

Sexual Assault

Janelle Koo and Robbyn K. Takeuchi

DEFINITION AND EPIDEMIOLOGY

The terms *sexual assault* and *rape* are often used interchangeably, although there are clear differences between them. *Rape* is a legal term and not a medical diagnosis. The legal definition of rape may vary among states, but the common components of the definition include a lack of consent, a threat or use of force, and penetration of a bodily orifice.[1] *Sexual assault* has a much broader definition. It is defined as any sexual act that is forced or coerced without the consent of the victim.[2] Rape and sexual assault are not sexually motivated acts; rather, they are motivated by rage, aggression, and the determination to dominate another human being.

According to the National Crime Victimization Survey, 204,370 rapes and sexual assaults were reported from 2003 to 2004.[3] Persons ages 12 or older experienced an annual average of 140,990 completed rapes, 109,230 attempted rapes, and 152,680 completed and attempted sexual assaults between 1992 and 2000.[4] Further surveys indicate that 1 out of 6 women in the United States experiences either a completed or attempted rape at some point in her lifetime.[5] The incidence of rape is about 10 times higher for women than men, although men are less likely to report the occurrence. (For the purpose of this chapter, the term *she* is used, although this information can also apply to men who have been victims of sexual assault.) As previously discussed, it is important to consider the differences between the terms *rape* and *sexual assault*, since these statistics account for only reported rape cases and do not indicate the incidence of sexual assault, which has a much broader scope.

There are no known risk factors for becoming a victim of sexual assault. In fact, anyone can be a victim regardless of age, race, gender, or socioeconomic status. However, sexual assault victims are predominantly female, and the perpetrators are almost always heterosexual males. Female victims are more likely to be assaulted by someone they know, and reports indicate that 3 out of 4 rape or sexual assault victimizations involve offenders with whom the victim had a relationship as a family member, intimate, or acquaintance.[5] Sexual assault can also occur in the context of any intimate partner relationship. This includes marital, nonmarital, gay, lesbian, or past relationships. However, this type of sexual assault often is recurring and is one of the symptoms of a larger domestic violence problem that needs to be addressed. Consequences for this type of ongoing sexual violence by an intimate partner are severe and require ongoing monitoring and attention by the health care provider. (See Chapter 264 for further information regarding evaluation and management.)

CLINICAL PRESENTATION

The physical presentation of the sexual assault victim in the clinic setting is immensely varied. Some patients may report a chief complaint of sexual assault to their health care provider, whereas others may not mention that a sexual assault has occurred. Likewise, the presentation of psychologic effects of trauma also varies among victims. Some patients may choose to disclose that a sexual assault occurred if asked by a trusted health care provider. However, other patients may deny that violence occurred despite the evidence of trauma. Whatever the reasons for the patient's denial, the health care provider must respect it and simply offer support.

It is not up to the provider to determine whether sexual assault has occurred; that must be left to the court to decide. Rather, it is often helpful for the provider to let the patient know that sexual assault is, unfortunately, a common experience, and that it is a problem the provider may be able to assist with. This may leave the door open should the patient decide in the future to disclose what happened. Unfortunately, in selected findings of a national study, most rape and sexual assault victims were not treated for their injuries.[4] According to these findings, only approximately 30% of victims received treatment, with 20% of this total receiving care at a physician's office or clinic.

INITIAL STABILIZATION AND MANAGEMENT AND PHYSICAL EXAMINATION

If the patient does disclose that she was sexually assaulted, the provider should further explore whether the patient desires to pursue legal action. The provider should defer a physical examination and refer the patient to the emergency department if the sexual assault occurred within the past 5 days and if the patient desires to pursue legal action. A referral to the emergency department will ensure that the appropriate measures are taken to collect evidence and comply with standardized protocol, which are integral to support the patient's desire for legal pursuits. Further, the emergency department will also be able to provide the patient with comprehensive and compassionate services, including crisis intervention, rape counseling, and referrals to appropriate community agencies.

The health care provider can prepare the patient for what to expect in the emergency department. It is not important that the provider request specific information about the assault, since this information will be gathered in the emergency department. Retelling the story can be traumatizing for the patient. Rather, providers can attentively listen and document what the patient desires to express. The health care provider should carefully note emotional responses (e.g., crying, restlessness, anxious behavior, shaking, withdrawal), since this would be useful in court as an adjunct to the emergency department records.

If the patient does not desire to pursue legal action, or if more than 5 days have passed since the assault, medical care can be managed in the office setting. The provider needs to obtain a detailed history and perform a physical and gynecologic examination. About 40% of rape victims suffered a collateral injury; 5% suffered a major injury such as severe lacerations, fractures, internal injuries, or unconsciousness.[6] Injuries were most common among victims ages 30 or older.[6] Possible gynecologic injuries include vaginal or anal tearing, rectal bleeding, bruising, or soreness. Other physical symptoms associated with trauma include gastrointestinal irritability, dysmenorrhea, pelvic pain, and urinary tract infection. (For specific treatment considerations, see chapters that address the specific injury, infection, and medical disorder.)

Potential consequences of sexual assault further include the risk of pregnancy, sexually transmitted diseases (STDs), and HIV/AIDS. If it has been more than 72 hours since the sexual assault, it is not feasible to offer pregnancy or STD prophylactics. A pregnancy test should be completed, with appropriate counseling pending the results. The patient should be tested for STDs (gonorrhea and chlamydia are the most prevalent), and standard treatment should be followed if the results are positive. The patient may express fears about having contracted HIV/AIDS; however, testing cannot be done until 3 to 6 months after the assault because of the length of time for seroconversion to occur. If the appropriate time has passed, patients should have pretest and posttest education and counseling. Education should include risks of acquiring the infection, potential transmission of the virus, and instruction about safe sex practices at least until testing is complete, or longer if the results are positive.

Clearly, appropriate referral needs to be made for any symptoms, illnesses, or injuries whose treatment is beyond the scope of the office setting. Patients may also commonly report psychosomatic complaints, including fatigue and tension headaches, with or without the report of sexual assault. These symptoms may need further exploration through a psychosocial assessment.

Primary Care Management

When a patient reports that she has been a victim of sexual assault and it has been determined that she will be treated in the primary care setting, it is important to assess more than the patient's physical well-being. Patients may seek care soon after the assault or after an extended period. The patient's account of the assault will aid the provider in understanding the patient's experience and what type of services may be of benefit.

Patients who seek care shortly after the assault may display a range of emotions. Some may appear frightened, shocked, or angry. Regardless of their demeanor, they are in need of understanding and support. The patient's emotional presentation is not indicative of the level of trauma that has been experienced. A review of the patient's home environment and support system is appropriate. Because of the stigma associated with sexual assault, it is sometimes difficult for victims to inform significant people in their life about their victimization. Some fear that their intimate partner or parent may seek physical revenge against the perpetrator, if the perpetrator is known to them. As a result, they may be reluctant or unwilling to disclose information in an effort to protect their partner or parent from potential legal problems. Unfortunately, some patients are afraid to inform someone about the assault because they think that no one will believe them or that they are to blame for the assault. This is especially true if the patient consumed alcohol or drugs before the assault or if she thought she was dressed in provocative attire. As a result, the patient may not receive adequate support.

The provider can assist patients in identifying people in their lives to whom they can disclose the assault and who can provide support. Patients may also benefit from a discussion of the various ways to talk with their family or partner about the assault. Patients may experience a high degree of fear over the potential for further harm and may be afraid to be alone or return home. They must be assisted in finding the means to appropriately address their fears.

Patients who initially seek care a while after the assault may be prompted to do so because of physical complaints, such as STDs or pregnancy, or because of psychologic difficulties. Some patients may experience symptoms of psychologic distress that are consistent with posttraumatic stress disorder (PTSD). One study revealed that almost one third of rape victims develop PTSD at some point after the rape; this rate is six times higher than the rate for women who have not been raped.[7]

Reactions of people who have been sexually assaulted vary depending on a variety of factors, including age, gender, and circumstances surrounding the assault. Regardless of when the patient seeks care after a sexual assault, it is important for the provider to gain an accurate understanding of the patient's concerns, level of functioning, and support system before developing an appropriate treatment plan. The health care provider's comfort level with the subject matter may affect the patient's willingness to disclose information that would provide insight into the patient's needs. The provider is in a pivotal role to aid the patient in identifying the need for additional services, including mental health services.

Documentation

Accurate and precise documentation of the patient's physical and emotional signs and symptoms of sexual assault are always necessary, but especially so when there is a possibility that the documentation will corroborate the patient's testimony in court. It is essential that health care providers use medical rather than legal terminology. For example, calling the assault the "alleged rape" should be avoided; rather, it should be described as the "reported sexual assault." Likewise, the word *patient* should be used rather than *victim*. The connotation of words must be considered. *Penetration* is a better word than *intercourse,* since the latter may sound as though the act were consensual. If the patient does not wish to have a certain part of the examination completed, it should not be documented as "refused," since this makes the patient sound uncooperative; rather, the provider should write that the patient "declined" the examination. Using the patient's own words in quotation marks whenever possible best captures the description of the incident and is extremely helpful in court. The provider should avoid writing "no weapons used" but should describe exactly what happened, since there may have been verbal or implied threats. It is also important to be wary of using medical terminology that could be misinterpreted. For example, if the patient appears calm and collected, it is better to document that than to say "no apparent distress." Documenting unnecessary history that is not related to the chief complaint (e.g., psychiatric history, substance abuse history) could be used in court to discredit the patient's testimony.

LIFE SPAN CONSIDERATIONS

Adolescents

Adolescents are also at risk for victimization, although studies indicate that young women are more likely to experience violence than young men. The National Survey of Adolescents found that 13% of female adolescents had experienced sexual violence at some point in their lives.[7] Adolescents also have a tendency not to seek services for a variety of reasons. They may feel responsible for the assault, concerned that their parents will find out, or that they will be further victimized if they disclose information. Adolescence can be a difficult period for patients as a result of developmental and social changes and of patients' attempts to define themselves as they mature. Being sexually assaulted may create numerous problems for an adolescent, including difficulty establishing trust and the development of psychiatric symptoms. For these reasons, adolescents should be referred to age-appropriate mental health services.

Older Adults

Older patients are particularly vulnerable because of age-related illness and an overall decrease in physical strength. They may sustain more injuries and specifically more genital injuries. Older women are also unlikely to report being sexually assaulted; they may feel extreme embarrassment, humiliation, and shame because they were raised during a time when issues related to sex were not discussed. Some patients may be concerned that reporting the assault will result in a loss of their independence.

SPECIFIC POPULATIONS

Male Patients

Although male victims represent a minority of sexual assault victims, it is critical that they be treated the same as female patients. Male victims may experience rectal or penile trauma, bleeding or discharge, infection, or trauma to the mouth and pharynx. The patient may receive frontal injuries from being in a prone position during the assault. Men are usually assaulted by other men. For many reasons, men are less likely than women to seek services after being sexually assaulted, although they commonly experience similar physical and emotional reactions. Men may feel that they are "less of a man," may experience shame about not being able to defend themselves, and may be confused about their sexuality. If the assailant was a woman, the patient may feel particularly weak or inferior. As with all victims of sexual assault, it is important for the patient to receive mental health services.

Immigrants

Many immigrants have difficulty accessing care because of limited resources, language barriers, and a lack of awareness regarding how to access services; however, additional concerns arise with respect to receiving services for sexual assault. Some patients may be afraid to report the sexual assault to authorities because they are concerned that it may have a negative impact on their immigration status, especially if the patient is an undocumented alien. They also may not understand that it is illegal for them to be assaulted and that they have a right to report the crime. Another significant factor for immigrants in accessing services to address sexual assault is their cultural beliefs. Some may think it is inappropriate for them to discuss intimate matters with a professional, although they may not have the means or methods to address their issues within a cultural context. It is important for health care providers to be aware of cultural factors when providing care, to modify their treatment to the extent that they are able, and to ensure that the patient is aware of his or her rights and the availability of services.

DISPOSITION AND REFERRAL

Under certain circumstances the victim of sexual assault may be treated in a primary care setting; however, it is preferable that the patient be treated in a specially equipped emergency department by trained staff if the examination occurs within several days of the assault. Because different facilities operate under different guidelines, it is imperative that the health care provider be aware of the guidelines for the facilities in the area so that appropriate referrals can be made. The patient should always be referred to mental health services that specifically address issues surrounding sexual assault. If the patient is treated in the primary care setting, an assessment must be made to determine his or her physical, mental health, and legal needs; level of functioning; and willingness to pursue additional services. The health care provider should use his or her influence to encourage patients to accept additional services as deemed appropriate based on the provider's assessment.

In specific circumstances providers are mandated to report the sexual assault to the proper authorities. Any sexual assault perpetrated on a victim who is under 18 years of age or on any adult who is physically dependent or cognitively impaired must be reported to the local child or adult protective agency. Health care providers are mandated to report any suspicion of sexual assault in these populations, regardless of whether the patient reports that sexual assault has occurred. Although it is not the provider's responsibility to prove that the violence occurred, it is his or her responsibility to act on the clinical evidence presented. Since laws vary among states, providers should become familiar with the laws within their area.

PREVENTION AND PATIENT EDUCATION

Sexual assault occurs in a variety of settings and may victimize people of all ages, races, religions, and socioeconomic backgrounds. Providers can give patients various tips to promote their general safety; however, there is no known prevention for sexual assault. The health care provider should educate the patient about the dynamics of sexual assault, including the fact that it is an act of violence, and encourage the patient to seek mental health services.

REFERENCES

1. US Department of Justice, Bureau of Justice Statistics: *Selected findings: violence against women: estimates from the redesigned survey,* Rockville, Md, Aug 1995, National Crime Justice Reference Services.
2. Massachusetts Department of Public Health in collaboration with Massachusetts Coalition Against Sexual Assault: *Supporting survivors of sexual assault,* ed 1, Boston, 1997, The Department.
3. US Department of Justice: *Criminal victimization,* Washington, DC, 2004, US Department of Justice Office of Justice Programs.
4. US Department of Justice: *Rape and sexual assault: reporting to police and medical attention,* Washington, DC, 2002, US Department of Justice Office of Justice Programs.
5. Macguire K, Pastore AL: *1994 Sourcebook of criminal justice statistics,* Washington, DC, 1995, US Department of Justice, Bureau of Justice Statistics.
6. US Department of Justice: *An analysis of data on rape and sexual assault,* Washington, DC, 1997, The Department.
7. Hodgson J, Kelley D: *Sexual violence: policies practices, and challenges in the United States and Canada,* Westport, Conn, 2002, Praeger.

CHAPTER 41

Syncope

Updated by Kathleen M. Benedetti

DEFINITION AND EPIDEMIOLOGY

Syncope is defined as a temporary loss of consciousness and postural tone that is followed by spontaneous complete recovery and does not require resuscitation. Presyncope or near-syncope is a sensation of light-headedness or faintness in which the patient senses that true syncope may be imminent but complete loss of consciousness never occurs.

The incidence of syncope in the general population is not known, although a study in the late 1990s revealed that annually syncope can account for up to 600,000 visits to the emergency department.[1] The closest estimates come from the Framingham study, in which approximately 3% of individuals experienced at least one syncopal episode over a 26-year period.[2,3] Among those who experienced syncope, the incidence of recurrence was approximately 30%.[2-5]

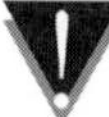

Immediate emergency department referral or physician consultation is indicated for syncope in a patient with a family history of sudden death or for syncope associated with exercise, chest pain, congestive heart failure (CHF), palpitations, acute hemorrhage, transient ischemic attacks, seizures, or an abnormal ECG or chest x-ray study. Patients with syncope and a medical history of anatomic heart disease or previous surgical repair of a cardiac lesion also require emergency department referral or physician consultation.

BOX 41-1

CAUSES OF SYNCOPE

CARDIAC

Mechanical or Obstructive Processes

- Cardiac valvular diseases
- Atrial myxoma
- Hypertrophic or obstructive cardiomyopathy
- Pulmonary hypertension
- Pulmonary embolism
- Pericardial disease
- Cardiac tamponade
- Myocardial infarction or ischemia

Arrhythmias

- Sick sinus syndrome
- Atrioventricular conduction disturbances
- Supraventricular or ventricular tachycardia
- Prolonged or shortened QT syndrome
- Pacemaker malfunction

NEUROLOGIC

Reflex or Neuromediated

- Vasovagal (common faint)
- Situational (micturition, cough, swallow, defecation)
- Carotid sinus hypersensitivity (primarily found in older adults)

Cerebrovascular

- Vertebrovascular transient ischemic attack

MISCELLANEOUS

- Hypoglycemia
- Psychiatric disease (panic disorder, hysteria, depression)
- Hypovolemia (especially in older patients who are taking antihypertensive medications)

PATHOPHYSIOLOGY

Syncope is a symptom of an underlying process (Box 41-1). There are two main pathophysiologic mechanisms by which syncope may occur. The first is through the deprivation of nutrients to the brain. In most cases this deprivation results from decreased blood flow to the brain secondary to hypovolemia, cardiac outflow obstruction, cardiac arrhythmias, or neurovascular etiologies. The second underlying mechanism is deprivation of oxygen delivery to the brain, which may be seen with hypoxia or anemia. True syncope needs to be distinguished from seizure disorders or other conditions that might result in altered levels of consciousness, such as iatrogenic syncope from medication therapy, drug or alcohol intoxication, concussions, amnesia, or metabolic causes such as hypoglycemia. It is important to note that seizurelike activity may be present with syncope; this is secondary to generalized cerebral hypoxia.

Cardiac causes need to be diagnosed early in the evaluation because these etiologies are associated with a 1-year mortality rate of 20% to 30% and an increased incidence of sudden death.[6,7] The cardiac causes consist of two major categories: (1) mechanical or ventricular outflow obstructive processes, and (2) arrhythmia. Possible mechanical or obstructive processes responsible for syncope include cardiac valvular disease, atrial myxoma, hypertrophic or obstructive cardiomyopathy, pulmonary hypertension, pulmonary embolism, pericardial disease or tamponade, acute myocardial infarction or ischemia, and possible prosthetic valve malfunction. Possible rhythm disturbances include sick sinus syndrome, atrioventricular conduction disturbances, supraventricular and ventricular tachycardias, long QT syndrome, and pacemaker system malfunction.

Neurovascular causes of syncope may be classified into reflex or neuromediated causes and cerebrovascular causes. Among the reflex or neuromediated causes of syncope are vasovagal causes (also known as the common faint), situational causes (including micturition, cough, swallowing, or defecation), and carotid sinus syncope (often associated with tight collars, shaving, head turning, and older adults). These neuromediated causes of syncope are thought to result from a poorly understood neural pathway in which neural signals sent from the medulla result in a vasodilatory response with venous pooling and cardioinhibition that results in bradycardia. In carotid sinus syncope and micturition syncope, the trigger sites are thought to be peripheral receptors that respond to mechanical stimuli. The main cerebrovascular type of syncope centers on the vertebrobasilar arteries through which the brainstem is perfused. The main causes of this type of syncope are transient ischemic attack, compression (i.e., cervical rib) of the vertebrobasilar circulation, and subclavian steal.

Several miscellaneous causes of syncope are not easily classified into any of the previously mentioned categories. Hypoglycemia is a possible metabolic case of syncope and is usually found in individuals with diabetes who have taken too much of a particular hypoglycemic agent. Hyperventilation is another possible cause. Several psychiatric causes, including depression, hysteria, and panic attacks, may subsequently result in hyperventilation, which can result in hypocarbia and cerebral vasoconstriction compounded by possible peripheral vasodilation. In approximately 38% to 50% of cases, no definitive etiology is found despite thorough evaluations.[8,9]

CLINICAL PRESENTATION

The history of present illness is essential to helping the health care provider determine whether a particular case should be treated on an outpatient or inpatient basis. The history needs to include a detailed account of the syncopal episode. In many cases a witness is needed to determine the specific details of the event. It should be established what the patient was doing before the syncopal episode and whether there were any preceding symptoms. A history of urinating, defecating, swallowing, coughing, shaving, turning the head, neck pressure, or pain before syncope is consistent with some form of neurally mediated syncope. Fainting just before a stressful event is consistent with vasovagal syncope. If the patient is able to relate the presyncopal or syncopal episode to a change from a horizontal to a vertical position, the episode may be a result of hypovolemia or orthostatic hypotension. Numbness and tingling in the face and hands suggest hyperventilation.

The patient may have felt some nausea, diaphoresis, or warmth just before losing consciousness. The presence of an aura, such as a peculiar smell, might be a clue to the presence of an underlying seizure disorder. Differentiating between a seizure and postsyncope, seizurelike activity can be difficult. A possible underlying cardiac etiology needs to be considered if the syncopal episode was sudden and without warning. The sudden onset of syncope is consistent with an arrhythmia, whereas the onset of syncope with exertion may be associated with a mechanical or obstructive process. The presence of chest pain, palpitations, syncope with exertion, and a positive family history of coronary artery disease also necessitates excluding a cardiac cause.[10]

How the patient acted while unconscious is important. Most syncopal events are brief; patients often recover once they are in the horizontal position, which allows the resumption of blood flow to the brain. The presence of seizure activity, urinary incontinence, fecal incontinence, and tongue biting may help differentiate a seizure from true syncope. Postictal symptoms during the recovery phase are more consistent with seizure.

Certain medications may be the underlying or contributing cause. Antihypertensive medications may aggravate orthostatic symptoms, especially in older adults. Antiarrhythmic drugs may have proarrhythmic side effects. It is important to know if the patient is being treated for a seizure disorder, any psychiatric disorders, or diabetes and if the patient has been taking medications as prescribed.

A thorough review of the patient's past medical history is also necessary. The social history should include alcohol use, possible illicit drug use, and the patient's occupation. In patients suspected of having an underlying cardiac problem, the presence of any cardiac risk factors for coronary artery disease should be determined. Risk factors include male gender, a family history of premature coronary artery disease, hypercholesterolemia, hypertension, smoking, and diabetes.

PHYSICAL EXAMINATION

After establishing that the patient is stable, the initial physical evaluation needs to focus on the cardiovascular system. Auscultation may reveal murmurs, gross rhythm disturbances, or extra heart sounds such as S_3 or S_4. The lungs should be auscultated for rales or crackles, which might indicate CHF, possibly secondary to an acute myocardial infarction or pulmonary disease. Other signs of CHF include jugular venous distention, hepatojugular reflux, and edema.

Orthostatic blood pressures (also known as *tilts*) should be measured to determine the presence of hypovolemia. These measurements are obtained by having the patient lie in the supine position for at least 5 minutes and then measuring the blood pressure and pulse. The blood pressure and pulse are checked while the patient is sitting up and then while standing. A drop in systolic pressure by at least 20 mm Hg, a drop in diastolic pressure by at least 10 mm Hg, or an increase in the pulse rate by at least 20 beats per minute when assuming a more upright position is considered a positive test.

Hypersensitive carotid sinus baroreceptors may be another underlying cause of syncope. If there are no carotid bruits, this baroreceptor response may be tested by a specialist. In this test, the patient is supine, IV access is established, and atropine is available, if needed. The patient's heart rhythm is observed on a cardiac monitor while carotid sinus pressure is applied. The monitor is checked for the presence of asystole for at least 3 seconds. The blood pressure should be measured to determine if the systolic blood pressure dropped at least 50 mm Hg.[10] Obviously this test should be reserved for a controlled setting in which possible deleterious consequences can be reversed. A complete neurologic examination, including a funduscopic examination, should also be performed on these patients. A rectal examination will help determine if gastrointestinal bleeding is present.

DIAGNOSTICS

Initial laboratory testing should include electrolytes, BUN, creatinine, glucose, and hematocrit. A chest x-ray study will help reveal any significant cardiac conditions that may result in CHF. Cardiomegaly is considered to be a heart shadow that takes up more than half of the chest cavity on the posteroanterior view. An ECG should be performed to help detect any possible arrhythmias. Cardiac enzymes should be drawn if the patient has cardiac risk factors, if the patient has a history of chest pain, or if physical findings are consistent with CHF. If a cardiac obstructive cause is suspected, an echocardiogram may be indicated. A pregnancy test should be performed on all female patients of childbearing age.[10]

DIFFERENTIAL DIAGNOSIS

The differential diagnosis of syncope includes vasovagal syncope, orthostatic hypotension, seizure disorder, alcohol abuse,

DIAGNOSTICS

Syncope

INITIAL
ECG
Orthostatic blood pressure
Pulse oximetry

LABORATORY
Serum electrolytes
BUN
Creatinine
Serum glucose
Cardiac isoenzymes if cardiac cause suspected
Brain natriuretic peptide

IMAGING
Echocardiogram*
CT scan or MRI of head*

OTHER
Holter monitor, event monitor, or implantable loop monitor*
Tilt-table test*
Exercise testing*
EEG*
Electrophysiology*

*If indicated.

cardiovascular disease with obstruction, cardiac arrhythmias, transient ischemic attack, concussion, hypovolemia, hypoglycemia, anemia, or hypoxia. In addition, syncope may be related to medication therapy or an anxiety attack.

INITIAL STABILIZATION AND MANAGEMENT

During a witnessed event, the patient should be placed in a supine position. Tight clothing should be loosened and the patient's head turned to the side. If the history and diagnostic testing indicate that an initial episode of syncope was not secondary to a cardiac pathologic condition, therapy can be directed at the underlying disorder. If the patient is unstable, the appropriate advanced cardiac life support and advanced trauma life support protocols need to be followed.

DISPOSITION AND REFERRAL

In the case of neuromediated syncope, and especially with recurring episodes, the patient should be referred to a neurologist for possible tilt-table testing and treatment, possibly with fludrocortisone, desmopressin, or pressor agents.[11] Cases of syncope with possible underlying cardiac causes need to be referred to an accepting physician as soon as possible for further evaluation. Patients who may have new-onset seizure disorder need to be referred for possible admission. Older patients deserve a thorough history to determine if some other problem in their home environment is preventing them from staying hydrated or taking their medications properly. These patients may need the help of a social worker or health benefits adviser.

All patients need to understand the importance of adequate hydration and need to avoid circumstances that might precipitate syncope. They should be told to return to the clinic if the syncope reoccurs. Depending on the suspected underlying cause, a referral to either a neurologist or cardiologist is appropriate at this time.

PREVENTION AND PATIENT EDUCATION

Patients and families should have careful explanation regarding the cause of the syncopal event. Prevention of injury is an important goal for the older population, where 30% of falls are due to syncope.[12] In the case of vasovagal, carotid sinus, and situational syncope, patients need to be made aware of the particular behaviors, activities, or circumstances that might result in syncopal episodes, and they should be given adequate avoidance strategies. Prevention of orthostatic changes necessitates that patients learn to rise slowly from the bed or chair, exercising the leg muscles before standing. Although syncope is often not recurrent, patients with syncope should be advised not to operate motorized equipment until the cause of the event is determined and treated.[13,14]

REFERENCES

1. Junaid A, Dubinsky IL: Establishing an approach to syncope in the emergency department, *J Emerg Med* 15(5):593-599, 1997.
2. Benditt DG, Lurie KG, Fabian WH: Clinical approach to diagnosis of syncope: an overview, *Cardiol Clin* 15(2):165-176, 1997.
3. Savage DD, Corwin L, McGee DL, and others: Epidemiologic features of isolated syncope: the Framingham study, *Stroke* 16:626-629, 1985.
4. Soteriades ES, Evans JC, Larson M, and others: Incidence and prognosis of syncope, *N Engl J Med* 347:878-885, 2002.
5. Kapoor WN, Kqarpf M, Wieand S, and others: A prospective evaluation and follow-up of patients with syncope, *N Engl J Med* 309:197-204, 1983.
6. Kapoor WN: Evaluation and outcome of patients with syncope, *Medicine* 69(3):160-175, 1990.
7. Silverstein MD, Singer DE, Mulley AG, and others: Patients with syncope admitted to medical intensive care units, *JAMA* 248(10): 1185-1189, 1982.
8. Linzer M, Yang EH, Estes NA, and others: Diagnosing syncope, part 2, Unexplained syncope, *Ann Intern Med* 127(1):76-86, 1997.
9. Kapoor WN: Evaluation and management of the patient with syncope, *JAMA* 268(18):2553-2560, 1992.
10. Linzer M, Yang EH, Estes NA, and others: Diagnosing syncope, part 1, Value of history, physical examination, and electrocardiography, *Ann Intern Med* 126(12):989-996, 1997.
11. Kaufmann H: Syncope: a neurologist viewpoint, *Cardiol Clin* 15(2):177-194, 1997.
12. Journal of the American College of Cardiology: *AHA/ACCF scientific statement on the evaluation of syncope*, Jan 30, 2006, retrieved from http://www.content.onlinejacc.org.
13. Bhatia A, Dhala A, Blanck Z, and others: Driving safety among patients with neurocardiogenic syncope, *Pacing Clin Electrophysiol* 22:1576, 1999.
14. Li H, Weitzel M, Easley A, and others: Potential risk of vasovagal syncope for motor vehicle driving, *Am J Cardiol* 85:184, 2000.

CHAPTER 42

Tachycardia

Terry Mahan Buttaro

DEFINITION AND EPIDEMIOLOGY

Tachycardia is described as a heart rate exceeding 100 beats per minute. Normal sinus tachycardia does not usually require medical intervention, but other tachyarrhythmias can result in hemodynamic compromise and warrant urgent treatment. A rapid assessment of airway, breathing, and circulation, as well as a complete history, physical examination, and 12-lead ECG, is indicated.

Asymptomatic individuals with tachycardia can have stable cardiac rhythms that do not require emergent treatment. Fever, nicotine, exercise, stimulants, medications, and anxiety can precipitate normal sinus tachycardia. Pregnancy, coronary heart disease, congestive heart failure, valvular heart disease, pulmonary embolus, pericardial disease, valvular disorders, ischemia, metabolic and electrolyte abnormalities, medications, toxins, infection, and volume depletion should be considered as possible precipitants identified with atrial and ventricular arrhythmias, as well as tachycardia.

Emergency department referral or physician consultation is indicated for new-onset atrial fibrillation, atrial flutter, ventricular tachycardia (VT), or supraventricular tachycardia (SVT).

PATHOPHYSIOLOGY

The pathology of tachycardia is varied. Sinus tachycardia is a normal physiologic response and should not be considered pathologic. Atrial fibrillation and flutter, the narrow-complex tachycardias (ectopic atrial tachycardia, multifocal atrial tachycardia, junctional tachycardia, and paroxysmal SVT tachycardia), the stable wide-complex tachycardias of unknown type, and monomorphic-polymorphic VT are tachyarrhythmias that can cause hemodynamic instability (see Chapter 124). In narrow-complex tachycardia, such as paroxysmal tachycardia, the heart rate increases suddenly and rapidly, then decreases suddenly. The attack may last seconds or days, during which time the ventricular rate is rapid and regular, usually between 150 and 225 beats per minute. This pathologic condition is most likely related to an aberrant reentry involving the arteriovenous (AV) node, although an obscure bypass tract near the AV node may cause the aberrant conduction (as in Wolff-Parkinson-White syndrome).

Atrial fibrillation and atrial flutter are rhythm disturbances characterized by rapid atrial stimulation and varied ventricular response. In flutter this can be a fleeting phenomenon. In fibrillation it can be related to stress. However, atrial arrhythmias are commonly related to varied disease states. These include coronary heart disease, rheumatic fever, mitral stenosis, thyrotoxicosis, infection, metabolic abnormalities, pulmonary embolism, and chronic lung disease.

Whether monomorphic or polymorphic, VT is a rhythm disturbance that arises in the ventricles. The arrhythmia is life threatening if the patient is pulseless, but the patient can be hemodynamically stable when VT is associated with a pulse.

CLINICAL PRESENTATION

Some tachyarrhythmias are well tolerated, but chest discomfort, anxiety, restlessness, shortness of breath, weakness, fatigue, dizziness, and palpitations are common presenting symptoms.[1] Any tachycardia associated with chest pressure, acute myocardial infarction or cardiac ischemia, an alteration in consciousness, hypotension or shock, shortness of breath, dyspnea on exertion, congestive heart failure, or dizziness requires emergency care. A careful history of the presenting event, past medical history, and review of allergies and medications can help determine whether an underlying pathologic condition is causing the tachycardia and will facilitate appropriate treatment.

PHYSICAL EXAMINATION

An ECG or "quick look' with a conventional or external defibrillator is necessary to determine the cardiac rhythm and presence of arrhythmias or ischemia.[1] Because tachycardia can precipitate hemodynamic instability, cardiac monitoring and assessment of vital signs (including temperature, blood pressure, heart rate, respirations, and oxygen saturation) should be continuous. The physical examination should be focused and exact. This will help elicit the precipitating pathologic condition, establish whether the patient is stable or unstable, and determine whether the tachycardia has precipitated serious signs and symptoms.

DIAGNOSTICS

Continuous assessment, cardiac monitoring, and a 12-lead ECG are necessary to identify the tachyarrhythmia and any deterioration in the patient's condition. A chest x-ray study and laboratory studies, including drug levels, electrolytes, CBC, and thyroid studies, may also be indicated, but are usually deferred until after emergency department evaluation.

DIAGNOSTICS

Tachycardia

INITIAL
ECG

LABORATORY
Drug levels*
Serum electrolytes (serum sodium, potassium, chloride, CO_2, and magnesium), BUN, and creatinine*
CBC and differential*
TSH*

IMAGING
Chest x-ray*

*If indicated.

DIFFERENTIAL DIAGNOSIS

Tachycardia

- Drug induced
- Hyperthyroidism
- Acute myocardial infarction
- Congestive heart failure
- Pulmonary embolus
- Hypotension
- Hypoxia
- Hypovolemia
- Infection
- Electrolyte disturbance

DIFFERENTIAL DIAGNOSIS

Atrial fibrillation, atrial flutter, narrow-complex tachycardias, stable wide-complex tachycardia of uncertain type, and VT are tachyarrhythmias with potentially serious consequences. The 2005 American Heart Association Guidelines for Emergency Cardiovascular Care recommend classifying patients as stable or unstable, identifying whether serious signs and symptoms are present, and determining whether the arrhythmia has caused these signs and symptoms.[1] Patients with unstable tachycardia may complain of chest discomfort, be hypotensive, or display cognitive changes or signs of shock.[1]

Identification of the tachycardia and its related pathologic condition is essential for appropriate treatment. To prevent inappropriate therapy, the patient's condition and the etiology of the tachycardia should be carefully considered before treatment is initiated. Medications, pregnancy, hyperthyroidism, acute myocardial infarction, congestive heart failure, pulmonary embolus, hypotension, hypoxia, hypovolemia, infection, electrolyte abnormalities, and other disorders may precipitate a rapid heart rate and its resultant symptoms. Treatment of the specific disorder may result in resolution of the tachycardia.

INITIAL STABILIZATION AND MANAGEMENT

Oxygen administration, a 12-lead ECG, and continuous monitoring of the patient's oxygen saturation and vital signs are critical. The ECG will permit identification of the tachycardia and enable appropriate treatment. IV access with a large-bore IV catheter and isotonic normal saline IV solution (with the IV fluid running at "keep open rate" to maintain catheter patency) is recommended. Suction, intubation, and defibrillation equipment should be readily available.

In healthy patients, urgent cardioversion is rarely necessary when the heart rate is less than 150 beats per minute, but for patients with coronary artery disease or other co-morbid illnesses, a lower heart rate may cause significant compromise. Immediate cardioversion is indicated if the patient is unstable because of the tachycardia.[1] *Consult with a physician experienced in advanced cardiac life support for synchronized cardioversion of unstable reentry SVT, unstable atrial flutter or fibrillation, unstable monomorphic VT, and polymorphic (irregular) tachycardia* (Box 42-1). If the patient is stable, certain medications can also be used to treat specific tachyarrhythmias (Box 42-2).

ACLS guidelines 2005 do not recommend treatment for tachycardia if the patient is stable and does not have chest pressure, acute myocardial infarction, change in mental status, hypotension, shortness of breath, congestive heart failure, or other signs and symptoms indicating instability.[1] The underlying precipitant of the tachycardia should be determined and appropriate treatment initiated.

BOX 42-1

CARDIOVERSION AND DEFIBRILLATION OF UNSTABLE PATIENTS WITH TACHYCARDIA

ATRIAL FIBRILLATION

- Synchronized cardioversion with monophasic waveform: 100-200 J*
- Synchronized cardioversion with biphasic waveform: 100-120 J

ATRIAL FLUTTER

- Synchronized cardioversion with monophasic waveform: 50-100 J*
- Synchronized cardioversion with biphasic waveform: no clear dosing recommendation†

MONOMORPHIC VENTRICULAR TACHYCARDIA

- Synchronized cardioversion with monophasic waveform: 100 J*
- Synchronized cardioversion with biphasic waveform: no clear dosing recommendations†

POLYMORPHIC VENTRICULAR TACHYCARDIA

- Treat as ventricular fibrillation with unsynchronized shocks
- If monophasic defibrillator: one shock at 360 J, then resume chest compressions and CPR for five cycles before checking rhythm and delivering a repeat shock
- If biphasic defibrillator: one shock at 120-200 J, then resume chest compressions and CPR for five cycles before checking rhythm and delivering a repeat shock‡

*If second shock is necessary, the number of joules can be increased as needed.
†Data from American Heart Association: Management of symptomatic bradycardia and tachycardia, *Circulation* 112(24):IV 67-77, 2005.
‡The effective electrical dose for monophasic and biphasic defibrillators is unclear. With biphasic defibrillators, the effective waveform dose can vary from manufacturer to manufacturer.

DISPOSITION AND REFERRAL

Ideally, symptomatic patients with tachycardia should be stabilized with initial management and transferred to the nearest emergency department. Immediate transfer by ambulance to an emergency department is indicated for patients requiring continued assessment and management.

PREVENTION AND PATIENT EDUCATION

Tachyarrhythmias often recur. Careful explanation of the specific disorder and how to recognize untoward symptoms is an important part of patient education. Because electrolyte disturbances and medications can precipitate some tachyarrhythmias, it is important that health care providers consider and review medication therapies regularly. Amiodarone or other antiarrhythmic medications, wearable defibrillators, implantable cardioverter-defibrillators, pacemakers, or ablation therapy may be indicated for the prevention of recurrent symptomatic tachycardia.[2,3]

BOX 42-2

MEDICATION THERAPY FOR PATIENTS WITH STABLE TACHYCARDIA

Sinus tachycardia: Treat underlying precipitant.

Narrow-complex QRS tachycardia (reentry supraventricular rhythm; narrow-complex QRS [<0.12 seconds] with or without P waves): If vagal maneuvers are unsuccessful, consider adenosine 6 mg rapid IV push. If rhythm continues, give adenosine 12 mg IV rapid push. Reentry supraventricular tachycardia (SVT) is probable rhythm if the rhythm converts to normal sinus rhythm (patient will require monitoring for recurrence). If rhythm does not convert with adenosine via rapid IV push, reevaluate rhythm (consider atrial flutter, ectopic atrial tachycardia, or junctional tachycardia and treat with nondihydropyridine calcium channel blocker or beta blocker [use cautiously if patient has history of lung disease or congestive heart failure]). Amiodarone* (150 mg IV over 10 minutes; can repeat every 10 minutes to maximum dose of 2.2 g) is also recommended for narrow-complex QRS tachycardias (reentry SVT rhythms) unresponsive to vagal maneuvers or adenosine.

Irregular narrow QRS tachycardia (atrial fibrillation, atrial flutter, or multifocal atrial tachycardia): Control rate with nondihydropyridine calcium channel blocker (diltiazem 0.25 mg/kg IV, or verapamil 2.5 to 5 mg IV over 5 minutes) or beta blocker (atenolol 5 mg IV over 5 minutes [may repeat in 10 minutes, if indicated] or metoprolol 5 mg IV over 5 minutes × three doses if well tolerated). Beta blockers should be used cautiously if there is a history of lung disease or congestive heart failure.

Regular stable wide-complex tachycardia (QRS >0.12 second): This is most likely ventricular tachycardia (VT) or SVT. If SVT, treat with adenosine (as in narrow-complex QRS tachycardia). If monomorphic VT, treat with synchronized cardioversion or amiodarone* 150 mg IV over 10 minutes (may repeat if needed up to 2.2 g/24 hr). An alternative medication for stable monomorphic VT is procainamide† 20 mg/min. Procainamide therapy is discontinued if the arrhythmia resolves, the QRS is prolonged more than 50% compared with the original QRS, the patient develops hypotension, or the maximum dosage is given (17 mg/kg).

Polymorphic (irregular) VT: Give amiodarone* 150 mg IV over 10 minutes (may repeat if needed up to 2.2 g/24 hr). Lidocaine‡ 0.5 to 0.75 mg IV q 5 min may be used (total dosing not to exceed 3 mg/kg) with preserved ventricular function or torsades de pointes. However, magnesium 1 to 2 g IV over 5 to 60 minutes is the preferred treatment for torsades de pointes.

Data from American Heart Association: Management of symptomatic bradycardia and tachycardia, *Circulation* 112(24):IV 67-77, 2005.

*Amiodarone: an IV infusion (1 mg/min for 6 hours, then 0.5 mg/min for 18 hours) is recommended after the initial IV bolus.[1]

†Procainamide: an IV infusion (1 to 4 mg/min in normal saline or D5W) is recommended after the initial IV bolus.[1]

‡Lidocaine: an IV infusion (1 to 4 mg/min) is recommended after the initial bolus.[1]

REFERENCES

1. American Heart Association: Management of symptomatic bradycardia and tachycardia, *Circulation* 112(24):IV 67-77, 2005.
2. Gretoratus G: Indications and recommendations for pacemaker therapy, *Am Fam Phys* 71(8):1563-1570, 2005.
3. Feldman AM, Klein H, Tchou P, and others: Use of a wearable defibrillator in terminating tachyarrhythmias in patients at high risk for sudden death: results of the WEARIT/BIROAD, *Pacing Clin Electrophysiol* 27(1):4-9, 2004.

CHAPTER 43

Thermal Injuries

Timothy J. Phillips

Extremes of environmental conditions often contribute to the development of heat- and cold-related injuries, including hyperthermia and hypothermia. A history of increased physical activity in the heat or prolonged exposure to cold temperatures may suggest thermal injury, but conditions such as alcohol or drug ingestion, trauma, psychiatric conditions, or medical conditions should also be considered.

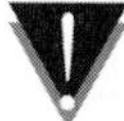

Immediate emergency department referral or physician consultation is indicated for patients with hypothermia, heatstroke, or heat exhaustion.

HEAT-RELATED INJURIES

DEFINITION AND EPIDEMIOLOGY

Heat stress and heat cramps are milder forms of heat-related injuries, whereas heatstroke and heat exhaustion are more severe. Heat injuries are differentiated not by specific temperature ranges but by symptoms and systemic changes that develop as body temperature increases. Some cases are too mild to be diagnosed, and some cases are not reported. Therefore it is difficult to estimate with accuracy the number of heat-related injuries. However, the Centers for Disease Control and Prevention estimated that 300 persons died of heat-related injuries in 2001.[1]

PATHOPHYSIOLOGY

Heat-related injuries occur when the metabolic demands of exercise raise the temperature of the body or when environmental heat stress is maximum. In warm environments, evaporation of sweat from the skin is the most important mechanism of heat dissipation.[2] Under certain conditions, however, an inadequate transfer of heat occurs and body temperature increases. Heat exhaustion is associated with a combination of conditions, including dehydration, loss of normal electrolyte balance, and respiratory alkalosis caused by exercise. Heatstroke caused by failure of the normal thermoregulatory mechanisms is believed to be related to dehydration complicated by a compensatory vasoconstriction of the peripheral vasculature.

CLINICAL PRESENTATION

Patients with heat stress usually exhibit mild changes in mental status and may also complain of dizziness and fatigue. Heat cramps are characterized by muscle spasms that may be accompanied by weakness, fatigue, nausea, and vomiting. More severe forms of heat injury, including heat exhaustion and heatstroke, are differentiated by worsening mental status changes. Heat exhaustion may be accompanied by a variety of symptoms, including nausea, vomiting, fatigue, irritability, headache, syncope, dyspnea, weakness, and increased sweating. Heatstroke may be characterized by vomiting, diarrhea, coma, seizures, and mental status changes.

PHYSICAL EXAMINATION

The spectrum of physical findings and presenting symptoms reflects the severity of the injury. Blood pressure and heart rate typically are elevated in patients with heat stress. Heart rate, blood pressure, and body temperature may be normal when heat cramps are present. In heat exhaustion, orthostatic vital signs and mental status changes may also be present, and core body temperature is typically less than 39° C (102.2° F). In addition to a core body temperature greater than 39° C (102.2° F), symptoms of heatstroke may include decreased blood pressure and mental status changes.

Heatstroke needs to be identified and treated immediately. Because outcome and resultant damage are related to the duration of hyperthermia, the core body temperature should be lowered quickly to 38° C (100.4° F) and monitored for maintenance. Simple, quick cooling measures include immersing the patient in ice water; covering the patient with an ice water cooling blanket; fanning; and placing ice packs in the groin, axillary, and neck areas. IV hydration should be started immediately, but rapid delivery of excessive fluids should be avoided. If other symptoms develop, specific therapy may be necessary for patients with coma, renal failure, coagulopathies, or acid-base abnormalities.

DIAGNOSTICS

Because the liver, kidneys, muscles, and coagulation systems are most susceptible to heat injury, laboratory assessment should include electrolytes, glucose, BUN, creatinine, liver function tests (LFTs), creatinine phosphokinase, and coagulation studies. A urinalysis should be obtained to assess kidney involvement. A variety of ECG changes may be observed. It is important to monitor patients with heatstroke for rhabdomyolysis, acute renal failure, and disseminated intravascular coagulation, which are well-known complications. Note that hepatic damage (elevated LFTs) is a consistent feature of heatstroke, and therefore an absence of this casts doubt on the diagnosis.

DIAGNOSTICS

Heat-Related Injuries

INITIAL
ECG

LABORATORY
Serum electrolytes
BUN
Creatinine
Creatinine phosphokinase
Serum glucose
LFTs
Coagulation studies (PT/PTT)
Urinalysis
CBC and differential

DIFFERENTIAL DIAGNOSIS

It is essential to recognize the seriousness of heat-related injuries. Heat stress, heat cramps, heat syncope, heatstroke, and heat exhaustion must be differentiated to ensure proper treatment. Presentation of the more emergent heat-related injuries may mimic other conditions, including systemic infections, dehydration, seizures, metabolic or neurologic abnormalities, cardiac arrhythmias, myocardial infarction, and

DIFFERENTIAL DIAGNOSIS

Heat-Related Injuries

- Heat stress, heat cramps, heatstroke, heat exhaustion, heat syncope
- Systemic infection
- Dehydration
- Seizures
- Metabolic or neurologic abnormality
- Cardiac arrhythmias
- Myocardial infarction
- Cocaine overdose

cocaine overdose. These should be considered if the patient does not respond to cooling measures.

INITIAL STABILIZATION AND MANAGEMENT

The degree of hyperthermia affects treatment. However, all patients with hyperthermia, regardless of severity, should be treated with rest, hydration, and cooling. Either oral or IV hydration can be used for minor heat cramps, but heat exhaustion requires IV hydration with either normal saline or lactated Ringer's solution at 250 ml/hr.

DISPOSITION AND REFERRAL

All patients with heat injuries should be assessed rapidly and treated initially with hydration, cooling measures, and rest. Transfer to an appropriate medical facility is indicated for significant dehydration, hyponatremia, or persistent mental status changes.[3]

PREVENTION AND PATIENT EDUCATION

Prevention of heat-related injuries includes physical conditioning and acclimatization. Daily exposure for 100 minutes a day results in near-maximum acclimatization in 7 to 14 days.[2] Patients should also understand the importance of drinking extra fluids during hot weather or if working or exercising in the heat, since individuals do not voluntarily drink as much as they lose with heavy exertion.

COLD-RELATED INJURIES

DEFINITION AND EPIDEMIOLOGY

Hypothermia is caused by decreased core body temperature. Unlike hyperthermia, it is categorized by specific ranges of core body temperatures. Frostbite injury results from exposure to cold temperatures and causes irreversible tissue damage. According to the Centers for Disease Control and Prevention,[4] an estimated 700 people died of hypothermia each year from 1979 to 1998. Frostbite, which usually affects the feet, occurs most commonly in adults between 30 and 49 years of age.[5]

PATHOPHYSIOLOGY

As core body temperature decreases, cardiac output, blood pressure, and heart rate initially increase, then decrease. An initial increase in respiratory rate is followed by a decrease in rate. The oxyhemoglobin dissociation curve is shifted to the left, with a subsequent decrease in oxygen delivery. This combination of decreased metabolic functioning leads to abnormalities in the functional capabilities of the pulmonary, cardiac, and central nervous systems.[6] When frostbite occurs, the tissue is damaged by the progressive effects of freezing, decreased oxygen, and the release of inflammatory factors into the tissue.

CLINICAL PRESENTATION

Mild hypothermia corresponds to a core body temperature of 32° to 35° C (89.6° to 95° F). Moderate hypothermia develops if cooling continues until the core body temperature reaches 28° to 32° C (82.4° to 89.6° F). Severe hypothermia results if the core body temperature decreases to less than 28° C (82.4° F).[7] Frostbite may have a varying degree of symptoms depending on the degree of local tissue injury; however, numbness is the presenting symptom 75% of the time.[8]

PHYSICAL EXAMINATION

In addition to the specific core temperature noted in patients with hypothermia, certain common symptoms are associated with each level of hypothermia. Symptoms associated with mild hypothermia often include shivering, tachycardia, tachypnea, and diuresis. Changes in skin color, balance, and memory may also be present in some cases. Shivering decreases, and mental status changes are noticeable with a further decrease of temperature to moderate hypothermia. With severe hypothermia, the provider may observe loss of reflexes; stupor or coma; and fixed, dilated pupils. Characteristic ECG changes depend on temperature. Above 35° C (95° F), sinus tachycardia is most common. Between 35° and 32° C (95° and 89.6° F), sinus bradycardia commonly occurs. Below 32° C (89.6° F), characteristic J waves may be seen. At 30° C (86° F), atrial arrhythmias are usual, whereas at 28° C (82.4° F), ventricular arrhythmias are more common. Asystole occurs at temperatures less than 20° C (68° F).[9]

Superficial frostbite is characterized by decreased sensation and erythema surrounding a central white area with or without blisters. Deep frostbite is characterized by hemorrhagic blisters or necrosis with tissue loss.[6]

DIAGNOSTICS

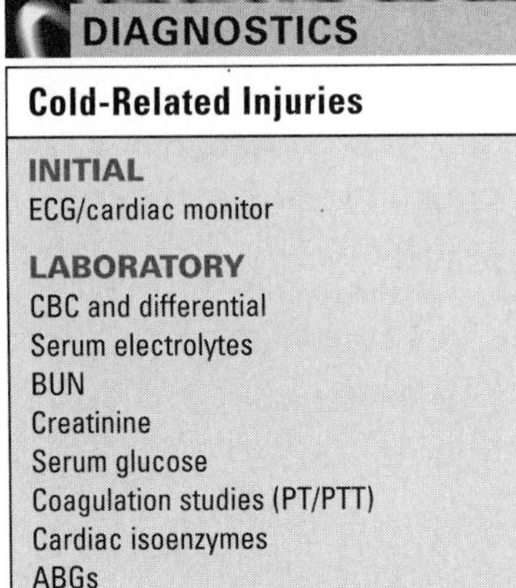

DIAGNOSTICS

Cold-Related Injuries

INITIAL
ECG/cardiac monitor

LABORATORY
CBC and differential
Serum electrolytes
BUN
Creatinine
Serum glucose
Coagulation studies (PT/PTT)
Cardiac isoenzymes
ABGs

Patients with hypothermia require cardiac monitoring and close observation for arrhythmias. Rectal temperature, preferably obtained with a continuous rectal probe, and vital signs are indicated. CBC, glucose, BUN, creatinine, serum electrolytes, coagulation studies (PT/PTT), cardiac isoenzymes, and arterial blood gases are also necessary.

DIFFERENTIAL DIAGNOSIS

Although the symptoms associated with hypothermia can be associated with other conditions, the core body temperature will indicate hypothermia. Further differentials should include the specific differences between mild, moderate, and severe hypothermia, as well as the difference between superficial and deep frostbite. This information will guide rewarming and treatment.

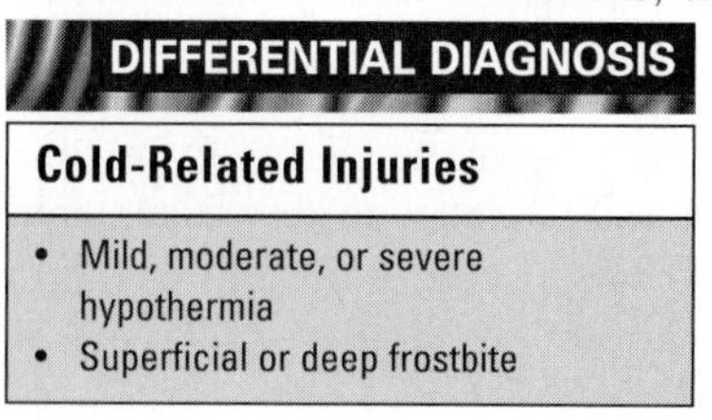
DIFFERENTIAL DIAGNOSIS
Cold-Related Injuries
• Mild, moderate, or severe hypothermia
• Superficial or deep frostbite

INITIAL STABILIZATION AND MANAGEMENT

Cold injuries require rewarming, and the method of rewarming is based on the clinical circumstances and availability of resources.[9] Regardless of the degree of cold injury, all patients with hypothermia should immediately have all cold or wet clothing removed and be covered with warm and dry blankets to prevent further heat loss. In addition, patients with moderate or severe hypothermia should be handled gently to prevent arrhythmias such as ventricular fibrillation. The care of patients in cardiac arrest necessitates rewarming because "death cannot be pronounced until the patient is warm and dead."[10]

Passive external rewarming includes placing these patients in a warm environment and covering them with warm, dry blankets. Active external rewarming includes warmed blankets, hot packs, warm bodies, or forced air rewarming.[9] Core rewarming includes perfusion of the body with warm IV fluids, administration of heated and humidified oxygen, and body cavity lavage with warm fluids. Hemodialysis and extracorporeal circulation are also considerations for rewarming.

Hypothermia precautions are also applicable to patients with frostbite. The injured part should be rewarmed as soon as possible with water between 37° and 40° C (98.6° and 104° F). Ibuprofen at a dosage of 12 mg/kg/day and topical aloe vera should be given to decrease the effects of inflammation.[11] Tetanus immunization status should be updated, and intravenous penicillin is recommended at a dosage of 500,000 units q 6 hr during the first 72 hours of treatment.[6] One precaution to follow is to not rewarm an affected extremity if there is a chance of refreezing before definitive treatment, since thaw-freeze-thaw creates tremendous tissue damage.

DISPOSITION AND REFERRAL

For mild symptoms that are resolved after rewarming, patients can be discharged. Other patients should be evaluated for hospitalization.[6] All patients with frostbite that exceeds the minimum symptoms should be hospitalized.

PREVENTION AND PATIENT EDUCATION

Hypothermia is preventable; however, nearly 700 people die each year from cold-related injuries.[12] Prevention of these injuries requires education regarding proper clothing and shelter. Layering of clothes to protect against extreme temperatures should also be advised. In addition, patients and families should understand that massaging the affected areas is contraindicated and that cold sensitivity is a common sequela of hypothermic injury. Advise patients to use the motto "comfortably cool" in cold environments to prevent sweating, since sweating can lead to hypothermia and frostbite later.

REFERENCES

1. Centers for Disease Control and Prevention: *Extreme heat,* retrieved Dec 7, 2006, from http://www.bt.cdc.gov/disasters/extremeheat/.
2. Yarbrough B, Vicario S: Heat illness. In Marx JA, Hockberger R, Walls R, editors: *Rosen's emergency medicine: concepts and clinical practice,* ed 5, St Louis, 2002, Mosby.
3. Glazer JL: Management of heatstroke and heat exhaustion, *Am Fam Phys* 71(11):2133-2140, 2141-2142, 2005.
4. Centers for Disease Control and Prevention: Hypothermia-related deaths—Philadelphia, 2001, and United States, 1999, *MMWR* 52(5):86-87, 2003, retrieved Dec 7, 2006, from http://www.cdc.gov/mmwr/preview/mmwrhtml/mm5205a3.htm.
5. Reamy BV: Frostbite: review and current concepts, *J Am Board Fam Pract* 11(1):34-40, 1998.
6. Tintinalli JE, Ruiz E, Krome RL, editors: *Emergency medicine,* ed 4, San Francisco, 1996, McGraw-Hill.
7. Gentilello LM: Advances in the management of hypothermia, *Surg Clin North Am* 75(2):243-256, 1995.
8. Danzl DF: Frostbite. In Marx JA, Hockberger R, Walls R, editors: *Rosen's emergency medicine: concepts and clinical practice,* ed 5, St Louis, 2002, Mosby.
9. Hanania NA, Zimmerman JL: Accidental hypothermia, *Crit Care Clin* 15(2):235-249, 1999.
10. Braun R, Krishel S: Environmental emergencies, *Emerg Med Clin North Am* 15(2):451-476, 1997.
11. Murphy J, Banwell P, Roberts A, and others: Frostbite: pathogenesis and treatment, *J Trauma* 48:171-188, 2000.
12. Hypothermia-related deaths: Utah, 2000 and United States, 1979-1998, *MMWR* 51(4):76-78, 2002.

PART 5

Evaluation and Management of Skin Disorders

JOANN TRYBULSKI, *Section Editor*

CHAPTER 44

Examination of the Skin and Approach to Diagnosing Skin Disorders

Margaret McAllister

DEFINITION AND EPIDEMIOLOGY

Skin problems occur in more than 25% of the general population and are the presenting complaint in 10% of primary care patients.[1] A large number of skin diseases manifest in similar ways. Factors such as age, ethnic and genetic makeup, risk factors, body habitus, skin surface, and self-care practices may complicate a diagnosis. Underlying systemic pathologic conditions may also contribute to the difficulty of making a definitive diagnosis of skin lesions.

OVERVIEW OF SKIN FUNCTION, ANATOMY, AND STRUCTURES

The primary functions of the skin include protection of the underlying body structures from ingress of microorganisms, control of body heat and elimination of body waste through perspiration, and prevention of injury to core body structures. The skin protects the body from infectious agents; protects against loss of body heat through conduction, convection, and radiation; and provides a first-line defense against mechanical, chemical, and thermal injury. Glands in the dermal layer of the skin secrete a substance that lubricates the body surface and assists with a variety of body functions. The peripheral sense receptors contained in the skin alert the body to pain, temperature changes, pressure, and touch.

The skin is composed of three layers: the epidermis; the dermis; and the hypodermis, or subcutis. The outer epidermal, or cuticle, layer is avascular and is divided into an outer horny layer (the stratum corneum) and an underlying horny layer (the stratum mucosum). The stratum corneum consists of keratinocytes—cells that originate in the basal cell layer of the epidermis and migrate upward to the stratum corneum and slough off as dead cells, called squames. As long as stratum corneum (the outer horny layer) is intact, normal skin bacteria are prevented from invading deeper skin and gaining access to the bloodstream. The lower layer of the epidermis contain the Langerhans' cells, which function as antigen-presenting cells that migrate to the lymph nodes and play an important role in the allergic skin response. Melanocytes found in the basal layer of the epidermis constitute the body's principal protection against ultraviolet (UV) radiation.[1]

The second layer of the skin, the dermis—also termed the *cutis, corneum*, or *true skin*—holds the epidermis in place. The dermis is composed of an outer papillary layer and an inner reticular layer that contains connective tissue and the blood supply, as well as lymphatic vessels, peripheral nerves, elastic tissue, and a reservoir of water and electrolytes. The dermal appendages are contained within the reticular layer and include the eccrine sweat glands that serve to control body temperature via evaporation, the sebum-producing sebaceous glands that lubricate the stratum corneum through openings in the skin (called pores), hair follicles, and the nail bed. Other appendages include apocrine glands attached to hair shafts located in the axillary, perianal, and genital areas. These glands respond to the increased hormone levels associated with puberty, adolescence, and young adulthood and decrease their activity with normal aging. A variation of the apocrine gland is the cerumen-producing glands lining the external auditory canal. The oily substance, cerumen, serves to protect the skin lining the ear canal from bacterial invasion.

A third layer of the skin, the hypodermis, or subcutis, functions to store fat, insulate the body from extremes in temperature, and provide a cushion against injury. It also contributes to the skin's mobility over underlying body parts.

CHANGES IN THE SKIN ASSOCIATED WITH AGING

With age, both structural and functional changes occur in the skin. These changes include a decrease in the number of Langerhans' cells; variation in size, shape, and staining of the keratinocytes; decrease in the thickness of the dermis; and loss of elastic tissue. There is a decrease in the number of sweat glands, hair follicles, and specialized nerve endings, as well as decreased vascularity and increased fragility of existing capillaries. Functional changes in the skin include a decreased inflammatory response; increased time for wound healing; thinning of the skin, resulting in increased fragility and risk of injury; decreased sweat capacity; and increased dryness secondary to reduced sebum production.[2,3]

ASSESSMENT

Formulating a differential diagnosis for skin lesions is based on an in-depth knowledge of various common skin disorders and their characteristic physical properties, including location and morphology. In addition, knowledge of the associated history typical of common rashes is essential. Variations in color, texture, and continuity of a patient's skin may be a normal genetic or ethnic variant, an indicator of local skin pathologic condition, or an indicator of an underlying systemic disease process. A proper assessment forms the basis for an appropriate care plan, patient education for self-care of acute and chronic skin lesions, and prevention of recurrence. Assessment begins with a careful history and physical examination. Additional investigative techniques, such as Wood's light examination, laboratory data, or microscopic skin scraping examination, may be necessary to ensure a definitive diagnosis.

Health History

Subjective components of a dermatologic history include taking a history from the patient or caregiver on the onset and progression of the rash, associated symptoms, any prior skin disorder, medications, social and occupational factors, and dietary practices. The health care provider inquires about self-care practices, such as homeopathic remedies, lotions, soaps, any change in laundry products, new clothing or fabrics, use of rubber gloves, cosmetics, sunbathing, tanning salons, and the humidity of the patient's typical ambient environment. In addition, a family or self-history of skin disorders, allergy, atopy, asthma, or eczema in childhood is reviewed.

Physical Examination

A hand-held magnifying lens (5× to 10×) is an important adjunct to the objective examination of skin lesions. Magnification affords the examiner the advantage of determining if the lesion is a disruption in the horny outer layer of the skin and can reveal changes in pigmentation throughout the lesion, such as in a melanoma. It can also be determined whether the lesion's borders are regular or irregular. The addition of oil to the skin further enhances the translucency of the stratum corneum and permits better visualization of skin fissures, hair follicles, and pores in the lesion.[4] The presence of scaling and inflammation can also be determined. A listing of primary and secondary lesions is provided in Figures 44-1 and 44-2.

Access to a freestanding light that can be adjusted to provide direct or oblique lighting is a necessary adjunct. Darkening the ambient lighting, allows for greater illumination and contrast of the involved lesion. Overillumination, however, may wash out important details of a lesion. Direct lighting with an intense penlight or the ophthalmoscope head with a halogen light permits visualization of closed vesicles or pustules and differentiation of fluid or cystic masses.

Another form of lighting is the Wood's light, or black light, which emits long wavelengths (>365 nm) of UV rays through a Wood's filter made of nickel oxide and silica, rendering UV rays harmless to the skin. The advantage is that, under this lighting method, skin diseases such as tinea versicolor fluoresce a white to yellow color, and erythrasma, a scaly skin condition caused by *Corynebacterium minutissimum*, fluoresces a bright coral red color.[5] Even small amounts of decreased melanin, such as vitiligo, are accentuated under the Wood's light and appear stark white. *Pseudomonas* infections appear yellow-green.[4]

Palpation of skin lesions provides information on the extent of the lesion below the skin surface, its consistency, its exact size, and associated pain. Certain lesions, such as dermatofibromas, will indent with lateral palpation, a distinguishing characteristic known as Fitzpatrick's sign. Dermatographism is a phenomenon that occurs when the skin of a person with urticaria has the skin lightly rubbed with a pointed object, such as the back of a fingernail. Histamine is released under the skin surface, and the skin becomes raised and red where the object touched it.

Diagnosis involves a close evaluation of the lesion's distribution or location, configuration, borders, size, shape, color, and surface characteristics or appearance. Documentation includes a description of the lesion's size, color, shape, surface characteristics, distribution, and configuration.

A discussion of skin examination techniques is provided in Box 44-1.

Quality of care is enhanced when providers develop strong interpersonal relationships with patients who come to see them with dermatologic problems. Patient satisfaction has been shown to be related to the provider's ability to teach patients about their condition and to show concern and caring for their problem. This in turn may lead to enhanced compliance and better treatment outcomes.[8]

Macules are localized changes in the skin color. They are flat and nonpalpable, but they may be scaly. Examples include freckles, lentigines (or "age spots"), actinic lentigines on sun-exposed areas, large macules of melasma seen in pregnancy, and the hypopigmented macular lesions of vitiligo and pityriasis alba. Oblique lighting may assist in determining if a macule is flat or raised, suggesting a papule.

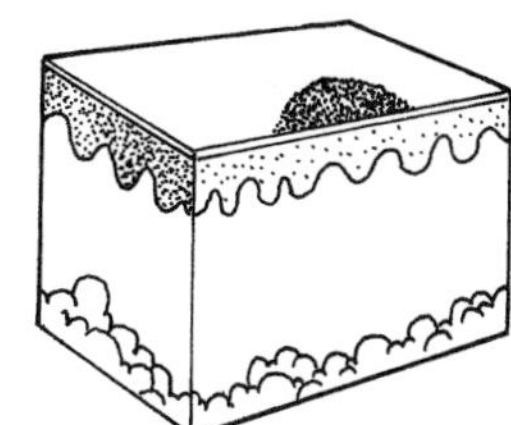

Papules can be solid or fluid-filled lesions that are elevated and are less than 5 mm in diameter. The size and shape of a papule can vary from pointed to flat-topped lesions. Examples of papules include atopic eczema or a viral exanthema that is a combined macular-papular rash.

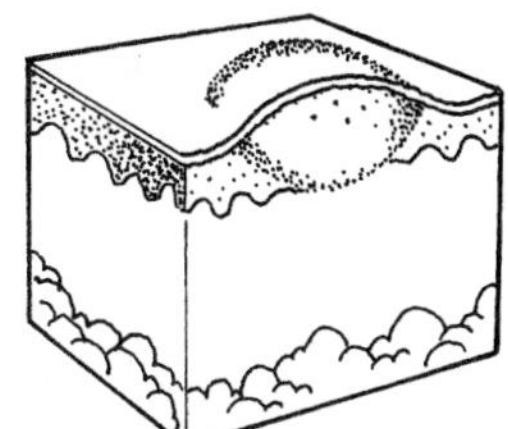

Nodules are both solid and elevated above the surface of the skin but usually originate deeper in skin layers. Nodules measure greater than 5 mm in diameter. Palpation assists in determining the depth of a nodule. If the skin slides over the nodule, it is beneath the dermis and in the subcutaneous layer. If the skin moves with the lesion, it is located in the dermis. A hemanginoma, a basal cell carcinoma, or melanoma may be termed a nodule.

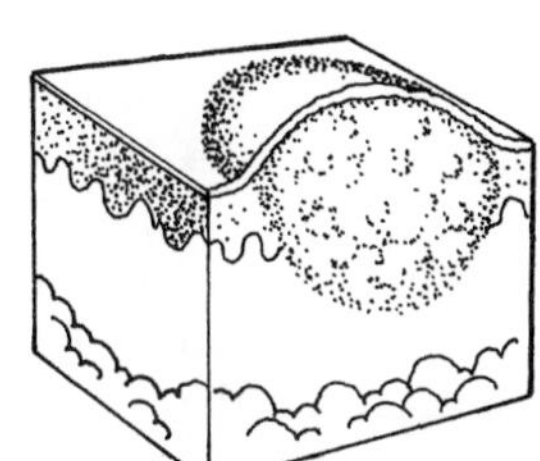

Plaques are elevated lesions larger than 5 mm in diameter. Like papules, they may take on a variety of shapes. A plaque is often a close grouping of multiple papules, such as is seen in seborrheic dermatitis, tinea corporis, tinea versicolor, or psoriasis.

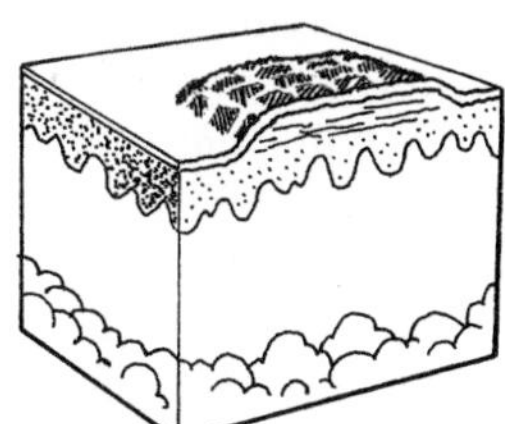

Vesicles and *bullae* are well-circumscribed, fluid-filled areas under the superficial layers of the skin. A vesicle can measure 5 mm in diameter. The covering over the vesicle is a thin layer of epithelium that is easily punctured. An example is the vesicle of herpes simplex or impetigo. Bullae are accumulations of fluid under the superficial layers of the skin that measure greater than 5 mm in diameter. Burns of the second degree constitute bullae, as do large impetigo lesions and the lesions of a fixed drug eruption.

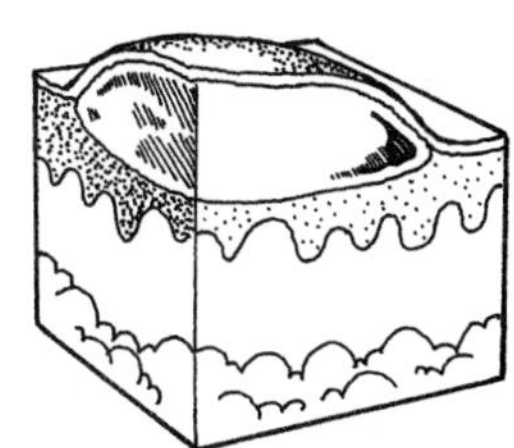

Wheals are an accumulation of fluid within the dermal layer of the skin that forms an edematous plaque. Wheals are localized edema of the skin, and they may appear in a variety of sizes and shapes. The color depends on the amount of fluid in the wheal. Examples of wheals include hives and angioedema.

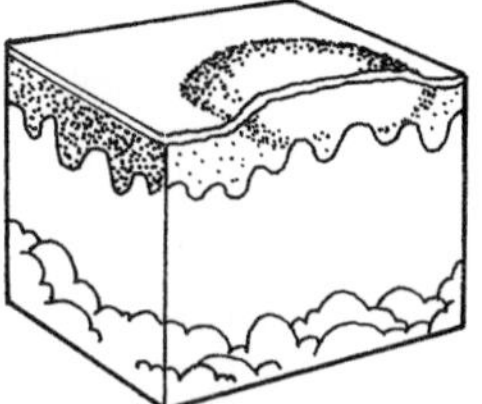

Pustules are abscessed lesions filled with pus. Furuncles and acne lesions are pustular and often respond to antibiotic and local therapy.

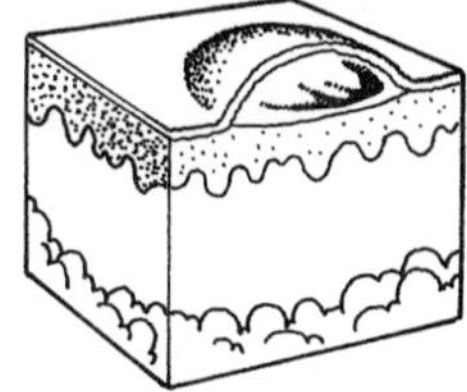

Figure 44-1

Primary lesions.

Scales are dried, thin, platelike lesions of cornified epithelium. These lesions are partially attached, partially separated from the epidermis, and commonly associated with exfoliative skin conditions. Scales are commonly seen with psoriasis or seborrheic dermatitis.

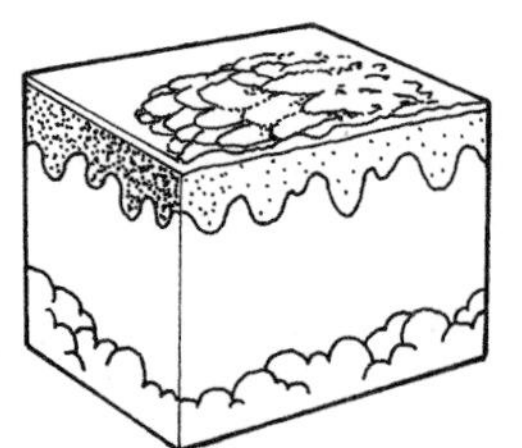

Crusts are hard, dried exudates that occur on the surface of ruptured vesicles or pustules. Crusted lesions and vesicles on an erythematous base are often seen in perioral herpes simplex or in herpes zoster.

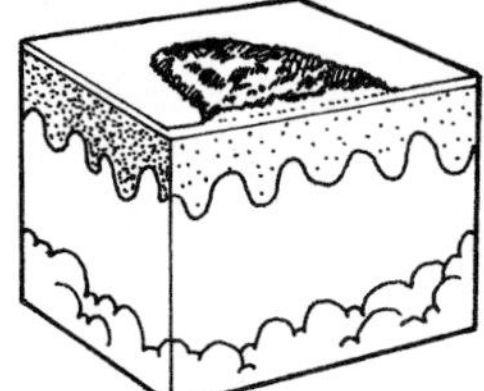

Erosions are skin injuries that may result from rubbing or shearing. This type of lesion is moist and may also result from a ruptured vesicular or pustular lesion.

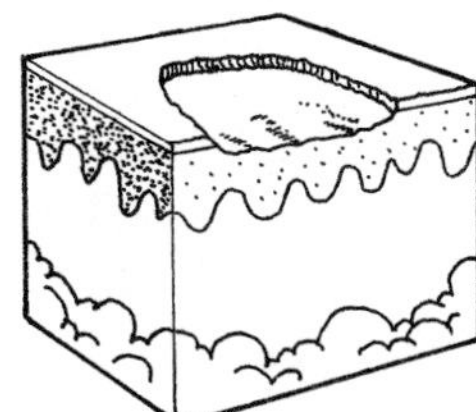

Fissures are slivered lesions that extend from the epidermis into the dermis. Fissures may occur from trauma but are also associated with inflexible, dried skin that cracks when stretched.

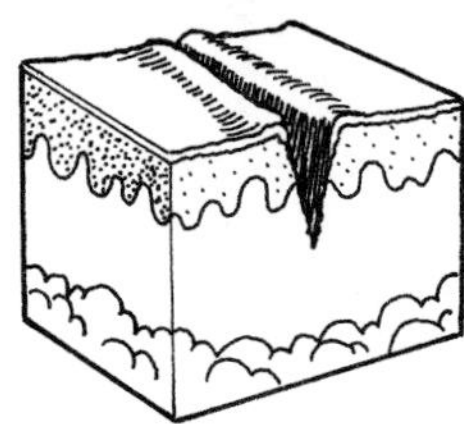

Atrophy is used to describe lesions that are inelastic and have lost characteristic rhomboid lines. In discoid lupus erythematosus, the lesions commonly seen on the scalp, face, arms, and torso have central atrophy but may have accompanying erythematous borders, scales, and telangiectasia.

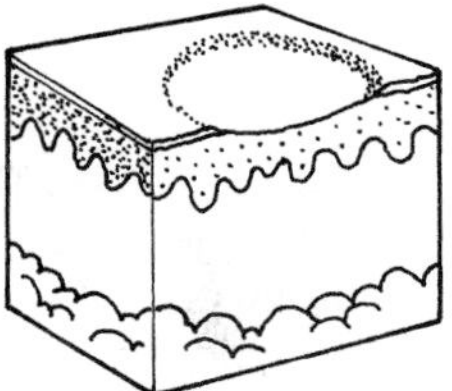

Ulcers are concave lesions with a sunken appearance. The result of trauma and/or poor circulation, ulcers extend from the epidermis into the dermis.

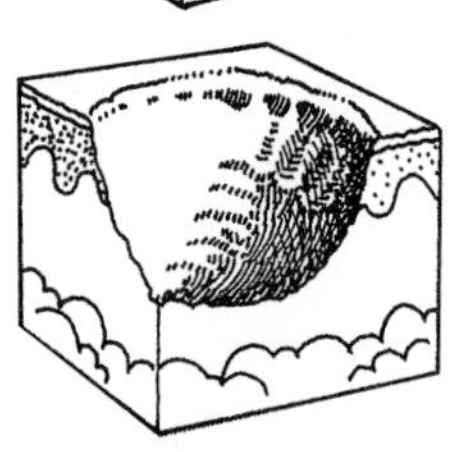

Scars are fibrous lesions that result from trauma to the skin. The appearance depends on the etiology of the injury, but new scars are generally hyperpigmented. As the lesion ages, the scar will fade and become hypopigmented.

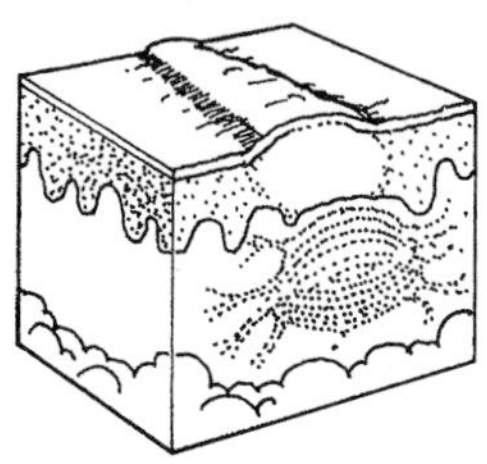

Figure 44-2

Secondary lesions. Secondary lesions are changes that occur in primary lesions as a result of environmental factors, self-care practices (such as scratching), inflammation of surrounding tissues, healing and scar formation, infection, and the use of topical medications such as steroids.

BOX 44-1

SKIN EXAMINATION TECHNIQUE

Diascopy can be performed using a flat microscope slide or other clear instrument, such as a magnifying glass. Blanching of blue to red lesions followed by a gradual refilling indicates blood in the capillaries; absence of blanching indicates blood leaching outside of the capillaries, as in petechiae.

Gram's stain of exudates from lesions is helpful in distinguishing the cause as either a gram-positive or gram-negative organism.

The Tzanck test with Wright's or Giemsa's stain can uncover multinucleated giant cells that are typical of herpes simplex or varicella zoster virus. The top of the vesicle must be removed to obtain fresh fluid from the base of the lesion.

A 10% to 30% potassium hydroxide (KOH) stain determines the presence of hyphae and spores consistent with candidiasis or uncovers the spaghetti-and-meatball appearance of tinea versicolor, caused by the skin fungus *Malassezia furur* and *Malassezia ovalis.*[5] Attempts should be made to obtain scrapings from the top of a lesion or from the advancing edge of a lesion. The skin lesion is aligned vertical to the microscopic slide, and a gentle scraping of the lesion with the side of a slide or a scalpel loosens skin debris collected on the slide below. KOH is applied directly to the scale debris and a coverslip is placed over the skin scraping, or the KOH is applied alongside the edge of the coverslip. KOH then gravitates to cover the specimen by capillary action. The specimen is then set under the microscope for examination, first using 10× power and then proceeding to 40× for finer detail. The examiner must be certain to close the condenser diaphragm and turn the condenser down to enhance the detail of hyphae that are embedded in the scaly debris.[6]

Culture for herpesvirus, streptococcus, staphyloccocus, or *Pseudomonas* organisms requires removal of the outer crust or cuticle of the lesion to obtain fluid for culturing. The fluid at the base of the lesion is most likely to be positive for the contributing organisms and free of contamination from the skin surface. A special viral culture–collecting device must be used in accordance with laboratory specifications. Bacterial cultures for streptococci and staphylococci can be collected with a regular throat culture–collecting swab. *Candida* organisms can be grown on Sabouraud's agar in a 2- to 6-day period, whereas dermatophytes take up to 2 to 4 weeks to grow on the same agar. The organisms of tinea versicolor grow only on special media.[6]

In *scabies preparation* a superficial skin shaving from a skin fold area is obtained from the top of a burrow and examined under oil immersion. Oil or KOH solution should be placed on the lesion first. With a scalpel the top is shaved off the lesion, and the debris is placed on a microscopic slide. Additional oil and a coverslip are added, and the specimen is examined under 10× magnification.[7] The presence of adult mites, eggs, or feces in the burrows is sufficient in the diagnosis of scabies.

REFERENCES

1. Greenberger N, Hinthorn DR: *History taking and physical examination: essentials and correlates*, St Louis, 1993, Mosby.
2. Goldsmith L, Lazarus GS, Tharp MD: *Adult and pediatric dermatology: a color guide to diagnosis and treatment*, Philadelphia, 1997, Davis.
3. Ebersol P, Hess P: *Towards healthy aging: human needs and nursing responses*, ed 5, St Louis, 1998, Mosby.
4. *Merck manual of geriatrics*, ed 3, Whitehouse Station, NJ, 2000, Merck.
5. Habif TP: *Clinical dermatology: a color guide to diagnosis and therapy*, ed 4, St Louis, 2004, Mosby.
6. Reeves JT, Maibach HI: *Clinical dermatology illustrated: a regional approach*, ed 3, Philadelphia, 1998, Davis.
7. Klauss W, Johnson RA, Suurmond R: *Fitzpatrick's color atlas and synopsis of clinical dermatology*, ed 5, New York, 2005, McGraw-Hill.
8. Renzi C, Abeni D, Picardi A, and others: Factors associated with patient satisfaction with care among dermatological outpatients, *Br J Dermatol* 145(4):617-623, 2001.

CHAPTER 45

Surgical Office Procedures

Eileen M. Deignan

As an external organ, the skin is accessible for diagnostic biopsies and therapeutic procedures. In the changing health care environment, more patients are seeing nondermatologists for skin problems. In fact, more nondermatologists than dermatologists receive visits for malignant skin tumors.[1,2] The diagnosis of malignant skin tumors by clinical examination and lesion biopsy is an important skill for a health care provider.

Skin biopsies are fundamental techniques in the diagnosis and management of neoplastic skin disease. With practice, they can be performed safely and with minimum scarring. However, these technical skills cannot substitute for clinical knowledge. Before performing a biopsy, the health care provider should always consider the diagnostic possibilities of the neoplasm, select the optimum biopsy site and technique, and determine if referral to a more experienced colleague is necessary. Inflammatory lesions that require a biopsy for diagnosis are probably best treated by a dermatologist.

INDICATIONS FOR BIOPSY

All suspicious neoplastic lesions should be biopsied. It is a greater error not to biopsy a suspicious lesion than to biopsy benign lesions too often. In a study of the ability of primary care residents to diagnose and manage possibly cancerous lesions, 33% did not recommend a skin biopsy in cases in which it was appropriate.[3] In many cases an excisional biopsy also serves as the treatment for some precancerous and malignant lesions.

A lesion that clinically appears to be an atypical nevus or malignant melanoma should be completely removed to the level of the subcutaneous fat with a punch or elliptical excision.[4] The thickness of a melanoma is the single most important criterion for predicting survival of patients with nonmetastatic melanoma.[5] In the event that the lesion is indeed a malignant melanoma, it is important that it be removed to the level of the subcutaneous fat so that its depth can be measured accurately. If a partial-thickness biopsy is performed on a melanoma, the true thickness of the lesion cannot be adequately evaluated.

BIOPSY REFERRAL

Patients with bleeding disorders, hematologic malignancies, and conditions that require anticoagulation therapy are more likely to develop complications from biopsies. Additionally, lower leg biopsies of patients with diabetes or vascular disease may be complicated by delayed wound healing. Thus these individuals should be referred to a dermatologist or surgeon for biopsy. If careful attention is given to hemostasis, patients who are taking aspirin can undergo biopsies in the health care provider's office.

Certain anatomic locations are more difficult to biopsy safely. The scalp, for example, is a particularly vascular area, and biopsies in this site often bleed profusely. The palms of the hands, soles of the feet, and lateral aspects of the fingers are also challenging areas to biopsy because of the underlying neurovasculature and fascia. Overall, the face is a cosmetically sensitive area; technically, the eyelids and nose are particularly challenging areas to biopsy. Patients requiring biopsies in any of these areas should be referred to an experienced dermatologist or surgeon.

SITE SELECTION

The goal of a biopsy is to obtain a specimen representative of the lesion. Small, suspicious lesions can be removed entirely with a punch or shave biopsy. For a larger lesion, often just a part is removed. In such cases the area that is thickest or has the most abnormal color should be sampled. These areas will be most likely to have a specific pathologic condition.

Melanocytic lesions are best approached with an excisional biopsy, in which the entire lesion is removed for histologic analysis. The punch biopsy can be used to sample part of a melanocytic lesion. It is important to remember that the sampled area may not include the most worrisome part of the lesion, and the result could be falsely reassuring.

TECHNIQUE CHOICE

Punch Biopsy

A punch biopsy is used to sample a lesion that appears to extend below the epidermis. As a diagnostic procedure, it is useful both to identify the disease process and to ascertain the depth of the process. For instance, the entire thickness of the epidermis should be sampled to diagnose a squamous cell carcinoma. If only part of the epidermis is sampled, neither the thickness of the epidermal abnormality nor the degree of invasion can be assessed. As a result, an actinic keratosis cannot be distinguished from a squamous cell carcinoma in situ or from an invasive squamous cell carcinoma (Table 45-1).

A punch biopsy is performed with a cylindric instrument called a *punch*. These instruments have a sharp circular edge to bore out a cylindric piece of tissue and are manufactured in diameters from 2 to 10 mm (0.08 to 0.4 inch). The 2-mm punch should be reserved for small lesions or cosmetically sensitive areas. It may not provide enough tissue for adequate analysis of most lesions. Depending on the location on the body, punches larger than 6 mm (0.25 inch) can have a cosmetic complication when the wound is repaired. The standing cutaneous horns ("dog ears") at the ends of a large oval wound closure can result in an unsightly scar. Instead of using a large punch, the health care provider should consider removing the lesion with an elliptic excision, thereby eliminating the standing cutaneous horns.

Shave (Parallel Plane) Biopsy

The shave biopsy is best for lesions that are elevated above the level of the epidermis or have a disease confined to the epidermis. Examples include superficial basal cell carcinoma, seborrheic keratosis, verruca vulgaris, and pyogenic

TABLE 45-1 Optimum Techniques for Biopsying Common Lesions

Lesion	Punch	Shave	Scissor	Ellipse
Suspicious pigmented lesion	Yes*	No	No	Yes
Basal cell carcinoma	Yes	Yes	No	Yes
Squamous cell carcinoma	Yes	No	No	Yes
Verruca vulgaris	No	Yes	Yes	No
Seborrheic keratosis	No	Yes	No	No
Pyogenic granuloma	No	Yes	Yes	No

*If lesion is small enough to be excised by punch.

granuloma (see Table 45-1). Because it is more superficial than a punch biopsy, a shave biopsy site usually heals more rapidly and with less scarring.

Scissor Excision

The scissor excision is useful for removing small exophytic or pedunculated growths such as acrochordons (skin tags), filiform warts, and polypoid nevi (see Table 45-1). A scissor excision that does not remove a significant amount of epidermis does not result in obvious scarring because of the superficial nature of the wound.

PREPARATION

The rationale for the biopsy and the wound care involved should be outlined for the patient, and informed consent should be obtained. The major complications of biopsies and scissor excisions are bleeding, infection, allergic contact dermatitis, and scarring. These possibilities should be stated before starting the procedure.

Shave biopsies leave a round or oval, depressed, and hypopigmented or hyperpigmented scar. Ideally, a sutured punch biopsy leaves a linear scar. A site left to close by secondary intention heals with a round, depressed scar.

The health care provider should inquire about the patient's tendency to form hypertrophic scars or keloids, which tend to occur on the deltoids and the chest. If a lesion on the chest or deltoid is to be biopsied, the patient should be counseled that a hypertrophic or keloid-type scar may form, even if there is no history of abnormal scarring.

Before the procedure, patients should be asked about medical conditions and medications that can predispose them to bleeding. Any sensitivities to the items used to care for the biopsy wound, such as antibiotic ointment or adhesive tape, should be ascertained. Immunosuppressive diseases or medications that could predispose the patient to infection or delay wound healing should be noted, and the patient should be advised.

BIOPSY PROCEDURE

Shave biopsies, punch biopsies, and scissor excisions are clean but not sterile procedures. Practitioners should wear gloves and eye protection, but masks and gowns are not necessary. A fenestrated drape will provide a clean field.

Materials

It may be helpful to assemble biopsy materials in one location. A complete set includes marking pens; alcohol pads; 1% or 2% lidocaine with and without epinephrine; 20-gauge (for drawing up) and 30-gauge (for injecting) needles; 3-ml syringes; gauze pads; fenestrated drapes; a selection of disposable punches; no. 15 blades; toothed forceps; scissors; needle drivers; 4-0, 5-0, and 6-0 nylon sutures; antibiotic ointment (bacitracin, not triple antibiotic with neomycin) or petroleum jelly; and adhesive bandages.

Anesthetic

The lesion should be marked with an indelible pen, since the lesion may not be visible after the injection of a local anesthetic as a result of the vasoconstrictive effect of lidocaine. The area is cleaned with alcohol, and 0.2 to 0.5 ml of 1% to 2% lidocaine with 1:100,000 epinephrine is infused (for patients with allergies to preservatives, a "preservative free" local anesthetic must be used). The lesion is raised by infusing anesthetic into and under the lesion; this facilitates the shave biopsy. Epinephrine causes local vasoconstriction, which decreases bleeding and prolongs the duration of anesthesia. Maximum vasoconstriction is achieved in 15 to 20 minutes. *Lidocaine without epinephrine is used if the area to be biopsied is the tip of the nose, the finger, the toe, or the penis.* The vasoconstrictive effect of epinephrine in these distal areas, which have limited blood supply, could result in necrosis.

Punch Biopsy

The skin is stabilized with the thumb and forefinger of one hand and is pulled perpendicular to the relaxed skin tension lines. The punch is held perpendicular to the skin and rotated into the skin with a firm, constant, circular motion (Figure 45-1). The punch is advanced until the tissue "gives" as the punch advances into the subcutaneous fat. The punch should be advanced cautiously in thin areas such as the fingers or face. The punch is removed, and either side of the wound is pressed gently. The core of tissue is grasped gently with the forceps and elevated out of the wound to expose the base. Care should be taken not to crush the specimen with the forceps. Scissors are used to sever the base of the sample from the underlying fat. The specimen is placed immediately in 10% neutral buffered formalin.

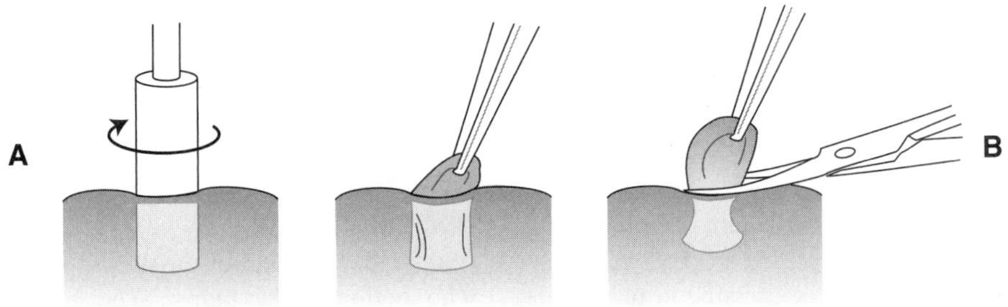

FIGURE 45-1

A, Punch biopsy. B, Scissor excision. (From Edmunds MW, Mayhew MS: *Procedures for primary care practitioners*, ed 2, St Louis, 2002, Mosby.)

Because of normal skin tension, the defect created by the biopsy will be oval. The defect is closed with monofilament nylon suture using a simple interrupted suture. One or two sutures should be sufficient. In general, 4-0 or 5-0 sutures can be used on the trunk and extremities; the finer 6-0 suture should be used for the face. Care should be taken while suturing to approximate and evert the wound edges for optimum healing.[5] The goal of suturing a punch biopsy is twofold: (1) hemostasis and (2) improved cosmetic result. Suturing requires more expertise and time, but the end result is often noticeably better than a wound that has been closed with Steri-Strips or allowed to heal by secondary intention.

Shave Biopsy

With a shave biopsy the area should be prepared and anesthetized in the same way as for a punch biopsy. The lesion is stabilized between the thumb and forefinger. A no. 15 blade is held parallel to the surface of the skin and stroked smoothly under the lesion, avoiding a sawing motion. To avoid creating a deep wound, strict attention should be given to keeping the blade parallel to the skin (Figure 45-2). The sample is grasped gently with forceps and placed immediately in 10% neutral buffered formalin.

Holding pressure on the wound for 5 minutes can usually control the small vessel bleeding created by the sampling. If needed, the field is blotted dry, and a cotton-tipped swab soaked in a chemical hemostatic agent (e.g., 20% aluminum chloride in absolute alcohol) is rolled across the field several times. Ferric subsulfate (Monsel's solution) and silver nitrate are also useful as hemostatic agents but should be avoided with cutaneous procedures. They are more corrosive than aluminum chloride and can tattoo the skin.

Scissor Excision

Because the pain of administering an anesthetic is often greater than the excision itself, very small lesions do not require an

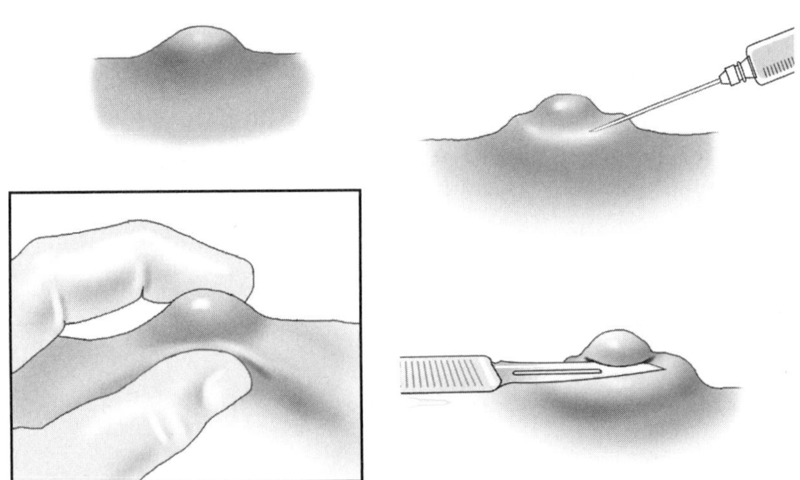

FIGURE 45-2

Shave biopsy. (From Edmunds MW, Mayhew MS: *Procedures for primary care practitioners*, ed 2, St Louis, 2002, Mosby.)

anesthetic. The lesion is held up with forceps and snipped at the base (see Figure 45-1). Aluminum chloride can be used for hemostasis. A bandage usually is not necessary.

WOUND CARE

The biopsy site will heal faster in a moist, occluded environment. Therefore the wound is dressed with an antibiotic ointment or petroleum jelly and an adhesive bandage. The patient should be instructed to leave the dressing in place for 12 to 24 hours. Thereafter the area is washed once a day with soap and water and covered again with an antibiotic ointment or petroleum jelly and adhesive bandage. Suture sites should be cleaned and dressed in this manner until the sutures are removed. Shave biopsy wounds, which heal by secondary intention, should reepithelialize in 7 to 10 days. After reepithelialization, no special care is needed in the area.

The timing of the biopsy suture removal is important for the cosmetic result. Sutures should be left in place long enough to prevent the wound from stretching or dehiscing but not so long that suture marks ("railroad tracks") remain at the wound edge. As a rule, sutures in areas not under tension (e.g., the face) should be removed in 5 to 7 days. Sutures in areas that are under tension (e.g., the trunk and extremities) should be left in place for 10 to 14 days.[6]

COMPLICATIONS

Infection, bleeding, scarring, and allergic reactions are the most common complications of biopsies. If a patient notes oozing of blood from the wound, he or she should place direct pressure on the site for 20 minutes. This intervention should be adequate to control small vessel bleeding. Immediate evaluation is essential if the wound continues to bleed. The sutures should be removed and the wound explored for a bleeding vessel.

Postbiopsy bacterial infections are usually caused by *Staphylococcus aureus* or group A streptococcus species.[7] Any purulent drainage should be cultured, and oral or topical antibiotic therapy should be considered. Biopsies on the hands and feet or in intertriginous areas such as the groin and axillae can become infected with *Candida* organisms. These infections usually respond well to topical antifungals.[8]

If erythema and pruritus develop around the wound site, a contact allergy to the antibiotic cream or dressing should be considered. The neomycin in triple-antibiotic cream is a notorious cause of contact allergy at biopsy sites. The alleged offending agent should be discontinued. Petroleum jelly is substituted if the reaction appears to be to the antibiotic ointment. A gauze pad held in place by paper tape is usually well tolerated by patients who react to adhesive bandages. Very exuberant reactions that vesiculate may require a short course of low-potency topical cortisone.[9]

DOCUMENTATION

Careful documentation is the responsibility of the provider who performs the biopsy. The age, gender, and pertinent history of the patient (e.g., duration of lesion, skin cancer risk factors, previous malignancies) are indicated on the pathology requisition sheet. A brief clinical description and the clinical diagnosis or differential diagnosis of the biopsied lesion should be provided for the pathologist.

The procedure is documented in the patient's chart. Along with the description and clinical diagnosis or differential diagnosis, the location of the lesion should be carefully described or drawn. It is particularly critical to identify the location of the lesion when a shave excision is performed. Otherwise, it may be difficult to locate the lesion should it require further treatment, since the scar may not be apparent after the wound has healed. Indications for the biopsy, informed consent, procedure, specimen disposition, dressing, wound care instructions, and follow-up plans should also be documented.

REFERENCES

1. Alguire PC, Mathes BM: Skin biopsy techniques for the internist, *J Gen Intern Med* 13(1):46-54, 1998.
2. Stern RS, Gardocki GJ: Office-based care of dermatologic disease, *J Am Acad Dermatol* 14(2 pt 1):286-293, 1986.
3. Gerbert B, Maurer T, Berger T, and others: Primary care physicians as gatekeepers in managed care: primary care physicians' and dermatologists' skills at secondary prevention of skin cancer, *Arch Dermatol* 132(9):1030-1038, 1996.
4. Bolognia JL: Biopsy techniques for pigmented lesions, *Dermatol Surg* 26(1):89-90, 2000.
5. Balch CM, Murad TM, Soong SJ, and others: Tumor thickness guide to surgical management of clinical stage I melanoma patients, *Cancer* 43(3):883-888, 1979.
6. Moy RL, Waldman B, Hein DW: A review of sutures and suturing techniques, *J Dermatol Surg Oncol* 18(9):785-795, 1992.
7. Haas AF, Grekin RC: Practical thoughts on antibiotic prophylaxis, *Arch Dermatol* 134(7):872-873, 1998.
8. Haas AF, Grekin RC: Antibiotic prophylaxis in dermatologic surgery, *J Am Acad Dermatol* 32(2 pt 1):155-176, quiz 177-180, 1995.
9. Gette MT, Marks JG Jr, Maloney ME: Frequency of postoperative allergic contact dermatitis to topical antibiotics, *Arch Dermatol* 128(3):365-367, 1992.

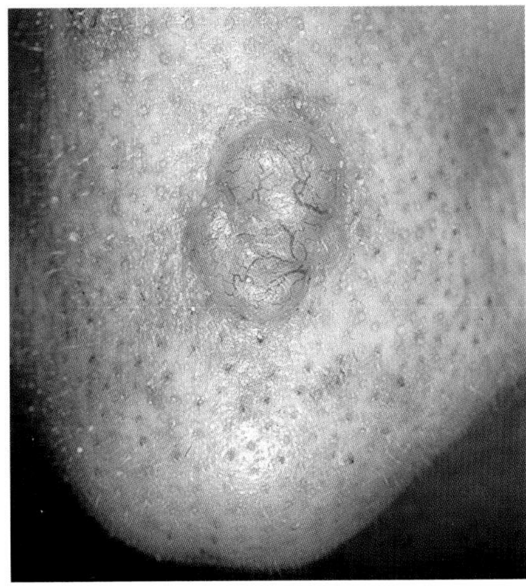

Plate 1 – Nodular basal cell carcinoma. (From Habif TP and others: *Skin disease: diagnosis and treatment,* St Louis, 2001, Mosby.)

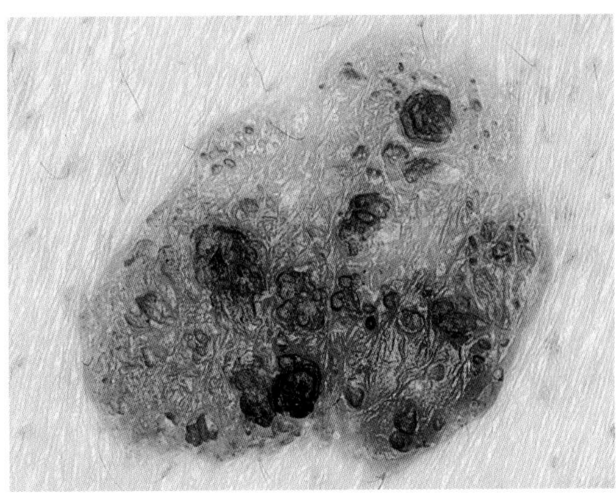

Plate 2 – Seborrheic keratosis (mimicking melanoma). (From Habif TP and others: *Skin disease: diagnosis and treatment,* St Louis, 2001, Mosby.)

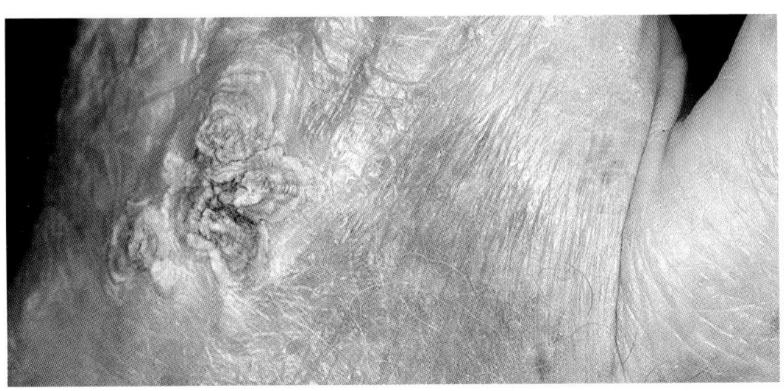

Plate 3 – Squamous cell cancer. (From Habif TP and others: *Skin disease: diagnosis and treatment,* St Louis, 2001, Mosby.)

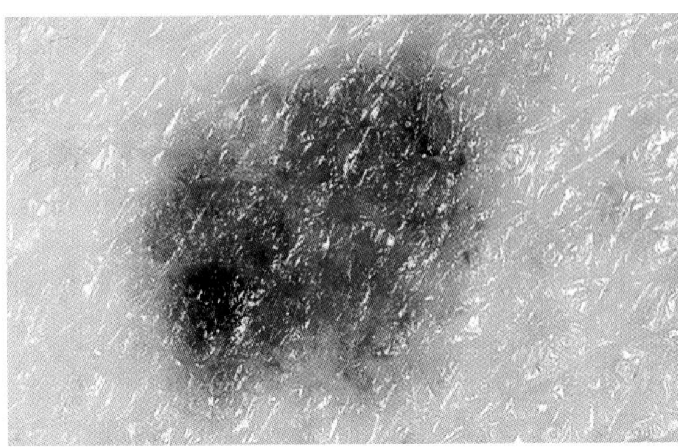

Plate 4 – Superficial spreading melanoma. (From Habif TP and others: *Skin disease: diagnosis and treatment,* St Louis, 2001, Mosby.)

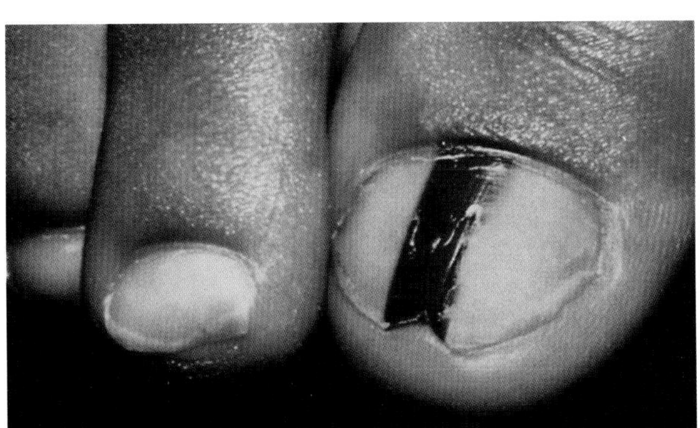

Plate 5 – Acral-lentiginous melanoma. It occurs most often on hands, feet, or nail beds of dark-skinned individuals. Very common in African Americans and Asian Americans. (From Habif TP and others: *Skin disease: diagnosis and treatment,* St Louis, 2001, Mosby.)

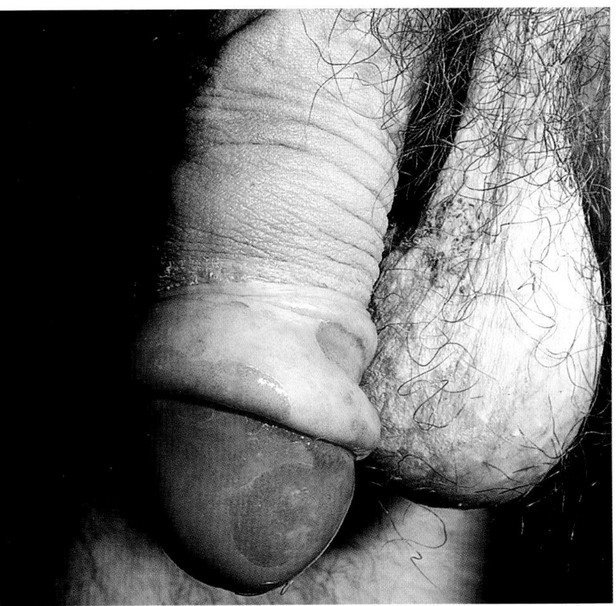

Plate 6 – Multiple syphilitic chancres. (From Fisher BK, Margesson LJ: *Genital skin disorders: diagnosis and treatment,* St Louis, 1998, Mosby.)

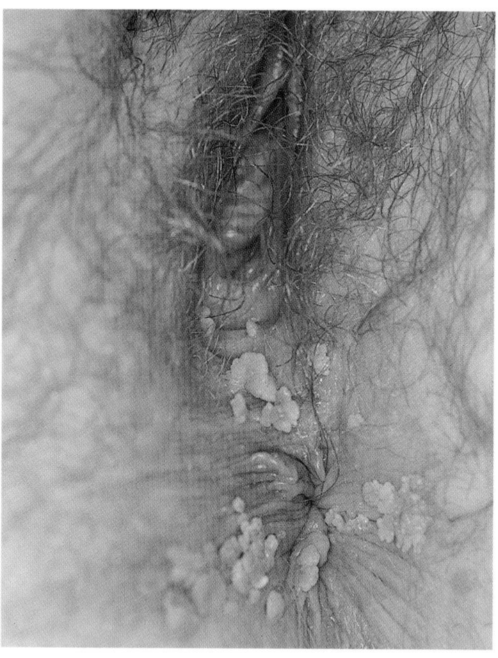

Plate 7 – Multiple condylomata in the perineum and perianal area. (From Fisher BK, Margesson LJ: *Genital skin disorders: diagnosis and treatment,* St Louis, 1998, Mosby.)

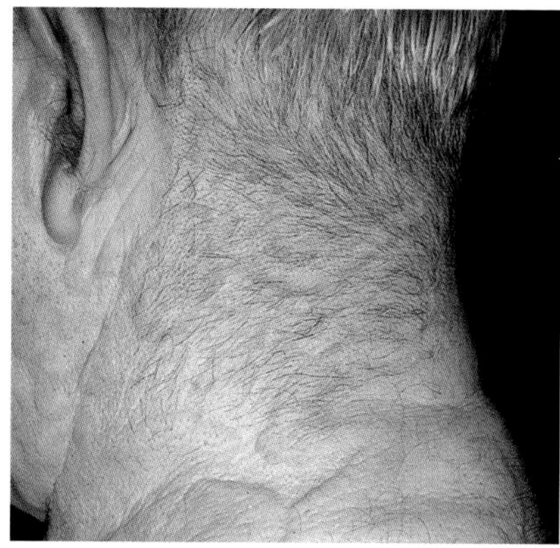

Plate 8 – Angioedema affects the face, lips, palms, soles, or a portion of an extremity. It may become confluent and cover wide areas. The color is uniform. Hives vary in color. (From Habif TP and others: *Skin disease: diagnosis and treatment,* St Louis, 2001, Mosby.)

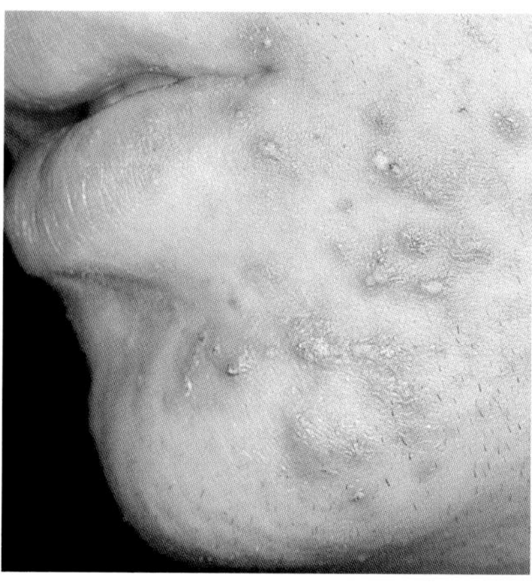

Plate 9 – Pustular acne. (From Habif TP and others: *Skin disease: diagnosis and treatment,* St Louis, 2001, Mosby.)

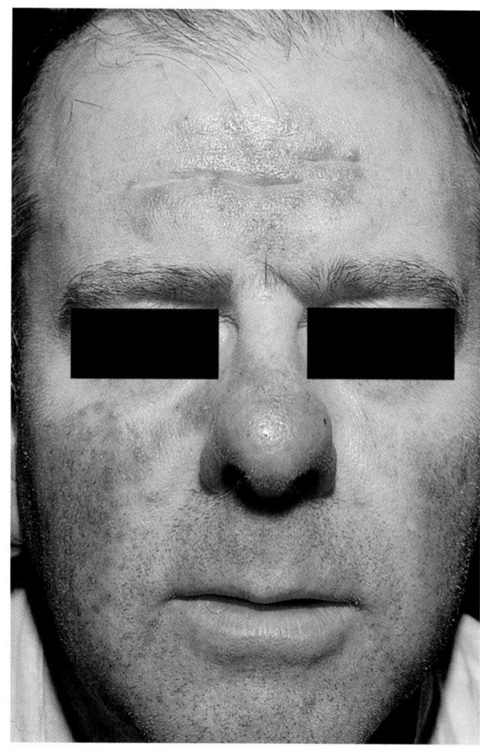

Plate 10 – Rosacea. (From Habif TP and others: *Skin disease: diagnosis and treatment,* St Louis, 2001, Mosby.)

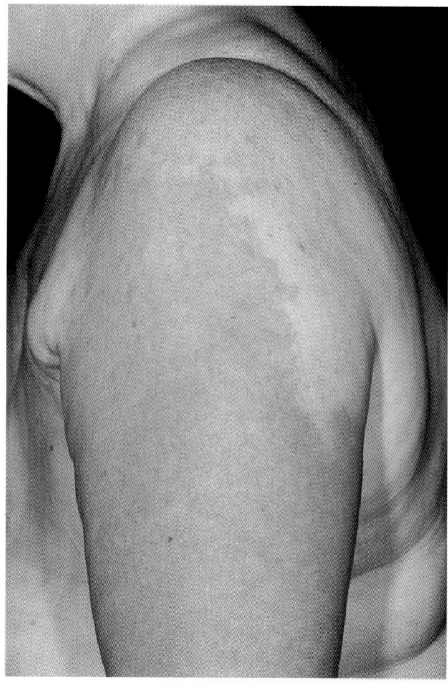

Plate 11 – Cellulitis. (From Habif TP and others: *Skin disease: diagnosis and treatment,* St Louis, 2001, Mosby.)

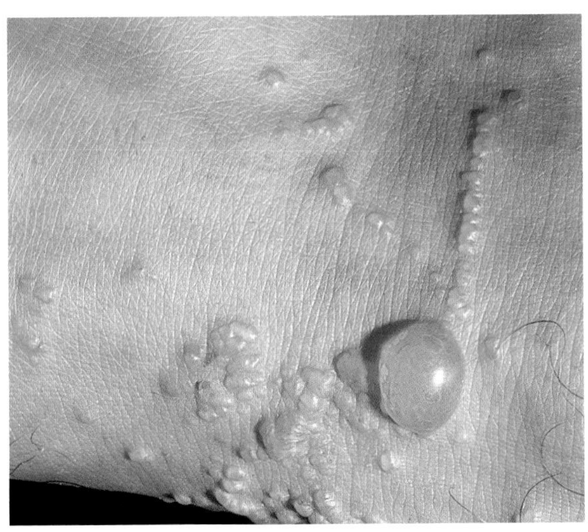

Plate 12 – Rhus dermatitis (poison ivy). (From Habif TP and others: *Skin disease: diagnosis and treatment,* St Louis, 2001, Mosby.)

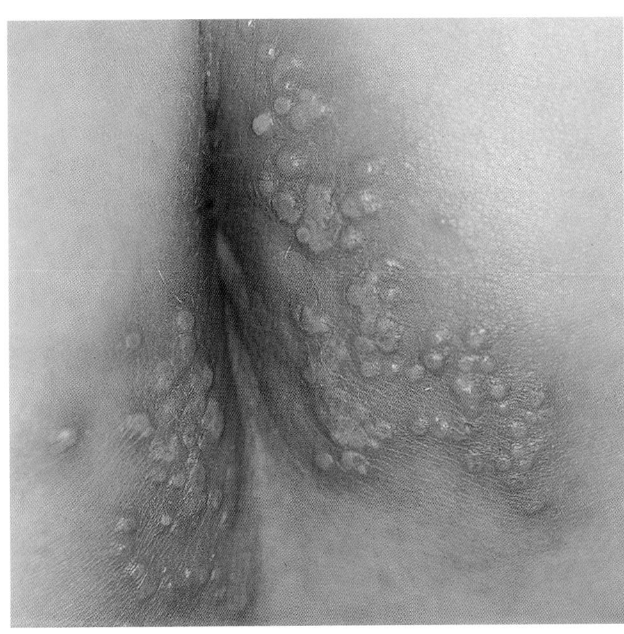

Plate 13 – Primary herpes simplex on the perineum and buttocks with groups of vesicles on a red base. (From Fisher BK, Margesson LJ: *Genital skin disorders: diagnosis and treatment,* St Louis, 1998, Mosby.)

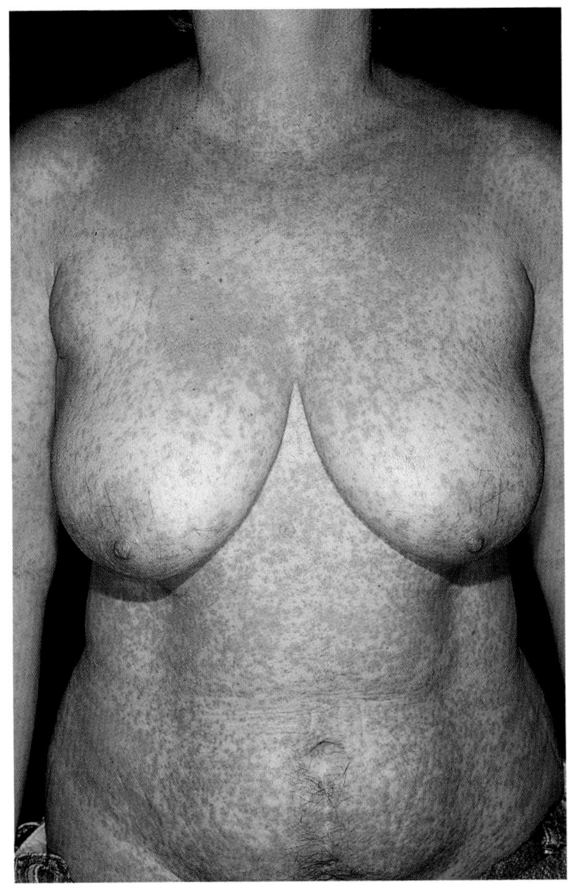

Plate 14 – Cutaneous drug reaction. (From Habif TP and others: *Skin disease: diagnosis and treatment,* St Louis, 2001, Mosby.)

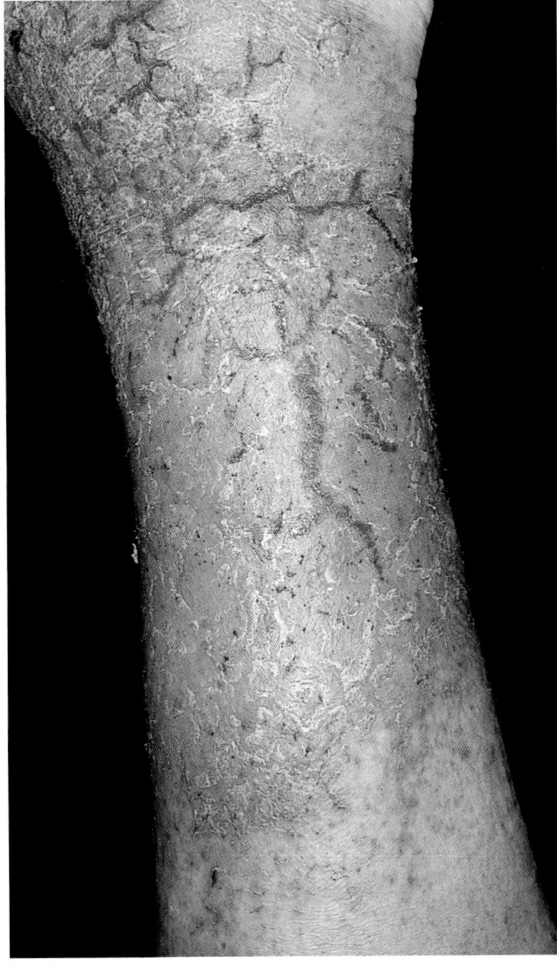

Plate 15 – Asteatotic eczema. (From Habif TP and others: *Skin disease: diagnosis and treatment,* St Louis, 2001, Mosby.)

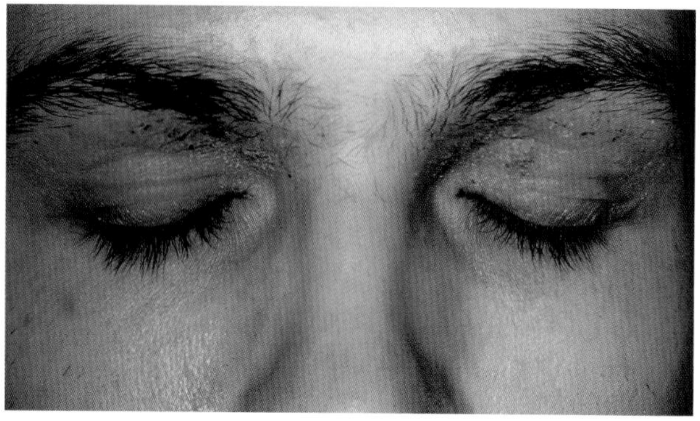

Plate 16 – Atopic dermatitis. (From Habif TP and others: *Skin disease: diagnosis and treatment,* St Louis, 2001, Mosby.)

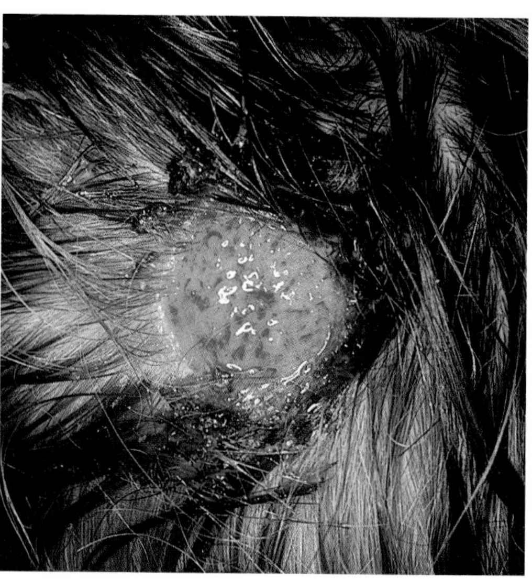

Plate 17 – Tinea capitus. (From Habif TP and others: *Skin disease: diagnosis and treatment,* St Louis, 2001, Mosby.)

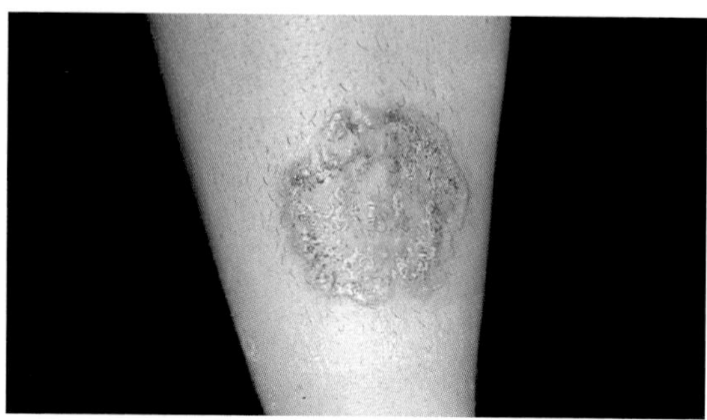

Plate 18 – Tinea corporis (ringworm of the body). (From Habif TP and others: *Skin disease: diagnosis and treatment,* St Louis, 2001, Mosby.)

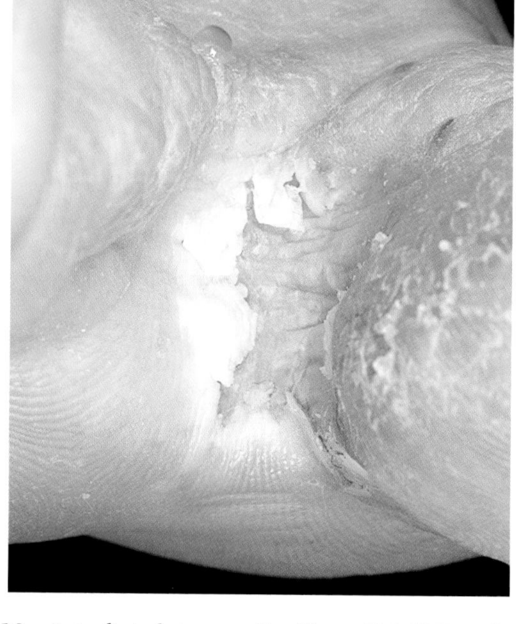

Plate 19 – Interdigital tinea pedis. (From Habif TP and others: *Skin disease: diagnosis and treatment,* St Louis, 2001, Mosby.)

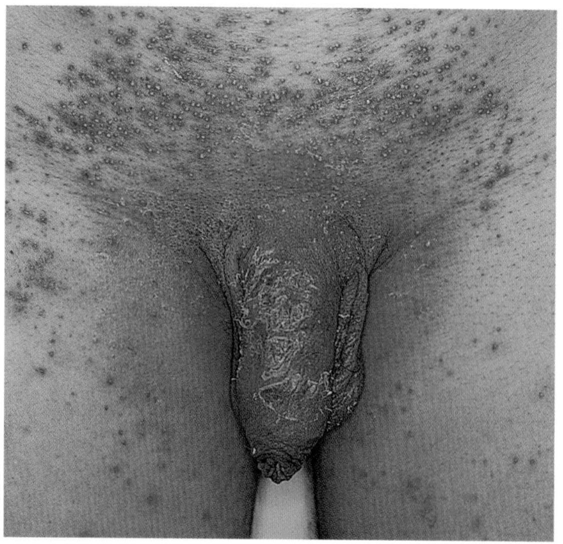

Plate 20 – Moniliasis (candidiasis). (From Fisher BK, Margesson LJ: *Genital skin disorders: diagnosis and treatment,* St Louis, 1998, Mosby.)

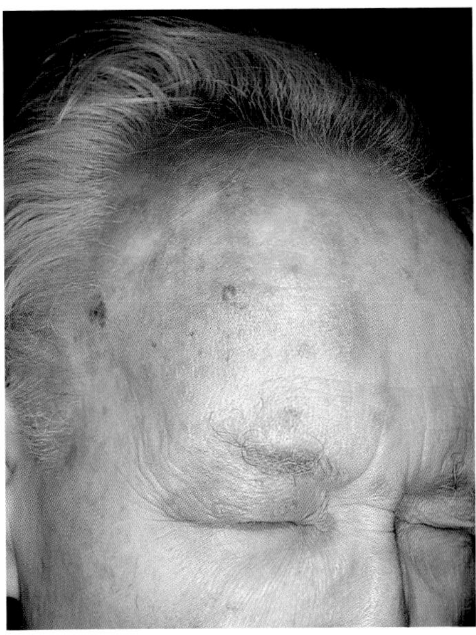

Plate 21 – Ophthalmic zoster. (From Habif TP and others: *Skin disease: diagnosis and treatment*, St Louis, 2001, Mosby.)

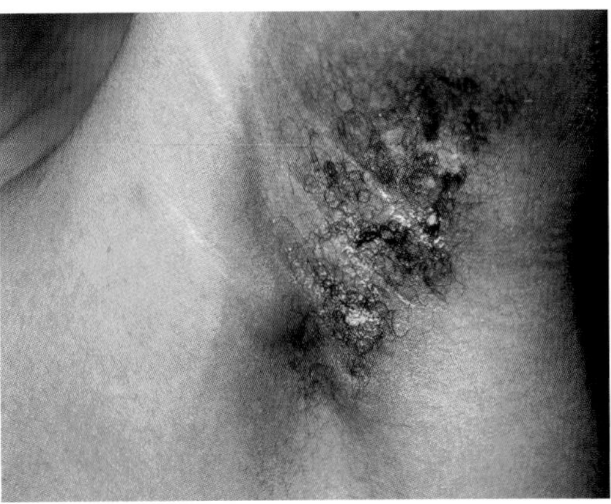

Plate 22 – Hidradenitis suppurative (acne inversa). Erythematous papules, cysts, nodules, and sinus tracts are seen in the axilla of this adolescent male. (From Paller AS, Mancini AJ: *Hurwitz clinical pediatric dermatology*, ed 3, Philadelphia, 2006, Elsevier.)

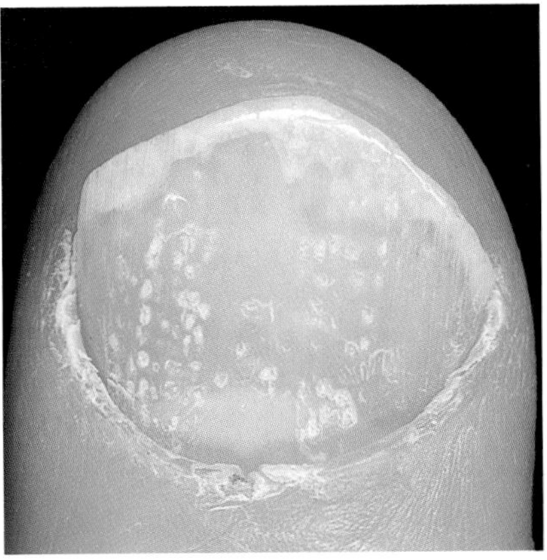

Plate 23 – Psoriasis of nails. (From Habif TP and others: *Skin disease: diagnosis and treatment*, St Louis, 2001, Mosby.)

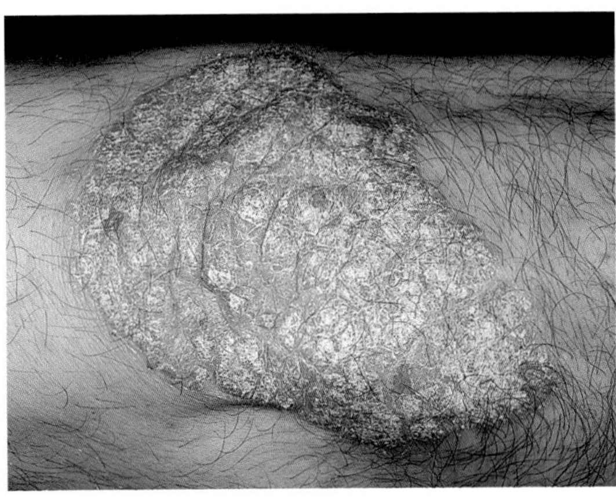

Plate 24 – Psoriasis. Thick, red plaques have a sharply defined border and adherent silvery scale. (From Habif TP and others: *Skin disease: diagnosis and treatment*, St Louis, 2001, Mosby.)

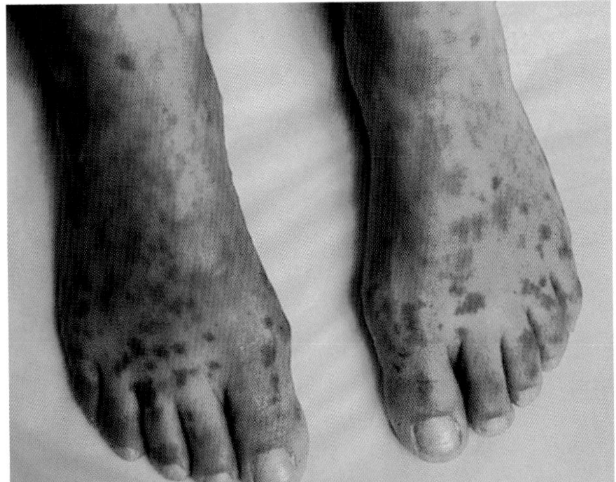

Plate 25 – Palpable purpura. (Reprinted from the *Clinical slide collection on the rheumatic diseases* © 1991, 1995. Used by permission of the American College of Rheumatology.)

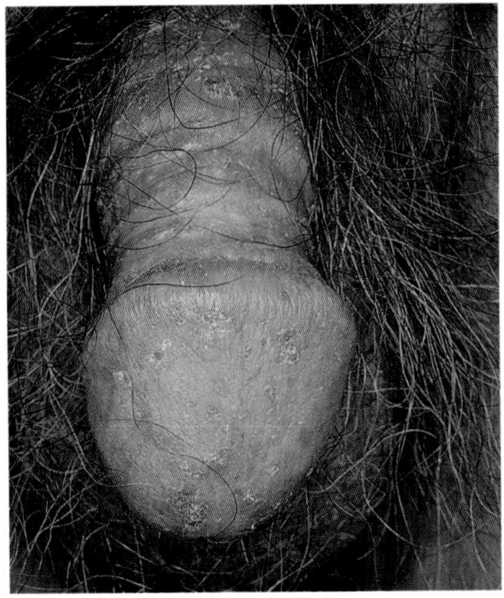

Plate 26 – Scabies. (From Fisher BK, Margesson LJ: *Genital skin disorders: diagnosis and treatment*, St Louis, 1998, Mosby.)

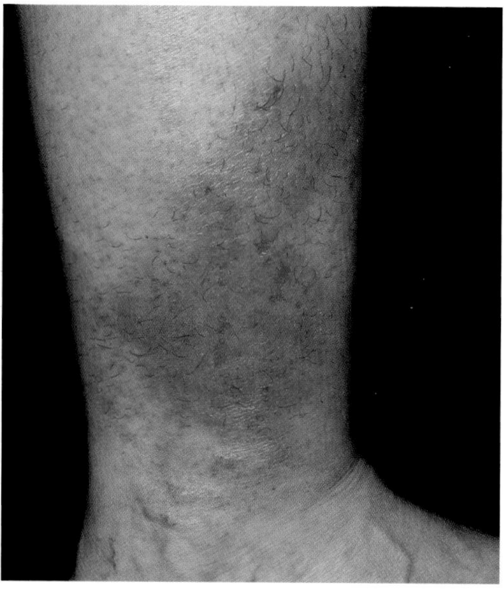

Plate 27 – Stasis dermatitis in early stage with erythema and erosions. (From Habif TP and others: *Skin disease: diagnosis and treatment,* St Louis, 2001, Mosby.)

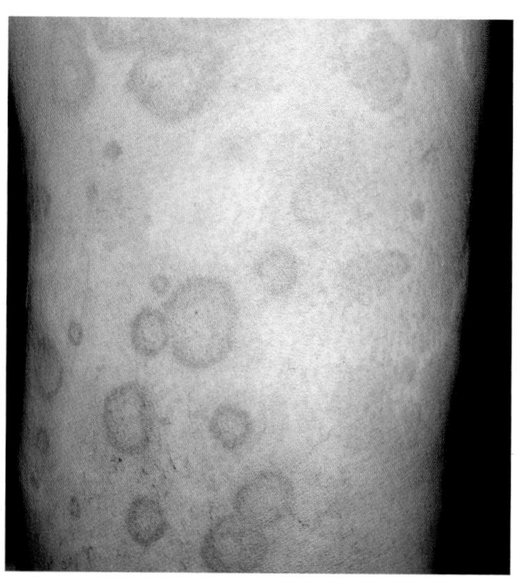

Plate 28 – Urticaria. (From Habif TP and others: *Skin disease: diagnosis and treatment,* St Louis, 2001, Mosby.)

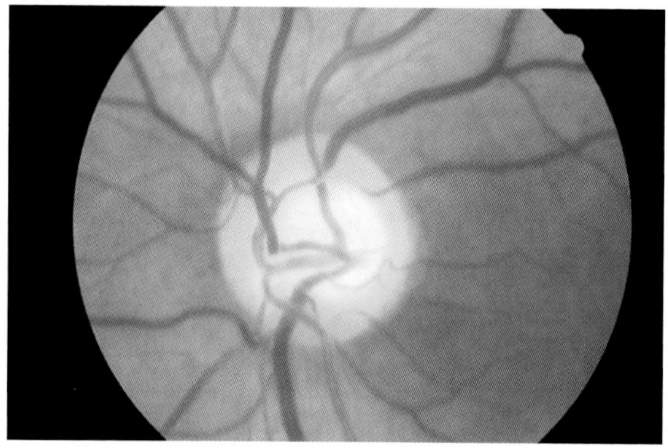

Plate 29 – Glaucoma with cupping. (Courtesy Buddy Crofton, CRA, COT.)

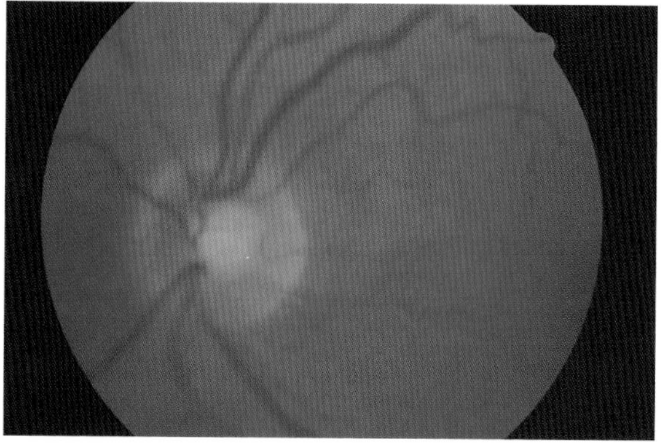

Plate 30 – Glaucoma. (Courtesy Buddy Crofton, CRA, COT.)

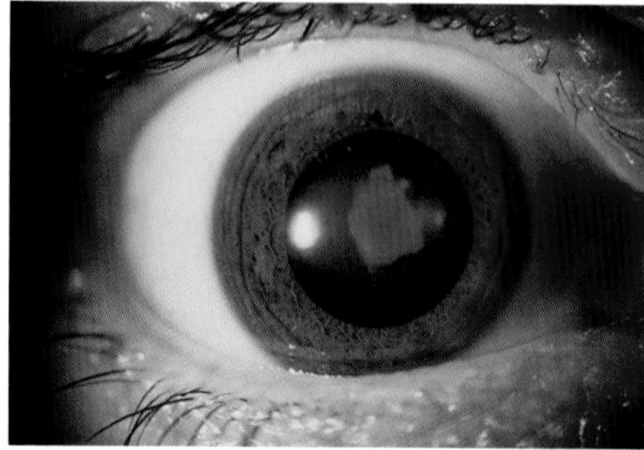

Plate 31 – Cataracts (dilated pupil). (Courtesy Buddy Crofton, CRA, COT.)

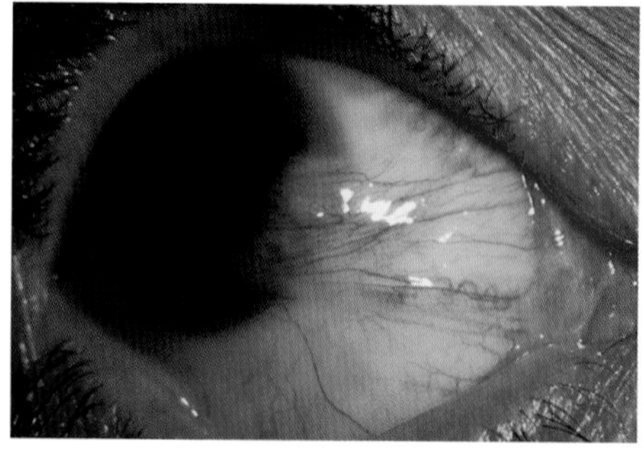

Plate 32 – Pterygium. (Courtesy Buddy Crofton, CRA, COT.)

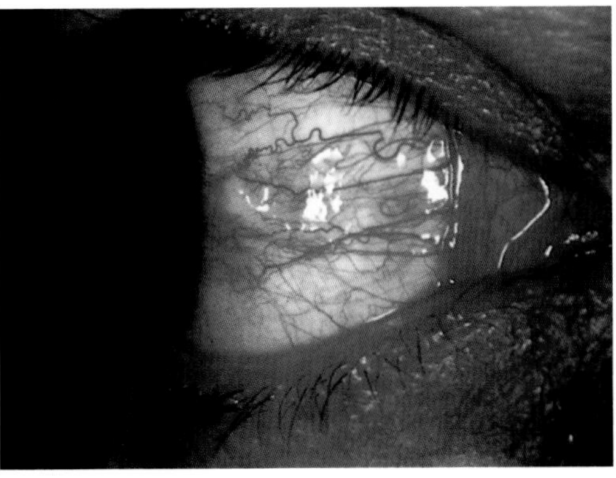

Plate 33 – Pingueculum. (Courtesy Buddy Crofton, CRA, COT.)

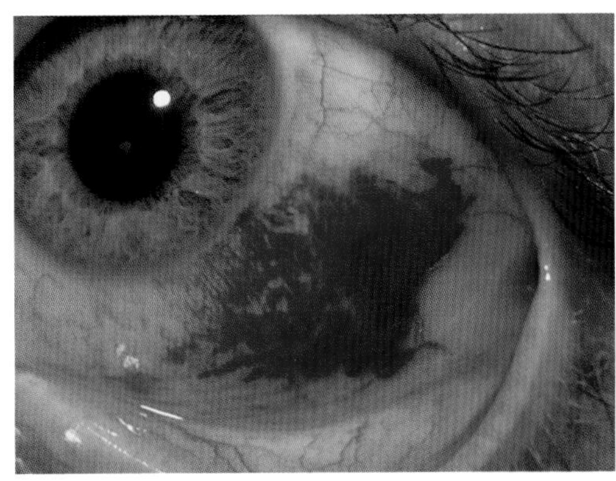

Plate 34 – Subconjunctival hemorrhage. (Courtesy Buddy Crofton, CRA, COT.)

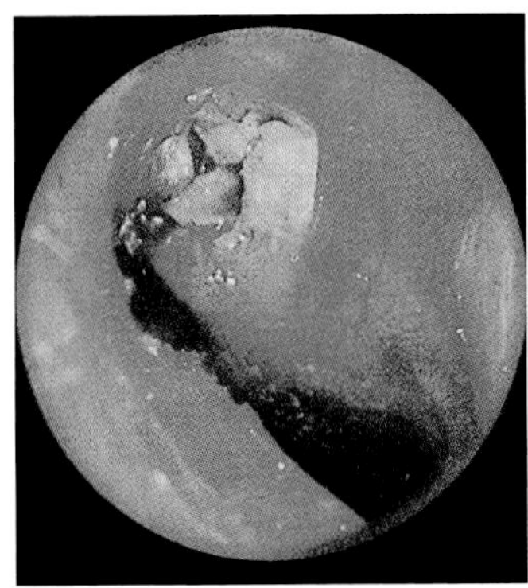

Plate 35 – Cholesteatoma. (From Malasanos L and others: *Health assessment,* ed 3, St Louis, 1986, Mosby; courtesy Richard A. Buckingham, MD, University of Illinois—Chicago.)

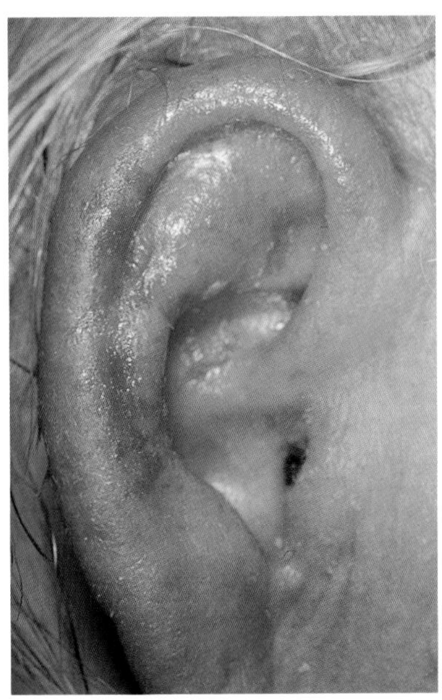

Plate 36 – Malignant otitis externa. (From Habif TP and others: *Skin disease: diagnosis and treatment,* St Louis, 2001, Mosby.)

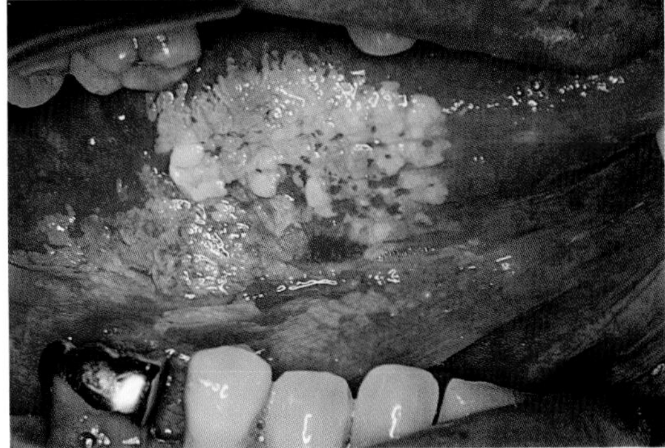

Plate 37 – Leukoplakia on the ventral aspect of the tongue. (From Eisen D, Lynch DP: *The mouth: diagnosis and treatment,* St Louis, 1998, Mosby.)

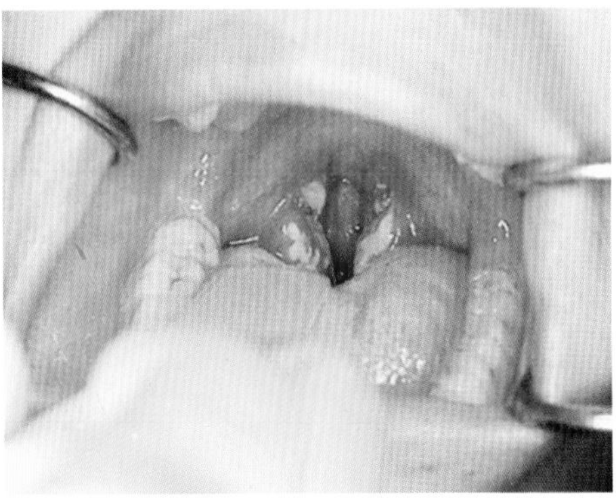

Plate 38 – Pharyngitis and tonsillitis. (From Barkauskas VH and others: *Health and physical assessment,* ed 2, St Louis, 1998, Mosby.)

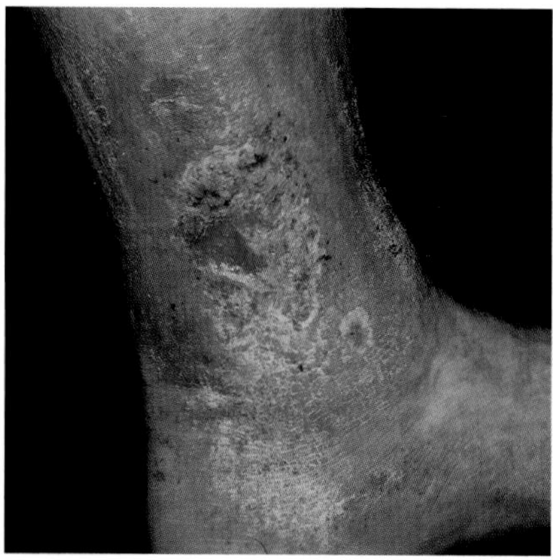

Plate 39 – Venous leg ulcers. (From Habif TP and others: *Skin disease: diagnosis and treatment,* St Louis, 2001, Mosby.)

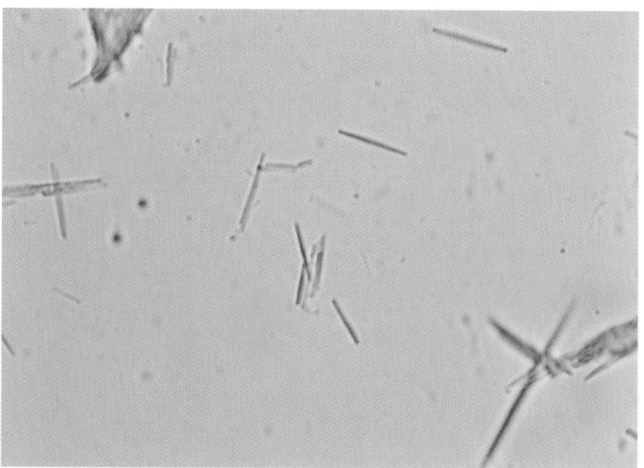

Plate 40 – Gout. Urate crystals in synovial fluid cause inflammation in the joint. (From Stevens ML: *Fundamentals of clinical hematology,* Philadelphia, 1997, Saunders.)

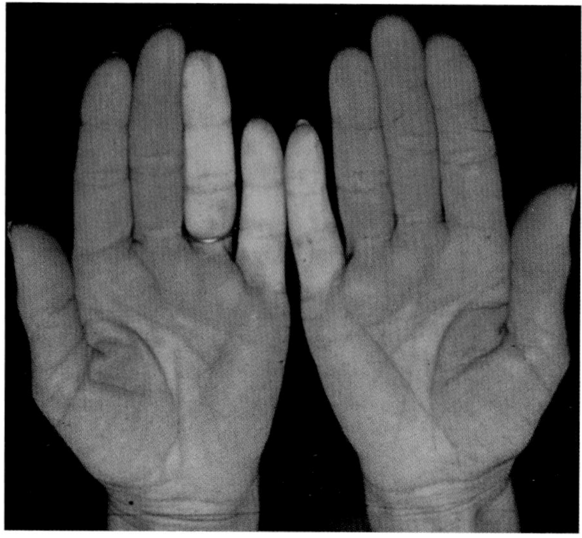

Plate 41 – Raynaud's disease. (From American College of Rheumatology.)

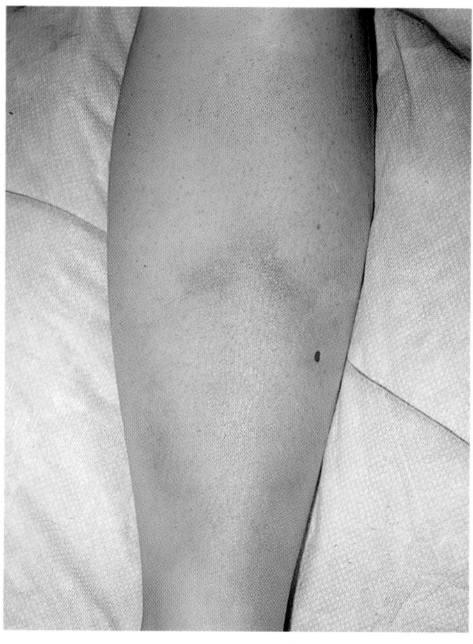

Plate 42 – Lyme disease (From Habif TP and others: *Skin disease: diagnosis and treatment,* St Louis, 2001, Mosby.)

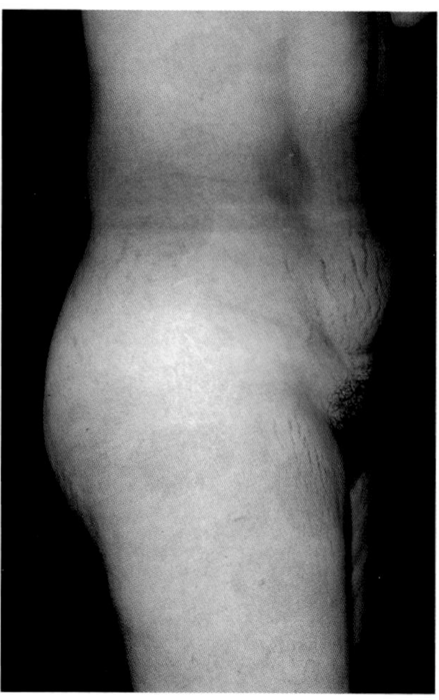

Plate 43 – Lyme disease (From Habif TP and others: *Skin disease: diagnosis and treatment,* St Louis, 2001, Mosby.)

CHAPTER 46

Principles of Dermatologic Therapy

Denise A. Vanacore

DEFINITION AND EPIDEMIOLOGY

The critical first step in treating any dermatologic condition is accurate diagnosis. Other important components are the type of lesion to be treated, the medication, the vehicle of the active medication, and the method used to apply the medication. A thorough history is the important step in the assessment of dermatologic problems.

In dermatologic therapy the type of lesion guides therapy. Moist, weeping lesions are treated with Burow's solution to hasten drying while providing soothing relief. In dry dermatitis, therapeutic agents incorporated into creams or ointments increase moisture in the skin and provide relief from pruritus.

SKIN STRUCTURE

The skin is the largest organ of the body. The primary function of the skin is to provide a barrier to substances from passage into the body. Three main layers form this barrier.[1] The stratum corneum is the most superficial section of the epidermis, or outer layer. The stratum corneum consists of enucleated keratinocytes, which are filled with keratin and an interfilamentous matrix. The middle layer is the dermis, which contains connective tissue and skin appendages. The innermost layer is the hypodermis, or subcutaneous layer, composed of adipose tissue.

The thickness and permeability of the stratum corneum vary on different areas of the body. When the stratum corneum is irritated and inflamed, the protective skin barrier is interrupted. These characteristics have clinical implications for dermatologic therapy because they affect drug absorption. The skin structure in older adults is dryer, thinner, and less elastic, which needs to be considered when prescribing for the elderly population.

MEDICATIONS

Variables to Consider When Prescribing

Several variables affect the pharmacologic response when dermatologic agents are applied to the skin.[2] The first variable is the regional variation in drug penetration, which is based on the thickness of the stratum corneum. There is an inverse relationship between the thickness of the stratum corneum and drug concentration. In areas such as the face, scalp, and scrotum, the stratum corneum is more permeable than others. In addition, there is increased permeability when the skin is inflamed. In addition, the concentration of the dermatologic medication affects its absorption in the skin. Finally, because the principal transport mechanism is passive diffusion, increasing the concentration gradient increases absorption.

Dermatologic Vehicles

The base in which the active medication is delivered (the vehicle) affects the drug's ability to permeate the skin. The vehicle may also provide important therapeutic effects to the skin, such as hydration. Drug absorption may be enhanced up to 10 times with the application of occlusive dressings.

The most common vehicles are combinations of powders, oils, and liquids in varying proportions. Powders aid in absorbing moisture, decrease friction, and help cover wide areas. Oils provide an emollient function and, because of their occlusive properties, often enhance drug absorption. Liquids provide a cooling, soothing sensation by evaporation while helping exudative lesions to dry. Some common pharmacotherapeutic preparations are described in Table 46-1.[3] The optimum vehicles for specific body sites are listed in Table 46-2. With variations in skin thickness, body hair, and type of lesion, it is important to choose the most appropriate vehicle.

Ointments. Ointments consist mainly of water suspended in oil and are an excellent lubricant. Goldstein and Goldstein stated that ointments are generally the most potent vehicles because of their increased occlusive effect[3]; however, they are not useful in hairy areas, and the greasiness of the product is not aesthetically acceptable to many patients. Ointments are best for dry, lichenified lesions because of the effects of lubrication and heat retention through decreased transepidermal water loss.

Creams. Creams are less potent than ointments but stronger than lotions. They consist of a semisolid emulsion of oil in water. Creams are a cosmetically appealing vehicle that can be washed off with water. They are used on nonhairy areas such as the palms and soles.[3]

Lotions. Lotions consist of a powder-in-water preparation and are a less potent vehicle.[3] Indications for the use of lotions include moist areas, dermatoses, pruritus, hairy areas, or large treatment areas. Lotions are commonly used to provide a cooling effect on the skin.

Solutions. Solutions consist of water in combination with various medications or substances. When used as bath soaks, solutions provide coolness and aid in drying exudative lesions.[3] Solutions are best for open or closed dressings, infected dermatoses, or hairy areas.

Gel. A gel is an oil-in-water, semisolid emulsion with alcohol in the base; it is transparent and colorless and liquefies on contact with the skin. Gels are an excellent vehicle for use on hairy body areas, and they combine the therapeutic advantages of ointments with the cosmetic advantages of creams.[3]

Topical Corticosteroids

Some of the most useful topical agents for treating a variety of dermatologic conditions are corticosteroids. The major effects of corticosteroids are the reduction of inflammatory response, vasoconstriction, and a decrease in collagen synthesis.[3] They are available in several classes based on

TABLE 46-1 Topical Pharmacotherapeutic Preparations

Category	Examples	Special Considerations
Lotions	Calamine, Valisone, lindane	Cools and dries as it evaporates; useful for treating moist or pruritic skin
Creams	Nivea, Purpose, most topical corticosteroids, antifungal agents	Helps retain water; cosmetically appealing; useful in high-humidity environments; easily washed off
Gels	Benzoyl peroxide, Erygel, Topicort, Lidex	Becomes liquid on contact; cosmetically appealing; avoid on acutely inflamed skin because alcohol base may cause stinging
Ointments	Petrolatum, Aquaphor, Eucerin, some topical corticosteroids	Helps retain water, hydrating; avoid use in exudative, infected lesions; may be greasy; complications include folliculitis, maceration, and miliaria
Emulsions	Cetaphil, Unibase	Water-in-oil preparations that are less occlusive than ointments
Pastes	Zinc oxide paste	Less greasy than ointments, with some drying action; good as protective barrier
Wet dressings		
Open	Apply 6-8 layers of gauze or a handkerchief, soaking wet, for 15 minutes 3 times daily	Antiinflammatory action and vasoconstriction helpful in decreasing edema and removing crust; offers relief of pruritus through evaporation and cooling
Closed	Same as for open, with plastic cover	Retains heat and causes maceration
Bath soaks	Aveeno, Alpha Keri	Temperature should be lukewarm, not hot; limit to 20-30 minutes; oils may make tub slippery
Powder	Zeasorb, Micatin, Tinactin	Promotes drying; increases surface area; decreases maceration and moisture; avoid in open wounds
Fixed	Unna's boot (zinc oxide gelatin boot)	Proper application aids in decreasing edema; leave the dressing in place for 1 week, then remove by soaking in warm water

From Goldstein B, Goldstein A: *Practical dermatology,* ed 2, Philadelphia, 1997, Mosby.

TABLE 46-2 Optimum Vehicle Selection for Specific Body Sites

Vehicle	Smooth, Nonhairy Skin; Thick, Hyperkeratotic Lesions	Hairy Areas	Palms, Soles	Infected Areas	Between Skin Folds; Moist, Macerated Lesions
Ointment	+++		+++		
Cream	++	+	++	+	++
Lotion		++		++	++
Solution		+++		+++	++
Gel		++		+	+
Spray: little clinical usefulness					

Modified from Goldstein B, Goldstein A: *Practical dermatology,* ed 2, Philadelphia, 1997, Mosby.
+, Infrequently used vehicle; *++,* acceptable vehicle; *+++,* preferred vehicle.

potency (Table 46-3), and they come in a variety of strengths and vehicles (Table 46-4).

Topical corticosteroids are exceptionally useful in treating various dermatologic diseases, but they are not without potential adverse effects. The higher the potency and the more prolonged the use, the higher the chance of developing adverse effects. Collagen synthesis is affected, which results in striae and tissue atrophy. These effects may be reversible when the drug is discontinued. Visible distended capillaries (telangiectasia) and purpura may result from a thinning of the epidermis. Corticosteroids in classes I to IV should never be used on the face or genitals. The health care provider should use caution when prescribing classes I, II, and III and should consider consultation with a physician. The health care provider should be familiar with several medication types in each class of corticosteroid for ease in prescribing.

When corticosteroids are used with occlusive dressings, there is an increase in drug penetration in the skin and an increased potential for adverse reactions. Learning a few drugs in each class will benefit the health care provider when prescribing topical corticosteroids.

PATIENT AND FAMILY EDUCATION

The first guideline of dermatologic therapy is to keep the treatment as simple as possible. Health care providers should prescribe enough medication to complete therapy, and the patient should discard any left over after the treatment. The amount of topical medication to dispense for adult use is listed in Table 46-5.

The provider should write out application procedures and ensure the patient fully understands the instructions. Important information to review with the patient includes

TABLE 46-3 Classes of Topical Corticosteroids

Class	Potency	Considerations	Examples	Indications
I	Ultra high	Consult physician	0.05% betamethasone dipropionate	Severe inflammatory dermatoses unresponsive to standard treatment
			0.05% clobetasol propionate	2-week use restriction; never use on the face or groin
II	Very high	Consult physician	0.05%-0.25% desoximetasone	Severe inflammatory dermatoses (e.g., psoriasis, severe atopic dermatitis, severe contact dermatitis)
			0.2% fluocinolone acetonide	
			0.5% triamcinolone acetonide	
III	High	Use with caution	0.025% betamethasone benzoate	Moderate cutaneous dermatoses
			0.025% fluocinolone acetonide	
			0.1% triamcinolone acetonide	
IV	Intermediate	Use with caution	0.025% triamcinolone acetonide	Moderate cutaneous dermatoses
			0.01% fluocinolone acetonide	
V	Low		2.5% hydrocortisone	Mild cutaneous dermatoses
			0.2% betamethasone	
VI	Very low		0.25%-1.0% hydrocortisone (i.e., OTC strengths)	Very mild, self-limiting dermatoses

Modified from Goldstein B, Goldstein A: *Practical dermatology*, ed 2, St Louis, 1997, Mosby.
OTC, Over-the-counter.

TABLE 46-4 Topical Corticosteroid Potency, Strongest (Class I) to Weakest (Class VI)

Brand Name	Generic Name	Preparation	Size
CLASS I (ULTRA HIGH)—UNRESPONSIVE SEVERE INFLAMMATORY DERMATOSES			
Cordran tape 4 mcg/cm^2	Flurandrenolide	Tape	2 × 3 inch, 24 × 3 inch, 80 × 3 inch
Diprolene 0.05%	Betamethasone dipropionate*	Cream, ointment, gel	15, 45 g
		Lotion	30, 60 ml
Diprolene AF 0.05%	Betamethasone dipropionate	Cream	15, 45 g
Psorcon 0.05%	Diflorasone diacetate	Cream, ointment	15, 30, 45, 60 g
Temovate E 0.05%	Clobetasol propionate*	Cream, ointment	15, 30, 45 g
		Lotion	25, 50 ml
		Gel	15, 30, 60 g
		Emollient cream	15, 30, 60 g
Ultravate 0.05%	Halobetasol propionate	Cream, ointment	15, 50 g
CLASS II (VERY HIGH)—SEVERE INFLAMMATORY DERMATOSES			
Aristocort 0.5%	Triamcinolone acetonide*	Cream, ointment	15, 240 g
Cyclocort 0.1%	Amcinonide	Cream, ointment	15, 30, 60 g
		Lotion	20, 60 ml
Diprosone 0.05%	Betamethasone dipropionate*	Cream, ointment	15, 45 g
		Aerosol	85 g
		Lotion	30, 60 ml
Florone 0.05%	Diflorasone diacetate	Cream, ointment	15, 30, 60 g
Halog 0.1%	Halcinonide	Cream, ointment	15, 30, 60, 240 g
		Solution	20, 60 ml
Lidex 0.05%	Fluocinonide*	Cream, ointment	15, 30, 60, 120 g
		Solution	20, 60 ml
		Gel	15, 30, 60, 120 g
Lidex E 0.05%	Fluocinonide	Cream	15, 30, 60, 120 g
Kenalog 0.05%	Triamcinolone acetonide*	Cream, ointment	20 g
Maxiflor 0.05%	Diflorasone diacetate	Cream	30, 60 g
		Ointment	15, 30, 60 g
Topicort 0.25%	Desoximetasone*	Cream	15, 60, 120 g
		Ointment	15, 60 g
		Gel 0.05%	15, 60 g

From Goldstein B, Goldstein A: *Practical dermatology*, ed 2, St Louis, 1997, Mosby.
*Available generically, but may not be as predictably effective. In most cases, however, it is much less expensive.

Continued

TABLE 46-4 Topical Corticosteroid Potency, Strongest (Class I) to Weakest (Class VI)—cont'd

Brand Name	Generic Name	Preparation	Size
CLASS III (HIGH)—MODERATE CUTANEOUS DERMATOSES			
Aristocort 0.1%	Triamcinolone acetonide*	Cream, ointment	15, 60, 240, 2520 g
Aristocort A 0.1%	Triamcinolone acetonide*	Cream	15, 60, 240 g
		Ointment	15, 60 g
Cutivate 0.05%	Fluticasone propionate	Cream	15, 30, 60 g
Cutivate 0.005%	Fluticasone propionate	Ointment	15, 30, 60 g
Dermatop 0.1%	Prednicarbate	Cream	15, 60 g
Elocon 0.1%	Mometasone furoate	Cream, ointment	15, 45 g
		Lotion	30, 60 ml
Kenalog 0.1%	Triamcinolone acetonide*	Cream	15, 60, 80, 240, 2520 g
		Ointment	15, 60, 80, 240 g
		Lotion	15, 60 ml
Synalar 0.025%	Fluocinolone acetonide*	Cream, ointment	15, 30, 60, 425 g
		Solution 0.01%	20, 60 ml
Synemol 0.025%	Fluocinolone acetonide*	Cream	15, 30, 60 g
Valisone 0.1%	Betamethasone valerate*	Cream	15, 45, 110, 430 g
		Ointment	15, 45 g
		Lotion	20, 60 ml
		Powder	5, 10 g
CLASS IV (INTERMEDIATE)—MODERATE CUTANEOUS DERMATOSES			
Aristocort 0.025%	Triamcinolone acetonide*	Cream	15, 60, 2520 g
Kenalog 0.025%	Triamcinolone acetonide*	Cream	15, 80, 240, 2520 g
		Lotion	60 ml
		Ointment	15, 80, 240 g
Locoid 0.1%	Hydrocortisone butyrate	Cream, ointment	15, 45 g
		Solution	30, 60 ml
Valisone 0.01%	Betamethasone valerate*	Cream	15, 60 g
Westcort 0.2%	Hydrocortisone valerate	Cream, ointment	15, 45, 60 g
CLASS V (LOW)—MILD CUTANEOUS DERMATOSES			
Aclovate 0.05%	Alclometasone dipropionate	Cream, ointment	15, 45, 60 g
Derma-Smoothe FS 0.01%	Fluocinolone acetonide	Oil120 ml	
DesOwen 0.05%	Desonide*	Cream	15, 60, 90 g
		Ointment	15, 60 g
		Lotion	60, 120 ml
FS Shampoo 0.01%	Fluocinolone acetonide	Shampoo	180 ml
Synalar 0.01%	Fluocinolone acetonide*	Cream	15, 30, 60, 425 g
		Solution	20, 60 ml
Tridesilon 0.05%	Desonide*	Cream, ointment	15, 60 g
CLASS VI (VERY LOW)—VERY MILD, SELF-LIMITING DERMATOSES			
Hytone 1%	Hydrocortisone*	Cream, ointment	30, 120 g
		Liquid	45, 75, 120 ml
		Lotion	120 ml
		Roll-on stick	14 g
Hytone 2.5%	Hydrocortisone*	Cream	30, 60 g
		Ointment	30 g
		Lotion	60 ml
Pramosone 1%	Hydrocortisone with pramoxine hydrochloride 1%	Cream	30, 60 g
		Ointment	30 g
		Lotion	60, 240 ml
Pramosone 2.5%	Hydrocortisone with pramoxine hydrochloride 1%	Cream	30 g
		Ointment	30 g
		Lotion	60, 120 ml

From Goldstein B, Goldstein A: *Practical dermatology*, ed 2, St Louis, 1997, Mosby.
*Available generically, but may not be as predictably effective. In most cases, however, it is much less expensive.

TABLE 46-5 Amount of Topical Medication to Dispense for Adult Use*

Body Area	b.i.d./1 week	t.i.d./2 weeks	b.i.d./4 weeks
Face and neck	15 g	45 g	60 g
Trunk	60 g	180 g	240 g
One arm	15 g	45 g	60 g
One leg	30 g	90 g	120 g
Hands and feet	15 g	45 g	60 g
Body	180 g	0.75-1 kg	1.25-2 kg

From Goldstein B, Goldstein A: *Practical dermatology*, ed 2, St Louis, 1997, Mosby.
*For children, use one third to one half these amounts.

whether to moisten the skin first, how much topical medication to apply, where to apply it, and whether the area can be occluded by a dressing. Patients should be instructed not to apply the dermatologic medication to areas other than where instructed. In addition, patients should be aware of possible adverse reactions and should know when to call the office and return for follow-up evaluation.

REFERENCES

1. DiPiro J, Talbert RL, Yee GC, and others: *Pharmacotherapy: a pathophysiologic approach*, ed 6, Stamford, Conn, 2005, Appleton & Lange.
2. Katzung B: *Basic and clinical pharmacology*, ed 9, Stamford, Conn, 2004, Appleton & Lange.
3. Goldstein B, Goldstein A: *Practical dermatology*, ed 2, St Louis, 1997, Mosby.

CHAPTER 47

Screening for Skin Cancer

Walter Elias, III
Updated by Denise A. Vanacore

DEFINITION AND EPIDEMIOLOGY

Although early detection and treatment of skin cancer can improve patient outcomes, evidence is insufficient to recommend for or against routine screening for early detection of skin cancer using a total-body skin examination.[1] Nevertheless, the purpose of skin cancer screening is to educate both the patient and the provider so they can identify the characteristic changes associated with skin cancer. These cancers include nonmelanomatous skin cancers (NMSCs) (e.g., basal cell carcinoma [BCC], squamous cell carcinoma [SCC]), and melanomatous (malignant melanoma [MM]) skin cancers.

It is known that 1 in 6 Americans develops skin cancer at some point.[2] Approximately 1.3 million cases of BCC or SCC are diagnosed each year. Between 1973 and 1995, the incidence of MM increased from 5.7 per 100,000 to 13.3 per 100,000.[1] An estimated 9600 persons died of skin cancer in 2000, with 7700 dying of MM and 1900 dying of other skin cancers.[3] In contrast to NMSC, which typically affects older adults, the frequency of MM peaks between 20 and 45 years of age.

The rising incidence of skin cancer over the past several decades may be primarily attributed to increased sun exposure associated with societal and lifestyle shifts in the U.S. population and to depletion of the protective ozone layer.[2] Ninety percent of all skin cancers are caused by the sun.[4]

Acute sunburns place the patient at increased risk, and the effects of sun damage are cumulative. Second-degree burns before age 18 years can double the incidence of NMSC and greatly increase the risk for MM.[5] Fair-skinned men and women older than 65 years, patients with atypical moles, and those with more than 50 nevi constitute known groups at substantially increased risk for developing melanoma.[2] In addition, skin cancers appear to have a hereditary component. Xeroderma pigmentosum is the prototype syndrome of genetically determined increased skin cancer risk. Warning signs for skin cancer include (1) an open sore that does not heal for 3 weeks; (2) a spot or sore that burns, itches, stings, crusts, or bleeds; and (3) any mole or spot that changes in size or texture; develops irregular borders; or appears pearly, translucent, or multicolored.

PATHOPHYSIOLOGY

Repeated and unprotected exposure to ultraviolet light causes photoaging of the skin over time. Normal skin aging begins by ages 30 to 35 years and is characterized by thinning, atrophy, decreased elasticity, and fragility that lead to wrinkling. Skin that is photoaged from sun damage may be coarse with yellow discoloration (solar elastosis), irregularly pigmented, rough, or atrophic with deep wrinkling. Reactive hyperplasia of melanocytes results in persistent hyperpigmentation or hypopigmentation of the hands, forearms, legs, chest, and back. Chronic exposure disrupts the maturation of the outer layer of the epidermis, resulting in scaling, roughness, seborrheic keratoses, actinic keratoses, and NMSCs[5-7]; heavy sun exposure is also a risk factor for MM.[1]

CLINICAL PRESENTATION

Providers and patients can reliably measure some risk factors for melanoma. Patients coming in for routine physical examinations should be queried concerning any changes in the appearance or size of skin lesions (Table 47-1). Questions about the patient's use of sunscreens, repeated sun exposure without protection, tendency to burn, outdoor employment, or family history of melanoma are beneficial to estimate the risk for NMSC or MM.[2,5]

PHYSICAL EXAMINATION

The most commonly advocated screening test for skin cancer is a complete and thorough total-body skin examination. With the patient disrobed, the examiner must systematically inspect the entire skin surface, including the nails and the soles of the feet.[1] Detection of a suspicious skin lesion such as BCC warrants biopsy or referral (Color Plate 1). NMSC lesions such as BCC may vary from a normal flesh-colored lesion to a slightly pigmented lesion (see Color Plate 1). These are characterized by a raised, shiny appearance, often with pearly borders. An SCC lesion is a roughened, scaling area that does not heal and readily bleeds when scraped (Color Plate 3). Keratinization of these can lead to a heaped-up appearance that flakes. MM is characterized by a lesion that is best described by the *ABCDE*s of MM (Color Plates 4 and 5).[1,2] These include *A*symmetry (of the entire lesion), *B*order (irregularities), *C*olor (variability within the lesion from a brown to black discoloration), *D*iameter (size greater than 6 mm [0.25 inch]), and *E*levation (recently raised). Additional symptoms suspicious for skin cancer include nonhealing skin areas, ulceration, bleeding, and weeping sores. In African Americans, Asian Americans, and dark-skinned individuals, abnormal lesions of the nails, hands, or feet should also be evaluated, since these are common sites for melanomas in these populations (see Color Plate 5).

DIAGNOSTICS

Skin biopsy is the definitive diagnostic test and is best performed by an experienced practitioner. A shave or punch biopsy technique is appropriate for diagnostic evaluation of suspected NMSC (see Chapter 45). Excisional biopsy (total removal) of suspicious MM lesions should be followed by a wider excision if MM is diagnosed.

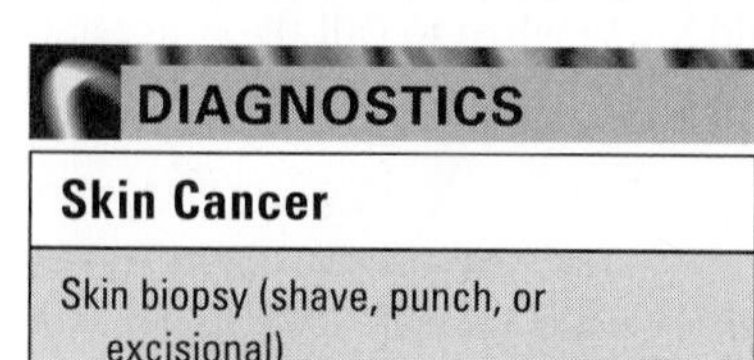
DIAGNOSTICS

Skin Cancer
Skin biopsy (shave, punch, or excisional)

TABLE 47-1 Signs Suggesting Malignancy in Pigmented Lesions

Sign	Implication
CHANGE IN COLOR	
Sudden darkening; brown, black	Increased number of tumor cells, the density of which varies within the lesion, creating irregular pigmentation
Spread of color into previously normal skin	Tumor cells migrating through epidermis at various speeds and in different directions (horizontal growth phase)
Red	Vasodilation and inflammation
White	Areas of regression or inflammation
Blue	Pigment deep in dermis; sign of increasing depth of tumor
CHANGE IN CHARACTERISTICS OF BORDER	
Irregular outline	Malignant cells migrating horizontally at different rates
Satellite pigmentation	Cells migrating beyond confines of primary tumor
Development of depigmented halo	Destruction of melanocytes by possible immunologic reaction and inflammation
CHANGES IN SURFACE CHARACTERISTICS THAT SHOULD PROMPT EVALUATION FOR SKIN CANCER	
Scaliness	
Erosion	
Oozing	
Crusting	
Bleeding	
Ulceration	
Elevation	
Loss of normal skin lines	
DEVELOPMENT OF SYMPTOMS THAT SHOULD PROMPT EVALUATION FOR SKIN CANCER	
Pruritus	
Tenderness	
Pain	

From Habif TP: *Clinical dermatology: a color guide to diagnosis and therapy*, ed 3, St Louis, 1996, Mosby.

DIFFERENTIAL DIAGNOSIS

Screening for skin cancer includes the evaluation of skin for all atypical-appearing lesions. Skin cancers may range from a seborrheic keratosis (Color Plate 2) to a premalignant solar (actinic) keratosis to a BCC, SCC, or MM. An actinic keratosis is a persistent or recurrent reddened and roughened area that scales or crusts. These lesions are effectively treated with liquid nitrogen using a freeze-thaw technique to obtain a 1- to 3-mm (0.04 to 0.12 inch) rim of freeze, which allows appropriately slow thawing over 20 to 40 seconds.[6]

DIFFERENTIAL DIAGNOSIS

Skin Cancer

- Actinic keratoses
- Basal cell carcinoma
- Squamous cell carcinoma
- Malignant melanoma
- Dysplastic nevi

MANAGEMENT

Treatment

BCC is treated with electrodesiccation and curettage. Definitive treatment of SCC is total excision. An experienced dermatologist or surgeon is best equipped to treat an MM lesion with a wide excision. If an NMSC or MM is recognized early by the patient or provider, surgical cure is close to 100%.

Co-Management with Specialists

An annual skin examination of sun-exposed areas is recommended for patients with the diagnosis of BCC or SCC. A family physician or dermatologist can accomplish this. A total annual skin examination by an experienced family physician or dermatologist is recommended for patients diagnosed with MM lesions.

COMPLICATIONS AND LIFE SPAN CONSIDERATIONS

Despite the tendency of NMSC lesions to be slow growing, failure to diagnose them can result in disfigurement. There is indirect evidence that the shift to screening and recognition of melanoma at earlier tumor stages may be associated with better clinical outcomes.[1] The survival rate at 5 years is inversely proportional to the depth of the MM at the time of diagnosis—the deeper the lesion at diagnosis, the lower the survival rate at 5 years. There are minimum risks from total-body skin examination; however, the examination may be embarrassing to some patients and could result in unnecessary treatment as a result of misdiagnosis or detection of lesions that might not have caused clinical consequences but were biopsied.[1]

INDICATIONS FOR REFERRAL OR HOSPITALIZATION

The identification of atypical-appearing skin lesions warrants referral or a biopsy. If the biopsy reveals an NMSC or MM, a trained family physician, dermatologist, or surgeon should provide the definitive treatment.

PATIENT EDUCATION AND HEALTH PROMOTION

The incidence of MM more than doubled between 1973 and 1995.[1] Knowing that damage to the skin caused by the sun is additive may help patients take precautions against sun exposure and thereby reduce their risk; 80% of lifetime sun exposure occurs before 18 years of age.[1] Precautions include avoiding the sun, wearing protective clothing, and using sunscreens to prevent solar damage to the skin, both for young children and adults. Prevention of sunburns, which carry a high risk of malignant transformation over time, is paramount. Education of patients at higher risk is crucial. (See the Clinical Presentation section for factors that place patients at higher risk.)

Sun exposure for longer than 15 minutes requires protection with a sunscreen that has a sun protection factor (SPF) of at least 15. Sunscreens should be applied before sun exposure and reapplied every 2 hours or after swimming.

It is important for patients to know they should seek medical attention for nonhealing sores (sores usually heal within 4 to 6 weeks) or for any lesion that changes in size, shape, texture, or color. Early identification of atypical-appearing skin lesions results in timely referral and effective treatment.

REFERENCES

1. US Preventive Services Task Force: Screening for skin cancer: recommendations and rationale, *Am J Prev Med* 20(3S):44-46, 2001, retrieved Dec 5, 2001, from http://www.ahrq.gov/clinic/ajpmsuppl/skcarr.htm.
2. Jerant AF, Johnson JT, Sheridan CD, and others: Early detection and treatment of skin cancer, *Am Fam Phys* 62(2):357-368, 2000.
3. American Cancer Society: *Cancer statistics*, retrieved Dec 6, 2006, from http://www.cancer.org/statistics/cff2000/selected_toc.html.
4. Fitzpatrick JE, Aeling JL: *Dermatology secrets in color*, ed 2, Philadelphia, 2001, Hanley & Belfus.
5. Kaminester LH: Current concepts: photoprotection, *Arch Fam Med* 5:289-295, 1996.
6. Cockerell CJ, Howell JB, Balch CM: Think melanoma, *South Med J* 86(12):1325-1333, 1993.
7. Habif TP: *Clinical dermatology: a color guide to diagnosis and therapy*, ed 3, St Louis, 1996, Mosby.

CHAPTER 48

Acne Vulgaris

Eileen M. Deignan and Bonnie Hooper

DEFINITION AND EPIDEMIOLOGY

Acne vulgaris is the most common dermatologic disorder in the United States. It is first observed in the pediatric age-group and can last well into the adult years. Although it is usually not a serious medical problem, acne should never be dismissed as a minor condition that will eventually be outgrown. The psychologic effects of prolonged acne and scars can be devastating. Advances in acne treatment enable management of this disease in many cases.

Acne vulgaris is a disorder of the pilosebaceous follicles. Its most prominent appearance during adolescence ("the peak of life") results in its name, which is derived from the Greek word *akmē*, meaning highest point or point.

Early lesions of acne develop in 40% of children 8 to 10 years old, and 85% of all adolescents develop some form of acne. Of adults in their thirties and forties, 10% continue to experience active lesions, and 6% to 10% of adults in their fifties have varying degrees of this disorder.[1,2] There appears to be a familial tendency toward acne, and it is more common in males than in females.

A dermatologic referral is indicated for isotretinoin (Accutane) therapy.

PATHOPHYSIOLOGY

The production of sebum appears to be directly related to androgenic stimulation. Before and during puberty, hormonal stimulation increases the production of the sebaceous glands in the pilosebaceous follicles. Abnormally adherent keratinocytes cause plugging of the pilosebaceous follicles, which contributes to the formation of the primary lesion (the comedone). Comedones include the open comedone (blackhead) and the closed comedone (whitehead). The open comedone is an obstruction at the follicular mouth, which is filled with plugs of stratum corneum cells. The black color is a result of compacted follicular cells, not dirt.[2] Closed comedones are a result of cystic swelling of the follicular duct below the epidermis. These closed comedones are the precursors of inflammatory papules and pustules (Color Plate 9). Inflammatory reactions to sebum, fatty acids, and *Propionibacterium acnes* lead to production of chemotactic factors and proinflammatory cytokines.[1,2] Inflammatory material around the comedone creates inflammatory papules and pustules.

Deeper lesions that develop in the lower portion of the follicle become nodulocystic lesions. Inflammatory acne may result in scars, most commonly from self-inflicted trauma from scratching and squeezing the lesions. These scars tend to be small pits. Rupture of cystic acne lesions also results in scar formation without any manipulation of the lesions. Another after-effect of acne is the formation of keloids, especially over the sternum and upper back. In patients with darker skin, inflammatory lesions often resolve with postinflammatory hyperpigmentation. Patients can be reassured that this "staining" is not scarring and usually clears spontaneously after several months.[3]

CLINICAL PRESENTATION AND PHYSICAL EXAMINATION

The duration of acne, past treatments, the use of topical products, medical abnormalities, menstrual history, family history of acne, and medications should be included in the patient's history. It is important to document how long previous treatments were used and any side effects. One frustrating fact of acne therapy is that most treatments require 6 to 12 weeks to take effect. If a therapy has been used for less than 6 to 12 weeks, it may not have been given an adequate trial.

In taking the history, the provider must consider that seasonal and hormonal factors affect acne flares. More severe lesions occur during the winter months when there is less sunlight, since acne is an inflammatory condition that responds to ultraviolet light. In addition, female patients typically report premenstrual acne flares.

A careful history should include an inquiry about exposure to cosmetic and hair styling products. Cosmetic acne can result from oil-based cosmetics, lotions, and hair products. It is usually worse in the areas in contact with the cosmetic. Similarly, pomade acne is seen on the forehead and neck as the result of oily lotions and creams used to style the hair.

Mechanical acne can result from friction from headbands, hats, helmets, chin straps, collars, and tight bras. Typically this presentation demonstrates acneiform lesions in the area where these devices contact the body, whereas other locations are spared. Acne excoriée is a subtype of acne in which the primary lesions have been scratched. Patients with acne excoriée must be encouraged to stop manipulating or scratching these lesions as an important part of successful therapy for this acne condition.[4]

Certain medications can induce or aggravate acne (Box 48-1).[2,3] In some cases of drug-induced acne, such as steroid-induced acne, the lesions are monomorphous. Typically, drug-induced acne has a rapid onset and may involve the usual acne areas as well as unusual areas such as the postauricular area, upper arms, lower back, abdomen, and legs.

BOX 48-1

DRUGS THAT INDUCE OR AGGRAVATE ACNE

- Androgens
- Adrenocorticotropic hormone
- Bromides
- Glucocorticoids
- Oral and fluorinated topical corticosteroids
- Hydantoins
- Iodides
- Isoniazid
- Lithium
- Phenobarbital
- Phenytoin
- Rifampin
- Trimethadione

A physical examination documents the type, location, and extent of acne lesions. The highest concentration of sebaceous glands occurs on the face, chest, back, and shoulders. Patients may be seen with a variety of lesions, including comedones, papules, pustules, and nodules. Surprisingly, the skin of a patient with acne will not necessarily be oily.

DIAGNOSTICS AND DIFFERENTIAL DIAGNOSIS

Acne is diagnosed by physical examination. Laboratory blood testing is necessary only if adrenal or gonadal dysfunction is a possible cause. Other conditions may be misdiagnosed as acne. These include milia, rosacea (Color Plate 10), the adenoma sebaceum lesions of tuberous sclerosis, nevus comedonicus, miliaria of the newborn, flat warts, and molluscum contagiosum.

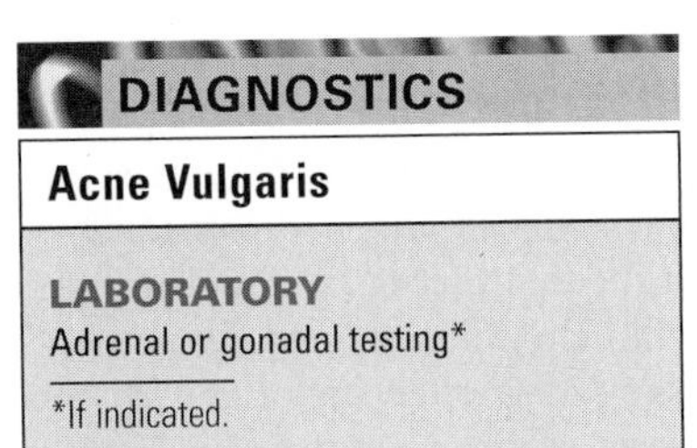

DIAGNOSTICS

Acne Vulgaris

LABORATORY
Adrenal or gonadal testing*

*If indicated.

MANAGEMENT

Therapy should be individualized according to the degree and severity of acne. Goals of treatment include (1) normalizing keratinization of the follicular epithelium, (2) decreasing sebum production, (3) reducing *P. acnes* proliferation, (4) reducing inflammation, and (5) minimizing scarring.

Mild cleansers and cleansing bars are helpful to remove sebum from the surface of the skin. They do not alter sebum production. Harsh soaps, astringents, "buff puffs," and grainy washes should be avoided because they may dry the skin or aggravate inflammatory lesions. Moisturizers, makeup, and hair products should be water based.

Excessive desquamation of the follicular epithelium, together with excess sebum production, contributes to comedone formation. Topical medications (keratolytics) that affect this process are tretinoin (Retin A), adapalene (Differin), tazarotene (Tazorac), azelaic acid (Azelex), and salicylic acid. These agents are applied to clean skin once daily, usually before bedtime. Side effects include erythema, dryness, and sun sensitivity. Systemic isotretinoin also decreases comedogenesis.

Several topical agents are available to decrease *P. acnes* proliferation and inhibit the production of inflammatory mediators. These agents include erythromycin, clindamycin, metronidazole, sulfonamide, azelaic acid, and benzoyl peroxide. There are also combination products of benzoyl peroxide and erythromycin or clindamycin. These are usually applied once or twice a day after cleansing. Although these agents may be used alone, they also work synergistically with keratolytics.

Oral antibiotics are effective in treating inflammatory acne by decreasing *P. acnes* and by reducing the concentration of free fatty acids, thereby inhibiting comedogenesis. Treatment for a minimum of 4 to 6 weeks is necessary to show improvement and may continue for several months. The most commonly used oral antibiotics include erythromycin, tetracycline, doxycycline, and minocycline.[5–8] Doxycycline and minocycline are strongly recommended by the American Academy of Dermatology (AAD) because there is strong evidence suggesting efficacy for these two antibiotic therapies, although minocycline is thought to be superior to doxycycline as well as to other antibiotics.[8] Less commonly used antibiotics include clindamycin, trimethoprim-sulfamethoxazole, azithromycin, cephalexin, ampicillin, and amoxicillin. Some patients require long-term treatment or intermittent courses of oral antibiotics until remission occurs. Doxycycline hyclate (Periostat), 20 mg b.i.d., a form of doxycycline initially used to treat periodontal infection and inflammation, has exhibited some success in moderate acne; however, Periostat is more expensive than plain doxycycline.[5] Because antibiotic resistance is increasing, the AAD recommends systemic treatment for moderate and severe cases.[8]

Systemic medications that cause sebaceous gland suppression include estrogen and spironolactone. They act by suppressing the androgenic stimulation of sebum production and may be beneficial to female patients with acne. The most effective estrogen dose is at least 50 mcg of ethinyl estradiol per day. Most combination oral contraceptives contain 35 mcg or less of ethinyl estradiol. Fortunately, these doses of estrogens can be effective in acne suppression when combined with a nonandrogenic progestin such as norgestimate or desogestrel. Spironolactone and drospirenone are antiandrogens that also reduce sebum production. Drospirenone is available as a combination oral contraceptive pill. Combination oral contraceptives and spironolactone are contraindicated in pregnant and lactating women and in the presence of thromboembolic disorders, renal impairment, and hyperkalemia.

Isotretinoin is restricted to the treatment of recalcitrant nodulocystic acne that has been unresponsive to standard therapies.[6] Its use is best managed by a dermatologist or dermatologic nurse practitioner. It is thought to inhibit sebum production, decrease follicular obstruction, and have an anti-inflammatory effect. Patients need monthly monitoring of triglycerides and hepatic function. Isotretinoin is potentially teratogenic, and careful contraceptive measures should be taken. Sexually active women of childbearing years must use two forms of birth control and be monitored for pregnancy monthly. Treatment usually lasts 4 to 6 months. Approximately 60% of patients who complete a course of isotretinoin therapy will experience a long-term remission. Of the other 40%, some require further courses of isotretinoin, but some have acne that is controllable with simpler forms of acne therapy.

Contrary to popular wisdom, acne does not appear to be related to certain foods. Therefore dietary restrictions are not indicated.

DIFFERENTIAL DIAGNOSIS

Acne Vulgaris

- Tuberous sclerosis
- Nevus comedonicus
- Flat warts
- Molluscum contagiosum
- Acne Rosacea

LIFE SPAN CONSIDERATIONS: ROSACEA

Sometimes called acne rosacea (see Color Plate 10), this condition is rare in children and occurs most often between 30 and 50 years of age. It often coexists with acne vulgaris and may closely mimic it. The hallmark or distinction, however, is that comedones do not occur in rosacea. Rosacea may arise de novo or may follow acne, sometimes by years. Occasionally rosacea is confused with perioral dermatitis, which is much more common in the younger population.

MANAGEMENT: ROSACEA

Neutral soaps are recommended. Plexion cleanser (sodium sulfacetamide 10% and sulfur 5%) has helped to reduce both erythema and papules. Patients do not need to avoid makeup. Topical steroids may cause acneiform eruptions or rebound flushing, although they may help with stinging and burning.

Persistent erythema and edema are difficult to treat but may be improved with lasers or Intense Pulsed Light. Transient flushing, especially of the central face, is also difficult to treat. Avoidance of trigger factors (e.g., alcohol, hot fluids, spicy foods) is essential. Papules and pustules are best treated with topical or oral antibiotics or topical azelaic acid. These medications help disrupt the link between flushing and papules.

Treatment usually begins with metronidazole 1% or 0.75% gel, cream, or lotion applied b.i.d. Topical antibiotics (e.g., erythromycin gel) may also be effective. Topical azelaic acid gel applied twice a day is also an effective first-line therapy. Oral antibiotics may be tried for cases in which control is inadequate. Tetracycline 250 to 500 mg PO b.i.d., doxycycline 100 to 200 mg q day, or minocycline 50 to 100 mg PO q day is the usual first line of therapy and should be continued for 2 to 3 months or until clearance occurs. Maintenance doses of tetracycline (250 to 500 mg q day) or minocycline (50 to 100 mg q day) may be required. Isotretinoin is occasionally used in recalcitrant or severe cases and is effective in low doses (0.1 to 0.2 mg/kg body weight/day). Telangiectasis, often the result of constant flushing, responds to a series of Intense Pulsed Light or laser treatments. Chronic granulomatous rosacea can result in a bulbous nose (rhinophyma). Surgical and ablative laser intervention are the most effective treatment modalities.

COMPLICATIONS

Acne-related facial scarring is the most obvious complication. A more common complication is hyperpigmentation, or staining, at the site of inflammatory lesions. Complications can also result from therapy. Serious side effects are associated with some systemic therapies, particularly isotretinoin, which is not only teratogenic but may also cause hypertriglyceridemia and hepatic dysfunction. In addition, serious social and psychologic effects are associated with severe acne.

The most serious medical complication of rosacea is the ocular form in which rosacea keratitis may develop, with resultant corneal ulcers. If this complication is suspected, the patient should be referred to an ophthalmologist.

INDICATIONS FOR REFERRAL OR HOSPITALIZATION

All patients with recalcitrant or severe nodulocystic acne should be referred to a dermatologist for treatment. Patients with issues related to depression and self-esteem should be referred to a mental health professional.

PATIENT AND FAMILY EDUCATION

Acne management and treatment take weeks to months before improvement is appreciated. Patience and understanding of the prescribed treatment regimen are crucial. Phone contact and periodic office visits will help evaluate improvement and compliance. This type of support is often important for this frustrating and often long-term or recurrent disorder. Patients with rosacea can contact the National Rosacea Society at http://www.rosacea.org for more information.

HEALTH PROMOTION

Patients are encouraged to gently wash their involved skin once or twice a day. An awareness that non–water-based cosmetic and hair products may cause acne is important. Patients may have jobs that require them to wear protective headgear and should be encouraged to maintain a careful face cleansing routine to minimize the occurrence of mechanical acne.

REFERENCES

1. Hurwitz S: *Clinical pediatric dermatology,* ed 2, Philadelphia, 1993, Saunders.
2. Weston WL, Lane AT, Morrelli JG: *Color textbook of pediatric dermatology,* ed 2, St Louis, 1996, Mosby.
3. Dershewitz RA: *Ambulatory pediatric care,* ed 2, Philadelphia, 1993, Lippincott.
4. Fox J: *Primary health care of children,* St Louis, 1997, Mosby.
5. Skidmore R, Kovach R, Walker C, and others: Effects of sub-antimicrobial dose doxycycline in the treatment of moderate acne, *Arch Dermatol* 139:459-464, 2003.
6. Leyden JJ: Therapy for acne vulgaris, *N Engl J Med* 336(16):1156-1162, 1997.
7. Johnson BA, Nunley JR: Use of systemic agents in the treatment of acne vulgaris, *Am Fam Phys* 62(8):1823-1830, 2000, retrieved Dec 13, 2006, from http://www.aafp.org/afp/20001015/1823.html.
8. American Academy of Dermatology: *Guidelines of care for acne vulgaris management,* retrieved Dec 13, 2006, from http://www.aad.org/NR/rdonlyres/FAD10239-F59B-486C-8082-28545B54F59A/0/Acne_Guideline.pdf.

CHAPTER 49

Alopecia

Eileen M. Deignan

DEFINITION AND EPIDEMIOLOGY

Alopecia is a term used to describe abnormal hair loss. There are multiple causes of hair loss, ranging from unusual congenital hair abnormalities to the commonly observed alopecia from androgenetic or pattern hair loss. Hair loss is a disturbing and highly emotional issue for many patients. The evaluation of the patient with alopecia involves a carefully elicited history, a physical examination, and sometimes laboratory studies or a biopsy of the scalp. The treatment of alopecia depends on the cause.

PATHOPHYSIOLOGY

Alopecia (except for congenital alopecia) can be divided into two types: scarring and nonscarring alopecia. The nonscarring alopecias, in which the hair follicles are still present, are usually a result of an abnormality of the hair cycle. The scarring alopecias, in which the hair follicles are absent or fibrosed, are usually the result of an intense inflammatory process of the scalp such as discoid lupus or kerion formation from tinea capitis.

A person is born with the 100,000 or so hair follicles that he or she will have throughout life.[1] Each hair follicle goes through a highly programmed cycle over and over again throughout its life.[2] The cycle of hair growth involves three phases: anagen, catagen, and telogen. The anagen (growth) phase varies depending on the location of the follicle on the body. This phase is longest on the scalp (producing long hairs) and much shorter on the eyebrows (producing short hairs). During the catagen phase, the hair involutes. This is the shortest of the three stages. During the telogen phase, the mature hair is shed. Most people lose 50 to 150 scalp hairs per day.

Three common types of hair loss are a result of anagen phase disturbance: androgenetic alopecia, anagen effluvium, and alopecia areata. Androgenetic alopecia, the most common type of hair loss, is the hereditary thinning of hair in susceptible men and women. Patterned thinning of the hair begins in men and women as early as the teenage years. Fifty percent of men and women have some androgenetic alopecia by age 50.[1] This condition results from the sensitivity of hair on certain portions of the scalp to androgens. Testosterone, an androgen, is converted to dihydrotestosterone (DHT) peripherally. DHT binds to receptors on scalp hair follicles, causing a series of events that leads to the shortening of the anagen, or growth, part of the cycle. As a result, hair follicles that previously produced thick, pigmented terminal hairs now make thin, vellus hairs. This process, called *miniaturization*, produces the fine hair seen in androgenetic alopecia, or pattern hair loss.

Anagen effluvium is the term used to describe the alopecia from the diffuse, rapid, and dramatic loss of anagen hairs. The most common cause is chemotherapy. Chemotherapeutic agents prevent the rapid division of the hair matrix cells. Hair production stops, and the hairs that are already present become frail, break off, and are shed. Normal hair production resumes when the antineoplastic medication is stopped.[2]

Alopecia areata is an autoimmune condition that results in well-demarcated areas of alopecia on the scalp or body. The condition is fairly common, affecting about 2% of the U.S. population.[1] In alopecia areata, there is an idiopathic inflammatory response around the hair bulb at the base of the hair. The inflammation forces the hair out of the anagen (growth) phase and into the telogen (shedding) stage. Spontaneous remission is common.

The transient shedding of telogen phase hairs is termed *telogen effluvium*. In this condition the hair prematurely enters the telogen phase. Multiple factors, including high fever, certain medications, endocrine abnormalities, anemia, childbirth, and malnutrition, can cause telogen effluvium.[1] The alopecia from telogen effluvium usually begins 4 to 6 weeks after the precipitating event and can persist for several months.

CLINICAL PRESENTATION

The history is a critical part of the evaluation of a person with alopecia. The provider should inquire about the duration and rapidity of the hair loss and about any symptoms that may be related to trichotillomania. Long and insidious hair loss is more indicative of androgenetic alopecia. It is important to ask whether the patient has had this type of hair loss before. Alopecia areata is often recurrent. The provider should also inquire about acute and chronic illnesses and current and past medications. An acute illness such as a high fever can trigger a telogen effluvium, as can hyperthyroidism or hypothyroidism. A family history of hair loss may represent a clue for androgenetic alopecia, sometimes a hereditary disorder. It is important to inquire about associated symptoms. Scalp itching, pain, or flaking points to an inflammation of the scalp from psoriasis or contact dermatitis from hair dye. These conditions inflame the scalp and can cause hair breakage with resultant alopecia. In addition, symptoms of scalp itching and flaking can indicate tinea capitis, a fungal infection of the scalp that weakens the hairs and produces alopecia.

PHYSICAL EXAMINATION

The physical examination begins with an evaluation of the pattern of hair loss. Androgenetic alopecia in males usually is seen as recession of the hair line at the temples and thinning in the frontal areas and the vertex. Women with androgenetic alopecia usually have diffuse thinning that is most pronounced in the frontal and parietal areas. A rim of hair along the frontal hairline is usually preserved.

Alopecia areata usually is initially seen as well-demarcated patches of hair loss. Singular, "exclamation point" hairs are sometimes visible. These exclamation point hairs are normal distally but are thinned proximal to the scalp. The scalp is not inflamed in alopecia areata. In addition, the eyebrows and eyelashes may be affected. Men may experience alopecia areata in the beard area. When the whole scalp is affected, the process is called *alopecia totalis*. If the whole body is involved, the process is called *alopecia universalis*.

Anagen effluvium tends to lead to a diffuse loss of hair, as does telogen effluvium. Scarring of the scalp suggests an inflammatory process such as lupus or lichen planus follicularis. Scaling on the scalp may suggest psoriasis or tinea capitis. Patchy hair loss with regrowing hairs of multiple lengths suggests trichotillomania, a condition in which the patient pulls or twists the hair.

DIAGNOSTICS

Findings from the history and physical examination guide diagnostic testing. If there is scaling on the scalp that is suggestive of tinea capitis, then several hairs or a scalp scraping is examined after preparation with potassium hydroxide (KOH). The presence of hyphae in the KOH preparation confirms the fungal cause for the alopecia.

DIAGNOSTICS

Alopecia

LABORATORY

KOH preparation
TSH
CBC
Serum glucose
Ferritin level*
VDRL*
DHEA-5*
Testosterone level*

*If indicated.

A hair pull test, in which a few dozen hairs are grasped firmly at the base and pulled, can help determine a telogen or anagen effluvium. The hair bulb from these pulled hairs is examined with a magnifying glass or under the microscope. Anagen and telogen hairs each have a characteristic appearance.

If telogen effluvium is suspected and there is no obvious cause, an underlying illness should be considered. Patients need an evaluation for hypothyroidism or hyperthyroidism. Iron deficiency anemia should be evaluated with hemoglobin, serum iron, iron-binding capacity, and ferritin tests.

A hormonal evaluation of a woman with androgenetic alopecia is not necessary unless she has other signs of a hormonal imbalance such as irregular menses, infertility, hirsutism, cystic acne, virilization, or galactorrhea.[1] In these women, evaluation for alopecia may include testosterone or dehydroepiandrosterone-5 (DHEA-5) levels, in addition to the other hormonal tests indicated by their symptoms.

Secondary syphilis is a cause of patchy alopecia. Patients suspected of having secondary syphilis should have a Venereal Disease Research Laboratory (VDRL) test performed. Finally, a scalp biopsy is sometimes helpful when the cause of the alopecia is not clear.

DIFFERENTIAL DIAGNOSIS

The differential diagnosis of hair loss is extensive. Table 49-1 can be used to differentiate among these conditions. The cause can usually be isolated with a careful history, physical examination, and some diagnostic tests.

MANAGEMENT

When an external factor is found with anagen or telogen effluvium, the key to the management of alopecia is removal of this causative factor. Anagen effluvium as a result of chemotherapy will reverse when the medication is stopped and the hair matrix is allowed to mature again. Telogen effluvium will also reverse when the causative factor or event is over or corrected and the hair cycle is allowed to return to normal.

Currently, androgenetic alopecia is most often medically treated with two medications: minoxidil and finasteride. Minoxidil is the only medication approved by the Food and Drug Administration for use by women. It is applied twice a day to the dry scalp. The side effects of the medication include dryness and irritation of the scalp. Hypertrichosis (excessive hair growth) occurs in 3% to 5% of women. This effect diminishes after a year of therapy.

Finasteride is an oral medication. It works by blocking the peripheral conversion of testosterone to DHT, the hormone responsible for causing the miniaturization of hairs in androgenetic alopecia. The medication is taken daily. Both minoxidil and finasteride should be used for 8 to 12 months to determine if they are effective.[2]

Many cases of alopecia areata resolve spontaneously; however, several treatment options are available. Therapies include topical and intralesional corticosteroids. Anthralin, an immunomodulating agent, and minoxidil are two topical agents that can be effective treatments. Topical immunotherapy, or contact sensitization, is an effective therapy but is not widely available.

TABLE 49-1 Diagnosis of Alopecia

Disease	Duration (years)	Scalp	Pattern	Pull Test
Alopecia areata	<1	Normal	Patchy; ! hairs	±
Anagen effluvium	Duration of chemotherapy	Normal	Diffuse	Hair breakage
Tinea capitis	<1	Scale, crust	Patchy	Hair breakage
Trichotillomania	>1	Normal to scarring	Patchy with stubble	—
Telogen effluvium	<1	Normal	Diffuse	↑ telogen
Androgenetic alopecia	>1	Normal	Pattern baldness	—
Systemic disease	<1	Normal	Diffuse	Normal/↑telogen
Hair breakage	<1	Normal	Patchy	Age appropriate

! hairs, Short, stubby, straight, "exclamation point" hairs.

DIFFERENTIAL DIAGNOSIS

Alopecia

GENERALIZED HAIR LOSS

- Telogen effluvium
- Acute blood loss
- Childbirth
- Inadequate protein intake
- High fever
- Medications (heparin, propranolol, vitamin A, warfarin, propylthiouracil, isotretinoin, lithium, beta blockers, amphetamines, acitretin)
- Stress
- Metabolic abnormalities (hypothyroidism, hyperthyroidism, diabetes)
- Severe illness
- Anemia
- Anagen effluvium
- Cancer therapy (chemotherapy, radiation)
- Poisoning (arsenic, thallium)
- Generalized patchy hair loss
- Secondary syphilis

LOCALIZED HAIR LOSS

- Androgenic alopecia (male or female pattern)
- Alopecia areata
- Atopic dermatitis
- Anemia
- Diabetes
- Pregnancy
- Thyroid disease
- Infection
- Stress
- Tick bite
- Lupus erythematosus
- Myasthenia gravis
- Vitiligo
- Hirsutism
- Scarring alopecia
- Developmental defects (aplasia cutis)
- Physical injury (burns, pressure)
- Infection (bacterial [folliculitis, furuncle], fungal [kerion], viral [herpes zoster])
- Neoplasms (metastatic cancer, sclerosing basal cell carcinoma)
- Lupus
- Lichen planus follicularis
- Cicatricial pemphigoid
- Scleroderma
- Traction alopecia
- Trichotillomania

COMPLICATIONS

Some types of hair loss are the result of systemic illness. Complications can result from these illnesses. In addition, complications can occur as a result of the psychologic effects that patients may experience with hair loss.

INDICATIONS FOR REFERRAL OR HOSPITALIZATION

Alopecia without a timely response to standard management options or cases in which the cause is unclear require consultation with a dermatologist. Patients should also be referred to a dermatologist or surgeon for consideration of hair transplantation. Patients with suspected trichotillomania may benefit from a mental health referral.

PATIENT AND FAMILY EDUCATION

Patients with androgenetic alopecia may be reassured to know that this is a common disorder. They should be reminded there are no restrictions on types of grooming products that they use. In addition, the frequency of hair washing will not affect the hair loss process.[1]

Patients with alopecia areata should know that spontaneous remissions and recurrences are common. They should also know that vitiligo, atopy (eczema, asthma, and hay fever), and thyroid disease are more common in people with alopecia areata.[3]

REFERENCES

1. Price VH: Treatment of hair loss, *N Engl J Med* 341(13):964-973, 1999.
2. Paus R, Costarelis G: The biology of hair follicles, *N Engl J Med* 341(7):491-497, 1999.
3. Arnold HL, Odom RM, James WD: *Andrews' diseases of the skin: clinical dermatology*, ed 8, Philadelphia, 1990, Saunders.

CHAPTER 50

Animal and Human Bites

Daniel W. O'Neill and Katherine E. Beben

DEFINITION AND EPIDEMIOLOGY

Approximately half of all Americans will suffer from an animal or human bite wound in their lifetime; and even though most of the 4.5 million bites annually are minor, there is a significant risk of injury and infection.[1] One million people seek medical attention annually, with an estimated health care cost of more than $100 million a year.

Domestic animals inflict the majority of bite wounds. Dog bites account for 80% to 90% of those bites which require medical care, but they have the lowest incidence of wound infection (2% to 13%).[2,3] These wounds most commonly affect the extremities, are seen more often in children and young adults, and are more frequent when the animal is provoked. Cat bites are the second most common type of mammalian bite, with an incidence of 400,000 per year. However, the infection rate is much higher (30% to 80%) as a result of the deep puncture wounds from the animal's sharp teeth.[1] The most common sites of injury include the arm, forearm, and hand.

Human bites account for 3% to 23% of bite wounds, have overall infection rates from 10% to 50%, and usually result from overly aggressive behavior.[4] The most common sites of infection include the nose, lip, and ear. Bites not located on the hand have an infection rate similar to that of routine lacerations, but the clenched-fist injury, or "fight bite," has a much higher complication rate because of the high penetrating force causing local tissue destruction and potentially osteomyelitis, tendonitis, and septic arthritis.

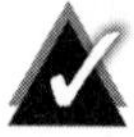

Physician consultation is indicated for suspected rabid animal bites; facial, hand, or extensive bites; tendon, bone, or joint involvement; or significant infectious complications.

PATHOPHYSIOLOGY

The morbidity and mortality associated with mammalian bites is mostly related to tissue injury or, more accurately, polymicrobial infection near the bite site. The pathogens involved reflect the oral flora of the culprit, the skin flora of the victim, and the environment in which the bite took place. Infections involving aerobes alone (24% to 44%) or mixed aerobes and anaerobes (54% to 66%) are the most common.[2] The risk factors for infection are listed in Box 50-1.

BOX 50-1

RISK FACTORS FOR BITE WOUND INFECTION

- Location on the hand or foot
- Puncture wounds
- Crush injuries
- Treatment delay of more than 12 hours
- Failure to irrigate and debride wound during initial management
- Age over 50 years
- Asplenia
- Immunocompromised state
- Alcoholism
- Diabetes mellitus
- Preexisting edema at the bite site
- Peripheral vascular disease

Animal bites can contain a variety of pathogens, both bacterial and viral. The most common aerobic bacteria are *Pasteurella, Streptococcus, Staphylococcus,* and *Corynebacterium* species.[1-4] *Bacteroides, Actinomyces, Porphyromonas,* and *Fusobacterium* species are common anaerobic isolates and may produce β-lactamase.[1-4] A rare but serious bacterial infection caused by *Capnocytophaga canimorsus* causes overwhelming sepsis, disseminated intravascular coagulation, and a 25% mortality rate in patients with predisposing conditions such as asplenia, liver disease, or immunosuppressive therapy.[1] Among viral diseases, rabies is the most common and well known. Animals such as bats, raccoons, skunks, and foxes are the most common carriers in the United States, whereas in other countries dogs and cats are the most predominant carriers. Other pathogens rarely transmitted through animal bites include those which cause tularemia, leptospirosis, cat-scratch disease, rat-bite fever, tetanus, plague, sporotrichosis, and blastomycosis.

Human bites are also polymicrobial, with similar pathogens; however, there are some important differences. *Pasteurella* and *Capnocytophaga* species are not transmitted through humans, but *Eikenella corrodens* is present in 30% of infected human bite injuries (particularly clenched fist), is often resistant to certain antibiotics, and can lead to a serious indolent infection.[2,4] Many of the isolates (24% to 43%) produce β-lactamase. Rare organisms from humans include herpes simplex 1 and 2, hepatitis B and C, and *Mycobacterium tuberculosis*. HIV has a biologic possibility of transmission through a bite wound, but there remains little evidence for this.[1]

CLINICAL PRESENTATION

A bite history must include the location and time of the bite; the breed and behavior of the animal; the domestication and rabies vaccine status of animal; whether the animal was provoked; drug allergies; current immunization status for tetanus and rabies; alcohol use; current medications; and past medical history with an emphasis on immunocompetence, history of splenectomy, chronic edema, or liver disease. The presence of infectious diseases in the biting human should be investigated. Patients may be unwilling to admit to human bite wounds, particularly in a clenched-fist injury.

PHYSICAL EXAMINATION

Physical examination should document the location, extent, and depth of the wound; type of wound (puncture, scratch, tear, or avulsion); and tenderness and other signs of infection (e.g., erythema, streaking, warmth, fluctuation, adenopathy, purulent discharge). There should be careful testing for involvement of underlying tendons, joints (range of motion), and nerves and for signs of compartment syndrome.

DIAGNOSTICS

DIAGNOSTICS

Animal and Human Bites

LABORATORY
Aerobic and anaerobic cultures of infected wounds only
Rabies status of suspicious animals
Hepatitis, HIV, and other transmissible disease status if human bite

IMAGING
X-rays for any bone or joint involvement or foreign body

Culturing fresh bite wounds offers no benefit, but wounds with signs of infection should be cultured for aerobic and anaerobic bacteria.[1,4] Blood cultures and CBC may be indicated if there are signs of systemic infection, but they have a low sensitivity.[1] C-reactive protein can be used to monitor response to treatment.[5] Radiographs are necessary if bone or joint involvement is possible or if a foreign body is present.[1,2,5]

DIFFERENTIAL DIAGNOSIS

None.

MANAGEMENT

After assessing for and treating life-threatening injuries, the provider should irrigate the wound with at least 150 ml of sterile saline solution.[1,2,4] Devitalized tissue, foreign bodies, and clots are cautiously debrided. Aggressive drainage, irrigation, and wound packing are necessary if cultures reveal an established wound infection. Most wounds do not develop signs of infection until 24 to 72 hours after the bite.[2] Most fresh dog bites and facial bites, whether of animal or human origin, can be sutured.[1-4] It is generally accepted that most cat and human bites, deep puncture wounds, clinically infected wounds, wounds over 6 to 12 hours old, and bites to the hand should be left open because of the high risk of infection.[1-5] These wounds can be closed by delayed primary closure or by secondary intention. Wounds involving the hand or foot should be immobilized and elevated for 1 to 3 days.[4,5] Close outpatient follow-up monitoring is recommended to track complications or treatment failures.

Infected bites require 7 to 14 days of targeted antibiotic therapy when soft tissue is involved or 21 days when infection involves bones or joints.[4] The selection of antibiotics is based on knowledge of the most common organisms encountered and on susceptibility testing of cultured organisms from infected wounds. Empiric therapy is most effective with amoxicillin–clavulanic acid 500 to 850 mg PO b.i.d. or cefoxitin 500 mg IV b.i.d.[1,2,4] In patients who are allergic to penicillin, doxycycline 100 mg b.i.d. or the combination of clindamycin with trimethoprim-sulfamethoxazole or ciprofloxacin can be used.[1,2,4] The newer quinolones (e.g., moxifloxacin) are active against all major bite wound pathogens.[2,4] Macrolides should be reserved for pregnant patients allergic to β-lactamase.[6]

Although antimicrobial therapy is obviously indicated in infected wounds, whether to treat fresh, uninfected wounds is still controversial. Some recommend that antibiotic prophylaxis should be given for all bite wounds except for patients who are seen 72 hours after injury with no signs of infection.[2] Others suggest that 3- to 5-day prophylaxis should be given only for high-risk wounds (see Box 50-1).[3,4]

Tetanus toxoid 0.5 ml IM should be administered to those who have not had a tetanus and diphtheria toxoid (Td) booster within the past 5 years.[3,4] Patients who have not completed a full primary series of three injections or whose vaccination status is unknown will require tetanus immune globulin 250 to 500 units IM with the first of three monthly doses of tetanus toxoid.[3,4]

The decision to provide postexposure antirabies treatment should be based on the guidelines of city or state public health departments, the Centers for Disease Control and Prevention, and the Advisory Committee on Immunization Practices. If rabies is suspected, the wound must be immediately washed with soap and water or 1% povidone-iodine solution, which significantly lowers transmission rates.[3] Every effort must be made with the help of public health authorities to make a decision regarding quarantine (isolation and observation) or sacrifice of the biting animal for pathologic brain examination. Postexposure prophylaxis consists of passive immunization with 20 to 40 IU/kg of human rabies immune globulin (HRIG), with half the dose injected around the wound and half given intramuscularly (gluteal or deltoid).[1,7] In addition, active immunization with 1 ml of human diploid cell rabies vaccine (HDCV) given intramuscularly (deltoid) on days 0, 3, 7, 14, and 28 is indicated.[1,3,7] Individuals with a preexposure HDCV vaccination history should receive an HDCV booster on days 0 and 3 but do not require HRIG.[8]

COMPLICATIONS

Infection is the most serious complication of bite wounds, resulting in cellulitis, lymphangitis, tenosynovitis, septic arthritis, and osteomyelitis. Rare complications include meningitis and death from sepsis. Patients with human bite and clenched-fist injuries are at particular risk for these complications. Other potential complications include hemorrhage, disfigurement, and decreased motor function or compartment syndrome. Hepatitis B or other systemic disease from human bites is an additional concern.

INDICATIONS FOR REFERRAL OR HOSPITALIZATION

Although most bite wounds can be handled on an outpatient basis, in a few cases (1% to 2% of patients) hospitalization is indicated: patients with systemic manifestations of infection (fever and chills), severe cellulitis, suspicion of noncompliance, and infected bites refractory to oral or outpatient therapy. Referrals would be necessary for the following: involvement of a joint, nerve, bone, or tendon or compartment syndrome (orthopedic referral); underlying illness such as poorly controlled diabetes, peripheral vascular disease, or an immunocompromised state (internal medicine or infectious disease referral); significant hand bites (hand surgery referral); extensive wounds requiring reconstructive surgery (plastic surgery referral); and head injuries (otolaryngologic or neurosurgery referral).[2,3]

PATIENT EDUCATION AND HEALTH PROMOTION

All patients should be encouraged not to provoke domestic animals or handle wild animals, especially raccoons, skunks, foxes, and bats. A rabies vaccine for pets (both dogs and cats) is mandatory in the United States but not in many foreign countries, including Mexico. Nervousness, aggressiveness, excessive drooling or foaming at the mouth, or fearlessness should raise the suspicion of rabid animals and prompt notification of the animal warden or health authorities.

Preexposure immunization with HDCV should be considered for high-risk groups such as animal handlers, veterinarians, certain laboratory workers, and persons living in or visiting countries with a significant rabies risk. The regimen would be 1 ml IM on days 0, 7, and 21 or 28 and a booster every 2 years.[7] A good source of patient education is http://www.intrepid.net/~twila/rabies.htm.

Td boosters should be given every 10 years routinely in all patients. Instructions to clean all bite wounds and seek medical care immediately should be given, especially for "fight bites" to the hand.

REFERENCES

1. Brinker D, Hancox JD, Bernardon SO: Assessment and initial treatment of lacerations, mammalian bites, and insect stings, *AACN Clin Issues* 14(4):401-410, 2003.
2. Brook I: Management of human and animal bite wounds: an overview, *Adv Skin Wound Care* 18:197-203, 2005.
3. Stefanopoulos PK, Tarantzopoulou AD: Facial bite wounds: management update, *Int J Oral Maxillofac Surg* 34:464-472, 2005.
4. Freer L: North American wild mammalian injuries, *Emerg Med Clin North Am* 22:445-473, 2004.
5. Lewis JA, Miller DR, Davies SG: Osteomyelitis complicating three types of traumatic hand wound, *J Wound Care* 13(7):281-283, 2004.
6. Goldstein EJC: Outpatient management of dog and cat bite wounds, *Fam Pract Recertification* 22(2):67-86, 2000.
7. Centers for Disease Control and Prevention: Human rabies—Florida, 2004, *MMWR* 54(31):767-769, 2005.
8. Advisory Committee on Immunization Practices: Human rabies prevention—United States, 1999, *MMWR* 48(RR-1):1-52, 1999.

CHAPTER 51

Burns (Minor)

Eileen M. Deignan and Gretchen Carrougher

DEFINITION AND EPIDEMIOLOGY

The skin is the largest organ of the body and functions as an excellent barrier against external injury. A burn can disturb this barrier function. A burn may be sustained from electrical, thermal, or chemical agents. Thermal burns constitute a large majority of these injuries; chemical burns make up a relatively small percentage.[1]

In the United States, approximately 2 million patients see their health care provider with burn injuries each year. Of these burns, 80% are minor and can be managed on an outpatient basis.[2]

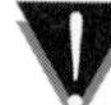

Immediate emergency department referral or physician consultation is indicated for burns that cause respiratory injury (inhalation or facial burns); burns of the hands, feet, genitals, or perianal area; full-thickness burns of more than 2% of the total body surface area (TBSA); minor burns of more than 10% TBSA in patients more than 50 years of age; or burns of more than 15% TBSA in patients 10 to 50 years of age.

PATHOPHYSIOLOGY

The temperature or heat content of the burning agent and the duration of exposure determine the extent of burn injury. A burn wound is best described by the zones of injury. Typically, three zones exist, with the innermost zone (zone of coagulation) representing the most damaged area. Cellular death and thrombosis of the blood vessels occur in this zone. The area of tissue adjacent to this zone is the zone of stasis, where blood flow is compromised. This zone may quickly progress to ischemia, or it may return to normal depending on several factors related to resuscitation. The outermost zone is the zone of hyperemia. This zone has received minimum damage, is characterized by increased blood flow, and will fully recover.[3]

A burn wound is defined by the size and depth of the wound. The size of the burn is quantified by the percentage of the TBSA burned. This percentage can be estimated in several ways. A very quick method assumes that the back of the patient's hand is approximately 1% of the patient's TBSA. Therefore the percentage of TBSA burned is the number of "hands" equal to the size of the burn.[3] Another method is the "rule of nines" (Figure 51-1).

The depth of a burn is described by the depth of skin injured and is either first, second, or third degree. First-degree (superficial) burns involve only the epidermis. Second-degree (partial-thickness) burns involve the dermis. Third-degree burns are full-thickness burns that extend to the subcutaneous fat. The hallmark of the third-degree burn is that the burn site is insensate.[3]

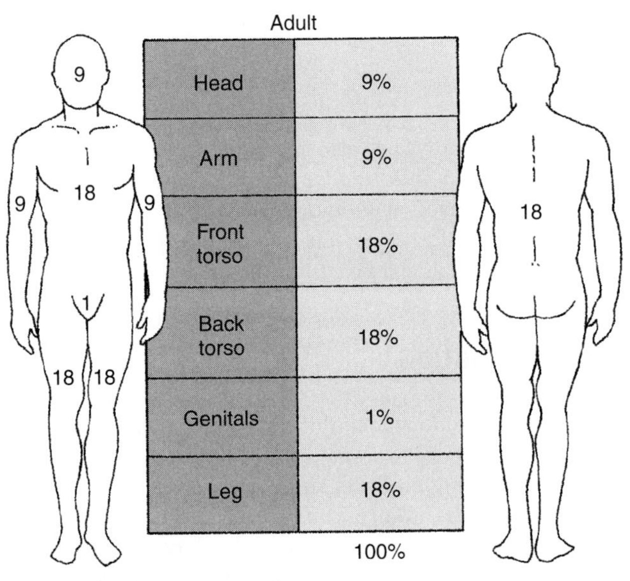

FIGURE 51-1

"Rule of nines" burn chart.

DIAGNOSTICS

Burns

LABORATORY (FOR SERIOUS BURNS)
CBC and differential
Serum electrolytes
Serum glucose
BUN
Creatinine
Urinalysis
Tissue cultures

IMAGING
Chest x-ray*

*If indicated.

DIFFERENTIAL DIAGNOSIS

Burns

- Chemical burns
- Electrical burns
- Thermal burns
- Ritter's disease
- Scalded skin syndrome

CLINICAL PRESENTATION

The health care provider must obtain a full history of the mechanism of injury. The type of thermal or chemical exposure, the duration of exposure, and the time since the injury are important details. This history will help determine any risk for associated traumatic, pulmonary, or ocular injury. A preexisting illness will affect the prognosis and disposition.[4]

PHYSICAL EXAMINATION

The physical examination of the burn victim should be methodic and thorough. Airway, breathing, and circulation should be assessed first; checking vital signs is also indicated. A circumferential burn in a limb may compromise circulation in the involved appendage. The depth, extent (percentage of TBSA burned), and location of the burn must be accurately determined and recorded. The examination should also include a search for any associated injuries.[4]

DIAGNOSTICS

The skin is a barrier, and infection and metabolic abnormalities can result when this barrier is disrupted. Simple thermal burns do not require diagnostic testing. For more serious injuries, CBC, glucose, electrolytes, BUN, creatinine, urinalysis, and tissue cultures may be necessary. A chest x-ray study is indicated for a suspected inhalation injury.

DIFFERENTIAL DIAGNOSIS

The differential diagnosis is determined primarily by history. Certain skin conditions (e.g., staphylococcal scalded skin syndrome, toxic epidermal necrolysis) can resemble a generalized burn.

MANAGEMENT

Management of the patient with burns depends on the classification of the burn. The severity, extent, and location of the burn guide the decisions for treatment. The American Burn Association classifies burns as major, moderate, and minor. Low-risk patients are those between 10 and 50 years of age. High-risk patients are those under 10 years of age and over 50 years of age. Poor-risk patients are those with underlying medical conditions such as heart disease, diabetes, or pulmonary problems. Minor burns involve less than 15% of TBSA in the 10- to 50-year age-group or less than 10% of TBSA in patients under 10 years of age or over 50 years of age. Minor full-thickness burns are less than 2% of TBSA in all age-groups.

Minor burns also have no other associated injuries and can be managed in the office or outpatient setting.[3] If the burn was caused by a chemical agent, the initial therapy is to remove the offending chemical and garments and begin aggressive irrigation. Otherwise, thermal and chemical burn management is similar.[1]

Minor burns are painful, and treatment should begin with analgesics. Ibuprofen, with its antiprostaglandin properties, is a good antiinflammatory and analgesic medication. Narcotic agents such as codeine are also appropriate analgesics. The burn wound needs to be cleaned with mild soap and water or saline; blisters should be debrided. Tetanus prophylaxis should be given as indicated.

Finally, a dressing must be applied. There are several ways to dress minor burns. The burn is usually covered with a thin layer of antimicrobial cream or ointment. The most common topical therapy used is silver sulfadiazine cream (Silvadene), but it cannot be used in patients with sulfa allergy. It should be used cautiously on the face, since the silver in the cream may be deposited in the skin, causing tattooing or staining. Bacitracin ointment is a good alternative. The wound should be washed and redressed twice daily. This regimen should continue for 7 to 10 days until the wound is healed. A burned extremity may require splinting and elevation.[3-5]

Some burns may require open dressings, in which a topical agent is applied without a dressing. The most common sites for open dressings are the face, neck, and perineum. The wound should be thoroughly washed two or three times a day and the topical agent reapplied.[4]

Alternative burn dressings include synthetic dressings such as DuoDERM, OpSite, Epigard, Epi-Lock, Biobrane, or Tegaderm. These biosynthetic dressings are applied to the fresh, clean, moist burn and are sized to approximate the outline of the burn with a slight amount of tension to achieve maximum adherence. These dressings are left in place until the wound heals (approximately 1 to 2 weeks). The dressing can be trimmed away as it spontaneously separates from the wound. Excessive fluid collection under the dressing must be aspirated, or the dressing should be changed. An outer dry dressing needs to be applied and changed daily.[3,4]

COMPLICATIONS

Complications of minor burns typically include local infection and inflammation. Treatment may include antibiotic therapy or a change in topical therapy. Serious complications are rare.

INDICATIONS FOR REFERRAL OR HOSPITALIZATION

Any burn injury larger than the American Burn Association's criteria for minor burns should be referred to the nearest emergency department for further evaluation and hospitalization as necessary. Burns that may result in functional or cosmetic impairment, have an associated injury, or involve high-risk patients require a referral for emergency evaluation. According to Hudspith and Rayatt,[6] burns that fail to heal within 2 to 3 weeks require further evaluation with a wound specialist. Consultation with a physiatrist or referral to physical therapy should be considered when appropriate.

PATIENT AND FAMILY EDUCATION

All burn patients should be seen in 24 hours for a wound check and for assessment of the depth and extent of the burn. Patients should be given clear discharge instructions that explain wound care. They also should be alerted for any signs and symptoms of infection or vascular compromise. If an extremity is involved, it should be elevated. Pain medications may be required. If pain medicine is prescribed, an explanation of how to use the analgesic and of the potential side effects is also necessary.

HEALTH PROMOTION

Home and work safety is the cornerstone of burn prevention. Manufacturer recommendations for protective equipment such as gloves, protective eyewear, and ventilation with certain household cleaning products and at the worksite can prevent chemical and inhalation burns. To prevent electrical burns, the electrical current must be turned off before attempting any electrical repairs, electrical outlets should have covers, and frayed electrical cords should be repaired or the fixture discarded. Lowering hot water temperatures will reduce the risk of scald injuries. Loose clothing should be restricted when cooking or when around open flames. Everyone should be familiar with the stop, drop, and roll technique if their clothes catch fire.

REFERENCES

1. Griglak MJ: Thermal injury, *Emerg Med Clin North Am* 10(2):369-383, 1992.
2. Schwartz LR: Thermal burns. In Tintinalli JE, editor: *Emergency medicine: a comprehensive study guide,* ed 4, New York, 1996, McGraw-Hill.
3. Jordan BS, Harrington DT: Management of the burn wound, *Nurs Clin North Am* 32(2):251-273, 1997.
4. Martin ML, Harchelroad FP: Chemical burns. In Tintinalli JE, editor: *Emergency medicine: a comprehensive study guide,* ed 4, New York, 1996, McGraw-Hill.
5. Monafo WW: Initial management of burns, *N Engl J Med* 335(21):1581-1586, 1996.
6. Hudspith J, Rayatt S: First aid and treatment of minor burns, BMJ 328:1487-1489, 2004.

CHAPTER 52

Cellulitis

Eileen M. Deignan

DEFINITION AND EPIDEMIOLOGY

Cellulitis is an acute skin infection that rapidly spreads and extends deeply from the dermis to the subcutaneous tissue. Cellulitis may progress to a more severe soft tissue infection.[1] The clinical presentation is characterized by erythema, induration, and pain.

Staphylococcus aureus and group A β-hemolytic streptococci are the most common causative agents of this cutaneous process in adults. *Haemophilus influenzae* type B cellulitis is found more commonly in children less than 3 years old.[2,3] Non–group A streptococcus is seen more commonly in patients with underlying abnormalities of the lymphatic system, such as lymphedema. In addition to the more common organisms, adults with co-morbid diseases such as diabetes mellitus or immunodeficiency may be infected with *Acinetobacter* organisms, *Clostridium septicum, Enterobacter* organisms, *Escherichia coli, H. influenzae, Pasteurella multocida, Proteus mirabilis, Pseudomonas aeruginosa,* and group B streptococcus.[2,4,5]

Physician consultation is indicated for patients with periorbital or orbital cellulitis, extensive cellulitis, and cellulitic infections that do not respond to antibiotic therapy within 24 to 48 hours.

PATHOPHYSIOLOGY

Cellulitis most often occurs after a break in the skin such as a laceration, ulceration, chronic dermatoses, or surgical wound. It may, however, develop after trauma to the skin or arise in apparently normal-appearing skin. The lower extremity is the most commonly affected site, but cellulitis may occur anywhere on the body. Areas of the body that have venous or lymphatic compromise from previous cellulitis, radiation treatments, or lymph node resection are more susceptible to recurrent cellulitis.[2]

CLINICAL PRESENTATION AND PHYSICAL EXAMINATION

The classic signs of cellulitis are erythema, induration, and pain (Color Plate 11). The borders of the infected area are usually sharply defined and may be slightly elevated. Blisters, abscesses, erosions, and necrosis may develop in the area of cellulitis. These signs may be accompanied by systemic symptoms, such as malaise, fever, and chills. The site of entry of the bacteria may be evident as breaks in the skin or ulcerations. Regional lymph nodes may be enlarged and tender.

Erysipelas is a superficial form of cellulitis that involves the lymphatic system. Erysipelas is characterized by a sharply demarcated, indurated border and lymphangitic “streaking” toward a regional lymph node. Typical areas involved include the lower legs, face, and ears. Facial erysipelas may follow a streptococcal infection of the upper respiratory tract.[6]

DIAGNOSTICS

The diagnosis of cellulitis is made primarily through the recognition of its distinctive clinical features (erythema, induration, and pain). Because the culture yield of aspirates and biopsy specimens is low, isolation of the etiologic agent is usually not attempted in healthy adults.[6,7] In adults with underlying disease, however, the results of cultures may be more helpful in selecting an appropriate antibiotic. The site most productive for needle aspirate for cultures has been found to be halfway between the leading edge and the center of the cellulitis.[8] Draining of wounds or abscesses provides a much higher culture yield and should be performed.[8] Draining abscesses also allows for more affective penetration of antibiotics into the infected area.

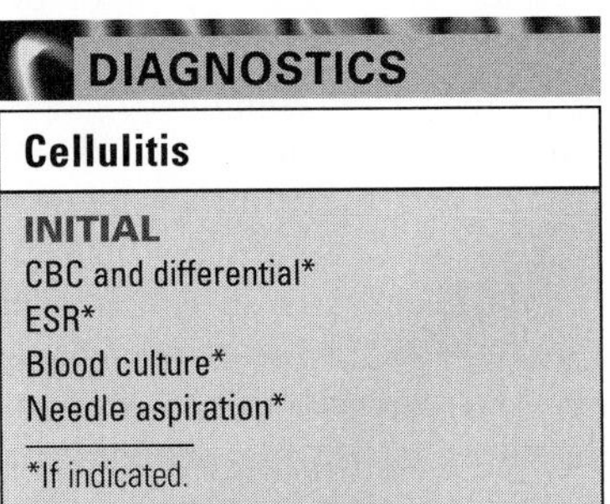

DIAGNOSTICS

Cellulitis

INITIAL
CBC and differential*
ESR*
Blood culture*
Needle aspiration*

*If indicated.

Patients with cellulitis typically have a mild leukocytosis and an elevated erythrocyte sedimentation rate (ESR). However, routine use of a CBC, ESR, and blood cultures is unwarranted in young, otherwise healthy adults.

DIFFERENTIAL DIAGNOSIS

The differential diagnosis of cellulitis includes erysipelas, stasis dermatitis, deep vein thrombosis, contact dermatitis, urticaria, erythema nodosum, erythema migrans, and early herpes zoster.[9] More severe, life-threatening infections, such as necrotizing fasciitis, staphylococcal scalded skin syndrome, and toxic epidermal necrolysis, must also be differentiated early from cellulitis. Cellulitis may also be superimposed on concurrent skin disease such as stasis dermatitis.

DIFFERENTIAL DIAGNOSIS

Cellulitis

- Erysipelas
- Atopic dermatitis
- Folliculitis
- Necrotizing fasciitis
- Scalded skin syndrome
- Toxic epidermal necrolysis

MANAGEMENT

In healthy adults, uncomplicated cases of cellulitis should be treated with antibiotics effective against staphylococcus and streptococcus, the presumptive etiologic agents.[6] A penicillinase-resistant penicillin such as dicloxacillin 500 mg PO q.i.d., or a cephalosporin such as cephalexin 250 to 500 mg PO q.i.d., for 7 to 10 days is appropriate. Erythromycin 250 to 500 PO q.i.d. is appropriate for those with a penicillin allergy. For more extensive but relatively uncomplicated infections, patients may receive an initial dose of a parenteral antibiotic such as cefazolin 1 g or ceftriaxone 1 g before leaving the office, followed by a full course of oral antibiotics. For patients with more severe symptoms (e.g., fever) or with underlying medical conditions that warrant closer monitoring, a once-daily dose of a long-acting parenteral antibiotic such as ceftriaxone 1 to 2 g or cefazolin with probenecid may be given until a good response is observed.[10] The patient may then be switched to an oral antibiotic to complete a total of

7 to 10 days of treatment. Initially, close follow-up monitoring of the patient is indicated to be certain the infection is responding to the antibiotic regimen.

In addition to rest, nonpharmacologic therapies such as the application of moist heat and elevation of the affected region should be advocated in all cases of cellulitis. In patients with abscess formation, incision and drainage are required.

COMPLICATIONS AND INDICATIONS FOR REFERRAL OR HOSPITALIZATION

In severe cellulitic infections or in patients who are unresponsive to previously mentioned therapies, referral for IV antibiotics is appropriate. Periorbital cellulitis is typically a result of sinusitis, upper respiratory tract infection, or eye trauma and is more common in children. Symptoms typically include erythema and edema of the eyelid, conjunctivitis, and chemosis (conjunctival edema). This condition is treated with warm soaks and aggressive antibiotic therapy such as nafcillin or oxacillin 1.5 g q 4 hr.

Far more uncommon is orbital cellulitis, in which there is exophthalmos, orbital pain, restricted eye movement, chemosis, and occasionally visual disturbances. This is an emergency and must be treated as such. Often the infection stems from an ethmoid or maxillary sinusitis and should be evaluated by a CT scan. Complications may include blindness, diplopia, brain abscess, and meningitis if the infection is not aggressively treated. IV antibiotics are indicated for all patients, with ceftriaxone 1 to 2 g IV q 12-24 hr being effective against most etiologic agents. Referral to an otolaryngologist is recommended for closer evaluation.

Soft tissue infections of the hands must be carefully evaluated to determine whether tendon sheaths, joint spaces, or muscle spaces are involved. Necrotizing soft tissue infections are a surgical emergency. The condition starts with redness and painful swelling of the deep tissues. A black eschar rapidly develops with necrosis of the underlying tissues. If necrotizing fasciitis, necrotizing cellulitis, or myonecrosis is suspected, immediate referral is indicated for prompt surgical debridement and IV antibiotics.[9,11]

Patients with diabetes mellitus need to be monitored closely, particularly when cellulitis involves the feet or hands. As a result of decreased circulation in the extremities from microvascular compromise, persons with diabetes are at a greater risk for developing ulcerations and osteomyelitis. Radiographs of the affected extremity are indicated to evaluate for bony involvement or the presence of air in the soft tissues.[11] Uncomplicated cases of nonulcerative cellulitis in patients with diabetes can be treated with amoxicillin-clavulanate or quinolones. These antibiotics are chosen because they cover gram-negative organisms and anaerobes that may infect patients with diabetes.[11,12] Ciprofloxacin 750 mg PO b.i.d. plus clindamycin 300 mg PO q.i.d. or metronidazole 500 mg PO q.i.d. may be used for mild cases of infected diabetic ulcers. More severe ulcerative infections or cases of osteomyelitis require IV antibiotics and referral to a surgeon for debridement.

PATIENT AND FAMILY EDUCATION

Patients and families need to be educated about the importance of avoiding skin infections. By carefully cleaning all skin wounds with a thorough washing and/or irrigation and covering wounds with dressings many skin infections can be prevented. Patients with diabetes should be encouraged to make a daily visual inspection of their feet to evaluate for pressure wounds and breaks in the skin. Underlying dermatoses such as tinea pedis, stasis dermatitis, and lymphedema should be treated aggressively, particularly in patients with diabetes, so the skin does not become a portal of entry for bacteria.[13]

REFERENCES

1. Lewis RT: Soft tissue infections, *World J Surg* 22(2):146-151, 1998.
2. Carroll JA: Common bacterial pyodermas: taking aim against the most likely pathogens, *Postgrad Med* 100(3):311-322, 1996.
3. Howe PM, Fajardo JE, Orcutt MA: Etiologic diagnosis of cellulitis: comparison of aspirates obtained from the leading edge and the point of maximal inflammation, *Pediatr Infect Dis J* 6:685-686, 1987.
4. Boddour LM, Bisno AL: Non–group A beta-hemolytic streptococcal cellulitis, *Am J Med* 79:155-159, 1985.
5. Kieflhofner MA, Brown B, Dall L: Influence of underlying disease process on the utility of cellulitis needle aspirates, *Arch Intern Med* 148:2451-2452, 1988.
6. Brogan TV, Nizet V, Waldhausen JH: Streptococcal skin infections, *N Engl J Med* 334(4):240-245, 1996.
7. Sachs MK: Cutaneous cellulitis, *Arch Dermatol* 127:493-496, 1991.
8. Epperly TD: The value of needle aspirate in the management of cellulitis, *J Fam Pract* 23(4):337-340, 1986.
9. Fitzpatrick TB: *Color atlas and synopsis of clinical dermatology: common and serious diseases,* ed 3, New York, 1997, McGraw-Hill.
10. Brown G, Chamberlain R, Goulding J, and others: Ceftriaxone versus cefazolin with probenecid for severe skin and soft tissue infections, *J Emerg Med* 14(5):547-551, 1996.
11. Elliot DC, Kufera JA, Myers RA: Necrotizing soft tissue infections: risk factors for mortality and strategies for management, *Ann Surg* 224(5):672-683, 1996.
12. Wood MJ, Logan MN: Ciprofloxacin for soft tissue infections, *J Antimicrob Chemother* 18(suppl D):159-164, 1986.
13. Swartz MN: Cellulitis, *N Engl J Med* 350:904-912, 2004.

CHAPTER 53

Contact Dermatitis

Eileen M. Deignan

DEFINITION AND EPIDEMIOLOGY

Irritant dermatitis, or nonallergic contact dermatitis, is an acute or chronic inflammatory reaction that results from a substance coming in contact with the skin. Common substances that create irritant dermatitis include acne preparations, harsh soaps, detergents, solvents, alkalis, and acids. Occlusion and sweating also contribute to irritant dermatitis.[1] Allergic contact dermatitis is the result of a delayed-type hypersensitivity reaction to an allergen coming in contact with the skin. Common causes of allergic contact dermatitis include poison ivy, poison oak, nickel, latex, rubber, and para-aminobenzoic acid (Table 53-1).[2,3]

PATHOPHYSIOLOGY

Irritant contact dermatitis results from prolonged exposure to an irritant that penetrates the epidermal barrier. The pathophysiology of allergic contact dermatitis differs. With the initial irritant exposure in cases of allergic contact dermatitis, epidermal Langerhans' cells absorb the irritant, or antigen. These specialized dendritic cells then present the antigen in the form of major histocompatibility complex (MHC) class II molecules to lymphocytic T cells. The T cells then proliferate and enter the circulation. A second exposure to the antigen elicits activation of the T lymphocytes to release inflammatory mediators, causing the skin reaction.[1-3]

CLINICAL PRESENTATION AND PHYSICAL EXAMINATION

A pruritic rash is a common presenting symptom with both irritant and allergic contact dermatitis. The rash of irritant contact dermatitis is sharply limited to the area of exposure. This dermatitis develops within a few hours of contact with the offending agent. Involved areas are initially erythematous and may develop vesicles, erosions, or crusting.

Allergic contact dermatitis also is usually sharply demarcated to the site of exposure, but the dermatitis may spread to areas that were not exposed. In some cases the eruption may become generalized. These lesions follow a similar pattern with initial erythema. Papules, vesicles, erosions, and crusts may develop[4] (Color Plate 12).

DIAGNOSTICS AND DIFFERENTIAL DIAGNOSIS

Irritant contact dermatitis may resemble atopic dermatitis or nummular dermatitis. The diagnosis of contact dermatitis is made when the location and pattern of the rash are consistent with the exposure history. Localization to the soles of the feet suggests a reaction to the insole of the shoe. Dermatitis around the neck suggests a reaction to a piece of jewelry. Impetigo, candidal infections, and dermatophyte infections may be confused with allergic contact dermatitis. A careful history or irritant exposure may confirm the correct diagnosis. Cultures and potassium hydroxide preparation can screen for infectious or fungal causes. Patch testing can sometimes help identify a contact allergen.

DIAGNOSTICS

Contact Dermatitis

LABORATORY

KOH preparation (to exclude tinea)*
Culture*
Patch testing to identify contact allergen*

*If indicated.

DIFFERENTIAL DIAGNOSIS

Contact Dermatitis

- Atopic dermatitis
- Dyshidrotic eczema
- Bacterial infections
- Candidal infections
- Phytophotodermatitis

TABLE 53-1 Contact Dermatitis: Distribution Diagnosis

Location	Material
Scalp and ears	Shampoo, hair dyes, topical medicines, metal earrings, eyeglasses
Eyelid	Nail polish (transferred by rubbing), cosmetics, contact lens solution, metal eyelash curlers
Face	Airborne allergens (poison ivy from burning leaves, ragweed), cosmetics, sunscreens, acne medications (e.g., benzoyl peroxide), aftershave lotion
Neck	Necklaces, airborne allergens (ragweed), perfumes, aftershave lotion
Trunk	Topical medication, sunscreens, poison ivy, plants (phototoxic reactions), clothing, undergarments (e.g., spandex bra, elastic waistband), metal belt buckles
Axillae	Deodorant (axillary vault), clothing (axillary folds)
Arms	Same as hand; watch and watchband
Hands	Soaps and detergents, foods, poison ivy, industrial solvents and oils, cement, metal (pots, rings), topical medications, rubber gloves in surgeons
Genitals	Poison ivy (transferred by hand), rubber condoms
Anal region	Hemorrhoid preparations (benzocaine, dibucaine [Nupercaine]), nystatin and triamcinolone (Mycolog II) cream
Lower legs	Topical medication (benzocaine, lanolin, neomycin), dye in socks
Feet	Shoes (rubber or leather), cement spilling into boots

From Habif TP: *Clinical dermatology*, ed 3, St Louis, 1996, Mosby.

Physician consultation is recommended for oral steroid use.

MANAGEMENT

Treatments for both irritant and allergic contact dermatitis involve avoidance of the offending agents. Gentle cleansing with mild soaps and cleansing creams followed by lubrication of the skin and application of mid- to high-potency topical glucocorticoid ointments two or three times a day will clear irritant dermatitis.[4] If the involvement of allergic contact dermatitis is extensive, the eruption may best be treated with oral glucocorticoids in consultation with a physician. The course of prednisone should start at about 1 mg/kg body weight. The dose should be tapered over 2 weeks.[5] A short course of oral steroids in the form of dose packs does not maintain the antiinflammatory effects adequately, and rebound is common.[2,3] If the lesions are vesicular and weepy, aluminum acetate (Domeboro) compresses two or three times a day for 1 or 2 days will help dry the lesions. Antihistamines can be used to help control the itching.

COMPLICATIONS

The most common complication of acute contact dermatitis is a superimposed bacterial infection. This can be treated with topical or systemic antibiotics, depending on the severity of involvement. If correctly treated, patients usually recover without serious sequelae.

INDICATIONS FOR REFERRAL OR HOSPITALIZATION

Referral to a dermatologist or dermatology nurse practitioner may be indicated for contact dermatitis. Specialty consultation is appropriate for widespread or recalcitrant contact dermatitis or when the exact diagnosis remains elusive.

PATIENT AND FAMILY EDUCATION

Patient education to avoid the offending antigen is crucial. Patients should understand the importance of continuing treatments for 2 to 3 weeks to prevent rebound. They should also be educated about proper application of steroid creams and their potential side effects. With oral corticosteroid use, patients must be told that the medications should be taken with food and only as prescribed, and they must be educated concerning the medications' potential side effects. In addition, patients must be able to recognize the signs and symptoms of infection.

REFERENCES

1. Dershewitz RA: *Ambulatory pediatric care,* ed 3, New York, 1998, Lippincott Williams & Wilkins.
2. Arndt K: *Manual of dermatologic therapeutics,* ed 6, New York, 2001, Lippincott Williams & Wilkins.
3. Weston WL, Lane AT, Morrelli JG: *Color textbook of pediatric dermatology,* ed 3, St Louis, 2002, Mosby.
4. Saary J, Qureshi R, Palda V, and others: A systematic review of contact dermatitis treatment and prevention, *J Am Acad Dermatol* 53(5):845, 2005.
5. Wolff K, Johnson RA, Suurmond R: *Fitzpatrick's color atlas and synopsis of clinical dermatology: common and serious diseases,* ed 5, New York, 2005, McGraw-Hill.

CHAPTER 54

Corns and Calluses

Margaret McAllister

DEFINITION

Corns and calluses are a painful reaction to pressure or friction on the underlying dermis covering the digital and plantar surfaces of the feet. Areas of excessive pressure or friction lead to hyperkeratotic, thickened skin that forms a padded area of protection for underlying skin structures. Corns, also termed *helomas*, are of two kinds: soft (heloma molle) and hard (heloma durum). Calluses (tylomas), although unsightly, are less bothersome than corns and are generally a reaction to friction on the metatarsal heads or other bony prominences and may be a response to body weight distribution.[1-3] Calluses are not well circumscribed and lack the central hyperkeratotic painful core that is found in corns.

PATHOPHYSIOLOGY

Soft corns stem from hyperkeratotic development in response to excessive pressure or friction. A soft corn is a spongy hyperkeratosis in the interdigital areas of the toes. The pain associated with soft corns is often extreme because the inflammation excites pressure on the nerve receptors in the dermis. Pressure on the skin over the heads and bases of the condyles of the metatarsals and phalanges results from extrinsic factors, including an improperly fitting toebox, short shoes, or shoes with stiff soles, or from intrinsic factors, such as arthritic changes, fractures, or congenital foot deformity. Both intrinsic and extrinsic factors contribute to the development of a compensatory response of the foot and toes. Downward pressure on the metatarsal heads and contracture of the phalanges set the stage for friction and pressure, leading to corn and callus formation. Both are hard and produce pain as the conical-shaped keratin points into the dermis, stimulating painful sensory nerve endings.[2] Pain is triggered by development of an underlying bursitis or adventitious bursa that acts as a buffer of protection for the underlying bone.[2]

CLINICAL PRESENTATION

Corns generally produce problems when symptoms interfere with the performance of daily activities. Obtaining a good occupational history and inspecting the style and fit of the patient's customary shoe are important. Inability to move the toes in the toebox or wearing pointed-toe or high-heeled shoes is frequently reported. Self-treatment by cutting or using over-the-counter plasters to remove the outer horny layer of tissue is common. Occasionally, soft corns are seen with evidence of maceration, inflammation, oozing, and severe pain. Secondary infections of interdigital soft corns are frequent and painful.

PHYSICAL EXAMINATION

Corns appear as well-circumscribed, translucent formations of keratin derived from the stratum corneum of the epidermis. Corns and calluses are located in areas of mechanical trauma.

The dorsolateral aspect of the fifth toe or the dorsal surface of the distal interphalangeal joints of the second, third, and fourth toes are the areas most commonly affected by pressure. Seed corns are small, localized lesions anywhere on the plantar surface; hard corns are located over bony prominences; soft corns occur between the toes, most often in the fourth web space; and "pump bumps" appear in adolescents as thickened soft tissue at the posterior aspect of the calcaneus secondary to wearing shoes that are too short.[4]

DIAGNOSTICS AND DIFFERENTIAL DIAGNOSIS

Inspection and examination are the only diagnostics generally indicated. Sometimes x-ray studies may be ordered to examine the bony structures of the feet. Hard corns are distinguished from warts by their slow onset, location over bony prominences, and painful response to direct pressure. Other factors include the lack of punctate bleeding when the corn is pared with a surgical scalpel, as well as evidence of furrowed skin lines on magnification that are not present in warts.[5] In some instances radiographs of the bony structures of the feet may be necessary to determine the intrinsic cause of corn and callus formation, such as arthritis, bony prominences, condylar projections, and malunion of an old fracture.[5,6]

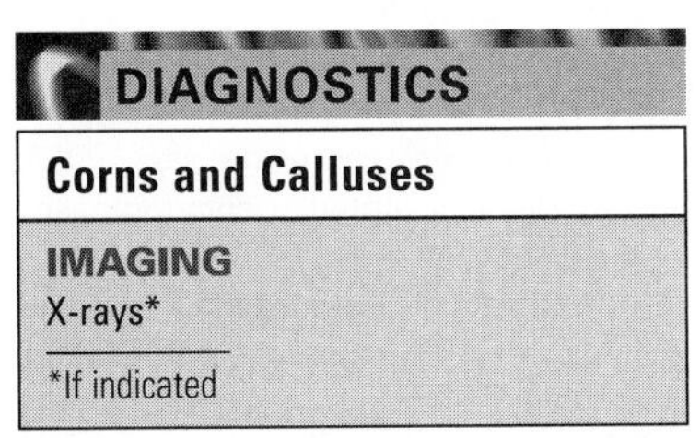
DIAGNOSTICS

Corns and Calluses

IMAGING
X-rays*

*If indicated

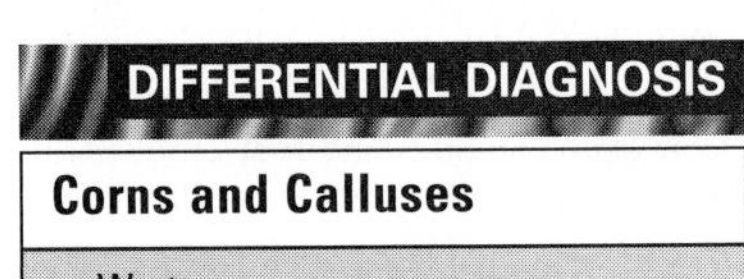
DIFFERENTIAL DIAGNOSIS

Corns and Calluses

- Warts
- Foreign body granuloma
- Porokeratosis plantaris discreta

MANAGEMENT

In general, patients should not apply caustic over-the-counter solutions to corns or calluses. An educated provider, however, can treat troublesome corns and calluses. Treatment begins by decreasing the size the callus or corn by gently paring the skin with a no. 15 scalpel blade. After the paring, the provider applies a 40% salicylic acid plaster cut to fit the size of the remaining lesion. Instructions to the patient after paring include keeping the area dry and leaving the acid plaster undisturbed for 48 to 72 hours. At the next visit, the provider pares the remaining skin and repositions the plaster patch. Tape is useful for keeping the patch positioned clear of normal skin. After the second paring, patients can use a metal nail file or a pumice stone to carefully remove the white "dead" skin before replacing the salicylic acid plaster themselves. Other instructions to the patient include discontinuing the patch once the lesion has cleared and returning to the provider should lesions fail to resolve within 1 to 2 weeks of treatment.

Providers should assess all patients for peripheral neuropathies and avoid the application of plasters in those affected with neuropathies because of risk for damage to normal skin if patients cannot feel foot pain that results from slippage of the patch onto normal skin. In lesions not amenable to the use of a plaster patch, providers can prescribe salicylic acid 10% to 20% in petrolatum (available in 30- to 45-g tubes). Patients failing treatment should be referred for foot x-ray studies to determine whether underlying bony abnormalities exist.[7]

Soft corn infections can be treated by twice-daily warm soaks and application of a topical antibiotic, such as mupirocin, that is effective against gram-positive organisms. If signs of cellulitis are present, additional oral medication should be started in the form of penicillinase-resistant penicillin, a first-generation cephalosporin, or erythromycin. After healing, the patient should be instructed to wear lamb's wool between the affected toes. The lamb's wool should be thick enough to prevent pain when the toes are juxtaposed. The patient also should be instructed to wear open-toed shoes if possible and purchase shoes that promote proper foot alignment plus provide room for movement of the toes in the toebox.

Treatment for calluses includes regular sanding with a pumice stone after softening the callus in warm water. Proper footwear, posture, and body habitus are further considerations in managing calluses.

General principles of treatment and prevention of corns and calluses include (1) provide pain relief, (2) discover and correct the cause for increased mechanical stress, (3) recommend appropriate footwear and orthotic devices, and (4) recommend surgery if conservative approaches fail.[3,6] Patients should be advised to wear shoes with extra depth to increase room for their toes. Padding may prove helpful in the form of toe crests and metatarsal pads that redistribute weight from the metatarsal head to the pad. Toe crests work well for patients with painful hammertoes but must be worn in conjunction with shoes with a sufficiently wide toebox. Other, more recent advances include a variety of shoe pads.

Co-Management with Specialists

Patients should be referred to a podiatrist or orthopedic surgeon who specializes in the care of feet if conservative treatments fail to relieve pressure and restore foot health. Patients with arthritis or hip deformities, those who bear weight on only one foot, and those who use assistive devices for ambulation are at greater risk for severe corns and calluses that do not respond to conservative treatment, since intrinsic factors are the underlying cause of the mechanical stress. These individuals are also more likely to develop painful hammertoes. Surgical remodeling of the toes can provide the patient with marked relief from painful pressure spots and enhance quality of life. Custom shoes are also a helpful adjunct.

LIFE SPAN CONSIDERATIONS

Adolescents and young adults are more likely to wear shoes that fit improperly to be fashionable or to make their feet look smaller. Foot inspection during annual physical examinations should focus on early detection of corns, calluses, and bunions that result from short, tight-fitting footwear. Studies indicate that women more commonly suffer from corns, calluses, bunions, and foot deformities than men.[8] Patients over 65 years old have more foot problems than the general population.[6] Foot pain associated with corns and calluses may prevent older adults from performing instrumental activities of daily living such as standing, shopping, and walking.[9]

Improperly fitted shoes are common in the elderly. Narrow shoes contribute to the development of toe corns, hallux valgus deformity, and foot pain in elderly patients.[10] Older adults are at increased risk for foot infections secondary to corn and callus formation, coupled with an increased incidence of poor circulation.

Working men and women who stand for long hours on the job are at greater risk for foot problems. Efforts should be made to assess their feet frequently and determine the adequacy of shoe fit for comfort and prevention of pressure points. Foot assessment should be included in the comprehensive physical examination of all patients as a means to evaluate foot health and provide necessary preventive education.

COMPLICATIONS

Secondary infections often occur in soft corns. Other complications are primarily in the form of irritation, self-inflicted injury from paring down the corns, and chemical burns from use of caustic over-the-counter keratolytic solutions.

INDICATIONS FOR REFERRAL OR HOSPITALIZATION

Hospitalization is generally not warranted except in cases of serious infection or when surgery is indicated for corns that fail to respond to conservative treatment. Diabetic patients with infected corns may require IV antibiotic treatment. Other indications for referral include custom fitting for orthotic shoes.[3,6] Patients with severe foot deformity who are unable to purchase commercially available shoes that do not put pressure on the feet and toes may benefit from custom-fit shoes; these are expensive but worth the investment for comfort and freedom from pressure-induced pain. Custom-fit shoes promote optimum balance and assist in the prevention of falls.

PATIENT EDUCATION AND HEALTH PROMOTION

Education focuses on prevention and treatment with properly fitting footwear that allows for sufficient toe space and an even distribution of body weight over the plantar surface of the foot.[6] Shoes should provide a shock-absorbing quality that absorbs pressure and friction rather than creating it. Gait and body habitus are other considerations.

REFERENCES

1. DeGowin RL, Brown DD: *DeGowin's diagnostic examination*, ed 7, New York, 2000, McGraw-Hill.
2. Robbins JM: Recognizing, treating, and preventing common foot problems, *Cleveland Clin J Med* 67(1):45-56, 2000.
3. Freeman DB: Corns and calluses resulting from mechanical hyperkeratosis, *Am Fam Phys* 65(11):2277-2280, 2002.
4. Silfverskklold JP: Common foot problems, *Postgrad Med* 89(5):183-188, 1991.
5. Singh D, Bentley G, Trevino SG: Fortnightly review: callosities, corns, and calluses, *BMJ* 312(7403):1403-1406, 1996.
6. Brainard BJ: Managing corns and plantar calluses, *Phys Sportsmed* 19(12):61-66, 1991.
7. Goldstein BG, Goldstein AO: *Benign neoplasms of the skin*, 2003, retrieved Nov 9, 2006, from http://patients.uptodate.com/topic.asp?file=pri_derm/7972.
8. Dunn JE, Link CL, Felson DT, and others: Prevalence of foot and ankle conditions in a multiethnic community sample of older adults, *Am J Epidemiol* 159(5):491-498, 2004.
9. Benvenuti F, Ferrucci L, Guralnik JM, and others: Foot pain and disability in older persons: an epidemiologic survey, *J Am Geriatr Soc* 43(5):479-484, 1995.
10. Menz HB, Morris ME: Footwear characteristics and foot problems in older people, *Gerontology* 51(5):346-351, 2005.

CHAPTER 55

Cutaneous Herpes

Joanne Marie Petrelli and
Maureen O'Hara Padden

DEFINITION AND EPIDEMIOLOGY

Cutaneous infections caused by the herpes simplex virus (HSV) can be of two serologic types: HSV-1, primarily oral lesions, and HSV-2, causing mainly genital infections (Color Plate 13). However, either virus can cause infection at either site. Oral HSV-1 infection recurs more frequently than oral HSV-2 infection; likewise, genital HSV-2 infection recurs more frequently than genital HSV-1 infection.[1] Both HSV-1 and HSV-2 are DNA viruses. Clinically, the lesions produced by each strain of the virus are indistinguishable.

There is a high prevalence of HSV-1 and HSV-2 throughout the world. Infection with the virus shows no seasonal variation. In the United States alone, 1 million people acquire genital herpes each year.[2] One third to one half of infected individuals lack clinical manifestations of infection.[3] Asymptomatic individuals can shed the virus in the absence of symptoms. In fact, transmission has been shown to occur most often in the setting of asymptomatic virus shedding. HSV shedding has been shown to be three times higher in genital secretions sampled between, rather than during, clinical recurrences.

Independent risk factors include multiple sexual partners, increasing age, female gender, low socioeconomic status, cocaine use, African American and Mexican American races, and HIV infection.[1,4,5]

PATHOPHYSIOLOGY

Transmission of HSV occurs by direct contact with active lesions or with secretions containing the virus. HSV is a double-stranded DNA virus that may enter the host through a skin disruption or intact mucous membranes. HSV-1 and HSV-2 share approximately 50% of their double-stranded DNA, and therefore infection with one form affords some protection against the other.[6] The virus attaches itself to epithelial cells, enters, and replicates, exploiting cellular components. Once infected, cells die and release clear fluid, causing the formation of vesicles and fusing to form multinucleated giant cells. During the infection process, the virus gains access to and infects regional, sensory, or autonomic nerves. The virus travels via the nerve axon to the ganglion, where it establishes a latent infection. Subsequently, the virus can reactivate and travel down the axon, where it causes a recurrent infection in the cutaneous area innervated by the affected root.[2]

CLINICAL PRESENTATION

HSV infection has three distinct phases: primary, latent, and recurrent infection. Lesions of the primary infection typically appear 2 to 12 days after inoculation, with a mean of 4 days.[1] Virus excretion in primary mucocutaneous infections can persist for up to 23 days. The occurrence of lesions may be preceded by a prodrome of burning or tenderness at the site of subsequent eruption. Multiple painful vesicles then appear at the site of infection and may be accompanied by tender lymphadenopathy in regional nodes. Fever, dysuria, vaginal discharge, or malaise may accompany the primary infection. Ulceration subsequently occurs, and lesions crust over and heal in immunocompetent patients within 2 to 3 weeks.

During the latent phase the virus remains dormant in the ganglion of the nerve that serves the affected dermatome. The recurrent phase is characterized by virus reactivation and the reappearance of lesions in the dermatome affected during the primary infection. The outbreak may not occur at exactly the same site. Reactivation of the virus can be caused by local or systemic stimuli such as immunodeficiency, trauma, fever, menses, ultraviolet light, and sexual intercourse. Although stress has been considered to be a trigger of HSV recurrence, recent evidence suggests that this may not be the case.[7] The primary infection may last 2 to 6 weeks, whereas recurrent infections are shorter (4 to 6 days) and are less severe, with markedly fewer lesions.

PHYSICAL EXAMINATION

The lesions of HSV infection are distinct. Grouped vesicles on an erythematous base appear on the lips, facial area, throat, or genital area (Color Plate 42). The fluid contained in the vesicles turns cloudy and the vesicles rupture, leaving erosions that subsequently crust over. Regional lymphadenopathy may be associated with primary or recurrent infections but is more common with primary infections. The various stages of lesions can often make diagnosis challenging.

DIAGNOSTICS

A diagnosis of HSV infection can be made clinically with a thorough history and physical examination. However, laboratory confirmation should be considered in patients with a newly diagnosed primary infection. In addition, it is important to elicit any history of HSV infection, HIV infection, or pregnancy. The definitive test for the diagnosis of cutaneous herpes simplex infections remains viral culture. Viral cultures can take 4 or 5 days with a sensitivity of 70% to 80%. Diagnosis may also be made using fluid obtained from a freshly unroofed vesicle for Tzanck preparation or using a direct fluorescent antibody (DFA) test. Both tests have lower sensitivity rates than culture. Viral cultures are most likely to be positive when fresh, moist lesions exist; however, the DFA test may still be positive in crusted, healing lesions.[8-11]

Serologic testing is available but often does not differentiate HSV-1 from HSV-2 and may only reveal previous exposure. Antigen detection tests are also of limited usefulness in primary infections, since antibody development may be delayed.[6-9] Polymerase chain reaction (PCR) tests are extremely sensitive and specific but are expensive and

> **DIAGNOSTICS**
>
> **Cutaneous Herpes**
>
> **LABORATORY**
> Viral cultures (diagnostic test of choice)
> Tzanck smear
> Direct fluorescent antibody*
>
> *If indicated.

are not indicated for mucocutaneous infections. PCR is most useful in the assessment of patients with suspected HSV encephalitis.[8]

DIFFERENTIAL DIAGNOSIS

DIFFERENTIAL DIAGNOSIS

Cutaneous Herpes

- Erythema multiforme
- Impetigo
- Varicella
- Herpes zoster
- Behçet's syndrome
- Herpes zoster
- Syphilis
- Coxsackievirus infection
- Herpangina
- Stevens-Johnson syndrome
- Aphthous stomatitis
- Ulcerative balanitis

The differential diagnosis of HSV infections is varied. Erythema multiforme, impetigo, varicella, Behçet's syndrome, coxsackievirus infection, syphilis, Stevens-Johnson syndrome, herpangina, aphthous stomatitis, and ulcerative balanitis should be considered. A thorough health history, appearance of lesions, and results of appropriate laboratory testing help with the differentiation among these diagnoses.

MANAGEMENT

Acyclovir remains the treatment of choice for most HSV infections (Table 55-1). Two newer precursor drugs, valacyclovir (which is converted to acyclovir) and famciclovir (which is converted to penciclovir), have been licensed for use and have been shown to have better bioavailability than acyclovir or penciclovir. However, they are considerably more expensive. Their clinical benefit is similar, and no evidence exists that one is better than the others. Their usefulness lies in the convenience of the dosing schedule, which may be important for patients with poor compliance. From a cost/benefit perspective, acyclovir is probably most useful in the management of herpes simplex infections, since it is now available in generic form.[10,11]

TABLE 55-1 Dosing Schedule for Mucocutaneous Herpes Simplex Infections

Drug	Dosage
INITIAL EPISODE	
Acyclovir	200 mg PO 5 times daily for 10 days
	5 mg/kg IV q 8 hr for 7 days
	400 mg PO t.i.d. for 10 days
Valacyclovir	1 g PO b.i.d. for 10 days
Famciclovir	250 mg PO t.i.d. for 10 days
RECURRENT EPISODES	
Acyclovir	400 mg PO b.i.d. for 5 days
Valacyclovir	500 mg PO b.i.d. for 5 days
Famciclovir	125-250 mg PO b.i.d. for 5 days
SUPPRESSION	
Acyclovir	400 mg PO b.i.d.
Valacyclovir	500 or 1000 mg PO q day or every other day; varies with HIV status, number of episodes per year, and creatinine clearance
Famciclovir	250 mg PO b.i.d.

Oral Gingivostomatitis

Evidence indicates that oral acyclovir suspension (200 mg five times per day or 400 mg three times per day for 5 days) significantly shortens the duration of oral lesions and reduces eating and drinking difficulties.

Primary Herpes Labialis

Evidence exists that initial orolabial infection with HSV should be treated with acyclovir 200 mg PO five times daily for 7 to 10 days.[11] Topical acyclovir has little efficacy and should not be used to treat mucocutaneous HSV infections.[12,13] However, the U.S. Food and Drug Administration (FDA) has approved penciclovir cream, applied every 2 hours (while awake) for 4 days, for treatment of herpes labialis. Limited evidence exists that penciclovir cream is useful in treating recurrent herpes labialis, with reduced pain and faster healing of lesions.[11-15]

Recurrent Herpes Labialis

Evidence of the benefit of treatment is unclear for recurrent herpes labialis. Only severe cases of recurrent herpes labialis should be treated. Recurrent outbreaks can be treated with the following acyclovir regimens: (1) 200 mg PO five times daily, (2) 400 mg PO t.i.d., or (3) 800 mg PO b.i.d. until lesions are crusted or for approximately 5 days.[11] Limited evidence exists regarding the benefit of a single stat dose of 800 mg acyclovir at the onset of prodrome to prevent recurrent outbreaks of HSV in some patients.[9,11-16]

Primary Genital Herpes

Evidence points to the benefit of treatment of primary genital herpes with either IV or oral acyclovir.[11-12] Patients may be treated with one of the following regimens: (1) 200 mg PO five times daily for 10 days, (2) 5 mg/kg IV q 8 hr for 7 days, or (3) 400 mg PO t.i.d. for 10 days.[1] Valacyclovir and famciclovir may also be used, but there is no evidence to suggest they are any more effective clinically, and they cost considerably more. They do offer the benefit of easier dosing, with valacyclovir given daily and famciclovir given three times daily. This may be important if compliance or ease of dosage schedule is an important consideration. The following dosing regimens may be used: (1) valacyclovir 1 g PO b.i.d. for 10 days, or (2) famciclovir 250 mg PO t.i.d. for 10 days.[11]

Recurrent Genital Herpes

Limited evidence exists for benefit of treatment of recurrent genital herpes labialis with acyclovir, famciclovir, or valacyclovir when started within 24 hours of onset.[11,17-20] However, medication only shortens the duration of lesions by 1 or 2 days and does not reduce the time until recurrence of infection. When drugs are given, the following regimens may be used: (1) acyclovir 400 mg PO b.i.d. for 5 days, (2) valacyclovir 500 mg PO b.i.d. for 5 days, or (3) famciclovir 125 to 250 mg PO b.i.d. for 5 days.[11]

Suppression of Frequent Recurrences

Some evidence indicates that patients with frequently recurring HSV infections (>6 per year) can benefit from suppression with acyclovir, famciclovir, or valacyclovir.[3,11-24] Patients may be treated with one of the following long-term suppressive therapy regimens: (1) acyclovir 400 mg PO b.i.d., (2) valacyclovir 500 to 1000 mg PO q day, or (3) famciclovir 250 mg PO b.i.d.[11] This reduces the number of recurrences and the frequency of asymptomatic shedding. It is important to understand that famciclovir and valacyclovir are no more effective than acyclovir for treating recurrent HSV infections.[11,22,23] Because of their cost, valacyclovir and famciclovir find greatest usefulness where compliance or convenience of dosing is an issue. The FDA has approved suppressive therapy with acyclovir for 12 months, although studies extending treatment to 5 years show no cumulative toxicity.[21] Patients with frequent orolabial HSV infection can be treated with similar regimens.

LIFE SPAN CONSIDERATIONS

Patients should understand that infection with HSV is lifelong and that there is no cure. There is currently no vaccination available; however, many vaccines are currently in different stages of development. These include vaccines made from proteins; peptides, or chains of amino acids; and the DNA virus itself.[3,25] The frequency and severity of attacks diminish in most individuals with time.

COMPLICATIONS

Complications of HSV are rare and typically occur in those who are already immunocompromised. Possible complications include aseptic meningitis, urinary retention, cutaneous dissemination, bacterial superinfection, erythema multiforme, and spontaneous abortion. A cesarean section is usually performed if the mother has active herpes lesions at or around the time of delivery. However, transmission rates to newborns from women who are antibody positive and have no symptoms at the time of delivery are less than 1%. Women who contract genital HSV-1 or HSV-2 in their third trimester of pregnancy are at high risk of infecting their newborns (30% to 50%).[4]

INDICATIONS FOR REFERRAL OR HOSPITALIZATION

Patients for whom a diagnosis of HSV is in question, who have superimposed HIV infection, who are on long-term suppressive therapy, or who fail to respond to routine therapy should be referred to a physician or specialist. Pregnant women also represent a special population and should be referred for evaluation by their obstetrician or family physician immediately.

Patients requiring large amounts of pain medication or patients who have severe disseminated infections, severe superimposed bacterial infections, an inability to void, or an inability to take anything by mouth should be considered for hospitalization.

PATIENT AND FAMILY EDUCATION

Patients must be made aware of their ability to transmit HSV even when they have no apparent lesions. The provider should encourage them to use condoms. The risk of neonatal transmission during pregnancy must be explained to both male and female patients. Patients should be encouraged to use lip balm with sunscreen when exposed to ultraviolet light to avoid precipitation of an outbreak.

Two types of counseling are required for those newly diagnosed with genital herpes: (1) medical counseling, dealing with clinical issues; and (2) emotional counseling concerning the impact of herpes on self-esteem, sexuality, and social interactions.[26] Patients may experience shame or depression because of their infection with HSV and should be referred to the National Herpes Hotline at (919) 361-8488 for available resources.

HEALTH PROMOTION

Patients can reduce their risk of acquiring genital herpes by limiting their lifetime number of sexual partners, by using condoms, and by becoming educated about transmission and shedding so they can avoid high-risk situations. The risk of orolabial herpes infection can also be reduced by limiting sexual partners and by avoiding direct contact with individuals with cold sores. Patients with orolabial and genital herpes must be counseled not to excoriate or rub the herpes lesions because of the risk for autoinoculation of other parts of the body.

REFERENCES

1. Centers for Disease Control and Prevention: 2002 sexually transmitted diseases treatment guidelines, *MMWR* 51:18-21, 2002.
2. Centers for Disease Control and Prevention: *Tracking hidden epidemics 2000,* retrieved Dec 11, 2006, from http://www.cdc.gov/std/Trends2000/herpes.htm.
3. Spruance SL,Tyring SK, De Gregorio B, and others: A large scale placebo-controlled, dose-ranging trial of perioral valacyclovir for episodic treatment of recurrent herpes genitalis: Valacyclovir HSV Study Group, *Arch Intern Med* 156(15):1729-1735, 1996.
4. Brown ZA, Walt A, Morrow A, and others: Effect of serologic status and cesarean delivery on transmission rates of herpes simplex virus from mother to infant, *JAMA* 289:203-209, 2003.
5. Ferri F: *Ferri's clinical advisor: instant diagnosis and treatment,* ed 8, St Louis, 2006, Mosby.
6. Annunziato PW, Gershon A: Herpes simplex virus infections, *Pediatr Rev* 17(12):415-423, 1996.
7. Green J, Kocsis A: Psychological factors in recurrent genital herpes, *Genitourin Med* 73:253-258, 1997.
8. Erlich KS: Management of herpes simplex and varicella-zoster virus infections, *West J Med* 166(3):211-215, 1997.
9. Leflore S, Anderson PL, Fletcher CV: A risk-benefit evaluation of acyclovir for the treatment and prophylaxis of herpes simplex virus infections, *Drug Saf* 23(2):131-142, 2000.
10. Cory L, Wald A, Patel R, and others: Once daily valacyclovir to reduce the risk of transmission of genital herpes, *N Engl J Med* 350:11, 2004.
11. Emmert DH: Treatment of common cutaneous herpes simplex virus infections, *Am Fam Phys* 61(6):1-12, 2000.
12. Review: topical acyclovir is of limited or no benefit to patients with recurrent herpes labialis, *ACP J Club* 15:6, 1991.
13. Worrall G: Topical acyclovir for recurrent herpes labialis in primary care, *Can Fam Phys* 37:92-98, 1991.
14. Whitley RJ: Acyclovir: a decade later, *N Engl J Med* 327:782-789, 1992.
15. Spruance SL: Penciclovir cream for the treatment of herpes simplex labialis, *JAMA* 277(17):1374-1379, 1997.
16. Shelley WB, Shelley ED: "Stat" single dose of acyclovir for prevention of herpes simplex, *Cutis* 57(6):453, 1996.
17. Reichman RC, Badger GJ, Mertz GJ, and others: Treatment of recurrent genital herpes simplex infections with oral acyclovir: a controlled trial, *JAMA* 251:2103-2107, 1984.
18. Famciclovir reduced lesion healing time in recurrent genital herpes, *ACP J Club* 125:69, 1996.
19. Diaz-Mitoma F, Sibbald RG, Sharon SD, and others: Oral famciclovir

for the suppression of recurrent genital herpes: a randomized controlled trial, *JAMA* 280:887-892, 1998.
20. Patel R, Bodsworth NJ, Woolley P, and others: Valacyclovir for the suppression of recurrent genital HSV infection: a placebo controlled study of once daily therapy, International Valacyclovir HSV Study Group, *Genitourin Med* 73(2):105-109, 1997.
21. Wald A, Zeh J, Barnum G, and others: Suppression of subclinical shedding of herpes simplex virus type II with acyclovir, *Ann Intern Med* 124:8-15, 1996.
22. Chosidow O, Drouault Y, LeConte-Veyriac F, and others: Famciclovir vs. acyclovir in immunocompetent patients with recurrent genital herpes infections: a parallel-groups, randomized, double blind clinical trial, *Br J Dermatol* 144(4):818-824, 2001.
23. Tyring SK, Douglas JM, Corey L, and others. A randomized, placebo-controlled comparison of oral valacyclovir and acyclovir in immunocompetent patients with recurrent genital herpes infections: the Valacyclovir International Study Group, *Arch Dermatol* 134(2):185-191, 1998.
24. Mertz GJ, Jones CC, Mills J, and others: Oral famciclovir for suppression of recurrent genital herpes simplex virus infection in women, *Arch Intern Med* 157:343-349, 1997.
25. National Institutes of Health: *Genital herpes, NIAID fact sheet,* retrieved Dec 11, 2005, from http://www.niaid.nih.gov/factsheets/stdherp.htm.
26. Warren T, Ebel C: Counseling the patient who has genital herpes or genital human papillomavirus infection, *Infect Disease Clin North Am* 19(2):459-476, 2005.

CHAPTER 56

Dermatitis Medicamentosa

Nancy W. Knee

DEFINITION AND EPIDEMIOLOGY

Dermatitis medicamentosa (drug eruption) is an eruption of the skin or mucous membranes that can occur up to 2 weeks after drug administration. These eruptions imitate almost all of the morphologic variations in dermatology, including exanthemas, urticaria, photosensitivity, fixed-drug reactions, palpable purpura, bullae, alopecia, onycholysis, acral erythema, lichenoid and acneiform lesions, toxic epidermal necrolysis, and erythema multiforme syndrome. Drug eruptions may occur at any age, are more common in women, and are the most common form of drug sensitivity reactions.[1]

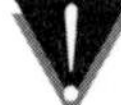

Immediate emergency department referral or physician consultation is indicated for anaphylaxis, severe erythema multiforme, or Stevens-Johnson syndrome.

PATHOPHYSIOLOGY

Drug eruptions are hypersensitivity manifestations of immunologic or nonimmunologic mechanisms stimulated by oral, topical, or parenteral drug administration.[2] Immunologic responses occur when specific antibodies or specifically sensitized lymphocytes to a drug develop during the sensitization period, which may be 4 or 5 days after initial exposure. Subsequent exposure to the drug results in a reaction that may occur within minutes, hours, or days.

Nonimmunologic responses, the most common, may be caused by accumulation of a drug, pharmacologic action of a drug, genetic factors, reaction of the drug with ultraviolet light, irritancy of topical solutions, and unknown factors.[2,3] Hypersensitivity reactions to antibacterial agents (mostly penicillin) and protease inhibitors (PIs) are examples of the latter, involving maculopapular rashes and urticaria.[2]

PIs may cause acute generalized exanthematous pustulosis (AGEP). AGEP manifests with onset of acute clinical symptoms, including fever higher than 38° C (100.4° F) and widespread exfoliative dermatitis following a pustular, morbilliform eruption that heals with discontinuation of the PI.[4]

CLINICAL PRESENTATION

Patients may come in for an office visit with a variety of skin reactions (itching, burning, pain), with or without rash[5] (Table 56-1). The most common is a confluent, maculopapular rash that may be pruritic (Color Plate 14). Knowledge about onset, progression of symptoms, fever, medication, and family history is essential. Onset can occur 7 to 10 days after starting the drug but may not occur until the course of medication is finished. The rash may last 1 to 2 weeks and then fades.[2] The rash may also be urticarial (always highly suspicious for drug reaction), or a fixed-drug reaction that occurs in the same area each time the drug is taken.[5]

TABLE 56-1 Skin Reactions

Dermatologic Types	Causative Agents	Manifestations
Exanthemas	Cillins, sulfonamides, barbiturates	Bright red scarlatiniform lesions, usually on trunk
Urticaria	Cillins, salicylates, erythromycin, carbamazepine	Typical, well-defined wheals on hands, feet, lips, generalized
Photosensitivity	Phenothiazines, tetracyclines, sulfonamides, artificial sweeteners	Dermatitis or gray-blue hyperpigmented areas on skin exposed to sun
Fixed-drug reactions	Phenolphthalein, tetracycline, sulfonamides	Dusky red or purple lesions that reappear in same area with repeated drug exposure
Purpura	Chlorothiazide, meprobamate, anticoagulants	Nonblanching purple lesions, usually generalized and on lower extremities
Bullae	Cillins, barbiturates, iodines, sulfonamides	Symmetric, erythematous, edematous, bullous lesions
Lichenoid lesions	Antimalarials, gold, thiazides, chlorpromazine	Angular papules that turn into scaly patches
Acneiform lesions	Corticosteroids, iodines, bromides, hydantoins	Acnelike but no comedones and with sudden onset
Toxic epidermal necrolysis	Barbiturates, hydantoins, cillins, sulfonamides	Areas of loosened, easily detached epidermis with a scalded appearance
Erythema multiforme	Cillins, barbiturates, sulfonamides	Vary from small vesicles or ulcers to widespread bullous lesions (Stevens-Johnson syndrome)

PHYSICAL EXAMINATION

Careful skin examination is indicated. The category of lesions and distribution should be noted. Further examination of the head, eyes, ears, nose, throat, and cardiopulmonary status may be necessary to exclude viral exanthema or anaphylaxis, a more severe, systemic reaction.

DIAGNOSTICS

No laboratory tests are available that can establish the diagnosis, although occasionally a CBC may reveal eosinophilia. Skin tests can evaluate sensitivity to penicillin. Diagnosis depends on a thorough drug history, including known allergies or hypersensitivities to all oral, topical, parenteral, over-the-counter, prescription, vitamin, and "natural" preparations and duration of symptoms.[6]

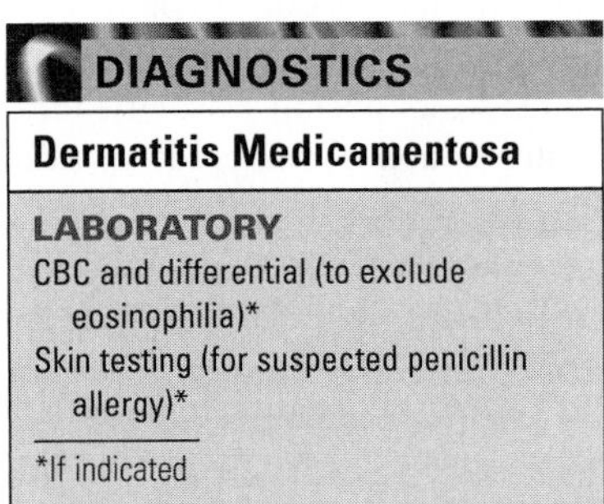
DIAGNOSTICS

Dermatitis Medicamentosa

LABORATORY

CBC and differential (to exclude eosinophilia)*

Skin testing (for suspected penicillin allergy)*

*If indicated

DIFFERENTIAL DIAGNOSIS

Other dermatologic processes must be excluded. These include urticaria, purpura, photosensitivity, bullous impetigo, contact or irritant dermatitis, acne vulgaris, rosacea, scarlet fever, staphylococcal infections, secondary syphilis, and viral rashes (e.g., herpes simplex mycoplasma).[6] Usually the sudden onset and symmetric nature of the eruptions (except in cases of topical administration of the offending product) establish the diagnosis as dermatitis medicamentosa. For example, urticaria-related drug reactions are seen as transient wheals in the skin caused by acute dermal edema. The more sudden and explosive the appearance of the urticaria, the more likely that a potent, life-threatening anaphylaxis may occur. Immediate discontinuation of the drug is imperative. Urticaria lesions are distinguished from erythema multiforme by the former's pruritic nature and will often "move" over 1 to 2 hours. Erythema multiforme lesions are not pruritic, are often painful, and may last 1 to 4 weeks.[6] Readministration of the pharmacologic preparation will confirm sensitivity; however, this may be life threatening, especially in immunologic responses.

DIFFERENTIAL DIAGNOSIS

Dermatitis Medicamentosa

- Urticaria
- Purpura
- Photosensitivity
- Impetigo
- Contact dermatitis
- Acne vulgaris
- Rosacea
- Scarlet fever
- Staphylococcal infection
- Syphilis
- Viral rashes

MANAGEMENT

Identification of the offending preparation and its removal will usually resolve the drug reaction, although the course of the reaction may progress for several days until the preparation is eliminated from the body.

Symptomatic treatment and hydration are advised. Cool compresses and tepid baths (e.g., Aveeno) may be soothing. For nonacute eruptions with dry, scaly, nonpruritic lesions, cooling lotions (e.g., Sarna Anti-Itch) may be applied.[2] Topical corticosteroid (group V[5]) ointment can be administered to a small area for more pruritic eruptions. If effective, the preparation may be applied to the entire eruption four times per day.[3] Oral antihistamines should also be administered to manage pruritus. For refractory cases oral corticosteroids may prove beneficial. For patients with severe reactions, including anaphylaxis, epinephrine 1:1000 (0.2 to 0.5 ml SQ) should be administered. Antihistamines should be used adjunctively.

COMPLICATIONS

Anaphylaxis is a potential life-threatening complication of reexposure to the offending preparation, especially in immunologic responses. Immunologic responses vary and may progress to Stevens-Johnson syndrome (epidermis peeling off in sheets), erythema multiforme (eruption of symmetric erythematous and edematous lesions of the skin or mucous membranes), myocarditis (inflammation of the myocardium), or other life-threatening conditions.

INDICATIONS FOR REFERRAL OR HOSPITALIZATION

Patients with erythema multiforme, Stevens-Johnson syndrome, or anaphylaxis require immediate referral. Any patient whose symptoms do not resolve in a timely manner should be referred for confirmation of the diagnosis and additional consultation.

CLINICAL INFORMATION RESOURCES

Online and other resources for drug interactions include PDR.net, MEDLINE (http://medline.cos.com), and Jerome Litt's Drug Eruption Global Database (http://www.drugeruptiondata.com).

PATIENT AND FAMILY EDUCATION AND HEALTH PROMOTION

Patients should be encouraged to wear medical alert bracelets or devices that list medication allergies. Home anaphylaxis or epinephrine kits should be prescribed, and both the patient and family should be instructed in their use. The patient's record should be flagged to alert other health care providers of the allergy, and all patients, including children, should be encouraged to tell providers about the allergy before any antibiotics or other medications are prescribed.

REFERENCES

1. Fitzpatrick T, Johnson R, Wolff K, and others: *Color atlas and synopsis of clinical dermatology,* ed 4, New York, 2001, McGraw-Hill.
2. Habif T, Campbell J, Quitadamo M, and others: *Skin disease: diagnosis and treatment,* St Louis, 2001, Mosby.
3. Beers MH, Porter RS, Jones TV: *The Merck manual,* ed 18, Rahway, NJ, 2006, Merck Research Laboratories.
4. Ward HA, Russo GG, Shrum J: Cutaneous manifestations of antiretroviral therapy, *J Am Acad Dermatol* 6:2, 2002.
5. Hebert AA, Ralston JP: Cutaneous reactions to anticonvulsant medications, *J Clin Psychiatry* 62(suppl 14):22-26, 2001.
6. Habif T: *Clinical dermatology: a color guide to diagnosis and therapy,* St Louis, 2004, Mosby.

CHAPTER 57

Dry Skin

Catherine E. Carter

DEFINITION AND EPIDEMIOLOGY

Dry skin is literally skin that lacks moisture or water. It is often characterized as rough or xerotic. Dry skin is common in dry climates and during the winter months. It is especially prevalent in older adults. Infants and children less than 2 years old have the same basic skin structure as adults; however, lack of maturity can make them more prone to the effects of drying. These effects lead to consequences in the vascular and nervous tissue within the skin layers. Teenage skin is susceptible to drying because of the hormonal changes of puberty. Teens are also susceptible because of application of chemical preparations such as makeup and cleansers. Older skin (over 60 years) is affected by the physiologic changes and the wear and tear of aging. Older skin is affected by hormone losses or decreases and the cumulative effect of years of sun exposure.

PATHOPHYSIOLOGY

Environments in which the humidity is below 30% cause dehydration of the stratum corneum layer of the skin. Cold air and heat in buildings, cars, and homes also contribute to skin dehydration, especially during the winter.

The stratum corneum of the epidermis is the primary protective layer of the skin. If this layer becomes too dry, the skin loses its ability to compensate and adequately protect the underlying structures from the outside elements. Moisture content of the skin contributes to its overall elasticity, tone, smoothness, and softness. Interruption of the epidermis can allow water to be lost, resulting in drying.

The stratum corneum layer is made up of lipids, water, proteins, and salts. The lipids come from sebaceous gland secretions in the form of sebum; the salts come from the sweat or apocrine glands. This lipid layer forms a natural emulsion of lipid and water. Depending on genetics and subject to age, climate, and time of year, this layer can be either more of oil in water emulsion or water in oil emulsion.[1] Hormones also play a role in this layer. Androgenic hormones tend to stimulate the layer, whereas estrogen, progesterone, and the corticosteroids tend to inhibit production of this layer.[1] Age also has a significant effect. Hormone production is relatively low during childhood, peaks during adolescence, decreases after age 35, and dramatically decreases after age 60. The decrease in sweat and sebum production from the glandular tissue leads to water loss through the skin. True deficiencies occur in old age because of structural and hormonal changes of the skin for which the body can no longer compensate.[1]

The thickness of the stratum corneum varies with location on the body. It averages 0.1 mm thick and is made up of flattened keratinocytes. These cells originate below the epidermal layer and migrate to the surface where they die and slough in the continual process of desquamation. The process of migration (from below the corneum) to the surface takes

28 days. The last 14 days are generally attributed to the process of protein (keratin) formulation as the cells change from living keratinocytes to a horny layer of dead cells.[1] The stratum corneum also contains by-products of keratin formation. These by-products contain substances that help bind water and assist in the natural moisturizing of the skin. These by-products consist of lactic acid, urea, urocanic acid, carbohydrates, and pyrrollidonecarboxylic acid.[1,2] The stratum corneum attempts to moisturize itself through the bodily process of perspiration. Drying that is sufficient to cause the stratum corneum to dry out and lose its ability to produce its own nonkeratin by-product substances causes the layer to lose its ability to bind water. Repeated exposure to solvents and soaps removes lipids from the skin. Natural skin oils are removed, and their protective nature is lost. Loss of water, lipids, or proteins alters the overall skin integrity and its ability to perform its protective functions.[1-4]

If the skin is working properly, the lipid layer and lower water barrier maintain the skin in a supple state. The lipid layer prevents water absorption by acting as a repellent. The lower water barrier prevents drying out and potential damage to lower skin structures in the dermis and subcutaneous layers.

CLINICAL PRESENTATION AND PHYSICAL EXAMINATION

Many individuals report having dry skin most of their lives, whereas others state that the problem developed with aging. Some report skin changes with the seasons or after an illness. In general, the dryness is initially seen as a rough patch that itches. Pruritus is worse on the lower extremities, which have less fat and muscle mass and less ability to replace the lipid layer elements. The hands and face are also common sites because of exposure to wind or air and hand washing. If moisture is not replaced, the skin becomes rough and occasionally loses its suppleness. It often becomes cracked and fissured.[5] Erythema craquele, an uneven diamond pattern with erythema at the edges, can develop (Color Plate 15).

DIAGNOSTICS AND DIFFERENTIAL DIAGNOSIS

Dry skin is a visual diagnosis. The differential diagnosis includes all other forms of dermatitis, including eczema, ichthyosis vulgaris, and scabies.[5,6] Secondary skin changes occurring as a result of scratching can complicate the appearance of the skin, making accurate diagnosis difficult.

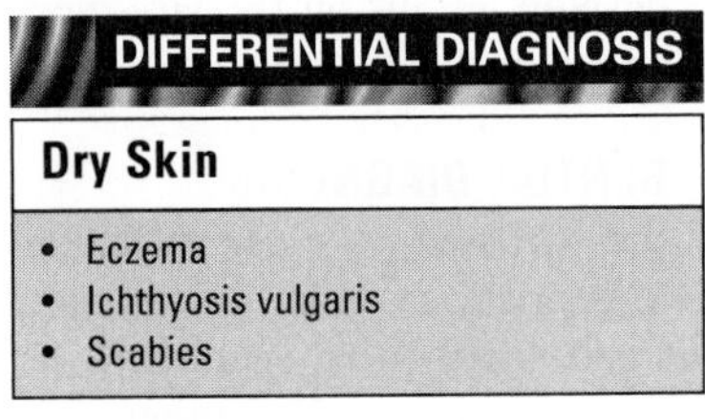
DIFFERENTIAL DIAGNOSIS

Dry Skin

- Eczema
- Ichthyosis vulgaris
- Scabies

MANAGEMENT

Xerotic skin is dry because of a lack of water. Treatment with lubricants and water-in-oil emulsions two or three times daily will restore moisture. Patients should be advised to take short baths with water that is not hot. For infants and even some older adults, bathing every other day and spot washing the axilla and groin can help minimize moisture loss. When toweling, the patient should pat the skin dry. Oils can be added to the skin immediately after toweling or just before rinsing. If applied before rinsing, the oil helps prevent the loss of moisture caused by rinsing and drying. If applied immediately after rinsing, the oils help prevent further loss of moisture and should be applied within 2 to 3 minutes of drying. Caution is advised; using oils can make the skin slippery. Infants can be at risk for being dropped, and all patients could be at risk for falls—a particular concern in older adults.

Antihistamines are often used to minimize scratching. Caution is advised, since the sedative effects of traditional antihistamines are potentially problematic. In older patients, interactions of the antihistamines with other medications or other disease entities are also a consideration (e.g., urinary retention secondary to benign prostatic hypertrophy may be exacerbated in older men). Creams and lotions containing the chemicals menthol and phenol can often help in the relief of pruritus and, based on the situation and severity, may be tried before systemic oral therapy. Treating dry skin early with moisturizers and emollients will help prevent secondary lesions resulting from scratching and irritation. Topical steroid creams can be applied to dry, itching skin. If moisturizers and emollients are used early enough, steroid creams may not be necessary. The steroid helps minimize the itch and secondary inflammation. The carrier cream, lotion, or ointment adds additional emollient to the skin to help retard further moisture loss. Steroid creams should be used with caution to prevent thinning of the skin. Patients are generally advised to use them for no more than a week and to use cautiously on the face, breasts, or genital areas. Good hygiene practices and attention to skin care are the mainstay in management and the prevention of dry skin.

COMPLICATIONS

Although complications are uncommon, they do occur. Infections and even cellulitis have occurred as a result of scratching. Scratching disrupts the epidermal barrier even further than drying. Penetration by exogenous toxins from surface staphylococcus, or in allergen-sensitive patients the introduction of allergic triggers, can exacerbate the dry skin and make it vulnerable to other dermatologic moieties. Other complications are generally secondary to treatment. Local reactions to perfumes in moisturizers can occur, as well as atrophy from long-term use of topical steroids.

INDICATIONS FOR REFERRAL OR HOSPITALIZATION

A dermatologic referral and hospitalization are not usually indicated. A referral to a dermatologist is warranted if the diagnosis is unclear.

PATIENT EDUCATION AND HEALTH PROMOTION

Patients with dry skin should understand the importance of keeping the room temperature comfortably low or as close to 20° C (68° F) as possible to help prevent the skin from drying. Humidifiers can help put moisture back in the air and are advisable for many patients. Patients who chronically use humidifiers require education on periodic cleaning with vinegar to minimize impurities. Bath water should be warm but not hot. Moisturizers should be applied just before rinsing or immediately after drying. Their use should include caution for slippage to prevent falls or injuries. Mild soaps or cleansers should be used sparingly. Low to medium potency topical corticosteroid ointments provides rapid relief for associated eczematous changes, but should be discontinued when symptoms have resolved. The patient should be cautioned against scratching; scratching leads to complications and exacerbates the skin irritation. Overall long-term management from year to year in appropriate patients can help prevent dry skin. The use of good skin care programs that can be modified seasonally can help control and prevent dry skin and its complications.

Travel increases during the winter and holiday months. Because air travel can significantly pull moisture from the air and lead to drying of the skin, patients should be instructed to keep well hydrated and use moisturizers as necessary. In addition, patients susceptible to dry skin should be cautioned to avoid extended use of high settings on car heaters, which can cause a loss of moisture from skin surfaces.

Patients should stay well hydrated. Soups and stews help replace water in the diet and are good sources of nutrients during the winter months. Older adults should be cautioned to limit their sodium consumption; however, the need for adequate hydration both externally and internally is important. Vitamins can be added to the daily regimen for patients who are not already taking a multivitamin or whose nutritional balance is of concern. This will help promote good skin integrity via overall nutritional health. It is important to encourage the basics: adequate nutrition, exercise, and rest. Medications added as needed will help prevent dry skin problems. Ideally emollients and moisturizers used at the slightest hint of skin drying should preclude the need for medication. Prevention of scratching is paramount to prevent further deterioration of the epidermal skin barrier through loss of moisture.

REFERENCES

1. Peters J: Caring for dry and damaged skin in the community, *Br J Commun Nurs* 6:12, 645-651, 2001.
2. Cork MJ: The importance of skin barrier function, *J Dermatol Treat* 8:S7-S13, 1997.
3. Bikowski J: The use of cleansers as therapeutic concomitants in various dermatologic disorders, *Cutis* 68:12-28, 2001.
4. Habif T: *Skin disease: diagnosis and treatment*, St Louis, 2001, Mosby.
5. Arndt K, Bowers KE, Alam M, and others: *Manual of dermatologic therapeutics*, ed 6, Philadelphia, 2001, Lippincott, Williams & Wilkins.
6. Weston WL, Lane AT, Morrelli JG: *Color textbook of pediatric dermatology*, ed 2, St Louis, 1996, Mosby.

CHAPTER 58

Eczematous Dermatitis (Atopic Dermatitis)

Eileen M. Deignan

DEFINITION AND EPIDEMIOLOGY

Eczematous dermatitis, or atopic dermatitis (AD), is a chronic disorder characterized by exacerbations and remissions of dry, itchy red skin. It is associated with an increased incidence of asthma, hay fever, or allergies. Patients with a tendency to develop these three conditions are called *atopics*. Many atopic patients also have a family history of atopy. From 30% to 80% of atopic patients experience eczematous flares throughout life.[1] AD is often called "the itch that rashes." Patients initially are bothered by itching, scratch an area, and then develop a rash at the site of scratching. Factors that aggravate AD include skin dryness, sweating, heat, and dry environments. Topical agents (e.g., harsh soaps and detergents) and wool also intensify AD. In addition, AD can be exacerbated by infections, stress, and allergies.

PATHOPHYSIOLOGY

Although the primary cause of AD remains unknown, patients with AD have elevated serum immunoglobulin E (IgE) levels and altered cell-mediated immunity. However, despite the correlation between elevated IgE levels and the severity of AD, not all patients with elevated IgE levels experience AD.[2]

CLINICAL PRESENTATION AND PHYSICAL EXAMINATION

AD is characterized by pruritic, erythematous, dry patches of skin, often with scale. Linear excoriations may be seen as a secondary change (Color Plate 16). The borders of eczematous lesions are not initially well defined. Crusting and oozing are common. Thickened skin with well-defined skin markings (lichenification) may develop in longstanding lesions as the result of scratching. In adults, eczema or AD may be generalized, with a tendency to develop lesions on the face, neck, flexural folds, wrists, and dorsa of the feet.

DIAGNOSTICS AND DIFFERENTIAL DIAGNOSIS

AD is a clinical diagnosis that is based on a careful history and examination. Seborrheic dermatitis can be differentiated from AD by its presentation and distribution. Seborrheic dermatitis typically manifests as nonpruritic, mildly erythematous plaques with waxy, yellow scale on the face, postauricular area, and scalp. Psoriasis is characterized by well-demarcated, intensely erythematous plaques with characteristic, overlying silvery scale. Areas of trauma such as the scalp, elbows, and knees are commonly involved.

Scabies typically is seen as a poorly defined pruritic eruption, often with linear burrows in the web spaces of the fingers. The breasts and genital areas are also often involved. The condition is commonly complicated by eczematous

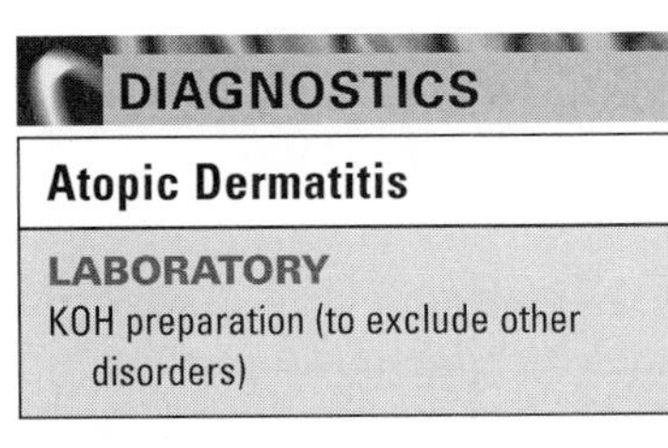

DIAGNOSTICS

Atopic Dermatitis

LABORATORY

KOH preparation (to exclude other disorders)

DIFFERENTIAL DIAGNOSIS

Atopic Dermatitis

- Seborrheic dermatitis
- Psoriasis
- Scabies
- Molluscum contagiosum
- Tinea

changes from scratching and rubbing. The diagnosis is confirmed by scraping a burrow and microscopically identifying mites, eggs, or fecal material in the scraped material.

Molluscum contagiosum lesions are small, dome-shaped papules with central umbilication. They are not easily confused with AD, but patients with molluscum often develop dermatitis in the area of molluscum lesions. In AD, dozens to hundreds of molluscum contagiosum lesions are some-times seen, usually around the eyes, axillae, and proximal extremities.[3]

Tinea (or superficial fungal infection) lesions have a sharply demarcated border with scale at the edge and central clearing. They are usually limited in number and sometimes form an arciform array. A scraping of the border of the lesion and treatment of the removed sample with potassium hydroxide (KOH) reveal hyphae on microscopic evaluation.

MANAGEMENT

Patient education is the cornerstone of AD treatment. The patient must learn to avoid rubbing and scratching the involved areas, since this only exacerbates the condition. With AD, it is said that "one scratch is too much and a thousand scratches is not enough." Therefore the goals of treatment are management of pruritus to prevent scratching and rubbing and skin hydration to prevent the primary disease.[4]

Antihistamines can control itching, allay anxiety, and induce sleep. Diphenhydramine and hydroxyzine are the drugs of choice, although nonsedating antihistamines may be preferred for daytime use.

Hydration through bathing in an oatmeal powder bath of tepid water can be soothing during an acute flare of AD. The bath should be immediately followed by the application of a bland emollient such as hydrated petrolatum.

Topical corticosteroid ointments are usually necessary to alleviate inflammation during an acute flare. These medications are applied to the erythematous areas two or three times per day. As the flare subsides, alternating the corticosteroids with lubricants will lessen the risks of prolonged steroid use.[2] Topical corticosteroids should be discontinued when the inflammation has subsided, whereas the use of lubricants and emollients should be continued.

The nonsteroidal calcineurin-inhibitor topical medications such as tacrolimus and pimecrolimus can be helpful for managing chronic AD. These medications are not indicated for patients under 2 weeks old. As with topical steroids, they should not be used chronically. They can be used both for eczema flares and intermittently for maintenance of conditions that are unresponsive to other therapies.[5]

People with AD should be aware of the drying effect of soaps. Mild soaps can be used to wash the body folds and genital area but should be avoided on other body parts.

Secondary bacterial infections should be treated with appropriate topical and systemic antibiotics. Systemic corticosteroids are seldom used in the treatment of AD and should be reserved for extreme cases that are not controlled with topical treatments. Phototherapy with narrow-band ultraviolet B light and photochemotherapy with psoralen plus ultraviolet A light may be helpful when standard therapies have failed.

COMPLICATIONS

Secondary bacterial infections are common from chronic excoriations. Group A β-hemolytic streptococci and staphylococci are the most common bacterial organisms. Bacterial secondary infection should be suspected, cultured for, and treated in patents with purulent or weepy lesions and in cases of AD that are slow to respond to standard therapies.

Patients with AD have a higher incidence of herpes simplex virus, molluscum contagiosum, and warts. These infections can be more frequent and widespread in patients with AD. Increases in cutaneous viral infections are related to defective cell-mediated immunity in the skin, as well as to the use of topical steroids and calcineurin inhibitors.

A particularly serious viral complication of AD is eczema herpeticum. A patient with this condition has an underlying skin disorder (usually AD) and develops a widespread eruption of vesicles and erosions when experiencing a primary herpes infection or herpes infection reactivation. A Giemsa-stained scraping of the base of a vesicle will reveal multinucleated giant cells. Eczema herpeticum should be treated with oral antiviral medications and supportive care.

INDICATIONS FOR REFERRAL OR HOSPITALIZATION

Failure to respond to topical treatments requires referral to a dermatologist or dermatology nurse practitioner for management. An eruption that is recalcitrant to treatment may resemble AD but actually be another disorder. For example, bullous pemphigoid and cutaneous T-cell lymphoma can sometimes resemble AD in their early stages.

In addition, evaluation and management by an allergist or allergy nurse practitioner may be needed for optimum care in a patient with known allergies or with suspicions for an allergic role in the disease.

Hospitalization may be required for intensive topical or systemic treatments. Hospitalization is also indicated for patients who are unresponsive to outpatient therapies.

PATIENT AND FAMILY EDUCATION

Patients should understand that AD has no cure. Weeks or months of control will be followed by sudden exacerbations. Patients should understand the proper use of antihistamines to control itching and the continuous use of lubricants and emollients to moisturize the skin. Patients require careful education on proper bathing and moisturizing and their role in decreasing the need for topical corticosteroids. Identification of aggravating factors such as stress, infections, weather change, dry skin, and contact sensitivity will aid in management.

REFERENCES

1. Arndt K: *Manual of dermatologic therapeutics,* ed 6, New York, 2001, Lippincott Williams & Wilkins.
2. Hanifin J: *Dermatologic therapy,* vol 1, Copenhagen, 1996, Munksgaard.
3. Weston WL, Lane AT, Morrelli JG: *Color textbook of pediatric dermatology,* ed 3, St Louis, 2002, Mosby.
4. Odom RB, James WD, Berger TG: *Andrew's diseases of the skin,* ed 9, Philadelphia, 2000, Saunders.
5. Simpson EL, Hanifin JM: Atopic dermatitis, *J Am Acad Dermatol* 53:115-128, 2005.

CHAPTER 59

Fungal Infections (Superficial)

Eileen M. Deignan

Superficial fungal infections are common problems. These fungal infections can cause a primary or secondary infection of the skin that may be difficult to accurately diagnose. Greater exposure to fungal pathogens is occurring in the healthy and fitness-minded population, in debilitated patients using systemic antibiotics, and in patients who are immunocompromised.

DERMATOPHYTE INFECTIONS

DEFINITION AND EPIDEMIOLOGY

A dermatophyte is a fungus that invades and proliferates within the nonviable keratinized tissues—the stratum corneum of the skin, hair, and nails. Three of the most common pathologic dermatophytes are *Trichophyton, Microsporum,* and *Epidermophyton* organisms. The infections produced by dermatophytes are known as tinea, dermatophytosis, or ringworm. The term *tinea* is derived from the Latin word for worm and was probably chosen because of the common presence of a migrating, circular pattern with the infection.[1]

PATHOPHYSIOLOGY

Fungal infections are usually transmitted through close contact with an infected person or animal. Indirect contact with fomites (infected towels, clothing) may also cause dermatophyte infections.

CLINICAL PRESENTATION AND PHYSICAL EXAMINATION

Tinea infections are transmitted by direct contact with organisms in the environment, animals, or other people. The infections are characterized and named according to their location. Tinea capitis (head/scalp) can be seen initially as patchy, scaly, nonscarring areas of hair loss (Color Plate 17). Depending on the infectious organism, the lesions may become inflamed, boggy, and pustular. Tinea corporis (body) appears on skin as erythematous plaques and papules in an annular or arciform pattern. Lesions often have slightly elevated borders with central clearing (Color Plate 18). Tinea cruris (jock itch) appears on the groin and upper inner thigh and extends to the gluteal folds as erythematous scaling patches with raised borders. The scrotum is often spared. Tinea pedis (athlete's foot) can occur as interdigital scaling, maceration, and fissuring (Color Plate 19). It can also appear as a mild erythematous scaling eruption that involves the sole and sides of the foot (moccasin distribution). Tinea manus (hand) is often a dry, diffuse, scaly eruption of the palms, with sharply marginated plaques on the dorsum of the hands. The feet are often also involved. Tinea unguium (nail), also called onychomycosis, most commonly manifests as the distal subungual type. The infection begins in the distal nail bed and spreads to infect the nail plate, causing the nail to appear thickened and yellowed, with subungual keratinous debris. Onychomycosis appears on lateral nail margins as a yellow discoloration. Increased nail thickness and distortion usually occur over time.

DIAGNOSTICS

The diagnosis of all fungal infections is based on clinical features and simple diagnostic procedures. The potassium hydroxide (KOH) microscopy preparation is a valuable, cost-effective tool that provides rapid confirmation of many types of fungal infections.[2] The key to a reliable KOH preparation includes properly obtaining an adequate specimen by scraping the active, leading border of a lesion. A no. 15 blade should be used to collect the scrapings on a glass slide. A 10% to 20% solution of KOH is placed directly on the collected scale, a coverslip is applied, the sample is gently heated, and a microscopic examination is performed. A negative KOH result does not always exclude dermatophyte infections. Fungal culture can be helpful to detect infection in the absence of a positive KOH result. Dermatophytes usually take a few weeks to grow in culture. Examination with long-wave ultraviolet light (Wood's lamp) is helpful for screening for tinea capitis caused by certain fungal species. *Trichophyton tonsurans*, the most common cause of tinea capitis in the United States, however, does not fluoresce.[3]

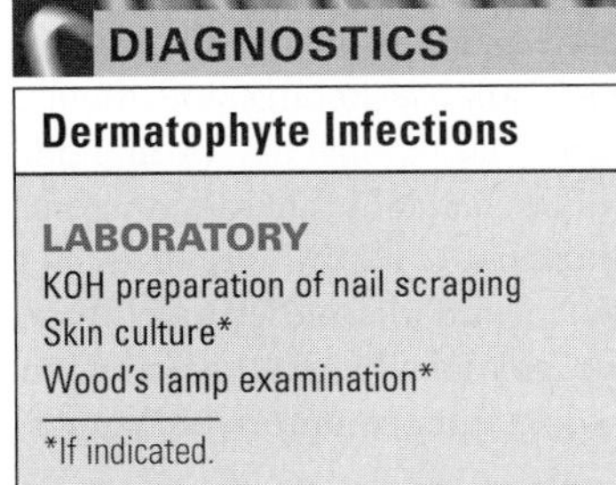

DIAGNOSTICS

Dermatophyte Infections

LABORATORY

KOH preparation of nail scraping
Skin culture*
Wood's lamp examination*

*If indicated.

DIFFERENTIAL DIAGNOSIS

See the Differential Diagnosis box.

DIFFERENTIAL DIAGNOSIS

Dermatophyte Infections

- Dermatitis
- Figurate erythemas
- Granulomatous dermatoses
- Papulosquamous eruptions
- Psoriasis
- Skin cancer
- Tinea
- Urticaria

MANAGEMENT

The treatment of tinea infections consists of removing the infecting organisms. Acute, exudative lesions are treated with drying agents such as aluminum sulfate (Domeboro) soaks. Topical antifungal solutions and creams reduce superficial scaling and organisms; keratolytic agents remove thick scales on the hands and feet, which allows topical antifungal agents to penetrate better. Several topical applications are available to treat tinea corporis: oxiconazole nitrate (Oxistat), clotrimazole (Lotrimin), econazole nitrate (Spectazole), ketoconazole (Nizoral), ciclopirox olamine (Loprox), or topical terbinafine hydrochloride (Lamisil) (Table 59-1). Treatment is usually continued 1 week past clearing to discourage recurrence; however, recurrence of tinea infections is common depending on the source.[4]

Systemic antifungal medications are used for widespread tinea or infections that involve the nails or scalp. A longstanding treatment for tinea capitis is griseofulvin for 2 to 4 months, or 2 weeks after negative KOH or culture results are obtained. Griseofulvin needs to be taken with high-fat food for complete absorption. Newer antifungal agents such as terbinafine and fluconazole (Diflucan) are effective with only 2 to 4 weeks of therapy.[5] The use of oral medications requires

TABLE 59-1 Examples of Cream Topical Treatment

Recommended Application to Affected Areas		Indicated For		
		Tinea (Pedis, Cruris, Corporis)	**Candidiasis**	**Tinea Versicolor**
Imidazoles				
Clotrimazole (Lotrimin)	Twice daily	X	X	X
Econazole (Spectazole)	Once daily for T and TV; twice daily for C	X	X	X
Miconazole (Monistat-Derm)	Twice daily for T and C; once daily for TV	X	X	X
Ketoconazole (Nizoral)	Once daily	X	X	X
Oxiconazole (Oxistat)	Once or twice daily	X		
Ciclopirox (Loprox)	Twice daily	X	X	X
Nystatin (Mycostatin)	Twice daily	X	X	
Terbinafine (Lamisil)	Twice daily	X		

GENERAL CONSIDERATIONS

Clinical improvement may be seen fairly soon after initiating treatment. Twice-daily applications, when indicated, should be done morning and evening. In general, all infections should be treated for 2 weeks to reduce the possibility of recurrence. Tinea pedis may require 6 weeks or more of treatment.

C, Candidiasis; *T*, tinea; *TV*, tinea versicolor.

careful dosing and monitoring for potential side effects. Treatment should not be considered complete until a follow-up negative fungal culture is obtained.[3]

Onychomycosis may be treated with oral terbinafine or with oral itraconazole (Sporanox). The oral dose of terbinafine is 250 mg daily—6 weeks for fingernail onychomycosis and 12 weeks for toenail involvement.[6-8] Terbinafine is not recommended for patients with a history of renal or liver dysfunction. Monitoring of liver function is required every 6 weeks or if the patient experiences nausea, anorexia, or fatigue during therapy. Neutropenia has been reported as a side effect of terbinafine therapy; therefore a CBC should be performed every 6 weeks or if there are symptoms suggestive of neutropenia.[8]

Varied dosing regimens are used with oral itraconazole. One regimen is 200 mg daily for 12 weeks for toenail involvement, and 200 mg twice daily for 1 week, then 3 weeks off, then 200 mg daily for 1 additional week for fingernail involvement.[8] The provider should monitor the patient for any suspicion of hepatic dysfunction. Itraconazole is metabolized by the cytochrome P450 3A4 (CYP3A4) system and affects the cytochrome P450 enzyme system; there are many drug interactions.[8] The provider should take a careful and complete drug history before initiating therapy.

Topical therapy for onychomycosis is relatively ineffective. Neither the oral nor the topical form of oral terbinafine or oral itraconazole is recommended for pregnant or nursing women. Unfortunately, the recurrence of onychomycosis is high, even with compliant therapy.

COMPLICATIONS

An uncommon complication of tinea capitis is the formation of a kerion, a boggy, exudative area on the scalp. It is a hypersensitivity reaction to the fungus. Kerion formations (tinea capitis) may result in permanent hair loss and scarring.[5] Fungal infections can also be complicated by bacterial superinfections. Other complications are associated with side effects and drug interactions with oral antifungal medications.

INDICATIONS FOR REFERRAL OR HOSPITALIZATION

Dermatophyte infections usually respond at least partially to treatment. Severe infections or infections that do not respond to treatment require a referral to a dermatologist. A referral to a dermatologist or dermatology nurse practitioner is recommended for treatment with oral antifungal medications.

PATIENT AND FAMILY EDUCATION

See the Patient and Family Education section under Candidiasis, p. 263.

CANDIDIASIS

PATHOPHYSIOLOGY

Candida albicans, a yeast, can normally be found on mucous membranes, in the gastrointestinal tract, in the vagina, and on the skin (Color Plate 20). *Candida* is usually an opportunistic organism. It is able to behave as a pathogen usually only in the presence of immunosuppression or in intertriginous areas. Predisposing factors to candidal infection include pregnancy; the use of birth control pills, antibiotics, or corticosteroids; malnutrition; diabetes and other endocrine diseases; or immunosuppressed conditions. A local environment that is warm, moist, macerated, or occluded favors the growth of this organism.

CLINICAL PRESENTATION AND PHYSICAL EXAMINATION

The clinical appearance of candidiasis depends on its location. Candidiasis of the mucous membranes is called *thrush*. Thrush appears as white or gray membranous plaques that are adherent to the buccal mucosa. If the plaques are scraped away, the base is macerated and brightly erythematous. The lesions can extend down the esophagus and to the lips and corners of the mouth. Perlèche, or angular cheilitis, is a fissuring and maceration of the corners of the mouth. The common causes of perlèche include candidal infection, bacterial infection, and irritant dermatitis.

Common sites of skin infection with *Candida* organisms are axillary, gluteal, perianal, and interdigital folds (see Color Plate 20). These intertriginous candidiasis lesions are usually pink or red moist patches bordered by a thin collarette of scale. They are sometimes surrounded by characteristic satellite pustules. Vaginal thrush causes intense itching and often a "cheesy" vaginal discharge. Candidal paronychia, or nail fold infection, is an inflammation of the nail fold. There is rounding and lifting of the nail fold, sometimes with a pus discharge. The nail can become thickened and discolored over time. Untreated severe candidiasis in any location has the potential to cause fungal septicemia in an immunocompromised patient.

DIAGNOSTICS

The diagnosis of candidiasis is based on clinical appearance, microscopic evaluation with a KOH preparation to look for budding yeast with or without hyphae, and/or a fungal culture. *C. albicans* grows readily on fungal media within 48 to 72 hours.

DIAGNOSTICS

Candidiasis
LABORATORY KOH preparation

DIFFERENTIAL DIAGNOSIS

The differential diagnosis depends on the affected area.

MANAGEMENT

The treatment of candidiasis is aimed at eliminating both the predisposing factors and the organism. A variety of agents—powders, vaginal douches, oral suspensions, creams, and tablets—are commonly used for the treatment of candidal infections (see Table 59-1). Superficial infections should usually be treated with topical therapy. If the infection is so widespread that the use of topical agents is impractical or too expensive, oral fluconazole or oral ketoconazole is appropriate.

COMPLICATIONS

The most serious complication of candidiasis is fungal septicemia, which may be seen in immunocompromised patients. Candidal esophagitis is a potential complication of antibiotic

DIFFERENTIAL DIAGNOSIS

Candidiasis

ORAL PHARYNX
- Aphthous ulcers, geographic tongue
- Leukoplakia

INTERTRIGINOUS AREAS
- Miliaria
- Bacterial infection

FEMALE GENITALS
- Bacterial vaginosis
- Trichomoniasis
- Allergic contact dermatitis
- Pediculosis pubis

MALE GENITALS
- Bacterial infection
- Psoriasis
- Tinea

NAILS
- Bacterial infection
- Tinea

From Dunn SA: *Mosby's primary care consultant,* St Louis, 1998, Mosby.

therapy or may be noted in patients who are severely immunocompromised, particularly patients with AIDS.

INDICATIONS FOR REFERRAL OR HOSPITALIZATION

Treatment is usually effective and a referral is not indicated. The differential diagnosis of candidal infection is large, however. Therefore infections recalcitrant to treatment require a physician or dermatologist referral to look for other causes for the eruption. Patients with yeast septicemia or other systemic manifestations or infection also require a physician consultation.

PATIENT AND FAMILY EDUCATION

Methods for reducing environmental factors that encourage heat, moisture, maceration, and trauma should be emphasized: drying thoroughly after bathing (especially in the axillae and toe webs and between and under the breasts), wearing absorbent materials such as cotton underwear and socks, changing socks frequently and avoiding constrictive clothing, not wearing the same shoes each day, and wearing sandals in warm weather.

During active infections or in the hope of preventing recurrence, a simple talc powder or antifungal powder (tolnaftate or miconazole [Zeasorb-AF]) should be applied to intertriginous or interdigital areas twice daily. With the reintroduction of many powders that contain cornstarch, it is extremely important to inform patients who are prone to fungal infections to avoid cornstarch-containing products because this substance encourages fungus growth.

Patients using oral steroid inhalers should understand the importance of rinsing the oral cavity after using these inhalers. Although there is no clearly documented benefit, some providers recommend that their patients eat yogurt daily while on antibiotic therapy to help prevent vaginal or oral yeast infections.

TINEA VERSICOLOR

DEFINITION AND EPIDEMIOLOGY

Tinea versicolor is a chronic, asymptomatic, and superficial fungal infection. This skin manifestation is common in young adults.

PATHOPHYSIOLOGY

The causative organism of tinea versicolor is *Malassezia furfur. Pityrosporum orbiculare* is the yeast form of the organism. The fungus is found on normal skin, and the infection is due to a change in the host's resistance to this organism. Tinea versicolor causes lesions in some individuals during periods of high heat and humidity. Thus the condition is more prevalent during the summer and in hot, humid regions. Exposure to sunlight often initiates an episode.

CLINICAL PRESENTATION AND PHYSICAL EXAMINATION

Lesions vary in color and are either white or light pink in the hypopigmented version, or tan or brown in the hyperpigmented version. They are slightly scaly and are round or oval coalescing papules and plaques. The usual sites for these lesions are the sternal region; the sides of the chest, abdomen, or back; the pubis; and the intertriginous areas. Hypopigmented lesions are more noticeable in darkly pigmented skin. Patients should be reassured that repigmentation will occur after treatment and with exposure to natural sunlight. However, this process can take several months.

DIAGNOSTICS

Diagnosis is by KOH examination, which reveals numerous short, straight hyphae and clusters of round, budding yeast; this configuration is commonly referred to as "spaghetti and meatballs." A KOH examination may be falsely negative if the patient has just showered.

DIAGNOSTICS

Tinea Versicolor

LABORATORY
KOH preparation

DIFFERENTIAL DIAGNOSIS

Vitiligo, pityriasis alba, pityriasis rosea, and small plaque parapsoriasis should be considered in the differential diagnosis. Lesions may resemble seborrheic dermatitis, but tinea versicolor most commonly affects the trunk, neck, and upper extremities, whereas seborrheic dermatitis affects hairy body areas. Although uncommon, secondary syphilis should be considered in the differential diagnosis.

DIFFERENTIAL DIAGNOSIS

Tinea Versicolor

- Pityriasis alba
- Pityriasis rosea
- Vitiligo
- Seborrheic dermatitis
- Secondary syphilis

MANAGEMENT

Common antifungal creams, such as the imidazoles, are useful in treating tinea versicolor (see Table 59-1). Medication is applied to the entire torso during active infections to eliminate inapparent lesions. Oral antifungal agents can also be used. Topical shampoos or suspensions containing selenium sulfide or pyrithione zinc are also effective in treatment or prophylaxis. Shampoos are applied to affected areas, allowed to dry, and rinsed away after remaining in place approximately 10 minutes. This treatment is repeated for 7 to 14 consecutive days during active infections, followed by periodic use of these shampoos or soaps if the patient is prone to frequent infections. Specific instructions should be reviewed with every product or drug.

COMPLICATIONS

Complications are unusual although drug-drug interactions are possible especially with the systemic antifungal medications.[9] Careful review of the patient's current medications is essential, particularly if fluconazole will be prescribed.[9] Some patients may develop *Pityrosporum* folliculitis, although this disorder usually resolves with topical therapy.

INDICATIONS FOR REFERRAL OR HOSPITALIZATION

A referral is not usually necessary. Rashes recalcitrant to treatment require a dermatology referral to reconsider the diagnosis.

PATIENT AND FAMILY EDUCATION

Patients should understand that tinea versicolor commonly recurs but is not a serious disorder. The regular use of any selenium sulfide shampoo for 10 minutes each day for a week followed by consistent weekly treatments will often prevent recurrences.

REFERENCES

1. Nicol NH, Huether SE: Alteration on the integument in children. In McCance J, Huether SE, editors: *Pathophysiology: the biologic basics for disease in adults and children*, ed 3, St Louis, 1998, Mosby.
2. Nicol NH, Black JM: Assessment of clients with integumentary disorders. In Black JM, Matassarin-Jacobs E, editors: *Medical-surgical nursing: clinical management for continuity of care*, ed 5, Philadelphia, 1997, Saunders.
3. Bradley BJ, Beck J, Mercurio MG, and others: Tinea capitis today: what nurses need to know about identifying and managing fungal infections of the scalp in the school setting, *J Sch Nurs* (suppl):1-16, 1996.
4. Rand S: Overview: the treatment of dermatophytosis, *J Am Acad Dermatol* 43(suppl 2):104-112, 2000.
5. Odom RB, James WD, Berger TG: *Andrews' diseases of the skin: clinical terminology*, ed 9, Philadelphia, 2000, Saunders.
6. Nicol NH, Black JM: Nursing care of clients with integumentary disorders. In Black JM, Matassarin-Jacobs E, editors: *Medical-surgical nursing: clinical management for continuity of care*, ed 5, Philadelphia, 1997, Saunders.
7. Elewski B, Weil M: Dermatophytes and superficial fungi. In Sams WM, Lynch P, editors: *Principles and practices of dermatologic therapy*, ed 2, New York, 1996, Churchill Livingstone.
8. *Nurse practitioner's prescribing reference*, New York, 2006, Prescribing Reference.
9. Yu DT, Peterson JF, Seger DL, and others. Frequency of potential azole drug-drug interactions and consequences of potential fluconazole drug interactions, *Pharmacoepidemiol Drug Saf* 14(11):755-767, 2005.

CHAPTER 60

Herpes Zoster (Shingles)

Eileen M. Deignan

DEFINITION AND EPIDEMIOLOGY

Herpes zoster (shingles) is caused by the varicella zoster virus, the same virus that causes chickenpox. After primary varicella infection (chickenpox) or vaccination, the virus lies dormant in the sensory root ganglion cells. The zoster eruption results from reactivation of the latent varicella infection in the dorsal root or cranial nerve ganglion cells.[1] The cause of reactivation is not known, but zoster is more common in older adults and immunosuppressed persons. Lesions appear over several days and last up to 7 weeks. The eruption can be painful and can result in significant residual pain, which is called *postherpetic neuralgia*.

Although zoster is self-limiting and common in adults, in some circumstances consultation is recommended.

Ophthalmologic consultation is indicated for ocular involvement. Physician consultation is recommended for lesions that involve multiple dermatomes or for cheek or nose involvement.

PATHOPHYSIOLOGY

After initial varicella infection, the virus lies dormant in the dorsal root ganglia. The causes of reactivation are not clear but may result from stress, trauma, reexposure to varicella, radiation therapy, or immunosuppressive therapy. Once reactivated, the virus replicates and travels down the sensory nerve into the skin.[2]

CLINICAL PRESENTATION AND PHYSICAL EXAMINATION

Zoster classically is seen as a unilateral eruption within one or a few dermatomes. It is common to have some lesions in the dermatome above and below the one primarily affected. The eruption is often preceded by pain in the affected dermatome. Because there is no accompanying eruption, the pain is sometimes mistaken for angina, renal colic, sciatica, or pleural pain. The eruption initially consists of erythematous papules and then, over the course of hours, develops into vesicles (Color Plate 21). New lesions may continue to develop over the course of several days. Healing time varies, ranging from 1 to 7 weeks. Low-grade fever and lymphadenopathy may be present. The most common areas of involvement are the thoracic, cranial (especially the trigeminal), and lumbar nerves.[3]

DIAGNOSTICS

Diagnosis is based on the clinical presentation of an eruption in a unilateral, dermatomal distribution. Patients may develop several lesions outside the primarily affected dermatome. Disseminated herpes zoster is a generalized eruption of lesions along with the typical segmental distribution.

A Tzanck test is a rapid way to confirm the diagnosis of zoster in the provider's office. Direct fluorescent antibody test is another rapid test that is available at some hospitals. Both

DIAGNOSTICS

Herpes Zoster

LABORATORY
Tzanck test (of lesion discharge)*
Antibody titer*
Direct fluorescent antibody test

*If indicated.

tests are preferred over a viral culture because they are more rapid and often more sensitive.

DIFFERENTIAL DIAGNOSIS

The pain associated with zoster can precede the eruption by 4 or 5 days. Depending on the distribution, the pain may mimic angina, renal colic, or pleuritic pain. Once the eruption is present, the cause of the pain is more obvious. Varicella is seldom confused with zoster because of the distribution of lesions. Herpes simplex infection can sometimes mimic zoster. A direct fluorescent antibody test or viral culture will differentiate the two. Coxsackievirus (hand-foot-and-mouth disease) is generally limited to the acral areas. Early vesicular eruptions of zoster can sometimes mimic contact dermatitis. The dermatomal distribution of zoster helps differentiate the two.

DIFFERENTIAL DIAGNOSIS

Herpes Zoster

- Varicella
- Hand-foot-and-mouth disease
- Rickettsialpox
- Dermatitis herpetiformis
- Contact dermatitis

MANAGEMENT

The treatment of uncomplicated herpes zoster is symptomatic treatment of lesions and prevention of secondary infection. Analgesic agents may be administered if necessary. Topical moist compresses and agents, such as calamine and aluminum sulfate (Domeboro) soaks, are soothing and will help dry vesicles. Antiviral therapy is an important part of zoster therapy. When started within the first few days of the eruption, it reduces zoster-associated pain. Antiviral treatment also is associated with faster healing of lesions. Acyclovir is effective in both localized and disseminated herpes zoster. If treatment with oral antiviral agents is started within 48 hours of onset, it can shorten the course and may reduce postherpetic neuralgia.

Acyclovir is dosed at 800 mg five times daily for 7 to 10 days. The newer antiviral agents valacyclovir and famciclovir are at least as effective as acyclovir, and perhaps more so because they achieve higher blood levels of medication. They are more expensive, but require less frequent medication dosing. They should be used with caution in patients with renal impairment. The use of antihistamines is helpful to reduce pruritus.[1,2]

COMPLICATIONS

Postherpetic neuralgia is the most common complication of zoster. Older adults tend to have more persistent pain after the zoster lesions have healed.[4] Postherpetic neuralgia is often difficult to control; some patients benefit from ibuprofen therapy. Other therapies include topical lidocaine preparations and topical capsaicin and oral gabapentin.[5]

Herpes zoster on the tip of the nose, around the eyes, and on the forehead requires immediate ophthalmologic examination. These findings signal possible involvement of the branch of the trigeminal nerve that innervates the cornea, which may cause ulceration on the cornea and result in permanent damage. Motor paralysis and facial palsy (Ramsay Hunt syndrome) may follow herpes zoster. Immunosuppressed individuals may develop dissemination, pneumonia, hepatitis, meningoencephalitis, and purpura fulminans.[1,2,6]

LIFE SPAN CONSIDERATIONS

Older adults are at risk for significant acute zoster-associated pain. Therefore older adults may benefit from concurrent antiviral and systemic corticosteroid treatment during the acute infection. In older adults, outbreaks of herpes zoster can occur in conjunction with other systemic illnesses.

INDICATIONS FOR REFERRAL OR HOSPITALIZATION

In ophthalmic zoster, ocular complications occur in approximately 50% of cases. Immediate referral to an ophthalmologist is indicated. Patients with generalized, disseminated zoster should be evaluated for malignancy, immunodeficiency, or AIDS.[2] Hospitalization is often necessary in patients with disseminated herpes zoster.

PATIENT AND FAMILY EDUCATION

Lesions of herpes zoster may contain varicella zoster virus, enabling transmission to susceptible individuals (including women of childbearing age who have not had the varicella vaccine or previous varicella infection). Herpes zoster itself is not transmissible, although care should be taken to avoid exposure to susceptible or immunosuppressed contacts; therefore patients with herpes zoster may continue to work and attend school.

Care should be taken to educate patients about the time course of zoster lesions and associated pain. They should also be given instructions about topical lesion care and pain relief.

There is now a vaccine available to decrease the morbidity and mortality associated with herpes zoster.[7] The herpes zoster vaccine (Zostavax) is a live vaccine that was shown to decrease the incidence of herpes zoster in persons older than 60 years. Now available, this vaccine can be considered as preventive therapy for appropriate patient populations.

REFERENCES

1. Arndt K: *Manual of dermatologic therapeutics,* ed 6, New York, 2001, Lippincott Williams & Wilkins.
2. Paller AS, Mancini AJ: *Hurwitz clinical pediatric dermatology,* ed 3, Philadelphia, 2005, Saunders.
3. Gilden DH, Kleinschmidt-DeMasters BK, LaGuardia JJ, and others: Neurologic complications of the reactivation of varicella-zoster virus, *N Engl J Med* 342:635, 2000.
4. Dershewitz RA: *Ambulatory pediatric care,* ed 3, New York, 1998, Lippincott Williams & Wilkins.
5. Gnann JW, Whitley RJ: Herpes zoster, *N Engl J Med* 347:340, 2002.
6. Odom RB, James WD, Berger TG: *Andrew's diseases of the skin,* ed 9, Philadelphia, 2000, Saunders.
7. Oxman MN, Levin MJ, Johnson GR, and others: A vaccine to prevent herpes zoster and post-herpetic neuralgia in older adults, *N Engl J Med* 352(22):2271-2284, 2005.

CHAPTER 61

Hidradenitis Suppurativa (Acne Inversa)

Margaret McAllister

DEFINITION AND EPIDEMIOLOGY

Hidradenitis suppurativa, now also referred to as acne inversa or cicatrizing perifolliculitis, has long been considered a disease of the apocrine glands. Histopathologic research indicates that the primary lesion is infundibulofolliculitis with secondary infection of the apocrine glands.[1,2] The presence of CD4 and CD8 lymphocytes indicates a cell-mediated cause for this disorder.[3] The disease is characterized by abscesses, draining sinus tracts, and comedones and may be found in association with severe nodulocystic acne and pilonidal sinuses.[4] The prevalence of hidradenitis is greater in females, with genitofemoral lesions being most common; axillary lesions are found equally in males and females, and anogenital lesions are found more commonly in males.[5,6] Case studies indicate that the onset of hydradenitis is associated with the production of adrenal androgens, dehydroepiandrosterone, and androstenedione at the time of adrenarche.[7] All ethnic groups are affected. A hereditary predisposition has been noted in females, with a mother-daughter transmission being most common,[5] and a familial autosomal dominant tendency exists.[1]

PATHOPHYSIOLOGY

The exact cause of hidradenitis is not known and is controversial. Theories of causation include keratin plugging of the apocrine ducts or a primary failure of the apocrine glands to drain effectively. An association with immunosuppression is cited in the literature.[2,4] With keratin plugging, the apocrine duct and hair follicle are occluded by keratin, which causes increased ductal pressure and inflammation. Bacteria cause the ducts to rupture and, with extension of infection, lead to cyst, sinus tract, and fistula formation. *Acne inversa* is proposed as a more appropriate name for this disease.[2] In a study of 41 patients with active hidradenitis suppurativa, bacteria isolated in 49% (20 of 41) of abscess lesions included *Staphylococcus aureus, Staphylococcus epidermidis,* and *Staphylococcus hominis.*[8] Other organisms implicated include *Escherichia coli, Proteus mirabilis, Pseudomonas aeruginosa,* and gram-negative organisms.[4-6]

CLINICAL PRESENTATION

The hallmarks of hidradenitis suppurativa are single or multiple areas of swelling, pain, and erythema accompanied by acute abscess formation. The active phase of the disease is preceded by the appearance of double or triple black comedones on the affected skin surface (Color Plate 43). The condition often progresses to a chronic state of pain, sepsis, sinus tract and fistula formation, purulent discharge, and keloids. Disfiguring scar formation marks longstanding hidradenitis. Patients usually give a history of multiple episodes of repeat abscesses that have been drained and treated with antibiotic medications over a period of years. Unlike acne, the disease is unrelenting and often progressive, leaving hypertrophic scars that form a basket-weave configuration accented by marked erythema beneath the breast and in the axillary, suprapubic, groin, and anogenital regions. Sinus tracts form under the skin in which connecting, inflamed, and plugged glands drain into each other and trap bacteria. Patients are concerned about the cause of the problem and may fear they have a malignant disease. Predisposing factors include obesity, a history of acne, and obstruction of the apocrine ducts.[5] Remissions of a spontaneous nature are noted in patients older than 35 years of age.[5]

PHYSICAL EXAMINATION

The lesions are palpated to determine their readiness for incision and drainage. The axillae, groin, perianal region, buttocks, chest, inframammary area, and back are examined to determine the involvement and extent of the disease.

DIAGNOSTICS

DIAGNOSTICS

Hidradenitis Suppurativa

LABORATORY
Culture and sensitivity of lesions with discharge

OTHER
Skin biopsy

The initial diagnosis is based on clinical observation. Lesions that are actively discharging are cultured, and sensitivity tests are performed. A skin biopsy is performed for patients with stubborn cases or suspicious lesions. Laboratory tests may be needed to exclude other, more serious underlying diseases.

DIFFERENTIAL DIAGNOSIS

DIFFERENTIAL DIAGNOSIS

Hidradenitis Suppurativa

- Bacterial folliculitis
- Bacterial furunculosis
- Scrofuloderma
- Granuloma inguinale
- Lymphogranuloma venereum
- Squamous cell carcinoma

The differential diagnosis for hidradenitis suppurativa includes bacterial folliculitis, furunculosis, scrofuloderma, granuloma inguinale, lymphogranuloma venereum, squamous cell carcinoma, sinus tracts, and fistulas associated with ulcerative colitis.[5,9-11]

MANAGEMENT

There are a variety of treatment measures, including the following topical, oral, and surgical interventions. A combination approach to treatment is advocated, including steroids, antibiotics, traditional surgery, carbon dioxide (CO_2) laser surgery, monoclonal antibody therapy, and isotretinoin.

Fluctuant abscesses in which the skin has become thin and the underlying mass is soft can be surgically incised and drained in the health care provider's office. A local anesthetic with 1% to 2% lidocaine with or without epinephrine is provided through a 30-gauge needle and a 1- to 3-ml syringe.

The sting of lidocaine can be buffered by preparing a mixture of 1 ml of sodium bicarbonate with 9 ml of lidocaine. A pointed, lance-shaped no. 11 surgical blade is recommended for incision. The blade is inserted parallel to the skin lines, cutting across the thin area of skin and creating an opening through which purulent material can drain. Pressure is applied to the surrounding tissue to facilitate drainage. A curette drawn back and forth through the abscess will loosen adhesions and aid in the removal of necrotic material. A semiocclusive sterile dressing with a thin film of topical bacitracin should then be applied. Care must be taken to cleanse the area daily with soap and water; the dressing is reapplied for 3 to 5 days.

Smaller nodules can be injected with triamcinolone acetonide 3 to 5 mg/ml diluted with lidocaine, followed by a course of oral antibiotics. Larger cysts can be injected with triamcinolone 3 to 5 mg/ml, directly into the wall of the lesion, and later incised. Low-grade inflammation is responsive to oral antibiotics, but long-term treatment is necessary before clinical remission is evident. Erythromycin 250 to 500 mg q.i.d., tetracycline 250 to 500 mg q.i.d., or minocycline 100 mg b.i.d. should be considered. Erythromycin 500 mg q.i.d. may be effective in a large adult during periods of active inflammation.[4] Topical isotretinoin cream 0.05% may be efficacious in relieving keratin plugging of the apocrine glands.[4] Isotretinoin 1 mg/kg/day for 20 weeks may be tried under co-management with a physician in the early stages of the disease or as an adjunct to surgical intervention.[4,5] Because of the teratogenic effects of this medication, all women must be screened for pregnancy before taking isotretinoin and protected against pregnancy while taking the medication. For severe pain and inflammation, a tapering dose of 70 mg of prednisone for 2 or 3 days and tapered over a 14-day period is prescribed.

Co-Management with Specialists

A referral to a dermatologist is recommended for patients with hidradenitis that is recalcitrant to traditional oral therapy or for patients with recurrent lesions following incision and drainage. Newer treatment approaches used by these specialists include CO_2 laser treatment and infliximab (Remicade), a chimeric, monoclonal antibody with high affinity for tumor necrosis factor α. Antiinflammatory drugs such as Aleve or Celebrex have also improved the condition.[12,13] Patients treated with oral isotretinoin 1 mg/kg/day for 20 weeks may be co-managed with a nurse practitioner or physician assistant for the purposes of determining treatment response and monitoring side effects (see Chapter 48 for precautions regarding isotretinoin therapy).

LIFE SPAN CONSIDERATIONS

Onset of hidradenitis suppurativa is usually between the second and fifth decades, with onset as early as puberty in some individuals.[9] Many cases of hidradenitis disappear after patients reach 35 years of age.

COMPLICATIONS

The health care provider should be aware of the impact of body image changes on patients with this disease, especially young adolescents. As with any chronic illness, an assessment for clinical depression and threats to self-esteem should be included as part of the ongoing care. Complications other than chronicity are rare, but fistulas from the groin area to the urethra and bladder have been reported.[5] Cases of reactive arthritis have been identified in the literature.[14] Vigilant follow-up monitoring is necessary to uncover those patients who fail to respond to treatment. Cases of anogenital squamous cell carcinoma have been diagnosed in patients with long-term hidradenitis.[10,11] Other complications are related to the treatment regimen. Patients taking large doses of erythromycin may experience damage to their auditory nerve and deafness.

INDICATIONS FOR REFERRAL OR HOSPITALIZATION

Surgical excision is recommended for patients with chronic, recurrent hidradenitis suppurativa that involves the sinus tracts and fibrotic scarring. Complete excision of the involved glands and skin grafting may be necessary. CO_2 laser treatments can be performed by a qualified dermatologist skilled in this technique. If surgery requires extensive surgical resection and reconstruction of the female genitals, the services of a gynecologic oncologist may be required.[6]

PATIENT EDUCATION

Patient education should explain that a clear cause for the disease is not known. Hypothetical causes of the disease process should be discussed. The average length of time for abscesses to heal is 6.9 days. Patients should be reassured that antiperspirants, shaving, other underarm deodorants, or depilatories are not implicated as a cause. Topical isotretinoin may cause skin irritation, and caution should be exercised to avoid excessive use. The provider should stress sun sensitivity with the use of isotretinoin and encourage patients to wear appropriate protective clothing while in the sun. Patients should be educated on the side effects of the prescribed antibiotics, including photosensitivity. Patients taking erythromycin must be advised to avoid concurrent ingestion of terfenadine, astemizole, and ketoconazole.

REFERENCES

1. Jansen I, Altmeyer P, Piewig GJ: Acne inversa (alias hidradenitis suppurativa), *Eur Acad Dermatol Venereol* 5(6):532-402, 2001.
2. Boer J, Weltevreden EF: Hidradenitis suppurativa or acne inversa: a clinicopathological study of early lesions, *Br J Dermatol* 135(5):721-725, 1996.
3. Boer J, Weltevreden EF: Hidradenitis suppurativa or acne inversa? A clinicopathological study of early lesions, *Br J Dermatol* 135(5):721-725, 1996.
4. Habif TP: *Clinical dermatology*, ed 4, St Louis, 2004, Mosby.
5. Wolff K, Johnson RA, Suurmond R: *Fitzpatrick's color atlas and synopsis of clinical dermatology*, ed 5, New York, 2005, McGraw-Hill.
6. Goldberg JM, Buchler DA, Dibbell DG: Advanced hidradenitis suppurativa presenting with bilateral vulvar masses, *Gynecol Oncol* 60(3):494-497, 1996.
7. Palmer RA, Keefe M: Early-onset hidradenitis suppurativa, *Clin Exp Dermatol* 26(6):501-503, 2001.
8. Jemec GB, Faber M, Gutschik E, and others: The bacteriology of hidradenitis suppurativa, *Dermatology* 193(3):203-206, 1996.
9. Barker R, Burton JR, Zieve PD: *Ambulatory care medicine*, ed 5, Baltimore, 1998, Williams & Wilkins.

10. Li M, Hunt MJ, Commens CA: Hidradenitis suppurativa, Dowling Degos disease and perianal squamous cell carcinoma, *Australas J Dermatol* 38(4):209-211, 1997.
11. Gur E, Neligan PC, Shafir R, and others: Squamous cell carcinoma in perineal inflammatory disease, *Ann Plast Surg* 38(6):653-657, 1997.
12. Sullivan TP, Welsh E, Kerdel FA, and others: Infliximab for hidradenitis suppurativa, *Br J Dermatol* 149(5):1046-1049, 2003.
13. Lapins J, Marcusson JA, Emtestam L: Surgical treatment of chronic hidradenitis suppurativa: CO_2 laser stripping–secondary intention technique, *Br J Dermatol* 131(4):551-556, 1994.
14. Bhalla R, Sequeira W: Arthritis associated with hidradenitis suppurativa, *Ann Rheum Dis* 53(1):64-66, 1994.

CHAPTER 62

Hyperhidrosis

Margaret McAllister

DEFINITION AND EPIDEMIOLOGY

Hyperhidrosis is a condition of excessive sweating marked by abnormal wetness, sweaty palms, excessive axillary sweating, gustatory-stimulated sweating, wet shoes, and offensive body odor. Most cases are idiopathic or primary in nature and only rarely indicate underlying secondary pathologic condition.[1-4]

PATHOPHYSIOLOGY

Perspiration is one of the body's mechanisms for thermal regulation and fluid and electrolyte balance. The center for body temperature regulation is located in the hypothalamus. Cooling perspiration is under hypothalamic control, whereas emotional perspiration is under cerebral control.[2,5] Sweat glands are located in the hypodermis of the skin. The eccrine duct opens directly onto the surface of the skin. Millions of sweat glands are located in the hypodermis throughout the body, with the largest concentration in the palms, soles, and axillae. Secretions from the eccrine glands function to cool the body. Neural control is anatomically sympathetic. However, sweating is subject to cholinergic control mediated by acetylcholine, not epinephrine.[2] Overactivity of the thoracic sympathetic ganglion may be the underlying cause for non–medically related excessive sweating.

The most common cause of generalized increased sweating is a decline in ovarian function. Changes in neurohumoral function lead to increased stimulation of the hypothalamic thermal regulatory center, leading to the hot flashes associated with menopause. Other factors include fever; underlying infection or malignancy; peripheral neuropathy or surgical damage to the autonomic nervous system; thyrotoxicosis; Parkinson's disease; and a variety of medications, including insulin, meperidine, pilocarpine, and alcohol abuse.[2]

CLINICAL PRESENTATION

The presentation of primary hyperhidrosis is excessive sweating unrelated to ambient heat or humidity. Areas most commonly affected include the palms, soles, and axillae, but the condition may involve any body surface or take on a unilateral distribution. Concern over the social consequences of this disorder (and its resulting body odor) and embarrassment may create a barrier to intimate relationships or affect the patient's choice of occupation. When the soles are involved, widespread fungal infections of the skin and nails are accompanied by foot odor. More generalized body sweating is associated with an underlying condition, whereas localized sweating confined to the palms, soles, and axillae is more often a response to anxiety or heat or is idiopathic. Episodic sweating may be associated with hypoglycemia. A history of medications, including oral hypoglycemic agents and selective serotonin reuptake inhibitors (SSRIs), and alcohol intake is an important consideration.

PHYSICAL EXAMINATION

Based on the history and presenting complaint, the health care provider should try to locate evidence of any underlying disease process. A complete history and physical assessment are done, searching for signs and symptoms of hyperthyroidism. Blood pressure should be measured to exclude high blood pressure associated with pheochromocytoma.[2] Heat intolerance associated with sweating in the upper half of the body and absence of sweating in the lower half of the body is evidence of diabetic peripheral autonomic neuropathy.[1]

In assessing the patient with generalized sweating, the examiner should look for miliaria rubra, an abnormal blocking of the sweat ducts. In this condition, sweat is trapped in the stratum corneum, creating tiny, pinpoint, clear papules that with pressure rupture the sweat ducts, creating an erythematous maculopapular rash. Other associated presentations include dyshidrotic eczema. This is a simple eczema promoted by the retention of sweat in the stratum corneum.

DIAGNOSTICS AND DIFFERENTIAL DIAGNOSIS

Thyroid and fasting blood glucose studies are indicated to exclude thyroid disease and diabetes. If night sweats are present, a purified protein derivative test is necessary to exclude tuberculosis. For perimenopausal women with hyperhidrosis, tests for follicle-stimulating hormone and luteinizing hormone are recommended to document menopause and provide patient reassurance. SSRIs may provoke night sweats. A different SSRI should be considered before changing drug classes.

The most common cause of excessive perspiration is a sympathetic-mediated response to stress. A careful history and examination will indicate the necessity to exclude hyperthyroidism with an ultrasensitive test for thyroid-stimulating hormone and thyroxine (T_4). A patient symptom diary of provoking factors, response to foods, body temperature, and amount and location of perspiration is a helpful adjunct in determining the cause of sweating. If infection or malignancy is suspected, a thorough evaluation is mandated. A tuberculin skin test should be performed for those with complaints of night sweats. A fasting blood glucose study is performed to exclude diabetes mellitus. In women with variations in the length and amount of menses, a search for accompanying symptoms of vasomotor hot flashes and objective evidence of ovarian failure is necessary. Symptoms of sweating and flushing accompanied by marked hypertension require an evaluation for pheochromocytoma. Evidence of central nervous system disease or autonomic peripheral neuropathy warrants referral to a neurologist.

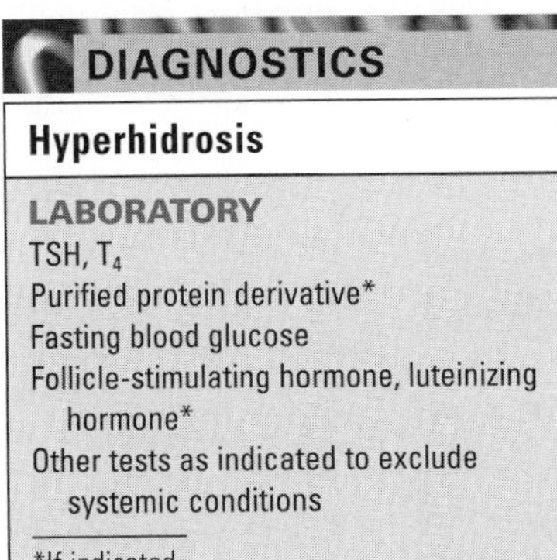
DIAGNOSTICS

Hyperhidrosis

LABORATORY
TSH, T_4
Purified protein derivative*
Fasting blood glucose
Follicle-stimulating hormone, luteinizing hormone*
Other tests as indicated to exclude systemic conditions

*If indicated.

DIFFERENTIAL DIAGNOSIS

Hyperhidrosis

- Hyperthyroidism
- Infection
- Malignancy
- Tuberculosis
- Diabetes mellitus
- Pheochromocytoma
- Alcoholism
- Central nervous system diseases
- Autonomic peripheral neuropathy
- Other hormonal imbalances

MANAGEMENT

Topical applications of 20% alcoholic solution of aluminum chloride hexahydrate (Drysol, Keralyt) can be effective in decreasing excessive perspiration on the hands, soles, and axillae. These treatments provide for a chemodenervation of the eccrine sweat glands.[6] A less potent solution of 6.25% aluminum chloride hexahydrate (Xerac) can be prescribed for patients who have more sensitive skin. The perspiring area is coated lightly with the solution and allowed to dry. An occlusive wrap is then applied, or vinyl gloves can be worn on the hands, and left on for 8 hours, followed by a complete soap-and-water wash of the affected areas. Applications are repeated every 2 or 3 days as tolerated. With satisfactory dryness, maintenance requires a once-weekly application.[2-4]

Liposuction of the axillary sweat glands has been effective,[7,8] as has surgical excision of axillary tissue.[9] Persistent primary palmar hyperhydrosis has shown a positive response to thoracic endoscopic surgery. Bilateral interruption of the upper dorsal sympathetic chain of D2 and D3 can provide a cure for primary hyperhydrosis.[10]

Co-Management with Specialist

Consultation with a dermatologist may be useful for patients who are refractory to topical treatments. The dermatologist may try a number of other remedies, including iontophoresis, in which an electrical current may be used to obstruct the sweat ducts.[2,4,11-13] Botulinum toxin has been found to be effective for hyperhidrosis affecting the axillae and palms and for gustatory sweating.[14,15] Liposuction has been shown to be effective for axillary hyperhydrosis.[7,8] Consideration of these and other treatments warrants consultation with an appropriate specialist. Sweating associated with anxiety or panic attacks warrants co-management with a mental health specialist or neuropsychiatrist.

COMPLICATIONS

Patients with hyperhidrosis may experience difficulty functioning in social or occupational situations as a result of this disorder, significantly affecting their quality of life. Other complications are rare, although patients with sensitive skin may develop reactions to the topical solutions prescribed for treatment. In most instances, decreasing the concentration of the solution will decrease skin irritation. Patients who undergo sympathectomy may experience compensatory sweating.

INDICATIONS FOR REFERRAL OR HOSPITALIZATION

Evidence of an underlying medical condition leading to secondary hyperhidrosis, such as pheochromocytoma, warrants referral. Primary hyperhidrosis refractory to topical treatments is referred for evaluation to a surgeon experienced in thoracoscopic sympathicolysis,[10] liposuction,[7,8] or axillary dissection.[9] Patients with excessive perspiration associated with anxiety or panic disorders can benefit from mental health counseling.

PATIENT AND FAMILY EDUCATION

Education is critical to assist patients in coping with and understanding this socially stigmatizing condition. A complete explanation of the etiology of primary hyperhidrosis and an explanation regarding sympathetic overactivity are provided. Patients need assurance that a search for an underlying pathologic reason for the disorder has been conducted. Results of laboratory tests must be provided. Support in the form of education for family members and significant others is an important aspect of comprehensive care. Good personal hygiene is encouraged for those with axillary sweating. Both open-toe and canvas shoes with cotton socks promote evaporation of foot perspiration while decreasing foot odor and preventing fungal infections of the feet. Occupational environments should be well ventilated and include air conditioning.

REFERENCES

1. Barker R, Burton JR, Zieve PD: *Ambulatory care medicine,* ed 6, Baltimore, 2003, Williams & Wilkins.
2. Gorroll AH, Mulley AG: *Primary care medicine,* ed 5, Philadelphia, 2005, Lippincott.
3. Rakel RE: *Textbook of family practice,* ed 6, Philadelphia, 2001, Saunders.
4. Rassner G: *Atlas of dermatology,* ed 3, Philadelphia, 1994, Lea & Febiger.
5. McArdle WD, Katch FI, Katch VL: *Exercise physiology,* Philadelphia, 1991, Lea & Febiger.
6. Benohanian A, Dansereau A, Bolduc C, and others: Localized hyperhidrosis treated with aluminum chloride in a salicylic acid gel base, *Int J Dermatol* 37(9):701-703, 1998.
7. Christ JE: The application of suction assisted lipectomy for the problem of axillary hyperhidrosis, *Surg Gynecol Obstet* 169(5):457-459, 1989.
8. Payne CM, Poe PT: Liposuction for axillary hyperhidrosis, *Clin Exp Dermatol* 23(1):9-10, 1998.
9. Naumann M, Lowe NJ, Kumar CR, and others: Botulinum toxin type A is a safe and effective treatment for axillary hyperhidrosis over 16 months: a prospective study, *Arch Dermatol* 139(6):731-736, 2003.
10. Drott C, Claes G: Hyperhidrosis treated by thoracoscopic sympathicotomy, *Cardiovasc Surg* 4(6):788-790, 1996.
11. Shen JL, Lin GS, Li WM: A new strategy of iontophoresis for hyperhidrosis, *J Am Acad Dermatol* 22(2):239-241, 1990.
12. Murphy R, Harrington CI: Treating hyperhidrosis: iontophoresis should be tried before other treatments [letter], *BMJ* 321(7262):702-703, 2000.
13. Kavanagh GM, Oh C, Shams C: BOTOX delivery by iontophoresis, *Br J Dermatol* 151(5):1093-1095, 2004.
14. Odderson IR: Hyperhidrosis treated by botulinum A exotoxin—treatment with botulinum toxin A, *Dermatol Surg* 24(11):1237-1241, 1998.
15. Heckmann M, Ceballos-Baumann AO, Plewing G, and others: Botulinum toxin A for axillary hyperhidrosis (excessive sweating), *N Engl J Med* 344:488-493, 2001.

CHAPTER 63

Intertrigo

Nancy W. Knee

DEFINITION AND EPIDEMIOLOGY

Intertrigo is a superficial mycotic infection that occurs between juxtaposed moist skin surfaces. Common sites include the inframammary folds, inner thighs, and axillary and perianal areas. Sweat retention, moisture, warmth, alterations in systemic immunity, systemic antibiotic therapy, and overgrowth of resident microorganisms are related factors.

Patients are susceptible to intertrigo at any age. Infants with thrush or diaper rash, women with vulvovaginitis, men with balanitis, individuals infected with HIV, and prolonged steroid users are particularly susceptible.[1] Other predisposing conditions and factors include psoriasis, eczema, diabetes, obesity, pregnancy, oral contraceptive use, and chemotherapy.[2]

PATHOPHYSIOLOGY

Intertrigo is caused by *Candida albicans.* This yeastlike fungus is normally found in the mouth, vagina, and gastrointestinal tract. Skin breakdown results from the release of toxins on the integumentary surface that subsequently cause irritation and result in maceration of cutaneous tissue.[3]

CLINICAL PRESENTATION AND PHYSICAL EXAMINATION

Intertrigo is initially seen as red, moist, and glistening plaques or patches, or moist, red papules and pustules. The borders are well defined, and the patches erode the epidermis, resulting in scaling. Pinpoint pustules outside the border are diagnostically important.[4]

DIAGNOSTICS

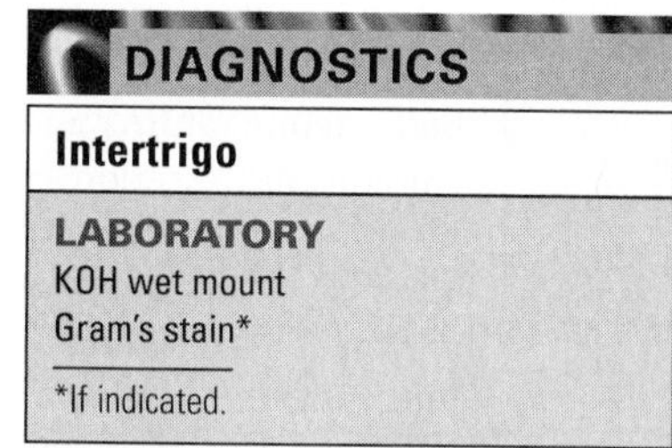
DIAGNOSTICS

Intertrigo

LABORATORY
KOH wet mount
Gram's stain*

*If indicated.

A potassium hydroxide (KOH) wet mount or gram-stained specimen with scrapings from the lesion is examined. A KOH preparation that is positive for pseudohyphae and budding spores confirms the diagnosis. Bacterial superinfection may be identified by culture.[2]

DIFFERENTIAL DIAGNOSIS

For intertriginous areas the differential diagnosis should include tinea, miliaria, psoriasis, seborrheic dermatitis, eczema, erythrasma, bacterial folliculitis, and contact dermatitis. Genital rashes may be caused by pediculosis pubis.[2] In females, bacterial vaginosis or trichomoniasis must be considered in the differential diagnosis.

MANAGEMENT

The site of the infection must be considered when selecting a medication. Topical nystatin, imidazole, or allylamine creams

DIFFERENTIAL DIAGNOSIS

Intertrigo

- Tinea
- Miliaria
- Bacterial infections
- Contact dermatitis
- Pediculosis pubis
- Bacterial vaginosis
- Trichomoniasis
- Psoriasis
- Seborrheic dermatitis
- Erythrasma
- Eczema

and powders may be applied two or three times daily for 7 to 14 days. Treatment should be continued several days after the skin clears. If antiinflammatory or antipruritic properties are needed, equal amounts of a low-strength hydrocortisone cream are added to the antifungal creams.[1] If the infection is recalcitrant or recurrent, nystatin oral suspension 100,000 units/ml, 5 ml swished and swallowed q.i.d. for 7 days, is indicated.[5] Oral ketoconazole can be effective, but the risk of hepatic toxicity and potential drug-drug interactions must be considered, and the patient must be carefully monitored. The infected area should be treated with a compress of cool water or Burow's solution applied for 20 minutes several times a day until the skin remains dry.[2] The affected area should be air dried frequently, and loose cotton clothing should be worn. An absorbent powder, not necessarily medicated, such as miconazole (Zeasorb), acting as a dry lubricant, may be applied after the inflammation subsides.[4]

LIFE SPAN CONSIDERATIONS

New parents should be counseled about the possibility of candidal rashes in the diaper area of infants. Women of childbearing age should be informed of the risk of these infections while taking oral contraceptives and during pregnancy.

COMPLICATIONS

A secondary bacterial infection may develop from scratching or other vehicles that may also affect skin integrity. Patients with frequent candidal infections should be evaluated for HIV, diabetes mellitus, or other immunocompromised states.

INDICATIONS FOR REFERRAL OR HOSPITALIZATION

Any patient who does not experience a resolution of symptoms of intertrigo within 2 weeks should be referred for additional consultation and confirmation of diagnosis. Immunocompromised patients require consultation with the appropriate specialist.

PATIENT AND FAMILY EDUCATION AND HEALTH PROMOTION

Assistance with weight reduction may be indicated for patients with intertrigo. Affected areas need to be exposed to light and air several times daily. A hair dryer set on cool can be effective for drying inframammary areas. Once the affected epidermis has healed, patients should be encouraged to keep prone areas clean and dry. Cornstarch- and talc-containing powders should be avoided. Wearing clean cotton underwear and avoiding tight clothing may also help reduce recurrence rates.

REFERENCES

1. Wolff K, Johnson RA, Suurmond R: *Fitzpatrick's color atlas and synopsis of clinical dermatology: common and serious diseases,* ed 5, New York, 2005, McGraw-Hill.
2. Habif T: *Skin disorders: diagnosis and treatment,* St Louis, 2004, Mosby.
3. Porth C: *Pathophysiology: concepts of altered health states,* ed 2, Philadelphia, 1986, Lippincott.
4. Habif T: *Clinical dermatology: a color guide to diagnosis and therapy,* Philadelphia, 2004, Mosby.
5. Beers MH, Porter RS, Jones TV: *The Merck manual,* ed 18, Rahway, NJ, 2006, Merck Research Laboratories.

CHAPTER 64

Nail Disorders

Nancy W. Knee

Immediate emergency department–surgical referral is indicated for paronychial infection of the tendon sheath.

HERPETIC WHITLOW

DEFINITION AND EPIDEMIOLOGY

Herpetic whitlow is an infection of the area between the fascial planes of the distal finger, usually surrounding the nail. This infection is most often seen in children with gingivostomatitis, in women with genital herpes, and in nurses.[1]

PATHOPHYSIOLOGY

The infecting pathogen is herpes simplex virus. The inoculation with the initial virus is often obscure. The virus remains dormant in the nerve ganglia; secondary eruptions may be related to stress, certain foods, sun exposure, and unknown precipitants.

CLINICAL PRESENTATION

Herpetiform vesicles or blisters erupt on the distal phalanx, sometimes after a short prodromal period of tingling or pruritus in the area of the eruption. Painful vesicles can be singular or coalescent, resemble a group of warts or a bacterial infection, and persist for 8 to 12 days; lesions then begin to dry, forming crusted fissures.[1] The course of the eruptions can persist for 21 days until resolution; healing may take longer in areas that remain moist. Persistent eruptions may cause scarring and atrophy.[2] In addition to the vesicles, the fingertip may be edematous, erythematous streaking may be evident on the forearm, and the axillary lymph nodes may become enlarged.[3]

PHYSICAL EXAMINATION

The nails should be inspected for shape, configuration, texture, and herpetiform vesicles. Axillary and epitrochlear nodes should be examined for lymphadenopathy.

DIAGNOSTICS AND DIFFERENTIAL DIAGNOSIS

Visualization of multinucleated giant cells using the Tzanck test confirms the diagnosis.[4] If the Tzanck test is negative, a herpes simplex culture should be obtained. The differential diagnosis should include a bacterial or candidal infection, such as paronychia.

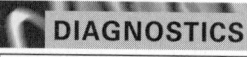

DIAGNOSTICS

Herpetic Whitlow
LABORATORY
Tzanck test
Herpes simplex culture*

*If indicated.

DIFFERENTIAL DIAGNOSIS

Herpetic Whitlow
Bacterial infection or warts

MANAGEMENT

Valacyclovir (Valtrex) may be given at 1 g b.i.d. for 10 days for initial episodes and 500 mg b.i.d. for 5 days for recurrent episodes. Chronic cases of herpetic whitlow may be treated with valacyclovir 500 mg to 1 g daily for up to 1 year. Creatinine clearance should be checked and the dose adjusted according to the creatinine clearance values if abnormal. L-Lysine is ineffective.[1] Cool water compresses can be used to decrease erythema and debride crusts, thus promoting healing.[1] Analgesia such as ibuprofen 800 mg t.i.d. may be administered for pain control; however, vesicular pain may require barbiturate analgesia.[4]

COMPLICATIONS

Secondary bacterial infection in conjunction with the viral syndrome is possible. However, there is little evidence that this is a concern.

INDICATIONS FOR REFERRAL OR HOSPITALIZATION

Physician referral is necessary if the virus is recalcitrant to treatment after 3 weeks. Hospitalization should not be required.

PATIENT AND FAMILY EDUCATION AND HEALTH PROMOTION

Patients require education regarding medication administration. Valacyclovir should be administered within 48 hours of the first prodromal signs. Patients should be advised to keep their infected digit(s) away from their mouth and eyes to prevent inoculation of these surfaces with the virus. If patients work in occupations in which they could infect other persons (e.g., nurse, manicurist), they should be advised to wear gloves when working. The provider should carefully explain signs and symptoms of infection and encourage the patient to call if complications develop.

PARONYCHIAL INFECTIONS

DEFINITION AND EPIDEMIOLOGY

Paronychial infections manifest as acute or chronic inflammation of the periungual tissues with an underlying bacterial or fungal infection. The microorganism can penetrate the periungual tissues through a split in the epidermis from trauma, a hangnail, irritation, or chronic exposure to water or irritants.[2]

Paronychial infections may be seen more often in women than in men; this may be related to manicures or the application of acrylic nails. Postmenopausal women may be at greater risk for chronic, candidal, paronychial infections because of diminished estrogen levels. An antiretroviral, indinavir, is also associated with paronychias because of interference with the alteration of retinoid metabolism.[5] Patients who work with chemicals are more at risk for infections because of the irritant nature of these substances and the risk of trauma.

PATHOPHYSIOLOGY

The causative organisms include *Pseudomonas, Proteus, Streptococcus,* and *Staphylococcus* organisms and *Candida albicans.*[2,4,6] The periungual tissues are inoculated via trauma, inert vehicles such as water, or soluble chemicals. Usually the infection follows the nail margin, or the infection may penetrate under the nail.

CLINICAL PRESENTATION AND PHYSICAL EXAMINATION

The nail folds, nail, and even digits are often described as throbbing. The nail may display distal onycholysis, discoloration, distortion, and ridging. Erythema and edema around the nail folds can be present. Force applied to the affected area releases purulent, often foul-smelling discharge.[4] Pyogenic granuloma–like lesions and granulation tissue are seen in the nail sulci in paronychias associated with indinavir.[5]

DIAGNOSTICS AND DIFFERENTIAL DIAGNOSIS

Potassium hydroxide (KOH) preparation will determine the presence of pseudohyphae and spores, which indicate candidal infection. Exudate can be cultured to determine the pathogen and to guide treatment.

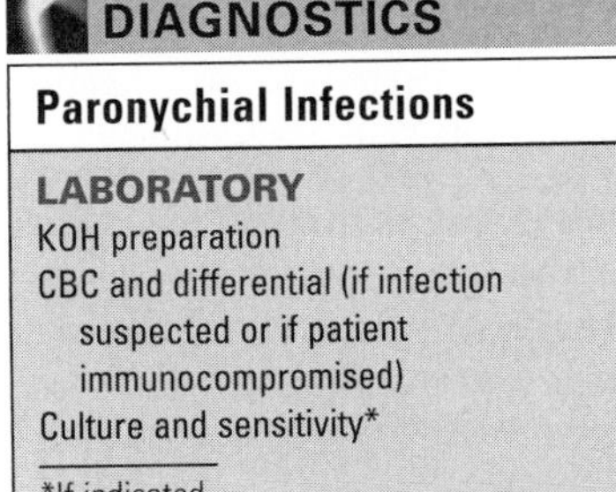

DIAGNOSTICS

Paronychial Infections

LABORATORY
KOH preparation
CBC and differential (if infection suspected or if patient immunocompromised)
Culture and sensitivity*

*If indicated.

The differential diagnosis includes herpetic whitlow and onychomycosis. However, paronychial infection is usually readily recognized.

MANAGEMENT

Treatment for acute infection includes hot compresses four times per day and systemic antibiotics if the pathogen is bacterial. Antibiotic therapy consists of a 7- to 10-day regimen of penicillin 25 to 50 mg/kg/day in divided doses q 6-8 hr, cephalexin 25 to 50 mg/kg/day in divided doses q 6-8 hr, or erythromycin 40 mg/kg/day in divided doses q 6 hr.[7] Ibuprofen or acetaminophen is used for analgesia. Any area with an accumulation of purulent secretions should be excised, drained, and cleansed with half-strength iodine twice per day.

DIFFERENTIAL DIAGNOSIS

Paronychial Infections

- Herpetic whitlow
- Onychomycosis

If *Candida* organisms are present, the affected area requires treatment with an antifungal lotion such as ciclopirox (Penlac), miconazole, or ketoconazole cream three times per day for 2 weeks.[2] The nail should be trimmed back to the juncture of the nail plate and nail bed. For chronic candidal infections, it is important to keep the hands dry and free of moisture. The patient should be treated with oral nystatin 500,000 units q.i.d. for 2 weeks because the likely source of infection is the mouth.

COMPLICATIONS

If untreated, the paronychial infection can invade deep into the digit, infecting the tendon and tendon sheaths. Infection along the tendon sheath requires immediate surgical intervention. Chronic mucocutaneous candidiasis can cause hyperkeratosis of the entire nail plate. These chronically infected nails can become distorted and may require excision.

INDICATIONS FOR REFERRAL OR HOSPITALIZATION

Physician referral is necessary if the infection continues after 2 weeks of treatment. Suspected infection of the tendons or tendon sheaths requires immediate referral to a physician or surgeon. Hospitalization may be required for surgical intervention.

PATIENT AND FAMILY EDUCATION AND HEALTH PROMOTION

It is imperative that patients understand the importance of keeping hands and nails as clean and dry as possible. Patient education should address the causative factors. Patients who have manicures or who wear acrylic nails should be advised to rest their nails and hands for 1 week every month.[4] Patients who deal with caustic chemicals and irritants are advised to wear protective gloves. The hands should be gloved when washing dishes or clothing by hand. Keeping the nails trimmed and dry will help prevent further infections.

ONYCHOMYCOSIS AND TINEA UNGUIUM

DEFINITION AND EPIDEMIOLOGY

The terms *onychomycosis* and *tinea unguium* are often used interchangeably; however, onychomycosis is any infection of the nails caused by a fungus, and tinea unguium, or ringworm, of the nail is defined as a dermatophyte infection of the nail plate. These infections cause thickening, roughness, and splitting of the nail, resulting in dystrophy of the nail and onycholysis. The distal component of the nail subsequently separates and then falls off.[2] Often ringworm of the toenails is seen in patients with longstanding tinea pedis. Both onychomycosis and tinea unguium are common in advancing age as a result of a reduction in blood flow.[4] Onychomycosis has a significant incidence of pain and can affect patients' lives physically and psychologically. This infection can interfere with walking, exercise, and social interaction. Trauma to the nail makes the nail susceptible to infection, which may be chronic.[8]

PATHOPHYSIOLOGY

The most common pathogens associated with tinea unguium are *Trichophyton rubrum* (most common in the general population and in patients with HIV), *Trichophyton mentagrophytes, Trichophyton interdigitale,* and *Epidermophyton floccosum.*[9] Onychomycosis caused by nondermatophytes is associated with *Candida* organisms.[4] There can be a genetic predisposition to *T. rubrum*; nail trauma may trigger nail invasion in adulthood.[8] Multiple organisms may be present in a single nail.[1]

CLINICAL PRESENTATION

Table 64-1 describes the physical presentation of nail dystrophies.

PHYSICAL EXAMINATION

Careful examination of the toes and fingers is essential. The color may be white or yellowed, and the texture powdery or thickened. Noting the condition of the subungual nail bed, that is, the degree of elevation and separation of nail from nail bed, and surrounding tissue is important to determine the presence of concurrent bacterial infection.

DIAGNOSTICS

Confirmation of the diagnosis is made via microscopic examination of nail scrapings with a KOH preparation or culture of nail debris.[10] It is essential to identify the invading organism as a dermatophyte or *Candida* for appropriate treatment. Histologic tests and periodic acid–Schiff staining are reliable for an accurate diagnosis to identify organisms susceptible to specific therapeutic agents.[1]

DIAGNOSTICS

Onychomycosis and Tinea Unguium

LABORATORY
KOH smear and culture
CBC and differential
LFTs*

*If indicated.

DIFFERENTIAL DIAGNOSIS

Pitting of the nail surface, a feature of psoriasis, is not characteristic of fungal infection. Leukonychia, white spots or bands that appear proximally, is most likely caused by minor trauma and may be mistaken for proximal subungual onychomycosis.[8] Conditions that must be excluded include psoriasis, eczema, trauma, lichen planus, onychogryposis, onycholysis, and leukonychia.[1] Psoriasis is often mistaken for dermatophyte and fungal infections, but the two may co-exist (Color Plate 22).[1]

DIFFERENTIAL DIAGNOSIS

Onychomycosis and Tinea Unguium

- Psoriasis
- Eczema
- Trauma
- Lichen planus
- Onychogryposis
- Herpetic whitlow
- Subungual malignant melanoma
- Peripheral vascular disease
- Pityriasis
- Medications
- Trophic changes
- Black nail paronychia
- Darier's disease
- Endocrine disorders

MANAGEMENT

Onychomycosis may be treated with terbinafine (Lamisil) 250 mg daily for 12 weeks for toenails, 6 weeks for fingernails. This medication has a low incidence of side effects. Intermittent terbinafine may also be used, 1 week a month for 11 months with monthly monitoring of proximal extension of nail bed lesion. Difficult cases may respond to ciclopirox with oral antifungals.[8] An alternative is itraconazole (Sporanox) 200 mg daily for 6 weeks, although failure rates and the risk of adverse drug interactions increase.[8] Liver function tests and CBC are checked before and at 6 weeks when starting terbinafine. Consistent, prolonged application of a topical antifungal agent after clinical response to an oral agent may prevent nail reinfection. Removing the infected nail affords better cure rates and longer remissions.[1]

TABLE 64-1 Nail Dystrophies

Nail Disorder	Clinical Presentation	Manifestations
Distal or lateral subungual onychomycosis	White to brownish yellow discoloration of nail	Subungual hyperkeratosis; separation of nail plate and nail bed lineal channels
White superficial onychomycosis	White, sharply outlined area on nail plate; nail surface soft, dry, and friable	Common in fingernails and toenails of HIV-infected patients Nail plate not thick; no separation of nail plate and nail bed
Proximal subungual onychomycosis (rare)	Leukonychia on proximal aspect of nail plate	None
Candidal infections	Thickening of nail plate Yellowish brown discoloration	Chronic mucocutaneous candidiasis Involves all nails Eventual disintegration of nail

COMPLICATIONS

Chronic dermatophytosis and infection result in hyperkeratosis. The nail plate separates from the nail bed, resulting in total dystrophic onychomycosis whereby the nail bed disappears, leaving behind a keratinized nail bed.[9]

INDICATIONS FOR REFERRAL OR HOSPITALIZATION

Patients with combinations of infection and underlying disease (e.g., psoriasis) would benefit from a referral. Discussion with the physician regarding recurrence or surgical or nonsurgical avulsion of nail dystrophy is also a consideration for a referral.

PATIENT AND FAMILY EDUCATION AND HEALTH PROMOTION

In many cases, nails do not become clear in 12 weeks. Patients should be assured that the medication remains in the nail plate for months and will continue to kill fungus.[1] These infections can be recalcitrant to treatment, which can take months or even years for complete resolution of the pathogens. To prevent recurrence, the patient can take ciclopirox two or three times a week, apply terbinafine cream in the nail area weekly, and avoid trauma to the tip of the nails from tight-fitting shoes. To prevent hyphae invasion into hyponychia, the patient should powder toe webs and soles, not shoes; avoid communal showers; and alternate several pairs of shoes for daily wear that maintain a dry, roomy environment for the feet. Patient education should be targeted toward causative factors. It is imperative that patients keep their hands and nails as dry as possible and avoid recurrence of tinea pedis. Footwear should be evaluated annually for size and suitability. The health care provider should review information concerning medication administration and instructions regarding signs of liver toxicity.

REFERENCES

1. Habif T, Campbell MJ, Quitadamo KA: *Skin disease: diagnosis and treatment,* St Louis, 2001, Mosby.
2. Beers MH, Porter RS, Jones TV: *The Merck manual,* ed 18, Rahway, NJ, 2006, Merck Research Laboratories.
3. Cauthorne-Burnette T, Estes ME: *Clinical companion for health assessment and physical examination,* Albany, NY, 1998, Delmar.
4. Wolff K, Johnson, RA, Suurmond R: *Fitzpatrick's color atlas and synopsis of clinical dermatology: common and serious diseases,* ed 5, New York, 2005, McGraw-Hill.
5. Ward HA, Russo GG, Shrum J: Cutaneous manifestations of antiretroviral therapy, *J Am Acad Dermatol* 46:284, 2002.
6. Murphy L: *Nurse practitioners' prescribing reference,* New York, 1998, Prescribing References.
7. White G: *Levene's color atlas of dermatology,* ed 2, London, 1997, Mosby-Wolfe.
8. Habif T: *Clinical dermatology: a color guide to diagnosis and therapy,* Philadelphia, 2004, Mosby.
9. Fenstermacher K, Hudson B: *Practice guidelines for family nurse practitioners,* Philadelphia, 1997, Saunders.
10. Mir A: *Atlas of clinical diagnosis,* Philadelphia, 1995, Saunders.

CHAPTER 65

Pigmentation Changes (Vitiligo)

Margaret McAllister

DEFINITION AND EPIDEMIOLOGY

Vitiligo is a skin disorder characterized by either a lifelong or a rapid disappearance of pigment-producing melanocytes in the epidermis and hair follicle. Lack of melanin leads to the appearance of progressive, symmetrically patterned, milky-white macules that merge to form larger depigmented areas. The macules give a variegated appearance to the skin that is similar to the white patches on a Holstein calf—hence the origin of the word from the Greek *vitelius,* which means "calf." The disease is psychologically troublesome, affecting the patient's self-esteem and interpersonal relationships. Although the disease shows no increased prevalence among dark-skinned racial groups, the variegated appearance of the skin proves to be especially traumatic for dark-pigmented populations. The appearance of vitiligo resembles leprosy, but the lesions of vitiligo do not have the anesthetic property of leprosy. However, the similarity in appearance to leprosy presents a social stigma for those patients with vitiligo living in leprosy-affected areas of the world.[1,2] The disease manifests itself in two forms: type A, a nondermatomal distribution; and type B, a segmental or dermatomal distribution (zosteriform) characterized by rapid spread.[1]

Vitiligo is seen in 1% to 2% of the general population without regard to race, ethnic origin, or gender.[1,3] Although some patients have no vitiligo in their family history, the condition has an inherited tendency, with 30% of cases reporting a family history of vitiligo in parents, offspring, or siblings.[2-4] Familial cases of vitiligo have been associated with autoimmune endocrine disorders; studies indicate that there is a genetic locus in affected individuals, but not in controls.[5,6] A family history of thyroid disease, diabetes mellitus, and vitiligo is associated with a risk for developing the condition.[3] Disease onset occurs between 10 and 30 years of age, with 50% of the cases occurring before age 20 and fewer cases reported in infancy and old age.[3,4,7]

PATHOPHYSIOLOGY

The exact cause of vitiligo is not known, although histologic studies point to an autoimmune pathologic condition directed at the melanocyte.[1,2] Except for the absence of melanocytes, skin function is normal. There is a progressive destruction of pigment-producing cells at the border of the dermis and epidermis. The nonsegmental (nondermatomal) variety of vitiligo is associated with a small risk of autoimmune-related disorders, such as type 1 diabetes mellitus and thyroid disease.[3]

Several theories exist to explain the phenomenon of vitiligo. The autoimmune theory proposes that there is a destruction of the cutaneous melanocytes with loss of the melanin-producing pigment. Histologic examination indicates that lymphocytes build up within the dermis and are involved in the destruction of the melanocytes. Coexisting diseases such as alopecia areata, autoimmune thyroid disorders, Addison's disease, atrophic gastritis, pernicious anemia, and type 1 diabetes underscore the relationship of dermatomal vitiligo to autoimmunity. Serum autoimmune antibodies against melanocytes, thyroid and adrenal tissue, islet cells, gastric parietal cells, and intrinsic factors have been demonstrated.

A second explanation, the neurogenic theory, supposes that a toxic substance is released by the peripheral nerve endings and interferes with the production of melanin. A third theory suggests a defect in the natural protective mechanism of melanin synthesis by melanocytes. Toxic substances accumulate during normal melanin production and later precipitate the destruction of the melanocytes.[1-4] The variation in presentation and progression of the two types of vitiligo indicates that the underlying pathologic condition for the two forms of disease may be distinctly different.

CLINICAL PRESENTATION

Vitiligo is characterized by a progressive and invasive hypopigmentation of the skin that is found on sun-exposed areas and extensor surfaces of the upper body. Most patients have no other clinical findings.[7] Vitiligo manifesting with well-defined areas of white hair is referred to as *poliosis*.[3] In general, the onset of vitiligo may follow stress; an injury to the skin such as a burn, bruise, or contusion (Koebner's phenomenon); and sunburn.[3] Vitiligo should not be confused with post-inflammatory hypopigmentation in which the skin has a faded pigment appearance rather than an absence of pigment.[2] Chemicals, including phenols, may cause depigmentation of the skin; therefore any history of a patient with vitiligo should include questions about chemical exposure.[2] In fair-skinned individuals the disease may go undetected until summer, when the sun-exposed areas tan and the melanin-free areas appear a contrasting chalky white.

PHYSICAL EXAMINATION

The extensor surfaces may have been traumatized previously; depigmentation first appears here in a symmetric fashion typical of the more common nondermatomal variety. The segmental variety is more often seen in children and follows a dermatomal distribution that progresses more rapidly. The dermatomal variety is not likely to be associated with autoimmune disorders or Koebner's phenomenon.[7] The border is not sharply demarcated but instead exhibits a tricolored, uneven appearance.[8] Box 65-1 indicates the usual presentation of the hypopigmented lesions of vitiligo. Since melanocytes are located in the eyes, ocular changes, such as uveitis and pigmentary changes in the fundus, can occur; other findings may include healed chorioretinitis or iritis.[2,9]

Vitiligo can best be described as a white, flat macule within the epidermis that varies in size from 5 mm to 5 cm (0.2 to 1.2 inches) with a convex outer edge. In the common non-segmental variety, the lesion is initially seen in a symmetric distribution on the body parts. Macules may eventually merge to cover the entire body in a condition termed *vitiligo universalis*. Variations of the disease presentation include smaller confetti-like lesions mixed with larger ones and the less common presentation of elevated, erythematous, pruritic lesions known as *inflammatory vitiligo*.[3,10] The segmental variety occurs in a band-type distribution on one side of the body. Confetti-sized hypomelanotic macules are common on sun-exposed surfaces of the arms.

BOX 65-1

HYPOPIGMENTED VITILIGO LESIONS

Bony surfaces—Back of hands and fingers, elbows and knees
Body orifices—Around the eyes, mouth, and nose
Body folds—Armpits and groin
Other areas—Legs, wrists, nipples, and genitals
Hair—Area within the affected path turning white

DIAGNOSTICS

The clinical presentation and physical examination are generally sufficient to make a diagnosis. In some instances, in lighter-skinned individuals and in underarm and genital regions, a Wood's light examination is necessary to make the diagnosis. A Wood's light will illuminate depigmented areas as chalky white. A skin scraping for a potassium hydroxide (KOH) examination fails to demonstrate hyphae or spores consistent with tinea versicolor, another common depigmenting lesion. Although not usually necessary, a skin biopsy will show an absence of melanocytes and melanin in the epidermis.

Vitiligo patients show an increased frequency of autoimmune disorders such as thyroid disease, type 1 diabetes, and pernicious anemia.[11] The patient should be assessed for signs and symptoms of thyroid disease; a screening for thyroid-stimulating hormone and thyroxine is recommended. However, the treatment of thyroid disease has no impact on the progression of vitiligo.[4] A fasting blood glucose is included in the initial diagnostic evaluation. A CBC with indexes is performed to detect the presence of macrocytosis, followed by an evaluation for vitamin B_{12} deficiency if indicated.

DIAGNOSTICS

Vitiligo

LABORATORY
Wood's lamp examination
KOH preparation
TSH, T_4
Fasting blood glucose
CBC and differential
Vitamin B_{12}

OTHER
Skin biopsy*

*If indicated.

DIFFERENTIAL DIAGNOSIS

Early or atypical lesions often require the exclusion of other hypopigmented conditions, including albinism, piebaldism, tuberous sclerosis, nevus anemicus, tinea, pityriasis alba, chemical skin exposure, and lichen sclerosis. Some of these disorders are associated with patchy depigmentation with inflammation and scaling or atrophy induration. A biopsy may be indicated to differentiate the underlying cause of depigmentation associated with these disorders.[2]

DIFFERENTIAL DIAGNOSIS

Vitiligo

- Albinism
- Piebaldism
- Tuberous sclerosis
- Nevus anemicus
- Chemical leukoderma
- Tinea versicolor
- Leprosy
- Pityriasis alba
- Lichen sclerosis
- Psoriasis
- Eczema

MANAGEMENT

Care of the patient with vitiligo involves the use of sunscreens (sun protection factor [SPF] 15 to 30) to protect the depigmented skin from burning and to reduce the tanning of melanin-producing areas of the adjacent skin. Extensive sunburn can produce a response similar to Koebner's phenomenon (trauma to the skin) and stimulate the depigmentation process to extend further. Cosmetic cover-ups assist the patient in managing the psychologic aspects of the disease and improve body image and coping mechanisms. A variety of cosmetic substances are commercially available, marketed under the names Covermark (Lydia O'Leary); Dermablend (Flori Roberts); Dermage; and C-Esta Make Up for Vitiligo. These products can be customized to match individual skin tones and are used by both sexes. Although these products do not come off in water, they do rub off and therefore may not sustain long periods of wear. Tanning creams containing dihydroxyacetone may be applied to induce the tanning of affected areas; these substances can be used for eyelids. Some patients desire no treatment aside from cosmetics and prefer to allow the disease to progress until all body parts are depigmented. However, it is difficult to judge how long this will take, which limits the usefulness of this approach in the treatment regimen.

After coexistent autoimmune disorders have been excluded, patients with vitiligo are generally referred to a dermatologist for treatment options. Therapy is directed toward either repigmentation therapy of the affected areas or depigmentation therapy of the unaffected areas. Repigmentation involving the use of high- to mid-potency class 3 and class 4 steroid creams applied twice a day to the affected areas is usually the first approach for patients with depigmentation involving less than 10% of the body and not involving the face. Another treatment approach with proven efficacy for patients with lesser involvement or more generalized vitiligo is treatment with narrow-band ultraviolet B (UVB); this approach, which involve the use of psoralens, has been found to be just as effective as psoralens plus ultraviolet light A (PUVA).[1,3,12,13] Recently occurring lesions and those of the facial and genital areas are the most responsive to topical steroid treatment.[3] Patients must be monitored every 2 months for evidence of skin atrophy. A response to treatment is indicated by the development of follicular pigmented spots that widen with time and persist. Areas with minimum hair follicles are slower to repigment. Oral corticosteroids have shown promise in patients with more aggressive forms of the disease; referral to a dermatologist is recommended.[13,14]

Efforts are in progress to develop guidelines in the management of vitiligo.[12] Meta-analysis of studies using class 3 corticosteroids and narrow-band UVB have shown these methods to be effective and safe for localized and generalized vitiligo, respectively.[1,3,15] However, steroid treatment failure is seen in nearly 20% of cases; failure is likely if no response is seen by the end of 2 months.[8] At this time, the patient should be referred back to the specialist for further evaluation and for treatment with PUVA, either topical or systemic. PUVA treatments should be performed by a qualified specialist. Close monitoring of the patient for response to treatment is necessary. Prevention of eye exposure to UV light must be strictly enforced by making certain that the patient wears glasses that filter all UV light. Up to 2 years of treatment may be necessary before repigmentation occurs.[8]

Another technique is chemical depigmentation to produce an artificially induced vitiligo universalis if more than 50% to 80% of the body is affected. Studies indicate that depigmentation treatments using monobenzone or a Q-switched ruby laser were equally effective.[12] The former involves the application of a monobenzone hydroquinone 20% (MEH) cream twice daily. The application produces an irreversible depigmentation that takes up to 2 to 3 months to begin and up to 9 to 12 months for a complete response. The depigmentation with MEH leads to chalk-white coloration of the skin like that of vitiligo macules.[3,4] The health care provider can monitor this treatment regimen if prescribed by the specialist. Patients are generally pleased with the outcome of this treatment.

COMPLICATIONS

Treatment with steroids may involve atrophy and striae formation, which increases the risk for easy bruising and infection. Steroid-induced glaucoma and cataracts are complications of steroid application around the eyes. Complications of PUVA treatment include a phototoxic reaction and ocular damage if appropriate UV-protective sunglasses are not used. Consultation with the specialist is necessary if evidence of skin atrophy, adrenal axis suppression, or steroid-induced glaucoma is seen.

INDICATIONS FOR REFERRAL

After coexistent autoimmune disorders have been excluded, patients with vitiligo are referred to a dermatologist for treatment options. Health care providers can assist with monitoring therapy, with a dermatology consultation for treatment questions. The involvement of eye pigment mandates a referral to an ophthalmologist for evaluation. A referral for mental health counseling may be indicated because this disorder can be psychologically stressful. In progressive forms of the disease the patient should be referred to a specialist for depigmentation therapy. Laser therapy is an option for those trained in the use of this technique. XTRAC is the first U.S. Food and Drug Administration–approved laser treatment for vitiligo.[1]

PATIENT AND FAMILY EDUCATION

Education includes teaching patients about the nature of the pigmentary changes and the lack of scientific knowledge concerning the true cause of the disease. Patients should be taught that the treatment response includes repigmentation that occurs first in areas with residual melanocytes. Vitiligo with late-life onset or longstanding lesions is less likely to respond to treatment. Risk factors associated with topical steroids include easy bruising, infection, and decreased vision. Patients are taught to observe their skin closely for the development of suspicious skin lesions suggestive of melanoma. The rule of fingertip units should be adhered to in prescribing and monitoring patients on topical steroids. One fingertip unit weighs 0.5 g and is the amount expressed from a tube applied to the fingertip. One half of a fingertip unit will cover the dorsum of the hand, and 2.5 fingertip units will cover the face. For lesions affecting the face, a 30-g tube should last for 10 days.[7] Patients should avoid using more steroid cream than directed and should avoid applying steroids around the eyes and moist genital areas, where thin skin enhances systemic absorption. Patients should avoid sunlight for 48 hours after each PUVA treatment.

Assessment of the patient's psychologic response to vitiligo includes body image adjustment, use of cosmetic coverings, and knowledge concerning the noncontagious nature of vitiligo. Family members should be included in the office visit for support and explanation concerning the benign nature of the disorder and the expected response to treatment. Instruction concerning the use of sunscreens to protect depigmented areas is critical.

REFERENCES

1. Huggins RH, Schwartz RA, Janniger CK: Vitiligo, *Acta Dermatovenerol Alp Panonica Adriat* 14(4):137-142, 144-145, 2005.
2. Goldstein BG, Goldstein AO: Vitiligo. In Rose BD, editor: *2006 UpToDate* (CD-ROM), Waltham, Mass, 2006.
3. Wolff K, Johnson RA, Suurmond R, editors: *Fitzpatrick's color atlas and synopsis of clinical dermatology,* ed 5, New York, 2005, McGraw-Hill.
4. Habif TP: *Clinical dermatology,* ed 5, St Louis, 2003, Mosby.
5. Alkhateeb A, Stetler GL, Old W, and others: Mapping of an autoimmunity susceptibility locus (AIS1) to chromosome 1p31.3-p32.2, *Hum Mol Gent* 11(6):661-667, 2002.
6. Arcos-Burgos M, Parodi E, Salgar M, and others: Vitiligo: complex segregation and linkage disequilibrium analyses with respect to microsatellite loci spanning the HLA, *Hum Genet* 110(4):334-342, 2002.
7. Schwartz RA, Janniger CK: Vitiligo, *Cutis* 60(5):239-244, 1997.
8. Reeves JT, Maibach HI: *Clinical dermatology illustrated: a regional approach,* ed 3, Philadelphia, 1998, Davis.
9. Biswas G, Barbhuiya JN, Biswas MC, and others: Clinical pattern of ocular manifestations in vitiligo, *J Indian Med Assoc* 101(8):478-480, 2003.
10. Verma SB: Inflammatory vitiligo with raised borders and psoriasiform histopathology, *Dermatol Online J* 11(3):13, 2005, retrieved March 17, 2006, from http://dermatology.cdlib.org/113/case_reports/vitiligo2/verma.html.
11. You-Min Y, Hong-Yong K: A study on the frequency of the autoimmune disorder in vitiligo patients, *Ann Dermatol* 13(4):218-221, 2001.
12. Njoo MD, Westerhof W, Bos JD, and others: The development of guidelines for the treatment of vitiligo: Clinical Epidemiology Unit of the Istituto Dermopatico dell'Immacolata–Istituto di Recovero e Cura a Carattere Scientifico (IDI-IRCCS) and the Archives of Dermatology, *Arch Dermatol* 135(12):1514-1521, 1999.
13. Seiter S, Ugurel S, Tilgen W, and others: Use of high-dose methylprednisolone pulse therapy in patients with progressive and stable vitiligo, *Int J Dermatol* 39(8):624-637, 2000.
14. Kim SM, Lee HS, Hann SK: The efficacy of low-dose oral corticosteroids in the treatment of vitiligo patients, *Int J Dermatol* 38(7):546-550, 1999.
15. Amercian Medical Association: The development of guidelines for the treatment of vitiligo, *Arch Fam Med* 9(10):954, 2000.

CHAPTER 66

Pruritus

Daniel W. O'Neill

DEFINITION AND EPIDEMIOLOGY

Pruritus is a sensation that leads to a desire to scratch. It is a common symptom that can be found in many dermatologic and systemic illnesses.

PATHOPHYSIOLOGY

Pruritus is characterized by the activation of a network of distinct free nerve endings situated at the dermoepidermal junction by local mediators such as histamine and/or numerous other peptides and proteases.[1] These impulses are carried by unmyelinated C fibers to the central nervous system, where the impulses are modulated by opioid peptides. Prostaglandins in the skin lower the threshold for itching. The exact pathophysiologic mechanisms leading to itching in systemic disease is ill defined. Scratching leads to symptomatic relief by temporarily destroying the nerve endings or stimulating pain fibers, but this often leads to the release of more mediators and the scratch-itch cycle, in which one scratch is too many and a million are not enough.

CLINICAL PRESENTATION AND PHYSICAL EXAMINATION

Dermatologic disorders can manifest with characteristic primary skin lesions; therefore, after obtaining a basic history of the present illness, the health care provider should perform a total skin examination to first identify or exclude dermatologic disorders.[1] Often the secondary skin lesions, such as excoriations (scratches), secondary infections (e.g., impetigo), hyperkeratotic skin changes, and lichenification (thickening, which indicates chronicity), obscure the primary lesion. If a diagnosis is not evident on initial examination, then a thorough history should include diurnal rhythms, character, severity, distribution, exacerbating and alleviating factors, and previous treatments. The history should also include medication use, alcohol use, past medical history, exposures (e.g., to people who are scratching, pets, soaps, detergents, dry air, chemicals), and a complete review of systems. A complete physical examination with emphasis on evaluation for organomegaly and adenopathy is then performed.

DIAGNOSTICS

If the symptoms persist and no dermatologic cause is discovered, screening laboratory examinations include a CBC with differential, serum glucose, aspartate and alanine transaminase, alkaline phosphatase, bilirubin, BUN, creatinine, thyroid panel, urinalysis, and chest radiograph. If indicated, a skin biopsy can be sent for pathologic examination (mycosis fungoides), immunofluorescence (pemphigoid and dermatitis herpetiformis), or special staining (mastocytosis). Serum ferritin, protein and immunoelectrophoresis, stool for ova and parasites, or other studies may also be indicated. Occasionally it is necessary to perform repeated evaluations in follow-up visits or to refer the patient for dermatologic or psychiatric evaluation.

DIAGNOSTICS

Pruritus

LABORATORY
CBC and differential
Serum glucose
LFTs
BUN
Creatinine
TSH
Urinalysis
Serum ferritin*
Protein and immunoelectrophoresis*
Stool cultures for ova and parasites*

IMAGING
Chest x-ray

OTHER
Skin biopsy

*If indicated.

DIFFERENTIAL DIAGNOSIS

Dermatologic disorders with pruritus as a predominant symptom are common. Some of these disorders are covered in detail in other chapters, and each has its own etiology, clinical presentation, and treatment considerations. Pruritus without diagnostic skin lesions that persists longer than 2 weeks and is undiagnosed after 2 weeks of evaluation is called *pruritus of undetermined origin* and may indicate a systemic disorder.[2] Medications are also an important cause of pruritus.

MANAGEMENT

The success of treatment for pruritus depends on identification of the underlying dermatologic or systemic cause. In addition to appropriate treatment of the cause, pruritus requires interventions to alleviate this annoying symptom, although often not completely. Medications that cause pruritus should be stopped. Taking steps to avoid irritants (e.g., wool or misguided topical therapy), reducing stress, and keeping the nails trimmed should be pursued. Cooling the skin by the use of light clothing; air conditioning; or frequent application of cool wet compresses, cooling lotions such as calamine, or aqueous creams is useful. A tepid bath before retiring can alleviate pruritus long enough for the patient to fall asleep. Decreased bathing frequency and emollients are effective for any condition in which dry skin (xerosis) is present. Disrupting the scratch-itch cycle by alleviating pruritus is a mainstay of therapy for dermatitis. Pramoxine hydrochloride (often combined with other topical agents) and 5% doxepin cream, a topical tricyclic antidepressant, have proved effective in several trials.[3] Topical and oral corticosteroids should be reserved only for cases of cutaneous inflammation. Topical antihistamines and anesthetics are sensitizers and therefore should be discouraged. Capsaicin works for localized pruritus.[4]

DIFFERENTIAL DIAGNOSIS

Pruritus

PRURITIC DERMATOLOGIC DISORDERS

Inflammatory Disorders

- Xerosis (asteatotic eczema)
- Atopic dermatitis (eczema, the "itch that rashes")
- Nummular eczema
- Dyshidrotic eczema
- Lichen simplex chronicus
- Contact dermatitis (chemical or allergic)
- Urticaria and dermatographism
- Lichen planus
- Psoriasis
- Aquagenic pruritus
- Rhus dermatitis (poison ivy and poison oak)
- Miliaria
- Neuropathic pruritus (nodular prurigo, brachioradial, or notalgia paresthetica)
- Bullous and prebullous pemphigoid
- Dermatitis herpetiformis
- Pruritic urticarial papules and plaques of pregnancy
- Polymorphic light eruption (and other photosensitive reactions)

Infectious Disorders

- Viral exanthema (e.g., varicella)
- Dermatophytes
- Folliculitis (hot tubs)
- Impetigo

Infestations

- Scabies
- Pediculosis
- Sea bather's eruption (jelly fish larvae)
- Insect bites (e.g., fleas, mites, bedbugs)
- Parasitic infections (e.g., onchocerciasis, echinococcosis, schistosomiasis)

Neoplastic Disorders

- Mycosis fungoides
- Mastocytosis

Environmental Disorders

- Sunburn
- Fiberglass dermatitis
- Pernio (chilblains)
- Winter itch (dry ambient environment, excessive bathing)
- Other (wool, hairs, fabric softeners, brighteners, other chemicals)
- Aquagenic pruritus (histamine mediated; lasts 1 hour after exposure to water)

SYSTEMIC DISORDERS COMMONLY ASSOCIATED WITH PRURITUS

Metabolic and Endocrine Disorders

- Diabetes mellitus (anogenital pruritus is more common)
- Postmenopausal estrogen withdrawal (anogenital and generalized)
- Adrenal insufficiency
- Carcinoid syndrome
- Hypothyroidism (secondary to dry skin in myxedema)
- Hyperthyroidism (secondary to elevated skin temperature)

Hematologic Disorders

- Polycythemia vera (typically water induced, or "bath itch")
- Iron deficiency anemia
- Paraproteinemia
- Waldenström's macroglobulinemia

Malignant Neoplasms

- Lymphoma (Hodgkin's) and leukemia
- Abdominal visceral carcinoma
- CNS tumors
- Multiple myeloma
- Mycosis fungoides

Hepatobiliary Disorders

- Primary biliary cirrhosis (from bile salts and associated substances)
- Biliary obstruction (cholestasis)
- Cholestasis of pregnancy

Renal Disorders

- Chronic renal failure (80% of patients on hemodialysis; can be from secondary hyperparathyroidism)

Parasitic Infestations

- Hookworm, onchocerciasis, ascariasis, trichinosis

Infections

- HIV (pruritus sometimes the primary presentation)

Psychologic States

- Delusions of parasitosis
- Neurotic excoriations (can be extensive)
- Psychogenic pruritus (anxiety induced)

MEDICATIONS THAT CAUSE PRURITUS

- Opiates and derivatives
- Aspirin
- Quinidine
- Phenothiazines*
- Tolbutamide*
- Erythromycin estolate*
- Hormones* (e.g., anabolic steroids, estrogens, progestins, testosterone)
- Vitamin B complex
- Psoralen plus ultraviolet A light
- Antimalarials
- Subclinical sensitivity to any drug

*Via cholestasis.

Oral therapy consists of H_1-antagonists such as diphenhydramine (25 to 50 mg q 6 hr) or hydroxyzine (25 to 50 mg q 4-6 hr), which can be beneficial, especially at bedtime. Sedative side effects are common, which may explain their therapeutic benefit. Nonsedating antihistamines have not been proven to be effective.[5] The oral tricyclic antidepressant doxepin (25 mg every night up to 300 mg daily [in divided doses]) is a potent H_1- and H_2-receptor blocker that has anxiolytic effects. Mirtazapine (15 to 45 mg nightly) or paroxetine (10 to 20 mg nightly) have been useful in case reports.[1] Opiate antagonists such as naltrexone (50 to 150 mg daily) have been used for various causes of pruritus with success.[6] Oral activated charcoal is a safe, effective therapy for uremic pruritus.[7] Cholestyramine (4 g once to three times daily) is effective for pruritus caused by cholestasis, but it can have untoward gastrointestinal side effects and should be taken with vitamin K and multivitamin supplements. Colestipol works similarly but is better tolerated. In refractory cases of cholestatic pruritus, ursodiol, phenobarbital, and rifampin have been used with good results.[3] Gabapentin (200 to 300 mg nightly) is effective for dialysis patients. Patients with liver disease should have diets high in polyunsaturated fatty acids. Thalidomide (50 to 200 mg daily) is used in some circumstances, but monitoring for neuropathy and thrombosis is necessary. Danazol is effective therapy for myeloproliferative disorders and other systemic disorders.[8] Aspirin or cyproheptadine (4 mg t.i.d.) have both been shown to help patients with pruritus from polycythemia vera. Ultraviolet B (UVB), sunlight, and topical clobetasol are all efficacious in pruritus associated with HIV disease.[4]

COMPLICATIONS

Secondary skin lesions from scratching and secondary infections are common. Other complications include an undiagnosed underlying systemic illness or untoward side effects from drug therapy.

INDICATIONS FOR REFERRAL OR HOSPITALIZATION

Consultation with a dermatologist should be considered for intractable cases of pruritus or when the cause remains unknown after the preliminary evaluation and follow-up. UVB phototherapy is effective for uremic pruritus (i.e., those receiving dialysis). Psoralen plus ultraviolet A, intralesional corticosteroid therapy, or other methods may be used. Other approaches include the use of acupuncture, transcutaneous electrical nerve stimulation, mechanical vibratory stimulation, or referral to a pain relief clinic. Psychotherapeutic interventions have been shown to be beneficial in some patients.[9] If a systemic disorder is discovered, referral to an endocrinologist, hematologist, oncologist, gastroenterologist, nephrologist, psychiatrist, or other subspecialist may be in order.

PATIENT AND FAMILY EDUCATION AND HEALTH PROMOTION

Lifestyle interventions to alleviate pruritus require a concerted effort at patient education to identify factors that provoke or worsen itching. Avoiding dry skin through the use of humidifiers, limited bathing, mild soaps, and emollients is critical. Elimination of wool and other clothing irritants, stress reduction measures, and instructions on medication side effects are also very helpful in the management of pruritus.

REFERENCES

1. Twycross R, Greaves MW, Handwerker H, and others: Itch: scratching more than the surface, *Q J Med* 96:7-26, 2003.
2. Hiramanek N: Itch: a symptom of occult disease, *Aust Fam Phys* 33(7):495-499, 2004.
3. Millikan LE: Treating pruritus: what's new in safe relief of symptoms? *Postgrad Med* 99:173, 1996.
4. Rupp JF, Kaplan DL: Pruritus: causes-cures, parts 1, 2, and 3, *Consultant* Nov:3157, 1999; Dec:3367, 1999; Feb:321, 2000.
5. Crownover BK, Jamieson B, Mott TF: Clinical inquiries: first- or second-generation antihistamines: which are more effective at controlling pruritus? *J Fam Pract* 53:742-744, 2004.
6. Wolfhagen FH, Sternieri E, Hop WC, and others: Oral naltrexone treatment for cholestatic pruritus: a double blind, placebo-controlled study, *Gastroenterology* 113:1264-1269, 1997.
7. Lugon JR: Uremic pruritus: a review, *Hemodial Int* 9(2):180-188, 2005.
8. Kolodny L, Horstman LL, Sevin BU, and others: Danazol relieves refractory pruritus associated with myeloproliferative disorders and other diseases, *Am J Hematol* 51:112-116, 1996.
9. Kimyai-Asadi A, Usman A: The role of psychological stress in skin disease, *J Cutan Med Surg* 5:140-145, 2001.

CHAPTER 67

Psoriasis

Catherine E. Carter

DEFINITION AND EPIDEMIOLOGY

Psoriasis is a papulosquamous eruption characterized by well-circumscribed erythematous macular and papular lesions with loosely adherent silvery white scale. It is a chronic, unpredictable disorder that is characterized by remissions and exacerbations throughout the life span. First episodes often appear in young adulthood, but they can appear later in life as well. Stress, anxiety, and illness often precede flares. Streptococcal pharyngitis (sore throat) and some drug therapies (beta blockers, antimalarial agents, systemic steroids, angiotensin-converting enzyme inhibitors)[1-3] may precipitate or exacerbate an outbreak. Time lost from school and work, as well as the emotional and financial constraints on families, mandates cost-effective and convenient treatments. Symptoms can be treated; however, as yet there is no cure. Remissions are common and can last for short periods or years, although in some persons the condition can be refractory.[4]

Psoriasis is an inflammatory disorder whose course is unpredictable. The exact cause is unknown; however, a genetic component appears to exist. The immune system triggers acceleration in growth and inflammation of skin cells. Although most patients experience localized plaques, extensive involvement may develop and cause the patient and family great social, psychologic, and economic distress.

From 1% to 3% of the population is affected by psoriasis, with 25% to 45% of cases beginning after age 10 years.[5] Psoriasis affects both sexes equally. Psoriasis is rare in infants; however, it does seem to be passed genetically and thus a familial tendency can increase risk. Interestingly, many individuals cannot recall family members who had the disease.

PATHOPHYSIOLOGY

Clinical trials performed around 1980 showed a link between the immune system and psoriasis. Bone marrow transplant patients who received the immunosuppressant drug cyclosporine showed dramatic clearing of any psoriasis.[3] More recent studies with monoclonal antibodies that target specific T-cell antagonists have also shown improvement in patients with severe psoriasis.[6]

Normal immune systems function in a protective manner. The body has antigen-presenting cells. These cells activate an immune response by T lymphocytes and dendritic cells to destroy antigens. T cells release cytokines. Cytokines are proteins that carry messages to activate the immune system and the body defenses against "invaders" or triggers.[3,7] Immune system disorders cause aberrant function in the body's fight against foreign proteins, viruses, and bacteria. In psoriasis this is reflected as increased proliferation of skin cells and the rapid deposition of dead cells on the skin surface, which form plaques. The normal 20- to 28-day skin cell life-to-death cycle increases rapidly to 3 or 4 days. Scaly papules and plaques form and collect on the surface in well-demarcated lesions. The lesions have an erythematous base with silvery white plaques that are adherent. The dermis is highly vascular, and tiny bleeding points are revealed if the scales are removed (Auspitz's sign).[2]

CLINICAL PRESENTATION AND PHYSICAL EXAMINATION

Psoriasis is a clinical diagnosis based on the characteristic silvery white scales (Color Plate 23). Common sites include the elbows, knees, scalp, genitals, and intergluteal cleft. In contrast to adult psoriasis, childhood psoriasis often involves the face. Many patients exhibit nail dystrophies (Color Plate 22), including pitting, yellowing of the distal portion, separation of the nail plate (onycholysis), and thickening of the entire nail (hyperkeratosis).

Cutaneous trauma can induce psoriasis 1 to 3 weeks after injury. This isomorphic response, also known as Koebner's phenomenon, occurs in a linear fashion along the lines of a scratch, abrasion, sunburn, or pressure.

Discrete scaly plaques that begin on the trunk and spread to the extremities, sparing the palms and soles, are indicative of guttate psoriasis. The word *guttate* is derived from the Latin word *gutta*, meaning "drop." Guttate psoriasis is seen after a streptococcal infection and is most common in adolescents. These patients are likely to develop psoriasis vulgaris (common, plaquelike psoriasis) later in life.

Erythroderma and pustular psoriasis are more serious forms of the disease. They are most common in patients older than 50 years and may be precipitated by infection and recent use of systemic steroids. Erythrodermic forms generally appear over a large portion of the body and can be precipitated by various treatments themselves. It can occur after treatment with systemic steroids or other toxic medication, emotional stress, or a severe illness.

Although most psoriatic lesions are asymptomatic, itching is variable. However, picking and scratching the lesions can produce Koebner's response, and the lesions worsen. Skin fold lesions tend to itch more than do common plaquelike lesions. The vulva is a common site for intense itching, or inverse psoriasis.[4]

In psoriatic arthritis, one or several joints are involved. Although rare in children, it is recognized with increasing frequency in patients younger than 16 years. It is most common in female patients, with the peak onset at age 9 to 12 years. The clinical presentation is similar to that of any inflammatory arthritis.[5,8] The rheumatoid factor is negative, and the distal interphalangeal joints are common sites for arthalgias.[2] Psoriatic arthritis in adults is slightly more prevalent in men.[5]

DIAGNOSTICS

The presence of silvery scales on red, erythematous plaques is characteristic; therefore the diagnosis is based on presentation.

DIFFERENTIAL DIAGNOSIS

In children the plaques of psoriasis are thinner and less scaly than in adults with psoriasis and are often confused with seborrhea and fungal infections. Seborrhea on the scalp tends to be patchy, red, and a bit oilier in appearance. Psoriasis is more plaquelike with thick scales. Psoriasis generally appears on extensor surfaces, whereas atopic dermatitis is found on most flexor surfaces. Lichen planus papules have more of a purple hue, and patients exhibit Wickham's striae (lacy, reticular, criss-crossed whitish lines) on many lesions. Flat warts do not have scale on the surface. Guttate psoriasis is often confused with pityriasis rosea; however, it lacks the characteristic herald patch, and the scale is thicker and more diffuse in psoriasis. Changes in the nails are often confused with onychomycosis. Culturing for the presence of fungus will help establish the diagnosis. Yellow discoloration is common in both fungal and psoriatic changes, as is nail separation. The nails in psoriasis are not well formed, since debris collects underneath, again because of rapid shedding of the skin layers. This debris leads to failure in the integrity of the nail and the onycholysis.

DIFFERENTIAL DIAGNOSIS

Psoriasis

- Lichen planus
- Flat warts
- Pityriasis rosea
- Rheumatoid arthritis
- Seborrheic dermatitis
- Atopic dermatitis
- Fungal infections (in nails)

MANAGEMENT

Good control can be achieved; however, it requires meticulous and consistent home care. Present therapy is aimed at reducing epidermal proliferation and decreasing inflammation. Topical corticosteroids produce rapid resolution of plaques. Moderate- to high-potency topical glucocorticosteroids applied two or three times per day produce maximum benefit in 2 to 3 weeks. This is less messy than some treatments and can reduce pruritus. Tolerance can develop, and atrophy can occur with continued use over time. Occlusion with moist wraps can hasten the therapy on large or thick plaques. Thin layers of DuoDERM alone can be placed and left for 5 to 7 days. Some providers prefer to start here, thinking initial corticosteroid use can make later use of the other modalities less effective.[2]

Intralesional injections with a corticosteroid suspension produce satisfactory results after one or two injections; this treatment requires a dermatology referral. Limitation of this therapy is atrophy and obvious discomfort from injections.

Phototherapy in the form of ultraviolet B light therapy and psoralen plus ultraviolet A light is highly effective for recalcitrant psoriasis. Therapy in the structured environment of a dermatologist's office is of more therapeutic value than sunbathing. Care must be taken to avoid sunburn and resultant Koebner's phenomenon. Long-term therapy is often required, and skin should be monitored for changes. Skin cancer risk increases, especially in fair individuals, and patients should be advised to shield the eyes to prevent cataract risk with any phototherapy modality.

Scalp psoriasis requires softening and removing the scales. A combination of 3% salicylic acid in mineral oil, glycerin, or olive oil, or a mixture of phenol and sodium chloride, should be massaged into the scalp and left on for several hours or overnight. An appropriate tar shampoo should then be used. Daily use of this therapy will remove the scale and allow penetration of a corticosteroid lotion to reduce inflammation.[9]

Coal tar preparations are an effective treatment and were a mainstay of therapy for many years. Newer preparations are more pleasant but are considered only moderately effective. Tar preparations can cause folliculitis and stain the skin and clothing. Their use has largely been replaced by topical corticosteroids. Anthralin can be irritating if not thoroughly washed off the skin, stains the skin and clothing, and is difficult to apply.

Topical vitamin D (calcipotriene [Dovonex]) and retinoid (tazarotene [Tazorac]) preparations, applied once daily, may be as effective as topical corticosteroid treatments and can be used in combination with steroids and phototherapy. These topical treatments reduce cell proliferation and induce remissions.

Oral retinoids (etretinate [Tegison], acitretin [Soriatane]) are useful for pustular and erythrodermic psoriasis. However, they have side effects similar to those of isotretinoin and should be used with caution in women of childbearing age because they are teratogenic. In addition, their effects on growing bones limit their use in children.

Methotrexate is an antimetabolite that is highly effective in treating severe, recalcitrant psoriasis and psoriatic arthritis. Its side effects include mucous membrane ulcers, lowered platelet and leukocyte counts, elevated liver enzyme levels, and gastrointestinal disturbances. It should be reserved for patients unresponsive to other therapies and for those with psoriatic arthritis.[10] Methotrexate and retinoid therapy should be co-managed with a dermatologist.

Cyclosporine is efficacious; however, it is also limited in use because of its potential nephrotoxicity. Relapse is also common once therapy is stopped. A dermatologist should manage patients who require cyclosporine therapy.

Combination therapy with topical agents, oral agents, and phototherapy is common. Even in patients maintained on topical treatments alone, it is useful to use multiple agents simultaneously for their synergistic effects. If more than 20% to 30% of the body is involved, generally the phototherapies and more systemic treatment are required. For smaller flares or chronicity, early treatment with combination therapies centered on topical treatments can manage the disease and minimize risk.

Guttate psoriasis should be treated with oral antibiotics to eliminate the streptococcal infection, in addition to topical preparations to reduce the scale and inflammation. Antistreptolysin levels should be monitored and elevations treated until remission.

Oral steroids should be used with caution because they can induce a pustular flare. They may be useful in controlling persistent erythroderma; however, they are not indicated in the treatment of psoriasis.

Newer classes of drugs are currently under study for use in psoriasis. Some of these classes are the monoclonal antibody drugs and the recombinant human tumor necrosis factor receptor formulations. Several are showing great promise; however, the side effects are still being studied and may limit usage.[3] Research is promising, but adherence to protocols and tracking of side effects to establish efficacy are important.

COMPLICATIONS

Complications are usually related to infection. Scratching can introduce bacteria from beneath fingernails into lesions. Guttate psoriasis, erythrodermic psoriasis, and pustular psoriasis are also potential complications. Both erythrodermic psoriasis and pustular psoriasis are rare; however, serious sequelae, including congestive heart failure and sepsis, are potential hazards. Other complications are generally secondary to treatment. These can include atrophy of skin with corticosteroid use, the risk with phototherapy of skin cancer and cataracts if the eyes are not protected, and the side effects on the metabolic profiles of strong antimetabolites or retinoids.

INDICATIONS FOR REFERRAL OR HOSPITALIZATION

A patient with recalcitrant or unresponsive psoriasis should be referred to a dermatologist for management with phototherapy and oral therapies. If a dermatology referral is not possible, an internist may be appropriate for oral therapy. Psoriatic arthritis often follows psoriasis by about 10 years. Early referral, close monitoring, and co-management with an internist or dermatologist can help identify appropriate patients to prevent the further debilitation to psoriatic arthritis in susceptible individuals. Referral to a rheumatologist or internist for patients with psoriatic arthritis is advised.

PATIENT AND FAMILY EDUCATION AND HEALTH PROMOTION

It is crucial for the patient and family to understand the chronic nature of psoriasis, as well as the genetic and environmental factors. Adherence to the prescribed regimen is necessary for effective treatment; however, this requires meticulous and consistent home care.

Patients should understand the use of moisturizers and lubricants to maintain control. Education regarding treatment modalities and emotional support for families, as well as patients, is an important part of treatment. Patients may contact the National Psoriasis Foundation (http://www.psoriasis.org), a not-for-profit organization dedicated to research, education, and support. Research is ongoing in the study of psoriasis. Patients and providers need to stay abreast of ongoing studies and treatment modalities and encourage ongoing collaborative practice across disciplines to meet the needs of these patients.

REFERENCES

1. Lehne R: *Pharmacology for nursing care,* ed 6, Philadelphia, 2006, Saunders.
2. Habif T: *Clinical dermatology: a color guide to diagnosis and therapy*, ed 4, St Louis, 2003, Mosby.
3. Gottlieb AB: Psoriasis: emerging therapeutic strategies, *Nat Rev Drug Discov* 4(1):19-34, 2005.
4. Tierney LM, McPhee SJ, Papadakis MA: *Current medical diagnosis and treatment 1997*, ed 36, Stamford, Conn, 1997, Appleton & Lange.
5. Vernon P: The heartbreak of psoriasis: no laughing matter, *J Pediatr Health Care* 11:32-33, 1997.
6. Bowcock A, Krueger J: Getting under the skin: the immunogenetics of psoriasis, *Nature Rev Immunol* 5(9):699-711, 2005.
7. National Psoriasis Foundation: *Immune system involvement,* retrieved Dec 12, 2006, from http://www.psoriasis.org/research/known/immune.php.
8. Paller AS, Mancini AJ: *Hurwitz's Clinical pediatric dermatology*, ed 3, Philadelphia, 2005, Saunders.
9. Arndt K, Bowers KE: *Manual of dermatologic therapeutics*, ed 6, Philadelphia, 2001, Lippincott Williams & Wilkins.
10. Weston WL, Lane AT, Morrelli JG: *Color textbook of pediatric dermatology*, ed 2, St Louis, 1996, Mosby.

CHAPTER 68

Purpura

Joanne Sandberg-Cook

DEFINITION AND EPIDEMIOLOGY

Purpura is a hemorrhaging into the skin. The size of the bleeding vessel determines the size of the lesion, which in turn may provide clues to the cause. Petechiae are lesions less than 3 mm (0.1 inch) in diameter; these indicate capillary bleeding. Lesions ranging from 3 mm to 1 cm (0.1 to 0.4 inches) are often referred to as *purpura*. Lesions larger than 1 cm are referred to as *ecchymoses*. All show a predilection for the limbs. Purpura is divided into two groups: inflammatory (palpable) and noninflammatory. Noninflammatory purpura is further divided into hemostatic defects, nonpalpable purpura, and nonhemostatic defects (vascular purpura).[1]

PATHOPHYSIOLOGY

Purpura is characterized by an extravasation of red blood cells into the dermis from small cutaneous vessels. Hemosiderin or hematoidin may be present if the purpura is chronic; this causes a characteristic red or brown discoloration. Purpura may be oval or round or irregularly outlined; it may be flat or raised (palpable) as a result of edema or induration.

Palpable purpura consists of raised, erythematous lesions, which do not blanch when the skin is pressed with a glass slide. Dilated superficial capillaries, in which the blood remains confined within the vessels, do blanch when pressed, thereby distinguishing them from true purpura.

Extravasation of blood from the vessel depends on the integrity of the blood vessel, which in turn depends on the strength of the vessel, the transmural pressure gradient that drives blood out of the vessel, and the competence of the mechanism that combats the basal level of vascular trauma.[1]

CLINICAL PRESENTATION

Because purpura is a symptom of many systemic diseases, these lesions seldom are seen without other symptoms. A review of systems should include an inquiry into other bleeding sites, abnormally heavy menstrual bleeding, trauma, recent infection (including sexually transmitted diseases), exposure to ticks or a tick bite, and recent travel to areas where Rocky Mountain spotted fever or Lyme's disease is endemic or epidemic. A complete medication history (including over-the-counter medications and allergies) should be taken. Any history of autoimmune disease or other serious illnesses such as leukemia or lymphoma should be noted. Recent complaints of fever, chills, arthralgias, and myalgias should be noted.

PHYSICAL EXAMINATION

The skin is the focus of the physical examination. The size, location, and shape of the lesions should be documented. Bullae and ulcerations can develop within any lesion larger than petechiae.[2] Lesions should be palpated for swelling (palpable purpura) or flatness against the skin. Palpable purpura is generally associated with inflammation of the vessel (Color Plate 24) (see Chapter 237). A glass slide pressed against the lesion determines whether it is blanchable, thereby differentiating it from erythema or dilated superficial capillaries.[1] Excoriation may imply pruritus.

The remainder of the general examination includes an oral examination to look for lesions of the gums or tongue and a joint examination to look for swelling, inflammation, or deformities that would suggest connective tissue disease. Fever, nuchal rigidity, organomegaly, or a new heart murmur may imply serious systemic disease or infection.

Observations of weight, nutritional status, or skin turgor may suggest nutritional deficiencies. Evidence of trauma (healing bruises, fractures) may indicate ongoing trauma as a cause.

DIAGNOSTICS

Laboratory studies help differentiate between inflammatory and noninflammatory purpura. (Inflammatory purpura [vasculitis] is discussed in Chapter 237.) A CBC with a platelet count (not an estimate) is most helpful. An erythrocyte sedimentation rate or C-reactive protein can be beneficial in excluding an inflammatory cause. A bleeding time, platelet count, prothrombin time, partial thromboplastin time, and International Normalized Ratio will determine the presence of coagulopathies. BUN, creatinine, and liver function tests are necessary to exclude organ disease. Immune studies to exclude autoimmune diseases such as lupus, rheumatoid arthritis, cryoglobulinemias, or scleroderma may be indicated depending on other physical findings and symptoms.

DIAGNOSTICS

Purpura

LABORATORY
- CBC and differential
- BUN
- Creatinine
- LFTs
- Platelet count
- ESR
- Bleeding time
- PT/PTT
- International Normalized Ratio
- Rheumatoid factor*
- Antinuclear antibodies*
- Antineutrophil cytoplasmic antibody*

*If indicated.

DIFFERENTIAL DIAGNOSIS

The differential diagnosis of purpura is extensive. Inflammatory and noninflammatory causes of purpura should be differentiated. Inflammatory purpura is most often palpable and is associated with the vasculitides. These syndromes can be life threatening and require prompt treatment in conjunction with a specialist (see Chapter 237). Causes of noninflammatory purpura include serious infectious diseases, medication hypersensitivity, trauma, vascular disorders, and bleeding disorders.

Systemic infections such as HIV/AIDS, cytomegalovirus, hepatitis B and C, herpes zoster, Lyme's disease (see Chapter 250), Rocky Mountain spotted fever, meningitis, syphilis, and gonococcemia have been associated with purpura.[2] Subacute bacterial endocarditis may manifest with fever, petechial skin rash, and a new heart murmur.

DIFFERENTIAL DIAGNOSIS

Purpura

INFLAMMATORY (PALPABLE)
Vasculitis
Cryoglobulinemia

NONINFLAMMATORY
Hemostatic Defects
Platelet abnormalities
Coagulation abnormalities

Nonpalpable Purpura
Increased pressure
- Venous stasis

Decreased vessel integrity
- Senile purpura
- Steroid excess
- Vitamin C deficiency
- Hormonal

Trauma
- Physical injury
- Solar injury

Infectious
- Bacterial (meningococcemia)
- Viral
- Rickettsial (Lyme's disease, Rocky Mountain spotted fever)

Embolic
Atheroembolic
- Cholesterol

Neoplastic
Leukemia
Lymphoma

Allergic
Medications
Contact

Thrombotic
Disseminated intravascular coagulation
Purpura fulminans
Antiphospholipid syndrome
Idiopathic thrombocytopenic purpura

Noninfectious presentations are often related to medications, including the long-term use of oral steroids and fluorinated topical steroids. Drug-induced vasculitis, also known as hypersensitivity vasculitis or leukocytoclastic vasculitis, is the most common cause of palpable purpura and can occur at any time during the course of the medication. These allergic reactions to medication may be associated with fever, arthralgia, and urticaria.[2] The most common causative agents are antibiotics, sulfonamides, thiazide diuretics, phenytoin, and allopurinol. Nonsteroidal antiinflammatory medications, including aspirin, can also cause petechial skin rashes.[3] Heparin, low–molecular weight heparin, and warfarin (Coumadin) can cause bleeding, which can result in purpura.

Trauma to blood vessels is initially seen as classic bruising, often involving the extremities, feet, hands (in the case of repetitive pounding), or face. The lesions associated with child abuse may involve bruising from pinching or grabbing or palpebral conjunctivae resulting from strangulation or smothering.[1] Senile purpura manifests as large ecchymoses on the extensor surfaces of the arms and hands of (usually) an older adult. Such lesions occur as a result of the skin thinning associated with age, sun damage, or prolonged steroid use in combination with minor trauma or shearing.[4] Laboratory studies are normal, and the patient should be reassured that the lesions are benign.

A variety of syndromes associated with vascular diseases can cause purpura. Atheroemboli secondary to cholesterol can cause petechiae, purpura, nodules, ulceration, and occlusion leading to gangrene. Fat emboli that occur 2 or 3 days after severe trauma can be seen with petechiae of the upper extremity, thorax, and conjunctivae.[1] Disseminated intravascular coagulation (DIC) demonstrates both thrombotic and hemorrhagic features. Purpura fulminans is a rare complication of DIC and results in hemorrhagic necrosis of the skin.[3] Palpable purpura may, rarely, be the initial presentation of a paraneoplastic syndrome, especially lymphoproliferative disease.[5]

Idiopathic thrombocytopenic purpura (ITP) is an acquired disorder of platelet aggregation in the microcirculation that can lead to bleeding. The bleeding associated with ITP can range from severe to only petechiae and easy bruising. Generally defined by a platelet count of less than 50,000/mm^3, this disorder can be seen in all age-groups. There is an association with von Willebrand's factor.[5] Treatment is usually reserved for those with a platelet count of less than 50,000/mm^3 who are at risk of bleeding. High-dose steroids either by mouth or intravenously are the first-line treatment. Some patients require IV immunoglobulins.[6] Splenectomy is reserved for those in whom medical treatment fails to raise platelet counts over 50,000/mm^3.[7]

Petechiae and ecchymoses are common.[3] Stasis dermatitis manifests with petechiae caused by capillary injury. This results from chronic venous stasis caused by valve incompetence. Later stages of chronic venous stasis are associated with an accumulation of hemosiderin, leading to the characteristic brown discoloration of the lower extremities.[3]

Miscellaneous causes of purpura include hemorrhagic gingivitis or stomatitis related to vitamin C deficiency (scurvy). Young girls occasionally tend to bruise easily because of hormonal changes. A tendency toward early stroke, multiple miscarriages, or thrombocytopenia may be associated with the presence of antiphospholipid antibodies, sometimes known as lupus anticoagulant. HIV/AIDS and cancers, including lymphomas and leukemias, can produce petechial or purpuric lesions.[2] Finally, defects in clotting factors or platelet abnormalities, including the quantity and quality of platelets, can lead to cutaneous bleeding (see Chapter 227).

MANAGEMENT

Treatment of purpura is directed toward the etiology. Patients with disorders of platelet count or function should be referred to a hematologist for possible bone marrow biopsy. Patients with palpable purpura should be advised that an extensive evaluation, including a skin biopsy, may be indicated. A referral to appropriate specialists, usually hematologists or rheumatologists, is indicated.

Patients with stasis dermatitis may benefit from the application of 1% hydrocortisone cream to help with the associated pruritus. A reassurance that the lesions are benign is needed for young women who bruise easily because of hormonal changes and for older patients with senile purpura.

LIFE SPAN CONSIDERATIONS

Purpura associated with hormonal change is most often seen in young women. Senile purpura is primarily a disease of older adults but can result from chronic steroid use. Antiphospholipid antibodies are most commonly found in women of childbearing years, but men and older women can also be affected. The vasculitides are most often seen in middle-aged patients, with several notable exceptions (see Chapter 237).

COMPLICATIONS

Complications of the skin lesions themselves include the formation of bullae, skin breakdown, and ulcer formation. Ulcers are slow to heal and can involve a large area. Necrosis of the skin, especially the fingertips, can be a complication of vascular lesions.

INDICATIONS FOR REFERRAL OR HOSPITALIZATION

Any patient with fever and a petechial skin rash should be hospitalized to exclude or evaluate life-threatening infection, systemic vasculitis, or neoplasm. This is especially necessary if the patient has a connective tissue disease such as lupus or rheumatoid arthritis, has a malignancy, or has been exposed to meningitis. Patients with acute bleeding disorders may require hospitalization to control bleeding and for transfusion (see Chapter 227). All patients with palpable purpura should be referred to a hematologist or rheumatologist for evaluation and treatment recommendations.

PATIENT EDUCATION AND HEALTH PROMOTION

Medications that may contribute to bleeding should be avoided unless the patient is advised to continue them as part of a treatment plan. Patients with stasis should be advised to avoid tight-fitting garments and prolonged standing. Chronic use of steroid creams or ointments should be discouraged because it leads to skin thinning and increased susceptibility to minor trauma.

REFERENCES

1. Lichtman MA, Beutler E, Kipps TJ, and others: *Williams hematology*, ed 7, New York, 2006, McGraw-Hill.
2. Braverman IM: *Skin signs of systemic disease*, ed 3, Philadelphia, 1998, Saunders.
3. Weedon D: *Skin pathology*, New York, 1997, Churchill Livingstone.
4. Soter N: Vasculitis. In Arnot KA, Wintroub BU, Robinson JK, and others, editors: *Primary care dermatology*, Philadelphia, 1997, Saunders.
5. Hunder GG: *Hypersensitivity vasculitis in adults*, retrieved Feb 3, 2006, from http://www.uptodate.com.
6. Tanoue K, Okita K, Akahoshi T, and others: Laparoscopic splenectomy for hematologic diseases, *Surgery* 131:S318, 2002.
7. George JN: *Treatment and prognosis of idiopathic thrombocytopenic purpura in adults*, retrieved Feb 3, 2006, from http://www.uptodate.com.

CHAPTER 69

Scabies

Eileen M. Deignan

DEFINITION AND EPIDEMIOLOGY

Scabies is an infection caused by infestation of the *Sarcoptes scabiei* mite. It can affect people of all ages and is more common in crowded living conditions and institutional facilities.

PATHOPHYSIOLOGY

The scabies mite is not visible to the unaided eye. The female mite is responsible for the infestations. The mite is oval and has four pairs of legs. It burrows into the stratum corneum and lays up to 38 eggs for 1 to 2 months before dying. The eggs hatch in approximately 1 week and reach maturity in 3 weeks, starting a new cycle.[1] The intense pruritus experienced with scabies infestation is a hypersensitivity reaction to the mites. It usually begins 2 to 4 weeks after infection in a person who was not previously sensitized. Pruritus may begin within a day of reinfestation in a previously sensitized person. Scabies is usually acquired through close personal contact, although the mite can survive off the human host for up to 3 days.

CLINICAL PRESENTATION AND PHYSICAL EXAMINATION

The clinical presentation of scabies is variable. Most commonly there are minimum findings in the setting of intractable pruritus. The skin lesions of scabies can be classified into two categories: lesions at the site of infestation and lesions secondary to hypersensitivity to the mite. Intraepidermal burrows are linear or serpiginous ridges that are produced by the infesting female mite. Common sites of burrows are the interdigital spaces of the hands, flexures of the wrists and arms, genitals, feet, buttocks, and axillae (Color Plate 25). A hypersensitivity reaction to the mites can be manifested as urticaria, eczematous dermatitis, and scabetic nodules. Excoriations, lichen simplex chronicus, and secondary infection may result from scratching.

DIAGNOSTICS

The classic burrow, a straight or S-shaped ridge 5 to 20 mm (0.2 to 0.8 inch) long, is present less than 20% of the time. Definitive confirmation is made with a "scabies prep." A drop of mineral oil is placed on a burrow, and the lesion is scraped with a no. 15 blade. The sample is viewed under a microscope and examined for mites, eggs, or feces.[2] There are usually only a few scabies mites on an infected patient. As a result, several areas may need to be sampled to get a confirmatory result.

DIAGNOSTICS

Scabies

LABORATORY
Microscopic examination for mites or eggs

DIFFERENTIAL DIAGNOSIS

Scabies may easily be mistaken for other skin disorders. The differential diagnosis should include contact dermatitis, asteatotic dermatitis, insect bites, animal scabies, seborrheic dermatitis, and psoriasis.

MANAGEMENT

Topical application of 5% permethrin cream (Elimite) is the treatment of choice. The cream should be applied from the neck down, giving attention to the interdigital webs, axillae, umbilicus, gluteal cleft, genitals, areas under the nails, and soles of the feet. Because scabies can infest the hairline of older adults, the product is massaged into the skin from head to toe in these patients. The medication should be left on for 8 to 12 hours and then washed off.[3,4] The treatment should be repeated in 1 week. This product can be safely used again in 1 week because it is rapidly metabolized.[3,4]

An important change in treatment guidelines is that lindane (Kwell) is no longer recommended for the treatment of scabies. Absorption of lindane is 10 times higher than that of permethrin. There have been reports of seizures with repeated exposure.

Persistent, pruritic papules and an eczematous dermatitis may result from both infestation and treatment. Lubrication and topical corticosteroids are used to treat the inflammation, and antihistamines are used to treat the pruritus. A secondary infection may result from scratching. Pustules, impetigo, and ecthyma should be treated with appropriate antibiotics.

Ivermectin is an antihelminthic medication useful for treating scabies. It is effective and relatively easy to use because it is administered orally. Because ivermectin is an oral medication that does not need to be absorbed by the skin, it is useful for patients with crusted scabies; however, at this time ivermectin is not FDA approved for treatment of scabies. The dose of ivermectin is 200 mcg/kg. The average adult dose is 12 to 18 mg, administered as a single, one-time dose. Some sources suggest administering a second dose 2 weeks later.[5,6]

DIFFERENTIAL DIAGNOSIS

Scabies

- Atopic dermatitis
- Insect bites
- Pediculosis
- Pityriasis rosea
- Animal scabies
- Seborrheic dermatitis
- Syphilis
- Contact dermatitis
- Psoriasis

COMPLICATIONS

Superinfection is a potential complication. Acute glomerulonephritis has been associated with streptococcal superinfection.

INDICATIONS FOR REFERRAL OR HOSPITALIZATION

Elimite is not approved by U.S. Food and Drug Administration for use in infants less than 2 months old. Whether permethrin is secreted in human milk is not known. Deaths have been associated with the use of ivermectin for scabies in older adults. Therefore this medication should be used with caution. Consultation with a physician or specialist is recommended if scabies is identified in these patients before a specific medication is chosen.[5]

PATIENT AND FAMILY EDUCATION

All household contacts should be identified and treated. All clothing and bedding must be washed in hot water and dried on the hot cycle, and stuffed sofas and chairs should be vacuumed. Materials that cannot be washed should be placed in a plastic bag for 1 week. Patients should be given written and verbal instructions. Recalcitrant infestation or persistent pruritus requires physician consultation.

REFERENCES

1. Weston WL, Lane AT, Morrelli JG: *Color textbook of pediatric dermatology,* ed 3, St Louis, 2002, Mosby.
2. Arndt K: *Manual of dermatologic therapeutics,* ed 6, New York, 2001, Lippincott Williams & Wilkins.
3. Paller AS, Mancini AJ: *Hurwitz's clinical pediatric dermatology,* ed 3, Philadelphia, 2005, Saunders.
4. Fox J: *Primary health care of children and adolescents,* ed 2, St Louis, 2002, Mosby.
5. Chouela E, Abeldano A, Pellerano G, and others: Diagnosis and treatment of scabies: a practical guide, *Am J Clin Dermatol* 3(1):9-18, 2002.
6. Chosidow O: Scabies, *N Engl J Med* 354:1718, 2006.

CHAPTER 70

Seborrheic Dermatitis

Eileen M. Deignan

DEFINITION AND EPIDEMIOLOGY

Seborrheic dermatitis is a chronic, common dermatosis. It is characterized by greasy, slightly erythematous scaling that occurs in areas with the highest concentration of sweat glands or sebaceous glands, including the scalp, face, and postauricular and intertriginous areas.[1]

PATHOPHYSIOLOGY

The cause of seborrheic dermatitis is unknown. Although an inflammatory reaction to *Malassezia furfur* has been postulated, it is possible that seborrheic dermatitis may be caused by yeast secondary to prolonged retention of sebum on the skin.[2,3]

CLINICAL PRESENTATION AND PHYSICAL EXAMINATION

Seborrheic dermatitis is seen in both young and old patients. In infants the most common presentation is yellow or brown scaling lesions on the scalp, which is called *cradle cap*. In adolescents and adults, another common presentation is dry, flaky scales on the scalp. This disorder is known as dandruff.

On the face and auricular area, seborrheic dermatitis is seen as greasy, erythematous, sharply marginated plaques. Polycyclic plaques are commonly seen on the sternal area. In the axillae and groin, the eruption manifests as more confluent plaques with a fine scale and less well-defined borders. This disorder may persist throughout life and may be worse during adolescence. Lesions are usually asymptomatic, although occasionally pruritus is present.[4]

DIAGNOSTICS AND DIFFERENTIAL DIAGNOSIS

The differential diagnosis is broad. More common diseases that can resemble seborrheic dermatitis include psoriasis, impetigo, dermatophytosis, tinea versicolor, intertriginous candidiasis, otitis externa, blepharitis, and systemic lupus erythematosus. Dermatophytosis, candidiasis, fungal otitis externa, and tinea versicolor can be differentiated from seborrhea with a potassium hydroxide scraping positive for hyphae. Psoriasis is often difficult to distinguish from seborrheic dermatitis. History and characteristic findings of psoriasis such as nail changes and lesions on the extensor surfaces help differentiate the two diseases.

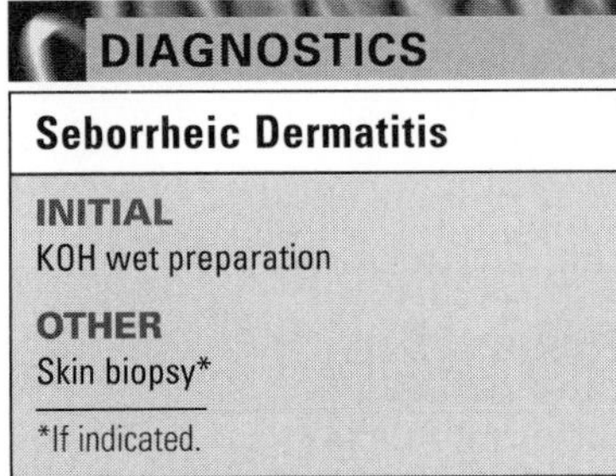

DIAGNOSTICS

Seborrheic Dermatitis

INITIAL
KOH wet preparation

OTHER
Skin biopsy*

*If indicated.

Less common diseases that can resemble seborrheic dermatitis include Langerhans' cell histiocytosis, acrodermatitis enteropathica, pemphigus foliaceus, and glucagonoma syndrome. If these disorders are considered, there should be consultation with a dermatologist.[2,5]

DIFFERENTIAL DIAGNOSIS

Seborrheic Dermatitis

- Dandruff
- Scabies
- Tinea
- Contact dermatitis
- Psoriasis
- Pemphigus
- Impetigo
- Dermatophytosis
- Candidal infection
- Langerhans' cell histiocytosis
- Acrodermatitis enteropathica
- Pemphigus foliaceus
- Glucagonoma syndrome

MANAGEMENT

Treatment depends on the location and severity of the disorder. In some cases, in patients who wash their hair only every week or less often, the condition will clear with more frequent washing. Antiseborrheic shampoos used three or four times a week will decrease eruptions or clear up the condition in some cases. Some patients may require a topical steroid in the form of a lotion, solution, or foam applied once a day after washing with an antiseborrheic shampoo. The topical steroid should be discontinued when the dermatitis improves. Mineral oil preparation massaged into the scalp and left to sit overnight will loosen the scales in the more severe, psoriasiform scalp seborrheic dermatitis.[4]

There are several options for therapy on the face. A simple solution is to use the lather of an antiseborrheic shampoo to wash the face on a daily basis. Alternatively, topical 2% ketoconazole cream or 10% sodium sulfacetamide wash can be used daily. If this intervention does not help, a mild topical steroid such as 1% or 2.5% hydrocortisone can be used daily until the eruption clears. The antiseborrheic shampoo, ketoconazole cream, or sodium sulfacetamide wash should be continued for maintenance. Similar therapies can be used for eruptions on the chest and in intertriginous areas.[6] Secondary bacterial or candidal infections should be treated with antibiotic or antifungal agents.

COMPLICATIONS

Secondary candidal infections and bacterial infections may occur, especially around the eyes and in intertriginous areas. These should be treated with appropriate antifungal or antibiotic medications. Periorificial dermatitis is a papular eruption that can occur around the eyes, nose, and mouth as a result of topical steroid overuse on the face. If this eruption occurs, topical steroids should be tapered off.

INDICATIONS FOR REFERRAL OR HOSPITALIZATION

Patients with unresponsive seborrheic dermatitis should be referred to a dermatologist for further workup. As indicated previously, several dermatoses can resemble seborrheic dermatitis but will not respond to the same therapies.

PATIENT AND FAMILY EDUCATION

Seborrheic dermatitis is chronic and recurrent. Proper use of antiseborrheic preparations several days per week will usually control the disorder.

REFERENCES

1. Paller AS, Mancini AJ: *Hurwitz's clinical pediatric dermatology*, ed 3, Philadelphia, 2005, Saunders.
2. Dershewitz RA: *Ambulatory pediatric care,* ed 3, Philadelphia, 1999, Lippincott-Raven.
3. Arndt K, Bowers KE: *Manual of dermatologic therapeutics*, ed 6, Philadelphia, 2001, Lippincott Williams & Wilkins.
4. Odom RB, James WD, Berger TG: *Andrew's diseases of the skin,* ed 9, Philadelphia, 2000, Saunders
5. Weston WL, Lane AT, Morrelli JG: *Color textbook of pediatric dermatology,* ed 2, St Louis, 1996, Mosby.
6. Gupta AK, Nicol K, Batra R: Role of antifungal agents in the treatment of seborrheic dermatitis, *Am J Clin Dermatol* 5(6):417-422, 2004.

CHAPTER 71

Stasis Dermatitis

Nancy W. Knee

DEFINITION AND EPIDEMIOLOGY

Stasis dermatitis is an eczematous eruption, inflammation, or chronic dermatitis of the skin of the lower extremities that may be acute, subacute, or chronic and recurrent.[1] The condition is usually associated with chronic venous insufficiency, and ulceration is a potential complication.[2] The condition is most often seen in persons over 50 years of age and is more common in women than in men.

PATHOPHYSIOLOGY

Stasis dermatitis is a recalcitrant condition related to venous incompetence associated with valve destruction. Valve leaflets become constricted and are unable to prevent venous regurgitation. This condition results in ischemia of the vasculature, skin, and supporting structures in the subcutaneous and dermal layers.[3] Perivascular fibrin deposits and small-vessel vasoconstriction may be contributing factors.[4]

CLINICAL PRESENTATION AND PHYSICAL EXAMINATION

The hallmark sign of stasis dermatitis is bronzing (hemosiderin staining) of the affected skin. The eruption can be unilateral or bilateral and is initially localized to the ankle (Color Plate 26). Edema, a common manifestation, progresses from distal to proximal, and varicose veins are often present.[1] The condition is often insidious; full manifestation of the signs and symptoms may take months. Patients may be initially seen with mild pruritus, xerosis, a scaly and erythematous rash, cutaneous atrophy, and bulla formation. The skin may be cyanotic when the extremity is in a dependent position. Secondary bacterial infection (usually staphylococcal) ensues, and painful ulceration eventually occurs.[4] Often there is a history of deep vein thrombosis.

DIAGNOSTICS

Doppler ultrasound and a venogram are used to diagnose venous insufficiency. Ulcers should be cultured for bacterial infection if indicated.

DIAGNOSTICS

Stasis Dermatitis

LABORATORY
Wound culture*

IMAGING
Doppler ultrasound or venogram for suspected deep vein thrombosis*

*If indicated.

DIFFERENTIAL DIAGNOSIS

Stasis Dermatitis

- Arterial insufficiency
- Carcinoma
- Sickle cell anemia
- Necrobiosis lipoidica
- Pyoderma gangrenosum
- Contact dermatitis

DIFFERENTIAL DIAGNOSIS

Other causes of ulceration should be considered. These include arterial insufficiency, carcinoma, sickle cell anemia, necrobiosis lipoidica, pyoderma gangrenosum, and contact dermatitis (i.e., neomycin).[5]

MANAGEMENT

Treatment for stasis dermatitis is based on the extent and acuity of the medical condition. The leg should be elevated above the heart for 30 minutes of rest at least four times a day to promote venous return and diminish or prevent edema. The patient should be fitted for graduated compression hose, and topical emollients should be applied daily. Maintenance of optimum skin integrity entails avoidance of trauma, including hot water in showers or baths, and irritants such as lanolin, wool, and alcohol.[1] Mild soaps (e.g., Dove, Neutrogena) and adequate fluid intake should be encouraged. Systemic antibiotics are necessary for any cellulitis. Occasionally topical corticosteroids are indicated for pruritic, nonulcerated areas. A midpotency steroid can be used for a short time, with gradual reduction to a low-potency steroid cream. However, steroids should not be used if there are any signs of infection.

In the ulcerative phase, wet-to-dry normal saline dressings should be applied two to four times per day. Silver sulfadiazine may be applied between wet-to-dry dressings provided there is no known sulfa allergy.[2] Cultures should be obtained to guide management if there is infection. The wound should be kept free of necrosis. In some instances Dakin solution no. 1 (a hypochlorite solution) may be indicated, but consultation with a wound care specialist is recommended before instituting anything other than normal saline wet-to-dry dressing.[2] In select instances (e.g., small ulcerative areas that do not inhibit ambulation), a zinc gelatin bandage, Unna's paste boot, or absorptive dressing such as calcium alginate under a compression bandage may be used.[4] These devices should be changed every 2 or 3 days initially, then once or twice a week when the edema diminishes and the ulcer begins to heal.[4] Group V steroids should be applied to the periphery of the ulcer only; otherwise healing will be compromised.[1] Elevation and compression bandages should be used in conjunction with these therapies.

COMPLICATIONS

Ulceration or cellulitis may progress to osteomyelitis or pyoderma gangrenosum. Either of these conditions can cause significant morbidity and may even be fatal in compromised hosts.

INDICATIONS FOR REFERRAL OR HOSPITALIZATION

Ulcerations that are recalcitrant to therapy or that penetrate past the dermal layer require referral to a general surgeon or plastic surgeon for partial-thickness grafting and/or recommended ulcer treatments. Hospitalization is indicated for patients who require surgical intervention, lack the ability to perform medical therapies at home, or have infections that require IV antibiotics.

PATIENT AND FAMILY EDUCATION AND HEALTH PROMOTION

Patients need to receive instruction and often closely monitored assistance regarding the application of compression hose, topical medications, colloid paste, or special dressings. The appropriate use, side effects, interactions, and contraindications of antibiotics should be carefully explained. Patients with chronic stasis dermatitis need to understand the importance of keeping the legs elevated as much as possible. The need for good nutrition, supplemental vitamins when indicated, and weight reduction should be discussed.

REFERENCES

1. Wolff K, Johnson RA, Suurmond R: *Fitzpatrick's color atlas and synopsis of clinical dermatology: common and serious diseases,* ed 5, New York, 2005, McGraw-Hill.
2. Habif T, Campbell MJ, Quitadamo KA: *Skin disease: diagnosis and treatment,* St Louis, 2001, Mosby.
3. Beers MH, Porter RS, Jones TV: *The Merck manual,* ed 18, Rahway, NJ, 2006, Merck Research Laboratories.
4. Fenstermacher K, Hudson B: *Practice guidelines for family nurse practitioners,* Philadelphia, 1997, Saunders.
5. Habif T: *Clinical dermatology: a color guide to diagnosis and therapy,* Philadelphia, 2004, Mosby.

CHAPTER 72

Urticaria

Susan R. Tussey and
Maureen O'Hara Padden

DEFINITION AND EPIDEMIOLOGY

Urticaria, also referred to as hives, is caused by a vascular reaction that occurs in the upper dermis of the skin. It is characterized by the development of wheals on the body surface (Color Plate 27). Acute urticaria is defined as episodes of hives lasting less than 6 weeks, whereas chronic urticaria is defined as hives persisting for more than 6 weeks.

Chronic urticaria can be categorized as idiopathic or autoimmune. On the continuum of urticaria, deeper release of vasoactive mediators into lower dermal and subcutaneous layers of the skin causes angioedema, and severe symptoms can result.[1]

Physical urticaria, which accounts for 20% to 30% of idiopathic cases,[2] is a distinct form of urticaria caused by exposure to physical triggers such as mechanical or thermal triggers, water, or cold. The hives associated with physical urticaria typically fade within an hour, except in the case of pressure urticaria, in which case the hives take longer to develop and subsequently take longer to fade. In some cases there is an association between thyroid autoimmunity and urticaria.[3] There may be an autoimmune component in some patients with chronic urticaria. Historically, it was believed that urticaria could be associated with an underlying malignancy such as lymphoma, leukemia, or colon cancer, but limited evidence suggests no association.[4] An association between *Helicobacter pylori* and urticaria also has been suggested and is currently being researched without promising results. However, it is not recommended that providers screen or treat for *H. pylori* colonization in patients without gastrointestinal complaints.[1]

Urticaria is a common disorder, affecting an estimated 10% to 20% of the population at some time during their life.[5] In most cases it is relatively mild in presentation, albeit frustrating for the patient. In other cases, however, it represents part of a continuum that includes anaphylaxis and can be life threatening. Two thirds of all cases occur between the ages of 20 and 40 years, and there appears to be no racial predilection.[6] *Acute* urticaria is more common in young adults, children, and atopic individuals. This form of urticaria is most often due to exposure to food allergens, food additives, medications, or radiocontrast media. *Chronic* urticaria is more common in middle-aged women, occurs twice as often in women as in men, and does not show the same predilection for individuals with atopy[6]; 75% of all cases are idiopathic. Only 50% of cases of chronic urticaria remit within a year, and up to 40% of cases lasting longer than 6 months persist for 10 years or more.[7]

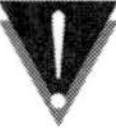

Immediate emergency department referral or physician consultation is indicated for urticaria patients with angioedema, respiratory failure, or hemodynamic compromise.

PATHOPHYSIOLOGY

Urticaria is an immediate hypersensitivity reaction that occurs after exposure to an allergen or antigen. Mast cells located in the loose connective tissue of the skin release histamine in response to the exposure. Histamine binds to H_1-receptors, leading to dilation of capillaries and vascular permeability. Arteriolar dilation leads to flaring around the lesions, and extravasation of fluid from the leaky capillaries leads to wheals, which are superficial itchy swellings in the skin. The histamine that is released causes the pruritus.[8] Deeper swellings of the skin and alimentary tract can occur in some cases; these swellings tend to be more painful than pruritic and are consistent with angioedema. Histamine also activates H_2-receptors, increasing gastric acid secretions.[9]

Mast cells can also be activated by IgE antibodies stimulated by foods, drugs, insect stings, latex, or animals. Alternatively, activation can occur directly from drugs, including opiates, NSAIDs, or radiocontrast media. Other cell mediators such as complement and neuropeptides (substance P) may be involved.

Recent laboratory research has implicated the complement system in chronic urticaria, particularly C5a, found on cutaneous cells but not pulmonary cells. This may explain the lack of pulmonary symptoms in chronic urticaria. Certain HLA class II associations are also being investigated as possible links to chronic autoimmune urticaria.[1,9]

CLINICAL PRESENTATION

Patients being seen with urticaria initially note pruritus followed by the development of hives. Lesions appear in crops that last for 2 to 3 hours and then disappear, only to flare up elsewhere later. They generally fade in less than 24 hours, leaving no trace. Episodes can occur as often as daily and in chronic urticaria can last for up to 2 years.

Important history can be simplified into the six *I*'s: *I*nfections, *I*ngestants (food), *I*njectants (drugs), *I*nsect stings, *I*nhalants (pollen), and *I*nternal disease. Latex allergy is an increasing cause of urticaria. Other historical factors to be elicited are exposure to heat, fever, or cold; exercise; change in menses; and emotional stress. In more severe cases of urticaria the patient may experience angioedema and complain of difficulty breathing.

Complementary and alternative medicine has increased use of "natural" herbal products that patients believe to be safe and may not mention in the history. Specific natural products identified in a voluntary Australian adverse drug reaction data base include echinacea, feverfew and willow, garlic, ginger, glucosamine, horseradish, royal jelly, valerian, and tea tree oil.[1,10]

PHYSICAL EXAMINATION

Physical examination reveals edematous pink or red wheals surrounded by a bright red flare. The center of the lesions may be clear or, rarely, may develop bullae. Lesions typically appear on the torso but may occur anywhere on the body. The patient with physical urticaria caused by exposure to some physical stimulus may show what is referred to as dermatographism on examination. Dermatographism is the development of a wheal-and-flare reaction when the skin is stroked with a pen or other physical stimulus. In severe cases of urticaria with angioedema, there may be swelling of the face or oropharynx and deeper swelling in the dermis.

DIAGNOSTICS

Laboratory tests are generally of little value unless the history or examination suggests that they are needed. In fact, most cases of urticaria require no laboratory investigation, especially if mild disease is responding to therapy. Tests may be helpful in cases of chronic urticaria where physical causative agents have been excluded. Typical laboratory workup would include a CBC, white blood cell differential, and erythrocyte sedimentation rate. Urinalysis, hepatitis panel, thyroid panel, thyroid antimicrosomal antibody, antinuclear antibody, rheumatoid factor, serum complement C3 and C4, cryoglobulin, serum IgE and immunoglobulin M (IgM), chest radiograph, and sinus series are less likely to be needed but may be ordered when indicated by history, physical examination, or consultation with a specialist. A skin biopsy may be done to assess for vasculitis if the sedimentation rate is increased or if hives are accompanied by arthralgia or burning sensation in the skin. Specific allergy or provocative tests may prove useful in certain patients (e.g., atopic individuals with severe urticaria) to establish sensitivity to certain foods that should be avoided.

DIFFERENTIAL DIAGNOSIS

There are many conditions that can be confused with urticaria. The following should be considered in the differential diagnosis: insect bites, vasculitis, pityriasis rosea, syphilis, bullous pemphigoid, systemic lupus erythematosus, urticaria pigmentosa, drug eruptions, and erythema multiforme.

MANAGEMENT

Identification of the responsible trigger and elimination would be ideal. However, most cases of urticaria are idiopathic, and providers often must turn to pharmacologic therapy.

DIAGNOSTICS

Urticaria

LABORATORY*

CBC and differential†
ESR†
Urinalysis†
LFTs†
TSH†
Thyroid antimicrosomal antibodies†
Antinuclear antibodies†
Rheumatoid factor†
Serum complement C3 and C4†
Cryoglobulin†
Serum IgE†
Serum IgM†
Hepatitis†

IMAGING

Chest x-ray†

*If no physical causes present.
†If indicated.

DIFFERENTIAL DIAGNOSIS

Urticaria

- Insect bites
- Vasculitis
- Pityriasis rosea
- Syphilis
- Bullous pemphigoid
- Systemic lupus erythematosus
- Urticaria pigmentosa
- Drug eruptions
- Erythema multiforme

Evidence exists for the benefit of treatment of acute and chronic urticaria with H_1-receptor antagonists, H_2-receptor antagonists, tricyclic antidepressants, leukotriene receptor antagonists, and, in some cases, steroids (Table 72-1).

Although older antihistamines such as diphenhydramine (Benadryl) and hydroxyzine (Atarax) were used commonly in the past, they have largely been replaced by newer, nonsedating H_1-blockers such as loratadine (Claritin), cetirizine (Zyrtec), fexofenadine (Allegra), and desloratadine (Clarinex). There is evidence for clinical benefit when these medications are used at higher doses.[11] Their efficacy combined with reduced sedation and anticholinergic side effects have made them first-line therapy in the treatment of urticaria. Because treating the symptoms of urticaria often requires higher doses of the H_1-blockers—doses that in most individuals would lead to significant sedation with the older H_1-blockers—the newer nonsedating H_1-blockers have found favor.[12] However, the addition of a sedating antihistamine (e.g., chlorpheniramine 4 to 12 mg or hydroxyzine 10 to 50 mg) at bedtime to the regimen of a patient already taking a nonsedating H_1-blocker

TABLE 72-1 Medications Used in Management of Urticaria and Angioedema

Medication	Dosage
H_1-RECEPTOR ANTAGONISTS	
Cetirizine HCl (Zyrtec)	Adults: 10-20 mg/day (tablet)
Loratadine (Claritin)	Adults: 10 mg/day (tablet)
Fexofenadine (Allegra)	Adults: 120 mg/day (capsules, tablets)
Desloratadine (Clarinex)	Adults: 5 mg/day (tablets, liquid)
H_2-RECEPTOR ANTAGONISTS	
Cimetidine (Tagamet)	300 mg q.i.d. (tablet, liquid)
Ranitidine HCl (Zantac)	150 mg PO b.i.d. (tablet, capsule, liquid, injection)
TRICYCLIC ANTIDEPRESSANTS	
Amitriptyline HCl (Elavil)	10-100 mg PO q day (tablet)
Doxepin (Sinequan)	10-100 mg PO q day (capsule, oral concentrate)
LEUKOTRIENE RECEPTOR ANTAGONISTS	
Montelukast sodium (Singulair)	Adults: 10 mg/day (tablet)
Zafirlukast (Accolate)	Adults: 20 mg PO b.i.d. (tablet)

HCl, Hydrochloride.

may help the patient sleep better. There is little evidence, however, that such an addition adds much to H_1-receptor blockade.

Evidence exists for clinical benefit when an H_2-blocker is added to an H_1-blocker in the case of urticaria that is refractory to H_1-blockade. An H_2-blocker such as cimetidine (Tagamet, 300 mg PO q.i.d.) or ranitidine (Zantac, 150 mg PO b.i.d.) can be added.[13] An H_2-blocker should only be used in conjunction with an H_1-blocker, since the evidence pertains to the benefit of H_2-blockers in cases of chronic urticaria that is refractory to treatment with H_1-blockers alone.[14-16] Evidence also exists for the benefit of treatment of refractory chronic urticaria with the tricyclic antidepressants.[17,18] Doxepin is the most potent H_1-blocker in the class and, when used, should be started at 25 mg PO h.s. and titrated to effect with a maximum dosage of 100 mg PO h.s. Alternatively, amitriptyline (Elavil) may be used at the same dosing interval of 10 to 100 mg PO h.s.

Recent limited evidence also suggests that the leukotriene inhibitors may be useful in some patients with chronic refractory urticaria, but in combination therapy with desloratadine.[19,20] Evidence exists for benefit of treatment of acute urticaria with oral corticosteroids such as prednisolone at a dosage of 50 mg/day for 3 days.[11] Long-term oral corticosteroids should not typically be used in chronic urticaria but may be used in select refractory cases under specialty consultation.[11]

Remember that cases of acute urticaria typically last no more than 5 to 7 days. Chronic urticaria is different. Individuals affected by chronic urticaria must try to modify their lifestyle to avoid the irritant that triggers the symptoms. Patients with a history of severe urticaria or angioedema should carry an epinephrine autoinjector for emergency use. Epinephrine 1:1000 0.3 ml SQ may be used in addition to the H_1-blocker if the patient exhibits any signs of angioedema or if urticaria is severe. A short course of oral corticosteroids may also be considered in the case of angioedema that affects the mouth.

COMPLICATIONS

Pruritus may lead to scratching, excoriation, and secondary infection. The most severe complication is angioedema or anaphylaxis accompanying the urticaria, which can lead to airway obstruction or cardiopulmonary arrest.

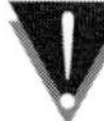

Immediate emergency department referral or physician consultation is indicated for patients with angioedema, respiratory failure, or hemodynamic compromise. Patients should be hospitalized if they require intubation or are at risk for airway compromise, severe anaphylaxis, or shock.

INDICATIONS FOR REFERRAL OR HOSPITALIZATION

Patients should be referred to a physician or specialist for further evaluation when the diagnosis is in question, when an underlying systemic disease is suspected or found, and when routine medical therapy is not effective.

PATIENT AND FAMILY EDUCATION AND HEALTH PROMOTION

Patients should be educated on the natural course and history of the disease, including the fact that the specific trigger may remain elusive. Surveillance should still be conducted in the form of diet or activity diaries. Patients and their families should be educated regarding signs and symptoms of anaphylaxis and angioedema and should understand the importance of avoiding known precipitants, since urticaria can plague them throughout their lives. Patients predisposed to severe urticaria, anaphylaxis, or angioedema should be educated in crisis management, including the use of subcutaneous epinephrine to avoid unnecessary morbidity or mortality. If patients have a history of anaphylaxis or angioedema, they should be provided with an injectable epinephrine preparation such as an EpiPen for emergency use. Both patient and family members should be educated in its use.

REFERENCES

1. Dibbern DA: Urticaria: selected highlights and recent advances, *Med Clin North Am* 90(1):187-209, 2006.
2. Dice JP: Physical urticaria, *Immunol Allergy Clin North Am* 24:225-246, 2004.
3. Leznoff A, Sussman GL: Syndrome of idiopathic chronic urticaria and angioedema with thyroid autoimmunity: a study in 90 patients, *J Allergy Clin Imunol* 84(1):66-71, 1989.
4. Lindelof B, Sigurgeirsson B, Walgren CF, and others: Chronic urticaria and cancer: an epidemiological study of 1155 patients, *Br J Dermatol* 123:453-456, 1990.
5. Mahmood T: Physical urticarias, *Am Fam Phys* 49(6):1411-1414, 1994.
6. Mahmood T: Urticaria, *Am Fam Phys* 51(4):811-816, 1995.
7. Greaves M: Chronic urticaria, *N Engl J Med* 332(26):1767-1772, 1995.
8. Sveum R: Urticaria: the diagnostic challenge of hives, *Postgrad Med* 100(2):77-84, 1996.
9. Habif TP: *Clinical dermatology*, ed 4, St Louis, 2004, Mosby.
10. Sheikh J: Advances in the treatment of chronic urticaria, *J Allergy Clin Immunol* 24:317-334, 2004.
11. Grattan C, Powell S, Humphreys F: Management and diagnostic guidelines for urticaria and angioedema, *Br J Dermatol* 144(4):708-714, 2001.
12. Goldsmith P, Dowd PM: The new H_1 antihistamines: treatment of urticaria and other clinical problems, *Dermatol Clin* 11(1):87-95, 1993.
13. Juhlin D, Landor M: Drug therapy for chronic urticaria, *Clin Rev Allergy* 10:349-369, 1992.
14. Singh G: H_2 blockers in chronic urticaria, *Int J Dermatol* 23(9):627-628, 1984.
15. Harvey RP, Schocket AL: The effect of H_1 and H_2 blockade on cutaneous histamine response in man, *J Allergy Clin Immunol* 65(2):136-139, 1980.
16. Phanuphak P, Schocket AL, Kohler PF: Treatment of idiopathic urticaria with combined H_1 and H_2 blockers, *Clin Allergy* 8(5):429-433, 1978.
17. Rao KS, Menon PK, Hilman BC, and others: Duration of the suppressive effect of tricyclic antidepressants on histamine-induced wheal and flare reactions in human skin, *J Allergy Clin Immunol* 82(5 pt 1):752-757, 1988.
18. Gupta M, Gupta AK, Ellis CN: Antidepressant drugs in dermatology: an update, *Arch Dermatol* 123:647-652, 1987.
19. Nettis E, Dambra D, D'Oronzio L, and others: Comparison of montelukast and fexofenadine for chronic idiopathic urticaria, *Arch Dermatol* 137(1):99-100, 2001.
20. DiLorenzo G, Pacor ML, Mansueto P, and others: Randomized placebo-controlled trial comparing desloratadine and montelukast in monotherapy and desloratadine plus montelukast in combined therapy for chronic idiopathic urticaria, *J Allergy Clin Immunol* 114(3):619-625, 2004.

CHAPTER 73

Warts

Eileen M. Deignan and Bonnie Hooper

DEFINITION AND EPIDEMIOLOGY

Verruca, or warts, are benign epidermal neoplasms. They are caused by various types of human papillomavirus (HPV), which are characterized as double-stranded DNA viruses that are members of the family Papovaviridae. Over 100 types of HPV have been identified on the basis of their DNA homology.[1-3] Although these genotypes can invade any anatomic site of the body, typically each has a predilection for a preferred body area. For example, HPV-1 and HPV-4 are usually identified in plantar, planus, and common warts. Thirty HPV types are genital types, including 15 subtypes that are associated with an increased risk for developing cervical cancers, including HPV types 16, 18, 31, 33, 35, 45, 51, 52, and 56.[4] (See the discussions of HPV in Chapters 21 and 176.)

The prevalence of warts in the general population has not been studied. Patients in the first and second decades of their lives bear a greater rate of occurrence.[5] It has been projected that at least 50% to 75% of sexually active men and women in the United States will acquire HPV infection at some point in their lives.[4] There is a decreased incidence of warts in African Americans and older adults.[2,6]

Individuals with decreased cellular immunity are particularly susceptible to HPV infection. In these patients warts can be extensive in terms of lesion size and area of involvement. Individuals previously infected with warts have three times the risk for reinfection.[6]

Certain environmental and occupational factors also increase the risk for developing warts. Periungual warts are much more common in butchers and in patients whose hands are exposed to chronic wet conditions, including chronic nail biters. Hyperhidrosis increases the chance for developing plantar warts.[7]

PATHOPHYSIOLOGY

Infection always originates from persons who harbor the host-specific HPV. It is postulated that infection occurs through breaks in the skin in contact with infected persons or their desquamated keratinocytes.[8] Once the virus gains access, it uses the host cell resources to coordinate its own gene expression and replicate. Although viral particles are found in the basal layer of infected tissue, replication occurs only in upper-level, differentiated epithelial cells. Autoinoculation can occur at sites of cutaneous trauma. Vertical transmission from infected mothers to their offspring (i.e., by ascending infection and passage through an infected birth canal) is a well-documented source of anogenital and laryngeal infection in infants.

Infection depends on the number of viral particles, the extent of contact, and the host's cellular immunity. Even though the virus confines itself to the epidermis, it generally spreads laterally for a considerable distance beyond the line that demarcates the wart from the normal skin. HPV may be actively replicating or may lie in a dormant, or latent, state. Lesions recur when the host's cell-mediated immunity can no longer hold the virus in check. Incubation periods range from 1 to 8 months.

CLINICAL PRESENTATION AND PHYSICAL EXAMINATION

HPV infection is usually asymptomatic. When it does result in clinical changes, it becomes manifest with several different morphologic characteristics. Verruca vulgaris, or common warts, are skin-colored, hyperkeratotic papules that occur most often on the backs of the hands, in periungual areas, and on the knees. Filiform warts are a variant of common warts and are distinguished by their fine, fingerlike projections. They usually occur on the face and occasionally may be tender. Verruca plana, or flat warts, are commonly seen on the face and extremities in crops of 1- to 2-mm papules that are smooth, flat, and skin colored to brown. Verruca plantaris, or plantar warts, are skin-colored papules or plaques on the plantar surface of the foot. They are often studded with black pinpoint-sized areas that represent thrombosed capillaries. These warts may be extremely tender and preclude weight bearing. The depth of plantar warts makes their treatment long and complicated.[7,8] Condyloma acuminata, or anogenital warts, are sexually transmitted and range from unobtrusive, small, skin-colored papules to large, cauliflower-like growths (Color Plate 7). Warts have also been described on the oral and nasal mucous membranes, conjunctivae, larynx, and cervix.

DIAGNOSTICS AND DIFFERENTIAL DIAGNOSIS

For women with genital warts, who may have increased risk for cervical cancer depending on the HPV type, recent advances in liquid-based technology have changed the concept of a traditional Pap test. HPV DNA testing was recently approved by the U.S. Food and Drug Administration (FDA) for use as an adjunct routine cervical cancer screening based on the use of liquid-based cytology. The FDA has approved HPV DNA testing as a screening test, but only among women over the age of 30 years as an adjunct to Pap smear testing. This age limitation is due to the concern that HPV screening amoung women younger than 30 years would result in an abundance of positive HPV results, a significant percentage of which resolve spontaneously or become undetectable within 2 years (see Chapters 21 and 176).

Diagnosis of some warts can be confirmed clinically by debriding the thickened hypertrophic epidermis with a scalpel or curette until the thrombosed capillary tips that rise perpendicular to the surface cause a speckled "seeds" appearance in the dermis.[5] The absence of skin lines within the lesion is considered a key diagnostic indicator. The differential diagnosis of warts includes keratoma, callus, lichen planus, squamous cell

DIFFERENTIAL DIAGNOSIS

Warts

- Keratoma
- Callus
- Lichen planus
- Squamous cell carcinoma
- Molluscum contagiosum
- Amelanotic melanoma
- Foreign body

carcinoma, molluscum contagiosum, amelanotic melanoma, and foreign body.

MANAGEMENT

Most warts are benign and asymptomatic and generally regress spontaneously over time. Fifty percent of all warts involute spontaneously by the end of 12 months, and 66% to 70% disappear within 24 months.[6,9] According to a task force of the American Academy of Dermatology's Committee on Guidelines of Care, indications for treatment include (1) the patient's desire for therapy; (2) the presence of pain, bleeding, itching, or burning; (3) lesions that are disabling or disfiguring; (4) large numbers or size of lesions; (5) prevention of spreading to unblemished skin; and (6) an immunocompromised state.[9]

Therapies are directed toward destruction of the lesions and include chemical destruction, cryotherapy, electrodesiccation, and laser ablation. Chemical destruction is done with a liquid agent or transdermal patches. Liquid preparations of salicylic acid, lactic acid, and dichloroacetic or trichloroacetic acid are used on common, flat, periungual, and plantar warts. Application once or twice a day, along with paring or filing of the lesion, has resulted in cure rates that exceed 60%.[9] A petroleum-based substance can be applied on the surrounding skin to protect it from chemical burn. Treatment may take up to 12 weeks. Cantharidin, applied every 2 to 3 weeks, is another option.[1,2] Daily use of topical tretinoin (Retin-A) has been advocated for flat warts. Imiquimod (Aldara) is U.S. Food and Drug Administration–approved for condyloma, but has been used also to treat plantar and common warts.[10] Podophyllum resin has a potential for systemic absorption, and serious adverse gastrointestinal and nervous system effects have been reported from this absorption.[1,6] Therefore podophyllum resin needs to be washed from the skin 1 to 4 hours after application, and it should never be used with patients who are pregnant.

Cryotherapy with liquid nitrogen is commonly used to treat warts. This therapy causes a stinging or burning sensation with application. Lesions usually heal in 1 to 2 weeks. Patients should be warned that this treatment can lead to hyperpigmentation, hypopigmentation, and scarring in the treated area. Treatment may be needed every other week to every third week until resolution. Nerve damage can occur if treatment is too vigorous in areas where the nerves are superficial, such as the lateral phalanges. Cryotherapy of periungual warts can affect the underlying nail matrix and cause nail dystrophy. Cryotherapy should be performed cautiously in patients with Raynaud's phenomenon. Cryotherapy used in combination with topical acids may produce a synergistic effect.[6]

Treatment with pulsed dye or other vascular laser destroys the blood supply to the wart, thereby decreasing nourishment to the virus and enhancing resolution. A temporary bruise will result at the treatment site.

More aggressive surgical techniques are available if topical agents and cryotherapy fail. Excision, curettage, and electrocautery increase the risk of scarring, and there is no evidence of improved success.[1,2,8] Administration of an anesthetic may cause a viral tract, which can potentially result in reinfection.

COMPLICATIONS

Plantar warts can be particularly painful and, if left untreated, may result in altered activity, abnormal gait, or foot deformities. Infections are rare, but autoinoculation from one area to another is common.

Genital warts (condyloma acuminata) are transmitted sexually and can be transmitted from mother to infant during childbirth. For both males and females, there is an increased risk of genital and rectal carcinoma.

INDICATIONS FOR REFERRAL OR HOSPITALIZATION

A referral to a dermatologist or podiatric surgeon is advised if all of the common techniques have failed or if the lesion is too large. Therapies include the use of intralesional bleomycin or *Candida* extract and laser ablation.[6,7] Cure rates with these more advanced techniques are not reported to be much higher than with the modalities used commonly in the past.

Several unconventional therapies may also be helpful adjuncts. Cimetidine (Tagamet) 25 to 40 mg/kg/day in three or four divided doses has been reported as benign and successful in approximately 80% of patients within 2 to 3 months.[11,12] Success rates appear higher in children, although this treatment method remains somewhat controversial and more recently has fallen out of favor. Hyperthermia water bath treatments may be an effective alternative in treating recalcitrant or extensive warts.[1,9,12] For this form of therapy to be effective, a temperature range of 45° to 48° C (113° to 118.4° F) needs to be maintained for at least 30 minutes per treatment session.[12]

PATIENT AND FAMILY EDUCATION

Patients and families should understand that most warts are benign, viral lesions that can spread from person to person (particularly in showers, locker rooms, or other public places) and may resolve spontaneously, although sometimes only after many years. Education should include self-treatment options and the side effects of all medications. Specific instructions (soaking and paring the wart before application of medicines) should be given regarding the proper use of over-the-counter treatments to enhance efficacy.

Patients and families should also be educated about a new vaccine, Gardasil, that helps protect against diseases caused by HPV types 6, 11, 16, and 18. Gardasil helps prevent diseases related to these HPV types but does not treat them, nor does it protect against HPV types to which there has been a prior exposure. Gardasil is a series of three immunizations given over a 6-month period and approved for girls and women 9 through 26 years of age. Education about the vaccine needs to emphasize that vaccination does not substitute for routine cervical cancer screening.

REFERENCES

1. Ordoukhanian E, Lane AT: Warts and molluscum contagiosum: beware of treatments worse than the disease, *Postgrad Med* 101(2):223-235, 1997.
2. Siegfried EC: Warts on children: an approach to therapy, *Pediatr Ann* 25(2):79-90, 1996.
3. Frasier LD: Human papillomavirus infections in children, *Pediatr Ann* 23(7):354-360, 1994.

4. Schiffman M, Castle PE: Human papillomavirus: epidemiology and public health, *Arch Pathol Lab Med* 127(8):930-1034, 2003.
5. Esterowitz D, Greer KE, Cooper PH, and others: Plantar warts in the athlete, *Am J Emerg Med* 13(4):441-443, 1995.
6. Kimble-Haas S: Primary care treatment approach to nongenital verruca, *Nurse Pract* 21(10):29-36, 1996.
7. Glover MG: Plantar warts, *Foot Ankle* 11(3):172-178, 1990.
8. Bolton RA: Nongenital warts: classification and treatment options, *Am Fam Phys* 43(6):2049-2056, 1991.
9. Landow K: Nongenital warts: when is treatment warranted? *Postgrad Med* 99(3):245-249, 1996.
10. Tyring SK: Human papilloma virus infections: epidemiology, pathogenesis, and host immune response, *J Am Acad Dermatol* 43(1 suppl):18-26, 2000.
11. Glass AT, Solomon BA: Cimetidine therapy for recalcitrant warts in adults, *Arch Dermatol* 132:680-682, 1996.
12. Kang S, Fitzpatrick TB: Debilitating verruca vulgaris in a patient infected with the human immunodeficiency virus: dramatic improvement with hyperthermia therapy, *Arch Dermatol* 130(3):294-296, 1994.

CHAPTER 74

Wound Management

Mary Young

DEFINITION AND EPIDEMIOLOGY

Tissue trauma accounts for significant morbidity and financial concern, with the cost of wound care estimated to be greater than $2 billion in the United States each year.[1-3] The incidence and prevalence of acute and chronic wounds vary with populations, geographic and demographic status, and general medical conditions. Acute wounds consist of lacerations, abrasions, avulsions, crush injuries, puncture wounds, insect or mammalian bites, traumatic or surgical wounds, burns, and skin tears. Chronic wounds consist of pressure ulcers, venous and arterial ulcers, diabetic foot ulcers, and nonhealing surgical or traumatic wounds.

Ulcers

Pressure ulcers affect 1.5 to 3 million Americans at any given time. In all, 60% to 90% occur in older adults, with 66% of older adults with hip fractures and 15% to 25% of persons admitted to long-term care facilities reportedly developing pressure ulcers. Acute care incidence is 2.7% to 29.5%, with prevalence at 3.5% to 29.5%.[4-11] Venous ulcers are present in 3.5% of persons over age 65 years; the recurrence rate is more than 70% as a result of chronic venous insufficiency. Arterial ulcers occur in a large percentage of patients with peripheral vascular disease. These ulcers are particularly difficult to heal as a result of poor perfusion, and revascularization is often needed to promote reperfusion and the hope of healing the ulcer.

Diabetic Foot Ulcers

Diabetic foot ulcers occur in approximately 15% of the more than 16 million people with diabetes. Ulcers precede amputation 85% of the time, with the cost of treatment exceeding $28,000 for the first 2 years after diagnosis. More than 50% of nontraumatic lower extremity amputations are performed on patients with diabetes.[12-17] Amputation and foot ulceration are the most common consequences of diabetic neuropathy and major causes of morbidity and disability in people with diabetes. Early recognition and management of independent risk factors can prevent or delay adverse outcomes.[12] The risk of ulcers or amputations increases in people who have had diabetes for more than 10 years; are male; have poor glucose control; or have cardiovascular, retinal, or renal complications (Boxes 74-1 and 74-2).[12]

Surgical Wounds

Surgical wounds are often treated in the outpatient setting secondary to rising costs of acute care management and reimbursement concerns. Wound infection and dehiscence preclude wound healing by secondary intention, with the health care provider and home health nurse managing these difficult-to-heal wounds.[3] A broad understanding of wound

BOX 74-1

RECOMMENDATIONS FOR FOOT CARE IN PERSONS WITH DIABETES

- Perform a comprehensive foot examination and provide foot self-care education annually on patients with diabetes to identify risk factors predictive of ulcers and the need for amputation.
- The foot examination can be accomplished in a primary care setting and should include the use of a monofilament, tuning fork, palpation, and visual examination.
- A multidisciplinary approach is recommended for individuals with foot ulcers and high-risk feet, especially those with a history of ulcer or amputation.
- Refer patients who smoke or have prior lower extremity complications to foot care specialists for ongoing preventive care and life-long surveillance.
- Initial screening for peripheral arterial disease (PAD) should include a history for claudication and an assessment of the pedal pulses. Consider obtaining an ankle-brachial index (ABI), since many patients with PAD are asymptomatic.
- Refer patients with significant claudication or a positive ABI for further vascular assessment and consider exercise, medications, and surgical options.

Data from Sumpio B, and others: Etiology and management of foot ulcerations. In Lee BY: *The wound management manual*, New York, 2005, McGraw-Hill.

BOX 74-2

FOOT-RELATED RISK CONDITIONS ASSOCIATED WITH INCREASED RISK OF AMPUTATION

- Peripheral neuropathy with loss of protective sensation
- Altered biomechanics (in the presence of neuropathy)
- Evidence of increased pressure (erythema, hemorrhage under a callus)
- Bony deformity
- Peripheral vascular disease (decreased or absent pedal pulses)
- A history of ulcers or amputation
- Severe nail pathologic condition

Data from Sumpio B, and others: Etiology and management of foot ulcerations. In Lee BY: *The wound management manual*, New York, 2005, McGraw-Hill.

healing physiology and general management principles will assist the provider in facilitating maximum wound repair.

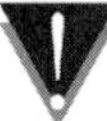

Immediate referral to a specialist is indicated for deep lacerations, especially when a fracture or tendon injury is suspected.

Immediate referral to a hand specialist is indicated for hand injuries.

Immediate referral to a plastic surgeon is indicated for facial and hand wounds because of the high priority for minimizing scarring and ensuring a return to normal motor function.[2]

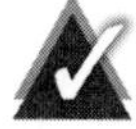

Physician consultation is indicated for deep puncture wounds of the foot, hand, chest, abdomen, and head.

Physician consultation is indicated for wounds requiring large amounts of debridement and wounds with continuous bleeding.

Classification of Wounds

Classification of wounds is unique to wound type, and reference to established classification systems is recommended.

Wounds involving only the epidermal layer are classified as superficial or partial thickness. Examples include simple lacerations, skin tears, first-degree burns, abrasions, and shallow ulcerations. These wounds usually heal easily within 2 to 6 days and require the least intervention. Full-thickness wounds involve the epidermis and dermis and may extend through subcutaneous tissue into muscle and bone. Examples include deep lacerations, second- and third-degree burns, various types of ulcers, and surgical or traumatic wounds.

Pressure ulcers may be partial or full thickness and are staged 1 through 4 according to the guidelines of the Agency for Healthcare Research and Quality (formerly the Agency for Health Care Policy and Research) (Box 74-3). Burns are classified as first, second, or third degree (Box 74-4) and require a unique approach. A referral is indicated when the burn is full thickness and/or occurs on the face, feet, hands, or perineum.[18]

BOX 74-3

PRESSURE ULCER STAGING (AHCPR GUIDELINES)

Stage I: Nonblanchable erythema of intact skin; the heralding lesion of skin ulceration.
Stage II: Partial-thickness skin loss involving epidermis and/or dermis. The ulcer is superficial and presents clinically as an abrasion, blister, or shallow crater.
Stage III: Full-thickness skin loss involving damage or necrosis of subcutaneous tissue that may extend down to, but not through, underlying fascia. The ulcer presents clinically as a deep crater with or without undermining of adjacent tissue.
Stage IV: Full-thickness skin loss with extensive destruction, tissue necrosis, or damage to muscle, bone, or supporting structures (e.g., tendon or joint capsule). NOTE: Undermining and sinus tracts may also be associated with stage IV pressure ulcers.

From Agency for Health Care Policy and Research: *Clinical practice guidelines: pressure ulcers in adults: prediction and prevention*, Rockville, Md, 1994, US Department of Health and Human Services, US Public Health Service, Agency for Health Care Policy and Research.

BOX 74-4

BURNS CLASSIFICATION

First degree: Superficial, involving only the epidermis. The skin appears dry and erythematous, without blisters, and is sensitive. The classic example is sunburn. Healing occurs in 5 to 10 days.
Second degree: Partial thickness, involving the epidermis and dermis. The skin appears pink, wet, and mottled and has blisters. The site is very painful, such as after a burn from boiling water. Healing occurs in 10 to 14 days.
Third degree: Full thickness, involving the epidermis and dermis, extending into subcutaneous tissue. The wound appears pale white, cherry red, or black. The tissue is very dry and often has necrotic areas to debride. This type of wound is anesthetic. Direct flames, electricity, or chemicals are common causative agents. Skin grafting is often required.

Modified from Wysocki A: Wound care management, *Nurs Clin North Am* 34(4):791, 1999.

BOX 74-5

PAYNE-MARTIN CLASSIFICATION SYSTEM FOR SKIN TEARS

CATEGORY I

- Skin tears without tissue loss.
- Linear type; epidermis and dermis have been pulled apart.
- Flap type; epidermal flap completely covers the dermis to within 1 mm of wound margin.

CATEGORY II

- Skin tears with partial tissue loss.
- Scant tissue loss; 25% or less of flap is lost.
- Moderate to large tissue loss; more than 25% of epidermal flap is lost.

CATEGORY III

- Skin tear with complete tissue loss.
- Epidermal flap is absent.

Modified from Baranoski S: Skin tears: the enemy of frail skin, *Adv Skin Wound Care* 13(3 pt 1):123-126, 2000.

Skin tears are a common occurrence in frail older adults, often occurring during routine daily activities such as washing and dressing. The shearing and friction forces against frail skin cause the tear, separating the epidermis from the dermis (partial thickness) or the dermis from underlying structures (full thickness). The Payne-Martin Classification System for grading tears is easy to use and is helpful in documentation[19] (Box 74-5). Diabetic foot ulcers and arterial and venous ulcers are determined by etiology and are usually full thickness. Several classification systems have emerged; Table 74-1 displays the University of Texas system for staging diabetic foot ulcers.

PATHOPHYSIOLOGY

Wound healing begins at the time of injury and proceeds over several months through the stages of inflammation, proliferation, and remodeling. Inflammation, which begins at the time of injury, is an essential first step in wound healing to provide local vasospasm and initiation of the clotting process. Neutrophils, oxygen, and nutrients are transported to the wound site, and proliferation begins. In this phase, epithelial cells migrate over the surface of the wound, collagen synthesis begins, and the wound begins to contract. Remodeling occurs over the next several months, with layering of collagen providing further contraction and tensile strength.[16,17]

Wound healing is affected by many internal and external factors. Internal factors include age, preexisting co-morbidities (i.e., diabetes mellitus, cardiovascular disease, autoimmune disorders), perfusion, oxygenation, nutrition, hydration, and some medications (especially steroids, immunosuppressants, and chemotherapeutic drugs). External factors include pressure; friction; shear; contamination with bacteria, debris, or necrotic tissue; and the wound environment (pH, moisture).[18,20]

Stages of wound healing may be interrupted by changes in the internal and external wound healing factors. Two common examples are the occurrence of anemia during wound healing, which slows the healing response as a result of decreased oxygenation, and pressure exerted over the site, which decreases perfusion and prolongs or delays wound healing.

Surgical wounds heal by primary, secondary, or tertiary intention. Primary intention implies that the wound edges are approximated and sutured, stapled, taped, or glued. Secondary intention implies that the wound edges are not approximated, usually because of failed primary intention (dehiscence) or infection. Secondary intention healing is prolonged and results in significant scarring. Delayed primary intention, or tertiary intention, refers to wounds that were not initially closed (usually because of infection, contamination, or wound stress) and are closed after some secondary intention healing has occurred.

CLINICAL PRESENTATION

Any break in skin integrity in the immunocompromised or diabetic patient warrants timely and complete evaluation. Early evaluation and intervention in this population of patients may prevent complications of healing, including infection.

Acute wounds are most often caused by accidental injury and include lacerations, abrasions, burns, bites, and puncture wounds. Patients with co-morbidities, especially diabetes mellitus and peripheral vascular disease, may be seen with lower extremity ulcers related to neuropathy and poor perfusion. Patients with decreased functioning resulting from brain injury, neurologic disease, or spinal cord injury often see their providers with complaints of pressure ulcers. Prevention, early identification, and appropriate management are of primary importance to avoid costly and irreversible tissue damage, especially in the medically compromised patient.

The patient's medication history is important to evaluate and guides management decisions. Immunosuppressive drugs, including chemotherapeutics and steroids, adversely affect wound healing by interrupting the inflammatory process, an important first step in mounting a healing response. Critical factors to elicit include the patient's age; allergies; employment; nutritional status; drug or alcohol use; smoking history;

TABLE 74-1 Diabetic Foot Ulcer Grades (University of Texas Classification System)

	0	1	2	3
A	Preulcerative or postulcerative lesion completely epithelialized	Superficial, not involving tendon, joint capsule, or bone	Penetrating to tendon or joint capsule	Penetrating to bone or joint capsule
B	With infection	With infection	With infection	With infection
C	With ischemia	With ischemia	With ischemia	With ischemia
D	With infection and ischemia	With infection and ischemia	With infection and ischemia	With infection and ischemia

Modified from *University of Texas classification system in diabetic foot exam,* retrieved Dec 15, 2006, from http://www.footandankle.com/DMfoot/start.html.

and immune status, including the last tetanus booster. Moreover, the provider must identify conditions that adversely affect wound healing, including diabetes mellitus, autoimmune disorders, malnutrition, positive smoking history, chronic respiratory disease, and peripheral vascular disease; these affect management plans.[17,21]

PHYSICAL EXAMINATION

Assessment of the wound must follow a thorough history. The nature and age of the wound, along with the patient's medical history, determine management strategies. Wound location, type, depth, previous treatments, and surrounding tissue assessment guide treatment decisions.

In addition to a thorough wound evaluation (including observation for tunneling, the presence and odor of exudate, and the appearance of all tissue in and around wound bed), a focused physical examination is important. In lower extremity wounds, perfusion is determined by pulse assessment and noninvasive diagnostic testing, if necessary. The absence or presence of peripheral perfusion and associated changes of edema, tissue color and warmth, and neurovascular status are essential to determine.[16]

Wounds that are healing or have the potential to heal will demonstrate pink or red tissue and the absence of excessive exudate, infection, and debris. The size of the wound, measured weekly, should slowly decrease. Healing wounds are pink, robust, and bumpy (granulation tissue), with pink to red healing edges that demonstrate migration by contact with the wound bed. Tissue is not healing if it is pale, nonblanchable, and flat and has raised hard edges.

DIAGNOSTICS

X-ray studies may be necessary in acute injuries to identify bone or tendon involvement. Separation, fracture, or dislocation usually requires referral to a specialist. Compound fractures, especially in hand injuries, require diligent management and antibiotic administration.

Noninvasive vascular studies are useful to determine arterial flow in patients with lower extremity ulceration. Bone scans or an MRI is helpful in diagnosing osteomyelitis; a bone biopsy is sometimes necessary for definitive diagnosis.[12]

CBCs are useful in detecting anemia, which can slow wound healing progression by decreasing perfusion and oxygenation. A slightly elevated WBC count may indicate the inflammatory response, whereas a WBC count that continues to rise may indicate an infection. Immunosuppressive disorders delay wound healing and may be first detected on CBC. A total lymphocyte count of less than 1500 cells/mm^3, coupled with an albumin level of less than 3.5 g/dl, is indicative of malnutrition, which delays wound healing. Patients with diabetes who have a hemoglobin A_{1c} level of greater than 8% are at increased risk of failed wound healing as a result of hyperglycemia.[12-14]

DIAGNOSTICS

Wound Management

LABORATORY
CBC and differential*
Hemoglobin A_{1c}
Albumin level*

IMAGING
X-ray*
Bone scan*
MRI*
Noninvasive vascular studies*

*If indicated.

DIFFERENTIAL DIAGNOSIS

The nature of injury and location of the wound determine diagnosis as well as treatment. Diagnosis and treatment of chronic wounds are determined by patient history, the presence of medical conditions, and the location and appearance of the wound.

Ulcers are chronic wounds that can be caused by several different underlying medical conditions. The diagnosis of the underlying cause is essential, since treatment of this condition affects ulcer recurrence rates. Most pressure ulcers occur over bony prominences, with 95% occurring over the sacrum, greater trochanter, ischial tuberosity, heel, or lateral malleolus.[16] Venous ulcers are typically located on the medial lower leg, above the medial malleolus. The wound is often large with irregular wound edges; the wound bed appears beefy red and granular, with moderate to heavy exudate. Associated skin changes include a brawny texture, edema, and hyperpigmentation. Venous ulcers are not usually painful.[15] Arterial ulcers occur most often over the pretibial area, on the tips of the toes, or over the lateral malleolus; they are painful, flat, and dry and have well-demarcated edges. The limb is traditionally thin, cool, pale or hyperemic, hairless, and shiny as a result of decreased perfusion. Diabetic foot ulcers appear most commonly on the plantar surface of the foot, often at the head of the first metatarsal joint of the great toe. They are often painless secondary to neuropathy, and they have dry, pale edges and wound bed and a black eschar cover.[16]

Thermal wounds are the most common type of burn. Eighty percent of these burns are handled in the outpatient setting; burn center referral is based on the American Burn Association's criteria for burn center referral.[22]

MANAGEMENT

The use of universal precautions is essential in wound assessment and treatment. The first step—establishing the type and nature of injury—guides wound management decisions. Referral to a specialist is indicated for deep lacerations, especially when a fracture or tendon injury is suspected. Facial and hand wounds are also best managed by specialists because of the high priority in minimizing scarring and ensuring a return to normal motor function. Regardless of wound type, the principles of wound healing guide management. Ensuring wound bed moisture, nutrition, perfusion, pH balance, freedom from infection and debris, and protection are imperative. Management of co-morbid conditions and reduction of risk factors, including careful blood glucose monitoring and control, smoking cessation, correction of malnutrition, and enhancement of perfusion, are important strategies. Ensuring intake of adequate protein and essential vitamins and minerals, especially vitamin C and zinc, may also enhance wound healing.[16,17]

Acute Wounds

Lacerations, Abrasions, Avulsions, Crush Injuries, Bites, Puncture Wounds, and Other Traumatic or Surgical Wounds. The primary management goals for all acute wounds are to control major hemorrhage, protect the patient and the wound, and promote comfort. After examining the wound, the health care provider must clean and debride it to remove dirt, debris, and foreign bodies. All traumatic wounds are considered contaminated and should be irrigated with normal saline solution (0.9%). The best method of irrigation is attaching a syringe and 22-gauge angiocatheter to 1 L of normal saline via IV tubing. This allows for extensive irrigation under pressure (5 to 15 psi is recommended), which is most effective for cleansing. (Use of a piston or bulb syringe alone does not generate enough pressure for adequate irrigation.) Sharp debridement of nonviable or necrotic tissue and complete hemostasis further decrease the risk for infection.

Decisions about wound closure depend on the wound type, location, and depth and tension of the wound edges. A wound with smooth edges that is not grossly contaminated (e.g., a laceration from a knife or razor) may be closed by approximating the wound edges and applying wound adhesive or Steri-Strips or suturing with appropriate material. Staples are an efficient closure medium but are usually used when closure must be quick and the wound is not located in an area where scarring is of concern. Wounds easily closed include small lacerations not over a joint; wounds with clean, even edges approximated without inversion or eversion; and lacerations in areas with no redundant tissue. Suturing guidelines are reviewed in Table 74-2. Abrasions, avulsions, crush injuries, bites, and puncture wounds are not usually closed. Tissue approximation, when appropriate, and the application of an antibiotic ointment covered by a sterile nonadherent dressing are standard practice. Keeping the wound out of water, observing for signs and symptoms of infection, and changing the dressing according to principles will aid wound healing.[20,23]

A dressing is applied after wound exploration, irrigation, cleansing, debridement, and closure (when appropriate). Dressings serve the purposes of protection, drainage absorption, insulation, maintenance of moisture and cleanliness, and facilitation of gaseous exchange. They should be easily removed without traumatizing tissue and are often multilayered. No single dressing may afford all these properties; several hundred wound care products are available to choose from.[19,24-27]

Selection of dressing is based on function, availability, cost, and comfort. The external layer is protective; several types of bulky gauze are available to choose from for this layer. Dressings may be secured with tape, stockinet, binders, or straps. Being mindful of minimizing tissue trauma can guide the choice of dressing security. For example, wounds that are large and highly exudative and require frequent changes should be secured with a binder, a stockinet, or Montgomery straps. This will decrease skin tearing and trauma from frequent tape removal.

The primary layer protects the wound edges and wound bed; it should not adhere to the wound and should be easily removed. Examples include Xeroform, Adaptic, and transparent dressings. The second layer should be highly absorptive and usually is thick cotton gauze. The final layer is used to hold the dressing in place and may be tape or loose gauze.

Tetanus immunization should be reviewed in all patients after any type of tissue trauma. Tetanus and diphtheria toxoid and tetanus immune globulin should be administered if immunization status is unknown or if the patient has received fewer than three lifetime doses. Immunization with tetanus-diphtheria toxoid is recommended for all patients with tetanus-prone wounds (including all contaminated wounds) if the previous immunization was more than 5 years ago[20] (Table 74-3 and Box 74-6).

Antibiotic prophylaxis with amoxicillin and clavulanate potassium (Augmentin 875/125) is recommended for all cat bite wounds because 80% become infected. Early prophylaxis

TABLE 74-2 Recommendations for Suturing

Location	Suggested Suture Size	Suggested Suture Removal
Scalp	Superficial closure: 4-5 Deep closure: 4	6-7 days
Trunk	Superficial closure: 4-5 Deep closure: 3-4	6-8 days
Arms	Superficial closure: 4-5 Deep closure: 3-4	Extensor surfaces: 10-14 days All others: 7-10 days
Legs	Superficial closure: 4-5 Deep closure: 3-4	Same as for arms
Hands: referral indicated, although simple lacerations may be repaired	Superficial closure: 5-6 Deep closure: 4	Palms: 7-10 days Extensor surfaces: 10-14 days
Feet (soles): referral indicated for tendon or nerve injury	Superficial or deep closure: 3-4	7-14 days
Facial (including eyelids, lips, ears): pressure dressing; referral indicated		3-5 days
Penis, scrotum: referral indicated		
Dog bites: bites >6 hours old and puncture wounds should not be sutured; consultation suggested for wounds <6 hours old		
Cat bites: puncture wounds should not be sutured		
Human bites: wounds should not be sutured		

TABLE 74-3 Tetanus Immunization*

Wound Type	Unknown Primary Immunization or Less Than Three Doses	Three or More Doses
Tetanus-prone wounds	Tetanus and diphtheria toxoid (Td) and tetanus immune globulin (TIG)	Td if >5 years since booster
Non–tetanus-prone wounds	Td	Td if >10 years since booster

Modified from Gilbert DN, Moellering RC, Eliopoulos GM, and others: *The Sanford guide to antimicrobial therapy,* Hyde Park, Vt, 2005, Antimicrobial Therapy.
*Dosages (for age 7 years or older): Td, 0.5 ml IM; TIG, 250 units IM.

BOX 74-6

TETANUS-PRONE VERSUS NON–TETANUS-PRONE WOUNDS

TETANUS-PRONE WOUNDS
- Puncture wounds
- Crush injuries
- Wounds more than 6 hours old
- Stellate wounds
- Wounds more than 1 cm (0.4 inch) long
- Wounds with devitalized tissue
- Obviously contaminated wounds

NON–TETANUS-PRONE WOUNDS
- Wounds less than 6 hours old
- Wounds with clean margins
- Wounds without devitalized tissue
- Wounds without organic contamination
- Wounds with clearly defined edges

(within 12 hours of the bite) is recommended for human and dog bite wounds, although the risk of infection is less. Clindamycin is an appropriate antibiotic for patients who are allergic to penicillin. Traumatic nonbite wounds should be treated prophylactically with cefazolin 1 g IV initially, followed by oral antibiotics. Contaminated wounds must be treated systematically (Table 74-4). Other wounds that require antibiotics are listed in Box 74-7.

Skin Tears. Skin tears should be gently cleansed with normal saline and patted dry or left to air dry; the skin should be as closely approximated as possible. Steri-Strips may be useful in holding the wound edges together, especially in a grade 2 or 3 tear. A dressing that requires infrequent changes while supplying moisture to the wound bed is recommended for treatment. A transparent dressing left in place 5 to 7 days is a good choice. Otherwise, a hydrogel or impregnated gauze such as Xeroform may be selected. Any dressing on a skin tear must be removed carefully to avoid interrupting the delicate tissue adherence.[19]

BOX 74-7

WOUNDS THAT REQUIRE ANTIBIOTIC THERAPY

- Wounds more than 8 hours old
- Crushing injuries
- Grossly contaminated wounds
- Fingertip avulsions with bone exposed
- Open fractures
- Tendon or joint involvement
- Mammalian bites
- Paronychia with pus
- Wound in a felon (soft tissue abscess in fingertip)
- Wounds in immunocompromised patients
- Wounds in patients with diabetes

Burns. Immediate treatment includes moving the patient away from the source of heat, removing jewelry or metal (which may continue to conduct heat), and applying cool compresses to decrease skin temperature. All burns should be cleansed with normal saline and gauze initially, necrotic tissue should be sharply debrided, and a topical antimicrobial cream or ointment should be applied. Ideally, the product should penetrate eschar, not interfere with healing; be minimally absorbed and nontoxic; and provide wide-spectrum antibiotic coverage. Silver sulfadiazine (Silvadene) is the most common choice. Mupirocin (Bactroban) can be used for patients who are allergic to sulfa. Application twice a day, with normal saline cleansing at each dressing change, is recommended. Excessive use can lead to a secondary infection of *Pseudomonas aeruginosa* or *Enterobacter cloacae,* and therefore its use should be limited to 14 to 21 days. Chemical burns should be emergently treated with rapid and copious irrigation with normal saline or water, then treated as described previously.[2]

Chronic Wounds

The principles of wound management guide treatment decisions, regardless of wound type. However, chronic wounds require specific intervention based on cause. The wound care

TABLE 74-4 Suggested Systemic Antibiotics for Contaminated Wounds

	Primary Antibiotics	Alternate Antibiotics
Infected wounds without sepsis	TMP-SMX (Bactrim) DS 1 tablet PO b.i.d. Clindamycin 300-450 mg PO t.i.d.	Minocycline, linezolid
Infected wounds; patient febrile Gram-positive (*Staphylococcus aureus,* MRSA) Wound culture and sensitivity should guide therapy	TMP-SMX DS 1 tablet PO b.i.d. Clindamycin 300-450 mg PO t.i.d. IV vancomycin or daptomycin	Minocycline, linezolid

Modified from Gilbert DN, Moellering RC, Eliopoulos GM, and others: *The Sanford guide to antimicrobial therapy,* Hyde Park, Vt, 2005, Antimicrobial Therapy.
MRSA, Methicillin-resistant *S. aureus; TMP-SMX,* trimethoprim-sulfamethoxazole.

product selection algorithm (Figure 74-1) can guide the selection of a dressing based on the appearance of the wound. The use of cytotoxic products, including povidone-iodine (Betadine), hydrogen peroxide, Dakin's solution (a sodium hypochlorite solution), and other bacteriostatic products previously thought to be beneficial, is not currently recommended. Antibiotic creams and ointments, including silver sulfadiazine, are appropriate for short periods in infected wounds and are prescribed for only 14 to 21 days. Normal saline 0.9% is the cleansing, irrigating, and wound packing product of choice in most wounds because it is isotonic, readily available, and inexpensive.

Pressure Ulcers. Pressure ulcers are treated by removing pressure and avoiding friction, shear, and moisture. The ulcers are cleaned twice daily with normal saline irrigation or a

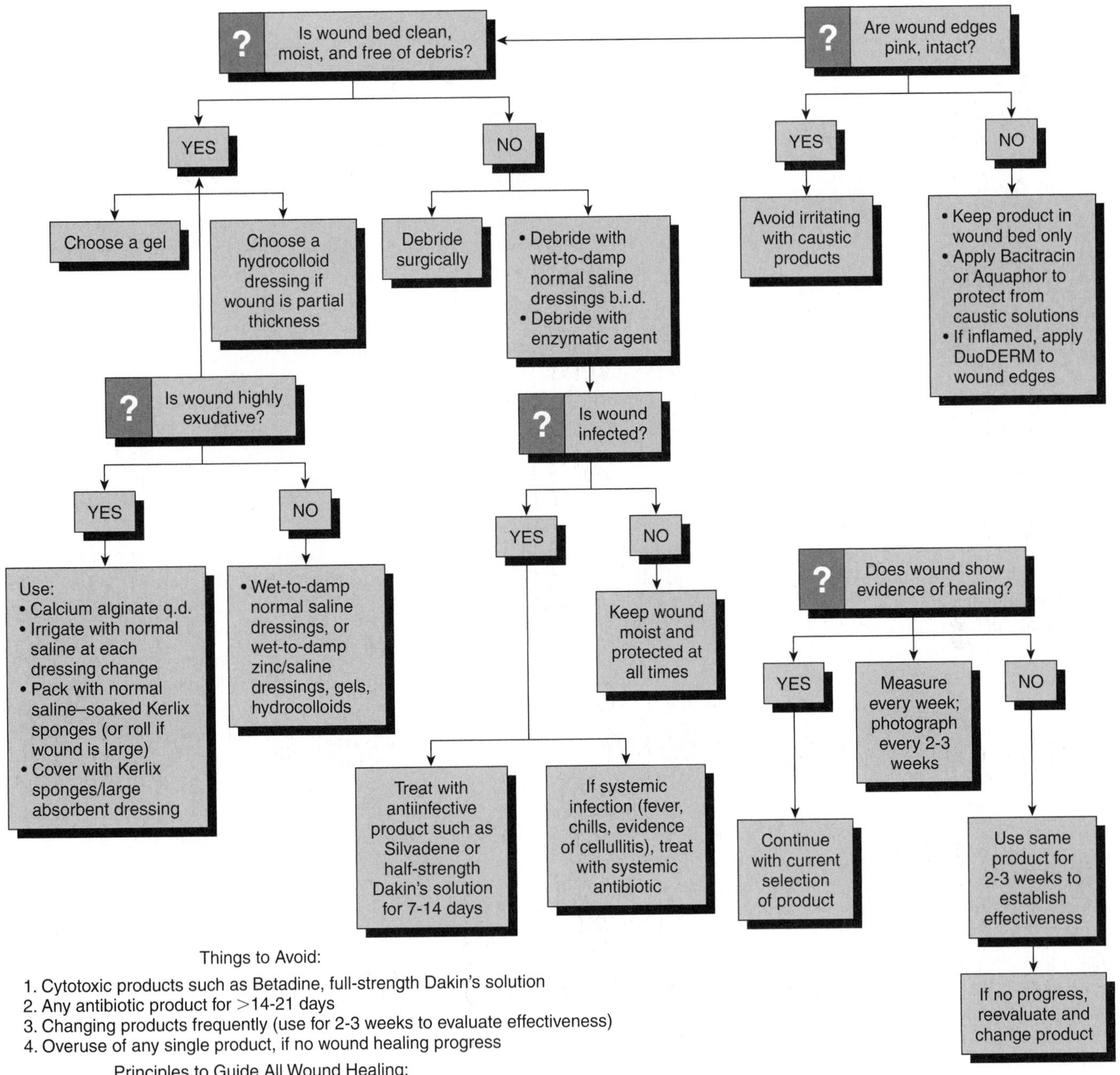

FIGURE 74-1

Algorithm for wound care product selection.

surfactant cleanser if fecal or urine contamination is a concern. Wound care products are selected to ensure protection, absorption of exudates, and gentle debridement. Stage 4 ulcers must be packed with a moist product, such as saline-impregnated gauze or a hydrogel; highly exudative wounds benefit from calcium alginate products. Stage 1 or 2 ulcers that are not infected may be treated with a hydrocolloid dressing, which may be left in place 5 to 7 days.

Venous Ulcers. Treatment of venous ulcers involves reducing edema with leg elevation, compression stockings, or graded compression devices. Unna's boot has been a useful dressing for many years; it provides compression and cannot be easily removed by the patient. However, it is not absorptive and therefore becomes less effective as the limb compresses over time.[15] Absorptive dressings (e.g., calcium alginate) combined with compression are more effective in venous ulcer care.

Arterial Ulcers. With arterial ulcers, perfusion is promoted by avoiding compression stockings or dressings and by encouraging dependent limb position most of the time. Four-inch wooden blocks placed under the head of the bed promote dependence while sleeping. Providing warmth to the lower extremities with cotton stockings and protecting from injury with well-fitting shoes can aid in prevention. Arterial ulcers should be gently cleansed with normal saline, and moisture may be provided with topical creams, hydrogels, or hydrocolloids. Saline dressings may macerate the surrounding tissue and are difficult to maintain. Unna's boot is inappropriate in the care of arterial ulcers because it dries an already dry wound bed and provides compression in a poorly perfused limb.

Diabetic Foot Ulcers. The high incidence and recurrence rate makes diabetic foot ulcers a common issue in diabetes care. Management of blood glucose is an essential component for foot ulcer prevention and healing. Additionally, specific ulcer management techniques include debridement to a clean ulcer base, treatment of any infection in the ulcer, consideration of modalities to promote wound healing, and the use of accommodative pressure-reducing devices such as custom-molded shoes or shoe inserts to off-load ulcer sites.

Debridement can be accomplished by surgical, mechanical, or autolytic methods. Surgical debridement is used to remove hyperkeratotic or necrotic tissue and should cause only minimum healthy tissue trauma and bleeding. Mechanical debridement involves the use of high-pressure water sprays. Whirlpool treatments are not recommended by some sources, since these treatments have a risk for skin burning and maceration in a patient population where there is impaired healing mechanisms (the diabetic population).[27] In the office setting a 30-ml syringe with an 18-gauge needle can be used for mechanical debridement. Autolytic debridement with film and hydrocolloid dressings allow leukocytes on the ulcer surface to degrade and release lysosomal enzymes that break down protein and mucopolysaccharide components of ulcer eschar; however, dressings that retain moisture are contraindicated in the presence of infection.[28,29]

Once the ulcer is debrided, prevention of infection is imperative to reduce risk of amputation; however, detection of infection is often difficult secondary to neuropathy and decreased inflammatory response. Dressings must be changed frequently, at least every 24 hours, and the ulcer is continually assessed for infection. Prolonged hyperglycemia may be the first indication of infection. Systemic antibiotics and assessment for osteomyelitis are essential to prevent amputation.[12-14]

There is evidence showing benefit for other treatment modalities such as cultured human dermis, hyperbaric oxygen therapy, total contact casting, electrical stimulation (E-Stim), and tissue growth factors.[27,28] Data continue to emerge in this area; however, some of these treatment modalities have high cost and are best used by a wound specialist. Graftskin, a bilayered skin substitute, has been used as a healing adjunct for full-thickness ulcers that do not have tendon, muscle, joint capsule, or bone exposure and have not responded to conventional therapy.[29]

Once ulcers are healed, patients require close, continuous monitoring to minimize recurrences. Pressure-relieving modalities (see Health Promotion, p. 305) may be used. Patients should be monitored daily, weekly, biweekly, and finally at 2-month intervals until stable, and then at least at 6-month intervals.[29,30]

Nonhealing Surgical or Traumatic Wounds. Wounds healing by secondary intention are often large and highly exudative. Wound packing with a hydrogel or calcium alginate to absorb exudate is often effective. The use of new technologic advances to enhance healing, such as vacuum-assisted closure, has promoted wound healing in large, open wounds.[24,31]

Adjunctive therapies are useful in chronic wounds; hyperbaric oxygen therapy is being used in treating diabetic foot ulcers with moderate success.[27] The V.A.C. System, developed by Kinetics Concepts, Inc., is useful to promote healing in chronic, moist, stage 3 or 4 pressure ulcers, as well as nonhealing surgical wounds and some lower extremity ulcers. Ultrasound, topical oxygen, and electrical stimulation may also be beneficial in certain wounds.[17,24,25,26,31]

Documentation must include the nature of the injury; wound type, location, and size in centimeters (length, width, depth); integrity of supporting structures (bone, wound, vasculature); and appearance of all exposed and surrounding tissue. A picture of the wound is most helpful, as is a drawing that demonstrates shape and where measurements were taken.[30] Depth is assessed with a sterile cotton swab placed into the deepest part of the wound, then measured (Box 74-8).

LIFE SPAN CONSIDERATIONS

Impaired skin integrity is common in older adults as a result of age-related skin changes, immobility, malnutrition, incontinence, immunocompromised status, polypharmacy, sensory deficits, and co-morbidities. Thinning of the epidermis, dermis, and subcutaneous tissue, coupled with decreased tensile strength and elasticity and poor epidermal-dermal adhesion, contributes to easy skin tears, pressure ulcers, and lower extremity ulcers.[19,32]

In addition, wound healing time is prolonged in older adults because of decreased oxygenation and perfusion and a decreased inflammatory response. Although the same principles of wound management apply in all populations, special

BOX 74-8

DOCUMENTATION OF WOUNDS

Wound
- Location
- Length
- Depth
- Edges

Presence of foreign bodies
Accompanying injuries
- Fractures
- Dislocations
- Tendon or ligament injuries
- Neurologic and cardiovascular findings

Diagnostic findings, radiologic conclusions
Treatments
Possible scar formation
Follow-up

diligence is recommended in caring for older adults. Consideration of the diminished ability to provide self-care and travel easily to and from medical facilities should prompt the provider to select appropriate dressings and to consider a referral to home health agencies for wound evaluation and care in the patient's setting. The risk of delayed wound healing contributes to infection, pain, and a decreased quality of life in patients who may already be compromised.[18,20]

COMPLICATIONS

Complications of wound healing include infection, dehiscence, delayed wound healing, extensive scarring, and sepsis. Serious infection of the face or hands and cellulitis that has not responded to oral antibiotic treatment require IV antibiotics and/or hospitalization.

INDICATIONS FOR REFERRAL OR HOSPITALIZATION

Referral decisions are guided by the location and nature of the wound; injury to bone, vasculature, or tendons; and the experience of the health care provider. Fractures; deep tissue, vascular, or organ damage; facial and hand injuries; or severely contaminated wounds require referral to a specialist. Large, open wounds or deep puncture wounds most likely require surgical intervention. Facial or hand wounds that are infected may require hospitalization and IV antibiotics. Chronic wounds such as ulcers may be best managed by referral to a wound care specialist who is part of an interdisciplinary team.

PATIENT AND FAMILY EDUCATION

Signs and symptoms of wound infection should be reviewed with the patient and family both verbally and in writing. Infection of the wound can greatly affect outcome and may impede wound healing and return of function. Demonstrating wound dressing techniques with the patient and family and observing a return demonstration when possible are helpful in ascertaining patient understanding. A patient teaching pamphlet or videotape with specific directions for wound cleansing and care reinforces teaching.

Reevaluation and follow-up evaluation for suture removal should be scheduled before discharge. Sutures are removed according to the location of the wound and the type of suture used. Referral for visiting nurses may be important for dressing changes, support in managing medications (especially antibiotics), and wound evaluation in the home. Follow-up monitoring of most wounds should occur within 7 to 10 days.

HEALTH PROMOTION

The cost of wound care in all populations exceeds $2 billion annually in the United States. Prevention of lower extremity ulcers and diligent foot care in patients with diabetes mellitus and peripheral vascular disease will prevent amputations, decrease the cost of multiple hospitalizations, and prolong and improve the overall quality of life. The use of pressure-relieving interventions such as callus removal, padded hosiery to reduce callus buildup, extra-depth shoes, and insoles to redistribute foot pressure have demonstrated some benefit in ulcer prevention.

Promoting healthy behaviors is an essential intervention in the prevention of traumatic wounds. Health care providers should encourage home safety and reinforce child safety practices. Other important health promotion issues to include in patient care encounters include promoting gun control and violence reduction, as well as encouraging automobile safety and seat belt use.

REFERENCES

1. Bryant R: *Acute and chronic wounds: nursing management*, St Louis, 2000, Mosby.
2. Hughes P: Wounds and wound management. In Sheehy S, Lenehan G: *Manual of clinical trauma care*, ed 3, St Louis, 1999, Mosby.
3. Kravitz M: Outpatient wound care, *Crit Care Nurs Clin North Am* 8(2):217-223, 1996.
4. Rainey J: *Wound care: a handbook for community nurses*, Philadelphia, 2002, Whurr.
5. Bostrom J, Mechanic J, Lazar N, and others: Preventing skin breakdown: nursing practices, costs and outcomes, *Appl Nurs Res* 9(4):184-188, 1996.
6. Bates-Jensen B: Pressure ulcers: pathophysiology and prevention. In Sussman S, Bates-Jensen B, editors: *Wound care: a collaborative practice manual for physical therapists and nurses*, ed 2, Philadephia, 2001, Lippincott Williams & Wilkins.
7. Rappl L: Management of pressure by therapeutic positioning. In Sussman S, Bates-Jensen B, editors: *Wound care: a collaborative practice manual for physical therapists and nurses*, ed 2, Philadephia, 2001, Lippincott Williams & Wilkins.
8. Registered Nurse's Association of Ontario: Risk assessment and prevention of pressure ulcers, retrieved Dec 15, 2006, from http://www.rnao.org/Page.asp?PageID=924&ContentID=816.
9. Bergstrom N, Allman RM, Alvarez OM, and others: *Treatment of pressure ulcers, clinical practice guidelines no 15*, AHCPR Pub No 95-0652, Rockville, Md, 1994, US Department of Health and Human Services, US Public Health Service, Agency for Health Care Policy and Research.
10. Mulder G: Evaluating and managing the diabetic foot: an overview, *Adv Skin Wound Care* 13(1):33-36, 2000.
11. National Pressure Ulcer Advisory Panel: *Pressure ulcers in America*, retrieved Dec 15, 2006, from http://www.npuap.org.
12. Sumpio B, and others: Etiology and management of foot ulcerations. In Lee BY: *The wound management manual*, New York, 2005, McGraw-Hill.
13. American Diabetes Association: Standards of medical care in diabetes—2006, *Diabetes Care* 29:S4-S42, 2006, retrieved Dec 15, 2006, from http://care.diabetesjournals.org/cgi/content/full/29/suppl_1/s4?maxtoshow=&HITS=10&hits=10&RESULTFORMAT=&f

ulltext=foot+ulcer&searchid=1139514046434_7642&FIRSTINDEX=0&volume=29&issue=suppl_1&journalcode=diacare#SEC15.

14. Effman N, Conlan J: Management of the neuropathic foot. In Sussman S, Bates-Jensen B, editors: *Wound care: a collaborative practice manual for physical therapists and nurses*, ed 2, Philadephia, 2001, Lippincott Williams & Wilkins.
15. NHS Center for Reviews and Dissemination: A systematic review of foot ulcers in patients with type 2 diabetes mellitus, part II, Treatment, *Database of Abstract and Reviews of Effectiveness*, 1(10), retrieved Dec 15, 2006, from http://www.unitedhealthfoundation.org/download/UHF%20Diabetes%20paper_all%20content_Aug11%2006.pdf.
16. Sieggreen M, Kline R: Arterial insufficiency and ulceration; diagnosis and treatment options, *Nurse Pract* 29(9):46-52, 2004.
17. Hess C: Management of the patient with a venous ulcer, *Adv Skin Wound Care* 13(2):79-83, 2000.
18. Boynton P, Jaworski D, Paustian C: Meeting the challenges of healing chronic wounds in older adults, *Nurs Clin North Am* 34(4):921-932, 1999.
19. Baranoski S: Skin tears: the enemy of frail skin, *Adv Skin Wound Care* 13(3 pt 1):123-126, 2000.
20. Bates-Jenson B: Chronic wound assessment, *Nurs Clin North Am* 34(4):799-839, 1999.
21. Wipke-Tevis D, Rantz MJ, Mehr DR, and others: Prevalence, incidence, management, and predictors of venous ulcers in the long-term-care population using the MDS, *Adv Skin Wound Care* 13(5):218-224, 2000.
22. Gordon M, Goodwin C: Initial assessment, management and stabilization of burns, *Nurs Clin North Am* 32(2):237-249, 1999.
23. Krasner D, Sibbald R: Nursing management of chronic wounds, *Nurs Clin North Am* 34(4):935-943, 1999.
24. Samson D, Lefevre F, Aronson N: *Wound-healing technologies: low-level laser and vacuum-assisted closure: summary, evidence report/technology assessment,* No 111, AHRQ Pub No 05-E005-1, Dec 2004, Rockville, Md, Agency for Healthcare Research and Quality, retrieved Dec 15, 2006, from http://www.ahrq.gov/clinic/epcsums/woundsum.htm.
25. Rolstad B, Ovington L, Harris A: Principles of wound management. In Bryant R: *Acute and chronic wounds: nursing management,* St Louis, 2000, Mosby.
26. Fowler E, Vesely N, Pelfrey M, and others: Wound care for persons with diabetes, *Home Health Nurse* 17(7):437-444, 1999.
27. Boykin J: The nitric oxide connection: hyperbaric oxygen therapy, becaplermin, and diabetic ulcer management, *Adv Skin Wound Care* 13:169-174, 2000.
28. Ladin D: Understanding dressings, *Clin Plast Surg* 25(3):433-441, 1998.
29. Ovington L: Wound care products: how to choose, *Home Health Nurse* 19(4):224-232, 2001.
30. Brill LR, Stone JA: New treatments for lower extremity ulcers, *Patient Care Nurse Pract* 4(120):9-20, 2001.
31. Niezgoda J, Schiby B: Negative-pressure wound therapy (vacuum-assisted closure). In Lee B: *The wound management manual*, New York, 2005, McGraw-Hill.
32. Nayduch D: Trauma wound management, *Nurs Clin North Am* 34(4):896-906, 1999.

PART 6

Evaluation and Management of Eye Disorders

CHAPTER 75

Evaluation of the Eyes

Kate Goldblum, Patricia Gillett,
Patricia A. Lamb, and Joyce Powers

Ocular assessment may focus on ocular health promotion, preventive vision care, or an episodic problem. Prevention includes regular eye examinations (especially after age 40 years) and the use of protective eyewear in sports, at work, and around hazardous materials. Early detection of ocular disorders and patient education about ocular symptoms requiring immediate evaluation are integral components of ocular health promotion. Episodic ocular problems require rapid examination. The provider should assess visual acuity in each eye (noting any differences in visual acuity between the two eyes or from previous measurements), ocular alignment and mobility, pupillary equality and reaction to light, gross visual fields, and the status of the optic discs.

Evaluation of the eyes may also provide further evidence of systemic disorders. Patients with diabetes or hypertension may have ocular fundus changes. Some neurologic disorders may initially be noticed as abnormalities on ocular examination. A thorough assessment can help identify patients with common vision-threatening problems such as cataracts, glaucoma, diabetic retinopathy, and age-related macular degeneration. Once identified, patients with these problems should be referred for appropriate evaluation and treatment.

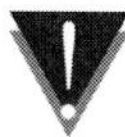

Immediate ophthalmology or emergency department referral is indicated for patients with sudden-onset vision loss not associated with an obvious disorder.

HISTORY

History of Present Illness

Careful identification and documentation of symptoms are crucial for diagnosis. It is important to consider the following elements in evaluating and documenting the symptom(s): location; severity; circumstances surrounding the onset; quality or character; aggravating, alleviating, or associated factors; duration; frequency; timing; and impact on activities of daily living. Identifying current or prior use of eye medications for the current problem and recent or current systemic illnesses, such as upper respiratory tract symptoms, is also important.

Past Medical History

A complete list of systemic and ocular medications helps identify disorders commonly associated with ocular manifestations such as diabetes and hypertension and may avoid adverse effects such as enhancement of systemic beta-blocker effects by ophthalmic beta agonists. In addition, many systemic medications have ophthalmic manifestations.[1] Identification of drug allergies and sensitivities is always important. Some of the more significant or common medical conditions with ocular manifestations include diabetes, hypertension, hyperthyroidism, lupus, AIDS, vascular disorders, migraine headache, von Recklinghausen's disease, Marfan's syndrome, sickle cell anemia, and rheumatoid arthritis.[2]

The ocular history should include glasses or contact lens wear, previous ocular injuries or surgeries, and patching or poor vision in childhood. A history of previous intraocular surgery is important in evaluating an abnormally shaped pupil. Knowing that patching occurred in childhood may be useful information in evaluating a difference in visual acuity between the right and left eyes in an adult because it could indicate that amblyopia, not some other disorder, is responsible for the discrepancy.

Family History

The presence of any of the following should be included in the ocular family history: glaucoma, cataracts, macular degeneration, retinitis pigmentosa, retinoblastoma, keratoconus, color blindness, nystagmus, albinism, choroideremia, and corneal dystrophies. Relevant medical family history includes rheumatoid arthritis, diabetes, cardiovascular disease (including hypertension), renal disease, and certain autoimmune disorders.

Social History

A general assessment of employment and leisure activities may identify concerns related to environmental hazards and the potential for ocular injury or trauma. This information is useful for patient education related to ocular injury prevention and the use of protective eyewear. Assessment of contact lens wear and hygiene practices may identify other ocular risks.

OCULAR EXAMINATION

Eye and Vision Screening

Screening for ocular problems, including visual impairment, is an important function in primary health care. Current guidelines suggest routine screening for amblyopia and strabismus in children during the preschool period[3] and routine visual acuity testing in older adults.[4] Other recommendations include screening in the pediatric population from birth throughout childhood with referral to an ophthalmologist for abnormal red reflex, structural abnormalities, inability to fixate on and follow an object, or unequal objection to covering each eye.[5] Routine vision screening should begin at age 3 years with referral for reduced visual acuity or a visual acuity difference greater than two lines on a vision chart.[6] Routine vision screening and ophthalmoscopic assessment of other age-groups may also be justified. In general, adults with no risk factors for an ocular problem should see an eye care professional every 1 to 10 years, depending on age. For individuals with risk factors, the frequency of evaluation increases.[4] Patients with diabetes need regular evaluation by an ophthalmologist.[7]

Visual Acuity Testing

The importance of measuring visual acuity in each eye before any further assessment, manipulation, or treatment cannot be overemphasized. It is imperative to assess and document visual acuity in each eye separately. This is important not only from a clinical standpoint but also from a medicolegal perspective, particularly in any situation involving ocular trauma. Visual acuity assessment and documentation provide evidence of the patient's visual acuity before diagnostic evaluation. This documentation provides an important clinical baseline and precludes subsequent allegations that vision loss was related to the examination technique or subsequent treatment.

Evaluation of both near and far vision in each eye separately, assessment with and without glasses, and avoidance of the pinhole effect obtained with squinting are important in accurately measuring visual acuity. A good standard of assessment is to always check the right eye first, lessening the likelihood of documentation errors. Results may vary as a result of motivation, attention, intelligence, and environmental variants. Visual acuity is determined by the smallest object that can be clearly seen and distinguished. Results of clinical visual acuity testing indicate foveal function, assuming the remainder of the visual system is normal.

The most common method of measuring visual acuity is a Snellen chart placed 20 feet from the patient, with results recorded as a fraction (e.g., 20/20 or 20/80). A measure of 20/80 means the person tested identifies letters at 20 feet that a person with average vision could identify at 80 feet. The individual with average vision sees 20/20. To determine visual acuity in preschoolers, mentally handicapped older children or adults, and illiterate adults, modified charts with numbers or a tumbling E may be used. Other charts, such as the HOTV or Allen figures, may also be used if the individual is unable to perform a more cognitively challenging test. The HOTV chart is a matching test in which the individual points to the letter on a hand-held chart that matches the letter on the distant chart. Allen figures are pictures of easily recognized objects such as a birthday cake or telephone. When using this chart, the examiner should know that cultural factors may interfere with correct recognition. For example, the Allen figure telephone does not look much like modern telephones with which most children today are familiar.

If the patient cannot identify the largest letter or object on the chart, the next level of visual acuity testing involves counting fingers at a certain distance. If the longest distance at which the patient can count fingers is 3 feet, the visual acuity is recorded as "CF at 3 feet." If the patient is unable to count fingers at any distance, the next measure is hand movement, again recorded as the longest distance that the patient can see the hand move (e.g., "HM at 6 inches"). If hand movement is not visible at any distance, the examiner uses a bright penlight to determine whether the patient has light perception. If the patient can see the light, the visual acuity is recorded as "LP." If not, "NLP" (no light perception) is recorded.

A Jaeger chart is used to measure near vision. The card is placed at 12 to 14 inches from the eyes, and results are recorded as the smallest line read (e.g., J_1 or J_{10}). J_1 is the level of near vision equivalent to 20/20 at distance and is equivalent to 4-point type. J_5 is 8-point type, and J_{10} is 14-point type. Standard newspaper print is 8-point type.

As noted previously, children who see better with one eye than the other should be referred to an ophthalmologist for evaluation for amblyopia. In most cases, if untreated before age 10 years, previously treatable amblyopia becomes a permanent vision loss.[5]

Pupil Evaluation

The pupil should be evaluated for dilation and constriction functions, equality, size, and shape. Pupillary response to light is either direct or consensual. Normal pupils are round and equal and react to light directly and consensually. An abnormal appearing pupil may indicate acute glaucoma, iatrogenic dilation, iritis, drug effects, congenital iris abnormalities, acquired iris abnormalities from trauma or prior surgery, or neurologic abnormalities. Physiologic, simple, or essential anisocoria is a normal finding in approximately 20% of the population.[8]

Extraocular Muscle Function

Extraocular muscle examination evaluates the movement of the six extraocular muscles innervated by three cranial nerves: III, IV, and VI. Hirschberg's test uses the corneal light reflex as a simple, practical evaluation of muscle balance. A light source is held midway between the patient's two eyes at a distance of 10 to 12 inches. The light is directed at the pupils as the patient looks straight ahead, and the light reflex is examined to determine if it is reflected symmetrically in each pupil. In the normal person both reflexes will be symmetric. If one eye is not straight, the light reflexes will be asymmetric when compared. Evaluation of the cardinal gaze positions is a further assessment of extraocular muscle function and is done by asking the patient to follow an object in each of the nine cardinal gaze positions.

The cover-uncover test also evaluates muscle function. One eye is occluded while the patient fixates on some object in primary gaze. The eye under the cover should be observed for movement as the occluder is removed. The second eye should be covered and the process repeated. There should be no movement in the uncovered eye. If the eye under the occluder deviates after the occluder is removed (while the opposite eye fixates), it is an indication that extraocular muscle function is compromised. This may occur as a result of abnormal innervation related to diabetic neuropathy or stroke. Abnormal extraocular muscle function may also result from a mechanical restriction such as in thyroid myopathy, muscle entrapment occurring secondary to orbital fractions, or an orbital neoplasm.

Visual Field Evaluation

The confrontation visual field examination evaluates visual function of the peripheral retina and identifies large visual field losses, which are usually accompanied by some functional impairment. Each eye should be tested separately, with the nontested eye covered and the patient's visual field compared with the examiner's visual field. Reasons for defects include advanced glaucoma, stroke, neoplasm, and retinal detachment. Visual field assessment depends on subjective patient replies. The results should be reproducible.

External Examination

The eyebrows, eyelids, eyelashes, and orbital rim should be inspected and palpated. The cornea, conjunctiva, iris, pupil, and anterior chamber should be inspected. The normal bulbar conjunctiva is translucent, moist, and membranous with rich vasculature. The cornea is a clear and avascular structure; the sclera is white. Anterior chamber depth can be assessed by shining a light obliquely across the eye. If the iris is abnormally close to the posterior corneal surface, the oblique light will not reach the opposite side of the eye. The irises are normally the same color. The symmetry of all structures should be noted. The eyelashes should be evenly distributed and curve outward. Normal lid margins are against the globe; lacrimal ducts are patent and without discharge. The skin should be intact and without redness, discharge, or lesions.

Intraocular Pressure Evaluation

Intraocular pressure can be measured in the primary care setting using a Tono-Pen or similar device. These devices are used after instillation of a topical anesthetic to the corneal surface. If a Tono-Pen or similar tonometer is not available, a gross estimation of intraocular pressure can be obtained by lightly palpating the globe through the closed upper lids. The normal eye should feel like a grape. This method can be especially useful in evaluating acute glaucoma, which usually is unilateral. In these patients a distinct difference in firmness between the involved eye and the uninvolved eye may be appreciated. An enlarged cup/disc ratio may be an indication that the patient has had a long period of elevated intraocular pressure (Color Plates 28 and 29).

Ophthalmoscopic Examination

Of all organs, the eye is most accessible to direct examination. The direct ophthalmoscope provides a magnified, upright image of the retinal structures. The ocular lens should be clear and centered behind the iris. The vitreous should be translucent and can normally contain floaters visible by ophthalmoscopic examination. If all the ocular media are clear, the retina should appear as a red reflex. The retina and optic disc should be examined. To facilitate a thorough retinal examination, the ophthalmoscope should be held stable at the pupil, and the patient should look in all four directions. The entry of the optic nerve into the globe forms the physiologic cup, which should be visible. The normal cup/disc ratio is less than 0.5. The macula lies 2 disc diameters from the optic nerve and somewhat superior to it. The macula is avascular and should be examined last because it is the most sensitive part of the retina.

SIGNS AND SYMPTOMS OF OCULAR DISEASE

Red Eye

Red eye is one of the most common ocular complaints in the primary care setting. Often the underlying disorder is self-limiting with minimum visual consequences, but it is important to recognize serious, vision-threatening conditions. The term *red eye* denotes hyperemia of the conjunctiva or sclera. It is also sometimes used to denote redness of the adnexal structures or periocular area.

The most common cause of red eye is conjunctivitis, which may be allergic, bacterial, or viral. Patients may also be seen with a red eye from episcleritis or scleritis. These are inflammatory conditions, although scleritis may rarely have a microbial cause. Episcleritis is almost always self-limiting and rarely requires topical antiinflammatory therapy. Scleritis is a more serious condition that can be vision threatening and is often related to an underlying autoimmune disorder. Patients with possible scleritis should be referred to an ophthalmologist.

The uveal tract of the eye consists of the iris, ciliary body, and choroid. Any or all of these structures may become inflamed, causing red eye. Iritis is an inflammation of the anterior uveal structure, the iris. Uveitis is an inflammation that also involves the posterior uveal structures. These inflammatory conditions are often associated with systemic disorders, many with an autoimmune component. Patients with iritis or uveitis should be referred to an ophthalmologist. Table 75-1 presents these and other ocular disorders that must be considered in the differential diagnosis of a patient seen with red eye.

Accurate diagnosis is critical in determining the appropriate therapy for red eye. For example, treating bacterial conjunctivitis with steroids may exacerbate the infection, and steroid use with a corneal abrasion or ulcer may lead to corneal melting and serious visual consequences. Conversely, treating herpetic keratitis with an antibiotic may delay appropriate therapy and lead to potentially serious consequences. Many ocular disorders can be difficult to accurately diagnose without a slit lamp. The health care provider should not hesitate to refer patients to an ophthalmologist in those situations when treatment does not produce the expected result or when the diagnosis remains obscure.

Vision Loss and Other Visual Disturbances

Visual disturbances can include decreased central or peripheral vision, metamorphopsia (distorted images), photopsia (light flashes), or vitreous opacities (floaters). It is critical to assess the vision of each eye individually. For the patient who normally wears corrective lenses, the visual acuity should be checked with glasses in place. If the glasses are unavailable, getting a pinhole acuity assessment will approximate a corrected acuity. If reduced visual acuity disappears with corrective lenses or pinhole testing, a refractive error is most likely.

It is also imperative to obtain a detailed history of the onset, duration, and other characteristics of symptoms. Visual loss may be unilateral or bilateral, may be transient or permanent, may occur suddenly or gradually, and may involve central or peripheral vision. Complaints of decreased peripheral vision are not common in the primary care setting because patients usually perceive only significant scotomas. "Sudden" vision loss must be distinguished from "suddenly noticed." A gradual vision loss in one eye may be "suddenly" noticed when the better eye is inadvertently occluded by a hand or some other object. Box 75-1 lists common causes of sudden and gradual vision loss. Table 75-2 presents the signs, symptoms, and management of sudden vision loss.

Amaurosis fugax is a transient, periodic visual loss. This condition may result from ophthalmic artery spasms in occlusive diseases of the internal carotid artery or from abnormalities of the aortic arch, both of which require referral for a cardiovascular evaluation. Amaurosis fugax may also result from temporal arteritis, which usually appears with accompanying tenderness or pain. These patients should be referred to an ophthalmologist for definitive diagnosis and management to prevent permanent vision loss. Transient visual loss,

TABLE 75-1 Red Eye: Differential Diagnosis and Management Guidelines

Disorder	Signs and Symptoms	Pain	Management
DISORDERS ASSOCIATED WITH OCULAR ADNEXA REDNESS			
Blepharitis	Ocular burning; eyelid margins red with scaling or crusting	Yes	Warm compresses; daily lid scrubs; erythromycin or bacitracin ophthalmic ointment for anterior blepharitis; see Chapter 77
Cellulitis			
Orbital	Vision sometimes affected; localized tenderness, erythema, edema; fever; proptosis	Yes	Referral to ophthalmologist for hospitalization, IV antibiotics; see Chapter 82
Periorbital	Vision usually not affected; localized tenderness, erythema, edema; fever sometimes present	Yes	Systemic, broad-spectrum antibiotics; office follow-up visit in 12-24 hours; see Chapter 82
Dacryocystitis	Chronic tearing; eyelash crusting; localized tenderness; circumscribed erythema, edema in the inferior medial canthal area; may be able to express purulent material from the nasolacrimal duct	Yes	Warm compresses; gentle massage; topical and/or systemic antibiotics; see Chapter 81
Eyelid lesions			
Chalazion	Nontender in chronic lesions; localized erythema, edema of eyelid(s)	No	Warm compresses; daily lid scrubs; lid massage; see Chapter 77
Hordeolum	Localized tenderness, erythema, edema of eyelid(s); internal lesions pointing to external or internal eyelid surface; external lesions pointing to eyelid margin	Yes	Warm compresses; lid scrubs for recurrent lesions; topical antibiotics; see Chapter 77
Soft tissue hemorrhage	Localized tenderness sometimes present; erythema, ecchymosis, edema of affected area	±	Cold compresses; if orbital floor fracture suspected, tomograms or CT scan
DISORDERS ASSOCIATED WITH OCULAR SURFACE REDNESS			
Angle-closure glaucoma	Severe pain; nausea, vomiting; halos around lights; photophobia; cornea cloudy with variable decrease in vision; conjunctival hyperemia; pupil middilated and fixed; firm globe; shallow anterior chamber	Yes	Emergent referral to ophthalmologist; consider pilocarpine 2% 1 drop q 15 min and/or acetazolamide 250-500 mg PO stat
Chemical exposure	Pain; conjunctival hyperemia, chemosis; corneal haze; decreased visual acuity	Yes	Immediate copious irrigation essential; emergent referral to ophthalmologist; see Chapter 84
Conjunctivitis			
Allergic	Pruritus; conjunctival hyperemia, chemosis; watery or stringy discharge	No	Avoiding allergens; cold compresses; topical and/or systemic medication; see Chapter 78
Bacterial	Photophobia with blepharospasm; mucopurulent discharge with eyelash mattering; edema, hyperemia; preauricular adenopathy only with hyperacute disorder	±	Topical antibiotic drops; systemic antibiotics necessary for gonococcal or chlamydial cause; see Chapter 78
Viral	Acute onset often associated with systemic illness; photophobia or foreign body sensation; preauricular adenopathy; hyperemia; chemosis; watery discharge; classic dendritic corneal lesion present with herpes simplex; periocular lesions present with herpes zoster ophthalmicus	±	Supportive treatment, including cool compresses, topical artificial tears; referral to ophthalmologist for herpetic conjunctivitis; see Chapter 78
Corneal foreign body, abrasion, or ulcer	Foreign body sensation with intense pain; photophobia; conjunctival hyperemia; may have decreased visual acuity; ulcers usually seen as white or opaque corneal lesion; immediate prior history of trauma common with abrasion but not erosion	Yes	Topical antibiotics (for prophylaxis) and systemic pain relievers in abrasions and after foreign body removal; no patching generally, *never* with ulcers or contact lens–related problems; urgent referral to ophthalmologist for erosions, emergent referral for ulcers; see Chapter 79
Dry eye	Sandy, gritty, foreign body sensation; burning; pruritus; conjunctival hyperemia; decreased visual acuity	±	Topical artificial tears; lubricating ointments at night; warm compresses; gentle eyelid massage; evaluation for systemic disorders; see Chapter 80
Episcleritis or scleritis	Mild to severe pain; circumscribed erythema of affected sclera; vision unaffected	Yes	Episcleritis usually self-limiting; with possible scleritis, referral to ophthalmologist
Hyphema	Microscopic or visible blood layering in anterior chamber usually after blunt trauma; often associated with other ocular symptoms	Yes	Urgent referral to ophthalmologist; see Chapter 84
Iritis or uveitis	Pain; photophobia; conjunctival hyperemia; pupil constriction; may have epiphora but no mucopurulent discharge	Yes	Urgent referral to ophthalmologist

Continued

TABLE 75-1 Red Eye: Differential Diagnosis and Management Guidelines—cont'd

Disorder	Signs and Symptoms	Pain	Management
DISORDERS ASSOCIATED WITH OCULAR SURFACE REDNESS—CONT'D			
Keratitis	Pain, photophobia; conjunctival hyperemia; corneal cloudiness with stromal involvement	Yes	Urgent referral to ophthalmologist
Pingueculum and pterygium	Ocular irritation or pain when inflamed; dry eye symptoms; fleshy lesion medial on conjunctiva; with pterygium, lesion extending onto cornea	Yes	Ocular lubricants; topical NSAIDs; with pterygium, routine referral to ophthalmologist; see Chapter 83
Subconjunctival hemorrhage	No subjective symptoms; bright red spot of blood visible under overlying conjunctiva; remainder of conjunctiva remaining white	No	Reassurance; no treatment necessary; see Chapter 84

BOX 75-1

VISION LOSS: DIFFERENTIAL DIAGNOSIS

SUDDEN
- Acute angle-closure glaucoma
- Central retinal vessel occlusion
- Hyphema or other trauma
- Endophthalmitis
- Iritis or uveitis
- Meningitis
- Migraine
- Optic or retrobulbar neuritis
- Retinal hemorrhage (macular area)
- Stroke
- Vitreous hemorrhage

GRADUAL
- Amblyopia
- Cataracts
- Corneal opacities
- Glaucoma
- Iritis or uveitis
- Macular degeneration
- Pituitary tumor
- Retinal detachment
- Vitreous opacities

photopsia, floaters, photophobia, metamorphopsia, or scintillating scotomas may accompany migraine headaches. Ocular symptoms common in migraines can occur without an associated headache. Unless the patient has a clear past history of ocular migraine, these patients should be referred to an ophthalmologist to rule out other potential problems such as retinal or vitreal detachment.

Metamorphopsia is commonly seen with macular degeneration and may also be a feature of central retinal vein occlusion. Any patient reporting new-onset visual distortion or a change in previously noted metamorphopsia should be referred to an ophthalmologist. Effective treatments are available for certain types of age-related macular degeneration.[9]

Photopsia (flashes or flickers of light) may result from a retinal problem or cortical stimulation. Photopsia from retinal problems may be another indication of an impending or actual retinal tear or detachment or a posterior vitreous detachment with retinal traction. Cortically induced photopsia may indicate migraine headache or occipital epilepsy.[10] Retinal detachment may also produce a persistent symptom described as a "curtain," "shadow," or "veil" falling over part of the visual field.

The vitreous is a thick, gel-like structure that degenerates and liquefies with aging. When this occurs, aggregates form vitreous floaters, which are perceived by the patient as gray or black shapes floating within the visual field. Depending on the size and number, floaters may be simply annoying or may cause visual disability. They are often absorbed. If floaters occur suddenly or increase in frequency or quantity, urgent referral to an ophthalmologist is necessary. These symptoms may indicate the presence of a posterior vitreous detachment, primary vitreous hemorrhage, retinal tear, or retinal detachment.

Ocular and Periocular Pain

Ocular or periocular pain can include any discomfort in or around the eye and may be described as burning, aching, throbbing, boring, stabbing, or irritating, as with a foreign body sensation. Any condition that stimulates the numerous pain receptors in the eyelids, cornea, conjunctiva, and uveal tract will cause ocular or periocular pain. Any inflammatory disorder of the conjunctiva, superficial layers of the cornea, or uveal tract can cause ocular irritation, burning, discomfort, or frank pain. Symptoms may be related to exposure to environmental irritants such as tobacco smoke or chemical fumes. Pain may also be referred from adjacent structures innervated by the ophthalmic division of cranial nerve V. Noninflammatory conditions affecting the optic nerve, retina, or vitreous do not usually result in pain.

Pain may occur coincidentally with other ocular symptoms, including decreased visual acuity, photophobia, ocular discharge, eyelid edema or erythema, ptosis, proptosis, or corneal cloudiness. Important history includes:

- Decrease in visual acuity
- Suddenness of onset
- Associated symptoms (including systemic symptoms such as nausea or vomiting)
- Contact lens use

TABLE 75-2 Sudden Vision Loss: Management Guidelines

Disorder	Signs and Symptoms	Management
Acute angle-closure glaucoma	See Table 75-1	See Table 75-1
Central retinal vessel occlusion	Arterial occlusion: vision loss typically more profound; cherry red macula seen against paleness of surrounding retina Venous occlusion: metamorphopsia; flame hemorrhages and dilated tortuous veins in ocular fundus	Urgent referral to ophthalmologist; with arterial occlusion, permanent vision loss possible in <2 hours; physician consultation to determine underlying cause
Hyphema or other trauma	See Table 75-1	See Table 75-1
Endophthalmitis	May or may not be associated with pain; lid edema; conjunctival injection; retinal hemorrhage	Emergent referral to ophthalmologist; visual prognosis dependent on immediate treatment
Iritis or uveitis	See Table 75-1	See Table 75-1
Meningitis	Systemic presentation of meningitis; see Chapter 214	See Chapter 214
Migraine	Scintillating scotomas; photopsia; headache; photophobia; phonophobia; see Chapter 213	See Chapter 213
Optic or retrobulbar neuritis	Variable vision loss; papilledema (present in optic neuritis, not in retrobulbar); pain on eye movement; sore globe	Referral to ophthalmologist within 24-48 hours
Retinal hemorrhage (macular area)	Central vision loss with no associated pain	Ophthalmologist or physician consultation; management dependent on cause
Stroke	Visual field defects; amaurosis fugax; hemianopsia; see Chapter 208	Immediate emergency department referral for all patients with suspected cerebrovascular accident
Vitreous hemorrhage	Ocular fundus possibly occluded in severe cases; if retina visible, examination may reveal signs of the underlying causative disorder (diabetic retinopathy, retinopathy of prematurity, retinal tear or detachment, vitreous detachment, trauma)	Ophthalmologist or physician consultation; management dependent on cause

- Exposure to ultraviolet light (such as outdoor activities or arc welding)
- Neurologic or systemic disorders
- Trauma

A complete ocular assessment should be performed in any patient with ocular pain. It is also important to examine the structures of the head and neck in any patient with a history of trauma. However, the eye should *never* be manipulated if there is any possibility of laceration or rupture of the ocular tissues. A shallow anterior chamber or abnormally shaped pupil may indicate a loss of aqueous humor secondary to a penetrating injury. Acute glaucoma should be excluded by measuring the intraocular pressure with a Tono-Pen or similar device, or by palpating the globes and comparing the affected eye with the unaffected eye. Patients with a painful eye from acute glaucoma usually have associated redness, nausea, and vomiting. The cornea and conjunctiva may be assessed to identify abrasions or ulcers by applying fluorescein dye and examining the external eye under fluorescent light. Applying a topical anesthetic such as proparacaine hydrochloride 0.5% (Ophthaine) or tetracaine hydrochloride 0.5% (Pontocaine) will help differentiate the superficial pain caused by corneal surface disorders from pain resulting from problems with the deeper structures.

It may be useful to approach the differential diagnosis of ocular pain by grouping possible causes according to accompanying symptoms. This approach is summarized in Table 75-3.

TABLE 75-3 Symptoms Associated with Ocular Pain and Possible Causes

Associated Symptom	Possible Causes
Photophobia	Acute glaucoma, migraine, corneal trauma, keratoconjunctivitis, iritis, uveitis, scleritis
Nausea and vomiting	Acute glaucoma, endophthalmitis
Itching	Chemical injury, severe dry eye, allergy
Pain on eye movement	Orbital pseudotumor, myositis, posterior scleritis, optic neuritis, trauma, orbital cellulitis
Foreign body sensation	Corneal ulcer or abrasion, conjunctivitis, overexposure to ultraviolet light, entropion, trichiasis, conjunctival or eyelid lesion (rule out actual corneal or conjunctival foreign body)

Other Ocular Signs and Symptoms

Chemosis is edema of the bulbar conjunctiva. The conjunctiva becomes balloon-like and translucent in appearance around the corneal limbus, making the cornea appear sunken. The most common cause is an allergic reaction. The history of onset and recent activities should help with diagnosis.

Epiphora is excessive tearing. Causes include obstruction of the normal tear drainage system and excessive production of tears caused by irritation or inflammation. Although persistent tearing of one or both eyes in an infant is a cardinal sign of congenital glaucoma, this is a rare condition. Tearing in infants is most often due to congenital nasolacrimal duct obstruction. The patient should be referred to an ophthalmologist when no underlying cause is apparent or if the epiphora worsens.

Ocular discharge may be clear, watery, purulent or mucopurulent, stringy, or ropy. The differential diagnosis of an ocular disorder may be aided by observing the nature of abnormal ocular secretions. Pus in the conjunctival sac causes the eyelashes to stick together and is most common in mucopurulent conjunctivitis. A profuse watery discharge with a burning or gritty sensation and pain may be present in viral conjunctivitis. Pruritus associated with a discharge varying from a watery to a stringy, mucuslike consistency may indicate allergic conjunctivitis.

Photophobia may occur for no known reason. However, almost any condition resulting in ocular irritation or inflammation may cause photophobia. Conditions to consider include iritis or uveitis, conjunctivitis, conjunctival or corneal foreign bodies, corneal abrasion, keratitis, congenital glaucoma in infants, and acute glaucoma in adults. Photophobia may also result from exposure keratitis. This condition occurs most commonly in arc welders, swimmers, or skiers who do not use lenses for protection from excessive direct or reflected ultraviolet light exposure.

Pruritus is the most common complaint in allergic conditions, including allergic conjunctivitis. The symptom is usually bilateral and may be seasonal with associated hay fever symptoms. Unilateral pruritus associated with erythema and chemosis may be iatrogenic or caused by an allergic reaction to topical ophthalmic preparations or, commonly, the preservative in the preparation. Patients with severe dry eye or a chemical injury may also experience pruritus.

REFERENCES

1. Tsiaras WG, and others: *Basic and clinical science course: update on general medicine*, San Francisco, 2005, American Academy of Ophthalmology.
2. Strochschein M: Systemic disorders with ophthalmic manifestations. In Goldblum K and Lamb P, editors: *Core curriculum for ophthalmic nursing*, ed 2, Dubuque, Iowa, 2002, Kendall Hunt.
3. US Preventive Services Task Force: *Screening for visual impairment in children younger than age 5 years: recommendation statement*, Rockville, Md, 2004, Agency for Healthcare Research and Quality, retrieved May 1, 2006, from http://www.ahrq.gov/clinc/3rduspstf/visionscr/vischrs.htm.
4. Mandelbaum S, Chew EY, Christman LM, and others: *Preferred practice pattern: comprehensive adult medical eye evaluation*, San Francisco, 2005, American Academy of Ophthalmology.
5. Bateman JB, Christman LM, Dankner SR, and others: *Preferred practice pattern: pediatric eye evaluations*, San Francisco, 2002, American Academy of Ophthalmology.
6. Committee on Practice and Ambulatory Medicine, Section on Ophthalmology: Eye examination and vision screening in infants, children, and young adults, *Pediatrics* 98(1):153-157, 1996, retrieved May 1, 2006, from http://www.aapos.org/associations/5371/files/visionscreeningpolicy.pdf.
7. Chew EY, Benson WE, Boldt HC, and others: *Preferred practice pattern: diabetic retinopathy*, San Francisco, 2003, American Academy of Ophthalmology.
8. Kline LB, and others: *Basic and clinical science course: neuro-ophthalmology*, San Francisco, 2005, American Academy of Ophthalmology.
9. Wormald R, and others: Photodynamic therapy for neovascular age-related macular degeneration (review), *Cochrane Database Syst Rev* (4):CD002030.pub2, DOI: 10.1002/14651858.CD002030.pub2, 2005.
10. Trobe JD: *The physician's guide to eyecare*, San Francisco, 2000, American Academy of Ophthalmology.

CHAPTER 76

Cataracts

Kate Goldblum, Patricia Gillett, and
Joyce Powers

DEFINITION AND EPIDEMIOLOGY

A cataract is an opacity in the crystalline lens of the eye. Although not all cataracts significantly affect visual acuity, they are a common cause of decreased visual acuity and the leading cause of preventable blindness in the United States for individuals over age 40 years.[1] Most cataracts occur in the aging population and can significantly affect the quality of life in older adults. Almost everyone will develop a cataract if he or she lives long enough. Between ages 65 and 74 years, 14% of men and 24% of women have visually significant cataracts. After age 75 years, these figures increase to 39% and 46%, respectively. The incidence of cataracts is higher in patients with diabetes. Age-related cataracts are usually bilateral but may develop at different rates. Congenital cataracts occur in approximately 1 in 2000 live births.[2] Congenital cataracts are an urgent ophthalmic problem because of the rapid development of amblyopia in the neonate.

PATHOPHYSIOLOGY

Cataracts form when altered metabolic processes affect the structure of the lens fiber. These changes are associated with aging, diabetes, trauma, heavy smoking, corticosteroid use, electrical shock, and exposure to ultraviolet light.

CLINICAL PRESENTATION

Initially the patient may complain of visual problems such as blurry vision or a "film" that obscures vision. The patient may also complain of glare from any source of bright light or altered color perception. Occasionally, a significant unilateral cataract will appear to cause a "sudden" loss of vision. The vision loss is not actually sudden; the patient notices it suddenly when the unaffected eye becomes obscured in some way. The history may include a gradual decrease in vision. Significant cataracts may cause a loss in the ability to continue usual leisure activities or to perform activities of daily living.

PHYSICAL EXAMINATION

The external ocular structures and the pupillary aperture should be examined. The red reflex may be dull. With an advanced cataract, the pupil will appear opaque because of the mature cataractous lens behind the iris (Color Plate 30). Ophthalmoscopic examination may reveal lens opacities and obscured retinal vasculature.

DIAGNOSTICS

None indicated.

DIFFERENTIAL DIAGNOSIS

The differential diagnosis includes any cause of decreased visual acuity, including macular degeneration and diabetic retinopathy. With advanced cataracts, the completely opaque lens may resemble an intraocular tumor that obscures the pupillary aperture.

DIFFERENTIAL DIAGNOSIS

Cataracts

- Macular degeneration
- Diabetic retinopathy
- Intraocular tumor
- Retinal detachment
- Scarring from previous trauma or irradiation

MANAGEMENT

A regular ophthalmic examination and changes in eyeglasses will temporarily improve the patient's ability to see as the cataract develops. Other mediating measures include using increased magnification and increased lighting to improve functional ability. It may be acceptable for the patient to make lifestyle modifications (e.g., ceasing nighttime driving), at least temporarily. The best clinical evidence to date supports that surgery will improve quality of life and is indicated when visual needs exceed the level of vision allowed by the cataract.[1]

LIFE SPAN CONSIDERATIONS

Congenital cataracts or cataracts that develop in children ages 10 years or younger must be urgently managed because of the certain risk of amblyopia. The morbidity attached to the extensive incidence of cataracts in older adults warrants referral for surgery even in individuals with multiple comorbidities. Advances in cataract surgery and management, including topical anesthesia, small incision surgery, and intraocular lenses, reduce the risks and hasten postoperative visual rehabilitation.[3] Even very old patients do well after cataract surgery.[4] Older patients with no deficits other than poor vision are 2.5 times more likely to experience a decline in functional ability than are patients with normal vision.[1] Visual deprivation from cataracts can affect cognitive function; cognition may improve with visual correction.[5]

COMPLICATIONS

Usually the only complication associated with cataracts is decreased visual acuity. In rare instances a cataract may cause phacolytic glaucoma or anterior uveitis and require immediate surgery. Mature cataractous lenses are more likely to dislocate. Mature cataracts may cause complete blindness, but surgery can still provide a good visual outcome.

INDICATIONS FOR REFERRAL OR HOSPITALIZATION

The patient should be referred to an ophthalmologist when visual acuity is reduced to a level that does not meet the patient's visual needs. The level at which this occurs varies from person to person, but with continuing improvements in surgical management and postoperative rehabilitation, there is no reason for patients who wish to see better to delay surgery.

PATIENT AND FAMILY EDUCATION

Larger-print materials, the use of magnifying devices, and increased lighting may allow adequate vision during the early phase of cataract development. Patients should be informed that cataracts are progressive and irreversible but surgical removal is safe and effective. Surgery is elective. Patients should be advised that only they can determine when their vision no longer meets their visual needs.

HEALTH PROMOTION

Patients should avoid known risk factors such as heavy smoking, ultraviolet radiation, and excessive alcohol consumption. Other risk factors over which patients may have some control include diabetes, corticosteroid use, electrical shock, and trauma.[6]

REFERENCES

1. Masket S, Chang DF, Lane SS and others: *Preferred practice patterns: cataract in the adult eye,* San Francisco, 2006, American Academy of Ophthalmology.
2. Rosenfeld SI, and others: *Basic and clinical science course: lens and cataract,* San Francisco, 2005, American Academy of Ophthalmology.
3. Solomon R, Donnenfeld ED: Recent advances and future frontiers in treating age-related cataracts, *JAMA* 290(2):248-251, 2003.
4. Syam PP, Eleftheriadis H, Casswell AG, and others: Clinical outcome following cataract surgery in very elderly patients, *Eye* 18(1):59-62, 2004.
5. Tamura H, Tsukamoto H, Mukai S, and others: Improvement in cognitive impairment after cataract surgery in elderly patients, *J Cataract Refract Surg* 30(3):598-602, 2004.
6. Goldblum K: Lens disorders. In Lamb P, Goldblum K, editors: *Core curriculum for ophthalmic nursing,* ed 2, Dubuque, Iowa, 2002, Kendall/Hunt.

CHAPTER 77

Chalazion, Hordeolum, and Blepharitis

Kate Goldblum, Patricia Gillett, and Joyce Powers

DEFINITION AND EPIDEMIOLOGY

Chalazia and hordeola are both inflammatory processes involving the glandular tissues of the eyelid, usually the upper eyelid. A hordeolum is also called a *stye*. An external hordeolum is an infection of the glands of Moll or Zeis, whereas an internal hordeolum is an infection of the meibomian gland. A chalazion also involves the meibomian gland but is a granulomatous inflammatory lesion rather than an infectious process. Although an acute infection of the meibomian gland is actually an internal hordeolum, it is sometimes referred to as an *acute chalazion*. These inflammatory lesions are often associated with blepharitis, an inflammatory condition of the eyelid margins. Blepharitis may be acute or chronic and is often categorized as anterior or posterior depending on the anatomic structures involved.[1] Anterior blepharitis involves the anterior lid margin surrounding the eyelashes and may extend to the posterior lid margin, conjunctiva, and cornea. When blepharitis is associated with *Staphylococcus aureus* infection, 80% of patients are women, probably related to use of contaminated eye makeup. Posterior blepharitis involves abnormal function of the meibomian glands, either hyperactive secretion or obstruction of the gland. These conditions are common ocular disorders seen in primary care.[2]

PATHOPHYSIOLOGY

The glandular structures involved in a chalazion or hordeolum become obstructed, leading to an inflammatory process. In the case of a hordeolum, a gland of Moll or Zeis becomes acutely inflamed and infected. The most commonly associated organism is *S. aureus*. In contrast, a chalazion involves a chronically inflamed meibomian gland without accompanying infection. Anterior blepharitis is most commonly associated with *S. aureus* infection but is also associated with other organisms. It may also involve abnormal sebaceous gland secretory function and is then termed *seborrheic blepharitis*. Excessive meibomian oil secretions or solidification of the oil with resultant blockage of the gland results in posterior blepharitis.

CLINICAL PRESENTATION

A chalazion or hordeolum may initially be seen with a localized erythematous swelling. A hordeolum is often tender on palpation, whereas chronic chalazia are normally nontender. There is usually no visual disturbance unless lid swelling is excessive. Larger lesions may press on the corneal surface and induce astigmatism, decreasing vision. An internal hordeolum typically points either externally to the skin or internally to the conjunctival surface. An external hordeolum

TABLE 77-1 Clinical Presentation of Blepharitis

	Crusting	Erythema, Edema	Loss of Eyelashes
Anterior	Hard	Yes	Yes
Anterior seborrheic	Oily	Yes	Rare
Posterior	±	Yes	No

is more superficial and points to the lid margin. A chalazion is usually located in the mid tarsus away from the lid margin and is usually a chronic lesion that is seen with or without acute inflammatory signs.

All forms of blepharitis may manifest with crusting and an erythematous lid margin. Alteration of the tear film layer may induce symptoms of dry eye (Table 77-1).

PHYSICAL EXAMINATION

The ocular adnexa, especially the lid margins, should be carefully inspected. Adequate lighting and some magnification are particularly helpful during this assessment. With blepharitis, the lid margins may be reddened and scaly. The lid should be palpated for swelling and masses, and the eyelid should be everted to examine the tarsal conjunctival surface for pointing. This maneuver may be difficult when the lid is swollen and painful. The sclera and conjunctiva should be inspected for erythema, edema, or exudate. Hordeola and chalazia may be initially indistinguishable. However, the initial acute manifestations of a chalazion will resolve within a few days, leaving a painless, slowly growing lid mass.

DIAGNOSTICS

None indicated.

DIFFERENTIAL DIAGNOSIS

Patients with multiple or recurrent chalazia or hordeola may have underlying diabetes mellitus. Benign or malignant tumors must be considered in patients with recurrent or atypical lesions. In addition to chalazia, hordeola, and blepharitis, the differential diagnosis for eyelid disorders includes cellulitis or abscess of the eyelid and acute dacryocystitis.[1]

DIFFERENTIAL DIAGNOSIS

Eyelid Disorders

- Hordeolum
- Blepharitis
- Benign or malignant tumors
- Chalazion
- Cellulitis
- Trauma
- Dermatitis
- Abscess
- Dacryocystitis

MANAGEMENT

Frequent application of warm, moist compresses to a hordeolum will often hasten the process of pointing and draining. If the hordeolum is associated with a specific eyelash, pulling the lash will also hasten draining. Topical antibiotics may be helpful and should be used four times daily for 1 week. These eyelid conditions are often caused by *S. aureus*, an organism with minimum susceptibility to neomycin-polymyxin B–gramicidin (Neosporin ophthalmic solution); this is not a good choice for treatment.[3] Tobramycin 0.3% (Tobrex ophthalmic solution) is a good choice for initial therapy. The more broad-spectrum topical antibiotics such as ofloxacin 0.3% (Ocuflox ophthalmic solution) or ciprofloxacin (Ciloxan ophthalmic solution) should be avoided unless the hordeolum recurs frequently or does not respond to other therapy. Ointments can be messy and blur the vision, and many patients prefer drops for these reasons.

Recurrent lesions require daily lid margin scrubs and topical antibiotics. Although commercial products for lid scrubs are available, an inexpensive and effective alternative is diluted baby shampoo (see Patient and Family Education). Patients with chronic or recurrent lesions may be co-managed with the ophthalmologist. Chronic chalazia may require steroid injection. If this is not effective, lesions must be surgically incised and removed by an ophthalmologist. Lid scrubs are also indicated for blepharitis management. Therapy for anterior blepharitis includes topical antibiotics. Table 77-2 summarizes the specific management of hordeola, chalazia, and the different forms of blepharitis.

LIFE SPAN CONSIDERATIONS

Hordeola are more common in children and adolescents and may occur in groups of lesions, since individuals in these age-groups tend to rub their eyelids and spread the infection. In contrast, chalazia are more common in adults.[4] In children a large lesion causing astigmatism or obstructing the visual axis may induce amblyopia. Younger children can develop significant amblyopia within weeks. Anterior blepharitis is more common in younger patients, and posterior blepharitis is more common in older patients.[5]

COMPLICATIONS

If left untreated, these lesions may progress to eyelid or periorbital cellulitis and require systemic antibiotics. Large lesions may induce astigmatism or mechanically restrict the visual field, but this is rare. Chronic blepharitis may result in scarring and the loss of protective eyelashes.

INDICATIONS FOR REFERRAL OR HOSPITALIZATION

Complicated cases may require referral to an ophthalmologist. Patients with recurrent or atypical lesions, lesions unresponsive to therapy, or unexplained vision loss should also be referred to an ophthalmologist. Blepharitis that does not respond to conservative management should be referred to an ophthalmologist for further evaluation and management, including possible systemic antibiotic therapy.

PATIENT AND FAMILY EDUCATION

Patients need instructions regarding good hygienic practices and daily lid scrubs. An inexpensive alternative to commercially available products for lid scrubs is 1 part baby shampoo diluted in 1 part water. The patient should be instructed to dip a clean, cotton-tipped swab in the solution and gently scrub the lid margins. A separate swab should be used for each eyelid. After the scrub, the patient should thoroughly rinse the area and pat it dry. Although it is an expensive recommendation, the patient with a hordeolum or blepharitis

TABLE 77-2 Management of Lid Disorders

Disorder	Compresses	Antibiotic	Steroid	Other
HORDEOLUM				
Internal: Zeis or Moll gland infection *External:* meibomian gland infection (sometimes referred to as *acute chalazion*)	Frequent warm, moist compresses to hasten pointing and drainage	Applied topically to prevent secondary infection from drainage; continue for 1 week; systemic doxycycline for recurrent lesions	None	Lid scrubs, especially if lesions recur; discarding of opened eye makeup to avoid reinfection
CHALAZION				
Meibomian gland inflammation (acute infection is more properly termed *external hordeolum*)	Frequent warm, moist compresses to liquefy glandular secretions	Not indicated	Intralesional injection sometimes effective in resolving lesion	Lid massage to help express impacted secretions; lid scrubs useful if associated with blepharitis
BLEPHARITIS				
Anterior	Daily or more frequent warm, moist compresses to help loosen crusts	Topical ophthalmic erythromycin or bacitracin ointment	None	Lid scrubs daily or more often to help remove crusts
Anterior seborrheic	Daily or more frequent warm, moist compresses to help loosen crusts	None	Occasional topical steroid if inflammation prominent	Lid scrubs daily or more often to help remove oily secretions
Posterior	Daily or more frequent warm, moist compresses to help liquefy secretions	None	None	Lid scrubs daily or more often to help remove oily secretions

associated with *S. aureus* infection should be instructed to discard all eye and face makeup, opened contact lens solutions, and used contact lens cases because of the risk of reinfection from contamination.

HEALTH PROMOTION

Good lid hygiene to control chronic blepharitis and prevent the recurrence of chalazia and hordeola is the primary consideration in health promotion.

REFERENCES

1. Matoba AY, Harris DJ, Meisler DM, and others: *Preferred practice pattern: blepharitis,* San Francisco, 2003, American Academy of Ophthalmology.
2. Pasternak A, Irish B: Ophthalmologic infections in primary care, *Clin Fam Pract* 6(1):19-33, 2004.
3. Levinson BA, Rutzen AR: New antimicrobials in ophthalmology, *Ophthalmol Clin North Am* 18:493-509, 2005.
4. Simon JW, Christman LM, Dankner SR, and others: *Basic and clinical science course: pediatric ophthalmology and strabismus,* San Francisco, 2005, American Academy of Ophthalmology.
5. Sutphin JE, and others: *Basic and clinical science course: external disease and cornea,* San Francisco, 2005, American Academy of Ophthalmology.

CHAPTER 78

Conjunctivitis

Kate Goldblum, Patricia Gillett, and
Joyce Powers

DEFINITION AND EPIDEMIOLOGY

Conjunctivitis is an inflammation or infection of the conjunctiva. Only the bulbar conjunctiva covering the sclera may be involved, or the inflammation may also involve the tarsal conjunctiva that lines the inside of the eyelids. The cornea may become involved with more severe inflammatory or infectious responses, in which case the condition is termed *keratoconjunctivitis*.

Conjunctivitis is a common ocular condition and can occur in all age-groups. Allergic conjunctivitis occurs seasonally or after ocular contact with sensitizing substances, such as in contact lens wearers who develop sensitivities to their lenses or the solutions used to care for them. Allergic conditions, which usually begin in childhood or adolescence, are more common in patients with a positive family history of allergy. Viral conjunctivitis is one of the most common ophthalmic conditions seen by health care providers; bacterial conjunctivitis is much less common.[1] Adenoviruses cause most cases of conjunctivitis and keratoconjunctivitis, including epidemic keratoconjunctivitis, which is highly contagious and is often spread via public swimming pools. Gonococcal and chlamydial infections are more likely to occur in the neonate or in patients at risk for sexually transmitted diseases. Chlamydial conjunctivitis, also called *inclusion conjunctivitis*, is becoming more common in the United States as a result of sexual spread of the causative organism.[2] The chlamydial organism may also be transferred from the mother's birth canal to infants during delivery. Toxic conjunctivitis occurs with exposure to noxious agents such as chlorinated water in swimming pools, hair sprays, other aerosol agents, and strong chemical fumes.

PATHOPHYSIOLOGY

Allergic conjunctivitis is an immunologically mediated response to a wide variety of allergens. Another noninfectious mechanism is a toxic response to various agents such as crab lice or to the benzalkonium chloride preservative in many topical medications. Bacterial conjunctivitis results from a variety of infectious organisms, including *Staphylococcus aureus*, streptococci, *Haemophilus influenzae*, *Neisseria gonorrhoeae*, *Proteus* organisms, and *Klebsiella pneumoniae*. Viral conjunctivitis commonly involves the adenoviruses, herpes simplex virus, and herpes zoster virus.

CLINICAL PRESENTATION

A variety of symptoms may be present depending on the cause and severity of the conjunctivitis. The most common sign of conjunctivitis is conjunctival hyperemia. Allergic conjunctivitis often causes generalized hyperemia, mild to severe itching, and an ocular discharge that may be clear and watery or stringy and mucoid. There may also be mild to severe chemosis. Severe edema may cause the cornea to appear sunken in the boggy conjunctiva. Vision is usually unaffected or mildly affected if there is significant tearing. Antecedent history of atopy is helpful in diagnosing allergic conjunctivitis.

Viral conjunctivitis has an acute onset and may be unilateral or bilateral with a watery discharge and preauricular or submandibular lymphadenopathy. It may be associated with fever and pharyngitis, especially in children. Viral conjunctivitis is usually self-limiting but may take weeks to completely resolve. Photophobia or a foreign body sensation may be present. Herpes simplex conjunctivitis manifests with a classic dendritic corneal lesion visible with fluorescein staining. Herpes zoster dermatitis may also involve the ocular structures, including the conjunctiva. In addition to the presence of a lesion on the tip of the nose (Hutchinson's sign), skin lesions on the inner corner of the eye and the side of the nose may also be helpful in identifying those patients with herpes zoster dermatitis who are at risk of ocular complications.[3]

In contrast, of the bacterial conjunctivitis entities, only hyperacute purulent bacterial conjunctivitis caused by gonococcal organisms or by the *Neisseria* species (primarily *N. gonorrhoeae* or, less commonly, *N. meningitidis*) cause preauricular lymphadenopathy.[4] Bacterial conjunctivitis has an acute onset and is not associated with systemic illness. Hyperemia, chemosis, photophobia with blepharospasm, and tearing may be present. Symptoms often begin in one eye and then involve the second eye. The patient may report that the eye is "stuck shut" with mucopurulent drainage on awakening. If a mucopurulent discharge is present in association with preauricular adenitis, a careful history should be obtained to determine whether there is an increased risk for other sexually transmitted disease, since chlamydia is found in up to one third of all patients with gonococcal conjunctivitis.[5]

PHYSICAL EXAMINATION

Although the history is the most helpful factor in making the correct diagnosis, the examination may provide additional clues or help exclude other causes of the patient's symptoms. The pupils should be observed for symmetry and response to light, and the eyelids should be examined for erythema, swelling, or hyperemia. The upper lids should be everted and the tarsal conjunctival surface checked for a cobblestone appearance, which indicates an allergic response. The possible presence of conjunctival foreign bodies should be evaluated using magnification. The sclera and conjunctiva should be observed for redness, edema, or discharge. The cornea should be evaluated for clarity. Herpetic lesions, foreign bodies, and ulcers should be excluded using magnification and an ultraviolet light source after fluorescein staining. The preauricular and submandibular glands should be palpated for the presence of lymphadenopathy.

DIAGNOSTICS

Patients with conjunctivitis should have corneal fluorescein staining to identify any possible corneal surface pathologic condition that may cause similar symptoms. Cultures are generally not necessary in the primary care setting. Exceptions include neonates with mucopurulent discharge and adolescents and adults at risk for sexually transmitted diseases. In

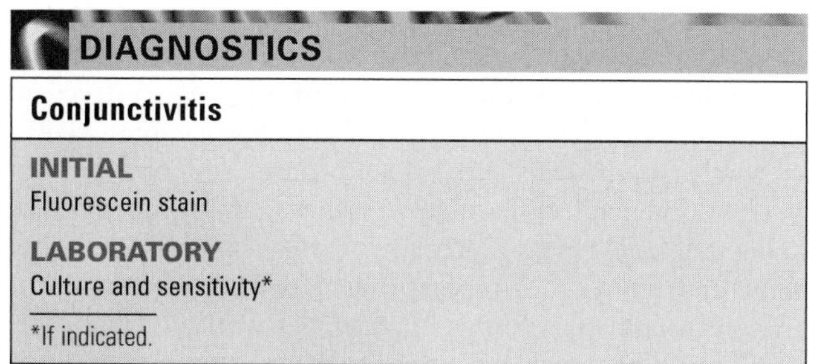

DIAGNOSTICS

Conjunctivitis

INITIAL
Fluorescein stain

LABORATORY
Culture and sensitivity*

*If indicated.

such cases the discharge must be cultured to determine whether the conjunctivitis is of gonococcal or chlamydial origin.[5]

DIFFERENTIAL DIAGNOSIS

DIFFERENTIAL DIAGNOSIS

Conjunctivitis

- Nasolacrimal duct obstruction
- Acute anterior uveitis
- Acute glaucoma
- Blepharitis
- Corneal abrasions or ulcers
- Corneal or conjunctival foreign bodies

Other causes of red eye include nasolacrimal duct obstruction, acute anterior uveitis, acute glaucoma, blepharitis, corneal abrasions or ulcers, and corneal or conjunctival foreign bodies. Further causes of red eye are listed in Table 75-1.

MANAGEMENT

Topical decongestant-antihistamine combinations such as naphazoline hydrochloride 0.025%–pheniramine maleate 0.3% (Naphcon-A) or naphazoline-antazoline (Vasocon-A) are available over the counter and may provide adequate relief for the symptoms of allergic conjunctivitis. The newer selective antihistamines levocabastine hydrochloride 0.05% (Livostin) and emedastine 0.05% (Emadine), as well as the antihistamine–mast cell stabilizers olopatadine 0.1% (Patanol) and azelastine 0.05% (Optivar), are very effective for relieving the symptoms of allergic conjunctivitis. NSAIDs such as ketorolac (Acular) or diclofenac (Voltaren) and the mast cell stabilizers lodoxamide tromethamine 0.1% (Alomide) or cromolyn sodium 4% (Crolom) can be helpful in allergic conjunctivitis. Severe allergic conjunctivitis may require topical steroid therapy, but such therapy can cause increased intraocular pressure (IOP) in susceptible patients and therefore should not be used unless the IOP can be checked periodically. Systemic antihistamines or other antiallergy agents may be helpful. Cold compresses may relieve itching and edema.

Although acute bacterial conjunctivitis is often self-limiting, topical antibiotics may hasten resolution.[6] Topical antibiotic drops such as sulfacetamide 10% (Bleph-10, Isopto Cetamide, or Sodium Sulamyd) or tobramycin (Tobrex) are effective in treating most uncomplicated cases of bacterial conjunctivitis. The second-generation fluoroquinolones, such as ciprofloxacin 0.3% (Ciloxan) or ofloxacin 0.3% (Ocuflox), or fourth-generation fluoroquinolones such as moxifloxacin 0.5% (Vigamox) or gatifloxacin 0.3% (Zymar), are appropriate in more severe cases, but those will be referred to an ophthalmologist in most situations. Chlamydial and gonococcal conjunctivitis must be treated with topical and systemic antibiotic therapy. The health care provider may manage the systemic antimicrobial therapy for gonococcal and chlamydial conjunctivitis. The ophthalmologist manages the ocular therapy and monitors the patient's progress.

Systemic penicillin and doxycycline therapy are the respective treatments of choice for gonococcal and chlamydial infections. Gentamicin 3 mg/ml (Garamycin Ophthalmic, Genoptic S.O.P., or Gentacidin), ofloxacin 0.3%, or norfloxacin (Chibroxin) ophthalmic drops may be used for gonococcal conjunctivitis. Tetracycline ophthalmic ointment (Terak) may be used for chlamydial conjunctivitis.

Viral conjunctivitis is usually self-limiting. Cool compresses may provide some symptomatic relief. Antiinfectives, steroids, and topical vasoconstrictors should not be used. Conjunctivitis of herpetic etiology should be referred to an ophthalmologist for antiviral therapy.

LIFE SPAN CONSIDERATIONS

Conjunctivitis can occur in all age-groups. During the first month of life, conjunctivitis is called *ophthalmia neonatorum*. Hyperacute purulent bacterial conjunctivitis is most common in neonates, adolescents, and adults because of its association with the *Neisseria* species and requires culture for confirmation. Overall, bacteria are less likely to be the cause of conjunctivitis in adults.[5] Viral conjunctivitis is more likely to be associated with fever and pharyngitis in children.

COMPLICATIONS

Severe allergic conjunctivitis can progress to vernal conjunctivitis and lead to corneal ulceration. Bacterial conjunctivitis can also involve the cornea, leading to keratitis and possibly ulceration. Infected corneal ulcers may result in intraocular infection and loss of the eye. Severe viral conjunctivitis may cause extensive scarring and cicatricial complications.

INDICATIONS FOR REFERRAL OR HOSPITALIZATION

Neonates with conjunctivitis should be referred to an ophthalmologist. All patients with suspected bacterial conjunctivitis should be referred to an ophthalmologist if the condition is unresponsive to antimicrobial therapy or if there is suspected corneal involvement. An ophthalmic referral is also necessary for complaints of significant ocular pain, decreased visual acuity, significant purulent discharge, recurrence, or a history of herpes simplex virus eye disease.[4] Steroid therapy for severe viral conjunctivitis is controversial and should be initiated by an ophthalmologist, as should treatment for herpetic viral keratoconjunctivitis.

PATIENT AND FAMILY EDUCATION

Patients should be instructed to use the prescribed medication for allergic conjunctivitis during the acute allergic periods and to avoid rubbing the eyes to prevent further irritation. Comfort measures such as cold compresses can be helpful. Patients should be warned to avoid the offending allergen whenever possible. Appropriate hygienic measures to prevent transmission to others are imperative with contagious conjunctivitis. Frequent and thorough hand washing is necessary for the patient and all close contacts. Patients should be advised not to share linens with others and to limit public contact during the acute phase when drainage occurs. In any case of infectious conjunctivitis, patients should be instructed to discard all opened eye makeup and to replace their contact lenses, cases, and opened solutions.

HEALTH PROMOTION

Eye makeup, ocular medications, and contact lens solutions and cases should not be shared with other individuals. They should also be replaced regularly to avoid possible ocular infections from contaminated items. Patients need to be informed that sexually transmitted diseases can infect the ocular structures through orogenital contact.

REFERENCES

1. Pasternack A, Irish B: Ophthalmologic infections in primary care, *Clin Fam Pract* 6(1):19-33, 2004.
2. Isada CM, Meisler DM: Gonococcal ocular disease. In Fraunfelder FT, Roy FH, Randall J, editors: *Current ocular therapy,* ed 5, Philadelphia, 2000, Saunders.
3. Zaal MJ, Volker-Dieben HJ, D'Amaro J: Prognostic value of Hutchinson's sign in acute herpes zoster ophthalmicus, *Graefes Arch Clin Exp Ophthalmol* 241:187-191, 2003.
4. American Academy of Ophthalmology Cornea/External Disease Panel (Matoba AY, and others): *Preferred practice pattern: conjunctivitis,* San Francisco, 2003, American Academy of Ophthalmology.
5. Sutphin JE, and others: *Basic and clinical science course: external disease and cornea,* San Francisco, 2005, American Academy of Ophthalmology.
6. Sheikh A, Hurwitz B: Antibiotics versus placebo for acute bacterial conjunctivitis, *Cochrane Database Syst Rev* (2):CD001211, DOI: 10.1002/14651858.CD001211.pub2, 2006.

CHAPTER 79

Corneal Surface Defects and Ocular Surface Foreign Bodies

Kate Goldblum, Patricia Gillett, and Joyce Powers

DEFINITION AND EPIDEMIOLOGY

The corneal surface may be disrupted by an abrasion, erosion, ulcer, or foreign body. An abrasion is a partial or complete defect in the epithelial layer of cells after some traumatic event or overexposure to ultraviolet (UV) light. An erosion is also a partial or complete defect in the epithelium but is not associated with trauma immediately preceding the symptoms. A corneal ulcer involves the underlying stromal layer in addition to the epithelial defect. This may or may not be infected. Ocular foreign bodies are any foreign matter that becomes lodged in the corneal or conjunctival tissues. Abrasions resulting from trauma may occur in any age-group. Foreign bodies are a common source of ocular injuries seen in primary care or emergency departments. Certain workers, such as mechanics, woodworkers, and other construction workers, have an increased risk of corneal abrasions or ocular foreign bodies if they do not use appropriate protective eyewear. Contact lens wearers are at increased risk for corneal abrasions. Extended contact lens wear increases the risk of corneal ulcers approximately fivefold over that of daily contact lens wear.[1] Erosions occur in patients with a history of prior corneal abrasion.

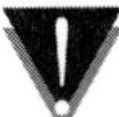

Immediate ophthalmology referral is indicated for all cornea ulcers and for all ocular foreign bodies that are penetrating, obviously impacted, associated with rust ring, or not readily removed by irrigation.

Immediate ophthalmology referral is indicated for ocular herpes simplex and ocular herpes zoster.

Urgent ophthalmology referral is indicated for corneal abrasions not resolved in 24 hours and for corneal lesions that are dendritic or punctate.

Urgent ophthalmology referral is indicated for suspected corneal erosions.

PATHOPHYSIOLOGY

An abrasion of the corneal epithelium may be caused by chemical or mechanical debridement resulting from trauma or UV radiation exposure. Corneal erosions occur if an abrasion disrupts Bowman's membrane. Decreased evaporation during sleep results in the formation of a fluid layer above the incompletely healed Bowman's membrane, below the epithelium. This allows repeated sloughing of the overlying epithelium when the patient awakens and opens the lid, removing the loose epithelial cells. Epithelial defects, whether abrasions or erosions, may allow bacterial, viral, or fungal organisms to invade the corneal stroma, resulting in an ulcer. Sterile corneal ulcers may also occur.

CLINICAL PRESENTATION

Because the cornea is highly innervated, any disruption in the corneal surface causes intense pain. Similar pain may be caused by a foreign body under the upper eyelid that rubs the corneal surface with each blink. Small disruptions in the corneal surface may initially produce a sandy or gritty sensation. With more extensive involvement, intense pain, ocular redness, tearing, photophobia, and often a foreign body sensation are present. A corneal ulcer usually appears as a white or opaque lesion. A clear history of trauma or excessive UV exposure usually precedes a corneal abrasion. The history may include contact lens wear or any recent ocular irritation that may have caused vigorous eye rubbing, resulting in an abrasion. In contrast, there may not be a clear history of exposure to an ocular foreign body when one is present. Corneal erosions are not immediately preceded by trauma. Careful questioning may elicit a history of prior corneal abrasion. There may or may not be decreased visual acuity depending on the extent and location of the pathologic condition.

PHYSICAL EXAMINATION

The upper lid of the involved eye should be everted and the tarsal conjunctival surface examined under magnification for the presence of foreign bodies. The cornea should be examined after the instillation of fluorescein. Corneal defects will stain and fluoresce when exposed to UV light, as will defects caused by foreign bodies. The conjunctiva should be examined for erythema and edema. The corneal surface should be evaluated, checking clarity and looking for areas of opacity or surface irregularity. An oblique light source can be used to assess anterior chamber depth and to identify hypopyon (pus in the anterior chamber). A perforated corneal ulcer or a penetrating foreign body may cause a flat anterior chamber, which is evident when the chamber is compared with the fellow eye.

DIAGNOSTICS

A corneal ulcer is an ophthalmic emergency, especially in the presence of hypopyon. Immediate culture and institution of antimicrobial therapy after an ophthalmology consult may be necessary when an ophthalmologist is not immediately available.

DIAGNOSTICS

Corneal Surface Defects and Foreign Bodies

INITIAL (CORNEAL ULCER)
Fluorescein stain

LABORATORY (CORNEAL ULCER)
Culture and sensitivity (if immediate ophthalmology consultation not available)

INITIAL (FOREIGN BODY)
Fluorescein stain

DIFFERENTIAL DIAGNOSIS

Corneal Surface Defects and Foreign Bodies

- Corneal lacerations
- Conjunctivitis
- Keratitis
- Blepharitis
- Dacryocystitis
- Inflamed pingueculum or pterygium
- Hordeolum (early)
- Chalazion (early)

DIFFERENTIAL DIAGNOSIS

The differential diagnosis includes corneal laceration, conjunctivitis, herpetic and other forms of keratitis, blepharitis, dacryocystitis, inflamed pingueculum or pterygium, and early hordeolum or chalazion.

MANAGEMENT

Minor corneal abrasions can be managed in the primary care setting. Antibiotic ointments such as tobramycin (Tobrex) or erythromycin (Ilotycin) are appropriate. Compliance may be better with a topical drop such as ciprofloxacin 0.3% (Ciloxan) or ofloxacin 0.3% (Ocuflox) because ointments blur vision. Patching does not hasten healing time, lessen pain, or decrease reports of blurred vision. In addition, compliance with the medication regimen is improved when the patient's eye is not patched.[2] A pain reliever is often necessary. Preparations with a steroid component should not be used because the steroid can slow healing and encourage bacterial growth.

If the abrasion is not healed within 1 or 2 days, or if there is a recurrence, the patient should be referred to an ophthalmologist.[3] All patients with apparent erosions should be urgently referred, and patients with corneal ulcer should be emergently referred to an ophthalmologist for evaluation and further therapy. If there is any delay in referral of a corneal ulcer, the lesion should be cultured, and broad-spectrum topical antibiotic drop should be started. Ciprofloxacin or ofloxacin should be used every 30 minutes until the patient is seen by the ophthalmologist.[4] The patient's tetanus immunization status should be determined.

Superficial corneal and conjunctival foreign bodies can be safely removed in the primary care setting. After application of a topical anesthetic, the health care provider can use a moist, cotton-tipped applicator to remove the foreign body. If the foreign body is superficially embedded, a 25-gauge needle may be necessary for removal if the provider is skilled in this procedure and has adequate magnification. Topical antibiotic therapy should be prescribed prophylactically. Clinical studies do not show any benefit in patching the eye in these patients.[2] In any case, *a firm patch should not be applied nor any medications instilled if there is any possibility or suspicion of a penetrating injury.* In addition, any patient with a contact lens–associated abrasion or ulcer should never be patched.

LIFE SPAN CONSIDERATIONS

Infants and children may not be cooperative, which makes careful examination and removal of foreign bodies too difficult in the primary care setting. These patients should be urgently referred to an ophthalmologist. The risk of corneal ulcer in patients who sleep in contact lenses is approximately five times that of patients who restrict lens wear to daytime. The former patients are more likely to be adolescents or young adults.

COMPLICATIONS

Corneal abrasions usually heal without complications but may result in a secondary bacterial keratitis. Corneal erosions and ulcers may cause corneal scarring with vision loss. Corneal ulcers may also result in endophthalmitis, an extensive ocular infection. Subsequent phthisis bulbi (wasting of the globe) and complete blindness may occur. Metallic foreign bodies produce a rust ring that must be completely removed using a slit lamp biomicroscope to prevent chronic problems. Cataract formation is common after any penetrating injury or ulcer.

INDICATIONS FOR REFERRAL OR HOSPITALIZATION

Referral to an ophthalmologist is necessary if a corneal abrasion (1) has not significantly improved within 24 hours, (2) has not completely resolved in 48 to 72 hours, or (3) shows any signs of infection. All patients with corneal ulcers should be emergently referred. Hospitalization may be required for IV antibiotic therapy. Any deeply embedded or centrally located corneal foreign body also requires referral to an ophthalmologist, as do metallic foreign bodies. All chemical injuries and any suspicion of ocular penetration require emergent referral to an ophthalmologist.

PATIENT AND FAMILY EDUCATION

It is imperative to instruct the patient to remove contact lenses immediately if there is any redness, ocular irritation, pain, or decrease in vision. Patients should be advised not to resume contact lens wear until 24 to 48 hours after a superficial abrasion has healed. Culture and subsequent disposal are necessary for all lens supplies and solutions if a corneal ulcer is present. Patients should dispose of any opened cosmetics because of the risk for contamination. Patients should be informed that corneal abrasions or surface defects that remain after foreign body removal can cause significant discomfort for 12 to 24 hours. They should be encouraged to use appropriate pain medications. Patients should be instructed to return before the scheduled follow-up examination if there is any purulent drainage, increased pain or redness, or decreased vision.

HEALTH PROMOTION

The use of proper protective eyewear is imperative during many work and leisure activities to prevent ocular injury. The health care provider should obtain information regarding such use by all patients in the primary care setting, and encourage patients to use appropriate protection.

REFERENCES

1. Sutphin JE, and others: *Basic and clinical science course: external disease and cornea*, San Francisco, 2005, American Academy of Ophthalmology.
2. Kaiser PJ: A comparison of pressure patching versus no patching for corneal abrasions due to trauma or foreign body removal: Corneal Abrasion Patching Study Group, *Ophthalmology* 102(12):1936-1942, 1995.
3. Wirbelauer C: Management of the red eye for the primary care physician, *Am J Med* 119:302-306, 2006.
4. Levinson BA, Rutzen AR: New antimicrobials in ophthalmology, *Ophthalmol Clin North Am* 18:493-509, 2005.

CHAPTER 80

Dry Eye Syndrome

Kate Goldblum, Patricia Gillett, and Joyce Powers

DEFINITION AND EPIDEMIOLOGY

Dry eye is a condition in which the ocular surface becomes desiccated. It affects the tarsal and bulbar conjunctivae and the cornea. The severity of the condition ranges from mild to severe, with more serious involvement resulting in extensive ocular surface changes. The term *keratoconjunctivitis sicca* has often been used interchangeably with dry eye. However, the current classification system separates cases of tear-deficient dry eye into non–Sjögren's syndrome and Sjögren's syndrome keratoconjunctivitis sicca. In addition to tear-deficient dry eye, the other major classification category is evaporative dry eye, mostly those patients with meibomian gland obstruction associated with blepharitis.[1] Dry eye occurs in the majority of patients with Sjögren's syndrome, a combination of dry eyes and dry mouth often linked with conditions mediated by the autoimmune system.[2] Dry eye is relatively common, affecting up to 15% of adults.[1]

PATHOPHYSIOLOGY

Dry eye may be caused by inadequate tear production, increased tear evaporation, abnormal tear composition, or abnormal tear spreading. These conditions can result from lacrimal gland dysfunction, mucin deficiency, environmental factors, lipid abnormalities, or inadequate tear film spread resulting from abnormal eyelid function or anatomic surface abnormalities. Dry eye is commonly associated with autoimmune diseases and other systemic disorders such as multiple sclerosis, lymphoma, and HIV.[2] Many medications may contribute to dry eye, including antihistamines, diuretics, tricyclics, atropine, isotretinoin, and many anticholinergics. Environmental factors such as low humidity and wind also play a role. Dry eye is a common problem in patients with abnormal lid function as a result of Bell's palsy.

CLINICAL PRESENTATION

The initial manifestations of dry eye may be redness; contact lens intolerance; visual blurring; and symptoms of ocular irritation such as burning, itching, scratchiness, foreign body sensation, or "sand in the eye." Symptoms worsen when environmental factors exacerbate tear evaporation or increase ocular irritation. Warmth, low humidity, fans, and secondhand smoke contribute to the symptoms. The bulbar conjunctiva may become erythematous and the periorbital skin may become dry and irritated if the patient rubs the eye in an effort to alleviate the symptoms. Conversely, excessive tearing may be the initial complaint if the tear film lacks adequate mucin or lipid. Important history includes exposure to environmental factors that contribute to dryness, medications, and previous injury. Symptoms that suggest autoimmune or other associated systemic disease such as lymphoma, sarcoidosis, or multiple sclerosis are also an important part of the clinical picture.[1]

PHYSICAL EXAMINATION

Careful external examination of the ocular surface and adnexa will identify conditions such as inadequate lid function or anatomic abnormalities that prevent normal tear distribution. Evaluation of the skin and joints is important to identify a systemic cause for dry eyes.

DIAGNOSTICS

Many diagnostic modalities exist to evaluate dry eye. Schirmer's tear testing can be done in the primary care setting. This test measures tear production using filter paper with or without prior instillation of a topical anesthetic. Without topical anesthesia, the normal eye will usually produce enough tears to wet the filter paper to at least 10 mm (0.4 inch) within 5 minutes.

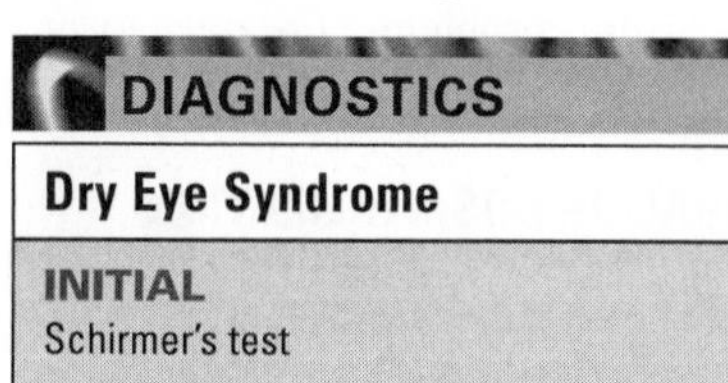
DIAGNOSTICS

Dry Eye Syndrome

INITIAL
Schirmer's test

DIFFERENTIAL DIAGNOSIS

Other causes of ocular irritation that may mimic the symptoms of dry eye include environmental irritants and ocular infection. Frequent use of preserved topical preparations may also cause or exacerbate ocular irritation.

DIFFERENTIAL DIAGNOSIS

Dry Eye Syndrome

- Ocular irritants (particularly preserved topical preparations)
- Environmental irritants
- Ocular infection

MANAGEMENT

Treating or controlling the underlying cause of dry eye is the basis of therapy. Topical therapy with ocular lubricants is often effective in alleviating symptoms. Artificial tears containing methylcellulose or polyvinyl alcohol (Celluvisc, Ocucoat, and HypoTears) are usually the most effective. However, there is great variation among individuals, and the patient should be encouraged to try several different preparations. Lubricating ointments may be helpful when used before sleeping, especially in patients with incomplete eyelid closure, but they are not appropriate for use during waking hours. Using preservative-free, unit-dose preparations helps prevent iatrogenic allergic responses, which greatly exacerbate the problem. Warm compresses and gentle eyelid massage may also be helpful in some cases.

LIFE SPAN CONSIDERATIONS

Dry eye is more common in older patients.[3]

COMPLICATIONS

Severe dry eye can result in corneal ulceration and extensive corneal scarring with subsequent visual disability. Conjunctival scarring with adhesions may also occur.

INDICATIONS FOR REFERRAL OR HOSPITALIZATION

Ocular lubricants and environmental control may not adequately relieve symptoms. In these situations, referral to an ophthalmologist for additional therapy is appropriate. Recent approval of a topical formulation of cyclosporine A (Restasis) gives the ophthalmologist an additional modality (besides topical steroids) to treat the inflammatory aspects of dry eye.[4] Systemic disorders associated with dry eye may require consultation and co-management with multiple specialists.

PATIENT AND FAMILY EDUCATION

Patients should be taught the importance of good hand washing before instilling ocular medications and the risks of sharing medications. Patients also need to be aware that frequent use of preserved artificial tears may worsen the problem by causing additional irritation. They should be taught appropriate technique for eyelid massage and warm compresses, which may help increase lipid in the tears.

HEALTH PROMOTION

Dry eye syndrome is a chronic condition. Knowledge of the environmental factors that exacerbate the condition and how to avoid or ameliorate those conditions is essential. Frequent or excessive use of preserved topical preparations may worsen symptoms and should be avoided.

REFERENCES

1. Sutphin JE, and others: *Basic and clinical science course: external disease and cornea,* San Francisco, 2005, American Academy of Ophthalmology.
2. Strochschein M: Systemic disorders. In Lamb P, Goldblum K, editors: *Core curriculum for ophthalmic nursing,* ed 2, Dubuque, Iowa, 2002, Kendall/Hunt.
3. Hogan RN: The eye in aging. In Albert DM, Jacobiec FA, editors: *Principles and practice of ophthalmology,* ed 2, Philadelphia, 2000, Saunders.
4. Tatlipinar S, Akpek EK: Topical cyclosporine in the treatment of ocular surface disorders, *Br J Ophthalmol* 89(10):1363-1367, 2005.

CHAPTER 81

Nasolacrimal Duct Obstruction and Dacryocystitis

Kate Goldblum, Patricia Gillett, and Joyce Powers

DEFINITION AND EPIDEMIOLOGY

Nasolacrimal duct obstruction (NLDO), also called dacryostenosis, is a congenital, acute, or chronic blockage that may be partial or complete. Abnormal duct patency and the resultant disruption of normal drainage may lead to dacryocystitis, an inflammation of the lacrimal sac. Approximately 5% of newborn infants have congenital dacryostenosis.[1]

PATHOPHYSIOLOGY

Congenital NLDO is usually caused by a mucosal membrane over the distal end of the duct.[2] Obstruction that is not congenital may result from involutional stenosis; trauma; neoplasia; or anatomic obstructions such as a deviated septum, polyps, or hypertrophied inferior turbinates. Chronic dacryocystitis may lead to scar tissue formation and NLDO in adult patients.

CLINICAL PRESENTATION

Infants with congenital dacryostenosis usually have chronic tearing or mucopurulent discharge and eyelash crusting. These symptoms usually appear within the first few weeks of life but occasionally occur later in early infancy. In most cases the obstruction clears spontaneously by 12 months of age. Spontaneous resolution after that time is unusual.[1] Adults often have similar symptoms, although the cause differs. Inadequate tear drainage results in an accumulation of tears in the palpebral fissure with eventual overflow down the cheeks. Mucopurulent discharge from the punctum may be present.

PHYSICAL EXAMINATION

The ocular adnexa and surface structures should be carefully examined for signs of inflammation, although the eye itself is not usually red unless there is an associated conjunctivitis. Palpation is an important part of the examination to assess for edema or tenderness. Pressing on the lacrimal sac may express discharge from the nasolacrimal punctum on the involved side. Fever and leukocytosis may be present in acute dacryocystitis.

DIAGNOSTICS

Diagnostics are usually not necessary. However, if purulent discharge is present, culture and sensitivity testing may be indicated, particularly in recalcitrant infections. A CBC may be indicated if fever is present.

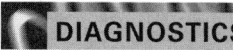

DIAGNOSTICS

Nasolacrimal Duct Obstruction and Dacryocystitis

LABORATORY

Culture and sensitivity (if purulent discharge is present)
CBC and differential (if fever is present)

DIFFERENTIAL DIAGNOSIS

DIFFERENTIAL DIAGNOSIS

Nasolacrimal Duct Obstruction and Dacryocystitis

- Conjunctivitis
- Blepharitis
- Glaucoma
- Corneal abrasion
- Corneal foreign body
- Tumor
- Foreign body
- Preseptal cellulitis

Tearing and ocular irritation may also indicate the presence of conjunctivitis, blepharitis, glaucoma, corneal abrasion, or a corneal foreign body. Mechanical obstruction should be considered, and the presence of a tumor, other neoplastic growth, or foreign body should be excluded. Dacryocystitis may be confused with or be a cause of preseptal cellulitis.[3]

MANAGEMENT

Because congenital NLDO clears spontaneously in most infants, the only treatment usually necessary is gentle daily massage over the lacrimal sac to promote drainage and encourage opening of the obstructing nasolacrimal duct membrane. Warm compresses over the involved eye will help loosen crusting on the eyelashes and may be most necessary after the infant awakens. Topical antibiotics may be prescribed for associated conjunctivitis or excessive mucopurulent drainage caused by *Streptococcus pneumoniae, Staphylococcus* organisms, *Pseudomonas* organisms, or *Haemophilus influenzae* (primarily in children). Infants with acute dacryocystitis should also receive systemic antibiotic therapy. Treatment for dacryocystitis in adults with an acute or chronic obstruction includes hot compresses and topical or systemic antibiotics. Antibiotic choice is based on Gram's stain.

Topical antibiotics include neomycin-polymyxin B–gramicidin (Neosporin), ciprofloxacin 0.3% (Ciloxan), or ofloxacin 0.3% (Ocuflox), 1 drop q 1-6 hr. Systemic therapy may include a first-generation cephalosporin such as cephalexin (Keflex) or erythromycin (Erythrocin), 500 mg q 12 hr. In the absence of mucopurulent drainage, prolonged use of topical antibiotics is not necessary in infants or adults.

Infants with congenital NLDO should be co-managed with a pediatric ophthalmologist if complications occur. Conservative management with massage and warm compresses is appropriate up to 12 months of age if no complications occur. Beyond age 12 months, nasolacrimal duct probing is indicated.

LIFE SPAN CONSIDERATIONS

Spontaneous clearing of congenital NLDO in infants occurs frequently. By 12 months of age, approximately 90% of cases have spontaneously resolved. Beyond 12 months of age, spontaneous resolution becomes much less likely, and there is an increased possibility of permanent consequences. Conversely, definitive treatment to relieve the obstruction is often necessary in adults.

COMPLICATIONS

NLDO usually precedes dacryocystitis, which can progress to abscess formation. The use of systemic antibiotics is necessary for abscess formation, ineffective topical antibiotic therapy, or recurrent dacryocystitis.

INDICATIONS FOR REFERRAL OR HOSPITALIZATION

After initial antibiotic therapy, adults with acute dacryocystitis should be referred to an ophthalmologist because the infection is secondary to obstruction and likely to recur without definitive treatment. The presence of dacryocystitis or abscess with systemic signs of fever, malaise, or leukocytosis may require hospitalization for IV antibiotic therapy.

PATIENT AND FAMILY EDUCATION

The parents or patient should receive instructions on warm compress application, nasolacrimal duct massage, and instillation of topical antibiotics. Patients should be told that antibiotics treat the infection but do not cure the obstruction. To avoid the unnecessary delay of definitive treatment when it is indicated, parents should be aware that nasolacrimal duct probing may be done in the ophthalmologist's office and does not require the use of a general anesthetic in that setting.

HEALTH PROMOTION

Immunizations should be encouraged to avoid potential complications of dacryocystitis resulting from *H. influenzae*.

REFERENCES

1. Simon JW, and others: *Basic and clinical science course: pediatric ophthalmology and strabismus*, San Francisco, 2005, American Academy of Ophthalmology.
2. Uphold CR, Graham MV: *Clinical guidelines in child health*, ed 3, Gainesville, Fla, 2003, Barmarrae Books.
3. Burns CE, Dunn AM, Brady MA, and others, editors: *Pediatric primary care: a handbook for nurse practitioners*, ed 3, St Louis, 2004, Saunders.

CHAPTER 82

Orbital and Periorbital Cellulitis

Kate Goldblum, Patricia Gillett, and Joyce Powers

DEFINITION AND EPIDEMIOLOGY

The orbital septum is a connective tissue structure that separates the anterior third of the orbit from the posterior two thirds. Orbital and periorbital cellulitis are bacterial infections involving the tissues of these areas. Periorbital cellulitis, also called preseptal cellulitis, involves the tissues anterior to the orbital septum; orbital cellulitis, also called postseptal cellulitis, involves the posterior tissues.

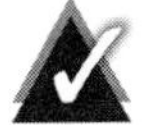

Ophthalmology consultation is recommended for periorbital cellulitis.

Ophthalmology referral is indicated for orbital cellulitis.

PATHOPHYSIOLOGY

The most common bacteria responsible for orbital and periorbital infections include *Staphylococcus aureus,* group A streptococcus, *Streptococcus pneumoniae,* and *Haemophilus influenzae.* Fungal infection should also be suspected, especially in immunocompromised patients. The mechanism of infection in orbital and periorbital cellulitis may involve the spread of infection from superficial lid infections, insect bites or other local trauma, impetigo, a foreign body, or respiratory infections. However, it most commonly occurs secondary to sinusitis.[1]

CLINICAL PRESENTATION

The initial presentation of periorbital or orbital cellulitis may include a history of trauma or insect bite to the periocular tissues. The most common signs and symptoms of periorbital cellulitis include erythema, warmth, and tenderness. Fever may or may not be present, and the eye is usually white with good mobility and vision. The patients may have pain with ocular movement. Orbital cellulitis usually is initially seen with similar signs and symptoms with the addition of proptosis, decreased ocular motility, fever, and leukocytosis. Vision and the pupillary response may or may not be decreased. Unilateral involvement is the most common presentation. All signs may be present in either periorbital or orbital cellulitis, but proptosis, restriction of eye movement, ocular redness, and decreased visual acuity are more suggestive of orbital cellulitis.

PHYSICAL EXAMINATION

The ocular tissues and adnexa should be carefully examined and palpated for erythema, warmth, edema, tenderness, drainage, restriction of extraocular muscle action, and proptosis. Evaluating the cranial nerves (CNs) involved in extraocular muscle movements (CNs III, IV, and VI) and assessing corneal sensitivity to identify potential involvement of CN V is important. The eye should be examined carefully for any sign of injury that may provide clues regarding the cause of the infection. The patient should be assessed for temperature elevation and other signs of systemic toxicity.

DIAGNOSTICS

A CBC with differential should be obtained. Any drainage should be cultured and blood cultures obtained if the signs and symptoms suggest a possible orbital cellulitis. In young children, blood cultures should be obtained in any case of cellulitis associated with fever.

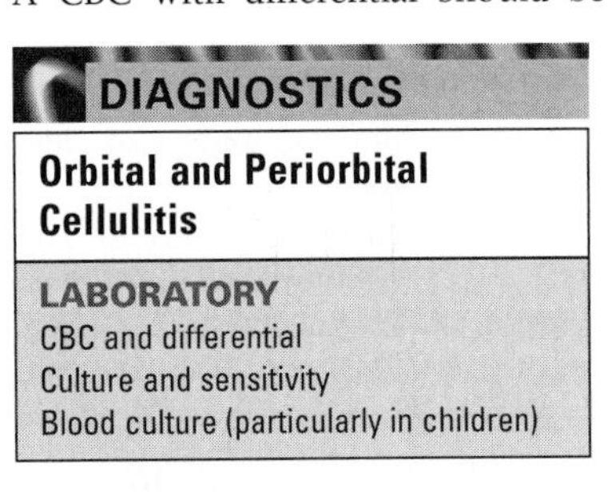

DIAGNOSTICS

Orbital and Periorbital Cellulitis

LABORATORY

CBC and differential
Culture and sensitivity
Blood culture (particularly in children)

DIFFERENTIAL DIAGNOSIS

Any disorder causing unilateral proptosis should be included in the differential diagnosis. Conjunctivitis with periocular tissue involvement, hordeolum, chalazion, dacryocystitis, or dacryoadenitis should be considered. Other considerations include pyoderma, insect bites, orbital tumor, pseudotumor, Graves' disease, and severe allergies.

MANAGEMENT

Periorbital cellulitis requires systemic, broad-spectrum antibiotic therapy. Follow-up evaluation in the office within 12 to 24 hours to monitor for signs of progression or lack of response to antibiotic therapy is important. Appropriate oral therapy for periorbital cellulitis includes broad-spectrum antibiotics such as cephalosporin or ampicillin–clavulanic acid.[2] Patients with significant systemic symptoms, periorbital cellulitis that fails to respond to oral antibiotics, or possible orbital cellulitis should be referred to an ophthalmologist or otolaryngologist for hospitalization and IV antibiotic therapy.[1] These patients should be monitored closely during the first 24 to 48 hours of hospitalization for lack of improvement or deterioration in condition.

LIFE SPAN CONSIDERATIONS

A primary concern in periorbital and orbital cellulitis is the patient's age. Neither orbital nor periorbital cellulitis is com-

DIFFERENTIAL DIAGNOSIS

Orbital and Periorbital Cellulitis

- Conjunctivitis
- Hordeolum
- Chalazion
- Dacryocystitis
- Dacryoadenitis
- Pyoderma
- Insect bite
- Orbital tumor
- Graves' disease
- Severe allergies

mon over the age of 20 years. Younger children are more likely to have periorbital rather than orbital cellulitis.[3] Any cellulitis in younger children or infants is potentially more serious.[2] *H. influenzae* type B is potentially life threatening in young children because it can lead to meningitis. This possibility should be a special concern in unvaccinated children.

COMPLICATIONS

Orbital cellulitis is a potentially fatal condition.[3] The possible complications of periorbital and orbital cellulitis can pose significant risk to the patient and include (1) meningitis; (2) cavernous sinus thrombosis; (3) central retinal artery or vein thrombosis; (4) subperiosteal, orbital, epidural, subdural, or brain abscess; and (5) optic nerve involvement with possible vision loss.[1]

INDICATIONS FOR REFERRAL OR HOSPITALIZATION

Patients with decreased visual acuity, systemic symptoms, or neurologic signs should be referred to an ophthalmologist. Patients with periorbital cellulitis that does not improve within 24 hours when treated with oral antibiotics should also be referred to an ophthalmologist. Patients with orbital cellulitis require hospitalization for initiation of IV antibiotics and other supportive therapy as indicated.

PATIENT AND FAMILY EDUCATION

When oral antibiotic therapy is prescribed, patients should be instructed to return before their scheduled follow-up visit (in 12 to 24 hours) if their symptoms increase in severity. They should also be reminded to complete the full course of antibiotic therapy and to return before the end of therapy if signs and symptoms do not continue to improve or if there is any worsening of the condition. Patients and families should be informed that fever, lethargy, and irritability are signs of possible sepsis or meningitis.

HEALTH PROMOTION

H. influenzae vaccination should be promoted in all children.

REFERENCES

1. Burns CE, Dunn AM, Brady MA, and others, editors: *Pediatric primary care: a handbook for nurse practitioners*, ed 3, St Louis, 2004, Saunders.
2. Simon JW, and others: *Basic and clinical science course: pediatric ophthalmology and strabismus*, San Francisco, 2005, American Academy of Ophthalmology.
3. Wald ER: Periorbital and orbital infections, *Pediatr Rev* 25(9):312-320, 2004.

CHAPTER 83

Pingueculum and Pterygium

Kate Goldblum, Patricia Gillett, and Joyce Powers

DEFINITION AND EPIDEMIOLOGY

Pinguecula and pterygia are degenerative lesions of the conjunctiva.[1] Pinguecula are often considered precursors of pterygia.[2] A pingueculum is confined to the bulbar conjunctiva, whereas a pterygium eventually extends onto the cornea, usually from the nasal aspect. These lesions occur most often in patients with a long history of outdoor activity.

PATHOPHYSIOLOGY

Pinguecula and pterygia result from epithelial hyperplasia secondary to degenerative changes. Chronic exposure to sunlight and other environmental irritants, such as wind, induce these changes.[3]

CLINICAL PRESENTATION

A pingueculum is characterized by an elevated, yellowish growth, almost always in the nasal aspect of the palpebral conjunctiva (Color Plate 32). When inflamed, the lesion is usually erythematous. Inflamed lesions produce mild to moderate ocular discomfort. Elevated lesions disrupt normal tear film distribution, resulting in symptoms of dry eye. A pterygium is characterized by a vascularized lesion that usually extends from the conjunctiva of the nasal palpebral fissure onto the nasal cornea (Color Plate 31). If the pterygium extends into the visual axis, vision loss occurs. Pterygia may also become inflamed and produce ocular discomfort. Contact lens wearers may experience discomfort and problems sooner.

PHYSICAL EXAMINATION

The ocular surface should be examined carefully, preferably under lighted magnification, looking for signs of inflammation such as edema and injection. Whether the lesion extends past the corneoscleral junction onto the cornea is important in determining the significance of the lesion.

DIAGNOSTICS

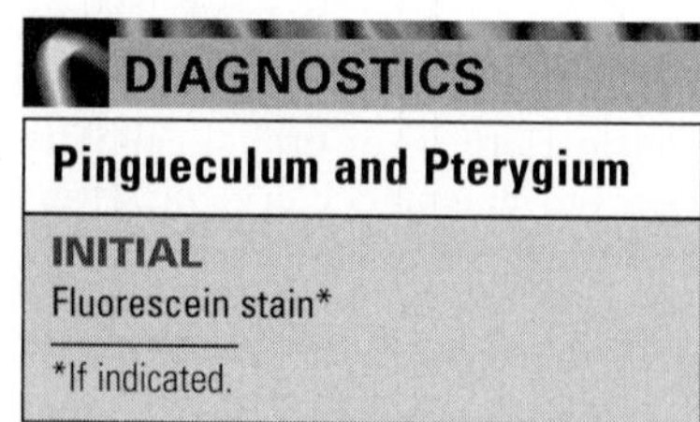
DIAGNOSTICS

Pingueculum and Pterygium

INITIAL
Fluorescein stain*

*If indicated.

The discomfort from a pterygium or pingueculum may mimic that of a corneal abrasion or erosion. If there is any question that a corneal lesion is present, fluorescein should be applied and the cornea carefully examined under fluorescent lighting.

DIFFERENTIAL DIAGNOSIS

Any ocular irritation may cause similar symptoms. The differential diagnosis includes episcleritis, scleritis, conjunctivitis, conjunctival dermoid, and corneal abrasion or erosion.

DIFFERENTIAL DIAGNOSIS

Pingueculum and Pterygium

- Episcleritis
- Scleritis
- Conjunctivitis
- Conjunctival dermoid
- Corneal abrasion or erosion

MANAGEMENT

Topical ophthalmic lubricants constitute initial therapy. Topical antiinflammatory agents such as ketorolac (Acular) and diclofenac (Voltaren) are useful in managing the mild inflammation of a pingueculum. More severely inflamed pinguecula may require topical steroid therapy. It is important to determine the intraocular pressure (IOP) before instituting topical steroids because they can raise the IOP. Some newer topical steroid preparations have less tendency to raise IOP than do many of the older topical steroids. Rimexolone (Vexol) or loteprednol (Alrex) ophthalmic solution 1 drop q.i.d. is less likely to cause a rise in IOP than is a steroid preparation such as prednisolone (Pred Forte). These medications should not be continued for longer than 1 week. It is also important to rule out the presence of corneal surface defects before prescribing topical steroids. In the primary care setting it is more difficult to exclude corneal ulcer or abrasion, but it is imperative to do so. If topical steroids are required, it is most appropriate to refer the patient to an ophthalmologist. Pinguecula may often be managed in the primary care setting, but co-management with an ophthalmologist is necessary if there are frequent or severe episodes of inflammation. An acutely inflamed pterygium may also require steroid therapy. Any lesion that begins to encroach on the cornea should be referred to an ophthalmologist for surgical evaluation.

LIFE SPAN CONSIDERATIONS

Because of the degenerative nature of pinguecula and pterygia, they do not occur in children, but they often occur in older adults who live in sunny or windy climates.

COMPLICATIONS

A pingueculum may evolve to a pterygium. As a pterygium extends onto the cornea and into the visual axis, it affects visual acuity. Surgical excision is necessary before this occurs, to avoid postoperative scarring in the central cornea with subsequent loss of visual acuity.

INDICATIONS FOR REFERRAL OR HOSPITALIZATION

Patients with inflamed pinguecula that do not respond to short-term topical antiinflammatory therapy should be referred to an ophthalmologist. All patients with pterygia approaching the corneoscleral border should be nonurgently referred for evaluation regarding the timing of surgical intervention. If topical steroid therapy is considered, physician consultation is recommended.

PATIENT AND FAMILY EDUCATION

Patients should be cautioned not to use over-the-counter vasoconstrictors for relief of redness. They may increase irritation and, if overused, can cause rebound conjunctival congestion.

HEALTH PROMOTION

The avoidance of excessive exposure to ultraviolet light and dry, windy environments may lessen the incidence of pterygia and pinguecula. Sunglasses with adequate blocking of ultraviolet A and ultraviolet B light should be recommended to all patients to help prevent these lesions.

REFERENCES

1. Sutphin JE, and others: *Basic and clinical science course: external disease and cornea,* San Francisco, 2005, American Academy of Ophthalmology.
2. Farah S, and others: Tumors of the cornea and conjunctiva. In Albert DM, Jakobiec FA, editors: *Principles and practice of ophthalmology* (CD ROM), ed 2, Philadelphia, 2000, Saunders.
3. Grossniklaus HE, and others: *Basic and clinical science course: ophthalmic pathology and intraocular tumors,* San Francisco, 2005, American Academy of Ophthalmology.

CHAPTER 84

Traumatic Ocular Disorders

Kate Goldblum, Patricia Gillett, and Joyce Powers

DEFINITION AND EPIDEMIOLOGY

Ocular trauma is a physical injury to the tissues of the eye or adnexa. It may be caused by any moving object that applies force to the eye or adnexal structures or even the head. Conversely, injury may be due to the individual moving into an external object, such as a tree branch or car dashboard. Such projectile trauma may result in either blunt or penetrating injuries. Not surprisingly, the amount of force exerted by a projectile is related to the type and extent of ocular injury.[1] Trauma may also occur with exposure of ocular tissues to toxic substances or extreme environmental conditions, including contact lens overwear.

Some examples of ocular trauma encountered in primary care include corneal or conjunctival foreign bodies, abrasions, lacerations, subconjunctival hemorrhages, hyphema, chemical exposure, traumatic miosis or mydriasis, orbital bone fractures, and thermal or radiation injuries. In addition to ultraviolet (UV) radiation, therapeutic radiation may also cause early or late ocular injuries to the ocular structures.[2] In the United States approximately 2 million eye injuries a year require treatment.[3] Many result in temporary or permanent visual disability. These ocular injuries represent a significant source of individual morbidity with both individual and societal economic impact.

PATHOPHYSIOLOGY

Trauma causing ocular injuries may involve the tissues of the globe itself, the ocular adnexa such as the eyelids or lacrimal apparatus, or the orbital bones. Blunt trauma often results in contusions or abrasions, but can also cause lacerations, penetrating injuries, or even globe rupture. A projectile object that fits within the orbital rim (e.g., a handball or fist) and directs energy into the orbit may cause a blow-out fracture of the bones of the orbital floor. The extraocular muscles can become trapped in these fractures, causing diplopia. Chemical trauma from exposure to acidic or alkaline agents can be visually devastating. Acidic chemicals cause protein precipitation that forms a barrier to deeper tissue penetration. In contrast, alkaline substances cause hydrolysis and cellular disruption, resulting in penetration of the chemical into the deeper ocular structures.[4] Consequently, exposure to alkaline agents often results in more severe damage to ocular tissues. Thermal burns from any hot object result in inflammation and may affect the ocular surface, the adnexa, or both. Radiation commonly affects the ocular surface, resulting in damage to the cells of the ocular surface, often causing a painful keratitis.[5]

A subconjunctival hemorrhage may result from a sudden increase in venous pressure that occurs during Valsalva's maneuver such as sneezing, coughing, or vomiting. The increased pressure causes a break in a conjunctival blood vessel, and blood leaks into the subconjunctival space. Gravity may cause the hemorrhage to shift location. Subconjunctival hemorrhages can also occur spontaneously, from rubbing the eye, or from other minor or major trauma to the eye. This type of hemorrhage may also be associated with hypertension, severe conjunctival inflammation, or any systemic condition that increases the risk of bleeding.[4]

CLINICAL PRESENTATION

Patients with an ocular problem secondary to trauma may manifest a wide variety of signs and symptoms and may or may not have an obvious history of the trauma. Common presenting signs and symptoms include ocular irritation, pain, redness, photophobia, edema or ecchymosis of the globe or ocular adnexa, or loss of vision. If there is a history of trauma, patients may be able to describe the circumstances surrounding the injury, providing clues to the type or extent of possible injury. Patients who are seen with abrasions and lacerations almost always relate some history of trauma. A subconjunctival hemorrhage manifests with a bright red spot of blood visible under the overlying conjunctiva (Color Plate 33). The rest of the conjunctiva remains white.

Although some signs of trauma, such as lacerations, ecchymosis, edema, and redness, are easily identified, a careful history can assist the health care provider in identifying more subtle results of trauma and avoiding the error of excluding a serious injury when, in fact, one exists. Penetrating injuries may be subtle, masquerading as less serious injuries and necessitating a high level of suspicion in all cases of trauma, particularly those arising from projectile force. It is often helpful to know the mechanism of injury and the specific source of injury. Table 84-1 lists common mechanisms of ocular injury and examples of sources that may be identified during the history. Other important history includes contact lens use, immunization status, history of glaucoma, previous eye injuries or surgeries, medications, and allergies.

PHYSICAL EXAMINATION

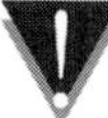

In any situation in which there is suspected or potential globe rupture, it is imperative not to touch or manipulate the eye.

If potential globe rupture is suspected, place a protective shield over the eye and refer the patient to an ophthalmologist immediately.

In all other cases of trauma, carefully examine the entire eye, including the ocular fundus. Always assess the visual acuity in both eyes, using the patient's usual correction, if possible. Inspect the adnexal ocular structures, ocular surface, anterior chamber, and ocular fundus carefully. Look for edema, erythema, ecchymosis, tenderness, discharge, foreign bodies, corneal abrasions, lacerations, hyphema (blood in the anterior chamber), dislocated or subluxed lens, ocular symmetry (particularly noting any enophthalmos or exophthalmos), and other signs of trauma. It is important to note that hyphema may be microscopic.

TABLE 84-1 Common Mechanisms of Ocular Trauma and Selected Sources

Mechanism	Possible Sources
Thermal energy	Curling irons Matches Hot grease or other liquids
Radiant energy	Ultraviolet (UV) radiation • Solar lamps • Sunlight • Arc welding Therapeutic ionizing radiation
Chemical agents	Detergents, disinfectants, or solvents Cosmetics Drain cleaners Fertilizers Battery acid Chlorine in pools Ammonia fumes
Projectile energy	Metal shavings Tree branches Fists, fingers, fingernails Fireworks Sports equipment (e.g., balls, rackets) Firearms, including BB guns Interior car parts (during vehicular crashes) Projectile matter from explosions Valsalva's maneuver (sudden venous congestion producing force)

Evaluate pupillary symmetry and function, and examine the ocular fundus for signs of hemorrhage. Assess extraocular muscle function in any situation in which there may be muscle entrapment. Evert the upper eyelid(s) in all patients with symptoms of foreign body or a history indicating this possibility. A foreign body can become embedded in the tarsal conjunctiva and will be missed if eyelid eversion is omitted from the examination.

DIAGNOSTICS

Examination of the ocular surface using fluorescein dye is helpful in determining whether the patient has a corneal abrasion or foreign body. If a slit lamp is available, slit lamp microscopy is also useful in the examination. X-ray studies, ultrasonography, CT, or MRI is necessary for suspected fractures, penetrating foreign bodies, or other occult trauma.

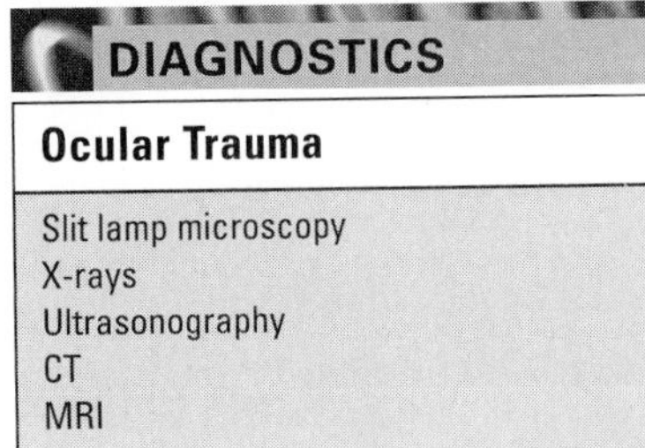

DIAGNOSTICS

Ocular Trauma

Slit lamp microscopy
X-rays
Ultrasonography
CT
MRI

DIFFERENTIAL DIAGNOSIS

The differential diagnosis in cases of trauma is extensive and ranges from minor disorders such as a superficial foreign body to extensive damage to the ocular structures that may result in loss of all vision or even the eye. It is important to determine whether a subconjunctival hemorrhage or hyphema is associated with a history of more serious systemic disorders that may increase the risk of spontaneous bleeding. In addition, patients with an atypical presentation of subconjunctival hemorrhage may have conjunctival Kaposi's sarcoma and should be evaluated for occult HIV.[6]

DIFFERENTIAL DIAGNOSIS

Ocular Trauma

- Foreign body
- Corneal abrasion
- Orbital fracture
- Globe rupture
- Hyphema
- Detached retina
- Thermal burns
- Radiation keratitis
- Chemical injury
- Subconjunctival hemorrhage

MANAGEMENT

In all cases of exposure to any form or type of chemical, the most important aspect of management is immediate, copious, and continuous irrigation of the ocular surface. It may be necessary to use a topical anesthetic and lid speculum to achieve adequate irrigation. Monitor the pH with litmus paper, and continue irrigation until the pH is normal. If unable to determine the pH (or if the pH remains abnormal), ensure that irrigation continues during transport to an ophthalmologist or emergency department. As previously noted, carefully shield any eye in which there is suspected or potential globe rupture without manipulating the eye. Control bleeding if it is possible to do so without putting pressure on the eye. Administer a tetanus booster if indicated.

Tetracaine 0.5% may be used to temporarily anesthetize the cornea for examination, but is not useful for pain relief because tachyphylaxis occurs with continued use. In addition, it is inappropriate for this purpose because it delays corneal healing. Practitioners skilled in the procedure may remove a superficially embedded foreign body from the conjunctiva or cornea using a 26-gauge needle. Normal saline irrigation is indicated to flush dirt or debris from the ocular surface and fornices. It may also be necessary to use a sterile cotton applicator moistened with normal saline to remove debris. A topical antibiotic such as tobramycin 0.3% (Tobrex) or ciprofloxacin 0.3% (Ciloxan) can be prescribed for infection prophylaxis. These ophthalmic drops are also appropriate in treating mild corneal abrasions. Patching following foreign body removal or for corneal abrasions is not mandatory. The primary advantages of patching are to prevent eyelid movement, which may continue to abrade the involved area, and to make the patient more comfortable. However, some patients are more comfortable without a patch. Abrasions associated with contact lens wear should never be patched.[4]

Keratitis resulting from exposure to UV light is painful, but usually resolves within 24 hours. Oral analgesics, lubricating ointment, and patching are appropriate therapy.[4] No treatment is necessary for a subconjunctival hemorrhage. The provider should simply reassure the patient that the lesion is benign and will resorb slowly, usually over 1 to 2 weeks.

LIFE SPAN CONSIDERATIONS

Children account for nearly half of all ocular injuries. If injuries result in permanent vision loss, children endure many more years of morbidity than do adults.[7] Health care providers should always consider the possibility of child or elder abuse when it is difficult to elicit a good history. In older patients who incur ocular trauma as the result of a fall, providers should determine whether an underlying disease process predisposed the patients to falling.

COMPLICATIONS

Patients with a history of corneal abrasion may later experience recurrent corneal erosions. Retinal detachment or other vision loss can follow any type of trauma. Extensive trauma to the ocular adnexa may result in loss of normal lid action or disruption of normal tear drainage. Chemical injuries can cause severe scarring of the cornea and conjunctiva that can disrupt normal ocular adnexal functions and reduce vision.

INDICATIONS FOR REFERRAL OR HOSPITALIZATION

Providers should refer all patients with chemical exposure, globe rupture, orbital fracture, hyphema, retinal detachment, or rust rings from metallic corneal foreign bodies to an ophthalmologist. If a corneal abrasion or UV keratitis has not healed in 24 hours, the patient should be referred to an ophthalmologist. Any unexplained loss of visual acuity following trauma requires referral to an ophthalmologist for definitive diagnosis and treatment; early treatment of traumatic optic neuropathy results in a greater rate of visual improvement.[8]

PATIENT AND FAMILY EDUCATION

Injury prevention should be the primary goal in patient education. All individuals should wear protective eyewear when using tools or chemicals or participating in sports.[9] Wearing UV protective eyewear during welding or outdoor activities can prevent UV keratitis. It is also important to provide basic first aid instructions in case of chemical exposure. Patients should understand that, after irrigation, they should seek follow-up care if there are any continuing signs or symptoms. Any patient with an eye patched should not drive with the patch in place because of the unaccustomed lack of depth perception. Providers should reassure patients with a subconjunctival hemorrhage that, although it is unsightly, it is not serious and will clear.

HEALTH PROMOTION

In addition to the prevention education discussed above, patients should be aware of the recommendations for routine eye care. This is especially important for patients who wear contact lenses, since misuse of these common devices can result in serious corneal compromise. Chapter 75 discusses current recommendations for routine eye care.

REFERENCES

1. Duma SM, Ng TP, Kennedy EA, and others: Determination of significant parameters for eye injury risk from projectiles, *J Trauma* 59:960-964, 2005.
2. Barabino S, Raghavan A, Loeffler J, and others: Radiotherapy-induced ocular surface disease, *Cornea* 24(8):909-914, 2005.
3. McGwin G, Xi A, Owsley C: Rate of eye injury in the United States, *Arch Ophthalmol* 123:970-976, 2005. [Erratum in *Arch Ophthalmol* 123:1285, 2005.]
4. Sutphin JE, and others: *Basic and clinical science course: external disease and cornea,* San Francisco, 2005, American Academy of Ophthalmology.
5. Wirbelauer C: Management of the red eye for the primary care physician, *Am J Med* 119:302-306, 2006.
6. Goldman L, Ausiello D: *Cecil textbook of medicine*, Philadelphia, 2004, Saunders.
7. Levine LM: Pediatric ocular trauma and shaken infant syndrome, *Pediatr Clin North Am* 50:137-148, 2003.
8. Rajiniganth MG: Traumatic optic neuropathy: visual outcome following combined therapy protocol, *Arch Otolaryngol Head Neck Surg* 130(8):1203-1206, 2003.
9. Rodriguez JO, Lavina AM, Agarwal A: Prevention and treatment of common eye injuries in sports, *Am Fam Phys* 67(7):1481-1488, 1494-1496, 2003.

PART 7

Evaluation and Management of Ear Disorders

CHAPTER 85

Auricular Disorders

Christell O. Bray and
Karen Koozer Olson

DEFINITION AND EPIDEMIOLOGY

Auricular disorders are those conditions which affect the external ear. The incidence and prevalence of the individual condition vary. The auricular disorder may be a secondary issue or may be discovered during the physical examination. Auricular disorders may be benign conditions associated with other disease processes, may be related to cultural practices such as body piercing, or may be a symptom of a serious illness that requires immediate referral and treatment.

Certain disease processes are associated with specific abnormalities of the auricle. Patients with Addison's disease may have calcification of the cartilage. The nodules of Hansen's disease may appear on the earlobe and be initially seen as multiple nodules on the ear and face. Patients with chronic arthritis may have hard nodules develop in the auricle. These rheumatoid nodules are usually accompanied by similar nodules on the hands, elbows, knees, or heels. Tophi are painless, hard or gritty, and irregular uric acid crystal deposits in the auricle. They form in relation to years of high uric acid levels. Pressure on these deposits may result in the expulsion of a white crystalline substance. A hematoma of the auricle occurs in response to blood disorders or trauma and manifests as a tender, blue, doughy mass that, if not drained, results in a deformity commonly referred to as "cauliflower ear."[1]

Common problems associated with piercing of the earlobes and the helix are local infection and tears from the pierced site. Keloids, which are firm masses of scar tissue that are not cosmetically acceptable but are otherwise benign, may also occur at the pierced site. Keloids occur more often in dark-skinned people. Multiple helix piercing can cause a perforation-like appearance.

Chondrodermatitis helicis is a chronic inflamed lesion, usually on the helix or antihelix, which most often affects older men. It is painful and may have crusting. A biopsy examination distinguishes it from carcinoma. Two types of skin cancer may be found on the auricle. Basal cell carcinoma is the most common form of skin cancer and the least deadly. It is a slowly growing cancer that is often found in areas exposed to the sun, such as the top of the auricle. This type of disorder is found in older persons, in fair-skinned patients, and in patients who have a history of sun exposure. The lesion appears as a shiny, irregular painless area. This form of cancer rarely metastasizes.

Squamous cell carcinoma (SCC) is also usually found in fair-skinned patients and in patients with a history of sun exposure. The typical lesion has a raised, crusted border around a center ulcer. SCC is a more serious form of skin cancer. It metastasizes to regional lymph nodes and can cause death. Skin cancer is probably the most common significant auricular disorder seen in primary care.

Malignant otitis externa is a severe form of otitis externa. It results in a severely swollen, erythematous, and tender auricle. It can lead to a life-threatening infection of the head and face. It is most likely to occur in patients with diabetes and in those who have compromised immune systems. The causative organism is usually *Pseudomonas aeruginosa.*[2]

PATHOPHYSIOLOGY

The auricle is the external ear structure that is composed chiefly of cartilage covered by skin. It is firm and elastic. It is divided into three parts: the top portion is the helix, the midsection is the antihelix, and the lower portion is the lobe. The function of the outer ear is to aid in receiving sound waves from the environment.

CLINICAL PRESENTATION

Often the patient is being seen for a general examination or follow-up. The complaint related to an auricular disorder is usually a minor issue. For tears and infection, the patient may be seen after a specific episode of trauma or with an erythematous, tender earlobe. Malignant otitis externa may manifest as a sequela to an infection or a respiratory illness and most often occurs in immunosuppressed or diabetic patients.

PHYSICAL EXAMINATION

The parameters of the auricular disorder should be noted; these include the onset, duration, and intensity of any symptoms. Any medications, treatments, or remedies that have been used on the auricle or systemically should also be documented, as should all related symptoms and past history of treatments and outcomes. A complete inspection and palpation of the auricle form the basis for evaluation. The examination should be modified to the individual findings.

The normal ears are placed level with the eyes. The ears of neonates are usually flat; however, in older infants this may indicate persistent side lying. Protruding ears should be examined to exclude edema from insect bites or infection. Normal earlobes are similar in size and placement and should move freely and painlessly. Infected pierced earlobes will be warm, tender, and erythematous and may have exudates. The lobes of older patients may be more prominent or pendulous. Dry or scaly skin of the external ear may indicate psoriasis or seborrhea. The external ear may also have skin breakdowns or erosions from prolonged pressure from eyeglasses or oxygen tubing. Cancerous or precancerous lesions are most often found on the top of the auricle. They may appear as shiny, irregular, painless lesions (basal cell carcinoma) or as raised, crusted lesions around a center ulcer (SCC).

DIAGNOSTICS

The diagnostic tests depend on the underlying disease process. A biopsy should be performed on any small, crusted, ulcerated or indurated lesion that does not heal properly. If the biopsy findings are positive, a complete cancer screening should be ordered. Rheumatoid arthritis profiles should be obtained in patients with rheumatoid nodules. If tophi are present, a uric acid chemistry profile is indicated. Calcification nodules related to Addison's disease indicate the need for endocrine studies.

DIAGNOSTICS

Auricular Disorders

LABORATORY
Culture and sensitivity*
Uric acid*
Rheumatoid arthritis*
Endocrine studies*

OTHER
Biopsy*

*If indicated.

DIFFERENTIAL DIAGNOSIS

The differential diagnosis includes all the diagnoses mentioned earlier.

MANAGEMENT

Infections of the earlobe or pinna that are a result of piercing can be treated with topical alcohol and antibiotic ointment or systemic antibiotic treatment such as ceftriaxone or cephalexin. Mild infections can be treated with cephalexin or dicloxacillin 500 mg PO q.i.d. for 7 to 10 days. Erythromycin is appropriate for penicillin-allergic patients. More severe infections should be treated with ceftriaxone 1 g IM or IV daily for 1 day or longer, depending on the severity of the infection. Oral antibiotic therapy should then be prescribed as previously noted.[2]

Most patients with malignant otitis externa require immediate referral to a physician or an otolaryngologist, admission to a hospital, and aggressive antimicrobial therapy. Patients with very early disease may be treated with ciprofloxacin (Cipro) 500 to 750 mg PO b.i.d. for 7 to 10 days with frequent follow-up.[2] A biopsy should be performed on any chronically inflamed lesion to ascertain whether it is malignant. An auricular hematoma should be drained using sterile technique and treated with topical antibiotic ointment or systemic antibiotics, depending on the extent of the wound. There is no clearly defined best treatment for acute auricular hematoma.[3]

LIFE SPAN CONSIDERATIONS

Life span considerations are related to the specific disease disorders. Complications from piercing are more likely in the young. Skin cancers are most likely to occur in middle-aged and older patients.

DIFFERENTIAL DIAGNOSIS

Auricular Disorders

- Cancer
- Rheumatoid arthritis
- Gout
- Addison's disease
- Infection

COMPLICATIONS

Complications are unusual but do occur. Trauma, if untreated, may result in painful nodules or a distorted cauliflower ear. Painless pinnal nodules may be a complication of Addison's disease, and any painless nodule may represent a carcinoma. Infections, if untreated, may spread systemically. Recurring pinnal infections should prompt concern for relapsing polychondritis, a degenerative cartilage disease that can cause tinnitus or deafness.

INDICATIONS FOR REFERRAL OR HOSPITALIZATION

Patients with torn earlobes are usually referred to a reconstructive surgeon for repair. Additionally, a trend that can lead to damage of the cartilage and subsequent deformity is high ear piercing in the pinna. If deformity and instability of the pinna are observed, a referral to a reconstructive surgeon is also recommended.[4,5] A biopsy should be performed on any cancerous or suspicious lesion. Malignant otitis externa requires immediate referral to a physician or hospital admission.

PATIENT AND FAMILY EDUCATION

Understanding the importance of sunscreen protection for the ears is essential. In addition, the signs of skin cancer—asymmetry, borders (irregular, ragged, notched, or blurred), color (irregular), and diameter (a lesion that is 6 mm [0.25 inch] or growing)—should be carefully explained.[6,7] The provider should stress the importance and correct way of cleaning and caring for the external ear canal and auricle. When selecting ear-piercing facilities, patients should look for facilities that employ licensed personnel and are inspected or approved by public health authorities. In addition, caution should be used when wearing heavy or dangling earrings, since the earring might be torn from the ear.

HEALTH PROMOTION

Health promotion is primarily related to the specific disease. Sunscreens and protective clothing are the best choice for the prevention of skin cancer.

REFERENCES

1. LeBlond RF, DeGowin RL, Brown DD: *DeGowin's diagnostic examination*, ed 8, New York, 2004, McGraw-Hill.
2. Gilbert DN, Moellering RC, Eliopoulos GM, and others: *The Sanford guide to antimicrobial therapy*, ed 35, Hyde Park, Vt, 2005, Antimicrobial Therapy.
3. Jones SE: *Interventions for acute auricular haematoma*, April 1, 2005, retrieved Dec 31, 2005, from http://www.medscape.com/viewarticle/486931_print.
4. Geneeskd NT: *Three patients with complications following piercing of the auricular cartilage*, 2004, retrieved Dec 16, 2005, from http://www.medscape.com/medline/abstract/15283028?prt=true.
5. Margulis A, Bauer BS, Alizadeh K: *Ear reconstruction after auricular chondritis secondary to ear piercing*, 2003, retrieved Dec 16, 2005, from http://www.medscape.com/medline/abstract/12560718?prt+true.
6. American Cancer Society: *Skin cancer facts*, April 5, 2005, retrieved Jan 6, 2006, from http://www.cancer.org/docroot/PED/content/ped_7_1_What_You_Need_To_Know_About.
7. American Cancer Society: *Skin cancer prevention and early detection*, Feb 3, 2005, retrieved Jan 6, 2006, from http://www.cancer.org/docroot/PED/content/ped_7_1_Skin_Cancer_Detection_What_You.

CHAPTER 86

Cerumen Impaction

Christell O. Bray and
Karen Koozer Olson

DEFINITION AND ETIOLOGY

Ceruminosis is a common cause of hearing deficit, especially in older individuals. Cerumen impaction occurs when increased amounts of hard cerumen either partially or completely occlude the external ear canal. Cerumen can become dry and immobile and occlude the canal for a variety of reasons. Although cerumen is an important defense against infection, many individuals think of a buildup of earwax as a sign of uncleanliness and make efforts to remove the wax, which compromises the integrity of the ear's defenses against infection and contributes to cerumen impaction. Dirt and other debris in the ear can contribute to the impaction. Cotton-tipped swabs used to clean the ear can push this material back into the canal; fibers from the swabs often complicate the situation.

PATHOPHYSIOLOGY

Cerumen is a soft, yellow, waxy, protective substance that is secreted by glands in the external ear canal. It is part of the mechanism used to protect the ear canal and tympanic membrane (TM) from dirt and debris. When cerumen is formed relatively close to the tympanic membrane, it is soft and fluid, colorless, and odorless. As the cerumen moves toward the distal part of the ear canal through the process of mandibular movement, it becomes drier and darker and develops its characteristic odor. If an individual uses a cotton swab to clean the ear canal, the harder cerumen that is not removed is pushed against the TM. This harder cerumen is more difficult for the natural processes to remove and therefore can contribute to the development of cerumen impaction. Additionally, excessive cerumen production, a narrow ear canal, or obstruction may predispose a patient to impaction. A recent research study implicates *Aspergillus flavus* as a possible contributing agent in chronic cerumen impaction.[1]

CLINICAL PRESENTATION

Patients with cerumen impaction typically complain of unilateral fullness or hearing loss. Itching, discomfort, tinnitus, cough, vertigo, and dizziness are also common complaints.

PHYSICAL EXAMINATION

The outer ear should be inspected for size, shape, color, and placement; the lobe, helix, and preauricular and postauricular lymph nodes should be bilaterally palpated. The body temperature and lymph nodes are usually normal. The normal ear should be inspected by having the patient tip his or her head toward the opposite shoulder. In adults the pinna is pulled gently up and backward; for young children and infants the ear is pulled downward. The largest speculum that will fit into the ear canal is gently inserted. Cerumen impaction may prevent the speculum from being fully inserted. The impaction will appear as a light-yellow to dark-brown mass that prevents or partially blocks visualization of the TM. Blood in the external ear canal appears as bright red to black and may be liquid or a solid mass. Sanguineous drainage often appears as honey-colored fluid.

DIFFERENTIAL DIAGNOSIS
Cerumen Impaction
• Foreign body

DIAGNOSTICS

No diagnostics are indicated.

DIFFERENTIAL DIAGNOSIS

The primary differential diagnosis is a foreign body in the external ear canal.

MANAGEMENT

If a ruptured TM is not suspected and there is no history of tympanostomy tubes or recent ear surgery, removal of the impaction is appropriate. If possible, a commercial wax softener or two or three drops of baby oil or mineral oil should be inserted in the affected ear daily for 3 to 5 days before removal is attempted. Removal with a cerumen spoon or curette is appropriate if direct visualization is possible, the cerumen is in the lateral third of the external ear canal, and the patient is able to remain still during removal. If the cerumen is deeper in the canal, tepid water irrigation with the Welch Allyn Ear Wash System, or a regular syringe with a flexible catheter, is required.

In addition to the previously mentioned contraindications for removal of the impaction, if vegetable matter such as a bean or pea is suspected, ear canal irrigation is contraindicated.[2] A ceruminolytic agent instilled in the canal for 15 to 20 minutes before the lavage will soften the cerumen and aid in removal. If a patient is known to have dry skin in the ear canal, ceruminolytics containing hydrogen peroxide should be avoided, since the peroxide can further dry the skin. Liquid docusate sodium has also been used successfully to soften cerumen.[3] These agents should not be used if infection or perforation is suspected, if the patient has a history of otologic surgery, or if the status of the TM is unknown. The irrigating solution should be at body temperature to minimize the chance of vertigo. If the patient is immunocompromised, a sterile solution should be used.[4] The auricle should be straightened as much as possible and the irrigant directed upward in the canal to minimize the pressure against the TM. The canal should be irrigated until clear unless the patient experiences pain or dizziness.

Limited evidence supports the efficacy of using curettes, cerumen spoons, or lavage.[5] In a Cochrane database exploration of the efficacy of ear drops for earwax removal, investigators found insufficient high-quality evidence to offer any specific recommendations on the effectiveness of ceruminolytics for the removal of symptomatic cerumen.[6]

The clinical indication for use of antibiotics and steroids after removal of a cerumen impaction is determined by the amount of excoriation and other conditions such as diabetes or an immunocompromised status. Frequently hydrocortisone–neomycin sulfate–polymyxin B sulfate (Cortisporin otic solution) or a mixture of white vinegar and rubbing alcohol in the canal every day for 2 or 3 days after the procedure can reduce the risk of otitis externa. Whenever cerumen impaction is noted in one ear, the other ear should be examined for ceruminosis.

LIFE SPAN CONSIDERATIONS

In older adults the glands that produce cerumen may become less productive, which can result in cerumen that is drier and more likely to collect in the canal and become impacted. Adults who work in noisy industries and are required to wear hearing protection may have an increased risk of cerumen impaction. Hearing aids, earplugs, swim molds, or other foreign bodies inserted into the external auditory canal can push the cerumen into the canal and predispose the patient to cerumen impaction.

COMPLICATIONS

Cerumen accumulation can decrease auditory acuity and cause pressure on and perforation of the TM. Removal of cerumen that has adhered to the wall of the external ear canal may leave an abraded or irritated area that can develop into otitis externa. Hearing loss and injury to the TM are other potential complications. Additionally, if the impaction is not completely removed, water retention behind the impaction can occur, predisposing the patient to infection.

INDICATIONS FOR REFERRAL OR HOSPITALIZATION

Patients with suspected perforation, chronic cerumen impaction, tympanostomy tubes, recent ear surgery, or pus or necrotic tissue in the ear canal should be referred to an otolaryngologist, as should patients who experience acute pain, dizziness, hearing loss, or damage to the external ear canal or TM during the ear lavage.

PATIENT AND FAMILY EDUCATION

Patients should be cautioned about the use of cotton-tipped swabs to clean the ear canal. The use of these swabs can push the cerumen further into the ear, and fibers from the swab can help to hold the cerumen in a mass. Soft cloths and soap and water should be used to clean the auricle. The external ear canal does not require cleaning. Patients must understand the importance of a medical evaluation if pain or discharge is noted.

HEALTH PROMOTION

Commercial ceruminolytics or baby oil, one or two drops in the ear canal once or twice a week, will help prevent cerumen from becoming hard and imbedded. Patients who wear hearing aids are more at risk for the development of ceruminosis and, if possible, should not wear the hearing aids while sleeping. Patients should be advised not to use any other home removal technique or device. Many of these home remedies have been shown to have adverse results.[7,8] A dangerous cerumen removal product advocated on selected websites is ear cones, which can result in burns to the tissue within the ear canal, perforation of the TM, external otitis, and temporary hearing loss.[4]

REFERENCES

1. Burkhart CN: *Aspergillus flavus* isolated in cerumen by scanning electron microscopy, *Infect Med* 17(9):624-626, 2000, retrieved Dec 15, 2006, from http://www.medscape.com/viewarticle/410088.
2. Rudy SF: *What precautions are necessary when irrigating the ear canals?* June 6, 2000, retrieved Dec 21, 2006, from http://medscape.com/viewarticle/413424_print.
3. Singer AJ, Sauris E, Viccellio AW: Ceruminolytic effects of docusate sodium: a randomized controlled trial, *Ann Emerg Med* 36:228-232, 2000.
4. Pray WS, Pray JJ: Earwax: should it be removed? *US Pharmacist* 30(5) 2005, retrieved Dec 21, 2005, from http://www.medscape.com/viewarticle/504788_print.
5. Dinces E: *Cerumen*, May 27, 2005, retrieved Dec 21, 2005, from http://www.utdol.com/application/topic/print.asp?file=genr_med/26969&type=A&selecte.
6. Burton MJ, Doree C: Ear drops for the removal of ear wax (review), *Cochrane Collab* (4), 2005, retrieved Dec 22, 2005, from http://www.thecochranelibrary.com.
7. Guest JF, Greener MJ, Robinson AC, and others: Impacted cerumen: composition, production, epidemiology and management, *QJM* 97:477-488, 2004.
8. Pulec JL, Dequine C: Traumatic perforation: Q-Tip injury, *Ear Nose Throat* 82:484, 2003.

CHAPTER 87

Cholesteatoma

Christell O. Bray and Chad J. Smith

DEFINITION

A cholesteatoma is an invasive growth of keratin-producing squamous epithelial cells typically found within the middle ear or mastoid air spaces. The term is actually a misnomer, since there is no cholesterol within the cyst.

PATHOPHYSIOLOGY

Cholesteatomas may be broadly categorized as congenital or acquired. Congenital cholesteatomas occur as nests of embryonic squamous epithelial cells in an ear without a history of tympanic membrane (TM) perforation or chronic infections. They are identified most frequently in early childhood (6 months to 5 years). As they grow, they can cause a retraction of the TM, fluid in the middle ear, and conductive hearing loss.[1] Most commonly, acquired cholesteatomas occur as squamous epithelial cells enter the middle ear after prolonged chronic negative pressure with a retraction pocket in the TM (primary) (Color Plate 34) or as a direct consequence of injury to the TM (secondary). Over time this tumor enlarges, producing proteolytic enzymes that cause destruction of the ossicles and erosion of inner ear structures, mastoid bone, and other cranial contents.[2] Chronic otitis media, drainage, mastoiditis, and disseminated infection may co-exist.

CLINICAL PRESENTATION

Congenital cholesteatomas are often asymptomatic and are usually identified behind an intact TM. Facial twitching can be a symptom of a primary cholesteatoma in a child with no other symptoms.[3] Acquired lesions, however, have histories of recurrent ear infections, pain, and drainage or TM retractions caused by eustachian tube dysfunction. Impaired hearing may be the first sign of middle ear destruction from a cholesteatoma. An uncommon although concerning symptom of cholesteatomas is dizziness. A cholesteatoma should be suspected in all cases of chronic draining ears, especially if there is no resolution after treatment with oral and topical antibiotics.[4] In more than 90% of cases a perforation, most commonly in the posterosuperior quadrant, of the TM is present, the exceptions being in cases of congenital cholesteaomas.[1]

PHYSICAL EXAMINATION

A complete otologic examination with attention to the ear canal, TM, and mastoid regions may reveal a white mass behind or perforating through the TM. Drainage indicates infection.

DIAGNOSTICS AND DIFFERENTIAL DIAGNOSIS

An audiogram can reveal conductive hearing loss. A CT scan and an MRI, if soft tissue involvement is suspected, aid in the diagnosis and determination of the extent of tumor involvement. The differential diagnosis should include all causes of conductive hearing loss.

DIAGNOSTICS

Cholesteatoma

INITIAL

Audiogram and tympanogram
CT scan*
MRI*

*If indicated.

DIFFERENTIAL DIAGNOSIS

Cholesteatoma

- Obstructive hearing loss
- Eardrum disorders
- Otosclerosis

MANAGEMENT

Referral to an ear, nose, and throat specialist is indicated, since cholesteatomas are destructive and are responsible for much of the morbidity associated with chronic otitis media. Cholesteatomas require surgical excision. Concurrent suppurative otitis media requires systemic antibiotic therapy and removal of debris from the canal.

COMPLICATIONS

Complications include deafness, mastoiditis, facial nerve paralysis, brain hernia or cerebrospinal fluid leakage, and disseminated infection.[3]

INDICATIONS FOR REFERRAL OR HOSPITALIZATION

All patients with a cholesteatoma must be evaluated and managed by an otolaryngologist. Surgical excision is the primary treatment. Even after appropriate surgical treatment, recurrence rates may be as high as 50%.[4]

PATIENT AND FAMILY EDUCATION

Patient education should include information about this condition and its association with chronic ear infections and TM perforations. The importance of documenting complete healing after TM perforations is stressed.

REFERENCES

1. Roland PS: *Cholesteatoma,* Jan 20, 2004, retrieved Dec 15, 2005, from http://www.emedicine.com/ped/topic384.htm.
2. Weber PC: *Etiology of hearing loss in adults,* May 27, 2005, retrieved Dec 27, 2005, from http://www.utdol.com/application/topic/print.asp?file=genr_med/20536&type=A&selecte.
3. Cummings CW, Haughey BH, Thomas JR, and others: *Cummings otolaryngology: head and neck surgery,* ed 4, St Louis, 2005, Mosby.
4. Rakel RE, editor: *Textbook of family practice,* ed 6, Philadelphia, 2002, Saunders.

CHAPTER 88

Impaired Hearing

Jane Leonard

DEFINITION AND EPIDEMIOLOGY

Impaired hearing is a defect in the proper identification of external sound. Impaired hearing affects both communication ability and personal safety and can also be a socially isolating experience. The prevalence of hearing loss increases with advancing age; it is a common condition for many aging adults. A complaint of hearing loss can reflect a wide variety of abnormalities and requires different considerations in children than in adults.

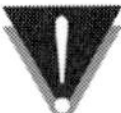

Immediate otolaryngologist or neurologist referral is indicated for patients with abrupt hearing loss.

PATHOPHYSIOLOGY

The ear is thought of in three segments: the outer ear, middle ear, and inner ear. Each section must function properly for hearing to occur normally. The outer ear is composed of the auricle and ear canal. The middle ear contains the tympanic membrane (TM), ossicles, and the middle ear space. Finally, the inner ear consists of the cochlea, semicircular canals, and internal auditory canals.[1]

Hearing loss may be classified into three types. A conductive loss involves any factor that limits the amount of external sounds from gaining access (being conducted) to the inner ear. A sensorineural loss involves the inner ear, especially the cochlea, or auditory nerves. Finally, a mixed hearing loss has both conductive and sensorineural components. A number of abnormalities may lead to hearing loss of each type. Conductive hearing loss is usually related to abnormalities of the outer or middle ear. Sensorineural hearing loss is related to a pathologic condition of the inner ear.[1]

In conductive hearing loss any component of the anatomic structures of the outer or middle ear can be involved. In the outer ear such factors include impacted cerumen, infection with edema, cholesteatoma, overgrowth of the bony wall, tumors, congenital atresia, and fibrotic stenosis from recurrent infection. Perforation, scar tissue, negative pressure from eustachian tube dysfunction, middle ear barotraumas, or any condition that impairs the mobility of the TM can impair hearing sensitivity. Causes of conductive loss from middle ear disease include acute otitis media, chronic serous otitis, and TM disorders. Otosclerosis, which is fusion of the stapes over the oval window, is a common cause of hearing loss in aging adults. Other conditions that interfere with the mechanical transmission of sound in the middle ear are trauma that damages the ossicles and congenital malformations.

Sensorineural hearing loss normally occurs from disorders of the inner ear. The cause may be associated with the cochlea, cranial nerve VIII (acoustic), the internal auditory canal, or the brain. Hearing loss that is congenital or hereditary occurs at or shortly after birth; it can indicate or result from such noninherited factors as maternal infections or medications or from inherited autosomal abnormalities. Sensorineural hearing loss can result from such factors as infections of the inner ear, Meniere's disease, inner ear barotraumas, trauma, and tumors.[1]

Presbycusis is a gradual degeneration within the cochlea that accompanies aging. There may also be degeneration of the mechanical structures and the central auditory connections. Multiple factors influence the rate at which hearing loss occurs: genetics, medications, infections, and exposure to noise. Noise trauma is a principal cause of cochlear damage. Persistent or repeated exposure to excessive noise causes stress, and mechanical damage occurs. High frequencies are affected initially, and then all frequencies are affected. A loud, explosive noise may cause severe and profound damage to these structures. In the United States the Occupational Safety and Health Administration (OSHA) has set standards and guidelines for noise exposure to protect workers. The OSHA standards limit the noise level exposure and state that protection must be worn (http://www.osha.gov).

Sensorineural hearing loss can also be caused by diseases that involve the endocrine, systemic, or metabolic systems; autoimmune disorders; iatrogenic factors; neurogenic disorders; and medications. Ototoxicity needs to be considered with sensorineural hearing loss. The prime suspects in ototoxicity include antineoplastics, salicylates, aminoglycosides, furosemide, and quinine-related drugs.

Mixed hearing loss combines elements of both conductive and sensorineural loss. Common causes of this loss include injury to the ear, infection, and congenital disorders.

CLINICAL PRESENTATION

The evaluation of hearing loss should determine whether the loss is acute, progressive, or fluctuating in nature. It is also important to determine whether the problem is unilateral or bilateral.

In addition to the nature of the hearing loss, associated symptoms of ear fullness, pain, vertigo, tinnitus, or cranial neuropathies should be documented. The medical history should incorporate current and past treatments with oral and IV medications or nonprescription drugs. Chronic illnesses, hospitalizations, and surgeries should be included in the history. A family history of hearing loss, neoplasms, renal disease, and imbalance disorders should be investigated. Finally, exposures to trauma and noise should also be noted.[2]

PHYSICAL EXAMINATION

A complete examination of the head, neck, and throat and an evaluation of cranial nerves and the auditory and vestibular system are essential. The pinna and external auditory canal should be inspected for malformations, lesions, exudates, and obstruction. Examination of the TM should assess for mobility (via pneumoscopy) and determine whether effusion, infection, perforation, or cholesteatoma is present.

Weber's and Rinne's tests help differentiate conductive and sensorineural hearing loss. Weber's test checks for lateralization of sound toward the ear with conductive loss. Rinne's test compares air and bone conduction. In normal hearing, air conduction (AC) is greater than bone conduction (BC) (AC > BC). In a conductive hearing loss, bone conduction is greater than air conduction (BC > AC), whereas in a sensorineural hearing loss air conduction remains greater than bone conduction, although reduced.

A screening audiogram is also necessary. A recent noise exposure history should be taken before administering a hearing test for more accurate results. Exposure to loud noises over the weekend, for example, may decrease hearing if tested on a Monday morning. Some say a mid-week test will result in better hearing.

DIAGNOSTICS

A formal audiogram, performed by an audiologist in a soundproof environment, is recommended if hearing is impaired on clinical examination. Formal testing consists of pure tone, air and bone conduction, and impedance audiometry. It can also include speech audiometry. Every audiologic workup should consist of a number of audiometric studies.

Laboratory tests should also be done to evaluate the patient for systemic or metabolic causes for the hearing loss. MRI or CT scans are indicated if tumors are suspected.[2]

DIFFERENTIAL DIAGNOSIS

The differential diagnosis of hearing loss is related to the nature of the presenting complaint: whether the loss was acute, gradual, fluctuant, or progressive.

Causes of acute hearing loss in adults can include sudden idiopathic sensorineural hearing loss, infections, perilymphatic fistula, ischemia of retrocochlear structures, multiple sclerosis, autoimmune diseases, trauma, chronic renal failure, and sickle cell anemia. Gradual hearing loss can be related to presbycusis, noise, familial factors, retrocochlear neoplasm, chronic otitis media, cholesteatoma, otosclerosis, hypothyroidism, diabetes, Paget's disease, chronic renal failure, and hyperlipoproteinemia. Differential diagnosis for fluctuating hearing loss includes perilymphatic fistula, Meniere's disease, multiple sclerosis, migraine headache, syphilis, autoimmune disorders, and sarcoidosis. Hearing loss that is rapidly progressive includes causes such as autoimmune inner ear disease, meningeal carcinoma, vasculitis, Lyme's disease, and ototoxic exposures.[3]

DIAGNOSTICS

Impaired Hearing

INITIAL

Audiogram

LABORATORY

CBC and differential (if anemia or infection is suspected)*
VDRL or RPR (to rule out syphilis)*
ESR, antinuclear antibodies, rheumatoid factor (if autoimmune cause is suspected)
TSH (if hypothyroid or hyperthyroid disorder is suspected)*

IMAGING

CT scan or MRI (if tumor is suspected)*

*If indicated.

DIFFERENTIAL DIAGNOSIS

Impaired Hearing

CONDUCTIVE HEARING LOSS

- Congenital atresia of the external auditory canal
- Cholesteatoma
- Foreign body
- Impacted cerumen
- Infection (otitis media, otitis externa)
- Otosclerosis
- Psoriasis or other dermatologic disease
- Trauma to external auditory canal
- Tumor
- Tympanic membrane perforation

SENSORINEURAL HEARING LOSS

- Acoustic neuroma
- Autoimmune hearing loss: polyarteritis nodosa, relapsing polychondritis, rheumatoid arthritis, systemic lupus erythematosus, Wegener's granulomatosis
- Barotrauma
- Congenital or hereditary factors
- Infection: meningitis, viruses
- Meniere's disease
- Metabolic abnormality: anemia, diabetes
- Neurologic disorder: multiple sclerosis, cerebrovascular accident, transient ischemic attack, Arnold-Chiari malformations, syphilis
- Ototoxic medications
- Paget's disease
- Presbycusis
- Trauma

MANAGEMENT AND CO-MANAGEMENT WITH SPECIALISTS

Conductive hearing loss associated with cerumen impaction or infection usually responds to impaction removal or resolution of infection (although hearing loss may lag behind clinical improvement of infection). Otolaryngology referral is indicated for patients with hearing deficit associated with trauma, congenital hearing loss, tumors, obstructions of the external auditory canal, nonhealing TM rupture, and otosclerosis. Tumors and obstructions of the external auditory canal must be surgically excised. Treatment for otosclerosis requires stapedectomy or sound amplification, whereas TM perforation may heal spontaneously or require a surgical patch or graft. Presbycusis and some other hearing impediments can be treated with hearing aids.

LIFE SPAN CONSIDERATIONS

Hearing loss is most often associated with aging, but hearing loss is possible in the first years of life, causing delays in speech, language, and cognitive development. Speech and language delays secondary to hearing loss are often preventable; thus early identification of hearing impairment is key to a child's success with communication.[4]

COMPLICATIONS

Impaired hearing may lead to social isolation, economic hardship, and accidents. Missed diagnoses may result in deafness.

INDICATIONS FOR REFERRAL OR HOSPITALIZATION

Referral to an otolaryngologist is appropriate when the diagnosis is unclear, when preliminary assessment indicates a serious condition, or when surgical intervention is an option. Referral to an audiologist is always appropriate for definitive testing. Abrupt hearing loss is cause for immediate referral to an appropriate specialist, usually an otolaryngologist or a neurologist.

PATIENT AND FAMILY EDUCATION

Patients should be aware that a sudden hearing loss, difficulty understanding what other people are saying, or a constant ringing in the ear requires further evaluation. They should receive a careful explanation about their particular type of hearing loss, as well as how medications, such as aspirin, NSAIDs, antibiotics, and diuretics, can cause hearing loss. Information about referral resources and options for management should also be presented to patients and their families. For patients considering hearing aids, careful explanation about the types of hearing devices available, their cost, and the fact that hearing loss cannot be completely restored is important to prevent any misunderstandings. Family members who live with a hearing-impaired person should understand the importance of decreasing background noise, facing the person when speaking so that the face and mouth are visible, and involving the hearing-impaired person in conversations.

HEALTH PROMOTION

Ototoxic medications should be monitored or, if possible, eliminated. Infants and children, especially those at high risk, should be considered for hearing screening. Adults should be questioned periodically about hearing impairment. Older adults need functional assessments done as needed. Ears should also be checked for cerumenosis and, if necessary, irrigated. Employees at risk for hearing loss from trauma or prolonged and elevated noise exposure are mandated by OSHA to limit their exposure and to wear protective equipment. Earplugs or protective equipment to reduce home, occupational, and recreational noise exposure should be encouraged to prevent any hearing loss.

REFERENCES

1. Weber PC: *Etiology of hearing loss in adults,* May 27, 2005, retrieved Dec 20, 2005, from http://www.utdol.com.
2. Weber PC: *Evaluation of hearing loss in adults,* Jan 6, 2005, retrieved Dec 20, 2005, from http://www.utdol.com.
3. Cummings C, Haughey B, Regan T, and others: *Cummings otolaryngology: head and neck surgery review*, ed 4, St Louis, 2005, Mosby.
4. Sanford B, Weber PC: *Etiology of hearing impairment in children*, Aug 11, 2005, retrieved Dec 20, 2005, from http://www.utdol.com.

CHAPTER 89

Inner Ear Disturbances

Christine A. Boodley

The third most common complaint of patients who are seen in an office or emergency department is lightheadedness, dizziness, unsteadiness, or disequilibrium.[1] This complaint, as well as those of hearing loss or tinnitus, may indicate an inner ear disturbance. Labyrinthitis, Meniere's disease, and tinnitus are three of the most common inner ear disturbances.

LABYRINTHITIS

DEFINITION AND EPIDEMIOLOGY

Labyrinthitis is an acute unilateral labyrinthine dysfunction, also called acute peripheral vestibulopathy or vestibular neuritis. The condition is characterized by brief severe vertigo, nausea, vomiting, and disequilibrium lasting a few days followed by vertigo and disequilibrium with rapid head movement that may last for weeks to months.[1] Approximately 20% of patients who come into a primary care setting or emergency department with complaints of vertigo have labyrinthitis.[2]

Vestibular neuronitis causes similar symptoms and is associated with a viral infection. However, although hearing may be affected in labyrinthitis, it is not affected in vestibular neuronitis. Treatment is the same for both conditions.[1]

PATHOPHYSIOLOGY

Labyrinthitis is most commonly caused by viral inflammation of the vestibular nerve; herpes simplex virus type 1 has been implicated in the disease.[3] Nerve inflammation is responsible for an asymmetry in the vestibular system that causes the sensation of vertigo.[2] Bacterial labyrinthitis, while rare, is more serious and may be a complication of otitis media or meningitis. Labyrinthitis may also be caused by irritation from chemical products associated with acute or chronic otitis media.[1]

CLINICAL PRESENTATION

Patients with labyrinthitis complain of severe vertigo, nausea, and vomiting aggravated by head movement. Tinnitus and hearing loss can be present. The most severe symptoms of vertigo usually subside within 48 to 72 hours, but they can last 4 or 5 days. Although most episodes resolve spontaneously, vertigo may recur for weeks or months when the head is turned suddenly.[1]

The history should include current medication use; history of head trauma; and the duration, episodic nature, and severity of the vertigo. Past medical history and recent infection, particularly in the respiratory tract, should be elicited. Precipitating or aggravating factors, including cough, sneeze, or change in head position, and associated symptoms should be ascertained to help determine the cause of the vertigo.

PHYSICAL EXAMINATION

A thorough ear, nose, and throat examination and a careful neurologic evaluation, including balance testing (Romberg's test), are recommended. A screening hearing examination usually reveals a unilateral hearing loss with labyrinthitis. Spontaneous nystagmus, horizontal or rotary, is often present with fast phases directed away from the affected ear. The nystagmus should decrease with visual fixation or increase with the use of Frenzel lenses (magnifying lenses that blur vision, making it hard to fix the gaze).[2] An abnormal neurologic examination suggests a more serious cause.

DIAGNOSTICS

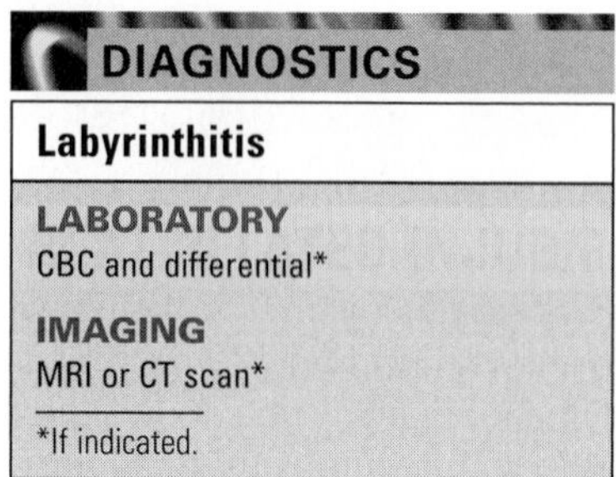
DIAGNOSTICS

Labyrinthitis

LABORATORY
CBC and differential*

IMAGING
MRI or CT scan*

*If indicated.

More definitive examinations to test hearing and to assess vertigo may be warranted. If bacterial labyrinthitis is suspected, a CBC with differential may be helpful. If a tumor is suspected, MRI or a CT scan is indicated.

DIFFERENTIAL DIAGNOSIS

Additional causes of peripheral vertigo and central vertigo must be considered. Benign positional vertigo is associated with changes in head position, especially when the patient is recumbent. Meniere's disease is associated with vertigo that recurs over months and years. Migrainous vertigo may occur with or without a headache.[4] Ramsay Hunt syndrome, caused by herpes zoster, includes hearing loss, facial palsy, and vertigo.[3] Central causes of vertigo, such as vascular disorders or tumors, are less common, have a more gradual onset, and usually have milder symptoms.[2] Multiple sclerosis, head trauma, barotrauma, and toxins such as drugs and alcohol can also cause similar symptoms.[5] Additional information about vertigo can be found in Chapter 206.

DIFFERENTIAL DIAGNOSIS

Labyrinthitis

- Benign paroxysmal positional vertigo
- Meniere's disease
- Migrainous vertigo
- Vascular disorders
- Trauma (head trauma, barotrauma)
- Toxins (medications, alcohol)
- Demyelinating disease (multiple sclerosis)
- Ramsay Hunt syndrome
- Tumors

MANAGEMENT

Bed rest may be indicated while the symptoms are severe. Antibiotics are appropriate if there is associated bacterial infection. Limited evidence exists that corticosteroids can help vestibular recovery.[6,7] Methylprednisolone can be given once daily for 22 days beginning with diagnosis. Recommended dosage is 100 mg on days 1 to 3, 80 mg on days 4 to 6, 60 mg on days 7 to 9, 40 mg on days 10 to 12, 20 mg on days 13 to 15, 10 mg on days 16 to 18, no medicine on days 19 and 21, and 10 mg on days 20 and 22.[7] Once the severe symptoms have passed, limited evidence exists that patients may benefit from vestibular enhancement exercises, which can be obtained through physical therapy services.[8,9] Evidence of benefit is unclear for offering symptomatic relief for several days using anticholinergics, antihistamines, long-acting benzodiazepines, or antiemetics. Anticholinergics and antihistamines are first-line agents; benzodiazepines are reserved for patients who cannot take drugs with anticholinergic effects. Meclizine 25 to 50 mg q 6 hr is commonly used and acceptable in pregnancy. Antiemetics may be added for relief of short-term severe vomiting.[2] These medications should be stopped after 3 days because continuing them may hamper vestibular recovery.[1]

LIFE SPAN CONSIDERATIONS

Medications for symptomatic relief of labyrinthitis can cause drowsiness and sedation. In older adults, lower doses of medications (e.g., 12.5 mg meclizine or less) should be considered to control sedation.

COMPLICATIONS

Sensorineural hearing loss can occur after inflammation of the inner ear. Suppurative otitis media or meningitis may be associated with labyrinthitis.[3]

INDICATIONS FOR REFERRAL OR HOSPITALIZATION

Consultation with an otolaryngologist is indicated if the diagnosis is unclear, the bacterial infection is severe, or symptoms do not resolve within 4 to 6 weeks. Associated suppurative otitis media or meningitis also necessitates referral. Severe dehydration indicates a need for IV rehydration and possible hospitalization.

PATIENT AND FAMILY EDUCATION

The provision of information about the disorder and reassurances will be helpful to patients and families. The importance of slowly changing positions should be discussed. In addition, adequate hydration and safety should be stressed. Patients, particularly older adults, may require assistance with activities of daily living or a walker or cane during the acute phase of the illness. Patients should avoid driving and operating heavy equipment while on sedatives or antihistamines.

Because the disorder usually resolves within 4 to 6 weeks, patients should understand the importance of notifying the health care provider if the symptoms continue or increase in severity. Follow-up evaluation should be scheduled to reassess the patient and ensure the vertigo is resolving.

MENIERE'S DISEASE

DEFINITION AND EPIDEMIOLOGY

Meniere's disease is a chronic condition of the inner ear characterized by recurrent vertigo and hearing loss. It is a complex of four symptoms that may or may not occur simultaneously: dizziness described as spinning vertigo, low-frequency sensorineural hearing loss, tinnitus, and a feeling of fullness in the affected ear. It is estimated that Meniere's disease affects 50 to 75 per 100,000 people.[10] Most patients acquire the disease after the fifth decade of life, although it can affect young children and the elderly. Forty-five percent of cases have bilateral involvement.[11]

PATHOPHYSIOLOGY

Meniere's disease involves excess fluid and pressure in the labyrinth of the inner ear that episodically distends the structures of the labyrinth and damages the vestibular and cochlear hair cells. There is no known cause, although immunologic mechanisms, genetic predisposition, anatomic variation, viral infection, and a vascular pathophysiology in common with migraine headaches have been suggested.[11]

CLINICAL PRESENTATION

Along with eliciting a careful symptom analysis, the health care provider should ask patients about a history of recurrent symptoms. Early in the disease process, patients have intermittent attacks of vertigo that last from minutes to hours, often associated with nausea and vomiting. These episodes are commonly accompanied by pressure in the ear, low-pitched tinnitus fluctuating in intensity, and hearing loss, usually in one ear. There can be long periods of remission. During later stages the attacks of vertigo may occur frequently, and the hearing loss is constant.

PHYSICAL EXAMINATION

Diagnosis is primarily based on symptom analysis, but Meniere's disease must be differentiated from other causes of vertigo. A thorough head and neck examination to exclude acute otitis media or other infectious process and a comprehensive neurologic examination are important. On physical examination, Weber's test will lateralize to the unaffected ear, and in Rinne's test, air conduction will be greater than bone conduction. Spontaneous nystagmus occurs during attacks and may not be present between attacks.[11]

DIAGNOSTICS

A definitive diagnosis of Meniere's can be made if the patients has had two episodes of spontaneous vertigo lasting at least 20 minutes each, audiometrically documented hearing loss, and tinnitus and/or aural fullness in one or both ears, and if other causes have been excluded.[12]

Basic testing for Meniere's includes an audiogram, MRI to rule out central nervous system (CNS) lesions,[10,11] thyroid-stimulating hormone, glucose, and fluorescent treponemal antibody absorption test to rule out other causes.[11] Additional testing, done by an otolaryngologist, may include vestibular testing; glycerine, urea, or sorbitol "stress" tests; electrocochleography; electronystagmography; and auditory brainstem testing.[11]

DIAGNOSTICS

Meniere's Disease

INITIAL
Audiogram

LABORATORY
TSH
Serum glucose
Fluorescent treponemal antibody absorption test

IMAGING
MRI (to rule out neuroma)

DIFFERENTIAL DIAGNOSIS

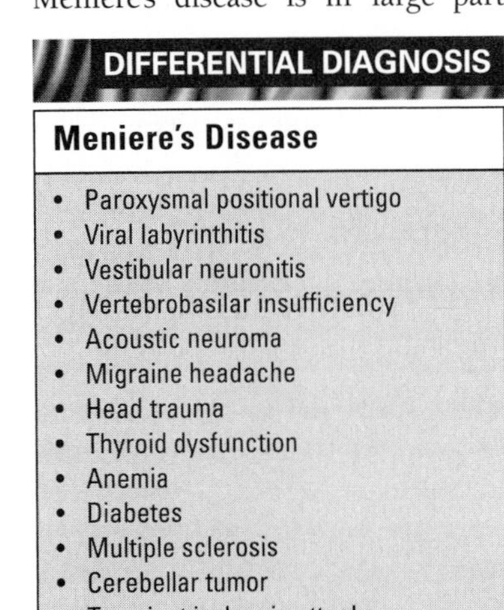

DIFFERENTIAL DIAGNOSIS

Meniere's Disease

- Paroxysmal positional vertigo
- Viral labyrinthitis
- Vestibular neuronitis
- Vertebrobasilar insufficiency
- Acoustic neuroma
- Migraine headache
- Head trauma
- Thyroid dysfunction
- Anemia
- Diabetes
- Multiple sclerosis
- Cerebellar tumor
- Transient ischemic attacks
- Cogan's syndrome

Meniere's disease is in large part diagnosed by excluding other disorders and is classified as idiopathic. Meniere's disease can be seen with only hearing loss or vertigo, both symptoms of many disorders. Conditions that must be considered and ruled out as part of a normal workup for the condition include acoustic neuroma, cerebellar tumors, diabetes, thyroid disease, and tertiary syphilis. Other differentials include benign paroxysmal positional vertigo, labyrinthitis, head trauma, vertebrobasilar insufficiency, multiple sclerosis, transient ischemic attack, migraine headache, anemia, and Cogan's syndrome.[11]

MANAGEMENT AND CO-MANAGEMENT WITH SPECIALISTS

If Meniere's disease is suspected, patients should be referred to an otolaryngologist for testing and management. There is no cure for the disease, and treatment can be difficult. The goals of therapy include managing the episodes of vertigo and arresting the disease process. Bed rest may be the most valuable recommendation during an acute episode. Restricting the intake of caffeine, alcohol, tobacco, and dietary sodium is also often suggested, although evidence of the benefit of such restrictions is unclear. Vestibular suppressants like meclizine and antiemetics like promethazine (Phenergan) may help for severe symptoms.[11]

Betahistine hydrochloride and diuretic therapy may reduce the severity of the attacks if they are not controlled by diet, but evidence of benefit is unclear.[13] In the United States generic betahistine hydrochloride can be obtained by prescription from a "compounding" pharmacist.[11] Recommended dosage is 8 to 16 mg t.i.d.[14] Limited evidence exists for benefit from vestibular rehabilitation.[8,9]

In severe cases, chemical labyrinthectomy with intracochlear gentamicin or surgical procedures such as labyrinthectomy, vestibular neurectomy, or decompression of the endolymphatic sac have been considered. These treatments are controversial, but may provide relief for patients with unrelenting symptoms.[11]

LIFE SPAN CONSIDERATIONS

Although Meniere's disease is more commonly diagnosed in middle-aged adults, older adults and children can also be afflicted.[11] The disorder can be particularly difficult to treat in pregnancy because medications are toxic to the fetus.

COMPLICATIONS

Hearing loss may be permanent. Injury from falls is a possible complication.

INDICATIONS FOR REFERRAL OR HOSPITALIZATION

Referral to an otolaryngologist or a neurootologist is indicated for diagnostic evaluation and management. Hospitalization is rarely indicated unless the patient becomes dehydrated or injured as a result of a fall. Hospitalization is necessary for surgical intervention.

PATIENT AND FAMILY EDUCATION

Patient information should include information about the disease pathology, expected course, and treatment choices. Reassurance will help to allay anxiety. Patient safety during acute episodes of vertigo and the sedative side effects of prescribed medications should be emphasized.

TINNITUS

DEFINITION AND EPIDEMIOLOGY

Tinnitus is defined as the perception of a sound when there is no sound in the environment.[10] It is usually a chronic, benign, but annoying ringing, buzzing, hissing, high-pitched screeching, whistling, or other noise in one or both ears that can be constant or intermittent. It can, however, herald a more serious disorder. It is estimated that as many as 50 million Americans have tinnitus. It worsens with age, affecting men more frequently than women.[15] A significant number of patients (approximately 15 million) seek medical assistance, and 2 million believe the tinnitus interferes with normal daily function.[16]

PATHOPHYSIOLOGY

The pathophysiology of tinnitus is not well understood, but current theories point to the CNS as the source of tinnitus, whatever the underlying cause.[15] Tinnitus has a wide range of causes, including somatic sounds, otosclerosis, presbycusis, toxins, noise trauma, barotrauma, eustachian tube dysfunction, acoustic neuroma, vascular abnormalities, and neuromuscular conditions, which complicate both diagnosis and treatment.

CLINICAL PRESENTATION

Patients with tinnitus have varying degrees of symptomatology and levels of debilitation, depending on the type and level of perceived sound. The history should include onset, duration, frequency, characteristics, and location of the sound, as well as past ear disease or injury, allergy history, noise exposure, hearing status, and medications. A description of the tinnitus can be helpful. High-pitched, continuous sounds are usually associated with sensorineural loss, low-pitched sounds with idiopathic tinnitus or Meniere's disease. Tinnitus described as pulsing or rushing is usually vascular in origin. Sounds similar to the ocean may result from eustachian tube dysfunction. Clicking sounds are usually somatic and may be caused by temporomandibular joint (TMJ) dysfunction or spasms of the muscular or middle ear structures. The spasms of ear structures may be symptomatic of an underlying neurologic disorder and warrant a thorough neurologic history and physical examination.[15] If the tinnitus is associated with hearing loss, any dizziness, vertigo, ear pressure, pain, or discharge should be noted. Tinnitus can either accompany or cause insomnia and depression, so the health care provider should inquire about both of these conditions.[15]

PHYSICAL EXAMINATION

The physical examination should include a complete ear, nose, throat, head, neck, and TMJ examination. If vascular tinnitus is suspected, the health care provider should include auscultation of preauricular areas, temples, orbits, and mastoids in various positions. The effects of positioning and jugular compression should be noted.[15] Hearing tests and a complete neurologic examination (including cranial nerves) are also indicated.

DIAGNOSTICS

A tinnitus handicap questionnaire is available to measure the degree of severity of tinnitus.[15] All patients with tinnitus thought to originate in the auditory system should receive a complete audiologic evaluation performed by an audiologist. Tests may include pure tone audiogram, tympanometry, auditory reflex testing, determination of speech discrimination abilities, and otoacoustic emissions testing. Patients believed to have vascular tinnitus should be evaluated by an otolaryngologist or neurologist. Laboratory testing may include a CBC and differential to rule out anemia and infection, erythrocyte sedimentation rate to rule out autoimmune disease, serum glucose, and thyroid function. If indicated, additional diagnostics include MRI or CT scan to rule out a CNS lesion.[15]

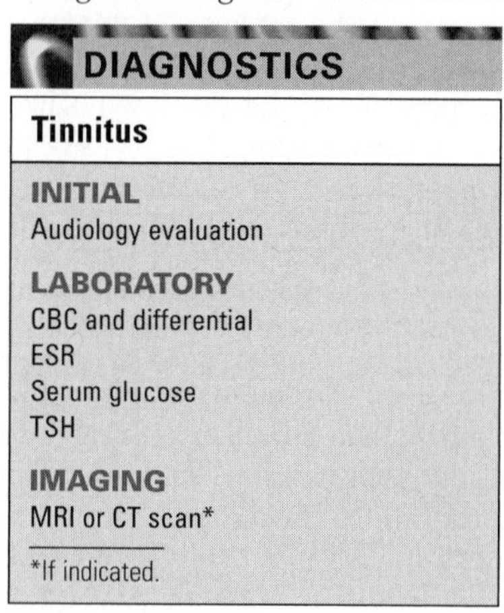
DIAGNOSTICS

Tinnitus

INITIAL
Audiology evaluation

LABORATORY
CBC and differential
ESR
Serum glucose
TSH

IMAGING
MRI or CT scan*

*If indicated.

DIFFERENTIAL DIAGNOSIS

The differential diagnosis should include those conditions which distinguish benign tinnitus from tinnitus caused by serious pathologic conditions. Excessive noise exposure and presbycusis are common causes of hearing loss and tinnitus. Medications, such as aspirin, can cause permanent or reversible tinnitus. Tinnitus of short duration is often caused by an acute process such as otitis, labyrinthitis, or noise exposure. Vascular disorders can cause pulsatile tinnitus and require in-depth evaluation by an otolaryngologist or neurologist. Spasm in the muscles of the ear or palate can be heard as an intermittent

DIFFERENTIAL DIAGNOSIS

Tinnitus

- Noise exposure
- Medication
- Presbycusis
- Labyrinthitis
- Otitis
- Somatic sounds, eustachian tube dysfunction
- Vascular disorders
- Meniere's disease
- CNS disorders (multiple sclerosis)
- Acoustic neuroma

tapping sound. Eustachian tube dysfunction causes a sound like the ocean. An acoustic neuroma is usually associated with unilateral tinnitus.[10] Meniere's disease is characterized by fluctuating tinnitus, hearing loss, aural fullness, or vertigo.

MANAGEMENT

Intermittent tinnitus is not usually considered serious, but unilateral tinnitus has been associated with an acoustic tumor; therefore consultation with the primary care physician is indicated to determine the need for MRI or CT scanning. Pulsatile tinnitus is also considered a serious symptom and necessitates evaluation by an otolaryngologist or neurologist. All ototoxic medications and excessive noise exposure need to be eliminated. Obvious local pathologic conditions should be treated (e.g., TMJ treatment or administration of antibiotics for infection).

Most patients with mild to moderate tinnitus adjust to the condition; although it is annoying, they do not find it debilitating. Patient education and reassurance are often all that can be offered. Other patients, with more severe tinnitus, find the condition disabling and should be referred to an otolaryngologist. If a sensorineural hearing loss is associated, referral for the application of other treatment modalities, such as hearing aids, sound masking, or cognitive behavioral therapy, may be indicated.[16] If no hearing loss is present, sound maskers alone, such as electronic noise-generating devices, mood tapes, or radio static, may diminish the intrusiveness of tinnitus.

The evidence of benefit is unclear for alternative therapies, including vitamins, herbal remedies, biofeedback, acupuncture, and electrical stimulation, but they may help individual patients. Antidepressants have proved somewhat helpful if depression or anxiety accompanies tinnitus. Treating insomnia in patients with tinnitus may decrease the severity of the tinnitus.[15]

COMPLICATIONS

No complications are associated with chronic, benign tinnitus. Missed diagnosis of tinnitus that is caused by serious underlying pathologic condition may lead to untreated disease and major complications.

INDICATIONS FOR REFERRAL OR HOSPITALIZATION

Consultation with the primary care physician is necessary when referral to an otolaryngologist or a neurologist is indicated. If there is a suspicion that the tinnitus is not benign or if pulsatile or unilateral tinnitus is present, the patient should be seen by the appropriate specialist.

PATIENT AND FAMILY EDUCATION

Information on the causes of tinnitus and hearing loss increases understanding for most patients. A discussion of treatment options and resources for treatment is beneficial. Reassurance about the benign and common experiences of tinnitus is also helpful. Resources about tinnitus can be obtained from the American Tinnitus Association (http://www.ata.org).

REFERENCES

1. Tusa RJ: Vertigo, *Neurol Clin* 19(1):23-55, 2001.
2. Barton J, and others: *Approach to the patient with vertigo,* retrieved Nov 19, 2005, from http://www.utdol.com/application/topic.asp?file=genneuro/2118.
3. Barton J: *Treatment of vertigo,* retrieved Nov 19, 2005, from http://www.utdol.com/application/topic.asp?file=genneuro/5875&type=A&selectedTitle=1~4.
4. Bajwa ZH, and others: *Pathophysiology, clinical manifestations, and diagnosis of migraine in adults,* retrieved Nov 22, 2005, from http://www.utdol.com.
5. Daroff RB, Carlson MD: Syncope, faintness, dizziness, and vertigo. In Kasper DL, Braunwald E, Fauci AS, and others, editors: *Harrison's principles of internal medicine,* ed 16, 2005, retrieved Dec 20, 2006, from http://www.accessmedicine.com/content.aspx?aID=52966.
6. Kitahara T, Kondoh K, Morihana T, and others: Steroid effects on vestibular compensation in humans, *Neurol Res* 25:287-289, 2003.
7. Strupp M, Zingler VC, Arbusow V, and others: Methylprednisolone, valacyclovir, or the combination for vestibular neuritis, *N Engl J Med* 351(4):354-361, 2004.
8. Strupp M, Arbusow V, Maag KP, and others: Vestibular exercises improve central vestibulospinal compensation after vestibular neuritis, *Neurology* 51(3):838-844, 1998.
9. Yardley L, Donovan-Hall M, Smith HE, and others: Effectiveness of primary care–based vestibular rehabilitation for chronic dizziness, *Ann Intern Med* 141(8):598-605, 2004.
10. Lalwani AK, Snow JB Jr: Disorders of smell, taste, and hearing. In Kasper DL, Braunwald E, Fauci AS, and others, editors: *Harrison's principles of internal medicine,* ed 16, 2005, retrieved Dec 20, 2006, from http://www.accessmedicine.com/content.aspx?aID=53859.
11. Dinces EA: *Meniere's disease,* retrieved Nov 22, 2005, from http://www.utdol.com/application/topic.asp?file=pri_neur/11845&type=A&selectedTitle=1~15.
12. Committee on Hearing and Equilibrium: Guidelines for the diagnosis and evaluation of therapy in Meniere's disease, *Otolaryngol Head Neck Surg* 113:181-185, 1995.
13. James AL, Burton MJ: Betahistine for Ménière's disease or syndrome, *Cochrane Database Syst Rev* (1):CD001873, DOI: 10.1002/14651858.CD001873, 2001.
14. *Betahistine: drug information,* retrieved Feb 15, 2005, from http://www.utdol.com/application/topic.asp?file=drug_a_k/163444&drug=true.
15. Dinces EA: *Tinnitus,* retrieved Nov 14, 2005, from http://www.utdol.com/application/topic.asp?file=genr_med/5223&type=A&selectedTitle=1~20.
16. American Tinnitus Association: *Frequently asked questions,* retrieved Dec 15, 2006, from http://www.ata.org/about_tinnitus/consumer/faq.html#2.

CHAPTER 90

Otitis Externa

Christine A. Boodley and
Karen Koozer Olson

DEFINITION AND EPIDEMIOLOGY

Otitis externa is commonly referred to as *earache* and is a superficial inflammation or infection of the external ear that usually is seen with unilateral pain in the external auditory canal. The disorder is often referred to as "swimmer's ear," although the causes are varied and can simply be related to skin damage from scratching the ear.

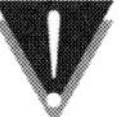

Immediate physician or otolaryngologist consultation is indicated for patients with malignant otitis externa (Color Plate 35).

PATHOPHYSIOLOGY

The superficial inflammatory process of the external auditory canal may have multiple precipitants, including cerumen impaction; trauma related to vigorous cleaning of the canal with cotton-tipped swabs; swimming in pools that are not properly maintained; or swimming in lakes, rivers, and oceans. The most common causative organisms are *Staphylococcus aureus* and *Pseudomonas, Candida,* and *Aspergillus* organisms.[1-3] Recent data indicate that community-acquired methicillin-resistant *S. aureus* (CA-MRSA) may be a causative agent in otitis. This appears to be more common after tympanostomy tube placement and in patients who do not respond to antibiotic therapy or have chronic or recurrent otitis.[2]

CLINICAL PRESENTATION

The usual presentation of otitis externa is unilateral pain in the ear canal. A feeling of fullness or itching may accompany the pain. Tenderness of the tragus may also be present, as may be mild lymphadenopathy and a low-grade fever.

PHYSICAL EXAMINATION

The physical examination may reveal a normal temperature and normal lymph nodes, but pain and tenderness are evident on palpation of the tragus and inspection of the external ear canal. The external ear canal may be erythematous and edematous. The tympanic membrane may be poorly visualized because of cerumen or edema and exudate in the auditory canal. Unilateral hearing deficits may be evident if the canal is markedly swollen or impacted with cerumen.

DIAGNOSTICS

Diagnostic testing is often unnecessary. However, a culture of canal drainage with antibiotic sensitivities is indicated for severe external otitis or for malignant otitis externa. The erythrocyte sedimentation rate may be elevated in malignant otitis externa. A CT scan or MRI is indicated if osteomyelitis of the temporal bone is suspected in patients with malignant otitis externa. As in any infectious process, the patient's immune status must be considered as part of the decision-making process.

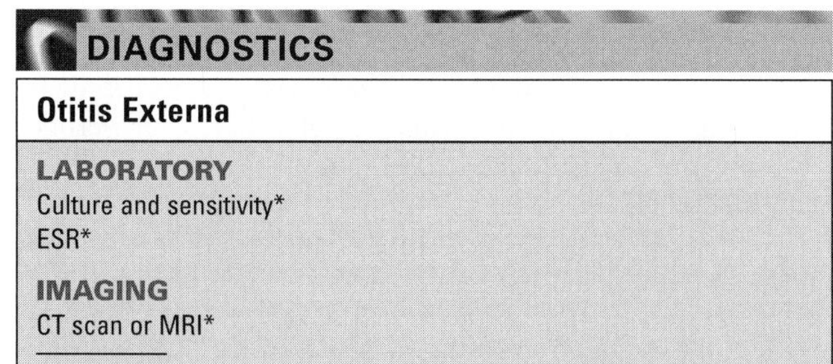

DIAGNOSTICS

Otitis Externa

LABORATORY
Culture and sensitivity*
ESR*

IMAGING
CT scan or MRI*

*If indicated.

DIFFERENTIAL DIAGNOSIS

The most common differential diagnoses are cerumen impaction and the presence of a foreign body in the external ear canal. Patients with recurrent episodes should be evaluated to determine whether the recurrent episode is a treatment failure or a new episode. CA-MRSA should be considered in patients who have had tympanostomy tube placement, who do not respond to antibiotic therapy, or who have chronic or recurrent otitis.[2]

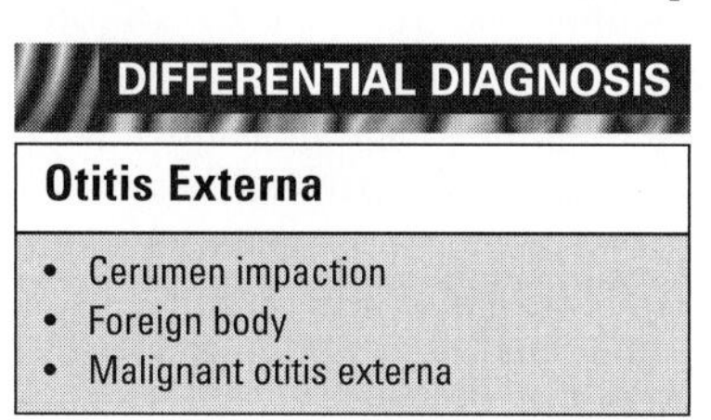

DIFFERENTIAL DIAGNOSIS

Otitis Externa

- Cerumen impaction
- Foreign body
- Malignant otitis externa

MANAGEMENT

Management of otitis externa depends on the complaint and the causative factors. Over-the-counter NSAIDs and complete cleaning and drying of the canal may be all that are necessary for mild inflammatory processes. Staphylococcal infections, which are characterized by yellow, crusty exudate, can be treated topically with an antibiotic-hydrocortisone compound (e.g., Cortisporin otic suspension [hydrocortisone–neomycin sulfate–polymyxin B sulfate] 4 drops b.i.d. to q.i.d. for 7 days in the external canal).[2] For acute disease, dicloxacillin 500 mg PO q.i.d. can be used for 7 to 10 days.[1] The insertion of a wick into the affected ear may enhance healing in particularly edematous and inflamed canals. *Pseudomonas* infections, which are often accompanied by a greenish exudate, also are treated with topical agents such as Cortisporin. A fine, white material on the affected skin may be indicative of fungal infections and is best treated with clotrimazole (Lotrimin) 1% 2 drops t.i.d. into the affected ear. CA-MRSA is often susceptible to sulfamethoxazole-trimethoprim (Bactrim DS).[1]

LIFE SPAN CONSIDERATIONS

Otitis externa is most common in young people and in swimmers; the incidence increases during the summer.

COMPLICATIONS

Complications of otitis externa are rare but include malignant otitis externa. This condition is usually caused by *Pseudomonas aeruginosa* and is most commonly seen in patients who have diabetes or are immunocompromised. It is associated with severe pain, necrosis, and osteomyelitis.

INDICATIONS FOR REFERRAL OR HOSPITALIZATION

Patients with suspected malignant otitis externa should be referred to an otolaryngologist or admitted to the hospital. Very early disease can be treated with ciprofloxacin (Cipro) 750 mg PO b.i.d. for 7 to 10 days with frequent follow-up.[1] In general, an erythematous, edematous, and tender auricle is indicative of virulent involvement of the deeper structures, which can progress to a life-threatening infection of the face and head. This condition requires immediate physician consultation and possible hospitalization for aggressive antimicrobial therapy. Patients who have diabetes or are immunocompromised may also require a referral for specialized care. Patients with severe otitis externa and frequent recurrences should be referred to an otolaryngologist.

PATIENT AND FAMILY EDUCATION

Patients need to be educated about medication management, the use of earplugs when swimming, and avoidance of the use of cotton-tipped swabs in the external ear. The importance of immediate follow-up if there is increased pain or increasing signs of infection should be stressed.

HEALTH PROMOTION

Swimmers should use earplugs, as well as a mixture of 1:2 white vinegar/rubbing alcohol drops in each ear after swimming, then antibiotic drops or a 2% acetic acid solution.[1]

REFERENCES

1. Gilbert D: *The Stanford guide to antimicrobial therapy*, ed 35, Hyde Park, Vt, 2005, Antimicrobial Therapy.
2. Estrada B: Will MRSA become a frequent cause of otitis? *Infect Med* 20(3):116, 2003, retrieved Dec 15, 2006, from http://www.medscape.com/viewarticle/451588.
3. Ferri F: *Ferri's clinical advisor: instant diagnosis and treatment*, St Louis, 2005, Mosby.

CHAPTER 91

Otitis Media

Christine A. Boodley and
Karen Koozer Olson

DEFINITION AND EPIDEMIOLOGY

Otitis media is an inflammatory or infective process of the middle ear that may be bacterial, fungal, or viral in origin and is most often associated with upper respiratory tract infections or allergies. Otitis media is the most frequent childhood infectious illness and accounts for a significant number of all antimicrobial prescriptions.[1] Acute otitis media has a rapid onset and short duration. Otitis media with effusion describes inflammation and infection of the middle ear with an accompanying accumulation of serous fluid that can last up to 3 weeks. Subacute otitis media is a middle ear effusion that lasts from 3 weeks to 3 months. If the effusion has persisted for more than 3 months, it is classified as chronic otitis with effusion. Recurrent otitis media is inflammation and infection of the middle ear that occurs frequently (two or more episodes in 6 months or three in 12 months) but resolves between episodes.[1]

PATHOPHYSIOLOGY

Otitis media is a dysfunction of the eustachian tube. The actual cause is unknown, but it may be sequelae of upper respiratory tract infections or allergies that result in edema of the eustachian tube. It may also result from reflux of the nasopharynx bacteria into the eustachian tube or obstruction.[2] Antecedent events may be infections or allergies that cause edema or congestion of the middle ear. Narrow eustachian tubes may predispose patients to episodes of otitis media. Exposure to cigarette smoke acts in several ways to increase the individual's risk for otitis media. Smokers are at higher risk for upper respiratory tract infections, plus the smoke may decrease the mucociliary functioning in the eustachian tube. When middle ear secretions accumulate in the eustachian tube, the opportunity for pathogen growth also increases. The most common pathogens are bacterial and viral. The most common bacterial causative agents are *Streptococcus pneumoniae* and *Haemophilus influenzae*. Chronic serous otitis is often associated with adenoidal hypertrophy, allergies, a deviated nasal septum, and the sequelae of upper respiratory tract infections and purulent otitis media.[3,4] Fifty-five percent of otitis infections are caused by bacteria; however, in 25% of cases no pathogen, either viral or bacterial, is discovered.[5] Clinical investigation has documented an increased incidence of otitis in which the causative agent is community-acquired methicillin-resistant *Staphylococcus aureus* (CA-MRSA).[6]

CLINICAL PRESENTATION

Clinical findings are related to the etiology. If the otitis media is related to allergic rhinitis, the clinical presentation will be significantly different than it would be if it were related to an upper respiratory tract infection. The patient with acute otitis media has an initial complaint of a painful ear and probably has other symptoms of illness, including warm, tender, and enlarged posterior auricular and cervical lymph nodes; rhinorrhea; vomiting; diarrhea; and fever. Patients with chronic otitis media or serous otitis may be asymptomatic or have mild pain. Vertigo, hearing loss, mild stuffiness, and a fullness or popping sensation in the ear are additional complaints.

PHYSICAL EXAMINATION

A history of ear infections, upper respiratory tract infections, allergies, smoke exposure, and any treatments and their effectiveness should be elicited. The development of the current illness, including the onset and duration of symptoms, ear pain or drainage, fever, irritability, hearing loss, tinnitus, or dizziness, should be noted. Associated symptoms, such as headache, nasal congestion, sore throat, or mouth pain, require investigation. Activities that involve barometric pressure changes, such as scuba diving and flying, may affect ear equilibrium. As with any infectious process, the patient's immune status must be considered. Temperature and vital signs may be within normal range, or the temperature may be elevated. The mouth, eyes, and nose examination may also be normal or may show signs and symptoms of upper respiratory tract infection. The frontal and maxillary sinuses are often tender on palpation and do not transilluminate. Mild to significant lymphadenopathy may be present. The tympanic membrane (TM) may be slightly erythematous or significantly inflamed and bulging. Bubbles seen behind the membrane indicate effusion.

The color of the TM may range from gray to red. Erythema of the TM is an inconclusive finding and may be related to crying or fever. In otitis media with effusion the TM is dull gray and may be injected. Fluid levels may be visible behind the membrane. A very white TM may be the result of scarring from previous infections or of pus behind the eardrum. Discharge in the canal suggests perforation. Purulent discharge in the ear canal may be cultured and used as a basis for antibiotic selection. Bullae between the TM layers are most often associated with *Mycoplasma pneumoniae.* In chronic serous otitis the TM may appear retracted with a diffuse light reflex. It has limited movement and bubbles or a fluid line may be seen behind the membrane.[3,4]

In acute otitis media the TM is red and bulging with obscure landmarks. Acute otitis media is often characterized by a throbbing, painful earache. Often there is fever. Hearing is usually impaired, and the patient may have nausea or dizziness. The disease is usually accompanied by cold or influenza symptoms. In serous otitis media there may be fullness and impaired hearing. Fluid levels or air bubbles may be seen behind the TM.

DIAGNOSTICS

Diagnosis is normally based on the otoscopic examination. Tympanometry may help with diagnosis if otoscopic examination cannot determine whether there is fluid in the middle ear.[5] Acoustic reflectometry, which is the use of sound waves to determine TM mobility, may also be helpful for diagnosis, although it is rarely used. The use of the pneumatic otoscope to determine whether the TM is mobile is the most commonly used technique. Weber's test and Rinne's test may be indicated to determine whether conduction and sensorineural hearing have been affected. Allergy testing should be considered in patients who have recurrent or chronic otitis symptoms and a history of allergies or allergic rhinitis. A sinus x-ray study or a CT scan of the sinuses may also be indicated for patients who have recurrent or chronic otitis media.

DIAGNOSTICS

Otitis Media

LABORATORY
CBC and differential*

IMAGING
Sinus x-ray or CT scan of sinuses*

OTHER
Allergy tests*
Tympanocentesis*
Culture and sensitivity*

*If indicated.

Immune status should be considered in patients with atypical otitis media or those who do not respond to therapy. Tympanocentesis may be indicated for recurrent otitis media to identify causative organisms. A CBC with differential should be ordered in immunocompromised patients.

DIFFERENTIAL DIAGNOSIS

DIFFERENTIAL DIAGNOSIS

Otitis Media

- Sinusitis
- Otitis externa
- Transient middle ear effusion
- Mastoiditis
- Temporomandibular joint disorder
- Mumps
- Dental disorders
- Tonsillitis
- Foreign body
- Head or ear trauma

Otitis externa, transient middle ear effusion related to barometric changes, mastoiditis, temporomandibular joint (TMJ) disorder, mumps, dental disorders, and tonsillitis should be considered. In addition, ear pain can result from a foreign body either in the nose or in the ear (more likely in young children) or from head or ear trauma.

MANAGEMENT

The management of bacterial otitis media has traditionally relied on the use of antibiotics (Table 91-1). However, many cases of otitis media can be treated symptomatically with

TABLE 91-1 Recommended Antibiotics for Adults with Acute Otitis Media (Bacterial)

Antibiotic	Dosage
Amoxicillin	500 mg to 1 g t.i.d. × 5-7 days
Trimethoprim-sulfamethoxazole (Bactrim DS)	1 tablet b.i.d. × 5-7 days
Erythromycin	333-500 mg t.i.d. × 5-7days
Amoxicillin-clavulanate (Augmentin XR)	2000/125 mg b.i.d. × 5-7 days
Cefuroxime (Ceftin)	250 mg b.i.d. × 5-7 days

Modified from Gilbert D: *The Sanford guide to antimicrobial therapy,* ed 35, Hyde Park, Vt, 2005, Antimicrobial Therapy.

acetaminophen or ibuprofen.[5] One fourth of all cases of otitis media have no bacterial component,[6] and many resolve without antimicrobial treatment.[4,6] Antibiotic therapy should be determined on an individual basis and depends on the history and presentation.

Amoxicillin continues to be the antibiotic of choice for the initial treatment of otitis media for patients who are not penicillin allergic. It is relatively easy to use, inexpensive, and effective. Clinical evidence supports the use of narrow-spectrum antimicrobial agents such as amoxicillin or sulfa drugs for initial treatment of acute onset otitis media.[7] Increasingly, however, a significant number of organisms, usually those which produce β-lactamase, are amoxicillin resistant. If initial therapy is not successful, a medication effective against these organisms, such as amoxicillin-clavulanate (Augmentin XR), should be considered. Other antibiotics commonly used are sulfonamides, cephalosporins, and macrolides.[3,5] CA-MSRA is generally treated using sulfamethoxazole-trimethoprim (Bactrim DS).[8] Providers need to distinguish between treatment failures (usually occurring within 14 days of antibiotic completion) and new episodes (occurring after 1 month of antibiotic completion) when selecting antimicrobial treatment.[9]

Prophylactic antibiotic use for the treatment and prevention of chronic or recurrent otitis media is still being debated. Prophylaxis is recommended after the occurrence of two or more otitis episodes in 6 months or 3 episodes in 12 months and is usually given for 3 months during the high-incidence winter and early spring months. The patient should be evaluated every 4 weeks. The prophylactic treatment for patients who are not allergic to penicillin is amoxicillin 20 mg/kg at bedtime.[6] Acetaminophen or ibuprofen for fever and discomfort is also recommended. The treatment of viral otitis media is symptomatic. Again, acetaminophen or ibuprofen is recommended for fever and discomfort. The use of antihistamines and decongestants has not been shown to be effective. However, they may be effective in the prevention of otitis media related to allergic rhinitis. Nasal sprays are recommended for symptomatic relief of otitis media with effusions or relief of serous otitis. The recommendation for adults is intranasal cromolyn sodium (NasalCrom) 1 spray in each nostril four to six times daily or beclomethasone dipropionate (Beconase AQ) 1 or 2 sprays in each nostril b.i.d.[4,6] Non-pharmacologic treatment for recurrent or chronic otitis media with effusion includes the use of myringotomy with tubes.

LIFE SPAN CONSIDERATIONS

Acute otitis media is primarily a disease of young children. In adults it most often occurs in smokers and in adults who are exposed to second-hand smoke. The elderly and Native Americans, especially Navajos and Alaskan Eskimos, are also at increased risk.[10]

COMPLICATIONS

Usually no long-term complications are evident. The most common short-term consequence is decreased conductive hearing loss. This may be a barrier to learning and may contribute to language developmental delays, especially if the problem is chronic and occurs in the preschool and early school-aged child. Eardrum perforation represents a common sequela of both acute otitis media and chronic otitis media with effusion. Hearing loss, perforation of the eardrum, cholesteatoma, acute mastoiditis, meningitis, and epidermal abscess are less common complications of otitis media.

INDICATIONS FOR REFERRAL OR HOSPITALIZATION

The patient with chronic or acute otitis media that does not respond to therapy in 2 or 3 days should be switched to an alternative therapy. If the patient does not respond to the alternative therapy, then referral to a physician or otolaryngologist is necessary. In addition, patients with chronic or recurrent otitis media warrant physician consultation.

PATIENT AND FAMILY EDUCATION

The risk of otitis media can be decreased by not smoking and by minimizing exposure to smoke. Smoking cessation should be encouraged (see Chapter 24). Otitis media is not contagious. However, patients may require careful explanation about symptomatic rather than antibiotic treatment of otitis media.

HEALTH PROMOTION

The best health promotion for patients to prevent otitis media is cessation of smoking and exposure to second-hand smoke. In children, recent research indicates that the pneumococcal conjugate vaccine may have a protective effect. In randomized clinical trials, immunized children had fewer episodes of otitis and fewer tube procedures.[11] Currently there is no clinical evidence to support home, complementary, or alternative remedies.

REFERENCES

1. Barclay L: *New clinical practice guidelines for acute otitis media,* 2004, retrieved Dec 16, 2006, from http://www.medscape.com/viewarticle/471768.
2. Goroll A, Mulley AG: *Primary care medicine: office evaluation and management of the adult patient,* ed 5, Philadelphia, 2000, Lippincott Williams & Wilkins.
3. Uphold C, Graham M: *Clinical guidelines in family practice,* ed 4, Gainesville, Fla, 2003, Barmarrae Books.
4. Ferri F: *Ferri's clinical advisor: instant diagnosis and treatment,* Philadelphia, 2005, Mosby.
5. Klein J: *Epidemiology; pathogenesis; diagnosis and complications of acute otitis media,* retrieved Jan 12, 2006, from http://www.utdol.com/application/topic.asp?file=pedi_id/2870%type=A&selectedTitle=2~7.
6. Gilbert D: *The Stanford guide to antimicrobial therapy,* ed 35, Hyde Park, Vt, 2005, Antimicrobial Therapy.
7. Shireman T, and others: Prescribing patterns and retreatment rates in patients with otitis media, *Clin Drug Invest* 22(5):303-311, 2002.
8. Estrada B: Will MRSA become a frequent cause of otitis? *Infect Med* 20(3):116, 2003, retrieved Dec 16, 2006, from http://www.medscape.com/viewarticle/451588.
9. Leibovitz E, Greenberg D, Piglansky L, and others: Recurrent acute otitis media occurring within 1 month from completion of antibiotic therapy: relationship to the original pathogen, *Pediatr Infect Dis J* 22(3):209-216, 2003, retrieved Dec 16, 2006, from http://www.medscape.com/viewarticle/450892.
10. Dunphy L, Winland-Brown JE: *Primary care: the art and science of advance practice nursing,* Philadelphia, 2001, Davis.
11. Fireman B, Black SB, Shinefield HR, and others: Impact of the pneumococcal vaccine on otitis media, *Pediatr Infect Dis J* 22(1):10-16, 2003, retrieved Dec 16, 2006, from http://www.medscape.com/viewarticle/448603.

CHAPTER 92

Tympanic Membrane Perforation

Updated by Jane Leonard

DEFINITION AND EPIDEMIOLOGY

Tympanic membrane (TM) perforation is an opening in the otherwise intact membrane that, as a mechanical component of hearing, separates the external from the middle ear. TM perforation results from a variety of conditions and is a cause of conductive hearing loss. Most perforations heal spontaneously without incident; however, some TM perforations may need referral to a specialist.

PATHOPHYSIOLOGY

Perforation can be caused by a variety of traumatic, infectious, and neoplastic processes. The TM can be lacerated or perforated by foreign objects in the external canal. Barotrauma, physical trauma, blast injury, or a fracture of the temporal skull can tear or perforate the TM. Occasionally the TM perforates with the pressure and inflammation of acute otitis media. Perforations often precede the development of a cholesteatoma.[1]

CLINICAL PRESENTATION AND PHYSICAL EXAMINATION

A thorough history will support the cause of the TM perforation. TM perforations are often discovered at the time of trauma or during the evaluation for middle ear infection. Perforation may also be observed in association with a cholesteatoma. Most patients with traumatic perforation experience pain and some degree of hearing loss. A thorough ear examination and an evaluation of hearing status should be included in the initial assessment.

DIAGNOSTICS AND DIFFERENTIAL DIAGNOSIS

After the perforation has healed, an audiogram is helpful in evaluating the presence or extent of hearing impairment. The differential diagnosis includes all causes of perforation, including trauma, infection, and neoplasm.

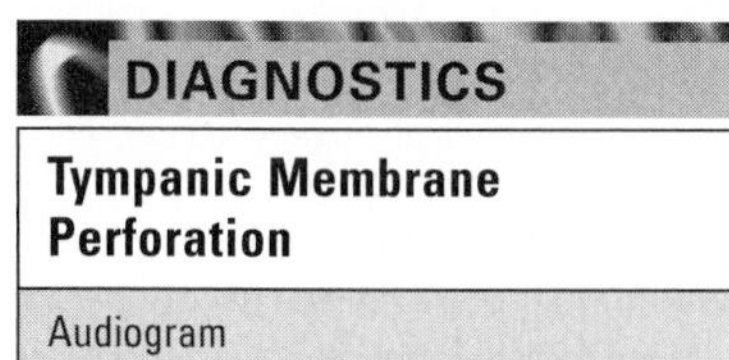

DIAGNOSTICS

Tympanic Membrane Perforation
Audiogram

DIFFERENTIAL DIAGNOSIS

Tympanic Membrane Perforation
• Barotrauma • Trauma • Blast injury • Infection • Neoplasm

MANAGEMENT

Most TM perforations heal spontaneously unless they become secondarily infected or are very large. Patients should keep water out of the ear until the perforation has healed. Antibiotic drops or systemic antibiotics are often necessary when infection is evident.

COMPLICATIONS AND INDICATIONS FOR REFERRAL OR HOSPITALIZATION

A middle ear infection, cholesteatoma, and impaired hearing are potential complications of a TM perforation. A referral to an otolaryngologist is appropriate for large perforations or for those which do not show evidence of timely healing. Also, TM perforations resulting from blast injury or major trauma should be referred to a specialist.[1] Blast injuries have been shown to cause inner ear trauma, as well as the obvious TM perforation, which can lead to profound hearing loss. Likewise, skull fractures can damage the inner ear structures, causing permanent damage.

PATIENT AND FAMILY EDUCATION

Patient education should include measures to protect the TM while it heals. Patients should not permit water to enter the ear until healing has occurred, and they should be encouraged to return for follow-up evaluation. The cause of the perforation should be determined so that repeat perforations are avoided. Special emphasis on the importance of not inserting objects (e.g., cotton-tipped applicators) into the external ear canal is also necessary.

REFERENCE

1. Weber PC: *Etiology of hearing loss in adults: tympanic membrane perforation,* May 27, 2005, retrieved Dec 20, 2005, from http://www.utdol.com.

PART 8

Evaluation and Management of Nose Disorders

TERRY MAHAN BUTTARO, *Section Editor*

CHAPTER 93

Chronic Nasal Congestion and Discharge

Updated by Elvi N. Rigby and
Patrice K. Nicholas

DEFINITION AND EPIDEMIOLOGY

It is estimated that 15% to 20% of the population experiences chronic or recurrent nasal congestion during their lifetime.[1] In fact, some people may experience chronic nasal congestion most of the time. These people may seek constant treatment because of the condition's profound effect on the quality of life. Lives are affected by constant discomfort and/or coughing, absenteeism from work, inability to participate in leisure activities, and the expense of treating the problem. Often the health care provider must be able to distinguish between the symptoms that indicate allergic rhinitis and those of an obstruction, inflammation, or vasomotor instability. Management of the condition can be achieved through the proper use of allergy testing and the effective use of antihistamines, decongestants, and topical corticosteroids.

PATHOPHYSIOLOGY

The pathology of chronic nasal congestion and discharge depends on the specific disease process that is causing the signs and symptoms. Acute nasal congestion is usually related to the common cold. Chronic rhinitis can be related to allergic and nonallergic rhinitis, medications, mechanical obstruction, pregnancy, hypothyroidism, and chronic inflammatory disease or to syphilis, rhinosclerosis, rhinosporidiosis, leishmaniasis, blastomycosis, histoplasmosis, and leprosy. The latter diseases are conditions that are initially seen with granuloma formation and destruction of soft tissue, cartilage, and bone.

CLINICAL PRESENTATION

The clinical presentation of chronic nasal congestion and discharge depends on the specific disease process that is causing the signs and symptoms. The most common causes include colds, medications, mechanical obstruction, chronic inflammatory disease, atrophic rhinitis, and hormonal changes. Other causes such as syphilis, rhinosporidiosis, leishmaniasis, blastomycosis, and histoplasmosis should also be considered. The clinical presentations of these diseases are found in Box 93-1.

BOX 93-1

CLINICAL PRESENTATION OF COMMON CAUSES OF CHRONIC NASAL CONGESTION AND DISCHARGE

SYPHILIS
- Secondary syphilis occurring about 6 to 8 weeks after exposure and the primary infection
- Characterized by a skin rash (macular, papular, or follicular), which often involves the palms and soles; may last 2 to 6 weeks
- Possible erosions of the mucous membranes
- Flulike symptoms: headache, generalized arthralgia, and malaise

RHINOSPORIDIOSIS
- Pedunculated polyps on mucous membranes
- Polyps possibly found on mucosa of the nose, larynx, eyes, penis, vagina, and sometimes skin

LEISHMANIASIS
- Localized cutaneous ulcers on the face
- Single or multiple, sharply demarcated, granulomatous, autoinoculable lesions of the face and mucous membranes

BLASTOMYCOSIS
- Signs and symptoms of bronchopneumonia
- A dry, hacking cough
- Chest pain, fever
- Nasal discharge

HISTOPLASMOSIS
- Nasal, oral ulcerations
- Lymphadenopathy, hepatomegaly, splenomegaly

DRUGS
- Nasal congestion
- Nasal mucosa erythema
- Atrophy of septal mucosa
- Septal perforation

HORMONAL CHANGES
- Nasal congestion
- Nasal obstruction

MECHANICAL OBSTRUCTION
- Visualization of polyps, tumor, deviated septum, or foreign body
- Unilateral obstruction, mild discomfort, and sneezing
- Unilateral purulent nasal discharge

CHRONIC INFLAMMATORY DISEASE
- Nasal ulceration
- Nasal obstruction

ATROPHIC RHINITIS
- Atrophic and sclerotic mucous membrane
- Abnormal patency of the nares
- Crust formation
- Foul odor

COLDS

PHYSICAL EXAMINATION

The patient should be asked to blow the nose with one side occluded to identify obstruction and then repeat with the other side. The nasal mucous membranes are inspected for erythema, pallor, atrophy, edema, crusting, and discharge. Any abnormalities, such as polyps, erosions, and septal deviations or perforations, should be noted. The vestibules should be inspected with a penlight while the patient's head is tipped back. A nasal speculum should be used for the examination to allow better visualization of the nasal cavity. The speculum blades should be inserted gently about 1.3 cm (0.5 inch) into the nostril. Control of the speculum can be increased by resting the index finger on the side of the patient's nose and steadying the patient's head with the nondominant hand. The blades should be opened gently to avoid pressure to the sensitive areas of the nose.

Inspection may be hampered by nasal congestion. In that case it may be necessary to shrink the nasal membranes with a topical vasoconstrictor (e.g., phenylephrine hydrochloride). When the medication is being instilled, the patient is asked to say "e" and to hold the sound. The technique occludes the upper airway and prevents the medication from running into the pharynx.[2]

DIAGNOSTICS

Selection of laboratory studies depends on the differential diagnosis and suspected disease process. Antigen challenge testing may be helpful in determining whether the symptoms are related to allergic or nonallergic disease. In vivo and in vitro testing methods are used for antigen challenge testing.

In vitro testing for allergen-specific immunoglobulin E (IgE) is the test of choice for the detection of allergen-specific IgE. The test involves skin testing for environmental allergens (dusts, molds, animal dander, and pollens). The testing is performed by introducing these potential allergens into the skin with needle pricks.

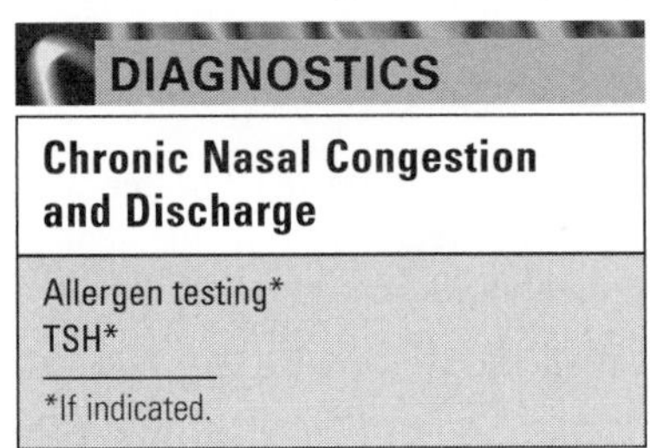

DIAGNOSTICS

Chronic Nasal Congestion and Discharge

Allergen testing*
TSH*

*If indicated.

Because a false-negative finding may result, antihistamines should not be taken for 12 to 24 hours before the testing. The size of the wheal and flare correlates well with the level of allergen-specific IgE.

DIFFERENTIAL DIAGNOSIS

Syphilis

In acquired syphilis, *Treponema pallidum* enters the body through the mucous membranes anywhere in the body. Although syphilis is classified as a sexually transmitted disease, structures of the mouth and nose can become infected. During the secondary stage of the disease, which immediately follows the primary stage, *T. pallidum* invades the skin and mucous membranes. It can mimic several skin disorders and cause erosions of the mucous membranes, including the nose.

DIFFERENTIAL DIAGNOSIS

Chronic Nasal Congestion and Discharge

- Syphilis
- Rhinosporidiosis
- Leishmaniasis
- Blastomycosis
- Histoplasmosis
- Medications, including street drugs (cocaine)
- Hormonal changes
- Mechanical obstruction
- Chronic inflammatory disease
- Atrophic rhinitis
- Leprosy

Rhinosporidiosis

Rhinosporidiosis is characterized by large, friable, sessile, or pedunculated polyps on the mucous membranes of the nose, eyes, larynx, penis, and vagina. It is apparently contracted by swimming in stagnant water and occurs mostly in boys and men from India and Ceylon. Spores can be found in biopsy material.

Leishmaniasis

Leishmaniasis is a disease caused by parasitic flagellate protozoa that are transmitted by the bite of a female sandfly. The lesions occur as ulcers principally involving mucous membranes of the nasopharyngeal and nasal cavity. Secondary infection producing nasal discharge may be the first sign of the infection. The infection is found in large part in people from developing countries.

Blastomycosis

An infectious disease caused by a fungus, blastomycosis primarily involves the lungs but can be spread (rarely) hematogenously to the oral and nasal mucosa. Initially the disease manifests with papulopustules; it progresses to a large lesion with an abruptly sloping, purple-red, abscess-studded border. Discharge may occur, particularly if a secondary infection is present. Blastomycosis is diagnosed by culture.

Histoplasmosis

Histoplasmosis is a fungal infection characterized by a primary pulmonary lesion with ulcerations of the oropharynx. The disseminated form is a defining disease for AIDS. Infection develops after the inhalation of dust that contains fungal spores. The majority of people who become infected live in the midwestern section of North America. The disease is diagnosed by culture.

Medications and Street Drugs

When nasal decongestants (e.g., oxymetazoline, phenylpropanolamine, pseudoephedrine) are overused, there may be a worsening of symptoms. After more than 3 days of continuous use, response to these agents becomes blunted (tachyphylaxis). Once the response to these medications has changed, the patient is likely to increase the number of times that the medication is used to obtain a therapeutic response. Cessation of the medication at this point may result in rebound nasal congestion. The congestion is believed to be a result of reflex vasodilation. The nasal mucosa appears to be erythematous.

Cocaine abuse is becoming a more common cause of nasal congestion in the primary care setting. Nasal snorting of cocaine results in nasal congestion and discharge. Cocaine is a potent sympathomimetic, and the reaction of the nasal passages is similar to that of nasal decongestant abuse. Recurrent nasal use of cocaine causes the nasal septal mucosa to become ischemic. This leads to tissue atrophy and telltale septal perforation.[1]

Hormonal Changes

The hormonal changes that occur during pregnancy and in hypothyroidism may cause the turbinate to become pale and edematous, leading to nasal congestion. Hypothyroidism may be subclinical except for nasal obstruction. The edema of the turbinates may be related histologically to the pathologic condition found in myxedema, which is a result of an alteration in the composition of the tissues. The connective fibers of certain structures become separated by an increased amount of protein and mucopolysaccharides. This complex binds to water, producing edema.[3] With pregnancy, the congestion is related to the fluid retention that normally occurs.

Mechanical Obstruction

Congestion, discharge, and recurrent episodes of sinusitis that are unilateral are the classic signs of mechanical obstruction. The obstruction can be due to a tumor, polyp, deviated septum, or foreign body in the nose. Neoplasms are rare, and polyps generally occur in association with allergic and idiopathic rhinitis, chronic sinusitis, aspirin-induced asthma, cystic fibrosis, and drug abuse.

Chronic Inflammatory Disease

Midline granuloma is a rare illness of unknown origin. The predominant sign of this disease is the development of ulceration that causes destruction of the upper respiratory tract. The ulceration may cause destruction of nasal structures. The presenting signs and symptoms include nasal stuffiness, crusting, and granulations. When this condition is found in patients older than 50 years, they may have a history of allergic rhinitis.

Atrophic Rhinitis

Atrophic rhinitis is characterized by an atrophic and sclerotic mucous membrane, abnormal patency of the nasal cavities, crust formation, and foul odor. The cause is unknown, and the disease appears primarily in women. The nasal turbinates are dry and atrophic, with crusts and fetid green nasal drainage, which is most likely a secondary infection. Anosmia is a common result of the disease process, as are frequent nosebleeds.

MANAGEMENT AND INDICATIONS FOR REFERRAL OR HOSPITALIZATION

Syphilis

Penicillin (penicillin G benzathine 2.4 million units IM) is the treatment of choice for primary, secondary, and early latent syphilis (<1 year's duration).[4] Patients who are allergic to penicillin may be treated with doxycycline 100 mg PO b.i.d. for 15 days or tetracycline 500 mg PO q.i.d. for 15 days.[4] Pregnant women who are allergic to penicillin can be treated with erythromycin 500 mg PO q.i.d. for 14 days.[4] Neurosyphilis or late latent syphilis requires a lumbar puncture and longer treatment regimens.

Rhinosporidiosis

This disease is rarely fatal unless the airway or other vital organs are compromised. However, the patient is at risk of developing secondary infections, which may be fatal. Complete excision of the early lesions is curative and is the treatment of choice for this disease.

Leishmaniasis

Healing occurs spontaneously in 2 to 18 months, leaving a depressed scar. Secondary infections must be treated with antibiotic-antiprotozoal agents. Patients who are suspected of having this disease should be referred to an infectious disease specialist. If the ulcers do not spontaneously resolve, treatment with sodium antimony gluconate, pentamidine, or amphotericin B is indicated.[5]

Blastomycosis

If untreated, blastomycosis is progressively fatal. Treatment should follow the guidelines of the Infectious Diseases Society of America (IDSA), although amphotericin B is usually effective.[6] Referral to a specialist in infectious diseases is indicated. Improvement begins in 1 week.

Histoplasmosis

The primary form of histoplasmosis is benign; however, it can be fatal in patients with AIDS. Referral to an infectious disease specialist is indicated. Treatment is based on IDSA guidelines, but both amphotericin B and itraconazole have been used effectively.[7]

Medications

When topical decongestants have been abused, the rebound nasal congestion will resolve 2 to 3 weeks after the medication is stopped. If cocaine has been abused, the septum will slowly heal once the drug is stopped.

Hormonal Changes

Nasal symptoms resolve with the correction of the hypothyroidism. The hormonal changes associated with pregnancy resolve after delivery.

Mechanical Obstruction

The nasal passages must be carefully cleared with suction. Care must be used to not push the object farther into the nose. Topical decongestants can shrink mucous membranes so that the object can be more easily visualized. One side of the nose can be occluded, and the patient is asked to blow forcefully. If this does not remove the object, an alligator forceps may be used to remove it. If the health care provider is unable to remove the object, referral to an emergency department or otolaryngologist is necessary.

Chronic Inflammatory Disease

The patient should be referred to an otolaryngologist for treatment.

Atrophic Rhinitis

The goals of treatment are reduction of crusting and the cessation of odor. Topical antibiotics, such as bacitracin, can be used, or topical or other estrogens and vitamins A and D may be effective.

COMPLICATIONS

Complications depend on the etiology; ulcerations, infection, and septal perforation may occur if the underlying disorder is undetected.

PATIENT AND FAMILY EDUCATION

The patient and family should understand the importance of following treatment recommendations. The patient should also be aware of the signs and symptoms of complications and recurring disease and know what to do if these signs and symptoms occur. Follow-up should be stressed.

HEALTH PROMOTION

Prevention of diseases such as syphilis, blastomycosis, and other protozoal or fungal infections will thwart the development of chronic nasal congestion. All patients should be educated about the dangers of decongestant abuse, cocaine, and exposure to chronic irritants and allergens.

REFERENCES

1. Goroll AH, Mulley AG: *Primary care medicine,* ed 5, Philadelphia, 2005, Lippincott, Williams & Wilkins.
2. Black J, Matassarin-Jacobs E: *Medical-surgical nursing: clinical management for continuity of care,* ed 5, Philadelphia, 1997, Saunders.
3. McCance K, Huether S: *Pathophysiology: the biological basis for disease in adults and children,* ed 5, St Louis, 2006, Mosby.
4. Hicks CB, Sparling PF: *Early syphilis,* retrieved June 22, 2006, from http://www.uptodate.com.
5. Leder K, Weller PF: *Treatment and prevention of leishmaniasis,* retrieved June 28, 2006, from http://www.uptodate.com.
6. Chapman SW: *Treatment of blastomycosis,* retrieved June 28, 2006, from http://www.uptodate.com.
7. Wheat J, Kauffman CA: *Diagnosis and treatment of pulmonary histoplasmosis,* retrieved June 15, 2002, from http://www.uptodate.com.

CHAPTER 94

Epistaxis

Updated by Elvi N. Rigby and
Patrice K. Nicholas

DEFINITION AND EPIDEMIOLOGY

Epistaxis (nosebleed) is a common problem experienced by most individuals at some point in their life. Estimates indicate that up to 60% of the population has had at least one episode of epistaxis throughout their lifetime; of this group, 6% seek medical care to treat epistaxis, with 1.6 in 10,000 requiring hospitalization.[1] Some individuals are more prone to nosebleeds because of the fragile mucous membranes. Predisposing factors include nasal trauma, rhinitis, drying of the nasal mucosa from low humidity, deviation of the nasal septum, alcohol use, and antiplatelet medications.

PATHOPHYSIOLOGY

Epistaxis may result from irritation, trauma, infection, or tumors. It can also be the result of systemic disease (e.g., hypertension, blood clotting disorders), systemic treatment (e.g., chemotherapy, anticoagulants), or nasal trauma (e.g., nose picking, foreign bodies, forceful nose blowing). Bleeding can occur from the anterior nares or posterior nares. Most nosebleeds occur within Kiesselbach's plexus, a vascular plexus on the anterior nasal septum, and are associated with irritated mucous membranes or trauma.[2] This plexus is particularly vulnerable and easily injured. Posterior nosebleeds occur within the posterior branches of the sphenopalatine artery, are idiopathic or associated with vascular disease, and can be difficult to control.[3]

CLINICAL PRESENTATION

Patients with epistaxis initially are seen with scant to copious amounts of blood emerging from the nares. Depending on the amount of bleeding, small clots may also emerge. Patients may report that the bleeding began spontaneously or that nasal trauma preceded the bleeding. A thorough history and elicitation of prescription or over-the-counter medication use, both oral and intranasal, are important to establish the cause of the bleeding and institute treatment.

PHYSICAL EXAMINATION

Vital signs and airway safety should first be determined, and the patient should be instructed to sit up straight, tilt the head forward, and apply firm, continuous pressure to the affected nostril. If the epistaxis is the result of trauma, the nose should be checked for fractures. An internal examination may be deferred until the blood flow has subsided, but if the bleeding does not readily subside, the nose should be examined with a nasal speculum. Good illumination and suction are necessary to locate the bleeding site. Topical 4% cocaine applied either as a spray or on a cotton strip serves both as an anesthetic and as a vasoconstricting agent. If this preparation is not available, a topical decongestant (e.g., oxymetazoline) can be used in conjunction with a topical anesthetic (e.g., tetracaine) to examine the nose.[4]

DIAGNOSTICS

DIAGNOSTICS

Epistaxis

LABORATORY
CBC and differential (if infection or large blood loss present)
Coagulation studies*

*If indicated.

It is important to consider any underlying condition that may have caused the epistaxis. Laboratory assessment of bleeding parameters may be necessary to exclude underlying disease, especially if the bleeding recurs without a clinical explanation. A CBC should be obtained if severe bleeding has occurred; prothrombin time/International Normalized Ratio (PT/INR) should be obtained if the patient is taking an anticoagulant.

DIFFERENTIAL DIAGNOSIS

Sudden epistaxis demands conscientious consideration. Although nasal trauma is the most common cause of nasal bleeding, it is critical to recognize other conditions that may result in bleeding from the nose. Other causes of recurrent epistaxis, such as hereditary hemorrhagic telangiectasia (Osler-Weber-Rendu disease) or tumor, should be considered.

MANAGEMENT

Most cases of epistaxis can be successfully treated with the application of direct pressure to the anterior portion of the nose for a minimum of 10 minutes. This technique is often successful because the most common source of epistaxis is the anterior part of the septum, where Kiesselbach's plexus is located. The patient should also be encouraged to sit in an upright position, since venous pressure is reduced in this position. The patient should also lean forward to decrease the swallowing of blood. Depending on the amount of bleeding, short-acting topical nasal decongestants (e.g., phenylephrine 0.125% to 1% solution, 1 or 2 sprays), which act as vasoconstrictors, may help stop the blood flow. If the bleeding area is noted anteriorly, the area can be dried and cauterized with a silver nitrate stick.[3]

If the bleeding site does not respond to direct pressure or cautery with the silver nitrate stick, *nasal packing with a nasal tampon or iodoform gauze must be placed by a practitioner skilled in this procedure.* The tampon or packing should be lubricated with petroleum jelly or bacitracin. Once in place, the pack is not removed for 48 to 72 hours.[3-5] If the bleeding continues, the opposite nostril should be packed in a similar fashion. Continued bleeding suggests there is a posterior rather than an anterior bleed and requires specialist consultation and possible hospitalization. Twice-daily oral amoxicillin-clavulanate (875/125 mg) or trimethoprim-sulfamethoxazole (double strength) is usually prescribed while the packing is in place.[3] Recent literature indicates that hemostatic sealants are increasingly used to limit epistaxis.[4,5]

DIFFERENTIAL DIAGNOSIS

Epistaxis

- Allergies
- Colds or other infectious processes
- Low humidity
- Medications (aspirin, NSAIDs, warfarin)
- High altitude
- Trauma
- Coagulation defect
- Hypertension
- Neoplasm
- Septal perforation
- Vascular abnormality
- Osler-Weber-Rendu disease

COMPLICATIONS

Complications are rare, since most nosebleeds are easily controlled. However, respiratory function can be compromised and patients may become hypotensive if bleeding is severe. Other complications are usually related to treatment and include abscess formation, septal perforation, or sinus infection. Toxic shock syndrome has also been reported as a complication of nasal packing[3]; thus appropriate antibiotic therapy is necessary while packing is in place.

INDICATIONS FOR REFERRAL OR HOSPITALIZATION

Occasionally a site of bleeding is inaccessible to direct control, or attempts to directly control the bleeding may be unsuccessful. In such cases, anterior and posterior nasal packing may be required. When the packing is in place in the posterior pharynx, the choanae (posterior nares) are occluded so that an anterior pack can be placed. The packing should be done in an operating room or specialist's office, since it is uncomfortable and the patient may become hypoxic.

Surgical intervention may be necessary if medical measures are not sufficient to eliminate epistaxis. Surgical techniques such as internal maxillary or ethmoid artery ligation may be considered by an otolaryngologist. This technique is certainly necessary when the bleeding becomes life threatening and other treatments have failed. The surgery is usually performed after posterior packing has failed to stop the bleeding.

PATIENT AND FAMILY EDUCATION AND HEALTH PROMOTION

After the bleeding has stopped, the patient is advised to avoid vigorous exercise and aspirin-containing medications for several days or weeks. The patient and family should also understand the importance of calling the health care provider if the bleeding recurs (particularly while packing is in place) and recognize the necessity of follow-up evaluation within 48 to 72 hours to ensure healing of the lesion.

Avoidance of tobacco and hot, spicy foods is also advisable because they may cause vasodilation. Avoidance of nasal trauma, including digital self-trauma, is an obvious necessity. Lubrication of the mucous membranes with petroleum jelly or bacitracin ointment may reduce nasal discomfort and reduce the need to manipulate the nasal passages. Home humidification may also prevent the nasal irritation that results from a dry environment. Patients should also understand how to treat nosebleeds at home by providing firm pressure to the nostrils for 10 to 30 minutes.

REFERENCES

1. Viehweg T, Roberson J, Hudson J: Epistaxis: diagnosis and treatment, *J Oral Maxillofac Surg* 64:511-518, 2006.
2. Alter H: *Approach to the patient with epistaxis*, retrieved May 2, 2006, from http://www.uptodate.com.
3. Mathiasen RN, Cruz RM: Prospective, randomized, controlled clinical trial of a novel matrix hemostatic sealant in patients with acute anterior epistaxis, *Laryngoscope* 115(5):899-902, 2005.
4. Bhatnagar RK, Berry S: Selective Surgigel packing for the treatment of posterior epistaxis, *Ear Nose Throat J* 83(9):633-634, 2006.
5. Jackler R, Kaplan M: Ear, nose, and throat. In Tierney L, McPhee S, Papadakis M, editors: *Current medical diagnosis and treatment*, Stamford, Conn, 2006, McGraw-Hill Medical.

CHAPTER 95

Nasal Trauma

Updated by Elvi N. Rigby and
Patrice K. Nicholas

DEFINITION AND EPIDEMIOLOGY

Nasal fractures are the most common trauma to the nose. The nasal bones are fractured more often than are other facial bones, and the nasal pyramid is the most commonly fractured bone in the body. Fractures of the nose may also include the ascending processes of the maxilla and the septum. Open nasal fractures are rare.[1] Nasal trauma, even if minor, can also cause septal hematomas.

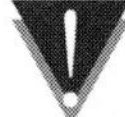

Immediate emergency department or neurologic referral is indicated for nasal trauma associated with leaking cerebrospinal fluid or a suspected dural tear.

PATHOPHYSIOLOGY

Nasal trauma is the result of a severe blow to the face. In adults, most facial blows are related to automobile accidents or sports injuries. However, falls and abuse are also associated with nasal and orbital trauma.

CLINICAL PRESENTATION

The mechanism of injury, medical history, allergies, and current medications should be discerned. Diplopia, visual changes, facial numbness, and other associated symptoms must also be determined. If the injury is recent, bleeding, which results from torn mucous membranes, can be profuse. Soft tissue swelling also develops promptly, may obscure the break, and can cause nasal obstruction. If the injury is older, edema may still be present and hematomas or ecchymosis visible.

PHYSICAL EXAMINATION

During inspection the health care provider should determine the presence of periorbital ecchymosis, edema, abrasions or lacerations, epistaxis, or cerebrospinal fluid leakage (blood-tinged liquid); trauma to the teeth, neck, or chest; and obvious deformity. Respiratory and cervical spine stability and vital signs should be assessed. Mouth breathing suggests the presence of a septal hematoma.

The dorsum (bridge) of the nose should be gently palpated for deformity, instability, crepitus, and point tenderness. It is also important to assess for a palpable step-off of the infraorbital rim, since this indicates a zygomatic complex fracture. Stability of the teeth and palate should also be evaluated. Intranasal examination is necessary to exclude septal hematoma, which appears as a widening of the anterior septum, visible just posterior to the columella. Septal fracture, displacement or deviation, hematoma, or laceration should be noted.[2] However, internal examination may be deferred until the blood flow has subsided. Epistaxis is almost always present when there has been trauma, and bleeding is a sign that the nose has been fractured.

DIAGNOSTICS

The diagnosis of nasal trauma begins with a history of a blow to the nose, usually with concurrent epistaxis. The classic signs and symptoms are tenderness, crepitation, or movement of nasal bones on palpation of the nose. Septal hematoma may be found on visual inspection. An x-ray examination may confirm the findings from the physical examination and identify any additional facial fractures. However, x-ray studies of the nasal bones seldom provide additional information and are not recommended unless there is suspicion of extensive trauma that extends beyond a simple nasal fracture. CT scan is necessary if cerebrospinal fluid leakage is noted or if more complex facial fractures are suspected.

DIAGNOSTICS

Nasal Trauma

IMAGING

X-ray study
CT scan*

*If indicated.

DIFFERENTIAL DIAGNOSIS

The differential diagnosis of nasal trauma is based on the force of the trauma. Frontal sinus fractures result from trauma to the forehead and, because of the location, may initially be seen as a nasal fracture. Brisk hemorrhage from the nasal cavity accompanies these fractures. Fractures of the posterior wall of the frontal sinus may cause dural tears and leakage of cerebrospinal fluid into the nasal cavity. Common injuries that should be included in the differential diagnosis include septal hematomas, other facial fractures, and orbital fractures.

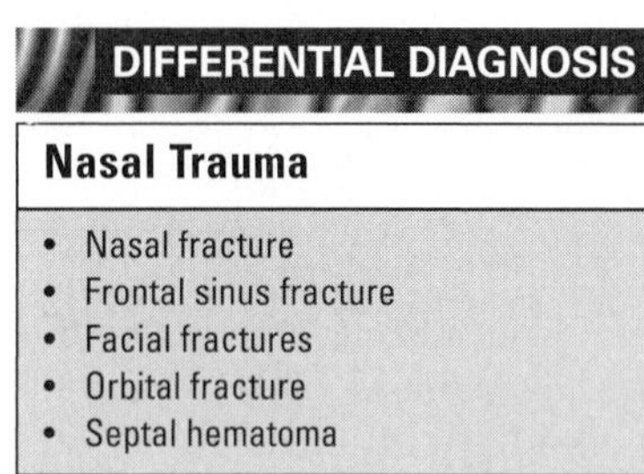

DIFFERENTIAL DIAGNOSIS

Nasal Trauma

- Nasal fracture
- Frontal sinus fracture
- Facial fractures
- Orbital fracture
- Septal hematoma

MANAGEMENT

Initial treatment consists of cool, local pressure to the affected area(s) to decrease edema and bleeding. A nasal fracture without deformity or septal hematoma may be treated with analgesia alone. Acetaminophen (Tylenol) with codeine or its equivalent is usually adequate. A simple laterally displaced fracture can be manually reduced. The patient should be given a topical intranasal anesthetic with codeine before reduction is attempted by a practitioner skilled in this procedure. The anesthetic is applied by inserting cotton pledgets that have been rolled into cylindric shapes into the nasal cavities. The pledgets are inserted with nasal forceps into the upper and lower nasal cavities and are left in place for 15 minutes. Topical anesthesia may be more effective if it is given with a local injected anesthetic. Nasal fracture reduction in children should be performed with the patient under general anesthesia.

A simple, laterally displaced fracture can be reduced by exerting thumb pressure on the nose in the direction opposite that of the initial fracture force. If the fracture has been reduced or if it is nondisplaced, otolaryngologic consultation within 3 days is indicated. Consultation is also recommended for suspected septal hematomas.

COMPLICATIONS

Septal hematomas may develop and can occlude the airway. Nasal trauma may result in a nasal hematoma that separates the septal cartilage from the adherent mucoperichondrium, which supplies the septum with nutrition.[1] A subperichondrial hematoma that remains untreated can result in the loss of nasal cartilage because the mucoperichondrium cannot reattach to the septum. Therefore the blood supply is lost and the septum becomes necrotic. The loss of nasal cartilage results in a saddle nose deformity. Failure to treat a hematoma may easily cause it to become infected. *Staphylococcus aureus* is the most likely organism involved because of its prevalence in the nose and on the skin.

Deviations of the nasal septum are often a complication of nasal trauma. The deviation may cause varying degrees of nasal obstruction and predispose the patient to sinusitis and epistaxis. This is a result of the loss of natural defenses such as the nasal cilia. Septal ulcers and perforations may occur after repeated trauma and even constant nose picking. In addition, nasal foreign bodies may mimic nasal trauma or fracture; this may occur as a result of trauma to the face in adults or introduction of a foreign body in the nasal cavity in the pediatric population.[3]

INDICATIONS FOR REFERRAL OR HOSPITALIZATION

If airflow obstruction develops in the nasal passages or if obvious deformity is present when the swelling subsides, consultation with an otolaryngologist within 3 to 5 days is warranted. Ideally, nasal fractures with deformity but no associated soft tissue swelling should be reduced immediately before edema develops. If edema develops, reduction should be delayed until the edema subsides, usually in 3 to 5 days. Reduction should not be delayed beyond 10 to 14 days. Any suspicion of leaking cerebrospinal fluid or a dural tear mandates immediate neurosurgical referral.

PATIENT AND FAMILY EDUCATION

The patient should understand the signs and symptoms of complications and whom to call if problems develop. In particular, the patient should return for evaluation if the pain becomes intense, if bleeding is profuse, and if nasal discharge becomes purulent with a foul odor. If packing has been placed, the patient should understand the importance of not removing the packing, that the health care provider will remove it. The patient should avoid any nose touching or picking, increase the degree of humidified air at home, and increase fluid intake. The dressings should not get wet, and swimming is not allowed until the dressings are removed and the health care provider gives permission to do so. Antihistamine use and smoking are contraindicated during the recovery period.

REFERENCES

1. Fermin S, Godinez D, Letterle S: Maxillofacial and neck trauma. In Stone CK, Humphries RL, editors: *Current emergency diagnosis and treatment*, New York, 2004, McGraw-Hill Medical.
2. Jackler R, Kaplan M: Ear, nose and throat. In Tierney L, McPhee S, Papadakis M, editors: *Current medical diagnosis and treatment*, Stamford, Conn, 2006, Appleton & Lange.
3. Maitra S, Hobbs CG, Evans KL: Foreign body mimicking a nasal bone fracture, *J Laryngol Otol* 19:1-3, 2006 [EPub], retrieved Dec 16, 2006, from http://www.ncbi.nlm.nih.gov/entrez/query.fcgi?cmd=search&db=pubmed&term=Evans+K[au]&dispmax=50.

CHAPTER 96

Rhinitis

Updated by Jena Beach

ALLERGIC RHINITIS

DEFINITION AND EPIDEMIOLOGY

Allergic rhinitis is an atopic process characterized by sneezing, rhinorrhea, nasal congestion, pruritus of the nose and eyes, popping of the ears, postnasal drip, throat clearing, and coughing. In more severe cases, systemic symptoms of fatigue, headache, and cognitive impairment may be present. It is caused by an immunoglobulin E (IgE)–mediated hypersensitivity response to foreign allergens and can affect any age-group. The hallmark of this condition is the temporal correlation of symptoms with exposure to allergens. The most common allergens are pollens, weeds, trees, grass, animal dander, dust mites, foods, insect stings, cockroach droppings, mold spores, and medications.

The prevalence of allergic rhinitis varies by location and depends on the type and quantity of airborne allergens. It has been estimated that as many as 20% of Americans are affected by allergic rhinitis.[1] Each year allergic rhinitis results in significant economic costs as well as unbearable symptoms for those afflicted.[2] Pharmacologic agents and surgical interventions to treat the symptoms are estimated to cost billions of dollars annually.[3]

PATHOPHYSIOLOGY

Symptoms of allergic rhinitis do not begin with primary exposure to the antigen. Instead, the initial exposure leads to antigen processing by helper T cells. With subsequent exposure to allergens, antibody production of B cells is stimulated, and the mast cells ultimately become coated with IgE antibodies. With repeated exposures, antibody cross-linking results in mast cell degranulation and the release of various mediators. These products, which include histamines and bradykinins, are responsible for the classic itching, sneezing, and rhinorrhea.

CLINICAL PRESENTATION

Allergic rhinitis should be suspected with seasonal or recurrent sneezing, disturbances of taste or smell, nasal congestion, dry mouth, postnasal discharge, and fatigue. Nasal discharge is thin and clear, and the patient may have nasal obstruction and facial discomfort. Watery, itchy, and puffy eyes commonly occur, but fever and chills are unusual. Typically, the patient has a personal or family history of asthma, eczema, or other atopic disease.

A detailed environmental exposure history is essential. Dust mites, animal dander, and indoor allergens should be suspected when winter symptoms predominate, since heating systems disseminate dust particles and aggravate symptoms during the winter months. Patients with seasonal symptoms are typically allergic to outdoor allergens such as pollen or ragweed. Symptoms that occur during late spring and early summer are generally triggered by grass pollens, whereas symptoms during late summer and early fall tend to be linked to weed pollens. Tree pollens tend to be associated with symptoms in late winter or early spring. These generalizations vary with geographic changes and daily fluctuations in allergen counts.

Because symptoms related to allergic rhinitis cause itching in the nose and throughout the upper respiratory tract, the pattern of symptoms is important. When is the patient asymptomatic? What medications has the patient been using? Where and when do symptoms occur? Is there associated itching and, if so, where?

The exact anatomic location of congestion should also be determined. Anatomic obstructions tend to cause unilateral nostril blockage, whereas nasal polyps generally cause bilateral obstruction.

PHYSICAL EXAMINATION

The physical examination can be performed with either a nasal speculum or an otoscope with an attached speculum. The classic boggy, swollen nasal turbinates with pale, bluish mucosa are often associated with bleeding, mucus, crusting, and other signs of inflammation. Common findings also include enlarged tonsils; postnasal drip; the "allergic salute," a crease across the nose from manipulating the tip of the nose; and conjunctival irritation.[4]

DIAGNOSTICS

The diagnosis of allergic rhinitis is generally based on the patient's history. However, nasal cytologic studies (Wright's stain) can determine the presence of neutrophils or eosinophils and determine whether the symptoms are related to allergic rhinitis or infection. Further diagnostic tests are typically performed by an allergist. The scratch test or patch tests are used to test for skin response to suspected allergens. Radioallergosorbent tests (RASTs) determine serum levels of allergen-specific IgE titers. Skin testing is less expensive and more sensitive and is therefore the preferred diagnostic.[5] However, RASTs are more specific and can be used in patients with dermatographism or equivocal skin tests or in patients who cannot discontinue antihistamines.[5]

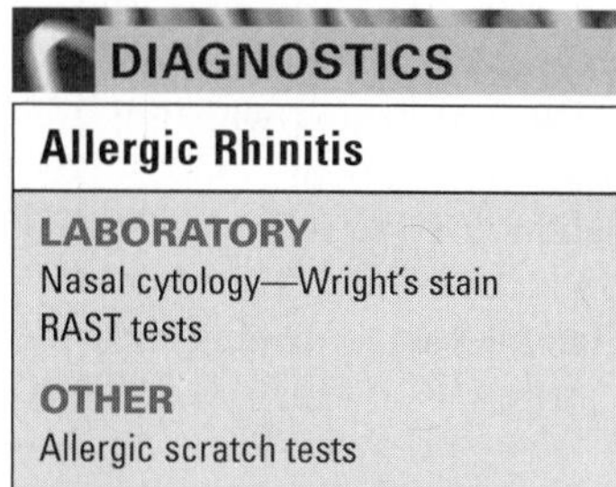

DIAGNOSTICS

Allergic Rhinitis

LABORATORY
Nasal cytology—Wright's stain
RAST tests

OTHER
Allergic scratch tests

DIFFERENTIAL DIAGNOSIS

Although many cases of rhinitis are allergic, other causes need to be considered, including idiopathic rhinitis and rhinitis medicamentosa. An infectious source is common and tends to be associated with fever, purulent sinus drainage, and other signs of infectious sinusitis. Causes of noninfectious rhinitis include aspirin sensitivity, anatomic blockage (nasal polyp, deviated nasal septum), hypothyroidism, and pregnancy. The use of reserpine, methyldopa, NSAIDs, and beta blockers has also been associated with rhinitis.[6]

DIFFERENTIAL DIAGNOSIS

Allergic Rhinitis

ALLERGIC
- Seasonal
- Perennial

INFECTIOUS
- Viral
- Bacterial

ANATOMIC
- Nasal polyps
- Deviated septum
- Neoplasm
- Adenoidal hypertrophy

IMMUNOLOGIC
- AIDS
- Primary ciliary dyskinesia
- Cystic fibrosis
- Humoral deficiencies

ENDOCRINE
- Hypothyroidism
- Pregnancy

IATROGENIC
- Rhinitis medicamentosa
- Aspirin
- Methyldopa
- Estrogen
- Reserpine
- Oral contraceptives
- Beta blockers

IDIOPATHIC

MANAGEMENT

Environmental Control

The most important way to control allergic rhinitis is through environmental control. Because the patient is typically allergic to several allergens, control of the indoor and outdoor environment is crucial.[6] Nonspecific irritants (e.g., smoke) and indirect contact (e.g., secondary contact of animal dander) can cause symptoms that are indistinguishable from those of allergies.[7] Although techniques to control environmental allergens are arduous, time consuming, and sometimes expensive, they are often essential for symptom control. In general, it tends to be the time commitment involved, not the costs, that makes environmental control difficult for patients.

If the allergen is outdoors, minimizing both direct and indirect exposure is recommended. Long-sleeved clothing and a mask may also be necessary to minimize direct contact. However, often it is the indirect contact—when the allergen is brought into the house—that proves to be most bothersome. Keeping the windows closed and bathing and changing clothes immediately after entering the home should minimize exposure.

Often an indoor allergen is the cause of complaints. House dust contains the waste products of dust mites that live in furniture, carpets, bedding, and mattresses. Stuffed animals are a significant problem for some patients. Pets, particularly cats and dogs, are also a major cause of allergic symptoms. Removing the pet is not an effective means of environmental control because many people are not willing to give up their animal. Effective strategies include keeping the pet out of the bedroom at all times; keeping the pet outdoors as much as possible; washing the pet and pet bedding weekly; ventilating the home frequently to promote air exchange; having a friend or family member who is not allergic clean regularly with a high-efficiency particulate air (HEPA) or double-bag vacuum; and minimizing carpeting, drapes, and upholstered furniture. If carpets cannot be removed, an acaricide powder can be used every other month to kill dust mites.[5] Carpeting should be made of synthetic and short-napped fibers. Rugs should be washable; all loose or old rugs should be removed. Curtains (which should be cotton and, preferably, washable) and furniture should be cleaned and wiped regularly; dust-catching blinds should be avoided.

Other recommendations include keeping closet doors shut; covering machine-washable polyester pillows and mattresses with allergy-free and zippered plastic covers; wet dusting; washing stuffed animals, sheets, and comforters in hot water (>54° C [130° F]) at least weekly; removing house plants and books; trimming bushes from the house; cleaning central heating and air-conditioning units; cleaning walls; using mold inhibitors when painting; reducing mold growth and humidity; and using a frost-free refrigerator. Although the efficacy of HEPA filters is unclear, HEPA furnace filters and room cleaners may also decrease allergen exposure.

In a closed environment the quality of the air has a significant impact on symptoms. Studies have suggested that sleeping in an allergy-free bedroom can be beneficial to symptom relief.[7] Smoking should not be allowed in the home. Humidification between 30% and 40% is optimum during the winter. High humidity can lead to mold growth, and therefore dehumidifying in the summer months is crucial. Any heating, humidifying, or air-conditioning device that depends on the delivery of forced air must have an effective air filter. There are two types of effective air filtration devices: (1) electrostatic filters, which depend on electrostatic precipitation of particulate matter as it is drawn through a charged field by a blower; and (2) HEPA filters, which depend on trapping particulate matter in a specially treated cellulose high-efficiency particulate air filter.[6] Electrostatic filters require that the particle-trapping device be washed, whereas HEPA filters often require that accessory filters be replaced on a regular basis. The accessory filters are needed to trap larger particles that would otherwise impair the efficiency of the unit. Keeping these units clean and free of dust should be a priority.

The provider-patient relationship is crucial in the control of environmental exposures. Recommendations should be reasonable and made with compassion and clarity.

Medications

Pharmacologic interventions are appropriate if strict environmental control has not worked sufficiently, but they should be used only when allergies significantly affect quality of life. Because pharmacologic agents may be used for extended periods, the safety, side effect profile, and cost-effectiveness of each agent must be considered carefully.

In the past, antihistamines were typically the first line of therapy for allergic rhinitis. However, a more recent meta-analysis of randomized, controlled trials revealed that antihistamines did not control symptoms as well as intranasal corticosteroids.[8] Nasally applied steroids alleviate nasal symptoms with fewer side effects and can be as effective for obstructive symptoms as the antihistamines and decongestants combined.[4] Formulations are equally effective and include beclomethasone, budesonide, flunisolide, fluticasone, and triamcinolone. Both aqueous and nonaqueous formulations are available. Patients with a dry, irritated nose tend to prefer the aqueous formulations, whereas those with naturally lubricated nasal passages tend to prefer the nonaqueous preparations.[4] Most nasal inhalers (except dexamethasone) can be safely used at the recommended dosage without concerns about systemic absorption. Once symptoms have been alleviated, the lowest dose that keeps the patient symptom free is recommended.

Burning, stinging, or epistaxis is occasionally reported with the use of nasal steroids, particularly in winter months. These problems are minimized by using proper technique, by applying a small amount of petroleum jelly to the nasal vestibules before using the nasal spray, and by also using a saline spray. Septal perforation is a rare complication; in fact, signs of atrophy of the mucosa are not commonly seen. Any such effects can be minimized by aiming the spray toward the lateral side of the nose, away from the septum. Patients over 60 years of age should be screened by an ophthalmologist before using nasal steroids, since reports have linked usage to open-angle glaucoma and cataracts in older adults.[4] The spray should be used regularly, but nasal steroids can take days or weeks to work. Antihistamine-decongestant combinations, although more effective if used before the exposure, can have more short-term benefits than steroid sprays. For patients with severe nasal obstruction, a short course of oral steroids can also be effective, although a combination of nasal steroids and antihistamines is safer.

Antihistamines directly minimize the allergic symptoms of rhinorrhea—itching, sneezing, conjunctival erythema, and tearing—by blocking the effects of histamines. These symptoms are mainly related to the early allergic response, and antihistamines are more effective if given before allergen exposure.[9] Antihistamines are much less effective at dealing with the late allergic response of nasal congestion.

The original first-generation antihistamines are available over the counter and are effective. However, they tend to be sedating and are not always practical for daytime use. Therefore first-generation antihistamines are best used at bedtime. Chlorpheniramine, diphenhydramine, and hydroxyzine are available in liquid form and reach peak levels in approximately 2 hours.[10] Diphenhydramine is particularly effective because its half-life is approximately 3.5 hours; however, caution should be used with older adults.

The sedating effect of the antihistamines varies by medication and is less problematic with the second-generation agents. Regimens that involve using a nonsedating, second-generation antihistamine in the morning and a sedating antihistamine before sleep have been useful for many patients.

The second-generation antihistamines are effective throughout the allergic cycle. They do not produce significant sedation and should therefore be considered a first line for treatment of allergic rhinitis before use of first-generation antihistamines[11] and for those who cannot tolerate inhaled nasal steroids. Additionally, they are indicated if benign prostatic hyperplasia is present, if narrow-angle glaucoma has been diagnosed, or if anticholinergic side effects are a problem.[12] Although more expensive than the first-generation agents, second-generation antihistamines can afford an improved quality of life and work performance that may dramatically offset the cost. Second-generation antihistamines include loratadine, cetirizine, acrivastine, fexofenadine, and levocabastine.

Agents such as loratadine and cetirizine have not precipitated cardiovascular arrhythmias (although astemizole, which is no longer available in the United States, did cause cardiovascular effects, particularly when used in combination with other drugs).[13] Although loratadine is metabolized by the CYP3A4 isoenzyme, it has a second, alternate pathway that uses the CYP2D6 isoenzyme; this alternate pathway can be activated if the primary pathway becomes overloaded. Thus increased drug levels do not occur with loratadine.

Although second-generation antihistamines are extremely effective, they tend not to alleviate nasal congestion. Therefore combination formulations with decongestants, such as fexofenadine and pseudoephedrine (Allegra-D) or loratadine and pseudoephedrine (Claritin-D), have become useful. Unfortunately, the decongestant component can cause sleeplessness, tachycardia, tremors, and other side effects. Antihistamines and decongestants are contraindicated for patients with hypertension, prostate enlargement, or narrow-angle glaucoma.

Other intranasal agents that can be helpful in controlling allergic rhinitis include azelastine (Astelin), cromolyn, and ipratropium bromide. Azelastine is an antihistamine spray, but it is expensive and can cause an unpleasant taste if not used correctly. Intranasal cromolyn affects the inhibition of mast cell degranulation; thus it affects local cytokine release. If taken regularly, cromolyn can prevent early- and late-phase allergic responses.[7] Unlike intranasal steroids, cromolyn is much less effective against nasal congestion; however, it is therapeutic for symptoms of sneezing, rhinorrhea, and itching.[4] The major problem is the dosing, which is four times daily. Nevertheless, its safety profile makes it an appealing choice for some patients.[4]

Intranasal ipratropium bromide, an anticholinergic agent, may also be effective for rhinorrhea and sneezing but is less useful for nasal congestion.[14,15] It is the treatment of choice for gustatory and skier's rhinitis and is often used to treat symptoms of the common cold.[4] It is generally safe and well tolerated. The most common drug-related problems are dryness and epistaxis.

Special consideration for patients who are pregnant includes use of chlorpheniramine and nasal cromolyn to alleviate symptoms. Intranasal beclomethasone may be used for intractable symptoms in place of oral therapy. Oral decongestants should be avoided during the first trimester.[2] As always, patients should inform their obstetrician/gynecologist of any medications they may be considering using for treatment.

Relief of nasal symptoms can also be achieved through the combined use of antihistamines and decongestants, topical nasal cromolyn, or topical nasal steroids.[4] For some patients, thick mucus secretions are a problem. Saline nasal sprays and high-dose guaifenesin can be helpful in thinning the discharge and improving symptoms.[4] Allergic rhinitis should not be treated with prolonged oral corticosteroid therapy; however, in some instances, short-term oral therapy of 5 to 7 days may be beneficial. Decongestant nasal sprays, if used, should be limited to 2 to 5 days of use to avoid rebound congestion.

Co-Management with Specialists

Immunotherapy is a long-term treatment for allergic rhinitis. Successful for patients with seasonal allergic rhinitis, immunotherapy also seems to be effective for other types of allergic rhinitis.[6,16] It may be effective if occupational exposures cannot be avoided and is generally considered if symptoms are present for more than 6 months, if symptoms are not relieved by environmental control and pharmacologic agents, and if the cost of immunotherapy is less than that of pharmacologic therapy. Injections are given every week in progressively increasing doses until a maintenance dose is achieved; after that, injections are given monthly.[17] Immunotherapy is not recommended for patients on beta-blocker therapy.

There is a risk of immediate and delayed reactions with immunotherapy. Generalized reactions tend to occur within 20 to 30 minutes, but more systemic reactions can be delayed. Although the risk of a severe reaction is small, the response can be fatal. Therefore patients should wait in the office for 30 minutes after the injection and carry an EpiPen if appropriate. The proper resuscitative equipment should be accessible if immunotherapy is offered, and a physician should be readily available.

COMPLICATIONS

Complications of allergic rhinitis are rare but potentially serious. Increased asthma exacerbations are related to rhinitis, and sleep apnea can be a problem in untreated rhinitis.[18,19] Thus treatment with medications and strict environmental control can be beneficial.

INDICATIONS FOR REFERRAL OR HOSPITALIZATION

Older adults with new-onset rhinitis may need a physician evaluation to exclude anatomic obstruction. However, most patients with new-onset rhinitis have been recently exposed to a new and offending agent and can be managed effectively without a referral. Some patients require a referral to an otolaryngologist. Any patient who sees a health care provider with new nasal complaints of congestion should have a nasal examination to assess for anatomic problems. Although nasopharyngeal neoplasms are rare, nasal polyps are common and often require surgical intervention. These patients can also have aspirin sensitivity and allergic asthma. A deviated septum can also produce symptoms that mimic classic rhinitis.

A second careful review of the patient's history, medication use, exposure to cigarette smoke and perfumes, and occupational exposures is indicated before making any referral. In addition, a home visit and review of inhaler technique are invaluable. Medications and medical problems that may be contributing to the symptoms should be investigated.[6] T-cell deficiencies (e.g., AIDS), cystic fibrosis, hypothyroidism, and humoral deficiencies should be considered. A referral to an allergist is indicated if the signs and symptoms continue and anatomic problems have been excluded.

Allergic rhinitis rarely requires hospitalization. Rare circumstances include anaphylaxis, a life-threatening hypersensitivity immune response, or the need for a surgical procedure (e.g., nasal polypectomy). Hospitalization is typically required for treatment and continued observation.

PATIENT AND FAMILY EDUCATION

Once the environmental allergens have been identified, recommendations can be made and a therapeutic regimen agreed on. Education is crucial in the management of allergic rhinitis. A dramatic improvement in symptoms is often noted when patients become experts on the triggers that activate symptoms. Therefore an allergy diary is often useful. Reducing exposure to dust mites, animal dander, molds, cockroaches, pollens, smoke, and other irritants is essential. Patients should also understand how to use nasal inhalers correctly and the importance of using inhalers regularly to promote their effectiveness. The side effect profile of these medications and of over-the-counter and prescription antihistamines and decongestants should also be discussed.

IDIOPATHIC, OR VASOMOTOR, RHINITIS

DEFINITION AND EPIDEMIOLOGY

Vasomotor rhinitis, which is now known as *idiopathic rhinitis*, is an important, often overlooked, nonallergic, noninfectious cause of perennial nasal congestion and rhinorrhea. Idiopathic rhinitis is not associated with itchiness of the eyes and nose or sneezing. It occurs in response to environmental triggers, such as cold air, strong smells, irritants, changes in weather, some medications (angiotensin-converting enzyme [ACE] inhibitors, beta blockers), stress, exercise, or certain foods.[10] In contrast to the symptoms of allergic rhinitis, which tend to be seasonal and periodic, vasomotor symptoms tend to be year-round and chronic.

PATHOPHYSIOLOGY

Symptoms of idiopathic rhinitis are provoked by environmental stimuli. It is distinguished from other types of rhinitis by its lack of purulent discharge. It has been postulated that the cause of idiopathic rhinitis involves an abnormal balance that favors parasympathetic control over sympathetic control of the nasal mucosa,[10] leading to intermittent vascular engorgement of the nasal mucous membranes. The underlying cause of this imbalance is unknown.

CLINICAL PRESENTATION

With idiopathic rhinitis, patients often report perennial nasal congestion but little discharge. Any discharge is generally described as watery. There are few, if any, symptoms on arising, but nasal congestion can begin shortly after getting out of bed. Exposure to cold bedrooms or bathrooms, stress, odors, spicy foods, sunlight, and other environmental factors are often cited as causes. These irritants appear to be nonspecific triggers for exaggerated physiologic responses.

One characteristic that distinguishes idiopathic rhinitis from allergic rhinitis is that itching, sneezing, and other irritative symptoms tend to occur with allergic rhinitis, whereas obstructive symptoms tend to occur with idiopathic rhinitis.[10] Tearing and itching of the eyes and sneezing are common in allergic rhinitis but uncommon with idiopathic rhinitis. Sneezing can occur at times with idiopathic rhinitis, usually in response to temperature changes.

PHYSICAL EXAMINATION

The physical appearance of the nasal mucosa often differs in allergic rhinitis and idiopathic rhinitis. Nasal polyps are often present in patients with allergic rhinitis (especially those with aspirin sensitivity); the presence of such polyps excludes a diagnosis of idiopathic rhinitis.[10] Moreover, the nasal mucosa is typically pale in allergic rhinitis but is often erythematous in idiopathic rhinitis.

DIAGNOSTICS AND DIFFERENTIAL DIAGNOSIS

Idiopathic rhinitis can be difficult to distinguish from allergic rhinitis. Although there is no definitive test, certain diagnostic tests can be useful. The appearance of nasal eosinophils is common in allergic rhinitis but is rarely seen with idiopathic rhinitis.[10] Skin testing is often positive in allergic rhinitis but not in idiopathic rhinitis.[10] Patients with idiopathic rhinitis demonstrate little correlation between positive skin tests and exposure history.[10] A positive skin test to a seasonal allergen in a patient with perennial symptoms is not clinically significant. Medication side effects, hypothyroidism, pregnancy, rhinitis medicamentosa, allergic rhinitis, aspirin sensitivity, infections, and nasal obstructions should also be considered in patients with symptoms of idiopathic rhinitis.

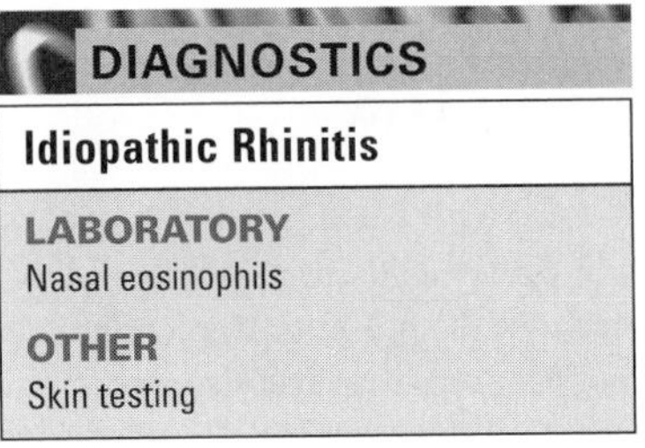

DIAGNOSTICS

Idiopathic Rhinitis

LABORATORY
Nasal eosinophils

OTHER
Skin testing

DIFFERENTIAL DIAGNOSIS

Idiopathic Rhinitis

- Allergic rhinitis
- Medication side effects
- Hypothyroidism
- Pregnancy
- Rhinitis medicamentosa
- Aspirin sensitivity
- Infections
- Nasal obstruction

MANAGEMENT

Unlike allergic rhinitis, idiopathic rhinitis does not usually respond to antihistamines. Oral decongestants are often effective and are best used around the clock.[6] Intranasal steroids can also be effective. As with allergic rhinitis, environmental avoidance is the best treatment; immunotherapy is often not effective. Idiopathic rhinitis is chronic, and avoidance of stimuli is important. Smoking, using perfumes or colognes, and eating spicy foods should be discouraged. Autonomic denervation of the nasal mucosa has been attempted, and some success has been achieved.[10] Otolaryngologists can also perform cryosurgery of the inferior turbinates, which can be helpful.[10]

COMPLICATIONS

Although little information is available on the long-term complications of idiopathic rhinitis, chronic problems can occur. Patients can suffer from sleep deprivation and a poor quality of life.

INDICATIONS FOR REFERRAL OR HOSPITALIZATION

Most patients can be managed effectively. A referral may be indicated if the diagnosis remains elusive, if treatments have not been effective, or if anatomic causes are being considered.

PATIENT AND FAMILY EDUCATION

It is important for the patient to understand that idiopathic rhinitis is a chronic condition and that the effectiveness of symptomatic treatment is limited. A detailed environmental history and minimization of potential exposures is most beneficial. Many of the measures that are effective for patients with allergic rhinitis will be effective for patients with idiopathic rhinitis. Regular use of topical decongestants should be avoided because of the potential for developing a tolerance to these agents.

OTHER CAUSES OF RHINITIS

INFECTIOUS

Upper respiratory tract infections typically are associated with rhinitis. A co-existent infection is present, and relatively prompt relief of symptoms occurs with resolution of the infection. Purulent discharge is common but not always present.

ANATOMIC

Anatomic causes of rhinitis include a deviated nasal septum, nasal polyps, and nasal tumors. In particular, neoplasms should be suspected in older adults. The most common cause of anatomic problems is nasal polyps, which can cause impressive obstructive symptoms. These are often found incidentally in patients with asthma who also have aspirin sensitivity. Symptoms can be perennial and difficult to differentiate from allergic rhinitis or idiopathic rhinitis. Treatment options include intranasal steroids or surgery.

RHINITIS MEDICAMENTOSA

Symptoms of nasal congestion may result from the chronic administration of sympatholytic drugs, NSAIDs, or topical decongestants. This most commonly develops with tolerance to topical decongestants. After the patient uses topical decongestants for approximately 1 or 2 weeks, the nasal mucosa suffers rebound engorgement through increased blood flow. Although these symptoms tend to continue for days or weeks, discontinuation of the offending drug is curative. A 1- to 2-week course of nasal steroids or, rarely, systemic steroids can be helpful during the withdrawal period.

PHARMACOLOGIC

Various medications, including beta blockers, ACE inhibitors, chlorpromazine, estrogen, and oral contraceptives, can cause symptoms that mimic those of allergic rhinitis. Treatment involves discontinuation of the medication.

FOOD- OR DRINK-RELATED RHINITIS

Symptoms of rhinitis may occur after ingestion of food or alcohol. The exact cause is unknown, but may be a cholinergic reaction or other mechanism.[1] If the rhinitis is caused by a food allergy, gastrointestinal, dermatologic, or systemic manifestations are usually present. Treatment involves avoidance of the trigger food or drink.

OTHER MEDICAL CAUSES

Pregnancy and hypothyroidism are common causes of rhinitis. Other causes include cocaine use and atrophic changes. Treatment is directed at the underlying medical problem.

REFERENCES

1. Sheikh J: *Rhinitis, allergic,* retrieved Dec 16, 2006, from http://www.emedicine.com/med/topic104.htm.
2. Schoenwetter WF, Dupclay L Jr, Appajosyula S, and others: Economic impact and quality of life burden of allergic rhinitis, *Curr Med Res Opin,* 2004, retrieved Dec 20, 2006, from http://www.medscape.com/viewarticle/472667_1.
3. Wood RP, Jafek BW, Eberhard R: Nasal obstruction. In Bailey BJ, editor: *Head and neck surgery: otolaryngology,* Philadelphia, 1993, Lippincott.
4. Ferguson BJ: Allergic rhinitis: options for pharmacotherapy and immunotherapy, *Postgrad Med* 101(5):117-131, 1997.
5. Ferguson BJ: Allergic rhinitis: recognizing signs, symptoms, and triggering allergens, *Postgrad Med* 101(5):110-116, 1997.
6. Martin D, Valentin MD: Allergies and related conditions. In Barker LR, Burton JR, Zieve PD, editors: *Principles of ambulatory medicine,* ed 4, Baltimore, 1995, Williams & Wilkins.
7. Georgitis JW, Kaiser HB, Kaliner M: Allergic rhinitis: taming the troubled nose, *Patient Care* 31:51-60, 1997.
8. Weiner JW, Abramson MJ, Puy RM: Intranasal corticosteroids versus oral H-1 receptor antagonists in allergic rhinitis: systematic review of randomized controlled trials, *Br Med J* 314:1624-1629, 1998.
9. Kause HF: Therapeutic advances in the management of allergic rhinitis and urticaria, *Otolaryngol Head Neck Surg* 111:364-372, 1994.
10. Stewart TW: Vasomotor rhinitis: neglected cause of nasal congestion, *Postgrad Med* 67(1):171-177, 1980.
11. Prenner BM, Schenkel E: Allergic rhinitis: treatment based on patient profiles, *Am J Med* 119(3):230-237, 2006.
12. Bousquet J, Bullinger F, Fayol C, and others: Assessment of quality of life in patients with perennial allergic rhinitis with the French version of the SF-36 Health Status Questionnaire, *J Allergy Clin Immunol* 94(2 Pt 1):182-188, 1994.
13. Corren J, and others: Emerging trends in the management of allergic respiratory disorders, *Clin Cour* 16(1):1-7, 1997.
14. Kaiser HB, Findlay SR, Georgitis JW, and others: Long-term treatment of perennial allergic rhinitis with ipratropium bromide nasal spray 0.06%, *J Allergy Clin Immunol* 95:1128-1132, 1995.
15. Georgitis JW: Nasal atropine sulfate: efficacy and safety of 0.050 percent and 0.075 percent solutions for severe rhinorrhea, *Arch Otolaryngol Head Neck Surg* 124:916-920, 1999.
16. Ross RN, Nelson HS, Finegold: Effectiveness of specific immunotherapy in the treatment of allergic rhinitis: an analysis of randomized, prospective, single or double blind, placebo-controlled studies, *Clin Ther* 22(3):342-350, 2000.
17. Varney VA, Gaga M, Frew AJ, and others: Usefulness of immunotherapy in patients with severe summer hay fever uncontrolled with antiallergic drugs, *Br Med J* 302:265-269, 1991.
18. McNicholas WT, Tarlo S, Cole P, and others: Obstructive apneas during sleep in patients with seasonal allergic rhinitis, *Am Rev Respir Dis* 126(4):625-628, 1982.
19. Dixon AE, Kaminsky DA, Holbrook JT, and others. Allergic rhinitis and sinusitis in asthma: differential effects on symptoms and pulmonary functions, *Chest* 130(2):429-435, 2006.

CHAPTER 97

Sinusitis

Updated by Jena Beach

DEFINITION AND EPIDEMIOLOGY

Sinusitis is defined as an inflammation of the mucosal surface of the paranasal sinuses. This common disorder develops in 20 million Americans per year, resulting in 18 million office visits and an average of 4 days of lost work per person per year.[1,2] Sinusitis has numerous subclassifications, but the most useful definitions include acute and chronic sinusitis. Acute sinusitis resolves with treatment within 2 to 3 weeks, whereas chronic sinusitis continues over an extended period. This is an important distinction, since treatment of chronic sinusitis is more complicated than treatment of acute sinusitis.

Acute sinusitis is an inflammatory process in the paranasal sinuses caused by viral, bacterial, and fungal infections or allergic reactions. The most common cause of acute sinusitis is a bacterial infection caused by *Streptococcus pneumoniae, Haemophilus influenzae,* or *Moraxella catarrhalis;* it is usually precipitated by an acute viral respiratory tract infection. Less common pathogens are *Chlamydia pneumoniae, Streptococcus pyogenes,* viruses, and fungi.

The symptoms of acute sinusitis are often confused with those of an upper respiratory tract infection. The presenting signs and symptoms include nasal congestion, purulent nasal discharge, and a headache that becomes more intense when the patient bends forward. Fever, fatigue, and other constitutional symptoms are common. The onset is abrupt, with infection in one or more paranasal sinuses. The benefit of antibiotic therapy in decreasing the symptoms and duration of illness has been documented.[3]

There is an association between sinusitis and asthma. The incidence of sinusitis in patients with asthma ranges from 40% to 75%. Treatment of the sinus infection results in improvement of asthma symptoms.[2]

Chronic sinusitis occurs with episodes of prolonged sinus infection (more than 8 weeks) that resist treatment or with recurrent acute infections that are inadequately treated and never resolve. The presentation of this disease is the frequent exacerbations of sinus infections that are caused by gram-negative rod or anaerobic microorganisms. In about 25% of cases chronic maxillary sinusitis is secondary to dental infection. The importance of the identification of an anaerobic infection is it can result in an anaerobic brain abscess that is hematologically spread from the sinuses. Gram-negative bacilli may cause sinusitis in patients who are intubated through the nose or who have a nasogastric tube placed in the nose. The trauma and obstruction caused by these tubes lead to a sinus infection.

Physician consultation is recommended when there is evidence of visual changes, periorbital cellulitis, mental status changes, high fever, or acute focal pain.

PATHOPHYSIOLOGY

Most sinus disease involves the maxillary and anterior ethmoidal sinuses. The maxillary sinus is the largest of the paranasal sinuses, and its ostium into the nose is superiorly placed, thereby failing to take advantage of gravity. These anatomic characteristics cause it to be the most commonly infected sinus. In community-acquired sinusitis, the sinus may fill with fluid during a viral infection, such as the flu or common cold; because the fluid is unable to drain, it becomes a good medium for bacterial growth. Bacterial sinusitis is most often a complication of a viral rhinosinusitis but is also associated with allergies, dental infection, or fluid introduced into the sinuses by diving and swimming. Sinusitis may also develop when fluid is trapped in the sinuses by anatomic abnormalities such as a deviated septum, adenoidal hypertrophy, neoplasms, or a foreign body. Patients with cystic fibrosis have thick mucosa that is not easily expelled by the normal mucociliary clearance mechanism and are at increased risk for sinusitis.

As the infection develops, the sinuses become inflamed; sensations of pain and pressure become intense and are the common symptoms of a sinus infection. Pain may be referred to the upper incisor and canine teeth via the branches of the trigeminal nerve, which traverse the floor of the sinus.

Chronic sinusitis is thought to result from an acute sinus infection that has not completely resolved with antibiotic treatment because the sinuses have not drained completely. Patients with chronic sinusitis may have an anatomic abnormality that inhibits normal mucus clearance and thus may not be able to completely recover from a sinus infection.

CLINICAL PRESENTATION

Acute sinusitis is characterized by nasal congestion, facial or dental pain, postnasal drip, headache, fever, and a yellow or green nasal discharge. Sensations of pain in the teeth and forehead are worse in the morning and when the patient bends forward from the waist. Acute frontal sinusitis usually causes pain and tenderness of the forehead. This pain can be elicited by palpation of the orbital roof just below the medial end of the eyebrow. Palpation here is more accurate than percussion of the supraorbital area.[4] An infection in the frontal sinuses produces pain and tenderness in the lower portion of the forehead and purulent drainage from the middle meatus of the nasal turbinates. Maxillary sinus infections produce pain and tenderness over the cheek area and may also cause erythema over the upper, lateral aspect of the check. The anterior ethmoid cells drain through the middle meatus, and the posterior cells drain through the superior meatus. Sphenoid sinusitis is rare but may cause pain behind the eyes or at the vertex, as well as facial pain. These sinuses drain through the superior meatus.

The common cold and allergic and idiopathic rhinitis are common antecedents to an acute sinus infection. A sore throat is common and may develop from the postnasal drip that is present with sinus infections. The drainage down the back of the throat may cause the sensation of material in the back of the pharynx, a need to swallow frequently to clear the throat, and a persistent cough when the patient is in a prone position. Gastrointestinal symptoms result from the swallowing of mucus.

Symptoms of chronic sinusitis may vary but typically involve one or more symptoms of acute sinusitis. Nasal congestion, discharge, and a cough that lasts for more than 30 days are common. Severe pain and headache are not usually present in chronic sinusitis. The pain that is present is usually a dull ache or pressure across the forehead or midface. Nasal drainage may be thick and green or yellow. A constant postnasal drip and chronic cough are present. Chronic sinusitis is thought to be one of the primary causes of reactive airway disease. Worsening of asthma is not unusual and may be a result of the sinobronchial reflex, mouth breathing, and postnasal drip containing inflammatory chemicals from the sinuses.[5] The patient with chronic sinusitis may also experience an increase in allergic symptoms, including nocturnal asthma, allergic rhinitis, and eczema.[5] When a patient is in a prone position, sinusitis symptoms worsen, especially at night.

PHYSICAL EXAMINATION

The presence of fever and vital signs should first be determined. Then evaluation of the nasal tract for nasal turbinate edema and erythema, as well as discharge in the nasal cavity and in the area of the turbinates, is necessary. The patency of both nares should be determined, and the nose inspected for septal deviation and polyps; however, examining the nose with a nasal speculum is often inadequate in evaluating sinusitis. Transillumination of the sinuses can in some instances provide helpful information, although transillumination does not differentiate between a viral or bacterial cause for the sinus inflammation. If the sinuses can be transilluminated, they are not likely to contain fluid; inability to transilluminate the sinuses suggests the presence of fluid in the sinuses. However, this test must be done with care, since improper technique can result in a false reading. Examination of the eyes, noting periorbital swelling, allergic shiners (dark circles under the eyes), and erythema, should precede percussion of the frontal and maxillary sinuses for tenderness—all of which indicate that a sinus infection is present. The pharynx should be examined for postnasal drip, erythema, and lymphoid hypertrophy. Because otitis media commonly occurs with sinusitis, otic examination is extremely important. The sinuses drain into the nasopharynx, and bacteria found in this discharge are easily transported to the eustachian tube, where they ascend to the middle ear, creating a middle ear infection.

The teeth should be examined for caries, and the gingivae examined for inflammation. Approximately 5% to 10% of patients with maxillary sinus infections have dental root infection; therefore the maxillary teeth should be tapped to determine if the teeth are infected.[3]

DIAGNOSTICS

Acute sinusitis can be diagnosed empirically from the history and physical examination. However, CT scanning may be indicated for patients with recalcitrant symptoms that have not responded to two or more courses of antibiotic therapy. An MRI may be necessary if the diagnosis is difficult and more information is required. These tests are highly sensitive, but it is important to remember that any upper respiratory tract infection can cause the CT scan to appear abnormal.[6]

DIAGNOSTICS

Sinusitis

LABORATORY
CBC and differential*

IMAGING
CT scan, or MRI (for recalcitrant infections)*

*If indicated.

DIFFERENTIAL DIAGNOSIS

DIFFERENTIAL DIAGNOSIS

Sinusitis

- Cold
- Dental abscess
- Trigeminal neuralgia
- Optical neuritis
- Atrophic, allergic, or idiopathic rhinitis
- Migraine or cluster headache
- Foreign body
- Tumor
- Nasal polyps
- Syphilis
- Rhinosporidiosis
- Leishmaniasis
- Blastomycosis
- Histoplasmosis

Other possible explanations for facial pain include dental abscess, trigeminal neuralgia, optic neuritis, viral rhinosinusitis, and migraine headache. Chronic rhinitis may occur in syphilis, rhinosporidiosis, leishmaniasis, blastomycosis, and histoplasmosis. These are all conditions characterized by granuloma formation and destruction of soft tissue, cartilage, and bone. Mechanical obstruction and atrophic rhinitis can also manifest with the same symptoms as chronic sinusitis and should be included in the differential diagnosis.

Dental Abscess

A dental abscess is an infection beside a tooth, usually near the root. The symptoms are localized or may radiate to the sinuses. An abscess is a collection of purulent material and is evidenced by inflammation, with fluctuation and pointing. Constitutional symptoms may be present. Fever, with chills and sweating, may progress to septicemia. If the abscess has been present for a long time, anemia may be present.

Trigeminal Neuralgia

Trigeminal neuralgia is degeneration of pressure on the trigeminal nerve, resulting in severe pain in and around that nerve. The pain is stabbing and radiates from the angle of the jaw along the branches of the nerve. Pain in the first branch is felt as lightning-like sensations along the eye and back over the forehead; it resembles the pain of a sinus infection.

Optic Neuritis

Optic neuritis is an inflammation that causes hyperesthesia, paresthesia, dysesthesia, or paralysis. The pain that results from optic neuritis can resemble the pain of sinusitis.

Viral Rhinosinusitis

The common cold often involves the paranasal sinuses. The common cold is an acute, afebrile infection of the respiratory tract, with inflammation of the upper airway, including the nose, parasinuses, throat, larynx, and often both bronchi.

Migraine Headache

A paroxysmal disorder characterized by recurrent attacks of headache, migraine can occur with or without associated visual and gastrointestinal disorders. The mechanism is thought to be related to episodic reductions in systemic serotonin concentrations, which in turn lead to the observed vasomotor changes. There may or may not be an aura. The pain begins after the aura subsides and may be unilateral or generalized. Migraines often resemble the headaches that are present with a sinus infection.

MANAGEMENT

Treatment of the rhinorrhea, sneezing, and coughing associated with viral rhinosinusitis consists of a first-generation antihistamine, an NSAID, and a decongestant or cough suppressant.[7] Antibiotics are not recommended for viral rhinosinusitis in healthy adults.[8] If symptoms continue for more than a week or are accompanied by *unilateral* facial pain, purulent nasal secretions, cough, or postnasal discharge, antibiotic therapy and decongestants are recommended.[7-9] Few studies document the efficacy of treatment of acute or chronic bacterial sinusitis. However, the Sinus and Allergy Health Partnership recommends using a 7- to 10-day course of high-dose amoxicillin-clavulanate or a fluoroquinolone such as levofloxacin (Levaquin) for acute bacterial rhinosinusitis to combat the most common pathogens, *S. pneumoniae, M. catarrhalis,* and *H. influenzae*.[1,10] Alternative antibiotic options include a second-generation cephalosporin, trimethoprim-sulfamethoxazole 160/800 mg (Bactrim DS) 1 tablet b.i.d., or doxycycline 100 mg PO b.i.d. Patients who do not respond to the initial antibiotic treatment can be given a different antibiotic for a longer period or referred to an otolaryngologist.

Topical therapy to reduce obstruction and mucosal inflammation is helpful in reducing the symptoms associated with sinusitis. Saline solutions may be used to liquefy secretions. Decongestants such as oxymetazoline (Neo-Synephrine) may decrease nasal congestion and edema, promoting drainage. Topical decongestants should not be used for more than 3 to 5 days to prevent rebound congestion. Nasal steroid preparations such as flunisolide (Nasalide) 2 puffs in each nostril b.i.d are beneficial in decreasing nasal congestion and in the long-term management of rhinitis. Intranasal steroids in acute sinusitis are not currently recommended, although symptomatic relief was documented in one study.[9,11] Nasal steroids are acceptable in the treatment of patients with chronic sinusitis.[9]

Oral decongestants can decrease nasal congestion and facilitate drainage. Pseudoephedrine (Sudafed) 30 to 120 mg b.i.d. (maximum adult dosage of 240 mg/day) is a major component of most oral decongestants and can be purchased over the counter.

COMPLICATIONS

In the antibiotic era it has become uncommon for sinusitis to become life threatening. However, a chronic infection may interfere with the quality of life, since chronic sinusitis can continue for extended periods, possibly years. The cost in time, pain, expense, and emotional stress is significant. Chronic sinusitis is also associated with asthma and may be a cause of chronic asthma.

Osteomyelitis of the frontal bone is a potential complication of sinusitis that has been increasing in the pediatric population.[12] If osteomyelitis develops, fever, pain, and edema over the involved bone will be present. The edema is called Pott's puffy tumor.[12]

An orbital infection is another possible complication of sinus infection because the orbit is surrounded on three sides by the paranasal sinuses. This complication occurs more often when the ethmoid sinuses are infected and the bacteria can extend through the lamina papyracea. The orbital infection may cause so much edema that the patient has difficulty with vision. Visual loss can also result from pressure on the optic nerve, which can cause a permanent loss of vision. In addition, if the optic nerve becomes infected, the infection can spread to the intracranial vault. Intracranial suppuration can develop, creating a brain abscess or meningitis. Patients with this condition are usually acutely ill and have an elevated temperature, severe headache, and symptoms of increased intracranial pressure.

Invasive fungal sinusitis is a rare but potentially fatal complication of chronic sinusitis in patients with a co-morbid immunologic disorder such as malignancy, HIV infection, diabetes, or drug-induced neutropenia.[13] Prompt recognition of the serious signs and symptoms (fever, facial pain, epistaxis, and cognitive or visual changes in an immunocompromised patient) associated with invasive fungal sinusitis is essential to prevent proliferation of the infection.[14] Invasive fungal sinusitis should not be confused with allergic fungal sinusitis, a benign but unremitting sinus infection more common in young people with asthma.[13]

INDICATIONS FOR REFERRAL OR HOSPITALIZATION

The patient who is not symptom free after the second treatment with antibiotics should be referred to an otolaryngologist or allergist. If the patient with chronic recurrent sinusitis has allergies, immunotherapy as indicated by skin testing may be necessary. Surgery may be indicated if the symptoms of sinusitis do not respond to medical therapy, chronic pain is present, or recurrent reactive airway disease develops. Endoscopic transnasal surgery has become more common and involves irrigation and suctioning of the sinuses. External approaches, such as the Caldwell-Luc operation, provide better visualization but can have severe complications such as optic nerve damage and blindness. In addition, the bone may be perforated and meningitis may result.[14]

Immediate physician consultation is indicated for immunocompromised patients with suspected fungal sinusitis and for patients with suspected acute bacterial sinusitis associated with visual changes, mental status changes, or periorbital edema.[13] Hospitalization for IV therapy and surgical consultation for biopsy or debridement are imperative.[12,13]

Scuba divers with chronic sinusitis can experience sinus barotraumas. Usually, this condition is not serious, but these patients can be at risk for neurologic compromise. For this reason, scuba divers with chronic sinusitis should be evaluated by an otolaryngologist.[15]

PATIENT AND FAMILY EDUCATION AND HEALTH PROMOTION

Patients should be aware that, although the symptoms of an upper respiratory tract infection and sinusitis are similar, antibiotic therapy is not beneficial in viral rhinosinusitis.[10,16] However, upper respiratory tract infections that increase in severity, do not resolve after 7 to 10 days, and are accompanied by symptoms suggestive of bacterial sinusitis do require treatment. The patient treated for sinusitis should be instructed to return for further evaluation if the symptoms have not improved in 48 to 72 hours. In addition, the patient must be able to recognize complications such as periorbital swelling and know to contact the health care provider immediately.

Patients with upper respiratory tract infections should understand the importance of blowing the nose gently to prevent the introduction of nasal fluid into the sinuses.[8] Patients should also know the signs and symptoms of viral respiratory infections and how to manage them with first-generation antihistamines, NSAIDs, and, if indicated, a decongestant or cough suppressant so that sinusitis can be controlled or at least treated early in the disease.[8]

If allergic rhinitis is a precursor to sinusitis, environmental control should be stressed. Humidified air and increased fluid intake are important to relieve nasal discomfort and liquefy secretions. Warm, moist air in the form of steam inhalation or warm compresses may relieve the feeling of pressure and headache, and any activity that might introduce fluid into the sinuses, such as swimming or diving, should be avoided. Smoking cessation and frequent hand washing are also strongly encouraged.

REFERENCES

1. Poole MD, Portugal LG: Treatment of rhinosinusitis in the outpatient setting, *Am J Med* 118(Suppl 7A):45S-50S, 2005.
2. Piccirillo JF, Mager DE, Frisse ME, and others: Impact of first-line vs. second-line antibiotics for treatment of acute uncomplicated sinusitis, *JAMA* 286:1849-1856, 2001.
3. Deferranti SD, Ioannidis JP, Lau J, and others: Are amoxicillin and folate inhibitors as effective as other antibiotics for acute sinusitis? A meta-analysis, *Br Med J* 317:632-637, 1998.
4. Jackler R, Kaplan M: Ear, nose and throat. In Tierney L, McPhee SJ, Papadakis M, editors: *Current medical diagnosis and treatment*, Stamford, Conn, 1997, Appleton & Lange.
5. Ticenor W: *Sinusitis for physicians*, 1997, retrieved Dec 16, 2006, from http://www.sinuses.com/md.htm
6. Gwaltney JM, Phillips CD, Miller RD, and others: Computerized tomographic study of the common cold, *N Engl J Med* 330:25-30, 1994.
7. Gwaltney JM: *Acute sinusitis*, retrieved Feb 2006 from http://www.uptodate.com.
8. Hickner JM, Bartlett JG, Besser RE, and others: Principles of appropriate antibiotic use for acute rhinosinusitis in adults: background, *Ann Intern Med* 134(6):498-505, 2001.
9. Gwaltney JM: *Acute sinusitis and rhinosinusitis*, retrieved Jan 14, 2006, from http://www.uptodate.com.
10. Brooke L: Microbiology and antimicrobial management of sinusitis, *J Laryngol Otol* 119(4):251-258, 2005.
11. Meltzer EO, Charous BL, Busse WW, and others: Added relief in the treatment of acute recurrent sinusitis with adjunctive mometasone furoate nasal spray: the Nasonex Sinusitis Group, *J Allergy Clin Immunol* 106:630-637, 2000.
12. Kombogiorgas D, Solanski GA: The Pott puffy tumor revisited: neurosurgical implications of this unforgotten entity. Case report and review of the literature, *J Neurosurg* 105(2):143-149, 2006.
13. Cox GM: *Perfect acute sinusitis*, retrieved Feb 2006 from http://www.uptodateonline.
14. Katz P: Wegener's granulomatosis. In Hurst J, editor: *Medicine for the practicing physician*, ed 4, Stamford, Conn, 1996, Appleton & Lange.
15. Parell GJ, Becker GD: Neurologic consequences of scuba diving with chronic sinusitis, *Laryngoscope* 110(8):1358-1360, 2000.
16. Gonzales R, Bartlett JG, Besser RE, and others: Principles of appropriate antibiotic use for treatment of acute respiratory tract infections in adults: background, specific aims, and methods, *Ann Emerg Med* 37(6):690-697, 2001.

CHAPTER 98

Smell and Taste Disturbances

Updated by Elvi N. Rigby and
Patrice K. Nicholas

DEFINITION AND EPIDEMIOLOGY

Disorders of smell and taste can be seriously debilitating to patients and are often diagnostic dilemmas for health care providers. Olfactory dysfunction can be described as the loss of the sense of smell (anosmia), smell distortion (parosmia, or dysosmia), or the diminished sense of smell (hyposmia). These dysfunctions can result from aging, tobacco, toxins, medications, malignancies, endocrine disorders, nasal inflammation, infection, malnutrition, head or facial trauma, Parkinson's disease, Alzheimer's disease, central nervous system disturbances, or varied other conditions.

Taste disorders include diminished taste (hypogeusia), unpleasant taste (aliageusia or phantogeusia), and any persistent taste (dysgeusia). Ageusia, or absent taste, does occur but is less common. Taste disorders are often related to olfactory dysfunction but can also be associated with anesthesia, malignancies, head and neck irradiation, surgical procedures, kidney or gastric dysfunction, metabolic or hepatic disorders, or psychiatric disturbances.

PATHOPHYSIOLOGY

During the process of smelling, odorant molecules are taken in through the nose; these molecules must pass through the nasal cavity to reach the cribriform area and become soluble in the mucus that lies over the dendrites of the olfactory receptor cells.[1] The inability of odorant molecules to reach the receptor cells of the olfactory nerve (cranial nerve [CN] I) is the most common cause of olfactory dysfunction. Therefore anosmia or hyposmia can by caused by any disease process that prevents the odorant molecules from reaching these receptor cells, including polyps, septal deformities, rhinitis, and nasal tumors. The olfactory dysfunction can also be associated with epithelial cell changes and can be either transient or permanent depending on the cause of the dysfunction. Approximately 20% of the dysfunction is idiopathic, usually developing after a viral illness.[1] An absent, diminished, or distorted sense of smell or taste can also be a sign of an endocrine disorder.

Any condition that causes the nasal mucus to be diminished, such as a drying of the nasal mucosa, can impair taste. Other conditions that can impair taste include heavy smoking, Sjögren's syndrome, radiotherapy of the head and neck, or peeling of the skin on the tongue. Ageusia also may result from disease of the chorda tympani or the gustatory fibers. Overuse of condiments and certain drugs can take away the sense of taste. Lesions involving sensory pathways to the taste centers of the brain, or diseases of the taste centers of the brain itself, can also interfere with the sense of taste.

CLINICAL PRESENTATION

Problems with taste and smell may or may not be associated with symptoms related to disorders that cause ageusia and anosmia. Most often, the presenting complaint is loss of taste or smell after an upper respiratory tract infection. In young adults the loss of smell often results from head trauma. If a patient has lost or experienced a decreased sense of smell, a thorough evaluation for intranasal and intracranial disease is required. A complete medical, occupational, smoking, and medication history is essential to diagnosis. Onset of symptoms (gradual versus acute) and associated symptoms should also be determined.

PHYSICAL EXAMINATION

The examination should confirm the patient's subjective complaint. Assessment for the loss of taste and smell focuses on the cranial nerves that provide information about taste and smell. The olfactory nerve (CN I) is a sensory nerve. Testing of this nerve begins with asking the patient to identify odors that are nonirritating and aromatic, such as coffee, isopropyl alcohol, and toothpaste. After testing CN I, the provider should inspect the nasopharynx for abnormalities (e.g., polyps), crusting, amount of mucus present, and any signs of upper respiratory tract problems. The pharyngeal examination should determine the presence of lesions, inflammation, or exudate.

The glossopharyngeal nerve (CN IX) is a mixed sensory-motor nerve. The sensory portion controls the taste sensation for the posterior third of the tongue. CN IX is tested along with the facial nerve (CN VII), which also is a mixed sensory-motor nerve. The sensory part of CN VII controls taste sensation for the anterior two thirds of the tongue. Each side of the tongue should be tested with sweet, salty, sour, and bitter flavors. The patient should protrude the tongue while identifying the taste and rinse the mouth before testing the other side. This process should be repeated with the posterior portion of the tongue.

After determining whether the complaint is related to olfactory or taste dysfunction, the provider should perform a more comprehensive examination, including weight; vital signs; and a conscientious ear, nose, throat, and neurologic evaluation.

DIAGNOSTICS

DIAGNOSTICS

Smell and Taste Disturbances

LABORATORY

CBC and differential
Electrolytes
Creatinine
LFTs
TSH
Antinuclear antibodies
ESR
Anti-Ro/SSA and anti-LA/SSB*

IMAGING

CT scan or MRI

*If indicated.

Assessment of odor and taste identification is an essential component of diagnostic testing for the loss of taste and smell. Both the University of Pennsylvania Smell Identification Test and the Threshold, Discrimination, Identification Test can be used in the primary care setting and can help assess smell disorders.[2] If these tests are unavailable, the patient should be referred to a specialist for specific assessment of smell and taste dysfunction. Laboratory testing should include a CBC, electrolytes, BUN, creatinine, liver function tests, thyroid-stimulating hormone, antinuclear antibodies, and erythrocyte sedimentation rate. If Sjögren's syndrome is suspected, antibodies to Ro/SSA and LA/SSB should be assessed.[2] An enhanced CT scan of the head or MRI may also be indicated to exclude neoplasms and unsuspected fractures of the floor of the cranial fossae. Further testing should be based on clinical presentation and physical findings.

DIFFERENTIAL DIAGNOSIS

The differential diagnosis for the loss of taste or smell includes disease processes that can affect the upper respiratory tract. The most common conditions are allergic and bacterial rhinitis, viral infections, head trauma, sinusitis, nasal polyps, and benign neoplasms. Anosmia can also be congenital or related to a meningioma, glioma, dementia, or aneurysm. Depression can be a cause of dysosmia. Aging, olfactory dysfunction, infection, radiotherapy, medications, malnutrition, Sjögren's syndrome, gastroesophageal reflux, endocrine disorders, trauma, cancer, and cancer therapy should be considered in the differential diagnosis of taste disorders.[3]

MANAGEMENT AND INDICATIONS FOR REFERRAL OR HOSPITALIZATION

The cause of a disrupted sense of taste or smell should be identified. It is particularly important to distinguish between olfactory and taste disturbance. Treatment of rhinitis, sinusitis, infection, gastroesophageal reflux disease, or anemia may restore the lost function. The diet should be reviewed and the overuse of condiments eliminated. If possible, medications that may be associated with this disorder should be discontinued or changed. Zinc therapy has been effective for some patients with taste disorders associated with head and neck cancer, malnutrition, and some other disorders, but the benefit of zinc and vitamin therapy for the treatment of smell and taste disorders is unclear.[2,4,5]

If such measures are unsuccessful, the patient should be referred to an otolaryngologist for a comprehensive nose and throat examination. If smell and taste testing cannot be performed in the primary care setting, the patient should be referred to a specialist for diagnostic evaluation. Suspected central nervous system disorders or conditions that cause destruction of the neuroepithelium or its central pathway require referral to a neurologist. Patients whose symptoms are related to allergies may benefit from consultation with an allergist, whereas those with dental disorders require referral to a dentist.

DIFFERENTIAL DIAGNOSIS

Smell and Taste Disturbances

- Viral infection
- Allergic or bacterial sinusitis
- Nasal polyps
- Benign neoplasms or tumors
- Sjögren's syndrome
- Endocrine disturbances
- Trauma
- Medications
- Irradiation
- Degenerative disorder
- Sinusitis
- Gastroesophageal reflux disease
- Cancer
- Malnutrition
- Depression

COMPLICATIONS

Complications of smell and taste disorders include a permanent loss of smell or taste. The loss of taste and smell can indicate a serious problem such as a brain tumor or degenerative nerve disease. The loss of these senses profoundly affects quality of life, and depression is a potential problem.[6] Patients may lose their appetite and lose weight. Olfactory dysfunction can also compromise safety.

PATIENT AND FAMILY EDUCATION AND HEALTH PROMOTION

If the sensory loss is permanent, the patient should be instructed to use more spices to season food. Patients who have lost the sense of smell should be counseled to install smoke detectors and to use electrical rather than gas appliances. The importance of continued personal hygiene and the avoidance of aggressively strong colognes should also be discussed.

REFERENCES

1. Hellerman D: Arthritis and musculoskeletal disorders. In Saunders C, Ho M, editors: *Current emergency diagnosis and treatment,* Stamford, Conn, 1997, Appleton & Lange.
2. Mann NM, Lafreniere D: *Evaluation of taste and smell disorders,* retrieved Feb 2006 from http://www.uptodate.com.
3. Johnson FM: Alterations in taste sensation: a case presentation of a patient with end-stage pancreatic cancer, *Cancer Nurs* 24(2):149-155, 2001.
4. Henkin RI, Martin BM, Agarwal RP: Efficacy of exogenous oral zinc in treatment of patients with carbonic anhydrase VI deficiency, *Am J Med Sci* 318(6):392-405, 1999.
5. Ripamonti C, Zecca E, Brunelli C, and others: A randomized, controlled clinical trial to evaluate the effects of zinc sulfate on cancer patients with taste alterations caused by head and neck irradiation, *Cancer* 82(10):1938-1945, 1998.
6. Welge-Luessen A, Hummel T, Stojan T, and others: What is the correlation between ratings and measures of olfactory function in patients with olfactory loss? *Am J Rhinol* 19(6):567-571, 2005.

CHAPTER 99

Tumors and Polyps of the Nose

Updated by Elvi N. Rigby and
Patrice K. Nicholas

NASAL TUMORS AND POLYPS

DEFINITION AND EPIDEMIOLOGY

Primary sites for malignant tumors can occur in the nose, nasopharynx, and paranasal sinuses. The broad spectrum of malignant lesions that occur in the nose and paranasal sinuses includes carcinomas, lymphomas, sarcomas, and melanomas. The most common, however, is squamous cell carcinoma.

The most common type of benign tumor is an inverted papilloma, which arises from the common wall between the nose and maxillary sinuses. A highly vascular benign tumor, the juvenile angiofibroma, is common in adolescent boys, bleeds easily, and can cause nasal obstruction. These tumors are nonmalignant, but they can cause considerable problems as they spread through the nasopharynx.[1]

Nasal polyps represent an inflammatory disorder of the nose and paranasal sinuses that can result in chronic nasal obstruction and a diminished sense of smell. The cause of these pale, edematous masses is unknown, but the lesions are commonly seen in patients with allergic rhinitis, which predisposes them to polyp formation, and in patients with acute or chronic infections. The presence of polyps in children may indicate the possibility of cystic fibrosis.

PATHOPHYSIOLOGY

The pathophysiology of benign and malignant tumors of the nasopharynx is varied and makes diagnosis difficult. However, a basic understanding of the different pathologic conditions can assist in diagnosis. Squamous cell carcinomas arise from the keratinocytes (the stratum germinativum and stratum spinosum layer) of the epithelium. This cancer develops in normal skin, in preexisting actinic keratosis, or in a patch of leukoplakia. The incidence is higher in men and is associated with smoking and heavy alcohol consumption. The inverted cell papillomas develop from the squamous cells in which the epithelium is invaginated into the vascular connective tissue stroma. They are invasive and behave in a locally malignant manner. Juvenile angiofibromas are vascular and may actually hemorrhage. They also act in a locally malignant manner. They spread from the nasopharynx to the nasal cavity, the sphenoid, and the parasinuses and may extend extradurally. Nasal polyps form at the site of massive dependent edema in the lamina propria of the mucous membrane, usually around the ostia of the maxillary sinuses.

CLINICAL PRESENTATION

Malignant tumors can occur in the nose, nasopharynx, and paranasal sinuses. Generally, these malignancies remain asymptomatic until late in their course. Early symptoms are nonspecific, mimicking those of rhinitis or sinusitis. Unilateral nasal obstruction and discharge accompanied by pain, recurrent hemorrhage, headache, or visual or olfactory changes suggest the presence of cancer. For this reason, any patient with unilateral or persistent nasal symptoms requires thorough evaluation.

Benign nasal tumors are associated with nasal obstruction, discharge, or facial swelling. These tumors can bleed easily and cause recurrent epistaxis. The tumor is usually easily visualized because of its growth and spread.

Symptoms of nasal polyps include nasal obstruction, hyposmia or anosmia, recurrent sinusitis, headache, and postnasal drip. In some patients, nasal polyps are accompanied by intrinsic asthma and intolerance to acetylsalicylic acid.[1] A developing polyp is teardrop shaped; when mature, it resembles a peeled seedless grape.

PHYSICAL EXAMINATION

A complete examination of the head and nasopharynx is essential. The vestibules should be inspected with a penlight while the patient's head is tipped back. Each naris should be inspected for erythema, edema, discharge, bleeding, or tumor. Further examination includes pharyngeal inspection and determination of lymph node involvement.

DIAGNOSTICS

Diagnostic testing for benign tumors and nasal polyps can include sinus x-ray studies for information about fluid levels and bone involvement, but CT scan or MRI is usually indicated if tumor is suspected. Endoscopic evaluation and biopsy are necessary for definitive diagnosis and treatment of suspected tumors. Complete blood studies are necessary to determine the presence of anemia or other hematologic disease.

DIFFERENTIAL DIAGNOSIS

Nasal Tumors and Polyps

- Benign or malignant polyps
- Wegener's granulomatosis

DIFFERENTIAL DIAGNOSIS

The differential diagnosis for tumors and polyps includes mucoceles; granulomas without systemic involvement; and Wegener's granulomatosis, a systemic vasculitis of unknown cause associated with granulomatous changes. Wegener's

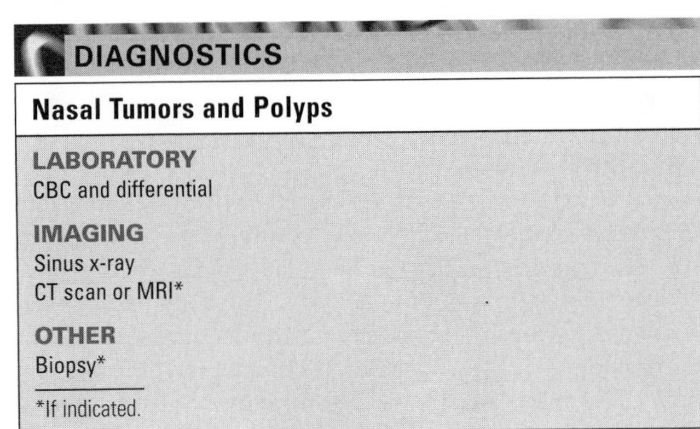
DIAGNOSTICS

Nasal Tumors and Polyps

LABORATORY
CBC and differential

IMAGING
Sinus x-ray
CT scan or MRI*

OTHER
Biopsy*

*If indicated.

granulomatosis is associated with glomerulonephritis and granulomatous lesions in the upper and lower respiratory tract. Other organ systems can also be affected.

MANAGEMENT AND INDICATIONS FOR REFERRAL OR HOSPITALIZATION

The successful treatment of small polyps involves the use of nasal steroid sprays. A short course of oral corticosteroid (e.g., prednisone, 6-day course of 21 5-mg tablets, with 30 mg on the first day and tapering by 5 mg each day) may also be therapeutic. When medical management is unsuccessful, evaluation by an otorhinolaryngologist is necessary. Polyps often require surgical removal. Benign and malignant tumors should be surgically excised; benign tumors can be removed endoscopically, but malignant tumors require a large surgical excision. If the tumor is malignant, chemotherapy and/or radiotherapy may be indicated. Patients with suspected Wegener's granulomatosis require specialist referral.

COMPLICATIONS

Complications of benign tumors and polyps include chronic nasal obstruction or olfactory dysfunction. Patients may have frequent recurrence of the tumors or polyps, necessitating frequent surgical procedures. A cancerous tumor may be terminal despite extensive therapy.

PATIENT AND FAMILY EDUCATION

Patients with benign or malignant tumors need to understand the importance of therapy. The patient should be aware of the signs and symptoms of complications or disease recurrence and the importance of continued follow-up monitoring.

WEGENER'S GRANULOMATOSIS

DEFINITION AND EPIDEMIOLOGY

Wegener's granulomatosis is a vasculitis characterized by glomerulonephritis plus granulomas of the nose and lung. The most destructive lesions of bone, cartilage, and soft tissue of the nose and paranasal sinuses are ultimately found on biopsy to be malignant neoplasms, such as lymphomas or carcinomas. The cause of this rare disorder is unknown. Without treatment Wegener's granulomatosis is invariably fatal; most patients survive less than a year after diagnosis.[2] However, the prognosis is good if the disease is diagnosed and treated early. The disease usually occurs in those older than 40 years, with equal frequency in men and women. It can also affect the skin; eyes; heart; and gastrointestinal, nervous, and musculoskeletal systems.

PATHOPHYSIOLOGY

A necrotizing vasculitis associated with autoimmunity, Wegener's granulomatosis is one of the many autoimmune diseases that occur when the immune system reacts against self-antigens and destroys host tissue. The body has a hypersensitive response; inflammation results and causes the destruction of healthy tissue. In this disease the probable self-antigen is unknown. The hypersensitivity results in chronic inflammation and causes the formation of a granuloma, a dense infiltration of lymphocytes and macrophages. If the macrophages cannot protect the body against tissue damage, the body attempts to wall off the infected site and a granuloma is formed.[3] In the vasculitis of Wegener's granulomatosis, immune complex is deposited in the blood vessel walls. Complement is activated, resulting in direct cellular injury and a decrease in the circulating levels of the complement components.[4] Once the process begins, the disorder usually develops over 4 to 12 months.[4]

CLINICAL PRESENTATION

Most patients with this condition initially complain of respiratory tract symptoms such as nasal congestion, nasal ulcerations, rhinitis, sinusitis, otitis media, otorrhea, hearing loss, gingival hypertrophy, cough, dyspnea, or hemoptysis.[2] Fever, weakness, malaise, weight loss, conjunctivitis, rashes or skin lesions, and polyarthralgias are other common complaints. The lungs are affected in 40% of newly diagnosed patients.[2] As the disease progresses, the percentage of lung involvement progresses, eventually reaching 80%, but patients with pulmonary involvement can be asymptomatic.[2] Renal disease is rarely apparent on initial presentation, although hematuria, red blood cell casts, and impaired renal function suggest renal involvement.[5]

PHYSICAL EXAMINATION

Physical findings may be absent initially despite numerous subjective complaints. If physical signs are present, they are usually associated with the upper respiratory tract and include nasal congestion and crusting, rhinorrhea, ulceration of the nasal septum, and epistaxis. The destruction of the nasal septum that results in saddle nose deformity, a characteristic sign of Wegener's granulomatosis, occurs late in the disease process. Infrequently there may be erosions through the skin that cover the nose and sinuses.[2] If there is pulmonary involvement, localized rales, rhonchi, and wheezing can be heard during auscultation. Other physical findings include unilateral proptosis, red eye, otitis media, symmetric polyarticular arthritis, and purpura.

DIAGNOSTICS

Routine laboratory studies add little to the diagnosis of Wegener's granulomatosis. Most patients have normocytic, normochromic anemia; leukocytosis; thrombocytosis; and elevated erythrocyte sedimentation rate. A urinalysis, plus BUN and creatinine, should be obtained to assess renal involvement.

A chest x-ray study is necessary to determine the presence of infiltrates, nodules, masses, and cavities, as well as sarcoidosis, tumor, or infection. Sinus x-ray studies may also be indicated to determine whether sinusitis or sinus destruction is present.

Most patients with Wegener's granulomatosis test positive for circulating antineutrophil cytoplasmic antibodies (cANCA), which are commonly found in this disorder.[2] Although a positive cANCA result suggests Wegener's granulomatosis, tissue biopsy of a suspicious lesion confirms

DIAGNOSTICS

Wegener's Granulomatosis

LABORATORY
Urinalysis
cANCA
CBC and differential*
ESR

DIAGNOSTICS
BUN
Creatinine

IMAGING
Chest x-ray
Sinus x-ray*

OTHER
Biopsy*

*If indicated.

diagnosis. Lung biopsy is preferred, although other sites can be used. The biopsy site depends on the severity of the illness, the risks of the surgical procedure, and the organ system involved.

DIFFERENTIAL DIAGNOSIS

The differential diagnosis for Wegener's granulomatosis includes other pulmonary-renal syndromes such as Goodpasture's syndrome, Churg-Strauss vasculitis, and systemic lupus erythematosus. Other vasculitides and rheumatic disorders should also be considered.

MANAGEMENT AND INDICATIONS FOR REFERRAL OR HOSPITALIZATION

A patient suspected of having Wegener's granulomatosis should be referred to a specialist as soon as the disease is suspected. In general, most patients will be hospitalized for diagnosis and the initiation of treatment. Currently, it is recommended that Wegener's granulomatosis be treated with immunosuppressive cytotoxic drugs such as cyclophosphamide (Cytoxan).[5] In most patients, therapy is started at a dosage of 1 to 2 mg/kg/day PO as a single dose. A response to this drug occurs within 2 weeks, and remission can be induced in up to 75% of patients[2]; however, most patients have relapses of the disease. Prednisone 1 mg/kg/day reduces the vascular edema and is given concurrently. After 2 or 3 weeks the steroids are slowly reduced to a maintenance dose; in some cases they may be discontinued after 4 months.[5] The cyclophosphamide is given for at least 1 full year and then is reduced by 25 mg every 2 to 3 months.[5] Treatment may differ for patients who have more critical pulmonary or kidney involvement, and in some instances other drug regimens may be indicated.[5]

The most serious side effect of cyclophosphamide is leukopenia; therefore the blood count needs to be checked on a routine basis. It is recommended that patients with Wegener's granulomatosis who are being treated with cyclophosphamide drink 1 to 2 quarts of liquid per day and empty the bladder frequently because of the risk of bladder cancer from the medication.

DIFFERENTIAL DIAGNOSIS

Wegener's Granulomatosis

- Goodpasture's syndrome
- Churg-Strauss vasculitis
- Systemic lupus erythematosus
- Vasculitic disorders
- Rheumatic disorders

COMPLICATIONS

The complication for this disease is the inability to create a remission. If the patient does not receive early treatment, the disease is generally fatal. Once proteinuria or hematuria develops, progression to renal failure can be rapid.[2] Morbidity may result from the disease or be related to toxicity from the treatment.

Pneumocystis carinii pneumonia related to immunosuppression is a potential treatment complication necessitating prophylactic therapy with trimethoprim-sulfamethoxazole.[6]

PATIENT AND FAMILY EDUCATION

Patients need to understand the necessity of adherence to therapy and frequent follow-up evaluation. Medication and side effects must be explained and understood. These patients should also be able to recognize the signs of renal, pulmonary, and other complications. In particular, they should be alert for the recurrence of nasal discharge, sinusitis, fever, and pulmonary changes.

REFERENCES

1. Jackler R, Kaplan M: Ear, nose and throat. In Tierney L, McPhee S, Papadakis M, editors: *Current medical diagnosis and treatment: ear, nose, and throat*, New York, 2006, McGraw-Hill Medical.
2. Bacon PA: The spectrum of Wegener's granulomatosis and disease relapse, *N Engl J Med* 352(4):330-332, 2005.
3. McCance K, Huether S: *Pathophysiology: the biological basis for disease in adults and children*, ed 5, St Louis, 2006, Mosby.
4. Puett D, Sergent B: Vasculitis. In Noble J, editor: *Textbook of primary care medicine*, ed 3, St Louis, 2001, Mosby.
5. Rose BD, King TE, Stone JH: *Treatment of Wegener's granulomatosis and microscopic polyangiitis*, retrieved April 26, 2006, from http://www.uptodate.com.
6. Chung JB, Armstrong K, Schwartz JS, and others: Cost-effectiveness of prophylaxis against *Pneumocystis carinii* pneumonia in patients with Wegener's granulomatosis undergoing immunosuppressive therapy, *Arthritis Rheum* 43(8):1841-1848, 2000.

PART 9

Evaluation and Management of Oropharynx Disorders

JOANN TRYBULSKI, *Section Editor*

CHAPTER 100

Dental Abscess

Debra S. Munsell

DEFINITION AND EPIDEMIOLOGY

Acute infection of the periapical tissue is commonly known as a dental abscess. These infections are often encountered in the general population and may resolve spontaneously.[1] However, they can cause chronic infections or life-threatening complications.

PATHOPHYSIOLOGY

Poor dental hygiene is one cause of dental abscesses. These abscesses arise as a result of infection by normal oral flora in a carious tooth or as a result of traumatized gingival mucosa.[1] Dental abscesses begin with necrosis of the tooth pulp, leading to bacterial invasion of the pulp chamber and deeper tissues. Deep cavities (caries) cause necrosis by initiating vasodilation and edema, which lead to pressure and pain in the rigid walls of the tooth. This pressure cuts off the circulation to the pulp, and the infection can invade the surrounding bone.

Multiple organisms, sometimes as many as five to 10, are usually found in abscesses. Initially, aerobic bacteria invade the necrotic pulp and create a hypoxic climate that favors the growth of anaerobic bacteria. Predominant organisms include *Bacteroides, Fusobacterium, Peptococcus,* and *Peptostreptococcus* organisms and *Streptococcus viridans*.

CLINICAL PRESENTATION

Abscesses usually occur in the setting of carious teeth or poor dental hygiene and cause localized pain, edema, and purulent discharge from the affected site. The site may be heat sensitive and friable. The tooth may be partially elevated out of the socket. The pain responds poorly to analgesic agents. If the abscess is minor, systemic signs may not be evident. More advanced infections may be associated with fever and lymphadenitis.

PHYSICAL EXAMINATION

Inspection of the gingiva surrounding the area of pain will reveal edema and erythema of the soft tissues and possibly a purulent discharge from a draining sinus tract. The tooth may be mobile and painful to manipulation. If the infection has progressed beyond the local area, orbital cellulitis, retropharyngeal space involvement, fascial plane invasion, or cavernous sinus thrombosis can occur. Signs of severe infection include trismus, airway compromise, and dysphagia. A patient unable to handle his or her own secretions or with involvement of the fascial spaces of the head and neck needs emergent care. Any patient who fails outpatient therapy should receive inpatient treatment.

DIAGNOSTICS

Physical examination remains the standard of diagnosis for a dental or periapical abscess. Routine radiologic screening is not recommended, since thickening of the periodontal membrane is the only finding visible before abscess formation, and abscesses develop rapidly. Chronic abscesses may reveal a radiolucent area at the tooth apex. A CBC may be indicated if cellulitis is suspected. Other diagnostics depend on complications.

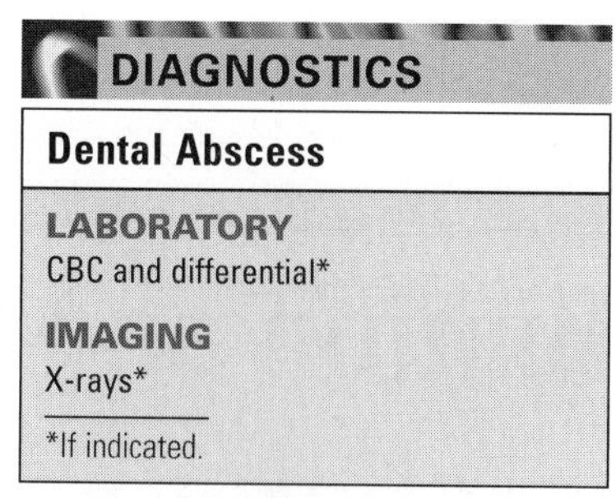

DIAGNOSTICS

Dental Abscess

LABORATORY
CBC and differential*

IMAGING
X-rays*

*If indicated.

DIFFERENTIAL DIAGNOSIS

All oral lesions must be evaluated for potential malignancy. If there is doubt about the lesion, a biopsy is necessary to exclude malignant disease, especially in populations predisposed to oral cavity cancer. Incidence of oral cavity cancer is approximately 3% to 4% per year, but a missed diagnosis significantly affects morbidity.

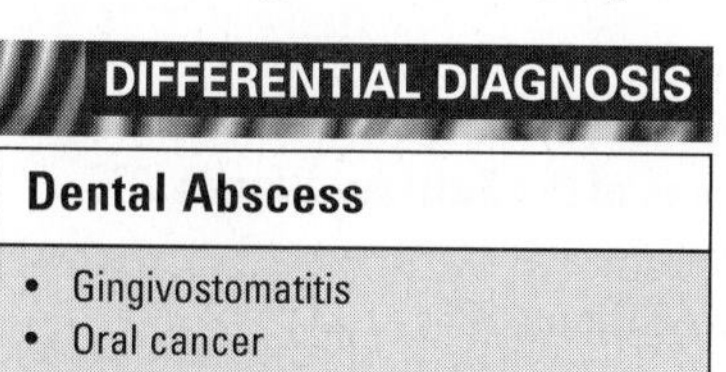

DIFFERENTIAL DIAGNOSIS

Dental Abscess

- Gingivostomatitis
- Oral cancer

MANAGEMENT

Management of a periapical abscess is primarily surgical. Dental extraction allows for the release of pressure and drainage of the abscess. Alternatively, many abscessed teeth are candidates for root canal therapy. Antibiotic coverage for both aerobic and anaerobic bacteria enhances infection resolution. Oral antibiotic therapy includes penicillin, clindamycin, and metronidazole. Metronidazole may be used in combination with penicillin but not alone. Amoxicillin with clavulanate is an alternative to penicillin. For patients who cannot take these antibiotics, erythromycin, cephalexin, sulfa, quinolones, and tetracycline are not as effective but may be used. If indicated, parenteral antibiotic therapy with penicillin, clindamycin, and metronidazole should be used. Cefazolin and cefoxitin are less effective. Gentamicin, chloramphenicol, tobramycin, amikacin, and any third-generation cephalosporin are not recommended because they fail to provide adequate protection, have adverse complications (chloramphenicol), are expensive, or are broader spectrum than necessary.[1]

Empiric therapy is usually indicated. Culture of the purulent discharge can result in a more specific bacterial diagnosis, and appropriate therapy can then be implemented. Analgesic therapy is instituted as an adjunct to antibiotic and surgical treatment. Hydration of the patient is necessary to ensure appropriate delivery of the antibiotic therapy chosen. Emergent surgery is indicated if there is a question of airway compromise or patient decompensation.

COMPLICATIONS

Complications arising from dental abscesses can range from minor to life threatening. Minor complications include the need for antibiotic therapy, dental extraction, or endodontic work (i.e., root canal). Major complications can include orbital cellulitis, fascial plane infections, osteomyelitis, dentocutaneous fistula, cavernous sinus thrombosis, and bacteremia with sepsis.[1] Up to 30% of deep neck space infections may be caused by dental abscesses.[1] In addition, the life-threatening complication of Ludwig's angina is a possibility. This infection of the deep mandibular space manifests with trismus, drooling, induration of the tongue and submandibular area, tachypnea, and dyspnea. Airway compromise can occur. Ludwig's angina is rare in children.[2]

INDICATIONS FOR REFERRAL OR HOSPITALIZATION

Dental abscesses are co-managed with dentists or endodontists to ensure adequate resolution of the initial infection, prevent complications, and institute preventive treatment. When signs and symptoms of bacteremia, orbital cellulitis, cavernous sinus thrombosis, or fascial plane involvement are present, prompt hospitalization and team management with a dentist or endodontist and an infectious disease consultant are indicated. Other indications for hospitalization include edema and erythema of the eyelids, exophthalmos, and conjunctival edema. Deep neck space infection is also an indication for hospitalization.

PATIENT AND FAMILY EDUCATION AND HEALTH PROMOTION

Early and proper dental care prevents most dental infections. Daily brushing, flossing, and appropriate dental hygiene are stressed. Early care of carious teeth can prevent future dental infections. Fluoride treatment of the local water supply or dietary fluoride supplements are excellent preventive measures.[2] Older adults and those with valvular disorders are strongly encouraged to practice good dental hygiene with early repair of carious teeth and prompt treatment of abscesses to prevent complications. The role of dental and gingival infection in myocardial infarction is an area currently under investigation.

REFERENCES

1. Cummings CW, Haughey BH, Thomas JR, and others: *Otolaryngology: head and neck surgery,* ed 4, St Louis, 2005, Mosby.
2. Schneider K, Segal G: *Dental abscess,* March 30, 2006, retrieved Dec 15, 2006, from http://www.emedicine.com/ped/topic2675.htm.

CHAPTER 101

Diseases of the Salivary Glands

Debra S. Munsell

DEFINITION AND EPIDEMIOLOGY

The salivary glands include the paired parotid glands, the submandibular and sublingual glands, and numerous minor salivary glands found in the upper aerodigestive tract. Diseases that affect the salivary glands are divided into neoplastic and nonneoplastic categories. The nonneoplastic category is further divided into infectious and noninfectious origins; neoplastic diseases can be either benign or malignant. Acute suppurative sialadenitis is covered in Chapter 104.

Salivary gland infections can be found in all age-groups and populations. Malignant neoplasms that involve the salivary glands account for approximately 5% of all head and neck tumors, not including skin cancers. The distribution of salivary tumors among men and women is virtually equal, with 1.2 per 100,000 for men and 0.7 per 100,000 for women. Warthin's tumor, a benign neoplasm, is more common in men than women. Salivary tumors in older adults most commonly affect the parotid glands. Several studies have identified an increased incidence of breast cancer in patients who have had mucoepidermoid carcinoma of the salivary glands, and an increase in minor salivary gland adenocarcinoma has been associated with occupational exposure to woodworking and to furniture, boot, and shoe manufacturing.[1]

PATHOPHYSIOLOGY

Recurrent parotitis, sialolithiasis (salivary gland stones), branchial cleft anomalies, Sjögren's syndrome, xerostomia, ptyalism (hypersalivation), sialosis, and benign lymphoepithelial lesion of Godwin are diagnoses classified as noninfectious salivary gland disorders. Sialectasis (dilation of a salivary duct, either acquired or congenital) can lead to recurrent parotitis. This dilation of the duct and gland can be produced by either stone formation or strictures. Sialolithiasis, which mainly affects the submandibular glands, refers to the formation of stones or calculi in the glands. These stones are predominantly hydroxyapatite, and there may be more than one.[1] The higher mucin content of the saliva produced in the submandibular glands, combined with an antigravity flow of saliva, contributes to stone formation.[2] The stagnant saliva in the gland also leads to the formation of stones. Elevated serum levels of calcium and phosphorus have not been associated with stone formation.[2] First branchial cleft anomalies also affect the salivary glands, primarily the paired parotid glands. Infected cysts and sinus tracts associated with these anomalies usually are initially seen in the preauricular area and can affect the facial nerve.[1]

Sjögren's syndrome is an autoimmune disorder that affects the salivary glands. On pathologic evaluation a lymphocytic infiltrate with acinar atrophy, ductal epithelial hyperplasia, and metaplasia can be found. Benign lymphoepithelial lesion of Godwin is an inflammatory condition often found in association with HIV infection. It can be confused pathologically with malignant lymphoma, metastatic carcinoma, sarcoidosis, or chronic sialadenitis.[3]

Xerostomia means dry mouth. Several diseases, as well as radiotherapy and drug therapy, can cause these symptoms. The production of excess saliva is called *ptyalism*; drug treatments and other medical conditions are usually the underlying causes. *Sialosis* refers to bilaterally recurring salivary gland edema. Acinar cell hypertrophy, interstitial edema, and striated duct atrophy may be present on pathologic examination. Alcoholism, metabolic disorders such as diabetes and various vitamin deficiencies, obesity, and malnutrition can also initiate enlargement of the salivary glands. Certain drugs, including the phenothiazines, heavy metals, thiourea, and iodide-containing substances, can cause salivary gland enlargement as a result of their cholinergic effects.

Infectious diseases that affect the salivary glands include mumps parotitis and other viral infections, syphilis, HIV, and granulomatous diseases. Granulomatous diseases affecting the salivary glands include tuberculosis, sarcoidosis, cat-scratch disease, uveoparotid fever (Heerfordt's syndrome), and actinomycosis.

Neoplastic changes also affect the salivary glands; 80% of salivary gland tumors involve the paired parotid glands.[4] Benign tumors that involve the salivary glands include pleomorphic adenoma, monomorphic adenoma, Warthin's tumor, and oncocytoma.

Malignant tumors of the salivary glands are more likely to be found in the minor salivary glands.[1] Parotid malignant tumors account for approximately one third of the malignant tumors of the salivary glands. These malignancies include mucoepidermoid carcinomas; acinic cell carcinomas; adenocarcinomas; and adenoid cystic, malignant mixed, and squamous cell carcinomas.[1] Mucoepidermoid carcinomas are the most common cancers of the major salivary glands and are most commonly seen in the parotid gland.[5]

CLINICAL PRESENTATION

The noninfectious entities that cause enlargement of the salivary gland usually are initially seen with painless swelling of the salivary gland. One exception is sialolithiasis, which is evidenced by painful edema of the affected gland and increased symptoms with meals. Sjögren's syndrome, associated with connective tissue diseases such as rheumatoid arthritis, polyarteritis nodosa, and systemic lupus erythematosus, manifests with the classic xerostomia, abnormal taste, keratoconjunctivitis sicca, dry tongue, and intermittent unilateral or bilateral swelling of the salivary gland. Bilateral salivary gland cysts characterize the benign lymphoepithelial lesion of Godwin, whereas a lack of saliva is associated with xerostomia; excess saliva production results in ptyalism. Some conditions associated with ptyalism include epilepsy, cerebral palsy, rabies, and stomatitis. Infectious diseases of the salivary glands usually cause a rapid onset of colicky pain with meals, edema, induration of the affected gland, malaise, and chills.[3] Mumps paramyxovirus infection peaks in the 4- to 6-year-old age-group and has an incubation period of 2 to 3 weeks. Fever, malaise, muscle aches, and headaches usually precede parotid swelling.

Benign and malignant processes of the salivary gland usually are seen initially as painless, unilateral masses. They may be cystic, as in Warthin's tumor. A prior history of radiation may be elicited. A small number of patients may complain of pain, and a few may have facial nerve paralysis or palsy.[1] Squamous cell carcinoma and malignant mixed tumors have a history of rapid growth and may manifest with facial pain and fixation of underlying structures. The salivary glands may also be the sites of metastatic spread of other malignancies of the head and neck, most commonly squamous cell carcinoma and malignant melanoma; the primary sites are found above the clavicles.[5] Primary malignant lymphomas have been reported but are rare.

PHYSICAL EXAMINATION

Nonneoplastic, noninfectious diseases of the salivary glands manifest as unilateral or bilateral swelling of the affected gland. In the case of sialolithiasis, a stone may be palpated in the corresponding duct. With Sjögren's syndrome, xerostomia and keratoconjunctivitis accompany unilateral or bilateral swelling of the salivary gland. Dry papillae on the tongue may be present. Menopausal women are most likely to be seen with this disease. Bilateral cystic masses may be palpated with a benign lymphoepithelial lesion of Godwin. Sialosis manifests as a bilateral, recurrent swelling of the affected glands.

Infectious diseases of the salivary gland result in inflammation, edema, and bilateral or unilateral involvement of the gland. Purulent discharge is present in acute bacterial infections. With a localized parotid abscess, pitting edema may be found. In viral infections such as mumps parotitis, a bilaterally and painfully enlarged gland and difficulty in opening the jaws (trismus) may be encountered.

Neoplastic diseases are usually distinguished by painless, firm masses that may be fast or slow growing. Patients seen late in the course of their disease may exhibit paralysis of the facial nerve, fixation of underlying structures, and possible skin involvement.

DIAGNOSTICS

Evaluation of salivary gland disease relies heavily on the patient's history and physical examination. A culture of purulent discharge from the affected duct may be performed if infectious entities are suspected. Fine-needle aspiration of the affected gland may be beneficial in diagnosing infectious agents, such as bacterial and granulomatous diseases. It is also indicted for patients with a chronic parotid lesion to exclude tuberculous parotitis, an uncommon disorder that should be included in the differential.[6] Anaerobic cultures are necessary to diagnose actinomycosis. Systemic evaluation of serum may be indicated to establish a diagnosis of HIV infection, mycobacterial disease, toxoplasmosis, and tularemia.[3] Skin testing may be useful in the diagnosis of tuberculosis and cat-scratch disease.

Viral titers may be requested if viral infections such as mumps paramyxovirus are suspected. Antibodies to the S and V antigen greater than 1:192 are expected. Mumps virus can be isolated in urine samples. A CT scan or ultrasonographic

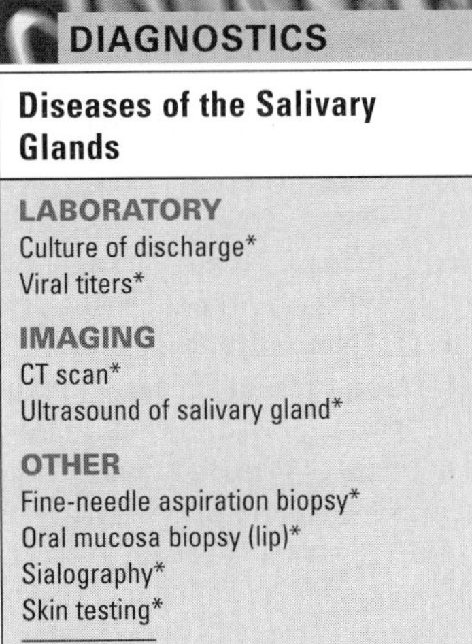

DIAGNOSTICS

Diseases of the Salivary Glands

LABORATORY
Culture of discharge*
Viral titers*

IMAGING
CT scan*
Ultrasound of salivary gland*

OTHER
Fine-needle aspiration biopsy*
Oral mucosa biopsy (lip)*
Sialography*
Skin testing*

*If indicated.

evaluations of the glands may be used if neoplastic disease is suspected. Sialography in conjunction with plain-tissue films can be used to diagnose sialolithiasis. Conventional radiography may be used to reveal submandibular gland stones, since 65% of these are radiopaque. Sjögren's syndrome is diagnosed by minor salivary gland biopsy, usually performed on the mucosal surface of the lip. Epinephrine should not be used in the procedure, since it interferes with the pathologic diagnosis. Rheumatoid factors, antinuclear factor, serum protein electrophoresis autoantibodies SSA and SSB, and other autoimmune studies should be initiated.

DIFFERENTIAL DIAGNOSIS

The differential diagnosis of noninfectious, nonneoplastic salivary gland disease includes drug therapy, sialolithiasis, branchial cleft anomalies, Sjögren's syndrome, xerostomia, ptyalism, and metabolic disorders such as diabetes. Infectious conditions that can affect the salivary gland are numerous and include HIV infection; viral infections such as mumps paramyxovirus, cytomegalovirus, and Epstein-Barr virus; bacterial infections, including *Staphylococcus aureus* and streptococci, tuberculosis, tularemia, actinomycosis, and cat-scratch disease; and parasitic diseases such as toxoplasmosis.[3]

Neoplastic involvement of the salivary glands includes both benign and malignant disease. Included in the differential diagnosis for benign lesions are pleomorphic adenoma, Warthin's tumor, monomorphic adenoma, and oncocytoma. Malignant tumors affecting the salivary glands include mucoepidermoid carcinoma, acinic cell carcinoma, adenocarcinoma, adenoid cystic carcinoma, malignant mixed tumors, and squamous cell carcinoma. The salivary glands can also be the site of metastatic disease to the head and neck. Included in these metastatic tumors are malignant melanoma, squamous cell carcinoma, and lymphoma. Primary malignant lymphoma of the salivary glands has been reported but is rare.[1]

DIFFERENTIAL DIAGNOSIS

Diseases of the Salivary Glands

- Infections (bacterial, viral, granulomatous, parasitic)
- Drug therapy
- Branchial cleft anomalies
- Sjögren's syndrome
- Benign or malignant tumors
- Sialolithiasis
- Xerostomia
- Ptyalism
- Metabolic disorders (diabetes)

MANAGEMENT

Management of many noninfectious diseases of the salivary gland is conservative. This should include pain management and hydration. Recurrent parotitis may be treated with surgical removal of the affected gland if the patient remains symptomatic. Sialolithiasis can be managed with warm compresses, analgesics, and sialagogues. Sialagogues are agents that stimulate the production and flow of saliva, such as lemon balls and chewing gum. Fluid and electrolyte replacement should be addressed. Many noninfectious, nonmalignant salivary gland problems are initiated by lack of adequate hydration. Surgical removal of the offending stone may be required. Branchial cleft anomalies are treated with surgical excision. Sjögren's syndrome is treated symptomatically with local and systemic therapy to address the xerostomia and xerophthalmia. Ptyalism may require surgical intervention, intraparotid injections of botulinum toxin A, or Nd:YAG laser treatment.[1]

Management of infectious diseases of the salivary glands depends on the cause of the disease. Management of acute suppurative parotitis is discussed in Chapter 104. Viral infection of the salivary glands, most commonly caused by the mumps paramyxovirus, requires conservative therapy that consists of adequate hydration, rest, and possibly diet modification. Hospitalization and consultation with infectious disease specialists may be necessary if infection progresses to involve other organs or structures. Infections that are suspected to be HIV infection should be evaluated by an HIV specialist; surgical intervention should be undertaken to evaluate appropriately for possible lymphoma, which has been associated with HIV salivary gland enlargement. Granulomatous infection of the salivary glands should be treated with the appropriate agents. Tubercular infections and nontubercular mycobacterial infections may require surgical removal because these infections may not respond to traditional therapies. Actinomycosis is treated with IV penicillin, followed by the oral form for several months. Surgical therapy may also be required. Clindamycin or erythromycin can be substituted if the patient is allergic to penicillin.[7] Cat-scratch disease can be treated symptomatically without antibiotic therapy. Toxoplasmosis can be treated with combination therapy that consists of pyrimethamine and trisulfapyrimidines, although in most cases this regimen is reserved for those who have systemic disease, are immunocompromised, or are pregnant.[3] Parenteral antibiotics, such as the aminoglycosides streptomycin or gentamicin, can be used for tularemia. Tetracycline has also been used for tularemia, but with mixed results.

Suspected benign or malignant salivary gland masses are managed surgically. With surgery of the parotid gland, preservation of the facial nerve is critical unless the nerve is already nonfunctional or has tumor involvement. A superficial parotidectomy is the surgical procedure of choice. Some surgeons propose that both the deep and superficial lobes of the parotid gland be treated with a total parotidectomy. Tumors of the minor salivary glands are treated with surgical excision. The extent of the procedure is dictated by the tumor site and the disease. Radiotherapy as a primary treatment modality is no longer recommended, although postoperative radiotherapy may be necessary for certain tissue types.[1] Neck dissection performed at the time of the surgical procedure may be indicated for tumors larger than 4 cm (1.6 inches), cancers that originate in the submandibular gland, and primary squamous cell carcinoma. If there is undifferentiated carcinoma or high-grade mucoepidermoid carcinoma, a neck dissection should also be performed at the time of the initial surgery.

LIFE SPAN CONSIDERATIONS

Mumps paramyxovirus is decreasing in incidence in the pediatric population because of routine immunization (measles-mumps-rubella [MMR]). Unimmunized children and adults are at risk for complications, including orchitis, encephalitis, meningitis, and cochleitis. Adults exposed to mumps paramyxovirus are more likely to develop serious complications such as mumps orchitis, pancreatitis, and nephritis. Adults who have not had the mumps are encouraged to have the MMR immunization. Older adults are at high risk for all types of salivary gland tumors. Sjögren's syndrome has a higher incidence in postmenopausal women because of the increased incidence of connective tissue disorders in this population. Pleomorphic adenomas are more common in people who have received prior radiation. Smokers have an increased rate of Warthin's tumors.[1]

COMPLICATIONS

Complications of diseases of the salivary glands include recurrent bouts of salivary gland swelling, pain, and stone formation, which may necessitate surgical intervention. Xerostomia produces serious dental caries because of the lack of saliva. Saliva has properties that aid in the prevention of caries. Dry mouth seriously affects the patient's quality of life, necessitating dietary changes and frequent sips of water. Infectious causes of salivary gland disease have a potential for sepsis. Encephalitis, orchitis, meningitis, and cochleitis are serious consequences of mumps paramyxovirus infection. On occasion, development of islet cell antibodies leading to acute onset of type 1 diabetes can occur. Bacterial infections and granulomatous diseases can be serious in patients who are immunocompromised. Patients diagnosed with Sjögren's syndrome have a significantly increased risk (relative risk = 44) for the development of non-Hodgkin's lymphoma and multiple myeloma.[1]

Benign tumors of the salivary gland rarely cause complications unless they are neglected and invade the facial nerve, underlying structures, or overlying skin. The recurrence rate is low for tumors excised appropriately and properly. However, malignant tumors of the salivary glands can be difficult to treat. Tumors such as adenoid cystic carcinoma, squamous cell carcinoma, and adenocarcinoma may metastasize to other local and regional sites. To ensure a good outcome, it is important to initiate appropriate surgical consultation if a tumor is suspected.

INDICATIONS FOR REFERRAL OR HOSPITALIZATION

Health care providers may manage many infectious and noninfectious diseases that affect the salivary glands. A team of qualified practitioners should manage acute suppurative parotitis (sialadenitis). Suspected benign and malignant masses should be referred to an appropriate head and neck surgeon for proper diagnosis and treatment. Sialolithiasis requires consultation with an otolaryngologist. Hospitalization may be required to manage the underlying condition causing salivary enlargement or to manage complications. Sjögren's syndrome may need to be managed by a specialist in autoimmune diseases.

PATIENT AND FAMILY EDUCATION

Patients should be encouraged to examine themselves for signs and symptoms of salivary gland disease. Painful or painless swelling of the salivary glands, xerostomia, ptyalism, and purulent discharge from salivary gland ducts are important conditions to investigate. Patients undergoing prolonged surgical procedures, especially gastrointestinal procedures, should maintain adequate hydration to avoid acute suppurative sialadenitis.

HEALTH PROMOTION

Important topics for health promotion include adequate hydration, attention to oral hygiene, and immunizations. In addition, it is important that the patient be taught to avoid risk factors such as radiation exposure and exposure to animals that may be vectors of disease.

REFERENCES

1. Lee KJ: *Essential otolaryngology: head and neck surgery*, ed 8, New York, 2003, McGraw-Hill.
2. Kennedy K, Driscoll B, O'Quinn F: Salivary gland diseases, *UTMB Grand Rounds*, Oct 30, 1996, retrieved Dec 15, 2006, from http://www.utmb.edu/otoref/Grnds/GrndsIndex.html.
3. Cummings CW, Haughey BH, Thomas JR, and others: *Otolaryngology: head and neck surgery*, ed 4, St Louis, 2005, Mosby.
4. Tierney LM, McRhee SJ, Papadakis MA: *Current medical diagnosis and treatment*, ed 44, New York, 2005, Lange Medical Books/McGraw Hill.
5. Myers E, Suen J: *Cancer of the head and neck*, ed 3, Philadelphia, 1996, Saunders.
6. Lee IK, Liu JW: Tuberculous parotitis: case report and literature review, *Ann Otol Laryngol* 114(7):547-551, 2005.
7. Gilbert DN, Moellering RC, Eliopoulos GM, and others: *The Sanford guide to antimicrobial therapy—2004*, ed 34, Hyde Park, Vt, 2004, Antimicrobial Therapy.

CHAPTER 102

Epiglottitis

Debra S. Munsell

DEFINITION AND EPIDEMIOLOGY

Epiglottitis (supraglottitis) is an acute inflammation of the epiglottis and surrounding structures. The inflammation is typically caused by a bacterial infection and less commonly occurs as a result of a viral illness or caustic and thermal injury to the epiglottis. Crack cocaine use has been increasingly associated with thermal injury to the hypopharynx.[1] Epiglottitis is a rare but serious life-threatening condition.

From the 1950s to the early 1990s epiglottitis typically was associated more often with children than with adults.[1] However, with the advent of vaccination for *Haemophilus* organisms, a dramatic decline in childhood epiglottitis has been noted. Epiglottitis is currently more common in the adult population than in children. Incidence is now decreasing in all age-groups, possibly as a result of a general decrease of *Haemophilus influenzae* type B (HIB) disease in the general population. Other pathogens associated with this disease include groups A, B, and C streptococcus; *Streptococcus pneumoniae; Klebsiella pneumoniae; Candida albicans; Staphylococcus aureus; Haemophilus parainfluenzae; Neisseria meningitidis;* varicella zoster; and various other viral pathogens.[2]

Male predominance has been reported with epiglottitis; however, male/female ratios have varied. The average age of adults with epiglottitis varies from 42 years to that age plus or minus 18.5 years.[3] One study noted an increase in cases during the summer months; however, most experts agree that there is not a predictable seasonal occurrence of epiglottitis.[4]

Epiglottitis among adults may follow an unpredictable clinical course, ranging from relatively benign disease to rapidly progressive disease with acute airway obstruction and possibly death.[3] The mortality rate for children is less than 1%, but the mortality rate for the adult population is in the range of 6% to 7%.[1] Delay in diagnosis is associated with a 9% to 18% mortality rate.[2]

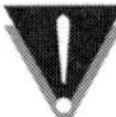

Immediate emergency department referral or physician consultation is indicated for patients with suspected epiglottitis.

PATHOPHYSIOLOGY

Epiglottitis can be caused by a variety of microorganisms. Two of the most common offending organisms are HIB and group A β-hemolytic streptococcus. In patients with underlying disease, *Aspergillus, Klebsiella,* and *Candida* organisms have been identified. A viral etiology has been postulated for some cases of adult epiglottitis, especially the milder cases.[5] Also, herpes simplex has been positively identified in adult epiglottitis.

CLINICAL PRESENTATION

Patients with epiglottitis are initially seen with severe sore throat, dysphagia, odynophagia, fever, and shortness of breath. Other complaints include the inability to swallow their own secretions, neck tenderness, lymphadenopathy, cough, drooling, stridor, respiratory distress, and hoarseness. The patient may adopt the tripod position, using accessory muscles for respiration. The onset and duration of symptoms before the patient's initial contact with the health care provider vary. Depending on the severity of symptoms, patients may seek treatment after having symptoms for less than 8 hours, or they may have had them for more than 4 days.

PHYSICAL EXAMINATION

Patients with epiglottitis may or may not have fever and a toxic appearance, depending on the severity of the infection. Physical findings by indirect laryngoscopy reveal an erythematous, edematous epiglottis with a narrow glottic opening. In patients experiencing respiratory distress, posturing in the upright "sniff" or tripod position with drooling may be noted. Substernal and supraclavicular retractions, tachycardia, tachypnea, and inspiratory stridor are common. With severe respiratory distress, changes in mental status, anxiety, pallor, cyanosis, and other signs of hypoxia may be present.

Precautions during the physical examination are required. If epiglottitis is suspected, the pharynx should not be examined, especially with a tongue depressor, since this may precipitate an airway emergency. Any inspection of the oral cavity requires that emergency airway management equipment be immediately available in case of laryngospasm.

DIAGNOSTICS

A definitive diagnosis of epiglottitis is made by indirect laryngoscopy with a flexible fiberoptic scope or a laryngeal mirror. Indirect laryngoscopy is considered a safe diagnostic tool in the adult population but not in children.

A lateral neck film can be useful but is not always diagnostic in the adult population. Findings on the lateral neck film suggestive of epiglottitis include a swollen epiglottis manifesting as a "thumbprint" sign. Because they have a fairly low sensitivity (true positives) rate, lateral neck films are not a true diagnostic tool.

DIAGNOSTICS

Epiglottitis

INITIAL
Airway stabilization mandatory before further diagnostic evaluation
Pulse oximetry

LABORATORY
CBC and differential
Blood cultures
Culture and sensitivity
ABGs

IMAGING
Lateral neck x-ray, chest x-ray

OTHER
Indirect laryngoscopy

A CBC often reveals leukocytosis with a shift to the left. Blood cultures may be obtained to exclude septicemia. A culture of the epiglottis is helpful in identifying the offending organism. Arterial blood gases may also be indicated. Fiberoptic endoscopy may reveal inhaled foreign substances such as the fibers from metal screens found in pipes used to smoke crack cocaine or other illicit drugs.[1]

DIFFERENTIAL DIAGNOSIS

Other conditions to consider in the differential diagnosis include Ludwig's angina, retropharyngeal and peritonsillar infections, tumor, caustic ingestions, allergic drug reactions, laryngeal trauma, uvulitis, bacterial tracheitis, angioedema, foreign body aspiration, and thermal injury. Signs and symptoms of Ludwig's angina, retropharyngeal abscess, and peritonsillar cellulitis or abscess are somewhat similar to those of epiglottitis, since all are seen with an infectious process. Ludwig's angina is an infection, or cellulitis, of the floor of the mouth, often involving the submental, sublingual, and/or submandibular spaces. Ludwig's angina typically results from a dental infection and can be easily diagnosed by CT scan. Retropharyngeal abscess can also be identified by CT scan and can be excluded by negative findings on physical examination. Peritonsillar cellulitis or abscess can be excluded by negative physical examination findings.

A tumor, trauma to the larynx, allergic drug reaction, or angioedema may be seen with signs similar to those of epiglottitis. A tumor or trauma to the larynx may cause sore throat, hoarseness, dysphagia, and respiratory distress; however, infectious findings are negative. Allergic drug reaction or angioedema typically manifests with respiratory distress and dermatologic findings. A history of illicit drug use or thermal injury should be elicited. Crack cocaine vaporizes at high temperatures, and the extreme heat of the inhaled vapors may incite acute inflammation of the epiglottis.

DIFFERENTIAL DIAGNOSIS

Epiglottitis

- Ludwig's angina
- Retropharyngeal and peritonsillar infections
- Tumor
- Trauma
- Allergic reaction
- Angioedema
- Illicit drug use
- Thermal injury

MANAGEMENT

Patients should be allowed to sit upright in a quiet environment with humidified oxygen. Treatment of epiglottitis consists of close observation for airway management, antibiotics, and, in some cases, steroids. The patient ideally should be hospitalized in the ICU for aggressive airway monitoring. Avoid sedation, racemic epinephrine, and inhaled medications.

Immediate consultation of trained ear-nose-throat or anesthesia personnel is mandatory. Isolation is sometimes recommended for the first 24 hours after the initiation of antibiotic therapy. Patients with an increased risk of airway obstruction (those with respiratory distress, tachycardia, tachypnea, or an increased WBC count) may require an artificial airway by intubation or tracheotomy. Continuous oxygen therapy and monitoring of oxygen saturation are necessary.

IV antibiotics should be initiated as soon as possible. In the past the usual treatment for epiglottitis was ampicillin and chloramphenicol; however, because of ampicillin-resistant *H. influenzae*, it is no longer recommended. Chloramphenicol is not often used because of the increased risk of aplastic anemia. A second- or third-generation cephalosporin (e.g., ceftriaxone IV or cefotaxime), ampicillin-sulbactam, clindamycin, or levofloxacin is the recommended treatment.[3,6] Although many experts advocate the use of steroids, it is not a universal standard of treatment. Randomized controlled trials proving benefit from steroid use are not available.

The use of rifampin as a prophylaxis against infection in close contacts is sometimes recommended, especially if *H. influenzae* type b is the suspected organism.[6] There have been cases of transmission of *Haemophilus* infection from children to adults and adults to children.[1]

LIFE SPAN CONSIDERATIONS

With the changes in the age of those affected by HIB infection, careful evaluation of all age-groups is suggested. A suspicion of epiglottitis should prompt an immediate referral to an emergency department capable of airway support. A careful history, including illicit drug use, should be documented.

COMPLICATIONS

Epiglottitis is a serious and potentially fatal condition. Death from airway obstruction may result. Other potentially fatal complications include septicemia and meningitis, resulting from the spread of infection. Other complications such as pulmonary edema, epiglottic abscess, vocal cord granuloma, and pneumomediastinum have been reported.

INDICATIONS FOR REFERRAL OR HOSPITALIZATION

All cases of epiglottitis or suspected epiglottitis require immediate referral. Hospitalization is necessary for close observation of the airway and initiation of appropriate antibiotic therapy.

PATIENT AND FAMILY EDUCATION

Explanation of all procedures is necessary to allay patient and family anxiety. The importance of the medical regimen should be stressed to enhance adherence. When steroids are prescribed, information on steroids and tapering of doses must be reviewed. If illicit drug use is documented, education and referral for counseling should be attempted.

HEALTH PROMOTION

Health promotion should include an age-appropriate immunization status review. Cases of thermal inhalation injuries resulting in epiglottitis have been documented in crack cocaine users. Caustic ingestions, foreign bodies, and other thermal inhalations have also resulted in signs and symptoms of epiglottitis.[7]

REFERENCES

1. Mayo-Smith M, Spinale J: Thermal epiglottitis in adults: a new complication of illicit drug use, *J Emerg Med* 15(4):483-485, 1997.
2. Park KW, Darvish A, Lowenstein E: Airway management for adult patients with acute epiglottitis, *Anesthesiology* 88:254-261, 1988.

3. Fairbanks DNF: *Pocket guide to antimicrobial therapy in otolaryngology–head and neck surgery,* ed 10, Alexandria, Va, 2001, American Academy of Otolaryngology–Head and Neck Surgery Foundation.
4. Hebert PC, Ducic Y, Boisvert D, and others: Adult epiglottitis in a Canadian setting, *Laryngoscope* 108:64-69, 1998.
5. Kass EG, McFadden EA, Jacobson S, and others: Acute epiglottitis in the adult: experience with a seasonal presentation, *Laryngoscope* 103:841-844, 1993.
6. Woods CR: *Epiglottitis,* 2006, retrieved Dec 20, 2006, from http://www.utdol.com/utd/store/index.do.
7. Shapiro J, Eavey RD, Baker AS: Adult supraglottitis: a prospective analysis, *JAMA* 259:563-567, 1988.

CHAPTER 103

Oral Infections

Debra S. Munsell

DEFINITION AND EPIDEMIOLOGY

Aphthous ulcers, stomatitis, and thrush are often encountered in primary care practice. Mechanical irritation, drug reactions, trauma, nutritional deficiencies, stress, and infection (bacterial, viral, or fungal) irritate and inflame the sensitive oral mucosa. These conditions may be localized to the oral mucosa or associated with systemic disease. Therefore it is important to accurately diagnose and appropriately care for these lesions.

Aphthous ulcers (recurrent aphthous ulceration, canker sores) are defined as shallow, painful, and often recurrent lesions of the oral mucosa. These are the most common oral mucosal lesions in North America. Children of lower socioeconomic status are more frequently affected than those with higher status.[1] Canker sores typically affect adolescents and young adults, with more females than males affected. Incidence has been noted to be 20% in the general population and up to 50% in students attending some professional schools.[1] Aphthous ulcerations of the oral mucosal surfaces have been reported on every populated continent.[1] Patients with known ulcerative colitis, Crohn's disease, or gluten-sensitive enteropathy may have aphthous ulcers as a feature of these diseases.

Stomatitis is a general term that refers to the inflammation of the soft tissues of the oral cavity. Chemical or heat injuries can initiate stomatitis; aspirin can cause an ulcerative lesion when used as a topical anesthetic on the oral mucosa. Burns sustained from hot food or liquids can also cause mucosal irritations. Certain food substances, chewing gum, oral mouth rinses, and dental products can induce painful lesions. Cinnamon flavoring has been implicated as a common culprit.[2]

Thrush, or candidal infection of the oral mucosa, is caused by the overgrowth of *Candida albicans,* bacteria that are normally found in the flora of the gastrointestinal tract. Immunocompromised hosts; patients with diabetes, ulcerative colitis, Crohn's disease, gluten sensitivity, vitamin deficiencies, or poor oral hygiene; patients who wear dentures; and others with poor general health are susceptible to oral mucosal lesions. These lesions may occur from infancy through maturity and can be a recurrent source of irritation.

PATHOPHYSIOLOGY

Aphthous ulcers are a common presenting problem for all age-groups. Although the exact etiology of these ulcers is not known, it is thought that cell-mediated hypersensitivity to the oral mucosa may be the cause. Other proposed etiologic factors include physical or emotional stress; trauma associated with physical, chemical, or local agents; deficiencies of vitamin B_{12}, folic acid, or iron; familial or genetic predisposition[1]; microbial agents; and hypersensitivity states (gluten-sensitive enteropathy). Generalized stomatitis may be caused by poor oral hygiene, ill-fitting dentures, nicotine abuse, mechanical trauma, chemical trauma from caustic substances, or hot foods. Thrush more typically occurs with underlying diabetes or with immunocompromised states. Parenteral antibiotic or steroid use has been implicated as a precursor to oral candidiasis.

CLINICAL PRESENTATION

Aphthous ulcers are painful, shallow ulcerations of the nonkeratinized oral mucosa and occur as solitary or multiple lesions. A prodrome of "burning or pricking" of the oral mucosa has been reported.[1] They are not typically found on the anterior hard palate or gingiva, and they may be recurrent. Ranging in size from 2 mm to several centimeters, aphthous ulcers may have a gray-yellow, pseudomembranous base surrounded by erythema. The disease itself is self-limiting, usually lasting 7 to 10 days.[1] Fever and lymphadenopathy are not usually present.

There are three categories of aphthous ulcers. Minor aphthous ulcers are generally the most common and range in size from 2 to 10 mm (0.08 to 0.4 inch); healing occurs over 10 to 14 days. Many people attribute these minor ulcers to stress, trauma, or even menses. Major aphthous ulcers may be seen as painful lesions that are 2 to 3 cm (0.8 to 1.2 inches) in diameter and are often in a state of cyclical eruption. Scarring is associated with these lesions. The third category is the herpetiform ulceration, which often is mistaken for lesions of the herpes simplex virus. These lesions are small (2 to 3 mm [0.08 to 0.12 inch]), are widely scattered or closely grouped, and may be recurrent. Viral cultures of these lesions are negative.

Stomatitis may be attributed to many different causes, most commonly denture irritation, poor oral hygiene, and nicotine abuse. Typically, stomatitis caused by denture irritation manifests as irritation of the soft tissue associated with denture contact. It is erythematous and painful.

Thrush usually appears as white, cottage cheese–like lesions that can be easily removed with a swab. The underlying tissue may bleed after manipulation.

PHYSICAL EXAMINATION

Aphthous ulceration can occur as a solitary lesion or multiple lesions. The usual presentation is a 2- to 10-mm (0.01 to 0.4 inch), ulcerative mucosal lesion that has a white-yellow central fibrinous pseudomembrane.[2]

Stomatitis lesions caused by poor oral hygiene and denture wearing are found underlying the denture or appliance, and they are erythematous and painful. Secondary candidiasis may also be associated with denture stomatitis.[3] Stomatitis from chemical or thermal injury manifests with a painful, sloughing, whitish mucosal surface, or the lesions may be erythematous with a white keratotic surface. Patients can usually report the inciting injury. Nicotinic stomatitis manifests as multiple, 1- to 2-mm (0.01 to 0.08 inch) papules on a background of white mucosa. The hard palate and anterior soft palate are most often involved, and the papules have erythematous centers. Inflammation of the openings of the minor salivary glands by thermal sources is the proposed cause.

DIAGNOSTICS

Aphthous ulcerations, as well as lesions of nicotinic and traumatic stomatitis, are diagnosed by clinical presentation and physical examination. Laboratory examinations may be performed to assess the patient's state of health and may include CBC, erythrocyte sedimentation rate, serum iron, folate and vitamin B_{12} levels, KOH examination, and Tzanck smear.[1] Candidal infections can also be diagnosed from the physical examination and presentation, but a microscopic examination of oral scrapings will reveal the classic findings of hyphae. Cultures on a mycologic medium (Sabouraud's dextrose agar, Pagano-Levin) may be obtained for confirmation.

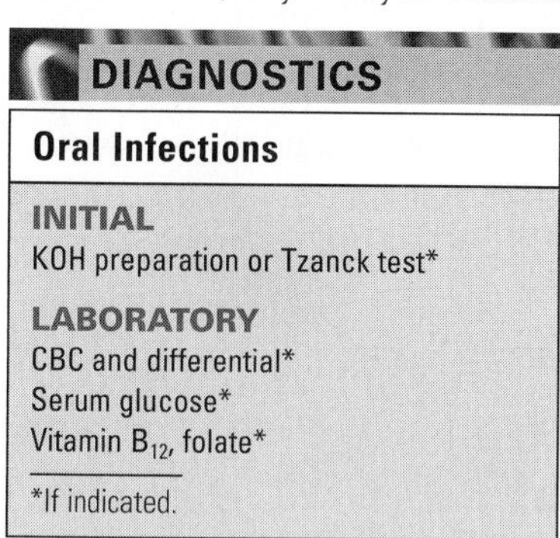
DIAGNOSTICS

Oral Infections

INITIAL
KOH preparation or Tzanck test*

LABORATORY
CBC and differential*
Serum glucose*
Vitamin B_{12}, folate*

*If indicated.

DIFFERENTIAL DIAGNOSIS

Carcinoma of the oral cavity should be suspected with oral erosive lesions that are slow to heal (greater than 2 weeks without resolution) or with thickened white patches that adhere to the oral mucosa. Although similar in appearance to aphthous ulcers, herpetic lesions are usually found only on the oral mucosa attached to bony structures. Additional causes of mucosal ulceration that are indicative of systemic disease include acute necrotizing ulcerative gingivitis (ANUG, Vincent's gingivitis), bullous pemphigoid, Behçet's syndrome, Crohn's disease, immune dysfunction, and hand-foot-and-mouth disease.

In ANUG, multiple ulcerative lesions occur with illness or stress and are associated with fetid odor, metallic taste, excessive salivation, and friable gingiva. In its most severe form, ANUG requires systemic antibiotic therapy to prevent septic sequelae, particularly with patients who are immunocompromised.

DIFFERENTIAL DIAGNOSIS

Oral Infections

- Aphthous ulcers
- Mechanical, chemical, thermal injury
- Drug reactions
- Nutritional deficiencies
- Infectious causes (bacterial, viral, fungal)
- Carcinoma
- Systemic disease (diabetes, Crohn's, Behçet's, acute necrotizing ulcerative gingivitis, hand-foot-and-mouth)
- Immune dysfunction

Bullous pemphigoid is a cutaneous disorder in which lesions commence as fixed urticarial plaques followed by clear bullae that appear on both normal and urticarial areas. This chronic eruption primarily affects flexor surfaces but may be generalized. The lesions occur in crops and transiently affect the oral mucosa.

Behçet's syndrome produces ulcerative lesions on oral and genital areas, with associated symptoms of uveitis and arthritis. Involvement of the central nervous system is less common; the ocular effects of Behçet's syndrome include retinal vasculitis and necrosis. Loss of vision can occur, even with aggressive treatment.

The lesions of Crohn's disease affect the mucosal surfaces of the gastrointestinal tract, including the oral cavity. Extensive or recurrent oral lesions necessitate careful evaluation for gastrointestinal symptoms, investigation of immune status, and screening for diabetes or other systemic disorders.

Hand-foot-and-mouth disease less commonly affects the buttocks and proximal extremities. This viral disease produces a mild, self-limiting illness. Inquiry concerning the sudden onset of gastrointestinal symptoms is helpful when clear vesicular lesions that ulcerate are found in the mouth and on the hands and feet.

MANAGEMENT

Aphthous stomatitis can be a vexing problem because recurrence is common. Treatment is directed at symptomatic relief. Methods of symptomatic relief with unclear benefit include the application of topical steroids (e.g., triamcinolone in Orabase, a dental paste) or a steroid mouth rinse with betamethasone syrup.[2]

Dexamethasone elixir 0.5 mg/ml, 5 ml swish and spit q.i.d., has been used in adults for severe or recurrent episodes. Current treatments that are likely to reduce the severity and duration of episodes, but not likely to affect recurrence rates, include (1) carbamide peroxide (Gly-Oxide) rinse, or bismuth subsalicylate (Kaopectate) and diphenhydramine (Benadryl) mixed in equal measures and applied to the irritated surfaces as a mouth rinse six times a day; and (2) avoidance of irritating, acidic, hot, or spicy foods. Other treatments with likely benefit are varied mouth rinse preparations. Viscous lidocaine is also used as a rinse, but careful observation is needed because this treatment may affect the swallowing and gag reflexes. Amlexanox oral paste, 0.25-inch of paste four times daily after oral care, is also indicated.[3] Several preparations or "mouthwash" recipes have been developed to assist in the relief of patients suffering from aphthous stomatitis.[4] One such compounded suspension consists of 30 ml diphenhydramine elixir and 60 ml Mylanta (aluminum and magnesium hydroxide), taken as a 5-ml swish and swallow three times daily and at bedtime.[5] Another compound is 60 ml Maalox (aluminum and magnesium hydroxide) and 4 g sucralfate used in the same manner.[5] Other treatments include the combination of diphenhydramine liquid, dexamethasone, nystatin suspension, and tetracycline (from capsules), swished and swallowed 1 teaspoon six times a day (after and between meals and at bedtime). Advice from a pharmacist should be obtained concerning this formulation. Acemannan oral gel or rinse p.r.n. can be used to sooth irritated tissue. For children and those in whom tetracycline is prohibited, amoxicillin-clavulanate can be substituted for the tetracycline.[6] However, severe eruptions may respond only to systemic steroids.

Nicotinic stomatitis can be treated by cessation of tobacco abuse. Denture stomatitis can be treated with thorough daily dental hygiene and removal of dentures at night. Secondary candidal infections, if suspected, should be treated appropriately. Trauma and chemical or thermal burns should be treated symptomatically with analgesics and baking soda–salt water rinses. If the offending agent is known, it should be avoided.

Candidal infections may be treated in several ways because antifungal agents are now supplied in many forms. A nystatin oral suspension, 100,000 units/ml, is a commonly used therapy; 5 ml of the suspension is swished and swallowed four times a day until 48 hours after the lesions have resolved. Lozenges of nystatin may also be prescribed. For patients with dentures, nystatin powder is applied to the dentures three or four times daily. Oral clotrimazole or nystatin troches are also widely prescribed. Antifungal creams may be applied under dental appliances. Some infections may respond only to systemic therapy with fluconazole 100 mg/day for 14 days.[3] In patients with diabetes, maintaining proper glucose levels is an important therapeutic component.

COMPLICATIONS

Aphthous stomatitis is usually a short-lived entity with few, if any, complications. Denture stomatitis and nicotine stomatitis are not thought to cause serious complications and are not associated with further development of oral carcinomas. Candidal infections of the oral cavity can be managed without complication in most instances. However, care should be taken to identify patients who may be immunocompromised or nutritionally at risk to adequately assess their needs.

INDICATIONS FOR REFERRAL OR HOSPITALIZATION

Aphthous stomatitis, dental and nicotinic stomatitis, and routine candidal infections rarely require referral. Severe cases of aphthous ulcers may need referral to assess the patient's immune status and need for systemic therapy. A physician or subspecialist in infectious diseases should be consulted if questions arise concerning possible carcinoma or if the patient is immunocompromised. Patients with routine eruptions are not candidates for hospitalization, but severely immunocompromised patients or patients with diabetes may need hospitalization for treatment of the underlying disease. Alcohol or tobacco use increases the risk for oral cancers, and patients with ulcers present for greater than 2 weeks without resolution or improvement should be referred for evaluation.

PATIENT EDUCATION AND HEALTH PROMOTION

Aphthous stomatitis is usually a recurrent eruption. Treatment of the underlying causes, if known, may alleviate future outbreaks. Crohn's disease; ulcerative colitis; stresses; deficiencies of vitamin B_{12}, iron, and folic acid; and estrogen sensitivity have been implicated in outbreaks. Avoidance of irritating food, beverages, and chemicals may alleviate some of the symptoms and decrease the number of recurrences. Proper oral hygiene and good denture care prevent most problems with denture-related stomatitis. Avoidance of excessively heated food and drink will prevent thermal stomatitis. Candidal infections can be anticipated in patients who are taking long courses of steroids and antibiotics; treatment for these patients should be started as soon as symptoms occur. Patients who are known to be immunocompromised should be monitored regularly for the signs and symptoms of developing candidal infections and treated accordingly. Patients with diabetes should be taught proper glycemic control measures and routine surveillance of skin and mucosal surfaces.

REFERENCES

1. Mirowiski GW, Nebesio CL: *Aphthous stomatitis*, retrieved Nov 29, 2005, from http://www.emedicine.com/derm/topic486.htm.
2. Cummings CW, Haughey BH, Thomas JR, and others: *Otolaryngology: head and neck surgery*, ed 4, St Louis, 2005, Mosby.
3. Rakel RE: *Conn's current therapy*, Philadelphia, 1998, Saunders.
4. *Tarascon pocket pharmacopoeia*, Loma Linda, Calif, 2005, Tarascon Publishing.
5. *MDACC 2004/2005 Pharmacy formulary and therapeutic index, division of pharmacy*, Hudson, Ohio, 2001, Lexi-Comp.
6. Fairbanks DNF: *Pocket guide to antimicrobial therapy in otolaryngology–head and neck surgery*, ed 11, Alexandria, Va, 2001, American Academy of Otolaryngology–Head and Neck Surgery Foundation.

CHAPTER 104

Parotitis

Debra S. Munsell

DEFINITION AND EPIDEMIOLOGY

An inflammatory reaction of the parotid gland, parotitis may be caused by bacterial, viral, fungal, or mycobacterial invasion. The most common infection is viral mumps. Since the advent of universal immunization for the mumps paramyxovirus, viral parotitis is becoming a rare occurrence in the United States. Acute suppurative parotitis is more likely to be encountered in the sixth to seventh decade of life in an equal male/female ratio.[1] This condition is also referred to as acute suppurative sialadenitis, surgical parotitis or surgical mumps, postoperative parotitis, or secondary parotitis.[1] Chronic illness, an immunocompromised host, recent surgical procedure, and hypovolemia are common precipitating factors.[1] Acute suppurative parotitis is also becoming a rare entity because of increased use of antibiotics in the perioperative setting and increased attention to perioperative hydration. Intrinsic factors such as medications (anticholinergics) and extrinsic factors such as radiotherapy may also precipitate an episode of parotitis. It is important to note that salivary gland enlargement can be the initial manifestation of HIV infection.[1,2]

PATHOPHYSIOLOGY

Multiple factors can contribute to the development of parotitis. Most commonly the infection begins with retrograde migration of oral cavity flora via Stensen's duct. Stasis of saliva, ductal obstruction, decreased stimulation of saliva (anorexia), decreased mastication, and poor oral hygiene contribute to retrograde migration.[3,4] Ill patients, recent surgical candidates, and those with acute or chronic hypovolemia (hemorrhage, diarrhea, emesis) exhibit factors that lead to stasis and retrograde migration. Although most of these infections occur in adults, neonates may exhibit parotitis, which is a life-threatening entity at this age.[2] In addition, parotid salivary secretions do not have great bacteriostatic properties, which can also augment inflammatory reactions.

CLINICAL PRESENTATION

The usual presentation consists of a rapid onset of localized pain, edema, and induration of the infected gland.[3] Systemic symptoms may include fever, chills, and malaise.[1] Viral inflammatory reactions most often are seen with edema (usually bilateral) and pain, which is exacerbated by mastication. Low-grade fever, arthralgias, malaise, and headache may also be present. Although parotitis is sometimes referred to as *surgical mumps*, it is not related to the viral syndrome mumps, which is caused by the mumps paramyxovirus. *Surgical mumps* refers to the similar appearance of glandular swelling seen in mumps and parotitis. Infection with HIV may produce bilaterally enlarged, painless parotid glands that gradually produce smaller amounts of saliva, resulting in complaints of xerostomia.[1]

PHYSICAL EXAMINATION

Bimanual palpation of the gland with attention to Stensen's duct should be performed. In parotitis, palpation of the gland elicits a suppurative discharge from Stensen's duct.[2,3] Bilateral edema is suggestive of viral infection, and a clear discharge is found on palpation of the duct. Suppurative discharge should be cultured. If the process has been present for several days, fluctuance of suppurative sialadenitis may not be palpable because of the anatomic septations in the parotid.[3]

DIAGNOSTICS

The diagnosis of parotitis is based on the clinical presentation and physical examination. A CBC with differential may reveal a leukocytosis with neutrophilia in suppurative cases.[1] Appropriate cultures and sensitivities should be obtained and fungal and mycobacterial studies requested when indicated. Radiographs or oblique soft tissue films are obtained if obstruction caused by calculus is suspected. CT scan, with contrast medium, is an excellent study to obtain, since it may delineate ductal stones or a suppurative process.[2]

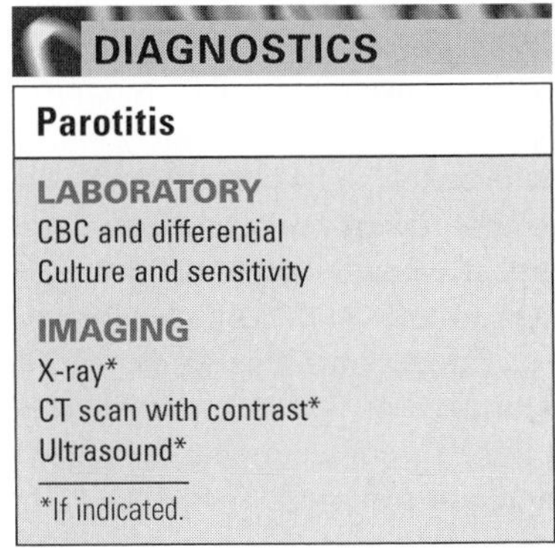

DIAGNOSTICS

Parotitis

LABORATORY
CBC and differential
Culture and sensitivity

IMAGING
X-ray*
CT scan with contrast*
Ultrasound*

*If indicated.

DIFFERENTIAL DIAGNOSIS

The differential diagnosis of parotitis should include bacterial, viral, mycobacterial, or fungal infections. In addition to paramyxovirus, identified agents of infection include cytomegalovirus, coxsackievirus, Epstein-Barr virus, and HIV. Mechanical or extrinsic factors such as radiotherapy or drug-induced parotitis should also be included in the differential diagnosis. Additionally, anticholinergic medications can initiate parotitis. Such medications include antiparkinsonian agents, atropine, dicyclomine hydrochloride, glycopyrrolate, scopolamine, and hyoscyamine sulfate. Many psychotropic medications have an atropine-like effect and can cause parotid swelling.[2]

DIFFERENTIAL DIAGNOSIS

Parotitis

Infection
- Bacterial
- Viral
- HIV
- Fungal
- Mycobacterial

Medications
Mechanical obstruction

MANAGEMENT

Nonsurgical treatments include parenteral antibiotics such as β-lactamase–resistant penicillins or cephalosporins. Recommended antibiotic therapy includes amoxicillin with clavulanate and clindamycin. Cefoxitin and nafcillin are suggested for refractory disease[5] (Box 104-1). Fluid and electrolyte replacement is necessary.[1] Attention to proper oral hygiene and the use of sialagogues, such as sugar-free hard candy and chewing gum, are also recommended. Sialagogues are agents that stimulate the production and flow of saliva. There is a questionable role for the use of steroids. Analgesics and local heat for relief of pain are beneficial. External bimanual massage (from distal to proximal) of the duct is also recommended.[1] Surgical drainage is appropriate if the infection is refractory for more than 3 or 4 days.[4,5] A CT scan or ultrasound examination of the parotid and neck is indicated if abscess formation has occurred after 3 or 4 days while the patient is taking aggressive parenteral antibiotics. Because of the usually debilitated states of patients predisposed to parotitis, a poor prognosis is associated with postoperative patients who develop parotitis. A 20% mortality rate is associated with the development of this infection.[1]

BOX 104-1

ANTIBIOTICS RECOMMENDED IN TREATMENT OF BACTERIAL PAROTITIS

- Amoxicillin with clavulanate (Augmentin)
- Ampicillin with sulbactam (Unasyn IV)
- Antistaphylococcal penicillin
- Clindamycin
- Cephalexin
- Cefoxitin
- Nafcillin
- Vancomycin IV and metronidazole

COMPLICATIONS

Complications include abscess formation and the need for surgical drainage.[2,4] The discomfort associated with this disorder may prevent the patient from eating and drinking, increasing the risk of hypovolemia and further compromising the patient. Suppurative parotitis is a rare occurrence postoperatively because of the routine use of preoperative and intraoperative antibiotic therapy. Chronic parotitis may develop as a result of an acute episode of suppurative parotitis.[2]

INDICATIONS FOR REFERRAL OR HOSPITALIZATION

Consultation with an otolaryngologist–head and neck surgeon is highly recommended. Patients who develop parotitis often require hospitalization for fluid replacement, careful monitoring, and IV antibiotics.

PATIENT AND FAMILY EDUCATION AND HEALTH PROMOTION

Preoperative attention to hydration and overall health status should be addressed if the patient is not a candidate for emergent surgery. After diagnosis, attention to hydration, parenteral antibiotics, oral hygiene, and sialagogue use should be addressed. Patients should be instructed in proper oral hygiene, which includes brushing and flossing the teeth and proper care of dentures and dental appliances. The side effects of medications should be discussed with the patient to determine whether medication is causing decreased salivary secretions.

REFERENCES

1. Cummings CW, Haughey BH, Thomas JR, and others: *Otolaryngology: head and neck surgery,* ed 4, St Louis, 2005, Mosby.
2. DeWeese DD: *Otolaryngology–head and neck surgery,* ed 7, St Louis, 1988, Mosby.
3. Templer JW: *Parotitis,* retrieved Nov 29, 2005, from http://www.emedicine.com/ent/topic600.htm.
4. Fattabi TT, Lyu PE, Van Sickels JE: Management of acute suppurative parotitis, *J Oral Maxillofac Surg* 60:446-448, 2002.
5. Way L: *Current surgical diagnosis and treatment,* ed 10, Norwalk, Conn, 1994, Appleton & Lange.

CHAPTER **105**

Peritonsillar Abscess

Debra S. Munsell

DEFINITION AND EPIDEMIOLOGY

A peritonsillar abscess (PTA) is an accumulation of pus located within the peritonsillar tissue. PTA is the most common deep infection of the head and neck.[1] The abscess usually occurs in patients with a history of recurrent, chronic, or improperly treated tonsillitis.[1] PTA may also develop in patients properly treated with penicillin. In such cases the abscess results from penicillin-resistant strains of bacteria.

Peritonsillar cellulitis and abscess formation are common occurrences in young adults.[2] It is seen most often in persons 20 to 40 years of age.[1,2] The incidence rate for PTA is approximately 30 per 100,000 person-years, or approximately 45,000 cases annually in the United States and Puerto Rico.[3,4] The relatively high incidence of PTAs reported raises the possibility that the decreasing rate of tonsillectomies might be increasing the risk for developing PTAs.[3]

Patients with a history of chronic tonsillitis are at risk for developing a PTA. The recurrence of PTA is reported to be variable—from 0% to 23%.[3] The risk of recurrence is higher if the patient is younger than 30 years of age.

Physician consultation is recommended for PTA.

PATHOPHYSIOLOGY

PTAs, which occur at the superior tonsillar pole, are caused by microorganisms that invade the tissue. Studies of tonsillitis have shown a high incidence of anaerobic organisms (principally bacteroids) and aerobic bacteria; group A β-hemolytic streptococci (GABHS) are commonly involved.[3] β-Lactamase production by anaerobes and some staphylococci results in ineffective treatment of pharyngitis, which can potentially precipitate a PTA.

The abscess formation results from the body's attempt to localize the infection. Erythema and swelling of the peritonsillar region result from increased blood supply and the collection of pus. The pus consists of cells, bacteria, and necrotic tissue. A group of salivary glands, Weber's glands, at the superior pole of the tonsils, also may play a role in the development of PTA. These glands are reported to assist in the removal of debris in the tonsil area. If these glands are obstructed by debris, inflammation, or pus, their function is impaired, leading to the development of PTA.[4]

CLINICAL PRESENTATION

Typically the presentation consists of fever, often 38.8° C (102° F) or higher; chills; fatigue; malaise; foul breath; and severe odynophagia. The patient may appear acutely ill and often complains of pain radiating to the ear of the affected side. Trismus (spasms of the masticatory muscles) is often noted. Drooling is typically present because of the inability to handle secretions. A "hot potato" (hoarse) voice is commonly noted.[1,4]

PHYSICAL EXAMINATION

With PTA there is marked edema and erythema of the peritonsillar tissue and soft palate; this tissue is often fluctuant and covered with exudate.[4] The findings are almost always unilateral, with the tonsil typically displaced downward and medially. The uvula is often edematous and displaced to the opposite side.[5] Other findings include tender cervical adenopathy, tachycardia, and signs of dehydration. Feelings of intense agitation and anxiety may be present, signaling an emergent airway disaster.

DIAGNOSTICS

PTAs are easily diagnosed on the basis of physical findings. A CT scan with contrast will confirm abscess formation and the presence of gas. Ultrasonography, either oral or cutaneous, in a cooperative, nonemergent patient can also be a useful diagnostic tool.[1] Pediatric patients usually are not cooperative enough to use this technique.

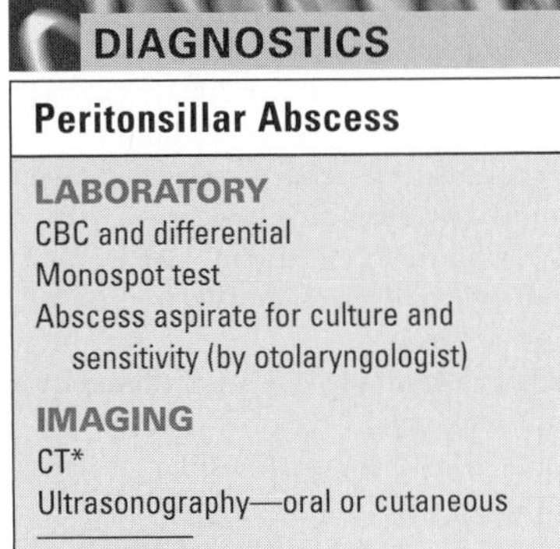
DIAGNOSTICS

Peritonsillar Abscess

LABORATORY
CBC and differential
Monospot test
Abscess aspirate for culture and sensitivity (by otolaryngologist)

IMAGING
CT*
Ultrasonography—oral or cutaneous

*If indicated.

A CBC often reveals leukocytosis. A Monospot test may be performed to exclude infectious mononucleosis. Aspiration of the abscess for culture and sensitivity typically reveals both aerobic and anaerobic bacteria.

DIFFERENTIAL DIAGNOSIS

When considering a diagnosis of PTA, the health care provider must exclude other conditions that manifest with similar signs and symptoms. These conditions include infectious mononucleosis; tumors; cervical adenitis; epiglottitis; retropharyngeal abscesses; aneurysms of the internal carotid artery; and dental, salivary gland, or mastoid infections.

Infectious mononucleosis can be excluded on the basis of clinical presentation, physical examination, and serologic findings. With mononucleosis, headache, malaise, fatigue, and anorexia are typically present before the sore throat. A tumor in the peritonsillar region is eliminated from diagnostic consideration by a lack of the physical findings usually present in an infectious process. A CT scan and, possibly, a biopsy are indicated if a tumor is suspected.

The signs and symptoms of PTAs are similar to those of epiglottitis, which is a potentially fatal condition if not diagnosed. Epiglottitis is less likely when there is peritonsillar swelling with preserved ability to swallow and no stridor auscultated over the larynx on physical examination. Indirect visualization of the epiglottis is a reliable method in the adult and may be necessary to exclude epiglottitis as a cause of symptoms.

DIFFERENTIAL DIAGNOSIS

Peritonsillar Abscess

- Infectious mononucleosis
- Tumors
- Cervical adenitis
- Epiglottitis
- Retropharyngeal abscess
- Aneurysm of internal carotid artery
- Dental, salivary, or mastoid infection

Cervical adenitis and retropharyngeal abscesses may be similar in their presentation. Both conditions reveal an ill or toxic patient, with signs of infection and neck pain. A retropharyngeal abscess can be identified with a CT scan. Dental, salivary, and mastoid infections can be excluded by observing the physical appearance of the oropharynx. Dental and salivary infections are more localized to the floor of the mouth, and mastoid infections are localized behind the affected ear. An absence of infectious signs and symptoms helps distinguish an aneurysm of the internal carotid artery from other causes. If an aneurysm of the internal carotid artery is suspected, an MRI or ultrasound is necessary.

MANAGEMENT

Oral antibiotic therapy is not sufficient for effective treatment of a PTA. Surgical intervention is required with needle aspiration, incision and drainage, or tonsillectomy. The majority of PTAs can be treated effectively with needle aspiration, antibiotics, and pain medication.[6] A tonsillectomy may be indicated in certain situations; it is rare to develop a PTA after tonsillectomy. Tonsillectomy is indicated for PTA associated with a history of chronic or recurrent tonsillitis or for an unusual presentation of the abscess.[1,2] Optimum hydration of the patient must be maintained, either orally or IV. A recent prospective study by Ozbek, Aygenc, Tuna, and others looked at the use of IV antibiotics plus a single high dose of IV steroids versus IV antibiotics alone in PTA patients.[7] The steroid dose was investigated to determine the possible relief of fever, pain, trismus, and dysphagia. The researchers concluded that steroid use before antibiotic therapy was more effective than antibiotic use alone.

As an adjunct to surgical intervention, the antibiotic regimen otolaryngologists prefer is cephalexin or another first-generation cephalosporin, with or without metronidazole, because of penicillin-resistant microorganisms. Alternative therapy includes the use of cefuroxime (with or without metronidazole); clindamycin; or, if mononucleosis has been excluded, amoxicillin-clavulanate.[8]

LIFE SPAN CONSIDERATIONS

Although PTA is an entity of the young, a high index of suspicion must be maintained in all age-groups. Early detection and treatment can prevent a life-threatening complication.

COMPLICATIONS

Serious and potentially fatal complications may result from a PTA. The abscess can result in airway obstruction from spread of the infection. Rupture of the abscess with aspiration of the infected material can cause severe and serious sequelae. If untreated, the infection may spread to involve the superior constrictor muscle, other deep spaces of the neck, and the mediastinum.[6] Necrosis of the muscle may result. Internal jugular vein thrombosis with septic pulmonary embolism can also occur.

Other complications of PTA include thrombophlebitis, chronic PTA, glottic edema, epiglottitis, septicemia, endocarditis, myocarditis, and hemorrhage. Poststreptococcal complications such as rheumatic fever and glomerulonephritis may result if the infected material consists of group A beta hemolytic streptococcus (GABHS). Thrombosis of the internal jugular vein (Lemierre's syndrome) is a rare sequela, usually the result of infection with *Fusobacterium necrophorum*. IV antibiotic therapy and surgical treatment of the abscess are required. Ligation or excision of the internal jugular vein is mandatory if septic emboli are noted. Anticoagulation therapy is a controversial issue for this syndrome.[2]

INDICATIONS FOR REFERRAL OR HOSPITALIZATION

After diagnosis of a PTA has been made, patients should be referred immediately to an otolaryngologist for an evaluation concerning surgical intervention and antibiotic therapy. Hospitalization may not be necessary, although the patient is usually hospitalized after aspiration and started on IV antibiotics. Patients may be discharged in 24 hours or less if symptoms subside and the abscess does not reappear. A follow-up visit with an otolaryngologist is necessary if tonsillectomy is indicated.

PATIENT AND FAMILY EDUCATION

Education concerning PTA as a complication of tonsillitis is important. PTA can recur, and therefore the signs and symptoms should be described to the patient and family. These include fever, chills, malaise, odynophagia, ear pain, inability to open the mouth, dysphagia, drooling, and a "hot potato" voice. The provider should also discuss the possible side effects of antibiotic therapy. These side effects may include nausea, vomiting, diarrhea, abdominal pain, lethargy, vaginitis, or a secondary yeast infection. Signs and symptoms of an allergic reaction, including urticaria, shortness of breath, wheezing, or tightness in the chest, indicate the necessity for immediate emergency treatment.

Patients should be informed that penicillin can decrease the effectiveness of oral contraceptives; therefore a back-up method of contraception is advised for the entire pill cycle in which antibiotic use occurs. In addition, penicillin is best absorbed on an empty stomach.

HEALTH PROMOTION

Patients with histories of recurrent tonsillitis, chronic tonsillitis, and inadequately treated tonsillitis should be monitored closely for signs of PTA. Consultation with an otolaryngologist is a must for these patients. The provider must stress that the patient complete any antimicrobial therapy regimen to minimize the development of resistant strains of bacteria.

REFERENCES

1. Steyer TE: Peritonsillar abscess: diagnosis and treatment, *Am Fam Phys* 65(1):93-96, 2002 [erratum in *Am Fam Phys* 66(1):30, 2002], retrieved Dec 16, 2006, from http://www.aafp.org/afp/20020101/93.html.
2. Shah UK: Tonsillitis and peritonsillar abscess, March 30, 2006, retrieved Dec 16, 2006, from http://www.emedicine.com.
3. Herzon FS: Peritonsillar abscess: incidence, current management practices, and a proposal for treatment guidelines, *Laryngoscope* 105(8 Pt 3 Suppl 74):1-17, 1995.
4. Kazzi AA, El-Sayed M: *Peritonsillar abscess*, Aug 7, 2004, retrieved Dec 16, 2006, from http://www.emedicine.com/.
5. Licamelli GR, Grillone GA: Inferior pole peritonsillar abscess, *Otolaryngol Head Neck Surg* 118:95-99, 1998.
6. Millan SB, Cumming WA: Supraglottic airway infections, *Prim Care* 23(4):741-758, 1996.
7. Ozbek C, Aygenc E, Tuna EU, and others: Use of steroids in the treatment of peritonsillar abscess, *J Laryngol Otol* 118:439-442, 2004.
8. Fairbanks DNF: *Pocket guide to antimicrobial therapy in otolaryngology–head and neck surgery*, Alexandria, Va, 2001, American Academy of Otolaryngology–Head and Neck Surgery Foundation.

CHAPTER 106

Pharyngitis and Tonsillitis

Debra S. Munsell

DEFINITION AND EPIDEMIOLOGY

Pharyngitis is a condition that encompasses infection or irritation of the pharynx and tonsils.[1] A common illness affecting both children and adults, pharyngitis is a common reason for people to seek health care.[2] Pharyngitis can manifest as an acute illness or a chronic condition. The causes are numerous and include both infectious and noninfectious agents.

Noninfectious causes of pharyngitis include referred pain, allergies, trauma from foreign bodies or burns, cancer, chemotherapy, radiation, psychosomatic illness, and irritation. Irritation of the pharynx may result from dust, smoke, dryness, or toxins, either inhaled or swallowed.

Infectious agents responsible for pharyngitis include viruses, bacteria, and, uncommonly, fungi or parasites. Viral infection is the most common cause of pharyngitis in all age-groups and can occur during any season.[3] The most common viruses, responsible for 6% to 20% of all cases, are the rhinovirus and adenovirus.[1] Other responsible agents include the Epstein-Barr virus, which causes mononucleosis; herpes simplex virus; influenza virus; parainfluenza virus; and cytomegalovirus.

The most common cause of bacterial infection is *Streptococcus pyogenes. S. pyogenes* includes groups A, C, and G β-hemolytic streptococcus. Group A β-hemolytic streptococcus (GABHS) is the most important to identify, since it is responsible for acute rheumatic fever (ARF) and poststreptococcal glomerulonephritis. GABHS typically peaks in the late winter and early spring, but it can be seen year round. Group C disease is more common among college students and adolescents. Community-wide and food-borne causes of pharyngitis have been connected to group G organisms.[1] Other offending agents include mycoplasmas, *Arcanobacterium haemolyticum,* chlamydiae, *Neisseria gonorrhoeae,* corynebacteria, and anaerobic bacteria.

Tonsillitis and pharyngitis are similar in clinical presentation, physical findings, diagnosis, and management (Color Plate 37). Tonsillitis is an acute or chronic inflammation of the tonsils and usually results from GABHS infection, although it may be caused by other bacteria or viruses. Tonsillitis may not be a concern unless the patient is symptomatic.

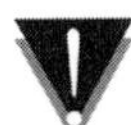

Immediate emergency department referral or physician consultation is indicated for pharyngeal abscess.

PATHOPHYSIOLOGY

The normal flora of the oral pharynx region consists of various and numerous microorganisms. These microorganisms are not harmful unless the immune system is weakened, resulting in increased susceptibility to illness. Pharyngitis or tonsillitis develops from exposure to a viral or bacterial agent, although some people can harbor or be colonized with pathogenic bacteria and remain free of infection.

Debate about the possibility of family pets acting as reservoirs for group A streptococcal infection is sometimes raised. At this point no credible evidence supports the idea of pets as reservoirs or as contributors to familial spread.[4]

CLINICAL PRESENTATION

The clinical presentation of pharyngitis or tonsillitis varies depending on the offending agent. Noninfectious pharyngitis has a somewhat different initial appearance from infectious pharyngitis. Typically, with noninfectious pharyngitis the patient reports a sore throat and dryness; if environmental allergens are the cause, symptoms often include rhinorrhea, watery eyes, and postnasal drip. Patients receiving radiation or chemotherapy may complain of pain, dryness, and dysphagia. Oropharyngeal candidiasis (thrush) may be present in these patients secondary to the immunosuppression.

The infectious causes of pharyngitis or tonsillitis are bacterial and viral. The presentation of symptoms can be similar. Viral causes are more common, and typically patients report the sudden onset of a sore throat, fever, malaise, cough, headache, myalgias, and fatigue. Patients may also report rhinitis, conjunctivitis (adenovirus), congestion, and a cough with sputum production.

One of the most common causes of bacterial pharyngitis or tonsillitis is GABHS. This disease is most prevalent in children under the age of 15 years. Patients may report a sudden onset of sore throat, painful swallowing, fever, chills, headache, nausea, vomiting, and abdominal pain.[1] With bacterial pharyngitis, rhinitis, cough, conjunctivitis, and myalgias are not typically present.

Other bacterial causes should be investigated if indicated, since *N. gonorrhoeae* and *Chlamydia* organisms can cause pharyngitis. Other bacteria such as group C and G streptococci, *M. pneumoniae,* and *A. haemolyticum* can be involved.[5] Often these patients report mild throat discomfort in addition to urethritis or vaginitis.

PHYSICAL EXAMINATION

In viral pharyngitis, findings include mild erythema with little or no pharyngeal exudate, although the pharynx may appear swollen, boggy, or pale.[6] Painful or tender lymphadenopathy is not typically present. Infectious mononucleosis typically produces pharyngeal erythema, tonsillar hypertrophy, white to gray-green exudate, petechiae at the junction of the hard and soft palate, and posterior cervical adenopathy. Hepatomegaly and splenomegaly may be identified in fewer than 50% of patients. Jaundice may be present, but that is unusual.[3]

In GABHS infection the physical examination reveals marked erythema of the throat and tonsils; patchy, discrete, white or yellowish exudate; and tender anterior cervical adenopathy (see Color Plate 37). Pressure on the tonsillar pillars may produce purulent drainage. The uvula may also be edematous, and fever greater than 38.3° C (101° F) is typical. Occasionally GABHS may be seen with an erythematous, persistent sore throat with little fever and no exudate.

DIAGNOSTICS

Although it is sometimes difficult to differentiate between viral and bacterial pharyngitis or tonsillitis, clinical presentation may indicate the diagnosis. No specific diagnostic test exists for viral pharyngitis.[3]

Diagnostic studies used to detect GABHS include a throat culture, rapid antigen detection test (RADT), and sometimes an antistreptolysin (ASO) titer. The ASO titer is not used during initial diagnostic screening but is obtained to identify or confirm a diagnosis of GABHS weeks to months after the infection. The RADT is often used because it is rapid and convenient. However, the RADT is less sensitive (true positives) than a throat culture. If the diagnosis of GABHS is suspected and the RADT result is negative, a throat culture is performed for confirmation. A CBC often reveals leukocytosis with GABHS.

Many studies have evaluated the efficacy of a clinical scoring system in the diagnosis of GABHS pharyngitis. Many medical societies have recommended various clinical indicators in an attempt to standardize diagnosis. The Centor criteria—tonsillar exudate; swollen, tender anterior cervical lymph nodes; and lack of cough and history of fever—have proven to be predictive of a positive diagnosis in adult patients.[7] Many other screening criteria can be located to address children and pharyngitis.

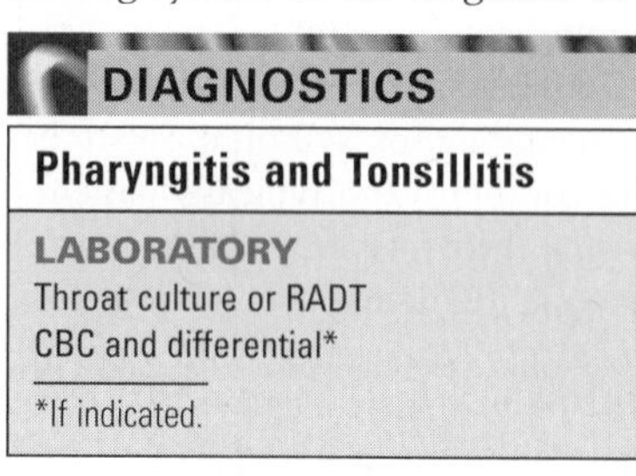

DIAGNOSTICS

Pharyngitis and Tonsillitis

LABORATORY

Throat culture or RADT

CBC and differential*

*If indicated.

DIFFERENTIAL DIAGNOSIS

The presence of an inflamed pharynx requires further investigation. The differential diagnosis should include infectious mononucleosis, allergies, thrush, peritonsillar cellulitis or abscess, pharyngeal abscess, epiglottitis, leukoplakia, and upper respiratory tract infection.

Infectious mononucleosis differs from pharyngitis or tonsillitis in clinical presentation, physical examination, and serologic findings. This diagnosis is seen more commonly in adolescents and young adults.[6] These patients usually are seen with headache, malaise, fatigue, and anorexia before the sore throat occurs. Hepatosplenomegaly may be noted during the physical examination. A CBC often reveals leukocytosis with atypical lymphocytes. A positive Monospot test reveals heterophil antibodies. The Monospot test is highly specific and sensitive, but it may take 1 to 2 weeks to produce a positive result. Therefore an initial false-negative finding may occur.

DIFFERENTIAL DIAGNOSIS

Pharyngitis and Tonsillitis

- Infectious mononucleosis
- Allergies
- Thrush
- Peritonsillar cellulitis or abscess
- Epiglottitis
- Upper respiratory tract infection
- Diphtheria
- Trauma
- Cancer
- Chemotherapy
- Radiation
- Irritation
- Viral, bacterial, fungal infection

Associated symptoms of teary, watery discharge from the eyes; pruritus; rhinitis; postnasal drip; pale, boggy nasal mucosa; and an erythematous pharynx with mucus are commonly seen with seasonal allergies. Thrush, a white, thick, cheese-like material that can be scraped off, is identified with a positive potassium hydroxide test result. Peritonsillar cellulitis differs from pharyngitis by the physical examination and the absence of pus on aspiration. Peritonsillar abscess can be diagnosed by presenting signs and symptoms and the aspiration of pus. Tonsillitis may be present with pharyngitis.

Although presenting signs and symptoms of an upper respiratory tract infection (URI) are similar to those of viral pharyngitis, a URI usually has associated symptoms such as cough, congestion, rhinitis, sneezing, injected conjunctiva, erythematous and edematous nasal mucosa, and an erythematous pharynx. Epiglottitis must be excluded by radiographic imaging or direct laryngoscopy once it is suspected; typically, however, patients with epiglottitis cannot effectively swallow even their own saliva.

Severe exudative pharyngitis or tonsillitis is usually present in mononucleosis. A thick, gray membrane over the tonsils and pharynx is indicative of diphtheria. Leukoplakia, a white patch, is a premalignant change that may arise anywhere on the oral mucosa (Color Plate 36). If it is suspected, a thorough history is warranted. If the lesion remains for more than 2 weeks, a biopsy is indicated.

MANAGEMENT

The most recent recommendations from the American College of Physicians in 2001 stressed the importance of not using antibiotic therapy unless there is strong evidence suggesting the presence of GABHS.[7] Criteria for treatment includes history of fever, exudative tonsillitis, anterior cervical lymphadenopathy that is tender, and absence of cough.[7] Antibiotic therapy (penicillin V 250 mg q.i.d. for 10 days) is indicated in GABHS pharyngitis to prevent complications. A one-time dose of benzathine penicillin, 1.2 million units IM, has also been proven effective. Penicillin is often prescribed because of the low cost, safety, and efficacy. Amoxicillin 250 mg t.i.d. to q.i.d. or 500 mg b.i.d. for 10 days is also appropriate. Erythromycin 250 mg q.i.d. for 10 days is indicated for patients with penicillin allergy.

A first- or second-generation cephalosporin is effective initially or for recurrent disease. There is a small chance, however, of cephalosporin allergy if the patient is allergic to penicillin. Clindamycin and amoxicillin-clavulanate have proven effective in recurrent episodes of GABHS pharyngitis. One of the macrolides, azithromycin, offers the convenience of once-a-day dosing for 5 days and has been proven effective, but it is expensive. The supportive measures described with viral pharyngitis also apply to GABHS pharyngitis or tonsillitis.

Treatment for non–group A streptococci is given for symptomatic relief, since the organisms are not linked to serious sequelae and do not produce a major antibody response.[1] Penicillin or erythromycin is effective, but the duration of treatment remains unclear.

Treatment of viral pharyngitis includes rest, fluids, humidification, voice rest, and warm saline gargles to ease discomfort. Acetaminophen or ibuprofen should be used for fever and general discomfort. Topical anesthetic sprays and throat lozenges are of benefit; however, they may produce further irritation in a small number of individuals.

Management of chronic pharyngitis or tonsillitis with GABHS infection may require tonsillectomy, although tonsillectomy is not done as often as in the past. Current recommendations suggest six or seven documented episodes of GABHS pharyngitis or tonsillitis within 1 year, five episodes a year for 2 consecutive years, or three episodes a year for 3 years before tonsillectomy is warranted.

LIFE SPAN CONSIDERATIONS

More than 40 million visits occur annually for pharyngitis in the adult population. More prescriptions are written for treatment of pharyngitis than any other respiratory infection, including pneumonia and otitis.[8] Reflux laryngitis is another cause for pharyngitis. Clearly, pharyngitis is an entity that affects all age-groups and populations. A comprehensive head and neck examination and history are required to accurately assess the situation and prescribe appropriate treatment. Pharyngitis that lasts more than 2 weeks in an adult smoker should be considered a cancer unless proven otherwise. Prompt and proper diagnosis of patients who truly have *S. pyogenes* infections can have a significant effect on the morbidity of the disease.[9]

COMPLICATIONS

Complications from chronic tonsillitis include upper airway obstruction, sleep apnea, and sleep disturbances. Peritonsillar cellulitis or abscess, retropharyngeal abscess, scarlet fever, ARF, and poststreptococcal glomerulonephritis may result if GABHS infections are untreated. Unfortunately, glomerulonephritis may result even with proper treatment. ARF can be prevented by prompt antibiotic therapy for the prescribed time.

INDICATIONS FOR REFERRAL OR HOSPITALIZATION

An evaluation by an otolaryngologist should be sought for recurrent GABHS infections or for complications that may result from pharyngitis. In addition, potential airway obstruction from pharyngitis or abscess requires immediate referral to an otolaryngologist and hospitalization. Peritonsillar abscess and retropharyngeal abscess require hospitalization for observation and IV antibiotics. Abscesses usually require incision and drainage. Patients with ARF and poststreptococcal glomerulonephritis may require hospitalization depending on symptoms. Patients diagnosed with ARF require antibiotic prophylaxis, although debate exists regarding the duration of prophylaxis.

PATIENT AND FAMILY EDUCATION

Education is extremely important, and adherence to antibiotic therapy must be stressed. Patients should understand that they are infectious until 24 hours after the start of antibiotic therapy and that a full course of antibiotics is needed to prevent reinfection or complications.

Education stresses adherence to prescribed therapy to ensure eradication of organisms. Possible side effects of antibiotic therapy, including allergic reaction, nausea, vomiting, diarrhea, abdominal pain, lethargy, vaginitis, and secondary yeast infection, should be explained. Signs and symptoms of an allergic reaction, such as urticaria (hives), shortness of breath, wheezing, or tightness in the chest, mandate immediate medical attention. Furthermore, since penicillin can decrease the effectiveness of oral contraceptives, additional contraception is recommended for the entire pill cycle in which the antibiotics are used. All patients with GABHS should be instructed to call the health care provider if symptoms escalate or if respiratory distress or difficulty swallowing develops. In general, patients should start to feel better 24 to 48 hours after the start of antibiotic therapy. Patients should be encouraged to use a new toothbrush 48 hours after antibiotic therapy is started to decrease the possibility of a recurrent infection. The old toothbrush should be discarded.

Education for the patient with viral pharyngitis is important. Supportive measures should be encouraged. Patients can expect symptom resolution of the pharyngitis over a 1- to 3-week period. Antibiotics are inappropriate in viral infections, but patients and families may require considerable teaching to understand the importance of avoiding antibiotic therapy when appropriate.

HEALTH PROMOTION

Health promotion involving pharyngitis covers many areas. Proper oral hygiene should be addressed with all age-groups at all visits. Education regarding the misuse of antibiotic therapy for viral entities should also be stressed. Of importance is teaching patients, families, and health care workers the importance and need for appropriate hand-washing technique. Limiting exposure to individuals with pharyngitis must also be included in patient teaching. Evaluation for age-appropriate immunization status should be stressed.

REFERENCES

1. Middleton DB: Pharyngitis, *Prim Care* 23(4):719-739, 1996.
2. Centor R, Meier F: Sore throat. In Dornbrand L, Hoole A, Pickard CG, editors: *Manual of clinical problems in adult ambulatory care,* Boston, 1992, Little, Brown.
3. Ruppert SD: Differential diagnosis of common causes of pediatric pharyngitis, *Nurse Pract* 21:38-48, 1996.
4. Bisno AL: Diagnosis and management of group A streptococcal pharyngitis: a practice guideline, *Clin Infect Dis* 25:574-583, 1997.
5. Dajani A, Taubert K, Ferrieri P, and others: Treatment of acute streptococcal pharyngitis and prevention of rheumatic fever: a statement for health professionals, *Pediatrics* 96(4 Pt 1):758-764, 1995, retrieved Dec 16, 2006, from http://www.americanheart.org/presenter.jhtml?identifier=1244.
6. Seller R: *Differential diagnosis of common complaints,* Philadelphia, 1993, Saunders.
7. Cooper RJ, Hoffman JR, Bartlett JR, and others: Principles of appropriate antibiotic use for acute pharyngitis in adults, *Ann Intern Med* 134(6):509-517, 2001.
8. Centor RM, Witherspoon JM, Dalton HP, and others: The diagnosis of strep throat in adults in the emergency room, *Med Decis Making* 1(3):239-246, 1981.
9. Stephenson KN: Acute and chronic pharyngitis across the lifespan, *Lippincotts Primary Care Pract* 4(5):471-489, 2000.

PART 10

Evaluation and Management of Pulmonary Disorders

PATRICIA POLGAR BAILEY, *Section Editor*

CHAPTER 107

Acute Bronchitis

Patricia Polgar Bailey

DEFINITION AND EPIDEMIOLOGY

Acute bronchitis is a transient inflammation of the trachea and major bronchi. Clinically, it is diagnosed on the basis of acute cough, with or without phlegm, and occasionally dyspnea and wheezing; it is usually associated with a generalized upper respiratory tract infection (URI).[1,2] The diagnosis is usually made in the autumn and winter months, when other URIs occur with frequency.[2]

Each year approximately 12 million episodes of acute bronchitis occur in individuals 18 years and older in the United States.[3] Acute URIs account for 70% of primary diagnoses made during ambulatory visits for cough-related illness.[1] In more than 90% of cases of acute bronchitis, the cause is associated with common cold viruses such as rhinovirus and coronavirus or with more invasive viruses such as influenza and adenovirus.[4,5] Less common nonviral causes of acute bronchitis include *Bordetella pertussis, Mycoplasma pneumoniae,* and *Chlamydia pneumoniae* (as distinguished from *Chlamydia trachomatis,* which causes pneumonia in neonates).

Despite evidence that viruses play a significant role in the development of acute bronchitis, it has been identified as one of the conditions for which antibiotics are most frequently overprescribed. Research indicates that 60% to 80% of adults with acute bronchitis receive antibiotic prescriptions, despite the fact that the vast majority of acute respiratory infections have a viral cause.[6] Studies of uncomplicated acute bronchitis in the general population demonstrate little benefit from antibiotic use, even with smokers. Any benefit demonstrated has been of questionable clinical significance (i.e., 0.5 days less of symptoms), which is offset by the risk of antibiotic use, including medication side effects, drug-drug interactions, financial burden, and the possibility of future antibiotic resistance.[7,8]

PATHOPHYSIOLOGY

Acute bronchitis causes edematous changes in the mucous membrane of the tracheobronchial tree and an increase in secretions. Destruction of the bronchial epithelium and loss of ciliary function is usually minimum with the common cold viruses but may be more extensive with *M. pneumoniae* and influenza viruses. Cigarette smoking and chemical irritants may increase the severity of the infection. Undiagnosed asthma may be a factor, but this can be difficult to establish because of the transient bronchial hyperresponsiveness (and abnormal spirometry results) that often accompany acute bronchitis.[2]

CLINICAL PRESENTATION AND PHYSICAL EXAMINATION

A cough with or without sputum production is the most common symptom reported with acute bronchitis. It begins early in the course of the URI. The sputum may be clear at the onset of the infection and become mucoid. The cough may also produce a burning substernal pain with inspiration. Nasal and pharyngeal symptoms subside after 3 or 4 days, but the cough usually remains prominent and progressive. A low-grade fever, wheezes, rhonchi, and coarse rales may be present. However, substantial abnormalities in vital signs are infrequent, especially in the elderly, even when symptoms have been present for a week or more.[6]

Because acute bronchitis is a clinical diagnosis, how providers assign the diagnosis varies. For example, some providers diagnose acute bronchitis only if a productive cough is present, whereas others make the determination based on the presence of purulent sputum.[2] Community-acquired pneumonia should be suspected if the patient's history includes dyspnea, high fever, tachycardia, evidence of consolidation on examination, or the presence of symptoms for 2 or more weeks.[5] Infection with *B. pertussis* should also be suspected in adults who have a paroxysmal cough lasting longer than 2 weeks, especially in the context of a community outbreak. Although infection with *B. pertussis* is not life threatening in adults, it is important that it be diagnosed because of the complications it can cause in older adults or in infants who have not been vaccinated against the disease.

DIAGNOSTICS

No diagnostic tests are necessary for acute bronchitis. Routine sputum cultures are not helpful because the nasopharyngeal area is colonized with bacterial flora. However, nasopharyngeal cultures should be obtained if *B. pertussis* or the influenza virus is suspected.

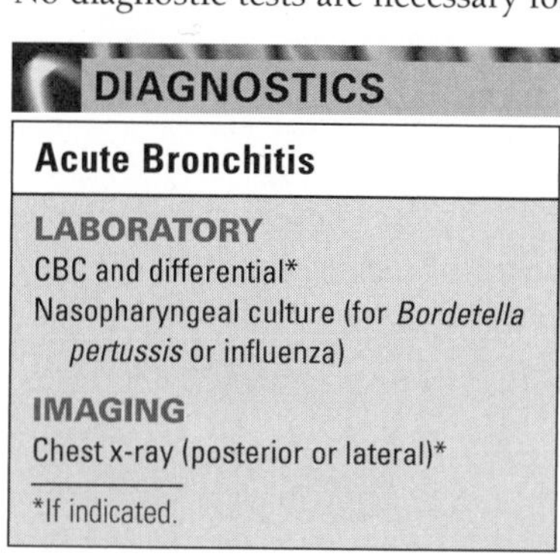

DIAGNOSTICS

Acute Bronchitis

LABORATORY

CBC and differential*

Nasopharyngeal culture (for *Bordetella pertussis* or influenza)

IMAGING

Chest x-ray (posterior or lateral)*

*If indicated.

A chest radiograph may be useful if the history and physical examination suggest the possibility of community-acquired pneumonia. A heightened suspicion of community-acquired pneumonia is reasonable in older adults because they may be seen initially with more subtle symptoms of lower respiratory tract infections.

DIFFERENTIAL DIAGNOSIS

DIFFERENTIAL DIAGNOSIS

Acute Bronchitis

- Asthma
- Chronic lung disease
- Foreign body aspiration
- Influenza
- Pertussis
- Pneumonia
- Rhinitis
- Severe acute respiratory syndrome (SARS)
- Sinusitis
- Tuberculosis
- Tumors

The vast majority of cases of acute bronchitis are viral.[5,6] Since pneumonia is the third most common cause of cough illness (following asthma) and potentially the most serious, the primary objective should be to exclude pneumonia, which is often bacterial in origin and requires antimicrobial therapy. Other differential diagnoses include rhinitis, sinusitis, foreign body aspiration, tuberculosis, tumors, and other chronic lung diseases.

MANAGEMENT

The mainstay of treatment in acute bronchitis is directed toward symptom reduction. Because most cases of acute bronchitis are viral, antibiotics are generally not warranted. Decreasing the cough with a dextromethorphan cough preparation (30 mg/5 ml, 1 to 2 teaspoons PO q 4 hr as needed; maximum of 4 doses/day) or benzonatate is reasonable. Codeine or hydrocodone may be useful at bedtime if the cough is severe. Antipyretics, bed rest, and increased fluid consumption to thin the secretions are also beneficial treatments. The use of β-adrenergic bronchodilators is a treatment option that may be beneficial, if wheezing is present.[7]

Reassurance and education are probably the most important modalities for treatment of acute bronchitis. For at least a decade, randomized, placebo-controlled trials have failed to demonstrate a role for antibiotic treatment of acute bronchitis. Based on this, in 1998 the U.S. Food and Drug Administration removed uncomplicated acute bronchitis as an indication for any additional trials of antimicrobial therapy. Since then, three published meta-analyses have reported no impact of antibiotic treatment on the duration of illness, activity limitation, and work loss associated with acute bronchitis.[2,5,8] Based on these data and the rapid emergence of antibiotic-resistant strains of bacteria, routine antibiotic treatment for acute bronchitis in adults is not justified.

Antibiotic therapy is recommended if pertussis is suspected. Pertussis is an acute bacterial infection of the respiratory tract caused by *B. pertussis*, a gram-negative bacterium. *B. pertussis* is transmitted primarily through aerosolized droplets of respiratory secretions or by direct contact with an infected person.[9] Studies indicate that pertussis may be present in 10% to 20% of patients with cough lasting longer than 2 weeks. Unfortunately, distinguishing pertussis from other sources of acute cough is difficult, since pertussis in adults with previous immunity does not lead to the classic features of whooping cough, which are seen in children. Suspicion of pertussis should be limited to individuals with a high probability of exposure, such as in community outbreaks.[1] Antimicrobial treatment of pertussis does not tend to improve symptoms unless it is started within 1 week of symptom onset, but it is thought to decrease shedding of the bacteria and in that way limit spread of the disease. Erythromycin has been the antimicrobial agent of choice for the treatment or postexposure prophylaxis of pertussis and is usually prescribed as 2 g/day in 4 divided doses for 14 days. Other macrolide antibiotics, including clarithromycin (1 g/day in 2 divided doses for 7 days) and azithromycin (500 mg on day 1, followed by 250 mg on days 2 to 5) can also be used.[9]

The most common pathogen isolated in acute bronchitis is influenza; therefore antiinfluenza agents, such as the neuroaminidase inhibiters, may be effective if influenza is diagnosed and treatment initiated within 48 hours after onset of symptoms (see Chapter 246). Since pneumonia is the third most common cause of cough illness, the presence of pneumonia should be excluded. Even though elderly persons may not always manifest the typical features of pneumonia, such as fever and other vital sign abnormalities, the predictive value of these simple clinical tools remains high and should not be neglected. For atypical manifestations of pneumonia in the elderly, such as diminished appetite, increased falls, and altered mental status, see Chapter 118.

Patients frequently expect to receive antibiotics for acute bronchitis, perhaps because they received antibiotics for similar symptoms in the past. Research indicates that patient satisfaction with an office visit for acute bronchitis does not depend on receiving antimicrobial therapy but rather is centered on the nature of the provider-patient relationship as experienced during that visit. Even though acute bronchitis is a common diagnosis that resolves on its own, patients' satisfaction is primarily related to how much time was spent explaining the illness and answering their questions.[2]

COMPLICATIONS

Although acute bronchitis is often viral and self-limiting, complications do occur. The development of a chronic cough, usually the result of postbronchitis reactive airway disease, can cause discomfort and sleep loss. Pneumonia results from bacterial superinfection and can cause dyspnea, chest pain, and anxiety in addition to other symptoms. If the cough lasts 3 weeks or longer, a chest x-ray study is indicated in the absence of other known causes.[2] Acute respiratory failure, although uncommon, is a potential sequela. Individuals with chronic bronchitis are more susceptible to superinfection and can develop exercise intolerance and hypoxia.

INDICATIONS FOR REFERRAL OR HOSPITALIZATION

Acute bronchitis that does not respond to symptomatic treatment and lingers longer than 2 weeks may require physician referral. Patients with progressive dyspnea, oxygen saturation less than 90%, and signs of sepsis require hospitalization for IV therapy, enhanced pulmonary therapy, and IV antibiotics.

PATIENT AND FAMILY EDUCATION

Education should include a realistic expectation of the duration of the cough (generally 10 to 14 days) and the general ineffectiveness of antibiotic therapy for this diagnosis. Rest, increased fluids, and breathing of moist air from a clean humidifier or warm shower should be encouraged. Patients should be counseled about smoking cessation and the need to avoid air pollution and irritants. An appropriate face mask can be helpful if work involves chemicals, dust, or other irritants. Patients should be encouraged to call their health care provider if the symptoms continue or increase in severity.

Additional patient education information can be obtained from the American Lung Association, 61 Broadway, 6th floor, New York, NY 10006; (800) 586-4872; http://www.lungusa.org.

REFERENCES

1. Wark P: Acute bronchitis, *Clin Evidence Concise* 14:465-466, 2005.
2. Snow V, Mottur-Pilson C, Gonzales R: Principles of appropriate antibiotic use for treatment of acute bronchitis in adults, *Ann Intern Med* 134(6):518-520, 2001.
3. Gonzales R, Sande M: Uncomplicated acute bronchitis, *Ann Intern Med* 133(12):981-991, 2000.
4. Stone S, Gonzales R, Maselli J, and others: Antibiotic prescribing for patients with colds, upper respiratory tract infections, and bronchitis: a

national study of hospital based emergency departments, *Ann Emerg Med* 36(4):320-327, 2000.
5. Gonzales R, Bartlett JG, Besser RE, and others: Principles of appropriate antibiotic use for treatment of uncomplicated acute bronchitis: background, *Ann Emerg Med* 37(6):720-727, 2001.
6. Steinman M, Sauaia A, Maselli J, and others: Office evaluation and treatment of elderly patients with acute bronchitis, *J Am Geriatr Soc* 52:875-879, 2004.
7. Irwin RS, Baumann MH, Bolser DC, and others: Diagnosis and management of cough executive summary. In American College of Chest Physicians: *ACCP Evidence-Based Clinical Practice Guidelines* 129:1S-23S, 2006, retrieved Dec 27, 2006, from http://www.chestjournal.org/cgi/content/full/129/1_suppl/1S.
8. Edmonds M: Antibiotic treatment for acute bronchitis, *Ann Emerg Med* 40(1):110-112, 2002.
9. Tiwari T, Murphy TV, Moran J, and others: Recommended antimicrobial agents for the treatment and postexposure prophylaxis of pertussis, *MMWR Recomm Rep* 54(RR-14):1-16, 2005.

CHAPTER 108

Asthma

Patricia Polgar Bailey

DEFINITION AND EPIDEMIOLOGY

Asthma is a chronic inflammatory disorder of the airways characterized by increased responsiveness of the tracheobronchial tree to various stimuli, resulting in episodic reversible narrowing and inflammation of the airways.[1,2] In susceptible individuals this bronchial inflammation causes recurrent episodes of wheezing, shortness of breath, chest tightness, and cough. These episodes are usually associated with widespread but variable airflow obstruction that is often reversible, either spontaneously or with treatment. The inflammation also causes an associated increase in the existing bronchial hyperresponsiveness to a variety of stimuli.[2,3]

Asthma attacks can vary from mild to life threatening and can be triggered by many factors, including allergens, infections, exercise, abrupt changes in weather, or exposure to airway irritants such as tobacco smoke.[2] The concept of asthma as a chronic and inflammatory process represents a change in the previous understanding of the disease and has important implications for its management.

Asthma is the most common chronic respiratory disorder among all age-groups, and the burden from asthma in the United States has increased over the past 2 decades.[1] In 2002, 30.8 million people (111 people per 1000) had been diagnosed with asthma during their lifetime, a prevalence of approximately 11%,[1] which represents an increase of 75% since 1980.[4] The current asthma prevalence is higher in children (8.9 million children <7 years of age affected) compared with adults (21.9 million affected); the prevalence rate is 12.2% for children compared with 10.6% for adults. Asthma affects more women than men (8.3% vs. 6.3%, respectively); women are about 7% more likely than men to ever have been diagnosed with asthma, but among children younger than 17 years of age, boys were more likely than girls to receive an asthma diagnosis (13.9% vs. 10.4%, respectively).[1,5] These statistics, as striking as they are, may still underestimate the actual prevalence of asthma. In a recent study of asthma in high school students, 18.9% self-reported lifetime asthma and 16.1% had current asthma.[5]

Among all racial and ethnic groups in the United States, Puerto Ricans have the highest rates of lifetime asthma (19.6%) and Mexicans the lowest (6.1%). Grouping all Hispanics masks the differences in asthma prevalence; compared with non-Hispanic Caucasians, Puerto Ricans are almost 80% more likely, and non-Hispanic African Americans and Native Americans are about 25% more likely, to have ever been diagnosed with asthma.[1]

Asthma attack prevalence refers to the number of people who had at least one asthma attack during the previous year and is a crude indicator of how many people have uncontrolled asthma or are at risk for a poor outcome, such as hospitalization.[1] In 2002 approximately 60% of those diagnosed with asthma reported having an asthma attack within the past year. Asthma attack prevalence decreases with age; 5.8% of children younger than 17 years of age had an asthma attack within the past year compared with 3.7% of adults. Women have a 35% higher asthma attack prevalence than men, but this pattern is reversed among children, in whom the attack prevalence for boys was 45% higher than the rate for girls.[1]

Asthma interferes with daily activities, including attending school and going to work. Among those who report having had one asthma attack within the past year, children younger than 17 years of age missed an average of 14.7 school days because of asthma, and employed adults (18 years of age and older) missed an average of 11.8 work days because of asthma.[1] Occupational asthma is currently the most common occupational ailment. Widespread exposure in the workplace environment to airborne dusts, gases, vapors, or fumes contributes to both the development of asthma and the worsening of asthma for those already afflicted. Lost work productivity is estimated at more than $1000 per person with asthma, or approximately $4.5 billion for all workers affected by asthma.[6]

Asthma is the sixth most common reason for visits in ambulatory settings, and two thirds of patients with asthma obtain their care from a health care provider in a primary care setting.[7-9] Nonetheless, asthma is still responsible for a disproportionate and increasing number of emergency department visits (2 million) and hospitalizations (0.5 million).[10,11] The type of medical setting in which persons receive health care for asthma differs for those with private health insurance and those without health insurance. Approximately 30% of asthma-related medical visits for persons without health insurance occurred in emergency departments, compared with only 6% of visits by those with private insurance.[12] Asthma is a condition that can be treated effectively in primary care, resulting in fewer emergency department visits, improved continuity of care, and decreased health care costs.

The mortality rate for asthma increased 118% from 1970 to 1995,[4] and the mortality rate from asthma remains high. In 2002, 4261 people died from asthma (1.5 per 100,000). Although the asthma prevalence is higher among children, asthma deaths in children are rare. Women have an asthma death rate about 40% higher than that of men.[1] High mortality rates are associated with high rates of hospitalization in impoverished urban areas. Asthma hospitalization rates have been highest among African Americans (19% higher incidence), women, and children; likewise, death rates have consistently been disproportionately higher among African Americans, especially those between 15 and 24 years of age.[3] Although prevalence is higher among racial and ethnic minorities, a more valid relationship may exist between socioeconomic status and increased asthma prevalence, morbidity, and mortality than between race and asthma prevalence. Asthma mortality has also been associated with poverty, urban living conditions, exposure to oxidant pollutants, and passive smoking.[8,13] Allergic asthmatic children exposed to high levels of indoor allergens, such as those associated with cockroaches, rodents, and mold, have more severe and more frequent episodes of asthma.[14]

The financial impact of asthma is considerable. At least 1% of all U.S. health care costs are spent on asthma. Direct and indirect asthma-related costs are estimated to be $12.7 billion per year, with emergency department visits and hospitalizations responsible for the majority of the cost.[11,15] Most of those hospitalized or seen in the emergency department had been there before, reflecting the fact that inadequate health care results in increased costs.[7,14]

Physician consultation is indicated for patients with Sa_{O_2} less than 90% on room air, peak flow less than 70%, and failure to improve with three nebulizer treatments or three epinephrine injections.

PATHOPHYSIOLOGY

It is now believed that the primary event in asthma is airway inflammation and that airway hyperresponsiveness and airflow obstruction are secondary and symptomatic features of the disease. Underlying airway inflammation (which involves cellular infiltration, edema, nerve irritation, and vasodilation) results in constriction of airway smooth muscle, increased mucus production, and airway hyperresponsiveness. Atopy, which is the genetic tendency for developing immunoglobulin E (IgE)–mediated hypersensitivity reactions in response to environmental antigens and allergens, is considered one of the strongest predisposing factors for the development of asthma. Certain stimuli induce asthma by causing or increasing airway inflammation, whereas other stimuli provoke bronchoconstriction in individuals who already have asthma or airway hyperresponsiveness. Inducers, stimuli that are known to increase inflammation, include inhaled allergens, low-molecular-weight sensitizers, viral or mycoplasmal respiratory infections, and high concentrations of noxious gases. Stimuli that trigger or cause bronchoconstriction include exercise, cold air, laughter, emotional upset, and inhaled irritants. Triggers of sudden severe bronchoconstriction include acetylsalicylic acid or NSAIDs, β-adrenergic blockers, food allergens, certain food additives, stings, bites, injections (e.g., allergy shots), and inhaled allergens.[16]

These stimuli set the stage for a cascade of cellular activation, which includes subsequent cytokine release and neurologic excitation. The antigenic response is limited by certain cellular processes such as mast cell activation through cytokines and infiltration by inflammatory cells, including neutrophils, eosinophils, and lymphocytes. The inflammatory cells are also the source of mediators, which induce bronchoconstriction, excess mucus production, airway edema, and further inflammatory cell influx, all of which lead to bronchial obstruction. The late-phase reaction, which generally occurs 3 to 8 hours after antigen exposure, is the result of new cellular infiltration and activation. Nocturnal and early morning bronchospasm, which occurs with relative frequency in persons with asthma, may be related to circadian variations in cortisol and epinephrine levels, vagal tone, and inflammatory mediators.[17]

One common, often overlooked, exacerbating factor of asthma is esophageal reflux of gastric contents. The incidence of gastroesophageal reflux in adults with asthma has been reported to range from 15% to 82% using pH monitoring.[18] Gastroesophageal reflux resulting in distal esophageal stimulation with acid may cause bronchoconstriction or may increase bronchial reactivity via vagal mechanisms. Although the potential mechanism exists for gastroesophageal reflux disease (GERD) to cause asthma symptoms and it is fairly well accepted that GERD may be an exacerbating factor, particularly in "difficult-to-control" asthma, it remains unclear whether there is a true causal relationship between reflux episodes and asthma symptoms. A recent study, involving the largest group of patients with difficult-to-control asthma to date, found that the identification and treatment of GERD failed to improve asthma outcome in the group as a whole. However, this study did not exclude the possibility that antireflux therapy does contribute to asthma control in persons with well-controlled asthma.[18]

Asthma is a disease that varies within and among individuals, but inflammation of the airways is a persistent feature, even in persons with mild asthma. Although asthma is considered to be a disease of reversible airflow obstruction, chronic airway inflammation can lead to progressive airway remodeling and airflow obstruction, eventually resulting in an irreversible deterioration of airway function.[12] At present asthma has no cure, but effective management can reduce its impact on quality of life and morbidity.

CLINICAL PRESENTATION

The clinical hallmarks of asthma include episodic wheezing associated with dyspnea, cough, and sputum production. Between episodes, symptoms may improve or completely resolve. Symptoms vary from mild to severe, with varying effects on activity. An increased index of suspicion for asthma is essential when respiratory symptoms, including cough, wheeze, shortness of breath, chest tightness, or soreness, persist or recur often.[14,19]

Although wheezing is probably the symptom most typically associated with asthma, the most common symptom of asthma and often the most troublesome is coughing. However, coughing is also the third most common presenting symptom in the ambulatory setting, with a corresponding long list of potential causes. Coughing is the only asthma symptom 7% to 57% of the time; this type of asthma is referred to as *cough-variant asthma.* Coughing is often treated symptomatically, which can easily result in a delayed or missed diagnosis of asthma. Asthma should be considered in the differential diagnosis of all patients with a cough, since it is such a common cause. Most persons with a cough do not have associated variable airflow obstruction; if obstruction is present and reversible with bronchodilator medication, the diagnosis of asthma is confirmed.[20]

In addition to chronic cough, asthma has several common clinical presentations. An acute asthmatic episode is characterized by airway obstruction, manifested by symptoms of breathlessness and anxiety, and often accompanied by wheezing and sometimes coughing. These symptoms may resolve within several hours if treatment is given or within 1 to 3 days, even without specific intervention, or they may progress to more severe airway obstruction and respiratory compromise if no therapy is provided. Between acute asthmatic episodes, airflow is normal and symptoms are absent. Several specific conditions are associated with acute asthma exacerbations.

Exercise-induced asthma refers to the development of airway obstruction in an individual after the cessation of exercise, even after brief periods of exercise. Symptoms usually begin 5 to 10 minutes after the completion of exercise and resolve within 1 to 4 hours. Certain forms of exercise, including skiing, ice hockey, and running in the cold, more commonly precipitate airway obstruction; other forms of exercise, such as swimming, less commonly precipitate airway obstruction, probably because of the warmer and more humid air being inspired. Cold or dry air often predisposes an asthmatic individual to airway obstruction, such as occurs, for example, when a person enters a dry, air-conditioned environment (such as an indoor mall) from the warmer, more humid outside air.

Common allergens that precipitate asthma include cat allergen (dander), house dust mite allergen, cockroach allergen, and tree and grass pollen. Viral illnesses can also induce airway obstruction in asthmatic individuals; symptoms may persist for weeks to months if therapy is not initiated. Occupational exposures are common asthma triggers. Early responses may occur within several hours; however, late responses may not occur for 8 to 12 hours after exposure. Often occupation-induced asthma symptoms may persist long after the individual has left the workplace; an important consideration is the differential diagnosis.

Approximately 1% to 10% of individuals with moderate to severe asthma have aspirin-induced asthma, which is characterized by symptoms of moderately severe airway obstruction, rhinorrhea, sneezing, tearing, dermal changes, and in some cases gastrointestinal symptoms (nausea, vomiting, cramping) when exposed to aspirin or other prostaglandin (H synthase type 1) inhibitors. The onset of aspirin-induced asthma occurs most often when patients are in their twenties and thirties. The diagnosis of aspirin-induced asthma is important for two reasons: aspirin-containing drugs should be avoided, since these drugs may induce life-threatening asthma attacks, and effective treatment is available specifically for this type of asthma.[21]

Acute severe asthma, although not pathologically distinct from acute asthma, represents a more severe and prolonged form of the illness. Acute severe asthma is often characterized by unremitting asthma symptoms (including shortness of breath, diminished exercise tolerance, and wheezing) for weeks with less than optimum response to therapy. Often asthmatic individuals develop prolonged severe asthma by inappropriately self-medicating with β_2-adrenergic agonist inhalers for weeks before seeking medical attention, at which point the risk of respiratory collapse and asphyxia may be great.[20]

Chronic stable asthma refers to asthma that is characterized by episodes of airway obstruction and airway symptoms. Although multiple asthma episodes may occur over a period of several months, most are of moderate severity and respond promptly to therapy. Asthma symptoms and exacerbations can generally be controlled through chronic medication use.[21]

Sample questions for the diagnosis and initial assessment of asthma have been developed by the National Institutes of Health (NIH)'s National Asthma Education and Prevention Program (NAEPP) (Box 108-1).[11] In addition to an assessment of symptoms, an individual's family history is helpful when a diagnosis of asthma is being considered. Often persons with

BOX 108-1

INITIAL ASSESSMENT OF ASTHMA

Consider asthma and performing spirometry if any of these indications are present.* These indications are not diagnostic by themselves, but the presence of multiple key indicators increases the probability of a diagnosis of asthma. Spirometry is needed to establish a diagnosis of asthma.

1. Wheezing—high-pitched whistling sounds when breathing out—especially in children. (Lack of wheezing and a normal chest examination do not exclude asthma.)
2. History of any one of the following:
   - Cough, worse particularly at night
   - Recurrent wheeze
   - Recurrent difficulty in breathing
   - Recurrent chest tightness
3. Reversible airflow limitation and diurnal variation as measured by using a peak flow meter, for example:
   - Peak expiratory flow (PEF) varies 20% or more from PEF measurement on arising in the morning (before taking an inhaled short-acting β_2 agonist) compared to PEF measurements in the early afternoon (after taking an inhaled short-acting beta2 agonist).
4. Symptoms occur or worsen in the presence of:
   - Exercise
   - Viral infection
   - Animals with fur or feathers
   - House-dust mites (in mattresses, pillows, upholstered furniture, carpets)
   - Mold
   - Smoke (tobacco, wood)
   - Pollen
   - Changes in weather
   - Strong emotional expression (laughing or crying hard)
   - Airborne chemicals or dusts
   - Menses
5. Symptoms occur or worsen at night, awakening the patient.

SUGGESTED ITEMS FOR MEDICAL HISTORY†

A detailed history of the new patient who is known or thought to have asthma should address the following items:

1. Symptoms
   - Cough
   - Wheezing
   - Shortness of breath
   - Chest tightness
   - Sputum production
2. Pattern of symptoms
   - Perennial, seasonal, or both
   - Continual, episodic, or both
   - Onset, duration, frequency (number of days or nights, per week or month)
   - Diurnal variations, especially nocturnal and on awakening in early morning
3. Precipitating and/or aggravating factors
   - Viral respiratory infections
   - Environmental allergens, indoor (e.g., mold, house-dust mite, cockroach, animal dander, or secretory products) and outdoor (e.g., pollen)
   - Exercise
   - Occupational chemicals or allergens
   - Environmental change (e.g., moving to new home; going on vacation; and/or alterations in workplace, work processes, or materials used)
   - Irritants (e.g., tobacco smoke, strong odors, air pollutants, occupational chemicals, dusts and particulates, vapors, gases, and aerosols)
   - Emotional expressions (e.g., fear, anger, frustration, hard crying or laughing)
   - Drugs (e.g., aspirin; beta blockers, including eye drops; nonsteroidal antiinflammatory drugs; others)
   - Food, food additives, and preservatives (e.g., sulfites)
   - Changes in weather, exposure to cold air
   - Endocrine factors (e.g., menses, pregnancy, thyroid disease)
4. Development of disease and treatment
   - Age of onset and diagnosis
   - History of early-life injury to airways (e.g., bronchopulmonary dysplasia, pneumonia, parental smoking)
   - Progress of disease (better or worse)
   - Present management and response, including plans for managing exacerbations
   - Need for oral corticosteroids and frequency of use
   - Co-morbid conditions
5. Family history
   - History of asthma, allergy, sinusitis, rhinitis, or nasal polyps in close relatives
6. Social history
   - Characteristics of home, including age, location, cooling and heating system, wood-burning stove, humidifier, carpeting over concrete, presence of molds or mildew, characteristics of rooms where patient spends time (e.g., bedroom and living room with attention to bedding, floor covering, stuffed furniture)
   - Smoking (patient and others in home or day care)
   - Social factors that interfere with adherence, such as substance abuse
   - Social supports and social networks
   - Level of education completed
   - Employment (if employed, characteristics of work environment)
7. Profile of typical exacerbation
   - Usual prodromal signs and symptoms
   - Usual patterns and management (what works?)
8. Impact of asthma on patient and family
   - Episodes of unscheduled care (emergency department, urgent care, hospitalizations)
   - Patient, parental, and spouse's or partner's knowledge of asthma and belief in the chronicity of asthma and in the efficacy of treatment
   - Patient perception and beliefs regarding use and long-term effects of medications
   - Ability of patient and parents, spouse, or partners to cope with disease
   - Level of family support and patient's and parents', spouse's, or partner's capacity to recognize severity of an exacerbation
   - Economic resources
   - Sociocultural beliefs

SAMPLE AND INITIAL ASSESSMENT OF ASTHMA

A "yes" answer to any questions suggests that an asthma diagnosis is likely.‡

In the past 12 months . . .

- Have you had a sudden severe episode or recurrent episodes of coughing, wheezing (high-pitched whistling sounds when breathing out), or shortness of breath?
- Have you had colds that "go to the chest" or take more than 10 days to get over?
- Have you had coughing, wheezing, or shortness of breath during a particular season or time of the year?
- Have you had coughing, wheezing, or shortness of breath in certain places or when exposed to certain things (e.g., animals, tobacco smoke, perfumes)?

Continued

BOX 108-1

INITIAL ASSESSMENT OF ASTHMA—CONT'D

SAMPLE AND INITIAL ASSESSMENT OF ASTHMA–CONT'D

- Have you used any medications that help you breathe better? How often?
- Are your symptoms relieved when the medications are used?

In the past 4 weeks, have you had coughing, wheezing, or shortness of breath . . .

- At night that has awakened you?
- In the early morning?
- After running, moderate exercise, or other physical activity?

From National Heart, Lung and Blood Institute; National Asthma Education and Prevention Program: *NAEPP Expert Panel Report guidelines for the diagnosis and management of asthma—update on selected topics 2002,* NIH Pub No 02-5075, Washington, DC, 2003, US Government Printing Office.

*Eczema, hay fever, or a family history of asthma or atopic disease are often associated asthma, but they are not key indicators.

†This list does not represent a standardized assessment or diagnostic instrument. The validity and reliability of this list have not been assessed.

‡These questions are examples and do not represent a standardized assessment or diagnostic instrument. The validity and reliability of these questions have not been assessed.

asthma have a family history of asthma or atopy. Also, family members are often able to identify specific exposures or circumstances that precipitate the patient's symptoms.[18] Sample questions for the follow-up assessment of patients with previously diagnosed asthma are listed in Box 108-2.

Asthma can be classified according to the frequency and severity of symptoms and the pattern of airflow limitation or according to the treatment steps necessary to decrease symptoms, improve lung function, and prevent exacerbations so as to allow for normal daily activities (Table 108-1). Asthma can have a variable course, and the degree of asthma control and the severity of asthma within an individual can change over time. Providers need to be aware of the difference between asthma control and severity. For example, severe asthma can be well-controlled, that is, few exacerbations with intensive pharmacotherapy and good self-management. On the other hand, an individual with mild asthma and little need of intensive treatment may still have periods of poor control. Persons with well-controlled asthma are still vulnerable to acute exacerbations, especially if exposed to factors that precipitate their asthma symptoms.[11]

There is increasing evidence that persons affected by problems of socioeconomic deprivation and psychosocial issues such as anxiety, depression, and stress are at increased risk for asthma exacerbations.[22] A study by Sandberg, Paton, Ahola, and others demonstrated that, even in children with asthma, psychosocial stress can worsen asthma control and increase the risk of an acute exacerbation.[23]

PHYSICAL EXAMINATION

The physical examination of the patient with asthma or suspected asthma can be divided into four objectives: (1) diagnosis and differential diagnosis, (2) assessment of asthma severity, (3) identification of adverse effects of medications, and (4) identification of concomitant medical problems. A complete physical examination is necessary if assessment of respiratory exertion or compromise is needed, co-existing medical conditions must be identified or evaluated, or the presentation is complex.[20]

The diagnosis of asthma is based on the history; physical examination; and certain diagnostic tests, particularly spirometry. The physical examination, although an essential part of the evaluation, may correlate poorly with objective measures of airway obstruction, such as pulmonary function tests (PFTs). In the asymptomatic patient the physical examination may be entirely normal. Nonetheless, assessing the severity of asthma and airway obstruction is the most important objective in evaluating a person with asthma. Wheezing may be detectable or elicited during forced expiration. In general, mild bronchospasm is associated with expiratory wheezing. As obstruction becomes more significant, wheezing is heard during both the inspiratory and expiratory phases, with a prolongation of the latter. With profound obstruction, wheezing may be heard only during the inspiratory phase or may be entirely absent. With severe obstruction the intensity of the breath sounds diminishes. As obstruction increases, accessory muscles of respiration are used; with significant obstruction, there may be evidence of hyperinflation with a low diaphragm and an increased anteroposterior diameter. Another rough measure of the degree of obstruction is pulsus paradoxus. An inspiratory decline in systolic blood pressure of greater than 10 mm Hg is abnormal, and one greater than 20 mm Hg generally reflects profound obstruction. However, this measure is crude and should not substitute for more direct measures of the degree of obstruction, such as spirometry.[24]

Severe asthma exacerbations are characterized by labored respirations, diaphoresis, anxiety, and breathlessness (inability to finish a complete sentence). A respiratory rate of 30 breaths per minute or more and a heart rate of 120 beats per minute or more suggest severe bronchospasm. Other signs and symptoms that often herald impending respiratory failure include agitation, confusion, somnolence, and cyanosis. Unilateral loss of breath sounds may reflect mucus plugging and secondary atelectasis, but pneumothorax must also be considered in this situation.[24] However, even a careful physical examination provides only a crude estimate of airway obstruction, and significant airway obstruction is possible even when the physical examination is entirely normal. Assessment of respiratory status is best accomplished through measurement of lung function with spirometry or peak flow meters.[25] The Global Initiative for Asthma's (GINA's) system of classifying the severity of asthma exacerbations is presented in Table 108-1. The physical examination is also important in identifying adverse effects of asthma medications. Side effects of β_2-adrenergic medications and theophylline include tachycardia and tremors. Inhaled corticosteroids can cause oral thrush and

BOX 108-2

COMPONENTS OF PRACTITIONER'S FOLLOW-UP ASSESSMENT: SAMPLE ROUTINE CLINICAL ASSESSMENT QUESTIONS*

MONITORING SIGNS AND SYMPTOMS

(Global assessment) Has your asthma been better or worse since your last visit?

(Recent assessment) In the past 2 weeks, how many days have you:

- Had problems with coughing, wheezing, shortness of breath, or chest tightness during the day?
- Awakened at night from sleep because of coughing or other asthma symptoms?
- Awakened in the morning with asthma symptoms that did not improve within 15 minutes of inhaling a short-acting inhaled β_2 agonist?
- Had symptoms while exercising or playing?

MONITORING PULMONARY FUNCTION

Lung Function

What is the highest and lowest your peak flow has been since your last visit?

Has your peak flow dropped below ___ L/min (80% of personal best) since your last visit?

What did you do when this occurred?

Peak Flow Monitoring Technique

Please show me how you measure your peak flow.

When do you usually measure your peak flow?

MONITORING QUALITY OF LIFE AND FUNCTIONAL STATUS

Since your last visit, how many days has your asthma caused you to:

- Miss work or school?
- Reduce your activities?
- (For caregivers) Change your activity because of your child's asthma?

Have you had any unscheduled or emergency department visits or hospital stays?

MONITORING EXACERBATION HISTORY

Since your last visit, have you had any episodes OR times when your asthma symptoms were a lot worse than usual?

- If yes—What do you think caused the symptoms to get worse?
- If yes—What did you do to control the symptoms?

MONITORING PHARMACOTHERAPY

Medications

What medications are you taking?

How often do you take each medication? How much do you take each time?

Have you missed or stopped taking any regular doses of your medications for any reason?

Have you had trouble filling your prescriptions?

How many puffs of your short-acting inhaled β_2 agonist (quick-relief medicine) do you use per day?

How many __________ (name short-acting inhaled β_2 agonist) inhalers (or pumps) have you been through in the past month?

Have you tried any other medicines or remedies?

Side Effects

Has your asthma medicine caused you any problems?

- Shakiness, nervousness, bad taste, sore throat, cough, upset stomach

Inhaler Technique

Please show me how you use your inhaler.

MONITORING PATIENT-PROVIDER COMMUNICATION AND PATIENT SATISFACTION

What questions have you had about your asthma daily self-management plan and action plan?

What problems have you had following your daily self-management plan? Your action plan?

Has anything prevented you from getting the treatment you need for your asthma from me or anyone else?

Have the costs of your asthma treatment interfered with your ability to get asthma care?

How can we improve your asthma care?

Let's review some important information:

- When should you increase your medications? Which medication(s)?
- When should you call me [your health care provider]? Do you know the after-hours phone number?
- If you can't reach me, what emergency department would you go to?

From National Institutes of Health, National Heart, Lung, and Blood Institute: *Highlights of the Expert Panel Report 2: guidelines for the diagnosis and management of asthma,* NIH Pub No 97-4051A, Washington, DC, 1997, US Department of Health and Human Services.

*These questions are examples and do not represent a standardized assessment instrument. The validity and reliability of these questions have not been assessed.

dysphonia. Adverse effects of oral (systemic) corticosteroids include central adiposity, hypertension, ecchymoses, cataracts, kyphosis, muscle weakness, and alterations in mental status.[25]

Co-existing medical problems can be conceptualized in two ways. Certain co-morbid conditions, such as nasal polyps, allergic rhinitis, sinusitis, and eczema, are commonly associated with asthma. In addition, some co-existing medical problems may be unrelated to asthma, but their identification and management have important implications for asthma therapy and control. Such possible co-morbidities include glaucoma, hypertension, gastroesophageal reflux, diabetes mellitus, arthritis, and a history of current malignancies.[25]

DIAGNOSTICS

A diagnosis of asthma is based on three components: (1) demonstration of episodic symptoms of airflow obstruction (e.g., wheeze, cough, shortness of breath), (2) evidence that airflow obstruction is at least partially reversible, and (3) exclusion of other conditions from the differential diagnosis.[3,25] A thorough history and physical examination are essential to making the diagnosis of asthma. Physical findings can be helpful in identifying significant obstruction as it occurs, but at best provide only a crude estimate of the degree of obstruction. However, significant obstruction may not be manifested as an abnormal physical finding; in addition, findings are likely to be completely normal between episodes. In fact, reduced expiratory flow rates (forced expiratory volume at 1 second, or FEV_1) and increased airway resistance may not be recognized as dyspnea until a 30% to 40% decline in FEV_1 has occurred.[24] Thus objective measures of pulmonary function, such as spirometry and peak flow meters, are essential in establishing the diagnosis of asthma and assessing its severity. Spirometry is now recommended (1) at the time of initial assessment to confirm the diagnosis of asthma, (2) after

TABLE 108-1 Severity of Asthma Attacks

Parameter*	Mild	Moderate	Severe	Respiratory Arrest Imminent
Breathless	Walking	Talking Infant: softer, shorter cry; difficulty feeding	At rest Infant stops feeding	
Talks in ...	Sentences	Phrases	Words	Drowsy or confused
Alertness	May be agitated	Usually agitated	Usually agitated	Paradoxical
Respiratory rate	Increased	Increased	Often >30/min	Paradoxical
GUIDE TO RATES OF BREATHING ASSOCIATED WITH RESPIRATORY DISTRESS IN AWAKE CHILDREN				
	Age	**Normal Rate (beats per minute)**		
	<2 months	<60		
	2-12 months	<50		
	1-5 years	<40		
	6-8 years	<30		
Accessory muscles and suprasternal retractions	Usually not	Usually	Usually	Thoraco-abdominal movement
Wheeze	Moderate, often only end-expiratory	Loud	Usually loud	Absence of wheeze
Pulse (beats per minute)	<100	100-120	>120	Bradycardia
GUIDE TO LIMITS OF NORMAL PULSE RATE IN CHILDREN				
	Age	**Normal Rate (beats per minute)**		
	Infants, 2-12 months	<160		
	Preschool, 1-2 years	<120		
	School age, 2-8 years	<110		
PEF after initial bronchodilator (% predicted or % personal best)	>80%	Approximately 60%-80%	<60% predicted or personal best (100 L/min adults) or response lasts <2 hours	
Pa_{O_2} (on air)†	Normal (test not usually necessary)	>60 mm Hg	<60 mm Hg; possible cyanosis	
and/or				
Pa_{CO_2}†	<45 mm Hg	<45 mm Hg	>45 mm Hg; possible respiratory failure	
Sa_{O_2}% (on air)†	>95%	91%-95%	<90%	
Hypercapnia (hypoventilation) develops more readily in young children than in adults and adolescents.				

From Global Initiative for Asthma: *Pocket guide for asthma management and prevention: a pocket guide for physicians and nurses,* updated 2005, NIH Pub No 02-3659, retrieved Sept 7, 2006, from http://www.ginasthma.org.
PEF, Peak expiratory flow.
*The presence of several parameters, but not necessarily all, indicates the general classification of the attack.
†Kilopascals are also used internationally; conversion would be appropriate in this regard.

treatment is initiated and symptoms and peak expiratory flow (PEF) have been stabilized, and (3) at least every 1 to 2 years.[3]

Although spirometry provides many measures, the most useful for evaluating asthma include the peak expiratory flow rate (PEFR), the FEV_1, the maximum mid-expiratory flow rate (MMEFR), and the forced vital capacity (FVC). Results are compared with expected values, derived from a population of healthy, nonsmoking adults, and are expressed as a percentage of the expected value.

Decreased rates of airflow throughout the vital capacity are the most common pulmonary function abnormality in mild asthma as reflected by abnormalities in the PEFR, the FEV_1, and the MMEFR (forced expiratory flow [FEF_{25-75}]). During bronchospasm, spirometry reveals obstruction with decreases in FEV_1 and MMEFR. The FEV_1/FVC ratio is also reduced. As obstruction increases, an increased residual volume and functional residual are noted. One of the diagnostic hallmarks of asthma is reversal of obstruction after the administration of a bronchodilator, which corresponds with both clinical improvement and improved spirometric values. In addition to helping establish the diagnosis of asthma, spirometry helps assess the adequacy of therapy, the need for further therapy and evaluation during emergencies, and the need for hospital admission. The severity of asthma attacks must be assessed by accurate and reproducible measures of airflow. Health care providers tend to underestimate the degree of airway obstruction in individuals with acute asthma, and knowledge of a person's pulmonary function has potentially important implications for treatment. For this reason, the NAEPP guidelines recommend the use of PFTs as part of the assessment and monitoring during the treatment of acute asthma.[20] During a severe asthma attack, recording of the entire spirogram may be difficult, but the FEV_1 can still be measured. As the asthma attack resolves, both the PEFR and the FEV_1 increase, whereas the MMEFR usually remains significantly diminished.[21]

Other laboratory tests that may be used to diagnose asthma or be included as part of the evaluation include airway responsiveness testing, arterial blood and other serum analysis, radiography, an ECG, and sputum cultures. Airway responsiveness testing measures the bronchoconstrictor response elicited by a standard stimulus. The FEV_1 is measured after inhalation of an aerosol containing graded amounts of a bronchoconstrictor agonist. The most common bronchoconstrictors used are methacholine and histamine.[21]

Individuals with asthma often have atopy, which is often reflected in blood eosinophilia as high as 4% to 8%. In addition, IgE serum levels are also often elevated. In fact, epidemiologic studies indicate that asthma is unusual in individuals with low IgE levels.[21]

Generally, the chest radiographs of individuals with asthma are normal. Therefore chest radiography is not indicated in the routine evaluation of patients with asthma unless physical examination findings are suggestive of infectious illness or respiratory complications such as pneumomediastinum or pneumothorax. If an asthma exacerbation is severe enough to warrant hospital admission, a chest x-ray film should be taken. The x-ray film may show hyperinflation (indicated by diaphragmatic depression) and abnormally translucent lung fields.[21]

Between asthma attacks, in the absence of respiratory infection, the sputum is usually clear. During an asthma attack, even in the absence of infection, the sputum may be yellow to green. This does not necessarily indicate infection; the color change may be from eosinophil peroxidase. Sputum cultures are generally not obtained unless there is suspicion of an acute contagious respiratory infection.[21]

An ECG is not part of the routine evaluation of a patient with asthma. If it is obtained during an asthma exacerbation, an ECG in the absence of cardiac disease is usually significant only for sinus tachycardia. In severe attacks, right-axis deviation, right bundle branch block, cor pulmonale, or even ST-T wave abnormalities may occur. If these abnormalities resolve as the asthma attack abates, no further cardiac evaluation is necessary. ECG findings should be monitored during asthma attacks for patients with significant cardiac disease to monitor for myocardial infarction, which can result from attack-induced stress.[24]

DIAGNOSTICS

Asthma

INITIAL
Peak flow meter
Pulse oximetry

LABORATORY
CBC and differential
IgE*

IMAGING
Chest x-ray*

OTHER
PFTs, airway responsiveness testing
ABGs*
ECG*

*If indicated.

DIFFERENTIAL DIAGNOSIS

The medical conditions most likely to be confused with asthma involve the upper respiratory system (e.g., croup, vocal cord dysfunction) and lower respiratory system (e.g., pneumonia, chronic obstructive pulmonary disease [COPD]), the cardiovascular system (e.g., valvular disease and cardiomyopathy), and the gastrointestinal system (e.g., GERD).[25]

Not all wheezing is due to asthma, and other causes should be excluded before a diagnosis of asthma is made. Spirometry can be used to help differentiate asthma from other possible conditions in the differential diagnosis. An FEV_1 of 80% of predicted or less with a reduced FEV_1/FVC ratio that normalizes or significantly improves with bronchodilator therapy raises the suspicion of asthma. Other causes of wheezing and upper airway obstruction include tracheomalacia, tracheal or bronchial masses, and laryngeal (vocal cord) dysfunction. The presence of stridor or focal wheezing on physical examination and with flow limitation on a flow volume loop is characteristic of tracheomalacia and tracheobronchial masses. Laryngeal dysfunction is caused by abnormal apposition of the vocal cords during the respiratory cycle and can generally be treated effectively by speech therapy. Laryngeal dysfunction is often initially misdiagnosed as asthma and often inappropriately treated with high-dose systemic steroids. Laryngoscopy is needed to confirm laryngeal dysfunction.[24]

DIFFERENTIAL DIAGNOSIS

Asthma

- Acute bronchiolitis (infectious, chemical)
- Airway obstruction by masses
- Central thoracic tumors
- Metastatic cancer
- Primary lung tumors
- Substernal thyroid tumors
- α_1-Antitrypsin deficiency
- Bronchiolitis obliterans organizing pneumonia
- Bronchial stenosis
- Carcinoid syndrome
- Cardiac failure
- Chronic obstructive pulmonary disease (chronic bronchitis or emphysema)
- Cystic fibrosis
- Endobronchial sarcoid
- Eosinophilia pneumonia
- Foreign body aspiration
- Interstitial fibrosis
- Pleural effusion
- Pulmonary emboli
- Systemic mastocytosis
- Systemic vasculitis (polyarteritis nodosa)
- Tracheomalacia

Persons with COPD, including emphysema and chronic bronchitis, may have acute episodes of airway obstruction and wheezing, especially during exacerbations of their disease. COPD is often accompanied by a history of smoking, reduced response to bronchodilator therapy, and irreversible PFT changes over time. In addition, COPD may be distinguished from asthma by signs of hyperinflation, such as diminished breath sounds, decreased heart sounds, and a flattened diaphragm. Chest wall deformities are suggestive of restrictive lung diseases. Dullness to percussion may indicate pneumonia or a pleural effusion. Foreign body aspiration should be considered if lateralizing wheezes are heard.[24,25]

α_1-Antitrypsin (AAT) deficiency is an inherited disorder, caused by an inborn error in the liver's production of AAT, which is the dominant protease in the lung and which protects alveoli from the destructive effects of serine proteases. AAT deficiency causes a syndrome of abnormalities, including neonatal jaundice, airflow obstruction, premature emphysema, and cirrhosis of the liver.[26,27] The primary respiratory effect of AAT deficiency is degradation of the protein elastin, a protein that is essential for the elastic recoil required for pulmonary expiratory function. As a result, chronic persistent airflow obstruction develops. AAT deficiency is a well-established cause of panacinar emphysema, but its role in the pathophysiology of asthma is less well understood. The prevalence of AAT deficiency is about 0.01% to 0.02% in those with emphysema; the prevalence of AAT deficiency among patients with asthma is not known.[26] Individuals with AAT deficiency often have symptoms similar to those of bronchial asthma; pulmonary function may be normal, especially among those who do not smoke. Hence a diagnosis of AAT deficiency is often missed or delayed. However, bronchopulmonary infections are common in persons with AAT deficiency, and their family history almost always includes lung disease. Asthmatic patients with AAT deficiency generally have more severe disease and often respond less to bronchodilators than do those without the disorder. Health care providers should have a high level of suspicion for AAT deficiency in young persons whose symptoms do not respond to appropriate asthma therapy, especially in the absence of smoking. Diagnosis of AAT deficiency is based on AAT serum levels but may also involve other diagnostic measurements, including PFTs, chest radiography, serum electrophoresis, and genotyping. Although management of AAT deficiency has some similarities to that of asthma, it also has important differences; diagnosis of AAT deficiency has critical implications for an individual's prognosis and quality of life.[27]

MANAGEMENT

Although the role of inflammation in the pathogenesis of asthma was recognized in the 1991 National Heart, Lung, and Blood Institute (NHLBI) guidelines on asthma management, asthma is now defined as a chronic inflammatory disease of the airways.[2] This new understanding of asthma pathology also suggests that much of asthma care will be provided by individuals and their families outside of and away from health care institutions and practitioners. In addition, inflammation is now understood to be one of the preeminent problems in asthma, which has shifted the focus of treatment from symptomatic to preventive therapy, including the need for antiinflammatory medications, environmental controls, and patient education.[11] GINA was created to increase awareness among health professionals, public health authorities, and the general public to improve the prevention and management of asthma through a concerted worldwide effort. GINA offers a framework for asthma management that can be adapted to local health care systems and resources.[7] Both the NAEPP of the NHLBI (NIH) and the GINA have identified six goals of asthma treatment, which differ only with regard to GINA's emphasis on preventing the possible sequelae of asthma, including irreversible airflow limitation and asthma-related death.[1,2] GINA's goals for successful asthma management are listed in Box 108-3.

BOX 108-3

GOALS FOR SUCCESSFUL ASTHMA MANAGEMENT

- Minimal or no symptoms, including nighttime symptoms
- Minimal asthma episodes or attacks
- No emergency visits to physicians or hospitals
- Minimal need for reliever medications
- No limitations on physical activities and exercise
- Nearly normal lung function
- Minimal or no side effects from medication

Global Initiative for Asthma: *Pocket guide for asthma management and prevention: a pocket guide for physicians and nurses,* NIH Pub No 02-3659, Washington, DC, updated 2005, US Government Printing Office.

The NHLBI Expert Panel for the Diagnosis and Management of Asthma and GINA use the same classification system of asthma severity, which is based on the frequency and severity of symptoms. Characteristics of each of these categories are presented in Tables 108-2 and 108-3. According to the guidelines, individuals should be assigned to the most severe asthma category in which any characteristic occurs. The major change from previous classification systems is the division of asthmatic patients into those with and those without mild persistent symptoms. This distinction has important clinical implications because, in general, the only persons not requiring antiinflammatory medications are those with intermittent symptoms.

Asthma pharmacotherapy is determined by the severity of the disease, and a summary of disease classification can also be found in Tables 108-2 and 108-3. The most effective medications for long-term control of asthma continue to be those with antiinflammatory effects, including the inhaled corticosteroids, mast-cell stabilizers such as cromolyn, long-acting β_2-adrenergic agonists, and the leukotriene modifiers. These medications are referred to in the Expert Panel Report (EPR)[2] as *long-term control medications* and in GINA as *controller* medications to emphasize their role in achieving and maintaining control of persistent asthma (Table 108-4). Relief of exacerbations and control of acute symptoms are achieved through the use of *quick-relief medications* (EPR) or *reliever* medication (GINA), chief among them being the short-acting β_2-adrenergic agonists, but also including anticholinergics and systemic glucocorticoids (Table 108-5). The new EPR guidelines also emphasize a stepwise management approach in which therapies should be initiated at higher levels (steps, not dosages) to establish control as quickly as possible (see Tables 108-2 and 108-3). After control has been achieved, therapy should be tapered for long-term management.[2]

Despite the fact that the approach to asthma therapy has been recommended by the NHLBI since 1991, studies indicate that asthma control, as defined by the asthma management guidelines, is not being achieved in the majority of patients.[12] There remains an overreliance on short-acting bronchodilators and underuse of antiinflammatory medications on the part

TABLE 108-2 Stepwise Approach to Managing Asthma in Adults and Children Older Than 5 Years of Age: Clinical Features

GOALS OF ASTHMA TREATMENT

- Prevent chronic and troublesome symptoms (e.g., coughing or breathlessness in the night, in the early morning, or after exertion).
- Maintain (near) "normal" pulmonary function.
- Maintain normal activity levels (including exercise and other physical activity).
- Prevent recurrent exacerbations of asthma and minimize the need for emergency department visits or hospitalizations.
- Provide optimal pharmacotherapy with minimal or no adverse effects.
- Meet patients' and families' expectations of and satisfaction with asthma care.

CLASSIFICATION OF SEVERITY OF ASTHMA

	Clinical Features Before Treatment*		
	Symptoms†	**Nighttime Symptoms**	**Lung Function**
STEP 4: Severe persistent	• Continual symptoms • Limited physical activity • Frequent exacerbations	Frequent	• FEV_1 or PEF ≤60% predicted • PEF variability >30%
STEP 3: Moderate persistent	• Daily symptoms • Daily use of inhaled short-acting β_2 agonist • Exacerbations affect activity • Exacerbations ≥2 times a week; may last days	>1 time a week	• FEV_1 or PEF 60%-80% predicted • PEF variability >30%
STEP 2: Mild persistent	• Symptoms >2 times a week but <1 time a day • Exacerbations may affect activity	>2 times a month	• FEV_1 or PEF ≥80% predicted • PEF variability 20%-30%
STEP 1: Mild intermittent	• Symptoms ≤2 times a week • Asymptomatic and normal PEF between exacerbations • Exacerbations brief (from a few hours to a few days); intensity may vary	≤2 times a month	• FEV_1 or PEF ≥80% predicted • PEF variability <20%

From National Heart, Lung, and Blood Institute: *Asthma statistics,* Bethesda, Md, 1997, National Institutes of Health, US Department of Health and Human Services, The Institute.

FEV_1, Forced expiratory volume measured in 1 second; *PEF,* peak expiratory flow.

*The presence of one of the features of severity is sufficient to place a patient in that category. An individual should be assigned to the most severe grade in which any feature occurs. The characteristics noted are general and may overlap because asthma is highly variable. Furthermore, an individual's classification may change over time.

†Patients at any level of severity can have mild, moderate, or severe exacerbations. Some patients with intermittent asthma experience severe and life-threatening exacerbations separated by long periods of normal lung function and no symptoms.

of both practitioners and persons with asthma. This suggests that the underlying pathophysiology of asthma and its implications for therapy are still not widely understood. As emphasized in the EPR stepwise approach, all patients except those with mild, intermittent asthma benefit from maintenance antiinflammatory medication. The use of antiinflammatory medications for maintenance (long-term control) of mild to moderate asthma results in fewer asthma exacerbations, fewer emergency department visits, decreased cost of care, fewer school or work days missed, and an improved quality of life.[19] Despite the guidelines, research suggests that asthma is often undertreated, both because of inappropriate prescribing or underprescribing by physicians and poor patient adherence to therapy.[28] In addition, research shows that patient adherence to asthma therapy is less than 50% and that patients most likely to be nonadherent to treatment are young patients who have had asthma for a short time—that is, those patients most likely to benefit from treatment.[29]

Adherence to the asthma management guidelines has been shown to lead to a reduction in health care utilization; the greatest gains were for those with moderate to severe disease.[30] Specifically, among both severe and less severe asthma groups, high use of inhaled short-acting beta agonists in the absence of inhaled corticosteroids (ICS) (inconsistent with the guidelines) has been associated with as much as a fourfold increase in hospitalization. The risk of hospitalization was progressively reduced with both low and high use of ICS. The protective effect of ICS on hospitalization has been reported in several studies, with the reduction rate ranging from 30% to 60%.[31]

In addition to long-term daily therapy to control symptoms and prevent exacerbations, asthma management guidelines also include strategies for classifying and managing exacerbations. Early introduction of oral corticosteroids and frequent use of short-acting beta agonists should be initiated as symptoms worsen. Table 108-1 includes parameters for assessing the severity of asthma attacks. Home and hospital treatment of asthma exacerbations are found in Box 108-4 and Figure 108-1.

An integral component of asthma management is the treatment of co-existing diseases, including rhinitis, sinusitis, and GERD. Evidence from clinical trials suggests no benefit from antibiotic therapy for asthma exacerbations, whether administered routinely or when the suspicion of bacterial

TABLE 108-3 Stepwise Approach to Managing Asthma in Adults and Children Older Than 5 Years of Age: Treatment*

	Long-Term Control	Quick Relief	Education
STEP 4: Severe persistent	Daily medications: • Antiinflammatory: inhaled corticosteroid (high dose). and • Long-acting bronchodilator: either **long-acting inhaled β_2 agonist,** sustained-release theophylline, or long-acting β_2 agonist tablets. and • Corticosteroid tablets or syrup long term (make repeat attempts to reduce systemic steroids and maintain control with high-dose inhaled steroids).	• Short-acting bronchodilator: **inhaled β_2 agonists** as needed for symptoms. • Intensity of treatment will depend on severity of exacerbation (see Table 108-1). Use of short-acting inhaled β_2 agonists on a daily basis, or increasing use, indicates the need for additional long-term-control therapy.	Steps 2 and 3 actions plus: • Refer to individual education/counseling.
STEP 3: Moderate persistent	Daily medication: Either • Antiinflammatory: inhaled corticosteroid (medium dose). or • Inhaled corticosteroid (low-medium dose) and add a long-acting bronchodilator, especially for nighttime symptoms; either **long-acting, inhaled β_2 agonist,** sustained-release theophylline, or long-acting β_2 agonist tablets. If needed • Antiinflammatory: inhaled corticosteroids (medium-high dose). and • **Long-acting bronchodilator,** especially for nighttime symptoms; either **long-acting inhaled β_2 agonist,** sustained-release theophylline, or long-acting β_2 agonist tablets.	• Short-acting bronchodilator: **inhaled β_2 agonists** as needed for symptoms. • Intensity of treatment will depend on severity of exacerbation (see Table 108-1). • Use of short-acting inhaled β_2 agonists on a daily basis, or increasing use, indicates the need for additional long-term-control therapy.	Step 1 actions plus: • Teach self-monitoring. • Refer to group education if available. • Review and update self-management plan.
STEP 2: Mild persistent	One daily medication: • **Antiinflammatory:** either **inhaled corticosteroid** (low doses) or **cromolyn** or **nedocromil** (children usually begin with a trial of cromolyn or nedocromil). • Sustained-release theophylline to serum concentration of 5-15 mcg/ml is an alternative, but not preferred, therapy. • Zafirlukast or zileuton may also be considered for patients ≥12 years of age, although their position in therapy is not fully established.	• Short-acting bronchodilator: **inhaled β_2 agonists** as needed for symptoms. • Intensity of treatment will depend on severity of exacerbation (see Table 108-1). • Use of short-acting inhaled β_2 agonists on a daily basis, or increasing use, indicates the need for additional long-term-control therapy.	Step 1 actions plus: • Teach self-monitoring. • Refer to group education if available. • Review and update self-management plan.

From National Heart, Lung, and Blood Institute: *Asthma statistics,* Bethesda, Md, 1997, National Institutes of Health, US Department of Health and Human Services, The Institute.
*Preferred treatments are in bold print.

NOTE:
- The stepwise approach presents general guidelines to assist clinical decision making; it is not intended to be a specific prescription. Asthma is highly variable; clinicians should tailor specific medication plans to the needs and circumstances of individual patients.
- Gain control as quickly as possible; then decrease treatment to the least medication necessary to maintain control. Gaining control may be accomplished by either starting treatment at the step most appropriate to the initial severity of the condition or starting at a higher level of therapy (e.g., a course of systemic corticosteroids or higher dose of inhaled corticosteroids).
- A rescue course of systemic corticosteroids may be needed at any time and at any step.
- Some patients with intermittent asthma experience severe and life-threatening exacerbations separated by long periods of normal lung function and no symptoms. This may be especially common with exacerbations provoked by respiratory infections. A short course of systemic corticosteroids is recommended.
- At each step, patients should control their environment to avoid or control factors that make their asthma worse (e.g., allergens, irritants); this requires specific diagnosis and education.
- Referral to an asthma specialist for consultation or co-management is *recommended* if there are difficulties achieving or maintaining control of asthma or if the patient requires step 4 care. Referral may be *considered* if the patient requires step 3 care (see Table 108-3).

TABLE 108-3 Stepwise Approach to Managing Asthma in Adults and Children Older Than 5 Years of Age: Treatment—cont'd

	Long-Term Control	Quick Relief	Education
STEP 1: Mild intermittent	• No daily medication needed.	• Short-acting bronchodilator: **inhaled β_2 agonists** as needed for symptoms. • Intensity of treatment will depend on severity of exacerbation (see Table 108-1). • Use of short-acting inhaled β_2 agonists >2 times a week may indicate the need to initiate long-term-control therapy.	• Teach basic facts about asthma. • Teach inhaler/spacer/holding chamber technique. • Discuss roles of medications. • Develop self-management plan. • Develop action plan for when and how to take rescue actions, especially for patients with a history of severe exacerbations. • Discuss appropriate environmental control measures to avoid exposure to known allergens and irritants (see Table 108-6).
↓Step down Review treatment every 1-6 months; a gradual stepwise reduction in treatment may be possible.		↑Step up If control is not maintained, consider step up. First, review patient medication technique, adherence, and environmental control (avoidance of allergens or other factors that contribute to asthma severity).	

TABLE 108-4 Glossary of Asthma Medications—Controller Medications

Names	Usual Doses	Side Effects	Comments
GLUCOCORTICOSTEROIDS (ADRENOCORTICOIDS, CORTICOSTEROIDS, GLUCOCORTICOIDS)			
Inhaled			
Beclomethasone Budesonide Flunisolide Fluticasone Mometasone furoate Triamcinolone	Beginning dose dependent on asthma severity (see Table 108-1) then titrated down over 2-3 months to lowest effective dose once control is achieved.	High daily doses may be associated with skin thinning and bruises, and rarely adrenal suppression. Local side effects are hoarseness and oropharyngeal candidiasis. Medium and high doses have produced minor growth delay or suppression (av. 1 cm) in children. Attainment of predicted adult height does not appear to be affected.	Potential but small risk of side effects is well balanced by efficacy. Spacer devices with MDIs and mouth washing with DPIs after inhalation decrease oral candidiasis. Preparations not equivalent on per puff or mcg basis (see Table 108-8).
Tablets or Syrups			
Hydrocortisone Methylprednisolone Prednisolone Prednisone	For daily control use lowest effective dose, 5-40 mg of prednisone equivalent in morning or q.o.d. For acute attacks 40-60 mg/day in 1-2 divided doses for adults or 1-2 mg/kg/day in children.	Used long term, may lead to osteoporosis, hypertension, diabetes, cataracts, adrenal suppression, growth suppression, obesity, skin thinning, or muscle weakness. Consider co-existing conditions that could be worsened by oral glucocorticosteroids (e.g., herpes virus infections, varicella, tuberculosis, hypertension).	Long-term use: alternate day am dosing produces less toxicity. Short term: 3-10 day "bursts" are effective for gaining prompt control.
SODIUM CROMOGLYCATE			
Cromolyn Cromones	MDI 2 or 5 mg 2-4 inhalations, 3-4 times daily. Nebulizer 20 mg 3-4 times daily	Minimal side effects. Cough may occur on inhalation.	May take 4-6 weeks to determine maximum effects. Frequent daily dosing required.

From Global Initiative for Asthma: *Pocket guide for asthma management and prevention: a pocket guide for physicians and nurses,* updated 2005, NIH Pub No 02-3659, retrieved Sept 7, 2006, from http://www.ginasthma.org.

Av, Average; *DPI,* dry powder inhaler; *MDI,* metered dose inhaler.

Continued

TABLE 108-4 Glossary of Asthma Medications—Controller Medications—cont'd

Names	Usual Doses	Side Effects	Comments
NEDOCROMIL			
Cromones	MDI 2 mg/puff 2-4 inhalations 2-4 times daily	Cough may occur on inhalation.	Some patients unable to tolerate the taste.
LONG-ACTING β_2 AGONISTS (β-ADRENERGIC SYMPATHOMIMETICS)			
Inhaled			
Formoterol (F) Salmeterol (Sm)	DPI—F: 1 inhalation (12 mcg) b.i.d. MDI—F: 2 puffs b.i.d. DPI—Sm: 1 inhalation (50 mcg) b.i.d. MDI—Sm: 2 puffs b.i.d.	Fewer and less significant side effects than tablets.	Always use as adjunct to antiinflammatory therapy. Combined with low-medium doses of inhaled glucocorticosteroid, is more effective than increasing the dose of inhaled glucocorticosteroids.
Sustained-Release Tablets			
Salbutamol (S) Terbutaline (T)	S: 4 mg q 12 hr T: 10 mg q 12 hr	May cause tachycardia, anxiety, skeletal muscle tremor, headache, hypokalemia.	As effective as sustained-release theophylline. No data for use as adjunctive therapy with inhaled glucocorticosteroids.
SUSTAINED-RELEASE THEOPHYLLINE			
Aminophylline Methylxanthine	Starting dose 10 mg/kg/day with usual 800 mg maximum in 1-2 divided doses	Nausea and vomiting are most common. Serious effects occurring at higher serum concentrations include seizures, tachycardia, and arrhythmias.	Theophylline level monitoring is often required. Absorption and metabolism may be affected by many factors, including febrile illness.
ANTILEUKOTRIENES			
Leukotriene modifiers Montelukast (M) Pranlukast Zafirlukast (Z) Zileuton (Zi)	**Adults**—M: 10 mg q.h.s. P: 450 mg b.i.d. Z: 20 mg b.i.d. Zi: 600 mg q.i.d. **Children**—M: 5 mg q.h.s. (6-14 years) M: 4 mg q.h.s. (2-5 years) Z: 10 mg b.i.d. (7-11 years)	Data are limited; no specific adverse effects to date at recommended doses. Elevation of liver enzymes with Z and Zi and limited case reports of reversible hepatitis and hyperbilirubinemia with Zi.	The position of antileukotrienes in asthma therapy is not fully established. They provide additive benefit when added to inhaled glucocorticosteroids, although not as effective as inhaled long-acting β_2 agonists.

From Global Initiative for Asthma: *Pocket guide for asthma management and prevention: a pocket guide for physicians and nurses,* updated 2005, NIH Pub No 02-3659, retrieved Sept 7, 2006, from http://www.ginasthma.org.
Av, Average; *DPI,* dry powder inhaler; *MDI,* metered dose inhaler.

infection is low. The NAEPP EPR recommendation is that antibiotics are not used in the treatment of acute asthma exacerbation except for the treatment of certain co-morbid conditions, such as fever and purulent sputum, evidence of pneumonia, and bacterial sinusitis.[3] Intranasal glucocorticoids may be helpful in the management of chronic rhinitis, whereas antibiotics are indicated for bacterial sinus infections.[3] Annual influenza vaccine is recommended for all persons with persistent asthma. For persons with GERD, acid-suppressive therapy may decrease asthma symptoms. Individuals with GERD often do not describe symptoms suggestive of GERD; approximately 25% to 30% of patients with asthma have clinically silent reflux.[32]

Given the known role of environmental triggers in the pathophysiology of asthma, it is essential that environmental interventions be implemented along with clinical approaches in the management of asthma. Interventions at the household level must include efforts to eliminate cockroaches, rodents, and mold. Individual efforts to sustain pest-free environments, especially in apartment complexes, will be effective only if efforts at the building, neighborhood, and city level are in place to bolster those efforts. Common asthma risk factors and actions to reduce exposure to them are listed in Table 108-6.[1]

Medications

Long-Term Control Medications

Corticosteroids. Corticosteroids are the most potent and effective antiinflammatory medications available for the treatment of moderate to severe asthma. Although the mechanism of action is not completely understood, they have been shown to reduce the synthesis of inflammatory mediators and to inhibit late responses to allergen (those occurring several hours after allergen exposure). Their ability to inhibit a wide variety of inflammatory responses probably accounts for their effectiveness in many types of asthma. ICSs are the most effective long-term therapy for persistent asthma and are recommended for every individual with persistent asthma symptoms. ICSs are generally well tolerated in low to moderate

TABLE 108-5 Glossary of Asthma Medications—Reliever Medications

Name	Usual Doses	Side Effects	Comments
SHORT-ACTING β_2 AGONISTS (ADRENERGICS, β_2 STIMULANTS, SYMPATHOMIMETICS)			
Albuterol Bitolterol Fenoterol Isoetharine Metaproterenol Pirbuterol Salbutamol Terbutaline	Differences in potency exist, but all products are essentially comparable on a per puff basis. For p.r.n. symptomatic use and pretreatment before exercise, 2 puffs MDI or 1 inhalation DPI. For asthma attacks 4-8 puffs q 2-4 hr; may administer q 20 min × 3 with medical supervision or the equivalent of 5 mg salbutamol by nebulizer.	Inhaled: tachycardia, skeletal muscle tremor, headache, and irritability. At very high dose, hyperglycemia, hypokalemia. Systemic administration as tablets or syrup increases the risk of these side effects.	Drug of choice for acute bronchospasm. Inhaled route has faster onset and is more effective than tablet or syrup. Increasing use, lack of expected effect, or use of >1 canister a month indicates poor asthma control; adjust long-term therapy accordingly. Use of ≥2 canisters per month is associated with an increased risk of a severe, life-threatening asthma attack.
ANTICHOLINERGICS			
Ipratropium bromide (IB)	IB—MDI 4-6 puffs q 6 hr or q 20 min in the emergency department. Nebulizer 500 mcg q 20 min × 3 then q 2-4 hr for adults and 250 mcg for children	Minimal mouth dryness or bad taste in the mouth. Other anticholinergic effects (e.g. urinary retention/difficulty, constipation, increased heart rate, GI upset)	May provide additive effects to β_2 agonist but has slower onset of action. Is an alternative for patients with intolerance for β_2 agonists.
Tiotropium (bromide monohydrate)	1 inhalation (18 mcg) using HandiHaler inhalation device only Not recommended for children	Mouth dryness of bad taste in the mouth (Same as IB)	May be helpful for long-term maintenance treatment of bronchospasm, especially if due to chronic bronchitis or emphysema.
Short-acting theophylline Aminophylline	7 mg/kg loading dose over 20 minutes followed by 0.4 mg/kg/hr continuous infusion.	Nausea, vomiting, headache. At higher serum concentrations: seizures, tachycardia, and arrhythmias.	Theophylline level monitoring is required. Obtain serum levels 12 and 24 hours into infusion. Maintain between 10-15 mcg/ml.
Epinephrine-adrenaline injection	1:1000 solution (1 mg/ml) 0.01 mg/kg up to 0.3-0.5 mg. Can give q 20 min × 3.	Similar, but more significant effects than selective β_2 agonist. In addition: hypertension, fever, vomiting in children, and hallucinations.	In general, not recommended for treating asthma attacks if selective β_2 agonists are available.

From Global Initiative for Asthma: *Pocket guide for asthma management and prevention: a pocket guide for physicians and nurses,* updated 2005, NIH Pub No 02-3659, retrieved Sept 7, 2006, from http://www.ginasthma.org.
DPI, Dry powder inhaler; *MDI,* metered dose inhaler.

BOX 108-4

MANAGEMENT OF AN ASTHMA ATTACK: HOME TREATMENT

ASSESS SEVERITY

- Cough, breathlessness, wheeze, chest tightness, use of accessory muscles, suprasternal retractions, and sleep disturbance.
- PEF less than 80% of personal best or predicted.

INITIAL TREATMENT

- Inhaled rapid-acting β_2 agonist up to three treatments in 1 hour.
- Patients at high risk of asthma-related death should contact physician promptly after initial treatment.

RESPONSE TO INITIAL TREATMENT

Good If . . .

Symptoms subside after initial β_2 agonist and relief is sustained for 4 hours.
PEF is >80% predicted or personal best.

Actions:

- May continue β_2 agonist every 3-4 hours for 1-2 days.
- Contact physician or nurse for follow-up instructions.

Incomplete If . . .

Symptoms decrease but return in less than 3 hours after initial β_2 agonist treatment.
PEF is 60%-80% predicted or personal best.

Actions

- Add oral glucocorticosteroid.
- Add inhaled anticholinergic.
- Continue β_2 agonist.
- Consult clinician urgently for instructions.

Poor If . . .

Symptoms persist or worsen despite initial β_2 agonist treatment.
PEF is <60% predicted or personal best.

Actions

- Add oral glucocorticosteroid.
- Repeat β_2 agonist immediately.
- Add inhaled anticholinergic.
- Immediately transport to hospital emergency department.

From National Institutes of Health, National Heart, Lung, and Blood Institute: *1997 Guidelines for the diagnosis and management of asthma: highlights of the Expert Panel Report 2,* Pub No 97-4051A, Washington DC, 1997, US Government Printing Office.
PEF, Peak expiratory flow.

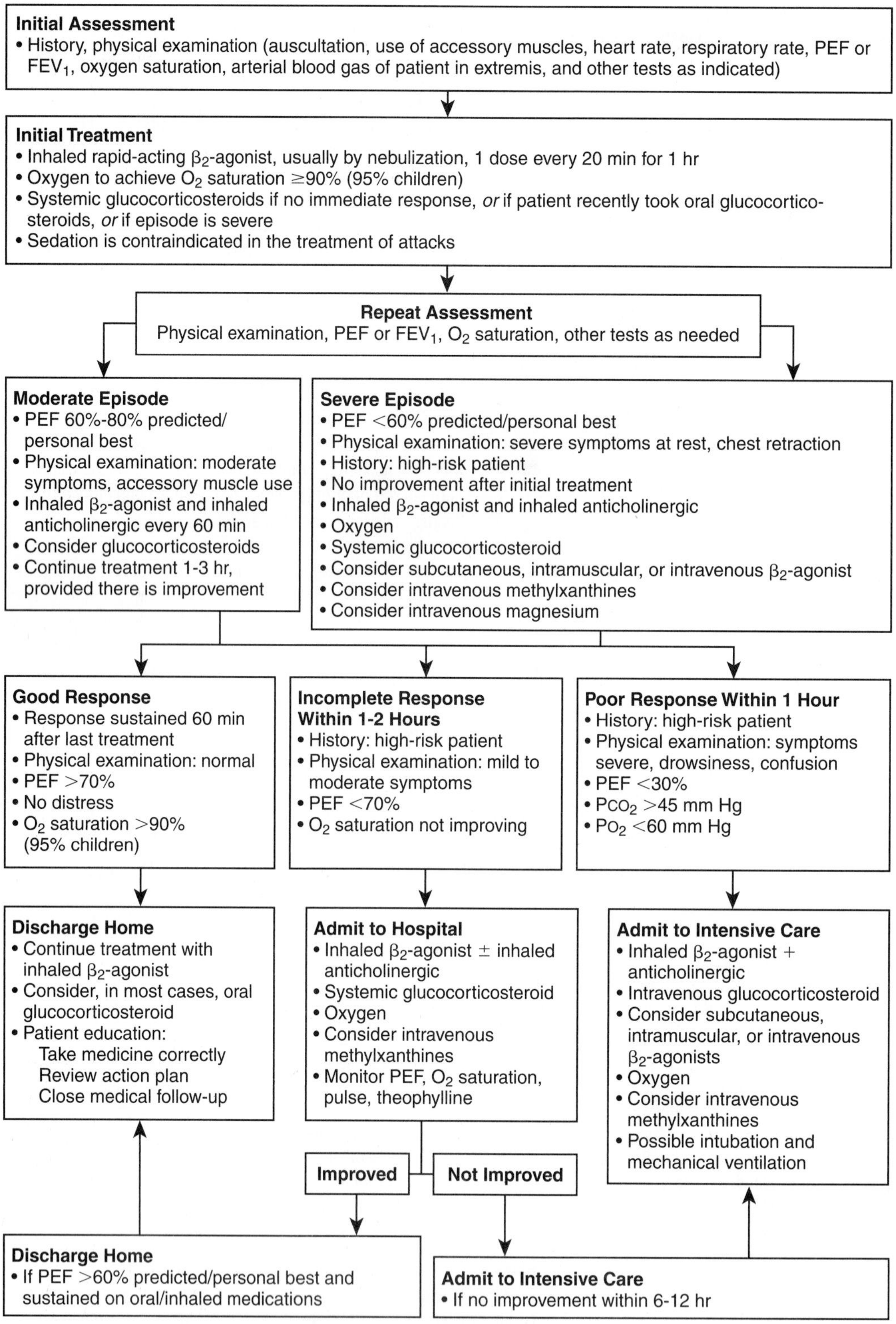

Initial Assessment
- History, physical examination (auscultation, use of accessory muscles, heart rate, respiratory rate, PEF or FEV_1, oxygen saturation, arterial blood gas of patient in extremis, and other tests as indicated)

↓

Initial Treatment
- Inhaled rapid-acting β_2-agonist, usually by nebulization, 1 dose every 20 min for 1 hr
- Oxygen to achieve O_2 saturation ≥90% (95% children)
- Systemic glucocorticosteroids if no immediate response, *or* if patient recently took oral glucocorticosteroids, *or* if episode is severe
- Sedation is contraindicated in the treatment of attacks

↓

Repeat Assessment
Physical examination, PEF or FEV_1, O_2 saturation, other tests as needed

Moderate Episode
- PEF 60%-80% predicted/personal best
- Physical examination: moderate symptoms, accessory muscle use
- Inhaled β_2-agonist and inhaled anticholinergic every 60 min
- Consider glucocorticosteroids
- Continue treatment 1-3 hr, provided there is improvement

Severe Episode
- PEF <60% predicted/personal best
- Physical examination: severe symptoms at rest, chest retraction
- History: high-risk patient
- No improvement after initial treatment
- Inhaled β_2-agonist and inhaled anticholinergic
- Oxygen
- Systemic glucocorticosteroid
- Consider subcutaneous, intramuscular, or intravenous β_2-agonist
- Consider intravenous methylxanthines
- Consider intravenous magnesium

Good Response
- Response sustained 60 min after last treatment
- Physical examination: normal
- PEF >70%
- No distress
- O_2 saturation >90% (95% children)

↓

Discharge Home
- Continue treatment with inhaled β_2-agonist
- Consider, in most cases, oral glucocorticosteroid
- Patient education:
  - Take medicine correctly
  - Review action plan
  - Close medical follow-up

Incomplete Response Within 1-2 Hours
- History: high-risk patient
- Physical examination: mild to moderate symptoms
- PEF <70%
- O_2 saturation not improving

↓

Admit to Hospital
- Inhaled β_2-agonist ± inhaled anticholinergic
- Systemic glucocorticosteroid
- Oxygen
- Consider intravenous methylxanthines
- Monitor PEF, O_2 saturation, pulse, theophylline

Improved → **Discharge Home**
- If PEF >60% predicted/personal best and sustained on oral/inhaled medications

Not Improved → **Admit to Intensive Care**
- If no improvement within 6-12 hr

Poor Response Within 1 Hour
- History: high-risk patient
- Physical examination: symptoms severe, drowsiness, confusion
- PEF <30%
- PCO_2 >45 mm Hg
- PO_2 <60 mm Hg

↓

Admit to Intensive Care
- Inhaled β_2-agonist + anticholinergic
- Intravenous glucocorticosteroid
- Consider subcutaneous, intramuscular, or intravenous β_2-agonists
- Oxygen
- Consider intravenous methylxanthines
- Possible intubation and mechanical ventilation

NOTE: Preferred treatments are inhaled β_2-agonists in high doses and glucocorticosteroids. If inhaled β_2-agonists are not available, methylxanthines may be considered.

FIGURE 108-1

Management of asthma attacks: hospital-based care. *FEV_1*, Forced expiratory volume in 1 second; *PEF*, peak expiratory flow. (From Global Initiative for Asthma: *Pocket guide for asthma management and prevention: a pocket guide for physicians and nurses*, updated 2005, NIH Pub No 02-3659.)

TABLE 108-6 Risk Factors and Actions to Reduce Exposures

Risk Factor	Actions
Domestic dust mite allergens (so small they are not visible to the naked eye)	Wash bed linens and blankets weekly in hot water and dry in a hot dryer or the sun. Encase pillows and mattresses in air-tight covers. Replace carpets with linoleum or wood flooring, especially in sleeping rooms. Use vinyl, leather, or plain wooden furniture instead of fabric-upholstered furniture. If possible, use vacuum cleaner with filters.
Tobacco smoke (whether the patient smokes or breathes in the smoke from others)	Stay away from tobacco smoke. Patients and parents should not smoke.
Allergens from animals with fur	Remove animals from the home, or at least from the sleeping area.
Cockroach allergen	Clean the home thoroughly and often. Use pesticide spray—but make certain the patient is not at home when spraying occurs.
Outdoor pollens and mold	Close windows and doors and remain indoors when pollen and mold counts are highest.
Indoor mold	Reduce dampness in the home; clean any damp areas frequently.
Physical activity	Do not avoid physical activity. Symptoms can be prevented by taking a rapid-acting inhaled β_2 agonist, a cromone, or a leukotriene modifier before strenuous exercise.
Drugs	Do not take beta blockers or aspirin or NSAIDs if these medicines cause asthma symptoms.

From Global Initiative for Asthma: *Pocket guide for asthma management and prevention: a pocket guide for physicians and nurses,* updated 2005, NIH Pub No 02-3659, retrieved Sept 7, 2006, from http://www.ginasthma.org.

doses and have fewer side effects for a given level of therapeutic effect than medications administered orally. There is no consensus on the specific type or dose of inhaled steroid to be used. In general, dosage begins with 2 to 4 puffs/day and is increased based on the individual's response. Each of the inhaled steroids has its own maximum number of doses per day as summarized in Table 108-7 (EPR).

High-potency ICSs, budesonide (Pulmicort) and fluticasone (Flovent), provide the same therapeutic effect as other ICSs but in fewer puffs. Both drugs come in preparations of different potencies; with the higher-potency inhalers, fewer puffs are necessary to deliver the same dose as compared with other types of steroid inhalers. The usual daily estimated comparative daily dosages for inhaled glucocorticoids and ICSs can be found in Table 108-8.

The major side effect of inhaled steroids is oral thrush, which can be prevented by good oral hygiene and the use of aerosol spacers during delivery. The safety of long-term

TABLE 108-7 Estimated Comparative Daily Dosages for Inhaled Corticosteroids

	Low Daily Dose		Medium Daily Dose		High Daily Dose	
Drug	Adult	Child*	Adult	Child*	Adult	Child*
Beclomethasone CFC 42 or 84 mcg/puff	168-504 mcg	84-336 mcg	504-840 mcg	336-672 mcg	>840 mcg	>672 mcg
Beclomethasone HFA 40 or 80 mcg/puff	80-240 mcg	80-160 mcg	240-480 mcg	160-320 mcg	>480 mcg	>320 mcg
Budesonide DPI 200 mcg/inhalation	200-600 mcg	200-400 mcg	600-1200 mcg	400-800 mcg	>1200 mcg	>800 mcg
Inhalation suspension for nebulization (child dose)		0.5 mcg		1 mcg		2 mcg
Flunisolide 250 mcg/puff	500-1000 mcg	500-750 mcg	1000-2000 mcg	1000-1250 mcg	>2000 mcg	>1250 mcg
Fluticasone MDI 44, 110, or 220 mcg/puff	88-264 mcg	88-176 mcg	264-660 mcg	176-440 mcg	>660 mcg	>440 mcg
Fluticasone DPI 50, 100, or 250 mcg/inhalation	100-300 mcg	100-200 mcg	300-600 mcg	200-400 mcg	>600 mcg	>400 mcg
Triamcinolone acetonide 100 mcg/puff	400-1000 mcg	400-800 mcg	1000-2000 mcg	800-1200 mcg	>2000 mcg	>1200 mcg

From Global Initiative for Asthma: *Pocket guide for asthma management and prevention: a pocket guide for physicians and nurses,* updated 2005, NIH Pub No 02-3659, retrieved Sept 7, 2006, from http://www.ginasthma.org.

CFC, Chlorofluorocarbon; *DPI,* dry powder inhaler; *HFA,* hydrofluoroalkane-134a; *MDI,* metered dose inhaler.

*Children ≤12 years of age.

TABLE 108-8 Usual Dosages for Long-Term Control Medications

Medication	Dosage Form	Adult Dose	Child Dose*
INHALED CORTICOSTEROIDS (See Table 108-7)			
SYSTEMIC CORTICOSTEROIDS		**(Applies to all 3 corticosteroids)**	
Methylprednisolone	2, 4, 8, 16, 32 mg tablets	7.5-60 mg/day in a single dose	0.25-2 mg/kg/day in single dose in AM or q.o.d. as needed for control
Prednisolone	5 mg tablets, 5 mg/5 cc, 15 mg/5 cc	Short-course "burst" to achieve control: 40-60 mg/day as single or 2 divided doses for 3-10 days	Short course "burst": 1-2 mg/kg/day, maximum 60 mg/day for 3-10 days
Prednisone	1, 2.5, 5, 10, 20, 50 mg tablets 5 mg/cc, 5 mg/5 cc		
LONG-ACTING INHALED β_2 AGONISTS†			
Salmeterol	MDI 21 mcg/puff	2 puffs q 12 hr	1-2 puffs q 12 hr
	DPI 50 mcg/blister	1 blister q 12 hr	1 blister q 12 hr
Formoterol	DPI 12 mcg/single-use capsule	1 capsule q 12 hr	1 capsule q 12 hr
COMBINED MEDICATION			
Fluticasone-salmeterol	DPI 100, 250, or 500 mcg/50 mcg	1 inhalation b.i.d.; dose depends on severity of asthma	1 inhalation b.i.d.; dose depends on severity of asthma
CROMOLYN AND NEDOCROMIL			
Cromolyn	MDI 1 mg/puff	2-4 puffs t.i.d.-q.i.d.	1-2 puffs t.i.d.-q.i.d.
	Nebulizer 20 mg/ampule	1 ampule t.i.d.-q.i.d.	1 ampule t.i.d.-q.i.d.
Nedocromil	MDI 1.75 mg/puff	2-4 puffs b.i.d.-q.i.d.	1-2 puffs b.i.d.-q.i.d.
LEUKOTRIENE MODIFIERS			
Montelukast	4-5 mg chewable tablet 10 mg tablet 10 mg q.h.s. (>14 years)	10 mg q.h.s.	4 mg q.h.s. (2-5 years) 5 mg q.h.s. (6-14 years)
Zafirlukast	10-20 mg tablet	40 mg/day (20 mg tablet b.i.d.)	20 mg/day (7-11 years) (10 mg tablet b.i.d.)
Zileuton	300 or 600 mg tablet	2400 mg/day (give tablets q.i.d.)	
METHYLXANTHINES‡			
Theophylline	Liquids, sustained-release tablets, and capsules	Starting dose 10 mg/kg/day up to 300 mg max; usual max 800 mg/day	Starting dose 10 mg/kg/day; usual max: <1 year of age: 0.2 (age in weeks) + 5 = mg/kg/day ≥1 year of age: 16 mg/kg/day

From National Heart, Lung, and Blood Institute: *Asthma statistics,* Bethesda, Md, Jan 1999, National Institutes of Health, US Department of Health and Human Services, The Institute.
DPI, Dry powder inhaler; *MDI,* metered dose inhaler.
*Children ≤12 years of age.
†Should not be used for symptom relief or for exacerbations. Use with inhaled corticosteroids.
‡Serum monitoring is important (serum concentration of 5-15 mcg/ml at steady state).

therapy with high-dose inhaled steroids has not been well established, and their use may be associated with untoward side effects, including adrenal suppression, bone loss, skin bruising, glaucoma, behavioral abnormalities, and the possibility of inhibited growth in children. It is still unknown whether the use of high-potency steroids increases the risk of adrenal suppression and other systemic side effects.[2,19]

Systemic corticosteroids are used in the management of asthma symptoms not responding to standard treatment. In general, a steroid "pulse" with initial dosages of prednisone of 40 to 60 mg/day tapering to 0 over the ensuing 1 to 2 weeks is prescribed. If symptoms worsen during this period, the dose is increased and the taper restarted. For persons not responding to a prednisone taper or with life-threatening symptoms, in-hospital treatment is necessary and IV methylprednisolone is often used.[2] Untoward side effects of systemic corticosteroids include hypothalamic–adrenal axis suppression, electrolyte imbalances, myopathy, osteoporosis, peptic ulcer, dermal atrophy, carbohydrate intolerance, increased intracranial pressure, and psychiatric disturbances.

Cromolyn and Nedocromil. Cromolyn sodium (Intal) and nedocromil sodium (Tilade) are antiinflammatory agents whose specific mechanism of action is not yet well understood. Both are used in the prophylaxis of mild to moderate asthma, rather than for the treatment of acute symptoms. Both agents are more useful when exposure to an identifiable factor (such as exercise, cold air, or animal dander) triggers symptoms.

These agents may be useful prophylactically when a known asthma trigger cannot be avoided. In such situations they may be good alternatives to inhaled steroids because they have a better safety and side effect profile. Both agents tend to be more useful in the pediatric population than in the adult population. In addition, if it is effective in controlling symptoms, nedocromil may be preferred to corticosteroid therapy during pregnancy for safety reasons. Nedocromil may also be particularly helpful in persons whose primary asthma symptom is cough. Nedocromil is the more potent of the two agents and has the advantage of twice-daily dosing. It is not well tolerated in some patients because of a perceived bitter taste or throat irritation.[2]

Xanthine Derivatives. Xanthine derivatives, such as theophylline, are used for long-term asthma management and sustained relief of symptoms. Theophylline and aminophylline have a long history of use in asthma and have been traditionally considered to be bronchodilators of moderate potency. These drugs also have an inotropic effect on the diaphragm and antiinflammatory activity, which may be beneficial in asthma. One of the major difficulties with using theophylline is its relatively narrow therapeutic index and the potentially significant variations in plasma levels, both in a single individual and within a population over time. A number of drugs affect the metabolism of theophylline, and careful monitoring of serum levels during treatment is recommended (Table 108-9). Acceptable therapeutic plasma levels are between 10 and 20 mcg/ml, although clinical improvement has been noted at subtherapeutic levels. Higher plasma levels are associated with gastrointestinal, cardiac, and central nervous system toxicity, including such symptoms as headache, nausea, vomiting, diarrhea, cardiac arrhythmias, and seizures.[21]

The use of theophylline in asthma management has declined with the availability of other maintenance medications that have fewer side effects and do not require monitoring of serum levels. Nonetheless, theophylline may be useful in certain situations (e.g., as an additional agent to ICS when better long-term control is still needed).

Leukotriene Modifiers. Currently four antileukotriene agents are on the market: montelukast, pranlukast, zafirlukast, and zileuton. These antiinflammatory agents target a single group of inflammatory mediators; they interfere with the effects of leukotrienes by either blocking the leukotriene receptor or reducing the activity of enzymes required for leukotriene synthesis. As inflammatory mediators, leukotrienes increase endothelial permeability, which increases airway edema and mucus secretion, further increasing airway obstruction. In addition, the leukotrienes directly potentiate bronchoconstriction mediated by leukotriene receptors on bronchial smooth muscle.[19,32] In persons with persistent asthma the leukotriene modifiers have been shown to increase persistent bronchodilation; reduce asthma symptoms, including nocturnal asthma symptoms; reduce medication use; and decrease the need for prednisone quick-relief therapy.[21] All leukotriene modifiers can increase prothrombin times in persons receiving anticoagulant therapy; prothrombin times should be monitored more closely in these cases.

Zafirlukast, montelukast, and pranlukast are oral leukotriene-receptor antagonists, which prevent the binding of leukotrienes at receptor sites. Zafirlukast has a relatively rapid onset of action, and its effects are additive with β-adrenergic bronchodilators. It has been shown to be helpful in reducing cold air–, exercise-, and allergen-induced bronchoconstriction and nocturnal asthma symptoms. Zafirlukast should be taken on an empty stomach. The other leukotriene-receptor antagonist, montelukast, is also rapidly absorbed after oral administration, with peak plasma levels achieved in 2.5 to 4 hours, depending on the dose. Montelukast is used in conjunction with other asthma therapies for the prophylaxis and chronic treatment of asthma. It should not be used as monotherapy for the treatment and management of exercise-induced bronchospasm and also should not be used for the treatment of acute asthma attacks. In clinical trials the most common adverse side effects were similar to those associated with zafirlukast. In addition, in rare cases montelukast therapy has been associated with systemic eosinophilia, although a causal relationship has not been established.[33]

Pranlukast, the newest leukotriene antagonist, is also indicated for the prophylactic treatment of chronic asthma in pediatric and adult patients. In limited clinical studies, pranlukast 225 mg b.i.d. appears to be as effective as montelukast 10 mg once daily and zafirlukast 40 mg b.i.d. in adults with mild to moderate asthma.[34] Pranlukast has also been shown to be effective in patients with mild to severe asthma. Gastrointestinal side effects and hepatic function abnormalities are the most commonly reported adverse side effects. Pranlukast can be used for monotherapy for the treatment of mild persistent asthma with as-required short-acting $beta_2$ agonists or in conjunction with ICS in the management of moderate or severe asthma.[34]

Zileuton is an oral leukotriene synthesis inhibitor with similar effects in clinical trials to those of the leukotriene receptor antagonists. Zileuton can be taken without regard to meals. In clinical trials zileuton therapy was associated with elevated liver enzyme levels in some subjects. For this reason, it is recommended that liver enzyme levels be obtained at baseline and monitored at regular intervals throughout the first year and periodically thereafter for persons receiving zileuton therapy. Its use is contraindicated in persons with active liver disease or with abnormal liver function tests. Zileuton also increases serum levels of theophylline, and in persons receiving concurrent theophylline therapy the dosage generally needs to be reduced by approximately 50%.[35] Several other antileukotriene agents are currently in clinical trials and are likely to receive U.S. Food and Drug Administration approval in the near future.

Because antileukotriene agents have only recently been approved for use in asthma management and because they are less potent than corticosteroids, specific guidelines for their use in asthma therapy have not yet been developed. Their use is recommended for the treatment of chronic persistent asthma. They may be helpful in reducing the quantity of inhaled or oral corticosteroids needed to control symptoms, which would be especially helpful for persons who experience troubling corticosteroid side effects. In addition, they may be effective alternatives to long-acting bronchodilators, such as

TABLE 108-9 Factors Affecting Serum Theophylline Concentrations*

Factor	Decreases Theophylline Concentrations	Increases Theophylline Concentrations	Recommended Action
Food	↓ Or delays absorption of some sustained-release theophylline (SRT) products	↑ Rate of absorption (fatty foods) products	Select theophylline preparation that is not affected by food.
Diet	↑ Metabolism (high protein)	↓ Metabolism (high carbohydrate)	Inform patients that major changes in diet are not recommended while taking theophylline.
Systemic, febrile viral illness (e.g., influenza)		↓ Metabolism	Decrease theophylline dose according to serum concentration level. Decrease dose by 50% if serum concentration measurement is not available.
Hypoxia, cor pulmonale, decompensated congestive heart failure, cirrhosis		↓ Metabolism	Decrease dose according to serum concentration level.
Age	↑ Metabolism (1- 9 years)	↓ Metabolism (<6 months, older adults)	Adjust dose according to serum concentration level.
Phenobarbital, phenytoin, carbamazepine	↑ Metabolism		Increase dose according to serum concentration level.
Cimetidine		↓ Metabolism	Use alternative H_2 blocker (e.g., famotidine or ranitidine).
Macrolides: TAO, erythromycin, clarithromycin		↓ Metabolism	Use alternative antibiotic or adjust theophylline dose.
Quinolones: ciprofloxacin, enoxacin		↓ Metabolism	Use alternative antibiotic or adjust theophylline dose. Circumvent with ofloxacin if quinolone therapy is required.
Rifampin	↑ Metabolism		Increase dose according to serum concentration level.
Ticlopidine		↓ Metabolism	Decrease dose according to serum concentration level.
Smoking	↑ Metabolism		Advise patient to stop smoking; increase dose according to serum concentration level.

From National Institutes of Health, National Heart, Lung and Blood Institute: *Highlights of the Expert Panel Report 2: guidelines for the diagnosis and management of asthma,* NIH Pub No 97-4051A, Washington, DC, 1997, US Department of Health and Human Services.
TAO, Triacetyloleandomycin.
*This list is not all inclusive; for discussion of other factors, see package inserts.

salmeterol (Serevent) and theophylline. They may also be helpful for persons with aspirin-induced asthma, since they offer some protection against a variety of environmental substances that often produce cross-reactions in persons with aspirin sensitivities.[35]

Long-Acting β_2-Adrenergic Agonists. Salmeterol is the only long-acting bronchodilator. It has an onset of action within 1 to 2 hours of administration and a duration of 10 to 14 hours. Because of its slow onset of action, salmeterol should never be used as a quick-relief medication for short-term relief of acute symptoms. The best use for long-acting β_2-adrenergic agonists has not yet been determined. Salmeterol has been used effectively in controlling nocturnal asthma symptoms. In addition, salmeterol may be effective in controlling anticipated exercise-induced asthma and may mitigate the need to use short-acting bronchodilators before each activity. When salmeterol is prescribed, patients need to be specifically instructed not to use this drug for relief of acute bronchospasm.[19,35]

Quick-Relief Medications

Short-Acting β_2-Adrenergic Agonists. Short-acting β_2-adrenergic agonists (bronchodilators) act as bronchodilators by relaxing airway smooth muscle that has become constricted as a result of stimuli in the environment (see Table 108-4). Short-acting bronchodilators may also provide effective prophylaxis against anticipated asthma triggers, including exercise, cold air, and certain allergens. Short-acting β_2-adrenergic agonists usually provide rapid relief of symptoms, but they do not affect the underlying inflammation associated with asthma. Short-acting β_2-adrenergic agonists are not approved as maintenance medications because their use does not improve long-term asthma control. An increase in the use of bronchodilator therapy indicates worsening asthma; in fact, the need for more than 2 puffs once or twice daily of bronchodilator (quick-relief) medication or the use of more than one canister per month is generally an indication that a person's asthma is inadequately controlled.[36] In such cases the asthma management plan should be reviewed, and anti-inflammatory medication should probably be added to the therapy or, if it is already being used, prescribed at an increased dose.[19] Short-acting β_2-adrenergic agonists are available in inhaled (metered-dose inhaler [MDI] or nebulizer), oral, and IV preparations. All β_2-adrenergic agonists used routinely for asthma therapy have an onset of action of 10 to 15 minutes and a duration of effect of 4 to 6 hours. Side effects of the short-acting bronchodilators include tachycardia, hypertension, tremors, nervousness, headache, dizziness, hyperactivity, insomnia, nausea, and muscle cramps.

Because these medications are generally administered by MDI, it is important that inhaler technique be reviewed on a regular basis. When bronchodilators do not promptly and completely resolve symptoms of bronchoconstriction, systemic glucocorticoid therapy is indicated for suppression and reversal of underlying airway inflammation.[37]

Anticholinergic Agents. Anticholinergic agents such as ipratropium bromide (Atrovent) are sometimes useful in reversing bronchoconstriction. Bronchial smooth muscle receptors, innervated by the vagus nerve, respond to acetylcholine, which induces bronchoconstriction. Anticholinergic agents have been shown to have a bronchodilator effect in persons with mild to moderate asthma, but the effect is generally not as significant as that of the short-acting β_2-adrenergic agents. They may be used as alternatives for symptomatic relief for those who have difficulty tolerating the side effects of the β_2-adrenergic bronchodilators.

Monitoring Therapy and Asthma Severity

Asthma management guidelines stress the importance of assessment of pulmonary function using PEFR meters rather than basing assessment on the individual's perception of dyspnea (POD). Studies have shown that in 60% of individuals there is no correlation between POD and simultaneous peak flow measurements and that the majority of individuals have a blunted POD (i.e., an underestimation of respiratory compromise), resulting in undertreatment of asthma, a delay in treatment changes, and perhaps even a predisposition to fatal asthma attacks.[38] Therefore it is recommended that all individuals with moderate to severe asthma learn how to monitor their PEF and have a flow meter at home. PEF monitoring during exacerbations should be encouraged for all those with moderate to severe, persistent asthma, and PEF should guide management. In addition, long-term daily peak flow monitoring is recommended for individuals with moderate to severe asthma to help maintain control of symptoms; however, if long-term monitoring is not done, periodic short-term monitoring is recommended for evaluating responses to therapy or assessing the effect of environmental exposures. All individuals with asthma who experience periodic severe asthma exacerbations may benefit from peak flow monitoring.[3]

Peak flow monitoring helps individuals follow the course of their disease, predict exacerbations, identify triggers, and assess their response to treatment.[19] PEF values, specifically the individual's personal best PEF, should be used as the basis for an action plan. An individual's personal best PEF can be estimated after a 2- to 3-week period during which the PEF is recorded at least once a day in the early afternoon. Additional measurements should be made after β_2-adrenergic inhalers are used for symptomatic relief. The personal best is usually achieved in the early afternoon after maximum effect of any therapy has stabilized or resolved the symptoms. The personal best should be reassessed periodically to account for progression of disease. A PEF value that is significantly higher than all the other measurements should be interpreted with caution; rather than reflecting a personal best, an outlying value may be due to spitting or coughing into the peak flow meter.[3]

A zone system similar to a traffic light has been successfully used to help patients interpret their symptoms and PEFR results. The use of this system is particularly helpful for asthmatic patients who are unable to recognize the severity of their asthma based on symptoms, which is estimated to be the case for more than 50% of patients. In addition, many studies have shown that asthma symptoms correlate poorly with the level of airway obstruction as determined by spirometry (FEV_1 and PEF). After treatment, subjective improvement in asthma symptoms may occur without a corresponding improvement in the degree of airway obstruction. For this reason, current guidelines recommend that airway obstruction be measured objectively when assessing patients with chronic asthma.[39]

The zone system consists of green, yellow, and red zones (or lights if the traffic light analogy is used). The green zone (or light) corresponds to a PEF measurement that is at least 80% of an individual's personal best or optimum control. For patients with irritable airways who decompensate quickly, the cutoff may be adjusted to 90%.[7] A measurement in the green zone reflects good asthma control and that it is *safe* to proceed. The yellow zone means *caution* and refers to a PEF measurement that is within 50% to 80% of the individual's personal best or optimum control. Some guidelines use a range of 60% to 80% for the yellow zone; the more conservative value of 60% promotes earlier intervention as the patient's condition begins to deteriorate. Symptoms that interfere with daily activities may be present; typical symptoms include cough, wheeze, chest tightness, shortness of breath, and nocturnal awakening. A measurement in the yellow zone indicates the need for a temporary increase in medication dose or frequency. The specific medication change is tailored to each individual and may include increased bronchodilator therapy, increased or added corticosteroid therapy, and a short course of oral corticosteroids.

In many ways the yellow zone is the key to the entire asthma action plan (AAP), since a measurement in this zone reflects worsening airway obstruction, which will usually continue to worsen if action is not taken. The written AAP should identify at what point the provider should be contacted; in general, patients should be instructed to contact their health care provider for mild to moderate symptoms that do not respond to treatment or for PEFs that remain within the yellow zone (50% to 80% of personal best). A PEF value or symptoms in the red zone mean *danger* and indicate the need for emergency treatment. A reduction in the PEF of 50% (or 40%) and dyspnea are the general criteria for the red zone. Other associated symptoms may include inability to blow into the peak flow meter, accessory respiratory muscle use, difficulty walking or talking because of asthma, and cyanosis. Immediately using inhaled rescue bronchodilator therapy and initiating or increasing oral corticosteroid therapy are necessary. If the PEFR does not improve after emergency treatment, the individual should be instructed to call 911 (or an emergency number) or proceed to the emergency department (or to his or her health care provider). The AAP should clearly state in the red zone portion when patients need to seek emergency care.[7,19]

The NAEPP has developed a self-management program for asthma exacerbations that is based on the zone system (see Tables 108-2 and 108-3). These asthma management guidelines emphasize the importance of teaching asthma self-management and prevention techniques to patients. This includes the provision of an individualized asthma action plan, accompanied by regular medical visits and reviews by a health care provider.[3]

It has been well established that improving asthma adherence can lead to better control. Despite growing awareness of the importance of asthma education, however, adherence to asthma treatment, including medications, the use of peak flow meters, and avoidance of environmental irritants, is still poor. The provider-patient relationship is central to improving adherence; all specific strategies aimed at improving adherence (such as simplifying medication regimens or using AAPs) must be developed in a therapeutic, trusting provider-patient relationship to be effective.[40] Studies have shown that asthma therapy based on influencing behavior and self-management of acute exacerbations results in improved control and decreased asthma morbidity.[7,41,42]

Current practice guidelines recommend follow-up visits at 1- to 6-month intervals, depending on the severity of asthma and the degree of control. Persons with mild asthma who, for example, experience occasional exacerbations only after exercise may need only an annual visit for asthma or have it addressed as part of an annual examination. On the other hand, persons with moderate to severe asthma with frequent exacerbations may need monthly visits to review PEFR readings and assess the effectiveness of medications and self-management.[35]

Co-Management with Specialists

The current NIH guidelines state that all patients who have had an asthma-related hospitalization (and thus, by definition, have chronic severe asthma) be evaluated by an asthma specialist. In addition, general reasons for consultation with a specialist include poorly controlled asthma, asthma that is unresponsive to appropriate therapy, the desire to obtain a second opinion, and periodic patient evaluation. Specific reasons for specialist consultation may include classification of asthma type and severity, interpretation of PFT results, assessment of possible occupational asthma, allergy skin testing, and advice about pharmacotherapy.[43] Evidence of poorly controlled asthma, including frequent missed days of work or school, dissatisfaction with the quality of life, and frequent emergency department visits and hospitalizations, may reflect lack of recognition of the disease severity by the patient or health care provider or treatment plans that are too simplistic. In such cases, referral to an asthma specialist is warranted and will likely improve control and the quality of life and decrease asthma-related morbidity and mortality.

LIFE SPAN CONSIDERATIONS

The preparation for pregnancy in women with asthma should, if possible, begin well in advance to achieve good asthma control before and during the pregnancy. In about equal proportions of women, the control of asthma will improve, worsen, or remain unchanged during pregnancy. Just as with any individual, unmanaged asthma in a pregnant woman may result in emergency department visits, hospitalizations, respiratory failure, and even death. In addition, poorly managed asthma has been associated with certain complications of pregnancy, including an increased incidence of preeclampsia, eclampsia, low birth weight, premature delivery, and infant death.[44] Given the potential for and possible consequences of asthma complications during pregnancy, it is vitally important that pulmonary function (minimally peak flow monitoring) be monitored throughout pregnancy. Because a 20% drop in peak flow often precedes the onset of symptoms, pregnant women need to be able to recognize when they fall 80% below their baseline. In addition, an appreciation of ability to improve or lack of improvement is essential so that appropriate prompt treatment can be initiated.

The basic management of asthma during pregnancy is similar to that in nonpregnant individuals. To minimize the need for medications, environmental and lifestyle controls assume an even more important role. No asthma therapy has been proved to be absolutely safe during pregnancy. For women who require only β_2-adrenergic agonists, metaproterenol is usually the drug of choice. For women requiring antiinflammatory medication, the use of beclomethasone or cromolyn is considered relatively safe. During more severe exacerbations of asthma, tapered regimens of oral prednisone are used, since the risks of anoxia to the fetus outweigh the possible risks of oral corticosteroid therapy.[17,24]

There has been a steady increase in the prevalence of asthma from adolescence to old age. Asthma tends to be less well recognized among older adults, since symptoms are often attributed to other respiratory ailments such as COPD, congestive heart failure, pulmonary aspiration, pulmonary embolism, and bronchogenic carcinoma. However, the tools usually used to diagnose asthma are still helpful in ruling out the differential diagnoses in this population. If the clinical picture is indistinguishable from either COPD or asthma, it is often useful to consider age of onset; asthmatics have generally experienced symptoms at an earlier age and had a clearer history during their younger years.[45,46]

In addition, subjective awareness and perception of symptoms tend to be poorer among older adults. For these reasons, asthma remains underdiagnosed and suboptimally treated in this population.[39] In older adults, chronic bronchitis may co-exist with asthma, which may affect management. Asthma medications may aggravate co-existing medical conditions, such as cardiac disease and osteoporosis; adjustments in the pharmacotherapy may need to be made. Certain drugs commonly used in older people, including aspirin and beta blockers, may adversely affect asthma. Finally, older adults may have particular difficulty with inhaler administration; their technique should be carefully reviewed, and devices such as spacers may be especially helpful in improving drug delivery in this population. Overall, asthma in older adults tends to be associated with poor overall health and reduced mobility, despite adjustment for living conditions, depression, cognition, visual or auditory impairment, and joint pain.[45]

Nonetheless, appropriate care in older individuals is achievable. Most adverse reactions to asthma drugs may require dose adjustment but are generally not significant enough to warrant discontinuation of the drug. The use of large-volume spacers improves the inhalation technique, and most older individuals prefer using this device to using the MDI alone.[45]

COMPLICATIONS

Complications of asthma include status asthmaticus and fatal asthma. Status asthmaticus is present when symptoms do not improve or remit with initial treatment of an acute exacerbation. During status asthmaticus, despite maximum therapy, respiratory failure may develop.[24] Signs and symptoms indicative of respiratory failure include paradoxical thoracoabdominal movement, absence of wheeze, bradycardia, and a deterioration in mental status. If an exacerbation is severe enough that respiratory failure seems possible, intubation should be performed sooner rather than later.[36]

The increasing rates of asthma morbidity and mortality are disturbing. The reasons for these increasing rates are unclear; however, certain risk factors for fatal asthma have been identified. Co-morbidity (such as from cardiovascular disease or COPD) and serious psychiatric disease or psychosocial problems increase the risk of fatal or near-fatal asthma. Difficulty perceiving airflow obstruction or its severity and a history of sudden severe exacerbations also increase the risk of fatal asthma. However, a period of 2 to 7 days of worsening asthma symptoms rather than a sudden deterioration often precedes hospitalizations, providing a window of opportunity to implement more aggressive therapy in an effort to prevent fatal or near-fatal events. Additional risk factors include hospitalization or emergency care for asthma within the past month, prior asthma-related ICU care, three or more emergency department visits or two or more hospitalizations for asthma during the past year, and prior intubation for asthma. Other risk factors include current use or withdrawal from systemic glucocorticoids and the use of three or more canisters of inhaled short-acting β_2-adrenergic agonists per month. Urban residence, low socioeconomic status, and illicit drug use also increase the risk for fatal asthma.[3,8,47] These risk factors affirm the need for interventions designed to prevent and control asthma, as well as therapy that includes the self-management of asthma symptoms during periods of exacerbation, especially for those at high risk.

Research has demonstrated that in comparison with other patient groups, adults with asthma who have lower socioeconomic status and less education are likely to receive care that has less continuity and is less intensive after hospital or emergency department discharge. In addition, a minority of these patients tend to have AAPs or adequate communication with their health care providers during the acute stages of the exacerbation. In addition, those most at risk for fatal asthma are more likely to depend primarily on the emergency department for management of exacerbations. In other words, those individuals who are at highest risk for complications of asthma are likely to receive the type of care that increases rather than mitigates the risk of future complications.[8,10,47-49]

INDICATIONS FOR REFERRAL OR HOSPITALIZATION

Referral to an asthma specialist for consultation or co-management is recommended if there are any difficulties achieving or maintaining control of asthma or if step 3 or 4 care is required. Hospitalization should be considered for all patients whose symptoms do not improve or remit with initial aggressive treatment of the acute exacerbation. The NHLBI's guidelines for the management of asthma exacerbations in the emergency department and hospital are included in Figure 108-1.

PATIENT EDUCATION

Patient education is both one of the most important and one of the most challenging aspects of asthma management. Asthma is a chronic disease and, like other chronic diseases, requires ongoing maintenance and prevention. Asthma that is treated only episodically when exacerbations occur will result in symptomatic relief at best. To achieve the other goals of asthma treatment (such as preventing symptoms, maintaining near-normal pulmonary function, minimizing the adverse effects of pharmacotherapy, and minimizing the need for emergency department visits and hospitalizations), patients and their families need to be well educated about the disease, its basis, and their role in monitoring symptoms and preventing exacerbations. Table 108-10 summarizes asthma education to be included as part of patient care visits.

Every patient with asthma should participate with his or her health care provider in setting up an individualized written asthma management plan, or AAP, that includes his or her own asthma triggers, a detailed description of relevant environmental control measures, instructions on the role and use of medications and delivery devices (e.g., spacers, nebulizers), monitoring techniques (e.g., PEFR meters), and instructions on how to tailor therapy to deal with changing symptoms. The use of peak flow meters and proper inhaler technique and use are described in Boxes 108-5 and 108-6, respectively. Patients should be taught how to recognize symptom patterns, interpret PEFR results, and increase treatment during exacerbations of asthma.[7,19] An AAP should be developed for each individual based on signs and symptoms and/or PEFR, with instructions on how and when to change pharmacotherapy and when to contact the health care provider. Emphasis should be placed on the long-term control medications (antiinflammatory medications) used to achieve and maintain control of persistent asthma and quick-relief medications (bronchodilators) used to treat acute symptoms and exacerbations.[3] In addition to allowing for the early recognition of symptoms and earlier initiation of treatment, which can minimize the severity of exacerbations, AAPs also increase confidence, security, and ability for self-control in individuals with asthma and their families.[11]

TABLE 108-10 Delivery of Asthma Education by Clinicians During Patient Care Visits

Assessment Questions	Information	Skills
RECOMMENDATIONS FOR INITIAL VISIT		
Focus on: • Concerns • Quality of life • Expectations • Goals of treatment	Teach in simple language.	Teach and demonstrate.
"What worries you most about your asthma?" "What do you want to accomplish at this visit?" "What do you want to be able to do that you can't do now because of your asthma?" "What do you expect from treatment?" "What medicines have you tried?" "What other questions do you have for me today?"	What is asthma? A chronic lung disease. The airways are very sensitive. They become inflamed and narrow; breathing becomes difficult. Asthma treatments: two types of medicines are needed: • Long-term control: medications that prevent symptoms, often by reducing inflammation • Quick relief: short-acting bronchodilator that relax muscles around airways Bring all medications to every appointment. When to seek medical advice. Provide appropriate telephone number.	Inhaler and spacer/holding chamber use. Check performance. Self-monitoring skills that are tied to an action plan: • Recognize intensity and frequency of asthma symptoms. • Review the signs of deterioration and the need to reevaluate therapy: Waking at night with asthma Increased medication use Decreased activity tolerance Use of a simple, written self-management plan and action plan
RECOMMENDATIONS FOR FIRST FOLLOW-UP VISIT (2-4 WEEKS OR SOONER AS NEEDED)		
Focus on: • Concerns • Quality of life • Expectations • Goals of treatment	Teach or review in simple language.	Teach or review and demonstrate.
Ask relevant questions from previous visit and also ask: "What medications are you taking?" "How and when are you taking them?" "What problems have you had using your medications?" "Please show me how you use your inhaled medications."	Use of two types of medications. Remind patient to bring all medications and the peak flow meter to every appointment for review. Self-evaluation of progress in asthma control using symptoms and peak flow as a guide.	Use of a daily self-management plan. Review and adjust as needed. Use of an action plan. Review and adjust as needed. Peak flow monitoring and daily diary recording. Correct inhaler and spacer/holding chamber technique.
RECOMMENDATIONS FOR SECOND FOLLOW-UP VISIT		
Focus on: • Expectations of visit • Goals of treatment • Medications • Quality of life	Teach or review in simple language.	Teach or review and demonstrate.
Ask relevant questions from previous visits and also ask: "Have you noticed anything in your home, work, or school that makes your asthma worse?" "Describe for me how you know when to call your doctor or go to the hospital for asthma care." "What questions do you have about the action plan? Can we make it easier?" "Are your medications causing you any problems?"	Relevant environmental control-avoidance strategies: • How to identify home, work, or school exposures that can cause or worsen asthma • How to control house-dust mites, animal exposures if applicable • How to avoid cigarette smoke (active and passive) Review all medications. Review and interpret peak flow measures and symptom scores from daily diary.	Inhaler/spacer/holding chamber technique. Peak flow technique. Use of daily self-management plan. Review and adjust as needed. Use of the action plan. Confirm that patient knows what to do if asthma gets worse.

TABLE 108-10 Delivery of Asthma Education by Clinicians During Patient Care Visits—cont'd

Assessment Questions	Information	Skills
RECOMMENDATIONS FOR SUBSEQUENT VISITS		
Focus on: • Expectation of visit • Goals of treatment • Medications • Quality of life	Teach or review in simple language.	Teach or review and demonstrate.
Ask relevant questions from previous visits and also ask: "How have you tried to control things that make your asthma worse?" "Please show me how you use your inhaled medication."	Review and reinforce all: • Educational messages • Environmental control strategies at home, work, or school • Medications Review and interpret from diary: • Peak flow • Symptom scores	Inhaler/spacer/holding chamber technique. Peak flow technique. Use of daily self-management plan. Review and adjust as needed. Use of the action plan. Confirm that patient knows what to do if asthma gets worse. Periodically review and adjust the written action plan.

From National Institutes of Health, National Heart, Lung, and Blood Institute: *Highlights of the Expert Panel Report 2: guidelines for the diagnosis and management of asthma,* NIH Pub No 97-4051A, Washington, DC, 1997, US Department of Health and Human Services.

BOX 108-5

PEAK FLOW METERS: USES AND TECHNIQUE

Lung function measurements assess airflow limitation and help diagnose and monitor the course of asthma.

To assess the level of airflow limitation, two methods are used. Peak flow meters measure peak expiratory flow (PEF), and spirometers measure forced expiratory volume in 1 second (FEV_1) and its accompanying forced vital capacity (FVC). The accuracy of all lung function measurements depends on patient effort and correct technique.

Several kinds of peak flow meters and spirometers are available, and the technique for use is similar for all. It is important to use a "low flow" peak flow meter for younger children. Appropriate ages for use are usually indicated by the manufacturer. To use a peak flow meter:

- Stand up and hold the peak flow meter without restricting movement of the marker.
- Make sure the marker is at the bottom of the scale.
- Take a deep breath, put the peak flow meter in your mouth, seal your lips around the mouthpiece, and breathe out as hard and fast as possible. Do not put your tongue inside the mouthpiece.
- Record the result. Return the marker to zero.
- Repeat twice more. Choose the highest of the three readings.

Daily PEF monitoring for 2 to 3 weeks is useful, when it is available, for establishing a diagnosis and treatment. If during 2 to 3 weeks a child cannot achieve 80% of predicted PEF (predicted values are provided with all peak flow meters), it may be necessary to determine the child's personal best value (e.g., by a course of oral glucocorticosteroid).

Long-term PEF monitoring is useful, along with review of symptoms, for evaluating a child's response to therapy. PEF monitoring can also help detect early signs of worsening before symptoms occur.

NOTE: Examples of available peak flow meters and instructions for use of inhalers and spacers can be found on http://www.ginasthma.org.

From Global Initiative for Asthma: *Pocket guide for asthma management and prevention in children,* updated 2005, retrieved Sept 20, 2006, from http://www.ginasthma.org/guidelineitem.asp??l1=2&l2=1&intld=49.

BOX 108-6

PROPER METERED-DOSE INHALER TECHNIQUE WITH AND WITHOUT A SPACER

1. Remove cap, hold inhaler upright, and shake inhaler well.
2. Tilting your head back slightly, exhale slowly and fully.
3. Place mouthpiece between lips, or open mouth widely and hold inhaler 1 to 2 inches from mouth.
4. Press down on inhaler once as you start to inhale slowly and deeply.
5. Continue to inhale slowly and deeply as long as you can.
6. Hold breath for 10 seconds (at least 4 seconds)
7. Exhale slowly through nose or pursed lips.
8. Repeat puffs as prescribed, waiting at least 1 minute between puffs.

Patients with asthma should have a copy of their AAP at home, work, and school, with all medications available at each location. In addition, they should be reminded and encouraged to plan ahead for vacations—to have an AAP with them and know emergency department locations and phone numbers.[6]

Persons with asthma and other household members need to be educated about the role of environmental triggers of asthma and efforts that they can take to reduce environmental hazards with the home and surrounding areas. Often cleaning crews require specialized training and equipment to decrease allergen levels in the environments they are servicing.

REFERENCES

1. Centers for Disease Control and Prevention: *Asthma prevalence, health care use and mortality, 2002,* National Center for Health Statistics, retrieved July 25, 2006, from http://www.cdc.gov/nchs/products/pubs/pubd/hestats/sathma/asthma.htm.
2. Global Initiative for Asthma: *Pocket guide for asthma management and prevention: a pocket guide for physicians and nurses,* updated 2005, NIH Pub No 02-3659.

3. National Heart, Lung and Blood Institute: *National Asthma Education and Prevention Program: NAEPP Expert Panel Report guidelines for the diagnosis and management of asthma—update on selected topics 2002*, NIH Pub No 02-5075, Washington, DC, 2003, US Government Printing Office.
4. National Heart, Lung, and Blood Institute: *Asthma statistics*, Bethesda, Md, Jan 1999, National Institutes of Health, US Department of Health and Human Services, The Institute.
5. Centers for Disease Control and Prevention: Self-reported asthma among high school students, *MMWR* 54(31):765-767, 2005.
6. Flaum M, Lung CL, Tinkelman D: Take control of high-cost asthma, *J Asthma* 34(1):5-14, 1997.
7. Hanania NA, David-Wang A, Kesten S, and others: Factors associated with emergency department dependence of patients with asthma, *Chest* 111(2):290-295, 1997.
8. Hartert TV, Windom HH, Peebles RS, and others: Inadequate outpatient medical therapy for patients with asthma admitted to two urban hospitals, *Am J Med* 100(4):386-394, 1996.
9. Vollmer WM, O'Hollaren M, Ettinger KM, and others: Specialty differences in the management of asthma: a cross-sectional assessment of allergists' patients and generalists' patients in a large HMO, *Arch Intern Med* 157(11):1201-1208, 1997.
10. Castro M, Schechtman KB, Halstead J, and others: Risk factors for asthma morbidity and mortality in a large metropolitan city, *J Asthma* 38(8):625-635, 2001.
11. Gillisen A: Managing asthma in the real world, *Int J Clin Pract* 58(6):592-603, 2004.
12. Centers for Disease Control and Prevention: Health-care visits for asthma, by medical setting and health insurance status—United States, 2003, *MMWR* 55(14):389-420, 2006.
13. Lang DM, Sherman MS, Polansky M: Guidelines and realities of asthma management: the Philadelphia story, *Arch Intern Med* 157(11):1193-2000, 1997.
14. Kinney PL, Northridge ME, Chew GL, and others: On the front lines: an environmental asthma intervention in New York City, *Am J Pub Health* 92(1):24-26, 2002.
15. National Heart, Lung, and Blood Institute; National Institutes of Health, National Heart, Lung, and Blood Institute: *Guidelines for the diagnosis and management of asthma: highlights of the Expert Panel Report 2*, Pub No 97-4051A, Washington, DC, 1997, US Government Printing Office.
16. Varner AE, Busse WW: Inflammation in asthma: why it's so important, *J Respir Dis* 17(7):605-616, 1996.
17. Kleerup EC, Tashkin DP: Outpatient treatment of asthma, *West J Med* 163(1):49-63, 1995.
18. Leggett J, Johnston B, Mils M, and others: Prevalence of gastroesophageal reflux in difficult asthma, *Chest* 127(4):1227-1231, 2005.
19. Keenan JM: Asthma management: the case for aiming at control rather than merely relief, *Postgrad Med* 103(3):53-69, 1998.
20. Irwin RS, Boulet LP, Cloutier MM, and others: Managing cough as a defense mechanism and as a symptom: a consensus panel report of the American College of Chest Physicians, *Chest* 114(2 Suppl Manag):113S-181S, 1998.
21. Drazen JM: Bronchial asthma. In Baum GL, Celli JDC, Karlinsky JB, editors: *Textbook of pulmonary diseases*, ed 6, Philadelphia, 1998, Lippincott-Raven.
22. Wright R, Steinbach S: Violence: an unrecognized environmental exposure that may contribute to greater asthma morbidity in high risk inner city populations, *Environ Health Perspect* 109:1085-1089, 2001.
23. Sandberg S, Paton JY, Ahola S, and others: The role of acute and chronic stress in asthma attacks in children, *Lancet* 356(9234):982-987, 2000.
24. Bigby TD: Asthma: clinical presentation and diagnosis. In Bordow RA, Moser KM, editors: *Manual of clinical problems in pulmonary medicine*, Boston, 1996, Little, Brown.
25. Li JTC, Sheeler RD: The asthma physical exam: what's valuable, what's not? *J Respir Dis* 17(9):735-738, 1996.
26. Blank CA, Brantly M: Clinical features and molecular characteristics of alpha$_1$-antitrypsin deficiency, *Ann Allergy Asthma Immunol* 72(2):105-120, 1994.
27. Pina JS, Horan MP: Alpha$_1$-antitrypsin deficiency and asthma: the continuing search for the relationship, *Postgrad Med* 101(4):305, 1997.
28. Sin D, Tu J: Underuse of inhaled steroid therapy in elderly patients with asthma, *Chest* 119:720-725, 2001.
29. Meng Y, Leung K, Berkbigler D, and others: Compliance with U.S. management guidelines and specialty care: a regional variation or national concern, *J Eval Clin Pract* 5:213-221, 1999.
30. Simonella L, Marks G, Sanderson K, and others: Cost-effectiveness of current and optimal treatment for adult asthma, *Intern Med J* 36:244-250, 2006.
31. Senthilselvan A, Lawson J, Rennie D, and others: Regular use of corticosteroids and low use of short-acting beta$_2$-agonists can reduce hospitalization, *Chest* 127:1242-1251, 2005.
32. Currie G, Lee K: Beneficial anti-inflammatory effects of leukotriene receptor antagonists in asthma, *Chest* 127:1458, 2005.
33. *Drug facts and comparisons: pocket version 2007*, St Louis, 2007, Facts & Comparisons.
34. Keam S, Lyseng-Williamson K, Goa K: Pranlukast: a review of its use in the management of asthma, *Drugs* 63:991-1019, 2003.
35. Fish JE, and others: Asthma care: new treatment strategies, new expectations, *Patient Care* 31(16):82-100, 1997.
36. Li JTC, Sheeler RD: Getting the most out of a 15 minute asthma visit, *J Respir Dis* 18(2):135-141, 1997.
37. Richman E: Asthma diagnosis and management: new severity classifications and therapy alternatives, *Clin Rev* 7(8):76-112, 1997.
38. Magadle R, Berar-Yanay N, Weiner P: The risk of hospitalization and near fatal and fatal asthma in relation to the perception of dyspnea, *Chest* 121(2):329-333, 2002.
39. Teeter JG, Bleecker ER: Relationship between airway obstruction and respiratory symptoms in adult asthmatics, *Chest* 113(2):272-277, 1998.
40. Bender B, Milgram H, Rand C: Nonadherence in asthmatic patients: is there a solution to the problem? *J Allergy Asthma Immunol* 79(3):177-185, 1997.
41. Taitel MS, Tses H, Bernstein IL, and others: A self-management program for adult asthma, part II, Cost-benefit analysis, *J Allergy Clin Immunol* 95(3):672-676, 1995.
42. Kotses H, Bernstein IL, Bernstein DI, and others: A self-management program for adult asthma, part I, Development and evaluation, *J Allergy Clin Immunol* 95(2):529-540, 1995.
43. Li JTC, Sheeler RD: Asthma specialty consultation: a two-way street, *J Respir Dis* 18(11):953-990, 1997.
44. Murdock MP: Asthma in pregnancy, *J Perinat Neonat Nurs* 14(4):27-36, 2002.
45. Quadrelli SA, Roncoroni A: Features of asthma in the elderly, *J Asthma* 38(5):377-389, 2001.
46. Parameswaran K, Hildreth AJ, Chadha D, and others: Asthma in the elderly: underperceived, underdiagnosed and undertreated: a community survey, *Respir Med* 92(3):573-577, 1998.
47. Turner MO, Noertjojo K, Vedal S, and others: Risk factors for near fatal asthma: a case-control study in hospitalized patients with asthma, *Am J Respir Crit Care Med* 157(6 Pt 1):1804-1809, 1998.
48. Haas JS, Cleary PD, Guadagnoli E, and others: The impact of socioeconomic status on the intensity of ambulatory treatment and health outcomes after hospital discharge for adults with asthma, *J Gen Intern Med* 9(3):121-126, 1994.
49. Gottlieb DJ, Beiser AS, O'Connor GT: Poverty, race, and medication use are correlates of asthma hospitalization rates: a small area analysis in Boston, *Chest* 108(1):28-35, 1995.

CHAPTER 109

Chest Pain (Noncardiac)

Clayton M. Smiley and Patricia Polgar Bailey

DEFINITION AND EPIDEMIOLOGY

Noncardiac chest pain is a recurrent substernal chest pressure or other chest discomfort believed to be unrelated to the heart after a reasonable cardiac evaluation. Because heart disease is the leading cause of death in the United States and because patients are commonly initially seen with chest pain in the primary care setting, it is important to be able to distinguish cardiac from noncardiac causes of chest pain.[1] Research indicates that it is possible to accurately differentiate between the two in the vast majority of cases. In a recent study of all patients initially diagnosed with noncardiac chest pain, 93.6% had no evidence of adverse cardiac events, 3.5% had possible evidence of adverse cardiac events, and only 2.8% had a definite cardiac event.[2]

Nevertheless, symptoms of chest pain are frightening to patients, and not all life-threatening causes of chest pain are of cardiac origin. Gastrointestinal and pulmonary causes of chest pain must also be considered.[1] According to one report, 67% of chest pain diagnoses in primary care patients were due to musculoskeletal, gastrointestinal, psychiatric, or pulmonary disorders. Only 16% were secondary to cardiac causes of all types, and another 16% were idiopathic.[3] Even in patients with chest pain undergoing cardiac catheterization, approximately 20% to 30% are found to have normal or insignificantly diseased coronary arteries.[4] In a recent study, 81% of moderate-risk women with chest pain syndrome were prospectively demonstrated to be experiencing noncardiac discomfort. Of the remainder, only 2.5% of women experienced cardiac events.[5]

The correct diagnosis for chest pain is most often obtained with a detailed history, supporting physical examination findings, and an ECG and/or chest x-ray study if indicated. Ruling out cardiac causes of chest pain or other noncardiac life-threatening conditions is an essential first step. The evaluation of cardiac chest pain is discussed separately in Chapter 126.

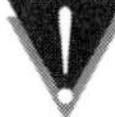

Immediate emergency department referral or physician consultation is indicated for hemodynamic instability or suspected pulmonary embolism, pneumothorax, esophageal rupture, or aortic dissection.

PATHOPHYSIOLOGY

The sympathetic chain, vagus, and phrenic nerves are responsible for carrying pain impulses in the thoracic cage. All the structures in the chest, including the chest wall, esophagus, lungs, heart, and diaphragm, have overlapping innervation. Thus pain from different organs, including those in the abdomen that abut the diaphragm (liver, spleen, stomach), may have similar referral patterns. In addition, patients may have a difficult time localizing pain from deep structures, whereas diseases involving more superficial structures such as the chest wall or pleura are more easily localized. Because there is no sensory innervation in the lung parenchyma, disease involving the alveoli or interstitium does not cause chest pain unless the pulmonary vasculature, bronchi, or pleura is involved.[6]

CLINICAL PRESENTATION

The history is crucial in determining the differential diagnosis and appropriate management in individuals complaining of chest pain. Careful questioning usually clarifies the cause. Some examples of questions are listed in Box 109-1. The following descriptions should be pursued when questioning the patient[7]:

Quality: Myocardial ischemia is more often a pressure that is vicelike or constricting. Sharp, stabbing, knifelike pain suggests a noncardiac cause.

Location: Pain that localizes to a small area of the chest suggests pleural or chest wall involvement.

Intensity: Aortic dissection, pneumothorax, or pulmonary embolism pain has an abrupt onset with the greatest intensity at the beginning. Ischemic chest pain is more gradual, and psychogenic causes of chest pain have a vaguer onset.

Duration: If the chest pain lasts only seconds or has been constant for weeks, it is not cardiac.

Aggravation: Symptoms related to eating such as dysphagia, odynophagia, and heartburn are more suggestive of esophageal chest pain, whereas chest pain that worsens with exercise is more classically like cardiac ischemia. Aggravation of the pain through position changes, deep breathing, or cough points to a musculoskeletal or pleural disorder.

Alleviation: Repeated palliation with antacids and food likely points to a gastrointestinal source. Esophageal and cardiac causes are both made better with sublingual nitroglycerin.

The patient's description of his or her symptoms should be viewed in the context of any history of cardiac, pulmonary, psychiatric, or musculoskeletal diseases. It is important to determine whether the patient has a history of similar symptoms or other illness, such as heart disease, pulmonary

BOX 109-1

SAMPLE QUESTIONS FOR PATIENTS WITH CHEST PAIN

- Where is the pain?
- How long have you had the pain?
- Do you have recurrent episodes of pain?
- How long does each episode last?
- What makes the pain better? Worse? (Breathing? Lying flat? Moving your arms, neck?)
- How would you describe the pain? (Burning? Crushing? Throbbing? Stabbing? Knifelike?)
- When does the pain occur? (With exertion? After eating? When moving your arms?)
- Is the pain associated with shortness of breath? (Cough? Palpitations? Nausea and vomiting? Fever? Leg pain? Coughing up blood?)

Modified from Swartz MB, editor: The heart. In *Textbook of physical diagnosis: history and examination,* Philadelphia, 1994, Saunders.

disease, and diabetes or a family history of heart disease. Other information to be elicited includes whether the patient has engaged in any recent unusual or strenuous physical activity. Has the patient experienced any heartburn, difficult or painful swallowing, or water brash? Does the patient tend to eat before bedtime? Has there been any blood in the stool or symptoms consistent with anemia? Has the patient had any recent emotional or psychologic stress? What is the daily caffeine intake, and are any street or illicit drugs being used? A thorough review of current medications, both over-the-counter and illicit, should be obtained, since this information may contribute to the decision-making process.[4]

Diagnosis of chest pain in the clinical setting has classically been based on some of the factors listed above, including location, description, and precipitants of the pain. This has led to a widely accepted classic *angina syndrome,* which has been shown to correlate well with underlying cardiac artery disease (CAD) in both men and women. However, research indicates that women with CAD often experience less typical symptoms, which can result in a missed diagnosis and improper treatment.[5] In addition, of the risk factors experienced by women, only the presence of diabetes mellitus proved to be significantly associated with adverse events or continuing symptoms.

PHYSICAL EXAMINATION

Examination of a patient with chest pain starts with an assessment of his or her general appearance and vital signs. The evaluation must begin with an exclusion of cardiac disease. The general appearance suggests the severity and possibly the seriousness of the symptoms. Abnormalities in vital signs point to an infectious, pulmonary, cardiac, or malignant process. Hemodynamic instability should prompt immediate referral to the emergency department. The majority of patients with noncardiac chest pain should have normal vital signs.

A general inspection of the chest may reveal a skin rash such as the unilateral rash of herpes zoster in a thoracic dermatome. Evidence of trauma either confirms a history of domestic violence or possibly indicates its existence, even if the patient did not discuss it.

The neck examination should focus on the presence of lymphadenopathy in the cervical chains or supraclavicular fossa. Elevation of the neck veins indicates volume overload and possible heart failure. Tracheal deviation points to a possible pneumothorax.

Palpation of the chest and range of motion of the upper body may cause chest pain in the presence of costochondritis, musculoskeletal disease, a rib fracture, or trauma. Dullness to percussion over a portion of the posterior chest indicates either a pleural effusion or a consolidative pulmonary process such as pneumonia.

Auscultation of the lungs may elicit asymmetric breath sounds, a pleural friction rub, wheezing, crackles, or absent or decreased breath sounds, all of which should prompt additional investigation with a chest x-ray study. The cardiac examination should evaluate for the presence of murmurs, extra heart sounds (S_3 or S_4), or friction rubs.

Examination of the abdomen may reveal tenderness in the epigastric area or right or left upper quadrants, causing irritation of the diaphragm and resultant referred chest pain. Finally, it should be remembered that many patients with noncardiac chest pain have a completely normal physical examination.

DIAGNOSTICS

The diagnostic testing options for chest pain are often limited in the primary care setting. If the patient's chest pain is considered cardiac in origin, a 12-lead ECG may demonstrate characteristic abnormalities. Although a normal ECG reduces the likelihood of an acute coronary syndrome by 70% to 90%, it does not completely rule it out. The ECG should be interpreted in the context of the patient's history and risk factors for heart disease.[8]

In individuals younger than 40 years of age, a normal ECG may be sufficient to rule out cardiac disease. However, in older patients or in those with risk factors (e.g., smoking, obesity, stress), an ECG, stress test, and/or coronary angiography may be necessary.[2] Noninvasive electroradiographic stress testing is less reliable in women than in men; in women it is associated with an increased frequency of false-positive results and frequent failure to achieve target heart rates. For these reasons, image-based stress testing has a strong predictive value and may be more helpful diagnostically in women than some noninvasive types of stress testing.[5]

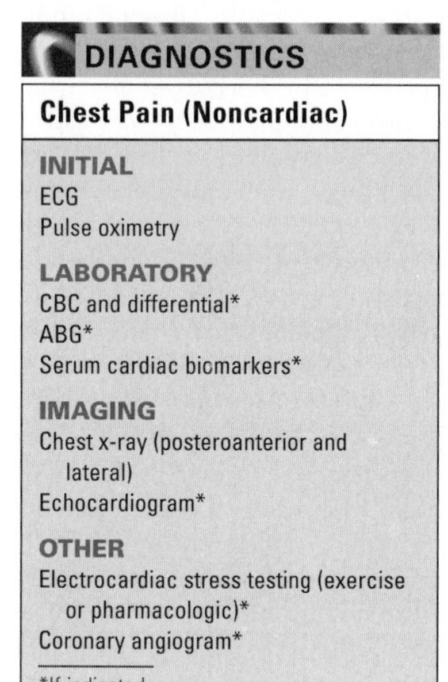

DIAGNOSTICS

Chest Pain (Noncardiac)

INITIAL
ECG
Pulse oximetry

LABORATORY
CBC and differential*
ABG*
Serum cardiac biomarkers*

IMAGING
Chest x-ray (posteroanterior and lateral)
Echocardiogram*

OTHER
Electrocardiac stress testing (exercise or pharmacologic)*
Coronary angiogram*

*If indicated.

The chest x-ray study is a useful diagnostic tool for detecting cardiac and pulmonary abnormalities. Pulse oximeters should be available to determine the oxygen saturation. Occasionally, other studies may be needed, such as an arterial blood gas or a CBC with differential. In most cases, however, a detailed history, physical examination, and possibly an ECG or chest x-ray study should give enough information to form a hypothesis regarding the cause of the symptoms.

DIFFERENTIAL DIAGNOSIS

The most common causes of noncardiac chest pain in the primary care setting are musculoskeletal, gastrointestinal, psychiatric, and pulmonary disease.[3] In a recent study, gastroesophageal disease accounted for approximately 42% of all cases of chest pain and was the most common cause in persons for whom myocardial infarction was ruled out.[1] The gastroesophageal causes of chest pain include gastroesophageal reflux disease (GERD), esophageal rupture or perforation (Boerhaave's syndrome), esophageal spasm, pill-induced esophagitis, peptic ulcer, pancreatitis, or cholescystitis. Symptoms highly suggestive of an esophageal disorder, especially reflux disease, include dysphagia, odynophagia, regurgitation, heartburn, and cough.[1,9] Clinical history alone cannot reliably differentiate between cardiac and esophageal chest pain. Chest pain associated with GERD may be triggered by exertion and may have characteristics similar to angina. However, esophageal-related pain is more likely to last for hours, occurs retrosternally without radiation, interrupts sleep, and is related to meals more often than cardiac chest pain. It is often more often related to other esophageal symptoms such as dysphagia and heartburn.

Esophageal perforation may be caused by instrument-induced damage; forceful vomiting; and diseases of the esophagus, such as esophagitis or neoplasm. The classic history for esophageal perforation is profound, sudden, severe, and constant pain from the neck to the epigastrium that is worsened by swallowing. Pain may occur after severe retching and vomiting.

Recent use of prescriptions such as doxycycline, NSAIDs, or alendronate might suggest pill-induced esophagitis. Although any pill, if not swallowed properly and with enough water, may cause esophagitis, alendronate has received the most attention, with recommendations to swallow the pill with at least 6 to 8 ounces of water and remain upright for at least 30 minutes after swallowing. Accidental ingestion of caustic substances can also cause chemical esophagitis.

Musculoskeletal conditions are a common cause of chest pain and in one study accounted for up to 28% of chest pain in patients for whom myocardial infarction was ruled out.[1] Musculoskeletal-related chest pain is often nagging and persistent, lasting anywhere from hours to weeks. Patients complain of superficial chest pain localized in a small area. The symptoms are aggravated by position, deep breathing, turning, or arm movement. Causes of musculoskeletal chest wall pain include costochondritis, routine muscle strains, rheumatologic diseases such as rheumatoid arthritis, ankylosing spondylitis, fibromyalgia, and other nonrheumatologic diseases such as neoplasms or fractures.

Herpes zoster can cause acute chest pain that is usually described as a burning sensation. The pain is generally located in a unilateral dermatomic distribution. Pain often occurs before the onset of vesicular lesions, so physical examination findings may not be present at the time of the initial complaint, making diagnosis difficult.[1]

Finally, the cause may be pulmonary if the vasculature, parenchyma, or pleural tissue is affected and the associated pain is frequently described as pleuritic in nature. Pulmonary embolism (PE) is a common and often missed diagnosis and is suggested by the onset of dyspnea; pleuritic chest pain; severe hypoxia; and the presence of risk factors such as recent surgery, underlying malignancy, and a sedentary lifestyle.[1] These symptoms are obviously nonspecific and require a high degree of clinical suspicion with special attention to known risk factors of PE, such as immobilization, history of previous venous thromboembolism, recent surgery, pregnancy, or malignancy. Another diagnosis that should be considered in patients with the sudden onset of sharp, stabbing chest pain is pneumothorax. Patients with primary pneumothorax are typically young tall men who smoke and have no history of lung disease.[6] Secondary spontaneous pneumothoraces occur in patients with cystic fibrosis, chronic obstructive pulmonary disease, and HIV and *Pneumocystis* pneumonia. Patients who have community-acquired pneumonia as the underlying cause of their chest pain are usually easily diagnosed based on the cough, fever, sputum production, and findings on physical examination and chest x-ray study.

Psychiatric diseases may underlie symptoms of chest pain in some primary care patients. In one study, patients with noncardiac chest pain and no abnormalities on upper endoscopy or other explanation for their symptoms had a higher prevalence of panic disorder, obsessive-compulsive disorder, and major depressive episodes.[9] These patients tend to be younger and female and have atypical symptoms and other diagnosed psychiatric illnesses.

DIFFERENTIAL DIAGNOSIS

Cardiac and Noncardiac Causes of Chest Pain

CARDIAC

Ischemic
- Angina
- Myocardial infarction
- Aortic stenosis
- Hypertrophic cardiomyopathy
- Coronary vasospasm

Nonischemic
- Pericarditis
- Aortic dissection
- Mitral valve prolapse

PULMONARY

Bronchitis
Malignancy
Pleurisy
Pneumonia
Pneumothorax
Pulmonary embolism

MUSCULOSKELETAL

Arthritis
Costochondritis
Compression radiculopathy
Rib fractures

GASTROINTESTINAL

Esophageal hyperalgesia
Gastritis
Reflux esophagitis
Referred gallbladder, pancreatic, hepatic, or splenic pain
Esophageal spasm
Esophageal perforation

DERMATOLOGIC

Herpes zoster

PSYCHIATRIC

Major depression
Panic disorder
Generalized anxiety disorder

MANAGEMENT

Management of patients with chest pain depends on the etiology of the disease process (Figure 109-1). Exclusion of CAD or other life-threatening noncardiac causes of chest pain is an essential first step.

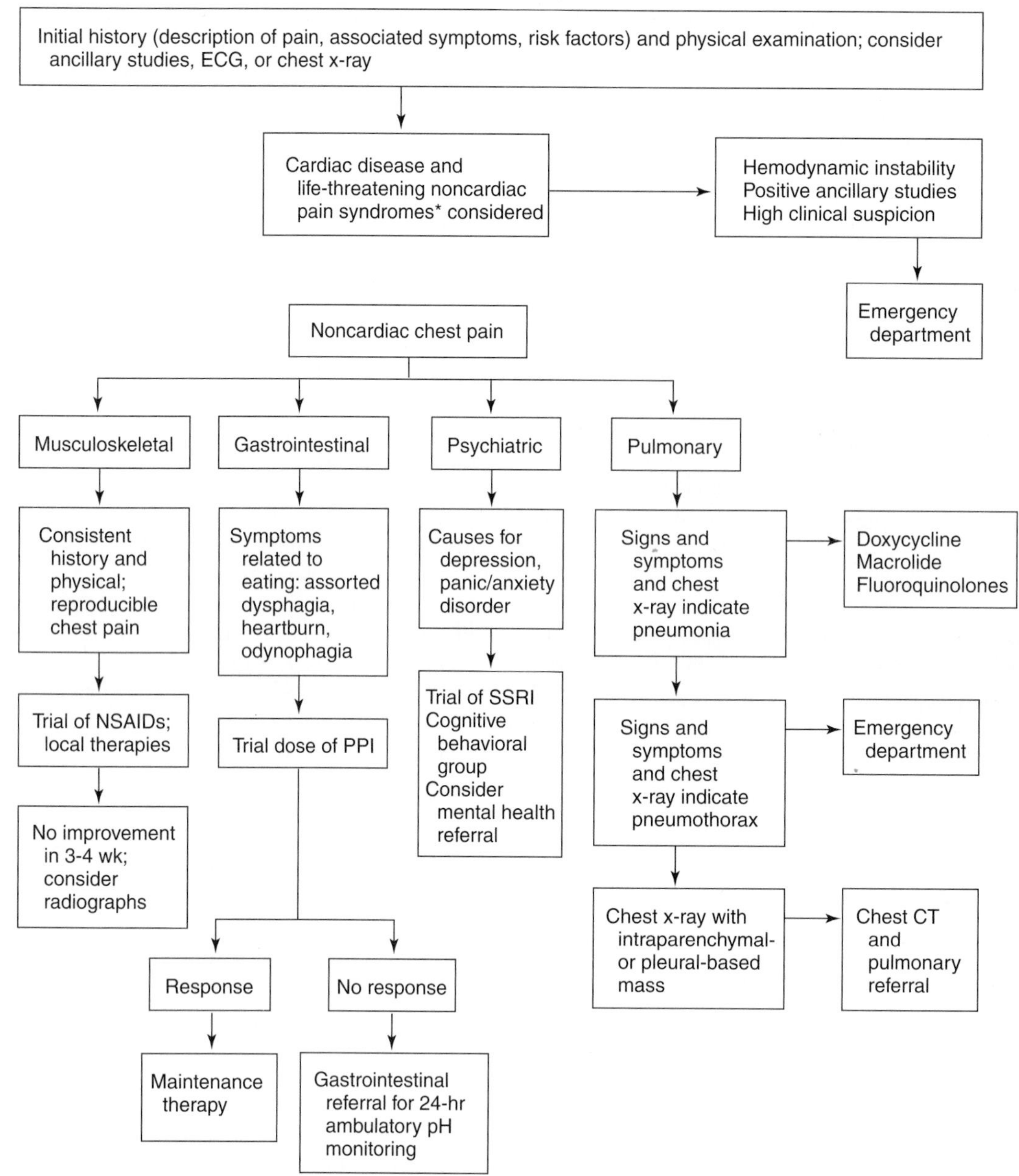

FIGURE 109-1

Approach to the patient with noncardiac chest pain. *PPI,* Proton pump inhibitors; *SSRI,* selective serotonin reuptake inhibitors. (Modified from Fang J, Bjorkman D: A critical approach to non-cardiac chest pain: pathophysiology, diagnosis, and treatment, *Am J Gastroenterol* 96:958-968, 2001.)

When the clinical picture suggests an esophageal source, the goal of therapy is to heal the esophagus, control symptoms, and prevent recurrence and complications. Mild to moderate GERD can be treated with H_2-receptor antagonists. Proton pump inhibitors are indicated for GERD refractory to H_2-antagonist medication. Persons with persistent symptoms should be referred to a gastroenterologist.

Musculoskeletal chest pain therapy includes the use of NSAIDs, rest, heat, or ice. For those patients who cannot tolerate traditional NSAIDs (older patients, those with a history of ulcer disease or previous gastrointestinal bleeding), a selective COX-2 inhibitor, such as celecoxib (Celebrex), may be indicated. However, there are continued concerns about the potential for cardiac events associated with Cox-2 inhibitors. Scheduled acetaminophen (Tylenol) 650 mg q 4-6 hr may also be helpful in these patients.

If a pulmonary disorder is suspected and the chest x-ray findings confirm suspicion, treatment will be self-evident. In the case of pneumonia, first-line treatment with antibiotics is indicated (see Chapter 118). A follow-up chest x-ray study should be done 6 to 8 weeks after treatment in all patients over the age of 50 years to document resolution of the infiltrate and to assess for an underlying cause of the process, such as a malignancy or another structural defect. Patients with a pneumothorax or suspected pulmonary embolism should be referred to the emergency department. An intraparenchymal or pleural-based mass causing chest pain deserves additional workup with a chest CT, pain management with analgesics, and a referral to a pulmonologist.

Psychiatric disease as a cause for noncardiac chest pain is common; however, it should always be a diagnosis of exclusion. If a diagnosis of panic disorder, depression, or generalized anxiety disorder is suspected, selective serotonin reuptake inhibitors are effective. One study even demonstrated a benefit of reducing noncardiac chest pain by 50% in those patients who did not meet DSM-IV criteria for panic disorder, major depressive disorder, or generalized anxiety disorder but did not otherwise have an explanation for their symptoms.[10] In addition, patients with these diagnoses have been shown to benefit from enrollment in cognitive behavioral therapy.[11]

LIFE SPAN CONSIDERATIONS

After cardiac and life-threatening noncardiac conditions are excluded, the patient's age is often an important factor in determining the diagnosis. Younger patients' chest pain is generally caused by more benign underlying conditions, whereas older patients with more risk factors and co-morbid conditions should be approached with caution. Regardless of the patient's age, cardiac and life-threatening noncardiac conditions should be ruled out first.

COMPLICATIONS

PE can be life threatening if diagnosis and treatment are delayed. Thus clinical suspicion of PE is important in all patients who are seen with respiratory or cardiac complaints. A pneumothorax can develop into a tension pneumothorax if it is not treated appropriately. With a tension pneumothorax, there is a mediastinal and tracheal shift to the contralateral side that causes hypotension and an increase in respiratory distress. This condition can be rapidly fatal if not diagnosed and treated. Pneumonia can proceed to respiratory failure even in young and otherwise healthy patients. Esophageal perforation leads to mediastinitis. Finally, acute aortic dissection can lead to cardiac valvular insufficiency, rapid hemodynamic collapse, and death if not addressed promptly.

INDICATIONS FOR REFERRAL OR HOSPITALIZATION

In patients with suspected reflux causing chest pain, a lack of response to high-dose proton pump inhibitor therapy should prompt a referral to a gastroenterologist. A pulmonologist should be consulted for any mass on chest x-ray film and for patients with recurring or nonresolving pneumonia, since these conditions may indicate an underlying malignancy or immune deficiency.

Emergency department referral or physician consultation is necessary when a cardiac origin of chest pain or a life-threatening noncardiac cause cannot be excluded.

PATIENT AND FAMILY EDUCATION AND HEALTH PROMOTION

Noncardiac chest pain can be a diagnosis with significant morbidity depending on the cause. Ensuring that patients are well informed about their diagnosis, its natural history, and possible complications improves the probability of a positive outcome. Patient education should emphasize how to recognize cardiac, pulmonary, or musculoskeletal chest pain and what to do when it occurs, including when to call 911 (or universal number). If the patient smokes, he or she should receive counseling on the importance of tobacco cessation at every visit. If any medications are prescribed, instructions should incorporate the correct administration of the drugs and their possible side effects.

REFERENCES

1. Karnath B, Holden M, Hussain N: Chest pain: differentiating cardiac from noncardiac causes, *Hosp Phys* 38:24-27, 38, 2004.
2. Miller C, Lindsell C, Khandelwai S, and others: Is the initial diagnostic impression of "noncardiac chest pain" adequate to exclude cardiac disease? *Ann Emerg Med* 44(6):565-574, 2004.
3. Klinkman MS, Stevens D, Gorenflo DW: Episodes of care for chest pain: a preliminary report from MIRNET: Michigan Research Network, *J Fam Pract* 38:345-352, 1994.
4. Gruber M: Patient with noncardiac chest pain, *Lippincott's Prim Care Pract* 2(4):432-435, 1998.
5. Sanfilippo A, Abdollah H, Knott C, and others: Defining low risk for coronary heart disease among women with chest pain syndrome, *J Women's Health* 14(3):240-247, 2005.
6. White P, and others: Common pulmonary problems: cough, hemoptysis, dyspnea, chest pain, and the abnormal chest x-ray. In Barker LR, Burton JR, Zieve PD, editors: *Principles of ambulatory medicine*, Baltimore, 1999, Williams & Wilkins.
7. Fang J, Bjorkman D: A critical approach to non-cardiac chest pain: pathophysiology, diagnosis, and treatment, *Am J Gastroenterol* 96:958-968, 2001.
8. Panju AA, Hemmelgarn BR, Guyatt GH, and others: The rational clinical examination: is this patient having a myocardial infarction? *JAMA* 280:1256-1263, 1998.
9. Ho KY, Kang JY, Yeo B, and others: Non-cardiac, non-esophageal chest pain: the relevance of psychological factors, *Gut* 43:105-110, 1998.
10. Varia I, Logue E, O'Connor C, and others: Randomized trial of sertraline in patients with unexplained chest pain of non-cardiac origin, *Am Heart J* 140:367-372, 2000.
11. Van Peski-Oosterbaan AS, Spinhoven P, van Rood Y, and others: Cognitive-behavioral therapy for non-cardiac chest pain: a randomized trial, *Am J Med* 106:424-429, 1999.

CHAPTER 110

Chronic Cough

Patricia Polgar Bailey

BOX 110-1

CHARACTERISTICS OF CHRONIC COUGH

- When did the cough start?
- Is it severe at night or during the day?
- Is it productive or dry?
- What characteristic does the sputum have?

DEFINITION AND EPIDEMIOLOGY

Cough, an important reflex action and respiratory defense mechanism, is designed to prevent the aspiration of foreign material into the lower respiratory tract and to clear excessive secretions, fluids, or foreign matter from the airway.[1,2] Although cough has a protective role, it can also transmit disease via airborne droplets and the contamination of objects, and it can be associated with complications, particularly when chronic. Excessive and chronic cough can result in numerous complications, including anxiety, fatigue, insomnia, myalgia, dysphonia, perspiration, urinary incontinence, and rib fractures. In addition, chronic cough may also be a symptom of underlying disease. For these reasons, a persistent chronic cough is a cause for concern for both the patient and health care provider.

Coughs may be classified as acute (lasting less than 3 weeks), subacute (lasting 3 to 8 weeks) and chronic (persisting beyond 8 weeks).[3] Most coughs are acute and self-limiting, with 90% being caused by viral respiratory tract infections. Therefore a cough that persists for more than 3 weeks and has failed initial treatment is defined as chronic (or subacute depending on the time frame) and should be investigated. Subacute cough is generally due to bacterial sinusitis or asthma but can also be caused by upper respiratory tract infections, including pertussis. Subacute coughs may also resolve without treatment depending on the cause.[3]

Overall, cough is the fifth most common symptom for which medical care is sought, accounting for 30 million visits annually and costing more than $2 billion each year in both prescribed and over-the-counter medications.[4-6] It is a common complaint of patients with smoking-related pulmonary disease, along with dyspnea and chest pain, but it also has an incidence of 20% among nonsmoking adults.[5,7] Although most smokers have a cough, they do not generally seek medical attention for the cough in particular.

Chronic cough can have many causes, but only a few diseases account for most cases. In adults the three most common causes of chronic cough are upper airway cough syndrome (previously referred to as *postnasal drip syndrome*), asthma, and gastroesophageal reflux disease (GERD). These have been referred to as the "pathogenic triad of chronic cough," accounting for almost all cases of cough in immunocompetent, nonsmoking adults who have normal chest radiographs and are not taking angiotensin-converting enzyme (ACE) inhibitors. Other common causes of cough include chronic bronchitis (primarily from cigarette smoking) and exposure to smoke and other irritants.

An understanding of the anatomic, physiologic, and pathophysiologic aspects of cough is important for diagnosis and appropriate treatment. The systematic, diagnostic protocol uses the anatomic characteristics of the cough reflex and enervation as a guide to finding the cause of the cough (Box 110-1).

PATHOPHYSIOLOGY

When a neural receptor along the respiratory tree is stimulated, an afferent signal is transmitted to the "cough center" of the brain, which is located in the medulla. From this center, via a complex reflex arc, the impulse is passed down the efferent pathway to the expiratory musculature.

The receptors of the afferent limb can be found anywhere along the respiratory tree. These include the vagus from the ears, larynx, trachea, bronchi, pleurae, and gastrointestinal tract; the trigeminal from the nose and the sinuses; the glossopharyngeal from the pharynx; and the phrenic from the diaphragm.

The efferent limb consists primarily of the phrenic and spinal nerves. After the stimulus reaches the cough center, the cough begins with a deep inspiration to approximately 50% of the vital capacity. This allows for maximum expiratory flow by increasing the lung elastic recoil and by decreasing airway frictional resistance. During this phase the glottis opens widely to allow rapid entry of large amounts of air into the lung. The glottis rapidly closes and the abdominal and intercostal muscles contract, increasing the intrapleural pressures to 100 to 200 mm Hg. In a fraction of a second, the glottis reopens, causing an explosive release of air. During this phase the tracheobronchial tree narrows, resulting in forces sufficient enough to strip mucus off the walls, creating sputum.

CLINICAL PRESENTATION

Studies have shown that a careful and detailed history will provide the diagnosis in 80% of all cases of cough.[4,8-10] Careful consideration of the various characteristics of cough may aid diagnosis (Figure 110-1). A cough that lasts for 3 consecutive months for more than 2 consecutive years is indicative of chronic bronchitis. A sudden onset of cough in the supine position with an associated sour taste in the mouth suggests esophageal reflux. A cough associated with constant throat clearing and thick mucus production, especially on rising from bed, is consistent with upper airway cough and sinusitis. Intermittent productive cough associated with wheezing is most probably asthma. A cough associated with rhinorrhea or sneezing may be a viral syndrome or the common cold. If it recurs annually at the same time of year, allergic rhinitis is possible. A loud hacking cough during the daytime that is nonproductive, leads to exhaustion, and is associated with emotional stress may suggest psychogenic cough. In addition, some authors have attributed certain sputum characteristics to a particular disease process (Box 110-2). Evaluation of these attributes may also aid in diagnosis.

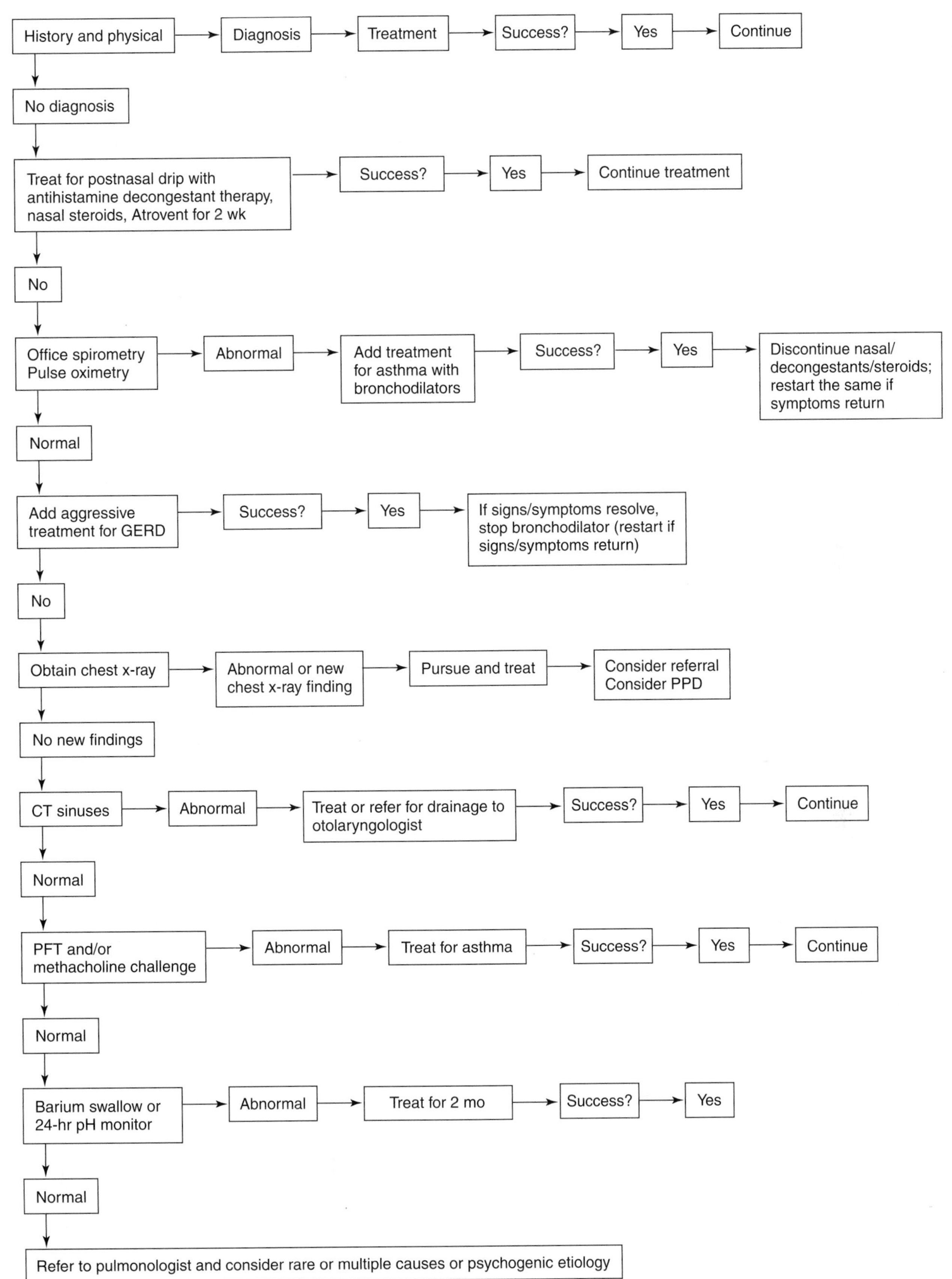

FIGURE 110-1

Diagnostic chronic cough protocol. *GERD*, Gastroesophageal reflux disease; *PPD*, purified protein derivative; *PFT*, pulmonary function tests.

BOX 110-2

SPUTUM CHARACTERISTICS OF VARIOUS PULMONARY DISORDERS

- Hemoptysis: bronchogenic cancer, pulmonary embolus, tuberculosis
- Yellow-green, purulent: bronchitis
- Pink frothy: pulmonary edema
- Fetid purulent: anaerobic infections
- Rust colored: pneumococcal pneumonia
- Foam, serous, mucopurulent layers: bronchiectasis

ACE inhibitors cause a nonproductive cough more often in women than in men. The cough may begin anytime after initiation of therapy and is not dose related. If ACE inhibitor related, the cough should subside within a few days to several weeks after discontinuation of the ACE inhibitor.[3]

PHYSICAL EXAMINATION

The physical examination has been reported to be diagnostic in 60% of cases.[10,11] Obvious findings include:

- Pharyngeal erythema with or without cobblestoning of the mucosa and purulent secretions, as seen in sinusitis, upper airway cough, or allergic disease
- Diffuse inspiratory crackles characteristic of pulmonary edema or fibrosis
- Expiratory wheezes as in asthma or chronic obstructive pulmonary disease
- Occasional hair rubbing against the eardrum or cerumen impaction in the canal

If the history and physical examination cannot establish the cause of the cough, a chest radiograph should be obtained, even though x-ray findings are diagnostic in only a minority of cases.[4,11] A normal chest x-ray film usually excludes malignancy, bronchiectasis, persistent pneumonia, sarcoidosis, and tuberculosis. The next step is to reconsider the most likely remaining causes of chronic cough, keeping in mind that chronic cough may fail to resolve because of inaccurate diagnosis or incorrect or insufficient therapy.[3]

DIAGNOSTICS

A chest radiograph will reveal the presence of a lung mass or parenchymal abnormalities, such as sarcoidosis, fibrosis, emphysema, and congestive heart failure. If chest films reveal abnormalities, further diagnostic studies may be indicated, possibly including bronchoscopy, pulmonary function tests (PFTs), CT scanning of the chest, barium esophagography, and cardiac studies. A bronchoscopy should be planned only for a specific diagnosis, keeping in mind that bronchoscopy has been shown to be of little diagnostic benefit when chest radiograph or CT findings are normal or nonlocalizing.[12] If the diagnosis is still not found, routine PFTs are indicated, and if these are negative, a methacholine challenge test is necessary.

At this point, up to 70% of the coughs will have been diagnosed. If the cause is still undetermined, however, a gastrointestinal evaluation with a barium swallow and a 24-hour pH esophageal monitoring should be considered. Further diagnostic tests include a CT scan of the sinuses or otolaryngologic evaluation. The majority of patients should now have a definite diagnosis. Undiagnosed cases of cough may include psychogenic cough, or the cause will be undetermined. Up to 25% to 50% of patients have multiple causes.[12]

DIAGNOSTICS

Chronic Cough

IMAGING
Chest x-ray*
Barium swallow*
Sinus CT*

OTHER
Bronchoscopy*
PFTs*
Purified protein derivative*
Methacholine challenge test*
24-hour esophageal pH monitoring*
Oxygen saturation level*

*If indicated.

Individuals with a compromised immune system require additional diagnostic testing as part of the initial workup. If a patient is immunocompromised, especially because of HIV infection, a chest radiograph and oxygen saturation level should be obtained earlier in the assessment. Chronic co-morbid conditions and acute critical illnesses can cause further depression of the immune system, thereby increasing the risk of infection.

DIFFERENTIAL DIAGNOSIS

The causes of cough are plentiful and diverse. Upper airway cough syndrome is believed to be the most common cause of chronic cough and should be one of the first conditions considered. In general, it occurs after viral upper respiratory tract infections. Other causes of upper airway cough syndrome include perennial rhinitis (e.g., rhinitis caused by seasonal allergens), irritants, drugs, vasomotor responses, and chronic sinusitis.[1] Alone, or in association with some other chronic condition, upper airway cough syndrome is the most common cause of chronic cough in immunocompetent nonsmoking adults who have a normal chest radiograph.[3] There are no signs and symptoms specific to the cough caused by upper airway cough syndrome; therefore it can be difficult to make the diagnosis based on the history and physical examination alone. Throat clearing and a cobblestone appearance on the posterior pharynx are features suggestive of, but not definite for, upper airway cough, since they can occur in other conditions. The diagnosis of upper airway cough syndrome is often made based on response to a trial of therapy.

Early asthma may manifest as chronic cough, and bronchial asthma is the second most common cause of chronic cough in immunocompetent adults. The cough may precede audible wheezes and is the only presenting symptom in up to 57% of asthma cases (cough-variant asthma). Given the high and increasing prevalence of asthma, it should always be considered as a possible cause of chronic cough, especially when persistent cough is exacerbated by cold or exercise or when the cough worsens at night. Airway hyperresponsiveness is suggestive of cough-variant asthma.[3] The degree and reversibility of obstruction is most accurately assessed by spirometry, which measures forced expiratory volume in 1 second (FEV_1). An FEV_1 that is less than 80% of predicted value and is strongly responsive to inhaled $beta_2$ agonist bronchodilators (an increase of at least 12% in the measured FEV_1) is strongly suggestive of asthma.[1]

If the PFT results are normal, an attempt to induce bronchospasm using a bronchoconstrictor such as methacholine should be tried. This is known as the methacholine challenge test and is diagnostic in 25% of patients.[13] A nebulized solution of methacholine is administered in a stepwise fashion, incrementally increasing the dose and repeating the spirometry after each dose. A 20% drop in FEV_1 from baseline is considered a positive result.[4] Other substances used as bronchoconstrictors include histamine, cold air exposure, and ultrasonic water mists.

Chronic bronchitis, from exposure to cigarette smoke and other irritants, accounts for between 5% and 12% of patients with chronic cough.[4,8,10] Although chronic bronchitis is a common cause of chronic cough, it accounts for only 5% of those who seek treatment, probably because many persons with "smoker's cough" do not seek medical care. Spirometry reveals an airflow obstruction that does not significantly respond to inhaled bronchodilators (or improvement in FEV_1 >12%). Smoking cessation is the most effective therapeutic intervention, since the majority of patients will have resolution or improvement of cough within 8 weeks. Unfortunately, the cough of persistent smokers is usually resistant to most, if not all, forms of therapeutic interventions, other than the elimination of tobacco smoke or other environmental irritants.

Bronchiectasis, another major airway disease, may also cause chronic cough. Responsible for only 4% of coughs, bronchiectasis is an enlargement of the peripheral airways that in the worst cases may give the lungs a "Swiss cheese" appearance on anatomic section.[4,8,10] Diagnosis depends on the history and recurrent episodes of purulent sputum, which, when left standing in a cup, may separate into three layers: frothy top, serous middle, and purulent bottom. The most efficient diagnostic modality is a high-resolution CT scan with characteristic finding of "tram tracking, saccules, and signet rings."

Gastroesophageal reflux accounts for 10% to 20% of all chronic coughs and is the third most common cause of cough in nonsmoking, immunocompetent adults who have normal chest x-ray films.[3-5] This cough can occur at any age, although it occurs most often in the middle to late sixties and occurs slightly more often in women. Most patients refer to concurrent abdominal complaints, such as dyspepsia or heartburn, although it is not unusual for patients to have no symptoms at all. The reflux material does not necessarily need to be aspirated or even reach the glottis to cause cough or bronchospasm. Studies commonly used for diagnosis include a barium swallow, esophagoscopy, manometry, and pH probe monitoring. Although the most sensitive and specific test for GERD is 24-hour esophageal pH monitoring, it is generally not recommended in the routine evaluation of GERD because of the inconvenience of this test. An alternative approach is to empirically treat patients diagnosed with GERD with antireflux medications such as proton pump inhibitors or H_2 histamines. If individuals do not respond well to medical therapy, additional diagnostic testing or surgery may be indicated.

Infectious causes such as pertussis and tuberculosis are reemerging and need to be considered as important differentials of chronic cough. Postinfectious cough syndrome constitutes between 10% and 20% of all cough complaints in the primary care setting.[14] It occurs after an upper respiratory tract infection and may cause a cough for 8 weeks or more. Most cases start with a viral syndrome; thus antibiotics are ineffective. Most coughs respond well to cough suppressants; some require inhaled steroids or a short course of oral prednisone. In nonsmokers some success has been reported with inhaled ipratropium bromide (Atrovent). Medication-induced cough affects 10% of patients receiving ACE inhibitors.[13,15] The mechanism is poorly understood and may affect patients early in the course of therapy or after several months or years. Cough usually resolves within 2 to 4 weeks of stopping the medication. All ACE inhibitors should then be avoided, and patients should be started on a different class of antihypertensives or an angiotensin II receptor blocker.

In adults of all ages and in children older than 1 year of age, upper airway cough syndrome, asthma, and GERD are the three most common causes of chronic cough. More often than not, chronic cough is a result of multiple causes.[1,4] Cardiac disease, particularly left ventricular failure, interstitial lung disease, bronchogenic carcinoma, sarcoidosis, foreign body aspiration, postradiation pneumonitis, and *metastatic* lung carcinoma, may all have a cough as the sole presenting symptom. (Although many health care providers are concerned about missing lung carcinoma, isolated chronic cough is a rare presentation of lung cancer.[16]) Other rare causes of cough include esophageal diverticulitis, stomach ulcer, pericardial effusion, and ear canal irritation.

The literature suggests that psychogenic cough is generally a loud, barking cough that is associated with high stress and typically does not occur at night. However, a cough that is not psychogenic can also be barking or honking, and most persons with chronic cough usually do not wake up during the night once they have fallen asleep. In addition to not coughing at night, patients with psychogenic cough are not awakened by cough and generally do not cough during enjoyable distractions.[3] Because a

DIFFERENTIAL DIAGNOSIS

Chronic Cough

MOST COMMON
- Upper airway cough (postnasal drip syndrome)
- Asthma
- Chronic bronchitis
- Gastroesophageal reflux disease
- Smoking and other irritants
- Angiotensin-converting enzyme inhibitors

LESS COMMON
- Bronchiectasis
- Medications
- Cardiac disease
- Postinfectious cough syndrome
- Sarcoidosis
- Foreign body aspiration
- Postradiation pneumonitis
- Psychogenic
- Ear canal irritation
- Gastrointestinal disturbances
- Eosinophilic bronchitis

RARE
- Tracheobronchial collapse
- Lung cancer
- Tuberculosis
- Occupational or environment induced
- Interstitial lung disease
- Hyperthyroidism
- Retrosternal goiter
- Carcinoid tumor
- Retained suture
- Hodgkin's disease
- Zenker's diverticulum
- Habit cough
- Pulmonary abscess
- Aspiration
- Psychogenic cough
- Irritable larynx
- Persistent pneumonia

psychogenic cough has no distinguishing features or diagnostic tests, it should remain a diagnosis of exclusion after all other possibilities have been eliminated. In a small percentage of cases, the cause will be undetermined.

MANAGEMENT

Therapy is either antitussive (to prevent, control, or eliminate cough) or protussive (to make cough more effective and productive). Antitussive treatment is indicated when the cough serves no useful purpose such as clearing the airway and can be specific or nonspecific. Specific treatment is directed at the mechanism directly responsible such as smoking cessation.[17] Nonspecific therapy is directed at the symptom and is meant to control the cough when specific therapy has failed or is not possible (e.g., inoperable lung cancer). Protussive treatment is indicated for patients for whom coughing serves a useful function, as with cystic fibrosis.[18]

Specific therapy is encouraged for the causative agent if a definitive diagnosis is found. Empiric therapy is appropriate when there is a reasonable suspicion of a specific diagnosis. Asthmatic patients should be treated with inhaled $beta_2$ agonists, inhaled corticosteroids, or inhaled nonsteroidal antiinflammatory medications such as cromolyn sodium or nedocromil sodium, and occasionally oral steroids.

Upper airway cough caused by sinusitis is treated with oral decongestants, nasal steroids, and possibly, but not necessarily, antibiotics. When upper airway cough is related to allergic or nonallergic rhinitis, an H_1 antihistamine is an appropriate alternative to antibiotic therapy. Antibiotics are indicated when there is purulent nasal drainage and sinus tenderness.

Chronic bronchitis is best treated with smoking cessation, an ipratropium bromide inhaler, and a $beta_2$ agonist inhaler. When purulent sputum is present, a 7- to 10-day course of antibiotics is indicated.

Management of GERD involves a trial of antireflux therapy. A proton pump inhibitor and possibly a prokinetic agent may relieve the GERD-associated cough in many cases.[19,20] However, it may take 6 months before the full benefit of therapy is realized. In addition, preventive lifestyle changes such as losing weight, stopping smoking, eating a diet low in acidic foods, and raising the head of the bed may help reduce the tone of the lower esophageal sphincter, thus mitigating symptoms.[1,20]

Demulcents are agents high in sugar content and are believed to coat the sensory receptors in the upper airways. They also promote swallowing, which may help suppress the cough reflex. Expectorants, such as guaifenesin, are believed to change the consistency of the sputum, thus making it easier to expectorate.

Opiates increase the latency threshold of the cough center. Codeine, oxycodone, and nonopiate dextromethorphan are standard therapy for severe nonproductive coughs. All are central nervous system depressants and, except for dextromethorphan, are addicting. Local anesthetics such as nebulized lidocaine are extremely effective and directly suppress the sensory nerve; however, these agents are difficult to administer.

COMPLICATIONS

Patients often develop costochondritis or hemoptysis as a result of strenuous coughing. Although usually not serious, these developments can be frightening for patients and families. Another recognized complication of cough is rib fracture, which occurs more commonly with chronic cough than acute cough. In at least one study, rib fracture occurred primarily in women.[21] Cough-induced rib fractures occur most often in ribs 5 through 9 and along the lateral aspect of the rib cage (similar to the anatomic distribution of rib fractures seen in rowers), likely related to the repetitive mechanical stress to the ribs caused by coughing. Reduced bone density is a risk factor for cough-related rib fractures, although such fractures also occur in individuals with normal bone density. Chest radiography has a relatively low sensitivity for detecting cough-induced rib fractures. Other complications of chronic cough include ruptures, emphysematous blebs, syncope, wheezing, dyspnea, and sleep interruption.

INDICATIONS FOR REFERRAL OR HOSPITALIZATION

All patients with coughs that do not respond to or resolve with treatment require physician consultation. Those patients with coughs related to cardiac disease, carcinoma, foreign body aspiration, or other suspected pathologic conditions require referral to the appropriate specialist with documentation of diagnostic evaluation, treatment, and treatment evaluation. Hospitalization may be indicated for wheezing and hypoxia, as well as for bronchoscopy or other therapeutic interventions (Box 110-3).

PATIENT AND FAMILY EDUCATION

Cough is a major concern for patients that usually requires medical attention. Diagnostic studies are rarely needed, and a systematic and logical approach generally affords relief for the vast majority of patients. Patients and families need to

BOX 110-3

INDICATIONS FOR REFERRAL

COMPLICATED COUGH WITH ANY OF THE FOLLOWING

- Cardiac causes
- Carcinoma: primary or metastatic
- Chronic aspiration (e.g., in patients with history of cerebrovascular accident)
- Foreign body in ear requiring evaluation
- Sinusitis requiring drainage

ABNORMAL TESTS REQUIRING SPECIALIST INTERVENTION

- Gastroesophageal reflux disease requiring 24-hour pH monitoring
- Any suspicion of allergy requiring bronchoprovocation testing
- Occupational exposure requiring legal intervention
- Suspicion of sarcoid, carcinoma, bronchiectasis, carcinoid, Zenker's diverticulum requiring bronchoscopy
- Retrosternal goiter requiring surgery
- Chronic obstructive pulmonary disease patients requiring home-oxygen supplementation
- Chest x-ray film suggestive of empyema

DANGER SIGNALS INDICATING COMPLICATED COUGH

- Hemoptysis
- Weight loss

Further testing or evaluation is indicated before concluding that the cough is psychogenic, a habitual cough, or a smoker's cough.

understand, however, that many coughs are viral in origin and that coughs may last 4 to 8 weeks. The health care provider should carefully explain the prescribed therapy, the need to use antibiotics only when indicated, and the signs and symptoms of serious cough-related illness.

REFERENCES

1. D'Urzo A, Jugovic P: Chronic cough: three most common causes, *Can Fam Phys* 48:1311-1316, 2002.
2. Duffy NC, Angus R: Casebook: chronic cough, *Practitioner* 246:84-96, 2002.
3. Holmes RL, Fadden CL: Evaluation of the patient with chronic cough, *Am Fam Phys* 69:2159-2166, 2169, 2004.
4. Irwin RS, Boulet LP, Cloutier MM, and others: Managing cough as a defense mechanism and as a symptom: a consensus panel report of the American College of Chest Physicians, *Chest* 114(2 Suppl):133S-181S, 1998.
5. Irwin RS, Curley FJ, Freanch CL: Chronic cough: the spectrum and frequency of causes, key components of the diagnostic evaluation, and outcomes of specific therapy, *Am Rev Respir Dis* 141:640-647, 1990.
6. Widdicombe J, Kamath S: Acute cough in the elderly, *Drugs Aging* 21(4):244-258, 2004.
7. Irwin RS, Madison M: Anatomical diagnostic protocol in evaluating chronic cough with specific reference to gastroesophageal reflux disease, *Am J Med* 108(Suppl 4A):126S-130S, 2000.
8. Irwin RS, Curley FJ: The treatment of cough: a comprehensive review, *Chest* 99:1477-1484, 1991.
9. Wartak JF, Sproule BJ, King EG: Differentiating causes of cough: an algorithmic approach, *J Respir Dis* 10:77-94, 1989.
10. Pratter MR, Bartter T, Akers S, and others: An algorithmic approach to chronic cough, *Ann Intern Med* 11:977-983, 1993.
11. Poe RH, Harder RV, Israel RH, and others: Chronic persistent cough: experience in diagnosis and outcome using an anatomic diagnostic protocol, *Chest* 95:723-728, 1989.
12. Barnes T, Afessa B, Swanson K, and others: The clinical utility of flexible bronchoscopy in the evaluation of chronic cough, *Chest* 126:268-272, 2004.
13. Boyards MC: Why is this patient still coughing? *J Respir Dis* 19:199, 1998.
14. Poe RH, Israel R: Evaluating and managing that nagging chronic cough, *J Respir Dis* 11:297-313, 1990.
15. Faller EW, Jackson DM: Physiology and treatment of cough, *Thorax* 45:425-430, 1990.
16. Irwin RS, Madison JM: Symptom research on chronic cough: a historical perspective, *Ann Intern Med* 134:809-814, 2001.
17. Rose VL: American College of Chest Physicians issues a consensus statement on the management of cough, *Am Fam Phys* 59(3):697-699, 1999.
18. Lawler WR: An office approach to the diagnosis of chronic cough, *Am Fam Phys* 58(9):2015-2022, 1998.
19. Kiljander T: The role of proton pump inhibitors in the management of gastroesophageal reflux disease–related asthma and chronic cough, *Am J Med* 115(3):65-71, 2003.
20. Irwin RS, Baumann MH, Bolser DC, and others: Diagnosis and management of cough executive summary. ACCP Evidence-Based Clinical Practice Guidelines, *Am Coll Chest Physicians* 129:1S-23S, 2006, retrieved Dec 27, 2006, from http://www.chestjournal.org/cgi/content/full/129/1_suppl/1S.
21. Hanak V, Hartman T, Ryu J: Cough-induced rib fractures, *Mayo Clinic Proc* 80(7):879-882, 2005.

CHAPTER 111

Chronic Obstructive Pulmonary Disease

Maureen B. Boardman

DEFINITION AND EPIDEMIOLOGY

Chronic obstructive pulmonary disease (COPD) refers to a cluster of disorders of the bronchi, the conducting airways, and the lung parenchyma. COPD is characterized by airflow limitation that is usually progressive, is not fully reversible, and is associated with an abnormal inflammatory response of the lungs.[1] *COPD* is the term used to describe two related lung diseases: chronic bronchitis and emphysema.[2,3] The terms *chronic obstructive airway disease* (COAD), *chronic obstructive lung disease* (COLD), *chronic airflow* or *airway obstruction* (CAO), and *chronic airflow limitation* (CAL) all refer to the same disorder.

Chronic bronchitis is defined clinically as a chronic, persistent cough and/or sputum production for 3 consecutive months each year for 2 consecutive years, with periodic acute exacerbations during which the symptoms worsen.[4] The pathologic features include inflammation of the cells lining the bronchial wall, hyperplasia of the mucous glands, and narrowing of the small airways.[5]

Emphysema is the permanent and abnormal enlargement of any part of the air spaces distal to the terminal bronchioles. Emphysema also involves destruction of the alveolar walls without fibrosis.[5]

The term *COPD* does not include other obstructive lung diseases such as asthma, even though asthma shares the same pathophysiologic common denominator as chronic bronchitis and emphysema, which is a slowing of the expiratory flow rate.[3] Asthma involves inflammation of the small airways. Although generally reversible, asthma can result in progressive airflow obstruction that over time becomes less and less reversible and resembles the obstruction seen with chronic bronchitis and emphysema. Persons with COPD can have a mix of emphysema, chronic bronchitis, and asthma that ranges from a "pure" emphysematous picture to a mixture of all three.

COPD is the fourth most common cause of death in the United States. According to Social Security disability statistics, it is second only to coronary heart disease in causing disability. COPD is projected to rank fifth in 2020 as a worldwide burden of disease.[6] According to the American Lung Association, the mortality rate of COPD has been increasing steadily over the past 20 years, while during this same period the mortality rates of many other chronic diseases have been in decline.[7,8] Approximately 10.7 million adults in the United States have been diagnosed with COPD.[9] However, close to 24 million U.S. adults have evidence of impaired lung function, indicating that COPD is likely greatly underdiagnosed, suggesting that the true prevalence of this disease is probably as high as 30 million to 35 million cases.[3,10,11] However, the proportion of U.S. population, ages 25 to 54, both male and female, with mild or moderate COPD has declined over the past quarter century, suggesting that the increase in hospitalizations and deaths caused by COPD may not continue.[1]

COPD is predominantly a smoker's disease that clusters in families and worsens with age. Approximately 80% to 90% of COPD deaths are caused by smoking.[12] A hereditary pattern caused by α_1-antitrypsin deficiency contributes to the "pure" emphysematous form of this disease.

The risks for COPD include genetic, behavioral, socioeconomic, and environmental factors (Box 111-1). Cigarette smoke and an occupation that involves regular exposure to a dusty environment are the two major external factors. Because smoking cessation slows the decline in the expiratory airflow, it is clear that smoking is a powerful factor in determining outcome.[13] When the disease is advanced, however, degeneration of lung function will probably continue even with smoking cessation. COPD is more common among individuals who are poor or undereducated. Cigarette smoking is also more common in these groups, but indigent populations still have worse lung function even when adjusted for smoking status. Other contributing factors include crowded living conditions with exposure to frequent viral infections, poorly ventilated homes, inadequate nutrition, exposure to passive cigarette smoke, and suboptimum care for childhood respiratory infections. It is possible that high levels of air pollution contribute to the development of chronic lung disease, but this has not been proven definitively.[14]

Morbidity and mortality rates from COPD are higher in Caucasians than in African Americans.[13] Mortality has always been higher in men than in women. However, recent data from the past 3 decades have demonstrated a gender shift in the number of smoking-related COPD cases being diagnosed each year. Data from the National Health and Nutrition Examination Survey showed significant increases in COPD mortality in 2000 compared with 1980, especially among women. During those 20 years, COPD death rates in the United States increased 13% but increased a dramatic 185% in women.[15] Because of the long latency period between smoking exposure and the development of clinical disease, deaths from this disease continue to increase despite the declining smoking rates in the United States.[16]

BOX 111-1

RISK FACTORS FOR DEVELOPING CHRONIC OBSTRUCTIVE PULMONARY DISEASE

- Cigarette smoking
- Airway hyperreactivity
- Childhood respiratory infections
- Occupational exposures
- Age
- Air pollution
- Passive exposure to smoke
- Poor nutrition
- Low socioeconomic status
- Crowded living conditions
- Family members with COPD
- α_1-Antitrypsin deficiency

Physician consultation is recommended for the initial diagnosis and management of patients with a significant change in condition or a failure to improve with prescribed therapies.

PATHOPHYSIOLOGY

The etiology of chronic bronchitis is not well understood, but chronic infection and airway hyperreactivity play important roles. The inflammatory process continues unabated even after withdrawing prolonged exposure to bronchial irritants such as smoke, dust, and fumes. Airway edema, airway wall thickening, excess mucus production, and loss of ciliary function result. Airflow is obstructed during both inspiration and expiration. Widespread bronchial narrowing with mucus plugging produces hypoxemia because of the mismatching of ventilation and perfusion. Hypercarbia results from the lack of ventilation. Chronic hypoxia and hypercarbia increase pulmonary arterial resistance and may lead to the development of pulmonary hypertension and, eventually, cor pulmonale. A sudden worsening of symptoms in severe chronic bronchitis can precipitate acute right-sided heart failure. Chronic bronchitis causes much less parenchymal damage than emphysema; therefore diffusing capacity, lung volumes, and compliance of lung tissue are not greatly altered.[5]

Enlargement of air spaces in emphysema is the result of alveolar wall destruction. This process is not completely understood but probably results from increased numbers of activated neutrophils that produce elastases—enzymes that destroy the elastin elements in the alveolar walls. Neutrophil-derived elastase is one of a group of destructive proteases contained in alveolar tissue. Usually a small amount of neutrophil elastase is inactivated by antielastases (also known as antiproteases), which are found in the serum and lung lining layer. The prime antielastase, which is present in the largest quantities, is α_1-antitrypsin.

Even though they account for fewer than 3% of cases, patients with a hereditary deficiency of α_1-antitrypsin have less inhibition of elastase and a much higher risk of developing emphysema.[5] The primary role of α_1-antitrypsin is to inhibit the function of several proteases, most notably human neutrophil elastase. Human neutrophil elastase degrades the protein elastin, which is key to the elastic recoil mechanism necessary for the lung's expiratory function. The lack of α_1-antitrypsin can lead to panacinar emphysema. Because the alveoli have lost their recoil mechanism, the driving force during respiration decreases and causes a chronic persistent airflow obstruction. In addition to inhibiting proteases, α_1-antitrypsin inhibits the function of lymphocytes, macrophages, and neutrophils.[17] Patients with a hereditary deficiency of α_1-antitrypsin have less inhibition of elastase and a much higher risk of developing emphysema.

Cigarette smoking also increases elastase activity by causing an influx of elastase-rich neutrophils into the alveoli and by causing the oxidative inactivation of antitrypsin. These processes result in a 30-fold increase in the risk of COPD.

Regardless of the mechanism, the end result of COPD is the destruction of alveolar architecture and the capillary bed lying within the alveolar wall. Initially, the reduction in size of the vascular bed parallels the fall in alveolar surface area.

Ventilation still roughly matches perfusion, and significant hypoxemia does not ensue. As the disease progresses, the elastic recoil of the airways is lost, and the poorly supported noncartilaginous airways collapse during expiration. Expiratory flow rates fall as a result, causing decreased airflow. Because this airflow obstruction is not uniform throughout the lung, there is uneven distribution of ventilation and blood perfusion. This uneven distribution causes arterial hypoxemia (decreased $Pa{O_2}$); decreased ventilation causes hypercarbia (increased $Pa{CO_2}$).

CLINICAL PRESENTATION

Diagnosing COPD requires a thorough patient history, physical examination, and diagnostic testing. The most common presenting complaint is dyspnea on exertion. This symptom develops late in the course of this disease, when irreversible changes may have already occurred.

COPD must be considered as a diagnosis in every patient who smokes, even in the absence of respiratory symptoms. Discussing smoking habits at every visit is an important strategy in the prevention of irreversible disease. Documentation should include onset of smoking, the average number of packs per day, and whether the patient has made any successful cessation attempts. Information about other respiratory symptoms, such as cough, sputum production, and exertional dyspnea, should be elicited and quantified.

The important medical history includes any recurrent or prolonged respiratory tract infections that have required antibiotic treatment. A childhood history of frequent respiratory tract infections and bronchitis and any history of asthma, recurrent sinus infections, or nasal polyps should be documented because such conditions are common in patients with COPD.

The family history, including allergies, tuberculosis, cystic fibrosis, COPD, and other chronic lung conditions, should be elicited. A detailed occupational history with special attention to exposure to noxious inhalants is essential.[13]

PHYSICAL EXAMINATION

Early in the disease process the physical examination is often normal. Even without the findings of advanced COPD, it is impossible to exclude the diagnosis in the person at risk. In fact, in a large autopsy series, only one in eight cases of emphysema had been diagnosed clinically.[18] However, if COPD is suspected based on the history and examination, it can be confirmed physiologically with simple spirometry.[1] In the late stages of COPD, the general physical findings include those resulting from hyperinflation. Inspection of the skin may show tobacco stains on the fingers and, occasionally, clubbing of the fingernails (convex nail plates). Chest inspection reveals an increase in the anteroposterior diameter, an increase in the intercostal spaces, and, in severe cases, abnormal retraction of the interspaces during inspiration. With inspiration there is diminished movement of the rib cage and increased movement of the abdominal wall. Abdominal and sternocleidomastoid muscles may be well developed but accompanied by diminished muscle mass in the thighs and legs. A forward-sitting posture with both hands on the knees to fix the shoulders, thereby permitting more effective use of the accessory cervical muscles, may be noted. Pursed-lip breathing with prolonged expirations is also characteristic of COPD.[19]

There is increased resonance on chest percussion. The diaphragm seems low and moves poorly with deep inspiration and expiration. Diminished transmission of breath sounds on auscultation is the most reliable finding; this indicates chronic airflow limitation. Early inspiratory crackles are commonly found. Wheezing may be elicited with forced expiration, but the presence of wheezing is more often found in reversible bronchospasm.[19]

Lung disease causes hypertrophy of the right ventricle of the heart, resulting in cor pulmonale. Therefore chronic cor pulmonale may be present in the advanced stage of COPD. The physical examination may reveal neck vein distention, peripheral edema, and hepatomegaly from an elevated right atrial pressure. Pulmonary hypertension and distention of the right ventricle cause a pronounced cardiac impulse in the epigastrium.

DIAGNOSTICS

Early detection of COPD is important for decreasing the associated morbidity and mortality. COPD can result in the loss of 40% to 50% of lung capacity before any problems are noticed.[16] During the presymptomatic period, laboratory measurements show airflow obstruction and can detect disease. A simple office maneuver may help determine if further testing is needed. After maximum inspiration, the patient exhales as forcefully as possible through the mouth. The practitioner auscultates the trachea over the upper sternum and measures the time between the first and last sound of forced expiration (forced expiratory time [FET]). An FET of 6 seconds or more is considered abnormal and suggests significant airflow obstruction.[20] An FET of less than 3 seconds makes significant airflow obstruction unlikely.

A prolonged FET should be confirmed with spirometric testing. The American Thoracic Society recommends providing screening spirometry in the office. Mild degrees of emphysema probably result in hyperinflation even before airflow abnormalities are present.[21] Spirometry should be performed at least once in every smoker over the age of 40 and in anyone who has cough, shortness of breath, or wheezing. Forced vital capacity (FVC), forced expiratory volume in 1 second (FEV_1), and the ratio of the two (FEV_1/FVC) are the primary spirometric measurements used for diagnosis.[13] Both FVC and residual volume increase with mild COPD (Box 111-2). Even slight decreases in FEV_1 or increases in FVC can lower the ratio below the normal 70% to 75%.[1] A low FEV_1/FVC ratio correlates with the early loss of ventilatory function and the early emergence of symptomatic COPD.[16] The severity of airflow obstruction is also reflected in the FEV_1.[13] Repeating these tests after patients use an inhaled bronchodilator may help identify a bronchospastic element of the disease. If the FVC or FEV_1 improves by 15% or more, bronchospasm is present. Even if flow rates do not respond to bronchodilators during the testing, some benefit may still be obtained from prolonged use.[19,22]

A posteroanterior and lateral chest x-ray study is useful for both the diagnosis of COPD and detection of its complications, such as pneumonia, pulmonary hypertension, and

BOX 111-2

CLASSIFICATION OF CHRONIC OBSTRUCTIVE PULMONARY DISEASE (COPD) BY SEVERITY

Stage 0: At risk—Chronic cough and sputum production. Lung function is still normal.

Stage I: Mild COPD—Mild airflow limitation (FEV_1/FVC <70% but FEV_1 >80% predicted), usually, but not always, chronic cough and sputum production. At this stage, the individual may not be aware that his or her lung function is abnormal.

Stage II: Moderate COPD—Worsening airflow limitation (50% <FEV_1 <80% predicted), and usually a progression of symptoms, with shortness of breath developing with exertion.

Stage III: Severe COPD—Further worsening of airflow limitation (30% <FEV_1 <50% predicted), increased shortness of breath, and repeated exacerbations. Exacerbations that have an impact on a patient's quality of life and prognosis are seen in patients with FEV_1 <50% predicted.

Stage IV: Very severe COPD—Severe airflow limitation (FEV_1 <30% predicted) or FEV_1 <50% predicted plus chronic respiratory failure. At this stage, quality of life is very impaired and exacerbations may be life threatening.

Adapted from Global Initiative for Chronic Obstructive Lung Disease: Global strategies for the diagnosis, management, and prevention of chronic obstructive pulmonary disease, *NHLBI/WHO Workshop Report,* Washington, DC, 2006, US Government Printing Office.

pneumothorax. The diagnosis of emphysema can be made if two or more of the following findings are present on the x-ray film: flattening of the diaphragm and blunting of the costophrenic angle on the posteroanterior view, enlargement of the retrosternal space on the lateral view, flattening or concavity of the diaphragmatic contour on the lateral view, or irregularity of lung field lucency.[13]

Pulse oximetry to estimate oxygen saturation can be helpful, but blood gas measurements are necessary to assess and manage patients during exacerbations and when oxygen therapy is indicated. The baseline measurement of blood gases is especially important when severe chronic bronchitis is present because it allows for a comparison with gases obtained during acute exacerbation.[13] Elevations of hematocrit and hemoglobin provide a measure of the severity of hypoxemia. Phlebotomy may become necessary if the elevation is severe. An ECG can indicate the severity of the lung disease and the presence of cor pulmonale. Significant findings include sinus tachycardia, multifocal atrial tachycardia, signs of right atrial enlargement (peaked P waves in leads II, III, and aV_F), signs of right ventricular hypertrophy (a tall R wave in lead V_1 and a deep S wave in lead V_6), and right-axis deviation.[8]

DIAGNOSTICS

Chronic Obstructive Pulmonary Disease

INITIAL

Spirometry (FVC and FEV_1)
Pulse oximetry

LABORATORY

CBC and differential*
ABGs*
α_1-Antitrypsin

IMAGING

Chest x-ray (posteroanterior and lateral)*

*If indicated.

Sputum is not routinely examined, but its inspection can help differentiate between a pulmonary infection and an exacerbation of reactive airways. The detection of neutrophils or eosinophils in the sputum will guide treatment between antibiotics or corticosteroids. Measurement of the α_1-antitrypsin levels is indicated if the patient has a strong family history of premature emphysema or α_1-antitrypsin deficiency.[13]

DIFFERENTIAL DIAGNOSIS

Distinguishing COPD from other causes of chronic cough or dyspnea is important for initial diagnosis and in acute exacerbations. A chronic cough could simply be secondary to chronic sinusitis or chronic rhinitis from allergies or post-infectious states. Gastroesophageal reflux, neoplasms, tuberculosis, interstitial lung diseases, and heart diseases (e.g., mitral stenosis or those causing chronic pulmonary edema) may cause chronic cough. Chronic coughs may also result from drugs such as angiotensin-converting enzyme inhibitors, beta blockers, and amiodarone.

Diseases that cause chronic dyspnea include COPD, chronic bronchitis, emphysema, cystic fibrosis, and asthma. Less common entities include diffuse interstitial lung disease, pulmonary vascular disease (including recurrent pulmonary emboli, pulmonary hypertension, and arteriovenous malfor-

DIFFERENTIAL DIAGNOSIS

Chronic Obstructive Pulmonary Disease

CHRONIC COUGH

- Chronic sinusitis
- Chronic rhinitis
- Gastroesophageal reflux
- Neoplasm
- Asthma
- Tuberculosis
- Interstitial lung disease
- Congenital heart disease
- Cardiac disease (mitral stenosis, congestive heart failure)
- Medications (angiotensin-converting enzyme inhibitors, beta blockers, amiodarone)

DYSPNEA

- Asthma
- Cystic fibrosis
- Interstitial lung disease
- Pulmonary embolism
- Pulmonary hypertension
- Arteriovenous malformation
- Other pulmonary vascular diseases
- Phrenic nerve dysfunction
- Neuromuscular disease
- Kyphoscoliosis or chest wall abnormalities
- Malignancy
- Anemia
- Obesity
- Ascites
- Metabolic acidosis
- Hyperthyroidism
- Congenital heart disease
- Abnormal hemoglobinopathies
- Hereditary emphysema (α_1-antitrypsin)

mation), and malignancies (including bronchogenic carcinoma and pulmonary metastatic disease). Phrenic nerve dysfunction or neuromuscular diseases can cause respiratory muscle weakness. Chest wall abnormalities, especially kyphoscoliosis, will cause chronic dyspnea. There are also nonpulmonary causes for dyspnea, including anemia, obesity, ascites, metabolic acidosis, hyperthyroidism, congenital heart disease, and abnormal hemoglobinopathies.

Some features are suggestive of COPD, rather than some of the most common pulmonary diseases that may share similar signs and symptoms. The onset of COPD is more likely to be in mid-life, with a long history of smoking and slowly progressing symptoms.[1] The onset of asthma is usually earlier in life, with varying symptoms occurring during the night and early morning. The patient often has a family history of asthma and may also have allergies, rhinitis, or eczema. The airflow limitations associated with asthma are largely reversible. Features suggestive of congestive heart failure include fine basilar crackles on auscultation and volume restriction versus airflow limitation on pulmonary function tests. A dilated heart and pulmonary edema may be noted on chest radiography. Bronchiectasis is associated with large volumes of purulent sputum and is commonly associated with bacterial infection. Coarse crackles may be noted on auscultation, and bronchial dilation and bronchial wall thickening may be seen on chest radiography or CT. Tuberculosis can occur at any age. Lung infiltrates are usually noted on chest radiography with microbiologic confirmation. It occurs most often when there is a high local prevalence of tuberculosis.[1]

MANAGEMENT

Certain therapeutic interventions for symptomatic COPD improve survival, and some improve symptoms. In the presence of hypoxemia, smoking cessation and oxygen therapy improve survival. Interventions that improve symptoms include pharmacotherapy, education, exercise, psychologic support, nutrition, and surgery.

The goals of treatment are to reverse or reduce airflow obstruction; control cough and secretions; prevent and eliminate infection; and control complications, including polycythemia, hypoxemia, and right-sided heart failure. It is important to relieve underlying depression and anxiety, maximize exercise tolerance, and educate patients about avoiding aggravating factors such as bronchial irritants.[23]

Smoking cessation is the single most important intervention to reduce the rapid decline of lung function in patients who smoke.[24] Treating tobacco use and dependence should be regarded as a primary and specific intervention. Smoking should be part of the routine evaluation of every health care visit, and every patient should be offered smoking cessation programs that involve multiple interventions that address the multifactorial causes of tobacco use.[1,25] In addition, providers should always express strong interest in helping their patients quit. Patients may be more inclined to stop smoking if they know their providers care that they stop smoking and if they understand that their smoking cessation is critical to preventing premature loss of lung function. The most comprehensive smoking cessation guidelines are available at http://www.surgeongeneral.gov/tobacco. Home oxygen is used in later stages of COPD because, unlike some pharmacotherapeutics, it improves survival in hypoxemic COPD. In fact, survival is related to the number of hours of supplemental oxygen used per day.[26] In one study, survival rates improved somewhat in patients who received oxygen 12 to 15 hours per day but improved most in those who received it 19 to 24 hours per day.[27] Other benefits of long-term oxygen include reduced polycythemia, reduced pulmonary artery pressures, reduced dyspnea, and improvement in neuropsychiatric testing. Another benefit may be the reduction of nocturnal arrhythmias, but it is unclear whether this translates into reduced mortality.

The Medicare criteria for 24-hour supplemental oxygen are $Pa{O_2}$ of 55 mm Hg or less or an oxygen saturation of 88% or less while breathing room air[25] (Box 111-3). Patients with cor pulmonale or erythrocytosis (hematocrit greater than 55%) and a $Pa{O_2}$ of 56 to 59 mm Hg or an $Sa{O_2}$ of 89% also qualify.[23] Patients with exercise-induced desaturation below 85% should use oxygen during exercise to reduce dyspnea and prevent hypoxemia. In the presence of daytime hypoxemia (a $Pa{O_2}$ of less than 55 mm Hg), a hematocrit greater than 50% to 55%, morning headaches, daytime sleepiness, and poor exercise tolerance are indications of oxygen desaturation during sleep.[28] Monitoring of oxygen saturation during the night may be indicated for these patients because sleep can cause hypoventilation and nocturnal hypoxemia. Oxygen therapy at night will reduce the incidence of nocturnal hypoxemia.[23]

The need for long-term oxygen therapy should be reassessed 30 to 90 days after an exacerbation for which oxygen was prescribed. Oxygen therapy may be discontinued if the patient no longer meets the blood gas criteria. The development of simpler and more portable oxygen tanks and devices has helped improve the quality of life and increase mobility for persons requiring long-term oxygen therapy.[25]

Pharmacotherapy

Currently there is no pharmacologic treatment that modifies the rate of decline of lung function or reduces or abolishes symptoms, but pharmacotherapy can improve exercise tolerance, reduce the number and severity of exacerbations, and improve lung function (Table 111-1). Pharmacotherapy should be based on the severity of disease and the patient's tolerance for certain drugs. In addition, a stepwise approach may be helpful.[25]

Inhaled bronchodilators relieve bronchospasm; methylxanthine therapy further enhances bronchodilation, albeit within a narrow therapeutic range; and corticosteroids reduce inflammation. Antibiotics will not treat exacerbations of COPD unless these exacerbations are precipitated by infections. Even though few patients with COPD actually have

BOX 111-3

CRITERIA FOR 24-HOUR SUPPLEMENTAL OXYGEN

- $Pa{O_2}$ of 55 mm Hg or less, or an oxygen saturation of 88% or less while breathing room air
- $Pa{O_2}$ of 56 to 59 mm Hg or an oxygen saturation of 89% or less with evidence of pulmonary hypertension, cor pulmonale, or erythrocytosis

TABLE 111-1 Pharmacologic Agents for COPD Therapy

Agent	Recommended Dose Range	Notes
ANTICHOLINERGICS		
Ipratropium bromide		
Metered-dose inhaler (MDI), 18 mcg/inhalation	2-4 puffs 4-6 times per day	Poorly absorbed systemically; few side effects; should be used regularly (not p.r.n.)
Solution for nebulization, 500 mcg/2.5 ml	3-4 times per day, separate doses by 6-8 hours	Precautions with narrow-angle glaucoma
β_2-ADRENERGIC AGONISTS		
Albuterol sulfate		
MDI, 90 mcg/inhalation	1-2 puffs q 4-6 hr	Use on p.r.n. basis preferable to a fixed-use schedule
Solution for nebulization, 0.5 ml of 0.5% solution	3-4 times per day	No more than 12 inhalations daily Relatively short-acting drug; avoid excessive use Caution with cardiac disease, hyperthyroidism, diabetes, seizure disorders
Bitolterol mesylate		
MDI, 370 mcg/inhalation	2 puffs at 1- to 3-minute intervals followed by a third puff if needed Maximum dose: 3 puffs	Same as albuterol
Solution for nebulization, 2 mg/ml; dilute to 2-4 ml	2-4 times per day	
Metaproterenol sulfate		
MDI, 650 mcg/inhalation	2-3 puffs q 3-4 hr	Same as albuterol
Solution for nebulization, 5.0% solution	0.2-0.3 ml of 5.0% solution in 2.5 ml of normal saline, 3-4 times per day	
Pirbuterol acetate, MDI, 200 mcg/inhalation	2 puffs q 4-6 hr	Same as albuterol
Terbutaline sulfate, MDI, 200 mcg/inhalation	2 puffs q 4-6 hr	Same as albuterol
Salmeterol xinafoate, MDI, 21 mcg/inhalation	2 puffs q 12 hr Maximum 2 doses/day	Same as albuterol Not for treatment of acute attacks May be helpful for nocturnal symptoms in COPD because it is a long-acting preparation
METHYLXANTHINES		
Theophylline		
Immediate-release tablets	10 mg/kg/day in 4 divided doses	Follow serum levels to regulate dose between 8 and 13 mg/day; reduce dose in patients with liver disease, cardiac disease, or seizures
Sustained-release tablets	10 mg/kg/day in 1-3 doses	Check for drug-drug interactions
ORAL CORTICOSTEROIDS		
Methylprednisolone	40-48 mg/day in divided doses for 3-4 days	Used to treat acute exacerbations
Prednisone	3- to 4-week tapering course: begin with 40-60 mg; taper by 10 mg q 4-5 days, ending with 4 or 5 days of 5 mg/day 2- to 3-week trial of steroids: 20-40 mg/day	Used to treat acute exacerbations Used for patients not responding to optimum doses of other drugs Steroid therapy associated with many side effects: osteoporosis, cataracts, hypertension, diabetes, peptic ulcers, psychic disorders, aseptic necrosis of hip, masking of infections, increased appetite, weight gain, and cushingoid effects Replace this form of steroid with inhaled form as soon as possible
INHALED CORTICOSTEROIDS		
Beclomethasone dipropionate, MDI, 42 mcg/inhalation	2 puffs 3-4 times per day or 4 puffs 2 times per day; maximum 20 puffs/day	Teach patients that inhaled corticosteroids are not bronchodilators; must be used regularly to be effective; mouth should be rinsed after use Side effects: hoarseness, dry mouth, oral fungal infections

TABLE 111-1 Pharmacologic Agents for COPD Therapy—cont'd

Agent	Recommended Dose Range	Notes
INHALED CORTICOSTEROIDS—CONT'D		
Flunisolide, MDI, 250 mcg/inhalation	2 puffs 2 times per day; maximum 8 puffs/day	Same as beclomethasone dipropionate
Triamcinolone acetonide, MDI, 100 mcg/inhalation	2 puffs 3-4 times per day, or 4 puffs 2 times per day; maximum 16 puffs/day	Same as beclomethasone dipropionate
Fluticasone-salmeterol, dry powder inhaler (DPI)	250 mcg/50 mcg/inhalation, 1 inhalation q 12 hr	Same as beclomethasone dipropionate
Budesonide, DPI	200 mcg/inhalation, 1-2 inhalations b.i.d.	Same as beclomethasone dipropionate
Fluticasone propionate, MDI	44, 110, or 220 mcg/puff; initial 88 mcg b.i.d., maximum 440 mcg b.i.d. 2-4 puffs b.i.d.	Same as beclomethasone dipropionate
MUCOACTIVE AGENTS		
Iodinated glycerol	60 mg 4 times per day	Prolonged use can lead to hypothyroidism 7-10 days of treatment needed before therapeutic effect occurs
Supersaturated potassium iodide solution (SSKI)	0.03-0.06 ml 3 times per day	Prolonged use can lead to hypothyroidism Most side effects are gastrointestinal

α_1-antitrypsin deficiency and the long-term efficacy of replacement therapy is unclear, its identification and treatment are important. Diuretics may also be useful in patients with cor pulmonale.

Bronchodilators. Bronchodilators can alleviate the symptoms of COPD, improve exercise tolerance, decrease the frequency of exacerbations, and improve the quality of life. With most bronchodilators, the preferred route is inhalation of long-acting agents. Some older patients may have difficulty effectively using a metered-dose inhaler (MDI), and the use of a spacer may facilitate inhalation.

Bronchodilators include β_2-adrenergic agonists and anticholinergics. Anticholinergics are a more effective first choice in patients with nonasthmatic COPD but are less effective than β_2-adrenergic agonists in patients with asthmatic COPD. In general, anticholinergics are considered to be agents of first choice unless symptoms are intermittent, in which case a β_2-adrenergic agonist should be the first choice.[24,27]

Anticholinergic Therapy. Anticholinergics are effective first-line therapy for patients with COPD. Stimulation of the cholinergic nerves to the bronchial smooth muscle causes bronchoconstriction. Decreased cholinergic stimulation lessens bronchoconstriction. The cholinergic receptors are plentiful in the proximal airways, and these are the ones which influence COPD. Adrenergic receptors are more plentiful in the distal airways, which play a larger role in asthma.

For persistent dyspnea and cough, anticholinergic treatment may be more effective than β_2-adrenergic agonists.[26] The effects of anticholinergics are slower in onset but are more prolonged and intense, making them more useful for patients with sustained symptoms. There are now two anticholinergics on the market in the United States. Ipratropium bromide has virtually no side effects because it is poorly absorbed systemically. The usual dose is 2 to 4 inhalations four to six times daily, with a recommended maximum of 12 inhalations daily. This medication should be used on a regular, not a p.r.n., basis. Tiotropium is a new long-acting anticholinergic; it is available in a dry-powder inhaler that has a duration of action of 24 hours.

β_2-Adrenergic Agonist Therapy. β_2-Adrenergic agonists (bronchodilators) cause bronchial smooth muscle dilation and can also improve mucociliary clearance. The major side effects include tachycardia and tremor from stimulation of β_1-receptors in muscle. Unfortunately, recommended dosages of these agents have been based on studies of patients with moderate, stable asthma. These dosages may not be appropriate for patients with COPD. As the severity of bronchospasm increase, the efficacy of β_2-adrenergic agonists decreases.

Some studies demonstrate that p.r.n. use of β_2-adrenergic agonists is superior to a fixed-use schedule.[29] Most agents in this class have a 4- to 6-hour duration. The dosage should not exceed 4 to 12 inhalations per day for the shorter-acting preparations (albuterol, pirbuterol acetate, metaproterenol sulfate, isoetharine, and terbutaline) or twice daily for the longer-acting preparations (salmeterol xinafoate, formoterol fumarate). The longer-acting inhaled preparations or the oral form of these medications may be more helpful in patients with nocturnal symptoms. Toxicity and drug-drug interactions must be avoided in older adults, especially those with co-existing heart disease.

Combination Therapy. The pairing of an anticholinergic and a short-acting beta$_2$ agonist in one MDI containing both ipratropium and albuterol has been shown in multiple studies to be superior in the treatment of COPD than either drug alone. The combination has also been shown to reduce exacerbations, lower cost, and improve lung function and quality of life.[30-32]

Methylxanthine Therapy. Theophylline is considered a third-line agent because its bronchodilatory effect is limited and its therapeutic range is narrow. Placebo-controlled studies have shown a significant positive effect of theophylline on spirometry, respiratory muscle strength, and resting blood gases. Other studies have shown that theophylline, in combination with bronchodilators, improves the subjective sensation of dyspnea and enhances quality of life.[33-36] Theophylline improves cardiac output, reduces pulmonary vascular resistance, and may have antiinflammatory effects. It may be used in patients who have not responded well to the first-line agents. Newer slow-release preparations have improved the problems related to its narrow therapeutic index and complex pharmacokinetics, leading to more stable plasma levels. Therapeutic levels should be measured and patients' levels kept on the lowest effective dose to maintain the recommended serum level of 8 to 13 mg/dl.[1] If levels rise, the risk of toxicity increases with little therapeutic gain. Theophylline is not recommended for patients receiving H_2-receptor blockers, fluoroquinolone, or macrolide antibiotics, since there is a likelihood of reduced theophylline clearance and a risk of toxicity.

Corticosteroids. Although oral corticosteroids improve airflow and gas exchange with acute exacerbations of COPD, their role in the management of COPD remains uncertain.[37,38] Complications, especially in older adults, make long-term therapy with oral corticosteroids problematic. These complications include skin damage, cataracts, diabetes, obesity, peptic ulcer disease, osteoporosis, and secondary infection. Oral steroids can be used to treat acute exacerbations. A 3- to 4-week tapering course of prednisone may be helpful. A dose of 40 to 60 mg of prednisone should be initiated and tapered by 10 mg every 4 or 5 days, ending with 4 or 5 days of 5 mg/day. Rebound bronchospasm can occur with faster tapers.

For patients who do not respond to optimum doses of other drugs, it is reasonable to try prednisone in doses of 20 to 40 mg/day. This trial of steroids should last 2 to 3 weeks. A 20% to 30% increase in FEV_1 must be demonstrated to justify continued use of oral steroids. Twice the lowest daily dose that maintains improvement should be prescribed on an every-other-day regimen to minimize side effects. If patients are taking long-term corticosteroids, other measures to improve symptoms of COPD should be considered. Lung volume reduction surgery and lung transplantation are two possible options.

The World Health Organization's Global Initiative for Chronic Obstructive Lung Disease (GOLD) guidelines suggest that inhaled corticosteroid use is only appropriate for COPD patients with an FEV_1 less than 50% predicted and repeated exacerbations. The GOLD guidelines go on to state, "Prolonged treatment with inhaled glucocorticosteroids may relieve symptoms in this carefully selected group of patients but does not modify the long term decline in FEV_1."[6]

Thus there is a place for inhaled corticosteroids in the stepwise approach to the treatment of symptomatic COPD. The FEV_1 should be rechecked after 3 to 4 months of therapy with inhaled corticosteroids. If the FEV_1 improves or stays the same, the same dosage should be continued. If the FEV_1 declines, discontinuation of the inhaled steroid should be considered. The side effects of inhaled corticosteroids are minimal. Oral candidiasis can be minimized by rinsing the mouth with water or mouthwash after every use or by using a spacer.[38]

Mucoactive Agents. Some patients with COPD form increased quantities of abnormal mucus. The value of mucopurative agents that decrease sputum viscosity and adhesiveness, which facilitates expectoration, has not been established in patients with COPD. Increasing hydration by the IV route, aerosolized route, or oral route does not decrease the thickness of secretions. Iodinated glycerol 60 mg q.i.d. may help. Another option for patients who have trouble coughing up thick, tenacious sputum is supersaturated potassium iodide solution 0.03 to 0.06 ml t.i.d. Patients may need to take this medication for 7 to 10 days before a therapeutic effect occurs.

Antibiotics. Viruses are probably responsible for at least half the exacerbations of COPD. Antibiotics have no value in the prevention or treatment of exacerbations of COPD unless there is evidence of a bacterial infection. Although antibiotics do reduce the severity and duration of these types of exacerbations, treatment is usually empiric because cultures of sputum are not cost-effective.[25,39] In a bacterial infection the most common pathogens include *Streptococcus pneumoniae, Haemophilus influenzae, Chlamydia pneumoniae,* and *Moraxella catarrhalis.*[25,26,39,40]

The antibiotic choice depends on several factors, including local resistance patterns and the cost of treatment. The mainstay antibiotics are broad-spectrum oral agents that the patient can keep at home to use at the first sign of an acute exacerbation. Typical choices are amoxicillin, ampicillin, cefaclor, doxycycline, and trimethoprim-sulfamethoxazole. Newer, more expensive antibiotics that extend the spectrum of coverage can be used for second-line therapy and include cefpodoxime, azithromycin, clarithromycin, levofloxacin, gatifloxacin, and moxifloxacin. Changing from a first- to a second-line antibiotic is necessary if the symptoms do not improve within 2 days, especially if persistent fever or purulent sputum is present.[39] If the patient is moderately ill or needs to be hospitalized, the antibiotic choice needs to be supported by sputum culture and sensitivity testing.[25]

Pulmonary Rehabilitation

Pulmonary rehabilitation has now become the treatment of choice for patients with COPD.[41,42] Pulmonary rehabilitation is a multidisciplinary team approach to care. It is designed to be highly individualized to meet the needs of each patient. The team makeup may vary from program to program but usually consists of a physician, a respiratory therapist, an exercise therapist and/or a physical therapist, an occupational therapist, psychosocial staff, and a dietitian-nutritionist. The two main objectives of pulmonary rehabilitation are (1) to control, alleviate, and in so far as possible reverse the symptoms and pathophysiologic processes contributing to respiratory compromise; and (2) to improve the quality and length of life for persons with COPD.[25] Instruction on nutrition, exercise, upper body weight training, and breathing techniques and guidance for maximizing energy reserves are critical components of any rehabilitation program. Pulmonary rehabilitation programs are also an excellent source of support for both patients and family members.

Exercise Training

Formal exercise programs are another cornerstone of pulmonary rehabilitation.[41-45] Programs emphasize lower extremity training, upper extremity training, and strength training. Most pulmonary rehabilitation exercise programs consist of 20- to 30-minute sessions three times a week for 6 to 8 weeks.[41] Participants are also taught breathing strategies such as pursed-lip breathing and controlled coughing to improve their ability to perform activities of daily living.

Immunizations

There is evidence that persons with COPD benefit from immunization against respiratory pathogens. A yearly immunization with the influenza vaccine is essential to decrease morbidity and mortality from influenza epidemics. Patients with COPD should also receive prophylaxis with the currently available polyvalent pneumococcal vaccine every 5 years.[25,39,40]

Psychologic Support

Patients with COPD may feel anxious, depressed, and fatigued. Counseling is recommended for those patients exhibiting signs and symptoms of major depression. Many of these problems improve when patients become involved in a pulmonary rehabilitation program. There is evidence that 15 to 20 rehabilitation sessions, including exercise, isolated physical therapy, and breathing techniques, are more effective in reducing anxiety than a similar number of counseling sessions. Sometimes an antidepressant is beneficial. Issues about sexuality should be discussed because most patients will not raise this sensitive issue themselves. If necessary, sexual counseling may be initiated.[26]

Nutrition

COPD often precipitates weight loss, since the increased work of breathing can double resting energy expenditures. This, along with decreased physical activity, tends to diminish fat and muscle stores. Weight loss is also aggravated by disease exacerbations or anorexia from medications or emotional issues. Severe dyspnea, coughing, and sputum production can interfere with eating. Caloric intake may need to be increased to 45 kcal/kg/day. Patients should be encouraged to eat frequent, small meals instead of a large meal; large meals cause abdominal distention, which impairs diaphragmatic function. Vitamin supplementation and commercially prepared drinks are convenient; easily digested; and high in protein, calories, and vitamins. Consultation with a registered dietitian is often necessary to plan for adequate nutrition.[25]

Surgery

Two types of surgery may be beneficial for some patients with COPD: lung volume reduction surgery (LVRS) and lung transplantation. The proposed benefit of LVRS is improved elastic recoil and diaphragmatic function, which is accomplished by reducing the volume of the lung and thereby decreasing hyperinflation.[11] Most patients will not benefit from LVRS, and optimum candidates have not been defined. Therefore, before any patient is considered for this surgery, all other conventional therapies must be exhausted without significant improvement in the patient's quality of life.

The recent development of nonsurgical volume reduction with intrabronchial one-way valves or sclerosing agents may be a viable option in the future. In the interim, lung transplantation is an option for younger patients who have end-stage COPD, are not candidates for LVRS, are highly symptomatic, and have diminished quality of life. Survival statistics vary significantly among centers. Costs associated with lung transplantation are very high, and donor availability is limited.[25,39]

COMPLICATIONS

Complications may be caused not only by the condition of COPD but also by the treatment. Drug effects should always be considered if there is a change in clinical condition. Long-term corticosteroids increase the risk for compression fractures because of accelerated osteoporosis. Some of these complications can be prevented by keeping the corticosteroid dose as low as possible, encouraging calcium supplementation, and prescribing biphosphonate therapy for patients who are unable to reduce their prednisone dose to less than 20 mg every other day.[8]

Theophylline toxicity should be considered in the presence of gastrointestinal symptoms, tremors, headache, or tachycardia. Other medications may affect the metabolism of theophylline. Corticosteroid or diuretic therapy may be responsible for hyperglycemia, hypokalemia, or azotemia.

Depression or marked anxiety often accompanies COPD. Patients with stable COPD tolerate antidepressant therapy, but most often depression improves when airflow obstruction improves; antiinflammatory therapy needs to be maximized during acute infections. Atypical mycobacterial disease should always be considered if chest radiographs show cavitary apical disease. Placement of an intermediate-strength purified protein derivative (PPD) skin test and a sputum examination for acid-fast bacilli are indicated.[13]

Fungal infections are important in the differential diagnosis of certain infiltrates in patients with COPD. Histoplasmosis is endemic in the Ohio and Mississippi river valleys. In the southwestern United States, coccidioidomycosis is endemic and can be seen in epidemic proportions after a dust storm. *Aspergillus* organisms are fungi that can be particularly dangerous in patients with COPD. Consultation is recommended before initiating specific antifungal therapy.[13]

Three other complications occur as a result of the disease process: sleep disorders, acute respiratory failure, and cor pulmonale. Although not always recognized, nocturnal oxygen desaturation in patients with COPD is fairly common. It is not usually caused by sleep apnea but by ventilation/perfusion abnormalities and short-term hypoventilation during rapid eye movement sleep. Patients who are not obese rarely develop co-existing upper airway obstruction. However, in some individuals who are obese, there is an added obstructive component to the usual mechanisms of transient hypoxemia. Sleep-related hypoxemia is suggested by an increased hematocrit in a patient who complains of morning headaches and daytime somnolence. Often the patient's significant other complains of intense snoring. Overnight home monitoring with pulse oximetry establishes the diagnosis. It is appropriate to prescribe home oxygen for nocturnal use if home monitoring with a pulse oximeter identifies an oxygen saturation of less than 88% and if symptoms of headache, fatigue, and poor exercise tolerance are present. Continuous positive airway pressure (CPAP) via a well-fitting nasal mask is helpful for patients with an obstructive component. If nocturnal oxygen desaturation is suspected, a referral should be made to a pulmonologist or sleep disorder specialist.[13]

Acute respiratory failure is the most severe complication of COPD. Acute worsening of arterial blood gases necessitates consultation and possible hospitalization.

Cor pulmonale is a severe complication of COPD and is an indication for consultation. Its pathologic definition is right ventricular enlargement, hypertrophy, or dilation secondary to lung disease.[13] Peripheral edema, elevation of the neck veins, and a congested liver reflect right-sided heart failure. In the presence of a significant degree of COPD and an elevated hematocrit with hypoxemia, the diagnosis of cor pulmonale as a complication of COPD can be made without further expensive tests other than an ECG. Standard therapy for cor pulmonale is to treat the underlying airflow obstruction and improve oxygenation. Restriction of salt intake to 2 g/day and a 24-hour diuretic can benefit those with mild heart failure. If decompensation continues, the addition of supplemental oxygen is indicated to achieve arterial oxygen saturation in the 90% to 95% range 24 hours a day. Hematocrit or hemoglobin levels should be monitored at 4- to 8-week intervals. If the patient is adequately oxygenated, the elevated hematocrit will resolve within that period. Persistent erythrocytosis reflects insufficient oxygen administration or the presence of desaturation during sleep despite the oxygen. A sleep study at this point may help determine whether additional therapy, such as CPAP, is needed during the night.

INDICATIONS FOR REFERRAL OR HOSPITALIZATION

Consultation is appropriate when (1) the disease progresses and the need for oral corticosteroids is evident, (2) presentation includes escalation of symptoms and fever, (3) hospitalization is indicated, (4) continuous or nocturnal oxygen is required, and (5) there is evidence of right-sided heart failure and cor pulmonale is present. Petty outlines 12 indications for consultation with a pulmonary specialist[13]:

1. Particularly severe disease, including persistent dyspnea with activities of daily living despite therapy and frequent recurrent exacerbations
2. Evaluation for and maintenance of oxygen therapy, including consideration of nocturnal oxygen therapy or transtracheal oxygen therapy
3. Inability to successfully taper the patient from systemic corticosteroids
4. Preoperative assessment for thoracic surgery or other surgery, which places the patient at high risk for pulmonary complications
5. Failure to respond after two courses of antibiotics for an acute exacerbation
6. Consideration of long-term intermittent or continuous antibiotic therapy
7. Persistent pulmonary infiltrate(s) on chest radiograph with no response to a course of antibiotics
8. Evaluation of sleep disturbances, including obstructive sleep apnea
9. Management of severe acute respiratory failure, especially if mechanical ventilation is a consideration
10. Cor pulmonale with clinical right-sided heart failure that is unresponsive to usual therapy
11. Consideration of new techniques in LVRS
12. Consideration of α_1-antitrypsin augmentation therapy

Hospitalization is based on the severity of the underlying respiratory dysfunction, the progression of symptoms, new or worsening cor pulmonale, or the existence of other comorbidities. Hypoxemia and hypercapnia are probably increasing if a patient does not respond adequately to treatment or is confused or unable to walk, eat, or sleep without aid. Hospitalization is warranted in these cases.

Some patients require admission to a specialized respiratory care unit. Issues that require admission include (1) severe dyspnea that does not respond to initial emergency therapy; (2) confusion, lethargy, or respiratory muscle fatigue characterized by paradoxical diaphragmatic motion; (3) persistent or worsening hypoxemia despite supplemental oxygen, or severe or worsening acidosis; and (4) the need for assisted mechanical ventilation.[23]

PATIENT AND FAMILY EDUCATION

Education has always been considered a cornerstone of pulmonary rehabilitation. However, until recently few studies unequivocally demonstrated the effectiveness of patient education, including behavior modification. Recently a structured education program, specifically designed for patients with COPD, demonstrated that self-management and behavior modification can be achieved, resulting in a substantial decrease in morbidity.[46] Patients can better recognize and treat the symptoms of COPD if they understand the nature of the disease and the implications of treatment. The importance of medication, oxygen therapy, smoking cessation, nutrition, exercise, breathing techniques to minimize dyspnea, and health promotion should be stressed. Patients and families need to understand that acute exacerbations of COPD may produce respiratory failure, a possible need for ventilatory support, and the possibility of death. Providers should help patients, during stable periods of health, and their family members think about advance planning and their preferences for end-of-life care. These discussions can help prepare patients with advanced COPD for a life-threatening exacerbation of the disease while also encouraging them to continue living and enjoying life.[1]

REFERENCES

1. Celli B, Macnee W: Standards for the diagnosis and treatment of patients with COPD: a summary of the ATS/ERS position paper, *Europ Respir J* 23:932-946, 2004.
2. Parmet S: Chronic obstructive pulmonary disease, *JAMA* 290(17): 2362, 2006.

3. American Lung Association: *Chronic obstructive pulmonary disease (COPD) fact sheet*, July 2005, retrieved July 5, 2006, from http://www.lungusa.org/site/pp.asp.
4. Celli BR, and others: The challenge of COPD: step by step through the workup, *Patient Care* 31(2):21-52, 1997.
5. Celli BR: Pathophysiology of chronic obstructive pulmonary disease, *Chest Surg Clin North Am* 5(4):623-633, 1995.
6. Global Initiative for Chronic Obstructive Lung Disease: Global strategies for the diagnosis, management, and prevention of chronic obstructive pulmonary disease, *NHLBI/WHO Workshop Report*, 2006, retrieved Jan 31, 2007, from http://goldcopd.com/Guidelineitem.asp?l1=2&l2=1&intId=989.
7. Hunter MH, Kim DE: COPD: management of acute exacerbations and chronic stable disease, *Am Fam Phys* 64(4):603-612, 2001.
8. American Lung Association: *Trends in chronic bronchitis and emphysema: morbidity and mortality*, New York, 2001, Epidemiology and Statistics Unit, The Association.
9. National Center for Health Statistics: *Report of final mortality statistics, 2002*, October 2006, retrieved Dec 7, 2006, from http://www.cdc.gov/nchs/pressroom/02facts/02facts.htm.
10. Mannimo D, Homa D, Akinbami L, and others: Chronic obstructive pulmonary disease surveillance—United States, 1997-2000, *MMWR* 51(SS06):1-16, 2001.
11. Petty TL: A new national strategy for COPD, *J Respir Dis* 18(4):365-369, 1997.
12. US Department of Health and Human Services: *The health consequences of smoking, a report of the surgeon general*, Washington, DC, 2004, The Department.
13. Petty TL: *Frontline treatment of COPD*, Denver, 2001, Snowdrift Pulmonary Foundation.
14. Bates DV, Sizto R: The Ontario air pollution study: identification of the causative agent, *Environ Health Perspect* 79:69-72, 1989.
15. Mannimo DM, Homa DM, Akinbami LJ, and others: Chronic obstructive pulmonary disease surveillance—United States, 1971-2000, *MMWR* 51:55-56, 2002.
16. Pina JS, Horan MP: Alpha$_1$-antitrypsin deficiency and asthma, *Postgrad Med* 101(4):153-168, 1997.
17. Goroll AH: Management of chronic obstructive pulmonary disease. In Coroll AH, May LA, Mulley AG, editors: *Primary care medicine: office evaluation and management of the adult patient*, ed 3, Philadelphia, 1995, Lippincott.
18. Bates B: *A guide to physical examination and history taking*, ed 5, Philadelphia, 1991, Lippincott.
19. Badgett RG, Tanaka DJ, Hunt DK, and others: Can moderate chronic obstructive pulmonary disease be diagnosed by historical and physical findings alone? *Am J Med* 94(2):188-196, 1993.
20. Petty TL, Silvers GW, Stanford RE: Mild emphysema is associated with reduced elastic recoil and increased lung size but not with airflow limitation, *Am Rev Respir Dis* 136(4):867-871, 1987.
21. American Thoracic Society: Lung function testing, selection of reference values, and interpretation strategies, *Am Rev Respir Dis* 144:1202-1208, 1991.
22. Celli BR, Cosentino A, Fiel S, and others: The challenge of COPD: therapeutic strategies that work, *Patient Care* 31(5):101-118, 1997.
23. Anthonisen NR, Connett JE, Kiley JP, and others: Effects of smoking intervention and the use of an inhaled anticholinergic bronchodilator on the rate of decline in FEV$_1$: the Lung Health Study, *JAMA* 272:1497-1505, 1994.
24. Celli BR: Current thoughts regarding treatment of chronic obstructive pulmonary disease, *Med Clin North Am* 80(3):589-609, 1996.
25. Cole C, Celli B: New treatment strategies for COPD, *Postgrad Med* 117(3):27-34, 2005.
26. Gross NJ: COPD management: options for patients with severe disease, *J Respir Dis* 17(6):494-501, 1996.
27. Celli BR, and others: The challenge of COPD: managing the special problems of chronic lung disease, *Patient Care* 31(7):87-98, 1997.
28. Petty TL: Developments in the early recognition and treatment of COPD, *Hosp Med* 32(8):13-20, 1996.
29. Van Schayck CP, Dompeling E, van Herwaarden CL, and others: Bronchodilator treatment in moderate asthma or chronic bronchitis: continuous or on demand? A randomized study, *BMJ* 303:1426-1431, 1991.
30. Gross N, Taskin D, Miller R, and others: Inhalation by nebulization of albuterol-ipratropium (dry combination) is superior to either agent alone in the treatment of chronic obstructive pulmonary disease, *Respiration* 65:354-362, 1998.
31. Campbell S: For COPD a combination of ipratropium bromide and albuterol sulfate is more effective than albuterol base, *Arch Intern Med* 159:156-160, 1999.
32. Dorinsky PM, Reisner C, Ferguson GT, and others: The combination of ipratropium and albuterol optimizes pulmonary function reversibility testing in patients with COPD, *Chest* 115:966-971, 1999.
33. Mahler DA, Matthay RA, Snyder PE, and others: Sustained-release theophylline reduces dyspnea in non-reversible obstructive airway disease, *Am Rev Respir Dis* 131:22-25, 1985.
34. McKay SE, Howie CA, Thomson AH, and others: Value of theophylline in the treatment of patients handicapped by chronic obstructive pulmonary disease, *Thorax* 48:227-232, 1993.
35. Pulmonary Rehabilitation Research NIH Workshop Summary: *Am Rev Respir Dis* 149:825-830, 1994.
36. Callahan CM, Dittus RS, Katz BP: Oral corticosteroid therapy for patients with stable chronic obstructive pulmonary disease: a meta-analysis, *Ann Intern Med* 114:216-223, 1991.
37. Thompson WH, Nielson CP, Carvalho P, and others: Controlled trial of oral prednisone in outpatients with acute COPD exacerbation, *Am J Respir Crit Care Med* 154:407-412, 1996.
38. Kerstjens HAM, Brand PL, Hughes MD, and others: A comparison of bronchodilator therapy with and without inhaled corticosteroids therapy for obstructive airway disease: Dutch Chronic Non-Specific Lung Disease Study Group, *N Engl J Med* 327:1413-1419, 1992.
39. Boyars MC: COPD: a step-care approach when FEV$_1$ is deteriorating, *Consultant* 37(6):1673-1687, 1997.
40. The debate over inhaled corticosteroid use in COPD, *J COPD Manage* 2(5):13-16, 2001.
41. Lacasse Y, Wong E, Guyatt GH, and others: Meta-analysis of respiratory rehabilitation in chronic obstructive pulmonary disease, *Lancet* 348:1115-1119, 1996.
42. Kharestan A: The role of pulmonary rehabilitation in the treatment of COPD patients, *J COPD Manage* 2(4):10-15, 2001.
43. Celli BR: Pulmonary rehabilitation for COPD: a practical approach for improving ventilatory conditioning, *Postgrad Med* 103:159-160, 167-168, 173-176, 1998.
44. Casaburi R: Exercise training in chronic obstructive pulmonary disease. In Casaburi R, Petty TL, editors: *Principles and practice of pulmonary rehabilitation*, Philadelphia, 1994, Saunders.
45. Cooper CB: Exercise in chronic pulmonary disease: aerobic exercise prescription, *Med Sci Sports Exer* 33(July Suppl):S671-S679, 2001.
46. Worth H, Dhein Y: Does patient education modify behavior in the management of COPD? *Patient Educ Couns* 52:267-270, 2004.

CHAPTER 112

Dyspnea

David Patrick Murphy

DEFINITION AND EPIDEMIOLOGY

Dyspnea is the clinical term for shortness of breath. The American Thoracic Society consensus panel defines dyspnea as "a term used to characterize a subjective experience of breathing discomfort that consists of qualitatively distinct sensations that vary in intensity. The experience derives from interactions among multiple physiologic, [psychologic], social, and environmental factors, and may induce secondary physiologic and behavioral responses."[1] Although breathlessness is expected after vigorous exercise, dyspnea is a cardinal manifestation of cardiopulmonary disease that warrants appropriate evaluation and treatment. It is also a common and disabling symptom of chronic lung disease, and measures of dyspnea are commonly used in evaluating outcomes in these diseases.[2]

PATHOPHYSIOLOGY

The mechanisms that trigger dyspnea are complex and vary by disease. It has been suggested that dyspnea occurs whenever sensory input from receptors in the airways, lung, and chest wall does not match up with respiratory drive.[3] These sensory receptors may respond to chemicals, stretch, irritation, or passive distention. For example, there appears to be a dissociation between sensory input and motor output in conditions that impose a mechanical load on the respiratory system by decreasing compliance of either the lung (e.g., pneumonia, pulmonary edema, fibrosis) or the chest wall (e.g., kyphoscoliosis, rib fractures, circumferential thorax burns) or by inhibiting airflow (e.g., asthma, chronic bronchitis, emphysema).[4] In addition, neuromuscular weakness or fatigue may cause dyspnea symptoms because of the inability of weakened muscles to generate an expected level of ventilation. Hypoxemia and hypercapnia stimulate chemoreceptors that may cause dyspnea through increased respiratory motor drive. Surprisingly, there is a poor correlation between dyspnea and blood gas abnormalities. Dyspneic patients are often perplexed to learn that they have adequate oxygen saturation or that supplemental oxygen administration does not relieve symptoms. It is important to understand that the perception of dyspnea varies greatly among patients and is influenced by various psychologic, social, and environmental factors.

CLINICAL PRESENTATION

Dyspnea is a common complaint, and the following dimensions are useful in elucidating the disease process that causes dyspnea: quality, timing, intensity, associated symptoms, and environmental exposures.

Quality

The descriptors patients use for dyspnea sensations may be diagnostically useful.[5-8] For example, patients with asthma tend to complain of "chest tightness" or "constriction." Diseases associated with an increased mechanical load (either resulting from decreased compliance or increased airway resistance) are often associated with feelings of excessive "work" or "effort." Patients with an increased drive to breathe (e.g., resulting from hypoxemia or hypercapnia) experience air hunger and may complain that they "can't get enough air in." Most pulmonary diseases probably activate multiple dyspnea mechanisms, leading to a composite of sensations that defy easy classification.

Timing

Although it is often impossible to pinpoint the precise onset of dyspnea, it is important to distinguish between acute and chronic symptoms. Sudden onset of dyspnea often heralds serious cardiopulmonary disease that requires immediate evaluation and treatment (e.g., pulmonary embolism, pneumothorax, myocardial infarction). Relative stability, intermittent exacerbations, or progressive debilitating symptoms may characterize chronic dyspnea. Patients who experience increasing symptoms or intermittent exacerbations should be carefully reevaluated for worsening disease or a new problem.

Intensity

Dyspnea severity is difficult to quantify, and therefore activity limitation is commonly used as a surrogate marker. Dyspnea is almost always first noticed with physical exertion and may progress to symptoms at rest. The degree of activity necessary to elicit symptoms may be quantified by asking questions such as, "How many flights of stairs can you climb?" or "How far can you walk on level ground?" One commonly used scale for classifying the severity of dyspnea was proposed and published by the Medical Research Council (Table 112-1).

Associated Symptoms

In addition to dyspnea, cardinal symptoms of pulmonary disease are chest pain, cough, hemoptysis, and wheezing.

TABLE 112-1 Dyspnea Scale

Grade	Degree	Defining Clinical Characteristics
0	None	Not troubled with breathlessness except with strenuous exercise
1	Slight	Troubled by shortness of breath when hurrying on level ground or walking up a slight hill
2	Moderate	Walks more slowly than people of the same age when on level ground because of breathlessness or has to stop for breath when walking at own pace on level ground
3	Severe	Stops for breath after walking about 100 yards or after a few minutes on level ground
4	Very severe	Too breathless to leave the house or breathless when dressing or undressing

From Medical Research Council Working Party: Long-term domiciliary oxygen therapy in chronic hypoxic cor pulmonale complicating chronic bronchitis and emphysema, *Lancet* 1:681-686, 1981.

Chest pain is one manifestation of ischemic heart disease but may also result from pneumothorax, pulmonary embolism, or rib trauma. Hemoptysis is a distressing symptom that may accompany dyspnea. Expectorated blood can originate from the nose, airways, or lung parenchyma. Cough is a common symptom of acute and chronic pulmonary disease. Persistent cough is most often caused by upper airway cough syndrome (previously referred as postnasal drip syndrome), gastroesophageal reflux, or asthma. Wheezing signifies airway diseases such as asthma and chronic obstructive pulmonary disease (COPD), or focal obstruction by a tumor such as a carcinoid lesion or aspirated foreign body. Patients who are initially seen with fever, chills, or night sweats should be evaluated for acute or chronic lung infections, including pneumonia, tuberculosis, and chronic bronchiectasis.

Dyspnea is often accompanied by fear and anxiety. A dyspnea-panic cycle has been described in which the sensation of breathlessness leads to anxiety, which creates muscle tension, which in turns leads to increased dyspnea and panic. Thus the anxiety associated with dyspnea can become a vicious cycle leading to future attacks of dyspnea.[9,10]

Exposures

The lungs are uniquely susceptible to various environmental hazards, including air pollution, dust, and smoke. A careful history of current and past tobacco use is essential in the evaluation of tobacco-related diseases such as asthma, chronic bronchitis, emphysema, spontaneous pneumothorax secondary to bullous disease, ischemic heart disease, respiratory bronchiolitis, and eosinophilic granuloma. In addition, many medications and therapeutic radiation are known to damage the lungs.

PHYSICAL EXAMINATION

The physical examination begins with careful assessment of the patient's vital signs. Normal respiratory rate in adults ranges from 12 to 20 breaths per minute, and a rapid or labored breathing pattern is often, but not always, evident in dyspneic patients. Many practitioners consider pulse oximetry a "vital sign," since it usually provides a reliable measure of arterial oxygen saturation. A normal oxygen saturation level, however, does not rule out carbon dioxide retention and ventilatory insufficiency; carbon dioxide levels must be directly measured with an arterial blood gas sample. Expiratory peak flow measurement may also be included in the initial assessment of patients with known airways disease or wheezing.

Breathing pattern and body position provide important clues to disease severity. The acutely dyspneic patient often sits upright and leans forward to optimize breathing mechanics. The inability to speak in full sentences and accessory respiratory muscle use indicate increased work of breathing. Patients with COPD often adopt a characteristic "pursed-lip" appearance. Shallow, rapid breathing or panting is characteristic of interstitial lung diseases in patients who have poor or decreased lung compliance. The skin may be diaphoretic, and the patient may appear anxious. Bluish discoloration of the skin and mucous membranes (cyanosis) results from increased amounts of deoxygenated hemoglobin. Central cyanosis, detected in the tongue and mucous membranes, is a more reliable indicator of oxygenation than peripheral cyanosis, which can also result from intense vasoconstriction of vessels in the extremities. Mental status may be depressed by either severe hypoxemia or hypercapnia. Digital or finger clubbing is an important finding often attributed to various lung diseases, but it is also seen in other disorders such as in inflammatory bowel disease and congenital heart disease.

The lung examination includes careful inspection of the thorax and abdomen. Chest wall deformities may limit lung expansion and contribute to dyspnea. During inspiration, normally the chest rises and the abdomen moves outward due to the contraction of the diaphragm (which moves downward). During inspiration in a patient with inspiratory muscle fatigue the chest rises (due to accessory muscle contraction) and the abdomen moves inward (due to upward movement of the diaphragm); this pattern of breathing is said to be *paradoxical* and indicates diaphragmatic weakness or fatigue. Palpation of the chest wall is useful in assessing tracheal position, symmetry of chest movement, areas of tenderness, and crepitus (subcutaneous air from pneumothorax or pneumomediastinum). Airless lung transmits sounds more efficiently than air-filled lung and is the basis for auscultatory consolidative findings, including bronchial breath sounds, egophony (E to A changes), and whisper pectoriloquy. The classic example of a disease that causes lung consolidation is pneumonia, although any process that fills (pus, water, blood, protein, cells) or collapses alveoli yields these findings. Abnormal, or *adventitious*, lung sounds are distinguished by whether they are continuous (high pitched equals wheezing, low pitched equals rhonchi) or discontinuous (crackles). Wheezing signifies bronchoconstriction or airway obstruction from secretions, tumor, or foreign body. Crackles are heard in a number of disease processes, including congestive heart failure and interstitial lung disease. Pleural friction rubs are grating sounds that may occur on inspiration or expiration as inflamed pleural surfaces rub against each other.

A detailed discussion of the cardiac examination is beyond the scope of this chapter, but is an important component of the evaluation of dyspneic patients. The pulse should be carefully analyzed for rate and rhythm. Atrial fibrillation is a common arrhythmia that can usually be diagnosed at the bedside by its "irregularly irregular" character. Left ventricular dysfunction and valvular heart disease also lend themselves to bedside diagnosis through palpation and auscultation. The extremities should also be assessed for pulse and edema.

In summary, the physical examination is an essential part of the workup of dyspneic patients and should be used to help direct the diagnostic evaluation. The absence of specific physical examination findings can be of greater diagnostic utility than positive findings in patients with chronic dyspnea. For example, interstitial lung disease and congestive heart failure are unlikely causes of dyspnea in a patient without crackles on lung examination.

DIAGNOSTICS

After a thorough history and physical examination are completed, further diagnostic studies may be necessary. A plain chest radiograph is helpful in elucidating many causes of dyspnea. Radiographic findings of hyperinflation, flattened hemidiaphragms, increased anterior clear space, and bullae support a diagnosis of COPD. Parenchymal infiltrates occur in many different disease processes but, in the context of an acute infectious syndrome, imply pneumonia. Congestive heart failure is recognized by cephalization of vessels, Kerley's B lines, and an enlarged cardiac silhouette. Frank pulmonary edema manifests with bilateral perihilar air space filling ("bat-wing" appearance) and pleural effusions. Pneumothorax and pleural effusion are generally easily detected on a plain chest radiograph, although small effusions may require decubitus views for confirmation. The chest radiograph is usually normal or reveals only subtle abnormalities in asthma and pulmonary embolism.

Spirometry is essential to the diagnosis and management of asthma and COPD. A decrease in the ratio of forced expiratory volume in 1 second to forced vital capacity (FEV_1/FVC) is the spirometric hallmark of obstruction. Bronchoprovocation testing with either methacholine or exercise may be necessary to diagnose asthma in patients with normal baseline spirometry. Proportionately reduced FEV_1 and FVC suggest restriction (a useful pneumonic for restrictive lung processes is *PAINT:* Pleural disease, Alveolar filling process, Interstitial lung disease, Neuromuscular disease, or Thoracic cage abnormalities), which should be confirmed with lung volume measurements. Diaphragmatic and respiratory muscle weakness may be detected with maximum inspiratory pressure and maximum expiratory pressure maneuvers, although these tests are neither sensitive nor specific.

The workup for pulmonary thromboembolic disease can be complicated and is often driven by the availability and expertise of local medical resources. An appropriate evaluation may initially include a ventilation/perfusion scan or CT angiogram. Symptomatic lower extremity clots (the source for most pulmonary emboli) are usually detected by ultrasound. Pulmonary angiography remains the definitive test for the diagnosis of pulmonary embolism.

Cardiac rhythm disturbances and hypertrophy may be noted on routine ECG, although intermittent arrhythmias may be detected only by long-term monitoring (e.g., telemetry, Holter, or event monitoring). Echocardiography is extremely useful in assessing left ventricular function, cardiac valve status, pericardial effusions, and, in some cases, pulmonary hypertension.

DIAGNOSTICS

Dyspnea

INITIAL
Peak flow
Pulse oximetry

LABORATORY
CBC and differential*
TSH*
BNP*

IMAGING
Chest x-ray (posteroanterior and lateral)*
CT scan*

OTHER
ABGs*
ECG*
Echocardiogram*
Exercise stress testing*
PFTs
V/Q scan or pulmonary angiogram*
Holter or event monitor*

*If indicated.

Other routine studies with utility in the evaluation of patients with dyspnea include hemoglobin level to exclude anemia, thyroid function tests to exclude hyperthyroidism, and brain natriuretic peptide (BNP) if heart failure is a consideration. More sophisticated testing such as formal cardiopulmonary exercise testing and cardiac catheterization obviously require referral to specialists.

DIFFERENTIAL DIAGNOSIS

Dyspnea is most commonly caused by cardiopulmonary disease, although anemia, neuromuscular weakness, gastroesophageal reflux, deconditioning, and psychogenic causes must be considered. The most common causes of acute dyspnea are asthma, bronchitis, pneumothorax, pneumonia, pulmonary embolism, chest trauma with rib fractures or pulmonary contusions, ischemic heart failure, psychogenic causes, and acute blood loss. The majority of patients with long-standing dyspnea have one of four causes: asthma, COPD, interstitial lung disease, or cardiomyopathy.[4]

DIFFERENTIAL DIAGNOSIS

Dyspnea

ACUTE
- Acute blood loss
- Airway obstruction
- Asthma
- Bronchitis
- Carbon monoxide poisoning
- Congestive heart failure or pulmonary edema
- Foreign body aspiration
- Ischemic heart disease
- Neuromuscular weakness
- Pleural effusion
- Pneumonia
- Pneumothorax
- Psychogenic causes
- Pulmonary contusions
- Pulmonary emboli
- Trauma (rib fractures or pulmonary contusions)

CHRONIC
- Anemia
- Asthma
- Cardiomyopathy
- Chronic obstructive pulmonary disease
- Congestive heart failure
- Cystic fibrosis
- Gastroesophageal reflux disease
- Interstitial pulmonary fibrosis
- Ischemic heart disease
- Obesity
- Pectus excavatum
- Pleural effusion
- Pulmonary hypertension
- Sarcoidosis
- Severe kyphoscoliosis
- Spondylitis

MANAGEMENT

The treatment of dyspnea entails treatment of the underlying disease process and symptomatic relief. Supplemental oxygen should be administered initially to all acutely dyspneic patients and to chronically dyspneic patients who are hypoxemic. The standard Medicare criteria for supplemental oxygen are as follows: $Pa{O_2}$ at rest of less than 55 mm Hg or oxygen saturation of 88% or less. Patients with a $Pa{O_2}$ of 56 to 59 mm Hg or an oxygen saturation of 89% or less warrant supplemental oxygen if they have underlying congestive heart failure or pulmonary hypertension. These criteria are based on two large studies that demonstrated improved survival in hypoxemic COPD patients treated with supplemental oxygen.[11,12] Patients who undergo desaturation during sleep or exercise also qualify for supplemental oxygen, although the data supporting these indications are not as strong. Administration of supplemental oxygen may worsen carbon dioxide retention in some patients with COPD. These patients require an arterial blood gas assessment to ensure adequate carbon dioxide elimination. Energy conservation strategies (e.g., walking slowly; periodically using resting positions, such as leaning forward while sitting in a chair; avoiding fatigue; and spacing chores at times when feeling good) and specific breathing techniques are often effective in patients with obstructive lung disease. Patients with difficulty mobilizing secretions (e.g., those with chronic bronchitis, bronchiectasis, cystic fibrosis) benefit from chest physiotherapy and airway clearance adjuncts such as the flutter device or vest airway clearance system. Anxiolytics and narcotics are sometimes effective in relieving dyspnea but must be used cautiously because of inherent respiratory depressant properties.

Formal pulmonary rehabilitation programs effectively incorporate dyspnea management therapies with nutrition and exercise. These programs have been shown to improve quality of life and may reduce unscheduled medical visits.[13-16]

COMPLICATIONS

Dyspnea limits a patient's activities of daily living. The consequences of uncontrolled dyspnea symptoms may include anxiety, depression, loss of job, and social isolation. Physical deconditioning results from decreased exercise and leads to a downward spiral of ever-decreasing activity.

INDICATIONS FOR REFERRAL OR HOSPITALIZATION

Patients with chronic dyspnea should be referred to a pulmonary specialist when the cause is not obvious from the history, physical examination, and screening studies, including CBC, chest radiograph, and spirometry. An echocardiogram and treadmill stress test may help differentiate between cardiac and pulmonary disease before the consultation.

The decision to hospitalize a patient depends initially on identifying the likely cause of respiratory distress. Conditions that need to be readily identified and mandate hospital admission include pulmonary embolism and myocardial infarction. Criteria for hospitalization of patients with other conditions such as pneumothorax, asthma, and COPD depend on the severity of the illness, response to treatment, and presence of co-morbid conditions.

PATIENT AND FAMILY EDUCATION AND HEALTH PROMOTION

Patients with chronic dyspnea need to be taught techniques that control symptoms and warning signs of the need for medical assistance. Pulmonary rehabilitation programs provide intense education for patients with severe pulmonary disease, but are expensive and not always available. All patients who use inhaled bronchodilators and corticosteroids should be regularly instructed in proper inhaler techniques, including the use of spacer devices. Asthmatic patients may benefit from home peak flow monitoring to detect worsening airflow obstruction, which offers an opportunity for early intervention. Smoking cessation is critical in the management of any cardiopulmonary disease, and providers play a pivotal role in educating their patients regarding the adverse effects of tobacco use and strategies to stop smoking.

REFERENCES

1. American Thoracic Society: Dyspnea: mechanisms, assessment, and management: a consensus statement, *Am J Respir Crit Care Med* 159:321-340, 1999.
2. Kaplan RM, Ries AL: Quality of life as outcome measures in pulmonary diseases, *J Cardiopulm Rehabil* 25:321-331, 2005.
3. Schwartzstein RM, Simon PM, Weiss JW, and others: Breathlessness induced by dissociation between ventilation and chemical drive, *Am Rev Respir Dis* 139:1231-1237, 1989.
4. Pratter MR, Curley FJ, Dubois J, and others: Cause and evaluation of chronic dyspnea in a pulmonary disease clinic, *Arch Intern Med* 149:2277-2282, 1989.
5. Harver A, Mahler DA, Schwartzstein RM, and others: Descriptors of breathlessness in healthy individuals: distinct and separable constructs, *Chest* 118:679-690, 2000.
6. Moy ML, Woodrow Weiss J, Sparrow D, and others: Quality of dyspnea in bronchoconstriction differs from external resistive loads, *Am J Respir Crit Care Med* 162(2 Pt 1):451-455, 2000.
7. O'Donnell DE, Chau LK, Webb KA: Qualitative aspects of exertional dyspnea in patients with interstitial lung disease, *J Appl Physiol* 84(6):2000-2009, 1998.
8. Mahler DA, Harver A, Lentine T, and others: Descriptors of breathlessness in cardiorespiratory diseases, *Am Respir Crit Care Med* 154:1357-1363, 1996.
9. Bailey PH: The dyspnea-anxiety-dyspnea cycle—COPD patients' stories of breathlessness: "It's scary when you can't breathe," *Qual Health Res* 14:760-778, 2004.
10. Periyakoil VS, Skultety K, Sheikh J: Panic, anxiety and chronic dyspnea, *J Palliat Med* 8:453-459, 2005.
11. Nocturnal Oxygen Therapy Trial Group: Continuous or nocturnal oxygen therapy in hypoxemic chronic obstructive lung disease: a clinical trial, *Ann Intern Med* 93:391-398, 1980.
12. Medical Research Council Working Party: Long-term domiciliary oxygen therapy in chronic hypoxic cor pulmonale complicating chronic bronchitis and emphysema, *Lancet* 1:681-686, 1981.
13. Fishman AP: Pulmonary rehabilitation research: NIH workshop summary, *Am Rev Respir Dis* 149:825-833, 1994.
14. Ries AL: Position paper of the American Association of Cardiovascular and Pulmonary Rehabilitation: scientific basis of pulmonary rehabilitation, *J Cardiopulm Rehabil* 10:418-441, 1990.
15. Pulmonary rehabilitation: joint ACCP/AACVPR evidence-based guidelines, *Chest* 112:1363-1396, 1997.
16. Oh E-G: The effects of home-based pulmonary rehabilitation in patients with chronic lung disease, *Int J Nurs Stud* 40:873-879, 2003.

CHAPTER 113

Hemoptysis

Patricia Polgar Bailey

DEFINITION AND EPIDEMIOLOGY

Hemoptysis refers to the expectoration of blood or blood-stained sputum from a site in the tracheobronchial tree, lung parenchyma, or pulmonary circulation as a result of bronchial or pulmonary hemorrhage. It can range from a small amount of blood-streaked sputum, which is commonly seen in bronchitis, to a massive hemorrhage, which is a medical emergency, since it rapidly causes death by asphyxiation. The classifications—nonmassive and massive—are based on the volume of blood loss; however, there are no uniform definitions for these categories. Hemoptysis is generally classified as nonmassive if the blood loss is less than 100 to 200 ml/day, whereas massive hemoptysis refers to more than this amount in 24 hours.[1,2] Massive hemoptysis is uncommon, occurring in less than 5% of patients with hemoptysis, but requires immediate attention because the reported mortality rate is 38% or higher.[2] Even slight bleeding may signify a serious condition, such as bronchogenic carcinoma or tuberculosis. Therefore blood loss volume is more helpful in directing management than in making a diagnosis.

The most common causes of hemoptysis in the United States are, in descending order, bronchitis, lung cancer, pneumonia, and tuberculosis. Similarly, these are the most common causes of hemoptysis seen in the primary care setting. However, tuberculosis is a leading cause of hemoptysis in developing countries and should be high on the list of differential diagnoses for patients who are from countries with a high prevalence of this disease or who have traveled to countries where tuberculosis is endemic.[2]

PATHOPHYSIOLOGY

For hemoptysis to occur, there must be some communication between the airways and the blood vessels of the lungs. The lungs receive blood from two relatively independent circulations: pulmonary and bronchial. The pulmonary circulation is characterized by lower pressures and higher volumes and is supplied with mixed venous blood via the pulmonary arteries. In contrast, the bronchial circulation supplies oxygenated blood in a high-pressure, low-volume circuit.

The bronchial arteries can become enlarged and more numerous in association with a variety of inflammatory or neoplastic diseases. Chronic inflammation, often associated with infectious processes, can lead to destruction of the connective tissue of blood vessels or result in erosion through the vessel wall. Angiographic studies have revealed that hemoptysis typically originates from disruptions of the branches of the bronchial arterial tree. This is presumably related to the connection of these arteries to the proliferative nests of small vessels often found in areas of inflammation and tumors.

CLINICAL PRESENTATION

It is common for patients to confuse hemoptysis with hematemesis or epistaxis. Patient history, including factors such as age, nutritional status, occupational and environmental exposures, and co-morbid conditions, can be useful in differentiating among the three conditions and can help narrow the differential diagnosis. Taking a thorough travel history is important, since tuberculosis and bronchiectasis appear to be decreasing as causes of hemoptysis in the United States, whereas they are still frequent causes of hemoptysis in other parts of the world.[3] Recent travel may have also increased the risk of parasitic infections, which can cause hemoptysis.

In addition, a description of the blood and accompanying symptoms can be helpful in differentiating between hemoptysis and hematemesis. Blood from the airways is usually bright red or pink, liquid or clotted in appearance, and frothy because of the presence of surfactant. The pH is alkaline, and it tends to be mixed with macrophages and neutrophils. Blood originating in the gastrointestinal tract is usually dark red, brown, or black; has a coffee ground appearance; and is rarely frothy. It is acidic and may be intermixed with food particles. Absence of nausea and vomiting and a history of lung disease raise the suspicion of hemoptysis, whereas the presence of nausea and vomiting and co-existing gastric or hepatic disease suggest hematemesis.[1]

It is important to carefully determine the chronology and volume of hemoptysis. Quantifying blood loss may be difficult, even in patients who are clinically stable, because they are often anxious and, as a result, usually overestimate the amount of blood loss. However, every effort should be made to determine the rate and volume of blood loss, which can include observing as the patient coughs and using a graduated container. Urgent evaluation and possible hospitalization are indicated if more than 50 ml of blood has been expectorated in the previous 24 hours. For smaller amounts of blood loss, a thorough diagnostic evaluation can be initiated in the primary care setting.

Mild hemoptysis, recurring sporadically over a few years, is common in smokers, who may have chronic bronchitis with intermittent flares of acute bronchitis. However, abrupt hemoptysis associated with cigarette smoking can also be seen with bronchogenic carcinoma. A long history of small-volume, recurrent hemoptysis with little or no sputum production is suspicious for processes such as bronchogenic carcinoma, bronchial adenoma, or vascular malformation. A history of chronic sputum production suggests an infectious cause such as bronchitis, bronchiectasis, lung abscess, or tuberculosis. Hemoptysis associated with bacterial pneumonia is suggested by an acute onset of fever, sputum production, and, commonly, pleuritic chest pain. Hemoptysis is commonly a late symptom of bronchogenic carcinoma and is preceded by a chronic cough, fatigue, and constitutional symptoms. Environmental exposure to asbestos, arsenic, chromium, nickel, and certain ethers can increase the risk of hemoptysis.[1]

PHYSICAL EXAMINATION

The presence of a fever is indicative of infection. A thorough examination of the ears, nose, and throat can detect upper airway sources of bleeding, such as laryngeal carcinoma lesions. Cervical, supraclavicular, or axillary adenopathy raises the suspicion of an intrathoracic malignancy. The presence of stridor or findings suggestive of chronic obstructive pulmonary disease, congestive heart failure, or pneumonia can be determined by auscultation of the chest.

Localized wheezing may indicate a local obstruction, foreign body, or bronchogenic carcinoma. A pleural friction rub may be the only sign of pulmonary infarction associated with a pulmonary embolism. Isolated crackles are nonspecific for the location of the primary disease because they may represent an inflammatory reaction to blood aspirated from another site.

Digital clubbing is suggestive of chronic lung disease, such as bronchiectasis or malignancy. Cardiac examination may help determine the presence of mitral stenosis. Localized adenopathy, especially a supraclavicular node, may be indicative of a lung malignancy. A bleeding disorder is suggested by the presence of petechiae or ecchymoses.

DIAGNOSTICS

A CBC and coagulation studies should be obtained, as well as a urinalysis if pulmonary-renal syndromes are suspected. A posteroanterior and lateral chest x-ray should be part of the routine workup. Comparing the chest radiograph with an earlier one is valuable in determining whether the lung process is acute or chronic. In addition, the chest x-ray study may be helpful in suggesting a source for the hemoptysis, such as pulmonary inflammatory disease or cancer. Important diagnostic findings include an air-fluid level of a lung abscess, the "crescent sign" of a mycetoma, a nodule that suggests a neoplasm, evidence of volume loss, or consolidation distal to an airway obstruction. Since a nondiagnostic chest x-ray film does not rule out serious disease, the decision to proceed with CT of the chest must be individualized according to the clinical situation.

High-resolution CT has become increasingly useful in the initial evaluation of hemoptysis, especially in the detection of bronchiectasis, parenchymal masses, and cavitary disease such as mycetoma. Chest CT and fiberoptic bronchoscopy have complementary roles in the evaluation of patients with hemoptysis, and the combination of these two tests has been shown to give a higher yield of specific diagnoses that either test alone. Fiberoptic bronchoscopy allows for direct visualization of the airways and localization of the bleeding source. Biopsy and lavage samples from the airways and alveolar spaces can be sent for cytologic and microbial studies. This procedure is relatively safe, is well tolerated, and can be performed on an outpatient basis. The proper timing for fiberoptic bronchoscopy is somewhat controversial. Most thoracic specialists prefer to perform bronchoscopy early in the course of hemoptysis. However, some believe bronchoscopy is indicated primarily if hemoptysis has been present for longer than 1 week or if the likelihood of cancer is greater because of systemic symptoms or risk factors such as male sex, age greater than 40 years, and a smoking history of more than 40 pack-years.[1,3]

Further evaluation of hemoptysis should be guided by clinical and radiographic findings. Lesions suggestive of cancer should be evaluated by sputum cytology, transthoracic needle aspiration, bronchoscopy, or open punch biopsy. Atypical cavitary disease with surrounding infiltrates suggests tuberculosis and should be evaluated by sputum acid-fast bacillus smears and cultures. If a pulmonary embolus is suspected, especially if there are risk factors for deep vein thrombosis and pulmonary thromboembolism, a ventilation/perfusion lung scan should be obtained.

DIAGNOSTICS

Hemoptysis

LABORATORY

CBC and differential*
Coagulation studies*
Sputum for acid-fast bacilli, Gram stain, culture and sensitivity
Sputum for cytology*
Urinalysis*

IMAGING

Chest x-ray
CT scan*
Ventilation/perfusion scan*

OTHER

Fiberoptic bronchoscopy*
Transthoracic needle aspiration*
Bronchoscopy or open punch biopsy*

*If indicated

DIFFERENTIAL DIAGNOSIS

Minor hemoptysis is generally not life threatening. Despite a thorough evaluation, many patients who are seen with hemoptysis do not receive a specific diagnosis, at least not

DIFFERENTIAL DIAGNOSIS

Hemoptysis

PULMONARY

- Bronchial adenoma
- Bronchiectasis*
- Bronchitis*
- Bronchogenic carcinoma
- Bronchopulmonary sequestration
- Cystic fibrosis
- Foreign body
- Fungal infections
- Lung abscess*
- Lung cancer*
- Metastatic tumor
- Mycetoma (aspergilloma or fungus ball)
- Noninvasive aspergillosis or mucormycosis
- Nontubercular mycobacteria
- Parasitic infection
- Pneumonia*
- Pulmonary contusion or trauma
- Pulmonary embolism*
- Pulmonary-renal syndromes (Goodpasture's syndrome, systemic lupus erythematosus, Wegener's granulomatosis)
- Tuberculosis*

CARDIOVASCULAR

- Arteriovenous malformation
- Bleeding diathesis
- Congestive heart failure*
- Mitral valve prolapse and mitral stenosis

MISCELLANEOUS

- Medications (anticoagulants, fibrinolytics, amiodarone)
- Pulmonary artery rupture caused by pulmonary arterial (Swan-Ganz) catheterization

*Common causes.

initially. The goal of further evaluation is to determine the cause, provide specific treatment (if available), and rule out underlying disease. The differential diagnosis is extensive and includes airway diseases, neoplasms, pulmonary vascular diseases, cardiovascular disease, and miscellaneous causes such as the use of anticoagulants or fibrinolytics. The most common cause of acute mild hemoptysis is bronchitis or infections such as pneumonia. Other common causes include lung cancer and lung abscesses, tuberculosis, bronchiectasis, and pulmonary thromboembolism. A history of recurrent pneumonia or hemoptysis with onset during adolescence suggests possible intralobular pulmonary sequestration, although the presentation may be mistaken for bronchiectasis or lung abscess.[4] Pulmonary embolism is an important diagnosis to consider when the presentation includes hemoptysis and pleuritic chest pain.[5]

MANAGEMENT

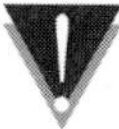

Immediate emergency department referral is indicated when the rate of bleeding qualifies as massive hemoptysis (a rate greater than 200 ml/day).

The overall goals of management include bleeding cessation, aspiration prevention, and treatment of the underlying cause. The most common presentation in primary care is acute mild hemoptysis caused by bronchitis. Antibiotics are indicated if the cause of hemoptysis is believed to be a bacterial infection, and cough suppressants, such as codeine and hydrocodone, can be helpful. Low-risk patients with normal chest x-ray films can be treated on an outpatient basis as indicated. If risk factors for lung cancer are present or hemoptysis is recurrent, outpatient fiberoptic bronchoscopy is recommended. A CT scan is indicated when there is a suspicion of malignancy and sputum cultures and bronchoscopy are not definitive or when peripheral or parenchymal disease is present on chest radiograph. If hemoptysis persists or the cause remains unclear, referral to a pulmonologist should be considered.

Patients with massive hemoptysis require rapid and decisive care. The immediate goal is to prevent asphyxiation, and therefore airway control should be ensured as rapidly as possible. Diagnosis and treatment must occur simultaneously. Airway maintenance is of utmost importance because asphyxiation, not exsanguination, is the primary cause of death. Supplemental oxygenation, localization, treatment of the bleeding site, and fluid therapy are essential.

The availability of typed and cross-matched blood is a necessity. Other temporizing measures include an endobronchial iced saline lavage and the application of fibrinogen-thrombin through the bronchoscope. If the patient does not respond to these measures or if the condition worsens, two major modes of therapy are available: surgical resection of the bleeding site and angiographic embolization. For patients who have localized lesions or intralobular sequestration, and who have adequate pulmonary function, surgical resection is generally the most effective therapy.[5]

COMPLICATIONS

Patients with hemoptysis resulting from noninfectious causes are at risk for frequent recurrences. Massive hemoptysis often recurs, both suddenly and without warning, and may be fatal. The most obvious complication is asphyxiation, which accounts for the majority of deaths from hemoptysis.

INDICATIONS FOR REFERRAL OR HOSPITALIZATION

Patients with hemoptysis are often referred to a pulmonary specialist for diagnostic evaluation unless their symptoms suggest infection and the hemoptysis responds to antibiotics. Specific indications for referral include consideration of CT scan or bronchoscopy, persistent or recurrent undiagnosed or recurrent hemoptysis, and massive or life-threatening hemoptysis. Hospitalization is rarely necessary unless hemoptysis is greater than 50 to 100 ml/24 hours or there is significant respiratory compromise.

PATIENT AND FAMILY EDUCATION

Hemoptysis is frightening for patients and may be a symptom of serious underlying disease. Education should include information about the diagnostic evaluation, that management is tailored to the underlying cause, and the importance of adhering to the prescribed treatment. The rate of recurrence in patients who smoke is likely to be high because common causes such as bronchitis and bronchogenic carcinoma are often related to smoking. Therefore it is imperative that patients be encouraged to quit smoking. Because hemoptysis can be particularly disconcerting, emotional support for the patient and family is especially important.

REFERENCES

1. Bidwell J, Pachner R: Hemoptysis: diagnosis and management, *Am Fam Phys* 72(7):1253-1260, 2005.
2. Johnson J: Manifestations of hemoptysis, *Postgrad Med* 112(4):101-113, 2002.
3. National Lung Health Education Program: Hemoptysis. In *Frontline assessment of common pulmonary presentations*, Denver, 2000, Snowdrift Pulmonary Foundation.
4. Behnia W, Catalano P, Brooks W: Hemoptysis in a 38-year-old-woman receiving an oral contraceptive, *Chest* 125:1944-1947, 2004.
5. Warburton M, Jackson M, Norton R, and others: Rare causes of haemoptysis in suspected pulmonary embolism, *BMJ* 329:557-558, 2004.

CHAPTER 114

Lung Cancer

Wendye DiSalvo

DEFINITION AND EPIDEMIOLOGY

Throughout the world, lung cancer continues to be the leading cause of cancer-related deaths. An average of 440 people die from lung cancer every day. There were approximately 160,000 deaths due to lung cancer in the United States in 2006—more than deaths due to breast, prostate, colon, kidney, melanoma, and liver cancers combined. Although cancer deaths overall have decreased recently, this is not true for lung cancer, which accounts for 30% of all cancer deaths. In fact, from 2006 to 2007, a 22% increase in lung cancer cases is expected.[1] The overall survival rate for all stages of lung cancer is 15% at 5 years. It is the most common cause of cancer-related death for both men and women. The number of newly diagnosed cases of lung cancer a year nearly equals the yearly mortality from the disease. More individuals die of lung cancer than breast, colorectal, and prostate cancer combined. In the United States there is an increased incidence of cancer in the African-American population in general and lung cancer specifically. Risk factors for lung cancer include tobacco use, environmental and occupational exposures, low socioeconomic status, decreased education, certain racial minorities, genetic predisposition, prior lung disease, dietary factors, and decreased physical activity.[2] The need to promote prevention, early detection, and treatment is urgent. Unfortunately, the population in need often has difficulty accessing health care.

Lung cancer research has focused on development of new and more effective treatment strategies, early identification of malignant transformation, genetic markers, early chemoprevention, and tobacco cessation strategies. Early identification of high-risk individuals, appropriate interventional studies, and implementation of prevention strategies are essential to reduce the number of new cases. No current recommended screening tests exist. Multiple trials during the past 50 years have been conducted using chest radiography (CXR), sputum cytology, and low–radiation dose spiral computed tomography (LDCT), either alone or in combination. To date there is no evidence that screening improves outcome in lung cancer. Results from previous studies showed that although CXR can detect early lung cancer, it also produces false-positive test results, causing needless extra tests.[3] This low positive predictive value makes CXR an unacceptable screening tool for lung cancer. The National Cancer Institute (NCI) is currently conducting a trial of 50,000 persons with a positive smoking history randomized to either a CXR or an LDCT study arm to help determine whether there are more efficacious ways to screen for lung cancer. Preliminary studies do suggest that LDCT is superior to CXR for screening lung cancers in high-risk individuals, although the cost-effectiveness of this screening technique is yet to be determined.[4,5]

PATHOPHYSIOLOGY

In the United States 80% to 90% of lung cancers are directly related to tobacco smoking. Risk factors related to the development of lung cancer in smokers include the degree of exposure from daily use of tobacco, pack-year history, extent of inhalation, use of filtered vs. unfiltered cigarettes, and age smoking commenced.[2] Exposure to environmental tobacco smoke is also associated with the development of lung cancer. The Cancer Protection Study II found an increased mortality of 20% in wives of smokers compared with women whose husbands did not smoke. Second-hand exposure to two or more packs of cigarettes a day demonstrated an increased risk; thus a dose-dependent relationship may be supported.[2,6]

The general pathologic features of lung cancer include genetic mutations, chromosomal translocations, gene amplification, microsatellite instability, and abnormal DNA methylation. Several chromosomal deletions are involved in the pathogenesis of lung cancer. The most common is the early loss of 9p and 3p, which can be found in the bronchial epithelium of former and current smokers. There is also activation of the *ras*, *Myc*, *Bcl-2*, *ErbB1*, and *ErbB2* oncogenes and loss of *p53*, *RB*, and *p16* tumor suppressor genes.[2,7]

The World Health Organization classification of lung cancer is accepted worldwide (Box 114-1). Approximately 80% of lung cancers are the non–small cell lung cancer (NSCLC) type. This major histologic type is divided into three major subtypes: adenocarcinoma (40%), squamous cell carcinoma/epidermoid (approximately 30%), and large cell carcinoma (15%). These histologic types are classified together, since there is a potential for cure through surgical resection when the tumor is localized. In the past, squamous cell carcinoma was the most common type of lung cancer; adenocarcinoma is now more common, especially in females.[8]

Classified as a subtype of adenocarcinoma, bronchoalveolar carcinoma represents 3% of lung carcinomas. Bronchoalveolar carcinoma is often seen in women and nonsmokers. The

BOX 114-1

WORLD HEALTH ORGANIZATION HISTOLOGIC CLASSIFICATION OF EPITHELIAL LUNG CANCER

I. Benign
II. Dysplasia and carcinoma in situ
III. Malignant
    A. Squamous cell
        1. Papillary cell
        2. Clear cell
        3. Small cell
    B. Small cell variants: combined small cell carcinoma
    C. Adenocarcinoma
        1. Acinar
        2. Papillary
        3. Bronchoalveolar
        4. Mucus secreting
    D. Large cell carcinoma
        1. Giant cell
        2. Clear cell

From Pass HI, Mitchell JB, Johnson DH, and others, editors: *Lung cancer: principles and practice*, ed 2, Philadelphia, 2000, Lippincott.

disease presentation is one of more diffuse lesions. Although the approach to treatment is the same as for other NSCLCs, a durable response may be seen with targeted therapies.[9] The second major type is small cell lung cancer (SCLC), which represents 20% of lung cancer cases. The histologic subtypes include small cell carcinoma (oat cell), mixed small cell–large cell, and combined small cell with squamous or glandular components. SCLC is classified as either limited (confined to one hemithorax that can be encompassed within a single radiographic port) or extensive stage (widely disseminated). Curative treatment in limited-stage disease is composed of the combined modality of chemotherapy and radiation. The only treatment for extensive-stage disease is palliative chemotherapy.[9]

CLINICAL PRESENTATION

Approximately 5% to 15% of all lung cancers manifest asymptomatically; thus a careful history to determine tobacco use or second-hand smoke exposure, previous asbestos exposure, or carcinogenic exposure is an essential component of the yearly physical examination.[10] Signs and symptoms depend on the location of the primary tumor, regional spread, and metastasis (Box 114-2). Symptoms may be classified according to the effect on the major airway, impingement of the tumor on extrapulmonary mediastinal structures, presence of paraneoplastic syndromes (most often seen in SCLC), effect of distant metastases, and presence or absence of systemic symptoms (e.g., weight loss).

The most common symptom of lung cancer is cough; it occurs in up to 75% of patients. Cough is widespread in cigarette smokers. The change in cough may be an insidious change from baseline. A persistent cough or change in cough warrants a CXR study and possibly further follow-up evaluation. Other clinical manifestations of lung cancer include dyspnea, hemoptysis, chest pain, wheezing, stridor, frequent upper respiratory tract infections, hoarseness, dysphagia, phrenic nerve paralysis, superior vena cava syndrome, pleural effusion, pericardial effusion, anorexia, weight loss, and upper extremity pain or edema.[2]

BOX 114-2

SIGNS AND SYMPTOMS OF LUNG CANCER DEPENDING ON TUMOR LOCATION

I. Location of tumor
   Central/endobronchial growth: Cough, dyspnea, hemoptysis, wheeze, bronchorrhea, stridor, pneumonia, atelectasis, chest pain
   Peripheral growth: pain from chest wall or pleural involvement, cough, dyspnea, signs and symptoms of lung abscess from a cavitating lesion
   Regional tumor impingement on extrapulmonary mediastinal structures: Tracheal obstruction, laryngeal nerve paralysis (hoarseness), dysphasia from esophageal compression, pleural effusion, pericardial effusion, superior vena cava obstruction, Horner's syndrome, Pancoast's syndrome, bone pain
II. *Extrathoracic metastatic disease:* Central nervous system (headache, seizures, spinal cord compression), bone (pain, fracture), liver metastases (jaundice, hepatomegaly), bone marrow (cytopenias), adrenal glands (adrenal insufficiency)
III. *Paraneoplastic syndromes:* Syndrome of inappropriate antidiuretic hormone, hypercalcemia, hypophosphatemia, hypertrophic pulmonary osteoarthropathy
IV. Systemic symptoms—anorexia, weight loss, fatigue, weakness, cachexia, anemia

Data from Houlihan N: *Lung cancer,* ed 1, Pittsburgh, 2004, Oncology Nursing Society.

PHYSICAL EXAMINATION

A comprehensive history and physical examination of a patient with risk factors or presenting symptoms suspicious for lung cancer should be conducted. History includes the reason for the office visit, past history (respiratory illness), smoking history and exposure to potential carcinogens (active and passive), and review of systems (including constitutional symptoms such as fatigue and weight loss). The physical examination should include but not be limited to inspection of head and neck (for cyanosis, swelling of the face, miosis, anhidrosis, and ptosis), chest (respiratory rate, use of accessory muscles, vascular markings), and extremities (swelling, clubbing). Palpation and percussion are used to determine if there are enlarged lymph nodes, dullness, discrepancy in lung expansion, and pain. Auscultation determines wheezing, egophony, decreased breath sounds, and muffled heart sounds.[2]

DIAGNOSTICS

In order for the health care provider to design appropriate treatment, diagnostic tests are performed to stage the patient's disease. General staging procedures and diagnostic staging include a complete and thorough physical examination and laboratory studies that include a CBC with differential; lactate dehydrogenase; a comprehensive metabolic profile that includes renal function, electrolytes, hepatic profile, and phosphorus; a CXR film that may show a definable mass; a CT scan of the chest; a positron emission tomography (PET) scan with or without CT to determine mediastinal or distant involvement; an abdominal CT scan to evaluate the liver and adrenal glands if not part of the chest CT (the adrenal glands are common sites of metastasis and are often asymptomatic); sputum cytology; bronchoscopy; mediastinoscopy; a bone scan if symptoms are present and a PET scan is not performed; ECG; and MRI of the brain if distant metastasis is suspected.[2]

DIAGNOSTICS

Lung Cancer

LABORATORY
CBC and differential
Electrolytes
Glucose
BUN
Creatinine
LFTs
Lactate dehydrogenase
Sputum cytology

IMAGING
Chest x-ray
CT scan of chest and abdomen
Bone scan if indicated
Positron emission tomography scan with or without CT

OTHER
Bronchoscopy
Mediastinoscopy
ECG
PFTs

Tissue diagnosis is essential for staging the patient's disease. Pretreatment prognostic factors include the size of the tumor, tumor histology, presence or absence of metastasis, performance status of the patient, presence or absence of weight loss, and presence of specific molecular markers.[10]

Staging of NSCLC refers to defining the size of the tumor (T), absence or presence of regional lymph node involvement (N), and absence or presence of metastases (M) (Table 114-1). The primary tumor is divided into four categories, T1 to T4 (depending on size, site, and local involvement). Lymph node spread is subdivided into three categories: N1 nodes (ipsilateral peribronchial and/or ipsilateral hilar lymph nodes, intrapulmonary nodes involved by direct extension of the primary tumor), N2 nodes (ipsilateral mediastinal nodes), and N3 nodes (contralateral or supraclavicular lymph node disease). Metastatic spread is present or absent.[8] Patients are

TABLE 114-1 International TNM Staging System for Lung Cancer

Stage	TNM Descriptions	5-Year Survival (%)
Occult carcinoma	TX, N0, M0	
0	Tis, N0, M0	
IA	T1 N0 M0	61
IB	T2 N0 M0	38
IIA	T1 N1 M0	34
IIB	T2-3 N0-1 M0	24
IIIA	T3 N0-1 M0	9
	T1-3 N2 M0	13
IIIB	T4 N0-2 M0	7
	Any T N3 M0	3
IV	Any T Any N M1	1
PRIMARY TUMOR (T)		
TX	Primary tumor cannot be assessed, or tumor proven by the presence of malignant cells in sputum or bronchial washings but not visualized by imaging or bronchoscopy	
T0	No evidence of primary tumor	
Tis	Carcinoma in situ	
T1	Tumor 3 cm or less in greatest dimension, surrounded by lung tissue or visceral pleura, without bronchoscopic evidence of invasion more proximal than the lobar bronchus* (i.e., not in the main bronchus)	
T2	Tumor with any of the following features of size or extent: >3 cm in greatest dimension Involves main bronchus, 2 cm or more distal to the carina Invades the visceral pleura Associated with atelectasis or obstructive pneumonitis that extends to the hilar region but does not involve the entire lung	
T3	Tumor of any size that directly invades any of the following: chest wall (including superior sulcus tumors), diaphragm, mediastinal pleura, parietal pericardium; or tumor in the main bronchus <2 cm distal to the carina, but without involvement of the carina; or associated atelectasis or obstructive pneumonitis of the entire lung	
T4	Tumor of any size that invades any of the following: mediastinum, heart, great vessels, trachea, esophagus, vertebral body, or carina; or separate tumor nodules in the same lobe; or tumor with malignant pleural effusion†	
REGIONAL LYMPH NODES (N)		
NX	Regional lymph nodes cannot be assessed	
N0	No regional lymph node metastasis	
N1	Metastasis to ipsilateral peribronchial and/or ipsilateral hilar lymph nodes, and intrapulmonary nodes, including involvement by direct extension of the tumor	
N2	Metastasis to ipsilateral mediastinal and/or subcarinal lymph node(s)	
N3	Metastasis to contralateral mediastinal, contralateral hilar, ipsilateral or contralateral scalene, or supraclavicular lymph nodes	
DISTANT METASTASES (M)		
MX	Distant metastasis cannot be assessed	
M0	No distant metastasis	
M1	Distant metastasis present	

Data from Kasper DL, Braunwald E, Fauci A, and others: *Harrison's principles of internal medicine,* ed 16, New York, 2005, McGraw-Hill; American Joint Committee on Cancer: *AJCC cancer staging manual,* ed 6, Chicago, 2002, The Committee.

*The uncommon superficial tumor of any size with its invasive component limited to the bronchial wall, which may extend proximal to the main bronchus, is also classified T1.

†Most pleural effusions associated with lung cancer are due to tumor. However, in a few patients multiple cytopathologic examinations of pleural fluid are negative for tumor. In these cases, fluid is nonbloody and is not an exudate. Such patients may be further evaluated by videothorascopy and direct pleural biopsies. When these elements and clinical judgment dictate that the effusion is not related to the tumor, the effusion should be excluded as a staging element and the patient should be staged T1, T2, or T3.

then classified as having stage IA or B, IIA or B, IIIA or B, or IV cancer.

DIFFERENTIAL DIAGNOSIS

Consider both pulmonary and extrapulmonary causes for presenting symptoms. Cough, dyspnea, hemoptysis, and wheezing are associated with a number of pulmonary conditions. When weight loss, cachexia, and anorexia are also present, serious illness is easily suspected. Moderate symptoms should not be overlooked, since early identification of lung cancer may enable long-term survival.[10]

DIFFERENTIAL DIAGNOSIS

Lung Cancer

- Cardiac (congestive heart failure, cardiomyopathy)
- Infection
- Interstitial pulmonary fibrosis
- Metastatic cancer—non–lung cancer primary
- Granulomatous diseases (sarcoidosis)
- Malignant lung tumor
- Mesothelioma
- Tuberculosis

MANAGEMENT

Treatment is either single or combined modality therapy that includes surgery, radiotherapy, chemotherapy, targeted therapies, or best supportive care. The intent of treatment is curative or palliative. A number of factors, including type of tumor, stage of the disease, patient age, functional status, and pulmonary status, guide appropriate interventions for each patient.[2]

Surgery in Non–Small Cell Lung Cancer

In the United States fewer than 25% of lung cancer patients will be diagnosed when their disease is at stage I or II. Regrettably, this early stage has the most potential for cure through surgical resection.[7] Overall survival at 5 years for stage I is 60% to 75%[11,12] and for stage II is 36% to 60%.[12] Surgical resection can be lobectomy (removal of lung lobe) or pneumonectomy (removal of the lung). Surgical techniques are aimed at sparing normal lung parenchyma and in stage I or II disease are the primary treatment modalities.[13] Several trials have been conducted to determine whether adjuvant chemotherapy after resection affects overall survival. The National Cancer Institute of Canada Clinical Trial Groups and the National Cancer Institute of the United States Intergroup JBR.[13] Trial Investigators conducted a study to determine whether adjuvant chemotherapy in resected early-stage lung cancer was of significant benefit. Patients (N = 482) were randomized to a regimen of vinorelbine plus cisplatin or to an observation arm. Evidence exists for benefit with an overall survival benefit of 15% at 5 years in the chemotherapy group.[11]

Stage III is divided into A and B. Stage IIIB disease is generally considered unresectable and is treated with a combination of chemotherapy and radiotherapy. Overall survival at 5 years is less than 5%. There is controversy over treatment of stage IIIA disease. The presence of N2 nodal disease has a poorer prognosis than stage IIIA disease with only a T3 tumor. New approaches to treatment of stages IIIA include neoadjuvant chemotherapy and/or radiotherapy followed by surgical excision. The treatment of stage IIIA patients is the subject of multiple clinical trials. Overall survival at 5 years is approximately 19%.[10]

Stage IV disease is not appropriate for surgical intervention, since it is disseminated at the time of diagnosis. Chemotherapy or palliative therapy is the primary management modality for stage IV disease. Overall survival at 5 years is less than 2%.[10] Surgery is not indicated in the treatment of SCLC except in a rare subset of patients with T1 N0 disease.[11]

Radiotherapy

Radiotherapy has undergone significant changes in recent years with respect to evolution of appropriate patient selection, technical innovation, and the use of multimodality therapy. The new developments include hyperfractionation (daily radiation dose divided into two treatments), continuous hyperfractionation (radiation administered in three fractions per day over 12 days), proton beam therapy, three-dimensional conformational radiotherapy, brachytherapy, and intensity-modulated radiotherapy.[2] The objective of employing new techniques is to improve patient outcome, spare healthy lung tissue, and decrease treatment-related side effects.

Radiotherapy is employed as treatment in inoperable stage I and II NSCLC or as palliation of symptoms for stage IV disease. In limited-stage SCLC, combined modality treatment with chemotherapy and radiotherapy is the standard of care.[10]

Chemotherapy

The use of chemotherapy in locally advanced (stage IIIB, IV) NSCLC and SCLC is standard. In NSCLC, four regimens (docetaxel, gemcitabine, paclitaxel, or vinorelbine) in combination with cisplatin are U.S. Food and Drug Administration–approved for first-line therapy. The goal of treatment is to prolong survival, palliate symptoms, and improve quality of life.[7] In limited-stage SCLC, a doublet of cisplatin and etoposide is used in combination with early concurrent radiotherapy. Overall survival is up to 13% at 5 years. There is a role for prophylactic cranial radiation with a 5% overall survival benefit at 5 years. In extensive-stage SCLC platinum-based therapy is at the core of treatment and may be combined with several agents, often etoposide. The duration of response is limited, and patients often succumb to their disease within 2 years.[14]

Side effects from chemotherapy are varied and specific to the agents used. Major hematologic side effects include neutropenia, anemia, and thrombocytopenia. However, the addition of colony-stimulating factors has had a positive effect on decreasing morbidity and mortality. To safely administer chemotherapy, evaluation of performance status, co-morbid conditions, and current medications is paramount at each office visit. Box 114-3 provides an outline for treatment according to stage.[10]

Targeted Therapies

Molecular targeted therapy research in relation to treatment of NSCLC is offering new hope. The mechanism of action varies, but essentially targeted therapies inhibit various functions that block signal transduction. The small molecules target a variety of receptors that control growth and other functions, especially when the receptors are overexpressed. This overexpression aids in the development and metastasis of cancer cells. The molecule approved for second-line therapy in the treatment of

BOX 114-3

SUMMARY OF TREATMENT APPROACH TO PATIENTS WITH LUNG CANCER

NON–SMALL CELL LUNG CANCER

Resectable (stages I, II, IIIA, and selected T3 N2 lesions)
- Surgery
- Radiotherapy for "nonoperable" patients
- Adjuvant radiotherapy and chemotherapy

Nonresectable (stages IIIB and IV)
- Combined modality therapy with radiation and chemotherapy or palliative chemotherapy
- Extrathoracic: radiotherapy to symptomatic local sites

SMALL CELL LUNG CANCER

Limited stage (good performance status)
- Combined modality of chemotherapy and radiotherapy
- Prophylactic cranial radiotherapy if complete response

Extensive stage (good performance status)
- Chemotherapy

Patients with poor performance status (all stages)
- Chemotherapy
- Palliative radiotherapy

ALL PATIENTS

Radiation for brain metastases, spinal cord compression, weight-bearing or painful lytic bony lesions (obstructive airway, hemoptysis in non–small cell lung cancer and in small cell cancer not responding to chemotherapy)

Diagnosis and treatment of other co-morbid issues and supportive care during treatment

Smoking cessation strategies

NSCLC is erlotinib (Tarceva). The medication is usually well tolerated, with the most common side effects being skin rash and diarrhea.[15]

Monoclonal antibodies are larger molecules that act outside the cell, interacting with receptors on the cell surface. The use of this therapy is being evaluated in ongoing clinical trials.

COMPLICATIONS

Complications are numerous and may be related to the treatment or to the disease process. Medications and particularly chemoradiotherapeutics may have significant side effects that may lead to death. Several oncologic emergencies are associated with the disease process. Prompt identification and treatment are paramount to decrease morbidity in the following events: superior vena cava syndrome, pericardial effusion, cardiac tamponade, spinal cord compression, thromboembolic events, neutropenic fever, and hypercalcemia.[2]

INDICATIONS FOR REFERRAL OR HOSPITALIZATION

Diagnostic evaluation and clinical staging are initiated by the health care provider. However, medical management of lung cancer is best provided by experienced oncologists. Lung cancer requires multidisciplinary collaboration among surgical, medical, and radiation oncologists. The role of the health care provider includes coordination of care among specialties, close supervision of other medical conditions, and supportive interventions. Hospitalization for surgical resection of the tumor is obvious. Hospitalization may also be appropriate if complications from radiation, chemotherapy, or the cancer itself occur.

PATIENT AND FAMILY EDUCATION

When a diagnosis of cancer is made, a careful explanation of the disease, staging, treatment, and side effects is critical. Pain management, bowel protocols, and evaluation for complications require continuous reinforcement and support.

HEALTH PROMOTION

Lung cancer is directly related to smoking. If smoking were eliminated, there would be up to a 90% reduction in lung cancer cases. Health care providers play an essential role in promoting smoking cessation strategies for patients and family members. Smoking cessation should be encouraged at every patient encounter. Advocacy related to education, legislation, and research is vital.

REFERENCES

1. Lung Cancer Alliance: Statistics courtesy of the Lung Cancer Alliance, Chicago, The Society of Thoracic Surgeons, retrieved Jan 18, 2006 from http://www.sts.org/documents/pdf/lung.cancer.stats.pdf
2. Houlihan N: *Lung cancer,* ed 1, Pittsburgh, 2004, Oncology Nursing Society.
3. National Cancer Institute: *Chest x-rays can detect early lung cancer but also can produce many false-positive results,* retrieved Jan 18, 2006, from http://www.cancer.gov/newscenter/pressreleases/PLCOLung Baseline.
4. Gohagan J, Marcus P, Fagerstrom R, and others: Baseline findings of a randomized feasibility trial of lung cancer screening with spiral CT scan vs chest radiograph: the Lung Screening Study of the National Cancer Institute, *Chest* 126(1):114-121, 2004.
5. Gohagan JK, Marcus PM, Fagerstrom RM, and others: Final results of the Lung Screening Study, a randomized feasibility study of spiral CT versus chest X-ray screening for lung cancer, *Lung Cancer* 47(1):9-15, 2005.
6. Samet J: Second hand smoke (*passive smoking*), retrieved Jan 19, 2007, from http://www.uptodateonline.com/utd/content/topic.do?topicKey=pri_pulm/5545&selectedTitle=1~29.
7. Pass HI, Mitchell JB, Johnson DH, and others, editors: *Lung cancer: principles and practice,* ed 2, Philadelphia, 2000, Lippincott.
8. Tazelaar HD. *Pathology of lung malignancies,* retrieved Jan 19, 2007, from http://www.uptodateonline.com/utd/content/topic.do?topicKey=lung_ca/11641&selectedTitle=26~341.
9. Devita VT, Hellman S, Rosenberg SA, editors: *Cancer: principles and practice of oncology,* ed 7, New York, 2004, Lippincott.
10. Kasper DL, Braunwald E, Fauci A, and others: *Harrison's principles of internal medicine,* ed 16, New York, 2005, McGraw-Hill.
11. Winston T: Vinorelbine plus cisplatin vs. observation in resected non-small cell lung cancer, *N Engl J Med* 23(352):2589-2597, 2005.
12. Straus G, Janne PA, Swanson S, and others: *Management of stage I and stage II non small cell lung cancer,* retrieved Jan 19, 2007, from http://www.uptodateonline.com/utd/content/topic.do?topicKey=lung_ca/9791&selectedTitle=3~3735.
13. Straus G, Schild SE: *Management of stage III non small cell lung cancer,* retrieved Jan 19, 2007, from http://www.uptodateonline.com/utd/content/topic.do?topicKey=lung_ca/2399&selectedTitle=9~341.
14. Kelly K: *Chemotherapy for small cell lung cancer,* retrieved Nov 21, 2005, from http://www.medscape.com.
15. Rigas JR, Dragnev KH: Targeted therapy with erlotinib prolongs survival in non–small cell lung cancer, *Community Oncology* 2(3):207-209, 2005.

CHAPTER 115

Occupational Respiratory Disease

Patricia Polgar Bailey

DEFINITION AND EPIDEMIOLOGY

Occupational respiratory disease results from work-related exposure to inhaled dusts, powders, solvents, gases, or fumes that adversely affect the upper and lower respiratory tract. Occupational respiratory diseases have been recorded since ancient history. Egyptian pictographs and the writings of Hippocrates document the role of occupational exposure in lung disease. Because many exposures do not result in acute symptoms, workers may be unaware that they have been exposed to potentially hazardous materials. The challenge for health care providers, especially those unfamiliar with occupational medicine, is to maintain a high index of suspicion that a symptom or cluster of symptoms may have a connection with a patient's job or work history. It is important to remember that work-related exposures do occur in occupations other than the obvious.[1]

Although the true scope of occupational lung disease is difficult to quantify, it is recognized that a small percentage of chronic occupational respiratory diseases is correctly associated with work-related exposures. Asthma is the most common type of occupational pulmonary disease in the industrialized world; an estimated 2% to 15% of all adult asthma cases are work related. Occupational asthma may be related to specific antigens in the workplace (e.g., psyllium or latex) or to chemical irritants.[2] Interstitial pulmonary fibrosis, which results from workplace exposure to asbestos and silica, persists throughout the world despite knowledge regarding the potential hazards of these substances and effective means for prevention. The death rate for silicosis declined by approximately 70% from 1982 to 2000, but it has increased nearly 400% for asbestosis, which is the only major pneumoconiosis to demonstrate increased mortality.[3] Approximately 65,000 workers in the United States have asbestosis; it is estimated that occupational asbestos exposure will contribute to 19,000 cases of mesothelioma and 55,000 cases of lung cancer by 2009. In the United States, 85,000 cotton mill workers are permanently or partially disabled as a result of exposure to cotton dust.[4] As many as 30% of coal miners (both active and retired) have coal workers' pneumoconiosis.[5] The prevalence of latex hypersensitivity, including latex-induced asthma, is as high as 14% among some groups of health care workers.[6]

Severe acute respiratory syndrome (SARS) is a newly emerging infectious disease that is largely spread by respiratory droplets. It is a specific atypical pneumonia that is highly contagious and is associated with significant morbidity and mortality. On March 12, 2003, the World Health Organization (WHO) issued a worldwide alert for SARS, and by July 31, 2003, a total of 8096 infected cases and 744 deaths were reported in 32 countries.[7] SARS was responsible for several well-documented nosocomial outbreaks in Canada, China, Hong Kong, Vietnam, and Singapore beginning in 2003 and involved the infection of 341 Hong Kong health care workers, including six deaths. More than 22% of SARS cases in Hong Kong were among health care workers.[8] In the United States, only eight persons had laboratory confirmation as SARS, and there were no SARS-related deaths. All eight persons with SARS had traveled to areas where SARS-coronavirus (CoV) transmission was occurring.[9]

The short- and long-term health effects of war-related exposures on military service personnel are a growing concern. Exposures to toxins during the past two decades have been different than those from previous wars. The Centers for Disease Control and Prevention (CDC) and other organizations such as the Agency for Toxic Substances and Disease Registry (ATSDR) have been studying the postservice morbidity and mortality of veterans who have served in the Vietnam, Gulf, and Iraq wars, as well as in the conflict in Afghanistan. There is some evidence that Gulf War veterans with previous respiratory illnesses, such as asthma, experienced more respiratory symptoms than veterans without a history of illness. However, this may not be unique to Gulf War veterans and may be similar to the experience of veterans of other wars, despite the exposure to spilled oil and smoke plumes unique to Gulf War veterans. At this point it is unclear whether there is a connection between war-related exposures and specific health outcomes that remain long after the exposure.[10,11]

Despite these significant statistics, the number of affected individuals captured in any occupational surveillance system remains a gross underestimate because the majority of cases are undiagnosed or are not attributed to workplace exposure.[3] Preventing the transmission of infectious diseases and mitigating the risk of other occupational illnesses pose a significant challenge. Incorporating the latest information of infection control and other work-related exposure and implementing the most effective and proven methods for prevention should be a high priority in all workplaces.

PATHOPHYSIOLOGY

Inhaled noxious substances affect the respiratory tract in several ways. Direct irritation results in increased mucus production; cough and airway hyperreactivity, which may cause bronchospasm; chest tightness or pain; dyspnea; pneumonitis; or pulmonary edema. The full effect of certain irritants may not be realized until 12 to 24 hours after the exposure. Small particles (≤5 μm) may remain in the lung to induce a fibrotic or granulomatous response. A latency period of 15 to 20 years between exposure and onset of clinical disease often obscures the causal relationship, which makes the diagnosis of occupational lung disease more difficult. Hypersensitivity and abnormal functioning of the immune system may contribute to the development of certain occupational respiratory diseases, including asthma, hypersensitivity pneumonitis, asbestosis, and chronic beryllium disease. The presence of certain host factors, such as cigarette smoking and exposure in the home environment (e.g., proximity to sources of pollutants), plays a role in the development of work-related lung disease. For example, cigarette smoking and asbestos exposure have a synergistic effect on the risk for lung cancer that is greater than the risk of either of these two exposures alone.[5]

Occupational respiratory diseases include obstructive airway diseases (asthma, byssinosis), interstitial lung disease (coal workers' pneumoconiosis, asbestosis, silicosis, acute and chronic beryllium disease, hypersensitivity pneumonitis), industrial bronchitis, cancer, and noncardiogenic pulmonary edema. Asthma, one of the most common types of occupational respiratory disease, has been associated with at least 250 specific workplace exposures. In comparison to many other occupational illnesses, asthma produces more persistent, even permanent, effects.[12] Byssinosis is another obstructive airway disease; it is associated with exposure to cotton, hemp, and flax processing, and is characterized by shortness of breath and chest tightness. Prolonged exposure can cause irreversible byssinosis, which is associated with fixed airway obstruction. Cigarette smoking significantly increases the risk of irreversible byssinosis.[4]

Many occupational toxins, including coal dust, asbestos, silica, and beryllium, contribute to the development of interstitial lung disease. The occurrence and extent of disease often depend on the level and chronicity of the exposure. Depending on the specific disease, fibrosis of the lung parenchyma, pleural thickening, and the formation of pleural plaques contribute to respiratory failure and increase the risk for the subsequent development of lung cancer and mesothelioma. Occupational exposures are associated with different types of pleuropulmonary malignancies—including laryngeal, bronchogenic, and oat cell carcinomas—as well as with mesothelioma, a tumor of the pleura and peritoneum.

Bronchitis is a common manifestation of airway irritation and inflammation that is associated with many occupational exposures, including irritant gases, welding fumes, and coal dust. *Chronic bronchitis* is defined as the presence of cough and sputum on most days for 3 months or longer per year and for 2 or more consecutive years.

Certain groups of health care professionals are at increased risk for occupational respiratory problems as a result of their exposure to specific pathogens and toxins. Occupational asthma (as well as latex-related dermatitis and life-threatening anaphylaxis) resulting from latex allergy is becoming an increasing problem among health care workers. Establishing a diagnosis of latex-related asthma is essential to avoid permanent respiratory compromise. With the resurgence of tuberculosis (TB) in this decade, increasing numbers of health care workers have become infected with TB. The risk for infection is compounded by the convergence of immunocompromised individuals in various settings staffed by health care workers, including long-term care facilities, hospitals, homeless shelters, correctional facilities, and drug treatment centers. Since 1990, a number of TB outbreaks have occurred in these settings, resulting in approximately 300 cases of TB. These outbreaks were characterized by transmission of both isoniazid-resistant TB and, in many cases, multidrug-resistant TB.[13]

There is some evidence that some Asian animals carry viruses similar to the virus that causes SARS, and they may have been the origin of the SARS virus that affects human. Transmission of SARS is largely by droplet route and appears to occur primarily from those who are symptomatic with the disease. The virus can also spread through contact with a SARS-CoV–contaminated surface or object and subsequent contact with the mouth, nose, or eyes.[9] There is also indirect evidence that the generation of aerosols and the lack of control of aerosols at the source has also been an important factor in the spread of SARS within hospital settings.[14] At least two cases of SARS transmission have been documented in workers in laboratories where SARS research was being done.[15,16]

CLINICAL PRESENTATION

Obtaining a thorough history from patients, including environmental and occupational exposure, smoking habits, and a careful review of respiratory symptoms, is important. The review of symptoms should include questions about onset of symptoms (rhinitis, conjunctivitis, cough, sputum production, wheezing, dyspnea, chest tightness or pain) and a history of allergies, asthma, and respiratory infections.[2] In addition, it is important to elicit the temporal relationship of symptoms to time spent at work. For example, an improvement of symptoms during periods away from work or intensification during periods at work might suggest an occupational exposure.

To accurately diagnose and manage occupational disease, health care providers must familiarize themselves with their patients' social and occupational environments. However, much more is involved than simply knowing an individual's work history. Detailed information about the jobs performed (including an outline of a typical workday), work habits, materials used (dyes, solvents, dusts, powders, acids, alkalis, gases, metals), and the use of protective equipment must be elicited. All workers should be asked about any safety or health concerns they might have. For many providers, some investigation and research are necessary before an accurate assessment of exposures is possible.

Exposure to noxious substances can cause various types of reactions in both the upper and lower respiratory tract. Acute symptoms of upper respiratory tract irritation include nasal and paranasal sinus irritation, sinus congestion, frontal headaches, rhinorrhea, and, occasionally, epistaxis. A dry cough and hoarseness may indicate pharyngeal and laryngeal inflammation, respectively. Mid–respiratory tract irritation and inflammation often result in bronchospasm, of which asthma is an example. Acute irritation of the deep respiratory tract causes pulmonary edema and pneumonitis.

Chronic respiratory exposure can result in various permanent pulmonary reactions. Chronic bronchitis is one of the most common pulmonary responses to long-term occupational exposure and results from excessive mucus production in the bronchi. Toxic workplace substances that can cause chronic bronchitis include mineral dusts and fumes (e.g., from coal, fibrous glass, asbestos, metal, and oils), organic dusts (e.g., from cotton, grains, and wood), gases (e.g., ozone and nitrous oxide), plastic compounds (isocyanates), acids, and smoke.

Fibrosis or pneumoconiosis (localized and nodular) is usually due to small particles of inorganic dust and produces symptoms that initially include a nonproductive cough and shortness of breath; in the later stages there is a productive cough, distant breath sounds, and right-sided heart failure. Pleural plaques and diffuse pleural thickening are manifestations of asbestos exposures. Emphysema-related changes, which include destruction of alveolar walls and air trapping, result from chronic exposure to coal dust or cadmium. The formation of pulmonary granulomas is a less common response to inhaled work-related exposures but can occur from chronic exposure to metal dust.[4] In addition, catastrophic exposures, such as occurred during the World Trade Center collapse, have been implicated in the development of granulomatous pulmonary disease.[17]

Most persons with SARS develop a fever of 38° C (100.4° F) or higher and may also report symptoms such as headache, shortness of breath, and cough. Other symptoms include body aches, rhinorrhea, malaise, and general discomfort. Approximately 10% to 20% of patients have diarrhea. After 2 to 7 days a dry, nonproductive cough may develop that eventually progresses to hypoxia. In some individuals these symptoms may progress quickly to severe shortness of breath and respiratory failure, requiring mechanical ventilation and high-dose steroids.[8]

PHYSICAL EXAMINATION

Many workplace exposures do not cause acute respiratory symptoms, and therefore the physical examination may be entirely normal. This is the one reason why occupational exposure is often not considered in the differential diagnosis and why the magnitude of occupational respiratory disease is grossly underestimated. However, it is important to always consider occupational asthma when an adult suddenly develops asthma.[2] The physical examination is most helpful when the results are abnormal because a normal physical examination does not negate the possibility of work-related respiratory disease. In fact, once an occupational exposure results in obvious acute symptoms, the disease may have already progressed to the point that symptomatic relief, rather than a cure, is all that is possible.

A thorough physical examination with special attention to the respiratory system is necessary. Auscultation can provide helpful diagnostic clues. Fine basilar crackles and a pleural friction rub are more common in certain interstitial lung diseases such as asbestosis. Wheezes, especially in association with a temporal relationship to work exposures, may raise the suspicion of asthma. Digital clubbing in a worker with a history of asbestos exposure might raise the suspicion of asbestosis, especially if other manifestations of the disease have already become apparent.

A cardiac examination is important; ventricular failure may reflect underlying lung disease; left ventricular failure may manifest as dyspnea, and right ventricular failure may denote severe and advanced lung disease.[12] In addition to assessing the respiratory and cardiac systems, the health care provider must perform a complete physical examination to identify manifestations of chronic or acute occupational exposure and to provide clues to the cause of the specific respiratory syndrome being evaluated.

DIAGNOSTICS

Important diagnostic tests include a chest radiograph and pulmonary function tests (PFTs). A chest x-ray examination can help identify early evidence and progression of parenchymal and pleural disease, including opacities, calcifications, and pleural thickening. In addition to a standard reading, chest x-ray studies should be interpreted according to the International Labor Organization (ILO) nomenclature and classification system. The ILO system provides a standardized set of comparison radiographs that can be used to classify x-ray films at one point in time or to follow an individual or group for changes over time.[12] Although chest x-ray studies do reveal evidence of abnormalities, they do not provide information about the degree of disability or impairment, nor do they provide an accurate assessment of lung function. For example, the chest x-ray film of an individual with severe obstructive lung disease might appear relatively normal.

PFTs are used to assess lung function. They are of value in determining the type and extent of lung disease, following the progression of disease for changes in severity or response to therapy, and fulfilling legal and compensatory purposes. The basic tests of ventilatory function can be performed with a spirometer, which can provide an accurate assessment of the relationship between chronic respiratory symptoms and diminished ventilatory capacity.[18] Although spirometry provides many measures, the most useful for evaluating work-related respiratory disease include forced vital capacity (FVC), forced expiratory volume in 1 second (FEV_1), and the ratio of these two measurements (FEV_1/FVC). FVC refers to the maximum volume of air that is exhaled after a maximum inspiration. FEV_1 is an estimate of the flow rate and is obtained by measuring the volume exhaled during the first second. Results are compared with expected values—which are derived from a healthy population of nonsmoking adults—and are expressed as a percentage of the expected value.[12]

Obstructive diseases such as asthma involve an obstruction in airflow without a reduction in lung volume. Therefore measurements of FVC remain within 80% to 120% of the population standard and are considered normal. However, measurements of both FEV_1 and FEV_1/FVC are decreased in asthma and other obstructive diseases. In contrast, restrictive disease, including silicosis, asbestosis, and coal worker's pneumoconiosis, is characterized by reductions in both FEV_1 and FVC, resulting in a normal or greater ratio of FEV_1/FVC. Mixed pulmonary conditions may also be present; this occurs when cigarette smoking or multiple environmental exposures co-exist with a given occupational exposure and may confuse the results of the PFTs. Nonetheless, PFTs are a useful instrument for considering the general characteristics of work-related lung disease. The response to bronchodilator inhalation is another method for differentiating between obstructive and restrictive airway disease.[12]

Additional PFTs include the measurement of residual volume, pulmonary diffusion lung capacity, arterial blood gases (Pa_{O_2}, P_{CO_2}, and pH), and exercise testing. Pulmonary compliance measures the distensibility of the lungs, which is reduced when lungs stiffen.

DIAGNOSTICS

Occupational Respiratory Disease

IMAGING
Chest x-ray
CT scan*
Other
PFTs
ABGs*
Skin testing*

*If indicated.

Skin testing can be helpful in identifying specific antigens.[2] A diagnosis of occupational asthma is a strong consideration if skin testing is positive and the patient has been having bronchospasms.

If SARS is suspected, a CBC, comprehensive metabolic panel, and chest radiograph should be obtained. The chest radiograph is important to help support the diagnosis of SARS. In one study 73% of patients with serologic confirmation of SARS also had chest films positive for pneumonia. Several laboratory tests, including a polymerase chain reaction, can be used to detect SARS-CoV. Serologic testing can also be performed to detect SARS-CoV antibodies produced after infection, and viral culture has also been used to detect SARS-CoV.[19]

DIFFERENTIAL DIAGNOSIS

Health care providers play a pivotal role in identifying occupational lung diseases and differentiating them from non–work-related respiratory disorders. More often than not, correctly diagnosed respiratory symptoms are incorrectly attributed to factors other than work because most health care providers are unfamiliar with their patients' jobs or job-related exposures.

Most symptoms related to occupational respiratory toxins are the same or similar to those associated with other respiratory illnesses, whether or not they are work related. Exploration of the work connection and recent travel history when obtaining patient histories, performing examinations, and evaluating symptoms is essential in the development of the differential diagnosis.[1] When triaging a person with any symptoms suggestive of SARS, it is important to ask about travel history, specifically to Hong Kong, Taiwan, or China, within the past 10 days before onset of symptoms. One must also inquire about friends or family members who may have traveled to these countries and been in contact with the patient.

DIFFERENTIAL DIAGNOSIS

Occupational Respiratory Disease

- Asthma
- Bronchitis
- Chronic obstructive pulmonary disease
- Emphysema
- Fibrosis
- Asbestosis
- Neoplasm
- Noncardiogenic pulmonary edema
- Pulmonary granuloma
- Respiratory tract irritants
- Severe acute respiratory syndrome

MANAGEMENT

The management of occupational respiratory diseases is a multifaceted process and should include general guidelines and specific instructions for modifying hazardous work conditions. Important steps include elimination of the exposure source, referral to a specialist, early diagnosis, effective treatment, and worker's compensation (if indicated).[18]

It is useful to distinguish between exposures that cause acute symptoms, those which may produce irreversible symptoms after prolonged exposure, and those which produce disease that is manifest only after a long latency period. Workers whose exposure produces airway changes that are acute or reversible once the exposure has been removed benefit the most from environmental controls (e.g., an exhaust system), alteration of work practices (e.g., wetting asbestos before removing it), and substitution of a nonhazardous substance for a hazardous one. Other preventive measures that benefit workers to a lesser extent include education regarding specific work hazards, use of personal protective equipment, administrative measures (e.g., job rotation), and screening for early detection of disease.

The management of occupational respiratory disease depends on the specific respiratory illness treated. It is essential that the patient be removed from the exposure as promptly as possible after symptoms have developed. For many occupational respiratory diseases the most important prognostic determinant is the length of exposure before diagnosis. The principles of managing occupational symptomatic asthma are the same as for nonoccupational asthma.[6] Treatment modalities specific to the disease and close monitoring of symptoms and lung function must be maintained for every individual with an occupational respiratory disease.

LIFE SPAN CONSIDERATIONS

Certain occupational respiratory toxins affect both the female and male reproductive processes, compromising the health of both the workers and their children. Information about pregnant women's work activities and those of their partner (including work done at home) and all related exposures should be obtained as part of the perinatal history. Although performed by more women in American society than in any other, household work is often forgotten as a source of potential respiratory toxins. Products used routinely in the home—including scouring powders, chlorine bleaches, furniture polish, drain cleaners, furniture or paint strippers containing organic solvents, glues, paints, epoxies, and pesticides— are all potential hazards, especially when used in a small or poorly ventilated area.[20]

Another important life span consideration related to occupational respiratory disease involves latency and older adults. Many occupational respiratory diseases are characterized by long asymptomatic periods from the time of exposure to clinical evidence of disease. The manifestation of certain cancers may not appear for 10 to 20 years or even longer after an occupational exposure. The screening of workers at risk for certain diseases such as cancer must take into consideration such latency issues. In addition, the differential diagnosis for a constellation of signs and symptoms must reflect occupational exposure that may have occurred many years before.

COMPLICATIONS

Complications of occupational respiratory disease depend on the specific disease process. TB or a fungal infection is a complication peculiar to silica pneumoconiosis. The increased risk of mortality associated with certain chronic respiratory exposures is now well recognized. For example, asbestos-related pleural thickening can cause respiratory failure. Multiple occupational exposures, including those to arsenic, chromium, vinyl chloride monomer, asbestos, and radiation, have been causally identified with respiratory tract cancers.

INDICATIONS FOR REFERRAL OR HOSPITALIZATION

Most health care providers are unfamiliar with occupational medicine. Patients should be referred to an occupational medicine specialist if a diagnosis is not clear or if symptoms are unresponsive to treatment. Chronic work-related respiratory tract illnesses are often best managed by an occupational medicine or pulmonary specialist. This includes the management of many respiratory diseases resulting from chronic exposures (e.g., asbestosis or byssinosis) and may also include the management of acute problems such as silicosis-related TB.

PATIENT AND FAMILY EDUCATION

Education must include an explanation of diagnostic tests and the specific treatment modalities being considered and used. The specifics depend on the specific respiratory disease involved. Occupational medicine is at its best preventive health care. Patients need to be educated about the relationship of their symptoms to workplace exposure, the consequences of continued exposure, and their rights and responsibilities as employees. Employers are required by law to maintain Material Safety Data Sheets (MSDSs), which describe toxic substances, their proper handling, and the symptoms that may arise from contact with them. However, many workers are unaware of the existence of MSDSs and need to be encouraged to read those which are relevant to their jobs. Education needs to include information about the importance of personal protective equipment and workplace hygiene. A list of resources, such as those offered through the Occupational Safety and Health Administration and the National Institute for Occupational Safety and Health, should be made available to the patient.

REFERENCES

1. Chester TJ, Fedoruk M, Langely R, and others: Caution: work can be hazardous to health, *Patient Care* Feb 1996.
2. Malo J-L, Lemiere C, Cartier A, and others: *Diagnosis and clinical assessment of occupational asthma,* retrieved Feb 1, 2007, from http://www.uptodateonline.com/utd/content/topic.do?topicKey=asthma/2403&selectedTitle=2~12.
3. Centers for Disease Control and Prevention: Changing patterns of pneumoconiosis mortality, United States, 1968-2000, *MMWR* 53(28):627-632, 2004.
4. Wang X-R, Eisen E, Zhang H-X, and others: Respiratory symptoms and cotton dust exposure: results of a 15 year follow-up observation, *Occup Environ Med* 60:935-941, 2003.
5. Oliver CL, Stoeckle JD: Prevention and evaluation of occupational respiratory disease. In Goroll AH, May LA, Mulley AG, editors: *Primary care medicine: office evaluation and management of the adult patient,* Philadelphia, 1995, Lippincott.
6. Burton AD: Latex allergy in health care workers, *Occup Med* 12:609-626, 1997.
7. World Health Organization: *Summary of probable SARS cases with onset of illness from 2002 to 31 July 2003,* retrieved July 5, 2006, from http://www.who.int/csr/sars/country/table2004_04_21/en/index.html.
8. Lau P, Chan C: SARS: reflective practice of a nurse manager, *J Clin Nurs* 14:28-34, 2005.
9. Centers for Disease Control and Prevention: *Severe acute respiratory syndrome (SARS),* 2003, retrieved July 5, 2006, from http://www.cdc.gov/ncidod/sars/faq.htm.
10. Centers for Disease Control and Prevention: *Veterans' health activities,* retrieved Jan 30, 2007, from http://www.cdc.gov/nceh/veterans/vet_hlth_actvy.pdf.
11. Agency for Toxic Substances and Disease Registry: *Congressional testimony: potential adverse effects of service in the Persian Gulf War,* retrieved Jan 30, 2007, from http://www.atsdr.cdc.gov/testimony/testimony-1992-09-16.html.
12. Wegman DH, Christiani DC: Respiratory disorders. In Levy BS, Wegman DH, editors: *Occupational health: recognizing and preventing work-related disease,* ed 2, Boston, 1988, Little, Brown.
13. McDiarmid MA: Tuberculosis in the health care industry, *Occup Med* 12:767-774, 1997.
14. Gamaage B, Moore D, Copes R, and others: Protecting health care workers from SARS and other respiratory pathogens: a review of the infection control literature, *Am J Infect Control* 33(2):114-121, 2005.
15. Heyman D, Aylward R, Wolff C: Dangerous pathogens in the laboratory: from smallpox to today's SARS setbacks and tomorrow's polio-free world, *Lancet* 363:1566-1568, 2004.
16. Gallaher S: Pathogenesis: SARS is born, *Dimens Crit Care Nurs* 24(2):51-54, 2005.
17. Safirstein B, Klukowicz A, Miller R, and others: Granulomatous pneumonitis following exposure to the World Trade Center collapse, *Chest* 123(1):301-304, 2003.
18. Kahan E, Weingarten MA, Appelbaum T: Attitudes of primary care physicians to the management of asthma and their perception of its relationship to patients' work, *Isr J Med Sci* 32:757-762, 1996.
19. Rainer T, Chan P, Ip M, and others: The spectrum of severe acute respiratory syndrome–associated coronavirus infection, *Ann Intern Med* 140:614-619, 2004.
20. Quinn MM, Woskie SR: Women and work. In Levy BS, Wegman DH, editors: *Occupational health: recognizing and preventing work-related disease,* ed 2, Boston, 1988, Little, Brown.

CHAPTER 116

Pleural Effusions

Patricia Polgar Bailey

BOX 116-1

POTENTIAL CAUSES OF PLEURAL EFFUSIONS

- Atelectasis
- Benign asbestos-related effusions
- Cirrhosis
- Congestive heart failure (most common cause)
- Drug-induced effusions
- Endocrine dysfunction
- Esophageal perforation
- Hepatic and splenic abscesses
- Infectious parasitic and fungal diseases
- Intraabdominal abscesses
- Malignancy (carcinoma, lymphoma, mesothelioma, leukemia)
- Nephrotic syndrome
- Pancreatic disease
- Peritoneal dialysis
- Pneumonia
- Pulmonary embolism
- Radiotherapy
- Rheumatoid arthritis
- Sarcoidosis
- Systemic lupus erythematosus and other connective tissue diseases
- Tuberculosis
- Viral illness, including HIV/AIDS

DEFINITION AND EPIDEMIOLOGY

A pleural effusion is an abnormal amount of fluid within the pleural space. The pleura, a serous, semitransparent, elastic membrane, covers the lung parenchyma, mediastinum, diaphragm, and rib cage and is divided into the parietal and visceral pleura. The parietal pleura lines the chest cavity, covering the chest wall, diaphragm, and mediastinum. It contains sensory nerves, and its blood supply comes from the systemic circulation and hence has hydrostatic pressure. The visceral pleura covers the entire surface of both lungs, including the interlobular fissures, and contains no pain fibers. Its blood flow is supplied by branches of the pulmonary circulation. The parietal and visceral pleurae are continuous at the hilum, where they are penetrated by both the pulmonary and bronchial vessels. The pleural space is an area approximately 10 to 20 μm in width, situated between the mesothelium of the parietal and visceral pleura.[1-3] Pleural fluid is normally produced in quantities just sufficient to lubricate the parietal and visceral surfaces. This small amount of fluid is constantly replenished and reabsorbed; absorption is principally via the lymphatic system.

The pleural space is referred to as one of the body's *potential spaces,* referring to the fact that normally only a very small amount of fluid volume is found within this space. Approximately 0.16 to 0.36 ml/kg of fluid is normally contained within the pleural space, with a total volume of less than 20 ml and total fluid flow of between 100 and 200 ml, unless some disease process or trauma has caused fluid or solid tissue to collect there. Pleural effusions are a common manifestation of many pulmonary and systemic diseases, most notably congestive heart failure (CHF), because of the elevation of pulmonary venous pressure. In addition, pleural effusions can result from a multitude of other diseases, including pulmonary tuberculosis, pulmonary embolus, and other lung diseases; chest injury or trauma; abdominal infections or pancreatitis; cancers, including lung, breast, and lymphoma; and connective tissue diseases such as rheumatoid arthritis and lupus. Pregnancy and certain types of surgery (e.g., heart, lung, abdominal, and organ transplantation) also increase the risk of developing pleural effusions. Medical therapeutics, including radiotherapy and some medications (e.g., nitrofurantoin and amiodarone), can also increase the likelihood of developing a pleural effusion.[3,4]

PATHOPHYSIOLOGY

An increased amount of fluid (an *effusion*) accumulates in the pleural space whenever the rate of fluid formation exceeds the rate of fluid absorption. Numerous conditions may lead to pleural effusions, including viral and bacterial infections, neoplasms, thromboemboli, cardiovascular dysfunction, and immunologic dysfunction (Box 116-1). Mechanisms that contribute to increased pleural fluid accumulation include (1) an increase in microvascular pressure (e.g., CHF), (2) a decrease in plasma osmotic pressure (e.g., hypoalbuminemia), (3) an increase in the permeability of microcirculation (e.g., pneumonia), (4) a decrease in pleural pressure (e.g., atelectasis), (5) impaired lymphatic drainage from pleural spaces (e.g., malignant effusions), and (6) movement of fluid across the diaphragm from the peritoneal cavity (e.g., inflammation from acute pancreatitis).[1] Parapneumonic effusions are the most common type of effusion and are associated with bacterial infections such as pneumonia, lung abscesses, and bronchiectasis.[4] Malignant pleural effusions are a common problem encountered in persons with advanced cancer, with breast, lung, and ovarian carcinomas and lymphoma accounting for more than 75% of all malignant pleural effusions.[5]

Pleural effusions are often categorized as transudates and exudates, based on the amount of protein detected in the pleural fluid. Exudative pleural effusions result primarily from pleural and lung inflammation (e.g., pneumonia) or impaired lymphatic drainage of the pleural space (e.g., malignancy). In fact, a variety of disease mechanisms, including pneumonia and other infections, malignant carcinomas, immunologic and lymphatic abnormalities, and iatrogenic factors, can cause exudates. Transudative effusions develop when systemic factors alter the formation or absorption of pleural fluid, rather than from pleuritic disease. They are produced by imbalances in hydrostatic and osmotic pressures across the pleural membrane and are usually bilateral. Transudates have a lower specific gravity and lower concentrations of protein and lactate dehydrogenase compared with exudative effusions.[3] CHF is probably the most common cause of transudative pleural effusions, but other disease processes that cause movement of fluid from the peritoneal space or retroperitoneal space, such as cirrhosis, nephrosis, or glomerulonephritis, can cause transudates.[4]

Age-related changes affecting the respiratory system play an important role in the development of pleural effusions. In addition to the expected changes related to aging, years of exposure to particulate matter, dust, occupational toxins, and episodic respiratory infections increase the risk of developing a pleural effusion.[4]

CLINICAL PRESENTATION

Persons with pleural effusions often are asymptomatic when initially seen. When symptoms do occur, the most common presenting complaints include dyspnea, nonproductive cough, pleuritic chest pain, and activity intolerance. Dyspnea is the most common complaint and often increases with recumbent positions.[4] Cough tends to worsen as the size of the effusion increases. Pleuritic pain is associated with inflammation of the parietal pleura and is caused by irritation of its sensory fibers.[1] This pain is often sharp, unilateral, and localized to the affected area, although it may also be experienced in the lower chest and ipsilateral shoulder or referred to the abdomen. Exacerbating factors include deep inspiration, cough, or other movement of the upper body.

Malignant tumors involving the parietal pleura generally cause steady, dull pain compared with the sharp, intermittent pain associated with an acute inflammatory process. Pleural effusions cause compression of adjacent lung tissue and reduce the amount of possible lung expansion, which may result in varying degrees of dyspnea, depending on the size and functional status of the underlying lung and the rate of fluid accumulation. However, dyspnea does not necessarily correlate with blood oxygen levels or the size of the pleural effusion but rather seems to be related to the increased thoracic cage size, which affects respiratory muscle function. Malignant pleural effusions in particular are often characterized by complaints of dyspnea that seem out of proportion to the size of the effusion.[6] The nonproductive cough is most likely due to lung compression and bronchial irritation.[4]

A thorough history is important and can be helpful in discriminating between the symptoms associated with the effusion and those of the primary underlying pathophysiologic process. Information about the presence of fever, cough, sputum production, dyspnea, or abdominal pain should be elicited. Past medical history, including systemic and chronic illnesses, previous surgeries, prior exposures (such as to tuberculosis and asbestos), and previous alcohol abuse, is important.

PHYSICAL EXAMINATION

Several findings on physical examination are suggestive of a pleural effusion; however, the clinical manifestations of the effusion may be overshadowed by the underlying disease process.[7] Common physical examination findings include decreased or absent breath sounds over the effusion, decreased respiratory excursion, dullness to percussion, reduced tactile fremitus, and decreased bronchial breath sounds, sometimes with egophony (E-to-A change) at the upper fluid borders. Pleural inflammation is often accompanied by a friction rub that is transitory and that generally disappears as fluid accumulates in the pleural space. Small effusions (<500 ml) may be associated with minimum or no findings. In situations where effusions are greater (>1500 ml) or pulmonary compromise is more substantial, the use of accessory muscles of respiration, inspiratory lag, cyanosis, bulging intercostal margins, mediastinal shift, and jugular vein distention may be evident. In addition to assessing the respiratory status, the provider needs to perform a complete physical examination to identify signs that may be manifestations of systemic or acute illness and suggest the cause of the effusion. For example, nonthoracic signs such as pedal edema, jugular venous distention, and an S_3 gallop might suggest CHF.[7]

DIAGNOSTICS

Once a pleural effusion is suspected, a chest radiograph should be obtained to confirm its presence and to look for other abnormalities that might help determine its cause. Normal amounts of fluid are not visible on chest x-ray films, which may fail to detect smaller effusions (<100 ml). Effusions that are detected (usually >100 ml) appear as blunting and medial displacement of the sharp costophrenic angle, pleural-based densities, infiltrates, hilar adenopathy, or signs of CHF. A subpulmonary effusion is suspected if the diaphragm is elevated. Chest radiographs do not attain 100% sensitivity until pleural effusions are more than 500 ml.[8] However, they can provide other diagnostic clues to the cause of the effusion. For example, large unilateral effusions usually shift the mediastinum to the contralateral hemithorax, and lack of such a shift with a large effusion may indicate a bronchial obstruction, lung tumor, mesothelioma, or fixed mediastinum from tumor or fibrosis.[9]

Although most pleural effusions are seen on chest films, chest ultrasound and CT are more reliable for detecting and localizing small pleural effusions. Smaller effusions should be confirmed by ultrasonography, which will detect effusions of 5 to 50 ml and are 100% sensitive for effusions of more than 100 ml.[4] In addition to their use in detecting smaller effusions, ultrasound examinations are used to guide diagnostic thoracentesis, resulting in improved yield and decreased complication rates.[9,10]

Once a pleural effusion has been discovered, identification of the disease process, procedure, or drug that caused the effusion is essential. Diagnostic evaluation relies heavily on examination of pleural fluid obtained by thoracentesis. In experienced hands, thoracentesis can be performed safely at the bedside and can be used to diagnose the cause of pleural effusions in 75% of cases.[1] Although a definitive diagnosis, such as the finding of malignant cells, can be established in only 25% of cases, relevant information (from fluid analyses, including cellular counts, chemistry profiles, cultures, and stains) that is useful for clinical decision making and for excluding certain causes of a pleural effusion is obtained in an additional 15% to 20% of cases.[4] In certain situations, where the clinical diagnosis and cause of the effusion are relatively secure and the clinical course is uncomplicated (e.g., uncomplicated CHF, small effusions after thoracic or abdominal surgery, postpartum effusion), therapy may be initiated and a thoracentesis performed only if the response to therapy is inadequate. However, whenever the cause of a pleural effusion is unclear, a diagnostic thoracentesis is generally warranted.[8]

Thoracentesis has no absolute contraindications. However, relative contraindications include a bleeding diathesis or systemic anticoagulation, a small volume of pleural fluid, mechanical ventilation, patient's inability to cooperate, and cutaneous disease such as herpes zoster infection at the needle entry site.[1,7,9] Preprocedure laboratory studies should include a CBC, prothrombin time, and partial thromboplastin time. The complication rate of thoracentesis is approximately 20% and includes pain at the puncture site, cutaneous and internal bleeding, pneumothorax, cough, empyema, and spleen or liver puncture; therefore obtaining informed consent before initiating the procedure is essential.[4]

DIAGNOSTICS

Pleural Effusions

LABORATORY
Pleural fluid analysis*

IMAGING
Chest x-ray
Ultrasound*
CT scan*
Thoracoscopy*

OTHER
Thoracentesis*
Fiberoptic bronchoscopy*
Pleural biopsy*

*If indicated.

Other tests needed to establish a definitive diagnosis may include a CT scan of the chest, thoracoscopy, fiberoptic bronchoscopy, and pleural biopsy. A chest CT scan is not obtained initially to confirm the presence of a pleural effusion; it is most useful after thoracentesis for further evaluation of suspected parenchymal or pleural abnormalities. Bronchoscopy and thoracoscopy are useful in the evaluation of exudative effusions whose cause is still unclear. Open pleural biopsy is required when other procedures have failed to provide a diagnosis.[8]

DIFFERENTIAL DIAGNOSIS

A number of diseases, including pneumothorax, pulmonary embolism, CHF, neoplasms, trauma, and tuberculosis, can cause symptoms similar to those characteristic of pleural effusions. Once a pleural effusion has been established, the differential diagnosis is based on the presence of transudative or exudative effusions, although a number of conditions can cause both. A transudative pleural effusion is generally associated with a systemic condition rather than a pleural disease. An exudate usually suggests a pathologic condition that specifically involves the pleural space. Pleural fluid characterized by high erythrocyte counts (>100,000/mm^3) is most often seen in cases of trauma, malignancy, and pulmonary embolism. Other laboratory evaluations, such as a pleural fluid eosinophil count, glucose concentration, and pH, can be used to help distinguish between the potential causes of the effusion.

DIFFERENTIAL DIAGNOSIS

Pleural Effusions

- Pneumothorax
- Pulmonary embolism
- Congestive heart failure
- Neoplasms
- Trauma
- Tuberculosis

MANAGEMENT

Management is based on treating the cause of the effusion, and a number of specialists may be needed, depending on the cause. In addition, symptomatic treatment is aimed at making the patient more comfortable, beginning when the evaluation is initiated and while the underlying cause is being treated. When an effusion is large, the removal of only 300 to 500 ml through thoracentesis may result in a marked decrease in dyspnea. Indomethacin is often used successfully to treat pleuritic pain and does not suppress respirations, as do narcotics. Malignant pleural effusions, especially in the face of advanced disease, are generally difficult to treat, and management often focuses on providing comfort measures. Some effusions are caused by viral infections and most often resolve without medical intervention.

COMPLICATIONS

Complications depend on the cause and extent of the effusion, accompanying respiratory or systemic compromise, co-morbid conditions, and the treatment modalities available. Malignant pleural effusions are a major cause of morbidity in cancer patients with advanced disease. Treatment is usually palliative, although treatment of the primary malignancy and temporizing symptomatic relief (e.g., repeated thoracentesis for recurrent effusions) may be helpful.

INDICATIONS FOR REFERRAL OR HOSPITALIZATION

The evaluation and treatment of a pleural effusion depend on the underlying disease process, degree of respiratory distress, and other contributory factors such as co-existing health problems. Persons without evidence of respiratory compromise can often be assessed and treated on an outpatient basis. Those with substantial respiratory compromise should be admitted to the hospital for further evaluation and treatment. Referral to a specialist is necessary to establish a definitive diagnosis and management plan.

PATIENT AND FAMILY EDUCATION

Education varies, depending on the cause of the pleural effusion. In all cases teaching must include an explanation of the diagnostic tests, such as thoracentesis, and the potential for chest tube placement and any additional surgical procedures. In addition, education should focus on relieving uncomfortable symptoms, such as dyspnea and pain, and helping patients deal with activity intolerance. Because multiple specialists are often involved in the evaluation of a pleural effusion, the health care provider's role in coordinating care and keeping the patient well informed and at the focus of decision making is essential.

REFERENCES

1. Sahn SA: Pleural anatomy, physiology, and diagnostic procedures. In Baum GL, Crapo JD, Celli BR, and others, editors: *Textbook of pulmonary diseases*, ed 6, Philadelphia, 1998, Lippincott-Raven.
2. Celli BR: Diseases of the chest wall. In Bennette C, Plum F, editors: *Cecil textbook of medicine*, ed 20, Philadelphia, 1996, Saunders.

3. Allibone S: Assessment and management of patients with pleural effusions, *Nurs Stand* 20(22):54-64, 2006.
4. Wing S: Pleural effusion: nursing care challenge in the elderly, *Geriatr Nurs* 25(6):348-354, 2004.
5. Patz EF: Malignant pleural effusions: recent advances and ambulatory sclerotherapy, *Chest* 113(1 Suppl):74S, 1998.
6. Light RW: Disorders of the pleura, mediastinum, and diaphragm. In Fauci AS, Braunwald E, Isselbacher KJ, and others, editors: *Harrison's principles of internal medicine,* ed 14, New York, 1998, McGraw-Hill.
7. Moser K: Pleural effusion. In Bordow RA, Moser KM, editors: *Manual of clinical problems in pulmonary medicine,* ed 4, 1996, Little, Brown.
8. Barrter T, Santarelli R, Akers SM, and others: The evaluation of pleural effusion, *Chest* 106(4):1209-1214, 1994 [erratum in *Chest* 107(2):592, 1995].
9. Rubins JB, Colice GL: Evaluating pleural effusions: how should you go about finding the cause? *Postgrad Med* 105(5):39-42, 45-48, 1999.
10. Diacon AH, Theron J, Bolliger CT: Transthoracic ultrasound for the pulmonologist, *Current Opin Pulmon Med* 11:307-312, 2005.

CHAPTER 117

Pleurisy

Patricia Polgar Bailey

DEFINITION AND EPIDEMIOLOGY

Pleurisy is an inflammation of the pleura, which is a two-ply membrane that lines each of the lungs and the chest cavity. The chest pain of pleurisy is caused by stimulation of the pain fibers in the parietal pleura; it is associated with inflammation of the pleural lining and can result from numerous localized and systemic disease processes.[1] Pleuritic pain is usually described as sharp or stabbing; is generally exacerbated by deep breathing, coughing, or sneezing; and is usually experienced over the lower portion of the chest.

PATHOPHYSIOLOGY

Pleurisy is caused by *pleuritis*, which is an inflammation of the pleural lining, with or without pleural effusion. The pleural layers are highly permeable and in close contact with microcirculation, which makes them responsive to local or systemic immunologic or inflammatory processes. Pleurisy has a variety of causes; it sometimes develops with excess fluid in the pleural cavity *(wet pleurisy)* and sometimes without *(dry pleurisy)*. Secondary pleurisy is the result of some other chest disease, such as pneumonia, tuberculosis, or a lung abscess, in which germs reach the pleura, as well as the lungs, and cause inflammation.

The most common causes of pleuritis include viral, bacterial, or tuberculosis infections, and pulmonary infarction or connective tissue diseases such as lupus erythematosus. Trauma to the chest wall is a less common cause of pleurisy, as is coronary bypass or valve replacement surgery (postpericardiotomy syndrome).[2]

Pleurisy is rarely caused by malignant processes; malignant tumors that involve the pleura generally cause a steady, dull pain compared with the sharp, stabbing, intermittent pain associated with pleural inflammation. Certain drugs, including nitrofurantoin, methotrexate, and procarbazine, have been associated with pleurisy.[3]

CLINICAL PRESENTATION

A thorough history is instrumental in determining the differential diagnosis for any type of chest pain. Pain on breathing (which may be minimum to severe depending on the degree of inflammation) and a stabbing or shooting chest pain are characteristics of pleurisy. Sometimes the pain may be felt in the shoulder. Milder pleurisy may be described as a "stitch in the side." Pleuritic pain is generally made worse by breathing, coughing, chest movement, sneezing, or talking. Often the most comfortable position for the patient is lying on the affected side, which limits expansion of the chest wall.[4]

PHYSICAL EXAMINATION

Pleuritic pain is usually located directly over the site of inflammation, and tenderness is increased with deep palpation. Rapid and shallow breathing may be associated symptoms, with limited chest wall expansion on the affected side. Percussion over the affected area may be dull if there is underlying consolidation or pleural effusion. Increased or diminished fremitus may also denote the presence or absence of consolidation. A pleural friction rub, which varies in intensity from a faint scratching sound to a loud creak, confirms the diagnosis of pleurisy. However, the absence of a pleural friction rub does not negate the presence of pleurisy because the presence of pleural fluid may mitigate or even nullify the rub.

A pleural friction rub may be heard during both phases of respiration but is often most pronounced at or near the end of inspiration. It disappears when patients hold their breath. A pleural friction rub may be localized or heard over a wider area and is generally most audible over the lateral and posterior regions of the inferior thorax. It is rarely heard over the upper thorax and lung apexes because of the limited movement of the lung in these areas compared with the lung bases. In general, a rub is heard only if the person takes a deep breath; a rub, even if present, is not audible during splinting or shallow breathing. Crackles can sometimes sound similar to a rub, but a cough usually diminishes crackles and has no effect on a rub. A sound similar to a pleural friction rub can be produced by sliding a stethoscope over the skin; firm pressure of the stethoscope on the skin should eliminate this "false rub" and intensify the sound of a real friction rub if present.[4]

Sometimes pleuritic inflammation can lead to pleural effusions, a collection of fluid between the pleura. Pleural effusions often ease the pain temporarily by providing a cushion between the inflamed membranes and, as a result, give a false sense of improvement when the situation is really getting worse. Large collections of pleural fluid can compress the lungs and further compromise respiration.

DIAGNOSTICS

Several laboratory tests, although themselves not diagnostic of pleurisy, may help elucidate the underlying cause. An elevated leukocyte count with a shift to the left suggests a bacterial infection such as pneumonia, an esophageal rupture, or an abscess. Leukopenia may reflect a viral process or lupus erythematosus. A chest x-ray examination may help diagnose bacterial pneumonia, pneumothorax, esophageal rupture, or problems below the diaphragm such as a subphrenic abscess or effusion. Thoracentesis and pleural fluid analysis can help identify the underlying cause once the existence of a pleural effusion has been established (see Chapter 116). If the cause of the pleurisy is still unclear, other studies, including a CT scan of the chest, a ventilation/perfusion scan, a pleural biopsy, or esophageal contrast studies, may be indicated.

DIAGNOSTICS

Pleurisy

LABORATORY
CBC and differential

IMAGING
Chest x-ray
CT scan*
V/Q scan*
Esophageal contrast studies*

OTHER
Thoracentesis, pleural fluid analysis*
Pleural biopsy*

*If indicated.

DIFFERENTIAL DIAGNOSIS

Problems that originate in other chest wall structures can produce pain similar to that of pleurisy; these conditions include pneumothorax, rib fractures, costochondritis, vertebral fractures, and nerve root pain from herpes zoster infection. The presence of a pleural friction rub confirms the pleuritis, but a patient history, physical examination, and pertinent diagnostic tests are still necessary to determine the most likely differential diagnosis.

Pleural effusion is a finding commonly associated with pleurisy and may be helpful in determining the diagnosis. Viral infections, rheumatic disease, and sarcoidosis often cause pleurisy in the absence of a pleural effusion. In contrast, pneumonia, *Mycobacterium* tuberculosis, lupus pleuritis, and postcardiac injury syndrome are generally associated with pleural effusions.[3,4]

The patient's history may be helpful in narrowing the differential diagnosis. For example, a recent leg fracture with casting raises the possibility of a pulmonary embolism. Occupational asbestos exposure might suggest asbestos pleurisy. A history of lupus erythematosus or sarcoidosis increases the suspicion of systemic connective tissue disease as the underlying cause of the pleurisy.[4]

Many types of pain experienced in the chest area are not pleuritic. Cardiac chest pain is often central and diffuse and is described as a pressing or squeezing rather than a sharp and intermittent pain. Cardiac pain (angina, acute myocardial infarction, dissecting aortic aneurysm) often radiates to the neck, jaw, or arms and worsens with exertion, which is not characteristic of pleurisy. Pericardial pain can be similar in character to pleuritic pain but is usually felt on the anterior side of the chest and back and is exacerbated by lying down. Chronic chest pain is not usually a result of parenchymal lung disease because the lung and visceral pleura are not innervated by pain fibers.

DIFFERENTIAL DIAGNOSIS

Pleurisy

- Pneumothorax
- Pleurodynia
- Pneumonia
- Myocardial infarction
- Angina
- Pericarditis
- Rib fracture
- Costochondritis
- Metastatic bone pain
- Cervical spine disease
- Musculoskeletal pain
- Pancreatitis
- Gallbladder disease
- Subphrenic abscess
- Peptic ulcer disease
- Esophageal disorder
- Tumor neuritis
- Myositis
- Aneurysm
- Thoracic outlet syndrome
- Herpes zoster

MANAGEMENT

The management of pleurisy is based on treatment of the underlying disease. Co-management with a specialist is necessary for all except the most benign causes of pleural inflammation. Drainage of the pleural space may be indicated if a pleural effusion is present (see Chapter 116). Certain systemic causes of inflammation, such as lupus erythematosus, respond well to corticosteroids. NSAIDs are used to provide symptomatic pain relief. Malignant diseases rarely cause pleurisy, and pleurisy generally resolves with appropriate and prompt treatment.[4]

COMPLICATIONS

The extent and complications of pleural inflammation depend on the underlying disease process. Some causes are self-limiting and have no chronic sequelae or complications. If the inflammation is chronic or pleural repair processes cause fibrosis, an inelastic membrane ("pleural peel") may form around the lung. This membrane causes lung entrapment and impairs respiratory function.[3]

INDICATIONS FOR REFERRAL OR HOSPITALIZATION

A referral is often necessary to determine or treat the underlying cause of the pleurisy. The requisite evaluation and management depend on the cause of the inflammation. Patients without evidence of respiratory compromise or acute illness can often be evaluated and treated on an outpatient basis. Patients with more significant respiratory compromise or highly contagious disease (e.g., active pulmonary tuberculosis) may need to be hospitalized for further evaluation and treatment.

PATIENT AND FAMILY EDUCATION

Patient education varies depending on the cause of the pleurisy. Teaching must include an explanation of and rationale for all diagnostic tests. Education should also focus on symptomatic relief. As in all cases in which multiple practitioners may be involved, the role of the health care provider is important in coordinating care and in keeping the patient well informed and at the focus of decision making.

REFERENCES

1. Marx J: *Rosen's emergency medicine: concepts and clinical practice*, ed 5, St Louis, 2002, Mosby.
2. Kelly B, Nicholas J, Chhablani R, and others: The postpericardiotomy syndrome as a cause of pleurisy in rehabilitation patients, *Arch Phys Med Rehabil* 81:517-518, 2000.
3. Kroegel C, Antony VB: Immunobiology of pleural inflammation: potential implications for pathogenesis, diagnosis, and therapy, *Eur Respir J* 10:2411-2418, 1997.
4. Sahn SA, Heffner JE: Approach to the patient with pleural disease. In Kelley WN, editor: *Textbook of internal medicine*, ed 3, Philadelphia, 1997, Lippincott-Raven.

CHAPTER 118

Pneumonia

Susan Harvey and Carol A. Whelan

DEFINITION AND EPIDEMIOLOGY

Pneumonia is an infection of the lower respiratory tract that is usually accompanied by cough, fever, malaise, and chest x-ray (CXR) abnormalities. Sputum production, dyspnea, fever, hypoxia, and hemoptysis may be present in some individuals with pneumonia, depending on the causative organism. The Infectious Disease Society of America (IDSA) defines community-acquired pneumonia (CAP) as an acute infection of the pulmonary parenchyma that is frequently associated with at least two symptoms of active infection, occurring in individuals who have not been hospitalized or resided in a long-term care facility for 14 days before the onset of symptoms.[1] In most cases of CAP, diagnosis is made by history and physical examination; identification of the etiologic agent is usually not necessary. Although the list of organisms causing CAP is long and increasing, relatively few organisms are responsible for most cases of pneumonia. In primary care practice, two of the most important issues related to pneumonia are awareness of the most common infectious pathogens and their treatment, and decisions regarding the appropriateness of outpatient treatment.

The treatment of pneumonia, both CAP and nosocomial, has been standardized to some degree by the publication of guidelines by the American Thoracic Society (ATS), with recent updates for CAP in 2001[2] and for nosocomial pneumonia in 2004.[3,4] The successful treatment of pneumonia depends on the correct empiric antibiotic selection and knowledge of its proven effectiveness in vivo. A working knowledge of the organisms that most commonly infect different age-groups and the habits or characteristics that put an individual at risk for specific etiologic agents is essential.

The most common cause of bacterial pneumonia is *Streptococcus pneumoniae*, estimated to be the cause of 20% to 60% of pneumonia cases.[2] Gram-negative organisms include *Haemophilus influenzae, Klebsiella pneumoniae,* and *Moraxella catarrhalis*. *M. catarrhalis* and *K. pneumoniae* infections are more commonly diagnosed when there is co-existent alcoholism. *Staphylococcus aureus* and *H. influenzae* infections often occur after a primary influenza infection. *M. catarrhalis*, a gram-negative organism not thought to be pathogenic, is most commonly found in those with chronic lung conditions such as chronic obstructive pulmonary disease (COPD). It is also found in patients with other underlying chronic lung conditions such as malignancy, with steroid use, and with diabetes.[5]

Another organism responsible for pneumonia is *Legionella pneumophila*. This organism was first implicated in 1976 after 182 people became ill in Philadelphia while attending an American Legion convention. The organism is a gram-negative bacillus that survives in water and soil. Contamination with the organism is acquired through inhalation of aerosolized droplets, thus making air-conditioning ventilating systems an obvious reservoir.

Finally, the atypical and nonbacterial organisms responsible for pneumonia include *Mycoplasma pneumoniae, Chlamydia pneumoniae* (the Taiwan acute respiratory [TWAR] strain), and multiple viruses. *Mycoplasma* organisms lack cell walls and cannot be stained and visualized by conventional methods. Infection with this organism causes a disease that is usually found in younger individuals and follows a milder course than that seen in patients with bacterial pneumonia. Chlamydial infection also manifests as a mild infection spread from person to person by aerosolized droplet secretions.

Pneumonia remains one of the leading causes of morbidity and mortality in the United States, especially in older adults and in those with underlying chronic disease. Pneumonia is the leading cause of death from infectious disease and the seventh most common cause of death in the United States.[6] It is estimated that 4 million episodes of pneumonia are diagnosed in the United States every year, with a total of 30 million days of disability.[7] These are surprising statistics given the advent of broad-spectrum antibiotics, a multivalent *Pneumococcus* vaccine, and sophisticated hospital care.

The elderly have the highest rates of CAP in the United States. Old age is associated with a variety of age-related declines in immune system function (immune senescence) and prevalent co-morbidities. As a result, the elderly constitute the largest immunocompromised population in the United States, putting them at risk for new infectious agents. Pathogens that are not typical causative agents of pneumonia must be considered as possible etiologic agents in the elderly. As a result, older adults are more likely to have CAP caused by resistant organism or tuberculosis and to require hospital admission.[8]

Clues to the specific cause of the pneumonia can be found in the patient's history. The CAPs include most of the organisms found in Table 118-1 except the enteric gram-negative bacilli, *Pseudomonas* organisms, and staphylococci, which are often found in patients who are hospitalized or live in nursing homes.

The incidence of some causes of pneumonia is linked to the season of the year and the geographic area. Influenza illness in the winter increases the prevalence of secondary *S. pneumoniae, S. aureus,* and *H. influenzae* pneumonias. *H. influenzae* is known to have a short incubation period and moves through communities rather quickly. Mycoplasmal infection usually moves through communities slowly because of a longer incubation period and lower communicability. *Legionella* organisms have been known to infect a large number of people simultaneously by infecting many within a group from a single reservoir.

PATHOPHYSIOLOGY

The lungs are usually a sterile environment maintained by a host of natural defenses. The airways act as a filtration and humidification system of inspired air. Epithelial cells line the entire respiratory tract and contain cilia that constantly beat upward toward the pharynx. This action is a physical means of elimination of foreign material. Also, an intact gag reflex prevents the entry of particles, mucus, and food debris. Finally, the immune system is responsible for defense mechanisms, such as the action of phagocytes, macrophages, neutrophils, complement, and immunoglobulins, which retard advancement of pathogenic organisms that do gain access to this normally sterile environment.

TABLE 118-1 Epidemiologic Characteristics Related to Specific Pathogens

Characteristics	Pathogen(s)
Alcoholism	Oral anaerobes *Streptococcus pneumoniae* Gram-negative bacilli
COPD, tobacco use	*Haemophilus influenzae* *S. pneumoniae* *Moraxella catarrhalis*
Nursing home resident	*S. pneumoniae* Gram-negative bacilli *H. influenzae* *Staphylococcus aureus*
Poor dental hygiene	Oral anaerobes
Recent exposure to contaminated plumbing or water	*Legionella* organisms
Exposure to birds	*Chlamydia psittaci* *Histoplasma capsulatum* (histoplasmosis)
HIV infection	*Pneumocystis carinii* *S. pneumoniae* *H. influenzae* *Mycobacterium tuberculosis*
Exposure to excreta of wild rodents	Sin nombre virus (hantavirus pulmonary syndrome)

Reprinted with permission from File TM, Tan JS, Plouffe JF: Community acquired pneumonia: what's needed for accurate diagnosis, *Postgrad Med* 99(1):102, 1996. ©1996 McGraw-Hill.

COPD, Chronic obstructive pulmonary disease.

In the healthy adult the above-mentioned host mechanisms prevent disease much of the time. However, a number of mechanisms allow pathogens to gain entry into the lungs; these mechanisms include an altered level of conscious from stroke, seizure, anesthesia, alcohol abuse, intoxication, and the sleep state. Epiglottic closure may be compromised in these situations and allow normal oral flora to gain entry.

Certain other conditions may predispose an individual to recurrent pneumonia; these include compromised immune function, cystic fibrosis, esophageal abnormalities, bronchial obstruction, and bronchiectasis.

CLINICAL PRESENTATION AND PHYSICAL EXAMINATION

The clinical presentation of pneumonia includes a history of fever, malaise, and cough with or without sputum production. The patient may also complain of hemoptysis, dyspnea, and pleuritic chest symptoms. The provider should focus on symptoms of bacterial, viral, and atypical pneumonia syndromes. Chest auscultation may reveal rales that do not clear with a cough, which may be found in both bacterial and atypical pneumonia. Consolidation, including dullness to percussion, bronchial breath sounds, and egophony (E-to-A changes), is found more commonly in the bacterial pneumonia syndromes. Chest radiographs are highly variable and may be normal in the early course of the disease. In addition, CXR films of patients with viral and mycoplasmal pneumonia may show large infiltrates with minimum outward symptoms. A prodrome of headache and sore throat is often associated with atypical pneumonia. Patients between the ages of 18 and 44 years are almost twice as likely to complain of pleuritic chest pain and have fever than those who are older than 75 years. Some patients, including the elderly, may show none of the classic signs of pneumonia but may have atypical complaints such as fatigue; lethargy; decreased appetite; increased falls; and mental status changes, such as confusion, stupor, or coma. In addition, older adults are more likely to be seen initially with tachypnea but less likely to have a cough or fever.

Bacterial Pneumonia Syndromes

Gram-Positive Bacteria. *S. pneumoniae* is the leading cause of pneumonia in any adult age-group with or without co-morbid conditions.[2,5,7,9] Pneumococcal pneumonia that is associated with bacteremia has a 20% mortality rate.[10] Those at risk for *S. pneumoniae* infection characteristically have some chronic condition, such as diabetes, COPD, asplenia, advanced age, cigarette smoking, congestive heart failure, dementia, alcoholism, or immunosuppression. From 20% to 60% of all hospitalized patients are infected with pneumococci.[2]

The history may include an abrupt onset of high fever with shaking chills, productive cough with purulent sputum, and possibly pleuritic-type chest pains. Physical examination may reveal signs of consolidation (egophony, increased fremitus, dullness to percussion, rales, and rhonchi), and CXR films reveal single or multiple lobar consolidation. Sputum analysis by Gram stain indicates gram-positive diplococci in pairs and short chains and large numbers of polymorphonuclear leukocytes.

S. aureus, although rarely a cause of CAP, must be considered, especially after a primary influenza infection, in older adults and in those with diabetes. From 2% to 10% of acute CAPs are due to staphylococci.[10] Suppurative conditions, including empyema, lung abscess, and pneumothorax, are common complications. Seeding to distant sites, such as bones, joints, liver, endocardium, and the meninges, may also occur.

Group A streptococci rarely cause CAP but have been found in epidemics among close groups that live together, such as military units. Symptoms may be similar to those of *S. pneumoniae,* and Gram stain reveals clumped spherical cocci, similar in appearance to a bunch of grapes.

Gram-Negative Bacteria. *H. influenzae,* another etiologic agent of CAP, is a small, gram-negative rod with a polysaccharide capsule. There are six serotypes, of which type b is the most severe and invasive (causing meningitis and sepsis). Some strains of *H. influenzae* are nonencapsulated and therefore cannot be typed. These are also capable of causing disease, but usually the disease is noninvasive and therefore less severe. These nontypeable strains of *H. influenzae* are usually found in acute bronchitis. Pneumonia caused by *H. influenzae* is usually caused by an encapsulated strain. Older adults and those with underlying chronic lung conditions are most susceptible to this bacteria.[11,12] The history usually includes an abrupt onset of fever, shaking chills, and cough with purulent sputum. The patient may describe pleuritic chest pain, and physical examination reveals signs of consolidation. A bronchopneumonia pattern is seen on the CXR film.

Aerobic gram-negative bacilli rarely colonize the upper airway in healthy individuals but are often found in people with an underlying disease such as alcoholism and in those who reside in health care facilities or nursing homes. Aspiration of the organisms is thought to be the mode of infection. *Pseudomonas* organisms, *K. pneumoniae,* and *Escherichia coli* may also become pulmonary pathogens. The mortality rate associated with gram-negative pneumonia is relatively high compared with other types of pneumonia.[13] Therefore a history of recent hospitalization or nursing home residency should heighten suspicion for a gram-negative pathogenesis. Polymicrobial infection is seen more often in older adults, and increased colonization of gram-negative bacilli of the upper airway is related to recent antimicrobial use, decreased activity, diabetes, and alcohol use.

M. catarrhalis is a β-lactamase–producing gram-negative aerobic diplococcus that was recently identified as a common pathogen found in individuals with COPD.[2,5] Often in patients with COPD, it is the only organism isolated from the lower respiratory tract. Other chronic conditions, such as alcoholism, steroid use, diabetes, and malignancy, increase the risk of *M. catarrhalis* infection. The highest incidence of this infection tends to be in the winter months.

Atypical Pneumonia Syndromes

Atypical pneumonia syndromes largely refer to pneumonias caused by nonbacterial organisms and by bacterial organisms that do not share the expected characteristics of most bacteria. *M. pneumoniae* is the most common offending organism in the majority of cases of pneumonia in those younger than 40 years of age.[5] It disproportionately affects older children and young adults. This "atypical" pneumonia syndrome is characterized by a prodrome of fever, headache, myalgias, and dry cough. These individuals usually appear less ill than do those with bacterial pneumonia. Symptoms may last up to 6 weeks and include a dry, hacking cough that may require a narcotic cough suppressant. Because of the long incubation period, mycoplasmal infection may spread slowly among family members. It should be viewed as a systemic disease with a pulmonary component.

The physical examination usually reveals fine rales with no signs of lung consolidation. A cutaneous manifestation may be present in the form of maculopapular eruptions. Rarely, examination of the tympanic membranes shows evidence of bullous myringitis, which can be very painful. CXR films reveal patchy alveolar densities or nonhomogeneous segmental infiltrates. The WBC count may be normal or only slightly elevated. Full recovery is expected with no residual effects in a previously healthy individual. However, the disease can be severe in those with sickle cell anemia, in older adults, and in those with immunosuppression.

C. pneumoniae (TWAR strain) is the etiologic agent for a common atypical pneumonia syndrome in younger individuals. Outbreaks occur in groups such as military units and college students. Symptoms are similar to those of mycoplasmal infection. Clinical presentation may include laryngitis, a hoarse voice, and nonexudative pharyngitis, in addition to the symptoms described above for mycoplasmal infection. Laryngitis is not present in any other atypical pneumonia syndrome. CXR films may show patchy consolidation, interstitial infiltrates, or funnel-shaped lesions. The WBC count is usually normal.

Multiple viruses, including adenoviruses, respiratory syncytial virus, and parainfluenza virus, may also cause pneumonia. Predilection for infection in children is most common. Cytomegalovirus and *Pneumocystis* may be the cause of pneumonia in the immunocompromised host. For years *Pneumocystis* has been referred to as *Pneumocystis carinii* pneumonia (PCP) and known to be the most common serious AIDS-defining opportunistic infection in the United States. Recent DNA analysis has demonstrated extensive diversity within the genus *Pneumocystis*, with different host species having different DNA sequences. In recognition of its genetic and functional distinctness, the organism that causes human PCP is now named *Pneumocystis jiroveci*.[14] Recently, infection with *Hantavirus* organisms has been recognized in the Southwestern United States. Fever, myalgias, and respiratory distress resembling acute respiratory distress syndrome are present.[2]

Three new pathogens can be added to the list of etiologic agents for CAP: the coronavirus (CoV) responsible for severe acute respiratory syndrome (SARS), human metapneumovirus (HMPV), and community-acquired methicillin-resistant *S. aureus* (CA-MRSA). The SARS-CoV was not documented in humans until 2002. It has been hypothesized that a previously unknown animal CoV may have mutated and infected humans. There is no specific treatment for SARS, and management is primarily supportive. SARS-CoV is highly contagious, so aggressive infection control measures are necessary to prevent spread of the disease.[15]

Another new pathogen of CAP is HMPV, a paramyxovirus first isolated in 2001 in children hospitalized with acute infections. Since then, HMPV has been reported in all age-groups, with varying stages of disease, from those who are asymptomatic to those with severe bronchitis and pneumonia. Like SARS-CoV, there is no specific treatment for HMPV.[15]

The third pathogen, CA-MRSA, is a combination of well-known health care–associated strains and newer isolates with distinctive genotypes. CA-MRSA is a virulent and resistant pathogen and causes outbreaks of serious infections, including skin and soft tissue infections and necrotizing pneumonia.[15]

Respiratory syncytial virus (RSV) is another important newly appreciated cause of pneumonia in older adults. Studies in which RSV was isolated by viral culture have demonstrated that it is common, occurring in 3% to 10% of older adults with pneumonia. The incidence was similar in high-risk and healthy seniors and about twice the incidence of influenza A.[15]

Legionnaire's Disease

L. pneumophila is the pulmonary pathogen responsible for legionnaire's disease. Symptoms of infection include dry cough; fever with a temperature between 38.3° and 38.8° C (101° and 102° F); altered mental status; relative bradycardia; headache; and gastrointestinal symptoms, including diarrhea.

Legionnaire's disease is caused by a gram-negative bacillus that is considered an atypical organism because it does not respond to the β-lactam antibiotics as do other gram-negative organisms. Suspicion for infection with *Legionella* organisms should be high, especially in older adults and in those with chronic underlying disease, who are most at risk for death. CXR films reveal rapid progression of asymmetric infiltrates without signs of consolidation. Serum titer levels for *Legionella* organisms can be obtained but are most often negative early in the disease. To be diagnostic, the titer must be greater than 1:256. Treatment with tetracycline and the macrolide antibiotics is recommended.

DIAGNOSTICS

Chest Radiography

The results of CXR films are most valuable when considered in the context of the history and physical examination. Currently, both IDSA and the ATS recommend a CXR for all patients diagnosed with pneumonia, to both establish the diagnosis and rule out complications,[3] although this may not always be feasible. Posteroanterior and lateral CXR films confirm pneumonia when new infiltrates are found on the films. However, a CXR film that is negative does not exclude the diagnosis of pneumonia. Dehydration and neutropenia may result in false-negative findings. Comparison of the current CXR films with old radiographs is always important to assess for changes. Bacterial patterns on the CXR films include lobar consolidation, cavitation, and large pleural effusions.

Sputum Analysis

Analysis of sputum can be helpful in identifying an etiologic agent in pneumonia; however, current guidelines from the ATS do not recommend this as routine for outpatients diagnosed with CAP.[3] Culture and Gram stain are excellent methods of identifying the pathologic agent when needed. A good sputum sample comes from the bronchial tree; it is not the same as saliva from the mouth. Although not usually available during the clinic visit, sputum produced on awakening in the morning is typically a good sample because of the strong reflex to cough when rising to an upright position. Sputum that contains less than 10 squamous epithelial cells and more than 25 neutrophils is considered an adequate sample. The patient is encouraged to rinse the mouth with water several times before trying to produce a sample. Inhalation of a warmed 3% to 10% saline solution may help the patient provide an adequate sample.

Other Tests

Multiple serologic and antigen studies are available to help identify the pathogen(s) responsible for the pneumonia. At least one study has examined the use of the rapid Binax NOW *S. pneumoniae* urinary antigen test for the diagnosis of pneumococcal infection in hospitalized patients.[16] Results are available in 15 minutes, and the test has a sensitivity and specificity of 82% and 97%, respectively.[12] These tests are not routinely used in the outpatient setting. Even after extensive

DIAGNOSTICS

Pneumonia

LABORATORY
Sputum analysis—culture and Gram stain*
CBC and differential*
Blood chemistries*
Blood cultures*
Complement fixation*
ABGs*
Viral culture*

IMAGING
Chest x-ray

OTHER
Bronchoscopy*

*If indicated.

diagnostic testing has been completed, many times the pathogen remains unidentified.

Current ATS diagnostic recommendations for CAP patients requiring hospital admission include assessment of gas exchange either by telemetry or arterial sampling, CBC with differential, blood chemistry, liver function tests, and two sets of blood cultures. Evidence for benefit of routine bronchoscopy does not exist.[3]

DIFFERENTIAL DIAGNOSIS

Multiple organisms must be considered in the differential diagnosis of pneumonia, as should syndromes that can mimic symptoms of the disease. These include pulmonary emboli, congestive heart failure, pulmonary tumors, and some inflammatory lung diseases.

DIFFERENTIAL DIAGNOSIS

Pneumonia

- *Streptococcus pneumoniae*
- *Mycoplasma pneumoniae*
- Respiratory viruses (including cytomegalovirus, hantavirus, respiratory syncytial virus)
- *Chlamydia pneumoniae* (TWAR strain)
- *Haemophilus influenzae*
- *Legionella pneumophila*
- *Staphylococcus aureus*
- Severe acute respiratory syndrome–coronavirus (SARS-CoV)
- Human metapneumovirus (HMPV)
- Community-acquired methicillin-resistant S. aureus (CA-MRSA)
- *Mycobacterium tuberculosis*
- Endemic fungi
- Aerobic gram-negative bacilli (e.g., *Pseudomonas aeruginosa*)
- Anaerobic infections
- Polymicrobial infections
- Pulmonary embolus
- Congestive heart failure
- Pulmonary tumors
- Inflammatory lung diseases
- Acute and chronic bronchitis

MANAGEMENT

Resistance patterns to all antibiotics are an increasing problem that is now more evident and widespread than at any other time in medical history. Careful, prudent use of antibiotics is absolutely necessary to curb this growing problem. The routine practice of trying to cover for all pathogens, especially gram-negative organisms, should be avoided; this only leads to increased resistance patterns. Initiation of antibiotic treatment in patients with CAP is empirically determined because the history and physical examination will not determine a specific cause for the disease.[17-20] Despite the use of sputum culture, Gram stain, and CXR studies, providers can accurately identify the causative organism only 40% to 70% of the time. Therefore the patient's age, the competency of the host immune system, underlying chronic conditions, patterns of resistance in the community, and knowledge of the most likely pathogens must be considered to accurately determine empiric antimicrobial therapy.

Recommendations for initial empiric antimicrobial therapy in the outpatient setting vary.[2,9] The recommendations for treatment of CAP are taken from the most recent guidelines and recommendations published by the ATS in 2001.[2] Since the last publication of these recommendations in 1993, there has been a shift in focus from age-groups and co-morbid conditions as the basis for drug selection to the most likely pathogens combined with modifying factors (Box 118-1) and/or co-existing cardiopulmonary disease (Table 118-2). Group I includes outpatients without cardiopulmonary disease and without modifying factors. Modifying factors include HIV infection, risk factors for infection with drug-resistant pneumococci, risk factors for gram-negative infection (including nursing home residence), and risk factors for infection with *Pseudomonas aeruginosa*. Group II includes outpatients with cardiopulmonary disease (congestive heart failure or COPD) and/or other modifying factors (risk factors

BOX 118-1

MODIFYING FACTORS THAT INCREASE THE RISK OF INFECTION WITH SPECIFIC PATHOGENS

- Penicillin-resistant and drug-resistant pneumococci
- Age over 65 years
- β-Lactam therapy within the past 3 months
- Alcoholism
- Immunosuppressive illness (including therapy with corticosteroids)
- Multiple medical co-morbidities
- Exposure to a child in a day care center
- Enteric gram-negative organisms
- Residence in a nursing home
- Underlying cardiopulmonary disease
- *Pseudomonas aeruginosa* infection
- Structural lung disease (bronchiectasis)
- Corticosteroid therapy (>10 mg/day of prednisone)
- Recent antibiotic therapy, especially broad-spectrum antibiotic therapy for more than 7 days in the past month
- Malnutrition

From Niederman MS, Mandell LA, Anzueto A, and others: Guidelines for the management of adults with community-acquired pneumonia: diagnosis, assessment of severity, antimicrobial therapy and prevention. *Am J Respir Crit Care Med* 163:1730-1754, 2001.

TABLE 118-2 Management of Pneumonia in Different Patient Groups

Organisms	Therapy
GROUP I: OUTPATIENTS, NO CARDIOPULMONARY DISEASE, NO MODIFYING FACTORS[a,b]	
Streptococcus pneumoniae *Mycoplasma pneumoniae* *Chlamydia pneumoniae* (alone or as mixed infection) *Haemophilus influenzae* Respiratory viruses Miscellaneous *Legionella* spp. *Mycobacterium tuberculosis* Endemic fungi	Advanced-generation macrolide: azithromycin or clarithromycin[c] *or* Doxycycline[d]
GROUP II: OUTPATIENTS, WITH CARDIOPULMONARY DISEASE AND/OR OTHER MODIFYING FACTORS[a,b]	
S. pneumoniae (including drug-resistant *S. pneumoniae* [DRSP]) *M. pneumoniae* *C. pneumoniae* Mixed infection (bacteria plus atypical pathogen or virus) *H. influenzae* Enteric gram-negatives Respiratory viruses Miscellaneous: *Moraxella catarrhalis*, *Legionella* spp., aspiration (anaerobes), *M. tuberculosis*, endemic fungi	[e]β-Lactam (oral cefpodoxime, cefuroxime, high-dose amoxicillin,[f] amoxicillin-clavulanate; or parenteral ceftriaxone followed by oral cefpodoxime) *plus* Macrolide or doxycycline *or* Antipneumococcal fluoroquinolone (used alone)
GROUP III: INPATIENTS, NOT IN ICU[a,g]	
Cardiopulmonary Disease and/or Modifying Factors (Including Being from a Nursing Home)	
S. pneumoniae (including DRSP) *H. influenzae* *M. pneumoniae* *C. pneumoniae* Mixed infection (bacteria plus atypical pathogen) Enteric gram-negatives Aspiration (anaerobes) Viruses *Legionella* spp. Miscellaneous: *M. tuberculosis*, endemic fungi, *Pneumocystis carinii*	[e]IV β-lactam[h] (cefotaxime, ceftriaxone, ampicillin-sulbactam, high-dose ampicillin) *plus* IV or oral macrolide or doxycycline[i] *or* IV antipneumococcal fluoroquinolone alone
No Cardiopulmonary Disease, No Modifying Factors	
S. pneumoniae *H. influenzae* *M. pneumoniae* *C. pneumoniae* Mixed infection (bacteria plus atypical pathogen) Viruses *Legionella* spp. Miscellaneous: *M. tuberculosis*, endemic fungi, *Pneumocystis jiroveci*	[e]IV azithromycin alone If macrolide allergic or intolerant: Doxycycline and a beta-lactam *or* Monotherapy with an antipneumococcal fluoroquinolone
GROUP IV: ICU-ADMITTED PATIENTS[a,g]	
No Risks for *Pseudomonas aeruginosa*	
S. pneumoniae (including DRSP) *Legionella* spp. *H. influenzae* Enteric gram-negative bacilli *S. aureus* *M. pneumoniae* Respiratory viruses Miscellaneous: *C. pneumoniae*, *M. tuberculosis*, endemic fungi	[e,j]IV β-lactam (cefotaxime, ceftriaxone)[h] *plus either* IV macrolide (azithromycin) *or* IV fluoroquinolone

Continued

TABLE 118-2 Management of Pneumonia in Different Patient Groups—cont'd

Organisms	Therapy
GROUP IV: ICU-ADMITTED PATIENTS[a,g]—CONT'D	
Risks for *Pseudomonas aeruginosa*	
All of the above pathogens plus *P. aeruginosa*	[e,j]Selected IV antipseudomonal β-lactam (cefepime, imipenem, meropenem, piperacillin-tazobactam)[k] *plus* IV antipseudomonal quinolone (ciprofloxacin) *or* Selected IV antipseudomonal β-lactam (cefepime, imipenem, meropenem, piperacillin-tazobactam)[k] *plus* IV aminoglycoside *plus either* IV macrolide (azithromycin) *or* IV nonpseudomonal fluoroquinolone

From Niederman MS, Mandell LA, Anzueto A, and others: Guidelines for the management of adults with community-acquired pneumonia: diagnosis, assessment of severity, antimicrobial therapy and prevention, *Am J Respir Crit Care Med* 163:1730-1754, 2001.
[a]Excludes patients at risk for HIV.
[b]In roughly 50%-90% of the cases no etiology was identified.
[c]Erythromycin is not active against *H. influenzae,* and the advanced-generation macrolides, azithromycin and clarithromycin, are better tolerated.
[d]Many isolates of *S. pneumoniae* are resistant to tetracycline, and it should be used only if the patient is allergic to or intolerant of macrolides.
[e]In no particular order.
[f]High-dose amoxicillin is 1 g every 8 hour; if a macrolide is used, erythromycin does not provide coverage of *H. influenzae,* and thus when amoxicillin is used, the addition of doxycycline or of an advanced-generation macrolide is required to provide adequate coverage of *H. influenzae.*
[g]In roughly one third to one half of the cases no etiology was identified.
[h]Antipseudomonal agents such as cefepime, piperacillin-tazobactam, imipenem, and meropenem are generally active against DRSP, but not recommended for routine use in this population that does not have risk factors for *P. aeruginosa.*
[i]Use of doxycycline or an advanced-generation macrolide (azithromycin or clarithromycin) will provide adequate coverage if the selected β-lactam is susceptible to bacterial β-lactamases.
[j]Combination therapy required.
[k]If β-lactam allergic, replace the listed β-lactam with aztreonam and combine with an aminoglycoside and an antipneumococcal fluoroquinolone as listed.

for drug-resistant *S. pneumoniae* or gram-negative bacteria). Group III includes inpatients not in the ICU, and group IV includes inpatients admitted to the ICU.[2]

Monotherapy generally is adequate treatment for outpatients with pneumonia but without co-morbid illness or modifying factors. Traditionally erythromycin was the most widely recommended antibiotic for this group of individuals. The most common pathogens in this group include *S. pneumoniae, M. pneumoniae,* respiratory viruses, *C. pneumoniae,* and *H. influenzae.* Other identified pathogens, including *Legionella* organisms, *Mycobacterium tuberculosis,* and endemic fungi, cause pneumonia to a lesser extent. The macrolide antibiotics, including erythromycin, azithromycin, and clarithromycin, are commonly used to treat this group. The ATS recommends an advanced-generation macrolide such as azithromycin or clarithromycin; both of these cover the expected organisms infecting group I. The ATS reports that the use of macrolides or doxycycline constitutes level III evidence, which includes case studies and expert opinion. The studies include in vitro antibiotic susceptibility. Erythromycin was dropped as a recommended treatment because of its lack of activity against *H. influenzae,* which often infects cigarette smokers. However, it remains a reasonable choice if cost or availability is a factor and the patient is not likely to be infected with *H. influenzae.* Azithromycin resistance may become a concern, in which case clarithromycin may be preferred in the treatment of CAP.

Doxycycline, a second antibiotic choice, offers predictable coverage against the atypical pathogens and *H. influenzae.* However, doxycycline is less likely to cover drug-resistant *S. pneumoniae,* which is an unlikely pathogen in this group. Doxycycline is inexpensive, offers twice-daily dosing, and has few gastrointestinal side effects.

Group II includes outpatients with cardiopulmonary diseases (congestive heart failure and COPD) or risk factors for drug-resistant *S. pneumoniae,* which include an age older than 65 years and nursing home residence. The pathogens are changed, but pneumococci remain the most likely cause of pneumonia for this group, especially pneumococci that are resistant to penicillin. Other organisms include *E. coli, Klebsiella* spp., and *P. aeruginosa.* Aspiration with anaerobes should be considered if there is poor dentition, neurologic illness, or impaired consciousness. Recommended initial therapy includes β-lactam drugs (penicillins and cephalosporins) as outlined in Table 118-2, with the addition of a macrolide or doxycycline. Second-line therapy could be monotherapy with an antipneumococcal fluoroquinolone; these include levofloxacin, moxifloxacin, and gatifloxacin. These recommendations from the ATS constitute level II evidence, which is supported by well-designed, controlled trials without randomization (including cohort, patient series, and case control studies).[2] Groups III and IV are not discussed here but are included to complete the recommendations by the ATS. A treatment algorithm is provided (Figure 118-1).

The duration of therapy is usually 7 to 14 days, depending on the severity of the illness, co-morbid illness, and resolution of the illness. The long half-life of azithromycin allows for a shorter duration of therapy, usually 5 days. Recent studies

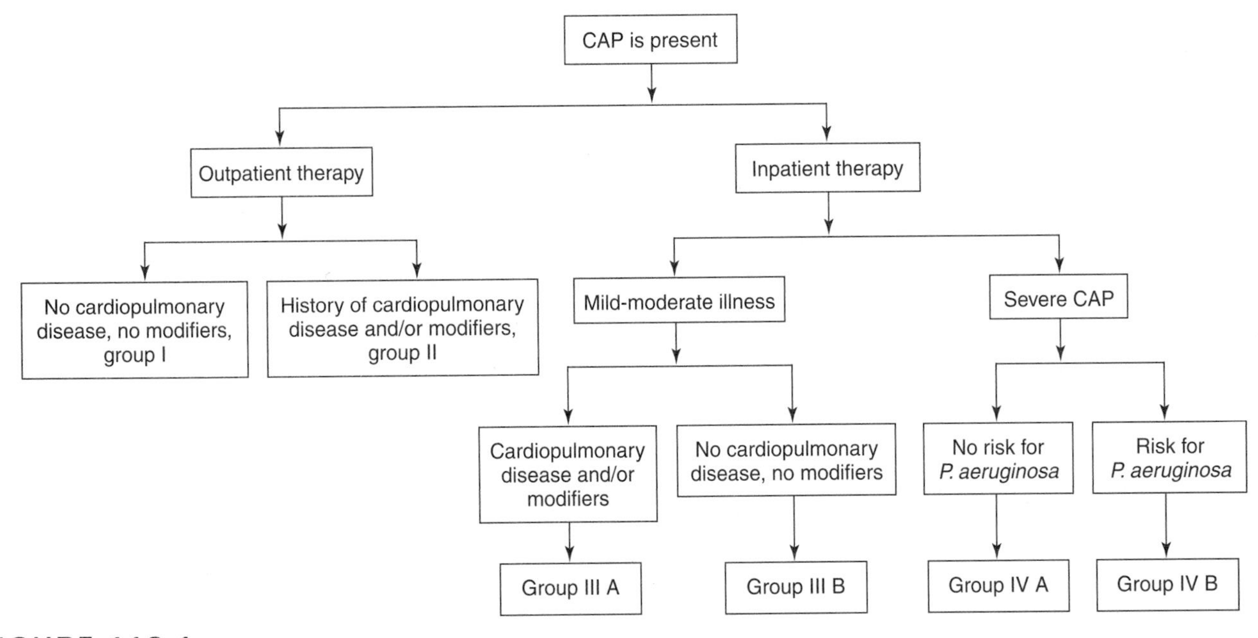

FIGURE 118-1

Treatment algorithm for pneumonia. For an explanation of group numbers, see Table 118-2. *CAP,* Community-acquired pneumonia. (From Niederman MS, Mandell LA, Anzueto A, and others: Guidelines for the management of adults with community-acquired pneumonia: diagnosis, assessment of severity, antimicrobial therapy and prevention, *Am J Respir Crit Care Med* 163:1730-1754, 2001.)

also support the use of higher-dose (750 mg) daily dosing of levofloxacin for shorter (5 days) treatment periods. In the immunocompromised patient, in general 50% additional time is needed for antibiotic therapy. Suspected mycoplasmal or chlamydial pneumonia requires 10 to 14 days. Infection with *Legionella* organisms, which takes the longest to resolve of all the CAPs, requires 14 or more days of antibiotic therapy.[2,7,9,11]

In addition, several new antibiotics are now available for treating CAP. Gemifloxacin is the newest in the class of fluoroquinolones and is active against gram-positive cocci, particularly streptococci, and against many anaerobes. Gemifloxacin is the most potent fluoroquinolone against drug-resistant *S. pneumoniae* and at this point is the least likely to be affected by resistant strains. Telithromycin is the first ketolide, a semisynthetic antibiotic, designed to overcome macrolide resistance in gram-positive cocci, particularly *S. pneumoniae*. The most significant advantage with telithromycin is its enhanced activity against macrolide-sensitive and macrolide-resistant *S. pneumoniae*. Its activity is similar or slightly increased compared with that of the macrolides against atypical organisms, such as *M. pneumoniae, C. pneumoniae,* and *L. pneumophila*. Finally, ertapenem is a β-lactam and a member of the carbapenem class of antibiotics. It has a relatively long half-life and broad spectrum of activity, which increases its effectiveness in patients with polymicrobial infections or patients with CAP who have been hospitalized.[15] Appropriate treatment for CA-MRSA includes vancomycin and linezolid and possibly trimethoprim-sulfamethoxazole and clindamycin. It has yet to be determined whether the addition of rifampin makes a difference. Linezolid is the first of a new class of antibiotics called the *oxazolidinones*. It is active against many gram-positive pathogens, including CA-MRSA, anaerobes, vancomycin-resistant enterococcus, and penicillin-resistant *S. pneumoniae*. The main concern with CA-MRSA is the necrotizing aspect of the infection. Many of the treatment options mentioned above have not yet been shown to decrease toxin production. Therefore linezolid may be the best choice.[15]

Older adults and those with co-existing illness are at increased risk of developing more virulent pneumonia, have longer healing times, need more supportive treatment, and require closer follow-up monitoring, especially with delayed resolution of pneumonia. Younger individuals without comorbid disease who are infected with pneumonia usually respond more quickly and have fewer complications.

With the increased prevalence of HIV/AIDS, the possibility of compromised immune function must be considered when there is delayed resolution of pneumonia or when a young individual seems to be more ill than would be expected with preserved immune function. A common cause of pneumonia in the patient with AIDS is *P. carinii,* which should be suspected despite the use of prophylactic antibiotic treatment before the onset of symptoms. Other common pathogens to consider include *S. pneumoniae, H. influenzae,* cytomegalovirus, and *M. tuberculosis*.

The choice of antibiotic therapy depends on careful consideration of the cost, the consequences of failing to respond to initial outpatient treatment and the need for hospitalization. Additional concerns include the likelihood of adherence to the treatment regimen, the existence of a supportive home environment, access to emergency department care if needed, the presence of an involved individual to identify significant changes in this illness should they occur, and the opportunity for follow-up in 24 to 48 hours.

Physician consultation is recommended for patients with oxygen saturation of less than 90% on room air, rigors, change in mental status, extremely abnormal vital signs, or co-morbid disease (e.g., diabetes, HIV, cancer, or COPD).

COMPLICATIONS

With minimum diagnostic testing and empiric antibiotic treatment, most patients will improve and show resolution of pneumonia. In most cases improvement is seen within 48 to 72 hours after initiation of antibiotics. Pneumonia that fails to resolve shows little clinical improvement after 4 weeks of therapy. Fever, cough, sputum production, and shortness of breath may still be present. CXR films also do not show improvement within this time frame.

When there is poor response to therapy, possibly the initial antibiotic choice was not correct, there was poor adherence to the oral antibiotic therapy, or the diagnosis of pneumonia was not accurate. Considerations should include the possibility of opportunistic fungal infections, *P. carinii*, tuberculosis, bronchogenic carcinoma, Wegener's granulomatosis, bronchiolitis obliterans with organizing pneumonia, and congestive heart failure. A diagnostic bronchoscopy, CT scan, and transthoracic needle aspiration and biopsy may be warranted to exclude these. If the diagnosis is still undetermined and there is no resolution, an open lung biopsy may be considered, and consultation with a pulmonologist is clearly warranted. Other complications of pneumonia include abscess, empyema, pulmonary vascular congestion, and pulmonary embolism.

INDICATIONS FOR REFERRAL OR HOSPITALIZATION

Delayed resolution of pneumonia and inpatient treatment generally require consultation. Pneumonia is the leading cause of death resulting from an infectious agent and, overall, the sixth leading cause of death in the United States. Therefore it is imperative to recognize patients who are not candidates for outpatient therapy. Indications for hospital admission are discussed in a similar fashion throughout the literature. Certain clinical criteria observed in the patient warrant hospitalization (Box 118-2). However, the health care provider's clinical judgment always supersedes written recommendations.

PATIENT AND FAMILY EDUCATION

Once the diagnosis of pneumonia has been made, patient education should include directions for use of the antibiotic and information on potential untoward effects of the drug. Follow-up instructions, depending on the clinical situation, may include 24-hour telephone contact or follow-up in the office after 24 to 48 hours. This will improve adherence to the prescribed therapy, provide an opportunity to address side effects of drug therapy, and allow progress to be monitored. The need for hospitalization should be assessed throughout the course of the illness. Education should include instructions to drink plenty of fluids and to use an antipyretic to control fever and myalgias when needed. Use of cough medicines should be avoided because the cough reflex and sputum expectoration enhance removal of thick secretions. However, in the event of a constant, nonproductive cough, as found especially with mycoplasmal infection, a narcotic such as codeine at night allows for more restorative sleep.

BOX 118-2

INDICATIONS FOR HOSPITALIZATION

Severe abnormality in vital signs:
- Heart rate >125 beats per minute
- Systolic blood pressure <90 mm Hg
- Respiratory rate >30 breaths per minute

Altered mental status

Oxygen saturation by pulse oximetry <90% on room air

Suppurative pneumonia-related infection (empyema, septic arthritis, meningitis, endocarditis)

Severe electrolyte imbalance or metabolic abnormality not known to be chronic:
- Sodium <130 mEq/L
- Hematocrit <30%
- Absolute neutrophil count <1000/mm^3 or WBC count <5000/mm^3
- BUN >50 mg/dl
- Creatinine >2.5 mg/dl

Acute co-existent medical condition requiring hospital admission that is independent of pneumonia

Failure to respond to outpatient treatment within 48 to 72 hours

From Niederman MS, Bass JB, Campbell GD, and others: Guidelines for the initial management of adults with community-acquired pneumonia: diagnosis, assessment of severity, and initial antimicrobial therapy, *Am Rev Respir Dis* 148(5):1418-1426, 1993.

HEALTH PROMOTION

Patients at risk for pneumonia should receive the pneumonia vaccination and should also be encouraged to receive a flu shot each year. Avoiding smoke and contact with persons who have a respiratory infection also decreases the risk of pneumonia. Daily exercise and eating healthy foods high in vitamins, nutrients, and fiber should also be encouraged.

REFERENCES

1. Barlett J, Dowell S, Mandell L, and others: Practice guidelines for the management of community-acquired pneumonia in adults, *Clin Infect Dis* 31:347-382, 2000.
2. Niederman MS, Manell LA, Anzueto A, and others: Guidelines for the management of adults with community-acquired pneumonia: diagnosis, assessment of severity, antimicrobial therapy and prevention, *Am J Respir Crit Care Med* 163:1730-1754, 2001.
3. American Thoracic Society: Guidelines for the management of adults with hospital-acquired, ventilator-associated, and healthcare associated pneumonia, *Am J Respir Crit Care Med* 171:388-416, 2005.
4. Kasper DL, Braunwald E, Fauci A, and others: *Harrison's principles of internal medicine*, ed 16, New York, 2004, McGraw-Hill.
5. Donowitz G, Mandell G: Acute pneumonia. In Mandell G, Bennett J, Dolin R, editors: *Principles and practice of infectious disease*, ed 5, New York, 1995, Churchill Livingstone.
6. Hoyert DL, Kung HC, Smith BL: Deaths: preliminary data from 2003. Death and death rates for the 10 leading causes of death in the United States, preliminary report 2003, *National Vital Statistics Report* 53(15):1-48, 2005, retrieved Jan 17, 2007, from http://64.136.148.48/7pdfs/nvsr53_15.pdf.
7. Mandell L: Antibiotic therapy for community-acquired pneumonia, *Clin Chest Med* 20(3):589-598, 1999.
8. High K: Pneumonia in older adults, *Postgrad Med* 118(4):18-27, 2005.
9. Bartlett J, Dowell SF, Mandell LA, and others: Guidelines from the Infectious Disease Society of America: practice guidelines for the

management of community-acquired pneumonia in adults, *Clin Infect Dis* 31:347-382, 2000.
10. Lieberman D: Atypical pathogens in community acquired pneumonia, *Clin Chest Med* 20(3):489-498, 1999.
11. Cunha B, Segreti J, Yaamauchi T: Community-acquired pneumonia: new bugs, new drugs, *Patient Care* 30(5):142-162, 1996.
12. Cunha B: Community-acquired pneumonia, *Med Clin North Am* 84(1):43-77, 2001.
13. Fagon JY, Chastre J, Hance AJ, and others: Nosocomial pneumonia in ventilated patients: a cohort study evaluating attributable mortality and hospital stay, *Am J Med* 94(3):281-288, 1993.
14. Stringer JR, Beard CB, Miller RF, and others: A new name (*Pneumocystis jiroveci*) for pneumocystis from humans, *Emerg Infect Dis* 8(9), 2002, retrieved Jan 19, 2007, from http://0-www.cdc.gov.mill1.sjlibrary.org:80/ncidod/EID/vol8no9/02-0096.htm.
15. Mandell L: Update on community-acquired pneumonia, *Postgrad Med* 118(4):35-46, 2005.
16. Smith M, Derrington P, Evans R, and others: Rapid diagnosis of bacteremic pneumococcal infections by using the Binax NOW *Streptococcus pneumoniae* urinary antigen tests: a prospective controlled clinical evaluation, *J Clin Microbiol* 41(7):2810-2813, 2003.
17. Miskovitch-Riddle L, Keresztes P: CAP management guidelines, *Nurse Pract* 31(1):43-55, 2006.
18. Farber M: Managing community-acquired pneumonia, *Postgrad Med* 105(4):106-114, 1999.
19. Heffelfinger J, Dowell SF, Jorgensen JH, and others: Management of community-acquired pneumonia in the era of pneumococcal resistance, *Arch Intern Med* 160:1399-1408, 2000.
20. Holten KB, Onusko EM: Appropriate prescribing of oral beta-lactam antibiotics, *Am Fam Phys* 62(3):611-620, 2000.

WEBSITE RESOURCES

Alliance for the Prudent Use of Antibiotics: http://www.tufts.edu/med/apua/
American Society for Microbiology: http://www.asm.org
American Thoracic Society: *Guidelines for the management of adults with community acquired-pneumonia*, retrieved Aug 12, 2002, from http://www.thoracic.org/sections/publications/statements/pages/mtpi/commacq1-25.html
Centers for Disease Control and Prevention: http://www.cdc.gov/drugresistance/
Infectious Disease Society of America: http://www.idsociety.org
Johns Hopkins ABX Guide: http://www.hopkins-abxguide.org
US Food and Drug Administration Center for Drug Evaluation and Research: http://www.fda.gov/cder

CHAPTER 119

Pneumothorax

Updated by Carol A. Whelan

DEFINITION AND EPIDEMIOLOGY

Pneumothorax is defined as the presence of air in the pleural space. It is caused by a variety of conditions, including disease processes and trauma. A spontaneous pneumothorax is one that occurs in the absence of thoracic trauma, and a primary spontaneous pneumothorax (PSP) occurs in the absence of either trauma or disease. A secondary spontaneous pneumothorax occurs in the presence of underlying lung disease, but in the absence of trauma.[1] A tension pneumothorax is one in which there is positive pressure in the pleural space throughout the respiratory cycle, and a traumatic pneumothorax results from trauma.[1]

The most common cause of PSP is spontaneous rupture of pleural apical blebs, lying in or just under the visceral pleura. PSP occurs most frequently in tall, thin, healthy men 30 to 40 years of age.[2] More than 90% of patients with PSP are smokers or ex-smokers. The incidence of PSP is 7.4 per 100,000 men and 1.2 per 100,000 women, for a total of 20,000 cases per year.[3] Secondary pneumothorax occurs in middle-aged adults and can result from chronic obstructive pulmonary disease,[1] systemic lupus erythematosus, sarcoidosis, emphysema, asthma, cystic fibrosis, and other pulmonary diseases.[2-5] Both penetrating and nonpenetrating trauma can cause traumatic pneumothorax and may occur at any age. There also are numerous iatrogenic causes, including the insertion of central lines or barotrauma related to surgery or resuscitation efforts. Tension pneumothorax results most frequently from mechanical ventilation or CPR. Tension pneumothorax is a medical emergency requiring immediate intervention, since the pressure is transferred to the mediastinum and results in decreased cardiac output and severely compromised ventilation.[1] Pneumothoraces have also occurred during pregnancy, labor, and the postpartum period. Approximately half of affected pregnant women have a previous respiratory infection, asthma, or previous pneumothorax.[6]

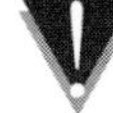

Immediate emergency department referral or physician consultation is indicated for patients with respiratory compromise.

PATHOPHYSIOLOGY

The loss of negative pressure when air enters the pleural space causes the lung or a portion of it to collapse. Air in the pleural space may occur spontaneously or may be caused by trauma, a ruptured bleb, or gas generated by microorganisms in empyema.

CLINICAL PRESENTATION

Although some patients with pneumothorax may be asymptomatic, the most common complaint is an acute onset of dyspnea, pain, and cough. The pain is sharp and is exacerbated by any type of movement. The pertinent history should include history of previous pneumothorax, trauma, or smoking; current medications; allergies; history of strenuous exercise; and other medical conditions.

PHYSICAL EXAMINATION

The physical findings depend on the size and nature of the pneumothorax. A tension or large pneumothorax is a medical emergency. Acute respiratory distress, diaphoresis, tachycardia, hypoxemia, tachypnea, tracheal deviation, cyanosis, neck vein distention, extreme anxiety, and impending cardiopulmonary arrest are unmistakable.[7] A smaller pneumothorax may cause dyspnea and discomfort, or the patient may be asymptomatic. Asymmetric chest excursion, absent breath sounds, and decreased tactile fremitus and hyperresonance on the affected side may be evident but depend on the size of the pneumothorax.

DIAGNOSTICS

Pulse oximetry should be determined. Chest x-ray studies, including anteroposterior and lateral views, are required. Expiratory or lateral decubitus films may be necessary to verify a small pneumothorax. A CT scan may be helpful in some cases.[6] Arterial blood gases, if available, should be obtained. Thoracoscopy also may be indicated.[4]

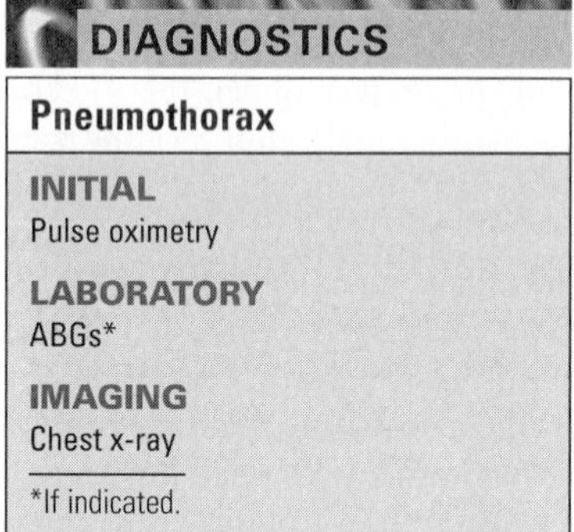

DIAGNOSTICS

Pneumothorax

INITIAL
Pulse oximetry

LABORATORY
ABGs*

IMAGING
Chest x-ray

*If indicated.

DIFFERENNTIAL DIAGNOSIS

Dyspnea and chest pain are identified with a large number of clinical problems. A history of lung diseases (e.g., emphysema, cancer, or a rare condition such as Marfan's syndrome) is important to note. Many pneumothoraces occur as a result of trauma, and therefore rib fractures, contusions, costochondral separation, and muscle strains need to be excluded. Other differential diagnoses to consider include pulmonary embolism, myocardial infarction, dissecting aortic aneurysm, pleurisy, pericarditis, and costochondritis. It is useful to remember that half of all patients with PSP have at least one recurrence.[1]

DIFFERENTIAL DIAGNOSIS

Pneumothorax

- Lung disease
- Trauma—blunt (contusion) or penetrating (fractured ribs)
- Pulmonary embolism
- Myocardial infarction
- Pericarditis
- Pleurisy
- Muscle strain, costochondritis
- Dissecting aortic aneurysm
- Diaphragmatic hernia

MANAGEMENT

A tension pneumothorax requires immediate intervention. To prevent death, a 16-gauge or larger-bore needle should be inserted into the pleural space at the midclavicular line of the second intercostal space on the affected side. Air is released immediately, but the needle must be left in place until a chest tube can be inserted.

No treatment is needed if the pneumothorax is small (<20% of the hemithorax) and the patient is asymptomatic. Spontaneous resolution occurs in 7 to 14 days.[8] Chest tube placement is vital in patients with symptoms; these patients should be referred for emergency care. The chest tube is left in place until the leak seals, which is usually 2 to 4 days. Ventilatory support is indicated in some cases.[2] Patients used to require a long hospital stay for pneumothorax treated with an indwelling chest tube. However, patients with chest tubes have recently been successfully managed on an outpatient basis. Options to prevent recurrences include the instillation of chemical sclerosing agents such as talc, doxycycline, tetracycline, or minocycline through a chest tube or thoracoscope; laser therapy; pleural abrasion; or thoracotomy.[2]

Secondary spontaneous pneumothorax usually requires more aggressive management because of the decreased reserve in patients with underlying disease. These patients should almost always be hospitalized for definitive treatment such as sclerosing therapy.[1]

LIFE SPAN CONSIDERATIONS

The frequency of recurrence is as high as 30% to 50%,[1,3] of which the complications may be more severe if there is concomitant respiratory or cardiac disease, especially chronic diseases that worsen with age. Efforts should be made to minimize and treat all possible exacerbating and complicating factors.

COMPLICATIONS

A large pneumothorax causes cardiac and ventilatory compromise, which may result in death. Chest tube placement can lead to numerous complications, including pulmonary edema, lung infarction, infection, trauma, bleeding, and subcutaneous emphysema.

INDICATIONS FOR REFERRAL OR HOSPITALIZATION

A patient with a large pneumothorax requires hospitalization for chest tube placement and resolution. Patients with secondary spontaneous pneumothorax and tension pneumothorax almost always require hospitalization, as do patients with respiratory compromise. Patients with PSP should be referred to a pulmonologist because the large (50%) incidence of recurrence and the possibility of subclinical lung disease. All patients with pneumothorax (other than simple traumatic) warrant evaluation by a pulmonologist both to rule out underlying lung disease and to define clinical management.

PATIENT AND FAMILY EDUCATION

Patient education should center on information regarding the cause, prevention, and treatment of a pneumothorax. Patients also need education regarding the care of chest tubes. If genetic testing is performed, patients and families need specific information and support.

Smoking cessation is an important educational issue with any lung problem and is an issue for patients with a pneumothorax, whatever the cause. If the patient has frequent, spontaneous recurrences, education regarding the importance of emergency care is necessary. Patients need to be cautioned against scuba diving and traveling to high altitudes. Health promotion is aimed primarily at the elimination of smoking in those at risk and the prevention of trauma.

REFERENCES

1. Kasper DL, Braunwald E, Fauci A, and others: *Harrison's principles of internal medicine,* ed 16, New York, 2005, McGraw-Hill.
2. Baum GL, and others: Diseases of the pleura and pleural space. In Baum GL, Crapo JD, Celli BR, and others, editors: *Textbook of pulmonary diseases*, ed 6, Philadelphia, 1998, Lippincott-Raven.
3. Fraser RS, and others: Pneumothorax. In Fraser RS, Muller NL, Colman N, and others: *Fraser and Pare's diagnosis of diseases of the chest,* ed 4, vol 4, Philadelphia, 1999, Saunders.
4. Baumann MH, Strange C, Heffner JE, and others: Management of spontaneous pneumothorax: an American College of Chest Physicians Delphi consensus statement, *Chest* 119(25):590-600, 2001.
5. Sood N, Paradowski LJ, Yankaskas JR: Outcomes of intensive care unit care in adults with cystic fibrosis, *Am J Respir Crit Care Med* 163:335-338, 2001.
6. Wallach SL: Spontaneous pneumothorax, *N Engl J Med* 343(4):300-301, 2000.
7. Golden PA: Thoracic trauma, *Orthoped Nurse* 19(5):37-46, 2000.
8. Richardson C, Baldwin D: Diagnosing acute shortness of breath in adult patients, *Practitioner* 244(5):478-482, 2000.

CHAPTER 120

Pulmonary Hypertension

Updated by Carol A. Whelan

DEFINITION AND EPIDEMIOLOGY

Pulmonary hypertension (PH) occurs when the pulmonary arterial (PA) pressure is inappropriately high for a given level of blood flow through the lungs.[1] In addition to sustained elevations of PA pressure, PH is characterized by right-sided heart failure, progressive dyspnea, and associated functional limitations.[2] The clinical definition is PA pressure of more than 25 mm Hg at rest or more than 30 mm Hg with exercise.[1,3] The causes of PH are diverse and may reflect increased filling pressures on the left side of the heart, increased pulmonary vascular resistance, or a combination of these factors. PH is usually a marker of advanced disease, regardless of the cause.

PH can be classified by etiology (primary or secondary) or by level of functional impairment (using the New York Heart Association [NYHA] classes I to IV). However, primary pulmonary hypertension (PPH) is clinically indistinguishable from PH by underlying causes, such as collagen vascular diseases, HIV infection, liver disease, drugs, and toxins.[2]

PPH is a rare clinical syndrome of PH that progresses rapidly to right ventricular failure and death.[1,3] The incidence of this process is small: 1 to 2 persons per 1 million worldwide.[3] PPH is generally considered to be a disease of younger people, with the greatest incidence between the ages of 20 and 45. PPH has been reported in older adults but is difficult to diagnosis because of the increased incidence of heart or lung diseases. In the PPH Registry, the ratio of women to men is 7:1, regardless of age at diagnosis.[1]

Secondary PH is defined as an increase within the pulmonary vascular bed attributable to an underlying disease. This increase may be due to hypoxia, hypertension, chronic obstructive pulmonary disease (COPD), mechanical obstruction of the pulmonary arteries, ischemic heart disease, valvular heart disease, or various other causes. The differential diagnosis of PH and its underlying cause is essential to facilitate treatment.

PATHOPHYSIOLOGY

A number of different conditions cause PH, which develops when flow or resistance to flow across the pulmonary vascular bed increases. During exercise, cardiac output increases three to fivefold, and the increased pulmonary blood flow raises the PA pressure. In a healthy person the vasculature accommodates the increase in flow through the distention of vessels. The increase in flow during exercise is usually temporary. However, with certain clinical conditions (lung disease, valvular heart disease, etc.), the increase in flow is sustained, which leads to a thickening of the vessels. When this remodeling of the vasculature occurs, PH may develop and may in fact seem out of proportion to the original disease.

Increased blood viscosity and decreased vessel radius may also increase vascular resistance. Causes include vessel destruction as seen in COPD, pulmonary fibrosis, or pulmonary embolus.[4]

The most common cause of increased pulmonary vascular resistance associated with chronic respiratory disease is hypoxia, which causes vasoconstriction, thickening of the vascular media (remodeling), and polycythemia.[4] The mechanisms responsible for hypoxic pulmonary vasoconstriction remain undefined, even after years of intensive study.[4] The cause of sustained PH is multifactorial, regardless of the original insult.[1] The variety of pathologic changes has given rise to a variety of treatment modalities.[4-6]

Recommendations include classifying PH into five categories that share pathogenesis and treatment paradigms: (1) pulmonary arterial hypertension (PAH), including idiopathic PAH associated with collagen vascular disease, congenital heart disease, portal hypertension, HIV infection, anorexiants, and others; (2) PH associated with left-sided heart and valvular disease; (3) PH associated with lung disease or hypoxemia such as COPD and sleep apnea; (4) central or distal thromboembolism; and (5) miscellaneous causes, including sarcoid and external compression, such as tumor.[7]

CLINICAL PRESENTATION

Patients are generally asymptomatic until the condition becomes severe. Sixty percent of patients are initially seen with dyspnea. Other associated symptoms include fatigue, angina, syncope, cough, hemoptysis, Raynaud's phenomenon, edema, and decreased exercise tolerance. Symptoms are insidious, and the average time for the onset of symptoms and diagnosis is 2 years.[1] A careful history is important because many conditions and some diet medications have been associated with PH.

PHYSICAL EXAMINATION

Physical findings initially may be subtle. Findings include a loud second heart sound (pulmonic component), decreased carotid pulse, evidence of right ventricular dilation (lifts or heaves), a murmur of tricuspid regurgitation, or pulmonic insufficiency. Signs of right ventricular failure with jugular vein distention, a loud S_3 on inspiration, cor pulmonale, increased liver size, ascites, and edema are signs of advanced disease. Lung fields are generally clear.

DIAGNOSTICS

A variety of noninvasive and invasive studies are necessary to evaluate PH. ECG changes include signs of right ventricular hypertrophy (an S wave in lead I and a Q wave and an inverted T wave in lead III may be the first changes; however, when these are seen, the condition is usually advanced). ECG changes suggestive of pulmonary embolism are the same as those in right ventricular hypertrophy and occur acutely. Chronic right ventricular pressure results in right-axis deviation and an R wave–to–S wave ratio of more than 1 in lead V_1.[1]

Chest x-ray examination may reveal pulmonary arteries that are increased in size. Although hypoxemia is a common finding, pulmonary function tests may demonstrate normal or only minimally restrictive elements. Arterial blood gases, ventilation/perfusion studies (to rule out an embolus), Doppler studies, and echocardiography are helpful, as are radionuclear diagnostics and CT or MRI. A typical blood gas study will show hypoxia and respiratory alkalosis. In certain cases a lung biopsy may be necessary to exclude interstitial lung disease.[1] Exercise studies may also be useful to evaluate response to treatment.[8] Pulmonary capillary wedge pressures are calculated during cardiac catheterization and are necessary for a definitive diagnosis. Serologic studies to screen for connective tissue diseases may also be indicated.[1] Brain natriuretic peptide (BNP) is recommended for patients with known pulmonary artery hypertension to aid in monitoring progress.[9]

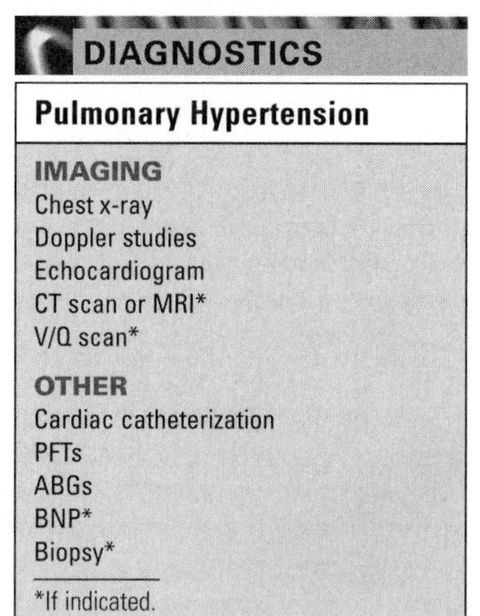

DIAGNOSTICS

Pulmonary Hypertension

IMAGING
Chest x-ray
Doppler studies
Echocardiogram
CT scan or MRI*
V/Q scan*

OTHER
Cardiac catheterization
PFTs
ABGs
BNP*
Biopsy*

*If indicated.

DIFFERENTIAL DIAGNOSIS

Although the diagnosis of PH is made simply by a measurement of PA pressure, the differential diagnosis of the underlying cause of the increased pressure is of utmost importance to identify the underlying problem and ensure proper treatment. Since PPH is a rare disease, diagnosis must be made by exclusion. The differential diagnosis includes restrictive, obstructive, and granulomatous lung disease; chronic liver disease; congenital, valvular, and myocardial heart disease; PA stenosis; pulmonary venous hypertension; thromboembolic disease; connective tissue disease (especially sarcoidosis); and sickle cell disease. Other causes to be considered include parasitic infection and IV drug use. Although rare in the United States, schistosomiasis is the leading cause of PH worldwide.[10]

DIFFERENTIAL DIAGNOSIS

Pulmonary Hypertension

- Restrictive lung disease
- Obstructive lung disease
- Sleep apnea
- Sickle cell disease
- Sarcoidosis
- Schistosomiasis
- Granulomatous lung disease
- Chronic liver disease
- Congenital heart disease
- Valvular heart disease
- Myocardial heart disease
- Pulmonary artery stenosis
- Pulmonary venous hypertension
- Thromboembolic disease
- Parasitic infection
- IV drug use
- Connective tissue disease
- Congenital heart disease (patent ductus arteriosus, ventricular septal defect)

MANAGEMENT

Recognition of the disease process is important for appropriate cardiac or pulmonary referral, particularly if an acute event such as pulmonary embolus is suspected. Oxygen therapy to maintain oxygen saturation greater than 92% aids in decreasing mortality.[11] Correction of acid-base imbalances, bronchodilation, treatment for emboli or mitral stenosis, antibiotics for infection, treatment for obstructive sleep apnea, and measures to improve left ventricular failure are all recommended.[1,5,12] Diuretics may help reduce right ventricular pressures and relieve peripheral edema, and digoxin can increase cardiac output. In PPH, anticoagulation is recommended to counteract thrombin deposition that occurs in the pulmonary circulation,[1,3,7,8,10,11]

Patients who respond with significant reductions in PA pressure to vasodilators at the time of cardiac catheterization are good candidates for high-dose calcium channel blockers, with doses twice the usual upper limit of normal being needed. Recent studies have shown that long-term therapy with prostacyclins is the optimum therapy for all patients with NYHA class III-IV disease status.[3,4,6,7,10] Epoprostenol (Flolan) is the best studied treatment of this class, with sustained improvement seen up to 10 years after initiation of treatment. Treatment is limited by the need for a permanent central venous catheter and an infusion pump, since the drug can only be given intravenously.[10] Aerosolized iloprost, a prostacyclin analog, may be an alternative therapy.[13]

Newer drugs are being developed, and the prostacyclin trepostinil is now U.S. Food and Drug Administration approved for PPH patients with NYHA class II-IV disease, who are unresponsive to conventional therapy. Trepostinil (Remodulin) improves survival and controls symptoms and does not require central venous access for administration, but it does need to be given subcutaneously via an infusion pump like those used for insulin administration.[13] Sildenafil is also being studied in the treatment of PH because of its mediation of nitric oxide, which lowers PA pressure.[10] In one small controlled study, sildenafil was efficacious in improving symptoms and exercise capacity in patients who received the medication vs. patients who received a placebo.[14] General treatment recommendations include regular physical activity, maintenance of ideal body weight, prevention of infection, avoidance of pregnancy, maintenance of adequate hemoglobin, oral anticoagulation, oxygenation, digoxin, diuretic with avoidance of orthostasis, and psychologic assistance.[7] Graded balloon dilation atrial septostomy may be indicated for patients with PPH that is unresponsive to vasodilator therapies.[11]

COMPLICATIONS

Complications of PH include the development of right and eventually left ventricular hypertrophy and death. PH is the most common cause of cor pulmonale, which is defined as right ventricular enlargement caused by pulmonary or cardiac disease.[10] Other complications include arrhythmias, both bradycardia and tachycardia; acute pulmonary embolism; pulmonary hemorrhage; and pneumonia. In addition to symptoms associated with PH such as dyspnea, other factors such as anxiety, depression, adverse effects of therapy, functional limitations, and social isolation may lead to impaired quality of life.[2] Most studies looking at the natural history of PH have focused on idiopathic PH (vs. PAH associated with another disease) and have found similar survival rates, including median survival of 2.8 years, with 1-year, 3-year, and 5-year survival rates of 68%, 48%, and 34%, respectively.[1,15] Hospitalization may be necessary for medication adjustment, monitoring, and imaging. The cause of death is usually right ventricular failure.[10]

INDICATIONS FOR REFERRAL OR HOSPITALIZATION

Because accurate diagnosis is crucial, referral to an appropriate specialist is recommended. Imaging, cardiac catheterization, pulmonary function testing, medication recommendations, and lung transplantation all require specialist referral.

PATIENT AND FAMILY EDUCATION

Patients with PH often require a tremendous amount of support from health care providers. Careful explanation of the disease process and the need for moderation during activity is important, since exercise may increase pulmonary vascular resistance and hypoxia. The side effects and adverse reactions of all medications should be carefully explained and understood by both patients and families.[3] The importance of a low-salt diet and the avoidance of over-the-counter medications (unless approved by the health care provider) should be stressed.[11]

For patients with end-stage PH, lung transplantation may be an option, although the waiting list for organ transplants is often long. Transplantation criteria include the patient's age, medical history, and overall condition at the time of transplantation. The risk management and complications of transplantation should be thoroughly explained.[4]

Although the incidence of familial PPH is approximately 6% of total cases of PPH (based on an NIH study done in the 1980s),[16] an estimated 300 new cases of PPH are diagnosed each year in the United States. Although this condition is inherited in an autosomal dominant pattern, most cases of PPH occur in individuals with no known family history.[17] Families need education and support if a genetic workup is chosen.

HEALTH PROMOTION

PPH is an uncommon disease process, occurring in approximately 1 to 2 per 1 million persons worldwide. The exact mechanisms of the disease are still undergoing study; however, the clinical course is deadly. Until recently patients and families had little hope for remission of this progressive disease.[3] Because secondary PH occurs as a complication of other disorders, such as COPD, sleep apnea, sickle cell crisis, connective tissue diseases, cardiac diseases, and thromboembolism, these disease processes must be monitored for the onset of complications. Lung diseases are the most common causes of PH, so the prevention of lung disease is a major challenge[3]; one of the major preventive measures for eliminating lung disease would be the prevention of smoking.

REFERENCES

1. Rounds S, Cutaia MV: Pulmonary hypertension: pathophysiology and clinical disorders. In Baum GL, Crapo JD, Celli BR, and others, editors: *Textbook of pulmonary medicine*, ed 6, Philadelphia, 1998, Lippincott-Raven.
2. Shafazand S, Doyle R, Gould M: Health-related quality of life in patients with pulmonary arterial hypertension, *Chest* 126:1452-1459, 2004.

3. Cheever KH, Kitzes B, Genther D: Epoprostenol therapy for primary pulmonary hypertension, *Crit Care Nurse* 19(4):20-27, 1999.
4. Russo-Magno PM, Hill NS: New approaches to pulmonary hypertension, *Hosp Pract* 36(3):29-32, 37-40, 2001.
5. Zhao L, Mason NA, Morrell NW, and others: Sildenafil inhibits hypoxia-induced pulmonary hypertension, *Circulation* 104(4):424-428, 2001.
6. Rich S: Medical treatment of pulmonary hypertension: a bridge to transplantation? *Am J Cardiol* 75:63A-66A, 1995.
7. Galie N, Torbicki A, Barst R, and others: Guidelines on diagnosis and treatment of pulmonary arterial hypertension: the Task Force on Diagnosis and Treatment of Pulmonary Arterial Hypertension of the European Society of Cardiology, *Eur Heart J* 25:2243-2278, 2004.
8. Sun XG, Hansen JE, Oudiz RJ, and others: Exercise pathophysiology in patients with primary pulmonary hypertension, *Circulation* 24(104):429-435, 2001.
9. Leuchte HH, Holzapfel M, Baumgartner RA, and others: Characterization of brain natriuretic peptide in long-term follow-up of pulmonary arterial hypertension, *Chest* 128(4):2368-2374, 2005.
10. Kasper DL, Braunwald E, Fauci A, and others: *Harrison's principles of internal medicine*, ed 16, New York, 2005, McGraw-Hill.
11. Berkowitz DS, Coyne NG: Understanding primary pulmonary hypertension, *Crit Care Nurse* 26(1):28-31, 2005.
12. Kessler R, Chaouat A, Schinkewitch P, and others: The obesity-hypoventilation syndrome revisited, *Chest* 120(2):369-376, 2001.
13. Leuchte HH, Schwaiblmair M, Baumgartner RA, and others: Hemodynamic response to sildenafil, nitric oxide, and iloprost in primary pulmonary hypertension, *Chest* 125(2):580-586, 2004.
14. Singh TP, Rohit M, Grover A, and others: A randomized, placebo-controlled, double-blind, crossover study to evaluate the efficacy of oral sildenafil therapy in severe pulmonary artery hypertension, *Am Heart J* 151(4):851, e1-5, 2006.
15. McLaughlin V, Doyle R, McCrory D: Prognosis of pulmonary hypertension, *Chest* 126:78S-92S, 2004.
16. Loscalzo J: Genetic clues to the cause of primary pulmonary hypertension, *N Engl J Med* 345(5):367-368, 2001.
17. Genetics Home Reference: *Primary pulmonary hypertension*, retrieved Dec 15, 2006, from http://ght.hlm.nih.gov/condition=primary pulmonaryhypertension.

CHAPTER 121 Sarcoidosis

Joanne Sandberg-Cook

DEFINITION AND EPIDEMIOLOGY

Sarcoidosis is a multisystem, inflammatory, granulomatous disease of unknown origin that commonly affects young and middle-aged adults. It involves the lungs and intrathoracic lymph nodes in more than 90% of affected patients, but it may essentially affect any organ (Table 121-1). More than 80% of patients are between 20 and 45 years of age; the disease is rare in children and older adults. The incidence may vary with geographic location. In Europe, the United Kingdom, Japan, and North America, incidence rates of 10 to 20 per 100,000 population have been cited. Reports of sarcoidosis appear to be rare in Africa, India, and Central and South America, probably because of the absence of mass screening programs and the presence of more common granulomatous diseases like tuberculosis.[1] No clear genetic basis has been established for sarcoidosis, but genetic factors may modulate its evolution and expression. Sarcoidosis is approximately four times more common in African Americans and is slightly more common in women; sporadic cases have been described in families.[2]

Physician consultation is indicated for all suspected cases of sarcoidosis.

PATHOPHYSIOLOGY

The characteristic pathologic feature of sarcoidosis is the non-caseating granuloma. The collection of macrophages and T cells that compose the granuloma release various chemokines and cytokines, including tumor necrosis factor-alpha.[2]

The granuloma is likely preceded by an alveolitis that involves the interstitium more than the alveolar spaces. Although the initial antigen is unknown, the alveolitis begins an accumulation of helper T lymphocyte (CD4) cells and

TABLE 121-1 Clinical Features of Sarcoidosis

Organ System	Symptoms or Presentation
Pulmonary	Dyspnea, cough, wheezing, chest pain
Upper airway	Dyspnea, nasal congestion, hoarseness, stridor, polyps
Dermatologic	Nodules, papules, plaques
Ocular	Photophobia, tearing, pain, decreased visual acuity, lacrimal gland enlargement, uveitis
Rheumatologic	Polyarthropathy, monoarthropathy, myopathy
Neurologic	Headache, hearing loss, paresthesias, seizures, cranial nerve palsy
Cardiologic	Syncope, dyspnea, arrhythmias, congestive heart failure, cardiac tamponade
Gastrointestinal	Dysphagia, abdominal pain, jaundice, hepatomegaly
Hematologic	Lymph node enlargement, hypersplenism
Renal	Kidney failure, calculi

macrophages. It is believed that activated macrophages may be responsible for the eventual development of fibrosis in some patients with sarcoidosis.

In the lung, granulomatous inflammation and fibrosis result in ventilation/perfusion imbalance and widening of the alveolar-arterial oxygen gradient. In the early stages, PaO_2 may be within the normal range at rest but decreases with exertion.

CLINICAL PRESENTATION AND PHYSICAL EXAMINATION

Sarcoidosis may affect almost any organ system and may appear in acute, subacute, or chronic form. Sarcoidosis is initially seen asymptomatically with an abnormal chest radiograph in approximately 50% of patients.[2] Patients who are symptomatic with this disorder have nonspecific features: dry cough, dyspnea, chest pain, fever, fatigue, anorexia, weight loss, and, occasionally, chills and night sweats. The nonspecificity of these symptoms delays diagnosis.[1] The symptoms and related organ involvement consistent with sarcoidosis are found in Table 121-1. Involvement of the upper airways and posterior pharynx may result in upper airway obstruction with worsening symptoms of dyspnea. Hoarseness and nasal obstruction may occur as a result of vocal cord and nasal mucosa granulomas (polyps). Hemoptysis is rarely seen; when present, it suggests mycetoma.

It is unusual to detect adventitious lung sounds on auscultation. Wheezing is occasionally audible in patients with advanced disease. Digital clubbing is rare. Dyspnea, dry cough, and chest pain occur commonly. Chest pain can be severe and difficult to distinguish from cardiac chest pain.[3]

Rheumatologic symptoms occur in 4% to 38% of patients with sarcoidosis.[4] These can manifest as an acute arthritis commonly involving the ankle, chronic polyarthritis, or myopathy.

Ocular lesions are seen in 20% of cases, with anterior uveitis seen most commonly. Symptoms may include redness, photophobia, and decreased visual acuity.[1] Other ocular lesions seen include posterior uveitis, retinal vasculitis, keratoconjunctivitis, and conjunctival follicles.[2]

Skin lesions are seen in 20% to 30% of cases. A maculopapular rash over the face and hairline is the most common subacute lesion.[2] Erythema nodosum is seen more commonly in women and, when seen in combination with hilar adenopathy, polyarthralgias, and fever, is referred to as Löfgren's syndrome.[3]

Clinical involvement of the central nervous system is unusual, but cranial nerve involvement can be seen. Asymptomatic granulomas can occur in any part of the female reproductive system, including the breast.

DIAGNOSTICS

Chest radiographs are abnormal in more than 90% of patients. In general, one of the following patterns is demonstrated: (1) bilateral hilar lymphadenopathy (BHL) (50% to 80% of cases), (2) parenchymal interstitial infiltrates (25% to 50%) with a predilection for upper- and mid-lung field distribution, or (3) both lymphadenopathy and interstitial disease. BHL is often the lesion that suggests the diagnosis of sarcoidosis.

Unless lymphadenopathy is present, the appearance of the chest radiograph may be indistinguishable from that of other interstitial lung disorders. Typically, radiographic lesions are bilateral and are distributed relatively symmetrically; asymmetric involvement is occasionally seen.

Staging systems based on the appearance of the chest radiograph have been in widespread use since 1957. The consensus now favors the following classification[3]:

Stage 0: Normal chest radiograph
Stage 1: BHL
Stage 2: BHL with pulmonary infiltrates
Stage 3: Pulmonary infiltrates without BHL
Stage 4: Pulmonary fibrosis

CT and high-resolution computed tomography (HRCT) of the chest are superior to a conventional chest x-ray study in defining the extent of parenchymal abnormalities in sarcoidosis. HRCT can help differentiate between reversible (mostly inflammatory) changes and irreversible (presumably fibrotic) alterations.

Hypergammaglobulinemia is seen in 30% to 80% of cases of sarcoidosis. Rheumatoid factor can be positive. The level of serum angiotensin-converting enzyme (ACE) is elevated in approximately 60% to 75% of patients with sarcoidosis; this level may be useful in following the course of the disease. Anemia occurs in 4% to 20% of patients.[3] Leukopenia, eosinophilia, and thrombocytopenia can be seen, although not commonly. The erythrocyte sedimentation rate is often elevated, but this can be a nonspecific finding. Hypercalcemia and hypercalciuria occasionally occur secondary to increased gastrointestinal absorption, abnormal vitamin D metabolism, and increased calcitriol production by sarcoid granulomas. Skin testing often reveals cutaneous anergy.

Pulmonary function tests may be normal or may reveal a restrictive pattern. This may be of most value in monitoring the course of the disease in individual cases. Radionuclide scanning reveals high uptake of gallium 67 (^{67}Ga) in pulmonary lesions of sarcoidosis. However, ^{67}Ga is also taken up by the lungs in patients with a large number of other diseases; therefore a high level of ^{67}Ga is not specific for sarcoidosis and not recommended as part of the routine evaluation.[2]

DIAGNOSTICS

Sarcoidosis

LABORATORY
CBC and differential
Electrolytes
Glucose
BUN
Creatinine
Calcium
Phosphorus
LFTs
ESR
Serum gamma globulin
Serum angiotensin-converting enzyme

IMAGING
Chest x-ray
CT scan

OTHER
PFTs
Bronchoscopy
Purified protein derivative

It is often reassuring to have a tissue diagnosis, and there are many techniques for this. The most specific location to biopsy for diagnosis is the lung. Bronchoscopy with transbronchial biopsies are positive in 50% to 60% of patients who do not have radiographic evidence of parenchymal disease. This positivity increases to 85% to 90% when there are radiographic abnormalities. A bronchoalveolar lavage performed at the time

DIFFERENTIAL DIAGNOSIS

Sarcoidosis

- Hypersensitivity pneumonitis
- Asbestosis
- Silicosis
- Infection, including tuberculosis, histoplasmosis, atypical mycobacterial infections, actinomycosis
- Malignancy: lymphoma
- Drug effects
- Vasculitis: Wegener's granulomatosis

of fiberoptic bronchoscopy retrieves inflammatory and immune effector cells from the lower respiratory tract that can also be diagnostic. Open lung biopsy via mediastinoscopy may yield tissue diagnosis where bronchoscopy has failed.[5] Biopsies can also be taken from other organ systems suspected to have sarcoid involvement (conjunctivae, skin, lymph nodes).

DIFFERENTIAL DIAGNOSIS

Many conditions can be seen with dyspnea, diffuse pulmonary infiltration, and granulomas. Hypersensitivity pneumonitis, asbestosis, silicosis, drug effects, bacterial or fungal infections, and malignancies should all be considered.

MANAGEMENT

The indications for treatment are not standardized, and there is no U.S. Food and Drug Administration–approved therapeutic agent. Response to therapy is variable. No treatment is recommended for asymptomatic patients with stage 1 or 2 disease. Those with fever or joint pains often respond to NSAIDs. Low-dose prednisone 15 to 20 mg/day may occasionally be needed to control symptoms that do not respond to NSAIDs. If symptoms of dyspnea or a cough develop, airway obstruction may be present and corticosteroid therapy is advisable. Oral corticosteroids are used cautiously with great respect for potential toxicity. In some cases inhaled corticosteroids may be effective.[2]

Patients with stage 2 disease who are symptomatic are treated with corticosteroids. Only observation is suggested for patients who are asymptomatic and have only mild impairment of lung function; treatment is needed for individuals who have progressive impairment of lung function. Patients with stage 3 or 4 sarcoidosis almost always require treatment with corticosteroids or another type of immunosuppressive treatment, but this is often unsatisfying. Sarcoidosis is very sensitive to corticosteroids. Typical regimens consist of a single daily dose of 20 to 40 mg of prednisone, which is gradually tapered over 6 months.[6] Some patients require a maintenance dosage of prednisone of approximately 10 to 15 mg/day, whereas others remain off prednisone indefinitely or for extended periods.

Alternatives to steroids are used for patients who develop severe side effects, do not respond to prednisone, or prefer not to take oral corticosteroids. Disease progression despite adequate corticosteroid therapy for longer than 1 year is also an indication for treatment with these agents.[6,7] Methotrexate, cyclophosphamide, and azathioprine have been used most extensively both as treatment and as steroid-sparing agents. All have shown modest efficacy in reducing symptoms. Thalidomide and chloroquine have also been used with modest effect.[7] The use of these agents is clearly valuable for selected patients, but there are no controlled studies of indications for use or efficacy. These agents along with antimalarial agents, including chloroquine and hydroxychloroquine, are also often used as the initial drug of choice in the treatment of chronic skin lesions from sarcoidosis. Recently studies have been conducted using infliximab, a tumor necrosis factor inhibitor, for patients who had failed to improve with first- or second-line therapies. In one study, 90% of patients treated with infliximab (N = 10) reported symptomatic improvement.[8] More and larger studies are required before recommending these drugs as part of the routine therapy for sarcoidosis.

LIFE SPAN CONSIDERATIONS

Sarcoidosis does not affect pregnancy but may flare after delivery. Sarcoidosis in children younger than age 15 showed the same organ distribution as in adults. The prognosis for children seems better than that for adults.[3] Patients older than 70 are more likely to be seen with systemic symptoms.[2]

COMPLICATIONS

Most complications of sarcoidosis, including osteoporosis, hyperglycemia, and gastric ulcers, occur as a result of corticosteroid therapy. Relapses are common and are determined by the reappearance of clinical signs and symptoms, chest radiograph abnormalities, and an elevated ACE level. In this situation a return to a previously high maintenance dose is sufficient to control recurrence.

Patients with sarcoidosis have demonstrated high levels of depression and stress as measured by health-related quality of life tests. This is likely because young people in the prime of their professional lives are most commonly affected by the disease or side effects of the medications. Those taking corticosteroids had lower scores than those who were not.[9]

INDICATIONS FOR REFERRAL OR HOSPITALIZATION

Sarcoidosis is a serious multisystem disease that requires physician consultation. Lung biopsies are usually necessary for diagnosis and require referral to a pulmonary specialist. If other biopsies are indicated, the appropriate specialist should be consulted. Therapy during the acute and chronic phases should be directed by the physician or specialist to ensure proper treatment. Hospitalization may be necessary for severe dyspnea and hypoxia or for severe cardiac dysfunction.

PATIENT AND FAMILY EDUCATION

The nature of the disease, including its varied presentation, must be carefully explained to patients. Medications, if indicated, and their side effects need to be discussed. It is important that patients understand the risk for worsening lung impairment or other organ damage if compliance with therapy is poor. It is important that patients be familiar with the clinical signs suggestive of possible recurrence of sarcoidosis.

REFERENCES

1. Aladesanmi O: Sarcoidosis: an update for the primary care physician, *Medscape* 6(1):e35, 2004, retrieved June 1, 2006, from http://www.medscape.com/viewarticle/470113.
2. King TE: *Overview of sarcoidosis*, retrieved June 1, 2006, from http://www.uptodate.com.
3. American Thoracic Society: Statement on sarcoidosis, *Am J Respir Crit Care Med* 160:736-755, 1999.
4. Abril A, Cohen M: Rheumatological manifestations of sarcoidosis, *Bull Rheum Dis* 49(3):2000, retrieved June 10, 2006, from http://www.arthritis.org/research/bulletin/vol.49/49_3.pdf.
5. Yanardag H, Caner M, Kaynak K, and others: Clinical value of mediastinoscopy in the diagnosis of sarcoidosis: an analysis of 68 cases, *Thorac Cardiovasc Surg* 54(3):198-201, 2006.
6. Shorr AF: *Corticosteroids for the treatment of chronic sarcoidosis: a pro-con debate, highlights of Chest 2003: 69th Annual Meeting of the American College of Chest Physicians,* retrieved June 10, 2006, from http://www.medscape.com/viewarticle/466526.
7. King TE: *Treatment of pulmonary sarcoidosis with alternatives to corticosteroids*, retrieved June 1, 2006, from http://www.uptodate.com.
8. Doty J, Mazur J, Judson M: Treatment of sarcoidosis with infliximab, *Chest* 127(3):1064-1071, 2005.
9. Cox C, Donahue J, Kataria Y, and others: Health related quality of life of persons with sarcoidosis, *Chest* 125:997-1004, 2004.

PART 11

Evaluation and Management of Cardiovascular Disorders

JOANN TRYBULSKI, *Section Editor*

CHAPTER 122

Cardiac Diagnostic Testing: Noninvasive Assessment of Coronary Artery Disease

Updated by Joanna D. Sikkema

DEFINITION AND EPIDEMIOLOGY

The accurate noninvasive assessment of the presence and severity of coronary artery disease (CAD) remains a major cause of concern for clinical practitioners. The current standard for noninvasive evaluation of CAD in patients with chest pain or with known CAD who see their health care provider for risk stratification is the exercise ECG, also called the *exercise tolerance test* (ETT). However, the exercise ECG has significant limitations in many patients, including those in whom the resting ECG is abnormal (Table 122-1) and those who are unable to exercise to an aerobic workload adequate to exclude provocable ischemia.

As a consequence of these and other limitations, it has become common to interface an imaging modality, such as myocardial perfusion imaging (MPI) or cardiac ultrasound, with the exercise ECG in an effort to improve the sensitivity and specificity of noninvasive CAD detection and thereby improve the ability to predict coronary heart disease. For patients who are at intermediate risk, either nuclear perfusion imaging or stress echocardiography is an acceptable choice.[1]

PATHOPHYSIOLOGY

To understand the application of exercise testing in patients with CAD, it is helpful to understand oxygen delivery to the myocardium. Unlike most other circulatory beds in the body, the coronary circulation allows for maximum oxygen extraction from the blood when the body is at rest. Increases in oxygen demand obligate an increase in myocardial blood flow. The healthy coronary circulation can increase flow approximately five times above the baseline level. The fundamental pathophysiology in CAD is a limitation of the ability of the coronary circulation to vasodilate appropriately. As a result, the ability to increase flow in the face of increased myocardial oxygen demand is limited.

In an ETT, patients are asked to perform incremental exercises based on standardized protocols. This results in positive chronotropic (rate) and inotropic (strength of contraction) stimulation of the cardiovascular system, which increases myocardial oxygen demand. The normal hemodynamic response to these stimuli is an increase in absolute coronary blood flow. However, this ability is reduced in the presence of CAD, which leads to an imbalance between oxygen supply and demand and results in myocardial ischemia.

EXERCISE TOLERANCE TEST

The standard first-line approach to provocative testing for CAD is the ETT, during which the patient (attached to a 12-lead ECG) is monitored continuously during graded exercise. The ECG response of normal hearts is maintenance of an "isoelectric" ST segment during exercise and recovery. By standard criteria, a positive test for CAD is defined by the development of horizontal or downsloping ST-segment depression of 1 mm measured 80 msec after the J point of the QRS complex (the junction between the QRS complex and the ST segment). ECG changes such as upsloping ST-segment depression or isolated T-wave changes have not demonstrated predictive value.

Because the interpretation of the test is based primarily on the development of characteristic ischemic ST-segment and T-wave changes, it is not surprising that resting ECG abnormalities can lead to a reduction in test sensitivity and specificity. The specificity of the routine ETT is reduced if the patient has had a prior myocardial infarction (MI) or if the patient has a resting bundle branch block conduction abnormality, since this produces persistent ST-segment and T-wave abnormalities.

A number of other factors can interfere with the sensitivity of the exercise test in detecting CAD. Because an increase in coronary blood flow is related to an increasing heart rate, clearly the sensitivity of the test is effort dependent. The standard is the peak heart rate achieved during exercise. Specifically, a test is considered negative for CAD only if the patient exercises to at least 85% of the age-predicted maximum heart rate without evidence of inducible ischemia (maximum heart rate = [220 − age]). If the patient fails to achieve this "target" heart rate, the test should be considered nondiagnostic, or insufficient to exclude ischemia. On the other hand, if there is evidence of ischemia (typical angina, ischemic ST changes) before the patient's target heart rate is reached, the test is considered strongly predictive of significant CAD. A second important predictor of more advanced CAD is exercise-induced hypotension (i.e., a fall in systolic blood pressure of at least 20 mm Hg at any point during exercise). It is helpful to correlate the ischemic leads on exercise ECG to the underlying coronary anatomy to roughly identify the culprit artery or arteries.

Medications such as beta blockers can attenuate the heart rate, making the rest of the exercise test less diagnostic. The decision to discontinue beta blockers 1 or 2 days before testing is influenced by the purpose of the exercise test. For ETTs ordered to detect angina, it is recommended that the cardiologist be consulted about withholding the medication before performing the test. ETTs performed to assess effectiveness of pharmacologic therapy require normal daily medication regimens. Imaging studies may be useful in patients who undergo a stress test during beta-blocker therapy.

Another potential contributor to the ETT's lack of sensitivity is derived from the limitations of the surface ECG related to the spatial distribution of the electrical abnormalities that occur in ischemia. This concept may be better understood if the ECG is considered as an imaging tool that examines the forces of cardiac depolarization and repolarization. To detect

TABLE 122-1 Exercise Testing Comparisons

Test	Benefits and Indications	Limitations
Treadmill exercise	Assesses ischemia, functional capacity, prognosis Equipment widely available Accuracy established in different populations	Sensitivity lower Poor specificity with females, resting ECG ST-T abnormalities, digoxin, LBBB, pacemakers No accuracy for site localization or extent of MI
Exercise myocardial perfusion imaging	Reproducible results Improved sensitivity and specificity over treadmill alone More accurately determines extent of CAD and prognosis Assesses myocardial viability	Increased cost Requires longer testing times Modest radiation exposure Specificity dependent on laboratory and image reading Artifacts from soft tissue (breast), diaphragm signal attenuation Requires additional equipment and personnel Low specificity with LBBB
Thallium	More extensive validation for detecting viable myocardium with rest-redistribution technique Assesses pulmonary uptake	
Sestamibi	Superior image with female or obese patients Measures left ventricular function	
Exercise radionuclide angiography	Well validated to identify patients with severe disease Risk stratification after MI Good images with obese or COPD patients Accurate information about ejection fractions	Limited availability and high expense Uses bicycle, not treadmill exercise Inaccurate when heart rate is irregular Reduced specificity with females, abnormal resting left ventricular function
Exercise echocardiography	Sensitivity and specificity comparable to those of exercise nuclear imaging Provides information on presence and extent of CAD Results immediately available Portable Less test time, lower cost than nuclear imaging Assesses multiple parameters: global and regional ventricular function, chamber size, wall thickness, valve function Accurate for diagnosis of CAD with resting ECG abnormalities, LBBB Detects left anterior descending coronary artery and multivessel disease	Interpretation nonstandardized and subjective Difficult to interpret with resting wall motion abnormalities Images possibly nondiagnostic because of poor image quality Prognostic potential uncertain because of a limited number of studies
Pharmacologic stress with dipyridamole or adenosine	Accurate assessments in patients unable to exercise Useful for preoperative risk assessment in patients with claudication or musculoskeletal limitations Relatively safe in selected patients (side effects rapidly reversible by ending infusion or administering aminophylline) More accurate than perfusion imaging in diagnosing CAD with LBBB	Cannot assess functional capacity ECG abnormalities less likely to occur than with exercise Contraindicated with hypotension, sick sinus syndrome, high-grade heart block, hyperreactive airways, oral dipyridamole therapy Must discontinue theophylline-containing medications for 72 hours and caffeine for 24 hours before testing Serial testing not possible to be used to assess therapy Possibility of dipyridamole inducing ischemia in 45% of patients with severe CAD Specificity reduced with right ventricular pacemakers
Dobutamine echocardiography	Accurate CAD assessments in patients unable to exercise Relatively safe in selected patients (side effects rapidly reversible by terminating infusion or administering a beta blocker) Detects threshold of myocardial ischemia Assesses myocardial viability More accurate than perfusion imaging in diagnosing CAD with LBBB	Cannot assess functional capacity ECG abnormalities less likely to occur than with exercise Contraindicated with hypotension, sick sinus syndrome, high-grade heart block, hyperreactive airways, oral dipyridamole therapy Must discontinue theophylline-containing medications for 72 hours and caffeine for 24 hours before testing Serial testing not possible to be used to assess therapy

Continued

TABLE 122-1 Exercise Testing Comparisons—cont'd

Test	Benefits and Indications	Limitations
Dobutamine echocardiography—cont'd	Establishes prognosis for LBBB, in absence of previous MI	Needs good echocardiographic windows Difficult with obese or COPD patients Requires extensive experience to read Labor intensive Can precipitate dangerous ventricular arrhythmias, especially with severe CAD, poor left ventricular function Contraindicated with aortic aneurysm

Data from Weiner DA: *Advantages and limitations of different exercise testing modalities,* retrieved Jan 9, 2002, from http://www.uptodate.com.
CAD, Coronary artery disease; *COPD,* chronic obstructive pulmonary disease; *LBBB,* left bundle branch block; *MI,* myocardial infarction.

ischemia, the repolarization phase of the cardiac cycle—the ST segment and T wave—is examined for abnormalities. ST-segment and T-wave changes in the surface ECG are related to both the extent and the severity of myocardial ischemia. As might be expected, the ETT is more sensitive for the detection of severe disease. Ischemia that is confined to the posterior and/or lateral segments of the left ventricle can be more difficult to detect.

Ischemic Cascade

Ischemic cascade can be described as follows:

Flow disturbance → Hypoperfusion → Diastolic dysfunction → Systolic dysfunction → ECG changes → Chest pain

The ST-segment and T-wave changes that are central to demonstrate ischemia on the ECG occur relatively late in the ischemic cascade.[2]

Imaging Adjuncts to the Exercise Tolerance Test

The various imaging modalities that can be used as adjuncts to the graded exercise test can be viewed in the context of the ischemic cascade. MPI is designed to detect the spatial distribution of myocardial blood flow (i.e., to define the regional heterogeneity of flow that characterizes regional ischemia). Cardiac ultrasound (two-dimensional echocardiography [2DE]) is designed to detect the abnormalities in regional wall motion that develop as a consequence of regional myocardial ischemia.

Examining the limitations of routine exercise testing from a historical perspective yields interesting information. The limitations detailed previously were clinically acceptable when the exercise study was performed principally as a binary diagnostic test (to determine whether CAD was present or absent) in patients with chest pain. The limited sensitivity of this test in a subgroup of patients with minimum CAD did not produce significant consequences. However, even with patients with minimum CAD, the use of the ETT did not yield significant answers about CAD status, primarily because these patients have a cardiovascular event rate of only 1% to 2% per year.

With the advent of effective coronary revascularization surgery, the ETT has assumed additional predictive clinical relevance. It is clear that powerful predictors of outcomes reside in clinical data and in ETT results independent of the ST-segment response, such as the hemodynamic response and the aerobic work capacity as reflected by exercise duration.

In contrast, the more recent expansion of interventional therapies to affect coronary revascularization has resulted in an important shift in the data that practitioners seek from provocative testing. For example, in patients with stable coronary syndromes, the judicious application of percutaneous coronary intervention requires that both the presence and territorial distribution of ischemia be defined. Further, in patients who have sustained prior myocardial injury, decisions regarding revascularization require a definition of ischemia both within and remote from the site of injury, as well as tissue viability within the zone of infarction.

It should also be emphasized that the usefulness of these adjunctive imaging modalities depends in part on the prevalence of disease in the patient population being studied. In general, these adjunctive modalities are most useful in patient populations with an intermediate pretest clinical probability of disease.

In the evaluation of patients with stable chest pain syndromes and normal surface ECGs, the conventional ETT typically provides adequate clinical information for diagnostic purposes. Similarly, in patients with known CAD and stable coronary syndromes, the ETT is typically adequate as a means of observing disease progression for purposes of prognostication and timing of revascularization procedures. However, with respect to the delineation of damaged myocardial regions and residual myocardial viability in zones of prior injury, it has become clear that adjunctive radiopharmaceutical and/or cardiac ultrasound imaging substantially improves test sensitivity and specificity (Box 122-1).

When considering ETT, health care providers should be aware of its relative contraindications. For these patients, consultation with a cardiologist is recommended. The following clinical alterations are relative contradictions to ETT: uncontrolled hypertension; significant ventricular arrhythmias; uncontrolled severe congestive heart failure; severe valvular heart disease consistent with aortic stenosis, mitral stenosis, or idiopathic hypertrophic subaortic stenosis; atrial fibrillation with an uncontrolled ventricular response; and a recent MI or unstable angina (may select modified testing 6 to 7 days after MI).

BOX 122-1

INDICATIONS FOR COUPLING NUCLEAR OR ULTRASOUND IMAGING TO STANDARD EXERCISE TOLERANCE TEST

- Left ventricular hypertrophy with ST-segment and T-wave abnormalities on resting ECG
- Abnormal baseline ST-segment and T-wave abnormalities on resting ECG for any reason
- Recent myocardial infarction, particularly with persistent rest ST-segment abnormalities
- Clinical use of digoxin
- Wolff-Parkinson-White syndrome
- Bundle branch block
- Ventricular pacemaker

MYOCARDIAL PERFUSION IMAGING

At present, thallium 201 chloride and technetium (Tc) 99m sestamibi are the radiopharmaceutical agents used for the detection of CAD in MPI. The distinctive properties of these two agents are well recognized. They appear comparable for CAD detection in patients with stable coronary syndromes; a number of sources have documented the clinical efficacy of sestamibi with thallium 201 chloride.[3-6]

Sestamibi imaging provides the capacity to "simultaneously" define left ventricular systolic function and myocardial perfusion. This offers a means to assess the impact of reperfusion therapies in patients with acute coronary syndromes.

The minimum redistribution of sestamibi, when combined with its protracted myocardial clearance (half life of approximately 5 hours), is well suited to the imaging of patients with acute coronary syndromes. Unlike thallium-based perfusion imaging, sestamibi image acquisition can be performed up to several hours after tracer injection. This allows for appropriate treatment and triage of patients with acute MI and unstable angina; the image acquired after such treatment will represent the status of myocardial perfusion at the time of tracer injection. Tracer injection can be repeated at a later time to assess myocardial salvage–residual viability in infarct patients or to define the presence, extent, and territorial distribution of ischemia in patients with unstable angina.

Researchers have found that sestamibi images performed in the emergency department may be useful in identifying low- vs. high-risk patients with suspected myocardial ischemia.[7] Furthermore, although MPI with thallium 201 chloride is typically coupled with exercise or pharmacologic stress, rest-redistribution imaging may provide valuable information in patients with unstable coronary syndromes, who are not suitable candidates for stress studies.

Because the diagnosis of perfusion defects requires the detection of decreased flow in one region relative to another, there will be occasional instances of false-negative scans in patients with severe three-vessel or left main CAD. These "balanced" flow disturbances (i.e., a decrease in coronary flow in more than two geographic territories) should be suspected in patients in whom clinical suspicion of severe CAD is high but whose MPI reveals uniform tracer uptake.

EXERCISE ECHOCARDIOGRAPHY

The practice of exercise echocardiography has expanded dramatically in recent years. Current data suggest that adjunctive echocardiographic imaging enhances the sensitivity and specificity of CAD detection to an extent comparable to that provided by nuclear techniques.[2] The 2DE evidence for ischemia includes an abnormal left ventricular ejection fraction (LVEF) response to exercise or the development of regional wall motion abnormalities.

As previously demonstrated in thallium imaging, the sensitivity of the 2DE technique for CAD detection is enhanced in patient subsets with multivessel CAD or prior MI. In addition, the sensitivity of exercise echocardiography is decreased in patients with resting wall motion abnormalities. In practical terms, patients in whom adequate ultrasound imaging views cannot be obtained (often including obese patients or those with severe emphysematous lung disease) should be considered for alternate imaging modalities.

COMPARISON OF MYOCARDIAL PERFUSION IMAGING WITH TWO-DIMENSIONAL ECHOCARDIOGRAPHY

Exercise 2DE with Doppler flow study is comparable to MPI for the detection of CAD. However, the respective modalities have relative strengths that merit comment. First, there is a greater accumulation of literature for MPI with respect to prognostication in patients with CAD. In addition, it appears that MPI may be preferable to 2DE for the recognition of incremental ischemia in myocardial regions characterized by abnormalities of resting wall motion. Further, quantification of myocardial perfusion data has been more extensively validated than comparable quantification of cardiac ultrasound; the latter technique has been limited by the technical difficulties attendant to endocardial border recognition. The majority of studies with exercise 2DE have been limited to qualitative visual assessment; it is also clear that the early 2DE data were acquired in patient groups with a relatively high incidence of significant CAD. Finally, MPI (e.g., rest-redistribution thallium 201 chloride scintigraphy and rest-injected Tc 99m sestamibi) is more amenable to the detection of ischemia in patients with unstable coronary syndromes in whom exercise is contraindicated. Serial rest 2DE images acquired in patients with unstable coronary syndromes may occasionally be useful if new or more extensive wall motion abnormalities can be detected during recurrent ischemia.

In contrast, 2DE offers access to the incremental information regarding left ventricular contractile performance that is analogous to that provided by exercise radionuclide ventriculography. LVEF response to exercise provides important prognostic information in patients with CAD; such information is available only inferentially by myocardial perfusion scintigraphy (i.e., pulmonary thallium uptake). Finally, with respect to viability assessment, it is to be emphasized that the detection of preserved contractile function in myocardial segments supplied by diseased coronary arteries is essential.

THREE-DIMENSIONAL AND DOPPLER FLOW ECHOCARDIOGRAPHY

Three-dimensional (3D) echocardiographic techniques are currently available that use MRI and computer-assisted 3D acquisition systems for 2DE. Three-dimensional technology is recently available and provides a unique view of structure and function within the heart. Current evidence-based guideline evaluations, however, center on 2DE with Doppler flow study.[8] Doppler flow studies are used to localize and quantify obstructions in the cardiovascular system. Primarily, the addition of a Doppler flow study to an echocardiogram enhances the ability to evaluate prosthetic valve function, detect and evaluate the blood shunting from a septal defect, and gauge the severity of valvular stenosis or regurgitation.[8]

CARDIAC MAGNETIC RESONANCE IMAGING AND ULTRAFAST COMPUTED TOMOGRAPHIC CARDIAC SCANS

Historically it has been difficult to image the moving structures of the heart and MRI has served as a less than reliable diagnostic tool. However, technology is rapidly advancing so that the MRI imaging techniques can present precise and detailed reflections of cardiac blood flow and tissue viability to assist with diagnosing CAD or the degree of damage from a heart attack. MRI has also been found to be useful in evaluating patients with a dissecting aortic aneurysm before surgery to determine the precise location and extent of dissection. Cardiac MRI is, with further technologic refinement, anticipated to provide accurate data to distinguish between stable and unstable plaque and to assist with quantifying CAD, replacing the diagnostic cardiac catheterization.[9]

Current investigations of 3D technology also involve ultrafast electron beam CT (EBCT). This emerging 3D technology performs a heart scan at a rapid rate, thus "freezing" cardiac motion. Coronary artery calcification is analyzed, and a total calcium score for a patient's coronary arteries is calculated based on the areas of calcification and the maximum CT calcium density.[10] Calcium generally does not appear in normal coronary arteries, so calcium deposits are determined to be a strong marker of atherosclerosis. However, EBCT does not define the location and extent of cardiac disease, and it does not image soft noncalcified plaque. A negative calcium score does not imply the presence of no plaque. With significant CAD (50% stenosis), only 2.5% of coronary segments have no detectable calcium on EBCT.[8] However, coronary calcium scoring has recently been proven to be accurate in predicting cardiovascular disease risk in apparently healthy middle-aged men in several studies.[11] EBCT scanning has also been found to be beneficial in motivating patients to adopt lifestyle changes and implement aggressive cardiovascular risk reduction strategies.

PHARMACOLOGIC STRESS TESTING

The clinical usefulness of adjunctive imaging modalities has been expanded by coupling such techniques to "pharmacologic" stress, an important advantage in patients who are unable to perform conventional treadmill or ergometer exercises. Pharmacologic agents currently in use are coronary vasodilators (e.g., dipyridamole [Persantine] and adenosine) or inotropic-chronotropic drugs (e.g., dobutamine).

The vasodilator drugs are applied to assess the effective coronary flow reserve (i.e., the ratio of maximum flow to basal flow). Because the extraction of tracer is proportional to blood flow, the coupling of vasodilators with MPI allows for the detection of regional flow disturbances. These regional perfusion abnormalities can be characterized as reversible (normal uptake at baseline, with decreased uptake after vasodilator) or fixed (indicative of prior infarction). The fact that vasodilators do not induce ischemia but simply unmask regional variations in flow reserve means that the ECG portion of the test will rarely demonstrate ischemic changes. However, on rare occasions ECG changes may be observed, and up to 20% of patients may experience angina. Ischemia may be caused by "coronary steal." The effects of dipyridamole can be reversed by IV aminophylline, and the effects of adenosine and dobutamine can be reversed by discontinuation of the infusion.

Another approach is to induce cardiac ischemia using a beta agonist such as dobutamine, which is administered in gradually increased doses until the goal heart rate is achieved (the provocation of ischemic chest pain or ST-segment changes may also lead to termination of the test). Dobutamine increases cardiac work, initially via an inotropic effect; a normal cardiac response to dobutamine is an increase in global left ventricular contractility. The chronotropic effects of this agent become apparent at higher infusion rates (20 to 50 mg/kg/min). Most commonly, inducible ischemia occurs at these higher infusion rates. Dobutamine is useful in patients who cannot tolerate the bronchoconstriction associated with adenosine administration.

As previously described, the development of regional wall motion abnormalities is often an early manifestation of ischemia. For this reason, dobutamine is most commonly coupled with 2DE (which is performed after each increase in dose) to determine regional abnormalities in left ventricular function or decreases in LVEF. The onset of new regional hypokinesis in a previously normally contracting segment is highly predictive of CAD in the artery supplying the dysfunctional segment. Alternatively, MPI can be coupled with dobutamine in patients with poor echocardiographic windows. The accuracies of dobutamine echocardiography and dobutamine MPI are comparable.

In a study by Sawada, Segar, Ryan, and others,[12] dobutamine echocardiography was shown to have comparable usefulness in patients with baseline normal wall motion (89% sensitivity and 85% specificity); however, the sensitivity was somewhat lower in patients with abnormal resting wall motion (81% sensitivity and 86% specificity). In another study, adenosine had similar sensitivity (86%) to dipyridamole when coupled with nuclear imaging but lower specificity (specificity 71% and accuracy 80%).[13] The poor performance of adenosine echocardiography (sensitivity 58%, specificity 87%, and accuracy 69%) underscores the importance of coupling vasodilators with perfusion imaging rather than with cardiac ultrasound, which requires the induction of ischemia to produce regional contractile dysfunction.

Another study found the sensitivity of dobutamine stress 2DE to be comparable to that of dobutamine single-photon emission CT (85% vs. 80%, respectively); the specificity of the two techniques was also comparable (82% vs. 74%, respectively), as were the predictive values.[13]

In summary, on the basis of these data, the following conclusions can be drawn:

- Vasodilator stress echocardiography is less sensitive for the detection of CAD than similar stress tests coupled with perfusion scintigraphy.
- Vasodilator stress echocardiography is less sensitive than exercise or dobutamine 2DE for disease detection.
- Vasodilator perfusion scintigraphy compares favorably with exercise–dobutamine scintigraphy or exercise–dobutamine 2DE with respect to CAD detection.

DIAGNOSTIC TESTING FOR CARDIOVASCULAR DISEASE IN WOMEN

Studies have documented the gender differences associated with cardiovascular disease.[14] Although cardiovascular disease is the leading cause of death in women, this disorder often is not diagnosed expeditiously. Unfortunately, studies investigating women and cardiovascular disease are limited. As a result, there is limited evidence to suggest the most appropriate cardiovascular diagnostic testing for women. To address this issue, the American Heart Association (AHA) reviewed existing studies and developed guidelines to aid primary care providers in choosing suitable diagnostic tests for women with suspected cardiovascular disease.[15]

All patients, even if asymptomatic, require risk stratification according to the Framingham risk score (low, intermediate, or high) to identify CAD risk equivalents.[15] At the present time, the American College of Cardiology (ACC)/AHA guidelines do not recommend stress tests for asymptomatic patients, unless the patient (men 45 years or older, women 55 years or older) is sedentary and wishes to begin exercising aggressively.[15] The exception is asymptomatic women with diabetes and peripheral arterial disease. These women are classified as high risk; diabetes and peripheral arterial disease are CAD risk equivalents. The recommendation for asymptomatic women with diabetes, peripheral vascular disease, and possible kidney disease is for secondary prevention strategies to prevent future cardiac events.[15]

For women who are symptomatic but who have a normal resting ECG, good exercise tolerance, and no coronary risk factors, an exercise stress test is appropriate; diagnostic imaging is not recommended for low-risk women who are asymptomatic.[15] For women who are symptomatic and have known CAD, an abnormal resting ECG, questionable exercise tolerance, or coronary risk factors (e.g., diabetes, peripheral arterial disease), stress test imaging is recommended.[15]

SUMMARY

The recognized limitations of the exercise ECG have resulted in the development of adjunctive, noninvasive imaging tests to evaluate patients with CAD. In particular, modalities that assess the contractile performance of the left ventricle and those which evaluate the status of regional myocardial perfusion have gained widespread application. Cardiac ultrasound and MPI are of comparable usefulness in detecting CAD. The data with respect to prognostication are most extensive for MPI techniques, but ultrasound-based prognostication data are accumulating.

Both functional studies and perfusion imaging have demonstrated clear usefulness in addressing the complex question of myocardial viability. These testing modalities are used to assess the presence of functional heart muscle in patients with ischemic heart disease and regional contractile dysfunction.

Although it is often inferred that ultrasound-based techniques and MPI techniques are competitive, it is clear that these modalities may in fact be complementary in the evaluation of selected patients with CAD. Recently, the ACC/AHA Task Force on Practice Guidelines suggested that exercise MPI or exercise echocardiography may be used as the initial test for diagnosis in patients with chronic stable angina who are able to exercise.[16] In addition, the ACC/AHA Committee on Clinical Application of Echocardiography recognizes that an exercise or a pharmacologic stress echocardiogram can be used to evaluate the presence or extent of ischemia where there is an underlying ECG abnormality that affects ECG interpretation (e.g., prior ischemia, left bundle branch block, Wolff-Parkinson-White syndrome).[8] There is conflicting evidence on whether echocardiographic techniques are preferable when there are no resting ECG abnormalities.[8] For asymptomatic patients at risk for CAD, it is unclear whether exercise testing is beneficial because there have been no clinical trials investigating exercise testing in this population.[17]

REFERENCES

1. Brown DA: Diagnosis and screening of coronary artery disease, *Primary Care* 32(4):931-946, 2005.
2. Schinkel AFL, Bax JJ, Geleijnse ML: Noninvasive evaluation of ischaemic heart disease: myocardial perfusion imaging or stress echocardiography, *Eur Heart J* 24(9):789-800, 2003.
3. Wackers FJ, Berman DS, Maddahi J, and others: Technetium-99m hexakis 2-methoxyisobutyl isonitrile: human biodistribution, dosimetry, safety, and preliminary comparison to thallium-201 for myocardial perfusion imaging, *J Nucl Med* 30(3):301-311, 1989.
4. Maisey MN, Lowery A, Bischof-Delaloye A, and others: European multicenter comparison of thallium-201 and technetium-99m methoxy isobutyl isonitrile in ischemic heart disease, *Eur J Nucl Med* 16:869, 1990.
5. Kiat H, Maddahi J, Roy LT, and others: Comparison of technetium 99m methoxy isobutyl isonitrile and thallium 201 for evaluation of coronary artery disease by planar and tomographic methods, *Am Heart J* 117(1):1-11, 1989.
6. Henkin RE, Levin DC, Bettmann MA, and others: Chronic chest pain without evidence of myocardial ischemia/infarction: American College of Radiology, ACR Appropriateness Criteria, *Radiology* 215(Suppl):85-88, 2000.
7. Kosnik JW, Zalenski RJ, Gryzbowski M, and others: Impact of technetium-99m sestamibi imaging on the emergency department management and costs in the evaluation of low-risk chest pain, *Acad Emerg Med* 8(4):315-323, 2001.
8. Cheitlin MD, Alpert JS, Armstrong WF, and others: ACC/AHA guidelines for the clinical application of echocardiography: a report of the American College of Cardiology/American Heart Association Task Force on Practice Guidelines (Committee on Clinical Application of Echocardiography), developed in collaboration with the American Society of Echocardiography, *Circulation* 95(6):1686-1744, 1997, retrieved Jan 4, 2007, from http://circ.ahajournals.org/cgi/content/full/95/6/1686.
9. Lima J, Desai M: Cardiovascular magnetic resonance imaging: current and emerging applications, *J Am Coll Cardiol* 44(6):1164-1171, 2004.
10. Laudon DA, Vukov LF, Breen JF, and others: Use of electron beam

computed tomography in the evaluation of chest pain patients in the emergency department, *Ann Emerg Med* 33(1):15-21, 1999.

11. Arad Y, Goodman KJ, Roth M, and others: Coronary calcification, coronary disease risk factors, C-reactive protein, and atherosclerotic cardiovascular disease events: the St. Francis Heart Study, *J Am Coll Cardiol* 46(1):158-165, 2005.
12. Sawada SG, Segar DS, Ryan T, and others: Echocardiographic detection of coronary artery disease during dobutamine infusion, *Circulation* 83(5):1605-1614, 1991.
13. Marwick T, Willemart B, D'Hondt AM, and others: Selection of the optimal nonexercise stress for the evaluation of ischemic regional myocardial dysfunction and malperfusion: comparison of dobutamine and adenosine using echocardiography and 99mTc-MIBI single photon emission computed tomography, *Circulation* 87(2):345-354, 1993.
14. Vaccarino V, Parsons L, Every NR, and others: Sex-based differences in early mortality after myocardial infraction, *N Engl J Med* 341(4):217-225, 1999.
15. Mieres JH, Shaw LJ, Arai A, and others. Role of noninvasive testing in the clinical evaluation of women with suspected coronary artery disease, *Circulation* 111:682-696, 2005.
16. Gibbons RJ, Chatterjee K, Daley J, and others: ACC/AHA/ACP-ASIM guidelines for the management of patients with chronic stable angina: a report of the American College of Cardiology/American Heart Association Task Forces on Practice Guidelines (Committee on Management of Patients with Chronic Stable Angina), *J Am Coll Cardiol* 33(7):2092-2197, 1999.
17. Lauer M, Froelicher ES, Williams M, and others: Exercise testing in asymptomatic adults: a statement for professionals from the American Heart Association Council on Clinical Cardiology, Subcommittee on Exercise, Cardiac Rehabilitation, and Prevention, *Circulation* 112(5):771-776, 2005.

CHAPTER 123

Abdominal Aortic Aneurysm

Updated by Janice D. Nunnelee

DEFINITION AND EPIDEMIOLOGY

Abdominal aortic aneurysm (AAA) is a progressive localized dilation of the abdominal aorta. With an AAA, the diameter of the suspicious area exceeds the normal diameter by 50% (1.5 times).[1] AAA develops in about 6% of men older than 65 years. The male/female ratio is 6:1.[2,3] Symptomatic aneurysms increase in number after age 70. Since the 1970s, the Western world has seen a dramatic rise in the incidence of aneurysms that remains valid even when better screening and access to health care are taken into effect.[3] Thus at least 1 million Americans have a clinically recognized AAA.

AAA is an important clinical diagnosis because it is associated with considerable risk of rupture and death as the aneurysm enlarges to a diameter of more than 5.0 cm (1.96 inches).[4] More than 30,000 people undergo elective aneurysm surgery in the United States each year. In 1991, 16,696 deaths in the United States were attributed to aortic aneurysms; aneurysms involving the infrarenal abdominal aorta accounted for 52% of deaths.[5] Overall, the rates of aortic aneurysm are higher for Caucasians than for African Americans and for men than for women.

Risk factors for AAA include atherosclerotic vascular disease, Caucasian race, male gender, advanced age, hypertension, smoking, chronic obstructive pulmonary disease (COPD), history of hernias, family history of AAA, and presence of other aneurysms.[4-6] Despite extensive investigation, the link between COPD and AAA remains elusive. Evidence suggests that the high prevalence of AAA in patients with COPD may be related to medications (oral steroids) and co-existing diseases, rather than a common pathway of pathogenesis involving plasma elastase or α_1-antitrypsin deficiency.[7] Another study suggests an association between AAA and elevated homocysteine plasma levels.[8] Homocysteine levels have been shown to be higher in patients with AAA than in control subjects without AAA. In addition, aneurysmal size has been shown to be larger in patients with hyperhomocysteinemia than in those with normohomocysteinemia. However, this may be explained by the increased prevalence of hyperhomocysteinemia in patients with atherosclerosis independent of the presence of an aneurysm.

The proposed causes of AAA include atherosclerosis, inflammation, mycotic infection, inheritable connective tissue disorders (Marfan's syndrome, type IV Ehrlos-Danlos syndrome), and trauma. Traditionally, atherosclerosis has been considered the most common cause of AAA. However, aneurysm formation is associated with atherosclerosis in only 25% of cases.

PATHOPHYSIOLOGY

AAA is a disease of the medial wall layer of the aorta. It is characterized by degeneration of the extracellular matrix proteins and the presence of an inflammatory cell infiltrate composed predominantly of T cells. Degradation of the cell wall proteins in the medial layer occurs as a result of complex interactions between genetic factors, inflammatory cytokines, matrix metalloproteinases (MMPs), tissue inhibitors of MMPs, and others. The consequences include dissolution and fragmentation of collagen and elastin, leading to expansion of the vessel wall.[9] When the aortic wall tension exceeds the tensile strength of the wall collagen and the wall can no longer withstand the repetitive force of systolic contraction, the aneurysm ruptures.

CLINICAL PRESENTATION

Although an AAA may cause symptoms as a result of the pressure on surrounding structures, about 75% are asymptomatic at initial diagnosis.[10] Asymptomatic AAAs are generally detected during an incidental radiologic or surgical procedure. Alternatively, in thin patients, a supine abdominal examination may readily show a pulsatile abdominal mass. Inflammatory AAAs may manifest with chronic abdominal pain or back pain and, sometimes, ureteral obstruction.[4] Other clinical symptoms may result from embolization or rupture of the aneurysm.

Thromboembolic phenomena may herald the presence of an AAA. Microembolic infarcts in the lower extremity of a patient with easily palpable pedal pulses may suggest either abdominal or popliteal aneurysm. Embolization of mural thrombus from an abdominal aneurysm may be seen with acute limb ischemia caused by femoral or popliteal occlusion.[10]

The classic diagnostic triad of hypovolemic shock, pulsatile abdominal mass, and abdominal or back pain is encountered in only a minority of patients with a ruptured AAA. Ruptured AAAs should be suspected in any patient who comes in with complaints of hypotension and atypical abdominal or back pain symptoms. In a patient with a history of aneurysm or pulsatile mass, the presence of abdominal pain must be considered to represent a rapidly expanding or ruptured aneurysm and must be treated accordingly. In the community setting the death rate from ruptured AAAs is almost 80%.

PHYSICAL EXAMINATION

Palpation of the abdomen for AAA is one of the few physical examination maneuvers that is an evidence-based recommendation in the periodic health examination of older men.[5,11,12] To detect AAA on physical examination, the patient is positioned supine with knees flexed to relax the abdominal wall. The examiner places the palm over the epigastrium to detect a transmitted pulsation. The examiner then places both hands on the abdomen with palms down and an index finger on either side of the pulsating area to measure the aortic width. An AAA is suspected when the aorta is judged to be at least 3.0 cm (1.2 inches) in maximum diameter.

Unfortunately, abdominal palpation has only moderate overall sensitivity for detecting AAAs (68%) and is highly dependent on the skill of the examiner.[11,12] The sensitivity of abdominal palpation increases with AAA diameter, from 61% for AAAs of 3.0 to 3.9 cm (1.2 to 1.5 inches), to 69% for AAAs of 4.0 to 4.9 cm (1.57 to 1.92 inches), and to 82% for AAAs over 5.0 cm (1.96 inches). The sensitivity of abdominal palpation also increases (91%) when the abdominal girth is less than 100 cm (40-inch waistline). When the girth is more than 100 cm and the aorta is palpable, the sensitivity is less (82%). Overall, when the girth is less than 100 cm and the AAA is more than 5.0 cm, abdominal palpation is highly sensitive (100%) for detecting AAA.

DIAGNOSTICS

Currently, ultrasound is the imaging study ordered most often for screening and initial confirmation of an aneurysm. This modality can provide a reasonably accurate measurement of initial size and be used for serial follow-up evaluation.[12,13] Some authors believe that screening men over age 65, particularly smokers, decreases mortality from rupture and is cost-effective.[14] The most accurate measurement of size by ultrasound is the anteroposterior diameter. (The transverse measurement may be larger due to distortion of the aorta.) High-resolution ultrasound allows the visualization of important anatomic markers, including the origin of the superior mesenteric artery, left renal vein indicating the level adjacent to the renal arteries, and the iliac arteries. Ultrasound also allows visualization of the halo effect of an inflammatory aneurysm. Duplex ultrasound illuminates aortoiliac occlusive disease.

CT with IV contrast is the most widely used imaging technique before aortic aneurysm repair. It permits the detection of inflammatory aneurysms, aneurysmal leakage, and penetrating aortic ulcers. It also delineates venous anomalies, periaortic lymphadenopathy, and horseshoe kidneys.[13]

The era of endoluminal repair of AAA necessitates selection of the proper endograft according to precise measurement of the size and length of both the proximal neck of the aneurysm and the common iliac arteries. This is best achieved by helical or spiral CT scanning, which allows the creation of three-dimensional images that can be rotated for viewing in any projection. This technique requires breath holding for 30 seconds. It also requires the administration of contrast medium (120 to 150 ml), which may be detrimental in patients with renal insufficiency.

DIAGNOSTICS

Abdominal Aortic Aneurysm

IMAGING

Abdominal ultrasound
Spiral CT with contrast*
MRI, MRA*

*If indicated.

Standard contrast aortography is the simplest method to define significant associated renal, visceral, or iliofemoral occlusive disease. Although no longer routinely recommended for all patients with AAA, preoperative aortography has selective indications, including suspicion of suprarenal extension, suspected visceral or renal artery disease, iliofemoral occlusive disease, horseshoe kidney, prior aortic or colonic surgery, and unusual aneurysms (e.g., mycotic, aortocaval fistula).[13]

MRI and magnetic resonance angiography (MRA) are alternative approaches to aortography.[13] Gadolinium-enhanced MRA images provide clear delineation of the renal and visceral vessels and occlusive disease of the iliofemoral vessels. In many centers, MRA has become the imaging study of choice for patients with renal insufficiency.

MRI and MRA have limitations, including inability to use on patients with pacemakers or other metallic hardware that would affect the magnetic field. In addition, for certain patients, claustrophobia or unstable medical conditions would preclude their being in the tube during the necessary acquisition time. In addition, MRA has not yet been validated as a method of sizing for endovascular aneurysm repair.

DIFFERENTIAL DIAGNOSIS

The differential diagnoses for AAA include conditions associated with abdominal pain or back pain. These conditions are listed in the Differential Diagnosis box.[14] CT is the most readily available method to rule out alternate causes of abdominal pain.

MANAGEMENT

The goal of AAA management is to prevent aneurysmal rupture while minimizing surgical risk. Thus the size of the aneurysm and the patient's medical status, life expectancy, and preference are critical factors in deciding the timing of elective AAA repair. AAA size is the best predictor of rupture risk. A fair amount of controversy persists about the best timing and method of AAA repair (operative or endoluminal) when considering preoperative risk factors and postoperative complications (Box 123-1).[15,16]

The majority of aneurysms expand slowly at a rate of 0.2 to 0.3 cm/year, or 10% of the diameter.[17] However, the risk of rupture increases significantly when an AAA exceeds 5.0 cm (1.96 inches) in diameter. This was demonstrated in an older population-based study in which the estimated risk of rupture based on the latest ultrasound study was 12% per year for an aneurysm 5.0 to 5.9 cm (1.96 to 2.32 inches) and 14% for aneurysms greater than 6.0 cm (2.36 inches) in those at higher risk or those referred for intervention.[18] In the United Kingdom Small Aneurysm Trial (UKSDAT) the relative risk of rupture was increased in females, those with AAAs of increased diameter, smokers, and patients with COPD.[18] Another factor found to be important in rupture risk is asymmetry in the aneurysm.[18,19]

Recent data from the UKSDAT[20] and the Veterans Administration Aneurysm Detection and Management Trial (ADAM)[18] help to guide decision making about the timing of surgical repair of small AAA (4.0 to 5.0 cm [1.57 to 1.96 inches]) vs. surveillance with serial ultrasound examinations or CT. These studies concluded that unless the aneurysm exceeds 5.5 cm (2.16 inches), there is no long-term survival advantage of early surgery over serial ultrasonographic surveillance at 6-month intervals. Elective repair is appropriately indicated for healthy patients with AAAs measuring 5.0 to 6.0 cm (1.96 to 2.36 inches).[4] During the 9-year follow-up of the UKSDAT, 74% of the surveillance group needed interventions, indicating that intervention is almost always necessary.

DIFFERENTIAL DIAGNOSIS

Abdominal Aortic Aneurysm

- Nephrolithiasis
- Myocardial infarction
- Esophageal rupture
- Perforated gastric ulcer
- Pancreatitis
- Bowel obstruction
- Cholelithiasis
- Diverticulitis
- Gastrointestinal bleed
- Appendicitis
- Pyelonephritis
- Ischemic bowel
- Back strain
- Arthritis
- Neoplasm
- Other causes of abdominal pain
- Other causes of back pain

BOX 123-1

FACTORS AFFECTING THE RISK OF ABDOMINAL AORTIC ANEURYSM RUPTURE

- Size (>6.0 cm [2.36 inches])
- Rapid expansion*
- Female gender
- Smoking
- Chronic obstructive pulmonary disease
- Family history of abdominal aortic aneurysm
- Asymmetrical abdominal aortic aneurysm

*It is difficult to predict the average expansion of an abdominal aortic aneurysm because intervention is planned in all but high-risk patients and those who refuse treatment.

Preoperative Cardiac Risk Stratification

Several older, large surveys have demonstrated that coronary artery disease is the most important underlying medical illness contributing to morbidity and mortality among individuals who undergo major vascular surgery, regardless of the type of peripheral vascular surgery, particularly when they are 70 years of age or older.[21-24] The American College of Cardiology (ACC) and the American Heart Association (AHA) developed guidelines to aid in cardiac risk stratification before noncardiac surgery.[25] According to the ACC/AHA guidelines,[25] aortic and other vascular procedures are considered high risk. Therefore patients should proceed to surgery without further cardiac evaluation only when they have no clinical predictors or minor clinical predictors (advanced age, abnormal ECG, cardiac rhythm other than sinus, low functional capacity, history of stroke, uncontrolled hypertension) with moderate or excellent functional capacity (≥4 METs, i.e., activities such as doing light housework like dusting and washing dishes or climbing a flight of stairs or a hill).[25-27] Preoperative noninvasive testing (pharmacologic stress testing) is indicated when patients are undergoing high-risk vascular surgery and they have two or more intermediate predictors of clinical risk (mild angina pectoris, prior myocardial infarction, compensated or prior congestive heart failure, diabetes mellitus, renal insufficiency) and poor functional capacity (≤4 METs). The results of noninvasive testing are then used to plan further perioperative management. This includes intensified medical therapy, cardiac catheterization, coronary revascularization, or, potentially, cancellation or delay of noncardiac surgery.

Other medical conditions may increase the mortality rate of aneurysm repair by twofold or threefold. They include chronic renal failure (serum creatinine level >3 mg/dl, or hemodialysis), COPD (FEV/FEV_1 <0.70), and liver cirrhosis with portal hypertension. These conditions increase the mortality rate from between 3% and 5% to between 8% and 10%.[4] In this Canadian North American study, the most significant predictors of mortality were ECG changes indicative of ischemia, COPD, and increased creatinine.[4]

Open Surgical Repair

Open surgical repair of an AAA is usually approached through a midline or a left flank retroperitoneal incision. Overall, these two approaches are generally interchangeable in the treatment of infrarenal aneurysm, although specific indications for the transperitoneal approach include right renal graft, right iliac artery aneurysm, prior left colectomy, and aneurysmal neck that turns to the right. Indications for the retroperitoneal approach include multiple prior laparotomies or abdominal surgeries, selected abdominal stoma, horseshoe kidney, inflammatory aneurysms, obesity, and juxtarenal and suprarenal aortic aneurysms.[28-30]

During open surgical repair of an AAA, the aneurysm is exposed and normal segments of the proximal and distal aorta are cross-clamped. The aneurysm is incised. Lumbar arteries, which back-bleed into the aneurysm, are oversewn. A prosthetic graft is positioned in the aorta, extending from a segment of normal aorta above the aneurysm to a segment of normal aorta below the aneurysm. If the aneurysm extends to the iliac arteries, a bifurcated prosthetic graft is used. The distal ends of the bifurcated limbs extend into the iliac or femoral arteries. The wall of the aneurysm is closed over the newly placed graft. The posterior peritoneum, and then the abdomen, is closed in the standard manner.

A number of advancements contributed to improved outcomes of open surgical repair. These include autotransfusion, balanced general and epidural anesthesia, and improved pain management with continuous epidural analgesia in the postoperative setting.

Today, most patients undergoing surgical repair of an AAA have their preoperative workups done on an outpatient basis. After restricting their dietary intake and managing their bowel evacuation at home on the day before surgery, these patients are admitted for same-day surgery. The surgery lasts 2 to 4 hours. Patients undergoing infrarenal AAA repair typically stay in the ICU for 1 night. They are transferred to the general care unit on postoperative day 1, when they get out of bed to move to a chair or walk. If the graft extends down to the femoral vessels, they are kept on bed rest until postoperative day 2. Also on postoperative day 2, the diet of patients who undergo AAA through a retroperitoneal approach is advanced to clear liquids and then diet as tolerated. If the operation is performed through a transperitoneal approach, return of bowel function may take a few days longer. Discharge to home with skilled nursing visits is projected for postoperative day 5, although it ranges from day 5 to 7. Home nursing care focuses on the incision, pain management, appetite and food intake, bowel function, and progression of activity.

Endovascular Stent Grafts

In 1991 Parodi, Palmaz, and Barone[31] reported the deployment of the first stent graft for the repair of AAA. A growing number of studies have documented the efficacy and generally satisfactory early results for a variety of transluminally placed endovascular grafts.[31-34]

Endoluminal AAA repair is associated with reduced length of hospital stay and decreased recovery time, accounting for its appeal to patients and physicians, as well as an upsurge of enthusiasm for the development and use of such devices.[32] It is appropriate in approximately 40% of AAA repairs.[14]

Endoluminal repair of AAA is achieved through exclusion of the aneurysm from the circulation by means of a prosthetic graft that is inserted from a remote site to the desired intraluminal location, under radiologic guidance, and then secured by an expandable stent attachment system. The devices may be commercially manufactured or custom made. They may consist of a bifurcated graft or a tube graft with a single limb (aortouniiliac). In addition, a modular product allows the creation of a variable bifurcated graft through the deployment and attachment of a contralateral limb and extensions. Also, if it is necessary to exclude the contralateral iliac artery but restore flow to the contralateral extremity, an aortouniiliac device has been combined with a standard operative femorofemoral bypass graft. When only tube grafts were available, endoluminal repair was rarely possible, but this rate has increased to less than 40% with the availability of bifurcated grafts and aortouniiliac grafts.[14] The development of the superspecialty of vascular therapy and the dissemination of skills have also increased the rate of usage.

The initial successful deployment of a stent graft has been reported in 95% to 97% of cases.[35] In most cases the procedure time is now less than 2 hours. Most procedures are performed with the patient under epidural anesthesia combined with conscious sedation. Only infrequently does an endovascular patient require an ICU stay. Patients are sent home after CT confirmation of graft placement and the absence of a leak at the attachment sites for the graft. The average length of hospital stay is now approximately 2.4 days, with more than 85% of patients discharged on their first or second postoperative day.[32]

The first routine follow-up visit with the vascular surgeon occurs 1 month after hospital discharge, at which time another CT scan is obtained to reaffirm the position of the graft, presence or absence of any leak, and evidence of sac shrinkage. It appears that smaller AAAs have fewer endoleaks than larger ones.[36,37] Thereafter CT scans are obtained every 6 months for several years. If the aneurysm and the prosthesis remain stable, the frequency of follow-up can be decreased to annual visits.

Patients report a return to a sense of preoperative health status 11 days after endoluminal repair vs. 47 days after open surgical repair.[32] However, as discussed later, long-term data about device durability and frequent endoleaks (leaks around the endovascular graft) preclude a universal shift from open surgical repair to endoluminal repair.

Ruptured AAAs present a unique challenge to endovascular repair. Because the first indication of their presence is often the back pain and hypotension associated with acute enlargement and rupture, the primary goal is patient stabilization. This is accomplished by gaining control of the rupture and preventing further hemorrhage. Once the patient is stabilized, repair of the aorta can be accomplished.

For elective repairs, grafts typically are chosen based on a series of measurements and often using three-dimensional reconstructions of CT scans and/or angiograms. The process can take several days, which is a luxury that is not available with an acute rupture. However, with increasing surgical experience and the availability of a range of graft sizes, this less invasive method of repair has been applied with some degree of success.[38-44] As the technology improves, this technique will play a wider role in the repair of ruptured AAAs. It is hoped that the dismal 80% to 90% mortality rate for ruptured AAAs will improve.

Laparoscopic and Laparoscopic-Assisted Aneurysm Surgery

The use of laparoscopic surgery for an AAA is still in the evaluation stage. It is offered in a few centers to those eligible for standard open repair. The results have not been compared with the other two methods of treatment.[5]

LIFE SPAN CONSIDERATIONS

In general, AAA is considered a disease of older, Caucasian men. However, AAA repair is often performed on young patients (≤50 years). Aneurysms are more commonly symptomatic in younger patients, although perioperative mortality and morbidity rates are not significantly different for young patients compared with older patients (≥65 years) with degenerative (atherosclerotic) AAAs.[40] Technique (open vs. endovascular) may be determined not by age but by the assessed risk to the patient and the size of the AAA. Those at risk of dying relatively soon because of a co-morbid condition may be chosen for endovascular repair.

COMPLICATIONS

Complications vary for surgical repair and endoluminal repair of AAAs. Mortality rates and short- and long-term graft complications are comparable for the two techniques.

In most large series the 30-day mortality rate for surgical repair is 3% to 5%.[6] If ECG changes of ischemia, COPD, and elevated creatinine are present, the mortality rate at 30 days is 50%. By comparison, patients with none of these factors have a perioperative mortality of less than 2%. Early surgical complications of arterial thrombosis, anastomotic rupture or bleeding, peripheral emboli, and limb loss are rare (1% to 3%) at centers with experience. In a recent 36-year population-based study of late graft complications, the 1-, 3-, and 5-year rates of survival free of graft complications were 97%, 95%, and 93%, respectively.[39] The primary cause of death was myocardial infarction. The rate of open conversion during endovascular repair is less than 5%. Further, the incidence of long-term complications is very low but includes anastomotic pseudoaneurysm (3%), graft thrombosis (2%), aortoenteric fistula (1.6%), graft infection (1.3%), anastomotic hemorrhage (1.3%), colonic ischemia (0.7%), and atheroembolism (0.3%).

The 30-day mortality rates for stent graft repairs are similar (3%) to those for standard surgical repair. However, for patients at high risk, mortality rates have been as high as 10% to 13%. The most common early complications include groin hematoma (6% to 7%), arterial thrombosis (2% to 3%), iliac artery rupture (1% to 1.5%), and thromboemboli (1% to 2%).[6]

Although long-term follow-up observations are limited, the most common long-term problem is endoleak.[5,37] An endoleak involves persistent filling of the aneurysm from either an anastomotic site or collateral blood vessels, most commonly caused by persistent bleeding from lumbar or inferior mesenteric artery branches in the AAA sac. Endoleaks occur in about one third of cases. Endoleaks close spontaneously in more than 50% of cases by 6 to 12 months after the procedure. Secondary catheter-based reinterventions are required to close an additional 10%. Surgical intervention has been required to treat 2% to 3% of long-term leaks. Aneurysm rupture occurs in 1% of patients within 1 to 2 years. Other common late complications include severe graft kinking (2%), graft migration (2%), and graft thrombosis (3%).[41]

INDICATIONS FOR REFERRAL OR HOSPITALIZATION

Patients with an AAA of 4.0 cm (1.57 inches) or larger should be referred to a vascular surgeon. Recent evidence suggests that outcomes for open repair of intact AAAs are better at large, urban institutions.[4,42] Therefore referral to a center with a vascular service experienced in treating AAAs is indicated with elective repairs. Using ultrasound examination, the vascular surgeon monitors expansion annually for aneurysms of 4.5 cm (1.77 inches) or less and every 6 months for aneurysms of 4.5 cm or greater. Although elective repair is usually considered when the AAA enlarges into the range of 5.0 to 6.0 cm (1.96 to 2.36 inches), repair of smaller aneurysms may occur if the patient cannot commit to the surveillance program. Rapid expansion beyond 10% of the diameter per year is also an indication for surgical repair. Finally, repair may be delayed until the diameter is 6 cm or larger in poor-risk patients.

If the aneurysm enlarges and is being considered for repair, a thin-slice CT scan may be performed for evaluating stent graft placement. However, indications for stent grafting vs. standard surgical repair have not yet been fully elucidated. Because the long-term outcomes of stent grafts are unknown, stent grafts are often reserved for older patients with limited life expectancy or for patients with other significant medical co-morbid conditions that make them a poor risk for open surgical repair.

PATIENT EDUCATION

During the period of surveillance of small aneurysms, patient education addresses modification of risk factors such as hypertension, smoking, and diabetes to slow AAA expansion; protocols for surveillance; options for elective treatment; indications for emergent evaluation; and surveillance of first-degree relatives. During the periprocedural phase, patient education focuses on the trajectory of care, including length of hospital stay, and postdischarge recovery, including of the care of the incision or catheterization site, resumption of usual activities of daily living, and long-term monitoring of graft patency and prevention or detection of subsequent aneurysms.

Hypertension and cigarette smoking are critical risk factors for expansion of AAA. Although beta blockade with propranolol has not demonstrated a significant difference in the rate of expansion of small AAAs or the need for surgery, treatment with beta blockers continues because of its effect on reducing coronary events.[4,18,43,44] Smoking cessation is likely to occur in only 15% to 25% of smokers but should be encouraged at every visit. However, smoking cessation does not preclude the development of AAA, nor will smoking cessation prevent expansion of AAA.

The frequency of surveillance depends on the size of the aneurysm at the most recent ultrasonographic study. Patients must commit to serial ultrasonographic examinations or consider early repair of a small aneurysm with the inherent risks and benefits of open surgical or endovascular repair.

Physicians and surgeons should describe both the standard open surgical procedure and endovascular stent graft procedure. The explanation should include early and late results of both types of procedures to inform the patient and assist in decision making.

After the detection of an AAA, patients should be counseled to report the new-onset symptoms of aneurysmal enlargement, such as abdominal or back pain, to their vascular surgeon. Symptoms of impending rupture, requiring immediate emergency care, include severe abdominal, flank, or back pain unrelieved by position change. The abdominal pain may be characterized as deep, boring, or tearing. Low back pain may be dull, radiating to the legs, similar to musculoskeletal pain. The flank pain may radiate to the groin and be associated with hematuria.

HEALTH PROMOTION

There is strong evidence to suggest a genetic predisposition to AAA.[4,45-47] Approximately 20% of patients with AAA will have a first-degree relative with AAA, suggesting the importance of periodic ultrasonographic screening after age 50 in these family members. This is most applicable to male siblings, who appear to be at highest risk.

There is also evidence suggesting the relationship between smoking and the development of AAA in men. For this reason, the U.S. Preventive Services Task Force recommends screening with ultrasonography for men older than 65 years with a past or current history of smoking.[48]

REFERENCES

1. Johnston KW, Rutherford RB, Tilson MD, and others: Suggested methods for reporting on arterial aneurysms, *J Vasc Surg* 13:452-458, 1991.
2. Drury D, Michaels JA, Jones L, and others: Systematic review of recent evidence for the safety and efficacy of elective endovascular repair in the management of infrarenal abdominal aortic aneurysm, *Br J Surg* 92:937-946, 2005.
3. Wassef M, Baxter T, Chisholm RL, and others: Pathogenesis of abdominal aortic aneurysms: a multidisciplinary research program supported by the National Heart, Lung, and Blood Institute, *J Vasc Surg* 34:730-738, 2001.
4. Brewster DC, Cronenwett JL, Hallett JW, and others: Guidelines for the treatment of abdominal aortic aneurysms: report of a subcommittee of the Joint Council of the American Association for Vascular Surgery and the Society for Vascular Surgery, *J Vasc Surg* 37(5):1106-1117, 2003.
5. Monely D, Given M, McGrath F, and others: The evolving rationale of elective treatment of abdominal aortic aneurysms, *Surgeon* 1:160-163, 2005.
6. Zarins CK, White RA, Schwarten D, and others: AneuRx stent graft versus open surgical repair of abdominal aortic aneurysms: multicenter prospective clinical trial, *J Vasc Surg* 29:292-308, 1999.
7. Lindholt JS, Heickendorff L, Antonsen S, and others: Natural history of abdominal aortic aneurysm with and without coexisting chronic obstructive pulmonary disease, *J Vasc Surg* 28:226-233, 1998.
8. Brunelli T, Prisco D, Fedi S, and others: High prevalence of mild hyperhomocysteinemia in patients with abdominal aortic aneurysm, *J Vasc Surg* 32:531-536, 2000.
9. Marian AJ: On genetics, inflammation, and abdominal aortic aneurysms: can single nucleotide polymorphisms predict the outcome? *Circulation* 103:2222-2224, 2001.
10. Thompson MM, Bell PR: ABC of arterial and venous disease: arterial aneurysms, *BMJ* 320:1193-1196, 2000.
11. Fink HA, Lederle FA, Roth CS, and others: The accuracy of physical examination to detect abdominal aortic aneurysm, *Arch Intern Med* 160:833-836, 2000.
12. Nunnelee JD, Spaner SD: The quality of research on physical examination for abdominal aortic aneurysm, *J Vasc Nursing* 22(1):14-18, 2004.
13. Hallett JW: What imaging studies does the surgeon really need before abdominal aortic aneurysm repair? In Abbott WM, editor: *Proceedings of current issues in vascular surgery*, Boston, 1999, Massachusetts General Hospital, Division of Vascular Surgery.
14. Daly KJ, Torella F, Ashleigh R, and others: Screening, diagnosis and advances in aortic aneurysm surgery, *Gerontology* 50(6):349-359, 2004.
15. Ketterling M: Abdominal aortic aneurysm: patients at peril, *Clin Rev* 11:59-64, 2001.
16. Cronenwett JL, Sargent SK, Wall WH, and others: Variables that affect the expansion rate and outcomes of small abdominal aortic aneurysms, *J Vasc Surg* 11:260-269, 1996.
17. Jones A, Cadill D, Gardham R: Outcome in patients with a large abdominal aortic aneurysm considered unfit for surgery, *Br J Surg* 85:124-128, 1998.
18. Lederle FA, Wilson SE, Johnson GR, and others: Design of abdominal aortic aneurysm detection and management (ADAM) study, *J Vasc Surg* 20:296-303, 1994.
19. UK Small Aneurysm Trial Participants: Mortality results for randomized controlled trial of early elective surgery or ultrasonographic surveillance for small abdominal aortic aneurysms, *Lancet* 352:1649-1655, 1998.
20. Lederle F, Wilson JE, Johnson GR, and others: Immediate repair compared with surveillance of small aortic aneurysms, *N Engl J Med* 346:1437-1444, 2002.
21. Plecha FR, Bertin VJ, Plecha EJ, and others: The early results of vascular surgery in patients 75 years of age and older: an analysis of 3259 cases, *J Vasc Surg* 2:769-774, 1985.
22. Fillinger MF, Raghavan ML, Marra SP, and others: In vivo analysis of mechanical wall stress and abdominal aortic aneurysm rupture risk, *J Vasc Surg* 36:589-597, 2002.
23. Goldman L: Cardiac risks and complications of non-cardiac surgery, *Ann Intern Med* 98:504-513, 1983.
24. Ashton CM, Petersen NJ, Wray NP, and others: The incidence of perioperative myocardial infarction in men undergoing noncardiac surgery, *Ann Intern Med* 118:504-510, 1993.
25. Roger VL, Ballard DJ, Hallett JW, and others: Influence of coronary artery disease on morbidity and mortality after abdominal aortic aneurysmectomy: a population-based study, 1971-1978, *J Am Coll Cardiol* 14:1245-1252, 1989.

26. Eagle KA, Berger PB, Calkins H, and others: ACC/AHA guideline update for perioperative cardiovascular evaluation for noncardiac surgery—executive summary: a report of the American College of Cardiologists/American Heart Association Task Force on Practice Guidelines (Committee to Update 1996 Guidelines on Preoperative Cardiovascular Evaluation for Noncardiac Surgery), *Circulation* 105(10):1257-1267, 2002 [erratum in *Circulation* 113(22):e846, 2006].
27. Hlatky MA, Boineau RE, Higginbotham MB, and others: A brief self-administered questionnaire to determine functional capacity (the Duke Activity Status Index), *Am J Cardiol* 64:651-654, 1989.
28. Fletcher GF, Balady G, Froelicher VF, and others: Exercise standards: a statement for healthcare professional from the American Heart Association Writing Group, *Circulation* 91:580-615, 1995.
29. Johnston KW: Multicenter prospective study of nonruptured abdominal aortic aneurysm, part II, *J Vasc Surg* 9:437-447, 1989.
30. Cambria RP, Brewster DC, Abbott WM, and others: Transperitoneal versus retroperitoneal approach for aortic reconstruction: a randomized prospective study, *J Vasc Surg* 11:314-325, 1990.
31. Parodi JC, Palmaz JC, Barone HD: Transfemoral intraluminal graft implantation for abdominal aortic aneurysms, *Ann Vasc Surg* 5:491-499, 1991.
32. Prinssen M, Verhoeven EL, Buth J, and others: A randomized trial comparing conventional and endovascular repair of abdominal aortic aneurysms, *N Engl J Med* 351:1607-1618, 2004.
33. Chuter TA, Risberg B, Hopkinson BR, and others: Clinical experience with a bifurcated endovascular graft for abdominal aortic aneurysm repair, *J Vasc Surg* 24:655-666, 1996.
34. Faries PL, Dayal R, Lin S, and others: Endovascular stent graft selection for the treatment of abdominal aortic aneurysms, *J Cardiovasc Surg (Torino)* 46(1):9-17, 2005.
35. Chuter TA, Barodi JC, Lawrence-Brown M: Management of abdominal aortic aneurysm: a decade of progress, *J Endovasc Ther* 11(Suppl 2):II82-II95, 2004.
36. May J, Woodburn K, White G: Endovascular treatment of infrarenal abdominal aortic aneurysms, *Ann Vasc Surg* 12:391-395, 1998.
37. Towne JB: Endovascular treatment of abdominal aortic aneurysms, *Am J Surg* 189(2):140-149, 2005.
38. Heikkinen MA, Arko FR, Zarins CK: What is the significance of endoleaks and endotension? *Surg Clin North Am* 84:1337-1352, 2004.
39. Ohki T, Veith FJ: Endovascular grafts and other image-guided catheter-based adjuncts to improve the treatment of ruptured aortoiliac aneurysms, *Ann Surg* 232:466-479, 2000.
40. Greenberg RK, Srivastava SD, Ouriel K, and others: An endoluminal method of hemorrhage control and repair of ruptured abdominal aortic aneurysms, *J Endovasc Ther* 7:1-7, 2000.
41. Cherr G, Edwards MS, Craven TE, and others: Survival of young patients after abdominal aortic aneurysm repair, *J Vasc Surg* 35:94-99, 2002.
42. Hallett JW, Marshall PM, Petterson TM, and others: Graft-related complications after abdominal aortic aneurysm repair: reassurance from a 36-year population-based experience, *J Vasc Surg* 25:277-284, 1997.
43. Huber TS, Wang JG, Derrow AE, and others: Experience in the United States with abdominal aortic aneurysm repair, *J Vasc Surg* 33:304-311, 2001.
44. Gadowski GR, Pilcher DB, Ricci MA: Abdominal aortic aneurysm expansion rate: effect of size and beta-adrenergic blockade, *J Vasc Surg* 19:727-731, 1994.
45. Poldermans D, Boersma E, Bax JJ, and others: The effect of bisoprolol on perioperative mortality and myocardial infarction in high risk patients undergoing vascular surgery, *N Engl J Med* 341:1789-1794, 1999.
46. Johansen K, Koepsell T: Familial tendency for abdominal aortic aneurysms, *JAMA* 256:1934-1936, 1986.
47. Tilson MD, Dang C: Generalized arteriomegaly: a possible predisposition to the formation of abdominal aortic aneurysms, *Arch Surg* 116:1030-1032, 1981.
48. US Preventive Services Task Force: Screening for abdominal aortic aneurysm: recommendations from the U.S. Preventive Services Task Force, *Ann Intern Med* 142(3):1-52, 2005.

CHAPTER 124

Cardiac Arrhythmias

Updated by Susan DiMattia

Cardiac arrhythmias vary widely in type and causality and occur in both the presence and absence of cardiac disease. They also vary in severity from trivial to life threatening. Classification is commonly accomplished by dividing the arrhythmias into two major subsets: tachyarrhythmias, or those producing heart rates of more than 100 beats per minute, and bradyarrhythmias, or those producing heart rates below 60 beats per minute. Arrhythmias may arise from conductive tissue anywhere within the atria, atrioventricular (AV) junction, or ventricles and are often further classified according to their place of origin. Patient symptoms are related to both the ventricular rate and the type of arrhythmia.

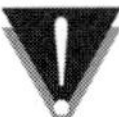

Emergency department referral or physician consultation is indicated for patients with life-threatening arrhythmias.

Physician consultation is indicated for new-onset rhythm disturbances and for arrhythmias associated with chest pain, syncope, dizziness, or treatment failure.

TACHYARRHYTHMIAS

DEFINITION AND EPIDEMIOLOGY

The majority of cardiac arrhythmias arise in or involve the atria. Atrial fibrillation, the most common sustained arrhythmia encountered in clinical practice, is estimated to occur in up to 2 million Americans.[1] It is more common among those over the age of 60 years.[2] Ventricular tachyarrhythmias, especially in the setting of serious, underlying organic cardiac disease, may predispose the patient to sudden death and increase mortality rates.[2,3] Although the true incidence of sudden cardiac death in the United States is unclear, current estimates suggest that sudden death accounts for 50% of cardiac deaths.[4] In the majority of cases, it is caused by ventricular fibrillation preceded by ventricular tachycardia (VT).[5] Risk factors for sudden death include ischemia, hypertrophic or dilated cardiomyopathy, and valvular or congenital heart disease.[3] Nonsustained VT develops in up to 10% of individuals after an acute myocardial infarction (MI).[3]

PATHOPHYSIOLOGY

The three major mechanisms responsible for most tachyarrhythmias are reentry, abnormal or enhanced automaticity, and triggered activity.[6] Reentry accounts for 80% to 90% of tachyarrhythmias and results from changes in the transmembrane potential of cardiac cells, which serve to alter the conduction pathways and refractoriness of cell membranes.[7]

Reentry

The mechanism for reentry involves the existence of two conduction pathways with nonhomogeneous refractory periods. They are connected both proximally and distally by conductive tissue, thereby creating a potential electrical circuit. Most typically, reentry is initiated into this system by a premature beat. The premature impulse, on finding one pathway still in its refractory period, travels along the pathway with the shorter refractory period, arriving at the distal portion of the circuit just as the other pathway becomes nonrefractory. The impulse is then conducted in retrograde fashion back to the proximal portion of the loop, finding the original pathway again ready to conduct. In this manner a circus movement is established whereby a single impulse is repeatedly conducted around the reentrant circuit.[6,7] The impulse escapes the loop at some point within each lap and depolarizes the rest of the myocardium, thereby creating a tachyarrhythmia.[6]

Abnormal or Enhanced Automaticity

Automaticity, or the ability to depolarize spontaneously, is a property common to all cardiac cells. Normally the automatic discharge of the sinus node proceeds at a rate faster than that of the remaining cardiac tissue, thereby establishing an orderly sequence of cardiac depolarization. However, a variety of factors, including ischemia, hypoxia, electrolyte imbalances, and drug effects, may enhance the automaticity of an ectopic focus, allowing it to depolarize more rapidly than the sinus node. Repeated discharge of an ectopic focus that exceeds the sinus node results in a tachyarrhythmia.

Triggered Activity

Triggered activity arises as a result of after depolarizations, or oscillations of membrane potential that attend or follow the action potential. When these oscillations depolarize the cell to threshold potential, they cause action potentials that result in extra systoles and tachycardia.[8] Triggered activity is thought to be the mechanism underlying the tachyarrhythmias associated with digoxin toxicity.[8,9] It may also be induced by antiarrhythmic agents and electrolyte imbalances.[8] Torsades de pointes (polymorphic VT associated with long QT intervals) is thought to be a triggered arrhythmia.[9]

CLINICAL PRESENTATION

Tachyarrhythmias may be entirely asymptomatic. Symptoms, when they do occur, are in large part related to the ventricular rate, the extent of underlying heart disease, ventricular function, and associated precipitating factors. Palpitations are the most common symptom caused by tachyarrhythmias. In patients with paroxysmal attacks, palpitations are usually regular and start and terminate abruptly. In patients with atrial fibrillation, palpitations are typically irregular and more sustained. Extra systoles may also cause palpitations or an awareness of isolated extra beats. The pause that follows an extra systole may be experienced as an actual cessation of the heartbeat.[10] Other causes of palpitations include thyrotoxicosis, hypovolemia, regurgitant valvular disease, anemia, hypoglycemia, pheochromocytoma, anemia, fever, and drugs (particularly digitalis, tricyclic antidepressants [TCAs], and antiarrhythmic agents).[10] Palpitations may also be a manifestation of an episode of acute anxiety.[5,10] Palpitations also commonly accompany the hot flashes of menopause.[11] Pertinent history includes the use of alcohol, tobacco, caffeine, sympathomimetics (commonly found in over-the-counter cold medicines), cocaine, theophylline, and thyroid medication because any of these may cause tachycardia and palpitations.[10] Any personal or family history of underlying heart disease or previous rhythm disturbance and its treatment are also relevant.

Because tachyarrhythmias tend to shorten diastole, ventricular filling is compromised, causing a drop in blood pressure, cardiac output, and coronary perfusion. Resultant symptoms may include lightheadedness, dizziness, syncope, fatigue, shortness of breath, and chest pain.[12-14] A serious tachyarrhythmia may result in hemodynamic decompensation, causing hypotension, chest pain, heart failure, change in level of consciousness, or even sudden cardiac death. It is important to assess both the arrhythmia and the patient's tolerance of it to determine the degree of urgency and the appropriate setting for intervention.

PHYSICAL EXAMINATION

The patient's general appearance, particularly color, evidence of diaphoresis, respiratory effort, and manifestations of anxiety, is important in evaluation of an arrhythmia. Indicators of the patient's hydration status, including skin turgor, status of mucous membranes, and orthostatic vital signs, are also relevant because dehydration and hypovolemia may cause a reflex tachycardia. Assessment of blood pressure, pulse, temperature, oxygen saturation, and mental status should accompany the initial assessment. Tachycardia with hypotension is indicative of cardiovascular compromise, requiring prompt intervention.

The examiner inspects and/or palpates the chest for parasternal lifts, heaves, and thrills. Auscultation of the heart for rate; rhythm; and the presence of murmurs, clicks, or extra heart sounds is essential. A benign systolic ejection murmur may accompany a tachycardia, whereas a murmur of any type may be associated with an underlying valve disorder. Absence of a murmur is not necessarily a significant finding, since rapid rates can often make accurate auscultation difficult. The patient should always be reexamined after the heart rate is controlled. An S_3 sound may warn of impending heart failure and is a significant finding. The "irregularly irregular" rhythm that is the hallmark of atrial fibrillation may also be the result of multiple extra systoles, whereas a regular tachycardia is more often associated with sinus tachycardia and other forms of supraventricular tachycardia (SVT). Alterations in pulse volume and irregularity may accompany ventricular ectopic beats, depending on the timing and force of ventricular contractions.

Assessment of the neck veins may provide information regarding atrial activity. An intermittent *a* wave may be observed. The *a* wave is absent with atrial fibrillation, since atrial systole is lost. A more prominent *a* wave than *v* wave may be observed with 2:1 AV block. Cannon *a* waves, or forceful, irregular expansions in the jugular pulse, may occur with AV dissociation as the atria contract against closed AV valves, causing a reflux of blood to the jugular veins.[8]

As part of the assessment, the examiner auscultates the lungs for rales, wheezes, or rhonchi and inspects the legs for edema. These may be present with associated cardiac failure as an indication that the rhythm is poorly tolerated by the patient. Other important findings include exophthalmos, an enlarged or nodular thyroid gland, or skin and hair changes commonly associated with hyperthyroidism.[8]

DIAGNOSTICS

12-Lead Electrocardiogram

The 12-lead ECG is indicated for initial evaluation of a suspected arrhythmia. This diagnostic tool has the notable limitation of providing only a brief view of the heart's electrical activity. Although sustained rhythms may easily be captured, paroxysmal rhythms may be elusive. However, even when the rate and rhythm are normal, the resting ECG may yield valuable information about the cause of an arrhythmia such as ventricular hypertrophy, MI, ischemia, drug effects, or electrolyte imbalance.[5] Indications of conduction abnormalities may also be present and include the widened QRS that accompanies intraventricular conduction delay; the shortened PR interval that accompanies preexcitation syndromes, such as Wolff-Parkinson-White (WPW); or the prolonged QT interval that may accompany idiopathic long QT syndrome or drug effects.[5,8] When abnormal rhythms are captured on the 12-lead ECG, the examiner needs to obtain a rhythm strip by allowing the tracing to continue for several minutes to fully evaluate the rhythm. With tachyarrhythmias, minor depressions of the ST segment and inversion of the T wave are commonly rate related and may be mistaken for indications of coronary disease.[10] These changes can be reevaluated once the rate is controlled.

Ambulatory Monitoring

Continuous ambulatory ECG (Holter monitoring) is a useful option for evaluating a suspected arrhythmia when symptoms are paroxysmal. Use of this portable device allows continuous recording of the heart's activity over a 24- to 48-hour period. The patient keeps a diary of activities and symptoms that can later be correlated with the tracing. The monitor is worn while patients go about their usual activities.

For the patient with infrequent symptoms, intermittent ambulatory ECG (event recording) may be more appropriate, since these devices can be worn for a long time. There are two types of these devices. The first type is worn externally and remains dormant until activated by the user at the onset of symptoms.[7] The second type is an implantable loop recorder. This device is implanted during a 20-minute procedure with the patient under local anesthesia by making a 2 cm (0.8 inch) incision under the skin. This device may stay in place for up to 14 months. It records activity during symptoms and can record an ECG when activated by an event. It can also track heart rate and rhythm; the data are stored and later can be played back for analysis.[15]

Provocative Testing and Electrophysiologic Studies

Provocative testing (e.g., the exercise ECG) may be helpful when the history suggests an arrhythmia in association with a specific activity. It is used for provocation of arrhythmias caused by ischemia or increased sympathetic activity. Exercise testing is also important to verify the absence of coronary ischemia before the use of type Ic antiarrhythmic agents.[16] Rhythms that put the patient at high risk for adverse events (very rapid SVT, WPW syndrome, complex ventricular ectopy, and VT) warrant referral to a specialist for electrophysiologic studies to properly identify and treat the problematic rhythm. Electrophysiologic studies (EPS) may also be indicated for investigating palpitations and syncope when noninvasive techniques have failed to definitively identify the problem.[17] EPS are invasive clinical techniques for the investigation and treatment of cardiac rhythm disorders. They permit a detailed analysis of the mechanism underlying the cardiac arrhythmia and precise location of the site of origin. Thus EPS can make an accurate diagnosis of an arrhythmia.[17]

Carotid Sinus Massage and Valsalva's Maneuver

Carotid sinus massage and Valsalva's maneuver may help differentiate one rhythm from another and are important diagnostic and therapeutic tools. Diagnostically, carotid sinus massage and Valsalva's maneuvers may cause transient AV block; this results in slowing of the ventricular response, enabling identification of the underlying rhythm. Therapeutically, these techniques may terminate rhythms for which the AV node is part of the reentry circuit, such as in AV nodal reentry tachycardia.[8]

Echocardiography

Two-dimensional transthoracic echocardiography should be performed during the initial workup of all arrhythmia patients to determine left atrial and left ventricular size, systolic function, and underlying structural heart disease. This is useful in guiding decisions regarding antiarrhythmic and antithrombotic therapy, particularly with regards to the patient with atrial fibrillation. Transesophageal echo is used to determine the presence or absence of left atrial thrombus before consideration of cardioversion.[1]

Other Diagnostics

Diagnostics, when appropriate, include a hemoglobin level to determine the presence of anemia, electrolytes to exclude hypokalemia and other electrolyte disturbances (e.g., hypomagnesemia), a thyroid-stimulating hormone (TSH) level if hyperthyroidism is suspected, a blood glucose determination if hypoglycemia is suspected, and a drug level for patients being treated with digoxin or other medications that might cause arrhythmia. Also chest x-ray studies are useful to identify structural disease, heart failure, or pneumonia.

DIAGNOSTICS

Tachyarrhythmias

INITIAL
ECG
Pulse oximetry

LABORATORY
Hemoglobin, hematocrit
Serum electrolytes
TSH
Blood glucose
Digoxin level*
Drug levels*

IMAGING
Echocardiography (to evaluate for underlying structural heart disease)

OTHER
Event monitor
Holter monitor
Provocative testing
Valsalva's maneuver*
Carotid sinus massage*

*If indicated.

DIFFERENTIAL DIAGNOSIS

Narrow QRS Tachycardia

Any rhythm with a QRS of 0.12 second or less is termed *supraventricular*, having originated at or above the AV node. The rhythms in the following paragraphs are included in this group and are described as they appear on the ECG.

Sinus Tachycardia

In sinus tachycardia a P wave precedes each QRS in a consistent 1:1 relationship. The rhythm is regular, the P waves are identical, the QRS complexes are normal and narrow, and the PR and QRS intervals are within normal ranges. The rate is over 100 beats per minute (Figure 124-1).

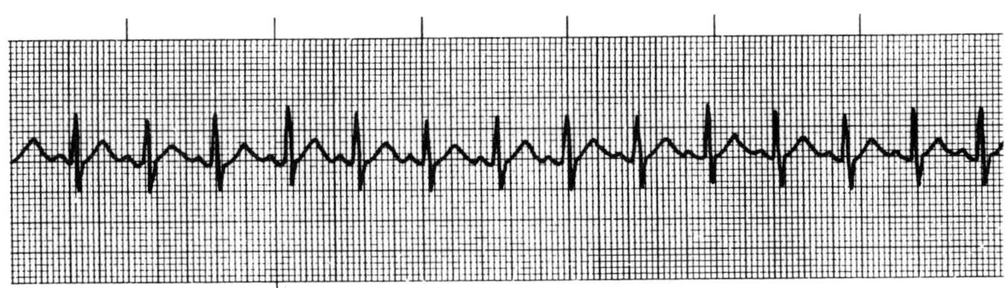

FIGURE 124-1

Sinus tachycardia. (From Andreoli KG, Fowkes VH, Zipes DP, and others: *Comprehensive cardiac care,* ed 2, St Louis, 1971, Mosby.)

Premature Atrial Contractions

Premature atrial contractions (PACs) do not, in and of themselves, constitute a tachyarrhythmia but are important in that they may initiate a tachyarrhythmia in the susceptible heart. Also, if they are numerous, they may cause the patient to complain of palpitations or a skipped or extra beat.[12] They are typically identified on the ECG within a prevailing sinus rhythm, which would be completely regular were it not for the premature beats. The PAC is a normal-looking beat in every way except that it occurs prematurely. Because its origin is outside the sinus node, the P wave, although normal, may appear different from the P waves of the prevailing rhythm. Because it is premature, the P wave may be buried or appear as a notch in the previous T wave. The PR interval may differ slightly from that of the prevailing rhythm, although it remains within the normal range. Because the beat depolarizes the sinus node, there is typically a partially compensatory pause before the next sinus beat (Figure 124-2).

Premature Junctional Contractions

Premature junctional contractions (PJCs) are another cause of irregularity in the heart rhythm. Also known as ectopic atrial contractions, PJCs are premature beats that originate in the AV node. They do not constitute a tachyarrhythmia but, like PACs, may initiate one in the susceptible heart. Because the impulse is carried to the ventricles along normal pathways, the resultant QRS complex is narrow and appears similar to the QRS complexes of the sinus rhythm. There may be retrograde conduction to the atria, yielding a P wave that can occur before, during, or after the QRS. If the P wave occurs before the QRS complex, the PR interval is less than 0.12 second. When a P wave is visible, it is typically negative in leads II, III, and aV_F.[8]

Multifocal Atrial Tachycardia

In multifocal atrial tachycardia the heart rate is usually 100 to 130 beats per minute and the rhythm is irregular. The P waves have three or more morphologic variations. The PP interval and the PR interval will be variable. This rhythm is usually seen in older patients with pulmonary, cardiovascular, or metabolic disturbances.

Paroxysmal Supraventricular Tachycardia

Paroxysmal supraventricular tachycardia (PSVT) is a rapid (140 to 240 beats per minute), generally regular rhythm that is typically initiated by a single beat and starts and stops abruptly. P waves may differ slightly in morphology compared with the sinus rhythm. The QRS is most typically narrow. P and QRS waves may exist in a 1:1 relationship, or variable AV block may alter this relationship. If the rate is very fast, P waves may be buried in the previous beat. Paroxysmal atrial tachycardia (PAT), particularly PAT with block, is often associated with digoxin toxicity.[8]

Atrioventricular Nodal Reentry Tachycardia

In AV nodal reentry tachycardia (AVNRT), the most common mechanism for PSVT, dual pathways within the AV node are responsible for the circus conduction. P waves, when they are visible, exist in a 1:1 relationship with the QRS. Often, in very fast rhythms, they are buried within the QRS and either are not visible or are seen as a distortion at the end of the QRS complex. This distortion appears as a pseudo–S wave in leads II, III, and aV_F and/or a pseudo–R′ wave in lead V_1.[8,18] The rate is usually 140 to 180 beats per minute and regular. The QRS is narrow and morphologically similar to that of the sinus rhythm. It is typically paroxysmal in nature and will terminate with Valsalva's maneuver or carotid sinus massage.

Atrioventricular Reentry Tachycardia

With AV reentry tachycardia (AVNT), the reentry occurs because of an accessory pathway between the atria and ventricles that bypasses the AV node. This mechanism is responsible for preexcitation syndromes such as Lown-Ganong-Levine syndrome and WPW syndrome. Typically there is a short PR interval. The QRS may be normal or wide. In WPW a delta wave, which is a slurred upstroke at the beginning of the QRS, may be seen. In orthodromic tachycardia the impulse is conducted first down the AV pathway and then back up via the accessory pathway. A narrow QRS results. In antidromic tachycardia the impulse conducts first down the accessory pathway and then back up through the AV pathway. The result is a wide QRS. Reentry rhythms conducted in this manner tend to be very fast because of the shorter refractory period of the accessory pathway.[5]

Atrial Flutter

In atrial flutter the atrial rate ranges from 250 to 350 beats per minute, producing a sawtooth appearance of the P waves. The atrial rate of 300 beats per minute usually has a 2:1 conduction to the ventricle, producing a QRS rate of 150 beats per minute.

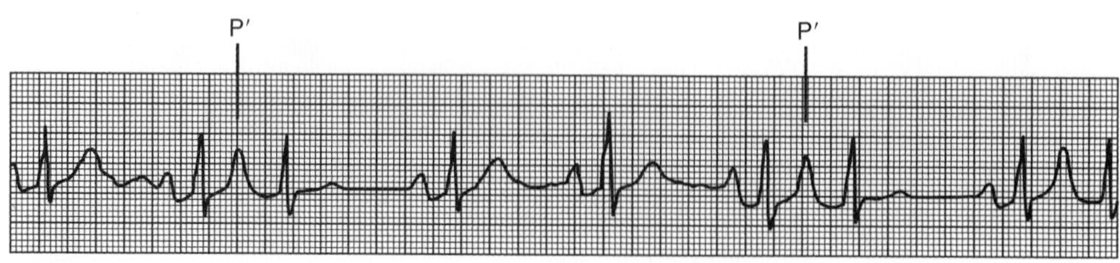

FIGURE 124-2

Premature atrial complexes hidden in T waves (lead II). (From Conover MB: *Understanding electrocardiography*, ed 7, St Louis, 1996, Mosby.)

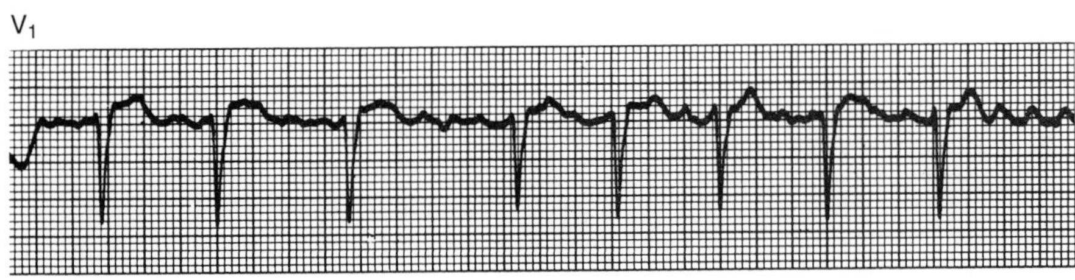

FIGURE 124-3

Atrial fibrillation. (From Conover MB: *Cardiac arrhythmias: exercises in pattern interpretations,* St Louis, 1974, Mosby.)

Atrial Fibrillation

Atrial fibrillation has the normal P wave replaced by fibrillatory F waves, producing a wavy baseline. The atrial rate is estimated to be between 350 and 650 beats per minute. There is an irregularly irregular ventricular response because the AV node will allow only a fraction of the atrial impulses to reach the ventricle (Figure 124-3).

Wide QRS Tachycardia

A QRS that is greater than 0.12 second may be SVT with aberrancy (a wide QRS produced by a refractory block of one of the bundle branches as the rapid impulses from the atria attempt to depolarize the ventricles), VT, or ventricular fibrillation. Differentiation between VT and SVT with aberrant conduction is often challenging but critical because treatment approaches differ significantly depending on the origin of the arrhythmia. A combination of leads is superior to one lead in making this differentiation.[19]

In SVT with aberrancy, the QRS is greater than 0.12 second wide but typically not greater than 0.14 second. Often a triphasic RSR′ right bundle branch pattern is seen in lead V_1. Because of the fast ventricular rate, the P wave may be buried in the previous beat or may be seen as a peaked or notched T wave in the previous beat. Carotid sinus massage may slow (and hence yield a 1:1 relationship of the P to the QRS) or even terminate the tachycardia.

Ventricular Tachycardia

VT is defined as three or more consecutive ventricular ectopic beats. The rhythm may be sustained or nonsustained, lasting more than or less than 30 seconds, respectively. The QRS width is greater than 0.12 second and often is greater than 0.14 second. It is usually fairly regular with a rate between 100 and 300 beats per minute. The most reliable criterion for correctly diagnosing VT is AV dissociation. P waves may be seen as distortions at different points in the ECG cycle. These are independent P waves that bear no relationship to the QRS. Other indicators that favor a diagnosis of VT over SVT are a QRS greater than 0.14 second; extreme right-axis deviation (between 180 and −90); concordance of the QRS pattern in all precordial leads (i.e., all positive or all negative deflections), particularly when concordance is negative; and a wide QRS pattern inconsistent with typical right or left bundle branch patterns.[8,9] This rhythm will not respond to carotid sinus massage (Figure 124-4).

Torsades de Pointes

The QRS morphologic pattern in VT may be uniform (monomorphic VT) or variable (polymorphic VT). A specific type of VT, torsades de pointes, deserves mention because the pharmacologic treatment for this disorder differs markedly from standard treatment for VT. Torsades de pointes is characterized by polymorphic QRS complexes that change in

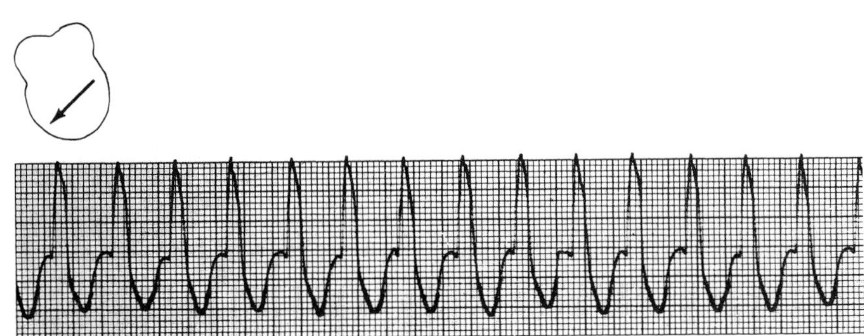

FIGURE 124-4

Ventricular tachycardia. (From Conover MB: *Understanding electrocardiography,* ed 5, St Louis, 1988, Mosby.)

DIFFERENTIAL DIAGNOSIS

Tachyarrhythmias

NARROW COMPLEX
- Sinus tachycardia
- Multifocal atrial tachycardia
- Paroxysmal atrial tachycardia
- Atrioventricular nodal reentry tachycardia
- Atrioventricular reciprocating tachycardia
- Atrial flutter
- Atrial fibrillation
- Premature atrial contractions
- Premature junctional contractions

WIDE COMPLEX
- Supraventricular tachycardia with aberrancy
- Ventricular tachycardia
- Ventricular fibrillation

amplitude and cycle length. It is associated with QT prolongation, which may be idiopathic or related to drug effects (antiarrhythmic agents of class Ia, IIc, and III; TCAs; and phenothiazines) or electrolyte imbalances (particularly hypokalemia or hypomagnesemia).[8,9]

Ventricular Fibrillation

Ventricular fibrillation is a rapid, disorganized electrical activity within the ventricles with no discrete QRS complexes. The heart is unable to contract, and the patient is in cardiac arrest.

Premature Ventricular Contractions

Premature ventricular contractions (PVCs) are extra premature beats that originate in the ventricle. They are characterized by wide (>0.12 second), bizarre QRS complexes that interrupt the prevailing rhythm. The P wave is typically absent, and the beat is most often followed by a full compensatory pause (the distance from the QRS preceding the PVC to the QRS that follows it is equal to twice the RR interval of the prevailing sinus rhythm). Typically, the T wave deflection is in opposition to that of the QRS complex.[7] Their description is included here because of their association with ventricular tachyarrhythmias (Figure 124-5).

MANAGEMENT

The decision to initiate long-term antiarrhythmic therapy depends on the severity and frequency of the arrhythmia and it hemodynamic consequences vs. the risks associated with the therapy itself. The need for long-term therapy must be carefully individualized to each patient, since the severity and importance of symptoms are highly variable, based on the clinical situation and the presence or absence of underlying coronary artery disease.[20]

Although many of the symptoms caused by arrhythmias are the result of the heart rate and the hemodynamic response, these can vary between patients and even between episodes in an individual patient. The effect of an arrhythmia on hemodynamics is not necessarily related to its cause, being largely dependent on the rate, nature, and severity of underlying heart disease; the presence or absence of AV synchrony; the ventricular activation sequence; and autonomic response and balance.

Results of clinical trials, such as the Cardiac Arrhythmia Suppression Trials (CAST I and CAST II), which demonstrated an increase in mortality in all treatment groups (patients with asymptomatic ventricular dysfunction after acute MI treated with encainide, flecainide, or moricizine) compared with a placebo group, have emphasized the need to critically analyze the need for antiarrhythmic therapy.[21] The concept of proarrhythmia, or antiarrhythmic agents inducing the very arrhythmias they are used to suppress, has radically altered antiarrhythmic therapy. The two general conditions for which antiarrhythmic therapy is appropriate are a potentially life-threatening arrhythmia and an arrhythmia that is significantly symptomatic.[7,8] The treatment of serious, recurrent, or potentially life-threatening arrhythmias requires referral to a cardiologist for aggressive management, possibly involving guided drug therapy based on electrophysiologic study results or use of implantable cardioverter-defibrillators (ICDs) or surgical (ablation) intervention.[6]

With these general principles in mind, the following discussion reviews general approaches to each arrhythmia. Pharmacologic agents are further outlined in Table 124-1.

For patients with atrial tachyarrhythmias who are hemodynamically unstable, immediate synchronized cardioversion may be recommended. Cardioversion is successful in 85% to 90% of cases.[12,14,22] Acute management may also be accom-

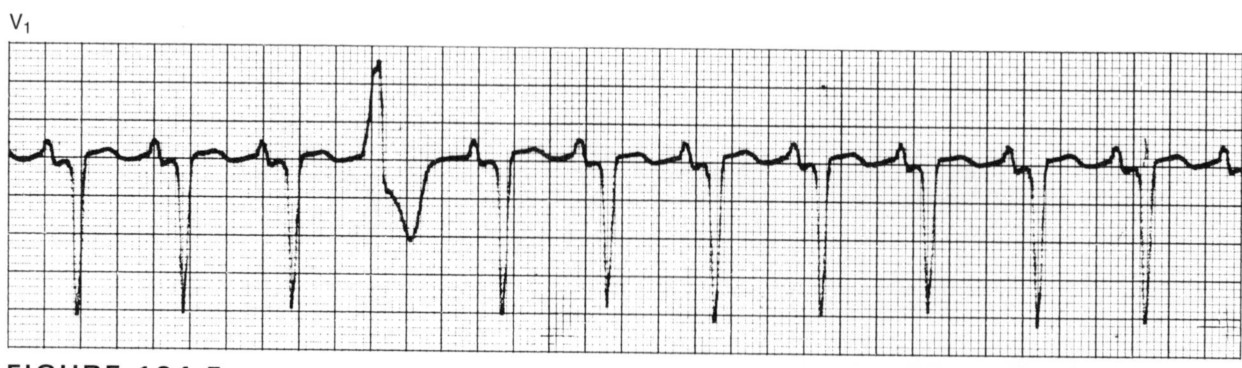

FIGURE 124-5

Premature ventricular contractions. (From Conover MB: *Pocket guide to electrocardiography*, ed 3, St Louis, 1994, Mosby.)

TABLE 124-1 Pharmacologic Arrhythmia Management

Agent	Dose	Cautions
CLASS I AGENTS*		
Ia		
Procainamide	IV: 20 mg/min; maximum: 15 mg/kg PO: 750-1250 mg q 12 hr	GI upset, hypotension, widening of QRS, lupuslike syndrome, anorexia, rash, proarrhythmia
Quinidine	IV: 6-10 mg/kg; rate of 0.4-0.5 mg/kg/min until arrhythmia suppressed or QRS complex widens, or hypotension or bradycardia occurs PO: 200-400 mg q 6 hr	GI upset, diarrhea, cinchonism, fever, rash, proarrhythmia, anorexia, tinnitus, increased digoxin and warfarin levels
Ib		
Lidocaine	IV: 1-1.5 mg/kg bolus, followed by infusion 1-4 mg/min; total: 3 mg/kg	Drowsiness, paresthesia, muscle twitching, lack of orientation, convulsions
Ic		
Flecainide	PO: 100-200 mg q 12 hr	Proarrhythmia, decreased left ventricular function, dizziness, visual disturbances, dyspnea, headache, nausea, fatigue, palpitation, chest pain, tremor, constipation; to be avoided in AV block or left ventricular dysfunction
Propafenone	PO: 150-300 mg q 8-12 hr	Proarrhythmia, unusual taste, dizziness, AV block, intraventricular conduction defect, constipation, headache, diplopia, fatigue; to be avoided in severe congestive heart failure (CHF), AV block, or chronic obstructive pulmonary disease (COPD)
CLASS II AGENTS†		
Esmolol	IV: 500 mcg/kg/min over 5-minute load; 50-200 mcg/kg/min infusion; not to exceed 48hr of 200 mcg/kg/min infusion	Nausea, vomiting, diarrhea, fatigue, weakness, CHF, hallucinations, insomnia, gait disturbance, mental status change, conduction abnormality, exacerbation of asthma; all beta blockers to be avoided in bronchospasm, CHF, and hypotension
Metoprolol	IV: 5 mg IV push q 5 min up to 15 mg PO: 50-450 mg/day in divided doses	
Propranolol	IV: 2 mg IV push; maximum: 0.1 mg/kg PO: 20-160 mg q 6 hr	
CLASS III AGENTS‡		
Sotalol	PO: 80-320 mg q 12 hr	Prolongation of QT, proarrhythmia, nausea, vomiting, dry mouth, diarrhea, retroperitoneal fibrosis, depression, fatigue, impotence, headache, bradycardia, AV block
Amiodarone	IV: 150 mg over 10- to 30-minute load; 1 mg/min ×6 hours; 0.5 mg/min up to 1 g/day PO: 800-1600 mg/day for 3-14 days; 100-400 mg/day maintenance	Corneal microdeposits, photosensitivity, liver and lung toxicity, hyperthyroidism, hypothyroidism, pulmonary fibrosis, proarrhythmia, AV block, increase in warfarin or digoxin levels, skin discoloration, prolonged elimination (half-life: 60 days)
Ibutilide	IV: 1 mg over 10 minutes, repeat ×1 in 10 minutes; 0.01 mg/kg for patient <60 kg	Proarrhythmia, AV block, bradycardia, nausea, headache
Bretylium	IV: 5-10 mg/kg up to 30 mg; infuse 1-2 mg/min	Hypotension, nausea, vomiting, bradycardia, initial catecholamine release with increase in heart rate and blood pressure
CLASS IV AGENTS§		
Verapamil	IV: 0.075-0.15 mg/kg over 2 minutes PO: 120-480 mg/day	Contraindicated in Wolff-Parkinson-White syndrome, sick sinus syndrome, excess beta blocker, procainamide, quinidine, or digoxin
Diltiazem	IV: 0.25-0.35 mg/kg over 2 minutes; 5-15 mg/hr constant ×24 hours PO: 120-480 mg/day	CHF, hypotension, nausea, edema, fatigue, conduction abnormalities, pain at injection site
MISCELLANEOUS AGENTS		
Adenosine	IV: 6- to 12-mg bolus	Facial flushing, dyspnea, chest pain, nausea, headache, lightheadedness, bronchospasm

AV, Atrioventricular; *GI,* gastrointestinal.
*Depress automaticity, increase refractoriness, and inhibit sodium channels.
†Beta-blocking effects.
‡Prolong the action potential and interfere with potassium-dependent repolarizing currents.
§Block inward calcium channels of sinoatrial and AV node.

Continued

TABLE 124-1 Pharmacologic Arrhythmia Management—cont'd

Agent	Dose	Cautions
MISCELLANEOUS AGENTS—CONT'D		
Digoxin	IV: 0.5-1 mg/24 hr in divided doses PO: 0.125-0.375 mg/day	Interactions with other agents (requiring reduction of digoxin), anorexia, nausea, vomiting, diarrhea, constipation, visual disturbances, psychiatric disturbances, all types of arrhythmias
Magnesium	IV: 1- to 2-g load over 1-2 minutes; 0.5-1 g/hr infusion	AV block, hypotension, flushing, sweating, depressed reflexes, respiratory paralysis, diarrhea
Epinephrine	IV: 1 mg q 3-5 min; 0.1 mg/kg for high dose	Ischemia with increased ventricular ectopy
Atropine	IV: 0.5-1 mg q 5 min; maximum: 0.04 mg/kg	Tachycardia; delirium; flushed, hot skin; ataxia; blurred vision; ischemia

plished with the IV administration of adenosine, antiarrhythmics such as amiodarone, calcium channel blockers, or beta blockers.[5]

Sinus Tachycardia

Sinus tachycardia is treated by removal or treatment of the underlying cause (e.g., fever, hypovolemia, hyperthyroidism, anxiety). Elimination of tobacco, alcohol, caffeine, or sympathomimetics (such as those found in over-the-counter cold medications and nose drops) may result in a return to normal heart rate.[8] Patients with inappropriate sinus tachycardia may require treatment with beta blockers or calcium channel blockers.[5]

PACs do not usually require treatment, but the cause may be investigated, particularly when the patient is aware of and bothered by them. In normal individuals PACs may be a result of various stimuli, including tobacco, alcohol, and caffeine. Their occurrence may diminish or disappear when these stimuli are withdrawn. PACs are also associated with ischemia, hypokalemia and hypomagnesemia, hypoxia, and myocardial stretch in early congestive heart failure. Correction of the underlying cause may halt the PACs.[8]

PJCs are not usually treated. If they initiate a tachyarrhythmia, treatment is directed toward controlling that rhythm.[8]

Multifocal Atrial Tachycardia

Multifocal atrial tachycardia occurs primarily in older patients with co-morbid disease. Sixty percent of these patients have significant pulmonary disease.[8,23] The diagnosis often occurs in the setting of congestive heart failure, exacerbation of the underlying pulmonary condition, or electrolyte imbalance. As with sinus tachycardia, therapy is directed toward correcting the precipitating factor (e.g., improving oxygenation, correcting electrolyte imbalance).[8]

Paroxysmal Supraventricular Tachycardia

Most cases of PSVT are reentrant and amenable to radiofrequency ablation when symptoms are significant and recurrent. Ablation is generally preferable to antiarrhythmic agents because of safety and tolerability concerns.[5] Pharmacologically, narrow-complex PSVT is treated by slowing AV conduction with digoxin, calcium channel blockers, or beta blockers and/or by suppressing atrial automaticity with class Ia, Ic, or III antiarrhythmic agents.[8]

Wide-complex PSVT must be managed with care in conjunction with a cardiologist. Electrophysiologic study with radiofrequency ablation is the treatment of choice. If pharmacologic management is instituted, care must be exercised because agents that increase the refractoriness of the AV node (digoxin, calcium channel blockers, and beta blockers), when used alone, may decrease the refractoriness of the accessory pathway and could cause a faster ventricular rate. Class Ia, Ic, and III agents are preferred because they increase the refractoriness of the bypass tract.

Atrial Fibrillation or Atrial Flutter

Management of the patient with atrial fibrillation or atrial flutter may be challenging because the best approach is often not clear and treatment must be highly individualized. The three therapeutic goals are rate control, restoration and maintenance of sinus rhythm, and prevention of thromboembolism. The risks and benefits of each treatment must be considered for each patient.[1]

When patients are seen with atrial fibrillation for the first time, a search for the cause should be undertaken. Common causes include rheumatic heart disease, mitral valve disease, hypertension (particularly with left ventricular hypertrophy), coronary heart disease, cardiomyopathy, hyperthyroidism, acute alcohol intoxication or withdrawal, stimulant ingestion (caffeine, amphetamines, theophylline), and acute pulmonary disease.[1]

A major decision to be made in treating atrial fibrillation is whether to attempt to restore and maintain sinus rhythm or to opt merely for ventricular rate control. Factors that contribute to this decision include duration of the atrial fibrillation and left atrial size. While not absolute, both left atrial enlargement and prolonged duration of atrial fibrillation can reduce the ability to maintain normal sinus rhythm.[20,24] Reasons for opting for restoration and maintenance of sinus rhythm include symptom relief, prevention of embolism, and prevention of cardiomyopathy.

Cardioversion can be accomplished via either electrical or pharmacologic means. Side effects and proarrhythmia are concerns with the use of antiarrhythmics. Flecainide, ibutilide, propafenone, amiodarone, and quinidine are the drugs of choice. Procainamide, sotalol, and digoxin may also be used. Both electrical and pharmacologic cardioversion carries the risk of thromboembolism.[1] When the rhythm has been sustained for longer than 48 hours, anticoagulation uninterrupted for 4 weeks before and for at least 4 weeks after elective cardioversion is necessary.[12,14,25]

A transesophageal echocardiogram (TEE) may also be obtained before cardioversion to exclude the presence of left atrial thrombus if the duration of atrial fibrillation is unclear and cardioversion is necessary. If atrial thrombus is present on TEE, the cardioversion is postponed for 4 more weeks of adequate anticoagulation and repeat TEE can be obtained.

One major consideration in determining treatment is the patient's tolerance of the lost atrial contraction that accompanies atrial fibrillation. Loss of AV synchrony and the irregularity of the ventricular rhythm both contribute to a decline in cardiac output that has been estimated to be about 15%.[1] Although patients without serious underlying disease may be able to tolerate this reduction without difficulty, a patient with limited cardiac reserve may decompensate quickly. The presence of mitral stenosis, restrictive or hypertrophic cardiomyopathy, pericardial disease, or ventricular hypertrophy increases the likelihood of hemodynamic deterioration with the onset of atrial fibrillation.[1] When the loss of atrial contraction is not as critical and the patient is hemodynamically stable, the decision is less obvious. Neither conversion to and maintenance of sinus rhythm nor rate control is clearly superior.[1] Information should be provided regarding the relative efficacy and potential side effects of antiarrhythmic agents. The duration of atrial fibrillation is an important determinant of success: the longer a patient experiences atrial fibrillation, the lower are the odds of maintaining sinus rhythm. The odds are very low, for instance, after 3 months of atrial fibrillation.[6]

Rate control is easier to achieve and is an acceptable goal in hemodynamically stable patients. Amiodarone, beta blockers, calcium channel blockers, and possibly digoxin are indicated for rate control alone.[1]

Thromboembolism is a major complication of recurrent or persistent atrial fibrillation. One third of these patients eventually experience strokes, of which 75% are thought to be embolic.[1] Anticoagulation greatly reduces this risk. Anticoagulation, when indicated, is accomplished with warfarin to maintain the International Normalized Ratio (INR) between 2 and 3 (see Chapter 227). For those who cannot take anticoagulants, aspirin 325 mg/day is an acceptable but less effective alternative.[1] Anticoagulation in low-risk patients—those younger than 60 years of age without heart disease—may be accomplished with aspirin. For all others, warfarin is preferred if not contraindicated.[1]

Finally, those with problematic or refractory atrial fibrillation may be candidates for nonpharmacologic approaches, including AV nodal ablation or modification and pacemaker implantation. The surgical maze procedure has been shown to be useful in controlling the tachyarrhythmia that occurs with atrial fibrillation.[1,26]

In some cases pulmonary vein isolation can be an effective and even curative approach to the management of atrial fibrillation. Research has shown that most atrial fibrillation signals come from the four pulmonary veins.[27] Blocking these impulses using pulmonary vein isolation enables the atria to pump more regularly. During pulmonary isolation, a physician inserts catheters into the blood vessels of the atria, allowing for the delivery of radiofrequency energy to the area of the atria that connects to the pulmonary vein. This produces a scar that blocks any impulses firing from within the pulmonary vein, thereby correcting the atrial fibrillation.[27]

Premature Ventricular Contractions

PVCs occur in both normal and diseased hearts. In the structurally normal heart PVCs are of no prognostic significance, and in the absence of severe symptomatology they require no treatment. However, complex ventricular ectopy (defined as >10 PVCs per minute over 24 hours or nonsustained VT) is rare in the normal heart, and the appearance of such should provoke an evaluation for underlying cardiac disease. The patient with cardiac disease (previous MI or depressed left ventricular ejection fraction) and complex ectopy is at increased risk for sudden death. However, antiarrhythmic therapy, although it may reduce the ectopy, has not been shown to decrease mortality; in the CAST studies, it was actually shown to increase the risk of sudden cardiac death.[8] When treatment is instituted, beta blockers are the drugs of choice.

Ventricular Tachycardia

Clinical management of nonsustained VT first includes identification and management of any underlying cause (e.g., digoxin toxicity, electrolyte imbalance, hypoxia, ischemia). In the absence of symptoms and underlying heart disease, treatment is rarely indicated. Patients with previous MI, structural heart disease, and low ejection fractions who have nonsustained VT, however, are at particularly high risk for adverse events, including sudden death. Beta blockers reduce these risks, but referral for electrophysiologic testing should be considered for this group, as well as for those with severe symptomatology.[6]

Sustained VT is typically an emergent situation requiring care at an acute care facility. Synchronized cardioversion with 100 to 360 J or appropriate biphasic dose is indicated for VT with hemodynamic compromise. Immediate defibrillation for ventricular fibrillation or VT without a pulse is required to prevent immediate death.[28]

Therapy to prevent recurrent sustained VT may include either pharmacologic management, ICD implantation, or a combination of the two. Those with significant left ventricular dysfunction are at particularly high risk for sudden death. Current evidence suggests that these patients are best managed with ICD implantation. In these patients with severe left ventricular dysfunction (ejection fraction <35%) simultaneous pacing of both ventricles (biventricular, or BiV, pacing) can help optimize cardiac pump function through synchronization of ventricular contraction. This approach, referred to as *cardiac resynchronization therapy*, can be achieved with a device designed only for pacing or can be incorporated into a combination device with an ICD.

For those with normal left ventricular function, a combination of amiodarone and a beta blocker may be used.[5] Electrophysiology study with radiofrequency ablation is appropriate for those with reentry VT.

COMPLICATIONS, INDICATIONS FOR REFERRAL OR HOSPITALIZATION, AND PATIENT AND FAMILY EDUCATION

See Complications, Indications for Referral or Hospitalization, and Patient and Family Education under Bradyarrhythmias.

BRADYARRHYTHMIAS

DEFINITION AND EPIDEMIOLOGY

Bradyarrhythmias may result from abnormalities in conduction between the sinus node and atrium, within the AV node, and in the intraventricular conduction pathways.[29] Sinus node dysfunction is most often found in older adults as an isolated phenomenon resulting from idiopathic fibrosis.[30] Interruption of blood supply to the sinus node from myocardial ischemia or infiltration of the structure as a result of collagen vascular disease, sarcoid, tumors, or amyloid will cause disruption of sinus node discharge. Sinus bradycardia may occur with hypothyroidism, advanced liver disease, hypothermia, or severe hypoxia and in patients taking calcium channel blockers or beta blockers. It may also occur normally in highly trained athletes.[30]

Idiopathic fibrosis is a major cause of AV block, particularly in older adults.[1] Diseases that can influence AV conduction include MI, coronary spasm, myocarditis, rheumatic fever, mononucleosis, Lyme's disease, sarcoidosis, amyloidosis, and neoplasms. Drugs such as digitalis, beta blockers, calcium channel blockers, and quinidine may also cause AV nodal conduction disturbances.[30]

Bundle branch block (BBB) may occur in the presence or absence of structural heart disease. It may be congenital or acquired, chronic or intermittent. It is often rate related and may be seen only when the heart exceeds some critical rate. Left bundle branch block (LBBB) is often a marker for ischemic heart disease, longstanding hypertension, severe aortic valve disease, or cardiomyopathy.[31]

PATHOPHYSIOLOGY

The sinus node is the cardiac conduction tissue with the highest intrinsic firing rate. It is the pacemaker of the normal heart. When sinus node discharge is suppressed or blocked by drugs or disease, bradycardia may result. The pacemaker function may be assumed by "escape" foci in the atrial tissue, the AV node, the His-Purkinje tissue, or the ventricular myocardium. The intrinsic rates of these areas are slower than in the sinoatrial (SA) node, resulting in bradycardia.

Conduction Blocks

Conduction blocks can also occur in the AV node or the His-Purkinje system. When the impulse is merely delayed, as with first-degree AV block or BBB, the heart rate may be unaffected. However, with higher degrees of block, significant bradycardia may occur. In second-degree AV block, impulse conduction through the AV node is intermittently blocked. An adequate ventricular rate may or may not be maintained. In third-degree, or complete, heart block, there is complete failure of AV conduction, and continuing ventricular activity depends on the emergence of an escape rhythm. Depending on where the escape rhythm originates, an adequate heart rate may or may not be maintained. The higher the level in the conduction system at which the block occurs, the faster is the escape rhythm. A block within the AV node, for instance, may result in an escape rhythm fast enough to prevent syncope. If both bundle branches are blocked, the ventricular escape rhythm may be too slow to maintain an adequate cardiac output, and syncope and death may result.

CLINICAL PRESENTATION

Symptoms accompanying bradycardia are largely dependent on the ventricular rate relative to metabolic demand and on the presence of underlying cardiac disease. Those with limited cardiac reserve would obviously tolerate a slow rate less well than would those with normal hearts. The American Heart Association recognizes two types of bradycardia: absolute and relative. Absolute bradycardia refers to any heart rate below 60 beats per minute. Relative bradycardia refers to a heart rate that is too slow to maintain normal blood pressure or cardiac output even if the rate is greater than 60 beats per minute.[29]

Bradycardia may be asymptomatic and may be an incidental finding on a routine ECG. In such cases it is most likely that the body's needs are being met despite the slow heart rate. Symptomatic bradycardia is defined as a documented bradyarrhythmia that is directly responsible for the development of frank syncope or near syncope, transient dizziness, or lightheadedness and confusional states resulting from cerebral hypoperfusion attributable to a slow ventricular rate.[32] Other symptoms include fatigue, exercise intolerance, and frank congestive heart failure. These symptoms may occur at rest or with exertion.[32]

Relevant aspects of the history include a careful review of all medications and identification of any underlying cardiac disease. It is important to discern whether the symptoms occur at rest or with exertion and whether there are any outstanding aggravating or alleviating factors. A vagal mechanism for bradycardia may be implicated, for instance, if the symptoms occur only with straining, such as with vomiting or moving the bowels.

PHYSICAL EXAMINATION

As with tachyarrhythmias, the focus of the physical examination for the patient with a suspected bradyarrhythmia is a thorough cardiopulmonary examination. Blood pressure and heart rate and rhythm are crucial, as are careful cardiac auscultation and respiratory assessment. Relevant findings include any murmurs, extra heart sounds, or signs of impending cardiac failure (rales, S_3, jugular vein distention, peripheral edema, or respiratory effort).

When the presenting complaint is syncope, near syncope, dizziness, or altered level of consciousness, a neurologic examination is necessary to explore the possibility of noncardiac causes. Orthostatic vital signs are also important to exclude orthostatic hypotension as a cause of syncope.

Finally, palpitations may be the presenting complaint when the bradyarrhythmia is a manifestation of sick sinus syndrome. This syndrome is often characterized by recurrent SVTs alternating with bradycardia (often called *tachy-brady syndrome*). The long pauses that often follow the termination of tachycardia may also cause symptoms, including syncope, dizziness, or confusion. Persistent bradycardia, sinus arrest, or SA exit block may also accompany sick sinus syndrome, with symptomatology similar to that of other forms of bradycardia.[5]

DIAGNOSTICS

Electrocardiography

As in any arrhythmia, the ECG is vital to accurate diagnosis. Ambulatory ECG (Holter monitoring, event recording) plays a special role in the diagnosis of bradyarrhythmias in that definite correlation of symptoms with a bradyarrhythmia is a requirement to fulfill the criteria of symptomatic bradycardia. Decisions about the need for a pacemaker are necessarily influenced by the presence or absence of symptoms that are directly attributable to bradycardia.[32] Ambulatory monitoring allows for this definitive correlation.

Provocative Testing

Provocative testing in the form of a tilt test may elicit bradyarrhythmias related to position change, such as malignant vasovagal syndrome, which is evidenced by exaggerated vagal response to emotional or painful stimuli. Carotid sinus massage during simultaneous ECG recording is useful for provoking symptomatic bradycardia in the carotid sinus syndrome, a disorder in which bradycardia occurs in response to carotid sinus hypersensitivity.

Other Diagnostics

Other tests may be necessary to exclude other causes of bradycardia. These include serum electrolytes to exclude hyperkalemia and other electrolyte imbalances, a digoxin level for patients being treated with digoxin, and a TSH level to exclude hypothyroidism.

DIAGNOSTICS

Bradyarrhythmias

INITIAL
ECG
Pulse oximetry

LABORATORY
Hemoglobin, hematocrit
Serum electrolytes
TSH
Blood glucose
Digoxin level*
Drug levels*

IMAGING
Echocardiography (if left ventricular dysfunction or valve disease is suspected)

OTHER
Event monitor
Holter monitor
Provocative testing

*If indicated.

DIFFERENTIAL DIAGNOSIS

Sinus Bradycardia

In sinus bradycardia the sinus node fires at a rate less than 60 beats per minute with a 1:1 relationship between each P wave and QRS complex. PR and QRS intervals are within normal range.

Sinoatrial Exit Block

SA exit block is the sudden cessation of sinus rhythm that results in long pauses. These pauses usually occur in a fixed pattern.

Atrioventricular Nodal Block

AV nodal block, in which conduction is delayed or blocked completely at the level of the AV node, may be transient, intermittent, or permanent. The block is termed *first, second,* or *third degree,* depending on the ability of the AV node to allow conduction of P waves to the ventricle.

First-Degree AV Block. In first-degree AV block the PR interval is greater than 0.20 second, but every P wave is conducted to the ventricle, resulting in a related QRS complex. First-degree block may occur in the presence or absence of bradycardia.

Second Degree, Type I. In second-degree, Mobitz type I AV block, there is progressive prolongation of the PR interval until a P wave is not conducted to the ventricle. The atrium/ventricle conduction ratio is usually 3:2 or 4:3, and a typical "group beating" of complexes occurs. This rhythm is also called Wenckebach's block (Figure 124-6).

Second Degree, Type II. In second-degree, Mobitz type II AV block, there is a constant PR interval until a P wave is simply not conducted (not followed by a QRS). This type of block is less common and more severe than Mobitz type I block and has a higher propensity to progress to complete heart block (Figure 124-7).

Third-Degree AV Block. In third-degree (complete) AV block, none of the atrial impulses are conducted to the ventricle. The P waves have no relationship to the QRS waves (AV dissociation). Typically, the pacemaker function is picked up by an escape focus, resulting in either a junctional or ventricular escape rhythm. Because these escape foci have lower intrinsic rates than the sinus node, bradycardia may result. A junctional escape rhythm is characterized by a slow rate (40 to 60 beats per minute) with QRS complexes of normal width, which are not related to P waves (P waves may be absent or may occur but bear no relationship to the QRS complexes whatsoever). A ventricular escape rhythm typically produces a bradycardia of less than 40 beats per minute and is characterized by wide QRS complexes (>0.12 second) that are not connected to P waves.

Bundle Branch Blocks

Once impulses pass across the AV node, conduction occurs rapidly to all sections of the ventricular muscle by way of the right and left bundle branches. In BBB, conduction is disrupted

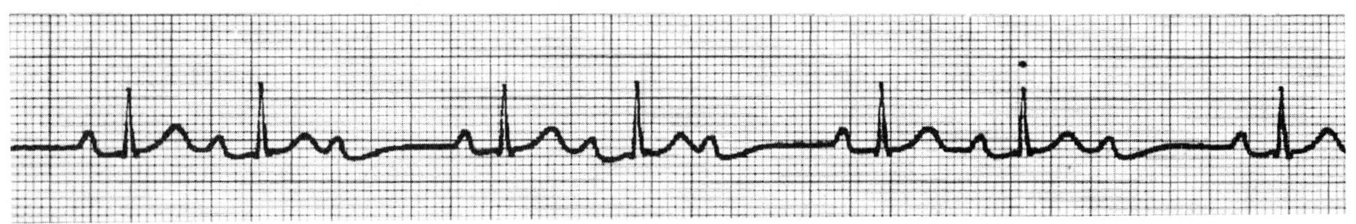

FIGURE 124-6

Second-degree atrioventricular block, Mobitz type I. (From Conover MB: *Understanding electrocardiography*, ed 7, St Louis, 1996, Mosby.)

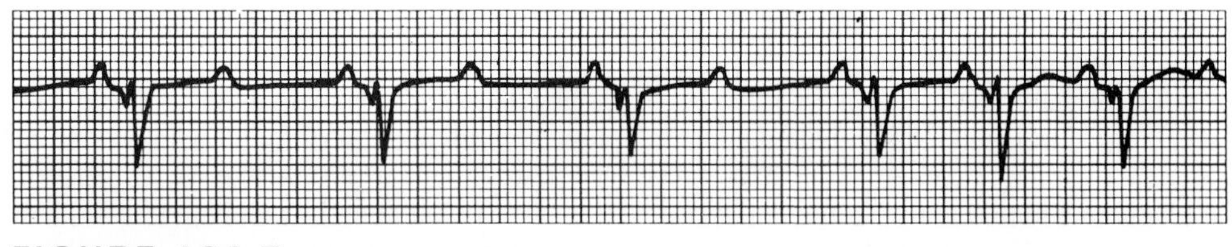

FIGURE 124-7

Second-degree atrioventricular block, Mobitz type II. (From Conover MB: *Cardiac arrhythmias: exercises in pattern interpretations*, St Louis, 1974, Mosby.)

down one or both of these branches, resulting in distortion and prolongation of the QRS complex. A QRS duration of 0.10 to 0.11 second results from incomplete BBB, whereas a QRS duration of 0.12 second or longer results from complete BBB. When conduction down the right bundle is blocked (right bundle branch block [RBBB]), the left bundle will conduct to the ventricle first. The ECG shows a small R wave, followed by an S wave and then a final R′ in lead V_1, whereas V_6 will show a deep, slurred S wave after initially normal Q and R waves. When conduction down the left bundle is blocked (LBBB), the right bundle will conduct to the ventricle first. The ECG shows a broad, slurred S wave in lead V_1 and an R′ in lead V_6.

Hemiblocks

The left bundle divides into the left anterior fascicle and the left posterior fascicle. When conduction is impaired in only one of the fascicles, a hemiblock occurs. A right-axis deviation will be noticed on the ECG with left posterior hemiblock, and a left-axis deviation will occur with left anterior hemiblock.

DIFFERENTIAL DIAGNOSIS

Bradyarrhythmias

Sinus bradycardia
Sinoatrial exit block
Atrioventricular nodal block
- First-degree atrioventricular block
- Second-degree atrioventricular block
  Mobitz type I
  Mobitz type II
- Third-degree (complete) atrioventricular block

Bundle branch block
- Right bundle branch block
- Left bundle branch block
  Left posterior hemiblock
  Left anterior hemiblock

MANAGEMENT

Emergent treatment of the patient with a bradyarrhythmia who is hemodynamically compromised consists of transcutaneous pacing (TCP). If a TCP is not available, IV atropine 0.5 mg may be administered (this dose can be repeated if necessary, but the total dose should not exceed 3 mg). However, atropine must be used with extreme caution in the setting of suspected MI because it may worsen ischemia or result in tachyarrhythmias.[31]

In the primary care setting, management of the patient with a bradyarrhythmia who is hemodynamically stable involves discerning whether the rhythm has a reversible or an irreversible cause. Many drugs may cause bradyarrhythmias. Withdrawal of the offending drug may be all that is required for restoration of an adequate ventricular rate. Correction of electrolyte imbalances, in particular hyperkalemia, may also result in resolution of the problem.

In general, patients with symptomatic bradycardia should be referred to a cardiologist unless a reversible cause can be identified and corrected. Patients with asymptomatic bradycardia may or may not require further intervention; this is determined in large part by the type of block, as described in the following paragraphs.

Sinus Bradycardia

Sinus bradycardia is treated only if the patient is symptomatic (e.g., lightheadedness or syncope occurs in the setting of a decreased heart rate). Withdrawal of drugs that produce an increase in vagal tone (i.e., edrophonium [Tensilon] or digitalis) or that decrease sympathetic tone (e.g., beta blockers, calcium channel blockers, amiodarone, or reserpine) may result in an increase in sinus node activity. A drug such as atropine, which blocks vagal tone, will increase the heart rate. A permanent pacemaker may be necessary for patients with chronic, symptomatic bradycardia.

Sinoatrial Exit Block

SA exit block is managed by removing the offending cause. Medications (e.g., quinidine, procainamide, or digitalis), ischemia, or excessive vagal tone may all induce this arrhythmia. In the absence of a reversible cause, the rhythm is managed as a sinus bradycardia, and treatment is not indicated unless the pauses are symptomatic.[10]

Heart Blocks

Heart block is treated by first correcting any underlying causes. First-degree AV block may be corrected by removing agents such as digitalis, beta blockers, calcium channel blockers, or class III agents (sotalol, amiodarone) or by treating hyperkalemia or ischemia after an MI. A pacemaker is generally not indicated. As with first-degree block, second-degree AV block is usually alleviated by correcting the underlying cause. Atropine may be given to increase the atrial rate, and a temporary or permanent pacemaker may be necessary. Virtually all patients with third-degree AV block will require a permanent pacemaker unless the block is suspected to be temporary (e.g., acute MI, drug effects). The rhythm may be treated emergently with atropine, epinephrine, or isoproterenol. The sudden development of a BBB requires treatment of the underlying cause, but a temporary pacemaker may be necessary in the presence of an MI.

LIFE SPAN CONSIDERATIONS

Older patients have the highest incidence of arrhythmias, as well as other co-morbid conditions.[22] Renal, hepatic, and cardiovascular disease will greatly affect left ventricular function, tolerance of the arrhythmia, and the ability for clearance of antiarrhythmic agents. Interactions with other agents must also be considered when treating an older patient for arrhythmias. Prescribing an agent such as amiodarone to a patient who is already taking warfarin or digoxin will, for example, increase the plasma levels of these drugs.

COMPLICATIONS

The most important determinants of mortality from an arrhythmia are the degree and nature of left ventricular dysfunction.[2] Sudden cardiac death is a real and present danger with complex ventricular arrhythmias, particularly in the setting of underlying cardiac disease. Exacerbation of cardiac ischemia or infarction or heart failure may also occur with tachyarrhythmias or bradyarrhythmias. Reduction in cardiac output will result in decreased perfusion to other vital organs (e.g., brain, kidneys). The risk of thromboembolism and stroke with atrial fibrillation has been previously discussed, as have the proarrhythmic effects of many of the antiarrhythmic agents. Lethal proarrhythmias occur in 1% to 2% of patients receiving antiarrhythmic therapy.[12,23,33,34]

INDICATIONS FOR REFERRAL OR HOSPITALIZATION

Obviously, any arrhythmia that produces hemodynamic decompensation (loss of pulse and blood pressure, syncope, chest pain) requires immediate hospitalization. Referral to an electrophysiologist is required if treatment for the arrhythmia will require nonpharmacologic agents, such as a pacemaker, catheter ablation, or ICD implantation. Electrophysiologic studies are required for guided pharmacologic therapy in the treatment of complex, potentially life-threatening arrhythmias. Electrophysiologic testing is also necessary if the patient is refractory to standard drug therapy or if the drug therapy itself produces life-threatening proarrhythmia.

PATIENT AND FAMILY EDUCATION

First, the provider should explain the nature of any particular arrhythmia. When the arrhythmia is harmless, this information may alleviate unnecessary fears and alterations in lifestyle. When a potentially serious arrhythmia does exist, a frank discussion of the problem and treatment options may enhance understanding and guide the decision-making process.

Discussion regarding the avoidance of any potential stimuli (e.g., alcohol, caffeine, cocaine, cigarettes) is important. Recommendations concerning steps to follow when the arrhythmia occurs should include a plan that addresses where and when to seek treatment. Careful medication teaching, including proper scheduling of doses, potential side effects, and interactions with over-the-counter medications, is essential.

For those who have a permanent pacemaker or automatic ICD, the provider reviews special precautions. The manufacturer is often able to provide excellent educational materials specific to any particular device.

Finally, the importance of involving family and significant others in teaching cannot be overemphasized. Depending on the nature of an arrhythmia, an individual may be rendered incapable of intervening on his or her behalf during an acute event. Family or others who are able to act in a timely and appropriate fashion may influence the outcome and survival of the affected individual. The families of patients with arrhythmias should learn CPR and develop an emergency plan.

REFERENCES

1. Fuster V, Rydén LE, Cannom DS: *ACC/AHA/ESC guidelines for the management of patients with atrial fibrillation 2006,* retrieved Jan 4, 2007, from http://circ.ahajournals.org/cgi/reprint/CIRCULATIONAHA.106.177031v1.
2. Singh B: Controlling cardiac arrhythmias: an overview with an historical perspective, *Am J Cardiol* 80(8A):4G-14G, 1997.
3. Banerji S, Kayser SR: Antiarrhythmic drug therapy, part IV, Ventricular arrhythmias, *Prog Cardiovasc Nurs* 12:32-36, 1997.
4. Zipes DP: Epidemiology and mechanisms of sudden cardiac death, *Can J Cardiol* 21(Suppl A):37A-40A, 2005.
5. Massie BM, Amidon TA: Heart. In Tierney LM, McPhee SJ, Papadakis MA, editors: *Current medical diagnosis and treatment,* ed 41, New York, 2001, Lange Medical Books/McGraw-Hill.
6. Fogoros RN: *Antiarrhythmic drugs,* Malden, Mass, 1997, Blackwell Science.
7. Canobbio MM: *Cardiovascular disorders,* St Louis, 1990, Mosby.
8. Conover MB: *Understanding electrocardiography,* ed 8, St Louis, 2003, Mosby.

9. Josephson ME, Zimetbaum P: The tachyarrhythmias. In Braunwald E, Fauci AS, Kasper DL, and others, editors: *Harrison's principles of internal medicine,* ed 15, New York, 2001, McGraw-Hill.
10. Lee TH: Chest discomfort and palpitation. In Braunwald E, Fauci AS, Kasper DL, and others, editors: *Harrison's principles of internal medicine,* ed 15, New York, 2001, McGraw-Hill.
11. Hacker NF, Moore JG: *Essentials of obstetrics and gynecology,* ed 2, Philadelphia, 1992, Saunders.
12. Sopher SM, Camm AJ: Atrial fibrillation: maintenance of sinus rhythm versus rate control, *Am J Cardiol* 77:24A-37A, 1996.
13. Ukani ZA, Ezekowitz MD: Contemporary management of atrial fibrillation, *Med Clin North Am* 79:1135-1149, 1995.
14. Morley J, Marinchak R, Rials SJ, and others: Atrial fibrillation, anticoagulation, and stroke, *Am J Cardiol* 77:38A-44A, 1996.
15. Solano A, Menozzi C, Maggi R, and others: Incidence, diagnostic yield and safety of the implantable loop-recorder to detect the mechanism of syncope in patients with and without structural heart disease, *Eur Heart J* 25(13):116-119, 2004.
16. Aschenberg W, Schluter M, Kremer P, and others: Transesophageal two-dimensional echocardiography for the detection of left atrial appendage thrombus, *J Am Coll Cardiol* 7:163-166, 1986.
17. Chen-Scarabelli C: Supraventricular arrhythmias: an electrophysiology primer, *Prog Cardiovasc Nurs* 20(1):24-31, 2005.
18. Tai CT, Chen SA, Chiang CE, and others: A new electrocardiographic algorithm using retrograde P waves for differentiating atrioventricular node reentrant tachycardia from atrioventricular reciprocating tachycardia mediated by concealed accessory pathway, *J Am Coll Cardiol* 29:394-402, 1997.
19. Kellen JC, Ettinger A, Todd L, and others: The Cardiac Arrhythmia Suppression Trial: implications for nursing practice, *Am J Crit Care* 5:19-25, 1996.
20. Miller J, Zipes D: Management of the patient with cardiac arrhythmias. In Braunwald E, Zipes D, Libby P, editors: *Heart disease: a textbook of cardiovascular medicine,* ed 6, Philadelphia, 2001, Saunders.
21. Kayser SR: Antiarrhythmic drug therapy, part I, General principles of drug selection, *Prog Cardiovasc Nurs* 11(2):33-37, 1996.
22. Kayser SR: Antiarrhythmic drug therapy, part III, Atrial fibrillation, *Prog Cardiovasc Nurs* 11(4):35-43, 1996.
23. Kastor JA: Multifocal atrial tachycardia, *N Engl J Med* 322:1713-1717, 1990.
24. Olgin J, Zipes D: Specific arrhythmias: diagnosis and treatment. In Braunwald E, Zipes D, Libby P, editors: *Heart disease: a textbook of cardiovascular medicine,* ed 6, Philadelphia, 2001, Saunders.
25. Schlicht JR, Davis RC, Naqi K, and others: Physician practices regarding anticoagulation and cardioversion of atrial fibrillation, *Arch Intern Med* 156:290-294, 1996.
26. Stevenson WG, Ellison K, Lefroy D, and others: Ablation therapy for cardiac arrhythmias, *Am J Cardiol* 80:56G-66G, 1997.
27. Wazni O, Marrouche NF, Martin DO, and others: Radiofrequency ablation vs antiarrhythmic drugs as first-line treatment of symptomatic atrial fibrillation: a randomized trial, *JAMA* 293:2634-2640, 2005.
28. American Heart Association: *Advanced life support,* Dallas, 1997, The Association.
29. American Heart Association: *Advanced cardiac life support provider manual,* Dallas, 2006, The Association.
30. Josephson ME: The bradyarrhythmias: disorders of sinus node function and AV conduction disturbances. In Braunwald E, Fauci AS, Kasper DL, and others, editors: *Harrison's principles of internal medicine,* ed 15, New York, 2001, McGraw-Hill.
31. Goldberger AL: Electrocardiography. In Braunwald E, Fauci AS, Kasper DL, and others, editors: *Harrison's principles of internal medicine,* ed 15, New York, 2001, McGraw-Hill.
32. Gregoratos G, Cheitlin MD, Conill A, and others: ACC/AHA guidelines for implantation of cardiac pacemakers and antiarrhythmia devices, *Circulation* 97:1325-1335, 1998, retrieved Jan 2, 2007, from http://circ.ahajournals.org/cgi/content/full/97/13/1325.
33. Antman EM, Beamer AD, Cantillon C, and others: Therapy of refractory symptomatic atrial fibrillation and atrial flutter: a staged approach with new antiarrhythmic drugs, *J Am Coll Cardiol* 15:698-707, 1990.
34. Campbell RW: Atrial fibrillation: steering a management course between thromboembolism and proarrhythmic risk, *Eur Heart J* 16(Suppl G):28-31, 1995.

CHAPTER 125

Carotid Artery Disease

Virginia Capasso, Erin Cox, and
Sharon M. Bouvier

DEFINITION AND EPIDEMIOLOGY

Stroke is the third leading cause of death in the United States.[1] Each year about 700,000 people suffer a new or recurrent stroke; about 500,000 of these are first attacks and 200,000 are recurrent attacks.[2] In the United States the overall death rate associated with stroke is 56.2%.[3]

The vast majority of strokes (88%) are ischemic strokes. Ischemic strokes result from oxygen deprivation to the brain as a result of partial or complete occlusion of an artery.[4] Atherosclerosis of the carotid artery, at the carotid bifurcation with involvement of the proximal internal carotid artery (ICA), is implicated in most ischemic strokes.[5] ICA stenosis of greater than 50% is present in about 4% to 8% of persons between the ages of 50 and 79 years.[6] Stenosis of the ICA is responsible for approximately 30% of ischemic strokes.[6] Atherosclerotic carotid artery stenosis is the most common cause of stroke in young adults.[7]

In short-term studies involving follow-up of 2 to 3 years, the annual stroke risk is approximately 1% to 3.4% among persons with asymptomatic carotid artery stenosis of between 50% and 99%.[8] In long term, 10-year and 15-year studies, respectively, the annual risk of ipsilateral stroke in asymptomatic patients with greater than 50% occlusion of the ICA (9.3% to 16.6%) is approximately twice that for individuals with less than 50% ICA occlusion (5.7% to 8.7%).[7] The risk of stroke in the territory of an asymptomatic carotid artery stenosis contralateral to the side of a symptomatic vessel varies with the degree of stenosis: 3.0% for 60% to 74% stenosis, 3.7% for 75% to 94% stenosis, 2.9% for 95% to 99% stenosis, and 1.9% for complete occlusion.[9,10]

In general, the risk factors for carotid stenosis are the same as for atherosclerotic cardiovascular disease. High systolic blood pressure, diabetes, high cholesterol levels, hypercoagulable states, and smoking have been specifically linked to an increased risk of carotid stenosis in older adults.[11] When compared with individuals 60 years of age or older, younger adults (50 years or younger) undergoing carotid endarterectomy (CEA) for carotid stenosis are significantly more likely to have a history of smoking, hypertension, and premature coronary artery disease and lower levels of high-density lipoprotein cholesterol.[7]

Elevated levels of plasma homocysteine may be another important risk factor for carotid stenosis.[12-17] Among individuals 55 to 74 years of age, hyperhomocysteinemia has been associated with thickening of the common carotid intima-media lining. Strong genetic links between carotid artery abnormalities and homocysteine levels have not been demonstrated in first-degree relatives of young adults with hyperhomocysteinemia. Unfortunately, in animal models, normalization of plasma homocysteine levels does not restore normal vascular function.

PATHOPHYSIOLOGY

Atherosclerotic carotid stenosis originates near the bifurcation of the common carotid artery in the region of the bulb.[5] Conditions near the bulb, including low shear stress, flow separation, and nonlaminar flow, increase the contact time between bloodborne particles, such as lipids, and the vessel wall. A fatty streak, consisting of mononuclear and foam cells, eventually develops into an atherosclerotic plaque. Blood flow to the brain can be reduced or interrupted by severe narrowing or occlusion of the ICA. In addition, turbulence may actually damage the atherosclerotic plaque, resulting in loss of intimal continuity or ulceration. Platelets and fibrin aggregate on the roughened intimal surface, and there is subsequent thrombosis. Fragments of a fractured plaque or thrombus may embolize to smaller distal arteries. Interruption of cerebral blood flow and cerebral infarction are the potential life-threatening sequelae.

CLINICAL PRESENTATION

Patients with carotid stenosis may be asymptomatic or symptomatic. Patients with severe carotid stenosis may be asymptomatic if the circle of Willis is competent and adequately perfuses the territory of the middle cerebral artery. In patients who are asymptomatic, a bruit may be detected on routine physical examination, suggesting that there is no correlation between the presence and absence of symptoms and bruits.

Patients with symptomatic carotid stenosis may be seen initially with transient ischemic attack (TIA) or stroke.[2] A TIA is a brief episode of neurologic dysfunction caused by a focal disturbance of brain or retinal ischemia with clinical symptoms typically lasting more than 1 hour and without evidence of infarction.[18] The 90-day risk of stroke is 10.5%.

Widespread use of modern brain imaging has led to a modification of the definition of stroke. A definition of stroke used for clinical trails has been adopted that requires neurologic "symptoms lasting >24 hours or imaging of an acute clinically relevant lesion in patients with rapidly vanishing symptoms."[2]

Symptoms derived from carotid artery occlusion, which develop gradually or in a stepwise pattern, include monocular blindness (amaurosis fugax) and contralateral motor and sensory deficits.[5] Global aphasia is present when the dominant hemisphere is involved. When the nondominant hemisphere is affected, the patient exhibits neglect of the opposite side of the body. The symptoms of carotid artery occlusion are differentiated from posterior circulation symptoms, which usually include binocular visual loss, vertigo, and "drop attacks."[5]

PHYSICAL EXAMINATION

The physical examination should include a complete cardiovascular and neurologic examination. Important components of the cardiovascular examination include palpation and auscultation of all bilateral peripheral pulses for bruits, as well as blood pressures in bilateral upper extremities in the lying and sitting position. The neurologic examination should include an examination of mental status, cranial nerves (including funduscopic examination), and motor and sensory function.

Although a carotid bruit is routinely listed as a clinical indicator of carotid stenosis, it has been shown to be a poor predictor of moderate to severe carotid stenosis[14] or stroke.[19] Other predictors of carotid stenosis include certain blood pressure characteristics. In a study of 187 older adults with isolated systolic hypertension, an elevated systolic blood pressure and increased pulse pressure were significant predictors of carotid stenosis.[15] In addition, an increased pulse pressure and decreased diastolic blood pressure were independent risk markers for carotid stenosis. The characteristic changes in blood pressure reflect compensation for reduced blood flow through the narrowed arterial lumen. Thus, when diastolic blood pressure drops, the pulse pressure widens as peripheral vascular resistance decreases to dilate the arterial lumen in the presence of worsening arterial occlusive disease.

DIAGNOSTICS

Digital subtraction angiography (DSA) is the definitive test for detection of vascular lesions, although it has inherent cost and risks, including risk of stroke in about 1% of cases and death in 0.1% cases.[20] Duplex ultrasound, which allows both assessment of the degree of stenosis and characterization of the plaque,[5] is now the primary diagnostic tool for carotid stenosis. A recent meta-analysis of studies of color duplex ultrasound demonstrated that, when the peak systolic velocity is greater than or equal to 130 cm/s, the sensitivity and specificity are very high, at 98% and 88%, respectively, in detecting stenotic internal carotid artery lesions of 50% or more. In the setting of a peak systolic velocity of more than 0 cm/s, the sensitivity and specificity of duplex ultrasound are 90% and 94%, respectively, in the detection of stenotic lesions of 70% or greater.[21] For recognizing carotid occlusion, duplex ultrasound has been shown to have a sensitivity of 96% and specificity of 100%.[22] Studies have demonstrated a high degree of agreement between duplex ultrasound and arteriography in the detection of more than 45% stenosis in the carotid artery.[16]

Magnetic resonance angiography (MRA) and CT angiography (CTA) with three-dimensional reconstruction are used increasingly to supplement duplex ultrasound and DSA in the diagnosis of internal carotid stenosis. In another recent meta-analysis, MRA had a sensitivity of 95% and a specificity of 90% in the diagnosis of stenotic lesions between 70% and 99% when compared with lesions of 70% or less.[22] MRA had a sensitivity of 98% and a specificity of 100% in detecting occlusion. Advantages of CTA include the capability of defining bone and soft tissue structures surrounding the diseased carotid arteries and tracing the course of a vessel that is tortuous or has a high bifurcation.[5] However, CTA may underestimate carotid stenosis as compared with rotational angiography. CTA may be helpful in screening symptomatic patients, although confirmatory MRA or DSA is still necessary.[23]

DIAGNOSTICS

Carotid Artery Disease

IMAGING
Duplex ultrasound
Digital subtraction angiography
Magnetic resonance angiography
CT angiography

DIFFERENTIAL DIAGNOSIS

The differential diagnosis of carotid artery disease depends on the presentation. In the presence of a carotid bruit, a negative duplex ultrasound necessitates further diagnostic evaluation. An echocardiogram will detect an intracardiac source of a murmur (e.g., valvular incompetence or septal defect) that is transmitted to the neck. An arteriogram of the aortic arch will demonstrate stenosis of extracranial vessels that are inaccessible to physical examination or noninvasive vascular testing.

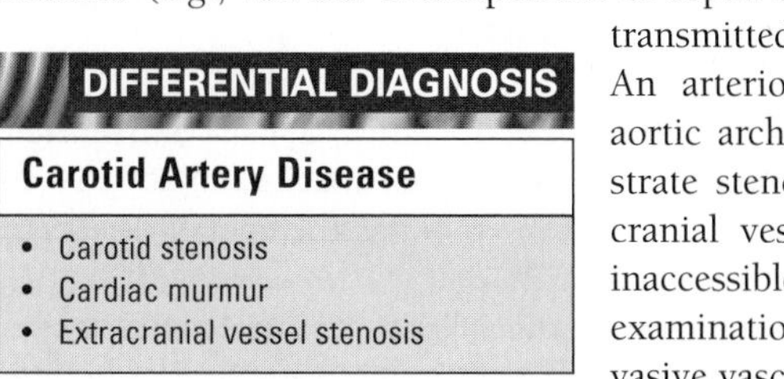
DIFFERENTIAL DIAGNOSIS

Carotid Artery Disease

- Carotid stenosis
- Cardiac murmur
- Extracranial vessel stenosis

MANAGEMENT

Management of asymptomatic and symptomatic carotid stenosis is based on guidelines developed from recent randomized trials.[20,24,25] Detection of a carotid bruit, development of transient ischemia, or a duplex ultrasound that reveals 60% or more occlusion of the ICA indicates the need for referral to a specialist (surgeon or neurologist). Carotid endarterectomy (CEA) is the definitive treatment for symptomatic and asymptomatic patients with severe carotid stenosis. Carotid angioplasty and stenting have been advocated as an alterative to surgical treatment with CEA.

Carotid Endarterectomy

CEA involves a neck incision and surgical removal of atheromatous material from the inside of the carotid artery.[4,26] Recommendations vary according to the presence or absence of symptoms and the degree of stenosis (Figure 125-1). CEA is recommended for asymptomatic individuals, with low surgical risk (<3%) and life expectancy greater than 5 years, who have high-grade stenotic lesion that reduces the diameter of the outflow tract by 60% or more.[9] The procedure should be performed by surgeons with low complication rates (<3%).[9] When comparing outcomes of surgical therapy with medical therapy, several trials have shown that the immediate and long-term risk of stroke or death is approximately 50% less among patients undergoing CEA.[25,27,28] The overall 5-year risk of any stroke or perioperative death also is almost 50% less for immediate endarterectomy (6.4%) as compared with deferred surgery (11.8%).[28] The benefit does not appear to be related to the degree of carotid stenosis. The surgical benefit is greater in men than women.[9]

Among symptomatic patients, CEA is beneficial for those who have had a TIA or nondisabling cerebrovascular attack within the previous 6 months. A recent *Cochrane's Systematic Review* revealed that, among patients with severe stenosis (European Carotid Surgery Trial [ECST], >80%, and North American Symptomatic Carotid Endarterectomy Trial [NASCET], >70%), surgery reduced the relative risk of disabling stroke or death by 48%. For patients with less severe stenosis (ECST, 70% to 79%, and NASCET, 50% to 69%), surgery reduced the relative risk of disabling stroke or death by

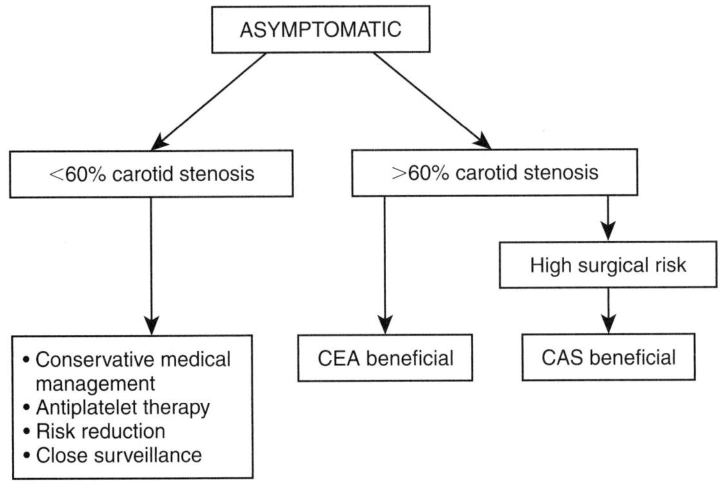

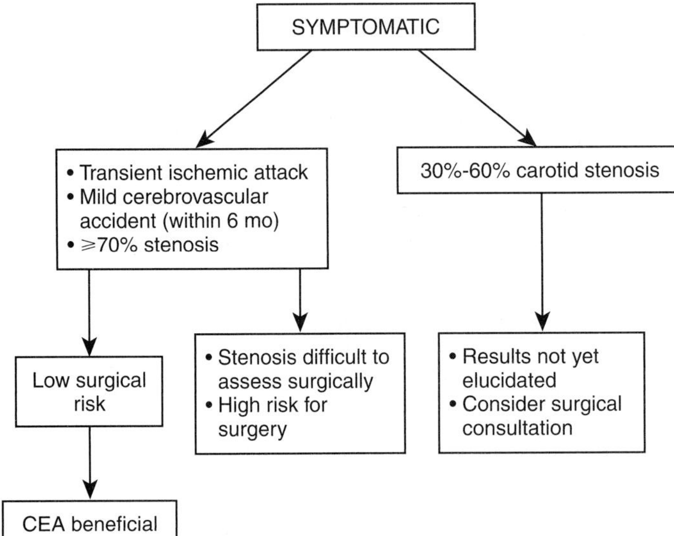

FIGURE 125-1

Guidelines for carotid endarterectomy *(CEA)*. *CAS*, Carotid angioplasty and stenting. (Adapted from Datillo JB: Peripheral vascular disease. In Hess ML: *Heart disease in primary care*, Philadelphia, 1999, Williams & Wilkins.)

27%.[4] Patients with less than 50% stenosis were "harmed" by surgery, that is, surgery increased the risk of disabling stroke or death by 20%.[4] When surgery is indicated for patients with TIA or stroke, surgery should be performed within 2 weeks rather than delaying surgery.[2]

For asymptomatic patients with less than 60% stenosis, the usual practice is watchful waiting. During this period, a duplex ultrasound may be repeated every 6 months and anticoagulants are prescribed for stroke prophylaxis. Although the prognostic and clinical value of serial duplex ultrasound imaging is considered low because of the low incidence of stroke in patients with asymptomatic ICA stenosis, the diagnostic value of serial duplex ultrasound imaging may increase among patients at high risk of disease progression and consequent disabling stroke as a result of the following risk factors: smoking, coronary artery disease, diabetes mellitus, peripheral arterial disease, hypertension, age, and increased levels of low-density lipoprotein cholesterol and fibrinogen.[6]

The anticoagulant regimen may include aspirin, warfarin, and clopidogrel. Preoperative and indefinite postoperative administration of daily aspirin, 75 to 325 mg, is recommended for patients undergoing carotid endarterectomy.[29] Lifelong administration of aspirin 75 to 162 mg is recommended for nonoperative patients with asymptomatic or recurrent carotid stenosis.[29]

Warfarin therapy may be beneficial for patients with concurrent atrial fibrillation or ventricular hypokinesis or a high risk for a thrombotic event. The initial approach is to anticoagulate to an INR (International Normalized Ratio) of 2.0 to 3.0.[9] In the absence of ischemic cerebral events, warfarin may be discontinued after another 3 months, and antiplatelet agents may be resumed.

Because of increased risk of side effects, ticlopidine no longer is used as a first-line agent. Ticlopidine may cause serious neutropenia. Therefore, clopidogrel is the drug of choice as an adjunct to aspirin.

Stroke prevention also includes the reduction of risk factors. The reduction of isolated systolic hypertension in people more than 60 years of age decreases the incidence of stroke by 36%.[30] Smoking cessation promptly reduces the risk of stroke by an amount proportional to the number of cigarettes smoked. The Scandinavian Simvastatin Survival Study reported a 30% reduction in fatal and nonfatal strokes in patients taking simvastatin; other studies of statin drugs used ultrasound and found a slowing of the progression of carotid atherosclerosis.[9,30-32] Blood pressure (<130/80 mm Hg) and blood lipids should be tightly controlled in patients with type 1 and type 2 diabetes.[9] Although heavy alcohol use is associated with an excessive risk of stroke, moderate use may serve a protective role by raising high-density lipoprotein cholesterol, thereby reducing the risk of atherosclerotic cardiovascular disease and consequent ischemic stroke. The role of postmenopausal estrogen replacement in stroke occurrence or prevention remains uncertain.[32]

Carotid Angioplasty and Stenting

Carotid angioplasty and stenting (CAS) involve insertion of a balloon-tipped catheter into a femoral artery in the groin, which is threaded retrograde through the arteries of the body to the location of the plaque within the carotid artery in the neck.[26] The balloon on the catheter is inflated and deflated rapidly, thereby compressing the plaque. A stent is then placed over the plaque and opened, thereby holding the artery open. The risk of distal embolization and stroke consequent to plaque fracture has been improved by the use of embolic protection devices.[26]

The Stroke Trials Registry lists 13 trials, of which four compare the outcomes of CEA and CAS.[33] Of the 13 studies, four have been completed and one is ongoing at the time of publication of this text (the Carotid Revascularization Endarterectomy Versus Stent Trial [CREST]).

The Stenting and Angioplasty with Protection in Patients at High Risk for Endarterectomy (SAPPHIRE) Trial compared the cumulative incidence of major cardiovascular event at 30 days and 1 year between symptomatic patients with 50% or greater stenosis and asymptomatic patients with 80% or greater carotid stenosis.[34] Approximately 70% of the enrolled patients had asymptomatic stenosis with rates of stroke, MI, and death, at 30 days and 1 year, respectively, of 5.4% and 10.2% for stenting and 9.9% and 21.5% for CEA. Of the 30% of enrolled patients who had symptomatic stenosis, the cumulative incidence of rates of stroke, MI, and death at 30 days or death or ipsilateral stroke between 31 days and 1 year was 5.8% for stenting and 12.6% for CEA. The study reportedly demonstrated that CAS was not inferior CEA, although the lower risk of MI for the stent compared with the high surgical risk in endarterectomy cases accounts for most of the benefit attributed to CAS.[9]

Alberts examined the rate of ipsilateral stroke, procedure-related death, or vascular death at 1 year among patients with symptomatic carotid artery stenosis (60% to 99%) who underwent CAS with a WALLSTENT endoprosthesis as compared with patients who underwent CEA for similar degrees of carotid stenosis.[35] The study showed that the primary endpoint occurred in 12% of patients who underwent CAS with a WALLSTENT endoprosthesis as compared with 3.6% among patients who underwent CEA. Thus, these studies suggest that carotid endarterectomy may have less stroke risk than CAS.

The Endarterectomy Versus Angioplasty in Patients with Symptomatic Severe Carotid Symptoms Stenosis (EVA-3S) Trial examined the efficacy of angioplasty and stenting with carotid endarterectomy in the secondary prevention of ischemic stroke among individuals less than 4 months after an ischemic stroke.[36] The 30-day risk of stroke was significantly higher in the stent group (9.6%) as compared with the CEA group (3.9%).

Given the wide range of results, the American Heart Association and American Stroke Association's recommended indications for CAS vary for the treatment of asymptomatic and symptomatic stenosis.[2,9] CAS may be a reasonable alternative to CEA in asymptomatic patients at high risk for surgical procedures.[9] CAS may be considered for patients with symptomatic severe stenosis (>70%) when the following conditions exist: "1) stenosis is difficult to access surgically, 2) medical conditions exist which greatly increase risk for surgery, 3) other specific circumstances exist such as radiation-induced stenosis or restenosis after CEA, [and 4) the procedure is] performed by operators with established periprocedural morbidity and mortality rates of 4% to 6%."[2]

Postprocedural care of the patient who has undergone CAS includes frequent neurologic and hemodynamic assessments. For 2 months after the procedure, the patient is treated with a daily dose of aspirin and clopidogrel. Patients who have undergone CAS are screened for restenosis with duplex ultrasound every 6 months for 2 years. CTA is performed for any evidence of significant restenosis. An angiogram is indicated if the patient develops any symptoms of restenosis, which may require subsequent angioplasty and stenting.

LIFE SPAN CONSIDERATIONS

According to the National Heart, Lung, and Blood Institute's Framingham Heart Study, 28% of people who suffer a stroke are under 65 years old.[1] For people over 55, the incidence of stroke more than doubles in each successive decade.[9] Stroke is more prevalent among men, who also have higher age-specific stroke incidence rates than women. Women have slightly higher age-specific stroke incidence among individuals 35 to 44 years and over 85 years. The higher incidence in women at younger ages (35 to 44 years) is attributed to increased risk of thrombogenesis associated with use of oral contraceptives and pregnancy. The higher incidence of stroke in women older than 85 years is attributed to the higher rate of cardiac-related deaths at earlier ages among men with cardiovascular disease.

Among individuals under the age of 45 years, CEA has been shown to be a safe procedure, with postoperative mortality, cerebrovascular accidents, and cardiac complications of less than 2%.[37] The 10-year disease-free interval may exceed 75%. However, when compared with groups of older patients undergoing CEA, the 10-year survival rate is lowest for patients under 45 years of age. The poor life expectancy is attributed to complications of atherosclerosis.

COMPLICATIONS

Complications of CEA include stroke (1% to 3%), hypertension (19% to 25%), hypotension (5% to 30%), MI (0.8% to 3%), bleeding (<1%), and cranial nerve injury (16%).[38] Most strokes (60%) are evident on awakening from anesthesia. Thrombotic strokes often occur 2 to 3 hours after surgery; embolic strokes, up to 2 days after surgery; and cerebral hemorrhages, 1 to 3 days after surgery. Hypertension, which may result from carotid sinus injury or increased baroreceptor activity, usually occurs 1 to 6 hours after surgery and may require the administration of IV antihypertensive medications. Hypotension, which occurs within 1.5 hours of surgery and may persist for 15 hours after surgery, may require low-dose phenylephrine infusion and, subsequently, precautions for orthostatic changes during mobilization of the patient.

Expanding hematomas in the neck pose a risk of respiratory compromise and require exploration. The most common cranial nerve injuries involve cranial nerve (CN) X (8%), CN XII (5% to 8%), and CN VII (2%). Injury to the recurrent laryngeal branch of the vagus nerve (CN X) causes hoarseness and ineffective cough, whereas injury to the superior laryngeal branch of the vagus nerve causes minor swallowing difficulty and an easily fatigued voice. Deviation of the tongue to the ipsilateral side provides evidence of injury to the hypoglossal nerve (CN XII). Drooping of the lip on the ipsilateral side and an inability to smile reflect injury to the marginal mandibular branch of the facial nerve (CN VII). Cranial nerve deficits are usually minor and transient, resolving in 4 to 6 weeks.

In addition to major complications of CAS, including stroke, MI, and death, which were discussed previously, systemic hypotension may occur for up to 36 hours after the procedure in response to stimulation of the carotid baroreceptors by balloon angioplasty and stenting.[39] After CAS, two distinct patterns of hypotension occur. The first is characterized by hypotension requiring vasopressor administration over a relatively acute period (i.e., ≤24 hours and usually ≤6 hours). These patients often have a history of previous MI, coronary artery disease, and unstable angina. The second pattern of hypotension is more protracted, necessitating vasopressor support and associated with intraprocedural hypotension and advanced age among women.

INDICATIONS FOR REFERRAL OR HOSPITALIZATION

All patients with suspected carotid artery disease resulting in ischemia should be referred for assessment whether or not a bruit is present. In most centers patients are referred to vascular surgeons for CEA, since surgical therapy with CEA is considered superior to medical therapy alone for treatment of severe carotid stenosis (>70%).[40-42]

CEA involves surgical atherectomy with or without a vein patch at the site of arteriotomy. CEA restores ipsilateral arterial blood flow in the common carotid artery, ICA, and middle cerebral artery, which renders cerebral blood flow less dependent on collateral flow through the basilar artery.[38]

Preoperative evaluation includes cardiac risk assessment for silent myocardial ischemia. Identification of positive predictive factors of perioperative cardiac events (advanced age, previous MI, and ventricular ectopic activity) indicates a need for exercise stress testing or pharmacologic nonstress testing and referral to cardiology. Unfortunately, most patients with peripheral arterial disease have intermittent claudication, which prevents adequate exercise stress testing. Silent ischemia is more effectively demonstrated by reversible defects on persantine-thallium or dobutamine-atropine scans. Extensive coronary disease necessitates coronary arteriography and intervention by cardiology. When indicated, CEA and coronary artery bypass grafts (CABG) may be performed sequentially during a single procedure. The most appropriate management of patients at moderate risk for perioperative events is less clear, and patients may benefit from involvement by a cardiac specialist. The addition of beta blockers to the therapeutic regimen is the only therapy shown to prevent perioperative MI.

CEA requires hospitalization after surgery and should be performed in a center with low rates of morbidity and mortality (<6%). Most patients undergoing elective CEA are admitted to the hospital on the morning of the procedure. Intake of all food and fluid is restricted after 12 AM. A general anesthetic is administered to most patients. A regional anesthetic may be used for high-risk patients, especially those with chronic respiratory diseases. The operative time is between 1 and 2 hours for an uncomplicated case. Patients are extubated and awake at the end of the case. They are transferred to the postanesthesia care unit (PACU) for 2 to 4 hours of observation before transfer to the general care unit. Infusion of IV fluid is discontinued in the PACU. Oral fluids may be started in the PACU, and the diet is advanced after transfer to the general care unit.

Most patients complain of only minor incisional discomfort, which is adequately managed with oral oxycodone with acetaminophen or acetaminophen alone. Other minor complaints include a sore throat (usually related to endotracheal intubation) and numbness of the ear and neck (related to nerve trauma by surgical retraction). In some centers, discharge occurs in the afternoon or evening of POD 1. Labile blood pressure during the postoperative period necessitates reevaluation of the patient's antihypertensive regimen before discharge; this is necessary to prevent syncopal episodes related to hypotension. In some institutions the treatment plan includes two home visits for blood pressure monitoring. The visits correspond with periods of high risk for bleeding resulting from reperfusion (POD 2 or 3 and POD 5 or 6).

PATIENT EDUCATION

Patient education focuses on preventing complications of CEA and secondary prevention of recurrent carotid stenosis. The importance of adhering to the antihypertensive regimen in preventing hyperperfusion syndrome and stroke is emphasized, as is the need for the patient to report transient loss of consciousness, severe headache, and transient or persistent neurologic deficit.[32]

Secondary prevention of recurrent carotid stenosis is directed at reducing risk factors. Because cigarette smoking is a risk factor for restenosis, efforts are directed at smoking cessation.[43] Elevated serum cholesterol may contribute to carotid stenosis, and therefore patients who have undergone CEA should be counseled and treated according to the guidelines of the Expert Panel on Detection, Evaluation, and Treatment of High Blood Cholesterol in Adults.[43,44] Heavy alcohol use is discouraged.

REFERENCES

1. American Heart Association: *2006 heart and stroke statistical update*, Dallas, 2006, The Association.
2. Sacco RL, Adams R, Albers G, and others: Guidelines for prevention of stroke in patients with ischemic stroke or transient ischemic attack, *Stroke* 37:577, 2006.

3. American Heart Association: *Heart disease and stroke statistics*—2006 update, retrieved Sept 3, 2006, from http://circ.ahajournals.org/content/full/113/6/e85/TBL2.
4. Cina CS, Clase CM, Haynes RB: Carotid endarterectomy for symptomatic carotid stenosis, *Cochrane Database Syst Rev* (3):CD001342, 2006.
5. Allain R, Marone LK, Meltzer J, and others: Carotid endarterectomy, *Int Anesthesiol Clin* 43:15-38, 2005.
6. Dodick DW, Meissner I, Meyer FB, and others: Evaluation and management of asymptomatic carotid artery stenosis, *Mayo Clin Proc* 79:937-944, 2004.
7. Levy PJ, Olin JW, Piedmonte MR, and others: Carotid endarterectomy in adults 50 years of age and younger: a retrospective comparative study, *J Vasc Surg* 25:326-331, 1997.
8. Nadareishvili ZG, Rothwell PM, Beletsky V, and others: Long-term risk of stroke and other vascular events in patients with asymptomatic carotid artery stenosis, *Arch Neurol* 59:1162-1166, 2002.
9. Inzitari D, Eliasziw M, Gates P, and others: The causes and risk of stroke in patients with asymptomatic internal-carotid-artery stenosis: North American Symptomatic Carotid Artery Trial Collaborators, *N Engl J Med* 342:1693-1700, 2000.
10. Barnett HJ, Gunton RW, Eliasziw M, and others: Causes and severity of ischemic stroke in patients with internal carotid artery stenosis, *JAMA* 283:1429-1436, 2000.
11. Goldstein LB, Adams R, Alberts MJ, and others: Primary prevention of stroke, *Stroke* 37:1583, 2006.
12. Mackey AE, Abrahamowicz M, Langlois Y, and others: Outcome of asymptomatic patients with carotid disease: Asymptomatic Cervical Bruit Study Group, *Neurology* 48:896-903, 1997.
13. Rockman CB, Riles TS, Lamparello PJ, and others: Natural history and management of the asymptomatic, moderately stenotic internal carotid artery, *J Vasc Surg* 25:423-431, 1997.
14. Wilson PW, Hoag JM, D'Agostino RB, and others: Cumulative effects of high cholesterol levels, high blood pressure and cigarette smoking on carotid stenosis, *N Engl J Med* 337(8):516-522, 1997.
15. Bots ML, Launer LJ, Lindemans J, and others: Homocysteine, atherosclerosis and prevalent cardiovascular disease in the elderly: the Rotterdam Study, *J Intern Med* 242(4):339-347, 1997.
16. De Jong SC, Stehouwer CD, Mackaay AJ, and others: High prevalence of hyperhomocysteinemia and asymptomatic vascular disease in siblings of young patients with vascular disease and hyperhomocysteinemia, *Arterioscler Thromb Vasc Biol* 17(11):2655-2662, 1997.
17. Lentz SR, Malinow MR, Piegors DJ, and others: Consequences of hyperhomocysteinemia on vascular function in atherosclerotic monkeys, *Arterioscler Thromb Vasc Biol* 17:2930-2934, 1997.
18. Albers GW, Caplan LR, Easton JD, and others: Transient ischemic attack: proposal for a new definition, *N Engl J Med* 347:1713-1716, 2002.
19. Rea T: The role of carotid bruit in screening for carotid stenosis, *Ann Intern Med* 127:657, 1997.
20. North American Symptomatic Carotid Endarterectomy Trial Collaborators: Beneficial effect of carotid endarterectomy in symptomatic patients with high-grade stenosis, *N Engl J Med* 325:445-453, 1991.
21. Jahromi AS, Cina CS, Liu Y, and others: Sensitivity and specificity of color duplex ultrasound in the estimation of internal carotid artery stenosis: a systematic review and meta-analysis, *J Vasc Surg* 41:962-972, 2005.
22. Nederkoorn PJ, van der Graaf Y, Hunink MG: Duplex ultrasound and magnetic resonance angiography compared with digital subtraction angiography in carotid artery stenosis: a systematic review, *Stroke* 34:1324-1332, 2003.
23. Berg M, Zhang Z, Ikonen A, and others: Multi-detector row CT angiography in the assessment of carotid artery disease in symptomatic patients: comparison of rotational angiography and digital subtraction angiography, *Am J Neuroradiol* 26:1022-1034, 2005.
24. European Carotid Surgery Collaborative Group: MRC European Carotid Surgery Trial: interim results for symptomatic patients with severe (70%-99%) or mild (0%-29%) carotid stenosis, *Lancet* 337:1235-1243, 2003.
25. Hobson RW, Weiss DG, Fields WS: Efficacy of CEA for asymptomatic carotid stenosis: the Veterans Affairs Cooperative Study Group, *N Engl J Med* 328:221-227, 1993.
26. *Carotid revascularization endarterectomy versus stenting trial*, retrieved Sept 9, 2006, from http://www.clinicaltrials.gov/ct/show/NCT00004732?order=1.
27. Executive Committee for the Asymptomatic Carotid Atherosclerosis Study: Endarterectomy for asymptomatic carotid artery stenosis, *JAMA* 273:1421-1428, 1995.
28. Halliday A, Mansfield A, Marro J, and others: MRC Asymptomatic Carotid Surgery Trial (ACST) Collaborative Group: prevention of disabling and fatal strokes by successful carotid endarterectomy in patients without recent neurological symptoms: randomised controlled trial, *Lancet* 363:1491-1502, 2004.
29. Clagett GP, Sobel M, Jackson MR, and others: Antithrombotic therapy in peripheral arterial occlusive disease: the Seventh ACCP Conference on Antithrombotic and Thrombolytic Therapy, *Chest* 126(3 Suppl):609S-626S, 2004.
30. Bruno A: Ischemic stroke, part 2, Optimal treatment and prevention, *Geriatrics* 48:37-54, 1993.
31. Mumma CM: Nursing role in management of stroke patient. In Lewis SM, Collier IC, Heitkemper MM, editors: *Medical-surgical nursing*, ed 4, St Louis, 1996, Mosby.
32. Ballard JL, Deiparine MK, Bergan JJ, and others: Cost-effective evaluation and treatment for carotid disease, *Arch Surg* 132:268-271, 1997.
33. The Internet Stroke Center: *Stroke trials*, retrieved Sept 9, 2006, from http://www.strokecenter.org/trails/TrialDetail.aspx?tid=208.
34. Yadav JS, Wholey MH, Kuntz RE, and others: Protected carotid-artery stenting versus endarterectomy in high-risk patients, *N Engl J Med* 351:1493-1501, 2004.
35. Alberts MJ: Results of a multicenter prospective randomized trial of carotid artery stenting vs. carotid endarterectomy, *Stroke* 32:325-d, 2001.
36. Mas JL, Chatellier G, Beyssen B: Carotid angioplasty and stenting with and without cerebral protection: clinical alert from the Endarterectomy Versus Angioplasty in Patients with Symptomatic Severe Carotid Stenosis (EVA-3S) trial, *Stroke* 35:e18-e20, 2004.
37. SHEP Cooperative Research Group: Prevention of stroke by antihypertensive drug treatment in older persons with isolated systolic hypertension: final results of the Systolic Hypertension in Elderly Program (SHEP), *JAMA* 265:3255-3264, 1991.
38. Randomized trial of cholesterol lowering in 4444 patients with coronary heart disease: the Scandinavian Simvastatin Survival Study (4S), *Lancet* 344:1383-1389, 1994.
39. Trocciola SM, Chaer RA, Lin SC, and others: Analysis of parameters associated with hypotension requiring vasopressor support after carotid angioplasty and stenting, *J Vasc Surg* 43(4):714-720, 2006.
40. Furberg CD, Adams HP Jr., Applegate WB, and others: Effect of lovastatin on early carotid atherosclerosis and cardiovascular events, *Circulation* 90:1679-1687, 1994.
41. Crouse JR, Byington RP, Bond MG, and others: Pravastatin, lipids and atherosclerosis in the carotid arteries (PLAC-II), *Am J Cardiol* 75:455-459, 1995.
42. Bettmann MA, Katzen BT, Whisnant J, and others: Carotid stenting and angioplasty: a statement for healthcare professionals from the Councils of Cardiovascular Radiology, Stroke, Cardiothoracic and Vascular Surgery, Epidemiology and Prevention, and Clinical Cardiology, American Heart Association, *Stroke* 29:336-338, 1998.
43. National Cholesterol Education Program: Summary of the second report of the NCEP Expert Panel on Detection, Evaluation, and Treatment of High Blood Cholesterol in Adults, *JAMA* 269(23):3015-3023, 1993.
44. Biller J, Feinberg WM, Castaldo JE: Guidelines for carotid endarterectomy: a statement for healthcare professionals from a special writing group of the Stroke Council, American Heart Association, *Circulation* 97:501-509, 1998.

CHAPTER 126

Chest Pain and Coronary Artery Disease

Updated by Joanna D. Sikkema

DEFINITION AND EPIDEMIOLOGY

Coronary heart disease remains the primary cause of death for both men and women in the United States. The American Heart Association (AHA) estimates that each year 7,100,000 Americans suffer a myocardial infarction (MI), mostly as a result of coronary thrombosis. Approximately 466,000 of these heart attacks are fatal. Nearly 335,000 people will die before ever reaching a hospital, primarily as a result of ventricular arrhythmias.[1] The majority of deaths among patients who do reach the hospital are attributable to left ventricular failure and cardiogenic shock within 96 hours after infarction.

Early reperfusion treatment of patients with an acute MI improves left ventricular systolic function and survival; therefore every effort must be made to minimize hospital delay. Although time is critical in the treatment of MI, patient delay, not transport or system inadequacy, has proved to be the biggest obstacle to obtaining timely medical treatment. Only one of five patients arrives at the hospital during that "golden hour," the time frame during which they would obtain the greatest benefits from reperfusion therapy. Many reasons exist for hospital delays, including the patient's lack of knowledge regarding heart attack symptoms. In random telephone surveys, 90% could identify chest pressure as a symptom of a heart attack, 67% could identify arm pain, 50% knew that shortness of breath could be related, and only 21% were aware that sweating could be a symptom. Overall the average patient interviewed could identify only two of the 11 heart attack symptoms.[2]

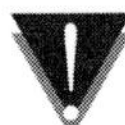

Immediate emergency department referral or physician consultation is indicated for patients with suspected MI.

Risk Factors for Coronary Artery Disease

It is currently believed that it is coronary artery plaque composition, morphology, and stability—not the degree of plaque stenosis—that determines the risk of cardiovascular events. Modification of controllable cardiac risk factors has been shown to decrease the frequency of cardiovascular morbidity and mortality.

Historically, risk factors have been subdivided into factors that are nonmodifiable, such as gender, age, and family history, and factors that are modifiable, such as smoking cessation, cholesterol levels, diabetes mellitus, and hypertension. It is now known that some cardiac risk factors are more predictive of coronary artery events than others. Pasternak, Grundy, Levy, and others have developed an evidence-based system whereby known and potential coronary risk factors are placed into a hierarchy based on four factors[3]:

- Risk factors for which there is a strong causal relationship to coronary artery disease (CAD) and for which interventions have been *proved* to reduce the incidence of CAD events (cigarette smoking, low-density lipoprotein [LDL] cholesterol, dietary factors, hypertension, thrombogenic factors)
- Risk factors that strongly suggest a causal relationship to CAD and for which interventions are *likely*, based on current pathophysiologic understanding and on epidemiologic and clinical trial evidence, to reduce the incidence of CAD events (diabetes, physical inactivity, high-density lipoprotein [HDL] cholesterol, obesity, postmenopausal status)
- Risk factors that are clearly associated with an increased CAD risk and for which modifications *might* lower the incidence of CAD events (psychosocial factors such as stress and depression, triglycerides, Lp(a) lipoprotein, homocysteine, oxidative stress)
- Risk factors associated with increased risk but ones that cannot be modified or whose modifications would be *unlikely* to change the incidence of CAD events (age, gender, family history) (Table 126-1)

However, updates to the 2001 recommendations and review of additional findings from lipid trials involving more than 500,000 patients have resulted in new therapeutic risk reduction targets. These are especially significant for high-risk patients and those with acute coronary syndrome (ACS). These aggressive recommendations are reviewed in Chapter 222.[4]

In addition to these risk factors, information is beginning to emerge that shows a relationship between sleep apnea and the development of coronary ischemia. Sleep apnea syndrome, irrespective of the type (obstructive, central, or mixed), leads to a cessation of airflow and a fall in oxygen saturation. When the oxygen saturation drops, often to profoundly low levels during sleep, disturbance in cardiac rhythm and elevation in pulmonary arterial pressure may occur as a consequence of hypoxia-induced pulmonary hypertension. Similar physiologic disturbances of hypoxia occur in the coronary arterial circulation. In the presence of critical coronary stenosis, hypoxia-induced coronary vasoconstriction as a result of impaired endothelial function may lead to coronary ischemia. The treatment of choice depends on the type of sleep apnea syndrome.

PATHOPHYSIOLOGY

Chronic Stable Angina

Chronic stable angina is precipitated by exertion and relieved by rest. A reduction in myocardial oxygen supply or increases in myocardial oxygen demand are the determinants of coronary ischemia. Although the pathology for unstable angina and the pathology for chronic stable angina both result from atherosclerotic lesions in the coronary arteries, the pathophysiology of each varies.

Under normal circumstances an increase in myocardial oxygen demand is balanced by an increase in myocardial oxygen supply. The three most important factors that determine myocardial oxygen demand are heart rate, systemic blood pressure (peripheral vascular resistance), and left ventricular wall tension. The heart rate and the systolic blood pressure exert independent influence on myocardial oxygen requirements, because both determine myocardial workload (Heart

TABLE 126-1 AHA/ACC Secondary Prevention for Patients with Coronary Artery Disease and Other Atherosclerotic Vascular Disease*

Risk Factors	Goal
Smoking	Complete cessation
Blood pressure control	<140/90 mm Hg <130/80 mm Hg if heart failure or renal insufficiency
Lipids	LDL <100 mg/dl as goal Reduce saturated fats to <7% calories Triglycerides < 200 mg/dl If triglycerides are ≥200 mg/dl, non-HDL should be <130 mg/dl Non-HDL = total cholesterol-HDL
Physical activity	30 minutes, 7 days per week (minimum 5 days per week)
Weight management	Body mass index of 18.5-24.9 kg/m^2 Waist circumference: men <40 inches, women <35 inches
Diabetes mellitus	Hemoglobin A_{1C} <7% is advised
MEDICATIONS	
ASA	75-162 mg PO daily; if ASA is contraindicated, use clopidogrel or warfarin. ASA is used alone or in combination with antiplatelet medications, depending on clinical situation.[18]
Beta blockers	All patients who have had myocardial infarction, acute coronary syndrome, or left ventricular dysfunction with or without heart failure symptoms, unless contraindicated
ACE inhibitors	All patients with left ventricular ejection fraction ≤40% and those with hypertension, diabetes, or chronic kidney disease, unless contraindicated
Influenza vaccine	All patients

From AHA/ACC guidelines for secondary prevention for patients with atherosclerotic cardiovascular disease: 2006 update, *Circulation* 113:2363-2372, 2006.
ACE, Angiotensin-converting enzyme; *ASA,* acetylsalicylic acid; *HDL,* high-density lipoprotein; *LDL,* low-density lipoprotein.
*Includes peripheral arterial disease, atherosclerotic aortic disease, and carotid artery disease.

rate × Systolic blood pressure = Myocardial workload). Therefore activities (e.g., exercise, hurrying, lifting) and increased metabolic demands (e.g., with fever, anemia, thyrotoxicosis) that increase the workload of the heart in the presence of a fixed and limited oxygen supply will increase myocardial oxygen requirements and thus precipitate ischemia and angina.

The coronary arteries exhibit changes in vascular tone (vasomotion). These changes play a significant role in the development of coronary ischemia. The endothelial lining is the innermost layer of the coronary artery. It is a monolayer, exocrine organ that actively participates in homeostasis and regulation of vascular tone by producing, secreting, and responding to a number of vasoactive substances, including prostacyclin, thrombin, histamine, serotonin, adenosine, endothelium-derived relaxing factor (EDRF), endothelin, and cholinergic agonists. Under normal circumstances the endothelium responds to vasoactive stimuli, such as mental stress, cold, and catecholamines, by releasing EDRF to maintain vasodilation.[5-7] In the presence of atherosclerosis, however, the endothelial function is impaired; hence the vasoconstrictive response is unopposed, leading to constriction at the site of atherosclerosis and adjacent areas. This results in a decrease in myocardial blood flow and induces coronary ischemia.

Silent Myocardial Ischemia

It has been recognized that asymptomatic occurrences of ischemia are more common than symptomatic episodes in patients with exertional angina symptoms. Silent myocardial ischemia occurs when there is objective evidence of ischemia in the absence of symptoms. Since the advent of continuous ambulatory ECG monitoring, many patients with typical stable angina have been found to have frequent episodes of asymptomatic ischemia.

The full clinical implications of silent ischemia are not well understood, but there is increased incidence of ischemia, MI, and sudden death in asymptomatic patients with positive exercise stress test results. In addition, patients with asymptomatic ischemia who have had an MI are at greater risk for a second coronary event. Ischemia can occur with or without evidence of increased myocardial oxygen demand (increased product of heart rate and blood pressure). Diabetic patients are at a twofold to fourfold greater risk of cardiovascular mortality compared with those without diabetes, and silent myocardial ischemia on stress testing occurs more often in patients with diabetes than in patients without diabetes.[8]

The pathogenesis of silent myocardial ischemia is not well understood, although several hypotheses exist. It has been suggested that some individuals have a higher endorphin level than others, which may play a role in the perception of pain. In addition, some patients have a higher ischemic pain threshold and greater tolerance of cold-induced ischemia. Finally, autonomic dysfunction, particularly in patients with diabetes, is thought to contribute to silent ischemia.

Microvascular Angina

The diagnosis of microvascular angina (syndrome X) is suspected when (1) there is a convincing history of angina chest pain with or without documented reversible ischemic ECG changes, (2) angiography fails to demonstrate obstruction or spasm of a major coronary artery, and (3) other conditions have been excluded from the differential diagnosis.

The etiology of microvascular angina is still not fully understood, although studies have demonstrated that some patients with this syndrome have an abnormal vasodilating response of their small or resistance vessels (diminished coronary reserve). Still other patients may have a low pain threshold or other noncardiac causes of pain. However, microvascular angina appears to have some gender significance as a presentation of ischemic heart disease in women. The Women's Ischemia Syndrome Evaluation (WISE) study showed that at least half of the women with clinical evidence of ischemia and open arteries have problems related to insufficient dilation of the arteries.[9]

Variant Angina (Coronary Artery Spasm, Prinzmetal's Angina)

In variant angina, coronary artery spasm should be suspected on the basis of the patient's history. Spasm can occur in any coronary artery; however, the right coronary artery and, to a lesser extent, the left anterior descending artery are more commonly affected. The spasm tends to be focal and reproducible at the same location. However, diffuse single-vessel coronary artery spasm may occur. Multivessel spasm is extremely rare; when it occurs, it is associated with intractable ventricular tachycardia. The cause of coronary artery spasm is abnormal endothelial cell function. This is especially true when injury to the endothelium results in decreased concentration of EDRF.

Unstable Angina and Non–ST-Segment Elevation Myocardial Infarction

The pathophysiology of acute MI has been controversial since Hippocrates first postulated that heart disease could cause sudden death. The causes of MI can be divided into those which decrease myocardial oxygen supply and those which increase myocardial oxygen demand. Atherosclerotic plaque results in a reduction of coronary blood flow, thereby reducing oxygen supply. These plaques reduce the cross-sectional area of coronary artery lumen, thus reducing coronary perfusion pressure. When a critical stenosis develops, coronary blood flow is adequate at rest but cannot increase to meet metabolic demands during exertion. The subendocardium blood reserve becomes much more limited than that of the subepicardium; therefore ischemia and infarction occur first in the subendocardial layer. When the infarction is limited to the subendocardial layer, the term *non–ST-segment elevation MI* or *non–Q wave MI* is applied.

The development of a vulnerable coronary artery lesion is multifactorial and depends on the biochemical and physical properties of that lesion. Unstable angina or non–ST-segment elevation MI is most commonly due to coronary artery narrowing caused by a nonocclusive thrombus that has developed from a ruptured atherosclerotic plaque. According to one theory, coronary atherosclerosis is initiated by oxidized LDLs, which are toxic to the endothelium of the coronary artery. A relatively new biomarker, $LpPLA_2$, has been found useful in risk stratification of patients for ACS. The enzyme $LpPLA_2$ is implicated in the formation of inflamed rupture-prone plaque, and its levels are not affected by an acute systemic inflammatory process (as is C-reactive protein [CRP]).[10] $LpPLA_2$ is produced primarily by macrophages and resides mainly in the LDL. Such toxicity initiates an inflammatory response, which stimulates chemotactic factors for circulating monocytes. Monocytes enter the vessel wall, transform into tissue macrophages, and ingest oxidized LDLs. Over time, lipid-filled macrophages (foam cells) die, creating an extracellular lipid pool with eventual formation of a fibrous cap. Proteolytic enzymes produced by activated macrophages erode the fibrous cap, producing areas that are fragile and prone to rupture. Increases in shear stress and vasomotor changes placed on this vulnerable lesion make it highly likely to rupture. Therefore the role of the inflammatory response as a trigger for plaque rupture cannot be overemphasized. Evidence is beginning to focus on the role of bacterial and viral infections and their effects on existing atheromatous lesions, making them more vulnerable and unstable with a predisposition to rupture and thrombose. A number of studies have shown the benefit of evaluating hs-CRP (high-sensitivity CRP) to determine cardiovascular risk.[11]

When plaque rupture occurs, the size of the resultant thrombus, whether a small mural or an occlusive thrombus, depends on several factors, including the amount of thrombogenic substrate that is exposed, the amount of local blood flow disturbances, and the actual thrombotic propensity of the vessel.

Therefore lesion disruption is a dynamic process that may lead to transient vessel occlusion and ischemia by a labile thrombus, resulting in unstable angina. These thrombotic occlusions often resolve spontaneously; however, they can recur within hours or days. In other cases, formation of a fixed thrombus and a more chronic occlusion may occur, resulting in acute MI.

Coronary artery narrowing of less than 80% generally does not induce development of collateral vessels. For this reason, smaller plaques that rupture are more likely to cause a significant clinical event during thrombotic occlusion of the vessel as a result of the absence of protective collateral flow.

Acute ST-Segment Elevation Myocardial Infarction

In most cases MI occurs when an atherosclerotic plaque ruptures, which serves as a nidus for thrombus formation with resultant coronary artery occlusion. The atherosclerotic plaque most likely to rupture is the nonocclusive plaque, which may rupture several times before producing MI. On each rupture, blood, fibrin, and platelet aggregates accumulate in the plaque, forming intraintimal or intraplaque thrombus and resulting in increases in plaque size, intraplaque pressure, and obstruction of the coronary lumen. When such a plaque ruptures, fissures, or ulcerates, MI and/or sudden death may occur. Plaque rupture with resulting thrombus formation is the common physiologic mechanism underlying unstable angina, MI, and sudden death. The amount of myocardial injury sustained is directly related to several factors, including the amount of thrombus present, the ability of the intrinsic lytic system to promote lysis, the impact of local vasoconstrictor substances on impeding blood flow, whether the vessel affected is partially or totally occluded, the presence or absence of collateral vessels and the quantity of blood they supply to the affected area, and the amount of myocardium supplied by the affected vessel.

The platelet is not only the smallest cell, it is also the most active in thrombus formation. The platelet consists of membranes, tubules, granules, and receptors. During activation the resting platelet undergoes a dramatic change that induces platelet-platelet interaction or aggregates. Such platelet aggregates play an important role in ACS and MI. Patients who died of unstable angina, MI, and sudden cardiac death have platelet aggregation, fibrin, and microthrombi as common findings. Because platelets are important in the pathophysiology of acute ischemic syndrome and MI, inhibiting platelet activation should be beneficial in reducing and preventing ACS.

CLINICAL PRESENTATION

Chronic Stable Angina

The patient with chronic stable angina demonstrates characteristic symptoms that occur with predictable frequency, severity, duration, and provocation. These symptoms occur with exertion, are relieved by rest or no more than one nitroglycerin tablet, and generally last for only 1 to 3 minutes. Chronic stable angina remains constant unless an acceleration of the disease process intervenes. The clinical presentation can best be evaluated by a detailed history of angina quality, location, radiation, severity, duration, and precipitating and relieving factors. Associative factors such as dyspnea, diaphoresis, nausea, vomiting, eructations, diarrhea, and fatigue should also be evaluated (Box 126-1).

William Heberden first defined the peculiar discomfort of myocardial ischemia as *angina pectoris*, which translated means a "strangling in the chest." The majority of patients do not refer to their angina symptoms as pain; thus questioning related to "chest pain" may prove misleading, and the diagnosis of angina pectoris may be missed. Discomfort originating from the chest may arise from many structures, including the skin, subcutaneous tissue, bone, muscle, vascular structures, nerves, pleura, lungs, pericardium, heart, esophagus, or gastrointestinal viscera.

Adjectives used to describe the *quality* of angina can be variable and are often conveyed as a pressure, heaviness, aching, constriction, tightness, squeezing, numbness, or burning sensation. Patients may demonstrate a clenched fist over the sternal area (Levine's sign) to further elucidate this feeling. The *location* of discomfort is predominantly behind the midsternum (retrosternal) or just to the left of the sternum, in an area approximately the size of a clenched fist. If the patient is able to localize the area of discomfort as being no larger than a fingertip, the sensation is seldom related to myocardial ischemia, and other causes should be considered. Myocardial ischemia can also encompass the territory between the epigastrium and the lower jaw, lower teeth, and hard palate, with sensations of tightness or constriction in the throat area.

Radiation symptoms are not uncommon and are related to involvement of the C8 to T4 spinal ganglia. These ganglia receive impulses from the heart and from peripheral dermatomes, which are transmitted to the spinal cord via afferent nerve fibers. When myocardial ischemia occurs, the sharing of these ganglia can produce discomfort to the other dermatomal areas. Thus stimulation of the dermatomes affecting the brachial plexus can result in discomfort or numbness anywhere along the medial surface of the left arm, including the fourth and fifth digits. Isolated wrist discomfort has also been reported. The right arm and lateral surfaces can be affected, although with less frequency.

Stimulation of the cervical plexus can result in suprascapular and intrascapular discomfort. Precipitating factors, including increased exertion, coitus, or emotion, tend to induce myocardial ischemia by increasing circulating catecholamine levels. This increases the metabolic oxygen needs of the heart in the setting of a limited oxygen supply, thereby producing angina symptoms. Eating a large meal may precipitate discomfort, as can increased metabolic demands from fever, chills, thyrotoxicosis, anemia, hypoglycemia, exposure to cold air, and the nicotine from cigarette smoking.

Relief of stable angina symptoms generally occurs within 1 to 3 minutes after the discontinuation of activity or with rest. When angina is related to emotional upheaval, it may take longer to decrease catecholamine levels, and angina symptoms may persist for a longer period. Nitroglycerin administration will usually provide relief within 5 minutes and is a useful diagnostic tool. When symptoms persist for longer than 20 minutes, the patient should no longer be considered to be having chronic stable angina and should be instructed to seek prompt medical attention.

Although cessation of activity generally produces relief of pain, it has been noted that some patients who develop angina with walking are able to continue walking, with eventual alleviation of the angina. These patients are able to "walk through" the angina event. There are several proposed hypotheses for the relief of angina during exercise. These include (1) dilation of functioning collateral blood vessels during exercise; (2) relief of coronary arterial spasm; and (3) vasodilation of systemic blood vessels with a corresponding decline in

BOX 126-1

HISTORY QUESTIONS FOR THE PATIENT WITH ANGINA

Chest pain information
- Precipitating factors (exertion, meals, stress, cold)
- Quality (pressure, squeezing, burning, stabbing)
- Radiation (shoulders, arm, wrist, neck, jaw, back)
- Relief measures (rest, nitroglycerin [hallmark], food)
- Severity (1-10 scale)
- Timing (activity, bedtime, meals, history of occurrence, duration)

Associative factors
- Dyspnea

Provoked by activity (chest pain first or dyspnea)
Orthopnea (how many pillows)
Paroxysmal nocturnal dyspnea (how soon after retiring to bed)
- Diaphoresis
- Gastrointestinal complaints (nausea, vomiting, diarrhea)
- Fatigue

Cardiac risk factors
Current medication profile

BOX 126-2

CANADIAN CARDIOVASCULAR SOCIETY CLASSIFICATION

Class I: Prolonged exertion evokes angina, without limits to normal activity.
Class II: Walking more than 2 blocks evokes angina, with slight limits to normal activity.
Class III: Walking less than 2 blocks evokes angina, with marked limits to normal activity.
Class IV: Minimal activity or rest evokes angina, with severe restrictions to activity.

systemic arterial blood pressure and heart rate, which in turn reduces myocardial oxygen demand.

The Canadian Cardiovascular Society Classification (CCSC) is a useful tool to determine the exercise tolerance of patients with stable angina pectoris and to determine the degree of disability that angina symptoms are imposing on the patient (Box 126-2).

Anginal Equivalents

For reasons that continue to remain unclear, myocardial ischemia can be experienced as dyspnea and/or fatigue rather than actual chest pressure; this is particularly true in women. Symptoms of dyspnea are generally noted to be stable when they occur with moderate exertion and unstable when they occur with minimum exertion or when they begin to awaken the patient during the night. The etiology of stable symptoms is related to increased myocardial demand, and the etiology of unstable symptoms is related to decreased myocardial supply. The dyspnea produced is due to myocardial ischemia resulting in diastolic dysfunction, which produces increased left-sided filling pressures. Fatigue often follows an activity and resolves within several minutes. The etiology is related to left ventricular dysfunction resulting in decreased cardiac output.

Microvascular Angina

The clinical presentation of microvascular angina is similar to that of classic angina, although atypical features are common, including rest pain, prolonged pain, and pain that is less responsive to nitroglycerin. Although there is no apparent gender difference in the perception of angina, the syndrome of microvascular angina is found predominantly in women. The authors of WISE, along with those of several other published reports, conclude that the vasculopathy in women leading to ischemic heart disease stems from a variety of factors unique to women—namely, smaller coronary vessels, more diffuse atherosclerosis, stiffer aortas, and more frequent microvascular dysfunction.[12]

Variant Angina

The sine qua non of variant angina pectoris is a history of spontaneous or unprovoked episodes of typical angina. Discomfort occurs predominantly at rest and is usually not provoked by exertion. Patients sometimes note that beta blockers exacerbate symptoms. The differential diagnosis on presentation should be unstable angina until it is proven otherwise.

Unstable Angina and Non–ST-Segment Elevation Myocardial Infarction

Diagnosis of unstable angina and non–ST-segment elevation MI depends predominately on a detailed patient history. The five most important factors from the initial history that enhance the likelihood of the patient experiencing an episode of ischemia are (1) the nature of symptoms, (2) prior history of CAD, (3) age greater than 75 years, (4) male sex, and (5) number of risk factors present for CAD. In addition, several factors may suggest an acceleration of the patient's chronic angina symptoms to an unstable or non–ST-segment elevation MI. These factors may include the angina event occurring with less provocation or at rest, a prolongation of the angina symptoms, an increase in the severity of symptoms, or newly associated findings with the chest discomfort. Physical examination findings of pulmonary edema, a new or worsening mitral regurgitation murmur, an S_3 heart sound, hypotension, bradycardia, or tachycardia suggest the patient is at high risk. A 12-lead ECG, preferably with and without chest pain, should also be obtained (Box 126-3).[13] It is particularly important to assess the duration of angina events and whether rest pain has been present to determine the patient's short-term risk of complications. Patients who are initially seen with prolonged chest pressure or an angina equivalent lasting longer than 20 minutes or in a crescendo pattern, coupled with ST-segment depression or T-wave inversion on the ECG, have a higher likelihood of suffering a non–ST-segment elevation MI as a result of an unstable angina event.[8] This is important because patients who develop a non–ST-segment elevation MI have a 70% higher risk of death and an 8.5% higher potential for reinfarction than those with unstable angina alone.[14]

Acute ST-Segment Elevation Myocardial Infarction

Classically, acute MI is diagnosed as a constellation of symptoms. Chest pain described as pressure, heaviness, squeezing, crushing, and aching is often associated with nausea, vomiting, diaphoresis, or dyspnea. Generally, the pain involves the sternum and/or epigastrium, and in many cases it may radiate to the arm, elbow, jaw, or neck. Any combination of these symptoms may occur in an individual patient. An unusual presentation may be cranial pain, which is usually different from a classic headache syndrome. Epigastrium pain secondary to acute MI may be misdiagnosed as indigestion, and referred pain to the shoulder on deep inspiration may be

BOX 126-3

UNSTABLE ANGINA PRESENTATIONS

- Angina while at rest within 1 week of presentation
- New-onset angina of Canadian Cardiovascular Society Classification (CCSC)
- CCSC class III or IV within 2 months of presentation
- Angina increasing to at least CCSC III or IV
- Variant angina
- Non–Q-wave myocardial infarction
- Post–myocardial infarction angina (>24 hours)

Data from US Department of Health and Human Services, Agency for Health Care Policy and Research: Diagnosing and managing unstable angina, *Clin Pract Guide* 10:2-18, 1994.

misdiagnosed as being splenic in nature. In the older patient, MI may manifest as a sudden onset of dyspnea, weakness, loss of consciousness, or confusion. Although chest discomfort may be the most common presenting symptom, it may be atypical or absent in some patients with ACS (silent acute MI). In addition, the chest discomfort of MI may be similar to that with causes of chest wall pain.

PHYSICAL EXAMINATION

Inspection of the chest may reveal the point of maximum impulse (PMI) to be downward or laterally displaced, suggestive of cardiomegaly, perhaps from hypertension. The PMI may also have a rocking quality, perhaps related to a left ventricular aneurysm from a previous MI. The thorax should be inspected to determine the presence of any rashes or vesicles, which may suggest a herpetic etiology. Inspection of the neck veins should be performed to assess the jugular venous pulse for any elevation. The contour of the internal jugular waveforms should also be noted. A funduscopic examination may reflect hypertension or diabetic retinopathy. Xanthomas or an early arcus senilis may be indicative of elevated cholesterol levels. The peripheral circulation should be assessed for any vascular lesions suggestive of arterial or venous disease.

Palpation during cardiac assessment is confined to assessing the upstroke of the carotid artery pulse and the PMI of the cardiac apex. The carotid upstroke should be brisk, yet not hyperdynamic. A prolonged carotid upstroke may indicate aortic stenosis, since ventricular emptying becomes delayed when ejected across a significantly stenotic valve. Conversely, a brisk carotid upstroke may indicate aortic regurgitation.

The PMI should be confined to the fifth intercostal space at the midclavicular line. With any downward or lateral displacement of the PMI, cardiomegaly should be considered. In a follow-up inspection, palpation of the PMI should confirm any aneurysm formation.

Auscultation of the chest may reveal a ventricular gallop (S_3) produced just after the second heart sound, which may be either physiologic or pathologic in nature. A physiologic S_3 may be heard in children and adults up to 35 to 40 years old. It may also be noted in women during their third trimester of pregnancy. A pathologic S_3 may be related to decreased myocardial contractility and is suggestive of heart failure caused by volume overload of the ventricles. This may be related to either mitral or tricuspid regurgitation.

An atrial gallop (S_4) may be noted just before the first heart sound and is produced by an increased resistance to ventricular filling caused by ventricular stiffness after atrial contraction. Left ventricular causes of an S_4 include cardiomyopathy, hypertension, MI, and aortic stenosis. Right ventricular causes include pulmonary hypertension and pulmonary stenosis. An S_4 may also be noted in trained athletes.

A pansystolic murmur audible at the apex during an episode of chest pain is most likely consistent with mitral regurgitation. It is often secondary to papillary muscle dysfunction as a result of left ventricular ischemia. A ventricular septal defect post-MI should also be considered and further evaluated with echocardiography.

Inflammation around the pericardium may produce a pericardial friction rub, which generally has one systolic and two diastolic components. The systolic component is produced when the ventricles contract in systole, whereas the diastolic components are produced in early and late diastole. The early diastolic component occurs as a result of rapid, passive ventricular filling, whereas the late diastolic component occurs with atrial contraction. The sound produced is very high and of a scratching or grating quality.

Adventitious breath sounds suggest heart failure. Their occurrence and the presence of any vascular bruits, indicating further vascular disease, should prompt further evaluation.

The physical examination is generally normal when the patient is not having episodes of variant angina; however, during episodes the patient may develop hypertension and tachycardia in response to the pain. In addition, the patient may have associated diaphoresis, nausea, and radiation of pain to the arm. Auscultation of the chest during an episode may reveal a gallop or transient systolic murmur originating from the mitral valve.

Approximately 90% of the diagnosis of an acute coronary event is made from the patient's history, ECGs, and laboratory data. The physical examination findings will support this diagnosis and help determine whether the patient is in heart failure or is manifesting evidence of a cardiac arrhythmia. The patient will understandably be anxious and on occasion will be diaphoretic. Generally, the pulse rate and blood pressure may be normal; however, with an extensive area of MI, the patient may have a compensatory tachycardia and be hypotensive (Box 126-4).

BOX 126-4

CARDIAC PHYSICAL ASSESSMENT

INSPECTION

Point of maximum impulse (PMI)—displaced downward and laterally, aneurysmal
Skin and extremities—color, edema, xanthomas, lesions
Neck veins—elevated jugular venous distention, contour of internal jugular pulse
Thorax—rashes, zoster
Funduscopic examination—evaluation for risk factors: diabetes mellitus, elevated cholesterol

PALPATION

Carotid upstroke—may be prolonged with aortic stenosis
PMI—may be diffuse with cardiac enlargement

AUSCULTATION

Ventricular gallop (S_3)—heart failure
Atrial gallop (S_4)—hypertension, myocardial infarction; caused by resistance of ventricular filling
Systolic mitral regurgitation murmur consistent with an ischemic papillary muscle
Pericardial friction rub—inflammation around the pericardial sac; may have one systolic and two diastolic components
Adventitious breath sounds
Carotid bruits—other vascular location

DIAGNOSTICS

Chronic Stable Angina

Electrocardiogram. In chronic stable angina the ECG can be useful for detecting cardiac ischemia during actual episodes of angina. During this period, ST-segment depressions with symmetric T-wave inversions in the affected leads may be noted. During pain-free intervals, however, the ECG will revert to normal limits. Other possible changes include evidence of a prior MI, left ventricular hypertrophy, and repolarization abnormalities.

Exercise Tolerance Testing (Stress Testing). Because of the nondiagnostic potential of the ECG in patients with intermittent episodes of chest pain, all patients who are suspected of having coronary ischemia should undergo an exercise tolerance test within 72 hours of presentation of symptoms. Stress testing, which may be pharmacologic or exercise based, is performed for diagnostic, prognostic, and management purposes.[15]

Stress testing for patients with a history of chest pain or angina-type symptoms should always be implemented with imaging. Imaging either with thallium or sestamibi should be added for those patients with uninterpretable resting ECGs resulting from the following conditions: (1) preexisting 1-mm ST-segment depressions, (2) left ventricular hypertrophy with strain, (3) left bundle branch block, (4) digoxin therapy, (5) ventricular pacing, or (6) Wolff-Parkinson-White syndrome.

The most commonly used definition for a positive exercise tolerance test result is the development of ECG changes consistent with ischemia. This ECG finding is a 1-mm or greater horizontal or downsloping ST-segment depression or ST-segment elevation that persists for at least 60 to 80 msec after the end of the QRS complex.

The ST-segment changes on a stress test are indicative of viable cardiac muscle being supplied by a narrowed coronary artery. The time frame in which symptoms or ECG changes appear should be noted, as should the hemodynamic response. Stress testing should not be performed in individuals with exacerbation of heart failure, uncontrolled cardiac arrhythmias, severe hypertension, unstable angina, an acute evolving MI, or critical aortic stenosis.

Coronary Angiography. The primary purpose of coronary angiography is to define the anatomy of the coronary arteries and evaluate for revascularization of occluded coronary arteries. Coronary angiography is currently the only method reliably available for defining the coronary vasculature. MRI and electron beam CT continue to be investigational tools in defining the coronary anatomy. Coronary angiography is used not only in diagnosis of CAD, but also in directing therapeutic interventions. It is important to note that coronary angiography does not provide information about the functional significance of a given coronary lesion, nor does it provide information regarding the patient's functional status and symptoms. Therefore coronary angiography in the setting of chronic stable angina should be reserved for those patients in whom the diagnosis is in doubt, whose symptoms are changing, who have failed to respond to medical therapy, and in whom an intervention is being contemplated. In patients with chronic stable angina, coronary angiography should be preceded by an exercise stress test with or without imaging as deemed appropriate.

Variant Angina

Electrocardiogram. Transient ST-segment elevation on a 12-lead ECG during an episode of variant angina is essential to make the diagnosis. ECG changes are usually observed in the leads related to the ventricular areas supplied by the affected vessels. On occasion, ECG changes may be dramatic but resolve readily with the use of sublingual nitroglycerin or nifedipine.

Echocardiogram. An echocardiogram obtained during a period of variant angina may reveal segmental wall motion abnormality, depending on the severity of the spasm and duration of the episode.

Exercise Tolerance Testing. An exercise tolerance test should be performed to exclude atherosclerotic disease. Most patients with noncritical CAD who have variant angina have a negative exercise tolerance test result.

Coronary Angiography. Patients with unprovoked chest discomfort at rest that is typical of angina may have variant angina. An exercise tolerance test should be the initial testing modality. On occasion, this test may be negative for ischemia, even though the patient is still experiencing chest discomfort. At that time, patients may undergo coronary arteriography to evaluate further for CAD. If variant angina is indeed suspected, all vasoactive medications should be discontinued at least 24 hours before coronary arteriography or any other provocative testing. Provocation of spasm with acetylcholine has been used to induce endothelial cell vasoreactivity. However, this practice has fallen out of vogue because of the potential to induce global spasm and hence lethal cardiac arrhythmias. Therefore diagnosis of variant angina is generally made from a patient history revealing nonexertional events that often are nocturnal.

Unstable Angina and Non–ST-Segment Elevation Myocardial Infarction

Electrocardiogram. The 12-lead ECG continues to be the principal diagnostic tool in the differentiation of an unstable angina and non–ST-segment elevation MI event. During an episode of angina discomfort the ECG findings depend on several factors, including the location of the involved vessel, amount of myocardium involved, duration of ischemia, and transient nature of the pathophysiologic process. During an episode of ischemia the electrical properties of the myocardial cells within and surrounding the area of ischemia are altered, producing changes on the surface ECG.

ST-segment depression, along with symmetrically inverted T waves, is generally present within minutes during an acute ischemic event. According to guidelines of the Agency for Healthcare Research and Quality (AHRQ), ST depressions more than 1 mm indicate a high likelihood of an unstable angina event, whereas ST depressions of 0.5 to 1 mm indicate an intermediate likelihood. These changes generally return to baseline once the ischemic event is resolved. As a rule, Q waves do not develop, and there is no distinct change in the R wave. Persistence of ST-segment depression for longer than 48 hours usually differentiates an unstable angina event from a non–ST-segment elevation MI. It should be emphasized that an absence of ST-segment or T-wave changes does not exclude the possibility of myocardial ischemia. In particular, ischemia affecting the left circumflex territory is not always demonstrated on the ECG.

Exercise Tolerance Testing. A standard low-level exercise stress test is considered the most reasonable test in patients able to exercise who have a resting ECG that is notable for ST-segment changes. Those patients with an ECG pattern that would interfere with test interpretation should have imaging performed.

Laboratory Data. Laboratory blood work for the patient with a potential unstable angina pattern should consist of hemoglobin and hematocrit levels to exclude anemia as a precipitating factor. Measurements of sodium, potassium, chloride, carbon dioxide, BUN, and creatinine should be obtained, along with a urinalysis. A fasting blood glucose level and fasting cholesterol profile should be obtained to identify potential coronary risk factors. Thyroid functions should be considered to exclude hyperthyroidism or hypothyroidism. Magnesium levels should be considered for repletion purposes. Cardiac markers (creatine phosphokinase [CPK], CPK-MB, and troponin levels) should be obtained to differentiate an unstable ischemic event from a non–ST-segment elevation MI (Table 126-2).[16] Samples for CRP analysis may also be drawn to determine the presence of an inflammatory response, which is gaining enhanced recognition as a precursor to plaque rupture.

Echocardiography. The echocardiogram is helpful during an acute ischemic event in several ways. Most important, it assists in detecting the location and extent of regional or global left ventricular dysfunction. Second, it assists in risk stratification before discharge. Finally, it is helpful for future evaluation of the remodeling and healing process. The ECG detects ischemia by evaluating the motion and thickening of the left ventricular walls. This becomes particularly helpful when the patient has chest pressure and nondiagnostic ECG findings.

Although there are many techniques to assess ventricular wall motion, the method most commonly used is the two-dimensional echocardiogram with M-mode. In acute coronary ischemia the two-dimensional echocardiogram with M-mode may demonstrate abnormal wall motion of the ischemic section, which occurs almost immediately. Wall motion abnormalities, however, can be influenced by any abnormalities in the adjacent muscle to which it is attached. Perhaps a more specific finding for ischemic cardiac muscle would be the inability of the affected myocardial muscle to thicken during systolic contraction. The nonischemic, or normal, region reveals normal motion and thickening toward the left ventricular cavity during systole. The M-mode echocardiogram is ideal for measuring wall thickness and chamber dimensions, whereas color Doppler is used in conjunction with the M-mode to assess a regurgitant lesion.

TABLE 126-2 Cardiac Markers

Cardiac Marker	Rises	Peaks	Normalizes
CPK-MB isoforms	3-12 hours	24 hours	48-72 hours
Myoglobin	1-3 hours	6 hours	24 hours
Troponin T and I	3-12 hours	3-4 hours	14 days

CPK-MB, Creatinine phosphokinase-MB.

Acute Myocardial Infarction

Electrocardiogram. ST-segment elevations are generally representative of myocardial injury but may also be seen with left ventricular hypertrophy, hypertrophic cardiomyopathy, Prinzmetal's angina, pericarditis, hyperkalemia, early polarization, and left bundle branch block. In addition, ST-segment and T-wave changes may be seen in a variety of disease processes, including infiltrative myocardial disease (neoplasm, sarcoidosis, amyloidosis, hemochromatosis), chest deformities, muscular dystrophy, electrolyte abnormalities, cerebrovascular accidents, pharmacologic treatments (digoxin, tricyclics), hyperventilation, and anxiety. Therefore the history and presenting symptoms remain the basis for the diagnosis of an acute or chronic coronary syndrome.

The initial ECG presentation during an acute MI may demonstrate "hyperacute" T-wave changes, which are demonstrated by their tall, peaked shape (Figure 126-1). Within minutes to an hour after the acute event, the ST segment becomes elevated in the leads reflecting the area of myocardium involved. Within hours to days, the T waves usually become inverted and Q waves may develop (Figure 126-2). Pathologic Q waves generally represent a Q-wave or transmural MI. A Q wave is best defined by a width of greater than 0.04 seconds and a height at least one third of the associated R wave, provided that the R wave exceeds 5 mm in height. Within 1 week the ST segment returns to baseline unless a left ventricular aneurysm develops. In this case ST-segment elevation will persist. It may take up to 1 or more months for the T wave to return to positivity. The occurrence of pericarditis after MI will be reflected by ST-segment elevation in all leads except aV_F and V_1, which will show ST-segment depression with a convex rather than concave curvature.

Reciprocal changes may be evident in the leads opposite the area of infarction, as opposed to those recorded by the leads facing the infarct zone. Reciprocal changes are evidenced by an abnormal Q wave being replaced by an abnormal R wave; an ST-segment elevation being replaced by an ST-segment depression; and deep, symmetric negative T waves being replaced by tall, symmetric positive T waves.

In many healthy individuals some degree of ST-segment elevation, especially in the precordial leads (V_2 to V_5), may be noted on the routine ECG. In most people the degree of elevation is minimal; however, it can vary from 1 to 4 mm in height. This phenomenon has been attributed to early ventricular repolarization. It can be differentiated from the

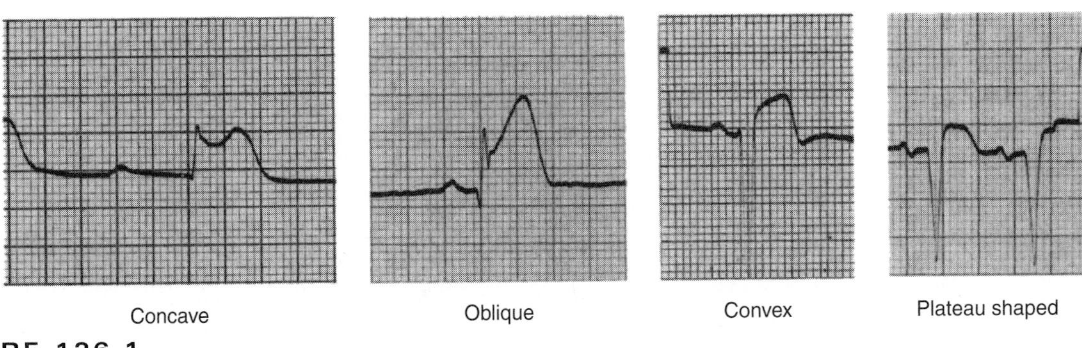

FIGURE 126-1

ST-segment elevations in acute myocardial infarction. (From Conover MB: *Understanding electrocardiography*, ed 7, St Louis, 1996, Mosby.)

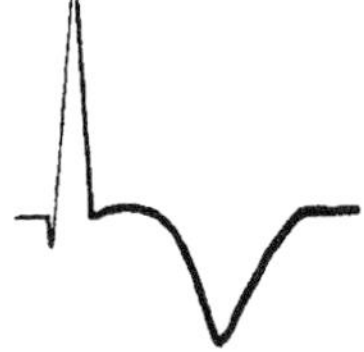

FIGURE 126-2

Typical coved ST segment and inverted T wave of evolving myocardial infarction. (From Conover MB: *Understanding electrocardiography*, ed 7, St Louis, 1996, Mosby.)

ST-segment elevation of an acute MI by the following: an upward concavity of the ST segment, an elevated takeoff of the ST segment at the J point (the junction of the end of the QRS complex and the beginning of the ST segment), and a distinct notching or slurring on the downstroke of the R wave.

Although the 12-lead ECG is useful in localizing the region of myocardial ischemia, it is limited in both the sensitivity and the specificity needed to distinguish the culprit coronary artery (Table 126-3 and Figures 126-3 to 126-5).

TABLE 126-3 Twelve-Lead ECG and Myocardial Infarction Territory

Lead	Territory
II, III, aV_F	Inferior wall
II, III, aV_F, V_5, V_6	Inferoapical wall
I, aV_L, V_5, V_6	Inferolateral wall
V_1-V_4	Anterior wall
I, aV_L, V_1-V_6	Anterolateral wall
V_1-V_3	Anteroseptal wall (ST-segment elevations)
V_5-V_6	Apical wall
I, aV_L, V_5-V_6	Lateral wall
V_1-V_3	Posterior wall (ST-segment depressions; tall, upright R wave)
V_1-V_2	Septal wall (ST-segment elevations)

Laboratory Data. For almost 30 years the creatine kinase (CK) and the CPK-MB levels have been used to detect myocardial cell injury. They were found to be moderately sensitive and specific. The American College of Cardiology (ACC) has recommended the use of myocardial markers such as the troponins and myoglobin. Troponin I and T are currently the new definitive diagnostic markers because of their high sensitivity and specificity. Like CPK-MBs, cardiac troponins become elevated within 3 to 4 hours. Troponin levels continue to be released for up to 11 days (7- to 14-day range) after a cardiac event. Thus troponin is a more useful diagnostic test than CPK-MB in predicting an acute coronary event and serving as a late cardiac marker. Myoglobin is found exclusively in both cardiac and skeletal striated muscle. It is released within 1 to 3 hours after a myocyte cell injury, which currently makes it the earliest marker of cell injury. Unfortunately, myoglobin lacks the cardiac specificity of the troponins. This can lead to false-positive results as a result of skeletal, renal, or other cardiac issues. Additionally, a mild leukocytosis of approximately 15,000/mm^3 may persist for up to 1 week.

When patients are seen with an acute MI caused by a known thrombotic lesion, there may be reason to suspect that they carry with them the additional burden of a hypercoagulable state. Therefore it may prove prudent to obtain a hypercoagulable panel for these patients.

Stress Testing. Myocardial perfusion imaging with thallium 201 or sestamibi, although very sensitive for the diagnosis of MI, cannot distinguish acute infarction from chronic scarring. Stress testing post-MI is often performed to determine the risk of future ischemic events and to provide an exercise prescription for cardiac rehabilitation.

Echocardiogram. Two-dimensional echocardiography can be of value in identifying wall motion abnormalities; estimating left ventricular ejection fraction; assessing for pericardial effusion, ventricular aneurysm, and left ventricular thrombus; and corroborating clinical and physical diagnosis of right ventricular infarction. Doppler echocardiography is useful in the detection of valvular regurgitant lesions, as well as ventricular and atrial septal defects. Echocardiography

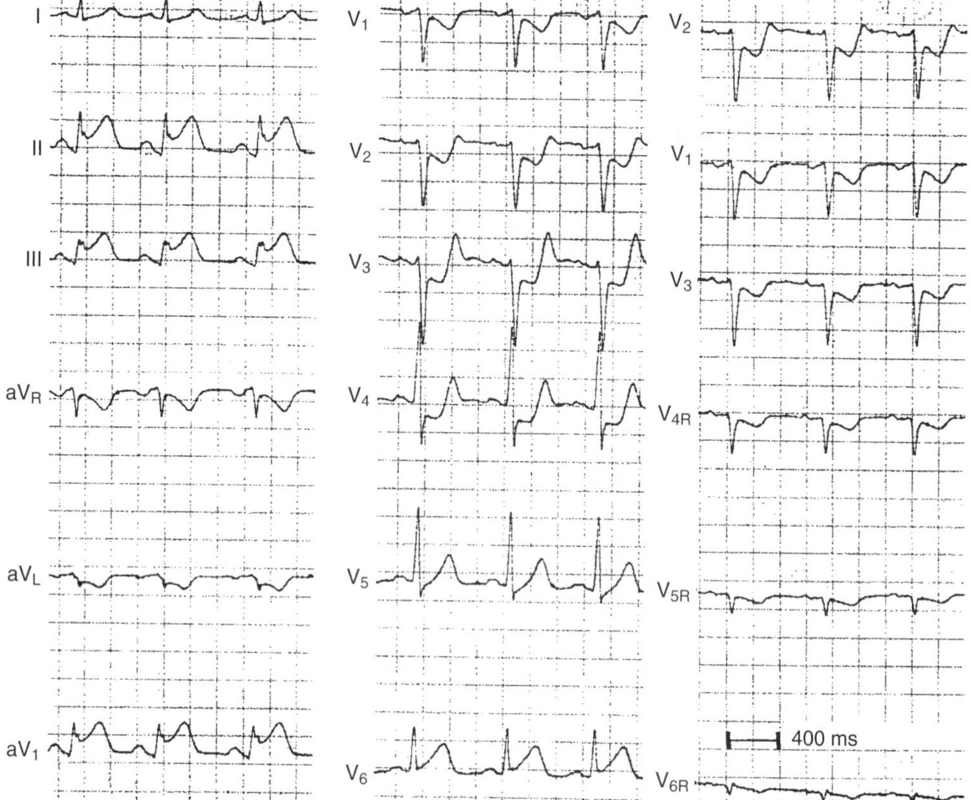

FIGURE 126-3

Acute inferior myocardial infarction caused by circumflex artery occlusion. Diagnosis was determined by the negative T wave in lead V_{4R} and the fact that the ST segment is higher in lead II than in lead III. (From Wellens HJJ, Conover MB: *The ECG in emergency decision making*, Philadelphia, 1991, Saunders.)

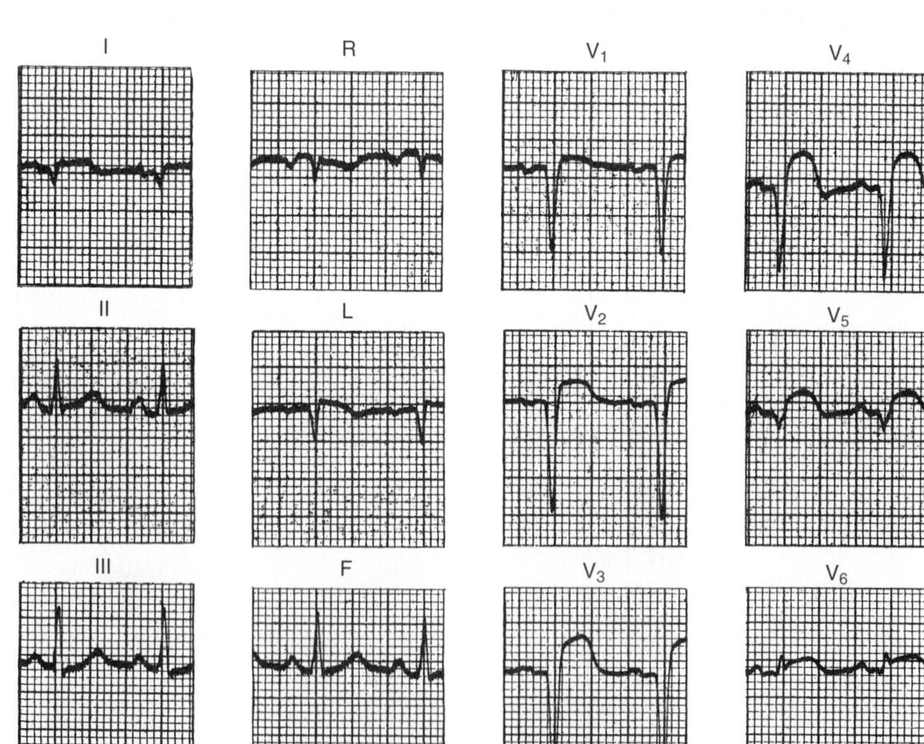

FIGURE 126-4

Anterolateral myocardial infarction. Diagnosis was made by the loss of the R-wave progression from lead V_1 to lead V_6 and the ST-segment elevation in those leads. (From Conover MB: *Understanding electrocardiography*, ed 7, St Louis, 1996, Mosby.)

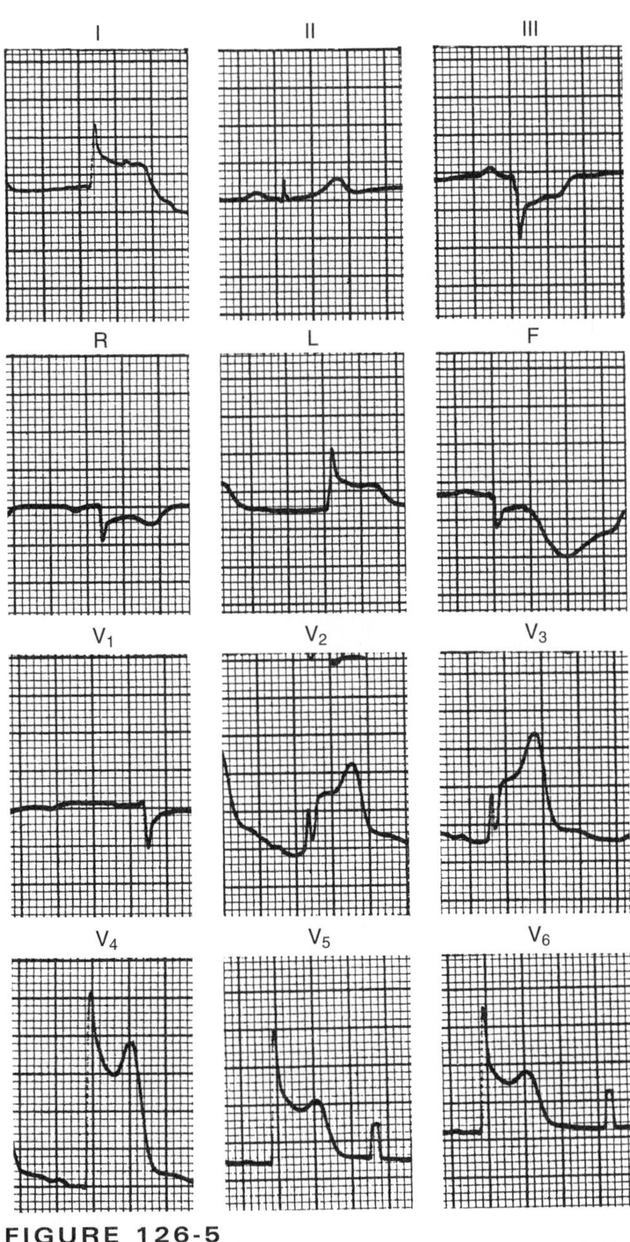

FIGURE 126-5

ECG showing massive anterolateral myocardial infarction. ST-segment elevation is evident in all superior leads. (From Conover MB: *Understanding electrocardiography*, ed 7, St Louis, 1996, Mosby.)

obtained early in the course of an evolving MI is helpful in diagnosis and can aid in the decision-making process. In addition, the echocardiogram can provide prognostic information regarding left ventricular function and identify patients who may be at risk for developing complications. Therefore serial echocardiograms are beneficial for future comparison.

DIFFERENTIAL DIAGNOSIS

The primary focus in the ambulatory care setting is to differentiate cardiac from noncardiac chest pain. Four chest pain syndromes have a particularly high mortality rate and therefore need to be expediently detected, diagnosed, and managed. These conditions are aortic dissection, MI, pulmonary embolus, and spontaneous pneumothorax. Conditions included in the differential diagnosis that have a lower mortality rate include gastrointestinal, pulmonary, valvular, inflammatory, integumentary, and psychologic disturbances (Table 126-4).

MANAGEMENT

Chronic Stable Angina

Treatment of chronic stable angina involves many modalities. Since this is a chronic disease, however, it is important to have a good provider-patient relationship and a means of objectively evaluating specific therapeutic interventions. Such an objective measure of evaluation and classification is the previously noted classification of the CCSC.

Patients should undergo baseline stress testing to determine their cardiac risk potential. The medication regimen should include acetylsalicylic acid, beta blockers, lipid-lowering agents based on a fasting cholesterol profile, and nitrates as needed. Risk factor modification is paramount to decrease the potential for disease progression.

Patients should be cautioned about specific angina triggers. For example, lifting a heavy load or performing arm exercise (isometric exercise) may precipitate angina symptoms because of an increase in myocardial oxygen demand. Walking in cold air may induce coronary vasoconstriction. It is advisable therefore to educate patients to cover their nose and mouth with a scarf when walking in cold air. Patients should be aware that sexual activity could precipitate angina and that this angina trigger is not position related. Finally, patients should be encouraged to exercise, since exercise appears to result in an eventual reduction in coronary blood flow for a given workload. As previously noted, patients should be aware of the "walk-through phenomenon," which is the relief of angina symptoms during exercise as exercise activity continues.

Silent Myocardial Ischemia

Few studies have evaluated whether pharmacologic intervention for silent myocardial ischemia has the same effect as that seen in patients who manifest symptoms of angina pectoris. It appears that the same principles apply and that all three classes of antiangina drugs may be beneficial. The use of aspirin in patients with asymptomatic ischemia after MI has been shown to reduce coronary events. Because vasoconstriction is thought to be a significant pathophysiologic component of this condition, a calcium channel blocker is recommended as first-line therapy. Beta blockers may also be used.

Management of patients with asymptomatic myocardial ischemia must be individualized. Treatment interventions should be based on (1) the degree to which the exercise stress test is positive, with particular attention to the stage at which ECG evidence of ischemia appears; (2) the magnitude and number of perfusion defects seen on thallium or sestamibi scintigraphy; (3) the ECG localization of ischemia; and (4) the change in left ventricular function documented on radionuclide ventriculography or echocardiography. Coronary arteriography is recommended in patients with evidence of severe ischemia on noninvasive testing. Asymptomatic patients with silent ischemia and significant left main CAD or three-vessel CAD and impaired left ventricular function are appropriate

TABLE 126-4 Differential Diagnosis: Chest Pain

Diagnosis	Symptoms	Physical Examination Findings
INTEGUMENTARY		
Herpes zoster	Prodromal symptoms of chest pressure Tingling, tenderness, and pain along involved dermatome(s)	Grouped vesicles along erythematous base
CHEST WALL DISCOMFORT		
Costochondritis	Anterior chest pain, sharply localized	Reproducible by pressure on costochondral junction
LUNGS		
Pneumonia	Pain when inflammatory process extends to pleura, resulting in chest pain that worsens with inspiration Fever, chills, cough, sputum production, dyspnea	Crackles or rales and/or decreased breath sounds over affected area Bronchial breath sounds with dense consolidation, increased fremitus, and egophony (E-to-A changes) Dullness to percussion
Pneumothorax	Sudden-onset, severe unilateral chest pain, generally pleuritic in nature Dyspnea	Diminished breath sounds on affected side Mediastinal emphysema may be present
Pneumothorax, tension	Same as pneumothorax, yet with substernal chest pressure with throat tightness	Same as pneumothorax, yet hypotension may be present Tracheal and mediastinal shift
Pulmonary embolus	Dyspnea Chest pain secondary to pulmonary infarction or inflammatory response (pleuritic)	Decreased breath sounds in affected area Hypotension with massive pulmonary embolus as a result of low cardiac output Hemoptysis, tachycardia, and hypoxia
Pulmonary hypertension	Mimics symptoms of ischemic chest pain Dyspnea	Prominent parasternal lift at lower left sternal border or xiphoid Pulmonic, tricuspid, or mitral regurgitation murmur(s) S_4 may be audible
HEART		
Aortic stenosis	Easy fatigability, dyspnea on exertion, syncope or near syncope, anterior chest pressure	Systolic murmur best heard over right base Delayed carotid upstrokes
Aortic dissections	Sudden onset of severe tearing, stabbing pain over anterior chest (proximal dissection) or interscapular-abdominal region (distal dissection) Diaphoresis, nausea, vomiting, near syncope	Hypertension in 50% of patients Pulses diminished or absent Neurologic symptoms (decreased cerebral-spinal cord perfusion) Aortic regurgitation murmur may be present as a result of aortic root dissection
Mitral valve prolapse	Sharp left anterior chest pain, generally occurring in response to stress or emotional events Chest discomfort lasting seconds to days Palpitations and dyspnea	Mitral valve click may be noted in systole at left lower sternal border
Pericarditis	Anterior chest pain that may radiate to shoulder area if diaphragmatic surface of pericardium is involved Sharp chest pain, which increases with inspiration or supine positioning (pleuritic), and lessens with forward positioning	Fever with bacterial or viral etiology Friction rub may or may not be present
GASTROINITESTINAL SYMPTOMS		
Reflux (gastroesophageal reflux disease)	Substernal burning, may radiate to neck, occurring 30 to 60 minutes after eating	
Acute cholecystitis	Right upper quadrant pain, epigastric pain Nausea, vomiting, and anorexia	Right upper quadrant tenderness plus Murphy's sign Fever may be present
PAIN DISORDERS		
	Intense anxiety that may last for several days Avoidance behavior because of inability to seek a safe refuge during an attack period Chest pain that is atypical Hypertension may be noted	

candidates for coronary artery bypass surgery. In the Asymptomatic Cardiac Ischemic Pilot Study, coronary revascularization significantly reduced the duration of silent ischemia and hospital readmissions over a 1-year period when compared with medical strategies.[17] Patients with silent myocardial ischemia require close follow-up monitoring with noninvasive testing to determine changes in left ventricular function and the time required for the exercise test to be positive, which indicates ischemia.

Microvascular Angina

Many patients with microvascular angina respond to beta blockers, calcium channel blockers, and nitrates; however, a large number of patients continue to have pain. The natural history of the disorder is variable. Many patients have resolution of symptoms with time but may have periods of exacerbation. Even in patients with persistent symptoms, there does not appear to be a risk for MI or sudden death. Patient reassurance is an important part of therapy.

Variant Angina

Acute treatment of the chest pain episode is generally sublingual nitroglycerin. Calcium channel blockers are the long-term treatment of choice for this condition. In most cases a single agent is sufficient, but in resistant cases combination therapy with a dihydropyridine calcium channel blocker such as nifedipine or amlodipine (Norvasc) coupled with a nondihydropyridine such as diltiazem or verapamil is useful. Continuous nitrate therapy is not recommended because of problems with tolerance, but targeted nitrates may be helpful in patients with a predictable pattern of pain. Beta blockers are contraindicated.

The natural history of spasm is one of periods of symptomatic exacerbation followed by periods of relative quiescence. Once a patient who is receiving therapy has been without symptoms for 6 to 12 months, medication withdrawal can be attempted. Patients with spasm without significant fixed coronary stenosis are not candidates for mechanical intervention.

Unstable Angina and Non–ST-Segment Elevation Myocardial Infarction

Early risk stratification should be performed to determine the likelihood of an acute cardiac ischemic event from a non–ST-segment elevation MI. The immediate management of this patient population consists of a detailed patient history, physical examination, 12-lead ECG, and cardiac markers. From this information the health care provider can generally classify the patient with chest pain in one of four categories: a noncardiac cause, a stable angina cause, a possible acute coronary artery syndrome, or a definite coronary artery syndrome.

Patients who have a low risk for adverse cardiac outcomes may be managed on an outpatient basis. These patients are seen with new-onset or worsening angina symptoms yet have not had a severe, prolonged, or at-rest event within the past 2 weeks. Their ECG is normal or unchanged during an episode of chest discomfort, and cardiac markers are within normal limits. Low-risk patients should be immediately started on aspirin therapy, 160 to 325 mg, unless contraindicated, along with daily beta-blocker therapy and sublingual nitroglycerin as needed. Identifiable precipitating clinical circumstances should be uncovered, as should any secondary causes (e.g., fever, anemia, hypotension, cardiomyopathy, aortic stenosis, thyrotoxicosis, or recent stressful events). Symptoms of unstable angina may resolve once the precipitating event is treated.

Low-risk patients should be seen for follow-up evaluation within a 72-hour period, at which time symptoms should be reevaluated for any further instability. Early exercise tolerance testing should also be performed. Patients should be educated regarding cardiac risk factors and aggressive plans for risk factor modification.

Patients in the intermediate- or high-risk category should be hospitalized for careful monitoring, risk stratification, and management. If the symptoms of ACS are identified in the office setting, immediate referral to an emergency department should be undertaken. The patient should be given sublingual nitroglycerin and chewable aspirin immediately. If chewable aspirin is not available, a regular aspirin tablet should be crushed and given to the patient. Once the patient is in the emergency department setting, beta-blocker therapy should be considered if the presenting hemodynamic profile permits, with the dose titrated to a heart rate of 50 to 60 beats per minute. Heparin should be given in a bolus of 80 units/kg of body weight and then infused at 14 units/kg/hr. The dosage is then titrated to achieve an activated partial thromboplastin time of 1.5 to 2.0 times the control. Low-molecular-weight heparin may also be considered in lieu of heparin therapy. A platelet glycoprotein IIb/IIIa receptor antagonist should be added to the regimen for patients with continuing ischemia or with other high-risk features and for patients for whom a percutaneous coronary intervention (PCI) is planned.

Acute ST-Segment Elevation Myocardial Infarction

Treatment goals for the patient with an acute MI are to restore blood supply to cardiac muscle, to relieve pain, and to decrease the incidence of complications (such as heart failure, myocardial rupture, valvular dysfunction, and fatal and nonfatal arrhythmias). Prevention of recurrent ischemia and infarction and efforts to decrease mortality should also be undertaken.

With these goals in mind, patients with an acute evolving ST-segment elevation MI should be transferred to a hospital with a dedicated chest pain center and interventional cardiac program, and the patients should be admitted to a specialized coronary unit, where continuous cardiac rhythm and hemodynamic monitoring can take place. Patients with a suspected MI who are considered at low risk for arrhythmias and hemodynamic compromise may be admitted to a telemetry unit where continuous arrhythmia monitoring is available.

The mortality rate of patients with an ST-segment elevation MI is higher than for those with a non–ST-segment elevation MI in the early phases of the acute event. However, recurrent infarction in the late hospital period is much higher in patients with a non–ST-segment elevation MI. When reinfarction occurs, it is associated with a high mortality rate. Thus the difference in long-term prognosis between an ST-segment and non–ST-segment elevation MI is not statistically significant.

Management of an acute ST-segment elevation MI has changed considerably in the past several years. The major area of interest has been the use of thrombolytic therapy, antiplatelet agents, and PCI to reestablish coronary artery patency and limit infarct size. The most crucial aspect of management is aimed at preserving the myocardium and reestablishing coronary flow within a critical time frame. Maximum benefit is achieved from lytic therapy when it is initiated within 1½ hours after the onset of symptoms. New ACC/AHA recommendations published in January 2006 now recommend that PCI be initiated within 90 minutes versus 120 minutes of hospital arrival and confirmation of an acute MI.[18] Modest benefit is attained when therapy is instituted 3 to 6 hours after the onset of infarction, and some benefit is possible when therapy is given up to 12 hours after the onset of infarction if chest pain is ongoing and ST-segment elevation is apparent in ECG leads that do not demonstrate new Q waves. General contraindications to lytic therapy include recent surgery or head trauma, active internal bleeding, suspected aortic dissection, pregnancy, diabetic hemorrhagic retinopathy, severe hypertension, and a history of cerebrovascular accident or allergic reaction to the thrombolytic agent. Hemorrhagic stroke is the most common complication. The rate increases with advancing age. Patients older than 70 years have strokes at twice the rate of younger patients; however, older patients may benefit from lytic therapy. Decisions about thrombolytic therapy must be made on a case-by-case basis in these patients.

Thrombus and platelet aggregation play an important role in the pathogenesis of acute MI. The use of heparin and aspirin to impede the process is indicated. Both heparin and aspirin have been shown to reduce the risk of fatal and nonfatal MI. Aspirin dosing of 75 to 162 mg should be started on all patients and continued indefinitely unless contraindicated. Clopidogrel (Plavix) 75 mg should be started in combination with aspirin and continued for up to 12 months in patients after ACS or PCI.[4] This treatment should be started immediately by having the patient chew an aspirin and should be continued indefinitely. Clopidogrel should be administered to all patients unable to take aspirin because of a hypersensitivity reaction. Heparin is generally administered by weight adjustment to keep the partial thromboplastin time 1.5 to 2 times normal. A glycoprotein IIb/IIIa receptor antagonist should be administered to patients with continuing ischemia, a planned coronary intervention, or other high-risk features.

Nitroglycerin paste or infusion is used if patients have ongoing ischemia. Nitroglycerin reduces systemic vascular resistance and pulmonary capillary wedge pressure and increases collateral coronary blood flow to the subendocardium, thereby protecting ischemic myocardium. When nitroglycerin is administered, an adequate coronary perfusion pressure should be maintained. (IV nitroglycerin 10 mcg/min initial dose and up to 300 mcg/min for the first 24 to 48 hours is usually administered, titrated according to the individual patient's response.)

The early use of IV beta blockers for patients with increased heart rates in the absence of contraindications (e.g., severe heart failure, hypotension, bradycardia, atrioventricular [AV] block) has been shown to reduce myocardial oxygen demand, infarct size, and ventricular fibrillation. In addition, beneficial effects of long-term beta blockers, without intrinsic sympathomimetic activity, have demonstrated reduction in mortality, reinfarction, and sudden death. Caution must be taken when administering beta blockers because of their occasional unpredictable hemodynamic effects. Metoprolol (Lopressor), 5 mg q 5 min for a total of 15 mg IV, continues to be the most commonly used beta blocker. For patients who tolerate the IV dosing, oral dosing should be initiated 15 minutes after the last IV dose at 25 to 50 mg q 6 hr for 48 hours. During this time the provider should periodically assess the patient for bradycardia and heart block on cardiac monitor and for evidence of bronchospasm on physical examination. If patients continue to tolerate this dosing regimen, they can be placed on 50 to 100 mg PO b.i.d.

The use of angiotensin-converting enzyme (ACE) inhibitors has improved the mortality rate and the prevention of heart failure and recurrent MI in patients with left ventricular function of 40% or less. If possible, ACE inhibitors should be started once the patient is hemodynamically stable. Renal issues should also be considered when starting ACE inhibitor therapy; renal artery stenosis is a contraindication to this therapy. Among lower-risk patients with normal left ventricular ejection fractions in whom cardiovascular risk factors are well controlled and revascularization has been performed, use of ACE inhibitors may be considered optional.[4]

Calcium channel blockers have been shown to be effective in acute and chronic stable angina, but there have been conflicting reports about their use for the patient with an acute MI. It is currently recommended that short-acting calcium antagonists not be used for patients with angina. Patients with continued post-MI ischemia caused by coronary vasospasm might benefit from a calcium channel blocker. Diltiazem has proven beneficial (for prevention of reinfarction and reduction in mortality) after non–Q-wave MI in patients who do not have heart failure.

Arrhythmias should be promptly diagnosed and treated to prevent further deterioration related to increased myocardial oxygen demands, decreased cardiac output, or electrical instability. The routine use of lidocaine is not recommended.

Pain relief is best remedied by enhancing coronary blood flow or by decreasing myocardial oxygen demand. With ongoing chest pain, morphine sulfate may be administered to decrease myocardial preload because of its vasodilatory effects. It should be noted that, as a narcotic, morphine may mask ischemic chest pain; thus the patient may be too sedated to communicate ongoing ischemic symptoms. Morphine may be dosed in 2-mg increments, with many patients requiring up to a total of 15 to 20 mg. Caution must be used in older patients and those with chronic obstructive pulmonary disease (COPD).

Pharmacologic Therapy for Coronary Artery Disease

Aspirin. Aspirin is effective in the treatment of CAD because of its effects on platelets and vascular endothelial cells. In platelets aspirin *irreversibly* inhibits the synthesis of cyclooxygenase, preventing the formation of thromboxane A_2, which is responsible for platelet aggregation. In vascular endothelial cells aspirin *temporarily* inhibits the synthesis of cyclooxygenase, which inhibits prostacyclin production and platelet aggregation. The clinical benefits of aspirin have been demonstrated at dosages of 75 to 325 mg/day. Although aspirin in doses of 75 mg has been demonstrated to inhibit platelet aggregation, its effectiveness in endothelial prostaglandin inhibition has yet to be determined.

Aspirin reaches appreciable plasma levels within 20 minutes and results in platelet inhibition within 60 minutes.[17] The antiplatelet effect of aspirin lasts for the 10-day life of the platelet; however, 10% of circulating platelets are replaced on a daily basis. Normal hemostasis can be achieved with only 20% of aspirin-free platelets. This becomes an important consideration in the timing of aspirin withdrawal for elective surgical procedures.

The Physicians' Health Study evaluated 22,071 male physicians receiving alternate-day doses of 325 mg of aspirin and found a 44% reduction in risk of first MI.[19] Findings for overall cardiovascular mortality were inconclusive because of an inadequate number of events. Although this study was encouraging, additional data on primary prevention are needed to assess the risk/benefit ratio of aspirin in a healthy population. Clinical judgment should be used for patients at risk for MI until further evidence becomes available.

Aspirin therapy has proven to benefit patients in the acute phase of an evolving MI and should be routinely administered with an initial loading dose of 162 mg PO unless an anaphylactic aspirin allergy is known.[20] Enteric-coated tablets should be chewed or crushed for more rapid absorption.

The most convincing evidence of the efficacy of aspirin therapy in an acute evolving MI came from the Second International Study of Infarct Survival.[21] In this trial, 17,197 patients came into see a health care provider within 24 hours of experiencing symptoms and were randomly assigned to receive aspirin (162 mg/day) or a placebo. After 5 weeks, patients who received aspirin therapy had a 23% reduction in mortality and a 49% reduction in nonfatal reinfarction when compared with the placebo group. In addition, the aspirin-treated group had no increase in gastrointestinal bleeding. For those patients with unstable angina, or those developing an acute MI who are unable to take aspirin because of a hypersensitivity reaction, clopidogrel should be administered.

Beta Blockers. Beta blockers have become the mainstay of therapy for patients with CAD. Beta blockers decrease myocardial oxygen consumption by decreasing the heart rate at rest and with exercise, by lowering the blood pressure, and by reducing myocardial contractility, thereby eliciting a negative inotropic effect. In contrast, these agents are not useful for vasospastic angina and may worsen the condition. Beta blockers have been shown to reduce total mortality, the rate of nonfatal infarction, infarct size, cardiovascular mortality, and sudden cardiac death.

Beta blockers can be classified according to their relative cardioselectivity and lipid solubility. Beta blockers may be "nonselective" (have an affinity for both β_1- and β_2-receptors) or "selective" (have an affinity for β_1-receptors). β_1-Receptors are located in the myocardium, with small amounts of β_2-receptors in the atrium. β_2-Receptors are primarily located in the bronchioles, peripheral vascular smooth muscles, and other specialized sites, such as pancreatic islet cells. Thus blockade of β_2-receptors may lead to bronchoconstriction or bronchospasm and peripheral vascular constriction, resulting in claudication. In addition, the mechanism whereby insulin-induced hypoglycemia is countered by stimulation of the liver to mobilize liver glycogen is β_2-receptor dependent. Thus blockade of β_2-receptors in a patient with diabetes may lead to an inappropriate response to hypoglycemia. This is important, since patients with CAD and asthma, COPD, diabetes, or intermittent claudication may benefit from a low dose of β_1-selective agents administered with caution. However, as the dose of such agents is increased, selectivity is lost, and both types of receptors become blocked (Box 126-5). Carvedilol, a newer generation of alpha- and beta-blocker combinations, has been found to significantly improve survival and complications of acute MI.[22]

Side effects of beta blockers include fatigue, impotence, cold extremities, bronchospasm, worsening claudication, bradycardia, and cardiac conduction disturbances. Central nervous system side effects are based on the agent's lipid solubility property. Agents that are lipid soluble readily cross the blood-brain barrier and are more likely to cause insomnia, depression, and nightmares; this may be seen in any patient but is commonly observed in older adults. Patients should be cautioned that sudden discontinuation of beta-blocker therapy may precipitate angina symptoms or lead to MI as a result of rebound tachycardia. Although much has been written about the beta-blocker withdrawal syndrome, the incidence is quite low. However, in discontinuing the drug, one should be prudent and taper the drug over several days. Some beta blockers have the capacity to stimulate either one or both β_1- and β_2-receptors, hence the term *intrinsic sympathomimetic activity*, as seen with pindolol. This property limits the efficacy of treating patients with angina because at higher doses the heart rate is not decreased and may even be increased. These agents may be beneficial in patients who have symptomatic sinus bradycardia when treated with other beta blockers. The

BOX 126-5

BETA-BLOCKER AGENTS

NONSELECTIVE BETA$_1$ AND BETA$_2$ BLOCKERS
- Propranolol (Inderal)
- Timolol (Blocadren)
- Nadolol (Corgard)
- Sotalol (Sotacar,* Betapace)
- Penbutolol (Levatol)

NONSELECTIVE, VASODILATORY
- Carteolol (Cartrol)
- Labetalol (Trandate, Normodyne)
- Pindolol (Visken)

CARDIOSELECTIVE—β_1-RECEPTORS ONLY
- Acebutolol (Sectral)
- Atenolol (Tenormin)
- Metoprolol (Lopressor, Betaloc,* Toprol-XL)

COMBINATION ALPHA$_1$ AND NONCARDIOSELECTIVE BETA BLOCKER
- Carvedilol (Coreg)

*Canada-only drugs.

major effect of beta blockers with sympathomimetic activity is lowering of blood pressure. Labetalol possesses both beta- and alpha-blocking actions. This drug can be used to treat patients with angina, as well as patients with significant hypertension.

Nitrates. Nitrates are recommended for the treatment of stable and unstable angina and the management of an acute MI. The clinical effectiveness of nitrates is in their ability to promote vascular smooth muscle relaxation, resulting in arteriolar and venous dilation. In smaller doses nitrates dilate the venous system, which causes peripheral pooling and decreased venous return to the heart (preload). This reduction in preload decreases the left ventricular size, ventricular filling pressures, and myocardial wall tension. In larger doses, nitrates dilate the arterial vasculature, lowering systemic blood pressure (afterload) and thereby decreasing the resistance to ventricular ejection, making it easier for the heart to contract. This overall reduction in left ventricular workload decreases myocardial oxygen consumption. The arteriolar dilating effect, however, may produce a reflex tachycardia, thereby increasing myocardial oxygen consumption. This effect may be attenuated by concurrent use of beta blockade. In addition, the combination of nitrates with calcium channel blockers should be undertaken cautiously, since postural hypotension may be a problem.

Coronary vasodilation is induced through the exogenous production of nitric oxide from nitrate metabolism, which is now known to be endothelium-derived relaxing factor (EDRF). In the coronary circulation, damage to the endothelial layer from atherosclerosis results in decreased availability of EDRF and hence a decreased vasodilatory response. Nitrates are endothelium-independent vasodilators and therefore do not require a functioning endothelium to deliver a vasodilating response. Nitrate administration results in the endogenous production of nitric oxide, which replaces the vasodilating effects of EDRF and promotes coronary vessel vasodilation.

Currently the three nitrate preparations available for use in the United States are nitroglycerin, isosorbide dinitrate (ISDN), and isosorbide mononitrate (ISMN) (Table 126-5).

Sublingual nitroglycerin tablets in doses of 0.4 mg are most useful for acute angina events because of the rapid course of action of sublingual nitroglycerin. Sublingual nitroglycerin is also recommended for prophylactic use before the patient engages in a physical activity or a stressful event that has historically precipitated an angina event. Sublingual nitroglycerin works within 3 to 5 minutes; however, antiischemic effects last for less than 30 minutes. Because of its short duration of action, sublingual nitroglycerin should be combined with oral nitrates for sustained effectiveness. Patients should be taught to take one nitroglycerin tablet every 5 minutes for a total of three tablets in a 15-minute period. Nitroglycerin is taken while the patient is seated to decrease preload by maximizing blood flow to the dilated peripheral circulation. If no relief is obtained after three nitroglycerin tablets, the patient should be transported by ambulance to the nearest medical facility. Nitroglycerin tablets retain their potency for up to 6 months after the bottle has been opened. Patients should be encouraged to keep nitroglycerin tablets in their amber-colored glass bottle, protected from moisture and extremes of temperature and light.

Nitroglycerin spray is particularly useful for patients with visual or neurologic impairments who may have difficulty handling a small tablet. The spray is delivered in a metered dose of 0.4 mg and should be applied to the surface of the tongue. Patients should be reminded not to inhale the spray. Each canister contains approximately 200 doses, and the canister will maintain its potency for up to 3 years.

Oral nitroglycerin is the nitrate of choice in the ambulatory population and can be taken as either ISDN (isosorbide dinitrate) or ISMN (isosorbide mononitrate). ISDN is extensively metabolized in the liver, where over half of it is converted to ISMN. Because of this bypass effect, ISDN is not effective for treating angina or enhancing exercise capacity in dosages of less than 20 mg q 4 hr. In 1991 the U.S. Food and Drug Administration approved ISMN, which does not undergo hepatic degradation, so that 100% of it is available after oral dosing. The main advantage of the ISMNs is that they can be administered once or twice daily, whereas ISDNs must be

TABLE 126-5 Nitrate Preparations*

Preparation	Starting Dose	Maximum Dose	Onset of Action	Duration of Action
Nitroglycerin (Nitrostat)	0.4 mg (1 tablet)	3 tablets in 15 minutes	1 minute	<30 minutes
Nitroglycerin (Nitrolingual)	0.4 mg (metered spray)	3 sprays in 15 minutes	1 minute	<30 minutes
ISDN (Isordil, Sorbitrate)	20 mg q 4-6 hr	60-80 mg q 4 hr	60-90 minutes	4-6 hours
ISDN-SR (Dilatrate-SR)	40 mg q 12 hr	80 mg b.i.d. or t.i.d.		
ISMN (Ismo, Monoket)	20 mg in am and 20 mg 7 hours later			
ISMN-SR (Imdur)	30-60 mg q day	120-240 mg q day		
Nitroglycerin ointment (2%) (Nitro-Bid, Nitrol)	0.5 inches q 4-6 hr	4-5 inches q 3-4 hr	30-60 minutes	3-6 hours
Nitroglycerin patch (Transderm-Nitro, Nitro-Dur, Nitrodisc, Deponit)	5 mg/24 hr (0.1 to 0.4 mg/hr)	2-3 patches of 15 mg in 24 hours	30 minutes	24 hours

ISDN, Isosorbide dinitrate; *ISMN,* isosorbide mononitrate.

*Dosing for nitrate preparations should include a dose-free interval each day to prevent refractory tolerance.

administered three or four times per day. The main disadvantage is the cost. ISMN preparations cost several times more than the generic ISDN, and this needs to be considered in prescribing practices. Aside from these two factors, there is no distinct advantage in using one of these preparations over the other.

Topical nitroglycerin is absorbed through the skin and can be administered either through a 2% ointment or through premeasured skin patches in dosages of 5, 10, 15, or 20 mg/day. The advantage of nitroglycerin ointment over other methods of administration is that the ointment can be removed promptly if any side effects develop. However, its disadvantages seem to outweigh its advantages in the ambulatory population. The ointment is messy to apply, can soil clothing, is seldom dosed consistently each time, and may produce a localized skin rash. The nitroglycerin patch produces a more controlled dosing and is generally favored over the ointment. Although initially topical nitroglycerin is effective, long-term usage can lead to nitrate tolerance and thus a decreased therapeutic effect. It is therefore recommended that topical nitroglycerin be removed from the skin for 8 to 12 hours daily.

Nitrate tolerance results from plasma nitrate levels sustained from continued nitrate administration. Nitrate tolerance is important to identify because it leads to a reduction in antiischemic benefits. The cause of nitrate tolerance is a complex, multifactorial phenomenon, and the mechanism remains elusive. However, the theory that is commonly associated with nitrate tolerance involves vascular depletion of sulfhydryl groups. The metabolism of nitrates requires the use of sulfhydryl to form intracellular nitric oxide from nitrates. This is the active molecule that stimulates guanylate cyclase to produce vasodilation. Continuous use of nitrates produces excess nitric oxide formation, thus depleting sulfhydryl groups. A sulfhydryl donor such as acetylcysteine has been used in experiments to counteract nitrate tolerance.

To avoid the effects of nitrate tolerance dosing, intervals free of nitrates must occur. For oral ISDN administration, a three-times-per-day dosing schedule (8 AM, 1 PM, and 6 PM) rather than a four-times-per-day schedule should be prescribed. With sustained-release ISDN administration, dosing at 8 AM and 2 PM would support nitrate-free intervals in the evening. Topical nitrates should be removed for 8 to 12 hours daily. This dosing schedule provides periods during the evening hours when the patient is without antiischemic therapy. For this reason, as well as the reflex tachycardia often seen with vasodilation in response to nitrate therapy, combination therapy with beta blockers or calcium channel blockers is recommended.

Calcium Channel Blockers. Calcium channel blockers are used in the treatment of hypertension and angina pectoris. They selectively inhibit the influx of calcium into the calcium L-channel in both smooth muscle and myocardial cells. All have a peripheral arteriolar and coronary vasodilating effect and a negative inotropic effect, although the latter is modest in the case of nifedipine. Two distinct classes of calcium channel antagonists have emerged on the basis of molecular structure: (1) the dihydropyridines (DHPs), with a chemical structure similar to nifedipine; and (2) the non-DHPs, such as verapamil (papaverine derivative) and diltiazem (benzothiazepine derivative).

The DHPs are more vascular selective; thus their dominant effect is peripheral and coronary vasodilation. They have minimum or no effect on the sinus and AV nodes. The rapid vasodilatory effects of these agents may lead to reflex tachycardia, exacerbation of heart failure, and stimulation of the renin-angiotensin system. These undesirable effects are more common among the short-acting DHPs, and as such should be avoided in the patient with an acute MI. Since the advent of truly long-acting agents (nifedipine XL, amlodipine, felodipine), there have been fewer side effects. In the PRAISE Trial, amlodipine had no detrimental effect on patients with ischemic class II or III heart failure.[23] The non-DHPs, which are less vascular selective than the DHPs, predominantly inhibit nodal tissue (decrease sinus rate) and myocardial contraction. These agents should be used with caution in patients taking beta blockers and in patients with left ventricular dysfunction. They may be safely used in appropriately selected patients without sinus node or AV node disease. Calcium antagonists have the ability to prevent coronary vasoconstriction. In general, verapamil or diltiazem is preferred over nifedipine and other DHPs for monotherapy, since agents in the latter group have the potential to cause a reflex tachycardia (Box 126-6).

Angiotensin-Converting Enzyme Inhibitors. The conical shape of the heart is designed for optimum efficiency in performance and energy utilization. MI induces alteration in the contour of the heart, leading to decreased left ventricular performance and increased energy requirement for a given workload. Preserving the contour of the heart after MI is essential for effective left ventricular performance and prevention of the development of left-sided heart failure. The consequences of poor left ventricular performance result in an increased 5-year mortality ranging from 26% to 75%.[24]

It is clear that stimulation of the renin-angiotensin-aldosterone system plays an important pathophysiologic role in the development of heart failure and poor left ventricular performance. ACE inhibitors can therefore inhibit or counteract the adverse hemodynamic and neurohumoral effects (increased preload, afterload, heart rate, sympathetic tone,

BOX 126-6

CALCIUM CHANNEL BLOCKERS

DIHYDROPYRIDINES

- Amlodipine (Norvasc)
- Isradipine (DynaCirc)
- Felodipine (Plendil)
- Nicardipine (Cardene)
- Nifedipine (Procardia, Adalat)
- Nisoldipine (Sular)

NONDIHYDROPYRIDINES

- Diphenylalkylamine derivative
- Verapamil (Calan, Covera HS, Isoptin, Verelan)

BENZOTHIAZEPINE DERIVATIVES

- Diltiazem (Cardizem, Dilacor, Tiazac)

catecholamines, and renin-angiotensin system activity) contributed by the system.

Several large trials have shown that administration of ACE inhibitors shortly after acute MI, once the patient is hemodynamically stable, has prevented the development of heart failure in patients with left ventricular dysfunction but without clinical heart failure.[25-27] In addition, ACE inhibitors reduced long-term mortality in patients with and without clinical evidence of heart failure through the inhibitors' ability to reverse the major hemodynamic and neurohumoral abnormalities associated with poor left ventricular performance.[28] Angiotensin-receptor blockers should be used in patients who are intolerant of ACE inhibitors and have heart failure or have had an MI with left ventricular ejection fraction of less than 40%.[4]

Anticoagulation. The use of anticoagulation with aspirin and heparin has significantly reduced the short-term risk of thromboembolic complications during an acute MI. However, the continuing use of a low-molecular-weight heparin beyond 1 week has not been shown to be effective in further risk reduction.[28] A significant percentage of patients with ACS experience major vascular events either during or within the first few months after their hospital stay. One alternative oral therapy to minimize cardiac complications is the use of the thienopyridine derivatives, the most promising of which is clopidogrel. This medication, in dosages of 75 mg/day in addition to aspirin therapy, was shown in the CURE trial to significantly decrease the incidence of nonfatal MI, strokes, in-hospital refractory ischemia or severe ischemic episodes, and heart failure events for up to 6 months.[29]

Cases where there is a mural thrombus represent another circumstance for anticoagulation. Ventricular mural thrombi are more common in patients with a large rather than small area of MI. Thrombi are often observed in the left ventricle, particularly in the apex, where aneurysm and pseudoaneurysm commonly form. On rare occasions, with extensive infarction, thrombus may be observed in the right ventricular apex. Warfarin (Coumadin) therapy is indicated in patients with a mural thrombus, especially in cases where the thrombus is mobile, has an irregular surface, and is protruding. Warfarin therapy is generally initiated for 3 to 6 months, after which time echocardiographic evaluation to assess the presence or absence of mural thrombus is performed. If the thrombus persists after warfarin therapy, it does not necessarily indicate continued embolic potential unless there is evidence of mobility. In addition, warfarin therapy is indicated in patients with severe left ventricular dysfunction and an ejection fraction of less than 20%.

The Coumadin Aspirin Reinfarction Study (CARS) was prematurely discontinued, because there was no difference between the combined therapy of warfarin plus aspirin and aspirin or warfarin alone.[30] This was a double-blind trial; however, there was difficulty in achieving an International Normalized Ratio (INR) of 1.5 or greater.

Cholesterol-Lowering Agents. Recent clinical trials have found that reductions in LDLs have reduced the risk of overall mortality, coronary mortality, major coronary events, coronary artery procedures, and strokes. Therefore an LDL cholesterol of less than 100 ml/dl is optimal, and it is recommended that further reduction to less than 70 mg/dl be achieved in high-risk patients.[4] A cholesterol profile should be obtained on hospital admission or within 24 hours. LDL cholesterol levels begin to decline in the first few hours after an event and may remain low for many weeks. Two major modalities of LDL-lowering therapy are therapeutic lifestyle changes (weight reduction, increased physical activity, and dietary reductions of saturated fats and cholesterol intake) and medication therapy. The drug of choice is usually a statin; however, a bile acid sequestrant or nicotinic acid may be used. After 12 weeks of drug therapy, the response to therapy can be reassessed. If the patient's goal has yet to be achieved, a more intensive drug therapy along with careful lifestyle analysis for compliance should be undertaken. Should the patient still have difficulty in achieving his or her goal, the patient should be referred to a specialist. Once the LDL goal has been achieved, the patient may be monitored every 4 to 6 months. Liver function tests and CPK levels should be periodically evaluated to detect any evidence of liver abnormalities or myositis.

Interventional Management of Coronary Artery Disease

Diagnostic Catheterization. The goal of the cardiac catheterization procedure is to provide detailed structural information to assess patient prognosis and to select an appropriate management strategy. According to ACC/AHA guidelines, patients considered for cardiac catheterization over ongoing medical therapy include those patients who (1) have recurrent symptoms that are not controlled with medical therapy; (2) are stratified into a high-risk group on noninvasive testing; (3) opt for early invasive strategy; (4) had prior angioplasty, bypass surgery, or MI; and (5) have significant heart failure and/or impaired left ventricular function and angina pectoris.[13]

Percutaneous Coronary Intervention. Percutaneous transluminal coronary angioplasty (PTCA) is a cardiac catheterization technique designed to decrease coronary artery obstruction, thus improving coronary blood flow. Since the inception of PTCA, its clinical and anatomic indications have expanded from the treatment of proximal single-vessel disease to multivessel disease and ACS. Although the use of PTCA has broadened, the mortality and emergency bypass rates have remained less than 1%. The low mortality rate can be attributed to improvement in medical therapy (clopidogrel, glycoprotein IIb/IIIa receptor blockers) and new adjunctive devices such as wire mesh stents, drug-eluting stents, atherectomy, and rotablation.

The general indications for PTCA and adjunctive therapy are related to the following high-risk indicators: (1) patients with recurrent angina or ischemia at rest or with low-level activities, (2) recurrent angina or ischemia with heart failure symptoms, (3) high-risk findings on noninvasive stress testing, (4) depressed left ventricular systolic function of less than 40% on noninvasive studies, (5) hemodynamic instability, (6) sustained ventricular tachycardia, (7) PCI within the past 6 months, and (8) a prior history of coronary artery bypass graft

(CABG) surgery. PTCA is contraindicated for significant left main CAD when the left main coronary artery is not protected by previous CABG.

No differences have been noted in the complication rates of death, MI, emergency need for CABG, abrupt vessel closure, or hemorrhage when comparing the early invasive treatment group with the noninvasive treatment group.[31] Stent restenosis has been significantly reduced with the advent of drug-eluting stents and the use of long-term antiplatelet agents. After PTCA, coronary artery stenting, and rotablation procedures, patients are generally discharged the next morning, with a follow-up cardiology appointment within 1 to 2 weeks. Medication therapy consists of aspirin (75 to 162 mg/day), beta-blocker therapy, cholesterol-lowering therapy as indicated, and nitroglycerin if needed. Clopidogrel, an antiplatelet medication, is prescribed daily at 75 mg in combination with aspirin for up to 12 month in patients after ACS or PCI with stent placement (>1 month for bare metal stents, >3 months for sirolimus-eluting stents, and >6 months for paclitaxel-eluting stents).[4] With the advent of these antiplatelet agents, the incidence of early stent thrombus has decreased to less than 1%. Subacute intracoronary stent thrombosis generally occurs 5 days after stent implantation, whereas endothelium restenosis generally occurs around the tenth to twelfth week. After any PCI, patients must be educated to seek immediate attention if angina symptoms should recur, indicating a potential vessel restenosis.

Coronary Artery Bypass Surgery. CABG is one of the most commonly performed surgical procedures in the United States. The indication for CABG is to improve the overall quality of life. Approximately 90% of patients have their symptoms relieved initially, with 70% of patients remaining free of symptoms at 1 to 3 years. When cardiac symptoms redevelop, they are generally associated with bypass graft occlusion. Overall, the occlusion rate for saphenous vein grafts is greater than that for left internal mammary artery grafts.

Because surgical treatment of ischemic heart disease is palliative, reoperative CABG is now common. The treatment of choice—reoperative coronary artery bypass, cardiology intervention, or medical therapy—depends on the patient's symptoms, medical history, coronary anatomy, and left ventricular function.

LIFE SPAN CONSIDERATIONS: WOMEN AND HEART DISEASE

Recently, the gender differences between men and women with respect to coronary anatomy, clinical presentation, and treatment modalities have been under investigation. The clinical presentation of women often does not typify the midsternal chest tightness with shoulder and arm radiation that men often experience. Instead, women may be seen initially with indigestion as their only symptom. Because the mortality rate from an MI is 44% in women compared with 27% in men, it is important that gender bias be eliminated from the clinical decision making and that the nuances of CAD in women be acknowledged.[32] Current data continue to show disparity in diagnosis and management of ACS and acute MI in women.[33]

The diagnosis of CAD in women has also proven difficult because of false-positive exercise tolerance testing in women. The ECG response to such testing in women has been shown to elicit an abnormal ischemic response in up to 67% of those tested, despite normal coronary arteries. Speculation in this area suggests women's lower hematocrit levels and higher circulating estrogen levels as plausible culprits. To provide greater test sensitivity and specificity, radionuclide testing may be performed. Despite the increased accuracy of this testing, a significant number of false-positive results still occur, mainly as a result of breast attenuation artifact, which may produce septal and anterior wall defects. Stress echocardiography may prove a more accurate method of noninvasive CAD testing in women.

COMPLICATIONS

The complications of ischemic heart disease and MI are potentially life threatening. Recurrent ischemia and reinfarction can increase the area of nonfunctioning myocardial tissue, creating mechanical complications such as papillary muscle rupture, ventricular aneurysm, or ventricular septal defect. Rhythm and conduction disturbances may arise without premonitory signs. Chest pain and anxiety associated with cardiac disease can produce hypertension, increasing afterload and oxygen demand. Heart failure, hypotension, and shock impair systemic perfusion and cardiac function.

INDICATIONS FOR REFERRAL OR HOSPITALIZATION

The patient whose condition is complicated by multiple co-morbid diseases (e.g., diabetes mellitus, hypertension, heart failure, hyperlipidemia, and peripheral vascular disease) should be referred to a cardiologist. Patients with chronic stable angina who develop a change in angina pattern should also be referred to a specialist. In addition, all patients with a documented history of coronary ischemic syndrome should be co-managed with a cardiologist. The patient's symptoms and co-morbid diseases should determine the frequency of visits to the specialist.

Ischemic CAD represents a spectrum of coronary insufficiency ranging from chronic stable angina, unstable angina, or non–Q-wave MI (subendomyocardial infarction) to transmural MI. Hospitalization is based on specific criteria.

Patients who have unstable angina pectoris, defined as new-onset angina (angina occurring within 1 month), angina occurring at rest and with minimum exertion, or crescendo angina should be admitted to the hospital. All patients who are suspected of having, or are having, an acute MI should be hospitalized.

PATIENT AND FAMILY EDUCATION

Considerations for patients with CAD include careful management of co-morbid illnesses, along with a thorough understanding of their disease process and prescribed medical regimen. Women who are candidates for hormone replacement therapy should be offered information about the risks and benefits of estrogen or hormone replacement therapy after menopause.

Patients need to be educated about CAD and heart attack warning signs. Angina symptoms are often present days to weeks before the onset of an acute MI. Therefore education to assist patients in recognizing cardiac symptoms and forming an early action plan should be undertaken. The National Institutes of Health suggest the use of a *TIME* method, which emphasizes *T*alking with patients about their risk of a heart attack, how to recognize symptoms, and an action step plan; *I*nvestigating their feelings about MI; *M*aking an action plan; and *E*valuating their understanding of the discussed recommendations and delay risks.[34]

It is well established that deaths occurring from acute MI occur within the first hour of onset. Therefore the importance of symptom education of an MI and rapid transport and early admission to a hospital cannot be overemphasized.

Both patients and families should understand the importance of calling 911 or an ambulance if the symptoms of a heart attack occur or are not relieved with sublingual nitroglycerin. These symptoms include chest pressure or discomfort; pain radiating to the arm, neck, or jaw; diaphoresis; nausea or vomiting; shortness of breath; dizziness; rapid or irregular pulse; and loss of consciousness. All families who have a family member with CAD should be encouraged to learn CPR.

HEALTH PROMOTION

Despite growing evidence from clinical trials establishing that risk factor modification can decrease coronary artery morbidity and mortality, the majority of patients still are not being treated. The AHA has developed a "Get with the Guidelines Program" to ensure patients are being discharged on appropriate medications and with risk factor counseling. These guidelines focus on smoking cessation, lipid lowering, ACE inhibitor use, beta blocker therapy, hypertension management, weight and exercise management, diabetes management, atrial fibrillation management, ASA or other antithrombotic medication, and alcohol and drug abuse management.[35]

REFERENCES

1. American Heart Association: *2005 heart and stroke statistical update*, Dallas, 2005, The Association.
2. Goff DC, Sellers DE, McGovern PG, and others: Knowledge of heart attack symptoms in a population survey in the United States: the REACT trial: Rapid Early Action for Coronary Treatment, *Arch Intern Med* 158:2329-2338, 1998.
3. Pasternak RC, Grundy SM, Levy D, and others: 27th Bethesda Conference: matching the intensity of risk factor management with the hazard for coronary disease events, Task Force 3, Spectrum of risk factors for coronary heart disease, *J Am Coll Cardiol* 27(5):978-990, 1996.
4. Smith SC, Allen J, Blair SN, and others: AHA/ACC guidelines for secondary prevention for patients with coronary and other atherosclerotic vascular disease: 2006 update: endorsed by the National Heart, Lung, and Blood Institute, *Circulation* 113:2363-2372, 2006.
5. Yeung AC, Vekshtein VI, Krantz DS, and others: The effect of atherosclerosis on the vasomotor response of coronary arteries to mental stress, *N Engl J Med* 325:1551-1556, 1991.
6. Nabel EG, Ganz P, Gordon JB, and others: Dilation of normal and constriction of atherosclerotic coronary arteries caused by the cold pressor test, *Circulation* 77:43-52, 1988.
7. Vita JA, Treasure CB, Nabel EG, and others: The coronary vasomotor response to acetylcholine relates to risk factors for coronary artery disease, *Circulation* 81:491-497, 1990.
8. Miller TD, Redberg R, Wackers WJ: Screening asymptomatic diabetic patients for coronary artery disease: why not? *J Am Coll Cardiol* 48(4):761-764, 2006.
9. Bairey Merz CN, Shaw LJ, Reis SE, and others: Gender differences in presentation, diagnosis and outcome with regard to gender-based pathophysiology of atherosclerosis and macrovascular and microvascular coronary disease, *J Am Coll Cardiol* 47(Suppl S):215-295, 2006.
10. O'Donoghue M, Morrow DA, Sabatine MS, and others: Lipoprotein-associated phospholipase A_2 and its association with cardiovascular outcomes in patients with acute coronary syndrome in the PROVE IT–TIMI Trial, *Circulation* 113:1745-1752, 2006.
11. Pearson TA, Mensah GA, Alexander RW, and others: Markers of inflammation and cardiovascular disease: application to clinical practice and public health practice: a statement for healthcare professionals from the Centers for Disease Control and Prevention and the American Heart Association, *Circulation* 107(3):499-511, 2003.
12. Lerman A, Sopko GL: Women and cardiovascular heart disease: clinical implications from the Women's Ischemia Syndrome Evaluation (WISE) study: are we smarter? *J Am Coll Cardiol* 47(Suppl S):595-625, 2006.
13. Braunwald E, Antman EM, Beasley JW, and others: ACC/AHA guidelines for the management of patients with unstable angina and non–ST-segment elevation myocardial infarction: executive summary and recommendations: a report of the American College of Cardiology/American Heart Association Task Force on Practice Guidelines (Committee on the Management of Patients with Unstable Angina), *Circulation* 102:1193-1209, 2000.
14. Cannon CP, Thompson B, McCabe CH, and others: Predictors of non–Q-wave MI in patients with acute ischemic syndrome: an analysis from the Thrombolysis in Myocardial Ischemia (TIMI) III trials, *Am J Cardiol* 75:977-981, 1995.
15. Fowler-Brown A, Pignone M, Pletcher M, and others: Exercise tolerance testing to screen for coronary heart disease: a systematic review for the U.S. Preventive Services Task Force, *Ann Intern Med* 140:W9-W24, 2004, retrieved Jan 9, 2007, from http://www.ahrq.gov/clinic/3rduspstf/chd/chdsum.pdf.
16. Puleo PR, Meyer D, Wathen C, and others: Use of a rapid assay of subforms of creatine kinase-MB to diagnose or rule out acute myocardial infarction, *N Engl J Med* 331:561-566, 1994.
17. Hirsh J, Dalen JE, Fuster V, and others: Aspirin and other platelet active drugs: the relationship between dose, effectiveness, and side effects, *Chest* 102(Suppl):327S-336S, 1992.
18. Smith SC, Feldman TE, Hirshfeld JW, and others: ACC/AHA/SCAI 2005 guideline update for percutaneous coronary intervention—summary article: a report of the American College of Cardiology/American Heart Association Task Force on Practice Guidelines (ACC/AHA/SCAI Writing Committee to Update the 2001 Guidelines for Percutaneous Coronary Intervention), *Circulation* 113:156-173, 2006.
19. Steering Committee of the Physicians' Health Study Research Group: Final report on the aspirin component of the ongoing Physicians' Health Study, *N Engl J Med* 321:129-135, 1989.
20. Harpaz D, Benderly M, Goldbourt U, and others: Effect of aspirin on mortality in women with symptomatic or silent myocardial ischemia, *Am J Cardiol* 78:1215-1219, 1996.
21. ISIS-2 (Second International Study of Infarct Survival) Collaborative Group: Randomized trial of intravenous streptokinase, oral aspirin, both, or neither among 17,197 cases of suspected acute myocardial infarction: ISIS-2, *Lancet* 2:349-360, 1988.
22. Dargie HJ: Effect of carvedilol on outcome after myocardial infarction in patients with left-ventricular dysfunction: the CAPRICORN randomized trial, *Lancet* 357:1385-1390, 2001.
23. Packer M, O'Connor CM, Ghali JK, and others: Effect of amlodipine on morbidity and mortality in severe chronic heart failure: Prospective Randomized Amlodipine Survival Evaluation Study Group, *N Engl J Med* 335:1107-1114, 1996.

24. Cowie MA: The epidemiology of heart failure, *Eur Heart J* 18:208-225, 1997.
25. SOLVD Investigators: Effects of enalapril on mortality and the development of heart failure in asymptomatic patients with reduced left ventricular ejection fractions, *N Engl J Med* 327:685-691, 1992.
26. McKelvie R, Benedic C, Yusuf S: Prevention of heart failure and management of asymptomatic left ventricular dysfunction, *BMJ* 318:1400-1402, 1999.
27. CONSENSUS Trial Study Group: Effects of enalapril on mortality in severe heart failure: results of the Cooperative North Scandinavian Enalapril Survival Study (CONSENSUS), *N Engl J Med* 316:1429-1435, 1987.
28. Fragmin and Fast Revascularization During Instability in Coronary Artery Disease (FRISC II) Investigators: Long-term low molecular-mass heparin in unstable coronary artery disease: FRISC II prospective randomized multicentre study, *Lancet* 354:701-707, 1999.
29. The Clopidogrel in Unstable Angina to Prevent Recurrent Events Trial Investigators: Effects of clopidogrel in addition to aspirin in patients with acute coronary syndromes without ST-segment elevations, *N Engl J Med* 345:494-503, 2001.
30. Coumadin Aspirin Reinfarction Study (CARS) Investigators: Randomized double-blind trial of fixed low-dose warfarin with aspirin after myocardial infarction, *Lancet* 350:389-396, 1997.
31. Boden WE, O'Rourke RA, Crawford MH: Outcomes in patients with acute non–Q-wave myocardial infarction randomly assigned to an invasive as compared with a conservative management strategy. Veterans Affairs Non Q Wave Infarction Strategies in Hospital (VANQWISH Trial Investigators), *N Engl J Med* 338:1785-1792, 1998.
32. McGrath D: Coronary artery disease in women, *Am J Nurse Pract* 2(6):7-23, 1998.
33. Jani SM, Montoye C, Mehta R, and others: Sex differences in the application of evidence-based therapies for the treatment of acute myocardial infarction: the American College of Cardiology's guidelines applied to practice projects in Michigan, *Arch Intern Med* 166:1164-1170, 2006.
34. US Department of Health and Human Services, National Institute of Health, National Heart, Lung, Blood Institute: *Act in time to heart attack signs: the T.I.M.E. method to help your patients make a heart attack survival plan,* Publication No. 01-3313, September, 2001, retrieved Jan 8, 2007, from http://www.nhlbi.nih.gov/health/prof/heart/mi/provider.pdf.
35. American Heart Association: *Get with the guidelines program,* retrieved Jan 8, 2007, from http://www.americanheart.org/presenter.jhtml?identifier=1165.

CHAPTER 127

Infective Endocarditis

Denise DeJoseph Gauthier and
Eric M. Isselbacher

DEFINITION AND EPIDEMIOLOGY

The clinical characteristics and bacteriologic evidence associated with infective endocarditis were recognized before the advent of antimicrobial therapy to combat the offending organisms. Before the discovery of antibiotics, endocarditis was a progressive and eventually fatal disorder. Even with diagnostic advancements and the availability of antimicrobial agents, infective endocarditis still carries a significant morbidity rate and can be life threatening. In addition, antibiotic resistance has significantly increased among many of the microorganisms. Although the overall incidence of infective endocarditis is relatively low, certain populations are at a higher risk. Primary prevention in these high-risk groups is of critical importance.[1-6]

Infective endocarditis refers to a microbial infection within the heart. These vegetations most often involve the heart valves, but they can occur on the intraventricular septum or mural endocardium. The majority of cases of endocarditis are the result of a bacterial infection; a few cases result from fungal organisms. Rarely, endocarditis may be the result of a rickettsial, spirochete, or chlamydial infection.[1-5]

Historically, endocarditis has been classified as acute or subacute according to its clinical course. Although classifications based on acuity are helpful, a more descriptive system has been introduced and is of greater therapeutic and prognostic value. Because the incidence of acute rheumatic heart disease is on the decline in developed countries, patients with mitral valve prolapse, prosthetic valve replacements, congenital heart abnormalities, or degenerative valve disease, as well as users of IV drugs, now account for the majority of patients diagnosed with endocarditis. Therefore endocarditis is currently classified according to the underlying valve anatomy together with the infectious etiology (e.g., native valve viridans streptococcal endocarditis).[3-5]

Native Valve Endocarditis

The majority of patients with native valve endocarditis who do not use IV drugs have a predisposing cardiac lesion. In the majority of cases the underlying cardiac lesion is mitral valve prolapse.[3-5] The patients at highest risk are men with a systolic murmur of mitral regurgitation, especially those over 45 years of age.[2,4] The overall incidence of native valve endocarditis in non–IV drug users is three times higher in men than in women.[3-5]

Endocarditis associated with rheumatic heart lesions is on the decline but still accounts for 30% of cases. Patients in this group tend to be middle aged or older, and the mitral valve is most often involved. Lesions associated with congenital heart disease are the underlying cause in 10% to 20% of patients.

Advances in the management of these structural abnormalities, including septal defects and patent ductus arteriosus, have significantly reduced the number of individuals at risk.[1,3]

Calcific degeneration of the valves is a predisposing factor in older adults. Previous endocarditis itself is a predisposing factor because of the valvular damage that results from the infection.[3] However, infective endocarditis can occur on valves that are morphologically normal; in recent years an increasing number of patients have no detectable predisposing cardiac lesion.[1,4]

Streptococcal species account for 50% to 70% of native valve endocarditis in non–IV drug users.[1,3] Viridans streptococci are normal inhabitants of the oropharynx and account for more than half of all streptococcal endocardial infections. Organisms in this group include *Streptococcus sanguis, S. salivarius, S. mutans,* and *S. mitis*. Viridans streptococci usually infect abnormal valves and are typically highly sensitive to penicillin.[1,4,7]

S. bovis, a group D streptococcus, is the causative organism in a small percentage of cases, but it is more common in individuals over 60 years of age and is strongly associated with a malignant or premalignant gastrointestinal lesions. Therefore patients with *S. bovis* endocarditis should be evaluated for an undetected gastrointestinal malignancy. *S. bovis* is a virulent microorganism, associated with significant valvular damage and resultant hemodynamic compromise, as well as a high risk of embolism. Although the microorganism is highly sensitive to penicillin, valvular destruction and persistent large vegetations are indications for surgical intervention.[3,6-9]

Group A β-hemolytic and group B streptococci account for fewer than 5% of cases; these organisms are capable of attacking normal valves, leading to rapid destruction and embolization of vegetative matter. Group B streptococci are normal flora of the gastrointestinal tract, oropharynx, vagina, and urethra. Co-morbid conditions associated with endocardial infection by these organisms include diabetes mellitus, carcinoma, osteomyelitis, malignancy, and hepatic failure. Penicillin alone may not be bactericidal; an aminoglycoside antibiotic may be necessary.[2,3,7]

Enterococci are indigenous to the gastrointestinal tract and urethra and are responsible for 10% of native valve endocarditis in non–IV drug users. *Enterococci faecalis, E. faecium,* and *E. durans* can attack normal or abnormal valves. Enterococcal endocarditis is usually seen in older men and young women who have a recent history of genitourinary surgery, trauma, or malignancy. Although rare, this condition may also occur in women who have undergone an abortion, a pregnancy, or a cesarean delivery. Enterococcal organisms are resistant to penicillin alone, and therefore an aminoglycoside is necessary to achieve eradication. The treatment of enterococcal endocarditis has become further complicated by β-lactamase–producing and aminoglycoside-resistant strains.[3,4,7]

Staphylococci are responsible for 20% to 25% of cases of native valve endocarditis, with most of these cases due to *Staphylococcus aureus* (coagulase-positive staphylococci). The majority of endocardial infections involving IV drug users can be attributed to this microorganism. *S. aureus* endocarditis is characterized by the rapid destruction of the involved valve with multiple metastatic abscesses; this often results in heart failure or death within days. Coagulase-negative species, such as *Staphylococcus epidermidis,* are uncommon pathogens in native valve endocarditis but are commonly associated with prosthetic valve involvement. Staphylococcal species are highly resistant to penicillin because of their ability to produce β-lactamase.[1,3,4,7]

Other potential pathogens in native valve endocarditis include the gram-negative organisms in the *HACEK* group (*Haemophilus, Actinobacillus, Cardiobacterium, Eikenella,* and *Kingella*), which are components of the oropharyngeal flora. These organisms account for approximately 5% to 10% of cases in non–IV drug users. Although the clinical course is typically subacute, these organisms are capable of producing large vegetations with a high risk of embolization. Unfortunately, the HACEK organisms are difficult to isolate from blood, which makes their diagnosis challenging.[2-4,7]

Fungal organisms are rarely responsible for native valve endocarditis in non–IV drug users. However, *Candida* and *Aspergillus* organisms can cause endocarditis in patients with IV catheters, especially if the patients are immunocompromised or are receiving broad-spectrum antimicrobial therapy. The course is subacute, but the prognosis is poor because of the relative ineffectiveness of current antifungal medications. Fungal infections result in large, friable vegetations that often embolize; therefore early surgical intervention is indicated.[3,4,10]

Prosthetic Valve Endocarditis

The overall risk of endocarditis in patients with prosthetic valves ranges between 1% and 4%, with the highest incidence within the first 12 months after surgery. The risk is increased 5% in patients who undergo valve replacement during active infection.[1,3,5,11-13] Although native valve endocarditis in non–IV drug users most often involves the mitral valve, there is no significant difference in infection rates between prosthetic aortic and prosthetic mitral valves. There also appears to be no significant long-term difference between bioprosthetic and mechanical implants. However, mechanical valves have a higher incidence of early prosthetic valve endocarditis (PVE). Other factors associated with an increased infection risk include advanced age, antecedent native valve infection, and a longer cardiopulmonary bypass time. Gender does not appear to alter the risks associated with mitral valve replacements.[5,12,13]

PVE is categorized as *early* when symptoms occur within 60 days of surgery or *late* when they occur after 1 year. The clinical presentation, microbiology, and morbidity and mortality rates differ. Early PVE is the result of perioperative seeding; it occurs either intraoperatively through direct contamination of the surgical field or postoperatively through contamination of central lines, pacemaker wires, or other indwelling sources. Despite prophylactic antibiotic therapy, the majority of early infections are the result of staphylococcal species, most commonly *S. epidermidis,* followed by *S. aureus.* Other pathogens include gram-negative bacilli, fungi (especially *Candida* organisms), streptococci, enterococci, and diphtheroids.[5,13]

Late PVE occurs after the new valve has endothelialized. The source of the infection is not related to the surgical procedure but may result from a transient bacteremia as a consequence of a dental, gastrointestinal, or genitourinary procedure, often in the setting of inadequate prophylaxis. The microbial isolates are similar to those seen in native valve endocarditis. Viridans streptococci account for the majority of cases that occur more than 1 or 2 years after implantation. Other streptococcal species, enterococci, staphylococci, gram-negative bacilli, fungi, and diphtheroids are more often involved within the first 18 months after surgery.[3,13]

Infections associated with early PVE usually result in rapid valvular dysfunction and destruction of the integrity of the suture line, thus heralding an acute and rapidly deteriorating course with a high mortality rate. Because late PVE is often caused by less virulent organisms, it often has a subacute course. However, if the offending organism is virulent, late PVE may also manifest as an acute, fulminant infection.[13]

Endocarditis in Intravenous Drug Users

Those who develop endocarditis associated with IV drug use tend to be younger (with a mean age in the thirties) and are most often male. The actual risk of infection among IV drug users is variable depending on the drugs injected, their method of preparation, and frequency of use. In this population, infection involving the tricuspid valve is most common. Right-sided endocarditis is otherwise rare; therefore IV drug use should be suspected when this type of endocarditis is discovered. Involvement of the aortic or mitral valve alone is seen in a small number of patients, whereas even fewer have a combination of left- and right-sided endocarditis. The majority of IV drug users who develop infective endocarditis have structurally normal valves before the infection; a significant minority, approximately 20%, have an underlying cardiac lesion from congenital disease or previous endocardial infection.[3,5]

Skin flora is the most common source of pathogenic microorganisms in users of IV drugs; contaminated drugs and drug paraphernalia are also bacterial sources. *S. aureus* is the most common offending organism; it is isolated in 60% of total cases and in 80% of cases involving the tricuspid valve. Various streptococcal and enterococcal species account for approximately 20% of total cases; gram-negative bacilli, particularly *Pseudomonas* and *Serratia* organisms, are responsible for an additional 10% of infections. Fungi, most often *Candida* organisms, are isolated only 5% of the time. More than one organism is isolated in approximately 5% of individuals.[1]

The majority of patients with right-sided endocarditis are noted to have pneumonia or septic pulmonary emboli as a result of direct embolization. These patients appear ill, with high fevers and shaking chills. Patients with a clinical syndrome consistent with tricuspid valve endocarditis should also be evaluated for a potential extracardiac source of the endovascular infection, such as septic thrombophlebitis. The overall mortality rate for right-sided endocarditis is approximately 10%.[1,5]

Endocarditis in Pregnancy

Endocarditis is a potentially serious complication of pregnancy; fortunately, it is uncommon. The overall incidence of endocarditis associated with pregnancy is declining as a result of a decreasing incidence of rheumatic heart disease, improvements in the management of complications during pregnancy and the postpartum period, and the legalization and standardization of abortion. Underlying cardiac lesions (which are present in the majority of women affected) and the use of illicit IV drugs are predisposing factors to endocarditis.[14,15]

Although dental procedures have been the most common means of bacterial entry, puerperal bacteremia can occur after a vaginal or cesarean delivery. Premature labor, prolonged rupture of the membranes, prolonged labor, or manual removal of the placenta may be predisposing factors. If these occur in the setting of an underlying cardiac lesion, the risk is substantial, and prophylactic antibiotics should be administered.[14,15]

PATHOPHYSIOLOGY

The development of endocarditis depends on the invasion of the bloodstream by a pathogen capable of attaching to an endothelial surface. The normal endothelium is not conducive to bacterial deposition. A high-velocity jet stream, a narrow valvular orifice, and a flow from a high- to a low-pressure chamber are hemodynamic features that predispose the patient to endocarditis. This forceful flow denudes the endothelium and allows for platelet and fibrin deposition. This layering of platelets and fibrin creates nonbacterial sterile vegetation, which in turn provides an ideal medium for bacterial adherence and growth. Virulent microorganisms, especially the staphylococcal species, are capable of attaching to even normal endothelium.[1,3,4]

Microorganisms typically attach just distal to the narrowed orifice of a turbulent jet, such as on the atrial surface of the mitral leaflets in mitral regurgitation or on the ventricular surface of the aortic cusps in the setting of aortic insufficiency. After colonization of the endothelial surface, bacteria begin the replication process. Further platelet and fibrin deposition over the bacteria provides insulation from phagocytic cellular defenses, which allows the microorganisms to thrive and form vegetations. Proliferation of the microorganism leads to local valvular destruction, tissue invasion, and possible embolization of the vegetative material.[1-4]

Morphologic characteristics of the vegetations depend on the offending organism and the duration of the infection. Lesions range from small, flat, or granular deposits to large, pedunculated, and friable formations. During the course of effective antimicrobial therapy, leukocytes and fibroblasts penetrate vegetations. This healing process results in fibrosis, occasionally with calcification, and eventual reendothelialization of the valvular surface.[12,16]

The signs and symptoms of infective endocarditis vary according to the causative organism and the degree of systemic involvement. Valvular infection can result in the disruption of valvular integrity, including perforation of a valve leaflet, rupture of chordae tendineae or papillary muscles, or leaflet prolapse. Penetration of bacteria into the adjacent myocardium can result in myocardial or perivalvular abscesses, which may result in conduction system disturbances and heart block. Further penetration of infection may produce fistulas between cardiac chambers. Large vegetations associated with fungal or *Haemophilus* infections can cause obstruction of the valvular orifice. Even after a bacterial cure has been achieved, fibrosis of the valve leaflets can result in hemodynamically significant valvular stenosis or regurgitation.[1,5,17]

Embolization of vegetative matter is not uncommon and most often involves the renal, splenic, coronary, or cerebral circulation. Myocardial infarction can be the result of embolization of the vegetative material down the coronary arteries. Pulmonary embolism is a complication associated with right-sided endocarditis in IV drug users or patients with fungal infections. Embolization of septic material can lead to abscess formation. Mycotic aneurysms occur as a direct result of septic invasion into the arterial wall or septic embolization, which weakens the vessel wall and predisposes it to rupture.[4,18,19]

Persistent bacteremia triggers an immune complex response of both the humoral and cell-mediated immune systems. As seen in many chronic infections, a generalized hypergammaglobulinemia develops. Immune complexes containing immunoglobulins G, M, and A (IgG, IgM, and IgA), along with complement, are deposited along the glomerular basement membrane of the kidney, precipitating glomerulonephritis. Peripheral manifestations of arthritic discomforts and cutaneous vasculitis may also be attributed to deposition of immune complexes in the joints and mucocutaneous vessels.[1,4,5]

CLINICAL PRESENTATION AND PHYSICAL EXAMINATION

The onset of symptoms usually occurs within days to weeks of the introduction of the microorganisms, but the symptoms may initially be nonspecific. Early symptoms of infection involving less virulent organisms such as viridans streptococci include generalized fatigue, malaise, night sweats, chills, and moderate weight loss. A highly pathogenic organism such as *S. aureus* may manifest with an abrupt onset that prompts the patient to seek early medical attention. The virility of the invading microorganism dictates the pace and severity of the disease course.[2,20]

Fever is present in the majority of patients but may be absent in older adults, immunocompromised hosts, or patients previously treated with antibiotics. The degree of fever depends on the causative microorganism; high-grade fevers are primarily associated with virulent infections.[1,2,4,5] The majority of patients become afebrile within 72 hours of initiating the appropriate antibiotic therapy. Persistent fever suggests an ineffective antimicrobial regimen or a myocardial or distant (metastatic) abscess formation.[17]

Heart murmurs are detectable in the majority of patients but may be absent early in the course or in patients with right-sided endocarditis. A new murmur of regurgitation or a true change in an existing murmur suggests an acute process and often heralds the development of congestive heart failure. The diagnosis of infective endocarditis must be entertained in any patient with a heart murmur and fever of unknown origin.[1,2,4]

Splenomegaly was commonly associated with endocarditis before the advent of antibiotic therapy, but it is now a rare finding.[1] Petechiae may be noted on the conjunctivae, palate, buccal mucosa, and extremities and are associated with a long-term infection. Splinter hemorrhages are linear, subungual hemorrhages that may appear in infective endocarditis. Both petechiae and splinter hemorrhages may represent embolic phenomena or vasculitis. Although sometimes seen in patients with infective endocarditis, they may also appear with other disease processes.[1,2,4,5]

Janeway's lesions and Osler's nodes are cutaneous lesions associated with endocarditis. Janeway's lesions are nontender, hemorrhagic macules (1 to 4 mm) on the palms and soles and are the result of septic embolization. Osler's nodes are painful nodules on the finger and toe pads that last hours to days. They have also been noted on the forearms, ears, and dorsa of the feet. Their pathogenesis is uncertain, but they are thought to be related to microembolization and subsequent inflammation or immune complex mediation. Osler's nodes are an uncommon finding and may also be associated with other disease processes.[1,2,4,5]

Roth's spots are retinal hemorrhages with a pale center located near the optic disc. They are an uncommon finding and can be associated with infective endocarditis or hematologic and connective tissue disorders.[1] Other ocular manifestations that have been documented include amaurosis fugax and painful blurring of vision.[2]

Evidence of neurologic involvement may be seen in approximately 20% to 40% of patients with infective endocarditis. Major embolization of the middle cerebral artery, the most commonly involved territory, manifests as hemiplegia. Mycotic aneurysms are potentially life-threatening complications that occur in 1% of patients, but they are most often associated with infections involving less virulent pathogens. They typically occur early in the course of the disease but can occur months or even years after a bacteriologic cure has been achieved. A severe unrelenting headache, transient neurologic changes, or signs of cranial nerve involvement suggest the possibility of an intracranial mycotic aneurysm. Brain abscesses, purulent meningitis, arteritis, transient ischemic attacks, embolic strokes, cranial nerve palsy, intracerebral bleeding, subarachnoid hemorrhage, and encephalomalacia have also been reported.[2,4,21]

Congestive heart failure is a serious complication and is the primary cause of death in patients with infective endocarditis. It may be secondary to valvular destruction, coronary embolization resulting in myocardial infarction, myocarditis, or myocardial abscess formation. Early recognition of cardiac decompensation and intensive intervention are critical. Failure of antimicrobial therapy or the development of refractory congestive heart failure is an indication for surgical intervention. Intracardiac complications requiring surgical intervention include valvular dehiscence, ruptured chordae tendineae, perforation of valve leaflets, and formation of an aneurysm or abscess. In these situations, surgical intervention may be lifesaving; therefore the presence of an active infection is not considered a surgical contraindication. Surgical intervention is also indicated in patients infected with brucellae or fungi and those with recurrent emboli, early PVE, or late PVE secondary to *S. aureus*.[10]

Renal involvement is another serious complication of infective endocarditis. Renal insufficiency is often the result of glomerulonephritis secondary to immune complex deposition on the glomerular basement membrane. It may also occur secondary to septic embolization, leading to renal infarction or abscess formation.[1]

Metastatic infections such as pyogenic meningitis, pyelonephritis, splenic abscesses, and osteomyelitis are most often noted in patients with *S. aureus* endocarditis. Metastatic infections are rarely seen in endocarditis involving less virulent microorganisms. Metastatic infections increase the risk of a relapse of infective endocarditis.[4]

Complaints of arthralgias and myalgias are common. Arthralgias tend to involve the proximal joints and lower extremities and may be monoarticular. Myalgias, often localized to the thigh or calf, are commonly unilateral and have no radicular pattern. These discomforts are often described at the time of presentation and may in part be a manifestation of elevated circulating immune complexes.[2,4]

Pulmonary embolism is most often associated with tricuspid valve endocarditis among IV drug users. It may also occur in patients with indwelling central venous catheters or in patients with left-sided endocarditis who have left-to-right shunting from a septal defect.[1,2]

DIAGNOSTICS

To establish the diagnosis of infective endocarditis, an effort should be made to isolate the pathogenic microorganisms from the blood. Three sets of blood cultures should be obtained from different venipuncture sites with samples drawn at least 30 to 60 minutes apart before initiating antimicrobial therapy. Cultures can be obtained at any time; a febrile state at the time of culture is not critical. There also is no particular advantage to drawing the culture from arterial blood rather than from venous blood.[2,5,22,23]

The first consideration when interpreting positive blood culture data is whether the bacteremia is sustained or transient. Intravascular infections such as endocarditis produce a sustained bacteremia, which is defined as the presence of the same microorganism in the blood for at least 1 hour. In contrast, transient bacteremia clears within 30 minutes or less. Consequently, only one blood culture in the series is likely to be positive in transient bacteremia, whereas all cultures are likely to be positive with sustained bacteremia. A single positive blood culture is most consistent with transient bacteremia (or contamination) but is not diagnostic for endocarditis, except for cultures positive for *Coxiella burnetii*.[23,24]

The next consideration is whether the identified pathogen is one typically associated with an intravascular infection or is more likely a result of another source of infection. Salmonellae, brucellae, and enteric gram-negative bacteria can produce sustained bacteremia yet are rarely pathogens in endocarditis. Organisms such as viridans streptococci and coagulase-negative staphylococci are common pathogenic organisms in endocarditis.

Other common abnormal laboratory findings in infective endocarditis include a normochromic, normocytic anemia, especially in infections of longer duration. The WBC count is usually within normal limits in less virulent infections, perhaps with a slight shift to the left. A marked leukocytosis with a shift to the left is a common finding in endocarditis caused by a virulent microorganism. The erythrocyte sedimentation rate is elevated, except in patients with cardiac or renal failure. A positive rheumatoid factor can be detected in half of the patients who have an infection lasting longer than 3 to 6 weeks. Circulating immune complexes are present in most patients; these levels decline as the infection is effectively treated. The serum complement level is usually decreased, especially in patients with glomerulonephritis.[1,2,5] The urinalysis result is most often abnormal, with proteinuria, microscopic hematuria, or pyuria. Serum creatinine may be elevated and reflects the degree of renal involvement secondary to glomerulonephritis or renovascular embolization.[1]

Echocardiography plays an important role in the evaluation of suspected or documented endocarditis. Vegetations appear as abnormal sessile or pedunculated echogenic masses attached to valve leaflets. Unfortunately, vegetations of less than 5 mm can be difficult to identify with transthoracic echocardiography; the sensitivity of this technique for native valve endocarditis is therefore only about 60%. With its greater resolution, transesophageal echocardiography can identify lesions as small as 2 to 3 mm and therefore has sensitivity as high as 90% to 100%.[19,25]

Identifying vegetations in the presence of a prosthetic valve is more difficult because the prosthesis causes acoustic shadowing of parts of the ultrasound image; in this setting the sensitivity of transthoracic echocardiography falls to approximately 20%.[26] Transesophageal echocardiography is capable of imaging prosthetic valves reliably, especially those in the mitral position; its sensitivity for vegetations in this setting falls only slightly to 86% to 94%.[27] Consequently, transesophageal echocardiography is preferred for evaluating suspected endocarditis in patients with valve prostheses.[19]

In addition to documenting the presence of vegetations in patients with endocarditis, echocardiography provides additional data of prognostic importance. First, the size, location, and mobility of vegetations as determined by echocardiography may be useful predictors of subsequent embolism. Second, echocardiography reliably identifies leaflet damage or associated valvular regurgitation that arises as a consequence of endocarditis. Finally, echocardiography can detect evidence of local invasion by an aggressive infection—such as an abscess or a fistula formation—that may be an indication for surgical repair.[12,16]

DIAGNOSTICS

Infective Endocarditis

LABORATORY
CBC and differential
ESR
Rheumatoid factor
Serum complement
Creatinine
Urinalysis
Blood cultures × 3 (30 minutes apart)

IMAGING
Transthoracic or transesophageal echocardiogram.

Clinical information, including the presenting signs and symptoms, findings on physical examination, laboratory and blood culture data, and echocardiographic findings, must be considered collectively by the provider when a diagnosis of infective endocarditis is considered. To help guide the diagnosis systematically, the new Duke criteria (Box 127-1) have become widely accepted.[26,28]

BOX 127-1

DUKE CRITERIA FOR DIAGNOSIS OF INFECTIVE ENDOCARDITIS

MAJOR CRITERIA

1. Positive blood cultures: one of the following:
   a. Typical organisms consistent with infective endocarditis from two separate cultures (viridans streptococci, *Streptococcus bovis,* HACEK group, *Staphylococcus aureus,* or community-acquired enterococci in the absence of a primary focus)
   b. Microorganisms consistent with infective endocarditis from persistently positive blood cultures (2 positive cultures >12 hours apart; or all of three or a majority of four or more separate cultures with the first and last sample at least 1 hour apart)
   c. Single positive blood culture for *Coxiella burnetii* or anti–phase 1 immunoglobulin G antibody titer >1:800
2. Evidence of endocardial involvement: echocardiogram demonstrating vegetation, abscess, new prosthetic valve dehiscence, or new valvular regurgitation (worsening or changing of preexisting murmur not sufficient). (Transesophageal echocardiography is recommended for prosthetic valves rated at least "possible infective endocarditis" by clinical criteria or complicated infective endocarditis, such as paravalvular abscess. Transthoracic echocardiography is the first approach in other patients.)

MINOR CRITERIA

1. Predisposition: Preexisting heart conditions
2. Fever: 38° C (100.4° F) or higher
3. Vascular phenomena: Arterial emboli, septic pulmonary emboli, mycotic aneurysms, intracranial hemorrhage, conjunctival hemorrhage, Janeway's lesions
4. Immune phenomena: Nephritis, Osler's nodes, Roth's spots, positive rheumatoid factor
5. Microbiologic: Positive blood cultures that do not meet major criteria, *or* serologic evidence of active infection with a microorganism consistent with endocarditis

DEFINITE INFECTIVE ENDOCARDITIS

1. Pathologic criteria
   a. Microorganisms: Documented by culture or histologic examination of vegetation, embolic material, or intracardiac abscess, or
   b. Pathologic: Presence of vegetation or intracardiac abscess, histologic confirmation of active endocarditis
   c. Clinical criteria: 2 major criteria, *or* 1 major and 3 minor criteria, *or* 5 minor criteria

POSSIBLE INFECTIVE ENDOCARDITIS

Presentation and findings that are consistent with diagnosis but fall short of *definite* criteria (but not *rejected*—1 major and 1 minor criterion or 3 minor criteria)

INFECTIVE ENDOCARDITIS REJECTED

1. Firm alternate diagnosis established *or*
2. Resolution of symptoms after 4 days or fewer of antibiotic therapy
3. No pathologic evidence at surgery or autopsy after 4 days or fewer of antibiotic therapy

Modified from Baddour LM, Wilson WR, Bayer AS, and others: Infective endocarditis: diagnosis, antimicrobial therapy, and management of complications: a statement for healthcare professionals, *Circulation* 111:e394-e434, 2005 [erratum in *Circulation* 112(15):2373, 2005]; and Li JS, Sexton DJ, Mick N, and others: Proposed modifications to the Duke criteria for the diagnosis of infective endocarditis, *Clin Infect Dis* 30:633-638, 2000.

DIFFERENTIAL DIAGNOSIS

The diagnosis of infective endocarditis must be considered in any patient with a cardiac murmur and a fever of unknown cause. The diagnosis should also be entertained in any febrile IV drug user, any patient with a prosthetic valve who is febrile or has evidence of valvular dysfunction, or any young person with a cerebrovascular accident.[1] The definitive diagnosis of endocarditis requires (1) the isolation of a pathogenic organism from the blood or embolic material, or (2) the demonstration of endocardial vegetations on echocardiography or at the time of surgery or autopsy.[26]

Other conditions can mimic the signs and symptoms of infective endocarditis, which makes a definitive diagnosis difficult at the time of initial presentation. A comprehensive diagnostic evaluation will usually yield an accurate diagnosis in a timely manner. Disease processes such as acute rheumatic fever, atrial myxoma, lymphoma, systemic lupus erythematosus, tuberculosis, thrombotic thrombocytopenic purpura, connective tissue disorders, sickle cell disease, and nonbacterial thrombotic endocarditis can produce a similar constellation of symptoms.[2,17]

DIFFERENTIAL DIAGNOSIS

Infective Endocarditis

- Acute rheumatic fever
- Atrial myxoma
- Systemic lupus erythematosus
- Thrombotic thrombocytopenic purpura
- Connective tissue disorders
- Sickle cell disease
- Nonbacterial thrombotic endocarditis

It is important to note that blood cultures obtained before the initiation of antimicrobial therapy will be positive in more than 95% of patients with infective endocarditis.[5] Therefore negative culture data should prompt further investigation into other possible causes of the fever and symptoms. If there is clinical suspicion of infective endocarditis in a patient with negative blood cultures, intensive efforts should be undertaken to identify fastidious microorganisms; these include prolonged incubation periods, culturing on special mediums, and serologic assessment. Microorganisms, including *C. burnetii* (Q fever), chlamydiae, *Tropheryma whippelii,* and *Bartonella* organisms, are difficult to isolate. Pathogens may potentially be isolated from embolized material or excised valve tissue.[5,23]

MANAGEMENT

The identification of the infecting organism and the institution of high-dose bactericidal therapy are the cornerstones of treatment. Parenteral administration of antibiotics is preferred to ensure predictably high serum levels. Throughout the prolonged course of treatment, ongoing assessment of the patient's response to therapy, as well as vigilance for the development of potential complications, is crucial. Clinical improvement with reduction of fever is usually seen within 1 week of appropriate antimicrobial therapy. Blood cultures should be rechecked and should become negative after several days of effective pharmacologic treatment. Persistent fevers should raise the suspicion of an intracardiac abscess, metastatic foci of infection, or inadequate antimicrobial therapy.[2,5,17]

The selection of antimicrobial agents and the duration of therapy vary depending on the microorganism isolated and the duration of infection. Infective endocarditis caused by highly penicillin-sensitive viridans streptococci can often be cured within 2 weeks with a dual regimen of penicillin G or ceftriaxone and an aminoglycoside. Intracardiac prostheses or infections of longer duration (which produce large vegetations) require a prolonged antibiotic course to achieve a successful cure. Table 127-1 summarizes the current treatment recommendations formulated by a consensus group of the American Heart Association.[19] Although these recommendaions do not include all subgroups or potential pathogens, they do provide treatment regimens for the most commonly encountered cases of infective endocarditis and incorporate recommendations for antibiotic resistance.[7,19]

Co-Management with Specialists

Infective endocarditis is a potentially life-threatening infection and should be managed collaboratively with a cardiologist. Any patient seen with fever and symptoms consistent with endocarditis should be hospitalized for immediate evaluation. Hemodynamic deterioration can be sudden, and IV antibiotic therapy should be initiated immediately after blood culture results have been obtained.

Cardiac surgery with replacement of the infected valve often becomes necessary in the treatment of patients who develop complications of infective endocarditis, most commonly as the result of a virulent pathogen. Surgery is indicated in the setting of refractory congestive heart failure secondary to valvular dysfunction or in the setting of multiple systemic emboli. Cardiac surgery is required for patients with PVE who show evidence of prosthetic instability or dehiscence. If the patient does not respond to appropriate and adequate antibiotic therapy, with the persistence of positive blood cultures, surgery may be necessary to eradicate the infection. Finally, an invasive infection that results in a perivalvular abscess or fistula often requires surgery to debride the necrotic tissue, repair the anatomic damage, and replace the infected valve. Infective endocarditis as a result of brucella or fungal infections can rarely be treated with antimicrobial therapy; therefore surgery is indicated in such cases.[5,10]

Primary Prevention

Because infective endocarditis is associated with significant morbidity and mortality, primary prevention for patients at risk is critical. The cardiac conditions believed to predispose patients to infective endocarditis are listed in Box 127-2. Identification and education of patients at risk are essential and are the responsibility of all providers. The American Heart Association's current recommendations for endocarditis prophylaxis are summarized in Box 127-3 and Tables 127-2 and 127-3. Prophylaxis is most effective when administered before the procedure. Recent data have demonstrated that adequate antibiotic blood levels are maintained for several hours after the initial dose; therefore single-dose therapy is now recommended.[27]

These guidelines are general. Practitioners must use their own clinical judgment in specific cases. For example, antibiotic prophylaxis is not generally recommended for patients undergoing colonoscopy. However, the gastroenterologist may choose to prescribe prophylaxis for high-risk patients.[29] Additionally, special consideration is required for patients with rheumatic heart disease who are receiving long-term penicillin therapy for the prevention of recurrent episodes of rheumatic fever. In this setting, oropharyngeal organisms may have become resistant to penicillin. Consequently, before the procedure these patients should receive prophylaxis with another appropriate antibiotic, such as clindamycin. One exception is rheumatic prophylaxis with monthly injections of benzathine penicillin. This regimen does not usually result in penicillin resistance, and therefore penicillin prophylaxis may be used safely.[27]

COMPLICATIONS

The acute complications associated with infective endocarditis are numerous, may involve all major organ systems, and are potentially life threatening. Cardiac complications are often the result of direct pathogen invasion, whereas metastatic complications result from septic embolization or immune complex deposition.

Another concern is the possibility of a relapse. After completion of the antibiotic course, blood cultures should be checked once or twice during the first 2 months. Relapses usually occur within the first few months, and blood cultures may become positive before clinical manifestation. Patients with a relapse in native valve endocarditis often respond to further antimicrobial treatment, but surgical intervention should be considered for patients with prosthetic valves or persistent enterococcal endocarditis.[5]

Occasionally it is impossible to completely eradicate the microorganism with antimicrobial therapy, and surgery may not be an option because of the high operative risk associated with co-morbid conditions. In this case, chronic suppressive therapy may help prevent the manifestations and complications of endocarditis.

INDICATIONS FOR REFERRAL OR HOSPITALIZATION

A diagnosis of infective endocarditis must be considered in any patient with a murmur and fever of unknown cause. This diagnosis must be considered in IV drug users or in patients with prosthetic valves who have a fever of unknown origin. Immediate consultation and hospitalization are warranted if the history, symptoms, and clinical findings raise a suspicion of infective endocarditis.

A diagnostic evaluation, including blood cultures and echocardiography, must be performed. After obtaining blood cultures, the early initiation of an IV antibiotic regimen is vital in minimizing the risks of valvular destruction and the metastatic complications associated with pathogenic invasion.

The availability of a wide assortment of infusion pumps and percutaneous central catheters has made home therapy an acceptable, cost-effective option for certain patients. Outpatient

Text continued on p. 550.

TABLE 127-1 Suggested Antibiotic Regimens

Antibiotic*	Dosage† and Route	Duration of Treatment	Comments
NATIVE VALVE ENDOCARDITIS CAUSED BY PENICILLIN-SENSITIVE VIRIDANS STREPTOCOCCI AND *STREPTOCOCCUS BOVIS*			
Penicillin G (Evidence exists for benefit)	12-18 million units/24 hr IV, either continuously or in 6 equal doses	4 weeks	Preferred in most patients over 65 years of age and in patients with impaired renal or cranial nerve VIII function.
or			
Ceftriaxone (Evidence exists for benefit)	2 g/24 hr IV or IM in 1 dose	4 weeks	
Penicillin G	12-18 million units/24 hr IV, either continuously or in 6 equal doses	2 weeks	
or			
Ceftriaxone	2 g/24 hr IV/IM in one dose	2 weeks	
plus			
Gentamicin (Evidence exists for benefit)	3 mg/kg/24 hr IV or IM in a single dose	2 weeks	Gentamicin dosing based on ideal body weight, not actual body weight.
Vancomycin (Evidence exists for benefit)	30 mg/kg/24 hr IV in 2 divided doses, not to exceed 2 g/24 hr unless serum levels monitored	4 weeks	Recommended for patients allergic to penicillin or ceftriaxone.
PROSTHETIC VALVE OR OTHER PROSTHETIC MATERIAL ENDOCARDITIS CAUSED BY VIRIDANS GROUP STREPTOCOCCI AND *STREPTOCOCCUS BOVIS*			
Penicillin-Susceptible Strains			
Penicillin G (Evidence exists for benefit)	24 million units/24 hr IV, either continuously or in 4-6 doses	6 weeks	
or			
Ceftriaxone (Evidence exists for benefit) with or without:	2 g/24 hr IV or IM in 1 dose	6 weeks	
Gentamicin†	3 mg/kg/24 hr IV or IM in 1 dose	2 weeks	The addition of gentamicin has not demonstrated higher cure rates compared with monotherapy.
Vancomycin‡ (Evidence exists for benefit)	30 mg/kg/24 hr IV in 2 divided doses, not to exceed 2 g/24 hr	6 weeks	Recommended only for patients allergic to penicillin or ceftriaxone.
Penicillin-Resistant Strains			
Penicillin G (Evidence exists for benefit)	24 million units/24 hr IV either continuously or in 4-6 doses	6 weeks	For relatively or fully resistant strains with MIC >0.12 mcg/ml.
or			
Ceftriaxone (Evidence exists for benefit)	2 g/24 hr IV or IM in 1 dose	6 weeks	
plus			
Gentamicin (Evidence exists for benefit)	3 mg/kg/24 hr IV or IM in 1 dose	6 weeks	
Vancomycin (Evidence exists for benefit)	30 mg/kg/24 hr IV in 2 divided doses, not to exceed 2 g/24 hr	6 weeks	Recommended only for patients allergic to penicillin or ceftriaxone.

Modified from Baddour LM, Wilson WR, Bayer AS, and others: Infective endocarditis: diagnosis, antimicrobial therapy, and management of complications: a statement for healthcare professionals, *Circulation* 111:e394-e434, 2005 [erratum in *Circulation* 112(15):2373, 2005].

MIC, Minimal inhibitory concentration.

*Desirable peak serum gentamicin level (1 hour after infusion) is approximately 3-4 mcg/ml. Desirable peak serum vancomycin level (1 hour after infusion) is 30-45 mcg/ml, for twice-daily dosing.

†Dosages recommended are for adults with normal renal function.

‡Cephalosporins should not be used in patients with immediate-type sensitivity reactions to penicillins (urticaria, angioedema, anaphylaxis).

TABLE 127-1 Suggested Antibiotic Regimens—cont'd

Antibiotic	Dosage and Route	Duration of Treatment	Comments
NATIVE VALVE ENDOCARDITIS CAUSED BY STRAINS OF VIRIDANS STREPTOCOCCI AND *STREPTOCOCCUS BOVIS* RELATIVELY RESISTANT TO PENICILLIN G			
Penicillin G *or*	24 million units/24 hr IV, either continuously or in 4-6 equal doses	4 weeks	Patients with penicillin-resistant strains (MIC >0.5 mcg/ml) should be treated with regimen recommended for enterococcal endocarditis (see below).
Ceftriaxone *plus*	2 g/24 hr IV or IM in a single dose		
Gentamicin (Evidence exists for benefit)	3 mg/kg/24 hr IM or IV in a single dose	2 weeks	Dose should be adjusted to achieve a peak concentration of 3-4 mcg/ml.
Vancomycin (Evidence exists for benefit)	30 mg/kg/24 hr IV in 2 equal doses, not to exceed 2 g/24 hr unless serum levels monitored	4 weeks	Vancomycin is recommended for patients allergic to penicillin or ceftriaxone.
ENTEROCOCCAL ENDOCARDITIS§			
Ampicillin (Evidence exists for benefit) *or*	12 g/24 hr IV in 6 doses	4-6 weeks	4 weeks if native valve and symptoms ≤3 months' duration; 6 weeks if symptoms >3 months; and a minimum of 6 weeks for prosthetic valve or prosthetic cardiac material.
Penicillin G *plus*	18-30 million units/24 hr IV, either c ontinuously or in 6 equal doses	4-6 weeks	4 weeks if native valve and symptoms ≤3 months' duration; 6 weeks if symptoms >3 months; and a minimum of 6 weeks for prosthetic valve or prosthetic cardiac material.
Gentamicin (Evidence exists for benefit)	1 mg/kg IV or IM q 8 hr	4-6 weeks	
Vancomycin *plus*	30 mg/kg/24 hr IV in 2 equal doses, not to exceed 2 g/24 hr unless serum levels monitored	6 weeks	Vancomycin is recommended for patients allergic to penicillin.
Gentamicin (Evidence exists for benefit)	1 mg/kg IM or IV q 8 hr	6 weeks	
ENTEROCOCCAL ENDOCARDITIS‡ (FOR STRAINS SUSCEPTIBLE TO PENICILLIN, STREPTOMYCIN, AND VANCOMYCIN, BUT RESISTANT TO GENTAMICIN)			
Ampicillin (Evidence exists for benefit) *or*	12 g/24 hr IV in 6 doses	4-6 weeks	4 weeks if native valve and symptoms ≤3 months' duration; 6 weeks if symptoms >3 months; and a minimum of 6 weeks for prosthetic valve or prosthetic cardiac material.
Penicillin G *plus*	24 million units/24 hr IV, either continuously or in 6 equal doses.	4-6 weeks	4 weeks if native valve and symptoms ≤3 months' duration; 6 weeks if symptoms >3 months; and a minimum of 6 weeks for prosthetic valve or prosthetic cardiac material.
Streptomycin (Evidence exists for benefit)	15 mg/kg/24 hr IV or IM in 2 doses	4-6 weeks (a minimum of 6 weeks for prosthetic valve or prosthetic cardiac material)	
Vancomycin *plus*	30 mg/kg/24 hr IV in 2 equal doses, not to exceed 2 g/24 hr unless serum levels monitored	6 weeks	Vancomycin is recommended for patients allergic to penicillin.
Streptomycin (Evidence exists for benefit)	15 mg/kg/24 hr IV or IM in 2 doses		

‡Cephalosporins should not be used in patients with immediate-type sensitivity reactions to penicillins (urticaria, angioedema, anaphylaxis).
§All enterococcal endocarditis must be tested for antimicrobial susceptibility.

Continued

TABLE 127-1 Suggested Antibiotic Regimens—cont'd

Antibiotic	Dosage and Route	Duration of Treatment	Comments
ENTEROCOCCAL ENDOCARDITIS‖ (FOR STRAINS RESISTANT TO PENICILLIN, BUT SUSCEPTIBLE TO AMINOGLYCOSIDE AND VANCOMYCIN)			
β-Lactamase–Producing Strain			
Ampicillin-sulbactam *plus*	12 g/24 hr IV in 4 doses	6 weeks	Unlikely that organism susceptible to gentamicin; if strain is gentamicin resistant, requires >6 weeks of ampicillin-sulbactam.
Gentamicin (Limited evidence exists for benefit)	1 mg/kg IM or IV q 8 hr	6 weeks	
Vancomycin *plus*	30 mg/kg/24 hr IV in 2 equal doses, not to exceed 2 g/24 hr unless serum levels monitored	6 weeks	Vancomycin is recommended for patients allergic to penicillin.
Gentamicin (Limited evidence exists for benefit)	1 mg/kg IM or IV q 8 hr		
Intrinsic Penicillin Resistance			
Vancomycin *plus*	30 mg/kg/24 hr IV in 2 equal doses, not to exceed 2 g/24 hr unless serum levels monitored	6 weeks	Infectious disease consultation recommended.
Gentamicin (Limited evidence exists for benefit)	1 mg/kg IM or IV q 8 hr		
ENTEROCOCCAL ENDOCARDITIS‖ (FOR STRAINS RESISTANT TO PENICILLIN, AMINOGLYCOSIDE, AND VANCOMYCIN)			
Enterococcus faecium			
Linezolid *or*	1200 mg/24 hr IV or PO in 2 doses	≥8 weeks	Use with infectious disease consultation. Bacteriologic cure with antimicrobial therapy is <50%. Reversible thrombocytopenia a risk with linezolid after 2 weeks of therapy
Quinupristin-dalfopristin (Limited evidence exists for benefit)	22.5 mg/kg/24 hr IV in 3 doses	≥8 weeks	Use with infectious disease consultation
Enterococcus faecalis			
Imipenem-cilastatin *plus*	2 g/24 hr IV in 4 doses	≥8 weeks	
Ampicillin (Limited evidence exists for benefit) *or*	12 g/24 hr IV in 6 doses		
Ceftriaxone *plus*	2 g/24 hr IV or IM in a single dose	≥8 weeks	
Ampicillin (Limited evidence exists for benefit)	12 g/24 hr IV in 6 doses		
STAPHYLOCOCCAL ENDOCARDITIS IN THE ABSENCE OF PROSTHETIC MATERIAL			
Oxacillin-Susceptible Strains			
Nafcillin or oxacillin (Evidence exists for benefit) *with optional*	12 g/24 hr IV in 4-6 doses	6 weeks	For uncomplicated right-sided infective endocarditis, 2 weeks.
Gentamicin¶	3 mg/kg/24 hr IV or IM in 2-3 doses	3-5 days	Benefit of additional aminoglycoside is unclear.

‖All enterococcal endocarditis must be tested for antimicrobial susceptibility.
¶Gentamicin should be given in close proximity to nafcillin, oxacillin, or vancomycin doses.

TABLE 127-1 Suggested Antibiotic Regimens—cont'd

Antibiotic	Dosage and Route	Duration of Treatment	Comments
STAPHYLOCOCCAL ENDOCARDITIS IN THE ABSENCE OF PROSTHETIC MATERIAL—CONT'D			
In Patients Who Are Penicillin Allergic (Nonanaphylactoid Type)			
Cefazolin (Evidence exists for benefit)	6 g/24 hr IV in 3 doses	6 weeks	Avoid cephalosporins in patients with anaphylactoid-type reactions to penicillin.
with optional			
Gentamicin¶	3 mg/kg/24 hr IV or IM in 2-3 doses	3-5 days	Benefit of additional aminoglycoside is unclear.
Oxacillin-Resistant Strains			
Vancomycin (Evidence exists for benefit)	30 mg/kg/24 hr IV in 2 doses	6 weeks	Adjust dosage to achieve peak serum concentration of 30-45 mcg/ml.
STAPHYLOCOCCAL ENDOCARDITIS IN THE PRESENCE OF PROSTHETIC MATERIAL			
Oxacillin-Susceptible Strains			
Nafcillin or oxacillin			
plus	12 g/24 hr IV in 6 doses	≥6 weeks	Vancomycin should be used in patients with anaphylactoid reactions to penicillin.
Rifampin	900 mg/24 hr IV or PO in 3 doses	≥6 weeks	
plus			
Gentamicin¶ (Evidence exists for benefit)	3 mg/kg/24 hr in 2-3 doses	2 weeks	
Oxacillin-Resistant Strains			
Vancomycin			
plus	30 mg/kg/24 hr in 2 doses	≤6 weeks	
Rifampin			
plus	900 mg/24 hr IV or PO in 3 doses	≤6 weeks	
Gentamicin¶ (Evidence exists for benefit)	3 mg/kg/24 hr IV or IM in 2-3 doses	2 weeks	
ENDOCARDITIS CAUSED BY HACEK MICROORGANISMS#			
Ceftriaxone (Evidence exists for benefit)	2 g/24 hr IV or IM in a single dose	4 weeks	Cefotaxime or other third- or fourth-generation cephalosporin may be substituted.
or			
Ampicillin-sulbactam (Limited evidence exists for benefit)	12 g/24 hr IV in 4 doses	4 weeks	
or			
Ciprofloxacin (Limited evidence exists for benefit)	1000 mg/24 hr PO or 800 mg/24 hr IV in 2 doses	4 weeks	Recommended only for patients unable to tolerate cephalosporin or ampicillin therapy. In patients with prosthetic valves, treatment recommended for 6 weeks.

#HACEK microorganisms include *Haemophilus parainfluenzae, Haemophilus aphrophilus, Actinobacillus actinomycetemcomitans, Cardiobacterium hominis, Eikenella corrodens,* and *Kingella kingae.*

BOX 127-2

ENDOCARDITIS RISK FACTORS

ENDOCARDITIS PROPHYLAXIS RECOMMENDED

High Risk

Prosthetic valves—mechanical, bioprosthetic, and homograft valves
Prior episode of infective endocarditis
Complex congenital heart disease (e.g., single ventricle, transposition of the great vessels, tetralogy of Fallot)
Surgically constructed pulmonary shunts

Moderate Risk

Congenital cardiac defects
Acquired valvular dysfunction (e.g., rheumatic heart disease)
Hypertrophic cardiomyopathy
Mitral valve prolapse with regurgitation and/or thickening of leaflets

ENDOCARDITIS PROPHYLAXIS NOT RECOMMENDED

Negligible Risk (No Greater Than the General Population)

Isolated secundum atrial septal defects
Surgically repaired atrial or ventricular septal defects or patent ductus arteriosus (without residua after 6 months)
Previous coronary artery bypass graft surgery
Mitral valve prolapse without regurgitation
Physiologic, functional, or innocent heart murmurs
Previous Kawasaki's syndrome without valvular dysfunction
Previous rheumatic fever without valvular dysfunction
Cardiac pacemakers or implanted defibrillators

Modified from Dajani AS, Taubert KA, Wilson W, and others: Prevention of bacterial endocarditis: recommendations by the American Heart Association, *JAMA* 227:1794-1801, 1997.

therapy may be considered for completing the prolonged antibiotic course only for patients who have demonstrated a response to treatment (negative blood cultures and afebrile state), are hemodynamically stable, are without complications such as congestive heart failure or embolic events, are reliable (non–IV drug users), and will comply with regular follow-up.[27]

PATIENT EDUCATION AND HEALTH PROMOTION

Education of patients and family members is crucial. The etiology and treatment of endocarditis, as well as the diagnostic tests, should be carefully explained. Patients should understand the importance of preventive therapy and current prophylaxis recommendations. Patients treated for infective

BOX 127-3

PROCEDURES AND ENDOCARDITIS PROPHYLAXIS

ENDOCARDITIS PROPHYLAXIS RECOMMENDED*

Dental Procedures

Prophylactic cleaning
Dental extractions or implant placement
Periodontal procedures
Root canal
Placement of subgingival antibiotic fibers
Initial placement of orthodontic bands but not brackets

Respiratory Tract Procedures

Tonsillectomy or adenoidectomy
Rigid bronchoscopy
Surgical procedures involving respiratory mucosa

Gastrointestinal Procedures†

Sclerotherapy for varices
Esophageal dilation
Endoscopic retrograde cholangiography with biliary obstruction
Biliary tract surgery
Surgery involving intestinal mucosa

Genitourinary Procedures

Cystoscopy
Urethral dilation
Prostate surgery

ENDOCARDITIS PROPHYLAXIS NOT RECOMMENDED

Dental Procedures

Restorative dentistry, including fillings
Local anesthetic injections (nonintraligamentary)
Postoperative suture removal
Orthodontic adjustment
Fluoride treatment and dental radiographs

Respiratory Tract Procedures

Endotracheal intubation
Flexible bronchoscopy with or without biopsy‡

Gastrointestinal Procedures

Transesophageal echocardiogram‡
Endoscopy with or without biopsy‡

Genitourinary Procedures

Vaginal hysterectomy‡
Vaginal delivery‡
Cesarean section
Involving uninfected tissue

- Urethral catheterization
- Dilation and curettage
- Therapeutic abortion
- Sterilization procedures
- Insertion and removal of intrauterine devices

Other Procedures

Cardiac catheterization, including angioplasty and intracoronary stent placement
Implantation of cardiac pacemakers and defibrillators
Incision or biopsy of surgically scrubbed skin
Circumcision

Modified from Baddour LM, Wilson WR, Bayer AS, and others: Infective endocarditis: diagnosis, antimicrobial therapy, and management of complications: a statement for healthcare professionals, *Circulation* 111:e394-e434, 2005 [erratum in *Circulation* 112(15):2373, 2005].
*Prophylaxis recommended for patients with high- and moderate-risk cardiac conditions.
†Prophylaxis recommended for high-risk patients; optional for moderate-risk patients.
‡Prophylaxis optional for high-risk patients.

TABLE 127-2 Antibiotic Prophylaxis for Dental, Oral, Respiratory Tract, or Esophageal Procedures

Patient Characteristics	Antibiotic	Dosage* and Route
Standard prophylaxis	Amoxicillin PO	2 g 1 hour before procedure
Inability to take oral medication	Ampicillin IM or IV	2 g within 30 minutes before procedure
Allergy to penicillin	Clindamycin PO	600 mg 1 hour before procedure
	or	
	Cephalexin† or cefadroxil PO	2 g 1 hour before procedure
	or	
	Azithromycin PO	500 mg 1 hour before procedure
	or	
	Clarithromycin PO	
Allergy to penicillin and inability to take oral medication	Clindamycin IV	600 mg within 30 minutes of procedure
	or	
	Cefazolin† IM or IV	1 g within 30 minutes of procedure

Modified from Dajani AS, Taubert KA, Wilson W, and others: Prevention of bacterial endocarditis: recommendations by the American Heart Association, *JAMA* 227:1794-1801, 1997.
*Dosages recommended are for adults with normal renal function.
†Cephalosporins should not be used in patients with hypersensitivity reactions to penicillins.

TABLE 127-3 Antibiotic Prophylaxis for Genitourinary and Gastrointestinal Procedures*

Patient Population	Antibiotic	Dosage† and Route
High-risk patients	Ampicillin *plus* Gentamicin‡	Ampicillin 2 g IV or IM *plus* gentamicin 1.5 mg/kg IV or IM within 30 minutes of procedure; then ampicillin 1 g IV or IM or amoxicillin 1 g PO 6 hours later
High-risk patients allergic to penicillin	Vancomycin *plus* Gentamicin†	Vancomycin 1 g IV over 1-2 hours *plus* gentamicin 1.5 mg/kg IV or IM; complete infusion or injection within 30 minutes of procedure
Moderate-risk patients	Amoxicillin *or* Ampicillin	Amoxicillin 2 g PO 1 hour before procedure, *or* ampicillin 2 g IV or IM within 30 minutes of procedure
Moderate-risk patients allergic to penicillin	Vancomycin	Vancomycin 1 g IV over 1-2 hours; complete infusion within 30 minutes of procedure

Modified from Dajani AS, Taubert KA, Wilson W, and others: Prevention of bacterial endocarditis: recommendations by the American Heart Association, *JAMA* 227:1794-1801, 1997.
*Excludes esophageal procedures.
†Dosages recommended are for adults with normal renal function. No second dose of vancomycin or gentamicin is recommended.
‡Gentamicin dose not to exceed 120 mg.

endocarditis should understand the risk of relapse and the importance of obtaining follow-up diagnostics and contacting the health care provider if there are any signs of illness.

REFERENCES

1. Bansal RC: Infective endocarditis, *Med Clin North Am* 79:1205-1240, 1995.
2. Cunha BA, Gill V, Lazar JM: Acute infective endocarditis: diagnostic and therapeutic approach, *Infect Dis Clin North Am* 10:811-834, 1996.
3. Korzeniowski OM, Chowdhury MH: Endocarditis of natural and prosthetic valves: treatment and prophylaxis. In Schlossberg D, editor: *Current therapy of infectious disease,* ed 2, St Louis, 2001, Mosby.
4. Wilson WR, Barasch E: Infective endocarditis. In Willerson JT, Cohn JN, editors: *Cardiovascular medicine,* ed 2, Philadelphia, 2000, Churchill Livingstone.
5. Mylonakis E, Calderwood SB: Medical progress: infective endocarditis in adults, *N Engl J Med* 345:1318-1330, 2001.
6. Cabell CH, Jollis JG, Peterson GE, and others: Changing patient characteristics and the effect on mortality in endocarditis, *Arch Intern Med* 162:90-94, 2002.
7. Wilson WR, Karchmer AW, Dajani AS, and others: Antibiotic treatment of adults with infective endocarditis due to streptococci, enterococci, staphylococci, and HACEK microorganisms, *JAMA* 274:1706-1713, 1995.
8. Kupferwasser I, Darius H, Muller AM, and others: Clinical and morphological characteristics in *Streptococcus bovis* endocarditis: a comparison with other causative microorganisms in 177 cases, *Heart* 80:276-280, 1998.
9. Pergola V, Di Salvo G, Habib G, and others: Comparison of clinical and echocardiographic characteristics of *Streptococcus bovis* endocarditis with that caused by other pathogens, *Am J Cardiol* 88:871-875, 2001.
10. Guerra JM, Tornos MP, Permanyer-Miraldo G, and others: Long term results of mechanical prosthesis for treatment of active infective endocarditis, *Heart* 86:63-68, 2001.

11. Gordon SM, Serkey JM, Longworth DL, and others: Early onset prosthetic valve endocarditis: the Cleveland Clinic experience 1992-1997, *Ann Thorac Surg* 69:1388-1392, 2000.
12. Di Salvo G, Habib G, Pergola V, and others: Echocardiography predicts embolic events in infective endocarditis, *J Am Coll Cardiol* 37:1069-1076, 2001.
13. Piper C, Korfer R, Horstkotte D: Prosthetic valve endocarditis, *Heart* 85:590-593, 2001.
14. Mueller SD, Willerson JT: Pregnancy and the heart. In Willerson JT, Cohn JN, editors: *Cardiovascular medicine,* ed 2, Philadelphia, 2000, Churchill Livingstone.
15. Mendelson MA, Lang RM: Pregnancy and cardiovascular disease. In Barron WM, Limdheimer MD, editors: *Medical disorders during pregnancy,* ed 3, St Louis, 2000, Mosby.
16. Vuille C, Nidorf M, Weyman AE, and others: Natural history of vegetations during successful medical treatment of endocarditis, *Am Heart J* 128:1200-1209, 1994.
17. Meine TJ, Nettles RE, Anderson DJ, and others: Cardiac conduction abnormalities in endocarditis defined by the Duke criteria, *Am Heart J* 142:280-285, 2001.
18. Oakley CM, Hall RJC: Endocarditis: problems—patients being treated for endocarditis and not doing well, *Heart* 85:470-474, 2001.
19. Baddour LM, Wilson WR, Bayer AS, and others: Infective endocarditis: diagnosis, antimicrobial therapy, and management of complications: a statement for healthcare professionals, *Circulation* 111:e394-e434, 2005 [erratum in *Circulation* 112(15):2373, 2005.
20. Netzer RO, Zolinger E, Seilder C, and others: Infective endocarditis: clinical spectrum, presentation and outcome: an analysis of 212 cases, 1980-1995, *Heart* 84:25-30, 2000.
21. Heiro M, Nikoskelainen J, Engblom E, and others: Neurologic manifestations of infective endocarditis: a 17-year experience in a teaching hospital in Finland, *Arch Intern Med* 160:2781-2787, 2000.
22. Eykyn SJ: Endocarditis: basics, *Heart* 86:476-480, 2001.
23. Shulman ST, Phair JP: Infective endocarditis. In Shulman ST, Phair JP, Peterson L, and others, editors: *The biologic and clinical basis of infectious diseases,* ed 5, Philadelphia, 1997, Saunders.
24. Li JS, Sexton DJ, Mick N, and others: Proposed modifications to the Duke criteria for the diagnosis of infective endocarditis, *Clin Infect Dis* 30:633-638, 2000.
25. Lindner JR, Case RA, Dent JM, and others: Diagnostic value of echocardiography in suspected endocarditis: an evaluation based on the pretest probability of disease, *Circulation* 93:730-736, 1996.
26. Durack DT, Lukes AS, Bright DK: New criteria for diagnosis of infective endocarditis: utilization of specific echocardiographic findings: Duke Endocarditis Service, *Am J Med* 96:200-209, 1994.
27. Andrews MM, von Reyn CF: Patient selection criteria and management guidelines for outpatient parenteral antibiotic therapy for native valve endocarditis, *Clin Infect Dis* 33:203-209, 2001.
28. Dajani AS, Taubert KA, Wilson W, and others: Prevention of bacterial endocarditis: recommendations by the American Heart Association, *JAMA* 227:1794-1801, 1997.
29. Hirota WK, Petersen K, Baron TH, and others: Guidelines for antibiotic prophylaxis for GI endoscopy, *Gastrointest Endosc* 58(4):475-482, 2003, retrieved Jan 13, 2007 from http://www.guideline.gov/summary/summary.aspx?ss=15&doc_id=4143&nbr=3179Quoting.

CHAPTER 128

Heart Failure

Roberta N. Regan

DEFINITION AND EPIDEMIOLOGY

Heart failure is the final pathophysiologic state in the progression of most cardiovascular disorders. Packer defines heart failure as a complex clinical syndrome characterized by abnormalities of left ventricular function and neurohormonal regulation accompanied by effort intolerance, fluid retention, and reduced longevity.[1] The spectrum of clinical presentation is wide, ranging from mild, effort-related signs and symptoms caused by fluid retention, to life-threatening arrhythmias and cardiogenic shock.

Etiology

The etiology of heart failure can be divided into three broad categories: (1) anatomic or functional abnormalities of the coronary vessels, myocardium, or cardiac valves; (2) biochemical and physiologic abnormalities that increase the myocardial workload or reduce myocardial oxygen delivery, thus impairing myocardial contraction; and (3) extracardiac factors that cause excessive demand on the cardiovascular system.[2] Treatment requires identification of the specific cause or causes and exacerbating factors for appropriate management and amelioration of precipitating factors.

With the widespread use of objective measures of myocardial function, such as echocardiography, it has become clear that there is a surprising variability in the degree of ventricular dysfunction despite a similar degree of clinical symptomatology. Left ventricular systolic dysfunction, present in the majority of patients with heart failure, is usually associated with symptoms when the left ventricular ejection fraction falls to less than 35%. Recent studies, including the V-HeFT II trial[3] and the SOLVD trial,[4] have shown that coronary artery disease is the most common cause of systolic dysfunction. At least 15% to 30% of patients with classic symptoms of heart failure have normal or minimally subnormal left ventricular ejection fractions. Most of these patients have primary left ventricular diastolic dysfunction. In this disorder left ventricular filling pressures are high, and during exercise there is a decreased stroke volume response. However, this is often asymptomatic, since the ejection fraction is normal (>50%).[5] The most common cause of heart failure resulting from primary diastolic dysfunction is hypertension.

Hypertension and valvular heart disease were considered the most common causes of heart failure 30 to 50 years ago. Today, in order of prevalence, the most common causes of heart failure are coronary artery disease, hypertension, alcohol, and idiopathic dilated cardiomyopathy. Most forms of chronic heart disease predispose the patient to heart failure over time, especially those disease processes which have the common pathophysiologic feature of left ventricular hypertrophy (Box 128-1).

BOX 128-1

CAUSES OF HEART FAILURE

CARDIOVASCULAR DISEASE

Ischemic heart disease
Toxic cardiomyopathy (e.g., alcohol, chemotherapeutic agents)
Idiopathic cardiomyopathies
- Dilated
- Hypertrophic
- Restricted

Hypertension
Valvular heart disease
Pericardial disease
Congenital defects
Chronic tachycardia

NONCARDIAC DISEASE

Endocrine or metabolic disorders (contractility not usually impaired; rather, metabolic demands are in excess of normal cardiac output; volume overload of the left ventricle)
Thyrotoxicosis
Anemia
Pregnancy
Fever, systemic infection
Arteriovenous fistulas
Vitamin B_1 deficiency (beriberi)

CONNECTIVE TISSUE DISEASES

Systemic lupus erythematosus
Polymyositis
Progressive systemic sclerosis (scleroderma)

PULMONARY DISEASES

Cor pulmonale secondary to chronic obstructive pulmonary disease
Pulmonary hypertension

From Moser DK, Cardin S: Heart failure. In Clochesy JM, Breu C, Cardin S, and others, editors: *Critical care nursing*, ed 2, Philadelphia, 1996, Saunders.

Incidence and Epidemiology

Heart failure is a leading cause of morbidity and mortality and represents a major public health problem in the United States. It is the only cardiovascular condition that is increasing in incidence in the United States. An estimated 4.6 million Americans carry the diagnosis of heart failure, and an estimated 400,000 new cases are identified each year. An estimated $20 billion was spent on care of patients with heart failure in 1999 alone.[6] Approximately 50% of persons with heart failure are symptomatic and over 65 years of age.[7]

The Framingham Heart Study enrolled more than 5000 people free of cardiac disease in a prospective observational study in the late 1940s. The study's data showed an increased incidence of heart failure with advancing age, with the incidence of heart failure doubling with each decade of life, especially in those who have a diagnosis of hypertension. There is a slightly higher incidence in men because of their greater vulnerability to coronary artery disease.[8] A total of 10% of Americans over 70 years old have been diagnosed with heart failure.[9]

Currently an average of 990,000 hospital admissions for heart failure occur annually in the United States, five times the number reported in 1971, validating the increasing prevalence of heart failure as the population ages. Hospitalizations for heart failure are increasing most rapidly in the over 65-year age-group.[1,10] In all, 60% of patients with heart failure carry a diagnosis of another serious, noncardiac co-morbid illness. In one study, subjects had a mean of three chronic conditions in addition to heart failure, with diabetes, chronic obstructive pulmonary disease (COPD), and anemia being the most common.[11] Because the prevalence of heart failure is expected to double in the twenty-first century, ambulatory and home care services for heart failure will have to increase as well.

A significant cause of death, heart failure has a 5-year survival rate of 24% in men and 38% in women. However, even in women only about 20% survive longer than 8 to 12 years. Thus heart failure is a more lethal condition than certain cancers.[12] Heart failure mortality increases with age, and the mortality rate is 50% higher in African Americans than in Caucasians and one third higher in men. The annual number of deaths directly attributable to heart failure has increased from 10,000 in 1968 to 42,000 in 1993, with another 219,000 deaths related to this condition.[13]

Physician consultation is indicated for new onset of heart failure in a patient with no previous history of cardiac disease. Physician consultation is recommended for patients with deterioration of previously stable congestive heart failure (CHF).

PATHOPHYSIOLOGY

Heart failure is in many ways a prototypical disorder of cardiovascular aging. Age-related cardiac changes combine with the high prevalence of cardiovascular disease in older adults in the United States, so that heart failure has become increasingly prevalent.[14] The etiology of heart failure can be multifactorial, resulting from ischemic heart disease, hypertension, cardiomyopathy, diabetes mellitus, metabolic syndrome, or hyperthyroidism. In this complex physiologic state, there is either a decline in the heart's ability to pump enough blood at a sufficient rate to sustain the body's physiologic functions, or the existence of elevated ventricular filling pressures. Thus, in general, heart failure has two distinct mechanisms: (1) diastolic dysfunction with increased ventricular stiffness and/or reduced ventricular compliance, and (2) systolic dysfunction with impaired ventricular contractility.[8,15]

Diastolic Dysfunction

With diastolic dysfunction the key problem is increased ventricular stiffness and reduced compliance, thus producing a rise in cardiac pressures during diastolic filling and the inability of the left ventricle to relax and accommodate a sufficient amount of oxygenated blood returning from the lungs. Left ventricular distensibility is reduced during part of or throughout the whole of diastole, and filling pressures must increase to maintain a constant ventricular volume. This condition in the left ventricle results in an increase in cardiac filling pressures during both rest and exercise, failure of the normal rise in cardiac output during exertion, and, occasionally, a reduction in cardiac output at rest. The heart attempts to compensate for this impaired distensibility through the "booster" effect of augmented atrial contraction. The most common causes of diastolic dysfunction are hypertension, ischemia resulting from coronary artery disease, aortic stenosis, and infiltrative or restrictive myocardial diseases.

Systolic Dysfunction

Systolic dysfunction remains the most common type of heart failure with a decrease in both the ejection fraction and cardiac output. In systolic dysfunction the three determinants of ventricular function—preload, contractility, and afterload—are usually all altered. Preload is the degree of myocardial fiber stretch at the end of ventricular filling. When the heart ejects subnormally, there is an increased volume of blood left in the ventricular chambers (increased left ventricular end-systolic volume). This excess volume leads to distention of the ventricles and increased interventricular pressure at the onset of diastole. Filling must then occur at higher pressures during diastole. At small increases of volume/pressure, nonfailing myocardial fibers have the intrinsic property of increasing their force of contraction in an attempt to "revert" the subsequent volume/pressure conditions of both heart ejection and filling back to normal. This intrinsic property also enables the heart to maintain cardiac output during states of pressure or volume overload.[2] However, in the failing heart, the failing myocardial fibers are both excessively overloaded and stretched beyond lengths commensurate with the normal reflex-increased force of contraction. Cardiac output eventually falls, precipitating symptoms and signs of either inadequate cardiac output or systemic or pulmonary congestion.

The ventricular dysfunction in heart failure is accompanied by a decrease in myocardial contractility, or force of contraction. This decline in contractility produces a reduction in ejection fraction and often stroke volume and cardiac output. Contractile force can be improved with the administration of positive inotropic agents, such as digoxin, and beta agonists, such as catecholamines. Physiologic states such as hypoxia and acidosis cause a reduction in contractility, as can both beta blockers and calcium channel blockers.

Afterload is the amount of left ventricular wall tension that develops during systole to eject blood. It is determined by both the size of the ventricular chamber (since wall tension must increase as the radius of the ventricle increases, according to Laplace's law) and the dynamic vascular resistance against which the heart contracts. Systolic blood pressure reasonably approximates afterload and is a clinically important indicator of myocardial load. Because afterload determines the ease or speed of ventricular contraction, the ejection fraction is a function of afterload. The ejection fraction is an afterload-dependent measure of contractility. The ejection fraction of a normal heart with normal contractility may, in fact, fall if the afterload is extremely high. Thus it is important to consider the degree of afterload elevation before deciding that contractility as measured by the afterload-dependent ejection fraction is truly abnormal. One must remember that each determinant of ventricular function is interrelated and may potentially contribute to ventricular systolic dysfunction. Eventually, ventricular dysfunction is evidenced by a decline in stroke volume and cardiac output.

Several systemic mechanisms exist for the body to compensate for the reduction in cardiac output. Early on, these compensatory mechanisms serve to increase cardiac output and tissue perfusion. In the long run, however, they lead to further cardiac injury and further decompensation.

Compensatory Mechanisms

Several interrelated compensatory mechanisms attempt to maintain normal ventricular contractility, ventricular pressures, cardiac output, and blood pressure. The three primary compensatory mechanisms include (1) increased sympathetic adrenergic activity with a resultant increase in circulating neurohormones, (2) neuroendocrine activation of the renin-angiotensin-aldosterone system, and (3) ventricular remodeling. To appreciate the mechanisms of heart failure, one must remember that these same three compensatory mechanisms are responsible for the deterioration of cardiac function as time passes.

Sympathetic Adrenergic Activity. Abnormalities of the baroreceptors and cardiac reflexes have been documented in heart failure.[16] Normally, stimulation of the baroreceptor reflex results in activation of the parasympathetic nervous system and an inhibition of the sympathetic nervous system, so that heart rate and systemic vascular resistance are reduced. The opposite occurs when the baroreceptors are inhibited in response to a reduction in blood pressure. In heart failure the baroreceptors are inhibited by the reduction in cardiac output and the activation of the sympathetic nervous system. As heart failure progresses, the baroreceptor function is depressed further, leading to even greater sympathetic overactivity despite intense vasoconstriction and volume retention.

In heart failure the reduction in cardiac output leads to tissue hypoperfusion and direct activation of the sympathetic nervous system. In turn, the activated sympathetic adrenergic system stimulates release of catecholamines from the cardiac adrenergic nerves and the adrenal medulla. Release of catecholamines causes not only direct stimulation of contractility and heart rate, but also vasoconstriction in less metabolically active organs (e.g., skin, kidneys). It also results in venoconstriction, which increases preload by increasing venous return. Catecholamines also affect the cardiac cells, producing an increased myocardial oxygen demand, hypertrophy of the cells themselves, and tissue necrosis. Over time, these cardiac myocyte effects can increase heart failure.

Moreover, as a result of sympathetic activation, plasma norepinephrine levels are elevated. The degree of plasma norepinephrine elevation correlates with the severity of heart failure and is predictive of mortality in heart failure. In addition, exposure of the myocardial β-receptors to high levels of circulating catecholamines produces a decrease in both the number of β-adrenergic receptors and their responsiveness to catecholamine stimulation. This elevation of circulating catecholamines and the sustained stimulation of the sympathetic nervous system can produce arrhythmias.

Neuroendocrine Activation. Two additional vasoconstrictor systems act as compensatory mechanisms and therefore are affected by heart failure: the renin-angiotensin-aldosterone system and arginine vasopressin. The renin-angiotensin-aldosterone system is activated as a result of a decline in blood pressure in the renal juxtaglomerular cells, which causes the release of increased renin, an enzyme. In fact, the degree of renin activity in plasma is related to the severity of heart failure. Renin acts on angiotensinogen, the plasma protein produced by the liver, to form angiotensin I. Angiotensin I is in turn converted into angiotensin II, a potent vasoconstrictor, through the action of angiotensin-converting enzyme (ACE), which is localized primarily in the lungs. This potent vasoconstrictor, angiotensin II, constricts the renal arterioles, thereby potentiating its own release. Other actions of angiotensin II are the stimulation of the thirst center, the release of aldosterone from the adrenal glands, and the trigger for the additional release of norepinephrine. In turn, aldosterone release promotes intravascular volume expansion by increasing sodium and water retention and stimulating potassium excretion. These multiple, synergistic mechanisms eventually place the failing myocardium at more risk by increasing preload and afterload, promoting electrolyte imbalance, and increasing the risk for ischemia and arrhythmias.

The other vasoconstrictor system involves arginine vasopressin, a substance released from the posterior pituitary gland. Of note, the serum levels of arginine vasopressin are proportional to the severity of the heart failure, since this substance is not released in all heart failure patients.[17]

In addition to the renin-angiotensin-aldosterone system and arginine vasopressin, endothelium-derived factors, such as endothelin, contribute to the vasoconstriction seen in heart failure. The contribution of these endothelium-derived factors has not been as well elucidated.[18]

During the course of neuroendocrine activity in heart failure, several vasodilators are also activated and serve as counterregulatory systems. In response to the increased atrial stretch that occurs during heart failure, atrial natriuretic factor, a peptide, is released into the circulation from atrial myocytes. This hormone attenuates the vasoconstrictor effects of the other constrictor hormones, inhibits the renin-angiotensin system, reduces aldosterone release, and suppresses the release of norepinephrine.[19] Other vasodilators, such as prostaglandins, bradykinin, kallidin, and dopamine, are also released, but these may be overwhelmed by the potent vasoconstrictor systems activated in heart failure.

Ventricular Remodeling. Yet another compensatory response to heart failure is ongoing remodeling of ventricular three-dimensional morphology. Both myocardial hypertrophy and dilation occur in varying degrees, depending on the cause of the heart failure. Dilation is an increase in the ventricular end-diastolic volume and represents an early compensatory response in volume overload in an attempt to increase contractility. In dilation, each individual myocyte lays down additional sarcomeres in series. Dilation preserves stroke volume and maintains cardiac output, but it also significantly increases wall stress. In turn, increased wall stress increases myocardial oxygen demand, a deleterious condition if significant coronary artery disease is present. Also, excessive wall stress may lead to myocyte loss and fibrosis of cardiac tissue.

Moreover, the condition of ventricular hypertrophy is a direct result of attempts to compensate for the increase in wall stress. Ventricular hypertrophy is an increase in the number of sarcomeres within each myocyte of ventricular heart muscle; these abnormal, large cells cannot contract as efficiently. Initially, myocardial hypertrophy distributes the greater degree of wall stress to a greater myocardial mass and thus "normalizes" the increased load per myocyte. Hypertrophy also increases the force of the ventricular contraction. Ultimately, however, ventricular remodeling in heart failure progresses to the point that it can no longer offer any compensatory advantage, especially when loading conditions remain abnormal or when myocardial disease causes myocyte loss.[19]

Escalating Heart Failure. At the onset of heart failure, all the compensatory mechanisms described are beneficial; however, over time, these compensatory mechanisms may themselves exacerbate heart failure. The fluid retention intended to enhance contractile force can cause pulmonary and systemic congestion. Arterial vasoconstriction can cause impaired tissue perfusion and increased afterload. Myocardial hypertrophy and the sympathetic activity can increase myocardial oxygen consumption. The result of all these responses is an increase in myocardial burden and an escalation in the degree of heart failure.

CLINICAL PRESENTATION AND PHYSICAL EXAMINATION

No single symptom, sign, or laboratory test can definitively diagnose heart failure. Therefore prudent clinical judgment and an understanding of the pathophysiology of heart failure are critical to evaluating the significance of an individual patient's presenting signs and symptoms, in conjunction with his or her medical history. The New York Heart Association (NYHA) functional classification is typically used to classify a patient's status; this classification expresses the relationship between the onset of symptoms (fatigue, dyspnea, palpitations, angina) and the degree of physical exertion (Box 128-2).

The American College of Cardiology (ACC) and American Heart Association (AHA) have devised a new classification system to complement, not replace, the NYHA classes. This new classification system grades patients in stages A through D.[20] Stage A designates patients at risk for development of failure: patients with hypertension, diabetes, coronary artery disease, myocarditis, use of cardiotoxic medications, or a family history of cardiomyopathy, but without symptoms of

BOX 128-2

NEW YORK HEART ASSOCIATION FUNCTIONAL CLASSIFICATION

Class I: No limitations. Ordinary physical activity does not cause undue fatigue, dyspnea, or palpitations.

Class II: Slight limitation of physical activity. Such patients are comfortable at rest. Ordinary physical activity results in fatigue, palpitations, dyspnea, or angina.

Class III: Marked limitation of physical activity. Although patients are comfortable at rest, less than ordinary activity will lead to symptoms.

Class IV: Inability to carry on any physical activity without discomfort. Symptoms of congestive heart failure are present even at rest. With any physical activity, increased discomfort is experienced.

From the American Heart Association: *Nomenclature and criteria for the diagnosis of diseases of the heart and great vessels,* ed 9, Dallas, 1994, The Association.

failure or evidence of structural heart damage. Stage B includes those patients with structural heart disease (previous myocardial infarction [MI], left ventricular systolic dysfunction, asymptomatic valvular disease) but without symptoms of failure. Stage C encompasses those patients with known structural heart disease and prior or current symptoms of failure. The final stage, stage D, is reserved for patients with refractory heart failure requiring specialized interventions: patients who have marked symptoms at rest, who are receiving maximum medication therapy, or who have had recurrent hospitalizations for failure.[20]

Dyspnea and Fatigue

Dyspnea and fatigue are the cardinal presenting symptoms of heart failure. The principal difference between exertional dyspnea in normal subjects and in the patient with heart failure is the degree of activity necessary to induce the symptom. Increasing heart failure is usually heralded by a change in the severity of dyspnea. Therefore it is necessary for the practitioner to ascertain whether changes have occurred in the extent of the exertion that actually causes the dyspnea. As the ventricular dysfunction advances, the intensity of the exertion needed to cause symptoms progressively declines. Interestingly, sedentary patients with heart failure may have a total absence of dyspnea.[21]

Fatigue that is seen with heart failure is a direct result of the generalized hypoxia of body tissues from the decrease in cardiac output and the resultant decrease in oxygen saturation of the blood. This results in easy fatigability, weakness, and dizziness. In addition, the loss of potassium induced by the increased levels of aldosterone can also cause muscle weakness. Compounding this muscle weakness is an alteration of the normal vascular response to exercise. Adequate vasodilation fails to occur during exercise, thereby reducing blood flow to the muscle and causing further muscle deconditioning. Recent studies have provided strong evidence that muscle deconditioning plays a more important role in fatigue than previously recognized.[21,22]

Orthopnea and Paroxysmal Nocturnal Dyspnea

Orthopnea is a common finding with heart failure. Orthopnea is shortness of breath that occurs while the patient is in the supine position and is typically relieved in part by the upright or sitting position. Although interstitial and alveolar pulmonary congestion are most likely present at all times, when a person is in an upright position, fluid in the lungs gravitates to the bases, making breathing somewhat easier. Paroxysmal nocturnal dyspnea is the onset of acute breathlessness at night. The exact cause of this symptom is unknown, but it is believed to be related to increased reabsorption of fluid from the periphery in the recumbent position, which leads to left ventricular overload, increasing the symptoms of failure.

Bronchospasm and Wheezing

In some patients, heart failure may cause reflex bronchospasm and wheezing. This condition, called *cardiac asthma*, results from pulmonary interstitial or alveolar edema present with CHF.[23] Typically, with cardiac asthma, patients have a nonproductive cough, especially in the recumbent position.

Crackles

Other adventitious lung sounds, crackles, may be heard on auscultation secondary to pulmonary fluid transudation; however, crackles are not always present with heart failure. In new-onset or acute escalation of heart failure, crackles are commonly present. When crackles are heard in early failure, they are at the lung bases because of the effects of gravity. In chronic heart failure, increased pulmonary fluid transudation may be accommodated by an increase in lymphatic drainage, so that the interstitial spaces and alveoli remain relatively dry and crackles may be absent.

Hemoptysis and Dysphagia

With more advanced heart failure, hemoptysis and dysphagia can be seen. Hemoptysis may result from bronchial vein bleeding resulting from venous distention, and dysphagia can occur as a result of esophageal compression from distention of the left atrium.

Pulmonary Edema

Perhaps the most dramatic clinical presentation of heart failure is acute pulmonary edema. This potentially life-threatening complication manifests as severe dyspnea, diaphoresis, and anxiety, with shallow, rapid breathing and, in a number of cases, pink, frothy sputum. Elevated blood pressure is common with pulmonary edema, probably because of an outpouring of endogenous catecholamines. Sinus tachycardia is also a component, although this finding may be absent in patients taking beta blockers, calcium channel blockers, or antiarrhythmic medications, all of which blunt heart rate response.

Abnormal Cardiac Examination Findings

Abnormalities in the cardiac examination are the presence of extra heart sounds, gallops (S_3, S_4) or murmurs, and the lateral displacement and abnormalities of the apical impulse. S_4 is the sound caused by the overdistention of the ventricles produced during late diastole as the stiffened ventricles expand further to accommodate the final diastolic filling volume of blood injected from the atria by atrial contraction (atrial kick). The presence of an S_3 indicates early diastolic rapid, turbulent left ventricular filling and is often evident when left ventricular systolic dysfunction is the mechanism of heart failure. These gallop sounds, S_4 and S_3, are best heard with the patient in the left lateral position. The presence of a loud S_4 gallop in the absence of an S_3 gallop suggests early failure or the presence of predominantly diastolic dysfunction, such as that resulting from hypertensive heart disease or hypertrophic or restrictive cardiomyopathy.

The location and character of the left ventricular apical impulse can provide important information regarding the mechanism of the heart failure. Displacement of the palpable apical impulse away from the midclavicular line toward the anterior axillary line indicates left ventricular enlargement. Furthermore, the palpable apical impulse should be a quick tap, narrow in distribution, not more than 1 to 2 cm (0.4 to 0.8 inch) in diameter. An impulse that is palpable with the palm of the hand, lasts longer, or is forceful indicates increased cardiac output or ventricular hypertrophy.

In addition, with increased cardiac volume or overload, a palpable impulse may be elicited with the palm placed on the sternum. This finding is a right ventricular tap or heave, indicating right ventricular enlargement and volume overload.

In all patients with heart failure a careful auscultatory examination is important to exclude acute or chronic valvular disease and other structural heart disease. A vigilant search for regurgitant or stenotic aortic and mitral valve murmurs is essential, since these conditions are an important yet potentially reversible cause of heart failure. In severe aortic stenosis the small-volume, but high-velocity, turbulent jet of blood flowing across the valve during systole creates a loud and harsh systolic murmur. In acute severe aortic or mitral regurgitation, on the hand, the large-volume, less turbulent jet of blood creates a softer murmur.

Jugular Venous Pressure, Hepatomegaly, and Peripheral Edema

The jugular veins provide a useful index of right atrial pressure and, thus, a guide to the presence of volume overload that can manifest as peripheral edema. Normal jugular venous pressure can be assessed by noting the upper limit of visible pulse undulation in the internal jugular veins with the patient supine and his or her head elevated at a 45-degree angle. With normal pressure, the upper level of jugular vein undulation is approximately 4 cm (1.6 inches) or less above the sternal angle. Ideally, the internal jugular vein is inspected, but since the external jugular venous system is more easily identified, it can also be used. The external jugular vein is compressed in the supraclavicular fossa, and as the examiner's finger strips the vein cephalad, blood rises in the more proximal portion of the vein; the height of this blood volume above the patient's clavicles reflects the central venous pressure. The height of the venous column normally falls during inspiration as a result of the accompanying decrease in intrathoracic pressure.

In patients with mild heart failure the jugular venous pressure may be normal at rest but rises quickly to abnormal levels with compression of the right upper quadrant, a sign known as the *hepatojugular reflex*. This sign is assessed by having the patient lie supine and semirecumbent at a 45-degree angle. The examiner exerts pressure with the hand on the patient's right upper quadrant and observes the jugular veins for distention. This maneuver causes a sudden increase in venous return, causing right ventricular end-diastolic and right atrial pressures to rise and remain elevated, which can be detected as jugular venous distention.

With heart failure, hepatomegaly (or liver enlargement) may be present and liver tenderness may be noted on abdominal palpation because of the stretching of the hepatic capsule. With chronic heart failure, however, liver tenderness is reduced, although liver enlargement persists. This enlargement of the liver is responsible for the anorexia, abdominal fullness, and/or nausea reported by patients with heart failure.

Although peripheral edema can be a common manifestation of heart failure, it does not correlate well with the level of systemic venous pressure and should not be used to estimate the degree of failure. In chronic heart failure, fluid volume may already be sufficiently expanded to cause edema in the presence of only slight elevations of systemic venous pressure.[24]

Peripheral edema, usually symmetric, is pitting, generally occurs in the dependent portions of the body, and is greatest at the end of the day. In advanced heart failure, generalized body edema, including ascites and anasarca, may be present.

Nocturia

Nocturia occurs as a result of nocturnal diuresis. This nocturnal diuresis lessens the degree of fluid retention. Nocturnal diuresis with nocturia results from fluid reabsorption and redistribution in the supine position, as well as a reduction in renal vasoconstriction that occurs at rest.

Altered Hemodynamics

As previously discussed, the major determinants of cardiac output are stroke volume and heart rate. Heart rate is altered by activation baroreceptors found in the carotid arteries by means of a complex feedback mechanism. Zucker has identified abnormalities in these baroreceptors in patients with heart failure that causes the abnormal activation of the sympathetic nervous system, the renin-angiotensin-aldosterone system, and vasopressin release and thus prevents an increase in heart rate in response to a reduction in pressure.[16] In advanced heart failure, however, sympathetic activation overwhelms the compensatory neurohormonal response and results in a resting tachycardia.

DIAGNOSTICS

The majority of patients with heart failure are initially seen with ventricular systolic dysfunction with a variable degree of diastolic dysfunction; however, a subset of patients has predominantly diastolic dysfunction. Because the clinical management of these two disease processes differs, a thorough diagnostic evaluation is critical. Table 128-1 reviews the history, physical examination, and diagnostic testing differences between systolic and diastolic dysfunction. The diagnostic evaluation should be limited to those studies necessary to (1) determine the type of ventricular dysfunction, primarily systolic or diastolic; (2) uncover correctable causes; (3) determine the prognosis; and (4) guide treatment.[25]

B Natriuretic Peptide

B (brain) natriuretic peptide (BNP) is a peptide synthesized and secreted almost exclusively by ventricular myocardial cells in response to elevations in end-diastolic pressure and volume. The V-HeFT trial confirmed this test as the strongest predictor of outcome in heart failure when compared with other neurohormones and clinical markers.[26] The BNP (Breathing Not Properly) Trial revealed this to be most helpful in differentiating cardiac from pulmonary etiologies, since values less than 100 have a 100% sensitivity and 97.1% specificity, making this extremely useful in ruling out CHF.[27] A BNP value of 400 has a high positive predictive value for determining CHF, and additional research shows values of 1000 to 4000 to be associated with CHF and values greater than 4000 to be directly related to CHF.[28] BNP is elevated in both diastolic and systolic dysfunction and therefore cannot be used to distinguish these two types of heart failure. Additionally, serial BNP levels can be measured over time and compared to steady-state levels to allow detection of trends that lead toward

TABLE 128-1 Systolic vs. Diastolic Dysfunction in Heart Failure: Differences in History, Physical Examination, and Diagnostic Tests*

Parameter	Systolic	Diastolic
HISTORY		
Coronary artery disease	++++	+
Hypertension	++	++++
Diabetes	+++	+
Valvular heart disease	++++	-
Paroxysmal dyspnea	++	+++
PHYSICAL EXAMINATION		
Cardiomegaly	+++	+
Soft heart sounds	++++	+
S_3 gallop	+++	+
S_4 gallop	+	+++
Hypertension	++	++++
Mitral regurgitation	+++	+
Rales	++	++
Edema	+++	+
Jugular venous distention	+++	+
CHEST X-RAY EXAMINATION		
Cardiomegaly	+++	+
Pulmonary congestion	+++	+++
ELECTROCARDIOGRAM		
Low voltage	+++	
Left ventricular hypertrophy	++	++++
Q waves	++	+
ECHOCARDIOGRAM		
Low ejection fraction	++++	–
Left ventricular dilation	++	–
Left ventricular hypertrophy	++	++++

From Young JB: Assessment of heart failure. In Colucci WS, editor: Heart failure: cardiac function and dysfunction. In Braunwald E, editor: *Atlas of heart disease*, vol 4, Philadelphia, 1995, Current Medicine.

*Plus signs indicate "suggestive" (the number reflects relative weight). Minus signs indicate "not very suggestive."

decompensation. Numerous studies have corroborated a significant correlation between echocardiographic findings and BNP values that may lead to more cost-effective diagnostic testing. Trials are ongoing to more accurately assess potential benefits.[27,28]

Urotensin

Human urotensin II is a newer potential diagnostic marker for CHF. This marker has potent vasoactive effects and stimulates myocardial expression of the natriuretic peptides. Levels are elevated in heart failure and may be a useful index in a similar way to BNP testing. Unlike the BNP, which correlates to NYHA class, urotensin levels are elevated in heart failure irrespective of age, sex, or NYHA class.[29] More testing is required to determine the cost-effectiveness of this diagnostic marker.

Chest X-Ray Examination

The size and shape of the cardiac silhouette and the presence of interstitial and alveolar edema comprise the radiologic evidence of heart failure. A common chest x-ray study finding in heart failure is cardiomegaly, with a cardiothoracic (size of heart to width of chest) ratio that is increased more than 50%. Normally, in the upright position, pulmonary blood flow is greater to the lung bases than to the apexes. This is evidenced on the plain chest x-ray film when the caliber of the vessels, particularly the veins, of the lower lung zones is compared with the caliber of the vessels of the upper lung zones. Patients with heart failure have a redistribution of pulmonary blood flow to the upper zones, so that the caliber of the upper zone vessels becomes equal to or greater than the caliber of lower zone vessels. This redistribution occurs because interstitial edema is more severe in lower lung fields as a result of gravity. The microvasculature is consequently compressed, and blood flow is shunted upward.

Another radiologic indicator of heart failure, interstitial pulmonary edema, occurs when the left atrial pressure is elevated above 20 mm Hg. The radiologic pattern of interstitial edema consists of varying combinations of septal, perivascular, and subpleural edema. Septal edema is manifested by Kerley's B lines, which are short, nonbranching lines seen at the periphery of the lower lung fields, extending to and perpendicular to the pleural surface. Perivascular edema is manifested both as central (hilar) haze and as loss of definition of lower zone vessels. Subpleural edema is indicated by a sharp pleural margin associated with a poorly defined density extending into the underlying lung. Interstitial edema may also be seen as peribronchial "cuffing" when airways are viewed in cross-section.

Alveolar edema, a third radiologic finding indicative of heart failure, occurs when the left atrial pressure is elevated above 30 mm Hg. This appears on the chest x-ray film as frank pulmonary opacification. The distribution of alveolar edema may be a typical central "bat wing" pattern, may be diffuse, or may be asymmetric, even unilateral. Opacification seen with alveolar edema is usually homogeneous but occasionally may be patchy, even mimicking pneumonia.

When left atrial pressure rises acutely, as in MI, providers should remember that a lag of several hours may occur before the appearance of radiologic pulmonary edema. In these patients crackles that suggest acute pulmonary edema are usually heard despite an unimpressive radiographic appearance. Conversely, when the left atrial pressure is rapidly lowered with therapy and crackles disappear, the edema may continue to be present on the chest x-ray film for several hours.

Echocardiography and Radionuclide Ventriculography

Measurement of ventricular performance is a critical step in the diagnostic evaluation. The combined use of history, physical examination, chest x-ray examination, and the ECG cannot be relied on to distinguish among major causes of heart failure. The use of echocardiography or radionuclide ventriculography can substantially improve the accuracy of differentiating between systolic and diastolic dysfunction when compared with clinical evaluation alone.[30]

The value of echocardiography cannot be overestimated in the diagnostic evaluation of known or suspected heart failure. It currently represents the single most effective tool in widespread clinical use for the assessment of heart failure.[31]

Approximately 70% of patients with heart failure have left ventricular systolic dysfunction, defined as a left ventricular ejection fraction of less than 40%.[21,31] Two-dimensional Doppler echocardiography provides information regarding biventricular systolic performance, wall thickness, and chamber dimensions. Segmental or regional wall motion abnormalities, chamber enlargement, and valvular disease can also be detected and quantified by echocardiography. Diastolic dysfunction can often be detected as well. Doppler echocardiography allows for the characterization of abnormal left ventricular filling in diastole. With significant diastolic dysfunction, this is seen as increased velocity, reduced volume, and delayed timing on the Doppler echocardiogram. The Advisory Council to Improve Outcomes Nationwide in Heart Failure and the ACC and AHA guidelines both recognize echocardiography as the preferred diagnostic tool for evaluating the cause of heart failure in patients.[21,31]

Radionuclide angiography is more accurate than echocardiography in the measurement of ejection fraction. In combination with exercise and a myocardial perfusion imaging agent (such as thallium or sestamibi), exercise radionuclide myocardial scintigraphy is a sensitive and specific diagnostic tool in the assessment of suspected or known coronary artery disease. The usefulness of radionuclide angiography as a diagnostic tool is limited by the inability to characterize valvular abnormalities, cardiac chamber volumes, wall thickness, and estimated intracardiac pressures.[21]

Exercise Testing

The exercise test, or stress test, provides important data on exercise and functional capacity, as well as prognostic information. Measurement of peak oxygen consumption during cardiopulmonary exercise testing is likely the single best predictor of survival in patients with advanced heart failure and currently determines the appropriateness and timing of heart transplantation.[30] Serial exercise testing with quantification of the workload achieved is helpful in determining the response to medical therapy. Exercise testing also permits the identification of suspected exercise-induced arrhythmias.

The use of submaximal exercise testing, such as the 6-minute walk test, is a viable option for those who do not have access to equipment to measure respiratory gases. The 6-minute walk test is a 100-foot self-paced walk during which the subject is asked to cover as much ground as possible.[32] The 6-minute walk test correlates well with peak oxygen consumption and predicts short-term survival in patients with advanced heart failure. Univariate and multivariate analysis found that the distance covered during the test was the strongest predictor of peak oxygen consumption and was equivalent to left ventricular ejection fraction in predicting mortality and hospital readmissions for heart failure.[33-35]

Cardiac Catheterization and Endomyocardial Biopsy

Clinical information gleaned from cardiac catheterization and measurement of hemodynamics is invaluable in patients with heart failure who have advanced symptoms or suboptimum response to medical therapy. Catheterization provides valuable information about the origin of congestive versus low-output symptoms through direct measurement of filling pressure and cardiac output, and it permits the direct measurement of systemic vascular resistance. Hemodynamic measurement provides an assessment of valvular dysfunction and identifies the presence of intracardiac shunts. From a therapeutic perspective, hemodynamic assessment can guide medical therapy in refractory cases, determine the need for circulatory support, and provide data for identifying the timing for valvular surgery.[36]

In addition, cardiac catheterization remains the best procedure for evaluating diastolic dysfunction properties because ventricular filling pressures can be measured directly. Although catheterization may not be beneficial for all heart failure patients, cardiac catheterization should be considered in patients with acute or acutely decompensated chronic heart failure not responding to treatment. Cardiac catheterization should also be considered in patients with angina or other signs of ischemia not responding to appropriate treatment.[21,31]

It has been established that during exercise radionuclide myocardial imaging, many patients with significant left ventricular dysfunction and dilation irrespective of cause have a positive myocardial redistribution study suggestive of coronary artery disease. Coronary artery angiography performed during cardiac catheterization is often necessary to diagnose the presence, extent, and severity of existing coronary artery disease. Furthermore, cardiac catheterization and coronary angiography are used with radionuclide imaging to assess viability of revascularization strategies for patients with ischemic cardiomyopathy.

Conversely, the role of right ventricular endomyocardial biopsy in the diagnostic evaluation is controversial. Biopsy is usually performed only in cases with a clear-cut acute

DIAGNOSTICS

Heart Failure

LABORATORY
CBC and differential
Glucose
Serum electrolytes
Magnesium
BUN, creatinine
LFTs
Cardiac enzymes
B natriuretic peptide
TSH*
Lipid profile*
Calcium*
$HgbA_{1c}$*

IMAGING
Chest x-ray
Radionuclide studies*

OTHER
ECG
Echocardiogram
Exercise testing*
IV ultrasound*
Cardiac catheterization, endomyocardial biopsy*

*If indicated.

symptomatic onset (within 6 months), with compelling clinical suspicion of infiltrative cardiomyopathy (such as amyloidosis, sarcoidosis, or metastatic cancer), or with suspected doxorubicin (Adriamycin) cardiotoxicity.

Intravascular Ultrasound

Intravascular ultrasound has proven extremely useful for three-dimensional image reconstruction and is now considered the definitive test for atherosclerosis imaging. Provision of cross-sectional images of the arterial wall and lumen, with the added benefit of excellent resolution, allows better assessment of atherosclerosis, vessel wall remodeling, and actual plaque burden. This surpasses the diagnostic capacity of angiography, where atherosclerotic burden and lesion composition cannot be accurately assessed.[37] Most helpful for determining the degree of atherosclerosis, this contributes to judging the prognosis of heart failure, since coronary artery disease is the primary cause.

Cardiac Magnetic Resonance Imaging

MRI is used to measure cardiac volumes, wall thickness, and left ventricular mass. Cardiac MRI also quantifies myocardial perfusion and function and detects pericardium thickening and degree of myocardial necrosis. Currently, use of MRI is not widespread and is recommended only if other imaging techniques are not diagnostically satisfactory.[31]

DIFFERENTIAL DIAGNOSIS

A variety of cardiac, pulmonary, and systemic disease states have dyspnea as a typical symptom and can be confused with heart failure on the basis of this symptom. Therefore systematic evaluation of dyspnea is critical to properly diagnose the underlying disease. The common disease processes leading to dyspnea can be broadly characterized as abnormalities in gas exchange, pulmonary circulation, respiratory mechanics, or cardiac function.

Chronic Pulmonary Conditions

The dyspnea of heart failure might be confused with chronic pulmonary conditions (Figure 128-1). The most common adult disorders of COPD, chronic bronchitis, asthma, exacerbated cystic fibrosis, and lung cancer are coincidentally seen in the same age range at risk for heart failure; however, these pulmonary conditions have physical examination findings that help distinguish them from heart failure. COPD represents a spectrum of disease severity and pathophysiology and is a common co-morbidity in patients with heart failure. In patients with underlying COPD and heart failure, it is often challenging to distinguish the dyspnea of pulmonary origin from the dyspnea of cardiac origin. Chronic dyspnea caused by COPD is often exacerbated by bending over forward (e.g., while putting on one's shoes), whereas dyspnea caused by heart failure is usually not aggravated by this. This simple maneuver may aid in the discernment of the origin of a patient's dyspnea.

Orthopnea (worsening dyspnea when the patient assumes a recumbent position) and paroxysmal nocturnal dyspnea (sudden waking from sleep with marked dyspnea) may result from either COPD or heart failure. These entities may be difficult to identify on the basis of symptom analysis; past medical history, risk for heart failure, and cardiac examination findings (S_3, S_4, jugular venous distention) in combination with other symptoms such as increased fatigue may help elucidate the cause as heart failure.

Asthma and Upper Respiratory Tract Infection

In clinical practice, new-onset heart failure is often mistaken for asthma or an upper respiratory tract infection (URI) because dyspnea is the predominant symptom. However, the duration of the dyspnea can be a clue to distinguish new-onset heart failure from asthma or URI. The asthmatic patient is usually free of chronic dyspnea but experiences episodic dyspnea, with prominent inspiratory and expiratory wheezing. Because pulmonary edema can trigger bronchospasm and wheezing, an acute asthma attack may mimic acute pulmonary edema, but usually airflow limitation and wheezing are more marked in acute asthma; in addition, the cardiac examination is notable for the lack of an enlarged apical impulse or an S_3 gallop.

Airway Obstruction

Aspiration with associated airway obstruction may produce acute dyspnea that can be mistaken for that of heart failure, as can the acute dyspnea associated with pneumonia or pneumothorax. However, a careful consideration of the entire clinical picture, with attention to the pulmonary examination indicating consolidation or absent breath sounds, helps the clinician distinguish heart failure from these pulmonary causes of dyspnea.

Pleural Effusions

Pleural effusions produce dyspnea of a more chronic nature that can be confused with heart failure. Dyspnea associated with effusions is usually gradual in onset and is nonexertional.[35] To further complicate this picture, clinicians must recall that pleural effusions may result from chronic heart failure or from other systemic conditions. Pleural effusions produce dyspnea through compression of underlying lung parenchyma and reduction in ventilated lung volume. Diminished breath sounds, dullness to percussion, and diminished tactile fremitus are noted on physical examination.

Pleural effusions are primarily transudative or exudative, both of which can help distinguish among the causes. Differentiation between transudative and exudative is based on the protein content and lactate dehydrogenase levels in the pleural fluid as compared with those levels in the serum. In all, 70% of transudative effusions are caused by heart failure because of abnormally high pleural capillary pressures. Transudative effusions can also result from liver failure, chronic renal failure, or hypoalbuminemia; however, these produce specific laboratory findings that can distinguish them from effusions caused by heart failure. Protein-enriched exudative effusions are primarily seen in malignancy, infection, and collagen vascular diseases.

Pulmonary Embolism

Pulmonary embolism may be initially seen with acute dyspnea and therefore be confused with heart failure. Symptoms of

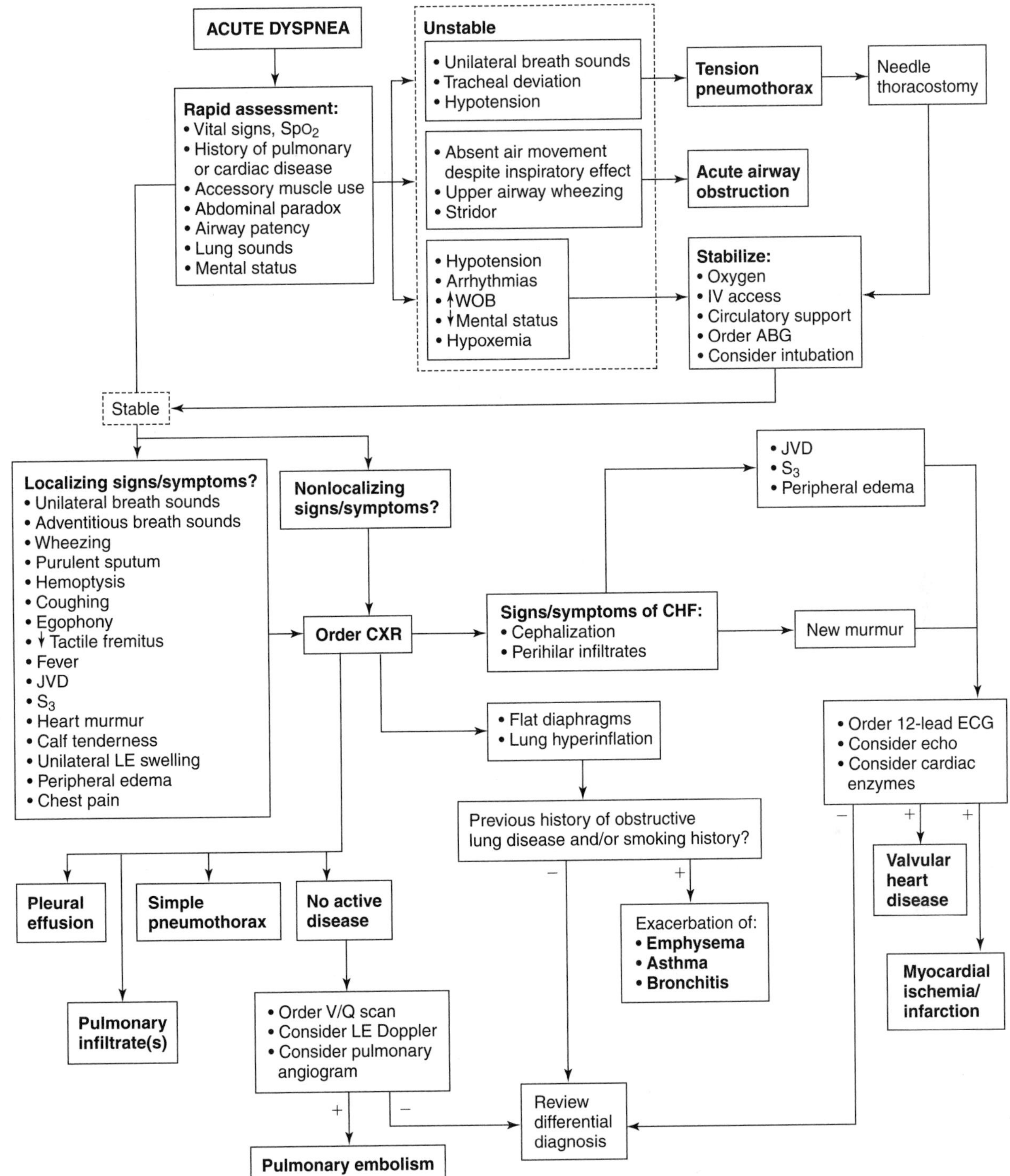

FIGURE 128-1

Acute dyspnea algorithm. *ABG,* Arterial blood gas; *BNP,* B natriuretic peptide; *CHF,* congestive heart failure; *CXR,* chest radiograph; *ECG,* electrocardiogram; *echo,* echocardiogram; *IV,* intravenous; *JVD,* jugular venous distention; *LE,* lower extremity; S_3, third heart sound; Spo_2, peripheral saturation of oxygen; *V/Q,* ventilation/perfusion ratio; *WOB,* work of breathing; ↑, increase; ↓, decrease; +, present; −, absent. (From Ferrin M, Tino G: Acute dyspnea, *AACN Clin Issues* 8(3):398-410, 1997.)

pulmonary embolism may be subtle and range from none, to mild dyspnea with pleuritic chest pain, to cardiac arrest. The most common cause of a pulmonary embolus, however, is a lower extremity deep vein thrombosis, which can cause unilateral leg pain and swelling that can suggest embolus as a cause for chest pain and dyspnea. In pulmonary embolus, arterial blood gas analysis may show hypoxemia; however, the best diagnostic test to identify a pulmonary embolus is the ventilation/perfusion scan, which exhibits ventilation/perfusion mismatch.

Neuromuscular Disorders

Neuromuscular disorders, such as myasthenia gravis and Guillain-Barré syndrome, can be differentiated from heart failure because the dyspnea from neuromuscular causes originate from respiratory muscle weakness, and other neurologic findings distinguish them from heart failure as well.

Anxiety

Finally, anxiety as the sole cause of dyspnea is uncommon and is always a diagnosis of exclusion. Clinicians must remember that anxiety is common with dyspnea of any cause, adds to the perceived severity, and prolongs the duration of the dyspnea.

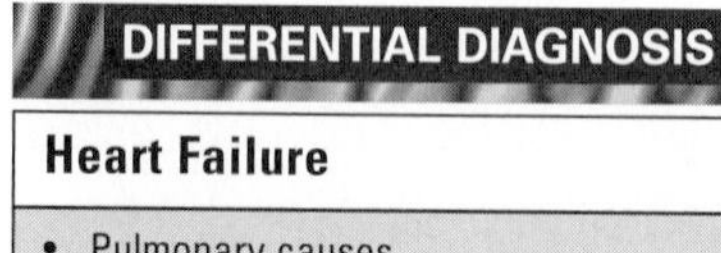

Heart Failure

- Pulmonary causes
- Cardiac causes
- Neuromuscular dysfunction
- Anxiety disorders

MANAGEMENT

Chronic or acute heart failure requires sufficient diagnostic testing to determine the specific cause. Coronary artery disease, valvular heart disease, and pericardial disease may be surgically treatable, mandating appropriate diagnostic studies. Once a specific diagnosis has been made, the first task in the treatment of heart failure is to treat specific reversible causes. Once reversible causes have been treated, management of the residual heart failure can be initiated. Heart failure caused by diastolic dysfunction must be differentiated from that caused by systolic dysfunction, since treatment options differ.

In general, the primary objectives in treatment of heart failure are fourfold: (1) prevention of further myocardial injury, (2) prevention of recurrence of clinical failure (congestive or low output), (3) relief of symptoms and signs, and (4) improvement in prognosis.[30] Correct selection and application of pharmacologic therapy require an understanding of the patient's pathophysiology and a careful history and physical examination.

The ACC/AHA classification stages represent a framework for management of left-sided heart failure. In stage A patients (risk, no symptoms, no structural abnormality), clear benefit exists for control of systolic and diastolic hypertension. Selected studies support treatment of lipid disorders, ACE inhibitor use in patients with diabetes and other cardiovascular risk factors, and control of tachycardic ventricular rates.[20] Benefits are unclear and are the result of expert consensus opinion for periodic evaluation for signs and symptoms of heart failure, smoking cessation, dietary salt reduction, nutritional supplements, avoidance of illicit drug use, limitation of alcohol consumption, or regular exercise.[20]

For stage B patients (those with structural heart disease, previous MI, left ventricular systolic dysfunction, and asymptomatic valvular disease, but without symptoms of failure), clear evidence exists for ACE inhibition and beta blockade, irrespective of the ejection fraction.[20] Evidence is unclear and is the result of consensus opinion for ACE inhibition or beta blockade for patients with reduced ejection fraction, valve replacement for hemodynamically significant stenosis or regurgitation, digoxin for patients with systolic dysfunction in sinus rhythm, or the recommendations made for stage A patients.[20]

Management for stage C patients (with known structural heart disease and with prior or current symptoms of failure) includes the health promotion measures previously mentioned in conjunction with daily weights, limitation of exercise during periods of acute decompensation, and close monitoring for decompensation. In these patients, nonadherence to medication and dietary regimens can precipitate rapid deterioration. Pharmacologic therapy in stage C typically involves four classes of medications: a diuretic, an ACE inhibitor, a beta blocker, and digitalis.[20]

In stage C patients, additional interventions have demonstrated value in selected patients. These include the use of aldosterone antagonists, angiotensin-receptor blockers, hydralazine, isosorbide dinitrate, and exercise training. Further interventions not currently recommended but under investigation include vasopeptidase inhibitors, endothelin antagonists, and cytokine antagonists. The value of synchronized biventricular pacing, external counterpulsation, and respiratory support techniques is being explored for patients with heart failure.[20]

Stage D patients with refractory heart failure require meticulous control of fluid balance. Clear evidence exits for benefit with both ACE inhibitors and beta blockers. It is important to recognize, however, that the increased role of neurohormonal factors in compensation of severe heart failure can place stage D patients at risk for hypotension and renal insufficiency with ACE inhibition, as well as at greater risk for increasing failure with beta blockade. Thus these agents should be used in small doses and with caution in these patients. Stage D patients are candidates for specialized interventions such as circulatory support measures, cardiac transplantation, and left ventricular assist devices.[20]

Pharmacologic Therapy Overview

Therapy for heart failure can be subdivided by pathophysiology (systolic vs. diastolic dysfunction) and by the level of symptomatic presentation defined by the NYHA classification. The NYHA subgroups are class I/II, without significant symptoms; class II/III, with mild to moderate signs and symptoms of clinical heart failure; and class III/IV, with persistent signs of disabling heart failure. Another way to view the overall management of systolic dysfunction (ejection fraction <40%) is based on the volume status. With no evidence of fluid excess, therapy with an ACE inhibitor (vasodilator) is begun.

Once the ACE dosage is stabilized, a beta blocker is added. A diuretic and/or digoxin can be added to manage new or persistent symptoms. With patients who have a fluid overload as evidenced by edema, pulmonary crackles, or jugular venous distention, therapy is initiated with a diuretic and an ACE inhibitor. When the patients are stabilized on these medications, digoxin may be added to reduce symptoms and increase exercise tolerance. Once the fluid overload is resolved, a beta-blocking agent may be added for persistent symptoms. Of course, a patient's renal status and other co-morbid conditions may affect decisions regarding therapy.

Vasodilators. Vasodilators reverse several of the characteristic physiologic compensatory mechanisms that accompany the development of heart failure. Vasodilators affect peripheral vasculature tone and have beneficial lowering effects on preload and afterload. Predominant venous vasodilators (such as nitroglycerin) increase venous compliance and redistribute blood volume to the venous capacitance vessels, thereby reducing ventricular filling volume and pressure. Predominant arterial vasodilators (such as ACE inhibitors) decrease arteriolar resistance, which reduces impedance to the left ventricular outflow, resulting in augmentation of the cardiac output and stroke volume. Vasodilators are an appropriate therapy for both systolic and diastolic dysfunction.

ACE Inhibitors. ACE inhibitors are the cornerstone of chronic management of symptomatic heart failure. The role of the ACE inhibitor emerged from the recognition that neurohormonal activation contributes to the pathogenesis of heart failure. By suppressing the production of angiotensin II, a potent vasoconstrictor, ACE inhibitors decrease systemic and pulmonary vascular resistance by preventing the release of aldosterone and norepinephrine while elevating the levels of the vasodilator hormone bradykinin.

ACE inhibitors should be considered a priority in all patients with left ventricular systolic dysfunction, unless absolutely contraindicated.[36] The following are potential contraindications: (1) history of compelling intolerance or adverse reaction to these agents, (2) serum potassium level greater than 5.5 mEq/L, or (3) symptomatic hypotension. Care should be used in patients who have a serum creatinine level greater than 3 mg/dl.[30] With the exception of these contraindications, ACE inhibitors should be used in all patients with left ventricular dysfunction and a left ventricular ejection fraction less than 40%, regardless of the level of symptoms.[38] ACE inhibitors have been shown to significantly reduce mortality, improve functional status, and reduce hospital admissions in patients with mild, moderate, and severe heart failure and left ventricular systolic dysfunction.[5,31,36-39] Concerns regarding side effects have been cited as a reason for the low usage of ACE inhibitors.[30] The average reduction in blood pressure and the abnormal alteration in serum chemistry values were quite small in the SOLVD trial, with only 2.2% of patients achieving a symptomatic reduction in blood pressure.[4] These results indicate that patients who begin ACE inhibitors should have their blood pressure, renal function, and serum potassium level monitored within 1 week. Maximum daily doses should be attempted in all patients (captopril 50 mg t.i.d., enalapril 20 mg b.i.d., lisinopril 40 mg q day).The ATLAS trial demonstrated more symptoms of heart failure and 25% higher neurohormonal levels patients receiving low vs. maximum doses of ACE inhibitors, indicating a significantly higher benefit with higher dosing.[38] Additional trials, including SMILE, TRACE, AIRE, SAVE, and CONSENSUS, have consistently demonstrated decreased mortality in heart failure patients after MI.[39] The HOPE trial revealed vasoprotective effects independent of blood pressure and remodeling effects. Additionally, a degradation product of angiotensin, the septapeptide angio IV, is thought to be involved in mediating states of hypercoagulability by stimulating release of plasminogen activator inhibitor, which would provide a plausible explanation for the beneficial effect of ACE inhibitors on risk of MI and other atherosclerotic events.[38,40] Despite the clear demonstration of benefits and nominal number of potential side effects, the EPICAL study notes continued underutilization of these drugs in daily practice.[41]

Angiotensin-Receptor Blocker Agents. Angiotensin-receptor blocking agents act directly on the angiotensin-renin-aldosterone system. These agents modify the effects of angiotensin II, the substance that promotes vasoconstriction, abnormal cell growth, and the release of aldosterone. All these responses, which are detrimental in heart failure, are mediated through the angiotensin I (AT1) receptor. Although ACE inhibitors decrease the conversion of angiotensin I to angiotensin II and prevent the breakdown of bradykinin, these agents do not completely suppress angiotensin II, which is formed by way of alternate pathways. Angiotensin-receptor blocker agents are selective for the AT1 receptor and thereby complete the process by interfering with the action of angiotensin II at the receptor level, shunting the angiotensin II to the AT2 receptor, which mediates vasodilation and decreased cell growth.[42] Recent evidence has shown that angiotensin receptor binders (ARBs) slow diabetic kidney failure and reduce worsening of renal function by 70% in type 2 diabetes.[43]

Losartan, irbesartan, valsartan, and candesartan (Atacand) are currently available in a variety of doses, which should be titrated with respect to blood pressure and laboratory monitoring when used alone or in conjunction with an ACE inhibitor.

Both the ELITE I and ELITE II trials compared losartan and captopril, revealing no significant difference in performance. The latter trial, however, revealed losartan to be better tolerated in terms of side effects. Subsequently, CHARM revealed a decrease in heart-related deaths and CHF hospital admissions when candesartan was added to standard therapy of beta blockers, ACE inhibitor, digoxin, diuretics, and aldactone. For those patients who cannot tolerate an ACE inhibitor, the CHARM-Alternative trial revealed a benefit from candesartan, which has led to U.S. Food and Drug Administration (FDA) approval for CHF for this medication alone. CHARM also showed a significant reduction in new-onset diabetes and a 9% reduction in relative risk in all-cause death.[44] It has been suggested that the addition of an ARB to an ACE inhibitor will provide more complete blockade of angiotensin II production, preventing more of the deleterious effects on the myocardium and the periphery. For this purpose, candesartan has been FDA approved for addition to ACE inhibitor therapy for NYHA class II to IV patients.[43-45]

Aspirin. Decreased risk of death has been demonstrated in patients with CHF taking aspirin with an ACE inhibitor vs. patients taking an ACE inhibitor alone.

Additional Options for Patients Unable to Tolerate ACE Inhibitors. Agency for Healthcare Research and Quality guidelines state that hydralazine combined with isosorbide dinitrate (Isordil) or isosorbide mononitrate (Imdur) is an appropriate alternative for patients who are unable to tolerate ACE inhibitors.[39]

Hydralazine is a direct arteriolar vasodilator, and isosorbide dinitrate is a venodilator. The combination of these agents results in an increase in cardiac output secondary to decreased impedance to ventricular ejection and decreased preload. The combination of hydralazine and isosorbide dinitrate improves survival and exercise tolerance in patients with heart failure.[4,46] These were the first medications to show improved survival in heart failure, but are currently not specifically recommended.[39] Side effects have been a significant problem in clinical trials, with 18% to 33% of patients discontinuing these medications because of headache, palpitations, and nasal congestion. Isosorbide dinitrate should generally be initiated at a dosage of 10 mg t.i.d. and increased weekly to 40 mg t.i.d. as tolerated. Hydralazine should be initiated at a dosage of 10 to 25 mg t.i.d. and increased weekly to 75 to 100 mg t.i.d. as tolerated. Therapy for hypotensive patients and those with severe heart failure should be initiated at lower doses. Three-times-per-day dosing is recommended to enhance compliance because poorer compliance and nitrate tolerance occur at four-times-per-day dosing.

Diuretics. Diuretics are important agents to relieve the signs and symptoms of systemic and pulmonary congestion caused by volume overload in heart failure. Many factors contribute to the sodium and water retention that causes volume overload in heart failure (Box 128-3). Diuretics promote sodium and fluid excretion, thus relieving both the symptoms (dyspnea, orthopnea, and paroxysmal nocturnal dyspnea) and the accompanying signs (crackles, S_3, jugular venous distention, hepatic engorgement, peripheral edema, and ascites) of volume overload.

Initial therapy with a thiazide diuretic is appropriate in mild heart failure, provided the creatinine clearance is greater than 30 ml/min. A loop diuretic, which is more potent, should be used with severe heart failure, renal insufficiency, or persistent edema, and can be used with a creatinine clearance of less than 30 ml/min.[30] If congestion does not resolve with a thiazide diuretic, a loop diuretic should be initiated to replace the thiazide diuretic. Symptoms of severe heart failure or significant renal dysfunction usually always require a loop diuretic agent. Loop diuretics are associated with acute and chronic distal tubular compensation and may be combined with a thiazide, thereby increasing diuretic potency by minimizing distal tubular compensation.[36] Diuretic dosing is summarized in Table 128-2. The standing dose of diuretic depends on the patient's body size, age, estimated glomerular filtration rate, renal function, amount of edema, and compliance with a low-sodium and fluid-restricted diet.

Intravascular volume depletion following diuretic administration reduces preload but has little effect on afterload. Excessive depletion of intravascular volume may actually increase afterload by causing reflex sympathetic stimulation and subsequent release of vasoconstrictors such as norepinephrine, epinephrine, renin, and angiotensin. Increased afterload may reduce cardiac output and lead to orthostatic hypotension, causing further activation of already augmented vasoconstrictive mechanisms. These diuretic-induced stimulatory effects on the renin-angiotensin-aldosterone system can be blocked to some extent by the concomitant administration of an ACE inhibitor.[47] Potent diuretics can cause serious electrolyte abnormalities such as hypokalemia and hypomagnesemia that require periodic measurement of serum potassium and magnesium. In instances of significant potassium wasting, potassium-sparing diuretics such as triamterene may be useful.

With disease progression the use of intermittent IV diuretics to overcome the significant neurohormonal responses that are antecedent to the increase in sodium and fluid retention may be necessary. A state of relative diuretic resistance is common in advanced heart failure or in long-term diuretic therapy. Metolazone, a potent oral thiazide-like agent, can be added to loop diuretics in such instances. Metolazone is usually effective with reduced renal function. Although the thiazide diuretics alone are usually ineffective in severe heart failure, the combination of a thiazide diuretic with a loop diuretic may be able to promote diuresis in refractory heart failure. Metolazone may be used in patients with renal failure, but should never be prescribed daily.

The RALES trial (Randomized Aldactone Survival Study) suggested a benefit in the addition of spironolactone in patients who had (1) symptoms of dyspnea at rest currently or within the past 6 months, or (2) "severe" or NYHA class IV heart failure.[36] This potassium-sparing diuretic and aldosterone antagonist is often helpful in promoting diuresis in patients taking high doses of loop diuretics and metolazone and has been shown to decrease both mortality and hospitalization rates in these patients. The blockade of aldosterone

BOX 128-3

FACTORS CONTRIBUTING TO EXCESS SODIUM AND WATER RETENTION IN HEART FAILURE

- Decreased cardiac output
- Decreased glomerular filtration rate secondary to reduced renal blood flow
- Redistribution of intrarenal blood flow to salt-conserving medulla
- Increased renal sympathetic nerve activity
- Increased arginine vasopressin (antidiuretic hormone) levels
- Activation of the renin-angiotensin-aldosterone system

From Moser DK, Cardin S: Heart failure. In Clochesy JM, Breu C, Cardin S, and others, editors: *Critical care nursing,* ed 2, Philadelphia, 1996, Saunders.

TABLE 128-2 Diuretics Used in Treatment of Chronic Heart Failure

Drug	Initial Dose (mg)	Recommended Maximum Dose (mg)	Potential Adverse Reactions
THIAZIDE DIURETICS			
Hydrochlorothiazide	25 q day	50 q day	Postural hypotension, hypokalemia, hyperuricemia
Chlorthalidone	25 q day	50 q day	
LOOP DIURETICS			
Furosemide	10-40 q day	240 b.i.d.	Same as thiazide diuretics
Bumetanide	0.5-1 q day	10 q day	
POTASSIUM-SPARING DIURETICS			
Spironolactone	25 q day	100 b.i.d.	Hyperkalemia (especially if given with ACE inhibitors), gynecomastia, rash
Triamterene	50 q day	100 b.i.d.	
Amiloride	5 q day	10 b.i.d.	
THIAZIDE-RELATED DIURETICS			
Metolazone (Zaroxolyn)	2.5 as single dose initially	20 q day	Same as with thiazide diuretics

From Konstam M, Dracup K, Baker D, and others: *Heart failure: evaluation and care of patients with left-ventricular systolic dysfunction,* Clinical Practice Guideline No 11, AHCPR Pub No 94-0612, Rockville, Md, 1994, US Department of Health and Human Services, Public Health Service, Agency for Health Care Policy and Research.
ACE, Angiotensin-converting enzyme.

receptors by spironolactone substantially reduced the risk of morbidity and death and improved symptoms as measured by NYHA class with benefits demonstrated in the first month after initiation of therapy.[47] Such diuretics promote hyperkalemia, however, and their use must be carefully monitored. Also, to date, no trials have assessed the safety or efficacy in patients with less severe heart failure.[36]

Digoxin. The cardiac glycosides, such as digoxin, have been used to treat heart failure for more than 200 years, but controversy still surrounds their use in heart failure.[48] Digoxin improves physical functioning and symptoms in patients with systolic dysfunction, but the addition of digoxin to diuretics and ACE inhibitors has not been clearly shown to reduce mortality.[36,49,50] There are three current recommendations for the use of digoxin in heart failure: (1) patients who have atrial fibrillation in conjunction with heart failure; (2) patients who have dyspnea at rest or a recent history of dyspnea at rest; and (3) those who remain symptomatic despite adequate dosages of diuretics, ACE inhibitors, and beta blockers.[36] In addition, the Digitalis Investigation Group trial revealed a trend toward excess mortality resulting from myocardial infarction and sudden death in those who likely had ischemic heart disease as the underlying cause of heart failure.[50]

Digoxin acts as a positive inotropic agent by increasing intracellular calcium in myocytes by altering calcium-sodium exchange (see Positive Inotropic Agents, p. 566, for further discussion). The increase in intracellular calcium available to actin-myosin filaments results in an increased contractile state of myocytes.[49] In addition, digoxin may resensitize baroreceptors that have been suppressed by increased neurohormonal sympathetic activity. Current evidence suggests that digoxin is an appropriate addition to ACE inhibitors and diuretics for the treatment of systolic dysfunction. Digoxin is not indicated in patients with primary diastolic dysfunction and preserved systolic function.[30,49]

Loading doses of digoxin are not necessary in heart failure. In the presence of normal renal function, the typical daily dose of 0.25 mg can be initiated. In patients with abnormal renal function, conduction defects, and small body size, as well as in older patients, digoxin dosing should be started at 0.125 mg/day and titrated on the basis of serum digoxin levels. There are numerous interactions between digoxin and other drugs, particularly amiodarone, quinidine, procainamide, diltiazem, verapamil, antibiotics, and anticholinergic agents. Patients taking these other agents should also be dosed with digoxin 0.125 mg/day.

There are no data to support regular measurement of serum digoxin levels. As a clinical rule of thumb, however, digoxin levels should be obtained when (1) heart failure worsens, (2) renal function deteriorates, (3) medications are added that affect digoxin levels, or (4) digoxin toxicity is suspected (Box 128-4). An adequately digitalized patient will have a serum digoxin concentration of 0.7 to 1.4 ng/ml; most patients with digoxin toxicity have elevated serum digoxin levels. Hypokalemia, hypomagnesemia, and hypercalcemia exacerbate digoxin toxicity.

Beta Blockers. One of the most important mechanisms responsible for progression of heart failure is activation of the sympathetic nervous system. This observation led to the

BOX 128-4

SIGNS OF DIGOXIN TOXICITY

- New arrhythmias
- Anorexia
- Nausea
- Confusion
- Visual disturbances

hypothesis that drugs that interfere with the actions of the sympathetic nervous system (e.g., beta blockers) may be beneficial in heart failure.[51] In several studies to date, beta blockers in carefully selected patients with heart failure have been shown to improve ventricular function, hemodynamics, functional status, and exercise tolerance, as well as reduce heart failure exacerbations.[52-57] In three published trials, as well as the COPERNICUS study (October 2002), treatment with carvedilol, metoprolol, or bisoprolol reduced mortality by at least 34% in patients with heart failure.[36] β-Adrenergic blocking agents exert their actions by occupying β-adrenergic receptor sites, which results in the inability of the beta agonists to exert their effects. Beta blockers reduce heart rate and thereby reduce myocardial oxygen consumption, inhibit the release of renin, and decrease the activation of the renin-angiotensin system.

Beta blockers are currently recommended for all patients with NHYA class II or III systolic heart failure. β-Adrenergic blockade is not recommended in those with heart failure who have bradycardia, significant heart block, or moderate to severe COPD and should be used with caution in patients with diabetes and at high risk for severe hypoglycemia. The benefits are especially well described for those patients with a history of MI and most patients with left ventricular dysfunction.[36]

Adjunctive Therapy

Anticoagulants. Many practitioners opt to anticoagulate patients with advanced systolic dysfunction (left ventricular ejection fraction <30% to 35%) because of the potential risk of systemic embolization. Review of a number of clinical trials has found that the risk is much lower than ordinarily thought, and data to date remain limited and controversial.[31,36,58] Further evidence suggests that the risks associated with anticoagulation may outweigh potential benefits in many patients with heart failure. Current recommendations are to avoid routine anticoagulation except in patients with heart failure who have a risk of embolization that is higher than baseline. Characteristics that place patients at a higher than baseline risk of cardiac thromboembolism include left ventricular ejection fraction of less than 30% to 35%, paroxysmal or chronic atrial fibrillation, or significant mitral regurgitation. There is no evidence to support use of anticoagulation in patients with sinus rhythm, even with a history of a previous vascular event or evidence of an intracardiac thrombus.[31]

Anticoagulation with warfarin with a target International Normalized Ratio (INR) of 2 to 3, along with close monitoring, is recommended. Close monitoring is especially important if right-sided heart failure and hepatic congestion worsen. Patients and their families need to understand the signs and symptoms of excess anticoagulation, as well as the need to take the appropriate dose of anticoagulant and to have blood work completed at the prescribed times.[30]

Antiarrhythmics. Between 35% and 50% of deaths resulting from heart failure are sudden and caused by presumed malignant tachyarrhythmias.[59] This observation has led to intense interest in the use of antiarrhythmic pharmacologic therapy and devices to reduce the risk of sudden arrhythmic cardiac death in patients with heart failure. Given the widespread availability of implantable cardioverter-defibrillators (ICDs) in particular, management of ventricular arrhythmias in patients with heart failure is rapidly evolving.

Frequent premature ventricular contractions (PVCs) and nonsustained ventricular tachycardia are common in heart failure as a result of elevated ventricular wall stress, focal myocardial fibrosis, electrolyte imbalances, effects of pharmacologic agents, high levels of circulating catecholamines, and myocardial ischemia. As the severity of heart failure progresses, nonsustained ventricular tachycardia is a nearly ubiquitous finding on Holter or telemetry monitoring. Although the presence of nonsustained ventricular tachycardia is a marker of a poorer prognosis, it is not necessarily a marker of a greater risk of sudden cardiac death.[60] There is no evidence to date that the suppression of asymptomatic PVCs or nonsustained ventricular tachycardia by antiarrhythmics is beneficial in patients with heart failure; however, a number of adverse factors are associated with the use of antiarrhythmic agents in patients with heart failure. Class I agents are considered to be proarrhythmic on the ventricular level, whereas class II agents have been associated with sudden death in heart failure.[31,61] On the basis of these facts, the routine use of antiarrhythmics in patients with heart failure who have brief, asymptomatic episodes of nonsustained ventricular tachycardia is not recommended.

Amiodarone. Two interventions that hold promise for patients with symptomatic or malignant arrhythmias and heart failure are amiodarone and the ICD. Amiodarone is effective against most supraventricular and ventricular arrhythmias and may restore sinus rhythm in patients with heart failure and atrial fibrillation. Amiodarone is the only antiarrhythmic drug without clinically significant negative inotropic effects. Data to date, however, do not show an improvement in overall mortality. In addition, potential side effects include hyperthyroidism or hypothyroidism, hepatitis, neuropathy, and pulmonary fibrosis. Careful monitoring is required with the use of amiodarone, and routine administration is not recommended in patients with heart failure.[31]

Implantable Cardioverter-Defibrillators. ICDs reliably detect and terminate malignant ventricular arrhythmias. In patients with reduced ejection fraction, prior MI, and inducible ventricular tachycardia, ICDs prevent sudden cardiac death. The role of ICDs in patients with reduced ejection fraction and prior myocardial and nonischemic cardiomyopathy is under investigation. As the cost, ease of implantation, and safety of ICDs improve, ICDs will likely be implanted more often in patients with significant depression of systolic function.

Positive Inotropic Agents. Positive inotropic agents increase the force of myocardial contraction. Despite the development of the newer generations of effective vasodilators, there is an ongoing search for a safe and efficacious orally administered positive inotropic agent. The long-term use of oral inotropic agents in clinical studies has been hampered by their risk of precipitating serious ventricular arrhythmias and increasing the risk of sudden cardiac death. To date, nearly every long-term orally administered inotropic agent has led to an increase in mortality from sudden cardiac death in patients with heart failure. There is as yet no safe, available oral inotropic agent other than digoxin.[62]

Long-term use of parenteral positive inotropic agents such as phosphodiesterase inhibitors (milrinone, amrinone, enoximone) and β-adrenergic agonists (dobutamine) has resulted in improved symptoms but increased rates of sudden cardiac death when patients receive therapy at home.[63,64] At present the use of continuous or intermittent parenteral positive inotropic agents is largely palliative in patients with end-stage heart failure. Such agents can be helpful, however, for patients with refractory volume overload or threatened end-organ dysfunction. Dobutamine directly stimulates β-adrenergic receptors of the heart, leading to an increase in heart rate and contractile force. The self-limited institution of an IV inotropic agent such as dobutamine can transiently improve systolic function, palliate low-output states, and improve end-organ dysfunction. Renal performance can also be improved with low-dose dopamine, which stimulates renal dopaminergic receptors, leading to renal vasodilation.[30] At higher doses dopamine may be deleterious by increasing myocardial oxygen demand and afterload. Because both dopamine and dobutamine at higher doses may cause vasoconstriction, the potent vasodilator nitroprusside may be necessary to counteract this vasoconstrictor effect.

Nesiritide, a synthetic BNP, has been under scrutiny by investigators and has proven safer than dobutamine when give parenterally in acutely decompensated heart failure. Cardiovascular dynamics improved much the same as with other vasodilators, inodilators, and inotropes in this condition, but nesiritide is better tolerated and is not shown to be a proarryhthmic.[40]

These results underscore the importance of factors other than myocardial contractility in determining the outcome of heart failure. To date, improvements in contractility have not led to improved outcomes. Continual pharmacologic modulation of myocardial preload and afterload, as well as pharmacologic inhibition of progressive myocyte hypertrophy and myocardial chamber dilation, are likely to be of more importance.

Vasopressin 2 Antagonist. In the ACTIV trial, tolvaptan, a new oral vasopressin receptor antagonist, was shown to reduce weight, decreasing reliance on diuretics, and normalize sodium in heart failure patients, who typically suffer from fluid retention and hyponatremia. This was not associated with acute or chronic changes in blood pressure, changes in serum potassium, or increases in BUN and creatinine and shows significant promise as an additional intervention. A large-scale trial, EVEREST, is currently underway to assess effects on mortality in patients hospitalized for CHF.[65]

Nonpharmacologic Therapy

The modern approach to the management of chronic heart failure is directed primarily at manipulating myocardial preload and afterload. Although pharmacologic therapy is the mainstay of treatment for patients with heart failure, several nonpharmacologic interventions are important and useful adjuncts to overall management.

Diet. Reduced-sodium diets have been recommended for the management of heart failure, although as yet no clinical studies have evaluated a specific sodium restriction. Volpe, Tritto, DeLuca, and others found that patients with mild heart failure exhibited impaired sodium excretion when given a high-sodium diet as compared with normal subjects.[66] In addition, patients with heart failure did not have an increase in atrial natriuretic factor in response to the oral sodium load, whereas in normal subjects atrial natriuretic factor increased by 40%. These findings underscore the susceptibility of sodium retention in patients with mild heart failure and indirectly support the usefulness of sodium restriction.

Diets restricted to 2 g of sodium are somewhat unpalatable for most patients, and the added cost of low-sodium foods makes adherence to them a challenge. However, patients with severe heart failure should try to adhere to a 2-g sodium diet whenever possible. Patients with mild to moderate heart failure should be advised to follow a 3-g sodium diet, which is a more reasonable and realistic goal for most patients and their families. This diet can be attained by avoiding foods with high sodium content, removing the salt shaker from the table, and not cooking with salt. Patients with heart failure require specific dietary instructions and guidelines on how to read the labels on all food packages. Involvement of family members who prepare the foods cannot be underestimated; these persons need to be included in all dietary education.

Alcohol consumption should be infrequent and modest. Alcohol should be completely prohibited in any patient with known or suspected alcohol-induced cardiomyopathy.[30]

Sudden increases in sodium intake in patients with well-compensated but relatively severe heart failure can lead to acute decompensation. Holidays and seasonal festivities are particularly problematic because of the alteration in food preparation, increased daily activity levels, and increase in emotional stressors during these times. Ethnic foods prepared during holiday seasons are often high in sodium. Careful selection and alterations in holiday eating patterns need to be discussed with patients and their families, and alternative food choices offered. Dietary referral may be beneficial.

Activity. Until recently, reduced activity, including occasional periods of bed rest, were considered a standard part of management for patients with heart failure. Bed rest is thought to promote diuresis in the short term, but in the long term the negative effects of bed rest likely outweigh its benefits.

The clinical benefits of exercise training result from the salutary effects of exercise on skeletal muscle rather than substantial improvements in myocardial function. Both bicycle ergometry and arm ergometry have been used for training programs, and improvements in patients who exercise at home have been noted.

Studies have demonstrated improvements in exercise tolerance and patient symptoms with varying modes, intensities, durations, and frequencies of exercise.[67,68] Therefore guidelines regarding exercise for patients with heart failure are not clear at present. It is necessary to adapt recommendations regarding exercise to the patient's current health status. Box 128-5 lists the relative criteria for initiating or increasing an exercise training program.

BOX 128-5

EXERCISE TRAINING GUIDELINES FOR PATIENTS WITH HEART FAILURE

Relative criteria for the initiation of an aerobic exercise training program in compensated heart failure
- Ability to speak without signs or symptoms of dyspnea (able to speak comfortably with a respiratory rate of <30 breaths per minute)
- Less than moderate fatigue
- Crackles (rales) present in more than half of the lungs
- Resting heart rate of <120 beats per minute
- Cardiac index of ≥1.8 L/min/m^2 (for invasively monitored patients)
- Central venous pressure of <12 mm Hg (for invasively monitored patients)

Relative criteria indicating a need to modify or terminate exercise training
- Marked dyspnea or fatigue
- Respiratory rate >40 breaths per minute during exercise
- Development of an S_3 heart sound or pulmonary crackles
- Increase in pulmonary crackles
- Increase in the sound of the second component of the second heart sound (P_2)
- Poor pulse pressure (<10 mm Hg difference between the systolic and diastolic blood pressure)
- Decrease in heart rate or blood pressure of >10 beats per minute or 10 mm Hg, respectively, during continuous (steady state) or progressive (increasing workload) exercise
- Increased supraventricular or ventricular ectopy
- Increase of >10 mm Hg in the mean pulmonary artery pressure (for invasively monitored patients)
- Increase or decrease of >6 mm Hg in the central venous pressure (for invasively monitored patients)
- Diaphoresis, pallor, or confusion

Modified from Cahalin L: Exercise training guidelines for patients with congestive heart failure, *Phys Ther* 76:516-533, 1997.

For most patients a regular walking program may be the most effective and functional mode of exercise. Most patients should begin with frequent, short walks and progress to less frequent, longer walks. Progression is based on individual prescriptions with adequate rest periods. Because dyspnea is the most common complaint, the level of perceived dyspnea is an acceptable method to define exercise intensity. Patients should exercise to a level that produces a moderate degree of dyspnea, with a rating of 3 on a scale of 1 to 10 (no dyspnea to dyspnea to the greatest degree).

Surgical Therapy

Mechanical Circulatory Support. For hospitalized patients with heart failure who have severe symptoms despite maximum medical therapy, including parenteral inotropic agents, mechanical circulatory support with intraaortic balloon pumps (IABPs) and ventricular assist devices (VADs) may provide a lifesaving bridge to cardiac transplantation.

Intraaortic balloon counterpulsation unloads the left ventricle and increases coronary artery perfusion. Myocardial ischemia is ameliorated, and left ventricular performance improves. The intraaortic balloon is positioned in the descending aorta, and it is inflated and deflated in synchrony with the mechanical events of the cardiac cycle. The usual role of the IABP in patients with heart failure is supportive while the patient is waiting for emergent cardiac transplantation.

VADs (e.g., external centrifugal pumps, extracorporeal membrane oxygenation systems, pulsatile short-term pumps, internal mechanical assist devices) were originally designed to support the left ventricle. Current VADs may also be used to support the right ventricle. Unlike the IABP, VADs completely unload either the right or left ventricle. The indication for VAD is cardiogenic shock refractory to conventional pharmacologic therapy and to IABP.[68]

Currently, the mean duration of mechanical circulatory support before transplantation is 50 days.[69] For this reason, considerable effort is made to support patients with portable left VADs outside the hospital. For portable VADs, the assist device pump or energy converter is implanted surgically, and the control or power source is worn externally. The control units and batteries are lighter (3.6 kg [8 pounds]) than those in the past and allow patients to be ambulatory.[70] Patients in whom a VAD has been implanted and who go on to transplantation have a long-term survival rate similar to that of patients who undergo routine transplantation.

Cardiac Transplantation. Cardiac transplantation is a reasonable therapeutic option for end-stage heart failure. For patients with severe symptoms and diminished life expectancy, cardiac transplantation may offer the only hope of improved quality of life and survival. After transplantation, survival is 85% at 1 year and 70% at 5 years.[71] In patients with severe symptoms almost refractory to medical therapy, the quality of life is clearly better for those who undergo cardiac transplantation.[23] Unfortunately, cardiac transplantation is an option for relatively few patients because of the limited supply of donor hearts. At any one time there can be 2800 people on the donor waiting list for a heart transplant.[72] Careful and expert medical management in selected patients may provide acceptable outcomes when cardiac transplantation is unavailable because of the shortage of donor hearts.

COMPLICATIONS

Arrhythmias

Studies have demonstrated a high prevalence of ventricular and atrial arrhythmias in patients with heart failure. Atrial fibrillation occurs in at least 20% of patients with heart failure and is associated with increased mortality.[73] Patients with rapid atrial fibrillation require rate control with either digoxin, a beta blocker, or in some cases a calcium channel blocker. At least one attempt at chemical or electrical cardioversion should be undertaken in most patients with heart failure and atrial fibrillation. Uncontrolled or new-onset atrial fibrillation can worsen heart failure or lead to acute decompensation. It is always prudent to try to convert new-onset atrial fibrillation to normal sinus rhythm. This often requires several weeks of anticoagulation and initiation of closely supervised antiarrhythmic therapy.

Low-dose amiodarone is an increasingly attractive option as an atrial stabilizing agent in patients with symptoms refractory to other agents. In rare instances, catheter ablation may be necessary to prevent uncontrolled, rapid ventricular rates,[24] especially in patients with hypertrophic cardiomyopathy or severe left ventricular failure.

Ventricular arrhythmias are present in nearly all patients with heart failure. Asymptomatic ventricular arrhythmias should not be treated. Because all antiarrhythmic agents can produce negative inotropic effects or proarrhythmia in patients with heart failure, initiation of therapy should occur in a hospital setting.

Progressive Dysfunction

It has been shown that recurrent exacerbations lead to hemodynamic alterations, including progressive ventricular dysfunction, subendocardial ischemia, change in left ventricular shape, and progression of remodeling.[74]

Metabolism

Longstanding severe heart failure may lead to anorexia as a result of hepatic and intestinal congestion. Occasionally there is impaired intestinal absorption of fat and protein.[75] The patient with heart failure may have an increase in total metabolism from an augmentation of myocardial oxygen consumption; excessive work of breathing; low-grade fevers; and elevated levels of tumor necrosis factor, a cytokine produced by monocytes.[76] The combination of reduced caloric intake and higher metabolism leads to a reduction in tissue mass that is often masked by the increase in fluid retention.

In heart failure, caloric malnutrition may be related to anorexia and early satiety, fat malabsorption may be due to congestion or altered hepatic management of lipids, and protein malnutrition may be related to changes in the bowel from elevated lymphatic production as a result of elevated systemic venous pressure. Medical therapy with vasodilators and diuretics tailored to normalize intracardiac pressures may decrease the prevalence of malnutrition in patients with heart failure.[75]

Vitamin supplements may be advisable for water-soluble vitamin loss associated with diuresis and problems with intestinal absorption of the fat-soluble vitamins. Frequent small snacks may also assist patients in meeting their caloric intake, and excessive fluid intake should be avoided.

INDICATIONS FOR REFERRAL OR HOSPITALIZATION

Patients with heart failure may benefit from cardiology consultation when symptoms appear to be refractory to the standard therapies of vasodilators, diuretics, ACE inhibitors, and digoxin. The onset of arrhythmias, coronary ischemia, or MI should prompt consultation as well. Cardiac transplantation may be considered for young patients failing to respond to maximum medical therapy.

Even with pharmacologic advances in heart failure management, the hospital readmission rate among older patients is between 29% and 47%.[77] This high readmission rate is related to inadequate symptom management by the patient, nonadherence to complex pharmacologic schedules and dietary regimens, social isolation, and the natural illness trajectory.[77]

Thus there has been increasing interest in developing disease management guidelines and strategies. Seven management strategies identified by a cardiology advisory board were (1) heart failure clinics, (2) home health advanced practice nurses, (3) community-based case managers, (4) patient telemanagement, (5) cardiac rehabilitation, (6) emergency department observation units, and (7) heart failure subacute care.[78]

Heart failure clinics have provided a mechanism for patients to be seen in a clinic for physical assessment, medication instruction, dietary education, and exercise training. For patients with heart failure who are unable to attend clinic sessions, the home health advanced practice nurse may be an appropriate referral. The advanced practice nurse with expertise in heart failure can see the patient at home three times per week for assessment of weight, vital signs, heart and lung sounds, and signs of peripheral edema. During the home visit the advanced practice nurse can continue patient teaching regarding medications, diet, and activity and develop a plan with the patient and family regarding emergency care and when to call the health care provider.

The use of telemedicine technology as a tool in disease management is expanding rapidly to meet the needs of patients in integrated health care delivery systems. A number of innovative attempts at telemedicine with patients with heart failure are underway and may be potential alternatives for management of these patients in their home.[79,80] Specifically, patients with heart failure are using telephone and computer technology to transmit data on vital signs, symptoms, and weight to a central repository where the health care providers can review trends.

Indications for hospitalization include suspicion of new-onset heart failure for diagnostic evaluation, clinical or ECG evidence of acute myocardial ischemia, pulmonary edema or severe respiratory distress, oxygen saturation below 90%, severe medical complications (e.g., pneumonia, renal failure), anasarca, symptomatic hypotension or syncope, heart failure refractory with maximal treatment program, and the need to evaluate home support for safe management in the community.[30]

In addition, hospitalization may be necessary for IV administration of diuretics such as metolazone to reduce interstitial edema, and for the institution of IV dobutamine to increase renal blood flow, or IV nesiritide to improve hemodynamics.[30,40]

LIFESPAN CONSIDERATIONS

Heart failure associated with normal left ventricle ejection fraction is more prevalent with increasing age.[81] Older women have a higher incidence of heart failure with a normal left ventricle ejection fraction than men.[81] Any co-morbidities should be treated in these patients with heart failure, particularly anemia, hyperthyroidism or hypothyroidism, and sleep apnea. Recommendations include managing systolic hypertension with diuretics, ACE inhibitors, and beta blockers; and using nitrates and beta blockers to treat myocardial ischemia.[81] In addition, nonsteroidal inflammatory medications should be avoided in elderly patients at risk for heart failure.[81]

EMERGING EVIDENCE

Our knowledge about the origins and mechanisms of and treatments for heart failure is continually evolving. Health care providers are advised to monitor specialty organizations, journals, and other guideline sources for timely information to make the best treatment decisions for their heart failure patients. One area of emerging evidence is the role of α-adrenergic receptors in heart failure and the therapeutic effect in treatment of heart failure with medications that are α-adrenergic receptor–blocking agents.[82]

Patients with heart failure many times have atrial fibrillation as a co-morbidity. A recent study demonstrated that candesartan reduced the occurrence of new onset atrial fibrillation in a population of patients with heart failure over a 37-month period.[83]

The use of aldosterone blockage is an area that potentially could have a large impact on the management of heart failure after acute myocardial infarction (AMI) with resulting systolic dysfunction. Results from the Eplerenone Post-Acute Myocardial Infarction Heart Failure Efficacy and Survival Study (EPHESUS) indicate that adding eplerenone to the standard therapy for heart failure in post-AMI patients demonstrated improvement in their outcomes. The recommendation from the researchers in this study is to conduct further investigations to guide the use of disease- and mechanism-targeted therapies, instead of the current symptom-focused approach to heart failure treatment.[84]

Statin medications are another therapy that has shown promise with heart failure patients in one study. Patients who had been diagnosed with heart failure were analyzed for use of statins and subsequent outcomes. Those patients who had not previously used statins but started them at the time of their heart failure diagnosis were found to have lower risks of subsequent hospitalization and death.[85]

These are exciting developments in the understanding and management of heart failure. Further investigations and consultations with cardiac specialists will guide use of these in individual heart failure patients.

PATIENT AND FAMILY EDUCATION

Many of the important concepts for managing heart failure are discussed in previous sections of this chapter. Patients and their families can take an active role in the management of this disorder if they understand the condition and its treatments. Support for weight reduction and smoking cessation, if applicable, may be helpful. Reinforcement of the importance of restricting salt, reducing stress, taking medications (and reporting side effects), and balancing rest with exercise is also of benefit. All patients should be weighed daily or every other day and should call the health care provider if they have a weight gain of more than 0.9 kg (2 pounds) in 2 days.

HEALTH PROMOTION

Prevention of CHF is linked to prevention of ischemic heart disease. Accordingly, all patients should be screened for heart disease risk and encouraged to reduce their risk by adopting a healthy lifestyle, including normalization of weight, low-fat diet, smoke exposure avoidance, and exercise. Interventions to screen for heart disease risk include a family history, blood pressure measurement, lipid screen, and blood glucose or hemoglobin A_{1C} to screen for diabetes. Patients should be encouraged to seek medical attention promptly for any heart attack signs or symptoms, unexplained fatigue, or dyspnea. Good control of blood pressure and diabetes is an essential component of prevention of CHF. Other cardiovascular diseases need close monitoring with timely intervention for any condition change.

REFERENCES

1. Packer M: Survival of patients with chronic heart failure and its potential modification by drug therapy. In Cohn JN, editor: *Drug treatment of heart failure,* ed 2, Secaucus, NJ, 1998, ATC International.
2. Braunwald E, Colucci WS, Grossman W: Aspects of heart failure: high-output failure: pulmonary edema. In Braunwald E, editor: *Heart disease,* ed 5, Philadelphia, 1997, Saunders.
3. Cohn JN, Johnson G, Ziesche S, and others: A comparison of enalapril with hydralazine-isosorbide dinitrate in the treatment of chronic congestive heart failure, *N Engl J Med* 325:303-310, 1991.
4. SOLVD Investigators: Effect of enalapril on survival in patients with reduced left ventricular ejection fractions and congestive heart failure, *N Engl J Med* 325:293-302, 1991.
5. Tajik A, Watson T: New Horizons in the management of cardiovascular disease, *Heart Views* 5(4):135-139, 2004.
6. Senni M, Rodeheffer RJ, Tribouilloy CM, and others: Use of echocardiography in the management of congestive heart failure in the community, *J Am Coll Cardiol* 33:164-170, 1999.
7. Kannel WB: Need and prospects for prevention of cardiac failure, *Eur J Clin Pharmacol* 49:S3-S9, 1996.
8. Kannel WB, Belanger AJ: Epidemiology of heart failure, *Am Heart J* 121:951-957, 1991.
9. Schocken DD, Arrieta MI, Leaverton PE: Prevalence and mortality rate of congestive heart failure in the United States, *J Am Coll Cardiol* 20:301-306, 1992.
10. Levy D: Heart and stroke statistics, 2003 update, *N Engl J Med* 347:1397, 2002.
11. Friedman MM: Older adults' symptoms and their duration before hospitalization for heart failure, *Heart Lung* 26:169-176, 1997.
12. Ho KK, Pinksy JL, Kannel WB, and others: The epidemiology of heart failure: the Framingham study, *J Am Coll Cardiol* 22(Suppl A):6A-13A, 1993.
13. National Heart, Lung, and Blood Institute: *National Institutes of Health data fact sheet,* Bethesda, Md, 1996, US Department of Health and Human Services, Public Health Services.
14. Rich MW: Epidemiology, pathophysiology, and etiology of congestive heart failure in older adults, *J Am Geriatr Soc* 45:968-974, 1997.
15. Goldsmith SR, Dick C: Differentiating systolic from diastolic heart failure: pathophysiologic and therapeutic considerations, *Am J Med* 95:645-655, 1993.
16. Zucker IH: Baro and cardiac reflex abnormalities in chronic heart failure. In Zucker IH, Gilmore JP, editors: *Reflex control of the circulation,* Boca Raton, Fla, 1991, CRC Press.
17. Benedict CR, Johnstone DE, Weiner DH, and others: Relation of neurohormonal activation to clinical variables and degree of left ventricular dysfunction: a report from the Registry of Studies of Left Ventricular Dysfunction, *J Am Coll Cardiol* 23:1410-1420, 1994.
18. Katz SD, Biasucci L, Sabba C, and others: Impaired endothelium-mediated vasodilatation in the peripheral vasculature of patients with congestive heart failure, *J Am Coll Cardiol* 19:918-925, 1992.
19. Opie LH: *The heart: physiology and metabolism,* New York, 1991, Raven Press.
20. American College of Cardiology/American Heart Association Committee: ACC/AHA guidelines for the evaluation and management of chronic heart failure in the adult, *Circulation* 104:2996-3007, 2001.
21. Wagoner A: Congestive heart failure and the role of two-dimensional Doppler echocardiography: a primer for cardiac sonographers, *J Am Soc Echocardiogr* 13:157-163, 2000.
22. Wilson JR, Mancini DM: Factors contributing to the exercise limitation of heart failure, *Circulation* 22(Suppl A):93A-98A, 1993.
23. Manning HL, Schwartzstein RM: Mechanism of disease: pathophysiology of dyspnea, *N Engl J Med* 333:1547-1553, 1995.

24. Stevenson LW, Perloff JK: The limited reliability of physical signs for estimating hemodynamics in chronic heart failure, *JAMA* 261:884-888, 1989.
25. Hunt SA, Abraham WT, Chin MH, and others: ACC/AHA 2005 Guideline Update for the diagnosis and management of chronic heart failure in the adult: report of the American College of Cardiology/American Heart Association Task Force on Practice Guidelines, *Circulation* 112:e154-e235, 2005.
26. Latini R, Masson S, deAngelis N, and others: Role of brain natriuretic peptide in the diagnosis and management of heart failure: current concepts, *J Card Fail* 8(5):288-299, 2002.
27. Villacorta H, Duarte A, Duarte NM, and others: The role of B-type natriuretic peptide in the diagnosis of congestive heart failure in patients presenting to an emergency department with dyspnea, *Arq Bras Cardiol* 79(6):569-572, 2002.
28. Waknine Y: *BNP test quick, useful for differential diagnosis of CHF,* Oct 8, 2004, retrieved Dec 1, 2005 from http://www.medscape.com/viewarticle/490981.
29. Ng LL, Loke I, O'Brien RJ, and others: Plasma urotensin in human systolic heart failure, *Circulation* 106(23):2877-2880, 2002.
30. Konstam MA, Dracup K, Baker D, and others: *Heart failure: evaluation and care of patients with left-ventricular systolic dysfunction*, Clinical Practice Guideline No 11, AHCPR Pub No 94-0612, Rockville, Md, 1994, US Department of Health and Human Services, Public Health Services, Agency for Health Care Policy and Research.
31. Remme WJ: Guidelines for the diagnosis and treatment of congestive heart failure, *Eur Heart J* 22:1527-1560, 2001.
32. Griffin BP, Shah PK, Diamond GA, and others: Incremental prognostic value of exercise hemodynamic variables in chronic congestive heart failure secondary to coronary artery disease or to dilated cardiomyopathy, *Am J Cardiol* 67:848-853, 1991.
33. Guyatt GH, Thompson PJ, Berman LB, and others: How should we measure function in patients with chronic heart and lung disease? *J Chronic Dis* 38:517-524, 1985.
34. Cahalin LP, Mathier MA, Semigran MJ, and others: The 6-minute walk test predicts peak oxygen uptake and survival in advanced heart failure, *Chest* 110:325-332, 1996.
35. Bittner V, Weiner DH, Yusuf S, and others: Prediction of mortality and morbidity with a 6-minute walk test in patients with left ventricular dysfunction, *JAMA* 270:1702-1707, 1993.
36. Chavey WE, Blaum CS, Bleske BE, and others: Guideline for the management of heart failure caused by systolic dysfunction, part II, Treatment, *Am Fam Phys* 64(6):1045-1054, 2001.
37. Arbab-Zadeh A, Demaria A, Penny WF, and others: Axial movement of the intravascular probe during the cardiac cycle: implications for three dimensional reconstruction and measurements of coronary dimensions, *Am Heart J* 150(5):994-999, 2005.
38. Brunner-La Rocca H, Weilenmann D, Kiowski W, and others: Within-patient comparison of effects of different dosages of enalapril on functional capacity and neurohormone levels in patients with chronic heart failure, *Am Heart J* 138(4):654-662, 1999.
39. Greenberg B, Quinones MA, Koilpalli C, and others: The effects of long term enalapril therapy on cardiac structure and function in patients with left ventricular dysfunction: results of the SOLVD echocardiography substudy, *Circulation* 91(10):2573-2581, 1995.
40. Tajik A, Watson T: New Horizons in the management of cardiovascular disease, *Heart Views* 5(4):135-144, 2003-2004.
41. Echemann M: Determinants of angiotensin-converting enzyme inhibitor prescription in severe heart failure with left ventricular systolic dysfunction: the EPICAL study, *Am Heart J* 139:624-631, 2000.
42. Miller AB: Angiotensin receptor blockers and aldosterone antagonists in congestive heart failure, *Cardiol Clin* 19:195-202, 2001.
43. Ramahi, T: Expanded role for ARBs in cardiovascular and renal disease? *Postgrad Med* 109(4):115-122, 2001.
44. Dunlap ME, Pfeffer MA, Probstfield JL, and others: *CHARM trial: heart failure drug saves lives, reduces hospitalizations,* Oct 19, 2004, retrieved Dec 1, 2005, from http://www.americanheart.org/presenter.jhtml?identifier=3025706.
45. Carson PE: Rationale for the use of combination angiotensin-converting enzyme inhibitor/angiotensin II receptor blocker therapy in heart failure, *Am Heart J* 140:361-366, 2000.
46. SOLVD Investigators: Effects of enalapril on mortality and the development of heart failure in asymptomatic patients with reduced left-ventricular ejection fraction, *N Engl J Med* 327:685-691, 1992.
47. Pitt B, Zannad F, Remme WJ, and others: The effect of spironolactone on morbidity and mortality in patients with severe heart failure: Randomized Aldactone Evaluation Study Investigators, *N Engl J Med* 341:709-716, 1999.
48. Cohn JM, Archibald DG, Ziesche S, and others: Effects of vasodilator therapy on mortality in chronic heart failure: results of a Veterans Administration Cooperative Study, *N Engl J Med* 314:1547-1552, 1986.
49. Captopril-Digoxin Multicenter Research Group: Comparative effects of therapy with captopril and digoxin in patients with mild to moderate heart failure, *JAMA* 259:539-544, 1988.
50. Kelly RA, Smith TW: Digoxin in heart failure: implications of recent trials, *J Am Coll Cardiol* 22(Suppl A):107A-112A, 1993.
51. Packer M, Gheorghiade M, Young JB, and others: Withdrawal of digoxin from patients with chronic heart failure treated with angiotensin-converting enzyme inhibitors: RADIANCE Study, *N Engl J Med* 329:1-7, 1993.
52. DiBianco R, Shabetai R, Kostuk W, and others: A comparison of oral milrinone, digoxin, and their combination in the treatment of patients with chronic heart failure, *N Engl J Med* 320:677-683, 1989.
53. Jaeschle R, Oxman AD, Guyatt GH: To what extent do congestive heart failure patients in sinus rhythm benefit from digoxin therapy? A systematic overview and meta-analysis, *Am J Med* 88:279-286, 1990.
54. Colucci WS, Packer M, Bristow MR, and others: Carvedilol inhibits clinical progression in patients with mild heart failure: US Carvedilol Heart Failure Group, *Circulation* 94:2800-2806, 1996.
55. Bristow MR: Pathophysiologic and pharmacologic rationales for clinical management of chronic heart failure with beta-blocking agents, *Am J Cardiol* 71:12C-22C, 1993.
56. Eichhorn EJ, Hjalmarson A: Beta-blocker treatment for chronic heart failure, *Circulation* 90:2153-2156, 1994.
57. CIBIS Investigators and Committees: A randomized trial of beta-blockade in heart failure: the Canadian Insufficiency Bisoprolol Study (CIBIS), *Circulation* 90:1765-1773, 1994.
58. Australia/New Zealand Heart Failure Research Collaborative Group: Randomised, placebo-controlled trial of carvedilol in patients with congestive heart failure due to ischaemic heart disease, *Lancet* 349:375-380, 1997.
59. Cohn JN, Benedict CR, LeJemtel TH, and others: Thromboembolism in left ventricular dysfunction, *Circulation* 86(Suppl I):252, 1992.
60. Podrid PJ, Fogel RI, Fuchs TT: Ventricular arrhythmias in congestive failure, *Am J Cardiol* 69:82G-98G, 1992.
61. Cleland J, Alamgir F, Nikitin NP, and others: What is the optimal medical management of ischemic heart failure? *Prog Cardiovasc Dis* 43:433-455, 2001.
62. Cleland JG, Dargie HJ, Findlay IN, and others: Clinical, haemodynamic and anti-arrhythmic effects of long-term treatment with amiodarone on patients in heart failure, *Br Heart J* 57:436-445, 1987.
63. Feldman AM, Bristow MR, Parmley WW, and others: Effects of vesnarinone on morbidity and mortality in patients with heart failure, *N Engl J Med* 329:149-155, 1993.
64. Packer M, Carver JR, Rodeheffer RJ, and others: Effect of oral milrinone on mortality in severe chronic heart failure: the PROMISE Study Research Group, *N Engl J Med* 325:1468-1475, 1991.
65. Gheorghiade M: Effects of tolvaptan, a vasopressor antagonist, in patients hospitalized with worsening heart failure, *JAMA* 291(16):1963-1971, 2004.
66. Volpe M, Tritto C, DeLuca N, and others: Abnormalities of sodium handling and of cardiovascular adaptations during high salt diet in patients with mild heart failure, *Circulation* 88(4 Pt 1):1620-1627, 1993.

67. Coats AJ, Adamopooulos S, Meyer TE, and others: Effects of physical training in chronic heart failure, *Lancet* 335:63-66, 1990.
68. Mancini DM, Henson D, La Manca J, and others: Benefit of selective respiratory muscle training on exercise capacity in patients with chronic congestive heart failure, *Circulation* 91:320-329, 1995.
69. Vargo RL: Bridging to transplant: mechanical support for heart failure, *Crit Care Nurs Clin North Am* 5:649-659, 1993.
70. Mehta SM, Aufiero TX, Pae WE, and others: Combined registry for the clinical use of mechanical ventricular assist pumps and the total artificial heart in conjunction with heart transplantation: sixth official report, 1994, *J Heart Lung Transplant* 14:585-593, 1995.
71. Moroney DA, Powers K: Outpatient use of left ventricular assist devices: nursing, technical, and educational considerations, *Am J Crit Care* 6:355-362, 1997.
72. OPTN, Organ Procurement Transplantation Network: *Overall by organ, current US waiting list retrieved,* Jan 13, 2007, from http://www.optn.org/latestData/rptData.asp.
73. Evans RW: The economics of heart transplantation, *Circulation* 75:63-75, 1987.
74. Jain P, Massie BM, Gattis WA, and others: Current treatment for the exacerbation of chronic heart failure resulting in hospitalization, *Am Heart J* 145(2 Suppl):S3-S17, 2003.
75. Carson OE, Johnson GR, Dunkman WB, and others: The influence of atrial fibrillation on prognosis in mild to moderate heart failure: the V-HeFT Studies: the V-HeFT Cooperative Study Group, *Circulation* 87(6 Suppl):VI102-VI110, 1993.
76. Berkowitz D, Croll MN, Likoff W: Malabsorption as a complication of congestive heart failure, *Am J Cardiol* 11:43-47, 1963.
77. Carr JG, Stevenson LW, Walden JA, and others: Prevalence and hemodynamic correlates of malnutrition in severe congestive heart failure secondary to ischemic or idiopathic dilated cardiomyopathy, *Am J Cardiol* 63:709-713, 1989.
78. Vinson JM, Rich MW, Sperry JC, and others: Early readmission of elderly patients with heart failure, *J Am Geriatr Soc* 38:1290-1295, 1990.
79. Cardiology Preeminence Roundtable: *Beyond four walls: cost effective management of chronic congestive heart failure,* Washington, DC, 1994, Advisory Board.
80. Williams RE, Keiler L, Sprang M, and others: Telemanagement of congestive heart failure: results of daily weights and symptom tracking, *J Am Coll Cardiol* 29(Suppl A):247A, 1997.
81. Aronow WS: ACC/AHA guideline update: treatment of heart failure with a normal left ventricular ejection fraction in the elderly, *Geriatrics* 61(5):16-20, 2006.
82. Shannon R, Chaudry M: Effect of alpha1-adrenergic receptors in cardiac pathology, *Am Heart J* 152(5):842-850, 2006.
83. Ducharme A, Swedburg K, Pfeffer MA, and others: Prevention of atrial fibrillation in patients with symptomatic chronic heart failure by candesartan in the Candesartan in Heart Failure: Assessment of Reduction in Mortality and Morbidity (CHARM) program, *Am Heart J* 152(1):86-92, 2006.
84. Greenberg B, Zannad F, Pitt B: Role of aldosterone blockade for treatment of heart failure and post-acute myocardial infarction, *Am J Cardiol* 97(10A):34F-40F, 2006.
85. Go AS, Lee WY, Yang J, and others: Statin therapy and risks for death and hospitalization in chronic heart failure, *JAMA* 296(17):2105-2111, 2006.

CHAPTER 129

Hypertension

Maryjane Giacalone and
Randall M. Zusman

DEFINITION AND EPIDEMIOLOGY

In 1972 the National Heart, Lung, and Blood Institute initiated a campaign to improve public awareness of the need for treatment of hypertension. The campaign has been successful in improving awareness and increasing treatment, but adequate control of hypertension still has not progressed to the same extent.[1]

Nearly 29% of Americans, or approximately 58 million people, have hypertension. Hypertension is a risk factor for coronary artery disease (CAD), heart failure, stroke, peripheral arterial disease, kidney disease, and retinopathy and therefore represents a significant public health threat. When hypertension is combined with other risk factors, its effect on the development of CAD is profound, contributing approximately 35% of the risk.[2-4]

In 2003 hypertension was directly responsible for 52,602 deaths (males 40.9%, females 59.1%) in the United States.[5] Research has shown that small gains in the control of hypertension can result in health improvements. Data extrapolated from the INTERSALT study have shown that an overall drop of 2 mm Hg in the distribution of blood pressure would result in a 6% annual reduction in stroke, a 4% reduction in CAD, and a 3% reduction in all-cause mortality.[6] The most recent data available reveal that, although 68.9% of Americans with high blood pressure are aware of it, only 58.4% are undergoing treatment, with only 31% having adequate blood pressure control.[1]

Blood pressure is that force in arterial structures created by an interplay of flow, volume, and constriction. High blood pressure, or hypertension, has been defined by determining the levels of blood pressure that cause target organ damage, morbidity, and mortality as arterial flow is delivered. It is known that 95% of all hypertension is primary, or essential, hypertension and has no known cause. The remaining 5% is termed *secondary hypertension* and is directly attributable to structural, circulatory, or chemical abnormalities. Published in 1997, the *Sixth Report of the Joint National Committee on Prevention, Detection, Evaluation, and Treatment of High Blood Pressure* (JNC 6) provided classifications for blood pressure values based on risk.[7] Subsequently, improved outcomes for diabetics with lower blood pressure values in the Hypertension Optimal Treatment (HOT) study prompted interest in modifying the JNC 6 classifications to recommend a lower target blood pressure of 130/80 mm Hg for diabetics.[8] Additionally, the cardiovascular and stroke risk associated with rising blood pressure values guided a decision to re-examine classifications for hypertension diagnosis and management. The *Seventh Report of the Joint National Committee on Prevention, Detection, Evaluation, and Treatment of High Blood Pressure* (JNC 7) has established new blood pressure parameters, including a category of prehypertension (Table 129-1).[9]

Incidence and Prevalence

Both systolic and diastolic blood pressures rise throughout childhood and early and middle adulthood; each is an independent predictor of cardiovascular disease, whether occurring alone or concurrently, in individuals younger than 50 years.[3,4] The rate of rise in diastolic blood pressure tends to level off or drop slightly in approximately the fifth decade of life. The resulting widened pulse pressure becomes equally important in predicting cardiovascular risk.[10] Systolic blood pressure continues to rise with advancing age, making isolated systolic hypertension more prevalent in the older adult. Three million individuals older than 60 years have isolated systolic hypertension.[9] More than half of individuals between ages 65 and 74 years and approximately three fourths of those 75 years and older have hypertension.[5]

There is a higher prevalence of hypertension among men until the fifth and sixth decade of life. After menopause, women have a higher incidence of this condition; by age 65, women have a higher overall prevalence of hypertension than men.[5,11]

In general, people of lower socioeconomic means and lower educational levels have a higher prevalence of hypertension. In these groups, poor diet, stress, and poor access to health care may play a role in the development of high blood pressure.[5]

Non-Hispanic blacks or African Americans have higher rates of hypertension than Caucasians. The baseline blood pressure in African-American children is higher than in Caucasian children and rises at a faster rate, producing higher rates of hypertension at younger ages. African Americans have a higher incidence of cardiovascular, stroke, and renal complications and have a higher mortality rate related to hypertension than do people of other ethnic backgrounds.[5,12-14] Enhanced renal sodium reabsorption occurs in 57% of African Americans as compared with 27% in other groups. This salt sensitivity—along with a generally poorer economic base, diet, and access to health care—contributes to the problem of high blood pressure among African Americans.

Risk Factors

Obesity, metabolic syndrome, a higher dietary intake of fat, a sodium intake in excess of sodium need, physical inactivity, and excessive alcohol intake are characteristics associated with Western culture and the development of hypertension.[2,6,9,12,13,15] Generally, the risk for hypertension is significant for both systolic and diastolic measurements. Prevention, detection, and treatment of hypertension should be public health priorities. The development of hypertension is probably multifactorial and therefore necessitates a coordinated, thoughtful, and individualized approach to diagnosis and treatment.

TABLE 129-1 Blood Pressure Classification

Category	Systolic Blood Pressure (mm Hg)		Diastolic Blood Pressure (mm Hg)
Normal	<120	*and*	<80
Prehypertension	120-139	*or*	80-89
Stage 1 hypertension	140-159	*or*	90-99
Stage 2 hypertension	>160	*or*	>100

From National Heart, Lung, and Blood Institute: *The seventh report of the Joint National Committee on Prevention, Detection, Evaluation, and Treatment of High Blood Pressure,* NIH Pub No 04-5230, Bethesda, Md, 2003, US Department of Health and Human Services.

PATHOPHYSIOLOGY

Blood pressure is the product of cardiac output (heart rate, myocardial contractility, and circulating volume and its impact on myocardial stretch) and peripheral resistance (vascular constriction and compliance). Anything that affects any part of this equation can affect blood pressure. In a properly functioning system, feedback loops maintain homeostasis.

Primary Hypertension

Sympathetic Nervous System. An increased heart rate can be caused by stimulation of the sympathetic nervous system in response to hypovolemia (baroreceptor response) or to physical or psychologic stressors (fever, anger, anxiety, exercise). An increased heart rate leads to an increase in cardiac output. The increase in blood pressure that follows is a normal response in these situations and is usually self-limiting because the heart rate response is caused by catecholamines or reduced by the parasympathetic response. Chronic stress may be an environmental factor that leads to the development of hypertension.

Excessive myocardial contractility (hyperkinesis) may also be the result of neurohormonal stimulation and has been suggested as a cause of mild hypertension, primarily in young adults. It has also been hypothesized that hyperkinesis is a cause of myocardial hypertrophy leading to hypertension, but there is no clear evidence to support this view. Hypertrophy is associated with hypertension but is usually considered a compensatory buildup of myocardial myofibrils to overcome high peripheral pressures.[16]

Sodium Balance and Salt Sensitivity. For years sodium has played a controversial role in the pathogenesis of hypertension.[14] Sodium's primary effect on blood pressure is related to excess circulating volume, but it may also affect contractility and vascular resistance.[16] Hypertension associated with salt sensitivity has been postulated to be caused by (1) an inability to normally excrete sodium via the kidneys (either through an upward shift in the arterial pressure required for sodium excretion or through a decrease in renal mass or filtration surface), resulting in an effectively increased circulating volume and a slight excess of total body sodium despite pressure natriuresis; (2) a resetting of the pressure-natriuresis curve, requiring higher blood pressures to maintain normal sodium and water balance; (3) abnormal electrolyte transport, resulting in disturbances in the cytosolic sodium/calcium balance and increased vasoconstriction; or (4) low renin levels, reduced numbers of nephrons, and modified sympathetic nervous system activity.[17-23]

Epidemiologic studies generally support a link between higher salt intake and the prevalence of hypertension.[6] Studies support some element of salt sensitivity among certain individuals, but there is no simple test to identify this sensitivity.[24] Some salt sensitivity has been linked to defects of the angiotensinogen gene.[25] Age, African-American heritage, diabetes, low renin levels, and nonmodulating hypertension often predict salt sensitivity.

Renin-Angiotensin System. Renin is an enzyme produced and released by the juxtaglomerular apparatus of the kidney in response to a low-flow state (reduced renal perfusion pressure or low circulating intravascular volume), sympathetic nervous system stimulation and/or catecholamine release, and hypokalemia. Once released, renin acts on angiotensinogen to create angiotensin I. In the pulmonary circulation, angiotensin-converting enzymes (ACEs) change angiotensin I to angiotensin II, a potent vasoconstrictor that over time and with prolonged production causes arterial stiffening and hypertrophy. Angiotensin II also causes aldosterone stimulation, which enhances sodium and water reabsorption from the renal tubules and effectively increases circulating volume. The resulting higher blood pressure should provide feedback to maintain homeostatic responses.

Feedback loops may not work properly in some individuals, allowing for higher circulating levels of renin and thus higher blood pressure. Unabated renin production may be related to undetectable arteriolar disease or ischemia that affects some nephrons. Renin levels are low in approximately 30% of individuals with hypertension, normal in 60%, and high in 10%.[25] One hypothesis suggests that individuals with high renin levels have hypertension related to vasoconstriction, whereas those with low renin levels have hypertension attributable to increased circulating volume and may be more responsive to diuretic therapy.[26]

Vascular Origin. In addition to the effect of angiotensin II, vascular hypertrophy may result from growth-enhancing substances, such as excessive levels of insulin, catecholamines, endothelins, natriuretic hormone, and growth hormone.[14,27-29] Also in consideration in the development of hypertension is the impact of capillary rarefaction, resulting in increased peripheral resistance, a depression of angiogenesis, or vessel regression.[30]

Obesity. There is a direct correlation between increasing weight and increasing blood pressure. Obesity, especially central obesity, has been linked to hypertension, metabolic syndrome, and cardiovascular mortality. Several theories have been advanced to explain the association between obesity and hypertension. One theory states that an increased sympathetic nervous system output results in activation of the renin-angiotensin-aldosterone system, thereby promoting sodium and water retention, increased circulating volume, increased cardiac output without increased peripheral resistance, and cardiac alterations. Other theories include those of metabolic anomalies, specifically hyperinsulinemia and insulin resistance.[25,29]

Approximately 25% to 30% of Americans are obese. Results from the Framingham Heart Study indicate that obesity accounts for 78% of hypertension in men and 65% of hypertension in women.[2] Benefits of weight loss include decreased insulin levels, improved insulin sensitivity, and decreased plasma norepinephrine levels. Other benefits not yet proven are decreased renin production and improved blood flow associated with a reduction in intracellular calcium levels.

Hypertension and obesity, glucose intolerance, or hyperlipidemia often occur together and greatly raise the risk for developing atherosclerotic cardiovascular disease. Research studies in central obesity, hyperglycemia, hyperinsulinemia, and insulin resistance have not yet shown that insulin-resistance syndromes have a pathogenic role in high blood pressure.

Other Dietary Influences. The Dietary Approaches to Stop Hypertension (DASH) study showed that blood pressure is decreased in response to a universally recommended diet that contains generous servings of fruits, vegetables, and low-fat dairy products with reduced saturated and total fat.[31]

Alcohol Intake. Excessive alcohol consumption is associated with hypertension and should be suspected in individuals who have been resistant to treatment. Alcohol may raise blood pressure by causing increases in sympathetic nervous system activity, activation of the renin-angiotensin system, or decreases in peripheral vascular tone and impairment of baroreceptor effectiveness.[23,24,29,32] Marked increases in blood pressure may occur with acute alcohol withdrawal but are unrelated to mechanisms of chronic hypertension. Overall reduction of alcohol intake results in a lowered blood pressure in hypertensive, heavy drinkers. Decreases in blood pressure are slow with alcohol restriction and peak in approximately 4 to 6 weeks.[33]

Exercise and Activity. Acute exercise can raise blood pressure in individuals with normotension and hypertension. The blood pressure rise is most dramatic and serious in those with uncontrolled hypertension. However, regular exercise can be beneficial if the person can adhere to an established exercise routine. The Centers for Disease Control and Prevention recommend regular exercise as an aid in lowering blood pressure. Regular isometric exercise has been shown to prevent the development of hypertension.[34] Regular aerobic exercise has been shown to reduce the incidence of cardiovascular events.[35]

Secondary Hypertension

Secondary hypertension can be ascribed to renal artery stenosis (RAS); pheochromocytoma; hyperaldosteronism; coarctation of the aorta; Cushing's syndrome; sleep apnea; thyroid disease; alcohol; and the use of steroids, oral contraceptives (hormone replacement therapy is an infrequent cause), or NSAIDs (Table 129-2). Although secondary causes account for approximately 5% of all hypertension cases, it is important to keep in mind that 5% translates to almost 3 million cases.

TABLE 129-2 Secondary Hypertension

	Clues			
	History and Physical	Screening	Diagnostic Testing	Treatment
CONDITION: ENDOGENOUS				
Renovascular condition (RAS)	Age <30 (fibromuscular) or >50 (atherosclerotic) History of atherosclerosis or risk factors Family history of RAS Abdominal bruits	Urinalysis Creatinine	Captopril flow scan Renal magnetic resonance arteriogram Renal arteriogram	Control hypertension: beta blockers Avoid ACE inhibitors Angioplasty Bypass surgery
Pheochromocytoma	*5 H's* (*H*ypertension, *H*eadache, *H*yperhidrosis, *H*ypermetabolic state, *H*yperglycemia) Hypertension after anesthetics, tricyclics Family history of endocrine disorders Hypertension after abdominal palpation Labile hypertension	Spot urine VMA 24-hour urine VMA and metanephrines	Spot urine VMA 24-hour urine VMA and 24-hour urine VMA and Plasma catecholamines (clonidine suppression test) CT scan of abdomen and pelvis Scintigraphy/MIBG imaging (to check for extrarenal and malignant masses)	Control hypertension: alpha blocker followed by beta blocker, or alpha-beta blocker Surgery
Hyperaldosteronism	Weakness Headache Fatigue Hypertension Hypokalemia	Unprovoked hypokalemia	Aldosterone levels before and after saline challenge Renin levels 24-hour urinary aldosterone 17-hydroxycorticosteroids CT scan of abdomen and pelvis Adrenal scintigraphy (if CT scan is negative) Adrenal vein catheterization (if CT scan and scintigraphy are negative)	If adrenal tumor: surgery If bilateral hyperplasia: potassium-sparing diuretics
Coarctation of the aorta	Young age Arm blood pressure > leg blood pressure Possible claudication Fatigue Late systolic murmur Apical heave	Chest x-ray	Echocardiogram Chest CT scan Aortogram	Surgery Angioplasty Stent
Thyroid disorder	Weight change Fatigue Metabolic change Temperature intolerance Edema Change in bowel habits Thyromegaly	Thyroid-stimulating hormone Weakness Muscle spasms Unprovoked hypokalemia	Triiodothyronine Thyroxine Thyroid-binding hormone	Treatment of underlying disorder Control hypertension in interim
Renal parenchymal disease: Polycystic kidney disease Glomerulonephritis Diabetic nephropathy Chronic renal failure Obstruction	Edema Nocturia Diabetes History of UTIs Pruritus Family history of polycystic kidney disease	Urinalysis Creatinine	24-hour urine: protein, creatinine, creatinine clearance Renal ultrasound IV pyelogram Diabetes testing	Depends on specific cause; control of volume intake, diuretics, and additional medical therapy; ACE inhibitor if diabetic (otherwise use with caution), control of glycemia, relief of obstruction

ACE, Angiotensin-converting enzyme; *MAO,* monoamine oxidase; *MIBG,* metaiodobenzylguanidine; *NSAIDs,* nonsteroidal antiinflammatory drugs; *RAS,* renal artery stenosis; *URI,* upper respiratory tract infection; *UTI,* urinary tract infection; *VMA,* vanillylmandelic acid.

Continued

TABLE 129-2 Secondary Hypertension—cont'd

	Clues			
	History and Physical	Screening	Diagnostic Testing	Treatment
CONDITION: ENDOGENOUS–CONT'D				
Cushing's syndrome	Hirsutism Edema Buffalo hump Moon facies Truncal obesity Red-purple striae	24-hour urine: free cortisol	Dexamethasone suppression test Pituitary MRI CT scan of thorax, abdomen	Surgery Control hypertension
Other: Anxiety Pregnancy Sleep apnea				
CONDITION: EXOGENOUS				
Alcohol	History of use			
Cocaine				Cessation of substance
NSAIDs	History of arthritis			Alternative treatment if necessary
Steroids	History of steroid-dependent conditions			
Sympathomimetics (over-the-counter cold remedies)	History of recent URI			
Weight control remedies				
Erythropoietin				
MAO inhibitors				

Renal Artery Stenosis. RAS results in hypertension when there is a 70% to 80% blockage of a renal artery,[36] often resulting in activation of the renin-angiotensin system.[37] Two different mechanisms have been shown to cause RAS. In individuals younger than 30 years, fibrodysplasia or fibromuscular dysplasia causes tight fibrous bands that alternate with normal or thin tissue along the renal artery, usually the medial portion. Fibrodysplasia affects more women than men. After age 50 years, atherosclerosis is the more likely cause of RAS and usually manifests in the proximal artery, extending from aortic plaque.[36-39] Hypertension from RAS can co-exist with essential hypertension; in elderly persons, RAS is likely to be a frequent contributor to hypertension. Angioplasty with or without stenting is the preferred treatment for fibrodysplastic RAS. Atherosclerotic RAS may also be treated with angioplasty with or without stenting; an ostial lesion is more difficult to resolve percutaneously. Surgical bypass of the renal artery is another option as long as the individual is healthy enough to undergo surgery.[39]

Pheochromocytoma. Pheochromocytoma is a catecholamine-producing tumor of the adrenal glands and is responsible for 0.1% to 1% of all cases of hypertension.[36,38] A small percentage of these tumors are malignant.[38] Hypertension seen with pheochromocytoma is constant in 50% of cases and labile in the other 50%.[38] Approximately 50% of cases involve the five *H*'s: *H*ypertension, *H*eadache, *H*yperhidrosis, *H*ypermetabolic state, and *H*yperglycemia. Bilateral headache, hyperhidrosis, and palpitations occur in 95% of the cases.[36]

Primary Hyperaldosteronism. Primary hyperaldosteronism is seen in fewer than 0.5% of all cases of hypertension and is more common in women. Adrenal adenoma accounts for 70% of all cases of primary hyperaldosteronism and is correctable by surgery. The other 30% result from bilateral adrenal hyperplasia, which must be managed medically. Primary hyperaldosteronism is suspected in patients with unprovoked hypokalemia.[36,38]

Coarctation of the Aorta. Coarctation of the aorta (a localized stricture of the aorta) is usually found in youth. It is typified by hypertension in the presence of claudication, delayed femoral pulses, decreased blood pressure in the lower extremities, and notching of ribs on chest x-ray films.[36,38] It is surgically correctable.

Cushing's Syndrome. Eighty percent of individuals with Cushing's syndrome have hypertension.[36] Cushing's syndrome is caused by hypersecretion of glucocorticoids by the adrenal cortex. This hypersecretion results from an adrenal tumor or overstimulation by the anterior pituitary.

Use of Certain Medications. The use of oral corticosteroids and anabolic steroids may also result in hypertension. All NSAIDs have been associated with hypertension.[40]

Obstructive Sleep Apnea. Obstructive sleep apnea, which affects 2% to 4% of the population,[41] is associated with hypertension and is thought to result from a hypoxia-driven sympathetic nervous system discharge.[42] Early studies show improvement in blood pressure with mechanically enhanced ventilation and avoidance of the supine position during sleep.[41] It may be more common in individuals with heart failure, end-stage renal disease, or central obesity. There is a possible association with leptin, which may be associated with the development of obesity, obstructive sleep apnea, and hypertension.[43]

Renal Parenchymal Disease. Renal parenchymal disease is associated with the development of hypertension and is also considered a result of hypertension. Renal insufficiency is apparent when creatinine levels rise higher than 1.5 mg/dl and the glomerular filtration rate falls to less than 50 ml/min. Renal parenchymal disease encompasses glomerular diseases (e.g., chronic renal failure, systemic lupus erythematosus, nephritis, diabetic nephropathy, glomerulonephritis, renal vasculitis) and interstitial diseases (e.g., polycystic kidney disease, chronic interstitial nephritis).[44]

The pathophysiology of renal parenchymal disease and hypertension likely involves factors that impair sodium excretion and lead to increased circulating volume. Over time, an increase in peripheral vascular resistance, which perpetuates blood pressure elevation, may result from changes in cytosolic electrolytes, heightened vascular reactivity, and proliferation of the smooth muscle cells. Increased activity of the renin-angiotensin system, which is more common in end-stage renal disease but is present in some cases of milder renal insufficiency, raises peripheral resistance by causing direct vasoconstriction and by increasing total available sodium.[45,46] Endothelins and the effects of reduced renal clearance of endothelium-derived relaxing factor inhibitors are potential areas for study and possible future treatment.

Genetics. Some studies have found a genetic link to some secondary causes of hypertension, such as hyperaldosteronism. No single significant association has been found for a genetic basis of essential hypertension, although a variety of genetic factors may contribute to the development of hypertension.[45]

CLINICAL PRESENTATION

Because most patients with hypertension are asymptomatic, the importance of screening cannot be overemphasized. Symptoms of high blood pressure usually occur only after the physical consequences of organ damage arise. Stroke, renal dysfunction, retinopathy, aortic dissection, and the sequelae of left ventricular hypertrophy are potential presenting conditions that result from longstanding undiagnosed hypertension. Secondary causes of hypertension are more likely to manifest with early symptoms reflective of the underlying cause, such as diabetic nephropathy and Cushing's syndrome. The JNC 7 therefore recommends that health care providers measure blood pressure at each patient visit.[9]

After obtaining an initial history and physical examination, the provider should schedule a follow-up evaluation on the basis of the systolic and diastolic blood pressure values obtained, the presence of concomitant cardiovascular risk factors, and evidence of end-organ dysfunction resulting from hypertension. On the basis of blood pressure alone, a systolic pressure greater than or equal to 180 mm Hg or a diastolic pressure greater than or equal to 110 mm Hg necessitates an urgent evaluation (Table 129-3) or immediate intervention if the patient exhibits signs of cardiac, cerebral, vascular, or renal complications.

The medical history, physical examination, and laboratory data obtained from a patient with high blood pressure should focus on eliciting the presence of cardiovascular risk factors, dysfunction of target organs, and evidence of possible secondary causes of hypertension.[9]

Cardiac risk factors are assessed in the medical history. The health risks associated with hypertension are compounded by tobacco use, hyperlipidemia, left ventricular hypertrophy, glucose intolerance, and a positive family history.[46] In addition, a complete cardiovascular, cerebrovascular, renovascular, endocrine, and family history is documented.

Any recent surgical, psychologic, social, environmental, or traumatic stress should be elicited. Such events may precipitate a temporary elevation in blood pressure or suggest a secondary

TABLE 129-3 Follow-up Based on Initial Blood Pressure Measurements for Adults Without Acute End-Organ Damage

Initial Blood Pressure (mm Hg)*	Follow-Up Recommended†
Normal (<120 systolic and <80 diastolic)	Recheck in 2 years
Prehypertension (120-139 systolic or 80-89 diastolic)	Recheck in 1 year‡
Stage 1 hypertension (140-159 systolic or 90-99 diastolic)	Confirm within 2 months†
Stage 2 hypertension (≥160 systolic or ≥100 diastolic)	Evaluate or refer to source of care within 1 month For those with higher pressures (e.g., >180/110 mm Hg), evaluate and treat immediately or within 1 week depending on clinical situation and complications

From National Heart, Lung, and Blood Institute: *The seventh report of the Joint National Committee on Prevention, Detection, Evaluation, and Treatment of High Blood Pressure,* NIH Pub No 04-5230, Bethesda, Md, 2003, US Department of Health and Human Services.
*If systolic and diastolic categories are different, follow recommendations for shorter time follow-up (e.g., 160/86 mm Hg should be evaluated or referred to source of care within 1 month).
†Modify the scheduling of follow-up according to reliable information about past blood pressure measurements, other cardiovascular risk factors, or target organ disease.
‡Provide advice about lifestyle modifications (use Lifestyle Modifications section).

cause of hypertension. For example, pheochromocytoma can adversely affect hemodynamic stability during surgery.

All over-the-counter and prescribed medications (both currently or formerly used by the patient) should be listed, including nicotine, herbal treatments, steroids, oral contraceptives, NSAIDs, sedatives, sympathomimetics, amphetamines, cyclosporine, erythropoietin, tricyclic antidepressants, monoamine oxidase inhibitors, and α- and β-adrenergic agonists.[47,48] The dosage, frequency, and duration of medications should be documented. A dietary assessment of sodium, cholesterol, fat, and alcohol intake must also be obtained.

The provider should elicit clues for potential secondary causes of hypertension, such as sleep apnea (loud snoring, erratic sleep, daytime somnolence), pheochromocytoma (severe headaches, diaphoresis, palpitations), aldosteronism (muscle cramps, weakness, polyuria, polydipsia, nocturia, rhabdomyolysis, paresthesias), mineralocorticoid alteration (licorice intake, chewing tobacco, oral steroid use), and renovascular conditions (hypokalemia).

Symptoms indicative of target organ damage must be sought. These symptoms can be neurovascular (transient weakness or blindness, loss of visual acuity, severe headache, confusion, lethargy, seizures), vascular (coarctation, impotence, claudication), cardiovascular (chest pain, dyspnea, palpitations, syncope), and renal (oliguria, hematuria, dysuria).

PHYSICAL EXAMINATION

Accurate assessment of blood pressure is crucial. The JNC 7 and the American Heart Association recommend that, to get an accurate reading, patients abstain from caffeine and nicotine for 30 minutes before measurement of blood pressure.[47,48] In addition, a cuff of the appropriate size (with the bladder of the cuff encompassing at least 80% of arm circumference) is applied 1 cm (0.4 inch) above the antecubital fossa. The patient's arm is positioned with support and is horizontal to the fourth intercostal space; the sphygmomanometer must be at the provider's eye level. The systolic value is the level at which the first Korotkoff sound appears; the diastolic value is the level at which sound disappears. An average of two measurements should be taken. Blood pressure and heart rate are measured in each arm while the patient is seated with feet on the floor; when warranted by concerns for orthostasis, these measurements are repeated after the patient has been standing for 2 minutes.[7]

Height and weight are recorded and guide weight management decisions. Other components of the physical examination gather evidence of end-organ impairment and secondary causes for hypertension.

Sustained hypertension produces a vascular effect. Retinal changes include arteriolar narrowing, arteriovenous nicking, exudates, hemorrhages, and, in severe cases, papilledema. The carotid arteries and aorta may have bruits, and impaired cerebral circulation may manifest as deficits on neurologic testing. Evidence of cardiac dysfunction (e.g., adventitious lung sounds, cardiac gallops, or displaced apical pulse) or left ventricular enlargement indicates complications of hypertension and affects treatment decisions. Pulse changes (diminished or absent) and skin changes (thinning, loss of extremity hair) point to peripheral circulatory impairment.

Hypertension produced as a result of other processes affects multiple organ systems. Striae, neurofibroma, or pruritic areas are important to note. Radial-femoral pulse delays and differences in blood pressure between arms or between arms and legs require further evaluation. Renal artery bruits or enlarged kidneys are evidence of kidney involvement. Thyroid findings of enlargement, bruits, or nodules necessitate additional testing.

DIAGNOSTICS

Because multiple factors may transiently increase or decrease blood pressure values, a diagnosis of hypertension is based on measurements obtained during at least three office visits.[9] Anxiety, oral contraceptives, nicotine, caffeine, and appetite suppressants are some of the more common causes of increased blood pressure.[47,48] Fluid loss and bed rest can decrease blood pressure.[49]

Routine evaluation of hypertension includes urinalysis, CBC, serum potassium, BUN, serum creatinine, fasting blood glucose, plasma lipoproteins, serum uric acid, and calcium. An ECG is obtained to assess evidence of ischemic heart disease or left ventricular hypertrophy (Figure 129-1). Left ventricular hypertrophy by ECG is manifested by a large S wave in V_1 and a large R wave in V_5. These two deflections will add up to more than 35 mm.[50]

DIFFERENTIAL DIAGNOSIS

The initial evaluation of a patient with hypertension should exclude the possibility of secondary hypertension. Diagnosis and treatment of an underlying secondary cause may ultimately resolve the hypertension. The more commonly noted

DIAGNOSTICS

Hypertension

LABORATORY

Urinalysis
CBC and differential
Serum glucose
Serum electrolytes
BUN
Creatinine
Fasting lipid profile
Calcium
Phosphorus
Uric acid
TSH*
24-hour urine cortisol (if Cushing's syndrome is suspected)
24-hour creatinine, catecholamines, and metanephrines (if pheochromocytoma is suspected)

IMAGING

Chest x-ray*
Abdominal ultrasound*
Renal angiogram*

OTHER

ECG
Echocardiogram*

*If indicated.

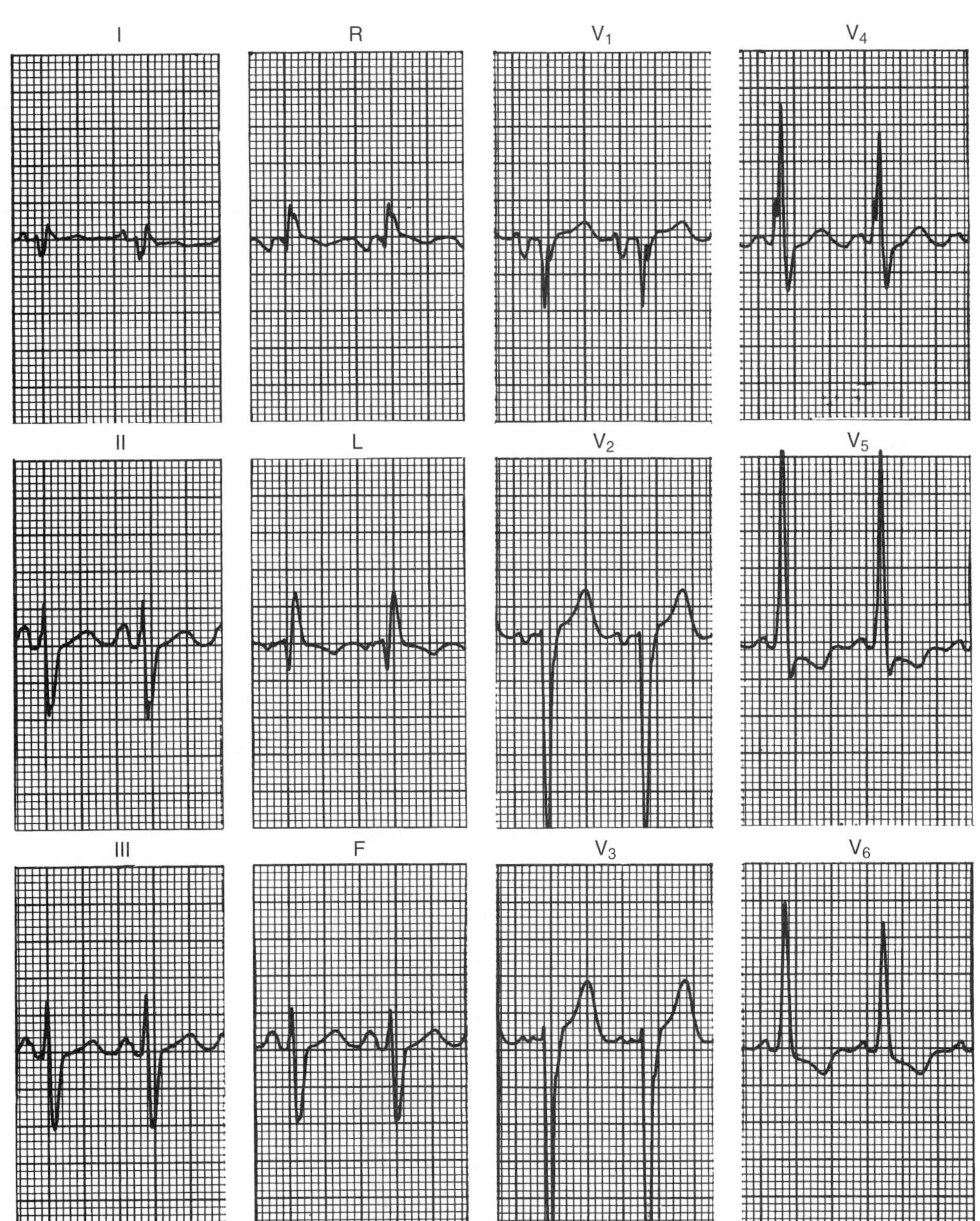

FIGURE 129-1

Left ventricular hypertrophy and strain with left atrial enlargement. (From Conover MB: *Understanding electrocardiography,* ed 7, St Louis, 1996, Mosby.)

DIFFERENTIAL DIAGNOSIS

Hypertension

- Primary hypertension
- Secondary hypertension
- Pheochromocytoma
- Cushing's syndrome
- Renal vascular disease
- Medications (see Table 129-2)
- Coarctation of the aorta
- Hypercalcemia caused by hyperparathyroidism
- Primary aldosteronism
- Alcohol
- Acromegaly
- Sleep apnea

secondary causes of hypertension, their symptoms, and diagnostic testing can be found in Table 129-2.

Among the differential diagnoses is "white coat hypertension," which is an elevated blood pressure related to the anticipation or anxiety of visiting a health care provider. When white coat hypertension is suspected, home or ambulatory blood pressure monitoring may be beneficial. Some cases of white coat hypertension are thought to be predictive of high blood pressure; in such cases patients may benefit from nonpharmacologic primary prevention techniques.[9]

MANAGEMENT

JNC 7 recommends using a risk stratification strategy for treatment on the basis of blood pressure, the presence of cardiac risk factors, and target organ damage[9] (Table 129-4). All

TABLE 129-4 Risk Stratification and Treatment of Hypertension

Blood Pressure Stages (mm Hg)	Risk Group A (No Risk Factors; No TOD/CCD)	Risk Group B (At Least One Risk Factor, Not Including Diabetes; No TOD/CCD)	Risk Group C (TOD/CCD and/or Diabetes, with or Without Other Risk Factors)
High-normal (130-139/85-89)	Lifestyle modification	Lifestyle modification	Lifestyle modification and drug therapy
Stage 1 (140-159/90-99)	Lifestyle modification (up to 12 months)	Lifestyle modification (up to 6 months)	Lifestyle modification and drug therapy
Stages 2 and 3 (≥160/≥100)	Drug therapy and lifestyle modification	Drug therapy and lifestyle modification	Drug therapy and lifestyle modification

Modified from National Institutes of Health: *The sixth report of the National Committee on Prevention, Detection, Evaluation, and Treatment of High Blood Pressure,* NIH Pub No 98-4080, Washington, DC, Nov 1997, The Institute.
TOD/CCD, Target organ damage/clinical cardiovascular disease.

individuals should adhere to nonpharmacologic recommendations for both primary prevention (limited evidence exists for benefit) and treatment (evidence exists for benefit). The methods include weight reduction, salt restriction, moderation of alcohol intake, exercise, and smoking cessation. Primary prevention is important because the risk of heart disease with hypertension is much greater than the risk reduction provided by secondary prevention of hypertension.[51]

Nonpharmacologic Therapy

Nonpharmacologic therapy is a key intervention for primary prevention; treatment of prehypertension; and treatment, along with pharmacologic therapy, of hypertension. Lifestyle interventions form the cornerstone of nonpharmacologic therapy.

Weight Reduction. A 4.5-kg (10-pound) weight reduction has been shown to result in lowered blood pressure; when necessary, a weight loss of more than 4.5 kg improves the results further.[31,52] Weight reduction is indicated if the patient is more than 110% of ideal body weight. Ideal body weight can be roughly calculated as 110 pounds for the first 5 feet of height plus 6 pounds for each inch over 5 feet (men), or 110 pounds for the first 5 feet of height plus 5 pounds for each inch over 5 feet (women). A typical daily caloric intake is estimated through a 24-hour diet recall by the patient. Calories may be reduced by 500 kcal/day to achieve a modest 0.45 kg (1 pound) per week weight reduction. Strategies for successful weight reduction include an emphasis on short-term weight reduction goals, avoidance of terms with negative connotations (e.g., "diet"), and follow-up visits for encouragement regarding reaching goals and maintaining healthy eating practices.

Salt Restriction and Healthy Eating Habits. Evidence in the DASH study has shown that a diet rich in fruits, whole grains, and vegetables, and low in red meats, saturated fat, cholesterol, and sugar-containing drinks lowered blood pressure.[31] In general, salt restriction has been shown to lower blood pressure among persons at all blood pressure levels, but especially in individuals who are salt sensitive.[23,24,33]

A subset of the DASH study looked at three levels of sodium intake, finding that the lower the salt intake, the lower the blood pressure, especially among African Americans. These blood-pressure lowering effects were in addition to those achieved with the overall healthier eating patterns in the DASH diet.[53] Maintaining a low-sodium diet can be difficult and is often marked by recidivism. Weight reduction may lead to decreased salt sensitivity, thereby obviating the need for salt restriction.[23]

Other Lifestyle Modifications. Additional important lifestyle recommendations involve exercise, limitation of alcohol use, stress management, and smoking cessation. Specific exercise recommendations and guidelines for alcohol use are found in Chapter 24 and under Patient and Family Education. Strategies for smoking cessation are found in Chapter 24.

Pharmacologic Therapy

The decision to start pharmacologic therapy should be individualized for each patient. The elements that factor into this decision include level of blood pressure and the presence of diabetes or renal disease.

Antihypertensives come in many different categories: diuretics, beta blockers, ACE inhibitors, angiotensin receptor blockers (ARBs), calcium channel blockers, and alpha blockers (Table 129-5). New antihypertensive drugs are currently under investigation. Each of the drugs in these categories has been shown to reach a certain level of efficacy in lowering blood pressure and therefore has been approved by the U.S. Food and Drug Administration (FDA). Diuretics and beta blockers have the advantage of being the most studied and have been proven effective in preventing stroke and reducing the risk of coronary disease. For this reason, they were recommended by the Joint National Commission on Hypertension as first-line pharmacologic treatments for uncomplicated hypertension in 1993 and, with some caveats, in 1997; JNC 7 recommends thiazide diuretics as first-line therapy in uncomplicated cases.[9] The recently completed ASCOT trial, however, suggests that a combination of calcium channel blockers and ACE inhibitor is more beneficial than a diuretic-beta blocker–based regimen.[54] Certain individuals have concomitant conditions that include specific indications for drugs other than diuretics or beta blockers. These patients should be started on the pharmacologic therapy most appropriate for their needs.[9]

In general, it is recommended to start with the lowest dose possible. Lower doses are associated with fewer side effects and are better tolerated so patients more readily adhere to a drug regimen. For better antihypertensive effects where needed, the dosage of an individual drug can be increased, or another drug (in a small dosage) can be added. Fixed-combination drugs for such treatment are on the market and are popular because they are often effective, have a low side effect profile, and are often less expensive than two separate pills.[55-57] If necessary (because of untoward effects or poor blood pressure control), another antihypertensive medication can be substituted. The majority of people require two medications for adequate blood pressure control.[8] For nonorthostatic patients whose blood pressures are equal to or greater than 160 mm Hg systolic or 100 mm Hg diastolic, two-drug therapy is suggested as initial pharmacologic treatment.[9]

Diuretics. Diuretics have been a mainstay of antihypertensive therapy and include thiazide, loop, and potassium-sparing diuretics. Because of their natriuretic nature, diuretics are especially effective in patients whose hypertension is typified by low sodium excretion and high circulating volume. Thiazide diuretics are preferred for initial therapy because of their potency and their long duration of action.[9] African Americans, older adults, and obese individuals often benefit from thiazides.[14] The ALLHAT study showed that diuretics were well tolerated and had good outcome profiles in comparison to ACE inhibitors and calcium channel blockers.[57] JNC 7 recommends thiazide diuretics as first-line therapy for hypertension without concomitant conditions such as CAD, renal disease, or diabetes.[9]

Mainly reserved for hypertension that is resistant to treatment or for patients with renal disease or heart failure, loop diuretics may be substituted when the glomerular filtration rate reaches approximately 60% or when the serum creatinine is greater than 1.7 mg/dl (150 μmol/L). Patients cannot be classified as "resistant" to treatment unless they remain hypertensive after a diuretic has been added to the regimen.[55]

By preventing some exchange of sodium for potassium in the distal tubule, potassium-sparing diuretics (e.g., triamterene, spironolactone, or eplerenone) are useful in combination with other diuretics to prevent hypokalemia. With a combination therapy such as hydrochlorothiazide with spironolactone, lower doses of each drug may produce better antihypertensive effects with better patient tolerance.

Patients should be monitored for efficacy of blood pressure control or for problems with side effects, cost, or adherence. Laboratory testing for glucose, potassium, lipid levels, and renal function should be performed shortly after starting therapy and several times during the first year of therapy to detect any possible adverse effects.

Problems with hypokalemia can be prevented or combated by advising a higher intake of potassium-rich fruits and vegetables,[14] such as bananas, greens, spinach, melon, raisins, apricots, and orange juice. Hypokalemia can also be controlled by adding a potassium supplement or adding an ACE inhibitor to antihypertensive therapy, if indicated. A potassium supplement should not be added to an ACE inhibitor unless the provider is certain that hypokalemia still exists; the potassium should be carefully checked at close intervals after the initiation of such therapy.

Beta Blockers. Beta blockers were mentioned by JNC 5 as first-line therapy for hypertension in individuals who have CAD, a high risk of CAD, or heart failure; JNC 7 maintains this recommendation.[9,58] Many beta blockers are now available with many different classifications: cardioselective vs. nonselective, with or without intrinsic sympathomimetic activity, lipophilic vs. hydrophilic, and combined alpha and beta blockers (Box 129-1). Beta blockers are inexpensive, well tolerated, and cardioprotective after myocardial infarction and improve outcomes in patients with heart failure.[59-63] Beta blockers are sometimes used for stage fright or for patients with hypertension and concomitant anxiety. A relative contraindication exists for individuals with diabetes and hyperlipidemia and for patients with peripheral vascular disease who have ischemia at rest.[59,60] Because beta blockers may produce bronchoconstriction, they are contraindicated in asthma and in other conditions with a bronchospastic component. Studies also suggest that beta blockers, when used as monotherapy in older adults, may not be effective.[63,64]

Angiotensin-Converting Enzyme Inhibitors. ACE inhibitors interrupt the conversion of angiotensin I to angiotensin II and are effective antihypertensive agents. Treatment with an ACE inhibitor improves triglyceride levels and insulin sensitivity and has a neutral or beneficial effect on other lipids and glucose levels in patients with diabetes.[65,66] ACE inhibitors are renoprotective, and there are documented improved survival rates in patients with heart failure caused by systolic dysfunction and regression of left ventricular hypertrophy.[65-68]

The JNC 7 recommends ACE inhibitor treatment of hypertension after first-line treatment unless special circumstances exist, such as patients with diabetes or heart failure with systolic dysfunction.[9] ACE inhibitor therapy is also recommended after acute anterior myocardial infarction with ST-segment elevation to prevent remodeling for patients with echocardiographic evidence of left ventricular systolic dysfunction (ejection fraction <40%) with or without symptoms.[60]

ACE inhibitors are contraindicated in pregnancy and are relatively contraindicated in hyperkalemia and with creatinine levels of more than 3.0 mg/dl. Laboratory testing for serum potassium and creatinine is indicated after initiation of therapy.

Angiotensin Receptor Blockers. ARBs received FDA approval for treatment of hypertension in 1995. These agents have a similar antihypertensive effect to ACE inhibitors. Definite evidence shows they are beneficial in patients with heart failure,[69] and they have had proven renoprotective benefits similar to those of ACE inhibitors in patients with type 2 diabetes.[70-73] The strength of the data would support the use of

Text continued on p. 586.

TABLE 129-5 Hypertensive Medications

Medication	Dosage	Compelling Indications	Effect on Co-Existing Conditions	
			Favorable	Unfavorable
DIURETICS		Heart failure; isolated systolic hypertension in older patients	Type 2 diabetes (low dose); osteoporosis (thiazides)	Type 1 and 2 diabetes (high dose); gout; renal insufficiency
Thiazide				
Chlorthalidone	12.5-50 mg/day			
Hydrochlorothiazide	12.5-50 mg/day			
Indapamide	1.25-5 mg/day			
Metolazone	2.5-10 mg/day			
Loop				
Bumetanide	0.5-4 mg divided b.i.d./t.i.d; up to 10 mg/day			
Ethacrynic acid	25-100 mg divided b.i.d./t.i.d.			
Furosemide	40-240 mg divided b.i.d./t.i.d.			
Torsemide	2.5-10 mg/day			
Potassium-Sparing				
Amiloride	5-10 mg/day			
Eplerenone	25 mg/day to 50 mg b.i.d.			
Spironolactone	25-100 mg/day			
Triamterene	25-100 mg/day			
ALPHA BLOCKERS		Hyperlipidemia; benign prostatic hypertrophy		
Doxazosin	1-16 mg/day			
Prazosin	2-40 mg/day divided b.i.d./t.i.d.			
Terazosin	1-20 mg/day			
BETA BLOCKERS		MI (nonintrinsic sympathomimetic activity)	Angina; atrial tachycardia and atrial fibrillation; essential tremor; migraine (noncardioselective); hyperthyroidism; preoperative hypertension	Bronchospasm; depression; diabetes types 1 and 2; hyperlipidemia; atrioventricular heart block; peripheral vascular disease
Acebutolol	200-800 mg/day			
Atenolol	25-100 mg/day-divided b.i.d.			
Betaxolol	5-20 mg/day			
Metoprolol	50-125 mg divided b.i.d.			
Metoprolol extended release	50-100 mg/day			
Toprol XL				
Nadolol	40-320 mg/day			
Pindolol	10-60 mg/day			
Propranolol	40-480 mg/day divided			
Timolol maleate	20-60 mg/day divided b.i.d.			
ALPHA-BETA BLOCKERS				
Carvedilol	12.5-50 mg b.i.d.		Heart failure	
Labetalol	200-1200 mg b.i.d.			Liver disease

Adapted from National Institutes of Health: *The seventh report of the Joint National Committee on Prevention, Detection, Evaluation, and Treatment of High Blood Pressure,* NIH Pub No 03-5233 Bethesda, Md, December 2003, The Institutes.

ACE, Angiotensin-converting enzyme; *AV,* atrioventricular; *CCBs,* calcium channel blocker; *COPD,* chronic obstructive pulmonary disease; *MI,* myocardial infarction; *NSAIDs,* nonsteroidal antiinflammatory drugs.

Efficacy		Side Effects		
ncrease	Decrease	Caution With	Short-Term Use	Possible
mbination diuretics with different sites of action	Steroids; NSAIDs; resin-binding drugs	Lithium (increased levels); potassium-sparing and ACE inhibitors may cause hyperkalemia	Increases cholesterol, blood glucose	Hyponatremia, hypokalemia (except in potassium-sparing), hypomagnesemia, hyperuricemia, hypercalcemia, hyperglycemia, sexual dysfunction
				Decreased clearance of verapamil with prazosin
ncomitant use of hepatically metabolized beta blockers; cimetidine; quinidine; food	NSAIDs; rifampin; phenobarbital; inducers of hepatic metabolism	Severe heart failure; asthma, bronchospastic COPD; diabetes (decreased hypoglycemic awareness); heart block; hypertriglyceridemia (associated with nonintrinsic sympathomimetic activity)		Bradycardia; fatigue; impaired circulation in extremities; sexual dysfunction; depression
				Postural hypotension; bronchospasm

Continued

TABLE 129-5 Hypertensive Medications—cont'd

Medication	Dosage	Compelling Indications	Effect on Co-Existing Conditions: Favorable	Effect on Co-Existing Conditions: Unfavorable
CALCIUM CHANNEL BLOCKERS		Isolated systolic hypertension (long-acting dihydropyridine)	Angina; cyclosporine-induced hypertension; diabetes type 1 and 2; nondihydropyridine: atrial tachycardia, atrial fibrillation, and migraine headache	Heart failure (except amlodipine) and second- and third-degree AV block (nondihydropyridine)
Dihydropyridines				
Amlodipine	2.5-10 mg/day			
Felodipine	2.5-10 mg/day			
Isradipine	5-20 mg/day			
Nicardipine	30-60 mg b.i.d. (long-acting only)			
Nifedipine (long-acting only)	30-120 mg/day			
Nondihydropyridines (Long-Acting Only)				
Diltiazem	120-360 mg*			
Verapamil	90-480 mg*			
ANGIOTENSIN-CONVERTING ENZYME INHIBITORS		Heart failure; diabetes type 1; MI with systolic dysfunction	Diabetes type 1; renal insufficiency (with creatinine <3 mg/dl)	Kidneys in renal artery stenosis; pregnancy
Captopril	25-100 mg divided b.i.d. or q.i.d.			
Enalapril	5-40 mg/day			
Fosinopril	10-40 mg/day PO*			
Lisinopril	5-40 mg/day			
Moexipril	7.5-30 mg/day PO			
Perindopril	4-8 mg/day PO			
Quinapril	10-80 mg/day			
Ramipril	2.5-20 mg/day PO			
Trandolapril	1-4 mg/day PO			
ANGIOTENSIN II BLOCKERS				
Candesartan	8-32 mg/day divided q day–b.i.d.			
Eprosartan	400-800 mg/day to b.i.d.			
Irbesartan	150-300 mg/day			
Losartan	25-100 mg/day			
Olmesartan	20-40 mg/day			
Telmisartan	20-80 mg/day PO			
Valsartan	80-320 mg/day			
VASODILATORS			Heart failure (with hydralazine along with nitrates when ACE inhibitors cannot be prescribed)	
Hydralazine	50-300 mg/day			
Minoxidil	5-100 mg/day			

*Frequency depends on formulation.

Efficacy		Side Effects		
Increase	**Decrease**	**Caution With**	**Short-Term Use**	**Possible**
Cimetidine or ranitidine with CCBs hepatically metabolized	Rifampin; phenobarbital; inducers of metabolism			**Dihydropyridines only:** Lower extremity edema, flushing, headache **L-channel nondihydropyridines only:** Conduction defects, heart failure, lower lithium levels (with verapamil); increased levels of quinidine, digoxin, sulfonylureas, and theophylline (competitive hepatic metabolism) with nondihydropyridines
With chlorpromazine	NSAIDs; antacids; food may decrease some absorption	Potassium-sparing diuretics Contraindicated in pregnancy		Cough; angioedema (rare); hyperkalemia; leukopenia; increased lithium levels
				Angioedema (isolated); hyperkalemia; less cough than with ACE inhibitors
		MAO inhibitors		Edema/fluid retention; tachycardia; lupus syndrome (hydralazine); hirsutism (minoxidil)

BOX 129-1

BETA BLOCKERS

Nonselective: propranolol, nadolol, sotalol, timolol, oxprenolol*
Cardioselective: atenolol, metoprolol, acebutolol
Intrinsic sympathomimetic activity: oxprenolol, celiprolol, pindolol, acebutolol
Lipid soluble: propranolol, metoprolol, pindolol
Lipid insoluble: atenolol, sotalol, nadolol
Alpha and beta blockers: labetalol, carvedilol

*May not be available in the United States.

ARBs as first-line therapy for people with type 2 diabetes and hypertension. Like ACE inhibitors, ARBs are contraindicated in pregnancy.

Calcium Channel Blockers. Calcium channel blockers perform by blocking calcium transport into cells, primarily the vascular and cardiac muscle cells. The calcium channel blockers consist of the dihydropyridines (e.g., nifedipine and amlodipine) and the nondihydropyridines (e.g., verapamil and diltiazem).

Calcium channel blockers are efficacious and well tolerated and have a relatively low side effect profile and a high adherence rate in comparison to other therapies.[73] They are metabolically neutral, which makes them advantageous for patients with diabetes or hyperlipidemia.[74] They are also effective antianginal medications.[40]

With the exception of amlodipine, calcium channel blockers may worsen heart failure and in general are contraindicated in patients with systolic dysfunction (ejection fraction <40%). In some patients, the dihydropyridines have been associated with leg edema unresponsive to diuretic therapy.

Calcium channel blockers can be used as first-line therapy in patients with hypertension and concomitant angina; long-acting formulations are preferred. Nondihydropyridines should be avoided in patients with sick sinus syndrome or bradycardia (heart rate <55 beats per minute) at rest. Caution is advised if these drugs are being combined with digoxin or a beta blocker.

α-Adrenergic Blockers. α-Adrenergic blockers have some favorable effects, which prompted the JNC 7 to recommend them in certain circumstances.[9] The doxazosin arm of the ALLHAT study[75] was discontinued prematurely because of higher rates of cardiovascular events and hospitalizations for heart failure among patients on doxazosin. Thus there is evidence that, despite its positive effect on benign prostatic hypertrophy and on lipids, doxazosin and α-adrenergic blockers in general should not be used as first-line pharmacologic treatment in hypertension. No studies have looked at α-adrenergic blockers as an added therapy. Therefore, although some sources recommend α-adrenergic blockers as additional therapy for patients with significant hyperlipidemia, patients with severe hypertension and hypertension related to renal disease may also benefit. However, there are no comparative data to support this use.[76]

Vasodilators (Minoxidil, Hydralazine). The direct vasodilators are recommended as second- or third-line medications for hypertension and are best used in combinations that control untoward effects such as edema or flushing.[9] Hydralazine is the most commonly used of these drugs and is most beneficial when used in combination with a diuretic to reduce compensatory volume expansion and with beta blockers to blunt the catecholamine response.[77] Hydralazine and nitrates can be used together in patients with hypertension and heart failure who do not tolerate ACE inhibitors or ARBs.[78] Hydralazine requires three or four times a day dosing, so adherence may be a problem for many patients. In high doses hydralazine may cause a lupuslike reaction. Minoxidil is less tolerated by women because of the possibility of facial hirsutism.

Monitoring

Follow-up strategy depends on the initial blood pressure (see Table 129-3). If blood pressure is not in good control, therapy can be advanced. If previously well-controlled blood pressure has risen, several areas should be explored. Poor adherence to the medical regimen because of a difficult dosage schedule, side effects, cost, or lack of understanding may be the cause. The patient history and physical examination should focus on possible secondary causes of hypertension. New conditions, such as renal parenchymal disease or RAS, can elevate a previously controlled blood pressure. Other causes may include new over-the-counter or mail-order herbal treatments, the use of NSAIDs, or excessive alcohol intake.[36,38]

Concomitant Conditions. In addition to the above, other conditions may raise other concerns. Patients with heart failure related to diastolic dysfunction are good candidates for diuretics (usually loop), ACE inhibitors, ARBs, calcium channel blockers, beta blockers, and long-acting nitrates. Caution should be used in starting or advancing antihypertensive therapy in patients with significant aortic stenosis, since lowering the blood pressure excessively can result in a decrease in coronary perfusion pressure.

Resistant Hypertension. Resistant hypertension is defined as blood pressure that is greater than or equal to 140/90 mm Hg despite treatment with a minimum of three drugs (including a diuretic) at maximum doses.

Co-Management with Specialists

Patients with concomitant diseases that are affected by or can cause hypertension may require collaborative management with a specialist in that field. An endocrinology consultation may be indicated for patients with diabetes. Nephrologists can provide collaborative care to patients with renal disease, and cardiologists can provide care to those with active CAD. Patients with autonomic failure, who have orthostatic hypotension but hypertension while supine, are challenging and would benefit from a consultation with a specialist in autonomic dysfunction or hypertension.[79]

LIFE SPAN CONSIDERATIONS

In general, systolic blood pressure rises with age, whereas diastolic blood pressure reaches a peak around 50 to 60 years of age and then may begin to decrease mildly. Isolated systolic hypertension is especially a problem for patients older than 60 years and is thought to result from aging, stiffening, and lack of compliance of the arteries. Isolated systolic hypertension responds well to most antihypertensive medications and especially to diuretics and calcium channel blockers. Advancing age does not preclude pharmacologic therapy. In fact, trials in older patients have shown beneficial outcomes in terms of stroke and total mortality in the treatment of systolic hypertension[11] and diastolic hypertension.[80] In this population, pharmacologic therapy may require gentle initiation and advancement to prevent excessive drops in blood pressure or orthostatic hypotension, which can result in falls.[81-83] Blood pressure goals are the same with older persons, however, and progress toward those goals has been associated with improved or preserved cognitive function.[84]

Secondary hypertension should be considered when hypertension develops before the age of 30 years (e.g., coarctation of the aorta or fibromuscular RAS) or after the age of 65 (e.g., atherosclerotic RAS). Hypertension during pregnancy (preeclampsia) is beyond the scope of this discussion.

COMPLICATIONS

Long-term complications of hypertension include left ventricular hypertrophy, heart failure, CAD, myocardial infarction, sudden death, aortic dissection, cerebrovascular disease, proteinuria, renal insufficiency, atherosclerotic conditions, retinopathy,[85,86] and hypertensive urgencies and emergencies.[87,88] Complications can result from long-term uncontrolled hypertension that assails target organs over time or from sudden surges of acute hypertension that result, for example, from acute glomerulonephritis or cocaine ingestion. A decline in cognitive functioning[89] and a higher incidence of dementia and Alzheimer's disease[90] have been associated with hypertension in older individuals.

Hypertensive Crises

Hypertensive emergencies are relatively rare events. Earlier and more pervasive diagnosis and treatment have reduced the incidence of malignant hypertension from untreated high blood pressure and have reduced mortality rates. A hypertensive crisis is present when blood pressure is high enough to threaten target organs acutely. JNC 7 differentiates between hypertensive emergencies and hypertensive urgencies as follows[9]:

Hypertensive Emergency Characteristics	Hypertensive Urgency Characteristics
Hypertensive encephalopathy	Upper levels stage 2 hypertension
Intracranial hemorrhage	Hypertension with optic disc edema
Unstable angina pectoris	Progressive target organ complications
Acute myocardial infarction	Severe perioperative hypertension
Pulmonary edema	
Dissecting aortic aneurysm	
Eclampsia	

The initial assessment of hypertensive crises should be aimed at two primary goals: (1) determining a threat to the most commonly affected target organs (fundi, brain, heart, and kidneys), and (2) finding a cause. Kaplan noted that, because various diagnostic options may be contaminated by drugs, blood and urine samples should be collected quickly before treatment but without delaying it.[91]

Drug	Interferes With
Labetalol	Catecholamine assays (alpha blocker)
Diuretics, potassium	Primary aldosteronism evaluation
Renin-suppressing drugs	Renovascular evaluation

Parenteral antihypertensive therapy is often indicated for hypertensive urgencies, but oral therapy may be appropriate. It may be advisable to coordinate the treatment of the cause (e.g., relief of pain in a postoperative patient) with the adjustment or initiation of medication. Observation of the patient for several hours after treatment to determine safety and efficacy is recommended.

Hypertensive emergencies require admission to an ICU and parenteral treatment (Table 129-6). The goal of treatment should be to reduce blood pressure slowly over a few hours, since rapid lowering of blood pressure can produce a shock effect in target organs. The brain maintains cerebral perfusion pressure by autoregulation, which balances perfusion via cerebral vasoconstriction or vasodilation in response to rises and falls in blood pressure. Normal autoregulation is easily maintained with blood pressure ranges of 70/40 to 190/130 mm Hg (allowing for some individual variation). However, the autoregulation curve skews to the right and upward in patients with chronic hypertension. If blood pressure exceeds the limits of autoregulation or if blood pressure drops precipitously, signs of cerebral hypoperfusion may be present.

Initially, patients with severe hypertension may appear with headache, dizziness, altered consciousness (lethargy, slowed

TABLE 129-6 Parenteral Medications for Severe Hypertension

Drug (Type)	Duration	Cautions and Comments
Nitroprusside (vasodilator)	1-10 minutes	Most rapid; use arterial monitoring; raises intracranial pressure
Nitroglycerin (vasodilator)	Minutes	Good for heart failure, coronary artery disease (CAD); tolerance may develop
Labetalol (alpha-beta blocker)	3-6 hours	Avoid in asthma; caution in heart failure
Esmolol (beta blocker)	<30 minutes	Avoid in heart failure and asthma
Nicardipine (calcium channel blocker)	3-6 hours	Prevents cerebral vasospasm; may cause ischemia
Furosemide (diuretic)	4 hours	Use with vasodilators
Hydralazine (diuretic)	>1 hour	Indicated for eclampsia; avoid in CAD, dissection
Fenoldopam (peripheral vasodilator and diuretic)	15 minutes	Contraindicated in glaucoma; may cause reflex tachycardia

mentation, confusion, agitation), and nausea.[92] Other target organs may produce profound symptoms in response to severe hypertension; pulmonary edema may occur in the setting of diastolic heart failure from excessively high afterload (peripheral resistance); retinal hemorrhage may occur. The physical examination, especially the retinal examination, should focus on target organ damage. Groups III and IV Keith-Wagener-Barker funduscopic changes may be the only or the initial sign of rapid deterioration with severe hypertension. Other possible changes may include blood pressure variation between the two arms resulting from coarctation or aortic dissection, ECG changes and chest pain consistent with unstable angina or myocardial infarction, and hematuria resulting from renal decompensation.

JNC 7 recommends initially reducing blood pressure gradually in the first 2 hours as dictated by co-morbid conditions.[9] The rate of fall should be tightly controlled. Effort should be made to control the pressure and avoid precipitous drops. For this reason, the prior practice of using sublingual, short-acting nifedipine is contraindicated.[9] Particular caution should be exercised with older adults, patients with chronic hypertension, patients who might have hypovolemia (diuretic use, recent loss of appetite, vomiting, or diarrhea), or patients who are taking vasoactive medications. In patients of all ages, overly aggressive therapy has been associated with adverse outcomes such as blindness, coma, and death.[87] The necessity of preventing permanent cerebral damage must be carefully achieved while lowering blood pressure enough to protect vital organs in circumstances such as acute heart failure, threatened myocardial infarction, or acute aortic dissection.

INDICATIONS FOR REFERRAL OR HOSPITALIZATION

A physician consultation is necessary when hypertension is resistant to therapy (failure of three full-dose antihypertensive drugs, including a diuretic) and when secondary causes attributable to lifestyle considerations or habits have been excluded. Certain secondary causes may be best diagnosed and managed collaboratively.

A patient who has known secondary hypertension caused by RAS should be referred to a hypertension specialist and a vascular radiologist or surgeon. Primary aldosteronism may require specialized input from an endocrinologist. As noted previously, patients with significant autonomic dysfunction may benefit from consultation with a hypertension or autonomic failure specialist.

Patients who have severe hypertension may require immediate treatment, consultation, referral, and, possibly, hospitalization. Both the degree of the blood pressure elevation and the presence of accompanying signs or symptoms of acute damage will dictate the next level of care.

Hospitalization is recommended for those with a blood pressure of 180/120 mm Hg and evidence of target organ dysfunction. Retinopathy may be the first presenting sign; grade 3 or 4 retinopathy with exudates and hemorrhage is a significant physical finding.[9,81,85,86] Target organ symptoms should be rapidly assessed. Neurologic symptoms include altered mental status, dizziness, blurred vision or loss of vision, focal neurologic deficits, and gastrointestinal symptoms. Cardiac symptoms include chest pain (or an anginal equivalent) or dyspnea accompanied by ECG changes, rales, and an S_3 on physical examination and possibly heart failure on chest x-ray study. Vascular symptoms may include tearing or burning chest pain or interscapular pain, with a variation in bilateral arm or leg blood pressure measurements, decreased pulses in lower extremities, or a widened mediastinum on the chest x-ray film. Renal signs may include oliguria, hematuria, proteinuria, or red cell casts by urinalysis.

PATIENT AND FAMILY EDUCATION

Topics that must be addressed include dietary instructions, exercise recommendations, risk factor modification, lifestyle issues, and the side effects associated with the medication prescribed. Patient comprehension is increased when handouts are given as references after the office visit.

General dietary recommendations include four servings of fruit, four servings of vegetables, and three servings of low-fat dairy products (DASH trial)[34]; reduction of cholesterol (<300 mg/day), saturated fat (<10% of total calories), and total fat (<30% of total calories) intake; control of blood glucose; and moderate alcohol intake (no more than 2 ounces 100 proof liquor, 8 ounces wine, or 34 ounces beer daily [half this amount for individuals smaller than the average male]). Total alcohol cessation may be necessary when hypertension is resistant to treatment.

Salt intake should be restricted to a maximum of 2.4 g/day. The DASH study showed that the lower the salt intake, the lower the blood pressure.[53] As noted previously, adherence may be difficult for many patients at extremely low income levels. Measures that help with salt restriction include avoiding adding salt to food, cooking with herbs, using fresh fruits and vegetables instead of canned, choosing fresh meats instead of deli or processed meats (e.g., bacon, sausage), and avoiding obviously salty foods (e.g., potato chips, pretzels, salted nuts). Labels showing sodium-free (5 mg/serving), very-low-sodium (<36 mg/serving), or low-sodium antacids (<141 mg/serving) should be selected.

Exercise recommendations are geared around provision of a specific exercise prescription (see Physical Activity, Chapter 24), with consideration of screening for CAD by physician consultation and/or stress testing in men older than 40 years and women older than 50 years.[93] The goal should be an established routine of exercise that is enjoyable and maintains interest with consistent progression of activity. Factors that need emphasis include adequate hydration, stretching, and warm-up and cool-down periods with more strenuous exercise.

Self-monitoring of blood pressure is a reasonable goal. If the patient agrees, family members should be provided with information concerning therapeutic recommendations. Individual knowledge concerning optimum level of blood pressure, factors affecting blood pressure, the necessity of treatment for control rather than cure of blood pressure, and dangers of quick weight loss programs is crucial. When a patient is prescribed medication, the dose, the medication's mechanism of action, monitoring required, and side effects are important topics to discuss to ensure patient understanding. Involvement of patients in the decision-making process, exploration of feelings concerning treatment regimens, exit interviews, and regular follow-up visits help the patient achieve therapeutic goals.

HEALTH PROMOTION

Health promotion involves risk factor modification that is directed toward cardiovascular disease and diabetes. Reduction to normal weight, smoking cessation, control of lipid levels, glycemic control, and stress management are key components of risk factor modification.

REFERENCES

1. Hajjar I, Kotchen TA: Trends in prevalence, awareness, treatment, and control of hypertension in the United States, 1988-2000, *JAMA* 290(2):199-206, 2003.
2. Kannel WB: Blood pressure as a cardiovascular risk factor, *JAMA* 275(24):1571-1576, 1996.
3. Whelton PK: Epidemiology of hypertension, *Lancet* 344:101-106, 1994.
4. Mortality after 16 years for participants randomized to the Multiple Risk Factor Intervention Trial, *Circulation* 94(5):946-951, 1996.
5. American Heart Association: *Statistical fact sheet*, 2004, retrieved Feb 5, 2006, from http://www.amhrt.org/presenter.jhtml?identifier=3000946.
6. Stamler R: Implications of the INTERSALT study, *Hypertension* 17(Suppl I):I16-I20, 1991.
7. National Heart, Lung, and Blood Institute: *The sixth report of the Joint National Committee on Prevention, Detection, Evaluation, and Treatment of High Blood Pressure,* NIH Pub No 98-4080, Bethesda, Md, 1997, US Department of Health and Human Services.
8. Curb JD, Pressel SL, Cutler JA, and others: Effect of diuretic-based antihypertensive treatment on cardiovascular disease risk in older diabetic patients with isolated systolic hypertension: Systolic Hypertension in the Elderly Program Cooperative Research Group, *JAMA* 276(23):1886-1892, 1996.
9. National Heart, Lung, and Blood Institute: *The seventh report of the Joint National Committee on Prevention, Detection, Evaluation, and Treatment of High Blood Pressure,* NIH Pub No 04-5230, Bethesda, Md, 2003, US Department of Health and Human Services.
10. Millar JA, Lever AF, Burke V: Pulse pressure as a risk factor for cardiovascular events in the MRC Mild Hypertension Trial, *J Hypertens* 17:1065-1072, 1999.
11. Materson BJ, Reda DJ, Cushman WC: Department of Veterans Affairs single-drug therapy of hypertension study: revised figures and new data, Department of Veterans Affairs Cooperative Study Group on Antihypertensive Agents, *Am J Hypertens* 8(2):189-192, 1995.
12. Kaplan N: Primary hypertension: pathogenesis. In Kaplan NM, editor: *Clinical hypertension,* ed 6, Baltimore, 1994, Williams & Wilkins.
13. Kaplan NM: Alcohol and hypertension, *Lancet* 345:1588-1589, 1995.
14. Ashida T, Kawano Y, Yoshimi H, and others: Effects of dietary salt on sodium-calcium exchange and ATP-driven calcium pump in arterial smooth muscle of Dahl rats, *J Hypertens* 10(11):1335-1341, 1992.
15. Kaplan NM: Ethnic aspects of hypertension, *Lancet* 344:450-452, 1994.
16. Midgley JP, Matthew AG, Greenwood CM, and others: Effect of reduced dietary sodium on blood pressure: a meta-analysis of randomized controlled trials, *JAMA* 275(20):1590-1597, 1996.
17. Campese VM, Karubian F, Chervu I, and others: Pressor reactivity to norepinephrine and angiotensin in salt-sensitive hypertensive patients, *Hypertension* 21:301-307, 1993.
18. Kaplan NM: Primary hypertension: from pathophysiology to prevention, *Arch Intern Med* 156:1919-1920, 1996.
19. Cowley AW, Roman RJ: The role of the kidney in hypertension, *JAMA* 275(20):1581-1589, 1996.
20. Navar LG: The kidney in blood pressure regulation and development of hypertension, *Med Clin North Am* 81(5):1165-1198, 1997.
21. Frohlich ED: Current clinical pathophysiologic considerations in essential hypertension, *Med Clin North Am* 81(5):1113-1129, 1997.
22. Pecker MS: Salt sensitivity in hypertensive patients: pathogenesis, identification, and treatment. In Laragh JH, Brenner BM, editors: *Hypertension: pathophysiology, diagnosis, and management,* ed 2, New York, 1995, Raven Press.
23. Reisin E: Nonpharmacologic approaches to hypertension: weight, sodium, alcohol, exercise, and tobacco considerations, *Med Clin North Am* 81(6):1289-1303, 1997.
24. Sullivan JM: Salt sensitivity: definition, conception, methodology, and long-term issues, *Hypertension* 17(Suppl I):I61-I68, 1991.
25. Oparil S, Calhoun DA: High blood pressure. In Dale DC, Federman DD, editors: *Scientific American medicine,* New York, 1997, Scientific American.
26. Massie BM: Systemic hypertension. In Tierney LM, McPhee SJ, Papadakis MA, editors: *Current medical diagnosis and treatment,* ed 36, Stamford, Conn, 1997, Appleton & Lange.
27. Mann SJ, Blumenfeld JD, Laragh JH: Issues, goals, and guidelines for choosing first-line and combination antihypertensive drug therapy. In Laragh JH, Brenner BM, editors: *Hypertension: pathophysiology, diagnosis and management,* ed 2, New York, 1995, Raven Press.
28. Forte P, Copland M, Smith LM, and others: Basal nitric oxide synthesis in essential hypertension, *Lancet* 349:837-842, 1997.
29. Haffner ST, Miettinen H, Gaskill SP, and others: Metabolic precursors of hypertension: the San Antonio heart study, *Arch Intern Med* 156:1994-2001, 1996.
30. Bobik A: The structural basis of hypertension: vascular remodeling, rarefaction and angiogenesis/arteriogenesis, *J Hypertens* 23:1473-1475, 2005.
31. Conlin PR, Chow D, Miller ER, and others: The effect of dietary patterns on blood pressure control in hypertensive patients: results from the Dietary Approaches to Stop Hypertension (DASH) trial, *Am J Hypertens* 13(9):949-955, 2000.
32. Ramsey LE, Yeo WW, Chadwick IG, and others: Non-pharmacological therapy of hypertension, *Br Med Bull* 50(2):494-508, 1994.
33. Alderman MH: Non-pharmacological treatment of hypertension, *Lancet* 344:307-311, 1994.
34. Blair SN, Goodyear NN, Gibbons LW, and others: Physical fitness and incidence of hypertension in healthy normotensive men and women, *JAMA* 252:487-490, 1984.
35. Paffenbarger RS, Hyde RT, Wing AL, and others: The association of changes in physical activity level and other lifestyle characteristics with mortality among men, *N Engl J Med* 328:538-545, 1993.
36. Adcock BB, Ireland RB: Secondary hypertension: a practical diagnostic approach, *Am Fam Phys* 55(4):1263-1270, 1997.
37. Safian RD, Textor SC: Renal-artery stenosis, *N Engl J Med* 344(6):431-442, 2000.
38. Ram CV: Secondary hypertension: workup and correction, *Hosp Pract* 29(4):137-150, 1994.
39. Schamess A, Bernik T, Tenner S: Refractory hypertension due to Conn's syndrome, *Postgrad Med* 95(4):199-203, 1994.
40. Pope JE, Anderson JJ, Felson DT: A meta-analysis of the effects of nonsteroidal anti-inflammatory drugs on blood pressure, *Arch Intern Med* 153:477-484, 1993.
41. Berger M, Oksenberg A, Silverberg DS, and others: Avoiding the supine position during sleep lowers 24-hour blood pressure in obstructive sleep apnea (OSA) patients, *J Hum Hypertens* 11(10):657-664, 1997.
42. Guilleminault C, Robinson A: Sleep-disordered breathing and hypertension: past lessons, future directions, *Sleep* 20(9):806-811, 1997.
43. Luft FC: Present status of genetic mechanisms in hypertension, *Med Clin North Am* 88:1-18, 2004.
44. Preston RA, Singer I, Epstein M: Renal parenchymal hypertension: current concepts of pathogenesis and management, *Arch Intern Med* 156:602-611, 1996.
45. Kaplan NM: Genetic factors in the pathogenesis of essential hypertension, retrieved Jan 15, 2007, from http://www.uptodateonline.com/utd/content/topic.do?topicKey=hyperten/20539.
46. McCarron D: High blood pressure. In Dale DC, Federman DD, editors: *Scientific American medicine,* New York, 1995, Scientific American.
47. Pentel P: Toxicity of over-the-counter stimulants, *JAMA* 252(14):1898-1903, 1984.
48. Freestone S, Ramsay LE: Pressor effect of coffee and cigarette smoking in hypertensive patients, *Clin Sci* 63:403, 1982.

49. Hossman V, Fitzgerald GA, Dollery CT: Influence of hospitalization and placebo therapy on blood pressure and sympathetic function in essential hypertension, *Hypertension* 3:113, 1981.
50. Dubin D: *Rapid interpretation of EKGs*, ed 4, Tampa, Fla, 1994, Cover Publishing.
51. Stamler J, Stamler R, Neaton JD: Blood pressure, systolic and diastolic, and cardiovascular risks: US population data, *Arch Intern Med* 153:598-615, 1993.
52. American Heart Association Subcommittee of Nutritionists: American Heart Association guidelines for weight management programs for healthy adults, *Heart Dis Stroke* 3(4):221-228, 1994.
53. Epstein M, Bakris G: Newer approaches to antihypertensive therapy: use of fixed dose combination therapy, *Arch Intern Med* 156:1969-1978, 1996.
54. Dahloff B, Sever PS, Poulter NR, and others: Prevention of cardiovascular events with an antihypertensive regimen of amlodipine adding perindopril as required versus atenolol adding bendroflumethiazide as required in the Anglo-Scandinavian Cardiac Outcomes Trial–Blood Pressure Lowering Arm (ASCOT-BPLA): a multicentre randomized controlled trial, *Lancet* 366:895-906, 2005.
55. Kaplan NM, Gifford RW: Choice of initial therapy for hypertension, *JAMA* 275(20):1577-1580, 1996.
56. Cushman WC, Ford CE, Cutler JA, and others: Success and predictors of blood pressure control in diverse North American settings: the Antihypertensive and Lipid-Lowering Treatment to Prevent Heart Attack, *J Clin Hypertens (Greenwich)* 4:393-404, 2002.
57. Lyons D, Petrie JC, Reid JL: Drug treatment: present and future, *Br Med Bull* 50(2):472-493, 1994.
58. The Fifth Report of the Joint National Committee on Detection, Evaluation, and Treatment of High Blood Pressure (JNC V): 1993, *Arch Intern Med* 153:154-183, 1993.
59. Rutherford JD, Braunwald E: Chronic ischemic heart disease. In Braunwald E, editor: *Heart disease: a textbook of cardiovascular medicine*, ed 4, Philadelphia, 1992, Saunders.
60. American College of Cardiology/American Heart Association Task Force on Practice Guidelines: ACC/AHA guidelines for the management of patients with acute myocardial infarction: a report of the American College of Cardiology/American Heart Association Task Force on Practice Guidelines (Committee on Management of Acute Myocardial Infarction), *Circulation* 28:1328, 1996.
61. Effect of metoprolol CR/XL in chronic heart failure: metoprolol CR/XL randomized intervention trial in congestive heart failure (MERIT-HF), *Lancet* 353(9169):2001-2007, 1999.
62. Packer M, Bristow MR, Cohn JN, and others: The effect of carvedilol on morbidity and mortality in patients with chronic heart failure, *N Engl J Med* 334(21):1349-1355, 1996.
63. Messerli FH, Grossman E, Goldbourt U: Are beta-blockers efficacious as first-line therapy for hypertension in the elderly? *JAMA* 279:1903-1907, 1998.
64. Staessen JA, Fagard R, Thijs L, and others: Randomised double-blind comparison of placebo and active treatment for older patients with isolated systolic hypertension: the Systolic Hypertension in Europe (Syst-Eur) Trial Investigators, *Lancet* 350:757-764, 1997.
65. Gifford RW: Antihypertensive therapy: angiotensin-converting enzyme inhibitors, angiotensin II receptor antagonists, and calcium antagonists, *Med Clin North Am* 81(6):1319-1333, 1997.
66. EUCLID study group: Randomised placebo-controlled trial of lisinopril in normotensive patients with insulin-dependent diabetes and normoalbuminuria or microalbuminuria, *Lancet* 349:1787-1791, 1997.
67. Consensus statement: Treatment of hypertension in diabetes, *Diabetes Care* 19(Suppl 1):S107-S113, 1996.
68. SOLVD Investigators: Effect of enalapril on survival in patients with reduced left ventricular ejection fractions and congestive heart failure, *N Engl J Med* 325:293-302, 1991.
69. Cohn JN, Tognoni G, Valsartan Heart Failure Trial Investigators: A randomized trial of the angiotensin-receptor blocker valsartan in chronic heart failure, *N Engl J Med* 345(23):1667-1675, 2001.
70. Brenner BM, Cooper ME, de Zeeuw D, and others: Effects of losartan on renal and cardiovascular outcomes in patients with type 2 diabetes and nephropathy, *N Engl J Med* 345:861-869, 2001.
71. Lewis EJ, Hunsicker LG, Clarke WR, and others: Renoprotective effect of the angiotensin-receptor antagonist irbesartan in patients with nephropathy due to type 2 diabetes, *N Engl J Med* 345:851-860, 2001.
72. Parving HH, Lehnert H, Brochner-Mortensen J, and others: The effect of irbesartan on the development of diabetic nephropathy in patients with type 2 diabetes, *N Engl J Med* 435:870-878, 2001.
73. Epstein M: The calcium antagonist controversy: the emerging importance of drug formulation as a determinant of risk, *Am J Cardiol* 79(10A):9-19, 1997.
74. Sowers JR: Effects of calcium antagonists on insulin sensitivity and other metabolic parameters, *Am J Cardiol* 79(10A):24-28, 1997.
75. ALLHAT Collaborative Research Group: Major cardiovascular events in hypertensive patients randomized to doxazosin vs chlorthalidone in the Antihypertensive and Lipid-Lowering Treatment to Prevent Heart Attack Trial (ALLHAT), *JAMA* 283:1967-1975, 2000.
76. Kaplan NM: Systemic hypertension: therapy. In Braunwald E, editor: *Heart disease: a textbook of cardiovascular medicine*, ed 4, Philadelphia, 1992, Saunders.
77. Frishman WH: Use of calcium antagonists in patients with ischemic heart disease and systemic hypertension, *Am J Cardiol* 79(10A):37-38, 1997.
78. Cohn J, Johnson G, Ziesche S, and others: A comparison of enalapril with hydralazine-isosorbide dinitrate in the treatment of chronic congestive heart failure, *N Engl J Med* 325:303-310, 1991.
79. Shibao C, Gamboa A, Diedrich A, and others: Management of hypertension in the setting of autonomic failure: a pathophysiologic approach, *Hypertension* 45:469-476, 2006.
80. Dahlof B, Lindholm LH, Hansson L, and others: Morbidity and mortality in the Swedish Trial in Old Patients with Hypertension (STOP-Hypertension), *Lancet* 338:1281-1285, 1991.
81. Glynn RJ, Brock DB, Harris T, and others: Use of antihypertensive drugs and trends in blood pressure in the elderly, *Arch Intern Med* 155:1855-1860, 1995.
82. Kaplan NM: Hypertension in the elderly, *Ann Rev Med* 45:27-35, 1995.
83. Sadowski AV, Redeker NS: The hypertensive elder: a review for the primary care provider, *Nurse Pract* 21(5):99-118, 1996.
84. Forette F, Seux ML, Staessen JA, and others: Prevention of dementia in randomized double-blind controlled Systolic Hypertension in Europe (Syst-Eur) trial, *Lancet* 352:1347-1351, 1998.
85. Chobanian AV, Alexander W: Exacerbation of atherosclerosis by hypertension, *Arch Intern Med* 156:1952-1956, 1996.
86. Arnett DK, Tyroler HA, Burke G, and others: Hypertension and subclinical carotid artery atherosclerosis in blacks and whites: the Atherosclerosis Risk in Communities Study, *Arch Intern Med* 156:1983-1989, 1996.
87. Thach AM, Schultz PJ: Nonemergent hypertension, *Emerg Med Clin North Am* 13(4):1009-1035, 1995.
88. Psaty BM, Smith NL, Siscovick DS, and others: Health outcomes associated with antihypertensive therapies used as first-line agents: a systematic review and meta-analysis, *JAMA* 277(9):739-745, 1997.
89. Elias MF, Wolf PA, D'Agostino RB, and others: Untreated blood pressure level is inversely related to cognitive functioning: the Framingham study, *Am J Epidemiol* 138(6):353-364, 1993.
90. Skoog I, Lernfelt B, Landahl S, and others: Fifteen-year longitudinal study of blood pressure and dementia, *Lancet* 347:1141-1145, 1996.
91. Kaplan NM: Management of hypertensive emergencies, *Lancet* 344:1335-1338, 1994.
92. Murphy C: Hypertensive emergencies, *Emerg Med Clin North Am* 13(4):973-1006, 1995.
93. Gibbons RJ, Balady GJ, Beasley JW, and others: ACC/AHA guidelines for exercise testing: executive summary, *Circulation* 96:345-354, 1997.

CHAPTER 130

Myocarditis

H. A. Morcos and JoAnn Trybulski

DEFINITION AND EPIDEMIOLOGY

Myocarditis, or inflammation of the myocardium, affects the myocardial cell, interstitium, or vascular components singularly or in combination, producing varied symptoms of variable duration.[1] The presentation of myocarditis may be subacute with minor symptoms that resolve spontaneously, or acute with severe, even life-threatening symptoms; moreover, symptoms may persist for an extended time in a chronic form of the illness.[1]

Myocardial inflammation is caused by myriad viruses, including HIV; in addition, fungi, rickettsiae, bacteria, spirochetes, protozoans, helminthes, medications, chemicals, systemic and metabolic disorders, pregnancy, radiation, physical agents (the most common is alcohol), hypersensitivity, or autoimmune reactions are precipitants (Box 130-1).[1,2] The incidence varies; epidemic outbreaks and clustering in families have been observed.[2]

Physician consultation is indicated for patients with suspected myocarditis.

PATHOPHYSIOLOGY

The origin of myocarditis can be multifactorial. Current explanations of pathogenesis center on two mechanisms: infectious and autoimmune or hypersensitivity. In infectious myocarditis the replication of the pathogen in myocardial tissue can damage myocardial cells by tissue toxins, which initiate a cellular and humoral immunologic response.[1,2] A maladaptive response produces myocardial damage by means of sensitized and hyperreactive T lymphocytes, resulting in autoimmune reactions of varying degrees and duration.[2] Factors that affect the immunologic response and cause the maladaptive response are toxic effects of the pathogen or substance on myocardial tissue in combination with host factors such as familial predisposition, peripartum state, hypoxia, exercise, nutritional status, ethanol intake, ionizing radiation, and exposure to temperature extremes.[3] The autoimmune response may be triggered by an infectious agent as explained previously or initiated as a reaction to a substance or condition. The common pathway seems to be the existence of cytokines, which are present in any T cell–mediated response.[3]

Recovery can be complete and without any damage, or the clinical course can be marked by progression to heart failure. Myocarditis has been found to be a precursor of cardiomyopathy, which may appear years after the initial inflammation.[4]

Three stages characterize viral myocarditis; each stage has different pathophysiology and manifestations. In phase 1, the viral phase, the virus enters the myocytes and triggers an immune response. This immune response modulates further replication of the virus but also enhances additional viral entry that may continue immune activation; this secondary immune response is predominant in the pathogenesis of mycocarditis.[5] Phase 2 includes triggering of an autoimmune response via T-cell activation, cytokine activation, and CD4 cell activation that produces autoreactive antibodies. The activated products destroy the virus-containing cells, in this case the myocytes, reducing the number of functional heart muscle cells.[5] This destruction of heart muscle cells over time produces dilated cardiomyopathy and represents the third phase of viral myocarditis. In one trial, patients with a more aggressive early immune response had a less severe course, whereas those with high levels of circulating $CD2^+$ T cells, indicating a greater late immune response and activation capable of mediating an autoimmune type of response, had an increased incidence of dilated cardiomyopathy and poorer survival statistics.[6]

CLINICAL PRESENTATION

Presenting symptoms range from none, with diagnosis an incidental finding on autopsy, to cardiomyopathy with end-stage heart failure. Brief cardiac inflammation is common with viral infections and may account for the transient weakness and transient exertional tachycardia early in viral illnesses.[1] These symptoms resolve after several days. Reports of continued fatigue, coupled with tachycardia associated with minimum exertion or palpitations, should prompt investigation for myocarditis.

Patients often recount accelerated pulse or palpitations in response to exercise. Stimulants such as caffeine or alcohol or even mildly exciting or stressful situations, such as watching a sporting event or movie or reading a tense book, may also precipitate palpitations or tachycardia. The clinical presentation may be characterized by various degrees of heart failure. Fever may be present,[2] as well as symptoms commonly found in the condition causing the myocarditis.

Acute chest pain mimicking myocardial infarction or the co-existence of pericarditis can occur with myocarditis.[1] Signs and symptoms of pulmonary and systemic embolism can co-exist as a complication.[1] Regrettably, sudden death secondary to arrhythmia or heart block or failure can be the initial presentation.[1,3]

PHYSICAL EXAMINATION

Tachycardia, either resting, with minimum exertion, or out of proportion to any fever, is a prominent feature.[7] Ectopy is often detected. Because the presentation of myocarditis ranges from asymptomatic to overt heart failure, the physical examination findings will reflect this spectrum. Some infectious agents such as coxsackievirus also affect the pericardium, producing pericardial pain, audible friction rub, or pleural effusion.[8]

Signs of heart failure vary with its severity. In myocarditis accompanied by heart failure, an S_3 or S_4 may be detected by cardiac auscultation. Milder cases may show only vascular redistribution of flow to upper lobes on chest x-ray film and no abnormal cardiac examination findings, whereas in more severe cases gallops, murmurs, peripheral edema, and an abnormal chest x-ray film showing an enlarged heart may be present.[1]

BOX 130-1

COMMON CAUSES OF MYOCARDITIS

INFECTIOUS

- Rickettsia (typhus, Q fever, Rocky Mountain spotted fever)
- Diphtheria
- Gonococci
- Typhoid fever
- Salmonella
- Streptococci
- Tuberculosis
- Meningococci
- Brucellosis
- Clostridia
- Staphylococci
- Psittacosis
- *Mycoplasma pneumoniae*
- Melioidosis
- Syphilis
- Leptospirosis
- Borelliosis
- Lyme disease
- Fungal (e.g., aspergillosis, candidiasis, coccidioidomycosis)
- Helminthic disease (e.g., trichinosis)
- Protozoan disease

VIRAL

- Coxsackievirus
- Echovirus
- HIV
- Cytomegalovirus
- Poliomyelitis
- Mononucleosis
- Hepatitis
- Rubeola
- Varicella
- Respiratory syncytial virus
- Herpes simplex virus
- Arbovirus
- Adenovirus
- Yellow fever
- Rabies

SYSTEMIC CONDITIONS

- Pregnancy
- Kawasaki's disease
- Collagen-vascular disorders (e.g., lupus)
- Infiltrative disorders (e.g., sarcoidosis)
- Hypereosinophilia
- Wegener's granulomatosis
- Thyrotoxicosis

DRUGS OR SUBSTANCES

- Hypersensitivity reactions
- Insect or snake bites
- Acetazolamide
- Alcohol
- *p*-Aminosalicylic acid
- Amphetamines
- Amphotericin B
- Antimony
- Arsenic
- Barbiturates
- Caffeine
- Carbamazepine
- Carbon monoxide
- Catecholamines
- Chloramphenicol
- Cocaine
- Diphenylhydantoin
- Diphtheria or tetanus toxoid
- Diuretics
- 5-Fluorouracil
- Heavy metals
- Horse serum
- Immunosuppressives
- Indomethacin
- Isoniazid
- Lithium
- Penicillins
- Phenothiazines
- Phenylbutazone
- Quinidine
- Rapeseed oil
- Smallpox vaccine
- Streptomycin
- Sulfonamides
- Sulfonylureas
- Theophylline
- Tetracycline

Modified from Rodenheffer R, Gersh B: Dilated cardiomyopathies and the mycarditides. In Guilani ER, Gersh BJ, McGoon MD, and others, editors: *The Mayo Clinic practice of cardiology,* St Louis, 1996, Mosby.

DIAGNOSTICS

Because myocarditis has varied presentations, the diagnosis is made either by clinical signs and symptoms or by pathologic cell biopsy criteria; these are neither uniformly sensitive nor specific.[9] Uniformly accepted diagnostic criteria are lacking.[10]

Initial laboratory evaluation includes CBC; cardiac enzymes; evaluation of renal and liver function; and appropriate titers, including viral or Lyme. Troponin I may be elevated after the onset of symptoms; this elevation is caused when lymphocytes infiltrate heart muscle.[11] In addition, other tests may be indicated to investigate suspected causes of myocardial inflammation.

A chest x-ray study is obtained; as mentioned previously, results are consistent with the degree of heart failure present. The ECG can be normal or reveal ST-segment and T-wave abnormalities. These abnormalities may vary, and the ECG may revert to normal on recovery.[2]

Atrial and/or ventricular arrhythmias with or without atrioventricular conduction blocks occur.[1] Twenty-four-hour cardiac monitoring is helpful when palpitations are reported to assess their clinical implications. An echocardiogram detects valvular, wall motion, and left ventricular output abnormalities.

If pulse oximetry is available in the office setting, it can be a useful modality to assist with diagnosis in mildly symptomatic cases with questionable tachycardia. The pulse oximeter is attached, and resting pulse rate and oxygen saturation in arterial blood (Sa_{O_2}) are recorded. The patient can then be asked to perform the maneuver that precipitated the tachycardia, such as walking a certain distance or climbing a flight of stairs, while pulse rates and SaO_2 are recorded. Tachycardia and mild desaturation have been observed. Of course, any findings of heart failure or reports of symptomatic palpitations or chest discomfort eliminate this as a recommended diagnostic aid.

The patient's clinical status and potential for deterioration in condition determine whether the initial evaluation is done on an outpatient basis or in the monitored hospital setting. Patients with severe cases of myocarditis may be evaluated with endomyocardial biopsy (EMB) to determine the diagnosis and to assess therapeutic response.[1] Whereas 80% to 90% of patients with clinical findings suggesting myocarditis have nonspecific histologic findings on EMB, the remaining 10% to 20% of these patients demonstrate histologic findings that are helpful for diagnosis. Histologic and histochemical stainings of EMB can be used to differentiate the various noninflammatory causes of ventricular dysfunction. In particular, positive findings on EMB can be used to differentiate between the diagnosis of acute myocardial infarction and acute myocarditis in cases where clinical findings overlap. EMB is also effective in distinguishing heart failure caused by giant cell myocarditis from other diseases.[12]

The low correlation of histologic evidence with clinical findings may be because of the difficulty of applying the Dallas criteria as accepted pathologic proof of myocarditis.[4] The Dallas criteria consider evidence of myocyte damage to be the presence of inflammatory infiltrate, T-cell lymphocytes only; there is also disagreement concerning the minimum number of T cells needed to meet criteria for diagnosis.[4] The Dallas criteria, established in 1984, exclude other evidence of inflammation such as cytokines, B cells, adhesion molecules, activated macrophages, and expressions of class II major histocompatibility antigens.[4]

The difficulty in establishing uniformly applicable diagnostic criteria may stem from the failure to define cellular markers or cell pathologic conditions indicative of myocarditis; or perhaps the multiple causes produce distinctly different clinical presentations.[6] Also, the infiltrative process of myocarditis may be transient, confounding biopsy results.[8]

Measurement of elevation in serum troponin I, a serum marker associated with cardiac injury that persists for up to 14 days, can be performed.[7] Cardiologists use nuclear imaging modalities such as antimyosin immunoscintigraphy.[9] The recently discovered diagnostic value of early- and delayed-perfusion cardiac MRI has produced adequate results for the diagnosis of acute myocarditis.[13] Laser microdissection is a new technique used primarily in clinical cardiovascular research to produce a molecular and genetic analysis of cardiac cells and differentiate between viral and autoimmune causes of myocarditis.[14]

There are an array of testing options, including some, like EMB, that are extremely invasive. The number of tests, coupled with the nonspecific findings on these tests in many cases of myocarditis, mandate that decisions about the specific diagnostic testing that an individual patient requires be made in consultation with cardiology.

DIAGNOSTICS

Myocarditis

INITIAL
Pulse oximetry*
Monitoring for palpitations

LABORATORY
CBC and differential
Cardiac enzymes
Troponin I
BUN
Creatinine
LFTs
Disease titers

IMAGING
Chest x-ray
MRI*
Early and delayed perfusion cardiac MRI

OTHER
Myocardial biopsy*
Echocardiogram
ECG
Holter or event monitoring
Endomyocardial biopsy

*If indicated.

DIFFERENTIAL DIAGNOSIS

Other causes for arrhythmia, heart failure, and poor exercise tolerance, including coronary artery, pulmonary, or valvular heart disease, must be excluded. Particularly, the existence of cardiomyopathy needs to be disproved. Cardiomyopathy is cardiac muscle disease, classified as dilated, hypertrophic, or restrictive.[1,15] If cardiomyopathy is suspected, appropriate testing to exclude reversible causes and evaluate cardiac function is required. Reversible causes of cardiomyopathy include metabolic and infiltrative diseases (e.g., hemochromatosis, amyloidosis, sarcoidosis, or glycogen storage disease), metabolic disorders (i.e., thyroid disease, acromegaly, Cushing's disease, or pheochromocytoma), toxic effects (i.e., alcohol, cocaine, antineoplastic agents, or amphetamines), radiation effects, nutritional deficiencies (i.e., thiamine or hypophosphatemia), collagen disorders, rheumatic fever, rheumatoid arthritis, neuromuscular disorders, septic shock, or transplant rejection.[1,10] An interesting cause of cardiomyopathy is Chagas' disease, a parasitic infection found predominantly in Central and South America, which may manifest with cardiomyopathy years after the initial infection.

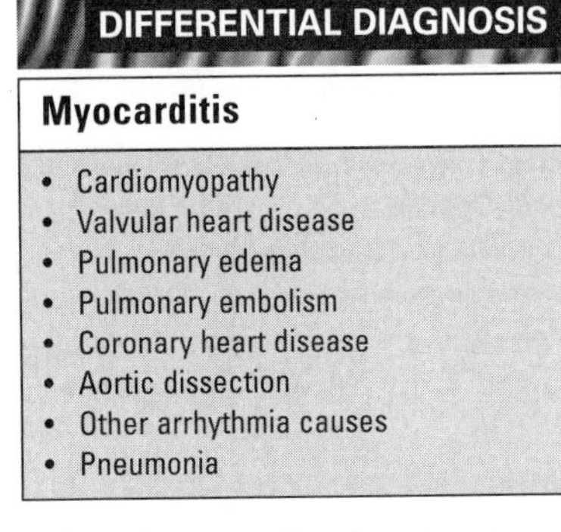
DIFFERENTIAL DIAGNOSIS

Myocarditis

- Cardiomyopathy
- Valvular heart disease
- Pulmonary edema
- Pulmonary embolism
- Coronary heart disease
- Aortic dissection
- Other arrhythmia causes
- Pneumonia

MANAGEMENT

Supportive therapy with bed rest; quiet environment; and restriction of smoking, alcohol, and caffeine is indicated for all patients. The decision to hospitalize is based on the patient's clinical status, the cause of the myocarditis, and the presence of arrhythmias or heart failure. Some patients with mild viral myocarditis and no heart failure or life-threatening arrhythmias may be managed as outpatients.

With viral myocarditis, an assessment of the phase of the disease is helpful, since recommendations have the potential to increase damage when the nonsteroidal agents are used at an incorrect stage of the disease. In phase 1, the viral replication phase, antiviral therapies are considered less helpful, since viral replication precedes development of the cardiac manifestations that characterize the condition, unless the specific viral agent has been identified or there is a known viral epidemic.[5] Immunosuppressive therapies are typically avoided at this stage. With infectious myocarditis, suppression of the early immune response with nonsteroidal antiinflammatory agents has shown increased viral replication and inflammation, producing more cardiac injury.[3] Therefore use of nonsteroidal agents should be restricted during the acute phase of the viral disease. Because studies have yielded inconsistent results with immunosuppressive therapies, only well-studied immunosuppressive drugs should be used and their use confined to patients with well-defined stage 2 disease.[5] One study points to the benefit of immunosuppressive therapy in patients with inflammatory dilated cardiomyopathy and active immune damage as demonstrated by the presence of human leukocyte antigen with myocardial biopsy.[16]

There is controversy over the role of prednisone alone or in combination with immunosuppressive agents in the treatment of myocarditis.[4,6] IV immune globulin (IVIG) remains controversial for the management of presumed viral myocarditis. Further randomized controlled trials are recommended to investigate the benefit of IVIG in patients suffering from myocarditis precipitated by a specific virus.[17]

Management of a patient with myocarditis is best achieved in consultation with a cardiologist. Immunosuppression may be recommended in patients with biopsy-proven myocarditis, patients not responding to conventional therapy, transplantation patients, patients with giant-cell myocarditis (severe symptoms with rapid disease progression), or patients with myocarditis as a sequela of systemic autoimmune disease.[18,19]

Antiarrhythmic medications are used to suppress life-threatening arrhythmias.[2] Cardiac failure is managed with conventional heart failure regimens, including angiotensin-converting enzyme inhibitors, diuretics, salt restriction, digitalis, beta blockers, vasodilators, aldosterone antagonists, and other modalities as determined by the patient's status.[20] Temporary or permanent pacing is indicated for symptomatic heart block.[2] Ventricular assist devices are currently being investigated. In one case report a ventricular assist device was successful in short-term use (20 days) with refractory ventricular fibrillation that was time limited.[21] Cardiac transplantation may be indicated in severe, irreversible cases. All management decisions are made with cardiology consultation.

LIFE SPAN CONSIDERATIONS

Young adults who are initially seen with chest pain and ECG changes suggestive of acute myocardial infarction should be investigated for nonrheumatic poststreptococcal myocarditis.[22] Myocarditis, leading to dilated cardiomyopathy, can be a complication of pregnancy, appearing in the last month or the first months after delivery.[2]

COMPLICATIONS

Sudden death from heart block, failure, or arrhythmia may occur.[1,3] Thromboembolic episodes can occur. Cardiomyopathy may occur immediately or years after apparent recovery.[3] Also, patients are at risk for continued cardiac symptoms in the chronic form of myocarditis.[1]

INDICATIONS FOR REFERRAL OR HOSPITALIZATION

Physician consultation is indicated during the initial evaluation and management and with follow-up evaluation of all patients with myocarditis. All patients suspected of myocarditis should have cardiology consultation to assist with their diagnosis and management and, if necessary, myocardial care biopsy.

All patients with myocarditis associated with heart failure or the potential for life-threatening arrhythmias should be hospitalized. In other patients the severity of the condition causing the myocarditis in association with the clinical status determines whether hospitalization is warranted.

PATIENT AND FAMILY EDUCATION

Patients with altered cardiac function are understandably anxious about their condition. A careful, sensitive explanation about the cause for the condition, rationale for testing, and realistic appraisal of their clinical status is vital for all patients with myocarditis.

Because stress has been found to cause tachycardia and palpitations in these patients, the importance of avoiding stimulating situations and substances such as caffeine, alcohol, chocolate, and cold medications should be emphasized. Rest with avoidance of any physical exercise, even housework or driving, is indicated in the acute phase. If patients are managed at home, family members should also be instructed regarding the importance of observing these restrictions.

Teaching about any medication is essential, as is reviewing the signs and symptoms that prompt immediate attention (i.e., fatigue, dyspnea, weight gain, swollen ankles, chest pain, mentation difficulty, unilateral leg pain, dizziness, or light-headedness in conjunction with palpitations). Patients should be instructed to "listen to their body" as they recover and resume activity gradually, while monitoring for elevated pulse rate and palpitations as indicators that an activity is still not tolerated. Frequent rest periods are indicated during the recovery period.

Work restrictions may be necessary for an extended period, even with mild cases. Patients should be seen regularly for support and guidance during the sometimes lengthy convalescent period. The importance of yearly vaccination against influenza is stressed with these patients. Continued support and explanations of the recovery process for family members are mandatory.

Anecdotally a mild, transient recurrence of palpitations and exertional tachycardia with subsequent infection has been observed. Patients recently recovered from myocarditis can be reassured about this occurrence, provided there are no symptomatic palpitations or signs of heart failure. However, it is not known whether this is a variant of or a marker for a chronic form of the disease.

All patients with a history of myocarditis should be assessed periodically for signs and symptoms of cardiomyopathy (e.g., dyspnea, exercise intolerance, and cardiac enlargement). The role of alcohol in the development of cardiomyopathy should be explained.

REFERENCES

1. Shah PM: Cardiomyopathies. In Stein JH, editor: *Internal medicine*, ed 5, St Louis, 1998, Mosby.
2. Rodenheffer R, Gersh B: Dilated cardiomyopathies and the myocarditides. In Guiliani ER, Gersh BJ, McGoon MD, and others, editors: *The Mayo Clinic practice of cardiology*, St Louis, 1996, Mosby.
3. Roddenheffer R, Gersh BJ, Kennel AJ: Myocarditis, dilated cardiomyopathy, and specific myocardial disease. In Guiliani ER, Gersh BJ, McGoon MD, and others, editors: *Cardiology: fundamentals and practice*, St Louis, 1991, Mosby.
4. McKenna WJ, Davies MJ: Editorial on immunosuppressive therapy for myocarditis, *N Engl J Med* 333(5):312, 1995.
5. Liu PP, Mason JW: Advances in the understanding of myocarditis, *Circulation* 104(9):1076-1082, 2001.
6. Mason JW, O'Connell JB, Herskowitz A, and others: A clinical trial of immunosuppressive therapy for myocarditis: the Myocarditis Treatment Trial Investigators, *N Engl J Med* 333(5):269-275, 1995.
7. Howes DS, Booker EA: *Myocarditis*, retrieved Jan 30, 2006, from http://www.emedicine.com/EMERG/topic326.htm.
8. Abelmann WH: Myocarditis. In Hurst JW, editor: *Medicine for the practicing physician*, Stamford, Conn, 1996, Appleton & Lange.
9. Smith SC, Ladenson JH, Mason JW, and others: Elevations of cardiac troponin I associated with myocarditis: experimental and clinical correlates, *Circulation* 95(1):163, 1997.
10. Khaw BA, Narula J: Non-invasive detection of myocyte necrosis in myocarditis and dilated cardiomyopathy with radiolabelled antimyosin, *Eur Heart J* 16(Suppl O):119-123, 1995.
11. Babuin L, Jaffe AS: Troponin: the biomarker of choice for the detection of cardiac injury, *CMAJ* 173(10):1191-1202, 2005.
12. Kingel K, Sauter M, Bock CT, and others: Molecular pathology of inflammatory cardiomyopathy, *Med Microbial Immunol (Berl)* 193(2-3):101-107, 2004.
13. Laissy JP, Hyafil F, Feldman LJ, and others: Differentiating acute myocardial infarction from myocarditis: diagnostic value of early- and delayed-perfusion cardiac MR imaging, *Radiology* 237:75-82, 2005.
14. Chimenti C, Pieroni M, Russo A, and others: Laser microdissection in clinical cardiovascular research, *Chest* 128:2876-2881, 2005.
15. Baughman KL, Kasper EK, Hershkowitz A: Myocardial and pericardial disease. In Noble J, editor: *Primary care medicine*, ed 2, St Louis, 1996, Mosby.
16. Wojnicz R, Nowalany-Kozielska E, Wojciechowska C, and others: Randomized, placebo-controlled study for immunosuppressive treatment of inflammatory dilated cardiomyopathy: 2 year follow-up results, *Circulation* 104:39-45, 2001.
17. Robinson J, Hartling L, Vandermeer B, and others: Intravenous immunoglobulin for presumed viral myocarditis in children and adults, *Cochrane Database Syst Rev* 1:CD004370, 2005.
18. Caforio AL, McKenna WJ: Recognition and optimum management of myocarditis, *Drugs* 52(4):515-525, 1996.
19. Feldman AM, McNamara D: Myocarditis, *N Engl J Med* 343(19):1388-1398, 2000.
20. Parrillo JE: Inflammatory cardiomyopathy (myocarditis): which patients should be treated with anti-inflammatory therapy? *Circulation* 104(1):4, 2001.
21. McGovern PC, Chambers S, Blumberg EA, and others: Successful explantation of a ventricular assist device following fulminant influenza type A–associated myocarditis, *J Heart Lung Transplant* 21(2):290-293, 2002.
22. Gill MV, Klein NC, Cunha BA: Non-rheumatic poststreptococcal myocarditis, *Heart Lung* 24(2):425, 1995.

CHAPTER 131

Peripheral Arterial Insufficiency

David R. Campbell

Peripheral arterial insufficiency is the condition that results when there is insufficient blood flow to the extremities. It is much more likely to occur in the lower extremities, although the increasing use of catheter interventions has made upper extremity problems more common. If the symptoms have been present for weeks or months, the condition is defined as chronic. If the symptoms develop over hours or days, it is referred to as acute.

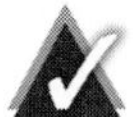

Immediate physician or vascular surgeon referral is indicated for suspected arterial occlusion or dissecting aneurysm.

CHRONIC ARTERIAL INSUFFICIENCY

DEFINITION AND EPIDEMIOLOGY

Chronic arterial insufficiency is one disease that has increasing prevalence as the population ages. Since the major cause is atherosclerosis, the risk factors for chronic arterial insufficiency are the same as those for coronary artery disease. Diabetes, hypertension, hyperlipidemia, and tobacco intake are all independent risk factors. Smokers are twice as likely to develop claudication.[1] Vascular disease is one of the most common complications of diabetes. Genetic factors have also long been recognized as being important, and recently an increased level of homocysteine was shown to be associated with premature atherosclerosis.[2] Even in younger patients, premature atherosclerosis is the most common cause of chronic arterial insufficiency, although rare causes include entrapment syndromes and adventitial cystic disease of the popliteal artery.

Numerous studies have confirmed that most patients with obstructive arterial disease have underlying coronary artery disease or diabetes and have on average a 10-year shorter life span.[1] The amputation rate is about 1% per year. However, the amputation rate is much higher in patients with diabetes and in active smokers.[1]

PATHOPHYSIOLOGY

The atherosclerotic plaque causing leg ischemia is identical to that seen in coronary artery disease and carotid disease. It is an intimal lesion that may affect any of the vessels of the lower extremity. The blockage may build up slowly, allowing collateral vessels to develop and thereby minimizing symptoms. Alternatively, intraplaque hemorrhage and thrombosis may lead to sudden expansion and acute symptomatology. The infrarenal aorta and iliac arteries are known as the *inflow arteries*, whereas the femoral, popliteal, and tibial vessels are the *outflow vessels*. Obstruction of the aortoiliac and femoral arteries is often seen in smokers, whereas tibial artery disease is much more common in patients with diabetes.

CLINICAL PRESENTATION

The classic symptom of peripheral arterial insufficiency is claudication. Claudication is a tightening or cramping pain usually in the calf muscles that is precipitated by exercise and is relieved by rest. With exercise there is an increased demand for blood that cannot be met. Subsequently lactic acid and other metabolites build up in the muscle, causing discomfort. The severity is assessed by how far a patient can walk before pain ensues. Although the distance may be reduced by an incline, cold weather, or a recent meal, it generally tends to be fairly consistent. Pain is always relieved immediately by stopping the activity and never occurs when the patient is at rest. Sometimes the thigh or buttock muscles are affected first. This is indicative of iliac artery obstruction (Leriche's syndrome). As the obstruction becomes more severe, the patient may develop pain at rest because circulation to the feet is impaired. Characteristically, the patient will go to bed and be awakened after a couple of hours by pain in the toes that is only relieved by gravity (e.g., getting out of bed or hanging the feet over the side of the bed). The patient may resort to sleeping in a chair to avoid the pain. Eventually, there is not enough blood to sustain viability, and gangrene ensues, usually beginning in the toes or heels. Ischemic rest pain is consistent; it occurs every night, unlike the intermittent leg cramps seen so often in older adults, which are not related to arterial insufficiency.

PHYSICAL EXAMINATION

On physical examination, muscle wasting, loss of hair, and reduced temperature in the affected limb may be noted. Careful pulse examination is important. Absent femoral pulses suggest inflow disease, whereas the absence of popliteal pulses implies isolated tibial disease. One physical sign that can be helpful in the diagnosis of peripheral vascular disease is dependent rubor. If the ischemic leg is elevated for 30 seconds, it becomes pale, since blood is unable to travel uphill. This renders the tissue ischemic, and the capillaries vasodilate. If the leg is then made dependent, blood travels down to those dilated capillaries, and a deep red color ensues. The longer the rubor takes to develop, the worse the ischemia. A careful history and physical examination will allow for a good assessment of the functional severity of the obstruction and the likely location.

DIAGNOSTICS

The most useful tool in assessing peripheral arterial insufficiency in the office is a portable Doppler instrument and a sphygmomanometer cuff. With these tools, it is possible to compare the systolic pressure at the brachial artery with that in the dorsalis pedis and posterior tibial arteries. This measurement is expressed as the ankle brachial index (ABI) and should be greater in the affected extremity than in the normal one. An ABI of 0.75 to 0.5 is consistent with claudication, and an ABI below 0.5 is consistent with rest pain or gangrene.

Patients with mild claudication may have palpable pulses at rest but lose them with exercise. This is best demonstrated in the vascular laboratory with an exercise noninvasive study. During this test the patient is placed on a treadmill and ABIs are measured at rest, while exercising, and on recovery.

Sometimes related medical conditions, such as obesity or peripheral edema, make it impossible to assess the pulse status. In these situations the pocket Doppler instrument may be invaluable. A normal pulse is triphasic but becomes increasingly monophasic with proximal obstruction. With practice it is relatively simple to distinguish these pulses. If Doppler ultrasonography reveals good triphasic pulses in the feet, there is unlikely to be significant ischemia. If the vascular status is unclear with physical examination, patients should be referred to the vascular laboratory for formal evaluation. Evaluation will provide the ABIs, the level at which the pulse becomes monophasic, and the pulse volume recording (a plethysmographic test that records the volume of the pulse in the extremity with each heartbeat). The forefoot tracing is helpful for the vascular surgeon to determine whether there is enough circulation to heal a foot lesion. This is particularly important in patients with diabetes, in whom ABIs are often inaccurate.

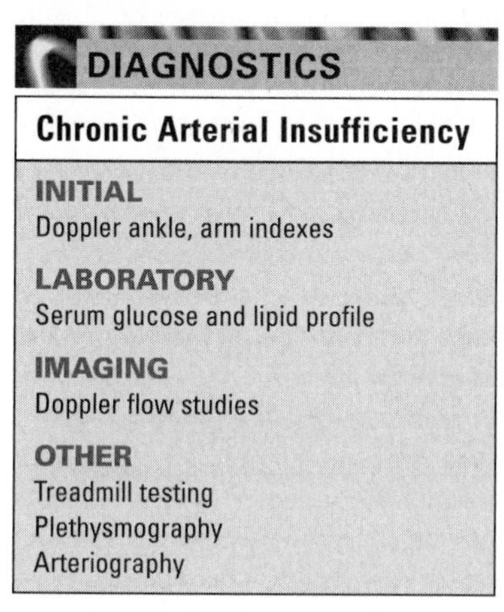

DIAGNOSTICS

Chronic Arterial Insufficiency

INITIAL
Doppler ankle, arm indexes

LABORATORY
Serum glucose and lipid profile

IMAGING
Doppler flow studies

OTHER
Treadmill testing
Plethysmography
Arteriography

Other tests are available but are used less often except in research protocols. Chief among these is the measurement of transcutaneous oxygen, which reflects the metabolic state of the target tissues. Unfortunately, variants such as ambient temperature make this test impractical as a routine test. Instead of a treadmill test, it is possible to use reactive hyperemia obtained after inflating a pressure cuff to suprasystolic pressure to produce vasodilation; however, this is somewhat uncomfortable and has not become routinely available.

DIFFERENTIAL DIAGNOSIS

The presence of peripheral neuropathy in diabetes makes the diagnosis of peripheral insufficiency difficult. Damage to the peripheral nerves may mask the symptoms of arterial insufficiency. Thus if patients have no feeling in their legs, they may simply complain that their legs get tired of walking. Without sensation, there may be no rest pain, and patients may be initially seen with painless gangrene. Other conditions that should be considered include cauda equina syndrome, Buerger's disease, leg cramps, and musculoskeletal disorders.

Cauda Equina Syndrome

Spinal stenosis causing pressure on the nerve roots may result in symptoms of claudication from the hip downward, which can easily be confused with Leriche's syndrome. This is becoming increasingly common as the population ages and progressive degenerative joint disease becomes more prevalent. The correct diagnosis can be made by ordering noninvasive exercise studies. In cauda equina syndrome there will be no pressure drop when the patient exercises on a treadmill.

Buerger's Disease

Buerger's disease is an inflammatory occlusive disease involving primarily the medium and smaller arteries of both the upper and lower extremities. Although less common in the United States, it is seen more often in the Middle East and Asia and appears to be directly related to the effects of smoking. Patients manifest the signs and symptoms of chronic arterial insufficiency, but apart from smoking have no other risk factors for atherosclerosis. Bypass surgery is rarely indicated because disease is more distal, but patients will experience remission if exposure to nicotine is avoided.

DIFFERENTIAL DIAGNOSIS

Chronic Arterial Insufficiency

- Acute peripheral arterial occlusion
- Peripheral neuropathy
- Cauda equina syndrome
- Buerger's disease
- Musculoskeletal condition
- Leg cramps

MANAGEMENT

Management of chronic arterial insufficiency depends on the severity of the symptoms. If the patient has stable claudication and is managing without much difficulty, then it is reasonable to treat the patient conservatively. Patients with mild, recent-onset claudication are likely to improve with conservative measures alone. These include lifestyle modifications as indicated, particularly tobacco cessation. Studies comparing exercise with angioplasty have shown that a daily exercise program involving walking to the point of pain as often as possible is as effective as angioplasty in providing relief of symptoms.[3] Because the ABI does not change, it is believed that this effect is produced by training the muscles rather than producing increased flow to the foot. Hypertension, hyperlipidemia, and diabetes must be treated aggressively.

Because these patients are at high risk for coronary artery disease, it is prudent to start them on a daily aspirin dosage as well. The literature on the role of aspirin, dipyridamole, and ticlopidine in peripheral vascular disease is extensive and confusing.[4] There is much disagreement as to whether aspirin confers benefit either preoperatively or postoperatively in patients with peripheral vascular disease. There is agreement, however, that low-dose aspirin (81 to 325 mg/day) reduces the incidence and mortality of subsequent myocardial infarction in patients older than 50 years. It makes sense therefore to initiate low-dose aspirin for all patients with peripheral vascular disease provided that there are no contraindications.

There has never been a study demonstrating a benefit to adding dipyridamole to that regimen. Ticlopidine, another antiplatelet agent, is at least as effective as aspirin, but it is expensive and has significant side effects. Clopidogrel (Plavix) is also more effective than aspirin and safer than ticlopidine, but it, too, is expensive and its role, if any, in the management of peripheral vascular disease remains to be determined.

Together with aspirin, most physicians now start their patients with peripheral vascular disease on a statin, whatever their cholesterol or low-density lipoprotein (LDL). It has been shown that statin therapy helps stabilize a plaque and lowers the LDL, and recent studies have suggested that bypasses are more durable if the patient is taking a statin.[5]

Pentoxifylline (Trental) has been shown to increase the distance that 30% of patients with claudication can walk, although the effect has been small. Recent trials of cilostazol (Pletal), a phosphodiesterase III inhibitor, have demonstrated significant improvement over both placebo and pentoxifylline in distance walked without symptoms for patients with claudication.[6] The main contraindication for cilostazol is a history of congestive heart failure. It is safe to say that neither of these drugs has had the hoped-for impact on the management of claudication.

COMPLICATIONS

Lower extremity ulcers may result from neuropathy, arterial insufficiency, infection, or a combination of these. Infection such as cellulitis or ulcers with extensive involvement may result in osteomyelitis. The presence of infection can also disturb blood glucose control, complicating diabetes management.

Associated with peripheral neuropathy is the development of calcification of the arteries. This is not related to the atherosclerotic lesion, which is an intimal lesion, but it does render the vessels relatively incompressible. This means that the ABI may be artificially elevated and less helpful in assessing the degree of ischemia. In these cases the pulse volume recording can be particularly helpful.

Thirty percent of patients with neuropathy also have an autonomic neuropathy, which is sometimes called an autosympathectomy. This condition results in diversion of blood from the nutrient vessels to the skin, making the skin unnaturally warm. Thus it is possible to see a diabetic patient with a minor skin lesion but with no symptoms and a warm foot that is critically ischemic. Failure to recognize this may result in further loss of tissue.

Diabetic Foot Ulcer

Diabetic neuropathy is a polyneuropathy and has a motor component. The paralysis of the intrinsic muscles results in clawing of the foot, and the patient tends to develop traumatic lesions over the metatarsal heads and on the tops of the toes. Healing may be impaired by relative arterial insufficiency.

Any infection requires treatment with appropriate debridement and antibiotics. Also, bed rest is indicated to minimize damage that may go undetected if neuropathy is present. If the ulcer is superficial, it can be treated on an outpatient basis, with non–weight bearing, dressing care, and a first-generation cephalosporin. If the ulcer is deep or has significant cellulitis, hospitalization is advised and broad-spectrum antibiotics instituted (see Chapter 71). Failure to heal with treatment suggests arterial insufficiency and merits referral to a vascular surgeon for possible arteriography.

INDICATIONS FOR REFERRAL OR HOSPITALIZATION

If patients are seen with severe claudication, rest pain, or gangrene, they should be referred promptly to a vascular surgeon for further evaluation. Once the extent of the severe ischemia has been identified, arteriography is indicated to demonstrate the extent and location of the obstruction.

Treatment may involve angioplasty and stent placement or surgery. Magnetic resonance arteriography (MRA) may be used in preference to standard arteriography in patients with abnormal renal function. MRA is also helpful in demonstrating arteries in the lower leg not seen on standard arteriography. In general, neither arteriography nor MRA should be ordered without vascular surgical consultation. Once the location and extent of the blockage have been identified, the surgeon and radiologist can collaborate to determine the appropriate therapy.

Endovascular procedures have been used in patients with localized iliac artery lesions and higher surgical risk.[7] More extensive and more distal disease is more likely to require bypass either with prosthetic material or with the patient's own saphenous vein. The use of endovascular procedures is determined best by discussion between the surgeon and the patient about the risks, benefits, and longevity of the repair, along with consideration of the anatomic location of the arterial lesions and of individual patient factors that affect surgical risk.[7]

Diabetic patients with neuropathy or arterial insufficiency require regular podiatry consultation. The podiatrist will determine the frequency of visits based on callus development. With appropriate shoes and care of calluses and nails, many patients with ischemia can avoid problems for long periods. Regular podiatry visits enable early recognition of potential problems and ensure expeditious referral and treatment.

Patients with superficial ulcers who do not improve with bed rest and treatment require referral to a vascular surgeon. More extensive ulcers require immediate vascular consultation.

PATIENT AND FAMILY EDUCATION

All patients should be advised to follow a low-fat diet, exercise regularly, and avoid all tobacco products. Patients over age 50 years without contraindications should understand the importance of low-dose daily aspirin. Patients with diabetes, particularly if neuropathy is present, should be instructed to visually inspect their feet daily and seek professional help for any foot lesion. Many patients with diabetes are terrified of amputation and should be reassured that, with good podiatric care and immediate attention to any problem, amputation can usually be avoided. All patients with arterial insufficiency should have their toenails cut by a podiatrist. In addition, patients should be given instructions about general foot protection measures, including wearing properly fitting shoes, avoiding synthetic materials in shoes that do not "breathe," and always wearing shoes or slippers. Direct contact with very hot or very cold substances or surfaces must be avoided. It is imperative to seek immediate medical evaluation for prolonged pain, sudden color changes, or a numb feeling in the extremities.

ACUTE ARTERIAL INSUFFICIENCY

DEFINITION AND EPIDEMIOLOGY

Acute arterial insufficiency is the sudden onset of the symptoms of ischemia. The incidence of acute arterial occlusion seems to be increasing.[7] This increase is partly related to better diagnosis and recognition, but also to the fact that patients with advanced heart disease are living longer and undergoing more invasive procedures. It is critical to make the diagnosis expeditiously to avoid loss of limb or life.

PATHOPHYSIOLOGY

Acute ischemia may result from an embolus from another source in a distal vessel. The most common source of an embolus is the heart. This may be the clot that forms on the ventricular wall after a myocardial infarction or a clot from the atrium in patients with atrial fibrillation. Rarely, a tumor in the heart such as atrial myxoma may break off and travel to the peripheral vessels.

Acute thrombosis of preexisting atherosclerotic lesions is the other major cause of acute ischemia. This type may be less severe than acute ischemia secondary to embolization, since collateral circulation has had time to develop. Aneurysms of the abdominal aorta or popliteal artery may cause acute ischemia secondary to acute thrombosis of the aneurysm. Once the embolus becomes lodged, the arteries and veins distal to the occlusion go into spasm. After a few hours, vasodilation occurs, and the thrombus begins to organize. At this point the ischemia becomes irreversible. It is generally accepted that if acute occlusion of the limb occurs and there is no collateral circulation, necrosis will begin after 6 hours unless the ischemia is relieved.

CLINICAL PRESENTATION

Classically, the patient will be seen with a history of sudden onset of pain in an extremity. A history of recent myocardial infarction or atrial fibrillation and the presence of normal circulation in the other limb suggest an embolus as the source. A previous history of peripheral vascular disease suggests acute thrombosis as the cause.

PHYSICAL EXAMINATION

On examination the limb is usually pale and pulseless with absent or diminished capillary refill. If there is loss of sensation or immobility of the foot, tissue loss is imminent. These signs and symptoms are often referred to as the five *P*'s: *P*ain, *P*allor, *P*ulselessness, *P*aresthesias, and *P*aralysis. Untreated, the limb becomes edematous, mottled, and eventually gangrenous. The sudden onset of pain with signs of acute ischemia and mottling from the waist down suggests acute aortic occlusion and demands immediate diagnosis and treatment if the patient is to survive.

DIAGNOSTICS

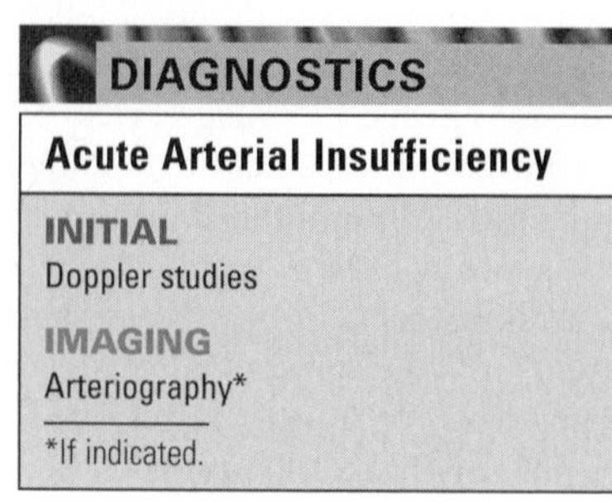
DIAGNOSTICS

Acute Arterial Insufficiency

INITIAL
Doppler studies

IMAGING
Arteriography*

*If indicated.

Diagnosis is generally based on the clinical presentation and examination. Doppler studies may be necessary to confirm the presence or absence of arterial pulses. Arteriography may be indicated in some circumstances.

DIFFERENTIAL DIAGNOSIS

The patient history usually suggests whether the ischemia is related to an embolus or thrombus. The most common error is misdiagnosing acute ischemia as an acute neurologic event. The consequent delay in treatment can result in limb loss or, in the case of acute aortic occlusion, death. Careful pulse examination at the time of presentation will avoid this problem. Other causes of acute arterial insufficiency or arterial occlusion include blue toe syndrome and aneurysms.

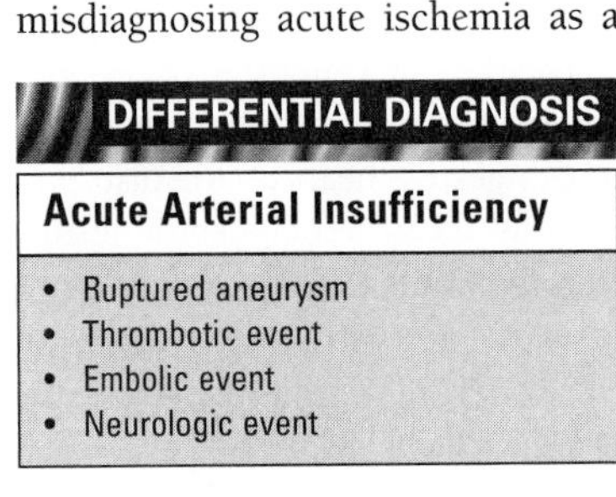

Blue Toe Syndrome

Bluish discoloration or localized gangrene of the feet without evidence of ischemia, infection, or peripheral neuropathy is known as *blue toe syndrome*. Blue toe syndrome results from microemboli from the heart, aorta, or peripheral arteries that are small enough to lodge in the capillaries. These emboli may be small thrombi from the heart or from an aortic or popliteal aneurysm. They may also be cholesterol emboli or atheroemboli from atherosclerotic plaques in the aorta, iliac arteries, or femoral arteries.

When blue toe syndrome is suspected, careful physical examination for the presence of an abdominal or popliteal aneurysm is mandatory. If there is no evidence of ischemia, infection, or peripheral neuropathy, a cardiac echocardiogram and abdominal ultrasound study should be obtained. If these are negative for a clot or abdominal aneurysm, antiplatelet therapy is begun and the patient is monitored closely. Consultation with a vascular surgeon is appropriate at this point. Usually, the lesion will improve over the next few weeks, but if it does not, or if emboli recur, a transesophageal echocardiogram and an aortogram of the thoracic aorta to the femoral arteries are indicated. If a localized lesion is discovered, it can be addressed, although diffuse atherosclerosis of the suprarenal aorta is often the source. In these cases recurrent embolization often leads to chronic renal failure and distal gangrene. Ligation of the iliac arteries with axillobifemoral bypass and preparation for dialysis are the current available therapies.

Aneurysm

An aneurysm is a localized enlargement of an artery that causes symptoms by expansion, rupture, or thrombosis. A true aneurysm is said to be present when the wall of the aneurysm is an arterial wall. If the wall is compressed connective tissue, however, then the rupture is a contained rupture, or false aneurysm.

Infrarenal aortic aneurysms are a common cause of death secondary to rupture. Often they are asymptomatic, although they may cause an acute onset of back or abdominal pain. If a pulsatile abdominal mass is discovered on physical examination, further evaluation with either abdominal ultrasound or a CT scan is indicated. If the presence of an aneurysm is confirmed, referral to a vascular surgeon is indicated. Femoral or popliteal aneurysms are less common but may be detected on physical examination and usually cause symptoms by expansion and thrombosis. They are often associated with aortic aneurysms, and an abdominal ultrasound should also be obtained if either of these is detected.

Patients with aneurysms should be advised that this condition is often congenital and that any blood relatives older than age 50 years should probably have an abdominal ultrasound.

MANAGEMENT

As soon as the diagnosis of acute arterial occlusion is made, a bolus of IV heparin (5000 units) should be given to prevent a clot from forming distal to the occlusion. Hospitalization and prompt referral to a vascular surgeon for evaluation with treatment are essential. Ideally, treatment, whether surgical or thrombolytic therapy, should be instituted within 6 hours of the occlusion.

COMPLICATIONS

Complications are less dependent on the effect of the acute occlusion than on the cause. Thus patients with an embolus at the time of a massive myocardial infarction will do poorly in comparison with those whose clot is from atrial fibrillation. Studies show a mortality rate with arterial occlusion of 22% to 39% and an amputation rate of 11% to 17%.[8,9]

INDICATIONS FOR REFERRAL OR HOSPITALIZATION

Immediate evaluation by a vascular surgeon is imperative. Acute arterial occlusion is an emergency in which treatment delay can impair limb viability or threaten life.

PATIENT AND FAMILY EDUCATION

Review of the signs and symptoms for acute arterial occlusion at regular intervals is indicated. For other educational points for review, see the Patient and Family Education section under Chronic Arterial Insufficiency, p. 598.

REFERENCES

1. Coffman JD: Peripheral vascular disease. In Noble J, editor: *Textbook of primary care medicine,* ed 3, St Louis, 2001, Mosby.
2. Molgaard J, Malinow MR, Lassvik C, and others: Hyperhomocyst(e)inaemia: an independent risk factor for intermittent claudication, *J Intern Med* 231:273-279, 1992.
3. Perkins JM, Collin J, Creasy TS, and others: Exercise training versus angioplasty for stable claudication: long and medium term results of a prospective randomised trial, *Eur J Vasc Endovasc Surg* 11(4):409-413, 1996.
4. Humphrey PW, Silver D: Antithrombotic therapy. In Rutherford RB, editor: *Vascular surgery,* Philadelphia, 1995, Saunders.
5. Abbruzzese TA, Havens J, Belkin M, and others: Statin therapy is associated with improved patency of autogenous infrainguinal bypass grafts, *J Vasc Surg* 39(6):1178-1185, 2004.
6. Dawson DL, Cutler BS, Hiatt WR, and others: A comparison of cilostazol and pentoxifylline for treating intermittent claudication, *Am J Med* 109(7):523-530, 2000.
7. Kanani RS, Garasic JM: Lower extremity arterial occlusive disease: role of percutaneous revascularization, *Curr Treat Options Cardiovasc Med* 7(2):99-107, 2005.
8. Brewster DC: Acute peripheral arterial occlusion, *Cardiol Clin* 9(3):497-513, 1991.
9. Baxter-Smith D, Ashton F, Slaney G: Peripheral arterial embolism: a 20-year review, *J Cardiovasc Surg* 29(4):453-457, 1988.

CHAPTER 132

Peripheral Edema

Debra Hobbins

DEFINITION AND EPIDEMIOLOGY

There is no standard clinical definition of peripheral edema.[1] Edema is commonly identified by the "pitting" that occurs when manual pressure is applied to various locations on the lower extremities. The physical appearance of edema is a sign of increased interstitial volume. There must be a significant increase in interstitial volume before edema becomes evident, and once present, small additional changes in interstitial volume can result in a disproportionate increase in the severity of the edema. Transient peripheral edema is common in the general population and is primarily related to posture, age, and climactic conditions.

Venous hypertension and impaired lymphatic function are two of the most important underlying pathomechanisms,[2] although peripheral edema can be a harbinger of a potentially serious disease. Early detection of the underlying disease process enables early treatment and prevents more serious complications. Peripheral edema is uncomfortable, sometimes intolerable, and causes considerable distress and disfigurement in patients.[3] Pedal edema may be ignored or missed completely because it is slow to develop; patients often will not complain until their shoes no longer fit. Interestingly, women are more likely than men to come forward with a complaint of edema.[4]

The implications of peripheral edema depend on a patient's health status and/or disease state. It can be an expected finding in a normal pregnancy as a result of the increase in total body water and increased peripheral venous pressure. It may also be a side effect of certain medications. However, disease states such as venous and arterial insufficiency, congestive heart failure, renal failure, and cirrhosis account for the majority of cases of peripheral edema.[5]

PATHOPHYSIOLOGY

All forms of edema are caused by excess interstitial fluid in the tissues—an imbalance between capillary filtration and lymph drainage. Described by Starling more than 100 years ago, edema results from an imbalance in the hydrostatic and colloid osmotic forces across the capillary wall, resulting in net transcapillary filtration that exceeds lymphatic flow.[4] The capillary wall is impermeable to plasma proteins, but freely permeable to water and low molecular solutes. Edema is described as trace, or barely detectable, to 4+ pitting.[1] Weight gain of 1.8 to 2.2 kg (4 to 5 pounds) usually precedes the visible signs of edema, and severe edema can cause tissues to be rocklike.

The amount of fluid in the interstitial space depends on several factors: capillary pressure and permeability, the interstitial and osmotic pressure that results from plasma colloids, lymphatic circulation, and total extracellular fluid. A change in any of these factors causes increased interstitial volume with resultant edema. Because of the effects of gravity, interstitial fluid tends to be first noted in the peripheral system; for example, an individual who remains predominantly in the supine position will first accumulate interstitial fluid in the sacral area.

The peripheral edema that results from congestive heart failure is produced by an elevation in venous pressure and capillary pressure. The resulting systemic venous congestion produces peripheral edema. Congestive heart failure also predisposes an individual to venous stasis. Venous stasis results from incompetent valves or a weakness in the venous walls themselves, causing dilation and valve failure with resultant reflux. Venous valves can also degenerate as a result of genetic factors, resolving thrombi, or advancing age.

With venous thrombi, obstruction of venous outflow causes an increase in pressure. As a result, fluid is pushed through the capillary membranes into the tissue space, which leads to edema.

The peripheral edema associated with cirrhosis or hypoalbuminemia results from decreased albumin. A decrease in plasma protein or an increase in the protein content of the interstitial fluid decreases oncotic pressure and results in fluid accumulation.

Electrolyte imbalance also plays a role in the development of peripheral edema. Edema is one of the most common manifestations of sodium excess. Whenever there is abnormal retention of salt in the body, water is also retained. The kidneys assume the major role in sodium balance. Reducing salt intake results in hypotonicity of the plasma with an increased loss of water via the kidneys. Many diuretics act directly on the kidney tubules to prevent sodium reabsorption.

Pharmacotherapy can result in peripheral edema, usually bilateral, with a cause-effect relationship suggested by elapsed time from the administration of a new drug to the onset of leg edema. A number of drug classes have been associated with peripheral edema in conjunction with weight gain: NSAIDs; cyclooxygenase-2 selective receptor inhibitors, such as celecoxib and rofecoxib; thiazolidinediones, such as rosiglitazone and pioglitazone[6]; pergolide[7] (treatment for Parkinson's disease, which was recently removed from the U.S. market); nonspecific vasodilators, such as hydralazine and minoxidil; beta blockers; central alpha agonists; peripheral alpha blockers; opiates; intrathecal opiate infusions; and calcium channel blockers (CCBs).[1] Drug-related edema should resolve completely on discontinuation of the drug, although this may take several days.

The edema that is observed with CCB treatment results from a decreased arteriolar resistance that is unmatched by the venous circulation and can differ in appearance from more traditional edema states. This edema results in lower extremity redness; warmth; and a nonblanching petechial rash, which is believed to occur as a result of red blood cell leakage from capillaries and can cause long-lasting discoloration. The incidence of edema with CCB therapy is medication and dose dependent and can range from 5% to as high as 70%. The incidence of edema related to the CCB therapy is higher in women than in men and related to upright posture and age.[3]

Peripheral edema also results from lymphedema, which may be caused by interference with the drainage of lymph from any part of the body. The function of the lymphatic vessels is to return to the bloodstream the water, protein, and products of cellular metabolism that cannot be reabsorbed by blood capillaries. The lymphatic channels drain the interstitial fluid. Blockage of the lymphatic system may be the result of an infection, malignant process, surgical procedure, or radiotherapy.

Edema resulting from sleep apnea is an uncommon form of peripheral edema. The right-sided pressure changes associated with sleep apnea can slow venous flow, promoting the onset of edema. This edema is not typically accompanied by other signs of volume excess and may wax and wane for reasons that may relate to the fluctuating nature of sleep apnea itself.[1]

CLINICAL PRESENTATION

The presence of edema does not necessarily mandate urgent treatment. A systematic approach is recommended to determine the underlying disease process. The patient may be seen with unilateral or bilateral swelling of the foot or leg. The color of the affected area may range from normal to pink, red, or brown. Pain and respiratory difficulties may or may not be present.

PHYSICAL EXAMINATION

Obtaining the past medical and current medication histories is critical. In addition, important factors related to the history of a patient with peripheral edema include location of the edema; unilateral or bilateral nature; history of acute trauma; any alteration in the fitting of clothing or shoes; the presence of a cough, progressive shortness of breath, or nocturnal dyspnea; and a report of the urine volume, color, and frequency.

During the physical examination, it is important to note the extent and severity of the edema. Because of the subjective nature of describing edema on the trace to 4+ scale, reporting the location of the edema, such as midshin or midthigh, provides more practical and reproducible information. Limb asymmetry is often evidence of chronic venous insufficiency.[1] Note the color and temperature of the skin and any breakdown or lesions. Also, the presence of any gait difficulty should be determined. The patient's current weight should be compared with previously recorded weights. During the cardiovascular examination, the presence of new gallops, murmurs, or jugular venous distention should be assessed. Ascites in the abdomen or rales on pulmonary auscultation should be determined, since these can indicate increased fluid volume.[8]

DIAGNOSTICS

A careful history and physical examination are helpful in determining the necessary screening tests to search for the cause of the peripheral edema. In unilateral edema with acute onset and pain a lower extremity ultrasound is obtained to exclude deep vein thrombosis. The ultrasound should be repeated in cases of persistent unilateral painful edema. A urinalysis is obtained to check for protein. Serum electrolytes, BUN, creatinine, total protein, albumin, and globulin may be measured to elicit the cause of the edema. With more generalized edema, liver function tests and a thyroid-stimulating hormone level are necessary. The presence of pelvic lymphadenopathy and peripheral edema necessitates an evaluation for a pelvic mass with appropriate radiographs, a CT scan, or an MRI of the abdomen and pelvis. Vascular or arterial studies are indicated if the lower extremities also show brawny skin color changes or symptoms suggesting venous or arterial insufficiency.

DIAGNOSTICS

Peripheral Edema

LABORATORY
- Urinalysis
- Serum electrolytes
- BUN
- Creatinine
- Total protein
- Glucose
- Serum albumin
- LFTs*
- 24-hour urine for albumin and creatinine*
- TSH*

IMAGING
- Chest x-ray*
- Doppler flow studies*
- Venogram*
- Abdominal, pelvic CT scan or MRI*
- Ultrasound*

*If indicated.

DIFFERENTIAL DIAGNOSIS

When there is evidence of lower extremity edema, the differential diagnosis ranges from idiopathic edema, stasis secondary to long periods of immobility and excessive sodium intake, and the Charcot's foot of diabetes; to serious entities such as renal failure, cirrhosis, pulmonary hypertension, HIV infection, or congestive heart failure.[9,10] The possibility of drug-induced peripheral edema should be investigated. A drug history is necessary to prevent unnecessary diagnostic testing or inappropriate treatment.[11] A history of phlebitis is important to note; postphlebitic syndrome is characterized by a chronically swollen limb and in some individuals can appear after 10 to 20 years because of incompetent veins.[12,13]

MANAGEMENT

Management of peripheral edema is dictated by the underlying cause. Restriction of sodium and frequent elevation of the affected extremities are helpful strategies; the use of support or compression stockings is a beneficial adjunct. These interventions may be all that is necessary when the edema is due to increased hydrostatic or decreased osmotic pressure. If the edema is a side effect of a drug, the medication may need to be changed, or a diuretic may need to be added to the regimen. When the underlying cause is cardiac failure, renal failure, or cirrhosis, treatment depends on the severity of the disease and the systems affected.

Co-Management with Specialists

In most cases the health care provider can manage the patient with peripheral edema. If the patient has significant renal or cardiac disease, the provider must initiate careful and ongoing communication regarding the choice of therapy and changes to the medication regimen. Home care nurses are a valuable

DIFFERENTIAL DIAGNOSIS

Peripheral Edema

- Idiopathic edema
- Renal failure
- Liver failure
- Cirrhosis
- Heart failure
- Cellulitis
- Trauma
- Sodium retention (increased intake or medication induced)
- Venous-arterial insufficiency
- Thrombophlebitis
- Lymphatic obstruction
- Allergic reaction
- Thyroid disease
- Pregnancy
- Menstruation
- Vasculitis
- Stasis
- Diabetes
- Pulmonary hypertension, HIV
- Sleep apnea

MEDICATIONS THAT MAY CAUSE PERIPHERAL EDEMA

- Calcium channel blockers
- Opiates (including intrathecal administration)
- Thiazolidinediones
- NSAIDs
- High-dose beta blockers
- Central alpha agonists
- Peripheral alpha blockers
- Cyclooxygenase-2 selective receptor inhibitors
- Pergolide

resource for patients with more complicated conditions. Diuresis can often be accomplished at home with a record of daily weights, determination of postural vital signs, and respiratory and cardiac assessment by the home care nurse in conjunction with monitoring of electrolytes and kidney function tests.

COMPLICATIONS

Complications of peripheral edema result from a failure to recognize the early warning signs and a delay in diagnosing a pathologic condition. Deep vein thrombosis can lead to embolization and life-threatening risks. Persistent peripheral edema may lead to tissue breakdown and resultant cellulitis.

Recent literature addresses an ECG syndrome—the attenuation of ECG voltage, mediated by a decrease in the electrical impedance of the body's volume conductor because of water overload and peripheral edema, regardless of the specific pathologic condition involved. The attenuation of ECG voltage affects the amplitude and duration of QRS complexes and P waves, resulting in serious clinical implications for patients with heart failure. ECG changes have been associated with masking both atrial abnormalities and the diagnoses of P pulmonale, P mitrale, and biatrial abnormality.[14,15] Also noted were the apparent conversions of complete intraventricular conduction delays or bundle branch blocks (BBBs) to incomplete BBBs, or vice versa.[16,17]

INDICATIONS FOR REFERRAL OR HOSPITALIZATION

Consultation with the appropriate specialist is appropriate for edema that results from cardiac, renal, or liver disease. The patient with significant venous insufficiency and persistent stasis ulcers may benefit from a vascular surgery consultation to discuss treatment options. Hospitalization and heparinization may be recommended for deep vein thrombosis. However, low-molecular-weight heparin (Lovenox) may enable a shorter hospital stay and closely monitored outpatient management for some patients.[18,19] Severe cellulitis often requires hospitalization.[12,18] In other circumstances hospitalization is recommended if the underlying pathologic condition (e.g., congestive heart failure) needs stabilization.

PATIENT AND FAMILY EDUCATION

The patient should understand the significant symptoms (e.g., increased weight in edema) that may indicate a deteriorating medical condition. The importance of good foot care, properly fitting footwear, rest, and elevation of the affected extremity should also be stressed. Patients should understand the importance of reporting any change in the appearance or sensation of the foot. The type of footwear can be observed during the office visit, and recommendations can be made if there is a problem. It is wise to ask the patient periodically if there has been a recent change in shoe size.

REFERENCES

1. Sica DA: Calcium channel blocker–related peripheral edema: can it be resolved? *J Clin Hypertens* 5(4):291-294, 297, 2003.
2. Friedli S, Mahler F: Venous and lymphatic reasons for edema—the swollen leg from the angiologist's point of view, *Ther Umsch* 61(11):643-647, 2004.
3. Weir MR: Incidence of pedal edema formation with dihydropyridine calcium channel blockers: issues and practical significance, *J Clin Hypertens* 5(5):330-335, 2003.
4. Chan CW, Carpenter JR, Rigamonti C, and others: Survival following the development of ascites and/or peripheral oedema in primary biliary cirrhosis: a staged prognostic model, *Scand J Gastroenterol* 40(9):1081-1089, 2005.
5. Treiman GS, Copland S, McNamara RM, and others: Factors influencing ulcer healing in patients with combined arterial and venous insufficiency, *J Vasc Surg* 33(6):1158-1164, 2001.
6. Page RL, Gozansky WS, Ruscin JM: Possible heart failure exacerbation associated with rosiglitazone: case report and literature review, *Pharmacotherapy* 23(7):945-954, 2003.
7. Bianchi M, Castiglioni MG: Refractory generalized edema: an infrequent complication of long-term pergolide treatment for Parkinson disease, *Clin Neuropharmacol* 28(5):245-246, 2005.
8. Sommer TC, Lee TH: Charcot foot: the diagnostic dilemma, *Am Fam Phys* 64(9):1591-1598, 2001.
9. Mehta NJ, Khan IA, Mehta RN, and others: HIV-related pulmonary hypertension: analytic review of 131 cases, *Chest* 118(4):1133-1141, 2000.
10. Rame JE, Dries DL, Drazner MH: The prognostic value of the physical examination in patients with chronic heart failure, *Congest Heart Fail* 9(3):170-175, 2003.
11. Aldrete JA, Couto da Silva JM: Leg edema from intrathecal opiate infusions, *Eur J Pain* 4(4):361-365, 2000.

12. Noble J, Greene H, Levinson W, and others: *Textbook of primary care medicine,* St Louis, 1996, Mosby.
13. Shah MG, Cho S, Atwood JE, and others: Peripheral edema due to heart disease: diagnosis and outcome, *Clin Cardiol* 29(1):31-35, 2006.
14. Madias JE: Peripheral edema masks the diagnoses of P pulmonale, P mitrale, and biatrial abnormality: clinical implications for patients with heart failure, *Congest Heart Fail* 12(1):20-24, 2006.
15. Madias JE: A comparison of 2-lead, 6-lead, and 12-lead ECGs in patients with changing edematous states, *Chest* 124(6):2057-2063, 2003.
16. Madias JE, Madias NE: Reversible attenuation of the ECG voltage due to peripheral edema associated with treatment with a COX-2 inhibitor, *Congest Heart Fail* 12(1):46-50, 2006.
17. Madias JE: Apparent amelioration of bundle branch blocks and intraventricular conduction delays mediated by anasarca, *J Electrocardiol* 38(4):415-416, 2005.
18. Levine M, Gent M, Hirsh J, and others: A comparison of low-molecular-weight heparin administered primarily at home with unfractionated heparin administered in the hospital for proximal deep-vein thrombosis, *N Engl J Med* 334(11):677-681, 1996.
19. Koopman MM, Prandoni P, Piovella F, and others: Treatment of venous thrombosis with intravenous unfractionated heparin administered in the hospital as compared with subcutaneous low-molecular-weight heparin administered at home: the Tasman Study Group, *N Engl J Med* 334(11):682-687, 1996.

CHAPTER 133

Peripheral Venous Insufficiency

David R. Campbell

Peripheral venous insufficiency occurs whenever there is obstruction to venous return in the superficial or deep veins of the upper or lower extremities. Important clinical syndromes related to venous insufficiency include deep vein thrombosis (DVT), venous stasis, varicose veins, stasis dermatitis, and leg ulceration.

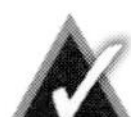

Physician consultation is indicated for all patients with deep vein thrombosis as documented by Doppler ultrasound.

DEEP VEIN THROMBOSIS OF THE LOWER EXTREMITY

DEFINITION AND EPIDEMIOLOGY

DVT is the development of a blood clot in the deep veins of the lower or, occasionally, the upper extremity. A DVT may include the iliac veins and the vena cava and is characterized by a relatively loose thrombotic attachment to the vein wall until the healing process starts.

Although the term *phlebitis* is often used to describe DVT, it should in fact be reserved for superficial phlebitis. Superficial phlebitis is an inflammation of the affected superficial veins as a result of local trauma, venous stasis, or infection; chemical injury may result from an IV injection. Because the clot is part of an inflammatory process that involves the vessel wall, there is no risk of pulmonary embolism unless the process extends to involve the deep system.

PATHOPHYSIOLOGY

The deep veins of the lower extremity are the main conduit by which the legs are emptied of blood. Blood travels back to the heart as a result of compression of the deep veins by leg muscles. Valves in the vein prevent reflux back down the vein because of gravity. Blood runs from the superficial system to the deep veins through perforator veins, which are also protected from reflux by the presence of valves. Any condition that produces stasis or hypercoagulability is likely to result in the formation of clots in the deep veins.[1] A major risk factor is surgery, particularly gynecologic operations or orthopedic procedures on the hip and knee. Bed rest produces stasis and may result in DVT. Long airplane or car rides are also risk factors.[2] Patients who have a tendency for hypercoagulation, particularly patients with malignancy, may be seen with DVT. A lesser but definite risk factor for DVT is use of estrogen preparations (e.g., contraceptives or hormone replacement therapy), and these should be considered in patients with other risk factors.[2]

A clot may form in any part of the deep venous system and may either propagate or remain localized. It may cause symptoms in two ways. First, there is a local effect in obstruction of blood flow, which rarely is so significant that it results in venous gangrene. Second, the clot may become detached and migrate to the lungs, forming an embolus. This is a common cause of death in at-risk patients.

CLINICAL PRESENTATION AND PHYSICAL EXAMINATION

A history of previous DVT, prolonged inactivity, estrogen use, or recent surgery or trauma should be obtained from the patient. The classic signs of DVT are leg edema and calf tenderness. Calf pain on dorsiflexion of the foot is known as Homans' sign. All these signs are relatively nonspecific; up to 50% of patients with DVT have no symptoms at all. Together, extensive thrombosis and extreme leg swelling have in the past been known as *phlegmasia alba dolens*.

The history and examination for superficial phlebitis differ from that for DVT. The patient may have a localized area of edema, erythema, and tenderness over a superficial vein, with increased temperature in the surrounding skin.

DIAGNOSTICS

The diagnosis of superficial phlebitis is based on the clinical findings; diagnostic tests are not usually needed. However, every patient with superficial phlebitis should have a duplex ultrasound to make sure he or she does not have a DVT as well. If a DVT is suspected on the basis of clinical signs or risk factors, the diagnosis can be made simply by duplex ultrasound of the legs.[3] Test results should document clot visualization, normal blood flow, compressibility of the veins, augmentation of flow with respiration, or reflux in the deep and superficial systems.

A newer test for evaluation of DVT is the D-dimer level. This is a global marker of coagulation activation and fibrinolysis and it has been suggested that in low-risk patients a low D dimer level may obviate the need for a duplex ultrasound. It may also be helpful in monitoring patients to avoid repeating the ultrasound. The exact role of D-dimer levels in the diagnosis of DVT remains to be clarified. Recent investigations have suggested there is variability in the sensitivity of the various D-dimer assays; additionally, the assays are less sensitive when patients have distal DVT and more sensitive when combined with assessment of pretest probability of DVT.[4,5] Soluble fibrin and total sialic acid measurements were investigated as serum markers for DVT in two recent, small-scale studies.[6,7]

The most common sites for DVT are the femoral veins; in this situation the duplex ultrasound is as accurate as venography. Isolated tibial or iliac vein thrombosis may be more difficult to diagnose; venography or magnetic resonance venography may be indicated if there is a high index of suspicion. Appropriate testing for malignancy, connective tissue disorders, or inherited autocoagulation deficiencies may be necessary. The need for further investigation is guided by the clinical presentation, past medical history, and family history.

DIFFERENTIAL DIAGNOSIS

It is not possible to diagnose DVT accurately on the basis of clinical presentation or physical examination alone. Other differential diagnoses that should be considered are superficial phlebitis, cellulitis, ruptured Baker's cyst, strained muscle, or a malignant neoplasm that is compromising the veins.

The possibility of an underlying malignancy or the existence of a connective tissue disorder must also be considered. Inherited deficiencies of protein C, protein S, or antithrombin III are important (albeit less common) causes, particularly in recurrent cases or in patients with a family history of DVT.

DIAGNOSTICS

Peripheral Venous Insufficiency

DEEP VEIN THROMBOSIS

Imaging

Duplex ultrasound*
Venography, magnetic resonance venography*

Laboratory

D-Dimer, protein C, protein S
Antithrombin III
Antiphospholipid antibodies
Factor V Leiden

CHRONIC VENOUS STASIS

None indicated

VARICOSE VEINS

Imaging

Duplex scan

VENOUS STASIS ULCERATION

Initial

Doppler ultrasound

*If indicated.

DIFFERENTIAL DIAGNOSIS

Peripheral Venous Insufficiency

DEEP VEIN THROMBOSIS

- Superficial phlebitis
- Cellulitis
- Ruptured Baker's cyst
- Strained muscle
- Malignant neoplasm

CHRONIC VENOUS STASIS

- Heart failure
- Malnutrition
- Lymphatic obstruction

VARICOSE VEINS

- Venous-arterial insufficiency
- Peripheral neuritis
- Arthritis

VENOUS STASIS ULCERATION

- Venous stasis ulceration
- Ischemic ulceration
- Neuropathic ulceration

MANAGEMENT

Management of superficial vein phlebitis consists of elevation of the leg and compression with an Ace bandage. NSAIDs and antibiotics are also indicated. It is important to note that superficial phlebitis may co-exist with DVT.

Management of DVT requires that heparin be initiated immediately to prevent a pulmonary embolism. Traditionally this has meant admission to the hospital for systemic heparinization. Typically a bolus of 5000 units is given, followed by a continuous infusion at 800 to 1400 units/hr (80 units/kg heparin bolus followed by an infusion of 18 units/kg/hr) to maintain a partial thromboplastin time (PTT) that is twice the normal rate. The PTT should be checked after 6 hours. The heparin infusion should be continued until the PTT has been in the therapeutic range for a minimum of 2 consecutive days. Warfarin (Coumadin) is started within the first 24 hours, and the patient is discharged once the International Normalized Ratio (INR) is between 2 and 3.[8] The regimen of warfarin is usually continued for 3 to 6 months.

Low-molecular-weight heparin (e.g., enoxaparin) given by subcutaneous injection has been shown in studies to be safe for at-home treatment of uncomplicated DVT.[9] These studies show the same or a lower incidence of complications when compared with standard heparin. Because enoxaparin has a long half-life, it can be given twice a day subcutaneously; its predictable anticoagulant response obviates the need for PTT monitoring. This has become the standard treatment in uncomplicated cases of DVT.

LIFE SPAN CONSIDERATIONS

DVT that is diagnosed during pregnancy should be managed on an individual basis after consultation with a vascular surgeon and the patient's obstetrician.[10] Heparin is generally safe during pregnancy and can be given to pregnant women to treat DVT. The use of warfarin is contraindicated during pregnancy. Any woman of childbearing age who is taking this medication should be advised of the risks of pregnancy. The introduction of enoxaparin has made the management of these patients much simpler.

A number of measures have been shown to be effective for DVT prophylaxis in patients undergoing surgery. Cuffs that provide intermittent leg pressure to reduce stasis are combined with subcutaneous heparin until the patient is mobile. Low-molecular-weight heparin has been approved for very-high-risk procedures (e.g., hip replacement) and is now being used instead of perioperative warfarin. Subcutaneous heparin twice a day is usually sufficient for medical patients who have been prescribed bed rest.

COMPLICATIONS

Pulmonary embolism is one of the major causes of postoperative morbidity and mortality.[11] In high-risk patients the key to prevention is appropriate surveillance for DVT with the duplex scan. Pulmonary embolism usually occurs within 2 weeks of DVT. After this time the clot is sufficiently organized to make detachment unlikely. Symptoms of a pulmonary embolus include the sudden onset of pleuritic chest pain and shortness of breath. The patient is noted to be hypoxic yet has a relatively normal chest x-ray film. Evidence of a clot in the leg by duplex scan combined with a positive lung scan is sufficient for diagnosis. A pulmonary arteriogram is indicated if the duplex scan is negative or if the lung scan is equivocal. Increasingly the lung scan and pulmonary angiography are being replaced by CT angiography, which is less invasive. If the patient's condition is critical, thrombolytic therapy can be started through the catheter used for the pulmonary arteriogram.

Postphlebitic syndrome is a chronic condition that may develop as a sequela to DVT. DVT can produce chronic changes in veins with loss of valve competence, and it is a cause of chronic venous stasis.[12]

All patients receiving heparin should have their platelet count checked every few days; a sudden drop in the count may be indicative of heparin-induced thrombocytopenia. If this occurs or if the patient has a known allergy to heparin, treatment with low-molecular-weight dextran should be used instead. Prophylactic placement of a vena cava filter to prevent pulmonary embolism should be considered if other medical conditions prevent the use of anticoagulation therapy.[13]

INDICATIONS FOR REFERRAL OR HOSPITALIZATION

A documented DVT in any patient requires a physician consultation, during which time the need for hospitalization and IV heparin vs. outpatient treatment with low-molecular-weight heparin can be determined. Vascular consultation is necessary for patients who may require placement of a vena cava filter.[14] If the inflammatory process continues despite treatment, excision may occasionally be indicated; in such cases a vascular consultation should be sought.

PATIENT AND FAMILY EDUCATION

Anticoagulant therapy should be carefully explained to patients and families, and the importance of routine laboratory testing to monitor therapy should be stressed. Patients should understand the necessity of contacting the health care provider if any abnormal bleeding occurs. In addition, patients should be familiar with the signs and symptoms of pulmonary embolism (e.g., chest pain, dyspnea) as indications for emergency care. A list of foods high in vitamin K and a careful explanation of how excess ingestion of these foods may decrease the action of warfarin are also necessary.

HEALTH PROMOTION

Other options for birth control should be discussed with patients, particularly those who smoke. High-risk patients should understand the risks associated with long plane and automobile journeys. They should also be advised to wear support stockings and to take an aspirin every day while traveling. Low-dose aspirin (81 to 365 mg) reduces the incidence and mortality of myocardial infarction in patients older than 50 years; it may be recommended in patients at risk for DVT who travel long distances. Adequate fluid intake, frequent rest breaks to stretch and exercise the legs, and passive intermittent contraction of the calf muscles enhance blood flow to the lower extremities during prolonged, confined travel conditions.

CHRONIC VENOUS STASIS

DEFINITION AND EPIDEMIOLOGY

Chronic venous stasis results from increased pressure in the deep veins. This condition produces edema, varicose veins, chronic skin changes, and ulceration.

PATHOPHYSIOLOGY

Human beings are relatively poorly adapted to walking on two legs for extended periods. The distribution of blood to the feet is accomplished by the heart in concert with gravity, but it is only the muscle pump and fragile venous valves that return the blood to the heart. Prolonged standing and a tall stature increase hydrostatic pressure on the valves. During pregnancy the hormone relaxin, which allows the pelvis to stretch, also causes the veins to distend and the valves to become incompetent. Resolution of this condition after pregnancy is often incomplete, resulting in increased venous stasis. Obesity and age-associated loss of tissue turgor are also factors that produce venous stasis.

Increased pressure may also result from proximal venous obstruction secondary to an old DVT or more commonly from reflux secondary to valvular incompetence. Valvular incompetence may result after recanalization after a DVT, or it may be primary in nature.

Even if the valves of the perforator and saphenous veins remain competent, deep venous hypertension affects the foot and ankle. The foot tends to swell, particularly if the patient stands much of the day. The point of maximum pressure is the ankle, and the skin becomes thickened and may react to the pressure with an eczematous reaction known as *stasis eczema*. Consequently, blood cells in the tiny venules break down under high pressure; hemosiderin is deposited under the skin to produce a characteristic brown staining that progresses with time.

CLINICAL PRESENTATION AND PHYSICAL EXAMINATION

The clinical appearance of chronic venous stasis varies depending on whether the superficial or deeper veins are affected. Chronic edema and skin discoloration on the legs and ankles may be present. Varicose veins, ulceration, and even cellulitis may result.

DIAGNOSTICS AND DIFFERENTIAL DIAGNOSIS

Diagnostic tests are unnecessary because the diagnosis is based on the clinical history and physical findings. The physical findings also guide the diagnosis. However, the peripheral edema associated with chronic venous stasis may also be caused by other disease entities. Medications, congestive heart failure, lymphatic obstruction, and malnutrition may all be associated with lower extremity edema (see the Diagnostics and Differential Diagnosis boxes, p. 604).

MANAGEMENT

Compression stockings and periodic leg elevation are the most important methods for controlling chronic venous insufficiency and preventing skin ulcers. Careful monitoring is important when venous ulcers occur. Normal saline wet-to-dry dressings or topical antibiotic therapies are indicated. Ulcer infections should be treated with the appropriate antibiotic.

COMPLICATIONS

Venous ulcers are the most common complication of chronic venous stasis. A superimposed infection and cellulitis are additional concerns. Severe edema may result in decreased mobility and an increased risk for falls or DVT.

INDICATIONS FOR REFERRAL OR HOSPITALIZATION

Venous ulcers or peripheral edema that does not respond to conventional therapies may require a referral to the appropriate specialist. Severe ulcers with extensive tissue loss may require evaluation by a plastic surgeon for possible grafting. Most patients can be successfully managed with careful outpatient follow-up visits. However, hospitalization may be indicated for severe edema, infection, or surgical valvuloplasty.

PATIENT AND FAMILY EDUCATION

The most effective treatment for leg swelling and stasis dermatitis is the use of support stockings.[15] Severe stasis eczema may require the use of 0.5% hydrocortisone cream in combination with compression. The hydrocortisone cream should be discontinued once the condition has resolved.

VARICOSE VEINS

PATHOPHYSIOLOGY

Varicose veins are caused by pathologic distention and proliferation of the superficial veins. Varicose veins include primary and secondary varicose veins as well as spider veins.

Primary varicose veins are usually familial. There is no previous history of DVT, and the varicosities are usually exacerbated by pregnancy. Progressive dilation of the superficial veins may be local or more extensive. Primary varicose veins result from incompetent perforators, which produce local varicosities, or from incompetence of the saphenous vein valves, which produces more generalized varicosities. Secondary varicose veins result from a previous DVT. Most commonly these are caused by incompetent valves following recanalization. When the deep venous system is totally occluded, these varicose veins may represent the main venous drainage from the leg; in this instance removal of the veins would be harmful. Telangiectasia or spider veins may result from increased pressure in the superficial veins. It is not clear why this condition is more predominant in some patients.

CLINICAL PRESENTATION AND PHYSICAL EXAMINATION

The pooling of blood in large varicose veins tends to produce symptoms of heaviness and discomfort in the legs while standing. Large varicose veins are unsightly and may produce severe anxiety and cause major lifestyle changes. Trauma to varicose veins may result in severe bleeding, particularly in older adults, since their skin may be atrophic and thereby provides less protection.

DIAGNOSTICS AND DIFFERENTIAL DIAGNOSIS

Diagnosis is based on inspection of the lower extremities when the patient is standing. Further differential consideration is usually unnecessary. The only important test indicated for varicose veins is the duplex scan to determine whether the deep system is patent and whether there is saphenofemoral reflux. Individual incompetent perforators in the leg may also be identified. If varicosities are not present, venous and arterial insufficiency, peripheral neuritis, and arthritis should be considered (see the Diagnostics and Differential Diagnosis boxes, p. 604).

MANAGEMENT

Asymptomatic varicose veins do not require treatment. There is no effective way to reduce venous pressure in the lower legs except with support stockings.

COMPLICATIONS

Occasionally a superficial varicosity will rupture, and significant bleeding may be noted. Topical compression and elevation of the extremity usually control the bleeding. Skin ulcerations are an additional complication of varicose veins.

INDICATIONS FOR REFERRAL OR HOSPITALIZATION

Referral to a vascular surgeon is indicated if support stockings are not effective in controlling symptoms or are poorly tolerated by the patient.

Treatment by a specialist may involve removal of the varicose veins or, alternatively, injection or laser treatment. Large veins are more appropriately removed in outpatient surgery, whereas smaller veins can be injected. Spider veins can be treated by either injection or laser treatment. Increasingly, obliteration of the long saphenous vein using a catheter and a radiofrequency generator or a laser have reduced the morbidity of saphenectomy; this can be done with the patient under local anesthesia in the office.[16]

PATIENT AND FAMILY EDUCATION

It is important to inform patients that none of the treatments for varicose veins eradicate the problem of high venous pressure. Therefore recurrence is the rule rather than the exception. This knowledge may affect a patient's decision to proceed with surgery. Patients should also understand that compression stockings and periodic leg elevation are beneficial.

VENOUS STASIS ULCERATION

DEFINITION AND EPIDEMIOLOGY

Venous stasis ulceration is the most severe complication of postphlebitic syndrome and rarely occurs without a history of DVT. With the introduction of heparin and the prompt diagnosis and treatment of DVT, venous stasis ulceration is now much less common.

PATHOPHYSIOLOGY

A number of factors contribute to venous ulceration. At first, peripheral edema increases as a result of incompetent valves in the venous system. This edema leads to capillary distention and the leakage of fluid and other substances into the surrounding tissue. If there is trauma to the skin of the affected extremity, oxygen and essential nutrients for healing are prevented from reaching the injured area. As a result, a superficial, irregularly shaped ulceration occurs. These ulcers can continue to erode, and cellulitis and superimposed infection can occur.

CLINICAL PRESENTATION AND PHYSICAL EXAMINATION

The patient with venous stasis ulceration typically is seen with an ulcer above the medial malleolus, and usually other signs of venous stasis are present (Color Plate 38). The ulcers have a distinctive presentation that permits differentiation from ischemic or diabetic ulcers (Box 133-1). At the time of presentation, the wound may be secondarily infected. Pulses may not be palpable because of local swelling or co-existent ischemia.

DIAGNOSTICS AND DIFFERENTIAL DIAGNOSIS

Diagnostic tests are usually unnecessary. A portal Doppler can be used to assess pulses if they are not readily palpable. The differential diagnosis should encompass all peripheral ulcers (see the Diagnostics and Differential Diagnosis boxes, p. 604).

MANAGEMENT

Management of venous stasis ulceration consists of bed rest. A wet-to-dry dressing may be tried; however, the ulcer should be debrided as indicated and oral antibiotics started, guided by aerobic and anaerobic cultures results whenever possible. A nonstick dressing may be less painful once the ulcer is clean. This treatment is accompanied by compression with an Ace wrap.

Compliance can be a real problem for many patients; some centers combat this by using a rigid dressing such as the Unna's paste boot, which provides compression and a dressing that needs to be changed only once a week. The Unna's paste boot should not be used if there is peripheral arterial disease. A referral is sometimes indicated for refractory cases.

COMPLICATIONS

Superimposed infection is a constant concern with venous stasis ulceration. Osteomyelitis is a potential hazard for ulcers that become infected.

BOX 133-1

CHARACTERISTICS OF LEG ULCERS BY CAUSE*

VENOUS STASIS
Occur around ankle, particularly medial side
History of phlebitis
Signs of venous stasis
Painful when secondarily infected
Improved by elevation

ISCHEMIC
Occur at tips of extremities or heel
History of claudication common
Very painful, but much worse on elevation
Absent pulses on physical examination
Secondary infection likely to spread very quickly

NEUROPATHIC (DIABETIC)
Occur at pressure points
Painless but co-existent neuritic pain possibly confusing
Often present after secondary infection

*More than one cause may be involved.

INDICATIONS FOR REFERRAL OR HOSPITALIZATION

A surgical referral is indicated if the ulcer fails to heal with the simple measures outlined previously. If the ulcer is clearly deteriorating, hospitalization may be required.

PATIENT AND FAMILY EDUCATION

Patient education is extremely important in preventing recurrence of this condition. Patients must understand the need to maintain compression and to be fitted with appropriate support stockings. In cases of severe edema an external pneumatic compression stocking may be necessary to reduce swelling at the end of the day.

Many patients fail to wear their prescribed support stockings because the wrong stockings are provided. In general, knee-high stockings are much better tolerated than any tight support that crosses the knee. The main exceptions are pregnant women and women with varicose veins in the thigh, who may find support pantyhose comfortable. When ordering stockings, the key factor is pressure (Table 133-1). The thick or fine-knit quality of the stockings affects only durability and patient acceptance.

TABLE 133-1 Recommendations for Support Stockings

Pressure (mm Hg)	Recommendations
0-10	Normal socks
10-20	Over-the-counter support stockings Recommended for individuals who are on their feet all day and for prophylaxis for DVT when traveling
20-30	Lowest pressure therapeutic stocking Good for individuals who are looking for more pressure than over-the-counter stockings or who cannot tolerate the higher pressures
30-40	Standard pressure for therapeutic stockings Instruct patients to shower in the evening so these stockings can be put on before getting out of bed; otherwise will be difficult for many patients, particularly older adults, to put on
40-50	Should be prescribed only for patients who do not get enough compression with 30-40 mm Hg Almost impossible to get on!

REFERENCES

1. Nordstrom M, Lindblad B, Bergqvist D, and others: A prospective study of the incidence of deep-vein thrombosis within a defined urban population, *J Intern Med* 232(2):155-160, 1992.
2. Lapostolle F, Surget V, Borron SW, and others: Severe pulmonary embolism associated with air travel, *N Engl J Med* 345(11):779-783, 2001.
3. Venous thrombotic disease and combined oral contraceptives: results of international multicentre case-control study: World Health Organization Collaborative Study of Cardiovascular Disease and Steroid Hormone Contraception, *Lancet* 346(8990):1575-1582, 1995.
4. Jennersjo CM, Fagerberg IH, Karlander SG, and others: Normal D-dimer concentration is a common finding in symptomatic outpatients with distal deep vein thrombosis, *Blood Coagul Fibrinolysis* 16(7):517-523, 2005.
5. Gardiner C, Pennaneac'h C, Walford C, and others: An evaluation of rapid D-dimer assays for the exclusion of deep vein thrombosis, *Br J Haematol* 128(6):842-848, 2005.
6. Ota S, Wada H, Nobori T, and others: Diagnosis of deep vein thrombosis by plasma-soluble fibrin or D-dimer, *Am J Hematol* 79(4):274-280, 2005.
7. Reganon E, Vila V, Martinez-Sales V, and others: Sialic acid is an inflammation marker associated with a history of deep vein thrombosis, *Thromb Res* 119(1):73-78, 2007 [Epub Feb 28, 2006].
8. Masuda EM, Kistner RL: Prospective comparison of duplex scanning and descending venography in the assessment of venous insufficiency, *Am J Surg* 164(3):254-259, 1992.
9. Schulman S, Rhedin AS, Lindmarker P, and others: A comparison of 6 weeks with 6 months of oral anticoagulant therapy after a first episode of venous thromboembolism: duration of Anticoagulation Trial Study Group, *N Engl J Med* 332(25):1661-1665, 1995.
10. Hirsh J, Siragusa S, Cosmi B, and others: Low molecular weight heparins in the treatment of patients with acute venous thromboembolism, *Thromb Haemost* 74:360-363, 1995.
11. Ginsberg JS, Brill-Edwards P, Burrows RF, and others: Venous thrombosis during pregnancy: leg and trimester of presentation, *Thromb Haemost* 67:519-520, 1992.
12. Quinn DA, Thompson BT, Terrin ML, and others: A prospective investigation of pulmonary embolism in women and men, *JAMA* 268:1689-1696, 1992.
13. Franzeck UK, Schalch I, Jager KA, and others: Prospective 12-year follow-up of clinical and hemodynamic sequelae after deep vein thrombosis in low-risk patients, *Circulation* 93(11):74-79, 1996.
14. Alexander JJ, Yuhas JP, Piotrowski JJ: Is the increasing use of prophylactic IVC filters justified? *Am J Surg* 168(2):102-106, 1994.
15. Abu-Own A, Shami SK, Chittenden SJ, and others: Microangiopathy of the skin and the effect of leg compression in patients with chronic venous insufficiency, *J Vasc Surg* 19:1074-1083, 1994.
16. Pichot O, Sessa C, Chandler JG, and others: Role of duplex imaging in endovenous obliteration for primary venous insufficiency, *J Endovasc Ther* 7(6):452-459, 2000.

CHAPTER 134

Valvular Heart Disease and Cardiac Murmurs

Updated by Terry Mahan Buttaro and JoAnn Trybulski

When a murmur is heard for the first time, it is important to determine whether it represents a pathologic condition and what type of condition it may represent. The generation of the sounds called *murmurs* is the same whether the cause is benign or a result of a severe pathologic condition, and therefore the cause is impossible to differentiate on the basis of the sound alone. What distinguishes benign from pathologic murmurs is often the associated physical findings or symptoms (Table 134-1). Some patients require referral for diagnostic testing, whereas the clinical assessment of others suggests that diagnostic testing is unnecessary.

A murmur is the relatively lengthy series of sounds produced by the turbulent flow of blood. Under normal conditions, blood flow is uniform or laminar within the vessel or chamber and is therefore free of audible vibration. When flow velocity is excessively high, or when normal flow occurs across an obstruction, turbulence and its resultant audible vibration occur. In a classic article on auscultation of the heart, Leatham noted that all murmurs were related to one of three factors[1]: (1) high rates of flow through a normal or abnormal valve; (2) forward flow through a constricted or irregular valve or into a dilated vessel; or (3) backward flow through a regurgitant valve, septal defect, or patent ductus arteriosus.

Murmurs may be characterized by a number of factors: location, intensity, pitch, radiation, and timing. Of these, timing is the most important factor. Timing delineates the critical division between systolic and diastolic murmurs, as well as the relationship to the heart sounds (S_1 and S_2; e.g., ending well before, right at, or continuing through S_2). As the heart rate increases, diastole shortens, and systole and diastole approach similar intervals. When this occurs, differentiating between S_1 (beginning of systole) and S_2 (beginning of diastole) on the basis of cadence alone becomes difficult. Palpation of the carotid pulse while simultaneously auscultating the heart at the base will easily permit the listener to focus and time S_1 (the onset of systole), which will occur slightly before the onset of the carotid pulse rise. Although the two components of S_2 (aortic, or A_2, and pulmonic, or P_2) are almost superimposed at end-expiration, with inspiration P_2 splits later, creating an easily audible gap. This will be best appreciated over the upper left sternal border. A systolic murmur that ends at or before A_2 will be a left-sided murmur (e.g., aortic stenosis [AS] or mitral regurgitation [MR]), whereas one that extends beyond A_2 will be emanating from the right side of the heart (i.e., pulmonic stenosis or tricuspid regurgitation).

Intensity, or loudness, which is related to the velocity of blood flow, describes how audible the murmur is. However, loudness does not equate with the severity of the underlying problem. Some of the loudest murmurs are due to a small muscular ventricular septal defect (VSD) in an adolescent, which is destined to close spontaneously. Murmurs are graded 1 (barely audible), 2 (faint but clearly heard), 3 (easily heard but without being able to palpate the vibrations on the chest wall), 4 (heard with a palpable thrill), 5 (heard with the stethoscope only partially in contact with the chest wall with a palpable thrill), or 6 (heard without a stethoscope with a palpable thrill). The location where a murmur is best heard is also generally noted (e.g., at the upper right sternal border [second intercostal space], upper left sternal border, lower left sternal border, or apical areas of the chest wall). These terms have largely superseded the earlier descriptors of aortic, pulmonic, tricuspid, and mitral locations because of the variable radiation or transmission of the sounds.

Systolic murmurs are classified into two general types: ejection type (midsystolic) and regurgitant type (pansystolic). In the ejection type the murmur is grade 1 or 2 and there is a period between S_1 (closure of the mitral and tricuspid valves) and the onset of the murmur. During this time the ventricle is generating pressure (isovolumetric contraction) to overcome the pressure in the great vessels (aorta and pulmonary artery) and open the aortic and pulmonic valves. The murmur builds in intensity as velocity increases, followed by a decrease in intensity, which occurs well before S_2 (closure of the aortic and pulmonic valves). Thus the murmur is diamond shaped, or crescendo-decrescendo. This murmur occurs with left ventricular outflow obstruction whether the obstruction is from rheumatic or calcific AS, idiopathic hypertrophic subaortic stenosis (IHSS) (also known as hypertrophic obstructive cardiomyopathy), or pneumonic stenosis. Most murmurs are of this type.

In contrast are the murmurs resulting from flow from a high-pressure chamber to a low-pressure chamber, which occurs in incompetent valves (mitral or tricuspid regurgitation) or with a VSD. As soon as pressure starts to develop, flow occurs throughout systole (pansystolic flow). The pressure gradient and therefore the intensity of the murmur are largely unchanged throughout systole. Such murmurs are described as plateau shaped. The murmurs of chronic tricuspid regurgitation or MR are the epitomes of the pansystolic murmur. However, when a significant gradient or differential of pressure does not exist between chambers, the murmurs will be truncated. Thus the murmur of severe acute MR may occur only during early systole because of rapid equalization of left atrial pressure with left ventricular pressure. Similarly, the classic murmur of a VSD, which may ordinarily be indistinguishable from that of chronic MR, may be truncated or even totally absent in the face of pulmonary hypertension (Eisenmenger's complex). The murmur of mitral valve prolapse is classically late systolic, often after a midsystolic click. Variation in intensity of the murmur with respiration is strongly associated with right-sided (pulmonic or tricuspid valve) abnormalities.[2]

Diastolic murmurs are related to regurgitation across either the aortic or the pulmonic valve, or to filling rumbles caused by flow across a normal (in exaggerated flow states) or obstructed mitral or tricuspid valve. Listening for the high-pitched diastolic murmur of aortic or pulmonic insufficiency

TABLE 134-1 Murmurs*

Diagnosis	Characteristic	Location, Radiation	Physical Examination Findings	Effect of Valsalva's Maneuver	ECG Findings	Chest X-Ray Findings
COMMON SYSTOLIC MURMURS						
Aortic stenosis	Harsh, crescendo-decrescendo	Right sternal border; radiation to neck	Delayed carotid upstroke; narrowed pulse pressure; systolic thrill at second right intercostal space	Decreased murmur	Left atrial enlargement; left-axis deviation; atrioventricular conduction delay; left ventricular hypertrophy	Aortic valve calcification; left ventricular hypertrophy
Mitral regurgitation	Pansystolic blowing	Apex; radiation to axilla	Laterally displaced, hyperdynamic apical impulse; brisk carotid upstroke	No change	Left ventricular hypertrophy	Left ventricular enlargement
Mitral valve prolapse	Mid- to late systolic; occasionally honking; may have midsystolic click; click and murmur can be intermittent	Lower left sternal border	May have scoliosis or pectus excavatum in connective tissue disorder	Murmur and/or click may move to later systole or disappear	Usually within normal limits; occasionally flat or inverted T in leads II, III, aV_F	Skeletal abnormalities, if present
Tricuspid regurgitation	Early, mid-, or late systolic or pansystolic	Lower left sternal border; radiation to right sternal border	Sustained precordial lift	Decreased murmur	Right atrial hypertrophy; right-axis deviation	Usually normal
Hypertrophic cardiomyopathy	Peaks midsystole	Left sternal border	Murmur decreased with change from standing to squatting; S_4 gallop may be present	Increased murmur	Left atrial enlargement; increased voltage; may have left ventricular hypertrophy	May have slight cardiac enlargement
Benign or innocent*	Early systolic; crescendo-decrescendo; changes intensity with rate	Variant	No underlying systemic findings; no findings of cardiac enlargement or failure; murmur disappears with breath holding	Murmur disappearing	Normal ECG	Normal findings
Ventricular septal defect	Pansystolic; louder in midsystole	Left sternal border; radiation to right sternal border	May have systolic thrill at lower left sternal border	Increased murmur	May have left atrial and ventricular enlargement	
COMMON DIASTOLIC MURMURS						
Aortic regurgitation	Loud, blowing, high pitched	Lower left sternal border	Widened pulse pressure; abrupt rise and fall in carotid upstroke	Increased murmur	Left ventricular hypertrophy; sinus tachycardia	Left ventricular hypertrophy; aortic valve calcification; ascending aortic dilation
Mitral stenosis	Low-pitched, diastolic rumble (mid)	Apex, left lateral position	Opening snap	No change or increased murmur	Left atrial enlargement; right-axis deviation	Left atrial enlargement; calcified mitral valve
Tricuspid stenosis	Decrescendo, low pitched	Fourth or fifth left intercostal space	Absent right ventricular impulse; diastolic thrill; lower left intercostal border may have opening snap at fourth left intercostal space	Decreased murmur	Height of P wave in lead II >2.5 mm; PR shortened; right atrial hypertrophy	Right atrial and vena cava shadows

*Assurance of whether a murmur is benign or innocent cannot be determined with 100% accuracy.

(regurgitation) is difficult and may require proper positioning of the patient. These murmurs are loudest early in diastole, when there is a large pressure gradient between the aorta and the left ventricle; they then fall in intensity as the pressure gradient falls, producing a decrescendo pattern of sound. They are best heard with the patient sitting, leaning forward, and exhaling—all of which minimize the distance from the stethoscope to the heart. The diaphragm of the stethoscope should be used because of the high-frequency response of the murmur.

The cause of the murmur cannot be discerned by the character of the murmur; however, it is generally acknowledged that aortic insufficiency murmurs heard best at the upper right sternal border are more likely related to dilation of the aortic root, in contrast to murmurs caused by damage to the aortic valve themselves. If the aortic insufficiency is acute and severe, the duration of the murmur may be truncated as a result of the rapid and premature equalization of pressures between the left ventricle and the aorta. Pulmonic insufficiency is usually found in the setting of pulmonary hypertension with dilation of the pulmonic artery and produces Graham Steell's murmur, which by clinical examination is almost indistinguishable from the murmur of aortic insufficiency. Low-pitched rumbles in diastole are caused by forward flow across a stenotic mitral or tricuspid valve. Such low-pitched murmurs are best appreciated using the bell of the stethoscope at the apical area with the patient lying slightly on the left side. Because the filling of the ventricles occurs primarily in early diastole (the rapid filling phase) and at the end of diastole (from atrial contraction), the murmur is loudest during these times. Therefore patients with atrial fibrillation will lack the presystolic accentuation of their diastolic rumbles, since they have no atrial contraction.

The duration, not the intensity, of the murmur correlates with the severity of the obstruction. Less severe stenosis will result in a shorter gradient across the stenotic valve, and a shorter murmur will result; more severe stenosis will result in a longer gradient across the stenotic valve, and a longer murmur (to the end of diastole) will result. Hyperdynamic states, such as anemia or fever, or the presence of atrial or ventricular septal defects producing shunting of blood from one chamber to the other during diastole, may produce murmurs in mid-diastole. Left atrial myxomas may obstruct flow across the mitral valve during diastole, producing a similar rumble, but one that is associated with a "tumor plop," instead of an opening snap.

Continuous murmurs begin in systole and extend at least partway into diastole. The classic continuous murmur is exemplified by the murmur associated with a patent ductus arteriosus. Intracardiac shunting between a high-pressure system (aorta) and a low-pressure system (pulmonary artery) exists throughout the cardiac cycle and may be heard in the region just beneath the left clavicle. Fistulas or localized arterial obstructions may also produce continuous murmurs. In addition, continuous murmurs are often associated with benign high-flow states. A continuous murmur, known as a venous hum and heard in the neck, is commonly noted in children and adolescents. It may be abolished by compression of the jugular vein. Similarly, women in the late stages of pregnancy, or lactating women shortly postpartum, may develop a continuous "mammary shuffle" over the breast that may be obliterated with firm pressure.

A group of murmurs that are not due to any pathologic obstruction to flow are termed *innocent, benign*, or *functional*. As noted previously, the acoustic-mechanical phenomena that create benign or innocent murmurs are the same as those which create pathologic conditions. The differentiation is based on the lack of other findings (e.g., abnormal carotid or peripheral pulses, associated symptoms). Several clues may help distinguish innocent murmurs from pathologic ones.[3] Murmurs that are due to an increased cardiac output (e.g., as a result of fever, thyrotoxicosis, anemia) may be termed *functional* because they are caused by excess flow across the outflow tract. Many older adults have decreased mobility of the aortic valves as a result of fibrosis and calcification (aortic sclerosis), which distorts the flow, without producing a significant gradient across the valve. Other older patients may have outflow murmurs that are due to ejection of blood into a kinked, tortuous aorta. A number of adolescents and young adults have ejection murmurs that mimic the flow murmur across the pulmonic valve as a result of an atrial septal defect. These patients have a narrowed anteroposterior chest dimension that is due to either a decreased curvature of the spine (straight back syndrome) or pectus excavatum.[3]

AORTIC STENOSIS

DEFINITION AND EPIDEMIOLOGY

Based purely on clinical findings, it is more difficult to assess the degree of severity of AS than it is to assess any other valvular abnormality. Valvular AS may be caused by rheumatic damage, congenital abnormality (bicuspid aortic valve), or degeneration caused by the aging process (calcific AS of older adults).[4] Over the past 3 decades, with the successful treatment of streptococcal pharyngitis, the etiology has shifted away from rheumatic to calcific. All such cases share a history of 20 to 30 years of repetitive mechanical trauma of the blood against the valve resulting in fibrosis, calcification, and eventually stenosis.

PATHOPHYSIOLOGY

Any reduction of the normal aortic valve orifice of approximately 3 cm^2 (1.2 square inches) will cause obstruction to the flow of blood from the left ventricle into the aorta during ventricular systole. A systolic pressure gradient develops between the left ventricle and the aorta. Left ventricular pressure rises, increasing systolic wall stress. The left ventricle hypertrophies as a compensatory mechanism to maintain adequate cardiac output. Valvular stenosis is generally considered to be significant when the valve area is reduced to 25% of normal. Therefore hemodynamically significant AS would be an aortic valve area of less than 0.75 cm^2 (0.3 square inches) in an adult, which is associated with a gradient of more than 50 mm Hg. A large pressure gradient across the aortic valve may be sustained for many years without a reduction in contractile function, with left ventricular dilation generally a very late manifestation. Persistent pressure overload to the left ventricle may eventually lead to left ventricular dilation, left atrial enlargement, and pulmonary hypertension.

CLINICAL PRESENTATION

Chest pain, syncope, and dyspnea are the classic symptoms associated with severe AS. With chronic AS there generally is a long latent period before the development of symptoms. Once symptoms develop, however, the progression to end-stage disease or death is precipitous, averaging 2 to 5 years.[5] Calcific AS has now become more predominant than rheumatic aortic stensosis,[6] and as a result the mean age of presentation is now in the sixties. Angina and syncope become manifest while the left ventricular function remains preserved; dyspnea indicates congestive heart failure (CHF) and left ventricular dysfunction.[6] Exertional angina occurs in about two thirds of patients with severe AS and may be due to coronary atherosclerosis or to the markedly increased myocardial oxygen demand. This may occur even in the presence of normal coronary arteries.[7,8]

Although uncommon, patients with severe AS have suffered sudden death, usually in association with exertion. Although the mechanism remains uncertain, a common hypothesis is an abnormal baroreceptor response, the Bezold-Jarisch reflex.[9] Dizziness or frank syncope occurs in 15% to 30% of patients and has been attributed to an abrupt fall in systemic vascular resistance in the presence of a fixed cardiac output, abrupt failure of the overloaded left ventricle during effort, or arrhythmia.[10] Left ventricular failure eventually occurs with symptoms of fatigue, cough, progressive dyspnea on exertion, orthopnea, and paroxysmal nocturnal dyspnea. If the problem is unrelieved, death is likely within 2 years in patients with heart failure, 3 years in those with syncope, and 5 years in those with angina.[11]

PHYSICAL EXAMINATION

No physical finding can reliably assess the severity of obstruction. Classically the carotid pulse has a slow rise with delayed peak and small volume (pulsus parvus and pulsus tardus). A notch or shudder in the upstroke (anacrotic notch) may be appreciated. The average examiner, however, is unable to distinguish a slow-rising pulse from a normal one.[12] Auscultation reveals a harsh crescendo-decrescendo systolic election murmur that begins after the first heart sound. The murmur of AS is loudest at the second right sternal edge and radiates to the left lateral sternal border and carotids. A thrill is often present. The murmur may become softer, or even inaudible, in patients with end-stage AS. Paradoxical splitting of the second heart sound (S_2) occurs as a result of delay in closure of the aortic valve. In severe stenosis the A_2 is often inaudible; therefore no splitting of S_2 is appreciated. An additional early systolic ejection sound or click may be heard, more commonly in younger patients with congenital or bicuspid AS. Left ventricular hypertrophy (LVH) produces a sustained thrust or heave of the apical impulse. Displacement of the apical impulse downward and to the left occurs after left ventricular failure develops and the ventricle dilates.

DIAGNOSTICS

The single most important fact concerning laboratory tests in patients with AS is that, with the exception of echocardiography, normal findings (e.g., lack of LVH or normal chest x-ray findings) do not exclude severe disease. The ECG demonstrates normal sinus rhythm with signs of LVH. Atrial fibrillation usually represents either end-stage disease with left ventricular decompensation or other associated disease. Conduction abnormalities, such as first-degree atrioventricular block, bundle branch block, and intraventricular conduction disturbances, are fairly common. The chest x-ray film may demonstrate rounding or prominence of the left ventricle as a result of concentric hypertrophy of the left ventricle, poststenotic dilation of the aorta, and calcification of the valve cusps, or the chest x-ray findings may be completely normal.

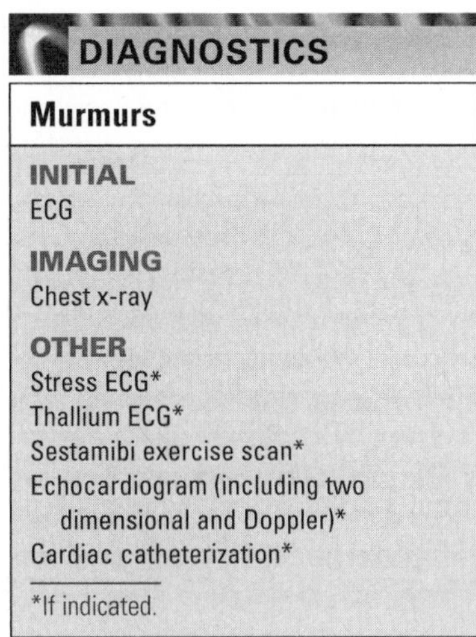
DIAGNOSTICS

Murmurs

INITIAL
ECG

IMAGING
Chest x-ray

OTHER
Stress ECG*
Thallium ECG*
Sestamibi exercise scan*
Echocardiogram (including two dimensional and Doppler)*
Cardiac catheterization*

*If indicated.

In contrast, a technically satisfactory, well-performed two-dimensional echocardiogram has the ability to exclude significant obstruction of the aortic valve. The Doppler portion of the examination is able to provide an assessment of the outflow gradient that closely approximates that obtained by cardiac catheterization. By combining Doppler ultrasonography and the echocardiogram, the examiner may make a reasonable calculation of the aortic valve area. Thickened, calcified, and immobile leaflets are readily noted by transthoracic two-dimensional echocardiography. The echocardiogram also demonstrates poststenotic dilation of the aorta and left ventricular wall thickening. Dilation of the left ventricle and/or reduced contractility (ejection fraction) occurs with myocardial failure. Equally important, additional valvular abnormalities (e.g., MR or mitral stenosis [MS]) are apparent, as are the findings of IHSS.

Cardiac catheterization can determine the severity of obstruction by recording the gradient across the valve and by calculating the valve area. Additional functional assessment of the left ventricle is possible. In the current era these findings often confirm those obtained by Doppler echocardiography. In adults the major indication for cardiac catheterization is to delineate the coronary anatomy. Even in patients without angina, approximately 50% will have significant coronary obstructions[7] (see the Diagnostics box above).

DIFFERENTIAL DIAGNOSIS

The major condition in the differential diagnosis for a systolic ejection murmur without valvular disease is the functional or innocent murmur (i.e., flow murmur without disease). The absence of symptoms or other physical abnormalities will generally lead to this diagnosis. In adults the major pathologic state that must be differentiated is IHSS, or hypertrophic obstructive cardiomyopathy. These patients may have similar symptomatology; however, the carotid upstroke is very brisk, with at times two distinct humps (pulsus bisferiens). The

DIFFERENTIAL DIAGNOSIS

Systolic Murmurs

EJECTION MURMURS
- Aortic stenosis
- Idiopathic hypertrophic subaortic stenosis
- Pulmonary stenosis

REGURGITANT MURMURS
- Mitral regurgitation or insufficiency
- Tricuspid regurgitation or insufficiency
- Ventricular septal defect

LATE SYSTOLIC MURMURS
- Mitral valve prolapse

CONTINUOUS MURMURS
- Patent ductus arteriosus
- Benign (innocent)
- Mammary shuffle

primary distinguishing characteristic is the murmur's response to maneuvers that increase or decrease the dynamic obstruction. Thus standing or the strain phase of Valsalva's maneuver decreases venous return, resulting in a smaller left ventricular outflow tract and an increase in the murmur intensity.

MANAGEMENT

Management of the patient with symptomatic AS is almost entirely surgical. Medications cannot increase the forward flow across a critically stenosed valve. Indeed, treatment of the symptomatic patient with high-grade AS is fraught with difficulties. Nitrates may decrease systemic vascular resistance and perfusion pressure. Calcium channel blockers and beta blockers may decrease left ventricular function and precipitate heart failure. Diuretics may result in hypovolemia and underperfusion similar to that with nitrates. Thus these medications must be used with great caution. However, patients with symptomatic AS and heart failure may benefit from angiotensin-converting enzyme inhibitors, diuretic therapy, and digoxin.[13] Digoxin may provide some benefit to a patient with AS who is symptomatic with atrial fibrillation or evidence of left ventricular dysfunction.[13] Medical therapy for the asymptomatic patient with AS consists of antibiotic prophylaxis for the prevention of infective endocarditis. Strenuous physical exertion should be avoided only by patients with high-grade lesions.

Co-Management with Specialists

Co-management with a specialist is reasonable for patients with AS to obtain a Doppler echocardiogram every 2 years for mild disease and annually for more severe disease. Patients with significant obstruction and modest symptoms, or those who are asymptomatic yet have severe obstruction, may require a Doppler echocardiogram every 6 months. It is recommended that medication therapy for patients with inoperable AS be discussed with the cardiologist.[13]

LIFE SPAN CONSIDERATIONS

Once patients with AS become symptomatic with angina or syncope, the average survival time is 2 to 3 years. Patients with CHF demonstrate an average survival time of 1.5 to 2 years.[5]

COMPLICATIONS

The initial symptoms associated with AS are generally angina and syncope or presyncope, as well as dyspnea and frank CHF, which, in the patient with just AS, are manifestations of a failing left ventricle. Atrial fibrillation occurs in less than 10% of patients with AS, and its occurrence should raise the possibility of concomitant mitral valve disease. If it occurs, prompt cardioversion is often required, since loss of atrial contraction may significantly impair left ventricular performance as a result of the markedly noncompliant left ventricle. Systematic calcium embolization to the retinal artery may result in partial visual loss and may be an additional indication for prompt surgical repair.[14]

INDICATIONS FOR REFERRAL OR HOSPITALIZATION AND PATIENT AND FAMILY EDUCATION

See Indications for Referral or Hospitalization and Patient and Family Education under Mitral Stenosis, p. 620.

AORTIC INSUFFICIENCY

DEFINITION AND EPIDEMIOLOGY

Aortic regurgitation occurs when the aortic valve fails to close completely, allowing blood to flow back into the left ventricle during ventricular diastole. This process may be either chronic or acute. It may occur as a result of involvement of the leaflets themselves or as a result of distortion of the aortic root. Pathologic processes that affect the aortic valve, leading to chronic aortic regurgitation, are inflammation (e.g., resulting from rheumatic fever, syphilis, rheumatoid arthritis), structural processes (e.g., unicuspid, bicuspid, aneurysm), disruptive processes (e.g., trauma, infective endocarditis, dissection), congenital conditions, or stress from hypertension, whereas acute aortic regurgitation most commonly occurs as a result of infective endocarditis, with dissecting aortic aneurysm and acute chest trauma being less common causes.

PATHOPHYSIOLOGY

Aortic regurgitation, or aortic insufficiency (AI), produces a volume overload to the left ventricle during diastole. The volume of blood regurgitated into the left ventricle determines whether the volume overload is mild, moderate, or severe. Regurgitant volume is determined by (1) the area of the regurgitant valve orifice, (2) the diastolic pressure gradient between the aorta and the left ventricle, and (3) the duration of diastole.[5] In chronic AI the left ventricle dilates, compensating with a gradual increase in end-diastolic volume. Initially, forward output is maintained as normal, and the ventricle may not ever have increased end-diastolic pressure, but wall stress is dramatically elevated. In acute aortic regurgitation there is no time for this adaptation to occur, and a dramatic increase in left ventricular end-diastolic pressure occurs with only minor increases in end-diastolic volume.

CLINICAL PRESENTATION AND PHYSICAL EXAMINATION

Patients with chronic aortic regurgitation may be asymptomatic for decades. When symptoms do occur, the patient usually complains of symptoms of CHF, especially dyspnea and fatigue. Patients may also complain of angina in the absence of significant coronary artery disease (CAD). Patients with acute aortic regurgitation are seen with symptoms of severe left-sided heart failure (dyspnea at rest, orthopnea, paroxysmal nocturnal dyspnea, fatigue, exhaustion) that have occurred suddenly. Symptoms of low forward cardiac output (fatigue and exhaustion) are overshadowed by symptoms of pulmonary congestion in patients with acute AI.

A number of physical findings differ between acute and chronic AI. In chronic AI the rate of rise of the peripheral pulse is rapid with quick collapse (Corrigan's, or water-hammer, pulse) as a result of the forceful ejection of blood in early systole and regurgitation during early diastole. The carotid pulse is often bisferious. Arterial blood pressure usually demonstrates a low diastolic pressure (Korotkoff's sounds may even be zero) with a normal systolic blood pressure, thus causing a widened pulse pressure in a patient with moderate or severe chronic AI. Patients with acute AI usually demonstrate a carotid arterial pulse with a sharp rise to a single, rapidly collapsing peak without a widened pulse pressure. A pulsus alternans may be present in severe acute AI, but it is unusual in patients with chronic AI. With chronic AI the apical impulse is displaced to the left and downward and is hyperdynamic.

Auscultation of the patient with AI often reveals an S_3. The diastolic murmur of chronic regurgitation is usually high pitched and blowing, with the duration correlating best with the severity of the insufficiency. In acute AI the murmur may be very short or even absent. A rumbling mid- or late diastolic murmur, the Austin Flint murmur, may be heard at the apex in the presence of at least moderate insufficiency. This represents functional MS of the mitral valve from the torrential regurgitant flow produced by the AI impinging on the anterior mitral valve leaflet. A loud systolic ejection murmur is common in both acute and chronic AI, even in the absence of valvular stenosis. In chronic AI, hepatomegaly and ascites may be present in patients with associated heart failure.

DIAGNOSTICS

The characteristic findings on the ECG for a patient with chronic AI is LVH, especially in the precordial leads. Conduction disturbances may occur with aortic regurgitation secondary to inflammatory processes. In severe acute AI the ECG is usually normal except for sinus tachycardia, without evidence of LVH.

As the severity of chronic aortic regurgitation increases, the left ventricular contour enlarges, producing a boot-shaped heart silhouette on the chest x-ray film. The aortic knob and ascending aorta become prominent with moderate to severe chronic AI. Patients with acute AI do not demonstrate cardiac enlargement but will exhibit increased venous redistribution to the upper lobes because of pulmonary venous and capillary hypertension secondary to an increased left ventricular end-diastolic pressure and left atrial pressure.

Echocardiography combined with color Doppler imaging has become the primary diagnostic tool for assessment of AI. Evidence of mild AI may be detected on Doppler imaging long before it is audible on auscultation. Transthoracic two-dimensional echocardiography may help identify possible causes for the regurgitation by documenting flail or prolapsing leaflets, a dilated aortic root, or evidence of vegetation. The greatest impact, however, is the ability of Doppler echocardiography to assess the severity of the regurgitation and assist in determining the optimum time for valve replacement, especially in the asymptomatic patient. Color Doppler imaging has been investigated for the ability to "quantify" the degree of regurgitation; however, not surprisingly, only a relative, "qualitative" assessment is possible, because the amount of regurgitation depends not only on the "size of the hole," but also on both the upstream and downstream pressures. However, echocardiography is able to quantify the ventricular dimensions and ventricular function (ejection fraction) well. Evidence of reduction in systolic function or marked and/or progressive ventricular dilation is an indication for surgery. Patients with a left ventricular end-systolic dimension of more than 55 mm (2.2 inches) have been found to have an increased risk of operative death or subsequent death from CHF[15] (see the Diagnostics box, p. 612).

DIFFERENTIAL DIAGNOSIS

The murmur of AI is an early diastolic murmur that must be differentiated from other early diastolic murmurs (pulmonary regurgitation and VSD). Most early diastolic murmurs are related to either pulmonary or aortic regurgitation. However, an early diastolic flow murmur can also sometimes be heard in patients with a VSD and a large left-to-right shunt.

DIFFERENTIAL DIAGNOSIS

Diastolic Murmurs

EARLY DIASTOLE
- Aortic insufficiency
- Pulmonary insufficiency
- Ventricular septal defect

MID- TO LATE DIASTOLE
- Mitral stenosis
- Tricuspid stenosis
- Austin Flint murmur

MANAGEMENT

Medical therapy for chronic aortic regurgitation consists of antibiotic prophylaxis to prevent infective endocarditis. Once left ventricular failure develops, digitalis glycosides, diuretics, and vasodilators are necessary to improve left ventricular function and reduce the aortic regurgitant fraction. Hydralazine and other vasodilators have been found to be useful in the asymptomatic or minimally symptomatic patient for reducing ventricular volumes, improving ejection fraction, and potentially delaying the need for surgery.[16,17]

The primary therapy for an incompetent valve, however, remains valve replacement. The critical issue is the timing of surgery. Surgery is advocated for symptomatic patients who have confirmed moderate to severe chronic AI or who have impaired or progressively worsening left ventricular function. Surgery is usually not indicated for asymptomatic patients with severe chronic AI who have good exercise tolerance and normal left ventricular function. The natural history of such patients has been excellent.[18] However, recent emphasis has been placed on distinguishing the patient with mild symptoms (New York Heart Association [NYHA] functional class II) from the truly asymptomatic patient, with strong consideration for early operation for the former.[19] Although the need for surgery at the onset of symptoms or ventricular dysfunction has been emphasized, even the patient with a grossly impaired left ventricular performance or severe symptoms may experience marked improvement in ventricular function and symptoms[20] and therefore should be considered as a candidate for valve replacement.

Co-Management with Specialists

Co-management with a specialist is considered when the patient with AI becomes symptomatic. Patients may live for years or decades with AI before the development of symptoms. However, as with AS, once symptoms develop, progressive deterioration will occur over the next few years unless surgical intervention occurs.

COMPLICATIONS

Other than progressive ventricular dysfunction and development of symptoms, the major complication is infective endocarditis. Patients who are nearing the time for consideration of valve replacement should undergo dental consultation.

INDICATIONS FOR REFERRAL OR HOSPITALIZATION AND PATIENT AND FAMILY EDUCATION

See Indications for Referral or Hospitalization and Patient and Family Education under Mitral Stenosis, p. 620.

MITRAL REGURGITATION

DEFINITION AND EPIDEMIOLOGY

Mitral insufficiency, or MR, may result from a disturbance of any of the functional components of the mitral valve or its supporting structures, which include the valve leaflets, papillary muscle, mitral valve annulus, chordae tendineae, or left ventricle itself. Rheumatic heart disease was generally the most common cause of chronic MR; however, with the reduction in the incidence of rheumatic fever, other causes such as ischemic heart disease and mitral valve prolapse have become the most common. Additional causes of MR, either acute or chronic, include congenital abnormalities, isolated rupture of the chordae tendineae, papillary muscle dysfunction, CAD, collagen vascular disease, and infective endocarditis.[13] Dilation of the left ventricle from any cause is likely to cause the mitral leaflets to fail to coapt. Acute regurgitation may occur as a result of spontaneous rupture of the chordae tendineae, blunt chest trauma, or necrotic disruption of a papillary muscle as a sequela of a myocardial infarction.

PATHOPHYSIOLOGY

The burden placed on the heart as a result of MR is dependent on the amount of reflux and the ventricular and atrial ability to compensate. During systole the left ventricle simultaneously ejects blood forward through the aortic valve or backward across an incompetent valve into the left atrium. The volume of mitral regurgitant flow in either chronic or acute MR therefore depends on the size of the regurgitant orifice and on the pressure gradient between the left ventricle and the left atrium. The latter is affected by the balance between the ease of regurgitation into the "low-pressure sump" of the left atrium and the flow out to the aorta. Regurgitant flow is decreased by any agent that decreases left ventricular size (such as diuretics) or shifts the balance toward forward output (such as afterload-reducing vasodilators). In contrast, regurgitation is increased by any factor that enlarges the left ventricle, depresses myocardial function, or increases resistance to forward flow (such as hypertension or AS). With chronic MR the increased volume of blood ejected back into the left atrium causes stretching and thinning of the atrial wall. The large, thin-walled atrium accommodates the large volume of blood ejected into it during ventricular systole. Although the pressure in the left atrium and pulmonary capillaries and veins is elevated during systole, the left atrial pressure decreases to near normal during ventricular diastole. The left ventricle dilates and becomes hypertrophied in response to the increased volume from the left atrium, so that sufficient cardiac output is maintained. Initially the additional volume to be ejected by the ventricle (increased preload) results in enhanced emptying. Therefore the ejection fraction is increased. "Normal" ejection fraction or other measures of cardiac systolic performance actually are likely to represent significantly abnormal ventricular function. Pulmonary hypertension rarely develops in the patient who has developed MR gradually over time.

In contrast, patients with acute MR develop a rapid increase in left atrial pressure as a result of the sudden volume overload into a normal, nondilated left atrium and ventricle. This results in sudden increased left ventricular end-diastolic, left atrial, and pulmonary venous pressure, producing interstitial edema that leads to pulmonary edema. Pulmonary hypertension may develop.

CLINICAL PRESENTATION AND PHYSICAL EXAMINATION

The patient with MR may remain asymptomatic for decades. Patients generally complain of fatigue and, later in the course of the disease, dyspnea on exertion. The former is a result of reduced forward cardiac output, whereas the latter occurs with the onset of left ventricular dysfunction. The severity of symptoms and clinical outcome of chronic MR depend not only on the degree of regurgitation, but also on associated additional valvular abnormalities, underlying ventricular dysfunction, and concomitant CAD. Palpitations are often noted, even in the patient without evidence of atrial fibrillation. Symptoms of CHF appear late in the course of chronic MR as a result of the gradual increase in volume overload. By the time symptoms appear, the degree of ventricular dysfunction may have progressed to such an extent as to be irreversible.

Those who develop acute MR have an abrupt onset of symptoms resulting from the sudden overload of the left atrium. A patient with rupture of a few chordae from subacute bacterial endocarditis or trauma usually complains of easy fatigue, dyspnea, pedal edema, and occasionally intermittent chest pain. A patient with a complete rupture of a papillary muscle generally has severe hypotension and florid pulmonary edema. With MR, palpation of the carotid pulse generally demonstrates a rapidly rising pulse. The apical impulse is hyperkinetic and displaces downward and to the left. Auscultation of the patient with chronic MR reveals a soft S_1. A loud P_2 or an accentuated pulmonic component of S_2 suggests the presence of pulmonary hypertension. An audible S_3 is present when there is hemodynamically significant MR; in combined MS and regurgitation, S_3 is indicative of predominant regurgitation. The hallmark murmur of MR is the pansystolic, blowing murmur best heard at the apex and radiating to the axilla or back. The murmur may radiate to other locations such as the back or sternum if papillary muscle dysfunction or partial rupture of supporting structures is present. Maneuvers that decrease left ventricular volume by decreasing impedance to left ventricular outflow or venous return (such as sudden standing or inhalation of amyl nitrite) will result in a decreased murmur, as will more chronically decreasing ventricular volume with diuresis. Increasing the impedance to left ventricular ejection (asking the patient to squeeze both fists in a handgrip) will increase regurgitation and thereby the intensity of the murmur.

DIAGNOSTICS

The ECG in chronic MR usually demonstrates normal sinus rhythm with left atrial hypertrophy in the early stage and atrial fibrillation later on. If the MR is secondary to underlying ventricular dysfunction and dilation, evidence of LVH is generally noted on the ECG. The chest x-ray film demonstrates an increase in both left ventricular and left atrial size.

Doppler echocardiography detects the high-velocity jet of regurgitant flow back into the left atrium. It permits sensitive detection of regurgitation of even a mild degree. Although the ability to quantify the degree of the regurgitation remains imprecise, the technique permits the more important prediction of clinical outcomes. The severity can be roughly estimated by the distance the jet goes into the atrium. Chronic MR usually produces a volume overload pattern and a large left atrium. Echocardiography can detect structural abnormalities such as flail leaflets; endocarditic vegetation; and thickened, rheumatic chordae. Determination of the end-systolic volume of the ventricle has proved to be a more reliable predictor of clinical prognosis.[21] Patients with dimensions greater than 50 mm (2 inches) had poor outcomes after surgery, in contrast to those with end-systolic diameters less than 40 mm (1.6 inches) (see the Diagnostics box, p. 612).

For patients with acute MR, a transesophageal echocardiogram may be indicated.[13] Coronary arteriography may be indicated for patients with severe MR accompanied by CAD.[13]

DIFFERENTIAL DIAGNOSIS

The murmur of MR or mitral insufficiency is a pansystolic murmur. Other pansystolic murmurs include the murmur of tricuspid regurgitation and VSD. On rare occasions the murmur of patent ductus arteriosus can be pansystolic also. Often, if the patient is tachycardic, these murmurs are difficult to distinguish from long systolic ejection murmurs. Because pansystolic murmurs are pathologic murmurs, differentiation is essential (see the Differential Diagnosis box, p. 613).

MANAGEMENT

Patients with acute MR related to bacterial endocarditis require IV antibiotic therapy with the appropriate antibiotic.[13] All patients with chronic MR, even those who are asymptomatic, should receive antibiotic prophylaxis before any dental or surgical procedure. If atrial fibrillation develops, digitalis glycosides are given to control the ventricular rate. Other agents such as calcium channel blockers or beta blockers may be less tolerated, given their potential to exacerbate the degree of regurgitation as a result of their negative contractile potential. Anticoagulation should be strongly considered to prevent systemic emboli. Dietary sodium restriction and diuretics will be useful for symptomatic patients. Agents that reduce afterload (hydralazine or angiotensin-converting enzyme inhibitors) will increase forward flow of blood and thereby improve symptoms, reverse hemodynamic alterations, and even delay the necessity for surgical intervention.[22] Investigations suggest the benefit of angiotensin-receptor blocker therapy for the patient intolerant of angiotensin-converting enzyme inhibitors.[23]

Co-Management with Specialists

Co-management with a specialist should be considered for patients with acute MR or once the patient with chronic MR becomes symptomatic and surgery is considered. Surgical therapy is aimed at improving symptoms, relieving severe pulmonary hypertension, and decreasing left ventricular volume and mass. The Department of Veterans Affairs Cooperative Study on Valvular Heart Disease has recommended surgery for significant MR or MS-MR before left ventricular ejection fraction is decreased to below 50%, the end-systolic volume index is increased to above 101 ml/m^2, or pulmonary hypertension develops, since left ventricular size and systolic function will likely be normal postoperatively and survival and functional class will be enhanced.[24,25] Other investigators have recommended using an ejection fraction cutoff of 60% as being indicative of significant ventricular dysfunction.[26]

Patients with marked left ventricular dysfunction may remain symptomatic even after surgical treatment. Such patients may show a decrease in ejection fraction and an increase in end-systolic volume immediately after surgery as the abolition of MR removes their "low-pressure sump," essentially increasing the afterload that the ventricle faces. These patients may require vasodilator treatment in the immediate postoperative period and in fact may be difficult to wean off bypass. Such patients may benefit from only partial repair of the valve, leaving some regurgitation.

Surgical techniques used to treat MR are valve repair or reconstruction and valve replacement. Valve repair or reconstruction repairs the disrupted functional component of the valve. Mitral valve repair retains the tethering effect of chordal attachments, which may prevent postoperative dilation of the left ventricle and decreases the chance of left ventricular dysfunction, which occurs after mitral valve replacement. A significant increase in exercise ejection fraction and stroke volume after mitral valve replacement has been found in patients in whom the chordae and papillary muscles were preserved.[26]

LIFE SPAN CONSIDERATIONS

Life span considerations for patients with MR depend on the degree of symptoms and the status of the left ventricular function. Patients with MR may remain asymptomatic for decades, with only a small percentage progressing to more severe MR requiring surgery.[27] Patients commonly may tolerate even significant MR for decades without development of symptoms.

COMPLICATIONS

Atrial fibrillation affects approximately 75% of patients with MR and is related to the size of the left atrium. Other complications include systemic embolization (generally in the presence of atrial fibrillation) and bacterial endocarditis.

INDICATIONS FOR REFERRAL OR HOSPITALIZATION AND PATIENT AND FAMILY EDUCATION

See Indications for Referral or Hospitalization and Patient and Family Education under Mitral Stenosis, p. 620).

MITRAL VALVE PROLAPSE

DEFINITION AND EPIDEMIOLOGY

A unique subset of patients with MR are those with mitral valve prolapse (MVP). Although the regurgitation is usually mild and often free of associated papillary muscle dysfunction, MVP appears to occur more often in patients with small ventricles resulting from thoracic deformities, such as the straight back syndrome or pectus excavatum. The syndrome seems to be most prevalent in young women between 20 and 40 years old, although it has been detected in males of all ages, with men over the age of 45 years at increased risk of developing complications of severe MR and endocarditis.[28]

PATHOPHYSIOLOGY

MVP is typically described as the posterior displacement or prolapse of one or both (more commonly the posterior) leaflets of the mitral valve into the left atrium during systole. This billowing back of the leaflet places stress on the chordae tendineae and papillary muscles, which may be the cause of the nonischemic chest discomfort. The myxomatous degeneration may, over time, result in thickened and redundant valves. As the valvular dysfunction progresses, insufficient coaptation will result in MR. The connective tissue changes may extend into the mitral annulus, enhancing the tendency for MR, and into the chordae tendineae, potentially resulting in sudden chordal rupture.

CLINICAL PRESENTATION AND PHYSICAL EXAMINATION

Most persons with MVP are asymptomatic. When symptoms do occur, the patient usually complains of chest discomfort, palpitations, mild dyspnea, fatigue, and anxiety. These symptoms are similar to those reported in the panic disorder syndrome. Both disorders may be a result of autonomic dysfunction.[29] The chest symptoms, along with the tremendous frequency of this disorder in the general population, mandate familiarity with its presentation. Although as many as 17% of healthy females may have auscultatory findings suggestive of this syndrome, a more valid estimate, relying on appropriate echocardiographic criteria, would place the frequency at 4% to 6%, or affecting more than 10 million males and females in the United States.[30,31]

MVP should probably be thought of as a continuum from the exaggeration of the normal, slight billowing of the mitral valve into the left atrium during systole; to a fully "floppy" valve; and finally to variable degrees of MR when the floppy, redundant leaflets no longer are able to coapt. At times the regurgitation may become severe, often as a result of the rupture of the chordae tendineae. Most commonly, the disorder exists by itself, generally in association with a characteristic pathologic myxomatous degeneration of the mitral valve. There appears to be a strong hereditary predisposition to the condition, although it may be associated with other conditions, some rare (e.g., Ehlers-Danlos syndrome) and others common (e.g., atrial septal defect). MVP has been noted in patients with CAD. The ischemic discomfort is usually described as brief attacks of severe, piercing pain localized to the apex. Palpitations are common and may result from a variety of arrhythmias.

Most cases of MVP are diagnosed on routine physical examination. Auscultation of the patient with MVP reveals a midsystolic click. This is a snapping extra heart sound heard best at the lower left sternal border or at the apex, and it may be only intermittently appreciated. The presence of an apical systolic murmur varies with the degree of MR. This systolic murmur is usually a late systolic crescendo-type that can be loud and musical. Maneuvers that decrease the left ventricular volume, such as standing, will both move the click earlier in systole and make the murmur longer. Pansystolic murmurs are usually an indication of pronounced MVP resulting in a more severe form of MR.

DIAGNOSTICS

Patients with MVP, most commonly those who are symptomatic, may demonstrate inverted T waves and nonspecific ST-segment changes in the inferior and left precordial leads of the ECG. These changes may be a manifestation of the ischemia to the papillary muscles resulting from the strain placed on these muscles by the prolapsed valve leaflets. Stress ECGs and thallium 201 or sestamibi exercise scans should be used when there is a need to differentiate MVP from CAD. This is especially important when the patient with suspected MVP complains of chest discomfort.

Supraventricular tachycardia is not uncommon in MVP. Other ventricular and supraventricular arrhythmias and conduction disturbances may also occur. There seems to be a slightly increased incidence of sudden death, presumably as a result of ventricular fibrillation, although this finding has not been firmly established.

Echocardiography, specifically two-dimensional echocardiography, is regarded by some as the single best technique to define this disorder. The echocardiogram shows the posterior mitral valve leaflet or both leaflets bowing or bulging back into the left atrium during systole. Such displacement, noted solely on the four-chamber view, is now recognized as a normal finding. Patients with thickened and redundant mitral valves form a higher-risk subgroup for subsequent complications.[31] Other echocardiographic findings include MR and flail leaflets in patients with ruptured chordae (see the Diagnostics box, p. 612).

DIFFERENTIAL DIAGNOSIS

The murmur of MVP is a late systolic murmur and is characterized by a midsystolic click. This click heralds the onset of the murmur. Because it is a murmur of mitral insufficiency, it should be differentiated from the pansystolic murmur of mitral insufficiency (see the Differential Diagnosis box, p. 613).

MANAGEMENT

Most persons with MVP are asymptomatic and require no intervention other than periodic clinical and echocardiographic follow-up evaluation every 3 to 5 years. Asymptomatic patients need reassurance that the condition is benign and usually uncomplicated, and that the prognosis is good. If a systolic murmur is present, however, the patient with MVP, even if asymptomatic, requires more frequent monitoring. Those with pansystolic murmurs are more likely to have more MR and require the same approach as noted for MR. However, even in the face of severe MR, many patients continue to do well.[27]

Antibiotic prophylaxis, although controversial, appears reasonable for MVP with evidence of MR. Patients with a history of palpitations or prolonged QT intervals should have 24-hour ambulatory monitoring. Beta-blocker therapy is often useful for palpitations or nonischemic chest pain. Patients with syncope or near syncope should be referred for more complete arrhythmia evaluation.

Co-Management with Specialists

Co-management with a specialist and life span considerations for MVP are related to the severity of the MR and are the same as previously described for MR. Surgical treatment of MVP is necessary when the MR has been progressive and severe. Mitral reconstruction with ring annuloplasty has been successful.

COMPLICATIONS

In addition to chordal rupture and progressive MR, endocarditis and sudden death have been associated with this disorder[32]; however, their incidence remains uncertain. Most reviews conclude that endocarditis and sudden death are rare. All of the complications are more common in older men or those with MVP and thickened leaflets.[28,31]

INDICATIONS FOR REFERRAL OR HOSPITALIZATION AND PATIENT AND FAMILY EDUCATION

See Indications for Referral or Hospitalization and Patient and Family Education under Mitral Stenosis, p. 620).

MITRAL STENOSIS

DEFINITION AND EPIDEMIOLOGY

MS is almost always caused by rheumatic heart disease. Thus, with the marked reduction of rheumatic carditis over the past 4 decades, the occurrence of MS has lessened. Less common causes of obstruction across the mitral valve that prevents normal emptying of the left atrium into the left ventricle during diastole include congenital stenoses; masses such as vegetation, clots, or benign tumors (atrial myxomas); and profound calcification of the mitral annulus. Damage to the mitral valve from rheumatic fever will cause the commissures of the leaflets themselves to fuse, the leaflets to thicken and fibrose, and the chordae to thicken and shorten, resulting in a thickened, scarred valve that is funnel shaped with a "fish mouth" appearance.

PATHOPHYSIOLOGY

The central pathophysiologic feature of MS is obstruction across the mitral valve during diastole. This results in a pressure gradient between the left atrium and the left ventricle. The increased left atrial pressure is transmitted to the pulmonary veins and capillaries, and eventually to the pulmonary arteries and right side of the heart. The normal mitral valve area is 4 to 6 cm^2 (1.5 to 2.3 square inches). There is usually no detectable pressure gradient across the normal mitral valve, even when flow is increased with exercise. As the valve area is reduced, the gradient across the valve increases. When the valve area is reduced to 25% of normal, hemodynamically significant stenosis is present. Critical MS occurs when the mitral valve opening is reduced to 1 cm^2 (0.4 square inch). With this degree of obstruction, the mean gradient, even at rest, is likely to be more than 20 mm Hg throughout diastole. With a further rise to 25 to 30 mm Hg, the left atrial pressure will exceed plasma oncotic pressure, and episodes of orthopnea or paroxysmal nocturnal dyspnea will develop. Chronic elevation of left atrial pressure produces a passive pressure load on the pulmonary vessel and causes hypertrophy and hyperplasia. In addition, there is a reactive vasoconstrictive aspect. Pulmonary hypertension may develop, which over time may produce right ventricular hypertrophy. In longstanding, severe MS, pulmonary hypertension may approach or exceed systemic levels.

A major advance in the ability to assess valvular obstruction was the derivation by Gorlin of a hydraulic formula for calculation of the cardiac valve area. An understanding of this formula helps in understanding the factors that result in increases in this gradient. This equation describes the relationship between the size of the opening (valve area) and how it relates to the flow rate across the valve and the pressure drop (gradient) across the valve. Thus, for any given valve area, an increase in flow volume (cardiac output) results in an increase in gradient. The "rate" aspect relates to the time available to get the blood across the valve (diastolic filling period). Increases in blood flow (resulting from hypervolemia or pregnancy) will increase the gradient. More dramatic is the effect of heart rate. As diastole, not systole, shortens with an increase in heart rate, fever or exercise may significantly elevate the gradient, especially because the gradient increases as a square of the increase in flow rate (i.e., a doubling of the heart rate will quadruple the gradient). Thus patients with mild to moderate MS who were previously asymptomatic may develop florid heart failure with the development of atrial fibrillation (which generally has a rapid ventricular response on initial occurrence).

CLINICAL PRESENTATION AND PHYSICAL EXAMINATION

The principal symptom of MS is dyspnea, which is graded according to the NYHA classification. Patients with asymptomatic MS are graded as functional class I. Patients with dyspnea that occurs with greater than ordinary exertion are graded as class II; patients with dyspnea that occurs with only mild exertion (less than ordinary activity) are class III; and those with dyspnea on minimum exertion, with episodes of orthopnea, paroxysmal nocturnal dyspnea, or pulmonary edema, are class IV.

Fatigue is also common with MS and in some cases may be more severe than the dyspnea. If atrial fibrillation develops, patients may also complain of palpitations. Hemoptysis may occur as a result of pulmonary hypertension and in rare instances may be massive. Hoarseness (Ortner's syndrome) may develop from compression of the left recurrent laryngeal nerve by a dilated left atrium. A small number of patients complain of angina-like chest pain, which may be due to concomitant CAD, pulmonary embolus, or pulmonary hypertension. Thromboembolism may be the presenting symptom in some patients.

Auscultation will typically reveal a loud S_1, an accentuated pulmonic component of S_2 (P_2) if pulmonary hypertension is present, and an opening snap heard with the diaphragm of the stethoscope. This snap is the snapping of the thickened mitral valve as it reaches the end of its maximum excursion during early diastole. This must be distinguished from an S_3 gallop sound, which is lower in pitch and occurs later in diastole (typically 0.12 second after S_2) than the opening snap, which occurs 0.04 to 0.10 second after S_2. The classic diastolic rumble of MS is heard with the bell of the stethoscope near the apex. It begins shortly after the opening snap and may have a presystolic accentuation in patients who are still in normal sinus rhythm. The murmur may be difficult to appreciate in the early stages of MS and can be better appreciated by listening with the patient in the left lateral decubitus position or by increasing the flow by having the patient perform mild exercise. As the severity of MS increases and valve leaflets become markedly calcified, the S_1 sound will decrease in intensity while the diagnostic rumble progresses to a pandiastolic murmur.

DIAGNOSTICS

The characteristic findings on the ECG are evidence of left atrial enlargement (widened, notched P wave in lead II with pronounced terminal negativity in V_1) in patients still in normal sinus rhythm, and evidence of right-axis deviation of the QRS or right ventricular hypertrophy. Atrial fibrillation is common. Chest x-ray examination may reveal a straightening of the left heart border or "double density" in the midportion of the cardiac silhouette, both of which are manifestations of left atrial enlargement. With chronic pulmonary hypertension the pulmonary vessels become prominent, and flow redistributes fluid in the upper lobes. Chronic accumulation of transudated fluid in the interstitial spaces of the lungs and lymphatic engorgement result in linear shadows perpendicular to the pleura, which are known as Kerley's B lines.

Probably no cardiac lesion has been so closely aligned with echocardiography as MS. Echocardiography has largely superseded cardiac catheterization as a means of quantifying the magnitude of the gradient and valve area; determining the presence of additional valvular lesions; and assessing ventricular function. Coronary arteriography still may be required in adults to exclude CAD. The M-mode echocardiogram is able to demonstrate the characteristic motion of the mitral valve, which resembles a square wave. In MS the anterior and posterior leaflets demonstrate *concordant* movement (both leaflets moving in concert anteriorly during diastole) as opposed to the normal *discordant* movement (leaflets moving in opposite directions). Two-dimensional echocardiography demonstrates the reduced excursion of the valve, with "doming" of the valve during diastole, and permits accurate assessment of the valve area by planimetry of the valve on the cross-sectional, or short-axis, view. In addition, dense echoes suggest calcification of the valve, which, along with assessment of the pliability, permits judgment as to the feasibility of commissurotomy vs. valve replacement.[33] Two-dimensional echocardiography will also assess the size of the left atrium and identify other causes for mitral obstruction, such as atrial myxoma. Doppler study not only documents the presence of regurgitation, but also permits another accurate method for estimating valve area, by means of either the "pressure–half-time" technique or the continuity equation. In the presence of tricuspid regurgitation, some degree of which is almost always present, pulmonary pressure can be estimated.

DIFFERENTIAL DIAGNOSIS

The murmur of MS is classified as a mid- to late diastolic murmur. Other mid- to late diastolic murmurs that should be considered in the differential diagnosis include an atrial presystolic murmur, the Austin Flint murmur, and the murmur of tricuspid stenosis. (See the Differential Diagnosis box, p. 614.)

MANAGEMENT

Treatment of the underlying obstructive lesion of MS is an operative procedure. Medical therapy aims include treatment of atrial fibrillation and prevention of recurrent episodes of rheumatic fever and systemic embolism. According to the American College of Cardiology/American Heart Association guidelines,[13] all patients with MS must receive antibiotic prophylaxis for infections, surgery, or any instrumentation procedure. Patients who have had one episode of rheumatic fever are at risk for a second episode. Recurrent episodes of rheumatic fever are dramatically reduced with secondary prophylaxis against streptococcal infections. Anemia or infections should be promptly treated because they increase the heart rate and therefore the gradient. Similarly, occupations that demand strenuous physical exertion should be avoided by patients with more than mild MS. Patients who are symptomatic should be treated with oral diuretics and sodium restriction.

Patients with MS who have atrial fibrillation should be treated with digoxin, beta blockers, and/or calcium channel blockers to slow the ventricular rate. Electrical cardioversion may be attempted in patients with mild MS and new-onset atrial fibrillation. Anticoagulation is required for 3 weeks before cardioversion to prevent emboli during conversion from atrial fibrillation to normal sinus rhythm. After cardioversion to normal sinus rhythm, antiarrhythmic therapy to maintain normal sinus rhythm may be indicated. The rate of successful cardioversion is low in patients who have been symptomatic for several years and who have a left atrium larger than 5 cm (2 inches) as documented by echocardiography; however, a single attempt is often worthwhile.

Anticoagulant therapy can help prevent venous thrombosis and pulmonary embolism and can reduce the frequency of systemic embolism in patients with MS who have experienced previous embolic episodes.[34] No benefit of anticoagulation has been shown for patients in normal sinus rhythm without a prior history of embolism. However, anticoagulation may be reasonable to consider for those patients found to have moderate MS by echocardiogram or those with symptoms, since systemic embolization is well recognized in these patients.

The primary determinant for surgical consideration is the degree of symptoms. Patients in NYHA class II/III would be considered surgical candidates. The onset of atrial fibrillation intensifies symptomatology and, even if the patient is successfully cardioverted, is a harbinger of impending need for intervention. Arterial thromboembolism increases the need for surgery.

Two surgical approaches are used: commissurotomy, either open (under direct visualization) or closed (using a dilator), and valve replacement. Commissurotomy is by necessity palliative, reducing the degree of obstruction, and is most successful in patients without huge atria or significant regurgitation calcification. Otherwise, patients require valve replacement. An alternative in selected cases is balloon mitral valvuloplasty. This technique has been demonstrated to be superior to closed commissurotomy and equivalent to open commissurotomy.[35] Given the lower costs and avoidance of open heart surgery, the balloon procedure should be considered the treatment of choice for pliable, stenotic valves. Suitable patients almost always would be considered earlier in their symptomatic natural history than they would be if full replacement were required.

Co-Management with Specialists and Life Span Considerations

Co-management with a specialist is necessary. Consultation should occur when the diagnosis is unclear or when cardioversion, surgery, or balloon valvuloplasty is being considered.

COMPLICATIONS

Patients with MS are at risk for thromboembolization. An additional complication is severe pulmonary hypertension. The clinical course of disease in these patients must be differentiated from that of patients with congenital heart disease. It is well recognized that the unfortunate patient with pulmonary hypertension caused by congenital heart disease (Eisenmenger's syndrome) has a very poor result after surgery. Initially it was believed that patients with mitral valve disease and marked pulmonary hypertension shared the same fate. However, a number of studies have demonstrated that, although they do have an increased operative mortality when compared with patients who are less severely affected, these patients demonstrate a striking and rapid improvement in pulmonary pressures.[36] For this reason, no such patient should be excluded from consideration as a surgical candidate.

INDICATIONS FOR REFERRAL OR HOSPITALIZATION

Any patient with valvular heart disease requires cardiology referral and hospitalization for cardiac catheterization, balloon angioplasty, or surgical intervention when necessary. Patients with acute bacterial endocarditis require IV antibiotics. Hospitalization may also be required for the management of complications such as heart failure or pulmonary edema.

PATIENT AND FAMILY EDUCATION

Patients with valvular disorders, whether from a stenotic valve or regurgitant valve, require basic knowledge of their condition to prevent complications. The medication regimen should be explained and its importance reinforced at every visit. Because antibiotic prophylaxis is required before any instrumentation procedure, this should also be explained and its importance reinforced periodically (see Chapter 127).

REFERENCES

1. Leatham A: Auscultation of the heart, *Lancet* 2(7049-7050):703-708, 757-766, 1958.
2. Lembo NJ, Dell'Italia LJ, Crawford MH, and others: Bedside diagnosis of systolic murmurs, *N Engl J Med* 318:1572-1578, 1988.
3. Castle RF: The innocent heart murmur, *J Colorado Med Soc* 69:45-48, 1972.
4. Rackley CE, and others: Aortic valve disease. In Hurst JW, Schlant RC, Rackley CE and others, editors: *The heart,* New York, 1990, McGraw-Hill.
5. Alpert JS: Chronic aortic regurgitation. In Dalen JE, Alpert JS, editors: *Valvular heart disease,* Boston, 1986, Little, Brown.
6. O'Rourke RA, Walsh RA: Recognition and treatment of acute aortic regurgitation, *J Intens Care Med* 1:33-46, 1986.
7. Julius BK, Spillman M, Vassalli G, and others: Angina pectoris in patients with aortic stenosis and normal coronary arteries: mechanisms and pathophysiologic concepts, *Circulation* 95:892-898, 1997.
8. Gould KL: Why angina pectoris in aortic stenosis? *Circulation* 95:790-792, 1997.
9. Mark A: The Bezold-Jarisch reflex revisited: clinical implications of inhibitory reflexes originating in the heart, *J Am Coll Cardiol* 1(1):90-102, 1983.
10. Seltzer A: Changing aspects of the natural history of valvular aortic stenosis, *N Engl J Med* 317:91-98, 1987.
11. Ross J, Braunwald E: Aortic stenosis, *Circulation* 38(1 Suppl):61-67, 1968.
12. Spodick DH, Sugiura T, Doi Y, and others: Rate of rise of the carotid pulse: an investigation of observer error in a common clinical measurement, *Am J Cardiol* 49(1):159-162, 1982.
13. ACC/AHA guidelines for the management of patient with valvular heart disease: a report of the American College of Cardiology/American Heart Association Task Force on Practice Guidelines (Committee on Management of Patients with Valvular Heart Disease), *J Am Coll Cardiol* 32(5):1486-1588, 2006, retrieved June 29, 2006, from http://www.acc.org/clinical/guidelines/valvular/jac5929fla16.htm#C.
14. Brockmeir LB, Adolph RJ, Gustin BW, and others: Calcium emboli to the retinal artery in calcific aortic stenosis, *Am Heart J* 101:32-37, 1981.
15. Henry WL, Bonow RD, Borer JS, and others: Observations on the optimal time for operative intervention for aortic regurgitation, part I, Evaluation of the results of aortic valve replacement in symptomatic patients, *Circulation* 61:471-483, 1980.
16. Greenberg B, Massie B, Bristow JD, and others: Long-term vasodilator therapy of chronic aortic insufficiency: a randomized double-blind, placebo-controlled clinical trial, *Circulation* 789:92-103, 1988.
17. Scognamiglio R, Rahimtoola SH, Fasoli G, and others: Nifedipine in asymptomatic patients with severe aortic regurgitation and normal left ventricular function, *N Engl J Med* 331:689-694, 1994.
18. Bonow RO, Rosing DR, McIntosh SL, and others: The natural history of asymptomatic patients with aortic regurgitation and normal left ventricular function, *Circulation* 68(3):509-517, 1983.
19. Klodas E, Enriquez-Sarano M, Tajik AJ, and others: Optimizing timing

of surgical correction in patients with severe aortic regurgitation: role of symptoms, *J Am Coll Cardiol* 130:746-752, 1997.

20. Stone PH, Clark RD, Goldschlager N, and others: Determinants of prognosis of patients with aortic regurgitation who undergo aortic valve replacement, *J Am Coll Cardiol* 3(5):1118-1126, 1984.
21. Wisenbaugh T, Skudicky D, Sareli P: Prediction of outcome after valve replacement for rheumatic mitral regurgitation in the era of chordal preservation, *Circulation* 89:191-197, 1994.
22. Greenberg B, Massie BM, Brundage BH, and others: Beneficial effects of hydralazine in severe mitral regurgitation, *Circulation* 58:273-278, 1978.
23. Dujardin KS, Serano ME, Seward JB, and others: A prospective trial on the effects of losartan on the degree of mitral regurgitation, *Circulation* 94:1-468, 1997.
24. Crawford M, Souchek J, Oprian CA, and others: Determinants of survival and left ventricular performance after mitral valve replacement: Department of Veterans Affairs Cooperative Study on Valvular Heart Disease, *Circulation* 81:1173-1181, 1990.
25. Enriquez-Sarano M, Tajik AJ, Schaff HV, and others: Echocardiographic prediction of survival after surgical correction of organic mitral regurgitation, *Circulation* 90:830-837, 1994.
26. David T, Burns RJ, Bacchus CM, and others: Mitral valve replacement for mitral regurgitation with and without preservation of chordae tendineae, *J Thorac Cardiovasc Surg* 88:718-725, 1984.
27. Rosen SE, Borer JS, Hochreiter C, and others: The natural history of the asymptomatic/minimally symptomatic patient with severe mitral regurgitation secondary to mitral valve prolapse and normal right and left ventricular performance, *Am J Cardiol* 74:374-380, 1994.
28. Devereux RB, Kramer-Fox R, Kligfield P: Mitral valve prolapse: causes, clinical manifestations, and management, *Ann Intern Med* 111:305-317, 1989.
29. Weissman NJ, Shear MK, Kramer-Fox R, and others: Contrasting patterns of autonomic dysfunction in patients with mitral valve prolapse and panic attacks, *Am J Med* 82:880-888, 1987.
30. Markiewicz W, Stoner J, London E, and others: Mitral valve prolapse in 100 presumably healthy young females, *Circulation* 53:464-473, 1976.
31. Marks AR, Choong CY, Sanfilippo AJ, and others: Identification of high risk and low risk subgroups of patients with mitral valve prolapse, *N Engl J Med* 320:1031-1036, 1989.
32. Mills P, Rose J, Hollingsworth J, and others: Long term prognosis of mitral valve prolapse, *N Engl J Med* 297:13-18, 1977.
33. Wilkins GT, Weyman AE, Abascal VM, and others: Percutaneous balloon dilatation of the mitral valve: an analysis of echocardiographic variables related to outcome and the mechanism of dilatation, *Br Heart J* 60:299-308, 1988.
34. Siegel R, Tresch DD, Keelan MH, and others: Effects of anticoagulation on recurrent systemic emboli in mitral stenosis, *Am J Cardiol* 60:1191-1192, 1987.
35. Ben Farhat MB, Ayara M, Maatouk F, and others: Percutaneous balloon versus surgical closed and open mitral commissurotomy: 7-year follow-up results of a randomized trial, *Circulation* 97:245-250, 1998.
36. Braunwald E, Braunwald NS, Ross J, and others: Effects of mitral-valve replacement on the pulmonary vascular dynamic of patients with pulmonary hypertension, *N Engl J Med* 273:509-514, 1965.

PART 12

Evaluation and Management of Gastrointestinal Disorders

TERRY MAHAN BUTTARO, *Section Editor*

CHAPTER 135

Abdominal Pain and Infections

Updated by Terry Mahan Buttaro

Whether in emergency departments or in primary care, abdominal pain is a common complaint.[1] The causes of abdominal pain are myriad, and often the patient's description of the pain is vague. Chronic abdominal pain may be intermittent or constant, organic or functional. In a previously well patient, the acute onset of severe abdominal pain for more than 6 hours usually indicates a condition requiring surgical evaluation and intervention.[2]

Frequently, the patient's description of the pain suggests the pathologic condition. With ulceration, pain is described as burning or gnawing. Hollow tube obstruction (bowel, biliary tree, ureters) has an intermittent colicky or wavelike quality, whereas the pain of peritoneal irritation is steady and increases with coughing, palpation, or movement. With metabolic disturbances or altered bowel motility, the pain may be crampy, and the distribution can be localized or generalized. In women, cyclical abdominal pain may be related to the menstrual cycle or have a gynecologic basis.[3] Vascular insufficiency is evidenced by a crampy discomfort or pain that occurs primarily in the midabdominal region but is related to meals (abdominal angina). Thrombosis produces a more progressive and severe pain. The pain associated with distention of an encapsulated structure (liver, kidney, spleen, ovary) is constant and aching. Nerve irritation can be severe and has a dermatome distribution. A dissecting aneurysm usually produces pain that is described as tearing.[2]

The location of pain may also suggest the source of the patient's discomfort. Pain localized to the right upper abdominal quadrant generally emanates from the chest cavity, liver, gallbladder, stomach, bowel, or right kidney or ureter. The most common diagnoses of pain in this area are cholecystitis and leaking duodenal ulcer.[2] Left upper quadrant pain is usually associated with the heart or chest cavity, spleen, stomach, pancreas (especially acute pancreatitis), left kidney, or ureter.[2] The source of left lower abdominal pain can include the bowel, left ureter, or pelvis and is most commonly associated with diverticulitis.[2] Right lower quadrant pain is associated with the appendix, bowel, right ureter, or pelvis, with the most common diagnosis being appendicitis. Cholecystitis or peptic ulcer perforation also must be considered.[3] Pain that migrates across several quadrants is typically associated with the bowel, whereas abdominal wall pain from trauma or inflammation can occur in any quadrant.

Abdominal pain can be subtle and the diagnosis obscure, particularly in older adults.[4] The older patient is less likely to mount a fever or pain response than is a young patient but is more likely to exhibit lethargy or mental status changes. In women of childbearing age, even those with a history of tubal ligation, it is imperative to exclude the possibility of ectopic pregnancy.

With acute abdominal pain, an accurate diagnosis is highly dependent on history, physical examination, and appropriate laboratory and radiologic procedures. Allergies, medication history (including over-the-counter drugs, vitamins, and supplements), surgical history, social and sexual history, last menstrual period, dietary history, last food or fluid ingested, and family history of abdominal pain are important considerations that should be elicited. Diseases that may cause acute abdominal pain include appendicitis, cholecystitis, diverticulitis, small bowel obstruction, perforated peptic ulcer, peritonitis, ruptured ectopic pregnancy, ruptured abdominal aortic aneurysm, hypercalcemia, superior mesenteric artery syndrome, and acute intermittent porphyria.[3] In female patients, it is important to obtain a sexual history and consider pelvic inflammatory disease. (Cholecystitis, diverticulitis, and ectopic pregnancy are discussed in Chapters 137, 141, and 171.) It is also essential to remember that acute diseases of the chest—including myocardial infarction, congestive heart failure, pulmonary infarction, and pneumonia—may mimic primary diseases of the abdomen.

Physician consultation is indicated for suspected gastrointestinal bleeding, bowel obstruction, postural vital sign changes, abnormal findings, jaundice, a positive pregnancy test, severe localized or unilateral lower abdominal pain, or a history of trauma.

APPENDICITIS

DEFINITION AND EPIDEMIOLOGY

Acute appendicitis is an inflammatory disease of the wall of the appendix that may result in perforation with subsequent peritonitis. In the United States, appendicitis occurs in approximately 7% of the population, but in other countries the incidence is lower and presumed to be related to increased dietary fiber.[5] This disorder is a common reason for emergency surgery, and the diagnosis is primarily based on the history and physical examination.

PATHOPHYSIOLOGY

Acute appendicitis is classified as simple, gangrenous, or perforated on the basis of operative findings. In simple appendicitis the appendix is viable and intact. Gangrenous appendicitis is characterized by necrosis of the appendiceal wall. Perforated appendicitis refers to disruption of the appendix. Acute appendicitis is thought to be secondary to obstruction of its orifice, with secondary bacterial infection.[6,7] Sixty percent of patients with appendicitis demonstrate lymphoid hyperplasia on pathologic examination. Lymphoid hyperplasia occurs most commonly after periods of dehydration and viral infection and is most common in the young. This may account for the increased incidence of appendicitis in younger populations.[8] One third of patients demonstrate a mechanical obstruction with solid fecal material.[6,8] Other causes of luminal obstruction include tumors, parasites, foreign bodies, and bacterial or viral agents.[6,7]

When the appendiceal lumen becomes obstructed, the mucosa continues to secrete fluid until the intraluminal pressure exceeds venous pressure. At this point, the appendix becomes hypoxic, the mucosa ulcerates, and bacteria invade the wall. Infection causes additional swelling and ischemia as a result of thrombosis of small intramural vessels. Gangrene and perforation usually develop in 24 to 36 hours. Perforation leads to a release of the luminal contents into the peritoneal cavity.

CLINICAL PRESENTATION

The most reliable historical feature in the diagnosis of acute appendicitis is the sequence of symptoms. Pain that starts in the epigastrium or periumbilical area, then localizes in the right lower quadrant is usually the initial symptom. The pain can be diffuse or occur at other sites in the abdomen, including the left lower quadrant.[1] The initial pain is described as colicky and not severe, but it reaches its peak in approximately 4 hours. The pain gradually subsides but reappears in the right lower quadrant, progressing to a severe ache that is exacerbated by movement. The exact location of pain may be variable and, though unusual, includes left lower quadrant pain. (This is due to the variable location of the diseased appendix: ascending, iliac, or pelvic.[2])

Anorexia, nausea or vomiting, constipation, or rarely diarrhea accompanied by low-grade fever follows the onset of pain. Not all patients will have every symptom; however, when the symptoms occur in any other order, the diagnosis of appendicitis should be questioned.

PHYSICAL EXAMINATION

The diagnosis of acute appendicitis requires a careful history and a thorough physical examination (including a pelvic examination for female patients). Usually a low-grade fever is present. Abdominal tenderness is elicited by asking the patient to cough. Localized tenderness is a valuable physical finding, and the patient can often specify the painful spot with one finger. By systematically palpating the abdomen with one finger, the practitioner confirms localized tenderness, usually in the right lower quadrant between the umbilicus and the anterosuperior iliac spine (McBurney's point). There may be signs of peritoneal irritation, including guarding, rebound tenderness, and obturator and psoas signs. The psoas sign is elicited by asking the supine patient to raise the straightened right leg against resistance by the practitioner. The obturator sign is elicited by passive rotation of the right leg with the patient supine and the right hip and knee flexed. A rectal examination may reveal tenderness or a mass.

DIAGNOSTICS

Most experts agree that the diagnosis of acute appendicitis is suggested by the history and physical examination. In fact, the rate of normal or perforated appendices at surgery has not changed since the addition of ultrasound or CT to the evaluation of suspected appendicitis, underscoring the importance of a careful clinical history and physical examination.[9] The health care provider should immediately refer a patient with suspected appendicitis for surgical consultation. Laboratory data in support of appendicitis include a WBC count that ranges from 10,000 to 16,000 cells/mm^3. A serum β-human chorionic gonadotropin (β-HCG) level should be obtained in women of childbearing age to assist in excluding a ruptured ectopic pregnancy. A normal C-reactive protein level in patients with abdominal pain for more than 24 hours suggests that the cause of the pain is not appendicitis. This finding is even more significant if the white blood cell count is normal and the neutrophil count is less than 75%.[5,10]

Imaging studies are not required in most cases of suspected appendicitis. However, imaging modalities may be necessary if the presentation is atypical or in patients at the extremes of age. Plain abdominal radiographs show nonspecific signs and are no longer recommended. Barium enema x-ray studies are safe and are thought to exclude a diagnosis of appendicitis if the appendix fills with barium. However, failure of the appendix to fill with barium does not necessarily indicate acute appendicitis; therefore other imaging modalities are generally used.

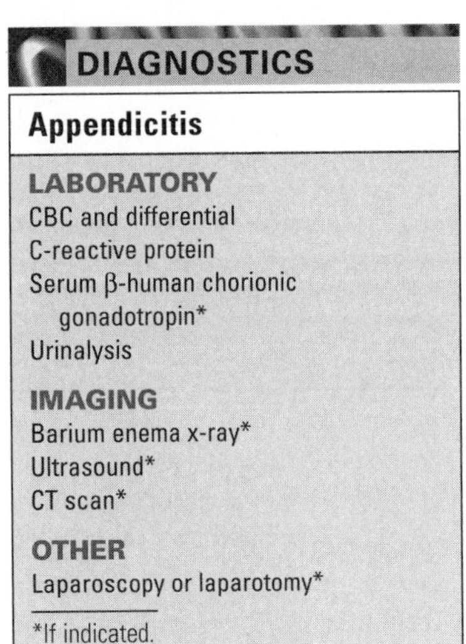

DIAGNOSTICS

Appendicitis

LABORATORY
CBC and differential
C-reactive protein
Serum β-human chorionic gonadotropin*
Urinalysis

IMAGING
Barium enema x-ray*
Ultrasound*
CT scan*

OTHER
Laparoscopy or laparotomy*

*If indicated.

Ultrasonographic evidence of appendicitis includes appendiceal wall thickening, luminal distention, and lack of compressibility.[5,11] Its usefulness is strictly limited by operator skill and interpretation. If the ultrasound is negative, clinical findings of acute appendicitis require intervention by laparoscopy or laparotomy. A CT scan is not usually justified in routine acute appendicitis unless the ultrasound is found to be normal or reliable ultrasound is not available.[8] CT is reliable in differentiating a periappendiceal phlegmon from an abscess.[7,12]

DIFFERENTIAL DIAGNOSIS

Other conditions that may mimic acute appendicitis include gastroenteritis, mesenteric lymphadenitis, acute salpingitis, mittelschmerz, ruptured ectopic pregnancy, ureteral colic, Meckel's diverticulitis, sigmoid diverticulitis, perforated peptic ulcer, cholecystitis, intestinal obstruction, cecal diverticulitis, intestinal ischemia, and perforated colonic carcinoma. Basilar pneumonia may also be confused with appendicitis.

MANAGEMENT

With appendicitis, a prompt appendectomy, preferably within 24 hours of symptom onset, is essential to prevent perforation and peritonitis.[2] Little preparation for surgery is required, but patients should have nothing by mouth. Intravenous fluid and electrolyte repletion is necessary. Older patients should be evaluated and treated for systemic disease. Perioperative systemic antibiotics such as metronidazole and ceftizoxime have been shown to prevent wound infection in simple appendicitis. If the appendix is perforated, triple antibiotic therapy with ampicillin, gentamicin, and clindamycin or monotherapy

DIFFERENTIAL DIAGNOSIS

Appendicitis

- Gastroenteritis
- Mesenteric lymphadenitis
- Acute salpingitis
- Mittelschmerz
- Ruptured ectopic pregnancy
- Ureteral colic
- Meckel's diverticulitis
- Sigmoid diverticulitis
- Perforated peptic ulcer
- Cholecystitis
- Intestinal obstruction
- Cecal diverticulitis
- Perforated colonic carcinoma
- Basilar pneumonia
- Pyelonephritis
- Intestinal obstruction
- Ureteral calculus
- Salpingitis, pelvic inflammatory disease
- Ruptured corpus luteum cyst
- Endometriosis
- Regional enteritis (Crohn's disease)

with a second-generation cephalosporin such as cefotetan is essential, as is fluid resuscitation with crystalloids followed by prompt appendectomy.[7,12] Antibiotics are also indicated for patients with suspected septicemia and patients scheduled for laparoscopic surgery.[5] Surgery for an appendiceal abscess may spread a localized infection to other parts of the peritoneal cavity; therefore percutaneous CT-guided drainage of an abscess is used to allow the acute inflammation to resolve before proceeding with elective appendectomy in 6 weeks to 3 months.[7]

COMPLICATIONS

Complications of appendicitis include gangrene, perforation with peritonitis, and abscess formation. Pylephlebitis, which is septic thrombophlebitis of the portal venous system, should be suspected in any patient with appendicitis who has shaking chills. Septicemia, urinary retention and infection, small bowel obstruction, and mesenteric thrombophlebitis may also occur. Common complications associated with appendectomy include wound infection, pneumonia, intraperitoneal abscesses, enterocutaneous fistulas, wound or inguinal hernias, and possibly minor bleeding.

INDICATIONS FOR REFERRAL OR HOSPITALIZATION

Immediate surgical referral or a transfer to the emergency department is indicated for suspected appendicitis or other acute abdominal pain. Hospitalization is indicated for monitoring and surgical care, if necessary.

PATIENT AND FAMILY EDUCATION

Abdominal pain may be a sign of serious illness or may be related to a chronic disorder. Patients should understand that localized abdominal pain or pain that increases in severity warrants discussion with the health care provider. Patients must also understand that abdominal pain accompanied by fever, chills, severe vomiting or diarrhea, significant rectal bleeding, black and tarry stools, weakness, or dizziness requires a visit to the health care provider. Families of older patients should understand that pain perception may be diminished; the associated delay in presentation results in more than 30% of older adults with appendicitis having perforation at presentation.[8] In older adults, any of the previously listed symptoms, even if unaccompanied by abdominal pain, should be evaluated by a medical professional.

SMALL BOWEL OBSTRUCTION

DEFINITION AND EPIDEMIOLOGY

Small bowel obstruction, a common cause of acute abdominal pain, is caused by a mechanical occlusion of the bowel lumen or paralysis (ileus) of the intestinal musculature.[13] As a result, fluid and gas accumulate proximal to the obstruction, causing nausea, vomiting, abdominal distention, and pain. It is essential to recognize bowel obstruction because it can cause vascular compromise, bowel ischemia, and peritonitis. Adhesions, hernias, and tumors are the most common causes of small bowel obstruction, although other conditions, such as fecal impaction, ischemia, abscesses, inflammatory bowel disease, volvulus, intussusception, strictures, and radiation enteritis, can also be responsible. Ileus is associated with trauma, a significant operative procedure, high-dose or frequent narcotic use, or an electrolyte abnormality.

PATHOPHYSIOLOGY

In a bowel obstruction, distention results in decreased absorption and increased secretions that cause further distention and fluid and electrolyte imbalances. Bacterial proliferation may occur as a result of stasis. Distention increases the risk of bowel perforation and diffuse peritonitis. Mechanical obstruction of the bowel lumen may occur from lesions (e.g., congenital, inflammatory, or neoplastic), polypoid tumors, intussusception, volvulus, gallstone ileus, impacted feces, or bezoar formation. Intussusception, often recognized as an abdominal mass on examination with a history of acute symptom onset, occurs when a bowel segment telescopes into the adjacent bowel, resulting in symptoms of intermittent bowel obstruction. Volvulus results from abnormal twisting of a bowel segment along its mesenteric axis.

CLINICAL PRESENTATION

Bowel obstruction manifests with intermittent and crampy abdominal pain, vomiting, obstipation, abdominal distention, and fever. The pain is usually relieved by vomiting, intestinal tube decompression, or the passage of intestinal contents through a partial obstruction. Pain that progresses in severity, localizes, or becomes constant demonstrates progression to a strangulated obstruction; this condition requires urgent surgery. Particular attention should be placed on the chronicle of the illness, the patient's medication history, last bowel movement, and presence of flatus. A prior history of bowel obstructions, abdominal irradiation, abdominal inflammation or cancer, or abdominal or pelvic operations should be identified, since these conditions are all associated with bowel obstructions.[13]

PHYSICAL EXAMINATION

Vital signs, including postural signs when possible, should be assessed. The presence of fever suggests an infectious process. Tachycardia and hypotension, when associated with a bowel obstruction, tend to be late symptoms and depend on the degree of hypovolemia that results from persistent vomiting or from toxemia caused by intestinal gangrene.[14]

A thorough physical examination is necessary to determine whether the patient's symptoms are related to a nonabdominal process (e.g., pneumonia, myocardial infarction).[13] The abdominal examination reveals a distended, tympanic abdomen. Peristaltic rushes and high-pitched tinkling sounds may be auscultated over the abdomen, although bowel sounds may be absent as the disorder progresses. Diffuse midabdominal tenderness is common; localized tenderness, abdominal guarding, rebound tenderness, and rigidity are concerning signs. The rectal examination may reveal stool, masses, tenderness, or occult blood. Particular attention needs to be placed on examination of potential hernial orifices, especially the area of the femoral ring because of its small opening and potential for bowel strangulation.[2]

DIAGNOSTICS

The radiographic evaluation should include upright and supine x-ray films of the abdomen and the upright chest. The upright abdominal film identifies a distended bowel proximal to the obstruction in addition to air-fluid levels. It may show free air if perforation has occurred. The supine radiograph may distinguish between ileus and obstruction. With an ileus the radiograph will show distended loops in both the large and small bowel; with an obstruction the segment proximal to the obstruction is distended, and the distal bowel loops are decreased in caliber.[14] The patient should also be evaluated for intraperitoneal masses; ascites; gallstones; renal calculi; foreign bodies; and gas within the bowel wall, portal venous system, or biliary tree.[14]

DIAGNOSTICS

Small Bowel Obstruction

LABORATORY

CBC and differential
Serum electrolytes, BUN, creatinine
Magnesium, calcium, TSH*
Serum β-human chorionic gonadotropin (in women of childbearing age)

IMAGING

Abdominal x-rays (upright and supine)*
Chest x-ray*
CT scan*
MRI*
Transabdominal ultrasound*

*If indicated.

Studies suggest that CT scanning after the administration of oral and IV contrast media may be the technique of choice in locating and identifying intestinal obstruction in the nonacute setting.[15] CT scanning is both specific and sensitive in diagnosing a bowel obstruction, but the MRI may be even more sensitive, and an MRI or transabdominal ultrasound can also identify small bowel obstruction without the use of contrast media.[16]

Other diagnostic studies include sigmoidoscopy if a rectal or distal sigmoid obstruction is suspected.[13] Contrast radiography (e.g., an upper gastrointestinal study, small bowel study, and barium enema) can be helpful in intermittent or suspected partial small bowel obstruction.

Laboratory data usually reflect a progressively increasing WBC count and electrolyte abnormalities. A thyroid-stimulating hormone, calcium, and magnesium level may be indicated if an ileus is suspected. Serum β-HCG should be measured to exclude pregnancy in women of childbearing age.

DIFFERENTIAL DIAGNOSIS

The differential diagnosis of small bowel obstruction includes gastroenteritis, paralytic ileus, intestinal perforation, ischemic colitis, idiopathic inflammatory bowel disease, mesenteric thrombosis, and retroperitoneal hemorrhage. Addison's disease, poisoning, diabetes mellitus, and tertiary syphilis may also mimic small bowel obstruction.

MANAGEMENT

Immediate hospitalization is required for the treatment of suspected bowel obstruction, and consultation with a surgeon is essential. Initial management of bowel obstruction includes restriction of all oral intakes, IV fluid therapy, electrolyte and acid-base correction, optimization of cardiopulmonary and renal function, and nasogastric decompression. Urgent laparotomy is required if the patient does not respond to supportive care or has advanced illness, ischemia, or perforation.[14] Otherwise, patients can be observed with serial physical examinations and radiographs. Patients with fecal impaction require disimpaction.[13] Antibiotic therapy is usually not indicated. However, broad-spectrum IV antibiotics are indicated in cases of strangulated bowel or as an adjunct to surgery.

COMPLICATIONS

A bowel obstruction may progress to bowel ischemia. Physical and diagnostic signs of ischemic bowel include fever, severe and continuous pain, hematemesis, peritoneal signs, hypotension, gas in the bowel wall or portal vein, abdominal free air, and acidosis.

DIFFERENTIAL DIAGNOSIS

Small Bowel Obstruction

- Gastroenteritis
- Paralytic ileus
- Intestinal perforation
- Ischemic colitis
- Idiopathic inflammatory bowel disease
- Mesenteric thrombosis
- Retroperitoneal hemorrhage
- Addison's disease
- Poisoning
- Diabetes mellitus
- Tertiary syphilis
- Neoplasm

INDICATIONS FOR REFERRAL OR HOSPITALIZATION AND PATIENT AND FAMILY EDUCATION

See Indications for Referral or Hospitalization and Patient and Family Education under Appendicitis, p. 626.

PERFORATED PEPTIC ULCER

DEFINITION AND EPIDEMIOLOGY

Peptic ulcer perforation is a life-threatening complication of peptic ulcer disease and is more common with duodenal ulcers than with gastric ulcers. Perforation may lead to a free perforation into the peritoneal cavity or perforation of an adjacent organ such as the pancreas, with resulting peritonitis or pancreatitis. Factors that predispose a patient to peptic ulcers are *Helicobacter pylori* infections, NSAIDs, tobacco abuse, and hypersecretory states such as Zöllinger-Ellison syndrome. Despite the advent of proton pump inhibitors and treatment modalities for *Helicobacter* infection, perforated peptic ulcers remain a significant cause of mortality.[17] The overall mortality rate for perforated gastric ulcers is approximately 10%.[6]

PATHOPHYSIOLOGY

Peptic ulcer perforations can be classified as (1) those in which the luminal contents freely escape into the peritoneal cavity, and (2) those in which the penetration is sealed by surrounding structures of peritoneum.[6] Because the anterior walls of the stomach and duodenum are not defended by contiguous tissue, ulcers in these locations are more likely to be complicated by free perforation, which leads to generalized peritonitis and the accumulation of air in the abdominal cavity.[6] Posterior gastric ulcers perforate into the lesser peritoneal sac, where the inflammatory reaction may be contained and form an intraabdominal abscess. Ulcers may also penetrate into the pancreas, liver, or greater omentum and cause intractable symptoms.

CLINICAL PRESENTATION

The most common presentation of a perforated peptic ulcer is the abrupt onset of severe abdominal pain followed rapidly by peritoneal signs. Pain begins in the epigastrium and spreads rapidly throughout the abdomen with frequent early radiation of pain to the scapular areas. Vomiting of coffee ground emesis, hematemesis, and/or melena or hematochezia occurs in some patients. The abruptness, severity, and rapid progression of symptoms lead the patient to seek prompt medical attention. Clinically, patients often demonstrate signs of improvement such as decreased pain and vomiting 6 to 12 hours after perforation. However, peritoneal signs remain, and the clinical improvement does not last long. By about 12 hours, the patient appears seriously ill, usually grunting with shallow respirations and the knees drawn up to the chest.

PHYSICAL EXAMINATION

In some patients, especially older adults, the pain may be absent or slight. Usually, the patient complains of severe upper abdominal tenderness, especially in the epigastric region. The pain is accompanied by boardlike rigidity of the abdomen. If it has been less than 24 hours since the perforation, a low-grade fever and tachycardia are often present, but hypotension is unusual.[12] Continued spilling of gastric and intestinal contents into the peritoneum causes chemical peritonitis and subsequent hypovolemia with the development of progressive hypotension and fever. Bowel sounds are absent in most cases.

DIAGNOSTICS

Perforation is suggested by the history and physical examination. The suspected diagnosis is confirmed by the detection of pneumoperitoneum on upright abdominal or chest x-ray films. If a pneumoperitoneum is absent, a water-soluble contrast examination may be used to demonstrate perforation.[12] A left lateral decubitus radiograph usually demonstrates air over the liver. When the diagnosis is suspected and the x-ray studies are negative, the diagnosis may be confirmed by endoscopy. Laboratory tests include a CBC with differential, serum electrolytes, BUN, creatinine, and serum amylase. A serum HCG is necessary for women of childbearing age.

DIAGNOSTICS

Perforated Peptic Ulcer

LABORATORY
CBC and differential
Serum electrolytes, BUN, creatinine
Serum amylase
Stool for occult blood
Type and crossmatch
Serum β-human chorionic gonadotropin (in women of childbearing age)

IMAGING
Abdominal x-ray (upright, left lateral decubitus)

OTHER
Endoscopy

DIFFERENTIAL DIAGNOSIS

The differential diagnoses of a perforated peptic ulcer include acute pancreatitis, acute cholecystitis, perforated acute appendicitis, colonic diverticulitis, intestinal obstruction, ruptured ectopic pregnancy, and postemetic esophageal rupture. Myocardial infarction may also mimic a perforated peptic ulcer.

MANAGEMENT

Immediate hospitalization and consultation with a surgeon are essential. Treatment of a perforate peptic ulcer is surgical in 95% of patients.[18] Management includes IV fluid resuscitation, correction of electrolyte abnormalities, and continuous nasogastric suction.[19] IV broad-spectrum antibiotics are also required. Blood transfusions may be necessary in the presence of hemorrhage. Early suspicion, recognition, and surgical repair are the keys to survival and decreased morbidity.

DIFFERENTIAL DIAGNOSIS

Perforated Peptic Ulcer

- Acute pancreatitis
- Acute cholecystitis
- Perforated appendix
- Colonic diverticulitis
- Myocardial infarction
- Intestinal obstruction
- Perforated colon

COMPLICATIONS

Despite the widespread use of H_2-blockers and proton pump inhibitors, the mortality rate of patients with perforated peptic ulcers continues to be significant, especially in older patients.[20] Vitamin deficiencies and dumping syndrome are possible surgical complications.[20]

INDICATIONS FOR REFERRAL OR HOSPITALIZATION AND PATIENT AND FAMILY EDUCATION

See Indications for Referral or Hospitalization and Patient and Family Education under Appendicitis, p. 626.

PERITONITIS

DEFINITION AND EPIDEMIOLOGY

Primary spontaneous bacterial peritonitis refers to a peritoneal infection in the absence of a clear precipitating factor such as a perforated viscus. The most common cause of spontaneous bacterial peritonitis in adults is cirrhosis complicated by portal hypertension and ascites.[6] *Secondary peritonitis* refers to spillage of gastrointestinal or genitourinary microorganisms into the peritoneal space. Secondary peritonitis is most commonly a result of pancreatitis, appendicitis, diverticulitis, cholecystitis, peritoneal dialysis, penetrating wounds of the bowel, or perforation of a gastric or duodenal ulcer.[21] In these instances a secondary infection may occur as either generalized peritonitis or localized abscesses.[22]

PATHOPHYSIOLOGY

Primary peritonitis is thought to result from a hematogenous and lymphogenous spread of bacteria through an intact gut wall from the intestinal lumen. The gut wall is thought to be more permeable to bacterial translocation because of wall edema from portal hypertension. In patients with cirrhosis, microorganisms removed from circulation by the liver may not be properly phagocytized by impaired liver macrophages and thus contaminate hepatic lymph and pass into the ascitic fluid. Portosystemic shunting also diminishes hepatic clearance of microorganisms, which perpetuates bacteremia and increases the potential for ascitic fluid infection.[20] Enteric microorganisms account for the majority of pathogens in patients with cirrhosis. *Escherichia coli* is the most commonly identified pathogen, followed by *Streptococcal pneumoniae; Klebsiella pneumoniae;* and other streptococcal species, including enterococci. Other organisms responsible for primary peritonitis may include *Neisseria gonorrhoeae, Chlamydia trachomatis, Mycobacterium tuberculosis,* and *Coccidioides immitis. Bacteroides fragilis* and *E. coli* are most commonly found when gastrointestinal perforation is the precipitating event.[22] Primary bacterial peritonitis is almost exclusively monomicrobial; if multiple organisms are identified, the diagnosis should be questioned and other sources for infection sought, such as perforated viscus.[22]

CLINICAL PRESENTATION

Many patients have a high fever and acute abdominal pain that can be diffuse, localized, or referred. In patients with cirrhosis, a temperature greater than 37.7° C (100° F) may be the only manifestation of peritoneal infection.[21] Additional complaints include diffuse abdominal pain, tenderness, nausea, vomiting, and diarrhea or constipation.

PHYSICAL EXAMINATION

With peritonitis, the physical examination may reveal abdominal distention, rigidity, diffuse abdominal tenderness, decreased bowel sounds, rebound tenderness, and guarding. Fever, tachycardia, tachypnea, and hypotension may also be present. Rectal examination may reveal tenderness if abscesses occur near this area.

DIAGNOSTICS

The diagnosis of peritonitis should be suspected on the basis of fever, abdominal pain and tenderness, and leukocytosis. Initially, a chest and abdominal x-ray study, CBC and differential, and serum electrolytes with a BUN and creatinine may be obtained in the primary care setting. Suspected peritonitis, especially that accompanied by decreasing bowel sounds, increasing tenderness, and rebound tenderness, warrants a laparotomy to confirm the diagnosis. Hospitalization and consultation with an internist, gastroenterologist, and surgeon are therefore required.

Patients with cirrhosis and spontaneous bacterial peritonitis should be diagnosed on the basis of the clinical appearance, presence of ascites, and ascitic fluid analysis, not a laparotomy.[23] Patients with ascites should undergo paracentesis in the hospital setting with peritoneal fluid analysis for cell count, differential, protein concentration, and a Gram stain and culture.[22] The diagnosis of primary bacterial peritonitis requires more than 250 to 500 white blood cells (WBCs) per cubic millimeter in the ascitic fluid, with more than 50% of them being polymorphonuclear neutrophils.[24] More than 500 WBCs per cubic millimeter indicates possible perforated viscus.[24] The ascitic fluid analysis will typically show a low protein concentration, pH of less than 7.35, and a lactate concentration of greater than 25 mg/dl.[22] In primary bacterial peritonitis, 30% to 50% of ascites fluid cultures are negative.[24] When a suspected intraabdominal abscess is present, CT- or ultrasound-guided aspiration is standard practice.[22]

DIAGNOSTICS

Peritonitis

LABORATORY
- CBC and differential
- Serum electrolytes
- BUN, creatinine
- Ascitic fluid analysis*
- Serum β-human chorionic gonadotropin (in women of childbearing age)

OTHER
- Chest x-ray
- KUB
- Laparotomy or endoscopy*
- Biopsy*
- CT scan
- Ultrasound-guided aspiration

*If indicated.

DIFFERENTIAL DIAGNOSIS

Diseases that may mimic peritonitis include pancreatitis, appendicitis, diverticulitis, gastroenteritis, salpingitis, and ischemic colitis. Secondary causes of peritonitis should also be considered, including perforated duodenal ulcer, perforated gastric ulcer, small bowel infarction or perforation, appendicitis,

DIFFERENTIAL DIAGNOSIS

Peritonitis

- Pancreatitis
- Appendicitis
- Diverticulitis
- Gastroenteritis
- Salpingitis
- Ischemic colitis
- Perforated duodenal ulcer
- Perforated gastric ulcer
- Small or large bowel perforation
- Cholecystitis
- Ruptured ectopic pregnancy
- Acute granulomatous peritonitis
- Chylous ascites
- Mesenteric lipodystrophy

large bowel perforation, and cholecystitis with or without perforation or pericholecystic abscess.

MANAGEMENT

With primary bacterial peritonitis, the peritoneal fluid Gram stain is often negative; therefore antibiotic therapy is usually empiric and is based on the most likely pathogens.[21] Cefotaxime 1 to 2 g IV q 6-8 hr or 500 to 1000 mg IV q 12 hr is proven treatment.[25] Third-generation cephalosporin antibiotics and the combination of ampicillin and an aminoglycoside have also proved to be effective.[22,26] Alternative antibiotic therapies include broad-spectrum penicillins, carbapenems, and β-lactam antibiotics combined with β-lactamase inhibitors.[22] Usual duration for therapy ranges from 3 to 7 days, but a recent meta-analysis of therapies has not shown a particular antibiotic or length of treatment to be most beneficial.[25,27] Antimicrobial therapy should be continued for cases in which peritoneal cultures are sterile but there is a strong suspicion of primary bacterial peritonitis.[22] Clinical improvement and a decline in the ascitic fluid leukocyte count (<250/mm^3) should occur after 24 to 48 hours of antimicrobial therapy; a failure to respond to therapy should prompt suspicion for other pathologic conditions. Fluid resuscitation, a nasogastric tube, and careful monitoring of vital signs and fluid balance are essential.

Preventive treatment in patients with cirrhotic ascites is recommended to reduce the incidence of spontaneous bacterial peritonitis. Oral norfloxacin 400 mg/day, ciprofloxacin once weekly, or double-strength trimethoprim-sulfamethoxazole administered daily for 5 days each week has been shown to reduce the incidence of peritonitis in these patients.[21,24,27] This reduction in rate of primary peritonitis does not change the mortality rate for cirrhotic patients, which is related to their underlying hepatic dysfunction.[22] Treatment of secondary peritonitis includes the use of appropriate antimicrobial therapy and surgical management as necessary.

COMPLICATIONS

Primary peritonitis is an ominous sign in the cirrhotic patient. After the first episode, only one third of patients will survive 1 year, and of these, one half will have a recurrence of peritonitis with a mortality rate of 50%.[28] These patients also have a high rate of umbilical and other abdominal wall hernias that can eventually lead to strangulation of contents and secondary peritonitis.

Nosocomial infections are common among patients with intraabdominal infections. Multiorgan failure occurs as a result of sepsis from intraabdominal infections and is the major cause of death in patients with intraabdominal infection.[29]

INDICATIONS FOR REFERRAL OR HOSPITALIZATION AND PATIENT AND FAMILY EDUCATION

See Indications for Referral or Hospitalization and Patient and Family Education under Appendicitis, p. 626.

RUPTURED AORTIC ANEURYSM

DEFINITION AND EPIDEMIOLOGY

An abdominal aortic aneurysm (AAA) is an abnormal dilation of the abdominal aorta that may rupture and cause exsanguination into the peritoneum. Fifty percent of patients with a ruptured AAA die before reaching a treatment facility, and 24% of those who do reach a facility die before reaching an operating room for attempted repair.[30] Most AAAs are atherosclerotic in origin; the remainder are caused by trauma, vasculitis, syphilis, or other infections.[31] Risk factors for AAA include atherosclerosis, hypertension, peripheral vascular disease, smoking (8:1 increased risk), male gender (4:1 increased risk), and advancing age.[8,32] AAA is a relatively common condition (30 to 66 per 1000 persons) and is increasing as the population ages.[30]

PATHOPHYSIOLOGY

The pathogenesis of most dissecting AAAs is atherosclerosis; the common underlying defect is vessel wall weakness secondary to a loss of elastin and collagen tissue in the aorta. The focal loss of elastic and muscle fibers in the media leads to cystic spaces filled with a metachromatic myxoid material. Weakening and replacement of elastin and collagen over time lead to increased aneurysm diameter and length. The initial event triggering the medial dissection is controversial, but more than 95% of cases show a transverse tear in the intima and internal media, and many postulate that a spontaneous laceration of the intima allows blood from the lumen to enter and dissect the media.[33] Alternatively, it has been postulated that a hemorrhage from the vasa vasorum into the media (which has been weakened by cystic medial necrosis) initiates stress on the intima, which leads to the intimal tear.[33]

CLINICAL PRESENTATION

A patient may be seen with a throbbing, aching back pain that can precede actual rupture. Conversely, a patient may come in for care days after a contained rupture.[2] In the majority of cases, however, the rupture of an AAA is accompanied by the sudden onset of severe abdominal pain that may be confined to the flank, low back, or groin with radiation to the back that brings the patients in urgently. Symptoms occur in this distribution because most AAAs rupture posterolaterally into the retroperitoneum.[30] Pain may worsen in the recumbent position and is relieved by sitting up or leaning forward. Faintness and syncope may occur as a result of blood loss and gradually worsen until shock finally supervenes.[12] It is not uncommon for a patient with a ruptured AAA to be initially seen with a chief complaint of angina from unrecognized blood loss that may actually delay full evaluation and definitive treatment.[2]

PHYSICAL EXAMINATION

During dissection, a pulsatile, painful mass can be palpated in the abdomen between the xiphoid process and the umbilicus. In AAAs the pulsations are felt directly over the mass and displace the examining fingers laterally. An aortic bruit may be present. Peripheral pulses may be unequal or absent but can be normal. Profound shock may rapidly ensue as a result of intraperitoneal leakage of blood.

DIAGNOSTICS

Additional diagnostic tests are not required if a ruptured AAA is suspected. The patient should be hospitalized immediately, with resuscitation and therapy in the operating room. If the diagnosis of rupture is in doubt and time allows, a CT scan is the standard for evaluation of an AAA because it can determine the extent of the aneurysmal process. Angiography is used preoperatively in elective repairs to demonstrate aortic and vascular anatomy and renal vessel involvement. An ultrasound can be a helpful screening tool in the early stages of the disease process or in the questionable emergency department patient. Abdominal plain x-ray films may show a soft tissue mass in the region of the abdominal aorta. A chest radiograph should also be obtained to evaluate the thoracic aorta. Laboratory tests should include a CBC, type and crossmatch, electrolytes, and renal function tests.

DIFFERENTIAL DIAGNOSIS

The most common misdiagnosis of ruptured AAA is myocardial infarction.[12] Other diseases or conditions that may mimic AAA include a perforated peptic ulcer, diverticulitis, appendicitis, peritonitis, acute pancreatitis, pyelonephritis, renal colic, renal infarct, and mesenteric ischemia.[32]

DIAGNOSTICS

Ruptured Aortic Aneurysm

LABORATORY
CBC and differential
Serum electrolytes
BUN
Creatinine
Serum β-human chorionic gonadotropin (in women of childbearing age)
Type and crossmatch

IMAGING
Chest x-ray
CT scan or MRI
Transthoracic echocardiography
Angiography
Ultrasound
Abdominal x-ray

OTHER
ECG

DIFFERENTIAL DIAGNOSIS

Ruptured Aortic Aneurysm

- Myocardial infarction
- Perforated peptic ulcer
- Diverticulitis
- Appendicitis
- Peritonitis
- Acute pancreatitis
- Pyelonephritis
- Renal colic or infarct
- Mesenteric ischemia

MANAGEMENT

When a rupture is strongly suspected, IV fluids should be initiated with no less than two large-bore peripheral IV sites; the patient should be crossmatched for blood, and an immediate laparotomy should be performed. Surgical excision of the aneurysm and prosthetic graft placement within the aneurysmal sac are urgently required.[31,32] The postoperative mortality rate is approximately 50%.[12]

COMPLICATIONS

Postoperative complications of ruptured AAA repair include colon infarction, sepsis, congestive heart failure, myocardial infarction, arrhythmias, liver dysfunction, renal failure, respiratory failure, pneumonia, and lower extremity ischemia.

INDICATIONS FOR REFERRAL OR HOSPITALIZATION AND PATIENT AND FAMILY EDUCATION

See Indications for Referral or Hospitalization and Patient and Family Education under Appendicitis, p. 626.

REFERENCES

1. Hou SK, Chern CH, How CK, and others: Diagnosis of appendicitis with left lower quadrant pain, *J Chin Med Assoc* 68(12):599-603, 2005.
2. Silen W: *Cope's early diagnosis of the acute abdomen,* ed 19, New York, 1996, Oxford University Press.
3. Buresh CT, Graber MA: Unusual causes of abdominal pain, *Emerg Med* 38(5):11-18, 2006.
4. Martinez JP, Mattu A: Abdominal pain in the elderly, *Emerg Med Clin North Am* 24(2):371-388, 2006.
5. Craig S: *Acute appendicitis,* retrieved Jan 13, 2007, from http://www.emedicine.com/EMERG/topic41.htm.
6. Rubin E, Farber JL: The gastrointestinal tract. In Rubin E, Farber JL, editors: *Pathology,* ed 2, Philadelphia, 1994, Lippincott.
7. Schrock TR: Acute appendicitis. In Sleisenger MH, Fordtran J, editors: *Gastrointestinal disease,* ed 5, Philadelphia, 2003, Saunders.
8. Liu CD, McFadden DW: Acute abdomen and appendix. In Greenfield LJ, Mulholland MW, Oldham KT, and others, editors: *Essentials of surgery: scientific principles and practice,* ed 2, Philadelphia, 1997, Lippincott-Raven.
9. Flum DR, Morris A, Koepsell T, and others: Has misdiagnosis of appendicitis decreased over time? A population-based analysis, *JAMA* 286:1748-1753, 2001.
10. Andersson RE, Hunagnder AP, Ghazi SH, and others: Diagnostic value of disease history, clinical presentation, and inflammatory parameters of appendicitis, *World J Surg* 23:133-140, 1999.

11. Karp SJ, Morris J, Soybel D: Small intestine and appendicitis. In Marino BS, editor: *Blueprints in surgery,* Malden, 1998, Blackwell Science.
12. Mulholland MW: Approach to the patient with acute abdomen. In Yamada T, editor: *Textbook of gastroenterology,* ed 2, Philadelphia, 1995, Lippincott.
13. Helton WS, Fisichella PM: Intestinal obstruction: assessment of intestinal obstruction, *ACS Surgery Online*, retrieved June 14, 2006, from http://www.medscape.com/viewarticle/535551.
14. Schuffler MD, Sinanan MN: Intestinal obstruction and pseudoobstruction. In Sleisenger MH, Fordtran JS, editors: *Gastrointestinal disease: pathophysiology, diagnosis, management,* ed 5, Philadelphia, 1993, Saunders.
15. Quigley EM, Hasler WL, Parkman HP: AGA technical review on nausea and vomiting, *Gastroenterology* 120:263-286, 2001.
16. Matsuoka H, Takahara T, Masaki T, and others: Preoperative evaluation by magnetic resonance imaging in patients with bowel obstruction, *Am J Surg* 183(6):614-617, 2002.
17. Towfigh S, Chandler C, Hines OJ, and others: Outcomes from peptic ulcer surgery have not benefited from advances in medical therapy, *Am J Surg* 68(4):385-389, 2002.
18. Lowe RC, Wolfe MM: Acid-peptic disorders, gastritis, and *Helicobacter pylori.* In Noble J, editor: *Textbook of primary care medicine,* ed 3, St Louis, 2001, Mosby.
19. Karp SJ, Morris J, Soybel D: Gallbladder. In Marino BS, editor: *Blueprints in surgery,* Malden, Mass, 1998, Blackwell Science.
20. Savanes C: Trends in perforated peptic ulcer: incidence, etiology, treatment, and prognosis, *World J Surg* 24(3):277-283, 2000.
21. Johnson CC, Baldessarre J, Levison ME: Peritonitis: update on pathophysiology, clinical manifestations, and management, *Clin Infect Dis* 24:1035-1045, 1997.
22. Lucey MR: Diseases of the peritoneum, mesentery, and omentum. In Goldman L, editor: *Cecil textbook of medicine,* ed 21, Philadelphia, 2000, Saunders.
23. Runyon BA: Surgical peritonitis and other diseases of the peritoneum, mesentery, omentum, and diaphragm. In Sleisenger MH, Fordtran JS, editors: *Gastrointestinal disease: pathophysiology, diagnosis, management,* ed 5, Philadelphia, 1993, Saunders.
24. Friedman SL: Alcoholic liver disease, cirrhosis, and its major sequelae. In Goldman L, editor: *Cecil textbook of medicine,* ed 21, Philadelphia, 2000, Saunders.
25. Guss DA: Disorders of the liver, biliary tract, and pancreas. In Rosen P, editor: *Emergency medicine: concepts and clinical practice,* ed 4, St Louis, 1998, Mosby.
26. Soares-Weiser K, Brezis M, Leibovici L: Antibiotics for spontaneous bacterial peritonitis in cirrhotics, *Cochrane Database Syst Rev* (3):CD002232, 2001.
27. Singh N, Gayowski T, Yu VL, and others: Trimethoprim-sulfamethoxazole for the prevention of spontaneous bacterial peritonitis in cirrhosis: a randomized trial, *Ann Intern Med* 122:595-598, 1995.
28. Garcia-Tsao G: The diagnosis of bacterial peritonitis: comparison of pH, lactate concentration, and leukocyte count, *Hepatology* 5:91-96, 1985.
29. Gorbach SL: Intraabdominal infections, *Clin Infect Dis* 17:961-965, 1993.
30. Brandt LJ, Boley SJ: Ischemic and vascular lesions of the bowel. In Sleisenger MH, Fordtran JS, editors: *Gastrointestinal disease: pathophysiology, diagnosis, management,* ed 5, Philadelphia, 1993, Saunders.
31. Blackbourne LH: Vascular surgery. In Blackbourne LH, editor: *Surgical recall,* Baltimore, 1994, Williams & Wilkins.
32. Goldstone J: Abdominal aortic aneurysms. In Greenfield LJ, Mulholland MW, Oldham KT, and others, editors: *Essentials of surgery: scientific principles and practice,* ed 2, Philadelphia, 1997, Lippincott-Raven.
33. Rubin E, Farber JL: Blood vessels. In Rubin E, Farber JL, editors: *Pathology,* ed 2, Philadelphia, 1994, Lippincott.

CHAPTER 136

Anorectal Complaints

Updated by Terry Mahan Buttaro

Anorectal complaints often encountered in the primary care setting include fecal incontinence, hemorrhoids, anal fissure, pruritus ani, anorectal pain, and anorectal abscess and fistula. However, other anorectal conditions such as a polyp, condyloma accuminata, malignancy, or a dermatologic disorder should be considered because these disorders often cause similar symptoms. A careful history and thorough physical examination are vital in making a correct diagnosis.

HEMORRHOIDS

DEFINITION AND EPIDEMIOLOGY

Hemorrhoids are masses of vascular tissue that, along with connective and muscular tissue, form a cushion in the submucosal layer of the anal canal. One of their functions is to help maintain closure of the anus. They are part of normal human anatomy, and therefore symptomatic hemorrhoids can potentially develop in all adults. External hemorrhoids lie below the dentate line and are covered by squamous epithelium. Internal hemorrhoids are located above the dentate line and are covered by columnar epithelium.

PATHOPHYSIOLOGY

The exact cause of hemorrhoids is not completely understood. However, it is thought that submucosal vascular cushions enlarge or prolapse as a result of increased pressure applied to the pelvic floor, causing external or internal hemorrhoids to develop.[1] Potential causes include pregnancy, straining, lifting, prolonged standing, poor fiber intake, and constipation or diarrhea.[1]

CLINICAL PRESENTATION

The most common presenting symptoms of hemorrhoids are bleeding, pruritus, protrusion, and pain. Internal hemorrhoids, which are usually painless, are associated with intermittent, painless, bright red rectal bleeding that occurs after defecation. The blood may be seen on the toilet paper, in the toilet water, or sometimes on the outside of the stool. Blood mixed in with the stool or dark-colored blood often indicates more proximal disease.

Internal hemorrhoids can be divided into four categories on the basis of severity: first-degree hemorrhoids may bulge but do not prolapse through the anal orifice; second-degree hemorrhoids prolapse during defecation but reduce spontaneously; third-degree hemorrhoids prolapse with defecation and require manual reinsertion; and fourth-degree hemorrhoids protrude permanently.[2] External hemorrhoids are less likely to bleed and are often asymptomatic unless thrombosis develops. The patient can also be seen with anal irritation, pruritus, or a palpable nodule. Symptoms of a thrombosed external hemorrhoid include edema and moderate to severe pain.[2]

PHYSICAL EXAMINATION

The entire perineum and perianal area should be inspected with the patient in a comfortable position (knee-chest, lithotomy, or left lateral prone). External hemorrhoids can be visualized around the anal orifice as the patient bears down, whereas internal hemorrhoids are best visualized using an anoscope as the patient bears down. An internal hemorrhoid is not palpable on rectal examination unless the hemorrhoid is thrombosed. Inflamed external hemorrhoids are erythematous and sensitive, whereas a thrombosed external hemorrhoid is tender and has a dark, bluish nodular appearance on one side of the anus.

Severe rectal pain is unusual, but if present suggests a gangrenous hemorrhoid.[1] Gangrenous hemorrhoids are fourth-degree internal hemorrhoids and require immediate surgical evaluation.

DIAGNOSTICS

If the history reveals heavy, prolonged bleeding, a CBC should be obtained to exclude anemia. To screen for bleeding from a more proximal site in the colon, the adult patient should be given stool cards for serial fecal occult blood testing once all hemorrhoidal bleeding has resolved. However, any patient who complains of rectal bleeding should undergo flexible sigmoidoscopy or colonoscopy to exclude malignancy.[2,3]

DIAGNOSTICS

Hemorrhoids

LABORATORY
Serial fecal occult blood testing
CBC and differential*

OTHER
Flexible sigmoidoscopy*
Colonoscopy*

*If indicated.

DIFFERENTIAL DIAGNOSIS

The differential diagnosis includes other anorectal conditions that can cause pain, bleeding, or protrusion. Examples are rectal prolapse, anal skin tags, hypertrophied anal papillae, rectal polyps or cancer, anal fissure, anal papillitis, inflammatory bowel disease, and condyloma or other sexually transmitted disease.

DIFFERENTIAL DIAGNOSIS

Hemorrhoids

- Rectal prolapse
- Anal skin tags
- Anal fissure
- Hypertrophied anal papillae
- Rectal polyps
- Anal papillitis
- Inflammatory bowel disease
- Condyloma acuminatum

MANAGEMENT

Guidelines for the treatment of hemorrhoids were published by the American Gastroenterological Association in 2004.[2] The treatment of hemorrhoids is based on the degree of the patient's symptoms. Most cases of hemorrhoids can be managed conservatively, and some patients require little or no treatment. A high-fiber diet and increased fluid intake are almost always recommended; according to an extensive literature review by Alonso-Coello, Mills, Heels-Ansdell, and others, fiber is an effective treatment for symptomatic hemorrhoids.[4] Fiber (20 to 30 g/day) absorbs water and helps soften the stool, thus preventing constipation and straining. Bulk-forming agents and stool softeners are sometimes used in addition to diet therapy to keep stools soft. Topical analgesics or hydrocortisone creams, suppositories, or foams (Table 136-1); frequent warm water sitz baths; and oral analgesics can help reduce inflammation and promote patient comfort.[1]

If a thrombosed external hemorrhoid is identified within 48 hours of onset, it can be evacuated by first infiltrating a local anesthetic into the base of the hemorrhoid. An elliptical incision is then made into the thrombus and the clot is expressed. Relief is immediate. This procedure can usually be carried out in the clinic setting by an *experienced* health care provider, but is not indicated in children or in patients who

TABLE 136-1 Topical Anorectal Antiinflammatory Preparations*

Preparation	Actions	How Supplied	Usual Dosage and Administration
ProctoCream-HC 2.5% (hydrocortisone acetate)	Antiinflammatory and antipruritic	Creams	Apply to affected area 2-4 times per day, depending on severity of condition.
Anusol-HC 2.5% (hydrocortisone)			
Analpram-HC 1%/1% and 2.5%/1% (hydrocortisone acetate and pramoxine)	Antiinflammatory and antipruritic, topical anesthetic		
Anusol-HC suppositories (hydrocortisone acetate)	Antiinflammatory and antipruritic	Suppositories	Place 1 suppository in rectum in morning and 1 at night for 2 weeks.
ProctoFoam-HC (hydrocortisone acetate and pramoxine)	Antiinflammatory and antipruritic, topical anesthetic	Aerosol container and anal applicator	Apply to affected area nightly for 2 weeks; may be used up to 3-4 times a day.

*Topical anal preparations containing hydrocortisone should not be used continuously for more than 2 weeks to avoid skin atrophy.

have bleeding disorders, are immunocompromised, or are pregnant.[1] Postoperative care includes a gauze pad applied to the site for 12 hours, followed by a sitz bath to remove the bandage and cleanse the area. Continued daily sitz baths and a minipad to protect clothing are recommended for several more days. If a thrombosed external hemorrhoid has been present for more than 48 hours or is not too painful, conservative measures, including mild analgesics, sitz baths, and topical anesthetic ointments, can be used.[1]

In one study, topical nifedipine (0.3% b.i.d.) was found to be helpful for acute thrombosed external hemorroids.[5] Another conservative treatment for thrombosed external hemorrhoids is the application of topical 0.5% nitroglycerin ointment.[6]

Patients with continued symptoms can require more aggressive therapy. Rubber band ligation, laser coagulation, sclerotherapy, bipolar diathermy coagulation, infared coagulation, or, if necessary, hemorrhoidectomy may be necessary to alleviate symptoms. A newer treatment, stapled hemorrhoidectomy, has been associated with less pain than a conventional hemorrhoidectomy, but current data indicate that this procedure can be associated with severe sequelae. In general, increased complications are associated with hemorrhoidectomies, and this procedure is recommended for only a small number of patients.[2] Cryotherapy is not recommended, since it was associated with significant complications.[2]

LIFE SPAN CONSIDERATIONS

Symptomatic hemorrhoids are a common disease entity. Although they can occur at any age in both sexes, they are more common in adults between 45 and 65 years of age.[1] The prevalence in the United States has been estimated to be as high as 75% of adults over the age of 50.[1]

COMPLICATIONS

Fourth-degree hemorrhoids are at risk for strangulation because they are irreducible. Strangulated hemorrhoids can become gangrenous, requiring immediate surgical intervention.[1,2]

Rubber band ligation has been associated with increased pain, infection, and sepsis. Hemorrhoidectomy has been associated with urinary tract infections, urinary retention, fecal impaction, delayed hemorrhage, and, rarely, infection. The newer stapled hemorrhoidectomy has been associated with some significant complications.[2]

INDICATIONS FOR REFERRAL OR HOSPITALIZATION

If conservative measures fail, patients should be referred to a gastroenterologist for infrared photocoagulation, electrocoagulation, or rubber banding before surgical hemorrhoidectomy is suggested. Surgery is often the treatment of choice for fourth-degree hemorrhoids, most third-degree hemorrhoids, strangulated hemorrhoids, or hemorrhoids that have not responded to other therapies. Emergent surgical evaluation is indicated for a gangrenous internal hemorrhoid.[1] Flexible sigmoidoscopy or colonoscopy should be performed on all patients with rectal bleeding to exclude a more proximal lesion, which could exist in addition to hemorrhoids.

PATIENT AND FAMILY EDUCATION

Patients should be instructed on how to increase dietary fiber and in the correct use of topical antiinflammatory agents; topical corticosteroids should be used judiciously to avoid atrophy. Patients should also be taught preventive measures, including increasing fluid intake, keeping the stool soft, avoiding straining during bowel movements, exercising regularly to help promote regular bowel movements, and keeping the anal area clean and dry. The patient should understand the importance of follow-up care, particularly if symptoms do not resolve with conservative measures.

ANAL FISSURE

DEFINITION AND EPIDEMIOLOGY

Anal fissures, painful linear cracks or tears in the lining of the anal canal, are a frequent cause of rectal bleeding and are common in children and middle-aged adults. A fissure present for less than 6 weeks is considered acute, whereas fissures present for longer than 6 weeks are designated as chronic.

PATHOPHYSIOLOGY

Anal fissures are sometimes seen in patients with Crohn's disease, tuberculosis, or leukemia.[7,8] However, most anal fissures are caused by trauma to the anal canal from passage of a large, hard stool. Other causes include frequent diarrhea, which can result in a chemical burn from severe alkalinity, and anal stenosis, which may predispose the patient to fissure formation. An acute fissure often resolves without intervention. However, a chronic ulcer surrounded by scar tissue may develop if the underlying sphincter goes into involuntary spasm, leading to diminished blood flow to the area.

CLINICAL PRESENTATION

Many patients seek treatment with the thought that they have hemorrhoids. Classic symptoms of an anal fissure are severe rectal pain during and after bowel movements and small amounts of bright red rectal bleeding seen on the toilet paper. Some patients avoid having a bowel movement because of the pain and thus produce even harder stools, which exacerbates the problem.[9]

PHYSICAL EXAMINATION

Because of the severe pain associated with an anal fissure, the physical examination should be done gently and with reassurance. The patient should be positioned in the left lateral decubitus position and a topical anesthetic applied to enable adequate visualization of the rectum and anus. The fissure is most easily visualized by spreading the buttocks to expose the anus. Ninety percent of fissures are located at the posterior midline, and the remainder are situated in the anterior midline.[1] A fissure located in a more lateral position usually indicates a sexually transmitted disease, tuberculosis, HIV infection, ulcerative colitis, Crohn's disease, malignancy, or other underlying disorder.[1] If the fissure is chronic, the examination may reveal a hypertrophied anal papilla proximal to the fissure and a sentinel pile or skin tag distal to the fissure at the anal verge. These findings are indicative of repetitive inflammation and healing with resultant formation of scar tissue and can lead to anal stenosis. If the fissure is extremely painful, digital rectal and anoscopic examination may be deferred. If the fissure is touched with a cotton-tipped applicator, the symptoms will often be reproduced, helping to confirm the diagnosis.

DIAGNOSTICS

There are no routine laboratory abnormalities.

DIFFERENTIAL DIAGNOSIS

Pain during bowel movements is not symptomatic of hemorrhoidal disease. Chronic anal fissures are often misdiagnosed as hemorrhoids because of the presence of a sentinel tag. Sometimes a large hypertrophied anal papilla can be mistaken for a polyp on digital rectal examination. Inflammatory bowel disease, carcinoma of the anus, leukemia, lymphoma, tuberculosis, syphilis, and other sexually transmitted diseases are also included in the differential diagnosis.

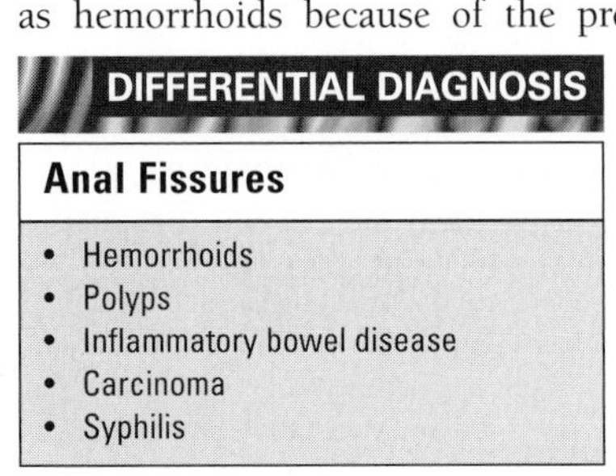
DIFFERENTIAL DIAGNOSIS

Anal Fissures

- Hemorrhoids
- Polyps
- Inflammatory bowel disease
- Carcinoma
- Syphilis

MANAGEMENT

Increased fiber and sitz baths are proven effective treatment for anal fissures.[7] Other therapies include the use of stool softeners and cream, suppositories, or foam containing anti-inflammatory agents (see Table 136-1). Topical anesthetic gel (lidocaine [Xylocaine] 2% jelly) applied before bowel movements can be helpful in reducing pain and spasm. Some evidence suggests that, by increasing blood flow and decreasing sphincter pressure, topical 0.2% glyceryl trinitrate ointment expedites healing.[7,10] Topical nifedipine is indicated for patients with sphincter spasm.[1] Botulinum toxin injection also has been shown to be effective for healing.[7,10] However, the studies involving nitroglycerin cream and botulinum injections were small, and fissures did recur in some patients.[10]

LIFE SPAN CONSIDERATIONS

Anal fissures are commonly seen in young and middle-aged adults but can occur at any age. Both sexes seem to be equally affected. Although they are common, the exact incidence of this disease is unknown.[9]

COMPLICATIONS AND INDICATIONS FOR REFERRAL OR HOSPITALIZATION

Patients with chronic or recurrent fissures that do not respond to conservative therapy should be referred for surgery. Lateral subcutaneous internal sphincterotomy reduces internal sphincter tone, allowing the fissure to heal. Complications of this procedure can include poor wound healing and rectal incontinence but are usually avoided.[9]

PATIENT AND FAMILY EDUCATION

Patients need to be informed that healing can take up to 6 weeks with conservative measures. They should be advised to return for follow-up if symptoms do not resolve or if they recur. Prevention includes keeping the stools soft with a high-fiber diet and adequate fluid intake and avoiding straining during bowel movements.

If topical nitroglycerin is prescribed, patients should understand how to use the preparation and be able to recognize the side effects associated with all nitrates. Nitrates are contraindicated in patients using sildenafil citrate.

PRURITUS ANI

DEFINITION AND EPIDEMIOLOGY

Pruritus ani, or itching of the anus and perianal skin, is a fairly common condition, affecting up to 5% of the population.[9] Although the true prevalence of this disorder is unknown, men are affected four times more often than women.[1,9,11]

PATHOPHYSIOLOGY

There are many different causes of pruritus ani. In many patients the condition has no identified cause. However, a recent study suggests that varied dermatologic conditions can cause the persistent itching that plagues some patients.[12] Other potential causes include hyperhidrosis, infections or infestations (i.e., scabies, pediculosis, fungus, or pinworms), medications, malignancies, and common systemic illnesses (e.g., renal insufficiency, liver disease, or diabetes).[1] Pruritus ani can also be related to improper hygiene or to the ingestion of certain foods or beverages. Common offenders include coffee, tea, soda, alcohol, tomatoes, citrus fruits, and chocolate.[11] These foods possibly affect the function of the internal anal sphincter, permitting the fecal soilage associated with pruritus ani.[11]

CLINICAL PRESENTATION

The patient often complains of an uncontrollable urge to scratch the anus. The symptoms tend to be worse at night or after a bowel movement. Sometimes the itching will involve the perianal area, buttocks, and vulva or scrotum. Scratching provides only transient relief and can lead to an itch-scratch cycle that exacerbates the condition.

PHYSICAL EXAMINATION

Diagnosis is made by a careful history and physical examination. The anus should be thoroughly inspected for obvious anorectal, infectious, or dermatologic disease. A digital rectal examination is also indicated. If the pruritus is chronic, the perianal skin may appear moist, excoriated, and macerated.

DIAGNOSTICS

Cultures may be useful if an infectious etiology is suspected. If the pruritus is primarily nocturnal, cellophane tape can be applied to the perianal skin in the early morning. The tape is then placed on a glass slide and examined under a microscope for pinworm eggs. For patients with intractable pruritus or a

DIAGNOSTICS

Pruritus Ani

LABORATORY
Cultures*
Microscopic examination for pinworm eggs*

OTHER
Biopsy*

*If indicated.

suspected dermatologic disease or malignancy, a biopsy sample obtained by a dermatologist can help confirm the diagnosis. Suspected sexually transmitted disease requires the appropriate workup to exclude chlamydia, gonorrhea, syphilis, or other diseases.

DIFFERENTIAL DIAGNOSIS

Psoriasis, malignancy, contact dermatitis, candidal infection, hidradenitis suppurativa, parasitic infection, sexually transmitted diseases, and anal fissures should be considered in the differential diagnosis.

DIFFERENTIAL DIAGNOSIS

Pruritus Ani

ANORECTAL DISEASES
- Diarrhea
- Fissures
- Fistulas
- Hemorrhoids
- Incontinence
- Skin tags
- Squamous cell cancer

DERMATOLOGIC DISEASES
- Atopic dermatitis
- Contact dermatitis
- Hidradenitis suppurativa
- Lichen planus
- Psoriasis

INFECTIONS OR INFESTATIONS
- Candidal infection
- Condyloma acuminatum infection
- Gonorrhea
- Herpes simplex
- Pinworms
- Scabies
- Pediculosis
- Syphilis

MALIGNANCIES
- Bowen's disease
- Paget's disease

OTHER CAUSES
- Dietary
- Idiopathic cause
- Overzealous hygiene
- Poor hygiene
- Psychogenic cause
- Warmth and moisture

MANAGEMENT

Any identified infectious or dermatologic disease should be treated. Once other pathologic causes of pruritus ani have been excluded, the patient's hygiene and dietary habits should be addressed. The anal area should be kept clean and dry, and overvigorous wiping or scratching should be avoided. Perfumed toilet paper, soaps, and hygiene products should not be used. A 1% hydrocortisone cream can be used initially but should be discontinued after 2 weeks to avoid skin atrophy.[11] Topical capsaicin has been used successfully for idiopathic pruritus that has not responded to the more commonly used therapies such as nonmedicated talcum powders or barrier creams (e.g., zinc oxide).[11,13,14] Patients should be encouraged to wear clean cotton underwear and avoid tight fitting clothing. Dietary restrictions of possible offending foods should be tried. A psyllium product can be used to bulk the stool in an attempt to prevent fecal soilage if loose stools are a problem.[11] Medications and foods that cause loose stools should be avoided if at all possible. If severe nocturnal itching is a problem, an antihistamine with antipruritic properties, such as hydroxyzine (Atarax), can help the patient sleep and assist in breaking the itch-scratch cycle. Relief of symptoms usually occurs in 4 to 6 weeks.[9]

LIFE SPAN CONSIDERATIONS

Pruritus ani is most common in the fourth, fifth, and sixth decades; however, this disorder can occur at any age.[9]

COMPLICATIONS

Scratching associated with pruritus ani can cause excoriations. These can become infected and require antibiotic therapy. Vaginal infections are also potential complications. Pruritus ani related to pinworm infestation can be easily spread to others, and reinfection is common.

INDICATIONS FOR REFERRAL OR HOSPITALIZATION

Referral to a specialist is rarely indicated for pruritus ani. If a dermatologic disease is suspected but not clearly identified, the patient should be referred to a dermatologist for further evaluation.[12] Suspicious lesions require biopsy, and any signs or symptoms suggesting bowel pathologic conditions require colonoscopy to exclude malignancy. If medical treatment has failed, referral to a gastroenterologist is indicated.[11]

PATIENT AND FAMILY EDUCATION

The patient should be educated about the possible cause of this condition. To help identify offending foods, the patient can be taught an elimination diet. The patient should be instructed about proper anal hygiene habits and to avoid scratching the area.

ANORECTAL ABSCESS OR FISTULA

DEFINITION AND EPIDEMIOLOGY

An anorectal abscess is an infection that occurs from obstruction of the duct of a perianal gland in the intersphincteric space. An anorectal fistula is the drainage of an abscess through an abnormal communication to the perianal skin. An abscess is the acute manifestation of an infection, and a fistula is the chronic manifestation. The incidence is higher in men than in women, with the most common ages being the third and fourth decades of life.[1]

PATHOPHYSIOLOGY

The most common cause of anorectal abscesses and fistulas is bacterial infection of the anal glands. These glands may become infected if obstruction with resulting stasis occurs from trauma, hard stools, foreign bodies, or diarrhea. Another common cause of anorectal abscesses or fistulas is Crohn's disease.[8]

CLINICAL PRESENTATION

Symptoms of an abscess include acute pain and swelling. The pain increases with movement, sitting, or bowel movements. Malaise and fever may also be present. The most common complaint of patients with an anorectal fistula is a persistent purulent drainage. A careful history is necessary to determine whether the patient has a history of immunocompetence, diabetes, Crohn's disease, or anorectal abscess or fistula.

PHYSICAL EXAMINATION

Inspection of the perineum may reveal erythema, heat, swelling, and tenderness. If the abscess is located higher in the anorectum, the perineum may be unrevealing, and the abscess may manifest as localized tenderness on rectal examination. On anoscopy, pus may be seen exuding from an opening into the anal canal. A fistula may be seen with pus oozing from a sinus or opening in the perineal skin. Inguinal lymph nodes may be enlarged.

DIAGNOSTICS

A CBC may reveal leukocytosis. With recurrent fistulas, a small bowel follow-through, colonoscopy, or barium enema may be indicated to exclude Crohn's disease.

DIFFERENTIAL DIAGNOSIS

With recurrent fistulas, Crohn's disease should be considered. Also included in the differential diagnosis are pilonidal sinus, hidradenitis suppurativa, anorectal malignancy, actinomycosis, sexually transmitted diseases, and lymphoma.

MANAGEMENT, COMPLICATIONS, AND INDICATIONS FOR REFERRAL OR HOSPITALIZATION

The treatment of an anorectal abscess or fistula is always surgical. Because of the risk of potentially fatal sepsis, medical management by itself is never indicated. When an anorectal abscess or a fistula is suspected, antibiotics should be started and tetanus immunization updated.[1] Surgery involves drainage of the abscess and fistulotomy, if indicated. The major complication of surgery for an abscess or a fistula is incontinence.

DIAGNOSTICS

Anorectal Abscess

LABORATORY
CBC and differential*

OTHER
Colonoscopy*
Barium enema*
Small bowel examination*

*If indicated.

DIFFERENTIAL DIAGNOSIS

Anorectal Abscess

- Crohn's disease
- Pilonidal sinus
- Hidradenitis suppurativa
- Carcinoma
- Actinomycosis
- Sexually transmitted diseases

PATIENT AND FAMILY EDUCATION

After surgery, the patient should be instructed to keep the stools soft with bulk-forming agents, a high-fiber diet, and stool softeners. Warm sitz baths can help with hygiene, promote healing, and provide comfort until healing is complete. The importance of follow-up visits to inspect the wound for proper healing should be emphasized.

REFERENCES

1. DeLashaw M, Foley K: Managing anorectal complaints, *Emerg Med* 38(5):44-50, 2006.
2. American Gastroenterological Association: American Gastroenterological Association medical position statement: diagnosis and treatment of hemorrhoids, *Gastroenterology* 126(5):1461-1462, 2004, retrieved June 9, 2006, from http://www.guideline.gov/summary/summary.aspx?ss=15&doc_id=5181&nbr=3563.
3. Bleday R, Breen E: *Treatment of hemorrhoids*, retrieved Jan 15, 2007, from http://www.uptodateonline.com/utd/content/topic.do?topicKey=gi_dis/12411&selectedTitle=1~3567.
4. Alonso-Coello P, Mills E, Heels-Ansdell D, and others: Fiber for the treatment of hemorrhoids complications: a systematic review and meta-analysis, *Am J Gastroenterol* 101(1):181-188, 2006.
5. Perotti P, Cavci J, Turci J: Conservative treatment of acute thrombosed external hemorrhoids with topical nifedipine, *Dis Colon Rectum* 44:405-409, 2001.
6. Gorfine SR: Treatment of benign anal disease with topical nitroglycerin, *Dis Colon Rectum* 38(5):453-456, 1995.
7. Breen E, Bleday R: *Anal fissures*, retrieved Jan 15, 2007, from http://www.uptodateonline.com/utd/content/topic.do?topicKey=gi_dis/13714&selectedTitle=1~33.
8. Bitton A, Belliveau P: *Perianal complications of Crohn's disease*, retrieved Jan 15, 2007, from http://www.uptodateonline.com/utd/content/topic.do?topicKey=inflambd/9003&selectedTitle=3~239.
9. Mazier WP: Hemorrhoids, fissures, and pruritus ani, *Surg Clin North Am* 74:1277-1292, 1994.
10. Jones M, Scholefield J: Anal fissures, *Clin Evidence* 6:330-335, 2001.
11. Bonis PAL, Breen E, Bleday R: *Approach to the patient with anal pruritus*, retrieved Jan 15, 2007, from http://www.uptodateonline.com/utd/content/topic.do?topicKey=gi_dis/15529&selectedTitle=1~20.
12. Dasan S, Neill SM, Donaldson DR, and others: Treatment of persistent pruritus ani in a combined colorectal and dermatological clinic, *Br J Surg* 86:1337-1340, 1999.
13. Anand P: Capsaicin and menthol in the treatment of itch and pain: recently cloned receptors provide the key, *Gut* 52(9):1233-1235, 2003.
14. Lysy J, Sistiery-Ittah M, Israelit Y, and others: Topical capsaicin—a novel and effective treatment for idiopathic intractable pruritus ani: a randomized, placebo controlled, crossover study, *Gut* 52(9):1323-1326, 2003.

CHAPTER 137

Cholelithiasis and Cholecystitis

Scott W. Shiffer

DEFINITION AND EPIDEMIOLOGY

Cholelithiasis and cholecystitis are worldwide disorders that result from inflammatory, infectious, neoplastic, metabolic, and congenital conditions. Gallbladder disease affects all cultures and is prevalent in most Western countries. From 20 million to 25 million Americans have cholelithiasis, and each year more than half of patients with newly diagnosed gallstone disease undergo a cholecystectomy.[1] In the United States, Native Americans have a high incidence of gallstones compared with other groups.[2] The highest incidence of acute cholecystitis is in adults ages 30 to 80 years; women have approximately twice the incidence of gallstones as men. Unfortunately, older men seem to be at risk for the development of acalculous cholecystitis, an uncommon condition that is being seen with increasing frequency.[3] Risk factors include age, ethnicity (Scandinavians and Pima Indians seem to have an increased incidence), family history, gender, medications, obesity, rapid weight loss, and hyperalimentation, as well as co-morbid disorders such as diabetes, Crohn's disease, alcoholic and biliary cirrhosis, and hyperparathyroidism (Box 137-1).[4]

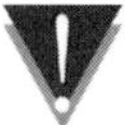
Physician consultation is indicated for acute cholecystitis.

PATHOPHYSIOLOGY

Gallstones are formed from bile constituent crystals and are divided into three primary types of stones: cholesterol, pigmented, and mixed.

BOX 137-1

RISK FACTORS FOR GALLSTONE FORMATION

Age: Increasing age*
Body habitus: Obesity, rapid weight loss
Childbearing: Pregnancy
Drugs: Fibric acid derivatives (or fibrates), contraceptive steroids, postmenopausal estrogens, progesterone, octreotide (Sandostatin), ceftriaxone (Rocephin)
Ethnicity: Pima Indians, Scandinavians
Family: Maternal family history of gallstones
Gender: Females
Hyperalimentation: Total parenteral nutrition,† fasting
Ileal and other metabolic diseases: Ileal disease (Crohn's disease), resection or bypass,* high triglycerides, diabetes mellitus, chronic hemolysis,* alcoholic cirrhosis,* biliary infection,* primary biliary cirrhosis, duodenal diverticula,* truncal vagotomy, hyperparathyroidism, low level of high-density lipoprotein cholesterol

From Ahmed A, Cheung RC, Keefe EB: Management of gallstones and their complications, *Am Fam Phys* 61(6):1673-1680, 1687-1688, 2000.
*Risk factors for pigment gallstone formation.
†Risk factor for cholesterol and pigment gallstone formation.

Cholesterol gallstones occur as a result of several conditions. First, a supersaturation of cholesterol in the bile must be present. Second, a "snowball" effect via nucleation of filamentous, helical, or tubular forms of nonhydrated cholesterol crystals must occur because there is either an excess of pronucleating factors or a lack of antinucleating factors.[5] Third, biliary sludge accumulates as a result of delayed gallbladder emptying and stasis.[6] Pregnancy and very-low-calorie diets leading to rapid weight loss are also associated with biliary sludge formation and lithogenesis.[1] Biliary proteins and lipids may act as co-factors in the cholesterol crystallization process, and there appears to be a link between an iron-deficient diet and cholesterol crystal formation.

Pigment gallstones result from excess unconjugated, insoluble bilirubin that precipitates into bilirubin crystals. This mechanism also can form the basis for a mixed type of stone associated with alcoholic liver disease and chronic hemolysis.[1] Black-pigmented gallstones remain in the gallbladder. Brown-pigmented gallstones and cholesterol stones can be found in the gallbladder, intrahepatic ducts, cystic duct, and common bile duct.

Small gallstones pass uneventfully through the common bile duct and do not cause distress. Larger stones may cause obstruction of the cystic or common bile duct, causing increased pressure to the ductal system that results in pain, nausea, and vomiting as a result of the contractile spasms of the smooth muscle. Because of the blockage, bile is prevented from entering the duodenum, reducing the body's ability to digest fat. The undigested fat passes from the small intestine into the large intestine, where bacteria convert the excess undigested fat into fatty acid derivatives. The fatty acid derivatives alter water absorption from the colon, which results in diarrhea and excess fluid loss. The obstruction also prevents bile secretion into the small intestine, resulting in jaundice.[2]

The gallbladder becomes inflamed as a result of various processes, including continued blockage of the cystic or common bile duct. This inflammation causes the release of prostaglandins and other chemicals that further inflame gallbladder tissue. In 75% of cases, bacterial infections contribute to the inflammatory response in acute cholecystitis.[6] HIV disease may lead to opportunistic infections of the biliary tract. The most common bacteria involved in biliary tract infections are *Escherichia coli, Klebsiella* organisms, and enterococci.[7] Gangrene of the gallbladder and possible perforation can result if the process is not stopped.

Cholecystitis can also occur in the absence of stones; this condition is labeled acute or chronic *acalculous cholecystitis.* Acalculous cholecystitis is classified as acute if the duration of symptoms is less than 1 month and as chronic if the symptoms have been present longer than 3 months. The pathophysiology of this condition is poorly understood. The inflammatory process is similar to that of cholecystitis except that gallstones are not present. A common cause of chronic acalculous cholecystitis is biliary dyskinesia. Risk factors associated with acute acalculous cholecystitis are outlined in Box 137-2.

CLINICAL PRESENTATION

Most patients with gallstones are asymptomatic.[8] However, patients with chronic cholecystitis often describe a recurrent,

BOX 137-2

RISK FACTORS ASSOCIATED WITH ACUTE ACALCULOUS CHOLECYSTITIS

Coronary artery disease
Previous myocardial infarction
Diabetes
Peripheral or cerebral vascular disease
Polyarteritis nodosa
Prolonged labor
Prolonged fasting
Immediate postoperative period
Hyperalimentation
Dehydration
Fibrosis of the gallbladder
Obstruction of the biliary or pancreatic ducts
Thrombosis of the cystic artery
Critical illnesses (e.g., bone marrow transplantation)
Severe illnesses
- Trauma
- Burns
- Sepsis

Major diseases
- AIDS
- Leptospirosis

mild to moderate, right upper quadrant and epigastric abdominal pain accompanied by nausea and vomiting. The pain may radiate to the region of the posterior right shoulder and scapula and is often associated with eating fatty foods.

Classically, symptomatic cholelithiasis manifests as biliary colic with intermittent or steady, right upper quadrant abdominal pain that radiates to the right posterior shoulder within an hour of eating any type of large meal.[9] The pain may be constant or intermittent and tapering, sometimes without complete relief. It is described as mild to severe and lasts from 1 to 6 hours. The biliary colic is accompanied by nausea and vomiting. There can be a history of these episodes, which increase in frequency.

Acute cholecystitis develops in a manner similar to symptomatic cholelithiasis, but biliary colic lasts longer than 6 hours. There usually is a history of intermittent colic consistent with chronic cholecystitis, and the patient may have anorexia, fever, and chills in addition to the nausea and vomiting observed in symptomatic cholelithiasis. As the gallbladder becomes progressively inflamed, the pain in the right upper quadrant becomes sharp. Charcot's triad of right upper quadrant abdominal pain, fever, and jaundice can be observed if a stone is lodged in the common bile duct.

Traditionally, patients with acute acalculous cholecystitis are critically ill and require hospitalization. Presentation includes generalized complaints, fever, nausea, vomiting, and loss of appetite. Often the patient has no significant medical history, although surgery, trauma, burns, and other disorders have been associated with acalculous cholecystitis. This condition should be considered in all patients who are seen with right upper quadrant pain in the absence of gallstones.[10]

PHYSICAL EXAMINATION

Depending on the severity of the condition, the physical examination in symptomatic cholelithiasis and chronic cholecystitis may be unremarkable. Right upper quadrant abdominal pain may be accompanied by tenderness. The diagnosis is based on the history, the exclusion of other disorders, and the results of the gallbladder ultrasound.

With acute cholecystitis, patients may have moderate distress from systemic toxicity, including tachycardia and fever. The right upper quadrant abdominal pain is associated with tenderness and muscle guarding or rigidity. The gallbladder is not commonly palpable, but a distended tender gallbladder confirms the diagnosis. Hypoactive bowel sounds and a positive Murphy's sign (an inability to take a deep breath during palpation beneath the right costal margin) may be noted. Dehydration is not uncommon. Jaundice is present in approximately 20% of patients and is the result of longstanding biliary obstruction or chronic hemolysis.[1,11]

The physical findings in acalculous cholecystitis are similar to those found in symptomatic gallstones: right upper quadrant pain, vomiting, fever, jaundice, and a positive Murphy's sign.

DIAGNOSTICS

Laboratory testing should be individualized, but a CBC with differential, urinalysis, liver function tests, and serum pancreatic enzymes are usually indicated (Table 137-1). A test for human chorionic gonadotropin is essential in women of childbearing age if potentially teratogenic clinical imaging studies are considered. An ECG is necessary if cardiac risk factors are present or if cardiac involvement is suspected.

Plain abdominal radiographs will demonstrate biliary air, marked hepatomegaly, and, in some cases, gallstones. A chest x-ray study will exclude right lower lobe pneumonia. Ultrasound is the most practical imaging study for evaluating the gallbladder and is considered accurate at least 95% of the time.[10] Pregnancy is not a contraindication for ultrasound examination.[12]

If further studies are required, scintigraphic imaging should follow ultrasonography. Biliary scintigraphy is the most accurate and specific test for diagnosing acute cholecystitis.

DIFFERENTIAL DIAGNOSIS

Cholecystitis has an extensive number of differential diagnoses. See the Differential Diagnosis box for a list of the more common ones.

DIAGNOSTICS

Cholelithiasis and Cholecystitis

LABORATORY
CBC and differential
LFTs (bilirubin, alkaline phosphate)

IMAGING
Ultrasound
Biliary scintigraphy

OTHER
Endoscopic retrograde cholangiopancreatogram*

*If indicated.

TABLE 137-1 Expected Laboratory Values in Biliary Tract Disease

	Serum Laboratory Tests						
	WBC	Bilirubin	Alkaline Phosphate	Aspartate Aminotransferase	Alanine Aminotransferase	Amylase	Lipase
Chronic cholecystitis	Normal	Normal	Normal	Normal	Normal	Normal	Normal
Symptomatic cholelithiasis	Normal	Normal or slight rise	Normal or slight rise	Normal	Normal	†	†
Acute cholecystitis	Normal or rise	Rise in 45% of patients	Rise in 23% of patients	Rise in 40% of patients	Normal	Rise in 13% of patients†	Normal
Acute acalculous cholecystitis	Rise	Slight rise	Slight rise	Slight rise	Slight rise	Normal	Normal
Chronic acalculous cholecystitis	Normal	Normal	Normal	Normal	Normal	Normal	Normal
Choledocholith	Rise	Rise	Rise	Rise*	Rise*	Rise†	Rise†

*A rise in the transaminases is associated with prolonged obstruction leading to hepatocellular destruction.
†A rise in the serum amylase and lipase is associated with pancreatitis secondary to ampulla of Vater stone obstruction.

DIFFERENTIAL DIAGNOSIS

Cholelithiasis and Cholecystitis

- Neoplasm
- Hepatitis or hepatic abscess
- Pancreatitis
- Gastritis
- Peptic ulcer disease
- Irritable bowel syndrome
- Appendicitis
- Fitz-Hugh–Curtis syndrome
- Pelvic inflammatory disease
- Pneumonia (right lower lobe)
- Pleuritis
- Pyelonephritis
- Myocardial ischemia or infarction
- Diverticulitis
- Herpes zoster
- Renal colic

MANAGEMENT

In general, asymptomatic gallstones do not require surgical intervention. However, there is a 20% chance of the development of symptoms, and gastroenterologists and surgeons will sometimes recommend prophylactic cholecystectomy.[1]

The initial management of symptomatic gallbladder disease begins with isotonic IV rehydration and correction of electrolyte abnormalities. Oral hydration is contraindicated during this time. Antispasmodic and antiemetic medications are used for uncomplicated cholelithiasis. In addition to an antiemetic, a nasogastric tube should be used for protracted vomiting to decompress the stomach. Pain should be managed with parenteral analgesics.[13] Meperidine is usually used because it causes less spasm of the sphincter of Oddi compared with other narcotics. An injectable nonsteroidal antiinflammatory prostaglandin inhibitor (ketorolac tromethamine) is also an effective pain reliever in nonbacterial gallbladder distention.[2]

With uncomplicated symptomatic cholelithiasis, discharge is appropriate once the condition has stabilized and oral hydration is maintained. Surgical consultation before discharge is advised. Acute cholecystitis should be suspected if the symptoms do not resolve within 4 to 6 hours; in this case, timely surgical referral for laparoscopic cholecystectomy is essential.[14] Prophylactic antibiotics may be indicated for patients with acute cholecystitis, but one small study revealed that prophylactic antibiotic therapy did not significantly decrease infection rates for patients undergoing elective cholecysectomy.[15]

Co-Management with Specialists

Medical dissolution, biliary lithotripsy, or surgical intervention requires further consultation to ensure optimum health care. Patients with diabetes and asymptomatic disease should have a consultation with a gastroenterologist or surgeon to determine whether further management is required.

After initial patient stabilization, treatment options for uncomplicated symptomatic cholelithiasis include medical dissolution therapy (oral or direct gallbladder irrigation), biliary lithotripsy, cholecystostomy (as an alternative surgical procedure), and open or laparoscopic cholecystectomy. Medical dissolution therapy of gallstones is attractive to patients who are poor surgical candidates or those who refuse surgery.[13]

The oral bile acid (chenodeoxycholic or ursodeoxycholic acid) method attempts to reduce the body's ability to create gallstones by limiting cholesterol saturation in the bile. This method is best for patients who have cholesterol stones smaller than 2 cm (0.8 inch) and have a functioning gallbladder. This therapy usually requires at least 9 months to 2 years to become effective; stones recur in 50% of patients within 5 years when the treatment is stopped.[1] The high cost of the medication may be a deterrent for this type of medical management.[1,9] Pending an improved long-term success rate, these drugs are best reserved for patients who may not be safe surgical candidates.

A second medical dissolution regimen involves direct gallbladder irrigation with ether-type solvents. This method dissolves small stones in approximately 2 to 4 hours. Unfortunately, stone recurrence is not unusual.

Biliary lithotripsy can be considered in 20% to 25% of patients with gallstones and is relatively safe. Energy waves are generated through a water bath and into the soft tissue and are transmitted into the stone. The relatively painless shock waves fracture the stones into smaller pieces that are then passed into the small intestine. The criteria for biliary lithotripsy are specific; in addition, it is an expensive therapy, and gallstone recurrence is reported at 50% by 5 years.[16]

Cholecystostomy is an alternative surgical procedure to open or laparoscopic cholecystectomy and is used if the patient has too much inflammation or is too ill for cholecystectomy. Either operatively or percutaneously, stones and bile are removed via the gallbladder fundus, and a tube is placed as an external drain.

An open cholecystectomy requires a subcostal surgical incision on the right side. The skin is separated with retractors, and the gallbladder is isolated from the liver. The cystic duct and cystic artery are ligated, and the diseased gallbladder is removed. This open surgical approach is necessary when there are relative contraindications for the laparoscopic method; these contradictions include coagulopathy, cirrhosis, portal hypertension, pregnancy, peritonitis, severe cardiopulmonary disease, and prior surgical adhesions.

Because of its safety, convenience, reduced postoperative pain, and shorter hospitalization (outpatient surgery at some facilities), laparoscopic cholecystectomy is the standard treatment for symptomatic gallbladder disease. Choledocholithiasis, or stones in the common bile duct, can also be managed through the laparoscopic approach, although in some instances this will be too difficult to manage safely. Some laparoscopic approaches require a conversion to the open cholecystectomy procedure—5% of patients undergoing treatment for chronic cholecystitis and 25% of patients with acute cholecystitis.[9]

In addition to the initial treatment of gallstone disease, perioperative antibiotics may be indicated. Bacteria associated with acute cholecystitis include *E. coli, Klebsiella pneumoniae, Clostridium welchii, Clostridium perfringens,* and *Streptococcus faecalis.* Therapeutic antibiotics are used for patients suffering from acute cholecystitis or cholangitis.[7]

When acalculous cholecystitis is recognized, an antibiotic regimen sensitive to gram-negative organisms is the first step to treating the infection. Surgical drainage or removal of the gallbladder is considered the definitive treatment. Laparoscopic cholecystectomy may be chosen to treat the condition. Ultrasound-guided percutaneous cholecystostomy under a local anesthetic agent is an excellent alternative and has a low mortality rate. Although symptoms of chronic acalculous cholecystitis and gallbladder dysfunction are relieved with cholecystectomy, caution is advised for this type of management pending further trials. Either a cholecystectomy or a cholecystostomy is required depending on the severity of the illness. Cholecystostomy is the treatment of choice with severe disease or extensive inflammation.[6]

COMPLICATIONS

Potential organ damage depends on the location of the gallstone obstruction in the biliary system. Patients with recurrent pain have twice the complication rate as patients without symptoms, and patients with symptomatic gallstones have a 70% chance of developing complications over their lifetime.[13] The most common complication is choledocholithiasis. In general, symptomatic gallstones require surgical intervention. If left untreated, the disease has potential complications, including a pus-filled gallbladder, which can lead to perforation. Local perforation can occur within 1 week after the onset of acute cholecystitis and can lead to the formation of a pericholecystic abscess. The mortality rate is 25% if a free perforation into the abdominal cavity occurs.[11] Should a large gallstone pass into the intestinal lumen, a small bowel obstruction is possible; this is called a *gallstone ileus.* Three times more common in men and associated with diabetes, gas-forming bacteria (*Clostridium* and coliform organisms) can lead to an emphysematous cholecystitis that further leads to gallbladder perforation.[11] The gallbladder may become gangrenous when extensive inflammation causes necrosis and thrombosis of the cystic artery. Stones lodged in the ampulla of Vater can cause gallstone pancreatitis. The porcelain gallbladder, an uncommon condition associated with cancer, is observed on plain radiographs. The porcelain appearance of the gallbladder rim is caused by calcification of the gallbladder.

The complication rate of gallstone disease varies and depends on the procedure chosen to manage the disease, the size of the gallstone, the patient's age, and co-morbid issues.

INDICATIONS FOR REFERRAL OR HOSPITALIZATION

Asymptomatic cholelithiasis does not require referral for surgical management except as previously discussed. Symptomatic gallstones or evidence of acalculous disease supported by ultrasound or oral cholecystogram requires further medical or surgical consultation for management and maintenance.

Acute cholecystitis requires hospitalization for IV antibiotics and fluid therapy. Nearly three fourths of patients who are medically managed have complete remission of their symptoms within 2 to 7 days of hospitalization.[1]

The postoperative course after a cholecystectomy varies according to whether the surgeon used the laparoscopic or the open approach. Laparoscopic cholecystectomy is the preferred procedure for elective cholecystectomy.[8] Laparoscopic cholecystectomy patients have a shorter hospitalization and return to work sooner (within 10 days).[17,18] Those who have undergone an open cholecystectomy may take much longer to return to unrestricted activities after surgery.[18]

Patients diagnosed with acalculous cholecystitis are admitted to the hospital. If a percutaneous catheter placement is used to drain the gallbladder, the catheter may be in place for 6 to 8 weeks; if no stones are present at postdrainage cholangiography, cholecystectomy may be unnecessary.[8]

PATIENT AND FAMILY EDUCATION

Patients who are obese should be counseled about the increased risk of gallstone formation. Patients should understand the importance of lifestyle dietary changes. Some risk factors have been implicated but not clearly demonstrated for cholelithiasis; still, it may be wise for patients to avoid excessive caffeine and alcohol intake and prolonged fasting. Although birth control pills may increase the possibility of gallstone disease during the first years of use, the clinical impact is not sufficient to avoid use, since pregnancy has the same physiologic effect and the low-dose oral contraceptives in current use are less likely to effect gallbladder disease.[19] An increase in the relative risk of stone formation is associated with thiazides; if possible, dosages should be reduced or the medication discontinued.

If gallstones are incidentally noted on x-ray, ultrasound, or other clinical imaging studies of the abdomen, reassurance that asymptomatic stones do not require surgery is needed. Patients seen with symptomatic gallbladder disease need an explanation of laboratory and imaging tests, referral, and management.

Many patients who are anticipating laparoscopic cholecystectomies underrate or have unrealistic expectations about postoperative pain and activity. Preparatory guidance in this area may be efficacious to ensure a more realistic understanding of the postoperative course. Older patients can expect to spend additional time in the hospital after a cholecystectomy.

REFERENCES

1. Greenberger NJ, Paumgartner G: Diseases of the gallbladder and bile ducts. In Kasper DL, Fauci AS, Longo DL, and others, editors: *Harrison's principles of internal medicine,* ed 16, New York, 2006, McGraw-Hill.
2. Aufderheide TP, Brady WJ: Cholecystitis and biliary colic. In Tintinalli JE, Ruiz E, Krome RL, editors: *Emergency medicine,* New York, 1996, McGraw-Hill.
3. Chung SC: Acute acalculous cholecystitis: a reminder that this condition may appear in a primary care practice, *Postgrad Med* 98(3):199-204, 1995.
4. Ahmed A, Cheung RC, Keefe EB: Management of gallstones and their complications, *Am Fam Phys* 61(6):1673-1680, 1687-1688, 2000.
5. Portincasa P, Van Erpecum KJ, Vanberge-Henegouen GP: Cholesterol crystallization in bile, *Gut* 41(2):138-141, 1997.
6. Neal DD, Moritz MJ, Jarrell BE: Liver, portal hypertension, and biliary tract. In Jarrell BE, Carabasi RA, editors: *Surgery,* ed 3, Baltimore, 1996, Williams & Wilkins.
7. Ahrendt SA, Pitt HA: Biliary tract. In Townsend CM: *Sabiston textbook of surgery*, ed 17, Philadelphia, 2004, Saunders.
8. Yusoff IF, Barkun JS, Barkun AN: Diagnosis and management of cholecystitis and cholangitis, *Gastroenterol Clin North Am* 32:1145-1168, 2003.
9. Giurgiu DI, Roslyn JJ: Treatment of gallstones in the 1990s, *Prim Care* 23(3):497-513, 1996.
10. Pinto KM: Acalculous cholecystitis: a case report, *Nurse Pract* 21(10):120-122, 1996.
11. DiMarino AJ: Gastrointestinal diseases. In Myers AR, editor: *Medicine,* ed 2, Philadelphia, 1994, Harwal.
12. Yates MR, Baron TH: Pregnancy and liver disease, *Clin Liver Dis* 3(1):131-146, 1999.
13. Dayton MT, and others: The biliary tract. In Lawrence PF, Bell RM, Dayton MT, editors: *Essentials of general surgery,* ed 2, Baltimore, 1992, Williams & Wilkins.
14. Stevens KA, Chi A, Lucas LC, and others: Immediate laparoscopic cholecystectomy for acute cholecystitis: no need to wait, *Am J Surg* 192(6):756-761, 2006.
15. Chang WT, Lee KT, Chuang SC, and others: The impact of prophylactic antibiotics on postoperative infection complication in elective laparoscopic cholecystectomy: a prospective randomized study, *Am J Surg* 191(6):721-725, 2006.
16. Schwesinger WH, Diehl AK: Changing indications for laparoscopic cholecystectomy: stones without symptoms and symptoms without stones, *Surg Clin North Am* 76(3):493-504, 1996.
17. Society of American Gastrointestinal Endoscopic Surgeons: Guidelines for the clinical application of laparoscopic biliary tract surgery, *Surg Endosc* 14:771-772, 2000.
18. Jatzko GR, Lisborg PH, Pertl AM, and others: Multivariate comparison of complications after laparoscopic cholecystectomy and open cholecystectomy, *Ann Surg* 221(4):381-386, 1995.
19. Benign gallbladder disease: newer data suggest little or no excess risk with oral contraceptive use, *Contraception Rep* 8(5):9-11, 1997.

CHAPTER 138

Cirrhosis

Updated by Terry Mahan Buttaro

DEFINITION AND EPIDEMIOLOGY

Cirrhosis is a serious, irreversible disease caused by exposure to persistent toxins that cause hepatocellular injury and compromise liver function. Although the most common causes of cirrhosis are alcohol and hepatitis B, D, and C, various drugs, including acetaminophen, amiodarone, chemotherapeutic agents, antibiotics, and carbon tetrachloride, are also associated with cirrhosis. The cause can be inherited or idiopathic, but primary and secondary biliary cirrhosis, infections, viruses, hemochromatosis, autoimmune hepatitis, nonalcoholic steatohepatitis (NASH), and other disorders also play a role in the development of cirrhosis (Box 138-1).

Cirrhosis is often classified by the underlying pathologic condition, but another common classification of cirrhosis is based on histologic findings. There are three types of cirrhosis: micronodular, macronodular, and mixed form.[1] Micronodular cirrhosis, often associated with ethanol and drug abuse, occurs when the repeated presence of an offending agent prevents the regeneration of normal tissue. As a result, the regenerating tissue produces small nodules that have limited functional abilities. Macronodular cirrhosis is often seen in hepatocellular carcinoma and is distinguished by larger nodules (2 to 3 cm [0.8 to 1.2 inches] in diameter) that may contain their own blood supply. The larger nodules resemble scar tissue and have limited functional abilities. Mixed-form cirrhosis consists of both macronodules and micronodules. This class or variety of cirrhosis has mixed characteristics, and the patient's liver functions are also varied.[1]

Child's classification is a functional tool that assesses the patient's nutritional and hepatic status (Table 138-1).[2] It is a fairly reliable prognostic indicator for patients with cirrhosis and end-stage liver disease. This classification demonstrates that patients with a combination of an albumin concentration of less than 3 g/dl, a serum bilirubin concentration of more than 3 g/dl, severe ascites, encephalopathy, and generalized wasting have a 50% operative mortality rate.[3] In established cases of cirrhosis with severe hepatic dysfunction, only 50% survive 2 years and 35% survive 5 years.[2]

BOX 138-1

DISEASES CAUSING CIRRHOSIS

- Metabolic disease (diabetes mellitus)
- Wilson's disease
- Hemochromatosis
- α_1-Antitrypsin deficiency
- Cardiac failure (congestive heart failure, myocardial infarction, valvular heart disease)
- Biliary tract obstruction
  - Primary obstruction (calculi)
  - Secondary obstruction (tumor)
- Venoocclusive disease (Budd-Chiari syndrome)
- Autoimmune disease (lupus erythematosus)

TABLE 138-1 Child's Criteria for Hepatic Functional Reserve

	A (Minimal)	B (Moderate)	C (Advanced)
Serum bilirubin	<2 mg/dl	2-3 mg/dl	>3 mg/dl
Serum albumin	>3.5 g/dl	3-3.5 g/dl	<3 g/dl
Ascites	None	Easily controlled	Poorly controlled
Neurologic disorders	None	Minimal	Advanced coma
Nutrition	Excellent	Good	Poor (wasting)

From Child CG, Turcotte J: The liver and portal hypertension. In Dunphy JE, editor: *Major problems in clinical surgery*, Philadelphia, 1964, Saunders.

The Model for End Stage Liver Disease (MELD) is a newer prognostic tool for cirrhosis. Based on the underlying cause of the cirrhosis and the serum creatinine, bilirubin, and International Normalized Ratio (INR), the MELD tool is used as a prediction tool for patients with cirrhosis and for prioritizing candidates for liver transplantation.[3,4]

The prognosis of cirrhosis depends on the cause and classification of the disease. If the cirrhosis is related to alcohol or hepatotoxic drugs, the major factor that determines survival is the patient's ability to stop drinking alcohol or taking hepatotoxic drugs. Progression of the disease can be halted if this occurs.

PATHOPHYSIOLOGY

Hepatocellular injury occurs when the liver is continually exposed to toxins or diseases that produce toxemia, inflammation, ischemia, and necrosis of the hepatic tissue. The persistent inflammation and necrosis stimulate hepatocellular regeneration, causing the development of fibrous (scar) tissue such as collagen by fibroblasts. As the regeneration process progresses, rigid nodules form, distorting the normal surrounding hepatic tissue. This deformation produces increased resistance to normal blood circulation, decreased blood flow, and even obstruction of normal portal venous flow, resulting in decreased liver functional abilities.[4] Portal hypertension results when increased hydrostatic pressure within the portal venous circulation develops as a result of inflammation and obstruction of blood flow. As cirrhosis progresses, the pressure in the portal circulation rises, increasing resistance to portal venous flow. Collateral circulation develops to bypass areas of obstruction and maintain adequate blood flow.[4] The collateral path to portal circulation occurs in many areas, most commonly the peritoneum, retroperitoneum, and thoracic cavities. Collateral circulation can also occur in the rectum, esophagus, and gastric areas. These collateral vessels contain varicosities susceptible to spontaneous rupture, hemorrhage, and subsequent death.

CLINICAL PRESENTATION

The onset of symptoms can be insidious, and patients with cirrhosis can be asymptomatic. In primary biliary cirrhosis

(PBC), fatigue is reportedly the most common symptom.[5] Fatigue is also one of the most common complaints in hereditary hemochromotosis.[6] Other complaints associated with cirrhosis are nonspecific and include weakness, malaise, pruritus, and weight loss. As the patient's condition weakens, anorexia is present and is often associated with nausea and vomiting. Hematemesis can also be a common presenting complaint. Abdominal pain, if present, is related to ascites and the stretching of the muscles around the enlarged liver. Chest pain caused by cardiomegaly has also been reported. Menstrual abnormalities, impotence, and sterility are other complaints. Neuropsychiatric symptoms such as difficulty concentrating, irritability, and confusion are associated with liver function failure.

A careful history, particularly a personal history of alcohol, toxic drug, or substance use and a specific review of the patient's social and work history, can identify high-risk behaviors such as IV drug use or a homosexual lifestyle. Additional information necessary to elicit includes a thorough review of all medications, including herbal and over-the-counter products; allergies; past medical history; and family history.[7] A history of recent blood transfusion or residence in an area of high hepatitis virus incidence also can suggest the diagnosis of cirrhosis.

PHYSICAL EXAMINATION

Bruising, hematemesis, melena, and hematochezia associated with clotting dysfunction may be the presenting signs of cirrhosis. Low-grade fever, anorexia, jaundice, or right upper quadrant pain can be present. The liver may be nodular, firm, enlarged, or shrunken (seen in late stages of cirrhosis), and the spleen may be enlarged. A fluid wave and increased abdominal girth will be evident if ascites are present. The presence of high pressures in the portal circulation often leads to the development of a venous hum (best heard over the epigastrium) and rectal and esophageal varices. As a result of the fluid shifts, peripheral edema is found in the feet, legs, and hands. Delirium, lethargy, and coma occur in the later stages of cirrhosis.

Other physical signs associated with cirrhosis include weight loss; tremors; cheilosis or glossitis; spider angiomas on the face, chest, and abdomen; palmar erythema; Dupuytren's contracture; nail changes (horizontal white bands on nail beds or distal whitening of the nails); gynecomastia in men; and changes in body hair distribution in women. Asterixis, or liver flap, can be elicited with severe cases of liver failure.

DIAGNOSTICS

Sometimes, in the early stages of cirrhosis, there are no significant diagnostic findings. At other times, it is the presence of laboratory abnormalities that suggests liver dysfunction. Although not found in all patients, hypoalbuminemia, elevated serum protein, hyperbilirubinemia, and elevated liver enzymes (aspartate transaminase and alanine aminotransferase) all indicate hepatocellular inflammation or injury. The alkaline phosphatase and γ-glutamyl transpeptidase levels are also often elevated.

Additional diagnostics depend on patient presentation, but it is important to determine the exact cause of the cirrhosis

DIAGNOSTICS

Cirrhosis

LABORATORY
CBC and differential
Serum electrolytes
Serum glucose
BUN
Creatinine
Serum protein
Albumin
Globulin
LFTs
Bilirubin
Alpha-fetoprotein*
Antimitochondrial antibodies
Anti–smooth muscle antibodies
Hepatitis screen
Fasting serum ferritin
Transferrin saturation
Total iron-binding capacity
*C282Y**
*H63D**
Serum protein electrophoresis*
Serum ceruloplasmin*

IMAGING
Ultrasound
CT scan
Doppler studies

OTHER
Liver biopsy
Esophagogastroscopy

*If indicated.

in newly diagnosed patients. Thus initial serologic workups should screen for antimitochondrial antibodies (a marker of PBC that distinguishes PBC from secondary biliary cirrhosis), antinuclear antibodies, anti–smooth muscle antibodies, antibodies to hepatitis C, hepatitis B surface antigen, and antibodies to hepatitis B core antigen and surface antigen. Fasting serum ferritin, transferrin saturation, and total iron-binding capacity should be obtained to exclude hereditary hemochromatosis.[8] If the transferrin saturation is significantly elevated (>45%), genetic testing for hereditary hemochromatosis (*C282Y* and *H63D*) is indicated.[6] Other suggested serologic workups include serum protein electrophoresis and, if Wilson's disease is a consideration (patient <50 years old), serum ceruloplasmin.

Other abnormalities in laboratory results are common. Pancytopenia, anemia (frequently macrocytic), thrombocytopenia, abnormal clotting mechanisms, and prolongation of prothrombin time all contribute to an increased potential for gastrointestinal bleeding.[8] Hyponatremia can indicate advanced illness, but other electrolyte abnormalities and renal insufficiency are also common. Ultrasound or CT scan can be used to confirm liver size, assess portal circulation, and determine the presence of occult ascites or tumor. Doppler studies can evaluate patency of hepatic, splenic, and portal veins, whereas upper endoscopy establishes the presence of esophageal and/or gastric varices.[9] However, liver biopsy, which may be contraindicated if coagulopathies are present, is the preferred diagnostic test to confirm cirrhosis and determine the cause of the liver dysfunction. Abdominal paracentesis and abdominal fluid analysis (to identify bacterial peritonitis or peritoneal carcinomatosis) are indicated in the presence of ascites. Upper endoscopy is recommended to diagnose esophageal varices.

DIFFERENTIAL DIAGNOSIS

Hepatocellular injury has varied causes, but it can be idiopathic. PBC is a chronic, progressive cholestatic disease of unknown etiology, although one recent study suggests environmental factors may play a role.[10] The nonsuppurative, granulomatous inflammatory destruction of the small interlobular bile ducts associated with PCB occurs within the liver and results in the development of cholestasis, liver failure, and cirrhosis.

Secondary biliary cirrhosis occurs when the disease is related to extrahepatic disease, as seen with cardiac failure, hemochromatosis, or Wilson's disease. Patients with neuropsychiatric symptoms should be evaluated for Wilson's disease. Uremia, nephrotic syndrome, metabolic disorders, pericarditis, various blood dyscrasias, biliary disease, and hepatitis are conditions that impair liver function and mimic cirrhosis. Thrombosis that is the result of cardiac or hematologic manifestations can obstruct blood flow and significantly alter liver function. The presence of a tumor (hepatocellular carcinoma or metastatic tumors) can be detected by imaging and is suspected if the serum alpha-fetoprotein concentration is elevated. The diagnosis of emphysema accompanied by liver dysfunction, especially in younger patients, suggests possible α_1-antitrypsin deficiency.[8] The presence of diabetes and endocrine disturbances in an older patient suggests hemochromatosis.[11] NASH, primary sclerosing cholangitis, or a parasitic infection such as *Schistosoma mansoni* should also be considered as a possible cause of hepatocellular injury.

DIFFERENTIAL DIAGNOSIS

Cirrhosis

- Primary biliary cirrhosis
- Secondary biliary cirrhosis
- Cardiac failure
- Hemochromatosis
- Wilson's disease
- Uremia
- Nephrotic syndrome
- Metabolic disorders
- Pericarditis
- Blood dyscrasias
- Biliary disease
- Hepatitis
- Thrombosis
- Tumor
- α_1-Antitrypsin deficiency
- Nonalcoholic steatohepatitis (NASH)
- Primary sclerosing cholangitis
- Parasitic infection
- Pancreatitis
- Common bile duct obstruction

MANAGEMENT

Cirrhosis is an irreversible disease process; however, careful management and early treatment of complications can improve survival. Thus the main focus of treatment involves the prevention of further liver dysfunction and the treatment of complications. Patients should be immunized with polyvalent pneumococcal vaccine, yearly influenza vaccine, and, unless already immune, both hepatitis A and B vaccines.[9,12] Reversible causes of cirrhosis such as alcohol or hepatotoxic medications such as NSAIDs must be eliminated (Box 138-2) because continued use will result in a limited life expectancy. Patients who have ongoing viral hepatitis B or C infection can have increased life expectancy with antiviral therapy, and those with autoimmune hepatitis benefit from corticosteroid therapy.[9,13] Other recommendations to prevent complications include yearly upper endoscopy to assess for the presence of esophageal varices and screening for liver cancer with a

BOX 138-2

HEPATOTOXIC DRUGS AND SUBSTANCES

ENVIRONMENTAL TOXINS

- Arsenic
- Fluorine
- Trichloroethylene
- Copper
- Vinyl chloride
- Toluene

DRUGS

- Isoniazid
- Folic acid analogs
- Sodium valproate
- Quinolone antibiotics
- Acetaminophen
- L-Asparaginase
- Purine antimetabolites
- Heavy metal chemotherapeutics
- Phenothiazines
- Ketoconazole
- Cytidine analogs
- Anthracenediones
- Megadose vitamin E
- NSAIDs
- Iron salts
- Gold sodium thiomalate
- Tetracycline
- Testosterone and derivatives
- Thioxanthenes
- Aspirin (high dose: >2 g/day)
- Nitrofurantoin
- Interleukins
- Inhaled anesthetics
- Retinoic acid and derivatives
- Estrogen antagonist and agonists
- Alkylating agents
- Hetastarch
- Flutamide, goserelin
- Griseofulvin
- Clozapine
- Butyrophenones
- Methyldopa
- Dantrolene

yearly liver ultrasound and serum alpha-fetoprotein every 6 months.[9,12,13]

Patients with portal hypertension require careful monitoring for complications such as ascites and varices. Paracentesis or the placement of a peritoneovenous shunt will help with fluid redistribution if a 2000 mg/day sodium diet, fluid restriction, and diuretic therapy are not successful (Box 138-3). Management of varices entails confirming the presence and location of varices. Although numerous drugs are currently being studied, only nonselective β-adrenergic blockers (e.g., propranolol and nadolol) have shown clear benefit in decreasing the risk of hemorrhage and death in patients who have large varices but have not yet had a variceal bleed.[9] Both these medications seem to provide some protection in preventing subsequent bleeding. For patients unable to take a beta blocker, isosorbide mononitrate 20 mg PO b.i.d. may be beneficial.[9] Somatostatin infusions for acute variceal bleeding seem to be effective and are associated with improved survival.[14] Bleeding varices can also be treated by balloon tamponade, injection sclerotherapy, endoscopic variceal band ligation, transjugular interhepatic portosystemic shunts (TIPS), portosystemic shunts, and/or periesophageal devascularization procedures[14,15] (Box 138-4). Endoscopic sclerotherapy and endoscopic band ligation have both been associated with improved survival.

Neurotoxin development is associated with severe liver disease and causes the cognitive defects of hepatic encephalopathy. Numerous factors, including infections, medications, gastrointestinal bleeding, and constipation, have been linked to the development of hepatic encephalopathy. The serum ammonia level may or may not be elevated. Oral lactulose 30 to 45 ml PO t.i.d. or q.i.d. to produce two or three daily soft stools helps treat and prevent hepatic encephalopathy, but the underlying cause should also be corrected. If the patient develops diarrhea, the dosage should be decreased to prevent fluid and electrolyte imbalance. Metronidazole and neomycin, an aminoglycoside, are sometimes used to treat hepatic encephalopathy. Neomycin should be used cautiously, especially if there is associated renal impairment.

BOX 138-3

MANAGEMENT OF ASCITES

DIETARY MANAGEMENT

- Restrict sodium to 2 g/day.
- Obtain dietary consultation.
- Protein: 1 to 1.5 g/kg/day.

FLUID MANAGEMENT

- Restrict fluid to 1500 ml when there is marked hyponatremia.
- Consider referral for large-volume paracentesis (5 to 6 L); admit for procedure.

PHARMACOLOGIC MANAGEMENT

- When sodium levels remain high, begin spironolactone 100 mg/day.
- Check sodium levels in 1 week, and if natriuresis and diuresis do not occur, increase daily dose by 100 mg every 4 to 5 days to a maximum of 400 mg/day. Monitor carefully for hyperkalemia.
- Adjust diuretic doses so that no more than 0.5 kg (1 pound) of fluid is lost per day. Consider furosemide in combination with spironolactone to promote diuresis.
- If patient has ascites and peripheral edema, no more than 1 kg of fluid loss is acceptable.
- Decrease dosage of diuretics by 50% if patient has signs and symptoms of hypovolemia.

LABORATORY TESTS

- Monitor weight, potassium, BUN, and creatinine every week or more often if patient's condition warrants it.

BOX 138-4

PREVENTION OF GASTROINTESTINAL BLEEDING

- Administer a beta blocker (propranolol) for prophylaxis in patients at increased risk for bleeding (because of ascites, encephalopathy, or confirmed presence of varices).
- Consider consultation with a gastroenterologist for patients to have sclerotherapy and shunt procedures for prevention of recurrent variceal bleeding.
- Monitor prothrombin time and platelet count. Although patients can have severe alterations in prothrombin time/partial thromboplastin time (PT/PTT), bleeding may not occur, and treatment is not indicated. To be certain that a vitamin K deficiency is not contributing to the alterations in PT/PTT, consider administering vitamin K 5 to 25 mg PO or 10 mg SQ or IM. May repeat in 12 hours if indicated.

Appropriate, regular diagnostic testing and attention to each patient's nutritional status are necessary to ensure management of iron deficiency, fluid and electrolyte balance, and protein-calorie malnutrition. The health care provider and nutritionist can design a patient-centered plan that will focus on consumption of a low-sodium diet, combined with protein 1 to 1.5 g/kg/day, with foods that meet the patient's physical, emotional, and cultural needs. Multivitamin supplementation each day is also advised. Patients with Wernicke's encephalopathy also require thiamine supplementation. The use of herbal medications has been studied, but these medications have not proved to be beneficial and, in some instances, may even be harmful.

The treatment of PBC is primarily palliative, although transplantation may be beneficial in severe cases. Current recommendations for the treatment of NASH include glycemic control, treatment for hyperlipidemia, and gradual weight loss when indicated. Small studies suggest that pioglitazone or metformin can decrease hepatic inflammation, but further research is necessary to provide conclusive evidence that these medications are, in fact, beneficial.[16-18]

Co-Management with Specialists

Management of the patient with cirrhosis is complex and requires coordinated efforts by specialists. For patients with drug or alcohol abuse, the first priority is to assist in eliminating the agent from use. Drug and alcohol treatment programs can help both the patient and the family. Collaboration with mental health specialists provides information about the patient's progress with alcohol or drug abuse and determines safe medication choices for patients if pharmacologic support for detoxification is needed.

The availability of social services is helpful in acquiring financial, physical, or psychologic assistance; attaining therapeutic home aides and home health nursing care; recommending support groups; or arranging transportation. If long-term care is needed, the social worker can provide information about available facilities that will meet the patient's and family's needs.

Endoscopic evaluation by the gastroenterologist is recommended to assess the presence of varices and or suspected variceal bleeding. Surgical consultation may also be indicated for surgical decompression of the portal system.

COMPLICATIONS

Ascites is often associated with cirrhosis and is produced by an imbalance between the formation and distribution of peritoneal fluid. Spontaneous bacterial peritonitis is a serious infection and a potential consequence of ascites. A recent study has shown an increased incidence of gram-positive cocci in bacterial peritonitis and an increased resistance to quinolone therapy.[19]

Endocrine abnormalities are common, and diabetes is often associated with cirrhosis, particularly when related to alcohol or hemochromatosis. Other complications associated with cirrhosis include hepatocellular carcinoma, portal hypertension, gastrointestinal bleeding, hepatorenal syndrome, pulmonary hypertension, hypoxemia, hepatic hydrothorax, coagulopathies, and splenomegaly or splenic hemorrhage.[20,21] Some patients can be severely immunocompromised and at risk for infection.

When hepatocellular damage is extensive, hepatic failure results. Hepatic encephalopathy, a neuropsychiatric syndrome typified by mental status changes and asterixis, is caused by high ammonia levels and rising toxic waste products (end products of metabolism). Hepatic encephalopathy can be chronic or acute and is often associated with gastrointestinal bleeding, increased dietary protein, fluid and electrolyte disorders, medications, or infection. Early recognition, correction of the underlying precipitant, careful monitoring, and treatment with lactulose or other medications to control ammonia production are essential (Box 138-5).

INDICATIONS FOR REFERRAL OR HOSPITALIZATION

Health care providers manage most patients with cirrhosis and monitor for complications. Prompt consultation and hospitalization are indicated for gastrointestinal bleeding, encephalopathy, increasing azotemia, peritoneal irritation, or unexplained fever.[21] Consultation with a gastroenterologist is indicated for ascites unresponsive to fluid and sodium restriction, diuresis, large-volume paracentesis (5 to 6 L), or gastrointestinal bleeding from varices. Patients with intractable ascites, variceal bleeding, progressive encephalopathy, Wilson's disease, end-stage liver disease, or hemochromatosis and candidates for liver transplantation are managed by a gastroenterologist. Consultation with a nephrologist is indicated for patients with oliguria, anuria, or azotemia.

BOX 138-5

HEPATIC FAILURE MANAGEMENT

1. Further restrict protein intake to 20 to 30 g/day.
2. Consult dietitian to ensure patient's intake of amino acids is adequate.
3. Monitor mental status; check asterixis by using a five-point star or signature testing.
4. Monitor ammonia levels.
5. Consider oral lactulose 15 to 30 ml q 4-6 hr, with subsequent adjustments in dosage to allow two or three soft stools per day. Consider adding oral neomycin 1 g b.i.d., or metronidazole 250 mg, if lactulose does not decrease ammonia levels.

BOX 138-6

PATIENT AND FAMILY EDUCATION

1. Eliminate use of alcohol and any hepatotoxic drugs.
2. Maintain strict dietary discipline.
    - Sodium restriction to 2 g/day
    - Protein restriction to 1 to 1.5 g/kg/day
    - Consult dietitian when in doubt about any phase of the diet.
3. Follow exercise plan.
    - Consult with physical therapist to determine plan for patient.
4. Participate in support group activities.
    - Alcoholics Anonymous
    - Al-Anon
5. Watch for signs of peripheral edema; call office for weight gain greater than 0.9 kg (2 pounds) per day.
6. Instruct patient's family to report any changes in patient's sensorium, posture, or gait.

PATIENT AND FAMILY EDUCATION

The patient and family should understand the benefits of the treatment plan. Dietary discipline, avoidance of hepatotoxic drugs (including NSAIDs), and support group activities are ways to achieve a successful outcome (Box 138-6). The importance of reducing the risk of gastrointestinal bleeding, recognizing the signs of variceal bleeding, and taking the appropriate course of action if bleeding occurs should be discussed.

Many patients with cirrhosis may be depressed. However, the use of antidepressant drugs is not usually indicated because of the high risk of oversedation and toxicity. Consultation with a psychopharmacologist could assist in designing a treatment regimen that could help the patient through this depression. Signs and complications of depression, as well as indications for immediate intervention, should be reviewed with the patient and family.

REFERENCES

1. Tobias M: Cirrhosis. In *Of the GI system and the liver*, Philadelphia, 1995, Lippincott.
2. Freidman L: Liver, biliary tract and pancreas. In Tierney LM, McPhee SJ, Papadakis A, editors: *Current medical diagnosis and treatment*, ed 44, Stamford, Conn, 2005, Appleton & Lange.
3. Goldberg E, Chopra S: *Overview of the complications, prognosis, and management of cirrhosis*, retrieved Jan 30, 2007, from http://www.uptodateonline.com/utd/content/topic.do?topicKey=cirrhosi/9247&selectedTitle=3~646.
4. Heuman DM, Abou-Assi SG, Habib A, and others: Persistent ascites and low serum sodium identify patients with cirrhosis and low MELD scores who are at high risk for early death, *Hepatology* 40(4):802-810, 2004.
5. Prince MI, James OF, Holland NP, and others: Validation of a fatigue impact score in primary biliary cirrhosis: towards a standard for clinical and trial use, *J Hepatol* 32:368-373, 2000.

6. Perlman BL: Hereditary hemochromatosis: early detection of a common yet elusive disease, *Consultant* 42:237-250, 2002.
7. Giboney PT: Mildly elevated liver transaminase levels in the asymptomatic patient, *Am Fam Phys* 71(6):1105-1110, 2005.
8. Portis R, Jacobs MA, Skerman JH, and others: HELLP syndrome: pathophysiology and anesthetic considerations, *AANA J* 65:37-47, 1997.
9. Riley TR, Bhatti AM: Preventive strategies in chronic liver disease, part II, Cirrhosis, *Am Fam Phys,* 2001, retrieved Jan 16, 2006, from http://www.aafp.org/afp/20011115/1735.html.
10. Prince MI, Chetwynd A, Diggle P, and others: The geographical distribution of primary biliary cirrhosis in a well-defined cohort, *Hepatology* 34:1083-1088, 2001.
11. Chalasani N, Horlander JC, Said A, and others: Screening for hepatocellular carcinoma in patients with advanced cirrhosis, *Am J Gastroenterol* 94:2988-2993, 1999.
12. Shiratori Y, Ito Y, Yokosuka O, and others: Antiviral therapy for cirrhotic hepatitis C: association with reduced hepatocellular carcinoma development and improved survival, *Ann Intern Med* 142(2):105-114, 2005.
13. Goldberg E, Chopra S: *Diagnostic approach to the patient with cirrhosis,* retrieved Jan 30, 2007, from http://www.uptodate.com.http://www.uptodateonline.com/utd/content/topic.do?topicKey=cirrhosi/6052&selectedTitle=1~646.
14. Moitinho E, Planas R, Banares R, and others: Multicenter randomized controlled trial comparing different schedules of somatostatin in the treatment of acute variceal bleeding, *J Hepatol* 35:712-718, 2001.
15. Pomier-Layrargues G, Villeneuve JP, and others: Transjugular intrahepatic portosystemic shunt (TIPS) versus endoscopic variceal ligation in the prevention of variceal bleeding in patients with cirrhosis: a random trial, *Gut* 48:390-396, 2001.
16. Nair S, Diehl AM, Wiseman M, and others: Metformin in the treatment of non-alcoholic steatohepatitis: a pilot open label trial, *Aliment Pharmacol Ther* 20:23, 2004.
17. Promrat K, Lutchman G, Uwaifo GI, and others: A pilot study of pioglitazone treatment for nonalcoholic steatohepatitis, *Hepatology* 39:188, 2004.
18. Sheth SG, Gordon FD, Chopra S: Review of nonalcoholic steatohepatitis, *Ann Intern Med* 126:137-145, 1997.
19. Fernandez J, Navasa M, Gómez J, Colmenero J, and others: Bacterial infections in cirrhosis: epidemiological changes with invasive procedures and norfloxacin prophylaxis, *Hepatology* 35:140-148, 2002.
20. Benvegnu L, Noventa FP, Gatta A, and others: Evidence for an association between the aetiology of cirrhosis and pattern of hepatocellular carcinoma development, *Gut* 48:110-115, 2001.
21. Kuper H, Ye W, Adami HO, and others: The risk of liver and bile duct cancer in patients with chronic viral hepatitis, alcoholism, or cirrhosis, *Hepatology* 34(4 Pt 1):714-718, 2001.

CHAPTER 139

Constipation

Terry Mahan Buttaro

DEFINITION AND EPIDEMIOLOGY

Constipation is one of the most common gastrointestinal complaints in the United States, resulting in more than 2.5 million primary care visits each year.[1] Hundreds of millions of dollars are spent to treat this chronic disorder, which especially affects children, women, and older adults. The causes of constipation are varied, but in older adults the increased incidence is possibly associated with age-related neuromuscular dysfunction.[2] Diminished vitality, decreased activity, and the consequences of many illnesses and medications are additional causes[3,4] (Box 139-1). Although not usually considered life threatening, constipation can be disconcerting and disabling and has been associated with urinary tract infections, impaction, and ileus.[2,3]

Constipation is usually defined as a decrease in the frequency of bowel movements. However, to fulfill the Rome II criteria for constipation, two of the following symptoms must have been present for at least 12 weeks in the past year: fewer than two bowel movements per week or the passage of hard or lumpy stools; a sensation of straining, a feeling of incomplete evacuation, and/or anorectal obstruction; and manual maneuvers to aid defecation in more than 25% of defecations.[5-7] Less than three stools per week is usually considered abnormal. Soft, easily passed stools are not indicative of constipation. A true clinical diagnosis is the finding of a large amount of feces in the rectal ampulla on digital examination and/or excessive feces in the colon, rectum, or both on the abdominal radiograph.

PATHOPHYSIOLOGY

The primary function of the large intestine is to store and concentrate fecal material before defecation. If the fecal contents remain in the large intestine for long periods, almost all water is absorbed, resulting in hard stools. Normal colonic motility depends on the integrity of the central nervous

BOX 139-1

MEDICATIONS ASSOCIATED WITH CONSTIPATION

- Amantidine
- Amitriptyline
- Antacids
- Anticholinergics
- Antihistamines
- Calcium channel blockers
- Calcium supplements
- Diuretics
- Iron supplements
- Narcotics
- NSAIDs

system, autonomic nervous system, gut wall innervation and receptors, circular smooth muscle, gastrointestinal neurotransmitters, and hormones. Healthy adults have normal gut transit time; total gut transit time is prolonged in patients with constipation.

Disordered colonic transit and pelvic floor or anorectal dysfunction (a failure to adequately empty the rectal contents) are the two primary causes of constipation.[8] Secondary causes include ignoring the urge to defecate; inadequate fiber or fluid intake; medications; pregnancy; Hirschsprung's disease; hypothyroidism; hypoparathyroidism; diabetes; hypokalemia; hypercalcemia; motility disorders; psychologic disturbances; and neurologic disorders such as Parkinson's disease, multiple sclerosis, and disorders of the peripheral or central nervous system. Fistulas, hemorrhoids, rectoceles, abscesses, neoplasms, and other functional abnormalities are also associated with constipation, but the cause can be idiopathic or even related to irritable bowel syndrome. Parasitic infections such as *Ascaris lumbricoides* (an intestinal nematode) have been identified with intestinal obstruction and should be considered in patients who travel to or live in endemic areas.[9]

CLINICAL PRESENTATION

Constipation is a subjective complaint and varies from one individual to another. Patients may complain of constipation and describe a feeling of nausea, bloating, and cramping and difficulty passing stools. The patient history should include when the change in bowel pattern occurred; the number of stools per day and week; the last bowel movement; the need to strain during defecation; the sensation of incomplete evacuation; and any episodes of fecal incontinence, diarrhea, abdominal pain, or blood or pain with defecation.[10,11] Possible systemic, neurologic, or other related symptoms should be elicited in addition to a past history of associated illnesses, a 24-hour dietary and fluid review, and complete medication review (including laxative and over-the-counter medication use).

PHYSICAL EXAMINATION

Although it is not uncommon to have normal findings, the physical examination is performed to exclude or verify the symptoms of constipation. Orthostatic hypotension or tachycardia implies dehydration; weight loss suggests anorexia or carcinoma. The oral examination may suggest poor dentition, ill-fitting dentures, lesions, or dehydration. Abdominal scars indicate a surgical history. Peristalsis and bowel sounds may be increased or decreased, suggesting a threatened obstruction or ileus. There may be increased dullness over areas of stool, and masses may be palpated. Rebound tenderness suggests a peritoneal inflammation. A gynecologic examination may demonstrate a rectocele. A rectal examination and anoscopy should determine anal abnormalities, sphincter tone and function, pain, lesions, rectal prolapse, impaction, hemorrhoids, or fissures. The neurologic examination may elicit autonomic dysfunction or neuropathy. Perineal descent is assessed by having the patient bear down while lying in the left lateral position (normal perineal descent while straining is 1 to 4 cm [0.4 to 1.6 inches]).

DIAGNOSTICS

Diagnostics exclude underlying pathologic conditions and metabolic disturbances. A CBC and differential and abdominal CT scan are indicated for acute-onset constipation to determine the existence of an intraabdominal infection or obstruction.[12] Abdominal x-ray studies and/or abdominal CT scan and CBC and differential are necessary in the presence of abdominal discomfort, nausea, or vomiting to exclude obstruction, ileus, megacolon, or volvulus. A recent change in bowel habits or the presence of abdominal pain or rectal bleeding mandates an evaluation for an obstructing neoplasm with colonoscopy or a barium enema. Abdominal radiographs or an abdominal ultrasound, plus a stool culture, is indicated if ascariasis is suspected.[9]

Other indicated diagnostics to evaluate chronic constipation include a stool sample for occult blood; thyroid-stimulating hormone; CBC; and chemistry profile, including calcium, potassium, and blood glucose. Although not necessarily indicated, a urinalysis and culture may reveal chronic cystitis, which is often related to constipation.

Further testing for chronic constipation that does not respond to therapeutic intervention includes balloon expulsion testing, barium enema, colonic transport, anorectal manometry, defecography, and electromyelography.[13,14]

DIFFERENTIAL DIAGNOSIS

It is critical to recognize the pathologic conditions that first manifest as constipation. Acute-onset constipation requires emergent evaluation to identify ileus, intraabdominal infection (e.g., appendicitis, diverticulitis), toxic megacolon, or obstructing lesion.[13] Causes of chronic constipation that must be considered include anxiety or other psychogenic disorder, colorectal carcinoma, colonic obstruction, ovarian cancer, hypothyroidism, hypopituitary disorder, hypokalemia, hypercalcemia, multiple endocrine neoplasia type 2, parasitic

DIAGNOSTICS

Constipation

LABORATORY
Urinalysis*
Stool for occult blood
TSH
CBC and differential
Chemistry profile (including calcium, potassium, serum glucose)
Stool culture*

IMAGING
Abdominal radiographs (KUB—flat plate and upright)*
Abdominal ultrasound*

OTHER
Barium enema*
Colonoscopy or flexible sigmoidoscopy*
Anorectal manometry*
Electromyelogram*
Colonic transport studies*

*If indicated.

DIFFERENTIAL DIAGNOSIS

Constipation

ACUTE CONSTIPATION
- Intraabdominal infection
- Ileus
- Toxic megacolon
- Obstructing lesion

CHRONIC CONSTIPATION
- Colon cancer
- Ovarian cancer
- Obstruction
- Endocrine disorder
- Electrolyte disorder
- Parasitic infection
- Motility disorders
- Neurologic disorders
- Psychologic disorder
- Rectal fissure
- Irritable bowel syndrome

infection, motility disorder, rectal fissure, and irritable bowel syndrome with alternating constipation and diarrhea.[15]

MANAGEMENT

Prevention and management of constipation depend on both the underlying cause and the individual patient. Volvulus and obstruction require immediate surgical evaluation. Ileus and pseudoobstruction can be medically managed with nasogastric suction and IV fluid.

Once a pathologic or life-threatening condition has been excluded, patients should be encouraged to keep a stool diary (noting frequency of stooling and associated symptoms) to both substantiate the constipation and aid in determining the effectiveness of interventions.[16] Although there is limited evidence specifying the correct management for constipation, the initial approach should include management of secondary causes, dietary measures, increased fluids to 1.5 to 2 L/day, periodic exercise, and bowel training.[3,17] An increase in fiber to 20 to 40 g/day over a period of weeks is appropriate. Often five prunes per day or 2 tablespoons of bran with meals followed by at least 8 ounces of liquid are adequate. If a patient is unable to consume the required diet, fiber supplements such as psyllium (Fiberall) or polycarbophil (FiberCon) combined with increased fluids are recommended. Initiating a moderate exercise program may help increase peristalsis, although exercise has not been proved to be an effective therapy. Patients should also be encouraged to develop regular bowel habits by allowing enough time for satisfactory bowel elimination and by attempting to defecate during a specific time period each day. Because the gastrocolic response is stimulated by eating, the patient should be encouraged to toilet 30 minutes after eating a meal.

Pharmacologic treatment is appropriate if there is no response to conservative measures. Although there is no evidence to suggest that fiber is superior to laxatives, there is moderate evidence to support the use of psyllium; thus, bulking agents such as psyllium or methylcellulose are suitable initially.[18] Docusate sodium may be added to soften the stool if bulk-forming agents are ineffective. For the flatulence and bloating associated with chronic constipation, probiotic beverages containing *Lactobacillus casei* strain Shirota may be helpful.

If straining is still present despite the addition of fiber and increased fluids, the American Gastroenterological Association (AGA) recommends Milk of Magnesia (MOM). MOM is readily available and inexpensive, but it has not been studied; therefore its true efficacy is unknown.[19] MOM should be used judiciously in patients with a history of congestive heart failure or renal insufficiency to avoid fluid and electrolyte abnormalities.[6,20] In the past there were few studies to recommend other laxatives, but recent evidence suggests that lactulose and polyethylene glycol (MiraLax) are effective.[21,22] Lactulose and polyethylene glycol are osmotic laxatives that are relatively safe (provided liquid intake is adequate) and can be titrated to produce a daily bowel movement.[23] Although not contraindicated, lactulose should be used cautiously in patients with diabetes. Tegaserod, a 5-HT_4 receptor partial agonist originally approved for constipation-related irritable bowel syndrome, has been taken off the U.S. market because adverse cardiovascular events were reported in some users.[24] The use of a stimulant laxative (senna or bisacodyl) every 3 days is also acceptable. The chronic use of castor oil, senna, cascara, or bisacodyl has been associated with intestinal mucosal damage and electrolyte abnormalities. The use of mineral oil has been associated with vitamin deficiency and therefore is not recommended.

A suppository, Fleet's enema, or tap water enema may also be used. Other medications, including colchicines, have shown efficacy in some studies but are not currently recommended.[25]

Patients with constipation related to pelvic floor dysfunction or neurologic injury may benefit from biofeedback training if a center that is equipped to provide electromyogram-guided biofeedback is available.[26-28] Surgical evaluation is necessary for patients with rectal prolapse and for those who require surgical intervention. The phases of constipation management are listed in Box 139-2.

COMPLICATIONS

Complications of constipation include the development of an ileus, ischemic bowel, megacolon, hernia, hemorrhoids, fecal impaction, or rectal or uterine prolapse. Laxative dependency is an added consequence.

INDICATIONS FOR REFERRAL OR HOSPITALIZATION

Nausea, vomiting, fever, and abdominal pain may indicate an ileus or ischemia and must be managed accordingly. Treatment is usually supportive and requires physician consultation when hospitalization is necessary to provide parenteral fluids and pain management. Referral to a gastroenterologist is indicated if a pathologic condition is suspected or if therapies are unsuccessful.

BOX 139-2

CONSTIPATION MANAGEMENT

PHASE 1

Lifestyle changes
- Exercise regularly.
- Develop regular bowel habits.

Dietary changes
- Increase dietary fiber to 20 to 40 g/day (prunes, bran, beans, broccoli, spinach, carrots, corn, potato, apple, and pears with skin).
- Decrease fats, particularly cheese.
- Increase fluids to 1.5 to 2 L/day.

PHASE 2

Use bulk-forming laxatives: methylcellulose (Citrucel) or psyllium (Metamucil), 1 teaspoon to 1 tablespoon one to three times daily in 240 ml water; or calcium polycarbophil (FiberCon), 2 tablets with 8 ounces of water one to four times daily, followed by a second glass of water; fluid intake should be increased.

PHASE 3

Use stool softeners.
- Dioctyl sodium sulfosuccinate: 100 mg PO t.i.d. followed by 8 ounces of water

PHASE 4

Use saline laxatives, if there are no contraindications.
- Milk of magnesia: 30 ml PO p.r.n. h.s.
- Magnesium citrate: 30 ml PO p.r.n. h.s.
- Fleet enema: one enema per rectum

PHASE 5

Use osmotic laxatives.
- Lactulose: 30 to 45 ml PO up to q.i.d., or 1 tablespoon every hour until bowel movement*
- MiraLax: 17 g in 8 ounces of water p.r.n. q. day*

Use stimulant laxatives.
- Bisacodyl: 5-15 mg PO q. day p.r.n.
- Senna (Senokot): 2 tablets PO p.r.n. h.s.
- Bisacodyl (Dulcolax) suppository: 1 per rectum q 3 days p.r.n.

PHASE 6

Severely constipated patients may require both oral laxatives and enemas or a suppository to alleviate constipation.

*These products may be expensive.

PATIENT AND FAMILY EDUCATION AND HEALTH PROMOTION

It is imperative that lifestyle changes be reinforced to establish consistent bowel habits. Patients should not delay in responding to the call to defecate and should be encouraged to sit on the toilet, with feet placed on a stool, at the same time each day for approximately 10 minutes; this should occur preferably after meals and/or the ingestion of a warm liquid to stimulate the gastrocolic reflex. The promotion of a low-fat, high-fiber diet and a minimum of 2 L of fluid per day is recommended. However, dietary fiber should be gradually introduced to avoid severe cramping and bloating. It is important that patients receive a careful explanation of medication side effects and understand the importance of avoiding laxatives when pregnant or unless necessary. Patients should also contact the health care provider for any change in bowel habits or if the constipation is associated with fever, bleeding, weight loss, and abdominal pain.

REFERENCES

1. Stewart WF, Liberman JN, Sandler RS, and others: Epidemiology of constipation (EPOC) study in the United States: relation of clinical subtypes to sociodemographic features, *Am J Gastroenterol* 94:3530-3540, 1999.
2. Camilleri M, Lee JS, Viramontes B, and others: Insights into the pathophysiology and mechanisms of constipation, irritable bowel syndrome, and diverticulosis in older people, *J Am Geriatric Soc* 48(9):1142-1150, 2000.
3. Abyad A, Mourad F: Constipation: common sense care of the older patient, *Geriatrics* 51(12):28-34, 1996.
4. Talley NJ, Fleming KC, Evans JM, and others: Constipation in an elderly community: a study of prevalence and potential risk factors, *Am J Gastroenterol* 91(1):19-25, 1996.
5. Robson K, Lembo T: Management of constipation in geriatric patients, *Long-Term Care Interface* 2(10):54-58, 2001.
6. Thompson WG, Longstreth GF, Drossman DA, and others: Functional bowel disorders and functional abdominal pain, *Gut* 45(Suppl 2):43-47, 1999.
7. American Gastroenterological Association: APA guideline: constipation, *Am J Gastroenterol* 119:1761, 2000.
8. Ashraf W, Park F, Lof J, and others: An examination of the reliability of reported stool frequency in the diagnosis of idiopathic constipation, *Am J Gastroenterol* 91(1):26-32, 1996.
9. Pfeifer J, Agachan F, Wexner SD: Surgery for constipation: a review, *Dis Colon Rectum* 39(4):444-460, 1996.
10. Wasadikar PP, Kulkarni AB: Intestinal obstruction due to ascariasis, *Br J Surg* 84(3):410-412, 1997.
11. Agachan F, Chen T, Pfeifer J, and others: A constipation scoring system to simplify evaluation and management of constipated patients, *Rectum* 39(6):681-685, 1996.
12. Basson MD: *Constipation, 2006*, retrieved Jan 20, 2007, from http://www.emedicine.com/med/topic2833.htm.
13. Koch A, Volderholzer WA, Klauser AG, and others: Symptoms in chronic constipation, *Dis Colon Rectum* 40(8):902-906, 1997.
14. Minguez M, Herreros B, Sanchiz V, and others: Predictive value of the balloon expulsion test for excluding the diagnosis of pelvic floor dyssynergia in constipation, *Gastroenterology* 126:57, 2004.
15. Richard ML, Carter SM, Pourmotabbed G: *Multiple endocrine neoplasia type 2*, 2005, retrieved Dec 20, 2005, from http://www.emedicine.com/med/topic1520.htm.
16. Bassotti G, Stanghellini V, Chiarioni G, and others: Upper gastrointestinal motor activity in patients with slow-transit constipation: further evidence for an enteric neuropathy, *Dig Dis Sci* 41(10):1999-2005, 1996.
17. Ashraf W, Pfeiffer RF, Park F, and others: Constipation in Parkinson's disease: objective assessment and response to psyllium, *Move Dis* 12(6):946-951, 1997.
18. Benton JM, O'Hara PA, Chen H, and others: Changing bowel hygiene practice successfully: a program to reduce laxative use in a chronic care hospital, *Geriatr Nurs* 18(1):12-17, 1997.
19. American College of Gastroenterology Chronic Constipation Task Force: An evidence-based approach to the management of chronic constipation in North America, *Am J Gastroenterol* 100:S1-S4, 2005.
20. Tramonte SM, Brand MB, Mulrow CD, and others: The treatment of chronic constipation in adults: a systemic review, *J Gen Intern Med* 12(1):15-24, 1997.
21. Ramkumar D, Rao SS: Efficacy and safety of traditional medical therapies for chronic constipation: systematic review, *Am J Gastroenterol* 100(4):936-971, 2005.
22. Migeon-Duballet I, Chabin M, Gautier A, and others: Long-term efficacy and cost-effectiveness of polyethylene glycol 3350 plus electrolytes in chronic constipation: a retrospective study in a disabled population, *Curr Med Res Opin* 22(6):1227-1235, 2006.
23. Verne GN, Davis RH, Robinson ME, and others: Treatment of chronic constipation with colchicine: randomized, double-blind, placebo-controlled, crossover trial, *Am J Gastroenterol* 98:1112, 2003.

24. US Food and Drug Administration, Center for Drug Evaluation and Research: *FDA public health advisory: tegaserod maleate (marketed as Zelnorm)*, retrieved April 23, 2007, from http://www.fda.gov/cder/drug/advisory/tegaserod.htm.
25. Emmanuel AV, Roy AJ, Nicholls TJ, and others: Prucalopride, a systemic enterokinetic, for the treatment of constipation, *Aliment Pharmacol Ther* 16:1347, 2002.
26. Clausen MR, Mortensen PB: Lactulose, disaccharides and colonic flora: clinical consequences, *Drugs* 53(6):930-942, 1997.
27. Ko CY, Tong J, Lehman RE, and others: Biofeedback is effective therapy for fecal incontinence and constipation, *Arch Surg* 132(8):829-833, 1997.
28. Van Outryve M, Pelckmans P: Biofeedback is superior to laxatives for normal transit constipation due to pelvic floor dyssynergia, *Gastroenterology* 131(1):333-334, 2006.

CHAPTER **140**

Diarrhea, Noninfectious

Terry Davies

DEFINITION AND EPIDEMIOLOGY

Worldwide, diarrhea accounts for more than 2 million deaths annually. In the United States, diarrhea accounts for more than 1 million physician visits; 250,000 hospital admissions; and 3000 deaths, mainly in older adults.[1-3] Diarrhea is defined as an increase in stool frequency of more than three stools per day, liquid stool, or at least 200 g of stool per day.[3] It can be further defined as infectious (inflammatory and noninflammatory) or noninfectious; and acute (less than 2 weeks' duration), persistent (2 to 4 weeks' duration), or chronic diarrhea (more than 4 weeks' duration).[1]

Diarrhea can range from a mild, self-limited episode to a severe life-threatening illness. Acute diarrhea accounts for 90% of cases and typically has an abrupt onset. Symptoms range from mild abdominal cramping to elevated fever, chills, nausea, and vomiting. Further evaluation is warranted if the diarrhea is profuse; grossly bloody; or associated with fever over 38.5° C (101° F), severe abdominal pain (especially in patients over 50 years of age), dehydration, or duration over 2 days. Diarrhea occurring in patients over 70 years or in immunocompromised patients also warrants evaluation by a health care provider.

In 10% of cases, acute diarrhea is related to medications, including antibiotics, cardiac antiarrhythmics, antihypertensives, NSAIDs, certain antidepressants, chemotherapeutic agents, laxatives, bronchodilators, and antacids.[2]

Persistent traveler's diarrhea is typically seen in patients with a recent history of travel. Chronic diarrhea can be intermittent or continuous or associated with a stool weight of 200 to 300 g/24 hr. Although chronic diarrhea is typically noninfectious, it warrants a further medical workup to exclude serious illness.[1,4,5]

Prompt medical evaluation is indicated if diarrhea is associated with fever, abdominal pain, dehydration, or bloody stool.

PATHOPHYSIOLOGY

Acute Infectious Diarrhea

The small intestine absorbs approximately 8.5 L of fluid daily, while the colon absorbs the remaining 1.5 L. An estimated 200 ml of fluid is lost in stool. Pathogens such as viruses, bacteria, or parasites can cause diarrhea. Viruses usually occur on a year-round basis but peak in the winter months. Bacterial illnesses are more common in the summer or early fall. Causes of acute infectious diarrhea are categorized as noninflammatory or inflammatory (Box 140-1). Infectious diarrhea, the most common type of diarrhea, is spread by food or water contamination, person-to-person contact, the fecal-oral route, or animals[1,2,6] (see Chapter 249).

Risk factors include travel, ingestion of certain foods (chicken, meat, fried rice, mayonnaise or cream, eggs,

BOX 140-1

CAUSES OF DIARRHEA

INFECTIOUS DIARRHEA

Noninflammatory Type

Viruses
- Rotavirus
- Norwalk-like virus

Bacteria
- Enterotoxigenic *Escherichia coli*
- *Clostridium perfringens*
- *Bacillus cereus*
- *Vibrio cholerae*

Parasites
- *Giardia lamblia*
- *Cryptosporidium organisms*

Inflammatory Type

Bacteria
- *Campylobacter jejuni*
- *Shigella* organisms
- Enterohemorrhagic *E. coli*
- *Clostridium difficile*
- *Vibrio parahaemolyticus*
- *Salmonella* organisms

Parasites
- *Entamoeba histolytica*

NONINFECTIOUS DIARRHEA

Medications (most common)
- NSAIDs
- Antihypertensives
- Antidepressants
- Chemotherapeutics
- Antacids (magnesium containing)
- Bronchodilators
- Laxatives (magnesium containing)
- Antibiotics
- Antiarrhythmic agents
- Diuretics

Lactose intolerance

Toxins, environmental
- Heavy metals; arsenic
- Organophosphates
- Insecticides
- Mushrooms

Endocrine disorders
- Thyroid disease
- Diabetes

Pernicious anemia

Irritable bowel syndrome

Inflammatory bowel disease

Crohn's disease

Malignancies

HIV disease

Tropical sprue

Celiac sprue

Scleroderma

Short bowel syndrome

Whipple's disease

seafood), and an immunocompromised state. Daycare employees, institutionalized persons, and patients with certain medical conditions (Reiter's syndrome, thyroiditis, pericarditis, and glomerulonephritis) may also be at increased risk for contracting infectious diarrhea.[6]

Inflammatory diarrhea occurs when the cells of the intestinal mucosa are destroyed by the offending pathogen. These pathogens affect the large intestine. Therefore the amount of diarrhea is minimum.[7] Symptoms include fever and bloody diarrhea (dysentery) along with left lower quadrant cramping, an urgency to defecate, and tenesmus. Fecal leukocytes may be present. Inflammatory diarrhea is usually caused by shigellosis, salmonellosis, *Campylobacter* or *Yersinia* organisms, amebas, or a toxin such as *Clostridium difficile* or *Escherichia coli* O157:H7 (see Box 140-1). Cytomegalovirus can cause intestinal ulceration with watery or blood diarrhea in the immunocompromised or HIV patient.[1,2]

Noninflammatory diarrhea does not invade the tissue but colonizes on the small bowel mucosa. This causes the small bowel to secrete excess fluid and electrolytes. Therefore there is little damage to the tissue.[7] Symptoms include massive volumes of diarrhea that is watery but not bloody. It is associated with cramping in the periumbilical region, bloating, nausea, or vomiting. This large amount of volume loss may quickly lead to dehydration associated with hypokalemia and metabolic acidosis. Noninflammatory diarrhea is usually caused either by a toxin-producing bacterium such as enterotoxigen *E. coli*, *Staphylococcus aureus*, *Bacillus cereus*, *Clostridium perfringens*, *Vibrio cholerae*, rotavirus, and Norwalk-like virus; or by parasites such as *Giardia lamblia* or *Cryptosporidium* organisms (see Box 140-1). If the diarrhea is caused by viral enteritis or *S. aureus*, food poisoning should be suspected.[1,5,6]

Acute Noninfectious Diarrhea

Approximately 10% of acute diarrhea is noninfectious, caused by medications, ischemia, and ingestion of certain toxins. Medications are the most common cause of acute diarrhea (see Box 140-1). Ischemic colitis and diverticulitis can produce large volumes of diarrhea. Toxins such as organophosphate insecticides (typically found in migrant farm workers), mushrooms, arsenic, and ciguatera and scombroid (environmental toxins found in fish) also cause diarrhea.

Noninfectious diarrhea should be considered when a specific pathogen has not been identified (see Box 140-1). Other causes include Whipple's disease, pernicious anemia, diabetes, malabsorption, scleroderma, or celiac sprue.[1,8]

Chronic Diarrhea

Chronic diarrhea is classified as osmotic, secretory, steatorrheal, inflammatory, dysmotile, and factitial.[1,5] Osmotic diarrhea occurs when solutes that are poorly absorbed and osmotically active disrupt the colon with an increase in liquid stools. Osmotic diarrhea stops with fasting or discontinuing the offending agent. Examples include osmotic magnesium-containing laxatives and carbohydrate malabsorption (lactase deficiency). Chronic diarrhea can also be caused by a secretory factor; defined as an imbalance in fluid and electrolytes. Clinically, there is a large volume of watery, painless stool that continues with fasting. Causes include medications, bowel resection, mucosal disease, or enterocolic fistulas. Rarer examples are hormones and congenital defects associated with ion absorption. Another cause of chronic diarrhea is steatorrheal, defined as a disruption of fat malabsorption. These conditions include intraluminal maldigestion, mucosal malabsorption, and postmucosal lymphatic obstruction. Chronic diarrhea can also be inflammatory and accompanied by pain, fever, and bleeding. Examples include inflammatory bowel disease, primary or secondary immunodeficiency, and eosinophilic gastroenteritis. Chronic diarrhea may also be related to dysmotility or hypermotility, which is usually secondary to another phenomenon. Lastly, factitial diarrhea includes those cases caused by deception or self-injury for secondary gain.[1,5]

CLINICAL PRESENTATION

The history is the most helpful factor in determining the cause of both acute and chronic diarrhea and assists in differentiating between acute infectious (inflammatory or noninflammatory), noninfectious, and chronic diarrhea. The initial history should include both clinical and epidemiologic aspects, as well as the patient's normal bowel pattern, when the diarrhea began, whether the onset was abrupt or gradual, and the character of the stool (watery, bloody, amount, frequency, and time). Particular attention should be given to bowel symptoms, including rectal discomfort; presence of bloody, mucoid, or purulent exudates in the stool; weight loss (gradual or acute); alternating patterns of diarrhea and constipation; nocturnal diarrhea; and any history of hemorrhoids. Associated symptoms, including nausea, vomiting, abdominal cramping, pain, fever, and chills (indicating dehydration or an inflammatory infection), must also be elicited. Other pertinent information includes increased thirst, dark or concentrated urine, oliguria, dizziness, and tenesmus. The patient should be questioned about current or previous medical conditions, including diabetes, thyroid disease, AIDS, and malignancies. All allergies and current medications (over-the-counter and prescription), including antibiotic treatment within the past 3 months, should be reviewed. The dietary history should include the use of any nutritional or dietary supplements or diet aids, especially sugar-free products that contain sorbitol or mannitol, which are poorly absorbed and may cause diarrhea.[1]

Epidemiologic concerns include travel to underdeveloped countries, consumption of unsafe food (raw meat, eggs, or shellfish; unpasteurized milk), swimming in or drinking untreated water, or a recent visit to a farm or zoo with reptiles or sick animals. Sexual habits, including anal or oral-anal intercourse, or an occupation as a food handler or caregiver is also pertinent.[1,2,8]

Family history should include any recent diarrheal illnesses in family members. Food poisoning should be suspected if others, either family members or close cohorts, have similar symptoms. Common causes of food poisoning include *S. aureus*, *C. perfringens*, and *B. cereus*.[1,2,8]

PHYSICAL EXAMINATION

The physical examination includes weight, temperature, and orthostatic vital signs (blood pressure and heart rate lying, sitting, and standing) to assess volume depletion (dry mucous membranes, decreased skin turgor, absent jugular venous pulsation). The patient's mental status should be noted along with a close assessment of skin color, temperature, rashes, or joint inflammation (Reiter's syndrome). The head and neck should be assessed for evidence of conjunctivitis (suggesting Reiter's syndrome), infection, thyromegaly, or lymphadenopathy.

A cardiovascular examination is indicated to determine the patient's response to the illness and to exclude the cardiac complications associated with some illnesses. During the abdominal examination particular care is necessary to determine abdominal distention, peristalsis, masses, organomegaly, tenderness, rigidity, rebound, guarding, fecal impaction, or bleeding. In the female patient with lower abdominal symptoms, a pelvic examination is imperative. In the geriatric patient, fecal impaction must be ruled out.[2,7,8]

DIAGNOSTICS

Acute Diarrhea

The cornerstone of diagnosis is stool analysis. For the patient who has mild, afebrile acute diarrhea, diagnostic evaluation is typically not indicated. This diarrhea is usually viral and considered benign. Symptoms usually resolve within 1 week, and a diagnosis is rarely documented.

For the patient with fever, abdominal pain, dehydration, protracted nausea and vomiting, diarrhea lasting longer than 1 week, blood in the stool, and an immunocompromised status, diagnostic testing should be more aggressive (Box 140-2).

BOX 140-2

EVALUATION OF ACUTE DIARRHEA

1. Symptomatic therapy
   a. Hydration (PO or IV)
   b. Diet modification
2. Symptoms persist: order fecal leukocytes
   a. Hypovolemia
   b. Bloody stools
   c. Fever
   d. >6 liquid stools per day
   e. >48 hours
   f. Severe abdominal pain
   g. Elderly (>70 years)
   h. Immunocompromised
3. Noninflammatory (giardiasis, drugs, *Clostridium perfringens*, *Staphylococcus aureus*, *Bacillus cereus*, Norwalk, rotavirus, inflammatory bowel disease)
   a. Continue symptomatic therapy
   b. Further medical evaluation if symptoms persist
4. Inflammatory (*Clostridium difficile; Escherichia coli; Shigella*, *Salmonella*, *Campylobacter* organisms; enterohemorrhagic diarrhea)
   a. Stool for ova and parasites and culture, *C. difficile* with antibiotic use (recent)
   b. Empiric therapy pending stool analysis or severe illness
5. Specific antibiotic therapy when pathogen identified

DIAGNOSTICS

Acute Diarrhea

LABORATORY
CBC and differential*
Serum electrolytes
Serum glucose
BUN
Creatinine*
Stool for occult blood and fecal leukocytes*
Stool for ova and parasites, culture for *Clostridium difficile**

IMAGING
KUB
Sigmoidoscopy
Colonoscopy
Abdominal CT scan
Upper endoscopy with small bowel biopsy

*If indicated.

A plain x-ray examination (kidney-ureters-bladder [KUB] and upright) of the abdomen is necessary if a small bowel obstruction or stool impaction with overflow incontinence is suspected. This usually is seen in older adults. If diarrhea continues after 2 weeks with no identified co-existing factors, bacterial causes such as giardiasis or infection with *Entamoeba* organisms or other pathogens should be considered to exclude inflammatory bowel disease and noninfectious acute diarrhea (colitis, diverticulitis, or bowel obstruction). Further diagnostics include a sigmoidoscopy, colonoscopy, or abdominal CT scan.[1-3,6,8]

Another consideration is lactose intolerance. Typically no diagnostics are indicated other than a trial of abstinence from foods or liquids that contain lactose. However, if the lactose-free diet trial fails to resolve the symptoms, a further workup is warranted.

Chronic Diarrhea

If the initial workup does not suggest a cause, further evaluation by a gastroenterologist is warranted. A 24-hour stool analysis for electrolytes, weight and quantitative fecal fat, and osmolality, along with a stool screen for laxatives, should be ordered. Routine laboratory tests include CBC, serum electrolytes, liver function tests, calcium, phosphorus, albumin, thyroid-stimulating hormone, β-carotene, and prothrombin time. Other laboratory tests may include immunoglobulin G and A antigliadin or tissue transglutaminase antibodies, serum vasoactive intestinal peptide, calcitonin, gastrin, and glucagon. Urine is sent to analyze 5-hydroxyindoleacetic acid (carcinoid), vanillylmandelic acid, metanephrine, and histamine.[5]

Plain abdominal radiography and CT scan will confirm pancreatitis and cancer of the pancreas. If Crohn's disease, lymphoma of the small bowel, or carcinoma and jejunal diverticula are suspected, a small intestinal barium study is indicated.[1,5] Sigmoidoscopy and/or colonoscopy with biopsy is useful to diagnose inflammatory bowel disease. If malabsorptive disorder (celiac sprue, Whipple's disease) is suspected, an upper endoscopy with small bowel biopsy is indicated. This procedure will also confirm *Cryptosporidium*, *Microsporida*, and *Mycobacterium avium-intracellulare* infection in AIDS patients.[1,5]

DIAGNOSTICS

Chronic Diarrhea

LABORATORY
CBC and differential
Serum glucose
BUN
Creatinine
LFTs
Calcium
Phosphorus
Albumin
TSH
β-Carotene
Prothrombin time
IgG and IgA
Serum vasoactive intestinal peptide
Calcitonin
Gastrin
Glucagons
Urine for 5-hydroxyindoleacetic acid
Vanillylmandelic acid
Metanephrine
Histamine

IMAGING
KUB
Abdominal CT
Barium study
Sigmoidoscopy
Colonoscopy with biopsy
Upper endoscopy with small bowel follow-through

DIFFERENTIAL DIAGNOSIS

Differential diagnoses to consider with acute diarrhea are classified as noninflammatory and inflammatory causes (see Box 140-2). The inflammatory pathogens usually affect the integrity of the lower intestinal mucosa. They manifest with fever and bloody stools. The noninflammatory pathogens usually affect the upper gastrointestinal tract (see Box 140-1). There may or may not be fever, but bloody diarrhea is not a common presenting symptom (see Chapter 249).

Differential diagnoses to consider with chronic diarrhea include medications, toxins, HIV, irritable bowel, impaction, diet (lactose intolerance), infection, malignancy, stress, acute diverticulitis, Crohn's disease, ulcerative colitis, and stress.

MANAGEMENT

Acute, Inflammatory, and Noninflammatory Diarrhea

Fluid and electrolyte replacement is the cornerstone of treatment for acute diarrhea. Initially, symptomatic therapy should be initiated. Oral fluid replacement should be initiated at home or in the office to manage a mild, uncomplicated episode of diarrhea. Sports drinks can be used in healthy adults to prevent dehydration. Sports drinks should be used cautiously in the pediatric population because the hypertonic solutions have a high carbohydrate and low electrolyte

DIFFERENTIAL DIAGNOSIS

Diarrhea

ACUTE DIARRHEA
- Amebiasis (usually associated with travel)
- *Staphylococcus aureus* (associated with contaminated food)
- *Campylobacter* organisms
- *Giardia lamblia* (associated with contaminated water)
- *Salmonella* organisms (associated with contaminated food)
- *Shigella* organisms
- Toxigenic *Escherichia coli* (traveler's diarrhea)
- Viral infection

CHRONIC DIARRHEA
- AIDS
- Colitis
- Crohn's disease
- Diet-related diarrhea (lactose intolerance)
- Impaction
- Irritable bowel syndrome
- Medication-related diarrhea
- Stress

content, which can intensify the diarrhea. A hyperosmolar solution containing glucose and electrolytes is advised to prevent future intestinal intraluminal fluid overload. Commercial preparations such as Pedialyte or Rehydralyte can be used. However, the American College of Gastroenterology recommends home-made solutions (Box 140-3). A cereal-based rehydrating solution, Ricelyte, which contains more calories than the glucose-based solution, may be used to decrease stool volume and the duration of the diarrhea. A home-made preparation can be made with 1 to 2 cups of rice cereal, 4 cups of water (boil if traveling), and ½ teaspoon of salt. If abdominal cramping is an associated symptom, fasting for 8 to 12 hours and applying moist heat to the abdomen as a comfort measure may help. If the patient fails to respond to oral rehydration, is worse, or has persistent symptoms, IV hydration may be indicated. Solid food products should be reintroduced as symptoms resolve and stools become more formed.

BOX 140-3

HOMEMADE ORAL REHYDRATING SOLUTIONS

- 8 oz orange or apple juice
- ½ tsp honey or corn syrup
- pinch of salt

Followed by
- 8 oz clear water
- ¼ tsp baking soda

or
- 4½ cups water
- ¼ tsp salt substitute (with potassium)
- ½ tsp baking soda
- ½ tsp salt
- 1-3 Tbsp sugar, honey, or corn syrup

In patients with a fever over 38.8° C (102° F), bloody diarrhea, abdominal pain, more than six unformed stools in a 24-hour period, profuse watery diarrhea, and dehydration, or in patients who are frail and elderly or immunocompromised (AIDS, transplant patients), a stool sample should be sent for fecal leukocyte testing (see Box 140-2).

Medications can be used for symptomatic relief of nausea and vomiting, abdominal cramping, and diarrhea. They are generally used in older children and healthy adults. Absorbents such as bismuth subsalicylate (e.g., Kaopectate, 4 tablespoons q 4 hours; or Pepto-Bismol, 2 to 4 tablespoons q 30 min not to exceed 8 doses/24 hr, or 1 to 2 tablets q 4-6 hr) and antispasmodic-anticholinergic-sedatives such as atropine sulfate–scopolamine hydrobromide–hyoscyamine sulfate–phenobarbital (Donnatal; 1 or 2 tablets t.i.d.) are used to decrease abdominal cramping. Antisecretory agents such as bismuth subsalicylate also have antiinflammatory effects and are commonly used if there is vomiting and abdominal cramping. These products may cause aspirin toxicity and should be used cautiously. Patients taking warfarin should be warned as well because anticoagulation will be affected. Also, Pepto-Bismol should not be used with HIV-positive or immunocompromised patients, who are at risk for encephalopathy. Concomitant use of Pepto-Bismol with antibiotics may decrease their effectiveness.[2]

Antimotility agents that are used in noninflammatory diarrhea include loperamide (Imodium; 4-mg caplets: 2 caplets initially, then 1 after each loose stool, not to exceed 16 mg/24 hr) and diphenoxylate hydrochloride–atropine sulfate (Lomotil [2.5-mg tablets], 2 tablets q 4-6 hr). Loperamide is preferred in children, pregnant women, and immunocompromised patients. If nausea is the main complaint, treatment with promethazine (Phenergan), prochlorperazine (Compazine), or another antiemetic is recommended.[2]

Empiric treatment with antibiotics should be considered if the patient has fecal leukocytes without a confirmed positive stool culture; if there is occult blood; if the patient has fever with profuse, watery diarrhea (>8 stools/day), appears dehydrated, has had symptoms for more than 1 week, and is immunocompromised; or if hospitalization is considered, since the most likely cause of the infection is *Salmonella*, *Shigella*, or *Campylobacter* pathogens. Ciprofloxacin (500 mg b.i.d. for 3 days) or norfloxacin (400 mg b.i.d. PO for 3 days) can be initiated until the stool culture results are verified, but should not be used in children or pregnant or lactating women. If the diarrhea persists for longer than 2 weeks, *Giardia* organisms may be suspected and metronidazole (250 mg q.i.d. PO for 7 days) can be initiated. Specific therapy is initiated once the pathogen is identified[2] (see Chapter 249).

Traveler's Diarrhea

Traveler's diarrhea is defined as the passage of two or more watery or unformed stools over a 24-hour period or the passage of any number of stools when associated with fever, vomiting, or abdominal cramps. The diarrhea can occur during or up to 10 days after travel.[9] It affects 20% to 50% of travelers to developing countries, including parts of the Caribbean, southern Asia, and Africa. Traveler's diarrhea lasts approximately 3 to 5 days. It is usually a self-limiting illness, and the patient rarely develops complications. The causative agents include enterotoxigenic *E. coli, C. jejuni,* salmonellae, and shigellae[2] (see Chapter 249 for more information on traveler's diarrhea, including treatment).

Chronic Diarrhea

Fluid and electrolyte replacement is an important treatment for chronic diarrhea. Depending on the specific cause of chronic diarrhea, treatment may be curative, suppressive, or empiric.

If the cause of the diarrhea is not known, treatment may include empiric use of a mild opiate such as loperamide 4 mg initially followed by 2 mg after each watery stool to a maximum of 16 mg/day, or diphenoxylate with atropine (Lomotil), one tablet 3 or 4 times a day.[1,5] Another option is codeine and deodorized tincture of opium (DTO). This agent is potentially habit forming and should be reserved for patients with chronic intractable diarrhea. It should be prescribed only in consultation with the physician and pharmacist. Clonidine 0.1 to 0.6 mg b.i.d. is an α_2-adrenergic agonist that inhibits intestinal electrolyte secretion. A clonidine patch 0.1 to 0.2 mg/day treats secretory diarrhea, diabetic diarrhea, or cryptosporidiosis.

Secretory diarrhea related to neuroendocrine tumors (vipomas, carcinoids) is treated with octreotide 50 to 250 mcg subcutaneous t.i.d. This agent is a somatostatin analog that stimulates intestinal fluid and electrolyte absorption and stops intestinal fluid secretions. Octreotide is also used to treat AIDS-related diarrhea.

For diarrhea caused by bile salts due to intestinal resection or ileal disease, cholestyramine (Questran) 4 g once daily or up to three times daily is recommended.[10] It should be noted that antimotility agents should not be used with inflammatory bowel disease.

COMPLICATIONS

Complications from diarrhea are usually a result of dehydration. Regardless of the cause, attention should be directed toward fluid and electrolyte replacement. Electrolyte disorders, particularly hypocalcemia, hypomagnesemia, and hypokalemia, are common in persistent diarrhea. Continuous diarrhea can require hospitalization for fluid and electrolyte replacement if the patient is unable to maintain hydration with oral fluid replacement. Sepsis and cardiovascular collapse are potential complications, and infants, older adults, and immunosuppressed patients are more susceptible to these complications. Refractory diarrhea is usually a symptom of a more serious illness and requires diagnostic evaluation and immediate physician consultation.[2,8]

INDICATIONS FOR REFERRAL OR HOSPITALIZATION

If dehydration is severe or protracted vomiting is present, IV fluids should be initiated. If symptoms of the illness persist beyond 3 weeks despite treatment measures, chronic lactose intolerance; giardiasis; malignancies; and disease states such as diabetes, thyrotoxicosis, lupus, HIV infection, or irritable bowel syndrome should be considered. Physician consultation is imperative in these cases.

HEALTH PROMOTION AND ILLNESS PREVENTION

Prevention of diarrhea should be the primary goal. Important information to convey to patients includes:

- Handwashing remains the best preventive measure. Always wash hands after handling chicken or other raw meats. Wash cutting boards frequently (plastic cutting boards that can be washed in a dishwasher are preferable). Change sponges and wash kitchen countertops frequently. Sponges should be washed and disinfected daily (by microwaving on high or placing in boiling water for 2 minutes).
- Use a meat thermometer to check temperature of roasts, chicken, and hamburger. When traveling, especially out of the country, drink and brush teeth with bottled water and eat only peeled fruits and vegetables. Avoid iced drinks, and never drink untreated water.
- Avoid high-risk foods, such as raw seafood, raw eggs, unpasteurized dairy products, and undercooked poultry and beef.
- Avoid foods that have sat out at room temperature for more than 2 hours, particularly foods not refrigerated or heated in buffets or food stands.
- Defrost meats in the microware (as directed) or refrigerator.
- Cook foods to the proper temperature.

PATIENT AND FAMILY EDUCATION

The following are some general recommendations that should be discussed with the patient and family.

- Practice good handwashing after each bowel movement to lessen the possibility of spread to other family members.
- Immunocompromised patients are at greater risk of severe infection and should be diligent about safe food handling and preparation.
- Drink frequent, small sips of fluids (water, tea, bouillon, flat cola, flat ginger ale, or sports drink) to avoid dehydration.
- Avoid foods and let your stomach rest for 12 hours (after the illness starts) or until you begin to feel better. Gradually add small amounts of food (e.g., crackers, toast, rice, bananas), but avoid those which will aggravate symptoms (e.g., dairy products, caffeine, high-fat or high-fiber foods, carbonated beverages, sugar-free products, and alcohol).
- It is better to avoid antidiarrheal products, since most cases of diarrhea are self-limiting.
- Rest.
- If symptoms persist or are accompanied by mental confusion, fever with temperature of more than 38.3° C (101° F), chills, vomiting, weakness (especially muscle weakness), dizziness, dry mouth, extreme thirst, little or no urinary output, severe abdominal discomfort, blurred vision, or black or bloody stools, immediately notify the health care provider.
- Some medications, particularly Pepto-Bismol, will cause stools to appear black.
- Children, daycare workers, or food handlers should remain at home until the diarrhea resolves.

REFERENCES

1. Ahlquist DA, Camilleri M: Diarrhea and constipation. In Kasper DL, Fauci AS, Longo DL, and others, editors: *Harrison's principles of internal medicine,* ed 16, New York, 2005, McGraw-Hill.
2. Dupont HL, and Practice Parameters Committee of the American College of Gastroenterology: Guidelines on acute infectious diarrhea in adults, *Am J Gastroenterol* 92(11):1962-1975, 1997.
3. Thielman NM, Guerrant RL: Acute infectious diarrhea, *N Engl J Med* 350(1):38-47, 2004.
4. Cheskin LJ: Constipation and diarrhea. In Barker LR, Burton JR, Zieve PD, editors: *Principles of ambulatory medicine,* Baltimore, 1999, Williams & Wilkins.
5. McQuaid K: Alimentary tract. In Tierney LM, McPhee SJ, Papadakis MA, editors: *Current medical diagnosis and treatment,* New York, 2006, McGraw-Hill.
6. Fauci A, Braunwald E, Isselbacher K, and others, editors: *Harrison's principles of internal medicine,* ed 14, New York, 1998, McGraw-Hill.
7. Bemmett RG: Acute gastroenteritis and associated conditions. In Barker LR, Burton JR, Zieve PD, editors: *Principles of ambulatory medicine,* Baltimore, 1999, Williams & Wilkins.
8. Guerrant RL, Van Gilder T, Steiner TS, and others: Practice guidelines for the management of infectious diarrhea, *Clin Infect Dis* 32:331-350, 2001.
9. Rao G, Allwalas MG, Slaymaker E, and others: Bismuth revisited: an effective way to prevent travelers' diarrhea, *J Travel Med* 11(4), 2004, retrieved Dec 19, 2005, from http://www.medscape.com/viewarticle/491696?src=search.
10. Leder K, Weller PF: *Giardiasis in adults,* 2006, retrieved Jan 20, 2007, from http://www.uptodateonline.com/appliation/topic/topic.

CHAPTER 141

Diverticular Disease

Louise P. Meyer

Diverticular disease is a common disorder of the colon occurring more often as life expectancy increases and as dietary practices include more refined foods. The disease manifests itself in a variety of clinical spectrums and in three different clinical patterns: (1) diverticulosis, or uncomplicated diverticular disease, the asymptomatic or symptomatic presence of noninflamed multiple colonic diverticula; (2) diverticulitis, or complicated diverticular disease associated with inflammation in one or more of the diverticula, with possible resultant perforation leading to abscess or fistula formation; and (3) hemorrhage, another complication of diverticular disease, often associated with a right-sided diverticulum or diverticula.

DIVERTICULOSIS

DEFINITION AND EPIDEMIOLOGY

Diverticulosis derives its name from the basic unit of diverticular disease, the diverticulum, which is an outpouching of mucosa through the colon wall. The occurrence of a single diverticulum is uncommon; hence the term *diverticulosis* is used to describe the condition of numerous diverticula in the colon. This term is an anatomic descriptor. Clinically, diverticulosis is an uncomplicated, asymptomatic or symptomatic disease without inflammation or bleeding.

The prevalence of colonic diverticulosis varies greatly in different geographic areas of the world. It is most common in the Western hemisphere and is rare in Africa, Asia, and many parts of South America. This disease is considered a deficiency disease of twentieth century Western civilization. Its emergence parallels a change in dietary habits that occurred during the Industrial Revolution of the 1850s, including the mechanical milling of crude cereal grain and wheat flour and the resultant loss of the nonabsorbable fiber content. At this time, there was also an increased consumption of white flour, refined sugar, conserves, and meat.[1]

Studies from less industrialized regions (e.g., Africa and Asia) document prevalence rates of diverticulosis of less than 0.2%.[1] The worldwide prevalence of diverticular disease is not truly known, but in the United States and other developed countries its prevalence approaches 10%.[2] In addition to geographic distribution, age is another important variable and is the key risk factor. Diverticulosis is rare before age 40 years, but occurs in later years, with an estimated incidence of 50% to 65% by age 80.[3-7]

PATHOPHYSIOLOGY

Colonic diverticula are defects of the large colon, especially the sigmoid, that develop with advancing age. They are saclike herniations of the mucosa through the muscularis propria and are actually pseudodiverticula because they do not contain the muscle layer.

The pathophysiologic changes common to all cases of diverticulosis of the colon are not entirely clear. Herniation of the muscular layer of the colon is the result of two factors: (1) an increased pressure gradient between the colonic lumen and the serosa, and (2) areas of relative weakness in the colonic wall.[8]

One commonly accepted hypothesis of diverticula formation is that low-fiber diets decrease the amount of intraluminal bulk in the colon, causing muscular hypertrophy as the colon tries to move the fecal matter along.[1] Lack of fecal bulk is thought to produce uncoordinated and irregular colonic peristalsis, which creates sacculations in the colon wall. There is increased pressure within these sacs, which results in diverticular outpouchings. These sacs occur at weak points, or natural breaks, in the muscle layer of the colon where the nutrient vessels, the vasa recta, pass through the muscularis propria into the submucosa. In addition, the colon wall, which is covered by connective tissue, loses its flexibility and tensile strength with age. A weakened bowel wall develops and may predispose an individual to formation of diverticula.

Therefore increasing fiber intake will reduce the incidence of diverticular disease.[7,9] This hypothesis is supported by another study in which vegetarians living in England had a 12% incidence of diverticular disease as compared with a 33% incidence among nonvegetarians who ingested half of the mean daily intake of dietary fiber.[10]

In terms of size and distribution, diverticula range from 1 or 2 mm to giant diverticula. In Western societies, diverticula occur predominantly in the sigmoid colon. In Asians who have adopted a Western diet, right-sided diverticula are more common.[7,11]

CLINICAL PRESENTATION

Patients with uncomplicated colonic diverticula, or diverticulosis, are often asymptomatic and rarely seek medical attention; at least 80% to 85% of these individuals are never seen with a clinical problem.[12] Symptomless diverticula are often noted when the colon is studied for another reason via a barium enema, colonoscopy, CT scan, or ultrasound.

By contrast, symptomatic patients may complain of irregular defecation, intermittent abdominal pain, bloating, or excessive flatulence. In general, there is a change in stool caliber, with descriptors that can range from flattened or ribbonlike to hard pellets. Associated complaints include urinary dysfunction, nausea, vomiting, and heartburn. Older individuals often relate recurrent bouts of steady or crampy pain (mostly in the left lower quadrant) in combination with constipation or alternating periods of diarrhea and constipation. They may also have abdominal distention that is relieved by the passage of flatus or stool. These symptoms can often mimic irritable bowel syndrome except that they are experienced at an older age. Those patients who are seen with right-sided pain tend to be younger, and their pain is easily mistaken for appendicitis.[6]

PHYSICAL EXAMINATION

For patients with uncomplicated symptoms the physical examination (both a pelvic and rectal examination) is usually normal. Fever is possible, but may not be present. The other vital signs are often normal, but in the presence of a massive diverticular bleed, tachycardia and hypotension are not uncommon. Most often, physical findings reveal mild, left lower quadrant tenderness with a thickened palpable sigmoid and descending colon. Isolated right lower quadrant tenderness also may be related to diverticulitis. Tenderness throughout the abdomen suggests perforation and peritonitis.[7] Rectal bleeding is infrequent, but painless bright red bleeding or maroon-colored stools suggest a diverticular bleed.[7]

DIAGNOSTICS

A CBC and urinalysis should be obtained. Screening laboratory values should be normal in uncomplicated diverticulosis; leukocytosis may be present in diverticulitis. A stool for occult blood is necessary, since uncomplicated diverticulosis is not known to cause occult rectal bleeding. Plain abdominal x-ray films will be normal and are unnecessary, although they are sometimes ordered to exclude the presence of free air in the abdomen. Rigid sigmoidoscopy usually cannot be performed beyond the rectosigmoid junction and for this reason is not particularly useful. The diagnosis of diverticulosis is most often established with a barium enema examination; this method is the best for determining the extent and severity of the disease. Although it is often used as a diagnostic tool, a colonoscopy is best used to assess the large bowel for a co-existing pathologic condition rather than for an actual diagnosis of diverticular disease.

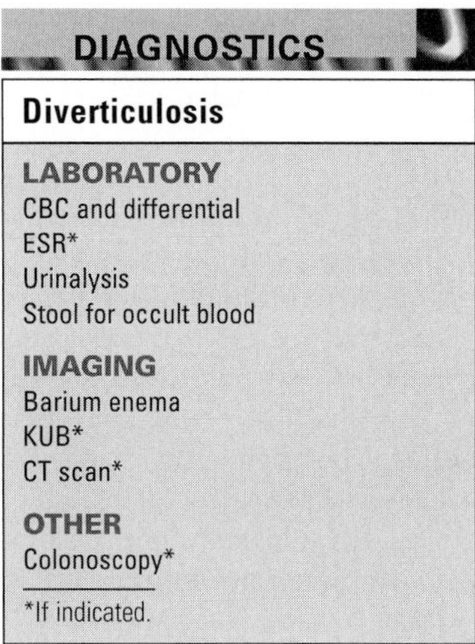

DIAGNOSTICS

Diverticulosis

LABORATORY
CBC and differential
ESR*
Urinalysis
Stool for occult blood

IMAGING
Barium enema
KUB*
CT scan*

OTHER
Colonoscopy*

*If indicated.

A CT scan is the preferred imaging study if acute diverticulitis is suspected. However, CT scan is not indicated for all patients, but should be considered if peritonitis, a diverticular abscess, or other complication is suspected.[7]

DIFFERENTIAL DIAGNOSIS

The hallmark of symptomatic diverticulosis is colicky abdominal pain in the absence of an inflammatory process. The cause of this pain is not fully understood but possibly is related to spasms in the sigmoid colon or an element of obstruction related to the spasms. This clinical entity must be differentiated from diverticulitis and any disease that causes abnormal intestinal motility.

The challenge is not so much in making the diagnosis as it is in distinguishing patients who have symptomatic diverticular disease from those who have diverticula plus other lesions that may be responsible for the symptoms. Irritable

DIFFERENTIAL DIAGNOSIS

Diverticulosis

- Diverticulitis
- Irritable bowel syndrome
- Cancer
- Cystitis
- Appendicitis
- Inflammatory bowel disease
- Crohn's disease
- Peritonitis
- Chronic ulcerative colitis
- Ischemic colitis
- Infectious colitis
- Radiation-induced colitis
- Gynecologic inflammatory or neoplastic diseases
- Vascular ectasia
- Ectopic pregnancy
- Anorectal disease
- Small or large bowel obstruction

bowel syndrome and colorectal cancer should be considered in the differential diagnosis. In patients with localized right-sided abdominal pain, appendicitis must be considered.

MANAGEMENT

Fiber is essential for normal intestinal function. Pioneering studies in the 1960s and 1970s revealed the relationship between colonic diverticulosis and low consumption of dietary fiber.[1,10] Earlier studies revealed that increased dietary fiber can provide symptomatic relief in patients with painful diverticulosis or recurrent diverticulitis.[13-15] A diet that includes 35 g of fiber may bring about significant change. In the United States adults consume approximately 11 to 23 g of fiber per day—half of the 27 to 40 g of daily fiber recommended by the World Health Organization and less than the 20 to 35 g proposed by the American Dietetic Association.[16,17]

Increased fiber intake can be achieved through the consumption of whole grains and cereals, fruits, vegetables, and legumes. These foods should be introduced gradually over a period of weeks to months to avoid excessive bloating and flatulence. Bran, a concentrated form of fiber, can be used as an adjunct to fiber consumption but should not be a replacement for other high-fiber foods. Some patients may need 2 g of bran three times a day to provide the bulk; it should be soaked or mixed in media such as hot cereal, applesauce, juice, or milk.

Fiber can also be given through commercially available high-fiber supplements or bulk formers such as psyllium hydrophilic mucilloid, methylcellulose, and calcium polycarbophil. These products work similarly to bran and must be taken with several glasses of fluid to be effective. They produce a softer, more frequent stool.

Current literature does not support the elimination of certain dietary foodstuffs in the management of diverticulosis. Nonetheless, patients should generally avoid popcorn, corn, nuts, and seeds.

Anticholinergic and antispasmodic agents have been used without substantiated evidence of their effectiveness. They may be used to relieve spasms. Care should be taken to avoid constipation. Surgical resection for pain relief, in the absence of documented inflammatory complications, is associated with a high rate of symptom recurrence and is therefore not recommended.[12]

LIFE SPAN CONSIDERATIONS

Diverticular disease is usually observed in adults older than 40 years, and incidence increases with age. Younger adults, however, can develop diverticular disease and associated complications such as diverticulitis and diverticular bleeding.

COMPLICATIONS

The majority of patients with diverticular disease have an uncomplicated course. However, several older studies have shown that 10% to 25% of individuals develop diverticulitis, with 5% eventually experiencing massive bleeding from a diverticulum.[3,18]

INDICATIONS FOR REFERRAL OR HOSPITALIZATION

Uncomplicated diverticular disease can be managed in the primary care setting. Questionable radiographic findings on any barium studies necessitate referral to a gastroenterologist for further evaluation. Patients with suspected diverticular abscess or rectal bleeding need further evaluation, and a referral or consultation is indicated.

Although the health care provider assumes responsibility for patient education, a referral to a dietitian may be beneficial for patients with recurrent, painful disease.

PATIENT AND FAMILY EDUCATION AND HEALTH PROMOTION

Patients' diet and symptoms should be reviewed at every session for prevention and health promotion. All patients need to be instructed about a nutritionally well-balanced diet that includes whole grain breads and cereals and fresh fruits and vegetables to attain the benefits of both types of fiber (see Figure 24-1).[17] The goal of 30 to 35 g of fiber per day requires the consumption of five fruits and vegetables (15 g), four high-fiber starches (8 g), and one high-fiber cereal (7 g).

It is important that patients be advised to increase their fiber intake gradually to prevent flatulence and abdominal discomfort. Patients can often tolerate 5- to 10-g increments every few weeks on the basis of symptoms. Bloating or flatulence resulting from bran intake usually resolves with continued use. If patients are taking pharmaceutical fiber supplements, it is especially important that they increase their fluid intake to at least eight 8-ounce glasses of fluid per day.

DIVERTICULITIS

DEFINITION AND EPIDEMIOLOGY

Diverticulitis, or complicated diverticular disease, is the most common complication of diverticulosis. An inflammatory condition that involves one or more colonic diverticula, diverticulitis is almost always symptomatic. Diverticulosis must be present before there can be an attack of diverticulitis.

The possibility of experiencing diverticulitis increases with the longer duration of diverticular disease and with increasing age. In one study approximately one fifth, or 20%, of all patients with radiologic evidence of diverticulosis developed diverticulitis in the sixth decade; this fraction increased to one third by the ninth decade.[3] A recent study by Marinella and Mustafa observed that, although rare, diverticulitis can occur in patients less than 35 years old.[19]

PATHOPHYSIOLOGY

The inflammation associated with diverticulitis is thought to result from the stagnation of fecal material in a single diverticulum. This produces a fecalith that leads to pressure necrosis of the mucosa and subsequent inflammation.[20] This inflammatory process progresses, and either a microperforation or a macroperforation ensues. A small perforation is easily contained by the pericolic tissues and becomes a localized phlegmon. A larger perforation may result in a walled-off pericolic abscess whose erosion may produce fistulas into adjacent structures such as the urinary bladder, vagina, small bowel, or anterior abdominal wall. If there is free perforation in the abdominal cavity, fecal peritonitis may occur.

CLINICAL PRESENTATION

The diagnosis of diverticulitis is often clinical, especially in a patient with known diverticula. Most patients with infection or localized inflammation have mild to moderate, colicky to steady, aching abdominal pain usually present in the left lower quadrant (93% to 100%) accompanied by fever (57% to 100%) and leukocytosis (69% to 83%).[2] Constipation or loose stools may or may not be present. There may be nausea and vomiting. Hematochezia is uncommon in diverticulitis and is more suggestive of other diagnoses. In some instances the patient is initially seen with complications of diverticulitis, such as recurrent urinary tract infections or feculent vaginal discharge resulting from fistulization. In other cases a patient may exhibit few or no symptoms and therefore does not seek medical attention for several days. Older patients or patients who are immunocompromised may have minimum abdominal pain, no fever, and a relatively benign physical examination, but still be septic.

PHYSICAL EXAMINATION

The physical examination of patients with diverticulitis may reveal mild distention. Bowel sounds are hyperactive if there is obstruction but are otherwise normal. Generally there is tenderness in the suprapubic region or over the involved colonic segment (often in the left lower quadrant). A mass may or may not be palpated. Pain in the right lower quadrant can be mistaken for acute appendicitis. There can be involuntary guarding and percussion tenderness localized in this area, indicating localized peritoneal inflammation. Patients who experience generalized abdominal pain and abdominal wall rigidity could have a perforated viscus. A rectal examination may reveal some tenderness in the pelvis, and occasionally a mass is palpated anteriorly. Stools are not usually positive for occult blood, but hematochezia is possible. In female patients a pelvic examination is a necessary component of the physical examination. Fever can be present, but a study found that 14% of patients were afebrile at presentation.[21]

DIAGNOSTICS

Initial laboratory studies may not be useful in diagnosing diverticulitis. Although a CBC is usually obtained, leukocytosis is not a requisite symptom of this condition. Urinalysis may reveal white blood cells if the inflammatory process is adjacent to the bladder or ureter. The presence of bacteria in the urine sample consistent with urinary tract infection is suggestive of a fistula. A pregnancy test is indicated for premenopausal and perimenopausal females.

Supine and upright plain x-ray films can be obtained to assess the presence of an ileus; a small or large bowel obstruction; or free abdominal air, which indicates perforation. A CT scan of the abdomen and pelvis has been used increasingly to evaluate patients with diverticulitis. It is the test of choice if diverticular complications are suspected because it gives a more accurate estimate of the degree of inflammation than do other studies.[22,23] Some authorities suggest that not all patients with acute diverticulitis require a CT scan for successful management, but recommend that it be performed under the following conditions: a questionable diagnosis, a suspected abscess or fistula, inadequate clinical improvement with medical treatment, as a diagnostic for patients who are immunocompromised (e.g., steroid dependent) where clinical evaluation is not a reliable indicator of their condition, or an unusual clinical situation such as right-sided diverticulitis.[12] A barium enema is not recommended with acute diverticulitis because of the risk of barium peritonitis.

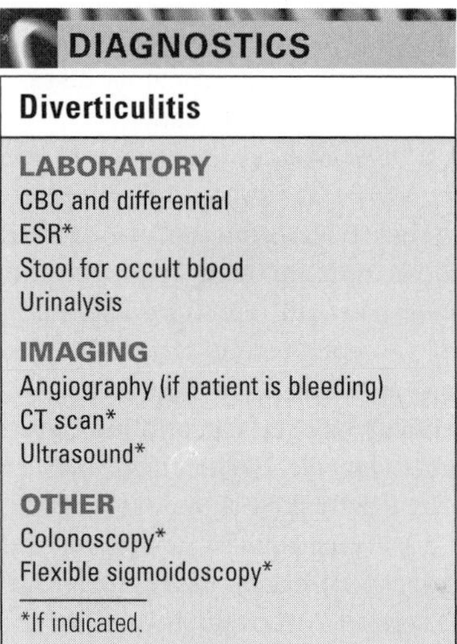
DIAGNOSTICS

Diverticulitis

LABORATORY
CBC and differential
ESR*
Stool for occult blood
Urinalysis

IMAGING
Angiography (if patient is bleeding)
CT scan*
Ultrasound*

OTHER
Colonoscopy*
Flexible sigmoidoscopy*

*If indicated.

Additional tests include ultrasound, flexible sigmoidoscopy, and colonoscopy. Ultrasonography is used to reveal extracolic fluid collections and to guide percutaneous drainage of pelvic and paracolic abscesses; however, ultrasonography is more operator dependent than CT scans. Patients may not be able to tolerate the external pressure, and imaging is limited in an obese patient.[6] Flexible sigmoidoscopy is often used during an episode of suspected diverticulitis. Its main usefulness arises in the event of colonic obstruction to differentiate an obstructing carcinoma from an obstructing diverticular mass. Colonoscopy is useful after the inflammatory process subsides.

DIFFERENTIAL DIAGNOSIS

Diverticulosis is sometimes associated with marked local tenderness and a palpable sigmoid loop and therefore may be mistaken for diverticulitis; however, fever and leukocytosis are generally absent with diverticulosis. Other differential diagnoses include acute appendicitis; peritonitis; cystitis; neoplasm; inflammatory bowel disease; ischemic colitis; radiation colitis; infectious colitis; small bowel obstruction;

DIFFERENTIAL DIAGNOSIS

Diverticulitis

- Diverticulosis
- Acute appendicitis
- Peritonitis
- Cystitis
- Neoplasm
- Inflammatory bowel disease
- Ischemic colitis
- Radiation colitis
- Infectious colitis
- Small bowel obstruction
- Pelvic inflammatory disease
- Endometriosis
- Ovarian cysts
- Ectopic pregnancy

and gynecologic disorders such as pelvic inflammatory disease, endometriosis, ovarian cysts, and ectopic pregnancy.

MANAGEMENT

The clinical spectrum of acute diverticulitis is diverse. Spontaneous resolution is common for many patients with low-grade fever, mild leukocytosis, and minimum abdominal tenderness. These patients do not require hospitalization. Treatment generally consists of taking clear liquids for 2 to 3 days, limiting physical activity, and taking oral antibiotics such as trimethoprim-sulfamethoxazole, (Bactrim DS) 160 mg/800 mg b.i.d., amoxicillin/clavulanate potassium (Augmentin), or ciprofloxacin 500 mg b.i.d. plus metronidazole 500 mg t.i.d. for 7 to 14 days.[6,23-25] As the patient begins to feel better, the diet is slowly advanced as tolerated. Mesalime in combination with antibiotic therapy or in combination with probiotics is one of the newer therapies that has been used successfully for diverticulitis.[26] According to Tursi, probiotics may help prevent recurrent diverticulitis for some patients.[26]

If fever and leukocytosis are absent, the patient may have only painful diverticular disease and not diverticulitis; for this condition antibiotics are withheld. The duration of treatment is determined by clinical response; generally treatment is discontinued when symptoms have resolved and the patient is afebrile. Pain medication is discouraged; symptomatic relief may be achieved with warm packs. Nonopiate analgesics may be used if necessary.

Immediately after an attack of diverticulitis, a short-term, low-fiber diet that consists of 15 g or less of dietary fiber is prescribed to reduce the volume of fecal material in the lower bowel and to prevent irritation to the colon. When the patient is asymptomatic, a gradual modification to a diet high in fiber (and free of seeds) may help reduce pressure inside the colon, thus reducing the chances of future attacks.[16] A colonoscopy is recommended after symptoms resolve to exclude carcinoma.[6]

At the opposite end of this spectrum are patients acutely ill with systemic peritonitis, sepsis, and hypovolemia. Any patient with a temperature of 38.5° C (101.3° F) or higher and with marked tenderness, signs of localized peritonitis, intestinal obstruction, or a suspected intraabdominal or pelvic abscess must be admitted to the hospital. Hospitalization is also recommended for diabetic or immunosuppressed patients, older adults, and patients with chronic renal failure in whom diverticulitis is suspected in the absence of the previously listed criteria. Hospital management includes assessment of fluid status and IV replacement, nasogastric suction if there is an obstruction or ileus, blood cultures, and broad-spectrum IV antibiotics that cover gram-negative anaerobes and gram-negative aerobes. Antibiotic selection might include metronidazole (anaerobic gram-negative bacilli) 750 to 1000 mg IV q 12 hr (15 mg/kg loading dose, then 7.5 mg/kg q 6 hr), plus a third-generation cephalosporin or an aminoglycoside such as gentamicin (aerobic gram-negative bacilli) 1.0 mg/kg IV q 8 hr (maximum dose 5 mg/kg/day in divided doses in life-threatening situations).[22,27,28] IV metronidazole plus IV levofloxacin and clindamycin are other options.[22,27,28] Other antibiotics appropriate for treatment of diverticulitis include ampicillin, piperacillin, or tazobactam.[26] Treatment time depends on symptom resolution and is usually maintained for 7 to 10 days. Variations of these treatments are based on patient needs. Only meperidine should be used for pain management. Morphine increases colonic spasm and may accentuate hypersegmentation.[6]

Further evaluation and management depend on patient assessment and response to initial treatment. If fever, abdominal signs, and leukocytosis have mostly resolved and bowel function has returned with the passage of flatus, a liquid diet can be started and slowly advanced to a low-fiber diet. When the patient is asymptomatic, a high-fiber diet can be gradually introduced. The patient is discharged with a regimen of oral antibiotics such as metronidazole 500 mg t.i.d. for 7 to 10 days. Studies such as a barium enema or colonoscopy should be performed 4 to 6 weeks after hospital discharge.

A CT scan is required if the patient fails to improve after 2 to 4 days of medical treatment; if the diagnosis is in doubt; or if a pelvic or abdominal abscess, fistula, or obstruction needs to be excluded. Occasionally, a peridiverticular abscess of more than 5 cm (2 inches) can be drained under CT guidance as long as the patient has adequate antibiotic coverage.[6]

Because most patients with uncomplicated diverticulitis recover with medical treatment and do not have recurrences of acute disease, surgery is not routinely recommended. However, surgical management is necessary in 15% to 30% of patients, since diverticulitis can recur despite medical management. Elective surgical intervention should be considered after the second episode. Urgent surgical intervention is also sometimes necessary. Younger patients especially may require more aggressive management; in these patients surgery is sometimes recommended after the first attack, although this approach is still somewhat controversial.[21,23,24] Elective surgical management generally consists of a single-stage procedure to decrease morbidity and mortality. A laparoscopic approach has been used for sigmoid resection. This approach decreases hospitalization time and shortens recovery.[6]

COMPLICATIONS

Complications of diverticulitis include free perforation with fecal peritonitis, suppurative peritonitis secondary to ruptured abscess, abdominal or pelvic abscess, fistula, or obstruction. It is estimated that 20% to 30% of patients will have recurrent diverticulitis; patients who experience a second episode have more than a 50% chance of having a third episode.[2] The chance of recurrence after the first episode is 90% within 5 years.[6]

Patients between 40 and 50 years old are at increased risk for developing complications.[21,27] Medical management may not be successful, recurrences with complications are common, and aggressive treatment with early surgery when the patient is stabilized is sometimes recommended.[27] Immunosuppressed patients are at especially high risk for complications because they may not experience a normal inflammatory response and subsequently can develop spontaneous colon perforation and perforated diverticula.[11,24] Aggressive management of these patients includes emergency surgical intervention.[8]

INDICATIONS FOR REFERRAL OR HOSPITALIZATION

The diagnosis of diverticulitis is, unfortunately, based on clinical findings that can be diagnostically nonspecific. The presentation, course of illness, and treatment plan can be challenging. Referral to a gastroenterologist is appropriate if the diagnosis is unclear, attacks are recurrent, or hospitalization is indicated. A surgical consultation is required for patients with suspected complications or those who are readmitted for a second episode of diverticulitis.

PATIENT AND FAMILY EDUCATION

During the convalescent period, patients require a low-fiber diet (<15 g/day) and careful diet instruction. Whole-grain breads and cereals, raw fruits and vegetables, nuts and seeds, and legumes should be avoided. Canned fruits and well-cooked vegetables are allowed in limited quantities. The diet can be liberalized as the patient's condition improves. Once stable and pain free, patients can reintroduce a high-fiber diet slowly, over several weeks, to avoid any abdominal distention or excessive flatulence. Symptoms often guide the treatment plan. A fiber preparation may be necessary for patients who are unable to follow a diet reasonably high in fiber. Regardless of fiber supplementation, 27% of patients who have had surgical treatments will continue to experience symptoms.[6]

Patients should avoid laxatives and enemas because these substances increase colonic pressure. It is important that patients establish a regular bowel movement pattern of once or twice a day to once every 2 or 3 days. With a high-fiber diet the stools should be softer and thus easier to pass.

In addition, patients should be aware of the importance of reporting recurrent pain promptly, especially if the pain is associated with chills or fever. Urgent hospitalization may be necessary.

DIVERTICULAR BLEEDING

DEFINITION AND EPIDEMIOLOGY

Severe bleeding is a less common complication of diverticulosis. Hemorrhage from a colonic diverticulum generally begins without warning in an older individual with otherwise asymptomatic diverticulosis. Painless rectal bleeding is associated with diverticulosis in 15% to 40% of patients and is usually self-limited.[2,29] Massive bleeding occurs in approximately 5% of patients and may be sufficient to require transfusion.[18]

PATHOPHYSIOLOGY

Bleeding arises from the rupture of one of the branches of the vasa recta adjacent to a diverticulum. The most common site for massive bleeding is the right colon, particularly in older adults.[29] It is important to remember that diverticular bleeding is neither chronic nor occult. Iron deficiency anemia associated with occult blood in the stool can never be attributed to diverticulosis without an appropriate diagnostic evaluation.

CLINICAL PRESENTATION

Diverticular bleeding usually occurs in an older patient with diverticulosis who has previously been asymptomatic or undiagnosed. The patient may or may not experience abdominal cramping and passes a large volume of bright red to dark maroon blood with or without signs of hypovolemia. The patient may have one or two more such movements and then no more, or the bleeding may continue for several days. Bleeding stops spontaneously in 80% of patients, with the rate of additional bleeding after one episode between 20% and 25%.[30] There are no distinctive features by which to distinguish diverticular bleeding from other causes of lower gastrointestinal bleeding.

PHYSICAL EXAMINATION

The physical examination is generally normal, although the digital rectal examination can reveal anorectal lesions as the source of bleeding. If blood loss is excessive, signs of hypovolemia with postural vital signs or shock may be present.

DIAGNOSTICS

A CBC will help determine not only the blood loss but also whether this bleeding has been ongoing. The initial assessment includes a rectal examination and a proctosigmoidoscopy, which may reveal bleeding from anorectal lesions, rectal cancer, or acute colitis. Upper gastrointestinal bleeding must be excluded by aspiration of gastric contents, and in some instances esophagogastroduodenoscopy is indicated.[29] A barium enema should never be the initial test in patients with diverticular bleeding because angiography or colonoscopy is precluded until the contrast material is evacuated. With slow bleeding, colonoscopy is the best approach, and a recent study suggests that colonoscopy is an effective diagnostic adjunct even in aggressive bleeding.[29] Scintigraphic or angiographic localization is necessary with brisk bleeding. Mesenteric angiography can be used as a diagnostic tool for localizing the bleeding site and as a

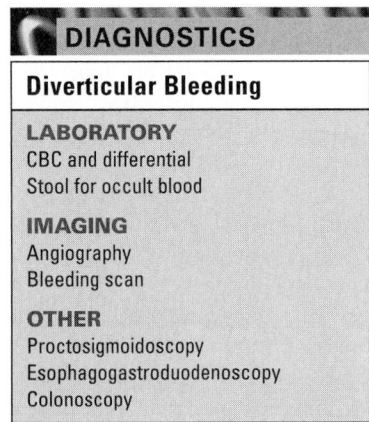

DIAGNOSTICS

Diverticular Bleeding

LABORATORY
CBC and differential
Stool for occult blood

IMAGING
Angiography
Bleeding scan

OTHER
Proctosigmoidoscopy
Esophagogastroduodenoscopy
Colonoscopy

therapeutic intervention in which vasoconstrictive drugs or an artificial blood clot can be infused to control the hemorrhage.

DIFFERENTIAL DIAGNOSIS

Diverticular bleeding is a diagnosis of exclusion. Patients who come in to see the health care provider with a massive hemorrhage often have no prior history of diverticular complications. Bleeding is characteristically sudden and brisk and is usually self-limited. Any gastrointestinal lesion that has the potential for massive hemorrhage (e.g., a duodenal ulcer or Meckel's diverticulum) can manifest in a manner similar to diverticular bleeding and must be excluded. Gastric aspiration is a crucial part of the evaluation. Lower tract sources (vascular ectasias; inflammatory diseases; and anorectal lesions such as hemorrhoids, fissures, lacerations, polyps, ulcers, and neoplasms) must be considered.

> **DIFFERENTIAL DIAGNOSIS**
>
> **Diverticular Bleeding**
>
> - Duodenal ulcer
> - Meckel's diverticulum
> - Vascular ectasia
> - Anorectal lesion
> - Inflammatory disease

MANAGEMENT

The prognosis for diverticular bleeding is generally favorable. Most bleeding stops spontaneously and does not recur. Therefore treatment of diverticular bleeding should begin with conservative medical management. Most patients can be observed without the need for urgent diagnostic or invasive therapeutic maneuvers. For those who do need intervention, the evaluation and treatment of diverticular bleeding are interrelated.

The primary interventions for diverticular bleeding are hemodynamic stabilization and resuscitation. Anal or rectal bleeding should first be excluded with a digital rectal examination and proctoscopy. Most cases of mild to moderate hemorrhage stop spontaneously with medical management that includes establishing IV access, placing a Foley catheter, and inserting a nasogastric tube to exclude an upper gastrointestinal source of bleeding. Laboratory tests should include electrolytes, CBC, coagulation studies, and blood type with crossmatch.

Patients, especially older patients, who have massive, active bleeding require observation in an ICU. As previously discussed, several diagnostic options are available, including radionucleotide scanning, angiography, and endoscopy. The patient with persistent diverticular bleeding also has several therapeutic options, including selective intraarterial infusion of vasopressin, angiographic embolization, or surgical resection.

Surgical intervention is required for massive and persistent bleeding that does not respond to medical treatment and interventional radiology. Surgery may also be recommended on an elective basis for patients with recurrent hemorrhages.

COMPLICATIONS

The complications of diverticular hemorrhage are related to hypovolemia and circulatory collapse. Older patients tolerate the hemorrhage poorly because of the ischemic risk to major organs with each bleeding episode.

INDICATIONS FOR REFERRAL OR HOSPITALIZATION

Massive bleeding is an urgent situation and requires collaboration and referral to a gastroenterologist. Surgical intervention may also be necessary. In older patients with bleeding, transient hypovolemia can be a serious problem for major organs, and immediate hospitalization must be considered.

PATIENT AND FAMILY EDUCATION

Careful patient education is essential because of the risk for recurrent bleeding after the first episode. It is important to advise patients to report symptoms in a timely fashion to avoid complications such as hypovolemia and circulatory collapse.

REFERENCES

1. Painter NS, Burkitt DP: Diverticular disease of the colon: a deficiency disease of western civilization, *Br Med J* 2(759):450-454, 1971.
2. Simmang CL, Shires GT: Diverticular disease of the colon. In Feldman M, Scharschmidt B, Sleisenger M, editors: *Sleisenger and Fordtran's gastrointestinal and liver disease pathophysiology/diagnosis/management*, ed 6, Philadelphia, 1997, Saunders.
3. Welch CE, Allen AW, Donaldson GA: An appraisal of the colon for diverticulitis of the sigmoid, *Ann Surg* 138:332, 1953.
4. Parks TG: Natural history of diverticular disease of the colon: a review of 521 cases, *Br Med J* 4(684):639-642, 1969.
5. Parks TG: Post-mortem studies on the colon with special reference to diverticular disease, *Proc R Soc Med* 61(9):932-934, 1968.
6. Ferzoco LB, Rapopoulos V, Silen W: Current concepts: acute diverticulitis, *N Engl J Med* 338(21):1521-1526, 1998.
7. Young-Fadok T, Pemberton JH: *Clinical manifestations and diagnosis of colonic diverticular disease*, 2006, retrieved June 24, 2006, from http://www.uptodateonline.com/utd/content/topic.do?topicKey=gi_dis/6375&selectedTitle=1~24.
8. Farthmann EH, Ruckauer KD, Harng RU: Evidenced-based surgery: diverticulitis—a surgical disease? *Arch Surg* 385:143-151, 2000.
9. Burkitt MD, Painter MS: Dietary fiber and disease, *JAMA* 229(8):1068-1074, 1974.
10. Gear JS, Ware A, Fursdon P, and others: Symptomless diverticular disease and intake of dietary fibre, *Lancet* 1(8115):511-514, 1979.
11. Stemmermann GN, Yatani R: Diverticulosis and polyps of the large intestine: a necropsy study of Hawaii Japanese, *Cancer* 31(5):1260-1270, 1973.
12. Pemberton JH, Armstrong DN, Dietzen CD: Diverticulitis. In Yamata T, Alpers DH, Owyang C, and others, editors: *Textbook of gastroenterology*, ed 2, Philadelphia, 1995, Lippincott.
13. Hyland JM, Taylor I: Does a high fibre diet prevent the complications of diverticular disease? *Br J Surg* 67(2):77-79, 1980.
14. Taylor I, Duthie HL: Bran tablets and diverticular disease, *Br Med J* 1(6016):988-990, 1976.
15. Leaky AL, Ellis RM, Quill DS, and others: High fiber diet in symptomatic diverticular disease of the colon, *Ann R Coll Surg Engl* 67(3):173-174, 1985.
16. The ins and outs of diverticular disease, *Dig Health Nutr* 1:1, 1997.
17. American Dietetic Association: Health implications of dietary fiber: technical support paper, *J Am Diet Assoc* 88(2):217-222, 1988.
18. McGuire HH, Haynes BW: Massive hemorrhage from diverticulosis of the colon: guidelines for therapy based on bleeding patterns observed in 50 cases, *Ann Surg* 175(6):847-855, 1972.
19. Marinella MA, Mustafa M: Acute diverticulitis in patients 40 years and younger, *Am J Emerg Med* 18(2):140-142, 2000.
20. McCarthy DW, Bumpers HL, Hoover EL: Etiology of diverticular disease with classic illustrations, *J Natl Med Assoc* 88(6):389-390, 1996.
21. Ambrosetti P, Robert JH, Witzig J, and others: Acute left colonic diverticulitis: a prospective analysis of 226 consecutive cases, *Surgery* 115(5):546-550, 1994.

22. Cho KC, Morehouse HT, Alterman DD, and others: Sigmoid diverticulitis: diagnostic role of CT: comparison with barium enema studies, *Radiology* 176(1):111-115, 1990.
23. Young-Fadok T, Pemberton JH: *Treatment of acute diverticulitis*, retrieved Jan 21, 2007, from http://www.uptodateonline.com/utd/content/topic.do?topicKey=gi_dis/7966&selectedTitle=1~4588.
24. Ouriel K, Schwartz SI: Diverticular disease in the young patient, *Surg Gynecol Obstet* 156(1):1-5, 1983.
25. Zarling EJ, Piontek F, Klemka-Walden L, and others: The effect of gastroenterology training on the efficiency and cost of care provided to patients with diverticulitis, *Gastroenterology* 112(6):1859-1862, 1997.
26. Tursi A: Acute diverticulitis of the colon: current medical therapeutic management, *Expert Opin Pharmacother* 5(1):55-59, 2004.
27. Salzman H, Lillie D: Diverticular disease: diagnosis and treatment, *Am Fam Physician* 72(7):1229-1234, 2005, retrieved Jan 21, 2007, from http://www.aafp.org/afp/20051001/1229.html.
28. Berk WA: *Detroit Receiving Hospital: emergency medicine handbook*, ed 5, Philadelphia, 2005, Davis.
29. Young-Fadok T, Pemberton JH: *Colonic diverticular bleeding*, retrieved Jan 21, 2007, from http://www.uptodateonline.com/utd/content/topic.do?topicKey=gi_dis/8520&selectedTitle=1~3379.
30. Schoetz DJ: Uncomplicated diverticulitis: indications for surgery and surgical management, *Surg Clin North Am* 73(5):965-974, 1993.

CHAPTER 142

Gastroesophageal Reflux Disease

Nancy D. Bolton

DEFINITION AND EPIDEMIOLOGY

Gastroesophageal reflux refers to the movement of gastric contents from the stomach to the esophagus. This occurs in virtually everyone several times a day without producing any symptoms or signs of damage. However, this normal physiologic process can be pathologic and can produce signs and symptoms of mucosal damage within the esophagus or in the pharynx, larynx, and respiratory tract. When mucosal damage occurs or when there are chronic symptoms, the individual is said to have gastroesophageal reflux disease (GERD).

GERD is one of the most prevalent and costly clinical conditions affecting the gastrointestinal tract. If the prevalence of GERD is based on heartburn, the disease is very common in Western countries. Every year more than 18 million Americans suffer from GERD.[1] An estimated $5.8 billion dollars is spent each year for antireflux medication, higher than that of all other gastrointestinal disorders.[2] GERD is slightly more common in males than in females and is more common in Caucasians than in African Americans.[3]

The most common symptom is heartburn and acid regurgitation. Three main types of GERD are defined as:

Nonerosive or endoscopic negative GERD: Heartburn without esophageal mucosal damage

Erosive GERD: Erosions or ulcers in the esophagus

Barrett's esophagus: A premalignant condition

The severity of symptoms is not always the best indicator of which type of GERD is present. Some contend that nonerosive GERD may be a separate entity and not part of a continuum, considering that symptoms may not progress over the spectrum.[4]

PATHOPHYSIOLOGY

No single mechanism explains all cases of GERD, but there are four probable factors in the pathogenesis of reflux:

- Transient lower esophageal sphincter (LES) relaxation
- Low resting pressure of the sphincter
- Poor esophageal clearance
- Defects in esophagogastric motility

Evidence suggests that the acid component of the refluxate is the cause of heartburn symptoms and erosion development.[4] Other factors include the duration of the acid reflux event on the esophageal mucosa and the extent and composition of refluxate.

The first factor, transient LES relaxation, has been shown to be the cause of most reflux events. LES relaxation allows the gastric contents to reflux back into the esophagus inappropriately, resulting in esophageal damage. In pregnancy, there is a 25% to 50% prevalence of reflux. This reflux results from the relaxant effects that circulating estrogen and progesterone have on the LES.[3]

The second factor, low resting pressure of the sphincter, has been demonstrated in a minority of patients with reflux esophagitis. It remains unclear whether low LES pressure is a cause or consequence of esophagitis, since chronic inflammation may also reduce the sphincter's ability to close. In addition, patients with chronic symptoms usually have a hiatal hernia. The hiatal hernia and reduced LES pressure appear to be co-factors that result in the greatest degree of reflux.[5] The presence of a hiatal hernia alone does not necessitate the presence of reflux esophagitis, since the majority of patients with hiatal hernias do not have any symptoms. The next pathogenetic factor is the esophagus's ability to clear itself of reflux material. Abnormalities in peristalsis increase the risk for esophagitis by failing to clear the refluxate, which increases contact time between mucosal acid and the esophagus. A decrease in esophageal peristalsis can be more pronounced in those with concomitant diseases such as diabetes mellitus or scleroderma, where the presence of neuromuscular dysfunction contributes to esophageal mucosal damage leading to esophagitis.

The last predisposing factor for the development of GERD is abnormal motility. This includes delayed gastric emptying in which the gastric contents are allowed to backwash into the esophagus as a result of their increased time in the stomach. This condition is seen with diabetes, postviral infections, and most commonly a functional disorder.

Defense mechanisms include salivary secretion, which plays an important role in buffering reflux material in the esophagus, and the secretion of alkaline fluid by the esophageal glands.[6] Salivation is decreased during sleep, which contributes to prolonged acid clearance and increased symptoms during the night. Abnormalities of salivary secretion, such as sicca syndrome, can diminish salivary production and lead to esophagitis.

CLINICAL PRESENTATION

The most common symptom of GERD is heartburn, which is usually described as a burning retrosternal discomfort. Other terms for heartburn include *indigestion, acid regurgitation, sour stomach,* and *bitter belching*. The hot sensation usually begins inferiorly and radiates up the entire retrosternal area to the neck, occasionally to the back, and, rarely, into the arms. The sensation may become so intense that it is described as pain. Heartburn is usually relieved with antacids, baking soda, or milk, but this remedy is often short lived. Heartburn is usually precipitated by food intake and occurs within 1 hour of eating, particularly after a large fatty meal.

Other foods that precipitate heartburn are foods high in fat or sugar, chocolate, coffee, and onions because they lower pressure in the LES (Box 142-1). Cigarette smoking and alcohol consumption may also lower pressure in the LES. Other foods that commonly cause heartburn are citrus products, tomato-based foods, and spicy foods. These foods do not affect LES pressure but instead are direct mucosal irritants. Other direct irritants include aspirin, NSAIDs, potassium, or just pills themselves.

BOX 142-1

FACTORS AFFECTING HEARTBURN

LOW PRESSURE ON LOWER ESOPHAGEAL SPHINCTER

Foods
- Fat
- Chocolate
- Onions
- Coffee
- Sugars

Medications
- Calcium channel blockers
- Progesterone
- Theophylline

Alcohol
Cigarettes

DIRECT MUCOSAL IRRITANT

Foods
- Citrus-based foods
- Tomato-based foods
- Coffee
- Spicy food

Medications
- NSAIDs
- Acetylsalicylic acid
- Tetracycline
- Potassium chloride
- Tablets

INCREASED INTRAABDOMINAL PRESSURE

Bending
Lifting
Straining
Exercise

Patients may also complain of heartburn that increases after going to bed, especially after eating late in the evening. This usually occurs within 1 to 2 hours of bedtime. In a study evaluating nighttime heartburn, 79% of patients with heartburn report symptoms at night, with 75% saying their sleep is affected and their ability to function the next day is impaired.[7] Several other maneuvers, including bending over, lifting, straining, or exercising, may also precipitate heartburn because of increased intraabdominal pressure. Unfortunately, the frequency or severity of heartburn is not predictive of the degree of esophageal tissue damage seen at endoscopy. Some patients with erosions are asymptomatic, whereas other patients with frequent and even severe symptoms can have overall normal tissue. However, patients with Barrett's esophagus have more predictive symptoms.[8]

Other symptoms of GERD include acid regurgitation, water brash, dysphagia, odynophagia, and chest pain. Acid regurgitation is the complaint of a bitter acidic fluid in the mouth that usually occurs at night or when bending over. This symptom should be differentiated from vomiting. Water brash is the appearance of salty-tasting fluid in the mouth because of stimulated saliva secretion. If delayed gastric emptying is the cause of GERD, abdominal fullness, nausea, and early satiety may be seen.

Dysphagia and odynophagia are more predictive of severe disease and should be considered alarm symptoms. Dysphagia is an impairment of swallowing food into the stomach and is experienced immediately after swallowing. Patients may say that the food "sticks," "hangs up," or "stops." Odynophagia is pain on swallowing; this type of pain usually occurs under the sternum and has a sharp quality. Odynophagia is more commonly associated with infectious esophagitis or pill ulceration.

Chest pain can mimic angina, which is not surprising because of the shared neural pathways. Esophageal disorders are probably the most common cause of noncardiac chest pain. Reflux is experienced by approximately 50% of patients with angina-type chest pain but normal coronary arteries.[9] Symptoms that are more suggestive of esophageal problems include pain that continues for hours; interrupts sleep; or is retrosternal without lateral radiation, meal related, or relieved with antacids. Pain that is not exercise induced is also suggestive of an esophageal disorder.

Other nonesophageal or atypical symptoms of GERD include sore throat, laryngitis, earache, gingivitis, poor dentition, chronic cough, hoarseness, bronchitis, asthma, sleep apnea, and aspiration pneumonia.[9]

PHYSICAL EXAMINATION

A careful history is probably more important than the physical findings. Epigastric tenderness or heme-positive stools may be the result of esophageal erosions, ulcerations, or even severe inflammation. Weight loss may be a concern, particularly in patients who have dysphagia. Respiratory wheezes and cough may be seen if there is associated asthma. An association between dental erosions and GERD has been found; thus an oral examination may suggest GERD in a patient with extensive loss of enamel and exposed dentin.[8]

DIAGNOSTICS

The combination of symptoms of heartburn and regurgitation, aggravated by recumbence or bending over and relieved by antacids, is generally diagnostic of GERD. Further diagnostic testing should be considered in patients with:

- Failed empiric therapy
- Sudden onset of symptoms and an age over 50 years
- Alarm symptoms suggesting complicated disease (anemia, dysphagia, bleeding, odynophagia)
- Longstanding symptoms of sufficient duration to put them at risk for Barrett's esophagus

The purpose of evaluating patients with long-term symptoms is to exclude complications of GERD. The practice guidelines of the American College of Gastroenterology (ACG) for 2005 recommend esophagogastroduodenoscopy (EGD), the technique of choice to identify Barrett's esophagus and diagnose GERD complications.[8] Barium radiography has poor specificity and sensitivity and should not be used as a screening test.[8]

Endoscopic biopsy is required to search for intestinal metaplasia diagnostic of Barrett's esophagus, a premalignant condition requiring surveillance in the coming years. With dysphagia, an upper endoscopy is always indicated initially because dilation of a possible stricture can occur at the same time as the diagnostic procedure.

A normal EGD in patients with GERD symptoms does not exclude the diagnosis. Up to 75% of patients will have a normal EGD but may well have pathologic amounts of acid reflux controlled by acid suppressants.[4] Ambulatory pH testing and esophageal manometry are of benefit in patients with refractory symptoms and before reflux surgery.[10] New advances in technology using a radiotelemetry capsule without the discomfort of a nasogastric tube may now allow increased use of this diagnostic tool.

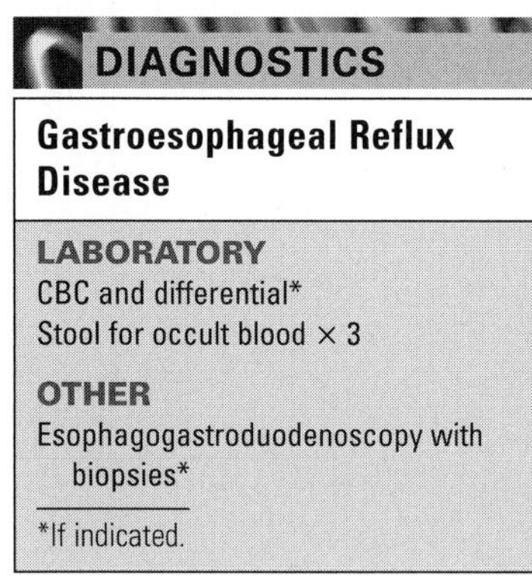
DIAGNOSTICS

Gastroesophageal Reflux Disease

LABORATORY
CBC and differential*
Stool for occult blood × 3

OTHER
Esophagogastroduodenoscopy with biopsies*

*If indicated.

Opinion is divided whether patients should be tested and treated for *Helicobacter pylori* before long-term proton pump inhibitor (PPI) therapy. This strategy is not seen in North America, where the prevalence of *H. pylori* is low and that of GERD is high.[10]

DIFFERENTIAL DIAGNOSIS

The symptoms of GERD can be similar to those of cholelithiasis, peptic ulcer disease, gastritis, angina, and esophageal motility disturbances. These disorders can be distinguished from GERD through the use of ultrasound, upper gastrointestinal x-ray studies, endoscopy, esophageal manometry, ECG, or coronary angiography. GERD may be the most common cause of esophagitis, but there are other causes, including cytomegalovirus, herpes, or *Candida* infections in patients who are immunocompromised. Medications such as tetracycline or potassium chloride, if dissolved in the esophagus, result in "pill esophagitis" (see Box 142-1). In unexplained cases of chest pain, cough, hoarseness, or asthma, GERD should be considered.

MANAGEMENT

The 2005 ACG practice guidelines address the management of GERD based on levels of evidence ratings of I to IV, with I having the strongest evidence. The goals of therapy are prompt and sustained symptom control; healing of the

DIFFERENTIAL DIAGNOSIS

Gastroesophageal Reflux Disease

- Cholelithiasis
- Peptic ulcer disease
- Gastritis
- Angina
- Esophageal motility disturbances
- Esophagitis secondary infection
- Tumor
- Esophageal infection
- Medication-induced "pill esophagitis"

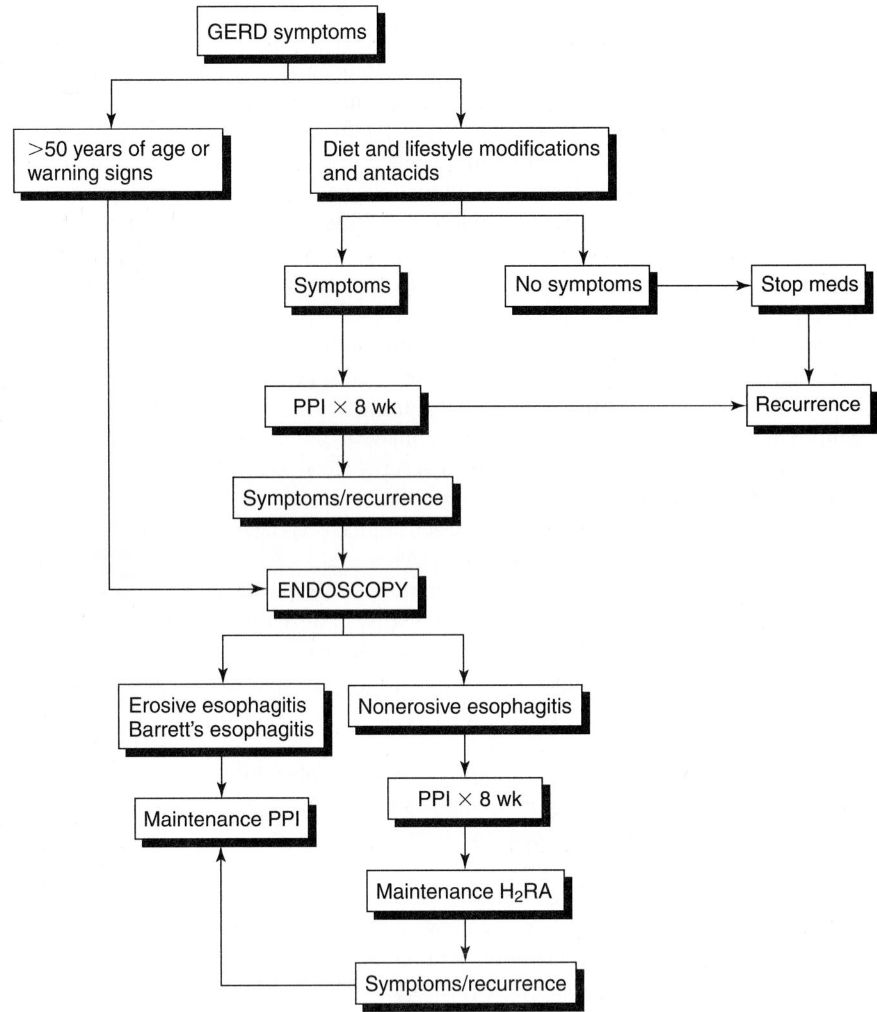

FIGURE 142-1

Gastroesophageal reflux disease *(GERD)* algorithm. *PPI,* Proton pump inhibitor; *H_2RA,* H_2-receptor antagonist.

injured esophageal mucosa; and prevention of complications, including stricture formation, Barrett's esophagus, and adenocarcinoma (Figure 142-1).[10]

Level of Evidence: IV

Besides empiric therapy with acid suppressants, lifestyle modification and patient-directed therapy are used initially. Many heartburn sufferers do not seek medical care and choose antacids and over-the-counter (OTC) acid suppressants. All four of the histamine$_2$ (H_2)–receptor antagonists approved for use in the United States are available OTC and do decrease gastric acid, particularly after a meal. They are often taken before an activity known to cause reflux symptoms. Antacids are helpful but have a shorter duration. Patients will also take OTC omeprazole, a PPI. Patients should seek medical advice if more than 14 days of treatment is required.

Lifestyle modifications may benefit patients with GERD, although these changes alone are unlikely to control symptoms (Box 142-2).[8] These steps include elevating the head of the bed, lowering fat intake, ceasing smoking, and avoiding recumbency for 3 hours after a meal. The true efficacy of these changes is lacking in the literature. Avoidance of chocolate, alcohol, peppermint, coffee, onion, and garlic can lower LES pressure. The potential negative effect of lifestyle changes on quality of life has not been studied. When symptoms persist, continued therapy is needed, or alarm symptoms develop, the patient should have further evaluation and treatment.

BOX 142-2

LIFESTYLE CHANGES FOR MANAGEMENT OF GASTROESOPHAGEAL REFLUX DISEASE

- Smoking cessation
- Reduced alcohol consumption
- Reduced dietary fat
- Decreased meal size

Level of Evidence: I

Acid suppression and maintenance therapy with PPIs are well documented as the treatment of choice for GERD. H_2-receptor antagonists in divided doses may be effective in a patient with mild GERD. In a meta-analysis of 33 randomized trials and more than 3000 patients with erosive GERD, symptomatic relief was seen in 27% of placebo-treated patients (only lifestyle modifications), 60% of those treated with H_2-receptor antagonists, and 83% of those treated with PPIs.[8] Healing rates were similar. Thus PPIs are superior to H_2-receptor antagonists (even in high doses multiple times a day) in controlling symptoms, healing esophagitis, and improving quality of life.

PPIs are safe and effective, and the benefit of chronic use outweighs any theoretic risk. PPIs should always be given before meals, usually breakfast. There is some evidence that nighttime heartburn may be better controlled by taking the medication before the evening meal.[8]

Twice daily PPI dosing is indicated for a diagnostic trial of noncardiac chest pain; empiric therapy for supraesophageal symptoms; partial response to standard prescription; and breakthrough symptoms, severe esophageal dysmotility, or Barrett's esophagus. The second dose should be given before the evening meal, not bedtime.

Because GERD is a chronic condition, continuous therapy to control symptoms and prevent complications is recommended in the ACG practice guidelines.[8]

GERD symptoms rapidly return in many patients once PPIs are discontinued. The goal of therapy is keeping symptoms under control and preventing complications. Up to 20% of patients may require only antacids and lifestyle modifications as maintenance therapy. A full dose of H_2-receptor antagonists given daily is not appropriate for GERD. Reduced dosages of PPIs such as alternative day or "weekend therapy" have been shown to be ineffective long-term prescriptions.[8] As needed and "on demand" use of PPIs is being evaluated.

Level of Evidence: II

Promotility agents may be used in selected patients as an adjunct to acid suppression. The currently available agents are not ideal for monotherapy. Nonerosive GERD patients more often need these and other agents despite PPIs. Laparoscopic fundoplication performed by an experienced surgeon is an option for the patient with well-documented chronic GERD. The best predictors for surgical success of GERD include:

- Less than 50 years old
- Typical reflux symptoms that completely resolve with medical therapy

Patients with atypical and supraesophageal symptoms or those who are refractory respond less effectively to surgery.[8]

Endoscopic Therapies

Several endoscopic techniques for GERD have been developed that are less invasive than laparoscopic fundoplication. As many as 80% of patients using these techniques have had their symptoms controlled with reduction or elimination of their antireflux medication.[10] The best candidates are those with well-documented diagnoses of GERD who respond to PPI therapy. Since these techniques are fairly recent, the long-term efficacy and cost-effectiveness are not known.

The Stretta System consists of a radiofrequency generation and a delivery catheter. The catheter is positioned and needles are deployed into the muscles of the gastroesophageal (GE) junction. Energy is delivered to create a series of thermal lesions.

EndoCinch is an endoscopic suturing system that places sutures to alter the anatomy of the GE junction by tightening the cardia of the lesser curve of the stomach.

Enteryx is a biopolymer that is injected along the muscle layer of the submucosal layer of the cardia.

The Gatekeeper involves submucosal placement of an expandable miniature hydrogel prosthesis in the area of the GE junction. After placement, the prosthesis will swell and bulk the GE junction. The advantage of this system is it can be removed if needed.

COMPLICATIONS

Complications of GERD include esophageal strictures, Barrett's esophagus, hemorrhage, and perforation. Strictures are bands of fibrous tissue in the distal esophagus, which can impede the progress of food from the mouth to the stomach. These bands develop over months to years and are characterized by dysphagia and a possible reduction in heartburn, since the stricture can act as a barrier to reflux. Initial treatment is with PPIs to reduce inflammation. Dilation may be necessary if symptoms are persistent and may need to be repeated months to years later.

In Barrett's esophagus the lower esophagus is lined with a simple columnar epithelium rather than with the normal stratified squamous epithelium.[3] This change results from chronic reflux—the columnar epithelium provides protection against acid. Although Barrett's esophagus is protective initially, it is a premalignant condition that can lead to the development of esophageal adenocarcinoma. Of the patients with esophagitis, 10% to 12% develop Barrett's esophagus, and approximately 10% of these patients develop adenocarcinoma.[6] Barrett's esophagus occurs more often in Caucasian men at an average age of 55 years.[1] The presentation is commonly heartburn or dysphagia. Biopsies are required to confirm the diagnosis. If Barrett's esophagus is present, periodic upper endoscopies with biopsies are recommended to assess the development of dysplasia or malignancy.

Surveillance endoscopy every 3 years is suggested for those patients who have GERD but not dysplasia. For patients with low-grade dysplasia, yearly endoscopy is recommended, whereas those with high-grade dysplasia should have endoscopy performed every 3 months.[11]

Hemorrhage and perforation are rare complications of ulcerative esophagitis. However, chronic bleeding and iron deficiency anemia can develop and may be the only sign of GERD.

INDICATIONS FOR REFERRAL OR HOSPITALIZATION

Although heartburn can be managed without a referral, it is important to identify patients who could profit from maximum long-term medical therapy or who have complications. Patients who initially received empiric treatment without success or whose symptoms recur when medications are stopped should have an upper endoscopy to determine whether esophagitis is present. A gastroenterology referral is indicated if the patient is more than 50 years of age or has the warning signs of dysphagia (both solid and liquid), odynophagia, unexplained iron deficiency anemia, weight loss, fecal occult bleeding, obstructive symptoms (nausea, vomiting, and early satiety), or anorexia.

PATIENT AND FAMILY EDUCATION

Education is imperative for patients with GERD. There is no one particular diet for patients with reflux. Patients should avoid fatty foods, chocolate, peppermint, and excessive alcohol consumption. Food that may elicit symptoms for one person may not necessarily produce symptoms in another; therefore selective avoidance of foods that precipitate symptoms is necessary. Lifestyle modifications are numerous and have been outlined previously. Taking the PPI 30 to 60 minutes before a meal is optimum, but only 36% of providers instruct patients on when to take the PPI.[12]

REFERENCES

1. Frank L, Kleinman L, Ganoczy D, and others: Upper gastrointestinal symptoms in North America: prevalence and relationship to healthcare utilization and quality of life, *Dig Dis Sci* 45:809-818, 2000.
2. Sandler RS, Everhart JE, Donowitz M, and others: The burden of selected digestive diseases in the United States, *Gastroenterology* 122:1500-1511, 2002.
3. Yamada T: *Textbook of gastroenterology*, ed 2, Philadelphia, 1995, Lippincott.
4. Tack J, Fass R: Review article: approaches to endoscopic-negative reflux disease: part of the GERD spectrum or a unique acid-related disorder? *Aliment Pharmacol Ther* 19(Suppl 1):28-34, 2005.
5. Sleisinger MH, Fortran JS: *Gastrointestinal disease*, ed 5, Philadelphia, 1993, Saunders.
6. Gallup Organization National Survey: *Heartburn across America*, Princeton, NJ, 1998, Gallup Organization.
7. Johnson DA, Orr WC, Carwley JA, and others: Effect of esomeprazole on nighttime heartburn and sleep quality in patients with GERD: a randomized, placebo-controlled trial, *Am J Gastroenterol* 100:1914-1922, 2005.
8. Devault K, Castell DO: Updated guidelines for the diagnosis and treatment of gastroesophageal reflux disease, *Am J Gastroenterol* 100:190-200, 2005.
9. Malagelada JR: Review article: supra-oesphageal manifestations of gastro-oesophageal reflux disease, *Aliment Pharmacol Ther* 19(Suppl 1):43-48, 2004.
10. Freston JW, Triadafilopoulos G: Review article: approaches to the long-term management of adults with GERD–proton pump inhibitor therapy, laparoscopic fundoplication or endoscopic therapy? *Aliment Pharmacol Ther* 19(Suppl 1):35-42, 2004.
11. Spechler SJ, Barr H: Review article: screening and surveillance of Barrett's oesophagus: what is a cost-effective framework? *Aliment Pharmacol Ther* 19(Suppl 1):49-53, 2004.
12. Howden CW, Chey WD: Gastroesophageal reflux disease, *J Fam Pract* 52:240-247, 2003.

CHAPTER 143

Gastrointestinal Hemorrhage

Margaret Costello

DEFINITION AND EPIDEMIOLOGY

Gastrointestinal (GI) bleeding is a common finding in the ambulatory care setting. Patients may report the symptoms as black tarry stools (melena), bright red stools (hematochezia), and even bright red vomitus (hematemesis).[1] GI hemorrhage can occur anywhere in the GI tract from the mouth to the anus and can be overt or occult[2] (Box 143-1). Overt GI bleeding is considered major when accompanied by hemodynamic instability and minor when it is not. Occult bleeding is not visible but can be detected by stool testing or indirectly suggested by iron deficiency anemia.

Pathologic processes that contribute to the incidence of GI bleeding vary from ulceration and inflammation to erosion of a blood vessel from a neoplasm.[3] Management of GI bleeding has remained constant over several decades. Hemodynamic stabilization of the patient, cessation of active bleeding, and prevention of recurrent bleeding have long remained the goals of medical management for this disorder, which occurs in approximately 100 cases per 100,000 per year.[4] Many of these patients require emergency treatment, hospitalization, and intensive care monitoring.

GI bleeding is subdivided into upper and lower GI bleeding according to its anatomic source. Patients with upper GI tract bleeding from a source proximal to the ligament of Treitz may be asymptomatic; have subtle signs of anemia and hypovolemia; or present dramatically with hematemesis, melena, or hematochezia.[5] The most common cause of upper GI bleeding is related to nonspecific mucosal abnormalities (42%). Peptic ulcer disease, previously a major factor in the incidence of upper GI bleeding, has been on the decline and is currently associated with only 21% of upper GI bleeding cases.

BOX 143-1

BLEEDING DEFINITIONS

Overt: Visible bright red or maroon-colored blood in feces or emesis.
Occult: No visible blood in feces or emesis.
Obscure: Patient may be seen with iron deficiency anemia (IDA) or have a positive fecal occult blood test (FOBT).
Obscure/Occult: IDA recurrent or persistent. FOBT positive. May or may not have visible bleeding. No bleeding source found at time of original endoscopy.
Obscure/Overt:

- IDA recurrent persistent. Positive FOBT. No visible blood in feces. No source identified.
- Blood visible in feces and emesis. Bleeding recurrent or persistent. No source found at original endoscopy.

Modified from Zuckerman GR, Prakash C, Askin MP, and others: American Gastroenterological Association practice guidelines, *Gastroenterology* 118(1):210, 2000.

Esophageal inflammation accounts for 15% of cases, and esophageal varices are implicated in 12% of cases of upper GI bleeding. Other causes—arteriovenous malformations, Mallory-Weiss syndrome, and tumors—accounted for less than 5% of all cases of upper GI bleeding. NSAIDs and aspirin are frequently implicated as a causative factor in the occurrence of upper GI bleeding and have been associated with a mortality rate reported between 21 and 24.8 cases per million people.[6,7] One third of these deaths were associated with low-dose aspirin use.[7] Other studies have also shown a significant relationship between low-dose aspirin and upper GI bleeding.[8,9] Upper GI bleeding has been estimated to cause more than 350,000 hospitalizations per year and has a 10% mortality rate.[10]

Lower GI tract bleeding from a source distal to the ligament of Treitz can cause occult blood loss or massive hematochezia and shock. The most common cause of lower GI bleeding is diverticulosis. Other common sources include cancer and polyps (19%); colitis and ulcers (18%); unknown (16%); angiodysplasia (8%); miscellaneous causes such as post-polypectomy, aortocolonic fistula, stercoral ulcer, and anastomotic bleeding (8%); and anorectal, hemorrhoids, fissures, rectal ulcers (4%).[11]

PATHOPHYSIOLOGY

The pathophysiology of GI bleeding can be associated with esophagitis, peptic ulcer disease, gastritis, *Helicobacter pylori,* esophageal or gastric varices, diverticulosis, gastric and colonic cancers, gastric and colonic polyps, and angiodysplasia.[2,4,5] Peptic ulcers are defects in the mucosa of the duodenum or stomach that are caused by a breakdown in the normal mucosal defenses. Bleeding from peptic ulcers occurs when the ulcer erodes into a blood vessel.[2,4,5] Contributing factors include alcohol, NSAIDs, excess stomach acid production, and *H. pylori.*

Gastritis causes bleeding from diffuse superficial lesions in the gastric mucosa that are usually caused by local irritants or that occur in association with *H. pylori.* NSAIDs inhibit cyclooxygenase, decreasing the synthesis of protective prostaglandins, and may have direct effects on the gastric mucosa, causing both irritation and superficial lesions. Alcohol ingestion causes the production of leukotrienes by the gastric mucosa, which may be responsible for vascular stasis, engorgement, and increased vascular permeability, which leads to hemorrhage.[12,13] Gastritis can also be caused by major physiologic stressors, including burns, sepsis, trauma, and long-distance running, secondary to decreased splanchnic blood flow and the resultant decrease in mucus production, bicarbonate secretion, and prostaglandin synthesis, all leading to a breakdown in the normal mucosal defenses.[12]

H. pylori has received a formidable amount of public attention and research since it was first described in 1984. This gram-negative spiral bacterium has adaptive mechanisms to survive in the human stomach, including the conversion of urea, water, and acid to ammonia and bicarbonate; the use of adhesions and toxins; its motility; and the fact that it is microaerophilic. Its importance is that nearly 100% of cases of chronic, superficial gastritis, 90% to 95% of duodenal ulcers, and 80% of gastric ulcers are believed to be caused by *H. pylori.*[12] Treatment of this organism has been shown to cure ulcer disease and decrease the incidence of ulcer recurrence and rebleeding.[14,15]

Esophageal varices arise from obstruction of the portal venous system, leading to increased portal pressure, which over time results in the development of dilated venous collaterals.[16] The most common cause of portal hypertension in the United States is cirrhosis from alcoholic and chronic active hepatitis; however, worldwide the most common cause is parasitic liver disease (particularly schistosomiasis).[14-17] Approximately one third of all patients with cirrhosis will bleed from varices; overall mortality is 30%.[5,18]

Diverticulosis is a significant factor in the incidence of acute lower GI bleeding.[4] Diverticula occur at the penetration site of nutrient vessels, with bleeding occurring as a consequence of arterial rupture into the diverticular sac.[12]

Angiodysplasias, small vascular tufts formed by capillaries, veins, and venules, representing an acquired arteriovenous malformation,[13] are the most common lesions found in the GI tract. A small percentage of these lesions are present at birth, but most angiodysplasias are detected in people older than 60 years.[19,20] Although massive bleeding is occasionally associated with these lesions, more often bleeding is slow, chronic, and occult.

CLINICAL PRESENTATION

Blood loss from the GI tract commonly manifests in varied ways. Hematemesis is bloody vomitus that is either fresh and bright red or older and "coffee ground" in appearance. Melena is stool that is black, shiny, and foul smelling as a result of blood degradation. Hematochezia is the passage of bright red to mahogany-colored blood from the rectum as pure blood, blood mixed with stool, blood clots, or bloody diarrhea. These manifestations are more overt or obvious, but occult blood loss is often more subtle. Occult blood loss can manifest as iron deficiency anemia or as a positive routine fecal occult blood test using a chemical reagent.[20] The presentation can include symptoms associated with blood loss, such as presyncope, dyspnea, angina, postural hypotension, and shock, with no overt bleeding source.

The history should include the amount, duration, and source of any bleeding, along with any associated symptoms, including dizziness, abdominal pain, chest pain, shortness of breath, diaphoresis, and weakness.[5] The patient should be questioned about prior episodes of bleeding and about other illnesses that can result in bleeding such as cirrhosis, cancer, coagulopathies, or connective tissue disease. All significant past medical and surgical conditions should be elicited and documented, as well as any allergies and medication usage, including alendronate, potassium chloride, anticoagulants, and over-the-counter preparations (especially aspirin and NSAIDs).[2] A careful history of alcohol, tobacco, and illicit drug use is also necessary.[2,5]

PHYSICAL EXAMINATION

The physical examination is brief and focused. The initial general appearance and a mental status evaluation of the patient should be noted. Vital signs should be obtained early and repeated frequently. The earliest sign of hypovolemia is tachycardia, with hypotension not occurring until volume loss approaches 40%.[21] The skin should be examined for color, temperature, turgor, moisture, and capillary refill. Cutaneous lesions on upper extremities, lips, and oral mucosa may reveal hereditary hemorrhagic telangiectasia or blue rubber bleb nevus syndrome. These can be related to a family history of GI bleeding.[2] Other cutaneous manifestations that should be noted on the physical examination include spider nevi, palmar erythema, scleral icterus, and parotid enlargement.

The cardiovascular examination should focus on the heart rate and the character of the peripheral pulses. Postural change in blood pressure should be immediately noted. Orthostasis suggests a blood volume loss of 15% to 20%.[21] If the blood pressure falls more than 10 to 15 mm Hg or the heart rate increases by more than 10 to 15 beats per minute when the patient stands from a supine position, consider immediate hospital admission.

The abdomen should be auscultated and palpated to identify a mass, tenderness, guarding, or rigidity. Abdominal pain, particularly cramping in the periumbilical area and abdominal distention, may indicate rapid intestinal transit of blood and indicate a major bleed.[22] A careful rectal examination can detect hemorrhoids, fissures, or rectal carcinoma. The stool should be examined for gross blood and melena and tested for occult blood.[23] After the patient is stabilized, a thorough physical examination should be performed in search of non-GI sources of bleeding such as increased or irregular menstrual bleeding in the presence of iron deficiency anemia.[24]

DIAGNOSTICS

The initial diagnostic step in the evaluation of GI bleeding should be insertion of a nasogastric (NG) tube, especially if the location of the bleeding is in question. An NG tube lavage that reveals blood or coffee ground–like material confirms the diagnosis of upper GI bleed,[22] although 16% of patients with actively bleeding lesions at endoscopy may not demonstrate blood in the aspirate.[23,24] The gastric lavage may not be positive for blood if the bleeding has ceased or if the bleeding is occurring beyond the closed pylorus.[22]

Laboratory evaluation of all patients with GI bleeding should include hemoglobin, hematocrit, and platelet count to assess baseline blood loss and platelet adequacy.[25] The patient's blood should be typed and crossmatched for 4 to 6 units of packed red blood cells, and laboratory studies for BUN, creatinine, glucose, calcium, liver function tests, prothrombin time, and activated partial thromboplastin time should be done.[5] An increased BUN level with normal creatinine is suggestive of an upper GI source.[14] Arterial blood gases may be helpful in both assessing oxygenation and clarifying the patient's acid-base status. An ECG should be obtained in all patients over 40 years old with chest or abdominal pain or a history of cardiac or pulmonary disease. Radiographic studies may include an acute abdominal series if there is suggestion of a perforated viscus or intestinal obstruction accompanying bleeding.

Screening for esophageal varices is recommended by the American College of Gastroenterology for the primary prevention of variceal hemorrhage.[26,27] Further diagnostic studies such as endoscopy, barium studies, bleeding scans, or angiography should be performed at the discretion of the consulting gastroenterologist or surgeon.[23-25,28]

DIAGNOSTICS

Gastrointestinal Bleeding

LABORATORY

Stool for occult bleeding
CBC with differential
Platelets
BUN
Creatinine
Serum glucose
Calcium
LFTs
Serum electrolytes
Amylase level
PT/PTT
ABGs
Helicobacter pylori
Type and crossmatch

IMAGING

Abdominal x-rays
Bleeding scans or angiography*
Upright chest x-ray (for severe abdominal pain)
CT of abdomen and surgical consult (if all other tests remain negative and patient continues to have severe abdominal pain with intestinal bleeding)

OTHER

Blood pressure tilts for orthostatic hypotension
ECG (if >40 years or with cardiac history)
Endoscopy*
Barium studies*
Air-contrast enema*
Nuclear scintigraphy*†
Selective mesenteric angiography*†
Enteroscopy*
Anoscopy†
Sigmoidoscopy†
Colonoscopy†

*If indicated.
†For evaluation of lower gastrointestinal bleeding.

DIFFERENTIAL DIAGNOSIS

The sources of GI bleeding may be categorized as inflammatory, mechanical, vascular, neoplastic, systemic, or anomalous. Patients with an upper GI source of bleeding generally are initially seen with hematemesis and/or melena, a bloody NG aspirate, an elevated BUN-creatinine ratio (>36), and hyperactive bowel sounds. Patients with a lower GI source of bleeding generally are seen with hematochezia, a clear NG aspirate, a normal BUN-creatinine ratio, and normoactive bowel sounds.[25]

The presence or history of black or red hematemesis confirms an upper GI source after bleeding from the nose and oropharynx is excluded. Melena represents an upper GI source 85% to 95% of the time, and hematochezia from a briskly

DIFFERENTIAL DIAGNOSIS

Gastrointestinal Bleeding

UPPER GASTROINTESTINAL BLEEDING (ORIGINATING ABOVE THE LIGAMENT OF TREITZ)

- Oral or pharyngeal lesions: swallowed blood from nose or oropharynx
- Swallowed hemoptysis
- Esophageal: varices, ulceration, esophagitis, Mallory-Weiss tear, carcinoma, trauma
- Gastric: peptic ulcer (including Cushing's and Curling's ulcers), gastritis, angiodysplasia, gastric neoplasms, hiatal hernia, gastric diverticulum, pseudoxanthoma elasticum, hereditary hemorrhagic telangiectasia (Rendu-Osler-Weber syndrome)
- Duodenal: peptic ulcer, duodenitis, angiodysplasia, aortoduodenal fistula, duodenal diverticulum, duodenal tumors, carcinoma of ampulla of Vater, parasites (e.g., hookworm), Crohn's disease
- Biliary: hematobilia (e.g., penetrating injury to liver, hepatobiliary malignancy, endoscopic papillotomy)

LOWER GASTROINTESTINAL BLEEDING (ORIGINATING BELOW THE LIGAMENT OF TREITZ)

Small Intestine

- Ischemic bowel disease (mesenteric thrombosis, embolism, vasculitis, trauma)
- Small bowel neoplasm: leiomyomas, carcinoids
- Hereditary hemorrhagic telangiectasia
- Meckel's diverticulum and other small intestine diverticula
- Aortoenteric fistula
- Intestinal hemangiomas: blue rubber bleb nevi, intestinal hemangiomas, cutaneous vascular nevi
- Hamartomatous polyps: Peutz-Jeghers syndrome (intestinal polyps, mucocutaneous pigmentation)
- Infections of small bowel: tuberculous enteritis, enteritis necroticans
- Volvulus
- Intussusception
- Lymphoma of small bowel, sarcoma, Kaposi's sarcoma
- Irradiation ileitis
- Arteriovenous malformation of small intestine
- Inflammatory bowel disease
- Polyarteritis nodosa
- Other: pancreatoenteric fistulas, Schönlein-Henoch purpura, Ehlers-Danlos syndrome, systemic lupus erythematosus, amyloidosis, metastatic melanoma

Colon

- Carcinoma (particularly left colon)
- Diverticular disease
- Inflammatory bowel disease
- Ischemic colitis
- Colonic polyps
- Vascular abnormalities: angiodysplasia, vascular ectasia
- Radiation colitis
- Infectious colitis
- Uremic colitis
- Aortoenteric fistula
- Lymphoma of large bowel
- Hemorrhoids
- Anal fissure
- Trauma, foreign body
- Solitary rectal or cecal ulcers
- Long-distance running

From Ferri F: *Ferri's clinical advisor 2002,* St Louis, 2002, Mosby.

bleeding upper GI source accounts for 10% of cases.[5] Vomiting, coughing, retching, or blunt abdominal trauma before bleeding suggests a Mallory-Weiss tear, the majority of which occur in the upper stomach. Painful upper GI bleeding is suggestive of peptic ulcer disease, gastritis, esophagitis, or duodenitis, with severe pain and peritoneal signs suggesting a perforated viscus. The bleeding of esophageal varices is suggested by a history of cirrhosis and painless bleeding.[5]

Lower GI sources of bleeding associated with abdominal pain include inflammatory bowel disease and aortoenteric fistula. Pain disproportionate to the physical findings is suggestive of ischemic bowel. Painless bleeding may be seen with diverticulosis, angiodysplasia, or hemorrhoids. Rectal pain may be associated with bleeding from anal fissures or hemorrhoids. Constipation may be a diagnostic clue for malignancy or hemorrhoids.

Inflammatory bowel disease or infectious diarrhea should not be overlooked in a patient with bloody diarrhea. Enterohemorrhagic *Escherichia coli* (especially *E. coli* O157:H7) is responsible for up to 20,000 infections per year in the United States alone.[25] This is commonly associated with the ingestion of undercooked ground meat, contaminated water, or unpasteurized milk. This particular strain of *E. coli* has been linked to 250 deaths per year in the United States.[29]

MANAGEMENT

The most important concept in the management of acute GI bleeding is that resuscitation and stabilization must precede diagnostic and therapeutic interventions. The initial priorities are the establishment of an adequate airway, ensuring oxygenation and ventilation, followed by restoration of the circulatory status to normal (Figure 143-1). All patients with hemodynamic instability (shock, orthostatic hypotension, decrease in hematocrit of at least 6%, or active bleeding) should be admitted to the ICU for resuscitation and close monitoring.[22]

Any patient thought to have significant bleeding should immediately have two large-bore IV lines or a central line placed. Fluid resuscitation should be vigorous and should consist of crystalloid infusions of either normal saline or lactated Ringer's solution at rates as rapid as the patient's cardiopulmonary system will allow to correct the volume deficit. Consideration of a central venous pressure line or a Swan-Ganz catheter should be given for patients with underlying cardiac, pulmonary, renal, or hepatic disease to prevent fluid overload.[5] A Foley catheter should be placed to assist with determining volume status, with a minimum urinary output of 30 to 50 ml/hr in the adult.

The blood product of choice initially is packed red blood cells for patients continuing to bleed, patients in shock, patients with very low hematocrit values, or patients who have symptoms related to poor tissue oxygenation (e.g., angina).[23] High-risk patients such as the elderly or those with severe comorbid conditions such as coronary artery disease should maintain hematocrit at greater than 30%. Young and otherwise healthy patients should maintain their hematocrit at greater than 20%.[22] For patients with massive blood loss, whole blood may be used. Close monitoring of coagulation parameters and

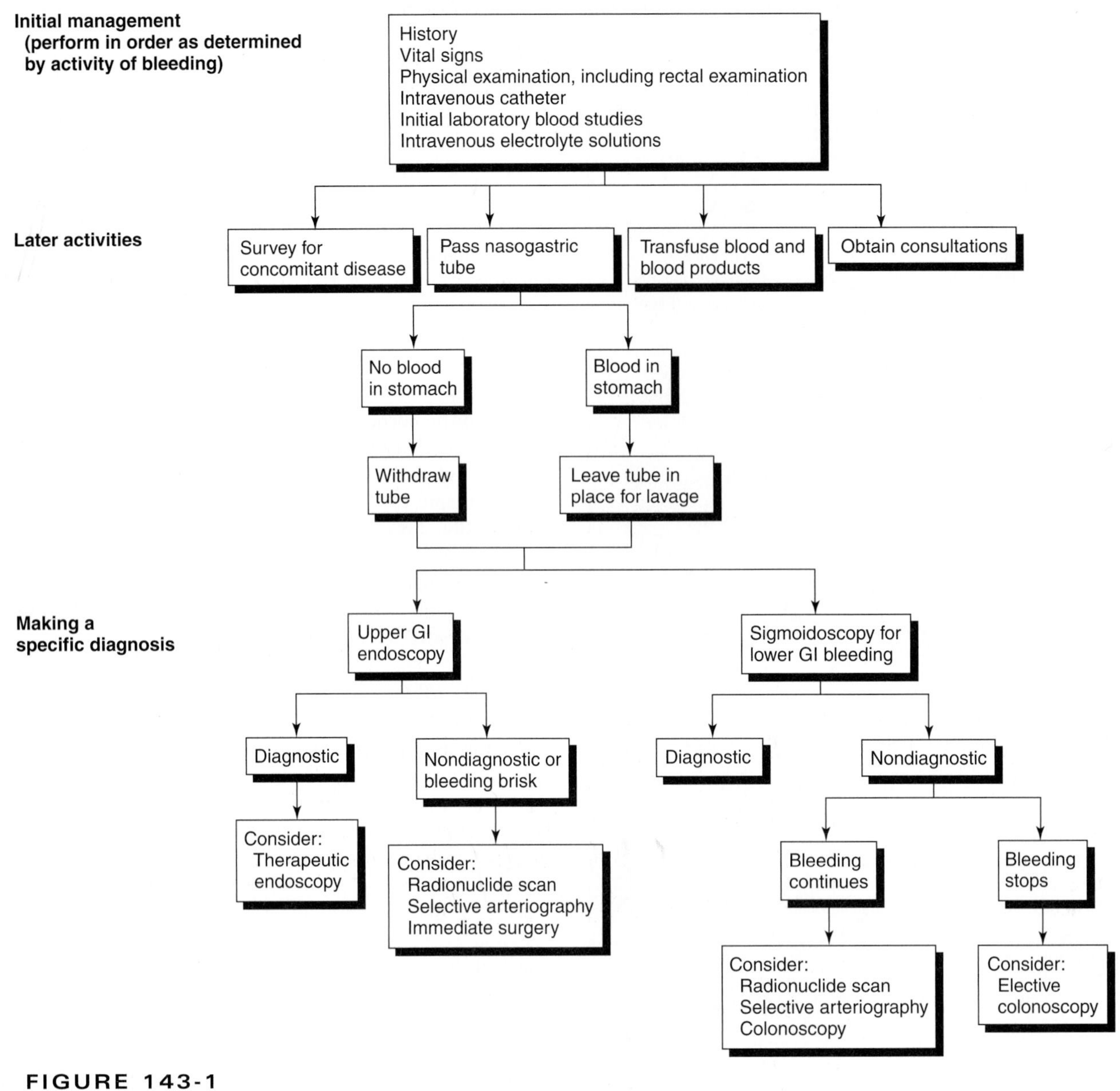

FIGURE 143-1

Management of gastrointestinal *(GI)* bleeding. (Modified from Stein JH, editor: *Internal medicine,* ed 5, St Louis, 1998, Mosby.)

serum calcium must accompany transfusion. Fresh frozen plasma may be used to correct coagulopathy (International Normalized Ratio [INR] >1.5) and should be given at a rate of 1 unit per every 5 to 6 units of blood transfused.[23] Patients with platelet counts less than 50,0000 μL should be transfused with platelets.[22]

The diagnostic test of choice in upper GI bleeding is endoscopy.[2,5,23] Endoscopy has the advantage of identifying patients with continued bleeding or high-risk lesions who will benefit from endoscopic therapy. Therapeutic endoscopy can achieve hemostasis once a bleeding lesion has been identified.[22] High-risk endoscopic findings include arterial bleeding, adherent clot, visible vessels, and varices. Those at risk for rebleeding, resulting in increased morbidity and mortality, are patients over age 60 years, those with coagulopathies and other concurrent illnesses, and anyone hospitalized at the time of bleeding.[23]

All patients with upper GI bleeding should be screened for *H. pylori* infection and treated appropriately.[27] In addition, treatment with PPIs is recommended for patients with upper GI bleeding.

Esophageal varices can cause large-volume GI bleeding because high portal pressures precipitate rupture of varices.[30] Octreotide, a long-acting analog of somatostatin, has become the vasoactive agent of choice for a patient experiencing acute GI bleeding. Octreotide decreases splanchnic and hepatic blood flow along with decreasing transhepatic and variceal pressures, thus reducing portal pressures. Octreotide is given with a 100-mcg IV bolus followed by a 50 mcg/hr continuous infusion.[23]

The most common definitive therapy for esophageal varices is endoscopic sclerotherapy or band ligation.[22] According to Sarin, Wadhawan, Agarwal, and others, endoscopic variceal ligation is as effective as propranolol for the prophylactic treatment of high-risk varices.[31] Endoscopic sclerotherapy involves either intravariceal or paravariceal injection of a sclerosing agent. It has proved to be more effective than balloon tamponade or medical therapy. Balloon tamponade such as the Sengstaken-Blakemore tube has a success rate of 70% to 80% but may cause severe complications, including aspiration, ulceration, and perforation, if used improperly.[4]

Diagnostic modalities available for the evaluation of lower GI bleeding include anoscopy, sigmoidoscopy, colonoscopy, nuclear scintigraphy, selective mesenteric angiography (with vasopressin infusion or selective embolization), enteroscopy, and operative therapy.[18] The evaluation of the patient with lower GI bleeding depends on the rate (moderate, severe) and frequency (continuous, recurrent) of the bleeding.[23] If there is clinical suspicion of an upper GI source, the patient should undergo NG lavage. Vigorous fluid resuscitation should precede any diagnostic evaluation. Since sigmoidoscopy in an unprepped patient may fail to produce the source of the bleeding, colonoscopy is now recommended for the evaluation of lower GI bleeding. If this fails to reveal a source of the bleeding, an endoscopy should be performed. Colonoscopy in this setting is the diagnostic procedure of choice because of its accuracy and therapeutic capability.[18,29] Barium studies are of little use in localizing acute lower GI bleeding and may actually yield misleading information.[4,32] Barium studies are usually reserved for high-risk patients who have contraindications to colonoscopy.

Radionuclide evaluation or a bleeding scan (red blood cell scan) is capable of detecting a hemorrhage as slow as 0.1 ml/min.[32] The tagged red blood cells circulate for 48 hours, and gamma camera scanning is then used to detect the tagged cells in the bowel's lumen, indicating lower GI bleeding. This test is positive 26% to 78% of the time.[4]

Enteroscopy, peroral or transnasal, is used for small bowel examination when both colonoscopy and endoscopy have not revealed a bleeding source. Causes of small bowel bleeding that can be detected by enteroscopy include large hiatal hernia sac erosions, peptic ulcer disease, and angioectasia.[33] Enteroscopy can also be used to evaluate suspected small bowel lesions, malabsorptive processes, and abnormal radiologic findings.

Indications for surgical management of lower GI bleeding include (1) transfusion of 4 or more units in 24 hours or more than 10 units overall, and (2) significant rebleeding that occurs within 1 week of initial cessation and in the presence of co-morbid disease.[4] Emergency surgery can be lifesaving but associated with high morbidity and mortality if the location of the lesion is not identified before the surgical procedure. Surgical resection can be associated with rebleeding in up to 30% of the cases.[2]

Co-Management with Specialists

Asymptomatic patients in whom GI bleeding is suggested during routine screening or hemodynamically stable patients with minor bleeding may be appropriately evaluated on an outpatient basis with specialty referral for endoscopy or radiologic studies.[23]

LIFE SPAN CONSIDERATIONS

Upper GI bleeding has an overall mortality of 5% to 10%.[4] Mortality is significantly higher in older adults, primarily a result of co-morbid disease. According to Fantry, peptic ulcer disease affects 4.5 million people in the United States each year.[34] Variceal bleeding occurs in more than 40% of patients with chronic liver disease; 30% to 50% of patients die from a variceal bleeding episode.

The patient with lower GI bleeding tends to be older than the patient with upper GI bleeding and hence has more co-morbid illness. The incidence of lower GI bleeding is unclear.[35] Acute lower GI bleeding is more common in men than women, and the incidence rises along with age. This increase may be related to the increased incidence of diverticulosis, angiodysplasia, and neoplasms in older adults.[4]

COMPLICATIONS

Many of the complications of GI bleeding are associated with the diagnostic or therapeutic modalities used in its treatment. Serious complications of endoscopy, bleeding scans, and angiography include bowel ischemia and infarction.[12] Perforation of the gut can occur with upper or lower endoscopy. Extraintestinal complications of angiography include local hematoma formation, dye allergy, and the potential for renal failure.

INDICATIONS FOR REFERRAL OR HOSPITALIZATION

All patients with acute upper GI bleeding require urgent consultation with a gastroenterologist.[5,32] Patients with hematochezia or signs of ongoing bleeding should also be immediately referred. A surgical consultation should be obtained for any patient who is hemodynamically unstable, has an abdominal aortic aneurysm or graft, or has a suspected perforation.[5,32]

Admission to the ICU is recommended for all high-risk patients with hemodynamically unstable GI bleeding or rebleeding and for patients who have (1) red hematemesis or grossly bloody gastric aspirate, (2) an abdominal aortic aneurysm or a graft, (3) any bleeding with severe anemia, (4) a large drop in hematocrit, or (5) unstable co-morbid disease.[5,32]

Hospitalization is recommended for patients with melena who are hemodynamically unstable or who have had recent bleeding with significant but stable co-morbid disease.[5] A select group of patients may be discharged home after urgent endoscopy, provided they are hemodynamically stable, have no co-morbid disease, and have no high-risk endoscopic findings.[5]

PATIENT AND FAMILY EDUCATION

Patients should understand that NSAIDs, alcohol, tobacco, diet, and stress can affect the disease. Substance abuse should be identified and patients actively encouraged to participate in alcohol or tobacco cessation programs. Stress management classes can be indicated for those patients whose lifestyles indicate that behavioral change in this area could be beneficial. General dietary guidelines should include (1) the need to avoid offending agents (generally spicy foods, alcohol, caffeine, chocolate); (2) the need to avoid late-night snacks in reflux disease; and (3) the fact that a low-fat, high-fiber diet has shown benefit in diverticular disease and in the prevention of colon cancer. All patients should have thorough education and demonstrate an understanding of all medication use, interactions, and possible side effects.

HEALTH PROMOTION

Screening colonoscopy is recommended for all men and women of average risk to begin at age 50 years. For those with a strong family history of GI bleeding or colon cancer, screening should begin at age 40 years.[36] EGD is suggested for patients with GERD unresponsive to treatment.

REFERENCES

1. Stedman TL: *Stedman's medical dictionary,* ed 26, Baltimore, 1995, Williams & Wilkins.
2. Zuckerman GR, Prakash C, Askin MP, and others: American Gastroenterological Association practice guidelines, *Gastroenterology* 118(1):201-221, 2000.
3. Rajan E, Ahlquist D: *Gastrointestinal bleeding,* 2003, retrieved Jan 7, 2006, from http://www.acpmedicine.com.
4. Fallah MA, Prakash C, Edmundowicz S: Acute gastrointestinal bleeding, *Med Clin North Am* 84(5):1183-1208, 2000.
5. McGuirk TD, Coyle WJ: Upper gastrointestinal tract bleeding, *Emerg Med Clin North Am* 14(3):523-545, 1996.
6. Jutabha R, Jensen D: *Major causes of upper gastrointestinal bleeding in adults,* retrieved Jan 23, 2007, from http://www.uptodateonline.com/utd/content/topic.do?topicKey=gi_dis/9702&selectedTitle=3~529.
7. Lanas A, Perez-Aisa MA, Feu F, and others: A nationwide study of mortality associated with hospital admission due to severe gastrointestinal events and those associated with nonsteroidal antiinflammatory drug use, *Am J Gastroenterol* 100(8):1685-1693, 2005.
8. Sapoznikov B, Vilkin A, Hershkovici M, and others: Minidose aspirin and gastrointestinal bleeding—a retrospective, case-control study in hospitalized patients, *Dig Dis Sci* 50(9):1621, 2005.
9. Nelson MR, Liew D, Bertram M, and others: Epidemiological modelling of routine use of low dose aspirin for the primary prevention of coronary heart disease and stroke in those aged, *BMJ* 330(7503):1306, 2005.
10. Eisen GM, Dominitz JA, Faigel DO, and others: An annotated algorithmic approach to upper gastrointestinal bleeding, *Gastrointest Endosc* 53(7):853-858, 2001.
11. Saab S, Jutabha R: *Etiology of lower gastrointestinal bleeding in adults,* retrieved Jan 23, 2007, from http://www.uptodate.com.http://www.uptodateonline.com/utd/content/topic.do?topicKey=gi_dis/14450.
12. Longstreth GF: Epidemiology and outcome of patients hospitalized with acute lower gastrointestinal hemorrhage: a population-based study, *Am J Gastroenterol* 92(3):419-424, 1997.
13. Yardley JH, Hendrix TR: Gastritis, duodenitis, and associated ulcerative lesions. In Yamada T, Alpers DH, Laine L, and others, editors: *Textbook of gastroenterology,* ed 3, Philadelphia, 1999, Lippincott.
14. Soll AH: Consensus conference: medical treatment of peptic ulcer disease: practice guidelines: Practice Parameters Committee of the American College of Gastroenterology, *JAMA* 275:622, 1996.
15. Hopkins RJ, Girardi LS, Turney EA: Relationship between *Helicobacter pylori* eradication and reduced duodenal and gastric ulcer recurrence: a review, *Gastroenterology* 110:1244, 1996.
16. Jutabha R, Jensen DM: Management of severe upper gastrointestinal bleeding in the patient with liver disease, *Med Clin North Am* 80:1035, 1996.
17. Brewer TG: Treatment of acute gastroesophageal variceal hemorrhage, *Med Clin North Am* 77(5):993-1009, 1993.
18. Smith JL, Graham DY: Variceal hemorrhage: a critical evaluation of survival analysis, *Gastroenterology* 82:968, 1982.
19. Gunnlaugsson O: Angiodysplasia of the stomach and duodenum, *Gastrointest Endosc* 31:251, 1985.
20. Peterson WL, Laine L: Gastrointestinal bleeding. In Fordtran JS, Sleisenger MH, editors: *Gastrointestinal diseases: pathophysiology, diagnosis, and management,* ed 5, Philadelphia, 1993, Saunders.
21. Cook JD, Skikne BS: Iron deficiency: definition and diagnosis, *J Int Med* 226:349, 1989.
22. Jutabha R, Jensen D: *Approach to the adult with upper gastrointestinal bleeding,* retrieved Jan 23, 2007, from http://www.uptodateonline.com/utd/content/topic.do?topicKey=gi_dis/15047.
23. Pianka JD, Affronti J: Management principles of gastrointestinal bleeding, *Prim Care Clin Office Pract* 28(3):557-575, 2001.
24. Ferri FF: Gastrointestinal bleeding. In Ferri FF, editor: *Ferri's clinical advisor 2002,* St Louis, 2002, Mosby.
25. Bono MJ: Lower gastrointestinal bleeding, *Emerg Clin North Am* 14(3):547-556, 1996.
26. Zaman A, Hapke RJ, Flora K, and others: Changing compliance to the American College of Gastroenterology guidelines for the management of variceal hemorrhage: a regional survey, *Am J Gastroenterol* 99(4):645-649, 2004.
27. Barkun A, Bardou M, Marshall JK: Consensus recommendations for managing patients with nonvariceal upper gastrointestinal bleeding, *Ann Intern Med* 139(10):843-857, 2003.
28. Oldfield EC, Wallace MR: The role of antibiotics in the treatment of infectious diarrhea, *Gastroenterol Clin North Am* 30(3):817-835, 2001.
29. Koutkia P, Mylonakis E, Flanigan T: Enterohemorrhagic *Escherichia coli* O157:H7: an emerging pathogen, *Am Fam Physician* 56(3):853-856, 1997.
30. Velayos F: Upper and lower gastrointestinal bleeding in the critically ill patient. In Parsons PE, Wiener-Kronish JP, editors: *Critical care secrets,* ed 3, Philadelphia, 2003, Hanley & Belfus.
31. Sarin SK, Wadhawan M, Agarwal S, and others: Endoscopic variceal ligation plus propranolol versus endoscopic variceal ligation alone in primary prophylaxis of variceal bleeding, *Am J Gastroenterol* 100(4):797-804, 2005.
32. Eisen GM, Dominitz JA, Faigel DO, and others: An annotated algorithmic approach to acute lower gastrointestinal bleeding, *Gastrointest Endosc* 53(7):859-863, 2001.
33. Eisen GM, Dominitz JA, Faigel DO, and others: Enteroscopy, *Gastrointest Endosc* 53(7):871-873, 2001.
34. Fantry GT: *Peptic ulcer disease,* 2005, retrieved April 2, 2006, from http://www.emedicine.com.
35. Cagir B, Cirincirone E: *Lower gastrointestinal bleeding: a surgical perspective,* 2005, retrieved April 2, 2006, from http://www.emedicine.com.
36. US Preventive Screening Task Force: Screening for colorectal cancer. In *Guide to clinical preventive services,* ed 2, Baltimore, 1996, Williams & Wilkins.

CHAPTER 144

Hepatitis

Wendy L. Biddle

DEFINITION AND EPIDEMIOLOGY

Hepatitis is a general term for inflammation in the liver. Hepatitis has numerous causes, including viruses, alcohol, medications, autoimmune disease, and metabolic defects. Inflammation that continues for 6 months is considered chronic liver disease and can eventually result in cirrhosis, characterized by scarring and death of hepatocytes. More than 5.5 million cases of chronic liver disease and cirrhosis occurred in the United States in 1998, for a rate of 2030 cases per 100,000 population. Chronic liver disease accounts for $1.4 billion in direct health care costs per year.[1]

Physician consultation and referral are indicated for patients with newly diagnosed hepatitis.

Viral Hepatitis

Viral hepatitis is attributed to five main groups of viruses that attack the liver: hepatitis virus A (HAV), B (HBV), C (HCV; previously known as non-A, non-B), D (HDV; previously known as delta and occurring only as co-infection with HBV), and E (HEV). The features of the viruses are described in Table 144-1. A sixth virus, G (HGV), has been isolated, but little is known about it.[2] Other viruses can cause a secondary hepatitis that never becomes chronic. Acute viral hepatitis can range in severity from a clinically asymptomatic infection to fulminant hepatic failure and death. Chronic viral hepatitis is considered to be the presence of virus 6 months from initial exposure and can range in severity from mild disease with minimum inflammation to cirrhosis, liver failure, and/or hepatocellular carcinoma.

HAV is an RNA virus in the Picornaviridae family. In developed countries, HAV accounts for up to one third of all cases of viral hepatitis. All strains of this virus belong to the same serotype; as a result, HAV immunoglobulin provides worldwide protection.[3] The virus can be inactivated by boiling for 1 minute or by exposure to formaldehyde, chlorine, or ultraviolet radiation. HAV occurs globally and is transmitted via the fecal-oral route, through person-to-person contact, and through the ingestion of contaminated food or water. Poor sanitation, poor personal hygiene, and overcrowding increase the transmission rate.

HAV can be found in liver cells, bile, stool, and blood. Hepatitis A has an incubation period of 2 to 6 weeks, with patients being most infectious in the late incubation period. The virus can be found in the stool 2 to 3 weeks before and up to 1 week after the development of clinical jaundice. Despite the presence of HAV in the liver, viral shedding in feces, viremia, and infectivity rapidly decrease once jaundice appears.[4] Therefore most patients are contagious when they are asymptomatic and are no longer contagious by the time they become diagnosed with jaundice. An important exception involves neonates, who can be infectious for up to 6 months after clinical jaundice develops.[3] HAV infection never progresses to chronic hepatitis.

Hepatitis B is endemic worldwide, especially in Asia, where the carrier rate is estimated to be 1:4. It is less prevalent in the United States, and new infections are decreasing, but the Centers for Disease Control and Prevention (CDC) estimated 60,000 new infections in 2004.[5] Approximately 1.2 million people were reported to have chronic hepatitis B from 1999 to 2002.[6] Hepatitis B is endemic among Alaskan Natives, with an estimated prevalence of 3% to 8%.[7]

HBV is a DNA virus that belongs to the Hepadnaviridae family. In Asia and Africa, HBV infection is seen mostly among newborns and young children and is spread via vertical transmission from mother to child. In North America and Europe, hepatitis B is more common among adolescents and young adults and is spread via sexual contact and percutaneous exposure. Each year in this country, 10,000 hospital admissions and 250 to 300 deaths are attributed to HBV infection. More than 1 million people in the United States are chronic carriers, and almost 5000 people die from HBV-related cirrhosis or hepatocellular carcinoma annually. The number of new cases of hepatitis B reported has declined each year since 1985. A safe and effective vaccine against HBV was introduced in 1982.[3]

Hepatitis B can present a clinical picture similar to that of the other subtypes, with a severity that can range from asymptomatic to fulminant and fatal liver failure; it can progress to chronic liver disease with cirrhosis and hepatocellular carcinoma.[4] HBV can be found in blood, tears, cerebrospinal fluid, breast milk, saliva, vaginal secretions, and seminal fluid. HBV is transmitted parenterally, via sexual contact, and perinatally. Heterosexual contact with a person infected with HBV is the most common mode of transmission, followed by IV drug use, homosexual activity, and, last, vertical transmission from mother to child at the time of birth. Transmission from blood transfusions is rare in the United States because of extensive screening processes. HBV is not transmitted via the fecal-oral route or by arthropod vectors. Compared with the general population, health care workers, especially surgeons, phlebotomists, and dialysis nurses, and the spouses of infected persons are at an increased risk for contracting HBV.

Hepatitis C, the number one reason for liver transplantation, has reached epidemic level in the United States, with an estimated 4 million people infected and anti-HCV seropositive (1% to 3% of the general population) and 2.7 million chronically viremic. These estimates are likely low, since this does not take into account the homeless, incarcerated, and hospitalized. Fortunately, new infections with HCV are uncommon; the primary cause of the approximately 38,000 new cases that occur per year is injection drug use.[8] Most infections occurred 10 to 30 years earlier. It is estimated that 20% to 40% of people with chronic hepatitis C will develop cirrhosis after 20 to 40 years. African Americans appear to have a slower disease progression with a lower incidence of cirrhosis than non–African Americans.[6,9]

HCV, first identified in 1989, is a single-strand RNA genome with a high rate of replication (10^{12} virions/day) and mutation. These characteristics lead to chronic infection, making it

TABLE 144-1 Features of Viral Hepatitis

	Hepatitis A	Hepatitis B	Hepatitis C	Hepatitis D	Hepatitis E
Incubation period	2-6 weeks	2-6 months	2-22 weeks	4-8 weeks	2-9 weeks
Onset	Usually acute	Usually insidious	Usually insidious	Usually acute	Usually acute
Symptoms					
Nausea and vomiting	Common	Common	Common	Common	Common
Fever	Common	Uncommon	Uncommon	Uncommon	Uncommon
Jaundice	50%	33%	25%	?	10%-20%
Arthralgias	Rare	Common	Rare	Rare	Rare
Diagnosis	IgM anti-HAV	HBsAg	Anti-HCV	IgM anti-HDV	Anti-HEV
Transmission					
Fecal-oral	Usual	Rare	No	?	Usual
Parenteral	Rare	Usual	Usual	Usual	No
Sexual	Yes	Yes	Yes	?	?
Perinatal	No	Yes	Yes	?	No
Sequelae					
Chronic carrier	No	5%-10%	Up to 75%	? Most	No
Chronic active hepatitis	No	Approximately 5%	75%	Up to 70%	No
Fulminant hepatitis	Approximately 0.1%	0.2%-1.0%	No	Up to 17%	2%-10%*
Recovery	99%	85%-90%	—	?	90%-98%*
Epidemiology					
Epidemics	Foodborne or waterborne	Contaminated blood products	IV drug abuse and contaminated blood products	Contaminated blood products	Foodborne or waterborne
Posttransfusion	Extremely rare	<5% of cases	85%-95% of cases	Possible	No
Prevention	ISG	HBIG vaccine	? ISG	Hepatitis B vaccine	? ISG from endemic areas

Modified from Stein JH: *Internal medicine*, ed 4, St Louis, 1994, Mosby.
IgM, Immunoglobulin M; *ISG*, human immune globulin; *HBIG*, hepatitis B immune globulin; *HbsAg*, hepatitis B surface antigen.
*10%-20% fatalities in pregnant women.

difficult to treat.[8] Currently six strains and multiple subtypes of the virus have been identified. Genotypes 2 and 3 respond better to treatment than does genotype 1, but 70% of people in the United States have genotype 1.

Once a person is infected, the body initiates humoral and cellular mechanisms. The Third National Health and Nutrition Examination Survey found that approximately 75% of patients with HCV develop chronic infection.[10] It is rare to see fulminant hepatic failure with acute HCV. The 25% believed to have cleared the virus may have a strong cellular immune response to HCV. Ineffective cellular immune responses lead to inflammation and damage in the liver. Extrahepatic manifestations of HCV occur when humoral immune responses are continually stimulated. These can involve the skin, kidney, and nerves. Factors associated with rapid disease progression and cirrhosis include older age at time of infection, alcohol abuse, male gender, and co-infection with HIV.[8]

HCV was transmitted via transfusions before July 1992, receipt of clotting factor concentrates produced before 1987, chronic hemodialysis, any injection of illegal drugs, and snorting of cocaine. No clinical trials have studied the possible risk factors of tattoos, manicures, and body piercings; however, theoretically these could be modes of transmission. These practices are not regulated and should be considered as possible risk factors, especially if there have been multiple exposures or the work was done in questionable environments. Health care workers and emergency medical personnel are at risk from needle sticks, sharps, or mucosal exposure to HCV-positive blood.[11] Sexual transmission is responsible for up to 20% of new cases, but the overall rate is believed to be less than 5%. Those with multiple partners have a two to five times higher risk of acquiring HCV through sexual contact. Long-term partners should be tested every 5 years. The rate of vertical transmission from mother to child during delivery is approximately 5%. Certain subgroups are believed to have an especially high rate: 20% of those on hemodialysis and even higher rates in prisoners.[8] Co-infection of HCV and HIV is becoming more prevalent, creating unique challenges in management. There is no evidence that arthropod vectors transmit HCV.

HDV is a DNA virus that requires co-infection with HBV for replication. It can be transmitted with HBV or may superinfect an individual who is already infected with HBV. It is transmitted parenterally through IV drug use and, rarely, via sexual contact. Perinatal transmission is rare and can be prevented through HBV prophylaxis. When seen in the Mediterranean region, HDV is endemic with HBV. In nonendemic areas such as the United States, HDV is associated with percutaneous exposure and blood transfusions. HDV is not transmitted through the fecal-oral route or by casual contact.

HEV is another RNA virus that has been identified as being responsible for some cases of non-A, non-B hepatitis. This virus has a short incubation period of 15 to 60 days and usually results in a self-limited disease. It is more common in children and young adults. Similar to HAV, HEV is enterically spread, most commonly via the ingestion of contaminated water. Areas endemic for HEV are Asia, Africa, and Central America. There have been no known cases in the United States, and international travelers are the only group at risk.[12] Infection during pregnancy can lead to liver failure, especially during the third trimester, with mortality rates as high as 30%.[3]

Alcoholic Hepatitis

Alcoholic hepatitis is a type of toxic liver injury associated with excessive alcoholic consumption on a chronic basis, usually 10 years or longer. It is estimated that 10% to 35% of heavy drinkers develop alcoholic hepatitis. Some controversy exists on the levels of alcohol that constitute heavy drinking, but an average of two or three drinks a day for a man and one or two drinks a day for a woman is recognized as increasing the risk of liver disease.[13]

Toxic Hepatitis

Toxic hepatitis, also known as *drug-induced hepatitis,* is usually not dependent on preexisting liver disease. The full range of severity may be expressed in any setting in which drugs are taken. Drug-induced liver disease accounts for between 1 in 600 and 1 in 3500 hospital admissions and between 2% and 3% of all hospital admissions resulting from adverse drug reactions. Between 500 and 1000 therapeutic agents have been implicated in the etiology of a broad spectrum of hepatic diseases. Drugs account for approximately 15% to 30% of all fulminant hepatic failures.[14] A thorough drug history should include information about recent and past exposure to therapeutic agents. Details about the patient's occupation and work environment, as well as the use of herbal preparations and "traditional" medications, should be obtained.[14]

Cirrhosis

Cirrhosis is one of the leading causes of death in the United States, killing approximately 25,000 people per year (9.3 deaths per 100,000), and alcohol is responsible for close to 50% of cirrhosis-related deaths.[15] Studies suggest a genetic predisposition to alcoholic liver disease, and some ethnic groups, such as Native Americans, are at higher risk. Heavy alcohol intake can affect nutritional status, producing primary or secondary malnutrition, which in turn can cause more liver damage.[16]

PATHOPHYSIOLOGY

Process of Inflammation and Development of Cirrhosis

The process of inflammation and development of scarring and cirrhosis is similar for all causes of hepatitis. The pathology of hepatitis involves inflammation and damage to the hepatocytes. Fibrosis and scarring with isolated hepatocyte injury and focal necrosis can develop. Mononuclear infiltration, which consists mostly of lymphocytes, invades the tissue, particularly around the portal triads. Cellular edema and death can occur. There may be a minor degree of periportal necrosis of hepatocytes around these triads, which gives the liver an appearance of piecemeal necrosis on microscopic examination. After the hepatocyte degenerates, its cytoplasm shrinks and condenses to form an acidophil body. The available space is then temporarily filled by monocytes. Although characteristic of acute viral hepatitis, these cytologic changes are not specific to this disease and can also be found with drug-induced injuries and other disease processes.[17]

The inflammatory and scarring processes can lead to "bridging" fibrosis between portal triads. This level of fibrosis and moderate inflammation is a sign that cirrhosis will develop if the damage continues. Increased numbers of liver cells begin to die, which may lead to more collapse and condensation of the liver stroma. This may occur over months in a severe acute injury but is more commonly seen in chronic infection, taking 10 or more years to develop.[17] Bridging necrosis and confluent necrosis can resolve, enabling complete regeneration and histologic recovery in acute hepatitis. Chronic hepatitis, however, can remain mild with little to no scarring ever developing. If scarring does develop, it is unlikely to improve without treatment. Over time, cirrhosis can lead to liver failure or hepatocellular carcinoma and death. Approximately 20% of people with cirrhosis from chronic hepatitis will develop a carcinoma.

Pathogenesis of Hepatitis

The exact pathogenesis of hepatitis A, C, D, and E is not clear. It seems that HBV involves immune complex–mediated tissue damage. Hepatitis B core antigen present on the hepatocyte cell membrane may act as a target for host antibody responses. Circulating immune complexes play an important role in explaining the extrahepatic diseases and serum sickness associated with HBV. These circulating complexes activate the complement system and can cause rash, fever, and angioedema when present as serum sickness or as other forms of immune complex disease such as glomerulonephritis and polyarteritis nodosa.[4]

Although the exact mechanism of alcohol damage to the liver is not known, there are several hypotheses. Ethanol is oxidized in the mitochondria, producing toxins that have harmful effects on lipid and carbohydrate metabolism. Acetylaldehyde is increased, causing hypoxia at the terminal veins in the liver, and oxygen-derived free radicals may cause damage of the liver cells. Proinflammatory cytokines are expressed, stimulating cells to produce collagen, which leads to fibrosis.

Liver damage from hepatotoxins, such as chlorpromazine, rifampin, and estrogens, is variable depending on the drug, dose, and individual hypersensitivity. Damage can appear quickly or may take weeks to months after beginning the medication. Proposed mechanisms include alteration of the membranes, interference with the hepatic uptake process, and free radicals causing lipid peroxidation.[16]

CLINICAL PRESENTATION

Most people are not aware when they develop acute hepatitis because the symptoms are similar to those of any other mild viral illness. Symptoms can include anorexia, fatigue, myalgias, nausea, fever, headaches, arthralgias, vomiting, and abdominal pain. Jaundice can occur, especially with HBV, but it is rare in other viral hepatitis illnesses.

Acute viral hepatitis occurs after an incubation period of varying lengths based on the specific virus. For HAV, the incubation period is 15 to 45 days; for HBV and HDV, 30 to 180 days; for HCV, 15 to 160 days; and for HEV, 14 to 60 days.[4] HDV infection can initially manifest as acute or chronic hepatitis and is dependent on HBV status; for HDV infection to occur, HBV must be present either chronically or simultaneously with HDV. These patients may have concomitant infection of both HBV and HDV acutely or a superimposed HDV infection with preexisting HBV. HBV and HDV are clinically indistinguishable from one another. The clinical suspicion for HDV infection should be high in patients who demonstrate fulminant hepatic failure and a history of positive hepatitis B surface antigen (HBsAg); in such cases an anti-HDV test should be ordered. Unfortunately, acute HEV is difficult to diagnose because no tests are commercially available. Suspicion of HEV should be increased in patients with clinical symptoms of hepatitis and a recent travel history to an underdeveloped country.[3]

People with alcoholic hepatitis commonly are seen with elevated liver function tests (LFTs) but can be asymptomatic. Often aspartate aminotransferase (AST [SGOT]) is higher than alanine aminotransferase (ALT [SGPT]), usually at a ratio of 2:1. Patients can have nonspecific symptoms such as nausea, vomiting, abdominal discomfort, or diarrhea. Those with advanced liver disease appear ill and malnourished and can be feverish.[13] There may be signs of cirrhosis such as jaundice, ascites, encephalopathy, and upper gastrointestinal bleeding.

The presentation of drug-induced liver disease can be a nonspecific febrile or viral-like illness. The diagnosis of chronic hepatitis can be challenging because patients often are not symptomatic until liver damage has progressed. Risk factors for the development of chronic hepatitis include a young age and immunosuppression.[3] Comparisons of the signs and symptoms of the hepatitis viruses are presented in Box 144-1.

BOX 144-1

SIGNS AND SYMPTOMS OF HEPATITIS

HEPATITIS A VIRUS
- May be asymptomatic
- Fever, jaundice, anorexia, nausea, malaise, myalgia
- Infectious 2 weeks before symptoms and 1 week after
- No carrier state or chronic illness

HEPATITIS B VIRUS
- May be asymptomatic
- Anorexia, nausea, myalgia, malaise, jaundice to fatal hepatitis
- Infectious 4 to 6 weeks before symptoms and for unpredictable time after symptoms
- Carrier state and chronic illness

HEPATITIS C VIRUS
- Patients may be asymptomatic
- Anorexia, nausea, malaise, rarely jaundice, myalgia
- Infectious 4 to 6 weeks before symptoms and unpredictable after symptoms
- 75% progress to chronic hepatitis

HEPATITIS D VIRUS
- May be asymptomatic
- Anorexia, nausea, malaise, jaundice, myalgia
- Infectious 4 to 6 weeks before symptoms and unpredictable after symptoms
- Occurs only with HBV as co-infection or as superinfection in chronic HBV infection

HEPATITIS E VIRUS
- May be asymptomatic
- Fever, jaundice, anorexia, nausea, malaise, myalgia
- Infectious 2 weeks before symptoms and 1 week after symptoms
- No carrier or chronic state

From Dunn SA: *Primary care consultant,* St Louis, 1998, Mosby.

PHYSICAL EXAMINATION

A low-grade fever with acute hepatitis is far more common with HAV and HEV, although patients with HBV can develop a serum sickness–like syndrome that can include fever, arthralgias, and rash. Dark-colored urine and clay-colored stools may precede the onset of clinical jaundice by 1 to 5 days. With the onset of jaundice, these constitutional symptoms usually diminish.[3]

On examination, patients with jaundice often have both hepatomegaly and splenomegaly. The onset of jaundice or the icteric phase can be observed when the serum bilirubin is greater than 2.5 mg/dl and is most easily observed in the sclera or under the tongue. Symptomatic hepatitis is difficult to miss, but half the patients with acute hepatitis do not develop jaundice. On the other end of the spectrum, a smaller portion of patients may develop fulminant hepatic failure.[3]

In alcoholic hepatitis the physical findings may be consistent with cholestasis. Fever, jaundice, and leukocytosis may be present. Skin rashes are common, and patients can have tender hepatomegaly, but splenomegaly is uncommon. Physical signs of alcoholic and nonalcoholic cirrhosis are similar, but it is believed that spider telangiectasia, especially on the trunk and upper extremities; parotid enlargement; gynecomastia; palmar erythema; and hepatomegaly are more common with alcoholic cirrhosis.[13]

The presence of extrahepatic manifestations can suggest toxic hepatitis. Fever, rash, and eosinophilia suggest drug hypersensitivity but are relatively nonspecific findings. Presenting signs may include pseudomononucleosis syndrome (phenytoin), systemic vasculitis (allopurinol and sulfonamides), and bone marrow suppression (NSAIDs).[14]

DIAGNOSTICS

The first sign of hepatitis may be the elevation of the serum aminotransferases: AST (SGOT) and ALT (SGPT). These enzymes increase proportionately during the prodromal phase of hepatitis and can reach 20 times normal. The ALT levels should not be used for diagnosis or assessment of severity of liver damage in chronic HCV infection. Although 60% to 70% of patients with chronic HCV infection have elevations of ALT levels, others may have normal or intermittently elevated levels.[18] One study suggests that people with normal ALT levels and HCV have mild chronic hepatitis and slow or absent disease progression to cirrhosis.[19]

The total bilirubin can continue to increase as the aminotransferases decline and may reach 20 mg/dl. There are equal proportions of direct and indirect bilirubin in patients with hepatitis, and bilirubin will also be present in urine. The prothrombin time (PT) is usually normal in patients with acute hepatitis but may become prolonged in patients with severe hepatitis; thus PT can be used as a marker of prognosis. If the PT is greater than three times normal (International Normalized Ratio [INR] 1.5), the patient should be evaluated for fulminant hepatic failure. The WBC count and hemoglobin-hematocrit are usually within normal limits. The platelet count is also normal but may be decreased in fulminant hepatic failure.[3]

Other laboratory tests that may be abnormal, indicating advancing liver damage, are platelet and albumin levels, which will be lower than normal. Anemia may be present. Lactate dehydrogenase and alkaline phosphatase levels are usually normal or mildly elevated. Alkaline phosphatase is not specific to the liver. An elevated alkaline phosphatase level can indicate a fatty liver or obstruction or disease in the bile ducts. If an elevated alkaline phosphatase level is documented, it is useful to determine how much of it is from the liver. Fractionation will show the percentages from the liver, bone, and intestines.

The elevation of aminotransferase levels does not seem to correlate with the histologic severity of the disease.[3] The only test that will provide information on the amount of inflammation and scarring in the liver is a biopsy. Scoring mechanisms can be used to provide a fairly standardized measure of the severity of liver disease.[20] Ultrasound and CT scan are equally useful in documenting tumors, fatty tissue, and size of the liver. The ultrasound is more cost-effective, providing screening information.

Hepatitis A should be suspected if hepatitis infection occurs after the ingestion of contaminated food or shellfish, after natural disasters, in institutionalized adults or children, in patients returning from travel to an endemic area, or in children or families of children in daycare facilities. Diagnosis can be confirmed by the presence of immunoglobulin M (IgM) anti-HAV during the acute illness. Eventually, the IgM anti-HAV decreases over several months, and immunoglobulin G (IgG) anti-HAV rises and persists indefinitely.[3]

The diagnosis of acute HBV depends on the presence of HBsAg and IgM antibodies to hepatitis B core antigen (antibody) (IgM anti-HBc, or HBcAb), which appear approximately the same time as the symptoms. The antibody to HBsAg (HBs antibody, or anti-HBs) develops after infection (approximately 4 to 5 months after exposure) and serves as an indicator of immunity. Anti-HBs is also detectable in individuals who have received the hepatitis B vaccination series or who have passive immunity secondary to hepatitis B immune globulin (HBIG). Anti-HBc indicates prior exposure or infection and lasts for a prolonged period. The presence of IgM anti-HBc indicates recent infection with HBV, typically within the previous 4 to 6 months.

If hepatitis Be antigen (HBeAg) is detected, the virus is undergoing active viral replication and the patient is highly infectious. Antibodies to HBeAg (anti-HBe) develop in most people with HBV and indicate decreases in infectivity and in replication of the virus (inactive phase).[3] Convalescence is suggested by normalization of elevated ALT; by loss of HBsAg, HBeAg, and HBV DNA; and by the development of anti-HBs. If this occurs within 6 months, the episode can be defined as acute hepatitis. Chronic infection occurs in approximately 2% to 5% of acutely infected individuals and is characterized by the persistence of HBsAg beyond 6 months and the presence of HBeAg and HBV DNA for months to years.[17]

Clinically evident acute hepatitis C infection occurs less often than HAV or HBV, and often patients are asymptomatic or only mildly ill. The first level of testing is the antibody to hepatitis C (HCVAb). If this is positive, the viral load should be tested by polymerase chain reaction (HCV RNA PCR). The sensitivity of this test has been greatly improved, and levels of virus are now detected from a few to more than several million international units/ml. If the viral load is detectable, the patient is considered to have chronic hepatitis C; the serology is not available to distinguish acute from chronic HCV. At least six different strains of the virus are known, and the genotype can be tested as well. The genotype is useful in determining potential response to treatment.[8]

HDV infection should be considered in patients with acute HBV infection who develop fulminant hepatic failure or in patients with chronic HBV who show evidence of deterioration. Anti-HDV can be detected to confirm the diagnosis of HDV infection. Patients co-infected with HDV have acute HBV and a positive anti-HDV test. Patients with chronic HBV and a positive anti-HDV test are superinfected. In patients who are superinfected, a high titer (>1:100) of anti-HDV indicates chronic hepatitis D.[3]

HEV infection should be considered in patients returning from travel to India, central and southeast Asia, and the Middle East. Unfortunately, no tests for HEV are commercially available in the United States. If there is epidemiologic evidence of acute HEV infection and if other causes have been eliminated, serum should be sent to the CDC, and an expert in hepatitis should be consulted.[3]

In general, if acute viral hepatitis is suspected, the appropriate serologic tests should include IgM anti-HAV, IgM anti-HBc, HBsAg, and anti-HCV. In patients known to have fulminant hepatic failure or previous infection with HBV, an anti-HDV test is reasonable. HBsAg, HBcAb, HBsAb, and anti-HCV are the appropriate serologic tests for patients with chronic hepatitis.[3]

DIAGNOSTICS

Hepatitis

LABORATORY

ALT, AST, alkaline phosphatase, bilirubin, IgM, protein, albumin, lactate dehydrogenase
CBC and differential, platelets
PT/INR
Hepatitis serologic tests
Genetic markers

OTHER

Abdominal ultrasound or CT scan
Biopsy*

*If indicated.

Typically, alcoholic hepatitis manifests as a cholestasis type of liver disease, with abnormalities seen as elevations in bilirubin and alkaline phosphatase levels. The ratio of AST to ALT is often greater than 2.0, which is considered diagnostic of this disease. Anemia is present in more than 90% of patients with alcoholic hepatitis, and leukocytosis is seen in 41% of patients. In more severe disease, PT may be prolonged, and the albumin concentration is often low. These two proteins are measures of the capacity of the liver to synthesize proteins.

Laboratory testing in the diagnosis of suspected drug-induced liver disease is helpful in excluding other causes of liver disease. Liver biopsy is indicated when the diagnosis remains unclear. Diagnosis depends on the history of exposure; consistent clinical, laboratory, and liver biopsy findings in select cases; and the resolution of liver injury after the presumed toxin has been removed.[14]

Noninvasive markers for hepatic fibrosis have been developed and show promise as adjuncts to diagnosis and management of liver disease.[21-23] Currently a blood test is available that indicates whether fibrosis is present, absent, or indeterminate. It is hoped that this first-generation test will result in more specific and sensitive testing for liver disease.

DIFFERENTIAL DIAGNOSIS

It is always important that patients be evaluated for other causes of liver disease. For instance, chronically elevated LFTs may be a result of alcoholic liver disease, drug- or toxin-induced hepatitis, hepatic steatosis, cholestatic conditions, metabolic diseases, granulomatous hepatitis, pericholangitis associated with inflammatory bowel disease, celiac sprue, or biliary or pancreatic disease. The most common cause of chronically elevated LFTs is fatty liver, affecting up to 20% of the general population. Fatty liver can progress to nonalcoholic steatohepatitis (NASH) and cirrhosis.

The most common drugs known to cause hepatitis are acetaminophen, isoniazid, methotrexate, methyldopa, nitrofurantoin, rifampin, and the cholesterol-lowering statins. Regular monitoring of LFTs is necessary because LFT elevation indicates the presence of liver inflammation. A secondary hepatitis can be caused by other viruses, such as Epstein-Barr virus, cytomegalovirus, HIV, herpes simplex virus, varicella-zoster virus, adenovirus, and coxsackievirus.

Hemochromatosis, increased levels of iron, is the most common inherited disorder in the United States. Testing of iron saturation and ferritin is used for screening. If elevated levels of iron are found, the gene for hemochromatosis can be sought with a test. Autoimmune hepatitis, seen primarily in young women, can be screened with antinuclear antibody testing. Wilson's disease, an autosomal recessive condition that results in toxic copper accumulation in the liver and other organs, must also be considered. Low levels of serum ceruloplasmin, elevated levels of urinary copper, and Kayser-Fleischer rings in the eyes can establish a diagnosis of Wilson's disease.[3] Sarcoidosis can affect the liver and is seen primarily in African Americans. Obtaining an angiotensin-converting enzyme level is used to screen for sarcoid.

DIFFERENTIAL DIAGNOSIS

Hepatitis

- Alcoholic liver disease
- α_1-Antitrypsin deficiency
- Autoimmune hepatitis
- Celiac sprue (gluten intolerance)
- Cholestatic conditions (primary sclerosing cholangitis, primary biliary cirrhosis)
- Granulomatous hepatitis (sarcoid)
- Hemochromatosis
- Hepatic steatosis
- Medication- or toxin-induced hepatitis
- Metabolic diseases
- Nonalcoholic steatohepatitis
- Wilson's disease

Celiac sprue has been known to elevate LFTs, which may be the only clinical sign of the disease. It occurs more frequently than previously thought and was probably missed frequently. It is recommended that a celiac disease panel that includes tissue transglutaminase antibody and antigliadin antibody be obtained. Small bowel biopsy is the definitive diagnostic test.

MANAGEMENT

The management of acute HAV and HBV consists primarily of treating the acute symptoms and providing supportive care. The vast majority of patients do well and experience no chronic sequelae. More than 99% of patients with HAV and up to 90% of patients with HBV recover without incident. Patients who recover from HAV infection do not develop chronic problems, whereas 6% to 10% of patients infected with HBV develop varying forms of chronic hepatitis.[3] If chronic hepatitis results from HBV infection, the HBsAg remains positive after the acute infection. In the acute, uncomplicated course the majority of patients do not require hospitalization, and only symptomatic care is needed. LFTs should be monitored every 2 weeks until normalization.

Before 1990 there was no effective treatment for chronic hepatitis. Interferon (IFN) alfa-2b has since been approved for the treatment of chronic HBV and HCV, with varying success. With the onset of the antiviral age associated with the new anti-HIV drugs, many new chronic hepatitis drugs are currently under investigation.

Chronic HBV infection in the active phase has three treatment options: IFN, lamivudine, and adefovir dipivoxil. IFN is the most expensive and is given as subcutaneous injections of 5 million units/day or 10 million units three times weekly for at least 16 weeks. A sustained response would be a disappearance of HBV DNA and normalization of ALT and AST that lasts at least 6 months after the completion of therapy. Sustained responses occur in approximately 37% of cases.[23,24] The side effect profile for IFN can be significant, including flulike symptoms, fatigue, injection site reactions, leukopenia, and rash.

Lamivudine is given orally for at least 1 year. If treatment is stopped too soon, viral replication recurs. A response of undetectable virus occurs in 17% of cases at 1 year but increases to 50% after 5 years of treatment. Resistance can develop and can cause viral loads to return to pretreatment levels. Adefovir is also an oral medication, and treatment is given for at least 1 year. Response rates of 21% at 48 weeks increase to 46% at 72 weeks. So far no resistance has been seen with adefovir at 1 year of treatment, but at 2 years there has been evidence of resistance developing. Both these medications are well tolerated with low side effect incidence.[23]

Currently, the most effective treatment for chronic HCV is pegylated IFN and ribavirin. Pegylation decreases clearance and breakdown of the drug, allowing the IFN to stay in the system longer. Side effects are more intense with pegylated IFN than regular IFN. Ribavirin is an antiviral medication that improves response rates when combined with IFN. Dosing depends on the product being used.[25] Recommended treatment time is 6 months for HCV genotypes 2 and 3 and 12 months for genotype 1. Several factors have been shown to have a significant impact on the response rate. These include the genotype and viral load, adherence to treatment regimen, and time to development of undetectable viral load. A sustained response is normalization of LFTs and undetectable viral load after treatment is stopped. Patients are monitored periodically after treatment to watch for resurgence of the virus. Patients who relapse can be retreated. Patients with HCV who did not respond to IFN therapy may respond to pegylated IFN and ribavirin retreatment.[26]

The mainstay of therapy for alcoholic hepatitis is alcohol abstinence. Involvement of family, friends, and support groups may be helpful. Malnutrition is a strong contributor to the morbidity and mortality associated with alcoholic hepatitis, and therefore assessment by a dietitian, adequate diet therapy, and vitamin replacement for deficiencies are essential. Parenteral vitamin B is preferred over oral therapy for better absorption in alcoholic patients. Multivitamin preparations that include folic acid, thiamine, vitamins A and D, and essential minerals are also important. In the absence of hepatic encephalopathy, a high-protein diet is recommended. Corticosteroid therapy in the treatment of alcoholic liver disease is controversial. Studies show that corticosteroids are beneficial for improvement in short-term survival in severe alcoholic hepatitis. However, if gastrointestinal bleeding, active infection, pancreatitis, or decompensated diabetes occurs, corticosteroids are contraindicated. Transplants are considered in patients with proven long-term abstinence, but recidivism is a concern.[13]

The most important principle in the management of toxic liver disease is removal of the suspected drug or offending agent. Supportive care of acute hepatitis and liver failure is provided as necessary. In the case of severe, drug-induced liver failure, urgent liver transplantation can be lifesaving. Currently the only specific treatment available is the administration of *N*-acetylcysteine for acetaminophen overdose. In general, corticosteroids have no value in the treatment of drug-induced liver disease.[14]

A new antibiotic, rifaximin, is promising in the treatment of hepatic encephalopathy. Standard treatment with lactulose requires a large enough dose to produce three loose stools a day. Compliance can be an issue. Rifaximin is a poorly absorbed antibiotic that has its effect in the intestinal tract and has a wide antibacterial spectrum. It helps reduce blood ammonia and therefore may be effective in managing hepatic encephalopathy. Research is ongoing.[27]

A variety of combination drugs are being studied to treat hepatitis B, such as lamivudine and IFN.[23] Multiple studies are ongoing to treat nonresponders, relapsers, and various subgroups (such as co-infected HIV/HCV patients and different ethnic groups) infected with chronic hepatitis C.[24,26]

LIFE SPAN CONSIDERATIONS

The liver is a remarkable organ that is capable of regeneration. The treatment of hepatitis has been shown to halt progression and improve liver histology. If hepatitis is treated and cirrhosis does not develop, patients can lead normal lives and their life span will be unaffected. If cirrhosis develops, the life span can be greatly reduced because cirrhosis is a leading cause of death.

Hepatitis is often insidious, and liver damage can be ongoing without the patient's knowledge. Often signs or symptoms do not appear for many years. Lifestyle becomes an important factor, but it is not the sole issue in deteriorating liver disease. Some patients have aggressive disease, and treatment is difficult. Thus it is imperative that health care providers screen for risk factors and routinely monitor LFTs. Abnormal LFT results should never be ignored. The sooner identification and treatment can begin, the better is the prognosis.

COMPLICATIONS

The most significant complications of hepatitis are cirrhosis, liver failure, and cancer. HAV is an acute, self-limiting disease that does not develop into a chronic carrier state. The majority of patients who contract HBV recover without difficulty, although chronic hepatitis and fulminant hepatic failure can occur with HBV. The greatest risk with chronic HBV is the development of hepatocellular cancer. Fulminant hepatic failure does occur in a small percentage of patients (<1%) with acute HAV and HBV. Rapid elevation of PT (more than three times normal), hyperbilirubinemia, and hepatic encephalopathy indicate fulminant hepatic failure. Hospitalization with rapid organ transplantation is the only treatment option; without transplantation, the mortality rate is very high.

The majority of people (75%) infected with chronic HCV do well, without complications. The most important factor in the progression of liver damage is alcohol intake. Those who drink regularly can increase their risk of developing cirrhosis to 50% in 5 years and their risk of cancer to 25%. Progression to cirrhosis can result in ascites, hepatic encephalopathy, peripheral edema, esophageal varices, and other complications of end-stage liver failure. Once cirrhosis is present, there is a risk for the development of hepatocellular carcinoma.

Alcoholic hepatitis has a significant risk of cirrhosis, liver failure, or cancer if the patient continues to drink alcohol. Physical and psychosocial problems and malnutrition are other complications associated with alcoholism.

The prognosis of toxic liver disease is highly variable and depends on the clinical circumstances and the etiologic agent involved. The overall fatality rate is approximately 5%. There is a much poorer prognosis with some agents because they induce acute hepatic necrosis or cause progressive chronic liver disease and cirrhosis.[17]

INDICATIONS FOR REFERRAL OR HOSPITALIZATION

Patients should be referred when abnormal LFT results are found (AST and/or ALT >40 units/L or elevated alkaline phosphatase). Interpretation of testing, need for liver biopsy, and management require specialist input. Even mild acute hepatitis should be referred, since there can be many complicating factors and long-term issues, management needs, and follow-up care. Patients with chronic HCV or HBV should be referred after initial testing. Any patients with signs of increasing liver failure or decompensation of cirrhosis should be emergently admitted to the hospital and gastroenterology or hepatology consult obtained.

PATIENT AND FAMILY EDUCATION

All patients with hepatitis require careful education about the infection, prevention, transmission, treatment options, and complications. The benefit of rest; diet; avoidance of hepatotoxic substances, especially alcohol; and medications should be emphasized.

Hepatitis A can be prevented. Contact with obviously contaminated food or water should be avoided, and infected individuals should not handle or prepare food. In addition, personal objects should not be shared, and hands should be washed thoroughly after patient contact. Health care workers should wear gloves when handling blood or body fluids. Travelers to underdeveloped countries should avoid eating uncooked shellfish, fruits, or vegetables or drinking water that could be contaminated.

Currently, the CDC recommends immune globulin for all travelers to developing countries where HAV is endemic. Hepatitis A immune globulin should be considered for travel that is going to be longer than 6 months. Prophylaxis against hepatitis A should be given as soon as possible after exposure (0.02 mg/kg IM), although it is of no benefit if not given within 2 weeks of exposure. Immunization with immune globulin lasts for 6 months. A hepatitis A vaccine is now currently available. The adult dose is 1.0 ml IM followed by a booster dose at 6 to 12 months. For children 2 to 18 years of age, 0.5 ml IM is given; a booster dose is required in 6 to 12 months. The vaccine is protective for many years, but the total duration of immunity is unknown.[3]

The current plan to eliminate hepatitis B involves routine screening of pregnant women, prophylaxis of infants born to infected women, and routine infant immunization. The hepatitis B vaccine should also be offered to persons at occupational risk, adolescents, IV drug users, recipients of multiple blood products, sexually active individuals, household contacts of HBV carriers, hemodialysis patients, and international travelers. Two vaccines are currently available in the United States: Recombivax HB and Engerix-B. The vaccines are given in a series of three injections: the first two doses 1 month apart, and the third dose given 6 months after the second dose. There are two dosing options for infants: (1) at birth, 1 to 2 months of age, then 6 to 18 months of age; or (2) at 1 to 2 months of age, 4 months of age, then 6 to 18 months of age. If doses are inadvertently missed, the second and third doses should be given 3 to 5 months apart. Antibodies to HBV develop in approximately 90% to 95% of vaccinated individuals but may be as low as 50% to 70% among individuals who are immunocompromised. Checking a titer after the series is completed can determine immune status. Vaccines should be administered in the anterolateral thigh for infants and in the deltoid for adults and children. The vaccine is safe to administer during pregnancy and along with other childhood immunizations.[3]

To prevent transmission, therapy should be initiated immediately after exposure to HBV. It is recommended that infants born to HBsAg-positive women receive HBIG (0.5 ml) and the first dose of the hepatitis B vaccination series within 12 hours of birth, with two more doses of vaccine at 1 and 6 months of age. The recommendations for prophylaxis after sexual exposure to HBV include HBIG (0.06 ml/kg IM) within 14 days of exposure and simultaneous hepatitis B vaccination, with the second and third injections at 1 and 6 months, respectively. The HBIG and hepatitis B vaccines should always be given at different sites.[3]

HBV and HCV are transmitted by blood; therefore patients need to understand the importance of not sharing razor blades, toothbrushes, or nail clippers. Partners of infected patients need to be tested because sexual transmission is possible. Barrier protection should be used, and partners should be told about the patient's hepatitis infection. Long-term monogamous partners can use their discretion if the partner is hepatitis negative, but all partners should be tested every few years to detect any seroconversion. Transmission from mother to baby during delivery is only about 5%, and it is controversial to test children until age 16 years. Household contacts have an extremely low risk. Patients with chronic hepatitis should clean up their blood spills with bleach and bag any bloodstained material before placing it in the trash.

All patients with liver disease should understand the significant risk of developing cirrhosis and cancer with alcohol ingestion. Patients should be counseled and resources provided to help them stop drinking. Referral to psychotherapy, substance abuse counselors, Alcoholics Anonymous, and support groups can be helpful. Family members and significant others need to be included in counseling and therapy.

Patients with chronic HBV and those with HCV with cirrhosis have a risk of developing hepatocellular carcinoma and need screening with ultrasound and alpha-fetoprotein tumor marker, on average every 6 months. Patients with chronic hepatitis should be vaccinated for both HAV and HBV as appropriate.

Treatment with IFN and peginterferon alfa-2b (Peg-Intron A) and ribavirin can cause leukopenia and anemia. Patients must follow up with scheduled appointments and blood tests. Patients must be taught how to administer the injections and need a full disclosure of the side effects of treatment, including depression.

A growing problem has been the incidence of fatty liver. Patients are at risk of developing NASH and eventually cirrhosis. All patients with fatty liver need education about diet, exercise and weight loss, risk of developing diabetes, and cirrhosis. Alcohol use should be minimal, and regular follow-up of LFTs at least yearly is needed. Periodic imaging may also be necessary, and at some point liver biopsy may be needed.[28]

HEALTH PROMOTION

Preventing hepatitis is possible with healthy lifestyles and avoidance of situations that increase risk. A healthy lifestyle includes alcohol and substance abuse avoidance, safe sexual practices, vaccinations, and regular checkups that include monitoring of LFTs.

Risk factors for hepatitis B and C include illicit IV drug use, intranasal cocaine use, tattoos, sexual contact with IV drug users and multiple sexual partners, blood transfusions before 1992, hemodialysis, occupational exposure to blood and needles, incarceration, and institutionalization.

Once hepatitis is diagnosed, complications and disease progression can be deterred by abstaining from alcohol and substance abuse, obtaining vaccinations, becoming knowledgeable about the disease, and maintaining regular follow-up with the health care provider.

REFERENCES

1. Sandler RS, Everhart JE, Donowitz M, and others: The burden of selected digestive diseases in the United States, *Gastroenterology* 122:1500-1511, 2002.
2. Linnen J, Wages J, Zhang-Keck ZY, and others: Molecular cloning and disease association of hepatitis G virus: a transfusion-transmissible agent, *Science* 271:505-508, 1996.
3. Noskin GA: Prevention, diagnosis, and management of viral hepatitis: a guide for primary care physicians, *Arch Fam Med* 4:923-934, 1995.
4. Dienstag JL, Isselbacher KJ: Acute and chronic hepatitis. In Isselbacher KJ, Braunwald E, Martin JB, and others, editors: *Harrison's principles of internal medicine,* ed 13, New York, 1994, McGraw-Hill.
5. Centers for Disease Control and Prevention: *Hepatitis surveillance,* retrieved Jan 26, 2007, from http://www.cdc.gov/ncidod/diseases/hepatitis/resource/PDFs/hep_surveillance_61.pdf.
6. Miller J, Finelli L, Bell BP: Incidence of acute hepatitis B—United States, 1990-2002, *MMWR* 52(51 & 52);1252-1254, 2004.
7. McMahon BJ, Holck P, Bulkow L, and others: Serologic and clinical outcomes of 1536 Alaska natives chronically infected with hepatitis B virus, *Ann Intern Med* 135:759-768, 2001.
8. Komanduri S, Cotler SJ: Hepatitis C: review, *Clin Perspect Gastroenterol* 4:91-99, 2002.
9. National Institutes of Health: *Consensus development conference statement,* Bethesda, Md, June 10-12, 2002, The Institutes.
10. Centers for Disease Control and Prevention: *Third national health and nutrition examination survey,* retrieved Jan 24, 2007, from http://0-www.cdc.gov.mill1.sjlibrary.org/nchs/data/nhanes/nhanes3/LAB2SE-acc.pdf.
11. Wiley TE, Brown J, Chan J: Hepatitis C infection in African Americans: its natural history and histological progression, *Am J Gastroenterol* 97:700-706, 2002.
12. Zimmerman RK, Ruben FL, Ahwesh ER: Hepatitis B virus infection, hepatitis B vaccine, and hepatitis B immune globulin, *J Fam Pract* 45:295-315, 1997.
13. Walsh K, Alexander G: Alcoholic liver disease, *Postgrad Med J* 76:280-286, 2000.
14. Zakim D, Boyer T: *Hepatology: a textbook of liver disease,* ed 3, Philadelphia, 1996, Saunders.
15. Park J, Akhtar RY, Dietrich DT: Chronic hepatitis C: latest diagnosis and treatment guidelines, *Consultant* 46(4):463-468, 2006, retrieved Feb 9, 2007, from http://www.consultantlive.com/article/showArticle.jhtml?articleID=184429289.
16. Persico M, Persico E, Suozzo R, and others: Natural history of hepatitis C virus carriers with persistently normal aminotransferase levels, *Gastroenterology* 118(4):760-764, 2000.
17. American Gastroenterological Association: *Hepatobiliary and pancreatic disorders in the burden of gastrointestinal diseases,* Bethesda, Md, 2001, The Association.
18. Tucker D: Normal and altered hepatobiliary and pancreatic exocrine function. In Bullock BA, Henze RL, editors: *Focus on pathophysiology,* Philadelphia, 2000, Lippincott Williams & Wilkins.
19. Ockner RK: Acute and chronic hepatitis. In Wyngaarden JB, Smith L, Bennett JC, and others, editors: *Cecil textbook of medicine,* ed 19, Philadelphia, 1992, Saunders.
20. Albanis E, Friedman SL: Noninvasive markers of hepatic fibrosis, *Clin Perspect Gastroenterol* 5:182-187, 2002.
21. Davis GL: Hepatitis B: diagnosis and treatment, *South Med J* 90:866-870, 1998.
22. Nunes D, Fleming C, Offner G: HIV infection does not affect the performance of noninvasive markers of fibrosis for the diagnosis of hepatitis C virus related liver disease, *J Acquir Immune Defic Syndr,* 2005, retrieved Jan 24, 2007, from http://x.medscape.com/viewarticle/517055_1.
23. Keefe EB, Dietrich DT, Han SB, and others: A treatment algorithm for the management of chronic hepatitis B virus infection in the United States, *Clin Gastroenterol Hepatol* 2:87-106, 2004.
24. Keefe EB, editor: Unanswered questions in the treatment of hepatitis C, *Gastroenterol Dis* 4(Suppl 1):2004.
25. Manns MP, McHutchison JG, Gordon SC, and others: Peginterferon alfa-2b plus ribavirin compared with interferon alfa-2b plus ribavirin for initial treatment of chronic hepatitis C: a randomised trial, *Lancet* 358:958-965, 2001.
26. Shiffman ML, Di Bisceglie AM, Lindsay KL, and others: Peginterferon alfa-2a and ribavirin in patients with chronic hepatitis C who have failed prior treatment, *Gastroenterology* 126:1015-1023, 2004.
27. Huang DB, DuPont HL: Rifaximin—a novel antimicrobial for enteric infections, *J Infect* 50:97-106, 2005.
28. American Gastroenterological Association: Medical position statement: nonalcoholic fatty liver disease and AGA technical review on nonalcoholic fatty liver disease, *Gastroenterology* 123:1702-1725, 2002.

CHAPTER 145

Inflammatory Bowel Disease

Wendy L. Biddle

DEFINITION AND EPIDEMIOLOGY

Inflammatory bowel disease (IBD) is a chronic inflammatory condition that affects approximately 1.4 million people in the United States and more than 2 million people in Europe.[1] There are two types of IBD: ulcerative colitis (UC) and Crohn's disease (CD). Both involve the intestinal tract and typically have periods of remission and exacerbation. Although UC and CD have many similarities, they also have significant differences.

UC is a chronic inflammation of the lining of the colonic mucosa. Beginning in the rectum, the inflammation is diffuse and continuous and may involve the entire colon (pancolitis) or only part of the colon. Disease involving only the rectum (proctitis) or involving the rectosigmoid colon accounts for approximately 40% to 50% of the cases of UC. An additional 30% to 40% of patients have disease extending proximally to the splenic flexure (left-sided UC). Twenty percent of patients with UC have pancolitis.[2]

CD is a chronic inflammation of all layers of the intestinal tract (transmural inflammation) and can involve any portion of the intestinal tract from the mouth to the anus. Approximately 30% to 40% of patients with CD have disease only in the small intestine (ileitis or regional enteritis). The terminal ileum is almost always involved, and 40% to 45% of patients have disease in the small and large intestines (ileocolitis). Approximately 15% to 25% of patients have disease only in the colon (Crohn's colitis, not to be confused with UC). CD occurs in the mouth, stomach, and duodenum in a very small percentage of patients.[3]

The transmural involvement in CD is responsible for many of the complications that occur. Although the inflammation can be patchy (unlike UC, which is nearly always continuous), the involvement of all layers of the bowel wall creates many problems. Fibrosis occurs from the inflammation and can partially or completely obstruct the lumen of the intestinal wall. Weakening of the intestinal wall from inflammation results in sinus tracts or fistulas. Fistulas can develop from bowel to bowel (enteroenteric), bowel to skin (enterocutaneous), bowel to bladder (enterovesical), or bowel to vagina (enterovaginal).

The annual incidences of UC and of CD are similar in both age of onset and worldwide distribution. The highest incidence of IBD is in North America, Europe, and Australia. The incidence in developing countries is much lower but has been increasing. The range of reported incidence per 100,000 population in Europe is approximately 10.4 for UC and 5.6 for CD. The prevalence in the United States is estimated to be 229 cases per 100,000 population for UC and 133 per 100,000 population for CD.[4,5] IBD affects men and women equally, but approximately 20% more men have UC and 20% more women have CD.[6] The peak age of onset is between 15 and 25 years, but IBD can appear at any age from infancy to older adulthood.

The cause of IBD is unknown, although there have been advances in our understanding. The current theory suggests some individuals are genetically predisposed. In these individuals their immune system is dysregulated, triggered by an environmental factor. These factors may include luminal bacteria, infection, or tobacco. There is indirect evidence that pathogenic bacteria may have a significant role as a trigger.[7]

For some persons with IBD, there seems to be a familial tendency in that these individuals have a first-degree relative with IBD. In these families most have the same form of IBD, although both UC and CD can occur in the same family. Persons of Jewish ethnicity originating in Europe have been shown to have a much higher risk of developing IBD.

Cigarette smoking has been shown to be one of the strongest environmental factors affecting IBD. Many studies have documented a higher risk of UC in former smokers.[8] Smoking may also affect the course of UC, demonstrating a protective role. The opposite relationship appears evident with CD. A history of *current* smoking is a risk factor for CD. Researchers have documented that smokers are twice as likely to develop CD.[9] Smoking also increases the likelihood of having ileal involvement and fistulizing or stenosing CD rather than colonic involvement and pure inflammatory CD. Continued smoking after surgery increases the risk of needing further surgery. Smokers are also more likely to need immunosuppressives and have a poor quality of life. The good news is that smoking cessation can reduce exacerbations and use of steroids and immunosuppressives.[8]

PATHOPHYSIOLOGY

It is thought that inflammatory and immune cells are responsible for UC and CD. A proposed mechanism of inflammation is an infection or other toxin that releases cell wall products that up-regulate macrophages and granulocytes. Macrophages and granulocytes activate circulating cells that migrate into the mucosa, releasing a variety of inflammatory factors such as cytokines, proteases, and oxygen-derived free radicals. These factors all promote inflammation, and the patient has no means of down-regulating the system to inhibit the inflammation. Either the tissue responds by resolving with scarring, or other secondary immune reactions continue to create irreversible damage.[7]

Advances in the genetics of IBD over the past decade have broadened the understanding of these diseases. It is now known that *CARD15* is a susceptibility gene for CD on chromosome 16q12 (IBD1). This established the genetics role in examining susceptibility to CD. Further studies have examined associations between genotype and phenotype. This knowledge is contributing to the further understanding of the clinical manifestations of IBD, such as disease location, behavior, natural history, and response to and side effects of medications.[10]

CLINICAL PRESENTATION

Both UC and CD can have similar presentations and can be difficult to distinguish. Approximately 10% of patients do not have a definite diagnosis, and the disease is known as *indeterminate colitis*. People may complain of symptoms for varying lengths of time, and it is not unusual to have someone report abdominal pain intermittently for years before other symptoms develop. Abdominal pain may be the only presenting complaint. The symptoms of abdominal pain and diarrhea are present in most persons with either disease. The abdominal pain may be diffuse (generalized lower pain) or localized to the right or left lower quadrants. The pain is usually a cramping sensation and can be intermittent or constant.

Tenesmus, or spasms in the rectum, and fecal incontinence may be reported. Stools are often loose or watery and may have blood. Rectal bleeding is usually present with colitis, either UC or Crohn's colitis. Patients may report blood seen only on the toilet paper after wiping, blood in the stool, or clots and large amounts of blood. With proctitis, rectal bleeding may be the only complaint, or constipation may be reported rather than diarrhea.

Other complaints may include fatigue, weight loss, anorexia, fever, chills, nausea, vomiting, joint pains, and mouth sores. CD may manifest with only vague complaints of fatigue and abdominal cramping, but it can be seen with intestinal obstruction and symptoms of vomiting, bloating, and no stool, as well as with perianal disease of anal fissures, perirectal abscess, or fistula.[11] Pertinent history includes recent antibiotic use or travel, the health of other household members, family history of IBD, previous history of abdominal pain or diarrhea, and medication review.

PHYSICAL EXAMINATION

The patient can appear quite ill or seem to be in no distress. Fever, more often seen in CD, and accompanying tachycardia can be present but often are not. All weight ranges can be seen, from underweight to obese. The young and the elderly can demonstrate significant weight loss, failure to thrive, and growth failure. Conjunctival inflammation or oral aphthous ulcers may be present. Abdominal examination usually reveals a tender lower abdomen, which may be more prominent on one side or the other, although the abdomen can be diffusely tender. Hyperactive bowel sounds and palpation of loops of bowel may be noted as a "fullness" in the lower abdomen. A mass, especially in the lower right quadrant, can signify ileocecal inflammation. Rectal examination for occult blood may be positive, with frank blood and tenderness. Perianal lesions, such as skin tags, anal fissure, and perianal fistula, are more suggestive of CD but can be seen in UC. Anal stenosis, abscess, or purulent drainage from a fistulous tract may be seen on rectal examination. The perianal disease is suggestive of IBD but can also be seen in healthy people. Joints do not usually appear red or edematous. Skin lesions (e.g., erythema nodosum, pyoderma gangrenosum, papulonecrotic skin lesions or rashes) may also be noted.

DIAGNOSTICS

Blood Tests

A CBC is useful to determine the presence of anemia. The platelet count will often be elevated in the presence of active inflammation or infection. The erythrocyte sedimentation rate can be elevated but is a nonspecific marker of inflammation. None of these tests is useful for diagnosis, although they have value in following a patient's progress. In addition, CD may result in malabsorption, especially after a small bowel resection. Monitoring electrolytes, glucose, BUN, creatinine, and the vitamin B_{12} level is necessary to determine and treat deficiencies in CD.

Genetic testing is now available as an adjunct to other diagnostics. Two markers, anti–*Saccharomyces cerevisiae* antibodies (ASCA) and perinuclear antineutrophil cytoplasmic antibodies (pANCA), have been developed for clinical use. Other markers being studied include OmpC immunoglobulin A (IgA) (predominant in human intestine) and I-2 IgA antibody (occurs in CD). The panel testing these three markers is commercially available and is highly sensitive, detecting approximately 94% of patients with IBD. From 60% to 80% of patients with UC and a subgroup of patients with UC-like CD are positive for pANCA. Sixty percent of patients with CD are positive for ASCA. IBD subtyping resulting in pANCA positive, ASCA negative, OmpC negative occurs in 14% of CD patients and 86% of UC patients. Several laboratories perform these tests, but the results vary. In general, detection of different pANCA antigens ranges in sensitivity from 0% to 63% and in specificity from 75% to 100%. For CD testing sensitivity is 44% and specificity is 87%. False-negative results can occur and should be considered. A positive test can be helpful for diagnosis, but does not obviate the need for other diagnostic testing. The IBD diagnostic markers are promising and will increasingly play a role in diagnosis of IBD as they are refined.[12]

Stool Tests

Initial presentation of diarrhea, as well as subsequent flares, should be evaluated for infection. Stool testing for ova and parasites should be performed three times to eliminate the most common pathogens. Testing for *Clostridium difficile* is important during flares, especially if the patient recently used antibiotics. Special cultures for other organisms can be requested. Fecal leukocytes can be tested in the stool specimen and are present with inflammation.

Radiography

The barium enema is of limited use in diagnosing IBD and is most useful in detecting colonic distention, obstruction, fistulas, strictures, or tumors. It can detect an abnormal terminal ileum (useful in diagnosing CD), but there are moderate false-positive and false-negative rates. A barium enema should not be used in patients with moderate to severe colitis because there is perforation risk when the colon is weakened from inflammation. MRI may be helpful in detecting fistulas and abscesses in patients with perianal CD.

Endoscopy

Flexible sigmoidoscopy examines the lower 76 cm (30 inches) of the colon and is useful to determine the source of bright red rectal bleeding. It is more useful for UC than for CD because UC almost always shows rectal inflammation; however, not all the inflamed tissue may be visible if the disease extends beyond the splenic flexure. Flexible sigmoidoscopy can be done with or without cleansing the bowels first, although usually a cleansing preparation is used. An enema can be administered just before the procedure to remove stool in the lower portion of the colon.

Colonoscopy is useful in differentiating UC and CD. Bowel cleansing is usually necessary for colonoscopy. Bowel preparations vary among institutions; many use a flavored osmotic salt solution that patients drink in large quantities (usually a gallon) the night before the colonoscopy. Patients with a history of congestive heart failure (CHF) or decreased kidney function (serum creatinine >1.5) should use the osmotic solutions. Polyethylene glycol (GlycoLax) is another nonabsorbed solution for bowel cleansing, which has no taste and is easier to drink. Those without CHF or kidney problems can use a phosphosoda liquid, which requires drinking only 3 ounces of the solution rather than a gallon. Large amounts of clear liquids the day before also help cleanse the colon.

Both UC and CD may have distinguishing features endoscopically that, if found, may help differentiate one from the other. On endoscopy, UC inflammation will be continuous with disease in the rectum, up to the point that the inflammation stops. CD can have "skip areas," sections of normal mucosa intermixed with inflamed mucosa. This skipping gives a cobblestone appearance to the mucosa. However, these distinguishing features may not be present, making the diagnosis difficult. Another useful endoscopic finding is an inflamed or abnormal terminal ileum that is almost exclusively present in CD. Newer endoscopic techniques have been developed, and technology continues to improve. A detailed explanation of new and promising techniques can be found in Hommes and Van Deventer's article.[13]

Mucosal biopsy samples, usually 3 to 4 mm, are especially helpful in diagnosis of IBD. Microscopically, acute and chronic inflammation can be seen. It may be difficult to distinguish UC from CD, and in these patients the disease may be labeled *indeterminate colitis* until a clear diagnosis can be made. UC can have cryptitis and crypt abscesses, whereas CD can show aphthous ulcers and granulomas.[2,3]

Virtual colonoscopy is an alternative to screening colonoscopy for colon cancer. This is done with a CT scan and requires the patient to be inflated with a large amount of air. The test is uncomfortable and costly and has a varying miss rate of polyps. It is not recommended as yet and has no role in diagnosing or managing IBD.

DIAGNOSTICS

Inflammatory Bowel Disease

LABORATORY

CBC and differential
Platelet count
ESR
Electrolytes
Serum glucose
BUN, creatinine
Vitamin B_{12}
Genetic testing
- Anti–*Saccharomyces cerevisiae* antibodies (ASCA)
- Perinuclear antineutrophil cytoplasmic antibodies (pANCA)

OmpC IgA and I-2 IgA antibody (new)
Stool tests*
- *Giardia* organisms
- *Campylobacter jejuni*
- *Clostridium difficile*
- *Yersinia enterocolitica*
- Salmonellae
- Shigellae

If immunocompromised:
- Cytomegalovirus
- *Cryptosporidium* organisms
- *Mycobacterium avium-intracellulare*

IMAGING*

MRI
Endoscopy
Flexible sigmoidoscopy
Colonoscopy
Barium enema

OTHER

Biopsy

*If indicated.

DIFFERENTIAL DIAGNOSIS

Several diagnoses should be excluded when a patient is seen with the common symptoms of IBD: abdominal pain, rectal bleeding, or diarrhea.

Rectal bleeding should never be ignored or assumed to be benign and should always be further evaluated. Bleeding may be from hemorrhoids, a fissure, or a colonic polyp. Abdominal pain in women may indicate endometriosis or pelvic inflammatory disease. Abdominal pain and diarrhea without bleeding may signify irritable bowel syndrome (IBS) or appendicitis. IBS is a chronic, benign condition with no organic disease present. The hallmarks of IBS are altered bowel habits and bloating and abdominal pain relieved by defecation.

Infectious causes of diarrhea need to be excluded. The most common pathogenic organisms to consider are *Giardia* organisms, *Campylobacter jejuni, C. difficile* (especially with a history of recent antibiotic use), *Yersinia enterocolitica,*

DIFFERENTIAL DIAGNOSIS

Inflammatory Bowel Disease*

- Infectious causes (e.g., cytomegalovirus, shigellae, *Campylobacter* organisms, *Clostridium difficile,* salmonellae, amebiasis, *Escherichia coli*)
- Irritable bowel syndrome
- Pelvic inflammatory disease and other gynecologic disorders
- Appendicitis
- Diverticulitis
- Microscopic, collagenous, or lymphocytic colitis
- Ischemic colitis
- Radiation enteritis or proctitis
- Lymphoma, adenocarcinoma, carcinoid tumor, metastatic cancer
- Systemic vasculitis and other vasculitides
- Medications (especially those causing chronic diarrhea)
- Bleeding from hemorrhoids, fissures, polyps

*Not inclusive.

salmonellae, and shigellae. If a host is immunocompromised, infections with such organisms as cytomegalovirus, cryptosporidia, and *Mycobacterium avium-intracellulare* should be excluded.[11]

Noninfectious causes include acute self-limited colitis, ischemic colitis (especially in patients over age 60 years), radiation enteritis or colitis (history of radiation to abdomen or pelvis; may be a late sequela), Behçet's syndrome, lymphoma, and systemic vasculitis. Over-the-counter medications that can be a source of diarrhea include antacids with magnesium, mints with sorbitol, and laxatives. Other medications that can cause diarrhea include metformin and proton pump inhibitors. Medications that can produce an inflammatory colitis include antibiotics, chemotherapeutic agents, NSAIDs, and gold.[11]

MANAGEMENT

5-Aminosalicylic Acid

First-line treatments for UC are the 5-aminosalicylic acid (ASA, mesalamine) products. Sulfasalazine has been used since the 1940s and has been proved to be safe and effective, even with long-term use.[14] Sulfasalazine is a sulfapyridine and a 5-ASA product connected by a bond. The 5-ASA has been shown to be the active ingredient, and the sulfapyridine is responsible for most of the side effects. Several 5-ASA products have become available during the past 10 years (Table 145-1). Studies have shown that 4 g/day in divided doses is effective in establishing remission in colitis. 5-ASA suppositories are effective for proctitis. Topical therapy, which includes suppositories and enemas, usually must be used on a long-term basis.

The 5-ASA products are also efficacious in treating UC and maintaining remission.[15] Rarely a patient may be allergic to 5-ASA; if so, the drug should be stopped. Patients will come to see their provider with a worsening of their colitis symptoms, which will improve with discontinuation of the medication. 5-ASA medications are most useful for UC and disease in the colon. The proposed mechanisms of action include inhibition of cyclooxygenase, lipoxygenase, platelet activating factor, interleukin-1, and other proinflammatory agents. They also scavenge reactive oxygen. They are indicated for mild to moderately active disease and maintenance of UC and active disease of CD. The 5-ASA products are also indicated for maintenance of CD in three circumstances: after 5-ASA induction, after steroid use, and postoperatively.

Corticosteroids

Oral and parenteral steroids are avoided if possible because of potential long-term side effects, including diabetes, osteoporosis, and cataracts. Currently steroids are the primary therapy for moderate to severe UC and for disease that is not responding to 5-ASA. Steroids have been shown to induce remission in mild to moderately active CD. Combinations with 5-ASA products are more effective. Budesonide is a newer steroid that is enteric coated and subject to high first pass metabolism, decreasing the side effects. It releases in the distal ileum and right colon and cannot be used for disease in the left colon. It is an alternative to steroids but has similar efficacy. Budesonide at 9 mg/day can induce remission in mildly to moderately active CD. At 6 mg/day it has been shown to prolong time to relapse at 6 months but not at 1 year. It is suggested as a first-line therapy for mild to moderate CD involving the ileum or ascending colon. If patients fail budesonide therapy, they can be treated with prednisone.[16]

Prednisone is usually started at dosages of 40 to 60 mg (0.25 to 0.75 mg/kg) PO q day, although occasionally higher dosages are used. Tapering to a lower dose is attempted within a few weeks. The tapering schedule depends greatly on the patient's response. A patient's symptoms may improve within a few days to a week of beginning prednisone. If a response is not immediate, the higher dose may be continued until a response is noted or the patient is hospitalized. The goal is to use a minimum dose of prednisone for a minimum amount of time. Once remission is achieved, patients are tapered off of steroids as soon as possible, although long, slow tapers may be necessary to prevent a flare.

Rectal steroids in the form of a retention enema or foam are useful for colitis and can provide relief of urgency and spasm in the rectum, in addition to healing the inflamed mucosa. Rectal steroids are used for a few weeks, usually until there is an improvement of rectal symptoms. There is some absorption

TABLE 145-1 Comparison of Medications for Ulcerative Colitis

Brand Name (Active Ingredient)	How Supplied	Route	Daily Dose for Active Disease*	Daily Dose for Maintenance of Remission*	Common Side Effects
Azulfidine (sulfasalazine)	500-mg tablets	Oral	4 g (8 pills)	2 g (4 pills)	Headache, nausea, allergy to sulfa
Asacol (mesalamine)	400-mg delayed-release tablets	Oral	2.4 g (6 pills)	1.6 g (4 pills)	Dyspepsia, abdominal pain
Dipentum (olsalazine)	250-mg capsules	Oral	1 g (4 capsules)	1 g (4 capsules)	Diarrhea
Pentasa (mesalamine)	500-mg capsules	Oral	4 g (8 capsules)	1.5 g (4 capsules)	GI upset, headache
Colazal (balsalazide)	750-mg capsules	Oral	2.4 g (9 capsules)	1.6 g (6 capsules)	GI upset, headache
Rowasa (mesalamine)	4 g/60 ml	Rectal Retention enema	4 g (1 enema)	Every other night or less often	Hemorrhoids, rectal pain
Rowasa (mesalamine)	500-mg suppositories	Rectal	1 g (2 suppositories)	500 mg (1 suppository)	Rectal irritation

*Oral medications should be taken 2-4 times daily as indicated.
GI, Gastrointestinal.

of the steroid systemically; thus long-term use (greater than a few months) is not routinely recommended.

Biologics

Biologics are the newest and most promising class of medications under development in the treatment of IBD. Infliximab, a tumor necrosis factor monoclonal antibody, is indicated for induction and maintenance of remission in CD. It is effective in treating fistulas, allowing patients to avoid or taper off steroids (steroid sparing), and recently obtained an indication for UC. It is administered intravenously at 2- to 3-month intervals. Serious adverse reactions include infection, infusion reactions, serum sickness–like reaction, and lupuslike syndrome. All patients must have a negative tuberculin test (purified protein derivative) before beginning therapy. Given alone or in combination with other immunomodulators, infliximab has induced remission in 25% to 35% and improvement in 45% to 54% of patients with refractory CD.[16] After several years of experience with infliximab, experts advise that the best treatment regimen is to give a dose at 0, 2, and 6 weeks and then every 8 weeks thereafter. Infusion reactions may be avoided by not extending the interval beyond 2 to 3 months and placing patients on immunosuppressives (azathioprine) before starting infliximab treatment.[17] Several other biologics are being developed.

Immunomodulators

There is a trend to use immunomodulators earlier in the course of disease than they have been used in the past. Azathioprine and 6-mercaptopurine (6-MP) may allow the patient to avoid steroids and are useful for steroid dependency. Some clinicians advocate using these medications as first-line treatment in CD.[18] These medications must be taken for 4 to 5 months before the full effect is seen. The initial dose of 6-MP is 50 mg. Phenotype and metabolite testing of 6-MP can determine those who are likely to become toxic and should not be started on the drug. The metabolite testing is done periodically during treatment to determine therapeutic level, which helps with dosing. It is recommended that a CBC, liver function tests (LFTs), amylase, and lipase levels be done initially as a baseline to monitor for bone marrow suppression, pancreatitis, and hepatotoxicity.[18] A CBC should be done weekly initially for 4 weeks, and then monthly along with periodic LFTs and amylase and lipase assessments.

The development of leukopenia or thrombocytopenia warrants immediate discontinuation of the drug. Other adverse reactions, such as pancreatitis and hepatotoxicity, can also occur, requiring termination of treatment. Pancreatitis usually occurs within the first 2 months, and patients usually are seen with a clinical picture of pancreatitis, complaining of abdominal pain. Hepatotoxicity is rare, but monitoring LFTs after the first month and then every 2 to 4 months is recommended. If an elevated liver enzyme level is found, the test should be repeated in 1 to 2 weeks. If the levels remain elevated or continue to rise, the drug should be discontinued and the patient referred to the gastroenterologist for further evaluation. Levels that are twice normal or higher are especially concerning and should prompt immediate referral to a gastroenterologist.

Genetic testing can be used to monitor and optimize therapy with 6-MP. Thiopurine methyltransferase (TPMT) genotyping determines the patient's ability to produce the TPMT enzyme. The testing can help identify those patients who would tolerate the drug and can also monitor drug metabolites to maximize the therapeutic effect.[18]

Parenteral methotrexate has been shown to be effective in CD, although fewer long-term data are available than with 6-MP or azathioprine. Methotrexate has been shown to induce and maintain remission in CD. CBCs and LFTs should be performed periodically. Monitoring for hepatotoxicity with liver biopsies is controversial, but needs to be done if LFTs remain elevated. There are no good data showing an association between methotrexate and malignancy.[19]

Miscellaneous Medications

Some data show induction of remission of CD with antibiotics, but patient tolerability can be a problem. Metronidazole is effective in treating perianal disease and in healing fistulas associated with CD. Other antibiotics such as ciprofloxacin are sometimes used, but sufficient data on efficacy are lacking. Research is ongoing on the use of antibiotics with IBD. Several studies use rifaximin, a new nonabsorbable antibiotic with wide-spectrum activity against intestinal pathogens, as a treatment for CD. Early reports are that rifaximin can be effective in mild to moderate CD and possibly in more severe disease.[7]

Cyclosporine has been studied for treatment of UC but has not been widely used. Antibiotics have not been shown to be as efficacious in UC compared with CD. Use of methotrexate, azathioprine, and steroids remains controversial, and debates continue about the best approach to treatment for the more refractory patients. Probiotics are gaining attention but are in early studies.

Surgery

Approximately 20% of patients with UC and 66% of patients with CD require surgery for refractory disease.[20] Patients with intractable disease are generally not responding to high doses of medications and may be systemically sick, with weight loss, anemia, nausea, and vomiting. Surgery is also indicated when dysplasia or cancer is found on biopsy. In UC a total colectomy is usually necessary. After surgery patients no longer have the colonic disease and can be taken off all IBD medications. Complications such as liver disease and ankylosing spondylitis may still be present, and treatment for these and other complications needs to be continued. Options for surgical treatment include an ileostomy and an ileal pouch–anal anastomosis (IPAA). With an IPAA the colon is removed except for some rectal tissue, the small intestine is anastomosed to the rectum, and an internal pouch is created to store stool. Patients have no external bag but have several loose stools a day and can develop complications.

In CD the average time from diagnosis to surgery is about 3 years. Surgery is indicated for medical therapy that failed, small bowel obstruction, fistulas, and abscesses. Up to 10% to 15% of patients are diagnosed with CD by surgery. A small bowel or colonic resection is the most common surgical procedure, although colectomy may be necessary in some patients. Many patients do well after surgery, but recurrence can occur in up to 80% of patients within 6 months.[21] Approximately one third of patients who had a resection will require a second procedure, and a smaller number of patients will require additional surgical procedures.

Many novel surgical techniques are being tried at various centers, which are constantly seeking better ways to help patients. Variations on ileoanal pouch procedures, stricture-plasties, and a multitude of other procedures continue to be advanced with the goals of preserving continence and repairing fistulas. Laparoscopic surgery now includes CD of the small bowel or terminal ileum and total colectomy for UC or CD. There is also an increase in the level of sophistication using robotic surgery.[22]

COMPLICATIONS

Studies have demonstrated an increased risk of colorectal cancer (CRC) in patients with IBD, especially those with pancolitis. The risk in UC begins to increase after 7 years of disease and continually rises.[23] A cumulative risk of CRC in a patient with UC is 2% at 10 years of disease and rises to 18% after 30 years of disease. Those patients with left-sided, limited colitis have less of an increase in risk (2.8%) than patients with pancolitis (14.8%) but still require regular surveillance. Initial CRC screening should begin at 7 to 8 years after disease onset and then annually or biannually after.

Patients with Crohn's colitis have a greater risk for CRC, similar to UC patients. Other issues with CD include the need for one or more surgeries, recurrence after surgery, and loss of small bowel. These can affect their health and quality of life.

A number of extraintestinal manifestations can occur with IBD. These primarily involve the eyes, mouth, peripheral joints, skin, and blood vessels. Some are related to the inflammatory activity of the bowel. They become active when the bowel inflammation is active and resolve when the IBD is in remission. These manifestations include aphthous stomatitis, iritis, uveitis, episcleritis, arthritis, and skin lesions (pyoderma gangrenosum, erythema nodosum).

Peripheral arthritis occurs in 10% to 12% of patients with UC and in up to 22% of patients with CD. Knees, ankles, and shoulders are most often affected. Between 1% and 26% of patients with UC and 3% to 16% of patients with CD develop ankylosing spondylitis. Treatment of the underlying IBD is the best management approach for the arthritis, although symptomatic treatment can be used. Caution should be used in treating with NSAIDs because they can trigger a flare of IBD.[24]

Other complications include liver disease (sclerosing cholangitis), gallstones, malabsorption (CD of the small bowel), renal disease (stones), and amyloidosis. Both men and women with IBD are at risk for osteoporosis, independent of steroid use. These complications are not associated with the inflammatory activity and need to be treated with standard management.

INDICATIONS FOR REFERRAL OR HOSPITALIZATION

The diagnosis of IBD can be difficult and requires physician consultation. Referral for diagnostic and follow-up endoscopy procedures, as well as management, is the best approach. Once a patient is on a treatment regimen, health care providers may be able to co-manage the IBD. Continual, close consultation with a gastroenterologist is necessary for optimum management and various treatment options.

Hospitalization is necessary at times for bowel rest, hydration, and parenteral medications. Patients who develop systemic symptoms such as weight loss, nausea, vomiting, severe abdominal pain, significant blood loss, or malnutrition should be evaluated and referred immediately.

PATIENT AND FAMILY EDUCATION

IBD has a significant impact on the quality of life for patients and their families. The stigma of a chronic bowel disease creates a unique set of problems. Patients may be afraid or unwilling to discuss their disease with loved ones, friends, and co-workers. Embarrassment about the symptoms and the need to be near a bathroom can prevent patients from participating in activities and outings. Fear of pain and diarrhea may keep them from eating, and they may become malnourished. Frequent visits and embarrassing, uncomfortable procedures may prevent them from seeking medical care when needed.

There is a great need for patient education for better disease management. Understanding the disease process, potential complications, medication side effects, and risks (such as cancer) is imperative. The need for regular health care visits and the importance of treatments and scheduled procedures should be emphasized. The patient should be educated about the need for a well-balanced diet and informed that there is no specific diet to follow for IBD. Written materials, videos, and educational meetings are available. The Crohn's and Colitis Foundation of America is a national patient organization that can provide information and support. Many local support groups also can provide a forum for learning and support for patients and their significant others.

When teaching patients with IBD, the provider should remember that they will be overwhelmed at first. Repetition is necessary to ensure that patients understand. Many visual aids are available that can help patients understand the disease and the procedures and tests that are necessary. In addition, because patients can obtain a great deal of misinformation from the media and well-meaning friends, relatives, and others, correction of misinformation and misconceptions will help. Above all, establishing a trusting, comfortable relationship and listening carefully to patients are vital to the long-term management of IBD.

HEALTH PROMOTION

IBD is a disease of remission and exacerbation. The cause is unknown. Family history plays a limited role; only 20% of IBD patients have a family member with IBD. Cigarette smoking tends to exacerbate CD, but smoking cessation increases the risk of developing UC. Still, all patients should be encouraged to stop smoking because the risks of smoking far outweigh any benefit.

IBD is a chronic disease with no known cure. Patients should be encouraged to maintain a healthy lifestyle, which should include stress management. Compliance with the prescribed treatment regimen and regular follow-up are the two most important strategies a patient can implement to maximize health. Maintenance of remission can be achieved with medications, with the right dose. People with IBD are at higher risk for colon cancer and need regular colon cancer surveillance. Maintaining regular follow-up with their health care provider and contacting their provider with early signs of a flare will minimize problems. Patients need to understand their medication regimen, the importance of not self-adjusting doses, and what monitoring is necessary. Family members need to be a part of the health care team as well. Health care providers can play a significant role in keeping the patient on track with their appointments, medications, and testing, ensuring the patient will obtain the highest level of wellness possible.

PATIENT INFORMATION

Crohn's and Colitis Foundation of America: http://www.ccfa.org, (800) 932-2423

National Digestive Diseases Information Clearinghouse: http://digestive.niddk.nih.gov, (800) 891-5389

REFERENCES

1. Loftus EV: Clinical epidemiology of inflammatory bowel disease: incidence, prevalence, and environmental influences, *Gastroenterology* 126:1504-1517, 2004.
2. Jewell DP: Ulcerative colitis. In Feldman M, Scharschmidt BF, Sleisenger MH, editors: *Sleisenger and Fordtran's gastrointestinal disease: pathophysiology/diagnosis/management,* ed 6, vol 2, Philadelphia, 1998, Saunders.
3. Kornbluth A, Sachar DB, Salomon P: Crohn's disease. In Feldman M, Scharschmidt BF, Sleisenger MH, editors: *Sleisenger and Fordtran's gastrointestinal disease: pathophysiology/diagnosis/management,* ed 6, vol 2, Philadelphia, 1998, Saunders.
4. Loftus EV, Silverstein MD, Sandborn WJ: Ulcerative colitis in Olmsted County, Minnesota, 1940-1993: incidence, prevalence, and survival, *Gut* 46:336-343, 2000.
5. Loftus EV, Silverstein MD, Sandborn WJ: Crohn's disease in Olmsted County, Minnesota, 1940-1993: incidence, prevalence, and survival, *Gastroenterology* 114:1161-1168, 1998.
6. Lashner BA: Epidemiology of inflammatory bowel disease, *Gastroenterol Clin North Am* 24(3):467-474, 1995.
7. Rubin DT, Kornbluth A: Role of antibiotics in the management of inflammatory bowel disease: a review, *Rev Gastroenterol Dis* 5(Suppl 3):S10-S15, 2005.
8. Loftus EV: Clinical epidemiology of inflammatory bowel disease: incidence, prevalence, and environmental influences, *Gastroenterology* 126:1504-1517, 2004.
9. Cosnes J, Carbonnel F, Carrat F, and others: Effects of current and former cigarette smoking on the clinical course of Crohn's disease, *Aliment Pharmacol Ther* 13(11):1403-1411, 1999.
10. Ahmad T, Tamboli CP, Jewell D, and others: Clinical relevance of advances in genetics and pharmacogenetics of IBD, *Gastroenterology* 126:1533-1549, 2004.
11. Sands BE: From symptom to diagnosis: clinical distinctions among various forms of intestinal inflammation, *Gastroenterology* 126:1518-1532, 2004.
12. Sandborn WJ: Serological markers in inflammatory bowel disease: state of the art, *Rev Gastroenterol Dis* 4:167-174, 2004.
13. Hommes DW, Van Deventer SJH: Endoscopy in inflammatory bowel disease, *Gastroenterology* 126:1561-1573, 2004.
14. Kornbluth A, Sachar DB: Ulcerative colitis practice guidelines in adults (update: American College of Gastroenterology, Practice Update Committee), 2004, retrieved Jan 26, 2007, from http://69.20.67.254/physicians/guidelines/UlcerativeColitisUpdate.pdf.
15. Hanauer SB: Medical therapy for ulcerative colitis 2004, *Gastroenterology* 126:1582-1592, 2004.
16. Sandborn WJ: Evidence-based treatment algorithm for mild to moderate Crohn's disease, *Am J Gastroenterol* 98(12 Suppl):S1-S5, 2003.
17. Navarro F, Hanauer SB: Treatment of inflammatory bowel disease: safety and tolerability issues, *Am J Gastroenterol* 98(12 Suppl):S18-S23, 2003.
18. Dubinsky MC: Azathiopurine, 6-mercaptopurine in inflammatory bowel disease: pharmacology, efficacy, and safety, *Clin Gastroenterol Hepatol* 2:731-743, 2004.
19. Feagan BG: Maintenance therapy for inflammatory bowel disease, *Am J Gastroenterol* 98(12 Suppl):S6-S17, 2003.
20. Platell C, Mackay J, Collopy B, and others: Crohn's disease: a colon and rectal department experience, *Aust NZ J Surg* 65(8):570-575, 1995.
21. Hanauer SB: Refractory Crohn's disease. In Prantera C, Korelitz BI, editors: *Crohn's disease,* New York, 1996, Marcel Dekker.
22. Fazio VW, Achkar E, editors: *The Cleveland Clinic Foundation: Digestive Disease Center outcomes, 2004,* Cleveland, 2005, Cleveland Clinic Foundation.
23. Itzkowitz SH, Harpaz N: Diagnosis and management of dysplasia in patients with inflammatory bowel disease, *Gastroenterology* 126:1634-1648, 2004.
24. Anderson M, Robinson M: Watching for—and managing—joint problems in inflammatory bowel disease, *J Musculoskel Med* Nov:28-34, 1996.

CHAPTER 146

Irritable Bowel Syndrome

Elizabeth Friedlander

DEFINITION AND EPIDEMIOLOGY

Irritable bowel syndrome (IBS) is a common gastrointestinal (GI) condition that is classified as a "functional" GI disorder because there are no identifiable organic or structural etiologies that explain its development.[1] According to the American Gastroenterological Association, IBS is defined as a combination of chronic or recurrent GI symptoms that are not explained by structural abnormalities; are attributed to the intestines; and are associated with symptoms of pain, bloating, or distention.[2]

IBS has been defined using the Manning criteria (symptom-based criteria widely used in clinical research) and, more recently, the 1989 Rome I and 1998 Rome II criteria.[3-5] The 1998 Rome II diagnostic criteria for IBS are listed in Box 146-1.[3] Additional features that support the diagnosis of IBS include abnormal stool passage (straining, urgency, or feeling of incomplete evacuation), passage of mucus, and bloating or feeling of abdominal distention.[6] In clinical practice, many providers use the diagnostic criteria of abdominal pain present at least 25% of the time during the previous 3 months, relieved by defecation, and associated with either a change in stool frequency or a change in stool consistency.[7]

In the past, IBS has been described in the literature according to a wide variety of names, including spastic colon, mucous colitis, nervous bowel, spastic colitis, and functional bowel. Although the term *functional bowel* is acceptable, the term *colitis* is inaccurate and misleading and should be avoided because inflammation is not part of the pathogenesis of IBS.[8]

Because of several factors, including the fluctuating nature of the illness, the reluctance of many persons to seek care for their symptoms, and the lack of sensitive diagnostic criteria, accurate estimates of worldwide IBS prevalence are difficult to make. Studies vary widely from 3% to 22%.[6] Most epidemiologic studies demonstrate that IBS is twice as common in females as in males and affects between 15% and 20% of the adult population in the United States.[2,4,7] Symptoms typically have their onset in late adolescence to early adulthood[9] with peak prevalence occurring in the third and fourth decades of life.[7] Although earlier studies suggested it was unusual to see an initial presentation of IBS in an individual older than 50 years, more recent studies have found high rates of IBS in elders.[6] The prevalence of IBS appears similar among Caucasians and African Americans but is lower among Hispanics.[10] Studies indicate that IBS is also common in non-Western regions, including Japan, China, South America, and India.[11]

Although as many as 75% of persons with complaints of IBS do not seek health care for their symptoms, IBS still accounts for 12% of visits to health care providers and 28% of gastroenterology referrals; this results in 2.4 million to 3.5 million provider visits per year in the United States.[2,4,7,9,12] Persons with IBS miss three times as many work days as do healthy individuals, see health care providers more often for GI and non-GI complaints, and incur an estimated $8 billion in annual health care costs in the United States.[2,4,12] In a recent study by Longstreth, Wilson, Knight, and colleagues, severity of abdominal pain and discomfort was a significant predictor of health care costs of IBS patients in a large health maintenance organization.[13] Total health care costs were 51% higher among patients with IBS when compared with patients without IBS. Patients with IBS filled an annual average of 40 prescriptions compared with 28 prescriptions for non-IBS patients.

To date, the approach to the diagnosis and management of IBS has been limited by an incomplete understanding of the pathogenesis, a lack of sensitive diagnostic criteria, and the absence of evidence-based treatment recommendations.[4] The goals of clinical management are twofold: (1) to exclude the presence of underlying organic disease while considering the risk and expense of a thorough diagnostic evaluation; and (2) to provide support, education, and reassurance to optimize the quality of life of those for whom IBS has become a chronic condition.

BOX 146-1

1998 ROME II DIAGNOSTIC CRITERIA FOR IRRITABLE BOWEL SYNDROME

Abdominal discomfort or pain with two of three features:

- Relief with defecation
- Onset associated with change in frequency of stool (less than three bowel movements per week or more than three bowel movements per day)
- Onset associated with change in appearance of stool (lumpy/hard or loose/watery)

These symptoms must be present at least 12 weeks in the past 12 months (not necessarily consecutive weeks).

Modified from Thompson WG, Longstreth GF, Drossman DA, and others: Functional bowel habits and functional abdominal pain, *Gut* 45(Suppl 2):1143-1147, 1999.

PATHOPHYSIOLOGY

Research over the past decade has dramatically improved our understanding of the etiology of IBS as a complex disorder involving a number of physiologic processes.[4,7] Recent studies have demonstrated that patients with IBS process sensory information from the gut differently than persons without IBS.[7] The signs and symptoms of IBS appear to be predominantly related to changes in central nervous system processing of sensory information; exaggerated normal intestinal motility patterns; and/or sensory abnormalities in the colon, rectum, or small intestine.[2,7] A number of theories have recently evolved regarding the mechanisms for altered intestinal motility and sensitivity.

Altered Motility

Although altered motility is often mentioned as a cause of IBS, much controversy remains regarding the exact electrical and contractile activity of the colon in IBS.[1] The types of motility patterns seen in the colon and small intestine of persons with

IBS are similar to the contractions seen in healthy persons, and there is a lack of agreement on the motility patterns responsible for the diarrhea and constipation associated with IBS.[4] Normal bowel motility predominantly consists of segmenting contractions that function to inhibit the transit of bowel contents. Any increase in segmenting contractions results in constipation, whereas a decrease in contractions results in more frequent stools.[8]

More consistently demonstrated in IBS is an exaggeration of normal colonic motility in response to external and enteric stimuli such as psychologic stress, anxiety, anger, various drugs, acute intestinal infection, and (more recently discovered) small bowel bacterial overgrowth.[1,4,14] Postinfectious IBS has been the topic of recent research, with a few studies demonstrating as many as 7% to 31% of post–acute gastroenteritis patients with previous normal bowel function developing long-term symptoms suggestive of IBS.[15] The exact cause of postinfectious IBS is unknown, but it could represent injury to the enteric nervous system, immune hypersensitivity, or chronic mucosal inflammation that results in an alteration of gut motility.[7] Proponents of the postinfectious theory speculate that as many as 25% of IBS patients are postinfectious and efforts should be directed toward measures to prevent food poisoning and traveler's diarrhea and to treat severe cases of acute gastroenteritis.[15] Further research into the use of antibiotics in acute gastroenteritis for the purpose of preventing IBS is currently being conducted.[15] Another area of developing research is the role of small bowel bacterial overgrowth in IBS symptomatology and the potential benefit of probiotics.[14]

Enhanced Visceral Sensation

Balloon distention studies of the sigmoid,[16] ileum, and colorectum demonstrate painful symptoms at significantly lower pressures and volumes in persons with IBS compared with healthy individuals.[1,4,7] This concept, known as *hyperalgesia,* suggests that altered visceral sensation plays a role in the pathogenesis of IBS.[4,7,16]

Research suggests that with IBS there is increased sensitivity to painful distention in the small bowel and colon, increased or unusual somatic referral of visceral pain, and increased sensitivity to normal intestinal functions. Several possible mechanisms of visceral afferent dysfunction have been suggested to explain the increased visceral sensitivity seen in IBS. These mechanisms include altered receptor sensitivity at the viscus, increased excitability of the dorsal horn neurons of the spinal cord, and altered central modulation of sensation.[1,4]

Role of Enteric Neurotransmitters

Evidence suggests that abnormalities in extrinsic autonomic innervation of the viscera occur with functional bowel disorders and that neuroimmune interactions may mediate stress-induced GI responses.[4,17,18] Research has focused on the role of enteric nervous system neurotransmitters, such as 5-hydroxytryptamine (5-HT [serotonin]), in controlling intestinal motility and visceral afferent (sensory) responses to normal stimuli (gas, sugars, bile acids, fatty acids) and noxious stimuli (allergens, infectious agents, balloon distention).[19] Ninety-five percent of the body's 5-HT is located in the gut, 3% is located in the brain, and 2% is located in platelets. 5-HT in the gut is manufactured and released from enterochromaffin cells located in the mucosa. Increases in intraluminal pressures result in the release of 5-HT. These neurotransmitters stimulate afferent fibers in the mucosa and initiate a peristaltic reflex, thereby enhancing GI motility and mediating visceral pain.[20] A preliminary study demonstrated increased plasma levels of postprandial 5-HT in women with IBS compared with healthy controls.[21] 5-HT may also play a role in mediating psychologic, stress-induced GI responses via the brain-gut axis.[7]

Psychosocial Factors

Studies of the relationship between psychosocial factors and IBS suggest that, although emotional responses to stress affect GI function and produce symptoms in all persons, these symptoms are produced to a greater extent in persons with IBS.[2,4] Although several studies report that persons with IBS have a greater incidence of psychiatric diagnoses and more psychosocial difficulties than healthy individuals, persons with IBS who do not seek health care for their GI complaints are psychologically similar to healthy individuals.[1] In addition, patients with IBS seen in a primary care setting have fewer psychologic disturbances than those who request to be seen by a gastroenterologist.[4,22] Therefore psychosocial factors do not seem to *cause* IBS symptoms but rather influence how the illness is interpreted and expressed by the individual.[1,22]

Several studies have suggested an increased reporting of childhood physical and sexual abuse among persons with IBS.[1,4,7,23-25] Although the adverse effects of abuse on health status are independent of GI function, psychosocial trauma often leads to poor illness adjustment and is associated with increased pain reporting, increased provider visits, increased medication use, referral to specialists, and an overall poor clinical outcome.[2,4,24] History of abuse is an important factor to consider in patients with IBS, although the timing of such a discussion is at the provider's discretion.[7]

Permanent remission of IBS is experienced by approximately 25% of patients; for the majority of patients IBS becomes a chronic illness.[7] As with any chronic illness, IBS has the potential to have an adverse impact on quality of life because it can lead to impairment of physical and psychosocial function, disability, work absenteeism, and increased provider visits.[2,4,26]

CLINICAL PRESENTATION

The symptoms of IBS usually begin in the late teens to twenties, are often gradual in onset, and are intermittent—lasting days, weeks, or months at a time.[1,8] After the exclusion of organic disease (especially in patients older than 50 years), the diagnosis is established according to the Rome II criteria (see Box 146-1), a set of symptom-based diagnostic criteria simplified from Rome I criteria.[2,3,27] Rome I criteria were derived from factor analysis that differentiated the symptoms of patients with IBS from those of healthy patients and patients with other GI disorders.[2-4,27]

Abdominal pain must be present for an IBS diagnosis.[7] The pain associated with IBS is usually described as nonradiating, intermittent, crampy pain in the lower abdomen (most commonly, the left lower quadrant). Some describe the pain as burning or sharp.[7] Although the frequency and intensity of abdominal pain may vary, the quality and location of the pain remain fairly constant over time for the individual.[8] The pain is typically worse 1 to 2 hours after meals; it is exacerbated by stress, often relieved by a bowel movement, and does not interrupt sleep.[8] Some patients report pain only with bowel movements.[7] Establishment of the absence of nocturnal symptoms is critical to the diagnosis of IBS as a functional GI disorder.[9]

Diarrhea, constipation, or a pattern of alternating diarrhea and constipation may be reported in conjunction with abdominal pain. It is often necessary to clarify what is meant by these complaints, since the normal pattern of defecation can range from three bowel movements per week to three bowel movements per day.[7] Mucus in the stool is sometimes reported. Complaints of abdominal distention and bloating are common and most likely reflect increased sensitivity to normal amounts of intestinal gas rather than an actual increase in gas.[8]

The likelihood of organic disease is indicated by an acute onset of GI symptoms or an onset of symptoms in patients older than 50 years. Nocturnal symptoms, bloody stools, weight loss, fever, arthralgias, myalgias, and fatigue are incompatible with a diagnosis of IBS and require immediate diagnostic evaluation or referral.[4,8,9] Although bleeding is not associated with IBS, it may occur secondary to an anal fissure or hemorrhoids aggravated by an alteration in bowel habits associated with IBS.[9] However, careful diagnostic evaluation is required before ascribing rectal bleeding to distal benign causes.

A complete health history should be elicited in the presence of abdominal pain with an alteration in bowel habits. The history should include a thorough investigation of the presenting symptoms, associated symptoms, and the presence of nocturnal symptoms. The patient should be questioned about previous diagnostic evaluations for similar symptoms. A past medical history and family history of GI problems, such as colon cancer, inflammatory bowel disease, and celiac disease, should be obtained. The patient should be asked about recent travel, GI infections, and the use of any prescription or over-the-counter medications that could cause diarrhea or constipation. A thorough review of diet, with particular emphasis on any food allergies or sensitivities such as lactose or fructose intolerance, should be undertaken. The review of symptoms should focus on the differential diagnoses for abdominal pain with an alteration in bowel habits. A menstrual history and gynecologic review of symptoms are essential in females to exclude urogenital sources of abdominal pain such as pelvic inflammatory disease (PID), ovarian cysts, uterine fibroids, or endometriosis. A sensitive psychosocial history should be elicited to determine sources of stress, coping mechanisms, support systems, reactions to stress in the past, and the use of psychologic counseling services to cope with past stressors. A history of physical or sexual abuse as a child or an adult should also be explored at some point.

PHYSICAL EXAMINATION

A thorough physical examination should be performed to exclude organic disease and to reassure the patient.[4,7] With IBS the physical examination is often unremarkable.[1,7] An abdominal, pelvic, and rectal examination should be performed. Increased tympany to percussion; a palpable, tender, cordlike sigmoid colon; and tenderness on rectal examination have been reported.[4,9] Significant abdominal tenderness or rectal tenderness, masses, or blood in the stool warrants further investigation.[7]

DIAGNOSTICS

The goals of testing patients with IBS are to establish an early diagnosis, exclude the presence of alternative or co-existing diagnoses, and avoid unnecessary testing.[7] When planning a diagnostic strategy for the patient with an alteration in bowel habits, the provider should consider several factors, including the duration and severity of symptoms, the demographic features, any family history of colon cancer, the nature and extent of psychosocial issues, and previous diagnostic evaluations for similar symptoms.[2,18] An initial approach should be based on the Rome II criteria in addition to a thorough history and physical examination and include a limited diagnostic screen aimed at excluding organic disease.[4,7] Few if any diagnostic tests are required in the young healthy patient who meets the symptom-based criteria for IBS and does not have "red flags" suggestive of organic disease uncovered during the history and physical examination.[4,7,18] A diagnosis of IBS with adequate initial evaluation is rarely associated with a need for additional diagnostics in the future.[4] Repeated testing should be avoided because it often leads the patient to question the reliability of the initial diagnosis.[9]

A limited screen for organic disease should include a CBC with differential, erythrocyte sedimentation rate, electrolytes, BUN, creatinine, glucose, thyroid-stimulating hormone, and a stool for occult blood and fecal leukocytes. If fecal leukocytes are positive, stool cultures for enteric pathogens, ova and parasites, and *Clostridium difficile* should be obtained. If occult blood is positive, the patient should be referred to a gastroenterologist for evaluation. Flexible sigmoidoscopy with or without a barium enema is generally recommended for young (<40 years), healthy patients with an acute change in bowel habits or rectal discomfort.[7] A colonoscopy should be performed for patients older than 50 years or patients with weight loss, anemia, occult blood, or risk factors for colorectal cancer.[2,4,7,27] Many patients with IBS are also lactose intolerant. Any patient with bloating, gas, distention, and diarrhea should undergo a 2-week trial of a lactose-free diet or a hydrogen breath test to exclude lactase deficiency.[7] Another alternative is to have patients drink a quart of milk. If they do not experience symptoms, it is unlikely they are lactose intolerant.[7] Liver function tests and an abdominal ultrasound to exclude gallstones may be required depending on the constellation of symptoms. Patients with persistent pain, diarrhea, and weight loss should undergo serologic testing for celiac disease.[7] Complaints of excess gas and bloating should be evaluated with a kidney-ureter-bladder scan of the abdomen.[4] Suspected urogenital causes of abdominal pain require further diagnostic testing or referral to a gynecologist.

If the initial diagnostic screen is negative, treatment of symptoms should be initiated and reevaluated in 3 to 6 weeks. This diagnostic strategy allows for a more conservative and cost-effective evaluation. If the initial treatment fails, addi-

DIAGNOSTICS

Irritable Bowel Syndrome

LABORATORY
CBC with differential
ESR
Serum electrolytes, BUN, creatinine, glucose
TSH
Stool for occult blood and fecal leukocytes (if fecal leukocytes positive, test for enteric pathogens, ova and parasites, and *Clostridium difficile*)
LFTs*
Serum transglutaminase antibody*
Hydrogen breath test*

IMAGING
KUB (flat plate and upright)*
Barium enema*
Abdominal ultrasound*

OTHER
Flexible sigmoidoscopy or colonoscopy*

*If indicated.

tional diagnostic studies or a referral to a gastroenterologist may be considered.[2,4] IBS patients older than 50 years with new or changed symptoms require a repeat evaluation.

DIFFERENTIAL DIAGNOSIS

A number of organic diseases have presentations similar to those of IBS. It is essential that they be considered in the diagnostic reasoning process. Colon cancer, inflammatory bowel disease, cholecystitis, pancreatic insufficiency, intestinal ischemia, intestinal parasites, lactase deficiency, fructose intolerance, malabsorption syndromes such as celiac disease, and viral gastroenteritis can cause abdominal pain or a change in bowel habits. Hypothyroidism can cause constipation, whereas hyperthyroidism and diabetes can cause diarrhea. Psychiatric conditions, including anxiety disorders, depression, and somatization, should be considered when evaluating the patient with a change in bowel habits.[1,2,8,9,24,28,29] Urogenital causes such as PID, endometriosis, ovarian cyst, and uterine fibroid should be considered in females with lower abdominal pain and gynecologic symptoms.[7]

DIFFERENTIAL DIAGNOSIS

Irritable Bowel Syndrome

- Colon cancer
- Inflammatory bowel disease (Crohn's disease and ulcerative colitis)
- Cholecystitis
- Pancreatic insufficiency
- Intestinal ischemia
- Intestinal parasites
- Lactase deficiency
- Fructose intolerance
- Malabsorption syndromes (celiac disease)
- Viral gastroenteritis
- Thyroid disease
- Diabetes-related diarrhea
- Anxiety disorders
- Depression
- Somatization
- Urogenital causes (pelvic inflammatory disease, endometriosis, ovarian cysts, uterine fibroids)

MANAGEMENT

The focus of IBS treatment is symptomatic and includes dietary modifications, medications, supportive and behavioral therapy, education, and reassurance. To date, no single therapy has proved to be more effective than another. One of the most important factors in the successful management of IBS appears to be the establishment of a therapeutic relationship.[1,27] A nonjudgmental, attentive approach is essential to assist patients in shifting their focus from finding a cause for their symptoms to finding a way to cope with them.[4] Health care providers must resist the urge to respond to chronic complaints with new or repeated diagnostic studies.[4,30]

Because both physiologic and psychosocial factors appear to play a role in the severity of symptoms and the expression of illness, both must be considered when developing a management plan.[4,27,31] Diagnosis and treatment of any underlying psychologic disorder, such as anxiety and depression, are essential.[9] Most patients (75%) with IBS have mild symptoms and can be managed in a primary care setting. They usually respond to education, reassurance, and dietary and lifestyle modifications.[4] A smaller number have moderate symptoms that are usually intermittent but can be disabling. They may have psychologic distress from their symptoms, but their symptoms correlate with gut physiology.[4] These patients often require gut-acting medications such as anticholinergic and antidiarrheal agents and, in some cases, psychologic counseling.[4] A very small number of patients have severe and refractory symptoms. They often report chronic, severe pain and psychosocial difficulties, and they require antidepressants, mental health referrals, and sometimes a pain management evaluation.[4] These patients require a team approach that includes co-management with gastroenterology.

Dietary Modification

Although true food allergies are uncommon, many patients with IBS report food intolerances.[7] In most cases it is not what the patient eats but rather the act of eating that precipitates symptoms.[7] Gas, bloating, distention, and a change in bowel habits are often attributed to the intake of certain foods (Box 146-2). Dairy products and gas-forming foods are the most common offenders.[1,8] Other foods and beverages that may cause or aggravate symptoms include items artificially sweetened with fructose or sorbitol, carbonated beverages, caffeine, alcohol, spicy foods, and fatty foods.[2,8]

Although care should be taken to avoid unnecessary dietary restrictions, since evidence of benefit is unclear, the initial recommendations should focus on eliminating foods suspected of causing or aggravating individual symptoms.[2] Use of a diary to record food intake and symptoms can help identify offending foods. Some patients may benefit from referral to a nutritionist.[10] Lactose intolerance should be excluded in all patients who initially are seen with symptoms of IBS.[1,7,32]

BOX 146-2

COMMON GAS-FORMING FOODS

- Beans, lentils, and other legumes
- Beer
- Broccoli
- Brussels sprouts
- Cabbage
- Carbonated beverages
- Cauliflower
- Coffee
- Grapes
- Plums
- Raisins
- Raw onions
- Red wine

Consideration should be given to hydrogen breath testing or recommendation of a 2- to 3-week trial of a lactose-free diet.[1,7,32] Fructose intolerance should likewise be excluded through a 7- to 10-day elimination of foods and beverages (fruit juices, sodas, sports drinks) containing a large amount of fructose.[7] Instructions should also include a recommendation to avoid medications that could aggravate symptoms, such as laxatives and antacids with laxative effects.[8]

The role of fiber therapy in IBS remains controversial.[33] Although it has been widely used in the treatment of IBS for many years, only three clinical trials have demonstrated benefit.[7] Fiber is likely to decrease constipation, but its role in relieving abdominal pain and diarrhea is less clear.[2] Clinical experience has demonstrated that many patients benefit from fiber after an initial period of bloating and abdominal discomfort. A trial of 20 to 30 g/day of fiber seems reasonable for the treatment of IBS.[1,8]

Synthetic fiber supplements are more soluble than natural fiber, cause less bloating, and may be better tolerated.[1] Slow introduction of the fiber load helps reduce gas and bloating. A number of commercial products are available as over-the-counter formulations. No one brand seems to have an advantage over another, although individual responses vary. Providers should instruct patients to try a different brand if one seems ineffective or produces side effects. Supplementation may be accomplished by giving 1 tablet, rounded tablespoon, or packet of psyllium (Metamucil) or calcium polycarbophil (FiberCon) with food or 8 ounces of liquid q. day to t.i.d. (according to response).[8] Another treatment option is methylcellulose (Citrucel) 1 scoop q. day to t.i.d. An alternative to synthetic fiber is a diet high in whole grains and natural fiber, a daily fluid intake of 64 ounces, regular exercise, and a set time each day to use the bathroom.[7] Simethicone may also be used to help relieve bloating.[7]

Pharmacotherapy

Antispasmodics. Despite a lack of clinical evidence to support benefit, antispasmodics seem to help those with meal-induced symptoms and tenesmus.[7] Anticholinergics act to reduce sigmoid motility in response to a fatty meal.[4,34] Medications such as dicyclomine (Bentyl) 10 to 40 mg q.i.d. p.r.n. may be tried by patients who experience postprandial abdominal pain, gas, and bloating.[1] To achieve maximum effectiveness, the medication should be taken 30 to 60 minutes before meals.[4] Hyoscyamine sulfate, the active ingredient in Levsin and Donnatal, is also an effective antispasmodic but has several side effects, including urinary retention, tachycardia, and dry mouth.[8] Clidinium, the active ingredient in Librax and Clindex, has fatigue as a common side effect.[7] Dicyclomine acts more selectively on the smooth muscle of the GI tract and may produce fewer side effects than the nonselective anticholinergics.[1] Analgesic medications, particularly narcotics, should be avoided if at all possible.[7]

Antidiarrheal Agents. Loperamide (Imodium) 2 to 4 mg q.i.d. p.r.n. decreases intestinal transit, enhances intestinal water absorption, and strengthens rectal sphincter tone, thereby improving the diarrhea, urgency, and fecal soiling in IBS patients with diarrhea.[4] Patients may take a maximum of 8 pills per day as needed to control symptoms. Polycarbophil can be added to help increase stool bulk. Pepto-Bismal, Kaopectate, and bile acid–sequestering agents, such as cholestyramine (Questran, Prevalite), should also be considered in the treatment of diarrhea-predominant IBS.[4] Randomized controlled trials have demonstrated benefit from alosetron (Lotronex), a 5-HT_3 receptor antagonist used for the treatment of abdominal pain, diarrhea, and bloating in women with IBS and diarrhea.[3] The U.S. Food and Drug Administration (FDA) withdrew alosetron from the market in 2000 because of several cases of ischemic colitis.[7] It is currently available under a limited-use program. Patients taking alosetron must be monitored closely for the development of constipation. Patients should be instructed to immediately stop the drug and notify their provider if constipation occurs. Cilansetron is a 5-HT_3 receptor antagonist similar to alosetron with indications for the treatment of IBS with diarrhea in both women and men.[7] Cilansetron has yet to receive FDA approval for marketing.

Anticonstipation Agents. Synthetic fiber is beneficial in treating constipation associated with IBS. In addition to fiber therapy, increasing fluids, and regular exercise, patients with constipation may benefit from stool softeners and osmotic laxatives such as lactulose and polyethylene glycol (MiraLax). Stimulant laxatives should be avoided whenever possible.

Psychotropic Agents. Antidepressants, including tricyclic agents and selective serotonin reuptake inhibitors (SSRIs), are often used to treat IBS, particularly in patients with severe or refractory pain and symptoms, impaired daily function, and associated depression or panic attacks.[4,28-30] The anticholinergic properties of the tricyclic antidepressants (amitriptyline, nortriptyline, desipramine) are believed to contribute to their effectiveness in treating the pain, gas, bloating, and frequent stools associated with IBS. Small clinical trials have shown benefit in alleviating abdominal pain.[7] Because of their tendency to cause constipation, the use of tricyclic agents should be avoided in IBS patients with constipation.

Because of the lower side effect profile of SSRIs, many providers are prescribing them instead of tricyclic agents, despite the fact that there are no clinical trials assessing their effect on patients with IBS.[4,7] These medications reduce depression, anxiety, and somatization rather than relieve abdominal pain per se.[7] A common side effect of SSRIs is diarrhea; therefore these drugs may prove most beneficial in treating IBS patients with constipation.

There is no clinical research to support the use of benzodiazepines in IBS; their use should be avoided because of their addictive potential.[1,4,9]

Alternative Therapies

Several alternative therapies have been studied in IBS, including cognitive-behavioral therapy, hypnosis, guided imagery, relaxation techniques, stress management, and acupuncture.[4,7,35,36] The data appear to support the value of alternative therapies in reducing anxiety and other psychologic symptoms and in decreasing GI symptoms.[4] Patients with underlying psychologic issues may benefit from a referral to a psychologist, mental health clinical nurse specialist, or psychiatric nurse practitioner. Patients with severe, refractory pain should be referred to a pain management program.[4]

Peppermint oil is a natural antispasmodic. With GI effects similar to those of calcium channel blockers, peppermint oil causes smooth muscle relaxation and can help with post-prandial pain and bloating. However, randomized controlled trials did not support this benefit.[7] Peppermint oil is also available in enteric-coated capsule form.

LIFE SPAN CONSIDERATIONS

IBS is a chronic recurrent disorder that frequently develops in late adolescence to early adulthood and continues throughout the life span. Exacerbations are common and often correlate with life stressors. Once thought to be a disease of young women, IBS is increasingly being recognized in men and older adults. An IBS diagnosis in an older person must be made cautiously and in consultation with a gastroenterologist to avoid missing a more serious diagnosis.

COMPLICATIONS

Although it is important to recognize that IBS is a chronic recurrent GI disorder in the majority of cases, serious complications from IBS are extremely rare. In some patients the chronic nature of symptoms leads to a reduced quality of life and clinical depression. Chronic constipation may also result in hemorrhoids, anal fissures, fecal impaction, and, rarely, intestinal obstruction.

INDICATIONS FOR REFERRAL OR HOSPITALIZATION

Nocturnal symptoms, bloody stools, fever, and weight loss are incompatible with a diagnosis of IBS and require immediate further diagnostic evaluation or referral (Box 146-3). Physician consultation and referral to a gastroenterologist are indicated if initial treatment of IBS fails, if organic disease is suspected or found, or if the patient is older than 50 years or has an established diagnosis of IBS and is reporting a change in the usual pattern of symptoms (Box 146-4). Gastroenterology specialists are also helpful in the co-management of a patient with complex IBS.[2,8,9]

BOX 146-3

EMERGENCY CRITERIA

Symptoms that are incompatible with irritable bowel syndrome and require immediate diagnostic evaluation or referral include:

- Nocturnal symptoms
- Bloody stools
- Fever
- Weight loss

BOX 146-4

INDICATIONS FOR REFERRAL

- Initial treatment failure
- Organic disease suspected
- Change in bowel habits in a patient older than 50 years
- Change in usual irritable bowel syndrome symptom pattern

PATIENT AND FAMILY EDUCATION

Dietary and lifestyle modifications such as the avoidance of foods that trigger symptoms, an increase in fluids and fiber, regular exercise, and alternative therapies should be discussed with patients.[9] Information regarding what constitutes "normal" bowel habits should be given. Bowel retraining should be encouraged by recommending sitting on the toilet (without straining) for 15 to 20 minutes each morning after breakfast.[9] Medications for symptom control should be reviewed, including a discussion regarding laxative abuse.[9]

Patients should be informed that the symptoms of IBS are very real. They should be taught that their symptoms are caused by an increased sensitivity and reactivity of the gut to stimuli, resulting in pain and/or abnormal motility.[4] They should understand that IBS is a chronic condition that does not lead to cancer or inflammatory bowel disease[9] and is characterized by periods of remission and exacerbation that often correlate with physical and psychologic stressors.[4] Reassurance has tremendous value in the treatment of IBS. Patients should be told that, although there is no cure, there is help, and the majority of patients learn to cope adequately with their symptoms and lead productive lives.[4]

HEALTH PROMOTION

The chronic nature of IBS symptoms may lead a patient with IBS to ignore a change in bowel habits resulting from an organic condition. Patients need to be instructed that, although IBS does not increase their risk for colorectal cancer, they should keep their screening current with recommended guidelines for colorectal screening in the general population, and they should immediately report a change in bowel habits that is atypical for their usual pattern of symptoms.

REFERENCES

1. Lynn RB, Friedman LS: Irritable bowel syndrome, *N Engl J Med* 329(26):1940-1943, 1993.
2. American Gastroenterological Association: Medical position paper: irritable bowel syndrome, *Gastroenterology* 112(6):2118-2119, 1997.

3. Thompson WG, Longstreth GF, Drossman DA, and others: Functional bowel disorders and functional abdominal pain, *Gut* 45(Suppl 2):1143-1147, 1999.
4. Drossman DA, Whitehead WE, Camilleri M: Irritable bowel syndrome: a technical review for practical guideline development, *Gastroenterology* 112(6):2120-2137, 1997.
5. Manning AP, Thompson WG, Heaton KW, and others: Toward positive diagnosis of the irritable bowel, *Br Med J* 2:653-654, 1978.
6. Talley NJ: Epidemiology, severity, and impact of irritable bowel syndrome, *Prac Gastroenterol* April(Suppl):4-12, 2005.
7. Lacy BE: Irritable bowel syndrome: an overview, *Gastroenterol Endoscopy News* Oct(Suppl):31-37, 2005.
8. Eastwood GL, Avundk C, editors: Irritable bowel syndrome. In *Manual of gastroenterology*, ed 2, Boston, 1994, Little, Brown.
9. Carlson E: Irritable bowel syndrome, *Nurse Pract* 23(1):83-93, 1998.
10. Zuckerman MJ, Guerra LG, Drossman DA, and others: Health-care-seeking behaviors related to bowel complaints: Hispanics versus non-Hispanic whites, *Dig Dis Sci* 41(1):77-82, 1996.
11. Thompson WG: Functional bowel disorders and functional abdominal pain. In Drossman DA, and others, editors: *Functional gastrointestinal disorders: diagnosis, pathophysiology and treatment,* McLean, Va, 1994, Degnon Associates.
12. Drossman DA, Li Z, Andruzzi E, and others: U.S. householder survey of functional gastrointestinal disorders: prevalence, sociodemography, and health impact, *Dig Dis Sci* 38:1569-1580, 1993.
13. Longstreth GF, Wilson A, Knight K, and others: Irritable bowel syndrome, health care use, and costs: a U.S. managed care perspective, *Am J Gastroenterol* 98(3):600-607, 2003.
14. Pimentel M, Chow EJ, Lin HC: Eradication of small intestinal bacterial overgrowth reduces symptoms of irritable bowel syndrome, *Am J Gastroenterol* 95(5):3503-3506, 2000.
15. Neal KR, Barker L, Spiller RC: Prognosis in post-infectious irritable bowel syndrome: a 6 year follow up study, *Gut* 51:410-413, 2002.
16. Munakata J, Naliboff B, Harraf F, and others: Repetitive sigmoid stimulation induces rectal hyperalgesia in patients with irritable bowel syndrome, *Gastroenterology* 112(1):55-63, 1997.
17. Heitkemper M, Jarrett M, Cain K, and others: Increased urine catecholamines and cortisol in women with irritable bowel syndrome, *Am J Gastroenterol* 91(5):906-913, 1996.
18. Mayer EA, Raybould HE: The role of visceral afferent mechanisms in functional bowel disorders, *Gastroenterology* 99(3):1688-1704, 1990.
19. Bueno L, Fioramonti J, Delvaux M, and others: Mediators and pharmacology of visceral sensitivity; from basic to clinical investigations, *Gastroenterology* 112(4):1714-1743, 1997.
20. Goyal RK, Hirano I: The enteric nervous system, *N Engl J Med* 334:1106-1115, 1996.
21. Bearcroft CP, Perrett D, Farthing MJG: Postprandial 5-hydroxytryptamine in diarrhea predominant irritable bowel syndrome: a pilot study, *Gut* 42:42-46, 1998.
22. Dewsnap P, Gomborone G, Libby G, and others: The prevalence of symptoms of irritable bowel syndrome among acute psychiatric inpatients with an affective diagnosis, *Psychosomatics* 37(4):385-389, 1996.
23. Drossman DA, and others: Psychosocial aspects of the functional gastrointestinal disorders, *Gastroenterol Int* 8:47-90, 1995.
24. Irwin C, Falsetti SA, Lydiard RB, and others: Comorbidity of post-traumatic stress disorder and irritable bowel syndrome, *J Clin Psychiatry* 57(12):576-578, 1996.
25. Drossman DA, Leserman J, Nachman G, and others: Sexual and physical abuse in women with functional or organic gastrointestinal disorders, *Ann Intern Med* 113:828-833, 1990.
26. Whitehead WE, Burnett CK, Cook EW: Impact of irritable bowel syndrome on quality of life, *Dig Dis Sci* 41(11):2248-2253, 1996.
27. Dalton CS, Drossman DA: Diagnosis and treatment of irritable bowel syndrome, *Am Fam Phys* 55(3):875-885, 1997.
28. Masand PS, Kaplan DS, Gupta S, and others: Irritable bowel syndrome and dysthymia: is there a relationship? *Psychosomatics* 38(1):63-69, 1997.
29. Zaubler TS, Katon W: Panic disorder and medical comorbidity: a review of the medical and psychiatric literature, *Bull Menninger Clin* 60(2 Suppl A):A12-A38, 1996.
30. Bonis PA, Norton RA: The challenge of irritable bowel syndrome, *Am Fam Phys* 53(4):1229-1236, 1996.
31. Lembo T, Fullerton S, Diehl D, and others: Symptom duration in patients with irritable bowel syndrome, *Am J Gastroenterol* 91(5):898-905, 1996.
32. Tolliver BA, Jackson MS, Jackson KL, and others: Does lactose maldigestion really play a role in the irritable bowel syndrome? *J Clin Gastroenterol* 23(1):15-17, 1996.
33. Bennett WG, Cerda JJ: Benefits of dietary fiber: myth or medicine? *Postgrad Med* 99(2):153-172, 1996.
34. Sullivan MA, Cohen S, Snape WJ: Colonic myoelectric activity in irritable bowel syndrome: effects of eating and anticholinergics, *N Engl J Med* 298:878-883, 1978.
35. VanDulmen AM, Fennis JF, Bleijenberg G: Cognitive-behavioral group therapy for irritable bowel syndrome: effects and long-term follow-up, *Psychosom Med* 58(5):508-514, 1996.
36. Houghton LA, Heyman DJ, Whorwell PJ: Symptomatology, quality of life and economic features of irritable bowel syndrome in hypnotherapy, *Ailment Pharmacol Ther* 10(1):91-95, 1996.

CHAPTER 147

Jaundice

Louise P. Meyer

DEFINITION AND EPIDEMIOLOGY

Jaundice, or icterus, is a yellow or greenish discoloration of the skin, sclerae, and mucous membranes caused by bile pigments of conjugated or unconjugated bilirubin.[1,2] There are multiple causes of jaundice, requiring determination of the underlying disorder.

Jaundice can be divided into three categories. The first type involves unconjugated hyperbilirubinemia, which results when the indirect fraction of bilirubin exceeds 80% of the total bilirubin.[3] Hemolytic jaundice is an example of this type. The second type, obstructive jaundice, is produced by conjugated bilirubin. Conjugated bilirubinemia develops when the direct fraction of bilirubin ranges from 20% to 60% of the total bilirubin.[3] Hepatocellular jaundice is the third category and is caused by failure of the liver cells to conjugate bilirubin.[1]

The causes of jaundice are categorized according to (1) symptoms (acute or chronic), (2) evidence of bile duct dilation, and (3) jaundice of the conjugated or unconjugated varieties.[1] Jaundice is common in newborns and occurs in 50% of term infants between the fourth and fourteenth day after birth.[4] In older children and young adults, common causes include viral hepatitis (accounts for 75% of jaundice in patients <30 years old), Gilbert's syndrome, drug-induced hepatitis, pregnancy, cirrhosis, and alcoholic hepatitis. In older patients, cirrhosis (accounts for 30% of jaundice in the 30- to 60-year-old age-group), pancreatic cancer, metastatic cancer to the liver, sepsis, common bile duct stone, and medication-induced hepatitis are the most common causes[2] (Box 147-1).

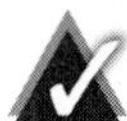
Physician consultation is indicated for patients with new-onset jaundice.

PATHOPHYSIOLOGY

The liver plays a major role in the metabolism of bile pigments. This process is divided into three distinct phases: (1) hepatic uptake, (2) conjugation, and (3) excretion.[1] A byproduct of hemolysis is bilirubin, which is produced through the breakdown of hemoglobin in red blood cells (RBCs).[5] There are two forms of bilirubin: indirect, or unconjugated, bilirubin (which is protein bound) and direct, or conjugated, bilirubin. The direct form circulates freely in the blood until it reaches the liver, where it is conjugated with glucuronide transferase and excreted into the bile.[1] An increase in unconjugated bilirubin is often associated with an increase in the destruction of RBCs. An increase in conjugated bilirubin is more likely seen with liver dysfunction or obstruction.[6] Disturbance in the passage of conjugated bilirubin from the liver to the intestine accounts for 60% of jaundice in patients older than 60 years.[2] With bile duct obstruction, bilirubin is conjugated by the hepatocytes but cannot flow into the duodenum.[1] Therefore bilirubin accumulates in the liver and enters the bloodstream, causing hyperbilirubinemia.

Extrahepatic obstructive jaundice develops if the common bile duct is occluded by gallstones or tumors, especially pancreatic carcinoma or strictures.[1,3] Because conjugated bilirubin is water soluble, it is excreted in the urine. This produces the characteristic orange urine with elevated conjugated bilirubin produced by inflammation.

Intrahepatic obstructive jaundice involves disturbances in hepatocyte function or obstruction of bile canaliculi. The uptake, conjugation, and excretion of bilirubin are affected, resulting in increased levels of conjugated and unconjugated bilirubin.[1]

Failure of liver cells to conjugate bilirubin causes hepatocellular damage, resulting in increased plasma concentrations of unconjugated bilirubin. In addition, bilirubin cannot pass from the liver to the intestine.[1] The causes of hepatitis include infections, medications, and genetic defects causing decreased enzyme production.

Hemolytic jaundice is caused by excessive hemolysis of RBCs. An increased amount of unconjugated bilirubin is formed through metabolism of the heme component of destroyed RBCs and exceeds the conjugation ability of the liver.[1] This causes the blood levels of unconjugated bilirubin to rise. Hemolysis can occur with blood transfusion reactions, after cardiopulmonary bypass, with sickle cell anemia, and with marrow or splenic destruction of RBCs. In sickle cell anemia, abnormal hemoglobin and a fragile cell membrane lead to hemolysis and an increase in the amount of free, unconjugated bilirubin.[1] Bone marrow development problems and defective erythropoiesis are conditions in which poorly manufactured

BOX 147-1

CLASSIFICATION AND CAUSES OF JAUNDICE

UNCONJUGATED HYPERBILIRUBINEMIA (PREDOMINANTLY INDIRECT-ACTING BILIRUBIN)

- Increased bilirubin production
- Hemolytic anemias (thalassemias, sideroblastic anemias, some pernicious anemias), hematoma, infarction
- Decreased hepatic uptake
- Posthepatitis, drug reactions, sepsis, prolonged fasting
- Decreased bilirubin conjugation (decreased hepatic glucuronosyltransferase)
- Hereditary transferase deficiency (Gilbert's syndrome, Crigler-Najjar syndrome)
- Acquired transferase deficiency: drug inhibition (e.g., chloramphenicol), breast milk, hepatocellular disease
- Neonatal jaundice

CONJUGATED HYPERBILIRUBINEMIA (PREDOMINANTLY DIRECT-ACTING BILIRUBIN)

- Impaired excretion: intrahepatic defects
- Familial defects (Dubin-Johnson syndrome, Rotor's syndrome), recurrent intrahepatic cholestasis, cholestatic jaundice of pregnancy
- Acquired disorders: viral or drug-induced hepatitis, cirrhosis, sepsis, postoperative complications, androgens, chlorpromazine, acetaminophen, sulfonamides, NSAIDs, aspirin, industrial poisons
- Impaired excretion: extrahepatic defects
- Gallstones, biliary malformation, infection, biliary or pancreatic tumors, chronic pancreatitis, pancreatic pseudocyst

erythrocytes are fragile and have a short life span. The result is an excess of unconjugated bilirubin that reaches the liver for conjugation.[1]

CLINICAL PRESENTATION

Jaundice is most commonly observed in the face, trunk, and sclera. Bilirubin is distributed uniformly in the sclera and is differentiated from the normal occurrence of the yellow subscleral fat that collects in the periphery.[1] In African Americans the mandibular frenum is a location to observe jaundice. Jaundice caused by carotene does not stain the sclera but rather is seen in the forehead, around the nasi, and in the palms and soles. The patient with jaundice may have pruritus, which often accompanies obstructive jaundice. The pruritus is caused by nerve injury in the skin by the bile pigments.[1] Cutaneous xanthomas may be seen in patients with jaundice from chronic cholestasis and suggest hypercholesterolemia. The presence of spider angiomas, palmar erythema, and ascites combined with malaise, anorexia, and right upper quadrant discomfort suggests chronic hepatocellular disease or cirrhosis. Colicky right upper quadrant pain, weight loss, and light-colored stools may be present in obstructive jaundice. Intermittent, colicky right upper quadrant pain before the onset of jaundice suggests choledocholithiasis.[3] Fever and chills may accompany biliary obstruction and virus- or drug-induced hepatitis. Occult blood in the stools suggests cancer as a cause for jaundice.

Appropriate history includes determining whether the jaundice is acute or chronic and ascertaining associated symptoms (e.g., fever, weight loss, anorexia, rash, pruritus, abdominal pain, or musculoskeletal aches and pains). In acute jaundice, inquiry focuses on hepatitis risks, including recent travel; transfusions; tattoos; IV drug use; alcohol intake; medications (prescription, herbals, or over the counter); food, toxin, animal, or infected person exposures; unsafe sexual practices; and symptoms of biliary tract disease. Chronic jaundice may suggest viral hepatitis, biliary tract disease, pancreatitis, or chronic alcohol intake. Weight loss, anorexia, malaise, and other symptoms of cancer are noted. In addition, a list of medications (including over the counter and herbal medications) taken by the patient and a complete family history, including cancer, Wilson's disease, hemochromatosis, and hereditary hemolytic anemias, provide vital information for an appropriate diagnosis. Exposure to toxins and the surgical history should also be elicited.

PHYSICAL EXAMINATION

Acute jaundice requires a complete examination to determine the cause of the illness. Determination of vital signs (including temperature); evaluation of the skin (including the palms and soles), sclera, and mucous membranes; assessment of the cardiovascular system for congestive heart failure; and evaluation of the abdomen for ascites, organomegaly, guarding, and tenderness are essential.[2,6] Fever and right upper quadrant tenderness are most often associated with choledocholithiasis, cholangitis, or cholecystitis. An enlarged, tender liver suggests acute hepatic inflammation or a rapidly growing hepatic tumor.[7] Splenomegaly suggests portal hypertension from acute or active chronic hepatitis, as well as cirrhosis.[5,6]

Chronic jaundice mandates evaluation for chronic liver disease. Gynecomastia, testicular atrophy, and splenomegaly are strongly associated with cirrhosis. In addition, palmar erythema, facial telangiectasia, and Dupuytren's contractures are associated with cirrhosis from chronic ethanol ingestion.[8] Lymphadenopathy suggests malignancy and can be related to a pancreatic tumor obstructing the splenic vein or to a metastatic lymphoma. When malignancy is suspected, the investigation should concentrate on determining the location of the primary tumor as indicated by heme-positive stool, abdominal masses, breast masses, thyroid nodules, or supraclavicular lymphadenopathy. Physical findings associated with specific liver diseases include distended neck veins and hepatojugular reflux (right-sided heart failure), xanthomas (primary biliary cirrhosis), and Kayser-Fleischer rings (Wilson's disease).[8]

DIAGNOSTICS

Liver function tests (LFTs)—including albumin, aspartate aminotransferase (AST), and alanine aminotransferase (ALT); total and direct serum bilirubin; serum alkaline phosphatase; stool guaiac; and urine bilirubin—are obtained, in addition to a CBC with platelet count and a prothrombin time (PT). Elevated ALT and AST levels result from hepatocellular necrosis or inflammation.[6] An AST level that is more than twice the ALT level is typical with alcoholic liver injury. Elevated alkaline phosphatase levels suggest cholestasis, primary biliary cirrhosis, or infiltrative liver disease (e.g., tumor, abscess, granulomas).[9] In obstructive liver disease the alkaline phosphatase may be more than three times the normal level.[3]

When the jaundice is not related to a biliary disorder or hepatic injury, the liver enzymes will be normal. A normal serum albumin suggests a more acute disease process than the chronic disease associated with low serum albumin.[10]

Unconjugated (indirect) hyperbilirubinemia suggests a hemolytic disorder, such as an autoimmune or microangiopathic hemolytic anemia. The most common cause of mild elevations of unconjugated bilirubin is Gilbert's syndrome, with physical stress, fever, fasting, or heavy alcohol ingestion as precipitants.[8]

Direct hyperbilirubinemia results from hepatocellular inflammation, cholestatic liver disease, or extrahepatic biliary obstruction. The presence of direct hyperbilirubinemia without liver enzyme abnormalities is uncommon but is seen in pregnancy, in sepsis, or after recent surgery.[8] Patients with elevated conjugated bilirubin should be evaluated for evidence of viral hepatitis, drug toxicity, or hepatic congestion. Serologic studies are used to diagnose hepatitis A, B, C, and D.[11] Common causes of toxic hepatitis include acetaminophen, allopurinol, androgenic steroids, aspirin and other salicylates, contraceptive steroids, chlorpromazine, erythromycin, glucocorticoids, mercaptopurine, methotrexate, plicamycin, NSAIDs, and sulfonamides.[12] Isolated conjugated direct hyperbilirubinemia is the primary symptom of two inherited disorders: Rotor's syndrome and Dubin-Johnson syndrome.[8,13]

In patients with chronic liver disease lacking a defined cause, serum iron, transferrin saturation, and ferritin should be measured to screen for hemochromatosis. In hemochromatosis the serum ferritin is substantially elevated. Plasma iron

DIAGNOSTICS

Jaundice

LABORATORY
LFTs
CBC and differential, platelets
PT/PTT
Hepatitis profile*
Serum iron, transferrin saturation, ferritin
Serum ceruloplasmin
Antimitochondrial antibodies
Antinuclear anti–smooth muscle and liver-kidney microsomal antibodies
α_1-Antitrypsin activity
Urine copper
Urine bilirubin

IMAGING
Ultrasonography
CT scan

OTHER
Endoscopic retrograde cholangiopancreatography or percutaneous transhepatic cholangiography*
Magnetic resonance cholangiopancreatography and endoscopic ultrasonography
Liver biopsy

*If indicated.

DIFFERENTIAL DIAGNOSIS

Jaundice

- Hepatitis
- Gilbert's syndrome
- Drug reaction
- Hemolytic anemia
- Hereditary syndromes
- Cirrhosis
- Cholestasis
- Postoperative jaundice
- Cholestatic jaundice of pregnancy
- Spirochete infection
- Infectious mononucleosis
- Sarcoidosis
- Lymphoma
- Toxins
- Cholangitis
- Tumor
- Choledochal cysts
- Choledocholithiasis
- Pancreatitis

may exceed 200 mcg/dl, and transferrin saturation exceeds 70%.[3] In patients younger than 30 years with abnormal LFT results or in patients with hepatitis who test negative for viruses A, B, C, and D and neurologic dysfunction, measurements of serum ceruloplasmin and urine copper levels are recommended to screen for Wilson's disease.[3] Other laboratory diagnostics to consider include antimitochondrial antibodies (for primary biliary cirrhosis), antinuclear anti–smooth muscle, and liver-kidney microsomal antibodies (for autoimmune hepatitis), and α_1-antitrypsin activity (for α_1-antitrypsin deficiency).[13]

Hepatobiliary imaging is recommended if the liver chemistry profile suggests cholestasis or extrahepatic obstruction. Ultrasound is greater than 90% specific and close to 90% sensitive in detecting obstruction. A CT scan is indicated in cases where ultrasound is unsatisfactory.[3,8] However, ultrasonography is an effective means of detecting stones in the gallbladder and is somewhat more sensitive than a CT scan.[3] Endoscopic retrograde cholangiopancreatography (ERCP) or percutaneous transhepatic cholangiography is indicated if extrahepatic obstruction is strongly suspected.[3] Newer imaging techniques to evaluate biliary obstruction and suspected malignancies include magnetic resonance cholangiopancreatography and endoscopic ultrasonography.[2] Percutaneous liver biopsy is the definitive study for determining the cause and extent of hepatocellular dysfunction or infiltrative liver disease, particularly if metastatic disease or a hepatic mass is suspected.[7]

DIFFERENTIAL DIAGNOSIS

The etiology of jaundice is multifactorial; consequently the presence of co-existing disease is an important aspect of the evaluation. The finding of unconjugated hyperbilirubinemia can be related to increased bilirubin production (hemolytic anemia) or impaired bilirubin uptake and storage (hepatitis sequelae, posthepatitis, Gilbert's syndrome, drug reactions). Hereditary syndromes such as Crigler-Najjar and Gilbert's syndromes (resulting from impaired glucuronosyltransferase activity) and Dubin-Johnson and Rotor's syndromes (resulting from faulty excretion of bilirubin) are examples of causes of unconjugated bilirubin.[8] Conjugated hyperbilirubinemia can be caused by hepatitis, cirrhosis, cholestasis, postoperative jaundice, spirochetal infections, infectious mononucleosis, sarcoidosis, lymphomas, and industrial toxins. Fever and chills suggest cholangitis. Causes of biliary obstructions include tumors, choledochal cysts, choledocholithiasis, pancreatitis, pancreatic neoplasms, and cholestatic jaundice of pregnancy. Jaundice during pregnancy is most commonly related to viral hepatitis.[6]

MANAGEMENT

The treatment of jaundice relates to the underlying disease process. Most patients with viral hepatitis can be treated symptomatically on an outpatient basis (see Chapter 144). When liver enzymes fail to return to normal levels within 6 months, liver biopsy is indicated.[3] Interferon alfa-2b may be useful in chronic hepatitis B and C after consultation with a gastroenterologist.[3] Cholangitis requires antibiotic therapy and surgical consultation. For patients with cholangitis, nonoperative biliary drainage can be performed via ERCP with transhepatically placed stents.[3] Surgical therapy is usually required for extrahepatic biliary obstruction. Gilbert's disease, Dubin-Johnson syndrome, and Rotor's syndrome beyond the neonatal period rarely require treatment to lower the bilirubin level. However, treatment for the primary disease process may require corticosteroids if the presentation of these diseases is complicated by hemolytic anemia.

The treatment for uncomplicated cirrhosis consists of voluntary restriction of activity if the patient has weakness and fatigue. The diet should be high in protein but low in sodium, and alcohol should be avoided. This regimen almost invariably results in improvement of hepatocellular function in patients with alcohol-induced cirrhosis.[8] Multivitamins and folic acid 1 mg/day may be given if the patient's diet is inadequate. Tranquilizers and sedatives should be avoided. When serum potassium falls below 3.5 mEq/L, the deficit of body potassium is approximately 300 to 500 mEq. This can be replaced over a few days with oral solutions of 10% potassium chloride, which provide 40 mEq of potassium/30 ml.[8] Protein can be restricted in stable cirrhotic patients to 45 g/day as long as there is a minimum of 400 g of carbohydrates ingested each day. Vegetable protein contains smaller amounts of ammonia, methionine, and aromatic acids and is better tolerated by these patients.[8] Lactulose is a nonabsorbable synthetic disaccharide that, when administered in dosages of 20 to 30 g t.i.d. to q.i.d., reduces blood ammonia and improves encephalopathy in the majority of patients. Patients with decompensated cirrhosis who are not responding to therapy should be considered for liver transplantation. A one-time dose of vitamin K, 5 to 25 mg PO or 10 mg SQ or IM, may improve prolongation of the PT. The dose may be repeated in 12 hours if necessary. An intravenous infusion of vitamin K is not recommended because of the risk of anaphylaxis.

Pruritus, which is commonly associated with jaundice, may be disabling to some patients, resulting in depression. Early treatment with agents such as cholestyramine three times per day and antihistamines three or four times daily is highly recommended.[3] Fragrance-free soaps, less frequent bathing, and use of emollients may also reduce the severity of pruritus.[5] Continued monitoring of LFTs; serologic tests; and hematologic studies of blood counts, platelets, and PTs as indicated are recommended for all patients with jaundice to detect complications.

COMPLICATIONS

The complications of jaundice are directly related to the underlying disease process. In cirrhosis, infection and gastrointestinal bleeding often precipitate decompensation. Potassium deficiency is common in cirrhosis and may contribute to hepatic encephalopathy.

Patients with hepatitis may experience one or two relapses during their recovery period. Complications of other underlying diseases associated with jaundice range from anemia to gastrointestinal infection, hepatocellular damage, encephalopathy, and postsurgical complications. The most serious complication of stenting is recurrent jaundice from stent occlusion and recurrent cholangitis.[14]

INDICATIONS FOR REFERRAL OR HOSPITALIZATION

The management of patients with jaundice is often a complex process because of the myriad underlying disease processes and the potential complications. The primary care physician is always consulted to determine the diagnosis and initial management plans. Consultation with a gastroenterologist, hepatologist, or surgeon is also often indicated.

Hospitalization of patients is indicated in cases of severe electrolyte imbalance or evidence of severe hepatocellular failure, ascites, and prolonged PT unresponsive to treatment.[3]

PATIENT AND FAMILY EDUCATION

It is imperative that patients understand the underlying disease process and prevention regimens. Appropriate levels of activity and rest, the importance of medication adherence, and the need for avoidance of over-the-counter medications that interfere with hepatic function should be emphasized. Appropriate dietary instruction is essential for patients with hepatic disease, and referral to a dietitian for instruction on specific diets is desirable.

REFERENCES

1. McCance KL, Huether SE: *Pathophysiology: the biological basis for disease in adults and children,* ed 3, St Louis, 1998, Mosby.
2. Barkun JS, Barkun AN: *Jaundice: approach to the jaundiced patient,* retrieved June 20, 2006, from http://www.medscape.com/viewarticle/535550.
3. Steiner GS, Lipsky MS: Jaundice. In Mengel MB, Schwiebert LP, editors: *Ambulatory medicine,* Norwalk, Conn, 1993, Appleton & Lange.
4. Seidel HM, Ball JW, Dains JE, and others: *Mosby's guide to physical examination,* ed 4, St Louis, 1999, Mosby.
5. Horrell CJ: Jaundice. In Camo-Sorrell D, Hawkins RA, editors: *Clinical manual for the oncology advanced practice nurse,* Pittsburgh, 2000, Oncology Nursing Press.
6. Guss DA: Disorders of the liver, biliary tract, and pancreas. In Rosen P, and others, editors: *Emergency medicine: concepts and clinical practice,* ed 4, St Louis, 1998, Mosby.
7. Lau W, Leung K, Leung TB, and others: A logical approach to hepatocellular carcinoma presenting with jaundice, *Ann Surg* 225(3):281-285, 1997.
8. Mezey E: Diseases of the liver. In Barker RL, Burton JR, Zieve PD, editors: *Principles of ambulatory medicine,* ed 4, Baltimore, 1995, Williams & Wilkins.
9. Driscoll CE, and others: *The family practice desk reference,* ed 3, St Louis, 1995, Mosby.
10. Kaplan MM: *Approach to the patient with abnormal liver function tests,* retrieved Jan 29, 2007, from http://www.uptodateonline.com/utd/content/topic.do?topicKey=hep_dis/14684&selectedTitle=14~1128.
11. Gentilini P, Laffi G, La Villa G, and others: Long course and prognostic factors of virus induced cirrhosis of the liver, *Am J Gastroenterol* 92(1):66-72, 1997.
12. Clark JF, Queener SF, Karb VB: *Pharmacologic basis of nursing practice,* ed 5, St Louis, 1997, Mosby.
13. Chowdhury NR, Chowdhury JR: *Diagnostic approach to the patient with jaundice or asymptomatic hyperbilirubinemia,* retrieved Jan 29, 2007, from http://www.uptodateonline.com/utd/content/topic.do?topicKey=hep_dis/8241&selectedTitle=1~1128.
14. Oran NT, Oran I, Memis A: Management of patients with malignant obstructive jaundice, *Cancer Nursing* 23(2):128-133, 2000.

CHAPTER 148

Nausea and Vomiting

Terry Davies

DEFINITION AND EPIDEMIOLOGY

Nausea, vomiting, and diarrhea account for more than 2 million office visits and 220,000 hospitalizations each year.[1] Causes of nausea and vomiting are varied and present a challenge to health care providers. Not only do the symptoms need to be controlled to provide patient comfort and prevent complications, but the underlying cause must be diagnosed to provide proper treatment.

Nausea is defined as an unpleasant or queasy sensation of being about to vomit. Vomiting may or may not occur. Vomiting is the expulsion of liquid or food from the stomach. It should be differentiated from retching (rhythmic contractions of the respiratory and abdominal muscles) and regurgitation (backward flow of food and liquids from the stomach to the mouth).[2,3]

Physician consultation is indicated if nausea and vomiting are accompanied by pain, dehydration, acute abdomen, fever, neurologic changes, or a metabolic imbalance.

PATHOPHYSIOLOGY

Vomiting is induced through stimulation of either the vomiting center (VC) or the chemoreceptor trigger zone (CTZ) of the central nervous system. Stimulation of the VC occurs through afferent vagal and sympathetic visceral pathways from delayed gastric emptying, distention, drugs, emotions, or ischemia. Irritation of the CTZ can occur with metabolic disorders, rapid changes in motion, or medications.

CLINICAL PRESENTATION

The presentation of nausea and vomiting varies from the gradual onset of symptoms noted with medication side effects, gastric retention, or early pregnancy to the acute episodes caused by viral gastroenteritis, food poisoning, increased intracranial pressure, or an acute abdominal emergency. Associated symptoms can include pain, headache, dizziness, tinnitus, diarrhea, fever, mental status changes, anxiety, and other symptoms associated with pregnancy. A thorough history should include the onset, duration, and severity of symptoms; associated symptoms; current medications; a history of medical problems (e.g., cancer, diabetes, irritable bowel syndrome); surgical history; and environmental exposures or therapies, including radiation or chemotherapy. The relationship of nausea and vomiting to food, the force of vomiting (projectile vs. retching), and the quality of the emesis (bile, undigested food) should be assessed. A 24-hour dietary review, with bowel symptoms (diarrhea vs. constipation) and the time of the last void, should also be determined.

Acute episodes of nausea and vomiting may be associated with viral gastroenteritis, food poisoning, or medication overdose. Acute emergencies such as acute pancreatitis, appendicitis, bowel obstruction, peritonitis, or cholecystitis may be accompanied by fever or pain. These symptoms also occur in acute episodes of Crohn's disease, colitis, and diverticulitis. Chronic or recurrent nausea and vomiting may be psychogenic or the result of radiation or chemotherapy, gastric disorders, migraine headaches, diabetic gastroparesis, or a metabolic or endocrine abnormality.

PHYSICAL EXAMINATION

A thorough examination should include weight, temperature, and orthostatic vital signs to assess volume status. The skin should be assessed for turgor, color, moisture, or rashes; the head and neck should be assessed for evidence of dehydration, acute infection, lymphadenopathy, rigidity, or thyromegaly. A cardiovascular examination is necessary to determine the patient's response to the illness or other signs of infection; abdominal and rectal examinations are crucial to assess for distention, peristalsis, tenderness, rigidity, rebound, masses, fecal impaction, and bleeding. Mental status, gait, and cranial nerve function are also essential components of the evaluation, particularly if increased intracranial pressure is suspected.

DIAGNOSTICS

The presentation of nausea and vomiting, as well as the physical findings, will guide testing. Laboratory tests may include urine for specific gravity, erythrocyte sedimentation rate, serum glucose, electrolytes, ketones, BUN, creatinine, amylase, liver function tests, and drug levels (if indicated). A serum human chorionic gonadotropin level should be obtained in women of childbearing age. Urinalysis with culture and sensitivity, CBC, thyroid-stimulating hormone, or further endocrine studies may be indicated in some cases.

DIAGNOSTICS

Nausea and Vomiting

LABORATORY
Urinalysis*
Serum electrolytes*
Serum glucose*
BUN*
Creatinine*
Serum ketones*
Amylase*
LFTs*
Drug levels*
Human chorionic gonadotropin*
CBC and differential*

IMAGING
Abdominal x-rays*
Ultrasound*
Barium swallow*
Endoscopic examination*
Head CT scan*

OTHER
EGG*

*If indicated.

Abdominal upright and plain x-ray films are necessary if an obstruction is suspected. An ultrasound, barium swallow, CT scan, or endoscopic examination may be indicated for masses, dysphagia, or suspected gastrointestinal bleeding or ulceration. If a cerebral hemorrhage or mass is suspected, a head CT scan should be ordered after physician consultation. An ECG is indicated if myocardial infarction is considered to be the cause of the nausea and vomiting.

DIFFERENTIAL DIAGNOSIS

Nausea and vomiting may be caused by an acute or chronic process. Differentiation of the cause will assist in treatment of the underlying disease and in patient education efforts.

MANAGEMENT

Management of nausea and vomiting involves correction of the underlying cause, control of symptoms, and prevention of complications. The possibility of intestinal obstruction or acute abdomen should be eliminated before initiating other treatment options. Uncomplicated viral gastroenteritis (without metabolic imbalance or dehydration) can be managed with increased fluid intake and diet restrictions. A clear liquid diet should be followed for 24 hours, followed by 24 hours of the BRAT (banana, rice, applesauce, and toast) diet. This regimen will provide the bowels sufficient rest. A bland diet is necessary the following week. Control of vomiting is important for patient comfort and prevention of complications. The use of antiemetics and/or IV hydration may be indicated. Antiemetic medications should be selected on the basis of the patient's medical history and the suspected cause of the nausea and vomiting (Box 148-1). Adequate fluid intake must be maintained to prevent dehydration, especially if the illness is prolonged or severe. Intake should exceed output by at least 500 ml in a 24-hour period. Assessment for hydration status should include postural vital signs along with the patient's ability to void every 2 to 3 hours. Oral hydration should be attempted in the office if the patient has postural hypotension and is able to tolerate fluid intake. If the patient is too nauseated or does not respond to oral fluid intake, IV hydration should be started. In general, 1 to 2 L of IV normal saline or lactated Ringer's solution over a few hours is well tolerated. Slower rates are recommended for older adults or patients who are debilitated. Physician consultation is recommended if postural hypotension is not corrected or if metabolic alkalosis or severe dehydration is present.

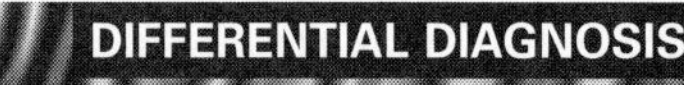

Nausea and Vomiting

ACUTE
- Acute abdomen (appendicitis, ischemic bowel, peritonitis, abdominal aortic aneurysm, volvulus)
- Acute labyrinthitis, Meniere's disease
- Cholecystitis
- Constipation
- Increased intracranial pressure
- Infection (viral, bacterial, or parasitic)
- Intestinal obstruction
- Medication (chemotherapy, toxic level of some medications, anesthesia, or side effect of medications)
- Metabolic disturbances (diabetic ketoacidosis, adrenal crisis)
- Migraine headache
- Motion sickness
- Myocardial infarction
- Pain
- Pregnancy
- Uremia

CHRONIC
- Achalasia
- Anorexia nervosa or bulimia
- Cancer
- Cirrhosis
- Crohn's disease
- Diabetic gastroparesis
- Diverticular disease
- Drug or alcohol use or withdrawal
- Hepatitis
- Irritable bowel syndrome
- Pancreatitis
- Peptic ulcer disease
- Psychogenic

Antiemetic medications are administered to treat or prevent nausea and vomiting. These medications can be given alone of in combination with other agents. Presently, the 5-hydroxytryptamine$_3$ (5-HT$_3$ [serotonin]) receptor antagonists are the cornerstone of antiemetic therapy and are used to treat postoperative emesis and chemotherapy-induced emesis (see Box 148-1).

A combination of a corticosteroid (dexamethasone 4 mg IV) and a dopamine antagonist (droperidol 1.25 mg IV) is highly effective for postoperative patients who received anesthesia and are experiencing nausea and vomiting.[4] Ondansetron (Zofran) 4 mg IV is also used successfully for controlling postoperative nausea and vomiting, but the combination therapy is less expensive than ondansetron.[2,3] In the past, butyrophenones (see Box 148-1) were also used before anesthesia and for postoperative nausea and vomiting, but they are rarely used now.[5]

The phenothiazines were initially used to prevent chemotherapy-induced emesis. The 5-HT$_3$ receptor antagonists are also used for the prevention of nausea and vomiting associated with chemotherapy (see Box 148-1). These agents used in combination with corticosteroids offer the greatest antiemetic treatment.[2,3] For the refractory nausea and vomiting associated with chemotherapy, the cannabinoids may be useful.

For the prevention of motion sickness, vertigo, and migraines, antihistamines and anticholinergics are excellent choices (see Box 148-1). These include diphenhydramine (Benadryl), meclizine (Antivert), dimenhydrinate (Dramamine), transdermal scopolamine, promethazine (Phenergan), and cyclizine (Marezine).[5] Acute labyrinthitis responds to a methylprednisolone tapered over 22 days.[2]

COMPLICATIONS

Complications of nausea and vomiting may be associated with the underlying condition. However, dehydration, hypokalemia, and metabolic acidosis are a concern. Although uncommon in

BOX 148-1

ANTIEMETIC MEDICATIONS

FOR GENERALIZED NAUSEA AND VOMITING

Bismuth Subsalicylate

For nausea with or without diarrhea

- **Pepto-Bismol:** 30 ml PO q 30-60 min; maximum 8 doses in 24 hours; available over the counter

Benzamides

Metoclopramide hydrochloride

For nausea related to diabetic gastroparesis: 10 mg PO 30 minutes before meals and at bedtime for 2-8 weeks, depending on response

For gastroesophageal reflux: 10-15 mg PO q.i.d. p.r.n. 30 minutes before meals and at bedtime; do not use for more than 12 weeks

For nausea and vomiting associated with chemotherapy: 1-2 mg/kg IV slowly over 1-2 minutes or infused over 15 minutes after diluting in 50 ml of D_5W, D5 1/2NS, normal saline, Ringer's solution, or lactated Ringer's solution; give first dose 30 minutes before chemotherapy, then q 2 hr p.r.n.; do not exceed 5 doses/day; may produce dystonic reaction when given IV; premedicate with diphenhydramine

Phenothiazines

Prochlorperazine (Compazine)

For severe nausea and vomiting: 5-10 mg PO t.i.d. or q.i.d., 5-10 mg IM q 3-4 hr p.r.n. (maximum 40 mg/day), or 25 mg rectal suppository q 12 hr p.r.n.; may give 2.5-10 mg IV at a rate not to exceed 5 mg/min; give IM injections in the upper outer quadrant of the gluteal muscle; use this drug when only a few doses are required for treatment

Promethazine hydrochloride (Phenergan)

For nausea: 12.5-25 mg PO, IM, or rectally q 4-6 hr p.r.n.; use cautiously in ambulatory patients because of possible pronounced sedative effects.

Trimethobenzamide hydrochloride (Tigan)

For mild to moderate nausea and vomiting: 250 mg PO t.i.d. or q.i.d., 200 mg IM t.i.d. or q.i.d., or 200 mg rectal suppository t.i.d. or q.i.d.; give IM injections in the upper outer quadrant of the gluteal muscle; for short-term treatment

FOR NAUSEA AND VOMITING ASSOCIATED WITH CHEMOTHERAPY

5-HT (Serotonin) Receptor Antagonists (also used for postoperative emesis)

For prevention of postoperative and chemotherapy-induced emesis

- Dolasetron (Anzemet): 100 mg or 1.8 mg/kg once daily IV, or 8 mg once daily PO
- Granisetron (Kytril): 1 mg or 0.01 mg/kg once daily IV, or 2 mg once daily PO
- Ondansetron (Zofran): 8 mg or 0.15 mg/kg once daily IV, or 8 mg t.i.d. PO
- Palonosetron (Aloxi): 0.25 mg IV

Dopamine Receptor Antagonists

Phenothiazines

For prevention of chemotherapy-induced events

- Prochlorperazine (Compazine): 5-10 mg PO q 6-8 hr, 5-10 mg IM, 2.5-10 mg IV q 3-4 hr, or 25 mg suppository q 12 hr
- Chlorpromazine (Thorazine): 10-25 mg PO q 4-6 hr, 25 mg IV q 3-4 hr, or 100 mg suppository q 6-8 hr

Butyrophenones

For nausea

- Droperidol (Inapsine): 1.25-5 mg IM

Benzamides

For nausea caused by cytotoxic drugs

- Metoclopramide (Reglan): 10-30 mg or 0.5 mg/kg IV q 6-8 hr or 10-20 mg PO q 6-8 hr
- Trimethobenzamide (Tigan): 250 mg PO q 6-8 hr or 200 mg IM or suppository q 6-8 hr

Cannabinoids

For chemotherapy-induced nausea and vomiting

- Dronabinol (Marinol): 5 mg/m^2 PO 1-3 hours before chemotherapy; repeated q 2-4 hr p.r.n. to maximum 6 doses daily[6]

Substance P/Neurokinin$_1$ Antagonists

For acute and delayed nausea and vomiting associated with chemotherapy

- Aprepitant (Emend): 125 mg PO 1 hour before chemotherapy, then 80 mg a day for 2 days. May be given with other agents (e.g., steroids, Zofran)

Benzodiazepines

For adjunct therapy to decrease anxiety and anticipatory emesis

- Alprazolam (Xanax): 0.5-1 mg once daily PO up to 3-6 mg/day
- Diazepam (Valium): 2-5 mg PO or IV q 4-6 hr
- Lorazepam (Ativan): 1-2 mg PO or IV q 4-6 hr

Antihistamines and Anticholinergic Agents

For motion sickness, vertigo, and migraines

- Diphenhydramine (Benadryl): 25-50 mg PO q 6 hr or 10-50 mg IV or IM
- Dimenhydrinate (Dramamine): 50 mg PO q 4 hr
- Cyclizine (Marezine): 50 mg PO or IM q 4 hr or 100 mg suppository q 4 hr
- Meclizine (Antivert): 25-50 mg PO q 24 hr
- Promethazine (Phenergan): 12.5-25 mg PO or IM q 4 hr or 12.5-25 mg rectally q 12 hr
- Transdermal scopolamine (Transderm-Scop): 1 patch 4 hr before travel, remove after 72 hours; postoperative, apply 1 patch the evening before surgery, remove 24 hours after surgery.
- Dolasetron is not indicated for adolescents or children and should not be used for the treatment of postoperative nausea/vomiting in adults.

alert patients, aspiration pneumonitis is a possibility in patients with decreased levels of consciousness. Continual vomiting may result in malnutrition and dental erosion. Forceful vomiting has been the cause of Mallory-Weiss syndrome and esophageal ruptures.

INDICATIONS FOR REFERRAL OR HOSPITALIZATION

Nausea and vomiting accompanied by pain, dehydration, acute abdomen, neurologic changes, or a metabolic imbalance may require hospitalization, and the primary physician should be consulted. Hospitalization may also be indicated if the patient is unable to maintain hydration status at home. Referral to an appropriate specialist may be necessary if the nausea or vomiting is not controlled by supportive measures such as hydration, diet change, and antiemetics; if the patient's condition worsens or does not respond to treatment; or if a psychologic component is present.

Metabolic disturbances, pregnancy, altered medication, and drug or alcohol levels should be managed in consultation with the primary physician. Consultation is required for emergencies such as acute myocardial infarction or for patients with neurologic changes. Prolonged or recurrent nausea or vomiting may indicate gastric paresis, irritable bowel, or pancreatitis and requires consultation with a gastroenterologist or appropriate specialist.

PATIENT AND FAMILY EDUCATION

Patients should be educated about adequate fluid intake, with special attention given to the types of fluid ingested. Oral rehydration solutions and broths are especially helpful in maintaining electrolyte balance. Dairy products and carbonated fluids should be avoided. A minimum of 96 to 120 ounces of fluid should be consumed each hour. An oral rehydration solution may be prepared by mixing 1 cup of orange juice, ¾ teaspoon salt, 1 teaspoon baking soda, 4 tablespoons of sugar, and 1 L of water.

Because dehydration can occur easily and cause persistent vomiting, patients should be instructed to notify their health care provider if:

- Vomiting persists despite antiemetic use.
- Vomiting is accompanied by fever, severe abdominal pain, severe headache, neck pain, or lethargy.
- Urinary output becomes dark, or the patient does not void at least every 2 hours during the day.
- Dizziness or lightheadedness occurs with or without position change.
- Patient is vomiting blood or fluid that has the appearance of coffee grounds.

HEALTH PROMOTION

Patients should be instructed in the proper handling and storage of food products to prevent contamination and possible food poisoning. Patients traveling abroad should receive the necessary vaccinations and treatments appropriate for the country visited. Guidelines are available from the Centers for Disease Control and Prevention or through local travel clinics.

REFERENCES

1. Hasker WL, Chey WD: Nausea and vomiting, *Gastroenterology* 125(6):1860-1867, 2003.
2. Longstreth GF: *Approach to the adult patient with nausea and vomiting*, 2006, retrieved Jan 20, 2007, from http://www.uptodateonline.com/utd/content/topic.do?topicKey=gi_dis/12029&selectedTitle=1~3485.
3. McQuaid KR: Alimentary tract. In Tierney LM, McPhee SJ, Papadakis MA, editors: *Current medical diagnosis and treatment*, New York, 2006, McGraw-Hill/Appleton & Lange.
4. Tramer MR: Treatment of postoperative nausea and vomiting, *BMJ* 327:762, 2003.
5. Longstreth GF, Hesketh PJ: *Characteristics of antiemetic drugs*, retrieved Jan 20, 2007, from http://www.uptodateonline.com/utd/content/topic.do?topicKey=gi_dis/12256&selectedTitle=5~3485.
6. Lehne RA: Other gastrointestinal drugs. In Lehne R, editor: *Pharmacology for patient care*, ed 6, St Louis, 2007, Saunders.

CHAPTER 149

Oropharyngeal Dysphagia

Talli McCormick

DEFINITION AND EPIDEMIOLOGY

Oropharyngeal dysphagia is a swallowing disorder that involves dysfunction of one or more stages in the normal sequence of swallowing. This type of dysphagia differs from upper gastrointestinal disorders in that the dysfunction involves oral, pharyngeal, and laryngeal structures. The dysphagia may be mild or severe, resulting in malnutrition, dehydration, choking, aspiration, pneumonia, and even death. Estimates of incidence in the community vary, but in nursing homes a significant number of residents may have feeding difficulties. Patients with aspiration are thought to have a 1-year mortality rate of 45%.[1]

PATHOPHYSIOLOGY

Dysphagia may be either oropharyngeal or esophageal. The etiology can be neurologic, neuromuscular, metabolic, pharmacologic, infectious, psychiatric, environmental, or structural. Identification of the causative agent or disease is paramount in the assessment and treatment of dysphagia. Structural causes are more common in esophageal dysphagia, and functional causes are more likely in oropharyngeal dysphagia (Box 149-1). Structural causes include trauma or surgery, tumor, webs, strictures or stenoses, diverticuli, infection, and, in some cases, cervical osteophytes or cricopharyngeal bars.[2]

To more fully understand dysphagia, it is essential to appreciate the anatomy and physiology of normal swallowing. Swallowing has three commonly described phases: oral, pharyngeal, and esophageal. In addition to these three phases, there are preparatory phases to the act of eating. Most of us decide when we are hungry and what we would like to eat. We prepare it or go to a restaurant. We decide with whom we will eat. These decisions involve autonomy, fairly intact cognition, and neuromuscular function. Nursing home residents and homebound older adults may have significant limitations or restrictions in this preparatory phase.[3]

During the oral phase, a multitude of sensory information is gathered about the food and the involved structures. Quantity, shape, consistency, and moisture content are determined, along with the temperature, taste, and location of the food. The touch and pressure exerted on the oral structures, especially the tongue and hard and soft palates, are transmitted to the brainstem for further action and distribution. This continuous assessment by the sensory system allows for precise communication with the muscles of mastication.

Chewing (mastication) involves cranial nerves (CNs) V (trigeminal), VII (facial), IX (glossopharyngeal), and XII (hypoglossal), in addition to the muscles of the jaw, cheeks, tongue, and palate. The lips remain closed during chewing, while the tongue and teeth prepare the food into a bolus of the

BOX 149-1

POTENTIAL CAUSES OF OROPHARYNGEAL DYSPHAGIA

IATROGENIC
- Medication side effects (e.g., xerostomia, chemotherapy, neuroleptics)
- Postsurgical muscular or neurogenic
- Radiation
- Corrosive (pill injury, intentional)

INFECTIOUS
- Diphtheria
- Botulism
- Lyme's disease
- Syphilis
- Mucositis (herpes, cytomegalovirus, Candida organisms, etc.)

METABOLIC
- Amyloidosis
- Cushing's syndrome
- Thyrotoxicosis
- Wilson's disease

MYOPATHIC
- Connective tissue disease
- Myasthenia gravis
- Myotonic dystrophy
- Oculopharyngeal dystrophy
- Polymyositis
- Sarcoidosis
- Paraneoplastic syndromes

NEUROLOGIC
- Brainstem tumors
- Head trauma
- Stroke
- Cerebral palsy
- Guillain-Barré syndrome
- Huntington's disease
- Multiple sclerosis
- Polio
- Postpolio syndrome
- Tardive dyskinesia
- Amyotrophic lateral sclerosis
- Parkinson's disease
- Dementia

STRUCTURAL
- Cricopharyngeal bar
- Zenker's diverticulum
- Cervical webs
- Oropharyngeal tumors
- Osteophytes and skeletal abnormalities
- Congenital (cleft palate, diverticula, pouches)

PSYCHIATRIC
- Grief
- Depression
- Globus

ENVIRONMENTAL
- Poor positioning
- Eating or being fed too quickly
- Eating or being fed too large a bolus
- Inappropriate consistency
- Poor oral health or hygiene
- Distractibility

Modified from Cook IJ, Kahrilal PJ: A technical review on management of oropharyngeal dysphagia, *Gastroenterology* 116(2):455-478, 1999; and Blackington E, McCormick T, Willson B, and others: Oropharyngeal dysphagia in the elderly, *Adv Nurse Pract* 9(7):45, 2001.

proper size and consistency. The soft palate descends to help hold the food within the mouth during chewing. The teeth close, the tongue places the bolus in its central groove, and the bolus is then rapidly pushed, or transferred, through the pillars (fauces) into the pharynx.

At this point, the bolus passes a ring of sensory receptors at the base of the tongue, pillars, soft palate, and posterior pharyngeal wall. The transmission of a sensory impulse indicating the presence of a bolus is sent via CN IX to the swallowing center in the brainstem, which then initiates the involuntary phase of the swallow.[3,4] Sensory input is also crucial to the pharyngeal stage. As the tongue pushes the bolus to the posterior pharynx, the soft palate flattens upward and backward (CN V), sealing off the nasopharynx. Simultaneously, the hyoid and larynx begin to move upward (CN X [vagus]), tipping back the epiglottis. The pillars lower, and the tongue presses against the posterior pharyngeal wall (CN IX) to block retrograde movement of the bolus into the oral cavity. Sensory fibers of CN X transmit information to the swallowing center in the brainstem. The impulse returns via the motor component of the vagus nerve and initiates peristalsis of the pharyngeal constrictors to propel the bolus toward the esophagus, passing the valleculae and piriform sinuses. The soft palate descends, the larynx continues to rise, and the epiglottis descends. As the epiglottis descends to block the laryngeal opening, the upper esophageal sphincter (UES) or cricopharyngeal sphincter opens to allow the bolus to pass into the esophagus.[3,4]

As the food bolus enters the esophagus, these processes begin in reverse. Once in the esophagus, the UES closes and peristalsis and gravity propel the bolus toward the stomach. The lower esophageal sphincter (LES) opens and the bolus enters the stomach. Normal transit time varies depending on bolus consistency but is generally 2 to 4 seconds.[3,4]

CLINICAL PRESENTATION

Dysphagic patients can be initially seen with malnutrition, weight loss, dehydration, or pneumonia. Problems in the oral stage include poor bolus control, spillage either from the lips or into the pharynx, dry oral membranes, pocketing or oral residue, and difficulty with chewing. Pharyngeal dysphagia often results from weakness or poor coordination of the pharyngeal muscles. This can cause delayed swallow, failure of airway protection, nasal or oral regurgitation, or residue remaining in the pharynx after swallow, manifested as coughing, choking, or gurgling.

Xerostomia (dry mouth), either intrinsic or extrinsic, can be a contributing factor in dysphagia. Globus, which is the sensation of a lump in the throat, can occur alone or co-exist with esophageal dysphagia, particularly when accompanied by chest pain or heartburn.[5] Globus alone is merely a sensory experience; swallowing itself is unimpaired.

A detailed history is the most important step in differential diagnosis. Because dysphagia can be associated with neurologic disease, a thorough neuromuscular history is also important. Obtaining an accurate history can be complicated by reduced alertness and cognitive and speech impairments, which can also affect the patient's ability to participate in examination, diagnostics, and treatment strategies.

Onset, progression, location, duration, and food consistency aid in diagnosis. A short duration associated with weight loss can indicate malignancy.[2] Abrupt onset associated with neurologic impairment suggests a cerebrovascular accident. Studies have estimated that one third to one half of new stroke patients will have dysphagia, and in 10% to 15% of these, the dysphagia will persist beyond 1 month. Swallowing thin liquids is often a problem after a stroke. Gradual progressive onset is more likely to be associated with Parkinson's disease, amyotrophic lateral sclerosis, sarcoidosis, myasthenia gravis, Alzheimer's disease, or other chronic diseases. Parkinson's disease is the most common movement disorder in older adults and leads to tongue rigidity and tremor, making bolus formation and transfer into the pharynx difficult. Difficulty swallowing only solids suggests a structural cause but not necessarily the location of the impairment. Ability to point to where the food "sticks" is useful for oropharyngeal obstructions and correlates well with radiographic studies.

Eating or being fed too rapidly may result in either oral or nasal regurgitation and choking. Coughing up food after meals can indicate a pharyngeal diverticulum.[2] Frequent swallowing can indicate oral or pharyngeal residue. Patient positioning, degree of distraction, companions or assistants, utensils used, food consistency, and likes and dislikes can all provide information useful not only in differential diagnosis but also in deciding on treatment strategies.

A complete review of all medications is necessary because some medications can cause or contribute to swallowing dysfunction, whereas others, such as alendronate sodium (Fosamax), NSAIDs, and potassium, can cause direct damage to the esophageal mucosa (Box 149-2). Xerostomia, altered esophageal sphincter pressure, and reduced alertness are other medication side effects that can affect swallowing.[1,3]

BOX 149-2

MEDICATION-RELATED CONDITIONS THAT CAUSE OROPHARYNGEAL DYSPHAGIA

XEROSTOMIA
- Antidepressants
- Antispasmodics
- Antihypertensives
- Anticholinergics
- Antihistamines
- Bronchodilators
- Sedatives

CENTRAL NERVOUS SYSTEM DEPRESSION
- Anticonvulsants
- Antianxiety agents (alprazolam, diazepam, chlordiazepoxide)
- Antispasmodics (dantrolene, baclofen)
- Antidepressants (trazodone, amitriptyline, desipramine)
- Neuroleptics (haloperidol, chlorpromazine, thioridazine)
- Sedatives

IMMUNOSUPPRESSION
- Antibiotics
- Cytotoxic agents

INCREASED SALIVATION
- Anticholinesterase
- Clonazepam
- Clozapine

NEUROMUSCULAR JUNCTION BLOCKADE
- Aminoglycoside antibiotics
- Botulinum toxin (Botox)

MYOPATHY
- Corticosteroids
- Lipid-lowering agents
- Colchicine
- L-Tryptophan

MUCOSAL INJURY
- Alendronate (Fosamax)
- Tetracycline
- NSAIDs
- Potassium
- Ferrous sulfate

LOWER ESOPHAGEAL SPHINCTER PRESSURE
- Theophylline
- Nitrates
- Calcium channel blockers
- Beta blockers
- Hormone replacement therapy
- Anticholinergics

PHYSICAL EXAMINATION

A thorough physical examination aids in the differential diagnosis, establishes the existence of deficits and impairments, and determines whether malnutrition or pneumonia is present.[2] A complete oral examination will reveal oral health and hygiene, including dentition, oral sensation, tongue strength, mobility, coordination, and specific CN function. Altered speech or voice, particularly nasal speech or a gurgling voice, should be noted. Nasal speech can indicate soft palate dysfunction, whereas a gurgling or wet voice is more indicative of weak pharyngeal constrictors. The presence or absence of the gag reflex is not predictive of swallowing dysfunction or risk of aspiration because the gag reflex may be absent in 20% to 40% of healthy adults.[6-8] Trial sips of water or spoonfuls of applesauce or pudding can reveal specific deficits. Observation and palpation of laryngeal elevation can detect delayed swallowing. The pharyngeal swallow should occur within approximately 1 second.

The complete neuromuscular examination includes CN function (particularly V, VII, IX, X, and XII) and assessment of muscle strength or weakness, muscle atrophy, or altered coordination. Involuntary movements, tremor, or gait disturbance should also be determined. A mental status assessment with particular emphasis on level of alertness and ability to concentrate and cooperate is important. Deformities of or past operations on the head, neck, or trunk may affect dysphagia or the ability to participate in diagnostic studies. Despite skillful and comprehensive physical examination, the risk for aspiration may not be fully appreciated without the use of radiographic study.[9]

DIAGNOSTICS

Videofluoroscopy, or modified barium swallow (MBS), is the most appropriate and commonly used imaging procedure. The primary purpose of the MBS is to determine if and to what degree aspiration occurs. Patients must be able to sit upright, hold still, and follow commands during the examination. Using contrast material, this radiographic study is designed to assess functional impairment of swallowing in four categories: delay in swallowing initiation, nasopharyngeal regurgitation, aspiration, and pharyngeal residue. Usually a variety of consistencies and bolus volumes are assessed during the MBS.

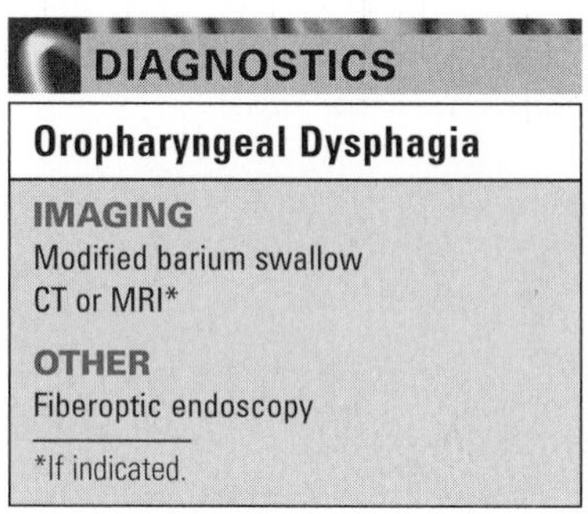
DIAGNOSTICS

Oropharyngeal Dysphagia

IMAGING
Modified barium swallow
CT or MRI*

OTHER
Fiberoptic endoscopy

*If indicated.

This study not only aids in diagnosis but also helps determine the effectiveness of various positions, consistencies, or maneuvers used in treatment.

If a structural, rather than functional, cause is suspected, nasoendoscopy should be considered. Nasoendoscopy permits direct visualization of the oral cavity, nasopharynx, pharynx, and larynx. Lesion biopsy samples can be obtained during the procedure.

If muscle weakness or problems with sphincter relaxation are suspected, manometry can measure intraluminal pressures during the swallow. Manometry can be synchronized with videofluoroscopy (manofluorography) to distinguish more subtle findings.[10]

The fiberoptic endoscopic examination of swallowing, ultrasound, electromyography, and electroglottography are other diagnostic procedures that can be appropriate, although these tests are more limited. CT or MRI of the head and neck can aid in diagnosis but does not describe the actual swallow mechanism.

DIFFERENTIAL DIAGNOSIS

See the Differential Diagnosis box, p. 711.

MANAGEMENT

Structural causes of dysphagia such as tumors, strictures, webs, or diverticuli are usually treated with surgery or dilation. Chemotherapy and/or radiation may be used for tumors. No randomized controlled trials have been conducted, but a number of case series indicate that webs and strictures are amenable to dilation. Cricopharyngeal myotomy is the most common surgical treatment for oropharyngeal dysphagia of structural origin, and consistent evidence of its benefit is available.[11,12]

Studies exploring the use of myotomy for dysphagia of neurogenic origin are very different. Data conflict and are often methodologically weak and sometimes qualitative. Nonetheless, myotomy may offer benefit to 50% of patients with neurogenic dysphagia.[2] It is suggested that patients who benefit may be those with a higher preoperative hypopharyngeal intrabolus pressure related to resistance of flow across the UES.[12] In patients with problems with coordination of UES or cricopharyngeal muscle and the pharynx, some improvement in swallowing has been shown with botulinum toxin (Botox) injections into the UES.[13-15] and with cricopharyngeal myotomy.[16,17] Other structural radiographic abnormalities exist, but their impact on swallowing is unclear.

The relationship of pharyngeal sensation, silent aspiration, and cough reflex was explored in a small Japanese study. Ebihara, Takahaski, Ebihara, and colleagues used a capsaicin troche at mealtimes with patients, with an improvement in latent swallowing time.[18] Oral nifedipine has also been used to improve swallowing in patients with Parkinson's disease.[19]

There is some support for the idea that the respiratory system may have a role in optimum swallowing. Gross, Atwood, Grayhack, and colleagues found that pharyngeal swallowing time was longer in subjects with residual lung volume than in persons with total lung capacity or functional residual capacity.[20] This implies a possible regulatory role of subglottic air pressure in optimum swallowing.

Intensive oral care and hygiene have been considered as a means of reducing pathogen load in aspirators, but Watando, Ebihara, Ebihara, and colleagues suggest oral care may have a role in improving cough sensitivity as well.[21]

Aspiration and Nonoral Feeding in Dysphagia of Functional Origin

Standard practice has been that patients found to have severe aspiration not treatable with dietary or positional modifications should receive nonoral feeding to prevent aspiration. It is clear that aspiration is evidence of severe swallowing dysfunction and that death is associated with aspiration pneumonia.[1,2] However, the relationship between aspiration and the risk of developing pneumonia is not as obvious. Smithard, O'Neill, Park, and others found that dysphagic stroke patients were at significant risk for chest infections, malnutrition, and death, but aspiration did not predict this risk.[22] Similarly, Johnson, McKenzie, and Sievers discovered that 29 of 60 dysphagic stroke patients developed pneumonia within 1 year.[23] However, this was not correlated with aspiration or pharyngeal pooling on videofluoroscopy. A recent study by Terpenning, Taylor, Lopatin, and others suggests an increased risk of aspiration pneumonia in patients who have chronic obstructive pulmonary disease or diabetes mellitus or who require assistance with feeding.[24] Aspiration pneumonia was also more common in subjects with oral *Porphyromonas gingivalis*, decayed teeth, and visible dental plaque. Although these authors hypothesized that poor healing associated with diabetes and poor pulmonary clearance could contribute to the development of pneumonia, they did not find an association with stroke.[24] Langmore, Terpenning, Schork, and others propose that patients with compromised functional capacity may be fed too quickly or with too large a bolus.[25] Croghan, Burke, Caplan, and others found that the 15 of 22 dysphagic patients who received feeding tubes were at a significantly higher risk of pneumonia and death than were the seven patients who did not receive them.[1] In summary, it appears that aspiration probably contributes to the risk of pneumonia but may not be the only important contributor; nonoral feeding

DIFFERENTIAL DIAGNOSIS

Oropharyngeal Dysphagia

MECHANICAL PROBLEMS

Acute inflammations
- Herpes simplex
- Tonsillitis, epiglottitis, pharyngitis, esophagitis
- Infectious and inflammatory bone and mucosal disorders

Chemical agents (aspirin, lozenges, gargles, alcohol)
Medications (see Box 149-2)
Skeletal anomalies
Muscle anomalies
Macroglossia
Pharyngoesophageal diverticulum
Carcinoma
Surgery
- Oral, palatal resections
- Glossectomy
- Supralaryngectomy; partial, total laryngectomy
- Tracheoesophageal puncture
- Chest surgery (coronary artery bypass graft)
- Endarterectomy
- Anterior cervical spine surgery

Irradiation
Cervical spine disease
Nasoenteric tubes
Tracheostoma tubes
Esophageal stenosis, webs, rings, stricture

NEUROGENIC PROBLEMS

Riley-Day syndrome
Acquired central nervous system disorders
- Stroke syndromes and vascular disorders
- Capsular infarct
- Pseudobulbar palsy
- Apraxias and agnosias
- Lacunar disease

Movement disorders
- Parkinson's disease
- Dystonias and dyskinesias
- Huntington's disease
- Palatal myoclonus

Poliomyelitis and other systemic infections
- Diphtheria
- Botulism
- Rabies
- Tetanus

Amyotrophic lateral sclerosis
Acquired peripheral nervous system disorders
Recurrent laryngeal neuropathies
Cranial nerve neuropathies
- Guillain-Barré syndrome
- Diabetes
- Leukemia
- Lymphoma
- Carcinoma
- Other neuropathies

Neurodevelopmental disorders
- Cerebral palsy
- Abnormal oral and pharyngeal reflexes
- Abnormal salivation
- Others

MYOGENIC PROBLEMS

Myasthenia gravis
Neuromuscular esophageal disorders
- Scleroderma
- Achalasia
- Diffuse spasm
- Others

OTHER CONDITIONS

Dementias
Multiple sclerosis
Tuberculosis
Syphilis
Neoplasms
Degenerative disorders
Psychopathology
Feeding phobias
Atypical parent-child interactions
Sensory deficits

may not reduce this risk in all patients, and in some patients it may increase this risk.

The goal of differential diagnosis is identification of the disease process causing the dysphagia, if present. For example, although there is little evidence that antiparkinsonian medications improve swallowing function in the long term, Thomas and Haigh offer case reports of a good response to antiparkinsonian medication.[26]

Swallowing Strategies and Therapies

Head positioning, swallowing maneuvers, and dietary textural modifications seem to demonstrate the clearest evidence of benefit in the treatment of functional dysphagia.[2] Table 149-1 provides data on swallowing therapy techniques, indications, and rationale. Many therapeutic measures require autonomy and fairly intact cognitive function for memory and learning. For patients with certain strokes, Alzheimer's disease, and some other neurologic diseases, this requirement may limit the usefulness of these techniques. Dietary modifications may be the best choice for many of these patients.

COMPLICATIONS

Complications associated with dysphagia include impaired quality of life, coughing, choking, aspiration, malnutrition, dehydration, pneumonia, and death. Gastrostomy tube placement may be necessary and appropriate for some patients.

INDICATIONS FOR REFERRAL OR HOSPITALIZATION

Dysphagic patients and/or their families should be offered dietary consultation. Other referrals will be dictated by the cause of the dysphagia. A gastroenterologist should be consulted for a suspected gastroesophageal problem. Structural abnormalities may require surgical intervention.

Moderate to severe cases of oropharyngeal dysphagia require referral to a speech therapist, particularly if therapeutic swallowing techniques are needed. Referral to a neurologist

TABLE 149-1 Swallowing Therapy Techniques, Rationales, and Indications

Technique	Execution (Rationale)	Indication
DIETARY MODIFICATION		
Thickened liquids	Reduced tendency to spill over tongue base	Disordered tongue function Preswallow spill or aspiration Impaired laryngeal closure
Thin liquids	Offers less resistance to flow	Weak pharyngeal contraction Reduced cricopharyngeal opening
MANEUVERS		
Supraglottic swallow	Breath hold, double swallow, forceful expiration (closes vocal folds before swallowing)	Aspiration: reduced or late vocal fold closures
Supersupraglottic swallow	Effortful breath hold (closes vocal folds before and during swallow) Increased anterior tilting of arytenoids	Aspiration (poor closure of laryngeal introitus)
Effortful swallow	Effortful tongue action (increases posterior motion of tongue base)	Poor posterior tongue base motion
Mendelsohn's maneuver	Prolong hyoid excursion guided by manual palpation (prolongs UES opening)	Poor pharyngeal clearance and laryngeal movement
POSTURAL ADJUSTMENTS		
Head tilt	Tilt posteriorly at swallow initiation (gravity clears oral cavity)	Poor tongue control
	Tilt laterally to unaffected side (directs bolus down stronger side)	Unilateral pharyngeal weakness
Chin tuck	Chin down (widens valleculae, displaces tongue base and epiglottis posteriorly)	Aspiration, delayed pharyngeal response, reduced posterior tongue base motion
Head rotation	Rotate head to affected side (isolates damaged side from bolus path, reduces LES pressure) on thyroid cartilage (increases adduction)	Unilateral pharyngeal weakness
	Rotate head to affected side with extrinsic pressure	Unilateral laryngeal dysfunction Unilateral pharyngeal dysfunction
Lying on side, elevation	Right or left lateral (bypass laryngeal introitus)	Aspiration, bilateral pharyngeal impairment or reduced laryngeal elevation
FACILITATORY TECHNIQUES		
Strengthening exercises	Various	Nonprogressive disease
Biofeedback	Augment volitional component	Poor pharyngeal clearance
Thermal stimulation	Cold, tactile stimulation to anterior faucial pillar	Delayed or absent swallow response
Gustatory stimulation	Sour bolus (facilitates swallow response)	Huntington's chorea, stroke

From Cook IJ, Kahrilas PJ: AGA technical review on management of oropharyngeal dysphagia, *Gastroenterology* 116(2):470, 1999.
LES, Lower esophageal sphincter; *UES,* upper esophageal sphincter.

is warranted for patients if the cause of the dysphagia is neurogenic. If oral health and hygiene are a concern, referral to a dentist for evaluation and treatment is indicated. Counseling or psychiatric consultation is necessary for patients experiencing grief or depression associated with the dysphagia.

Other co-morbid illnesses or conditions may affect dysphagia or contribute to the development of pneumonia. Pulmonary rehabilitation may be indicated for patients with concurrent lung disease. Suspected pneumonia should usually be evaluated at the hospital, especially if gastric fluid is thought to be the aspirate. Malnutrition or dehydration may require hospital admission.

PATIENT AND FAMILY EDUCATION

The most important aspects of education include patient feeding, positioning, maneuvers, and dietary textural modifications. Speech therapists can teach patients and families positioning and maneuvers to improve swallowing efficacy. The Silver Spoons program, a volunteer program, was designed to facilitate safe feeding and can also assist family members or institutional staff.[27] Paying careful attention to bolus size and consistency, allowing plenty of time for meals, and ensuring proper patient positioning for meals improves safety.

Discussion concerning the risks and benefits of feeding tubes in specific disease entities is important for patients, families, and, often, staff. Feeding tubes may not seem appropriate for patients with severe dementia.[28] Cultural and religious preferences must be respected. Other concurrent illnesses may be important considerations. More research is needed, but for any given patient the decision to place a feeding tube must remain individualized and carefully considered.

HEALTH PROMOTION

Regular health screenings and recommendations regarding diet, exercise, and smoking cessation can prevent or delay the onset of disease, particularly in those with a strong family history of stroke. Once dysphagia is established, good oral hygiene, dental care, careful attention to positioning and swallowing techniques, and management of co-morbid illnesses, particularly respiratory illnesses and diabetes, can help to prevent pneumonia. Counseling can be beneficial for patients with a family history of hereditary neurologic or myopathic disorders associated with dysphagia. Support for families caring for dysphagic members may also help reduce caregiver stress.

REFERENCES

1. Croghan JE, Burke EM, Caplan S, and others: Pilot study of 12-month outcomes of nursing home patients with aspiration on video-fluoroscopy, *Dysphagia* 9:141-146, 1994.
2. Cook IJ, Kahrilas PJ: AGA technical review on management of oropharyngeal dysphagia, *Gastroenterology* 116(2):455-478, 1999.
3. Blackington E, McCormick T, Willson B, and others: Oropharyngeal dysphagia in the elderly, *Adv Nurse Pract* 9(7):42-49, 2001.
4. Perlman AL, Christensen J: Topography and functional anatomy of the swallowing structures. In Perlman AL, Schulze-Delrieu K, editors: *Deglutition and its disorders: anatomy physiology, clinical diagnosis and management,* San Diego, 1997, Singular.
5. Moser G, Vacariu-Granser GV, Schneider C, and others: High incidence of esophageal motor disorder in consecutive patients with globus sensation, *Gastroenterology* 101:1512-1521, 1991.
6. Leder SB: Gag reflex and dysphagia, *Head Neck* 18:138-141, 1996.
7. Leder SB: Videofluoroscopic evaluation of aspiration with visual examination of the gag reflex and velar movement, *Dysphagia* 12:21-23, 1997.
8. Davies AE, Kidd D, Stone SP, and others: Pharyngeal sensation and gag reflex in healthy subjects, *Lancet* 345:487-488, 1995.
9. Splaingard ML, Hutchins B, Sultan L, and others: Aspiration in rehabilitation patients: video-fluoroscopy vs bedside clinical assessment. *Arch Phys Med Rehabil* 69:637-640, 1988.
10. Jacob P, Kahrilas PJ, Logemann JA, and others: Upper esophageal sphincter opening and modulation during swallowing, *Gastroenterology* 97:1469-1478, 1989.
11. Shaw DW, Cook IJ, Jamieson GG, and others: Influence of surgery on deglutitive upper esophageal sphincter mechanics in Zenker's diverticulum, *Gut* 38:806-811, 1996.
12. Bhattacharyya N: *Cricopharyngeal myotomy*, 2005, retrieved April 4, 2006, from http://www.emedicine.com.
13. Ali GN, Wallace KL, Laundl TM, and others: Predictors of outcomes following cricopharyngeal disruption for pharyngeal dysphagia, *Dysphagia* 12:133-139, 1997.
14. Murry T, Wasserman T, Carrau RL, and others: Injection of botulinum toxin A for the treatment of dysfunction of the upper esophageal sphincter, *Am J Otolaryngol* 26(3):157-162, 2005.
15. Zaninotto G, Marchese Rgaona R, Briani C, and others: The role of botulinum toxin injection and upper esophageal myotomy in treating oropharyngeal dysphagia, *J Gastrointestinal Surg* 8(8):997-1006, 2004.
16. Kelly JH: Management of upper esophageal disorders: indications and complications of myotomy, *Am J Med* 6(108 Suppl 4a):43S-46S, 2000.
17. Born LJ, Harned RH, Rikkers LF, and others: Cricopharyngeal dysfunction in Parkinson's disease: role in dysphagia and response to myotomy, *Mov Disorders* 11(91):53-58, 1996.
18. Ebihara I, Takahaski H, Ebihara S, and others: Capsaicin troche for swallowing dysfunction in older people, *J Am Geriatr Soc* 53(5):824-828, 2005.
19. Perez I, Smithard DG, Davies H, and others: Pharmacologic treatment of dysphagia in stroke, *Dysphagia* 13(1):12-16, 1998.
20. Gross RD, Atwood CW, Grayhack JP, and others: Lung volume effects on pharyngeal swallowing physiology, *J Appl Physiol* 95(6):2211-2217, 2003.
21. Watando A, Ebihara S, Ebihara T, and others: Daily oral care and cough reflex sensitivity in elderly nursing home patients, *Chest* 126(4):1066-1070, 2004.
22. Smithard DG, O'Neill PA, Park C, and others: Complications and outcome after acute stroke: does dysphagia matter? *Stroke* 27:1200-1204, 1996.
23. Johnson ER, McKenzie SW, Sievers A: Aspiration pneumonia in stroke, *Arch Phys Med Rehabil* 74:973-976, 1993.
24. Terpenning MS, Taylor GW, Lopatin DE, and others: Aspiration pneumonia: dental and oral risk factors in an older veteran population, *J Am Geriatr Soc* 49:557-563, 2001.
25. Langmore SE, Terpenning MS, Schork A, and others: Predictors of aspiration pneumonia: how important is dysphagia? *Dysphagia* 13:69-81, 1998.
26. Thomas M, Haigh RA: Dysphagia, a reversible cause not to be forgotten, *Postgrad Med J* 71:94-95, 1995.
27. Musson ND, Frye GD, Nash M: Silver Spoons: supervised volunteers provide feeding of patients, *Geriatr Nurs* 18(1):18-19, 1997.
28. Braun UK, Kunik ME, Rabeneck L, and others: Malnutrition in patients with severe dementia: is there a place for PEG tube feeding? *Ann Long-Term Care* 9(9):47-55, 2001.

CHAPTER 150

Pancreatitis

Margaret Costello

Physician consultation is indicated for patients with suspected pancreatitis.

ACUTE PANCREATITIS

DEFINITION AND EPIDEMIOLOGY

Acute pancreatitis is a severe inflammatory condition of the pancreas. The patient with acute pancreatitis typically is seen with severe abdominal pain and an elevation of pancreatic enzymes. The clinical course can range from mild disease to life-threatening multiorgan failure, sepsis, and possibly death. Acute pancreatitis can be divided into two broad categories: edematous (or mild) pancreatitis and necrotizing (or severe) pancreatitis. Interstitial pancreatic edema and mild peripancreatic fat necrosis are present in edematous pancreatitis. Necrotizing pancreatitis, on the other hand, is characterized by extensive necrosis, hemorrhage, and widespread peripancreatic and intrapancreatic fat necrosis.

The cause of pancreatitis is varied. A number of factors have been implicated as precipitants (Boxes 150-1 and 150-2). The most common cause of pancreatitis is gallstones, responsible for 45% of all cases of pancreatitis in the United States.[1] Toxins are another cause of acute pancreatitis, with ethyl alcohol the precipitant implicated in 35% of pancreatitis cases.[1] Other causes of pancreatitis include trauma from injury or surgery, which may cause disruption of the ductal system or damage to the pancreas.[1] Conditions that cause hypercalcemia such as hyperparathyroidism are also implicated in the development of pancreatitis. However, the reasons for this are not clearly understood. Hyperlipidemia associated with lipid levels greater than 1000 mg/dl is known to increase the risk of pancreatitis.[1] Parasites and viral infections such as HIV have been implicated in the development of pancreatitis. Some medications are associated with pancreatitis. The exact relationship is unknown, but may be related to a hypersensitivity reaction, which results in pancreatic injury. Some medications implicated in the development of acute pancreatitis are thiazide diuretics and furosemide (Lasix). Lesions that result in pancreatic ductal obstruction such as tumors also may cause pancreatitis.

For unknown reasons, the incidence of acute pancreatitis has been increasing.[2] The overall incidence of pancreatitis in the United States over the past 20 years increased nearly 60% despite reduced alcohol ingestion in the same time period.[3]

PATHOPHYSIOLOGY

The exact mechanism of pancreatitis is not well understood, but the most common explanation is related to autodigestion of the pancreas. For reasons unknown, the pancreatic enzymes are activated in the pancreas rather than the intestine. Trypsinogen, an inactive enzyme produced by the pancreas, is normally released into the intestines by the pancreatic ducts and activated by trypsin. In pancreatitis the trypsin is present in the pancreas and not only digests the pancreas but also activates other enzymes such as elastase and phospholipase A. Elastase and phospholipase A are also involved in the autodigestion of the pancreas. Elastase causes hemorrhage through break down of the elastic fibers of the blood vessels. Phospholipase A has been implicated in fat necrosis.[4]

Although most patients typically experience minimum organ dysfunction as a result of pancreatitis, approximately 10% to 15% develop systemic inflammatory response syndrome (SIRS). SIRS appears to be caused by the activation of an inflammatory cascade mediated by cytokines, immunocytes, and the complement system. The inflammatory cytokines cause macrophages to migrate to the lungs, kidneys, and other tissues distant from the pancreas. SIRS leads to a fulminant course with pancreatic necrosis and multiorgan failure.[5]

CLINICAL PRESENTATION

The main presentation of acute pancreatitis is the sudden onset of constant, knifelike, poorly localized abdominal pain, which radiates to the back in about 50% of patients. The pancreas is in a retroperitoneal location, and signs of peritoneal irritation such as rebound tenderness are frequently absent.

PHYSICAL EXAMINATION

Early recognition of pancreatitis in clinical practice is of utmost importance. However, the physical examination frequently misses the diagnosis, since the presenting symptoms are nonspecific and may be mistaken for a variety of other disease processes. The most common presentation is intense abdominal pain so severe that the patient is reluctant to take a deep breath. This results in hypoventilation and contributes to the increased incidence of respiratory complications such as atelectasis; therefore crackles may be present in lungs on examination. The pain is worse in the supine position and often increases in severity with time. Many patients are initially seen with symptoms of dehydration from nausea and vomiting. Abdominal distention caused by the leakage of fluid into the retroperitoneum is common and results in protrusion of abdominal contents forward. Upper abdominal palpation of a mass may suggest the presence of a pancreatic pseudocyst. Evidence of retroperitoneal hemorrhage, although rare, may be observed. Cullen's sign (bruising of the periumbilicus) or Grey Turner's sign (bruising of the flank) is consistent with the hemorrhagic findings in acute severe pancreatitis. Both Cullen's and Grey Turner's signs are specific for pancreatitis, but their occurrence is rare and associated with increased mortality. Jaundice, an uncommon finding, also may occur and is related to compression of the common bile duct by the edematous head of the pancreas. Clinical conditions such as tachycardia, orthostatic hypotension, shock, and peritonitis are late signs associated with severe acute pancreatitis, which is associated with a grave prognosis.[6]

DIAGNOSTICS

Serum amylase is the most common test used to diagnose acute pancreatitis. Rising 6 to 12 hours after the onset of

BOX 150-1

FACTORS ASSOCIATED WITH ACUTE PANCREATITIS

MOST FREQUENT CAUSES

Gallstones
Alcoholism
Idiopathic (may be related to diverse causes)

FREQUENT CAUSES

Toxins
- Ethyl alcohol
- Methyl alcohol
- Organophosphorous insecticides
- Scorpion venom

Medications
- Angiotensin-converting enzyme inhibitors
- Acetaminophen
- Aminosalicylates
- Asparaginase (Elspar)
- Azathioprine (Imuran)
- Chlorthalidone
- Cimetidine
- Corticosteroids
- ddI (2′,3′-dideoxyinosine: associated with concurrent pentamidine treatment)
- Erythromycin
- Estrogens (identified with type IV or V hyperlipidemia)
- Ethacrynic acid
- Furosemide (rare)
- Iatrogenic hypercalcemia
- IV lipids
- L-Asparaginase
- Methyldopa (rare)
- Metronidazole (rare)
- Nitrofurantoin
- Nonsteroidals
- Olsalazine 5-ASA (rare)
- Pentamidine (rare)
- Phenformin (rare)
- Ranitidine
- Sulindac
- Sulfonamides (rare)
- Tetracycline (rare)
- Thiazide diuretics
- Valproic acid

Blunt abdominal trauma
Crohn's disease of the duodenum
End-stage renal failure
Iatrogenic trauma: cardiopulmonary bypass, endoscopic retrograde cholangiopancreatography, endoscopic sphincterotomy, manometry of the sphincter of Oddi, organ transplant, postoperative pancreatitis following abdominal or thoracic surgery
Hyperparathyroidism associated with hypercalcemia
Infection
- Parasitic: *Ascaris* worms, clonorchiasis
- Viral: coxsackievirus, cytomegalovirus, mumps, and fulminant viral hepatitis
- Bacterial: *Campylobacter jejuni, Mycoplasma pneumoniae, Salmonella* organisms, microlithiasis

Lipid abnormalities (hypertriglyceridemia)
Metabolic abnormalities: hypercalcemia associate with excessive doses of vitamin D, parathyroid adenoma, familial hypocalciuric hypercalcemia, hypercalcemia associated with total parenteral nutrition
Pancreatic divisum
Pancreatic outflow obstruction:
- Afferent loop obstruction, annular pancreatitis

Penetrating peptic ulcer
Pregnancy
Surgery (endoscopic retrograde cholangiopancreatography)
Trauma
Tumor: primary and metastatic

LESS FREQUENT CAUSES

Hereditary
Pancreatic cancer
Periampullary duodenal diverticulum
Refeeding after fasting
Rheumatologic disorders: systemic lupus erythematosus, mixed connective tissue disorders, scleroderma
Thrombotic thrombocytopenic purpura
Vasculitis

BOX 150-2

FACTORS ASSOCIATED WITH ACUTE PANCREATITIS IN HIV-POSITIVE PATIENTS

INFECTION

Cytomegalovirus
- Cryptococcus
- Cryptosporidia
- *Mycobacterium avium* and *Mycobacterium tuberculosis*
- *Toxoplasma gondii*

MEDICATIONS

Didanosine
Pentamidine
Trimethoprim-sulfamethoxazole

symptoms, serum amylase levels usually return to normal within 3 to 5 days in uncomplicated cases. For unknown reasons this elevation is not always seen in alcoholic or hypertriglyceridemia-associated pancreatitis. Serum amylase elevation is considered a nonspecific finding, since the serum amylase may be elevated for other conditions such as diseases of the salivary glands, which also produce amylase. The serum lipase level is more diagnostic, especially in patients seen several days after the acute attack and is elevated in both alcoholic and nonalcoholic pancreatitis.[7] Serum and urinary trypsinogen-2 and trypsinogen activation peptide can be elevated in acute pancreatitis.[8] Urinary trypsinogen-2 test strip may offer rapid and reliable diagnosis for acute pancreatitis.

Hemoconcentration, hyperglycemia, electrolyte abnormalities, and leukocytosis are commonly seen. Hypertriglyceridemia, hyperbilirubinemia, and transient hypocalcemia may also be present. Elevated liver enzyme levels combined with increased bilirubin and serum alanine aminotransferase indicate the probability of biliary pancreatitis, whereas an elevated C-reactive protein level indicates the possibility of pancreatic necrosis. A C-reactive protein greater than 150 mg/dl at 48 hours distinguishes mild from severe disease.

Abdominal radiographs are useful in the exclusion of other causes of abdominal pain such as bowel obstruction or perforated bowel but are not diagnostic for pancreatitis. Chest x-ray studies are recommended and may show pneumonia, left lower lobe atelectasis, or effusion. Although ultrasonography offers the most sensitive estimate of gallstone-induced pancreatitis, it may not be reliable because of abdominal distention caused by gas, which obscures the pancreas. Contrast-induced CT scanning is the most useful imaging technique, not only for diagnosis but also for detecting a pseudocyst (collection of fluid around or within the pancreas) and recognizing pancreatic necrosis. MRI and magnetic resonance cholangiopancreatography (MRCP) are used in the diagnosis of acute pancreatitis. MRI is considered more useful in the effort to categorize acute fluid collections and is more sensitive in diagnosing milder forms of pancreatitis. MRCP is better able to delineate the pancreatic and bile ducts.[9]

In 30% of patients diagnosed with pancreatitis, the etiology is unknown. The majority of these patients will have no further episodes. Those patients with recurrent pancreatitis may benefit from endoscopic retrograde cholangiopancreatography (ERCP) to assist in determining the cause.[10]

DIFFERENTIAL DIAGNOSIS

The patient who is seen with abdominal pain requires meticulous assessment. Many disease processes manifest with abdominal pain. A thorough history of the pain, including location, time of onset, severity, and quality, in addition to associated symptoms, will assist in determining the diagnosis. Questions regarding gastrointestinal function such appetite, nausea, vomiting, and the presence of blood in the stool will be useful. The possibility of gynecologic conditions also must be considered in women with abdominal pain.[11]

DIAGNOSTICS

Acute Pancreatitis

LABORATORY

CHEM-7 (electrolytes, BUN, creatinine)
Fasting lipid profile*
Serum and urinary trypsinogen-2
Trypsinogen activation peptide
C-reactive protein*
TSH*
Serum human chorionic gonadotropin (in women of childbearing age)

IMAGING

CT scan
Ultrasound
KUB
Chest x-ray
HIDA (hepatoiminodiacetic acid [lidofenin]) scan*

OTHER

ECG
Endoscopic retrograde cholangiopancreatography*

*If indicated.

DIFFERENTIAL DIAGNOSIS

Acute Pancreatitis

- Myocardial infarction
- Bowel obstruction
- Acute cholecystitis
- Biliary or renal colic
- Peptic ulcer disease
- Ruptured aortic aneurysm or acute aortic dissection
- Gynecologic conditions
- Pneumonia
- Diverticulosis
- Pulmonary embolus
- Mesenteric ischemia or infarction

MANAGEMENT

Recognition of underlying abdominal emergencies and the need for quick surgical intervention is essential. Treatment of pancreatitis is generally aimed at decreasing pancreatic inflammation and correcting any predisposing factors such as removing gallstones in gallstone pancreatitis. No oral medications, food, or fluids should be ingested, and precipitants of the attack, such as alcohol or medications, should be eliminated. The patient may accumulate a great deal of fluid in the injured pancreas. Monitoring fluid status is critical. Hospitalization is usually indicated for analgesia and IV rehydration, as well as to monitor vital signs, volume status, and electrolytes.

Pain is typically treated with opioid analgesia. Meperidine is used cautiously because of the propensity of its metabolites to accumulate in and cause neuromuscular irritation and possibly seizures. Morphine has been shown in human studies to cause an increase in pressure of the sphincter of Oddi; however, there is no evidence that this has a negative effect on the pancreas's condition. Fentanyl is sometimes used but can cause respiratory depression.

Antibiotic therapy for acute pancreatitis is controversial but is appropriate if secondary infection or necrotizing pancreatitis is present.[12]

Pain cessation, plus normalization of vital signs, radiographic studies, and laboratory values, indicates resolving pancreatitis. Liquids can be resumed and small amounts of food gradually added once pain has subsided if serum amylase and lipase levels have also normalized. The recurrence of pain indicates the need to repeat serum amylase and lipase determinations and to again restrict oral intake. For patients with protracted attacks of pancreatitis, enteral feedings or total parenteral nutrition may be required, although a study by Abou-Assi, Craig, and O'Keefe suggests that hypocaloric enteral feeding may be safer than resting the bowel for patients with acute pancreatitis.[13] A second study by Marik and Zaloga also suggests the benefit of enteral nutrition for patients with acute pancreatitis.[14]

CT scanning to determine the presence of necrosis or other complications is indicated for patients who do not respond to supportive measures. ERCP may be necessary for gallstone pancreatitis, whereas surgical intervention may be necessary for necrotizing pancreatitis or infection.[15]

COMPLICATIONS

Unfortunately, patients who have recovered from acute pancreatitis are at significant risk for recurrence. Continued pain, malabsorption, or new-onset diabetes mellitus signals the potential development of chronic pancreatitis and warrants immediate investigation. The majority of patients will recover with supportive therapy, although approximately 25% of patients will have complications. These complications include hypocalcemia and other metabolic abnormalities, blindness (Purtscher's retinopathy), localized abscesses, phlegmons, pseudocysts, necrosis, hemorrhage, and multisystem organ failure. The majority of deaths are caused by pulmonary failure or sepsis.[16]

INDICATIONS FOR REFERRAL OR HOSPITALIZATION

The treatment of acute pancreatitis is primarily supportive and requires physician consultation. Hospitalization for careful observation, frequent assessment of vital signs, laboratory analysis, IV fluid replacement, normalization of electrolytes and glucose, and parenteral analgesia is indicated for all patients. Nutritional gastroenterology and surgical consultations are also recommended.

Hemodynamic monitoring, ERCP, or surgical intervention may be indicated for patients with cholangitis, worsening jaundice, a pseudocyst larger than 5 cm (1.9 inches), pancreatic hemorrhage, abscess, or necrosis. Although surgical debridement for pancreatic necrosis is indicated, the benefits of ERCP, surgery, antibiotics, and peritoneal lavage remain controversial.[5]

PATIENT AND FAMILY EDUCATION AND HEALTH PROMOTION

Patients should understand that severe abdominal pain with or without radiation, nausea, vomiting, or diaphoresis requires immediate evaluation. It is also important that patients understand the risk of repeated attacks of pancreatitis, the need to avoid possible precipitants, and the importance of adherence to prescribed therapy. Patient education regarding contributing factors such as alcohol use must be discussed. Because the mortality rate from alcoholic pancreatitis is high, alcohol must be avoided. A low-fat diet, weight loss, exercise, and normalization of triglycerides should be the goal for patients with pancreatitis associated with hypertriglyceridemia. Medications that may have caused the pancreatitis should also be avoided.

CHRONIC PANCREATITIS

DEFINITION AND EPIDEMIOLOGY

Chronic pancreatitis, an inflammatory condition of the pancreas, is characterized by morphologic and histologic changes in the pancreas. Chronic pancreatitis differs from acute pancreatitis in that acute pancreatitis is nonprogressive, whereas the inflammatory changes in chronic pancreatitis permanently impair the exocrine and endocrine function of the gland. The prevailing opinion regarding the parenchymal injury in acute pancreatitis such as that induced by a passage of a gallstone is that it is both pathologically and morphologically different from the injury that occurs in chronic pancreatitis.

Chronic pancreatitis is a disease of multiple causes such as alcoholism, duct obstruction from tumors, strictures, hypercalcemia, hyperlipidemia, genetic mutations, and possibly dietary or environmental causes (Box 150-3). In a substantial number of cases no identifiable cause can be found. Approximately 10% to 20% of cases are idiopathic. Recently, an autoimmune chronic pancreatitis with a similar presentation to those of acute pancreatitis and pancreatic malignancy was identified.[17]

Alcohol is a major factor in both acute and chronic pancreatitis. Alcohol abuse accounts for 70% to 80% of cases of chronic pancreatitis.[3] Although the exact pathogenesis is not clearly understood, the risk appears related to the duration and amount of alcohol consumed rather than the type of alcohol or the pattern of consumption.[18] Heredity is the cause of pancreatitis in a small group of people. Mutations occurring on the trypsin gene interfere with its activation and permit autodigestion of the pancreas. Pancreatic duct obstruction from trauma, calcific stones, or tumors can result in chronic pancreatitis. Tropical pancreatitis is a common cause of pancreatitis in parts of India and the tropics. Systemic diseases such as lupus erythematosus and cystic fibrosis have been linked to chronic pancreatitis as well. Malnutrition or consumption of sorghum may play a role in the development of chronic pancreatitis in southern India, Indonesia, and central Africa and South Africa. Uncommon causes of chronic pancreatitis include severe malnutrition, hemochromatosis, trauma, sicca syndrome, radiation injury, gastric surgery, and tuberculosis.

In patients older than 40 years, the finding of pancreatic dysfunction mandates an evaluation for pancreatic cancer. Pancreatic dysfunction in adults ages 20 to 40 years should

BOX 150-3

CAUSES OF CHRONIC PANCREATITIS

- Alcohol abuse
- Hereditary pancreatitis
- Ductal obstruction
- Tropical pancreatitis
- Autoimmune disease
- Cystic fibrosis
- Hyperparathyroidism
- Hypertriglyceridemia
- Hereditary pancreatitis (mutation of trypsinogen gene)
- Idiopathic pancreatitis (associated with atherosclerotic disease)
- Nutritional deficiencies (of antioxidants, such as selenium or vitamin C or E)

From Freedman SD, Bishop MD: *Etiology and pathogenesis of chronic pancreatitis,* retrieved Jan 14, 2007, from http://www.uptodateonline.com/utd/content/topic.do?topicKey=pancdis/5929&selectedTitle=2~74.

trigger an investigation for cystic fibrosis, since 85% of patients with cystic fibrosis have some pancreatic insufficiency. Fifty percent of patients with chronic pancreatitis die within 25 years of diagnosis, with 15% to 20% of those deaths related to complications. The remainder die of disease associated with chronic alcohol abuse.[19]

PATHOPHYSIOLOGY

The pathophysiology of chronic pancreatitis is multifactorial and not completely understood. One possible explanation is that the increased secretion of pancreatic plugging causes proteinaceous plugs to form within the interlobular and intralobular ducts, causing obstructions of ducts and subsequent scarring and damage because of inflammatory changes.[20] Other considerations include autoimmune disorders or genetic abnormalities.

CLINICAL PRESENTATION

Pain and pancreatic insufficiency characterize chronic pancreatitis. The pain of chronic pancreatitis may be absent or severe, recurrent or constant. The pain is typically epigastric and may be referred to the upper back, anterior chest, or flank. Nausea and vomiting may accompany the pain. Usually, the discomfort is not relieved by food or antacids and intensifies with alcohol or fatty food. Pain often occurs 15 to 20 minutes after eating. Weight loss, diarrhea, and oily stools may be reported as a result of fat malabsorption. When the destruction of pancreatic function results in diabetes, the typical symptoms of polyuria, polydipsia, and polyphagia may be observed. Glucose intolerance occurs frequently in the disease process, and typically the patient requires insulin as the disease progresses. Patients with severe pancreatic dysfunction have difficulty digesting complex foods or absorbing products of digestion. Significant protein and fat deficiencies occur when more than 90% of pancreatic function is lost.[20,21]

PHYSICAL EXAMINATION

Even in the presence of severe pain, physical examination may reveal few overt findings. Slight fever, weight loss, or abdominal tenderness may be present. Jaundice, signifying common bile duct obstruction, is less common. If pancreatic dysfunction results in severe malabsorption, signs of malnutrition will be evident.[21]

DIAGNOSTICS

Laboratory data are useful to exclude other causes of abdominal pain and to determine whether pancreatic insufficiency exists. In contrast to acute pancreatitis, elevated serum amylase and lipase levels are not typically present. There is a minimal (if any) increase in pancreatic enzymes in the blood because of significant fibrosis, which results in decreased concentration of these enzymes within the pancreas. CBC and liver function tests are typically normal. Increased bilirubin and alkaline phosphatase levels can indicate compression of bile ducts and should prompt investigation for fibrosis, edema, or tumor. The presence of pancreatic insufficiency is indicated by elevated blood glucose or steatorrhea. Steatorrhea can be diagnosed with Sudan stain of the feces and examination of fecal fat stool content. The patient typically eats 100 g of fat daily, and stool is collected over a 72-hour period. A fecal fat level of greater than 7 g is diagnostic of malabsorption.[21]

The secretin stimulation test is considered the definitive test in assessing pancreatic function. This diagnostic involves measurement of the bicarbonate concentration of duodenum fluid after the administration of secretin. Secretin causes the secretion of bicarbonate-rich fluid from the pancreas. A peak bicarbonate concentration of less than 80 mEq/L is consistent with chronic pancreatitis. Other laboratory tests include serum bilirubin and alkaline phosphatase. Elevations of these suggest compression of the intrapancreatic portion of the bile duct by edema, fibrosis, or pancreatic cancer. Erythrocyte sedimentation rate, IgG4, rheumatoid factor, antinuclear antibodies, and anti–smooth muscle antibody titer are elevated in autoimmune chronic pancreatitis.[21]

Imaging studies and pancreatic function tests complement one another. Abdominal radiographs, endoscopic ultrasound (EUS), CT scan, MRI, ERCP, and MRCP are diagnostic imaging studies that are useful in chronic pancreatitis. In one third of patients, abdominal radiographs (kidney-ureter-bladder [KUB]) may demonstrate pancreatic calcifications, thereby supporting the diagnosis.[3] Abdominal ultrasound may expedite early diagnosis because pancreatic enlargement and calcifications can be seen earlier than on abdominal radiographs. Similar findings occur with pancreatic cancer. CT has been determined to have a test sensitivity of 90%. Evidence of ductal dilation with focal enlargement, fluid collections, or calcifications on CT scanning or MRI indicates chronic pancreatitis. When there are no calcifications or evidence of pancreatic exocrine dysfunction (steatorrhea), ERCP demonstrates beading of the main pancreatic duct and ectatic side branches in chronic pancreatitis; the results of ERCP may be normal in early disease. With normal ERCP results and continued suspicion of chronic pancreatitis, pancreatic enzyme testing or EUS is the next step for evaluation. EUS requires a skilled endosonographer; stone formation on EUS is the most predictive feature of chronic pancreatitis. Other EUS findings include visible side branches, cysts, lobularity, irregularity or dilation of a main duct, hyperechoic foci, hyperechoic strands, and a main duct with hyperechoic margins. The severity of chronic pancreatitis correlates with the number of EUS findings observed. MRCP is useful in assessing the pancreatic ducts, which may not be visible with ERCP. MRCP is also increasingly being studied for use in evaluating pancreatic exocrine function and in the early diagnosis of chronic pancreatitis.[20]

DIAGNOSTICS

Chronic Pancreatitis

LABORATORY
- CBC and differential
- Serum amylase
- Serum lipase
- Serum bilirubin
- Serum glucose
- Serum alkaline phosphatase
- Stool for steatorrhea (fecal fat)

IMAGING
- CT scan
- KUB,* abdominal ultrasound*

OTHER
- Endoscopic retrograde cholangiopancreatography*
- Secretin stimulation test*

*If indicated.

DIFFERENTIAL DIAGNOSIS

A strong history of alcoholism suggests the diagnosis of chronic pancreatitis in the patient with abdominal pain. However, pseudocysts, pancreatic cancer, peptic ulcer disease, cholelithiasis, biliary tract obstruction, irritable bowel syndrome, and pancreatic stones should be excluded when considering the diagnosis of chronic pancreatitis.

In addition, because pancreatic cancer may manifest with signs and symptoms similar to those of chronic pancreatitis, patients may require ERCP or EUS for diagnosis. Pancreatic cancer should be suspected as a cause of chronic pancreatitis–like pain when a patient is older, has a negative history of alcohol use, has recent weight loss, has an extended duration of symptoms, and exhibits other constitutional signs and symptoms (e.g., fatigue, insomnia, anorexia). Consistent with the diagnosis of pancreatic cancer is a pancreatic duct stricture more than 10 mm (0.4 inch) long on ERCP. Tumor markers (carcinoembryonic antigen, CA 19-9) may be normal or abnormal with pancreatic cancer.[21]

Normal results on the D-xylose absorption test exclude the possibility of intestinal malabsorption. Angiography is used to exclude mesenteric vascular disease as the origin of chronic abdominal pain. Finally, the health care provider must recognize that chronic pancreatitis can occur in the setting of autoimmune diseases such as Sjögren's syndrome, systemic lupus erythematosus, and primary biliary cirrhosis and use appropriate testing to exclude associated conditions as warranted by the patient's history and presentation.

DIFFERENTIAL DIAGNOSIS

Chronic Pancreatitis

- Pseudocysts
- Pancreatic cancer
- Peptic ulcer disease
- Cholelithiasis
- Biliary tract obstruction
- Pancreatic stones
- Narcotics
- Pancreatic cancer
- Intestinal malabsorption
- Mesenteric vascular disease

MANAGEMENT

The treatment of pancreatic dysfunction, pain control, and correction of symptomatic pancreatic structural abnormalities are the goals of chronic pancreatitis treatment. These management modalities require medical and possibly surgical intervention.

Pain Control

The strong relationship between alcohol consumption and pancreatitis underscores the importance of alcohol abstinence to prevent further damage and reduce pain. The intense pain of chronic pancreatitis, coupled with inconsistent pain relief, is a risk factor for narcotic addiction. A short course of opiates with low-dose amitriptyline and nonsteroidal medication may break the pain cycle. Nerve blocks have not been found to provide long-term pain relief in the treatment of chronic pancreatitis. Studies have found that the celiac nerve block provides relief of pain for 2 to 4 months, if at all, and poses a risk of irreversible nerve damage.[21] Other pancreatitis pain management strategies include referral to a pain clinic and relaxation techniques.

Nutritional Interventions

Dietary interventions include fasting or small meals with decreased fat content. The administration of octreotide, a pancreatic secretion inhibitor, has yielded variant results for symptom relief.[20] In chronic pancreatitis, patients experience nutritional deficiencies and chronic pain. Steatorrhea and diarrhea are produced by exocrine dysfunction; these are managed with a low-fat diet (<20 g/day), inhibition of gastric acid secretion with H_2 blockers to reduce the pancreatic secretions, and pancreatic enzyme replacement. Pancreatic enzyme supplements suppress the feedback loops in the duodenum that regulate the release of cholecystokinin (CCK). CCK stimulates digestive enzyme release from the pancreas and is deactivated by trypsin, which is decreased in chronic pancreatitis. Oral administration of trypsin can correct this problem, decreasing the CCK-mediated stimulation of the pancreas. Enzyme supplementation is recommended for those patients who continue to have pain that has not responded to other conservative measures. Current recommendations of supplements are pancrelipase (Viokase), 6 tablets with meals. Each Viokase 16 tablet contains 16,000 units of lipase, 30,000 units of protease, and 30,000 units of amylase.[21] A proton pump inhibitor or H_2 receptor blocker is also recommended.[21] Additional nutritional support with supplementation of fat-soluble vitamins may be necessary.

Surgical Interventions

When a patient has pain nonresponsive to medical therapies, surgical interventions may be necessary. Extracorporeal shock wave lithotripsy can be helpful in relieving the obstruction of pancreatic secretions in the 22% to 60% of patients with chronic pancreatitis who have pancreatic duct stones. Endoscopic therapy may provide pain relief in some patients by decompressing an obstructed pancreatic duct. Endoscopic placement of stents within the pancreatic ducts relieves recurrent or persistent pain associated with chronic pancreatitis. Pancreatic duct sphincterotomy with stone extraction has been found to provide relief of pain. However, studies have shown that the presence or absence of stones does not correlate with the existence of pain.[21]

Surgical options for chronic pancreatitis include denervation procedures, which involve interruption of the nerve fibers passing through the celiac ganglion and splanchnic nerves from the pancreas. The benefit of this procedure lasts approximately 2 years before the pain recurs. Another surgical intervention involves decompression and drainage of the pancreatic duct. Gastric and biliary drainage may be necessary as well because of obstruction or strictures of the bile duct or duodenum. Resection of a portion of the pancreas may be an option for those patients with ongoing pain who are not considered candidates for drainage procedures. Resection of the pancreatic head may provide pain relief in up to 85% of patients. Patients who have undergone pancreatectomy may have exocrine and endocrine dysfunction. Pancreatic insufficiency can result with extensive resection, and severe diabetes can ensue. Autologous islet cell transplantation after entire gland resection is a topic under current exploration. Total pancreatectomy is a last resort in patients who fail all other treatments. Despite the availability of these techniques, the criteria for surgical intervention is not agreed on. Consultation with a gastroenterologist is advised for diagnostic verification and collaborative management. Invasive studies may be indicated as the patient's condition changes or as complications follow.[20]

LIFE SPAN CONSIDERATIONS

Steatorrhea, diabetes, and pancreatic calcifications are complications commonly experienced by older adults with long-standing chronic pancreatitis. Also, idiopathic senile chronic pancreatitis may occur in adults older than 60 years. Two variants of senile chronic pancreatitis have been identified. In the first type, patients exhibit the typical symptoms of steatorrhea, weight loss, or diabetes; there is no pain. Primary inflammatory pancreatitis, the second and less common version, occurs primarily in women and manifests with weight loss, steatorrhea, atypical or absent pain, fever, hypergammaglobulinemia, or chronic hepatitis. Other causes of malabsorption in older adults should be considered. Celiac disease, small bowel contamination, and pancreatic cancer must be excluded.

COMPLICATIONS

Chronic pancreatitis can be associated with a variety of complications. The most common complications are pseudocyst formation and mechanical obstruction of the duodenum and common bile duct.[22] Diabetes, exocrine insufficiency, malnutrition, pancreatic ascites, pleural effusion, splenic vein thrombosis, gastric varices, and pain are other complications associated with chronic pancreatitis.[22] The development of extrahepatic biliary obstruction is signified by serum alkaline phosphatase levels that are twice the normal level for longer than 2 months. Portal hypertension may occur as a result of thrombosis in the splenic or portal veins, pancreatic abscess, common bile duct obstruction, peptic ulcer, pseudoaneurysm of adjacent arteries, gastrointestinal bleeding, ascites from a leaking pseudocyst or damaged duct, and pancreatic cancer.

INDICATIONS FOR REFERRAL OR HOSPITALIZATION

The primary care or collaborating physician is consulted for the initial diagnosis and management. Subsequent deterioration or complications in patient status warrant continued physician guidance. Initial testing for stable, uncomplicated patients can be accomplished in the outpatient setting. Hospitalization is required for the management of serious complications and for surgical drainage or resection procedures.

PATIENT AND FAMILY EDUCATION

It is vital that patients and families understand the recurrent, chronic character of the disease. Careful explanation of each individual's etiologic factors and the need for alcohol abstinence is necessary. Patients with endocrine insufficiency should receive diabetic education because they are susceptible to macrovascular and microvascular complications. Patients with exocrine insufficiency must understand the origin of steatorrhea, the purpose and dosing of dietary supplements, components of a low-fat diet, and supplementation with fat-soluble vitamins and calcium. Guidelines for follow-up care, pain management, and symptoms requiring immediate attention are important to clarify and update.

PANCREATIC PSEUDOCYST

DEFINITION AND EPIDEMIOLOGY

Pseudocysts develop in approximately 10% of patients with chronic pancreatitis. Pancreatic pseudocysts contain blood, tissue, fluid, pancreatic digestive enzymes, and cellular debris accumulated in a cystlike mass. The prefix *pseudo* is used because this localized collection of material does not have an epithelial lining, a hallmark for a true cyst.

Pseudocysts form as sequelae of acute pancreatitis or in association with chronic pancreatitis. Other, less common causes include gallbladder disease, surgery, and trauma. Pseudocysts, occurring singularly or as multiple lesions, develop primarily in the body or tail of the pancreas but are found outside the pancreas.

PATHOPHYSIOLOGY

Pseudocysts develop as a result of ductal disruptions and contain a large concentration of pancreatic enzymes. Pseudocysts may be single or multiple, small or large, and may be located in or outside of the pancreas. The walls of the pseudocyst are formed by adjacent structures such as the stomach, transverse megacolon, gastrocolic omentum, and pancreas. An absence of epithelial tissue distinguishes pseudocysts from pancreatic cysts.[22]

CLINICAL PRESENTATION

Most pancreatic pseudocysts are asymptomatic. When symptoms occur, the presenting symptoms are typically related to the location and extent of the fluid collection. Abdominal pain may be a presenting symptom related to expansion of the pseudocyst. Other symptoms associated with pseudocyst formation include low-grade fever, jaundice, diaphragm inflammation, pleural effusion, and ascites. Pseudocyst expansion may also contribute to duodenal or biliary obstruction, vascular occlusion, and fistula formation into adjacent viscera. Gastrointestinal bleeding can result when a pseudoaneurysm forms from adjacent vessel necrosis and bleeds into a pancreatic duct.[23]

DIAGNOSTICS

Diagnostics include pancreatic imaging by CT, MRI, or ultrasonography. With pleural effusion or ascites, the thoracentesis or paracentesis fluid has amylase levels above 1000 international units/L when there is a pseudocyst.[23] Biopsy samples and CEA levels of cystic fluid from suspicious cystic lesions exclude premalignant growths or malignancies.[24,25] This is accomplished by CT-guided percutaneous needle biopsy. ERCP before surgery is indicated to determine ductal and pseudocyst anatomy. Serologic analysis includes amylase, glucose, alkaline phosphatase, and bilirubin. Elevations of blood glucose and amylase are common. Increased serum alkaline phosphatase or bilirubin levels indicate compression of the common bile duct as it passes through the pancreas from extrahepatic biliary obstruction. With pancreatic pseudocyst,

DIAGNOSTICS

Pancreatic Pseudocyst

LABORATORY
CBC and differential
Serum amylase
Serum glucose
Alkaline phosphatase
Bilirubin

IMAGING
CT scan, MRI, or ultrasound

OTHER
Endoscopic retrograde cholangiopancreatography, biopsy

a CBC may show decreased hemoglobin or an elevated WBC count.

DIFFERENTIAL DIAGNOSIS

The presence of pancreatic fluid masses requires investigation. Pseudocysts can be confused with and should be distinguished from pancreatic abscesses, malignant cystadenomas, cystadenocarcinomas, retention cysts, congenital conditions, and desmoids. Concerns that a fluid collection is not a pseudocyst are prompted by a patient having no prior history of acute pancreatitis, chronic pancreatitis, or pancreatic trauma; the absence of inflammatory changes on CT scan; and the presence of internal septae in the cyst.[23] EUS with fine needle aspiration is used to exclude malignancy in cystic lesions, since pancreatic neoplasms may be cystic.

DIFFERENTIAL DIAGNOSIS

Pancreatic Pseudocyst

- Pancreatic abscesses
- Malignant cystadenomas
- Cystadenocarcinomas
- Retention cysts
- Congenital conditions
- Desmoids

MANAGEMENT

The decision process for pseudocyst management contains several steps. First, alternative diagnoses, particularly the possibility that the cyst may represent a neoplasm, are excluded. Next, the provider considers whether a complication of pseudocyst, a pseudoaneurysm, is present. This complication occurs in approximately 10% of patients with a pancreatic pseudocyst[23] (see Complications, below). In patients without discomfort, neoplasm, or pseudoaneurysm, conservative management may be possible and the pancreatic pseudocyst safely monitored.[23] Currently there are several drainage options for pseudocysts, based on cystic location and patient symptoms. These options are multiple internal drainage procedures, percutaneous catheter drainage, or endoscopic approaches. Indications for drainage include rapid enlargement, compression of surrounding structures, pain, or signs of infection.

Co-Management with Specialists

Initial evaluation, laboratory tests, and imaging studies can be performed in the primary care setting. Complications, invasive diagnostics, and evaluation for surgery require collaboration with specialists in radiology, surgery, and gastroenterology.

COMPLICATIONS

Occasionally confused with pancreatic abscesses, infected pseudocysts cause severe pain, a fever with a high temperature, chills, and leukocytosis. On ultrasound or CT scan, infection is viewed as a diffuse area of necrosis, whereas an abscess is seen as a well-defined area of purulence. Furthermore, pseudocysts may erode and perforate structures, resulting in rupture into the peritoneal cavity or gastrointestinal tract. Stomach perforation can manifest with few symptoms and require no treatment; peritoneal perforation necessitates surgical intervention and can be fatal. Colon perforation is seen with abdominal pain and self-limited bloody diarrhea. Pseudocysts can also erode blood vessels, creating a pseudoaneurysm and producing hemorrhage and shock. Three clinical findings are associated with pseudoaneurysm formation: gastrointestinal bleeding, sudden pseudocyst enlargement, and an unexplained decrease in hematocrit.[24] Elevated serum amylase levels and ascitic fluid containing amylase and protein suggest a leaking pseudocyst.

INDICATIONS FOR REFERRAL OR HOSPITALIZATION

If a pseudocyst or another complication is suspected, the collaborating physician is consulted during the initial visit. Long-term management requires careful and continued collaboration with the primary care physician.

PATIENT AND FAMILY EDUCATION

Patients at risk for pseudocyst formation should be educated about the symptoms of a pseudocyst and the necessity to contact their health care provider for increased or persistent pain. Patients with known pseudocysts should receive instruction concerning the etiology of their condition, complications and their symptoms, and indications to seek medical attention.

REFERENCES

1. Bowyer M: In Parsons P, Weiner-Kronish J, editors: *Critical care secrets*, ed 3, Philadelphia, 2003, Hanley & Belfus.
2. Munoz A, Katerndahl DA, Al-Kawas F: Acute pancreatitis: diagnosis and management, *Am Fam Phys* 62:164-174, 2000.
3. Fioranti J: Incidence of acute pancreatitis on the rise, *Internal Medicine News*, June 15, 2004, retrieved Jan 15, 2007, from http://www.accessmylibrary.com/coms2/summary_0286-5117631_ITM.
4. Cole L: Unraveling the mystery of acute pancreatitis, *Nursing* 31:58, 2001.
5. Mitchell RM, Byrne MF, Baillie J: Pancreatitis, *Lancet* 36(9367):1447-1455, 2003.
6. Mergener K, Baillie J: Acute pancreatitis, *Br J Med* 316(7124):44-48, 1998.
7. Baillie J: Acute pancreatitis, *Emerg Med* 33(8):12-19, 2001.
8. Johnson CD, Lempinen M, Imrie CW, and others: Urinary trypsinogen peptide as a marker of severe acute pancreatitis, *Br J Surg* 91(8):1027-1033, 2004.
9. Balthazar EJ: Acute pancreatitis: assessment of the severity with clinical and CT evaluation, *Radiology* 223:603-613, 2002.
10. Chari S, Swaroop VS: *Clinical manifestations and diagnosis of acute pancreatitis*, 2006, retrieved Jan 14, 2007, from http://www.uptodateonline.com/utd/content/topic.do?topicKey=pancdis/7667&selectedTitle=2~132.

11. Rhoads K, Varma M: The acute abdomen. In Parsons P, Weiner-Kronish J, editors: *Critical care secrets*, ed 3, Philadelphia, 2003, Hanley & Belfus.
12. Mayerle J, Simon P, Lerch MM: Medical treatment of acute pancreatitis, *Gastroenterol Clin North Am* 33(4):855-869, viii, 2004.
13. Abou-Assi S, Craig K, O'Keefe SJ: Hypocaloric jejunal feeding is better than total parenteral nutrition in acute pancreatitis: results of a randomized comparative study, *Am J Gastroenterol* 97(9):2255-2262, 2002.
14. Marik PE, Zaloga GP: Meta-analysis of parenteral nutrition versus enteral nutrition in patients with acute pancreatitis, *Br Med J* 328(7453):1407, 2004.
15. Chari S, Swaroop VS: *Treatment of acute pancreatitis*, 2006, retrieved Jan 14, 2007, from http://www.uptodateonline.com/utd/content/topic.do?topicKey=pancdis/11212&selectedTitle=1~132.
16. Steinberg W, Tenner S: Acute pancreatitis, *N Engl J Med* 330(17):1198-1210, 1994.
17. Kim KP, Kim MH, Song MH, and others: Autoimmune chronic pancreatitis, *Am J Gastroenterol* 99(8):1605-1616, 2004.
18. Freedman SD, Bishop MD: *Etiology and pathogenesis of chronic pancreatitis*, retrieved Jan 14, 2007, from http://www.uptodateonline.com/utd/content/topic.do?topicKey=pancdis/5929&selectedTitle=2~74.
19. Grendell JH, Cello JP: Chronic pancreatitis. In Sleisenger MS, Fordtran JS, editors: *Gastrointestinal disease: pathology, diagnosis, management*, ed 5, Philadelphia, 1993, Saunders.
20. Warshaw AL, Banks PA, Fernandez DC: AGA technical review: treatment of pain in chronic pancreatitis, *Gastroenterology* 115:765-766, 1998.
21. Freedman SD, Bishop MD: *Clinical manifestations and diagnosis of chronic pancreatitis in adults*, retrieved Jan 14, 2007, from http://www.uptodateonline.com/utd/content/topic.do?topicKey=pancdis/6795.
22. Freedman SD, Bishop MD: *Complications of chronic pancreatitis*, retrieved Jan 14, 2007, from http://www.uptodateonline.com/utd/content/topic.do?topicKey=pancdis/6466&selectedTitle=1~74.
23. Howell DA, Shah RJ, Parsons WG, and others: *Diagnosis and management of pseudocysts of the pancreas*, retrieved Jan 14, 2007 from http://www.uptodateonline.com/utd/content/topic.do?topicKey=pancdis/7294&selectedTitle=1~21.
24. Rosenfeld AT: The evaluation of pancreatic cysts, *J Clin Gastroenterol* 20:94-95, 1995.
25. Lim SJ, Alasadi R, Wayne JD, and others: Preoperative evaluation of pancreatic cystic lesions: cost-benefit analysis and proposed management algorithm, *Surgery* 138(4):672-679, 2005.

CHAPTER 151

Tumors of the Gastrointestinal Tract

Louise P. Meyer

Tumors of the gastrointestinal tract may be benign or malignant. It is essential that malignant tumors be identified as early as possible and treated appropriately. This chapter focuses on the common malignancies of the esophagus, stomach, small intestine, and colon; common benign tumors of the gastrointestinal tract are also mentioned.

TUMORS OF THE ESOPHAGUS

DEFINITION AND EPIDEMIOLOGY

Esophageal carcinoma most commonly occurs during the sixth decade of life, and in the United States this particular cancer accounts for 10,000 or more deaths each year.[1] In the past, most esophageal malignancies were squamous cell carcinomas. However, in the United States there has been a significant increase in the incidence of adenocarcinoma that arises from the columnar cells found in Barrett's esophagus.[1] Worldwide, squamous cell carcinoma is the cause of most esophageal cancers, with an incidence ranging from 30 to 800 per 100,000 in varied parts of the world.[1] Endemic areas include regions of northern China, South Africa, the Normandy and Brittany provinces of France, northern Iran, India, and areas of Asia.[2,3]

Risk factors for the development of esophageal cancer include chronic smoking; primary squamous cell carcinoma of the head and neck; alcohol consumption; thermal injury from the ingestion of hot liquids; and exposure to aflatoxin, asbestos fibers, and nitrosamines.[3,4] Nutritional deficiencies of riboflavin; niacin; zinc; protein; and vitamins A, E, and C have also been implicated.[3-6] The major risk factors for squamous cell esophageal carcinoma are chronic smoking and alcohol consumption, celiac sprue, Plummer-Vinson syndrome, and tylosis.[3,6-8] The single most important risk factor for the development of adenocarcinoma of the esophagus is esophageal reflux leading to the premalignant condition of Barrett's esophagus.[4,6,7,9]

PATHOPHYSIOLOGY

Squamous cell carcinomas of the esophagus involve the middle third of the esophagus in 50% of cases and can be polypoid, ulcerative, or infiltrative.[3] Polypoid tumors are the most common and may project into the lumen, causing obstruction. Ulcerating tumors may penetrate into the mediastinum, causing hemorrhage rather than obstruction. Infiltrative tumors may have circumferential involvement, causing thickening and stenosis of the esophageal wall.[3] Esophageal adenocarcinomas arise in Barrett's esophagus—a metaplasia of the distal esophagus occurring in association with long-term gastroesophageal reflux. Its extensive lymphatic system allows cancers of the esophagus to spread locally and into adjacent mediastinal structures regardless of tumor type.[5]

CLINICAL PRESENTATION

Dysphagia is the classic presenting symptom of esophageal carcinoma. This symptom indicates that the esophageal lumen has been reduced by at least half of its normal diameter.[4] Other symptoms include anorexia, weight loss, and odynophagia with radiation to the back. Hoarseness results from tumor involvement of the recurrent laryngeal nerve, and a tracheoesophageal fistula may produce a chronic cough.[3,4] The clinical features of esophageal adenocarcinoma are similar to those of squamous cell carcinoma but may also produce early satiety, nausea, vomiting, and bloating because of tumor encroachment into the stomach.

PHYSICAL EXAMINATION

Fixed supraclavicular, cervical, and axillary lymphadenopathy are signs of advanced disease. Both hepatomegaly secondary to metastatic disease and superior vena cava syndrome indicate a poor prognosis.[4,5]

DIAGNOSTICS

New-onset dysphagia should prompt an evaluation for an esophageal tumor. Diagnostic evaluation of the patient with a suspected esophageal carcinoma is a two-step procedure that begins with a barium esophagram and is followed by an upper gastrointestinal endoscopy with biopsy and cytologic tests.[4-6,10] The barium esophagram and endoscopy are used in evaluating the primary tumor. Endoscopic ultrasound will help determine the extent of disease locally.[6] A clinical examination, biochemical assay, chest x-ray examination, CT scan, radionuclide bone scan, ultrasonography, and biopsy of suspicious lesions may be useful in the metastatic evaluation.[4-6,10]

DIAGNOSTICS

Esophageal Tumors

IMAGING

Contrast radiographs
Chest x-rays*
CT scan*
Radionuclide bone scans*
Ultrasound*

OTHER

Barium esophagram
Upper gastrointestinal endoscopy with biopsy and cytologic tests

*If indicated.

DIFFERENTIAL DIAGNOSIS

In the adult patient with a new onset of progressive, solid dysphagia, the differential diagnosis includes esophageal squamous cell carcinoma, esophageal adenocarcinoma, adenocarcinoma of the gastric cardia, benign peptic stricture, corrosive stricture, and esophageal motor disorders such as achalasia or scleroderma. Symptoms of dysphagia, especially in a patient older than 45 years, mandate a complete evaluation to exclude esophageal carcinoma.

DIFFERENTIAL DIAGNOSIS

Esophageal Tumors

- Benign esophageal leiomyoma
- Esophageal carcinoma
- Esophageal adenocarcinoma
- Adenocarcinoma of the gastric cardia
- Benign peptic stricture
- Corrosive stricture
- Esophageal motor disorders

MANAGEMENT

Gastroenterologic, oncologic, and surgical consultations are critical for the evaluation of esophageal tumors. A total thoracic esophagectomy with gastric pull-up or colon interposition is usually required for surgical intervention in esophageal carcinoma.[10] Although somewhat controversial, concurrent radiation and chemotherapy before surgery may provide the best potential for cure in locally advanced disease.[5,6] However, palliation for dysphagia may be the only realistic goal because most patients have incurable disease at the time of diagnosis. Palliation can be accomplished by peroral stenting through the stenosis and transendoscopic ablation of obstructing tumors by laser photocoagulation. For advanced disease, esophagectomy provides superb palliation.[7] Radiotherapy may provide palliation for patients who are not candidates for surgery.[7] Postoperative elevation of serum carcinoembryonic antigen (CEA) levels may be the first objective sign of recurrent disease and should prompt additional therapy such as surgery or chemotherapy.[8,11]

COMPLICATIONS

Because of the distensibility of the esophagus, esophageal carcinoma tends to be silent until late in its course. Complications are usually related to mediastinal extension or esophageal narrowing and may include obstruction, hemorrhage, perforation, and fistula formation. Because the esophagus lacks a true serosa, cancer is often not contained at the time of diagnosis. The lungs and liver are the most common sites of hematogenous metastasis. Complications of esophageal resection include torsion or gangrene of the gastric, colonic, or jejunal pull-up; anastomotic leak; anastomotic stricture; subphrenic abscess; hemorrhage; wound infection and dehiscence; sepsis; dumping syndrome; and reflux esophagitis.

PATIENT AND FAMILY EDUCATION

Dietary instructions should be consistent with the degree of dysphagia experienced. Patients who have responded to therapy but continue to use alcohol and tobacco products during treatment demonstrate a poor response to treatment and an increased rate of local recurrence.[9] Therefore patients should be encouraged to discontinue the use of these products and should be provided with therapeutic interventions for alcohol and tobacco cessation.[7,9]

HEALTH PROMOTION

Patients should be regularly questioned about the presence of heartburn or other signs of gastroesophageal reflux so that appropriate diagnostics and treatment can be initiated. Primary prevention of esophageal cancer includes avoidance of all tobacco products and of heavy alcohol consumption. It is also important to consume a diet that is rich in fruits and vegetables and to maintain a normal weight. With obesity, there can be increased acid reflux, thus multiplying the risk for adenocarcinoma of the lower esophagus and stomach.[7,9]

TUMORS OF THE STOMACH

DEFINITION AND EPIDEMIOLOGY

Over the past 50 years the incidence of gastric cancer in the United States has dramatically declined.[3] This decrease has been attributed to improved refrigeration and the reduced consumption of preserved foods.[3] However, in other parts of the world, gastric carcinoma is the second most common cause of cancer-related death.[12] In Japan and Chile the incidence of gastric cancer is seven to eight times higher than in the United States.[3] In this country, gastric carcinoma occurs more often in African Americans, Hispanics, and Native Americans.[8] Common benign tumors of the stomach include leiomyomas and epithelial polyps.

Risk factors for gastric adenocarcinoma include *Helicobacter pylori* gastritis, chronic atrophic gastritis, pernicious anemia, and gastric polyps.[3,8] Dietary risk factors include a decreased consumption of fruits and vegetables and an increased intake of salt, nitrates and nitrites, and smoked and poorly preserved foods.[3,8] Genetic factors linked to gastric carcinoma include hereditary nonpolyposis colorectal cancer, familial polyposis, and first-degree relatives of patients with gastric cancer. A partial gastrectomy for peptic ulcer disease is also associated with an increased risk of gastric carcinoma.

PATHOPHYSIOLOGY

Gastric cancer is divided into intestinal and diffuse types. The intestinal type of gastric adenocarcinoma has distinct, large glands lined by columnar cells with a well-defined brush border; this type tends to occur in the distal stomach and may be polypoid or ulcerated.[13] The diffuse type of gastric cancer extends widely without distinct margins and infiltrates and thickens the stomach wall without forming a mass. Gastric carcinomas spread via direct extension, lymphatic spread, hematogenous metastasis, and peritoneal seeding.

CLINICAL PRESENTATION

Weight loss, abdominal pain, anorexia, nausea, and vomiting are the most common symptoms of advanced gastric carcinoma.[3,8,14] The abdominal pain begins as insidious upper abdominal discomfort that ranges in intensity from a vague sense of postprandial fullness to a severe, steady pain.[15] Other symptoms include a change in bowel habits, dysphagia, melena, anemic symptoms, and hemorrhage.[8,16]

PHYSICAL EXAMINATION

Patients with advanced gastric cancer may be initially seen with cachexia, small bowel obstruction, epigastric mass, ascites, hepatomegaly, or lower extremity edema. Metastases may also manifest as an enlarged left supraclavicular lymph node (Virchow's node) or an enlarged left anterior axillary lymph node, enlarged periumbilical lymph nodes (Sister Mary Joseph's node), an enlarged ovary (Krukenberg's tumor), or a mass on Blumer's shelf on rectal examination.

DIAGNOSTICS

An upper gastrointestinal endoscopy is the imaging modality of choice for stomach tumors because it allows direct visualization and biopsy of the tumor.[17] A minimum of four biopsies of the lesion should be made; diagnostic accuracy approaches 100% with 10 biopsies.[17] After diagnosis, staging is performed to determine the presence of local spread or distant metastasis. The metastatic evaluation includes liver biochemical assays, abdominal CT scanning, and biopsy of suspected nodes.[8] Blood studies may reveal hypochromic, microcytic anemia secondary to iron deficiency. The stool is often positive for occult blood.

DIAGNOSTICS

Stomach Tumors

LABORATORY
LFTs
CBC and differential
Stool for occult blood

IMAGING
Contrast radiographs
CT scan of abdomen

OTHER
Endoscopy and biopsy

DIFFERENTIAL DIAGNOSIS

The differential diagnosis for tumors of the stomach includes gastric lymphoma; leiomyosarcoma; and gastric metastasis from the lung, breast, and melanoma. Kaposi's sarcoma of the stomach, which may be present in patients with AIDS, and hypertrophic gastropathy (Meniere's disease) are also included in the differential diagnosis.

DIFFERENTIAL DIAGNOSIS

Stomach Tumors

- Gastric lymphoma
- Leiomyosarcoma
- Gastric metastasis
- Kaposi's sarcoma of the stomach
- Hypertrophic gastropathy

MANAGEMENT

Gastroenterologic, surgical, and oncologic consultations are essential for a patient with gastric cancer. Complete resection of the gastric carcinoma and adjacent lymph nodes offers the only chance for cure. A palliative resection should be considered for patients with advanced lesions who are initially seen with obstruction or bleeding. Obstruction and dysphagia from large carcinomas of the gastric cardia can be managed by laser coagulation, which results in recanalization of the lumen and the relief of obstructive symptoms.[18]

Because gastric cancers are radioresistant, adequate control of the tumor requires doses of radiation that exceed the tolerance of the surrounding structures.[13] Therefore moderate doses of radiation are used only for symptom palliation. Adjuvant chemotherapy in gastric cancer appears to offer no advantage for survival after a curative resection.[8,15]

COMPLICATIONS

Gastric carcinomas are detected at an advanced stage, and the prognosis of this neoplasm remains poor. Ovarian metastases occur in approximately 10% of gastric cancers and may be associated with ovarian dysfunction such as virilization.[13] Intraperitoneal dissemination of the tumor may occur with involvement of the omentum, peritoneum, and serosa of the intestine.

PATIENT AND FAMILY EDUCATION

Although gastric tumors and small colon tumors may be associated with aging, cancer can affect younger patients. Weight loss, anorexia, difficulty swallowing, abdominal pain, a change in bowel habits, and blood in the stool are all signs of gastrointestinal cancers. Patients should be reminded to notify their health care provider if any of these symptoms occurs. In addition, patients should routinely be asked about a family history of gastrointestinal or other cancers.

HEALTH PROMOTION

A well-balanced diet rich in fruits and vegetables is important for overall good health. Such a diet will provide sufficient vitamins and antioxidants to maintain health. Consumption of smoked and highly salted, nitrated food should be avoided or severely limited. Only food that is refrigerated and kept under safe conditions should be consumed. Avoidance of all tobacco products is strongly recommended.[9,19]

Because infectious agents have been associated with gastric cancer, it is important to practice good hygiene. Diagnosis of *H. pylori* infection and subsequent treatment also contribute to a reduction in the incidence of gastric cancer.[19]

Exposure to glycol ethers, hydraulic fluids, and leaded gasoline should also be limited. Education of the public along with increasing protection and surveillance in the workplace will limit or eliminate exposure to these products.[19]

TUMORS OF THE SMALL INTESTINE

DEFINITION AND EPIDEMIOLOGY

Cancer of the small bowel is not as common as other gastrointestinal cancers, although small bowel cancers may be more difficult to diagnose.[20] Adenocarcinomas of the small intestine account for 40% to 50% of malignancies of the small bowel.[5,17,20] After resection of small bowel adenocarcinomas, there is a 5-year survival rate of 20%.[21] The peak incidence of symptomatic tumors is in the sixth decade of life.[21] The highest rate of small bowel adenocarcinoma occurs in African-American men.[21] Other malignant neoplasms of the small intestine include carcinoid tumors, lymphomas, and leiomyosarcomas.[3] All carcinoid tumors should be considered malignant. Metastasis occurs in up to 90% of patients with carcinoid tumors larger than 2 cm (0.8 inch).[22] More than 95% of all gastrointestinal carcinoids occur in the appendix, rectum, and small intestine.[23]

The three most common benign tumors of the small intestine are adenomas, leiomyomas, and lipomas.[3,21] Multiple adenomas may occur in the small intestine in Peutz-Jeghers syndrome and are considered benign; however, in 2% to 3% of these patients, adenocarcinoma develops.[3]

Risk factors for adenocarcinoma of the small bowel include Crohn's disease, sprue, ileostomy stomas, pouches and conduits, familial adenomatous polyposis, and Peutz-Jeghers syndrome.[8,23] Patients with Crohn's disease have a 100-fold increased risk of developing carcinoma of the small bowel, and adenocarcinoma develops 10 years earlier than expected for this malignancy.[3]

PATHOPHYSIOLOGY

Adenocarcinomas of the small intestine may be polypoid, ulcerative, or annular and stenosing. The tumors infiltrate through the bowel wall and invade adjacent organs. Venous invasion of the lymph nodes occurs via either metastasis or direct extension of the tumor.

Carcinoid tumors are well-differentiated endocrine tumors that arise from the enterochromaffin cells at the base of Lieberkühn's crypts. These cells give the tumor its most clinically distinctive feature—its ability to secrete tumor products that induce the carcinoid syndrome.[3,21,23] Serotonin is believed to be the humoral mediator responsible for the diarrhea that occurs with carcinoid syndrome.[3] Serotonin is deaminated by monoamine oxidase to 5-hydroxyindoleacetic acid (5-HIAA), which is excreted in the urine.[3] The right side of the heart is exposed to the effects of tumor products that have been released into the vena cava from hepatic metastases. Endocardial fibrosis may occur as a result, forming plaques on the tricuspid and pulmonic valves, the endocardium of the right cardiac chambers, the vena cava, the coronary sinus, and the pulmonary artery.[3]

CLINICAL PRESENTATION

With both benign and malignant small bowel tumors, abdominal pain is the most common symptom. Other symptoms include nausea, vomiting, cramping abdominal pain, abdominal distention aggravated by eating, and weight loss. Unless patients manifest the carcinoid syndrome—characterized by flushing, diarrhea, wheezing, and sweating—no specific signs or symptoms suggest the diagnosis.[17]

PHYSICAL EXAMINATION

A palpable abdominal mass may be present in up to 40% of patients with a small bowel malignancy.[23] Duodenal adenocarcinomas that involve Vater's ampulla may cause obstructive jaundice or pancreatitis.[3,21] Hepatomegaly, ascites, and jaundice indicate advanced metastatic disease. Pulmonic stenosis may cause a systolic murmur in patients with carcinoid syndrome.[3]

DIAGNOSTICS

In the evaluation of small bowel tumors, the stool should be tested for occult blood. However, the diagnostic modality of choice is a small bowel follow-through (SBFT), an extension of the conventional barium meal in which the barium is ingested orally.[23] Enteroclysis, synonymous with a small bowel enema, may be performed by infusing approximately 1 L of barium until bowel distention occurs and the barium reaches the terminal ileum.[23] Enteroclysis is superior to SBFT in the diagnosis of small bowel disease, except for lesions of the terminal ileum.

Additional studies after barium radiology may be indicated and include CT scanning, arteriography, serotonin and metabolite levels, scintigraphy, endoscopy, and possibly capsule endoscopy.[23,24] Endoscopy is indicated for duodenal lesions that are accessible with gastroduodenoscopy and for terminal ileal lesions accessible with colonoscopy. A CT scan is indicated to determine metastasis, including hepatic involvement, by possible malignant tumors. Arteriography is indicated in cases of obscure gastrointestinal bleeding. Measurement of serotonin and metabolites (5-HIAA), as well as scintigraphy, may be necessary for suspected carcinoid tumors.[23] A

DIAGNOSTICS

Small Intestine Tumors

LABORATORY
CBC and differential
Stool for occult blood
Serotonin and metabolites (5-HIAA)*

IMAGING
Small bowel follow-through
Enteroclysis
Endoscopy*
Capsule endoscopy*
Arteriography*
Scintigraphy*
CT scan*

OTHER
Laparotomy*

*If indicated.

laparotomy may be necessary when the diagnostic modalities are insufficient.

DIFFERENTIAL DIAGNOSIS

Small bowel tumors may be considered one of the less common causes of intestinal obstruction, occult gastrointestinal blood loss, weight loss, and unexplained abdominal pain. The diagnosis of a small bowel tumor often is not made before laparotomy. Therefore the differential diagnosis includes adhesions, hernias, intussusception, volvulus, intraabdominal abscesses and hematomas, endometriosis, pelvic inflammatory disease, Crohn's disease, ischemia, hematoma associated with oral anticoagulant therapy, radiation enteritis, amyloidosis, ingested foreign bodies, gallstones, bezoars, and worms.

MANAGEMENT

Gastroenterologic, oncologic, and surgical consultations are essential to provide optimum care for patients with small bowel tumors. These cancers are managed surgically, which offers the only hope for cure. Because adenocarcinomas metastasize early to regional lymph nodes, a wide resection is undertaken.[23] If the lesions cannot be resected for cure, a palliative resection of the main lesion is recommended. Chemotherapy and radiotherapy yield minimum benefit.[23] The 5-year survival rate for adenocarcinoma of the small bowel is not greater than 20%, even after curative resection.[23]

Because carcinoid tumors greater than 1 cm (0.4 inch) in diameter are capable of metastasizing, a wide resection should be undertaken. Nonresectable intestinal and hepatic metastatic carcinoids should have aggressive debulking to alleviate symptoms of the carcinoid syndrome and possibly prolong survival.[23] Carcinoid syndrome may be treated with injections of octreotide (a synthetic somatostatin analog that is a serotonin antagonist) to provide symptomatic relief until surgical management of the carcinoid tumor can be performed.[17,22,23] Hepatic artery embolization with combination chemotherapy and interferon-γ may control symptoms of carcinoid syndrome.[22]

DIFFERENTIAL DIAGNOSIS

Small Intestine Tumors

- Adhesions
- Hernias
- Intussusception
- Volvulus
- Intraabdominal abscess or hematoma
- Endometriosis
- Pelvic inflammatory disease
- Crohn's disease
- Ischemia
- Hematoma associated with oral anticoagulant therapy
- Radiation enteritis
- Amyloidosis
- Foreign body, bezoars, worms
- Gallstones
- Malignant tumors (including lymphoma)
- Benign tumors

INDICATIONS FOR REFERRAL OR HOSPITALIZATION

Large lesions of the small intestine may produce partial or intermittent obstruction, bleeding, intussusception, and volvulus. Carcinoid tumors spread locally to regional lymph nodes, the liver, other intraabdominal organs, and the lung. Small carcinoid tumors normally do not invade or obstruct the bowel lumen but can penetrate the muscle layer and lead to adhesions, bowel kinking, angulation, and obstruction. Massive fibrosis of the mesenteries, omentum, and peritoneum may result from the leakage of serotonin and other vasoactive substances. High serum levels of 5-HIAA may cause endocardial fibrotic plaques that stiffen and fix the tricuspid and pulmonic valves, which may lead to right-sided heart failure.[3]

PATIENT AND FAMILY EDUCATION

Patient and family education for tumors of the small intestine is the same as for tumors of the stomach, p. 724.

HEALTH PROMOTION

Please see the Health Promotion section for Tumors of the Colon, p. 725.

TUMORS OF THE COLON

DEFINITION AND EPIDEMIOLOGY

Colorectal cancer is the third most common cancer in the United States and is the second leading cause of cancer deaths.[8,25,26] Approximately 55,000 men and women in the United States die each year from colorectal cancer.[27] Adenocarcinomas account for more than 95% of all malignant tumors of the large bowel.[8] Risk factors for the development of colorectal cancer include prior colorectal cancer; ulcerative colitis; hereditary and genetic factors; familial polyposis syndromes; history of breast or female genital cancer; and a high-fat, low-bulk diet. Benign tumors of the colon include polyps and polyposis syndromes.

PATHOPHYSIOLOGY

Colorectal adenocarcinomas may be polypoid, ulcerating, or infiltrative. Adenocarcinomas of the colon form well-differentiated glands and secrete large amounts of mucin.[25] Signet-ring cells, in which a large vacuole of mucin displaces the nucleus to one side, may be present in some tumors.[3,22,25] Colorectal carcinoma can spread intraluminally or via direct extension, hematogenous spread, lymphatic dissemination, or transperitoneal seeding.

Genetic alterations in malignancy include deletions, amplifications, and single-nucleotide mutations; *ras* point mutations are observed in almost half of all colon cancers and in approximately one third of patients with familial adenomatous polyposis. The *ras* genes encode for proteins located on the inner surface of the plasma membrane, bind guanine nucleotides, and are involved in signal transduction from the cell membrane to the nucleus.[22] Mutations located at critical positions in the gene alter the *ras* protein so that signal transduction is unregulated, which leads to additional cell growth. A mutation at just one of three codons—12, 13, and 61—of the *Kras2* gene is the mechanism via which the *ras* oncogene is activated in many colorectal neoplasms.[28]

The gene most responsible for malignant conversion of benign colonic neoplasms appears to be *p53*. The tumor suppressor *p53* gene prevents nuclear replication after injuries that are likely to damage the DNA. In the presence of damaged DNA the level of *p53* protein rises in the cell, and progression into the cell cycle is prevented.[22] The cell then repairs the damage, or programmed cell death ensues. Inactivation of the *p53* gene permits mutated DNA to be replicated and removes the restraint on abnormal cell behavior. Mutations of the *p53* gene are probably some of the most common and most powerful tumor-causing genetic lesions.

Other genetic abnormalities in malignant colonic tumors include the high expression of the *c-Myc* oncogene, deletion of the *DCC* ("deleted in colon cancer") gene, and mutation of the *MCC* ("mutated in colon cancer") gene.[3,28] The loss of heterozygosity, which refers to the deletion of one chromosomal allele, has been observed in colon carcinoma on the genes of chromosomes 17 and 18.[28] The *MCC* gene has shown mutations in colon cancer and is located on chromosome 5 in the same region as the familial adenomatous polyposis gene.[3]

CLINICAL PRESENTATION

The symptoms of colon carcinoma depend on the location of the tumor. Cancers of the proximal colon usually attain a larger size before becoming symptomatic compared with cancers of the left colon and rectum. Fatigue; shortness of breath; angina caused by hypochromic, microcytic anemia; and a melanotic, liquid stool may be the principal means of presentation of right-sided colonic masses. Abdominal discomfort may be present as the tumor increases in size. Obstruction is uncommon because of the large diameters of the cecum and ascending colon. The left colon has a smaller lumen than the proximal colon, and therefore obstructive symptoms may occur. Left-sided symptoms include cramps, gas pain, and a decrease in the caliber of the stool. Carcinomas of the descending and sigmoid colon are often circumferential and may also cause obstruction.

Patients with colon carcinoma may experience colicky abdominal pain, especially after meals, and a change in bowel habits. Constipation may alternate with an increased frequency of defecation. Hematochezia may be present with distal rather than proximal lesions, and bright red blood passed via the rectum may be seen with cancers that involve the left colon and rectum. Approximately half of patients with colon cancer experience anorexia and weight loss.

PHYSICAL EXAMINATION

Patients may initially be seen with a palpable abdominal mass and signs of distention or intestinal obstruction. Supraclavicular nodes may be positive with left-sided cancer, and the liver may be enlarged because of metastasis.[3,22]

DIAGNOSTICS

Visual inspection and digital examination of the anus and distal rectum are important in the evaluation of colorectal tumors to permit palpation of a possible tumor and to obtain stool to test for occult blood. A CBC should also be obtained. The air-contrast barium enema is used initially to detect polyps and cancers of the colon.[17,28] However, the sensitivity of the barium enema is directly related to the diligence of the radiologist. If the air-contrast barium enema is negative, a colonoscopy must be performed.[28] A colonoscopy, as well as flexible sigmoidoscopy, allows for direct visualization and biopsy of the colon.[17] Virtual colonoscopy, which is a high-resolution CT scan, is a promising new screening tool that is in trial.[29] However, there are continued concerns that virtual colonoscopy may not detect small tumors. The CEA is not a useful screening test but is a valuable marker for recurring cancer.[10] The metastatic evaluation includes a CT scan, a chest x-ray study, and liver function tests.[5,17]

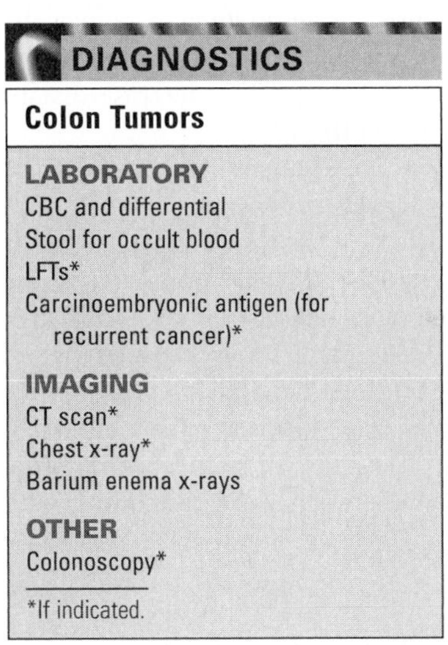

DIAGNOSTICS

Colon Tumors

LABORATORY
CBC and differential
Stool for occult blood
LFTs*
Carcinoembryonic antigen (for recurrent cancer)*

IMAGING
CT scan*
Chest x-ray*
Barium enema x-rays

OTHER
Colonoscopy*

*If indicated.

DIFFERENTIAL DIAGNOSIS

The differential diagnosis of colon carcinoma includes benign tumors, diverticulitis, ulcerative colitis, Crohn's disease, tuberculosis, amebiasis, fungal masses, schistosomiasis, viral lesions such as cytomegalovirus, feces, lymphoid polyps and lymphoma, carcinoid tumors, metastatic lesions, and Kaposi's sarcoma. Obstructing lesions may include strictures from inflammation, radiation and ischemic colitis, and volvulus. In addition, extrinsic compression may occur from endometriosis and pancreatitis.

MANAGEMENT

Gastroenterologic, oncologic, and surgical consultations are necessary to provide optimum care for patients with colorectal

DIFFERENTIAL DIAGNOSIS

Colon Tumors

- Benign tumors
- Diverticulitis
- Ulcerative colitis
- Crohn's disease
- Tuberculosis
- Amebiasis
- Fungal masses
- Schistosomiasis
- Viral or metastatic lesions
- Feces
- Lymphoid polyps, lymphoma
- Carcinoid tumors
- Kaposi's sarcoma
- Inflammatory bowel disease
- Strictures
- Extrinsic compression from endometriosis or pancreatitis

tumors. The primary treatment of colorectal cancer is surgical intervention with wide resection (hemicolectomy) and removal of regional lymph nodes.[28] Adjuvant chemotherapy for colon cancer has been used in an attempt to reduce the recurrence rate of metastatic disease.[28] It has been shown to decrease the recurrence rate by 30% and to decrease distant metastasis by 50% in stage II and III disease.[30]

The use of radiotherapy as an adjunctive treatment is not beneficial for colon cancers outside of the rectum.[28] The CEA sample should be drawn before removal of a primary tumor because not all cancers produce this glycoprotein. If the preoperative value is not elevated, the test is not informative in the postoperative period. If the CEA is elevated before surgery, the CEA should be repeated 1 month after surgery for tumor recurrence (if the physician and patient are willing to undertake repeat surgery).[28] Detection of recurrence by serial CEA has been shown to occur between 1 and 18 months, with a median of 3 months.[31]

COMPLICATIONS

Colorectal cancer may cause large bowel obstruction or perforation in cancers that reach an advanced stage.[3] Rate of recurrence within the abdominal cavity, including liver metastasis, is high.[31] Distant metastases, which are thought to be disseminated via hematogenous spread, may occur to the lungs, adrenal glands, bones, and brain.[31] Weight loss, fatigue, rectal bleeding, abdominal and pelvic pain, coughing, a change in bowel habits, and bone pain may signal recurrent disease.

PATIENT AND FAMILY EDUCATION

Because 10% of tumors are palpated rectally, annual digital rectal examinations should be started at 40 years of age.[10] Annual testing for fecal occult blood should also start at age 40. Also recommended is a sigmoidoscopy at age 45, or 8 years younger than the youngest family member afflicted with colon cancer, and then every 3 years thereafter. In patients with familial polyposis of the colon, colorectal cancer is inevitable 10 to 15 years after the onset of polyposis, and elective complete colectomy is required. Other family members must be screened for the dominant inheritance pattern.[8] The American Cancer Society recommends that routine screening for colon cancer begin at 50 years of age with annual fecal occult blood testing, a sigmoidoscopy every 5 years, and a colonoscopy every 10 years.[32,33] If polyps are present, a repeat flexible sigmoidoscopy is indicated in 3 years. However, the guidelines may differ for older patients.[34]

Individuals at high risk for the development of colon carcinoma, such as those with familial polyposis syndrome, prior adenomatous colonic polyps or cancer, or longstanding ulcerative colitis involving the entire colon, may require screening before age 40 and more frequent periodic screening tests (including examination of the entire colon) (see Chapter 20).[8,33]

Healthy diets with increased fiber and decreased fat intake may help prevent colon cancer. Therefore these diets should be explained and encouraged routinely.

To detect the postoperative recurrence of colorectal carcinoma, patients should be evaluated every 3 months for 2 years with history, CEA, and physical examination and then every 6 months for 2 more years.[10] A screening colonoscopy should also be performed 1 year after surgery and, if normal, then every 3 years.[10]

HEALTH PROMOTION

Promotion of a healthy lifestyle is essential in the prevention of colorectal cancer. Patients should be encouraged to exercise on a regular basis—30 minutes at least three times weekly. More vigorous exercise may provide more benefit. A diet that provides five servings of fruits and vegetables and is low in red meat will help minimize the risk of colorectal cancer. It is important to limit the fat intake to 25% to 30% of the total caloric intake and to increase the amount of fiber to 20 to 30 g/day. These recommendations will help maintain a normal body weight. Avoidance of tobacco products and heavy alcohol consumption is also important.[9]

REFERENCES

1. Patti M, Tedesco P: *Esophageal cancer*, 2005, retrieved June 29, 2006, from http://www.emedicine.com/med/topic741.htm.
2. Kirby TJ, Rice TW: The epidemiology of esophageal carcinoma: the changing face of a disease, *Chest Surg Clin North Am* 4(2):217-225, 1994.
3. Rubin E, Farber JL: The gastrointestinal tract. In Rubin E, Farber JL, editors: *Pathology*, ed 2, Philadelphia, 1994, Lippincott.
4. Reid BJ, Thomas CR: Esophageal neoplasms. In Yamada T, editor: *Textbook of gastroenterology*, ed 2, Philadelphia, 1995, Lippincott.
5. Fox JR, Kuwada S: Today's approach to esophageal cancer: what is the role of the primary care physician? *Postgrad Med* 107(5):109-114, 2000.
6. Quinn KL, Reedy A: Esophageal cancer: therapeutic approaches and nursing care, *Semin Oncol Nurs* 15(1):17-25, 1999.
7. Brooks-Brunn J: Esophageal cancer: an overview, *Med Surg Nurs* 9(5):248-254, 2000.
8. Barron T, and others: Gastrointestinal disease. In Andreoli TE, Plum F, Bennett CJ, and others, editors: *Cecil essentials of medicine*, ed 4, Philadelphia, 1997, Saunders.
9. Byers T, Nestle M, McTiernan A, and others: American Cancer Society guidelines on nutrition and physical activity for cancer prevention: reducing the risk of cancer with healthy food choices and physical activity, *Cancer* 52(2):92-119, 2002, retrieved Jan 13, 2006 from

http://www.ncbi.nlm.nih.gov/entrez/query.fcgi?db=pubmed&cmd=Search&itool=pubmed_AbstractPlus&term=%22American+Cancer+Society+2001+Nutrition+and+Physical+Activity+Guidelines+Advisory+Committee%22%5BCorporate+Author%5D.

10. Blackbourne LH: Thoracic surgery: esophageal carcinoma. In Blackbourne LH, editor: *Surgical recall,* Baltimore, 1994, Williams & Wilkins.
11. Clark GWB, Ireland AP, Hagan JA, and others: Carcinoembryonic antigen measurements in the management of esophageal cancer: an indicator of subclinical recurrence, *Am J Surg* 170(6):597-600, 1995.
12. Mehta VK, Fisher G: *Gastric cancer*, 2006, retrieved June 29, 2006, from http://www.emedicine.com/med/topic845.htm.
13. Davis GR: Neoplasms of the stomach. In Sleisenger MH, Fordtran J, editors: *Gastrointestinal disease,* ed 5, Philadelphia, 1993, Saunders.
14. Orringer MB: Complications of esophageal surgery. In Zuidema GD, editor: *Shackelford's surgery of the alimentary tract,* ed 4, Philadelphia, 1996, Saunders.
15. Hermans J, Bonenkamp JJ, Boon MC, and others: Adjuvant therapy after curative resection for gastric cancer: meta-analysis of randomized trials, *J Clin Oncol* 11(8):1441-1447, 1993.
16. Albert C: Clinical aspects of gastric cancer. In Rustgi AK, editor: *Gastrointestinal cancers: biology, diagnosis, and therapy,* Philadelphia, 1995, Lippincott-Raven.
17. Karp SJ, Morris J, Soybel D: Esophagus. In Marino BS, editor: *Blueprints in surgery,* Malden, Mass, 1988, Blackwell Science.
18. Fuchs CS, Mayer RJ: Gastric carcinoma, *N Engl J Med* 333(1):32-41, 1995.
19. Christian TK, Stadlander H, Waterbor JW: Molecular epidemiology, pathogenesis and prevention of gastric cancer, *Carcinogenesis* 20(12):2195-2207, 1999.
20. Chandra RV, Miller JA, Jones IT, and others: Small bowel malignancy, an elusive diagnosis, *MJA* 180:182-183, 2004, retrieved July 2, 2006, from http://www.mja.com.au/public/issues/180_04_160204/cha10429_fm.pdf.
21. Greager JA, and others: Neoplasms of the small intestine. In Zuidema GD, editor: *Shackelford's surgery of the alimentary tract,* ed 4, Philadelphia, 1996, Saunders.
22. Marshall JB, Bodnarchuk G: Carcinoid tumors of the gut: our experience over 3 decades and review of the literature, *J Clin Gastroenterol* 16(2):123-129, 1993.
23. Lance PL: Tumors and other neoplastic diseases of the small bowel. In Yamada T, editor: *Textbook of gastroenterology,* ed 2, Philadelphia, 1995, Lippincott.
24. Costamagna G, Shah SK, Riccione ME, and others: A prospective trial comparing small bowel radiographs and video capsule endoscopy for suspected small bowel disease, *Gastroenterology* 123:999-1005, 2002.
25. Bresalier RS, Kim YS: Malignant neoplasms of the large intestine. In Sleisenger MH, Fordtran JS, editors: *Gastrointestinal disease: pathophysiology, diagnosis, management,* ed 5, Philadelphia, 1993, Saunders.
26. El-Diery WS: *Colon cancer, adenocarcinoma*, 2006, retrieved June 29, 2006, from http://www.emedicine.com/med/topic413.htm.
27. Winawer SJ: New colorectal cancer screening guidelines, *Gastroenterology* 124(2):544-560, 2003.
28. Boland CR: Malignant tumors of the colon. In Yamada T, editor: *Textbook of gastroenterology,* ed 2, Philadelphia, 1995, Lippincott.
29. Kuwada S: Colorectal cancer 2000, *Postgrad Med* 107(5):96-107, 2000.
30. Stefanik DC, Muscari E: Colon cancer, *Am J Nurs* April(Suppl):36-40, 2000.
31. Averbach AM, Sugarbaker PH: Use of tumor markers and radiologic tests in follow-up. In Cohen AM, Winawer SJ, editors: *Cancer of the colon, rectum, and anus,* New York, 1995, McGraw-Hill.
32. Ransohoff DF, Sandler RS: Screening for colorectal cancer, *N Engl J Med* 346(1):40-44, 2002.
33. American Cancer Society: *American Cancer Society guidelines for the early detection of cancer,* retrieved Jan 13, 2007 from http://www.cancer.org/docroot/PED/content/PED_2_3X_ACS_Cancer_Detection_Guidelines_36.asp.
34. Lin OS, Kozarek RA, Schembre DB, and others: Screening colonoscopy in very elderly patients: presence of neoplasia and impact of life expectancy, *JAMA* 295:2357-2365, 2006.

CHAPTER 152

Ulcer Disease

Donna M. Glynn

DEFINITION AND EPIDEMIOLOGY

Peptic ulcer disease is a pathologic, destructive, chronic disorder characterized by ulceration of the gastric and duodenal mucosa. The two common causes of peptic ulcers in the United States are *Helicobacter pylori* infection and NSAID use. Gastric and duodenal ulcers have had a serious impact on the economics of health care and society because of recurrence, increased office visits, medication costs, diagnostic costs, and patient quality-of-life concerns. Therefore it is essential to obtain a thorough health history, identify potential risk factors, and provide a cost-effective diagnosis and treatment plan.

Ulcer disease may be defined as an imbalance both in the amount of acid-pepsin production and in the ability of the gastric and duodenal lining to protect itself. Peptic ulcer disease affects 6.5 million individuals in the United States. *H. pylori*, a gram-negative rod first identified by Warren and Marshall in 1983, is a major causative organism in the development of ulcer disease.[1] The prevalence of *H. pylori* in the United States is approximately 30% of the population. *H. pylori* infection is a benign condition in many individuals and manifests as the causative agent in the development of peptic ulcer disease and gastric cancer in others. The second most common cause of ulcer disease is NSAID usage. NSAIDs are a commonly prescribed medication and account for more than 70 million prescriptions per year. It is estimated that 14 million to 20 million patients take an NSAID or aspirin daily, which increases the risk of mucosal damage. Approximately 15% of all patients using NSAIDs will suffer a gastrointestinal injury, resulting in 70,000 hospitalizations and 10,000 to 20,000 deaths per year.[2] COX-2 inhibitors are generally considered safer to the gastrointestinal tract; however, this class of medications commonly prescribed for arthritis pain can also cause gastric or duodenal ulcer formation and has been related to adverse cardiovascular events.

Other risk factors for the development of ulcer disease include family history, cigarette smoking, chronic obstructive pulmonary disease, caffeine ingestion, alcohol, cirrhosis, and stress. Certain conditions and genetic factors have also been identified as risk factors for the development of peptic ulcer disease. Zollinger-Ellison syndrome, a condition that causes increased acid production, results in ulcer disease. Genetic risk factors include first-degree relatives with ulcer disease, blood group O, elevated levels of pepsinogen I, the presence of HLA-B5 antigen, and decreased red blood cell acetylcholinesterase.[3]

PATHOPHYSIOLOGY

The function of the gastrointestinal tract is the digestion of food and absorption of nutrients. This process is achieved by high concentrations of acid and pepsin that are secreted from the parietal cells of the stomach. The surface of the mucosa secretes alkaline mucus that protects the mucosa from self-digestion. However, when this system is interrupted, the protective tissue is damaged and erosion or ulcer formation occurs. Gastric ulcers are commonly found distal to the junction between the antrum and the acid secretory mucosa. Duodenal ulcers are primarily located in the duodenal bulb or within 3 cm (1.2 inches) of the pyloric duodenal junction and are usually less than 1 cm (0.4 inch) in diameter. Reducing the production of acid and pepsin is key to the promotion of healing and prevention of recurrence.

H. pylori, a spiral-shaped flagellated organism, is acquired via the orofecal route. Once ingested, *H. pylori* attaches to the gastric mucosa and produces local tissue injury, resulting in the release of cytotoxins and proteases.[4]

CLINICAL PRESENTATION

Although some patients are asymptomatic, the most common presenting chief complaint is epigastric pain. This discomfort is often described as a sharp, burning, aching, gnawing pain occurring 1½ to 3 hours after meals or in the middle of the night. The patient will report that the pain is usually relieved with the ingestion of food or antacids; however, the symptoms are recurrent, with episodes lasting from hours to days to months. Changes in the intensity, duration, or location of the pain may indicate penetration or perforation of an ulcer. Symptoms of nausea and vomiting are rare. Ironically, weight gain is not uncommon because the ingestion of food alleviates the pain.

PHYSICAL EXAMINATION

Inspection, auscultation, and percussion generally yield negative findings. In rare presentations, auscultation may reveal a succession splash 4 hours or longer after meals, which would indicate a duodenal or pyloric channel ulcer, causing gastric outlet obstruction. Palpation may produce epigastric tenderness midline between the umbilicus and xiphoid process. If a perforation has occurred, the patient will have a rigid abdomen and generalized rebound tenderness. Rectal examination should be included with testing for melena.

DIAGNOSTICS

A CBC will exclude anemia. Serum culture for *H. pylori* is also indicated initially. C-urea breath testing is a noninvasive method for identifying *H. pylori*. It is important to determine the use of over-the-counter proton pump inhibitors (PPIs), since the breath test will be inaccurate if the patient has used this treatment during the past 2 weeks. Fecal urea testing can distinguish current infection from past infection, similar to the breath testing.[5]

DIAGNOSTICS

Ulcer Disease

LABORATORY
CBC and differential
Helicobacter pylori testing
Serum
- C-urea breath test
- Fecal urea testing

Stool for occult blood

OTHER
Endoscopy*

*If indicated.

Patients over age 50 with ulcer symptoms should have an upper endoscopy to exclude malignancy and obtain biopsies for *H. pylori*.[6] For younger patients who respond to treatment expeditiously, endoscopy is not indicated.

DIFFERENTIAL DIAGNOSIS

DIFFERENTIAL DIAGNOSIS

Ulcer Disease

- Cholecystitis
- Diverticulosis
- Irritable bowel syndrome
- Nonulcer dyspepsia
- Gastroesophageal reflux disease
- Pancreatitis
- Malignancy
- Zollinger-Ellison syndrome

Differential diagnosis for peptic ulcer disease is based on the symptoms reported and the location of the pain. Cholecystitis manifests as right upper quadrant abdominal discomfort. Vague abdominal pain with reports of diarrhea or constipation may be associated with diverticulosis, irritable bowel syndrome, or nonulcer dyspepsia. Gastroesophageal reflux disease, pancreatitis, and malignancy should also be considered. Zollinger-Ellison syndrome is a condition of excessive acid production. This should be considered if the individual does not respond to the traditional diet, smoking cessation, and pharmacologic therapy.

MANAGEMENT

First-line treatment of peptic ulcer disease is a 2-week trial of antiulcer therapy. If NSAID or COX-2 inhibitor use is documented, the medications should be discontinued. **If objective findings include anemia, gastrointestinal bleeding, rigid abdomen, weight loss, or new-onset dyspepsia in an individual older than 50 years of age, an immediate physician consultation is indicated.** If symptoms persist after the 2-week course of therapy, referral to a gastroenterologist for endoscopy is appropriate. Recent studies support endoscopy over barium-contrast radiography as having higher rates of detecting pathologic conditions, including *H. pylori*, through direct observation and biopsy.[7]

Treatment options of peptic ulcer disease include H_2-receptor antagonists (H_2RA), PPIs, and prostaglandin therapy. The H_2RAs include cimetidine, famotidine, nizatidine, and ranitidine. These preparations inhibit gastric acid secretion by blocking the H_2-receptors of the parietal cells. H_2RA therapy is associated with 75% to 98% healing rate over a 4- to 6-week period in documented peptic ulcer disease. Therapy needs to be continued with maintenance dosing at bedtime for 1 year to prevent recurrence. H_2RA therapy is available over the counter, which presents new challenges for health care providers. Again, an in-depth history that includes over-the-counter medication use is extremely important when contemplating treatment options.

PPIs are the most potent and most expensive treatment option for peptic ulcer disease. Omeprazole, lansoprazole, rabeprazole, and esomeprazole are effective in blocking the production of acid secretion. Daily dosing eliminates acid production and also improves patient compliance. Investigation of over-the-counter medication use is once again required, since omeprazole is available for purchase without prescription.

Prostaglandin therapy protects the gastric-duodenal mucosa and should be considered for individuals with documented peptic ulcer disease who are unable to discontinue NSAID use. Misoprostol is the only available agent for the prevention of NSAID-induced gastric ulcers. It inhibits acid production and prevents duodenal damage. The therapeutic dose has been shown to produce transient side effects of cramping and diarrhea, which can be eliminated with a lower dose. Sucralfate is also indicated for treatment of active duodenal ulcer and maintenance of healed duodenal ulcers.

Treatment options for *H. pylori* eradication continue to be closely evaluated for efficacy and compliance. Bismuth, once widely used, is now considered only for cases refractory to treatment. No one regimen has been proved to be more effective than any other, but current studies support the use of two-antibiotic preparations, which produce higher efficacy and coverage for resistant organisms.[8] Although there are other appropriate treatment regimens (Box 152-1), one that is

BOX 152-1

HELICOBACTER PYLORI TREATMENT OPTIONS

1. Bismuth 2 tablets q.i.d.
   Metronidazole 250 mg t.i.d. or q.i.d.
   Tetracycline 500 mg q.i.d.
   Omeprazole 20 mg b.i.d.
   Duration: 1 week
   Cost: $
   Efficacy 94%-98%
2. Bismuth 2 tablets q.i.d.
   Metronidazole 250 mg t.i.d. or q.i.d.
   Tetracycline 500 mg q.i.d.
   H_2-receptor antagonist therapy as directed for 1 month
   Duration: 2 weeks
   Cost: $
   Efficacy >90%
3. Bismuth 2 tablets q.i.d.
   Tetracycline 500 mg q.i.d.
   Clarithromycin 500 mg t.i.d.
   H_2-receptor antagonist h.s.
   Duration: 2 weeks
   Cost: $$$
   Efficacy >90%
4. Bismuth 2 tablets q.i.d.*
   Tetracycline 500 mg q.i.d.
   Metronidazole 500 mg t.i.d.
   Omeprazole 20 mg b.i.d.
   Duration: 1 week
   Cost: $
   Efficacy >90%
5. Bismuth 2 tablets q.i.d.
   Clarithromycin 500 mg t.i.d.
   Tetracycline 500 mg q.i.d.
   Duration: 1-2 weeks
   Cost: $ 1 week
   $$ 2 weeks
   Efficacy >90%
6. Ranitidine bismuth citrate 400 mg b.i.d. for 1 month
   Clarithromycin 500 mg t.i.d. for 2 weeks
   Durations: As above
   Cost: $$
   Efficacy 82%

Modified from NIH Consensus Development Panel on *Helicobacter pylori* in Peptic Ulcer Disease: NIH consensus conference: *Helicobacter pylori* in peptic ulcer disease, *JAMA* 272, 1994.

Cost: $, $100; $$, $100-$200, $$$ >$200.

*Requires 3 days of pretreatment with omeprazole before antibiotic therapy.

frequently used consists of a PPI, amoxicillin 1 g PO b.i.d., and clarithromycin, 500 mg PO b.i.d. for 2 weeks.[8] For penicillin allergic patients, metronidazole 500 mg PO b.i.d. is recommended.[9] An alternate regimen proposed by the American College of Gastroenterology consists of a PPI, bismuth 525 mg PO q.i.d., metronidazole 500 mg PO q.i.d., and tetracycline 500 mg PO t.i.d. for 2 weeks.[9] PPI therapy has documented improved efficacy over the H_2RAs, but cost and adherence must be considered before initiating therapy.[10]

COMPLICATIONS

Perforation of gastric or duodenal ulcers is a life-threatening complication of chronic ulcer disease. This is most common in older patients and requires emergency care. Other complications include hemorrhage, gastric ulcer obstruction, and ulcers refractory to treatment.

INDICATIONS FOR REFERRAL OR HOSPITALIZATION

Gastroenterology referral is indicated for endoscopy if bleeding is suspected or for examination of the mucosal lining. Surgical referral is indicated for emergency intervention and in cases of prolonged refractory ulcer disease.

PATIENT AND FAMILY EDUCATION

Patient education involves the identification and modification of risk factors, specifically cigarette smoking. Once a diagnosis of ulcer disease has been established, education should also include the signs and symptoms of hemorrhage, perforation, gastrointestinal bleeding, and anemia. In addition, the consequences of medication nonadherence related to the treatment of peptic ulcer disease and *H. pylori* infections should be carefully reviewed.

REFERENCES

1. Everhart JE: Recent developments in the epidemiology of *Helicobacter pylori*, *Gastroenterol Clin North Am* 29:559-578, 2000.
2. Smalley WE, Griffin MR, Fought RL, and others: Excess costs from gastrointestinal disease associated with nonsteroidal anti-inflammatory drugs, *J Gen Intern Med* 11:461-466, 1996.
3. Soll AH: Consensus conference: medical treatment of peptic ulcer disease: practice guidelines, *JAMA* 275(8):622-629, 1996.
4. Damianos AJ, McGarrity TJ: Treatment strategies for *Helicobacter pylori* infection, *Am J Gastroenterol* 55(8):2765-2786, 1997.
5. Vaira D, Nimish V, Menegatti M, and others: The stool test for detection of *Helicobacter pylori* after eradication therapy, *Ann Intern Med* 136:280, 2002.
6. National Guideline Clearinghouse: *Peptic ulcer disease,* retrieved Jan 13, 2007, from http://www.guideline.gov/summary/summary.aspx?ss=15&doc_id=7406&nbr=4376.
7. Culter AF, Havstad S, Ma CK, and others: Accuracy of invasive and noninvasive tests to diagnose *Helicobacter pylori* infection, *Gastroenterology* 109:136-141, 1995.
8. Peura DA: *Treatment regimens for* Helicobacter pylori, 2006, retrieved Jan 13, 2007, from http://www.uptodateonline.com/utd/content/topic.do?topicKey=acidpep/10778&selectedTitle=3~3590.
9. Howden CW, Hunt RH: *Guidelines for the management of* Helicobacter pylori *infection,* retrieved Jan 13, 2007, from http://www.acg.gi.org/physicians/guidelines/ManagementofHpylori.pdf.
10. Suerbaum S, Michetti P: *Helicobacter pylori* infection, *N Engl J Med* 347:1175-1186, 2002.

PART 13

Evaluation and Management of Genitourinary Disorders

PATRICIA POLGAR BAILEY, *Section Editor*

CHAPTER 153

Male Sexual Dysfunction

Laura Stempkowski and
Patricia Polgar Bailey

DEFINTION AND EPIDEMIOLOGY

Sexual dysfunction refers to disorders in which people cannot respond normally in key areas of sexual function, including difficulty or inability to enjoy sexual intercourse.[1] Sexual dysfunction affects a significant number of both men and women; as many as 31% of men and 43% of women may suffer from sexual dysfunction at some point in their lives.[2] Sexual dysfunction is often distressing for those involved and can lead to sexual frustration, guilt, loss of self-esteem, and interpersonal problems.[3]

The human sexual response can be described as a cycle with four phases: desire, excitement, orgasm, and resolution. Sexual dysfunction affects one or more of the first three phases. Resolution is simply the relaxation and reduction in arousal after orgasm. Resolution to the preexcitement phase occurs more rapidly with age, although this is most noticeable in older men. The amount of time that must pass before a man is capable of another ejaculation increases as men age.

The desire phase of the cycle consists of an urge to have sex, sexual fantasies, and sexual attraction to others. Hypoactive sexual desire is a lack of interest in sex or sexual activity, although the actual sexual experience may be normal.[1] The perception or stereotype of men in our culture is that they want sex as often as they can get it; however, hypoactive sexual desire affects as many as 16% of men, and during the past decade the number of men seeking treatment for it has increased.[2] There is an important distinction between people who have normal sexual desires but choose as part of their lifestyle not to engage in sexual relations vs. people with hypoactive sexual desire. Hypoactive sexual desire is also different from sexual aversion, which refers to people who find sex distinctly unpleasant or repulsive.

Disorders of the excitement phase of the sexual response cycle are marked by physical changes such as general physical arousal: increases in heart rate, blood pressure, the rate of breathing, and muscle tension. Erectile dysfunction (ED) affects the excitement phase. ED is the consistent inability to achieve and maintain a firm erection for satisfactory sexual activity.[4] Since the National Institutes of Health Consensus Conference in 1988, the term *erectile dysfunction* has replaced the term *impotence*.[5] ED is now recognized as a medical problem with potential psychologic consequences that may interfere with a man's quality of life, self-esteem, and interpersonal relationships.

In the United States, approximately 10 million to 20 million men, or about 10% of the general male population, suffer from ED.[2,6] The percentage of men suffering from ED increases with age, and the majority of men with this problem are over 65 years of age. These data are consistent with those of the Massachusetts Male Aging Study, conducted between 1987 and 1989 on middle-aged and elderly men, which found an overall rate of ED of 52%.[4] The probability of ED was 39% at age 40 and 67% at age 70. Men with ED are often embarrassed about discussing their problem openly with health care providers; consequently, most men seek treatment only after being referred by a family physician. Embarrassment and lack of adequate information are the two most commonly cited reasons for failing to seek treatment.[4] The advent of new pharmacologic agents for treating ED and their associated publicity have increased the awareness of the scope of this problem and resulted in an increased number of men seeking treatment.

During the orgasmic phase of the sexual response cycle, an individual's sexual pleasure peaks, sexual tension is released, and the man's semen is ejaculated. Male sexual dysfunctions during this phase include premature ejaculation and male orgasmic disorder. A man suffering from premature ejaculation persistently reaches orgasm with little sexual stimulation, before, on, or shortly after penetration and before he wants to. About 29% of men in the United States experience premature ejaculation; most commonly these are young, sexually inexperienced men, typically under 30 years of age.[2] Premature ejaculation is generally believed to be due to inexperience (e.g., a man's first sexual encounter), although some have suggested that it might also be related to anxiety, hurried masturbation experiences, or lack of insight into one's own sexual arousal.[7] However, at this point there is inconsistent clear clinical research to support these theories. *Male orgasmic disorder* refers to a man who cannot reach orgasm or is delayed in reaching orgasm after normal sexual excitement. This disorder affects 8% of the male population and typically is frustrating and upsetting.[2]

Men are often hesitant to discuss sexual problems with their providers, and in general consult them for health-related problems less frequently than do women. In addition, the emphasis in health care visits, particularly for men, tends to be on cardiovascular diseases and other common chronic illnesses, such as hypertension and diabetes, while ignoring conditions that may be of a more sensitive nature, thereby reducing the opportunity for the recognition and treatment of problems that substantially affect the quality of life.[8] Men also tend to seek help for specific problems rather than general health concerns and often do not report complaints directly to the provider but wait for the provider to find out why they are really there. In addition, the female partner in a relationship significantly influences a man's health-seeking behavior. Men who do not have a supportive partner or who feel particularly vulnerable or fearful or are in denial are less likely to seek help for issues related to sexual dysfunction.[8]

Although sexual dysfunction affects a sizable portion of the male population, a lack of discussion of the condition prevents a significant number of affected men from receiving treatment. Health care providers have become well versed in asking questions about patients' sexual practices when screening for sexually transmitted diseases (STDs) and HIV, but are less experienced and more uncomfortable when it comes to investigating sexual satisfaction among patients and their partners.[9] It is important for health care providers to include sexual assessment as a component of routine health care surveillance and become comfortable in eliciting the information that will help identify sexual dysfunction, give insight into its etiology, and guide further intervention. Health care providers are in a unique position to address sexual and relationship issues that exist between their patients and their partners. In addition to providing more holistic care, discussing and addressing sexual health concerns may uncover underlying co-morbid conditions, improve quality of life and self-esteem, foster a better patient-provider relationship, and increase patient satisfaction.[9]

PATHOPHYSIOLOGY

Disorders of Desire

The etiology of disorders of desire is multifactorial and a combination of biologic, psychologic, and sociocultural factors. Several hormones combine to produce sexual desire, and lower levels of them can lower the sex drive. In men and women, sexual desire is linked to levels of androgen, testosterone, and dehydroepiandrosterone (DHEA). In men testosterone levels begin to decline in the fifth decade and continue to decline throughout life. DHEA levels begin to decline in the thirties and continue steadily until reaching a low by age 60.[8] Chronic physical illness, as well as stress, pain, or depression related to the illness, directly affects the desire to have sex. The sex drive can also be lowered by some pain medications; certain psychotropic drugs; and a number of illegal drugs such as cocaine, marijuana, and amphetamines. In addition, low levels of alcohol can enhance the sex drive by reducing inhibitions, but at high levels alcohol can reduce sex drive. Circumstances and social pressures such as job stress, marital discord and divorce, death in the family, and infertility difficulties can affect one's desire to have sex.

Disorders of Excitement

Erectile function is a neurovascular event that is initiated by cognitive or tactile stimulation that is processed in the brain. Chemical mediators cause the essential relaxation of tissue and perfusion of the corpora cavernosum and corpus spongiosum. Nitric oxide and cyclic guanosine monophosphate (cGMP) are the primary noncholinergic and cholinergic mediators responsible for the neurogenic aspect of erection. Engorgement of the corpora and corpus spongiosum, in turn, compresses the veins to prevent the venous outflow of blood. This is how the erection is maintained and accounts for the vascular component of erection.[10] Any factor that interferes with this process may lead to ED.

The etiology of ED may be clearly identified (e.g., a radical prostatectomy) or may be multifactorial, requiring comprehensive assessment. Although in the past ED was believed to be psychogenic, it has now been shown that more than 70% of cases have a physiologic origin.[10] Alterations in vascular supply, hormonal changes, neurologic dysfunction, or medications and associated systemic disease may contribute to ED.

Psychogenic. Psychologic factors that may be of etiologic significance include performance anxiety, guilt, and strict religious constraints. Life events, such as a business failure, loss of health, or deterioration in the partner relationship, may also contribute to ED because of their impact on mood, anxiety, self-esteem, and depression. Developmental vulnerabilities, such as a history of child abuse, may have a profound effect on sexual function.[11] Psychologic issues, when combined with physiologic problems, can result in significant erectile difficulties.

Hormonal. Testosterone deficiency may be caused by hypothalamic or pituitary tumors or treatment aimed at suppressing testosterone, such as hormonal therapy in the treatment of prostate cancer. Although the primary effect of testosterone deficiency is decreased libido, ED may result as well. Other conditions that may precipitate decreased libido or ED because of their hormonal effects include hyperprolactinemia, hyperthyroidism, hypothyroidism, Cushing's syndrome, and Addison's disease.[11]

Angiogenic-Neurogenic. Angiogenic-neurogenic disorders that cause ED may be related to the stage of erection—a failure to initiate erection, a failure to achieve erection, or a failure to sustain erection. Potential causes of angiogenic-neurogenic ED and the major associated conditions are listed in Box 153-1.

Pharmacologic Risk Factors. The major classes of drugs that affect erectile function include antihypertensives, antidepressants, and major tranquilizers. ED may result from pharmacologic effects on the central nervous system, vascular system, hormone levels, and libido (Box 153-2). Other medications that have been associated with ED include hormonal agents (e.g., antiandrogens), protease inhibitors,[12] and cytotoxic agents.[13]

BOX 153-1

CAUSES OF ERECTILE DYSFUNCTION

NEUROGENIC
- Multiple sclerosis
- Peripheral neuropathy
- Radical prostatectomy
- Spinal cord injury
- Stroke

ANGIOGENIC
- Cardiovascular or peripheral vascular disease
- Congestive heart failure
- Cigarette smoking
- Diabetes mellitus
- Trauma to perineum or pelvis

HORMONAL
- Decreased testosterone or luteinizing hormone or increased prolactin

PSYCHOGENIC
- Anxiety
- Depression
- Stress

MEDICATIONS
- See Box 153-2

Data from Albaugh J, Lewis J: Insight into the management of erectile dysfunction, part I, *Urol Nurs* 19(4):242, 1999.

BOX 153-2

DRUGS THAT MAY CAUSE ERECTILE DYSFUNCTION

ANTIHYPERTENSIVES
- Beta blockers: propranolol, atenolol
- Diuretics: hydrochlorothiazide, amiloride, chlorthalidone, spironolactone
- Angiotensin-converting enzyme inhibitors: enalapril, lisinopril
- Centrally acting agents: clonidine, methyldopa
- Peripherally acting agents: guanethidine
- Miscellaneous: labetalol, reserpine

ANTIDEPRESSANTS
- Tricyclics: amoxapine, imipramine, clomipramine
- Miscellaneous: bupropion, tranylcypromine, venlafaxine

OTHER DRUGS
- Antipsychotics: chlorpromazine, fluphenazine, lithium, thioridazine, sulpiride
- Antianxiety: chlordiazepoxide
- Antiarrhythmics: digoxin, phenytoin
- Anticonvulsants: acetazolamide, carbamazepine, phenytoin, phenobarbital, primidone
- Anticholinergics: atropine, dicyclomine, ipratropium, scopolamine
- Histamine$_2$ agonists: cimetidine, ranitidine, famotidine
- Miscellaneous medications: clofibrate, dichlorphenamide, fenfluramine, ketoconazole, methadone, methazolamide, norethindrone, thiabendazole
- Illicit and abused drugs: alcohol, amphetamines, cocaine, marijuana, tobacco

Data from Albaugh J, Lewis J: Insight into the management of erectile dysfunction, part I, *Urol Nurs* 19(4):242, 1999.

Surgical Risk Factors. ED may occur after major surgery that potentially alters either the innervation or blood flow to the penis. These procedures may also affect a man's body image and self-perception of masculinity. Examples of such procedures are the radical prostatectomy, radical cystectomy, and abdominal-perineal resection. Nerve-sparing techniques minimize this risk and may result in the preservation of erectile function.

Other Factors. Pelvic radiotherapy (e.g., to treat prostate cancer) may damage nerves and blood vessels, potentially resulting in ED.

Disorders of Orgasm

Male orgasmic disorders (i.e., problems with ejaculation) can be due to low testosterone levels, certain neurologic diseases, and some head and spinal cord injuries. Certain drugs, including hypertensive medications, antidepressants, anxiolytics, antipsychotics, and alcohol, can slow down the sympathetic nervous system and can also affect ejaculation. For example, fluoxetine (Prozac) and other selective serotonin reuptake inhibitors (SSRIs) appear to interfere with ejaculation in as many as 40% of men who are taking them.[14] An important psychologic cause of male orgasmic disorder seems to be performance anxiety and the spectator role. If a man focuses on reaching orgasm, he stops being an aroused participant and instead has a tendency to be a self-critical and fearful observer.

CLINICAL PRESENTATION

Men may not readily offer information about sexual dysfunction, even though it may be the reason for the visit. Because men often avoid routine visits and are known to underuse primary care in general, the provider could suspect that a man with vague somatic complaints might actually be in the office because of concerns about sexual dysfunction. The interactions between the provider and patient are vital in establishing rapport, and it is important to remember that the patient's anticipation of the discussion or concern about bringing up the issue may be the source of considerable anxiety or stress.[9] Thus, sensitively introducing the subject of sexual health may help create a more comfortable atmosphere and facilitate discussion.

Providers should obtain a broad history, which includes not only sexual concerns, but also relationships and life events. Open-ended questions help elucidate the onset of concerns, course over time, and factors that may improve or worsen symptoms. It is helpful to start by asking general questions about sexual activity and interest and then relate this to healthy "masculine" intimacy, rather than by directly asking questions about sexual function. It is important to keep in mind the impact that physical, psychologic, and relationship issues can have on sexual health. Compassionate and normalizing statements can be helpful, such as "It is common for men who have had prostate cancer to notice changes in their interest in sexual activity."

In obtaining a history from the patient or partner, the provider may find it useful to identify three types of factors that can contribute to sexual dysfunction: predisposing factors (e.g., restrictive upbringing, disturbed relationships, traumatic sexual experiences), which might make a man more susceptible to sexual dysfunction; precipitating factors (e.g., dysfunction in the partner, discord in the relationship, depression or anxiety, co-morbid medical conditions), which may have triggered the onset of the problem; and maintaining factors (e.g., performance anxiety, relationship issues, impaired self-image, poor communication), which sustain the problem.[9]

Specific inquiries about ED should include questions that address the onset of ED (gradual or abrupt); if there is difficulty achieving or maintaining an erection, or both; and the presence and quality of nocturnal erections. In addition, the onset of ED, particularly if associated with a specific event (e.g., stress), should be determined. A urologic questionnaire, such as *The Sexual Health Inventory for Men,*[15] may be helpful in obtaining information of such a personal nature. The clinical history should include current health problems; a review of systems; and current medications, including nonprescription drugs and herbal formulations.

In eliciting information regarding sexual health, the provider also must consider generational issues. The sexual behaviors and interests of aging Baby Boomers are now beginning to emerge through surveys, such as those conducted by AARP. For example, Baby Boomers appear to hold traditional values regarding extramarital relationships but are more willing than former generations to experiment with new activities, such as watching pornography with their partners and trying new sexual positions.[8] Another issue to consider is the growing population of divorced and single adults who engage in sexual relationships and may be at risk for STDs, including HIV.[9] Relationship issues are a major factor in the decline in sexual activity among older adults.

Relatively little research has been done on the needs and interests of sexual minority patients, but it is important to consider that homosexual men may be reluctant to disclose their sexual orientation or discuss sexuality because of the negative associations with being gay. Maintaining a nonjudgmental and accepting attitude can increase the comfort level of a patient who finds it difficult to discuss issues related to sexual identity.

PHYSICAL EXAMINATION

The history will guide the physical examination, which, if indicated, also focuses on detecting signs of endocrine, vascular, or neurologic deficits and penile abnormality. Testicular atrophy, gynecomastia, or signs of hypothyroidism or hyperthyroidism may indicate hormonal abnormalities. Vascular assessment includes checking pulses in the lower extremities and observing for vascular skin changes in the lower extremities (e.g., hair loss). Neurologic assessment is focused on testing for genital reflexes (bulbocavernosus, cremasteric, scrotal, sphincter tone) and light touch discrimination.[11] During the genital examination, it is important to palpate for penile plaques, which may indicate Peyronie's disease. Plaques in the tunica albuginea limit penile distensibility, causing a bend in the penis with erection. This may interfere with sexual activity by making penetration difficult.[16]

Although approximately 75% of patients complaining of ED have an organic cause (resulting from vascular, neuronal, or endocrine factors), psychosocial, cognitive, and interpersonal variables, often related to illness or disease, play in exacerbating or maintaining ED. Assessment of these issues is essential in the evaluation of ED and other types of sexual dysfunction.

DIAGNOSTICS

The history and physical examination will determine which diagnostic and laboratory tests are indicated. Detecting underlying medical problems is essential in the evaluation of sexual dysfunction, and appropriate diagnostic testing is indicated. This section discusses specific diagnostic tests for ED.

Initially, nocturnal penile tumescence is evaluated to determine whether ED is attributed to a psychogenic or organic condition.[17] The Snap-Gauge, a Velcro band with three colored films arranged parallel to each other, is fitted around the penis. Each film ruptures to correspond with the intracavernosal pressures found in erection. Response is gauged by the number of films broken, with 0 to 1 indicating absent rigidity and 2 to 3 indicating rigid erections. Studies have shown the Snap-Gauge results to be inaccurate up to one third of the time.[17]

The Rigi-Scan (Dacomed Corporation, Minneapolis) is a more sophisticated device that provides continuous tumescence monitoring and can distinguish functional from inadequate erections in the majority of cases.[17]

Studies to evaluate penile vasculature include the intracavernosal injection of a vasoactive drug (e.g., alprostadil) or color duplex Doppler ultrasound (CDDU). CCDU evaluates anatomic abnormalities and measures both penile inflow and outflow.[18]

In the absence of a reliable test, the clinician must rely on the patient's history, physical examination, and laboratory testing—thyroid-stimulating hormone, luteinizing hormone, serum electrolytes, serum glucose, BUN, creatinine, serum testosterone, prolactin, and cholesterol—to determine the etiology of ED.

DIAGNOSTICS

Erectile Dysfunction

LABORATORY

CBC and differential
Serum glucose and/or HbA_{1c}
Serum electrolytes
BUN and creatinine
Cholesterol
TSH
Prolactin
Serum testosterone
Luteinizing hormone

OTHER

As indicated (see Diagnostics section.

DIFFERENTIAL DIAGNOSIS

See Differential Diagnosis box.

MANAGEMENT

Research supports a multidisciplinary approach to the treatment of sexual dysfunction. Health care providers need to determine their own comfort level with discussions about sexuality and sexual dysfunction. In addition, health care providers need to determine whether the patient's major issues are psychogenic, relational, or organic (often all three are involved) and whether referral to a psychologist, marriage counselor, or sex therapist might be helpful. Relationship counseling (or referral) may be appropriate to help the patient and partner with any emotional and communication barriers to sexual success. Effective communication is essential, and the provider can recommend some excellent self-help books and videos.

Anxiety reduction techniques have been a prominent part of psychologic approaches for sexual dysfunction. These techniques are based on the principle that, by removing the source of the anxiety (e.g., by forbidding intercourse and permitting only nondemand caressing), men can overcome performance anxiety and inhibitions. Providers can help

DIFFERENTIAL DIAGNOSIS

Erectile Dysfunction

- Decreased libido
- Anorgasmia
- Ejaculatory dysfunction

alleviate the anxiety by encouraging sensuality, extended foreplay, and a focus on pleasure rather than arousal. It is important to remind the persons involved that treatment often takes time to be fully effective and be comfortably integrated into their sex lives.[8]

Cognitive restructuring techniques can be used to overcome sexual ignorance and to challenge unrealistic expectations that couples may have about sexuality. Sexual dysfunction, such as ED, and associated anxiety can sometimes lead to the cessation of all sexual activity. In these situations, couples can be coached to give and receive pleasure in other ways such as manual or oral stimulation. Increased stimulation may also be necessary for the male partner to achieve an erection and thus can augment pharmacologic therapy.[8]

An important first step in management is determining where in the sexual response cycle the problem lies. For example, loss of sexual desire can be the result of life stressors, which may begin or worsen at midlife and can subsequently result in feelings of failure and low self-esteem. Supplemental testosterone has been shown to improve libido in older men with low testosterone levels. A causal relationship between testosterone supplementation and prostate cancer has not been demonstrated.[9]

Treatment options specifically for ED depend on the cause and patient-partner preference. The range of options includes psychotherapy, medication, sexual counseling, and surgery. Patients usually choose the least invasive treatment first and progress to more invasive treatments until an acceptable method is found.[6]

Psychotherapy is the preferred treatment for psychogenic ED. Sexual counseling can enhance communication, ease some of the stress associated with ED, and dispel myths. For instance, men may not realize they do not have to have an erection to have an orgasm and may believe intercourse to be their only means of sexual expression. In mixed psychogenic and organic ED, psychotherapy may relieve anxieties and increase the success of medical or surgical intervention.

For men whose only difficulty is maintaining an erection, a constriction band (e.g., ACTIS venous flow controller) applied at the base of the penis after erection is achieved, may be all that is needed.[19] Vacuum devices are associated with an 80% to 90% success rate and are among the least invasive and least expensive of the current treatment options. They produce an erection by creating a vacuum around the penis that triggers passive blood flow into the corpora cavernosa. Erection is then maintained by a constriction band applied at the base of the penis.

5 Phosphodiesterase (PDE-5) inhibitors are a class of oral medications that facilitate erection by enhancing the effects of nitric oxide and blocking the degradation of cGMP. Currently three PDE-5 inhibitors are available in the United States: sildenafil (Viagra), vardenafil (Levitra), and tadalafil (Cialis). They are similar in their action and efficacy. Common to all three drugs is the need for sexual stimulation to effect the release of nitric oxide. Evidence has shown the PDE-5 inhibitors to be effective in a wide range of patients with ED.[20] They are not the preferred option for men with neurogenic ED and are absolutely contraindicated in patients who are taking nitrates (Table 153-1).

Although PDE-5 inhibitors have a similar mechanism of action, there are significant differences between the agents in terms of pharmacokinetics; the ones that most directly affect patient preference are onset and duration of action. Both sildenafil and vardenafil have a rapid onset of action, and both remain effective for a short time. In addition, both drugs are more effective if taken on an empty stomach; eating high-fat meal before taking either drug reduces the peak plasma concentration. Tadalafil has a longer median half life than the other two drugs, resulting in a period of responsiveness for 24 to 36 hours. In addition, neither the consumption of a high-fat meal nor the timing of the dosing (morning or evening) has an effect on changes in plasma concentration or time to maximum response.[21]

By facilitating a sexual response, PDE-5 inhibitors may help couples return to a more satisfying sexual lifestyle.[21] However, even with these agents, other underlying or unresolved issues may require counseling or other types of psychologic intervention.[9]

Sexual dysfunction is a common side effect of some antidepressant medications, particularly SSRIs and other potent serotonin reuptake inhibitors (SRIs) such as venlafaxine (Effexor) and clomipramine (Anafranil). Sexual dysfunction associated with these medications is a reason commonly cited for discontinuing them.[22] In a recent study, patients taking bupropion sustained-release (Wellbutrin SR), in addition to their existing SSRI antidepressant, reported an increased desire to engage in sexual activity and frequency of sexual activity when compared with a group taking placebo.[22] The combination of bupropion and an SSRI result in a few adverse side effects, including irritability, dry mouth,

TABLE 153-1 5 Phosphodiesterase Inhibitors

Drug	Sildenafil (Viagra)	Vardenafil (Levitra)	Tadalafil (Cialis)
Dose	25-100 mg on an empty stomach	5-20 mg	5-20 mg
Peak time	1 hour	42-54 minutes	2 hours
Gone from body	8-12 hours	8-12 hours	36 hours
Contraindications	Nitrates (Caution with alpha blockers)	Nitrates (Caution with alpha blockers)	Nitrates (Caution with alpha blockers other than tamsulosin [Flomax])
Side effects	Headache, flushing, nasal congestion, abnormal vision	Headache, flushing, nasal congestion, abnormal vision (rare)	Headache, flushing, nasal congestion, abnormal vision, back or muscle pain (8%)

and headache. The authors of the study concluded that "improvements in sexual function and residual depressive symptoms when bupropion SR is added to an SSRI may improve quality of life in patients with SSRI-induced sexual dysfunction."[23]

Alprostadil (prostaglandin E_1) is indicated for the treatment of ED related to angiogenic, neurogenic, psychogenic, or mixed etiologies. Alprostadil is available as a urethral suppository (Muse) or as a solution for intracavernosal injection (Caverject, Edex).[19] The dose is highly individualized and requires the patient to have a test dose in the clinical setting. For this reason, patients wishing to pursue this option are usually referred to a urologist.

Only 5% to 10% of ED is caused by hormonal imbalance, such as low levels of testosterone or high levels of prolactin.[19] Testosterone replacement therapy is available by injection or transdermal patch with the goal of keeping the serum testosterone level within normal limits.

Surgical management includes vascular surgery or implantation of a penile prosthesis. The goal of vascular surgery is to increase arterial inflow to the corpora cavernosa and increase venous outflow resistance. Candidates are selected only after careful vascular examination, measurement of intracavernous pressures, and observation of the patient's response to certain pharmacologic agents. Younger men with discrete lesions, usually sustained from pelvic or perineal trauma, seem to be the best candidates for vascular surgery.

Penile prostheses may be malleable, mechanical, or inflatable devices and provide girth and rigidity; they do not increase length. The decision to proceed with implant therapy often comes after treatment when the less invasive options have failed. Complications of penile implants are infection, erosion, and component failure. Because of improvements in design and more durable materials, the complication rate has significantly decreased over the past few years, and patient-partner satisfaction has been shown to be 80% to 90%.[19]

Current research may lead to the development of new oral agents for ED and offer insight into combination therapy that may lead to successful therapy when single-agent treatment has failed.

COMPLICATIONS

Unfulfilled or even destroyed relationships, lack of self-esteem, and depression are common complications of sexual dysfunction. Often difficulties related to sexual health cause the cessation of all sexual activity. This withdrawal of affection can lead to diminished sexual desire and can exacerbate whatever distance or conflict already exists in the relationship.

INDICATIONS FOR REFERRAL

Underlying or refractory medical problems should be referred to the appropriate specialist. Persistent sexual dysfunction requires consultation with a urologist who has subspecialty in sexual dysfunction. Patients with hormonal abnormalities should be referred to an endocrinologist or urologist. Referral for sexual counseling or psychotherapy should be considered when appropriate. Modern sex therapy is short-term and instructive, typically lasting 15 to 20 sessions. It centers on specific sexual problems and includes assessment and conceptualization of the problem, education about sexuality, recognition of mutual responsibility and attitude change if necessary, elimination of performance anxiety, and help with improving sexual and general communication skills to change destructive lifestyle or marital interactions. Sex therapy does not deal with broad personality issues and does not take the place of psychologic counseling if that is indicated.[1]

PATIENT AND PARTNER EDUCATION

Patient education is essential to the success of treatment for sexual dysfunction. The health care provider must take the necessary time to counsel patients regarding the available options appropriate to their individual needs. It is important to remember that sexual dysfunction is a couple's problem and to include the partner whenever possible. The patient and partner should have realistic expectations of treatment and understand their role in its success.

Whether patients are using a vacuum device, taking an oral medication, using a urethral suppository, or undergoing penile injection therapy, it is important that they are instructed in its use. If the patient has elected injection therapy, it is important that the patient and partner feel comfortable with the injection process and are able to demonstrate accurate administration. Instructions should be provided in writing along with numbers to call should they have further questions or problems. Follow-up is important to determine if further intervention is needed. Patients appreciate knowing that their providers are concerned about their sexual health and are open to discussing these issues with them.

HEALTH PROMOTION

Early detection and screening for patients at high risk for sexual dysfunction should be considered in the primary care setting. Such patients include those with a history of heavy cigarette use; chronic medical problems such as hypertension, diabetes, or cardiovascular disease; psychologic issues; and unresolved life stressors. Sexual dysfunction may be the first indication of underlying cardiovascular disease or serious comorbidity. Health promotional behaviors such as smoking cessation, daily exercise, low-fat diet, and stress reduction can minimize risk for sexual dysfunction.

REFERENCES

1. Comer R: *Abnormal psychology,* ed 5, New York, 2004, Worth.
2. Heiman J: Sexual dysfunction: overview of prevalence, etiological factors and treatments, *J Sex Res* 39(1):73-78, 2002.
3. Basson R, Berman J, Burnett A, and others: Report of the International Consensus Development Conference on Female Dysfunctions: definitions and classifications, *J Sex Marital Therapy* 27(2):83-94, 2001.
4. Mulhall JP, Goldstein I: Epidemiology of erectile dysfunction. In Mulcahy JJ, editor: *Diagnosis and management of male sexual dysfunction,* New York, 1997, Igaku-Shoin.
5. NIH Consensus Conference: Impotence: NIH Consensus Development Panel on Impotence, *JAMA* 270(1):83-90, 1993.
6. Lue TF: Physiology of penile erection and pathophysiology of erectile dysfunction and priapism. In Walsh PC, Retik A, Vaughan ED Jr, and others, editors: *Campbell's urology,* ed 7, vol 2, Philadelphia, 1998, Saunders.
7. Westheimer R, Lopater S: *Human sexuality: a psychosocial perspective,* Baltimore, 2002, Williams & Wilkins.

8. Nusbaum M, Lenahan P, Sadovsky R: Sexual health in aging men and women: addressing the physiologic and psychologic sexual changes that occur with age, *Geriatrics* 60(9):18-23, 2006.
9. Dunn M: Restoration of couple's intimacy and relationship vital to reestablishing erectile function, *JADA* 104(3 Suppl 4):56-60, 2004.
10. Albaugh J, Lewis J: Insights into the management of erectile dysfunction, part I, *Urol Nurs* 19(4):241-245, 1999.
11. Maurice WL: *Sexual medicine in primary care,* St Louis, 1999, Mosby.
12. Schrooten W, Colebunders R, Youle M, and others: Sexual dysfunction associated with protease inhibitor containing highly active antiretroviral treatment, *AIDS* 15:1019, 2001.
13. Lewis RW: Epidemiology of erectile dysfunction, *Urol Clin North Am* 28:209, 2001.
14. Clayton A, Pradko J, Croft H, and others: Prevalence of sexual dysfunction among new antidepressants, *J Clin Psychiatr* 63(4):357-366, 2002.
15. Rosen RC, Cappelleri JC, Smith MD, and others: Development and evaluation of an abridged, five-item version of the International Index of Erectile Function (IIEF-5), as a diagnostic tool for erectile dysfunction, *Int J Impot Res* 11:319, 1999.
16. Carson CC: Peyronie's disease: etiology, diagnosis, and treatment. In Mulcahy JJ, editor: *Diagnosis and management of male sexual dysfunction,* New York, 1997, Igaku-Shoin.
17. Daitch JA, Lakin MM, Montague DK: Nocturnal penile tumescence monitoring. In Mulcahy JJ, editor: *Diagnosis and management of male sexual dysfunction,* New York, 1997, Igaku-Shoin.
18. Brodereick GA: Noninvasive arterial evaluation of the patient complaining of erectile dysfunction with color duplex Doppler ultrasound. In Mulcahy JJ, editor: *Diagnosis and management of male sexual dysfunction,* New York, 1997, Igaku-Shoin.
19. Albaugh J, Lewis J: Insights into the management of erectile dysfunction, part II, *Urol Nurs* 20(1):29-36, 53, 2000.
20. Burnett AL: Erectile dysfunction, *J Urol* 175:S25-S31, 2006.
21. Nusbaum M: Therapeutic options for patients returning to sexual activity, *JADA* 104(3 Suppl 4):52-55, 2004.
22. Clinical update: bupropion SR for SSRI-induced sexual dysfunction, *Brown Univ Pharmacol Update*, March 2004, p 5.
23. Clayton A, Warnock J, Kornstein S, and others: A placebo-controlled trial of bupropion SR as an antidote for selective serotonin reuptake inhibitor–induced sexual dysfunction, *J Clin Psychiatr* 65(1):62-67, 2004.

CHAPTER 154

Hypokalemia and Hyperkalemia

Carol A. Whelan

DEFINITION AND EPIDEMIOLOGY

The amount of potassium present in the average human body is approximately 50 mEq/kg. Of this, 90% is found in intracellular fluid, 8% in skin and bones, and 2% in extracellular fluid.[1-5] The maintenance of this relatively small amount of extracellular potassium is critical; small changes can cause serious clinical consequences.

The definitions of *hypokalemia* and *hyperkalemia* are stated in terms of extracellular (or serum) potassium. Normal values for serum potassium depend on individual laboratories, but the usual range for normal values is approximately 3.5 to 5 mEq/L. Potassium imbalances can be defined as acute or chronic and can be further defined by the degree of severity.

Chronic hypokalemia and hyperkalemia develop in a minimum of weeks to months, and acute hypokalemia and hyperkalemia occur over hours to days. Mild hypokalemia occurs at serum levels of 3.5 to 4 mEq/L; moderate hypokalemia, 3 to 3.5 mEq/L; and severe hypokalemia, below 3 mEq/L. Mild to moderate hyperkalemia is defined as a serum level of 5.5 to 6.9 mEq/L, and severe hyperkalemia as a serum level of 7 mEq/L or greater.

Levels of potassium in the intracellular and extracellular fluids do not always correlate, as seen in diabetic ketoacidosis. Severe depletion of intracellular potassium (termed *potassium deficiency*) as a result of osmotic diuresis (which leads to increased renal loss of potassium), despite normal or even elevated extracellular (serum) levels of potassium, is caused by insulin deficiency.[6] Once exogenous insulin is administered, clinical hypokalemia may develop rapidly.[6]

In the vast majority of cases, hypokalemia is drug induced; approximately 30% of all patients who are treated with non–potassium-sparing diuretics develop low serum potassium levels.[5] Most cases of chronic hyperkalemia are caused by renal failure; however, the increased use of spironolactone after the publication of the Randomized Aldactone Evaluation Study has resulted in a marked increase in morbidity and mortality from hyperkalemia, with an estimated 50 excess hospital admissions per 1000 additional prescriptions for spironolactone.[7]

Physician consultation is indicated for serum potassium levels lower than 3 or higher than 6 mEq/L.

PATHOPHYSIOLOGY

Potassium balance is affected by intake, excretion, and internal potassium regulation.[1-3] The minimum daily requirement for potassium intake in the normal adult is approximately 40 to 50 mEq.[1-3] Excretion occurs primarily in the kidneys and gastrointestinal tract, with a small amount excreted in perspiration. Internal potassium regulation depends on acid-base balance, plasma insulin levels, plasma catecholamine levels, and aldosterone activity.[3]

Because the kidneys are normally able to conserve potassium efficiently, hypokalemia is rarely a result of inadequate intake. The main causes of hypokalemia are increased renal loss from exogenous drug administration; primary or secondary hyperaldosteronism; and internal shifting of potassium from the extracellular to the intracellular space, which can occur with insulin administration or catecholamine excess (Box 154-1). Although vomiting may cause hypokalemia, it is not because of a loss of potassium from the gastrointestinal tract but rather because of secondary hyperaldosteronism related to volume depletion[8] or, more rarely, metabolic alkalosis from loss of gastric secretions.[5]

The kidneys' ability to maintain potassium homeostasis is preserved until the glomerular filtration rate (GFR) falls below 10 ml/min.[8] Therefore chronic hyperkalemia in patients with GFRs exceeding 20 ml/min is most likely caused by either drug therapy, a defect in mineralocorticoid activity, or a lesion within the cortical collecting system.[2] Causes of hyperkalemia are listed in Box 154-2.

BOX 154-2

CAUSES OF HYPERKALEMIA

Pseudohyperkalemia
- Traumatic venipuncture
- Severe leukocytosis

True hyperkalemia
- Renal failure
- Angiotensin-converting enzyme inhibitors
- Potassium-sparing diuretics
- NSAIDs
- Trimethoprim-sulfamethoxazole
- Heparin
- Beta blockers
- Hypoaldosteronism
- Type 4 renal tubular acidosis
- Adrenal insufficiency (Addison's disease)
- Sickle cell anemia
- Systemic lupus erythematosus
- Insulin deficiency
- Acidosis
- Familial hyperkalemic periodic paralysis
- Rhabdomyolysis
- Tumor lysis syndrome

CLINICAL PRESENTATION

The prevention of clinically significant hypokalemia and hyperkalemia is essential. In the absence of early detection and treatment, hypokalemia can cause serious complications and even death. The major symptoms are associated with skeletal muscle.[2,4] Hypokalemia causes hyperpolarization, which decreases impulse conduction and muscular contraction.[2] Flaccid paralysis, beginning in the extremities and moving centrally, can eventually lead to respiratory paralysis. Possible cardiac complications include ventricular arrhythmias. Typical ECG findings include ST-segment depression, flattening and inversion of the T wave, and a prominent U wave.[2,4] The appearance and severity of these ECG abnormalities do not correspond to the degree of hypokalemia and should not be used as a substitute for monitoring serum levels.[4]

BOX 154-1

CAUSES OF HYPOKALEMIA

- Non–potassium-sparing diuretics
- Antibiotics
- Alcoholism
- Osmotic diuresis
- Primary hyperaldosteronism
- Secondary hyperaldosteronism
- Glucocorticoid-induced hypertension
- Malignant hypertension
- Renovascular hypertension
- Renin-secreting tumor
- Liddle's syndrome
- 11β-Hydroxysteroid dehydrogenase deficiency
- Excessive licorice ingestion
- Congenital adrenal hyperplasia
- Type 1 renal tubular acidosis
- Type 2 renal tubular acidosis
- Bartter's syndrome
- Gitelman's syndrome
- Hypomagnesemia
- Exogenous insulin administration
- Catecholamine excess
- Familial periodic hypokalemic paralysis
- Thyrotoxic hypokalemic paralysis
- Leukemia
- β-Adrenergic agonists
- Trauma

Clinical manifestations of hyperkalemia are chiefly cardiac, although neuromuscular complications can also occur.[2] ECG changes associated with hyperkalemia include peaked T waves (often the first ECG finding), ST-segment depression, widening of the QRS and PR intervals, and loss of the P wave.[2] A late ECG sign is the appearance of a sine-wave pattern,[2,4] which usually indicates impending ventricular fibrillation and asystole.[2]

Although cardiac manifestations are obviously the most dangerous sequelae of hyperkalemia, neuromuscular complications, including paresthesias and fasciculations in the extremities, may be seen. Peripheral paralysis can occur, but paralysis of the respiratory muscles is rare.[2]

PHYSICAL EXAMINATION

A thorough history is the most important part of the physical examination. Any history of diuretic use, laxative use, vomiting, diarrhea, abnormal urinary output, diabetes mellitus, or hypertension, as well as a thorough diet and medication history, should be elicited. The physical examination should include a full assessment of vital signs (including orthostatic blood pressures); assessment of volume status[5]; and examination of the neuromuscular system, including assessment of muscular strength and reflexes.

DIAGNOSTICS

Diagnostics should assess the degree of the potassium imbalance, as well as the cause. Serum electrolytes, BUN, serum creatinine, serum glucose, a 12-lead ECG, and urinary electrolytes should be obtained.

Hypokalemia

Persons whose hypokalemia is not iatrogenic (i.e., drug induced) or the result of vomiting, diarrhea, alcoholism, or excessive licorice ingestion should be evaluated to determine the underlying cause of the hypokalemia. To effectively organize the diagnostic evaluation, those with hypokalemia may be subdivided into three groups: those with increased renal potassium excretion (>20 mEq/L) and hypertension, those with increased renal potassium excretion but without hypertension, and those with normal or decreased renal potassium excretion.

With concomitant hypertension, plasma renin activity (PRA) and plasma aldosterone levels should be measured but only *after* the hypokalemia has been corrected. Primary hyperaldosteronism is suggested if the PRA is suppressed and the plasma aldosterone levels are elevated. Secondary hyperaldosteronism will result in both a high PRA and a high plasma aldosterone level. Liddle's syndrome will also cause hypokalemia and hypertension, but both PRA and plasma aldosterone levels will be suppressed.[3]

When blood pressure is normal, measurement of serum bicarbonate helps further the differential diagnosis.[5] Low serum bicarbonate levels are consistent with diabetic ketoacidosis, metabolic acidosis, or renal tubular acidosis (RTA).[5] Hypokalemia associated with hyperchloremic metabolic acidosis is suggestive of type 1 RTA; a morning urinary pH should be checked. Levels higher than 6 are consistent with type 1 RTA.[3]

High serum bicarbonate levels in normotensive patients are consistent with Bartter's syndrome.[5] Bartter's syndrome will also result in high PRA and plasma aldosterone levels, but this is quite rare and is usually seen only in children or young adults. In addition to the abnormal laboratory findings, patients with Bartter's syndrome typically are of short stature, have muscle weakness, and are normotensive.[3]

Hypokalemia and normal serum bicarbonate levels in normotensive patients may also be caused by magnesium deficiency.[3] Individuals undergoing chemotherapy and those with a history of alcoholism and malabsorption syndrome are at risk for developing magnesium deficiency.[3]

Occasionally hypokalemia is not due to increased renal loss; these patients will have low urinary potassium (<20 mEq/L).[5] The differential diagnosis is fairly limited and generally involves some sort of gastrointestinal loss, through laxative abuse, villous adenoma, or severe diarrhea.[5] Patients previously treated with non–potassium-sparing diuretics who are potassium depleted will also have low urinary potassium.[5] Catecholamine excess, whether endogenous (as seen in acute myocardial infarction) or exogenous (as in β-adrenergic agonist administration), may also cause transient hypokalemia because of an increased cellular uptake of potassium.[5]

If the cause of the hypokalemia is still unknown after thorough investigation of past medical history, medication profile, and evaluation, referral to an endocrinologist is indicated.

Hyperkalemia

In cases of hyperkalemia, renal status should be determined. Individuals with chronic renal failure (CRF) who previously had normal potassium levels should have a 24-hour urine collection to assess for creatinine clearance and be questioned thoroughly regarding any diet changes; infection; trauma; and the use of NSAIDs, spironolactone, and other medications. Numerous cases of trimethoprim-sulfamethoxazole–induced hyperkalemia have been reported. Individuals with preexisting renal impairment or disturbances in potassium excretion or with HIV infection and those treated with angiotensin-converting enzyme (ACE) inhibitors, angiotensin receptor blockers (ARBs), and spironolactone appear to be most at risk.[9]

Persons without renal failure and hyperkalemia should be assessed for adrenocortical insufficiency (Addison's disease), which almost always results in hyponatremia, hypertension, hypovolemia, and renal insufficiency.[3] A cosyntropin stimulation test (with referral to an endocrinologist) should be performed if Addison's disease is suspected.

DIAGNOSTICS

Hypokalemia

LABORATORY
Serum electrolytes
BUN
Creatinine
Serum glucose
Serum magnesium
Plasma osmolality*
Urinary potassium—random
24-hour urine collection for potassium*
Urine osmolality*
Early-morning urinary pH*
Plasma renin activity*
Plasma aldosteronism*

OTHER
ECG*
ABGs

*If indicated.

DIAGNOSTICS

Hyperkalemia

LABORATORY
Serum electrolytes
BUN
Creatinine
Serum glucose
24-hour urine collection for creatinine clearance*
Plasma aldosterone*
Cosyntropin stimulation test*

OTHER
ECG
ABGs*

*If indicated.

Hyperkalemia may also result from hypoaldosteronism and is twice as common in patients with diabetes mellitus.[3] PRA and plasma aldosterone levels are diagnostic. Secondary hypoaldosteronism can result from the prolonged use of heparin, but in general the hyperkalemia is mild.[3] ACE inhibitors and ARBs also decrease aldosterone levels and can cause hyperkalemia. Tubular unresponsiveness to aldosterone may also cause hyperkalemia and may be seen in sickle cell disease, systemic lupus erythematosus, and amyloidosis.[3]

DIFFERENTIAL DIAGNOSIS

Hypokalemia and hyperkalemia are caused by a variety of disorders. Hypokalemia is usually related to one or more of the following: extracellular-to-intracellular potassium shift or renal and extrarenal potassium losses. Inadequate potassium intake is a relatively uncommon cause of hypokalemia. Hyperkalemia is related to inadequate potassium excretion, excessive potassium intake, or an intracellular shift of potassium from tissue to serum.

MANAGEMENT

The management of hypokalemia and hyperkalemia begins with identification of the underlying cause. Except for patients who are surreptitiously inducing vomiting or using large amounts of diuretics or laxatives, the cause of the potassium imbalance is usually readily apparent.[3] Most cases are a result of either diuretic use or renal failure. Hyperkalemia can also be a pseudohyperkalemia, which may be caused by traumatic venipuncture or, rarely, leukocytosis in the setting of leukemia.[3]

All at-risk patients should be frequently screened using laboratory analysis. When diuretics are being prescribed, the patient's serum potassium concentration should be checked before initiation of treatment and then 1 and 4 weeks after the initiation of therapy.[5]

In persons with chronic hyperkalemia, any use of ACE inhibitors, ARBs, NSAIDs, potassium-sparing diuretics, or salt substitutes (those containing potassium chloride) should be reassessed and most likely discontinued.[3]

Acute Hypokalemia

The treatment of acute hypokalemia involves the administration of oral or IV potassium supplements. If life-threatening arrhythmias or neuromuscular symptoms are present, IV potassium supplementation should be initiated.[3] IV potassium concentration should not exceed 40 mEq/L. IV potassium is usually infused at a rate of less than 10 mEq/hr.[10] Cardiac monitoring and frequent serum potassium assessment (every 3 to 6 hours) are essential. Once all cardiac arrhythmias or neuromuscular symptoms have disappeared, the patient may be switched to oral replacement. The normal dosage for oral potassium is 20 to 40 mEq b.i.d. to q.i.d.[3]

> **DIFFERENTIAL DIAGNOSIS**
>
> **Hypokalemia and Hyperkalemia**
>
> **HYPOKALEMIA**
> - Inadequate dietary intake
> - Extracellular-to-intracellular potassium shift
> - Renal and extrarenal potassium loss
>
> **HYPERKALEMIA**
> - Inadequate potassium excretion
> - Excessive potassium intake
> - Intracellular shift of potassium to serum

Chronic Hypokalemia

The primary goal of treatment of chronic hypokalemia is identification of the underlying cause. In cases of drug-induced hypokalemia the medication should be changed, if possible. If the clinical status prohibits this, then treatment depends on the degree of hypokalemia. Some controversy exists as to whether individuals with mild hypokalemia (3.5 to 4 mEq/L) should be aggressively treated[3,5]; however, they can certainly benefit from dietary teaching. In patients with potassium levels lower than 3.5 mEq/L, oral supplementation should be given, with normal dosages ranging between 20 and 80 mEq/day. Persons with hyperaldosteronism should be referred to an endocrinologist and may be successfully managed with spironolactone or eplerenone; eplerenone has been associated with fewer side effects because of its low affinity for sex hormone receptors.[11] If an aldosterone-secreting tumor is identified, surgical removal may be preferred.

Acute Hyperkalemia

Treatment of acute hyperkalemia with life-threatening symptoms (generally seen at potassium levels ≥7 mEq/L) is accomplished by the administration of IV calcium.[2-4] The usual recommended dose is 10 ml of a 10% calcium solution such as calcium chloride. The ECG should be monitored while the calcium is administered. Calcium should be administered only when ECG changes such as a widening QRS have occurred.[3,4] Calcium does not correct the underlying hyperkalemia; it only counters the adverse neuromuscular effects of hyperkalemia.[4] Calcium infusion should always be followed by specific therapy aimed at lowering the plasma potassium level (i.e., insulin and glucose infusion).

The administration of IV glucose and insulin is the quickest way to treat acute hyperkalemia that has not yet resulted in life-threatening sequelae.[3,4] This results in a shift of extracellular potassium into the cell.[4] Care should be taken in diabetic patients with hyperkalemia, since glucose infusion that is not accompanied by a matching infusion of insulin can actually result in increased hyperkalemia because of extracellular hyperosmolarity.[2]

When the individual is able to safely take medication orally and life-threatening sequelae have not developed, treatment with sodium polystyrene sulfate (Kayexalate) in sorbitol solution may be used. This may be the treatment of choice in outpatients who are stable but have potassium levels in the 5.5 to 6.9 mEq/L range. In patients unable to tolerate oral administration, polystyrene sulfate may be given rectally.[3]

Sodium bicarbonate is occasionally used in the treatment of hyperkalemia, both to treat the acidosis that may accompany hyperkalemia and to correct the hyperkalemia itself by causing a pH-dependent shift of potassium from the extracellular to the intracellular space.[4] Sodium bicarbonate should be used with caution, and care should be taken not to cause sodium overload or metabolic alkalosis.[3]

Chronic Hyperkalemia

The most common cause of chronic hyperkalemia is renal failure; therefore the most common management of chronic hyperkalemia is dialysis. It is rare for intake alone to account for hyperkalemia because renal excretion increases with increased intake in patients with normal renal function. Diet modification is essential, however, in persons with renal failure and chronic hyperkalemia. Referral to a dietitian can be helpful.

The treatment of chronic hyperkalemia caused by hypoaldosteronism may be accomplished with oral polystyrene sulfate or furosemide, but the preferred treatment is fludrocortisone acetate (Florinef).[3] If Addison's disease is diagnosed, treatment with replacement hydrocortisone should correct the hyperkalemia.

COMPLICATIONS

Potassium abnormalities are potentially life threatening. Cardiac conduction defects, arrhythmias, ileus, paralysis, muscle weakness, increased blood pressure, and renal injury are consequences of hypokalemia. Hyperkalemia also causes cardiac arrhythmias, heart block, ventricular fibrillation, muscle weakness, and paralysis.

INDICATIONS FOR REFERRAL OR HOSPITALIZATION

Any patients found to have an underlying metabolic disorder as a cause of hypokalemia or hyperkalemia and patients in whom the cause of the hypokalemia or hyperkalemia is unknown should be referred to an endocrinologist. Individuals with hyperkalemia and renal disease should always be referred to a renal specialist. All persons with life-threatening symptoms of hypokalemia or hyperkalemia should be evaluated for possible hospitalization. Also, those with hyperkalemia and acute renal failure should be urgently hospitalized.

PATIENT AND FAMILY EDUCATION

Patient education for hypokalemia or hyperkalemia should center on diet education and awareness of the importance of continued chronic supplementation therapy and laboratory monitoring. Education regarding potential drug effects on hypokalemia or hyperkalemia is also important. Chronic laxative use should be avoided because this has been associated with potassium loss. Individuals with chronic hypokalemia should avoid large amounts of licorice, which have also been associated with hypokalemia. Those taking potassium supplements should be advised not to crush the potassium tablets and to swallow the tablet with a large glass of fluid. If untoward effects of potassium occur, the patient should be advised to call or see a health care provider.

HEALTH PROMOTION

Since hyperkalemia is usually secondary to renal failure and hypokalemia is usually the result of diuretic use, health promotion should focus on the prevention of renal failure and hypertension. When prevention is no longer possible, patient education regarding the need for monitoring and prevention of complications is paramount.

REFERENCES

1. Brenner BM: *The kidney,* ed 5, Philadelphia, 1996, Saunders.
2. Levine DZ: *Caring for the renal patient,* ed 3, Philadelphia, 1997, Saunders.
3. Mandal AK: Hematuria and hypokalemia, *Med Clin North Am* 81(3):641-652, 1997.
4. Kasper D, Braunwald E, Fauci A, and others: *Harrison's principles of internal medicine,* ed 16, New York, 2005, McGraw-Hill.
5. Barker RL, Burton JR, Zieve PD: *Principles of ambulatory medicine,* ed 4, Baltimore, 1995, Williams & Wilkins.
6. Whelan CA: Chronic renal failure: nondialysis care, *Am J Nurse Pract* 2(7):21-31, 1998.
7. Juurlink DN, Mamdani MM, Lee DS, and others: Rates of hyperkalemia after publication of the Randomized Aldactone Evaluation Study, *N Engl J Med* 351:543-551, 2004.
8. Greenberg A: *Primer on kidney diseases,* ed 2, New York, 1994, Academic Press.
9. Perazella MA: Trimethoprim-induced hyperkalaemia: clinical data, mechanism, prevention and management, *Drug Safety* 22(3):227-236, 2000.
10. Kruse JA, Carlson RW: Rapid correction of hypokalemia using concentrated intravenous potassium chloride infusion, *Arch Intern Med* 150(3):613-617, 1990.
11. Weinberger MH, White WB, Ruilope LM, and others: Effects of eplerenone versus losartan in patients with low-renin hypertension, *Am Heart J* 150(3):423-433, 2005.

CHAPTER 155

Incontinence

Kelley Hamill Lemay

DEFINITION AND EPIDEMIOLOGY

Urinary incontinence is the involuntary transient or persistent loss of urine (Box 155-1). It is experienced by 30% to 50% of women and 17% of men over the age of 60 and by up to 50% of elderly nursing home residents.[1] Incontinence is considered to be one of the major causes of institutionalization in the geriatric population, but incontinence is not limited to the elderly. Twenty percent to 30% of young community dwellers are also afflicted by this disorder.[1] Urinary incontinence should not be considered normal at any age and is not an expected outcome of aging. Impaired mobility, pelvic floor weakness, pelvic trauma, benign prostatic hypertrophy, medications, bowel status, and conditions related to aging may all contribute to incontinence.[2,3]

The annual cost of managing incontinence for all age-groups was nearly $20 billion dollars in 2000.[2] However, despite its financial tax on society, incontinence is rarely addressed by patients with their health care providers.[2] Thus it behooves health care providers to identify patients who could benefit from therapeutic regimens to minimize the overall impact of incontinence.

PATHOPHYSIOLOGY

Urinary incontinence is usually the symptom of an underlying bladder or sphincter condition, but may also be related to an extrinsic problem that can be easily treated. There are five main types of urinary incontinence: stress incontinence, urge incontinence, mixed incontinence, overflow incontinence, and functional or transient incontinence. Bladder dysfunction in relation to incontinence can be classified as follows.

Stress Incontinence

Stress urinary incontinence (SUI) is leakage of urine with stress maneuvers that increase intraabdominal pressure (coughing, sneezing, etc.) and subsequently elevate bladder pressure.[4] Elevated bladder pressure can overcome the sphincter pressure, which opens the urethra and causes leakage.[4] Stress incontinence is seen in those who have either or both of the following issues:

Anatomic SUI: Previously termed *genuine stress incontinence*, anatomic incontinence refers to hypermobility of the bladder neck (vesicourethral junction). Generally, the sphincter is competent at rest, but once intraabdominal pressure rises, the bladder neck and urethra rotate below the pelvic floor muscles. Once below the pelvic floor, the sphincter is overcome and leakage occurs.[5]

Intrinsic sphincter deficiency (ISD): ISD indicates an open bladder neck at rest. Even a mild increase in intraabdominal pressure in individuals with ISD can result in leakage.[5] Although ISD can occur naturally, patients who have had radical pelvic surgery may also experience a compromise of their intrinsic sphincter, predisposing them to incontinence.

BOX 155-1

PERSISTENT INCONTINENCE

Stress incontinence: Loss of urine associated with activities that increase intraabdominal pressure

Urge incontinence: Involuntary loss of urine preceded by a strong, unexpected urge to void

Overflow incontinence: An involuntary loss of urine associated with incomplete emptying

Mixed incontinence: Urge and stress incontinence together

Urinary Urge Incontinence

Urge is the most common cause of incontinence in older adults and manifests as the sudden, often uncontrollable sensation to void.[6] This urge can then lead to urinary urge incontinence (UUI).[4] However, in patients with severe urge, incontinence may not be realized until actual leakage occurs. *Overactive bladder* (OAB) is a newer term used to describe the phenomenon of urgency and frequency with or without UUI.[7] The sensation of urge can be attributed to either detrusor overactivity (DO) or poor bladder compliance as indicated below.

Detrusor Overactivity. DO is instability of detrusor muscle during bladder filling as a result of:

Idiopathic causes: When no defined contributor can be identified, DO is idiopathic. Prominent theories for DO include increased stimulation of α_1-receptors in the bladder, disruption of somatic and autonomic nervous systems that help regulate voiding, disruption of afferent and efferent pathways, and increased activation of muscarinic (M2 and M3) receptors in the bladder.[8]

Neurogenic causes: Patients who have spinal cord injuries below T11-L1,2 or neurologic conditions, such as multiple sclerosis, diabetes mellitus, and spina bifida, can have a disruption in voluntary micturation control. Reflex micturation often results, leading to bladder hyperactivity and urge incontinence.[9]

In both idiopathic and neurogenic DO, bladder pressures surpass sphincter and urethral pressures, causing the bladder neck to open and incontinence to occur.

Poor Bladder Compliance. Normal bladder compliance allows large amounts of urine to be stored with minimum changes in bladder pressure.[10] With poor compliance, large bladder pressures are seen with small increases in volumes.[10] This can be due to the loss of viscoelasticity in detrusor muscle and/or changes in neuroregulatory activity.

Mixed Incontinence

Stress and urge incontinence can occur together, with contributing factors as previously discussed.

Overflow Incontinence

Incomplete emptying of urine often results in passive loss of small amounts of urine when bladder pressures elevate, either episodically or continuously, as the bladder fills beyond capacity. Overflow incontinence is seen in patients with either urethral obstruction or poor detrusor contractility.[4] Bladder pressure surpasses sphincter and urethral pressure, which allows "overflow" of urine to occur. This is more commonly seen in men than women, and causes include benign prostatic hyperplasia (BPH), other radical pelvic surgery, detrusor inactivity, neurologic issues, and certain medications.[5]

Functional or Transient Incontinence

Pathologic conditions external to the urinary tract can also cause incontinence. Such factors are indicated in Resnick's *DIAPPERS* pneumonic (Box 155-2).[11] Reversal of these conditions may treat the incontinence.

CLINICAL PRESENTATION

The presentation of incontinence can vary depending on etiology. A careful history and physical examination should exclude causes of transient incontinence that can be easily treated. SUI, UUI, mixed, and overflow incontinence may manifest similarly, so careful history taking may help delineate the type of incontinence experienced. A history should include a detailed review of symptoms related to incontinence, bowel habits, and medications; medical, surgical, and genitourinary histories; history of pelvic trauma; and neurologic issues.[5] The onset, precipitants, duration, characteristics (frequency, timing, amount, etc.), alleviating factors, and treatments tried should all be documented. Alterations in bowel or bladder habits, number of pads used, and the response to previous treatments should be noted as well.

PHYSICAL EXAMINATION

The physical examination should not only evaluate for the presence of edema, neurologic conditions, and functional ability, but also depict current abdominal or flank, pelvic, rectal, and genital status. Mental status, mobility, and social evaluations should be performed, especially in older adults, since they may indicate functional incontinence. Other types of incontinence must first be considered, though, before making a diagnosis of functional incontinence.

The physical examination for SUI includes abdominal, pelvic, and rectal components. Observation for urine loss with or without bladder neck hypermobility via Valsalva's and cough maneuvers should occur while the patient is in the supine position. If no incontinence is seen supinely with these maneuvers, the examination may be repeated with the patient standing. Bladder neck hypermobility can also be determined with the Q-Tip test.[12] If, when inserted superficially into the urethra, the Q-Tip moves more than 30 degrees from a horizontal plane, lack of urethral support is delineated.[12] Furthermore, pelvic organ prolapse and effectiveness of the patient's ability to perform Kegel exercises (contract the pelvic floor) should be noted. General observation of pelvic anatomy should be made and any abnormalities, including atrophy, documented. The relationship between estrogen and incontinence in perimenopausal and menopausal women has not been well defined. However, lack of estrogen and subsequent vaginal atrophy may contribute to symptoms of stress incontinence.[13]

UUI may not be detectable on physical examination. Subjective complaints may be most beneficial in detecting urge and urge incontinence. However, examination of pelvic anatomy and pelvic floor strength may reveal contributors to bladder symptoms, such as constipation and vaginal atrophy. Urinary tract infections must be excluded in this patient population.

Mixed incontinence requires a physical examination to assess for SUI and UUI. This should be performed as previously discussed.

Finally, overflow incontinence can often be determined through abdominal and vaginal examinations. Bladder distention may be easily palpated abdominally or vaginally. Evaluation of general pelvic anatomy should also occur.

BOX 155-2

RESNICK'S DIAPPERS PNEUMONIC

*D*elerium/confusional state
*I*nfection—urinary (only symptomatic)
*A*trophic urethritis, vaginitis
*P*harmaceuticals
*P*sychologic, especially severe depression (rare)
*E*xcess urinary output (e.g., congestive heart failure, hyperglycemia)
*R*estricted mobility
*S*tool impaction

From Resnick NM: Urinary incontinence. In Cassel CK, Cohen HJ, Larson ER, and others, editors: *Geriatric medicine,* ed 3, New York, 1997, Springer.

DIAGNOSTICS

A urinalysis is performed to exclude hematuria, pyuria, glucosuria, or proteinuria. Hematuria, defined as more than 3 red blood cells per high-powered field on urinalysis,[13] warrants further workup with cytology, upper tract imaging, and bladder cystoscopy. Urine cytologic studies should also be obtained in patients with gross hematuria, risk factors for bladder cancer, or irritative symptoms.[14] A urine culture is necessary to exclude a urinary tract infection in patients with pyuria or irritative symptoms. BUN and creatinine levels should be obtained if compromised renal function is suspected, especially with overflow incontinence. If polyuria is suspected, serum glucose and calcium tests are also recommended.

DIAGNOSTICS

Incontinence

LABORATORY
Urinalysis
Urine culture and sensitivity
BUN
Creatinine
Serum glucose*
Calcium*
Urine for cytology*

OTHER
Postvoid residual
Urodynamic testing

*If indicated.

A postvoid residual (PVR) is helpful to exclude incomplete emptying and can be obtained through either pelvic ultrasound or catheterization. Generally, a PVR of less than 50 ml is considered normal,[15] whereas residuals of more than 100 ml are considered abnormal and require further evaluation.

Additional testing is usually not necessary for the basic evaluation of urinary incontinence unless onset is sudden, symptoms are severe, or suprapubic pain or hematuria is present. The patient should be referred to a urologist if further diagnostic testing (e.g., simple cystometry, urodynamics) is necessary or if the diagnosis is uncertain.[16] The health care provider should refer the patient if an effective care plan cannot be devised, if hematuria is present without infection, if surgical intervention is being considered, or if therapy has failed.

DIFFERENTIAL DIAGNOSIS

If incontinence is believed to be functional, the first step in treatment is to manage the underlying condition. This may be as simple as moving a commode to the bedside of a newly immobile patient recovering from orthopedic surgery. Medical conditions that may exacerbate incontinence should be treated, and conditions that contribute to incontinence should be minimized or discontinued if possible. When all nonurologic causes of incontinence have been ruled out, the type of incontinence—based on history and physical and diagnostic data—can be determined. Once identified, a management plan for the type of incontinence afflicting the patient can be initiated.

DIFFERENTIAL DIAGNOSIS

Incontinence

- Stress urinary incontinence (SUI)
  - Anatomic SUI
  - Intrinsic sphincter deficiency
- Urge incontinence
  - Detrusor overactivity (idiopathic or neurogenic)
  - Poor bladder compliance
- Mixed incontinence
- Overflow incontinence
- Functional or transient incontinence
- Increased urinary production
- Lower urinary tract conditions
- Medications

MANAGEMENT

The treatment of incontinence varies according to cause, but behavioral and pharmacologic therapies are generally first-line therapies in the treatment of urinary incontinence. Surgical therapies may be indicated in some individuals (Box 155-3).

Stress Incontinence

Behavioral Therapies. Behavioral therapies used to treat SUI include timed voiding, double voiding, smoking cessation, weight loss, pelvic muscle exercises (PMEs), pessary placement, and bowel management. Timed voiding, or voiding every 2 hours during the day, allows adequate time for the patient's bladder to fill but not overdistend. This will minimize the amount of urine in the bladder to leak when a stress maneuver does occur.[17] Use of a bladder diary may be beneficial to map voiding occurrences so the patient and health care provider can review these to identify bladder habits.

Double voiding is used for patients who empty incompletely. It consists of having the patient change position on the toilet, get up and sit back down, or just allow a few extra minutes for the bladder to empty fully while on the toilet. Having a patient sit with her knees apart on the toilet to relaxing the pelvic floor muscles will facilitate this process. In a patient with stress incontinence and poor emptying, improved emptying may allow for improved control.

BOX 155-3

MANAGEMENT OF INCONTINENCE

STRESS INCONTINENCE

- Behavioral therapies: timed or double voiding, smoking cessation, weight loss, pelvic muscle exercises with or without a physical therapist, pessary, bowel management
- Medical therapies: α-adrenergic agonists, anticholinergics, tricyclic antidepressants, estrogen
- Surgical therapies: injectables, suspensions, slings, artificial sphincters

URGE INCONTINENCE

- Behavioral therapies: as above with bladder training, scheduled voiding, and bladder irritant minimization
- Medical therapies: anticholinergic-antimuscarinics
- Surgical therapies: neurosacral modulation, bladder augmentation

MIXED INCONTINENCE

- Combination of therapies for stress and urge incontinence

OVERFLOW INCONTINENCE

- Behavioral therapies: timed or double voiding, clean intermittent catheterization, pessary
- Medical therapies: alpha$_1$ blockers, 5α-reductase inhibitors
- Surgery to relieve urethral obstruction or reduce prolapse

FUNCTIONAL OR TRANSIENT INCONTINENCE

- Treat underlying cause

Smoking cessation helps minimize events that increase intraabdominal pressure, since smokers are often more likely to cough because of respiratory side effects and infections.[17] Tobacco is also a bladder irritant and can increase the sense of urgency.[18] Weight loss, too, can help minimize SUI, since increased abdominal girth may apply more pressure to the bladder when stress maneuvers occur.[19]

PMEs, or Kegels, strengthen the pelvic floor. These exercises are beneficial because, when performed correctly, pelvic floor contraction can help prevent stress incontinence by occluding the urethra during physical activities that may cause symptoms.[17,20] They may also improve resting pressure in the urethra and increase bulk around the urethra, which may prevent stress and urge incontinence.[17] Kegels are performed by tightening only the pelvic floor muscles as if controlling defecation or urination. Contraction of abdominal, thigh, and gluteal muscles should be avoided. Appropriate technique is best assessed by placing a finger in the vagina so the appropriate muscles can be isolated. Contractions should be held for up to 10 seconds followed by a period of relaxation. Exercises should be performed as three sets of 10, three times a day, for 6 months, even though benefit may be seen by 4 to 8 weeks.[17]

Referral to a physical therapist (PT) is often beneficial for patients who are unable to appropriately isolate the pelvic floor muscles or are unsure they are performing Kegels correctly. The PT may use adjuncts such as biofeedback or electrical stimulation to further improve the patient's ability to contract the pelvic floor. Biofeedback is used to augment Kegels in patients with stress or urge incontinence because it increases awareness of pelvic floor function and helps change responses in an attempt to improve urination.[17] One of the simplest forms of biofeedback is the use of vaginal weights.[17] Patients are instructed to insert a weight intravaginally and retain it during ambulation via contraction of the pelvic floor muscles.[17] Vaginal weights range from 20 to 100 g (0.7 to 3.5 ounces), and exercises should start with light weights and gradually increase.

Electrical stimulation of the pelvic floor muscles may also be effective in treating stress, urge, and mixed incontinence. Electrical stimulation must be performed by a professional skilled in this procedure.[17]

Pessary placement may be helpful in patients with bladder or pelvic organ prolapse. There are also pessaries specifically designed for incontinence that work by elevating the bladder neck. Referral to a skilled pessary fitter for appropriate fitting and management is important, since patients may need to try a variety of types and sizes before getting a good fit.

Bowel management is important in minimizing incontinence. Stool impaction can increase external pressure on the bladder and increasing the likelihood of irritability, and excessive straining with defecation may also contribute to denervation of the external anal sphincter and pelvic floor muscles.[21] This denervation is thought to result in bladder symptoms.[21] Ideally, the goal is moderation of the gastrointestinal tract so one large, soft bowel movement per day or every other day is achieved.

Medical Therapies. α-Adrenergic agonists, such as pseudoephedrine (Sudafed), increase urethral pressure and outlet resistance to decrease incontinence.[22] Although not curative or approved for this indication, α-adrenergics may improve symptoms.[22]

Estrogen replacement may be helpful in treating postmenopausal stress incontinence in women who have signs of vaginal atrophy, although controversy still exists about whether estrogen therapy provides benefit, since many studies have not found symptom improvement with estrogen use.[23] However, adequate trials have still not been done. It is generally believed, though, that estrogen may be worth trying in women who have no contraindications to estrogen therapy.[22] Given the results of the Women's Health Initiative and other recent studies, woman must be counseled about the risks vs. benefits of hormone replacement therapy.[24,25]

Conjugated estrogen may be given orally, and risks in relation to benefit should be thoroughly discussed before it is started. If oral estrogen is started in a woman with an intact uterus, oral progesterone should also be given.[23,26] Periurethral estrogen creams have a very low incidence of systemic levels and can be administered daily for 2 weeks, then twice weekly thereafter.

Imipramine or other tricyclic antidepressants may be recommended, especially in younger patients, if other therapies have proved ineffective. At dosages of 10 to 25 mg PO b.i.d., imipramine has both alpha agonist and anticholinergic effects, which make it useful for patients with SUI or mixed incontinence.[22,26] In general, these drugs should be used carefully in older adults because of potential adverse effects, mostly cardiac and anticholinergic. Orthostatic hypotension with an increased risk of falls may be more likely in the elderly, as could dizziness, fatigue, dry mouth, and constipation.[26]

Surgical Therapies. Surgery should be considered if treatment regimens are ineffective or if patients are not able to adhere to other treatment plans. Stress incontinence is the most common type of incontinence treated with surgery. Surgery is done to either lift or provide support to the urethra or bladder neck. Choices include retropubic suspensions, a variety of sling procedures, urethral bulking agents, and artificial urinary sphincters. Referral to a urologist or urogynecologist is recommended if surgery is being considered. The type of surgery performed depends on patient anatomy, urodynamic findings, and patient expectations.

Urge Incontinence

Behavioral Therapies. Behavioral methods for treating UUI also include timed and double voiding, use of a voiding diary, pelvic floor exercises with or without a PT, weight reduction, smoking cessation, and bowel management. However, bladder training, scheduled voiding, and overall minimization of bladder irritants can also be recommended.

With UUI, a voiding diary documenting time and amount of each void and the time of any incontinent episode will help illustrate which treatments could be most beneficial. The patient who routinely has urge incontinence on the way to the toilet after waiting 4 to 5 hours to void may need to incorporate something as simple as timed voiding every 2 hours into his or her daily routine.

Bladder training is of benefit to the patient who voids frequently (every 30 minutes to 1 hour) during the day, but can sleep through the night and void 300 ml in the morning. Bladder training requires the patient to postpone voiding, resist the sense of urgency, and void on a predetermined schedule. Intervals of 10 to 15 minutes should be added to the current voiding pattern and then gradually increased so the patient can reach a goal of voiding every 2 to 3 hours. The bladder should be emptied at the scheduled intervals, and voiding should be delayed if urge occurs. "Quick flicks," or four or five quick repetitions of Kegel exercises, work to counteract bladder spasms, buying the patient more time to get to the bathroom without rushing or leaking.[20]

Scheduled or prompted voiding by a caregiver may be effective when a patient cannot use the toilet independently.[17] Assistance with toileting should be provided every 2 to 4 hours during the day and night to minimize incontinence. Habit training, another method for decreasing incontinence in dependent patients, occurs when a toileting schedule is developed in accordance with the patient's past voiding habits.[17] Based on a record of incontinence, a schedule can be developed to minimize episodes of incontinence.[17]

Regulating bladder irritants can help decrease urgency and UUI. Spicy, acidic, and caffeinated foods tend to irritate the bladder and increase the sense of urgency.[18] Chocolate, tomatoes, citrus fruits or juices, most nuts, coffee, tea, dark sodas, alcohol, and tobacco can all contribute to irritative symptoms.[18] Furthermore, moderation of overall fluid intake to between 48 and 64 oz/day can help maintain hydration while moderating frequency. A voiding diary may be beneficial to determine this.

Medical Therapies. Medications are generally helpful in moderating urge incontinence.[27] Anticholinergic-antimuscarinic agents are the cornerstone of medical therapy, since they work to block impulses to muscarinic acetylcholine receptors (M2, M3) found in the bladder.[23] In turn, the number and strength of involuntary bladder contractions decrease and urinary frequency is moderated. Anticholinergic agents can have side effects of dry mouth, confusion, constipation, dizziness and blurred vision, and tachycardia.[26]

Tolterodine tartrate (Detrol) and oxybutynin chloride (Ditropan) are examples of antimuscarinics.[27] These agents can be used safely for both younger and older patients with overactive bladder.[26] Oxybutynin, once used extensively, has greater anticholinergic side effects than other anticholinergics and may be reserved for younger patients. Ditropan XL, an extended release formulation of oxybutynin, and Oxytrol, transdermal oxybutynin, have been shown to produce less anticholinergic side effects than regular oxybutynin.[22] Newer anticholinergics continue to be developed with an effort to increase efficacy while reducing side effects. Trospium (Sanctura) is a quanternary amine and, in theory, has less ability to cross the blood brain barrier. Darifenacin (Enablex) and solifenacin (Vesicare) are selective for M3 receptors, which may increase efficacy and decrease M2-mediated side effects.[27] However, since all these drugs have the potential to cause side effects in the frail geriatric patient, they should be started at low doses and gradually titrated until either symptoms improve or nontolerability indicates further medication trials.

Tricyclics may be helpful for certain patients with UUI. Again, low doses of these drugs should be used in the elderly because of the potential for adverse effects.

Surgical Therapies. Surgical therapies may be indicated in some patients with severe urge incontinence. Surgical therapies, done to counteract bladder contractions or increase bladder capacity, include neurosacral modulation and bladder augmentation. Referral to a urologist should occur if surgery is being considered.

Mixed Incontinence

After careful diagnostic evaluation, the patient may be found to have mixed incontinence. Treatment using a combination of previously described behavioral or medical therapies is warranted.

Overflow Incontinence

Overflow incontinence can be managed with timed and double voiding, but also with clean intermittent catheterization (CIC), a pessary, medical therapies, or surgical options. CIC is recommended for patients who have poor emptying secondary to poor detrusor function or for patients with urethral obstruction who are poor surgical candidates. This should be done often enough that CIC amounts, if the patient does not void volitionally, or total void plus CIC amounts remain less than 500 ml with each cath-void event.

A pessary may be helpful for prolapse that causes partial urethral obstruction. A pessary provides support to the vaginal canal so the bladder can empty more completely. However, when it is placed, another type of incontinence may become more prevalent once the bladder is in proper anatomic position.

Medications are used to relieve overflow incontinence in relation to BPH. $Alpha_1$ blockers tamsulosin hydrochloride (Flomax) and terazosin (Hytrin), as well as 5α-reductase inhibitors, such as finasteride (Proscar) and dutasteride (Avodart), can be used in this case. There is no role for these medications in women.

Surgery is often indicated to relieve urethral obstruction caused by BPH or a nonreducible prolapse. Referral to a urologist should occur if surgery is being considered.

Functional Incontinence

Functional incontinence can be resolved through treatment of the underlying cause. Behavioral therapies may be beneficial as well.

LIFE SPAN CONSIDERATIONS

Incontinence can occur at any age, but is more prevalent in the older adult. Changes in the urinary tract that occur with aging can contribute to the development of incontinence. Bladder capacity, contractility, and the ability to postpone voiding are thought to decline with age. Prostate size, urethral obstruction, involuntary bladder contractions, and PVRs, on the other hand, may increase.[28] These changes, as well as increased chronic health conditions and medications that affect the urinary tract, explain why incontinence is so prevalent in the geriatric population.

COMPLICATIONS

Incontinence can contribute to medical morbidities, including perineal candidal infections, pressure ulcers, urinary tract infections, urosepsis, falls, and sleep interruption.[29,30] At the same time, incontinence can contribute to poor self-esteem, social withdrawal, depression, and sexual dysfunction secondary to embarrassment.[29] Because of this, patients in the home environment may try to limit fluid intake in an effort to control incontinence. By minimizing fluid intake, patients may put themselves at risk for dehydration and its sequelae.

CONSIDERATION FOR REFERRAL

Again, consultation with a physician is important when there is difficulty determining the type of incontinence or when traditional treatment regimens provide inadequate relief of symptoms. Incontinence that does not respond adequately to initial treatment may be managed more effectively in collaboration with a PT; continence nurse; and urologist, urogynecologist, or specialized nurse practitioner.

A urology referral is indicated with incontinence and an abnormal PVR, a prostate examination that suggests prostate cancer, a neurologic condition, symptomatic pelvic prolapse, recurrent symptomatic urinary tract infections, a history of radical pelvic or incontinence surgery, or persistent symptoms of difficult or incomplete bladder emptying. Further testing is warranted when the diagnosis is uncertain, when hematuria without infection is present, when surgical intervention is being considered, or when therapy of reasonable duration has failed.

PATIENT EDUCATION

Effectiveness of behavioral strategies in the treatment of incontinence depends on the education and adherence of patients, families, and caregivers to the treatment plan agreed on. Plans for behavioral interventions should be realistic and meet the needs of patients and caregivers. Regular follow-up visits will help reinforce therapeutic options, support efforts to obtain treatment goals, and allow care-plan modification so optimum outcomes can be obtained.

REFERENCES

1. Hunskaar S, Burgio K, Clark A, and others: Epidemiology of urinary and fecal incontinence and pelvic organ prolapse. In *Incontinence: Third International Consultation on Incontinence, vol 1, Basic evaluation,* Paris, 2005.
2. Hu TW, Wagner TH, Bentkover JD, and others: Costs of urinary incontinence and overactive bladder in the United States: a comparative study, *Urology* 63:461, 2004.
3. Brundage DJ, Linton AD: Age-related changes in the genitourinary system. In Matteson MA, McConnell ES, Linton AD, editors: *Gerontological nursing,* Philadelphia, 1997, Saunders.
4. Abrams P, Cardozo L, Fall M, and others: The standardization of terminology of lower urinary tract function: report from the Standardization Sub-committee of the International Continence Society, *Neurourol Urodynamics* 21:167, 2002.
5. Wein AJ, Rovner ES: Voiding function and dysfunction. In Hanno PM, Malkowicz SB, Wein AJ, editors: *Clinical manual of urology,* New York, 2001, McGraw-Hill.
6. Newman DK, Giovannini D: The overactive bladder: a nursing perspective, *AJN* 102(6):36-44, 2002.
7. Lai HH, Gross M, Boone TB, and others: Pharmacologic and surgical management of detrusor instability. In Vasavada SP, Appel RA, Sand PK, and others, editors: *Female urology, urogynecology, and voiding dysfunction,* New York, 2005, Taylor & Francis.
8. Zderic SA, Chacko S, Disanto MD, and others: Voiding function and dysfunction. In Gillenwater JY, Grayhack JT, Howards SS, and others, editors: *Adult and pediatric urology*, Philadelphia, 2002, Lippincott Williams & Wilkins.
9. Wein AJ: Neuromuscular dysfunction of the lower urinary tract. In Walsh PC, Retic AB, Stamey TA, and others, editors: *Campbell's urology,* ed 8, Philadelphia, 2002, Saunders.
10. Bruenenfelder J, McGuire EJ: Videourodynamics. In Vasavada SP, Appel RA, Sand PK, and others, editors: *Female urology, urogynecology, and voiding dysfunction,* New York, 2005, Taylor & Francis.
11. Resnick NM: Urinary incontinence. In Cassel CK, Cohen HJ, Larson ER, and others, editors: *Geriatric medicine,* ed 3, New York, 1997, Springer.
12. Rosenberg MT, Dmochowski RR: Overactive bladder: evaluation and management in primary care, *Cleveland Clin J Med* 72:149-156, 2005.
13. Klausner AP, Vapnek JM: Urinary incontinence in the geriatric population, *Mt Sinai J Med* 70:54-61, 2003.
14. Rosen MT: A primary care approach to overactive bladder and urinary incontinence. In *Overactive bladder: management guide,* Montvale, NJ, 2005, Tomson PDR.
15. Dambro MR: Urinary incontinence, hematuria. In Dambro MR, editor: *Griffith's 5-minute clinical consult, 2004,* Philadelphia, 2003, Lippincott Williams & Wilkins.
16. Penn C, Lekan-Rutledge D, Joers AM, and others: Assessment of urinary incontinence, *J Gerontol Nurs* 22(1):8-19, 1996.
17. Newman D: Behavioral treatments. In Vasavada SP, Appel RA, Sand PK, and others, editors: *Female urology, urogynecology, and voiding dysfunction,* New York, 2005, Taylor & Francis.
18. Interstitial Cystitis Association: *Treatment options: IC and diet,* retrieved Jan 11, 2006, from http://www.IChelp.org/treatmentandselfhelp/ICanddiet.html.
19. Subak LL, Whitcomb E, Shen H, and others: Weight loss: a novel and effective treatment for urinary incontinence, *J Urol* 174:190, 2005.
20. Burgio KL: Behavioral treatment options for urinary incontinence, *Gastroenterology* 126:S82-S89, 2004.
21. Lubowsk DZ, Swash M, Nicholls RJ, and others: Increase in pudendal nerve terminal motor latency with defaecation straining, *Br J Surg* 75:1095, 1988.
22. Wein AJ, Rovner ES: Pharmacologic management of incontinence. In Vasavada SP, Appel RA, Sand PK, and others, editors: *Female urology, urogynecology, and voiding dysfunction,* New York, 2005, Taylor & Francis.
23. Moehrer B, Hextall A, Jackson S: Oestrogens for urinary incontinence in women (review), *Cochran Rev* (4), 2005, retrieved Jan 16, 2006, from http://www.mrw.interscience.wiley.com/cochrane/clsysrev/articles/CD001405/pdf_fs.html.
24. Rossouvw JE, Anderson GL, Prentice RL, and others: Risks and benefits of estrogen plus progestin in healthy menopausal women, *JAMA* 288:321-333, 2002.
25. Langer RD: Postmenopausal hormone therapy: what's appropriate today, *CME Bulletin* 4:1-10, 2005.
26. Blaivas JG, Broutz A: Urinary incontinence: pathophysiology, evaluation and management overview. In Walsh PC, Retic AB, Stamey TA, and others, editors: *Campbell's urology,* ed 8, Philadelphia, 2002, Saunders.
27. Staskin DR, Wein AJ, Andersson KE, and others: Overview consensus statement, *Urology* 60(Suppl 5a):1-6, 2002.
28. Resnick NM, Yalla S: Geriatric incontinence and voiding dysfunction. In Walsh PC, Retic AB, Stamey TA, and others, editors: *Campbell's urology,* ed 8, Philadelphia, 2002, Saunders.
29. Ouslander JG, Zarit SH, Orr NK, and others: Incontinence among elderly community-dwelling dementia patients: characteristics, management and impact on caregivers, *J Am Geriatr Soc* 38:440, 1990.
30. Brown JS, Vittinghoff E, Wymann JF, and others: Urinary incontinence: does it increase risk for falls and fractures? *J Am Geriatr Soc* 48:721-725, 2000.

CHAPTER 156

Infectious Processes: Urinary Tract Infections and Sexually Transmitted Diseases

Marilyn Bleiler Green and
Patricia Polgar Bailey

Physician consultation is recommended for newly diagnosed syphilis.

Physician-obstetric consultation is indicated for pregnant women with suspected pyelonephritis.

URINARY TRACT INFECTIONS

DEFINITION AND EPIDEMIOLOGY

Urinary tract infection (UTI) is a broad term used to describe bacterial infection or inflammation of the bladder (cystitis), urethra (urethritis), or renal pelvis and kidneys (pyelonephritis) and microbial colonization of the urine. All these structures, as well as adjacent structures such as the epididymis and prostate, are at risk of acquiring infection from the common urinary stream. A lower UTI is an infection or inflammation of the bladder or urethra. Upper or ascending UTIs include infections of the ureters and kidneys. Simple or uncomplicated UTIs are infections experienced by women with no significant history of UTIs and characterized by recent onset of mild to moderate symptoms. All other UTIs are considered complicated or nonsimple. In addition, UTIs can be due to acute or chronic infections.

Infection of the urinary tract is a common problem, second in frequency only to respiratory infections. Approximately 10% of women are diagnosed with UTIs in the United States yearly, and this is associated with direct medical costs of $1.6 billion per year.[1] UTIs are responsible for more than 8 million office visits yearly in the United States.[2]

UTIs are a particular problem in certain patient groups. Young, sexually active women are disproportionately affected. The incidence of cystitis among premenopausal sexually active women is 0.5 to 0.7 infections per person-year (7 million to 8 million cases yearly), and an estimated 50% of women will experience cystitis at some point in life. Of those, up to 50% develop recurrent infections, mostly as a result of reinfection (rather than relapse).[2] Approximately 3% to 5% of women have multiple recurrences over many years.[3] UTIs remain a significant problem in older women, in terms of both asymptomatic bacteriuria and symptomatic infections.[4,5]

UTIs are unusual in men less than 50 years old with normal urologic structures. During the mid-1950s and 1960s, the incidence of UTIs increased, largely as a result of prostate hypertrophy and obstruction of the urinary tract. Additional common reasons for UTIs in men include instrumentation, anatomic and functional abnormalities, suppressed host defense mechanisms, and anal intercourse. After age 65 years, the incidence of UTIs in men begins to equal that in women because of benign prostatic hyperplasia.[5]

PATHOPHYSIOLOGY

Most UTIs in women are secondary to ascending infection from the periurethral or perianal area. Cystitis in women is more common than in men because of the proximity of the urethral opening and vagina to the perianal area. Bacteria reach the bladder through the urethra and may ascend to the kidneys through the ureters.[1] Colonization of the vaginal introitus plays an important role in recurrent infections.

A relatively narrow spectrum of microorganisms causes the majority of UTIs; the most prominent pathogens include *Escherichia coli* (approximately 28% of cases); gram-negative organisms, including *Klebsiella, Proteus, Enterobacter*, and *Serratia* organisms (approximately 40%); and gram-positive cocci such as enterococci and staphylococci (approximately 20%). Approximately 95% of simple lower UTIs are caused by autoinoculation with Enterobacteriaceae from the bowel. *E. coli* is the causative bacterium in approximately 90% of cases of uncomplicated, acute cystitis (i.e., healthy females with anatomically normal urinary tract) and 30% of nosocomial infections in men and women. *Staphylococcus saprophyticus* is also common in young women in ambulatory settings and can account for as much as 10% to 20% of UTIs, especially during the summer months.[6,7]

Complicated UTIs may be due to a number of infectious agents other than *E. coli*. Common aerobes include *Klebsiella pneumoniae, Proteus mirabilis, Pseudomonas aeruginosa*, and *Enterococcus* species. Enterococci are particularly common in nosocomial UTIs of either sex.[6] Most UTIs in women are not due to complicating conditions or serious problems. Sexual intercourse, diaphragm use with spermicidal agents for contraception, impaired voiding, and age (likely due to the hypoestrogenic state with vaginal mucosal atrophy) increase the risk of UTIs, as do certain medical conditions such as diabetes, obesity, urinary tract calculi, sickle cell trait, and frequent or indwelling bladder catheterization.[1] Factors not associated with UTIs include direction of wiping the perineum after defecation; tampon use; bubble baths; douching; tight clothing; and intake of carbonated beverages, coffee, or tea.[8]

Because UTIs are uncommon in men less than 50 years old, they are considered complicated infections in men.[4] The incidence is higher in newborns, infants, and older men, all of whom are more likely to have anatomic abnormalities of the urinary tract. Some data suggest that lack of circumcision may contribute to the increased incidence of UTI among young men; however, this was not confirmed in subsequent studies in which the majority of men with acute cystitis had been circumcised.[9] Homosexuality has been identified as a risk factor for UTI in men, and heterosexual anal coitus may also increase the risk of UTI in young, healthy men. Prostatic hypertrophy significantly increases the risk of UTI in older adults.[9] Risk factors for UTIs in women and men are listed in Box 156-1.

BOX 156-1

RISK FACTORS FOR URINARY TRACT INFECTIONS

WOMEN

- Inherent anatomic risk (4-cm female urethra vs. 20-cm male urethra)
- Fecal contamination
- History of recent urinary tract infection
- Decreased fluid intake
- Irregular bladder emptying
- Vaginal pH >4.5
- Sexual intercourse
- Failure to void within 10 to 15 minutes of coitus
- Diaphragm or spermicide use
- Symptomatic partner
- Pregnancy
- Menopause
- Hyperuremia
- Neurogenic bladder
- Kidney disease
- Urologic abnormalities
- Instrumentation
- Immunosuppression

MEN

- Urologic abnormalities
- Neurogenic bladder
- Instrumentation
- Benign prostatic hyperplasia
- Anal intercourse
- Immunosuppression

CLINICAL PRESENTATION

UTIs can be subdivided into several distinct types of infection: acute uncomplicated UTIs, recurrent UTIs, complicated UTIs, urethritis, pyelonephritis, and asymptomatic bacteriuria, with different characteristics associated with each of these syndromes.

Acute uncomplicated UTIs are characterized by signs and symptoms of bladder irritation: increased frequency, urgency, dysuria, and occasionally hematuria. The term *uncomplicated infection* implies that this is a relatively uncommon occurrence in the affected individual who is also otherwise healthy, that there are a small number of responsible pathogens that are susceptible to first-line narrow-spectrum antimicrobial agents, and that there are no underlying urologic or gynecologic abnormalities. A more acute presentation, including high fever, chills, flank pain, costovertebral angle (CVA) tenderness, nausea, and vomiting, is suggestive of pyelonephritis or urosepsis.

Approximately 50% of women who have UTIs will experience recurrent infections.[3] There are two basic patterns of recurrence: relapse and reinfection. *Relapse* refers to infection caused by bacterial persistence—infection by the previously treated pathogen, which was not completely eradicated by the course of antimicrobial therapy. *Reinfection* refers to recurrence of infection by introduction of a new bacterial strain. In the majority of women, recurrent UTIs are due to reinfection rather than relapse.

Groups often bothered by recurrent infections include sexually active women who report a temporal relationship of urinary symptoms to intercourse, those with compromised host defenses because of underlying systemic illness or immunosuppressive therapy, those with a history of upper UTIs, and pregnant women. Infections caused by relapse are usually caused by certain pathogens including *Klebsiella, Pseudomonas, Proteus*, and *Enterococcus* organisms.

Complicated UTIs are those which occur in patients with underlying urologic or gynecologic abnormalities or which are caused by pathogens that have developed antimicrobial resistance. UTIs are also considered complicated when comorbidity or other factors increase the risk of persistence, recurrence, or treatment failure. Common causes of complicated infections include functional or anatomic abnormalities of the urinary tract (e.g., a history of polycystic renal disease, nephrolithiasis, neurogenic bladder), underlying disease (e.g., diabetes mellitus, AIDS, or any other immunocompromising illness), use of immune-modifying drugs, pregnancy, the presence of an indwelling catheter, recent instrumentation (e.g., catheterization or cystoscopy), and older age.[10] However, these complicating factors are not always immediately apparent and do not necessarily predict the initial presentation, which can range from a mild cystitis to an acutely toxic presentation. Differentiating between types of UTI and underlying causes is important in determining effective treatment regimens. UTIs in men are uncommon and often represent underlying abnormalities; therefore they are considered at least partially complicated.

Pyelonephritis refers to bacterial infection of the upper urinary tract, which includes the kidneys and the ureters, and usually results from ascending infection. A sustained bladder infection and reflux increase the risk of ascending infection. High fever, chills, flank pain, CVA tenderness, nausea, and vomiting in the presence of urinary symptoms are suggestive of pyelonephritis. However, kidney infection may also manifest with only bladder irritation and the absence of any of the classic signs or symptoms. The presence of white blood cell (WBC) casts on microscopy is considered pathognomonic for pyelonephritis. *E. coli* accounts for more than 80% of acute uncomplicated cases of pyelonephritis.[4] Pyelonephritis in male patients suggests an underlying urologic structural abnormality. Renal calculi and embolic infarction can also cause flank pain and hematuria, mimicking pyelonephritis. However, unlike the case with UTIs, urine cultures are sterile and no bacteria are seen on Gram's stain.

Urethritis is characterized by an inflammation (mechanical, chemical, or bacterial) of the urethra alone. Infection of the urogenital tract by sexually transmitted diseases (STDs), especially chlamydia, has reached epidemic proportions. Prevalence is highest among sexually active adolescents and young adults. Urethritis is generally classified as gonococcal or nongonococcal in etiology. Nongonococcal urethritis (NGU) is most common, with *Chlamydia* being the most frequent causative organism. Other urethral pathogens include *Ureaplasma urealyticum, Mycoplasma hominis*, and, in women, *Trichomonas vaginalis* and *Gardnerella vaginalis*. Symptoms are usually mild and gradual in onset. Women may experience vaginal discharge or bleeding from concomitant cervicitis and lower abdominal pain. Signs and symptoms of urethritis may include dysuria and irritative symptoms, frequency, urethral discharge, and pruritus at the distal end of the penis. Urinalysis often demonstrates pyuria and, less commonly, hematuria.

Urine cultures generally show a colony count of less than 100/ml. A low colony count in the presence of the aforementioned symptoms is suggestive of urethritis. Approximately 1% to 2% of women have urethritis, and in postmenopausal women urethritis and atrophic vaginitis are common causes of lower urinary tract symptoms.[11]

Asymptomatic bacteriuria refers to a colony count of at least 100,000/ml in the absence of symptoms. Asymptomatic bacteriuria is more common in women; increases in both sexes with advancing age; and is found in as many as 40% of older men and women, especially those living in nursing homes. In addition to advancing age and nursing homes, asymptomatic bacteriuria is also associated with a history of indwelling catheterization, instrumentation, urinary incontinence, multiple medical illnesses, and impaired functional and mental status. It is several-fold more common in women with diabetes mellitus.[12] However, the prevalence of asymptomatic bacteriuria in sexually active young women is still quite high, at 5% to 6%, similar to the prevalence in pregnancy.[1] Screening for asymptomatic bacteriuria is recommended only for pregnant women and before urologic surgery. Treatment of asymptomatic bacteriuria before urologic surgery decreases the risk of postsurgical complications. Treatment of pregnant women with asymptomatic bacteriuria, particularly during the first trimester, reduces the risk of acute pyelonephritis and the risks of prematurity and low birth weight in their infants.[13] Some authorities have recommended using a colony count of 10,000/ml or greater to increase the sensitivity of the test. However, most clinicians use 100,000/ml as a clinically significant parameter, particularly in asymptomatic women, and thus require treatment at that level.[14,15]

PHYSICAL EXAMINATION

Important history to elicit from the woman with a complaint of UTI symptoms includes urinary frequency; nocturia; dysuria or burning on urination; pruritus; fever or chills; hematuria; vaginal or pelvic signs and symptoms; last menstrual period; and any prior history of UTIs, cervicitis, or pelvic inflammatory disease (PID). Patients should be queried about medical history, specifically immunocompromising disease, use of immune-modifying drugs, and recent instrumentation. It is worth noting that most women know when they have a UTI; women with a history of UTI correctly diagnosis (as confirmed by urine culture) themselves as having a UTI more than 90% of the time.[5]

Vaginal symptoms, external irritation on urination, and dyspareunia are helpful in sorting out vaginal etiologies from those referable to the urinary tract. Male patients should be assessed for urethral discharge, penile lesions, a history of UTIs or STDs, and prior treatment, if any. It is important to ask all patients about sexual history and risk factors for gonorrhea or chlamydia, including new or symptomatic sex partners.

The physical examination should include assessment of vital signs, signs and symptoms of acute illness, and dehydration. An examination of the female patient should include a pelvic examination if there is any indication that infection is not solely associated with the urinary tract. The vulva, vagina, cervix, periurethral area, and perianal area should be assessed for discharge, excoriations, tenderness, and ulcerations. In male patients the penis should be checked for discharge, lesions, ulcerations, and swelling. The prostate should be checked for tenderness, swelling, masses, or nodules.

The pace, extensiveness, and order of the evaluation are largely dictated by the clinical presentation. The diagnosis of UTI is suggested by the history and physical examination and confirmed by examination of the urine.

DIAGNOSTICS

The urinalysis is the most important initial study. A urine dipstick is a reasonable rapid diagnostic aid. A clean-voided specimen minimizes contamination from vaginal and labial sources. Leukocyte esterase reflects the presence of WBCs in the urine. However, not all UTIs are associated with WBCs in the urine. The nitrite test reflects the presence of urinary nitrite, which is reduced from urinary nitrate by certain bacteria, although not all bacteria reduce nitrate to nitrite. If both the nitrite test and the leukocyte esterase test are positive, then a UTI is present more than 90% of the time.

In addition to the information obtained from the dipstick, urine can be examined microscopically, which allows for easier detection of red blood cells, WBCs, bacteria, and WBC casts. Correlation with subsequent culture is approximately 90%. Uncentrifuged urine can be examined under a coverslip with an oil immersion lens. A WBC count of less than 7/mm^3 on low power is abnormal, although not specific for infection. A WBC count of 7/mm^3 suggests that infection is not present. A count of greater than 5 WBCs per high-powered field of spun urine is suggestive of a UTI. Sheets of numerous crystals suggest calculi, and the presence of WBC casts (a renal cylindric plug of tightly packed leukocytes) are considered proof positive of kidney involvement (either stones or infection). Abnormalities for pH, protein, and blood are nonspecific with respect to UTIs. In the presence of symptoms but a negative dipstick, direct demonstration by microscopy or culture should be done before excluding the possibility of infection.

Urine culture is the definitive test and should be obtained in all patients who are febrile, are seriously ill, have a history of frequent UTIs, or have recently been hospitalized or for whom empiric treatment has failed. Infections in pregnant women should always be cultured.[16] In addition, cultures should be obtained in young men because infections are unusual and suggestive of underlying problems. If prostatitis is suspected in men, segmental urine and expressed prostatic secretions should be obtained, viewed microscopically, and cultured. There are differing views regarding the need for urine cultures in otherwise healthy women with mild to moderate symptoms. A 100,000/ml colony count is no longer considered a useful parameter for symptomatic women; this traditional criterion for infection provides for high specificity but poor sensitivity (as low as 50% in young women). A colony count as low as 10,000/ml can cause symptomatic infections in some people, and most experts agree that UTIs can even occur with bacterial counts as low as 100/ml. Some of these individuals, if untreated, may tend to return with even more severe infections at even higher colony counts.[4,17]

The bacterial species identified by the culture is as important as the colony count. The presence of multiple species suggests contamination of the specimen, except in the case of catheterization or other special circumstances. Small numbers of certain pathogens, including *Klebsiella* organisms and *E. coli*, should be regarded as suspicious. Large numbers of skin flora, such as *Staphylococcus epidermidis*, diphtheroids, and β-hemolytic streptococci, can usually be ignored. Anaerobic bacteria do not usually cause UTIs; their presence suggests communication with the bowel. *Candida* organisms usually suggest vaginal contamination.

Sterile pyuria is defined as a negative urine culture despite a positive urinalysis (e.g., positive leukocyte esterase). This condition requires further investigation, since the absence of pathogens on culture does not imply the absence of infection. Some infectious organisms, such as those causing NGU, do not grow on standard laboratory media. Cultures specific for these organisms, such as antigen and DNA detection techniques, should be considered if the history and physical examination suggest a chlamydial or nongonococcal cause. However, many patients with urethral syndrome do not have a demonstrable infectious agent even when special culture media are used. Gram-negative intracellular diplococci on Gram's stain are diagnostic for gonococcal urethritis. Renal tuberculosis, systemic illness, vaginal contamination, and kidney stones can also cause leukocytosis in the absence of a positive culture.[18]

"Test of cure" urine cultures should be obtained in men and whenever there is suspicion that an infection may not have been eradicated. Routine "test of cure" cultures are generally not indicated unless a persistent (as opposed to a recurrent) UTI is suspected. The recurrence of a UTI within 2 weeks is suggestive of a persistent UTI. One posttreatment urinalysis may be helpful to exclude hematuria, since persistent hematuria requires further diagnostic evaluation to exclude renal calculi and tumors.[8]

Persistent UTIs require more extensive urologic evaluation. Renal ultrasonography is a quick, noninvasive way to evaluate renal function; it can detect kidney size, scarring, calculi, renal tumors, and hydronephrosis. Indications for evaluating patients with UTIs with ultrasound include frequent recurrent UTIs in female patients or failure to eradicate infection despite appropriate therapy; acute pyelonephritis in male patients; recurrent pyelonephritis in female patients; or acute infection with systemic symptoms, palpable bladder or renal mass, and signs and symptoms suggestive of renal calculi or *Proteus* infection (e.g., pH >7, posttreatment pyuria).[8,19]

IV pyelogram (IVP) scanning and CT scanning may be useful if the ultrasound examination is noninformative or nonspecific. Both can provide additional details to help guide treatment. CT scans are better than either ultrasound or IVP for imaging certain conditions, including lymphadenopathy and renal abscesses and masses. MRI provides even sharper imaging but at considerably greater expense. Radioisotope scans of the kidney may be required to further define anatomic abnormalities.[6] Cystoscopy involves a visual examination of the interior of the bladder by means of a cystoscope and is used to exclude bladder disease. A voiding cystourethrogram is the study of choice for demonstrating and determining the degree of vesicourethral reflux (i.e., the retrograde flow from the bladder to the ureters). Retrograde flow is associated with, but not necessarily the cause of, infection.

DIAGNOSTICS

Urinary Tract Infections

LABORATORY
Urinalysis (clean-voided specimen)
Urine culture and sensitivity*
Sexually transmitted disease cultures*
Segmented urine and expressed prostatic secretions in men*

IMAGING
Renal ultrasound*
IV pyelography*
CT scan, MRI*
Radiography of kidney*

OTHER
Cystoscopy*
Voiding cystourethrogram*

*If indicated.

DIFFERENTIAL DIAGNOSIS

The differential diagnosis of an acute uncomplicated UTI includes urethritis, vaginal infections (e.g., *Gardnerella* organisms, *Candida albicans*, or *Trichomonas* organisms), STDs that may lead to cervicitis or PID (e.g., *Chlamydia trachomatis*, *Neisseria gonorrhoeae*), and other STDs (e.g., herpes simplex virus) that may mimic symptoms of UTI but are considered distinct from UTIs.[11] The diagnosis is usually made on the basis of the history, presenting signs and symptoms, and findings on urinalysis and other laboratory work. In the case of a negative urine dipstick in the presence of urinary symptoms, microscopic evaluation or culture should be performed before deciding that a UTI is not present. A pelvic examination should be considered in a female patient if the history is suggestive of vulvovaginitis from candidiasis, trichomoniasis, or another infection such as herpes simplex. Chlamydial and gonorrheal cultures should be obtained in a sexually active women to exclude urethritis. The combination of cervical discharge, cervical motion tenderness, and adnexal tenderness suggests cervicitis or PID. Atrophic vaginitis should be considered in a postmenopausal woman not using topical estrogen therapy. A woman who is initially seen with one or more symptoms of UTI has a probability of infection of at least 50%. Specific combinations of symptoms (e.g., dysuria and frequency without vaginal discharge) substantially increase the likelihood of UTI. In contrast, the history and physical examination are less reliable in accurately excluding UTI in women with urinary symptoms. A urine culture and pelvic examination should be considered in women who demonstrate symptoms of UTI but whose history and physical examination are essentially negative.[10]

Clinical syndromes in women that mimic UTIs include acute urethral syndrome (also referred to as symptomatic abacteriuria) and interstitial cystitis. Clinical presentation is characterized by bladder irritation, frequency, urgency, and dysuria. The urinalysis is often unimpressive, with few leukocytes and no bacteria. Urine cultures show no significant colony counts, and urethral cultures are often negative. Studies have shown that some women have bacterial infection with

DIFFERENTIAL DIAGNOSIS

Urinary Tract Infections

ACUTE INFECTIONS
- Urethritis
- Vaginitis
- Cervicitis
- Pelvic inflammatory disease
- Herpes simplex
- Acute urethral syndrome
- Interstitial cystitis

CHRONIC INFECTIONS
- Structural abnormalities
- Neurologic dysfunction
- Renal calculi or masses
- Intrarenal or perirenal abscess
- Bladder tuberculosis
- Prostate enlargement

very low colony counts; these women respond to the standard therapy for an uncomplicated UTI.[20] Approximately 30% of these women have no pyuria and no detectable infection. A subset of these women may have interstitial cystitis, which may be an advanced stage of infection of the lower urinary tract resulting from either conventional pathogens or organisms established earlier in the urethra and tissues below the bladder as a result of repeated and prolonged administration of antibiotics. No treatment has been found to be effective once the histologic changes have become established.[21] Symptoms include suprapubic discomfort, especially with a full bladder, and symptoms are often relieved with voiding. Urinalysis is often normal, but hematuria may be present. Urine cultures are sterile. The cause of the symptoms is difficult to diagnose; if hematuria is present and persists, other causes of hematuria, such as bladder cancer, should be excluded. No definitive therapy for interstitial cystitis has been developed. It is hoped that improved diagnosis and management at initial stages of infection or inflammation will decrease the prevalence of this chronic condition. Tricyclics may provide some symptomatic relief for women with interstitial cystitis.[21]

The differential diagnosis for recurrent UTIs includes structural abnormalities (such as obstructive uropathy, congenital anomalies, urinary tract fistulas), neurologic dysfunction, renal calculi and renal masses, intrarenal and perirenal abscesses, bladder tuberculosis, and prostate enlargement in men. Patients with recurrent UTIs or infections that do not respond to standard antimicrobial therapy should be referred to the urologist to exclude underlying causes.[19]

MANAGEMENT

A wide range of antibiotic agents are effective in treating UTIs; nonetheless, drug selection must be made carefully. Common and avoidable reasons for treatment failure include inappropriate antibiotic selection, adverse reactions, subtherapeutic dosing, and inadequate treatment duration. The choice of antibiotics should be determined by the criteria listed in Box 156-2. Antibiotics used to treat routine UTIs include trimethoprim-sulfamethoxazole (TMP-SMX), ampicillin, cephalosporins, fluoroquinolones, and nitrofurantoin. Based on the criteria listed in Box 156-2, however, certain antibiotics may not be appropriate in all situations.

TMP-SMX is bacteriolytic and relatively inexpensive and therefore considered the drug of choice for the treatment of community-acquired acute uncomplicated cystitis. Reported bacterial eradication and cure rates are higher than 85% to 90%. Most of the side effects and allergic reactions to this drug combination are due to the sulfa component. There is some evidence that trimethoprim alone provides antimicrobial coverage that is comparable to that of the combination and therefore can also be used alone.[22] Acute uncomplicated UTIs should usually be treated with an antibiotic for 3 days; 3-day regimens have been shown to give the same cure rate as traditional 7- to 10-day courses in at least 90% of women.[3] Single-dose treatment of an uncomplicated UTI is less effective than a 3-day course.[17]

BOX 156-2

CRITERIA FOR ANTIBIOTIC SELECTION FOR URINARY TRACT INFECTIONS

- Type of urinary tract infection (acute uncomplicated, complicated, recurrent)
- Microorganism susceptibility (culture and sensitivity)
- Likelihood of bacterial resistance
- Adequate antimicrobial concentration achieved in urine
- Toxicity
- Side effects
- Renal function
- Concomitant conditions

There is, however, an increasing prevalence of antimicrobial resistance among women with community-acquired infections, 17% to TMP-SMX, 38% to ampicillin, and 1.9% to 2.5% to fluoroquinolones.[20] Therefore TMP-SMX is not recommended as the empiric drug for UTI treatment in areas where 10% to 20% of strains demonstrate antimicrobial resistance.[23]

Additional first-line antimicrobial agents (both effective and inexpensive) include ampicillin, amoxicillin, and amoxicillin-clavulanate. However, TMP-SMX–resistant organisms are often resistant to multiple drugs, including ampicillin, amoxicillin, and first-generation cephalosporins. In fact, *E. coli* resistance to these drugs exceeds 30% in most locations. Resistance to amoxicillin-clavulanate is only slightly lower than resistance to amoxicillin alone and is often independent of β-lactamase activity.[22-24]

Fluoroquinolones (e.g., ciprofloxacin, ofloxacin, norfloxacin, levofloxacin) are an appropriate alternative to TMP-SMX. They provide good coverage and tend to be well tolerated; however, they are generally significantly more expensive than other commonly used drugs. At present, the *E. coli* strains that cause community-acquired infections are still susceptible to fluoroquinolones, although there are reports of increased fluoroquinolone resistance.[20] More widespread use of these drugs will likely result in increasing antimicrobial resistance, which is the basis for reserving this class of drugs for treatment of complicated infections. Fluoroquinolones are also generally effective against Enterobacteriaceae, as well as staphylococci, *P. aeruginosa*, *Mycoplasma* organisms, chlamydiae, and some streptococci.

Additional treatment options include the cephalosporins and nitrofurantoin. Cephalosporins (e.g., cefuroxime) are also effective in treating typical pathogens but tend to be relatively expensive. Their side effect profile is similar to that of the aminopenicillins.[20] Nitrofurantoin (50 to 100 mg q 12 hr) is a synthetic antibacterial agent and is indicated for the treatment of acute uncomplicated UTIs caused by susceptible strains of *E. coli* or *S. saprophyticus*, as well as several other gram-positive aerobes such as *S. epidermidis* and *Staphylococcus aureus*. It is also effective for prophylaxis of recurrent UTI. Side effects of nitrofurantoin are relatively rare but significant, including pulmonary complications and hepatitis. Although nitrofurantoin is pregnancy category B during the first trimester, it is category X at term because of the increased risk of CPD6 anemia. Table 156-1 includes a list of antibiotics effective in treating UTIs.

Suboptimum candidates for short-course therapy include those with diabetes mellitus, a history of relapses or more than three UTIs during the past year, and an immunocompromised status. Such patients require more conventional antimicrobial therapy of 10 to 14 days for what are considered complicated UTIs. In addition, men should be treated with a 7- to 10-day course of therapy because all UTIs in men are considered complicated.

Given the global problem of increasing antimicrobial resistance, the use of broad-spectrum antibiotics for uncomplicated UTIs should be avoided if possible. Broad-spectrum antibiotics such as the fluoroquinolones should be reserved for the treatment of infections caused by resistant gram-negative pathogens, where their use has been shown to decrease hospitalization time and the need for IV therapy.[25]

Phenazopyridine (Pyridium), a urinary tract analgesic, is sometimes used in patients with dysuria. It is often prescribed alone or concurrently with an antimicrobial agent. A dosage of 200 mg t.i.d. for 48 to 72 hours may relieve dysuria in true UTIs; however, the use of phenazopyridine and an antibiotic has not been proven to be more effective or provide more rapid relief of symptoms than the use of an antibiotic alone. Phenazopyridine is a dye (urine will turn orange and can stain fabric) and can accumulate in older adults or in anyone with impaired renal function, precipitating renal failure. It should be avoided in persons with hepatitis and hemolytic anemia and is contraindicated in all those with glucose-6-phosphate dehydrogenase deficiency.

TABLE 156-1 Antibiotic Treatment for Urinary Tract Infections

Antibiotic	Drug Category	Dosage
Trimethoprim-sulfamethoxazole	C*	160/800 mg b.i.d.
Trimethoprim	C*	100 mg b.i.d.
Ampicillin	B	250-500 mg t.i.d. or q.i.d.
Amoxicillin	B	250-500 mg t.i.d. or q.i.d.
Amoxicillin-clavulanate	B	250-500 mg t.i.d. or q.i.d.
Erythromycin	B	250-500 mg q.i.d.
Cefuroxime	B	125-250 mg b.i.d.
Cephalexin	B	250 mg b.i.d.
Nitrofurantoin	B (1st trimester) X (at term)	50-100 mg b.i.d.
Ciprofloxacin	C	250-500 mg, b.i.d. or q.i.d.
Levofloxacin	C	250 mg q day
Norfloxacin	C	400 mg b.i.d.
Ofloxacin	C	300 mg b.i.d.

*Should not be prescribed for pregnant women in the third trimester.

The effectiveness of specific nonpharmacologic therapies, especially cranberry juice, is still unclear, although the consensus in the lay public is that cranberry juice is helpful in treating and preventing UTIs. A Cochrane review (2000) found insufficient evidence to recommend the use of cranberry juice to manage UTI.[26] However, more recent studies suggest that both cranberry and lingonberry juice may have some beneficial effect in the management and prevention of UTIs and have a variable effect in their treatment.[3] The assumption has been that cranberry juice's acidification of urine is responsible for its antibacterial effect; however, increased urine acidification does not appear to play a role. Rather, the inhibition of bacterial adherence to uroepithelial cells seems to explain the beneficial effect of cranberry or lingonberry juice supplementation. Dosages of 200 to 750 ml or equivalent concentrated tablets daily have been found to be effective.[9] In addition, at least two studies have shown that drinking cranberry juice daily reduces the recurrence rate of UTIs compared with ingestion of *Lactobacillus* organisms and placebo.[27-30]

Recurrent UTIs should be treated as outlined in the preceding paragraphs and documented by at least one urine culture. If recurrences are frequent, such as three or more in a year, the urinary tract should be evaluated for abnormalities; patients with structural problems should be referred to the appropriate specialist, usually a urologist or gynecologist. Three or more infections per year in the absence of urologic abnormalities are an indication for antibiotic prophylaxis. Recurrent cystitis can be managed by one of several strategies: continuous prophylaxis, postcoital prophylaxis, or therapy initiated by the patient. Of the prophylactic regimens that have been used, continuous low-dose prophylaxis is the most well established. This type of regimen consists of daily or three times a week subtherapeutic doses of an antibiotic known to be effective in the treatment of UTI. In addition, these antibiotics can also be taken after intercourse, or they can be initiated by the patient on experiencing symptoms. Patient-initiated therapy may be prescribed in the form of multiple 3-day courses of antibiotics to be started at the onset of UTI symptoms; such treatment has been found to be both cost-effective and safe with respect to drug toxicity.[20] The most commonly used agents for continuous prophylaxis include TMP-SMX 40 to 200 mg (half a single-strength tablet), trimethoprim 40 to 80 mg, nitrofurantoin 50 to 100 mg, norfloxacin 200 mg, or cephalexin 250 mg. Postmenopausal women who experience recurrent UTIs may find symptomatic relief with topical estrogen cream. Studies on oral estrogen therapy and its effect on recurrent UTI symptoms are inconclusive.[8]

Complicated UTIs are those which occur in patients with urologic abnormalities or other co-morbidities that increase the risk of infections caused by pathogens resistant to antibiotics. These complications may not be completely obvious and do not necessarily predict the severity of infection on presentation. The clinical spectrum ranges from a mild cystitis to an acute pyelonephritis with systemic complications, but can also include long periods of asymptomatic bacteriuria. Treatment of complicated UTIs should be extended for at least 7 days and must be based on urine culture and susceptibility testing. TMP-SMX is a reasonable empiric first choice while results of the culture and sensitivity are pending. A posttreatment test of cure is not necessary as long as symptoms have completely resolved. If culture-directed therapy fails, a repeat urine culture and further evaluation are indicated.[17]

Diabetes mellitus is one of the most common primary care problems associated with a significant increased risk of developing complications of UTI or unusual forms of infections. Individuals with diabetes are also more likely to develop rare complications, such as emphysematous cystitis and pyelonephritis, abscess formation, and renal papillary necrosis, compared with those who do not have diabetes mellitus. In addition, the prevalence of urinary tract anatomic or physiologic abnormalities seems to be greater among those with diabetes. The most common pathogen is *E. coli*, but unusual pathogens and fungal infections, particularly *Candida* species, are more common among persons with diabetes. For these reasons, the initial choice of antibiotic therapy should be based on the Gram's stain of the urine and on results of recent urine cultures, if available. Fungal infection should also be considered if there is a history of prior fungal infection, recent instrumentation, or broad-spectrum antibiotic use. The majority of pathogens in this population are still sensitive to the fluoroquinolones, and reasonable empiric first choices include ciprofloxacin, levofloxacin, and gatifloxacin. Additional options include imipenem, ticarcillin-clavulanate, and piperacillin-tazobactam. Therapy should be continued for 7 days or possibly longer depending on individual circumstances.[31]

Asymptomatic bacteriuria should be treated in pregnancy and before urologic surgery. Antimicrobial therapy should be based on urine culture and antibiotic susceptibility. Most infections respond to 3-day courses of amoxicillin, TMP-SMX (contraindicated in third trimester of pregnancy), an oral cephalosporin, or nitrofurantoin (contraindicated at term). In most other adults, asymptomatic bacteriuria does not cause symptomatic infection, renal failure, urosepsis, or increased mortality; therefore routine screening and treatment in other adult groups are not recommended.[4]

Treatment of urethritis depends on suspicion, if not confirmation, of the causative agent. Diagnosis of urethritis is confirmed by culture, but treatment is often empiric, based on the history, symptoms, and a urine culture significant for sterile pyuria. The most common cause of urethritis is *C. trachomatis*, which responds to doxycycline 100 mg PO b.i.d. for 7 days, azithromycin 1 g in a single dose, and ofloxacin 400 mg PO q 12 hr for 5 days. These drugs are usually also effective against *Ureaplasma* organisms. Pregnant women, for whom these drugs are contraindicated, can be treated with erythromycin base 500 mg PO q.i.d. for 7 days (erythromycin estolate is contraindicated in pregnancy). Less common causes of urethritis include *N. gonorrhoeae*, which requires a dose of ceftriaxone (Rocephin) 250 mg IM. Treatment of *N. gonorrhoeae* should include simultaneous treatment of NGU with both ceftriaxone and doxycycline or ofloxacin as a single agent. Infection with *Trichomonas* organisms, if identified, should be treated with metronidazole 250 mg PO t.i.d. for 1 week.

Treatment of pyelonephritis depends on the acuity and severity of symptoms, complicating risk factors, susceptibility of the pathogen to oral antimicrobial agents, and the patient's social supports. Antimicrobial therapy is based on Gram's stain and antibiotic susceptibility. Patients who are otherwise healthy can be treated on an outpatient basis with 10 to 14 days of oral antibiotics, provided that the patient is reliable, can take oral antibiotics, and has a phone and means of transportation should signs and symptoms worsen. Older adults and those with acute, severe symptoms and possibly urosepsis are candidates for hospitalization and often require parenteral therapy. A history of diabetes mellitus, sickle cell anemia, nephrolithiasis, or excessive analgesic use increases the risk of renal papillary necrosis and subsequent obstruction and can be considered an indication for hospitalization.

Co-Management with Specialists

Patients with frequent recurrent or relapsing UTIs should be referred for further evaluation, especially if underlying urologic or gynecologic abnormalities have not been excluded. Those with underlying functional, metabolic, or structural urologic abnormalities, which increase the risk of UTIs, should be managed in conjunction with a specialist. Patients with co-morbidity that does not affect the risk of UTIs but that increases the severity of infection once contracted may benefit from collaboration with a specialist.

LIFE SPAN CONSIDERATIONS

Asymptomatic UTIs are more prevalent in pregnant women; screening for and treatment of infection are indicated in these women to decrease the risk of acute pyelonephritis, premature delivery, and low birth weight. Refer to Table 156-1 for a list of treatment options during pregnancy.

UTIs are the most common cause of bacterial infection in older adults but are often not accompanied by the classic signs and symptoms. Symptoms are often subtle and may include a vague change in mental status, decreased appetite, lethargy, and increased falls (sustained during efforts to get to the bathroom). UTIs are also the most common cause of sepsis, the second most common cause of bacteremia in the geriatric population, and an important cause of morbidity and mortality in nursing facilities.[32]

COMPLICATIONS

The most common complication of UTI is pyelonephritis, a bacterial infection of the kidney resulting from ascending untreated or inadequately treated lower UTI. Pyelonephritis can be treated effectively on an outpatient basis, and clinical response should occur within 48 to 72 hours of starting therapy. If no improvement is noted or if the patient's condition worsens, aggressive investigation for complications of renal infection or urinary obstruction should be undertaken, which generally requires hospitalization. Acute pyelonephritis is the most common serious medical complication of pregnancy, and 1% to 2% of pregnant women are admitted for this condition despite perinatal screening and treatment for bacteriuria.[1] Urosepsis is a potentially life-threatening systemic complication of UTI that requires high-dose parenteral antimicrobial therapy.

INDICATIONS FOR REFERRAL OR HOSPITALIZATION

Any patient who appears acutely ill or with signs and symptoms of obstruction or urosepsis requires immediate hospitalization. Specific signs and symptoms requiring consideration for hospitalization or referral include rigors, high fever, flank pain, nausea, and vomiting.

PATIENT AND FAMILY EDUCATION

Nonpharmacologic measures have been demonstrated to prevent episodic or recurrent UTIs. Sexual intercourse and failure to void within 10 to 15 minutes after coitus are the two factors most consistently associated with UTIs. In discussing the association between these two factors and UTIs with a patient, the provider must distinguish between UTIs and STDs. Explanations and suggestions must be offered in a way that is nonjudgmental and does not imply guilt. There is no basis for suggesting changes in a patient's sex life; however, recommending that a woman void within 10 to 15 minutes after coitus to decrease the frequency of UTIs is reasonable. Drinking plenty of fluids (64 to 80 ounces), urinating frequently, wiping from front to back, and avoiding feminine hygiene products (for the genital area) that contain deodorants may also be helpful in preventing UTIs.[33,34] Women who have had previous UTIs should be encouraged to seek treatment as soon as symptoms are recognized.

Women who use a diaphragm or spermicide may wish to consider an alternative form of birth control to avoid UTIs. This discussion must include the risks and benefits of other contraceptive options. Given the other options, some women may prefer to continue diaphragm use along with antibiotic prophylaxis as a way to minimize recurrent infections.

Women who suffer from recurrent UTIs should be educated about the possible benefits of antimicrobial suppression or postcoital prophylaxis, depending on the situation. Intravaginal estrogen cream may be helpful for postmenopausal women who suffer from recurrent UTIs. Daily ingestion of cranberries, whether in juice, concentrate, cocktail formulation, or capsule supplementation, may have a beneficial role in preventing UTIs, especially in women experiencing recurrent infections.[2]

Other behavioral changes commonly recommended, such as avoiding tight or synthetic underwear, vaginal douching, and tampon use, have not been substantiated. Providers should refrain from suggesting lifestyle changes that may be more reflective of their biases than of clinical research.

SEXUALLY TRANSMITTED DISEASES

DEFINITION AND EPIDEMIOLOGY

The term *sexually transmitted disease* encompasses more than 25 infectious organisms that are transmitted through sexual activity and the dozens of clinical syndromes associated with these organisms. Excluding the human immunodeficiency virus (HIV), the most common STDs in the United States are chlamydia, gonorrhea, genital herpes, human papillomavirus, trichomoniasis, and bacterial vaginosis.[35]

STDs are almost always transmitted from person to person by sexual intercourse. STDs are spread most efficiently by anal or vaginal intercourse and less effectively by oral intercourse. Pregnant women infected with an STD may infect infants in utero, during birth, or through breastfeeding.[36] Women are more vulnerable to STDs because they are more biologically susceptible to certain STDs than men and are more likely to have asymptomatic infection.

The management of STDs is often confounded by the inclusiveness of the term itself. A number of different organisms may be associated with different syndromes; for example, genital ulcers can result from herpes, chancroid, syphilis, or other infections.

Over the past 10 to 15 years the epidemiology of STDs has changed dramatically. As a group, STDs are considered to be at epidemic proportions.[36] Five of the top 10 reportable infectious diseases in the United States are STDs (chlamydial infection, gonorrhea, HIV/AIDS, primary and secondary syphilis, and hepatitis B virus infection).[37] There are approximately 19 million new cases of STDs annually in the United States.[35] Rates of many STDs, particularly viral STDs (genital herpes, HIV, and human papillomavirus), are higher now than they were 3 decades ago. Syphilis continues to remain a problem in the United States, with rates reaching epidemic proportions in the mid-1980s and early 1990s.[38] Although the incidence of syphilis declined to a record low in 2000, the incidence of primary and secondary syphilis began increasing again in 2003 to 2004. Most increases were observed only among men. Female numbers did not increase, and the rate of congenital syphilis decreased.[35]

STDs affect persons of all racial, cultural, and socioeconomic groups, but with wide discrepancies among these groups. The rate of gonorrhea in African-American adolescents is more than 30 times the rate in Caucasian adolescents and 11 times higher than rates among Hispanics.[35,39] The rate of primary and secondary syphilis in African Americans is nearly 23% times that in Caucasians.[35] Rates continue to remain considerably higher for African Americans and Hispanics than for Caucasians. However, the racial gaps are narrowing due in part to declining rates in African Americans and increases in syphilis in Caucasian men in recent years.[35]

Adolescents and young adults are at the greatest risk of acquiring an STD. Approximately 3 million teenagers acquire an STD each year. The incidence of gonorrhea and chlamydia is highest in 15- to 19-year-olds. Young men and women under age 25 account for two thirds of all cases of chlamydia and gonorrhea in the United States. Sexual behavior that includes multiple partners, inconsistent use of condoms, and endocervical ectopia in female patients contributes to the higher risk in this age-group.[35,36,40-42]

CLINICAL PRESENTATION

A significant number of persons with STDs have no apparent signs or symptoms. More than one site may be infected simultaneously (e.g., cervix plus urethra), and symptoms may overlap and involve more than one pathogen. Diseases are tentatively classified into syndromes to narrow the field of possible pathogens.[43,44]

Because STDs do not always manifest with distinct clinical features, determining which patients are at risk necessitates a thorough sexual history. Practitioners are advised to adopt a standardized approach to anyone at risk for an STD. Eliciting

BOX 156-3

SEXUAL HISTORY QUESTIONS

- Condoms—consistency of use, and for what sexual practices
- Previous sexually transmitted diseases
- Medication allergies
- Most recent sexual encounter and number of partners in past 2 months and past year
- High-risk behaviors, including use of drugs and alcohol (or use by partners), including which drugs, how often, and what route
- Does patient have sex with men, women, or both?
- Do partners have sex with men, women, or both?
- Travel and location
- Dysuria, frequency, hematuria
- Adenopathy
- Fatigue, weight loss, night sweats, unexplained diarrhea, fever

ADDITIONAL HISTORY FOR WOMEN

- Vaginal discharge, bleeding, color
- Skin rash, lesions, sores; location
- Pruritus (vulvar, anal, oral, other)
- Pain (abdominal, vaginal, vulvar, anal, headache, joints)
- Rectal discharge, pain, blood
- Birth control methods, consistency of use
- Last menstrual period, description, changes

ADDITIONAL HISTORY FOR MEN

- Penile discharge
- Lesions (penis, scrotum, oral cavity, other)
- Skin rash
- Pruritus (urethra, anus, skin)
- Pain (testes, joints, headache, anal)
- Adenopathy
- Rectal discharge, bleeding, constipation

a history for an STD needs to be routine, standardized, and guided by the individual's age. An effective sexual history is critical for diagnosis and for counseling individuals with regard to risk-reduction behaviors. Sexual orientation and sexual behavior can be sensitive topics. Questions are best phrased in an open-ended, nonjudgmental, and nontechnical format and must address pertinent data (Box 156-3). Consideration of age-related developmental characteristics, particularly those associated with adolescence, is critical. It is not uncommon for female adolescents to protect themselves against pregnancy with oral contraceptives yet forgo condoms.[45,46]

With few exceptions, adolescents in the United States can be provided with confidential diagnosis and treatment of STDs without parental consent or knowledge. In many states adolescents can be provided with HIV counseling and testing without parental consent or knowledge.[40]

PHYSICAL EXAMINATION

The physical examination for an STD incorporates the same principles as the history. It is routine; standardized; and sensitive to the patient's age, individual needs, and cultural heritage. Consistently examining all areas reduces the chance of a missed diagnosis. Minimum physical examination procedures for women and men are listed in Box 156-4.

BOX 156-4

MINIMUM PHYSICAL EXAMINATION FOR SEXUALLY TRANSMITTED DISEASES

WOMEN

- Examination of the mouth
- Examination of the lymph nodes
- Examination of the skin on the thorax, abdomen, limbs, palms, soles
- Examination of the anogenital area
- Pelvic examination, including speculum examination and bimanual examination
- Assessment for cervical motion tenderness
- Palpation for inguinal and femoral adenopathy

MEN

- Examination of the mouth
- Examination of the lymph nodes
- Examination of the skin of the thorax, abdomen, limbs, palms, soles
- Examination of the external genitals and anus

Every effort should be made to allay anxiety. All steps of the examination should be explained before beginning. Female patients normally void before the examination. However, when collecting specimens, it is important to follow manufacturer's recommendations to ensure proper specimen collection technique. Female patients may or may not void before examination depending on the diagnostic test used.

DIAGNOSTICS

After completing the routine screening history and examination, the health care provider may be able to classify the patient in one of several clinical syndromes. This narrows the field of possible pathogens that cause the syndrome and guides treatment. If the patient is asymptomatic, therapy is determined by the laboratory results. Partners of persons with identified STDs are evaluated and treated on the basis of their last sexual encounter and the particular STD in question. Early, specific diagnosis and treatment of symptomatic and asymptomatic persons will prevent further transmission of disease to their partners. However, appropriate diagnosis of an STD often requires multiple specific diagnostic tests because of the variety of STDs. "Syndromic diagnosis," which uses the patient's history, results of physical examination, and laboratory test results, can be used for the diagnosis of clinical syndromes.[36] Nucleic acid amplification tests (NAATs) are critical new tools used to diagnose chlamydia and gonorrhea. They are more sensitive and permit urine testing, which reduces the dependence on invasive procedures.[41] Table 156-2 outlines the STDs and their associated pathogens and syndromes, appropriate diagnostics, and differential diagnoses.

MANAGEMENT

The major curable syndromes in adults include urethritis in men; vaginal discharge, cervicitis, and PID in women; and genital ulcers in both men and women. In the United States it is common to initiate treatments effective against all common bacteria causing these syndromes while laboratory results are pending. Co-infection with more than one organism is common. It is not useful for mild or asymptomatic infection.

TABLE 156-2 Treatment Profile for Sexually Transmitted Diseases

Pathogen, Differential Diagnosis	Clinical Presentation	Diagnosis	Consultation, Co-Management	Complications	Management
CHLAMYDIA					
Chlamydia trachomatis **Differential diagnosis:** Pelvic inflammatory disease (PID); gonorrhea	Often asymptomatic **Female:** Endocervical mucus (yellow or green), cervical ectopy, or edema **Male:** dysuria, mucoid purulent discharge, itching	Ligase chain reaction (LCR) swab Polymerase chain reaction (PCR) swab DNA probe Direct fluorescent antibody (DFA) Enzyme immunoassay (EIA), enzyme-linked immunosorbent assay (ELISA) Urine LCR Leukocyte esterase test (LET)	Treatment failure HIV-positive patients	PID Perihepatitis Reiter's syndrome Chronic conjunctivitis Chronic pelvic pain Infant infection Epididymitis	Collect specimen for chlamydia. Treat presumptively in patients with PID, nongonococcal urethritis (NGU), gonococcal infection, epididymitis in men <35 years old. Perform syphilis serology. Offer HIV counseling and testing.
GONORRHEA					
Neisseria gonorrhoeae **Differential diagnosis:** NGU; PID	Purulent urethral discharge Dysuria Pruritus Anorectal burning Skin lesions **Female:** Frequently asymptomatic; dysuria; leukorrhea; abnormal uterine bleeding; cervical motion tenderness; vaginal discharge; pharyngeal edema or erythema	Gram's stain Direct culture LCR PCR swab Gen-Probe EIA LET (requires confirmation)	Treatment failure Complications	Prostatitis Epididymitis Cystitis PID Disseminated gonorrhea Gonococcal conjunctivitis	Treat presumptively for chlamydia. Specimen testing for gonorrhea should occur before other testing. Partners are evaluated and treated. Perform syphilis serology. Offer HIV counseling and testing.
NONGONOCOCCAL URETHRITIS					
C. trachomatis (23%-55% of cases) *Ureaplasma urealyticum* (20%-40% of cases) *Trichomonas vaginalis* (25% of cases) Herpes simplex virus **Differential diagnosis:** Gonorrhea	Dysuria Mucoid or purulent discharge Pruritus Hematuria Frequency Urgency Endocervical exudate, friability	Gram's stain Wet mount Tests for gonorrhea and chlamydia	Treatment failure Complications	Epididymitis Penile edema Reiter's syndrome Tenosynovitis	If microscopic tests are not available, treat for both gonorrhea and chlamydia.

TABLE 156-2 Treatment Profile for Sexually Transmitted Diseases—cont'd

Pathogen, Differential Diagnosis	Clinical Presentation	Diagnosis	Consultation, Co-Management	Complications	Management
PRIMARY SYPHILIS					
Treponema pallidum **Differential diagnosis:** Genital herpes; chancroid; lymphogranuloma venereum; balanitis, excoriation of nonulcerative lesions; squamous cell carcinoma	Painless chancre at site of inoculation Discrete, enlarged, painless regional lymph nodes Incubation: 10-90 days, average 21 days	Dark-field microscopy Nontreponemal serology (rapid plasma reagin [RPR], Venereal Disease Research Laboratory [VDRL]) Confirm with treponemal serology (MHA-TP, FTA-ABS) Sequential serologic testing; use same testing method and laboratory	Positive diagnosis of disease All HIV-positive patients	Secondary syphilis Meningitis Cardiovascular or neurologic disease Facilitates HIV transmission Left untreated, can cause perinatal death or congenital syphilis in infants	Systemic disease: average incubation is 3 weeks. Chancre is unnoticed in 15%-39% of cases. Perform nontreponemal serology and clinical follow-up at 6 and 12 months. Note fourfold drop in titer; evaluate for HIV infection. Treatment failure: retreatment and consultation with specialist are indicated; patients may need lumbar puncture.
SECONDARY SYPHILIS					
T. pallidum **Differential diagnosis:** All undiagnosed mucocutaneous skin eruptions (e.g., drug eruption, pityriasis rosea, scabies)	Ulcerations: symmetric papillosquamous eruption on palms, soles, mucous membranes, trunk Appears 2-8 weeks after appearance of chancre Generalized adenopathy Malaise, arthralgias Oral mucous patches Condylomata lata Hepatosplenomegaly Symptoms of urinary tract infection	As with primary syphilis	As with primary syphilis	As above	Increased incidence is associated with crack cocaine and illicit drug use. At 6 and 12 months follow-up, assess for fourfold drop in titer. A fourfold increase in titer at any time may represent treatment failure or reinfection.
LATENT SYPHILIS (EARLY LATENT, LATE LATENT)					
T. pallidum	Positive serology without evidence of clinical disease Evaluate for aortitis, neurosyphilis iritis	Reactive VDRL or RPR Reactive FTA-ABS or MHA-TP	All cases managed with specialist	Progression of disease	Latent syphilis is diagnosed as probable on the basis of documented seroconversion or on a fourfold increase in titer of nontreponemal test. History of symptoms or exposure to partner during previous 12 months.

Continued

TABLE 156-2 Treatment Profile for Sexually Transmitted Diseases—cont'd

Pathogen, Differential Diagnosis	Clinical Presentation	Diagnosis	Consultation, Co-Management	Complications	Management
CHANCROID					
Haemophilus ducreyi **Differential diagnosis:** Genital herpes; primary syphilis; lymphogranuloma venereum; infected or traumatic lesions	One or more painful genital ulcers with tender inguinal adenopathy May have supportive inguinal adenopathy and undermined ulcer borders	Isolation of *H. ducreyi* Most cases diagnosed on clinical grounds Painful ulcers 4-7 days after exposure Usually coronal sulcus in men Prepuce in women	Treatment failure	Successful treatment cures infection In extensive cases, scarring despite successful therapy	Reexamine patients at 3-7 days. Larger ulcers heal more slowly. No evidence of *T. pallidum* appears on dark-field examination or by serology. Culture is negative for herpes simplex virus. Partner contact: examine and treat within 10 days. Perform syphilis serology. Offer HIV counseling.
GENITAL HERPES (PRIMARY, RECURRENT)					
Herpes simplex virus 2 (HSV-2) and sometimes HSV-1 **Differential diagnosis:** Primary syphilis; chancroid; fixed drug eruption; folliculitis	Primary: Vesicular lesions on erythematous base **Male:** Penis shaft, glans, urethra, rectum **Female:** Vulva, vagina, anus, cervix Lesions painful, with malaise, fever, painful adenopathy Lesions ulcerative to superficial ulcers **Recurrent:** Clinical prodrome—pain, itching, burning, tingling Constitutional symptoms rare Vesicles Superficial ulcers	History and physical examination with confirmation by viral culture Moist swab of unroofed or weeping vesicle from base of ulcer Tzanck smear of scrapings from lesion looking for multinucleated giant cells Testing for HSV routine in all atypical and all undiagnosed genital ulcers	Secondary infection Ocular infection Persistent constitutional symptoms Urinary retention Primary or recurrent infection during pregnancy HIV-positive patients	Secondary infection Ocular infection Neonatal infection Premature delivery Spontaneous abortion Intrauterine growth retardation Fetal infection	Treatment is symptomatic. Infection may recur. HSV may be transmitted to sex partners even when no lesions are present. Support groups are available. Many educational resources are available.

Antimicrobial therapy is available for all bacterial STDs, as well as those caused by protozoa and ectoparasites. Drugs for viral STDs are largely limited to symptom alleviation because they cannot eradicate the organism. The standards published by the Centers for Disease Control and Prevention (CDC) in 2006 use the regimens listed in Box 156-5.[44] For most STDs the partners of patients should be examined. According to the standards published by the CDC,[44] when exposure to a treatable STD is considered likely, appropriate antimicrobial agents should be administered, even though clinical signs of infection are not evident and laboratory tests are not yet available. Evidence suggests that the regimens recommended by the CDC are beneficial for specific STDs.[44,47] In many states the local state or health department can assist in partner notification for selected STDs (e.g., HIV infection, syphilis, gonorrhea, hepatitis B, and chlamydia).

Co-Management with Specialists

All pregnant and HIV-positive patients should be co-managed with a specialist or collaborating physician. All treatment failures necessitate management with a specialist. Consultation or co-management with a specialist is necessary for all cases of syphilis (see Table 156-2).

LIFE SPAN CONSIDERATIONS

Adolescents or young adults under 20 years of age are at the highest risk for acquiring an STD. They are more likely than other groups to have unprotected sex and multiple sex partners, and young women may also choose partners older than themselves. In addition, young women are biologically more susceptible to chlamydia, gonorrhea, and HIV. Screening of asymptomatic high-risk patients, with sensitivity to age-related developmental and cultural characteristics, is required.

BOX 156-5

TREATMENT OF SEXUALLY TRANSMITTED DISEASES

TREATMENT OF DISEASES CHARACTERIZED BY URETHRITIS OR CERVICITIS

Uncomplicated Gonococcal Infections

Recommended Regimens

A single dose of:

- Cefixime 400 mg PO, *or*
- Ceftriaxone 125 mg IM, *or*
- Ciprofloxacin 500 mg PO,* *or*
- Ofloxacin 400 mg PO,* *or*
- Levofloxacin 250 mg PO*

Plus a regimen effective against co-infection with *Chlamydia trachomatis,* such as:

- Azithromycin 1 g PO in a single dose, *or*
- Doxycycline 100 mg b.i.d. for 7 days

Chlamydia

Recommended Regimens

Azithromycin, 1 g PO in a single dose, *or*
Doxycycline, 100 mg PO b.i.d. for 7 days

Alternative Regimens

Erythromycin base 500 mg PO q.i.d. for 7 days, *or*
Erythromycin ethylsuccinate 800 mg PO q.i.d. for 7 days, *or*
Ofloxacin 300 mg PO b.i.d. for 7 days *or*
Levofloxacin 500 mg PO once a day for 7 days

Nongonococcal Urethritis

Recommended Regimens

Azithromycin 1 g PO in a single dose, *or*
Doxycycline 100 mg PO b.i.d. for 7 days

Alternative Regimens

Erythromycin base 500 mg PO q.i.d. for 7 days, *or*
Erythromycin ethylsuccinate 800 mg PO q.i.d. for 7 days, *or*
Ofloxacin 300 mg PO b.i.d. for 7 days *or*
Levofloxacin 500 mg PO for 7 days

TREATMENT OF DISEASES CHARACTERIZED BY GENITAL ULCERS

Genital Herpes: First Clinical Episode

Recommended Regimens

Acyclovir 400 mg PO t.i.d. for 7-10 days, *or*
Acyclovir 200 mg PO five times daily for 7-10 days *or*
Famciclovir 250 mg PO t.i.d. for 7-10 days, *or*
Valacyclovir 1 g PO b.i.d. for 7-10 days

Genital Herpes: Recurrent Episodes

Recommended Regimens

Acyclovir 400 mg PO t.i.d. for 5 days, *or*
Acyclovir 800 mg PO t.i.d. for 2 days, *or*
Acyclovir 800 mg PO b.i.d. for 5 days, *or*
Famciclovir 125 mg PO b.i.d. for 5 days, *or*
Famciclovir 1000 mg PO b.i.d. for 1 day
Valacyclovir 500 mg PO b.i.d. for 3 days, *or*
Valacyclovir 1 g PO daily for 5 days

Primary, Secondary, or Latent Syphilis of Less Than 1 Year's Duration

Recommended Regimens

Benzathine penicillin G, 2.4 million units IM in a single dose

If Allergic to Penicillin

Doxycycline 100 mg b.i.d. for 14 days *or*
Tetracycline 500 mg PO q.i.d. for 14 days

Early Latent Syphilis

Recommended Regimens

Benzathine penicillin G 2.4 million units IM in a single dose

Late Latent Syphilis of More Than 1 Year's Duration or Unknown Duration

Recommended Regimens

Benzathine penicillin G 7.2 million units total, administered as 3 doses of 2.4 million units IM each, at 1-week intervals

Chancroid

Recommended Regimens

Azithromycin 1 g PO in a single dose, *or*
Ceftriaxone 250 mg IM in a single dose, *or*
Ciprofloxacin 500 mg PO b.i.d. for 3 days, *or*
Erythromycin base 500 mg PO t.i.d. for 7 days

From Centers for Disease Control and Prevention: Sexually transmitted diseases treatment guideline, 2006, *MMWR* 55(RR-11):1-94, 2006. Consult these guidelines for more detailed recommendations, including guidelines for treatment of pregnant patients, HIV-infected patients, allergic patients, and other specific groups.

*Quinolones should not be used for infections in men who have sex with men or in those with a history of recent foreign travel or who have partners with a recent history of foreign travel, infections acquired in California or Hawaii, or infections acquired in other areas with increased quinoline-resistant *Neisseria gonorrhoeae* prevalence.[44]

STD prevention should be initiated before sexual activity begins, with education about healthy, safe sexual practices and continual reinforcement throughout the life span. Additional life span considerations relate to the development of PID in women, with possible consequences of infertility, ectopic pregnancies, and chronic pelvic pain.

Prevention of viral STDs requires the adoption of lifelong healthy sexual behaviors to help avoid acquisition and spread of infection. The prevalence of herpes increases with age because the disease, once acquired, stays within the body. The rates of new infections of herpes and human papillomavirus are typically highest in the late teens and early twenties.[35] Factors related to the spread and acquisition of STDs often include other high-risk behaviors, such as multiple partners, use of illicit drugs, excessive alcohol use, and unsafe sexual practices such as inconsistent use or no use of condoms. Prevention of reinfection often necessitates other lifestyle behavior changes that address these specific risk factors.[36,41]

DISEASES CHARACTERIZED BY CERVICITIS AND URETHRITIS

Urethritis, or inflammation of the urethra, is caused by an infection characterized by the discharge of mucoid or purulent material and by burning during urination. Urethritis is the most common STD syndrome in men. Asymptomatic infections are common.[44] Urethritis is classified as gonococcal if caused by *N. gonorrhoeae* (gonorrhea) or as NGU if *N. gonorrhoeae* is not detected. The frequency of gonococcal urethritis and NGU varies by population studies.[35,36,40]

GONORRHEA

Definition and Epidemiology

Gonorrhea is a reportable disease caused by the gram-negative diplococcus *N. gonorrhoeae*. It primarily involves mucocutaneous surfaces of the genitourinary tract, pharynx, conjunctiva, and anus. In men it is often characterized by a purulent urethral discharge, whereas in up to 80% of women it is asymptomatic. The causative agent, *N. gonorrhoeae*, was discovered in 1879 by Albert Neisser.[35,40,44,48-50] Left untreated, it can result in a range of complications from acute salpingitis in female patients, perihepatitis (Fitz-Hugh–Curtis syndrome), and disseminated gonococcal infections, to ophthalmia neonatorum in newborns. Infections caused by gonorrhea are a major cause of PID, ectopic pregnancy, and chronic pelvic pain in the United States.[36,43] In untreated men, gonorrhea can cause epididymitis, a painful condition of the testicles that can result in infertility.[35]

Gonorrhea is the second most commonly reported infectious disease in the United States with more than 330,000 cases reported in 2004. This represented a 76% decline in gonorrhea rates since 1975 and was the lowest recorded level since reporting began in 1941.[35] Populations at risk for gonorrhea include young, sexually active individuals (such as teenagers); non-Caucasian urban poor; and other individuals who engage in high-risk behaviors such as use of illegal drugs or prostitution.[35] African-American men remain the group most affected. Drug resistance is becoming an increasing concern in the treatment and prevention of gonorrhea. In 2004 6.8% of gonorrhea isolates demonstrated resistance to fluoroquinolones, a leading class of antibiotics used to treat this disease. Resistance is eight times higher among men who have sex with men than in heterosexuals. Providers are urged to check with their state health departments for state-reported cases of resistance to fluoroquinolones. Carriers with no symptoms or those who have ignored symptoms usually spread gonorrhea.[48] Up to 50% of persons with gonorrhea have a co-existent chlamydial infection.[35,36]

Pathophysiology

N. gonorrhoeae is a human pathogen that infects mucus-secreting columnar and transitional epithelium. The portal of entry can be the genitourinary tract, eyes, oropharynx, anorectum, or skin. Transmission by vaginal or anal intercourse is more efficient than orogenital transmission. Autoinoculation of the organism to the eyes is possible. Neonates can acquire the infection during passage through the birth canal. The incubation period is 1 to 14 days after exposure, with a peak of 2 to 5 days in male patients. Longer intervals between exposure and the onset of symptoms are common. Some men never develop symptoms. In women the infection typically becomes evident 2 to 7 days after exposure. The infection generally begins in the anterior urethra, accessory urethral glands, Bartholin's or Skene's glands, and the cervix. If untreated, gonorrhea spreads from its initial sites upward into the genital tract, prostate, and epididymis in men and into the fallopian tubes in women. Pharyngitis may develop after orogenital contact. The organism may also invade the bloodstream, leading to bacteremic involvement of other tissues, including joint spaces, heart valves, meninges, and other tissues. Menstruation increases the risk of intraluminal ascent from the cervix and predisposes the patient to gonococcal bacteremia.[44]

Clinical Presentation

Although customarily categorized as gonococcal urethritis or NGU, cases of gonococcal urethritis in one fourth of male patients may occur with simultaneous chlamydial infection.[40,43] Signs and symptoms of infection with *N. gonorrhoeae* include urethritis, with purulent urethral discharge (drip) in 75% of men, as well as dysuria and pruritus. Urethral discharge can range from clear to purulent and copious. Discharge with gonococcal urethritis is most often purulent, whereas that with NGU tends to be clear or mucoid. It is impossible to distinguish between the two on clinical grounds alone. Less commonly seen is hematuria, frequency, or urgency. Asymptomatic infections can occur but are less typical with gonococcal infections than with NGU. Pharyngeal infection usually occurs in association with anogenital gonorrhea. The majority of pharyngeal infections are asymptomatic. Infection may be transmitted to genital sites through oral sex or progress to disseminated gonococcal infection. Anorectal infection may manifest with anorectal burning, mucopurulent discharge, and painful bowel movements.[41,49,51] Fewer than 5% of men have no symptoms.[36]

In female patients gonorrheal infection is often asymptomatic in the early stage of disease (up to 80% of cases) and may not be detectable until the disease is more advanced. Initial symptoms in women (2 to 7 days after exposure) include dysuria, leukorrhea, lower abdominal discomfort, abnormal uterine bleeding, and dysuria. Later signs may include adnexal tenderness, cervical motion tenderness, purulent vaginal discharge, elevated temperature, right upper quadrant pain, joint pain or swelling, skin lesions, nausea, and vomiting. Signs of disseminated disease occur most often when gonorrhea is acquired during menses or pregnancy and include tenosynovitis, skin lesions, fever, and polyarthralgias.[51,52] Pharyngitis can occur with orogenital contact, and anorectal signs may be present with rectal involvement.

Diagnostics

Laboratory diagnosis of gonorrhea depends on the setting and on the availability of diagnostic laboratory facilities. Microscopic examination of gram-stained urethral or cervical specimens can detect infection with *N. gonorrhoeae*. The sensitivity of Gram's stain is higher in symptomatic men (90% to 95%) than in asymptomatic men (70%). Gram's stain is less sensitive for cervical infections in women (30% to 65%) and is not useful in diagnosing pharyngeal and rectal infections.[41]

Culture testing has been the reference standard against which all other tests have been compared. The most sensitive and specific test for detecting gonococcal infection is direct culture from sites of exposure (urethra, endocervix, throat, rectum). Nonculture screening tests are increasingly available, and the newer NAATs are substantially more sensitive than the first generation of nonculture tests.[41]

In clinical settings where handling and storage of culture media are difficult, nonculture methods of testing are popular. Because chlamydia and gonorrhea cause similar symptoms and often occur simultaneously, diagnostic and screening tests for the two infections are usually performed together, using the same swab or urine specimen. Nonculture tests do not provide information on susceptibility.

Testing for gonorrhea and chlamydia in females is possible by coupling the test with routine liquid-based Papanicolaou's (Pap) tests. NAAT urine tests greatly facilitate routine screening of high-risk populations (adolescents) during periodic well-visit examinations. No matter what test is used, the provider is cautioned to refer to the manufacturer's directions.

CHLAMYDIA

Definition and Epidemiology

Chlamydia is an STD caused by an intracellular, parasitic organism, *C. trachomatis*. Currently there are at least 15 recognized serotypes of *C. trachomatis*. Clinical syndromes associated with certain *C. trachomatis* serotypes include NGU, mucopurulent cervicitis, PID, lymphogranuloma venereum (LGV), acute urethral syndrome in female patients, ocular infections, proctocolitis, epididymitis, and Reiter's syndrome in adults. *C. trachomatis* may be acquired by infants through an infected birth canal, causing pneumonia and conjunctivitis in newborns.[52]

Chlamydia is the most commonly reported infectious disease STD in the United States. Each year, an estimated 2.8 million new cases of genital infection caused by *C. trachomatis* occur in the United States at a cost of $2.4 billion.[35,36] Chlamydial infection is especially prevalent among adolescents. In the past 2 decades, genital chlamydial infection has been identified as a major public health problem because of its association with several disease syndromes, including NGU, mucopurulent cervicitis, and PID.[52]

In female patients these infections often result in serious reproductive tract complications. A number of factors limit documentation of the incidence and prevalence of genital chlamydial infection, including large numbers of asymptomatic persons in whom infection can be detected only through screening.[35]

Pathophysiology

C. trachomatis can be serologically divided into types A, B, and C, which are associated with trachoma; types L1, L2, and L3, which are associated with LGV; and types D through K, which are associated with genital infections and their complications.[52] The organism infects the genital tract of women most commonly at the transition zone of the endocervix.[41] Chlamydia should be suspected in female patients with probable cervicitis on the basis of mucopurulent discharge from the cervical os, easily induced bleeding, and edema in the area of ectopy.[8] In male patients symptoms often resemble those of gonorrhea. Up to 85% of women and 25% of men with chlamydia are asymptomatic (see Table 156-2).[36]

Diagnostics

Chlamydia organisms, which are obligate and intracellular, are found within urethral, cervical, and rectal epithelial cells, but not in exudate or pus. Because a specimen containing purulent discharge is inadequate for identification of the organism, if the provider is using an endocervical swab, the cervical os must be cleaned to remove debris and secretions. NAATs are quickly becoming the preferred method of testing because of their high sensitivity and ease of use and transport. NAATs are used for both endocervical swabs and urine-based test for chlamydia. As with the tests for gonorrhea, the chlamydia test can be coupled with liquid-based Pap smears during routine well-visit examinations in high-risk populations. Regardless of the method used, it is important to closely follow the manufacturer's instructions for specimen collection and transport.[35]

DISEASES CHARACTERIZED BY GENITAL ULCERS

In the United States most young, sexually active patients who have genital ulcers have genital herpes, syphilis, or chancroid. More than one of these diseases can be present in a patient who has genital ulcers. Each has been associated with an increased risk of HIV infection.[44] Other causes of genital ulcers include LGV and HIV. Noninfectious causes include trauma, Behçet's syndrome, neoplasms, and fixed drug eruptions.

SYPHILIS

Definition and Epidemiology

Syphilis is a complex systemic STD caused by *Treponema pallidum*. Syphilis has been classified by the CDC into several stages, depending on the length of infection (Box 156-6).[39] Patients may be initially seen with signs and symptoms of primary infection (ulcer or chancre at the infection site; see Color Plate 6), secondary infection (rash, mucocutaneous lesions, and adenopathy), or tertiary infection (cardiac, neurologic, ophthalmic, auditory, or gummatous lesions).[44]

The reemergence of syphilis between 1987 and 1990 was most notable among populations that included illicit drug

BOX 156-6

STAGES OF SYPHILIS

- Primary syphilis
- Secondary syphilis
- Latent syphilis
- Early latent syphilis
- Late latent syphilis
- Latent syphilis, unknown duration
- Neurosyphilis
- Late syphilis
- Syphilitic stillbirth

users, particularly crack cocaine users and their sex partners.[36,38] The rate of primary and secondary syphilis declined in the 1990 and reached a record low in 2000. However, rates are once again rising. Between 2003 and 2004 the national rate of primary and secondary syphilis rose 8%. These increases were observed only among men. The rate among females remained stable, and the rate of congenital syphilis declined.[35]

Pathophysiology

Syphilis is usually spread through contact with infectious lesions; the infection can enter the host during sexual activity through sites where the epithelium has been disrupted from minor trauma. Sexual contact with a partner who has early syphilis is associated with the highest risk of developing the disease. The mean time from exposure to the development of active infection (chancre formation) is 21 days (range 7 to 60 days). At this time the individual becomes actively infectious.[46]

Chancres typically develop at the site of inoculation. Since syphilitic lesions are painless, in contrast to lesions associated with chancroid, some patients may not be aware of them. Secondary syphilis, the hematogenous dissemination of *T. pallidum*, causes more widespread findings, including macules and papules on the trunk, neck, palms, and soles. Condylomata lata, which are raised, flat, broad, grayish papular lesions, may occur in moist areas such as the anus, scrotum, and vulva. Mucous patches (small, asymptomatic, shallow ulcerations) may occur in the oral or genital mucosa or at the angles of the mouth.[40,46-48]

The signs of primary and secondary syphilis may resolve spontaneously even without treatment. The patient then enters the latent stage of the disease, in which there are generally no clinical signs or symptoms of infection and diagnosis is made on the basis of serology. A pregnant woman with latent disease can infect her fetus.[46]

Tertiary syphilis manifests after a variable period of latency in approximately one third of patients who fail to receive treatment. Late-stage syphilis may occur 10 to 20 years after initial infection. It may appear as gummatous disease (rubbery lumps or lesions found in subcutaneous tissue), cardiovascular disease, or neurosyphilis in one third of untreated patients. Neurosyphilis can occur in all stages of syphilis, and the diagnosis is based on clinical findings and examination of the serum and cerebrospinal fluid.[46]

Diagnostics

Dark-field examinations and direct fluorescent antibody tests of lesion exudate or tissue are the definitive methods for diagnosing early syphilis. Serologic testing using nontreponemal tests (e.g., Venereal Disease Research Laboratory [VDRL] and rapid plasma reagin) and treponemal tests (e.g., fluorescent treponemal antibody absorbed and microhemagglutination assay for antibody to *T. pallidum*) is done for presumptive diagnosis. The use of one test alone is not sufficient. The nontreponemal test, the initial screening test, correlates with disease activity and is reported quantitatively. The treponemal test is used to confirm the diagnosis,[52] since false-positive nontreponemal test results are associated with hepatitis, viral pneumonia, pregnancy, infectious mononucleosis, and other viral infections. Chronic false-positive findings are associated with connective tissue diseases such as systemic lupus erythematosus.[46] Patients treated for early syphilis whose nontreponemal test either shows an increase or fails to show a fourfold decline in *T. pallidum* within 6 months should be retreated. Further evaluation may also be indicated.

GENITAL HERPES

Definition and Epidemiology

Herpes simplex virus (HSV) infection is a condition characterized by primary infection of the genital or anal area with visible, painful genital or anal lesions or grouped vesicles at the site of inoculation and regional lymphadenopathy. Recurrent HSV infections are characterized by a normal course of recurring outbreaks of vesicles at the same site. Both HSV-1 and HSV-2 can infect the genitals, but recurrences are much less frequent with HSV-1 infection than genital HSV-2 infection. For these reasons clinical diagnosis of genital herpes should be confirmed with type-specific laboratory testing.

HSV-2 causes the majority of cases of genital herpes infections. Up to 30% of first-episode cases of genital herpes are caused by HSV-1. It is estimated that 16% (approximately 1 in 5) of the U.S. adult population is HSV-2 seropositive.[53] The prevalence of HSV-2 in the United States is estimated at approximately 21.9% with projections of an additional 1 million people becoming infected each year. Of those infected, as many as 70% or more could be unaware of infection or be asymptomatic.[53]

Spread of genital herpes is by direct contact, with transmission by infected secretions. Transmissibility is higher with active lesions, but asymptomatic shedding of virus with transmission is also probable. Asymptomatic shedding occurs more often during the first 3 months after primary infection.[50,53] Most neonatal HSV-2 infections occur during delivery in women who have acquired HSV-2 during pregnancy. Neonatal HSV infections range from mild and localized infection to fatal and disseminated disease. One fourth of HSV-infected neonates develop disseminated disease, and one third have encephalitis. Even with treatment, the mortality rate is 57% among infants with disseminated disease and 15% among those with encephalitis.[41]

Pathophysiology

After an inoculation onto a mucosal surface, the virus undergoes primary replication, resulting in the production of the characteristic lesion (a thin-walled vesicle on an erythematous base). With primary infection the HSV travels along sensory nerves and establishes latency within sensory nerve fibers for life. Reactivation occurs via spread down peripheral sensory nerve pathways, with further replication occurring at cutaneous sites corresponding to distributions of the sensory nerves. Reactivation can be symptomatic or asymptomatic. The sexual contacts of individuals with either symptomatic or asymptomatic disease are at risk of becoming infected.[50]

Diagnostics

Diagnosis of HSV is often a clinical decision based on the patient's history and the morphologic characteristics of the lesions. Isolation of HSV in cell culture is the preferred virologic test. Some tests do not distinguish between HSV-1 and HSV-2. Unfortunately healing lesions affect the sensitivity of virologic testing. Recently several serologic tests have been developed based on antibody to HSV glycoproteins G1 and G2, which have antigenic specificities to HSV-1 and HSV-2. The CDC recommends that any serologic testing for herpes simplex use type-specific assays. A number of other products are now available for serologic testing, including the HerpeSelect 1 or HerpeSelect 2 enzyme-linked immunosorbent assay (ELISA) immunoglobulin G. Antibody response occurs 2 to 12 weeks after infection and is lifelong. Serologic testing will not be positive at the time of the primary outbreak.[44,54]

CHANCROID

Definition and Epidemiology

Chancroid is an STD characterized by painful genital ulceration and inflammatory inguinal adenopathy. The disease is characterized by infection with *Haemophilus ducreyi*.[39] From 1987 to 1995, cases of chancroid in the United States have steadily declined, with approximately 3500 cases reported in 1991 and 606 cases reported in 1995. Only 31 cases were reported in 2001.[35]

Clinical Presentation

Chancroid is a genital ulcer disease characterized by one or a few painful ulcers that develop after an incubation of 4 to 7 days. The most distinguishing feature is deep, raw, painful ulcerations. Painful inguinal adenopathy, often unilateral, develops in 50% of patients 1 to 2 weeks after the primary lesion. Buboes occur and may drain spontaneously.[40]

Diagnostics

Diagnosis is often clinical. Confirmation is based on isolation of *H. ducreyi* from a clinical specimen.[49]

OTHER ULCERATIVE DISEASES

LGV and granuloma inguinale are two other causes of genital ulcers. These genital ulcers are rare in the United States, but endemic to certain tropical areas. Granuloma inguinale is characterized by painless progressive ulcers and regional lymphadenopathy. The lesions bleed easily on contact. The causative agent is difficult to culture, and diagnosis requires staining.[44]

LGV is a systemic STD caused by a variety of *C. trachomatis*. It rarely occurs in the United States. In 2004 a rise of LGV cases was noted in the Netherlands, where fewer than five cases per year are normally reported; 92 cases were reported in 2004. A primary lesion that is a small, nonpainful genital papule that can ulcerate after an initial 3- to 30-day incubation period characterizes LGV. Symptoms include tender, unilateral or bilateral inguinal and/or femoral adenopathy and hemorrhagic proctitis. Providers in the United States should be aware of this infectious disease, especially if caring for men who have sex with men.[51] Suspicion of either of these conditions requires consultation and often referral to a practitioner skilled in the diagnosis of STDs.

INDICATIONS FOR REFERRAL OR HOSPITALIZATION

It is not common for patients with STDs to require hospitalization. Indications include signs and symptoms of systemic disease not appropriate for outpatient treatment, ineffective outpatient treatment, or complications related to an STD such as PID. Referral to a specialist in infectious disease is indicated for all cases of LGV, syphilis, or granuloma inguinale, as well as for all treatment failures.

PATIENT AND FAMILY EDUCATION

Patient education efforts need to focus on preventing the establishment of high-risk behaviors before sexual activity is initiated. The general public is largely unaware of the health consequences of STDs because many infections are asymptomatic; major health consequences, such as infertility and chronic disease, occur years after initial infections; and the stigma associated with STDs often inhibits frank and open discussion about STDs and their consequences. Population-specific educational efforts and screening for specific STDs must be established to help curb this hidden epidemic.[36]

HEALTH PROMOTION

Efforts to prevent the STDs include promotion of healthy sexual practices, including targeting other high-risk behaviors often associated with the acquisition of an STD. These behaviors include excessive alcohol intake, substance abuse, and high-risk sexual practices such as inconsistent or no condom use and multiple sex partners. Patients who are sexually active, regardless of age, should be educated on the risk of transmitting or acquiring the different STDs and on the various transmission modes. Sensitivity to the patient's age, culture, religion, and setting are integral to successful health promotion and disease prevention activities.

Many resources for patient education are available. Adolescents are at higher risk for certain, often asymptomatic STDs. Efforts targeting this age-group must include an awareness of peer pressures and self-esteem, which may affect the patient's health behavior patterns. Sex education can become a controversial issue for patients, families, and schools. This age-group with few exceptions is able to consent to confidential diagnosis and treatment of STDs. This provides the opportunity for promotion of healthy sexual practices in a non-threatening environment.

A great deal of information is available on the Internet for both the health care provider and the patient. For patients and families who may be uncomfortable discussing these topics, the Internet offers a number of reputable and informative resources. The CDC, Division of STD Prevention, has not only the current treatment guidelines, but also STD fact sheets and valuable links to other sites. For more information, contact:

Centers for Disease Control and Prevention: Division of STD Prevention, http://www.cdc.gov/std

CDC National STD Hotline: (800) 232-4636 (24 hours/day, 7 days/week)

American Social Health Association (ASHA): *http://www.ashastd.org*

Sexually Transmitted Infections Hotline (ASHA): (919) 361-8488

REFERENCES

1. Sheffield J, Cunningham F: Urinary tract infection in women, *Obst Gynecol* 106(5):1085-1092, 2005.
2. Foxman B, Barlow R, D'Arcy H, and others: Urinary tract infection: self-reported incidence and associated costs, *Ann Epidemiol* 10(8):509-515, 2000.
3. Fihn S: Clinical practice: acute uncomplicated urinary tract infection in women, *N Engl J Med* 349:259-266, 2003.
4. Hooton TM: Recurrent urinary tract infection in women, *Int J Antimicrob Agents* 17(4):259-268, 2001.
5. National Center for Health Statistics, Centers for Disease Control and Prevention, US Department of Health and Human Services: Ambulatory care visits to physician offices, hospital outpatient departments, and emergency departments: United States, 1997, *Vital Health Statistics Series* 13(143), 1999.
6. Hooton TM, Scholes D, Hughes JP, and others: A prospective study of risk factors for symptomatic urinary tract infections in young women, *N Engl J Med* 335(7):468-474, 1996.
7. Stamm WE: Towards control of urinary tract infections, *Lancet Infect Dis* 2(2):120-122, 2002.
8. National Nosocomial Infections Surveillance Systems: *Data summary from October 1986–April 1998: a report from the NNIS System*, Atlanta, 1998, Centers for Disease Control and Prevention.
9. Krieger JN, Ross SO, Simonsen JM: Urinary tract infections in healthy university men, *J Urol* 149:1046-1048, 1993.
10. Campbell J, Felver M, Kamarei S: "Telephone treatment" of uncomplicated acute cystitis, *Cleveland Clin J Med* 66(8):495-501, 1999.
11. Bent S, Nallamothu BK, Simel DL, and others: Does this woman have an acute uncomplicated urinary tract infection? *JAMA* 287(20):2701-2710, 2002.
12. Raz R, Gennesin Y, Wasser J, and others: Recurrent urinary tract infection in post-menopausal women, *Clin Infect Dis* 30:152-156, 2000.
13. Ronald A, Ludwig E: Urinary tract infections in adults with diabetes, *Int J Antimicrob Agents* 17:287-292, 2001.
14. Wilson M, Gaido L: Laboratory diagnosis of urinary tract infections in adult patients, *Clin Infect Dis* 38:1150-1158, 2004.
15. McNair R, MacDonald S, Dooley S, and others: Evaluation of the centrifuged and Gram-stained smear, urinalysis, and reagent strip testing to detect asymptomatic bacteriuria in obstetric patients, *Am J Obstet Gynecol* 182:1076-1079, 2000.
16. Delzell JE, Lefevre ML: Urinary tract infection during pregnancy, *Am Fam Phys* 62:713-720, 2000.
17. Leiner S: Recurrent urinary tract infections in otherwise healthy women: rational strategies for work-up and management, *Nurse Pract* 20(2):48-56, 1995.
18. Stapleton A, Stamm WE: Prevention of urinary tract infection, *Infect Dis Clin North Am* 11(3):719-733, 1997.
19. Hassay K: Effective management of urinary discomfort, *Nurse Pract* 20(2):36-44, 1995.
20. Mehnert-Kay S: Diagnosis and management of uncomplicated urinary tract infections, *Am Fam Phys* 72(3):451-456, 2005.
21. Gantz NM, Noskin GA: Complicated UTI: targeting the pathogens, *Patient Care* 31(7):212-223, 1997.
22. Maskell R: Broadening the concept of urinary tract infection (letter), *Br J Urol* 76:5, 1995.
23. Kunin CM: *Urinary tract infections: detection, prevention and management*, ed 5, Baltimore, 1997, Williams & Wilkins.
24. Raz R, Chazan B, Kennes Y, and others: Empiric use of trimethoprim-sulfamethoxazole (TMP-SMX) in the treatment of women with uncomplicated urinary tract infections, in a geographical area with a high prevalence of TMP-SMX resistant uropathogens, *Clin Infect Dis* 32:1165-1169, 2002.
25. Stapleton A: Prevention of recurrent urinary tract infections in women, *Lancet* 353:7-8, 1999.
26. Jepson R, Mihaljevic L, Craig J: Cranberries for treating urinary tract infections, *Cochrane Database Syst Rev* (2):CD001322, 2000.
27. Gupta K, Sahm DF, Mayfield D, and others: Antimicrobial resistance among uropathogens that cause community-acquired urinary tract infections in women: a nationwide analysis, *Clin Infect Dis* 33:89-94, 2001.
28. Lowe FC, Fagelman E: Cranberry juice and urinary tract infections: what is the evidence? *Urology* 57:407-413, 2001.
29. Triezenberg DJ: Can regular intake of either cranberry juice or a drink containing *Lactobacillus* bacteria prevent urinary tract infection (UTI) recurrence in women after an initial episode? *J Fam Pract* 50(10):841, 2001.
30. Kontiokari T, Sundqvist K, Nuutinen M, and others: Randomised trial of cranberry-lingonberry juice and *Lactobacillus* GG drink for the prevention of urinary tract infections in women, *BMJ* 322(7302):1571, 2001.
31. Stapleton A: Urinary tract infections in patients with diabetes, *Am J Med* 133(1A):80S-84S, 2002.
32. Yoshikawa TT, Nicolle LE, Norman DC, and others: Management of complicated urinary tract infection in older patients, *J Am Geriatr Soc* 44:1235-1241, 1996.
33. JAMA patient page: urinary tract infections, *JAMA* 283(12):1646, 2000.
34. Patient information: urinary tract infections, *Cleveland Clin J Med* 66(8):502, 1999.
35. Centers for Disease Control and Prevention: *STD surveillance 2004: trends in reportable STDs in the United States 2004*, retrieved Jan 2006 from http://www.cdc.gov/std/stats/trends2004.htm.
36. Institute of Medicine, Committee on Prevention and Control of Sexually Transmitted Diseases: *The hidden epidemic: confronting sexually transmitted diseases*, Washington, DC, 1997, National Academy Press.
37. Centers for Disease Control and Prevention: Summary of notifiable diseases, United States, *MMWR* 52(54):1-85, 2005.
38. Hook EW, Marra CM: Acquired syphilis in adults, *N Engl J Med* 326(16):1060-1066, 1992.
39. Centers for Disease Control and Prevention: Case definitions for infectious conditions under public health surveillance, *MMWR* 46(RR-10):34-37, 1997.
40. Fitzpatrick TB, Johnson RA, Polano MK, and others: *Color atlas and synopsis of clinical dermatology*, ed 3, New York, 1997, McGraw-Hill.
41. Centers for Disease Control and Prevention: Screening tests to detect *Chlamydia trachomatis* and *Neisseria gonorrhoeae* infections—2002, *MMWR* 51(RR-15):1-27, 2002.
42. Gunn RA, Veinbergs E, Freidman LS: Adolescent health care providers: establishing a dialogue and assessing sexually transmitted disease prevention practices, *Sex Trans Dis* 24:90-93, 1997.
43. Holmes KK, Morse SA: Gonococcal infections. In Fauci AS, Braunwald E, Isselbacher KJ, and others, editors: *Harrison's principles of internal medicine*, ed 14, New York, 1998, McGraw-Hill.
44. Centers for Disease Control and Prevention: Sexually transmitted diseases treatment guidelines, *MMWR* 55(RR-11):1-94, 2006.
45. History taking. In STD/HIV Prevention Training Center of New England: *Home study module, 3-day intensive course*, 1997.
46. Larson S, Steiner B, Rudolph A: Laboratory diagnosis and interpretation of tests for syphilis, *Clin Microbiol Rev* 8(1):1-19, 1995.
47. Barton S: *Clinical evidence 4*, London, 2001, British Medical Journal Publishing Group.
48. Fiumara NJ: *Pictorial guide to sexually transmitted diseases*, New York, 1989, Reed.
49. Felenstein D: Syphilis 1996. In STD/HIV Prevention Training Center of New England: *Home study module, 3-day intensive course*, 1997.

50. Cowan FM: Testing for type specific antibody to herpes simplex virus: implications for clinical practice, *J Antimicrob Chemother* 45(Suppl T-3):9-13, 2000.
51. Centers for Disease Control and Prevention: Lymphogranuloma venereum among men who have sex with men—Netherlands, 2003-2004, *MMWR* 53(42):985-988, 2004.
52. Mehring PC: Sexually transmitted diseases. In Porth CM, editor: *Pathophysiology: concepts of altered health states*, ed 4, Philadelphia, 1994, Lippincott.
53. Leone PA, Fleming DT, Gilsenan AW, and others: Seroprevalence of herpes simplex virus-2 in suburban care offices in the United States, *Sex Trans Dis* 31:311-316, 2004.
54. US Preventive Services Task Force: *Screening for genital herpes*, March 2005, retrieved Feb 10, 2006, from http://ahrq.gov/clinic/uspstf/herpes/herpesup2.htm.htm.

CHAPTER 157

Obstructive Uropathy

Kelley Hamill Lemay

DEFINITION AND EPIDEMIOLOGY

Obstructive uropathy refers to structural or functional changes in the urinary tract that impair urine flow. Left untreated, obstruction can result in progressive renal damage and potential renal failure.[1] The degree, duration, and location of obstruction determine the extent of functional and pathologic alterations in the kidney.

Obstructive uropathy is relatively common, can occur at any age, and can be seen anywhere in the urinary tract from the urethral meatus to the renal tubules.[2] It can be classified by cause (congenital or acquired), duration (acute or chronic), degree (partial or complete), and level (upper or lower urinary tract).[1] In children, congenital disorders are seen most commonly. For adults, acquired disorders are more prevalent, with urolithiasis being the most common disorder in young adults.[2] In individuals over the age of 60, men are generally more afflicted than women, and benign prostatic hyperplasia (BPH) and prostate carcinoma are the most prevalent culprits in this age-group.[2]

PATHOPHYSIOLOGY

Obstruction of urine flow can result from intrinsic or extrinsic mechanical blockage, as well as from functional defects not associated with a fixed occlusion. Lesions causing mechanical obstruction can occur at any level of the upper or lower urinary tract.[1] When the lesion is above the level of the bladder, unilateral dilation of the ureter and kidney (hydronephrosis) can occur. However, when the lesion is below the level of the bladder, bilateral involvement of the kidneys occurs, unless there is a solitary kidney. Forms of mechanical obstructions are listed in Box 157-1.

Obstruction of urine flow causes urinary retention and increased pressure proximal to the obstruction.[2] A significant or prolonged pressure increase can lead to considerable renal tissue damage with resultant renal insufficiency or failure.[1,2]

Functional impairment of urine flow can also result from disorders that involve both the ureter and bladder. Neurogenic bladder dysfunction, an example of this, can be caused by upper neuron damage or lower spinal cord injury. Upper neuron damage may produce involuntary micturition against a closed bladder neck or external sphincter, whereas lower spinal tract injury can cause the bladder to become atonic.[3] In many cases a significant urinary residual may occur, resulting in increased bladder pressure and subsequent upper tract pressures.[1,2] This may or may not be accompanied by reflux of urine into the ureters. Ischemia of the upper tracts can occur when pressures are elevated, which can then lead to substantial renal injury and even tissue death.[2]

BOX 157-1

COMMON CAUSES OF OBSTRUCTIVE UROPATHY

INTRINSIC CAUSES

Intraluminal
- Stones
- Papilla
- Clots
- Fungal balls

Structural
- Stricture
- Tumors, polyps
- Infection: granuloma
- Anatomic defects
- Valve or sphincter abnormalities

Functional
- Vesicoureteral reflux
- Adynamic ureters
- Neurogenic bladder

EXTRINSIC CAUSES

Abdominal
- Ileum, left colon, duodenum
- Aneurysms

Pelvic
- Prostatic hypertrophy
- Cysts, tumors of the uterus, ovaries
- Endometriosis
- Pregnancy
- Phimosis, meatal stenosis

Retroperitoneal
- Fibrosis
- Tumor, lymphoma

CLINICAL PRESENTATION

The presentation of obstructive uropathies can vary depending on cause. The health care provider should obtain a history with detailed review of symptoms, including onset, duration, location, aggravating and alleviating factors, characteristics of symptoms, changes in voiding or bowel patterns, and management therapies previously tried. Further inquiry should address current medications, medical and surgical histories, genitourinary history, family history (especially related to urologic issues), and history of pelvic trauma or neurologic issues.

In acute obstruction, pain is generally the most common presenting symptom.[2] Flank pain occurring in a crescendo-decrescendo pattern radiating to the lower abdomen, testes, or labia is not uncommon in acute obstruction. Flank pain that occurs only with urination is pathognomonic of vesicoureteral reflux, although reflux can also be asymptomatic.[4,5]

Chronic (slowly developing) obstructive lesions may be asymptomatic. Polyuria with resultant nocturia can be seen in chronic partial obstruction, whereas anuria and acute renal failure can be seen in total complete bilateral obstruction or obstruction of a solitary kidney. A pattern of oliguria or anuria alternating with polyuria or sudden onset of anuria suggests the presence of some type of obstructive uropathy.[2]

Bladder outlet obstruction, when incomplete, is often accompanied by other lower urinary tract symptoms, including frequency, nocturia, urgency, urge incontinence, hesitancy, poor stream, straining to initiate a urinary stream, postvoid dribbling, and overflow incontinence.[1,2] Noting changes in the pattern of urinary output, abrupt alterations vs. gradual changes, and fluctuation in urinary symptoms is important. Recurrent urinary tract infections (UTIs) can also be seen with chronic partial obstructions, so UTIs should be ruled out in patients with urologic symptoms.[1]

PHYSICAL EXAMINATION

A general physical examination should be performed on all patients. Blood pressure measurement is critical, since both acute and chronic hydronephrosis can be accompanied by severe hypertension.[2] Signs of azotemia (pallor, skin changes, dizziness, and lethargy) should be monitored if kidney function is thought to be disrupted.[6] A fever may indicate infection. Palpation and percussion of the abdomen can often reveal bladder distention. An enlarged, tender kidney may be noted, especially in thin patients, and may manifest as a flank mass or increased abdominal girth. Costovertebral angle, or flank, tenderness can be related to urolithiasis or infection.[1]

In men a digital rectal examination will help determine the size of the prostate gland and the presence of nodules. Prostate size does not directly correlate with intensity of lower urinary tract symptoms. However, symptoms are related to the degree of obstruction caused by the prostate.[7] The penis should be inspected for evidence of meatal stricture or phimosis.

In women a pelvic examination should occur. Careful inspection of the external genitals, vaginal and uterine cavities, and the rectum may reveal contributors to urinary obstruction. It may also yield information about anatomy, such as prolapse, that might contribute to obstruction.

DIAGNOSTICS

Several in-office diagnostic studies may be helpful in making a diagnosis. A postvoid residual provides information about the residual urine in the bladder. Catheterization provides a sterile urine specimen for analysis, and a urine culture should be done to exclude infection. Urinalysis is necessary for all patients for whom obstructive uropathy is suspected. This assesses for pyuria, microscopic hematuria, and abnormalities in urine pH as may occur with a stone or infection.[2] Gross hematuria is often seen in acute obstruction and is generally due to calculi or bladder tumor, but can be due to infection as well.[1] Uric acid crystals in the urine sediment raise the suspicion of uric acid nephropathy or calculi.

Routine blood studies are nonspecific. CBC and electrolytes may be helpful in identifying anemia and alterations in fluid status. BUN and creatinine will be helpful in determining alterations in renal function if renal insufficiency is suspected.[1,2] Blood glucose or hemoglobin A_{1c} can help assess for diabetes. Further workup depends on results from the above-mentioned tests and the cause of symptoms suspected.

In patients with flank pain, renal calculus must be excluded (refer to Chapter 164). A stone protocol noncontrast CT scan is the best test to detect a stone and obstruction without using contrast.[2] If stones are not suspected, a diagnostic ultrasound evaluation is the preferred procedure for visualizing the renal pelvis and diagnosing hydronephrosis.[2] Urodynamics may be helpful in diagnosing lower tract obstruction like bladder outlet obstruction. Other procedures useful in determining

DIAGNOSTICS

Obstructive Uropathy

INITIAL
Postvoid residual
Urine dip for leukocytes, nitrites, blood

LABORATORY
CBC and differential
Serum electrolytes
BUN
Creatinine
Serum glucose
Urinalysis
Urine cultures*
Blood cultures*

IMAGING
KUB
IV pyelogram
Ultrasound
CT scan
Antegrade and retrograde pyelography

OTHER
Whitaker's test
Cystoscopy
Urodynamics

*If indicated.

the site of obstruction include antegrade or retrograde pyelography.[1,2] In patients for whom upper tract obstruction is suspected, pressure flow studies (i.e., Whitaker's test) may be required.[2] This provides direct visualization of the bladder, urethra, prostate, and ureteral openings, providing anatomic evaluation but no functional information.

DIFFERENTIAL DIAGNOSIS

Voiding difficulty, recurrent infection, pain, or changes in urinary pattern are common in individuals of all ages. Causes of obstruction—congenital, acquired intrinsic, or acquired extrinsic—can occur at any level of the urinary tract, but are most commonly seen at the level of the ureter, bladder outlet, or urethra (see Box 157-1).

DIFFERENTIAL DIAGNOSIS

Obstructive Uropathy

- Appendicitis
- Ectopic pregnancy
- Gallbladder disease
- Aortic or renal aneurysm
- Vascular, glomerular, or tubulointerstitial disease

In individuals with flank pain, abnormalities of adjacent structures and referred pain should be considered. These can include appendicitis, ectopic pregnancy, gallbladder disease, aortic aneurysm, and renal aneurysm. In the presence of renal insufficiency, other causes of renal failure must be considered, including vascular, glomerular, and tubulointerstitial diseases.[8]

MANAGEMENT

Treatment to relieve partial obstruction is indicated when the patient has recurrent infections, significant symptoms, urinary retention, and impaired renal function. Urinary tract obstruction complicated by infection should be relieved as soon as possible to prevent development of sepsis, preserve renal function, normalize blood pressure, correct fluid and electrolyte imbalances, and treat pain. Acute treatment of lower tract obstruction is catheterization.[2]

Obstruction caused by BPH is not always progressive, and the patient need not be treated unless there is retention, recurrent infection, or unacceptable symptoms. Irritative symptoms often include frequency, nocturia, difficulty initiating a urinary stream, dribbling, or incontinence. Chronic urinary retention because of prostatic hypertrophy may respond to $alpha_1$ blockers such as terazosin (Hytrin) or doxazosin (Cardura).[9] There are at least three subtypes of $alpha_1$ receptors, with the 1a subtype being most predominant in the prostate.[9] Alpha blockers specific for the 1a subtype include tamsulosin hydrochloride (Flomax) or alfusolin (Uroxatral).

5α-Reductase inhibitors, such as finasteride (Proscar) or dutasteride (Avodart), can be effective for relieving symptoms of BPH by reducing prostate size, thereby increasing urinary flow (refer to Chapter 159).[9]

The decision to undertake surgical or instrumental procedures for the relief of obstruction depends on the location of obstruction, presence of infection, and status of renal function. Relief of complete obstruction should occur as soon as possible after diagnosis. Infection in the face of an acute obstruction requires emergent treatment, since relief of obstruction and antibiotics are both essential in treating the infection. Furthermore, antibiotics are given before any surgical intervention used to relieve obstruction. In cases of chronic incomplete obstruction, like BPH, ideally surgery is done only when the urine is sterile.

LIFE SPAN CONSIDERATIONS

Obstructive uropathy can occur at any age. Prenatal ultrasound has made it possible to diagnose obstruction in the fetus during pregnancy. In the young adult, acute obstruction is most likely a result of calculi. In women, pelvic cancer is an important cause of obstruction, and in men, the most common culprits are BPH and prostate cancer.

COMPLICATIONS

Complications of untreated urinary tract obstruction include azotemia, life-threatening sepsis, and obstructive nephropathy that can lead to chronic renal insufficiency or renal failure. Complications of surgical procedures include infection, sepsis, bleeding, voiding difficulty, and pain.

Profound and prolonged diuresis, known as *postobstructive diuresis*, can follow relief of complete obstruction.[2] This diuresis—characterized by marked losses of water and solutes such as sodium, potassium, and magnesium—is usually self-limited. However, loss of solutes can often result in hypovolemia, hyponatremia, hypokalemia, and hypomagnesemia. Careful fluid replacement, weight, and serum and urine electrolyte monitoring should occur in these patients.[2]

INDICATIONS FOR REFERRAL OR HOSPITALIZATION

Renal calculi greater than 5 to 7 mm usually do not pass spontaneously and should be treated surgically.[10] These patients, as well as those with other obstructive symptoms, should be referred to a urologist for consultation and initiation of an appropriate care plan. In cases of anuria and acute renal failure, a nephrology referral should occur for appropriate management, since hospitalization or dialysis may be needed.

PATIENT EDUCATION

Patients with urinary tract obstruction are frequently uncomfortable and often frightened. Every effort should be made to alleviate discomfort and provide information and reassurance. All patients with obstruction should be taught the signs and symptoms of infection and how to take their temperature. In cases where obstruction is due to calculi, they need to understand that the likelihood of recurrence is high. Adequate daily fluid intake may help prevent recurrence. Dietary modification, depending on the type of stone, may be indicated as well.[10] Patients with BPH taking nonselective alpha blockers need to be advised of the potential for postural hypotension and confusion, especially if elderly. Finally, all patients need to know how to access the health care system in an emergency situation, whether they are at home or traveling.

REFERENCES

1. Tanagho EA: Urinary obstruction and stasis. In Tanagho EA, McAninch JW: *Smith's general urology*, ed 16, New York, 2004, McGraw-Hill.
2. Klahr S: Obstructive uropathy. In Goldman L, Ausiello D: *Cecil textbook of medicine*, ed 22, Philadelphia, 2004, Saunders.
3. Wein AJ: Neuromuscular dysfunction of the lower urinary tract and its management. In Walsh PC: *Campbell's urology*, ed 8, Philadelphia, 2002, Saunders.
4. Tanagho EA: Vesicoureteral reflux. In Tanagho EA, McAninch JW: *Smith's general urology*, ed 16, New York, 2004, McGraw-Hill.
5. Atala A, Keating MA: Vesicoureteral reflux and megaureter. In Walsh PC: *Campbell's urology*, ed 8, Philadelphia, 2002, Saunders.
6. Post TW, Rose BD: *Clinical manifestations and diagnosis of volume depletion in adults*, retrieved Feb 20, 2007, from http://www.uptodateonline.com/utd/content/topic.do?topicKey=fldlytes/13927&anchor=30.
7. Cunningham GR, Kadmon D: *Diagnosis of benign prostatic hyperplasia*, retrieved Feb 20, 2007, from http://www.uptodateonline.com/utd/content/topic.do?topicKey=genr_med/34741&selectedTitle=11~.
8. Garrick R: Obstructive nephropathy. In Hurst JW, editor: *Medicine for the practicing physician*, ed 4, Stamford, Conn, 1996, Appleton & Lange.
9. Cunningham GR, Kadmon D: *Management of benign prostatic hyperplasia*, retrieved Feb 20, 2007, from http://www.uptodateonline.com/utd/content/topic.do?topicKey=genr_med/36528.
10. Menon M, Resnick MI: Urinary lithiasis: etiology, diagnosis and medical management. In Walsh PC: *Campbell's urology*, ed 8, Philadelphia, 2002, Saunders.

CHAPTER 158

Renal Disease and Pregnancy

Patricia Polgar Bailey

DEFINITION AND EPIDEMIOLOGY

The concerns of pregnancy with chronic renal insufficiency are twofold: the effects of the pregnancy on renal function and the effects of the renal insufficiency on the pregnancy. The effect of renal dysfunction on pregnancy depends on several factors, including the degree of maternal renal impairment at the time of conception, the presence of hypertension at the time of conception and during pregnancy, the type of underlying renal disease, and maternal co-morbidity.[1] Advances in the management of pregnancy in women with renal disease during the past 2 decades have resulted in remarkably improved maternal and neonatal outcomes. Fetal survival rates in women with mild renal insufficiency are approximately 95%. In women with more serious renal disease, fetal survival rates are as low as 50% to 75%, with a high proportion of premature deliveries and low-birth-weight infants. Pregnancy in women with end-stage renal disease (ESRD) occurs rarely; only approximately 1% of women of childbearing age on dialysis become pregnant. The overall success rate of pregnancies in women with ESRD averages 50%.[2]

Physician consultation is indicated for the pregnant woman with underlying renal disease, deteriorating renal function, and suspected pyelonephritis.

PATHOPHYSIOLOGY

During a normal pregnancy, renal function changes significantly. Kidney weight and size increase, and renal length increases by approximately 1 cm (0.4 inch). However, the most significant changes occur in the collecting system, where dilation of renal calyces, pelvis, and ureters may be observed in the initial trimester and persist 3 to 4 months postpartum.[3] Maternal extracellular fluid, especially plasma volume, increases by 30% to 50% to provide adequate blood supply to the fetoplacental unit. Renal plasma flow increases by 50% to 70%, and this change is most pronounced in the first two trimesters. This is one of the factors that leads to an increased glomerular filtration rate (GFR), which increases by 50% from the first trimester, peaks at about the thirteenth week of a normal pregnancy, and can reach levels up to 150%.[3,4] As a result of these changes, serum creatinine falls to approximately 0.7 mg/dl and BUN falls to 9 mg/dl. Blood pressure also drops during pregnancy to an average of 105/60 mm Hg. There is an increase in kidney size of 1 to 1.5 cm (0.4 to 0.6 inch). High plasma levels of progesterone contribute to dilation of the ureters and renal calyces, which is referred to as *hydronephrosis of pregnancy*. There is an increased risk of developing bacteriuria because of the sluggish urine flow through the dilated renal tubules.

These changes remain throughout pregnancy and return to baseline values at the end of the pregnancy. Attempts to identify renal disease in pregnancy must take into consideration the normal physiologic changes during pregnancy, since what might be considered normal blood pressure and renal function values in many adults are clearly elevated values in pregnant women.[2,5]

The effect of pregnancy on the course of chronic renal disease has not been clearly established. However, many of the normally occurring physiologic changes during pregnancy, including an increase in GFR and renal plasma flow, put a pregnant woman with renal disease at increased risk for poor maternal and fetal outcome. In women with primary glomerulonephritis and mild renal insufficiency (serum creatinine <1.4 mg/dl) at the time of conception, pregnancy may induce an increase in serum creatinine and increasing hypertension. However, renal function generally returns to baseline postpartum. In general, fetal survival rates for women with mild renal insufficiency are good, approaching 95% in most studies.[4] However, complications, including SGA infants, preterm labor, and stillbirth, are increased even in women with mild renal insufficiency.[4] In women with more advanced renal disease, pregnancy may induce an acceleration in renal failure and a worsening fetal outcome.[2,5] This group of woman may continue to experience a decrease in renal function postpartum.[4]

It is generally accepted that the fetal prognosis is not determined by the type of glomerular disease; rather it is determined by the presence or absence of risk factors associated with the nephropathy, including the degree of proteinuria, hypertension, and renal function impairment at the time of conception. Women are considered in terms of the following three categories: (1) preserved or only mildly impaired renal function (serum creatinine 1.4 mg/dl) and no hypertension, (2) moderate renal insufficiency (serum creatinine 1.3 mg/dl [some use 2.5 mg/dl as the cut-off]), and (3) severe renal insufficiency (serum creatinine 3.0 mg/dl or higher). For women in the first category, maternal outcome is usually good and perinatal mortality is now less than 5%. However, this may not hold true for certain specific diseases, such as scleroderma, periarteritis nodosum, and other disorders associated with hypertension.[3]

In women with primary nonglomerular kidney disease, maternal and fetal morbidity correlates most significantly with the level of renal function at the time of conception. In certain diseases such as autosomal dominant polycystic kidney disease (ADPKD), pregnancy outcomes are generally uncompromised because the majority of women with ADPKD of childbearing age have normal renal function. In contrast, fetal and maternal outcomes are at greater risk in women with diabetes who have overt nephropathy and impaired renal function.[5]

The cause of accelerated renal impairment in some pregnant women is not clear. Worsening hypertension increases the risk for poor outcomes and probably contributes directly to worsening renal function. Urinary tract infections in this population are common and suggest a further decline in renal function. Proteinuria, which almost always decreases during pregnancy if there is underlying renal impairment, may further damage the kidneys.[4]

In women with renal impairment because of systemic disease, pregnancy can be problematic, with poor maternal and fetal outcomes. Disease activity may worsen during the pregnancy; in addition, the sequelae associated with the multisystem disease may add to those risk factors specific to the renal disease.[5] Data on outcomes for women with moderate or severe kidney dysfunction is more limited. Fetal outcome in the former group is still good (excluding first trimester abortions), but less than 40% of pregnancies in women undergoing dialysis are successful. However, the greatest concern in this group of women has to do with maternal outcome. About one third of women with moderate to severe renal impairment experience worsening, sometimes even life-threatening hypertension, and approximately one fourth of these women suffer from a decrease in GFR, which continues to worsen after the delivery.[3]

Lupus nephritis deserves special consideration. Systemic lupus erythematosus (SLE) is an autoimmune disease that commonly strikes women during childbearing years and is a common cause of renal insufficiency in these women. Nephritis is one of the most serious complications of SLE, and exacerbations increase the risk of renal failure.[6] Approximately half the women with SLE experience an exacerbation of lupus during pregnancy, although this occurs less commonly in women who have been in remission for at least 6 months. With new and better immunosuppressive drugs to manage SLE, the number of pregnancies is increasing several fold.[7]

CLINICAL PRESENTATION AND PHYSICAL EXAMINATION

Irregular menses are common among women with renal disease; as renal impairment progresses to ESRD, increasing numbers of women do not ovulate and are amenorrheic. However, during the past decade there have been significant advances in medical therapies for women with renal disease. Recombinant human erythropoietin therapy—a therapy that, in addition to its effects on hypothalamic function, may also improve sexual interest and function—has been introduced. In addition, increasing percentages of women with advanced renal disease are menstruating compared with earlier reports (approximately 40% compared with 10% a decade ago). A significant percentage of women who are sexually active report not using any method of birth control, perhaps because of their misperception regarding infertility.[8]

Women with renal impairment may assume that missed menses are due to the menstrual irregularity associated with their disease. Increasingly, women with renal disease are able to conceive; thus all sexually active women of childbearing age with renal impairment who come to their health care provider because of missed menses should have a serum human chorionic gonadotropin (HCG) sample drawn to exclude pregnancy. However, serum HCG can be elevated in women with severe renal disease (and increased serum creatinine), so ultrasound may be necessary to determine viable pregnancy.[6] Menstrual irregularities and amenorrhea occur most often in women with higher serum creatinine levels. After renal transplantation, menstrual irregularities may improve. Providers should maintain a high index of suspicion that amenorrhea may be due to pregnancy in women with milder renal insufficiency and in those with kidney transplants. The history and physical examination should include a careful review of all current medications as well as the standard prenatal evaluation and renal function tests.

In some women renal disease first manifests itself during pregnancy. A presentation that includes proteinurea, hypertension, and an elevated serum creatinine level is suspicious for renal disease. Such a constellation of signs also mimics preeclampsia, especially when it occurs during the latter half of pregnancy, and accurate diagnosis depends on further evaluation.

DIAGNOSTICS AND DIFFERENTIAL DIAGNOSIS

Urinalysis and renal function should be monitored regularly. Because anemia is associated with both pregnancy and renal disease, the hemoglobin and hematocrit should be checked at regular intervals to determine the need for erythropoietin. Pregnancy in women with lupus nephritis requires screening for lupus anticoagulant activity.

MANAGEMENT

For pregnant women with renal disease, multidisciplinary management is essential, preferably in a tertiary care facility, with close coordination among a specialist in high-risk obstetric care, an attendant in a neonatal intensive care unit, and a nephrologist. Referrals should be made at the beginning of gestation, and close multidisciplinary care should continue throughout the pregnancy.[2] Women with known renal disease should be examined by their obstetricians at biweekly intervals until 32 weeks' gestation and weekly thereafter.[4]

Many medications used to treat renal disease are contraindicated in pregnancy. According to August, Vella, and Sayegh, ACE inhibitors, angiotensin II receptor blockers, and certain immunosuppressants should be discontinued as soon as pregnancy is determined.[6] Discussion with the nephrologist and obstetrician is necessary to provide appropriate substitute medications.

Maternal renal function and blood pressure control are the two most important determinants of fetal outcome. There is general agreement that high blood pressure in pregnant women with renal disease should be treated more aggressively than in patients with isolated essential hypertension. What constitutes optimum blood pressure control in these women is still being debated; however, research suggests that the diastolic blood pressure maintained between 80 and 90 mm Hg may be a useful criterion.[3] In general, the blood pressure goal should be less than 120/80 mm Hg to preserve renal function.

Monthly monitoring of renal status for asymptomatic bacteriuria, proteinuria, and preeclampsia are also important components of management.[5] Progress in obstetric and neonatal care has increased the probability that women with impaired renal function will be able to give birth to living infants, albeit often premature infants of low birth weight, without a prohibitive risk of worsening the mother's renal function. Crucial to the best possible maternal and fetal outcome is closely coordinated care between the obstetrician and the nephrologist and optimum blood pressure control.[9]

ESRD, requiring dialysis, is associated with a significant decrease in fertility. However, pregnancy occurs in approximately 1% of patients, usually within the first few years of starting dialysis. Generally, the fetal outcome is poor, with infants surviving in only 23% to 55% of pregnancies; of these, many have significant morbidities. Approximately 85% are born prematurely and up to 28% are small for gestational age. Maternal complications, including death and worsening hypertension, occur in more than 80% of cases. In general, pregnancy is considered contraindicated while on dialysis.[4]

DIAGNOSTICS

Pregnancy in Renal Disease

LABORATORY
Hemoglobin and hematocrit
Serum human chorionic gonadotropin
Urinalysis*
24-hour urine for proteinuria*
BUN, creatinine*

IMAGING
Ultrasound, as determined by obstetrician

*As determined by nephrologist.

COMPLICATIONS

The two most significant complications of pregnancy in women with chronic renal disease are an acceleration of maternal renal disease and poor fetal outcome. Maternal morbidity is due primarily to the increased risk of preeclampsia, hypertension, or both. Fetal morbidity is principally related to the increased risk of preterm delivery and intrauterine growth retardation (IUGR).[2]

The effect of pregnancy in women with renal disease depends on several factors, including whether renal impairment is the primary disease or is associated with a systemic process, and the level of renal function at the time of conception.[5] Pregnancy in women with renal insufficiency, but with preserved renal function and normal blood pressure at the time of conception, generally does not result in a worsening of the maternal renal condition.[4] However, IUGR is seen even with mild renal disease (serum creatinine <1.4 mg/dl).[2] In contrast, if renal function is significantly impaired or there is co-existing hypertension at the time of conception, the probability of poor maternal and fetal outcome is significantly increased. An accelerated deterioration of maternal renal function during pregnancy has been reported in one third or more of women with significantly compromised renal function. In addition, the fetal loss rate is as high as 16% to 33% (not including first-trimester abortions), and a high proportion of premature deliveries and low-birth-weight infants has been reported in this population.[9]

Pregnancy in women with ESRD on maintenance dialysis is rare. Fertility is decreased in these women as a result of uremia-associated hypothalamopituitary dysfunction, which results in ovarian dysfunction and anovulatory cycles.[2] The diagnosis of pregnancy can be difficult and is generally made late. The perinatal course is generally complicated, with a poor fetal outcome. In addition, the high risk of an unsuccessful outcome can precipitate an emotional crisis in women who are already experiencing significant stress in association with their chronic illness. However, with improvements in dialysis efficacy and in the general condition of patients on dialysis, fertility has been augmented, and there is reason to have a more optimistic view about the course of pregnancy. Appropriate contraception is necessary for all women with renal dysfunction who are of childbearing age to prevent unplanned or unwanted pregnancies.[2,5]

INDICATIONS FOR REFERRAL OR HOSPITALIZATION

Pregnant women with underlying renal disease or women who develop renal dysfunction during pregnancy require careful management by specialists. All pregnant women with underlying renal disease or deteriorating renal function should be referred to a nephrologist and a specialist in high-risk obstetric care. Because the risk of fetal death is significantly higher for these women, hospitalization in a tertiary care facility is advised for delivery or for any other problems associated with the pregnancy.

PATIENT AND FAMILY EDUCATION

Women with preexisting renal disease who are considering pregnancy should have preconception counseling about their prospects for a successful pregnancy and the effect of pregnancy on their underlying disease. Pregnancy in all women with renal disease should, insofar as possible, be planned so that conception takes place at a time when risks are minimal. Patients with primary renal disease and normal or near-normal renal function have few contraindications to pregnancy. The best time for patients with systemic renal disease, such as systemic lupus erythematosus, to conceive is after stable remission of the disease process for at least 1 year. Diabetic women with nephropathy should achieve optimum glycemic control before conceiving. Women with diabetes and hypertension are at particularly high risk for poor pregnancy outcomes. These higher risks should be discussed when counseling women who are considering childbearing. In addition, women should be counseled about the importance of blood pressure control and close follow-up from the time of conception and throughout the pregnancy.[1,4]

REFERENCES

1. Holley JL, Bernardini J, Quadri KHM, and others: Pregnancy outcomes in a prospective matched control study of pregnancy and renal disease, *Clin Nephrol* 45(2):77-82, 1996.
2. Clark EC, Sterns RH: Chronic renal disease. In Leppert PC, Howard R, editors: *Primary care for women,* Philadelphia, 1997, Lippincott-Raven.
3. Lindheimer M: *Renal disease and pregnancy*, Geneva Foundation for Medical Education and Research, retrieved July 13, 2006, from http://www.gfmer.ch/Endo/lectures.
4. Agraharkar M: *Renal disease and pregnancy*, May 17, 2006, retrieved July 13, 2006, from http://www.emedicine.com/med/topic3253.htm.
5. Jungers P, Chauveau D: Pregnancy in renal disease, *Kidney Int* 52(4):871-875, 1997.
6. August P, Vella J, Sayegh MH: *Pregnancy in women with underlying renal disease,* retrieved Feb 23, 2007, from http://www.uptodateonline.com/utd/content/topic.do?topicKey=renldis/5345&selectedTitle=1~4143&source=search_result.
7. Tanden A, Ibenez D, Gladman D, and others: The effect of pregnancy in lupus nephritis, *Arthritis Rheum* 50(12):3941-3946, 2004.
8. Holley JL, Schmidt RJ, Bender FH, and others: Gynecologic and reproductive issues in women on dialysis, *Am J Kidney Dis* 29(5):685-690, 1997.
9. Jungers P, Chauveau D, Choukroun G, and others: Pregnancy in women with impaired renal function, *Clin Nephrol* 47(5):281-288, 1997.

CHAPTER 159

Prostate Disorders

Carol A. Whelan

BENIGN PROSTATIC HYPERPLASIA

DEFINITION AND EPIDEMIOLOGY

Benign prostatic hyperplasia (BPH), an almost ubiquitous phenomenon among the elderly, is a noncancerous enlargement of the prostate gland. BPH is present in up to 90% of all men by the eighth decade of life.[1]

PATHOPHYSIOLOGY

The prostate gland undergoes its first growth spurt during puberty and attains an average size of 20 g (0.7 ounce) by age 20. The gland then undergoes a second growth spurt during the fifth decade of life. This growth is characterized by localized proliferation in the periureteral region, leading to glandular compression, which may cause ureteral compression.[1]

The development of the prostate gland depends on androgen secretion, and both the presence of testes and advancing age are necessary for the development of BPH.[1] Dihydrotestosterone (DHT) is the main mediator of the growth and secretory function of the prostate and is the active metabolite that results from testosterone conversion.[2] BPH seems to be related to a complex interaction between androgen and estrogen secretion; abnormal serum elevations of androgen and estrogen stimulate prostatic growth. Other factors that contribute to prostatic enlargement appear to be related to the elaboration of certain growth factors, the formation and maintenance of DHT levels, and the functioning of androgen receptors.[2]

CLINICAL PRESENTATION

The symptoms of BPH are either obstructive or irritative in character. The term *lower urinary tract symptoms* is often used to describe any of the symptoms of BPH, although this term is not specific to BPH. Obstructive symptoms include urinary hesitancy, decreased caliber and force of the stream, and postvoid dribbling. These symptoms are related to bladder outlet obstruction. Irritative symptoms include frequency, urgency, and nocturia and occur as a result of decreased functional bladder capacity and instability or infection. Occasionally, hematuria accompanies BPH. Episodic symptoms may be present over many years with a gradual increase in the intensity of symptoms over time.

A thorough history is important. Current over-the-counter and prescription medication use should be explored to determine the presence of anticholinergics, which can impair bladder contractility, or sympathomimetics, which increase outflow resistance. Diuretics, which can cause an increased output of urine, may lead to urinary retention, especially in the presence of partially decompensated detrusor muscle.

BPH symptoms may be quantified using a symptom index developed by the American Urological Association to aid in classifying symptom severity and in developing a treatment plan[3] (Table 159-1). Symptoms are rated according to frequency of occurrence.[4]

PHYSICAL EXAMINATION

A digital rectal examination (DRE) and a focused neurologic examination assessing sacral nerve roots are recommended to evaluate for rectal or prostate malignancy, to determine neurologic problems that may result in bladder symptoms, and to evaluate anal sphincter tone. A lower abdominal examination is necessary to ascertain bladder distention from urinary retention. Prostatic nodules or induration should be noted on rectal examination because these findings suggest prostate cancer. The normal prostate is heart shaped and measures approximately 4 × 3 × 2 cm (1.6 × 1.2 × 0.8 inches). With BPH there may be uniform or focal enlargement of the prostate. The size of the prostate does not always correlate with symptom severity, however, and should not direct therapy. The median sulcus is often obliterated in BPH, and it is often difficult to palpate over the base of the prostate because of the gland's enlarged size in advanced stages. With BPH the gland is nontender and should be rubbery and smooth in consistency.

DIAGNOSTICS

A urinalysis should be performed to exclude a urinary tract infection or hematuria. Determination of the creatinine level is no longer considered necessary to assess renal function, although it may be prudent to obtain a baseline serum creatinine. According to American Urological Association guidelines (2006), measurement of serum prostate-specific antigen (PSA) is appropriate for men with a greater than 10-year life expectancy for physical findings suspicious of prostate cancer (abnormal DRE) and if 5α-reductase inhibitor therapy is planned.[4] The PSA test is a less specific indicator of prostate cancer in men who have BPH, but men should be advised that they have a 10% to 15% risk of having coexistent prostate cancer and that the PSA test is available for screening.[5] Assessment of free PSA and PSA velocity (the rate of rise per year) may help increase specificity for prostate cancer. Noncancerous prostate growth rarely results in a PSA velocity greater than 0.75 ng/ml/year.[1] It should be noted that the use of finasteride may result in a 50% reduction of baseline PSA levels, which may result in a delay in diagnosing prostate cancer.

> **DIAGNOSTICS**
>
> **Benign Prostatic Hyperplasia**
>
> **LABORATORY**
> Urinalysis
> Serum creatinine
> PSA*
>
> **IMAGING**
> At discretion of urologist
>
> *If indicated.

DIFFERENTIAL DIAGNOSIS

Symptoms of bladder outlet obstruction mandate evaluation for bladder calculi, urethral stricture, cancer of the prostate, and bladder neck contracture. Bladder cancer (as well as renal cancer) should be a consideration in a male patient with unexplained hematuria. Urinary tract infection must be excluded if there are complaints of irritative voiding symp-

TABLE 159-1 American Urological Association Symptom Index for Benign Prostatic Hyperplasia

Questions to Be Answered	Not at All	Less Than 1 Time in 5	Less Than Half the Time	About Half the Time	More Than Half the Time	Almost Always
Over the past month, how often have you had a sensation of not emptying your bladder completely after you finish urinating?	0	1	2	3	4	5
Over the past month, how often have you had to urinate again less than 2 hours after you finished urinating?	0	1	2	3	4	5
Over the past month, how often have you found you stopped and started again several times when you urinated?	0	1	2	3	4	5
Over the past month, how often have you found it difficult to postpone urination?	0	1	2	3	4	5
Over the past month, how often have you had a weak urinary stream?	0	1	2	3	4	5
Over the past month, how often have you had to push or strain to begin urination?	0	1	2	3	4	5
Over the past month, how many times did you most typically get up to urinate from the time you went to bed at night until the time you got up in the morning?	0 (None)	1 (1 time)	2 (2 times)	3 (3 times)	4 (4 times)	5 (5 times)

From Barry MJ, Fowler FJ Jr, O'Leary MP, and others: The American Urologic Association symptom index for benign prostatic hyperplasia. The Measurement Committee of the American Urological Association, *J Urol* 148(5):1549-1557, 1992.
A score of 0 to 7 indicates mild symptoms; 8 to 19, moderate symptoms; and 20 to 35, severe symptoms.

toms. If abnormalities are found on neurologic examination and problems with urinary retention are present, neurologic disease must be considered.[6] Prostate cancer should be considered when an asymmetric enlargement, nodule, or induration is palpated on rectal examination.

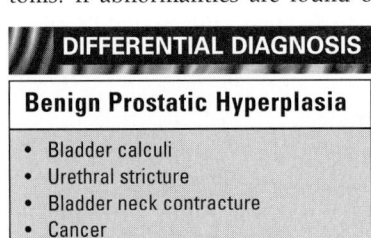

DIFFERENTIAL DIAGNOSIS

Benign Prostatic Hyperplasia

- Bladder calculi
- Urethral stricture
- Bladder neck contracture
- Cancer
- Urinary tract infection
- Neurologic disorder

MANAGEMENT

The traditional management goal for treatment of BPH has been relief of symptoms. Publication of the Medical Treatment of Prostatic Symptoms (MTOPS) study in 2002 has led some clinicians and researchers to classify BPH as a progressive disease, the progression of which can be slowed by the aggressive use of finasteride and alpha blockers.[7] Regardless of how one views BPH, the treatment options include watchful waiting, 5α-reductase enzyme inhibitor (finasteride or dutasteride) therapy, α_1-adrenergic antagonist therapy, combination drug therapy, balloon dilation, or surgery.[4] The benefits and risks associated with each treatment should be explained. It is important to advise the patient that, if he chooses watchful waiting, other treatment approaches can be considered at any time if symptoms increase.

α-Adrenergic antagonists have long been the main treatment for BPH. They work by lowering bladder neck and ureteral resistance. Finasteride shrinks prostatic glandular hyperplasia by decreasing tissue DHT levels.[1] The MTOPS study (funded by the National Institute of Diabetes and Digestive and Kidney Diseases) concluded that treatment with a combination of finasteride and doxazosin resulted in a 67% risk reduction of BPH symptoms, vs. 34% for finasteride alone and 39% for doxazosin alone.[7] The study authors also argued that combination therapy should become the standard of care because it decreased the incidence of urinary retention and the need for invasive procedures when compared with other therapies. The publication of this study had a powerful impact on prescribing patterns, and given its large size (N = 3047) and lengthy average follow-up time (4.5 years), it was widely regarded as ushering in a new era of combination therapy for BPH.[7] Just a few months later, however, the results of the Prospective European Doxazosin and Combination Therapy (PREDICT) trial disputed these findings.[8] The study investigators found that the addition of finasteride to doxazosin resulted in no additional benefit, but they did suggest that finasteride may be of some benefit in patients with prostate size greater than 40 g (1.4 ounces).[8] The PREDICT study involved 1007 men who were monitored for a 52-week trial.[9] Although there is no true consensus on the optimum treatment of symptomatic BPH, consideration of combination therapy in patients with large prostate volumes appears warranted.

Controversy also exists on whether the use of nonspecific alpha blockers such as doxazosin should be replaced with specific alpha blockers such as tamsulosin. Specific alpha blockers have the benefit of being blood pressure neutral, since they act only on the smooth muscle of the prostate, and not the vasculature. This may be of benefit in the elderly, who may experience postural hypotension, especially during the night when rising to void.

Limited evidence exists regarding the benefit of using saw palmetto extract in the treatment of mild BPH. Therapy with saw palmetto extract does appear to be safe with little or no adverse effects.[10,11]

Balloon dilation reduces symptoms in the short term, but long-term follow-up of the procedure has not been adequately studied. Transurethral resection of the prostate, transurethral incision of the prostate, and open prostatectomy are surgical procedures that are effective for severe BPH.

COMPLICATIONS

Urinary tract infection and urinary retention are common sequelae of BPH. In addition, urinary retention can result in renal problems if not detected early.

INDICATIONS FOR REFERRAL OR HOSPITALIZATION

Referral to a urologist is necessary for surgical intervention. Indications for surgery include urinary retention; intractable symptoms related to obstruction; recurrent or persistent urinary tract infection; recurrent prostatic bleeding; significant postvoid residual; changes in the kidneys, ureters, or bladder caused by prostatic obstruction; an abnormally low urinary flow rate; or bladder calculi. IV urography, filling cystometry, uroflowmetry, urethrocystoscopy, pressure-flow studies, and measurement of postvoid residuals may be helpful in individual situations, and their need can best be determined by a urologist. They are not recommended as standard tests for the evaluation of BPH.[4]

Acute urinary retention with a distended bladder confirmed by palpation or catheterization increases the risk of infection and renal complications, and hospitalization may be indicated.

PATIENT AND FAMILY EDUCATION

Patients should understand the advantages and risks of each treatment option so that they can make informed decisions. Patients should be advised of the importance of monitoring symptom progression and reporting any abrupt change in symptom pattern, which may indicate a complication or another pathologic process.

PROSTATITIS

DEFINITION AND EPIDEMIOLOGY

Prostatitis, or inflammation of the prostate gland, is a common problem in the adult male population. There are four basic types of prostatitis: acute bacterial, chronic bacterial, nonbacterial, and prostatodynia. Accurate diagnostic differentiation of these is a prerequisite for effective management.

The prostate gland, through which the urethra passes, is an organ located adjacent to and at the inferior aspect of the bladder. Bacterial prostatitis (both acute and chronic) is caused by bacterial inflammation. However, nonbacterial prostatitis, for which there is no identifiable cause, is the most common cause of prostatic inflammation. Prostatodynia is characterized by symptoms of prostatic inflammation but without signs of inflammation on physical examination. It has been estimated that 25% of male primary care visits with genitourinary complaints are related to prostatitis.[12]

PATHOPHYSIOLOGY

The organisms responsible for acute and chronic prostatitis are usually gram-negative organisms and include *Escherichia coli* and *Klebsiella, Pseudomonas, Proteus*, and *Enterobacter* organisms, with *E. coli* being the most common.[13] Other enterococci that are normally found in feces can also cause prostatitis. A zinc-containing antibacterial factor present in normal prostatic fluid aids in resisting infection. Abnormally low levels of this factor have been associated with bacterial prostatitis.[2]

Acute bacterial prostatitis results from the ascent of organized, colonized bacteria from the lower urethra to the prostate. The urethral bacteria may be a result of infection or normal fecal flora. Increases in intraurethral pressure as a result of intercourse can result in bacterial deposition into the prostate. Difficulty in bacterial eradication increases the risk of chronic infection. Urologic instrumentation is another common cause of acute bacterial prostatitis.

The cause of nonbacterial prostatitis is less clear. *Ureaplasma urealyticum* and *Chlamydia, Gardnerella*, and *Mycoplasma* organisms have occasionally been found on urine and prostatic secretion cultures and are considered potential causative agents. However, their actual significance is unknown. Nonbacterial prostatitis may have a noninfectious inflammatory etiology that is possibly related to autoimmune dysfunction.[6]

The cause of prostatodynia is also unknown. There is some evidence that it may be related to a neurologic disorder that results in voiding dysfunction and in dysfunction of the pelvic floor musculature.[6,14]

CLINICAL PRESENTATION

Fever, chills, malaise, myalgias, and arthralgias are common with acute bacterial prostatitis. Genitourinary symptoms include hesitancy, frequency, urgency, nocturia, dysuria, and a sensation of incomplete bladder emptying. Accompanying complaints may be low back pain, perineal pain, or suprapubic pain. PSA levels are often markedly elevated and should not be checked in the acute stages of prostatitis because they are not reliable indicators of either infection or cure.

The presentation of chronic prostatitis tends to be more varied than that of acute prostatitis and may include a history of recurrent urinary tract infection (usually with the same organism) and complaints of urinary frequency, urgency, and burning on urination. Perineal, inguinal, or suprapubic pain may be present.[15]

Nonbacterial prostatitis is characterized by prostatic pain or vague discomfort of the suprapubic, scrotal, inguinal, lower back, or perineal areas. Pain on ejaculation may also occur. Urinary symptoms such as hesitancy, a decrease in the urinary stream, frequency, urgency, and burning on urination may also be present.

Symptoms suggestive of prostatodynia include pain and discomfort in the pelvic area and problems related to urinary flow such as hesitancy, an interrupted flow, postvoid dribbling, and decreased flow. Frequency, urgency, and nocturia may be present. Penile and urethral pain, as well as discomfort in the lower back, suprapubic area, testicles, groin, and perineum, is often reported. The patient usually has no history of urinary tract infection, but may have a lifetime history of voiding difficulties.

PHYSICAL EXAMINATION

Abdominal and rectal examinations are important components of the physical examination for symptoms related to the prostate. The abdominal examination should exclude bladder distention, and the prostate gland should be examined for size, consistency, and tenderness. Normally, the prostate is heart shaped and measures approximately 4 × 3 × 2 cm (1.6 × 1.2 × 0.8 inches).

In acute bacterial prostatitis the prostate is typically enlarged, with tenderness and induration. The prostate examination should be performed gently without excessive manipulation to avoid inducing bacteremia. Urinary retention and fever may be present.

The prostate examination in chronic bacterial prostatitis may be nonspecific or may reveal a tender or boggy prostate. In nonbacterial prostatitis the prostate examination is usually normal, but occasionally a soft, boggy prostate with tenderness may be present. Physical examination in prostatodynia is unremarkable with the exception that increased anal sphincter tone and paraprostatic tenderness may be present.

DIAGNOSTICS

The history and physical examination are often adequate to diagnose prostatitis. Examination of expressed prostatic secretions (EPS) may be helpful to both diagnose and determine the type of prostatitis, but it should not be done if acute prostatitis is suspected. Segmented urine specimens representing the urethral (voided bladder [VB] 1), bladder (VB2), EPS, and postprostatic massage (VB3) contents are obtained and viewed for the presence of white blood cells (WBCs). More than 10 WBCs per high-power field on the EPS or spun VB3 is suggestive of bacterial prostatitis. Cultures of the EPS and VB3 specimens should show significant growth of colonies (>5000/ml) with bacterial prostatitis.

The segmented urine specimens are collected after foreskin retraction and cleaning of the glans penis. The first 10-ml specimen is labeled VB1. A midstream urine specimen is labeled VB2. The practitioner should then ask the patient to bend over while the patient is retracting the foreskin and holding a specimen container in front of the meatus. The practitioner should press on the lateral lobe of the prostate and slide the examining finger toward the midline six or seven times on each side of the prostate. Milking the secretions by applying gentle pressure on the bulbous urethra may be necessary to obtain the EPS. The VB3 specimen is the 5 to 10 ml of urine passed immediately after prostatic massage. Because bacterial prostatitis is almost always caused by gram-negative organisms, many clinicians choose to initially treat suspected prostatitis empirically based on history and physical examination.

If acute bacterial prostatitis is suspected, prostatic massage should be avoided to minimize a risk of bacteremia. In acute bacterial prostatitis the urinalysis results may reveal pyuria, bacteriuria, and varying degrees of hematuria, with urine culture necessary for organism identification. A CBC is significant for increased numbers of leukocytes with a left shift.

In chronic bacterial prostatitis the urinalysis is normal unless there is a co-existent cystitis. However, both the EPS and VB3 specimens show increased numbers of leukocytes. Culture of the organisms in the VB3 specimen is necessary for diagnosis.

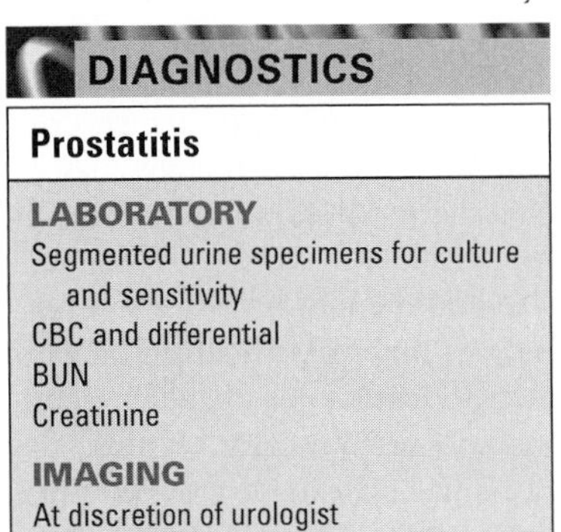
DIAGNOSTICS

Prostatitis

LABORATORY
Segmented urine specimens for culture and sensitivity
CBC and differential
BUN
Creatinine

IMAGING
At discretion of urologist

Urine cultures are negative with nonbacterial prostatitis, but increased numbers of leukocytes are seen in the EPS specimen. In prostatodynia the urine and EPS specimens are normal. Urodynamic testing may show signs of dysfunctional voiding.

DIFFERENTIAL DIAGNOSIS

The diagnosis of acute prostatitis is usually made on the basis of the clinical presentation and the markedly tender prostate on physical examination. It can be distinguished from acute pyelonephritis, acute epididymitis, and acute diverticulosis by a careful history, physical examination, and urinalysis. Prostatic enlargement from BPH or prostate cancer causing urinary retention can usually be distinguished from acute bacterial prostatitis on rectal examination.

Chronic bacterial prostatitis can be differentiated from chronic urethritis and cystitis with segmented urine cultures. Other common causes of urinary outflow problems, such as BPH, urethral stricture, and prostate cancer, need to be considered. Bladder carcinoma, sphincter dyssynergia, and neurogenic bladder also can cause lower urinary tract irritative symptoms.[16] Rectal examination should help exclude anal disease, such as tumors, which may manifest similarly to chronic prostatitis.

The primary condition to be considered in the differential diagnosis of nonbacterial prostatitis is chronic bacterial prostatitis. The absence of positive cultures and a negative history of urinary tract infection support the diagnosis of nonbacterial prostatitis. A urinary cytologic examination and cystoscopy are indicated to exclude bladder cancer in the older

DIFFERENTIAL DIAGNOSIS

Prostatitis

- Acute or chronic bacterial prostatitis
- Acute pyelonephritis
- Acute epididymitis
- Acute diverticulitis
- Prostatic cancer or bladder cancer
- Benign prostatic hyperplasia
- Urethral stricture
- Sphincter dyssynergy
- Neurogenic bladder
- Interstitial cystitis
- Obstructive calculus

man with irritative voiding symptoms and negative cultures.[6] Interstitial cystitis and carcinoma in situ of the bladder may be seen with similar symptoms in the younger man.

MANAGEMENT

Many patients with acute prostatitis are severely ill and require broad-spectrum antibiotic therapy. Depending on the severity of the illness, hospitalization and IV antibiotic therapy may be indicated. Research has shown the use of fluoroquinolones to be beneficial.[17] A patient who is afebrile for 24 to 48 hours should be switched from IV to oral therapy.

Those who are less acutely ill may be treated on an outpatient basis with oral antibiotics. Trimethoprim-sulfamethoxazole and fluoroquinolones are effective in treating the illness,[18] but penicillins and cephalosporins do not penetrate the prostatic epithelium. The length of appropriate treatment ranges from 2 to 6 weeks. In general, acute bacterial prostatitis requires antibiotic therapy for a minimum of 3 weeks to prevent the development of chronic bacterial prostatitis.[13,16,19] Follow-up segmented urine cultures, including prostatic secretions, are necessary after treatment is completed. Local measures may be helpful in reducing discomfort. Sitz baths, three times per day, may reduce perineal pain. Analgesics, antipyretics, stool softeners, and bed rest may also be beneficial.

The treatment of chronic bacterial prostatitis is more complex because of the difficulty in attaining therapeutic intraprostatic antibiotic levels in a noninflamed prostate. The antibiotics that have demonstrated the highest effectiveness include trimethoprim-sulfamethoxazole, the fluoroquinolones, and erythromycin. Trimethoprim-sulfamethoxazole for 4 to 16 weeks generally provides effective treatment.[19] Fluoroquinolones have good prostatic penetration and are effective against most of the causative organisms. Treatment length is often 3 weeks to 4 months.[19] It is recommended that a segmented urine culture be conducted on all men being treated with antibiotics 4 weeks into treatment. If the urine is not sterile at that time, treatment should be changed.[14]

Curing chronic bacterial prostatitis may be difficult. A cure is demonstrated by negative segmented urine cultures 6 months after completion of therapy.[20] However, the WBC count may remain elevated long after a cure. If a relapse occurs, a longer course of antibiotic therapy is necessary. If a cure is not achieved, a low dose of antibiotics may be prescribed to prevent symptomatic infection. Commonly used medications include trimethoprim-sulfamethoxazole DS (160 mg/800 mg, 1 tablet/day or q.o.d.) or nitrofurantoin (50 to 100 mg/day).

Supportive measures such as warm water baths may be helpful in the treatment of chronic bacterial prostatitis. Beverages that produce rapid bladder expansion, such as coffee, tea, and alcohol, should be avoided. The use of medications that impair bladder function (e.g., anticholinergics, sedatives, antidepressants) should be assessed.

The treatment of nonbacterial prostatitis is controversial because of the inability to isolate a causative organism. If *Ureaplasma* or *Chlamydia* organisms are suspected, doxycycline, erythromycin, or a fluoroquinolone should be prescribed for 2 to 4 weeks.[13] If the patient does not respond to treatment, antibiotic therapy should be discontinued and the emphasis shifted to symptomatic relief. Supportive measures as described previously may be helpful, including warm tub baths and the use of NSAIDs. Normal sexual activity is not contraindicated. If patients complain of irritative voiding problems, a trial of anticholinergic medications, such as oxybutynin chloride, may be effective. If spicy foods, alcohol, or caffeine aggravates symptoms, they should be avoided.

The treatment of prostatodynia includes the use of alpha-blocking agents that relax the muscles of the bladder neck. To minimize the risk of hypotension, therapy should be initiated with a low dose. The use of biofeedback, referral to a mental health professional for stress and emotional problems, and the use of sitz baths and NSAIDs may also be helpful in prostatodynia.

LIFE SPAN CONSIDERATIONS

The risk of sexually transmitted diseases, which can be difficult to identify by culture and may need to be treated empirically, should be assessed. In the older man, the possibility of co-existent BPH or prostate cancer, which can potentiate the signs and symptoms of prostatitis, should be considered.

COMPLICATIONS

A prostatic abscess rarely occurs as a complication of acute bacterial prostatitis except in immunocompromised patients. The symptoms are similar to those of acute bacterial prostatitis, but on rectal examination there is a fluctuance of the affected lobe. Diagnosis can be confirmed with transrectal ultrasound (TRUS). The treatment usually includes surgical drainage and antibiotics. Other complications of acute bacterial prostatitis may include pyelonephritis, epididymitis, seminal vesiculitis, and bacteremia.

INDICATIONS FOR REFERRAL OR HOSPITALIZATION

Because of the severity of the illness associated with acute bacterial prostatitis and the potential chronicity of bacterial and nonbacterial prostatitis and prostatodynia, co-management with a urologist is often indicated. Urologic referral is indicated for severe cases of acute bacterial prostatitis, when co-morbidity increases the risk of sequelae or signs of urinary retention are present. Refractory chronic prostatitis in the presence of prostatic stones also requires urologic referral. If symptoms do not resolve after the treatment of nonbacterial prostatitis or prostatodynia, a urologic referral is necessary to exclude cystitis[21] or bladder cancer and to confirm the original diagnosis.

Hospitalization is indicated for acute illness. If prostate enlargement results in urinary retention, urinary catheterization is contraindicated and a percutaneous suprapubic tube is necessary until the prostatic enlargement subsides.

PATIENT AND FAMILY EDUCATION

Education regarding the cause of patients' symptoms and treatment is necessary. The long duration of antibiotic treatment in several of these conditions requires that patients understand the necessity of maintaining an adequate therapeutic level for the duration of therapy. The importance of follow-up care should be stressed, as well as the importance of using condoms to prevent the reintroduction of bacteria into the urethra with sexual intercourse. Anal intercourse should be avoided with acute bacterial prostatitis.

PROSTATE CANCER

DEFINITION AND EPIDEMIOLOGY

Cancer of the prostate is the most common malignancy in men in the United States and the second leading cause of cancer death in men over the age of 55.[1] In the United States in 2004, 230,000 new cases were diagnosed and 29,000 known deaths occurred from prostate cancer, making it the second leading cause of cancer death in men.[22] Risk factors for prostate cancer include advancing age, African-American race, and a positive family history of prostate cancer. As a result of effective screening and the aging of the U.S. population, the number of prostate cancer cases diagnosed has increased; however, deaths due to prostate cancer have decreased significantly in the past 5 years, and the majority of men diagnosed with prostate cancer (eight of nine) do not die of the disease.[1,23]

Eighty percent of cases are diagnosed in men over age 65, with incidence rates being 66% higher in African-American men than in Caucasian men.[24,25] The mortality rate of African-American men is estimated to be twice that of Caucasian men,[24] and both tumor size and tumor precursors are increased in African-American men. The 5-year survival rate for prostate cancer is greater than 80% when it is detected at an early stage.[26]

PATHOPHYSIOLOGY

The most common type of prostate cancer is adenocarcinoma. It develops in the acinar glands located in the posterior peripheral zone of the prostate. Histologic grading is an important predictor of prognosis. The Gleason system incorporates clinical and physiologic parameters for grading of the malignancy[27] (Table 159-2). Tumors can arise in one or both lobes of the prostate and can spread within the prostate, through the prostatic capsule, and through the seminal vesicles or the base of the bladder, with metastasis occurring via the lymphatic and circulatory systems.[26]

CLINICAL PRESENTATION

Presenting symptoms of prostate cancer may include urinary hesitancy, urgency, nocturia, and frequency, although in early stages of the disease the patient is usually asymptomatic. Symptoms tend to increase in intensity over a 1- to 2-month period, which is different from the slow, gradual progression in symptoms that occurs in BPH. In more advanced disease, presenting symptoms may include back pain, impotence, and other bone pain that suggests metastasis. Other symptoms of metastasis include weight loss; constipation; malaise; hematuria; and rectal pain or symptoms related to nerve root compression, such as paresthesias or extremity weakness.

PHYSICAL EXAMINATION

A firm nodule on rectal examination; induration; or a stony, asymmetric prostate is suspicious for prostate cancer. In the early disease stage the prostate examination will generally be normal. Routine DRE is recommended for men over the age of 50. The American Cancer Society recommends that African-American men older than age 45 and men over the age of 40 with a family history of prostate cancer be screened annually for prostate cancer with a DRE.[23]

TABLE 159-2 Gleason Grading Scale

Stage	Description
A1	Clinically undetectable, lesion is confined to one lobe of prostate; well-differentiated local adenocarcinoma found on pathologic examination
A2	Clinically undetectable, diffuse or multifocal distribution of well-differentiated tumor found on pathologic examination
B1	May be palpable on rectal examination; limited to one lobe of prostate; confined within prostate capsule; nodule <1.5 cm; metastasis to lymph nodes in 10%-20% of patients
B2	Involves both lobes of prostate; metastasis to lymph nodes in 15%-40%; nodules >1.5 cm
C	Local extension outside of prostate capsule into vesicles or surrounding tissue; lymph node metastasis in 40%-80%; no metastasis to other sites
D1	Metastatic involvement of pelvic lymph nodes; lesions may extend into bladder, rectum or pelvis
D2	Distant metastases

From Vetrosky DT, Gerdom L, White GL: Prostate cancer: pathology, diagnosis, and management, *Clin Rev* 7(5):79-100, 1997.

DIAGNOSTICS AND DIFFERENTIAL DIAGNOSIS

Measurement of the PSA combined with DRE is considered the most sensitive and specific screening method for prostate cancer. The PSA is a protease enzyme secreted by the prostate gland, and levels may be elevated in benign and malignant conditions of the prostate. A PSA level below 5 mcg/L is considered normal; however, algorithms exist that adjust normal values for age and race. Values between 5 and 10 mcg/L may be seen in early prostate cancer and other benign conditions, and values over 10 mcg/L suggest prostate cancer. Values above 80 mcg/L may indicate advanced or metastatic disease. The PSA test has a 96% sensitivity and 95% specificity for the detection of early prostate cancer.[23] The use of the free PSA test and determination of PSA velocity (rate of rise) may increase specificity for prostate cancer. A rate of rise of more than 0.75 ng/ml/yr is considered highly sensitive for prostate cancer.[1]

An alternative method of considering normal ranges for the PSA test is according to age:

AGE (years)	PSA: NORMAL RANGE (mcg/L)
40-49	0-2.5
50-59	0-3.5
60-69	0-4.5
70-79	0-6.5

Studies suggest that different age-specific reference ranges should be considered for African-American men because many cases in this population would be missed using the traditional reference ranges. For the test to have 95%

DIAGNOSTICS

Prostate Cancer

LABORATORY
PSA
CBC and differential*

OTHER
Needle biopsy

*If indicated.

sensitivity in African-American men, the following reference ranges are suggested[28]:

AGE (years)	PSA: NORMAL RANGE (mcg/L)	SPECIFICITY (%)
40-49	0-2.0	93
50-59	0-4.0	88
60-69	0-4.5	81
70-79	0-5.5	78

If the PSA is greater than 4.0 ng/ml or DRE is abnormal, TRUS of the prostate with a TRUS-guided biopsy is recommended. The TRUS allows for guided biopsy of suspicious hypoechoic areas.

In cases with a positive biopsy of the prostate and a PSA above 10 mcg/L, a radionuclide bone scan may be necessary to determine the presence of bone metastases. A CT scan or MRI of the abdomen and pelvis is important to assess the regional lymph nodes. A chest x-ray study can exclude metastasis to the lungs. An elevated alkaline phosphatase level suggests bone metastasis, and an elevated acid phosphatase level is correlated with extension outside the prostatic capsule.[23] The differential diagnosis includes BPH and prostatitis when there is an abnormal DRE and PSA test.

DIFFERENTIAL DIAGNOSIS

Prostate Cancer

- Bladder outlet obstruction
- Urinary tract infection
- Prostate calculi
- Benign prostatic hyperplasia
- Prostatitis

MANAGEMENT

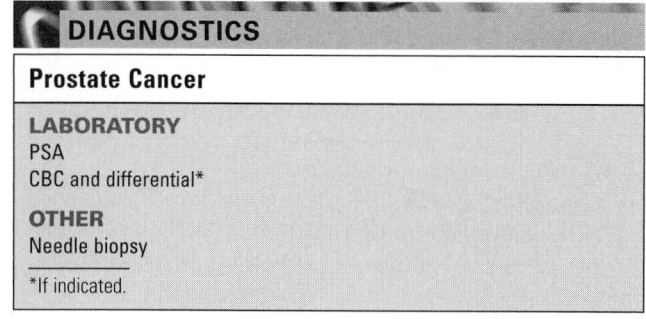

Treatment decisions are based on the stage at diagnosis; prognostic features of the tumor; and the patient's age, medical condition, and treatment preference. Decisions regarding therapy are complex and controversial. The current therapy with disease classified as stage A or B is radical prostatectomy or radiotherapy. Long-term survival rates are 80% to 90% with either treatment.[29] Cryotherapy is being used more commonly in localized prostate cancer.

Hormonal therapy has been used for symptomatic patients with advanced disease, but evidence does not clearly show whether androgen suppression improves long-term outcome.[30] Hormone treatments include oral estrogens, orchiectomy, luteinizing hormone–releasing hormone (LHRH) agonists, antiandrogens, and progestational agents. LHRH agonists act by initially stimulating pituitary gonadotropin production and later inhibiting it.

Pain management is often an important treatment issue in more advanced disease. Palliative treatment with radiation and medication may help relieve the pain.

LIFE SPAN CONSIDERATIONS

PSA screening is not recommended for men over the age of 70 with limited life expectancy[31] because of the typically slow progression of the disease and because men over the age of 70 are generally less likely candidates for radical prostatectomy. Early hormonal treatment for asymptomatic disease is still controversial. Treatment options, including risks and benefits, should be discussed with older patients who have asymptomatic, localized disease.

COMPLICATIONS

The major complication of prostate cancer is metastatic disease. Risks of surgery include hemorrhage or injury to the obturator nerve, ureter, or rectum. The long-term complications of surgery include incontinence and impotence.[23] Problems associated with radiotherapy include urinary problems, intestinal sequelae, impotence, and transient edema. Intestinal problems include diarrhea, fecal incontinence, rectal bleeding, intestinal obstruction, rectal strictures, mucus discharge, and tenesmus. Potential urologic problems include cystitis, hematuria, frequency, dysuria, and urethral stricture. The main complications of cryotherapy include urethral stricture, irritative symptoms, urinary incontinence, impotence, rectourethral fistula, bladder neck contracture, and urinary retention.

INDICATIONS FOR REFERRAL OR HOSPITALIZATION

A referral should be made to a urologist when a suspicious finding is found on DRE or the PSA is elevated (after discussing options and implications for treatment with the patient, some patients may decline referral). After treatment, the health care provider can offer follow-up care that includes monitoring the PSA levels. After radical prostatectomy, the PSA level should fall to less than 0.2 mcg/L. PSA levels also fall after radiotherapy and continue to decrease for 12 months after completion of therapy. PSA levels should be tested at 6 and 12 months after treatment and annually thereafter. An increase in PSA should be evaluated with a TRUS and biopsy. Hospitalization may also be necessary in the case of advanced metastatic disease.

PATIENT AND FAMILY EDUCATION

Education includes the importance of screening for prostate cancer, the strengths and limitations of PSA screening, and the implications of an abnormal prostate examination or PSA test.

HEALTH PROMOTION

Patient education is an important aspect of maintaining good prostate health. Fortunately, many new resources are available, although Web-based information varies in accuracy and content. Simply making patients aware of the symptoms of prostate disorders via waiting room literature may help increase their willingness to discuss prostate symptoms. To help prevent prostate cancer, limited evidence for benefit exists for diets high in lycopene (found in tomatoes) and low in fat.[1,32,33]

REFERENCES

1. Kasper DL, Fauci AS, Longo DL, and others: *Harrison's principles of internal medicine,* ed 16, New York, 2005, McGraw-Hill.
2. Kelley WN, editor: *Essentials of internal medicine,* Philadelphia, 1994, Lippincott.
3. Barry MJ, Fowler FJ Jr, O'Leary MP, and others: The American Urological Association symptom index for benign prostatic hyperplasia. The Measurement Committee of the American Urological Association, *J Urol* 148(5):1549-1557, 1992.
4. Kaplan SA: Update on the American Urological Association Guidelines for the Treatment of Benign Prostatic Hyperplasia, *Rev Urol* 8(Suppl 4):S10–S17, 2006, retrieved March 2, 2007, from http://www.pubmedcentral.nih.gov/articlerender.fcgi?artid=1765043.
5. Goodson JD, Barry MJ: Management of benign prostatic hyperplasia. In Goroll AH, May LA, Mulley AG, editors: *Primary care medicine: office evaluation and management of the adult patient,* ed 3, Philadelphia, 1995, Lippincott.
6. Presti JC, Stoller ML, Carroll PR: Urology. In Tierney LM, McPhee SJ, Papadakis MA, editors: *Current medical diagnosis and treatment,* ed 34, Norwalk, Conn, 1995, Appleton & Lange.
7. Holtgrewe HL, Mebust WK, Dowd JB, and others: The American Urological Association symptom index for benign prostatic hyperplasia, *J Urol* 167(2):265, abstract 1042, 2002.
8. Lepor H, Williford WO, Barry MJ, and others: The efficacy of terazosin, finasteride, or both in benign prostatic, *N Engl J Med* 335:533-539, 1996.
9. Kirby RS, Roehrborn C, Boyle P, and others. Efficacy and tolerability of doxazosin and finasteride alone or in combination, in treatment of symptoms of BPH: the prospective European doxazosin and combination therapy (PREDICT) trial, *Urology* 61:119-126, 2003.
10. Marks LS, Partin AW, Epstein JI, and others: Effects of saw palmetto herbal blend in men with symptomatic benign prostatic hyperplasia, *J Urol* 163:1451-1456, 2000.
11. Gerber GS: Saw palmetto for the treatment of men with lower urinary tract symptoms, *J Urol* 163:1408-1412, 2000.
12. Meares EM: Prostatitis, *Med Clin North Am* 75(2):405-424, 1991.
13. Criste G, Gray D, Gallo B: Prostatitis: a review of diagnosis and management, *Nurse Pract* 19(7):32-38, 1994.
14. Denman SJ, Murphy PA: Genitourinary infections. In Barker LR, Burton JR, Zieve PD, editors: *Principles of ambulatory medicine,* ed 4, Baltimore, 1995, Williams & Wilkins.
15. Krieger JN, Egan KJ, Ross SO, and others: Chronic pelvic pains represent the most prominent urogenital symptoms of chronic prostatitis, *Urology* 48(5):715-722, 1996.
16. Goodson JD: Management of acute and chronic prostatitis. In Goroll AH, May LA, Mulley AG, editors: *Primary care medicine: office evaluation and management of the adult patient,* ed 3, Philadelphia, 1995, Lippincott.
17. Chow RD: Prostatitis: work-up and treatment of men with telltale symptoms, *Geriatrics* 56:32-36, 2001.
18. Berg D: *Handbook of primary care medicine,* Philadelphia, 1993, Lippincott.
19. Donovan DA, Nicholas PK: Prostatitis: diagnosis and treatment in primary care, *Nurse Pract* 22(4):144-156, 1997.
20. Berger PE, Hanno PM: A spectrum of prostatitis syndromes, *Patient Care* 24(99):95-111, 1990.
21. Miller JL, Rothman I, Bavendam TG, and others: Prostatodynia and interstitial cystitis: one and the same? *Urology* 45(4):587-590, 1995.
22. Lee JJ: Design considerations for efficient prostate cancer chemoprevention trials, *Urology* 58(Suppl 1):205-212, 2001.
23. Pinto HA: Prostate cancer. In Fishman MC, Hoffman AR, Klausner RD, and others, editors: *Medicine,* ed 4, Philadelphia, 1996, Lippincott-Raven.
24. American Cancer Society: *Cancer facts and figures—1997 and addendum,* Atlanta, 1997, The Society.
25. Nicoll LH, Carroll P: The prostate, *Lippincott Health Promotion Lett* 2(1):1-8, 1997.
26. Vetrosky DT, Gerdom L, White GL: Prostate cancer: pathology, diagnosis, and management, *Clin Rev* 7(5):79-100, 1997.
27. Gleason DF, Melligor GT: Prediction of prognosis of prostatic adenocarcinoma by combined histologic grading and clinical staging, *J Urol* 111:58-64, 1974.
28. Tewari A, and others: Prostate neoplasms. In Lonergan ET, editor: *Geriatrics: a Lange clinical manual,* Norwalk, Conn, 1996, Appleton & Lange.
29. Berger RE, Hanno PM: The fine points of prostatitis care, *Patient Care,* Sept 15, pp 91-107, 1992.
30. Theyer G, Hamilton G: Current status of intermittent androgen suppression in the treatment of prostate cancer, *Urology* 52:353-359, 1998.
31. Walter LC, Bertenthal D, Lindquist K, and others: PSA screening among elderly men with limited life expectancies, *JAMA* 296:2336-2342, 2371-2373, 2006.
32. Arab L, Steck S: Lycopene and cardiovascular disease, *Am J Clin Nutr* 72:1691S-1695S, 2000.
33. Moyad MA: Fat reduction to prevent prostate cancer: waiting for more evidence? *Curr Opin Urol* 11:457-461, 2001.

CHAPTER 160

Proteinuria and Hematuria

Carol A. Whelan

Proteinuria and hematuria are relatively common findings on routine urinalysis. However, these findings can also be signs of serious disease or neoplasm, and therefore a careful, systematic evaluation is essential.[1-5]

PROTEINURIA

DEFINITION AND EPIDEMIOLOGY

Approximately 15 kg of protein are filtered through the adult kidney each day, with normally less than 150 mg excreted.[1,3,4] Proteinuria is generally defined as urinary protein excretion of more than 150 mg/day (10 to 20 mg/dl) and is the hallmark of renal disease. The term *microalbuminuria* is defined as the excretion of 30 to 150 mg/day of protein and is a sign of early renal disease, particularly in patients with diabetes.[6] The term *macroalbuminuria* is occasionally used to describe rates of more than 300 mg/day.

Proteinuria can be classified as transient or persistent. Transient proteinuria is caused by a temporary change in glomerular hemodynamics, which causes the excess of protein. These conditions are usually of a benign or self-limiting nature and include orthostatic (postural) proteinuria, dehydration, fever, exercise, and emotional stress. Congestive heart failure and seizures can also cause transient proteinuria.[6] Persistent proteinuria is defined as 1+ protein on a standard dipstick (which corresponds to approximately 30 mg/dl) two or more times over a 3-month period.[7] Persistent proteinuria indicates a pathologic process, and the etiology must be investigated. Some common causes of persistent proteinuria are listed in Box 160-1.

Although isolated proteinuria is not necessarily associated with excess morbidity and mortality, it is often a sign of serious systemic disease. In the United States, diabetes is the leading cause of end-stage renal disease (ESRD), and in both type 1 and type 2 diabetes, microalbuminuria is the first sign of deteriorating renal function.[8] As kidney function declines, microalbuminuria becomes full-fledged proteinuria. Hypertension is the second leading cause of ESRD. ESRD has a yearly mortality rate of 20%, and nephrotic syndrome carries a high risk of morbidity and mortality.

Urinary albumin excretion has also been shown to predict blood pressure progression in nondiabetic, nonhypertensive individuals and appears to precede progression to higher blood pressure stages.[9] Therefore proteinuria may be a useful biomarker for identifying individuals who are at risk for developing hypertension.[9] In addition, persistent proteinuria in excess of 1 g/day has been associated with increased cardiac morbidity and mortality.[10]

Certain population groups, including African Americans, Native Americans, Hispanic Americans, and Pacific Islanders, are at increased risk for developing proteinuria. Aging and obesity are also risk factors for developing proteinuria.[8]

BOX 160-1

COMMON CAUSES OF PROTEINURIA

DRUG INDUCED
- Lithium
- Cyclosporin
- Cisplatin
- NSAIDs

HEREDITARY
- Polycystic kidney disease
- Medullary kidney disease

IMMUNE
- Drug allergies
- Collagen vascular disorders
- Immunoglobulin A nephropathy
- Sarcoidosis

INFECTION
- Bacterial, fungal, or parasitic infection
- Tuberculosis

METABOLIC
- Hyperuricemia
- Hypercalcemia
- Amyloidosis

VASCULAR
- Diabetes mellitus
- Hypertension
- Sickle cell disease
- Radiation nephritis

INCREASED PRODUCTION
- Multiple causes

PATHOPHYSIOLOGY

Normal urine proteins are composed of approximately 40% to 50% Tamm-Horsfall proteins, 30% to 40% albumin, and 20% to 30% various plasma proteins.[3,4] Protein excretion is affected by three factors: (1) prevention of excretion by the glomerular capillary wall, (2) reabsorption and catabolism by the proximal tubule cells, and (3) production of low-molecular-weight proteins.[3,4] Therefore proteinuria is classified as either glomerular, tubular, or overflow in origin.[1,3] Glomerular proteinuria is the most common type of persistent proteinuria, and albumin is the primary urinary protein.[6] Tubular proteinuria results when malfunctioning tubule cells no longer metabolize or reabsorb the protein that has been normally filtered. In this condition, low-molecular-weight proteins are the predominant type of protein, and the amount rarely exceeds 2 g/day. Overflow proteinuria occurs when low-molecular-weight proteins overwhelm the ability of the tubules to reabsorb filtered proteins.[6]

CLINICAL PRESENTATION

The clinical presentation of the patient with proteinuria can vary from healthy young adults with functional proteinuria related to prolonged exercise to seriously ill diabetic patients with nephrotic syndrome. Therefore all individuals should be screened for proteinuria by routine dipstick testing. Especially important is the routine screening of pregnant women. Proteinuria before 24 weeks' gestation indicates a likely glomerulonephritis, whereas proteinuria after 24 weeks' gestation is usually a sign of preeclampsia.[5]

Persistent proteinuria in patients with diabetes is usually a result of diabetic nephropathy. However, uncontrolled diabetes mellitus may cause transient proteinuria, most likely as a result of hyperfiltration and decreased tubular reabsorption.[11]

PHYSICAL EXAMINATION

With proteinuria, a complete and thorough history is essential. Specific areas of focus should include recent acute or chronic illness, surgery, diagnostic procedures (especially those requiring contrast media), urinary frequency or symptoms suggesting infection, risk factors for HIV infection, medications taken (including over-the-counter medications), a family history of renal disease or diabetes, and recent physical activity (especially exercise or cold-weather activities). The physical examination should be comprehensive and thorough; in the case of co-existent diabetes, the severity of the diabetes should be assessed to determine whether it correlates with the severity of proteinuria. Diabetic retinopathy is often present in patients with diabetic renal disease.[1]

DIAGNOSTICS AND DIFFERENTIAL DIAGNOSIS

Proteinuria is usually detected on routine dipstick testing, and any value of 1 or greater on two or more occasions should be investigated. Limitations of dipstick testing include false-negative results caused by dilution, an inability to detect microalbuminuria (although ultrasensitive dipstick tests are now available that can measure low rates of microalbuminuria), false-positive results caused by certain medications, and an inability of dipstick reagents to detect light-chain proteins.[1]

Once proteinuria has been identified, unless the cause is readily identified (e.g., preeclampsia or diabetes), the urine should be tested for Bence Jones proteins (the presence of which suggests multiple myeloma).[1] In addition, a full blood chemistry panel with fasting blood glucose, a lipid profile, urine culture and sensitivity, and CBC with differential are indicated. Further evaluation of persistent proteinuria usually includes determination of 24-hour urinary protein excretion or spot urinary protein/creatinine ratio, microscopic examination of urinary sediment, urinary protein electrophoresis, and additional assessment of renal function.[6] A diagnostic flowchart for the evaluation of proteinuria is provided in Figure 160-1.

It is important to determine whether the proteinuria is persistent or transient.[1] Transient proteinuria in an otherwise healthy patient that is secondary to an identifiable cause (e.g., exercise, fever, congestive heart failure) may be classified as functional proteinuria and does not require further diagnostic testing or evaluation.[1,3]

Persistent proteinuria that cannot be classified as functional proteinuria requires further investigation. Investigation should begin with a 24-hour measurement of urine protein and creatinine clearance to determine the urinary protein excretion and the protein/creatinine ratio.[4] If the excretion rate is 3.5 g/day or more, the patient by definition has nephrotic syndrome,[4] which is usually accompanied by hypoalbuminemia, hyperlipidemia, and edema. Nephrotic syndrome mandates a nephrologist's evaluation. It is important to remember that diabetes is the leading cause of nephrotic syndrome and accounts for 75% of all cases.[1]

If the 24-hour urinary protein excretion rate is less than 3.5 g/day, patients should be classified as having normal or abnormal renal function. Proteinuria in the presence of normal renal function is defined as "isolated" proteinuria; in these patients the next step is to determine whether the proteinuria is orthostatic or nonorthostatic.[1] Urinary protein excretion can increase after prolonged standing, and therefore three early-morning voids should be checked for protein. If all the results are negative, a diagnosis of orthostatic proteinuria can be made, and no further diagnostic tests are necessary.[1] However, referral to a renal specialist is also appropriate because this is a poorly understood, although generally benign and self-limited, condition.[1,3]

Patients with nonorthostatic proteinuria and normal renal function and without an elevation in Bence Jones proteins

DIAGNOSTICS

Proteinuria

LABORATORY
Urine dipstick
Urine for Bence Jones proteins
CBC and differential
Serum electrolytes
Serum glucose
BUN
Creatinine
Serum albumin
Calcium and phosphorus
Lipid profile
Urinalysis
Urine culture and sensitivity*
24-hour urine for volume, protein, and creatinine clearance*
Three early morning urines for protein*
Serum protein electrophoresis*
Urine protein electrophoresis*
ESR, antinuclear antibodies, lupus preparation (if collagen disease is suspected)*
Antistreptolysin O titer, complement (C3, C4) (if glomerulonephritis is suspected)
Hepatitis B surface antigen (if hepatitis vasculitis is suspected)

IMAGING
Renal ultrasound
IV pyelogram*

OTHER
Renal biopsy*

*If indicated.

DIFFERENTIAL DIAGNOSIS

Proteinuria

- Transient proteinuria
- Persistent proteinuria
- Orthostatic proteinuria or nonorthostatic proteinuria
- Glomerulonephritis
- Diabetic nephropathy
- Nephrotic syndrome
- Vasculitis
- Medications

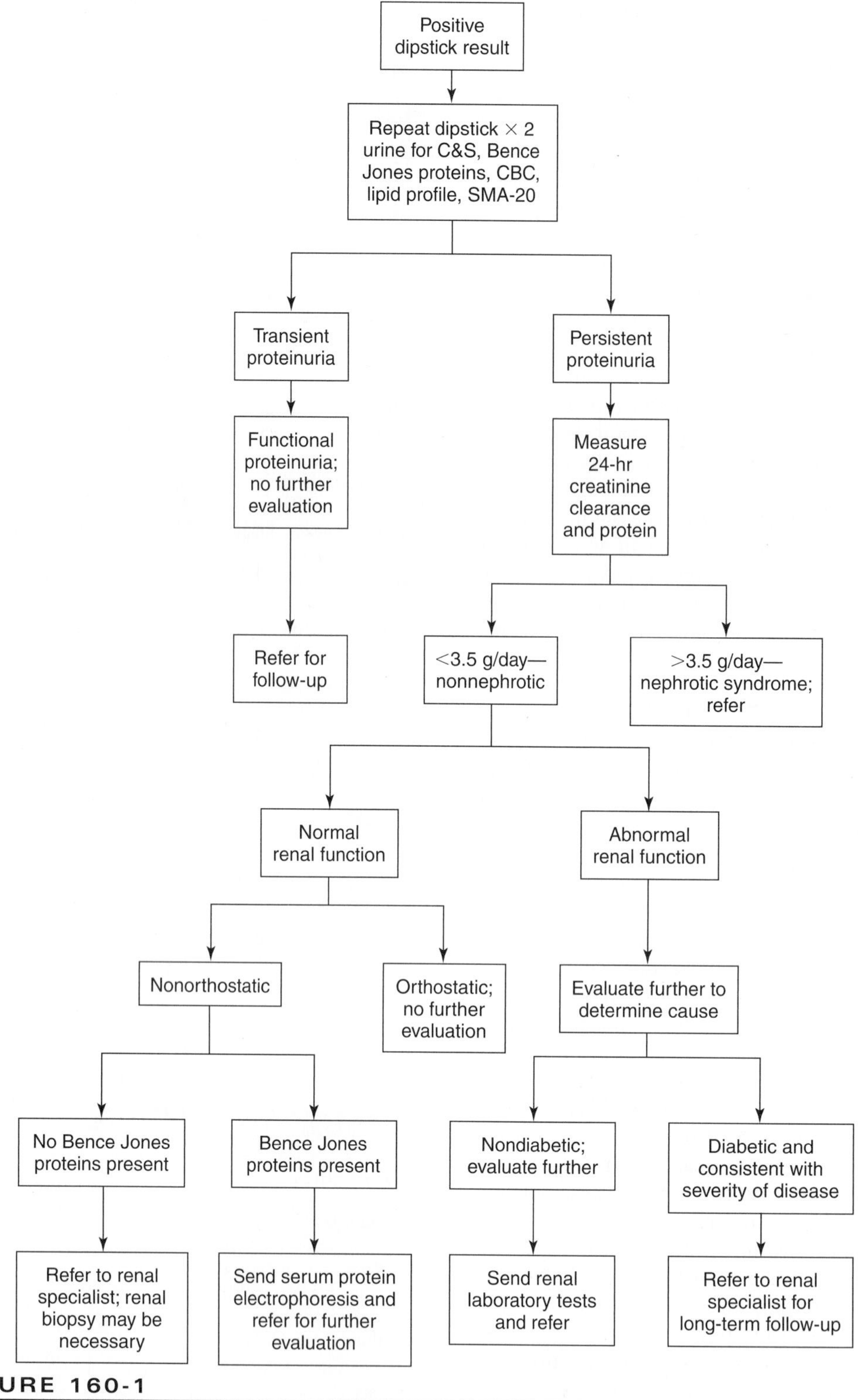

FIGURE 160-1

Evaluation of proteinuria. *C&S*, Culture and sensitivity; *SMA-20*, sequential multiple analysis of 20 chemical constituents.

should be referred to a renal specialist. A renal biopsy may be needed to determine the cause of the proteinuria. The presence of Bence Jones proteins warrants a serum protein electrophoresis and a referral for further evaluation to exclude multiple myeloma.

Other diagnostic tests depend on presentation and differential diagnosis. Collagen disease, glomerulonephritis, hepatitis-induced vasculitis, urate-related renal disease, diabetes, and other systemic disease or structural abnormalities should be considered in the evaluation of proteinuria.[5]

MANAGEMENT

Management of proteinuria obviously depends on the underlying cause, but some general principles apply. A careful medication review should be performed, and any medications implicated in proteinuria should be discontinued. Angiotensin-converting enzyme (ACE) inhibitors and angiotensin-receptor blockers (ARBs) have been found to reduce proteinuria, most likely by decreasing interglomerular pressure, and thus may be indicated.[1] Diabetes and hyperlipidemia, if present, should be aggressively managed; blood pressure control is also important. Patients with chronic renal failure should be managed aggressively to help prevent or delay the onset of ESRD (see Chapter 161). Sodium- and protein-restricted diets may be indicated for some patients. No matter what the cause, persistent proteinuria should be aggressively managed, both by controlling the underlying disease and by directing specific therapy (usually ACE inhibitors or ARBs) aimed at reducing protein excretion. The goal for treatment is protein excretion rates (as measured by collecting a 24-hour urine sample for total protein) of 1 g/day or less, since rates higher than this have been shown to increase cardiovascular disease.

COMPLICATIONS

Nephrotic syndrome with associated edema, hypoalbuminemia, and extrarenal complications is a potential consequence of proteinuria. Cardiovascular morbidity and mortality, immobilization, hyperlipidemia, hypercoagulability, and electrolyte disturbances are additional complications.

INDICATIONS FOR REFERRAL OR HOSPITALIZATION

All patients with renal disease or abnormal renal function should be referred to a renal specialist for consultation and management guidance. Referrals for patients with isolated orthostatic proteinuria should be based on a thorough risk assessment and evaluation of their general health, life span considerations, and concerns for aggressive management.

Any patients seen with nephrotic syndrome, acute renal failure, renal failure of unknown origin, or unstable vital signs should be urgently referred for hospitalization. New-onset proteinuria in pregnant women should be considered a medical emergency, and urgent referral to exclude eclampsia is indicated.

PATIENT AND FAMILY EDUCATION

Patient education depends on the cause of proteinuria, but diet education, diabetic teaching for patients with diabetes, and education concerning blood pressure management are usually necessary. Especially critical is that the patient and family understand the importance of diagnostic testing and regular follow-up care.

HEMATURIA

DEFINITION AND EPIDEMIOLOGY

Hematuria is generally defined as three or more red blood cells (RBCs) per high-powered field (HPF).[2,3] Transient hematuria is defined as hematuria that occurs on one occasion, whereas persistent hematuria is defined as hematuria that occurs on two or more consecutive occasions.[1,6] Exercise-induced hematuria in healthy young adults is not associated with any known morbidity or mortality, but both transient and persistent hematuria can be signs of serious disease. Common causes of hematuria are listed in Box 160-2.

The rates for hematuria in the general population vary with gender and age. One study of 1000 men ages 18 to 33 years documented rates of transient hematuria of 38.7%, with virtually all patients found to have no serious disease.[3] Other studies have documented rates of transient hematuria up to 13% in postmenopausal women, with again relatively no

BOX 160-2

COMMON CAUSES OF HEMATURIA

GLOMERULAR
- Glomerulonephritis
- Lupus nephritis
- Interstitial nephritis
- Pyelonephritis
- Vasculitis
- Alport's syndrome

NONGLOMERULAR
- Infection
- Neoplasm of the bladder, ureter, prostate, or kidney
- Renal or bladder calculi
- Polycystic kidney disease
- Sickle cell (disease or trait)
- Trauma
- Increased bleeding time
- Hemorrhagic cystitis
- Schistosomiasis
- Nutcracker phenomenon

MISCELLANEOUS
- Drug induced
- Exercise
- Endometriosis

PSEUDOHEMATURIA
- Menstrual contamination
- Hemoglobinuria
- Myoglobinuria
- Porphyrins
- Red food dyes
- Dilantin
- Quinine
- Phenothiazines
- Rifampin

serious pathologic conditions identified.[1] However, in men over 50 years old, even transient hematuria is often an indication of more serious disease, with up to 2.4% of this population having urinary tract malignancy.[1] Gross hematuria in older men denotes a significant risk of malignancy, with documented rates as high as 20%.[3]

PATHOPHYSIOLOGY

Normal urinary excretion of RBCs is 2 million/day, which results in 2 to 3 RBCs/HPF.[5] Isolated hematuria (hematuria unaccompanied by any other abnormal urine components) can result from bleeding anywhere from the renal pelvis to the urethra but is rarely caused by systemic disease.[5] Hematuria related to renal disease enters the tubular field along the nephron and produces RBC casts that are indicative of the renal origin.[2,4,5] Bacterial infections are a common cause of hematuria, and the presence of bacteria on urinalysis is suggestive of an infectious cause. Acute cystitis or urethritis can cause gross hematuria and is more common in women than in men.[2,12] The presence of proteinuria and hematuria is suggestive of glomerular or interstitial nephritis.[4]

The nutcracker phenomenon is a rare but important cause of hematuria. The left renal vein normally passes between the superior mesenteric artery and the aorta. However, in the nutcracker phenomenon, the left renal vein is compressed in the angle created by the two arteries, resulting in increased venous pressure and the development of collateral veins. The increased venous pressure causes minute ruptures in the thin wall of the septum separating the veins from the collecting system. In addition to hematuria, signs and symptoms include flank and abdominal pain, orthostatic proteinuria, vulvar varices in women, and varicocele in men.[13]

CLINICAL PRESENTATION

Hematuria is often accompanied by clinically significant symptoms or by abnormalities in the urinalysis that can aid in identifying the source of bleeding. The patient's age, gender, and level of physical activity should always be considered (long-distance runners have been documented to have rates of hematuria as high as 18%).[5] Hematuria associated with pyuria suggests an infectious process, whereas colicky flank pain suggests pain originating from a ureter.[5] A prostatic or urethral source is likely when bleeding occurs only at the beginning or end of micturition.[4,14] The presence of hemoptysis, acute renal failure, and hematuria is highly suggestive of Goodpasture's syndrome.[2] Glomerulonephritis is signified by hematuria accompanied by edema, hypertension, and a sore throat or skin infection,[3,12] although patients often may not report any recent signs or symptoms of infection.

PHYSICAL EXAMINATION

A thorough patient history should be obtained, including urinary patterns, urine color, timing of hematuria (beginning, end, or throughout micturition; transient or persistent), flank pain, history of renal calculi, urinary tract infections (UTIs), hemoptysis or bloody nasal secretions, recent acute or chronic illness, medications (including over-the-counter and illicit drugs), history of sexually transmitted disease, risk for HIV infection, or a history of travel to areas with endemic schistosomiasis (the leading cause of hematuria worldwide).[2] A complete family history specifically related to renal disease, sickle cell disease or traits, and congenital deafness (indicating Alport's syndrome) is also necessary. A comprehensive physical examination, including a pelvic examination in women and a prostate examination in men, is warranted.

DIAGNOSTICS AND DIFFERENTIAL DIAGNOSIS

The most important diagnostic element for hematuria is the urinalysis (Figure 160-2).[2] A urinalysis with RBC casts indicates hematuria originating from the renal parenchyma.[2] Further evidence of a renal source is significant proteinuria (>1 g/24 hr), dysmorphic RBCs, cola-colored urine, or renal insufficiency.[2-5] One major limitation of dipstick testing is that it detects the perioxidase activity of erythrocytes, not RBCs, in the urine. However, myoglobin and hemoglobin will also catalyze this reaction, so a positive test may indicate hematuria, myoglobinuria, or hemoglobinuria. If the dipstick is positive for heme but no increased numbers of RBCs are seen by microscopic examination, the urine should be tested for myoglobinuria and hemoglobinuria.[14]

Hematuria can be divided into glomerular, renal (i.e., nonglomerular), and urologic causes. Glomerular hematuria is

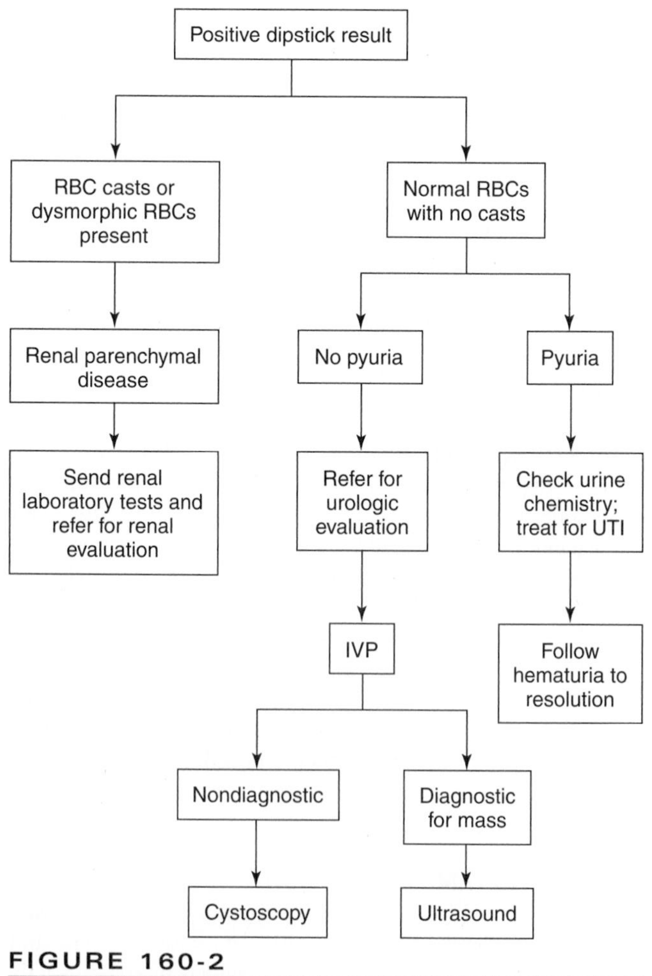

FIGURE 160-2

Evaluation of hematuria.

typically associated with significant proteinuria, erythrocyte casts, and dysmorphic RBCs. However, 20% of patients with biopsy-proven glomerulonephritis are seen with hematuria alone. Berger's disease (immunoglobulin A nephropathy) is the most common cause of glomerular hematuria.[6] Nonglomerular or renal hematuria is due to tubulointerstitial, renovascular, or metabolic disorders. As with glomerular hematuria, there is often co-existing proteinuria but no dysmorphic RBCs or erythrocyte casts. The evaluation of glomerular and nonglomerular hematuria requires an assessment of renal function and 24-hour urine or spot urinary protein/creatinine ratio. Urologic causes of nonglomerular hematuria include tumors, calculi, and infections. It is distinguished from other types of hematuria by the absence of proteinuria, dysmorphic RBCs, and erythrocyte casts. Up to 20% of patients with gross hematuria have a urinary tract malignancy, so a full workup, including cystoscopy and imaging of the upper urinary tract, needs to be done.[6]

In addition, an attempt to localize the source of the hematuria can be made by the three glass test or segmented urine specimens (see Chapter 159). Hematuria in voided bladder 1 (VB1) indicates anterior urethral lesions or urethritis as the source; hematuria only in VB3 may be produced by lesions in the posterior urethra, bladder neck, or trigone. Hematuria in all three specimens (VB1, VB2, VB3) is consistent with a cause at or above the bladder.

DIAGNOSTICS

Hematuria

LABORATORY
Urinalysis
Urine culture and sensitivity*
Urine for cytology*
CBC and differential*
Serum glucose*
Serum electrolytes*
BUN*
Creatinine*
PT/PTT*
Antinuclear antibodies
Immunoglobulins, cryoglobulins
Cytoplasmic-antinuclear cytoplasmic antibodies*
Antiglomerular basement membrane antibodies*
Antistreptolysin O titer*
Serum protein electrophoresis*
Venereal Disease Research Laboratory (VDRL) tests*
24-hour urine for calcium, uric acid*

IMAGING
Ultrasound of kidney, ureters, bladder*
IV pyelogram*
CT scan, MRI*
Retrograde pyelography*
Arteriography*

OTHER
Cystoscopy*
Renal biopsy*

*If indicated.

A referral to a urologist is indicated when a renal origin is suggested. Antinuclear antibodies, immunoglobulins, cryoglobulins, cytoplasmic-antinuclear cytoplasmic antibodies, antiglomerular basement membrane antibodies, serum electrolytes, serum glucose, BUN, creatinine, antistreptolysin O titer, serum protein electrophoresis, and Venereal Disease Research Laboratory (VDRL) tests[2,11] are indicated.

When hematuria originates from the lower urinary tract, intact and uniform RBCs should be present.[2,3,13] The presence of intact RBCs, white blood cells (WBCs), and bacteria suggests hematuria resulting from a UTI. The decision to obtain a urine culture and sensitivity should be guided by the patient's age and gender and the presence of resistant organisms in the local population. After treatment has been completed, a repeat urinalysis is necessary to ensure that the hematuria has resolved. Failure to follow hematuria to resolution may result in failure to diagnose a serious condition (which in fact may have contributed to the development of the original UTI). If symptoms are suggestive of a UTI despite a negative urine culture, a diagnosis of chlamydia or tuberculosis should be investigated.[4,5]

DIFFERENTIAL DIAGNOSIS

Hematuria

- Urinary tract infection
- Sexually transmitted disease
- Tuberculosis
- Malignancy
- Renal calculi
- Exercise, medication, or food induced
- Glomerular disease
- Bladder outlet obstruction

If the hematuria resolves after treatment of the UTI, no further diagnostic testing is indicated, although the presence of repeat UTIs in low-risk populations such as young men should always be fully investigated. If hematuria fails to resolve despite resolution of the UTI, referral for a urologic evaluation is required.[2]

In the absence of RBC casts or bacteria and WBCs, a urologic evaluation should be performed, usually with IV pyelography (IVP).[2,3,5,11] If the IVP is diagnostic for a mass, an ultrasound or CT scan to determine if the mass is cystic or solid is suggested. A solid mass should either be further evaluated by arteriography or referred to a urologic surgeon for excision and pathologic testing. If the IVP is nondiagnostic, the next step in the evaluation is cystoscopy, which includes inspection, biopsy, and culture of the bladder tissue. Cystoscopy is highly diagnostic for uroepithelial neoplasms. If the cystoscopy is nondiagnostic, the urologist may request a retrograde pyelography, arteriography, or renal biopsy (see Figure 160-2).

MANAGEMENT

Management of hematuria consists mainly of identification, diagnosis, and referral. Further management considerations are based on the underlying pathologic condition, not on the presence of the hematuria itself.

COMPLICATIONS

Complications of hematuria depend on the underlying pathologic condition. Urinary obstruction, renal failure, anemia, infections, and hydronephrosis are potential complications.

INDICATIONS FOR REFERRAL OR HOSPITALIZATION

Isolated, transient hematuria or hematuria related to a UTI does not require a urology consultation. Referral to a renal or urology specialist is indicated to evaluate other causes of hematuria. Patients with large amounts of frank hematuria, severe flank pain suggestive of renal calculi, unstable vital signs, signs of urologic obstruction, or acute renal failure should be referred for urgent evaluation and possible hospitalization.

PATIENT AND FAMILY EDUCATION

Patient education largely depends on the cause of the hematuria; advice and educational material specific to the underlying pathologic process are appropriate. One of the major goals of education in asymptomatic hematuria is to reinforce the importance of the diagnostic evaluation. Other guidance should focus on the explanation of tests, medications, untoward effects, and the need for careful follow-up evaluation when indicated.

REFERENCES

1. Hassan A: Proteinuria, *Postgrad Med* 101(4):173-180, 1997.
2. McCarthy JJ: Outpatient evaluation of hematuria, *Postgrad Med* 101(2):125-131, 1997.
3. Ahmed Z, Lee J: Asymptomatic urinary abnormalities: hematuria and proteinuria, *Med Clin North Am* 81(3):641-652, 1997.
4. Isselbacher KJ, Braunwald E, Wilson JD, and others: *Harrison's principles of internal medicine,* ed 13, New York, 1994, McGraw-Hill.
5. Barker RL, Burton JR, Zieve PD: *Principles of ambulatory medicine,* ed 4, Baltimore, 1995, Williams & Wilkins.
6. Simerville J, Maxted W, Pahira J: Urinalysis: a comprehensive review, *Am Fam Phys* 71(6):1153-1162, 2005.
7. Castner D, Douglas C: Chronic kidney disease, *Nursing 2005* 35(12):58-63, 2005.
8. National Institute of Diabetes and Digestive and Kidney Diseases: *Proteinuria,* NIH Pub No 05-4732, Bethesda, Md, Aug 2005, National Institutes of Health, retrieved March 2, 2007, from http://kidney.niddk.nih.gov/kudiseases/pubs/pdf/proteinuria.pdf.
9. Wang T, Evans J, Meigs J, and others: Low-grade albuminuria and the risks of hypertension and blood pressure progression, *Circulation* 111:1370-1376, 2005.
10. Dell'Omo G, Penno G, Giorgi D, and others: Association between high-normal albuminuria and risk factors for cardiovascular and renal disease in essential hypertensive men, *Am J Kid Dis* 40:1-8, 2002.
11. Mandal AK, Jennette JC: *Diagnosis and management of renal disease and hypertension,* Philadelphia, 1988, Lea & Febiger.
12. Gambrell RC, Blount BW: Exercise induced hematuria, *Am Fam Phys* 53(3):905-912, 1996.
13. Hokama A, Oshiro Y: A thin 43-year-old woman with gross hematuria, *CMAJ* 173(3):251, 2005.
14. Levine DZ: *Caring for the renal patient,* ed 3, London, 1997, Saunders.

CHAPTER 161

Renal Failure

Carol A. Whelan

DEFINITION AND EPIDEMIOLOGY

Renal failure is a complex and challenging health issue that demands the involvement of both specialists and health care providers. Defined as a glomerular filtration rate (GFR) of less than 50% of normal, renal failure consists of two distinct types: chronic renal failure (CRF) and acute renal failure (ARF).[1,2]

CRF is defined as a reduction in GFR that has been present for at least 2 to 3 months.[1-3] However, CRF should not be viewed in simple mathematic terms but rather as an ongoing process of renal injury that causes compensatory hyperfiltration in less-affected glomeruli, which eventually leads to the destruction of those glomeruli as well.[1] This ongoing destruction results in a steady and predictable decline in renal function, which eventually affects every organ system in the body.[1,2]

ARF is defined as an increase in serum creatinine of 0.5 mg/dl or more within 24 hours or as a loss of renal function that has occurred over a period of hours or days. ARF can be classified either by the physiologic cause (prerenal, intrarenal, or postrenal) or by the amount of urine produced (anuric, oliguric, or nonoliguric).[4]

Mild renal failure is usually defined as a GFR of approximately 35% to 50% of normal, whereas moderate renal failure is defined as a GFR of approximately 20% to 35% of normal.[1] Severe renal failure occurs at a GFR of 10% to 20% of normal, with rates below 10% being classified as end-stage renal disease (ESRD).[1] Patients with GFRs of 51% to 79% of normal may be classified as having chronic renal insufficiency (CRI). It is important to identify all patients with impaired renal function to prevent or slow the onset of CRF.

Although exact statistics regarding the prevalence of mild to moderate renal failure are not available, the epidemiology of ESRD has been widely documented by the U.S. Renal Data System (USRDS), which collects statistics on all Medicare patients on dialysis. Since 1974, the United States has extended Medicare coverage to virtually all patients on dialysis in the United States; therefore these data are highly representative of the current dialysis population. According to the USRDS, more than 100,000 new patients began treatment for ESRD in 2003, with a current dialysis population of almost 325,000.

The two leading causes of ESRD are diabetes mellitus (44.8%) and hypertension (27.1%). Other causes of ESRD include glomerulonephritis (8.5%), interstitial nephritis (3.6%), cystic kidney disease (3.5%), and collagen vascular disease (2.2%). Diabetic ESRD continues to increase, but the rate of growth has slowed in recent years, especially among Caucasians. Statistically, non-Caucasians are four times more likely to require dialysis, and although African Americans make up 13% of the U.S. population, they represent 30% of patients with ESRD. The cost of treating ESRD was $14.1 billion in 2001, and this figure is expected to continue to rise.[5] The USRDS data may be accessed at http://www.usrds.org.

ARF is primarily an iatrogenic disease of hospitalized patients. It is estimated that up to 5% of all hospitalized patients will develop some degree of ARF.[4]

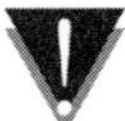

Immediate emergency department referral or physician consultation is indicated for patients with ARF.

Nephrology consultation is indicated for patients with CRF.

PATHOPHYSIOLOGY

The basic pathophysiology of CRF is that of renal injury and loss of functioning nephrons (the mechanism of which depends on the underlying cause). This results in hyperfiltration in the surviving glomeruli (in an attempt by the body to increase GFR), which then causes ongoing glomerular stress and renal injury, resulting in glomerular destruction.[1,3] The result is a decrease in GFR and a continuance of the hyperperfusion destruction syndrome. If this process is allowed to progress, it leads to uremic syndrome (a constellation of symptoms that occurs in severe renal failure).

The pathophysiology of ARF depends on the site of occurrence. Prerenal ARF, the most common type of ARF, is caused by renal hypoperfusion and does not result in structural kidney damage.[4] Intrarenal ARF, the result of damage to the renal parenchyma, may be a result of prolonged prerenal ARF (which leads to acute tubular necrosis), toxins, interstitial nephritis, or acute glomerulonephritis.[4] Postrenal (obstructive) ARF results from physical obstruction of urine outflow and may be caused by neoplasm, prostatic enlargement, bladder dysfunction, or nephrolithiasis.[4,6]

BOX 161-1

MAJOR COMPLICATIONS OF CHRONIC RENAL FAILURE

CARDIOVASCULAR COMPLICATIONS

- Atherosclerosis
- Congestive heart failure
- Hypertension
- Pulmonary edema
- Pericarditis

METABOLIC COMPLICATIONS

- Hyperkalemia
- Metabolic acidosis
- Alterations in vitamin D, calcium, and phosphorus metabolism and absorption
- Hyperparathyroidism
- Renal osteodystrophies
- Hyperlipidemia
- Nausea, vomiting
- Anorexia

PSYCHOSOCIAL COMPLICATIONS

- Depression
- Insomnia
- Suicide
- Sexual dysfunction
- Impoverishment
- Unemployment

HEMATOLOGIC COMPLICATIONS

- Anemia
- Leukopenia
- Erythropoietin deficiency

CLINICAL PRESENTATION

The clinical presentation of CRF is often subtle, and symptoms are uncommon with a GFR above 35%. Therefore suspicion for mild renal disease should be based on recognition of the primary pathologic mechanism responsible for renal injury, particularly in patients with diabetes mellitus and hypertension.

Once the GFR falls below 35%, a variety of metabolic, psychiatric, hematologic, cardiovascular, and acid-base regulatory problems occur. Clinical presentation at this point depends on the particular complication and on the underlying cause of renal failure (Box 161-1).[1-3,6,7]

The usual clinical presentation of ARF is that of prerenal ARF in a hospitalized patient who has undergone surgery, been exposed to radiocontrast dye, received aminoglycoside antibiotics, or developed sepsis.[4] Most of these patients have identifiable risk factors, such as CRI, CRF, advanced age, liver disease, diabetes, or vascular disease.[4] Therefore it is essential to identify those at high risk *before* ARF develops. It is equally important to begin early screening for all the complications of renal disease to prevent morbidity and to establish a credible baseline for the individual patient.

PHYSICAL EXAMINATION

The physical examination should include both a focused examination to identify pathologic processes caused by the primary disease entity (e.g., diabetes mellitus or hypertension) and a broader examination that attempts to identify the effects of progressive renal failure. Areas of importance include assessment of vital signs (including measurement of bilateral and orthostatic blood pressure); funduscopic evaluation for signs of arteriovenous nicking, diabetic retinopathy, and papilledema; assessment of volume status by determination of jugular vein distention; auscultation of lung sounds; assessment for edema or ascites; and assessment of heart sounds to screen for volume overload and pericarditis. A full abdominal examination should include auscultation for renal artery bruits; examination of the skin for ecchymosis, rashes (especially those suggesting collagen vascular disorders), or uremic frost; percussion of the bladder (to exclude distention); rectal examination; and evaluation of the prostate (to exclude obstruction) in male patients.[6] Formal and informal mental status examinations should be included to screen for depression and other psychiatric complications.

DIAGNOSTICS

The most important diagnostic tool in monitoring both patients with known renal failure and those at risk for renal failure is dipstick urinalysis, which should be performed at virtually every office visit. The presence of proteinuria should alert the clinician to perform a full 24-hour urine analysis for protein and creatinine clearance. Furthermore, all diabetic patients who are negative for protein on dipstick testing should have laboratory testing for microalbuminuria. This testing should be initiated at time of diagnosis for type 2 diabetics and 2 years after diagnosis for type 1 diabetics.

DIAGNOSTICS

Renal Failure

LABORATORY
Urinalysis and urine osmolality
24-hour urine collection for volume, protein, creatinine clearance
CBC and differential
Serum electrolytes
Serum glucose
BUN
Creatinine
Calcium, ionized calcium
Albumin
Total protein
Phosphorus
Magnesium
Uric acid
PTH
Serum complement levels (C3 and C4)*
Antinuclear antibodies*
Rheumatoid factor*
Cryoglobulins*
Antistreptococcal antibodies*
Antineutrophil cytoplasmic antibodies*
Hepatitis B*
HIV*

IMAGING
Ultrasound
CT or MRI

OTHER
Renal biopsy
ECG

*If indicated.

In addition to urinalysis, a baseline should be established for all renal patients by obtaining a full chemistry panel, including electrolytes, fasting blood glucose, magnesium, phosphorus, ionized calcium, total protein and serum albumin, BUN, creatinine, liver enzymes, lipid profile, CBC, and intact parathyroid hormone (PTH). Further studies include renal biopsy and nuclear imaging. However, the risks associated with arteriography compel consultation with a nephrologist before subjecting the patient to potential complications.

Although imaging studies are not particularly useful in diagnosing the extent of renal disease, renal ultrasound is recommended to determine the presence of cysts or obstruction and to document the size of the kidneys.[6,7] This is necessary, since CRF characteristically results in smaller than average kidneys, whereas ARF is characterized by normal or even enlarged kidneys. Asymmetry may be a result of unilateral renal artery stenosis.[7]

DIFFERENTIAL DIAGNOSIS

The main issue in the diagnosis of CRF is exclusion of ARF. ARF is a potentially reversible, life-threatening condition, and all patients with ARF should be hospitalized and managed by specialists. The most common type of ARF seen in primary care is prerenal ARF (caused by renal hypoperfusion) related to volume depletion, hypotension, aminoglycoside antibiotic use, and radiocontrast dye exposure.[4] Often these patients have preexisting risk factors, such as CRI, CRF, advanced age, liver disease, diabetes, or vascular disease.[4] In addition, some patients with CRF have a small degree of reversible prerenal ARF caused by hypovolemia or alterations in renal hemodynamics that result in renal hypoperfusion (e.g., from NSAIDs or angiotensin-converting enzyme [ACE] inhibitors).

DIFFERENTIAL DIAGNOSIS

Renal Failure

- Acute renal failure
- Prerenal failure
- Intrarenal failure
- Postrenal failure
- Chronic renal failure

Urinalysis is highly diagnostic in differentiating between ARF and CRF. Prerenal ARF is usually accompanied by urine osmolality of more than 500 mosm/kg, specific gravity of more than 1.020, and hyaline casts. Intrarenal ARF results in a urine osmolality of around 300 mosm/kg; a specific gravity of around 1.010; tubular casts; tubular cells; and a distinctive brownish, muddy appearance that is due to brown granular casts.[4,7]

Occasionally outpatients will be seen with postrenal obstructive ARF. A distended bladder, flank pain, and prostatic enlargement are potential causes. Ultrasound imaging virtually always detects obstruction.[7]

If, after a thorough history and physical examination, ARF is still considered a potential diagnosis, the patient should be urgently referred to a renal specialist. Renal ultrasound evaluation or biopsy may be necessary for a definitive diagnosis.

Vigilance is necessary to determine any underlying correctable pathologic process that may be causing renal failure. Renal vascular hypertension should always be considered when renal function deteriorates rapidly with the initiation of ACE inhibitors or when abdominal bruits are heard on auscultation.

MANAGEMENT AND COMPLICATIONS

Mild to Moderate Chronic Renal Failure

In January 2000 the National Kidney Foundation (NKF) launched the Kidney Disease Outcomes Quality Initiative (KDOQI), whose purpose is to develop and publish evidence-based clinical practice guidelines. These guidelines are available on the NKF's website at http://www.kidney.org.

Although mild to moderate CRF produces relatively few symptoms, interventions to decrease morbidity and mortality, as well as interventions to slow or even halt the progression of renal failure, are most effective at this stage. Therefore the first goal of treatment is the identification of patients with mild to moderate CRF via screening tools such as urinary dipstick testing for protein, the measurement of urinary albumin excretion (rates greater than 30 mg/24 hr are considered abnormal and have been shown to be a precursor for diabetic nephropathy), and the measurement of urinary creatinine clearance via timed urine collection (preferably a 24-hour collection).[8] Evidence exists for the benefits of lowering urinary protein excretion rates below 1 g/day; reduction of proteinuria is both renal protective and cardiovascular protective. ACE inhibitors and ARBs should be used aggressively, and these drugs may be prescribed concurrently. These drugs can be beneficial when used in combination; the COOPERATE Trial documented that the combination led to a decrease in progression to ESRD (11% vs. 23%) and a greater reduction in proteinuria (76% vs. 43%).[9] Serum potassium levels must be monitored, and the use of a mild diuretic (such as hydrochloride thiazide) may help normalize levels.

Progression of CRF should be monitored via 24-hour urine measurements of creatinine clearance, since the provider should not rely solely on estimates of renal function based on serum creatinine. The urine should also be regularly examined by dipstick and microscopic analysis, with measurement of specific gravity, proteinuria, hematuria, pyuria, and sediment. When a 24-hour urine sample is being collected for creatinine clearance, measurement should also be made of total protein.

If the patient has diabetes, glycosylated hemoglobin should be monitored; levels within 10% of normal are ideal. Once the hematocrit falls below 32%, erythropoietin (EPO) levels should also be obtained. The clinical decision as to how often the previously mentioned laboratory values should be monitored depends on the severity of the renal disease and the presence of abnormalities in laboratory values.

Cardiovascular Management and Complications. Cardiovascular complications are the leading cause of death among patients with ESRD, accounting for more than 50% of deaths in the first year of dialysis.[10] The current mortality rate for U.S. patients with ESRD is more than 20% per year.[10] Therefore prevention of cardiovascular complications is of the utmost priority. Unfortunately, 70% of patients who begin dialysis treatment already have left ventricular hypertrophy and 40% have congestive heart failure (CHF).[10,11]

Once CRF has been identified, management of hypertension (if present) is extremely important. Adequate blood pressure control has been proven beneficial.[10] Ideally, the patient's blood pressure should be reduced to 130/80 mm Hg. The United Kingdom Prospective Diabetes Study showed benefit of even lower systolic pressures, with reduction in complications continuing to at least a systolic pressure of 114 mm Hg.[12] The use of ACE inhibitors and ARBs has also been shown to be beneficial in patients with diabetic nephropathy and for those with nondiabetic renal disease and proteinuria.[9,13-16] ACE inhibitors and ARBs must be used cautiously in patients at risk for hyperkalemia and should not be used in patients with renal artery stenosis unless prescribed by a renal specialist, in which case close monitoring of renal function is absolutely essential.[7,8] It is necessary to repeat a serum potassium, BUN, and serum creatinine measurement 1 week after initiation of ACE inhibitor and ARB therapy. In addition, careful blood pressure monitoring is important, both to ensure control of hypertension (with a maximum blood pressure of 130/80 mm Hg) and to guard against hypotensive responses to ACE inhibitor therapy.

Hyperlipidemia is both a complication of CRF and a potential factor in the progression of the disease.[17] Lowering low-density lipoprotein (LDL) cholesterol in patients with coronary artery disease (CAD) is recommended.[18] A wide variety of agents are available for the treatment of lipid disorders, although most have dosing limitations dependent on the degree of CRF present. When appropriate lipid goals are being determined, any patient with diabetes and CRF should be viewed as having CAD; therefore secondary prevention goals (i.e., LDL <70 mg/dl) should be sought.

Dietary Management and Metabolic Complications. An essential component of management is diet modification (Table 161-1). Dietary referral is beneficial for optimum care. This is especially true in patients with underlying diabetes and in patients who are under or over ideal body weight, since the dietary recommendations must be modified for these patients. American Dietetic Association (ADA) guidelines for renal failure diets are available in the *Manual of Clinical Dietetics*.[19]

Although protein restriction is widely recommended, the issue of how much to restrict protein remains controversial. A protein restriction of approximately 0.6 to 0.8 g/kg/day is widely recommended, but it is important to monitor nutritional status via measurement of serum albumin and total protein.[2,6,19] A statistical correlation has been established between increased mortality rates and patients who are seen for initiation of dialysis and who have low serum albumin and total protein levels.[20] Although this relationship has been established only as a temporal and not a causal relationship, maintaining serum albumin and protein levels within normal limits would appear to be prudent management.[19]

Studies have shown the benefits of tight glycemic control in halting or slowing the progression of diabetic renal disease.[2,6,7,20-22] Glycosylated hemoglobin levels within 10% of normal have been shown to be highly protective and associated with a lack of target organ damage.[7,8,22]

Although hyperkalemia is not usually a major issue in mild to moderate renal failure, monitoring of serum potassium (especially in patients taking ACE inhibitors or ARBs) is mandatory. Patients receiving ACE inhibitor therapy may require decreased dosages to maintain serum potassium within normal limits. Some patients may not tolerate ACE inhibitor–induced hyperkalemia, and the medication will have to be discontinued. Most patients should be instructed to avoid potassium-containing salt substitutes, particularly since many hypertensive patients are told to restrict salt and may use salt substitutes without realizing that these substitutes contain almost pure potassium. Dietary potassium can also be restricted to less than 60 mEq/day. If necessary, sodium polystyrene

TABLE 161-1 Dietary Recommendations for Adult Patients with Chronic Renal Failure Who Are Not on Dialysis

	Recommendation
Protein	0.6-0.8 g/kg/day
Calories	35 kcal/kg/day
Phosphorus	8-12 mg/kg/day
Calcium	1.2-1.6 g/day
Sodium	1-3 g/day
Potassium	Not restricted unless serum potassium level is elevated or urinary output is <1 L/day

Data from American Dietetic Association: *Manual of clinical dietetics*, ed 5, Chicago, 1996, The Association.

(Kayexalate) should be prescribed to maintain serum potassium levels below 6 mEq/L.

Control of serum phosphorus and calcium is crucial in preventing metabolic complications, and many patients with CRF ultimately develop secondary hyperparathyroidism and renal osteodystrophy, even though these are often preventable entities. In addition, diets low in phosphorus (0.8 to 1 g/day) have been shown to delay the progression of renal failure, probably as a result of the prevention of deposition of phosphate and calcium in the interstitium of the kidney.[19]

In addition to limiting intake of phosphorus, patients with renal failure require supplemental calcium. Calcium taken with meals helps decrease absorption of phosphorus, and calcium taken between meals helps raise serum calcium levels.[6] A normal starting dosage of calcium is usually 600 mg PO b.i.d. with meals; this can be adjusted on the basis of ionized calcium values, intact PTH, and serum phosphorus. Patients with CRF should receive 800 IU of vitamin D per day, and serum levels should be monitored. Use of aluminum or magnesium antacids should be avoided, since these can cause aluminum or magnesium toxicity.

Because of alterations in metabolism and renal function, many drugs must be avoided or adjusted on the basis of renal function. When any drug is prescribed for a patient with CRF, manufacturer's recommendations regarding use in CRF should be determined and creatinine clearance should be estimated:

$$\text{Creatinine clearance} = (140 - \text{Age}) \times \text{Weight [kg]}/72 \times \text{Serum creatinine (mg/dl)} \times 0.85 \text{ (if the patient is female)}$$

A partial listing of drugs requiring dosing adjustments is presented in Box 161-2. Recently, a newer calculation to estimate GFR from serum creatinine has been developed that accounts for race, age, and gender. Although the calculation is complex, many diagnostic laboratories are offering to list the result automatically when measuring serum creatinine. For more information and to view the calculation, see http://www.kidney.org/professionals/KLS/gfr.cfm. It should be noted that the equation is less useful at estimating GFRs above 60%.[23]

BOX 161-2

DRUGS REQUIRING DOSAGE ADJUSTMENT IN CHRONIC RENAL FAILURE*

- Antibiotics
- NSAIDs
- Digoxin
- Phenobarbital
- Narcotics
- Antiarrhythmics
- Antihypertensives
- Antifungals
- Antivirals
- Librium
- Lithium carbonate

*Always consult the manufacturer's instructions when prescribing any drugs for patients with chronic renal failure.

Hematologic Management and Complications. EPO production is usually normal, with GFR rates above 20%. However, the CBC should be monitored, and if the hematocrit level falls below 32% (the level at which EPO production is stimulated), serum EPO levels should be monitored to determine if this is the cause of the anemia. If serum EPO is low despite the presence of anemia, exogenous EPO should be given. To avoid transfusion-related hepatitis B, immunization should be given to those patients who are antibody negative.

Psychosocial Management and Complications. Although the medical management of CRF may seem overwhelming to even veteran health care providers, it is often devastating to the victim of CRF. Therefore it is essential to provide adequate social and psychiatric support. Referral to a social worker is often advantageous to help provide social support and assist the patient in applying for financial assistance and entitlement programs. Even with Medicare coverage, the cost of medical care can be devastating, and many patients with CRF are unable to continue working because of medical complications.

Severe Renal Failure

When GFR falls below 20%, the progression to ESRD is virtually inevitable. Therefore, since prevention of progression is improbable, prevention of complications becomes paramount. Although continued control of hypertension, hyperglycemia, hyperlipidemia, and serum potassium, phosphorus, magnesium, and calcium is important, the goals become more difficult as the GFR approaches 10%. Consultation with a renal specialist aids in management.

Cardiovascular Management and Complications. Despite careful management, complications and management issues may develop. The onset of CHF and pulmonary edema may indicate the need for dialysis. Hypertension may escalate, and increasingly higher doses of both diuretics and antihypertensive medications may be needed. However, at this point ACE inhibitors and ARBs may not be tolerated, and if hyperkalemia is present, these drugs should probably be discontinued.

Dietary Management and Metabolic Complications. The NKF's KDOQI lists guidelines for advanced CRF patients treated without dialysis. The guidelines state that evidence *suggests* that low-protein diets "may retard the progression of renal failure or delay the need for dialysis therapy."[24] The protein guidelines call for approximately 0.60 g/kg/day. The guidelines acknowledge that confusion remains within the nephrology community as to the role of protein restriction, partly because of the previously mentioned correlation with lower serum albumin levels and higher mortality rates. The guidelines further suggest that maintenance of adequate caloric intake (35 kcal/kg/day) may help maintain nutritional status.

The maintenance of calcium and phosphorus values within as normal a range as possible is also important. Nausea and vomiting may become problematic, and the use of high-calorie supplements may be necessary. Although restriction of salt and potassium may not have been previously necessary, these elements now must be restricted. Intact PTH levels should be monitored; levels two to three times normal can be expected, but levels above this range indicate the need for endocrinology referral.

Hematologic Management and Complications. Anemia will become apparent, and endogenous EPO production will likely be inadequate. If EPO therapy is required, the KDOQI recommends a target hematocrit of 33% to 36%. EPO is available in vials of 10,000 units/ml. Given subcutaneously, the drugs should be given in dosages calculated on the basis of the patient's weight (50 units/kg/week). Monthly hematocrit measurements are necessary during therapy so that the dosage can be appropriately increased if necessary. Measurements of serum iron and ferritin levels are recommended before initiating EPO therapy and periodically to indicate whether iron therapy should be initiated.

Psychosocial Management and Complications. One of the major tasks to be accomplished during this phase is planning for dialysis. This may be traumatic for the patient but is crucial for the prevention of major complications. A referral to a nephrologist is now indicated if one has not already been made. The type of dialysis should be determined and the appropriate type of access established (arteriovenous fistulas take up to 3 months to heal and therefore should be placed well in advance). If continuous ambulatory peritoneal dialysis (CAPD) is elected, training is required and should be started as early as possible. Patients should visit the dialysis unit that will be managing their care to familiarize themselves with both the routine and the staff.

Depression and suicide are major considerations, and every effort should be made to provide psychosocial support. Selective serotonin reuptake inhibitor antidepressants can be used, and the dosage does not have to be adjusted for CRF. If transplantation is a possibility, discussions regarding this issue can begin.

End-Stage Renal Disease

Cardiovascular Management and Complications. Hypertension and hyperlipidemia should continue to be aggressively managed. Whereas the renal specialist may be concerned with fluid and electrolyte balance, the health care provider should consider the potential for cardiovascular complications, since these are leading causes of death in patients with ESRD.[2] Hypertension should be aggressively managed.

Pulmonary edema and CHF are major concerns in ESRD. If the patient is unstable, hospitalization and urgent dialysis may be necessary. All episodes of CHF and pulmonary edema should be reported to the renal specialist so adjustments can be made in the dialysate fluid to compensate for fluid overload.

Dietary Management and Metabolic Complications. Dietary management should be aimed at control of electrolytes (including calcium, phosphorus, and potassium), prevention of malnutrition, and maintenance of acceptable fluid volume status.[17] Daily dietary requirements for patients with ESRD depend on the type of dialysis chosen (CAPD vs. hemodialysis). Current ADA guidelines for patients on CAPD or hemodialysis are outlined in Table 161-2. All patients with ESRD should be referred to a dietitian for optimization of nutritional status.

Hematologic Management and Complications. EPO replacement therapy will be necessary. EPO given subcutaneously is more effectively absorbed than EPO given intravenously (or into extracorporeal blood during hemodialysis).

Psychosocial Management and Complications. The stress of dealing with severe chronic illness can be psychologically devastating. Patients with ESRD (especially patients on hemodialysis) are known to suffer from high rates of depression, insomnia, and anxiety.[8] Often ignored, sexual dysfunction occurs at high rates in both male and female patients with ESRD.[8] The treatment of these and other psychiatric complications should begin before the onset of ESRD.

INDICATIONS FOR REFERRAL OR HOSPITALIZATION

All patients with CRF should be referred as early as possible to a renal specialist for consultation. If a dietitian is available, referral should be made as soon as CRF is identified.

Hospitalization should be considered for any acute, life-threatening disorder, and potential problems are innumerable. More common causes include acute fluid and electrolyte disorders, acute hypertensive emergency, pulmonary edema, acute CHF, pericarditis, and metabolic acidosis.

PATIENT AND FAMILY EDUCATION

Patient education in renal failure is highly complex. CRF and ESRD require carefully coordinated care. Enrollment in diabetic classes when appropriate, renal diet cooking classes, and support groups can be of tremendous benefit. By gradually

TABLE 161-2 Dietary Recommendations for Adults with End-Stage Renal Disease (Based on Dialysis Method)

	Recommendation for Hemodialysis	Recommendation for Peritoneal Dialysis
Protein	1.1-1.4 g/kg/day	1.2-1.5 g/kg/day
Calories	30-35 kcal/kg/day	25-35 kcal/kg/day
Phosphorus	<17 mg/kg/day	<17 mg/kg/day
Calcium	1.0-1.8 g/day	1.0-1.8 g/day
Fluid	Daily urinary output + 500-750 ml/day	2-3 L/day based on weight and blood pressure
Sodium	2-3 g/day	3-4 g/day based on weight
Potassium	40 mg/kg	Unrestricted unless elevated

Data from American Dietetic Association: *Manual of clinical dietetics*, ed 5, Chicago, 1996, The Association.

introducing different educational materials and enabling the patient to help control the course of the disease, the health care provider can help restore a sense of independence and confidence in the patient.

REFERENCES

1. Kasper DL Braunwald E, Fauci A, and others: *Harrison's principles of internal medicine,* ed 16, New York, 2005, McGraw-Hill.
2. Malhotra D, Tzamaloukas AH: Non-dialysis management of chronic renal failure, *Med Clin North Am* 81:749-766, 1997.
3. Barker RL, Burton JR, Zieve PD: *Principles of ambulatory medicine,* ed 4, Baltimore, 1995, Williams & Wilkins.
4. Mindell JA, Chertow GM: A practical approach to acute renal failure, *Med Clin North Am* 81:731-748, 1997.
5. National Institutes of Health, National Institute of Diabetes and Digestive and Kidney Diseases: *US renal data system, USRDS 2005 annual data report: atlas of end-stage renal disease in the U.S.*, Bethesda, Md, 2005, The Institutes.
6. Levine DZ: *Caring for the renal patient,* ed 3, Philadelphia, 1997, Saunders.
7. Avram MM, Klahr S: *Renal disease progression and management,* Philadelphia, 1996, Saunders.
8. Bennett PH, Haffner S, Kasiske BL, and others: Screening and management of microalbuminuria in patients with diabetes mellitus: recommendations to the Scientific Advisory Board of the National Kidney Foundation from an ad hoc committee of the Council on Diabetes Mellitus of the National Kidney Foundation, *Am J Kidney Dis* 25(1):107-112, 1995.
9. Lewis EJ, Hunsicker LG, Clarke WR, and others: Renoprotective effect of the angiotensin-receptor antagonist irbesartan in patients with nephropathy due to type 2 diabetes, *N Engl J Med* 345(12):851-860, 2001.
10. Eknoyan G, Levey AS, Levin NW, and others: The national epidemic of chronic kidney disease, *Postgrad Med* 110(3):23-29, 2001.
11. London GM: Left ventricular alterations and end-stage renal disease, *Nephrol Dial Transplant* 17(1 Suppl):S29-S36, 2002.
12. UK Prospective Diabetes Study (UKPDS) Group: Efficacy of atenolol and captopril in reducing risk of macrovascular and microvascular complications in type 2 diabetes, *BMJ* 317:703-713, 1998.
13. Parving HH: Benefits and costs of antihypertensive treatment in incipient and overt diabetic nephropathy, *J Hypertension* 16(1 Suppl):S99-S101, 1998.
14. Bernadet-Monrozies P, Rostaing L, Kamar N, and others: The effect of angiotensin-converting enzyme inhibitors on the progression of chronic renal failure, *Presse Med* 31(36):1714-1720, 2002.
15. Porush JG: Hypertension and chronic renal failure: the use of ACE inhibitors, *Am J Kidney Dis* 31(1):177-184, 1998.
16. Mogensen CE: Preventing end-stage renal disease, *Diabetic Med* 15(Suppl 4):S51-S56, 1998.
17. Degroot PJ, Kenler SR, Dwyer JT: Optimizing dialysis: past, present and future, *Nutr Today* 32:30-36, 1997.
18. Stein EA: Managing dyslipidemia in the high risk patient, *Am J Cardiol* 89(5A):50C-57C, 2002.
19. American Dietetic Association: *Manual of clinical dietetics,* ed 5, Chicago, 1996, The Association.
20. Hood VL, Gennari FJ: End stage renal disease: measures to prevent or slow its progression, *Postgrad Med* 100:163-176, 1996.
21. Owen WF: *Primary care of patients with chronic renal failure,* Unpublished manuscript, 1997.
22. Diabetes Control and Complications Trial Research Group: The effect of intensive treatment of diabetes on the development and progression of long-term complications in insulin-dependent diabetes mellitus, *N Engl J Med* 329:977-986, 1993.
23. Levey AS, Bosch JP, Lewis JB, and others: A more accurate method to estimate glomerular filtration rate from serum creatinine: a new prediction equation, *Ann Intern Med* 130(6):461-470, 1999.
24. National Kidney Foundation Disease Outcome Quality Initiative: *Clinical guidelines*, 2000, retrieved Feb 28, 2007, http://www.kidney.org/professionals/kdoqi/guidelines_ckd/toc.htm.

CHAPTER 162

Testicular Disorders

Updated by Patricia Polgar Bailey

DEFINITION AND EPIDEMIOLOGY

Scrotal pain may be a symptom of an underlying pathologic condition of the scrotum or testis. The pain may be described as sharp, dull, aching, uncomfortable, or tender; and it is characterized as mild, moderate, or severe. The pain may be sudden in onset, remitting, or progressively escalating in severity. Scrotal pain may be the chief complaint or an incidental finding during the history and physical examination. It is necessary to determine the cause of the pain to evaluate the need for emergent referral or intervention and to exclude potentially life-threatening conditions.

Scrotal masses may be nodules or cystic changes on the skin of the scrotum; may involve intrascrotal contents such as the testis, epididymis, spermatic cord, or tunica vaginalis; or may be the result of abdominal structures herniated into the scrotal sac. Palpation may reveal single or multiple nodules of varying sizes with consistencies that range from soft to firm. The mass may be freely movable or fixed and may range from nontender to extremely painful to touch or manipulation. Masses are found during testicular self-examination (TSE) or are discovered during examination and palpation of the scrotum by a health care provider. The mass may go undetected if it is small, if enlargement is gradual, or if discomfort is minimum or absent.

Scrotal swelling, or edema, may involve only one scrotum (left or right hemiscrotal edema) or both scrota (bilateral scrotal edema) and may indicate the presence of an underlying pathologic condition. Edema caused by a hydrocele may be benign, whereas swelling related to testicular torsion or a malignant tumor of the testis may be potentially life threatening. The clinical presentation of testicular cysts and dysplasias is enlarged testes, and both are clinically interpreted as neoplasms until otherwise evaluated.[1] Testicular tumors are usually malignant and account for approximately 1% of all malignancies in men.

The epidemiology of scrotal pain, masses, and swelling depends on the etiology of the disorders that manifest these symptoms. Specific disorders may occur more often in certain age-groups. The causes of scrotal pain, masses or tumors, or swelling discussed in this chapter are limited to those most commonly encountered in primary care: varicocele, epididymitis, epididymoorchitis, spermatocele, hydrocele, torsion of the spermatic cord, trauma, scrotal hernia, and testicular tumors.

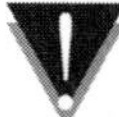

Immediate emergency department referral or physician consultation is indicated for patients with sudden-onset unilateral scrotal pain or testicular torsion.

Physician consultation is indicated for trauma, epididymitis, or right varicocele.

PATHOPHYSIOLOGY

A varicocele is caused by incompetent valves within the veins arising from the pampiniform plexus. This condition allows the reflux of blood from the spermatic vein, which results in dilated, tortuous varicose veins in the spermatic cord.[2] The incidence of varicocele is approximately 20% in young men and most often affects the left side.[3,4]

Epididymitis is an acute or chronic inflammation of the epididymis. The cause may be bacterial, viral, parasitic, chemically induced, or related to trauma,[5] and it is further categorized as a nonspecific or specific infection or traumatic injury.[5] Nonspecific infections are caused by gram-negative rods, gram-positive cocci, or anaerobic bacteria associated with a group of diseases with similar symptoms.[6] Inflammation of the epididymis is occasionally caused by trauma or urinary reflux from the urethra through the vas deferens.[6] The two most common causes, especially in younger men, are *Chlamydia trachomatis* and *Neisseria gonorrhoeae*. Other causative agents include *Escherichia coli, Haemophilus influenzae*, tuberculosis, cryptococci, or *Brucella* organisms in men who engage in unprotected anal intercourse. Epididymitis has several nonsexually transmitted causes, including Enterobacteriaceae and *Pseudomonas aeroginosa*, which are associated with urinary tract infections and prostatitis.[7] In men over 35 years old, epididymitis is most often associated with gram-negative rods or urologic procedures such as transurethral resection of the prostate or urethral catheterization. Epididymal inflammation may result as an asymptomatic complication of secondary syphilis, whereas tubercular epididymitis results from involvement of the prostate. Epididymitis can also occur in conjunction with inflammation of the testis (epididymoorchitis) as a result of reflux of urine from straining, although the exact cause is unclear.[2]

Orchitis is a systemic, bloodborne infection that results in an acute inflammation of the testis. It may co-exist with epididymitis; be a consequence of a systemic viral infections such as mumps; or be a complication of syphilis, mycobacterial infections, or fungal infections.[2] Epididymoorchitis is a complication in 20% to 35% of adolescent boys and young men with mumps[6] and can occur as a complication of many infectious diseases.[2,6] A hydrocele may also accompany the inflammation.[4]

A spermatocele is a painless sperm-filled cyst of the epididymis located between the head of the epididymis and the testes, and arising from the tubules that connect the right testis to the head of the epididymis. Spermatoceles are most frequently located superior and posterior to the testes.[4] The cause of this condition is unclear. Spermatoceles are usually small but can enlarge to several centimeters.[3]

A hydrocele is an accumulation of fluid within the tunica vaginalis as seen in adults; it may also result from a patent processus vaginalis at birth. In adults a hydrocele is often the result of trauma, a hernia, or a testicular tumor or a complication of epididymitis.

Similar to a hydrocele, a hematocele is a collection of fluid in the tunica vaginalis of the testes and manifests as a mass. However, a hematocele is a collection of blood (rather than serous fluid), which usually is precipitated by trauma and can be painful and tender on palpation.[4]

Testicular torsion is an obstruction of blood flow to the testes because of a twisting of the arteries and veins in the spermatic cord. Torsion of the spermatic cord is most often seen in the left testis. The left spermatic cord is longer and becomes twisted twice as often as that on the right side. Trauma may be the precipitating factor in young males. The torsion can be intermittent or complete and at times may resolve spontaneously. This condition results in congestion of venous blood flow and concomitant edema of the testis. If not resolved spontaneously or surgically, torsion can result in complete venous obstruction and necrosis of the testicular tissues.[4,8]

Trauma to the scrotum can be caused by burns or blunt force, or it may be penetrating and involve the testicle. Although only 2% to 3% of male patients coming in for medical care have genitourinary trauma injury, most of these injuries involve the scrotum and/or testis. Approximately 6% of testicular torsions are trauma induced, but they may be overlooked in the face of a hematoma or bruising.[9] A scrotal hernia results when a segment of the bowel slips through the internal inguinal ring, where it may remain in the inguinal canal or pass into the scrotal sac.[2] The hernia may spontaneously reduce by digital manipulation or when the patient lies supine, or it may become strangulated and require surgical reduction.

The origin of testicular tumors can be divided into three primary categories: germ cell origin, gonadal sex cord or stromal origin, and miscellaneous origin. On the basis of the histologic and genetic origin of the tumor, neoplasms of germ cell origin may be further divided into seminomas, nonseminomas, and non–germ cell tumors.[10]

Testicular malignancies are relatively uncommon in the general population, occurring in only two or three men per 100,000 each year.[11] The most common age of occurrence is between 15 and 35 years,[12] although these tumors have also been reported in infants and in older men.[13] The risk for testicular cancer in Caucasian men is more than five times that of African-American men and more than double that of Asian men.[14] There is a 35 times greater incidence in men who have a history of cryptorchism,[15] and a man with undescended testicles has up to a 32-fold increased risk for developing cancer, especially if the cryptorchism is not corrected before age 11 years.[14] The reason for this association is unclear, although it is theorized that the elevated temperatures of the testes may be carcinogenic or that some men may have a genetic predisposition to cryptorchism and testicular cancer.[4] Seminomas are the most common type of testicular tumor and account for 90% to 95% of all primary malignancies.[11,12] Testicular nonseminomas are often associated with serum tumor marker products, particularly alpha-fetoprotein (AFP) and human chorionic gonadotropin (HCG). These markers are sensitive to changes in body tumors and can be used for diagnosis, prognosis, and monitoring of treatment response.

Although the exact cause of testicular tumors is unknown, tumors have been associated with scrotal trauma, atrophy, cryptorchism, and exogenous estrogen exposure.[10] Approximately 50% of patients diagnosed with a malignant testicular tumor have a history of cryptorchism, and 10% to 15% of patients have a history of scrotal trauma.[15,16] Studies also support an increased risk of tumor development in the sons of women exposed to diethylstilbestrol, estrogen, or estrogen-progestin combinations in the first 2 months of pregnancy.[10] In 10% of the cases studied the development of testicular cancer has been linked with metastatic disease elsewhere in the body.[15] Studies also suggest a link between the development of testicular cancer and exposure to toxic chemicals or viruses.[10,12]

The development of testicular tumor cells is believed to occur during embryonic germ cell development within the testes. During normal male embryonic development, germ cells become spermatocytes. Tumor cells develop when embryonic germ cells undergo an abnormal pattern of differentiation. Germ cell tumors represent approximately 90% to 95% of all testicular tumors; nongerminal cell tumors such as Leydig's and Sertoli's cell tumors represent fewer than 5% of all testicular tumors.[10] Leydig's cell tumors are the most common and occur in both children and young adults. Metastasis from testicular tumors occurs primarily via the lymphatic system to other parts of the body.[11]

Elephantiasis is caused by a filariasis that affects the scrotum causing massive scrotal lymphedema. Filariasis includes a group of diseases caused by threadlike roundworms, called filaria, which are transmitted by various mosquitoes, flies, and biting midges. Testicular filariasis is due most often to *Wuchereria bancrofti*. Although this is a rare cause of testicular problems in the United States, it should be considered in the differential diagnosis in persons who have recently traveled to tropical areas or in health care workers involved in humanitarian missions. People who live in the tropics, including sub-Saharan Africa, Egypt, southern Asia, the Western Pacific Islands, the northeastern coasts of South and Central American, and the Caribbean Islands, are at increased risk for filariasis.

CLINICAL PRESENTATION

With testicular disorders, the history and presenting symptoms often suggest the underlying pathologic condition. Because some disorders may not cause significant discomfort, however, all male patients should be queried about changes in testicular size or the presence of nodules, pain, or penile discharge. The following disorders may be identified by the presenting complaint:

Varicocele: There are usually no visible outward signs other than a blue color through light-colored scrotal skin. The patient may complain of a dull pain or ache in the affected hemiscrotum or may be asymptomatic.[2] Men may complain of an enlarged testicle that decreases when supine.[4]

Epididymitis: The patient is seen with history of sudden onset of severe pain that is partially relieved by elevating the scrotum (Prehn's sign). Accumulation of scrotal edema is rapid and accompanied by fever.[2] Complaints may also include dysuria, a penile discharge, or flank pain.

Orchitis: The patient has a history of sudden onset of acute or moderate pain, testicular swelling, and fever; the patient may have a concomitant hydrocele.[2]

Spermatocele: A spermatocele is most often found on examination and is usually asymptomatic, but any discomfort is usually relieved with scrotal elevation.[4] Enlarged and movable, a spermatocele may feel like a third testis or be mistaken for a hydrocele.[2]

Hydrocele: The patient may report a gradual enlargement that has become bothersome as a result of bulk in the scrotum.[2] There is marked edema, which may be uncomfortable because of the added weight. Hydroceles are usually painless and may be present for long periods, partially resolve, and recur before the patient seeks medical attention. A hydrocele may occur secondary to a tumor when excess serous fluid accumulates in the scrotal sac. A large scrotal mass that develops after minimum trauma to the testicles may suggest rupture of a testicular neoplasm.

Hematocele: The patient may report a painful scrotum that is tender to palpation, which began after recent trauma.

Torsion of the spermatic cord: This condition is sudden in onset, is extremely painful, and may awaken the patient from sleep or be trauma induced. In addition to testicular pain, the patient may experience abdominal pain, nausea, and vomiting with no fever.[2]

Trauma: There may be a history of blunt or penetrating injury to the scrotum that may involve the scrotal contents. Bruising, bleeding, or edema may be visible. Depending on the type and extent of the injury, the patient may be in excruciating pain or have little pain other than extreme tenderness to manipulation. If the trauma results in injury and inflammation of the epididymis, fever may also be present.

Scrotal hernia: Scrotal swelling and pain on straining are common complaints.[2] The edema is increased after standing in an erect position but decreases when the patient is recumbent.

Testicular tumors: The patient generally seeks medical care for evaluation of an abnormal mass found during self-examination. Approximately 10% of patients complain of pain or discomfort in the testicles. Rarely, infertility is the presenting complaint.[5] The most common symptom or finding associated with a testicular tumor is the presence of a palpable mass that is often accompanied by edema or a sensation of fullness or heaviness in the scrotum. Patients may complain of scrotal pain; on rare occasions, an abdominal mass may be palpable. Other complaints such as back or abdominal pain, nausea, anorexia, or bowel and bladder symptoms may occur with retroperitoneal lymph node involvement.[5,6] Systemic endocrine effects may cause gynecomastia; as a result, associated lymph nodes may be enlarged and tender.

Elephantiasis: This condition leads to massive scrotal lymphedema and may or may not be accompanied by urticaria.[4]

PHYSICAL EXAMINATION

Examination begins with inspection of the scrotum. Scrotal size can change with temperature variations because of the cremaster muscle mechanism. Asymmetry is expected because the left hemiscrotum is normally lower than the right. The skin of each hemiscrotum should be inspected carefully, spreading the rugae between the fingers. Care should be taken to inspect both the anterior and posterior surfaces to detect any lesions. It is common to find multiple sebaceous cysts on the scrotal skin; these are small, firm, nontender, and white to yellowish in color.[2]

Each hemiscrotum should be palpated with the thumb and first two fingers of both hands. The scrotal contents should be easily movable in a sliding fashion. The testes should be oval, smooth, equal, and firm but rubbery. The normal epididymis is softer than the testis, nontender, and smooth. To palpate the spermatic cord, the provider should slide the fingers and thumb up from the epididymis. The cord should feel smooth and nontender. Documentation should include any tenderness or pain, discoloration, edema, or abnormal findings, such as those seen in the following conditions:

Varicocele: Bluish color shows through the scrotal skin; when the patient stands, palpation of the soft mass reveals a "bag of worms" on the proximal spermatic cord.[2] Right varicoceles may indicate venous obstruction or renal cancer. Varicoceles decrease when the patient is supine.

Epididymitis: The scrotum is red, enlarged, and extremely tender. The epididymis may be enlarged and difficult to distinguish from the testis. The scrotal skin over the affected area may be edematous and thickened. Tubercular epididymitis manifests as a characteristic beading of the vas deferens. A history of prostatitis may be a precursor to the development of epididymitis.

Orchitis: As with epididymitis, testicular edema may be so pronounced that it is difficult to distinguish the testes from the epididymis. Palpation may reveal swollen, very tense testes that are painful, and the patient may be febrile. The onset of unilateral or bilateral erythema, edema, and scrotal tenderness occurs 3 to 4 days after onset of infection. A hydrocele may accompany the inflammation.[4]

Spermatocele: The spermatocele is palpated as a small, nontender, freely movable mass above and behind the testis. The mass may arise from the vasa efferentia (tubules that connect the rete testis to the epididymis), the epididymis, or cystic structures on the upper pole of the testis.[2] Transillumination of the mass in a darkened room may help visualize the mass.

Hydrocele: Palpation reveals a nontender mass that transilluminates easily, unless there is an underlying inflammatory process such as an epididymal infection.

Hematocele: Palpation reveals scrotal swelling that transilluminates and may be tender to palpation.

Torsion of the spermatic cord: The scrotum may be edematous and erythematous, and the affected scrotum may be higher because of shortening that occurs as a result of rotation. Torsion usually occurs in the left hemiscrotum. The spermatic cord is swollen and extremely tender, and the epididymis may be felt anteriorly. The cremaster response is absent on the affected side.[2]

Trauma: Bruising, bleeding, and edema may be present. Inspection should include careful comparison of coloration to determine the extent of bruising or expanding hematoma. A ruptured testis should be suspected if there is evidence of increasing hematoma, edema, and pain.

Palpation should include external skin and scrotal contents. Documentation includes the time and date of injury, type of trauma, and any change in signs or symptoms since the time of injury.

Scrotal hernia: Inspection reveals an enlarged hemiscrotum that may spontaneously reduce when supine. Palpation reveals an enlarged mass in the scrotum that may spontaneously reduce when the patient is reclining. The provider will not be able to move the fingers above the mass, which should be soft and mushy but painless unless incarcerated and ischemic. Scrotal hernias do not transilluminate. Auscultation of bowel sounds over the mass is significant for the diagnosis of bowel in the scrotal sac.

Testicular tumor: Inquiry should focus on previous trauma to the scrotum or perineal area and the history or presence of cryptorchism, pain, swelling, or sensations in the scrotum. The physical examination should include inspection and palpation of the abdomen, perineal area, scrotal sac, testes, and surrounding lymph nodes. Palpation should be performed using both hands to assist in differentiating between a mass located on the body of the testicle and a mass located on or within the epididymis. The location, size, mobility, and degree of tenderness of normal structures, as well as any abnormal findings, should be noted.

Elephantiasis: This condition is characterized by massive scrotal lymphedema.

Any solid, firm mass within the body of the testicle should be considered a tumor unless proven otherwise. A painless mass in one or both hemiscrotums with or without a hydrocele suggests malignancy.[11] Supraclavicular, scalene, and inguinal nodes are often enlarged.[11] Back pain may be present if masses are located in the retroperitoneal area. Scrotal transillumination performed in a darkened room may be used to visualize abnormalities and detect solid vs. fluid-filled masses.[12]

DIAGNOSTICS

Many testicular disorders are readily recognized at the time of presentation and do not require further evaluation. In general, clinical presentation and physical examination guide the choice of appropriate diagnostics:

Varicocele: Semen analysis may reveal oligospermia or azoospermia but can be normal.

Epididymitis: Doppler ultrasound may show increased sound waves caused by hyperemia.[5] Laboratory tests reveal white blood cells and bacteriuria.[2]

Orchitis: Doppler ultrasound may show increased sound waves caused by hyperemia.[5]

Spermatocele: A mass is located at the proximal aspect of the spermatic cord. Transillumination of the mass is expected.

Hydrocele: A hydrocele will transilluminate in a darkened room. (A cystic mass transilluminates; a tumor does not.)

Hematocele: Ultrasonography is used to evaluate blood flow. Surgical exploration may be necessary to rule out cancer.

Torsion of the spermatic cord: Doppler ultrasound may show diminished sound waves caused by ischemia.[5]

Trauma: The patient demonstrates visible bruising. Ultrasonography may be used to determine if the testis is intact.

Scrotal hernia: A scrotal hernia does not transilluminate.

Testicular tumor: The diagnosis of testicular cancer is generally confirmed through direct surgical exploration of the testes. Serum tumor markers, HCG, AFP, and lactate dehydrogenase may be used to support the history and physical examination findings. Tumor markers elevate when disease is present and return to normal during recovery.[16] A negative marker does not necessarily exclude disease, but an elevated marker is considered clinically significant.[12] High levels of HCG are seen in both seminomatous and nonseminomatous tumors, whereas AFP levels are elevated only in seminomas.[10] Ultrasonography is useful in detecting nonpalpable testicular masses and in confirming the size and location of palpable tumors. Differentiation of intratesticular masses from extratesticular masses may also be accomplished using ultrasound.[17] Abdominopelvic CT or other x-ray studies may be necessary to determine the extent and location of metastasis.

Elephantiasis: The only definite way to make the diagnosis of lymphatic filariasis is by detecting the parasite itself,

DIAGNOSTICS

Testicular Disorders

VARICOCELE
Laboratory
Semen analysis

EPIDIDYMITIS
Laboratory
Urinalysis
CBC and differential

Imaging
Doppler ultrasound

ORCHITIS
Imaging
Doppler ultrasound

TORSION OF SPERMATIC CORD
Imaging
Doppler ultrasound

TRAUMA
Imaging
Ultrasound

TESTICULAR TUMOR
Laboratory
HCG
AFP
Lactate dehydrogenase
Serum tumor markers
Clinical staging

Imaging
Ultrasound
CT scans

either the adult worms or the microfilariae. The microfilariae can sometimes be detected by microscopic examination of a blood sample, but often people with chronic infection do not have the microfilariae in their blood. In such cases, the urine, hydrocele fluid, or other clinical tests are necessary. Blood samples should be obtained during the night, when microfilariae are more numerous in the bloodstream. Detecting the adult worms is more difficult because they often exist deep in the lymphatic system.

To assist practitioners in assessing the extent of testicular disease, various clinical staging systems have been developed and are based on surgical findings and histologic examination of retroperitoneal lymph nodes: stage I, tumor confined to testis; stage II, tumor spread to regional lymph nodes; stage III, tumor spread beyond retroperitoneal nodes.[10] Numerous other staging systems have been developed and are useful for describing and standardizing the clinical stages of testicular tumors.

DIFFERENTIAL DIAGNOSIS

The differential diagnosis for any testicular disorder should first exclude the possibility of a testicular tumor. It is often difficult to differentiate between epididymitis and orchitis because the symptoms are similar. A varicocele is more discernible than other scrotal masses because on palpation this mass classically resembles a bag of worms. However, many of the other conditions may have hydrocele development as a symptom.

> **DIFFERENTIAL DIAGNOSIS**
>
> **Testicular Disorders**
>
> - Tumor
> - Cysts
> - Testicular torsion
> - Epididymitis
> - Orchitis
> - Hydrocele
> - Hematocele
> - Varicocele
> - Hernia
> - Hematoma
> - Spermatocele
> - Elephantiasis

The differential diagnosis for testicular tumors includes cysts, testicular torsion, epididymitis, or epididymal orchitis. A hydrocele, hernia, hematoma, or spermatocele may also mimic a testicular tumor.[16] The presence of a testicular mass is suggestive of a tumor and indicates the need for immediate referral.

Various diagnostics such as urine culture, urinalysis, Doppler ultrasound, and nuclear scan may be indicated to determine the cause of pain, mass, or edema. The history is probably as valuable as the physical examination in making a definitive diagnosis of the condition on the basis of signs, symptoms, precipitating factors, and length of time these have been present (or if they have changed over time).

MANAGEMENT

Management of testicular disorders depends on the specific type of disorder.

Varicocele: Treatment is ligation of the spermatic vein by a surgeon. However, recent review of the literature found insufficient evidence that ligation of the varicocele improves pregnancy rate in couples with unexplained fertility, whereas several studies in this review demonstrated improvement in semen quality after varicocele treatment.[18,19]

Epididymitis and orchitis: Antiinfective therapy is recommended, with guidance by sensitivity reports. The following antibiotic regimens are effective against the most common causes of epididymitis: single dose ceftriaxone 250 mg and doxycycline 250 mg b.i.d. for 10 days (or ofloxacin 300 mg b.i.d. for 10 days or levofloxacin 500 mg/day for 10 days). In severe cases it may be necessary to use parenteral antibiotics.[5] With tubercular epididymitis, an epididymectomy may be performed to eradicate the condition.[5] Antipyretics should be used to reduce discomfort and fever, and an antiinflammatory agent should be prescribed. An antiemetic can also be prescribed for nausea and vomiting. Bed rest and scrotal elevation are also recommended for epididymitis. Hot or cold compresses may be helpful for orchitis.

Spermatocele: No treatment is required unless the patient complains of discomfort or concern because of the increasing size of the mass. Treatment, if warranted (i.e., if the mass is painful), is excision of the mass.

Hydrocele: Active treatment is not warranted unless complications are present. If indicated, the hydrocele should be drained surgically and the hydrocele sac reanastomosed. Unfortunately, hydroceles may recur.[3] Some recent investigations for treatment have included sclerosing hydroceles to reduce recurrence rates.[20]

Torsion of the spermatic cord: Treatment is immediate surgical exploration (within 6 hours) and intervention to prevent ischemia and restore blood flow.

Trauma/hematocele: If all scrotal contents are intact, trauma injuries can be treated symptomatically with ice and elevation. However, if there is concern that the testicle has been ruptured or penetrated, or if other contents are not palpated as intact, immediate surgical exploration and intervention should be undertaken. Consultation with the primary care physician or urologist is recommended.

Scrotal hernia: If the herniated bowel is reducible, surgical referral for possible future repair is indicated. However, pain may indicate incarceration of the bowel, in which case immediate emergency department referral and surgical consultation are indicated.

Testicular tumor: Prompt evaluation is essential. Surgical exploration and intervention are indicated if a mass in or adjacent to the testis cannot be satisfactorily evaluated with physical examination, transillumination, and ultrasonography. Primary treatment for seminomas involves radical orchiectomy followed by irradiation of the retroperitoneal lymph for low-stage seminomas and chemotherapy for more advanced stage seminomas. Nonseminomas are also treated with radical orchiectomy followed by retroperitoneal lymphadenectomy. Chemotherapy may be used for more advanced stage nonseminomas.[10] Follow-up visits should include a thorough physical examination, a chest x-ray study, and measurement of serum tumor markers monthly for the first year, every 2 months for the second year, and every 3 to 6 months for up to 5 years.

Elephantiasis: The recommended treatment for *W. bancrofti* is diethylcarbamazine. This medicine can be obtained from the CDC Parasitic Drug Service, (404) 639-3670.

After a malignancy has been confirmed, the patient with testicular cancer may be placed on chemotherapy. In addition, the use of NSAIDs and other analgesic agents may be necessary to relieve pain and inflammation.

LIFE SPAN CONSIDERATIONS

Four issues should be considered in the assessment and treatment of conditions involving the scrotum or testes: threat to life, immediate pain or discomfort, potential for infertility or impotence, and quality of life. Treatment success may depend on the patient's overall health, available treatment options, and age-related issues affecting treatment decisions. Although the patient's age may influence concerns regarding fertility, the potential loss of potency should not be disregarded in men of advanced age.

Surgical intervention for testicular tumors may result in body image disturbances and altered sexuality in adolescence and later life. After an orchiectomy, counseling may be indicated to assist in coping with loss related to alterations in the genitals and reproductive system. Education related to chemotherapy and surgical intervention is important to promote understanding and acceptance of the disorder and treatment.

COMPLICATIONS

Varicoceles can cause infertility because sperm concentration and motility are decreased in 65% to 75% of patients. The condition can be reversed if the varicocele is surgically corrected.[3] Infertility is also the most serious complication of epididymitis, orchitis, and spermatocele. In orchitis, testicular atrophy may develop in 50% of patients; on palpation, the testes are small and soft.[5] If a hydrocele is large, bowel herniation is likely and should be considered. Testicular tumors and epididymitis should be excluded. Unless complications such as diminished blood supply to the testis or hemorrhage resulting from trauma are present, active therapy for hydrocele is not required.[3]

Torsion of the spermatic cord is a medical emergency and should be surgically explored and relieved as quickly as possible to prevent the development of gangrene. A delay in treatment could result in testicular infarction and loss of the affected testicle. In scrotal trauma the most pressing concern is whether the testis has been ruptured or the blood supply compromised from trauma-induced torsion of the spermatic cord. A referral to a urologist is required to verify that the testis and other scrotal contents are intact, with the injury treated symptomatically. Scrotal hernia with pain may indicate incarceration of the bowel and danger of ischemia, necrosis, and subsequent gangrene.

Testicular tumors are the most common malignancy and the third leading cause of death in young men.[15] Unlike other cancers, testicular cancer is potentially curable, even in an advanced stage. Improvements in diagnostic techniques and treatments over the past 25 years have resulted in an increased survival rate of approximately 90%.[16] The occurrence of testicular cancer in men over age 60 years is uncommon.[16] Prognosis with treatment may depend on the presence of other age-related or chronic health conditions at the time of treatment.

INDICATIONS FOR REFERRAL OR HOSPITALIZATION

Patients suspected of having a testicular mass, torsion of the spermatic cord, or an incarcerated scrotal hernia require immediate referral. Epididymitis and minor scrotal trauma can be managed by the health care provider unless complications are present or the testis is involved in a traumatic injury. A spermatocele should be referred for possible excision, as should the hydrocele that is expanding, is causing pain, or may be caused by a scrotal tumor.

Hospitalization should be considered if the pain is unremitting, if a testicular mass is suspected, or if edema from testicular involvement cannot be excluded. Decisions regarding treatment alternatives may require in-depth discussion and consideration.

PATIENT AND FAMILY EDUCATION

Diagnosis, treatment options, potential outcomes, and the need for follow-up care should be carefully explained to patients. All patients should be encouraged to discuss their concerns or fears regarding the diagnosis and treatment or treatment options. These concerns and fears should be addressed truthfully regarding potential complications and the severity of the condition.

Patients with testicular masses require ongoing education and support from the time of diagnosis through all phases of treatment. Whenever possible, the spouse or significant other should be educated about the disease process, prognosis, treatment, and effects of treatment on relationships and sexuality. The patient and family should be encouraged to verbalize feelings and to support each other throughout the process.

HEALTH PROMOTION

Male patients, from adolescents to older adults, should be instructed on the correct method of TSE, asked to do a return demonstration, and encouraged to teach other males (including teenagers) in their family the method and importance of the examination, since this is the beginning of the age range for testicular cancer. The TSE should be performed monthly and is best performed after a warm bath or show when the skin of the scrotum is relaxed.[21] Patients should see their health care provider if any abnormalities are detected.

REFERENCES

1. Peterson RO: Testicular neoplasms. In Caputo GM, Wight A, editors: *Urologic pathology,* ed 2, Philadelphia, 1992, Lippincott.
2. Jarvis C: Male genitalia. In Jarvis C, editor: *Physical examination and health assessment,* ed 2, Philadelphia, 1996, Saunders.
3. McAninch JW: Disorders of the testis, scrotum, and spermatic cord. In Tanagho EA, McAninch JW, editors: *Smith's general urology,* ed 14, Norwalk, Conn, 1995, Appleton & Lange.
4. Mullen B: Testicular complaints in the young man, *J Am Acad Nurse Pract* 16(11):490-495, 2004.
5. Gray M: Scrotal inflammation. In Gray M, editor: *Genitourinary disorders,* St Louis, 1992, Mosby.
6. Meares EM: Nonspecific infections of the genitourinary tract. In

Tanagho EA, McAninch JW, editors: *Smith's general urology*, ed 14, Norwalk, Conn, 1995, Appleton & Lange.

7. Robinson K, McCance K: Alterations of the reproductive system. In McCance K, Heuther S, editors: *Pathophysiology: the biologic basis for disease in adults and children*, ed 14, Philadelphia, 2002, Mosby.
8. Sugar EC, Hoyler-Grant C: Disorders of the external genitalia in children. In Karlowizc KA, editor: *Urologic nursing: principles and practice*, Philadelphia, 1995, Saunders.
9. Lrhorfi H, Manunta A, Rodriguez A, and others: Trauma induced testicular torsion, *J Urol* 168(6):2548, 2002.
10. Klimaszewski AD, Karlowicz KA: Cancer of the male genitalia. In Karlowicz KA, editor: *Urologic nursing: principles and practice*, Philadelphia, 1995, Saunders.
11. Gray MR: Testicular tumors. In Gray M, editor: *Genitourinary disorders*, St Louis, 1992, Mosby.
12. Kleier J: Testicular cancer hits below the belt, *Nurs Spect* 13:685-692, 2003.
13. Rowland RG, Fosta RS, Donohue J: Scrotum and testis. In Gillenwater JY, Howards SS, Grayhack JT, and others, editors: *Adult and pediatric urology*, ed 3, St Louis, 1996, Mosby.
14. Herrinton L, Zhao W, Hussen G: Management of cryptorchism and risk of testicular cancer, *Am J Epidemiol* 157(7):602-605, 2003.
15. Spirnack JP: Adult scrotal mass. In Resnick MI, Caldamone AA, Spirnack JP, editors: *Decision making in urology*, ed 2, Philadelphia, 1991, Decker.
16. Richie JP: Detection and treatment of testicular cancer, *CA Cancer J Clin* 43(3):151-175, 1993.
17. Comiter CV, Benson CJ, Capelouto CC, and others: Nonpalpable intratesticular masses detected sonographically, *J Urol* 154(4):1367-1369, 1995.
18. Centers for Disease Control and Prevention: Filariasis lymphatic, *Health information for international travel, 2005-2006*, Atlanta, 2005, US Department of Health and Human Services, Public Health Service.
19. Evers JLH, Collins JA, Vandekerckhove P: Surgery or embolisation for varicocele in subfertile men, *Cochrane Database Syst Rev* (3), 2002, retrieved Sept 2, 2002, from http://gateway2.ovid.com/oviedweb.cgi.
20. Yilmaz U, Ekmeckcioglu O, Tatlisen A, and others: Does pleurodesis for pleural effusions give bright ideas about agents for hydrocele sclerotherapy? *Int Urol Nephrol* 32(1):89-92, 2000.
21. Cleveland Clinic: *Disorders of the testes*, retrieved July 14, 2006, from http://www.clevelandclinic.org/health/health.

CHAPTER 163

Tumors of the Genitourinary Tract (Kidneys, Ureters, Bladder)

Laura Stempkowski

DEFINITION AND EPIDEMIOLOGY

Tumors of the genitourinary tract may be benign or malignant. Benign renal tumors include adenomas, oncocytomas, and angiomyolipomas and are often incidentally found on imaging studies. Adenomas are small tumors of the renal cortex and are most often asymptomatic. Oncocytomas are adenomas of the renal collecting tubule and represent 1% to 14% of renal tumors. Although considered benign, on rare occasions they have demonstrated malignant potential. Angiomyolipomas, as the name implies, contain vascular tissue, smooth muscle cells, and fatty elements. Because of the potential for hemorrhage, they may become symptomatic, manifesting with pain, hematuria, or hypertension.[1]

Renal cell carcinoma (RCC) is the most prevalent malignant renal tumor in adults and constitutes more than 90% of all adult renal cancers. Wilms' tumor is a childhood renal tumor affecting approximately 1 in 10,000 children under the age of 15 years.[2]

Cancer of the bladder is the second most common cancer of the genitourinary tract.[3] The male/female ratio is 3:1, and the average age at diagnosis is 65 years.[4] As the population ages, the incidence of bladder cancer is increasing, but the incidence of advanced bladder cancer and the mortality rate are decreasing.[4] The etiology is unknown, but known risk factors include cigarette smoking and occupational exposures to chemicals, dyes, rubber, petroleum, leather, and printing chemicals. Chronic infection has been associated with bladder cancer, secondary to neurogenic bladder, stones, or long-term indwelling catheter use.[5]

PATHOPHYSIOLOGY

Renal Cell Carcinoma

In all, 85% of renal tumors are parenchymal tumors; the remainder have a uroepithelial origin or arise from supporting structures. RCC is an adenocarcinoma of the kidney that most frequently originates from the proximal tubule.[6] Evidence of metastasis is present in one third of patients at the time of diagnosis. The most common site of metastasis is the lungs.[6] RCCs are often associated with paraneoplastic syndromes, which may produce the initial symptoms (e.g., fever, anemia, cachexia, hypercalcemia, erythrocytosis, hypertension, hepatic dysfunction).[6] Occasionally, a kidney cancer may be initially seen as a fever of unknown origin.[7]

RCC occurs with equal frequency in either kidney and may occur in the upper, middle, or lower poles. Tumor size at presentation varies from 1 to 10 cm (0.4 to 4 inches) or larger, and tumor size has been inversely correlated with survival.[1] Prognosis and treatment recommendations are based on the stage of disease. Two systems are commonly used to define the extent of disease: Robson's staging system and the TNM (tumor-nodes-metastasis) classification for kidney cancer.[6]

Wilms' Tumor

Wilms' tumor is unilateral in 95% of cases and is associated with several congenital anomalies, including cryptorchism, ureteral duplication, and hypospadias.[6] Acquired von Willebrand's disease has been associated with Wilms' tumor and should be considered in children with coagulation abnormalities or bleeding symptoms.[2]

Wilms' tumor may be familial or sporadic in occurrence and is associated with chromosomal abnormalities. The familial type is thought to be inherited by autosomal dominant transmission.[3]

Wilms' tumors are usually large and multilobulated with focal areas of hemorrhage and necrosis. Metastasis (e.g., lungs, liver) is present in 10% to 15% of cases at the time of diagnosis.[3] Staging of Wilms' tumor is based on the National Wilms' Tumor Study staging system and consists of five stages. The range is from stage I (tumor limited to kidney and completely excisable) to stage IV (hematogenous metastasis to lung, liver, bone, and brain) and stage V (bilateral renal involvement).[3]

Bladder Cancer

Bladder cancer develops within the urothelium, the lining of the urinary tract. The urothelium is composed of three to seven layers of transitional cells that cover the muscular layers of the bladder wall. Proliferative changes of the transitional cells may result in cancer, which may remain superficial or progress to invasive or metastatic disease.

Urothelial carcinoma (transitional cell carcinoma [TCC]) accounts for approximately 90% of all bladder cancers and may appear as papillary lesions or, less commonly, as sessile or ulcerated lesions.[3] A papilloma or papillary tumor is a less aggressive transitional cell tumor. Nontransitional cell carcinomas include adenocarcinomas, squamous cell carcinomas, undifferentiated carcinomas, and mixed carcinomas. Squamous cell carcinomas account for 2% to 5% of bladder cancers and are more resistant to treatment.[8] They may be seen with high-grade urothelial carcinomas in which squamous differentiation has occurred or as a result of chronic infection, bladder stones, long-term indwelling urethral catheter use, or schistosomiasis.[7]

Carcinomas of the bladder are graded and staged in an effort to define the aggressiveness and extent of disease. Staging defines the depth of invasion within the bladder and progression of disease: stage 0 (mucosal changes) to stage D (lymph node involvement). The depth of invasion into muscle layers and perivesical fat increases the risk of metastasis.[4] Grading refers to the degree of cellular differentiation from normal urothelium. Transitional cell carcinomas are graded on a numeric scale from 1 to 4, with the higher grade tumors being more invasive and aggressive in behavior.

It is important to remember that TCC can progress to, or initially appear as, upper tract lesions. At least 90% of malignancies arising within the renal pelvis and ureter are TCCs. TCC of the upper tract is seen in nearly 5% of patients who have had bladder cancer.[9] Conversely, at least 50% of patients first seen with upper tract urothelial carcinoma have or develop bladder cancer.[10]

CLINICAL PRESENTATION

The average age at diagnosis of RCC is 55 to 60 years, with a male/female ratio of 2:1.[3] The classic triad of flank pain, hematuria, and renal mass occurs in less than 10% of patients, and consequently RCC is often not diagnosed until metastasis has occurred. A significant number of RCCs are found incidentally on imaging for other clinical problems.

Wilms' tumor affects children, with the mean age at diagnosis being 3½ to 4 years.[2] In Wilms' tumor, the prevalent feature is an abdominal mass. Abdominal pain, which may suggest an acute abdomen, occurs in 30% to 40% of these patients.

More than 70% of bladder cancer patients are first seen with intermittent painless gross hematuria that is often described as continuing throughout urination. Irritative voiding symptoms (e.g., urgency, frequency, dysuria) may or may not be present.[5] The presence of microhematuria also may herald a urothelial malignancy and requires further investigation.

PHYSICAL EXAMINATION

The majority of genitourinary tract tumors are not associated with specific findings on physical examination. However, approximately 80% of children with Wilms' tumor will have a large, smooth, firm flank mass that often extends across the midline.

DIAGNOSTICS

A hematuria workup should include a cystoscopy and an imaging study of the upper tracts. An IV pyelogram is being used less frequently in favor of the spiral CT (CT urogram) for imaging the kidneys, ureters, and bladder.[7]

DIFFERENTIAL DIAGNOSIS

See Differential Diagnosis box.

MANAGEMENT

Renal Cell Carcinoma

The prognosis for RCC is poor unless it is diagnosed and treated before metastasis occurs. Surgical intervention for localized disease offers the only potential for cure.[11] Surgical options include a radical nephrectomy, which may be done as a laparoscopic procedure or as an open procedure. A nephron-sparing partial nephrectomy may be an option in select situations.[12]

Preoperative renal artery embolization may be used to minimize blood loss or to minimize pain or hematuria in the event of a nonresectable tumor.[11] For patients with disseminated disease, radiotherapy is used for palliation of metastatic lesions (e.g., to the brain, bone, or lungs). RCC has shown limited response to biologic response modifiers (e.g., interferons, interleukin). Interleukin-2 has been the most effective of these for treating metastatic RCC. Clinical trials investigating vaccine therapy are promising and ongoing.[13]

DIAGNOSTICS

Genitourinary Tumors

RENAL CELL CARCINOMA

Laboratory
Urinalysis
Urine cytology*
CBC and differential
LFTs
Calcium

Imaging
IV pyelogram
Ultrasound
CT scans, MRI
Renal angiography*
Retrograde pyelography*

Other
Cystoscopy

WILMS' TUMOR

Laboratory
Urinalysis
CBC and differential
BUN, creatinine
Coagulation screening

Imaging
Ultrasound
CT scan
Chest x-ray*

BLADDER CANCER

Laboratory
Urine for cytology

Imaging
Spiral CT (CT urogram)
Ultrasound
IV pyelogram
CT scan

Other
Cystoscopy with biopsies

*If indicated.

DIFFERENTIAL DIAGNOSIS

Genitourinary Tumors

RENAL CELL CARCINOMA

- Simple cyst
- Angiomyolipoma
- Renal abscess
- Arteriovenous malformations
- Renal lymphoma
- Transitional cell carcinoma of renal pelvis
- Adrenal cancer
- Oncocytoma

WILMS' TUMOR

- Neuroblastoma
- Hydronephrosis
- Mesoblastic nephroma
- Fecal mass
- Renal tumor, non-Wilms' tumor

BLADDER CANCER

- Urinary tract infections
- Interstitial cystitis
- Hemorrhagic cystitis
- Fibrous polyp
- Endometriosis
- Hematoma
- Bladder calculi

Over the past few years, as more has been learned about the molecular aspects of disease progression, kidney cancer research has turned toward targeted therapies for the treatment of advanced disease. In placebo-controlled trials, targeted therapies have demonstrated significant increases in progression-free survival. Recently the U.S. Food and Drug Administration approved two oral tyrosine kinase inhibitors, sorafenib (Nexavar) and sunitinib (Sutent) for use as single-agent therapy for metastatic RCC.[14] The study of targeted therapies continues to be an important aspect of kidney cancer research, offering new hope to those with metastatic disease.

Wilms' Tumor

For the child with Wilms' tumor, multimodality therapy has been successful, with cure rates currently approaching 90%.[2]

Bladder Cancer

Transurethral resection of the bladder tumor is usually the initial treatment of superficial bladder cancer. In cases of less aggressive cancer, follow-up surveillance may include interval urine cytologic studies and repeat cystoscopy with transurethral resection as necessary. Adjuvant intravesical therapy (e.g., bacillus Calmette-Guérin, mitomycin-C, thiotepa, doxorubicin) may be used for tumors with unfavorable prognostic features (e.g., frequent recurrence, multifocal tumors, carcinoma in situ).[11] For muscle-invasive bladder tumors, a radical cystectomy with urinary diversion remains the standard therapy. Options for urinary diversion include ileal conduit, continent diversion, and orthotopic neobladder. Bladder conservation therapy, with combined modality therapy with radiation and chemotherapy, may be an option for some patients.[15]

COMPLICATIONS

See Box 163-1.

INDICATIONS FOR REFERRAL OR HOSPITALIZATION

A history and clinical presentation suspicious for genitourinary tumors mandate specialist referral and consultation. Hospitalization may be indicated for cases of acute illness or advanced disease.

BOX 163-1

COMPLICATIONS OF COMMON GENITOURINARY TUMORS

RENAL CELL CARCINOMA

- Complications of metastasis
- Anemia
- Pain
- Hypercalcemia
- Erythrocytosis
- Hypertension
- Hepatic dysfunction

WILMS' TUMOR

- Treatment-related morbidity
- Metastasis-related morbidity
- Complications of associated congenital anomalies

BLADDER CANCER

- Bladder perforation
- Hematuria
- Clot retention
- Metastasis
- Treatment-related morbidity
- Obstruction

PATIENT EDUCATION

Patient education regarding tumors of the genitourinary tract should include information regarding prevention, the disease process, diagnostic and staging procedures, treatment options, prognosis, and symptom management. The importance of lifelong surveillance and follow-up must be emphasized.

HEALTH PROMOTION

There currently are no screening tests for cancers of the kidneys, ureters, or bladder. Urine cytologic testing may be done, but it is important to remember that it is most sensitive and specific in high-grade urothelial cancers. Urine cytology may be falsely negative in as many of 50% to 75% of cases of low to moderate grade urothelial cancers.[7]

Cigarette smoking remains the greatest risk factor for bladder cancer. Health promotion that emphasizes no smoking or smoking cessation is a critical aspect of prevention.

REFERENCES

1. Langdon DR, Liang BA, Harris RD: Imaging of renal tumors. In Ernstoff MS, Heaney JA, Peschel RE, editors: *Urologic cancer,* Cambridge, Mass, 1997, Blackwell Science.
2. Williams JA, Greenwald CA, Rao BN: Wilms' tumor. In Vogelzang NJ, Scardino PT, Shipley WU, and others, editors: *Genitourinary oncology,* ed 2, Philadelphia, 2000, Lippincott Williams & Wilkins.
3. Carroll PR: Urothelial carcinoma: cancers of the bladder, ureter, and renal pelvis. In Tanagho EA, McAninch JW, editors: *Smith's general urology,* ed 14, Norwalk, Conn, 1995, Appleton & Lange.
4. Hudson MA, Catalona WJ: Urothelial tumors of the bladder, upper tracts, and prostate. In Gillenwater JY, Howards SS, Grayhack JT, and others, editors: *Adult and pediatric urology,* ed 3, vol 1, St Louis, 1996, Mosby.
5. Hawkins CA: Diagnosis of and screening for urothelial cancer. In Ernstoff MS, Heaney JA, Peschel RE, editors: *Urologic cancer,* Cambridge, Mass, 1997, Blackwell Science.
6. McDougal WS, Garnick MB: Clinical signs and symptoms of renal cell carcinoma. In Vogelzang NJ, Scardino PT, Shipley WU, and others, editors: *Genitourinary oncology,* ed 2, Philadelphia, 2000, Lippincott Williams & Wilkins.
7. Droller MJ: Primary care update on kidney and bladder cancer: a urologic perspective, *Med Clin North Am* 88:309-328, 2004.
8. Flynn SD, Kacinski B, Peschel RE: Pathology and staging of urothelial cancer. In Ernstoff MS, Heaney JA, Peschel RE, editors: *Urologic cancer,* Cambridge, Mass, 1997, Blackwell Science.
9. Heney NM: Management of tumors in the renal pelvis and ureter. In Ernstoff MS, Heaney JA, Peschel RE, editors: *Urologic cancer,* Cambridge, Mass, 1997, Blackwell Science.
10. Keeley FX, Bibbo M, Bagley DH: Ureteroscopic treatment and surveillance of upper tract TCC, *J Urol* 157:1560-1565, 1997.
11. Dreicer R, Williams RD: Renal parenchymal neoplasms. In Tanagho EA, McAninch JW: *Smith's general urology,* ed 14, Norwalk, Conn, 1995, Appleton & Lange.
12. Franklin JR, deKernion JB: Surgical approaches to renal cell carcinoma. In Ernstoff MS, Heaney JA, Peschel RE, editors: *Urologic cancer,* Cambridge, Mass, 1997, Blackwell Science.
13. Gorsch SM, Ernstoff MS: Biologic therapy of renal cell carcinoma. In Ernstoff MS, Heaney JA, Peschel RE, editors: *Urologic cancer,* Cambridge, Mass, 1997, Blackwell Science.
14. Tucker S: Targeted therapy of renal cell carcinoma, *Commun Oncol* 3(7):419-420, 2006.
15. Heaney JA: Future directions in urothelial cancer. In Ernstoff MS, Heaney JA, Peschel RE, editors: *Urologic cancer,* Cambridge, Mass, 1997, Blackwell Science.

CHAPTER 164

Urinary Calculi

Carol A. Whelan

DEFINITION AND EPIDEMIOLOGY

Urinary calculi, or urolithiasis, refers to calcifications or "stones" that form in the urinary system, primarily in the kidneys (nephrolithiasis) or ureter (ureterolithiasis); they may also form in or migrate to the lower urinary system (bladder or urethra).[1] The problem of urinary calculi has been documented as far back in history as the Egyptian mummies.[2] The majority of stones are found within the kidney, but stone formation may also occur in the ureter, bladder, and urinary diversion structures (e.g., ileal conduit, orthotopic bladder). Although many questions about stone formation remain unanswered, understanding of the causes has improved in recent years. As a result, greater emphasis is directed at the prevention of stone formation.

Urolithiasis is the third most common disorder of the urinary tract,[3,4] with a prevalence rate of up to 10% to 12%.[5,6] The incidence of stone formation may be related to geography, climate, season, age, gender, and heredity.[5] Kidney stones and upper ureter stones are more common in the United States than in other parts of the world and may be related to the dietary preferences for foods high in animal protein. The lifetime risk of kidney stones is highest in the adult Caucasian man and is close to 20%. This incidence is three times greater than the average incidence in females. Caucasian women have the next highest incidence of stones (5% to 10%), followed by African-American women and men. However, African-America men demonstrate a higher incidence of stones associated with urinary tract infections caused by urea-splitting bacteria.[7]

Kidney stones are most prevalent between the ages of 20 and 40, although it is not unusual for the first stone to occur before the age of 20.[8] The peak age in men is 30 years. Women have a bimodal age distribution, with peaks at 35 and 55 years. In the United States, stone disease in children is usually related to metabolic alterations or a tendency to develop stones after urinary diversion.

The recurrence rate for stone formation is approximately 5% in the first year and as high as 50% within the first 5 years after the initial stone.[7,8] Fifty-five percent of those with recurrent stones have a family history of stones, which increases the risk of stone formation threefold.[9] Nonetheless, the genetic predisposition to stones is controversial, except for stones resulting from enzyme deficiencies (e.g., cystinuria and xanthinuria). In addition to a family history of kidney stones, other risk factors include insulin-resistant states, a history of hypertension or gout, primary hyperparathyroidism, chronic metabolic acidosis, and surgical menopause. Obesity is associated with insulin resistance and compensatory hyperinsulinemia, both of which can contribute to stone formation. In addition, body mass index and waist circumference have been positively associated with kidney stone formation in both men and women. Larger body size, irrespective of obesity, may result in the increased secretion of uric acid and oxalate, which are risk factors for calcium oxalate kidney stone formation.[10]

Excessive ingestion of substances that produce stones, such as purines (e.g., seafood, organ meats), oxalates (e.g., colas, chocolate), calcium (e.g., dairy products), and phosphate, increases the incidence of stone formation. Other predisposing factors include occupation (e.g., sedentary activity, risks of dehydration) and medications (e.g., acetazolamide, antacids, ascorbic acid in dosages of 2 g or more daily, hydrochlorothiazide, and indinavir [Crixivan]).

Environmental factors such as exposure to drinking water high in minerals may contribute to stone formation. Geographic variables such as a tropical climate may be a factor. Stone formation is somewhat greater in mountainous and high desert areas.[7] In the United States the incidence of stone formation is highest in the Southeast, but it is also prevalent in the Northwest and Southwest. Symptoms of complications related to urolithiasis tend to occur more often during the summer season.[2]

PATHOPHYSIOLOGY

The formation of urinary calculi is a multifaceted process. The natural sequence of urine changes leading to stone development include urine saturation, urine supersaturation, formation of crystalline materials, crystal nucleation, aggregation, retention of crystals by the urothelium, and continued growth of the stone on retained crystals.[6] Reduced urinary flow is the most common abnormality, and the most important factor to correct, with kidney stones. Any factor that reduces urinary flow, causes obstruction, or reduces urinary volume (e.g., dehydration or inadequate fluid intake) increases the risk of kidney stones.[7] The entire process is influenced by multiple chemical, physical, physical-chemical, biochemical, and physiologic events. The components of urinary stones include calcium oxalate, calcium phosphate, bacteria, purines, or cystine; the majority of stones are mixtures of two or more components.

The various types of stones include calcium, uric acid, struvite (magnesium ammonium phosphate [MAP]), cystine, and xanthine.[4] Calcium stones are the most common type and account for approximately 70% of all stones formed.[4] Approximately 26% of these stones are composed of pure calcium oxalate; 7% are pure calcium phosphate; and the remainder are a combination of calcium oxalate and calcium phosphate, a few of which may contain a uric acid core.[4] Calcium stones are radiopaque, tend to be limited to 1 cm (0.4 inch) in size, and differ in etiology. Urine levels of oxalate, normally a metabolic by-product, may increase as a result of the ingestion of foods high in oxalate such as rhubarb, nuts, cocoa, tea, beans, lime peel, and green leafy vegetables; this condition is termed *hyperoxaluria*. Hyperoxaluria may also develop with certain malabsorptive small bowel disorders, including Crohn's disease, jejunoileal bypass, celiac sprue, chronic pancreatitis, and biliary obstruction. The ingestion of ethylene glycol, a major component of antifreeze, can also result in hyperoxaluria. Primary hyperoxaluria, an enzyme deficiency, is one of the most severe of the diseases causing stone formation.[4] Urine saturation with uric acid, known as hyperuricosuria, may result in urate crystals that serve as a nidus for calcium oxalate nucleation. Hypocitraturia, in which citrate in the urine forms a highly soluble complex with calcium, is an important inhibitor of stone formation.

Conditions that cause reduced citrate excretion include distal renal tubular acidosis (RTA), diarrheal disorders, infection, exercise, starvation, and androgen and magnesium deficiency. RTA results in metabolic acidosis, defective urinary acidification, hypokalemia, and reduced urinary citrate concentrations. Metabolic acidosis increases bone resorption, resulting in increased calcium and phosphate concentration. Favorable conditions for calcium phosphate stone formation are high urine pH, reduced citrate excretion, and increased urinary concentration of calcium and phosphate. Stone formation is also encouraged by anatomic abnormalities that reduce urine flow or cause stasis, including horseshoe kidney, genitourinary diverticula, obstructive disorders, and medullary sponge kidney.

Uric acid stones account for 5% to 10% of all stones and are more prevalent in men. Uric acid is an end product of purine metabolism; increased uricosuria is often due to dehydration and excessive purine intake. Other risk factors include a consistently low urine pH, gout, myeloproliferative disorders, cytotoxic drugs, and conditions that predispose a patient to concentrated urine. Uric acid stones are radiolucent and appear as filling defects on the x-ray study.[4] Prevention involves reducing dietary purines, administering allopurinol to reduce uric acid excretion, and maintaining a urine volume of more than 2 L/day and a urinary pH of more than 6.0.[3] Alkalization of urine may help prevent and dissolve stones.

Struvite stones, composed of MAP, are also referred to as *infection stones*. Struvite stones account for approximately 10% to 15% of all stones, are more prevalent in women, and are often manifest as renal staghorn calculi. Struvite stones grow rapidly and recur frequently. Urease, a bacterial enzyme, precipitates urea splitting and results in high ammonium concentration and alkaline urine (pH range of 6.8 to 8.3). This elevated pH causes the MAP crystals to precipitate, creating the struvite stone. Struvite does not form in the absence of infection; the urinary infection is usually from *Proteus* organisms.

Cystinuria is a genetic abnormality in which there is an excessive urinary excretion of the amino acids cystine, ornithine, lysine, and arginine. The low solubility of cystine results in stone formation, accounting for 1% to 2% of all stones. Cystine stones are radiopaque and tend to be round. The peak incidence of cystine stones is in the second and third decade of life. Cystinuria should be suspected with stone formation in children.

Xanthinuria is caused by a congenital deficiency of the enzyme xanthine oxidase, which results in stone formation and increased excretion of xanthine. These stones are radiolucent and are often mistaken for uric acid stones.

CLINICAL PRESENTATION

Symptoms vary and depend on the size and location of the stones. Generally, symptoms include acute renal or ureteral colic, hematuria (microscopic or occult blood in the urine), urinary tract infection, or vague abdominal or flank pain.[7] Persons with renal colic often are initially seen with severe flank pain that may migrate anteriorly and into the groin as the stone moves from the kidney toward the bladder. Renal or ureteral colic is a result of the stone obstruction of the urinary tract. This obstruction is usually in one or more of five locations: (1) the calyx; (2) the ureteropelvic junction; (3) at or near the pelvic brim, where the ureter begins to arch over the iliac vessels; (4) the posterior pelvis, where the ureter is crossed anteriorly by the pelvic blood vessels and the broad ligament; and (5) the ureterovesical junction, which is the most constricted area.[4] Renal or ureteral colic is often associated with nausea and vomiting, gross hematuria, and dysuria. Fever may be present if infection occurs with the stone. Patients are often extremely restless as they attempt to find a comfortable position. Less often there may be persistent microhematuria or intermittent dull pain that extends over weeks or months. Once a stone enters the bladder, dysuria, frequency, and urgency may be the only symptoms. Once the stone passes out of the bladder, symptoms resolve.

PHYSICAL EXAMINATION

A careful medical history should be obtained and should include stone history, medical problems, medications, family history, occupation, diet, and fluid intake. The physical examination includes assessment of systemic symptoms; meticulous abdominal examination to exclude other sources of pain is essential. Typical examination findings include fever, tachycardia, diaphoresis, and costovertebral angle tenderness.

DIAGNOSTICS

Proper evaluation can identify the underlying cause of stone formation in up to 97% of patients.[11] Furthermore, up to 50% of all first-time stone formers will have a recurrence.[11] The cornerstone of diagnostics is a detailed history and physical, after which the appropriate laboratory work can be ordered.

Urinalysis and culture and sensitivity are essential to determine pH and to identify the presence of bacteria, crystals, and red blood cells. Hematuria may be microscopic or gross and occur with or without infection. An increase in the urine pH and the presence of crystals may give clues as to whether the stone is alkaline or acidic.[7] In addition, the urine should be strained for stone analysis. A CBC, a complete metabolic panel (SMA-20), serum calcium, and an intact parathyroid hormone (PTH) level should be obtained. If the cause is still unknown, a 24-hour urine sample with the patient on his or her usual diet should be obtained and measured for calcium, oxalate, citrate, magnesium, sodium, and sulfate.[7]

Urine pH above 6.5 suggests infection, and a follow-up culture is necessary.[11] Urine pH below 5.4 associated with metabolic acidosis is almost always RTA, whereas the presence of benzene crystals is diagnostic of cystinuria.[11] Elevated intact PTH levels and hypercalcemia are the result of either hyperparathyroidism (primary or secondary) or sarcoidosis.[11]

An abdominal x-ray study (flat plate) of the kidneys, ureter, and bladder will identify renal stones that are radiopaque and is helpful in documenting the number, size, and location of the stones in the urinary tract. A flat plate is also helpful in identifying nephrocalcinosis, hyperparathyroidism, primary hyperparathyroidism, primary hyperoxaluria, RTA, or sarcoidosis.[7]

A renal ultrasound will aid in diagnosis and can be used as a screening tool for hydronephrosis or stones within the

DIAGNOSTICS

Urinary Calculi

LABORATORY

Urinalysis and culture and sensitivity
CBC and differential
Complete metabolic panel
PTH
24-hour urine (for calcium oxalate, citrate, magnesium, sodium, and sulfate)*
Urine culture*

IMAGING

Abdominal x-rays (flat plate) of KUB*
Renal ultrasound
Cystoscopy*
IV pyelogram and intramuscular pyelogram with tomography*
CT scan*
Retrograde pyelography*

OTHER

Urine strain for stone analysis

*If indicated.

DIFFERENTIAL DIAGNOSIS

Urinary Calculi

- Gastroenteritis
- Salpingitis
- Ovarian cyst
- Peptic ulcer disease
- Aortic abdominal aneurysm
- Incarcerated inguinal hernia
- Acute appendicitis
- Ectopic and unrecognized pregnancy
- Diverticular disease
- Biliary stones
- Epididymitis
- Acute back strain
- Colitis
- Bowel obstruction
- Acute renal artery embolism
- Orchitis

kidney or renal pelvis. Renal ultrasonography can also determine the amount of renal parenchyma involved in an obstructed kidney.

The IV pyelogram (IVP) has long been considered the primary diagnostic tool for identifying urinary tract calculi, since it provides anatomic and functional information and can identify the size and location of the stone, the presence and severity of obstruction, and any renal and ureteral abnormalities.[7] However, it is important to remember that the IVP is contraindicated in patients with sensitivity to radiologic dye.

The CT scan (usually noncontrast) is thought to be the best radiographic tool for acute renal colic, since it creates images of the urinary tract and shows delayed penetration of IV contrast through the obstructed kidney, which is the hallmark of an acute urinary obstruction.[7,8] CT findings indicative of acute urinary obstruction because of a stone include renal enlargement, hydronephrosis, ureteral dilation, perinephric stranding, and periureteral edema.[12] For many reasons the CT is considered superior to an IVP in detecting renal ureteral calculi and is routinely performed on most patients in whom a diagnosis of urolithiasis is suspected.[7]

DIFFERENTIAL DIAGNOSIS

Urolithiasis can mimic other causes of visceral pain. Therefore it is essential to consider other causes of abdominal and flank pain such as appendicitis, cholecystitis, peptic ulcer, pancreatitis, ectopic pregnancy, and dissecting aortic aneurysm in persons with abdominal symptoms. Other diagnoses to consider are listed in the Differential Diagnosis box.

MANAGEMENT

Nonpharmacologic means of treatment should be used initially for all patients regardless of stone type. All patients with recurrent stones should have stone analysis to plan appropriate treatment. Stone management guidelines depend on the size and location of the stone, the presence or absence of associated infection, the presence of one or two kidneys, and the severity of symptoms. Most stones pass spontaneously without any residual damage. Urinary calculi 4 mm (0.16 inch) or less in diameter pass spontaneously in approximately 90% of patients. Stones 4 to 6 mm (0.16 to 0.24 inch) pass spontaneously in approximately 50% of patients, whereas stones larger than 6 mm (0.24 inch) pass without intervention in only 20% of patients. Stones larger than 8 mm (0.3 inch) pass in only 20% of patients and usually require surgical intervention.[12]

Larger stones were considered a major problem before the 1980s, when extensive surgical procedures were often needed. The morbidity associated with stone disease has been greatly reduced with the advent of extracorporeal techniques for stone treatment and with the refinement of endoscopic surgery. The three major endourologic procedures are extracorporeal shock wave lithotripsy (ESWL), percutaneous nephrolithotomy (PCNL), and ureteroscopy. ESWL is the least invasive treatment and the treatment of choice for 80% to 85% of stones.[13] It is indicated for stones that cannot be passed spontaneously, can be visualized on x-ray film, are located in the proximal ureter or kidney, and are less than 2.5 to 3 cm (1 to 1.2 inches). PCNL is the treatment of choice for renal and proximal ureteral stones larger than 2 to 3 cm (0.8 to 1.2 inches). Ureteroscopy, an emergency procedure, may be performed to relieve obstruction, to allow basket extraction of stones, or to allow lithotripsy of stones in the distal ureter.

Calcium stones are the most complex of all stones in their causes and treatments. The accepted theory of etiology is an imbalance between urinary excretion of insoluble salts and water, which results in an environment of supersaturation.[13] Therefore treatment is aimed at raising urine flow rate and reducing excretions of stone-forming salts. Stone formation associated with idiopathic hypercalciuria can be decreased with a twice-daily dose of thiazides and a low-calcium, low-protein, low-sodium diet. The use of thiazides has been shown to be beneficial in preventing renal stones, since thiazide diuretics decrease urinary calcium excretion by augmenting tubular reabsorption of calcium, but do not decrease intestinal absorption in absorptive hypercalciuria. However, the effect may be mitigated after 2 or more years of treatment.[8] Although the role of allopurinol is not well understood in the prevention of calcium stones, it has proven effectiveness in such cases. Calcium stones associated with hyperparathyroidism are best prevented by treatment of the underlying condition; referral to endocrinology is indicated. Administration of oral citrate or alkali replacement decreases the chances for stone formation.

The main cause of hyperoxaluria seems to be related to diet and is most easily regulated by omitting foods high in oxalate, such as colas, chocolate, and peanuts. Management of hyperoxaluria related to malabsorption syndromes is multifaceted and may include improvement of bowel function, reduced fat and oxalate intake, and the administration of calcium and cholestyramine. Pyridoxine, a co-factor in the alanine-glycoxylate pathway, may reduce the production of oxalate by reducing enzyme activity. In an observational study, high intake of vitamin B_6 (>40 mg/day) was inversely associated with oxalate stone formation in women.[8]

Hyperuricosuria, which is associated with calcium oxalate stones, is most simply managed by reducing the intake of foods that cause elevated uric acid excretion. Persistent stone formation may be treated with allopurinol, to inhibit uric acid synthesis and decrease urinary uric acid excretion. Potassium citrate should also be given to increase urine pH, since uric acid precipitates in acidic urine.[8]

Uric acid stones are managed most practically by maintaining a urinary output greater than 2 L/day and alkalinizing the urine.[14] Maintaining a urinary pH above 6.0 increases the solubility of urate ions, thereby decreasing stone formation. Avoidance of excessive purine intake may be beneficial. Commonly used alkalinizing agents are sodium bicarbonate and potassium citrate,[14] but limited evidence exists for their benefit.[15] Allopurinol, which inhibits the formation of uric acid, is commonly used when the patient fails to respond to diet control and alkalinizing agents, but again, only limited evidence exists for its benefit.[15]

Management of MAP (struvite) stones may require medical or surgical interventions. Antimicrobial therapy to sterilize the urine is necessary to treat infection.[8] It may also be necessary in the long term to slow the growth of stones or prevent the formation of new stones. It is not itself definitive therapy but may be valuable adjunctive therapy. Urease inhibitors may be used to prevent struvite formation or to slow the growth of existing calculi.[16] The most commonly used urease inhibitor is acetohydroxamic acid. Hydroxyurea, once thought to be a potent inhibitor, is no longer considered effective and also has demonstrated high toxicity rates. Irrigation with chemical solutions to dissolve the stone or stone fragments, called *chemolysis*, is no longer considered effective because of the risks of treatment and the length of time necessary for stone dissolution.[16] Surgical options include nephrolithotomy, ESWL, and PCNL. The American Urological Association Nephrolithiasis Guidelines Panel recommends that PCNL or a combination of PCNL and ESWL be the first-line treatment for struvite calculi.[16,17] ESWL is considered appropriate for small (2 cm [0.8 inch]) struvite calculi, and nephrolithotomy is an acceptable option for complex struvite calculi.

Prevention of cystine stones includes reduced intake of protein-rich foods and high intake of fluids (3 L/day). Alkalinization of urine (pH >7.0) may be of limited value given its tendency to precipitate the formation of calcium stones. D-Penicillamine or tiopronin (Thiola) may be prescribed to reduce stone formation. Among the more common side effects of long-term D-penicillamine therapy is vitamin B_{12} deficiency. Tiopronin has fewer side effects but still poses some risk for hematologic changes, fever, proteinuria, and rash. Prevention of xanthine stones includes high fluid intake and urinary alkalinization.

COMPLICATIONS

Renal calculi are associated with an increased risk of urinary tract infection with the potential for progression to pyelonephritis and sepsis.[7] Hydronephrosis, which is associated with partial or complete obstruction of the renal pelvis or ureter, is another possible complication. Additional potential sequelae include renal tissue damage and renal failure as a result of obstruction or stone movement and nephrocalcinosis as a result of deposition of calcium phosphate in the renal parenchyma.[5] If stones are bilateral, they can cause renal scarring and damage, which can result in acute and chronic renal failure.[7]

INDICATIONS FOR REFERRAL OR HOSPITALIZATION

Management of kidney or urinary tract stones often requires both medical and surgical intervention. Specific treatment depends on a number of factors, including stone type and location. The presence of infection or obstruction is an indication for urologic referral. Patients with persistent pain, gross hematuria, fever, or chills should be referred. Severe obstruction, infection, pain, and serious bleeding may require hospitalization.

PATIENT AND FAMILY EDUCATION

Patients suspected of having stones should be instructed to increase fluid intake, strain all urine, and use analgesics as necessary. An emphasis on healthy lifestyle habits such as regular exercise, generous fluid intake (2 to 4 L/day), and a balanced diet high in fiber is integral to stone prevention. Effective stone prevention depends on the stone type and identifying risk factors for stone formation. Therefore specific patient education is based on individual risk factors, the type of stone produced by the patient, a prescribed medical regimen, and co-morbidities. Research has demonstrated that obesity is a significant factor in stone formation with aging, since the majority of weight gain is from fat and not bone or muscle.[10] This increased risk may be greater in women than in men. Therefore the importance of exercise and weight management must be emphasized in any prevention program.

REFERENCES

1. Bernier F: Management of clients with urinary disorders. In Black J, Hawks J, editors: *Medical surgical nursing: clinical management for positive outcomes*, ed 7, St Louis, 2005, Mosby.
2. Wolf J: *Nephrolithiasis*, retrieved July 10, 2006, from http://www.emedicine.com/MED/topic1600.htm.

3. Stoller ML, Bolton DM: Urinary stone disease. In Tanagho EA, McAninch JW, editors: *Smith's general urology,* ed 14, Norwalk, Conn, 1995, Appleton & Lange.
4. Monk RD: Clinical approach to adults, *Semin Nephrol* 16(5):375-388, 1996.
5. Bruton DS, and others: Urinary calculi. In Karlowicz KA, editor: *Urologic nursing: principles and practice,* Philadelphia, 1995, Saunders.
6. Menon M, Parulkar BG, Drach G: Urinary lithiasis: etiology, diagnosis and medical management. In Walsh PC, Retik A, Vaughan ED Jr, and others, editors: *Campbell's urology,* ed 7, vol 2, Philadelphia, 1998, Saunders.
7. Colella J, Kochis E, Galli B, and others: Urolithiasis/nephrolithiasis: what's it all about? *Urol Nurs* 25(6):427-475, 2005.
8. Techman J: Acute renal colic from ureteral calculi, *N Engl J Med* 350:384-393, 2004.
9. Parmar M: Kidney stones, *Clin Rev* 328:1420-1424, 2004.
10. Taylor E, Stampfer M, Curhan G: Obesity, weight gain, and the risk of kidney stones, *JAMA* 293(4):455-462, 2005.
11. Rivers K, Shetty S, Menon M: When and how to evaluate a patient with nephrolithiasis, *Urol Clin North Am* 27(2):203-213, 2000.
12. Tanagho E, McAninch J: *Smith's general urology*, ed 16, Norwalk, Conn, 2004, Appleton & Lange.
13. Lingerman JE: Lithotripsy and surgery, *Semin Nephrol* 16(5):487-498, 1996.
14. Parks JH, Coe FL: Pathogenesis and treatment of calcium stones, *Semin Nephrol* 16(5):398-411, 1996.
15. Pearle MS, Roehrborn CG, Pak CY: Meta-analysis of randomized trials for the prevention of calcium oxalate nephrolithiasis, *J Endourol* 13(9):679-685, 1999.
16. Asplin JR: Uric acid stones, *Semin Nephrol* 16(5):412-425, 1996.
17. Meng M: *Struvite and staghorn calculi*, retrieved Feb 28, 2006, from http://www.emedicine.com/med/topic2834.htm.

PART 14

Evaluation and Management of Gynecologic Concerns

PATRICIA POLGAR BAILEY, *Section Editor*

CHAPTER 165

Amenorrhea

Marie Elena Botte

DEFINITION AND EPIDEMIOLOGY

Amenorrhea is the absence or abnormal cessation of menstrual bleeding.[1] Primary amenorrhea has been defined as the absence of both spontaneous uterine bleeding and secondary sexual characteristics (delayed puberty) at age 14 or by 2 years after sexual maturation,[2] or the absence of menarche at age 16 regardless of the presence of secondary sexual characteristics.[3,4] Secondary amenorrhea refers to the absence of menstrual bleeding by 18 months after menarche,[2] for 12 months, or three cycle lengths, in a woman with prior oligomenorrhea,[4] and the cessation of menstrual bleeding for 6 months in a woman with prior regular menses. Although the average age for menarche in the United States is 12.7 years[5] (12.8 years for Caucasian adolescents and slightly earlier, 12.6 years, for their African-American counterparts), there is a range of 9 to 16 years, and factors besides race such as nutritional status, body fat, and maternal age at menarche are also contributory.[2]

Primary amenorrhea has an estimated prevalence of between 0.1% and 0.3%.[4] Secondary amenorrhea is much more common, affecting between 1% and 3% of women of reproductive age in the general population.[6] Higher prevalence has been noted in specific subgroups of women, such as college students, endurance athletes (particularly runners[7,8] and elite athletes in sports that emphasize thinness or a specific weight, such as ballet),[9-11] and women who are obese.[12] The risk of amenorrhea seems to be highest in younger women who are more educated and older at menarche, as well as in users of oral contraceptives.

Up to 25% of female athletes experience exercise-induced amenorrhea.[13] The female athlete triad involves the combination of amenorrhea, osteoporosis, and disordered eating,[14,15] and in female college athletes disordered eating is estimated to be between 15% and 62%.[16] Women with systemic lupus erythematosus receiving pulse cyclophosphamide therapy are at increased risk of sustained amenorrhea, and women diagnosed with type 1 diabetes mellitus before menarche have an increased probability of delayed menarche and menstrual disturbances, including amenorrhea.[17] Approximately 2.5% of healthy adolescents will experience pubertal delay.[3]

PATHOPHYSIOLOGY

Aside from physiologic amenorrhea resulting from constitutional delay, pregnancy, lactation, or menopause, the pathophysiologic mechanisms for amenorrhea generally involve disorders of the sex chromosomes, hypothalamic-pituitary-ovarian axis, and related hormone production; the responsiveness of the uterine endometrium to various hormones; and the patency of the outflow tract. Because normal ovarian development depends on the presence of at least two X chromosomes, abnormalities involving X and Y chromosomes can result in gonadal failure, agonadism, gonadal dysgenesis, and androgen resistance (testicular feminization).[18] Problems with hypothalamic synthesis or release of gonadotropin-releasing hormone (GnRH) can result in hypogonadotropic hypogonadism. Müllerian agenesis, obstruction of the vaginal outflow tract (such as with an imperforate hymen), cervical stenosis, or transverse vaginal septa are structural causes for primary amenorrhea. Physiologic lesions such as tumors or adenomas,[19] systemic illness, or total-body and nodal irradiation may also contribute to the problem.[20-23]

Disorders of the hypothalamic-pituitary-ovarian axis can cause primary or secondary amenorrhea. Hypothalamic causes for dysfunction have been linked to weight loss, intensive exercise,[24] starvation, eating disorders, and psychogenic stress[25,26] in nonathletic, normal weight women, and can result in pubertal delay or secondary hormonal insufficiency. Some authors have proposed that a central signal related to a deficit in energy results in a reduction of mean and pulsatile gonadotropin secretion and diminished estradiol concentration in the early follicular phase of affected women.[11] Recent studies indicate that leptin, a hormone secreted by adipocytes whose main function is to signal energy availability in energy-deficient states, may have a major role in the regulation, synthesis, and secretion of sex steroids, gonadotropins, and GnRH.[27-29]

The physiologic mechanism resulting in amenorrhea and hypothalamic dysfunction associated with anorexia nervosa has yet to be fully elucidated, but it is believed that altered neuroregulation of neuropeptides, including leptin and neuropeptide Y, may contribute to persistent amenorrhea even after weight gain in anorexics with low initial body mass index (BMI).[30] Persistent amenorrhea has also been correlated with a longer duration of eating disorders and the presence of a concomitant anxiety disorder.[31] The majority of young women with amenorrhea are estrogen deficient; a minority have normal estrogen levels that are unopposed by progesterone secondary to anovulation.[6]

One study found that among anorectic and bulimic women, those with amenorrhea had a mean percent of ideal body weight, as defined by Metropolitan Life Insurance Company criteria, of 74% ±1%, compared with 102% ±19% for those who were menstruating.[31] Another study found no statistically significant association between amenorrhea and BMI but did note an association between amenorrhea and fasting or purging behaviors in normal and above-weight teenagers that was most evident in the heaviest subjects.[32] Neurotransmitter abnormalities (central dopaminergic and opioid activity) may modulate the response of luteinizing hormone (LH) to GnRH.[33] Amenorrhea can also be seen in obese patients; reduction of body fat can bring about return of regular menstrual flow.

Prolactinemia associated with amenorrhea following normal puberty may be caused by breastfeeding, microadenomas or macroadenomas of the pituitary, renal failure, or the use of medications (e.g., psychoactive drugs such as haloperidol, amitriptyline, benzodiazepines, cocaine). Studies have suggested that (1) suppression of normal ovarian cyclic activity in women with pituitary microadenomas may be mediated by hyperprolactinemia, which blocks the action of gonadotropin at the ovarian level, and (2) that anovulation associated with hyperprolactinemic amenorrhea is primarily caused by both impaired gonadotropin pulsatility and derangement of the estrogen-positive feedback effect on LH in the face of a continued ovarian response to gonadotropin.[34,35] In polycystic ovary syndrome, a low ratio of progesterone to estrogen is associated with menstrual irregularity[36] and amenorrhea.

Certain drugs, such as chemotherapeutic agents[37] or thalidomide,[38] may affect menstruation. Transient amenorrhea can also result from administration of leuprolide (Lupron) in the treatment of fibroids or endometriosis, from elicit heroin use,[39] or from gabapentin.[40] Autoimmune disorders, such as Addison's disease, hypothyroidism, and toxic thyroiditis, have also been associated with amenorrhea, perhaps as a result of connections between genes controlling reproductive function and genes associated with autoimmune conditions on a segment of the major histocompatibility complex.[41] In thalassemic patients with secondary amenorrhea, severe and progressive damage to the hypothalamic-pituitary axis has been demonstrated by gonadotropin pulse abnormalities, marked reduction in GnRH-stimulated gonadotropin levels, and even apulsatility.[42]

CLINICAL PRESENTATION

Relevant history in the evaluation of amenorrhea includes a thorough menstrual history (age at menarche, frequency, duration, flow, last menstrual period, history of missed menses). A complete sexual history (number of partners; date of last intercourse; method of birth control and percentage of use; number of pregnancies, abortions, miscarriages, or ectopic pregnancies; and surgical history), as well as the age at menarche and menopause for family members and any family history of infertility, is also necessary.

Probable signs of past ovulatory cycles include breast tenderness, cyclic abdominal pain or bloating, and changes in the cervical mucus. The past medical history should be examined specifically for autoimmune disorders, childhood onset of type 1 diabetes mellitus, previous irradiation or chemotherapy, frequent fractures or osteoporosis, and thyroid or adrenal dysfunction. A complete medication history regarding prescribed, over-the-counter, and illicit drug use should be obtained. Nutritional and exercise factors, including disordered eating behavior, recent weight loss or gain, and athletic training, are evaluated, along with endocrinologic markers of growth and development (growth charts and the presence or absence of secondary sexual characteristics, specifically breast development and pubic hair).

A review of systems may reveal indications of systemic illness such as thyroid dysfunction, headaches, or visual disturbances (possibly indicating a cranial mass in the area of the pituitary or hypothalamus), galactorrhea, or signs of hyperandrogenism (hirsutism, truncal obesity, deepening of the voice) or hypoestrogenism (hot flashes, vaginal dryness, headaches, depression, dyspareunia, decreasing breast size). A social history may indicate substance abuse or stressful life events (e.g., going away to college, entering religious life or the armed forces, sudden changes in the environment, death or divorce in the family), which have been linked with amenorrhea.[20,22]

PHYSICAL EXAMINATION

In addition to an evaluation of general growth and development (congenital short stature together with neck webbing and a pigeon chest suggests Turner's syndrome), the physical examination may reveal signs of androgen excess (hirsutism, acne, male pattern hair loss, truncal obesity, clitoromegaly >1 cm [0.4 inch]), androgen insensitivity (complete absence of axillary and pubic hair), hyperprolactinemia (galactorrhea on breast examination), decreased estrogen status (pale, dry vaginal mucosa; scant cervical mucus), or eating disorders (cachexia, hypothermia, lanugo hair, decreased blood pressure, bradycardia, dry skin, tooth decay, chipmunk cheeks, Chvostek's sign). Assessment of visual acuity and a funduscopic examination are important because vision changes or retinal abnormalities may reflect an intracranial mass. The thyroid is palpated for masses or nodules. A pelvic examination assesses estrogen status via vaginal epithelium and cervical mucus; may identify an imperforate hymen; and also provides a gross evaluation of the cervix, uterus, and ovaries. Presumptive signs of pregnancy include breast tenderness, a bluish cervix (Chadwick's sign), fatigue, nausea, vomiting, and urinary frequency. Probable signs of pregnancy are an enlarged uterus, a positive pregnancy test, and softening of the lower uterine segment (Goodell's and Hegar's signs). Enlarged ovaries are palpable in 60% of women with polycystic ovary syndrome[22] and, in combination with acne, obesity, and acanthosis nigricans, suggest this diagnosis. Abdominal striae on nulliparous women may be indicative of hypercortisolism, and skin tags, fissures, and fecal occult blood may indicate inflammatory bowel disease.

DIAGNOSTICS

The possibility of pregnancy or lactation-induced amenorrhea must be excluded in all women before any other diagnostic evaluation is initiated. Next, follicle-stimulating hormone (FSH) and LH should be checked to detect anovulation, thyroid-stimulating hormone (TSH) to evaluate for hypothyroidism, and prolactin levels to check for hyperprolactinemia or possibly for an early presentation of acromegaly, which produces excess prolactin and growth hormone. The best time to obtain a prolactin level is early in the morning after a 12-hour fast. There should be no stimulation of the breasts before the serum level is drawn. If prolactin levels are elevated, a CT scan of the sella turcica to identify microadenomas and macroadenomas is necessary. If these tests are normal, a progesterone challenge test, which classically consists of 10 mg of medroxyprogesterone administered daily for 5 to 7 days, can be used to further evaluate estrogen status. Any vaginal bleeding within 2 to 7 days after the cessation of progesterone signals a positive progesterone challenge, indicating both adequate estrogen stores and patency of the outflow tract. A negative progesterone challenge (i.e., no bleeding 2 to 7 days after cessation of progesterone) indicates either inadequate estrogen stores or an obstruction of the outflow tract. To further differentiate hypoestrogenism from obstruction, the test can be repeated after daily administration of 2.5 mg of estrogen for 21 days, followed by 10 mg of progesterone for the next 5 days. If there is still no withdrawal bleeding, investigation into structural or outflow reasons for the amenorrhea should ensue.

If amenorrhea is secondary to anovulation, potential causes include Cushing's syndrome, adrenal or ovarian tumors, premature ovarian failure, or, more commonly, polycystic ovary syndrome. An FSH level elevated beyond 20 IU/L after repeated measurements is indicative of ovarian failure. An elevated LH/FSH ratio (>0.2) is suggestive of polycystic ovary syndrome; an FSH greater than 30 mIU/ml indicates menopausal status.

To differentiate between pituitary and hypothalamic amenorrhea, an LH-releasing hormone test is generally performed in conjunction with imaging of the sellar region by CT or MRI. Research shows that long-term administration of pulsatile GnRH can indicate hypothalamic amenorrhea by an ovulatory response within two treatment cycles and confirms the diagnosis in an area where diagnosis has generally been made by exclusion.[43] In the absence of an ovulatory response, a pituitary cause for the amenorrhea should be suspected.

DIAGNOSTICS

Amenorrhea

LABORATORY
Serum human chorionic gonadotropin
Thyroid profile
Thyroid antibodies*
Luteinizing hormone
Follicle-stimulating hormone
Prolactin
DHEA
Serum electrolytes
Serum glucose
BUN
Creatinine
ESR
Urinary free cortisol*
Glucose tolerance test*

IMAGING
CT or MRI*

OTHER
Clomiphene challenge test

*If indicated.

MRI has been shown to be an effective and accurate tool for evaluating the cause of primary amenorrhea and planning for surgery, particularly when this involves congenital disorders of sexual differentiation and localization of the gonads.[44] MRI of the sellar region is also important in the assessment of pituitary adenomas and is more effective than CT in detecting empty sella syndrome.[43] A hysterosalpingogram or sonohystogram can be used to outline the uterine cavity if a bicornuate uterus or double cervix is suspected.

Other diagnostic tests that may be useful in particular situations include the clomiphene challenge test, which may provide information necessary to make an early diagnosis of waning ovarian function in hypergonadotropic amenorrhea.[45] Increased serum dehydroepiandrosterone (DHEA) (>700 mg/dl) indicates an adrenal origin for androgens in women with hirsutism, and elevated plasma testosterone levels (>90 ng/dl) suggest tumors of adrenal and ovarian origin or congenital adrenal hyperplasia; levels above 200 ng/dl are found in the rare Sertoli-Leydig cell tumors.[46] The level of sex hormone–binding globulin, which binds potent androgens such as testosterone and thereby controls the level of active androgens in circulation, may also provide useful clinical information.

Chemistry profiles (including serum electrolytes, serum glucose, BUN, and creatinine), urinary free cortisol, thyroid antibodies, an erythrocyte sedimentation rate, and a glucose tolerance test can help differentiate possible causes of autoimmune-related amenorrhea, such as Addison's disease, diabetes mellitus, thyroiditis, and hypoparathyroidism. This is especially important considering that 20% to 40% of cases of premature ovarian failure are associated with autoimmune disease.[4] The diagnosis of premature ovarian failure in a young woman (generally under age 25 or 30 years) warrants karyotyping to exclude the presence of a Y chromosome.

DIFFERENTIAL DIAGNOSIS

Primary Amenorrhea

Physiologic primary amenorrhea may be attributable to constitutional delay, although 97% to 99% of young women experience menarche by age 16 years[22,47] and 95% by 14.5 years.[5] Failure of the gonads to develop normally accounts for half of all cases of primary amenorrhea.[48] Other possible causes include Turner's syndrome (45,X)[49]; mosaicism; abnormal X chromosomes; the presence of an intact or fragmented Y chromosome; complex chromosomal rearrangement[50]; chromosomal deletions[51]; pure gonadal dysgenesis (may manifest with hyperandrogenism); and the rare 17α-hydroxylase deficiency, which is seen with hypernatremia, hypokalemia, and hypocortisolism.[48]

Additional causes of primary amenorrhea include structural abnormalities (imperforate hymen, transverse septum, congenital absence of the uterus or vagina), premature ovarian failure (may be idiopathic or secondary to radiation or chemotherapeutics), malnutrition, systemic illness, tumors (ovarian, hypothalamic, parasellar, or adrenal), and any of the disturbances in the hypothalamic-pituitary-ovarian axis that also cause secondary amenorrhea. In one retrospective study the most common causes of primary amenorrhea were hypergonadotropic amenorrhea secondary to ovarian failure and congenital absence of the uterus and vagina.[52]

Rare causes of primary amenorrhea include gonadal dysgenesis caused by chromosomal translocation, mutations in the beta subunit of FSH, vaginal inversion and uterus acollis, multiple endocrine neoplasia, progesterone-producing adrenal adenoma, increased melatonin secretion from a cystic pineal lesion, and childhood trauma.

Secondary Amenorrhea

Pregnancy is the most common cause of secondary amenorrhea; lactation and early menopause are other physiologic possibilities. Transient amenorrhea may occur in the first 2 postmenarchal years, after discontinuation of oral contraceptives, and in the majority of women who receive medroxyprogesterone (Depo-Provera) for contraception.[22,53] Aside from these causes, secondary amenorrhea is most often linked to disordered functioning somewhere along the hypothalamic-pituitary-ovarian axis.

Other causes of secondary amenorrhea include premature ovarian failure and chronic anovulatory disorder (polycystic ovary syndrome, obesity-related disorder, idiopathic disorder). Less common conditions include pituitary tumors, hyperprolactinemia, Sheehan's syndrome (postpartum pituitary necrosis), hypogonadotropic hypogonadism, thyroid disease, tuberculosis, and late-onset 21-hydroxylase deficiency. For the

DIFFERENTIAL DIAGNOSIS

Amenorrhea

PRIMARY AMENORRHEA

- Structural abnormalities
- Premature ovarian failure
- Malnutrition
- Systemic illness
- Tumors: ovarian, hypothalamic, parasellar, or adrenal
- Disturbance of hypothalamic-pituitary-ovarian axis
- Gonadal dysgenesis (chromosomal translocation)
- Vaginal inversion
- Uterus acollis
- Multiple endocrine neoplasia
- Trauma
- Cystic pineal lesion
- Turner's syndrome
- 17α-Hydroxylase deficiency

SECONDARY AMENORRHEA

- Pregnancy
- Lactation
- Menopause and perimenopause
- Medications (oral contraceptives, reserpine, metoclopramide, medroxyprogesterone)
- Disorder of hypothalamic-pituitary-ovarian axis
- Premature ovarian failure
- Chronic anovulatory disorder (polycystic ovary syndrome, obesity-related disorder, idiopathic disorder)
- Sheehan's syndrome
- Hypogonadotropic hypogonadism
- Thyroid disease
- Tuberculosis
- Late-onset 21-hydroxylase deficiency
- Pituitary tumor
- Hyperprolactinemia

majority of women a clinical history; physical examination; and laboratory determination of TSH, LH, FSH, and prolactin levels are sufficient for diagnosis.

Categorization of amenorrhea by etiology (hyperprolactinemic, hyperandrogenic, hypergonadotropic, and hypogonadotropic) provides a helpful framework for consideration of the differential diagnosis, evaluation, and management.

Hyperprolactinemic amenorrhea can be caused by drugs (including reserpine, phenothiazines, oral contraceptives, metoclopramide, and α-methyldopa), prolactin-secreting tumors of the pituitary, or systemic illnesses such as acromegaly or hypothyroidism. Physiologic causes for increased prolactin levels include lactation and nipple stimulation. For this reason, prolactin levels are most helpful when drawn before a clinical breast examination.

Hyperandrogenic amenorrhea is seen most commonly in women with polycystic ovary syndrome[54] (also called hyperandrogenic chronic anovulation or Stein-Leventhal syndrome) but may also be caused by obesity, Cushing's syndrome, hyperprolactinemia, thyroid disease, adrenal disease (hyperplasia, adenoma, carcinoma), androgen-secreting ovarian tumors, or drug abuse.[4,21]

Hypergonadotropic amenorrhea affects about 1% of women under the age of 40 years. The differential diagnosis for ovarian failure includes chromosomal (mosaicism and gonadal dysgenesis), autoimmune (Hashimoto's thyroiditis, Addison's disease, diabetes mellitus, hypoparathyroidism), metabolic (ovarian enzymatic defects), familial, infectious (mumps), idiopathic, or iatrogenic (irradiation, chemotherapy) causes, as well as resistant ovary syndrome.[55]

Hypogonadotropic amenorrhea can be a result of emotional or physical stress (including athletic training), depression, nutritional deficiency, weight loss, eating disorders, thyroid or adrenal dysfunction, isolated gonadotropin deficiency (Kallmann's syndrome), or hypothalamic or pituitary lesions (craniopharyngiomas, germinomas, pituitary adenomas, endodermal sinus tumors, pituitary apoplexy, empty sella syndrome, postpartum ischemia, necrosis of the pituitary gland).[4,55] Amenorrhea is one of the cardinal features of anorexia nervosa. Head injuries (especially head-on automobile collisions resulting in whiplash) and external irradiation can damage the hypothalamus[56]; infections (tuberculosis, HIV) can disrupt pituitary function.[57]

In addition to disorders of the hypothalamic-pituitary-ovarian axis, secondary amenorrhea can be due to uterine pathologic conditions, including endometrial hyperplasia, postpartum uterine adhesions, or iatrogenic Asherman's syndrome. Rare causes of secondary amenorrhea include hydrocephalus, Pendred's syndrome, onchocerciasis, inhibin-secreting ovarian tumors,[58] Sjögren's syndrome,[59] and neurosarcoidosis.

MANAGEMENT

Women with eating disorders, such as anorexia nervosa, are best managed in collaboration with psychiatric or other specialized eating disorder services. Evidence of anatomic or endocrinologic abnormalities mandates co-management with the appropriate specialist. In amenorrhea caused by systemic illness or endocrinopathy, treatment of the underlying cause, such as diabetes mellitus or hypothyroidism, generally resolves the amenorrhea as a result of renewed ovarian function.[2] Spontaneous recovery of menses after diagnosis of premature ovarian failure,[60] after prolonged irradiation-induced ovarian failure from treatment of Hodgkin's disease, and in cases of chemotherapy-induced ovarian failure also occurs[23,57,61]; there is evidence to suggest that taxane, as an adjuvant agent, may help prevent chemotherapy-related amenorrhea[37] and that the use of oral contraceptives during chemotherapy may also decrease posttreatment amenorrhea.[61] Gonadal function should be reassessed periodically in these women, and oral contraceptives are a good choice for hormone replacement in women not desiring pregnancy.[57]

Menses generally return between 6 and 14 months after a last injection of medroxyprogesterone and within 6 months after stopping oral contraceptives in post–oral contraceptive amenorrhea. Eventual return of menstruation has been shown, after a variable interval, for less than half of women with medically refractory menorrhagia after endometrial ablation and uterine resection.[62] In perimenopausal women amenorrheic intervals are common and do not require any treatment aside from adequate contraception when pregnancy is not desired; in these women unplanned pregnancy is possible unless FSH levels have been consistently elevated (>30 mIU/ml) and the amenorrhea has been present for more than 1 year.[63]

Complete recovery of gonadal function in hypothalamic amenorrhea depends on restoration of the hypothalamic-pituitary-adrenal and the hypothalamic-pituitary-thyroidal axes,[64,65] and so psychologic interventions that focus on changing behaviors and attitudes[66] and pharmacologic interventions that target the resultant hormonal dysfunction are often necessary. Several studies have demonstrated the effectiveness of lifestyle modifications, including diet and exercise, for the recovery of regular menses,[67] and multidisciplinary approaches to treatment are generally encouraged.[15] Whereas women with anorexia or other eating disorders and endurance athletes have benefited from increased caloric intake and decreased exercise,[21] some overweight and hirsute women with hyperandrogenism may recover normal menses with control of excess body weight via caloric restriction.[4] One study found that menses returned at approximately 90% of standard body weight and that 86% of women who attained this weight gain experienced menstrual return within 6 months.[65] Another study stressed the individual nature of weight targets and noted that these can often be predicted by the weight at which previous menstrual function ceased.[67]

Recombinant human leptin has been used in research settings in women with hypothalamic amenorrhea,[27,68] resulting in normalization of levels of reproductive hormones, follicular development, and menstrual cyclicity.[28] GnRH administration on alternate days has been used to increase FSH levels, reinstate LH pulsatility, and, in conjunction with clomiphene therapy, induce ovulation in women with weight loss–associated amenorrhea.[69] Naltrexone hydrochloride, an oral antiopioid, has also been studied as an agent in the management of amenorrhea resulting from hypogonadotropic syndromes.[66]

Estrogen, the current standard of pharmacologic care, does not address the underlying infertility or neuroendocrine dysfunction associated with hypothalamic amenorrhea, but use of oral contraceptives by these women has been shown to improve lumbar spine and total body bone mineral density.[70] Supplemental estrogen and progesterone (as with oral contraceptives) have been recommended for the prevention of further bone loss and subsequent fracture development in women with decreased estrogen levels,[71] although normalizing body weight is the single most important factor in regaining bone density.[72] Irreversible bone loss can occur after 3 years of amenorrhea, and although scant direct evidence supports the use of hormone replacement therapy in amenorrheic women,[16] there is some evidence that taking long-term triphasic oral contraceptives can increase total lumbar spine bone mineral density in women with hypothalamic amenorrhea and osteopenia[73] and improve both endothelial function and dyslipidemia in amenorrheic athletes.[74] Adequate calcium and, if indicated, vitamin D intake or supplementation plus weight-bearing exercise should be encouraged in women who are amenorrheic for any reason to help maintain bone density.

Administration of estrogen and progesterone is also necessary after hysteroscopic adhesiolysis to reestablish a functional endometrium in women with Asherman's syndrome.[6] No treatment is required if women maintain normal estradiol and prolactin levels in post–oral contraceptive amenorrhea.[75] Amenorrhea caused by onchocerciasis has been reversed with ivermectin,[76] and amenorrhea caused by heroin use has been reversed with methadone maintenance.[39]

Bromocriptine has been widely studied with demonstrated effectiveness for promoting menstrual bleeding and ovulation and for years has been the drug of choice for hyperprolactinemic amenorrhea and the syndrome of galactorrhea-amenorrhea.[75,77] In case of relapse, this treatment should be resumed and continued. More recently, cabergoline has been shown to be more effective and better tolerated than bromocriptine, with fewer gastrointestinal symptoms.[78-80] Subcutaneous pulsatile GnRH therapy combined with human chorionic gonadotropin has also been proposed as a method of ovulation induction if these women should desire pregnancy.[35]

LIFE SPAN CONSIDERATIONS

The prognosis regarding present or future fertility is a major concern of many women with amenorrhea and will guide the treatment plan in most instances. For women with hypothalamic amenorrhea resulting from stress, weight loss, or exercise, reassurance regarding the reversible nature of the problem after requisite lifestyle modification may be all that is necessary. For other women, such as those with premature ovarian failure or structural or chromosomal abnormalities incompatible with achieving a natural pregnancy, alternatives such as adoption, egg donation, or surrogacy may need to be considered.

COMPLICATIONS

Untreated amenorrhea is associated with significant long-term morbidity, especially when it occurs in younger women.[6] Loss of body weight is adversely related to pituitary-ovarian function, and in 20% to 30% of women with weight loss–related amenorrhea no restoration of function is attained despite recovery of body weight.[69]

Hypoestrogenemic amenorrhea has been associated with an increased risk of osteoporosis and fractures.[16,81,82] One study found that the bone density of women with primary amenorrhea was significantly lower than the bone density of women with secondary amenorrhea and that 21 out of 27 patients studied had osteopenia, a higher rate than that reported for postmenopausal women.[71] Another study of women with amenorrhea found hypoestrogenism and lower spine, wrist, and metatarsal bone mineral density, which remained below control levels despite a return of menses in some subjects.[81] Although some improvements in bone mineral density have been observed with appropriate treatment for amenorrhea, this recovery in bone mass has not been substantial,[83] again emphasizing the importance of early diagnosis and treatment.[14]

The hypoestrogenemic state has also been associated with endothelial dysfunction, unfavorable lipid profiles, and a significantly increased risk of cardiovascular events.[84,85] Anovulatory amenorrhea puts women at increased risk for endometrial hyperplasia and endometrial carcinoma. Women with polycystic ovary syndrome have a threefold increased risk of developing hypertension and a sixfold increased risk of developing type 2 diabetes mellitus; a sevenfold increased risk for coronary heart disease is seen in women with chronic hyperandrogenic anovulation.[4]

INDICATIONS FOR REFERRAL OR HOSPITALIZATION

Suspected or confirmed genetic abnormalities that result in primary or secondary amenorrhea warrant referral to a specialist for more thorough evaluation. Young women with either Y chromosome fragments or an entire Y chromosome will need to have their gonads removed after pubertal development is complete because of the increased risk of malignant gonadoblastoma.[48] Referral to an infertility specialist is particularly indicated for women with ovarian reserve factors, anovulatory cycles, hyperprolactinemia, and genetic or structural factors.

Hospitalization may be necessary for women with anorexia nervosa who have lost more than 30% of their desired body weight and fail to gain weight, as well as for those with suicidal ideation.[53] Inpatient surgical care may be indicated for women with tumors or adenomas associated with amenorrhea.

PATIENT AND FAMILY EDUCATION AND HEALTH PROMOTION

Women will have varying educational needs depending on the cause of their amenorrhea, but all women should receive basic nutritional counseling with an emphasis on obtaining sufficient calcium via either food sources or supplementation. Women should also be reminded that pregnancy can occur in the presence of amenorrhea; sexually active women not desiring pregnancy, especially adolescents, should receive appropriate contraceptive counseling. Women with genetic or congenital abnormalities may wonder about their ability to become pregnant and need to be apprised of their reproductive potential. The necessity for gonadectomy to prevent future malignancies should be discussed with women who have Y chromosome fragments or a Y chromosome.

The reversible nature of most cases of hypothalamic amenorrhea resulting from stress, weight changes, or exercise, as well as the temporary (6 months or less) duration of post–oral contraceptive amenorrhea, can be stressed when relevant. When counseling athletes, the health care provider should remind them, as well as trainers and coaches, that amenorrhea can be an indication of overtraining and can contribute to future performance deficits, especially in light of the long-term health consequences, such as fractures and osteoporosis.[13,86,87] As with hypoestrogenemic women, women with androgen excess are at increased risk of lipid abnormalities and coronary artery disease.[13] Counseling may be required in an effort to reduce other contributing risk factors, such as obesity.

REFERENCES

1. Practice Committee of the American Society for Reproductive Medicine: Current evaluation of amenorrhea, *Fertility Sterility* 82(1):266-272, 2004.
2. Pletcher J, Slap G: Adolescent gynecology, part 1, Common disorders, *Pediatr Clin North Am* 46(3):505-518, 1999.
3. Rosen D, Foster C: Delayed puberty, *Pediatr Rev* 22(9):309-315, 2001.
4. Kiningham RB, Apgar BS, Schwenk TL: Evaluation of amenorrhea, *Am Fam Phys* 53(4):1185-1194, 1996.
5. Mitan L, Slap G: Adolescent menstrual disorders, *Med Clin North Am* 84(4):851-868, 2000.
6. Schachter M, Shoham Z: Amenorrhea during the reproductive years: is it safe? *Fertility Sterility* 62(1):1-16, 1994.
7. Fogelholm M, Van Marken Lichtenbelt W, Ottenheijm R, and others: Amenorrhea in ballet dancers in the Netherlands, *Med Sci Sports Exerc* 28(5):545-550, 1996.
8. Klock SC, DeSouza MJ: Eating disorder characteristics and psychiatric symptomatology of eumenorrheic and amenorrheic runners, *Int J Eat Disord* 17(2):161-166, 1995.
9. Torstveit MK, Sundgot-Borgen J: Participation in leanness sports but not training volume is associated with menstrual dysfunction: a national survey of 1276 elite athletes and controls, *Br J Sports Med* 39(3):141-147, 2005.
10. Stokic E, Srdic B, Barak O: Body mass index, body fat mass and the occurrence of amenorrhea in ballet dancers, *Gynecol Endocrinol* 20(4):195-199, 2005.
11. Stafford DE: Altered hypothalamic-pituitary-ovarian axis function in young female athletes: implications and recommendations for management, *Treat Endocrinol* 4(3):147-154, 2005.
12. Linne Y: Effects of obesity on women's reproduction and complications during pregnancy, *Obesity Rev* 5(3):137-143, 2004.
13. Warren MP: Clinical review 77: evaluation of secondary amenorrhea, *J Clin Endocrinol Metab* 81(2):437-442, 1996.
14. Goodman LR, Warren MP: The female athlete and menstrual function, *Curr Opin Obstet Gynecol* 17(5):466-470, 2005.
15. Waldrop J: Early identification and interventions for female athlete triad, *J Pediatr Health Care* 19(4):213-220, 2005.
16. Hobart J, Smucker D: The female athlete triad, *Am Fam Phys* 61(11):3357-3364, 3367, 2000.
17. Yeshaya A, Orvieto R, Dicker D, and others: Menstrual characteristics and women suffering from insulin-dependent diabetes mellitus, *Int J Fertil Menopausal Stud* 40(5):269-273, 1995.
18. Warren MP, Hagey AR: The genetics, diagnosis and treatment of amenorrhea, *Minerva Ginecologica* 56(5):437-455, 2004.
19. Page LK, LeMaire WJ: Prolactin-producing pituitary adenomas, *J Microsurg* 1(3):182-186, 1979.
20. Tolis G, Diamante E: Distress amenorrhea, *Ann NY Acad Sci* 771:660-664, 1995.
21. Epp SL: The diagnosis and treatment of athletic amenorrhea, *Phys Assist* 4(3):129-144, 1997.
22. Chikotas N: Secondary amenorrhea, *J Am Acad Nurse Pract* 7(9):453-460, 1995.
23. Halyard MY, Cornella JL, Grado GL, and others: Prolonged amenorrhea associated with total nodal irradiation for Hodgkin's disease, *J Natl Med Assoc* 88(6):391-393, 1996.
24. Punpilai S, Sujitra T, Ouyporn T, and others: Menstrual status and bone mineral density among female athletes, *Nurs Health Sci* 7(4):259-265, 2005.
25. Genazzani AD: Neuroendocrine aspects of amenorrhea related to stress, *Pediatr Endocrinol Rev* 2(4):661-668, 2005.
26. Fioroni L, Fava M, Genazzani AD, and others: Life events impact in patients with secondary amenorrhoea, *J Psychosom Res* 38(6):617-622, 1994.
27. Chan JL, Mantzoros CS: Role of leptin in energy-deprivation states: normal human physiology and clinical implications for hypothalamic amenorrhoea and anorexia nervosa, *Lancet* 366(9479):74-85, 2005.
28. Welt CK, Chan JL, Bullen J, and others: Recombinant human leptin in women with hypothalamic amenorrhea, *N Engl J Med* 351(10):987-997, 2004.
29. Ahima RS: Body fat, leptin, and hypothalamic amenorrhea [comment], *N Engl J Med* 351(10):959-962, 2004.
30. Oswiecimska J, and others: Prospective evaluation of leptin and neuropeptide Y (NPY) serum levels in girls with anorexia nervosa, *Neuroendocrinol Lett* 26(4):301-304, 2005.

31. Copeland PM, Sacks NR, Herzog DB: Longitudinal follow-up of amenorrhea in eating disorders, *Psychosom Med* 57(2):121-126, 1995.
32. Selzer R, Caust J, Hibbert M, and others: The association between secondary amenorrhea and common eating disordered weight control practices in an adolescent population, *J Adolesc Health* 19(1):56-61, 1996.
33. Golden NH, Shenker IR: Amenorrhea in anorexia nervosa: neuroendocrine control of hypothalamic dysfunction, *Int J Eating Dis* 16(1):53-60, 1994.
34. Luboshitzky R, Lavi S, Thuma I, and others: Nocturnal melatonin and luteinizing hormone rhythms in women with hyperprolactinemic amenorrhea, *J Pineal Res* 20(2):72-78, 1996.
35. Matsuzaki T, and others: Mechanism of anovulation in hyperprolactinemic amenorrhea determined by pulsatile gonadotropin-releasing hormone injection combined with human chorionic gonadotropin, *Fertility Sterility* 62(6):1143-1149, 1994.
36. Doi SA, and others: Irregular cycles and steroid hormones in polycystic ovary syndrome, *Hum Reprod* 20(9):2402-2408, 2005.
37. Davis AL, Klitus M, Mintzer DM: Chemotherapy-induced amenorrhea from adjuvant breast cancer treatment: the effect of the addition of taxanes, *Clin Breast Cancer* 6(5):421-424, 2005.
38. Dharia SP, Steinkampf MP, Cater C: Thalidomide-induced amenorrhea: case report and literature review, *Fertility Sterility* 82(2):460-462, 2004.
39. Schmittner J, and others: Menstrual cycle length during methadone maintenance, *Addiction* 100(6):829-836, 2005.
40. Berger JJ: Amenorrhea in a patient after treatment with gabapentin for complex regional pain syndrome type II, *Clin J Pain* 20(3):192-194, 2004.
41. Jin K, and others: Reproductive failure and the major histocompatibility complex, *Am J Hum Genet* 56(6):1456-1467, 1995.
42. Chatterjee R, and others: Prospective study of the hypothalamic-pituitary axis in thalassaemic patients who developed secondary amenorrhea, *Clin Endocrinol* 39(3):287-296, 1993.
43. Grana M, and others: Long-term administration of pulsatile gonadotropin-releasing hormone for exploration of pituitary functionality in amenorrheic patients, *Gynecol Endocrinol* 11(2):91-99, 1997.
44. Reinhold C, and others: Primary amenorrhea: evaluation with MR imaging, *Radiology* 203(2):383-390, 1997.
45. Lin J, Yu C: Hypergonadotropic secondary amenorrhea: clinical analysis of 126 cases, *Chung-Hua Fu Chan Ko Tsa Chih (Chinese J Obstet Gynecol)* 31(5):278-282, 1996.
46. Tsai CC, Collins SH, Swanger SJ: Ovarian Sertoli-Leydig cell tumor in an amenorrheic hirsute patient, *Chang Keng i Hsueh (Chang Gung Med J)* 19(2):191-195, 1996.
47. Aloi JA: Evaluation of amenorrhea, *Compr Therapy* 21(10):575-578, 1995.
48. Mishell DD, and others: *Comprehensive gynecology*, St Louis, 1997, Mosby.
49. Jabbar S: Frequency of primary amenorrhea due to chromosomal aberration, *JCPSP (J Coll Phys Surg Pakistan)* 14(6):329-332, 2004.
50. Hernando C, and others: Primary amenorrhea in a woman with a cryptic complex chromosome rearrangement involving the critical regions Xp11.2 and Xq24, *Fertility Sterility* 82(6):1666-1671, 2004.
51. Gersak K, and others: A novel 30 bp deletion in the FOXL2 gene in a phenotypically normal woman with primary amenorrhoea: case report, *Hum Reprod* 19(12):2767-2770, 2004.
52. Seshadri L, and others: Endocrine profile of women with amenorrhea and oligomenorrhea, *Int J Gynaecol Obstet* 45(3):247-252, 1994.
53. McGee C: Secondary amenorrhea leading to osteoporosis: incidence and prevention, *Nurse Pract* 22(5):38-45, 48, 51-52, 57-58, 63-64, 1997.
54. Guttmann-Bauman I: Approach to adolescent polycystic ovary syndrome (PCOS) in the pediatric endocrine community in the U.S.A., *J Pediatr Endocrinol* 18(5):499-506, 2005.
55. Warren M, Freid J: Hypothalamic amenorrhea, *Endocrinol Metab Clin North Am* 30(3)611-629, 2001.
56. Yen SSC: Female hypogonadotropic hypogonadism, *Endocrinol Metab Clin North Am* 22(1):29-57, 1993.
57. Nasir J, and others: Spontaneous recovery of chemotherapy-induced primary ovarian failure, *Clin Endocrinol* 46(2):217-219, 1997.
58. Kurihara S, and others: Inhibin-producing ovarian granulosa cell tumor as a cause of secondary amenorrhea: case report and review of the literature, *J Obstet Gynaecol Res* 30(6):439-443, 2004.
59. Haga HJ, and others: Reproduction and gynaecological manifestations in women with primary Sjögren's syndrome: a case-control study, *Scand J Rheumatol* 34(1):45-48, 2005.
60. Vital-Reyes V, and others: Spontaneous pregnancy in a woman with premature ovarian failure: a case report, *J Reprod Med* 49(12):989-991, 2004.
61. Behringer K, and others: Secondary amenorrhea after Hodgkin's lymphoma is influenced by age at treatment, stage of disease, chemotherapy regimen, and the use of oral contraceptives during therapy: a report from the German Hodgkin's Lymphoma Study Group, *J Clin Oncol* 23(30):7555-7564, 2005.
62. Seeras RC, Gilliland GB: Resumption of menstruation after amenorrhea in women treated by endometrial ablation and myometrial resection, *J Am Assoc Gynecol Laparosc* 4(3):305-309, 1997.
63. North American Menopause Society: Clinical challenges of perimenopause: consensus opinion of the North American Menopause Society, *Menopause* 7:5-13, 2000.
64. Berga SL, Loucks TL: The diagnosis and treatment of stress-induced anovulation, *Minerva Ginecologica* 57(1):45-54, 2005.
65. Golden NH, and others: Resumption of menses in anorexia nervosa, *Arch Pediatr Adolesc Med* 151(1):16-21, 1997.
66. Manieri C, and others: Naltrexone must not be considered a real therapy in functional hypothalamic amenorrhea: the results of a double blind controlled study, *Panminerva Medica* 35(4):214-217, 1993.
67. Swenne I: Weight requirements for return of menstruations in teenage girls with eating disorders, weight loss and secondary amenorrhoea, *Acta Paediatrica* 93(11):1449-1455, 2004.
68. Musso C, and others: The long-term effect of recombinant methionyl human leptin therapy on hyperandrogenism and menstrual function in female and pituitary function in male and female hypoleptinemic lipodystrophic patients, *Metab Clin Exper* 54(2):255-263, 2005.
69. Kotsuji F, and others: Alternate-day GnRH therapy for ovarian hypofunction induced by weight loss: treatment of six patients who remained amenorrhoeic after weight gain, *Clin Endocrinol* 39(6):641-648, 1993.
70. Hergenroeder AC, and others: Bone mineral changes in young women with hypothalamic amenorrhea treated with oral contraceptives, medroxyprogesterone, or placebo over 12 months, *Am J Obstet Gynecol* 176(5):1017-1025, 1997.
71. Ulrich U, and others: Osteopenia in primary and secondary amenorrhea, *Hormone Metab Res* 27(9):423-435, 1995.
72. Seidenfeld ME, Rickert VI: Impact of anorexia, bulimia, and obesity on the gynecologic health of adolescents, *Am Fam Phys* 64(3):367-368, 2001.
73. Warren MP, and others: Effects of an oral contraceptive (norgestimate/ethinyl estradiol) on bone mineral density in women with hypothalamic amenorrhea and osteopenia: an open-label extension of a double-blind, placebo-controlled study, *Contraception* 72(3):206-211, 2005.
74. Rickenlund A, and others: Oral contraceptives improve endothelial function in amenorrheic athletes, *J Clin Endocrinol Metab* 90(6):3162-3167, 2005.
75. Karaman AS, Uran B, Erler A: Serum prolactin levels in postpill amenorrheic patients, *Int J Gynaecol Obstet* 43(2):177-180, 1993.
76. Anosike JC, Abanobi OC: Reversal of amenorrhoea after Mectizan treatment, *Trop Geograph Med* 47(5):222-224, 1995.
77. Tartagni M, and others: Long-term follow-up of women with amenorrhea-galactorrhea treated with bromocriptine, *Clin Exper Obstet Gynecol* 22(4):301-306, 1995.
78. Pascal-Vigneron V, and others: Hyperprolactinemic amenorrhea: treatment with cabergoline versus bromocriptine: results of a national

multicenter randomized double-blind study, *Presse Medicale* 24(16):753-757, 1995.
79. Webster J, and others: Comparison of cabergoline and bromocriptine in the treatment of hyperprolactinemic amenorrhea, *N Engl J Med* 31:904-909, 1994.
80. Biller B, and others: Treatment of prolactin secreting macroadenomas with once weekly agonist cabergoline, *J Clin Endocrinol Metab* 81:2338-2343, 1996.
81. Jonnavithula S, and others: Bone density is compromised in amenorrheic women despite return of menses: a 2-year study, *Obstet Gynecol* 81(5 Pt 1):669-674, 1993.
82. Borer KT: Physical activity in the prevention and amelioration of osteoporosis in women: interaction of mechanical, hormonal and dietary factors, *Sports Med* 35(9):779-830, 2005.
83. Gulekli B, Davies MC, Jacobs HS: Effect of treatment on established osteoporosis in young women with amenorrhea, *Clin Endocrinol* 41(3):275-281, 1994.
84. Rickenlund A, and others: Amenorrhea in female athletes is associated with endothelial dysfunction and unfavorable lipid profile, *J Clin Endocrinol Metab* 90(3):1354-1359, 2005.
85. O'Donnell E, De Souza MJ: The cardiovascular effects of chronic hypoestrogenism in amenorrhoeic athletes: a critical review, *Sports Med* 34(9):601-627, 2004.
86. Dueck CA, and others: Treatment of athletic amenorrhea with a diet and training intervention program, *Int J Sport Nutr* 6(1):24-40, 1996.
87. Rumball JS, Lebrun CM: Use of the preparticipation physical examination form to screen for the female athlete triad in Canadian Interuniversity Sport universities, *Clin J Sport Med* 15(5):320-325, 2005.

CHAPTER 166

Bartholin's Gland Cysts and Abscesses

Marie Elena Botte

DEFINITION AND EPIDEMIOLOGY

The Bartholin's glands, also known as the greater vestibular or vulvovaginal glands, were first discovered by the French anatomist Joseph Guichard du Verney in the late seventeenth century[1]; their physiology was described by the Danish anatomist Gaspard Bartholin in 1677.[2] These paired glands, homologous to the male bulbourethral glands in structure, placement, and function, have ducts about 2.5 cm (1 inch) long that open into the vestibule just distal to the hymenal ring at the 5-o'clock and 7-o'clock positions.[3] The glands continuously secrete mucus, which lubricates the vulva, and are generally not palpable unless a cyst or abscess develops.[4] Bartholin's gland cysts are generally noninfectious enlargements of the gland related to ductal obstruction,[5] which can occur as a result of inflammation, mucus, or congenitally narrowed ducts.[6] Bartholin's gland abscesses, also called bartholinitis or Bartholin's adenitis,[7] are the result of acute infection followed by obstruction.[8]

Bartholin's gland cysts occur most often during women's reproductive years[2,4,9]; one study found that 83% of patients were between 20 and 50 years.[2] Clinicians are likely to encounter cysts of this gland in approximately 2% to 3% of new gynecologic patients and once per 46 pelvic examinations.[10]

PATHOPHYSIOLOGY

Cysts of the Bartholin's gland are related to obstruction of the duct orifice.[5,9] They are most commonly the result of trauma, parturition, or episiotomy[11] and can be the result of inflammatory scarring, epithelial metaplasia, or inspissated secretions that accumulate.[9] In the presence of an infectious process, inflammation of the gland's acinus may lead to abscess.[6,8] Most cases are self-limiting but can be severely discomforting.[7]

Any opportunistic genital or genitourinary organism can be the cause of an acute inflammation, and there is increasing evidence for the involvement of organisms typically responsible for respiratory disease, such as *Streptococcus pneumoniae* and *Haemophilus influenzae*, including resistant strains.[12,13] Studies have demonstrated the presence of *Chlamydia trachomatis*, *Neisseria sicca*,[13-16] and *Brucella melitensis*[17]; *Bacteroides* species have been detected in cultures from abscess formations in HIV antibody–positive women. Capnophilic bacteria[18]; pure gram-negative cultures (*Escherichia coli* and *Proteus* organisms); *Neisseria gonorrhoeae*; and polymicrobial flora, including gram-negative and gram-positive anaerobes, have also been cultured. Aerobic and facultative organisms have also been implicated in abscess formation.[8] A study from Japan found that *E. coli* was the most frequently isolated organism,[12] and another study, emphasizing the polymicrobial nature of Bartholin's gland abscess, found an average of 2.6 isolates per specimen[19]—1.7 anaerobic (mostly *Bacteroides* species with some peptostreptococci) and 0.9 aerobic and facultatives (*E. coli* and *N. gonorrhoeae*).

CLINICAL PRESENTATION

Bartholin's gland cysts are often asymptomatic,[10] generally unilateral,[7] and range in size from 1 to 3 cm (0.4 to 1.2 inches)[20]; they can be chronic or recurrent. Associated pain is generally a sign of an infectious process and development of an abscess, which can often grow large and rapidly over 2 to 4 days. Women may be seen with pain, especially while walking or standing; swelling; dyspareunia; or tenderness. Specific inquiry into recent history of infectious process may yield clues to etiology. A recent vaginal delivery or history of localized trauma can be explored.

PHYSICAL EXAMINATION

Physical examination includes vital signs, visualization of the affected area, and assessment of accompanying inguinal node involvement. Patients usually exhibit a unilateral, erythematous, edematous mass located lateral to the vestibule that ranges from tender to extremely painful. The size may vary, and discharge is usually present. A speculum or bimanual examination may be too painful until the cyst or abscess has been treated.

DIAGNOSTICS

Culturing of cystic contents and the cervix for sexually transmitted diseases has been recommended to ensure adequate treatment of women and their sexual contacts.[21] A CBC can identify leukocytosis.

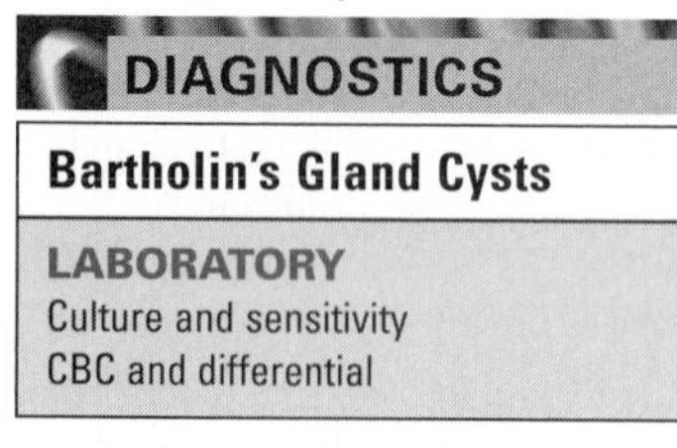

DIAGNOSTICS
Bartholin's Gland Cysts
LABORATORY
Culture and sensitivity
CBC and differential

DIFFERENTIAL DIAGNOSIS

Cysts or abscesses of the Bartholin's gland represent the majority of cysts in the vulvar region[10] and are the most common diseases of the gland.[11] Although solid benign tumors,[22,23] adenocarcinomas,[24-27] high-grade squamous intraepithelial neoplasias,[28] neuroendocrine carcinomas,[29] adenoid cystic carcinomas,[30,31] mixed tumors, leiomyomas, adenofibromas, mucinous cystadenomas, papillary tumors, mucocele-like changes, endometriosis, and malacoplakia all can originate in (or, in the case of endometriosis, infiltrate[32]) Bartholin's gland,[10] these presentations are rare. Carcinoma of Bartholin's gland, which can be primary,[33] accounts for less than 1% of all female genital neoplasms.[34] Tuberculosis of Bartholin's gland is also rare (vulval and vaginal infections account for less than 2% of genital tuberculosis) but should be considered if swelling does not resolve after excision.[35] Primary neuroendocrine carcinoma (Merkel's cell carcinoma) of the vulva can both originate in Bartholin's gland[36] and mimic a Bartholin's gland abscess.[37]

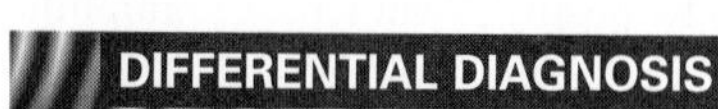

Bartholin's Gland Cysts

- Tumors
- Genital tuberculosis

MANAGEMENT

The goal of management is to preserve the gland and its function if possible,[4] and many options are available, including antibiotics and office procedures such as catheter placement for drainage.

Antibiotics

When initiated early, empiric antibiotic treatment can potentially prevent full-blown abscess formation and should focus on both aerobic and anaerobic organisms as potential sources of infection.[7] Treatment is generally initiated with broad-spectrum antibiotics to decrease the chance of abscess formation or the need for surgical intervention. Erythromycin 250 mg q.i.d. for 10 days is a usual first-line therapy, followed by doxycycline 100 mg b.i.d. for 10 days (not for pregnant women) or cephalexin 250 mg q.i.d. for 10 days for those who are allergic to or cannot tolerate erythromycin. Follow-up evaluation after antibiotic therapy is recommended at 7 to 10 days or sooner if there is fever or increased pain.

Surgical Treatments

A variety of surgical options to treat Bartholin's gland cysts and abscesses have been cited in the literature, ranging from simple incision and drainage techniques (with or without the insertion of a catheter) to visualization and expression of cyst contents using ultrasound imaging,[38] and the application of silver nitrate or carbon dioxide (CO_2) lasers. Adequate pain control is an important issue for all women who have surgical intervention for Bartholin's cysts and abscesses. Because sufficient local anesthesia is often difficult to obtain for cyst drainage, the pudendal block, which anesthetizes the lower vagina and posterior vulva, has been recommended as an adjunct for regional anesthesia.[39]

Incision and Drainage. Incision and drainage followed by packing with gauze are a commonly used management strategy for Bartholin's cysts and abscesses and were once the mainstay of treatment.[3] The procedure requires minimum surgical skill but is not without disadvantages. Although the procedure is effective for temporary relief of symptoms, the recurrence rate is high.[3] Weekly follow-up monitoring is recommended after placement of a drain.

Excision of Bartholin's Gland. Removal of the entire gland, once standard procedure,[5] is now recommended only when there is suspicion of malignancy[2] or for recurrent abscess.[20] Current surgical practices emphasize preservation of the gland's function.

Marsupialization and Window Operation. Both these treatments seek to create and maintain a patent fistula for drainage of the cyst or abscess. The techniques differ significantly only in that the cyst is excised in the marsupialization procedure whereas a "window" is cut unto the cyst or abscess in the latter procedure. In both marsupialization and window techniques, pudendal or local anesthesia is used and the edges of the opened cyst cavity are sutured to the adjacent labial skin to make a permanent opening. The gland remains functional after both procedures,[3,9] and the size of the fistulas created gradually decreases over time. Recurrence rates for marsupialization are between 2% and 24%,[3] and there is one case in the literature of a pregnant woman who became septic after marsupialization.[40] Recommended follow-up care after marsupialization is 4 to 6 weeks.

Catheter or Drain Placement. The goal of catheter or drain placement is the creation of a fistula through which the gland can continue to drain. The drain can be placed after a simple stab wound or a marsupialization procedure and generally is left in place for 6 to 8 weeks to ensure fistula patency.[3,11] Recurrence rate is about 24%.[11] Both the Word catheter[41] and the rubber Jacobi ring have been used effectively; the Jacobi ring may be better tolerated than the Word catheter.[42]

Carbon Dioxide Laser Therapy. With the patient under local anesthesia, the CO_2 laser is used first to create a defect from the vulvar skin to the cystic cavity as near as possible to the original duct tract. Mucus is released from the cyst on entering the cavity, and the gland is gently massaged to express the remaining free mucus. The neostoma that is created allows for continued drainage after the procedure without the presence of sutures or mechanical devices such as catheters or drains and allows an epithelial-lined tract to form. Glandular function is maintained, sexual function is not impaired after a 2-week healing period, and the size of the created defect is substantially reduced with complete healing (shrinking from approximately 1.5 to 0.2 cm [0.6 to 0.08 inch]).[5]

In a second type of procedure done with the patient under general anesthesia, the CO_2 laser is used to vaporize the internal capsule of the cystic formation after a simple incision.[2,43] Both procedures take about 10 minutes or less,[5,43] and healing generally occurs without scarring. A disadvantage of these approaches is that the laser equipment is expensive to install and maintain.

Silver Nitrate. Insertion of silver nitrate into a scalpel-formed incision has been shown in several studies to be a simple and inexpensive option for treatment,[44,45] as effective as traditional excision techniques and with fewer complications.[44,46] However, chemical burning of the vulva has been observed.[44] There is evidence to suggest that alcohol sclerotherapy to Bartholin's gland cysts or abscesses is as effective as silver nitrate and is associated with fewer complications.[47]

LIFE SPAN CONSIDERATIONS

Bartholin's gland cysts and abscesses are most common in women of reproductive age, yet, when adequately treated, women maintain function without reproductive or other sequelae such as dyspareunia.

COMPLICATIONS

Incision and drainage are often followed by cyst recurrence,[43] and gland excision may be accompanied by hemorrhage, hematoma formation, trauma to surrounding tissues, scarring, a long healing process, and subsequent dyspareunia from loss of vaginal lubrication.[3,43,44] Toxic shock syndrome, a very rare complication, has been noted in the literature,[48] both before and after corrective surgical procedures.[8] True necrotizing fasciitis has been noted in one case after an abscess that drained spontaneously[49] and in another after incision and drainage of a gland abscess.[50]

INDICATIONS FOR REFERRAL OR HOSPITALIZATION

Health care providers not comfortable managing Bartholin's cysts and abscesses are encouraged to refer these cases to experienced surgeons for appropriate therapy. Bartholin's gland cysts or abscesses are generally managed successfully on an outpatient basis, but systemic infection or other complications remain valid indications for hospitalization.

Women who have been treated by surgeons for Bartholin's gland cysts or abscesses should have continued follow-up care with their health care providers. Providers can also check for possible sequelae to treatment, including dyspareunia, in the course of routine gynecologic or other primary care provision.

PATIENT AND FAMILY EDUCATION

Explaining to patients the basic physiology of the Bartholin's gland and the pathophysiology involved in cyst or abscess may help demystify the condition and the treatment experience. Women may also benefit from an explanation of what to do and expect after a treatment strategy is used. After CO_2 therapy, for example, patients are instructed to refrain from sexual intercourse for 2 weeks; potential postoperative discomfort is managed with salt water soaks.[5] Women should be counseled to expect drainage of mucus for 2 or 3 days after certain procedures while the cyst or abscess resolves. Proper hygiene, sitz baths or soaks, and condom use are also helpful in the treatment and prevention of future Bartholin's gland cysts and abscesses.

REFERENCES

1. Bouchet A, Gaspard II: Bartholin et la glande vulvovaginale, *Ann Chirurgie* 125(5):483-488, 2000.
2. Heah J: Methods of treatment for cysts and abscesses of Bartholin's gland, *Br J Obstet Gynaecol* 95:321-322, 1988.
3. Downs MC, Randall HW: The ambulatory surgical management of Bartholin duct cysts, *J Emerg Med* 7(6):623-626, 1989.
4. Omole F, Simmons BJ, Hacker Y: Management of Bartholin's duct cyst and gland abscess, *Am Fam Phys* 68(1):135-140, 2003.
5. Davis GD: Management of Bartholin duct cysts with the carbon dioxide laser, *Obstet Gynecol* 65(2):279-280, 1985.
6. Quint E, Smith Y: Adolescent gynecology, part 1, Common disorders, *Pediatr Clin North Am* 46(3):593-606, 1999.
7. Cunha B: Bartholin's gland abscess, *Emerg Med* 26(5):85-86, 1994.
8. Lopez-Zeno JA, Ross E, O'Grady JP: Septic shock complicating drainage of a Bartholin gland abscess, *Obstet Gynecol* 76(5):915-916, 1990.
9. Cho JY, Myoung OA, Cha KS: Window operation: an alternate treatment method for Bartholin gland cysts and abscesses, *Obstet Gynecol* 76(5 Pt 1):886-888, 1990.
10. Enghardt MH, Valente PT, Day DH: Papilloma of Bartholin's gland duct cyst: first report of a case, *Int J Gynecol Pathol* 12(1):86-92, 1993.
11. Yavetz H, Lessing JB, Jaffa JA, and others: Fistulization: an effective

treatment for Bartholin's abscesses and cysts, *Acta Obstet Gynecol Scand* 66:63-64, 1987.

12. Tanaka K, Mikamo H, Ninomiya M, and others: Microbiology of Bartholin's gland abscess in Japan, *J Clin Microbiol* 43(8):4258-4261, 2005.
13. Mikamo H, Tamaya T, Tanaka K, and others: [Two cases of Bartholin's gland abscesses caused by *Streptococcus pneumoniae* and *Haemophilus influenzae*], *Jpn J Antibiot* 58(4):375-381, 2005.
14. Hoosen AA, Nteta C, Moodley J, and others: Sexually transmitted diseases including HIV infection in women with Bartholin's gland abscesses, *Genitour Med* 71(3):155-157, 1995.
15. Van Bosterhaut B, Buts R, Veys A, and others: *Haemophilus influenzae* bartholinitis, *Eur J Clin Microbiol Infect Dis* 9(6):442, 1990.
16. Berger SA, Gorea A, Peyser MR, and others: Bartholin's gland abscess caused by *Neisseria sicca*, *J Clin Microbiol* 26(6):1589, 1988.
17. Peled N, David Y, Yagupsky P: Bartholin's gland abscess caused by *Brucella melitensis*, *J Clin Microbiol* 42(2):917-918, 2004.
18. Quentin R, Pierre F, Dubois M, and others: Frequent isolation of capnophilic bacteria in aspirate from Bartholin's gland abscesses and cysts, *Eur J Clin Microbiol Infect Dis* 9(2):138-141, 1990.
19. Brook I: Aerobic and anaerobic microbiology of Bartholin's abscess, *Surg Gynecol Obstet* 169(1):32-34, 1989.
20. Schroeder B: Vulvar disorders in adolescents, *Obstet Gynecol Clin* 27(1):35-48, 2000.
21. Bleker OP, Smalbraak DJ, Schutte MF: Bartholin's abscess: the role of *Chlamydia trachomatis*, *Genitour Med* 66(1):24-25, 1990.
22. Foushee JHS, Reeves WJ, McCool JA: Benign masses of Bartholin's gland, *Obstet Gynecol* 31(5):695-701, 1968.
23. Mandsager NT, Young TW: Pain during sexual response due to bilateral Bartholin's gland adenomas: a case report, *J Reprod Med* 37(12):983-985, 1992.
24. Hastrup N, Andersen ES: Adenocarcinoma of Bartholin's gland associated with extramammary Paget's disease of the vulva, *Acta Obstet Gynecol Scand* 67(4):375-377, 1988.
25. Ferrandina G, Testa AC, Zannoni GF, and others: Skull metastasis in primary vulvar adenocarcinoma of the Bartholin's gland: a case report, *Gynecol Oncol* 98(2):322-324, 2005.
26. Balepa L, Baeyens L, Nemec E, and others: First detection of sentinel node in adenocarcinoma of Bartholin's gland, *J Gynecol Obstet Biol Reprod (Paris)* 33(7):649-651, 2004.
27. Kokcu A, Cetinkaya MB, Aydin O, and others: Primary-adenocarcinoma of Bartholin's gland: a case report, *Eur J Gynaecol Oncol* 25(5):651-652, 2004.
28. Sidra LM, Maresh M: High grade squamous intraepithelial neoplasia in a Bartholin's cyst, *J Obstet Gynaecol* 25(1):88-89, 2005.
29. Jones MA, Mann EW, Caldwell CL, and others: Small cell neuroendocrine carcinoma of Bartholin's gland, *Am J Clin Pathol* 94(4):439-442, 1990.
30. Kiechle-Schwarz M, Kommoss F, Schmidt J, and others: Cytogenetic analysis of an adenoid cystic carcinoma of the Bartholin's gland: a rare, semimalignant tumor of the female genitourinary tract, *Cancer Genet Cytogenet* 61(1):26-30, 1992.
31. Amichetti M, Aldovini D: Primary adenoid cystic carcinoma of the Bartholin's gland: a clinical, histological and immunocytochemical study of a case, *Eur J Surg Oncol* 14(4):335-339, 1988.
32. Gocmen A, Inaloz HS, Sari I, and others: Endometriosis in the Bartholin gland, *Eur J Obstet Gynecol Reprod Biol* 114(1):110-111, 2004.
33. Obermair A: Primary Bartholin gland carcinoma: a report of seven cases, *Aust NZ J Obstet Gynaecol* 41(1):78-81, 2001.
34. Copeland LJ, Sneige N, Gershenson DM, and others: Bartholin gland carcinoma, *Obstet Gynecol* 67(6):794-801, 1986.
35. Dhall K, Das SS, Dey P: Tuberculosis of Bartholin's gland, *Int J Gynecol Obstet* 48:223-224, 1995.
36. Khoury-Collado F, Elliott KS, Lee YC, and others: Merkel cell carcinoma of the Bartholin's gland, *Gynecol Oncol* 97(3):928-931, 2005.
37. Pawar R, Vijayalakshmy AR, Kahn S, and others: Primary neuroendocrine carcinoma (Merkel's cell carcinoma) of the vulva mimicking as a Bartholin's gland abscess, *Ann Saudi Med* 25(2):161-164, 2005.
38. Eppel W: Ultrasound imaging of Bartholin's cysts, *Gynecol Obstet Invest* 49(3):179-182, 2000.
39. Anderson GV: The forgotten block, *J Emerg Med* 8(4):505-506, 1990.
40. Miller NR, Garry DJ, Klapper AS, and others: Sepsis after Bartholin's duct abscess marsupialization in a gravida, *J Reprod Med* 46(10):913-915, 2001.
41. Owen JW, Koza J, Shiblee T, and others: Placement of a Word catheter: a resident training model, *Am J Obstet Gynecol* 192(5):1385-1387, 2005.
42. Gennis P, Li SF, Provataris J, and others: Jacobi ring catheter treatment of Bartholin's abscesses, *Am J Emerg Med* 23(3):414-415, 2005.
43. Lashgari M, Keene M: Excision of Bartholin duct cysts using the CO_2 laser, *Obstet Gynecol* 67(5):735-736, 1986.
44. Mungan T, Urgur M, Yalcin H, and others: Treatment of Bartholin's cyst and abscess: excision versus silver nitrate, *Eur J Obstet Gynecol Reprod Biol* 63(1):61-63, 1995.
45. Ergeneli M: Silver nitrate for Bartholin gland cysts [letter], *Eur J Obstet Gynecol Reprod Biol* 82(2):231-232, 1999.
46. Bulatovic S: Therapy of inflammatory changes in Bartholin's glands, *Medicinski Pregled* 53(5-6):289-292, 2000.
47. Kafali H, Yurtseven S, Ozardali I: Aspiration and alcohol sclerotherapy: a novel method for management of Bartholin's cyst or abscess, *Eur J Obstet Gynecol Reprod Biol* 112(1):98-101, 2004.
48. Shearin RS, Boehlke J, Karanth S: Toxic shock-like syndrome associated with Bartholin's gland abscess: case report, *Am J Obstet Gynecol* 160(5 Pt 1):1073-1074, 1989.
49. Frohlich EP, Schein M: Necrotizing fasciitis arising from Bartholin's abscess: case report and review of the literature, *Israel J Med Sci* 25(11):644-647, 1989.
50. Kdous M, Hachicha R, Iraqui Y, and others: Necrotizing fasciitis of the perineum secondary to a surgical treatment of Bartholin's gland abscess, *Gynecol Obstet Fertil* 33(11):887-890, 2005.

CHAPTER 167

Breast Disorders

Cynthia J. Gantt and Patricia Polgar Bailey

Evaluation of breast complaints and screening for breast cancer account for a significant number of primary care visits. The most frequent breast complaints include breast pain, breast lumps, and nipple discharge. Most breast lumps and other breast complaints are due to benign conditions, but breast disease can also be an important risk factor for cancer.[1] Studies have shown that women with certain kinds of benign breast disease have a relative risk for breast cancer of 1.35 to 1.6 compared with women in the general population.[2,3] In addition, chest wall pain, which may be felt as breast pain, can have causes that are not related to the breast, including ischemic heart disease and gallbladder disease. For these reasons, accurate evaluation and appropriate follow-up are essential. In addition, many women fail to be reassured about their breast symptoms after a benign diagnosis, which heightens the need for appropriate support for women with breast symptoms.[1]

Surgical referral is indicated for patients with persistent symptoms of mastitis (despite antibiotic therapy), unilateral spontaneous nipple discharge, or a dominant mass.

BREAST PAIN AND INFECTIONS

DEFINITION AND EPIDEMIOLOGY

Breast pain is often referred to as mastalgia or mastodynia. The incidence of mastalgia is estimated to be as high as 70%, the most common breast problem encountered in primary care.[4] Although increased awareness and overestimation of breast cancer risk may prompt women to be more inclined to seek medical treatment for breast concerns, mastalgia is generally underreported.[3] Premenstrual, or cyclic, breast pain is the most common type of mastalgia and usually occurs during the late luteal phase of the menstrual cycle, in association with the premenstrual syndrome or independently, and resolves after menses.[5,6] Cyclic breast pain is common. In a recent study of healthy women in the United States, 11% had moderate to severe cyclic breast pain and 58% had mild discomfort.[7]

Noncyclic mastalgia involves constant or intermittent pain that is unrelated to the menstrual cycle.[3,6] It is less common than cyclic mastalgia and occurs most frequently in women 40 to 50 years old. It accounts for about 31% of women being seen for mastalgia.[3] Noncyclic mastalgia may result from pregnancy, mastitis, thrombophlebitis, macrocysts, benign tumors, fibrocystic breast changes, or cancer; however, these conditions explain only a minority of noncyclic mastalgia cases. Most noncyclic mastalgia occurs for unknown reasons, but it is thought to be related more often to an anatomic cause than a hormonal one. Noncyclic breast pain usually resolves spontaneously without treatment.[3] Breast infections are generically known as *mastitis*. Mastitis is overwhelmingly associated with lactation but must always be differentiated from inflammatory breast cancer.

Raynaud's phenomenon of the nipple was first described in 1970 as nipple vasospasm but was ascribed to psychosomatic concerns. The term *psychosomatic sore nipples* was used to describe women with "some fear or unhappy association connected with breasts or breastfeeding." In 1992 Coates suggested that nipple vasospasm might be related to Raynaud's phenomenon, and since then it has been recognized by many lactation experts as a treatable cause of painful breastfeeding.[8] Raynaud's phenomenon occurs more frequently in women than men, affecting up to 20% of women of childbearing age.[8] It was originally thought to affect the distal parts of extremities but now has been described as occurring in many other vessels, including coronary, gastrointestinal, penile, and placental, in addition to the nipple.[8]

PATHOPHYSIOLOGY

Although the breasts are hormonally influenced, little is known about the mechanisms of action and interaction of hormones and their effect on breast tissue.[5] Reports of response to bromocriptine, a prolactin inhibitor and dopamine agonist, in alleviating mastalgia seem to implicate prolactin, even in women with normal laboratory findings. Furthermore, women during menarche and perimenopause have a high incidence of breast problems. A decreased ratio of progesterone to estrogen, which is seen in physiologic anovulatory cycles during these periods, has also been suggested, but not proven.[5] Fluid retention has not been shown to correlate with mastalgia.[9] Breast pain is not related to breast size, weight, or fluid retention. Mastalgia is sometimes associated with a solitary cyst or diffuse fibrocystic changes, yet no specific histologic findings differentiate women who do from women who do not experience breast pain.[5,10,11]

In lactational, or puerperal, mastitis, organisms enter the breast ductal system from the infant through the nipple and cause infection in a segment of the breast where milk drainage is poor. Breast milk provides a good culture medium for these microorganisms. Puerperal mastitis is most commonly caused by *Staphylococcus aureus*; however, other organisms also have been implicated in puerperal mastitis. Nonpuerperal mastitis is rare and can have several origins, including squamous metaplasia of the lactational ducts, periareolar abscesses, and cellulitis.[12]

Histologic findings associated with fibrocystic breast changes include macrocysts, microcysts, proliferation of epithelial tissue, duct hyperplasia, and connective tissue fibrosis.[13]

Raynaud's phenomenon is characterized by vasospasm of the arterioles, which causes intermittent ischemia of the affected body part, manifested as pallor and followed by cyanosis as the venous blood is deoxygenated. This is followed by reflex vasodilation, at which point there is subsequent erythema of the area, manifested as a triphasic color change and usually associated with pain, burning, and paresthesias. The initial vasospasm is usually precipitated by cold but can be induced by a number of factors, including emotional stress.

CLINICAL PRESENTATION

Cyclic mastalgia usually starts in the luteal phase of the menstrual cycle, increases in intensity until menses begins, and then dissipates, although pain may be present during the entire cycle with increased intensity premenstrually.[3] Cyclic mastalgia usually begins in the third or fourth decade of life. It is usually bilateral and poorly localized, although it typically involves the upper outer breast area and radiates to the upper arm and axilla. Women will describe the pain as dull, heavy, or aching. Symptoms tend to persist with intermittent relapses, but remission can occur with hormonal events such as pregnancy or menopause. Only 14% of women with cyclic mastalgia experience spontaneous resolution of symptoms, whereas 42% experience resolution at menopause.[3] In contrast, noncyclic mastalgia is often unilateral, localized, and described as a sharp, burning pain. Mastalgia is the sole presenting symptom of breast cancer approximately 7% of the time.[4] There may be an association between breast pain and anxiety, depression, emotional distress, somatization, and a history of emotional abuse. Women with breast pain may experience greater cyclic fluctuations in anxiety and depression, but it remains unclear whether there is any kind of causal or consequential relationship between breast pain and psychologic distress.[3]

Puerperal mastitis is usually unilateral and most commonly develops during the second to fourth week after delivery, but may occur any time during lactation.[12] Women with puerperal mastitis often are seen with breast engorgement and tenderness, fever, chills, anorexia, headache, and malaise. Erythema is usually confined to the area of a single breast lobule. A discrete mass is suggestive of abscess formation. The axillary lymph nodes may be tender and enlarged. Nonpuerperal mastitis is a rare condition most often seen in women who are immunocompromised (e.g., women with diabetes or who have undergone radiation treatment) and those with autoimmune disorders. Nonpuerperal mastitis may also be accompanied by nipple discharge (see Nipple Discharge and Galactorrhea, pp. 829-834).

Pain and erythema involving the entire breast, accompanied by increased breast firmness and size, are suggestive of inflammatory breast carcinoma and require immediate referral. Some patients with inflammatory carcinoma are initially seen with a red, swollen breast with thickened, edematous skin (peau d'orange), with or without a palpable mass.

The breast pain associated with Raynaud's phenomenon is usually severe and throbbing and is often mistaken for *Candida albicans* infection. Poor positioning and poor attachment may cause blanching of the nipple and pain during breastfeeding; the nipple pain can be so severe that it causes women to stop breastfeeding.

Several well-established risk factors, primarily age and female sex, are associated with the development of breast cancer. A history of breast cancer in a first-degree relative (mother, sister, daughter) is highly significant, especially if the cancer was diagnosed before menopause. Women with first-degree relatives with premenopausal breast cancer have a threefold to fourfold increased risk of developing breast cancer. Early menarche and late menopause may also increase the risk of breast cancer by increasing lifetime exposure to hormones. Similarly, women who gave birth to their first child after age 30 years or who never became pregnant are also at increased risk. Apparently, this is due to an increase in female reproductive hormones accelerating cell division in breast tissue, which in turn augments the risk of mutations. A history of atypical hyperplasia on biopsy (see Breast Masses, pp. 832-834) or a history of benign breast disease requiring at least two breast biopsies increases the chance of a breast mass being cancerous. Other risk factors identified for developing breast cancer include a high socioeconomic status, Caucasian race, and history of exposure to ionizing radiation. It is important to note that most women with breast cancer do not have any identifiable risk factors.[14] Generally, the pain associated with breast cancer is unilateral, constant, and intense.[3]

A thorough history and breast cancer risk assessment should be obtained from every woman who comes into her health care provider with a breast complaint. The provider should elicit current symptoms such as nipple discharge, breast mass, change in mass with the menstrual cycle, mass in axilla, skin dimpling, ulceration, inflammation, and noncyclic pain; current medications, including hormone therapy; history of previous breast cancer or other breast problems; history of breast implants or breast reduction; age at menarche and menopause; history of trauma; history of other types of cancer; and, in premenopausal women, pregnancy and lactation history. Breast cancer screening history should include the date and results of the last clinical breast examination (CBE) and mammography.[11]

Only an estimated 7% of breast cancers are hereditary. A woman with a *BRCA1* mutation is estimated to have a 56% to 87% lifetime risk of developing breast cancer. Half of women with the *BRCA1* mutation are diagnosed with breast cancer by age 41. (For a discussion of the involvement of the *BRCA1* gene in ovarian cancer, see Chapter 173.) A recent study found that the risk of breast cancer is significantly lower for those with the *BRCA2* mutation. The increased risk of breast cancer was 15% at age 50 years and 35% at age 70 years, compared with 2% and 8% at these ages in noncarriers. *BRCA2* mutations also increase the risk of male breast cancer.[14]

PHYSICAL EXAMINATION

A thorough history and breast examination must be performed on every woman who is seen with a breast problem and must be directed at identifying and characterizing breast-related symptoms. Breast examination must be methodical and carefully executed to include all breast tissue. The breasts should be inspected for differences in size, skin changes, retraction or dimpling of the skin or nipple, prominent venous patterns, pain, lesions, and signs of inflammation. The axillary, supraclavicular, and infraclavicular areas should be palpated with the woman in the sitting position. Examination of the breasts should be performed with the woman both sitting and supine, with her hands behind her head. The examiner should use the flat surface of the fingertips to palpate all of the breast tissue against the chest wall. In women with a history of nipple discharge, the nipple-areolar complex is compressed very gently in the horizontal and vertical directions. If this technique does not elicit discharge, firm, equal pressure should be applied from the periphery toward the nipple. To distinguish multiple from single discharges, pressure must be distributed evenly so that the duct system is milked for each number on the clock. Skin changes that may signify carcinoma include erythema, retraction, dimpling, and nipple excoriation or crustiness.

Quantifying breast pain may be difficult because it is often variable. However, assessment of pain using a pain-rating instrument or scale can be particularly useful in evaluating cyclic breast pain and response to treatment.

DIAGNOSTICS

Noncyclic breast pain is initially investigated with a bilateral mammogram in postmenopausal women, although the likelihood of an abnormal finding is low. An ultrasound is often performed alone to evaluate persistent, noncyclic mastalgia in young women and as an adjust to mammography in older women.[3] Mammography is not indicated in young women with cyclic breast pain in the absence of focal pain, suspicious findings, or risk factors, or in lactating women with an initial presentation of mastitis. However, a mammogram should be considered in women ages 30 to 35 years or older who have a family history of breast cancer or other risk factors for breast cancer.[3] In addition, a mammogram should be considered in any woman with a breast infection that does not respond to appropriate antibiotic therapy within 3 to 7 days. Ultrasound may detect abscess formation in a lactating woman with suspected mastitis but is not required. Laboratory studies are generally not useful, but a pregnancy test should be done for a woman of reproductive age if the history or physical examination suggests that pregnancy is possible. Other hormone levels, such as estrogen, progesterone, and prolactin, are usually within normal limits in women with breast pain and therefore are not indicated as part of the workup.[3]

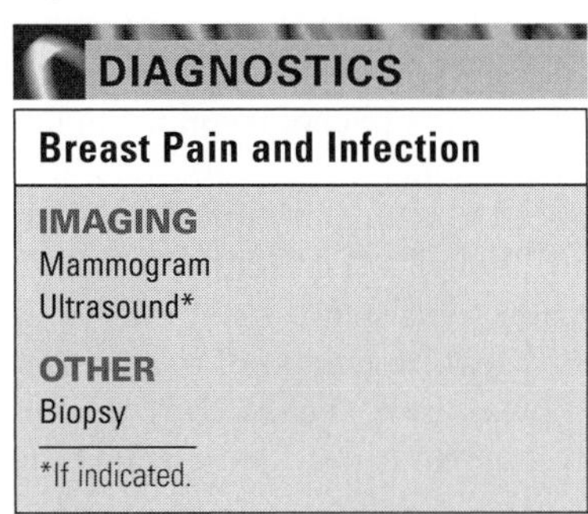

DIAGNOSTICS

Breast Pain and Infection

IMAGING
Mammogram
Ultrasound*

OTHER
Biopsy

*If indicated.

Diagnosis of inflammatory breast cancer cannot be made with radiographic examination alone; pathologic examination is required for confirmation. A skin biopsy reveals dermal lymphatics congested with cancer cells.

DIFFERENTIAL DIAGNOSIS

The differential diagnosis of breast pain includes a normal physiologic event, a hematoma or fat necrosis often related to past trauma, a ruptured cyst, a nonruptured cyst under tension, infection, a tumor, and an idiopathic condition.

Chest wall or nonbreast pain accounts for about 7% of women seen with complaints of mastalgia. Pain that is limited to a particular area and characterized by a burning or knifelike sensation may be chest wall pain. There are several distinct types of chest wall pain, including localized or diffuse pain; radicular pain from cervical arthritis; slipping and cracking ribs; and pain from Tietze's syndrome, also known as costochondritis.[3] This is an inflammation of the costochondral junction that can occur spontaneously or after radiotherapy.[5]

DIFFERENTIAL DIAGNOSIS

Breast Pain and Infection

NONBREAST CAUSES	BREAST CAUSES
• Achalasia	• Hormone therapy
• Angina	• Macrocysts
• Cervical radiculopathy	• Fibrocystic breast changes
• Cholecystitis	• Sclerosing adenoma
• Cholelithiasis	• Duct ectasia
• Costochondritis (Tietze's syndrome)	• Mastitis
• Fractured rib(s)	• Pregnancy
• Hiatal hernia	• Postpartum engorgement
• Systemic infections (including tuberculosis, syphilis, fungal infections)	• Trauma
• Myalgia	• Thrombophlebitis
• Neuralgia	• Breast cancer
• Peptic ulcer disease	
• Pleurisy	
• Trauma (nonbreast)	

The pain can be reproduced with pressure over the costal cartilage rather than the more generalized pattern of mastalgia. Movement may also precipitate chest wall pain, and there is no relationship to the menstrual cycle.[4,6] Chest wall syndromes can occur even in the absence of a clear precipitating event, which sometimes heightens the woman's concern that the pain is due to a suspicious or malignant cause.[3]

In lactating women the differential diagnoses for mastitis include breast engorgement, which is usually bilateral unless only one breast is being used for feedings, and the rare inflammatory carcinoma. In nonlactating women, acute mastitis must be differentiated from inflammatory breast cancer, which represents only 0.5% of all breast cancers.[10] In inflammatory breast cancer the erythema and induration are usually more diffuse and skin changes are more common. The principal indication of cancer, however, is the failure to respond to appropriate antibiotic therapy. Other differential diagnoses include mammary duct ectasia (also known as plasma cell mastitis and nonlactational chronic breast abscess), unrecognized gross cystic disease, other extrinsic infections, numerous skin diseases, and other thoracic diseases such as metastatic lung cancer and lung granulomas.[5]

MANAGEMENT

After a thorough history, evaluation, and risk assessment, reassurance will be all that is needed for 85% of women with cyclic mastalgia. For the 15% of the women not helped with reassurance alone, use of a pain chart for at least two cycles may elucidate any patterns of mastalgia. Patients can also be reassured that breast pain has a high spontaneous remission rate (60% to 80%).[6] Relief of symptoms may come for these women after some hormonal event such as pregnancy, menopause, or the use of oral contraceptives.[5] Management of cyclic mastalgia should also include reevaluation of the breast pain at a different time during the menstrual cycle, preferably soon after the menses.

Proven benefits for the treatment of cyclic mastalgia are few. Because of the extreme variability in mastalgia, only treatments that have been tested in randomized, controlled trials (RCTs) can be confidently considered. Danazol (Danocrine), an antigonadotropin, is the only drug labeled by the U.S. Food and Drug Administration for the treatment of mastalgia. RCTs have demonstrated a response rate of 50% to 75% in women with cyclic breast pain who received danazol 100 to 400 mg/day PO in two divided doses. Approximately 75% of women with noncyclic pain responded to the drug.[9] Typically, the initial dosage is 200 mg daily, eventually tapering to lower doses, with alternate-day or luteal-phase administration. However, initial dosages of 50 to 400 mg/day have been described. Unfortunately side effects plague 30% of women, eventually resulting in discontinuation of the drug in approximately 15% of women, even when breast pain is improved. Adverse effects are primarily dose related and androgenic, including acne, hair loss, lowered voice pitch, weight gain, headache, nausea, rash, anxiety, and depression.[3] The severe side effect profile and teratogenic potential of danazol support referral or collaboration before initiation of treatment.

Other pharmacologic agents used to treat mastalgia include dopamine agonists, such as bromocriptine, since one of the hormonal abnormalities detected in women with mastalgia has been an increase in thyrotropin-induced prolactin secretion. Although clinical improvement occurs in 47% to 88% of symptomatic women, up to 29% of women in some studies have stopped taking the medication because of side effects.[3]

The selective estrogen receptor modulator tamoxifen is used to prevent and treat breast cancer but has also been effective in reducing pain in 71% to 96% of women with cyclic mastalgia and 56% of women with noncyclic mastalgia. Tamoxifen has a serious potential side effect profile, including deep vein thrombosis and endometrial cancer, as well as the more benign side effects of hot flashes, nausea, menstrual irregularity, vaginal dryness, and weight gain. Tamoxifen compares favorably with danazol and bromocriptine with regard to efficacy and adverse effects, and tamoxifen has become increasingly familiar because of the large numbers of premenopausal women in breast cancer prevention trials. But like the other hormonal agents, use of tamoxifen for breast pain should be reserved for women with severe mastalgia that is not responding to other forms of therapy.[3]

For puerperal mastitis, empiric treatment with dicloxacillin 500 mg q 6 hr for 7 to 10 days, or clindamycin 300 mg q 6 hr for penicillin-allergic patients, is appropriate. The woman should be encouraged to continue nursing during therapy, since adequate drainage of the infected area is important.[15] Improved drainage and emptying of the breast may be accomplished by altering positions while breastfeeding. Breast emptying by manual expression or hand pump, breast massage, and hot showers may also improve drainage, thereby decreasing discomfort. Cool compresses after breastfeeding may decrease inflammation. Women should be discouraged from weaning at this time, since the resulting breast engorgement can increase the severity of the mastitis. Reevaluation should be performed 3 days after initiation of treatment if significant improvement has not been seen during that interval.[12]

In the older, nonlactating woman with suspected mastitis, outpatient antibiotic therapy for 7 or more days with clindamycin 300 mg q 6 hr, amoxicillin-clavulanate (Augmentin) 500 mg q 12 hr, or cephalexin 500 mg q 6 hr is indicated.[15] The increased risk of inflammatory carcinoma in this population mandates close follow-up monitoring. Failure to fully respond to antibiotics requires immediate referral. Overall prognosis and survival from inflammatory breast cancer are directly affected by timely diagnosis and treatment. Therefore prompt referral for a definitive tissue diagnosis is required.

Supportive bras can be helpful. Some women report some temporary relief with NSAIDs and acetaminophen.[10] Pharmacologic treatment options without significant adverse reactions include oral contraceptives (which, if thought to be a contributing factor to cyclic mastalgia, may be discontinued or changed to an alternative agent with a lower estrogen and higher progesterone content). In both puerperal and nonpuerperal mastitis, acetaminophen or NSAIDs and moist heat may be beneficial.

Treatment options for Raynaud's phenomenon include methods to prevent or decrease cold exposure, avoidance of vasoconstrictive drugs such as nicotine that could precipitate or exacerbate symptoms, and pharmacologic measures. Nifedipine, a calcium channel blocker, has vasodilatory effects and has been used to treat Raynaud's phenomenon, including Raynaud's phenomenon of the nipple.[8]

Caffeine avoidance has been a popular treatment measure in women with breast pain, although a therapeutic benefit for caffeine restriction has not been consistently demonstrated in controlled studies. Vitamin E supplementation has also been advocated as a treatment for breast pain. However, two double-blind, placebo-controlled RCTs demonstrated no benefit to this approach.[9] Diuretics; salt restriction; pyridoxine; reduced dietary fat, increased fiber, and soy isoflavone; and smoking cessation, although often recommended, have not been proven to be effective.[16] Other reported treatment options for Raynaud's phenomenon include aerobic exercise, biofeedback, calcium and magnesium supplementation, vitamin B_6 supplementation, and use of evening primrose oil and fish oil.[8]

LIFE SPAN CONSIDERATIONS

Benign breast symptoms generally occur in women during the menstruating years, with a mean age of 39 years and a range of 16 to 67 years.[5] Because the incidence of carcinoma increases with age, any breast complaint in a postmenopausal woman is worrisome. Puerperal mastitis is by far the most common type of mastitis and often exacerbates the fatigue, discomfort, and stress normally associated with the postnatal period.

COMPLICATIONS

Mastalgia may be associated with a benign macrocyst (see Breast Masses, pp. 832-834). Mastitis may either be initially seen with or progress to include abscess formation. An abscess occurs in approximately 10% of puerperal mastitis cases. Abscess formation is also a risk in nonpuerperal mastitis and requires referral. If the patient's symptoms do not respond to appropriate antibiotic therapy within a few days, the possibility of a breast abscess or inflammatory breast cancer must be considered.[10,12]

INDICATIONS FOR REFERRAL OR HOSPITALIZATION

Treatment of cyclic mastalgia with antigonadotropic agents should be managed by, or in consultation with, a specialist because of the severity of the side effect profile and the teratogenicity of this class of drugs.

Surgical intervention for incision and drainage is also needed when a fluctuant mass, suspicious for an underlying abscess, accompanies mastitis. IV antibiotics may be required to treat acute mastitis unresponsive to oral agents. In-home IV therapy or hospitalization is required for administration of appropriate antibiotics. Surgical referral is also indicated when inflammatory breast cancer is suspected. The diagnosis is made after an incisional skin biopsy.

Because the only currently available reputable form of primary prevention is bilateral prophylactic mastectomy, a family history that includes a first-degree relative who was diagnosed when premenopausal and/or diagnosed with bilateral disease, or two or more family members who have been affected by breast cancer, suggests possible familial clustering. In such cases referral for possible genetic counseling and gene mapping should be discussed.

PATIENT EDUCATION

Many women are initially seen with mild forms of mastalgia, fearful that they have cancer. Premenopausal women who experience breast pain should receive a thorough CBE and education and should be reassured that pain is rarely a presenting symptom of breast cancer.. Lactating women should also be reassured that mastitis is a common complication of lactation, the nutrition of the breast milk is unaffected by the infection, and a history of mastitis is not associated with an increased risk of breast cancer.

Research shows that even after a benign diagnosis, up to one third of women report that they are either unsure or not reassured about their breast symptoms. A significant percentage of women who undergo evaluation and receive a benign diagnosis for their breast symptoms remain anxious about the possibility of breast cancer or sinister breast disease.[1] A recent study found that women who were not reassured were more likely to have only a high school education and have more perceived stress compared with the general population of women.[1] The type of diagnostic test done did not have any impact on reassurance, nor did the woman's perceived cancer risk. Identifying women who are less likely to feel reassured is important so that additional support can be offered at an early stage in the diagnosis process.

Although women themselves first detect 70% to 90% of masses, there is much debate over whether routine breast self-examination (BSE) screening reduces the risk of mortality from breast cancer. Yet for women who have come to their provider with a breast complaint, encouraging self-monitoring is often an important part of follow-up care. Menstruating women should be advised to perform BSE during the week after menses.[10]

NIPPLE DISCHARGE AND GALACTORRHEA

DEFINITION AND EPIDEMIOLOGY

Nipple discharge most often involves a benign process. Nipple discharge has been reported in 10% to 15% of women with benign breast disease and is found in 2.5% to 3% of women with breast cancer. Nipple discharge encompasses all breast secretions, both spontaneous and those requiring manual expression. Galactorrhea includes spontaneous, nonpuerperal, and nonlactational nipple discharge that is either grossly milky or composed of fat droplets identified microscopically. Galactorrhea is usually caused by stimulation of the breast by elevated prolactin secretions from the pituitary. Galactorrhea is not a symptom of breast cancer.[10] Nipple discharge is considered pathologic and requires referral if it is spontaneous, unilateral, and persistent and contains new or occult blood.[6]

Bilateral nipple discharges usually have physiologic causes (such as hyperprolactinemia associated with infertility that may lead to galactorrhea), but can occur in bilateral breast disease such as mammary duct ectasia. Mammary duct ectasia is a benign condition occurring in postmenopausal women, characterized by dilation of the ducts, nipple secretions (may be spontaneous or nonspontaneous), and periductal inflammation.[11] Nipple secretions associated with mammary duct ectasia are multicolored, sticky, and heme negative.[10]

Pathologic nipple discharges occur spontaneously, are unilateral, come from a single duct opening on the nipple, and are serous or bloody. This type of discharge is most commonly associated with a benign intraductal papilloma. An intraductal papilloma is a neoplastic growth within a major breast duct.[5,10]

Galactorrhea may be physiologic, idiopathic, a side effect of certain medications, or related to neoplasms or central nervous system (CNS) disorders, but it is most commonly associated with several drugs or, secondly, with pituitary or CNS lesions. Hormonal agents, primarily oral contraceptives, are the most common pharmacologic cause of nipple discharge. Galactorrhea is often associated with pregnancy and can persist for 1 to 2 years postpartum, but it may also co-exist with anovulatory syndromes.

PATHOPHYSIOLOGY

Most nipple discharge is physiologic in nature and is not symptomatic of any pathologic condition. The breast of a nonlactating woman secretes fluid into the ductal system of the breast. Usually this fluid is absorbed into the blood and lymphatic systems.[10] Stimulation of estrogen, progesterone, and prolactin, as well as the presence of growth hormones, insulin, and adrenal hormones, may initiate nipple discharge. When the physiologic fluid is secreted through the nipple, it is generally bilateral, serous, arising from multiple ducts, and not spontaneous.

The most common cause of pathologic nipple discharge is intraductal papilloma, followed by duct ectasia. The presence of an associated palpable mass increases the likelihood of cancer.[9] The most common causes of occult blood in nipple discharge are, in order of frequency, intraductal papilloma, mammary duct ectasia, fibrocystic changes, and carcinoma.[5]

Prolactin is a stress hormone known to transform mammary epithelial cells from a presecretory to a secretory state. Because lactogenesis can occur in breast tissue that is metabolically stimulated by various hormones such as estrogen, progesterone, corticosteroids, insulin, growth hormone, and thyroid hormones, disruptions of any of these underlying systems can result in galactorrhea.[17]

CLINICAL PRESENTATION

The first step in evaluating nipple discharge is to determine whether it is physiologic or pathologic. Nipple discharges are considered pathologic if they are spontaneous, bloody, or associated with a mass. Pathologic discharges are usually unilateral and involve a single duct. Physiologic nipple discharges are characterized by discharge only with compression and by multiple duct involvement. These discharges are often bilateral. With either pathologic or physiologic discharges, the fluid may be clear, yellow, white, or dark green.[9] The duration of the discharge and any personal or family history of breast cancer must also be elicited.

A complete medication and past medical history, including endocrine and reproductive histories, should be obtained to exclude lactational discharge. Although it is not common, lactational secretions may persist for years after weaning if the breasts continue to be manually stimulated.

Mammary duct ectasia often manifests with dark green, brown, or blackish multiple duct discharge. It is seen in the perimenopausal period. Pituitary prolactinomas are associated with elevated prolactin levels. Clinical signs and symptoms in addition to galactorrhea include headache; amenorrhea; defects in peripheral vision; hirsutism; acne; and hypogonadism appearing as decreased libido, decreased fertility, or decreased bone density.[10,17]

PHYSICAL EXAMINATION

A thorough breast examination as previously described should be performed to assess for an underlying breast mass and should include gentle compression of the nipple-areolar complex between the thumb and index finger. Milking the ducts with equal pressure from various directions is required to determine the origin of the discharge from either a single duct or multiple ducts.

In the presence of galactorrhea, funduscopic examination to exclude papilledema, as well as evaluation of visual acuity, visual fields by confrontation, and extraocular movements, is indicated to detect a bitemporal field defect and asymmetry of field loss, which are common in parapituitary lesions. Neurologic and thyroid examinations should also be performed.

DIAGNOSTICS

Nipple discharge should be tested for occult blood. Cytologic studies are not recommended because the absence of malignant cells does not exclude malignancy or distinguish intraductal from invasive cancer. A diagnostic mammogram should be obtained in the evaluation of unilateral, spontaneous, clear, serous, or bloody discharge to discern nonpalpable masses or calcifications. Any mammographic abnormality should correspond to the quadrant of the breast from which the discharge originates to be considered relevant to the cause of the discharge. Most of these mammograms are normal, but this should not deter referral to a specialist for further evaluation.[11]

Pregnancy should be excluded by obtaining a human chorionic gonadotropin level in all premenopausal women experiencing amenorrhea and galactorrhea. Serum prolactin is the single most important test that can establish a lesion of pituitary or CNS origin. The serum prolactin level may be artificially elevated if measured after breast stimulation, including clinical examination, and is more accurate when obtained in the fasting state. If serum prolactin is only marginally elevated, repeat or serial testing should be performed to document accurate results. The majority of women with hyperprolactinemia have microadenomas of the pituitary. Serum prolactin may be normal or only slightly elevated when galactorrhea is drug related. Thyroid profiles should also be obtained, since primary hypothyroidism can cause elevation of serum prolactin and galactorrhea.

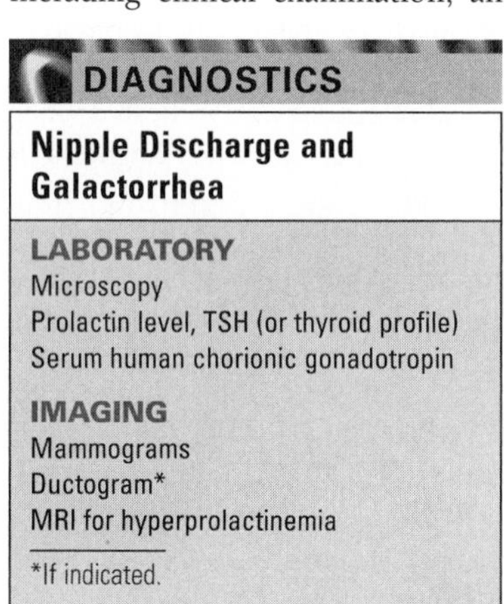
DIAGNOSTICS

Nipple Discharge and Galactorrhea

LABORATORY
Microscopy
Prolactin level, TSH (or thyroid profile)
Serum human chorionic gonadotropin

IMAGING
Mammograms
Ductogram*
MRI for hyperprolactinemia

*If indicated.

MRI of the brain is indicated for the patient with symptoms suggestive of an intracranial mass, galactorrhea with amenorrhea, or an elevated prolactin level (>20 ng/ml). An MRI may be obtained when galactorrhea is associated with amenorrhea or oligomenorrhea even with a normal prolactin level, since the risk of pituitary adenoma is still significant.[17]

DIFFERENTIAL DIAGNOSIS

Duct ectasia, nonpuerperal mastitis, intraductal papilloma, and breast cancer must be considered in the presence of a nonmilky nipple discharge. Pseudonipple discharges can be caused by inverted nipples, eczema, or infection (see Breast Abnormalities, pp. 835-836).

The differential diagnosis of galactorrhea includes pituitary adenomas, neurologic disorders, hypothyroidism, numerous medications, breast stimulation, chest wall irritation (e.g., clothing, breast implants, postreduction), and physiologic causes.[18]

MANAGEMENT

Treatment of underlying infection, as previously described, is required if nipple discharge is related to acute mastitis. When a chemical origin for galactorrhea is suspected, discontinuation or substitution with a comparable pharmacologic agent may be attempted when possible. Restoration to the euthyroid state is indicated if hypothyroidism is present. Minimum intervention is required for galactorrhea of idiopathic, drug related, or physiologic origin.

Mammary duct ectasia is self-limited and not related to neoplasms. Treatment is not necessary unless the patient insists, and then the only effective treatment is surgical removal of all

DIFFERENTIAL DIAGNOSIS

Nipple Discharge and Galactorrhea

BREAST-RELATED CAUSES
- Duct ectasia
- Nonpuerperal mastitis
- Intraductal papilloma
- Breast cancer

CHEMICAL AGENTS
- Amphetamines
- Anesthetics
- Arginine
- Atypical antipsychotics (clozapine, loxapine, risperidone)
- Benzamides (metoclopramide, sulpiride*)
- Benzodiazepines
- Butyrophenones (haloperidol)
- Cimetidine
- Danazol
- Dronabinol
- Estrogen
- Flunarizine*
- Isoniazid
- Methyldopa
- Monoamine oxidase inhibitors
- Opiates
- Oral contraceptives
- Phenothiazines
- Progestins
- Rauwolfia alkaloids
- Reserpine
- Selective serotonin reuptake inhibitors
- Thioxanthenes
- Thyrotropin-releasing hormone
- Tricyclic antidepressants
- Verapamil

IDIOPATHIC CAUSES
- Conditions related to abnormal dopamine secretion

MEDICAL (NONMALIGNANT) CONDITIONS
- Addison's disease
- Ahumada–del Castillo syndrome†
- Chiari-Frommel syndrome†
- Chronic renal failure
- Chest wall lesions
- CNS lesions (involving hypothalamus or pituitary)
- Cushing's disease
- Endocrine anovulatory syndromes
- Forbes-Albright syndrome
- Hand-Schüller-Christian disease
- Head trauma
- Liver failure
- Multiple sclerosis
- Polycystic ovaries
- Postencephalitis
- Primary hypothyroidism
- Renal failure
- Sarcoidosis
- Thoracic herpes zoster

MEDICAL (MALIGNANT) CONDITIONS
- Adrenal carcinoma
- Breast carcinoma (rare)
- Bronchogenic carcinoma
- Chest wall lesions
- CNS lesions (involving hypothalamus or pituitary)
- Ovarian cystic teratoma
- Renal adenocarcinoma

PHYSIOLOGIC CONDITIONS
- Cyclic menstrual hormone variations
- Pregnancy (after first trimester)
- Postlactation (few months to 5 years)
- Nipple stimulation
- Stress

SURGICAL PROCEDURES‡
- Implantation of breast prostheses
- Postthoracotomy
- Reduction mammoplasty

PSEUDODISCHARGES
- Atopic dermatitis
- Herpes simplex
- Infected Montgomery's glands
- Inverted nipples
- Lactiferous sinuses
- Molluscum contagiosum
- Nipple trauma
- Paget's disease
- Sebaceous cysts of the nipple

*Not available in the United States.
†May be associated with pituitary tumors.
‡Procedures that may result in irritation to the afferent arc.

the involved ducts. Because intraductal papillomas usually manifest with a spontaneous bloody discharge, excision is required to exclude carcinoma.[10]

Co-Management with Specialists

In the past, bromocriptine was routinely used to treat galactorrhea, including the treatment of pituitary microadenomas. However, increased concern has been raised related to the use of bromocriptine. Increased rates of hypertensive crises and stroke have been documented in postpartum women who used the drug.[10] Therefore this medication, if used at all, should be used in consultation with a specialist.

Controversy also exists regarding the frequency of follow-up care for pituitary microadenomas. Repeat MRI examinations are often recommended until the growth of the lesion is established, and these should be performed in conjunction with the consulting specialist.

LIFE SPAN CONSIDERATIONS

Most women are concerned about getting breast cancer, and nipple discharge usually heightens concerns about possible malignancy. Although nipple discharge is not commonly associated with cancer, care must be taken to ensure that a complete workup is conducted. Galactorrhea is more common in premenopausal women, and duct ectasia is seen more often in perimenopausal and postmenopausal women.

INDICATIONS FOR REFERRAL OR HOSPITALIZATION

All patients with spontaneous or unilateral nipple discharge, regardless of color, should be referred for surgical evaluation. Intraductal papillomas require surgical biopsy and excision.[9] Galactorrhea accompanied by decreased visual fields, deterioration in visual acuity, papilledema, progressive headache, and nausea or vomiting should be promptly discussed and referred to a neurologist, endocrinologist, or neuroendocrinologist. When idiopathic galactorrhea is suspected, referral to a specialist for confirmation of the diagnosis is also indicated.

PATIENT AND FAMILY EDUCATION

Patients should be reassured that most causes of breast discharge are nonmalignant. In the presence of a normal prolactin level and menses, women with galactorrhea should be informed of its normal physiologic association with nipple and breast stimulation. Patients with pituitary adenoma should be reassured of the generally favorable response to treatment. Accurate and clear information, support, and close follow-up monitoring will help minimize the anxiety that often accompanies the presence of breast discharge.

BREAST MASSES

DEFINITION AND EPIDEMIOLOGY

Although a breast mass is the most common presentation of breast cancer, 90% of breast masses are caused by benign lesions such as cysts, fibroadenomas, and fibrocystic changes.[6] Breast masses are different entities in women who are less than 30 years of age, 31 to 50 years of age, or older than 50 years of age. Nine of 10 new masses in premenopausal women are benign.[6] Nonetheless, every woman, regardless of age, who develops a breast mass should be evaluated and monitored to exclude or establish a diagnosis of cancer. The average lifetime risk of breast cancer is 12%, or approximately 1 in 8 women. The decision to evaluate a palpable breast mass should not depend on the presence or absence of risk factors. More than 75% of women with newly diagnosed breast cancer have no identifiable risk factors.[13]

The breast undergoes substantial morphologic changes between early adolescence and menopause, ranging from a predominance of ducts, lobules, and interlobular stroma to fibrous change and cyst formation, formerly referred to as *fibrocystic disease of the breast*. The term *fibrocystic changes* is now preferred, since 50% to 60% of women without breast disease may have fibrocystic changes, such as breasts with nondiscrete nodules, which entail no increased risk of breast cancer and are distinguished from those which confer a small increase in relative risk.[6]

Benign gross cysts are the most common type of dominant lump and are characterized as a distinct entity consisting of a palpable, fluid-filled sac within the breast tissue. Although gross cysts may be found in younger women, they are most commonly found in women between 35 and 50 years old. Cysts are rare in postmenopausal women not on hormone replacement therapy (HRT) and should be viewed as breast cancer until proven otherwise. Fibroadenomas are the most common benign solid lesion of the female breast. Characteristically, fibroadenomas are painless, well-circumscribed, freely movable masses with a rounded, lobulated, or discoid configuration. They usually have a rubbery feeling, but may appear hard, especially if calcified. Fibroadenomas occur most often in women in their twenties and thirties but may occur anytime after puberty, and even during menopause. They are hormonally responsive and may increase in size toward the end of the menstrual cycle.

It is impossible to distinguish between fibroadenomas and cysts on CBE alone; therefore imaging (ultrasound and/or mammography) and tissue sampling (e.g., fine needle aspiration [FNA]) are required for diagnosis. This combination of diagnostic measures is referred to as the *triple test*. Fibrocystic changes include a compilation of nondiscrete breast masses that are often accompanied by breast pain. Fibrocystic changes tend to occur most commonly in women in their twenties and thirties. Tissue diagnosis and imaging are required less often in these women.[5]

PATHOPHYSIOLOGY

Breast cysts are fluid filled and are thought to arise from dilation or obstruction of collecting ducts. Rarely, a cyst with an irregular wall may signify intracystic carcinoma or a carcinoma adjacent to the cyst.[12] Debate continues about any increased risk of developing breast cancer in women with a history of breast cysts. Evidence exists associating some forms of atypical hyperplasia found on breast biopsy with an increased risk of later breast cancer development.[10] Therefore women with a history of cystic breasts who are seen with a dominant mass should not be ignored or labeled as having "just another cyst."

Fibroadenomas occur when periductal stromal connective tissue proliferates within the lobules of the breast. Estrogen receptors are present in fibroadenomatous tissue. Exogenous estrogen, progesterone, pregnancy, and lactation can stimulate the growth of fibroadenomas.[5] The relationship between fibroadenomas and breast cancer is complicated. Histologically, when a mass is composed of microscopic elements beyond the basic glandular tissues that make up simple fibroadenomas, the lesion is labeled a *complex fibroadenoma*. Simple fibroadenomas do not appear to increase the risk of developing breast cancer. One third of fibroadenomas are thought to be complex and, in the presence of a family history of breast cancer, seem to increase the risk of future breast cancer development.[10]

CLINICAL PRESENTATION

A discrete, palpable mass is three dimensional, different from surrounding tissues, and usually asymmetric compared with normal glandular tissue that is generally mirrored in the contralateral breast. Clinical signs that suggest (but are not diagnostic of) a benign condition include a mass that is soft or rubbery and mobile. Features suggestive of malignancy include a mass that feels firm or hard, has an irregular shape, is solitary, and feels different from surrounding breast tissue. Occasionally breast cancers are fixed and associated with other signs such as skin retraction, dimpling, erythema, nipple discharge, nipple retraction, and skin changes.[10,12]

Cysts are dominant, discrete masses that are fluid filled and round and usually change cyclically on a monthly basis, with enlargement and pain occurring before menses. Pain associated with breast cysts often occurs in the upper outer quadrants and radiates to the axilla. Cysts are most commonly found in women between 35 and 50 years old.[5] Fibroadenomas are solid, encapsulated, and usually nontender masses. They are most commonly found in the upper outer quadrant and tend to be unilateral, although they can exist anywhere in either breast and more than one can be present at a time. Although they can enlarge cyclically before menses, they tend to be uniform in size over time or increase in size at a gradual rate. They are most commonly found in women in their twenties, although they can be present anytime from puberty through menopause.[10]

Fibrocystic changes manifest as prominent, rubbery, thickened, symmetric plaques of glandular breast tissue that lack discreteness and blend into the surrounding breast tissue. Pain is the most common complaint and can be cyclic. The pain is often bilateral; is poorly localized; and extends to the shoulder, axilla, or arm.[5]

PHYSICAL EXAMINATION

Key historical features in the evaluation of a breast lump are the length of time the mass has been present, pain, change in size or texture over time, relationship to menstrual cycle, and nipple discharge. Risk factors for breast cancer (see Breast Pain and Infections, pp. 825-829) should be assessed. Also important is pathologic information on any previous breast cyst aspirations, including a personal history of atypical hyperplasia, which can increase the risk of breast cancer three to five times and double that in women with a strong family history of breast cancer.[5]

CBE of a woman with a complaint of a dominant breast mass should include assessing for a symmetric finding in both breasts, the consistency or texture of any mass, mobility, size, and shape.[11] Nipple discharge should also be assessed if reported (see Nipple Discharge and Galactorrhea, pp. 829-832).

DIAGNOSTICS

CBE is a method of detection, not an independent diagnostic test. Diagnostic mammography usually is the initial test for a palpable mass in women 35 to 40 years. A negative mammogram should not deter follow-up evaluation, since 15% to 18% of mammograms appear negative in the presence of a palpable cancer. Mammography is usually performed, since hematoma formation secondary to biopsy procedures may obscure radiographic findings. For younger women the dense glandular tissue lowers the sensitivity of mammograms, and ultrasound directed at the area of concern is the preferred imaging study.[5] In diagnosing any dominant mass, the provider usually performs FNA to determine whether the mass is cystic or solid. If the lesion is cystic, the fluid is aspirated and the cyst collapsed. If no fluid is obtained or an underlying mass is palpated after aspiration, it is assumed that it is a solid lesion requiring open biopsy.[5] FNA also has the potential benefit of decreasing the size of the cyst and relieving any accompanying pain. Cysts require surgical biopsy only if the aspirated fluid is bloody, the palpable abnormality does not resolve completely after aspiration of fluid, or the same cyst recurs multiple times in a short time period.[10]

DIAGNOSTICS

Breast Masses

IMAGING
Mammogram
Ultrasound

OTHER
Biopsy

DIFFERENTIAL DIAGNOSIS

The differential diagnosis of a dominant breast mass includes invasive breast cancer, macrocyst (clinically evident cyst), and fibroadenoma. In addition, prominent areas of fibrocystic change, fat necrosis as a result of surgical or extraneous trauma, and a galactocele (a milk cyst in a lactating woman) may be seen as a breast mass.[9]

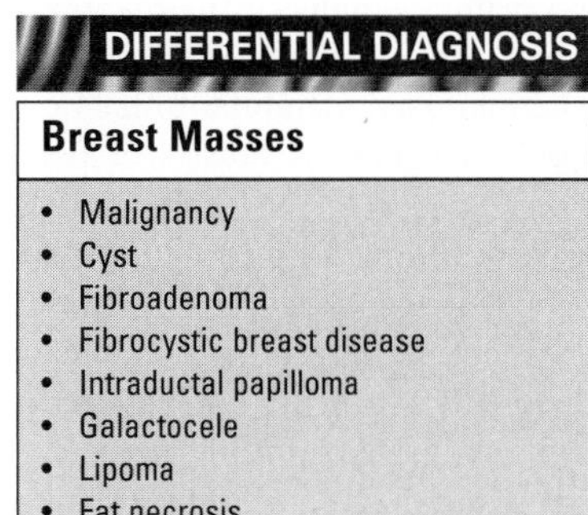
DIFFERENTIAL DIAGNOSIS

Breast Masses

- Malignancy
- Cyst
- Fibroadenoma
- Fibrocystic breast disease
- Intraductal papilloma
- Galactocele
- Lipoma
- Fat necrosis

MANAGEMENT

Management of the patient with a breast mass varies according to age, clinical history, and clinical findings. Detection of a breast mass usually creates significant anxiety in a woman and her family and requires sensitive communication.[10] If a cyst is detected, aspiration is often offered and requested by women for both diagnosis and relief of pain.

Cysts require cytologic analysis of aspirate fluid and surgical biopsy only if the aspirated fluid is bloody, the palpable abnormality does not resolve completely after the aspiration of fluid, or the cyst recurs. This approach has been supported by large studies of benign-appearing cyst fluid aspirates.[9] No cancers were ultimately identified in 6782 aspirates of low-probability samples. Patients with a solitary breast cyst must be reexamined 4 to 6 weeks after cyst aspiration to determine whether the cyst has recurred.[9]

Noncystic masses in premenopausal women that are different from the surrounding breast tissue require histologic sampling by FNA, core cutting, or needle or excisional biopsy. Observation for one or two menstrual cycles is appropriate only for vague asymmetry or nodularity when it is unclear that a dominant breast mass is present.[9]

The accuracy for FNA alone is high. One review of 4943 FNAs reported 87% sensitivity for carcinoma. In another review of 3545 such procedures a 9.6% false-negative rate was reported. When the triple test approach—CBE, imaging (ultrasound or mammography), and FNA—indicates benign breast disease, one review found that the likelihood of cancer was only 0.6%.[9]

Routine practice has been to excise fibroadenomas. However, there is increasing support for observation in women younger than 35 to 40 years when the lesion can be diagnosed by nonsurgical procedures: CBE, ultrasonography, and FNA.[10,13]

LIFE SPAN CONSIDERATIONS

Approximately 78% of women are over age 50 years when breast cancer is diagnosed. Approximately 22% of breast cancers are diagnosed in women under 50 years of age. An estimated 7% of invasive breast cancers are diagnosed in women younger than 40 years.[13] Because the risk of breast carcinoma increases with age, any dominant mass or asymmetric thickening in postmenopausal woman should raise the index of suspicion for malignancy. Therefore abnormalities detected on physical examination in women over 40 years old should be regarded as possible cancers until they are documented as benign.[10]

Physical examination and mammography of the breasts of young premenopausal women can be challenging because of breast lumpiness from the increased glandular-to-fat ratio when compared to the more homogeneous breasts of postmenopausal women.[12]

Cystic findings become less common after menopause, although cysts, pain, and discharge can be found in women taking HRT.[11] Fibrocystic symptoms may remain stable or worsen until menopause. Up to 20% of women may experience spontaneous resolution.[13] Approximately 1 in 3000 pregnant women will develop invasive breast cancer.[13] Any breast mass discovered during pregnancy or lactation must be thoroughly evaluated as suggested for all premenopausal women.

INDICATIONS FOR REFERRAL OR HOSPITALIZATION

A palpable solid mass in all women, regardless of age, requires both consultation by a specialist and referral for surgical evaluation. Women should be referred for mammography or ultrasound and FNA so that triple testing, including CBE, is provided. The triple test helps make a decision about whether further studies (e.g., open surgical biopsy) are needed in the workup to avoid delays in the diagnosis and treatment of breast cancer.[10] Even when fibrocystic changes are suspected, surgical evaluation of a persistent, palpable dominant mass or lump is required. Tissue diagnosis alone will provide a definitive diagnosis and determine the presence of atypical hyperplasia.

Women with a strong family history of breast cancer may be candidates for genetic testing for *BRCA* mutations. Increased surveillance and prophylactic mastectomies are the current approaches for women with these genetic mutations. This raises many psychosocial and ethical issues. In addition, women with increased risk of breast cancer and certain types of benign breast lesions can be offered tamoxifen as a preventive strategy. The risk of breast cancer is determined with the use of certain models, such as the Gail and Claus models, and the evaluation of the benefits compared with the risks of tamoxifen.[6] Risk factors not included in either of these models include the degree of breast density, plasma levels of free estradiol, bone density, weight gain after menopause, and waist-to-hip ratio. Current recommendations suggest that women with a 5-year relative risk of breast cancer of more than 1.67% and no contraindications to tamoxifen should be informed about the option of taking tamoxifen for 5 years.[6] A recent overview of breast cancer prevention trials showed a reduction of 50% in the relative risk of cancer with tamoxifen, but this benefit may be offset by the relative risks, including thomboemboli, endometrial cancer, and cataract maturation associated with the drug.[19]

PATIENT AND FAMILY EDUCATION

Most women are worried about developing breast cancer. Women need reassurance regarding the benign nature of breast lesions that wax and wane with hormonal variation, as well as the rationale behind conservative vs. surgical management. Education must also focus on the need for prudent breast evaluation of all breast symptoms and lesions regardless of the improbability of malignancy.

BREAST ABNORMALITIES

DEFINITION AND EPIDEMIOLOGY

Paget's disease of the nipple (PDN) is a superficial manifestation of an underlying breast carcinoma most often of ductal origin. PDN is believed to represent 1% to 3% of all breast cancers. PDN is rare in men but is associated with a poorer prognosis in men.[20]

Gynecomastia is an enlargement of the male breast caused by the proliferation of glandular tissue and should prompt investigation for a cause. Gynecomastia is an almost universally benign finding among boys in middle to late puberty.[21]

PATHOPHYSIOLOGY

Controversy exists regarding the origin of the malignant cells seen in PDN. They may represent malignant breast ductal epithelial cells, which then migrate into the epidermis of the nipple.[20]

Gynecomastia in the older man is associated with an altered ratio of estrogen to androgens in a number of conditions, including aging, malnutrition, testicular pathologic condition, hypogonadism, cirrhosis, and thyrotoxicosis. Hormonal secretions from neoplasms in the testis or adrenal glands may cause gynecomastia. Other tumors may secrete ectopic hormones such as those from bronchogenic carcinoma or hepatoma.[5] Drugs most commonly implicated in causing gynecomastia include digoxin, cimetidine, ketoconazole, flutamide, estrogen, and related drugs and anabolic steroids.[21] Pubertal gynecomastia may be related to an estradiol-testosterone imbalance.[5]

CLINICAL PRESENTATION

Clinically, PDN appears as a unilateral, well-demarcated, erythematous, scaly plaque first appearing on the nipple and subsequently spreading to the areola. The surrounding skin is usually spared. Serous or sanguineous discharge, pain, crusting, pruritus, burning, epithelial thickening, erythema, ulceration, nipple retraction, and an underlying breast mass (in up to 60% of patients) may be seen. A small vesicular lesion on the nipple, persistent soreness, pain, or pruritus of the nipple-areolar complex in the absence of other clinical symptoms should be evaluated thoroughly because these may be early manifestations of PDN.[20]

Men with gynecomastia are seen with asymmetric or symmetric breast enlargement. Gynecomastia is a common clinical condition, with peak prevalence in the forties to seventies and an incidence that ranges from 30% to 55% in adult men. In benign gynecomastia of adolescence, the breast tissue is usually asymmetric and often tender.[21]

PHYSICAL EXAMINATION

A thorough breast examination as described previously must be conducted. PDN may be seen solely with scaling of the nipple, but it may also be accompanied by erythematous and excoriated, retracted nipples. The erosion of the areolar tissue may produce copious clear or viscous yellow exudate. As the disease steadily progresses, the excoriated surface of the nipple may result in a bloody discharge and associated adenopathy.

A detailed history, including medication and alcohol use, is essential in assessing gynecomastia. The breast area is palpated while the patient lies supine. The presence of a rubbery mass below the areola usually indicates the presence of mammary tissue, not just fatty tissue. Any dominant firm, fixed, unilateral mass should raise suspicion for breast carcinoma.[16]

DIAGNOSTICS

If PDN is suspected, punch biopsy of the nipple either may be performed as an office procedure or referred to a surgeon. As with all breast abnormalities, mammography is indicated, but should not delay referral to a specialist.

To evaluate gynecomastia, the provider must initiate a history; physical examination; and laboratory studies to determine signs of thyroid excess, liver disease, lung cancer, and hypogonadism. This evaluation usually indicates the possible cause of gynecomastia. If no cause is found, further evaluation may involve testing for serum human chorionic gonadotropin, testosterone, estradiol, and luteinizing hormone to exclude other causes of hormonal disruption.[21]

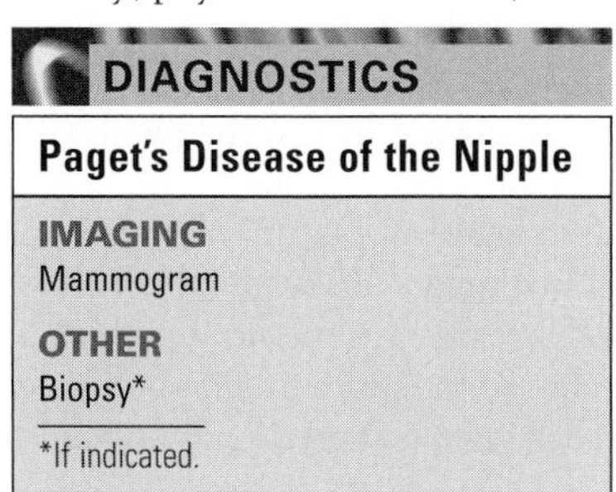

DIAGNOSTICS

Paget's Disease of the Nipple

IMAGING
Mammogram

OTHER
Biopsy*

*If indicated.

DIFFERENTIAL DIAGNOSIS

For patients with lesions involving the nipple, PDN should be suspected until proven otherwise. This is true even for a lesion that has healed spontaneously, since patients have been identified with healed nipple lesions that were subsequently diagnosed as PDN. PDN is most commonly misdiagnosed as eczema (Table 167-1). Eczema involving the nipple (vs. the areola) is rare and, when present, is usually bilateral. The differential diagnosis of PDN includes psoriasis, contact dermatitis, tinea, basal cell carcinoma, Bowen's disease, and benign intraductal papilloma of the nipple.

DIFFERENTIAL DIAGNOSIS

Paget's Disease of the Nipple

- Eczema
- Psoriasis
- Contact dermatitis
- Lichen sclerosus
- Nevoid hyperkeratosis of areola
- Malignant melanoma
- Bowen's disease
- Carcinoma
- Intraductal papilloma
- Herpes
- Tinea versicolor

TABLE 167-1 Eczema vs. Paget's Disease of the Nipple

Eczema	Paget's Disease of the Nipple
Usually bilateral	Unilateral
Intermittent history with rapid progression	Continuous history with slow progression
Moist initially	Moist or dry
Indistinct border	Irregular but distinct border
Areola involved, nipple may be spared	Nipple always involved and disappears in advanced cases
Itching common	Itching common

Direct spread of invasive carcinoma from the underlying breast may be considered after PDN is excluded.[20]

Male breast cancer, although uncommon (fewer than 1% of male cancers), must be excluded in men 40 years and older with a unilateral breast mass. The risk of breast cancer in patients with Klinefelter's syndrome with gynecomastia is increased approximately twentyfold.[21] True gynecomastia needs to be differentiated from pseudogynecomastia, the enlargement in the area of the breasts caused by excess fatty tissue, which is due to obesity, not iatrogenic factors.

MANAGEMENT

PDN is treated with mastectomy or breast conservation surgery and may be followed with radiation treatments.[20] If there is suspicion that the gynecomastia is related to a medication, the suspected agent should be discontinued and the breast reassessed for resolution of the gynecomastia.

INDICATIONS FOR REFERRAL OR HOSPITALIZATION

Because histologic diagnosis of PDN is required, surgical referral for skin biopsy or excisional biopsy of the underlying mass is indicated. Biopsy-proven PDN should be viewed as an invasive breast cancer and must be referred to an oncologist for management.[20]

Patients seen with gynecomastia should be referred when breast cancer is suspected or when concern exists for other serious disease processes (e.g., alcoholism, liver disease).

PATIENT AND FAMILY EDUCATION

Patients undergoing evaluation for PDN require the same accurate information, support, and well-coordinated care that all patients anticipating a possible diagnosis of cancer deserve.

Men should be advised that gynecomastia associated with chemical agents should resolve when the agents are stopped. Men may need reassurance because of the altered body image issues that may accompany gynecomastia. Gynecomastia of adolescence typically resolves spontaneously within 2 years.[5]

REFERENCES

1. Meechan G, Collins J, Moss-Moris R, and others: Who is not reassured following benign diagnosis of breast symptoms? *Psycho-Oncol* 14:239-246, 2005.
2. Hartmann L, Sellers T, Frost M, and others: Benign breast disease and the risk of breast cancer, *N Engl J Med* 353:229-237, 2005.
3. Smith R, Pruthi S, Fitzpatrick L: Evaluation and management of breast pain, *Mayo Clin Proc* 79:353-372, 2004.

4. Padden DL: Mastalgia: evaluation and management, *Nurse Pract Forum* 11(4):213-218, 2000.
5. Johnson C: Benign breast disease, *Nurse Pract Forum* 10(3):137-144, 1999.
6. Santen R, Mansel R: Benign breast disorders, *N Engl J Med* 353:275-285, 2005.
7. Adler D, South-Paul J, Adera T, and others: Cyclic mastalgia: prevalence and associated health and behavioral factors, *J Psychosom Obstet Gynecol* 22:71-76, 2001.
8. Anderson J, Held N, Wright K: Raynaud's phenomenon of the nipple: a treatable cause of painful breastfeeding, *Pediatrics* 113(4):360-363, 2004.
9. Morrow M: The evaluation of common breast problems, *Am Fam Phys* 61(8):2371-2378, 2000.
10. McCool WF, Stone-Condry M, Bradford HM, and others: Breast health care: a review, *J Nurse Midwifery* 43(6):406-430, 1998.
11. Clinical Breast Protocols Workgroup, California Department of Health Services: *Breast diagnostic algorithms for primary care clinicians,* Davis, Calif, 2000, University of California–Davis.
12. Apantaku LM: Breast cancer diagnosis and screening, *Am Fam Phys* 62(3):929-934, 2000.
13. Pruthi P: Detection and evaluation of a palpable breast mass, *Mayo Clin Proc* 76(6):641-648, 2001.
14. Shepherd JE, Muto MG: Testing for genetic susceptibility to ovarian and breast cancer, *Patient Care* 34(11):131-153, 2000.
15. Gilbert DN, Moellering RC, Sande MA: *The Sanford guide to antimicrobial therapy,* Vienna, Va, 2001, Antimicrobial Therapy.
16. Horner NK, Lampe JW: Potential mechanisms of diet therapy for fibrocystic conditions show inadequate evidence of effectiveness, *J Am Diet Assoc* 100(11):1368-1380, 2000.
17. Whitman-Elia GF, Windham NQ: Galactorrhea may be clue to serious problem, *Postgrad Med* 107(7):165-171, 2000.
18. Pena KS, Rosenfeld, JA: Evaluation and treatment of galactorrhea, *Am Fam Phys* 63(9):1763-1770, 2001.
19. Cuzick J, Powles T, Veronesi U, and others: Overview of the main outcomes in breast cancer prevention trials, *Lancet* 361:296-300, 2003.
20. Whitaker-Worth DL, Carlone V, Susser WS, and others: Dermatologic diseases of the breast and nipple, *J Am Acad Dermatol* 43(5 Pt 1):733-751, 2000.
21. Bakshi S, Miller DK: Assessment of the aging man, *Med Clin North Am* 83(5):1131-1149, 1999.

CHAPTER 168

Chronic Pelvic Pain

Cynthia M. Williams and Elizabeth C. Sensenig

DEFINITION AND EPIDEMIOLOGY

Chronic pelvic pain (CPP) is a continuous or episodic, nonmenstrual pain that persists for more than 6 months, occurs below the umbilicus, and is severe enough to cause functional disability or require treatment.[1] The pain is considered chronic when one of these conditions is met: (1) it is refractory to medical management, (2) there is impairment of physical functioning (including sexual), (3) signs of depression are present, and (4) the pain becomes the highest priority for both the patient and her family.[2]

CPP is one of the most common medical problems affecting women today. The prevalence of CPP is 12% to 25% at any point in time; CPP affects 33% to 39% of women during their lifetime, with a higher prevalence found in health care settings than in the general population.[3] It has been estimated that approximately 10% of all referrals to gynecologists are for CPP, and it is a common indication for diagnostic and therapeutic surgery.[1] CPP is considered the principal indication for 40% of gynecologic laparoscopies and 20% of all hysterectomies performed for benign disease done annually in the United States.[4,5] Recent studies suggest that women with CPP have a lower quality of life than women without CPP, and as might be expected, the use of analgesics is common in some women with CPP.[6] CPP is not unique to women. Men also experience CPP, not caused by prostate problems, which is characterized by pain in the groin area; urinary problems, including discomfort; low back pain; and erectile dysfunction[7] (see Chapter 153).

Research indicates that women with CPP use three times more medications of any type, have four times more nongynecologic surgeries, are four times more likely to have a hysterectomy, and have reduced quality of life compared with women without CPP.[3] Based on the demographic profiles of large surveys, women with CPP are no different from women without CPP in terms of race, age, ethnicity, education, socioeconomic status, or employment status.[8,9]

Potential visceral sources of CPP include the reproductive, genitourinary, and gastrointestinal tracts; potential somatic sources include the pelvic bones, ligaments, muscles, and fascia. CPP may result from psychologic disorders or neurologic diseases, both central and peripheral.[10] CPP may be caused by one disorder, or it can be the end result of several diagnoses with each contributing to the generation of pain and requiring management. The distinction between acute and chronic pain is significant. In acute pain, the pain is often a symptom of underlying tissue damage, but with chronic pain, the pain itself becomes the disease. CPP is itself the diagnosis.[11] Women with diagnoses that involve more than one organ system have greater pain than women with only one system involved.[9]

Populations at Increased Risk of Chronic Pelvic Pain

Physical and Sexual Abuse. A significant association exists between physical and sexual abuse and CPP. Up to 40% to 50% of women with CPP disclose a history of physical and/or sexual abuse.[12-14] Evidence suggests that abuse may result in biophysical changes. One study found, after controlling for psychiatric disturbance, that adult survivors had lower thresholds for pain.[15] If a history of abuse is obtained, it is important to ensure that the woman is not currently being abused or in danger.

Pelvic Inflammatory Disease. Approximately 18% to 35% of all women with acute pelvic inflammatory disease (PID) develop CPP.[16,17] The mechanisms by which CPP results from PID are not known. Whether acute PID is treated with inpatient or outpatient regimens does not appear to alter the odds of developing subsequent CPP (34% with outpatient therapy vs. 30% with inpatient therapy).[16,17]

Endometriosis. Endometriosis is the most common diagnosis made at the time of gynecologic laparoscopy for the evaluation of CPP. Endometriosis is diagnosed laparoscopically in approximately 33% of women with CPP. In practices specializing in the treatment of endometriosis, 70% or more of patients with CPP are diagnosed with endometriosis.[10]

Interstitial Cystitis. Interstitial cystitis is a chronic inflammatory condition of the bladder. It is clinically characterized by voiding symptoms of urgency and frequency in the absence of evidence of another disease that could cause the symptoms.[18,19] Pelvic pain is reported by up to 70% of women with interstitial cystitis and occasionally is the presenting symptom or chief complaint.[19]

Irritable Bowel Syndrome. Approximately one third of women with CPP have irritable bowel syndrome (IBS).[9] IBS is a functional gastrointestinal disorder characterized by intermittent or chronic abdominal pain that is associated with bowel symptoms such as bloating, urgency, diarrhea, and constipation. IBS is associated with certain gynecologic problems such as endometriosis, dyspareunia, and dysmenorrhea.[3] Women with both CPP and IBS are more likely to have screening and diagnostic procedures done and are less likely to have improvement after laparoscopy compared to women with only CPP.[3]

Musculoskeletal Disorders. Faulty posture such as lumbar lordosis and thoracic kyphosis (called "typical pelvic pain posture") may account for up to 75% of cases of CPP.[20] Faulty posture may contribute to weak and deconditioned muscles, which allow for imbalances in the pelvis with formation of trigger points and hypertonicity and, as a result, pelvic pain.[10] Other musculoskeletal disorders such as trigger points, lumbar vertebral disorders, pelvic floor myalgia, and fibromyalgia may cause or contribute to pelvic pain.

Postsurgical Pain. Chronic pain has been reported after several types of surgical procedures, including after cholecystectomy and groin hernia repair in less than 30% of patients and after cesarean section in 6% of patients. A recent study also found a 48.4% incidence of CPP in patients up to 5.6 years after surgery for pelvic fracture.[6]

PATHOPHYSIOLOGY

Chronic pain is a dynamic interaction of the combined influences of the mind and nervous system on the body. In addition to the organ system where the pain originated, other organ systems become involved and, in addition, emotional changes occur with the long-term tension of CPP. For example, pain can cause muscle tension, which can in turn cause changes in the muscles of the pelvis, the adjacent urinary tract (bladder, urethra), the bowel, connective tissue, and even skin of the area. Often these secondary changes become more significant than the original cause of the pain and also may overshadow the original disease process, making it harder to diagnose.

There are different theories regarding the development of chronic pain. According to an older theory of pain, called the cartesian theory, neurons carry pain signals from the damaged areas through the spinal cord directly to the cortex of the brain, where the pain is perceived. This theory is now thought to be an oversimplification of the development of chronic pain.

A newer theory, the gate control theory, posits that pain signals arise from the injured or adversely affected tissues and travel through specialized nerve cells to the spinal cord, where they can be intensified, reduced, and even blocked before they are transmitted to the brain. The spinal cord acts a functional "gate" with respect to the pain signals. This gate is influenced by local factors such as nerve inputs in the spinal cord and by descending signals from higher brain centers. Thus internal influences, other than the pain itself, and external environmental factors all affect the nature of the pain's impulse transmission. If the gates are damaged by chronic pain, they may remain open even after the tissue damage has resolved or been controlled. In other words, the pain remains despite the fact that the original cause of the pain has been treated; this type of pain is referred to as *neuropathic pain*, a key factor in CPP.[11]

CLINICAL PRESENTATION

The evaluation of CPP can require many office visits and become a highly frustrating experience for both patient and provider. A complete and thorough history and physical examination are crucial in developing a rational approach to women with CPP. It is important that the patient understand early on that visits are not only for evaluation and treatment but also for the formation of a continued therapeutic relationship between patient and provider.[21,22]

The history should include a description of the nature, intensity, distribution, radiation, location, and daily pattern of the pain. Associated events, including complaints of fever, sweats, fatigue, anorexia, nausea, vomiting, and constipation, should be elicited. The relationship of the pain to posture, meals, bowel movements, voiding, menstruation, intercourse, and medications, as well as any factors that aggravate or alleviate the pain, should be determined. Past surgeries, pelvic infections, and a history of infertility are important diagnostic clues to the origin of the pain.[23]

BOX 168-1

CHRONIC PELVIC PAIN QUESTIONNAIRE (SAMPLE QUESTIONS)

- How and when did the pain begin?
- What actions or activities make it better or worse?
- Does it vary based on time of day, week, or menstrual cycle?
- Does it affect your sleep?
- Has it spread beyond where it first was noted?
- Is it associated with abnormal skin sensations, muscle or joint pain, or back pain?
- Do you have any urinary pain or problems, constipation, diarrhea, or other bowel complaints?
- Has it affected your daily routine at home and at work?
- Has it led to emotional changes such as anxiety or depression?
- What have you personally done to attempt to alleviate the pain?
- What has your physician done?
- Have these been successful to any degree?
- What medications are you currently using?
- What do you think is causing your pain?
- What concerns you most about your pain?

Adapted from the International Pelvic Pain Society: *Chronic pelvic pain: a patient education booklet*, 1999, retrieved March 7, 2007, from http://www.pelvicpain.org/pdf/Patients/CPP_Pt_Ed_Booklet.pdf.

It is helpful to obtain an understanding from the women of the past and present status of her pain, the chronology, and how it developed. It can be helpful to have a woman complete a detailed pain questionnaire before her first visit. Box 168-1 includes some questions that should be included on a CPP questionnaire.

PHYSICAL EXAMINATION

The physical examination should be thorough, complete, and guided by the history. It will differ from a standard gynecologic examination, since it is designed to provide information beyond the condition of the female genitals. The initial part of the examination should begin with observation of the patient's general demeanor during the interview. The five major sources that contribute to pelvic pain should be completely evaluated: gynecologic, gastrointestinal, psychologic, musculoskeletal, and urologic.

The abdomen should be examined to elicit a point or area of tenderness. It is important that the patient be allowed to indicate the location of the pain and the depth of palpation necessary to elicit the discomfort. If pain is experienced during palpation of the abdomen, a trigger point, hernia, endometriosis, or hematoma is likely. Costovertebral angle tenderness should also be elicited if there is tenderness with suprapubic palpation. The groin should be evaluated for inflamed lymph nodes and hernias.

The back should be examined for lordosis; scoliosis; and any tenderness over the paraspinal musculature, sacroiliac joints, or spine prominence. Range of motion should be evaluated. By having the patient lie in the lateral decubitus position, the examiner can accomplish passive thigh extension, which may reveal psoas muscle tenderness.

The pelvic examination should be performed in a gentle, stepwise manner. Attention should be given to any evidence of a vulvar pathologic condition. Pelvic relaxation should be evaluated by having the patient bear down while the practitioner separates the labia and observes for a significant cystocele, rectocele, enterocele, or cervical or uterine prolapse.

A single-digit transvaginal examination (monomanual) is necessary to elicit any tenderness in the adnexa, cervix, or posterior vagina; along the vaginal side walls; or near the base of the bladder or urethra. Special attention during palpation of the levator ani muscles, piriform muscles, and coccyx is important, because all have been implicated as a cause of CPP and discomfort.

A careful speculum examination is performed to visualize the cervix and vagina and to inspect for neoplasms, prolapse, or infections. This examination may reveal vaginismus, with involuntary spasms of the vaginal musculature that make insertion of the speculum difficult.

The bimanual examination and rectovaginal examination complete the genitourinary evaluation. Particular attention should be given to areas of tenderness. Cervical motion tenderness has been associated with endometriosis, pelvic adhesive disease, inflammatory bowel disease (IBD), and ureteral colic. A fixed retroverted uterus or an enlarged boggy uterus, the hallmark of adenomyosis, may be noted. Uterine fibroids do not classically cause pain unless they are degenerating or infarcting, but their enlargement may cause a feeling of heaviness and pressure on nerve endings in the lower abdomen and pelvis. Finally, the rectovaginal examination may reveal nodularity in the cul-de-sac that is associated with endometriosis. The examination may also help identify any rectal masses, and the piriform muscle can be evaluated for spasms and tenderness.

DIAGNOSTICS

Laboratory studies should be based on the history and physical findings. The usual evaluation for CPP should include vaginal and cervical cultures, urinalysis, a urine culture, CBC, and sedimentation rate. A transvaginal ultrasound may be beneficial if the bimanual examination was difficult; if it revealed adnexal tenderness, a mass, or uterine enlargement; or if irregularity was noted.

Laparoscopy is generally indicated, especially if the pelvic examination is abnormal. Commonly found abnormalities include endometriosis, adhesions, and chronic PID. Thus this modality is appropriate in the diagnosis and treatment of CPP.[23,24]

DIAGNOSTICS

Chronic Pelvic Pain

LABORATORY
Cervical cultures*
CBC and differential
Serum human chorionic gonadotropin
ESR
Urinalysis*
Culture and sensitivity*

IMAGING
Transvaginal ultrasound
Renal ultrasound
MRI or CT scan

OTHER
Laparoscopy*
Trigger point injection*

*If indicated.

Another technique that is diagnostic for CPP is trigger point injection. This technique is also therapeutic for patients whose pain is caused by abdominal wall trigger points. The trigger point can be injected with 1% lidocaine

(Xylocaine) or 0.25% bupivacaine with a 25-gauge, 1.5-inch needle.[2] After eliminating the abdominal trigger point, the pelvic examination can be repeated to identify any pelvic pathologic condition. Other locally tender points such as the vaginal cuff have been successfully injected for pain management.

DIFFERENTIAL DIAGNOSIS

The differential diagnosis is extensive for CPP. From a primary care perspective, a good history and physical examination aid in the differential diagnosis. The most common cause of CPP is probably gastrointestinal.[4,17] Irritable bowel syndrome (IBS) is believed to account for 50% of all cases of CPP.[13] IBS is a chronic functional bowel disorder that is often accompanied by gynecologic complaints and labeled as CPP. IBS consists of a constellation of symptoms, including abdominal pain or discomfort that is relieved with defecation; it is usually associated with alternating constipation and diarrhea. The pain of IBS is usually worse around the time of menstruation and may be associated with dyspareunia.

CPP and IBS share many of the same psychosocial factors, including a high prevalence of depression and somatization and a history of physical or sexual abuse.[17] A diagnosis of IBS should be included in any differential diagnosis of CPP. As with any other gastrointestinal complaint, more serious disease entities need to be excluded, including IBD, diverticulitis, and malignancy.

Urinary tract problems may manifest as CPP. Because the gynecologic and urinary systems share embryologic origins, differentiating the source of pain can be difficult. A pathologic condition of the urinary tract can demonstrate a constellation of symptoms, including pelvic pain, dysuria, urgency, hesitancy, dyspareunia, postcoital voiding difficulties, and incontinence. Urethral syndrome, chronic urethritis, interstitial cystitis, and bladder spasms should be considered in the differential diagnosis.[18]

Musculoskeletal diseases are also associated with CPP. These conditions include postural problems, herniated disc disease, chronic pelvic tilt, degenerative joint disease, and myofascial trigger points. Levator ani muscle spasms and piriform muscle spasms are two conditions that are easy to evaluate on physical examination and may be a source of pain and discomfort.

Levator ani muscle spasms are perhaps one of the most overlooked causes of CPP.[25] They usually are initially seen as sacral pain. The pain is caused by contraction and spasm of the levator ani muscles. Palpation of this muscle group reveals tenderness and increasing pain with voluntary contraction. Teaching the patient to relax these muscles and the vaginal muscles will help alleviate the discomfort.

Piriform syndrome or spasms of the piriform muscle during external rotation of the leg can be reproduced by contraction of the externally rotated leg against resistance. Because the piriform muscle can be palpated transvaginally, tenderness along the muscle should be evaluated during bimanual examination. Physical therapy is usually indicated to help relieve the spasms.

A gynecologic source of pain should always be considered. Although a pathologic condition is more likely with acute pain, certain entities are more commonly seen with CPP.

DIFFERENTIAL DIAGNOSIS

Chronic Pelvic Pain

MUSCULOSKELETAL
- Myofascial
- Coccygodynia
- Low back pain
- Scoliosis and other postural problems
- Spasm of the pelvic floor

GASTROINTESTINAL
- Irritable bowel syndrome
- Diverticulosis or diverticulitis

UROLOGIC
- Interstitial cystitis
- Chronic pyelonephritis
- Stones

GYNECOLOGIC
- Dysmenorrhea
- Pain with ovulation
- Chronic pelvic inflammatory disease
- Adhesions
- Endometriosis
- Adenomyosis
- Endometritis
- Uterine fibroids

PSYCHOLOGIC
- Depression
- Abuse
- Opiate dependency
- Somatization

Endometriosis is a chronic condition often seen during laparoscopy for CPP.[25] Endometriosis is caused by the development of implants outside the endometrium. Because these implants can be found anywhere and are responsive to the cyclic hormonal cycle, the point source of the pain can be elusive. On physical examination, either tenderness in the cul-de-sac or along the uterosacral ligaments (early finding) or nodularity in the same locations (late finding) may be noted. The diagnosis should be confirmed by laparoscopy.

Adhesions are scar tissue that can form between any two abdominal organs, usually after surgery or intraabdominal infections such as PID. The pain occurs because of the stretching of usually mobile structures that are now scarred. Patients usually complain of a substantial positional component to the pain. The diagnosis can be confirmed by laparoscopy.

Other gynecologic origins of CPP include pain with ovulation, dysmenorrhea, functional ovarian cysts, ovarian torsion, chronic PID, pelvic congestion of the reproductive organ venous system, adenomyosis, and leiomyomas.

If no other pathologic entity or explanation can be found for the pain, a psychiatric component such as clinical depression or somatization disorder should be considered. Screening for depression and referral to a psychiatrist can assist in this area.

MANAGEMENT

Information for evidence-based management of CPP is not widely available. Success in treating women with CPP is greatly facilitated by winning their trust and confidence. In general, positive reinforcement and general psychologic support are important in the early diagnostic phase of CPP. Women suffer for years, and many are told the problem is psychosomatic. Consideration of depression and sleep disorders is important, since treatment of these conditions enhances management of the chronic pain syndrome. If a cause for the pain is identified, appropriate management should be undertaken with the assistance of the appropriate physician specialist.

During the diagnostic evaluation, the pain component should be treated effectively and promptly. NSAIDs can be prescribed to address the discomfort and pain. These medications should be given on a routine schedule, not on an as-needed basis. Menstrual cycle suppression with oral, transdermal, or subcutaneous contraceptives (medroxyprogesterone [Depo-Provera]) may be helpful.

Recently a protocol was developed at Stanford University, now referred to as the Stanford protocol, to treat CPP in both women and men. The Stanford protocol methodology consists of two essential elements: paradoxic relaxation and pelvic floor trigger point release. This protocol involves applying trigger point release therapy to approximately 40 trigger points related to CPP. Patients are taught external and internal trigger point therapy. Paradoxic relaxation involves encouraging patients to relax when they feel pain, based on the theory that accepting the tension helps to relax it. The Stanford protocol is conducted in a 6-day intensive immersion clinic, involving approximately 30 hours of treatment. During the clinic, patients are trained in paradoxic relaxation, receive daily physical therapy, are educated in self-administration of the Stanford protocol trigger point release, and are taught specific stretches and physical therapy techniques. The goal of the clinic is for patients to self-administer most of the protocol without reliance on additional treatments and for patients to resolve their symptoms without dependency on drugs. In a recent study involving 138 men with CPP, nearly three fourths of the volunteers indicated at least moderate improvement. However, this study had no control group, and the benefits could have been due to the placebo effect. More research needs to be done using the Stanford protocol. For more information, contact the Stanford University School of Medicine or http://www.pelvicpainhelp.com.[7,26]

Regardless of the treatment used, regular office visits are important for patients with CPP. These visits enable discussion of the progress of the diagnostic process and assessment of therapy, and they provide reassurance and support during the evaluation period.[23,24]

LIFE SPAN CONSIDERATIONS

CPP usually occurs during a woman's late twenties and early thirties but can be seen across the reproductive life span. This can be a stressful period in a woman's life. She may be married, considering pregnancy or raising children, and involved in a career. CPP can profoundly affect a woman's personal and professional life. An open mind and the pursuit of appropriate diagnostics, as well as support of the patient's fears, anxieties, and stresses, can have a profound impact on the understanding of CPP and ultimate pain control.[26]

COMPLICATIONS

Numerous pathologic conditions have been identified with CPP, and the potential for complications is incalculable. Many women suffer great frustration associated with the diagnosis and treatment of this disorder. In addition, there is often a psychogenic component to the disorder that is not easily addressed.

INDICATIONS FOR REFERRAL OR HOSPITALIZATION

The etiology of CPP is often complex and multifaceted, and treatment may involve several specialists. A coordinated multidisciplinary approach has been advocated.[23,24] Prompt referral to physical therapy, gastroenterology, urology, and pain management programs as indicated should be considered. Consultation with a physician is appropriate to ensure coordination of care with appropriate referrals to specialists when indicated.[27]

PATIENT AND FAMILY EDUCATION

Reassurance that the causes of CPP, although real and concerning, tend to be less urgent than the causes of acute pelvic pain can be helpful. In addition, it is important that the patient understand that additional diagnostic testing may not be indicated. Education should include information about the possible sources of pain and an explanation that the alleviation of pain may be best achieved by a combination of therapies, including medical, psychologic, and behavioral treatments.

HEALTH PROMOTION

Helping a woman understand her body and the sources of possible pain can assist her in coping. As always, a healthy diet, regular exercise, moderation of alcohol intake, and relaxation techniques can go a long way toward improving a woman's management of the stress and anxiety associated with CPP.

REFERENCES

1. Reiter C: A profile of women with chronic pelvic pain, *Clin Obstet Gynecol* 33:130-136, 1990.
2. Steege J: Office management of chronic pelvic pain, *Clin Obstet Gynecol* 40(3):554-563, 1997.
3. Williams R, Hartmann K, Sandler R, and others: Recognition and treatment of irritable bowel syndrome among women with chronic pelvic pain, *Am J Obstet Gynecol* 192:761-767, 2005.
4. Mathias S, Kuppermann M, Liberman R, and others: Chronic pelvic pain: prevalence, health related quality of life, and economic correlate, *Obstet Gynecol* 87:321, 1996.
5. Howard F: The role of laparoscopy in chronic pelvic pain: promise and pitfalls, *Obstet Gynecol Surv* 48:357, 1993.
6. Meyhoff C, Thomsen C, Rasmussen L, and others: High incidence of chronic pain following surgery for pelvic fracture, *Clin J Pain* 22(2):167-172, 2006.
7. Medical matters: new treatment for chronic pelvic pain syndrome, *Consumer Rep Health*, Jan 2006, p 10.
8. Farquhar C, Steiner C: Hysterectomy rate in the United States 1990-1997, *Obstet Gynecol* 99:229, 2002.
9. Zondervan K, Yudkin P, Vessey M, and others: Chronic pelvic pain in the community—symptoms, investigations, and diagnoses, *Am J Obstet Gynecol* 184:1149-1155, 2001.
10. Howard F: *Chronic pelvic pain*, ACOG Technical Bull No 51, Washington, DC, 2004, American College of Obstetricians and Gynecologists.
11. Wenof M, Perry C: Chronic pelvic pain. In *The International Pelvic Pain Society patient education booklet*, 1999, retrieved July 27, 2006, from http://www.pelvicpain.org/pdf/Patient/CPP_Pt_ED_Booklet.pdf.
12. Rapkin A, Kames L, Dark L, and others: History of physical and sexual abuse in women with chronic pelvic pain, *Obstet Gynecol* 76:92-96, 1990.

13. Reiter RC, Gambone JC: Demographic and historic variables in women with idiopathic chronic pelvic pain, *Obstet Gynecol* 75:428-432, 1990.
14. Jamieson DJ, Steege JF: The association of sexual abuse with pelvic pain complaints in a primary care population, *Am J Obstet Gynecol* 177:1408-1412, 1997.
15. Scarinci IC, McDonald-Haile J, Bradley LA, and others: Altered pain perception and psychosocial features among women with gastrointestinal disorders and history of abuse: a preliminary model, *Am J Med* 97:108-118, 1994.
16. Ness R, Soper D, Holley L, and others: Effectiveness of inpatient and outpatient treatment strategies for women with pelvic inflammatory disease: results from the Pelvic Inflammatory Disease Evaluation and Clinical Health (PEACH) Randomized Trial, *Am J Obstet Gynecol* 186:929-937, 2002.
17. Westrom L: Effects of acute pelvic inflammatory disease on fertility, *Am J Obstet Gynecol* 21:707-713, 1975.
18. Summitt R: Urogynecologic causes of chronic pelvic pain, *Obstet Gynecol Clin North Am* 20:658-698, 1993.
19. Ramahi A, Richardson D: A practical approach to the painful bladder syndrome, *J Reprod Med* 35:805-809, 1990.
20. King P, Myers C, Ling FW, and others: Musculoskeletal factors in chronic pelvic pain, *J Psychosom Obstet Gyneco*l 12(Suppl):87-98, 1991.
21. Ryder R: Chronic pelvic pain, *Am Fam Phys* 54:225-232, 1996.
22. Price J, Blake R: Chronic pelvic pain: the assessment as therapy, *J Psychosom Res* 46:7-14, 1999.
23. Smith R: *Chronic pelvic pain*, ACOG Technical Bull No 223, Washington, DC, 1996, American College of Obstetricians and Gynecologists.
24. Roseff SJ, Murphy AA: Laparoscopy in the diagnosis and therapy of chronic pelvic pain, *Clin Obstet Gynecol* 33:137-144, 1990.
25. Zondervan K, Yudkin P, Vessey M, and others: Prevalence and incidence of chronic pelvic pain in primary care: evidence from a national general practice database, *Br J Obstet Gynecol* 106:1149, 1992.
26. Wise D: *Plenary address to the National Institutes of Health, Scientific workshop on prostatitis/chronic pelvic pain syndromes*, Baltimore, Oct 21, 2005, retrieved Aug 2, 2006, from http://www.pelvicpainhelp.com/ph_address.html.
27. Lipscomb G, Ling F: Chronic pelvic pain, *Med Clin North Am* 49:505-507, 1995.

CHAPTER 169

Dysmenorrhea

Patricia Polgar Bailey

DEFINITION AND EPIDEMIOLOGY

The term *dysmenorrhea,* from the Greek word meaning "difficult monthly flow," refers to painful menstruation. Dysmenorrhea is classified as either primary or secondary. Primary dysmenorrhea is defined as painful menses despite normal pelvic anatomy and ovulation. It usually occurs within 6 to 12 months after menarche begins and ovulatory cycles are established.[1] However, it can begin as late as 1 to 3 years after menarche.[2] It usually begins during adolescence and is characterized by cramping pelvic pain beginning just before, or with the onset of, menstrual flow and typically lasting 1 to 3 days. Secondary dysmenorrhea usually appears later in life, after some years of painless menstruation, and generally has an organic cause such as endometriosis, uterine fibroids, adenomyosis, pelvic inflammatory disease, other pelvic pathologic conditions, or an intrauterine contraceptive device (IUD).[3]

Dysmenorrhea is one of the most commonly encountered gynecologic disorders and at one time was considered to be a psychologic problem. Researchers estimate that up to 90% of adolescents and 25% of all women in the United States experience dysmenorrhea.[2,4] The peak incidence of dysmenorrhea is during the late teenage years and early twenties.[5] Approximately 10% to 15% of women who experience dysmenorrhea have discomfort that interferes with normal daily activity for 1 to 3 days each month. Dysmenorrhea is the greatest single cause of lost work and school hours in females.[2] It is difficult to estimate the economic burden of missed work from dysmenorrhea, but clearly it accounts for significant lost wages and diminished quality of life. Nevertheless, many women choose to "suffer silently" and do not discuss dysmenorrhea with any health care provider. Providers should be aware of the possibility of improving the quality of a woman's life by reducing or relieving the discomfort of dysmenorrhea. In addition, the willingness to discuss this common but possibly sensitive issue may pave the way to a more satisfying patient-provider relationship.[3]

PATHOPHYSIOLOGY

Primary dysmenorrhea has been attributed to uterine contractions or ischemia, psychologic influences, and cervical factors. Contractions in the menstruating uterus and pain have been attributed to the production of prostaglandins, specifically PGF_{2a} and PGE_2.[2] The prostaglandins also cause the nausea and diarrhea associated with dysmenorrhea. Current evidence shows that the menstrual fluid of women with primary dysmenorrhea has higher than normal levels of these prostaglandins.[1] Normal menstruation produces contractions of 50 to 80 mm Hg, lasting 15 to 30 seconds, that help to expel the menstrual fluids. The resting uterine pressures are normally 5 to 15 mm Hg. However, in women with primary dysmenorrhea, contractions may exceed 400 mm Hg and last longer than 90 seconds, with resting pressures as high as 80 to 100 mm Hg.[5]

This prostaglandin hypothesis can also explain the extragenital symptoms of primary dysmenorrhea. It has been shown that IV injection of prostaglandins causes nausea, vomiting, diarrhea, headache, and syncope, which are symptoms often seen in severe primary dysmenorrhea.[6] Anovulatory cycles are associated with lower levels of prostaglandins and as a result usually no dysmenorrhea.[2]

However, despite the supporting evidence for a link between higher prostaglandin levels and dysmenorrhea, it is likely that the explanation for menstrual pain is not as simple as the cyclic production of one hormone. Women with dysmenorrhea may have complex alterations in hormonal patterns that exist throughout the cycle and affect a number of factors such as higher basal body temperature and disrupted sleep patterns.[3] Vasopressin may also play a role by increasing uterine contractility and causing ischemic pain as a result of vasoconstriction. Elevated vasopressin levels have been reported in women with primary dysmenorrhea.[1] In addition, women have differing perceptions of pain, and this may affect how they experience dysmenorrhea.[3]

There is no convincing evidence that mechanical cervical obstruction or severe uterine flexion causing obstructed uterine flow is present in patients with primary dysmenorrhea,[7] although heavy menstrual flow is associated with dysmenorrhea. Some studies have suggested that young age and nulliparity are associated with dysmenorrhea, but the correlation with age was not substantiated in other studies once parity and other factors were controlled for.[1] There is no evidence to support an association between tubal sterilization and the prevalence of dysmenorrhea.[1,4]

Behavioral risk factors for dysmenorrhea have long been of interest because of the possibility of effective intervention. Several studies have found an association between smoking and dysmenorrhea.[8,9] Associations between dysmenorrhea and being overweight, physical activity, and alcohol consumption have been inconsistent, although an association between poor self-rated overall health and dysmenorrhea has been noted.[1] Studies have shown an association between stress and risk for dysmenorrhea, which is biologically plausible, although the mechanisms linking the two are not yet completely understood.[10] Stress may indirectly affect prostaglandin synthesis and concentrations through the release of corticotropin-releasing hormone. Prostaglandins affect uterine muscle and vascular tone, and an imbalance of prostaglandins has been linked to the occurrence of dysmenorrhea.[10] Other psychologic problems have not been convincingly demonstrated to be the initial cause of primary dysmenorrhea, but depression, anxiety, and disruption of social supports have been associated with menstrual pain.[11,12] There have been no consistent associations between socioeconomic status and dysmenorrhea.[1,4]

Cultural and family influences may have a profound effect on how a woman experiences dysmenorrhea. The attitudes a woman has towards menstruation are often formed early in life and may be influenced by many factors, including her culture, religion, family, friends, and sexual partners. Additional emotional influences may be due to perceptions of fertility, ability to bear children, or the relationship with the sexual partner. Many women begin menstruating with little or no accurate information, and menstrual sensations and discomfort may be distressing, frightening, or viewed as punishment. A woman's beliefs regarding menstruation may directly affect the way she experiences it and her willingness to report any problems to her provider or seek treatment.[3]

Secondary dysmenorrhea is caused by a pathologic process that affects the uterus, fallopian tubes, ovaries, or pelvic peritoneum. These processes can cause pain by altering pressures in or around pelvic structures, changing or restricting blood flow, or irritating the pelvic peritoneum. They can occur with the normal physiology of menstruation or act completely independently, with symptoms appearing during specific points in the menstrual cycle.[5]

Dysmenorrhea (primary and secondary) is a distinct and separate entity from premenstrual syndrome (PMS), and the two should not be confused. The term *PMS* is used to describe a predictable set of physical and affective symptoms that occur cyclically during the luteal phase and resolve quickly on or near the onset of the menstrual cycle. The etiology of PMS is not known, but it is a relatively uncommon disorder during adolescence, in contrast to primary dysmenorrhea, which affects the majority of adolescent girls.[2]

CLINICAL PRESENTATION

The diagnosis of primary dysmenorrhea is based on clinical features. The initial onset of symptoms is usually within 6 to 12 months of menarche, with 90% of girls with primary dysmenorrhea experiencing symptoms within 2 years of menarche. Girls will complain of recurrent sharp, cramplike, or spasmodic lower abdominal pain that is usually over the suprapubic area. The pain will often radiate to the back, sacrum, or inner thighs. The pain usually begins a few hours before or just after the onset of menstruation and lasts the first 1 to 3 days of menstruation; it can be associated with nausea, vomiting, diarrhea, low back pain, or headache. Some young women also have associated systemic symptoms, including nausea, vomiting, loose bowel movements, or dizziness.[2]

A history of pain that is inconsistent with the kind of low anterior pelvic pain described above (i.e., beginning in adolescence and associated specifically with menstrual cycles) is suggestive of secondary dysmenorrhea. The signs and symptoms of secondary dysmenorrhea are determined by the underlying pathologic process. A clue that may distinguish primary dysmenorrhea from secondary dysmenorrhea is the age of onset. Secondary dysmenorrhea usually occurs in women 30 or 40 years of age. The pain is often not limited to the menses and is less related to the first day of flow. There may be an array of associated symptoms, which include dyspareunia, infertility, and abnormal bleeding. The history should include age at menarche, menstrual history, last menstrual period, location and severity of discomfort, associated symptoms (headache, dizziness, nausea, vomiting, diarrhea, dyschezia), amount of school or work missed, medications, method of birth control, and whether it is being used correctly. Abdominal and pelvic pain not related to the menstrual cycle should also be explored.

PHYSICAL EXAMINATION

Physical examination findings are normal in primary dysmenorrhea. The diagnosis is based on a careful history. When the history or physical examination suggests secondary dysmenorrhea, the evaluation should follow accordingly and is based on the suspicion of underlying pathologic condition.

The physical examination for secondary dysmenorrhea must include a thorough abdominal, pelvic, and rectovaginal examination. Clues to diagnosis may be asymmetric enlargement of the uterus or adnexa (indicating myomas or other tumors), symmetric enlargement (indicating adenomyosis), painful nodules in the posterior cul-de-sac together with restricted motion of the uterus (indicating endometriosis), cervical stenosis (suggesting retrograde menstruation), or restricted motion of the uterus together with thickened adnexal structures (indicating pelvic scarring or adhesions).[5]

DIAGNOSTICS

No diagnostic studies are needed for the diagnosis of primary dysmenorrhea. However, if the diagnosis of primary vs. secondary dysmenorrhea is not clear, certain diagnostic tests may be helpful. Laboratory evaluation may include a CBC, erythrocyte sedimentation rate, and genital cultures for pathogens. Radiologic evaluation may include pelvic ultrasound or hysterosalpingography. If the final diagnosis is still unconfirmed, the patient may require a laparoscopy, hysteroscopy, or dilation and curettage.

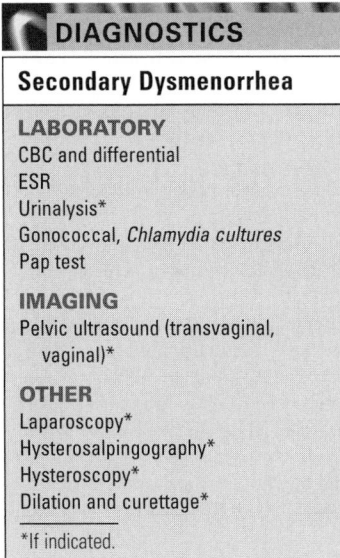

DIAGNOSTICS

Secondary Dysmenorrhea

LABORATORY
CBC and differential
ESR
Urinalysis*
Gonococcal, *Chlamydia cultures*
Pap test

IMAGING
Pelvic ultrasound (transvaginal, vaginal)*

OTHER
Laparoscopy*
Hysterosalpingography*
Hysteroscopy*
Dilation and curettage*

*If indicated.

DIFFERENTIAL DIAGNOSIS

Although the diagnosis of primary dysmenorrhea is made by a careful history and clinical presentation, the cause of secondary dysmenorrhea can be difficult to determine, and it is important to be aware of the possible causes. These causes can be broadly classified as intrauterine or extrauterine. Intrauterine causes include myomas, adenomyosis, polyps, an IUD, infection, cervical stenosis, and cervical lesions. Extrauterine causes include endometriosis; tumors (myomas or malignant); inflammation; adhesions; psychogenic causes such as pelvic congestion syndrome; and nongynecologic causes, which include urologic, gastrointestinal, musculoskeletal, and psychiatric conditions.[5]

MANAGEMENT

The mainstay of treatment for primary dysmenorrhea includes NSAIDs, which are antiprostaglandins, and oral contraceptives. NSAIDs are the best-established initial therapy for dysmenorrhea. They inhibit prostaglandin synthesis and thereby provide pain relief. They decrease the volume of menstrual flow, which may mitigate the dysmenorrhea.[1] Many studies have shown NSAIDs, including the cyclooxygenase-2 inhibitors, beneficial in the treatment of dysmenorrhea, although no studies have clearly determined which NSAIDs are the most efficacious.[3] Typical examples of NSAIDs that are approved by the U.S. Food and Drug Administration for treating primary dysmenorrhea are listed in Box 169-1. The choice for any particular drug may be determined by a woman's preference based on individual experience, dosing patterns, side effects, or cost.[3] NSAIDs may be the most effective when therapy is started before the onset of menstrual pain and flow, and they need not be continued for the entire menstrual cycle.[1]

Treatment of dysmenorrhea is a well-recognized "off-label" use for oral contraceptive pills.[13] Although more studies need to address the efficacy of oral contraceptives in the management of dysmenorrhea, it is theorized that oral contraceptives reduce prostaglandin release during menstruation, reduce and shorten the length of menstrual flow, and inhibit ovulation, thus reducing the pain of primary dysmenorrhea.[1,3] If the discomfort of primary dysmenorrhea is not controlled with NSAIDs or oral contraceptives, further diagnostic evaluation is indicated to exclude pelvic pathologic condition.

Other approaches used in the management of dysmenorrhea include calcium channel blockers (such as nifedipine or diltiazem), tocolytic agents (such as albuterol [Salbutamol]),

DIFFERENTIAL DIAGNOSIS

Dysmenorrhea

INTRAUTERINE CAUSES	Fibroids
Myomas	Inflammation
Adenomyosis	Adhesions
Polyps	Imperforate hymen
Intrauterine contraceptive device	Psychogenic causes
Infection	• Pelvic congestion syndrome
Cervical stenosis	Nongynecologic causes
Cervical lesions	• Urologic conditions
EXTRAUTERINE CAUSES	• Gastrointestinal conditions
Ectopic pregnancy	• Musculoskeletal conditions
Endometriosis	• Psychiatric conditions
Tumors	

BOX 169-1

EXAMPLES OF NSAIDs FOR TREATING DYSMENORRHEA

- Ibuprofen 400-800 mg PO q 6 hr for 3 days
- Naproxen 500 mg as initial dose, then 250 mg q 6-8 hr for 3 days
- Naproxen sodium 550 mg as initial dose, then 275 mg q 6-8 hr for 3 days
- Mefenamic acid 500 mg as initial dose, then 250 mg q 4-6 hr for 3 days
- Meclofenamate 100 mg as initial dose, then 50 to 100 mg q 6 hr (not to exceed 400 mg/day) for 3 days

progestogens, transcutaneous electrical nerve stimulation (TENS), acupuncture, herbal remedies, exercise, low-fat vegetarian diet, increased dietary fiber, castor oil packs to the abdomen, vitamin E (500 IU for 2 days before and 3 days after the onset of menses), fish oil supplement, psychotherapy, and hypnosis. TENS units, vitamin E, and exercise have proven beneficial in some studies, but more and larger studies are necessary to determine the effectiveness of other treatments.[1,14]

IUDs have historically been a relative contraindication in women with preexisting dysmenorrhea. However, there is some evidence that the frameless levonorgestrel-releasing IUD (Mirena) may reduce dysmenorrhea, since the progestin may act directly on the endometrium to reduce endometrial proliferation, as well as reduce menstrual flow and pain. This IUD has been introduced in Europe for the management of primary and secondary dysmenorrhea but is not currently labeled for this use in the United States.[1,3] Another option that may be available in the near future includes a vasopressin-receptor antagonist.

Presacral neurectomy and uterosacral ligament division were used in the past to treat dysmenorrhea but are rarely performed today.[1,3]

Narcotic analgesics should not be used for the typical level of discomfort associated with dysmenorrhea. Not only do narcotics raise issues related to prescription drug abuse, but the side effects of narcotics, such as sedation, and potential drug interactions may further affect a woman's ability to fully participate in daily life activities.[3]

These treatments for primary dysmenorrhea may also assist in the treatment of secondary dysmenorrhea. However, successful treatment of secondary dysmenorrhea depends on an accurate diagnosis of the cause of the pelvic pain.[3,5] In the absence of a clear diagnosis, nonacute pain can be treated empirically for a short time with some of the interventions described above.

COMPLICATIONS

Dysmenorrhea may be a difficult and frustrating condition to treat in some patients. If patients diagnosed with primary dysmenorrhea do not respond to conventional treatment, the diagnosis may need to be reassessed.

INDICATIONS FOR REFERRAL OR HOSPITALIZATION

Patients with recalcitrant primary dysmenorrhea and no apparent secondary causes found by physical examination, laboratory studies, and radiologic studies need to be referred for gynecologic evaluation for possible surgical diagnostic evaluation and treatment. Referral is also necessary if a secondary cause is found and requires surgical intervention. In difficult cases psychologic factors must be considered, and mental health referral may be warranted.

PATIENT AND FAMILY EDUCATION

Women with dysmenorrhea must be educated about the disorder and the rationale for certain treatments. Women on NSAID therapy should understand the potential gastrointestinal adverse effects associated with NSAIDs. One study has shown that risk factors for dysmenorrhea include early age at menarche, long menstrual periods, smoking, alcohol intake, and weight greater than the 90th percentile.[15] Given the possible association between stress and dysmenorrhea, stress reduction may be an effective preventive strategy for some and should be included in education regarding a healthy lifestyle.

REFERENCES

1. French L: Dysmenorrhea, *Am Acad Fam Phys* 71:285-291, 292, 2005.
2. McEvoy M, Chang J, Coupey S: Common menstrual disorders in adolescence, *Am J Maternal Child Nurs* 29(1):41-49, 2004.
3. Durain D: Primary dysmenorrhea: assessment and management, *J Midwif Women's Health* 49(6):520-528, 2004.
4. Weissman A, Hartz A, Hansen M, and others: The natural history of dysmenorrhoea: a longitudinal study, *Br J Obstet Gynaecol* 111:345-352, 2004.
5. Maxson WS, Rosenwaks Z: Dysmenorrhea and premenstrual syndrome. In Copeland LJ, editor: *Textbook of gynecology*, Philadelphia, 1993, Saunders.
6. Proctor M, Farquhar C: Dysmenorrhea. In Barton S, editor: *Clinical evidence*, London, 2001, BMJ Publishing Group.
7. Eden JA: Dysmenorrhea and premenstrual syndrome. In Hacker NF, Moore JG, editors: *Essentials of obstetrics and gynecology*, ed 2, Philadelphia, 1992, Saunders.
8. Harlow SD, Park M: A longitudinal study of risk factors for the occurrence, duration and severity of menstrual cramps in a cohort of college women, *Br J Obstet Gynecol* 103:1134-1142, 1996.
9. Parazzini F, Tozzi L, Mezzopane R, and others: Cigarette smoking, alcohol consumption, and risk of primary dysmenorrheal, *Epidemiology* 5:469-472, 1994.
10. Wang L, Wang, X, Wang W, and others: Stress and dysmenorrhoea: a population based prospective study, *Occup Environ Med* 61(12):1021-1026, 2004.
11. Zang T, Wang L, Xu X: Stress and dysmenorrhea: a population based prospective study, *Occup Environ Med* 61:1021-1026, 2004.
12. Alonso C, Coe C: Disruptions of social relationships accentuate the association between emotional distress and menstrual pain in young women, *Health Psychol* 20:411-416, 2001.
13. Davis A, Westhoff C, O'Connell K, and others: Oral contraceptives for dysmenorrhea in adolescent girls, *Obstet Gynecol* 106(1):97-104, 2005.
14. Nagata C, Hirokawa K, Shimizu N, and others: Associations of menstrual pain with intakes of soy, fat and dietary fiber in Japanese women, *Eur J Clin Nutr* 59:88-92, 2005.
15. Kennedy S: Primary dysmenorrhea, *Lancet* 349(9095):1116, 1997.

CHAPTER 170

Dyspareunia

Marie Elena Botte

DEFINITION AND EPIDEMIOLOGY

Dyspareunia is defined as recurrent or persistent genital pain associated with sexual intercourse.[1] The condition is not unique to women; men can have dyspareunia from a variety of causes, including dermatologic infections, structural abnormalities,[2] and anodyspareunia in men who have receptive anal sex.[3] However, it is much more commonly encountered in women and is therefore almost exclusively described as a women's health issue. Dyspareunia can develop secondary to other vulvar problems such as vulvar vestibulitis, vaginismus, or vulvodynia. *Vulvar vestibulitis* refers to severe pain on vestibular contact or with attempted vaginal entry, tenderness to pressure within the vestibule, and vulvar erythema.[4] *Vaginismus* is involuntary spasm of the muscles surrounding the outer third of the vagina brought on by real, imagined, or anticipated attempts at vaginal penetration.[5] *Vulvodynia* refers to chronic vulvar discomfort that may involve complaints of rawness, burning, stinging, or irritation; it is not necessarily related to sexual activity.

Dyspareunia is a common gynecologic complaint,[6] with an estimated prevalence of between 12.8% and 60%.[7-10] Factors influencing dyspareunia include spontaneous and postabortive pelvic inflammatory disease; early postpartum or perimenopausal status; a history of sexual abuse or cervical cancer[11-14]; and psychosocial factors such as rigid religious upbringing, low physical and emotional satisfaction, decreased general happiness, or previous painful sexual experience. Dyspareunia has not been consistently associated with factors such as age, parity, marital status, race, income, or education.[8] Hormonal and sexual history factors (oral contraception use before age 17 years and first intercourse before age 15 years) have been proposed as causes for vulvar vestibulitis syndrome.[15] Other studies have found that women with vulvar vestibulitis had a lower pain threshold, a higher magnitude estimation of pain, higher trait anxiety, increased somatization, poorer body image than controls, hypervigilance for coital pain, and a selective attentional bias toward pain stimuli.[16,17]

PATHOPHYSIOLOGY

Although the *Diagnostic and Statistical Manual of Mental Disorders* currently classifies dyspareunia as a sexual pain disorder,[18] a debate rages as to whether dyspareunia reflects a predominant psychopathology, a condition of sexual dysfunction, or a physical pain syndrome.[19,20] However it is classified academically, there is evidence of high levels of psychologic distress in some women with dyspareunia, particularly those with vulvar vestibulitis[21] and vulvodynia.[22] Various etiologies for dyspareunia are noted in the literature, including inflammatory and infectious processes (human semen carries the irritating toxin in ciguatera), nonalcoholic liver disease (by decreasing vaginal lubrication), chemotherapy, trauma (horseback riding, sexual abuse, genital mutilation), and genital manifestations of other systemic diseases such as discoid lupus erythematosus.[23-27]

Structural abnormalities that can cause dyspareunia include glomus tumors; leiomyomas of the uterus and urethra[28]; vaginal, urethral, and hymenal abnormalities; postobstetric or postoperative vulvar outlet stenosis; and stenosing lichen planus. Women with deep infiltrating endometriosis of the uterosacral ligament can have severe impairment of sexual function,[29-31] and many have had deep dyspareunia for their entire sex lives.[32] Aortoiliac or atherosclerotic disease can diminish pelvic blood flow and lead to vaginal wall and clitoral smooth muscle fibrosis.[1] Pelvic floor surgery can either ameliorate preexisting dyspareunia or cause it.[33-35] Episiotomies, particularly those involving the mediolateral technique and glycerol-impregnated chromic catgut, have been tied to significant increases in dyspareunia.[36-39] Obstetric instrumentation and perineal trauma during delivery contribute to postpartum dyspareunia.[36,40,41]

Dyspareunia is often due to inadequate vaginal lubrication. This can often be attributable to either insufficient stimulation or arousal during sexual activity or can be related to decreased estrogen, a condition noted in postmenopausal women, women taking tamoxifen for chemoprevention of breast cancer,[42] and breast cancer survivors.[43,44] Superficial dyspareunia has been associated with factitious urticaria,[45] vulvovaginal candidal infection and recurrent candidiasis,[46] urinary tract infections,[27] urinary incontinence,[47] occlusion of Bartholin's gland duct,[48] Bowen's disease, interstitial cystitis, and focal vestibulitis.

Tiny mucosal tears have been implicated in focal vulvitis,[38] and perivascular inflammation has been proposed as a mechanism causing dyspareunia in women with Sjögren's syndrome.[23] Dyspareunia after a normal pelvic examination has been linked with overexertion of the levator ani muscles and subsequent myalgia after the initiation of Kegel exercises.[34] When the levator ani muscles are hypertonic, vaginismus can result.[1,49]

One study found a group of women with progressively worsening dyspareunia who had been treated unsuccessfully for nonspecific vulvitis and vaginitis whose external genitals appeared normal on close visual inspection but under magnification revealed erythema around the Bartholin's duct openings.[50] In another study of 21 women treated surgically for dyspareunia and vulvodynia, stricture of the vaginal introitus secondary to membranous hypertrophy of the posterior fourchette was noted.[51] In addition to histologic findings of chronic nonspecific inflammation in many of the women and two with changes suggestive of human papillomavirus infection, 80% of these women had erythema and tenderness of the vestibule.

In vulvar vestibulitis syndrome a conditioned, protective, muscle-guarding response has been proposed leading to a pelvic floor pathologic condition. In one recent study, women with vulvar vestibulitis had significantly more vaginal hypertonicity, decreased vaginal muscle strength, and a restriction of the vaginal opening, compared with controls.[49] Recent data suggest that vaginismus cannot easily be distinguished from vestibulitis by vaginal spasm and pain alone, but that women with vaginismus demonstrate significantly greater vaginal and pelvic muscle tone and lower muscle strength, have a higher frequency of defensive and avoidant distress behaviors during pelvic examinations, and recall past attempts at intercourse with more affective distress.[52]

CLINICAL PRESENTATION

Health care providers need to take an active role in inquiring specifically about discomfort during or after sexual intercourse and not simply assume that women will raise the issue if it is a problem. Women often will not voice this concern even if it is the main reason for their visit.[38,53] Research has shown that, although some women will discuss dyspareunia with their partner, far fewer consult a health care provider for the problem. Of women who seek medical help, only 15% receive a specific diagnosis or effective treatment.

A thorough symptom analysis will guide the physical examination and should specifically include questioning about the onset of the discomfort and its relationship to particular partners; positions; times in the menstrual cycle; contraceptive devices and substances (such as latex condoms, spermicides, or lubricants); and products such as douches, soaps, tampons, or detergents. Women may report pain with tampon use or pelvic examinations. Important information to gather includes number of pregnancies and type of delivery, surgical history, history of rape or sexual abuse, and menopausal signs and symptoms. Knowing whether the pain is on entry, postcoital, generalizable to the entire vulva, felt only with deep thrusting, or localized to a particular anatomic structure or area is helpful in determining the cause of the discomfort. Several symptom-related scales have been proposed, such as the Female Sexual Function Index,[54] but are not widely used in clinical practice.

PHYSICAL EXAMINATION

A thorough pelvic examination is necessary for all complaints of dyspareunia. The experience can be educational for the woman and more informative for the provider if the patient sits somewhat upright and holds a small hand mirror; this allows the woman to see what is happening and feel more in control.[55] It is important to correlate the discomfort elicited during the pelvic examination with specific physical findings whenever possible. In addition, clarification should be sought regarding pain elicited to determine whether it is similar to what the woman has been experiencing during intercourse, since many women find pelvic examinations generally uncomfortable.

The external genitals should be examined for erythema, pigment changes, lesions (including herpes and condyloma), and indications of trauma or abuse. Touching the vestibule and the hymen with a moistened cotton swab may elicit the pain of vulvar vestibulitis, a condition in which there is exquisite tenderness to pressure at specific sites, often accompanied by erythema.

A finger inserted gently into the introitus and gradually pressed in a posterior direction may elicit the spasms of vaginismus; conscious control of the pelvic floor musculature can be evaluated by asking the woman to squeeze and relax the muscles around the examiner's finger. The Bartholin's glands, which are normally not palpable, may be tender and enlarged. A narrow, well-lubricated speculum should be used to evaluate the vagina. A bimanual examination can assess for uterine and ovarian size, fibroids, ovarian cysts, other pelvic masses, cervical motion tenderness (seen with pelvic inflammatory disease), and the position of the uterus. Hemorrhoids or prolapse of the uterus, bladder, or rectum may be evident. A rectal or rectovaginal examination is generally not necessary.

DIAGNOSTICS

Wet mounts, potassium hydroxide prep and cultures of vaginal discharge, endocervical Papanicolaou's smear, and *Chlamydia trachomatis* and *Neisseria gonorrhoeae* cultures will help rule out infection as a cause for either superficial or deep dyspareunia.[38] A CBC and erythrocyte sedimentation rate can help identify inflammation and infection; a urinalysis evaluates for urinary tract infection, and a human chorionic gonadotropin can exclude ectopic pregnancy.

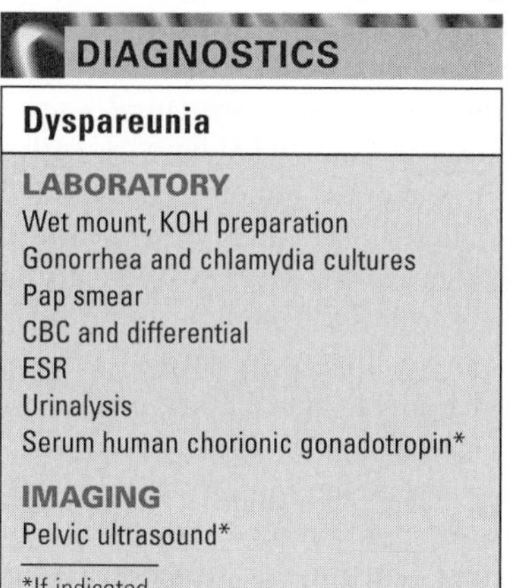

DIAGNOSTICS

Dyspareunia

LABORATORY
Wet mount, KOH preparation
Gonorrhea and chlamydia cultures
Pap smear
CBC and differential
ESR
Urinalysis
Serum human chorionic gonadotropin*

IMAGING
Pelvic ultrasound*

*If indicated.

DIFFERENTIAL DIAGNOSIS

Potential causes for dyspareunia include both psychologic and pathophysiologic etiologies. Most cases are probably a combination of both. A problem that is initially physical often has a continued and escalating psychologic impact. Potential causes for dyspareunia are listed in the Differential Diagnosis

DIFFERENTIAL DIAGNOSIS

Dyspareunia

SURFACE (OCCURS WITH PENETRATION)
- Insufficient arousal
- Hypoestrogenic mucosa
- Vaginitis
- Vaginismus
- Hymenal abnormalities
- Dermatopathology
- Postherpetic neuralgia

FOCAL
- Vulvar vestibulitis
- Bartholin's gland cyst or abscess
- Episiotomy scar
- Residual sutures
- Introital tear
- Herpetic lesions
- Urethral problems

DEEP (OCCURS WITH PENILE THRUSTING)
- Pelvic inflammatory disease
- Fibroids
- Endometriosis
- Hemorrhoids
- Inflammatory bowel disease
- Retroverted uterus
- Uterine prolapse
- Pelvic adhesions or masses

POSTCOITAL
- Urinary tract infection
- Vulvodynia

IRRITANTS
- Contraceptive devices
- Spermicides
- Douches
- Feminine hygiene products
- Soaps

PSYCHOSOCIAL FACTORS
- Anxiety
- Prior painful sexual experience
- Rigid upbringing

box and are arranged according to the phase of intercourse during which the symptom is experienced.

MANAGEMENT AND HEALTH PROMOTION

Women with dyspareunia resulting from insufficient lubrication may benefit significantly from education regarding the physiology of female arousal and the importance of allowing adequate time before vaginal penetration for the vascular engorgement of genital tissues that results in glandular secretions. If the problem is estrogen-insufficient vaginal dryness, national guidelines suggest topical estrogen cream or hormone replacement therapy (HRT) as the most effective way to build up the vascularity of the vaginal epithelium and thereby induce physiologic lubrication.[56-60] Women need to be informed about the risks of HRT before any decisions are made about treatment. Alternative vaginal lubrication (water-based products such as glycerin [Astroglide]) for those women using condoms or diaphragms) is suggested for those women for whom supplemental estrogen is contraindicated. Alternative sexual positioning (female astride to control penetration) or position changes can alleviate the pain of dyspareunia for some women, as can nonsteroidal agents, topical application of lidocaine, or a warm bath before sex.[61]

Dyspareunia secondary to endometriosis has been treated successfully during therapy and for 6 months afterward with both gonadotropin-releasing hormone (GnRH) analogs (nafarelin acetate) and danazol[62,63]; options studied include using a danazol-loaded intrauterine device.[64] Add-back therapy (combining the GnRH agonist with other agents such as estrogens, progestins, or bisphosphonates) improves pain control with reduced bone mineral density loss.[63] Treatment of vaginismus-related dyspareunia focuses on helping the woman regain voluntary control of the muscles of the pelvic floor.[5] Treatments for vulvodynia include a low-oxalate diet and calcium citrate supplementation to neutralize urinary oxalates and tricyclic agents.[65,66] Behavioral approaches are most often used and often involve pelvic floor contraction-relaxation exercises and using fingers or dilators to progressively desensitize the woman to vaginal penetration. Surgical intervention is rarely required and may be detrimental to the resolution of vaginismus.[5]

Behavioral treatment is first-line therapy for vulvar vestibulitis syndrome; research documents no statistical difference in effect between this option and corrective surgery.[67] Vulvar vestibulitis has been treated successfully with pelvic floor surface electromyography biofeedback,[68] the manual techniques of pelvic floor physical therapists,[49] topical estrogen cream applied twice a day for 4 to 8 weeks, intralesional injections of interferon,[65] and local application of capsaicin cream.[69] Recent research suggests that treatment strategies for vulvar vestibulitis would be prudent to address fear, anxiety, and physiologic sensory systems.[17] Surgical intervention such as a modified vestibulectomy[70] and vaginal apex repair[71] can be effective in cases refractory to more conservative approaches.

LIFE SPAN CONSIDERATIONS

Dyspareunia affects sexually active women of all ages but may become increasingly evident at times of major transition in a woman's life, including onset of sexual activity, childbirth, and menopause.

COMPLICATIONS

Dyspareunia is known to have a detrimental effect on relationships and can continue unacknowledged and unaided for years in the absence of clinician inquiry and therapeutic involvement. Although the morbidity associated with dyspareunia varies widely with its attendant cause, the impact on a woman's quality of life can be profound and should not be underestimated.

INDICATIONS FOR REFERRAL OR HOSPITALIZATION

Women with dyspareunia related to severe psychologic distress or anxiety may be best managed in collaboration with psychiatric or other counseling services. For severe vulvar vestibulitis unresponsive to conservative behavioral-based therapies, perineoplasty or posterior vestibulectomy can be performed as a last resort[4,72] and involves a crescent-shaped posterior vestibular excision followed by vaginal advancement. Surgery is less successful if there is concomitant vaginismus (unless the vaginismus is treated first),[4] in dyspareunia present since first intercourse, and in women with associated persistent vulvar pain.[73]

One treatment guideline suggests that hysterectomy may be indicated for women with documented pelvic adhesions unresponsive to lysis or for women over 30 years old with more than 6 months of moderate to severe idiopathic dyspareunia unresponsive to nonsteroidal drugs and/or HRT who do not desire further children, but only after other potential causes have been excluded by laparoscopy or laparotomy, colonoscopy and barium enema, cystoscopy and IV pyelography, and psychologic evaluation.[74] For some women in whom dyspareunia is related to prior hysterectomy, surgical excision of the vaginal apex has been a successful surgical procedure.[75]

PATIENT AND FAMILY EDUCATION

Education is central in the management of dyspareunia, particularly when the cause of discomfort is attributable to insufficient sexual arousal time and lubrication, spasms of vaginismus, control of concomitant infections, or the use of irritating or allergenic products. Taking the time to educate individuals about their bodies and the particular strategies necessary to attain or resume sexual activity without discomfort is an important aspect of comprehensive, holistic primary care.

REFERENCES

1. Berman J, Goldstein I: Female sexual dysfunction, *Urol Clin North Am* 28(2):405-416, 2001.
2. Shechet J, Tannenbaum B, Freid S: Male dyspareunia in the uncircumcised patient, *Am Fam Phys* 60(1):54, 56, 1999.
3. Damon W, Rosser BR: Anodyspareunia in men who have sex with men: prevalence, predictors, consequences and the development of DSM diagnostic criteria, *J Sex Marital Therapy* 31(2):129-141, 2005.
4. Abramov L, Wolman I, David MP: Vaginismus: an important factor in the evaluation and management of vulvar vestibulitis syndrome, *Gynecol Obstet Invest* 38(3):194-197, 1994.
5. Biswas A, Ratnam SS: Vaginismus and outcome of treatment, *Ann Acad Med Singapore* 24(5):755-758, 1995.

6. Munday P, Green J, Randall C, and others: Vulval vestibulitis: a common cause of dyspareunia? *BJOG* 112(4):500-503, 2005.
7. Ponholzer A, Roehlich M, Racz U, and others: Female sexual dysfunction in a healthy Austrian cohort: prevalence and risk factors, *Eur Urol* 47(3):366-374, discussion 374-375, 2005.
8. Heim L: Evaluation and differential diagnosis of dyspareunia, *Am Fam Phys* 63(8):1535-1544, 2001.
9. Jamieson DJ, Steege JF: The prevalence of dysmenorrhea, dyspareunia, pelvic pain, and irritable bowel syndrome in primary care practices, *Obstet Gynecol* 87(1):55-58, 1996.
10. Glatt AE, Zinner SH, McCormack WM: The prevalence of dyspareunia, *Obstet Gynecol* 75(3 Pt 1):433-436, 1990.
11. Heisterberg L: Factors influencing spontaneous abortion, dyspareunia, dysmenorrhea, and pelvic pain, *Obstet Gynecol* 81(4):594-597, 1993.
12. Connolly A, Thorp J, Pahel L: Effects of pregnancy and childbirth on postpartum sexual function: a longitudinal prospective study, *Int Urogynecol J* 16(4):263-267, 2005.
13. Avis NE, and others: Correlates of sexual function among multi-ethnic middle-aged women: results from the Study of Women's Health Across the Nation (SWAN) [see comment], *Menopause* 12(4):385-398, 2005.
14. Bergmark K, and others: Synergy between sexual abuse and cervical cancer in causing sexual dysfunction, *J Sex Marital Therapy* 31(5):361-383, 2005.
15. Bazin S, and others: Vulvar vestibulitis syndrome: an exploratory case-control study, *Obstet Gynecol* 83(1):47-50, 1994.
16. Granot M, Lavee Y: Psychological factors associated with perception of experimental pain in vulvar vestibulitis syndrome, *J Sex Marital Therapy* 31(4):285-302, 2005.
17. Payne KA, and others: When sex hurts, anxiety and fear orient attention towards pain, *Eur J Pain* 9(4):427-436. 2005.
18. American Psychiatric Association: *Diagnostic and statistical manual of mental disorders*, ed 4 (text rev), Washington, DC, 2000, The Association.
19. Binik YM: Should dyspareunia be retained as a sexual dysfunction in DSM-V? A painful classification decision [see comment], *Arch Sex Behav* 34(1):11-21, 2005.
20. Basson R: Recent advances in women's sexual function and dysfunction, *Menopause* 11(6 Pt 2):714-725, 2004.
21. Green J, Hetherton J: Psychological aspects of vulvar vestibulitis syndrome, *J Psychosom Obstet Gynecol* 26(2):101-106, 2005.
22. Wylie K, Hallam-Jones R, Harrington C: Psychological difficulties within a group of patients with vulvodynia, *J Psychosom Obstet Gynecol* 25(3-4):257-265, 2004.
23. Skopouli FN, and others: Obstetric and gynaecologic profile in patients with primary Sjögren's syndrome, *Ann Rheum Dis* 53(9):569-573, 1994.
24. Krychman ML, and others: Chemotherapy-induced dyspareunia: a case study of vaginal mucositis and pegylated liposomal doxorubicin injection in advanced stage ovarian carcinoma, *Gynecol Oncol* 93(2):561-563, 2004.
25. Wallis L: When rites are wrong, *Nurs Stand* 20(4):24-26, 2005.
26. Engman M, Lindehammar H, Wijma B: Surface electromyography diagnostics in women with partial vaginismus with or without vulvar vestibulitis and in asymptomatic women, *J Psychosom Obstet Gynecol* 25(3-4):281-294, 2004.
27. Jones MA, and others: Small cell neuroendocrine carcinoma of Bartholin's gland, *Am J Clin Pathol* 94(4):439-442, 1990.
28. Goto K, and others: Leiomyoma of the female urethra: urodynamic changes after surgical intervention, *Int Urogynecol J* 16(2):162-164, 2005.
29. Chapron C, and others: Presurgical diagnosis of posterior deep infiltrating endometriosis based on a standardized questionnaire, *Hum Reprod* 20(2):507-513, 2005.
30. Jones G, Jenkinson C, Kennedy S: The impact of endometriosis upon quality of life: a qualitative analysis, *J Psychosom Obstet Gynecol* 25(2):123-133, 2004.
31. Denny E: Women's experience of endometriosis, *J Adv Nurs* 46(6):641-648, 2004.
32. Ferrero S, and others: Quality of sex life in women with endometriosis and deep dyspareunia, *Fertility Sterility* 83(3):573-579, 2005.
33. Helstrom L, Nilsson B: Impact of vaginal surgery on sexuality and quality of life in women with urinary incontinence or genital descensus, *Acta Obstet Gynecol Scand* 84(1):79-84, 2005.
34. DeLancey JOL, Sampselle CM, Punch MR: Kegel dyspareunia: levator ani myalgia caused by overexertion, *Obstet Gynecol* 82(4):658-659, 1993.
35. Abramov Y, and others: Do alterations in vaginal dimensions after reconstructive pelvic surgeries affect the risk for dyspareunia? *Am J Obstet Gynecol* 192(5):1573-1577, 2005.
36. Klein MC, and others: A comparison of urinary and sexual outcomes in women experiencing vaginal and Caesarean births, *J Obstet Gynaecol Canada* 27(4):332-339, 2005.
37. Bex PJ, Hofmeyer GJ: Perineal management during childbirth and subsequent dyspareunia, *Clin Exper Obstet Gynecol* 14(2):97-100, 1987.
38. Sarazin SK, Seymour SF: Causes and treatment options for women with dyspareunia, *Nurse Pract* 16(10):30, 35-38, 41, 1991.
39. Grant A: Dyspareunia associated with the use of glycerol-impregnated catgut to repair perineal trauma: report of a 3-year follow up study, *Br J Obstet Gynecol* 96(6):741-743, 1989.
40. Signorello L: Postpartum sexual functioning and its relationship to perineal trauma: a retrospective cohort study of primiparous women, *Am J Obstet Gynecol* 184(5):881-890, 2001.
41. Hicks TL, and others: Postpartum sexual functioning and method of delivery: summary of the evidence, *J Midwifery Women's Health* 49(5):430-436, 2004.
42. Melnikow J, and others: Preferences of Women Evaluating Risks of Tamoxifen (POWER) study of preferences for tamoxifen for breast cancer risk reduction, *Cancer* 103(10):1996-2005, 2005.
43. Loprinzi CL, and others: Phase III randomized double blind study to evaluate the efficacy of a polycarbil-based vaginal moisturizer in women with breast cancer, *J Clin Oncol* 15(3):969-973, 1997.
44. Schultz PN, and others: Breast cancer: relationship between menopausal symptoms, physiologic health effects of cancer treatment and physical constraints on quality of life in long-term survivors [see comment], *J Clin Nurs* 14(2):204-211, 2005.
45. Lambris A, Greaves MW: Dyspareunia and vulvodynia are probably common manifestations of factitious urticaria, *Br J Dermatol* 136(1):140-141, 1997.
46. Rylander E, and others: Vulvovaginal candida in a young sexually active population: prevalence and association with oro-genital sex and frequent pain at intercourse, *Sexually Trans Infect* 80(1):54-57, 2004.
47. Handa VL, and others: Sexual function among women with urinary incontinence and pelvic organ prolapse, *Am J Obstet Gynecol* 191(3):751-756, 2004.
48. Sarrel PM, and others: Pain during sex response due to occlusion of the Bartholin gland duct, *Obstet Gynecol* 62(2):261-264, 1983.
49. Reissing ED, and others: Pelvic floor muscle functioning in women with vulvar vestibulitis syndrome, *J Psychosom Obstet Gynecol* 26(2):107-113, 2005.
50. Lopez-Zeno JA, Ross E, O'Grady JP: Septic shock complicating drainage of a Bartholin gland abscess, *Obstet Gynecol* 76(5):915-916, 1990.
51. Barbero M, and others: Membranous hypertrophy of the posterior fourchette as a cause of dyspareunia and vulvodynia, *J Reprod Med* 39(12):949-952, 1994.
52. Reissing ED, and others: Vaginal spasm, pain, and behavior: an empirical investigation of the diagnosis of vaginismus, *Arch Sexual Behav* 33(1):5-17, 2004.
53. Jarvis GJ: Dyspareunia, *Br Med J* 288:1555-1556, 1987.
54. Masheb RM, and others: Assessing sexual function and dyspareunia with the Female Sexual Function Index (FSFI) in women with vulvodynia, *J Sex Marital Therapy* 30(5):315-324, 2004.
55. Steege JF, Ling FW: Dyspareunia: a special type of chronic pelvic pain, *Obstet Gynecol Clin North Am* 20(4):779-793, 1993.

56. North American Menopause Society: Clinical challenges of perimenopause: consensus opinion of the North American Menopause Society, *Menopause* 7(1):5-13, 2000.
57. North American Menopause Society: A decision tree for the use of estrogen replacement therapy or hormone replacement therapy in postmenopausal women: consensus of the North American Menopause Society, *Menopause* 7(2):76-86, 2000.
58. US Preventive Services Task Force: *Postmenopausal hormone prophylaxis*, Baltimore, 1996, Williams & Wilkins.
59. American Association of Clinical Endocrinologists: AACE medical guidelines for clinical practice for management of menopause, *Endocrine Pract* 355-366, 1999.
60. National Institutes of Health: National Institutes of Health State-of-the-Science Conference statement: management of menopause-related symptoms, *Ann Intern Med* 142(12 Pt 1):1003-1013, 2005.
61. Phillips N: Female sexual dysfunction: evaluation and treatment, *Am Fam Phys* 62(1):127-136, 2000.
62. Adamson GD, Kwei L, Edgren EA: Pain of endometriosis: effects of nafarelin and danazol therapy, *Int J Fertility Menop Studies* 39(4):215-217, 1994.
63. Zupi E, and others: Add-back therapy in the treatment of endometriosis-associated pain, *Fertility Sterility* 82(5):1303-1308, 2004.
64. Cobellis L, and others: A danazol-loaded intrauterine device decreases dysmenorrhea, pelvic pain, and dyspareunia associated with endometriosis, *Fertility Sterility* 82(1):239-240, 2004.
65. Metts J: Vulvodynia and vulvar vestibulitis: challenges in diagnosis and management, *Am Fam Phys* 59(6):1547-1556, 1999.
66. Quint E, Smith Y: Adolescent gynecology, part 1, Common disorders, *Pediatr Clin North Am* 46(3):593-606, 1999.
67. Weijmar Schultz WC, and others: Behavioral approach with or without surgical intervention to the vulvar vestibulitis syndrome: a prospective randomized and non-randomized study, *J Psychosom Obstet Gynaecol* 17(3):143-148, 1996.
68. Rosenbaum TY: Physiotherapy treatment of sexual pain disorders, *J Sex Marital Therapy* 31(4):329-340, 2005.
69. Steinberg AC, and others: Capsaicin for the treatment of vulvar vestibulitis, *Am J Obstet Gynecol* 192(5):1549-1553, 2005.
70. Lavy Y, and others: Modified vulvar vestibulectomy: simple and effective surgery for the treatment of vulvar vestibulitis, *Eur J Obstet Gynecol Reprod Biol* 120(1):91-95, 2005.
71. Lamvu G, and others: Vaginal apex resection: a treatment option for vaginal apex pain, *Obstet Gynecol* 104(6):1340-1346, 2004.
72. Berville S, Moyal-Barracco M, Paniel BJ: Treatment of vulvar vestibulitis by posterior vestibulectomy: 12 case reports, *J Gynecologie Obstetrique Biologie Reproduc* 26(1):71-75, 1997.
73. Bornstein J, and others: Predicting the outcome of surgical treatment of vulvar vestibulitis, *Obstet Gynecol* 89(5 Pt 1):695-698, 1997.
74. Group OCD: *Hysterectomy*, Lexington, Mass, 1997 (rev 1999).
75. Sharp H: The role of vaginal apex excision in the management of persistent posthysterectomy dyspareunia, *Am J Obstet Gynecol* 183(6):1385-1388, 2000.

CHAPTER 171

Ectopic Pregnancy

Marie Elena Botte

DEFINITION AND EPIDEMIOLOGY

Ectopic pregnancy occurs when a fertilized ovum implants anywhere outside of the uterus. Occurring in 1 out of 100 pregnancies,[1] ectopic pregnancy is the second leading cause of maternal mortality[2] and the leading cause of pregnancy-related death in the first trimester.[3,4] The rate of ectopic pregnancy in the United States rose dramatically in the past few decades[5]; prevalence rose sixfold since 1970, peaking in the late 1980s,[4] perhaps because of an attendant increase in sexually transmitted diseases, increased frequency of sterilization procedures, and delayed childbearing[6]; the incidence possibly plateaued around the turn of the twenty-first century.[7] The rate of ectopic pregnancy has been found to increase dramatically after the age of 30, especially beyond the age of 35.[8] The mortality rate related to ectopic pregnancy is still high (6% of pregnancy-related deaths in one recent study[9]), and for African Americans it is still much higher than for Caucasian women[4,9]; among adolescents of minority race the rate is five times that of their Caucasian counterparts, a difference not entirely explained by the difference in prevalence between these groups.[10]

Risk factors for ectopic pregnancy include tubal pathologic conditions; prior tubal surgery; a prior ectopic gestation; in vitro fertilization[11] (embryo transfer and assisted hatching[12]); and use of intrauterine devices (IUDs), particularly progesterone-only devices.[13]

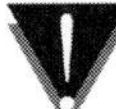

Immediate emergency department referral or physician consultation is indicated for female patients with a positive test for serum human chorionic gonadotropin (HCG), abdominal pain, and vaginal bleeding.

PATHOPHYSIOLOGY

Proposed pathophysiologic explanations for ectopic pregnancy include abnormal embryogenesis[14,15] (with serious chromosomal aberration in one third of cases[16]), ascending *Chlamydia trachomatis* infection that scars the fallopian tubes,[17] and luteal phase defects.[18] History of or current pelvic inflammatory disease (PID) and in utero diethylstilbestrol (DES) exposure may also result in ectopic gestation. Cases have been reported that involve clear cell hyperplasia of the fallopian tube[19] and development in a cesarean section scar.[20] Although implantation can occur anywhere on the cervix, in the abdomen, or on the ovary, 95% of ectopic pregnancies implant in the fallopian tube.[2]

Cervical pregnancy, which accounts for less than 1% of all ectopic pregnancies, has been associated with cervicouterine instrumentation[14]; ovarian pregnancy has been associated with ovulation induction and intrauterine insemination.[21] Persistent ectopic pregnancy involves residual trophoblastic activity and a beta-HCG level that rises or plateaus, whereas chronic ectopic pregnancy contains no active trophoblastic tissue and results in an HCG level that is low or absent.[22] One retrospective study found that chronic ectopic pregnancy accounts for as much as 20.3% of all ectopic pregnancies.[23]

CLINICAL PRESENTATION

Risk factors for ectopic pregnancy should be elicited for any woman when pregnancy is suspected, although identifiable factors may be absent in many women with ectopic pregnancies.[24] Risk factors that interfere with fallopian tube function include past or current history of the following: sexually transmitted infections and PID,[25,26] including recurrent chlamydial infection[27]; pregnancy occurring while on oral contraceptives (because of the mechanism of action of the birth control pill on the ciliary movement of the fallopian tube); previous history of ectopic pregnancy[24,28]; history of infertility[24]; in utero DES exposure[28]; documented tubal pathologic condition[28]; prior appendectomy or pelvic operation[24]; cesarean section[29]; prior tubal sterilization or operation[24,28,30,31]; history of in vitro fertilization[2]; and congenital malformation of the fallopian tubes.[2] Cigarette smoking,[2,32] vaginal douching,[33,34] multiple sexual partners, and early age at first intercourse have weaker evidence for association. Although IUDs per se do not increase the risk for ectopic pregnancy, pregnancies that occur with these devices in place are more likely to be ectopic.[35] Previous induced abortion has not been associated with subsequent ectopic pregnancy.[36,37]

Symptoms of unruptured ectopic pregnancy can be vague and subacute. The most common symptom of ectopic pregnancy is abdominal pain, which may manifest in isolation or in combination with vaginal bleeding or spotting, dizziness, and shoulder pain[38] (which suggests blood irritating the diaphragm); symptoms generally appear between 6 and 12 weeks' gestation. Amenorrhea for 1 to 2 months and the usual early signs of pregnancy (nausea, fatigue, breast heaviness) are often part of the initial presentation. Women can also be seen with generalized or unilateral pelvic or abdominal pain described as sharp, cramping, continuous, or intermittent. Less common presenting symptoms include acute urinary retention[39] and abnormal dark, scant vaginal bleeding. Painless vaginal bleeding is the most common presentation for cervical pregnancy.[40] Pain that radiates to the shoulder is more common in a ruptured ectopic pregnancy. Acute syncopal episodes and hypotension are possible secondary to rupture-induced peritoneal hemorrhage. Chronic ectopic pregnancy generally appears as a pelvic mass, with minimum symptoms such as intermittent pain and a low or absent HCG titer.[23,41]

PHYSICAL EXAMINATION

Any suspicion of ectopic pregnancy requires a thorough physical examination, although the history and physical examination, with a combined sensitivity of 50%, can neither exclude nor confirm an ectopic pregnancy. Postural vital signs and temperature are essential to indicate the presence of hypotension or infection. Speculum examination may reveal a bulging cul de sac (indicative of hemoperitoneum in rupture), a bluish coloration of the cervix (a normal finding in any pregnancy), and vaginal bleeding. Uterine enlargement occurs in roughly one fourth of women with ectopic pregnancy, but its size may be less than expected according to dates (generally smaller than 8 weeks' size). Approximately 75% of women with ectopic pregnancies have abdominal tenderness,[2] but the abdominal examination may be normal if the ectopic pregnancy has not ruptured; cervical motion tenderness may also be present. An adnexal mass and peritoneal signs, although uncommon, are highly predictive of ectopic gestation.

The pelvic examination may also reveal signs that suggest a cause other than ectopic pregnancy as the source of the bleeding, such as hemorrhoids, urethral irritation, cervical lesions, or condyloma. Although tissue at the os is a sign of spontaneous abortion and an open os and heavy vaginal bleeding are predictive of an abnormal intrauterine pregnancy, absence of these signs does not differentiate ectopic from intrauterine gestation.[42]

DIAGNOSTICS

Pregnancy tests have become increasingly sensitive in recent years and are the first step in the diagnosis of any suspected ectopic pregnancy. The slope of a rising HCG titer has been found to be a useful determinant of early ectopic pregnancy below the ultrasonographic discriminatory zone.[43,44] In normal pregnancy, this titer doubles every 1.4 to 3.5 days,[6] with a minimum of 66% increase suggesting viable pregnancy in clinical practice; a titer that plateaus or falls suggests either ectopic pregnancy or miscarriage, although some ectopic pregnancies (and nonviable intrauterine pregnancies) do have abnormally rising HCG levels. Recent evidence suggests that declining HCG levels in spontaneous abortions can be distinguished from those in ectopic gestation; ectopic gestation (or retained trophoblastic tissue) has a rate of decline that is less than 21% at 2 days or 60% at 7 days.[45] Because nearly all ectopic pregnancies have HCG titers less than 50,000 mIU/ml, a single value above this level can help rule out ectopic pregnancy.

Initial diagnostic tests also include a CBC, since women with ectopic gestation are often anemic, and a blood type and Rh determination. Serum progesterone is a useful marker of viable pregnancy[1,6,46]; levels over 25 ng/ml are highly predictive of successful intrauterine pregnancy and correlate with low risk of ectopic pregnancy,[47] and levels less than 5 ng/ml indicate nonviable pregnancies with nearly 100% sensitivity. Other potential markers for ectopic pregnancy include leukemia inhibitory factor (involved in the implantation process), vascular endothelial growth factor, and smooth muscle heavy-chain myosin (implicated in smooth muscle destruction), but at present none of these indexes is sufficiently discriminatory to be useful in clinical practice.[48-50]

Ultrasonography is particularly useful for demonstrating viable intrauterine pregnancy and ectopic gestation[51,52]; spontaneous heterotopic pregnancy (co-existent uterine and ectopic gestation) is so rare that detection of intrauterine pregnancy on ultrasound essentially rules out ectopic gestation.[6,53] Transvaginal ultrasound can detect ectopic pregnancy in one third of women with beta-HCG levels less than 1000 mIU/ml,[54] and 3 weeks after missed menses, virtually all viable intrauterine pregnancies, half of nonviable intrauterine and viable ectopic pregnancies, and one fourth of nonviable ectopic pregnancies can be detected with this method.[55] At low HCG levels, ultrasound is often nondiagnostic, but when HCG levels are greater than 1800 mIU/ml, sonography is helpful in establishing the location and viability of the pregnancy and is an essential investigation for all women requesting termination of pregnancy.[56] When HCG levels are 2000 mIU/ml or more and the mean sac diameter is 3 mm or more, the sensitivity for diagnosing an intrauterine pregnancy is increased.[51] The lack of independent movement of an adjacent mass and ovary and the intradecidual sign on ultrasound have been strongly associated with the absence of ectopic gestation,[51,57] while a trilaminar pattern (specific but not sensitive in ectopic pregnancy) and the thickness of the endometrium (it is thinner in ectopic gestation) have also been studied as ways to differentiate ectopic from viable uterine gestations on ultrasound.[58]

Many clinicians therefore advocate the combined use of transvaginal sonography and beta-HCG levels, citing an ability to detect earlier and smaller ectopic pregnancies without the attendant risks of a surgical procedure.[1,6,43,59,60] At HCG levels of 1500 to 1800 mIU/ml, a gestational sac should be visible[35]; at more than 5000 mIU/ml, a yolk sac is visible.[61] When ultrasound findings are indeterminate, diagnostic laparoscopy is considered by many to be the definitive test for diagnosis of ectopic pregnancy.[60] However, the advent of new strategies, particularly very sensitive pregnancy tests and ultrasonography, contributes to "near perfect" noninvasive diagnostic acumen[2,28] and permits medical management of the condition in carefully selected instances.

DIAGNOSTICS

Ectopic Pregnancy

LABORATORY

Serum human chorionic gonadotropin (HCG) (beta-HCG)
CBC and differential
Type and crossmatch*
Rh titers*

IMAGING

Pelvic ultrasound
Pelvic CT or MRI*

*If indicated.

DIFFERENTIAL DIAGNOSIS

Ectopic pregnancy must be considered a likely possibility in any woman of childbearing age with abdominal pain (or bleeding) until proved otherwise.[62] Other possible differential diagnoses include appendicitis, salpingitis, cholecystitis, PID, intrauterine pregnancy with inaccurate dates, corpus luteum cyst, gestational trophoblastic neoplasm, incomplete or missed spontaneous abortion, endometriosis, pelvic mass, ureteral calculi, and adnexal torsion. A twisted cystic teratoma[63] or a ruptured malignant ovarian tumor[64] may appear similarly to a ruptured ectopic pregnancy.

DIFFERENTIAL DIAGNOSIS

Ectopic Pregnancy

- Appendicitis
- Salpingitis
- Cholecystitis
- Pelvic inflammatory disease
- Intrauterine pregnancy
- Corpus luteum cyst
- Gestational trophoblastic neoplasm
- Incomplete abortion
- Endometriosis
- Pelvic mass
- Ureteral calculi
- Adnexal torsion
- Cystic teratoma
- Ruptured malignant ovarian tumor

MANAGEMENT

Spontaneous resolution is not uncommon, occurring in up to 88% of cases that are less vascular and less advanced (1 to 3.5 cm [0.4 to 1.4 inches]) and in which declining HCG levels are initially low (<200 mIU/ml).[6,65] The likelihood of successful expectant management can be predicted by the HCG level at presentation and is significantly lower (3216 mIU/L vs. 15,900 mIU/L in one study of interstitial gestation) in cases of successful conservative treatment.[65] During the course of resolution, associated beta-HCG levels become undetectable in 3 to 45 days (mean, 15.8 days).

Surgical laparoscopy or laparotomy remains the only treatment choice for ruptured ectopic pregnancy,[2] and laparoscopy is the cornerstone of treatment in most cases of ectopic gestation.[66,67] Although laparoscopy is the standard treatment for all ectopic pregnancies,[68] attendant risks include perioperative and postoperative complications (24% in one study),[69] including uncontrollable hemorrhage, adhesion formation,[2] subcutaneous emphysema and pneumothorax,[70] and reduced subsequent fertility.[2]

Methotrexate therapy, with or without leucovorin rescue or accompanying mifepristone, has been widely used as a nonsurgical intervention for unruptured ectopic pregnancies smaller than 3.5 cm (1.4 inches).[2,71,72] A folic acid antagonist that inhibits purine and pyrimidine synthesis, methotrexate interferes with DNA synthesis and cellular multiplication. Rapidly growing tissues such as fetal and trophoblastic cells are most susceptible. Various dosage strategies have been explored,[73,74] with decreased occurrence and severity of side effects observed in single, low-dose intramuscular injections.[2] Methotrexate or potassium chloride has also been used in ultrasound-guided local injections, equally successfully, in unruptured live ectopic pregnancies.[75]

Methotrexate has been used successfully to decrease the incidence of persistent ectopic pregnancy after salpingostomy,[76] in cervical pregnancy,[77] and in women eligible for expectant management.[78] Uterine embolization with methotrexate for elected cases of early interstitial gestation may decrease the risk of hemorrhage.[79] Appropriate candidates for methotrexate therapy should be hemodynamically stable, have no active renal or hepatic disease, and have no evidence of thrombocytopenia or leukopenia. Initial HCG levels in this population should be low, the gestational sac should be small (<3.5 cm [1.4 inches]) or absent,[80] and there should be no discernible fetal cardiac activity on ultrasound. Methotrexate therapy has a 94% success rate as long as the woman fits the appropriate criteria. Methotrexate 50 mg/m^2 is given intramuscularly, followed by a repeat HCG and symptom assessment on day 4 and another HCG on day 7. For women whose HCG titers do not decline significantly (by 15%), a second injection of methotrexate is indicated; this is more likely to be necessary if a yolk sac was visualized on ultrasound.[80] If a woman's HCG titer declines by the seventh day, she should be monitored weekly until it is undetectable. Side effects of treatment with methotrexate include diarrhea, nausea, perioral irritation, and transient transaminase elevations. Similar tubal patency rates have been shown after both methotrexate treatment and expectant management.[81]

LIFE SPAN CONSIDERATIONS

All sexually active women of reproductive age are theoretically at risk for ectopic pregnancy, especially if they have one or more of the risk factors mentioned earlier. Women in their twenties are more likely to have ectopic gestation, but adolescents and perimenopausal women are also at risk.[26] Women, including those for whom infertility is an issue, may require the provider's support in expressing and grieving the loss of the pregnancy and the baby who was expected.[82]

COMPLICATIONS

Ruptured ectopic pregnancy can result in acute, massive bleeding and poses an immediate threat to life.[2] Rupture is more likely at higher presenting levels of HCG and multiple ovulation or ovulation induction.[82] Misdiagnosis, which occurs in as many as 12% of cases, can result in sudden death secondary to internal hemorrhage and infection. Nonfatal sequelae of delayed diagnosis include infection and an increased rate of salpingectomy, potentially affecting future fertility.[83] Missed or delayed diagnoses and subsequent ruptures occur more often in women previously treated with therapeutic abortions when ectopic pregnancies were not suspected. In addition, the risk of a missed or delayed diagnosis is higher in women considered to be less at risk for an ectopic pregnancy, including those with no history of ectopic pregnancy, those with at least one child, and those who have a history of tubal ligation.[38,84,85]

Methotrexate has adverse effects, including mucositis, abdominal cramping, and malaise.[86] Its administration has been associated with cases of anaphylaxis,[86] alopecia,[87] and life-threatening neutropenia[88]; high doses can cause bone marrow depression, hepatotoxicity, stomatitis, pulmonary fibrosis, and photosensitivity.[2] The risk of persistent ectopic pregnancy ranges from 3% to 20% after conservative surgical therapy and 9.8% for treatment with methotrexate.[89] Research has shown a significantly reduced fertility rate postoperatively for some women after ectopic pregnancy[90] and a relationship between advancing age, prior ectopic pregnancy, and declining future pregnancy rates.[91]

INDICATIONS FOR REFERRAL OR HOSPITALIZATION

All women with suspected ectopic pregnancy should be referred immediately to an attending physician or a gynecologist for evaluation because the consequences for missed or delayed diagnosis can be dire. Ruptured ectopic pregnancy is a surgical emergency and requires immediate admission and attention. Suggestive HCG levels (<1000 mIU/ml) and an indeterminate vaginal ultrasound necessitate further evaluation, preferably as an inpatient.[92] Although transient abdominal pain is common in the second week after methotrexate administration and generally resolves within 24 hours,[71] severe pain is an indication for hospital-based observation because it may indicate tubal rupture.

PATIENT AND FAMILY EDUCATION

All women should be apprised of their subsequent risk of reduced fertility and recurrent ectopic pregnancy. Condom use should be encouraged to reduce the likelihood of infection and PID, since declining rates of chlamydial infection have been associated with declining rates of ectopic pregnancy.[93] Women on birth control pills should be reminded to take them as directed. Women at risk for ectopic pregnancy should alert their provider when they become pregnant. Women who have received methotrexate therapy for unruptured ectopic pregnancy need to refrain from sexual activity and consuming alcohol or vitamins containing folic acid until after resolution of the ectopic pregnancy. These women should also be alerted to the possibility that they may experience increased abdominal pain 5 to 10 days after therapy. Further clinical evaluation would be necessary at this point because severe pain may indicate tubal abortion and rupture. One study indicated good subsequent fertility rates in women who had received methotrexate for ectopic pregnancy (more than half conceived within 1 year of attempting pregnancy) and suggested that fertility in these cases depends more on prior medical history than on the treatment for the ectopic pregnancy.[94]

REFERENCES

1. Eisinger S: Early pregnancy bleeding: a rational approach, *Clin Fam Pract* 3(2), 2001.
2. Maiolatesi CR, Peddicord K: Methotrexate for nonsurgical treatment of ectopic pregnancy: nursing implications, *J Obstet Gynecol Neonat Nurs* 25(3):205-208, 1996.
3. Centers for Disease Control and Prevention: Ectopic pregnancy—United States, 1990-1992, *MMWR* 44(3):46-48, 1995.
4. Calderon JL, Shaheen M, Pan D, and others: Multi-cultural surveillance for ectopic pregnancy: California 1991-2000, *Ethnicity Dis* 15(4 Suppl 5):S5-20-4, 2005.
5. Morgan A: Adnexal mass evaluation in the emergency department, *Emerg Med Clin North Am* 19(3):799-816, 2001.
6. Carr R, Evans P: Ectopic pregnancy, *Primary Care Clin Office Pract* 27(1):169-183, 2000.
7. Van Den Eeden SK, and others: Ectopic pregnancy rate and treatment utilization in a large managed care organization, *Obstet Gynecol* 105(5 Pt 1):1052-1057, 2005.
8. Coste J, and others: Incidence of ectopic pregnancy: first results of a population-based register in France, *Hum Reprod* 9(4):742-745, 1994.
9. Anderson FW, Hogan JG, Ansbacher R: Sudden death: ectopic pregnancy mortality, *Obstet Gynecol* 103(6):1218-1223, 2004.
10. Bernstein J: Ectopic pregnancy: a nursing approach to excess risk among minority women, *J Obstet Gynecol Neonat Nurs* 24(9):803-810, 1995.
11. Tulandi T, Al-Jaroudi D: Interstitial pregnancy: results generated from the Society of Reproductive Surgeons Registry, *Obstet Gynecol* 103(1):47-50, 2004.
12. Jun SH, Milki AA: Assisted hatching is associated with a higher ectopic pregnancy rate, *Fertility Sterility* 81(6):1701-1703, 2004.
13. Basu A, Candelier C: Ectopic pregnancy with postcoital contraception—a case report, *Eur J Contracep Reprod Health Care* 10(1):6-8, 2005.
14. Ushakov FB, and others: Cervical pregnancy: past and future, *Obstet Gynecol Surv* 52(1):45-59, 1997.
15. Toikkanen S, Joensuu H, Erkkola R: DNA aneuploidy in ectopic pregnancy and spontaneous abortions, *Eur J Obstet Gynecol Reprod Biol* 51(1):9-13, 1993.
16. Karikoski R, Aine R, Heinonen PK: Abnormal embryogenesis in the etiology of ectopic pregnancy, *Gynecol Obstet Invest* 36(3):158-162, 1993.
17. Lan J, and others: *Chlamydia trachomatis* and ectopic pregnancy: retrospective analysis of salpingectomy specimens, endometrial biopsies, and cervical smears, *J Clin Pathol* 48(9):815-819, 1995.
18. Guillaume AJ, and others: Luteal phase defects and ectopic pregnancy, *Fertility Sterility* 63(1):30-33, 1995.
19. Tziorttziotis DV, and others: Clear cell hyperplasia of the fallopian

tube epithelium associated with ectopic pregnancy: report of a case, *Int J Gynecol Pathol* 16(1):79-80, 1997.
20. Godin PA, Bassil S, Donnez J: An ectopic pregnancy developing in a previous caesarian section scar, *Fertility Sterility* 67(2):398-400, 1997.
21. Bontis J, and others: Intrafollicular ovarian pregnancy after ovulation induction/intrauterine insemination: pathophysiological aspects and diagnostic problems, *Hum Reprod* 12(2):376-378, 1997.
22. Dunn RC, Taskin O: Chronic ectopic pregnancy after clinically successful methotrexate treatment of ectopic pregnancy, *Int J Gynaecol Obstet* 51(3):247-249, 1995.
23. Turan C, and others: Transvaginal sonographic findings of chronic ectopic pregnancy, *Eur J Obstet Gynecol Reprod Biol* 67(2):115-119, 1996.
24. Garrett AM, Vukov LF: Risk factors for ectopic pregnancy in a rural population, *Fam Med* 28(2):111-113, 1996.
25. Coste J, and others: Sexually transmitted diseases as a major cause of ectopic pregnancy: results from a large case-control study in France, *Fertility Sterility* 62(2):289-295, 1994.
26. Ramirez NC, Lawrence WD, Ginsburg KA: Ectopic pregnancy: a recent 5-year study and review of the last 50 years' literature, *J Reprod Med* 41(10):733-740, 1996.
27. Hillis SD, and others: Recurrent chlamydial infections increase the risks of hospitalization for ectopic pregnancy and pelvic inflammatory disease, *Am J Obstet Gynecol* 176(1 Pt 1):103-107, 1997.
28. Ankum WM, and others: Risk factors for ectopic pregnancy: a meta-analysis, *Fertility Sterility* 65(6):1093-1099, 1996.
29. Hemminki E, Merilainen J: Long-term effects of cesarean sections: ectopic pregnancies and placental problems, *Am J Obstet Gynecol* 174(5):1569-1574, 1996.
30. Peterson HB, Xia Z, Hughes JM, and others: The risk of ectopic pregnancy after tubal sterilization: findings from the U.S. Collaborative Review of Sterilization Working Group, *N Engl J Med* 336(11):762-767, 1997.
31. Napolitano PG, Vu K, Rosa C: Pregnancy after failed tubal sterilization, *J Reprod Med* 41(8):609-613, 1996.
32. Saraiya M, and others: Cigarette smoking as a risk factor for ectopic pregnancy, *Am J Obstet Gynecol* 178:493-498, 1999.
33. Kendrick JS, and others: Vaginal douching and the risk of ectopic pregnancy among black women, *Am J Obstet Gynecol* 176(5):991-997, 1997.
34. Zhang J, Thomas AG, Leybovich E: Vaginal douching and adverse health affects: a meta-analysis, *Am J Pub Health* 87(7):1207-1211, 1997.
35. Tenore J: Ectopic pregnancy, *Am Fam Phys* 61(4):220, 222, 225, 2000.
36. Skjeldestad FE, Atrash HK: Evaluation of induced abortion as a risk factor for ectopic pregnancy: a case-control study, *Acta Obstet Gynecol Scand* 76(2):151-158, 1997.
37. Altrash HK, and others: The relation between induced abortion and pregnancy, *Obstet Gynecol* 89(4):512-518, 1997.
38. Diamond MP, and others: Failure of standard criteria to diagnose nonemergency ectopic pregnancies in a noninfertility patient population, *J Am Assoc Gynecol Laparosc* 1(2):131-134, 1994.
39. David P, Gianotti A, Garmel G: Acute urinary retention due to ectopic pregnancy, *Am J Emerg Med* 17(1):44-45, 1999.
40. Acosta DA: Cervical pregnancy—a forgotten entity in family practice, *J Am Board Fam Pract* 10(4):290-295, 1997.
41. Abramov Y, and others: Doppler findings in chronic ectopic pregnancy: a case report, *Ultrasound Obstet Gynecol* 9(5):344-346, 1997.
42. Dart R, Kaplan B, Varalkis K: Predictive value of history and physical examination in patients with suspected ectopic pregnancy, *Ann Emerg Med* 33(3):283-290, 1999.
43. Dart R, Mitterando J, Dart L: Rate of change of serial beta-human chorionic gonadotropin values as a predictor of ectopic pregnancy in patients with indeterminate transvaginal ultrasound findings, *Ann Emerg Med* 34(6):703-710, 1999.
44. Gronlund B, Marushak A: Serial human chorionic gonadotrophin determination in the diagnosis of ectopic pregnancy, *Aust NZ J Obstet Gynaecol* 33(3):312-314, 1993.
45. Barnhart K, and others: Decline of serum human chorionic gonadotropin and spontaneous complete abortion: defining the normal curve, *Obstet Gynecol* 104(5 Pt 1):975-981, 2004.
46. Condous G, and others: Human chorionic gonadotrophin and progesterone levels in pregnancies of unknown location, *Int J Gynaecol Obstet* 86(3):351-357, 2004.
47. Buckley R, King KG, Disney JD, and others: Serum progesterone testing to predict ectopic pregnancy in symptomatic first-trimester patients, *Ann Emerg Med* 36(2):95-100, 2000.
48. Birkhahn R, Gaeta TJ, Suzuki T, and others: Serum levels of smooth muscle heavy-chain myosin in patients with ectopic pregnancy, *Ann Emerg Med* 36(2):101-107, 2000.
49. Wegner N, Mershon J: Evaluation of leukemia inhibitory factor as a marker of ectopic pregnancy, *Am J Obstet Gynecol* 184(6):1074-1076, 2001.
50. Daponte A, and others: The value of a single combined measurement of VEGF, glycodelin, progesterone, PAPP-A, HPL and LIF for differentiating between ectopic and abnormal intrauterine pregnancy, *Hum Reprod* 20(11):3163-3166, 2005.
51. Chiang G, and others: The intradecidual sign: is it reliable for diagnosis of early intrauterine pregnancy? *AJR* 183(3):725-731, 2004.
52. Condous G, and others: The accuracy of transvaginal ultrasonography for the diagnosis of ectopic pregnancy prior to surgery, *Hum Reprod* 20(5):1404-1409, 2005.
53. Durston W, and others: Ultrasound availability in the evaluation of ectopic pregnancy in the ED: comparison of quality and cost-effectiveness with different approaches, *Am J Emerg Med* 18(4):408-417, 2000.
54. Dart RG, Kaplan B, Cox C: Transvaginal ultrasound in patients with low beta-human chorionic gonadotropin values: how often is the study diagnostic? *Ann Emerg Med* 30(2):135-140, 1997.
55. Popp LW, Colditz A, Gaetje R: Diagnosis of intrauterine and ectopic pregnancy at 5-7 postmenstrual weeks, *Int J Gynaecol Obstet* 44(1):33-38, 1994.
56. Sinha P, Pradhan A, Chowdhury V: Value of routine transvaginal ultrasound scan in women requesting early termination of pregnancy, *J Obstet Gynaecol* 24(4):426-428, 2004.
57. Blaivas M, Lyon M: Reliability of adnexal mass mobility in distinguishing possible ectopic pregnancy from corpus luteum cysts, *J Ultrasound Med* 24(5):599-603, 605, 2005.
58. Hammoud AO, and others: The role of sonographic endometrial patterns and endometrial thickness in the differential diagnosis of ectopic pregnancy, *Am J Obstet Gynecol* 192(5):1370-1375, 2005.
59. Farquhar CM: Ectopic pregnancy, *Lancet* 366(9485):583-591, 2005.
60. Atri M, and others: Role of endovaginal sonography in the diagnosis and management of ectopic pregnancy, *Radiographics* 16(4):755-774, 1996.
61. Scroggins K, Smucker W, Krishen A: Spontaneous pregnancy loss, *Primary Care Clin Office Pract* 27(1):153-167, 2000.
62. Gaeta TJ, Raderos M, Izquierdo I: Atypical ectopic pregnancy, *Am J Emerg Med* 11(3):233-234, 1993.
63. Pothula V, Matseoane S, Godfrey H: Gonadotropin-producing benign cystic teratoma simulating a ruptured ectopic pregnancy, *J Natl Med Assoc* 86(3):221-222, 1994.
64. Riley GM, Babcock C, Jain K: Ruptured malignant ovarian tumor mimicking ruptured ectopic pregnancy, *J Ultrasound Med* 15(12):871-873, 1996.
65. Cassik P, and others: Factors influencing the success of conservative treatment of interstitial pregnancy, *Ultrasound Obstet Gynecol* 26(3):279-282, 2005.
66. Hajenius P, and others: Interventions for tubal ectopic pregnancy, *Cochrane Library* (4):CD000324, 2005.
67. Hsu S, and others: Laparoscopic management of tubal ectopic pregnancy in obese women, *Fertility Sterility* 81(1):198-202, 2004.
68. Buster JE, Carson SA: Ectopic pregnancy: new advances in diagnosis and treatment, *Curr Opin Obstet Gynecol* 7(3):168-176, 1995.
69. Clasen K, and others: Ectopic pregnancy: let's cut: strict laparoscopic approach to 194 consecutive cases and review of literature on alternatives, *Hum Reprod* 12(3):596-601, 1997.

70. Perko G, Fernandes A: Subcutaneous emphysema and pneumothorax during laparoscopy for ectopic pregnancy removal, *Acta Anaesthesiol Scand* 41(6):792-794, 1997.
71. Gazvani M, Emery S: Mifepristone and methotrexate: the combination for medical treatment of ectopic pregnancy, *Am J Obstet Gynecol* 180(6):1599-1560, 1999.
72. Barnhart K, Esposito M, Coutifaris C: An update on the medical treatment of ectopic pregnancy, *Obstet Gynecol Clin North Am* 27(3):653-667, 2000.
73. Erdem M, and others: Single-dose methotrexate for the treatment of unruptured ectopic pregnancy, *Arch Gynecol Obstet* 270(4):201-204, 2004.
74. Lipscomb GH, Givens VM, Meyer NL, and others: Comparison of multidose and single-dose methotrexate protocols for the treatment of ectopic pregnancy, *Am J Obstet Gynecol* 192(6):1844-1848, 2005.
75. Monteagudo A, and others: Non-surgical management of live ectopic pregnancy with ultrasound-guided local injection: a case series, *Ultrasound Obstet Gynecol* 25(3):282-288, 2005.
76. Graczykowski JW, Mishell DR: Methotrexate prophylaxis for persistent ectopic pregnancy after conservative treatment by salpingostomy, *Obstet Gynecol* 89(1):118-121, 1997.
77. Kung F: Efficacy of methotrexate treatment in viable and nonviable cervical pregnancies, *Am J Obstet Gynecol* 181(6):1438-1444, 1999.
78. Korhonnen J, Stenman UH, Ylostalo P: Low-dose oral methotrexate with expectant management of ectopic pregnancy, *Obstet Gynecol* 88(5):775-778, 1996.
79. Deruelle P, and others: Management of interstitial pregnancy using selective uterine artery embolization, *Obstet Gynecol* 106(5 Pt 2):1165-1167, 2005.
80. Bixby S, Tello R, Kuligowska E: Presence of a yolk sac on transvaginal sonography is the most reliable predictor of single-dose methotrexate treatment failure in ectopic pregnancy [see comment], *J Ultrasound Med* 24(5):591-598, 2005.
81. Elito J, Han KK, Camano L: Tubal patency after clinical treatment of unruptured ectopic pregnancy, *Int J Gynaecol Obstet* 88(3):309-313, 2005.
82. Job-Spira N, Fernandez H, Bouver J, and others: Ruptured tubal ectopic pregnancy: risk factors and reproductive outcome: results of a population-based study in France, *Am J Obstet Gynecol* 180(4):938-944, 1999.
83. Robson SJ, O'Shea RT: Undiagnosed ectopic pregnancy: a retrospective analysis of 31 "missed" ectopic pregnancies at a teaching hospital, *Aust NZ J Obstet Gynaecol* 36(2):182-185, 1996.
84. Li L, Smialek JE: Sudden death due to rupture of ectopic pregnancy concurrent with therapeutic abortion, *Arch Pathol Lab Med* 117(7):698-700, 1993.
85. Saxon D, and others: A study of ruptured tubal ectopic pregnancy, *Obstet Gynecol* 90(1):46-49, 1997.
86. Straka M, Zeringue E, Goldman M: A rare drug reaction to methotrexate after treatment for ectopic pregnancy, *Obstet Gynecol* 103(5 Pt 2):1047-1048, 2004.
87. Trout S, Kemmann E: Reversible alopecia after single-dose methotrexate treatment in a patient with ectopic pregnancy, *Fertility Sterility* 64(4):866-867, 1995.
88. Isaacs JDJ, McGehee RP, Cowan BD: Life-threatening neutropenia following methotrexate treatment of ectopic pregnancy: a report of two cases, *Obstet Gynecol* 88(4 Pt 2):694-696, 1996.
89. Yao M, Tulandi T: Current status of surgical and nonsurgical management of ectopic pregnancy, *Fertility Sterility* 67(3):421-433, 1997.
90. Korell M, Albrich W, Hepp H: Fertility after organ preserving surgery of ectopic pregnancy: results of a multicenter study, *Fertility Sterility* 68(2):220-223, 1997.
91. Al-Nuaim L, and others: Reproductive potential after an ectopic pregnancy, *Fertility Sterility* 64(5):942-946, 1995.
92. Kaplan BC, and others: Ectopic pregnancy: prospective study with improved diagnostic accuracy, *Ann Emerg Med* 28(1):10-17, 1996.
93. Egger M, and others: Screening for chlamydial infections and the risk of ectopic pregnancy in a county in Sweden: ecological analysis, *Br Med J* 1(1):22-23, 1999.
94. Gervaise A, and others: Reproductive outcome after methotrexate treatment of tubal pregnancies, *Fertility Sterility* 82(2):304-308, 2004.

CHAPTER 172

Fertility Control

Patricia Polgar Bailey

DEFINITION AND EPIDEMIOLOGY

In the United States, 95% of sexually active women have used contraception at some time in their lives. Many of these women have tried more than one method of contraception. In 2002 the most frequent contraceptive method among women ages 15 to 44 years was oral contraception (OC) (31%). Other leading methods were female sterilization (27%) and the male condom (18%). A small but significant number of women (9%) were using the new, long-acting hormonal methods, including injectables, implants, and the patch.[1]

Many of the women currently using some method of fertility control express concern over the potential side effects and health risks associated with contraceptive use.[2] Approximately 49% of pregnancies in the United States are unintended; in 2002, 35% of births were unintended.[3,4] Given the frequency of unintended pregnancy in the United States, it is essential that health care providers educate and counsel women and their partners on the variety of feasible options. It is imperative that the woman (and her partner if desired) be involved in the care plan rather than be merely a recipient of the provider's expertise and advice. Discussion should include information about the risks and benefits of contraceptive options, their potential side effects, their rate of efficacy, and effects on future fertility.

In addition to the possible emotional and health care cost associated with unintended pregnancies, one financial analysis found that, compared with pregnancy and abortion, contraception saves an estimated $9000 to $14,000 in health care costs per woman of childbearing age over a 5-year period. Although some methods of contraception have side effects, morbidity and mortality rates are higher for pregnancy and childbirth than for any single contraceptive measure.[5]

HORMONAL CONTRACEPTION

Oral Contraceptives

The oral contraceptive pill (OCP) is a highly effective means of preventing pregnancy and has played an important role in contraception since its approval by the U.S. Food and Drug Administration (FDA) in 1960. The terms *birth control pill*, *combined oral contraceptive*, and *oral contraceptive* generally refer to pills containing both estrogen and progestin. In this chapter, these terms are not used to refer to progestin-only pills, also known as *minipills*. OCPs prevent pregnancy by blocking follicle-stimulating hormone (FSH) and luteinizing hormone (LH) surges, thereby inhibiting ovulation. They also thicken the cervical mucus to hamper the ability of the sperm to reach the egg, accelerate ovum transport through the fallopian tube, and alter the endometrium in a way that makes it unreceptive to the implantation of a fertilized egg. Thus, should ovulation take place, the risk of pregnancy remains minimal.[6]

Two synthetic estrogens are commonly used in OC formulations in the United States: (1) ethinyl estradiol, which is pharmacologically active; and (2) mestranol, which is approximately 50% less potent than ethinyl estradiol and requires metabolism in the liver to become pharmacologically active.[6] The dose of estrogen used in combination OCPs has decreased dramatically since OCPs first became available; common doses of ethinyl estradiol in OCs range from 20 to 50 mcg, with those most widely prescribed containing 30 to 35 mcg, whereas mestranol is found commercially only in a dose of 50 mcg in one OC combination (including one brand and two generic versions).[6] The lower dose formulations have the same rate of efficacy but fewer adverse effects.[2] OCPs also contain one of several progestins, including norethindrone, levonorgestrel, norgestrel, norethindrone acetate, ethynodiol diacetate, norgestimate, and desogestrel. The latter two progestins, norgestimate and desogestrel, are less androgenic progestins; the OCP formulations that use them are referred to as third-generation contraceptives.

Several different types of OCPs are available and vary according to the dose of hormones and the formulations within each cycle pack. Monophasic OCPs have a constant dose of estrogen and progestin in each of the 21 active tablets of the cycle pack. Phasic OCPs have altering doses of progestin and, in some cases, estrogen throughout the cycle. The aim of manufacturers in lowering the total monthly exogenous hormone dose while trying to simulate a woman's normal menstrual cycle is to reduce the metabolic side effects associated with OCP use.

Finally, studies on the length of time that active pills are given have contributed to more options for OCP users. The FDA recently approved the use of levonorgestrel–ethinyl estradiol (Seasonale) in an extended OCP regimen consisting of 84 days of active pills and 7 days of nonhormonal pills.[5]

With perfect use, OCPs are 99.5% to 99.9% effective in preventing pregnancy. However, with typical use in the United States, the rate of efficacy drops to 95% to 97%.[6,7] (All efficacy rates are based on a 1-year time frame.) An important reason for the decreased efficacy of OCPs is that it depends on daily adherence. Research shows that close to 50% of OCP users fail to take one or more pills per cycle, and almost 25% fail to take two or more pills.[5] In addition, the reduced efficacy of OCPs is due to the high rate of women who discontinue taking the pill, the reasons for which are multifactorial.[5] For some women, spotting or other side effects contribute to pill failure; others misunderstand the importance of taking the pill on a regular basis.[8] Approximately 50% of women discontinue OCP or other reversible contraception use within 1 year.[9] Because of these high rates of discontinuation, it has been recommended that all women who are prescribed OCPs be provided an additional method of birth control.

The regimen of OCPs should be initiated on either the first day of menses or on the first Sunday after menses begin. Women should be encouraged to take OCPs at the same time every day and to associate pill taking with a certain daily habit or ritual if that facilitates compliance. Daily compliance is essential to ensuring efficacy. Women who miss one or two tablets should take two tablets for each of the missed days. Women who miss more than 2 days should continue taking the pills as prescribed but use an additional form of birth control for the remainder of the cycle. Women who often miss doses of OCPs should be encouraged to consider a form of fertility control that does not depend on daily compliance.[2]

The side effects of OCPs are a major reason for noncompliance and discontinuation. Just over half of all OCP users are satisfied with the method. Of the dissatisfied users, 94% mention side effects that include nausea, headaches, weight gain, mood alteration, mastalgia, and menstrual problems.[10] The extent and type of side effect differ slightly between individual OCPs because of variations in the amount and kind of estrogen and progestin contained within each product. Nausea and breast tenderness resulting from the estrogen component of OCPs are common side effects. OCPs cause an increase in blood pressure, which should be monitored once or twice a year in all women and more often in women with a history of hypertension. Menstrual changes, including intermenstrual (breakthrough) spotting or bleeding, occur in 25% of women during the first 3 months of OCP use and decrease significantly during subsequent use. Women with persistent intermenstrual bleeding after 3 months of OCP use should be evaluated for possible causes of bleeding unrelated to OCP use, including infection or neoplasia.[2] Amenorrhea may also occur, especially in women who have been using OCPs for a prolonged period. Other possible side effects include a decreased libido (decreased interest in sex or in the ability to have an orgasm), fluid retention, leukorrhea, pruritus, and headaches. Tension headaches are not considered to be related to OCP use and should be evaluated and managed accordingly. Migraine headaches are known to either improve or worsen while taking OCPs. Women who experience "classic migraines" and women who experience increased frequency or intensity of migraines while taking OCPs should be advised to use some other form of fertility control.

Some of the "short-lived" side effects associated with OCPs tend to dissipate by the third or fourth cycle. Specific side effects can be attributed to the estrogen or progestin components. Once the responsible component has been identified, it can then be determined whether the side effect is caused by an excess or deficiency of that component, and the provider can discuss OCP options that may lead to increased satisfaction.

Substantial contraceptive and noncontraceptive benefits are associated with OCPs. Menstrual improvements associated with OCPs include more regular and predictable menses, a 25% reduction in anemia resulting from menorrhagia, less dysmenorrhea, fewer days for menses, a reduced flow, and the restoration of regular menses in anovulatory women. There is a 50% decrease in functional ovarian cysts among OCP users, with a 75% reduction in functional cyst-related hospital admissions. Additional gynecologic benefits include a decrease in the incidence of gynecologic cancers, including epithelial ovarian cancer (20% to 80% reduction) and endometrial adenocarcinoma (40% reduction when used for at least 2 years and 60% reduction when used for at least 4 years), and the prevention and treatment of endometriosis (30% reduction). Certain conditions occur less often in women taking OCPs; there is a 50% combined reduction in breast fibroadenoma and fibrocystic changes, a 50% reduction in pelvic inflammatory disease (PID) (with the exception of infections caused by *Chlamydia trachomatis*), and a 90% reduction in ectopic pregnancies. Additional benefits may include suppression of acne, maintenance of or increased bone mineral density, a decreased risk of atherosclerosis and severe rheumatoid arthritis, and enhanced sexual enjoyment.[2,6,7,11]

OCPs also have significant health risks and disadvantages, including a lack of protection against HIV infection—a greater threat to the health of many sexually active individuals than an unplanned pregnancy. To protect against HIV infection, barrier methods (e.g., condoms) must be used in conjunction with OCPs. Other possible untoward side effects resulting from the estrogen component in pills includes increased breast size (ductal and fatty tissue), stimulation of breast neoplasia, cervical erosion or ectopia, thromboembolic complications, pulmonary emboli, cerebrovascular accidents, hepatocellular adenomas and cancer, the growth of leiomyomas, telangiectasia, and a rise in the cholesterol concentration in gallbladder bile.[7]

The risk of cardiovascular disease (CVD) associated with OCP use has been a concern since the first cases were reported among pill users. The relative risk of myocardial infarction (MI) among current users of all combination OCPs has not been found to be statistically significant compared to nonusers in the Myocardial Infarction and Oral Contraceptive Study (MICA).[12] The risk of MI in combination OC users is highest among smokers and those taking formulations containing at least 50 mcg of estrogen. Cigarette smoking is the most prominent risk factor for MI in combination OC users. A fourfold to fortyfold increase in MI risk has been demonstrated in women on OC who smoke at least 25 cigarettes per day.[13] This increased risk has not been demonstrated in healthy nonsmokers, and it has been difficult to determine the true risk in smokers receiving a low-dose formulation (estrogen <50 mcg).[13]

Studies also suggest that, in women using OCPs containing the second-generation progestins levonorgestrel and norethisterone, there is an excess risk of 4 to 10 cases of venous thromboembolism per 100,000 women; this results in one to two extra deaths per million women per year. The risk seems to double with pills containing the third-generation progestins desogestrel (and gestodene, which is not available in the United States) compared with the second-generation progestin levonorgestrel.[13] Despite the scare in 1995 regarding these newer progestins, the risk attributable to them is still relatively small given the excess mortality of only 1 to 2 per million per year. This increased risk of thromboembolism is still less than the risk associated with high-dose estrogen OCPs. There is also tentative evidence that these less androgenic progestins do not carry the increased risk of MI seen with levonorgestrel, a second-generation progestin.[12,14,15]

Studies on stroke and OCPs have demonstrated no increase in risk or an increased risk of only 0.5 per 100,000 woman-years for low-dose pill users less than 35 years of age who have no cardiovascular risk factors. In addition, the type of progestin does not seem to influence the risk. Thus, in the absence of risk factors, low-dose pills may carry no excess risk of stroke. For women using high-dose pills, the excess risk for cerebrovascular accidents is 8 per 100,000; in low-dose pill users older than 35 years, the risk is 2 per 100,000. Evidence suggests that the use of OCPs raises the risk of acute MI by less than 1 per 100,000 woman-years, which translates into fewer than three additional cases per year. The risk may be greater in older women who smoke. Appropriate screening, particularly of blood pressure, before initiating and during OCP use will likely reduce this risk.[14]

The potential impact of OCP use on breast cancer is a concern for a great number of women interested in this form of fertility control. Epidemiologic data suggest that current OCP users have an increased relative risk of breast cancer of 1.0 to 1.24[16]; this risk seems confined largely to tumors localized to the breast. Women who begin taking OCPs before age 20 years have a somewhat higher risk than those who start later. For women who use the pill when older, for example, up to the age of 40 years, the estimated cumulative incidence is 199 per 10,000 women at age 50 years (an excess of 19 cases per 10,000) and 394 per 10,000 women at age 60 (an excess of 14 cases per 10,000). The patterns of breast cancer risk seem similar for both progestin-only and combined OCPs, with no difference between oral and injectable preparations.[14] Pattern of OC use such as any current or past use, interval since last use, and dose of estrogen did not appear to be associated with an increased risk of breast cancer.[16]

Both the estrogen and progestin components of OCPs may potentially increase breast tenderness, headaches, hypertension, and the risk for MI. The androgenic effects of the progestin in OCPs may be associated with increased appetite and weight gain, depression, fatigue and tiredness, decreased libido and sexual pleasure, acne and oily skin, increased breast size (alveolar tissue), an increase in low-density lipoprotein cholesterol, a decrease in high-density lipoprotein (HDL) cholesterol, glucose intolerance, and decreased carbohydrate tolerance.[7]

OCPs should not be prescribed for women with the following conditions: a history of thrombophlebitis or thromboembolic disorder, cerebrovascular accident, coronary artery or ischemic heart disease, breast cancer or suspected breast cancer, suspected estrogen-dependent neoplasia, pregnancy or suspected pregnancy, concomitant hepatic adenoma or liver cancer, and markedly impaired liver function. Caution should be used in prescribing OCPs to women older than 35 years old who smoke more than 15 cigarettes per day; women who develop migraines after the initiation of OCPs; or women with blood pressure greater than 140/90 mm Hg, diabetes mellitus, obesity with a body mass index of 30 kg/m^2, immobilization pending within the next 4 weeks, undiagnosed vaginal or uterine bleeding, sickle cell disease or sickle cell–hemoglobin C disease, lactation, gestational diabetes, active gallbladder disease, congenital hyperbilirubinemia, a history of cardiac or renal disease, family history of hyperlipidemia, or death of a parent or sibling from MI before age 50 years. In addition, caution should be used when considering OCPs for women before the third postpartum week or for those older than age 50 years.[7,16]

The warning signs to teach OCP users can be summarized with the acronym *ACHES*, which refers to *A*bdominal pain (severe); *C*hest pain (severe), cough, or shortness of breath; *H*eadaches (severe), dizziness, weakness, or numbness; *E*ye problems (vision loss or blurring) or speech problems; and *S*evere leg pain (calf or thigh). Women who experience any of these signs or symptoms or who develop depression, jaundice, or a breast lump should discontinue taking the pill and consult their provider. OCP users who smoke should be encouraged to quit smoking; if quitting is not possible, they should consider discontinuing the use of OCPs after age 35 years and definitely by age 40 years.[7]

Progestin-Only Pills (Minipills). Progestin-only pills were introduced approximately 10 years after OCPs appeared on the market. Several types of progestins have been used in OC products and are often referred to by generation: first, second, third, and now fourth. The progestins found in OCs differ based on their estrogenic, antiestrogenic, progestational, and androgenic properties.[6] Progestin-only pills prevent pregnancy mainly by thickening the cervical mucus to slow sperm motility and interfering with or preventing sperm penetration. Progestins may also work by inhibiting ovulation; creating a thin, atrophic endometrium; and promoting luteolysis.[6] Progestin-only pills are taken on a daily basis, with no pill-free days. Progestin-only pills are most effective if ovulation is inhibited and are generally considered less effective than OCPs. Failure rates vary from 1.1% to 13.2% during the first year of use. Because of their lack of an estrogen component, minipills are preferred in women who are lactating[6]; their efficacy rate for these women is close to 100%. Progestin-only pills are also useful for women who wish to use an OCP but have contraindications to combined pills.

The structural similarity of the progestins to testosterone largely determines their androgenic activity. This androgenic activity is often associated with the side effects of progestins, which may include menstrual cycle disturbances, weight gain, breast tenderness, an increase in functional ovarian cysts, ectopic pregnancy, interactions with anticonvulsants, and bone density decrease.[5,7] Because of their lack of estrogen, minipills are not associated with some of the same potential side effects of combination OCs, such as thromboembolic disorders (e.g., MI and cerebrovascular disease) and gallbladder disease. Minipills are associated with a higher incidence of ectopic pregnancy when compared with other contraceptive measures.[6]

Spironolactone Analogs. Drospirenone (3 mg) is the newest progestin and has been combined with ethinyl estradiol (30 mcg) to form a new monophasic oral contraceptive (Yasmin). Drospirenone is a spironolactone analog with antimineralcorticoid and antiandrogenic properties. A 3 mg/day dosage displays antimineralcorticoid activity similar to that of 25 mg of sprironolactone, which may be a good choice in women who experience significant sodium and water retention during their cycle.[6] Hyperkalemia is a potential adverse effect related to the potassium-sparing effects of drospirenone. Consequently this product should not be given to women with conditions that might predispose them to elevated potassium levels (e.g., renal impairment, hepatic dysfunction, adrenal sufficiency) or in combination with medications that can increase potassium levels such as angiotensin-converting enzyme inhibitors, potassium supplements, or potassium-sparing diuretics.[6] Pregnancy should be excluded before this oral contraceptive is started.

Injectable Contraception

One injectable form of contraception available in the United States is medroxyprogesterone acetate (MPA) (Depo-Provera). MPA prevents pregnancy by inhibiting ovulation and is used by more than 14 million women worldwide.[11] A 150-mg injection of MPA suppresses ovulation for 14 weeks. With a prescribed dose given every 3 months, contraceptive efficacy is 99.7%. The recommended time to initiate MPA is within 5 days of the onset of menses, partly to ensure that the woman is not pregnant but also because administration at this time prevents ovulation during the first month of use. MPA injections should be administered every 12 weeks, which provides a 2-week "grace" period given the 14-week duration of action. The possibility of pregnancy should first be excluded for any woman who is more than 2 weeks late for her MPA injection.[2] Side effects include irregular menses and reversible bone loss.

MPA–estradiol cypionate suspension (Lunelle [MPA/E_2C]) is the first monthly injectable contraceptive to be prescribed in the United States. Administered into the deltoid, gluteus maximus, or anterior thigh, a 0.5 ml IM injection is given within 5 days of the onset of the menstrual period and every 28 to 30 days thereafter. Amenorrhea, common in MPA, is not associated with MPA/E_2C. There seems to be a high level of satisfaction with MPA/E_2C, and studies have shown it to be highly effective (in a 12-month study no pregnancies occurred).[8] Unfortunately, manufacturing problems have affected the availability of Lunelle. It is expected, however, that it will be available in the future.

Menstrual changes occur in almost all women who use MPA and are the most common cause for dissatisfaction and discontinued use of this form of fertility control. Irregular bleeding usually resolves within the first month of use. Amenorrhea is the most common menstrual change with persistent use of MPA. Women for whom menstrual irregularities are disconcerting should be counseled regarding alternative contraceptive choices. Other side effects of MPA include headache, abdominal or breast bloating, fatigue, depression, decreased libido, and a 0.4- to 1.4-kg (1- to 3-pound) weight gain.[2] MPA is a reversible form of contraception, but a return to fertility is often delayed after discontinuation of MPA. Within 10 months of the last injection, 50% of women who discontinue MPA to become pregnant are able to conceive, but in others fertility may not be restored for as long as 18 months.[2]

MPA is associated with certain noncontraceptive benefits, such as a reduction in or elimination of premenstrual symptoms, a reduced risk of PID, a decreased risk of endometrial cancer, hematologic improvement in women with sickle cell disease, and reduced seizures in women with seizure disorders. MPA-induced amenorrhea may make MPA a good contraceptive choice for women with menorrhagia, dysmenorrhea, and iron deficiency anemia, as well as for women with mental deficits who have menstrual hygiene problems.

Both MPA and MPA/E_2C are associated with certain health risks. As is the case with OCPs, MPA and MPA/E_2C provide no protection from many sexually transmitted diseases (STDs), including HIV. Currently no data suggest that either of these products is associated with an increased risk of breast, endometrial, ovarian, or cervical carcinoma. HDL cholesterol levels tend to fall in women using MPA.[7] Decreased bone density has been noted among some MPA users, but this was reversed with discontinuation of MPA.[11]

Women should be counseled to use an additional form of contraception for the first 2 weeks after the first MPA or MPA/E_2C injection. Women who are at risk for STDs should use a barrier method of contraception, preferably condoms. Women who become concerned about their menstrual irregularities on MPA or who develop signs or symptoms of infection should consult their health care provider. Women need to be informed about the likely delay in fertility after discontinuation of MPA. MPA is not the best choice for women who wish to become pregnant within the next 1 to 2 years; these women should be counseled regarding alternative contraceptive options. MPA/E_2C has not seemed to delay fertility.

Contraceptive Implants

The contraceptive implant levonorgestrel (Norplant), which consisted of six progestin-coated Silastic implants filled with 36 mg of crystalline levonorgestrel, is no longer being manufactured. Seven years ago, the manufacturer announced that any implant distributed after October 1999 may not be effective and recommended backup contraception or implant removal. It is unlikely that any women still have a Norplant contraceptive implant. However, if a woman presents with a Norplant contraceptive implant, the risk of pregnancy should be reiterated, and a pregnancy test should be obtained if amenorrhea develops. Implant removal is a minor office procedure that should be performed by a practitioner specifically trained in the procedure.

A single-rod implant (Implanon) was recently approved by the FDA for use by women in the United States.[5] Implanon is a thin, flexible plastic rod, approximately 4 cm long, that delivers ethylene vinyl acetate impregnated with 68 mg of etonogestrel (the same drug used in the contraceptive vaginal ring). The rod delivers an average of 40 mcg of etonogestrel every day, inhibiting ovulation and thickening cervical mucus. It prevents pregnancy for 3 years and does not interfere with fertility once the rod is removed. Menstrual periods usually return to normal in 1 month after removal of the rod.[17] The rod is typically inserted into the inside portion of the upper arm. A provider trained in Implanon insertion can perform this procedure in the office. The most common side effect is irregular menstrual bleeding.[18]

Another implant, levonorgestrel (Jadelle), is a two-rod implant also approved by the FDA, although it is still unavailable in the United States. It is widely used in other countries and provides more significant birth control than many other types of birth control in women of normal weight.[18]

Contraceptive Patch

Norelgestromin–ethinyl estradiol transdermal system (Ortho Evra) is the first contraceptive patch available in the United States. The patch delivers 20 mcg of ethinyl estradiol and 150 mcg of norelgestromin daily and is 99% effective, with a method failure rate of 0.7 pregnancies per 100 woman-years. It inhibits ovulation in much the same way as OCPs. Each cycle consists of a contraceptive patch applied to the lower abdomen, buttocks, upper outer arm, or upper torso (excluding the breasts) once a week for 3 weeks. After the third week the patch is removed for a contraceptive-free week during which withdrawal bleeding occurs.

The contraceptive patch may be less effective in women weighing more than 90 kg (198 pounds), but reported advantages include ease of use, improved adherence, reversibility, and steady-state hormonal levels. During the first 2 months of patch use, spotting rates can be higher than with OCP use, but spotting rates were similar for both methods in subsequent cycles. Additional side effects include breast discomfort, headache, nausea, dysmenorrhea, and skin irritation at the patch site. In at least one study, compliance was significantly greater with the patch than with OCP use.[19]

In November 2005, the FDA issued a warning that the birth control patch could be associated with an increased risk of thromboembolism. Studies are ongoing, but this form of birth control is not advised for patients at risk for thromboembolism (e.g, women over age 35 and women with a previous history of blood clots, hypertension, or diabetes).[18] The patch should also not be prescribed for women who smoke. All patients starting on the contraceptive patch or hormonal birth control should understand the risks of thromboembolism and the importance of stopping the medication and calling the healthcare provider immediately if they develop a severe headache, chest pain or pressure, shortness of breath, abdominal pain, or leg pain.

Postcoital Contraception

Postcoital contraception, also referred to as emergency contraception or the "morning-after pill," is intended for women who have experienced a single episode of unprotected intercourse within a given menstrual cycle. Postcoital contraception can also be used in cases of sexual assault.[1,11,14] Emergency contraceptives contain the hormones estrogen and progestin (levonorgestrel), either separately or in combination. Several contraceptive regimens have been used for this purpose (Table 172-1). The FDA has approved two products for prescription use for emergency contraception, Preven (approved in 1998) and Plan B (approved in 1999).[20] All these methods prevent implantation, but to be effective, they must be taken within the first 72 hours after unprotected intercourse.

The side effects of all emergency contraceptive regimens include nausea and vomiting, breast tenderness, dizziness, menorrhagia, and abdominal pain. The combination method (ethinyl estradiol and norgestrel [Ovral]) uses a relatively lower steroid dose than others, thus mitigating the side effects but retaining a demonstrated efficacy rate of 98%. In 2006, the FDA approved Plan B as a nonprescription form of postcoital contraception for women 18 years of age and older.[20] In most states, women under the age of 18 need a prescription for Plan B. Women should be educated about the availability of postcoital contraception to prevent unplanned or unwanted pregnancies in the event an emergency occurs.

BARRIER METHODS

Barrier methods of fertility control are so named because they act as mechanical barriers and prevent pregnancy by blocking the passage of sperm through their surfaces. In addition, they prevent or reduce contact with genital lesions, discharges, or secretions.

Condoms

Most condoms made in the United States are manufactured from latex; approximately 5% are made from animal skin (usually lamb intestine). Although both types of condoms interfere with the passage of sperm, only latex condoms protect against STDs (including HIV) and viral infections (hepatitis B and herpes simplex). Failure rates with condoms are as low as 3% with perfect use and as high as 12% with typical use (based on 1 year of use).[2,7] A polyurethane female condom (Reality) is now available and has the benefit of affording women direct control of contraception and disease prevention. However, failure rates for the female condom are significantly higher (5% with perfect use, 21% with typical use) than for male condoms. Among women using some form of fertility control during the past decade, male condom use has increased from 15% in 1988 to 20% in 1995. Condoms are the only immediately reversible method of contraception for men.

TABLE 172-1 Postcoital Contraceptive Regimens

Drug	Trade Name	Dosage
Ethinyl estradiol	*	2.5 mg PO b.i.d. for 5 days
Norgestrel and ethinyl estradiol	Ovral	2 doses PO q 12 hr
	Lo/Ovral	4 doses PO q 12 hr
Ethinyl estradiol plus levonorgestrel†	Nordette, Levlen, Triphasil Tri-Levlen (yellow pills only)	4 doses PO q 12 hr
	Preven	2 tablets within 72 hours of unprotected intercourse; 2 or more tablets 12 hours later
Levonorgestrel 0.75 mg	Plan B	1 tablet within 72 hours of unprotected intercourse; second tablet 12 hours later

*Not available in the United States as a single preparation.
†Considered to be 75% effective.

Patient education regarding condom use should include information about how to put on and remove a condom, the need to leave a receptacle at the tip of the condom to avoid breakage, what to do in case of condom slippage or damage, and the importance of avoiding oil-based products (e.g., petroleum jelly, cold cream) when extra lubrication is needed.

Diaphragms and Cervical Caps

Diaphragms and cervical caps are female barrier methods of contraception. Both must be individually fitted to be effective; even with correct use, failure rates are as high as 5% to 9% for nulliparous users and 5% to 26% for parous users during the first year of use. Diaphragm use has steadily decreased during the past 15 years. At this point it is one of the least commonly used forms of contraception. Both the diaphragm and the cervical cap are used with spermicidal cream or jelly.

The diaphragm is a dome-shaped rubber cap that comes in a variety of sizes. It fits into the vagina, covering the cervix and the anterior vagina from the pubic symphysis to the posterior fornix. The diaphragm should remain in place for at least 6 hours after intercourse, but no more than 24 hours (to minimize the risk of toxic shock syndrome). Once in position, the diaphragm provides effective contraception for 6 hours, after which fresh spermicide must be applied if additional contraceptive protection is desired. A weight gain of more than 25% requires a refitting.

The cervical cap is a deep, soft rubber cup that covers the surface and fits snugly around the base of the cervix. The cap provides continuous contraceptive protection over 24 hours regardless of how often intercourse occurs. Additional spermicide or jelly is not needed for repeated intercourse.

Advantages of the female barrier methods include a lack of dependence on partners for contraception and none of the side effects of systemic hormones. With the exception of the female condom, all female vaginal barrier methods are used in conjunction with spermicides. Some protection against HIV is afforded if the spermicide contains nonoxynol-9. On the other hand, research has demonstrated that vaginal irritation caused by nonoxynol-9 may *increase* HIV susceptibility. Reduction in the risk of other STDs, including gonorrhea and chlamydia, varies from 10% to 50% depending on the study. Risks associated with the use of diaphragms and cervical caps include latex allergy, toxic shock syndrome, and recurrent urinary tract infections.[2,7]

Spermicides

A variety of over-the-counter spermicidal products are available in the United States and include foams, creams, gels, suppositories, and films. The active ingredient in all spermicides available in the United States is nonoxynol-9 or a similar agent that destroys the membrane of the sperm cell. Spermicides can be used alone but, as noted earlier, are also essential for the effective functioning of diaphragms and cervical caps. Effectiveness varies with the type of usage and compliance; failure rates vary from 20% with typical use to 10% with educated, motivated couples.[2]

One major advantage of spermicides is that they are available over the counter. Many women also appreciate that there is no partner involvement with this method. Spermicides provide some protection against gonorrhea and chlamydia. Side effects include allergic reactions to the active ingredient or to the particular spermicide base or vehicle, which generally manifests itself as vulvar pruritus or a rash. Women who are prone to yeast infections may notice an increased frequency of this problem when spermicides are used. Although women do not need to consult a health care provider to use spermicides, it is nonetheless important for this option to be discussed in any family planning session.

Cervical Sponge and Lea Contraceptive

These two forms of barrier birth control are now available without a prescription. The sponge is moistened with water and inserted into the vagina. It should be removed within 24 hours as it has been associated with toxic shock syndrome.[18] The Lea contraceptive is reusable silicone device inserted over the vagina before intercourse.[18] It is used with a spermicide cream and should not remain in the vagina longer than 48 hours.[18] When removed it must be washed and dried.

Intrauterine Devices

Intrauterine contraceptive devices currently available in the United States include (1) the copper T380A, a T-shaped, polyethylene device with a stem and cross arms partly covered by copper wire and tubing; (2) the progesterone-releasing IUD (Progestasert), a plastic, T-shaped device that releases 65 mcg of progesterone per day for at least 1 year; and (3) the levonorgestrel-containing IUD (Mirena), a recently approved, slow-releasing pump device that releases 20 mcg of levonorgestrel per day and provides effective contraception for at least 5 years.[2,8]

Copper IUDs prevent fertilization primarily by creating a spermicidal environment. The IUD causes the endometrium to initiate a foreign body reaction, which results in sterile inflammation and inhibits sperm from reaching the fallopian tube. As the inflammatory response is heightened, local prostaglandin response is increased, and endometrial enzyme production is inhibited. Progesterone-releasing IUDs thicken the cervical mucus, reduce sperm penetration, and inhibit sperm survival and implantation. The copper T380A, with a failure rate of only 0.5% to 0.8% during the first year of use, is more effective in preventing pregnancy than Progestasert, which has a failure rate of approximately 3% during the first year of use. IUD use has declined significantly in the last two decades due to the availability of other forms of contraception. The IUDs currently in use are associated with far fewer complications than the early copper-containing IUDs (including the Dalkon Shield) of the 1980s. Copper-containing IUDs can increase bleeding and dysmenorrhea, whereas the levonorgestrel system lessens these symptoms. Possible disadvantages to and complications of IUD use include an increased risk of PID, although recent data indicate that copper IUDs are associated with lower rates of PID than was previously thought. Evidence suggests that the risk of PID is even lower with the levonorgestrel system.[5] Insertion-related infection may be prevented by administering 200 mg doxycycline to the woman 1 hour before insertion. Women who develop asymptomatic gonorrhea or chlamydia infections may be treated with the IUD in place. Removal of the IUD is recommended if the infection does not respond to therapy or if actual PID develops as a result of the infection. It is unclear whether IUDs increase the rate of transmission of HIV. IUDs may increase uterine lining bleeding, making transmission of the virus easier, but this has not been demonstrated by research. Other potential side effects include increased dysmenorrhea, bleeding, or spotting; 10% of IUDs are removed for these reasons.

Of the pregnancies that do occur with IUDs in place, 50% result in spontaneous abortion. In contrast to the older-generation IUDs, the copper T380A decreases rather than increases the overall risk of ectopic pregnancy by 90% as compared with the risk for noncontraceptive users. On the other hand, the progesterone-releasing IUD has an ectopic pregnancy rate that is 50% to 80% *higher* than that for women not using contraception. Reduction of ectopic pregnancies is greatest with contraceptive methods that inhibit ovulation. When an IUD user does become pregnant, there is an increased ratio of ectopic to intrauterine gestations.[2]

IUDs should not be prescribed for women with a history of ectopic pregnancy; nulliparous women; or women with active, recent, or recurrent pelvic infections, including postpartum endometriosis or infection after an abortion or known or suspected pregnancy. Caution should be exercised if an IUD is being considered for a woman with risk factors for PID or STDs; undiagnosed irregular, heavy, or abnormal vaginal bleeding; a cervical or uterine malignancy; or an unresolved Papanicolaou's (Pap) test. Additional precautions include a history of previous problems with IUDs (e.g., pregnancies, expulsion, perforation, pain, or heavy bleeding), a history of vasovagal reactivity or fainting, valvular heart disease (e.g., aortic stenosis), uterine anatomic abnormalities, and a history of anemia.

For most nulliparous women there are better contraceptive options than an IUD; nulliparous women tend to tolerate IUDs less well than women who have carried at least one pregnancy to term. There may also be a slightly increased risk of infertility in women with a history of IUD use.[7] Patient education should include information about checking for the IUD string as well as the signs and symptoms of possible complications, including pain, bleeding, odorous discharge, fever, or missed menses.[2]

Vaginal Ring

Etonogestrel–ethinyl estradiol vaginal ring (NuvaRing) is a vaginal contraceptive ring that delivers 15 mcg ethinyl estradiol and 120 mcg of etonogestrel each day. The flexible, circular ring is inserted in the vagina by the woman and kept in for 3 weeks. Unlike the diaphragm, the vaginal ring does not have to be in a specific position, since the hormones can be absorbed anywhere in the vagina.[5] If for some reason the ring is out of the vagina for more than 3 hours, back-up contraception should be used until the ring has been back in place for 7 days. After 3 weeks, the ring is removed for 1 week. Withdrawal bleeding usually begins within 2 to 3 days of the ring-free week. To prevent pregnancy, a new ring must be inserted after the ring-free week (7 days). In a study of 1145 women monitored through 12,109 cycles, six pregnancies occurred.[18] The vaginal ring provides contraception using lower hormonal doses than other contraceptive methods, is readily reversible, and is easy for patients to use. Headache, nausea, and vaginal discomfort have been reported in 15% of patients.[18] Studies show that 90% of women are able to use the device correctly.[5]

SURGICAL STERILIZATION

Methods of surgical sterilization include tubal sterilization and vasectomy. Sterilization is the most commonly reported method of fertility control; in the United States in 2002, it was the method used by 27% contraceptive users ages 15 to 44 years.[1] Advantages of both male and female sterilization include its permanence, high rate of efficacy (0.4% failure rate for women and 0.15% for men), cost-effectiveness, lack of significant long-term side effects, and lack of need for partner compliance. Permanence is also a disadvantage of sterilization; sometimes the procedures can be reversed, but this is difficult and expensive. In addition, sterilization provides no protection against STDs, including HIV.[7]

NATURAL FAMILY PLANNING

Natural family planning (NFP) includes any method of family planning that is based on observations of the signs of fertility rather than on interference with physiologic function. It is important for health care providers to suggest NFP to their patients because it may be an attractive option for many women who might otherwise be unaware of its benefits. The two major forms of NFP practiced in the United States are the ovulation method and the symptothermal method (STM).

Conscientious application of the principles of NFP is an effective method of family planning, with failure rates of 3% for the ovulation method, 2% for the STM, and 1% when intercourse is confined to the postovulation period.[7] Undoubtedly, abstinence is a major stumbling block for many couples when first considering NFP. Nevertheless, couples who choose NFP grow to appreciate abstinence as a significant avenue for personal growth in their relationship by fostering emotional intimacy and encouraging balance within the sexual relationship.

Ovulation Method

The ovulation method is based on a single fertility sign: the changes in the mucus secreted by a woman's cervix. Hormonal changes cause the cervical mucus to vary in appearance and consistency throughout the menstrual cycle, forming a recognizable pattern that corresponds to her fertility. During menstruation, estrogen and progesterone levels are at their lowest. This low hormonal level allows the pituitary gland to release FSH, thus initiating the growth of several ova. The follicles release estrogen as they develop. Estrogen causes the endometrium to thicken in anticipation of the possibility of pregnancy, and it also influences the characteristics of the cervical mucus. When the level of estrogen is low, a woman will experience vulvar dryness; an opaque, sticky mucus appears as estrogen increases. Fertile mucus forms channels within itself to allow for the passage of sperm. By contrast, the opaque sticky mucus seen before and after ovulation has a closely woven microstructure that hinders the passage of sperm and forms a plug in the cervical os. In absence of fertile cervical mucus, sperm can live in the vaginal tract for only 30 minutes to 24 hours. In the presence of cervical mucus, sperm remain viable for up to 5 or 6 days.[21]

With the ovulation method, the average cycle is divided into four phases: (1) menstruation, (2) the postmenstrual infertile days, (3) the fertile period, and (4) the 2-week infertile period of postovulation. Any day of bleeding is considered a fertile period because bleeding may mask the presence of mucus, but most women do not secrete cervical mucus until several days after menstruation has ended. As long as cervical mucus is not present, intercourse can occur every other evening in the postmenstrual period. Intercourse is confined to the evening because the absence of cervical mucus must be ensured if pregnancy is to be avoided. The absence of mucus in the morning might be a postural effect rather than a true absence. Intercourse is further restricted to every other evening because semen can take 24 hours to leave the vaginal area and can mask the presence of mucus.

Cervical mucus can be checked and examined by wiping a toilet tissue across the vaginal opening either before or after urination. Cervical mucus, if present, remains on top of the tissue without being absorbed; it should be examined for elasticity and translucence. At the first sign of mucus the couple should abstain from sexual intercourse and genital-to-genital contact of any type. The period of abstinence extends until the evening of the fourth day after the appearance of clear, stretchy, lubricating mucus (peak mucus), at which time intercourse is not restricted again until menstruation. Ovulation typically occurs within 1 day before, during, or after the appearance of peak mucus.[7]

Symptothermal Method

The second method of family planning, STM, is similar to the ovulation method but uses two other fertility signs besides cervical mucus: basal body temperature and the position, shape, and consistency of the cervix. STM is the most widely used method of NFP in the United States. Advocates of this method place particular emphasis on the cooperation of man and woman in fertility regulation.

With STM, the menstrual cycle is separated into three phases. The relatively infertile phase lasts from the beginning of menstruation to the onset of any mucus. The fertile phase lasts from the first sign of mucus until the beginning of the third phase. The third phase, known as the postovulatory infertility phase (or the absolute infertility phase), begins on the fourth day of a temperature elevation and the fifth day of the drying of the cervical mucus.[21] A basal thermometer (useful for measuring subtle variations in body temperature between 35.5° and 37.7° C [96° and 100° F]) is used to record morning body temperatures. Typically, a biphasic curve is observed over the course of the menstrual cycle, with low temperatures recorded before ovulation and slightly higher temperatures recorded after ovulation. A typical postovulatory elevation ranges between 0.4° and 1° F above the average of the last 6 ovulatory days.[22] The temperature rise is caused by the presence of progesterone, which is released by the empty follicle after ovulation. At least 3 days of elevated temperatures must be recorded before the postovulatory infertile phase begins on the evening of that third day. Basal body temperature does not give any advance warning of ovulation but indicates when ovulation has passed.

Palpation of the cervix is performed as an adjunct to the other signs of fertility. During the infertile period the cervix is firm and low in the vagina, and the cervical os is closed. As ovulation approaches, the cervix softens and elevates until it is almost out of reach, and the cervical os opens. Some women find this to be a helpful sign; others do not. In some cycles these signs provide information as to when the woman is capable of conceiving. Couples who wish to avoid pregnancy should wait to have intercourse until all signs indicate that the fertile time has passed.

CONTRACEPTIVE VACCINES

The contraceptive choices available to women at this time include steroid contraceptives, IUDs, barrier methods, spermicides, NFP, male and female sterilization, and, more recently emergency contraception. However, the world's population is still growing at a tremendous rate, and unintended pregnancies continue to be a major public health issue. Contraceptive vaccines may prove to be a valuable alternative and, if viable, may be more acceptable than the currently available methods of contraception because of the possibility of high specificity, limited side effects, low cost, and infrequent administration. Several targets are being explored for the development of contraceptive vaccines, including gamete production (gonadotropin-releasing hormone, FSH and LH), gamete function (zona pellucida and sperm), and gamete outcome (human chorionic gonadotropin).[23]

REASONS FOR CONTRACEPTIVE NONUSE

In the United States, where contraception is generally widely available, it is surprising that almost 50% of pregnancies are still considered unintended. Unintended pregnancy may occur for many reasons, including nonuse of contraception; failure to use contraceptive methods consistently and correctly; and, far less frequently, method failure.[24] Studies show that reasons for nonuse differ by event and by age at the time of the event. Concern about parents finding out was the most common reason that young women did not use contraception at first sex or first unintended pregnancy. On the other hand, older women who had been pregnant previously and who had presumably already attained their sexual and reproductive health independence reported problems related to accessing contraception, discontinuation of contraception, and a general ambivalence about contraception.[24] This heightens the need for improving contraceptive counseling and designing education programs for women, parents, and providers.

REFERENCES

1. Centers for Disease Control and Prevention: Primary contraceptive methods among women aged 15-44 years—United States, 2002, *MMWR* 54(6):141-164, 2005.
2. Kaunitz AM, Illions EH, Jones JL, and others: Contraception: a clinical review for the internist, *Med Clin North Am* 7(6):1377-1409, 1995.
3. Henshaw S: Unintended pregnancy in the United States, *Fam Plan Perspect* 30(1):24-29, 46, 1998.
4. Abma J, Martinez G, Mosher W, and others: Teenagers n the United States: sexual activity, contraceptive use and childbearing, *Vital Health Stat* 23(24):35, 2004.

5. Herndon E, Zieman M: New contraceptive options, *Am Fam Phys* 69:853-860, 2004.
6. Edwards L: An update on oral contraceptive options, *Formulary* 39:104-121, 2004.
7. Hatcher RA, Trussell J, Stewart F, and others, editors: *Contraceptive technology*, ed 16, New York, 1994, Irvington.
8. Moore A: Adherence issues with contraceptive regimens: old problems, added options, *Women's Health Care* 1(4):9-14, 2002.
9. Jolly J: New age of contraceptives, *Drug Facts Comparisons NEWS* 3:83-85, 2003.
10. Rosenfeld A, Zahorik PM, Saint W, and others: Women's satisfaction with birth control, *J Fam Pract* 36(2):169-173, 1993.
11. Kubba AA: Contraception: a review, *Int J Clin Pract* 52(2):102-105, 1998.
12. Dunn N, Thorogood M, Faragher B, and others: Oral contraceptive use and myocardial infarction results of the MICA case-control study, *BMJ* 318:1579-1584, 1999.
13. Pymar H, Creinin M: The risks of oral contraceptive pills, *Semin Reprod Med* 19:305-312, 2001.
14. Mazza D: Recent advances in contraception, *Aust Fam Phys* 27(5):347-352, 1998.
15. Chasan-Taber L, Stampfer MJ: Epidemiology of oral contraceptives and cardiovascular disease, *Ann Intern Med* 128(6):467-477, 1998.
16. Marchbanks P, McDonald J, Wilson H, and others: Oral contraceptives and the risk for breast cancer, *N Engl J Med* 346:2025-2032, 2002.
17. Women's Health Information: *Contraceptive implants—information for women,* April 18, 2006, retrieved March 4, 2007, from http://www.rwh.org.au/womnensinfo/factsheets.cfm?doc_id=7191.
18. Zieman M: *Overview of contraception*, retrieved March 5, 2007, from http://www.utdol.com/utd.
19. Audet M, Moreau M, Koltun W, and others: Evaluation of contraceptive efficacy and cycle control of a transdermal contraceptive patch vs. an oral contraceptive: a randomized controlled trial, *JAMA* 285:2347-2354, 2001.
20. US Food and Drug Administration: *FDA's decision regarding Plan B: questions and answers,* May 2, 2004, retrieved July 28, 2006, from http://www.fda.gove/bbs/topics/NEWS/2006/NEW01436.html.
21. Hamilton K: The symptothermal method of natural family planning, *Phys Assist* 8(11), 1984.
22. Geerling JH: Natural family planning, *Am Fam Phys* 52(6):1749-1760, 1995.
23. Naz R: Contraceptive vaccines, *Drugs* 65(5):69, 593-603, 2005.
24. Iuliano A, Speizer I, Santelli J, and others: Reasons for contraceptive nonuse at first sex and unintended pregnancy, *Am J Health Behav* 30(1):92-102, 2006.

CHAPTER **173**

Genital Tract Cancers

Denise T. Bynum and Patricia Polgar Bailey

Gynecologic malignancies include vulvar, vaginal, cervical, endometrial, ovarian, and fallopian tube cancers; endometrial, ovarian, and cervical cancers are the most commonly diagnosed. In the United States genital tract cancers account for approximately 18% of the total cancer incidence in women 10 to 44 years of age.[1] Cervical and endometrial cancers have a high cure rate because of several factors, including (1) premalignant changes that lead to early diagnosis (especially with cervical cancer) and (2) metastatic spread that is local and regional in the early stages (in cervical and endometrial cancer). In addition, these cancers are sensitive to radiation (cervical and endometrial cancer) and chemotherapy (choriocarcinoma and, sometimes, ovarian cancer). The terminology for cervical dysplasia and carcinoma in situ has changed to *cervical intraepithelial neoplasia* (CIN). Similarly, the terminology for preinvasive vulvar and vaginal lesions has changed to *vulvar intraepithelial neoplasia* (VIN) and *vaginal intraepithelial neoplasia* (VAIN), respectively.[2]

All suspicious lesions in the genital tract require referral to a gynecologist for biopsy. Surgical management is usually the initial treatment and is often curative, particularly in the early stages.[2] If cancer is confirmed, a gynecologic oncologist should be consulted. The gynecologic oncologist has extensive surgical experience and expertise in radiation and medical oncology.

VULVAR CANCER

DEFINITION AND EPIDEMIOLOGY

Approximately 4000 cases of vulvar cancer were diagnosed in 2003.[3] Vulvar cancer accounts for 4% of all female genital tract cancers and 0.6% of all cancers in women.[4] Lymph node status is the most significant prognostic factor. The 5-year survival rate is 90% for women without nodal involvement and decreases to 30% to 55% for women with positive nodes.[4]

PATHOPHYSIOLOGY

Risk factors for vulvar cancers include cigarette smoking, human papillomavirus (HPV) infection, HIV infection or other conditions that cause immunosuppression, low socioeconomic status, VIN, chronic vulvar inflammation, other genital tract cancers, genital herpes infections, lichen sclerosus, chronic granulomatous disease, and syphilis. Malignant melanomas of the vulva and vagina represent a group of rare malignancies that have been historically difficult to treat and have a high mortality rate.[5] Persons with a family history of melanoma or atypical moles have an increased risk of this type of genital cancer.

There are several types of vulvar cancers. Squamous cell carcinomas account for the majority of invasive cancers.

Verrucous carcinoma is a subtype of invasive squamous cell that causes cauliflower-like growths similar to genital warts.[4] Paget's disease is a lesion of unknown cause that arises from the apocrine-bearing part of the vulvar skin. Paget's disease manifests with pruritus, soreness, erythematous skin, and hyperkeratotic plaques and may be confused with candidiasis. Bartholin's gland carcinoma is a carcinoma of the mucin-secreting glands on either side of the lower vagina. The tumor may initially be seen as a unilateral deep mass and is often diagnosed as a cyst or an abscess. Bartholin's gland carcinoma accounts for 2% of vulvar malignancies and occurs in a younger age-group than vulvar squamous cell carcinoma.[2] Adenocarcinoma cells are found within the epidermis and skin appendages.

CLINICAL PRESENTATION

Most patients have a history of vulvar irritation, burning or pain, pruritus, local discomfort, excoriation, fissuring, painful irritation, bleeding and discharge, and/or a painful vulvar lump. The lesion may be white, raised, hyperkeratotic, or pigmented. Invasive cancers may manifest with a foul discharge. Many tumors are detected late and may be seen initially with rectal bleeding, urethral obstruction, or large involved inguinal lymph nodes.

PHYSICAL EXAMINATION

Early diagnosis in vulvar cancer is important. The initial lesion may appear as a small raised area or as an ulceration that will not heal, or it may be associated with a secondary infection. The cancer spreads along the labia. Regional lymph nodes require examination because the cancer will metastasize freely as a result of the many lymph channels in that area. The presence of palpable lymph nodes usually represents malignant spread.

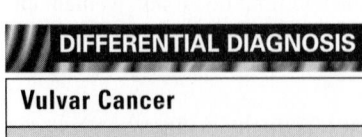

DIAGNOSTICS AND DIFFERENTIAL DIAGNOSIS

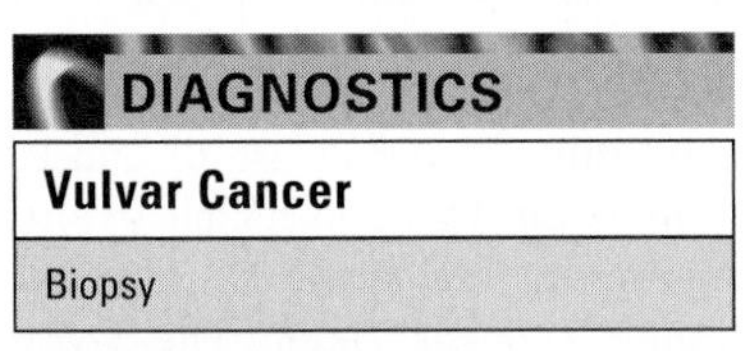
DIAGNOSTICS

Vulvar Cancer

Biopsy

DIFFERENTIAL DIAGNOSIS

Vulvar Cancer

- Carcinoma
- Dermatitis
- Syphilis
- Granuloma inguinale
- Eczema
- Crohn's disease

Vulvar carcinoma can be mistaken for other conditions, including eczema or dermatitis, ulcerative lesions such as syphilis, or granuloma inguinale. The definitive diagnosis requires a biopsy. Metastatic disease may increase serum calcium levels. Crohn's disease can manifest as an ulcerative area on the vulva, and a lesion, on rare occasion, could be a metastasis from a distant site.

MANAGEMENT AND INDICATIONS FOR REFERRAL OR HOSPITALIZATION

All patients with a suspicious lesion of the vulva require referral for biopsy. Treatment is primarily wide surgical excision, vulvectomy, or pelvic exenteration. Treatments for preinvasive lesions include local chemotherapy or laser therapy. Cystoscopy and sigmoidoscopy are often indicated to exclude invasive disease. During the past 20 years, treatment has changed from radical vulvectomy with inguinal and deep pelvic lymphadenectomy to a much less extensive vulvectomy and selective groin resection. Pelvic lymphadenectomy is rarely done.[6]

LIFE SPAN CONSIDERATIONS

Invasive vulvar cancer occurs most often between the ages of 65 and 70, with noninvasive vulvar cancer occurring most often in women ages 20 years or younger. Seventy-five percent of vulvar cancers occur in women older than 50.[3] The preinvasive lesions can occur at any age but are more common in younger patients and are associated with HPV infection.

COMPLICATIONS

Complications after genital tract cancer depend on the stage of the cancer and method of treatment. Usual complications include those associated with radiation, chemotherapy, or surgery. Metastasis can occur if the cancer is invasive. (For further information, see Chapter 257.)

PATIENT AND FAMILY EDUCATION

All patients should understand the necessity of screening to ensure early detection of vulvar and vaginal cancer. Screening methods include an annual pelvic examination and Papanicolaou's (Pap) test, monthly genital self-examination, and prompt reporting of unusual symptoms.[7] As is true for all forms of genital cancer, access to information about the disease, its treatment, and consequences is clearly important. However, it is likely that many providers underestimate their patients' desire for information while possibly overestimating their desire to make decisions. Opportunities to discuss the diagnosis and receive appropriate information seem to be the key to effective practice, whether or not patients want to be actively involved in making treatment decisions.[8]

VAGINAL CANCER

DEFINITION AND EPIDEMIOLOGY

Vaginal cancer is an uncommon tumor that accounts for 3% of genital tract cancers.[4] More than 1 million women have been exposed to diethylstilbestrol (DES), which was commonly used between 1940 and 1971 for the prevention of spontaneous abortions.[4] The incidence of vaginal cancer in exposed daughters is estimated at 1:1000.[4] The prognosis for vaginal cancer depends on the stage and involvement of lymph nodes. The 5-year survival rate is 96% for stage 0, 73% for stage I disease, 58% for stage II disease, 36% for stage III/IV disease, and 14% for melanoma.[4]

PATHOPHYSIOLOGY

Squamous cell carcinomas account for 85% of tumors, with the remaining 15% consisting of adenocarcinomas, sarcomas, leiomyosarcomas, and melanomas.[2] Squamous cell carcinomas arise from surface epithelial cells, adenocarcinomas arise from glandular cells, sarcomas arise from connective tissue,

BOX 173-1

RISK FACTORS FOR VAGINAL CANCER

- Human papillomavirus infection
- Sexually transmitted diseases (genital herpes simplex)
- Prior irradiation of pelvis
- Smoking
- Immunosuppressive therapy
- Chemotherapy for other malignancy
- Prolonged use of pessary
- Previous malignancy of uterus, cervix, or vulva
- Diethylstilbestrol exposure in utero
- Advanced age
- Vaginal adenosis or irritation

and melanomas arise from melanocytes. Non–clear cell adenocarcinoma is very rare, occurs predominantly in postmenopausal women, and has a worse prognosis than squamous cell carcinoma.[7] Clear cell adenocarcinoma is usually associated with DES exposure in utero. VAIN occurs in the upper third of the vagina and is detected with an abnormal Pap test. Primary vaginal tumors are rare. If the tumor is primary, it is usually a squamous cell carcinoma. However, these are usually extensions from endometrial, ovarian, vulvar, renal, or colorectal cancers. Primary adenocarcinoma of the vagina is rare and most often related to DES exposure. These cancers were diagnosed more often in the 1970s and 1980s.[2] Box 173-1 presents risk factors for vaginal cancer.

CLINICAL PRESENTATION

Twenty percent of vaginal carcinomas are asymptomatic and found on a routine pelvic examination. The most common symptom is abnormal bleeding; however, the patient may also complain of vaginal, back, leg, or pelvic pain; dyspareunia; dysuria; constipation; or vaginal discharge or mass. A patient with an advanced tumor usually complains of continuous pain or urinary or bowel problems. The most common site for a primary tumor is the upper third of the vagina.

PHYSICAL EXAMINATION

The tumor can develop anywhere but is most often found on the lower anterior and lateral vaginal wall. Late-stage signs, such as leg edema or lymph node involvement, are found with adenocarcinoma in more than 95% of cases.[2]

DIAGNOSTICS AND DIFFERENTIAL DIAGNOSIS

The patient should be referred for colposcopy (the study of the transformation zone using a microscope with low magnification) and to exclude primary disease elsewhere. The Pap test has a low sensitivity for detecting clear cell carcinoma; thus DES-exposed women without symptoms should be seen by a gynecologist for inspection of the vagina and cervix, biopsy, and colposcopy. The differential diagnosis includes VAIN, a metastatic lesion, and, if the woman is of childbearing age, trophoblastic disease.

DIAGNOSTICS

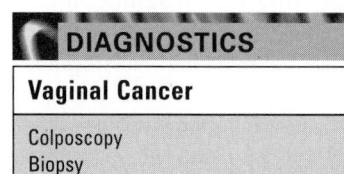

Vaginal Cancer

Colposcopy
Biopsy

DIFFERENTIAL DIAGNOSIS

Vaginal Cancer

- Vaginal intraepithelial neoplasia
- Metastatic lesion
- Trophoblastic disease

MANAGEMENT AND INDICATIONS FOR REFERRAL OR HOSPITALIZATION

Patients with suspicious lesions require colposcopy and biopsy. Wide excision with the patient under anesthesia, as well as cystoscopy and sigmoidoscopy, may be necessary to ensure that the cancer is not invasive. The treatment depends on the type and stage of the disease and may include radiation or pelvic exenteration. Vaporization with a carbon dioxide laser or intravaginal application of 5-fluorouracil may be used for premalignant lesions. Chemotherapy has not been proved effective for vaginal cancer.[3]

LIFE SPAN CONSIDERATIONS

Age is a risk factor for squamous cell cancer of the vagina. Most patients with this type of cancer are older than age 50. In contrast, clear cell adenocarcinoma has a patient age range of 7 to 29 years, with the average age at diagnosis of 19. The peak incidence is between 14 and 20 years and is associated with DES exposure in utero. With most of the women exposed to DES now between the ages of 30 and 60, the number of new cases of this type of cancer has decreased.[4]

COMPLICATIONS

Complications after genital tract cancer depend on the stage of the cancer and method of treatment and include those associated with radiation, chemotherapy, or surgery. (For further information, see Chapter 257.)

PATIENT AND FAMILY EDUCATION

After vaginal cancer, follow-up includes a pelvic examination and Pap test every 3 months for 2 years and then every 6 months for 3 years, with a chest x-ray study annually. Patients with vaginal cancer require a careful explanation that they are more likely to develop a malignancy in the cervix or vulva. Even after a hysterectomy, a Pap test should be done at least every 1 to 2 years. DES-exposed women should be vigilantly monitored with yearly Pap tests. Female patients exposed to DES in utero who have symptoms should be examined despite their age, and beginning at age 14 (or menarche) these patients should have examinations twice a year or more often if epithelial changes are present.

CERVICAL CANCER

DEFINITION AND EPIDEMIOLOGY

Approximately 12,000 cases of invasive cervical cancer were diagnosed in 2003. However, it is estimated that noninvasive cervical cancer (CIN) is nearly four times more common than invasive cervical cancer.[3] A Pap test is a widely used cancer screen and is considered to be largely responsible for the sharp decline in the mortality rates due to cervical cancer. This cancer is the easiest to cure if found early. The incidence of invasive cancer of the cervix has decreased, but that of CIN has increased.

The mortality rate has decreased in African-American women but is still more than twice that of Caucasian women (6.7% compared with 2.5%). The mortality rate has decreased with the use of Pap tests and colposcopy. Cervical cancer has a 5-year survival rate of 100% for preinvasive cancer, 92% for localized cancer, and 70% for all stages.[4]

In 2006 the first HPV vaccine (Gardasil) was approved by the U.S. Food and Drug Administration. This is the first vaccine developed to prevent cervical cancer, precancerous cervical lesions, and genital warts due to human papilloma virus (HPV). The vaccine is highly effective against four types of the HPV, including two that account for about 70% of cervical cancer. The vaccine is currently recommended for women 11 to 26 years of age but can be given to girls as young as 9.[9]

BOX 173-2

RISK FACTORS FOR CERVICAL CANCER

- Early sexual activity (younger than ages 16 to 18 years)
- Multiple sexual partners (four or more)
- Young age at first pregnancy
- Short intervals between pregnancies
- Sexually transmitted diseases (including human papillomavirus and herpes simplex)
- Low socioeconomic status
- Cigarette smoking
- Oral contraceptive use
- HIV infection
- Immunosuppression
- Increased parity
- Poor personal hygiene
- Uncircumcised partner
- Promiscuous male partners
- Diethylstilbestrol exposure
- Advanced age

PATHOPHYSIOLOGY

Squamous cell carcinomas account for 85% to 90% of cervical cancers.[1] Adenocarcinoma can also occur in the cervix. This cancer arises from precursor lesions that begin with atypical cervical cells and gradually progress to CIN and eventually to invasive cancer of the cervix. These precursor lesions can regress or progress into malignancy.[2] As mentioned earlier, the terminology for noninvasive cervical squamous epithelial lesions has changed from carcinoma in situ and dysplasia to CIN. The CIN system grades the lesion according to the involvement of the epithelial thickness:

CIN grade I (mild dysplasia): Lesion well differentiated; involves initial third of the epithelial layer

CIN grade II (moderate dysplasia): Less differentiated; involves one third to two thirds of the epithelial layer

CIN grade III (severe dysplasia): Undifferentiated two thirds, full-thickness (carcinoma in situ) involvement

Cervical cancer has a long latency during the preinvasive period. The immature transformation zone of the cervix is particularly sensitive to viral infections. This may explain why those who are sexually active early have an increased incidence of cervical cancer.[2] Box 173-2 presents risk factors for cervical cancer.

CLINICAL PRESENTATION

Early symptoms include abnormal uterine bleeding (postmenopausal, postcoital, after douching, or intermenstrual) or foul vaginal discharge. Bleeding usually begins as light and serosanguineous and becomes heavier and more persistent as the tumor enlarges. Late symptoms include pain, leg edema, and urinary and rectal symptoms.

PHYSICAL EXAMINATION

A vaginal examination may reveal an enlarged cervix, friable tumor on the cervix, or ulcerative lesion that bleeds easily on contact. A Pap test will detect precancerous and cancerous lesions on the cervix or within the endocervix even if the cervix appears normal. The Pap test should include a scraping from the cervical os and a brushing from the endocervical canal. The specimen should be sent for interpretation by an experienced cytopathologist. The patient should be assessed for anemia if she has persistent heavy bleeding. A lesion on the cervix requires biopsy even if the Pap test is negative.

DIAGNOSTICS AND DIFFERENTIAL DIAGNOSIS

Epithelial cell abnormalities require diligent follow-up. If an infection is likely, the infection should be treated and the test repeated in 3 months. If an infection is unlikely, the test should be repeated in 3 months. If atypical cells continue at that point, the patient should be referred for colposcopy, endocervical curettage, or cone biopsy to locate the lesion. Atypical cells are always significant and require intervention. High-grade changes on the Pap smear require immediate referral for colposcopy. The differential diagnosis includes severe cervicitis, a cervical polyp, carcinoma of the endometrium with cervical extension, and metastatic carcinoma.

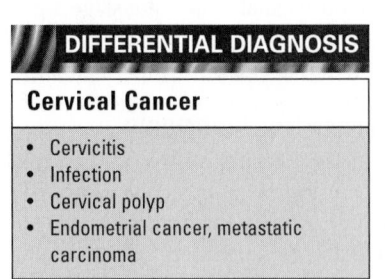

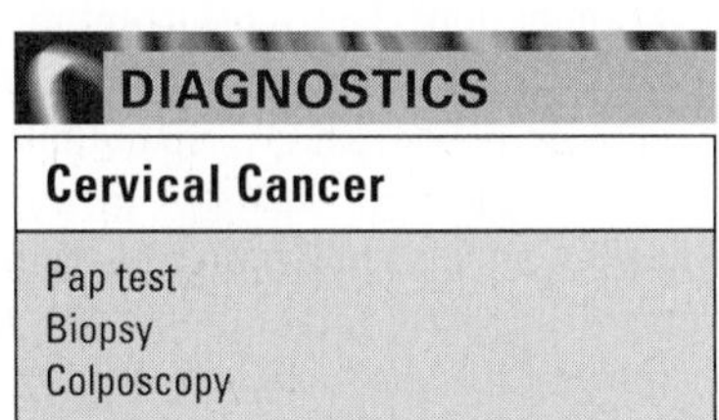

DIAGNOSTICS

Cervical Cancer

Pap test
Biopsy
Colposcopy

DIFFERENTIAL DIAGNOSIS

Cervical Cancer

- Cervicitis
- Infection
- Cervical polyp
- Endometrial cancer, metastatic carcinoma

MANAGEMENT AND INDICATIONS FOR REFERRAL OR HOSPITALIZATION

The patient should be referred for radiation, electrocautery, cryotherapy, conization, or hysterectomy. The treatment choices are based on the size, location, and histologic characteristics of the lesion and the patient's age, parity, and reliability for follow-up.

LIFE SPAN CONSIDERATIONS

The NCI reports that women 65 years old and older account for 24% of all cases and 41% of deaths.[3] Lower screening rates are viewed as the cause. Some sources recommend that screening can cease after age 65 if there is a history of regularly obtained negative smears and the patient has no high-risk characteristics. There is debate about this because of the number of malignancies seen in older adults. Pap tests should be performed annually if not performed regularly before age 65 years or if the smear has been abnormal. The incidence of CIN peaks between the ages of 20 and 30 years. After age 25 years, the cases of invasive cervical cancer increase with age, along with the chance of dying from the disease.[3]

COMPLICATIONS

Complications from genital tract cancer depend on the stage of the cancer and method of treatment and include those associated with radiation, chemotherapy, or surgery. (For further information, see Chapter 257.)

PATIENT AND FAMILY EDUCATION

The American Cancer Society recommends cervical cancer screening within 3 years for sexually active women and at age 21 for all women. Annual Pap smears and pelvic examinations are then recommended until age 30. At that time, if the woman has never had an abnormal cytology report or has had three consecutive normal cytology reports, the Pap test and pelvic examination can be performed every 3 years.[4] Women with a history of cervical cancer or history of diethylstilbestrol (DES) exposure will require continued annual Pap smears and pelvic examinations.[4] Immunocompromised women require annual screenings, but in some instances, more frequent screenings are indicated.[4] Women age 70 or older with an intact cervix and history of three consecutive satisfactory examinations with cytology-negative reports within the past 10 years can defer further testing.[4] Women age 70 who have never had a Pap smear or who have an unclear Pap smear history should have continued screenings. Careful monitoring for vulvar or other genital cancers is advised.

ENDOMETRIAL CANCER

DEFINITION AND EPIDEMIOLOGY

Endometrial cancer is the most common female genital tract cancer and the fourth most common malignancy in women.[2] Approximately 40,000 new cases of endometrial cancer were diagnosed in 2003.[10] Providers need to be aware of risk factors, diagnostic tests, pertinent history, and symptoms. The American Cancer Society notes the 5-year survival rate for all cases to be 84%.[4] The survival rate for Caucasian women exceeds that for African-American women by 15% at each stage.[3]

PATHOPHYSIOLOGY

Excess estrogen is the biggest risk factor for endometrial cancer. Most women who develop endometrial cancer have a history of exposure to abnormal estrogen levels. The risk of taking estrogen is neutralized with the addition of progestin. The risk is increased among first-degree relatives of patients with endometrial cancer and is associated with breast and colon cancer. Unopposed estrogen causes the endometrium to become thicker and more vascular (hyperplasia). Endometrial hyperplasia is divided into three groups: simple, complex, and atypical. Endometrial carcinoma develops in 20% to 30% of women with untreated atypical hyperplasia.[1] Without progesterone, the structural support needed to sustain vascularity is not present and spontaneous superficial random hemorrhages occur.[11] Box 173-3 presents risk and protective factors associated with endometrial cancer.

CLINICAL PRESENTATION AND PHYSICAL EXAMINATION

The symptoms of endometrial cancer often appear while cure is still possible. Patients may be seen with painless postmenopausal bleeding, discharge, painful or difficult urination, dyspareunia, or pelvic pain. Later signs of uterine cancer include cramping, pelvic discomfort, postcoital bleeding, lower abdominal pressure, and enlarged lymph nodes. A detailed history of menstruation, dyspareunia, pelvic pain, fever, trauma, and intrauterine contraceptive device use should be elicited, and risk factors for endometrial cancer reviewed. The physical examination includes a bimanual pelvic examination; Pap test; and assessment for abdominal masses, signs of bleeding disorders, and thyroid abnormalities.

BOX 173-3

ENDOMETRIAL CANCER: RISK AND PROTECTIVE FACTORS

RISK FACTORS

- Obesity
- Menstruation span
- Early menarche
- Late menopause
- No children
- Age (greater than 50)
- Polycystic ovary syndrome (Stein-Leventhal syndrome)
- Ovulation failure, infertility
- Estrogen-secreting tumors
- Other endocrine disorders
- Hypertension
- Diabetes mellitus
- Immunodeficiency
- Endometrial hyperplasia
- Diet high in animal fat
- Ovarian cancer
- Breast cancer
- Caucasian race
- Estrogen replacement therapy without progesterone (long term, high doses)
- Tamoxifen therapy
- Sequential oral contraception
- Hormonal therapy
- Previous radiotherapy (pelvic)
- Diethylstilbestrol exposure
- History of inherited form of colorectal cancer

PROTECTIVE FACTORS

- Combined oral contraception
- High parity

DIAGNOSTICS

The Pap test is not usually effective in detecting endometrial cancer. If endometrial cancer is suspected or if the patient is at high risk for its development, referral for a pelvic examination, transvaginal ultrasound, endometrial biopsy, hysteroscopy, and/or dilation and curettage (D&C) is necessary. Endometrial aspiration is a more direct sampling of the uterine cavity and is less painful than a D&C. If endometrial cancer is suspected, the following tests are required: serum human chorionic gonadotropin (if the patient is of reproductive age), CBC, BUN, creatinine, platelet count, cultures to exclude infection, saline and potassium hydroxide preparations of vaginal secretions, clotting studies, and hormone levels to detect menopausal status.[3,12]

DIAGNOSTICS

Endometrial Cancer

LABORATORY

Serum human chorionic gonadotropin (if of reproductive age)
CBC and differential, platelets
Cultures
Vaginal wet preparations and cultures
Coagulation profile
BUN
PT/PTT*
Creatinine
Hormone levels*

OTHER

Biopsy (endometrial)
Hysteroscopy and/or dilation and curettage
Transvaginal ultrasound

*If indicated.

DIFFERENTIAL DIAGNOSIS

Benign causes of bleeding include atrophic vaginitis, cervicitis, cervical polyps, ovarian cysts, inflammation, infection, endometriosis, uterine fibroids, uterine prolapse, polyps, erosions, pelvic inflammatory disease (PID), trauma (foreign body, sexual abuse, tampon), and complications of pregnancy (retained products of conception). In addition, systemic diseases (bleeding, thyroid, liver, renal disorders) and medications (oral contraceptives, steroids, anticoagulants, neuroleptics, major tranquilizers) can cause bleeding.

MANAGEMENT AND INDICATIONS FOR REFERRAL OR HOSPITALIZATION

An endometrial biopsy is essential for any patient with postmenopausal bleeding. Women at risk because of hormonal therapy require an annual endometrial sampling and other diagnostic interventions. Surgery is the treatment of choice for endometrial cancer except in late-stage disease. Treatment also includes radiation, hormonal therapy, and chemotherapy and depends on the type and stage of cancer and the patient's overall medical condition.

DIFFERENTIAL DIAGNOSIS

Endometrial Cancer

- Atrophic vaginitis
- Cervicitis
- Cervical polyp
- Ovarian cyst
- Inflammation
- Infection
- Endometriosis
- Systemic disease
- Uterine fibroids
- Uterine prolapse
- Uterine polyp
- Pelvic inflammatory disease
- Trauma
- Medications
- Pregnancy

LIFE SPAN CONSIDERATIONS

The average age for the diagnosis of endometrial cancer is 60, and the incidence increases with advancing age. When endometrial cancer occurs before the age of 40 years, it is usually associated with chronic obesity or anovulation.[12]

COMPLICATIONS

Complications after genital tract cancer depend on the stage of the cancer and method of treatment and include those associated with radiation, chemotherapy, or surgery. (For further information, see Chapter 257.)

PATIENT AND FAMILY EDUCATION

Patients should understand that the use of estrogen plus progesterone for postmenopausal hormone replacement therapy does not increase the risk of endometrial cancer. It is also necessary that women understand the importance of evaluation for unusual bleeding.

OVARIAN CANCER

DEFINITION AND EPIDEMIOLOGY

Ovarian cancer has a high fatality rate and is the sixth leading cause of death from cancer in women, with approximately 25,000 new cases diagnosed in 2003.[3] The National Ovarian Cancer Coalition notes that ovarian cancer accounts for 4% of all cancers among women. The death rates have not changed significantly in the past 50 years, with only 25% of ovarian cancers found early.[13] The 5-year survival rate is 90% for stage I, 70% for stage II, and 15% to 20% for stage III or IV.[13]

PATHOPHYSIOLOGY

The risk of developing ovarian cancer is influenced by genetic, hormonal, and environmental factors. Approximately 5% to 10% of women have a genetically acquired risk of ovarian cancer because of inherited mutations in the *BRCA1* and *BRCA2* tumor suppressor genes. The overall risk of developing ovarian cancer is 20% to 60% for those with *BRCA1* mutations and 10% to 35% for those with *BRCA2* mutations.[14] Some data suggest that women with *BRCA* mutation–mediated ovarian cancer may have better survival rates than woman with sporadic ovarian cases. This may be due to improved tumor response to platinum-based chemotherapy in those with *BRCA*-related cancer.[14]

Tumors primarily arise from the epithelial cells; however, they can also arise from the germinal or stromal cells of the ovary. Increased age and family history are risk factors, with family history being the best predictor of risk. One second-degree relative with ovarian cancer increases the lifetime risk to 2.9%; one first-degree relative with ovarian cancer increases the lifetime risk to 4% to 5%; and two or more affected first-degree relatives increases the risk to 30% to 50%.[11] The *BRCA1* gene, identified in 1994, has been linked to breast and ovarian cancer.[15] However, these hereditary syndromes occur in few

BOX 173-4

EPITHELIAL OVARIAN CANCER: RISK AND PROTECTIVE FACTORS

RISK FACTORS
- Advancing age
- Northern European or North American descent
- Nulliparity*
- Personal history of breast,* endometrial, or colon cancer
- Family history of ovarian cancer
- Infertility*
- Fertility drugs
- Dietary fat consumption*
- Milk product consumption
- Coffee consumption
- Perineal talc usage*
- Menstrual history (more periods* = increased risk)

PROTECTIVE FACTORS
- Pregnancy
- Tubal ligation or hysterectomy
- Oral contraceptives

Data from Griffiths CT, Silverstone A, Tobias J, and others: *Gynecologic oncology,* London, 1997, Mosby-Wolfe.
*Each of these risk factors increases the lifetime risk by 2%.

cases of ovarian cancer. Box 173-4 presents risk and protective factors associated with ovarian cancer.

CLINICAL PRESENTATION

If the patient comes in to see her health care provider with signs and symptoms of ovarian cancer, metastasis has occurred in 75% of the cases.[2] Only 25% of ovarian carcinomas are diagnosed at a time when they are curable.[2,4] There are no early warning symptoms. Early-stage disease is usually diagnosed from an asymptomatic mass noted on a routine pelvic examination. The usual presenting symptoms are the result of advanced disease and include abdominal pain, distention, bloating, nausea, pelvic discomfort, pressure or pain, weight loss, urinary frequency, leg pain, bleeding between periods or after menopause, and shortness of breath.

PHYSICAL EXAMINATION

A pelvic examination for an adnexal mass should be done but is not sensitive for detecting ovarian cancer. The assessment should include all possible conditions in the differential diagnosis.

DIAGNOSTICS

CA_{125} is an antigenic determinant on a serum glycoprotein that is elevated in most women with epithelial ovarian cancer. CA_{125} is also elevated in late-stage endometrial cancers and in about 60% of pancreatic cancers. A value above 35 units/ml is abnormal but nonspecific. Elevations may be the result of cervical, endometrial, or fallopian tube carcinoma or pregnancy; benign ovarian cysts; PID; endometriosis; or uterine leiomyoma.[2,11] Elevated CA_{125} levels may require transabdominal or transvaginal ultrasound evaluation. Invasive diagnostic evaluation, often including laparotomy, may be necessary.

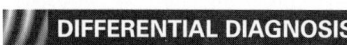

DIAGNOSTICS

Ovarian Cancer

LABORATORY
CA_{125}

IMAGING
Ultrasound (abdominal, vaginal)

OTHER
Laparoscopy
Biopsy

DIFFERENTIAL DIAGNOSIS

Other conditions can manifest as a pelvic mass. These include sigmoid diverticulitis; pregnancy; a distended bladder; a low-lying distended cecum; stool in the sigmoid colon; a pelvic kidney; and a fallopian tube, uterine, or gastrointestinal tumor.[2] Carcinoma of the fallopian tube is so rare (0.3% of gynecologic cancers) that it is considered an appendage of ovarian cancer.[2] It should be suspected with atypical presentations (i.e., women with abnormal vaginal bleeding that does not respond to hormone therapy after a D&C).[16]

DIFFERENTIAL DIAGNOSIS

Ovarian Cancer

- Sigmoid diverticulitis
- Pregnancy
- Distended bladder
- Distended cecum
- Stool in sigmoid colon
- Pelvic kidney
- Fallopian tube, uterine, or gastrointestinal tumor

MANAGEMENT AND INDICATIONS FOR REFERRAL OR HOSPITALIZATION

All patients with suspected ovarian carcinoma are referred for surgery, radiation, and/or chemotherapy. Older female patients with gastrointestinal symptoms need an evaluation for ovarian cancer if a gastrointestinal cause for the symptoms is not isolated.

LIFE SPAN CONSIDERATIONS

Advancing age correlates with increased incidence of the disease and its virulence. The survival rate for women older than 65 years is half that for younger women.[1]

COMPLICATIONS

Complications after genital tract cancer depend on the stage of the cancer and method of treatment and include those associated with radiation, chemotherapy, or surgery. (For further information, see Chapter 257.)

PATIENT AND FAMILY EDUCATION

Patients with a familial history of the rare hereditary form of ovarian cancer should be referred to a gynecology specialist to determine appropriate screening and follow-up. Patients with a family history of sporadic ovarian cancer may benefit from screening and should be referred for consultation. Routine screening of the population is not necessary.

REFERENCES

1. O'Leary M, Sheaffer J, Finkelstein J, and others: Female genital tract cancer. In Bleyer A, O'Leary M, Barr R, and others, editors: *Cancer epidemiology in older adolescents and young adults 15 to 29 years of age, including SEER incidence and survival: 1975-2000 (SEER AYA Monograph)*, NIH Pub No 06-5767, Bethesda, Md, 2006, National Cancer Institute, pp 163-172.
2. Griffiths CT, Silverstone A, Tobias J, and others: *Gynecologic oncology*, London, 1997, Mosby-Wolfe.
3. Ohio State University Medical Center: *Gynecological health at a glance*, retrieved March 4, 2006, from http://medicalcenter.osu.edu/patientcare/healthinformation/otherhealthtopics/GynecologicalHealth/StatisticsGynecologicalHe4423/index.cfm.
4. Smith RA, Cokkinides V, Eyre HJ: *American cancer society guidelines for the early detection of cancer*, 2006, retrieved March 5, 2007, from http://caonline.amcancersoc.org/cgi/content/full/56/1/11.
5. Rodriguez A: Female genital tract melanoma: the evidence is only skin deep, *Curr Opin Obstet Gynecol* 17:1-4, 2005.
6. Echt ML, Finan MA, Hoffman MS, and others: Detection of sentinel lymph nodes with lymphazuria in cervical, uterine and vulvar malignancies, *South Med J* 92(2):204-208, 1999.
7. Bynum DT: Vaginal carcinoma: a rare but treatable cancer, *J Soc Gynecol Nurse Oncol* 6:24-36, 1996.
8. Booth K, Beaver K, Kitchner H, and others: Women's experiences of information, psychological distress and worry after treatment for gynecological cancer, *Patient Educ Counsel* 56:225-232, 2005.
9. Immunization Action Coalition: *Ask the experts: human papillomavirus*, retrieved March 3, 2006, from http://www.immunize.org/catg.d/p2021q.htm.
10. Dolinsky C: *Endometrial cancer: the basics*, 2006, retrieved March 5, 2007, from http://www.oncolink.com/types/article.cfm?c=6&s=18&ss=137&id=8227.
11. Driscoll CE, Bope ET, Smith CW, and others: *The family practice desk reference*, ed 3, St Louis, 1996, Mosby.
12. Elliott JL, Hosford SL, Demopoulos RI, and others: Endometrial adenocarcinoma and polycystic ovary syndrome: risk factors, management, and prognosis, *South Med J* 94(5):529-531, 2001.
13. National Ovarian Cancer Coalition: *Understanding ovarian cancer*, retrieved Aug 12, 2002, from http://www.ovarian.org.
14. Karlan B, Markman M, Eifel P: Ovarian cancer, peritoneal carcinoma, and fallopian tube carcinoma. In DeVita V, Hellman S, Rosenberg S, editors: *Principles and practice of oncology*, ed 7, Philadelphia, 2005, Williams & Wilkins.
15. Olopade OI: Genetics in clinical cancer care: the future is now, *N Engl J Med* 335:1455-1456, 1996.
16. Raychaudhuri K, Hirsh PJ: Atypical presentation of primary fallopian tube carcinoma, *J Obstet Gynaecol* 17(4):403-406, 1997.

CHAPTER 174

Infertility

Marie Elena Botte

DEFINITION AND EPIDEMIOLOGY

Infertility is defined as a couple's inability to conceive after 1 year of unprotected intercourse[1-4] or to carry a pregnancy to live birth.[5] Infertility affects 1 couple in 6, and prevalence increases dramatically with both paternal and maternal age.[1,2,6] In this chapter, infertility is contrasted with *sterility*, a term that applies to those members of a population for whom there is no possibility of attaining a natural pregnancy.[7] Although as many as 12% to 28% of couples experience transient or persistent infertility at some point in their lives[6] and 1 in 10 couples seeks medical help for the problem of subfertility,[8] 10% to 50% of involuntarily childless people never seek professional help.[9] The recent increase in the numbers of individuals who see health care professionals for help with infertility is most likely attributable to a combination of factors, including an increasing number of women delaying the birth of their first child[10] and widespread media attention regarding new reproductive technologies. An estimated 15% of all couples experience infertility, and half these couples remain unable to have a biologic child of their own.[4]

PATHOPHYSIOLOGY

Physiologic dysfunction in men accounts for approximately 20% to 50% of all cases of infertility[3,9,11]; ovulatory dysfunction in women contributes to 25% of infertility cases; and tubal factors (20%), endometriosis (5%), and unexplained causes (between 10% and 25%) are other factors. Multiple factors contribute to infertility in 40% of couples,[3] and combined male and female factors occur in about 30%.[9] In 10% to 25% of cases, no specific factor can be identified.[4,9,12] The odds of delivering a healthy infant drop 3.5% per year after age 30 years. For women younger than 25, the rate of impaired fertility is 11.7%; this rate rises to 42.1% for women older than 35 years.

Male-factor infertility can generally be attributable to chromosomal or structural defects or to endocrine abnormalities of the hypothalamic-pituitary-testicular axis.[13,14] Contributing hypothalamic-pituitary disorders include congenital gonadotropin-releasing hormone (GnRH) deficiency (Kalmann's syndrome); hemochromatosis; pituitary and hypothalamic tumors; infiltrative disorders (tuberculosis, sarcoidosis); hormonal disturbance (androgen, cortisol, and estrogen excess; hyperprolactinemia); or systemic disorders such as chronic illness, obesity, and nutritional deficiencies.[15] Structural causes include cryptorchism, aplasia or obstruction in the male genital tract, varicoceles (generally only a problem when accompanied by other factors such as abnormal semen analysis), congenital bilateral absence of the vas deferens (which can indicate partial expression of a gene mutation for cystic fibrosis), impotence, or ejaculatory dysfunction. Factors influencing spermatogenesis or motility include inflammation or infection (postpubertal mumps, gonorrhea, chlamydial infection); direct injury or trauma (including postoperative); radiation; chemotherapy; heat; medications; toxic exposures; and abuse of substances, including alcohol,[16] cocaine, steroids, and marijuana. Male-factor infertility can involve a low sperm concentration (oligospermia), poor sperm motility (asthenospermia), abnormal sperm morphology (teratospermia), or, more commonly, a constellation of all three variables (oligoasthenoteratozoospermia).[17]

Environmental exposures,[11,18] possibly in an occupational setting, to solvents,[19,20] pesticides,[20,21] heavy metals,[22] pharmaceuticals, anesthetic gases, ionizing radiation, heat, and lead[23-25] are established reproductive hazards for both men and women. Occupational exposures in male workers can affect the male reproductive system, leading to sperm abnormalities, hyperestrogenism, impotence, infertility, or increased spontaneous abortions in their partners.[26-28] Use of anabolic steroids can also contribute to male-factor infertility.[29] Cigarette smoking is associated with infertility in both women and men.[26,30,31] In women, shift work, obesity,[32] and occupational exposure to chemotherapeutic drugs have also been associated with an increased subsequent risk of infertility.[33] Health care providers can consult websites of the National Institute for Occupational Safety and Health (http://www.cdc.gov/niosh/homepage.html) and the Occupational Safety and Health Administration (http://www.osha.gov) for further information on reproductive hazards and their management.

Tubal infertility has been associated with lower family income.[34] Ovulatory dysfunctions range from congenital absence of the ovaries and premature ovarian failure to various disruptions in the hypothalamic-pituitary-ovarian axis and other metabolic or endocrine conditions such as hypothyroidism and hyperthyroidism.[35] Uterine and fallopian pathologic conditions include current or past pelvic inflammatory disease resulting in salpingitis, endometriosis, iatrogenic Asherman's syndrome after overly vigorous curettage, fibroids, bicornuate uterus, and postinfectious or operative tubal scarring and adhesions. Preembryonic developmental problems and implantation problems have been postulated as possible causes for idiopathic infertility.[36]

Pathophysiology involved in infertility includes theories relating to energy deficits inhibiting GnRH/luteinizing hormone (LH) secretion,[37] interference with circadian rhythms, and the temporal pattern of endocrine functions in shift work.[38] In addition, endogenous opioid-mediated inhibition of the hypothalamic GnRH pulse generator has been implicated in hypothalamic ovarian failure.[39] The link between infertility and various autoimmune disorders may be related to the fact that the segment of the major histocompatibility complex that contains genes that affect reproduction also contains genes associated with various autoimmune disorders.[40] Diabetes mellitus has been linked at least in part to a functional deficit of hypothalamic noradrenergic neurons,[41] and cystic fibrosis has been connected to congenital bilateral absence of the vas deferens.[42]

CLINICAL PRESENTATION

Ideally, both members of the couple are present for the initial interview; this is invaluable not only for the comprehensiveness of the medical history but also for providing insight into the couple's communication and decision-making style, emotional status, ability to support each other, coping strategies, and current level of functioning.[43] Subsequent interviews with either partner alone may reveal information (e.g., previous pregnancies, abortions, or infections) that the individual is not comfortable disclosing otherwise. Essential components of relevant history to elicit include duration of the couple's infertility, previous pregnancy or siring of children, and age, since these factors have been consistently demonstrated to affect the prognosis.

Other relevant historical information includes a thorough obstetric and gynecologic history (contraceptive use, prior pregnancy, therapeutic abortion, miscarriage, infection, pathologic conditions, or procedures). Particular attention is given to the menstrual history for cues related to ovulatory cycles, including midcycle discomfort, regular menses, premenstrual symptomatology, and periods that occur every 27 to 30 days.[2] The past medical history focuses on infections, surgeries, medications, and systemic and autoimmune disorders. Family history is assessed for relatives with infertility or early menopause, autoimmune disorders such as lupus, and maternal diethylstilbestrol (DES) exposure. A review of systems may reveal weight changes; signs of estrogen deficiency or excess; signs of thyroid imbalance; hyperandrogenism or virilism; hyposmia (which may be related to Kallmann's syndrome); or signs of galactorrhea, headaches, or visual disturbances (which are possibly suggestive of pituitary pathologic condition).

Social history should include patterns of smoking, alcohol or other substance use such as caffeine; exercise patterns; level of stress and coping strategies; potential eating disorders; and frequency of intercourse. Occupational history may reveal a host of potential reproductive threats, including the prolonged waiting time to pregnancy observed in female shift workers.[38] Laboratory workers, health care workers (including anesthetists, dental assistants, and hospital personnel), farmers, painters, and construction workers may be exposed to reproductive toxins such as lead, nitrous oxide, and solvents; domestic exposures include recent home renovation, contaminated air or ground water, and domestic pesticide use.[24] Various population-based studies have failed to find a correlation between consanguinity (uncle-niece, first cousins, and first-degree cousins once removed) and primary sterility.[44] Infertility has also been shown not to be related to prior cervical laser surgery.[45]

PHYSICAL EXAMINATION

Examination of the male partner includes inspection of the genitals for abnormalities, including phimosis, varicocele (the most commonly identified genital abnormality in subfertile men), and hypospadias. The bilateral presence of the vas deferens is established, and the testes are palpated for maldescent, consistency, and size. Decreased testicular size is related to impaired spermatogenesis; the length of the testes (measured in a warm room, after the patient has been standing for several minutes) should be more than 4 cm (1.6 inches) and the volume more than 20 ml by orchidometry.[46]

Physical examination of the female partner includes palpation of the thyroid; a breast examination to check for galactorrhea; and evaluation of signs of hypoestrogenic status (dry, pale vaginal mucosa), androgen excess (hirsutism, male pattern hair loss, acne, obesity), or virilization (changes in body fat distribution, a lowering of the voice, or clitoromegaly). A pelvic examination also provides a gross indication of the state of the reproductive organs and may detect enlarged ovaries or other masses such as uterine fibroids. Changes in visual acuity or visual fields may be indicative of a cranial (pituitary) mass.

DIAGNOSTICS

Considerable debate surrounds the selection and interpretation of diagnostic studies in the context of a basic fertility workup[7,47] because of the difficulty in establishing cutoff points for "abnormal" in investigations such as semen analysis and the demonstrated inability of many analyses to differentiate between fertile and infertile individuals.[48,49] Complicating the issue is the likelihood that many couples represent a constellation of factors, such as varicoceles and low-normal sperm count; although each may be relatively insignificant in isolation, they combine synergistically to produce clinical infertility.

According to World Health Organization guidelines, semen analysis should be performed early on in the evaluation, after 36 to 48 hours of abstinence.[7] National guidelines from England[50] and the U.S. Institute for Clinical Systems Improvement[51] suggest a repeat semen analysis after 4 months if the first test was normal and there has been no intervening pregnancy. If semen analysis indicates oligospermia, a follicle-stimulating hormone (FSH) and testosterone level should be obtained before referral to a male infertility specialist; if the serum testosterone level is low or the patient has other symptoms of hypogonadism (decreased libido and/or potency), a prolactin level should also be obtained. Testicular volume assessment with an orchidometer combined with basal serum FSH level can also be used to estimate future fertility in individuals who are long-term survivors of malignancy in childhood or adolescence.[52] The postcoital test (PCT) has received mixed reviews in the literature and is generally not recommended.[50,51] It can be useful to confirm that intercourse has taken place, but it has poor sensitivity, specificity, positive predictive value, and negative predictive value.[2]

Although the only definitive proof of ovulation in a particular cycle remains a subsequent pregnancy, ovulatory assessment has traditionally been done with basal body temperature charting.[53] A biphasic curve demonstrating a consistently raised temperature in the later half of the cycle is one of the simplest, most inexpensive, and most practical ways to assess ovulatory function,[54] but the resultant curves can be difficult to interpret. Plasma midluteal progesterone concentration[7] (a level >3 ng/ml is confirmatory but cannot assess the quality of the luteal phase) and home kits for measuring the LH surge in urine can be useful to help confirm ovulation.[3] All female patients merit a rubella titer (if indicated), cervical cytology (Papanicolaou's test), and *Chlamydia* culture or serum antibody (found in 73% of patients with distal tubal occlusion and in no patients with normal fallopian tubes in one study of women undergoing an infertility evaluation).[3,7] Evaluation of tubal patency is most commonly done by hysterosalpingography and can even be therapeutic in that women have been known to conceive soon after this procedure.[3,55] For women more than 35 years of age, a day-3 FSH level and an estradiol level are indicated to assess ovarian reserve (elevated day-3 FSH levels indicate a poorer outcome with assisted reproductive technologies).

Additional laboratory assessment is indicated by the patient's history and physical examination and is *not* warranted for all women concerned about their fertility, especially those with regular menstrual cycles. These tests include prolactin and thyroid assays,[50] testosterone, and dehydroepiandrosterone (DHEA) and 17-hydroxyprogesterone tests where indicated, and clomiphene challenge or day-3 FSH to evaluate ovarian reserve.[56] Anticardiolipin antibody, antiphospholipid antibody, and antinuclear antibody assessments can be performed to exclude lupus.

DIAGNOSTICS

Infertility

MEN
Laboratory
Semen analysis
Follicle-stimulating hormone
Testosterone level*
Prolactin level*
Hepatitis screen
HIV

Other
Testicular volume assessment

WOMEN
Laboratory
Rubella titer*
Pap smear
Chlamydia culture or serum antibody
Gonococcal culture
Follicle-stimulating hormone
Luteinizing hormone
TSH
Rapid plasma reagin*
CBC and differential
Purified protein derivative
Antiphospholipid antibody*
Antinuclear antibody*
Clomiphene stimulation test
DHEA
ESR*
Hepatitis screen
HIV

Other
Hysterosalpingography

*If indicated.

DIFFERENTIAL DIAGNOSIS

A wide range of conditions can contribute to infertility and early pregnancy loss, including genetic, structural, and endocrine disorders; acquired infections[57] (*Trichomonas, Chlamydia* organisms); treatment of other conditions with radiation or chemotherapy; body mass index; personal behaviors like alcohol consumption and maternal cigarette smoking; medications; sexual dysfunction; antisperm antibodies; previous genital or pelvic surgery; exposure to reproductive toxins; and other chronic medical diseases, such as thyroid dysfunction,[35,58] celiac disease, inflammatory bowel disease, and hemochromatosis.[59] Congenital causes include gonadal dysgenesis; chromosomal mosaicism; congenital bilateral absence of the vas deferens or the uterus; Klinefelter's syndrome (small hard testes, gynecomastia); Turner's syndrome (short stature, pigeon chest, webbed neck); deletions in the Y chromosome genes; and isolated corticotropin deficiency,[60] which is rare but treatable. Male factors contributing to infertility are generally determined by semen analysis.

DIFFERENTIAL DIAGNOSIS

Infertility

- Genetic disorder
- Structural disorder
- Endocrine disorder
- Co-morbid illness
- Infection
- Body mass index
- Medications (including chemotherapy)
- Alcohol
- Smoking
- Antisperm antibody
- Sexual dysfunction
- Chemical exposure
- Radiation

Ovulatory dysfunction can be attributable to hyperprolactinemia; hypogonadotropic hypogonadism (these women have decreased serum estradiol levels and no withdrawal bleeding after a progesterone challenge); hypergonadotropic hypogonadism (elevated FSH levels indicating premature ovarian failure and possible presence of Y chromosome in young women); and normogonadotropic anovulatory conditions, including polycystic ovary syndrome (a hyperandrogenic condition often seen with acne, weight gain, hirsutism, or acanthosis nigricans when hyperinsulinemia is also contributing), luteal phase defects, and multifollicular ovaries.

MANAGEMENT

Although the provision of infertility services is beyond the scope of practice of most health care providers, they nevertheless perform an important initial exploration of historical, physical examination, and selected diagnostic factors that can facilitate expedient and timely referral to appropriate specialists when indicated. Health care providers can also intervene early in terms of improving modifiable lifestyle risk factors, improving coping mechanisms, providing basic preconceptual education and care, and improving overall health for all patients who are attempting conception. General health-promoting interventions for the couple include normalizing weight; improving nutritional status; providing folate supplementation; reducing stress[61]; and eliminating potential detrimental factors such as cigarette smoking,[62,63] caffeine and alcohol intake, illicit drug use, and exposure to potential reproductive toxins.[18] These interventions, which may increase a couple's chances of attaining pregnancy, might also improve their psychologic health.[64]

Of all couples diagnosed as infertile, 15% to 60% will experience pregnancy without treatment of any kind within 1 year, and 25% to 80% will be successful within 2 years.[3,7] Prognosis in these instances is more encouraging if the duration of infertility has been less than 3 years, if the woman is younger than 32 years, and if the couple has previously conceived a child.[65] Prognosis is worse for situations involving endometriosis, male-factor infertility, and tubal pathologic conditions or multiple factors.[7,65] Individuals warranting an expedited workup and referral to a specialist include women without periods, with irregular periods, or with bleeding between periods, as well as those who have pain with intercourse and a history of abdominal surgery, ruptured appendix, or upper genital tract infection.[2] Men for whom similar expedited workup and referral is appropriate include those with difficulty sustaining an erection; an inability to ejaculate during intercourse; and a history of testicular injury, infection, or maldescension.[2]

It is essential from the outset to reinforce with any couple seeking treatment that appropriately directed therapy, excluding advanced reproductive technologies, is unsuccessful up to 50% of the time.[3,7] More elaborate assisted reproductive technologies (ARTs) such as in vitro fertilization (IVF) and the newer intracytoplasmic sperm injection along with donor gametes and surrogacy may provide hope for pregnancy otherwise unattainable through more conventional means. However, these approaches can be expensive and risky, and they often raise moral and ethical dilemmas regarding their use.[66]

Any treatment plan should follow a full discussion regarding all possible treatment options, including adoption, child-free living without intervention of any kind, and the possibility of stopping at any time in the treatment process. Discussion must address attendant benefits, risks, time required for participation, and costs, along with reasonable estimations of probability for achieving pregnancy based on relevant infertility factors both with and without treatment.[67] Ongoing counseling for the couple should be offered and encouraged. Counseling may help the couple discontinue treatment when appropriate, solicit second opinions, participate in support groups, establish a (necessarily arbitrary) time limit for treatment, and take time off from treatment to give them a sense of control and balance in their lives. Patients are referred to a specialist for evaluation and management of ARTs.

Pharmacologic Therapy

When infertility is due to hypothalamic-pituitary insufficiency in the male partner (as is the case in 1% to 2% of couples with male-factor infertility), these men often respond well to gonadotropin or GnRH therapy.[15] Induction of ovulation according to a variety of protocols involving gonadotropins has been used for hypogonadotropic hypogonadism in women.[68-70] Chronic opiate agonist administration (naltrexone) can normalize ovarian function for women with hypothalamic ovarian failure.[39,71] Another approach, which requires referral to a specialist, entails pulsatile administration of GnRH, specifically at frequencies of 90 or 120 minutes, which more reliably induce follicular development, ovulation, and normal luteal function.[71,72] Bromocriptine or other, newer dopamine agonists such as cabergoline are indicated in the treatment of hyperprolactinemia.

Antiestrogens such as clomiphene citrate or tamoxifen are used for the induction of ovulation in women with polycystic ovary syndrome.[7,73] Estrogen replacement for women with hypergonadotropic hypogonadism is important to prevent osteoporosis; ovulation-inducing therapies are neither useful nor indicated for these women. For women with chemotherapy-induced ovarian failure, ovarian function should be reassessed periodically, since spontaneous recovery has been noted.[74] Clomiphene, human menopausal gonadotropin, and various ART procedures are often used empirically for unexplained infertility.

ARTs include such technologies as gamete intrafallopian transfer (GIFT), IVF, direct intraperitoneal injection of sperm, intrafollicular injection of sperm, and preimplantation genetic diagnosis.[75] The induction of superovulation is often followed by artificial insemination of some kind; success is highly influenced by the woman's age, with cycle fecundity dropping from an average of 0.23% to 0.05% after age 40 years.[76]

Women or men being managed by specialists for infertility still require basic primary care services. This enables the health care provider to assess and intervene on behalf of the couple's functional, emotional, and psychospiritual responses to continuing therapy. Somatization is a common manifestation of the psychologic stress of infertility,[9] as are sexual problems; depressive reactions; emotional instability; relationship difficulties; reduced self-confidence and self-esteem; and feelings of anger, guilt, grief, isolation, and anxiety.

LIFE SPAN CONSIDERATIONS

A cultural tendency to delay childbearing[10] combined with the fact of decreased fecundability with increasing age necessitates prompt investigation into infertility in certain cases.[77] According to the American Society of Reproductive Medicine, an infertility evaluation is warranted after 1 year of coital exposure for couples in which the woman is younger than 35 years and after 6 months when she is older than 35 years.[78]

COMPLICATIONS

Women with polycystic ovary syndrome do not generally respond as well to ovulation induction as do women with other ovulatory disorders and have an increased risk of ovarian hyperstimulation and spontaneous abortion when they do respond.[7,79] Women with fibroids have a lower implantation rate with ART,[80] women with endometriosis have a decreased pregnancy rate after ART procedures than do controls,[81] and women age 40 or older have a higher risk for cesarean delivery after infertility treatment that is independent of other risk factors.[82] Other infertility treatment–related complications include a controversial association between fertility drugs and ovarian cancer[7,83] and the protracted psychic anguish that can accompany successive failed treatment cycles.

The incidence and risks of multiple gestation associated with ARTs have been well documented in the literature,[84-87] and even resultant singleton pregnancies represent obstetric risks, given an increased incidence of pregnancy-induced hypertension, placenta previa, elective cesarean, and preterm labor; an increased risk for major malformation[88]; and a lower mean birth weight than controls.[89,90] Twins that are the result of IVF also have an increased rate of preterm birth compared with spontaneously conceived twin controls.[91] (For all initial numbers of fetuses in an ART-induced multifetal pregnancy, including twins, reduction to a lower number decreases subsequent fetal loss, prematurity, and infant morbidity and mortality.[92]) Although the medical problems associated with ART-assisted multiple gestations have been widely emphasized in the medical literature, several studies note a desire among fertility patients for multiple births[93]; one study found that 67% to 90% of infertile couples expressed a desire for twins, and the majority of these couples rejected concerns about multiple gestations.[94] In another study a significant proportion (41%) of fertility patients considered multiple birth an ideal treatment outcome.[95] This clearly indicates a need for additional education about the risks and complications associated with ARTs.

INDICATIONS FOR REFERRAL OR HOSPITALIZATION

Referral to a reproductive urologist is indicated for male factors identified on semen analysis.[3] Referral to a reproductive endocrinologist or fertility specialist is indicated for an abnormal PCT, for a basic infertility workup that does not disclose the source of the problem, or for any of the various ART procedures should they be a couple's only hope for conception. Couples interested in exploring complementary therapeutic options may find some success with acupuncture.[96] Pathologic conditions, including adhesiolysis and various testicular, uterine, or tubal conditions, may require surgical repair. In addition, complications from therapy (moderate to severe ovarian hyperstimulation syndrome) may require hospitalization.

PATIENT AND FAMILY EDUCATION

Infertility and its often unsuccessful medical treatment present a conglomerate of stresses and losses with which the couple must contend,[43] including the loss of biologic children and the experiences of pregnancy and breastfeeding. Individuals endure the stresses of complicated, expensive, and invasive treatment interventions, which can be experienced as humiliating, embarrassing, frustrating, and disappointing for women and their partners.[97] Adjusting to infertile status is easier for individuals with positive self-esteem, an internal locus of control, and higher socioeconomic status, whereas increased anxiety and distress have been associated with advancing age, undifferentiated sex-role identity, and low self-esteem.[98] Several studies have supported the contention that perceptions about motherhood, identity development, personal happiness, and well-being are involved in many women's desires for having children[99]; this desire for children often remains strong after many years of infertility.

Motives for medical consultation by infertile couples, in addition to the desire to have a child, include a desire for education and understanding regarding the cause of the infertility.[100] Health care providers should be aware of research indicating a disparity between the medical diagnosis and the perception of the diagnosis in 38% of infertile persons,[101] along with a tendency for patients to blame themselves for the infertility. Basic education for infertile persons includes advising them to have intercourse about twice a week[3] and to avoid lubricants that may be spermicidal such as K-Y Jelly, petroleum jelly, and Surgilube. In contrast, raw egg white and vegetable oil do not seem to affect sperm motility.[46] The provider should also encourage cessation of alcohol or illicit drug use, smoking cessation,[102,103] proper nutrition, normalization of body mass index (especially for women), and strategies for stress reduction. Health care providers can also provide an initial infertility workup that focuses on explaining the various diagnostic procedures and addressing couples' concerns and questions as they arise. The American Society of Reproductive Medicine website (http://www.asrm.org) is a good source of patient information.

It is particularly important to provide couples with an accurate estimation of the success rates that are expected by various procedures and the concordant risks, discomforts, and expenses.[104] Unfortunately, there have been fewer randomized clinical trials in the area of infertility management than in other branches of medical science, and many studies have small sample sizes, inappropriate design, and pseudorandomization.[105] For couples who are able to conceive with treatment, providers of primary care can stress the normalcy of the pregnancy and help the couple through the normative developmental processes of pregnancy and parenthood.

Many providers emphasize helping couples to determine their own end point and timeline for intervention attempts,[67] since there always seems to be some promising or potential development around the corner.[53] Some research has indicated increased social support and greater contentment over time for infertile couples,[5] but continuing interventions can also have a detrimental effect on the well-being of individuals and the couple,[106,107] with one study finding a greater psychologic than physiologic burden sustained when undergoing infertility treatment with IVF.[108]

Because the length of time that a woman has been infertile is related to her future fecundability[109] and because fertility decreases exponentially with increasing age,[69] many infertile individuals confront the necessity of redefining their expectations and goals related to establishing a family. Providers play an important role in facilitating the grieving process for the many losses sustained throughout the experience of diagnosis and treatment.[110] This process is important because it constitutes the experiential prerequisite to acceptance and is essential for the couple to move on with their lives. Clinician support can enforce an "unsuccessful" couple's eventual realization that they have been thorough and have tried sufficient therapeutic intervention and that cessation of such interventions is reasonable and advisable. Couples can then be supported in their efforts to plan their lives in ways that may include consideration of adoption or child-free living as valid alternatives to biologic parenthood.

REFERENCES

1. Frey KA, Patel KS: Initial evaluation and management of infertility by the primary care physician, *Mayo Clin Proc* 79(11):1439-1443, 2004.
2. Penzias A: Infertility: contemporary office-based evaluation and treatment, *Obstet Gynecol Clin* 27(3):473-486, 2000.
3. Morell V: Basic infertility assessment, *Primary Care Clin Office Pract* 24(1):195-204, 1997.
4. Templeton A: Infertility: epidemiology, aetiology and effective management, *Health Bull* 53(5):294-298, 1995.
5. Hirsch AM, Hirsch SM: The long-term psychosocial effects of infertility, *J Obstet Gynecol Neonat Nurs* 24(6):517-522, 1995.
6. De La Rochebrochard E, Thonneau P: Paternal age > or = 40 years: an important risk factor for infertility, *Am J Obstet Gynecol* 189(4):901-905, 2003.
7. Infertility revisited: the state of the art today and tomorrow: the ESHRE Capri workshop, European Society for Human Reproduction and Embryology, *Hum Reprod* 11(8):1779-1807, 1996.
8. De Kreser D, Baker H: Infertility in men: recent advances and continuing controversies, *J Clin Endocrinol Metab* 84(10):3443-3450, 1999.
9. Himmel W, Ittner E, Kochen MM, and others: Management of involuntary childlessness, *Br J Gen Pract* 47(415):111-118, 1997.
10. Baird DT, and others: Fertility and ageing, *Hum Reprod Update* 11(3):261-276, 2005.
11. Pasqualotto FF, and others: Effects of medical therapy, alcohol, smoking, and endocrine disruptors on male infertility, *Revista do Hospital das Clinicas; Faculdade de Medicina Da Universidade de Sao Paulo* 59(6):375-382, 2004.
12. Organization WH: Towards more objectivity in diagnosis and management of male fertility, *Int J Androl* 7(Suppl):1-53, 1997.
13. Griffin DK, Finch KA: The genetic and cytogenetic basis of male infertility, *Hum Fertil* 8(1):19-26, 2005.
14. Dohle GR, and others: Genetic risk factors in infertile men with severe oligozoospermia and azoospermia, *Hum Reprod* 17(1):13-16, 2002.
15. Khorram O, and others: Reproductive technologies for male infertility, *J Clin Endocrinol Metab* 86(6):2373-2379, 2001.
16. Tsujimura A, and others: Effect of lifestyle factors on infertility in men, *Arch Androl* 50(1):15-17, 2004.
17. Isidori A, Latini M, Romanelli F: Treatment of male infertility, *Contraception* 72(4):314-318, 2005.
18. Sheweita SA, Tilmisany AM, Al-Sawaf H: Mechanisms of male infertility: role of antioxidants, *Curr Drug Metab* 6(5):495-501, 2005.
19. Cherry N, and others: Occupational exposure to solvents and male infertility, *Occup Environ Med* 58(10):635-640, 2001.
20. Oliva A, Spira A, Multigner L: Contribution of environmental factors to the risk of male infertility, *Hum Reprod* 16(8):1768-1776, 2001.
21. Petrelli G, Figa-Talamanca I: Reduction in fertility in male greenhouse workers exposed to pesticides, *Eur J Epidemiol* 17(7):675-677, 2001.
22. Podzimek S, and others: Sensitization to inorganic mercury could be a risk factor for infertility, *Neuro Endocrinol Lett* 26(4):277-282, 2005.
23. Frazier L: Workplace reproductive problems, *Primary Care Clin Office Pract* 27(4), 2000.
24. Solomon GM: Reproductive toxins: a growing concern at work in the community, *J Occup Environ Med* 39(2):105-107, 1996.
25. Sallmen M: Exposure to lead and male fertility, *Int J Occup Med Environ Health* 14(3):219-222, 2001.
26. Chia SE, Tay SK: Occupational risk for male infertility: a case-control study of 218 infertile and 227 fertile men, *J Occup Environ Med* 43(11):946-951, 2001.
27. Baranski B: Effects of the workplace on fertility and other related reproductive outcomes, *Environ Health Perspect* 101(Suppl 2):81-90, 1993.
28. Petrelli G, Mantovani A: Environmental risk factors and male fertility and reproduction, *Contraception* 65(4):297-300, 2002.
29. Lombardo F, and others: Androgens and fertility, *J Endocrinol Invest* 28(3 Suppl):51-55, 2005.
30. Mallampalli A, Guntupalli KK: Smoking and systemic disease, *Med Clin North Am* 88(6):1431-1451, x, 2004.
31. Jensen MS, and others: Lower sperm counts following prenatal tobacco exposure, *Hum Reprod* 20(9):2559-2566, 2005.
32. Pender JR, Pories WJ: Epidemiology of obesity in the United States, *Gastroenterol Clin North Am* 34(1):1-7, 2005.
33. Valanis B, and others: Occupational exposure to antineoplastic agents and self-reported infertility among nurses and pharmacists, *J Occup Environ Med* 39(6):574-580, 1997.
34. Collins JA, Burrows EA, Willan AR: Occupation and the clinical characteristics of infertile couples, *Can J Pub Health* 85(1):28-32, 1994.
35. Poppe K, and others: Thyroid dysfunction and autoimmunity in infertile women, *Thyroid* 12(11):997-1001, 2002.
36. Martin JS, and others: The pregnancy rates of cohorts of idiopathic infertility couples gives insights into the underlying mechanism of infertility, *Fertility Sterility* 64(1):98-102, 1995.
37. Wade GN, Jones JE: Neuroendocrinology of nutritional infertility, *Am J Physiol* 287(6):R1277-R1296, 2004.
38. Bisanti L, and others: Shift work and subfertility: a European multicenter study: European Study Group on Infertility and Subfertility, *J Occup Environ Med* 38(4):352-358, 1996.
39. Wildt L, and others: Treatment with naltrexone in hypothalamic ovarian failure: induction of ovulation and pregnancy, *Hum Reprod* 8(3):350-358, 1993.

40. Jin K, and others: Reproductive failure and the major histocompatibility complex, *Am J Hum Genet* 56(6):1456-1467, 1995.
41. Bitar MS: The role of catecholamines in the etiology of infertility in diabetes mellitus, *Life Sci* 61(1):65-73, 1997.
42. Lissens W, and others: Cystic fibrosis and infertility caused by congenital absence of the vas deferens and related clinical entities, *Hum Reprod* 11(Suppl 4):55-78, 1996.
43. Boxer AS: Images of infertility, *Nurse Pract Forum* 7(2):60-63, 1996.
44. Edmond M, De Braekeleer M: Inbreeding effects on fertility and sterility: a case-control study in Saguenay-Lac-Saint-Jean (Quebec, Canada) based on a population registry 1838-1971, *Ann Hum Biol* 20(6):545-555, 1993.
45. Spitzer M, and others: The fertility of women after cervical laser surgery, *Obstet Gynecol* 86(4 Pt 1):504-508, 1995.
46. Spitz A, Kim E, Lipshultz L: Contemporary approach to the male infertility evaluation, *Obstet Gynecol Clin North Am* 27(3):487-516, 2000.
47. Puttermans P, Ombelet W, Brosens I: Reflections on the way to conduct an investigation of subfertility, *Hum Reprod* 10(Suppl 1):80-89, 1995.
48. Guzick DS, and others: Infertility evaluation in fertile women: a model for assessing the efficacy of infertility testing, *Hum Reprod* 9(12):2306-2310, 1994.
49. Guzick DS: Do infertility tests discriminate between fertile and infertile populations? *Hum Reprod* 10(8):2008-2009, 1995.
50. Royal College of Obstetricians and Gynaecologists: *The initial investigation and management of the infertile couple,* London, 1998, The College.
51. Institute for Clinical Systems Improvement: *Diagnosis and management of infertility*, Bloomington, Minn, 2000 (updated April 2001), The Institute.
52. Muller HL, and others: Gonadal function of young adults after therapy of malignancies during childhood or adolescence, *Eur J Pediatr* 155(9):763-769, 1996.
53. Mastroianni LJ: Forty years of infertility management: exponential progress and a demanding future, *Nurse Pract Forum* 7(2):87-91, 1996.
54. Ayres-de-Compos D, and others: Inter-observer agreement in analysis of basal body temperature graphs from infertile women, *Hum Reprod* 10(8):2010-2016, 1995.
55. Baramki TA: Hysterosalpingography [see comment], *Fertility Sterility* 83(6):1595-1606, 2005.
56. Macklon NS, Fauser BC: Ovarian reserve, *Semin Reprod Med* 23(3):248-256, 2005.
57. Soper D: Trichomoniasis: under control or undercontrolled? *Am J Obstet Gynecol* 190(1):281-290, 2004.
58. Poppe K, Velkeniers B: Female infertility and the thyroid, *Best Pract Res Clin Endocrinol Metab* 18(2):153-165, 2004.
59. Bradley RJ, Rosen MP: Subfertility and gastrointestinal disease: "unexplained" is often undiagnosed, *Obstet Gynecol Surv* 59(2):108-117, 2004.
60. Atkin SL, Masson EA, White MC: Isolated adrenocorticotropin deficiency presenting as primary infertility, *J Endocrinol Invest* 18(6):456-459, 1995.
61. Schneid-Kofman N, Sheiner E: Does stress effect male infertility? A debate, *Med Sci Monitor* 11(8):SR11-SR13, 2005.
62. Mallampalli A, Guntupalli KK: Smoking and systemic disease, *Med Clin North Am* 88(6):1431-1451, 2004.
63. Practice Committee of the American Society for Reproductive Medicine: Smoking and infertility, *Fertility Sterility* 81(4):1181-1186, 2004.
64. Galletly C, and others: A group program for obese, infertile women: weight loss and improved psychological health, *J Psychosom Obstet Gynecol* 17(2):125-128, 1996.
65. Moran, and others: Prognosis for fertility analyzing different variables in men and women, *Arch Androl* 36(3):197-204, 1996.
66. Baird PA: Ethical issues of fertility and reproduction, *Ann Rev Med* 47:107-116, 1996.
67. Paulson RJ, Sauer MV: Counseling the infertile couple: when enough is enough, *Obstet Gynecol* 78(3 Pt 1):462-464, 1991.
68. Balen AH, and others: Cumulative conception and live birth rates after the treatment of anovulatory infertility: safety and efficacy of ovulation induction in 200 patients, *Hum Reprod* 9(8):1563-1570, 1994.
69. Fox R, Ekeroma A, Wardle P: Ovarian response to purified FSH in infertile women with long-standing hypogonadotropic hypogonadism, *Aust NZ J Obstet Gynecol* 37(1):92-94, 1997.
70. Messinis IE: Ovulation induction: a mini review, *Hum Reprod* 20(10):2688-2697, 2005.
71. Leyendecker G, Waibel-Treber S, Wildt L: Pulsatile administration of gonadotropin-releasing hormone and oral administration of naltrexone in hypothalamic amenorrhea, *Hum Reprod* 8(Suppl 2):184-188, 1993.
72. Letterie GS, and others: Ovulation induction using s.c. pulsatile gonadotropin-releasing hormone: effectiveness of different pulse frequencies, *Hum Reprod* 11(1):19-22, 1996.
73. Homburg R: Clomiphene citrate—end of an era? A mini-review, *Hum Reprod* 20(8):2043-2051, 2005.
74. Nasir J, and others: Spontaneous recovery of chemotherapy-induced primary ovarian failure, *Clin Endocrinol* 46(2):217-219, 1997.
75. Kearns WG, and others: Preimplantation genetic diagnosis and screening, *Semin Reprod Med* 23(4):336-347, 2005.
76. Lobo RA: Unexplained infertility, *J Reprod Med* 38(4):241-249, 1993.
77. Gnoth C, and others: Definition and prevalence of subfertility and infertility, *Hum Reprod* 20(5):1144-1147, 2005.
78. Stansberry J: The infertile couple: an overview of pathophysiology and diagnostic evaluation for the primary care provider, *Nurse Pract Forum* 7(2):76-86, 1996.
79. Wang JX, Davies MJ, Norman RJ: Polycystic ovarian syndrome and the risk of spontaneous abortion following assisted reproductive technology treatment, *Hum Reprod* 16(12):2606-2609, 2001.
80. Benecke C, and others: Effect of fibroids on fertility in patients undergoing assisted reproduction: a structured literature review [see comment], *Gynecol Obstet Invest* 59(4):225-230, 2005.
81. De Hondt A, and others: Endometriosis and subfertility treatment: a review, *Minerva Ginecologica* 57(3):257-267, 2005.
82. Sheiner E, and others: Infertility treatment is an independent risk factor for cesarean section among nulliparous women aged 40 and above, *Am J Obstet Gynecol* 185(4):888-892, 2001.
83. Ness RB, and others: Infertility, fertility drugs, and ovarian cancer: a pooled analysis of case-control studies, *Am J Epidemiol* 155(3):217-224, 2002.
84. Wilson EE: Assisted reproductive technologies and multiple gestations, *Clin Perinatol* 32(2):315-328, 2005.
85. Armour KL, Callister LC: Prevention of triplets and higher order multiples: trends in reproductive medicine, *J Perinat Neonat Nurs* 19(2):103-111, 2005.
86. Fauser BC, Devroey P, Macklon NS: Multiple birth resulting from ovarian stimulation for subfertility treatment [see comment], *Lancet* 365(9473):1807-1816, 2005.
87. Filicori M, and others: Impact of medically assisted fertility on preterm birth, *BJOG Int J Obstet Gynaecol* 112(Suppl 1):113-117, 2005.
88. Ludwig M: Risk during pregnancy and birth after assisted reproductive technologies: an integral view of the problem, *Semin Reprod Med* 23(4):363-367, 2005.
89. Tanbo T, and others: Obstetric outcome in singleton pregnancies after assisted reproduction, *Obstet Gynecol* 86(2):188-192, 1995.
90. Shiota K, Yamada S: Assisted reproductive technologies and birth defects, *Congen Anom* 45(2):39-43, 2005.
91. McDonald S, and others: Perinatal outcomes of in vitro fertilization twins: a systematic review and meta-analyses, *Am J Obstet Gynecol* 193(1):141-152, 2005.
92. Evans MI, and others: Update on selective reduction, *Prenat Diagnosis* 25(9):807-813, 2005.
93. Ryan GL, and others: The desire of infertile patients for multiple births, *Fertility Sterility* 81(3):500-504, 2004.

94. Gleicher N, and others: The desire for multiple births in couples with infertility problems contraindicates present practice patterns, *Hum Reprod* 10(5):1079-1084, 1995.
95. Child TJ, Henderson AM, Tan SL: The desire for multiple pregnancy in male and female infertility patients, *Hum Reprod* 19(3):558-561, 2004.
96. Xiaoming M, and others: Clinical studies in the mechanism for acupuncture stimulation of ovulation, *J Trad Chinese Med* 13(2):115-119, 1993.
97. Cwikel J, Gidron Y, Sheiner E: Psychological interactions with infertility among women, *Eur J Obstet Gynecol Reprod Biol* 117(2):126-131, 2004.
98. Koropatnick S, Daniluk J, Pattinson HA: Infertility: a non-event transition, *Fertility Sterility* 59(1):163-171, 1993.
99. Van Balen F, Trimbos-Kemper TC: Involuntarily childless couples: their desire to have children and their motives, *J Psychosom Obstet Gynaecol* 16(3):137-144, 1995.
100. Van Balen F, Verdurmen J, Ketting E: Choices and motivations of infertile couples, *Patient Educ Counsel* 31(1):19-27, 1997.
101. Van Balen F, Trimbos-Kemper T, Verdurmen J: Perception of diagnosis and openness of patients about infertility, *Patient Educ Counsel* 28(3):247-252, 1996.
102. Hughes EG, Brennan BG: Does cigarette smoking impair natural or assisted fecundity? *Fertility Sterility* 66(5):679-689, 1996.
103. Bolumar F, Olsen J, Boldsen J: Smoking reduces fecundity: a European multicenter study on infertility and subfecundity: the European Study Group on Infertility and Subfecundity, *Am J Epidemiol* 143(6):578-587, 1996.
104. Stovall DW, Guzick DS: Current management of unexplained infertility, *Curr Opin Obstet Gynecol* 5(2):228-233, 1993.
105. Vandekerckhove P, and others: Infertility treatment: from cookery to science: the epidemiology of randomised controlled trials, *Br J Obstet Gynaecol* 100(11):1005-1036, 1993.
106. Van Balen F, Trimbos-Kemper TC: Factors influencing the well-being of long-term infertile couples, *J Psychosom Obstet Gynaecol* 15(3):157-164, 1994.
107. Berg BJ, Wilson JF: Patterns of psychological distress in infertile couples, *J Psychosom Obstet Gynaecol* 16(2):65-78, 1995.
108. Van Balen F, Naaktgeboren N, Trimbos-Kemper TC: In vitro fertilization: the expense of treatment, pregnancy, and delivery, *Hum Reprod* 11(1):95-98, 1996.
109. Jansen RP: Relative infertility: modeling clinical paradoxes, *Fertility Sterility* 59(5):1041-1045, 1993.
110. Alesi R: Infertility and its treatment—an emotional roller coaster, *Aust Fam Phys* 34(3):135-138, 2005.

CHAPTER 175

Menopause

JoNell Efantis Potter and Trudi Simon

DEFINITION AND EPIDEMIOLOGY

Menopause is defined as the permanent cessation of menstruation resulting from the loss of ovarian follicular activity. Natural menopause is recognized to have occurred after 12 consecutive months of amenorrhea for which there is no other pathologic or physiologic cause. Menopause occurs with the final menstrual period, which is known with certainty only in retrospect a year or more after the final menses.

Currently approximately 30 million U.S. women are now menopausal; another 6 million or more will reach this stage of life in the next decade.[1] The number of women older than 65 years is also expected to increase from 18 million in 1990 to more than 25 million in 2020. Most women will live one third of their lives beyond menopause.

Natural Menopause

Natural menopause occurs when a woman has not had a menstrual period for 1 full year and experiences a cessation of ovulation. Most women in Western countries experience this event between the ages of 45 and 55 (median age, 50 to 52). The only two factors that are known to consistently influence age at natural menopause are smoking status and genetics. Women who smoke generally reach menopause 2 years earlier than nonsmokers, suggesting that smoking adversely effects ovarian function. Women may experience menopause at the same time that their mothers and sisters did. There is no known relationship between a woman's age at menarche and her age at menopause.

Induced Menopause

Women who experience an abrupt menopause because of bilateral salpingo-oophorectomy or chemotherapy are considered to have induced menopause. Induced menopause poses special challenges for women because of the abrupt cessation of ovarian function, with significant decreases in estradiol, testosterone, and dehydroepiandrosterone. Women who have experienced induced menopause tend to have increased vasomotor symptoms. This represents a radical change in a woman's life, and it is important to assess both her ability to cope with this change and her future health concerns, including cardiovascular health, bone health, and overall well-being.

Premature Menopause and Premature Ovarian Failure

Natural menopause that occurs before age 40 is considered premature. It can result from genetic or autoimmune factors, but there is often no known explanation. Premature ovarian failure (POF) is defined as the full or intermittent loss of ovarian function in women younger than 40 years.[2] This condition affects approximately 1% of women under 40, and half of these women may still experience some ovarian function. Therefore POF should not be equated with menopause. Various factors such as genetics, autoimmune diseases, and surgery or chemotherapy have been found to trigger the onset of POF.[3]

Perimenopausal Transitional Years

A transitional state known as *perimenopause* occurs when hormone levels are fluctuating and women begin to experience physical changes before the last menstrual cycle. The perimenopause transitions usually begin in a woman's forties. The median age at onset of the perimenopause ranges from 45 to 47 years, but onset may occur as early as 35 years. Therefore there is still a risk of unintended pregnancy during perimenopause. The endocrine changes and signs and symptoms associated with perimenopause may extend over a period of several years and end with complete cessation of menses (menopause). Characteristic perimenopausal changes include a change in the amount or duration of menstrual flow, a change in length of menstrual cycle, and skipping of menstrual cycles. Although most of these changes result from erratic hormonal levels due to anovulatory cycles, women need to be carefully evaluated for potential disease (neoplasia) and pregnancy.

Climacteric

According to the Council of Affiliated Menopause Societies, *climacteric* refers to the phase in a women's aging process marking the transition from the reproductive to the nonreproductive state, thus making climacteric a process rather than a point in time.[4]

PATHOPHYSIOLOGY

The endocrine changes that occur during the perimenopausal transition are complex, involving changes in levels of follicle-stimulating hormone (FSH), luteinizing hormone (LH), estradiol, estrone, and adrenal steroids. The perimenopause transition is characterized by a decrease in the number of functional ovarian follicles and significant fluctuations in hormone levels from one cycle to the next. Both central nervous system (CNS) control mechanisms and decline of follicles within the ovary contribute to the initiation and progression of the perimenopausal transition. Despite the declining number of functional follicles, ovarian estrogen production may reach or exceed midreproductive levels during some of perimenopause. During the late reproductive stage, elevation of FSH (>10 IU/L) in the early follicular stage (days 2 to 5 of the menstrual cycle) is the first measurable sign of reproductive aging. Eventually, the accelerated loss of follicles and resultant decline of inhibin B lead to elevated FSH levels.

The ovaries contain the maximum number of germ cells during fetal development, and follicular loss begins in utero. Women are born with 1 million to 2 million follicles. By menopause they have only a few hundred to a few thousand remaining. Most follicular loss results from atresia (cell death and degeneration), not ovulation (<500 follicles over a lifetime). The rate in the fall in the number of follicles is linear until approximately age 37, after which there is a steeper decline until menopause. The rate of atresia varies from woman to woman. As the number of ovarian follicles declines, levels of inhibin B fall, allowing FSH to rise and, for a time, sustain follicular development and ovulatory function. The higher levels of FSH recruit relatively more follicles per cycle, which might contribute to accelerated follicular atresia after age 37. Overproduction of estradiol by this enlarged cohort of recruited follicles may be responsible for common perimenopausal symptoms: bloating, irritability, mastalgia, menorrhagia, growth of uterine fibroids, vasomotor symptoms, insomnia, migraines, and premenstrual syndrome (PMS) dysphoria. The perimenopausal woman is not totally protected from an unplanned pregnancy until amenorrhea greater than 1 year occurs or consistently elevated levels of FSH (greater than 30 mIU/ml) can be demonstrated.

In the early 1970s estrogen was believed to be primarily a reproductive hormone, with effects limited to the uterus and mammary glands. Current concepts of estrogen action, however, are extraordinarily complex. Evidence now indicates that estrogen exerts effects on tissues such as bone, brain, eyes, teeth, vasomotor system, heart, breast, colon, and urogenital tract. At least two distinct estrogen receptors (ERs) have been identified: alpha and beta. ER-α is found in the reproductive system (uterus, breast) and liver. ER-β is found in bone, blood vessels, lungs, and urogenital tract. Both ER-α and ER-β are found in the ovary and the CNS.

A greater understanding of the ER mechanism allows us to understand how mixed agonist-antagonists drugs can have selective actions on specific target tissues. New agents are being developed in an effort to isolate desired actions from unwanted side effects. The first of a new generation of synthetic target tissue–specific drugs has now become available. These selective estrogen receptor modulators (SERMs) have both estrogen agonist and estrogen antagonist activity. SERMs can give women the benefit of estrogen without some of the risks. SERMs bind to the estrogen receptors and exert site-specific estrogenic or antiestrogenic effects in different target tissues.

CLINICAL PRESENTATION

Clinical concerns for perimenopausal or menopausal women include:

- Irregular bleeding, the most frequently reported perimenopausal symptom.
- Bleeding that is heavier and prolonged, or cycles that are shorter or longer than usual. Intermenstrual spotting and postcoital spotting should be evaluated for pathologic causes.
- Vasomotor hot flashes, the second most frequent perimenopausal symptom.
- Urogenital atrophy.

The loss of estrogen associated with menopause is accompanied by many short-term and long-term physical changes. These changes can be divided into early symptoms, intermediate physical changes, and later in life chronic diseases like cardiovascular disease (CVD) and osteoporosis and fractures.

Early Symptoms

Vasomotor symptoms are characterized by vasomotor instability, hot flashes, day sweats, and night sweats. The vasomotor flush is viewed as the hallmark of the female climacteric, experienced to some degree by most (85%) of postmenopausal women. The physiology of the hot flash is still not completely understood. It is not strictly accurate to say that hot flashes are caused by low or fluctuating estrogen levels, although estrogen administration has been shown to diminish the frequency of hot flashes. The term *hot flash* is descriptive of a sudden onset of reddening of the skin over the head, neck, and chest, accompanied by a feeling of intense body heat and concluded by profuse perspiration. The duration varies from a few seconds to several minutes. Flashes are more frequent and severe at night or during times of stress. For the majority of women, hot flashes dissipate on their own within an average of 4 years. Mild to moderate hot flashes can be managed with lifestyle changes such as wearing light, layered clothing; lowering the thermostat; avoiding spicy foods, caffeine, and alcohol; and engaging in relaxation exercises.[5]

Insomnia involving early morning waking is a troublesome symptom that is responsive to estrogen therapy (ET). Insomnia may occur in association with or independent of hot flashes. Women on hormone therapy (HT) have shorter sleep latency and more frequent and prolonged rapid eye movement (REM) sleep. Irritability is often associated with insomnia and may respond to the sleep induced by ET.

Intermediate Physical Changes

The anatomic and hormonal changes associated with aging combine to affect the genitourinary system, resulting in many changes. Decreased endogenous estrogen levels cause changes to the vaginal epithelium that result in reduced lactic acid production, increased pH, thinning of the vaginal mucosa, reduced vaginal secretions, and reduced compressibility of the urethral mucosa. Potential urogenital changes that occur at midlife and beyond include dryness and irritation of the vagina, itching and irritation of the vulva, discomfort during sexual activity, urinary urgency or the need to urinate more frequently, urinary tract infections, and urine leakage when coughing or sneezing (incontinence). It is believed that a significant number of women age 45 to 64 have urinary incontinence and that many of these women endure incontinence for 3 to 7 years before discussing the problem with a health care provider, most often because they believe that incontinence is normal for women or older people.

Decline in sexual activity during these years is influenced more by culture and attitudes than by nature and physiology. The single most significant determinant of sexual activity for older women is the availability or unavailability of a partner. Given the availability of a partner, the same general high or low rate of sexual activity can be maintained throughout life. Individuals who are sexually active earlier in life can continue to be sexually active into old age.

Disease Associated with Postmenopausal Women

CVD, osteoporosis, dementia of the Alzheimer's type, and cancers are of the most concern to health care providers of menopausal women.

Cardiovascular Disease. The significance of CVD in women was not understood before the late 1980s. CVD is the leading cause of mortality in women in the United States.[6] More than 2.5 million women in the United States are hospitalized for CVD annually. More than a half a million die from CVD yearly, primarily as a consequence of myocardial infarction.[6] Although breast cancer is the disease most feared by women, approximately 1 in 3 will die of coronary heart disease (CHD), whereas 1 in 25 will die of breast cancer.

In some women with CHD the initial manifestation of the disease is chest pain. However, women also tend to have pain at rest, shortness of breath, and fatigue as the presenting manifestations. Women and their health care providers may discount cardiac complaints, perhaps because of a longstanding perception of CHD as a man's disease or perhaps because cardiac symptoms in women are often vague or dissimilar to those symptoms experienced by men. For this reason, it is important that health care providers not dismiss a woman's complaint of chest pain, fatigue, or shortness of breath as benign or noncardiac in nature.

Osteoporosis. Osteoporosis is a silent disease that has become recognized as a major public health problem for women in the United States. It is characterized by low bone mass and microarchitectural deterioration of bone tissue. The clinical significance of osteoporosis is an increased risk for fractures, which subsequently increases disability and mortality. Osteoporosis is a "silent" risk factor for fracture, just as hypertension is for stroke. Osteoporosis is a serious and disabling but preventable disease. The incidence of osteoporosis is expected to rise as the population over age 50 grows. Currently, 28 million to 30 million Americans have low bone mass (osteopenia) or osteoporosis, resulting in an estimated total health care cost of $14 billion per year.[7] Of the 1.5 million osteoporotic fractures that occur each year, 80% occur in women. Twenty percent of non-Hispanic white and Asian women age 50 and older are estimated to have osteoporosis, and 52% are estimated to have low bone mass. Non-Hispanic black women have a decreased risk—5% and 34% for osteoporosis and low bone mass, respectively—but Hispanic women have slightly higher risks—10% and 49%, respectively. One of every two Caucasian woman will experience an osteoporosis-related fracture.[7]

Bone mineral density (BMD) testing provides information regarding the risk for fractures related to osteoporosis. Dual-energy x-ray absorptiometry (DEXA) is the technical standard for measuring BMD and can measure BMD at the spine and hip. Other tests to evaluate BMD include single-energy x-ray absorptiometry, radiographic absorptiometry, quantitative computed tomography, and ultrasound densitometry. However, these tests should be used only when DEXA is not available. BMD testing should be undertaken by all postmenopausal women under age 65 who have one or more additional risk fractures for osteoporotic fracture (besides menopause); all women ages 65 and older regardless of additional risk factors; postmenopausal women with fractures (to confirm diagnosis and determine severity).; women who are considering therapy for osteoporosis, if BMD testing would facilitate the decision; and women who have been on HT for prolonged periods.

Osteoporosis can be defined by BMD:

Normal: BMD within 1 SD of a "young normal" adult (*t*-distribution above -1).

Low bone mass (osteopenia): BMD between 1 and 2.5 SD below that of a "young normal" adult (*t*-distribution between −1 and −2.5).

Osteoporosis: BMD more than 2.5 SD below that of a "young normal" adult (*t*-distribution below −2.5). Women in this group who have already experienced one or more fractures are deemed to have severe or established osteoporosis.

PHYSICAL EXAMINATION

Annual physical examinations are recommended and should occur more frequently based on chronic conditions or acute presentation of symptoms. During an annual examination, screening tests based on the woman's age and health history are indicated.

The U.S. Department of Health and Human Services and the U.S. Preventive Services Task Force, the leading independent panel of private sector experts in prevention and primary care, provide recommendations for screening women in midlife.[8] These recommendations are considered the definitive guidelines for preventive services delivered in the clinical setting, although these guidelines may differ slightly from the guidelines issued by other organizations. The task force conducts rigorous scientific assessments of the effectiveness of a broad range of clinical preventive services and updates recommendations based on these findings. Providers should refer to these guidelines available at http://www.ahrq.gov to guide screening during physical examinations based on the patient's age and disease history to determine which women will need certain screening tests earlier, or more often, than others.

The task force[9] has made the following general recommendations, based on scientific evidence, about which screening tests women in the midlife should have:

- Mammograms every 1 to 2 years
- Papanicolaou's (Pap) smears every 1 to 2 years if sexually active
- Cholesterol checks starting at age 45
- Blood pressure at least every 2 years
- Colorectal cancer tests starting at age 50

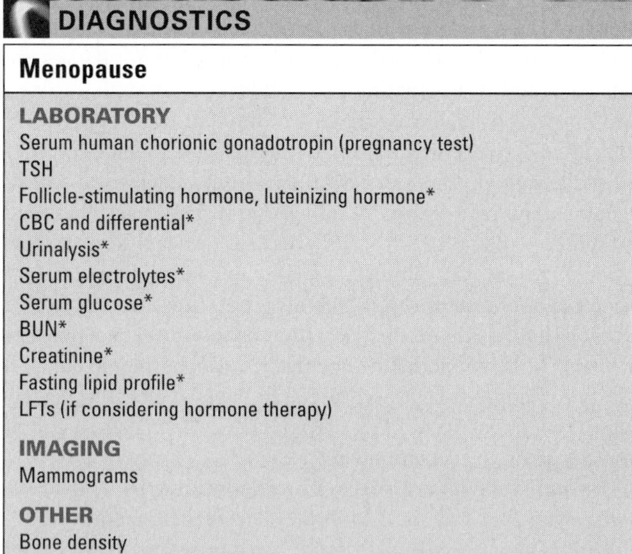

DIAGNOSTICS

Menopause

LABORATORY

Serum human chorionic gonadotropin (pregnancy test)
TSH
Follicle-stimulating hormone, luteinizing hormone*
CBC and differential*
Urinalysis*
Serum electrolytes*
Serum glucose*
BUN*
Creatinine*
Fasting lipid profile*
LFTs (if considering hormone therapy)

IMAGING

Mammograms

OTHER

Bone density
ECG

*If indicated.

DIAGNOSTICS

There is no one test of ovarian function currently available to either predict or confirm menopause. Health care providers must rely on careful use of hormone testing to establish that it has been reached. When the clinical situation is not clear, estrogen deficiency as the cause of hot flashes should be documented by elevated FSH level. It is generally accepted that menopause has been reached when FSH levels are consistently greater than 30 IU/L. The difficulty in using FSH levels as a marker for menopause is that these levels may decrease back to their premenopausal ranges for a temporary period.

Additional diagnostic testing is often necessary to rule out other differential diagnoses if the diagnosis of menopause is not clear, to determine the need for additional evaluation, and to guide management. A CBC should be done to assess for anemia, which may result from prolonged menorrhagia. A complete chemistry profile, including serum electrolytes, serum glucose, BUN, creatinine, fasting glucose, fasting lipid profile, and liver enzymes (including lactate dehydrogenase and alkaline phosphatase), should be obtained, particularly if HT may be considered. A thyroid-stimulating hormone level to exclude hypothyroidism as a cause of menstrual irregularity or other symptoms and urinalysis to detect microscopic hematuria or proteinuria are necessary. Additional screening tests such as a mammogram should be ordered in accordance with current recommendations. For women at risk for osteoporosis, a baseline BMD measurement is necessary to predict the extent of intervention needed to prevent osteoporosis. An ECG may be necessary to exclude cardiac abnormality for women experiencing palpitations.

DIFFERENTIAL DIAGNOSIS

Not all hot flashes are due to estrogen deficiency. Flushing and sweating can be secondary to diseases, including pheochromocytoma, leukemias, thyroid abnormalities, and psychosomatic symptoms.

Mood disturbances are another common concern during this time. Midlife and menopause are times of multiple life changes, and all women may have some degree of increased risk for depression, anxiety, and other mental health problems. There is reason to associate the middle years with negative life experiences. The events that come to mind are impressive: onset of a major illness or disability in self or spouse, death of a spouse, divorce, retirement from employment, financial insecurity, the need to provide care for very old parents, and separation from children. Feelings of depression, irritability, confusion, and impaired memory are often associated with insomnia and therefore may respond to HT. (Current evidence does not link estrogen levels during menopausal transition to major depressive disorder.[10])

Women's sexual function can be influenced by many potential factors other than menopause and estrogen deficiency, including previous attitudes, age-related changes, body

DIFFERENTIAL DIAGNOSIS

Menopause

- Amenorrhea
- Cardiac abnormality
- Menstrual irregularity
- Pregnancy
- Thyroid disorder
- Hypothalamic dysfunction
- Uterine outlet obstruction
- Polycystic kidney disease
- Pheochromocytoma
- Leukemia and other cancer
- Psychosomatic illness

image and poor self-esteem, health status and medical complications, incontinence, sleep disturbance, family stress, medications, male sexual dysfunction, and decreased androgen levels.

The differential diagnosis of chest pain in women should include consideration of angina pectoris, pericarditis, esophageal reflux or spasm, pulmonary embolism, pneumonia, gastritis, peptic ulcer, costochondritis, mitral valve prolapse, and hyperventilation. Given the complexity of the diagnosis and treatment of chest pain, this condition is best referred to a cardiologist.

MANAGEMENT

Lifestyle Changes

A discussion with a health care provider is the first step in determining a woman's best treatment options. Modifying lifestyle choices can have a significant and positive impact on health. The cessation of substance use (including tobacco and illicit drugs); the decrease in alcohol and caffeine intake; the initiation of an adequate exercise plan; a balanced, healthy diet; weight management; and stress reduction are all measures that can be incorporated into a comprehensive therapeutic plan.[11]

Nonprescriptive Therapies

In addition to modifying lifestyle choices, various over-the-counter products may help alleviate some minor problems associated with menopause. However, a woman's health care provider should be involved in the decision to use nonprescriptive products, since no therapy is without risk. A daily multivitamin and mineral supplement would also be of benefit to most women. If adequate calcium cannot be obtained from the diet, a separate calcium supplement may be required to reach the recommended level of 1200 to 1500 mg/day of calcium. Vaginal lubricants and vaginal moisturizers are some of the products available to help solve minor vaginal moisture problems. No vaginal lubricant or moisturizer treats the cause of menopause-related vaginal dryness and atrophy. This condition is attributed to the lack of estrogen and can be improved with prescription ET, which has been approved by the U.S. Food and Drug Administration (FDA) for treating vaginal atrophy.

Prescription Therapies

According to the North American Menopause Society, an individual risk profile is essential for every woman contemplating any regimen of estrogen-progestin therapy (EPT) or ET. Treatment of menopause symptoms such as vasomotor instability, sleep disturbance, and urogenital changes remains the primary indication for EPT and ET. The only menopause-related indication for progestin use appears to be endometrial protection from unopposed estrogen therapy. No EPT or ET regimen should be used for primary or secondary prevention of CHD.[12-16] Many EPT and ET products are FDA approved for the prevention of postmenopausal osteoporosis. However, because of the risks associated with these forms of therapy, alternatives should also be considered, weighing the risks and benefits of each. Use of EPT or ET should be limited to the shortest duration consistent with treatment goals. Lower than standard doses of EPT and ET should be considered, and alternative routes of EPT may offer advantages, although the long-term benefit/risk ratio has not been demonstrated.[17]

Numerous therapeutic options for postmenopausal women are available for ET. The most effective ET regimen includes the lowest dose needed to prevent bone loss, minimize cardiovascular-related risk factors, minimize side effects, and minimize postmenopausal symptoms. Unopposed ET is prescribed for patients who have undergone surgical removal of the uterus. Combination ET plus a progestin (HT) is required for a woman with a uterus to reduce the risk of endometrial adenocarcinoma, which is significantly increased in women using unopposed estrogen. Systemic ET is prescribed as oral tablets, transdermal patches, or a vaginal ring. Local estrogen is available in vaginal creams, vaginal tablets, or a vaginal ring.[9,18]

Hormone Therapy Regimens

All postmenopausal women should be counseled about HT with an initial evaluation that encompasses history and complete physical examination, including pelvic and breast examination; family history; dietary history; lifestyle evaluation; and accurate height, weight, blood pressure, fasting lipid profile, and other laboratory values. HT should be used only after verification of absence of contraindications.

Research. In the 1980s, combined estrogen-progestin was the standard of care for women who had not had a hysterectomy.[19] Before that, estrogen alone had been the dominant hormone until the increased risk of endometrial cancer led to the addition of progestins for women with an intact uterus.

Although HT has been approved for the relief of menopausal symptoms and prevention of osteoporosis, long-term use had been widely accepted to prevent a range of chronic conditions, especially CHD.[20] This relationship was of great public health importance, since CVD is the leading cause of death and a major cause of disability in women.

The majority of observational epidemiologic studies that examined the role of HT-ET in women without established CHD have consistently demonstrated a lower incidence of CHD events among users of ET alone, with similar results observed for HT. A recent meta-analysis showed an approximate 35%

to 50% reduction in CHD events among users of ET alone, with similar results for HT.[17]

There appears to be a biologic basis for a role of ET-HT in the prevention of CVD. Well-established lipid alterations are associated with ET such as decreased levels of low-density lipoprotein (LDL) cholesterol and increased levels of high-density lipoprotein (HDL) cholesterol, both by about 10% to 15%. Oral ET shows an increase in triglyceride levels by about 20%, although the clinical significance of this has not been established. It is important to note that the efficacy in lipid reduction varies by route of delivery. Oral ET provides greater lipid reductions than transdermal delivery. When ET is combined with medroxyprogesterone acetate (MPA), there is a small attenuation of the beneficial HDL-raising effects. This attenuation is decreased when ET is combined with natural progesterone. Beneficial vascular effects of ET-HT include the prevention of arterial spasms, improvement of arterial blood flow, increase in nitric oxide production, and promotion of coronary vasodilation. ET-HT also favorably affects other risk markers for CVD, including fibrinogen, plasma viscosity, insulin sensitivity, homocysteine, platelet aggregation, and endothelial cell activation. This information lends support to the role of HT in the primary prevention of CVD. However, bias cannot be ruled out, since observational studies suffer from "healthy user" bias. Women who are receiving ET-HT are more likely to be of a higher socioeconomic status, to be healthier, to seek medical care, and to exercise.

Clinical Trials. The Heart and Estrogen/Progestin Replacement Study (HERS) and the Women's Health Initiative (WHI) have provided new information that questions longstanding clinical practice and prescribing patterns for estrogen and progestin therapy. HERS was a randomized, blinded, placebo-controlled trial of continuous-combined estrogen-progestin therapy in postmenopausal women with documented CHD (N = 2763).[21] HERS was designed to determine whether the combination of conjugated equine estrogen (CEE) and MPA alters the risk for CHD events in postmenopausal women with established coronary disease. The initial study ended after 4.1 years because an analysis suggested a possible higher risk of coronary events during the first year. Because the study showed an increased risk after 1 year, but possibly a reduced risk after 3 to 5 years, the study was extended in a follow-up study, HERS II (N = 2321). The net effect for the entire study was that the investigators could not show that hormones were cardioprotective. The results of HERS II showed that HT did not provide cardiac protection in women who had previously diagnosed heart disease.

WHI is a National Institutes of Health–sponsored, multicenter study begun in 1993.[22] The study consisted of three interrelated clinical trials and an observational study in apparently healthy women ages 50 to 79 years. The planned duration of the trial was 8½ years. The purpose of the trial was to assess the major benefits and risks of ET-HT with regard to specific outcomes: CHD, venous thrombotic events, breast cancer, colon cancer, and fractures. WHI's randomized, blinded, placebo-controlled hormone study had an arm of continuous combined estrogen-progestin therapy for women with a uterus (N = 16,608) and an estrogen-only arm for women who had undergone a hysterectomy (N = 10,739). Women in this trial were randomly assigned to either hormone therapy or placebo. The combined HT arm of the study was terminated in July 2002 after an average 5.2 years of follow-up because the overall risks exceeded benefits.

The trial results are reported primarily in terms of relative risk, which is appropriate for studies of cause. When applying the results to clinical practice, providers must translate them into absolute risk. The WHI data describe the increased risk for an entire population—not the increased risk for an individual woman. The absolute risk of harm to an individual woman is very small. There was no difference in the number of deaths between the estrogen-progestin group and the placebo group. The increased risk of breast cancer for each woman in the WHI study who was taking HT was less than $\frac{1}{10}$ of 1% per year. However, if you apply that increased risk to an entire population over several years, the number of women affected increases dramatically and becomes an important public health concern. The slight increase in invasive breast cancer occurred earlier than anticipated from observational studies (within 5 years). In the WHI data the increase was significant at year 4, with a trend to a later decline in number of events. This would appear to confirm that HT provides a growth-promoting rather than a causative role in breast cancer. With the premature termination of this study, this question was not answered.

Hormone Therapy Guidelines

In women who have had a hysterectomy, it is advised that HT should be initiated with estrogen alone. In women with a uterus, progestin is usually added to ET to reduce the risk of endometrial hyperplasia and cancer associated with ET. In this case the provider should initiate sequential HT with a separate estrogen and progestin to titrate to a woman's symptoms and avoid unpredictable bleeding in the early postmenopausal period. The progestin is taken for 12 days per cycle, and the provider should consider switching to a continuous regimen after symptoms have stabilized. The woman should use transdermal estrogens if there is concern about thrombotic or inflammatory effects or hepatic function. Statins should be used concurrently when indicated. The provider must monitor for breast disease, changes in lipid profile, and fasting glucose levels in women at above-average risk for CVD, and monitor clinically significant unexpected uterine bleeding.[23]

Cyclic Hormone Therapy. Estrogen is used for 25 days each month, with progestin added the last 10 to 14 days, followed by 3 to 6 days of no therapy. This most closely mimics the normal premenopausal ovulatory cycle. Disadvantages are that 80% of women have withdrawal bleeding when the progestin is stopped. Vasomotor symptoms may occur during the therapy-free interval.

Continuous-Cyclic Hormone Therapy (Sequential). Estrogen is used continuously every day of the month, with progestin added for 10 to 14 days each month. Uterine bleeding occurs in about 80% of women when progestin is withdrawn. An advantage is that there is no estrogen-free period during which vasomotor symptoms can occur.

Continuous-Combined Hormone Therapy. Estrogen and progestin are taken every day. An advantage is that the monthly cumulative dose of progestin is decreased. Eighty percent of women on this regimen experience no bleeding. Also, compliance is improved. The two most common reasons why women discontinue or do not start HT are fear of cancer and vaginal bleeding, so going from 80% to 90% of women experiencing withdrawal bleeding (as with other types of HT) to 80% experiencing no bleeding represents a major accomplishment.

On the other hand, when bleeding does occur, it is unpredictable in timing. When bleeding persists after several months of continuous-combined therapy, an endometrial biopsy or transvaginal ultrasound is warranted to rule out abnormal pathologic conditions.

Screening Parameters for Postmenopausal Bleeding for Women Using Hormone Therapy or Estrogen Therapy. For women using cyclic HT (estrogen plus progestin), endometrial evaluation should be considered if bleeding occurs at any time other than the expected time of withdrawal bleeding, or if heavier or more prolonged withdrawal bleeding occurs.

For women using continuous-combined HT, endometrial evaluation must be considered when irregular bleeding persists more than 6 months after beginning therapy, or earlier if other risk factors are present. Earlier biopsy can be considered on the basis of individual circumstances, including:

- Risk factors for endometrial cancer
- Past history of unopposed ET
- Clinician anxiety
- Patient anxiety

Persistent vaginal bleeding in a postmenopausal woman, whether on or off HT, requires evaluation with an endometrial biopsy or dilation and curettage, despite transvaginal ultrasound findings.

Management of Osteoporosis

Estrogen has been used for decades in the treatment of women with osteoporosis. Estrogens (oral and transdermal preparations) decrease bone loss, reduce the incidence of fracture, and prevent height loss. Most menopause-related bone loss occurs during the first 3 to 6 years after the onset of menopause. However, some bone loss caused by low estrogen levels may continue for as long as 20 years. If begun soon after menopause, ET or HT prevents this early phase of bone loss and decreases the incidence of subsequent osteoporotic fractures by 50%. ET or HT is also effective in women with established osteoporosis: it increases mean vertebral bone mass by more than 5% and decreases fracture incidence by 50% or more.[24] However, there are concerns about the potentially serious adverse effects associated with ET or HT and there are alternative treatment options for osteoporosis.

Alendronate (Fosamax), a biphosphonate, has been approved for both the treatment and prevention of postmenopausal osteoporosis. Treatment reduces incidence of fracture by 50% in patients with osteoporosis.

Risedronate (Actonel) and ibandronate (Boniva) are other biphosphonates approved for the treatment and prevention of postmenopausal osteoporosis. Gastrointestinal side effects from risedronate may not be as common as with alendronate.

Tamoxifen was approved by the FDA in 1997 as a therapeutic agent for advanced breast cancer. In 1998 it was approved for the primary prevention of breast cancer in high-risk women. Tamoxifen can also promote increased bone density, but vasomotor symptoms are common with tamoxifen. Serious side effects include endometrial cancer, pulmonary embolism, deep vein thrombophlebitis, and cataract formation. Tamoxifen also has beneficial effects on BMD and serum lipid levels in postmenopausal women.[25]

Raloxifene (Evista) is a SERM approved by the FDA for the prevention and treatment of osteoporosis. Raloxifene may also have cardioprotective benefits. It was found to have no proliferative effect on the uterus or breast tissue, and its effects on lipid profile are similar to those of estrogens. Side effects include hot flashes, leg cramps, and blood clots. For this reason, it is contraindicated if the woman has had a previous history of thromboembolism. Clinical trials suggest raloxifene may reduce breast cancer risk and it is currently being compared with tamoxifen in a large randomized study.[26] Neither tamoxifen nor raloxifene is appropriate for treating the vasomotor symptoms associated with menopause.

Salmon calcitonin is a hormone that inhibits bone resorption. It is considered the least effective of the pharmacologic agents for osteoporosis.

Management of Vasomotor and Genitourinary Symptoms

Short term HT is still appropriate for the management of vasomotor symptoms and genitourinary atrophy in many perimenopausal and menopausal women. The lowest effective dose regimen as described above should be used.

For vaginal atrophy, topical estrogen cream (e.g., conjugated estrogen [Premarin] 0.625 mg/g intravaginally for 3 weeks of every month) can be used short term. For women bothered by hot flashes but opposed to using HT or in whom HT is contraindicated, other therapies can be considered to promote sleep and well-being. Low-dose contraceptive therapy is acceptable for nonsmoking women before age 50. Clonidine, gabapentin, and some antidepressants (e.g., venlafaxine [Effexor] and paroxetine [Paxil]) are helpful for vasomotor symptoms.[27] Herbal or alternative therapies have not been proven to be effective and, in fact, may be harmful.[27]

LIFE SPAN CONSIDERATIONS

As women make the transition through midlife, important physical and psychologic changes occur that may affect their everyday lives. Children age and leave the home; parents age and become dependent; and chronic health conditions develop that limit physical activity, affecting daily living and financial status. Providers must be cognizant of these issues and their impact on women in midlife. Psychosocial distress, anxiety, and depression are important conditions to assess and treat in addition to the multiple physical changes women experience during this stage of life.[28]

COMPLICATIONS

Many EPT and ET products are FDA-approved for the prevention of postmenopausal osteoporosis. However, because of the risks associated with these forms of therapy, alternatives should also be considered, weighing the risks and benefits of each.

When considering treatment of osteoporosis with bisphosphonates such as alendronate, providers should discuss side effects with the patient, including upper gastrointestinal tract disturbance, esophageal symptoms (chest pain, heartburn, dysphagia), and rarely esophageal ulceration.

When treating the vasomotor symptoms associated with ET and HT, the risks and side effects should be carefully explained to the patient. ET side effects include breast tenderness, nausea, and headaches. Progestin-related adverse effects encompass menses and withdrawal bleeding, bloating, mood changes, and rash. Recent studies have shown a twofold to fourfold increase in the risk of venous thromboembolism (VT) in users of ET and HT.[29] This risk must be weighed against documented benefits of hormone use. VT carries with it a low risk of mortality, around 1%. Caution must be used in women with preexisting risk factors for VT: family history of VT, gross obesity, past history of VT, and intercurrent illness associated with immobilization. Risk is generally present in the first year of treatment only.[29]

The most clearly documented adverse consequence of estrogen treatment is a twofold to threefold increase in the risk of endometrial cancer in women with an intact uterus. The risk of endometrial cancer is not increased in women who also take progestins. Women who use a combined estrogen and progestin regimen after menopause have a lower risk for endometrial cancer than untreated women do. The principal factor that predisposes women to the development of endometrial cancer is chronic, unopposed exposure to estrogen, whether endogenous or exogenous. Factors conferring this risk are early menarche, late menopause, obesity, chronic anovulation, estrogen-secreting ovarian tumors, ingestion of unopposed estrogen (the increased risk persists after discontinuation of estrogen), possibly hypertension and diabetes (although this may be related to obesity), a history of breast or ovarian cancer, and use of tamoxifen. The presenting symptom of endometrial cancer is abnormal uterine bleeding. Endometrial cancer should be suspected in postmenopausal women who have any bleeding and in perimenopausal women who have menstrual abnormalities characterized by an increased menstrual flow, a decreased menstrual interval, or intermenstrual bleeding.[30]

Breast surveillance with conscientious clinical examinations and annual mammography is important for all women in this age-group and is especially important for women taking hormones. With research results in conflict and the pathophysiology of breast cancer unknown, it is not possible to speculate with confidence about the role that estrogen plays in breast cancer risk.[31,32] HT is generally contraindicated in women with breast cancer unless the decision to treat follows an informed discussion and is managed with an oncology consultation.

Endometrial cancer within 5 years is another contraindication for HT. For higher grades or stages of endometrial cancer, therapy is generally contraindicated unless the decision to treat follows an informed decision. For grade I, stage I, cautious use of therapy after a hysterectomy is advised. ET should be used with progestins, even in the woman who has had a hysterectomy.

Other contraindications to HT include unexplained vaginal bleeding, acute liver disease, chronic severe hepatic dysfunction (aspartate aminotransferase greater than twice normal), and recent or active thrombophlebitis or thromboembolic disorders. For some women with familial mixed hyperlipidemia or hypertriglyceridemia (triglycerides ≥300 mg/dl), ET may increase triglycerides. Nonoral routes of administration should be considered. ET may also exacerbate endometriosis. Cautious use of HT should be undertaken in women with a history of leiomyomas, atraumatic thrombophlebitis or thromboembolic event, gallbladder disease and no cholecystectomy, seizure disorders, and migraine headaches.[33]

Conditions that do not represent contraindications for HT include controlled hypertension, diabetes mellitus, and elevated cholesterol.

INDICATIONS FOR REFERRAL OR HOSPITALIZATION

Women who are experiencing menopausal symptoms that interfere with activities of daily living may need further evaluation. Referral to a provider who is an experienced menopausal specialist, endocrinologist, or gynecologist is indicated.

PATIENT AND FAMILY EDUCATION

All postmenopausal women should be counseled about the use of ET and HT.[34] This is especially true for women with premature menopause or induced menopause. In the absence of contraindications, ET and HT can be offered to treat specific menopausal symptoms. Each woman's health profile should be reviewed and a program of preventive care encouraged. In particular, the risks of osteoporosis, CVD, CNS disorders, cancer (breast, colon, endometrial), and deep vein thrombosis should be addressed. Both the risks and benefits associated with HT should be discussed.

Discussing the risk interventions in Table 175-1 with menopausal women and adhering to the recommendations is strongly suggested for the prevention of CVD in this group.

HEALTH PROMOTION

Menopause and perimenopause provide health care professionals with an opportunity to recommend healthy lifestyle changes (e.g., increased exercise and, if indicated, weight reduction and smoking cessation). Risk factors associated with CVD and osteoporosis (Box 175-1) should be identified and treatment options discussed with the patient. The best protection against postmenopausal osteoporosis is prevention (Box 175-2). Calcium supplementation (1200 to 1500 mg/day) is also encouraged. For additional information about osteoporosis prevention, refer to Chapter 196.

TABLE 175-1 Risk Interventions and Recommendations for Cardiovascular Disease Prevention

Risk Intervention	Recommendations
Smoking Goal: complete cessation	Ask about smoking status as part of routine evaluation. Provide counseling, nicotine replacement, drug therapy, and formal cessation programs.
Blood pressure control Goal: <140 mm Hg systolic, <90 mm Hg diastolic Blood pressure goals vary according to risk factors.	Measure blood pressure in all adults at least every 2 years. Promote lifestyle modifications. Follow medication guidelines from National Institutes of Health.*
Cholesterol management Optimal values (depends on number of risk factors and 10-year absolute CHD risk): LDL <100 mg/dL: optimum TC <200 mg/dL: desirable HDL ≥60: high	Complete lipoprotein profile (TC, LDL, HDL, and triglycerides) is the preferred initial test. Measure in all adults ages 20 years or older every 5 years. Follow guidelines from the third report of the National Cholesterol Education Program.[†]
Weight management Goal: achieve and maintain desirable weight (BMI 21-25 kg/m^2; desirable waist-to-hip ratio <0.8)	Measure patient's weight and height, BMI, and waist-to-hip ratio as part of routine evaluation. Start weight management and physical activity as appropriate.
Physical activity Goal: exercise regularly 5 times per week for 30 minutes	Ask about physical activity status and exercise habits as part of routine evaluation. Advise medically supervised programs for those with low functional capacity or co-morbidities.
Estrogens	Do not initiate HT for the sole purpose of primary or secondary prevention of CVD. Limit use of estrogens to prevention of osteoporosis and treatment of menopausal symptoms.
Alcohol intake	Counsel to limit intake to no more than 0.5 ounces of ethanol per day.
Sodium intake	Counsel to reduce intake to <100 mmol/day (<2.4 g of sodium or <6 g of sodium chloride).
Calcium and magnesium	Counsel to maintain adequate amounts for general health.
Potassium intake	Counsel to maintain adequate potassium intake (approximately 90 mmol/day).
Fats	Counsel to reduce intake of dietary saturated fat and cholesterol for overall cardiovascular health.
DASH diet (DASH study) The results of this trial demonstrate that the DASH diet substantially lowers blood pressure and may help prevent and control hypertension.	Advise patients to follow Dietary Approaches to Stop Hypertension (DASH) diet, a diet rich in fruits, vegetables, low-fat dairy foods, dietary fiber, potassium, calcium, and magnesium and low in saturated fats and cholesterol. (See JNC 7 guidelines.[‡])
Still-experimental primary intervention	Aspirin prophylaxis, megavitamins, antioxidant supplementation.

BMI, Body mass index; *CHD,* coronary heart disease; *CVD,* cardiovascular disease; *HDL,* high-density lipoprotein; *HT,* hormone therapy; *LDL,* low-density lipoprotein; *TC,* total cholesterol.

*National Institutes of Health: *The seventh report of the Joint National Committee on Prevention, Detection, Evaluation and Treatment of High Blood Pressure,* Washington, DC, 2003, The Institutes.

†National Cholesterol Education Program; National Heart, Lung, and Blood Institute: *Third Report of the Expert Panel on Detection, Evaluation, and Treatment of High Blood Cholesterol in Adults (Adult Treatment Panel III),* Bethesda, Md, 2002, National Institutes of Health.

‡National High Blood Pressure Education Program; National Heart, Lung, and Blood Institute: *The Seventh Report of the Joint National Committee on Prevention, Detection, Evaluation, and Treatment of High Blood Pressure (JNC 7),* Bethesda, Md, 2003, National Institutes of Health.

BOX 175-1

RISK FACTORS FOR POSTMENOPAUSAL OSTEOPOROSIS

MEDICATIONS

- Corticosteroids (7.5 mg/day or more of prednisone or equivalent for ≥6 months)
- Long-term use of certain anticonvulsant medications (e.g., phenytoin)
- Anticoagulant agents (e.g., heparin, warfarin)
- Immunosuppressive drugs (e.g., cyclosporin)
- Levothyroxine
- Intramuscular medroxyprogesterone in premenopausal women
- Lithium
- Tamoxifen (premenopausal use)

GENETIC FACTORS

- Advanced age
- First-degree relative with low-trauma fracture
- Caucasian or Asian race
- Slender physical frame

ENVIRONMENTAL FACTORS

- Cigarette smoking
- Excessive alcohol use (>7 drinks weekly)
- Sedentary lifestyle, prolonged immobilization
- Diet low in calcium
- Excessive use of caffeine

MENSTRUAL STATUS

- Early menopause without estrogen or hormone therapy
- Premenopausal hypogonadism
- Previous amenorrhea (e.g., because of anorexia nervosa or exercise-induced amenorrhea)
- Hyperprolactinemia

DISEASE STATES

- Osteoporotic fracture as an adult
- Primary hyperparathyroidism
- Thyrotoxicosis
- Cushing's syndrome
- Multiple myeloma
- Rheumatoid arthritis
- Malabsorption syndromes (e.g., celiac disease, Crohn's disease)
- Chronic obstructive pulmonary disease
- Anorexia nervosa
- Chronic liver disease
- Chronic renal disease

BOX 175-2

POSSIBLE PREVENTION AND TREATMENT INTERVENTIONS FOR OSTEOPOROSIS

WEIGHT-BEARING EXERCISE

- Early in life, promotes higher peak bone mass
- Weight bearing and strength training (most beneficial for bone health)
- Increases muscle mass and strength.
- Exercise programs for elderly to increase muscle strength and reduce the risk of falls

NUTRITION

- Calcium: ≥1200 mg/day (<600 mg/day in typical American diet)
- Vitamin D: 400 to 800 IU/day (enhances intestinal absorption of calcium)

SMOKING CESSATION

- Smoking leads to lower bone mass and fractures.

REFERENCES

1. Smith P: Menopause: assessment, treatment and patient education, *Nurse Pract* 30:33-43, 2005.
2. Speroff L: Managing the patient with premature ovarian failure, *Council Hormone Educ* 3(4):1-12, 2005.
3. Nelson LM, and others: An update: spontaneous premature ovarian failure is not an early menopause, *Fertil Steril* 83(5):1327-1332, 2005.
4. North American Menopause Society: *Menopause core curriculum study guide*, ed 2, Mayfield Heights, Ohio, 2002, The Society.
5. American College of Obstetricians and Gynecologists: *Frequently asked questions about hormone therapy,* October 2004, retrieved March 8, 2007, from http://www.acog.org/from_home/publications/press_releases/nr10-01-04.cfm.
6. Expert Panel Writing Group: Evidence-based guidelines for cardiovascular disease prevention in women, *Circulation* 109:672-693, 2004.
7. Miller R: Osteoporosis in post-menopausal women: therapy options across a wide range of risk for fracture, *Geriatrics* 61:24-30, 2006.
8. US Department of Health and Human Services, Agency for Healthcare Research and Quality: *Women: stay healthy at any age,* AHRQ Pub No APPIP03-0008, Jan 2004, retrieved March 8, 2007, from http://www.ahrq.gov/ppip/healthywom.pdf.
9. US Preventive Services Task Force: Postmenopausal hormone replacement therapy for the primary prevention of chronic condition, *Am Fam Phys* 67:358-364, 2003.
10. Harvard Women's Health Watch: Perimenopause: rocky road to menopause, *Harvard Health Publications* 12(12):1-4, 2005.
11. North American Menopause Society: *Menopause guidebook: helping women make informed healthcare decisions through perimenopause and beyond*, Mayfield Heights, Ohio, 2001, The Society.
12. Langer RD: Hormone replacement therapy and coronary heart disease in light of the PEPI Trial, *Int J Fertil Womens Med* 44:136-141, 1999.
13. Langer RD: Hormone replacement and the prevention of cardiovascular disease, *Am J Cardiol* 89(12 Suppl):36E-46E, 2002.
14. Langer RD: Legend meets reality: estrogen plus progestin and coronary heart disease in the Women's Health Initiative, *Menopaus Med* 10:5-7, 2003.
15. Manson JE, and others: Estrogen plus progestin and risk of coronary heart disease, *N Engl J Med* 349:523-534, 2003.
16. Herrington DM, and others: HERS Study Group: statin therapy, cardiovascular events, and total mortality in the Heart and Estrogen/Progestin Replacement Study (HERS), *Circulation* 105:2962-2967, 2002.
17. North American Menopause Society: Recommendations for estrogen and progestogen use in peri- and postmenopausal women, *Menopause* 11(6):589-600, 2004.
18. American College of Obstetricians and Gynecologists Task Force for Hormone Therapy: Hormone therapy, *Obstet Gynecol* 104(4 Suppl):1S-131S, 2004.
19. Anderson GL, and others: Women's Health Initiative Steering Committee: effects of conjugated equine estrogen in postmenopausal women with hysterectomy, *JAMA* 291:1701-1712, 2004.
20. North American Menopause Society: Treatment of menopause-associated vasomotor symptoms, *Menopause* 11:11-33, 2004.

21. Hulley S, and others: Randomized trial of estrogen plus progestin for secondary prevention of coronary heart disease in postmenopausal women, *JAMA* 280:605-613, 1998.
22. Rossouw JE, and others: Risks and benefits of estrogen plus progestin in healthy postmenopausal women, *JAMA* 288:321-333, 2002.
23. Langer RD: Postmenopausal hormone therapy: what's appropriate today, *CME Bull* 4:1-10, 2005.
24. Riggs BL, and others: The prevention and treatment of osteoporosis, *N Engl J Med* 327:620-627, 1992.
25. Collaborative Group on Hormonal Factors in Breast Cancer: Breast cancer and hormone replacement therapy: collaborative reanalysis of data from 51 epidemiologic studies of 52,705 women with breast cancer and 108,411 women without breast cancer, *Lancet* 350:1047-1059, 1997.
26. Cummings SR, and others: The effect of raloxifene on risk of breast cancer in postmenopausal women, *JAMA* 281:2189-2197, 1999.
27. Santen RJ: Patient information: alternatives to postmenopausal hormone therapy, retrieved March 7, 2007, from http://www.uptodate.com.
28. Wilcox S, and others: Knowledge and perceived risk of major diseases in middle-aged and older women, *Heath Psychol* 18:346-353, 1999.
29. Zegura B, and others: Double blind, randomized study of estradiol replacement therapy on markers of inflammation, coagulation and fibrinolysis, *Atherosclerosis* 168:123-129, 2003.
30. Langer RD: Progestins: pharmacologic characteristics and clinically relevant differences, *Int J Fertil* 45(Suppl):63-72, 2000.
31. Ross RK, and others: Effect of hormone replacement therapy on breast cancer risk: estrogen versus estrogen plus progestin, *J Natl Cancer Inst* 92:328-332, 2000.
32. Harvie M, and others: Association of gain and loss of weight before and after menopause with risk of postmenopausal breast cancer in the Iowa women's health study, *Cancer Epidemiol Biomarkers Prev* 14(3):656-661, 2005.
33. Apgar BS, and others: Hormone therapy: continuing discussion and debate, *Am Fam Phys* 67:1444, 1446-1449, 2003.
34. Hays J, and others: Effects of estrogen plus progestin on health-related quality of life, *N Engl J Med* 348:1839-1854, 2003.

CHAPTER 176

Pap Smear Abnormalities

Cathy Cramer Bertram

DEFINITION AND EPIDEMIOLOGY

The Papanicolaou's (Pap) smear is a screening test for cervical cancer that involves collection of exfoliated cervical cells for cytologic staining and examination. Among the 50 million Pap smears obtained annually in the United States, approximately 3.5 million (7%) reveal cytologic abnormalities requiring follow-up.[1] Cervical cancer is the second most common cancer among women worldwide, with an incidence of approximately 450,000 new cases per year.[2] However, in countries such as the United States, where Pap smear screening is offered, the cervical cancer rates are much lower. In 2006, there were 9700 new cervical cancer cases and 3700 deaths from cervical cancer.[3] Cervical cancer mortality has decreased by 70% since the introduction of the Pap smear 50 years ago. However, health disparity research has revealed that poor women and particular ethnic minorities have a higher incidence of cervical cancer mortality within the United States, with rates higher in African-American and Hispanic women than in Caucasian women.[3]

It is now known that particular strains of human papillomavirus (HPV) are involved in the etiology of cervical cancer. Papillomaviruses are small, double-stranded DNA viruses. Among the more than 100 types of HPV, 30 are genital subtypes. Of these, 15 high-risk HPV types have been identified as etiologic agents in cervical carcinogenesis. HPV 16 accounts for approximately 50% of cervical cancers worldwide.[4] Low-risk HPV subtypes, such as HPV 6 and HPV 11, are associated with genital warts and are not implicated in the etiology of malignant cervical disease.[2,5] HPV is the most common sexually transmitted infection in the United States with an estimated 5.5 million new cases per year. This amounts to a prevalence of approximately 20 million women and men currently infected with some form of genital HPV. It is estimated that more than 6 million sexually active women are infected with HPV each year, and that by age 50, at least 80% of sexually active women will have acquired HPV infection.[6] Despite this high incidence of HPV infection, cervical cancer rates remain low. This is explained by the finding that a majority of HPV infections resolve spontaneously, and only persistent infection with high-risk viral types are associated with the development of a high-grade cervical lesion, or dysplasia, a precursor to cervical cancer.[4]

PATHOPHYSIOLOGY

Although the natural history of HPV is only partially understood at this time, researchers have suggested that high-risk HPV type, HPV persistence, and environmental co-factors are required for cervical carcinogenesis. The factors that determine persistence are poorly understood at this time. Host factors associated with risk of cervical cancer in the presence of

HPV include older age, nutritional status, immune function, and smoking.[7]

HPV contains genes that encode for proteins with particular functions in the virus's life cycle. Among high-risk HPV types, the role of E6 and E7 proteins is unique, allowing HPV to successfully take control of an infected host cell for its own replication and survival. A normal host cell contains two important tumor suppressor genes (*p53* and *pRb*) that act as the guardians of the cell. Among high-risk HPV types, such as HPV 16, E6 and E7 proteins interfere with the *p53* and *pRb* host cell tumor suppressor genes, disrupting the normal cell life cycle. In a normal nonreplicating cell, *pRb* is bound to another protein, E2F, which is required for DNA replication. When HPV viral protein E7 displaces the connection between *pRb* and E2F, the usual control that *pRb* exerts over cell replication is disabled. Unbound E2F causes a normally nonreplicating cell to begin the complex sequence of cell replication necessary for the survival and reproduction of HPV. Usually, if *pRb* is dysfunctional, the other guardian of the cell, *p53*, recognizes this dysfunction and initiates a mechanism that suspends the cell cycle processes in order to repair the damage. Normally, when *p53* recognizes that the damage is not reparable, it triggers apoptosis (programmed cell death), preventing the damaged cell from future replication. However, HPV also disables *p53*, thereby allowing damaged cells to escape death and HPV to thrive. This aberrant replication process increases susceptibility to gene mutation. An unstable genome gives rise to carcinogenesis.[8-11] This process provides definitive evidence for the mechanism by which HPV can cause cervical cancer under the necessary conditions.

HPV enters the cervix presumably through microtrauma during sexual intercourse. The virus passes through the cervical epithelium to the basal cell layer, where it enters the normally replicating basal cell.[9] HPV does not kill its host cell. The virus exploits the replicating machinery of the basal cell to establish itself and begins to reproduce insidiously. It then accompanies the host cell through natural epithelial cell maturation until it is detectable in the normally nonreplicating suprabasal cells and surface epithelium. It has been suggested that HPV might exist as a latent infection for 1 to 8 months.[8,9] After latency, it enters its productive phase. At this stage the virus produces a protective capsid that allows it to survive attached to superficial and exfoliated squamous cells. This protective capsid makes HPV highly infectious and sexually transmittable. It has also been suggested that a productive infection usually lasts 3 to 6 months,[9] although further studies are required to confirm this.[8]

Persistent HPV under the necessary conditions gives rise to cervical dysplasia, also described as cervical intraepithelial neoplasia (CIN). Low-grade lesions detected by Pap smear and confirmed by cervical biopsy frequently resolve spontaneously. The probability of regression of CIN I reportedly is 57%.[12] However, high-grade lesions detected by Pap smears and confirmed by cervical biopsy are more likely to progress to cervical cancer. In women who are immunocompromised as a result of HIV infection, there is a higher likelihood that cervical disease will ultimately progress.

CLINICAL PRESENTATION AND PHYSICAL EXAMINATION

Although frank cervical cancer may appear as a visible cervical lesion or a visible benign condyloma on the cervix, most cervical lesions detected as Pap smear abnormalities are not visible by routine speculum and pelvic examination.

DIAGNOSTICS: CERVICAL CANCER SCREENING

Two techniques are currently available for Pap smear specimen collection. The traditional Pap smear involves collection of endocervical cells with a cytobrush or cotton swab, and collection of ectocervical cells using a wooden or plastic spatula. A slide is prepared and fixative applied immediately after specimen collection. A more recent technology for Pap smear specimen collection and processing uses a liquid-based medium (SurePath, ThinPrep). The examiner uses a cervical brush or broom for collection of both endocervical and ectocervical cells, by rotating the collection device 360 degrees, five times within the transformation zone, and placing it in a liquid-filled vial for processing. The laboratory centrifuges the specimens, allowing the separation of cervical cells from blood, mucus, and cellular debris. When liquid-based cytology is used in the collection of a Pap smear, additional testing for gonorrhea, chlamydia, and HPV can be performed from the same specimen.

HPV DNA testing has been approved by the U.S. Food and Drug Administration (FDA) as an adjunct to Pap smear testing when atypical squamous cells (ASC-US), a low-grade Pap smear abnormality, is detected. The FDA has also approved HPV DNA testing as a screening test, but only among women over the age of 30 as an adjunct to Pap smear screening. This age limitation is based on the concern that the high prevalence of inconsequential, transient HPV infections among women under the age of 30 would result in an abundance of positive HPV results, resulting in unnecessary procedures and psychosocial concerns. HPV infection among women 18 to 25 is more commonly transient and appears to frequently resolve spontaneously or become undetectable within a period of 2 years.[4] Women over age 30 with a normal Pap smear and negative high-risk type HPV DNA test can extend Pap smear screening intervals to every 2 to 3 years rather than annually.

The accuracy of Pap smear screening depends in part on proper specimen collection technique. Optimally, a Pap smear should not be obtained during menses. Health care providers should be aware that the Pap smear sample should be obtained from the area known as the transformation zone of the cervix. The normal ectocervix (external surface of the cervix) is covered by stratified squamous epithelium. The endocervix (internal surface of the cervix) contains mucus-secreting columnar epithelium. A normal physiologic process (metaplasia) transforms columnar epithelium into squamous epithelium. The borderline between the columnar epithelium and squamous epithelium is called the *squamocolumnar junction*. The region of the cervix where columnar epithelium transform into modified squamous epithelium is aptly named the *transformation zone*. The location of the squamocolumnar junction and the transformation zone varies according to a woman's age and hormonal influences. It may be located on the ectocervix, at the cervical os, or on the endocervix. During adolescence, pregnancy, and in some women taking oral contraceptives, the squamocolumnar junction is visible on the ectocervix. In menopausal women the squamocolumnar junction is usually located higher in the endocervix, which is less visible.[8,10]

DIFFERENTIAL DIAGNOSIS

Causes of Pap smear abnormalities are shown in the Differential Diagnosis box.

MANAGEMENT

In 2001 new consensus guidelines were developed for the management of abnormal Pap smears based on a revision of the Bethesda system (Box 176-1), a classification system for the reporting of abnormal cervical cytologic findings. Atypical squamous cells (ASC-US, ASC-H) or low-grade squamous intraepithelial lesions (LSIL) are classified as low-grade lesions. High-grade squamous intraepithelial lesions (HSIL), carcinoma in situ (CIN), and cervical cancer are classified as high-grade lesions. High-grade lesions represent precursor lesions for the development of squamous cell carcinoma of the cervix. Atypical glandular cells, which are less frequently reported, may represent a precursor lesion for adenocarcinoma of the cervix.

The Pap smear is considered a screening test, whereas the biopsy is considered the definitive test for diagnosis. Further clinical decision making is based on the result of the biopsy. If there is no evidence of biopsy-proven cervical dysplasia, or CIN, then surveillance can be done by repeating the Pap smear at particular intervals. If the biopsy reveals CIN I, patients can be managed conservatively by repeating surveillance at particular intervals. In some cases of persistent low-grade lesions, patients are given the option of surveillance vs. treatment with an ablative procedure such as cryotherapy or with an excisional procedure such as loop electrosurgical excision procedure (LEEP). If the biopsy reveals CIN II, CIN III, or more advanced abnormalities, treatment is needed.[1]

The 2001 consensus guidelines indicate at what point to begin Pap smear screening, at what age Pap smear screening can be stopped, appropriate screening intervals, when to use adjunctive HPV DNA testing, and when to refer for further evaluation or treatment.[13] The guidelines offer more than one management strategy depending on the strength of evidence to support practice. Practices with considerable evidence to support one strategy compared with another strategy are classified as "preferred." A practice is classified as "acceptable" if there is either evidence that another approach is superior or there is a lack of available evidence to favor competing strategies (Table 176-1).[13]

DIFFERENTIAL DIAGNOSIS

Abnormal Pap Smear

For a low-grade or high-grade lesion associated with high-risk human papillomavirus
- Condyloma
- Cervical cancer
- Normal transformation zone variation
- Cervical polyp
- Nabothian cyst

BOX 176-1

THE 2001 BETHESDA SYSTEM (ABRIDGED)

SPECIMEN ADEQUACY

Satisfactory for evaluation
Unsatisfactory for evaluation

GENERAL CATEGORIZATION

Negative for intraepithelial lesion or malignancy
Epithelial cell abnormality
Other

INTERPRETATION/RESULT

Negative for Intraepithelial Lesions or Malignancy

Organisms identified
- *Trichomonas vaginalis*
- Fungal organisms consistent with *Candida* species
- Shift in flora suggestive of bacterial vaginosis
- Bacteria consistent with *Actinomyces* species
- Cellular changes consistent with herpes simplex virus

Other nonneoplastic findings may include:
- Reactive cellular changes associated with inflammation
- Atrophic changes

Epithelial Cell Abnormalities

Squamous cell abnormalities
- Atypical squamous cells of undetermined significance (ASC-US)
- Atypical squamous cells, cannot exclude HSIL (ASC-H)
- Low-grade squamous intraepithelial lesion (LSIL) encompassing HPV, mild dysplasia, CIN I
- High-grade squamous intraepithelial lesion (HSIL) encompassing moderate and severe dysplasia, CIN, CIN II, CIN III
- Squamous cell carcinoma

Glandular cell abnormalities
- Atypical glandular cells (AGC)
- Atypical glandular cells favor neoplastic (AGC)
- Endocervical adenocarcinoma in situ (AIS)
- Adenocarcinoma

Other (List Not Comprehensive)

Endometrial cells in a woman over 40 years of age

Adapted from Solomon D, Davey D, Kurman R, and others: The 2001 Bethesda system: terminology for reporting results of cervical cytology, *JAMA* 287(16):2114-2119, 2002.

LIFE SPAN CONSIDERATIONS

Pap smear screening should begin at age 21 or within 3 years of the initiation of sexual intercourse. Pap smears and pelvic examinations are then recommended yearly until age 30. At that time, if the woman has never had an abnormal cytology report or has had three consecutive normal cytology reports, the Pap test and pelvic examination can be performed every 3 years.[14] Immunocompromised women and women with a history of cervical cancer or diethylstilbestrol (DES) exposure will require continued annual Pap smears and pelvic examinations, although some of these women will require more frequent screenings when indicated.[14] Elderly women who have had at least three normal Pap smears for the past 10 years can discontinue screening at age 70. Women who have had a

TABLE 176-1 2001 Consensus Guidelines for Management of Women with Cervical Cytologic Abnormalities

Pap Smear or Biopsy Result	Acceptable Approach	Preferred Approach
Atypical squamous cells (ASC-US)	Repeat Pap in 4-6 months × 2.	Test HPV DNA.* If +, do colposcopy. If −, repeat in 12 months.
ASC-US in postmenopausal women if atrophy present	Treat with intravaginal estrogen cream. Repeat Pap 1 week after therapy. *or* Test HPV DNA. If +, do colposcopy. If −, repeat in 12 months. *or* Colposcopy	
ASC-H		Colposcopy
Low-grade squamous intraepithelial lesions (LSIL)		Colposcopy
LSIL in postmenopausal women with no prior abnormal Pap and low-risk history	Repeat Pap 4-6 months × 2. *or* Treat with intravaginal estrogen cream and repeat Pap in 1 week. *or* Test HPV DNA 12 months after index Pap. If +, do colposcopy. If −, repeat Pap in 12 months.	
LSIL in adolescents	Colposcopy *or* Repeat Pap in 6 months × 2. *or* Test HPV DNA 12 months after index Pap. If +, do colposcopy. If −, repeat Pap in 12 months.	
High-grade squamous intraepithelial lesions (HSIL)		Colposcopy
Atypical glandular cells		Colposcopy with endocervical and endometrial sampling
Management of biopsy-confirmed CIN I and satisfactory colposcopy	Do Pap smear and colposcopy at 12 months. *or* Treat using ablation (cryotherapy) or excision (LEEP). If recurrent CIN I, LEEP is preferred over cryotherapy.	Do not treat.† Repeat Pap in 6 months × 2. *or* Test HPV DNA in 12 months. If +, repeat colposcopy. If −, repeat Pap annually.
Management of biopsy-confirmed CIN II and III and satisfactory colposcopy	Perform either excision or ablation of transformation zone.† Then repeat Pap in 4-6 months × 3. *or* Repeat Pap and colposcopy in 4-6 months. *or* Test HPV DNA at least 6 months after treatment. If +, do colposcopy. If −, perform annual Pap.	

From American Society for Colposcopy and Cervical Pathology: *Consensus guidelines for the management of women with abnormal cervical cytology, algorithms,* 2002, retrieved March 6, 2007, from http://www.guideline.gov/summary/summary.aspx?ss=15&doc_id=3286&nbr=2512.
CIN, Cervical intraepithelial lesion; *HPV,* human papillomavirus; *LEEP,* loop electrosurgical excision procedure.
* + HPV DNA hereafter indicates positive high-risk HPV viral subtypes such as HPV 16.
†Management may vary if pregnant, immunosuppressed, or adolescent.

total hysterectomy (including removal of the cervix) do not need Pap smears unless the hysterectomy was performed because of a precancerous or cancerous condition.

INDICATIONS FOR REFERRAL

Colposcopy involves an office procedure in which the cervix and vagina are viewed directly under magnification and a cervical biopsy is obtained. According to the consensus guidelines for the management of abnormal Pap smears, most women with abnormal Pap smears should be referred to a trained physician or nurse practitioner colposcopist for further evaluation.[13] Exceptions include patients with ASC-US, and adolescents or postmenopausal women under certain circumstances. Patients with ASC-US lesions with a concurrent positive HPV DNA test and those with LSIL should be referred for colposcopy. Formerly, it was common practice to delay colposcopy and repeat the Pap smear in 3 months after an initial ASC-US or LSIL Pap smear result. Although the strategy of repeating the Pap smear in 4 to 6 months remains acceptable, the preferred strategy for the management of ASC-

US is to obtain an HPV DNA test. If it is positive for high-risk viral types, then the patient is referred for colposcopy and biopsy. For LSIL, patients are referred for colposcopy. An HPV DNA test is not done with LSIL, since most LSILs involve HPV. All patients with HSIL and ASC-US should be referred for colposcopy.

If a clinician notes a visible cervical lesion, particularly an erythematous, exophytic lesion, the patient should be referred for further evaluation by colposcopy regardless of the Pap smear result, since some frank cervical cancers may not be detected by Pap smear.

PATIENT AND FAMILY EDUCATION

If HPV is discussed during disclosure of an abnormal Pap smear, patient education should include information that places the risk of cervical cancer in perspective, including the commonality of HPV and the possibility that HPV infection is likely to resolve within a 2-year period, particularly among younger women. It is important for patients to understand that Pap smear testing remains the primary test of persistent or recurrent cervical disease, and that treatment decisions are made based on both Pap smear (cytology) and biopsy (pathology) results, not on isolated HPV DNA testing. Reassurance that cervical cancer is preventable when precancerous lesions are detected and treated is appropriate.

In 2006, the first vaccine designed to prevent HPV was approved by the FDA. The vaccine, Gardasil, is the first vaccine developed to prevent cervical cancer, precancerous genital lesions, and genital warts due to HPV. The vaccine is highly effective against four types of the HPV virus, including two (16 and 18) that cause about 70% of cervical cancers. The vaccine is currently recommended for women aged 11 to 26 but can be given to girls as young as 9. Gardasil is licensed as a three-dose series given at 0, 2, and 6 months. The vaccine is given intramuscularly in the deltoid muscle.[6]

HPV vaccine recipients who have not acquired HPV will get benefit from the vaccine. Women previously infected with one of the HPV types prevented by the vaccine will not benefit from that part of the vaccine but can still obtain protection from one of the other vaccine virus types. Ideally, the vaccine should be administered before the onset of sexual activity, but sexually active woman should still be vaccinated.

Because the presence of HPV, a sexually transmitted virus, combined with the fear of potential cervical cancer often produces considerable psychologic distress, it remains important to offer adequate counseling and information regarding the nature of HPV and abnormal Pap smears when giving abnormal Pap smear results to women. Women may express concerns about future fertility, the stigma of having exposure to a sexually transmitted virus, or how to appropriately talk about HPV with their partner or supportive others. They may be afraid of diagnostic or treatment procedures or may have misconceptions about HPV or about medical jargon often used to describe their condition. Extensive information or counseling can be obtained by referral to a women's health nurse practitioner, nurse, or physician with expertise in the management of abnormal Pap smears. Excellent resources for patient education and support regarding abnormal Pap smears and HPV include the Association of Reproductive Health Professionals, http://www.arhp.org; the American Social Health Association, http://www.ashastd.org; and the National Women's Health Resource Center, http://www.healthywomen.org.

HEALTH PROMOTION

Women should be advised to have regular Pap smear screening. Although condom use does not prevent transmission of HPV to the external genitals, it appears to afford protection against cervical HPV infection. Healthy lifestyle habits, including good nutrition and avoidance of smoking, should be encouraged.

REFERENCES

1. Wright TC, Cox JT, Massad LS, and others: 2001 Consensus guidelines for the management of women with cervical cytological abnormalities, *JAMA* 287(16):2120-2129, 2002.
2. Anhang R, Goodman A, Goldie S: HPV communication: review of existing research and recommendations for patient education, *CA: Cancer J Clin* 54:248-259, 2005.
3. American Cancer Society: *Surveillance research*, 2006, retrieved March 6, 2007, from http://www.seer.cancer.gov/cgi-bin/csr/1975_2003/search.pl#results.
4. Schiffman M, Castle PE: Human papillomavirus: epidemiology and public health, *Arch Pathol Lab Med* 127(8):930-1034, 2003.
5. Douglas JM, Stone KM, St. Louis ME, and others: *Prevention of genital HPV infection and sequelae: report of an external consultants' meeting*, Department of Health and Human Services, Centers for Disease Control and Prevention, Division of STD, 1999, retrieved March 7, 2007, from http://www.cdc.gov/nchstp/dstd/Reportspublications/99HPVReport.htm.
6. Immunization Action Coalition: *Ask the experts: human papillomavirus*, retrieved Feb 9, 2007, from http://www.immunize.org/catg.d/p2021q.htm.
7. US Preventive Services Task Force: *Guide to clinical preventive services*, ed 2, Washington, DC, 1996 with updates 2005, US Department of Health and Human Services, Office of Disease Prevention and Health Promotion, retrieved March 7, 2007, from http://www.ahrq.gov/clinic/pocketgd/gcps2.htm#Cervical.
8. Bertram CC: Evidence for practice: oral contraception and risk of cervical cancer, *J Am Acad Nurse Pract* 16(10):455-461, 2004.
9. Cox T, Buck HW, Kinney W, and others, editors: *Human papillomavirus and cervical cancer*, ARHP Clinical Proceedings, Washington, DC, March 2001, Association of Reproductive Health Professionals.
10. Stern PL, Stanley MA, editors: *Human papillomavirus and cervical cancer*, Oxford, 1994, Oxford Medical Publications.
11. ZurHausen H: Papillomavirus and cancer: from basic studies to clinical application, *Nature* 2:342-350, 2002.
12. Unger ER, Duarte-Franco E: Human papillomaviruses: into the new millennium, *Obstet Gynecol Clin* 28(4):653-666, 2001.
13. American Society for Colposcopy and Cervical Pathology: *Consensus guidelines for the management of women with abnormal cervical cytology, algorithms*, 2002, retrieved March 6, 2007, from http://www.guideline.gov/summary/summary.aspx?ss=15&doc_id=3286&nbr=2512.
14. Smith RA, Cokkinides V, Eyre HJ: *American Cancer Society guidelines for the early detection of cancer*, 2006, retrieved March 5, 2007, from http://www.caonline.amcancersoc.org/cgi/content/full/56/1/11.

CHAPTER 177

Pelvic Inflammatory Disease

Patricia Polgar Bailey

DEFINITION AND EPIDEMIOLOGY

Pelvic inflammatory disease (PID) refers to a spectrum of inflammatory disorders of the upper genital tract in women. It can include any combination of endometritis, salpingitis, tubo-ovarian abscess (TOA), and pelvic peritonitis.[1] Although acute signs and symptoms are often moderately severe, the long-term sequelae resulting from fallopian tube damage and scarring can be serious, including ectopic pregnancy, recurrent episodes of PID, chronic pelvic pain, and infertility.[2,3]

PID is the most common gynecologic reason for emergency department (ED) visits and hospitalizations in the United States, affecting more than 8% of all reproductive-age women and 11% of African-American reproductive-age women.[2,3] Although the number of PID-related ED visits and hospitalizations remains high, more than three fourths of women treated for PID in the United States are now treated as outpatients, a trend that has been increasing over the past 2 decades.[2] Based on research looking at trends in PID from 1985 to 2001, cases of PID (based on hospital discharges and estimated ambulatory cases) have decreased significantly, but the annual estimate of acute and unspecified PID cases diagnosed in the United States is greater than had previously been published.[3] Based on these data, clinically evident PID remains an important public health concern for women and health care providers, especially those working in outpatient settings.

Direct costs for care of acute PID and its sequelae are estimated at $2 billion yearly. Indirect costs related to PID, which include productivity loss and losses related to premature death, are much higher, at an estimated $10 billion yearly.[3] The high financial and social costs related to PID are important to consider if the full impact of this disease is to be appreciated.

Risk factors for PID include being younger than 25, having multiple sexual partners, not currently or consistently using contraception, and living in an area with a high prevalence of sexually transmitted diseases (STDs). There is a strong correlation between the incidence of STDs and PID in any given population. Other risk factors for PID include penetration of the cervical mucus barrier during medical procedures, including the insertion of an intrauterine contraceptive device, and vaginal douching. A woman's risk for PID is decreased if she uses barrier contraception, takes oral contraceptives, or has had a tubal sterilization.

The risk of PID in young women is significant; 75% of all cases of PID occur in women under the age of 25, and 20% of cases are in the adolescent age-group.[1,4] In 2003, almost half of all U.S. high school students had engaged in sexual intercourse, and 14.4% had four or more partners, making STDs a major public health problem for adolescents.[4] Contact with multiple sexual partners, inconsistent use of contraception, and biologic vulnerability can account for the increased incidence of STDs in women younger than 25, although it does not fully account for the increased incidence of PID. Younger women with chlamydial infections of the cervix have a higher incidence of upper genital tract infection than do older women.[5]

Previous diagnosis of PID is a risk factor for subsequent episodes, with approximately 15% to 25% of all women with PID experiencing more than one episode.[5] These subsequent infections are generally new, primary attacks of PID, not flares of latent or chronic infection.[5] Reinfection is often related to contact with untreated sexual partners. In addition, one third of women with PID will suffer from chronic pelvic pain.[6]

PATHOPHYSIOLOGY

PID is usually a polymicrobial infection, caused by organisms that ascend from the vagina and cervix along the mucosa of the endometrium to infect the mucosa of the fallopian tubes. The most common organisms implicated in PID (one third to three quarters of cases) include *Neisseria gonorrhoeae* and *Chlamydia trachomatis;* however, microorganisms that can be part of the normal vaginal flora (e.g., anaerobes, *Gardnerella vaginalis, Haemophilus influenzae,* enteric gram-negative rods, and *Streptococcus agalactiae*) can also cause PID.[1,2] *Mycoplasma hominis* and *Ureaplasma urealyticum* are also possible etiologic agents.[1] The mildest form of salpingitis involves tubal hyperemia, edema of the tubal wall, and exudate on the tubal surface and fimbriated ends.[7] If salpingitis is left untreated, further inflammatory changes of the pelvic organs occur, including tubal adhesions, pyosalpinx, or TOA.

The Fitz-Hugh–Curtis syndrome (FHCS) involves perihepatic inflammation that is due to the transperitoneal, lymphatic, or vascular spread of *N. gonorrhoeae* or *C. trachomatis.* There is inflammation of the liver capsule without parenchymal involvement.[7] FHCS develops in 5% to 10% of women with PID.[5] Chronic FHCS is characterized by adhesions between the anterior liver surface and the parietal peritoneum beneath the diaphragm. The treatment is the same as for PID.

The increased incidence of PID in young women may be explained by a larger cervical squamocolumnar junction, allowing for easier colonization with *N. gonorrhoeae* or *C. trachomatis,* and by a decreased antibody response.[5] However, PID is uncommon in pregnancy because of the physiologic changes in the uterus. The uterotubal junction is closed as early as the seventh week of gestation, and the chorioamnion covers the endocervix around the twelfth to fifteenth week. An ascending infection before the twelfth week often leads to endometritis and spontaneous abortion. After the twelfth week, it results primarily in chorioamnionitis.

Rarely, PID can result from secondary extension of infection of adjacent organs, as in appendicitis or diverticulitis. It may also result from hematogenous dissemination of tuberculosis or as a rare complication of a tropical disease such as schistosomiasis. The following discussion refers only to ascending infections resulting in PID.

CLINICAL PRESENTATION

The clinical presentation of PID varies widely. Although some women are truly asymptomatic, others remain undiagnosed because of their mild or nonspecific signs and symptoms.

These can include abnormal vaginal bleeding, dyspareunia, and vaginal discharge. Lower abdominal and pelvic pain of less than 2 weeks' duration is the most common presenting symptom. It is usually described as dull and constant and is worsened by movement and sexual intercourse. The onset of symptoms occurs most commonly in the first half of the menstrual cycle. Complaints of fever or abnormal vaginal discharge may also be present.

PID caused by gonococci is usually associated with a more intense inflammatory reaction in the tubal lumen than the reaction caused by chlamydial infection. Therefore the woman with a gonococcal PID may have a more acute presentation, often requiring hospitalization. It is estimated that 15% of women with *N. gonorrhoeae* show signs of acute PID, compared with 10% with chlamydia-related cervicitis.[3]

Women with FHCS are initially seen with right upper quadrant pain, pleuritic pain, and tenderness on liver palpation. These symptoms are often mistaken for cholecystitis or pneumonia.

PHYSICAL EXAMINATION

The clinical diagnosis of acute PID is imprecise, and no single history, physical, or laboratory finding is both sensitive and specific for the diagnosis of acute PID. According to the Centers for Disease Control and Prevention (CDC), the following three minimum clinical criteria for PID must be met before antibiotic therapy should be initiated: (1) lower abdominal tenderness, (2) adnexal tenderness, and (3) cervical motion tenderness. In addition, no other cause for the illness should be evident (e.g., diverticulitis, ectopic pregnancy, or appendicitis). The following additional criteria support a diagnosis of PID:

- Oral temperature over 38.3° C (101° F)
- Abnormal cervical or vaginal mucopurulent discharge
- Presence of white blood cells (WBCs) on saline microscopy of vaginal secretions
- Elevated erythrocyte sedimentation rate
- Elevated C-reactive protein
- Laboratory documentation of cervical infection with *N. gonorrhoeae* or *C. trachomatis*

Most women with PID have either mucopurulent cervical discharge or WBCs on microscopic evaluation of vaginal fluid. If the cervical discharge appears normal and no WBCs appear on the wet mount, the diagnosis of PID is unlikely.[1]

DIAGNOSTICS

Acute PID is difficult to diagnose because of the wide variation in signs and symptoms. The clinical diagnosis of symptomatic PID has a positive predictive value for salpingitis of 65% to 90% of what is predicted with laparoscopy.[1] A pregnancy test should be obtained immediately to assess for the possibility of ectopic pregnancy, although a negative result is not conclusive. Pelvic ultrasound evaluation is indicated when TOA is suspected. Additional studies to consider include syphilis (rapid plasma reagin) and HIV serologic studies. PID can be diagnosed clinically and empiric therapy initiated based on some of the findings listed above. However, a diagnostic evaluation that includes some more extensive diagnostic studies may be necessary if the diagnosis is unclear.

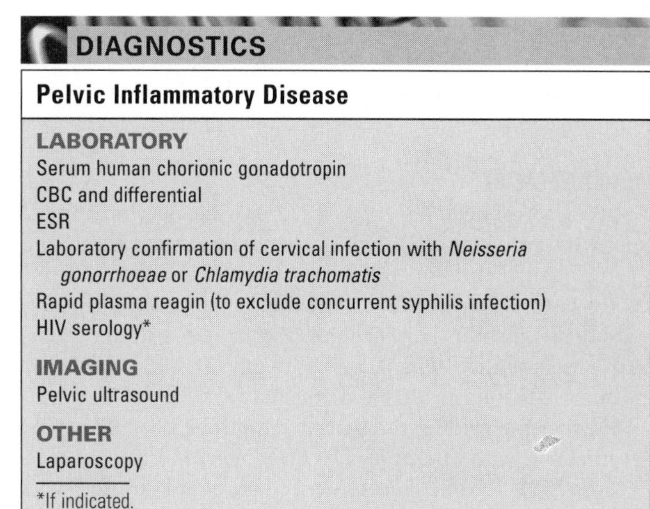

DIAGNOSTICS

Pelvic Inflammatory Disease

LABORATORY

Serum human chorionic gonadotropin
CBC and differential
ESR
Laboratory confirmation of cervical infection with *Neisseria gonorrhoeae* or *Chlamydia trachomatis*
Rapid plasma reagin (to exclude concurrent syphilis infection)
HIV serology*

IMAGING

Pelvic ultrasound

OTHER

Laparoscopy

*If indicated.

The most specific criteria for diagnosing PID include[1]:

- Endometrial biopsy with histopathologic evidence of endometritis
- Transvaginal sonography or MRI techniques showing thickened, fluid-filled tubes with or without free pelvic fluid or tubo-ovarian complex
- Laparoscopic abnormalities consistent with PID

An accurate diagnosis of PID is difficult, given the wide variation in symptoms on presentation. However, the potential damage to the reproductive health of women with even mild or atypical PID is well documented.[1] Diagnosis and management of other causes of lower abdominal pain are unlikely to be affected by the initiation of empiric therapy for PID.

DIFFERENTIAL DIAGNOSIS

The most important conditions in the differential diagnosis for PID are ectopic pregnancy, acute appendicitis, ovarian torsion, and ovarian cyst. Other conditions to consider include endometriosis, corpus luteum bleeding, pelvic adhesions, benign ovarian tumor, irritable bowel syndrome (IBS), diverticulitis, pyelonephritis, and cystitis.

It is well recognized that women with IBS often are seen in gynecology practices, since both IBS and PID can give rise to lower abdominal pain. A study comparing the symptomatology of IBS with that of laparoscopically confirmed PID and endometriosis found that, in patients seen with lower abdominal pain, the presence of concomitant gastrointestinal symptoms, such as bowel symptoms, was more consistent with a gastrointestinal disorder such as IBS than with gynecologic disease.[8] Since IBS affects 15% of the population, it is important to consider that a significant percentage of

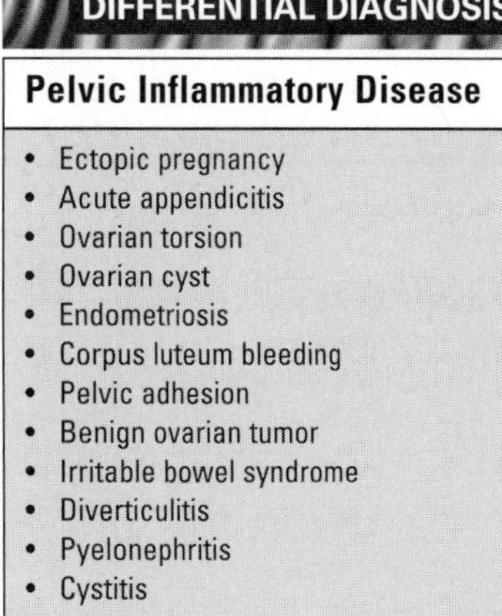

DIFFERENTIAL DIAGNOSIS

Pelvic Inflammatory Disease

- Ectopic pregnancy
- Acute appendicitis
- Ovarian torsion
- Ovarian cyst
- Endometriosis
- Corpus luteum bleeding
- Pelvic adhesion
- Benign ovarian tumor
- Irritable bowel syndrome
- Diverticulitis
- Pyelonephritis
- Cystitis

women may have co-existing PID and gastrointestinal disease. For example, in the study cited above, 30% of women with gynecologic pathologic conditions also had symptoms suggestive of IBS.[8]

MANAGEMENT

Treatment regimens for PID must provide empiric, broad-spectrum antimicrobial coverage, including anaerobic coverage. No single antibiotic agent is adequate; thus combination therapy is necessary. In choosing a therapy, the provider should consider availability, cost, patient acceptance, and antimicrobial susceptibility. The CDC provides periodic treatment recommendations for PID and other STDs.

Estimates regarding the percentage of cases of PID caused by infection with *C. trachomatis* or *N. gonorrhoeae* vary from 16% to 75%.[2] Nonetheless, most women are treated with antibiotics directed toward these bacteria.[9] However, in a recent study of women with clinically suspected PID, gram-negative and anaerobic gram-positive bacteria were also isolated and strongly associated with endometriosis.[9] For this reason, it has been recommended that all women with PID be treated with medication regimens that include metronidazole. This approach may reduce some of the frequency of potential PID sequelae, including recurrent PID, ectopic pregnancy, chronic pelvic pain, and infertility. Current guidelines from the CDC for treatment of PID include the addition of metronidazole for full coverage against anaerobes and bacterial vaginosis.[9]

Oral and parenteral therapy for PID is outlined in Box 177-1.[1] Patients receiving oral therapy should be reevaluated within 72 hours. Clinical improvement is indicated by defervescence; reduction in direct or rebound abdominal tenderness; and reduction in uterine, adnexal, and cervical motion tenderness. If significant clinical improvement is not seen within 72 hours after initiating therapy, the patient should be reevaluated to confirm the diagnosis and initiate parenteral

BOX 177-1

ORAL AND PARENTERAL THERAPY FOR PELVIC INFLAMMATORY DISEASE

PARENTERAL REGIMEN A

Cefotetan 2 g IV q 12 hr *or*
Cefoxitin 2 g IV q 6 hr
plus
Doxycycline 100 mg PO or IV q 12 hr

NOTE: Because of pain associated with infusion, doxycycline should be administered orally when possible, even when the patient is hospitalized. Both oral and IV administrations of doxycycline provide similar bioavailability.

Parenteral therapy may be discontinued 24 hours after a patient improves clinically, and oral therapy with doxycycline (100 mg b.i.d.) should continue to complete 14 days of therapy. When tubo-ovarian abscess is present, many health care providers use clindamycin or metronidazole with doxycycline for continued therapy rather than doxycycline alone because the combination provides more effective anaerobic coverage.

PARENTERAL REGIMEN B

Clindamycin 900 mg IV q 8 hr
plus
Gentamicin loading dose IV or IM (2 mg/kg of body weight) followed by a maintenance dose (1.5 mg/kg) q 8 hr. Single daily dosing may be substituted.

NOTE: Parenteral therapy can be discontinued 24 hours after a patient improves clinically; continuing oral therapy should consist of doxycycline 100 mg PO b.i.d. or clindamycin 450 mg PO q.i.d. to complete a total of 14 days of therapy. When tubo-ovarian abscess is present, clindamycin may be preferable to doxycycline because clindamycin provides more anaerobic coverage.

ALTERNATIVE PARENTERAL REGIMENS

Levofloxacin 500 mg IV q day* *or*
Ofloxacin 400 mg IV q 12 hr*
with or without
Metronidazole 500 mg IV q 8 hr *or*
Ampicillin-sulbactam 3 g IV q 6 hr
plus
Doxycycline 100 mg orally or IV q 12 hr

NOTE: Levofloxacin is as effective as ofloxacin and may be substituted; its single daily dosing makes it advantageous from a compliance perspective. Ampicillin-sulbactam plus doxycycline has good coverage against *Chlamydia trachomatis, Neisseria gonorrhoeae,* and anaerobes and is effective for patients who have tubo-ovarian abscess.

ORAL REGIMEN A

Levofloxacin 500 mg PO q day for 14 days* *or*
Ofloxacin 400 mg PO b.i.d. for 14 days*
with or without
Metronidazole 500 mg PO b.i.d. for 14 days

ORAL REGIMEN B

Ceftriaxone 250 mg IM in a single dose *or*
Cefoxitin 2 g IM in a single dose and probenecid 1 g PO administered concurrently in a single dose *or*
Other parenteral third-generation cephalosporin (e.g., ceftizoxime or cefotaxime)
plus
Doxycycline 100 mg PO b.i.d. for 14 days
plus
Metronidazole 500 mg PO b.i.d. for 14 days

NOTE: The optimum choice of a cephalosporin for regimen B is unclear; although cefoxitin has better anaerobic coverage, ceftriaxone has better coverage against *N. gonorrhoeae.* Clinical trials have demonstrated that a single dose of cefoxitin is effective in obtaining short-term clinical response in women who have PID; however, the theoretic limitations in its coverage of anaerobes may require the addition of metronidazole to the treatment regimen. Metronidazole also will effectively treat bacterial vaginosis, which is often associated with PID.

ALTERNATIVE ORAL REGIMENS

There are data to suggest that amoxicillin-clavulanate plus doxycycline is effective in obtaining short-term clinical response; however, gastrointestinal symptoms might limit compliance with this regimen.

From Centers for Disease Control and Prevention: 2006 Sexually transmitted diseases treatment guidelines, *MMWR* 55(RR-11):1-100, 2006.

*Quinolones should not be used in persons with a history of recent foreign travel or partner's travel, infections acquired in California or Hawaii, or infections acquired in other areas with increased quinolone-resistant *Neisseria gonorrhoeae* (QRNG) prevalence.

therapy and/or surgical intervention. Patients should be tested for cure of infection with *C. trachomatis* and *N. gonorrhoeae* 4 to 6 weeks after the completion of therapy.

Patients receiving parenteral therapy should show substantial improvement within 72 hours after therapy is initiated. Those who do not receive parenteral therapy usually require further diagnostic evaluation or surgical intervention.

Since the trend has been toward outpatient treatment for PID, concerns have been raised that outpatient treatment may be less effective than inpatient treatment at preventing some of the complications of PID, such as recurrent PID or infertility. However, studies comparing the inpatient and outpatient treatment regimens of the CDC have found no differences between inpatient and outpatient treatment groups in the rates of pregnancy, time to pregnancy, recurrence of PID, chronic pelvic pain, or ectopic pregnancy among women with mild to moderate PID.[10] In at least one subsequent study comparing the effectiveness of inpatient and outpatient treatments among women with suspected PID, ectopic pregnancy was found to occur rarely and more frequently in the outpatient group, but this difference was not significant.[6] Currently, the CDC recommends hospitalizing women based on health care provider discretion and in certain situations (see Indications for Referral or Hospitalization).

Despite documented effective outpatient care for PID, recent studies have demonstrated that adolescents treated in outpatient settings, specifically academic pediatric ambulatory care settings and the ED, do not consistently receive adequate evaluations, medications, and self-care instructions at discharge.[11,12] For example, treatment for adolescents with PID was fully compliant with CDC guidelines in only 35% of cases, and adolescents tended not to be admitted to the hospital at the recommended time. In one recent study, 40% of the adolescent girls treated in the ED did not have either health insurance or an identified primary provider or medical home for follow-up care.[11] This is particularly problematic, since one of the premises of outpatient PID management is that patients have follow-up within 48 to 72 hours. Given the significant risk of future health problems associated with PID, efforts to adhere to recommended practice guidelines and ensure patient adherence to care are critical in this high-risk population.

Treatment of sexual partners of women with PID is imperative because of the risk for re-infection of the patient and the high incidence of urethral gonococcal or chlamydial infections in the male sexual partner. Partners who had sexual contact with the patient during the 60 days preceding the onset of symptoms should be treated empirically with regimens effective against *C. trachomatis* and *N. gonorrhoeae*, regardless of the apparent etiology of PID or pathogens isolated from the patient.[1] Sexual abstinence should be recommended until both partners have completed treatment.

COMPLICATIONS

Sequelae of PID include a significantly increased risk of tubal factor infertility, ectopic pregnancy, and chronic pelvic pain. A small number of deaths annually result from a ruptured TOA. Furthermore, the duration, severity, and number of episodes of PID are proportional to the prevalence of long-term sequelae.

INDICATIONS FOR REFERRAL OR HOSPITALIZATION

Referral for hospitalization of the patient with PID is indicated if:

- Surgical emergencies, such as appendicitis or ectopic pregnancy, cannot be excluded.
- The patient is pregnant.
- The patient has failed to respond clinically to outpatient therapy.
- The patient is unable to follow or tolerate an outpatient regimen.
- The patient has severe illness, nausea and vomiting, or a high fever.
- The patient has a TOA.
- The patient is immunodeficient (e.g., HIV-positive with a low CD4 count or receiving immunosuppressive therapy).

In early observational studies, HIV-infected women with PID were more likely to require surgical intervention.[1] A subsequent and more comprehensive study showed that despite a more severe clinical presentation, HIV-infected women with PID responded equally well to standard parenteral therapies.[1]

Gynecologic or surgical consultation is indicated when the diagnosis is unclear. Unilateral pelvic pain or a mass is a strong indication for laparoscopy.

PATIENT AND FAMILY EDUCATION

Patient education is an extremely important component in the treatment of the woman with PID. It must include clear information regarding the diagnosis, including transmission and sequelae. The need for completion of therapy regardless of symptoms, timely follow-up, and partner treatment cannot be overemphasized. It is also helpful to encourage the patient in appropriate medical care–seeking behavior, including seeking care immediately when symptoms recur. The behaviors that increase the risk of PID also increase the risk for HIV infection. Rates of recurrent PID, chronic pelvic pain, and infertility have been shown to be highest among nonpersistent condom users.[13] Referral for HIV testing and counseling is recommended. Finally, information regarding prevention of future infections must be reviewed and repeated at all follow-up visits.

REFERENCES

1. Centers for Disease Control and Prevention: 2006 Sexually transmitted diseases treatment guidelines, *MMWR* 55(RR-11):1-100, 2006.
2. Ness R, Trautmann G, Richter H, and others: Effectiveness of treatment strategies of some women with pelvic inflammatory disease, *Obstet Gynecol* 106(3):573-580, 2005.
3. Sutton M, Sternberg M, Zaidi A, and others: Trends in pelvic inflammatory disease hospital discharges and ambulatory visits, United States, 1985-2001, *Sexually Trans Dis* 32(12):778-784, 2005.
4. Centers for Disease Control and Prevention: Youth risk behavior surveillance—United States, 2003, *MMWR* 53(SS-4):19-22, 2004.
5. Mishell DR, Droegemueller W: *Comprehensive gynecology*, ed 3, St Louis, 1997, Mosby.
6. Haggerty C, Peipert J, Weitzen S, and others: Predictors of chronic pelvic pain in an urban population of women with symptoms and signs of pelvic inflammatory disease, *Sexually Trans Dis* 32(5):293-299, 2005.
7. Soper DE: Pelvic inflammatory disease. In Rock JA, Faro S, Gant NF, and others, editors: *Advances in obstetrics and gynecology*, vol 1, St Louis, 1994, Mosby.

8. Lea R, Bancroft K, Whorwell P: Irritable bowel syndrome, chronic pelvic inflammatory disease and endometriosis: a comparison of symptomatology, *Eur J Gastroenterol Hepatol* 16:1269-1272, 2004.
9. Haggerty C, Hillier S, Bass D, and others: Bacterial vaginosis and anaerobic bacteria are associated with endometriosis, *Clin Infect Dis* 39:990-995, 2004.
10. Ness RB, Soper DE, Holley RL, and others: Effectiveness of inpatient and outpatient treatment strategies for women with pelvic inflammatory disease: results from the Pelvic Inflammatory Disease Evaluation and Clinical Health (PEACH) randomized trial, *Am J Obstet Gynecol* 186:929-937, 2002.
11. Trent M, Ellen J, Walker A: Pelvic inflammatory disease in adolescents, *Pediatr Emerg Care* 21(7):431-436, 2005.
12. Beckman KR, Melzer-Lange MD, Gorelick MH: Emergency department management of sexually transmitted infections in US adolescents: results from the National Hospital Ambulatory Medical Care Survey, *Ann Emerg Med* 43(3):333-338, 2004.
13. Ness R, Randall H, Richter H, and others: Condom use and the risk of recurrent pelvic inflammatory disease, chronic pelvic pain or infertility following an episode of pelvic inflammatory disease, *Am J Pub Health* 94(8):1327-1330, 2004.

CHAPTER 178

Preconception Care

Debra Hobbins

DEFINITION AND EPIDEMIOLOGY

Preconception care has been proposed as an innovative, preventive strategy of identifying and modifying a woman's risks or behaviors through appropriate education, management, or referral to increase the proportion of intended pregnancies, reduce reproductive risks before conception, improve the mother's long-term health, and decrease rates of both maternal and infant morbidity and mortality.[1-3] It is estimated that 40% to 60% of all births are unintended at conception, with 95% teen pregnancies unplanned. For the past 80 years the two leading causes of infant mortality in the United States have been congenital malformations and disorders related to short gestation and low birth weight. These statistics emphasize the need to incorporate preconceptional health promotion into each encounter, with every reproductive-age woman, at an age-appropriate level, in whatever setting she may be seen.[4-9] The critical phase of organogenesis occurs during days 17 to 56 after conception—before most women know they are pregnant.[10] Optimum prenatal care is initiated through preconceptional health promotion.

Traditionally, women's health care has been segmented, with childbearing separated from women's overall health promotion and management of chronic health issues. Pregnancy has been viewed as a discrete event, with little relationship to a woman's health before or after. The paradigm is shifting! Nursing has long promoted the concept of integrated health care for women, of which preconceptional health promotion is a critical element. Integrated health care for women recognizes that women receive care on a continuum, from menarche through menopause, and that links exist between childbearing and a woman's health across her life span.[11] Research indicates that much of what happens during pregnancy has implications for the later life of the woman, her immediate offspring, and her descendents for generations to come.[12]

PARTNER INVOLVEMENT

Partner involvement in preconceptional health promotion contributes to the couple's emotional well-being; is important for family, genetic, and psychosocial histories; and provides an opportunity to educate the woman and her partner equally about the potential influences of their lifestyle and health status on a future pregnancy.[13-15] Smoking and alcohol use by the father are implicated in low birth weight and subfertility. Advanced paternal age is associated with autosomal dominant disease caused by new single-gene mutations, such as neurofibromatosis; X-linked diseases; and disorders of nondisjunction, such as Down's syndrome (trisomy 21). Paternal chemical or substance exposures may contribute to adverse reproductive outcomes and affect the maternal environment, contributing to subfertility or infertility, spontaneous abortion, and low birth weight.[16] Partner promiscuity, IV drug use, or bisexuality puts the woman and fetus at risk for all sexually transmitted diseases.[1,17,18] It is critical to speak to the woman alone about her reproductive, sexually transmitted disease, and abuse history.

The partner of a lesbian should be involved, when requested, in discussions about health care, especially pregnancy and childbirth. Between 2% and 23% of all women are lesbians, with 30% having experienced pregnancy and 16% having birthed children.[19] Increasing numbers of lesbian couples are choosing to bear children, with two related issues most pronounced: finding a lesbian-sensitive health care provider and deciding how to conceive.[20]

HEALTH ASSESSMENT AND INTERVENTIONS

Maternal Health and Risks

Advanced maternal age is becoming more common. Women older than 35 years are at increased risk for subfertility because of medical illness, premature menopause, anovulation and endometriosis, chromosome abnormalities, chronic illness, pregnancy complications, cesarean birth, and fetal death.[21,22] Teenage mothers have an increased risk of low-birth-weight infants, preterm infants, infants who die at birth, and infants who die before 1 year of age.[23]

There is current evidence linking maternal birth weight with the subsequent development of ischemic heart disease, hypertension, and diabetes.[24] However, women who have given birth to infants weighing less than 2500 g (5.5 pounds), when compared with women whose babies weighed more than 3500 g (7.7 pounds), were at significantly greater risk of death from ischemic heart disease. Women who were small for gestational age (SGA) are at increased risk for birthing infants who are SGA, and the daughters of these women are at increased risk for continuing the pattern and having infants who are SGA. Women who weighed 3625 g (8 pounds) or more at birth are at increased risk for birthing babies weighing more than 4000 g (8.8 pounds). Fathers of low-birth-weight babies are at increased risk of coronary heart disease, hypertension, and diabetes.[24,25]

The provider needs to determine the woman's underweight or overweight status, eating disorders, pica, and vegetarian eating habits. Neural tube defects (NTDs) occur in the first 17 to 30 days after conception.[26] Obesity at conception is linked to an increased risk of birth defects[27]; NTDs, independent of folic acid intake; difficulty conceiving; and pregnancy complications such as gestational diabetes, thrombophlebitis, hypertension, preterm birth, induction of labor, prolonged labor, difficult birth, and emergent cesarean birth. In addition, obese women have two to five times the risk of pregnancy-related mortality than women of normal weight.[28,29] Infants born to overweight women are predisposed to obesity later in life. Women who are underweight at conception are at an increased risk for preterm and low-birth-weight infants.[7,30,31]

In a woman with significant medical problems, the provider must assess the potential risk to the woman and her fetus (Box 178-1). This is especially necessary if the woman's life expectancy could be markedly reduced by pregnancy or if the fetus could have a high likelihood of complications. Maternal conditions that pose this risk include congenital heart disease, Marfan's syndrome, cardiomyopathy, renal insufficiency, coarctation of the aorta, and hypertension.[14,32] Diabetic teratogenesis is related to first-trimester hyperglycemia.[33] Women with diabetes need to be educated about the importance of developing and continuing good general health practices and maintaining optimum glycemic control before conception and throughout pregnancy. Glycosylated hemoglobin (HbA_{1c}) is an excellent marker of glycemic control for the prior 6 weeks. Because only one third of women with diabetes seek preconceptional care, contraceptive management and preconceptional health promotion should occur at each visit.[34,35]

Chronic illnesses need to be under control before conception[14,15,18] (see Box 178-1). Exposure or immunity to infectious diseases, including sexually transmitted diseases, needs to be investigated; strategies to treat these diseases or to minimize the risks should be discussed with the couple[4,11,15,36] (Box 178-2; see also Box 178-1).

Hyperthermia and temperatures of greater than 38.8° C (102° F) during the first weeks of pregnancy have been associated with NTDs.[18] Factors that have contributed to previous poor pregnancy outcomes or that could affect future pregnancies and may be amenable to intervention are identified before conception[37] (see Box 178-1). A list of both prescription and over-the-counter drugs, including homeopathic remedies, should be obtained from the couple. Couples must be informed about medications with teratogenic potential (see Box 178-1) to enable them to plan carefully for pregnancy. The woman may be able to modify, substitute, or eliminate these drugs before conception.[36]

Reproductive and Family History

Elements of a woman's reproductive history, such as number, dates, outcomes of prior pregnancies, and infant weight and method of birth, are important to identify as factors that may have contributed to earlier poor pregnancy outcomes but may be amenable to intervention.[38] Interpregnancy intervals of less than 17 months and more than 59 months have been associated with increased risk for low-birth-weight, preterm, and SGA infants.[39]

All individuals are estimated to carry five to seven lethal recessive genes.[40] Preconceptional education regarding genetic conditions provides the couple with information for understanding the opportunities for antenatal diagnosis, its limitations, and the risks involved. The couple can use this information to consider their reproductive options and to make knowledge-based decisions about the reproductive risks they are willing to take or whether they should avoid a pregnancy.[1,41] Questioning all couples about personal or family histories of birth defects, mental retardation, consanguinity, and genetic diseases is critical.[7,41] Ethnic background has also emerged as a component of genetic screening[1,14,23] (see Box 178-1).

Socioeconomic Factors

Housing, home environment, family and social support, and safety need to be addressed. It is estimated that 17% to 37% of pregnant women experience domestic abuse; this abuse is more common than gestational diabetes, hypertension, and birth defects.[42] Victims of domestic abuse are at increased risk

BOX 178-1

HEALTH ASSESSMENT: HISTORY

DEMOGRAPHICS
- Age less than 15 or over 35 years
- Birth weight

FAMILY HISTORY
- Birth defects
- Consanguinity
- Cystic fibrosis
- Down's syndrome
- Duchenne's muscular dystrophy
- Fragile X syndrome
- Hemoglobinopathies
- Hemophilia
- Mental retardation
- Phenylketonuria
- Sickle cell disease
- Tay-Sachs disease

ETHNIC BACKGROUND: CARRIER TESTING
- α-Thalassemia: African, Southeast Asian, Filipino
- β-Thalassemia: African, Mediterranean, Southeast Asian, Indo-Pakistani, Asian, African American
- Cystic fibrosis: Caucasian
- Sickle cell anemia: African, African American, Middle Eastern, Indo-Pakistani, Latino, Mediterranean
- Tay-Sachs disease: Ashkenazi Jew, French Canadian, Cajun

SOCIAL HISTORY
- Alcohol and tobacco use
- Cultural beliefs and issues
- Employment
- Family and social support
- Financial concerns
- Home environment and safety
- Housing
- Life stresses
- Violence

NUTRITION HISTORY
- Anorexia, bulimia, pica
- Body mass index
- Caffeine intake
- Diet and supplements
- Exercise
- Folic acid
- Vitamin D
- Weight for height

MEDICAL HISTORY
- Anemia
- Asthma
- Chronic hypertension
- Depression
- Diabetes
- Heart disease
- Marfan's syndrome
- Pulmonary hypertension
- Recurrent urinary tract infections
- Renal disease
- Seizure disorder
- Surgery, trauma
- Cancer
- Systemic lupus erythematosus, autoimmune disease
- Thromboembolic disease
- Thyroid disease
- Tuberculosis
- Visual impairment

INFECTIOUS DISEASE HISTORY
- Immunization status
- Cytomegalovirus
- Hepatitis B
- Hepatitis C (particularly IV drug users)
- Human parvovirus B19 (fifth disease)
- Listeriosis
- Rubella, proven immunity
- Toxoplasmosis, outdoor cat
- Tuberculosis
- Varicella-zoster

SEXUALLY TRANSMITTED DISEASES
- Chlamydia
- Gonorrhea
- Hepatitis B
- Herpes simplex virus
- HIV/AIDS
- Human papillomavirus
- Syphilis

TOXIC EXPOSURES
- Alcohol
- Recreational or IV drugs
- Hyperthermia
- Illegal substances, drug abuse
- Tobacco
- Home: oven cleaners, paint, bleach, wood finishing items, well water, methyl mercury (fish)
- Work: pesticides, cytotoxics, heavy metals, gases, ethylene oxide, polychlorinated biphenyls, solvents, vinyl chloride, radiation, vibrating machines, persistent organic pollutants

REPRODUCTIVE HISTORY
- Birth of child less than 2500 g (5.5 pounds) or more than 4080 g (9 pounds)
- Birth-related complications
- Cervical abnormality
- Cesarean birth
- Contraceptive method
- Diethylstilbestrol exposure
- Gestational diabetes
- Menstrual dysfunction
- NICU or neonatal death
- Pelvic infections
- Preeclampsia
- Preterm birth
- Previous child with birth defect
- Prior fetal losses
- Subfertility
- Uterine malformations

BOX 178-1

HEALTH ASSESSMENT: HISTORY—CONT'D

MEDICATION HISTORY

Prescription Teratogens

- Androgenic steroids
- Angiotensin-converting enzyme inhibitors
- Carbamazepine (Tegretol)
- Cytotoxics
- Diuretics
- Divalproex sodium, valproic acid (Depakote)
- Etretinate (Tegison)*
- Fluoxetine (Prozac)
- Gold
- Hormonal contraceptives
- Isotretinoin (Accutane)
- Lithium
- Paroxetine (Paxil)
- Phenobarbital
- Phenytoin (Dilantin)
- Primidone
- Trimethadione (Tridione, Trimedone)*
- Warfarin (Coumadin)

Over-the-Counter Teratogens

- Aspirin
- Ibuprofen
- Loratadine
- Teas
- Vitamin A (>10,000 IU/day)

*No longer available in the United States.

BOX 178-2

INTEGRATED HEALTH CARE FOR WOMEN: PHYSICAL EXAMINATION AND LABORATORY TESTS

PHYSICAL EXAMINATION

In All Patients

- Height
- Weight
- Blood pressure
- Pulse
- Thyroid examination
- Cardiac examination
- Respiratory examination
- Breast examination
- Pelvic examination
- Pelvimetry

As Indicated

- Ophthalmoscopic
- Neurologic
- Lower extremities

LABORATORY TESTS

In All Patients

- Blood type, Rh factor
- Antibody titer (direct Coombs' test)
- Hemoglobin, hematocrit
- Rubella titer
- Syphilis (rapid plasma reagin)
- Dipstick or urinalysis
- Culture and sensitivity (asymptomatic bacteriuria)
- Pap test
- Chlamydia
- Gonorrhea
- Wet mount of vaginal discharge (bacterial vaginosis)
- Hepatitis B surface antigen
- HIV

As Indicated

- Cytomegalovirus titer
- Drug screen
- Genetic testing
- Glycosylated hemoglobin (HbA_{1c})
- Hemoglobin electrophoresis
- Hepatitis C antibodies
- Herpes simplex
- Lead level
- Thyroid function studies
- Toxicology screen
- Toxoplasma titer
- Tuberculosis (purified protein derivative)
- Varicella-zoster titer

for placental separation; perinatal hemorrhage; rupture of the uterus, liver, or spleen; and preterm birth.[14] Screening for domestic violence must be incorporated into a routine history taking (see Chapter 24).[43] Cultural and extended family issues surrounding childbearing deserve exploration and may alert the health care provider to potential marital problems, parenting issues, beliefs of grandparents, and influences that may affect the woman's psychosocial situation.

Employment and financial concerns need to be discussed preconceptionally. Long work hours, work-related stress, strenuous physical work, and prolonged standing contribute to preterm births.[44] Ascertaining the nature of employment provides clues about exposure to environmental toxins and work hazards. Toxic exposures may result in infertility, spontaneous abortions, or congenital malformations in offspring. The toxic, mutagenic, teratogenic, and carcinogenic effects may not become apparent until childhood or adulthood in the form of behavioral disorders and neoplasms.[45,46]

Pregnancy and childbirth are often the first major medical expenses that couples incur, and these costs are often underestimated. It is critical that the health care provider initiate dialogue regarding childbearing costs, insurance coverage, and family leave policies.[1,14,15]

Substance Abuse

Fetal alcohol syndrome is more prevalent than both Down's syndrome and spina bifida and is the leading cause of mental retardation. Because alcohol is a known teratogen and no amount has been proved safe, many health care providers advocate alcohol abstinence during attempts for conception and during pregnancy.[14,23] Alcohol use is associated with stillbirth, low birth weight, and spontaneous abortion.

Smoking, the leading preventable cause of low birth weight, increases the risk of spontaneous abortion, preterm labor, upper respiratory tract infections in infants, and deaths from sudden infant death syndrome.[47]

Recreational and IV drug use carries an overall increased risk of nutritional deficiencies. Marijuana use may contribute to low birth weight, preterm birth, and congenital malformations.[1,9] Cocaine or crack use can lead to placental abruption, preterm birth, intrauterine growth restriction, congenital malformations, and dysfunction of the central nervous system in newborns; heroin or methadone use can cause neonatal withdrawal syndrome.[1,9,15,23] In addition, IV drug use increases the risks for infection with HIV, hepatitis viruses B and C, and skin abscesses.[15,23]

Limiting caffeine to 300 mg/day (the amount in 2 cups of coffee) is recommended.[14]

HEALTH PROMOTION

Every woman capable of becoming pregnant should consume 0.4 mg/day of folic acid to reduce the risk of NTDs and orofacial clefts in offspring.[48-50] Risk of NTDs can be reduced by 50% to 85% with maternal folic acid intake. Folic acid is now added to all enriched cereal grain products.[51] Folic acid supplements provide greater elevation in serum folate levels than dietary food intake.[52] Women who have birthed a fetus affected by an NTD should consume 4.0 mg/day. Green tea has been implicated in causing NTDs; women double their risk for an NTD in their fetus if they consume one or two cups of tea per day within 3 months of conception and during the first trimester.[53]

Supplements of elemental iron, 30 to 60 mg/day, are appropriate for women with anemia.[54] Prenatal vitamins are often prescribed preconceptionally because of the difficulty of determining a patient's nutritional status. However, their routine use is not recommended.[55,56] Research suggests that periconceptional ingestion of folic acid–containing multivitamin supplements reduces the occurrence of the first NTD, urinary tract and cardiovascular congenital abnormalities, and congenital limb deficiencies more than does folic acid alone.[57] Health promotion education should also include healthy nutrition, regular exercise, and adequate sleep.

Preconceptional health promotion seeks to improve health outcomes for the woman, her offspring, and future generations by identifying risks, providing education to facilitate knowledge-based decision making, and instituting appropriate interventions (Box 178-3).

BOX 178-3

PERICONCEPTIONAL COUNSELING AND INTERVENTIONS

EDUCATION

- Menstrual cycle and calendar
- Fertile period, sexuality
- Plans for childbearing
- Family planning methods
- Discontinuing method
- Intercourse frequency and timing
- Subfertility evaluation if no conception after 12 months (or 6 months if older than 37 years)
- Control of chronic illness
- Medication changes as indicated
- Risk factors for sexually transmitted diseases, pelvic inflammatory disease
- Lifestyle and employment risks
- Substance abuse risks
- Environmental exposures
- Employment exposures
- Healthy diet
- Health insurance, benefits, family leave policies
- Partner, family, social support
- Hyperthermia risks

LIFESTYLE CHANGES

- Smoking cessation
- Elimination of alcohol, illicit drugs
- Limiting of caffeine to 300 mg/day
- Limiting of over-the-counter medications
- Folic acid 0.4 mg/day (supplement)
- Prenatal vitamins and vitamin D as indicated
- Calcium supplement 1200 mg/day
- Iron 30 to 60 mg/day
- Regular exercise 15 to 30 minutes, interspersed with rest, water
- Avoidance of hot tub or sauna
- Treatment of fever
- Avoidance of teas

IMMUNIZATION INFORMATION

- Contraindicated in pregnancy: measles, mumps, rubella (MMR); varicella; polio; avoid conception for 3 months after immunization
- Not contraindicated: tetanus-diphtheria (Td); booster every 10 years
- If indicated: hepatitis B

POSSIBLE REFERRAL

- Cooperative extension services
- Genetic counseling
- Management of chronic illness
- Nutrition counseling to attain appropriate weight or treat an eating disorder
- Specialists as indicated
- Substance abuse counseling
- Substitution or elimination of teratogenic medications
- Woman, Infants and Children program referral
- Dentist
- Laboratory studies
- Domestic violence assistance or counseling
- Financial or medical assistance

Integrated health care for women emphasizes health promotion and disease prevention for every woman. The current expectation is that in every visit the health care provider offers preconceptional health promotion, in some form, to every woman capable of conceiving and documents this in the medical record.[58,59] Most babies are born healthy. Fetal, neonatal, and maternal complications can occur under the best of circumstances. Preconceptional health promotion does not guarantee a good pregnancy outcome, but it does assist families in maximizing resources and minimizing risk.[60]

REFERENCES

1. Cefalo RC, Bowes WA, Moos MK: Preconception care: a means of prevention, *Baillieres Clin Obstet Gynaecol* 9:403-416, 1995.
2. Schrander-Stumpel C: Preconception care: challenge of the new millennium? *Am J Med Genet* 89:58-61, 1999.
3. Moos MK: Preconception care, *JOGNN* 32(4):514-515, 2003.
4. Centers for Disease Control and Prevention: State-specific pregnancy and birth rates among teenagers—United States, 1991-1992, *MMWR* 44:676-684, 1995.
5. Hobbins D: Full circle: the evolution of preconception health promotion in America, *JOGNN* 32(4):516-522, 2003.
6. Institute of Medicine: *The well-being of children and families*, Washington, DC, 1995, National Academy Press.
7. American Academy of Pediatrics, American College of Obstetricians and Gynecologists: *Guidelines for perinatal care*, ed 4, Elk Grove Village, Ill, 1997, The Academy.
8. Adams MM, and others: Pregnancy planning and pre-conception counseling: the PRAMS Working Group, *Obstet Gynecol* 82:955-959, 1993.
9. Morrow CE: Preventive care in pregnancy, *Prim Care* 22:775-784, 1995.
10. Leavitt C: Preconception health promotion, *Prim Care* 20:537-549, 1993.
11. Walker LO, Tinkle MB: Toward an integrative science of women's health, *JOGNN* 25:379-382, 1996.
12. Hobbins D: Every woman, every time: state-of-the-science, state-of-the-art, *J Perinat Neonat Nurs* 20:43-45, 2006.
13. Hobbins D: *Preconception care: maximizing the health of women and their newborns*, AWHONN Practice Monograph, Washington, DC, 2001, Association of Women's Health, Obstetric and Neonatal Nurses.
14. Cheng D: Preconception health care for the primary care practitioner, *Md Med J* 45:297-304, 1996.
15. Swan LL, Apgar B: Preconceptual obstetric risk assessment and health promotion, *Am Fam Phys* 51:1875-1885, 1995.
16. Frazier LM, Jones TL: Managing patients with concerns about workplace reproductive hazards, *J Am Med Women's Assoc* 55:80-83, 105, 2000.
17. Summers L, Price RA: Preconception care: an opportunity to maximize health in pregnancy, *J Nurse Midwifery* 38:188-198, 1993.
18. Olsen ME: Preconception evaluation and intervention, *South Med J* 87:639-645, 1994.
19. Cashatt CL: *Queer and expecting: lesbian, bisexual, and transgender women in the childbearing literature* (senior thesis), Seattle, June 2003, Department of Women's Studies, University of Washington.
20. National Women's Health Information Center: *Frequently asked questions—lesbian health*, Office on Women's Health, retrieved from http://www.WomensHealth.gov.
21. Van Montfrans JM, and others: Are elevated concentrations in the preconceptional period a risk factor for Down's syndrome pregnancies? *Hum Reprod* 16:1270-1273, 2001.
22. Parnell T: Fertility, conception, and childbirth in women of mature reproductive age: new hope through NaProTECHNOLOGY. In Hilgers TW: *The medical and surgical practice of NaProTECHNOLOGY*, Omaha, 2004, Pope Paul VI Institute Press.
23. Leuzzi RA, Scoles KS: Preconception counseling for the primary care physician, *Med Clin North Am* 80:337-369, 1996.
24. Das UD, Sysyn GD: Abnormal fetal growth: intrauterine growth retardation, small for gestational age, large for gestational age (review), *Pediatr Clin North Am* 51(3):639-654, viii, 2004.
25. Smith GC, and others: Pregnancy complications and maternal risk of ischaemic heart disease: a retrospective cohort study of 129,290 births, *Lancet* 357(9273):2002-2006, 2001.
26. Centers for Disease Control and Prevention: Knowledge and use of folic acid among women of reproductive age—Michigan, 1998, *MMWR* 50(10):185-189, 2001.
27. US Department of Health and Human Services: Progress review on maternal, infant, and child health. In *Healthy People 2010*, 2003, retrieved March 6, 2007, from http://www.cdc.gov/hchs/about/otheract/hpdata2010/fa16/mich.htm.
28. Moos MK: *A snapshot of preconceptional health: thoughts on what we know... and what we don't*, presentation at National Summit on Preconception Care, Atlanta, June 21, 2005.
29. Levine L: *Interconceptional education and counseling: for Florida's healthy start high risk women*, presentation at National Summit on Preconception Care, Atlanta, June 21-23, 2005.
30. Werler MM, and others: Prepregnant weight in relation to risk of neural tube defects, *JAMA* 275:1089-1092, 1996.
31. Siega-Riz AM, Adair LS, Hobel CJ: Maternal underweight status and inadequate rate of weight gain during the third trimester of pregnancy increases the risk of preterm delivery, *J Nutr* 126:146-153, 1996.
32. Arafeh JMR, Baird SM: Cardiac disease in pregnancy, *Crit Care Nurs* 29(1):32-52, 2006.
33. Rodgers BD, Rodgers DE: Efficacy of preconception care of diabetic women in a community setting, *J Reprod Med* 41:422-426, 1996.
34. American Diabetes Association: Preconception care of women with diabetes, *Diabetes Care* 20(Suppl 11):840-843, 1997.
35. Holing EV: Preconception care of women with diabetes: the unrevealed obstacles, *J Matern Fetal Med* 9:10-13, 2000.
36. Centers for Disease Control and Prevention: US Public Health Service recommendation for human immunodeficiency virus counseling and voluntary testing for pregnant women, *MMWR* 44(RR-7):1-15, 1995.
37. Cefalo KC, Moos MK: *Preconceptional health care: a practical guide*, ed 2, St Louis, 1995, Mosby.
38. In Hilgers TW: *The medical and surgical practice of NaProTECHNOLOGY*, Omaha, 2004, Pope Paul VI Institute Press.
39. Zhu BP: Effect of interpregnancy interval on birth outcomes: findings from three recent US studies, *Int J Gynecol Obstet* 89(Suppl 1):S25-S33, 2005.
40. Vogel F, Jotulsky AG: *Human genetics*, ed 3, New York, 1995, Springer.
41. Eng CM, and others: Prenatal genetic carrier testing using triple disease screening, *JAMA* 278:1268-1272, 1997.
42. McFarlane J, and others: Assessing for abuse during pregnancy, *JAMA* 267:3176-3178, 1992.
43. American Medical Association, Council on Scientific Affairs: Violence against women: relevance for medical practitioners, *JAMA* 267:3184-3189, 1992.
44. Luke B, and others: The association between occupational factors and preterm birth: a United States Nurses Study, *Am J Obstet Gynecol* 173:849-862, 1995.
45. Postlethwaite D: Preconception health counseling for women exposed to teratogens: the role of the nurse, *JOGNN* 32(4):523-532, 2003.
46. Berkowitz GS, Marcus M: Occupational exposures and reproduction. In Lee RV, editor: *Current obstetric medicine*, St Louis, 1993, Mosby.
47. Houston TK, and others: Active and passive smoking and development of glucose intolerance among young adults in a prospective cohort: CARDIA study, *BMJ* 332(7549):1064-1069, 2006.
48. US Preventive Services Task Force: *Guide to clinical preventive services: report of the U.S. Preventive Services Task Force*, ed 2, Baltimore, 1996, Williams & Wilkins.
49. Hurren C, and others: Folic acid and prevention of neural-tube defects, *Lancet* 350:664, 1997.
50. Shaw GM, and others: Risks of orofacial clefts in children born to women using multivitamin-containing folic acid periconceptionally, *Lancet* 346:393-396, 1995.

51. Centers for Disease Control and Prevention: Knowledge and use of folic acid by women of childbearing age—United States 1997, *MMWR* 46:721-723, 1997.
52. Elkin AC, Higham J: Folic acid supplements are more effective than increasing dietary folate intake in elevating serum folate levels, *Br J Obstet Gynecol* 107(2):285-289, 2000.
53. Green tea not for moms-to-be, *Am Baby* 20:3 2005.
54. Freightner JW: *Routine iron supplementation during pregnancy: the Canadian guide to clinical preventive health care,* Ottawa, 1994, Publications Canada, Canadian Task Force on the Periodic Health Examination.
55. Kolasa KM, Weismiller DG: Nutrition during pregnancy, *Am Fam Phys* 56:205-212, 1995.
56. Yu SM, and others: Preconceptional and prenatal multivitamin mineral supplement use in the 1988 National Maternal and Infant Health Study, *Am J Pub Health* 86:240-242, 1996.
57. Czeizel AE: Primary prevention of neural-tube defects and some other major congenital abnormalities: recommendations for the appropriate use of folic acid during pregnancy, *Paediatr Drugs* 2:437-439, 2000.
58. Morrison EH: Preconception care, *Prim Care* 27:1-12, 2000.
59. Bernstein PS, and others: Improving preconception care, *J Reprod Med* 45:546-552, 2000.
60. Stanford JB, Hobbins D: Obstetric risk assessment, section A, Preconception risk assessment. In Ratcliffe SD, and others, editors: *Family practice obstetrics,* ed 2, Philadelphia, 2001, Hanley & Belfus.

CHAPTER 179

Sexual Dysfunction, Female

Cynthia M. Williams and
Patricia Polgar Bailey

DEFINITION AND EPIDEMIOLOGY

Human sexual expression is complex, is a crucial part of our development and daily functioning, and changes throughout the life cycle. Sexual activity is connected to the satisfaction of our basic needs and associated with our self-esteem.[1] It is strongly influenced by culturally defined roles, religious beliefs, and the physical and emotional health of the individual.[2] Sexual dysfunction has no singular explanation; it is influenced by both internal and external forces. However, a useful definition for sexual dysfunction is any sexual behavior or problem that makes sexual expression difficult or constantly dissatisfying to the individual or partner.[3] It may also be useful to define sexual dysfunction by what it is not, rather than by what it is. Most health care providers would agree that there is no sexual dysfunction if a woman reports being satisfied with her sex life and denies any problems or distress related to sexual issues. But the difficulty in diagnosis arises if a woman reports having "a little bit of a problem" or "somewhat of a problem." At what point does having a less than perfect sex life become diagnosed as sexual dysfunction?[4] Rather than thinking of sexual health as a perfect sex life, the provider can more broadly conceptualize it as the ability to enjoy sexual activity without emotional or physical discomfort.

A recent consensus development conference on female sexual dysfunction (FSD) further classified sexual dysfunction into four major categories: (1) sexual desire disorders, including hypoactive sexual desire and sexual aversion; (2) sexual arousal disorder; (3) orgasmic disorders; and (4) sexual pain disorders, including dyspareunia, vaginismus, and noncoital sexual pain.[5]

Sexual problems probably exist in one form or another throughout a woman's life. For many reasons, including their own attitudes and beliefs, personal comfort, experience, and knowledge, health care providers may be reluctant to make inquiries into the sexual health of their patients.[6,7] The epidemiologic studies of FSD are few and flawed. The prevalence of sexual dysfunction among all women ranges between 25% and 63%.[8] In a recent analysis of the National Health and Social Life Survey (NHSLS) the prevalence of sexual dysfunction was found to be 43% for women younger than 60 years.[8,9]

Estimates on the prevalence of sexual dysfunction in postmenopausal women varies from 68% to 86.5% depending on where the study was done.[10] A recent study by Addis, Van Den Eden, Wassel-Fyr, and others found that nearly three fourths of middle-aged women (mean age 55.9 years) were sexually active; of this group, approximately two thirds were at least somewhat satisfied, and 33% reported a problems with sexual function.[10] Data from the Addis study showed that higher socioeconomic status (higher education and higher income) was correlated with increased sexual activity, but that increased education status was also correlated with increasing sexual dysfunction. In addition, better mental health was correlated with increased sexual satisfaction, whereas increased body mass index was associated with less sexual satisfaction.[10]

Data from the NHSLS indicated that sexual dysfunction is more prevalent in women (43%) than in men (31%) and that prevalence is affected by a variety of factors, including race, history of traumatic sexual experience, and deteriorating social position. Poor physical and emotional health, negative sexual experiences, and overall well-being greatly influenced FSD.[8] The diagnosis and treatment of cancers, such as breast cancer, can have a detrimental effect on sexual health because of changes in body image, fertility, physical well-being, and emotional distress. The maintenance of sexual health is an important quality-of-life issue for people with cancer.[11]

FSD is associated with many of the same disease processes that are associated with male erectile dysfunction, including aging, hypertension, atherosclerotic disease, cigarette smoking, and pelvic operations.[5] The most commonly encountered sexual concerns range from painful intercourse, misinformation, psychosexual dysfunction, failure to achieve orgasm, extramarital sex, and organic sexual dysfunction to sexual abuse to sexual preference concerns.[12]

PATHOPHYSIOLOGY

Insight into sexual problems and dysfunction depends on an understanding of the human sexual response cycle.[13] The sexual response cycle includes the desire, arousal (vascular), orgasm (muscular), and resolution (in men) phases. Desire is the factor that initiates the overall sexual response cycle. Others have stressed the need for a different model to explain the sexual response cycle in women.[14] The classic sexual response model first defined by Masters and Johnson may not fully explain the underpinnings of a woman's sexual health, including the concepts that women have a lower biologic urge to be sexual for release of sexual tension; the motivation, or "drive," to be sexual may be tied to nonsexual gains or rewards; sexual arousal is a subjective mental excitement; and, finally, orgasmic release of sexual tension may or may not occur in every sexual encounter.[15,16] An understanding of sexual dysfunction should recognize that any of the above may overlap in a positive or negative manner and affect further sexual encounters.

Several etiologies should be considered in the evaluation of FSD. Vasculogenic impotence in men may be analogous to clitoral and vaginal vascular insufficiency in women. Any problem that affects blood flow, such as cardiovascular disease and kidney failure or damage to the neurologic system (e.g., diabetes), can result in this problem.[17] In addition, certain medications and substance abuse (e.g., alcohol, smoking) can contribute to this problem. Spinal cord injury or any diseases of the central or peripheral nervous system can result in neurogenic FSD, especially as it concerns lubrication and orgasm. Any dysfunction of the hypothalamic-pituitary axis from either surgical or medical castration, natural menopause, premature ovarian failure, or chronic birth control use can result in hormonally based FSD. Finally, psychogenic issues, with or without organic disease, can lead to FSD. This also includes medications used to treat depression, especially the selective serotonin reuptake inhibitors (SSRIs).[18,19] Sociocultural factors, such as marital stress, have been tied to sexual dysfunction.[20]

CLINICAL PRESENTATION

The sexual history is an important component of care, but neither patients nor health care providers should be forced to discuss sexuality.[6,7] Providers need to be comfortable with their own sexuality and willing to discuss the subject. An open, understanding, nonjudgmental attitude and a willingness to explore sexual health will allow the patient to discuss sexual concerns.

A brief sexual history should include the gynecologic history, sexual activity, number of partners, homosexual or heterosexual relationships, difficult or abusive sexual experiences, and satisfaction with sexual experiences. Problems with desire, arousal, lubrication, orgasm, pain, bleeding, or lesions; sexually transmitted disease exposure; and the need for contraception should also be reviewed. In addition, exploration of recent life events (e.g., divorce, separation, or recent losses) and cultural attitudes toward sexual activity should be considered. Because medications can affect all phases of the sexual cycle, a drug review is imperative.

When a sexual problem is elicited, the history should include a detailed description of symptoms and the onset, course, patient's perception of the disorder, past medical history, and past treatments and outcomes. It is also important to determine the patient's expectations and goals for treatment.

PHYSICAL EXAMINATION

A complete physical examination is indicated, with particular attention to the genitourinary, vascular, and neurologic systems. The examination should determine the presence of galactorrhea and nipple erection; vulvar lesions, anomalies, or tenderness; labial thickness or thickening; and any notable rectocele or cystocele. The clitoris, hymen, vagina, and cervix should be examined for signs of infection, injury, atrophy, adhesions, or discharge. Evaluation of the bulbocavernosus reflex demonstrates integrity of the S2 to S4 sacral nerves, part of the neurologic foundation of the sexual response cycle. A bimanual examination is necessary to palpate the vagina, cervix, uterus, and adnexa. Vaginal muscle tone can be evaluated by inserting fingers in the vagina and having the patient squeeze them; a lack of tone may indicate vaginismus.

DIAGNOSTICS

Specific laboratory tests are indicated for physiologic phase disorders, although no one battery of tests is recommended.[6,7] Diagnostic studies are guided by the history and physical examination and may include cultures, a thyroid panel, CBC, hormonal studies, serum corticosteroids, fasting glucose, and renal and liver function studies. Screening for depression may also be indicated.

DIAGNOSTICS

Sexual Dysfunction

LABORATORY

- Luteinizing hormone
- Follicle-stimulating hormone
- CBC and differential
- Thyroid profile
- Liver enzymes
- Prolactin
- Testosterone
- Serum estradiol
- Hemoglobin A_{1c}
- Fasting glucose
- BUN
- Creatinine
- Vaginal cultures for *Chlamydia* organisms and gonorrhea

DIFFERENTIAL DIAGNOSIS

Psychosocial difficulties; depression; posttraumatic stress disorder; hormonal imbalance; thyroid, adrenal, liver, and kidney disorders; diabetes; infection; injury; substance abuse; arterial insufficiency; and neurologic disease or injury should be considered in the differential diagnosis. In addition, many common diseases and medications can affect sexual functioning (Table 179-1).[6]

MANAGEMENT

Over the past 35 years major changes have occurred in the treatment of sexual dysfunction.[1] Still, management of FSD can be challenging and frustrating for the woman and her provider. When sexual dysfunction is caused by a medical problem, such as disease, injury, medication, or substance abuse, the health care provider is in a pivotal position to address those issues. Not all complaints of FSD are psychologic, but the clinical and basic science of the study of FSD is in its infancy. Currently no medication therapies for FSD are approved by the U.S. Food and Drug Administration (FDA), but many medications used for the treatment of male erectile dysfunction are being used in clinical protocols with women.[18]

DIFFERENTIAL DIAGNOSIS

Sexual Dysfunction

DISEASES AND OTHER FACTORS THAT AFFECT SEXUAL FUNCTION

- Diabetes
- Thyroid disease
- Coronary artery disease
- Congestive heart failure
- Vascular disease
- Dementia
- Chronic obstructive pulmonary disease

PSYCHOLOGIC FACTORS THAT DECREASE LIBIDO

- Depression
- Anxiety
- Posttraumatic stress disorder
- Fatigue

CONDITIONS THAT CAUSE PAINFUL OR UNCOMFORTABLE INTERCOURSE

- Inadequate vaginal lubrication
- Introital dyspareunia
- Scarring
- Thick or intact hymen
- Vaginismus
- Clitoral hyperstimulation
- Endometriosis
- Ovarian cysts
- Arthritis
- Psychogenic pain from previous trauma

TABLE 179-1 Common Medications Causing Sexual Dysfunction

Class of Drugs	Example
Antihypertensives	Thiazide diuretics, clonidine, methyldopa, captopril, beta blockers
Antidepressants	Amitriptyline, imipramine, trazodone, monoamine oxidase inhibitors, selective serotonin reuptake inhibitors
Hormonal agents	Estrogen, progesterone
Anticholinergics	Atropine, hydroxyzine
H_2-receptor antagonists	Cimetidine
Antipsychotics	Chlorpromazine, thiothixene, haloperidol
Sedatives	Alcohol, barbiturates
Anxiolytics	Diazepam

Estrogen replacement therapy can improve clitoral sensitivity, increase libido, and decrease pain with intercourse. In addition, local or topical estrogens (estrogen vaginal cream and the vaginal estradiol ring) can relieve symptoms of vaginal dryness, burning, and urinary frequency and urgency.

Methyl testosterone has been used in postmenopausal women for symptoms ranging from lack of desire to lack of vaginal lubrication. Potential benefits of therapy included increases in clitoral sensitivity, vaginal lubrication, libido, and arousal. The potential side effects of weight gain, clitoral enlargement, increased facial hair, and hypercholesterolemia may outweigh the benefits.

Sildenafil (Viagra), a selective type V phosphodiesterase inhibitor, appears to improve both subjective and physiologic parameters in a small study of women who were administered sildenafil.[21] Sildenafil also appears to benefit women with SSRI-precipitated sexual dysfunction.[22]

Phentolamine (Vasomax), an α-adrenergic blocker that causes vascular smooth muscle relaxation, has been studied in men. A small pilot study in menopausal women with sexual arousal disorder noted an improvement in lubrication and pleasurable sensations in the vagina.[23]

Recently the FDA approved a vacuum therapy device to enhance clitoral engorgement.[24] The Clitoral Therapy Device (EROS-CTD) was effective, especially in postmenopausal women, in increasing genital sensation and lubrication, enabling the women to achieve orgasm, and improving overall sexual satisfaction. More research is needed to evaluate long-term and prophylactic use of this device.

COMPLICATIONS

Many sexual concerns involve pregnancy issues. Methods of contraception may influence a woman's sexual response and cause problems or dysfunction. Hormonal contraception may affect desire, libido, or performance, although many women discover enhanced sexuality, knowing pregnancy is unlikely. For women desiring pregnancy, the stress and timing of intercourse may interfere adversely with both pleasure and communication.

INDICATIONS FOR REFERRAL OR HOSPITALIZATION

Many sexual concerns and dysfunctions can be treated with good anticipatory guidance and education about sexuality and sexual health. For some patients the underlying medical condition is treated. For those who may require extensive general or sex therapy, referral to a reputable, certified sex therapist is warranted. In addition, if it is available, evaluation in a women's sexual health clinic may allow for a better elucidation of the problem, validate the individual, and lead to a more comprehensive treatment approach.[18]

Modern sex therapy is short-term and instructive, typically lasting 15 to 20 sessions. It generally focuses on specific problems, rather than broad personality issues. Modern sex therapy generally includes the following principles and techniques, which are applied in almost all cases, regardless of the dysfunction, and which may be helpful to incorporate, at least to some degree, in the primary care setting:

Assessing and conceptualizing the problem: The focus is on gathering information about past life events and how current factors are contributing to the dysfunction.[25]

Sharing mutual responsibility: Both partners in the relationship share the sexual problem, regardless of who has the actual dysfunction, and treatment will be more successful when both are in therapy.[25]

Educating about sexuality: Lack of education about the physiology and techniques of sexual activity often contributes to sexual dysfunction. Education in the form of discussions, instructional books, and videotapes may be helpful.[26]

Changing attitudes: Beliefs and attitudes about sexuality resulting from past traumatic events, family attitudes, and cultural ideas may be preventing sexual arousal and pleasure. Examining and changing some of these beliefs may be helpful.[19]

Eliminating performance anxiety and the spectator role: Nondemand pleasuring (sensual acts other than intercourse or reaching orgasm) and building back up to sexual intercourse can be a way of eliminating or reducing performance anxiety.

Increasing sexual and general communication skills: Training in how best to communicate and how to give instructions in a nonthreatening and informative manner can be helpful.[20]

Changing destructive lifestyles and marital interactions: Couples may be encouraged to change aspects of their lifestyle or take steps to improve a situation that is having a destructive effect on their relationship.[20]

Addressing physical and medical factors.

PATIENT AND FAMILY EDUCATION AND HEALTH PROMOTION

The opportunity to explore sexual concerns through an open dialogue is the most therapeutic approach. Education should be directed toward understanding normal sexual response and the stages associated with the sexual response cycle. The importance of diet, exercise, and adequate sleep cannot be overstated because stress and fatigue are significant factors that affect sexual desire. Promoting cholesterol reduction, tobacco cessation, and blood pressure and glycemic control may go a long way in the prevention of potential vasculogenic causes of FSD.

The following resources can assist patients with sexual dysfunction:

- Barbach L: *For yourself: fulfillment of female sexuality*, New York, 2000, Signet.
- Berman JL: *For women only: a revolutionary guide to overcoming sexual dysfunction and reclaiming your sex life*, New York, 2001, Henry Holt.
- Butler R, Lewis M: *The new love and sex after sixty*, New York, 2002, Ballantine.
- Kaplan HS: *The illustrated manual of sex therapy*, New York, 1988, Brunner/Mazel.
- American Association of Sexuality Educators Counselors and Therapists, http://www.aasect.org
- American Psychological Association, http://www.apa.org
- Kinsey Institute for Research in Sex, Gender, and Reproduction, http://www.indiana.edu/~kinsey

REFERENCES

1. Comer R: *Abnormal psychology*, New York, 2004, Worth.
2. Bullard DG, Caplan H: Sexual problems. In Feldman MD, Christensen JF, editors: *Behavioral medicine in primary care*, Stamford, Conn, 1997, Appleton & Lange.
3. Klingman EW: Office evaluation of sexual function and complaints, *Clin Geriatr Med* 7:15-39, 1991.
4. Gierhart B: When does a "less than perfect" sex life become female sexual dysfunction? *Obstet Gynecol* 107(4):750-751, 2006.
5. Basson R, Berman J, Burnett A, and others: Report of the International Consensus Development Conference on Female Sexual Dysfunction: definitions and classifications, *J Urol* 163(3):888-893, 2000.
6. Phillips NA: Female sexual dysfunction: evaluation and treatment, *Am Fam Phys* 62:127-136, 141-142, 2000.
7. MacLaren A: Primary care for women: comprehensive sexual health assessment, *J Nurse Midwif* 40:104-119, 1995.
8. Laumann EO, Paik A, Rosen RC: Sexual dysfunction in the United States: prevalence and predictors, *JAMA* 281:537-544, 1999.
9. Heiman JR: Sexual dysfunction: overview of prevalence, etiologic factors, and treatments, *J Sex Res* 39(1):73-78, 2002.
10. Addis I, Van Den Eden S, Wassel-Fyr C, and others: Sexual activity and function in middle-aged and older women, *Obstet Gynecol* 107(4):755-764, 2006.
11. Bakewell R, Volker R: Sexual dysfunction related to the treatment of young women with cancer, *Clin J Oncol Nurs* 9(6):697-702, 2005.
12. Driscoll CE: Assisting patients with sexual problems. In Taylor RB, editor: *Family medicine*, New York, 1994, Springer-Verlag.
13. Berman JR, Goldstein I: Female sexual dysfunction, *Urol Clin North Am* 28:405-415, 2001.
14. Basson R: The female sexual response: a different model, *J Sex Marital Ther* 26:51-65, 2000.
15. Masters WH, Johnson VE: *Human sexual response*, Boston, 1966, Little Brown.
16. Masters WH, Johnson VE: *Human sexual inadequacy*, Boston, 1970, Little Brown.
17. Frohman E: Sexual dysfunction in neurologic disease, *Clin Neuropharmacol* 25(3):126-132, 2002.
18. Berman JR, Berman L, Goldstein I: Female sexual dysfunction: incidence, pathophysiology, evaluation and treatment options, *Urology* 54:385-391, 1999.

19. Gitlin MJ: Psychotropic medications and their effects on sexual function: diagnosis, biology, and treatment approaches, *J Clin Psychiatr* 55:406-413, 1994.
20. Metz M, Epstein N: Assessing the role of relationship conflict in sexual dysfunction, *J Sex Marital Ther* 28(2):129-164, 2002.
21. Berman JR, Berman LA, Lin H, and others: Effect of sildenafil on subjective and physiologic parameters of the female sexual response in women with sexual arousal disorder, *J Sex Marital Ther* 27(5):411-420, 2001.
22. Rosen RC, Lane RM, Menza M: Effects of SSRI on sexual dysfunction: a critical review, *J Clin Psychopharmacol* 19:67-85, 1999.
23. Rosen R, Phillips NA, Gendrano NC 3rd, and others: Oral phentolamine and female sexual arousal disorder: a pilot study, *J Sex Marital Ther* 25(2):137-144, 1999.
24. Billups KL, Berman L, Berman J, and others: A new non-pharmacological vacuum therapy for female sexual dysfunction, *J Sex Marital Ther* 27:435-441, 2001.
25. Bach A, Wincze J, Barlow DH: Sexual dysfunction. In Barlow DH, editor: *Clinical handbook of psychological disorders: a step-by-step treatment manual,* ed 3, New York, 2001, Guilford.
26. Westheimer R, Lopater S: Human sexuality: *A psychological perspective*, Baltimore, 2002, Lippincott Williams & Wilkins.

CHAPTER 180

Unplanned Pregnancy

Patricia Polgar Bailey

DEFINITION AND EPIDEMIOLOGY

The term *unplanned pregnancy* is defined as a pregnancy that is undesired at the time of conception or that is mistimed (occurs earlier than desired).[1,2] However, using a single term to refer to unplanned pregnancies masks some of the differences between women with mistimed pregnancies and those with unwanted pregnancies. Women with unwanted or unintended pregnancies are more likely to have health risks that could negatively affect pregnancy outcomes. Unintended pregnancies are associated with greater unfavorable maternal behaviors and increased health risks for both mother and child than mistimed pregnancies. Therefore clarifying the difference between mistimed and unintended pregnancy may help guide clinicians as they provide direct services to women and infants.[2]

When pregnancies are unintended, women are more likely to receive little or no preconception, prenatal, and preventive care.[3] In addition, babies born to mothers who did not intend to become pregnant are at an increased risk for exposure to harmful substances, including tobacco and alcohol, which in turn increases the risks for low birth weight and infant and childhood morbidity.[4]

Estimates of unintended pregnancy prevalence in the United States are as high as 50% to 60%; slightly more than one third (35%) of live U.S. births are the result of an unintended pregnancy.[1,5] Approximately 13% of unintended pregnancies end in miscarriage. There are no official statistics kept on the number of children adopted each year, but estimates range from 1% to 3% of unplanned pregnancies.[6]

The high prevalence of unintended pregnancy is surprising given that contraception is widely available in the United States. However, one study indicated that only 51% to 63% of adults discuss contraception with a health care provider.[7] In addition, reasons for contraceptive nonuse differ depending on the age of the woman and the circumstances surrounding the event. For example, contraceptive nonuse at first intercourse and hence unintended pregnancy were most often related to concerns that parents would find out about sexual activity. Older women with a second or higher-order pregnancy were more likely to discontinue contraception because of its side effects and medical complications.[1] This has important implications for provider education related to contraception and family.

Adolescent women have the highest proportion of unintended pregnancies, with at least 75% of pregnancies to women less than 19 years of age unintended.[1] About half of unintended pregnancies end in abortion. The U.S. abortion rate fell by 17% from 1992 to 2000 (from 25.7 to 21.3 abortions per 1000 women 15 to 44 years of age), reaching its lowest level since the 1970s.[8]

The decline in abortion rate varies significantly by subgroup. The greatest rate of decline has occurred among high-income women, college-educated women, and teenagers. In contrast, the abortion rate has increased among low-income women and low-income teenagers. The ethnic differences in abortion rates diminish when income is controlled for.[9] In 2000 the abortion rate for low-income women was nearly double that for wealthy women. The economic disparities in U.S. abortion rates mirror the growing differences in access to care among the rich and the poor in this country.[10]

CLINICAL PRESENTATION

A positive pregnancy test can generate a variety of responses. For some patients, the news brings joy and excitement; for others, the news can be a crisis of varying proportion. Although many personal and socioeconomic factors may affect a woman's individual reaction, one common denominator is ensured: the woman's life is changed.

The health care provider is often the patient's first confidante in the first few minutes surrounding the news of an unplanned pregnancy and is in a unique position to assist her in meeting her total health and wellness needs. For women for whom the pregnancy represents a crisis, several types of reactions can occur. With an unplanned pregnancy, the health care provider's response is critical in establishing and maintaining an environment that feels safe and supportive to the patient. The provider's initial role is to listen; both verbal and nonverbal communications provide information that is useful in developing the care plan. The patient needs to be allowed time to express her feelings.

Patients feel especially vulnerable and pressured to find a quick and easy solution. Many report feeling as though they are racing against the clock, and they look to the significant people in their life for support and advice. Support may be lacking, or advice from these sources may differ from what the patient desires. A study by Joyce, Kaestner, and Korenman found that the parents' disagreement over the pregnancy was the most important predictor of instability in the mother's intention regarding the pregnancy.[11] In addition, a woman's intentions regarding the pregnancy are not fixed and may change depending on where she is on the continuum from preconception to postpartum.

In many cases the pregnancy is not the only issue that concerns the patient. In fact, the patient's reaction to the pregnancy may conceal her real concerns—finances, domestic violence, sexual abuse, or other issues. Assessing these concerns is essential in the decision-making process.

MANAGEMENT AND COUNSELING

Counseling a woman with an unplanned pregnancy can be challenging and emotionally difficult for both the health care provider and the woman involved. This challenge is accentuated by the personal feelings that each provider may have about unplanned pregnancy, the options available, and by the fact that an unplanned pregnancy can be a crisis in a woman's life.[6] Health care providers need to understand and accept that a woman's perspective, goals, and way of achieving them may conflict with their own. Before a provider can put aside his or her own beliefs and biases about reproductive choices and options, he or she needs to thoughtfully reflect on what those beliefs might be and how they might influence the education and counseling provided to a woman with an unplanned pregnancy. It is virtually impossible for a provider to rid himself or herself of personal values and biases, but the provider must be committed to and vigilant about keeping those biases out of the interaction with the woman and other people involved in the situation.

Every woman has the right to factual and unbiased information about reproductive choices, in order to make an informed decision about the pregnancy. Based on this, it is important for the provider to keep in mind that the woman is responsible for defining how the unplanned pregnancy is a problem for her, and she is responsible for her own exploration, assessing her options and ultimately making a decision and acting on it. The provider's role is to actively listen to the woman, provide information and support, and help the woman assess her options. The solution to the unplanned pregnancy lies with the woman.[6]

After the patient has expressed herself, the health care provider can assist with prioritizing the patient's concerns and needs by focusing on one issue at a time. By exhibiting a willingness to listen and help, the provider helps build the patient's confidence. An exploration of the patient's feelings about pregnancy, the child, abortion, and abortion alternatives provides an opportunity to further process the situation. It is also helpful for the provider to know whether the patient has previously experienced an unplanned pregnancy or whether she knows anyone who has dealt with an unplanned pregnancy and the decision to either have an abortion, raise the child, or surrender the child for adoption. A critical piece of information concerns the woman's support system and the role of the child's father in the woman's life and in the decisions about this pregnancy. Although patients seek a rapid solution to the crisis of an unplanned pregnancy, the provider should encourage the patient to take the time necessary to make an informed decision regarding this life-changing situation, since even a decision to end the pregnancy can have long-term effects.

Patients may need time to process their emotions and discuss the pregnancy with the significant people in their lives. A scheduled follow-up visit provides an opportunity to further discuss with the patient her reactions and their effect on decision making, as well as to provide information and available support services. These initial meetings play an important role in how patients react to their pregnancy and assist with the decision-making process.

The health care provider should inform the patient of the full range of available options. For someone experiencing an unplanned or a crisis pregnancy, abortion is often viewed as the only solution. However, other viable options do exist. Referrals to crisis pregnancy centers can provide patients with the expertise of trained staff and can broaden their options. If the patient does not want to go to a crisis pregnancy center or if one is not accessible to her, a referral to a professional counselor is appropriate. The more informed the patient is, the less likely it is that she will regret the eventual decision.

Regardless of the decision, continued and unconditional acceptance of and compassion toward the patient will contribute to her overall wellness at this critical time.

Counseling a patient who is experiencing a crisis pregnancy can be very challenging. The following framework, which contains lists of questions for the health care provider to ask the patient, may help make this interaction fruitful for both patient and provider:

Focus on the patient. There is often a great deal of conversation about and concern for the infant. However, it is the woman who is experiencing the crisis, and it is she who ultimately makes the most adjustments.

Inquire about the patient's feelings. The health care provider should ask some of the following questions:

- How are you feeling about this pregnancy? or What does the pregnancy mean to you?
- Before finding out that you were pregnant, what were your feelings about abortion? Adoption? Parenting?
- Under what circumstances do you believe abortion (adoption, parenting) is okay? Not okay? Why?
- Under what circumstances would you like to become a parent?
- Who knows that you are pregnant?
- What is your relationship with the father of the baby? How involved is he in the decision making? How supportive will he be of your decision?
- Who is your support system?
- Are you considering an abortion?
- Would you consider alternatives to abortion?

Make abortion real. If a patient is considering an abortion, it is important that she have as much accurate information as possible about the procedures involved, the risks, and the possible complications:

- Have you ever been pregnant before?
- Have you ever had an abortion?
- What does abortion mean to you?
- Do you know how abortions are performed?
- Do you know the physical risks of having an abortion?
- Do you know anyone who has had an abortion?
- What were your opinions about abortion before you learned you were pregnant?

Make the infant real. To make an informed decision, the patient needs to learn about the development of the fetus. The health care provider should be prepared to discuss the different stages of fetal development:

- Do you know the present physical development of your baby?

Focus on the woman and her future. The health care provider should ask:

- Under what circumstances would you like to become a parent?
- How would you feel if this was your only pregnancy?
- What are your goals for the next year? The next 5 years? How would each alternative help or hinder the achievement of these goals?
- What part of your circumstances is the most frightening or challenging?
- What is the worst thing you think might happen?
- How would you like for things to turn out for you ideally?

Remind the patient that she has time to make her decision. The provider should discuss the hormones of pregnancy and how they affect the decision-making process, especially during the first few months.

Use caution when mentioning adoption as an option. The word *adoption* can generate negative or even painful feelings. When counseling patients, it is helpful to listen for any hints as a guide to the patient's feelings about this topic. Both the health care provider and the patient need to remember that adoption is an option. It is not a quick decision, but rather a process to work through.

Develop a care plan. For patients who are committed to continuing the pregnancy, a care plan needs to be developed and should cover the following topics:

- Referral to an obstetrician for prenatal care
- Prenatal vitamins for the patient to take while awaiting her first prenatal visit
- Information on diet and healthy lifestyle
- Financial resources
- Type of aid available to the patient, if needed, before and after birth
- Plans with regard to work or school
- Type of housing arrangements available during the pregnancy and after delivery
- The patient's relationship with the father of the baby
- Marriage
- Single-parenting issues
- Adoption (Even if the patient plans to keep her infant, she needs to consider the issues involved in adoption and the impact of adoption on herself and the infant.)
- Child support
- Day care
- Support from family and friends

For the patient who has decided to have an abortion, the complexities involved should be realistically reviewed. For example, a woman who is being pressured by the father of the child to have an abortion runs the same risk of being abandoned after the abortion as if she keeps the child. A woman who has repeated abortions needs to consider the possibility of future gynecologic, obstetric, and psychologic complications. It is not uncommon for women who have had an abortion to experience a subsequent miscarriage, ectopic pregnancy, placenta previa, abruptio placentae, or premature birth. Psychologic problems can include guilt, remorse, anger, eating disorders, addictions, and spiritual alienation. These manifestations are categorized under a condition called *postabortion stress syndrome* and may be similar to those of posttraumatic stress disorder (see Chapter 264).

The health care provider should provide factual information and be understanding as the patient makes plans and considers her options. The provider should avoid exerting pressure or being judgmental. The decision must be made by the patient; preparation is directed toward helping the patient make a decision that she can live with in the future.

If the patient plans to place the infant for adoption, assistance should be provided to establish future life goals. Professional counseling and support services are critical to prepare for the legal termination of parental rights and to assist the woman with some of the psychologic aspects of releasing her infant. The patient should be encouraged not to view adoption as an indication of lack of love for her infant or as an indication that she is any less of a mother than a woman who keeps her infant. The choice of adoption can be viewed as providing both the patient and the infant with opportunities not otherwise possible.

Attempts should be made to thoroughly explore the possibilities of keeping the infant. Failure to go through this thinking and feeling process may contribute to future regrets concerning this decision.

LIFE SPAN CONSIDERATIONS

Research on unintended pregnancies indicates, as expected, that the age of the mother is strongly associated with intention. Recent studies show that more than 80% of mothers under the age of 18 indicated that they did not intend to become pregnant. In contrast, only 19% to 22% of women in their early thirties report that they did not intend to become pregnant. Although a significant number of older women may not intend to become pregnant, the percentage is still considerably lower than in the under 18 group.[5] Given this profile of unintended pregnancy, it is important for providers to ask all women of childbearing age about their plans for having children and to discuss the potential risks inherent in unplanned pregnancy and the benefits of planning.

COMPLICATIONS

Unplanned pregnancy has different associated risks depending on whether the pregnancy was unwanted or untimed. According to a recent study comparing the mood states and parental attitudes of mothers with unplanned pregnancies, women with unplanned pregnancies demonstrate greater mood disturbances during their last month of pregnancy and during the first year postpartum than women with planned pregnancies. In particular, during the last month of pregnancy, women with unintended pregnancies had greater levels of anxiety, depression, irritability, weariness, and confusion compared with women with planned pregnancies.[12]

INDICATIONS FOR REFERRAL

Referrals are based on a woman's decision regarding her pregnancy. Providers need to be aware of resources in the community to support a woman's choices.

PATIENT EDUCATION

Health care providers are in a unique position to provide pregnancy options counseling for women experiencing the crisis of an unplanned pregnancy. This type of counseling is based on a commitment to respecting patient autonomy, providing accurate information, and supporting women in their choices.

RESOURCE FOR HEALTH CARE PROVIDERS

Brown SS, Eisenberg L, editors: The best intentions: unintended pregnancy and the well-being of children and families, Washington, DC, 1995, Institute of Medicine, National Academy Press, http://www.nap.edu/catalog.php?record_id=4903#toc.

RESOURCES FOR WOMEN CONSIDERING ADOPTION

Brown SS, Eisenberg L, editors: The best intentions: unintended pregnancy and the well-being of children and families, Washington, DC, 1995, Institute of Medicine, National Academy Press, http://www.nap.edu/catalog.php?record_id=4903#toc.

Concerned United Birthparents, http://www.Cubirthparents.org

Child Welfare Information Gateway, http://www.childwelfare.gov

Gilman L: *The adoption resource book,* ed 4, New York, 1998, Harper Collins.

Melina LF: *Raising adopted children,* New York, 2001, Harper Collins.

Pavao J: *The family of adoption,* Boston, 2005, Beacon Press.

Romanchik B: *Being a birth parent: finding our place,* Royal Oak, Mich, 1999, R-Squared Press (an open adoption pocket guidebook).

Romanchik B: *Your rights and responsibilities: a guide for expectant parents pondering adoption,* Royal Oak, Mich, 1999, R-Squared Press (an open adoption guidebook).

RESOURCES FOR WOMEN CONSIDERING ABORTION

Baker A: *Abortion and adoptions counseling: a comprehensive reference,* Granite City, Ill, 1995, Hope Clinic for Women.

Runkle A: *In good conscience: a practical emotional and spiritual guide to deciding whether to have an abortion,* San Francisco, 1998, Jossey-Bass.

National Abortion Federation: *Unsure about your pregnancy? A guide to making the right decision for you,* http://www.prochoice.org/pubs_research/publications/downloads/are_you_pregnant/pregnancy_guide_english.pdf.

REFERENCES

1. Iuliano A, Speizer I, Santelli J, and others: Reasons for contraceptive nonuse at first sex and unintended pregnancy, *Am J Health Behav* 30(1):92-102, 2006.
2. D'Angelo D, Gilbert B, Rochat R, and others: Differences between mistimed and unwanted pregnancies among women who have live births, *Perspect Sex Reprod Health* 36(5):192-197, 2004.
3. Husley T: Association between early prenatal care and mother's intention of and desire for the pregnancy, *J Obstet Gynecol Neonat Nurs* 30:275-282, 2001.
4. Orr S, Miller C, James S, and others: Unintended pregnancy and preterm birth, *Pediatr Perinat Epidemiol* 14:309-313, 2000.
5. Aquilino M, Losch M: Fertility across the lifespan: desire for pregnancy at conception, *Matern Child Nurs* 30(4):256-262, 2005.
6. Singer J: Options counseling: techniques for caring for women with unintended pregnancies, *J Midwif Women's Health* 49(3):235-242, 2004.
7. Delbanco S, Lundy J, Hoff T, and others: Public knowledge and perceptions about unplanned pregnancy and contraception in three countries, *Fam Plan Perspect* 29:70-75, 1997.
8. Finer L, Henshaw S: Abortion incidence and services in the United States in 2000, *Perspect Sex Reprod Health* 35:6-15, 2003.
9. Jones R, Darroch J, Henshaw S: Patterns in the socioeconomic characteristics of women obtaining abortions in 2000-2001, *Perspect Sex Reprod Health* 34:226-245, 2002.
10. Lesnewski R: Preventing unintended pregnancy: implications for physicians, *Am Fam Phys* 69(12):2779-2780, 2782, 2004.
11. Joyce T, Kaestner R, Korenman S: The stability of pregnancy intentions and pregnancy-related maternal behaviors, *Matern Child Health J* 4:171-178, 2000.
12. Grussu P, Quatraro R, Nasta M: Profile of mood states: comparing women with planned and unplanned pregnancies, *Birth* 32(2):107-114, 2005.

CHAPTER 181

Vulvar and Vaginal Disorders

Patricia Polgar Bailey

NONNEOPLASTIC EPITHELIAL DISORDERS

DEFINITION AND EPIDEMIOLOGY

Benign vulvar disorders, although an infrequent cause of primary care visits, account for significant patient concern. Signs and symptoms include pruritus, pain, burning, irritation, and a mass or growth, with pruritus often being the chief patient complaint. Women have often tried various nonprescription remedies before coming to a provider.[1]

Vulvar pruritus is a common vulvar symptom that may be unrelated to vaginitis, sexually transmitted diseases (STDs), Bartholin's duct cysts, or neoplasms. Proper treatment of vulvar pruritus depends on an accurate diagnosis. Women with vulvar pruritus often receive multiple treatments in the absence of a correct diagnosis; women are commonly prescribed therapy over the phone without ever having been examined, even if symptoms have been recurrent.[2]

In examining women with vulvar pruritus, the provider is advised to ask about and inspect other areas of the body; many conditions affecting other organ systems, including tuberculosis, Crohn's disease, and endometriosis, can have vulvar manifestations. For example, vulvar psoriasis may have an unusual presentation, but more typical psoriatic lesions are often seen simultaneously elsewhere on the body and may provide a diagnostic clue.

The visual inspection is essential in identifying vulvar changes. A handheld microscope, or in some cases a colposcope, may allow for more detailed inspection. Vaginitis, cervicitis, and other STDs should be excluded. Some of the other common vulvar conditions causing pruritus are presented in this chapter.

Nonneoplastic epithelial disorders were formerly referred to as *vulvar dystrophies*. They were renamed under a classification scheme adopted in 1987 by the International Society for the Study of Vulvovaginal Disease to include the following:

- Lichen sclerosus (LS)
- Squamous hyperplasia
- Other dermatoses

LICHEN SCLEROSUS

Pathophysiology

LS (formerly lichen sclerosus et atrophicus) is no longer thought to be an atrophic disease, but the etiology of this chronic condition remains unknown. Some theories suggest that LS may be triggered by an infectious process, excessive friction, an autoimmune process, abnormal hormonal levels (especially testosterone), or genetic predisposition.[3,4]

Although primarily seen in perimenopausal and postmenopausal Caucasian women, LS occurs in females of all ages, including young girls. It affects males but at rates much lower than in females. LS is primarily found in the anogenital region, but it can be seen elsewhere on the body, such as the neck and shoulders.

Clinical Presentation and Physical Examination

Although it is sometimes asymptomatic, LS often results in severe vulvar pruritus or dyspareunia. Affected areas include the labia minora, vulvar vestibule, perineum, and clitoris; the vagina is usually spared. Early LS can be particularly difficult to diagnose. On examination white papules can be seen, and the epithelium may appear normal or thin, resembling parchment. There is also typically decreased tissue elasticity, and edema may be present, depending on the disease stage. Fissures and secondary infections may develop, especially with sexual activity or scratching, which may make diagnosis especially difficult.[5] With disease progression, papules develop into large, hypopigmented, symmetric plaques, often hourglass or keyhole shaped, on the labia minora and vulva, which can resemble hyperplasia. If these are not treated, there is eventual loss of vulvar architecture such that the labia minora are no longer seen, and introital stenosis may develop, resulting in dyspareunia, ecchymoses, fissures, and telangiectases.[1,5,6]

Diagnostics and Differential Diagnosis

The differential diagnosis for LS includes lichen planus, which is more likely to involve erosive lesions in the vagina, or vitiligo, which has similar white plaques but no epithelial thinning.[5] The diagnosis is made by examination, and although vulvar biopsy may not be needed in clear-cut cases, it is important to exclude atypia or mixed diagnoses.[7] Findings on histologic examination include hyperkeratosis, epithelial thinning, cytoplasmic vacuolation of the basal layer of cells, follicular plugging, homogenization of the subepithelial layer, and inflammatory cell infiltration consisting of lymphocytes with few plasma cells. In addition, chronic fungal and allergic causes should be considered. Thyroid studies are recommended because approximately one third of women with LS are hypothyroid, although this relationship is unclear.[6]

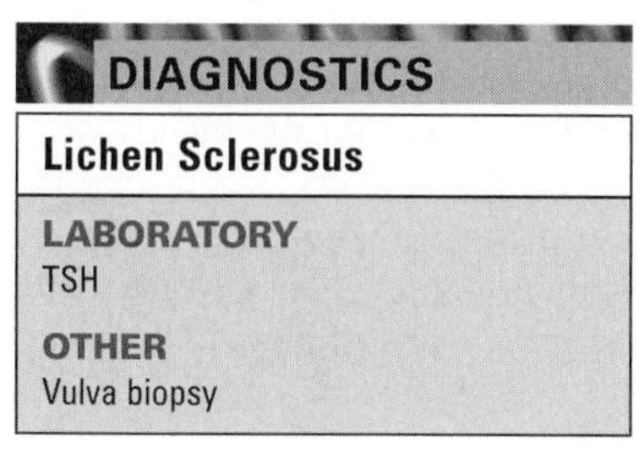

DIAGNOSTICS

Lichen Sclerosus

LABORATORY
TSH

OTHER
Vulva biopsy

DIFFERENTIAL DIAGNOSIS

Lichen Sclerosus

- Lichen planus

Management

Management has evolved over the years, and currently potent corticosteroids provide the best outcomes. The current treatment of choice is clobetasol propionate 0.05% (Cormax, Temovate), which is the most studied and has been shown to improve histologic changes. It provides short-term relief and long-term control in most women. It can be applied as an ointment twice daily for 1 to 3 months, with the dose gradually tapered.[8-11] Maintenance therapy may require as few as one or two applications per week.[1] If lesions recur, treatment can be reinstated. Long-term sequelae of topical steroids have not been noticed with this disorder.[11] Contact dermatitis is a rare but reported side effect of this medication. Subsequent LS recurrences are managed by reinstating the clobetasol therapy.[11] Long-term sequelae of potent topical corticosteroids (atrophy and thinning of skin and subcutaneous tissues) have not been clinically significant in this disorder.[11] Hydroxyzine 25 to 50 mg h.s. may also help relieve pruritus associated with LS.

Until recently, standard treatment for LS was testosterone propionate 2% in petroleum applied to the vulva or affected area two to three times per day for 2 to 6 months, followed by tapering to less frequent applications for maintenance therapy.[6] Recent studies show that testosterone is only slightly more effective than placebo. Increased serum androgens are seen in adults after 4 weeks of using testosterone, and many develop symptoms of clitoromegaly, acne, hair loss, voice changes, and increased libido, requiring cessation of medication.[12,13] Despite these known side effects, this regimen is still commonly prescribed.

Complications and Indications for Referral or Hospitalization

If there is any question of hyperplasia or a mixed diagnosis, a gynecologic referral for a biopsy to exclude atypia is indicated, especially in older women. LS is often seen in combination with hyperplasia and requires closer follow-up monitoring.[6] Prophylactic surgery, previously recommended to prevent conversion to cancer, is no longer considered appropriate management.[3,4,14] The role of surgery is quite defined in LS and should be limited to repair of introital stenosis or confirmed malignant disease.[4,12] Although surgery is sometimes advocated for management of recalcitrant symptoms, it should be remembered that women are still at risk for LS recurrence even after vulvectomy.

Patient and Family Education

The likelihood of recurrence of LS should be discussed; however, connections between childhood LS and future outbreaks or increased risk of neoplastic changes are unclear.[4] Adherence to treatment regimens and follow-up visits should be encouraged. The affected area should be kept as clean and dry as possible, and application of a thin layer of petroleum jelly to the affected area to limit moisture loss may be helpful. The patient should be taught vulvar self-examination and to report early symptoms so that recurrences may be controlled with the lowest-potency medication possible.

SQUAMOUS CELL HYPERPLASIA

Pathophysiology

Generally, squamous cell hyperplasia is the result of repetitive surface trauma from irritants that cause scratching or rubbing—a perpetual itch-scratch cycle. Squamous cell hyperplasia is characterized histologically by epithelial thickening and hyperkeratosis, lengthening and thickening of the rete pegs, and an inflammatory reaction in the dermis. It manifests, as do most of the nonneoplastic epithelial disorders, as pruritus, which may be secondary to degeneration and inflammation of terminal nerve fibers. The diagnosis is one of exclusion, and because the condition is often thought to be the equivalent to lichen simplex chronicus, there is some diagnostic confusion.[1]

Clinical Presentation and Physical Examination

The affected woman may complain of pain, limitation of movement because of strictures, and dyspareunia. Squamous cell hyperplasia has a varied gross appearance, since it may be affected by moisture, scratching, or medications. The skin may look red or white depending on the amount of hyperkeratosis.

It may affect the labia majora, intralabial sulci, outer aspect of the labia minora, and clitoris. The skin may exhibit thickening, fissures, or excoriations. Lesions may be localized or poorly defined.

Diagnostics and Differential Diagnosis

It can be difficult to differentiate among the nonneoplastic epithelial disorders. A biopsy should be performed for histologic diagnosis; a punch biopsy, using adequate local analgesia, is generally the easiest type. Suturing of the biopsy site is rarely needed, since adequate hemostasis can be achieved with silver nitrate. The most important areas from which biopsy specimens should be taken are those of fissuring, ulceration, induration, or thick plaques. An additional reason for performing a biopsy is to exclude koilocytotic atypia, since both LS and squamous cell hyperplasia have a risk of carcinogenic transformation of 1% to 5%.[4]

Management

Treatment, as with LS, is aimed at relieving the itch-scratch cycle. General attention to proper hygiene is important. If the skin is moist or macerated, 5% Burow's solution applied three or four times daily for 30 to 60 minutes is beneficial.[1] Systemic antihistamines or tricyclic antidepressants, especially taken at bedtime, may help. The treatment of choice is application of a potent corticosteroid cream. Clobetasol propionate 0.05% and betamethasone have both been studied.[3] Unlike in LS, close monitoring for signs of long-term, adverse sequelae is essential.[1] For refractory lesions, intralesional injections of triamcinolone acetonide may be used.[1] Surgical treatment should be avoided, if possible, because the recurrence rate can be 40% to 50%.[1] Complications, considerations for referral, and patient education are the same as for LS.

CONTACT OR ALLERGIC DERMATITIS

The description of symptom onset can distinguish contact dermatitis from allergic dermatitis.[9] Contact dermatitis occurs when there is an immediate irritation of the area after exposure to an offending substance. Allergic responses, on the other hand, develop several days after exposure. The diagnosis of these conditions is made by history and physical examination findings that include erythema or edema. Both these conditions are relieved when the triggering substance is identified and eliminated. The list of possible irritants is extensive. Women should be asked about treatments to the vulva (either prescribed or over-the-counter medications) and use of feminine hygiene products such as douches, sprays, and deodorants; tampons or pads; condoms; spermicides; lubricants; laundry detergents; soaps; and shampoos. Burow's compresses, sitz baths, or emollients may improve symptoms. Allergic dermatitis usually takes a long time to resolve after exposure is terminated; resolution may be facilitated by a short course of topical steroids.

ECZEMA

Like eczema elsewhere on the body, vulvar eczema is typically a result of persistent scratching or aggravation of an area after an allergic trigger and can be an acute or chronic condition. The typical presentation includes severe pruritus lasting several weeks or more. A red rash or erythema without distinct borders is usually observed on examination and, if left untreated, can progress to the thickened scaly plaques seen in squamous cell hyperplasia.[6] The diagnosis is made by the symptom history, vulvar examination, and presence of eczema on other parts of the body; biopsies are not beneficial. Psoriasis and seborrhea are often confused with eczema, and any diagnosis will be hampered if the area has been scratched. The provider should be alert to the possibility of secondary infection with continued dermal irritation.[6]

Treatment of pruritus includes cold compresses, Burow's solution, and antihistamines. In addition, acute exacerbation of symptoms can be treated with an oral prednisone taper, which can be followed by topical betamethasone 0.1% b.i.d. to t.i.d. for 2 weeks, and then tapered. Less potent topical steroids, such as triamcinolone cream 0.1%, may also provide relief. Triamcinolone acetonide injections can be used for recalcitrant eczema. Secondary infections must also be treated. Any known triggers should be avoided. The use of mild soaps and a moisturizer to improve skin hydration may be helpful.

PSORIASIS

Often seen on the knees or elbows, psoriasis is an inherited chronic condition that appears as a pruritic, red and scaly, or thick white fissured plaque with clear-cut borders. It is often exacerbated by stress and occurs simultaneously on various parts of the body. In addition, new psoriatic lesions may develop at an injury site (referred to as Koebner's phenomenon). Biopsies are rarely useful for diagnosis, but candidiasis, eczema, seborrhea, and Paget's disease should be excluded.[6]

Treatment for psoriasis is aimed at symptom relief. Calcipotriene ointment (Dovonex), a topical vitamin D_3 preparation, is effective without the risk of skin atrophy.[1] Low-potency corticosteroid creams can be used but are seldom effective by themselves. Ultraviolet treatments are used to treat psoriasis; efficacy for vulvar lesions may be limited. Tar preparations are irritating to the vulvar skin and should be avoided.[1] Referral should be made to a gynecologist or dermatologist for recalcitrant symptoms, when steroid injections, methotrexate, retinoids, or cyclosporine therapy may be helpful.[15] Patient education should include stress management, which may reduce recurrence.

LICHEN PLANUS

Lichen planus can be an acute or chronic dermatosis affecting the skin, mucous membranes, or both. The cause is uncertain, but evidence suggests that it is immunologically mediated.[16] In the genital area the appearance ranges from delicate, white, reticulated papules to an erosive, desquamating process. Large denuded areas may lead to profuse leukorrhea or can become adherent, causing stenosis of the vaginal introitus. Diagnosis is confirmed by biopsy.

Initial treatment consists of topical high-potency corticosteroid ointments or intralesional corticosteroid injections for symptomatic relief. Short courses of systemic corticosteroids may be needed for severe symptoms or flares of disease.[17,18]

OTHER NONNEOPLASTIC EPITHELIAL DISORDERS

Other nonneoplastic epithelial disorders include the "dark lesions" of lentigo melanosis (a frecklelike concentration of melanocytes), nevi, carcinoma, and melanoma and result from stimulation of the number or function of the melanocytes. Paget's disease, a red, scaly, localized eczematous lesion, is characterized by nests of clear cells at the tips of the rete pegs and hyperkeratosis. Early in the disease the gross appearance is characterized as "velvety" and then later as "mottled." Paget's disease has a 20% to 30% risk of transformation to cancer.[14]

VULVAR PAIN

In 1983 the International Society for the Study of Vulvovaginal Disease recommended that the term *vulvodynia* be used to describe burning vulvar pain.[19] Although burning vulvar symptoms can be attributed to conditions such as vaginitis, human papillomavirus (HPV), or dermatoses such as those described in this chapter, the term is generally reserved for conditions such as vulvar vestibulitis syndrome (VVS) and dysesthetic (essential) vulvodynia (DV), which have no known cause. It is hoped that increased understanding of these conditions will be accompanied by more precise nomenclature. Vulvodynia is a chronic vulvar pain of uncertain etiology that affects up to 16% of women in the general population.[20]

VULVAR VESTIBULITIS SYNDROME

Definition and Epidemiology

VVS is a chronic inflammatory condition of the vulvar vestibule that is characterized by burning pain on touch, which can persist for several days after the touch is removed. In 1987 Friedrich defined the condition and included three criteria for diagnosis: (1) severe pain on vestibular touch or attempted vaginal entry, (2) tenderness to pressure localized within the vulvar vestibule, and (3) physical findings confined to vestibular erythema of various degrees.[21] Although VVS is now better understood, the etiology and most appropriate treatment of this condition remain unknown.

Vulvar vestibulitis is found almost exclusively in women of reproductive age who are or have been sexually active. The true prevalence is unknown. The majority of affected women are Caucasian (97%) and nulliparous (75%).[22] Primary (no identifiable initial trigger or time of onset) and secondary (such as after HPV or vaginitis treatment or postpartum) categories of VVS have been suggested.

Pathophysiology

For reasons that are unclear but that may suggest a genetic cause or selection bias, VVS is predominantly seen in Caucasian women, many of whom report having a relative who experienced similar symptoms or at least difficulty with tampon insertion.[23,24]

Causes of VVS, including HPV and a *Candida*-triggered autoimmune response, have been suggested but not supported in the literature. In fact, treatments for HPV, such as topical acid or laser therapy, can lead to secondary VVS. A causal association between VVS and *Candida* organisms has not been established, but as more women treat themselves repeatedly with over-the-counter vaginal fungicides, sensitivity to ingredients in these preparations may develop, increasing the risk of developing VVS. Other theories include an association between VVS and interstitial cystitis, both of which are inflammatory conditions of tissues that share embryologic origins. Many of these women have overlapping urinary and vulvar symptoms.[25,26] VVS may also be associated with a sympathetically maintained pain feedback loop that is perpetuated by an underlying pelvic floor muscle instability or hypertonicity that is initially triggered by a superficial tissue insult.[27,28]

The association between VVS and oral contraceptives remains controversial. It has been suggested that oral contraceptives down-regulate receptors enough to cause epithelial thinning, but research has not demonstrated a clear association between oral contraceptives and the incidence of VVS. Although reports include exacerbation of symptoms related to the menstrual cycle or pregnancy, no mechanism has been identified.[23] In addition, various hormonal creams have been shown to be generally ineffective in treating VVS.[15]

Given the lack of obvious clinical findings, VVS was long thought to be a result of sexual dysfunction, childhood trauma, or some other psychologic disorder, theories now recognized as fallacious. A chronic pain syndrome that heavily affects sexual relationships and daily activities is apt to be, not surprisingly, accompanied by anxiety or depression. These issues should be addressed, but to assume a causal link with VVS is inappropriate.

Clinical Presentation

A thorough history is essential to managing VVS. Presentation commonly includes complaints of severe, burning vulvar pain during introital penetration with sexual intercourse or tampon use, during bicycle or horseback riding, or when wearing tight or bulky clothing. Pain may last a few minutes or as long as a few days after the trigger has been removed. Symptoms have often been present for months or years, resulting in a long history of frequent consultations. The history should include information about the initial onset of symptoms (if an initial onset can be identified), along with symptom characteristics, duration, and frequency. The impact of symptoms on sexual function should be determined, including how often intercourse is attempted and how often it is stopped because of pain. Assessment should also be made as to the impact of symptoms on daily activities and how often thoughts are distracted by symptoms during the course of a day. The presence of back pain, muscle soreness, and bowel and urinary patterns may be helpful in identifying related disorders. Previous ineffective treatment should be documented. Prior management has often included repeated treatment for yeast or bacterial infections; determining whether treatment was empiric or culture based is essential. A review of previous medical records can be helpful. Women should also be asked if they have developed any techniques of their own to ease discomfort.

Physical Examination and Diagnostics

Generally, visual examination of the vulva and introitus is unremarkable, although erythema near the vestibular glands may be present. The most revealing test is the use of a water- or saline-moistened cotton-tipped applicator to test for sensitivity to touch. This is done by simply touching with the applicator in multiple locations around the labia minora, vestibule, clitoris, and urethra to determine any areas of tenderness, to elicit burning, and to rate the degree of discomfort. With VVS, tenderness or burning is usually triggered near Bartholin's glands, near the posterior fourchette, and to either side of the urethral opening. Use of the smallest speculum possible and a gentle, unhurried examination with extra lubrication will be better tolerated. Colposcopic evaluation of the involved areas, although advocated by some, is generally not appropriate unless physical findings suggest HPV or vulvar intraepithelial neoplasia. Vulvar biopsies typically show inflammation and should be performed only if a pathologic condition is suggested by the physical examination.[29]

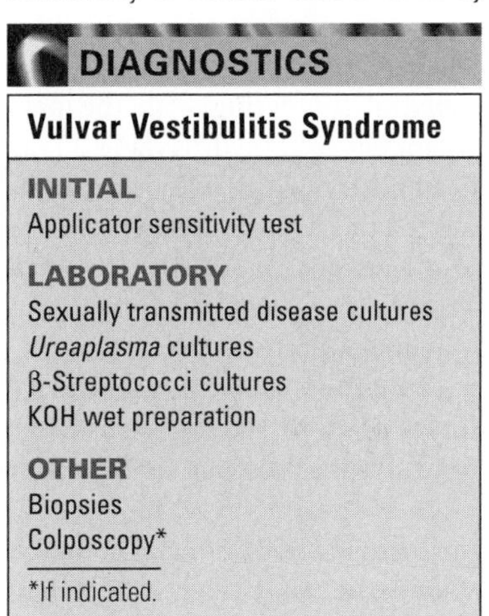
DIAGNOSTICS

Vulvar Vestibulitis Syndrome

INITIAL
Applicator sensitivity test

LABORATORY
Sexually transmitted disease cultures
Ureaplasma cultures
β-Streptococci cultures
KOH wet preparation

OTHER
Biopsies
Colposcopy*

*If indicated.

Differential Diagnosis

STDs should be excluded and cultures performed for β-streptococci and *Candida* and *Ureaplasma* organisms.[30,31] The diagnosis of VVS is made on the basis of the history, positive physical examination findings, and negative cultures.[21]

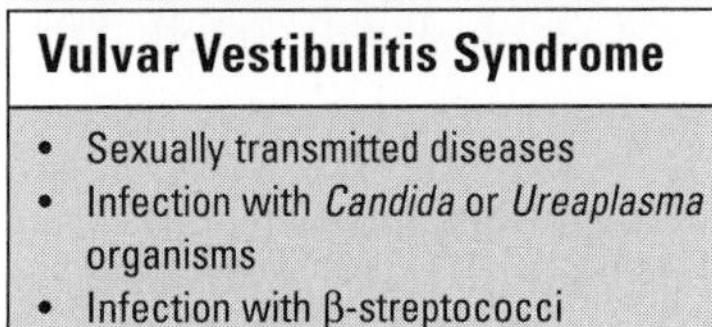
DIFFERENTIAL DIAGNOSIS

Vulvar Vestibulitis Syndrome

- Sexually transmitted diseases
- Infection with *Candida* or *Ureaplasma* organisms
- Infection with β-streptococci

Management

Although spontaneous resolution of symptoms is possible, treating VVS is often a matter of trial and error and requires a solid provider-patient relationship.[32] Although many treatments are aimed at what is thought to be the underlying problem, the fact that the primary symptom is pain cannot be forgotten. Reassurance that this condition is real and that the concerns are legitimate is important. Women should be informed that partial symptom relief is likely, but that it will take time for adequate treatment trials. Realistic goals and time frames should be established and extra time planned for appointments.[33] Each woman should be involved as much as possible and should keep a daily symptom log, noting any possible pain triggers and rating the severity and duration of symptoms. Decisions to seek alternative forms of treatment, such as acupuncture, should be supported and incorporated into the overall management plan.

Treatment of VVS is dictated by the woman's history. If recurrent candidiasis is suspected, the provider could institute a trial of fluconazole 150 mg weekly for 2 months, then biweekly for another 2 months, followed by one dose monthly. Liver function tests generally do not need to be performed, but careful evaluation for possible drug interactions (e.g., oral hypoglycemics, anticoagulants) is required.[22] Topical antifungal creams such as terconazole, miconazole, and clotrimazole may further irritate the vestibule.

Other oral treatments aimed at interfering with the pain feedback loop include antihistamines (e.g., hydroxyzine 25 mg h.s.) or antidepressant medications. Low-dose antidepressants have long been used to manage pain, and it should be carefully explained that this is the indication for which the antidepressant is being prescribed. Suggested antidepressant regimens include oral amitriptyline or nortriptyline 10 mg h.s., with a gradual increase every 2 to 4 weeks (while monitoring for side effects) to a total dosage of 75 to 100 mg h.s.[34] Often patients will notice improvement with a dosage of 50 mg or less every day.

Another noninvasive approach involves education about calcium oxalate restriction and calcium citrate supplementation. Many common foods, such as peanut butter, are high in calcium oxalates, and although restricting intake may be difficult, some have found it helpful. Symptom reduction has been achieved with calcium citrate and a low-oxalate diet.[35] Additional information on low-oxalate diets can be obtained from national VVS groups.

Complications

Patients with vulvar pain may be reticent to discuss physical and sexual concerns and reluctant to have pelvic examinations. The disorder may be embarrassing and frustrating and may prohibit some patients from enjoying life or an intimate sexual relationship. These patients require considerable support and understanding and often will benefit from psychologic counseling.

Indications for Referral or Hospitalization

Consultation with a physical therapist is helpful to evaluate for pelvic asymmetry and problems with the pelvic floor musculature, which typically shows instability and increased resting tone in patients with VVS.[27,28] Trigger point physical therapy for myofascial release may be therapeutic, especially for patients complaining of back pain or persistent muscle soreness.[35,36] Continued pelvic floor muscle dysfunction may perpetuate the sympathetically maintained pain feedback loop. Twice-daily biofeedback exercises may help reestablish muscle stability over the course of many months and provide significant, if not complete, symptom relief.[27]

If the response to any of the aforementioned interventions has been inadequate, referral should be made to a gynecologist knowledgeable about different treatment options, such as interferon injections, laser surgery, and vestibulectomy.[37] Interferon therapy involves vestibular injections three times a week for 4 weeks. Mixed results have been realized with both interferon therapy and laser surgery.[38,39] Vestibulectomy remains the final option and has a success rate of 50% to 60% (complete symptom relief), which is thought to improve with the use of newer surgical methods and appropriate screening of patients.[40] Counseling and preoperative or postoperative treatment of vaginismus using dilators have been shown to improve surgical outcomes.[40,41]

Patient and Family Education

The impact of VVS on intimate relationships is significant, and the woman's partner should be included in discussions when possible and appropriate. Counseling referrals should be offered with the understanding that the health care provider does not believe symptoms are psychogenic in nature, but rather that there are real emotional challenges to living with a chronic pain syndrome; the provider should also acknowledge that hope often gives way to disappointment before symptom relief is experienced. Local peer support groups can be found in some areas, and women can contact national groups for more information (Box 181-1).

BOX 181-1

PATIENT EDUCATION AND RESOURCES

1. Wear loose, soft clothing as much as possible, such as skirts without underwear while at home. Avoid spandex and stockings, or try thigh-high or shorter stockings.
2. Wear all-white, all-cotton underwear always (not just cotton crotch panel).
3. Use only white, unscented toilet paper.
4. Use mild laundry detergent and rinse underwear a second time in hot water.
5. When bathing, use mild soap and carefully rinse vulvar area with plain water. Ensure all soaps and shampoos are completely rinsed from area.
6. Avoid deodorant tampons and pads; instead of panty liners on light days, wear old underwear that can get stained. Another option is reusable cotton menstrual pads, available from GladRags, PO Box 12648, Portland, OR 97212; (800) 799-4523; http://www.gladrags.com.
7. Avoid douches and deodorant sprays or powders in the groin area.
8. Use pure vegetable oil or mineral oil for lubrication with sex; avoid other commercial lubricants and spermicides.
9. Maintain as much nonpenetrating sexual activity as possible.
10. Rinse vulva after voiding with plain water spray bottle.
11. Keep detailed symptom diary that includes at least the following: characteristics of symptoms, their severity and duration, and triggering event if identified.
12. Contact national resources for local support groups, additional information, and newsletters:
    VP (Vulvar Pain) Foundation
    PO Drawer 177
    Graham, NC 27253
    (336) 226-0704 http://www.vulvarpainfoundation.org
    National Vulvodynia Association
    PO Box 4491
    Silver Spring, MD 20914
    (301) 299-0775
    http://www.nva.org

When discussing treatment options, providers should first counsel women to avoid vulvar irritants and implement the self-care measures described in Box 181-1. Many topical treatment options have been tried, including estrogen and progesterone creams and topical anesthetics such as lidocaine 2% jelly. Although some women may respond to these therapies, others will experience an exacerbation of symptoms with any topical medication.[32]

DYSESTHETIC (ESSENTIAL) VULVODYNIA

DV is characterized by spontaneous and constant vulvar pain without the focal tenderness typically seen in VVS. In DV, pain is not confined to coital attempts or other known triggers. Complaints of concomitant urethral, rectal, or back pain are more common than with VVS.[34] This condition may represent a neuropathic process such as a reflex sympathetic dystrophy or pudendal neuralgia.[42] Other than more widespread symptom distribution, physical findings on examination are similarly unremarkable, as with VVS.

The goal of treatment in DV is pain management. If initial attempts at treating symptoms are not successful, consultation with a pain management specialist may be helpful. As with VVS, attention should be given to pain and the emotional impact chronic pain can have on a person's life. Counseling referrals should be offered. Topical or oral estrogen may be useful in some cases, but women with DV are more likely than those with VVS to respond well to antidepressant therapy.[34] Dosages are the same as those used for VVS. If antidepressants are unsuccessful, anticonvulsants such as phenytoin or carbamazepine may be helpful, but their use requires strict monitoring of blood levels. A 50% success rate with nerve blocks of three to six injections has been demonstrated. Surgery is a final option and is thought to be more effective for DV than laser surgery or alcohol injections.[34] Alternative forms of chronic pain management, such as guided imagery or acupuncture, may be useful as well, but outcome data are not yet available.

GENITAL HUMAN PAPILLOMAVIRUS

DEFINITION AND EPIDEMIOLOGY

Genital HPV is a group of at least 30 HPV types that have an affinity for the anogenital region. Clinical genital HPV infections are well known as genital warts, or condylomata acuminata; these are benign tumors often caused by HPV types 6 and 11, which have a low risk for oncogenicity. Infections with HPV types 16 and 18, with a high risk for oncogenicity, have been associated with high-grade intraepithelial neoplasia and genital cancers, particularly cervical cancer.

Genital HPV is the most common viral STD. The exact prevalence and incidence of HPV infections are unknown. However, it has been estimated that at any given time approximately 1% of sexually active women have external genital warts and that 20% to 50% have subclinical or latent genital HPV infection.[39] Approximately 50% to 80% of men who have sexual intercourse with women with HPV will develop HPV infection.[40]

PATHOPHYSIOLOGY

The pathophysiology of genital HPV infection is not clearly understood.[41] It seems, however, that HPV enters the genital epithelium through an area of microtrauma. Patients exposed to genital HPV may develop clinical, subclinical, or latent infections. Clinical infection results from productive infection in which the cells have altered differentiation and/or transit time and the development of warts. In subclinical infection, HPV viral proteins and infectious particles are present, but there is no overtly visible change in the skin. In latent infection, HPV DNA is in the cell, but the complete viral particles are not assembled. The vast majority of latent HPV infections are transient and self-limiting.[42]

As indicated previously, genital HPV is considered an STD. It is most often spread by genital skin–to–genital skin contact. Although the incidence is infrequent, nonsexual routes of transmission, including autoinoculation and vertical and perinatal transmission, are also possible. Infection with HPV may be followed by a latency period ranging from 2 weeks to several years. The long latency or incubation period makes it challenging to determine the origin of the virus and its mode of transmission. The degree to which transmission is possible in latent and subclinical infection is not known; however, researchers have proposed that individuals with HPV are less infectious when they are free of visible warts.[43] Although much remains unknown about the specifics of infectivity, condom use is encouraged. Female condoms may be more helpful than male condoms during heterosexual intercourse because, when used properly, they substantially decrease the area of exposed genital skin.[44]

CLINICAL PRESENTATION

Genital Warts

Genital warts, also known as condylomata acuminata, are benign tumors that often have a pointed, irregular, fissured appearance. Their appearance ranges from single, small, painless, smooth, flat, skin-colored warts to fleshy papules that may become confluent cauliflower-like growths (Color Plate 7). Although they are often asymptomatic, genital warts can be associated with pruritus, burning, pain, and bleeding. They usually regress spontaneously but may last anywhere from a month to several years.

Genital warts in women occur most often on the vulva, but they may also be seen on the introitus, vagina, perineum, perianal area, urethra, and cervix. In men genital warts often occur on the distal third of the penis and on the urethral meatus, urethra, scrotum, and perianal area. Some men with urethral lesions have hematuria. Rarely, genital warts can be found on the oral mucosa, larynx, trachea, rectum, or bladder.

Intraepithelial Neoplasia

HPV infection can lead to intraepithelial lesions, which are dysplastic changes of the anogenital epithelium. HPV is most often associated with the development of intraepithelial lesions of the cervix, referred to as *cervical intraepithelial neoplasia*; however, it is also associated with intraepithelial lesions of the vulva, vagina, anus, and penis. The vast majority of HPV infections will not become malignant even if left untreated.[45]

DIAGNOSTICS

The diagnosis of genital warts is usually made during visual inspection on the basis of the typical clinical appearance. A biopsy and histologic examination should be performed when patients have frequent recurrences or resistant, large, or pigmented warts. The threshold for biopsy should be lowered in patients who are immunosuppressed, since these patients are at greater risk of developing squamous cell carcinoma. Because of the risk of developing anal cancer associated with the presence of intraanal warts, anoscopy may be considered for patients who have genital warts and a history of anal-receptive intercourse. All women with genital warts should have a Papanicolaou's (Pap) test performed to screen for cervical HPV infection. Screening for syphilis (rapid plasma reagin), other STDs, and HIV should be offered.

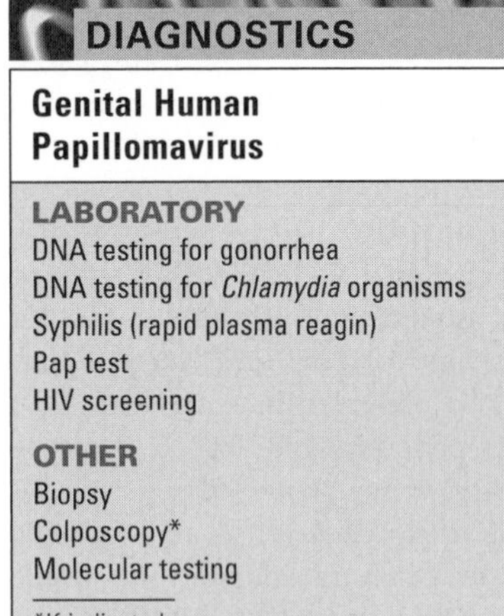

DIAGNOSTICS

Genital Human Papillomavirus

LABORATORY
DNA testing for gonorrhea
DNA testing for *Chlamydia* organisms
Syphilis (rapid plasma reagin)
Pap test
HIV screening

OTHER
Biopsy
Colposcopy*
Molecular testing

*If indicated.

The application of 3% to 5% acetic acid causes most tissue infected with HPV to whiten. This is called acetowhitening. However, acetic acid application is not a specific test for HPV infection, and the specificity and sensitivity of this procedure for screening have not been defined. Therefore routine use of this procedure for screening to detect HPV infection is not recommended.[46] Magnification (often with a colposcope) and directed biopsy allow practitioners to diagnose subclinical HPV infection. Histologic evidence of HPV infection is characterized by koilocytosis.

Latent genital HPV infection can be diagnosed by way of molecular testing and typing of genital HPV DNA. The utility of HPV DNA testing and typing in clinical practice is currently under debate, and it is not yet routinely recommended.[46]

DIFFERENTIAL DIAGNOSIS

See the Differential Diagnosis box.

DIFFERENTIAL DIAGNOSIS

Genital Human Papillomavirus

- Condylomata lata
- Molluscum contagiosum
- Herpes simplex virus
- Nevi
- Skin tags
- Folliculitis
- Vestibular papillae
- Seborrheic keratosis
- Sebaceous cysts
- Benign pearly penile papules
- Lichen planus
- Psoriasis
- Bowenoid papulosis*
- Intraepithelial neoplasm*
- Malignant melanoma*

*Bowenoid papulosis, malignant melanoma, and giant condyloma (Buschke-Löwenstein tumor) are neoplasms that, if suspected, require biopsy.[48]

MANAGEMENT

Current treatment for clinical HPV infection is aimed at removal of genital warts. Although wart-free periods are often achieved, recurrences are common with all therapies. The topical treatments considered first-line agents for most genital wart infections are discussed in Box 181-2. If a patient has extensive, large, vaginal, urethral, cervical, or rectal warts, or if treatment with the agents in Box 181-2 is ineffective, then another method of treatment should be tried and the patient referred to a facility experienced with modalities such as the loop electrosurgical excisional procedure, carbon dioxide laser, electrodesiccation, electrocauterization, surgical excision, intralesional interferon-α, or topical 5-fluorouracil cream.

LIFE SPAN CONSIDERATIONS

Genital warts tend to grow faster and larger during pregnancy; however, elective cesarean delivery is not recommended for women with genital HPV unless warts present mechanical obstruction. Vertical or perinatal transmission occurs infrequently. There is an association between genital warts in the mother and the development of juvenile laryngeal papillomatosis and external anogenital, nasooral, respiratory, and conjunctival warts in the child. In addition to vertical transmission from infected mothers, possible modes of HPV transmission in children include autoinoculation, casual social contact, and sexual abuse.

BOX 181-2

COMMON TOPICAL TREATMENTS FOR GENITAL WARTS

Cryotherapy with liquid nitrogen or probe: Applied weekly or biweekly to wart and 1-mm area of surrounding skin until warts are cleared. Some pain may be experienced during and after therapy.

Podofilox 0.5% (Condylox): Approved for self-treatment of external genital warts; applied to warts twice a day for 3 days, followed by a 4-day period of no treatment. This cycle can be repeated four times if necessary. Health care provider applies first treatment to teach technique. There is mild to no discomfort with treatment. It is contraindicated in pregnancy.

Podophyllum 10% to 25%: In a compound or tincture of benzoin. Applied to warts and washed off in 1 to 4 hours. The treatment can be repeated weekly if necessary. Discomfort may be mild. It is contraindicated in pregnancy and is not to be used on the cervix, vagina, or urethra. Systemic reactions have occurred with extensive use.

Trichloracetic acid (TCA) 80% to 90%: Applied to warts (normal tissue should be carefully avoided) and powdered with talc or baking soda to remove excess acid. Treatment can be repeated weekly if necessary. Sharp pain is common and may be decreased by applying lidocaine jelly or spray to skin around the wart.

Imiquimod 5% (Aldara): Self-applied cream for treatment of external and perianal genital warts. Applied to affected area, rubbed in completely, three times a week for a maximum of 16 weeks. Patient should avoid intercourse on nights cream is applied and wash off cream 6 to 10 hours after application. The cream can weaken condoms and diaphragms. Side effects of erythema, flaking, and edema may occur.

Modified from Centers for Disease Control and Prevention: 2006 Sexually transmitted diseases treatment guidelines, *MMWR* 55(RR-11):1-100, 2006.

COMPLICATIONS

The development of cervical cancer remains the largest threat of all HPV-associated neoplasias. (See Chapter 176 for further discussion.)

INDICATIONS FOR REFERRAL OR HOSPITALIZATION

A biopsy should be performed on any lesions that appear atypical, pigmented, or persistent to exclude malignancy. Pathologists interpreting biopsies need to be informed of previous treatment of affected areas, since podophyllum and 5-fluorouracil can cause atypical-appearing cells that could be falsely diagnosed as advanced intraepithelial neoplasia or cancer. If extensive warts are present or the presentation is uncertain, referral to an obstetrician/gynecologist is indicated.

PATIENT AND FAMILY EDUCATION

Diagnosis and treatment of HPV can be traumatic, negatively affecting relationships, employment, self-concept, self-esteem, sexuality, and mental health. Because of the potential psychosocial and psychosexual sequelae of HPV infection, the health care provider should assess the disease's personal impact on the lives of patients.

Information related to the nature of the virus, potential recurrences, modes of transmission, and treatment, as well as the benefits of follow-up care, should be presented to patients verbally and in written format. Sexual practices and safer sex should be discussed in an open and nonjudgmental manner. Anticipatory guidance or role playing with patients to help them disclose their HPV status to future or current partners may also be helpful. Encouraging patients and their partners to perform genital self-examination is suggested as well.

HEALTH PROMOTION

Health-promoting practices, such as limiting alcohol consumption, eating a well-balanced diet, quitting smoking, getting regular sleep and exercise, and reducing stress, help decrease the progression and recurrence of HPV infections. The American Social Health Association* has a quarterly newsletter, *HPV News,* designed to address the concerns of people with genital HPV infection.

VAGINITIS AND VAGINOSIS

DEFINITION AND EPIDEMIOLOGY

Vaginitis and vaginosis are disorders of the vagina that are characterized by vaginal discharge, odor, or vulvovaginal irritation. Vaginitis involves inflammation, whereas vaginosis does not. Both have historically been grouped under the term *vaginitis*. They result from an imbalance in the vaginal ecosystem, which may be caused by bacterial, fungal, protozoan, or viral infection[47]; hypoestrogenic states; foreign bodies; contact dermatitis; or allergy. Recurrent vaginitis is defined as four or more episodes within a year.

Affecting women of all ages, vaginitis is the most common gynecologic problem encountered by health care providers. Bacterial vaginosis (BV) is the most common cause of vaginitis, with an incidence of 15% to 65%, depending on the location of practice.[48] Approximately 50% of the women meeting the diagnostic criteria for BV are asymptomatic.[45] A common cause of vaginitis is vulvovaginal candidiasis (VVC), with an estimated 1.3 million cases annually in the United States.[45,47] An estimated 75% of all women will experience at least one episode of VVC in their lifetime, and 40% to 45% will experience more than one episode.[46] The third most common cause of vaginitis is trichomoniasis, which is also commonly asymptomatic.

*American Social Health Association, PO Box 13827, Research Triangle Park, NC 27709; (919) 361-8400; http://www.ashastd.org.

BACTERIAL VAGINOSIS

Pathophysiology

BV is characterized by the replacement of the normal, hydrogen peroxide–producing *Lactobacillus* organisms in the vagina with high concentrations of anaerobic bacteria, *Gardnerella vaginalis, Mycoplasma hominis*, and *Bacteroides* and *Mobiluncus* organisms.[45-47] BV is the most common cause of vaginitis symptoms among women of childbearing age. It is also referred to as nonspecific vaginitis or *Gardnerella* vaginitis.[47]

In the presence of BV infection, protective hydrogen peroxide–producing lactobacilli are significantly reduced. These changes are accompanied by an elevated pH, which facilitates the growth of the pathogenic organisms and their adherence to vaginal epithelia, seen as "clue" cells on a saline wet mount. The anaerobes facilitate the release of amines, which produce the characteristic "fishy" odor, especially on alkalinization of the vaginal discharge. BV is the most common cause of vaginal discharge or malodor; however, more than 50% of women with BV are asymptomatic.[45] The cause of microbial alterations in BV is not fully understood. It is associated with sexual activity, since women who have never been sexually active rarely get BV and women with multiple male sexual partners are at higher risk. See Box 181-3 for other suspected risk factors for BV. However, it cannot be strictly classified as an STD. The principal argument against sexual transmission of BV is the reported lack of benefit from treating male partners.[44,45]

Clinical Presentation

Symptoms of BV most often include an increased quantity of malodorous vaginal discharge, most noticeable after intercourse and during menses because of the alkaline nature of

BOX 181-3

SUSPECTED RISK FACTORS FOR BACTERIAL VAGINOSIS

- New sexual partner in the past month
- Multiple sexual partners
- Presence of a sexually transmitted disease
- Oral receptive sex
- Lesbian sexual relationship
- Early first coitus
- Douching
- Intrauterine contraceptive device use
- Cigarette smoking

semen and blood.[48] Some patients experience mild to moderate vulvovaginal irritation. On examination the vaginal discharge is often thin, homogeneous, and adherent to the vaginal walls and cervix. The fishy amine odor may be present, and rarely there is vaginal inflammation.

Physical Examination

The physical examination begins with visual inspection of the pubic area and vulva, and vaginal examination. Assessment of the skin turgor and elasticity; the presence of normal or sparse pubic hair; and whether the labia are full, atrophic, or dry is important. Any vulvovaginal erythema, lesions, discharge, or prolapse should be noted. A speculum examination is necessary to determine the color, consistency, viscosity, and odor of any vaginal or cervical discharge. In addition, the pH of any vaginal fluid should be tested. Erythema, lesions, erosion, or friability of the cervical surface or vaginal walls can be helpful in determining the diagnosis. A bimanual examination is done to assess for cervical motion tenderness and for uterine or adnexal masses or pain.

Diagnostics

The diagnosis of BV can be made by clinical or Gram's stain criteria. Clinical criteria require the presence of three of the following[45,46]:

1. Homogeneous, white, noninflammatory discharge that adheres to the vaginal walls
2. The presence of clue cells on microscopic examination
3. pH of vaginal fluid over 4.5
4. Vaginal discharge with a fishy odor before or after the addition of 10% potassium hydroxide (KOH) (positive whiff test)
5. The relative concentration of the bacterial morphotypes characteristic of BV (as determined with Gram's stain), which will be increased 100-fold to 1000-fold (Culture is not recommended because it is not specific.)

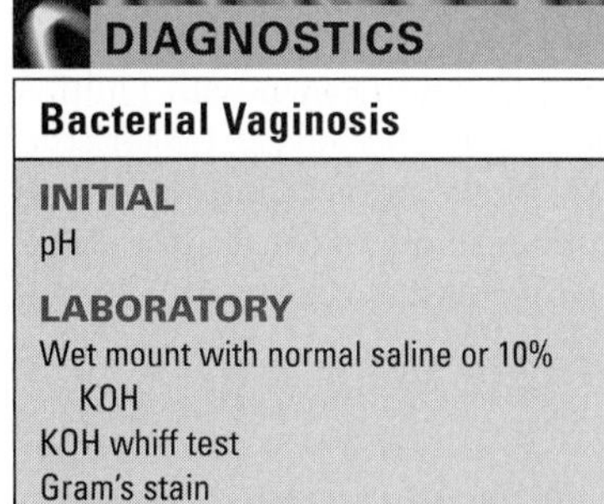

DIAGNOSTICS

Bacterial Vaginosis

INITIAL
pH

LABORATORY
Wet mount with normal saline or 10% KOH
KOH whiff test
Gram's stain

Differential Diagnosis

See the Differential Diagnosis box.

DIFFERENTIAL DIAGNOSIS

Vaginitis and Vaginosis

- Bacterial vaginosis
- Trichomoniasis
- Candidiasis
- Gonorrhea
- Chlamydia
- Cytolytic vaginosis
- Viral infections
- Foreign bodies
- Cervicitis
- Hypersensitivity
- Physiologic discharge

Management

Treatment options for BV are outlined in Box 181-4. The most common side effect of oral metronidazole is gastrointestinal upset. Patients taking metronidazole should be advised to avoid the use of alcohol during treatment and for 24 hours thereafter to avoid a disulfiram-like reaction (severe nausea and vomiting). Oral clindamycin has been shown to be as effective as oral metronidazole, but it is more expensive and may cause diarrhea.[45] Metronidazole 2 g single-dose therapy has the lowest efficacy for BV and is no longer a recommended or alternative therapy.[45] Metronidazole extended release (Flagyl ER) 750 mg once daily has been approved by the U.S. Food and Drug Administration (FDA) for treatment of BV, although data regarding clinical equivalency or comparing these regimens with other regimens have not been published. The results of clinical trials indicate that a woman's response to therapy and the likelihood of relapse or recurrence are not affected by treatment of a woman's sex partner. Therefore routine treatment of sexual partners is not recommended.[46]

Treatment of BV in pregnancy is of particular importance because of its association with adverse pregnancy outcomes, including preterm, low-birth-weight deliveries; intraamniotic infection; postpartum endometriosis; and postcesarean wound infection.[45] Treatment should use one of the oral therapies outlined in Box 181-4 to penetrate the chorion, amnion, and decidua.[46] Intravaginal clindamycin is not recommended in pregnancy because of an increased risk of preterm delivery.[45] Although metronidazole was previously contraindicated in the first trimester, multiple studies and meta-analyses have not demonstrated an association between metronidazole use during pregnancy and teratogenic or mutagenic effects in newborns.[45,48] The lower recommended doses further limit fetal exposure. Treatment in pregnancy should be followed by a test of cure 1 month after completion of therapy and by retreatment if necessary. Screening of the asymptomatic pregnant woman for BV remains controversial, although most agree that women at high risk for preterm delivery should be screened and treated in the early second trimester.[45,48] Several clinical trials have been done and more are under way to clarify

BOX 181-4

TREATMENT OF BACTERIAL VAGINOSIS

STANDARD TREATMENT
Metronidazole 500 mg PO b.i.d. for 7 days *or*
Clindamycin cream 2%, 1 full applicator (5 g) intravaginally h.s. for 7 days, *or*
Metronidazole gel 0.75%, 1 full applicator (5 g) intravaginally q day for 5 days

ALTERNATIVE REGIMENS
Clindamycin 300 mg PO b.i.d. for 7 days *or*
Clindamycin ovules 100 g intravaginally q.h.s. for 3 days

TREATMENT IN PREGNANCY*
Metronidazole 500 mg PO b.i.d. for 7 days *or*
Metronidazole 250 mg PO t.i.d. for 7 days *or*
Clindamycin 300 mg PO b.i.d. for 7 days

Modified from Centers for Disease Control and Prevention: 2006 Sexually transmitted diseases treatment guidelines, *MMWR* 55(RR-11):1-100, 2006.
*See text for discussion.

the benefits of therapy for BV in pregnancy.[45] Some studies in which oral clindamycin was used demonstrated a reduction in preterm birth. However, in other trials, where intravaginal clindamycin cream was administered at 16 to 32 weeks' gestation, there was an increase in adverse events (e.g., low birth weight and neonatal infection). Therefore intravaginal clindamycin cream should be used only during the first half of pregnancy.[45]

BV recurs within a month in about 30% of women.[49] Persistence of pathogens, an unidentified host factor, failure of lactobacilli to recolonize the vagina, and reinfection from a male partner are possible explanations. The provider should consider performing a routine test of cure (vaginal pH, whiff test, and a saline wet mount) 2 to 3 weeks after therapy to ensure that infection is resolved and to confirm regrowth of lactobacilli. For recurrent BV infections, defined as three or more episodes yearly, the provider can use alternative first-line agents and suggest prophylactic use of intravaginal metronidazole, twice a week for 3 to 6 months.[50]

Complications

Once considered benign, BV is now associated with many serious gynecologic and obstetric complications (Box 181-5). Perhaps of greatest concern is the possible link between BV and infection with HIV, as supported by several recent studies.[51-55] The shift in vaginal pH from acidity to alkalinity associated with the presence of semen may favor male-to-female transmission of HIV, and HIV infection is consistently associated with reduced levels of vaginal lactobacilli.[56]

The bacterial flora of BV have been implicated in pelvic inflammatory disease (PID) and have also been associated with endometritis, PID, and vaginal cuff cellulitis after invasive procedures. Evidence supports the screening and treatment of BV before therapeutic abortion,[45] and hysterectomy should be considered for patients at high risk for preterm labor.

Indications for Referral or Hospitalization and Patient and Family Education

See Indications for Referral or Hospitalization, p. 922, and Patient and Family Education, p. 923.

BOX 181-5

COMPLICATIONS ASSOCIATED WITH BACTERIAL VAGINOSIS

GYNECOLOGIC

- Increased risk of HIV
- Recurrent cystitis
- Pelvic inflammatory disease (PID), including postabortion and subclinical PID
- Cervicitis
- Abnormal Pap smears
- Postsurgical gynecologic infections

OBSTETRIC

- Early spontaneous abortion
- Preterm labor
- Premature rupture of membranes
- Chorioamnionitis
- Postpartum endometritis

VULVOVAGINAL CANDIDIASIS

Pathophysiology

VVC is caused by growth of the fungus *Candida* in the vagina. Most infections involve *Candida albicans*, although up to 17% may be caused by nonalbicans species.[57] The most common nonalbicans species involved in VVC are *Torulopsis glabrata* and *Candida tropicalis*, which may manifest atypically and be more resistant to standard therapies. Women with HIV infection or recurrent VVC are twice as likely to have nonalbicans VVC.[57] An estimated 75% of women will have at least one episode of VVC, and 40% to 45% will have two or more episodes.[45]

Several factors may trigger the change from colonization to proliferation, which results in the development of symptomatic VVC. These include changes in the vaginal ecosystem and possible phenotypic changes in the *Candida* organism. Symptomatic VVC involves candidal tissue invasion, causing inflammation, mucosal swelling, erythema, and exfoliation of epithelia. Factors that cause an increased susceptibility to VVC include antibiotic therapy, pregnancy, uncontrolled diabetes mellitus, use of oral contraceptives (especially high-dose formulations), immunosuppression, and occlusive synthetic clothing.[46]

Recurrent VVC is defined as four or more documented episodes of VVC in 1 year. The pathophysiology of recurrent or chronic VVC remains controversial. It affects less than 5% of women annually, and the majority have no predisposing condition, such as diabetes or immunosuppression. Earlier theories on the cause of recurrent VVC have included reinfection from an intestinal reservoir; sexual transmission; and the "vaginal relapse theory," which proposes that incomplete eradication of *Candida* organisms occurs after treatment and that the small numbers of *Candida* organisms present then multiply and result in recurrence. More recent theories propose deficiencies in the normal protective vaginal flora; a deficiency in antigen-specific, cell-mediated immunity to *Candida* organisms; and a possible local hypersensitivity to *Candida* organisms, predisposing the patient to recurrences.

Clinical Presentation

Typical symptoms of VVC include pruritus and vaginal discharge. Other symptoms may include vulvar burning, dyspareunia, vulvar dysuria, and vaginal irritation. Vaginal discharge is not always present, and there may only be a small amount. The thick whitish gray discharge is typically described as cottage cheese–like, although it can vary from thin to thick.[46] It is important to assess for recent use of over-the-counter preparations.

Physical Examination

On physical examination the vulva and vagina may be hyperemic and edematous. Vulvar excoriation may be present. The vaginal discharge is usually whitish, curdlike, and adherent to the vaginal walls. Variations in the vaginal discharge are possible, although care must be taken to exclude concurrent infections.

Diagnostics

The diagnosis of VVC can be made on demonstration of pseudohyphae or yeast on a 10% KOH wet mount or Gram's

DIAGNOSTICS

Vulvovaginal Candidiasis

INITIAL
pH

LABORATORY
Wet mount with normal saline or 10% KOH
Gram's stain
Culture

stain, or by culture. Use of KOH in microscopy improves visualization by disrupting cellular material, which may obscure the yeast forms. The vaginal pH in VVC is normal (4 to 4.5). Identification of yeast in the absence of symptoms is not an indication for treatment.

Differential Diagnosis

See the Differential Diagnosis box, p. 918.

Management

Treatment options for VVC are outlined in Box 181-6. The single-dose topical therapies should be reserved for mild VVC because of their slightly lower effectiveness. Multiday regimens are more appropriate for moderate to severe VVC, and the use of a cream is preferred in the presence of vulvar symptoms. Use of terconazole is more effective in nonalbicans VVC. The choice of an oral vs. topical therapy can be based on patient preference. However, increased cost and a small risk of liver toxicity cause some health care providers to reserve oral fluconazole for recurrent or recalcitrant VVC. Treatment of VVC in pregnancy should use one of the topical azoles, preferably for 7 days.[45] Treatment of sexual partners is not indicated except in cases of symptomatic balanitis or penile dermatitis.

BOX 181-6

RECOMMENDED REGIMENS FOR TREATMENT OF VULVOVAGINAL CANDIDIASIS

INTRAVAGINAL AGENTS

Butoconazole 2% cream, 5 g intravaginally for 3 days,* *or*
Butoconazole 2% cream, 5 g (butoconazole sustained release), single intravaginal application, *or*
Clotrimazole 1% cream, 5 g intravaginally for 7 to 14 days,* *or*
Clotrimazole 100-mg vaginal tablet for 7 days *or*
Clotrimazole 100-mg vaginal tablet, 2 tablets for 3 days, *or*
Clotrimazole 500-mg vaginal tablet, 1 tablet in a single application, *or*
Miconazole 2% cream, 5 g intravaginally for 7 days,* *or*
Miconazole 100-mg vaginal suppository, 1 suppository for 7 days,* *or*
Miconazole 200-mg vaginal suppository, 1 suppository for 3 days,* *or*
Miconazole 1200-mg vaginal suppository, 1 suppository for 1 day, *or*
Nystatin 100,000-unit vaginal tablet, 1 tablet for 14 days, *or*
Tioconazole 6.5% ointment, 5 g intravaginally in a single application,* *or*
Terconazole 0.4% cream, 5 g intravaginally for 7 days, *or*
Terconazole 0.8% cream, 5 g intravaginally for 3 days, *or*
Terconazole 80-mg vaginal suppository, 1 suppository for 3 days

ORAL AGENT

Fluconazole 150-mg oral tablet, 1 tablet in a single dose

Modified from Centers for Disease Control and Prevention: 2006 Sexually transmitted diseases treatment guidelines, *MMWR* 55(RR-11):1-100, 2006.
*Over-the-counter preparations.
NOTE: The creams and suppositories in this regimen are oil based and may weaken latex condoms and diaphragms.

In recurrent VVC it is necessary to assess for predisposing conditions and to confirm the diagnosis by culture. Evaluation should include a fasting glucose in nonpregnant patients or a glucose tolerance test if the patient is pregnant. Routine HIV testing is not indicated in patients without identifiable risk factors.[45]

An optimum treatment strategy for recurrent VVC has not been defined. Treatment must be individualized based on a comparison of effectiveness, convenience and ease of use, potential side effects, comorbidities, and cost. If a woman has infrequent recurrences, the simplest and most cost-effective regimen probably involves self-diagnosis and early initiation of topical therapy. For established diagnoses of recurrent VVC, maintenance therapy needs to be given frequently enough to prevent vaginal regrowth, but the optimal interval has not been established. Ketoconazole administered orally once daily, clotrimazole administered intravaginally twice weekly, terconazole administered intravaginally once weekly, and itraconazole administered orally once monthly have been relatively effective in reducing the recurrence of VVC.[58] In a randomized, prospective placebo-controlled study, weekly fluconazole administered during a six-month period reduced the frequency of recurrent VVC by more than 90%.[59] Patients taking oral antifungal agents should have their liver function tests monitored regularly.

Complications

Complications are uncommon. Superficial lesions and lacerations may occur in the vagina and vulva. Severely immunosuppressed patients may develop systemic infection. Patients with type 2 diabetes who are taking oral hypoglycemic medications and are being treated with fluconazole may develop severe hypoglycemia. Interactions of fluconazole with other drugs, particularly warfarin, are potentially serious.

Indications for Referral or Hospitalization and Patient and Family Education

See Indications for Referral or Hospitalization, p. 922, and Patient and Family Education, p. 923.

TRICHOMONIASIS

Pathophysiology

Trichomoniasis results from vaginal infection with the flagellated protozoan *Trichomonas vaginalis*, which is predominantly sexually transmitted. Transmission through contact with fomites may occur rarely.

Clinical Presentation and Physical Examination

Symptoms of trichomoniasis include vulvovaginal irritation, increased vaginal discharge, and occasional dysuria. On examination the discharge can be yellow-green, copious, and frothy. Vaginal inflammation is present, and punctate hemorrhages on the cervix are occasionally seen, producing the so-called strawberry cervix.

Diagnostics

In trichomoniasis the vaginal pH is greater than 4.5. Motile, flagellated trichomonads and leukocytes are seen on a saline wet mount. Diagnosis by wet mount has approximately 30% to

DIAGNOSTICS

Trichomoniasis

INITIAL
pH

LABORATORY
Wet mount with normal saline or 10% KOH
Culture
Pap test
Direct immunofluorescent antibody staining*

*If indicated.

70% sensitivity.[46] Diagnosis by culture is more sensitive and should be considered if there is suspicion of trichomoniasis but the wet mount is negative. Polymerase chain reaction testing is also available, although it is not commonly used at this time. The diagnosis can also be made incidentally if the organisms are found on a Pap test.

Differential Diagnosis

See the Differential Diagnosis box, p. 918.

Management

Treatment options for trichomoniasis are outlined in Box 181-7. Concurrent treatment of sexual partners is necessary, and the patient and her partner(s) should refrain from sexual activity until all have completed treatment and are symptom free. Patients and their partners must be instructed to avoid alcohol during treatment with metronidazole and for 24 hours after its completion to avoid a disulfiram-type reaction (severe nausea and vomiting). Recommended regimens include metronidazole 2 g orally in a single dose or tinidazole 2 g orally in a single dose. An alternative regimen is metronidazole 500 mg b.i.d. for 7 days.[46]

Patients with culture-documented trichomoniasis who do not respond to treatment as outlined in Box 181-7 and in whom reinfection has been excluded should be managed with expert consultation, including metronidazole susceptibility testing, which is available through the Centers for Disease Control and Prevention.[46]

BOX 181-7

TREATMENT OF TRICHOMONIASIS

RECOMMENDED REGIMEN
Metronidazole 2 g PO in a single dose *or*
Tinidazole 2 g PO in a single dose

ALTERNATIVE REGIMEN
Metronidazole 500 mg PO b.i.d. for 7 days

IN THE EVENT OF TREATMENT FAILURE
Retreat the patient and her partner(s) with metronidazole 500 mg PO b.i.d. for 7 days.

IF TREATMENT IS AGAIN UNSUCCESSFUL
Retreat patient with metronidazole 2 g PO q day for 3 to 5 days.

Modified from Centers for Disease Control and Prevention: 2006 Guidelines for treatment of sexually transmitted diseases, *MMWR* 55(RR-11):1-100, 2006.

Complications

Trichomoniasis in pregnancy has been associated with such adverse outcomes as premature rupture of membranes, preterm delivery, and low birth weight. The use of metronidazole in pregnancy has been controversial because of safety concerns. As discussed in the Bacterial Vaginosis section, this stance has been increasingly challenged. More conservative sources recommend waiting until the second trimester to treat with metronidazole, 2 g PO in a single dose, whereas some newer data suggest that waiting is not necessary.[57] If waiting until the second trimester to treat is preferred, clotrimazole can be used intravaginally for symptomatic relief. A test of cure should follow treatment of trichomoniasis in pregnancy.

Indications for Referral or Hospitalization and Patient and Family Education

See Indications for Referral or Hospitalization, p. 922, and Patient and Family Education, p. 923.

ATROPHIC VAGINITIS

Pathophysiology

Atrophic vaginitis is caused by reduced endogenous estrogen levels. This is most commonly found in the postmenopausal patient, although lactation, antagonistic medications, and ovarian failure resulting from disease processes also induce hypoestrogenic states. The lower estrogen level causes the vaginal epithelium to become thin and fragile, with a decreased glycogen content. There is an increased pH as a result of decreased lactic acid production, leading to an environment prone to an overgrowth of pathogenic organisms and to a lowered concentration of lactobacilli. Despite these changes, most women with vaginal atrophy are not symptomatic.

Clinical Presentation and Physical Examination

Women with atrophic vaginitis are seen with complaints of vaginal soreness, vulvovaginal dryness, occasional vaginal discharge or spotting, and dyspareunia. The vulvar skin is thin, with decreased subcutaneous tissue and variable pubic hair loss. The vaginal walls are pale with decreased or absent rugae, with occasional petechiae. Vaginal discharge can be thick, watery, or blood tinged.

Diagnostics

The vaginal pH in atrophic vaginitis is usually 5.5 to 7. The saline wet mount reveals increased leukocytes and small, round epithelia. If unexplained vaginal bleeding is present,

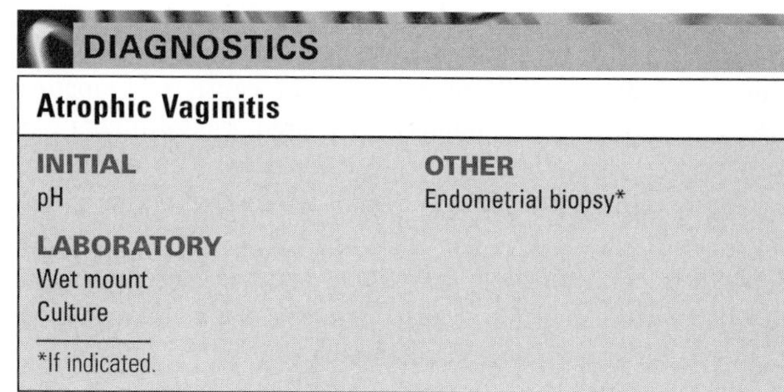

DIAGNOSTICS

Atrophic Vaginitis

INITIAL	OTHER
pH	Endometrial biopsy*
LABORATORY	
Wet mount	
Culture	

*If indicated.

endometrial biopsy is necessary. Similarly, if vulvar pruritus is present, a biopsy is indicated to exclude vulvar dystrophy or carcinoma. Cultures to exclude concurrent infections are done as indicated.

Differential Diagnosis

Although the majority of patients with vaginitis have one of the conditions outlined in the preceding material, other important, although less common, conditions should be considered in the differential diagnosis. See Differential Diagnosis box, p. 918.

Cytolytic Vaginosis. Cytolytic vaginosis (CV) is an important condition to consider in the differential diagnosis for recurrent atrophic vaginitis. It is caused by an overgrowth of *Lactobacillus* organisms in the vagina, which causes a decreased pH. This increased acidity is believed to be responsible for the irritative symptoms. Patients are seen with vulvovaginal pruritus, dyspareunia, clumpy white discharge, and vulvar dysuria. There tends to be an increase in symptoms during the luteal phase of the menstrual cycle. Most patients have tried numerous antifungal therapies to treat their symptoms, with only limited relief.

The diagnosis of CV is primarily by saline wet mount. There is an absence of trichomonads, "clue cells," and *Candida* organisms. There is an increase in lactobacilli, which may adhere to the epithelial cells, producing a "false clue cell." There may be bare or "naked" nuclei, the products of cytolysis. The pH is generally 3.5 to 4.5.

Treatment of CV involves raising the vaginal pH. The patient should be encouraged to discontinue all antifungal treatments. The use of tampons should be discontinued, thus allowing the alkaline menstrual blood to bathe the vaginal walls.[53] Baking soda sitz baths can decrease the irritative vulvar symptoms by neutralizing the acidic secretions. The patient can add 2 to 4 tablespoons of baking soda to 1 to 2 inches of warm bathwater for the sitz bath. Finally, if these conservative measures do not provide relief, the patient can use baking soda douches once or twice a week as needed.[60] These can be prepared using 1 to 2 teaspoons of baking soda in a pint of warm water.

Viral Infections. Viral infections such as herpes simplex virus (HSV) and HPV can also cause vaginal complaints. HSV can affect the cervix, causing profuse vaginal discharge, along with pain and ulceration. HPV can produce exophytic vaginal lesions, and larger condylomas can produce vaginal discharge, postcoital bleeding, and pruritus. The diagnosis and treatment of these viruses are outlined elsewhere in this text.

Foreign Body. Vaginal foreign bodies can cause inflammatory reactions leading to malodorous discharge, risk of ulceration, and fissures secondary to pressure necrosis. The symptoms generally resolve with the removal of the foreign body.

Cervicitis. Mucopurulent cervicitis is another cause of vaginal discharge that may also cause irritative vaginal symptoms. Cultures for gonorrhea and chlamydia should be performed.

Hypersensitivity. Allergy and contact dermatitis are possible causes of vaginitis symptoms. A thorough history can help identify any offending agents, especially spermicides, latex, bubble baths, feminine hygiene products, and soaps. Latex sensitivity should be suspected if the patient's symptoms are reproduced with a gynecologic examination using latex gloves. The elimination of the offending agent, short-term use of a mild corticosteroid cream, cool compresses, and use of a bland emollient such as mineral oil should provide relief of the symptoms. Avoidance of latex can be challenging. Use of nonlatex condoms or the female condom should be recommended, although nonlatex male condoms are less protective for HIV. The patient's chart should be labeled in cases of latex sensitivity to avoid future use of latex gloves or other products during examinations. Referral is indicated if symptoms do not resolve within 1 to 2 weeks and other causes cannot be identified.

Physiologic Discharge. Finally, the patient seen with increased vaginal discharge in the absence of malodor or irritative symptoms may simply need education regarding physiologic discharge and the cyclic variations that are possible.

Management

Treatment of atrophic vaginitis involves estrogen therapy, which causes maturation of the epithelium, reversing the changes that resulted in the vaginitis. Treatment usually involves topical estrogen cream, tablets, or vaginal rings. Recommended regimens include estradiol cream 0.1%, 2 to 4 g intravaginally every day for 1 to 2 weeks, then 1 to 2 g intravaginally every day for 1 to 2 weeks, then 1 g intravaginally one to three times per week for maintenance; or conjugated estrogen cream, 2 to 4 g intravaginally every day for 1 to 2 weeks, then 2 to 4 g intravaginally every other day for 1 to 2 weeks. The conjugated estrogen cream is then tapered and discontinued. A pill form of estradiol is also available and is used intravaginally every day for 1 to 2 weeks, then twice weekly for 2 to 4 weeks, then tapered and discontinued. A vaginal estrogen ring is available that is placed in the vagina and remains in place for 90 days.

An effort to taper and discontinue any regimen should be attempted after 3 months, since continued therapy may not be necessary. If treatment continues for more than 3 months, the addition of periodic progestin therapy is indicated in the patient with an intact uterus (e.g., medroxyprogesterone acetate 10 mg PO q day for the first 7 days of each month). Patients with atrophic vaginitis in whom estrogen is contraindicated may benefit from the use of lubricants or acidifying agents, although success has been limited.

Indications for Referral or Hospitalization

Consultation with a gynecologist is indicated in cases of treatment failure, as previously indicated. Postmenopausal women with unexplained vaginal bleeding or vulvar pruritus require referral for appropriate biopsy. Gynecologic consultation is also indicated in cases with an unusual presentation or in which the etiology is unknown or unclear.

Patient and Family Education

Thorough patient education is necessary regarding diagnosis, transmission, treatment, prevention, need for treatment of sexual partners, need for test of cure, and the sequelae of remaining untreated. Anticipatory guidance regarding medication side effects is essential. Furthermore, patients need counseling regarding the time by which relief can be expected and the indications for reevaluation. HIV testing and counseling should be considered in patients whose sexual activities have put them at higher risk.

REFERENCES

1. Larrabee R, Kylander J: Benign vulvar disorders: identifying features, practical management of nonneoplastic conditions and tumors, *Postgrad Med* 109(5):151-164, 2001.
2. Nunns D, Mandel D: The chronically symptomatic vulva: prevalence in primary health care, *Genitourin Med* 72:343-344, 1996.
3. Meffert L, Davis B, Grimwood R: Lichen sclerosus, *J Am Acad Dermatol* 32(3):393-416, 1995.
4. Thomas R, and others: Anogenital lichen sclerosus in women, *J Royal Soc Med* 89:694-698, 1995.
5. Leibowitch M: Lichen sclerosus, *Semin Dermatol* 15(1):42-46, 1996.
6. Wilkinson E, Stone K: *Atlas of vulvar disease,* Baltimore, 1995, Williams & Wilkins.
7. O'Keefe R, and others: Audit of 114 non-neoplastic vulvar biopsies, *Br J Obstet Gynaecol* 102:780-786, 1995.
8. Bracco G, and others: Clinical and histologic effects of topical treatments of vulvar lichen sclerosus: a critical evaluation, *J Reprod Med* 38(1):37-40, 1993.
9. Bornstein J, and others: Clobetasol dipropionate 0.05% versus testosterone propionate 2% topical application for severe lichen sclerosus, *Am J Obstet Gynecol* 178:80-84, 1998.
10. Lorenz B, and others: Lichen sclerosus: therapy with clobetasol propionate, *J Reprod Med* 43(9):790-794, 1998.
11. Sinha P, and others: Lichen sclerosus of the vulva: long-term steroid maintenance therapy, *J Reprod Med* 44(7):621-624, 1999.
12. Zellis S, Pincus S: Treatment of vulvar dermatoses, *Semin Dermatol* 15(1):71-76, 1996.
13. Joura E, and others: Short-term effects of topical testosterone in vulvar lichen sclerosus, *Obstet Gynecol* 89(2):297-299, 1997.
14. Abramov Y, and others: Surgical treatment of vulvar lichen sclerosus: a review, *Obstet Gynecol Surv* 51(3):193-199, 1996.
15. Kaufman RH, Faro S: *Benign diseases of the vulva and vagina,* ed 4, St Louis, 1994, Mosby.
16. Fitzpatrick TB, and others: Disorders of cell kinetics and differentiation. In *Color atlas and synopsis of clinical dermatology: common and serious disease,* ed 5, New York, 1997, McGraw-Hill.
17. Hopkins MP, Snyder MK: Benign disorders of vulva and vagina. In Curtis MG, Hopkins MP, editors: *Glass's office gynecology,* ed 5, Baltimore, 1999, Williams & Wilkins.
18. Lewis FM: Vulvar lichen planus, *Br J Dermatol* 138(4):569-575, 1998.
19. Lynch P: Vulvodynia: a syndrome of unexplained vulvar pain, psychologic disability and sexual dysfunction: the 1985 ISSVD presidential address, *J Reprod Med* 31(9):773-780, 1986.
20. Arnold L, Bachmann G, Rosen R, and others: Vulvodynia: characteristics and associations with comorbidities and quality of life, *Obstet Gynecol* 107:617-624, 2006.
21. Friedrich EG: Vulvar vestibulitis syndrome, *J Reprod Med* 32:110-114, 1987.
22. Davis G, Hutchison C: Clinical management of vulvodynia, *Clin Obstet Gynecol* 42(2):221-233, 1999.
23. Goestch M: Vulvar vestibulitis: prevalence and historic features in a general gynecologic population, *Am J Obstet Gynecol* 164(6):1609-1616, 1991.
24. Furlonge C, and others: Vulvar vestibulitis syndrome: a clinico-pathological study, *Br J Obstet Gynaecol* 98:703-706, 1991.
25. Fitzpatrick C, and others: Vulvar vestibulitis and interstitial cystitis: a disorder of urogenital sinus-derived epithelium? *Obstet Gynecol* 81(5):860-861, 1993.
26. Foster D, Robinson J, Davis K: Urethral pressure variation in women with vulvar vestibulitis syndrome, *Am J Obstet Gynecol* 169(1):107-112, 1993.
27. Glazer H, and others: Treatment of vulvar vestibulitis syndrome with electromyographic biofeedback of pelvic floor musculature, *J Reprod Med* 40(4):284-290, 1995.
28. White G, Jantos M, Glazer H: Establishing the diagnosis of vulvar vestibulitis, *J Reprod Med* 42(3):157-160, 1997.
29. Mann M, and others: Vulvar vestibulitis: significant clinical variables and treatment outcomes, *Obstet Gynecol* 79(1):122-125, 1992.
30. Bazin S, and others: Vulvar vestibulitis syndrome: an exploratory case-control study, *Obstet Gynecol* 83(1):47-50, 1994.
31. Sjöberg I, Lundqvist E: Vulvar vestibulitis in the north of Sweden: an epidemiologic case-control study, *J Reprod Med* 42(3):166-168, 1997.
32. Foster D, and others: Long-term outcome of perineoplasty for vulvar vestibulitis, *J Women Health* 4(6):669-675, 1995.
33. Julian T: Essential "dysesthetic" vulvodynia: (1) diagnosis and evaluation; (2) a rational approach for management, *Adv Colposcopy* 1-8, 1994.
34. McKay M: Dysesthetic ("essential") vulvodynia: treatment with amitriptyline, *J Reprod Med* 38(1):9-13, 1993.
35. Edwards L: Vulvodynia: an addendum by Libby Edwards, MD, *Fitzpatrick's J Clin Dermatol* 3(5):10-12, 1995.
36. Solomons C, Melmed M, Heitler S: Calcium citrate for vulvar vestibulitis: a case report, *J Reprod Med* 36(12):879-882, 1991.
37. Pomerantz E: Vulvodynia: etiology and treatment strategies, *J Ob/Gyn Patient* 18(3):10-12, 1994.
38. Spadt S: Suffering in silence: managing vulvar pain patients, *Contemp Nurse Pract* 51:32-38, 1995.
39. Marinoff S, and others: Intralesional alpha interferon: cost-effective therapy for vulvar vestibulitis syndrome, *J Reprod Med* 38(1):19-24, 1993.
40. Reid R, and others: Flashlamp-excited dye laser therapy of idiopathic vulvodynia is safe and efficacious, *Am J Obstet Gynecol* 172(6):1684-1701, 1995.
41. Abramov L, Wolman I, David M: Vaginismus: an important factor in the evaluation and management of vulvar vestibulitis syndrome, *Gynecol Obstet Invest* 38:194-197, 1994.
42. Schover L, Youngs D, Cannata R: Psychosexual aspects of the evaluation and management of vulvar vestibulitis, *Am J Obstet Gynecol* 167(3):630-636, 1992.
43. Jones K, Lehr S: Vulvodynia: diagnostic techniques and treatment modalities, *Nurse Pract* 19(4):34-46, 1994.
44. Wakamatsu MM: Vaginitis. In Carlson KJ, Eisenstat SA, editors: *Primary care of women,* St Louis, 1995, Mosby.
45. Colli E, and others: Treatment of male partners and reoccurrence of bacterial vaginosis: a randomized trial, *Genitourin Med* 73:267-270, 1997.
46. Centers for Disease Control and Prevention: 2006 guidelines for treatment of sexually transmitted diseases, *MMWR* 55(RR-11):1-100, 2006.
47. National Institute of Allergy and Infectious Disease: *Vaginitis due to vaginal infections,* Oct 2004, National Institutes of Health, retrieved Aug 4, 2006, from http://niaid.nih.gov/factsheets.vaginitis.htm.
48. Mead PB, and others: Screening for lower genital tract pathogens in the OB patient, *Contemp Ob/Gyn* 42(5):126-145, 1997.
49. Burtin P, and others: Safety of metronidazole in pregnancy: a meta-analysis, *Am J Obstet Gynecol* 172:525-529, 1995.
50. Hay P: Recurrent bacterial vaginosis, *Curr Infect Dis Rep* 2:506-512, 2000.
51. Sobel JD, Leaman D: Suppressive maintenance therapy of recurrent bacterial vaginosis utilizing 0.75% metronidazole gel, *Int J Gynaecol Obstet* 67(Suppl):41, 1999.

52. Taha TE, and others: Bacterial vaginosis and disturbances of vaginal flora: association with increased acquisition of HIV, *AIDS* 12:1699-1706, 1998.
53. Royce RA, and others: Bacterial vaginosis associated with HIV infection in pregnant women from North Carolina, *J AIDS Hum Retrovirol* 20:382-386, 1999.
54. Taha TE, and others: HIV infection and disturbances of vaginal flora during pregnancy, *J AIDS Hum Retrovirol* 20:52-59, 1999.
55. Martin HL, and others: Vaginal lactobacilli, microbial flora and risk of human immunodeficiency virus type 1 and sexually transmitted disease acquisition, *J Infect Dis* 180:1863-1868, 1999.
56. Tevi-Benissan C, and others: In vivo semen-associated pH neutralization of cervicovaginal secretions, *Clin Diagn Lab Immunol* 4:367-374, 1997.
57. Spinillo A, and others: Prevalence of and risk factors for fungal vaginitis caused by non-albicans species, *Am J Obstet Gynecol* 176:138-141, 1997.
58. Ringdahl EN: Treatment of recurrent vulvovaginal candidiasis, *Am Fam Phys* 61:3306-3312, 3317, 2000.
59. Sobel JD, Wiesenfeld HC, Martens M, and others: Maintenance fluconazole therapy for recurrent vulvovaginal candidiasis, *N Engl J Med* 351:876-883, 2004.
60. Secor RMC: Cytolytic vaginosis: a common cause of cyclic vulvovaginitis, *Nurse Pract Forum* 3(3):145-148, 1992.

PART 15

Evaluation and Management of Musculoskeletal and Arthritic Disorders

JOANNE SANDBERG-COOK, *Section Editor*

CHAPTER 182

Ankle and Foot Pain

Marie-Eileen Onieal

The foot contains 26 bones. Twelve of these bones are components of the medial and lateral longitudinal arches. In conjunction with the ankle, the foot plays a major role in supporting the body and providing locomotion. These functions can cause painful conditions of the foot that develop in the heel, arch, or forefoot. Improper or ill-fitting footwear is often the culprit.

In the United States, foot and ankle problems are the reason for more than 5.3 million visits every year to health care providers. Approximately 1.6 million visits are for ankle sprains, and 950,000 visits are for ankle fractures.[1] Sports injuries are often the cause, but even activities of daily living stress the foot and ankle. Walking alone puts up to 1.5 times the body weight on the foot. The average person logs roughly 1000 miles yearly. During 1 hour of strenuous exercise, feet cushion up to 1 million pounds of pressure.

The specific functions of the ankle and foot predispose them to injuries and disorders that can result in chronic problems if not identified quickly and managed properly.

ANKLE SPRAINS

DEFINITION AND EPIDEMIOLOGY

The uniaxial ankle joint, or ankle joint, is the most primitive joint in the body and is crucial to walking, running, and the performance of all sports. The limited motion of the ankle gives it stability. The ankle joint consists of three major bones: the tibia, fibula, and talus. The tibia and fibula form the ankle mortise, and the talus fits into this mortise. The talus, which has no muscle or tendon attachment, gives the ankle its hinge motion. The talus also bears the entire weight of the extremity during walking. The deltoid, anterior talofibular, calcaneal fibular, and the posterior talofibular ligaments hold the ankle bones in the mortise.

Ankle sprains occur at all ages and are the most common problem encountered by health care providers. A sprain is a ligamentous injury caused by an abnormal motion, a sudden change in direction, or a misstep on an uneven surface. Even a minor ankle sprain can jeopardize joint stability. The severity of the physical findings determines the sprain category (Table 182-1). The categories define the management of the injury, but the category parameters are indistinct. Previous ankle sprains can increase the potential for injury recurrence. Early diagnosis, treatment, and rehabilitation decrease the recurrence of a sprain in a previously injured ankle.

TABLE 182-1 Classification and Treatment of Ankle Sprains

First Degree	Second Degree	Third Degree
PATHOLOGY		
Stretching or minor tearing of ligament fibers	Partial tearing of ligament fibers	Complete tearing of ligament fibers
FINDINGS		
Minimum pain	Mild to moderate pain	Severe pain
Mild swelling	Moderate swelling	Significant swelling*
Mild ecchymosis	Moderate ecchymosis	Severe ecchymosis*
Full range of motion (ROM)	Painful, slightly limited motion	Loss of function
Mild point tenderness	Point tenderness over joint	Severe pain (difficult examination)
Stable joint	Mild joint laxity with stress	Abnormal joint movement
Ability to bear weight	Painful to bear weight (may be unable to do so)	Inability to bear weight
TREATMENT		
RICE; active ROM exercises	RICE; active ROM exercises as tolerated	Referral to orthopedic surgeon (may require surgery)
Non–weight-bearing activity (swimming, stationary bike)	Partial weight bearing (crutches, cane) as tolerated Gradual progression to full weight bearing	Cast for 4-6 weeks No weight bearing Gradual progression to full weight bearing
Return to sports in 2-3 weeks	Return to sports in 4-8 weeks with ankle support (Aircast or taping)	Rehabilitation before returning to sports with ankle support (Aircast or taping)
SEQUELAE		
Tends to recur in first month if not fully rehabilitated	Recurrent sprains, joint instability, traumatic arthritis	Persistent instability (nonsurgical treatment), traumatic arthritis

Created by Marie-Eileen Onieal, PhD, MMHS, RNC, PNP, FAANP.
RICE, Rest, ice, compression, and elevation.
*Occurs rapidly, usually within the first 30 minutes.

PATHOPHYSIOLOGY

Two types of injuries cause an ankle sprain. The most common is the inversion injury, in which the foot plantar flexes and internally rotates as the ankle inverts. The "roll" of the ankle injures the lateral ligaments and can also cause a lateral avulsion fracture. The less common eversion injury occurs when the ankle sustains an external rotation mechanism. Eversion stress injures the medial structures of the ankle, damaging the deltoid ligament or the syndesmosis.

CLINICAL PRESENTATION

The most common presentation of an ankle sprain is a swollen and painful joint. Ecchymosis and decreased range of motion are generally present. In many instances, weight bearing causes pain; some patients are unable to bear any weight on the affected joint.

When obtaining the history, it is important to determine whether the patient heard any audible sounds at the time of injury. An audible "snap" or "pop" indicates the potential for a more serious injury. Immediate swelling or ecchymosis raises the suspicion of a fracture or the amount of joint involvement. Patients also commonly report a sensation of lightheadedness, nausea, or diaphoresis immediately after the injury.[2]

PHYSICAL EXAMINATION

With a sprain, the ankle joint is often swollen and ecchymotic, and the edema can create an illusion of deformity. Limited active and passive motion and point tenderness at the site of injury are common. Joint laxity is present in more severe sprains. Muscle spasm often prevents accurate testing of strength and stability. If the injury is not acute, swelling and ecchymosis at the lateral aspect of the foot and the toes are common. With severe ankle sprains, tenderness may extend up the extremity. The entire lower limb should always be palpated.

DIAGNOSTICS

Although guidelines for radiographs are controversial, plain radiographs are necessary for severe injuries. An x-ray study of the lower leg should also be performed if there is tenderness at the fibular head. With less severe injuries, radiographs are used to exclude an avulsion injury. More extensive radiologic examinations such as stress films, CT scans, and MRIs are considered in consultation with an orthopedic surgeon.

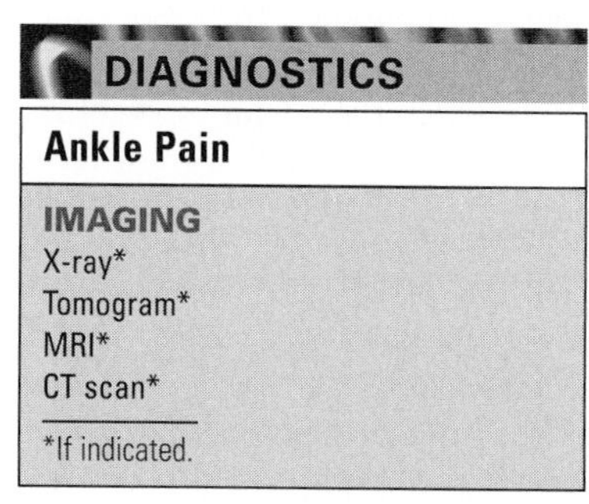
DIAGNOSTICS

Ankle Pain

IMAGING
X-ray*
Tomogram*
MRI*
CT scan*

*If indicated.

DIFFERENTIAL DIAGNOSIS

Ankle injuries range from simple strains to severe injuries. The possibility of associated fibula fracture, stress fracture, avulsion fracture, or dislocation should be considered. Bursitis and tendinitis should be included in the differential diagnosis.

DIFFERENTIAL DIAGNOSIS

Ankle Pain

- Trauma, fracture
- Strain
- Sprain (first, second, or third degree)
- Bursitis
- Dislocation or subluxation
- Tendinitis
- Achilles tendonitis
- Achilles bursitis

MANAGEMENT

The severity of the sprain dictates the management (see Table 182-1). TED (thromboembolic disease) hose provide support to the entire lower limb, aid circulation, and are less bulky than ankle splints or braces. All sprains require rehabilitation to restore the ankle to a stable and pain-free state. It is important for patients to understand that the treatment and recovery process will take weeks. Rehabilitation should begin as soon as possible after the injury and should include range-of-motion and strengthening exercises.[3,4] Even a severely edematous ankle can be mobilized with the simple exercise of "writing the alphabet" with the affected foot. A program of active and passive resistive exercises progresses as range of motion and strength improve. Patients can return to sports when they are pain free and able to balance on the injured leg. The patient with a second- or third-degree sprain should wear an external ankle support such as the Aircast stirrup for the remainder of the season.[3,4]

COMPLICATIONS

Most ankle sprains tend to recur within the first month if the ankle has not been fully rehabilitated. Second- and third-degree sprains carry with them an increased risk of joint instability and traumatic arthritis. A weak ankle joint is at risk for fracture when stressed.

INDICATIONS FOR REFERRAL OR HOSPITALIZATION

Fractures, dislocations or subluxations, and third-degree sprains require an orthopedic referral. Physical therapy may also be indicated to promote rehabilitation and a safe return to sports or work-related activities.

PATIENT AND FAMILY EDUCATION

Patients need to understand the importance of RICE (rest, ice, compression, and elevation), as well as the necessity of preventing weight bearing on the injured ankle. Patients and family members should also be instructed in medication dosages and side effects, proper elastic bandage wrapping technique, cast care, and crutch usage. The recuperative process and the risk of recurrence also require explanation.

ACHILLES TENDINITIS

DEFINITION AND EPIDEMIOLOGY

The Achilles tendon is posterior to the ankle joint and is responsible for flexion and extension of the ankle. It attaches the gastrocnemius and the soleus muscles of the calf to the calcaneus muscle, and it is palpated from the distal pole of the calf to the calcaneus.[5] The two most common injuries of the Achilles tendon are tendinitis and rupture.

Achilles tendinitis is a painful inflammation with or without swelling around the Achilles tendon. Unlike other tendons, the Achilles tendon does not have a synovial sheath but instead has a paratenon, which has a similar function. Except for severe cases, true Achilles tendinitis primarily affects the paratenon.[6] A nodule of mucoid degeneration forms in the body of the tendon in severe or chronic Achilles tendinitis.[7]

PATHOPHYSIOLOGY

Improper training, running up hills, or wearing shoes with soles that are too rigid often causes Achilles tendinitis. Shoes or boots with a high back can also irritate the tendon, causing inflammation. Wearing shoes with heels that maintain plantar flexion for long periods causes the tendon to shorten. Changing to flat or running shoes then increases stress on the tendon. Occasionally, Achilles tendinitis is caused by an anatomic abnormality such as excessive foot pronation or tight hamstrings or gastrocnemius muscles.[4,7]

CLINICAL PRESENTATION

Patients with Achilles tendinitis may have intermittent symptoms and may describe a pain that subsides during exercise but increases in severity while at rest. Morning stiffness or severe pain when climbing stairs is also common. Most patients have an abnormal gait. Some limp, and some walk on their toes to avoid the heel-strike phase of walking.

PHYSICAL EXAMINATION

Localized swelling may be present around the tendon. A palpable nodule and crepitus may be present in severe or chronic cases.[8]

DIAGNOSTICS

Radiologic or laboratory tests are usually unnecessary, but the appropriate diagnostic tests should be guided by the history. MRI may be useful in diagnosing a ruptured tendon.

DIFFERENTIAL DIAGNOSIS

Heel pain may have varied causes. Sprains, infection, fracture, plantar fasciitis, and partial tendon rupture should be considered in the differential diagnosis of Achilles tendinitis.

MANAGEMENT

Treatment of the acute phase of Achilles tendinitis begins with the cessation of all sports activities and exercise. Tendon rest is imperative to avoid further injury. In severe tendinitis, crutches and partial weight bearing are indicated. NSAIDs and an ice massage for 20 minutes three or four times a day help to decrease inflammation and pain. A simple shoe insert that raises the heel approximately 2 cm (0.8 inch) also helps ease strain on the tendon. In more severe or chronic cases, ultrasound is an adjunct therapy. Regular follow-up visits to assess progress and to discourage the patient from returning to activity prematurely are necessary. Resolution of acute tendinitis can take 8 weeks or longer. A program of stretching and strengthening begins when pain and swelling have subsided. To prevent recurrence or rupture, it is essential that patients do stretching exercises before engaging in any exercise.

COMPLICATIONS

Achilles tendon rupture is the most common complication of Achilles tendinitis. Shortening of the tendon, chronic tendinitis, and injuries as a result of the commonly associated abnormal gait also may result from acute tendinitis.

INDICATIONS FOR REFERRAL OR HOSPITALIZATION

Patients with severe tendinitis or suspected tendon rupture require immediate referral to an orthopedic surgeon. In addition, patients who fail conservative therapy or who have significant tightness in the hamstrings or gastrocnemius require referral.

PATIENT AND FAMILY EDUCATION

Achilles tendinitis can be a frustrating, slowly resolving, and recurrent problem. Patients with this condition need support during rehabilitation and need to be educated about proper retraining and stretching programs. During the rehabilitative phase, alternative activities such as swimming or cycling can be pursued as long as participation does not cause pain.

ACHILLES TENDON RUPTURE

DEFINITION AND EPIDEMIOLOGY

Achilles tendon rupture is a sudden event that results from a forced stretch on an already degenerating tendon; it is a soft tissue emergency. Although Achilles tendon ruptures are not common, there is an increased risk for this injury in poorly conditioned athletes more than 30 years old. In all, 80% of those injured are men; moreover, because most right-handed people begin their gait with their left foot, there is a higher incidence of left tendon ruptures.[9]

PATHOPHYSIOLOGY

Despite being the thickest and strongest tendon in the body, the Achilles tendon is the one most commonly ruptured, possibly as a result of underlying tendon degeneration or weakness that predisposes the tendon to rupture. In persons over age 30 years, there is a decreased blood supply to the area where the tendon most often ruptures. Often the offending event is a jump, a sudden change in direction, or simply a push off in stride. The pop of a tendon rupture is audible to others nearby.

CLINICAL PRESENTATION

The classic comment by patients with an Achilles tendon rupture is, "I thought I was shot in the calf." There is sudden weakness in the ankle. It is impossible to rise up on the toes, and most people limp; pain, however, is not common.

PHYSICAL EXAMINATION

There is a visible and palpable "gap" overlying the tendon where the rupture occurred, usually about 4 cm (1.5 inches) above the calcaneal prominence. The definitive evaluation is Thompson's test, which is performed with the patient kneeling on a chair or prone with the knee in flexed position. The tendon is intact if the foot plantar flexes when the calf is squeezed (negative Thompson). If there is no movement, the tendon is ruptured (positive Thompson). Thompson's test can be negative if the tear is partial.

DIAGNOSTICS

Radiologic examinations are not helpful because tendons are not radiopaque. MRI will demonstrate the rupture and can be used if indicated.

DIFFERENTIAL DIAGNOSIS

The classic presentation and physical findings that characterize a ruptured Achilles tendon simplify the diagnosis. However, the diagnosis may be more complex with a partial tear. Achilles tendinitis or Achilles bursitis is not usually associated with a sudden onset.

MANAGEMENT

There are two accepted treatments for the ruptured Achilles tendon. The conservative, nonsurgical approach requires a long-leg cast with the foot in a plantar-flexed position. The cast stays on for approximately 6 weeks, allowing the tendon to heal by scar formation. Wearing a heel lift for 2 months helps prevent undue stress on the new scar after casting. Unfortunately, this method has multiple disadvantages. The tendon heals longer in length, which weakens the calf muscle and the push-off power. Calf muscles also atrophy in a cast (usually about 20%), which adds to the decreased strength and size. In addition, 20% of the tendons allowed to heal in this manner rupture again once activities resume.[10] Patients with chronic pain who are not surgical candidates may benefit from an ankle-foot orthosis.

The second method of treatment for a ruptured Achilles tendon is surgical repair. The patient is in a long-leg cast for 6 weeks after surgery; then the patient wears a short-leg, walking cast for an additional 4 weeks.[11] As in the nonoperative method, a heel lift is used to prevent undue stress on the tendon. The surgical method is superior to the nonoperative method because it restores 95% of the normal power of the calf muscle.[10]

COMPLICATIONS

Weakened or atrophied muscles are a common complication of tendon ruptures. Close attention to rehabilitation and muscle strengthening after the injury helps reduce the magnitude of these complications.

INDICATIONS FOR REFERRAL OR HOSPITALIZATION

An Achilles tendon rupture is a soft tissue emergency. Immediate referral to an orthopedic surgeon is required.

PATIENT AND FAMILY EDUCATION

The most important education regarding Achilles tendon rupture is preventive. Patients who are beginning to exercise should be instructed to follow a simple, gentle stretching program beforehand. For example, patients can stand on a slanted board or on the edge of a step and let their heels drop below the level of the step. They hold this stretched position for 10 to 15 seconds, then repeat the exercise for 10 to 15 minutes. If patients cannot feel a pull on the Achilles tendon, they are not doing the stretch properly. Bouncing is counterproductive.

OSTEOCHONDRITIS DISSECANS

DEFINITION AND EPIDEMIOLOGY

With osteochondritis dissecans, a small fragment of bone underlying the articular cartilage becomes avascular and necrotic. In some cases, this necrotic area dislodges from the surface. Repeated stress on the joint causes a separation of the articular surface of the joint. Osteochondritis dissecans is seen more in adolescents and young adults and usually in males. It is common in athletes who participate in activities that place great stress on the ankle (ballet dancers, runners, basketball players). This condition also occurs at the knee and elbow.

PATHOPHYSIOLOGY

The etiology of this condition is unknown. Several theories have suggested various causes, including trauma, nonunion of a fracture line, and ischemic necrosis. Additionally noted are a familial tendency, certain skeletal abnormalities, or endocrine abnormalities.[12]

CLINICAL PRESENTATION

The usual presentation of osteochondritis dissecans is chronic pain and swelling that develops gradually over months. Activity increases the swelling and the pain, which intensifies as the ankle stiffens. Rest relieves the symptoms. Occasionally, the athlete will recall a trauma event.

PHYSICAL EXAMINATION

Range of motion is usually normal, and the joint is stable. Because the damaged area is within the joint, it is often difficult to palpate an area of tenderness.

DIAGNOSTICS

Radiologic examination alone provides the definitive diagnosis. Plain x-ray films of the ankle occasionally reveal a loose bone fragment or an area of sclerotic bone. Tomograms or MRIs help better define the lesion and the staging of the injury.

DIFFERENTIAL DIAGNOSIS

As in any joint, trauma or fracture should be considered. Tendinitis and recurrent sprain should also be considered.

MANAGEMENT

Osteochondritis dissecans warrants close observation by an orthopedic surgeon. The injured area has decreased or no capacity to heal itself; therefore surgery is often necessary. In the younger child with a shorter duration of pain, immobilization in a cast for 4 to 6 weeks may resolve the problem. Older patients, patients with a longer duration of injury, or patients with a loose bone fragment require surgery.

COMPLICATIONS

Degenerative arthritis, decreased range of motion, and chronic pain are all potential sequelae of this condition.

INDICATIONS FOR REFERRAL OR HOSPITALIZATION

Osteochondritis dissecans is a potentially serious condition. Orthopedic consultation is recommended to prevent complications.

PATIENT AND FAMILY EDUCATION

The exact cause of osteochondritis dissecans is unknown. Therefore it is important that patients and families understand that any joint pain that occurs during exercise or interferes with normal activities of daily living requires medical assessment. Careful explanation of the potential sequelae of this condition, including degenerative arthritis, decreased range of motion, and chronic pain, is also necessary.

PLANTAR FASCIITIS

DEFINITION AND EPIDEMIOLOGY

Plantar fasciitis is a painful disorder that involves the plantar aspect of the heel. It can be acute or chronic and is characterized by pain in the bottom of the foot—along the arch and the heel bone. A dense fibrous tissue, the plantar fascia, extends from the calcaneal tuberosity to the metatarsal heads. The fascia can become irritated from overuse, trauma, or shoes with poor arch support. People with flat or cavus feet are especially vulnerable to this condition.

PATHOPHYSIOLOGY

The plantar fascia supports the arch and the sole of the foot. High impact or stress, such as running and jumping, increases the pressure exerted on the fascia by spreading the toes or flattening the arch; this tears the fascia. Four common causes of fascia tears or inflammation are a sudden turn that places increased pressure on the sole of the foot, shoes with inadequate support, shoes with stiff soles, and feet that pronate excessively. Patients commonly have heel spurs. The pain is gradual in onset and increases as the inflammation worsens or as the tear extends.

CLINICAL PRESENTATION

Patients with plantar fasciitis complain of pain with weight bearing the first thing in the morning or after periods of rest. High-impact activities, running, and rising up on toes aggravate the pain or make it unbearable. Occasionally patients limp or avoid planting the heel when walking.

PHYSICAL EXAMINATION

With plantar fasciitis, there is point tenderness at the insertion of the fascia to the calcaneus. The patient may have fullness along the arch and pain along the body of the fascia, at the medial and lateral aspects of the heel, or at the metatarsal heads.

DIAGNOSTICS

X-ray studies are indicated to rule out any bony abnormality or other underlying causes such as a foreign body. Radiographs often reveal a bone spur that points forward from the heel.

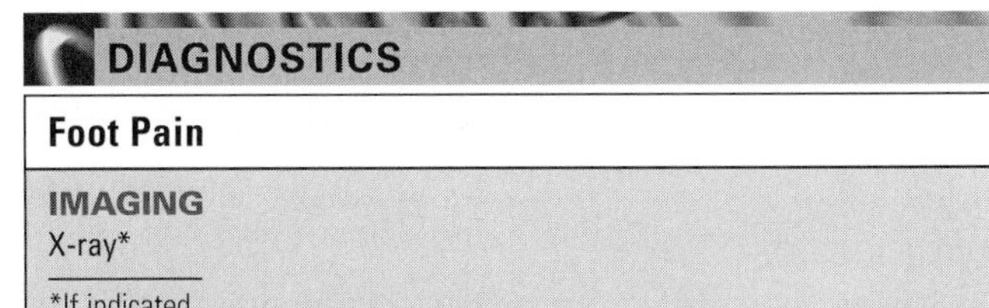
DIAGNOSTICS

Foot Pain

IMAGING
X-ray*

*If indicated.

DIFFERENTIAL DIAGNOSIS

A history of early morning heel discomfort that resolves after several minutes but returns later in the day is usually clinically diagnostic of plantar fasciitis. However, other causes of heel pain, including calcaneal fracture, retrocalcaneal or infracalcaneal bursitis, gout, infection of the calcaneal fat pad, arthritis, Reiter's syndrome, plantar warts, and tarsal tunnel syndrome, should be considered.

MANAGEMENT

A conservative approach to managing this condition begins with complete rest from high-impact activities. All shoes should have good arch support, which can be achieved with commercially available arch supports. Some patients do well with a heel cup or heel pad that raises the heel approximately $\frac{1}{4}$ inch. NSAIDs and ice massage help reduce inflammation and pain. A key component of treatment is a program of exercises that stretch the heel cord and plantar fascia.

COMPLICATIONS

Usually no complications are associated with plantar fasciitis. However, an alteration in gait can cause other musculoskeletal problems such as hip or back pain. Plantar fasciitis can be a lingering problem that frustrates both the patient and provider.

INDICATIONS FOR REFERRAL OR HOSPITALIZATION

Any patient who fails to respond to conservative therapies should be referred to an orthopedic surgeon or a podiatrist. Ultrasound treatment by a physical therapist helps in severe cases; some patients benefit from custom-made orthotics, whereas others require cortisone injections. In rare cases, the fascia is surgically released.

DIFFERENTIAL DIAGNOSIS

Foot Pain

HEEL	FOREFOOT PAIN
• Plantar fasciitis	• Morton's neuroma
• Calcaneal fracture	• Fracture
• Retrocalcaneal or infracalcaneal bursitis	• Infection
• Gout	• Ganglion
• Infection	• Ledderhose's syndrome
• Reiter's syndrome	• Flat feet
• Tarsal tunnel syndrome	• Corn
	• Bunion
	• Peripheral neuritis

PATIENT AND FAMILY EDUCATION

Rest is the first treatment for plantar fasciitis. Patients are advised to keep weight off the foot until the inflammation goes away. Ice to the sore area for 20 minutes three or four times a day can be helpful to relieve symptoms. Often the health care provider will prescribe nonsteroidal antiinflammatory medication such as ibuprofen. Custom orthotics and/or night splints that keep the foot in dorsiflexion can be helpful. A program of home exercises to stretch the Achilles tendon and plantar fascia are the mainstay of treating the condition and lessening the chance of recurrence.[13]

MORTON'S NEUROMA

DEFINITION AND EPIDEMIOLOGY

A neuroma is a nerve tumor that can result from external pressure on a nerve. Morton's neuroma is a result of perineural fibrosis of the plantar nerve at the point where the medial and lateral branches of the plantar nerve converge. This condition is seen primarily in women, with the most common cause being tight or high-heeled shoes.[14] This condition can also develop in people with claw toes and bunions.

PATHOPHYSIOLOGY

Compression of the interdigital plantar nerves causes repeated trauma, which in turn causes fibrosis of the nerve. Tight, pointed-toe shoes aggravate the irritation once the neuroma has formed.

CLINICAL PRESENTATION

Patients with Morton's neuroma complain of severe pain and burning in the region of the third web space. Going barefoot and foot massages relieve the discomfort. Elevation of the foot aggravates the condition.

PHYSICAL EXAMINATION

With Morton's neuroma, there is point tenderness and often edema over the third web space—between the third and fourth metatarsals. Compressing the metatarsals toward the midline of the foot reproduces the pain. Occasionally, paresthesia occurs at the reciprocal surfaces of the toes. The examination is otherwise unremarkable.

DIAGNOSTICS

Radiographs are indicated in the absence of a clear-cut history. X-ray studies occasionally reveal a narrowing of the space between the metatarsals, which creates the underlying cause.[13]

DIFFERENTIAL DIAGNOSIS

The plantar surface of the foot should be smooth and nontender. Calluses and plantar warts on the ball of the foot may be tender, rough, and nodular. Ganglions are cystlike in appearance, whereas infectious processes classically have edema, erythema, warmth, and tenderness. Ledderhose's syndrome is characterized by a painless, thickened palmar fascia and is often associated with Dupuytren's contracture (see Chapter 188) and Peyronie's disease. The presence of edema and tenderness between the third and fourth metatarsal heads strongly suggests Morton's neuroma; however, stress fractures should be considered in the differential diagnosis.

MANAGEMENT

Conservative treatment can resolve this condition. Wider toed shoes, separation of the toes with a small pad, and NSAIDs all help reduce the inflammation. In persistent cases, injection with steroids is often effective.

COMPLICATIONS

Removal of the neuroma causes the toes to become permanently numb.

INDICATIONS FOR REFERRAL OR HOSPITALIZATION

If conservative treatment and steroid injections are not effective, a referral for excision of the neuroma is advised.

PATIENT AND FAMILY EDUCATION

Patients should be encouraged to wear properly fitting shoes that have adequate toe room, good arch support, and a low or flat heel. Shoes should be bought at the end of the day, when feet are bigger, and should be replaced when support wears out. Shoes should be fitted to ensure proper size. Metatarsal arch pads, if used correctly, may ease the discomfort associated with Morton's neuroma and metatarsalgia.

OTHER COMMON FOOT PROBLEMS

Bunions, bunionettes, corns, calluses, hammertoes, hallux rigidus, hallux valgus, plantar warts, and ingrown toenails are discussed in Table 182-2, along with their differential diagnoses and management.

TABLE 182-2 Other Common Foot Problems*

Problem	Presentation	Examination and Diagnostics	Differential Diagnosis and Management
BUNION			
An inflammatory deformity of the first metatarsophalangeal (MTP) joint related to flat feet or laxity of the first toe and first metatarsal bone	Intense pain over the first MTP joint	Edema, deformity, and tenderness of the first metatarsal head; may have joint crepitus on palpation **Diagnostics:** If gout is suspected, uric acid levels and joint aspiration are considered; x-ray studies are not diagnostic.	**Differential diagnosis:** Gout **Management:** Warm packs or soaks, NSAIDs, and well-fitted shoes with adequate toe space Podiatry referral indicated for custom-made protective shield or foot mold Orthopedic/podiatry referral necessary for surgical correction if conservative management does not control pain
BUNIONETTE			
Pressure over the bony prominence on the fifth metatarsal head that results in bursa or ulceration	Painful, edematous lesion on the MTP joint of the fifth toe	Edema and erythema over the lateral aspect of the MTP of the fifth toe; may be accompanied by a cystlike, fluid-filled lesion	Properly fitting shoes with adequate toe room, bunion padding Filing down of hard lesions
CORN			
Hard corn (heloma durum): Hyperkeratotic lesions caused by pressure or friction; usually found on the toes or other bony prominence *Soft corn (heloma molle):* Macerated, interdigital, and painful; caused by pressure	Painful lesion between toes or on dorsal surface of toes	Erythematous, painful lesion; may also have hammertoes	Avoidance of tight-fitting shoes, use of corn pads to relieve pressure, routine paring of corns with file or scalpel Powder and lambswool or soft cotton between toes to prevent excessive moisture Referral to orthotics for customized orthotic device Surgical repair for accompanying hammertoe or arthroplasty p.r.n. Vigilant care for patients with diabetes or peripheral vascular disease (PVD) to prevent corns or calluses and ulceration or infection
CALLUS			
Hypertrophied area of skin on sole of foot related to excessive supination, pronation, or other abnormality	Usually asymptomatic	Dried, hypertrophied epidermal layer; may surround or protect a plantar wart or foreign body	Daily skin cream or lanolin, use of pumice stone by patient Debridement of painful calluses with a scalpel to relieve pressure Orthotic device as indicated For patients with diabetes or PVD, see Corn
HALLUX FLEXUS (HAMMERTOE OR CLAW TOE)			
Dorsiflexion of proximal joint of second toe while middle joint is plantar flexed	Painful corn the most common complaint	Dorsal flexion of first phalanx of second toe (either foot), with plantar flexion in second phalanx; may be accompanied by painful callus on metatarsal head and/or at nail end, as well as painful corn on dorsal surface of the proximal interphalangeal joint	See Corn Referral to podiatrist or orthopedic surgeon for surgical repair
HALLUX RIGIDUS			
Inflexible great toe, usually a result of arthritic changes	Pain with ambulation, climbing stairs	Immobile, fixated first MTP joint; may be slightly edematous with accompanying irregularity of joint edges related to osteophyte formation; diminished active and passive range of motion caused by immobility and pain **Diagnostics:** X-ray (anteroposterior, lateral views)	NSAIDs for pain Podiatry or orthopedic referral for surgical repair

*Because of the classic presentation of these disorders, diagnostic testing and differential diagnoses are noted only when indicated.

TABLE 182-2 Other Common Foot Problems—cont'd

Problem	Presentation	Examination and Diagnostics	Differential Diagnosis and Management
HALLUX VALGUS, HALLUX VARUS			
Hallux valgus: Great toe laterally displaced toward other toes *Hallux varus:* Great toe medially displaced away from other toes	Painful bunion of first MTP joint	*Hallux valgus:* Great toe laterally displaced with possible accompanying bunion, hammertoe; may have extension of second toe over great toe *Hallux varus:* Great toe medially displaced	Bunion care as described under Bunion Surgical or podiatry referral as indicated
PLANTAR WARTS			
Warty growth on plantar surface caused by viral infection	May be asymptomatic or may be complaints of pruritic, painful lesion on sole of foot; increasing pain with weight-bearing activities	Callus possibly obscuring wart, which commonly is 1 mm to 1 cm in size Paring of callus revealing rough lesion with numerous small, black spots in center of lesion	***Differential diagnosis:*** Porokeratotic lesion, foreign body **Management:** May resolve spontaneously For patients without diabetes or PVD: daily debridement with pumice stone, application of salicylic acid solution nightly to affected area, and gentle debridement of lesion each morning with an emery board Reminder to patients that lesions can spread, so debrided tissue must be carefully discarded Referral to podiatry indicated if conservative measures fail
ONYCHOCRYPTOSIS (INGROWN TOENAIL)			
Usually related to poor nail trimming or tight-fitting shoes	Pain and edema of great toe	Tender, edematous, erythematous area at corner of distal nail bed; lateral nail bed usually involved and obscured by hypertrophied tissue Evidence of purulent discharge Careful examination for lymphangitis and range of motion	For minimum ingrown toenail, wedge removal of nail edge to relieve discomfort If infection is present, patient is immunocompromised, or nail is severely ingrown, podiatry or surgical consult for nail excision and possible matricectomy Treatment of infection with appropriate antibiotic; patient instructed to soak foot in warm water several times daily, elevate foot, apply bandage, and wear open-toed shoes or soft slippers Further instruction regarding nail care

REFERENCES

1. American Academy of Orthopaedic Surgeons: *Fact sheet: the foot and ankle,* retrieved Oct 2005 from http://orthoinfo.aaos.org/fact/thr_report.cfm?thread_id=100&topcategory=Foot.
2. Mercier LR: The ankle and foot. In *Practical orthopedics,* Chicago, 1980, Mosby.
3. American Academy of Orthopaedic Surgeons: The foot. In *Athletic training and sports medicine,* ed 2, Park Ridge, Ill, 1991, The Academy.
4. American Academy of Orthopaedic Surgeons, American Academy of Pediatrics; Griffin LY editor: *Essentials of musculoskeletal care,* ed 3, Rosemont, Ill, 2005, American Academy of Orthopaedic Surgeons.
5. American Academy of Orthopaedic Surgeons: Physiology of tissue repair. In *Athletic training and sports medicine,* ed 2, Park Ridge, Ill, 1991.
6. Southmayd W, Hoffman M: The foot. In *Sports health: the complete book of athletic injuries,* New York, 1989, Quickfox.
7. Harwood-Nuss A, Wolfson A, Linden C, and others: *The clinical practice of emergency medicine,* ed 5, Philadelphia, 2005, Lippincott.
8. American Academy of Orthopaedic Surgeons: The ankle. In *Athletic training and sports medicine,* ed 2, Park Ridge, Ill, 1991, The Academy.
9. Onieal ME: Ankle sprains (question and answer), *J Am Acad Nurse Pract* 5(5):226-227, 1993.
10. Hoppenfeld S, editor: Physical examination of the foot and ankle. In *Physical examination of the spine and extremities,* New York, 1976, Appleton-Century-Crofts.
11. Brody DM: Running injuries, *Clin Sympos* 32(4):1-36, 1980.
12. Graham J: Injuries to the knee and leg. In McLatchie BR, editor: *Essentials of sports medicine,* New York, 1993, Churchill Livingstone.
13. American Academy of Orthopedic Surgeons: *Fact sheet: plantar fasciitis,* retrieved Feb 6, 2007, from http://orthoinfo.aos.org/fact/thr_report.cfm?thread_ID=144.
14. Southmayd W, Hoffman M: The ankle. In *Sports health: the complete book of athletic injuries,* New York, 1989, Quickfox.

CHAPTER 183

Bone Tumors

Henry DeGroot III

DEFINITION AND EPIDEMIOLOGY

Bone tumors are defined as a growth of benign or malignant neoplastic tissue within bone. In addition, destructive or symptomatic lesions can occur in bone as a result of abnormal growth of normal or nonneoplastic tissues, such as pigmented villonodular synovitis, osteochondroma, and aneurysmal bone cyst. Cancers that originate in connective tissues such as bone, tendons, or muscles are classified as sarcomas. Osteosarcoma, the most common bone sarcoma, originates from primitive mesenchymal bone-forming cells. Ewing's sarcoma originates from cells that arise in the embryonic neural crest. Chondrosarcoma develops in primitive mesenchymal cartilage-forming cells.[1]

The incidence of benign bone tumors is difficult to estimate, since many are left untreated and others are never discovered. The most common benign bone tumor is osteochondroma, which may account for 30% to 40% of all benign bone tumors.[2] Nonossifying fibroma is estimated to occur in 30% to 40% of all children over the age of 2 years, but many of these benign, self-limiting tumors are probably never discovered.[3] In persons ages 20 to 40, giant cell tumor and enchondroma are the most commonly diagnosed benign bone tumors.

The most common malignant tumor that originates in bone is multiple myeloma, within incidence of 2 or 3 per 100,000. African Americans have twice the risk of multiple myeloma as Caucasian Americans, and Asian Americans have one half the risk. Multiple myeloma is diagnosed in 15,000 persons in the United States per year. The average age at diagnosis is 66 years, and only 2% of patients are younger than 40 at diagnosis.[4]

The primary malignant tumors that develop within the bones are called sarcomas. Osteosarcoma is the most common of these. The incidence of osteosarcoma is estimated to be 1 in 1 million. After osteosarcoma, chondrosarcoma and malignant fibrous histiocytoma are the most common varieties of sarcoma. Approximately 3000 primary bone sarcomas are diagnosed each year in the United States.

In adults the most common malignant tumor that occurs in bone is a metastasis from a primary adenocarcinoma. Approximately 70% of patients with advanced breast or prostate cancer will develop bone metastasis. Approximately 15% to 30% of patients with kidney, lung, uterine, thyroid, stomach, rectal, bladder, or colon cancer will develop metastatic cancer in the bones. Approximately 350,000 people die with bone metastasis each year in United States. New treatments have resulted in increased survival for cancer patients, which paradoxically creates a larger population of individuals who are at risk for metastasis from cancer.[5]

PATHOPHYSIOLOGY

In most cases, bone tumors arise from a molecular abnormality of the DNA in the tumor cells. This abnormality is most often caused by a somatic mutation, which results in the deletion, addition, or rearrangement of the nuclear DNA. The growth of the tumor is caused by the activation of a tumor promoter gene or by the inactivation of a tumor suppressor gene. More than one genetic event or mutation may be necessary for the development of cancer. The severity or nature of the bone tumor can be more precisely defined by analyzing the DNA makeup of the tumor cells. Unfortunately, the wealth of new knowledge about tumor genetics has not brought dramatic improvements in treatment or survival for most sarcoma patients.

Some bone cancers arise from an inherited tumor gene. One example is the retinoblastoma, or *Rb,* gene. The cells of normal individuals have two intact *Rb* genes on chromosome 13. Families with the retinoblastoma trait inherit one defective copy of the gene. As the child grows, an additional mutation that inactivates the second, normal copy of the gene must occur to initiate formation of a retinoblastoma tumor. These individuals are also at increased risk for osteosarcoma, small cell lung cancer, and synovial sarcoma.[6]

Some malignant bone tumors are caused by chronic disease states. Approximately 5% of patients with widespread Paget's disease of bone (see Chapter 197) develop sarcoma in the affected bones, usually osteosarcoma. Patients with longstanding infection in the bone (see Chapter 197) are at risk of developing a malignant tumor, including squamous cell carcinoma, in the site of the draining infection. Occupational exposure to chemicals and other toxins has not been definitively linked to the development of bone sarcoma.

CLINICAL PRESENTATION

Some benign, nonaggressive bone tumors are discovered as incidental findings. Adults with shoulder pain and children who injure a knee or an ankle in sports can have an incidental tumor discovered during an x-ray study of the painful area. After an appropriate evaluation by a tumor specialist, further evaluation and treatment of these tumors may not be necessary.

Benign, locally aggressive and destructive tumors in adults such as giant cell tumor, fibrous dysplasia, and osteoblastoma are initially seen with gradually increasing pain and sometimes with pathologic fracture. Adult patients who have prolonged, gradually worsening pain following what was thought to be a muscle sprain or contusion should have a plain x-ray examination to rule out a bone tumor.

The most common malignancy in the bones of adults is a metastasis from a primary adenocarcinoma in some other site. Patients with cancers of the breast, prostate, lung, thyroid, kidney, and some gastrointestinal sites have an increased risk of bone metastasis and should receive regular follow-up monitoring for bone lesions. Patients with a new or persistent pain and a history of one of these cancers should be investigated for metastasis.

The most common sarcoma in adults is chondrosarcoma. This tumor manifests with gradually increasing pain, often in the hip or pelvis area, and this pain can be mistaken for arthritis. Chondrosarcoma may not appear overly aggressive on the x-ray film, and this may unfortunately lead to misdiagnosis and mistreatment.

Patients with chordoma, a type of sarcoma that has a predilection for the sacrum, may come to their health care provider with persistent low back pain, constipation, or even difficulty with defecation. Digital rectal examination reveals a mass growing out of the sacrum, which can block the rectum.

The location of some tumors depends on the cell type of the lesion. Chondroblastoma, a benign but locally destructive cartilage-forming tumor, occurs almost exclusively in the epiphysis of the bones. Adamantinoma, a low-grade malignant tumor, occurs almost exclusively in the tibia and fibula. Other tumors occur in areas of rapid bone growth. Accordingly, the distal femur, the proximal tibia, and the proximal femur are common locations for bone tumors.

In adults, metastatic tumors are more likely to occur in areas where active hematopoietic marrow (red marrow) persists, such as the proximal long bones, vertebral bodies, skull, sternum, and ribs. In other cases of metastasis the pattern of cancer spread follows the path the cancer cells take as they become separated from the main tumor and flow through the veins to become lodged in the new location. American otolaryngologist Oscar Vivian Batson (1894-1979)[7] observed a system of valveless veins, now called Batson's plexus, that connects the breast, the kidney, and the prostate with the vertebral bodies and bones of the pelvis. Movement of cancer cells through this plexus of veins is responsible for the frequency of metastasis in the spine and pelvis.

MEDICAL HISTORY AND PHYSICAL EXAMINATION

The evaluation of a bone tumor begins with a thorough history and physical examination. In addition to the general medical history, the patient's personal cancer history must be thoroughly elicited. Some patients who have had cancer in the past eventually consider themselves cured, and they may not reveal their cancer history unless carefully prompted. Discovery of the patient's history of cancer may be all that is necessary to establish the origin of the bone tumor.

In taking the history, the provider must establish the precise chronology of the pain. Often patients will ascribe the pain from a bone tumor to a minor injury or accident that happened around the time the pain developed. However, closer questioning will often reveal that the pain gradually developed before the accident.

A careful and complete examination depends on access to the entire area of the body involved in the problem. The shoulder, hip, and knee cannot be fully examined with the patient's clothing left on, and an incomplete examination may contribute to delay in making the correct diagnosis. The area needs to be examined for the presence of a mass. The general examination will reveal a systemic condition that might lead to bone deformity, such as a growth disturbance, nutritional imbalance, or metabolic deficiency.

DIAGNOSTICS

Laboratory tests can be helpful but not diagnostic. For example, a patient with suspected multiple myeloma, who has multiple lytic bone lesions on x-ray studies, should have a CBC and a serum and urine protein electrophoresis test to identify secretion of tumor paraproteins. A patient with a history of prostate cancer who has a new bone lesion in the pelvis should have his prostate-specific antigen levels measured to help confirm the diagnosis of prostate cancer metastasis.

In benign bone tumors, laboratory examinations are usually not helpful. If the bone lesion seen on the x-ray film is caused by infection, the patient may have an elevated or normal WBC count, with an elevated erythrocyte sedimentation rate and elevated C-reactive protein level. In sarcoma, no diagnostic blood tests exist. Elevated serum levels of alkaline phosphatase have been shown to be a negative prognostic factor in osteosarcoma.

After the history and physical examination have been completed, the best next step is a plain x-ray examination. Advanced imaging such as MRIs and bone scans are not recommended at this stage. Depending on the features on the plain x-ray film, the differential diagnosis can be constructed. Benign bone lesions are usually well circumscribed and may have a prominent sclerotic margin on plain x-rays films. Benign but locally aggressive lesions may also be well to moderately well circumscribed. There may be expansion or even focal destruction of the bone cortex. There may be some expansion into the soft tissue. Aggressive bone lesions are usually poorly circumscribed. There may be permeative destruction of the bone, where the bone appears to be moth eaten. The lesion may aggressively destroy the nearby cortex, or it may pass directly out of the bone into the soft tissue without destroying the cortex. A large soft tissue mass may be seen.[8]

Advanced imaging should be coordinated with a specialist. CT scans are most helpful for lesions that form bone or lesions that occur in complex bones such as the pelvis and spine. CT scan is the best imaging modality to determine the extent of bone destruction and to determine the exact extent of the bony lesion. Data from CT scans can be used to quantitate the risk of pathologic fracture from a lesion.[9]

MRI scan is the best imaging modality for finding soft tissue lesions or non-bone-forming bone tumors, and for determining the status of the nearby anatomy for surgical planning. MRI scans will detect bone tumors, such as early metastasis from breast cancer, that may be invisible on other scanning studies. MRI scan is extremely valuable for planning surgery on bone tumors.

Radionucleotide bone scans are helpful for detecting lesions that may be invisible on plain x-ray studies. An abnormal finding on a radionucleotide bone scan is not diagnostic of a tumor, since the abnormality may be caused by an old fracture, arthritis, or other factors. Positron

DIAGNOSTICS

Bone Tumors

LABORATORY

Serum and urine protein immunoelectrophoresis
CBC and differential
ESR
Prostate-specific antigen (if indicated)
Urinalysis
Alkaline phosphatase
Calcium
Uric acid
5-Hydroxyindole acetic acid
Carcinoembryonic antigen
CA_{125}
Phosphorus
LFTs

IMAGING

X-ray—2 plane
Bone scan
CT scan, MRI

OTHER

Bone biopsy

emission tomography (PET) scans may detect tumors that might otherwise be missed. PET scans can be used to assess the effectiveness of treatment for bone tumors. Ultrasound scans and angiograms were formerly used to locate and diagnose bone tumors. However, ultrasound has been superseded by MRI scans, and angiograms have been superseded by magnetic resonance angiography.

Role of Biopsy

Biopsy, either by traditional incisional methods, by core needle methods, or by fine needle aspiration methods, is the technique of sampling the cells of the tumor for pathologic diagnosis. A biopsy should be the last procedure after all the imaging studies, examinations, and other necessary investigations have been completed.

Biopsy of bone tumors has been associated with numerous complications and problems. Although biopsy is technically a straightforward procedure, the complications resulting from a poorly planned or poorly executed biopsy may have a profound impact on the patient's treatment and prognosis. Therefore most tumor specialists recommend that the biopsy of the bone tumor be performed only by the surgeon who will be performing the definitive surgical treatment of the lesion.[10]

The interpretation of bone tumor pathology is a complex and difficult task, and typically referred to specialized pathologists who have wide experience in bone tumor diagnosis. It is essential for the bone tumor surgeon, the radiologist, and the pathologist to work together in a cooperative manner to diagnose a bone tumor.

DIFFERENTIAL DIAGNOSIS

The differential diagnosis is based on the patient's age, the location of the lesion, the radiographic appearance, and other information such as laboratory examinations. Once a short list of possibilities has been formulated, a biopsy is performed to narrow the list down to the correct diagnosis.

In addition to a primary bone tumor, other lesions need to be considered such as metabolic, infectious, congenital, posttraumatic, and degenerative lesions. Common diseases such as gout and less common metabolic abnormalities such as Gaucher's disease can cause significant bone lesions that appear to be tumors. In children and adults, infection causes localized bone destruction, swelling, and pain and can be hard to distinguish from bone cancer. Tuberculosis can affect bones and joints and appears to be an aggressive, destructive process on x-ray films. Locally aggressive processes such as pigmented villonodular synovitis can cause bone lesions adjacent to the hip, knee, and ankle.

DIFFERENTIAL DIAGNOSIS

Bone Tumors

- Arthritis (monoarticular and polyarticular)
- Avascular necrosis and bone infarcts
- Bursitis
- Cellulitis
- Deep vein thrombosis
- Ganglion and epidermoid cysts
- Gaucher's disease
- Heterotopic ossification
- Infections (tuberculosis)
- Leukemia
- Neurogenic arthropathy (Charcot's joint)
- Osteomyelitis
- Paget's disease
- Pigmented villonodular synovitis
- Stress fracture

MANAGEMENT

Benign Bone Tumors

Treatment of benign bone tumors depends on their biologic behavior. Latent bone lesions, such as nonossifying fibroma, enchondroma, and fibrous dysplasia, may require no treatment. These benign tumors do not represent a significant risk to the patient's health. Once a bone tumor specialist has examined these tumors and determined that there is no increased risk of pathologic fracture, the tumor may be observed without biopsy. X-ray studies to verify that the tumor is not growing or changing are recommended every 3 to 6 months for 2 or 3 years. In some circumstances, when there is a risk of pathologic fracture, the tumor is removed by curettage and the bone is strengthened with a plate or an intramedullary implant.

Benign, locally aggressive tumors, such a giant cell tumor, chondroblastoma, and chondromyxoid fibroma, require local treatment. After the workup and diagnosis, the lesions are normally removed by complete curettage. To reduce the chance of local recurrence, phenol, liquid nitrogen, or a mechanical bur may be used to additionally treat the site of the tumor and remove or kill any residual cells. The bone defect is filled with acrylic bone cement or bone graft, and a plate or screws may be added according to the surgeon's preference.

Malignant Tumors and Sarcoma in Bone

Multiple myeloma is treated by chemotherapy, orthopedic stabilization of bone lesions that are at risk of creating pathologic fractures, and bisphosphonates. Monitoring for hypercalcemia, anemia, dehydration, and infection is necessary.

The treatment for primary malignant bone tumors varies by tumor type and stage. Low-grade malignant tumors, such as many chondrosarcomas, adamantinoma, and epithelioid hemangioendothelioma, are treated by surgery alone. The goal of surgery in these cases is to remove the entire tumor, including a cuff of surrounding normal tissue to ensure that there is no local recurrence. Chemotherapy and radiotherapy are usually not used in low-grade sarcomas.

High-grade malignant sarcomas are treated with multimodality treatment, including surgery, chemotherapy, and radiotherapy. Osteosarcoma and Ewing's sarcoma are treated with preoperative (neoadjuvant) multiagent chemotherapy, followed by complete surgical removal of the tumor with reconstruction of the bone defect, followed by more chemotherapy. In Ewing's sarcoma, if the surgical treatment does not result in a wide margin, radiotherapy is used to reduce the risk of local recurrence. Patients undergoing treatment for sarcoma also require bisphosphonate medications, such as pamidronate or etidronate, to prevent unnecessary loss of bone calcium during treatment.

Metastatic Cancers in Bone

Metastatic tumors are treated based on location, symptoms, tumor type, and expected patient survival. Most patients with cancer metastasis in bone cannot be cured, but function, quality-of-life, and survival can be dramatically enhanced by aggressive and appropriate medical and surgical treatments. Patients with known metastatic lesions in bone should be systematically monitored for additional metastatic lesions so that they may be treated before they become advanced and cause complications. Once a lesion is discovered, it should be evaluated by an orthopedic surgeon to estimate the risk of pathologic fracture. Pathologic fracture risk is calculated based on the size, radiologic features, pain characteristics, and skeletal location of the lesions. Metastatic lesions in the proximal femur around the hip have the highest risk of pathologic fracture.[11]

Lesions in weight-bearing bones such as the femur are frequently stabilized with orthopedic plates or rods to relieve pain, prevent fracture, and maintain and maximize patient's ability to ambulate fully and remain independent. Treatment for impending pathologic fracture results in easier treatment, shorter operating time, lower blood loss, and more rapid recovery for the patient. After orthopedic stabilization, radiation is sometimes used to prevent or delay the local recurrence of the tumor. Once pathologic fracture has occurred, orthopedic stabilization is helpful in restoring functional ability and relieving pain. Orthopedic stabilization of metastatic lesions will help maintain the patients' independence, dignity, and self-worth and minimize their dependency, need for institutional care, and dependency on narcotic drugs. Surgical treatment of a bone tumor does not result in spread of the tumor, as is commonly supposed.

For small metastatic lesions in non-weight-bearing bones, such as the ribs or scapula, radiation is typically used. The radiation slows or blocks the growth of tumor cells in a dose-dependent fashion. Radiation has also been shown to give effective pain control in the majority of patients. The radionucleotides strontium 89 and samarium 153 have been shown to be effective for generalized bone pain in cases with widely disseminated metastatic deposits.[12]

Every patient with new or recurrent metastatic cancer in the bones should be treated with bisphosphonate medications to prevent unnecessary loss of bone calcium. These medications have been shown to decrease the risk of an additional metastatic event and may increase survival.[13] Zoledronic acid is the current drug of choice, but pamidronate, clodronate (currently not available in the United States), and ibandronate are also used. Additional complications of skeletal metastasis that can be reduced with bisphosphonates include hypercalcemia of malignancy, bone pain, and pathologic fracture.

Pain Management

Patients with bone tumors require a comprehensive pain management program. Benign bone tumors typically cause moderate pain, and surgical treatment results in a temporary increase in pain that can be easily managed with conventional modalities.

Patients with malignant or metastatic tumors in bone require more advanced pain control modalities than those with benign tumors. Long-acting pain medicines, transdermal delivery systems, pain medicine pumps, and multidrug protocols using controlled-release narcotics coupled with short-acting narcotics for breakthrough pain have been successfully used in the management of cancer pain. All patients should be given bisphosphonate medications such as pamidronate, clodronate, ibandronate, or zoledronic acid, which can decrease pain by preventing the growth and development of new and existing bone lesions. Although it is tempting to place patients with metastatic bone lesions on activity restriction to prevent pain, this may unintentionally accelerate bone damage because of disuse atrophy and calcium loss. Maintenance of normal activity levels should be the goal wherever possible.

Postsurgical pain and phantom limb pain can be significant challenges in sarcoma patients. Gabapentin, amitriptyline, and benzodiazepine drugs, as well as physical therapy, counseling, and counterirritant therapy such as transcutaneous electrical nerve stimulation (TENS) units, are helpful adjuncts in complex pain control situations. Severe or chronic postoperative or postcancer pain is often managed by pain control specialists.

PROGNOSIS AND SURVIVAL

Primary Benign and Malignant Bone Tumors

Most benign bone tumors have no impact on patient prognosis or survival. Aggressive bone tumors may result in local damage to bones and joints and result in loss of mobility or function. Some severe multifocal bone tumors, such as hereditary multiple exostosis, can lead to severe limitation of mobility, deformity, and chronic pain.

The prognosis for malignant sarcoma in bone is strongly related to the stage of the tumor, rather than the cell type of the tumor. Low-grade sarcomas without metastasis are classified as stage I. These tumors are associated with a good to excellent long-term survival (approximately 90% survival at 10 years). However, tumor recurrence and complications can occur even years after treatment.

High-grade sarcomas without metastasis are classified as stage II. Typical survival for patients with these lesions is between 50% and 70% at 5 years, and between 40% and 60% at 10 years. Survival for children with osteosarcoma without metastasis is 70% at 5 years. Patients with metastatic lesions at presentation have a 20% 5-year survival.[13] Unfortunately, stage-specific survival in high-grade sarcoma has not changed dramatically over the past few decades, despite the discovery of enhanced diagnostic and therapeutic modalities, new chemotherapeutic agents, and new surgical techniques.[14]

Metastatic Bone Tumors

The prognosis for patients with metastatic cancer in the bone depends strongly on the cell type. In breast cancer an estimated 30% of patients will have micrometastasis in the bone marrow at the time of diagnosis. Micrometastasis is a significant negative prognostic factor in survival. Patients with larger tumors, positive lymph nodes, or hormone receptor–negative tumors are at risk for micrometastasis.

For prostate cancer the median survival after bone metastasis is 3 years. However, there is wide variation, and survival predictions for any individual patient should be viewed with some skepticism. Elevated levels of serum markers of bone resorption or bone osteoclast activity, visceral involvement, and poor performance status have been shown to have negative prognostic significance.[15]

Lung cancer that has metastasized to bone is associated with a relatively short median survival, approximately 6 months. However, palliative radiation treatment, stabilization of impending pathologic fractures, and effective pain management are still useful in maintaining quality of life and independent function.

LIFE SPAN CONSIDERATIONS

Bone cancers have a strong predilection for certain age ranges. Children under the age of 5 years are at risk for metastatic neuroblastoma in the bone. After age 8, the risk of Ewing's sarcoma begins to increase, and at age 12 to 15, the risk of osteosarcoma increases. The risk of bone sarcoma increases around the time of the child's growth spurt. In children and teenagers under 20 years of age, the incidence of malignant bone tumors is 8.7 per million. Adults older than 40 are at increasing risk of metastatic cancers to the bone, and the incidence of chondrosarcoma peaks around age 60. The incidence of multiple myeloma peaks around age 55. Benign bone tumors are uncommon in children under 10. Between ages 10 and 20, osteochondroma, osteoid osteoma, Langerhans' cell histiocytosis, and fibrous dysplasia are common benign bone tumors.

INDICATIONS FOR REFERRAL OR HOSPITALIZATION

The number of different bone tumors and the complexities of their treatment make it difficult for health care providers to ensure the best treatment for patients with suspected bone tumors. Early and prompt referral of these patients to an orthopedic oncologist for evaluation, diagnostic workup, and possible treatment is the best course of action. It is preferable to refer patients before advanced imaging studies have been performed, or to schedule the advanced imaging studies in cooperation with the orthopedic oncologist. In this way, necessary imaging studies can be performed in a timely fashion while avoiding wasteful and unnecessary tests. In virtually every case, biopsy should be performed only by the surgeon who will be performing the definitive tumor treatment.

Delay in diagnosis of bone cancer and bone tumors has been the cause of a significant amount of malpractice litigation against physicians and health care providers of all types. Many factors contribute to delay in diagnosis. The patient may fail to appear in a timely fashion for an evaluation or may miss a scheduled follow-up appointment. The physician or health care provider may fail to appreciate the significance of the patient's complaints, perform an incomplete examination, or fail to schedule tests in a timely manner. Bone tumors sometimes are seen with symptoms that mimic minor musculoskeletal injuries, which can lead to an incorrect diagnosis. The common perception that patients with cancer have cachexia, night pain, weight loss, or other severe systemic symptoms is false and misleading. Patients with sarcoma may appear perfectly healthy on initial presentation. Fortunately, a complete history, a careful examination, and a plain x-ray study are usually more than sufficient to establish the correct diagnosis.

PATIENT AND FAMILY EDUCATION

Since the discovery of a bone tumor always brings the specter of bone cancer, the patient and family should receive complete and comprehensive information about the condition as soon as it is available. If the referring health care provider is not able to determine the nature and health risk associated with the tumor, it is preferable not to speculate about the possible outcomes, since this may only increase anxiety and stress.

The treatment of benign and malignant bone tumors may have a significant impact on the patient's quality of life or function. Therefore the patient and his or her family should participate to the greatest extent possible in selecting the appropriate treatment. They should receive complete information about treatment alternatives, including benefits and potential complications. This allows the patient to understand the process and come to a cooperative decision about the best treatment based on the health care provider's recommendation. Patients with cancer who have a strong support network have been shown to have better survival rates than patients who are isolated and lack support.[16] The initial diagnosis can be emotionally devastating to the patient and to a family; compassion, support, and excellent communication are necessary. The patient and family should be encouraged to join a support group or participate in family or individual counseling.

REFERENCES

1. Mirra JM, editor: *Bone tumors: clinical, radiologic, and pathologic correlations*, Philadelphia, 1989, Lea & Febiger.
2. Samartzis D, Marco RA: Osteochondroma of the sacrum: a case report and review of the literature, *Spine* 31(13):E425-E429, 2006.
3. Smith S: *Fibrous cortical defect and nonossifying fibroma*, updated 2003, retrieved Feb 4, 2006, from http://www.emedicine.com/radio/topic283.htm.
4. Ries LAG, Eisner MP, Kosary CL, and others, editors: *SEER cancer statistics review, 1975-2002*, Bethesda, Md, 2005, National Cancer Institute, retrieved Feb 4, 2007, from http://seer.cancer.gov/csr/1975_2002.
5. Manabe J, Kawaguchi N, Matsumoto S, and others: Surgical treatment of bone metastasis: indications and outcomes, *Int J Clin Oncol* 10(2):103-111, 2005.
6. Hayden JB, Hoang BH: Osteosarcoma: basic science and clinical implications, *Orthop Clin North Am* 37(1):1-7, 2006.
7. *Dorland's medical dictionary*, Philadelphia, 2004, Saunders.
8. DeGroot H III: *The good, the bad, and the ugly: how to begin the work-up of a bone tumor*, retrieved Jan 31, 2006, from http://www.bonetumor.org/tumors/pages/page8.html.
9. Snyder BD, Hauser-Kara DA, Hipp JA, and others: Predicting fracture through benign skeletal lesions with quantitative computed tomography, *J Bone Joint Surg* 88(1):55-70, 2006.
10. Mankin HJ, Mankin CJ, Simon MA: Members of the Musculoskeletal Tumor Society: the hazards of the biopsy, revisited, *J Bone Joint Surg* 78(5):656-663, 1996.
11. DeGroot H III: *Evaluation of the risk of pathologic fractures secondary to metastatic bone disease*, Oct 2001, retrieved Jan 31, 2006, from http://www.bonetumor.org/tumors/pages/pathFX.htm.
12. Falkmer U, Jarhult J, Wersall P, and others: A systematic overview of radiation therapy effects in skeletal metastases, *Acta Oncol* 42(5-6):620-633, 2003.
13. Radford M, Gibbons CL: Management of skeletal metastases, *Hosp Med* 63(12):722-725, 2002.
14. Bruland OS, Pihl A: On the current management of osteosarcoma: a critical evaluation and a proposal for a modified treatment strategy, *Eur J Cancer* 33(11):1725-1731, 1997.
15. Coleman RE: Skeletal complications of malignancy, *Cancer* 80(8 Suppl):1588-1594, 1997.
16. Thaxton L, Emshoff JG, Guessous O: Prostate cancer support groups: a literature review, *J Psychosoc Oncol* 23(1):25-40, 2005.

CHAPTER 184

Bursitis

Scott W. Shiffer

A bursa is a sac lined with synovial fluid, which provides lubrication and facilitates smooth movement between tissues of an extremity. Bursitis is a pathologic inflammatory disorder of the bursae caused by varied acute or insidious processes. These processes may include overuse or acute trauma, autoimmune diseases, crystal deposits, acute or chronic pyogenic infection, or hemorrhage.[1,2] Bursitis can result in mild pain or become a disabling condition. There are numerous bursae throughout the body, but only a few ever become inflamed or problematic. The most commonly affected bursae are located at the shoulder, hip, knee, elbow, and heel.

SHOULDER BURSITIS

DEFINITION AND EPIDEMIOLOGY

The four major bursae around the shoulder include the subacromial (subdeltoid), subcoracoid, subscapularis, and scapular bursae. The subacromial bursa is located between the deltoid muscle and rotator cuff and extends under the acromion and coracoacromial arch. Subacromial bursitis is the most common type of bursitis and is commonly seen in older adults and in athletes less than 25 years of age.[1,3] This condition is generally caused by mechanical irritation resulting from overhead activities, and it leads to rotator cuff tendinitis. If left untreated, the condition progresses into an irreversible impingement condition.[3]

CLINICAL PRESENTATION AND PHYSICAL EXAMINATION

Anterior or lateral shoulder pain with acute or insidious onset is the most common presenting complaint of shoulder bursitis. The pain is exacerbated by overhead activities, and there may be a deep aching that interrupts sleep at night.[4,5] Increased pain with active abduction and internal rotation of the arm, plus tenderness below the acromion, is demonstrated. Weakness can often be established with internal rotation. A complete neuromuscular examination with careful palpation and passive and active range of motion should be performed. The Neer's and Hawkins' impingement signs are diagnostic and indicate inflammation of the subacromial bursa and rotator cuff (Box 184-1).[3,4]

DIAGNOSTICS AND DIFFERENTIAL DIAGNOSIS

Plain radiographs are often normal in the early stages of shoulder bursitis.[1,3,6] X-ray studies may demonstrate a hooked acromion, calcification of the supraspinatus tendon, osteopenia of the humerus greater tuberosity, and a distance of less than 5 mm between the acromion and humerus.[4] MRI is useful in the later stages of the disease.[1] If the condition is related to an autoimmune or inflammatory process, serologic tests may reveal an elevated erythrocyte sedimentation rate, a positive rheumatoid factor, or antinuclear antibodies. If a septic cause is suspected, a Gram's stain and culture of the bursa fluid should be obtained. If an aseptic condition is the cause of the bursitis, crystals may be observed in the bursa aspirate (Box 184-2).[4] The differential diagnosis includes tubercular effusion, infection, arthritis, hemarthrosis, gout, and pseudogout.

The impingement injection test is one method of differentiating between impingement and other shoulder disorders.[3,7] With this test, 10 ml of 1% lidocaine (Xylocaine) is injected into the subacromial space; after 5 to 10 minutes, the tests for impingement are repeated. If the pain is reduced 50%, the shoulder pain is secondary to subacromial bursitis and tendinitis.[3,5]

BOX 184-1

NEER'S AND HAWKINS' IMPINGEMENT SIGNS

NEER'S IMPINGEMENT SIGN

- Raise and pull on straightened arm forcibly from the side to full abduction above the head.
- A positive test will cause pain.

HAWKINS' IMPINGEMENT SIGN

- Flex the elbow to 90 degrees, and raise the upper arm to 90 degrees abduction (parallel to the floor). Then rotate the arm internally across the front of the body causing compression of the rotator cuff and subacromial bursa between the head of the humerus and coracoacromial ligament.
- A positive test will cause pain.

Data from Neer CS: Impingement lesions, *Gen Orthop* 173:70-77, 1983; and Hawkins RJ, Kennedy JC: Impingement syndrome in athletes, *Am J Sports Med* 8:151-157, 1980.

DIAGNOSTICS

Bursitis

LABORATORY
CBC and differential*
ESR*
Rheumatoid factor*
Uric acid*
Antinuclear antibody*
Culture and sensitivity (of bursa fluid)*
Gram's stain (of bursa fluid)*
Analysis of bursa aspirate for crystals*

IMAGING
X-ray
Ultrasound
MRI

OTHERS
Joint aspiration

*If indicated.

DIFFERENTIAL DIAGNOSIS

Shoulder Bursitis

- Fracture or dislocation
- Trauma
- Arthritis (osteoarthritis or rheumatoid arthritis)
- Adhesive capsulitis
- Rotator cuff tendinitis or tear
- Strain
- Referred pain
- Subacromial spur
- Neoplasm

BOX 184-2

GUIDELINES FOR BURSA ASPIRATION AND INJECTION

PURPOSE

The purpose of bursa aspiration and injection is to evaluate the bursa fluid to determine the cause of the inflammation and to drain abnormal fluid accumulation to relieve pain. Local anesthetics such as lidocaine or corticosteroids may be introduced into the bursa for symptomatic management of inflammation. Subacromial, trochanteric, anserine, and prepatellar bursitis are conditions that improve with local corticosteroids injection.

CONTRAINDICATIONS

Contraindications to aspiration and injection include cellulitis at the injection site, primary coagulopathy or uncontrolled anticoagulant therapy, septic effusion of a bursa or periarticular structure, more than three previous injections at the same site in the previous 12 months or lack of improvement after two prior injections, suspected bacteremia from another site, unstable joints (for corticosteroid injection), tumors, fractures, joint prosthesis, or inaccessible joints.

PATIENT EDUCATION AND CONSENT

Patient education and consent are necessary before the procedure. The risks and benefits of bursa aspiration should be explained. Adverse effects of introducing a needle into the bursa include infection, bleeding, and pain. Potential complications of corticosteroid therapy include postinjection flare (increased pain for 1 or 2 days), arthropathy, tendon rupture, facial flushing, skin atrophy and depigmentation, transient paresis, hypersensitivity reaction, pericapsular calcification, and acceleration of cartilage attrition.

TECHNIQUE

Aseptic technique for bursa aspiration and injection begins by prepping the site for aspiration or injection with povidone-iodine and draping accordingly. The appropriate needle for the procedure is selected: an 18- or 20-gauge needle for aspiration, and a 22- or 25-gauge 1½-inch needle for injection. A 5- or 10-ml Luer-Lok syringe is recommended. Figures 188-1 to 188-7 demonstrate techniques for aspirating and injecting bursae.

A variety of corticosteroid preparations are available in different potencies. The three common corticosteroid local injection therapies used to treat bursitis are hydrocortisone acetate 25 or 50 mg/ml, which is short acting (use 8 to 40 mg); triamcinolone acetonide 40 mg/ml, an intermediate-acting preparation (use 4 to 10 mg); and long-acting dexamethasone sodium acetate 8 mg/ml (use 1.5 to 3 mg).

Lidocaine is combined with the steroid of choice to disperse the steroid in the injection site. A history of lidocaine allergy must first be obtained. Lidocaine 5 ml is combined with the steroid for subacromial, trochanteric, or calcaneal bursae. For smaller bursae, such as the olecranon and prepatellar, up to 3 ml of lidocaine combined with the chosen steroid is recommended.

FOLLOW-UP

Procedure after-care includes applying a bandage over the aspiration-injection site and explaining to the patient that the procedure is provided in addition to other conservative measures and is not a cure in itself. Oral NSAIDs are continued if there is no contraindication. Symptoms of infection should be reported immediately.

Data from Pfeninger JL: Joint and soft tissue aspiration and injection. In Pfeninger JL, Fowler GC, editors: *Procedures for primary care physicians,* St Louis, 1994, Mosby.

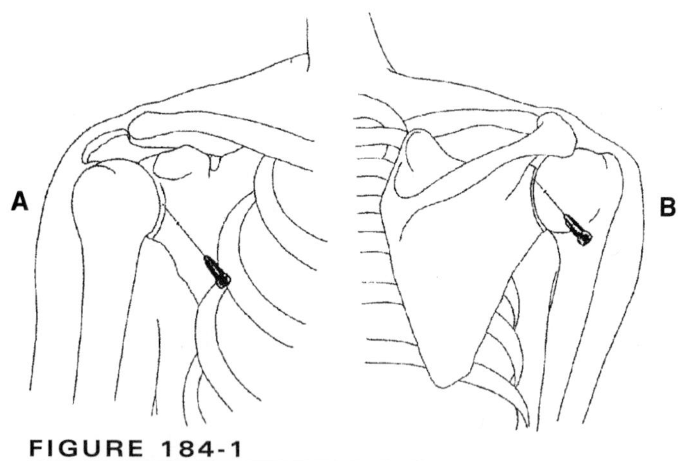

FIGURE 184-1

Arthrocentesis of the shoulder. **A**, Anterior approach. **B**, Posterior approach. (From Noble JP: *Textbook of primary care medicine,* ed 3, St Louis, 2001, Mosby.)

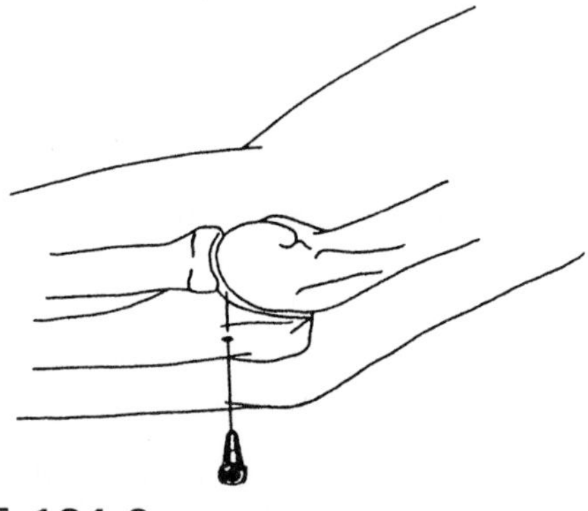

FIGURE 184-2

Arthrocentesis of the elbow. (From Noble JP: *Textbook of primary care medicine,* ed 3, St Louis, 2001, Mosby.)

MANAGEMENT

Except for autoimmune and septic shoulder conditions, treatment is directed at rehabilitating the rotator cuff. More than 90% of patients with subacromial bursitis respond to periodic gentle range-of-motion joint activities, avoidance of activities that exacerbate the pain, thermal modalities, either heat or ice, and NSAIDs. Additional pain relief may be provided by scheduled doses of acetaminophen. Stronger analgesics are occasionally necessary, especially at night.[3,4] Immobilization should be avoided, since it may worsen the condition by causing adhesions.[3] Severe cases of shoulder bursitis may be managed with corticosteroid injections, which are limited to three injections in a 12-month period no fewer than 30 days apart.[4,8] Physical therapy for appropriate exercises, ultrasound, and electrical stimulation are also appropriate methods of treatment. A demonstrated rotator cuff tear or subacromial fibrosis warrants an orthopedic referral.[3,9]

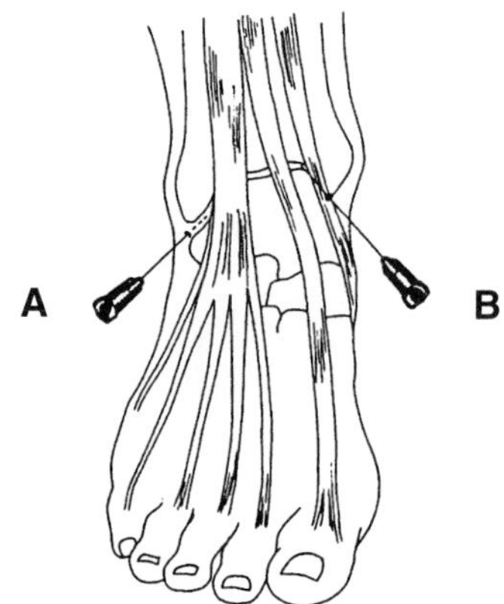

FIGURE 184-3

Arthrocentesis of the ankle. **A**, Medial approach. **B**, Lateral approach. (From Noble JP: *Textbook of primary care medicine,* ed 3, St Louis, 2001, Mosby.)

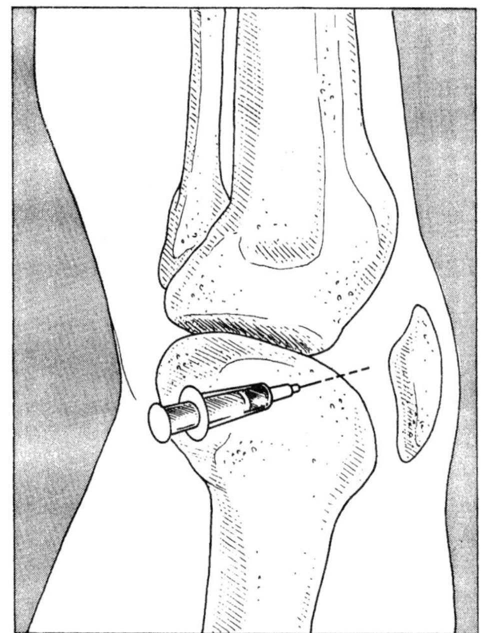

FIGURE 184-4

Arthrocentesis of the knee. (From Noble JP: *Textbook of primary care medicine,* ed 3, St Louis, 2001, Mosby.)

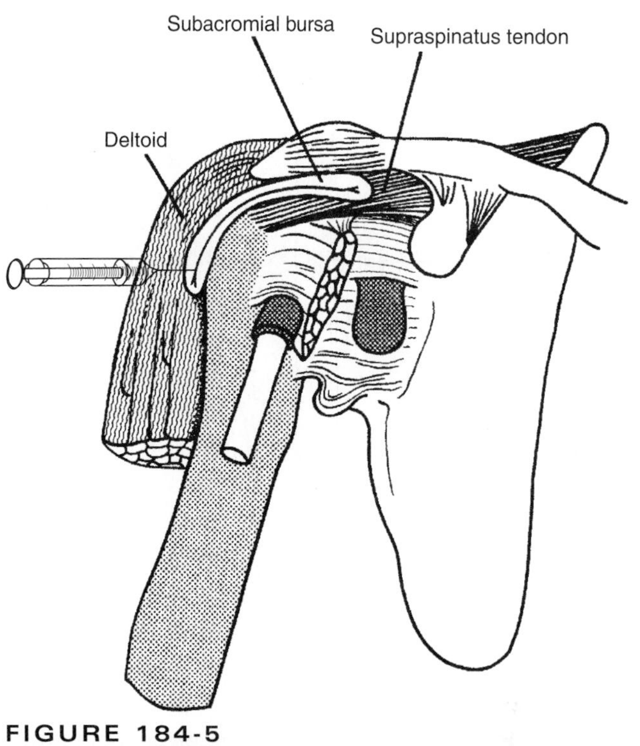

FIGURE 184-5

Injection of the subacromial bursa. (From Noble JP: *Textbook of primary care medicine,* ed 3, St Louis, 2001, Mosby.)

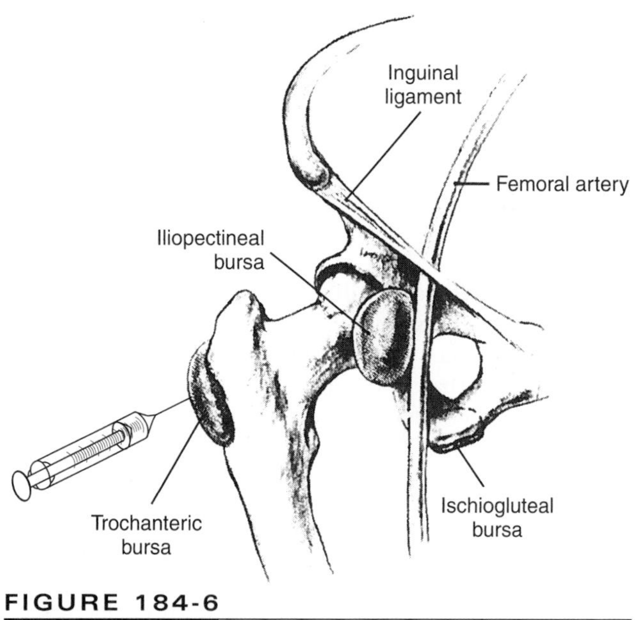

FIGURE 184-6

Injection of the trochanteric bursa. (From Noble JP: *Textbook of primary care medicine,* ed 3, St Louis, 2001, Mosby.)

ELBOW (OLECRANON) BURSITIS

Located on the posterior, extensor aspect of the elbow, olecranon bursitis is the most common type of elbow bursitis. The bursa is swollen and tender, but no elbow motion is lost. Olecranon bursitis may be chronic or acute and septic or aseptic. Most cases result from trauma; chronic olecranon bursitis is related to repetitive trauma that results in thickening of the bursa wall. Antibiotics should be started while awaiting culture results if septic bursitis is suspected (*Staphylococcus aureus* account for the majority of septic cases).[10] Other common causes include trauma, rheumatoid arthritis, gout, and pseudogout. For a more thorough discussion of elbow bursitis, see Chapter 185.

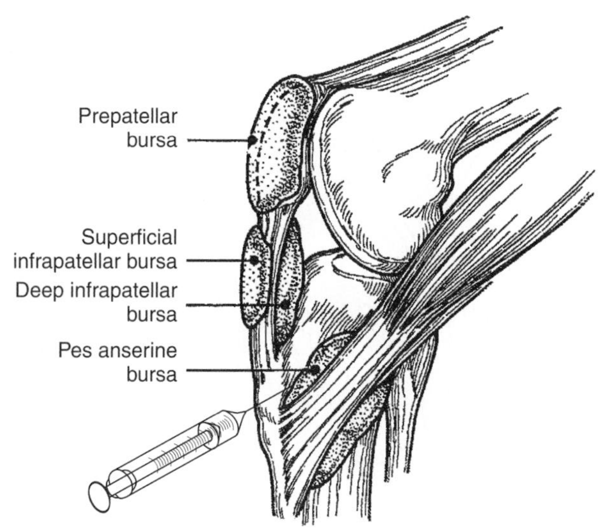

FIGURE 184-7

Injection of the anserine bursa. (From Noble JP: *Textbook of primary care medicine,* ed 3, St Louis, 2001, Mosby.)

DIFFERENTIAL DIAGNOSIS

Elbow (Olecranon) Bursitis

- Septic bursitis
- Gout
- Arthritis (osteoarthritis or rheumatoid arthritis)
- Tendinitis
- Effusion
- Fracture
- Epicondylitis
- Sprain
- Trauma

HIP BURSITIS

DEFINITION AND EPIDEMIOLOGY

Hip bursitis is a common disorder that results from acute or recurrent trauma, musculotendinous overuse, degenerative changes, biomechanical abnormalities, or systemic disease. The trochanteric, iliopsoas, and ischiogluteal groups are the major structures of bursae around the hip. Trochanteric bursitis is a common disorder, affecting women somewhat more often than men (Table 184-1). Conditions that can contribute to trochanteric bursitis include osteoarthritis (OA) of the spine, leg length discrepancy, and scoliosis.

DIFFERENTIAL DIAGNOSIS

Hip Bursitis

- Arthritis (osteoarthritis and rheumatoid arthritis)
- Sciatica
- Aseptic arthritis
- Fracture
- Peripheral neuropathy
- Avascular necrosis
- Referred pelvic pain
- Trauma
- Lumbar spine disease
- Thrombophlebitis
- Sacroiliitis
- Neoplasm

CLINICAL PRESENTATION

Hip bursitis is characterized by pain over the affected bursa. The pain may be sudden or gradual in onset and results from overuse or trauma. Depending on which bursa is inflamed, the pain can have a pseudoradicular quality with radiation down the lateral thigh to the knee or anteriorly to the groin. Pain is often worse at night. Passive joint mobility is usually not affected, although guarding may limit active mobility.

MANAGEMENT

Hip bursitis is managed with NSAIDs, rest, heat, and ice application. A steroid injection may be helpful if more conservative treatment is unsuccessful. Physical therapy with ultrasound treatments will optimize the rehabilitation regimen.

KNEE BURSITIS

DEFINITION AND EPIDEMIOLOGY

Numerous bursae are found around the knee. Anserine bursitis is commonly seen in middle-aged to older women with larger legs. It often follows new weight-bearing activities. Pain is characteristically located over the medial aspect of the knee, about 5 cm (2 inches) below the knee margin. The prepatellar bursa is located between the skin and the patella and is one of the most common sites of pyogenic bursitis. Prepatellar

TABLE 184-1 Hip Bursitis

	Hip Bursae		
	Trochanteric	**Ischiogluteal**	**Iliopsoas**
Location of pain	Lateral hip to lateral thigh and buttock	Ischial tuberosity into posterior thigh; worse with sitting	Groin, with radiation to anterior hip
Examination	Pain worse with hip rotation; may be soft tissue swelling	Tenderness over the ischial tuberosity	Pain worse with resisted hip flexion and hyperextension
Diagnostics	X-rays are usually normal and noncontributory for hip bursitis; a bone scan may be helpful only in refractory conditions.		
Differential diagnosis*	Fracture of the greater trochanter	Fracture	Hip arthritis

Data from Steinberg GG: Hip, pelvis, and proximal thigh. In Steinberg GG, Akins CM, Baron DT, editors: *Ramamurti's orthopedics in primary care,* ed 2, Baltimore, 1992, Williams & Wilkins.
*Consider herniated disc, avascular necrosis, or systemic disease.

DIFFERENTIAL DIAGNOSIS

Knee (Prepatellar) Bursitis

- Effusion
- Arthritis (osteoarthritis or rheumatoid arthritis)
- Fracture
- Gout
- Sprain
- Ligament or meniscus injury
- Retropatellar bursitis
- Pes anserine bursitis
- Osteochondritis dissecans
- Referred pain
- Overuse syndrome
- Chondromalacia
- Patellofemoral joint instability
- Trauma
- Septic bursitis

bursitis is sometimes referred to as *housemaid's knee* and commonly results from activities that require excessive kneeling, such as carpentry, wrestling, or carpet laying.[2,11]

CLINICAL PRESENTATION AND PHYSICAL EXAMINATION

Except in infectious cases, severe pain is unusual in prepatellar bursitis.[12] There is, however, tenderness over the anterior knee that is accompanied by localized edema over the lower half of the patella and upper body of the patellar ligament (prepatellar bursitis) or on both sides of the patellar ligament (infrapatellar bursitis). Often there is bursa thickening that feels rough, like nodules or bone chips. Although the inflamed bursa causes swelling, the edema is different from that noted when there is fluid in the knee joint. The ballottement test may be used to evaluate for knee effusion by applying firm downward pressure to the patella (Figure 184-8). If a click is felt when the patella reaches the femoral condyle, an effusion is likely present. Because knee effusion is absent, a ballottement test for a floating patella will be negative. A pyogenic prepatellar bursitis may appear cellulitic. Anserine bursitis is exquisitely tender to palpation and often associated with OA of the knee, especially if the patient has a valgus (knock-knee) deformity.

The differential diagnosis includes tubercular effusion, infection, arthritis, hemarthrosis, gout, and pseudogout.

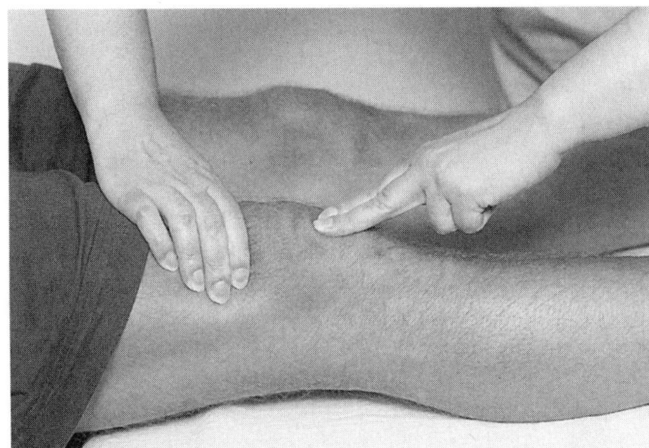

FIGURE 184-8

Ballottement of the knee. (From Barkauskas VH: *Health and physical assessment,* ed 2, St Louis, 1998, Mosby.)

MANAGEMENT

Acute and chronic knee bursitis is best managed initially with conservative treatment, including rest, physical therapy, and NSAIDs. Acute bursitis may also respond to ice application and aspiration of the affected site and injection of steroids. Septic prepatellar bursitis, commonly caused by *S. aureus*,[11] often responds well to immobilization, one or two daily aspirations, and appropriate antibiotic coverage.[12]

HEEL (CALCANEAL) BURSITIS

DEFINITION AND EPIDEMIOLOGY

Two clinically significant bursae are located in the posterior heel. The retrocalcaneal bursa lies between the calcaneus and the Achilles tendon and is usually associated with systemic inflammatory diseases such as the spondyloarthropathies, rheumatoid arthritis, and gout.[13] The posterior calcaneal bursa is located between the Achilles tendon and the skin. Calcaneal bursitis is the result of local mechanical irritation to the posterior heel and affects ice skaters (primarily female) and long-distance runners.[12]

CLINICAL PRESENTATION AND PHYSICAL EXAMINATION

The usual presentation of calcaneal bursitis includes a history of poorly fitting shoes. This causes the heel to rub on the back of the shoe and results in heel pain.[14] Physical findings include a palpable, swollen bursa that is tender at the Achilles tendon insertion site at the posterior heel. There may also be erythema of the affected area.

DIAGNOSTICS AND DIFFERENTIAL DIAGNOSIS

Reiter's syndrome, fracture, os trigonum syndrome, loose bodies, or calcaneal apophysitis are possible causes of calcaneal pain. In addition, tubercular effusions, infection, inflammatory arthritis, hemarthrosis, gout, and pseudogout should be considered. Achilles tendinitis and osteomyelitis can both cause heel pain.

MANAGEMENT

Conservative management of calcaneal bursitis requires rest, NSAIDs, and the avoidance of poorly fitting shoes. Application of heat and cold may alleviate some pain. Physical therapy for Achilles tendon stretching and ankle flexion-extension exercises may also be helpful. In some cases, a corticosteroid injection to the affected bursa is beneficial.[8] However, caution is advised to avoid injecting and subsequently weakening the Achilles tendon.[12] An ultrasound-guided steroid injection may be beneficial if a nonguided ultrasound injection is not successful.[15]

DIFFERENTIAL DIAGNOSIS

Heel (Calcaneal) Bursitis

- Trauma, fracture
- Achilles tendinitis
- Plantar fasciitis

LIFE SPAN CONSIDERATIONS

With aging, tendons become less elastic, making them more susceptible to injury. Also with aging or disuse atrophy, the muscles become weaker, exhibit less bulk and endurance, and are less able to absorb mechanical forces. Some patients may have a genetic predisposition to these syndromes related to inherited variations in anatomy resulting in altered biomechanics. Bursitis has no impact on longevity.

COMPLICATIONS

The pain of bursitis can be disabling for many patients. Some patients with shoulder or elbow bursitis stop using the affected extremity, resulting in increased disability; others do not bear weight on the affected extremity to avoid pain. Unfortunately, recurrent episodes of acute bursitis can develop into chronic bursitis. The adjacent tissue may be compromised in cases of severe bursal swelling, and it may be difficult to determine the true cause of the patient's discomfort. Infection of the bursa or surrounding tissue is not uncommon. Oral antibiotic therapy may be sufficient for some patients with septic bursitis, but many patients require IV antibiotic therapy, hospitalization, and daily aspiration of the bursa fluid.

INDICATIONS FOR REFERRAL OR HOSPITALIZATION

Patients with suspected septic bursitis should be referred to a physician or orthopedic specialist expediently. Aspiration of the infected bursa for fluid analysis and antibiotic therapy are indicated. Hospitalization may be required for some patients, particularly those who have diabetes or are immunosuppressed.

A referral to an orthopedist or a rheumatologist is appropriate for patients who do not respond to conservative measures within a reasonable period. Physical therapy often expedites recovery, minimizes pain, and prevents joint immobility.

PATIENT AND FAMILY EDUCATION

Because bursitis is related to repetitive activities, such as the kneeling associated with prepatellar bursitis, recurrence is possible. Patients should understand this and try to avoid activities that may exacerbate the disorder. Patients with prepatellar bursitis should use knee pads. Rest is indicated during the acute process, but gentle stretching and range-of-motion exercises should begin as soon as possible and continue indefinitely to prevent stiffness and maintain mobility. Ice or heat plus NSAIDs help decrease joint inflammation. A joint that becomes erythematous, tender, and swollen with associated fever requires assessment by a health care provider. If corticosteroid injections are necessary, the risks and benefits should be discussed before injection.

REFERENCES

1. Reveille JD: Soft tissue rheumatism: diagnosis and treatment, *Am J Med* 102(1A):23S-29S, 1997.
2. Dlabach JA: Nontraumatic soft tissue disorders. In Canale ST: *Campbell's operative orthopedics*, ed 10, St Louis, 2003, Mosby.
3. Hunter DM: Shoulder pain. In Tintinalli JE, Ruiz E, Krome RL, editors: *Emergency medicine,* New York, 1996, McGraw-Hill.
4. Salzman KL, Lillegard WA, Butcher JD: Upper extremity bursitis, *Am Fam Phys* 56(7):1797-1806, 1997.
5. Belzer JP, Durkin RC: Common disorders of the shoulder, *Prim Care* 23(2):365-388, 1996.
6. Bureau NJ, Dussault RG, Keats TE: Imaging of bursae around the shoulder joint, *Skeletal Radiol* 25(6):513-517, 1996.
7. Pfeninger JL: Joint and soft tissue aspiration and injection. In Pfeninger JL, Fowler GC, editors: *Procedures for primary care physicians,* St Louis, 1994, Mosby.
8. Larson HM, O'Connor FG, Nirschl RP: Shoulder pain: the role of diagnostic injections, *Am Fam Phys* 53(5):1637-1647, 1995.
9. Green A: Arthroscopic treatment of impingement syndrome, *Orthop Clin North Am* 26(4):631-641, 1996.
10. Deu RS, Carek PJ: Common sports injuries: upper extremity injuries, *Clin Fam Pract* 7(2):249-265, 2005.
11. Valeriano-Marcet J, Carter JD, Vasey FB: Soft tissue disease, *Rheum Dis Clin North Am* 29:77-88, 2003.
12. Butcher JD, Salzman KL, Lillegard WA: Lower extremity bursitis, *Am Fam Phys* 53(7):2317-2324, 1996.
13. Liu NYN, Canoso JJ: Periarticular rheumatic disorders. In Noble JP, editor: *Textbook of primary care medicine,* ed 3, St Louis, 2001, Mosby.
14. Quirk R: Common foot and ankle injuries in dance, *Orthop Clin North Am* 25(1):123-133, 1994.
15. Cunnane G, Brophy DP, Gibney RG, and others: Diagnosis and treatment of heel pain in chronic inflammatory arthritis using ultrasound, *Semin Arthritis Rheum* 25(6):383-389, 1996.

CHAPTER 185

Elbow Pain

Denise A. Vanacore

DEFINITION AND EPIDEMIOLOGY

A hinged joint that allows flexion and rotation of the forearm, the elbow provides a wide, stable arc of motion for the hand.[1] Microtears of the muscles, ligaments, and tendons from inflammation and trauma are common causes of acute and chronic elbow pain.

Most elbow injuries result from overuse during high force and/or repetitive motion activities. Two groups of people seem to be at increased risk for elbow disorders. The first is high-performance athletes, especially in racket and throwing sports such as baseball, tennis, and basketball. The second group includes those with jobs that require forceful or repetitive wrist and elbow rotation, lifting, gripping, or torquing motions. High-risk occupations include factory workers, laborers, carpenters, and grocery checkers. The prevalence of occupational epicondylitis is as high as 5%.[2] In the general population, injuries may occur from pursuing recreational hobbies. Improper preparation, lack of strength or conditioning, or overzealousness can all contribute to elbow pain.

The elbow is also vulnerable to inflammatory arthritides, including rheumatoid arthritis and the spondyloarthropathies.

PATHOPHYSIOLOGY

The elbow is formed by the articulations of the humerus, radius, and ulna. The humeroulnar articulation is a hinge joint and allows elbow flexion and extension. The humeroradial and radioulnar articulations are partially ligamental; their flexibility allows rotation of the radius and pronation-supination of the forearm.

Stability of the elbow is accomplished through bones, ligaments, and muscles. The humeroulnar joint is the main stabilizer for flexion-extension of the elbow. Rotational stability is divided into valgus and varus stabilizers. A valgus stress is a force on the medial elbow from throwing or axial compression. Primary valgus stabilizers are the medial (ulnar) collateral ligaments and their supporting muscles. A varus stress is a force on the lateral elbow. The lateral (radial) collateral ligaments stabilize for varus stress.

Elbow injuries may be classified as acute or chronic. Acute injuries result from a single high force, such as a fall or direct blow, that is greater in strength than the tendon, ligament, or bone affected.[1,3] However, the vast majority of injuries are chronic. Chronic injuries occur from repetitive, submaximum forces that overload the elbow's ability to adequately heal, causing recurrent pain.

CLINICAL PRESENTATION

Elbow pain may be traced to a specific activity or chain of events or may appear insidiously, with no identifiable trigger. Once an injury has occurred, everyday activities such as picking up groceries, reaching, or pulling can cause pain. A thorough history, including occupational and recreational activities and any prior elbow injury, is essential. A history of other joint pain or swelling is also needed to exclude rheumatoid arthritis, psoriasis, crystal arthropathies, or other systemic diseases.

PHYSICAL EXAMINATION

Physical examination is performed on both elbows to assess for alteration in carrying angle, posture, strength, and range of motion. Bony and soft tissue landmarks should be assessed for asymmetry, malalignment, erythema, swelling, and tenderness. Bony landmarks to examine are the medial and lateral epicondyles of the humerus and the olecranon process of the ulna. Range of motion testing includes flexion and extension, and pronation and supination. Normal flexion and extension are 0 to 135 degrees. The elbow can rotate from 0 to 180 degrees. Normal range of motion effectively rules out involvement of the elbow joint itself. Functional range of motion for normal activities of daily living is 30 to 130 degrees of flexion, with the greatest strength and greatest stress on the elbow at 70 degrees.[3] Extraarticular pathologic conditions, including epicondylitis or olecranon bursitis, rarely affect elbow range of motion.[4]

The extensor tendons at the lateral epicondyle and the flexor tendons at the medial epicondyle are palpated for tenderness. Several confirmatory tests or maneuvers may be helpful. Resisted wrist extension or flexion may help diagnose lateral or medial epicondylitis, respectively. A local anesthetic block can be placed near the suspected involved tendon. Relief of pain with this injection is confirmatory.[4]

Posteriorly, the olecranon bursa overlies the olecranon process. The olecranon bursa is inspected and palpated for swelling, chronic thickening, or both.

The ulnar nerve sits in a groove between the medial epicondyle and the olecranon process.[5] Tinel's sign is positive when tapping over the ulnar groove reproduces pain or numbness felt in the fourth and fifth fingers. Muscles for wrist flexion and pronation originate via tendons from the medial epicondyle, then spread out along the palmar surface of the forearm.

Physical examination should include the wrist, shoulder, and neck, since pathologic conditions at theses sites may cause referred pain to the elbow. Location and radiation of the pain are critical for accurate assessment.

DIAGNOSTICS

Testing is based on the mechanism of injury or duration of symptoms. X-ray studies of the elbow are the most commonly ordered tests. Standard x-ray studies include an anteroposterior film with the elbow fully extended and supinated and a lateral view with the elbow flexed at 90 degrees and the forearm supinated. Oblique views may be needed to better study the radial head and shaft, the humeral condyles, and the coronoid process of the ulna.[6] Laboratory testing is based on the clinical history. A CBC, erythrocyte sedimentation rate, rheumatoid factor, antinuclear antibody test, Lyme's titer, or elbow joint aspiration may be indicated to exclude infection or systemic disease. Joint aspirate should be evaluated with a culture and Gram's stain and examined for crystals.

DIAGNOSTICS

Elbow Pain

LABORATORY
CBC and differential*
ESR*
Rheumatoid factor*
Antinuclear antibodies*
Lyme's titer*

IMAGING
X-ray* (anteroposterior, lateral, and oblique)

OTHER
Joint aspiration*

*If indicated.

DIFFERENTIAL DIAGNOSIS

The most common causes of elbow pain are sprains, fractures, bursitis, and epicondylitis. Lateral epicondylitis is called *tennis elbow*; medial epicondylitis is called *golfer's elbow*. Medial collateral ligament instability and ulnar neuritis can also cause pain (Table 185-1). Elbow pain is often due to local injury but may result from a referred, external condition. Based on the

DIFFERENTIAL DIAGNOSIS

Elbow Pain

- Arthritis (rheumatic or osteoarthritis)
- Brachial plexus disease
- Bursitis
- Cardiovascular disease
- Cervical disc disease
- Cubital tunnel syndrome
- Diabetes
- Digital biceps tendon rupture
- Dislocation
- Epicondylitis, lateral (tennis elbow)
- Epicondylitis, medial (golfer's elbow)
- Fracture
- Gout
- Impingement
- Lyme disease
- Osteochondrosis
- Osteophytes
- Overuse injuries
- Peripheral nerve entrapment
- Pseudogout
- Psoriatic arthritis
- Radicular pain
- Septic joint
- Sprain
- Tendinitis
- Thoracic outlet syndrome
- Triceps rupture
- Ulnar neuritis

TABLE 185-1 Common Elbow Ailments*

Ailment	Presentation	Examination	Differential Diagnosis and Management
EPICONDYLITIS			
Inflammatory condition characterized by pain at tendon origin of muscle groups at medial (golfer's elbow) or lateral (tennis elbow) aspects of elbow; usually self-limiting, but may take several months for full recovery	Gradual or acute onset of pain along affected epicondyle, with or without radiation; possible history of heavy lifting, hammering, screwing, or gripping	Local tenderness over or just distal to affected epicondyle; possible tenderness of flexor and extensor muscles; range of motion (ROM) and distal neurovascular examination within normal limits *Lateral epicondylitis:* Pain at or around lateral epicondyle reproduced by resistive wrist extension (examiner applying pressure to force wrist into flexion while patient extends wrist) *Medial epicondylitis:* Pain exacerbated by resistive wrist flexion	**Differential diagnosis:** Carpal tunnel syndrome, cervical radiculopathy, rotator cuff tendinitis, lateral or medial collateral ligament sprains, osteoarthritis, or avulsion fracture **Management:** Conservative treatment: NSAIDs, tennis elbow splint, "palms-up" lifting, toning exercises of wrist extensors; steroid injection if above treatment is unsuccessful; orthopedic referral for surgical evaluation if treatment fails
SPRAINS			
Tearing or stretching of lateral or medial collateral ligaments from varus or valgus stretch	Pain after throwing, overhead, or weight-bearing activity (medial) or fall onto extended elbow (lateral)	Tenderness of overlying affected ligaments; medial tenderness a maximal of 2 cm (0.8 inch) distal to epicondyle, with pain and/or instability with valgus stretch at 30 degrees of elbow flexion; lateral tenderness vague, reproduced only with arm extended and supinated	**Differential diagnosis:** Epicondylitis, radial or ulnar nerve irritation, avulsion fracture, or ligament tear **Management:** RICE; may use sling and splint for 48 hours if significant pain and edema

*Created by Terry Mahan Buttaro, MS, RN, CS, CEN, CCRN, ANP, GNP.
RICE, Rest, ice, compression, elevation.

TABLE 185-1 Common Elbow Ailments*—cont'd

Ailment	Presentation	Examination	Differential Diagnosis and Management
RADIAL HEAD FRACTURES			
Usually caused by fall onto outstretched hand; commonly involves superior portion of radial bone	Affected arm usually cradled at 90 degrees; pain decreasing 30 minutes after injury, then recurring several hours later because of bleeding in joint	Local or diffuse edema; tenderness over radial head; ROM limited, rotation quite painful; grasp strength diminished; intact radial pulse and normal neurologic examination of hand and wrist	**Differential diagnosis:** Acute lateral epicondylitis, capsular tears, cartilage injury, subluxation or dislocation of radial head, fracture of olecranon or humerus **Management:** Ice, immobilization with posterior splint or sling with elbow flexed at 90 degrees; surgical repair often required for displaced or complicated fractures
ULNAR NEURITIS			
Also called cubital tunnel syndrome Compression of ulnar nerve causing numbness or tingling in nerve's distribution	May be complication of rheumatoid arthritis, ganglion, elbow fracture, repeated irritation, or medial ligament sprain; pain usually localized to medial elbow; may radiate down forearm or cause clumsiness of hand; numbness and tingling replacing pain in severe cases	Tenderness of ulnar groove; sensory loss of fifth digit; diminished motor strength of fourth and fifth digits; positive Tinel's sign (tingling sensation down forearm and hand in ulnar distribution when tapping over ulnar groove); in severe cases may be forearm motor weakness and muscle atrophy **Diagnostics:** electromyographic studies	**Differential diagnosis:** Medial epicondylitis, cervical disc disease, thoracic outlet syndrome **Management:** Rest of affected hand; elbow pads; wrist-elbow splint, support in neutral position; ice, NSAIDs, physical therapy; conservative treatment rarely effective; referral to orthopedics or neurology appropriate
OLECRANON BURSITIS			
Swelling of bursal sac underlying olecranon process; may be acute, chronic, septic, or aseptic and associated with history of trauma, rheumatoid arthritis, or gout	After acute injury, development of painful, edematous elbow; in chronic inflammation, soft, edematous nontender elbow; ROM often intact	Edema, possible tenderness over posterior elbow; full ROM and normal neurologic examination; in chronic bursitis, rough nodular consistency noted; if secondary infection, fever, warmth, erythema, and tenderness present	**Differential diagnosis:** Consider tendinitis; synovitis if edema is diffuse with limited elbow extension; infection; fracture with history of trauma; gout if extremely tender and erythematous; osteophytes; osteochondrosis **Management:** X-rays if indicated; aspiration of bursal fluid for diagnosis; hospitalization of patients with septic bursitis for aspiration, IV antibiotics p.r.n.; otherwise, RICE, NSAIDs, antibiotics if indicated; steroid injection p.r.n.; orthopedic referral if no response to treatment in 1 week

*Created by Terry Mahan Buttaro, MS, RN, CS, CEN, CCRN, ANP, GNP.
RICE, Rest, ice, compression, elevation.

history, the differential diagnosis for referred pain should include cervical disc or nerve root problems; thoracic outlet or brachial plexus disease; radicular pain from shoulder, neck, or wrist overuse injuries; diabetes; cardiovascular disease; and peripheral nerve entrapment syndromes.[4,6] Acute injuries are most often related to overuse, direct trauma, or fractures. Systemic diseases that may cause elbow pain, such as rheumatoid arthritis (Chapter 235), osteoarthritis (Chapter 194), psoriatic arthritis (Chapter 232), Lyme's disease (Chapter 250), and infection, should also be considered. Based on examination, with neurologic findings, an electromyogram and nerve conduction studies may be indicated to rule out nerve entrapment.

MANAGEMENT

Ideally, treatment begins before injury occurs. Injury prevention strategies include flexibility, strength, and endurance training; warm-up and cool-down stretching exercises; and avoidance of fatigue by limiting total activity time. Proper equipment, body mechanics, and ergonomics are also important to prevent injuries.

Once injury occurs, general goals of treatment are pain management, healing of microtears, and prevention of reinjury. RICE therapy (rest, ice, compression, and elevation) and activity modification should be initiated to protect the elbow from further injury and to reduce pain and swelling. NSAIDs can be used to reduce pain and tissue inflammation. After 2 weeks of conservative treatment, corticosteroid injection may be considered to provide further improvement in the condition.[7] Steroid injections may provide temporary relief that allows the patient to fully participate in rehabilitation activities.[8] Splinting that keeps the wrist in 30 to 45 degrees of extension may be useful for lateral epicondylitis.[8] Physical therapy with ultrasound or electrical stimulation can be used acutely, followed by rehabilitation exercises and a gradual return to activity. Changes in technique, equipment, and ergonomics should also be implemented to prevent injury recurrence.[8]

Management of arthritis includes antiinflammatory medications, balanced rest and exercise, joint conservation techniques, and avoidance of pain-generating activities. Occupational therapy can be helpful to these patients.

COMPLICATIONS

Recurrent epicondylitis or tendinitis may cause cumulative weakening of those tissues, resulting in impairment of grip function or lifting ability and nerve entrapment of the arm.[6,7] Limitation of elbow range of motion, arthritis, and chronic elbow pain may be caused by improper diagnosis or failure to treat the underlying elbow disorder.

CONSIDERATION FOR REFERRAL

Acute trauma resulting in fracture, dislocation, and vascular or neurologic clinical findings should be referred to an orthopedist. Recurrent injury, failure to improve with basic management, chronic pain with activity, complaints of arm weakness, or complaints of pain or swelling in other joints should also be referred. Both physical and occupational therapists can be extremely helpful with both treatment and education. Vocational counseling may be indicated for those patients with repetitive stress injuries causing elbow pain and disability.

PATIENT EDUCATION

Injury prevention and early recovery are assisted by teaching about proper stretching and conditioning exercises, the need for rest at early symptoms of pain, use of ergonomic redesign (in rackets, workplace, power tools), and proper body mechanics for sports and repetitive motion activities. Individuals with recurrent injury or any change in elbow function or mobility should be advised to seek prompt medical attention to minimize complications.

REFERENCES

1. Caldwell GL, Safran MR: Elbow problems in the athlete, *Orthop Clin North Am* 26(3):465-485, 1995.
2. Hales TR, Bernard BP: Epidemiology of work-related musculoskeletal disorders, *Orthop Clin North Am* 27(4):679-710, 1996.
3. Safran MR: Elbow injuries in athletes: a review, *Clin Orthop* 310:257-277, 1995.
4. Anderson B, Anderson R: *Evaluation of the patient with elbow pain*, retrieved May 16, 2006, from http://www.utdol.com/utd/content/topic.do?topicKey=ad_orth/6626.
5. Hoppinfield S: *Physical examination of the spine and extremities*, Norwalk, Conn, 1976, Appleton-Century-Crofts.
6. Mercier LR: *Practical orthopedics*, ed 4, St Louis, 1995, Mosby.
7. Cardone D, Talia A: Diagnostic and therapeutic injection of the elbow region, *Am Fam Phys* 66:2097-2100, 2002.
8. Sellards R, Kuebrich C: The elbow: diagnosis and treatment of common injuries, *Clin Office Pract* 32:1, 2005.

CHAPTER 186

Fibromyalgia and Myofascial Pain Syndrome

Lin A. Brown

DEFINITION AND EPIDEMIOLOGY

Fibromyalgia syndrome (FMS) is a disorder usually included with rheumatologic conditions that is characterized by symptoms of widespread musculoskeletal pain, fatigue, nonrestorative sleep, depression, headaches, and gastrointestinal complaints (irritable bowel syndrome). FMS gained acceptance as a disorder in 1990 after the American College of Rheumatology developed classification criteria for the disorder (Box-186-1).

Fibromyalgia is defined as more than 3 months of musculoskeletal pain present above and below the waist bilaterally, associated with pain on palpation of tender points. No other source of pain is identified (see Box 186-1 and Figure 186-1). The pain is usually accompanied by profound fatigue and sleep

BOX 186-1

AMERICAN COLLEGE OF RHEUMATOLOGY 1990 CRITERIA FOR CLASSIFICATION OF FIBROMYALGIA*

- **History of widespread pain.** Pain is considered widespread when all of the following are present: pain on the left side of the body, pain on the right side of the body, pain above the waist, and pain below the waist. In addition, axial skeletal pain (cervical spine or anterior chest or thoracic spine or low back) must be present. In the definition, shoulder and buttock pain is considered as pain for each involved side. "Low back" pain is considered lower segment pain.
- **Pain in 11 of 18 tender point sites on digital palpation.** Digital palpation should be performed with an approximate force of 4 kg. For a tender point to be considered "positive," the subject must state that the palpation was painful. "Tender" is not to be considered "painful." Pain on digital palpation, must be present in at least 11 of the following 18 tender point sites:

  Occiput: bilateral, at the suboccipital muscle insertions
  Low cervical: bilateral, at the anterior aspects of the intertransverse spaces at C5-C7
  Trapezius: bilateral, at the midpoint of the upper border
  Supraspinatus: bilateral, at origins, above the scapula spine near the medial border
  Second rib: bilateral, at the second costochondral junctions, just lateral to the junctions on upper surfaces
  Lateral epicondyle: bilateral, 2 cm distal to the epicondyles
  Gluteal: bilateral, in upper outer quadrants of buttocks in anterior folds of muscle
  Greater trochanter: bilateral, posterior to the trochanteric prominence
  Knee: bilateral, at the medial fat pad proximal to the joint line

From Wolfe F, Smythe HA, Yunus MB and others: The American College of Rheumatology 1990 criteria for the classification of fibromyalgia: report of the multicenter criteria committee, *Arthritis Rheum* 33(2):160-172, 1990.

*For classification purposes, patients are said to have fibromyalgia if both criteria are satisfied. Widespread pain must have been present for at least 3 months. The presence of a second clinical disorder does not exclude the diagnosis of fibromyalgia.

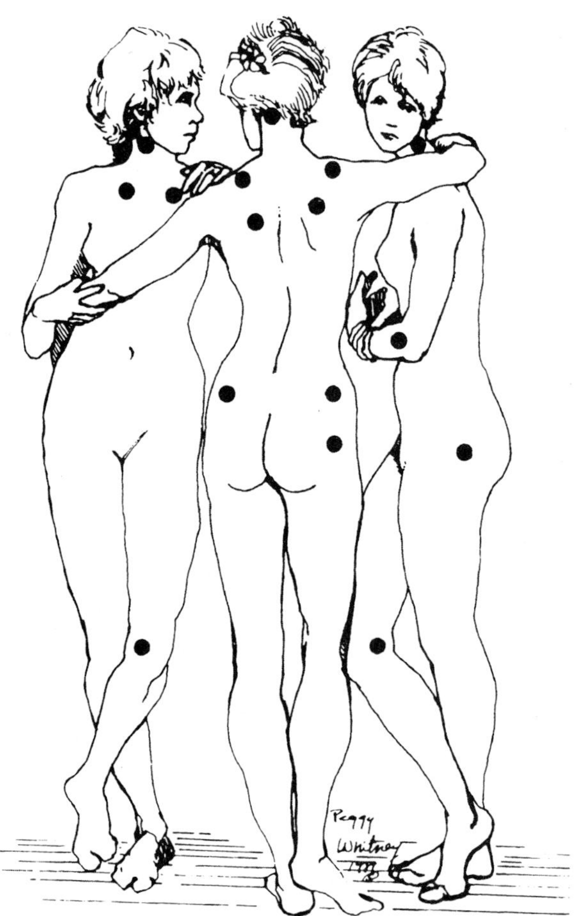

FIGURE 186-1

Tender point locations for the 1990 classification criteria for fibromyalgia. (From Wolfe F, Smythe HA, Yunus MB, and others: The American College of Rheumatology 1990 criteria for the classification of fibromyalgia: report of the Multicenter Criteria Committee, *Arthritis Rheum* 33(2):160-172, 1990.)

disturbance (nonrestorative sleep). Fibromyalgia may occur in the presence of other rheumatologic disorders such as lupus and rheumatoid arthritis.[1] Most patients with chronic fatigue syndrome also meet diagnostic criteria for FMS. Myofascial pain syndrome is a more limited expression of the condition (e.g., shoulder and neck, upper back).

FMS is eight to nine times more prevalent in women than men in all age-groups, with an onset generally at 40 to 50 years of age. FMS rarely begins after the age of 55. Approximately 2% of the total population is affected, and incidence increases with age to 8% in women 60 to 69 years old.[2] FMS affects 3 million to 6 million Americans, accounting for 2% of all primary care visits, 10% of all internal medicine referrals, and up to 20% of rheumatology referrals.[1,2] Symptoms start gradually in adulthood or rarely, in childhood, and wax and wane in intensity.[1]

PATHOPHYSIOLOGY

Although the cause of FMS is unclear, new research has implicated central nervous system dysfunction and not muscle disease, autoimmune disease, or viral disease. Pain beginning in the periphery is processed in the spinal cord and transmitted to the brain. For unclear reasons, some pain becomes heard "louder" at the level of the spinal cord and brain, a condition called *central sensitization*. The brain responds with pain recognition at a lower threshold and over a wider area than that originally involved.[3] In addition, neuroendocrine disturbances at the level of the hypothalamus and/or pituitary, involving decreased levels of growth hormone (GH), insulin-like growth factor (IGF), and possibly prolactin, have been found in FMS patients.[4] These hormones are released during the stages of sleep, specifically GH in stages 3 and 4 of non–rapid eye movement (REM) sleep. In sleep studies, patients with FMS have disturbances with non-REM sleep and difficulty progressing to stage 3 and 4 sleep, resulting in morning fatigue. One third of FMS patients have low IGF, an indication of low GH secretion, lending credence to disturbed stage 4 sleep as important in FMS. Treatment with GH increases IGF levels; improves pain and sleep; and reduces overall symptoms, although the cost is prohibitive.[3,4]

Other neuroendocrine abnormalities include elevation of cerebrospinal fluid substance P levels and dysregulated cortisol production. FMS patients have three times the levels of substance P, which is significant because this neurotransmitter plays a role in enhanced pain perception. This may be the reason for the heightened pain perception experienced by fibromyalgia patients. Alteration in the hypopituitary-adrenal axis with low production of cortisol, perhaps secondary to chronic stress response, contrasts with depression, where high production of cortisol is found. These results suggest that the etiology of FMS may be a product of disturbances in the autonomic and endocrine stress response systems.[3] In addition, serotonin levels are low in the brain and in the platelets of fibromyalgia patients.

Although the above theories explain part of the pathogenesis of FMS, the primary cause of the central dysregulation is unknown. FMS frequently follows trauma, viral illness, and stress.

CLINICAL PRESENTATION

Persistent widespread pain is the hallmark of the syndrome, along with chronic fatigue. Patients have a variety of other somatic complaints, include nonrestorative sleep; cognitive difficulties; auditory, vestibular, and ocular complaints; chronic rhinitis or "allergies"; migraines; palpitations; irritable bowel syndrome; subjective sense of joint swelling; and mood disorders.[5] With such generalized complaints, it is clear how the patient's complaints can be confused with an autoimmune disease such as lupus.

PHYSICAL EXAMINATION

With fibromyalgia, muscle strength is normal (although may be affected by pain), and there is no evidence of synovitis or soft tissue inflammation. Making the diagnosis depends on findings from the history and physical examination. FMS should be considered with any musculoskeletal pain not explained by a clearly defined anatomic lesion.

The American College of Rheumatology developed criteria characteristic of FMS symptoms[6] (see Box 186-1). Pressure point evaluation of sites is accomplished using 4 kg (8.8

pounds) of pressure, with the report of pain, not tenderness, at 11 of the 18 sites; widespread pain on the left and right side; and pain above and below the waist. (A pressure of 4 kg is achieved by digital palpation with the thumb, using enough pressure to blanch the thumbnail.) Shoulder and buttock pain qualifies for the definition of pain on each side, and low back pain must be present. Pain of the cervical spine, anterior chest, and thoracic spine (axial skeletal pain) also is required for diagnosis. However, these criteria were not meant to be rigid, and some patients who do not exhibit 11 tender points still fit the diagnosis of FMS. Trigger point scores may be a marker of greater stress or anxiety (see Figure 186-1).

DIAGNOSTICS

An in-depth history and physical examination reduce the need for extensive and expensive objective tests. Typically laboratory values and electromyography findings are normal. CBC, erythrocyte sedimentation rate, rheumatoid factor, antinuclear antibodies, and thyroid-stimulating hormone are of value in excluding underlying autoimmune disorders such as rheumatoid arthritis and lupus. Sleep studies may be warranted for some patients, especially those with characteristics of obstructive sleep apnea (OSA). OSA is characterized by daytime *sleepiness*, as opposed to daytime *fatigue*. Patients find themselves falling asleep during daytime activities such as driving. Radiographs are of limited value.

DIFFERENTIAL DIAGNOSIS

Symptoms of fibromyalgia often overlap with those of myofascial pain syndrome, chronic fatigue syndrome, hypothyroidism, bursitis or tendinitis, depression, and anxiety. Connective tissue diseases that should be included in the differential diagnosis include rheumatoid arthritis, systemic lupus erythematosus, polymyalgia rheumatica, and polymyositis.

MANAGEMENT

Treatment of FMS does not fit a specific algorithm or paradigm and is as much of an art as a science. The goal of therapy should be patient empowerment to control pain, enhance sleep, and maintain mobility. Education allows the patient opportunities to individualize treatment and reduce symptoms. Treatment may incorporate pharmacologic therapies, cognitive behavioral therapy, exercise, and alternative therapies.[7]

Pharmacology

Low doses of tricyclic drugs have been studied, particularly amitriptyline 10 mg taken 2 to 3 hours before bedtime, allowing peak sedative effect and reducing sedation on awakening. Cyclobenzaprine, also a tricyclic, can be used as well, at 5 to 10 mg at night (Table 186-1). Dosages should start low and increase slowly. Selective serotonin reuptake inhibitors, such as fluoxetine (Prozac) 20 mg, have also been studied, but dufloxatine (Cymbalta), a dual serotonin-norepinephrine reuptake inhibitor, may work better.

Other medications that have proved helpful for pain include gabapentin (Neurontin) and pregabalin (Lyrica). Trazodone (Desyrel) and zolpidem (Ambien) may help sleep but do not increase time in stage 4. NSAIDs and acetaminophen can be tried and are commonly prescribed, although

TABLE 186-1 Pharmacologic Therapy for Fibromyalgia

Medication	Proposed Action
Amitriptyline 10-20 mg q.h.s., gradually increasing to 70 mg	Restoration of sleep
Cyclobenzaprine 10 mg t.i.d. p.r.n. or in combination with amitriptyline	Pain relief
Selective serotonin reuptake inhibitor: fluoxetine (Prozac) 20 mg, alone or in combination with amitriptyline	Antidepressant and pain relief
Venlafaxine 75 mg PO b.i.d. or t.i.d.	Augment central adrenergic response to decrease pain
Gabapentin 300 mg t.i.d.	Pain relief
Trazodone 50 mg PO q.h.s.	Pain relief
Zolpidem tartrate (Ambien) 5-10 mg PO q.h.s.	Improve sleep
Lidocaine 1% 2-3 ml equal parts IM in tender point areas	Pain relief for recalcitrant tender point pain
Dufloxatine (Cymbalta)	Antidepressant and pain relief

NSAIDs have not been proved effective. Identifying pain generators such as osteoarthritis of the knee, spinal stenosis, restless leg syndrome, or diabetic neuropathy can result in treatment of these conditions, which may play a role in reducing sleep disturbances and pain.[3,7]

Chronic Opioid Analgesic Therapy

Chronic opioid analgesic therapy (COAT) should be avoided, although controlled clinical trials show COAT to be effective in non-cancer-related pain. If it is used, patients need to be aware of the high dependency possibility and be closely monitored.[7] The provider should sign a contract with any patient started on a narcotic medication so that dysfunctional behavior can be avoided.

Cognitive Behavioral Therapy

Cognitive behavioral therapy uses different approaches to integrate coping skills, relaxation training, activity pacing, visual imagery techniques, and goal setting to allow the patient control to improve function and pain.[4,7] It has been shown in multiple studies to be effective in treating FMS by reducing pain and increasing a sense of well-being.[8]

The Arthritis Foundation (http://www.arthritis.org) and other websites can help direct patients to self-help books and classes.

Exercise

Aerobic exercise can improve pain and have an antidepressant effect.[9] Usually patients with fibromyalgia have not been active physically and experience increased pain when they begin an aerobic exercise program. Gentle stretching is a must before engaging in a low-impact activity such as biking, swimming, and walking. Massage aids in relaxation and produces physiologic benefits. Encouragement to continue the exercise program is needed to combat the continued muscle wasting often associated with fibromyalgia, as well as to alleviate patients' perception that pain is inevitable. Patients should consider a one-on-one therapist or exercise partner for any program to improve success.[10] Exercise and cognitive behavioral therapy are clearly beneficial.

Alternative Therapies

Acupuncture, chiropractic manipulation, and trigger point injections have been studied and are reported to be effective adjuncts to a treatment regimen. The judicious use of trigger point injections with lidocaine (Xylocaine) or bupivacaine (Marcaine) has been attempted for symptoms not controlled with other medications, with some success.[11] Any treatment that is not effective should be discontinued.

Multidisciplinary Approach

Group therapy programs are based on cognitive behavioral therapy approaches for living day to day effectively and increasing endurance and strength. An evidence-based clinical review evaluated seven trials and found insufficient evidence that these programs are effective by themselves; rather, they worked better as an adjunct to a primary provider. The studies were of low quality, and variables tested were so different, it was difficult to standardize the trials for comparison. More research needs to be done to establish the effects of a multidisciplinary approach to treatment for FMS.[12]

COMPLICATIONS

Disability is a difficult issue in FMS, since it is often difficult to document or receive compensation. Other complications include depression, insomnia, muscle atrophy, misdiagnosis, and drug-seeking behavior.

INDICATIONS FOR REFERRAL OR HOSPITALIZATION

FMS patients should be managed in primary care, where there is a partnership and willingness for creativity in treatment plans, perhaps including alternative treatments. Pain management clinics for pain control and transcutaneous electrical nerve stimulation (TENS) units have been effective for chronic pain. Psychologists, physiologists, physical therapists, and chiropractors may aid in symptom control. Hospital admissions are not required.

PATIENT AND FAMILY EDUCATION

Education is imperative for improved patient understanding of fibromyalgia and the development of individual strategies to cope with the pain, fatigue, and chronic nature of the syndrome. The importance of regular exercise and adequate rest should be emphasized. Family members are affected and should be involved in education to understand the disorder and to maximize support for these patients. Support groups can be invaluable. Information abounds on the Internet, so careful evaluation is required. Available resources include:

Arthritis Foundation
1330 West Peachtree St., Suite 100
Atlanta, GA 30309
(404) 872-7100
http://www.arthritis.org

National Institute of Arthritis and Musculoskeletal and Skin Diseases
National Institutes of Health
http://www.niams.nih.gov

Fibromyalgia Network
PO Box 31750
Tucson, AZ 85751
(800) 853-2929
http://www.fmnetnews.com

HEALTH PROMOTION

FMS is a syndrome that requires empowering patients with the tools needed for improving activities of daily living. Healthy diet, weight control, support systems, stress reduction through meditation or counseling, and improved self-esteem are all within the patient's control.

REFERENCES

1. Wolfe F: The fibromyalgia problem (editorial), *J Rheumatol* 24(7):1247-1249, 1997.
2. Wolfe F, Ross K, Anderson J, and others: The prevalence and characteristics of fibromyalgia in the general population, *Arthritis Rheum* 38(1):19-28, 1995.
3. Chen H: Contemporary management of neuropathic pain for the primary care physician, *Mayo Clin Proc* 79:1533-1545, 2004.
4. Landis CA, Lentz MJ, Rothermel J, and others: Decreased nocturnal levels of prolactin and growth hormone in women with fibromyalgia, *J Clin Endocrinol Metab* 86(4):1672-1678, 2001.
5. Millea P: Treating fibromyalgia, *Am Fam Phys* 62(7):1572-1582, 1587, 2000.
6. Wolfe F, Smythe HA, Yunus MB, and others: The American College of Rheumatology 1990 criteria for the classification of fibromyalgia: report of the Multicenter Criteria Committee, *Arthritis Rheum* 33(2):160-172, 1990.
7. Winfield J: Pain management in the rheumatic diseases, *Rheum Dis Clin North Am* 25:55-79, 1999.
8. Bennett R, Nelson D: Cognitive behavioral therapy for fibromyalgia, *Nature Clin Pract Rheumatol* 2(8):416-424, 2006.
9. Littlejohn GO: Balanced treatments for fibromyalgia, *Arthritis Rheum* 50:2725-2729, 2004.
10. Goldenberg DL: Management of fibromyalgia syndrome, *JAMA* 292:2388-2395, 2004.
11. Karper WB, Hopewell R, Hodge M: Exercise program effects on one woman with dermatomyositis, *Rehabil Nurs* 26(4):129-131, 158-159, 2001.
12. Berman B: The evidence for acupuncture as a treatment for rheumatologic conditions, *Rheum Dis Clin North Am* 26(1):103-115, 2000.
13. Bennett R: Multidisciplinary group programs to treat fibromyalgia patients, *Rheum Dis Clin North Am* 22(2):351-367, 1996.

CHAPTER 187

Gout

Naomi Schlesinger

DEFINITION

Gout is a systemic metabolic disease. Gout has been considered through the centuries as a disease of the wealthy, associated with rich food and wine. Humans do not express the enzyme urate oxidase (uricase) because of a mutation of the uricase gene during evolution, which converts urate to the more soluble and easily excreted compound allantoin. This may lead to hyperuricemia. Hyperuricemia has four clinical stages[1]: asymptomatic hyperuricemia, acute gouty arthritis, intercritical gout (intervals between acute attacks), and chronic tophaceous gout. Inflammatory arthritis in patients with gout is caused by crystals of monosodium urate (MSU) that form as a result of chronically elevated levels of urate in plasma and extracellular fluids. Gout is a common disease affecting more than 1% of the population. The incidence is rising worldwide in both men over 40 and older women.[2]

The asymptomatic hyperuricemia stage is when the patient has elevated levels of serum urate (SU), but no previous episode of an acute flare or other clinical indication of the disease. During this phase, however, MSU crystals may "silently" deposit in the tissues and joints and result in "hidden damage," which can occasionally occur over time even in the absence of clinical gout. Often hyperuricemia is present for prolonged periods in the absence of clinical signs of gout. Acute flares occur as a result of the deposition of urate crystals and activation of an inflammatory response. This causes symptoms such as inflammation and intense pain. Over time, or with the help of agents to terminate the acute flare, the flare will subside. At that point, even though the patient is not experiencing a flare, he or she is still considered to have gout and is in the intercritical stage until another flare occurs. Uncontrolled hyperuricemia and resultant gout can eventually evolve into the advanced stage of the disease: chronic tophaceous gout.

The serum uric acid (SU) level is the single most important risk factor for developing gout.[3] The SU level is elevated when it exceeds 6.8 mg/dl, the limit of solubility of MSU in serum at 37° C (98.6° F). It is important to note that a sustained elevation of SU is virtually essential for the development of gout but by itself is insufficient to cause the disease.

The risk of damage beyond the musculoskeletal system from protracted hyperuricemia or recurrent attacks of gout is small. Urolithiasis is uncommon, with the annual incidence being approximately 1% in gout and 0.3% in otherwise asymptomatic hyperuricemia.

EPIDEMIOLOGY

Incidence

Little data exist on the incidence of gout. It is difficult to accurately measure incidence and prevalence of a disease that is episodic and recurrent. In Sudbury, Massachusetts, the estimated annual incidence of gout in the 1960s was 1 in 1000.[4] Campion, Glynn, and DeLabry, using data from the Normative Aging Study, prospectively studied the incidence of gouty arthritis in relation to SU level.[3] More than 2000 healthy men born between 1884 and 1945 were included in this study and followed for a mean of 14.9 years. When SU levels were greater than 9 mg/dl, the annual incidence of gout was 4.9% and the cumulative incidence of the first gouty attack was 22% in 5 years. For those with SU levels of 7 to 8.9 mg/dl, the cumulative incidence was 3% at 5 years.

Prevalence

Gouty arthritis is the most common inflammatory arthritis in men over 40.[2] The National Health Interview Survey (NHIS) from 1983 to 1985 determined the prevalence rate of self-reported gout to be 13.6 cases per 1000 men and 6.4 cases per 1000 women, but the more recent NHIS data suggest the combined prevalence for both men and women to be 8.4 cases per 1000.[5]

The prevalence of gout in different geographic regions has been well documented. The results suggest that environmental, racial, and hereditary differences may influence the development of gout. It has recently become clear that gout is most common in the spring.[6] The seasonal variation in acute gout attacks is remarkably similar around the world, in geographic areas that differ widely and over many years.[6]

PATHOPHYSIOLOGY

Uricase, an end product of purine metabolism, is an enzyme that converts uric acid to allantoin and is lacking in humans. The solubility of MSU is a direct function of temperature. At 37° C (98.6° F) the maximum solubility of urate in physiologic saline is 6.8 mg/dl, but at 30° C (86° F) it is only 4.5 mg/dl. If SU concentration is increased for a sustained period, MSU will come out of solution to form crystals. Microtophi will subsequently form, particularly in the cooler parts of the body such as distal extremities, olecranon bursa, and ears. Sustained hyperuricemia is a risk factor for acute gouty arthritis, tophaceous gout, and uric acid nephrolithiasis. However, most patients with hyperuricemia will never have an attack of gout, and no treatment is required, although it is prudent to determine the cause of hyperuricemia and correct it if possible.

Uric acid production is increased in males after puberty and in females after menopause. The predominant cause of hyperuricemia in most patients is undersecretion of urate by the kidneys. Lower clearance of urate is seen in all gout patients compared with normal controls.[7]

CLINICAL PRESENTATION

Acute gouty arthritis is characterized by rapid onset and build-up of pain. The first attack often begins at night and wakes the patient up from sleep. During an acute gouty attack the patient endures exquisite pain associated with warmth, redness, swelling, and decreased range of motion of the affected joint. The initial episode is usually monoarticular. The first metatarsophalangeal joint is the initial one involved in approximately half the patients. Acute synovitis of the first metatarsophalangeal joint of the big toe is referred to as *podagra*. Other joints involved (in decreasing order of frequency) are insteps, heels, knees, wrists, fingers, and elbows.[8]

In his classic description of the onset of an acute gouty attack, Thomas Sydenham, London, 1683, a long-time sufferer from gout, writes: "The victim goes to bed and sleeps quietly. About two in the morning he is awakened by a pain in the great toe; rarely in the heel, ankle or instep. The pain resembles that of a dislocated bone.... [It] becomes so exquisitely painful as not to endure the weight of clothes nor the shaking of the room by a person walking in."[9]

Systemic symptoms and signs of fatigue, fever, and chills may accompany the acute arthritis. The natural course of untreated gouty arthritis varies from episodes that last several hours to several weeks.

Chronic tophaceous gout usually develops after 10 or more years of acute intermittent gout, although rarely patients are seen with tophi as their initial manifestation of the disease. In transplant patients tophi are more common and may occur within 5 years or less of renal transplantation.[10] Tophi appear as firm swellings. They may appear at any site. Most common sites for the tophi to appear are digits of the hands and feet and in the olecranon bursa. Tophi of the helix or antihelix of the ear are classic but less common. Tophi may be associated with a destructive deforming arthritis and may ulcerate, in which case secondary infection may be a problem.

Acute flares of gout occur more often in the presence of precipitating factors, but also may occur when these factors are not present. Local trauma and binges of alcohol, overeating, or fasting have been implicated as factors that precipitate an acute flare. In the hospital setting, acute flares of gout often occur postoperatively or are associated with severe acute medical illnesses. Changes in the SU levels in the body also can precipitate a disease flare because homeostatic mechanisms mobilize the deposited crystals. This is commonly seen in patients newly initiated on urate-lowering therapy and can be mitigated by slowly titrating the dose upward and adding concomitant prophylactic therapy such as NSAIDs or colchicines.[11] Finally, seasonal factors, such as increased attacks of gout in the spring, have been noted to relate to acute flares.[6]

DIAGNOSIS

During the 1960s McCarty and Hollander described the currently accepted method for establishing a definitive diagnosis of gout: needle aspiration of the acutely inflamed joint or suspected tophus[12] (Color Plate 39). Even when clinical appearance strongly suggests gout, diagnosis has to be confirmed by needle aspiration.[13] MSU crystals can be observed in more than 95% of patients experiencing attacks of acute gouty arthritis.[14] In some asymptomatic patients, MSU crystals are also detected in joints in which there is no inflammation,[15,16] and this is also believed to confirm the diagnosis.

In 1977 the American College of Rheumatology published criteria for the classification of gout for use in either clinical settings or population-based epidemiologic studies.[17] One needs 6 out of 13 minor criteria, or 1 major criterion (MSU crystals in synovial fluid or tophus) to make the diagnosis of gout by these preliminary criteria (Box 187-1).

BOX 187-1

1977 CRITERIA FOR CLASSIFICATION OF ACUTE ARTHRITIS OF PRIMARY GOUT

1. More than one attack of acute arthritis
2. Maximum inflammation developed within 1 day
3. Monoarthritis attack
4. Redness observed over joints
5. First metatarsophalangeal joint painful or swollen
6. Unilateral first metatarsophalangeal joint attack
7. Unilateral tarsal joint attack
8. Tophus (proven or suspected)
9. Hyperuricemia
10. Asymmetric swelling within a joint on x-ray
11. Subcortical cysts without erosions on x-ray
12. Monosodium urate monohydrate crystals in joint fluid during attack
13. Joint fluid culture negative for organisms during attack

One needs 6 out of 13 minor criteria or 1 major criterion (MSU crystals in synovial fluid or tophus) to make the diagnosis of gout by these preliminary criteria.

From Wallace SL, Robinson H, Masi AT, and others: Preliminary criteria for the classification of the acute arthritis of primary gout, *Arthritis Rheum* 20(3):895-900, 1977.

Demonstrating the presence of MSU crystals in the joint fluid or tophus is still the definitive standard for the diagnosis of gout today. Supportive data necessary for the diagnosis of gout include a typical clinical history of a sudden and severe exquisitely painful joint, most classically in the first metatarsophalangeal joint (toe) that may wake the patient up. The patient may have renal disease or be on medications that can elevate SU. Other data that can support the acute arthritis being a gouty flare include an elevated SU, radiologic evidence of punched out erosions on plain x-ray studies, and a favorable response to treatment with colchicine or an NSAID (e.g., indomethacin [Indocin]) and topical ice.

DIFFERENTIAL DIAGNOSIS

Difficulties in the clinical diagnosis of gout occur because the disease can be polyarticular and chronic, especially in the elderly. Atypical joint involvement can also occur, such as Heberden's nodes, especially in women. It can cause diagnostic confusion with rheumatoid arthritis. However, gouty arthritis tends to be less symmetric than typical rheumatoid arthritis. Tophi sometimes tend to be confused with rheumatoid nodules, and therefore, when in doubt, needle aspiration should be done to look for MSU crystals.

It is sometimes difficult to determine whether the patient with acute arthritis has gout or pseudogout. Calcium pyrophosphate dihydrate (CPPD) deposition disease has two main forms. One is chronic arthritis, and the other is known as *pseudogout* because its clinical presentation of an acute arthritic attack, taking place in one or a few joints, is similar to the gout presentation. Almost half of acute attacks of CPPD crystal deposition disease affect the knees, but the wrists, metacarpophalangeal joints, elbows, and shoulders may be involved. However, under compensated polarized light, the difference between the two types of crystals is evident and the correct diagnosis can be made. The CPPD crystals are rhomboid shaped and have weakly positive birefringence.

MANAGEMENT

There are three stages in the management of gout: (1) treating the acute attack, (2) lowering excess stores of uric acid to prevent flares of gouty arthritis and to prevent tissue deposition of urate, and (3) providing antiinflammatory prophylaxis to prevent acute flares. Current treatments for both acute and chronic gout are based more on practitioners' experience than on evidence-based medicine.[1]

Nonpharmacologic Management

Gout is a metabolic disorder. It is influenced by dietary factors (including overeating, obesity, alcohol abuse, and hyperlipidemia) and insulin resistance syndrome. Avoiding factors that may contribute to the development of gout among asymptomatic hyperuricemic patients may reduce gouty attacks. Avoiding diuretics, weight gain, and alcohol consumption may lead to a decrease in the number of gouty arthritis attacks and its prevalence.

The main approaches to dietary measures in gout are the traditional low-purine, low-protein, alcohol-restricted diet, as opposed to a diet focused on weight reduction with unlimited purines, limited calories, and restricted carbohydrates but increased proportional intake of protein and unsaturated fat. In an observational study monitoring gouty patients on a diet moderately decreased in calories and increased in protein, the mean SU decreased by 18% after 4 months of dietary intervention.[18] This was accompanied by a 67% reduction in monthly gouty attack frequency. The authors advocate limitation of carbohydrate intake, an increased proportional intake of protein, and the use of unsaturated fat, since they all enhance insulin sensitivity and therefore may promote a reduction in SU.

An alcohol-restricted diet in gouty patients is of importance because alcohol consumption is closely associated with hyperuricemia and gout. It is estimated that half of gout sufferers drink excessively.[19]

Joint motion may increase inflammation because of gouty arthritis, whereas rest of affected joints may aid in its resolution.[20] Less medication is needed if the patient can rest the afflicted joint for 1 or 2 days.[21] Cold applications may also be a useful adjunct to treatment of acute gouty arthritis.[22]

Pharmacologic Management

Treatment of Acute Gout. The options available for the treatment of acute gouty attacks are NSAIDs, colchicine, corticosteroids, adrenocorticotropic hormone (ACTH), and intraarticular corticosteroids. In a patient without complications, NSAIDs are the preferred therapy (Box 187-2).

The most important determinant of therapeutic success is not which NSAID is chosen, but rather how soon NSAID therapy is initiated. In more than 90% of patients, the attack completely resolves within 5 to 8 days of initiation of therapy. Unfortunately, the use of NSAIDs is limited by side effects. NSAID therapy should be avoided in patients with peptic ulcer disease, low creatinine clearance, liver disease, and poorly compensated congestive heart failure and in patients receiving anticoagulation therapy. Side effects of NSAIDs are also more pronounced in elderly patients.

BOX 187-2

TREATMENT OF ACUTE GOUT

- Ideally, confirm diagnosis by joint aspiration: intracellular monosodium urate crystals in synovial fluid. (This can be difficult in the primary care setting, especially where access to rheumatologists is limited or nonexistent.)
- Initial treatment is with NSAIDs, unless there are risk factors for their use: age over 65 years (relative risk), creatinine clearance less than 50 ml/min, poorly controlled congestive heart failure, history of or active peptic ulcer disease, anticoagulant therapy, or hepatic dysfunction. NSAIDs should be used early in the attack. Higher doses need to be used in first 24 to 48 hours. It does not matter which NSAID is used.
- If one or two joints are involved, intraarticular corticosteroid treatment maybe beneficial.
- In severe oligoarticular or polyarticular gouty attack or when NSAIDs are not tolerated or are contraindicated, use systemic corticosteroids (7 to 14 day taper). Parenteral, intramuscular, or IV (corticosteroids or adrenocorticotropic hormone) medications may be helpful, especially in patients with renal failure.
- Oral colchicine should be used within 24 to 48 hours of onset of an acute attack. Colchicine should be used cautiously because of its toxicity. IV colchicine should probably not be used for treatment of acute gout.
- Do not treat hyperuricemia during the acute attack.

Colchicine is the classic medication for gout but has the smallest benefit-to-toxicity ratio of the drugs that are used in the management of gout.[23] It is most effective during the first 12 to 24 hours of an attack, and its effectiveness declines with the duration of inflammation. Colchicine should not be used if the glomerular filtration rate (GFR) is less than 10 ml/min, and the dose should be decreased by at least half if the GFR is less than 50 ml/min. Colchicine also should be avoided in patients with hepatic dysfunction, biliary obstruction, or an inability to tolerate diarrhea.

A clinical response to colchicine is not pathognomonic for gout; it can also be seen with pseudogout, sarcoid arthropathy, psoriatic arthritis, and calcific tendinitis.

Intraarticular corticosteroids are currently accepted as beneficial when only one or two joints are actively inflamed.[24] Patients with polyarticular gout who demonstrate suboptimum or delayed response to oral NSAIDs or who have contraindications to usual NSAIDs may also benefit from adjunctive corticosteroid injections into joints with persistent synovitis.[25] Ensuring that the joint is not infected before injecting intraarticular corticosteroids is particularly important.

Corticosteroids can be given to those patients who cannot use NSAIDs or colchicine. Steroids can be given orally, intravenously, intramuscularly, intraarticularly, or indirectly via ACTH. Prednisone can be given at a dose of approximately 30 mg for 1 to 3 days and then tapered over 1 to 2 weeks. Tapering more rapidly can result in a rebound flare. Using parenteral corticosteroids confers no advantage unless the patient cannot take oral medications.

Randomized long-term prospective, placebo-controlled trials are needed to evaluate the therapeutic role of colchicine vs. NSAIDs as well as that of corticosteroids and ACTH in the treatment of acute gout.

Treatment of Chronic Gout. Long-term control of hyperuricemia to prevent gouty attacks and sequelae of longstanding hyperuricemia such as chronic tophaceous gout, urate nephropathy, and uric acid stones is important. Optimum treatment requires longstanding reduction in SU (Box 187-3). Maintaining the SU level at less than 6 mg/dl and not just within the "normal range" helps to ensure resolution of tophi and eventual cessation of acute gouty attacks.

The evidence on when to start urate-lowering drugs is conflicting. Because the initial attacks of gout are infrequent, self-limiting, and easily treated, chronic therapy is many times not indicated. Cost-effectiveness of urate-lowering therapy has been studied, with the conclusion that therapy is cost saving in patients who have two or more attacks a year.[26]

In all cases, the risks and benefits need to be judged based on the individual patient. For instance, in an elderly patient with multiple medical problems and renal insufficiency, the risks of therapy to lower uric acid levels may outweigh the benefits.

Urate-lowering drugs should not be started during an acute attack, since it could lead to a more intense and prolonged attack. Typically, they should be started 6 to 8 weeks after the attack has resolved.

Urate-lowering drugs include the uricostatic drugs, which are xanthine oxidase inhibitors that decrease UA synthesis and include allopurinol, febuxostat (investigational), and oxypurinol (investigational); the uricosuric drugs that inhibit UA reabsorption in the proximal tubule, which include probenecid, sulfinpyrazone (not available in the United States), and benzobromarone (not available in the United States); losartan and fenofibrate, which have a small uricosuric effect; and the uricolytic drugs, such as uricase (investigational), which catalyzes conversion of UA into allantoin.

Allopurinol is the most commonly prescribed urate-lowering agent, primarily because of its once a day dosing and its great efficacy.[27] It can be given in a single morning dose of 300 mg initially and increased to 800 mg if needed. Dosage adjustments are necessary in patients with impaired creatinine clearance; in patients with renal failure the initial dosage would be 50 to 100 mg every day or every other day. (The final dosage in a patient with a creatinine level of 2 mg/dl will be half of the dosage given a patient with normal renal function.[28,29])

Probenecid is the most widely used uricosuric agent available in the United States. The maintenance dosage of probenecid ranges from 500 mg to 3 g/day, administered b.i.d. or t.i.d.

Febuxostat, which is in development, may become a leading choice of xanthine oxidase inhibitors. Uricosuric drugs such as probenecid are the urate-lowering drugs of choice in allopurinol-allergic patients, underexcretors with normal renal function, and patients with no history of urolithiasis. Recombinant uricase's use in patients with chronic gout is limited by the need for parenteral administration, potential antigenicity, and production of antiuricase antibodies and declining efficacy.

BOX 187-3

TREATMENT OF CHRONIC GOUT

- Start urate-lowering drugs only in patients who have two or more attacks a year.
- Urate-lowering drugs should not be started during an acute attack.
- Uricosuric drugs are the urate-lowering drugs of choice in allopurinol-allergic patients, underexcretors with normal renal function, and patients with no history of urolithiasis.
- Use allopurinol in patients with renal calculi, renal insufficiency, concomitant diuretic therapy, cyclosporine therapy, or urate overproduction.
- Use concomitant colchicine prophylaxis until uric acid has been at desired level for some months and no recent gouty attacks have occurred (6 to 12 months).
- Monitor serum urate (SU) and aim for uric acid <6 mg/dl. Check SU every 3 to 6 months and adjust the urate-lowering drug dose accordingly.

Prophylaxis

Prophylactic treatment is not recommended unless one is also prescribing a urate-lowering agent. Prophylactic use of colchicine or an NSAID may block the acute inflammatory response but will not alter crystal deposition. With continued deposition, but without the warning signs of recurrent bouts of acute arthritis, tophi will develop, and joint tissue destruction can advance without notice.

Small daily doses of colchicine or an NSAID can be used effectively to prevent acute attacks of gout,[30,31] but maintaining SU below 6 mg/dl is what ultimately decreases the incidence of gouty attacks.

If a patient with tophaceous gout is given an initial prescription for a urate-lowering medication and lacks both significant renal impairment (a serum creatinine level ≥2 mg/dl or measured/estimated creatinine clearance ≤50 ml/min) and peptic ulcer disease, then a prophylactic antiinflammatory agent (colchicine or NSAID) should be given concomitantly because prophylactic antiinflammatory therapy may reduce the risk of rebound gout attacks, which frequently follow the initiation of urate-lowering therapy.

Prophylaxis usually is continued until the SU value has been maintained at less than 6 mg/dl and not just within the normal range and there have been no acute attacks for 3 to 6 months. It is important to warn patients that discontinuation of the prophylactic medication may be followed by an exacerbation of acute gouty arthritis and advise them what to do should that occur.

COMPLICATIONS

The main extraarticular complications of gout are renal complications. These include nephrolithiasis and gouty nephropathy.

Nephrolithiasis occurs in approximately 10% to 25% of patients with primary gout.[32] The solubility of uric acid crystals increases as the urine pH becomes more alkaline. Acidic urine saturated with uric acid crystals may result in spontaneous stone formation. Other types of stones may also develop, since uric acid can act as a nidus for calcium oxalate or phosphate stones.

Long-term deposition of crystals in the renal parenchyma can cause chronic urate nephropathy. The formation of microtophi causes a giant cell inflammatory reaction. This results in proteinuria and inability of the kidney to concentrate urine.

Other complications may be related to gouty arthritis therapy. The two main medications leading to complications are colchicine and allopurinol. Severe side effects of colchicine include bone marrow suppression, renal failure, alopecia, disseminated intravascular coagulation, hepatic necrosis, diarrhea, seizures, arrhythmias leading to complete heart block, and death. Neuromuscular toxicity related to colchicine therapy is also a well-recognized complication. Acute rhabdomyolysis with myoglobinuria and renal failure is most commonly seen in individuals concomitantly taking an HMG-CoA reductase inhibitor (statin) or cyclosporine.

About 20% of patients who take allopurinol report side effects, with 5% of patients discontinuing the medication. More common side effects include gastrointestinal intolerance and skin rashes. Other adverse reactions include fever, toxic epidermal necrolysis, alopecia, bone marrow suppression with leukopenia or thrombocytopenia, agranulocytosis, aplastic anemia, granulomatous hepatitis, jaundice, sarcoid-like reaction, and vasculitis. The most severe reaction is the allopurinol hypersensitivity syndrome, which consists of a constellation of findings that may include fever, skin rash, eosinophilia, hepatitis, progressive renal insufficiency, and death. This is most likely to develop in individuals with preexisting renal dysfunction and those taking diuretics.

INDICATIONS FOR REFERRAL OR HOSPITALIZATION

The rheumatologist should be consulted to establish a diagnosis of gout by joint aspiration and crystal identification; if the treatment is effective but drug toxicity or intolerance occurs, a rheumatology consultation is warranted as well. This could occur if the patient is still having attacks of gout on the maximum tolerated treatment, the diagnosis is in doubt, or the patient is unable to use or tolerate his or her medication.

Hospitalization is rarely necessary unless there is confirmed or suspected bacterial arthritis in a patient suspected of having gout; a severe drug reaction occurs (such as allopurinol hypersensitivity); or drug therapy worsens a co-morbidity the patient suffers from (e.g., such as when a patient with diabetes mellitus is given corticosteroids and blood glucose levels are hard to control).

PATIENT AND FAMILY EDUCATION

Health care providers should educate patients with gout and their families on the following points:

- Gout can be accurately diagnosed by identifying the characteristic crystals.
- There are three types of treatment for gout: medications to control the attacks of joint pain (e.g., NSAIDs, colchicine, and corticosteroids); medications for prophylaxis to prevent further attacks (e.g., colchicine and NSAIDs); and medications that will help lower the level of uric acid in the body over time so the attacks occur less frequently or not at all.
- People with chronic gout often require lifetime treatment with drugs to lower the uric acid body pool.
- Lifestyle changes, such as controlling weight, limiting alcohol consumption, and limiting meals with meats and fish rich in purines, are helpful in controlling gout.

The following websites may also be helpful:

American College of Rheumatology, http://www.rheumatology.org/public/factsheets/gout_new.asp?aud=pat

Arthritis Foundation, http://www.arthritis.org

National Institute of Arthritis and Musculoskeletal and Skin Diseases, http://www.niams.nih.gov

REFERENCES

1. Schlesinger N: Management of acute and chronic gouty arthritis: present state-of-the-art, *Drugs* 64:2399-2416, 2004.
2. Choi HK, Curhan G: Gout: epidemiology and lifestyle choices, *Curr Opin Rheumatol* 17(3):341-345, 2005.
3. Campion EW, Glynn RJ, DeLabry LO: Asymptomatic hyperuricemia: risks and consequences in the Normative Aging Study, *Am J Med* 82:421-426, 1987.
4. Wernick R, Winkler C, Campbell S: Tophi as the initial manifestation of gout: report of six cases and review of the literature, *Arch Intern Med* 152:873-876, 1992.
5. Lawrence RC, Helmick CG, Arnett FC, and others: Estimates of the prevalence of selected arthritis and selected musculoskeletal disorders in the United States, *Arthritis Rheum* 41(9):778-799, 1998.
6. Schlesinger N, Gowin KM, Baker DG, and others: Acute gouty arthritis is seasonal, *J Rheumatol* 25(2):342-344, 1998.
7. Perez-Ruiz F, Calabozo M, Erauskin GG, and others: Renal underexcretion of uric acid is present in patients with apparent high urinary uric acid output, *Arthritis Rheum* 47(6):610-613, 2002.
8. Grahame R, Scott JT: Clinical survey of 354 patients with gout, *Ann Rheum Dis* 29:461, 1970.
9. Weede RP: *Poison in the pot: the legacy of lead*, Carbondale, Ill, 1984, Southern Illinois University Press.
10. Bacethge BA, Work J, Landreneau MD, and others: Tophaceous gout in patients with renal transplantation treated with cyclosporine A, *J Rheumatol* 20:718-720, 1993.
11. Schlesinger N, Baker DG, Schumacher HR: Gout: how well have diagnostic tests and therapies been evaluated? *Curr Opin Orthoped* 11:71-76, 2000.
12. McCarty DJ, Hollander JL: Identification of urate crystals in gouty synovial fluid, *Ann Intern Med* 54:452-460, 1961.
13. Lally EV, Zimmerman B, Ho G, and others: Urate mediated inflammation in nodal arthritis: clinical and roentgenographic correlations, *Arthritis Rheum* 32:86-90, 1989.
14. Reginato AJ, Schumacher HR: Crystal associated arthropathies, *Clin Geriatr Med* 4:295-322, 1988.
15. Weinberger A, Schumacher HR, Agudelo CA: Urate crystals in asymptomatic metatarsophalangeal joints, *Ann Intern Med* 92:56-57, 1979.
16. Bomalaski JS, Lluberas G, Schumacher HR: Monosodium urate crystals in the knee joints of patients with asymptomatic non-tophaceous gout, *Arthritis Rheum* 29:1480-1484, 1986.
17. Wallace SL, Robinson H, Masi AT, and others: Preliminary criteria for the classification of the acute arthritis of primary gout, *Arthritis Rheum* 20(3):895-900, 1977.
18. Dessein PH, Shipton AE, Stanwix AE, and others: Beneficial effects of weight loss associated with moderate calorie/carbohydrate restriction, and increased proportional intake of protein and unsaturated fat on serum and lipoprotein levels in gout: a pilot study, *Ann Rheum Dis* 59:539-543, 2000.
19. Sharpe CR: A case-controlled study of alcohol consumption and drinking behaviour in patients with acute gout, *Can Med Assoc J* 131:563-567, 1984.
20. Agudelo CA, Schumacher HR, Phelps P: Effect of exercise on urate crystal–induced inflammation in canine joints, *Arthritis Rheum* 15:609-616, 1972.

21. Schumacher HR: Crystal induced arthritis: an overview, *Am J Med* 100(Suppl 2A):46-52, 1996.
22. Schlesinger N, Baker DG, Beutler AM, and others: Local ice therapy during bouts of acute gouty arthritis, *J Rheumatol* 29:331-334, 2002.
23. Paulus HE, Schlosstein LH, Godfrey RC, and others: Prophylactic colchicine therapy in intercritical gout, *Arthritis Rheum* 17:609-614, 1987.
24. Gordon GV, Schumacher HR: Management of gout, *Am Fam Phys* 10:62-66, 1969.
25. Gray RG, Tenenbaum J, Gottlieb NL: Local corticosteroid injection treatment in rheumatic disorders, *Semin Arthritis Rheum* 10:231-254, 1979.
26. Emmerson BT: The management of gout, *N Engl J Med* 334:455-551, 1996.
27. Schumacher HR, Moreno Alvarez JM: Clues to common crystal induced arthropathies, *IM* 14:35-47, 1993.
28. Singer JZ, Wallace SL: The allopurinol hypersensitivity syndrome: unnecessary morbidity and mortality, *Arthritis Rheum* 29:82-87, 1986.
29. Hande KR, Noone RM, Stone WJ: Severe allopurinol toxicity: description and guidelines for prevention in patients with renal insufficiency, *Am J Med* 76(1):47-56, 1984.
30. Cheng TT, Lai HM, Chiu CK, and others: A single-blind, randomized, controlled trial to assess the efficacy and tolerability of rofecoxib, diclofenac sodium, and meloxicam in patients with acute gouty arthritis, *Clin Ther* 20:399-406, 2004.
31. Winkler Prins VJ, Weismantel AM: How effective is prophylactic therapy for gout in people with prior attacks? *J Fam Pract* 53(10):837-838, 2004.
32. Yu TF: Nephrolithiasis in patients with gout, *Postgrad Med* 63:164-170, 1978.

CHAPTER 188

Hand and Wrist Pain

Karin C. Dieselman

DEFINITION AND EPIDEMIOLOGY

Hand disorders may result from recreational or work-related activities or inflammatory or degenerative disease. Fractures, strains and sprains, and arthritis of the hands and fingers are problems commonly seen in primary care (see Chapter 199). Job specialization, repetitive tasks, and workplace demographics have contributed to an increased incidence of cumulative hand and wrist injuries. In 1992, 60% of new work-related disorders were associated with repetitive movement.[1,2] These injuries, which are also known as cumulative trauma disorders (CTDs), account for 56% of occupational injuries and are defined as muscle, tendon, osseous, or neurologic conditions produced or exacerbated by repetitive movements.[3] A study of workers' compensation claims in Washington state from 1987 to 1995 demonstrated an incidence rate of hand and wrist disorders of 98.2 cases per 10,000.[4] Many other factors, including sports activities, age, and various medical conditions, contribute to the development of hand and wrist pain.

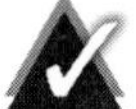

Immediate orthopedic referral is indicated if the finger cannot be passively extended (trigger finger).

PATHOPHYSIOLOGY

CTDs usually result from microtrauma that, over time, affects the tendons, tendon sheaths, and connective tissues. The exact pathologic mechanism is not clearly understood.[1,5] In the past, it was thought that overuse syndromes represented an inflammatory process, but more recent studies have shown no identifiable inflammation or tissue damage.[1,6] Sports injuries of the hand and wrist are common, including injuries to the palm from swinging a baseball bat or golf club or injury to the thumb from the strap of a ski pole. Other causes of hand and wrist pain include trauma and fracture, which can lead to avascular necrosis, especially of the scaphoid and hamate bones, and arthritis, both inflammatory and degenerative.[4] Patients with diabetes and pregnant women have a higher incidence of carpal tunnel syndrome (CTS).

CLINICAL PRESENTATION

Localized pain, numbness, tingling, weakness, and immobility are the common reasons that patients with hand or wrist disorders seek care.[7] The symptoms may be intermittent or constant and often affect quality of life. The diagnosis of any hand or wrist disorder is facilitated by a comprehensive medical, recreational, and occupational history. The precise anatomic location of the problem, as well as onset, quality, intensity, radiation, evolution, and exacerbating and relieving factors, should be documented. It is usually helpful to have the patient draw a hand diagram and document the areas of numbness, tingling, pain, or sensory loss. The history should include work environment, job tasks, dominant hand, history of injury, co-morbid illnesses, recreational activities, hobbies, allergies, and current medication use. If the patient is a woman of childbearing age, the date of the last menstrual period should be noted.

Trigger finger, or stenosing tenosynovitis, is a disorder of the flexor tendons of the fingers or thumb. This condition, which may be more prevalent in patients with diabetes, occurs when a nodule or thickening in the tendon catches on the edge of the tendon sheath as the tendon attempts to glide during movement. This thickening narrows the fibro-osseous canal, which impedes tendon movement. The pulley action is impaired, causing a painful locking or triggering of the affected digit or thumb during extension. Although any digit may be affected, the middle or ring finger is most commonly involved.

Chronic stenosing tenosynovitis of the wrist, or de Quervain's disease, is typically encountered in occupations that require repetitive wrist and thumb movements. Initially the patient may describe a catching sensation as thumb extension is attempted after flexion. As the condition progresses, the thumb may become locked in flexion.

Dupuytren's contracture, or palmar fibrosis, may be a hereditary process that initially develops as a painless nodule on the palmar fascia at the base of a digit. An inflammatory fibrosis subsequently expands into a bandlike cord under puckered skin and causes a flexion contracture. Although any finger (and both hands) may be affected, the resultant contracture most often affects the ring finger. The little finger may also be involved.

CTS is one of many nerve entrapment neuropathies and results from compression of the median nerve in the carpal tunnel of the wrist. An opening under the carpal ligament on the palmar side of the carpal bones, the carpal tunnel is the passageway for the nine digital flexor tendons, blood vessels, and the median nerve of the hand. Pregnancy, menopause, arthritis, diabetes, hypertension, hypothyroidism, trauma, and a history of occupational or sports-related activities are some of the conditions that affect these structures and result in nerve entrapment. The tendons swell with overuse, which decreases the cross-sectional area in the tunnel. Synovial fluid increases to decrease friction, but the resultant pressure in the small tunnel causes pressure on the median nerve. Conduction is impeded, muscle strength is decreased because of the disturbance in motor fibers, and pain and paresthesia occur because of the disturbance in the sensory fibers.[8]

Intermittent wrist pain with numbness and tingling that radiates from the palm to the thumb, index finger, middle finger, or ring finger are common presenting complaints of CTS. Additionally, the patient may awaken during the night with numbness, may complain of pain and tightness at the wrist and forearm that increases with activity, and may describe an inability to hold objects or a tendency to drop things. If the compression continues, the motor component of the median nerve is affected, and the ability to grasp with the thumb and index finger may be lost.

Cubital tunnel syndrome is a nerve entrapment neuropathy that results from ulnar nerve compression below the notch of the elbow. Pain that radiates from the elbow to the ring or little finger, numbness, and tingling are characteristics of this syndrome. A diminished grasp indicates motor dysfunction (see Chapter 185).

Trapeziometacarpal arthritis is a common site of arthritis in women. Common complaints include pain at the base of the thumb and weakness and pain with pinching. Arthritis in this area can also be seen with osteoarthritis of the distal interphalangeal (DIP) and proximal interphalangeal (PIP) joints, referred to as Heberden's (DIP) and Bouchard's (PIP) nodes (see Chapter 194).

PHYSICAL EXAMINATION

Muscle wasting, arm shortening, edema, point tenderness, deformity, pulses, and skin color and temperature should be noted when examining patients with hand or wrist pain. Passive and active range of motion, muscle strength, and sensory and motor testing are also necessary. Additional specific tests may be indicated. Physical findings seen in common causes of hand and wrist pain include the following.

Trigger Finger

The PIP joint of the affected finger or thumb is flexed at 90 degrees. The digit can usually be extended, but there may be considerable pain with extension. With trigger thumb, resisted thumb extension can exacerbate the pain over the affected tendons. The nodule may be palpable.

Tenosynovitis

On inspection, there may be a palpable nodule at the base of the thumb. Edema and tenderness may be present over the radial stylus. A positive Finklestein's test is confirmed if pain over the radial stylus is reproduced when the patient folds the thumb across the palm, flexes the fingers over the thumb, and then the clinician deviates the hand in the direction of the ulna. Grip and pinch strength should also be assessed.

Palmar Fibrosis

Contracture may be evident on one or both hands, as well as on the feet, and may interfere with function. Painless edema along the nodule is also present.

Carpal Tunnel Syndrome

Atrophy of the thenar eminence may be evident, but generally edema is not present. Tenderness, motor strength (including grip and pinch), and sensory deficits must be determined. Phalen's maneuver and Tinel's sign may reproduce symptoms (Figures 188-1 and 188-2).

Trapeziometacarpal Arthritis

Pain is elicited by adducting the first metacarpal and hyperextending the first metacarpal phalange. The grind test will also elicit pain. This is a degenerative form of arthritis and is often seen with other manifestations of degenerative arthritis of the hands, including Heberden's and Bouchard's nodes (see Chapter 194).

DIAGNOSTICS AND DIFFERENTIAL DIAGNOSIS

An x-ray study may be indicated if bony abnormalities are suspected. Laboratory studies are rarely necessary. However, serum glucose, thyroid-stimulating hormone (TSH), erythrocyte sedimentation rate (ESR), antinuclear antibodies (ANA), and rheumatoid factor may be indicated. Cyclic citrullinated peptide, a new serologic marker for rheumatoid arthritis (RA),

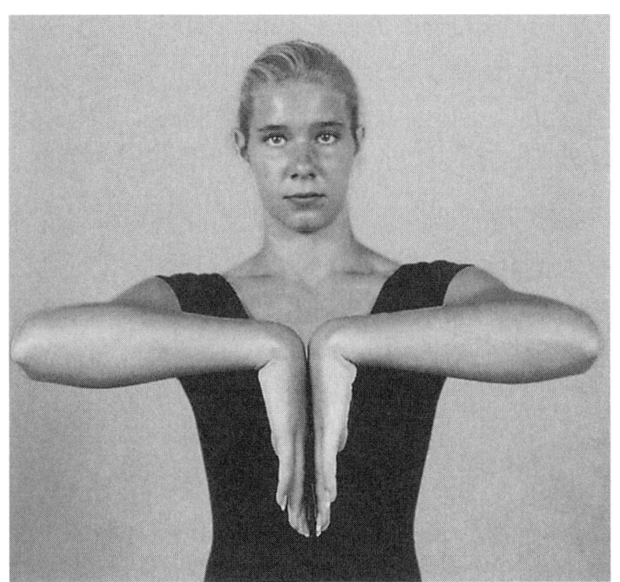

FIGURE 188-1

Phalen's maneuver for carpal tunnel syndrome. (From Barkauskas VH: *Health and physical assessment,* ed 2, St Louis, 1998, Mosby.)

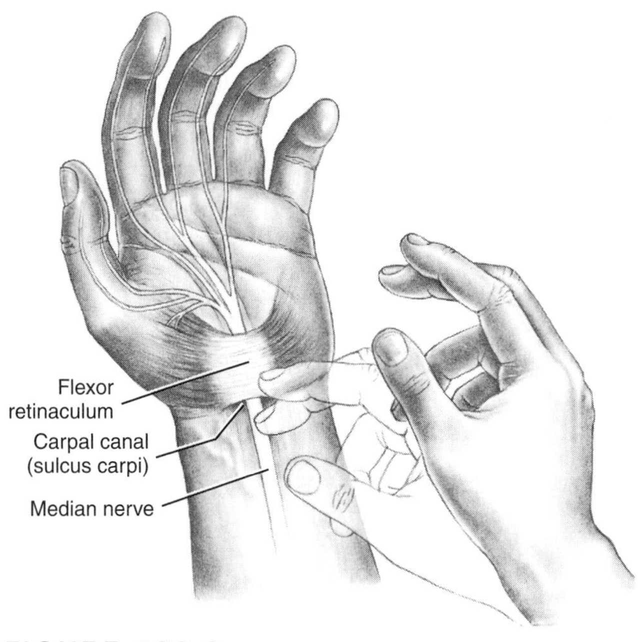

FIGURE 188-2

Eliciting Tinel's sign. (From Barkauskas VH: *Health and physical assessment,* ed 2, St Louis, 1998, Mosby.)

may be helpful in the differential diagnosis to determine whether the patient's symptoms are related to RA or another autoimmune disorder.[9] An electromyogram (EMG) may be ordered by a specialist.

Trigger Finger

Diagnostic tests are not indicated unless associated conditions are suspected. The differential diagnosis should include joint arthrosis, rheumatoid arthritis, flexor tendon rupture, tendon sheath cysts, and Dupuytren's contracture. Associated conditions include diabetes, rheumatoid arthritis, and occupational or recreational vibration exposure.

Tenosynovitis

X-ray studies are indicated to exclude fracture or arthritis. CBC, ESR, ANA, and rheumatoid factor may also be measured if rheumatoid arthritis is suspected. The differential diagnosis includes stenosing tenosynovitis of the thumb, fracture, or arthritis.

Palmar Fibrosis

Dupuytren's contracture has a classic appearance. The diagnosis is based on a history of painless swelling plus inspection and palpation of the nodule. Diagnostic tests and a differential diagnosis are usually unnecessary.

Carpal Tunnel Syndrome

An x-ray study of the wrist is recommended to exclude bony abnormalities; cervical films are used to exclude cervical radiculopathy. Electrodiagnostic studies, such as EMG and nerve conduction studies, may be necessary for both CTS and cubital tunnel syndrome if symptoms do not respond to conservative treatment. Laboratory studies are rarely indicated, but serum glucose, CBC, ESR, ANA, rheumatoid factor, and TSH may be required for certain patients. The differential diagnosis includes cervical radiculopathy, basal joint arthritis of the thumb, thoracic outlet syndrome, and polyneuropathy.[8]

Trapeziometacarpal Arthritis

X-ray studies are indicated to exclude fracture. The differential diagnosis should also include infection, radial bursitis, tenosynovitis, and sprain.

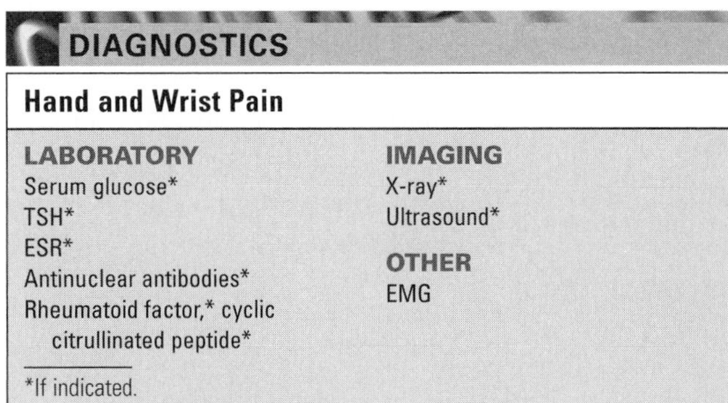

DIAGNOSTICS

Hand and Wrist Pain

LABORATORY	IMAGING
Serum glucose*	X-ray*
TSH*	Ultrasound*
ESR*	**OTHER**
Antinuclear antibodies*	EMG
Rheumatoid factor,* cyclic citrullinated peptide*	

*If indicated.

DIFFERENTIAL DIAGNOSIS

Hand and Wrist Pain

- Fracture
- Sprain
- Strain
- Ganglion
- Stenosing tenosynovitis
- de Quervain's disease
- Dupuytren's contracture
- Carpal tunnel syndrome
- Cubital tunnel syndrome
- Trapeziometacarpal arthritis
- Rheumatoid arthritis
- Osteoarthritis
- Raynaud's syndrome

MANAGEMENT AND INDICATIONS FOR REFERRAL OR HOSPITALIZATION

Treatment should be expedient and interdisciplinary to avoid prolonged disability. Reduction of risk factors, prevention of further injury, management of pain, restoration of function, and strengthening of muscle should be the primary goals of treatment.[1,5,7] Referral to physical and occupational therapists can be extremely helpful. Vocational counseling may be needed.

Trigger Finger

Immediate orthopedic referral is indicated if the finger cannot be passively extended. Treatment of an associated condition, rest, NSAIDs, and splinting of the PIP of the affected finger are appropriate interventions. A thumb spica splint should be applied to affected thumbs. If there is no improvement after 2 weeks, an orthopedic evaluation is indicated for possible corticosteroid injection or surgical release of the tendon.

Tenosynovitis

Ice, NSAIDs, and continuous immobilization in a padded gutter splint are initially indicated; cortisone injection of the nodule may offer the greatest relief. An orthopedic referral is necessary if there is no improvement after 2 weeks.

Palmar Fibrosis

If contractures are interfering with function, a referral to a hand specialist for surgical excision of the fascia may be warranted. Passive extension, NSAIDs, and cortisone injections have had less than impressive results and are not recommended.

Carpal Tunnel Syndrome

Treatment consists of neutral wrist splints, NSAIDs, ice, and work-home modification (Box 188-1). If there is no improvement in 3 weeks, a referral to a hand specialist is indicated for steroid injection or surgical evaluation.

Trapeziometacarpal Arthritis

The use of splinting and NSAIDs for 3 weeks is appropriate initially. If relief is not achieved, a referral to an orthopedist for steroid injection is warranted.

COMPLICATIONS

Contractures and pain are significant complications of hand and wrist disorders. In addition, nerve compression can jeopardize the sensory function, motor function, and reflexes of the affected hand. These problems affect quality of life, work, and recreational activities. Although surgery is indicated for hand disorders that are not responsive to conservative therapies, there is an inherent risk in any surgical procedure. Continued symptoms, reflex sympathetic dystrophy, nerve damage, and disfigurement are additional hazards associated with any surgical procedure of the hand or wrist.

BOX 189-1

TREATMENT OF CARPAL TUNNEL SYNDROME

- Rest or reduce activity
- Ice or cold packs to affected area
- NSAIDs (if no contraindications)
- Splinting at night
- Physical or occupational therapy
- Orthopedic, neurosurgical, or plastic surgery referral, if persistent symptoms
- Ergonomic adaptations to the work environment

PATIENT AND FAMILY EDUCATION

Patients should understand the importance of hourly 10-minute rest periods during activities that require repetitive hand movements. Splints that keep the wrist straight or slightly extended should be worn at night and, if necessary, during the day. Careful explanation of splint use is important because patients often remove the splint during activity, which results in further inflammation and a prolonged recovery period. Wrist splints can also be worn while sleeping to relieve discomfort during the night.

The use of cold packs and NSAID therapy should also be explained. Hand weakness, symptoms that increase in severity, or symptoms not relieved by conservative therapies should be reported to the health care provider.

HEALTH PROMOTION

Avoiding overexertion of the hand and wrist can prevent many cases of injury. Warming up and stretching these muscles before activity may help decrease the risk of injury.[10] The use of proper body mechanics may also reduce the risk of injury. It may be necessary to arrange the work environment to allow for more comfort and less strain on the body.[10] Taking frequent rest breaks during repetitive activities and doing strengthening exercises may help as well. Joint protection and energy-conservation techniques and the use of adaptive equipment may be necessary for painful or arthritic hands.

REFERENCES

1. Mooney V: Overuse syndromes of the upper extremity: rational and effective treatment, *J Musculoskel Med* 15(8):11-18, 1998.
2. Silverstein BA, Stetson DS, Keyserling WM, and others: Work-related musculoskeletal disorders: comparison of data sources for surveillance, *Am J Ind Med* 31(5):600-608, 1997.
3. Melhorn JM: Cumulative trauma disorders and repetitive strain injuries. The future, *Clin Orthop Relat Res* Jun(351):107-126, 1998.
4. Forman T, Forman S, Rose N: A clinical approach to diagnosing wrist pain, *Am Fam Phys* 72(9):1753-1759, retrieved Feb 14, 2006, from http://www.aafp.org/afp/20051101/1753.html.
5. Higgs PE, Young VL: Cumulative trauma disorders, *Clin Plast Surg* 23(3):421-433, 1996.
6. Barbe MF, Barr AE: Inflammation and the pathophysiology of work-related musculoskeletal disorders, *Brain Behav Immun* 20(5):423-429, 2006.
7. Sheon RP: Repetitive strain injury, part 2, Diagnostic and treatment tips on six common problems: the Goff Group, *Postgrad Med* 102(4):72-78, 1997.
8. LoBuano C: Identifying entrapment and compression neuropathies, *Patient Care Nurse Pract* 2(12):28-36, 1999.
9. Vallbracht I, Rieber J, Oppermann M, and others: Diagnostic and clinical value of anti-cyclic citrullinated peptide antibodies compared with rheumatoid factor isotypes in rheumatoid arthritis, *Ann Rheum Dis* 63:1079-1084, 2004.
10. Farnsworth EM: Diagnosis and management of repetitive strain injury, *Adv Nurse Pract* 9(8):32-38, 2001.

CHAPTER 189

Hip Pain

Ann S. Bruner-Welch

DEFINITION AND EPIDEMIOLOGY

Hip pain is a common complaint in primary care and a major source of discomfort and functional limitation, especially among older adults. Considering that hip pain is a symptom of an underlying pathologic process and not a disease in and of itself, numerous underlying causes may be described.[1] An accurate diagnosis and appropriate management are important in reducing the burden for both the patient and the family.

The patient who is seen with a chief complaint of hip pain may be a diagnostic challenge for the health care provider. The anatomy of the hip encompasses a large area, so the patient may have difficulty localizing the specific area of discomfort. Hip pain may be broadly defined as any sensation of pain immediately surrounding or within the pelvic girdle. It may be accompanied by limitation of range of motion, which may be exacerbated by activity or weight bearing.

Because hip pain is a symptom and not a specific disease entity, there is no epidemiologic pattern that describes the prevalence and incidence. Major causes of hip pain differ across age-groups and may be categorized as traumatic or nontraumatic (Table 189-1).

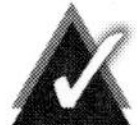

Orthopedic consultation is indicated for patients with suspected hip dislocation, fracture, sepsis, end-stage degenerative joint disease that is failing conservative care, or osseous abnormalities that are seen radiographically.

PATHOPHYSIOLOGY

Understanding the mechanisms of hip pain requires a review of the anatomy of the hip joint and structures of the pelvic girdle. The hip, like the shoulder, is a ball and socket and is classified as a diarthrodial, or synovial, joint. A fibrous capsule of ligaments and cartilage covers the points at which the bones articulate. A membrane that secretes synovial fluid provides lubrication for motion. Spaces between the tendons, ligaments, and bones, called *bursae,* permit ease of motion and reduce friction.

The ball and socket of the hip joint itself is made up of the head of the proximal femur and the acetabulum, which is formed by the ischium, pubis, and ilium. Strong ligaments form the capsule that covers the entire hip joint. Completely lining the capsule and extending down the neck of the femur is the synovial membrane.

The primary functions of the hip are weight bearing and locomotion. The muscles of the hip are essential in maintaining upright stability and gait. The muscles of the hip may be classified into five functional groups according to their action: the abductors, flexors, adductors, extensors, and rotators. Musculotendinous pain of the hip may contribute to distortions of gait, which may produce a limp.

The underlying cause of the pain determines the actual pathophysiology. Arthralgia secondary to degenerative joint disease results from the breakdown and loss of cartilage at the points of stress and motion in the joint.[2] Bursitis is caused by inflammation of the bursae surrounding and protecting the joint capsule.[3] Inflammation may be the result of prior or repetitive trauma or an extension of an inflammatory process such as rheumatoid arthritis. Avascular necrosis is loss of blood supply and subsequent death of subchondral bone tissue, often related to trauma or the use of corticosteroids. It can occur in a number of sites in the body, including the femoral head. The cartilage remains intact; however, the bone beneath it becomes flattened and misshapen.[4]

TABLE 189-1 Causes of Hip Pain and Age-Groups Commonly Affected

Age-Group	Traumatic Cause*	Nontraumatic Cause
Adolescents and young adults	SCFE[†] Stress fracture Sprains, strains	SCFE Juvenile arthritis
Adults	Stress fracture Sprains, strains	Bursitis Neuropathy Fasciitis Rheumatoid arthritis or osteoarthritis
Older adults	Hip fracture Dislocation	Osteoarthritis Bursitis Neuropathy Fasciitis Spinal stenosis

*Avascular necrosis should *always* be ruled out for hip pain caused by trauma.
[†]Slipped capital femoral epiphysis *(SCFE)* may occur with or without trauma.

CLINICAL PRESENTATION

For the patient who comes to see a health care provider with a chief complaint of hip pain, a careful history must be obtained with particular attention to the history of the present illness. Any history of joint replacement and recent or old trauma to the hip and lower back or history of cancer should be obtained. Pertinent questions related to location, onset, duration, severity, setting, associated manifestations, and aggravating or alleviating factors will be useful in narrowing the diagnosis.

For most patients with hip pain, the pain is increased with activity. Pain at rest may indicate inflammatory, infectious, or neoplastic disease. With degenerative joint disease (osteoarthritis [OA]), the pain will become progressively more severe with activity and can occur in the groin, buttock, anterior or lateral thigh, or knee. Often the patient may not be able to determine the exact location of the pain, as synovitis, muscle spasm, and capsular contracture progress. The pain is often accompanied by stiffness on first arising in the morning and after long periods of inactivity (gel phenomenon). The duration of stiffness with OA is usually short, lasting only 5 to 30 minutes. Walking or prolonged standing will tend to aggravate the pain, and rest relieves it. When OA is the cause, pain may also occur in other joints of the body, especially the knees and the joints of the hands.

Bursitis, another common cause of hip pain in adults, is seen with point tenderness and focal pain over the bursa. Any of the three major bursae surrounding the hip may be affected. Patients with trochanteric bursitis will complain of pain in the lateral hip posterior to the greater trochanter with frequent radiation down the lateral thigh to the knee.[3] Ischiogluteal bursitis is seen as pain over the ischial tuberosity with radiation to the posterior thigh. Pain in the groin with radiation to the anterior thigh may indicate iliopsoas bursitis. Pain will be aggravated with walking (see Chapter 184).

The patient with septic or infectious arthritis of the hip may be seen after an incident of trauma or after surgery. A contiguous site of bacterial infection may also create a route for bacterial invasion of the joint. High fever, excruciating pain, and limited range of motion may be present. In the adolescent and young adult, *Neisseria gonorrhoeae* is the most common causative organism. In adults of all ages *Staphylococcus aureus* is the usual source of infection, although other pathogens may be implicated.[5]

Avascular necrosis, often associated with trauma, alcohol abuse, corticosteroids, protease inhibitors, rheumatoid arthritis, or systemic lupus erythematosus, can be bilateral. The patient will report a gradual onset of dull aching or throbbing pain in the groin, lateral hip, or buttock.[4]

An insidious onset of moderate to severe hip, thigh, or knee pain associated with a limp or an acute onset of hip pain after injury, especially in an adolescent, should raise the suspicion of slipped capital femoral epiphysis (SCFE).[6] SCFE is also associated with obesity; more than half of affected adolescents exceed the 95th percentile for weight and age. Delayed sexual maturity may also be evident.

PHYSICAL EXAMINATION

Two tests of hip function during physical examination are essential: gait and range of motion. The gait may be affected by a limp (antalgic gait) that is characterized by an exaggerated swaying motion of the upper body toward the painful hip while walking (Trendelenburg's gait). Motion restrictions of abduction and internal rotation are usually more pronounced than restriction of adduction and external rotation. Pain, muscle spasm, and guarding are noted with passive and active range of motion. Inspection may reveal a flexion-contracture of the hip and atrophy of the musculature of the buttocks. Crepitus of the joint may be felt or heard with palpation and movement.

Pain on palpation that is well localized (point tenderness) and possibly accompanied by redness, warmth, and swelling may indicate bursitis. Hip flexion and internal rotation may exacerbate the pain. In the older patient, fracture may be suspected if there is a history of a fall or rotational injury to the hip. The patient will complain of hip, groin, or thigh pain and will be unable to bear weight or move the leg. The affected extremity will usually be shortened and externally rotated. In the adolescent patient with SCFE, significant muscle spasm and restricted internal rotation will be evident.[6]

DIAGNOSTICS

The diagnosis of hip pain is often made on the basis of clinical examination of the patient. However, diagnostic testing is warranted if there has been trauma or to exclude more serious causes of hip pain, such as avascular necrosis of the femur. X-ray studies should include an anteroposterior (AP) view of the pelvis, frog-leg and AP views of the hip, and two views of the lumbosacral spine. Weight-bearing films are important to assess the extent of joint degeneration and joint space narrowing. If avascular necrosis is suspected, MRI is the diagnostic test of choice. MRI is not as sensitive in identifying cartilaginous changes of the joint. If rheumatic causes are suspected, a CBC, erythrocyte sedimentation rate, and rheumatic factor analysis should be obtained. With radiographic evidence of effusion, joint aspiration, performed under fluoroscopic guidance, is indicated. Aspirate is sent for culture and sensitivity, a cell count with differential, and identification of crystalline deposits.[3,4,7,8]

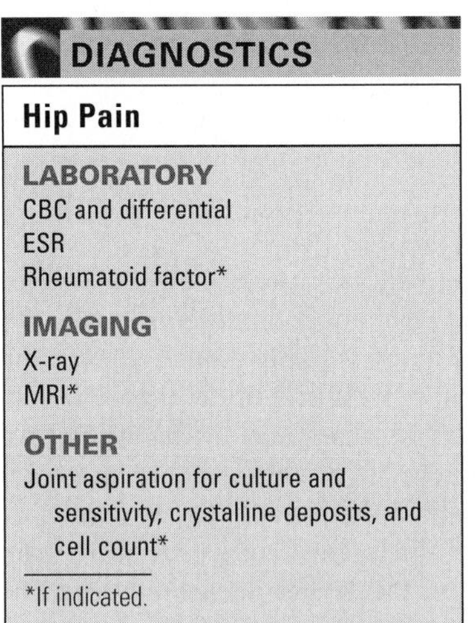
DIAGNOSTICS

Hip Pain

LABORATORY
CBC and differential
ESR
Rheumatoid factor*

IMAGING
X-ray
MRI*

OTHER
Joint aspiration for culture and sensitivity, crystalline deposits, and cell count*

*If indicated.

DIFFERENTIAL DIAGNOSIS

Although the most common cause of hip pain in the adult is OA, other diagnostic possibilities should be considered if there is no relief of symptoms with standard treatment. Fractures, dislocations, inflammatory conditions, rheumatoid arthritis, infections, and avascular necrosis are other important causes of hip pain.[1,4,7]

Minimum force applied to the hip joint may produce a fracture, especially in the older woman with osteoporosis. In patients who are runners or who participate in sports, a femoral stress fracture should also be considered as a hip pain etiology.

Traumatic dislocations are more often seen in young patients who engage in activities with a risk for violent injury. Joint infection or avascular necrosis should be excluded for any patient who has a history of trauma to the hip or risk factors such as alcohol abuse, a suppressed immune system, corticosteroid use, HIV, or IV drug use.[4]

Extraarticular causes of hip pain include referred pain from degenerative discs, spinal stenosis, sacroiliac dysfunction, leg length discrepancies, bursitis, bone diseases such as osteoporosis, malignancy, Paget's disease, and osteomyelitis. Neuropathic pain of diabetes, alcoholism, and vitamin B_{12} deficiency, as well as vascular diseases such as atherosclerosis, diabetes, and vasculitis, need to be considered.

Infection of the hip joint is rare in adults, although this should be considered in children or adults with a prosthetic hip and new-onset hip pain. Patients in whom septic arthritis of the hip develops are typically immunocompromised because of corticosteroids or chemotherapeutic agents. IV drug users are also at increased risk for joint infection. Antibiotic-resistant microorganisms such as methicillin-resistant *S. aureus* (MRSA) are becoming a community-acquired phenomenon in addition to nosocomial infection (see Chapter 243). Either way, these organisms can be invasive and difficult to treat.[8]

DIFFERENTIAL DIAGNOSIS

Hip Pain

• Rheumatoid arthritis	• Septic sacroiliitis
• Osteoarthritis	• Osteomyelitis
• Septic arthritis	• Cellulitis
• Joint infection	• Gout
• Malignancy	• Pseudogout
• Sprain	• Sickle cell disease
• Strain	• Avascular necrosis
• Stress fracture	• Osteoporosis
• Traumatic dislocation	• Paget's disease
• Bursitis or tendinitis	• Neuropathy
• Fasciitis	• Vascular disease

An important cause of hip pain in the adolescent is SCFE, which may or may not be associated with trauma.[6] Although the underlying cause is unclear, SCFE is most likely to be seen during the growth spurt between the ages of 10 and 15 years. The typical patient is an obese male adolescent. Juvenile arthritis is another important consideration in the adolescent age range, since it can lead to joint destruction and failure with the need for subsequent replacement in early adulthood.[9]

MANAGEMENT

Hip pain is a symptom of an underlying pathophysiologic process. Although hip pain has the potential to produce functional limitations and to impair quality of life, the management should be directed toward identifying and treating the underlying cause of the pain.[1] Evidence-based practice in treating the adult patient with hip pain is focused on the various causes of the hip pain such as OA (see Chapter 194). Pain management is a major issue for patients with OA involving the hip. Although most randomized controlled trials have focused on OA of the knee, some have demonstrated benefits of using NSAIDs and acetaminophen analgesics in relief of hip pain.[2,8,10] Both classes of analgesics have been shown to reduce pain secondary to OA. There is no clear evidence that either class of analgesic is superior in reducing OA pain. Capsaicin, an over-the-counter topical analgesic, has also been shown to provide short-term pain relief and has fewer side effects than oral agents. The adverse effect most commonly reported for topical agents is local skin irritation. For pain related to bursitis, tendinitis, or traumatic injury, NSAIDs will likely be more effective in controlling the pain and promoting mobility.

Nonpharmacologic measures are aimed at restoring and maintaining function of the joint as an adjunct to pharmacologic therapy. Recommendations for complete rest or inactivity of the joint should be given only after careful weighing of the risk vs. benefit. Muscular atrophy and weakness may result and contribute to the primary problem. Evidence for benefit does exist for exercise and education in reducing pain, with the strongest evidence pointing to the benefits of exercise.[11] Exercise also improves functional status and provides a sense of well-being. Range of motion and low-stress, low-impact exercises should be prescribed. An aquatic exercise program, as recommended by the Arthritis Foundation, may promote mobility while relieving mechanical weight bearing on the joint.[12] Use of heat before and ice after exercise can also alleviate pain.

COMPLICATIONS

Complications of hip pain depend on the cause. Osteoporosis of the hip may result in a spontaneous fracture with or without trauma. Degenerative joint disease and the various inflammatory and traumatic conditions that are accompanied by loss of function and mobility may result in falls with injury and the numerous cardiovascular effects of deconditioning. Older patients in particular should be monitored for gastrointestinal irritation if taking NSAIDs. An adolescent with SCFE has a guarded long-term prognosis for repeat injury and complications. Avascular necrosis of the femoral head may occur in approximately 30% of patients with SCFE. Premature development of degenerative arthritis may occur with or without avascular necrosis.

INDICATIONS FOR REFERRAL OR HOSPITALIZATION

Hip pain requires an ongoing assessment of the patient's functional capabilities and relief of painful symptoms. A multidisciplinary approach involving a physical therapist or an occupational therapist is indicated. Physical therapy improves joint mobility and prevents the complications of joint disuse. Occupational therapists may assist patients with limitations of function in adapting activities of daily living for optimum independence. Referral to an orthopedic surgeon is indicated for patients suspected of having joint infection or avascular necrosis or for those with progressive loss of function or refractive chronic pain. Urgent referral is required for patients with hip fracture and dislocation.

PATIENT AND FAMILY EDUCATION AND HEALTH PROMOTION

Chronic joint pain can be mentally and physically wearing on the patient. A multidisciplinary approach to care with the patient as an active participant in the decision-making process may prove more satisfactory for the patient and provider over the long term. The patient is entitled to an explanation regarding the source of the pain and whether it is likely to be temporary or chronic. Facilitating patient understanding of anticipated outcomes and prognosis is extremely beneficial in strengthening the patient-provider relationship.

Health-promoting activities should be directed toward maintaining and preserving function of the joint. The management of a painful hip may include range-of-motion and muscle strengthening exercises, as recommended by the physical therapist. Maintenance of optimum weight should be encouraged because the excess weight places tremendous stresses on the hip. The patient taking NSAIDs should take these medications with food and be knowledgeable of the signs and symptoms of gastrointestinal irritation. Because the risk of falls may be increased with hip pain, especially among older adults, an assessment of the home environment and the need for ambulatory assistive devices is warranted.

REFERENCES

1. Cluett J: Hip pain: common conditions and treatment, *Orthopedics,* retrieved March 26, 2006, from http://orthopedics.about.com/cs/hipsurgery/a/hippain.htm.
2. Simon L: *Update in osteoporosis and osteoarthritis,* retrieved Feb 5, 2007, from http://www.medscape.com/viwearticle/550598.
3. American Academy of Orthopaedic Surgeons: *Hip bursitis,* Sept 2005, retrieved March 26, 2006, from http://orthoinfo.aaos.org.
4. National Institute of Arthritis and Musculoskeletal and Skin Diseases: *Questions and answers about osteonecrosis (avascular necrosis),* retrieved from March 26, 2006, from http://www.niams.nih.gov/hi/topics/osteonecrosis/index.htm.
5. American Geriatrics Society: AGA clinical practice guideline: the management of persistent pain in older persons, *J Am Geriatr Soc* 50(6):1-20, 2002.
6. American Academy of Orthopaedic Surgeons: *Slipped capital femoral epiphysis* (review), June 2004, retrieved March 26, 2006, from http://orthoinfo.aaos.org/fact/thr_report.cfm?Thread_ID=160&topcategory=Hip.
7. *Bone and joint infections,* retrieved March 26, 2006, from http://www.mayoclinic.com/health/bone-and-joint-infections/DS00545.
8. *Study questions greater GI safety of COX-2 inhibitors,* retrieved March 26, 2006, from http://www.medscape.com/viewarticle/518295.
9. Szer IS: *Juvenile rheumatoid arthritis and pediatric Sjögren's syndrome,* American College of Rheumatology 64th annual scientific meeting, Oct 29–Nov 2, 2000, retrieved March 26, 2006, from http://www.medscape.com/viewarticle/420526.
10. Cluett J: *Which nonsteroidal anti-inflammatory medication is best? Glucosamine and chondroitin and nonsteroidal anti-inflammatory pain medication,* retrieved March 26, 2006, from http://orthopedics.about.com./cs/paindrugs/a/bestnsaids.
11. Fransen M, McConnell S, Bell M: Exercise for osteoarthritis of the hip or knee, *Cochrane Database of Systematic Reviews* 2:CD004376, 2001.
12. The Arthritis Foundation: *Exercise and arthritis,* retrieved Feb 7, 2007, from http://www.arthritis.org/conditions/exercise/default.asp.

CHAPTER 190

Infectious Arthritis

Kevin D. Kerin

DEFINITION AND EPIDEMIOLOGY

Inflammation of a joint is called *arthritis* and is an observable finding, whereas pain in a joint is called *arthralgia* and is a subjective description. One important type of arthritis is infectious arthritis. The term *septic arthritis* is most commonly used to describe bacterial arthritis. An infectious cause of joint inflammation needs to be considered even when a non-infectious inflammatory arthritis (rheumatoid arthritis, gout) has been previously diagnosed. Infectious arthritis may be caused by a large number of organisms, including bacteria, fungi, viruses, and filariae. Bacterial and viral arthritis usually are seen acutely with systemic symptoms. Lyme disease and mycobacterial, fungal, filarial, and some bacterial arthritis *(Neisseria gonorrhoeae, Neisseria meningitidis)* may be chronic and relatively indolent. Infectious arthritis is seen in all age-groups, although the highest incidence is in children and the elderly.[1]

PATHOPHYSIOLOGY

Synovial joints such as the knee or hip are particularly susceptible to infection. One explanation is that synovial tissue is highly vascularized, lacks a basement membrane, and is thus susceptible to the hematogenous spread of infectious organisms from a locus of infection.[2] Other avenues of infection of the joint space include extension of infection from osteomyelitis, adjacent soft tissue infection, or direct inoculation from penetration of a foreign body.[3] A joint infection is a medical emergency and can be a rapid, severely destructive process. Once a bacterial infection is established in a joint space, a complex cascade of events follows, including changes in synovial tissue; migration of acute and chronic inflammatory cells to the joint space; release of inflammatory cytokines, proteases, and collagenases; changes in intraarticular fluid volume and pressure; and chondrocyte changes.[4] *Staphylococcus aureus* is the most common cause of acute bacterial arthritis across all age-groups.[2]

It is no accident that *S. aureus* is the most common cause of infectious arthritis. Its predilection for joints can be explained in part by the structure of the microbe, which elaborates certain surface and secreted proteins (e.g., microbial surface components recognizing adhesive matrix molecules, or MSCRAMM)[5] and may facilitate colonization of tissue. This organism also has receptors for glycoproteins found in joints and has frequent access to hematogenous seeding from minor wounds and abrasions.[6] Streptococci are also normal skin flora, second only to *S. aureus* as etiologic agents of infectious arthritis. *N. gonorrhoeae* is the most common cause of infectious arthritis from a sexually transmitted bacterium and is mostly seen in sexually active adults under 30 years old.[7] This is not unexpected given the ease with which *N. gonorrhoeae* invades the bloodstream during menses or parturition and after acute urethritis. Gram-negative bacilli cause approximately 10% of cases of septic arthritis, often in older adults and neonates, and are associated with a better outcome than gram-positive infections.[8] Anaerobes are an uncommon cause of infectious arthritis and are associated with human bites, intraabdominal abscesses, and periarticular decubitus ulcers.

CLINICAL PRESENTATION

Septic arthritis usually is seen with the acute onset of a painful, red, swollen joint, which is warm to the touch. An important and distinguishing historical point is that the affected joint is painful at rest as well as with motion and weight bearing. The pain of arthritis from other causes usually is relieved with rest.[9] Fever is usually present but may be low grade or absent (especially in the elderly). Rigors caused by bacteremia may also be present. Fever and rigors have low sensitivity and specificity in the diagnosis of septic arthritis, since these findings may be seen in acute crystal-induced arthritis.[3] Any joint may be involved, yet the knee and hip are the most commonly affected. Septic arthritis in an unusual location such as the sternoclavicular or sacroiliac joint should raise the suspicion of injection drug use. The sudden onset of monoarticular arthritis is the usual presentation of nongonococcal arthritis, although approximately 12% of the time there is a polyarticular presentation.[10] A polyarticular septic arthritis is sometimes seen with streptococcal or staphylococcal infections but usually affects only two or three joints.

Infectious arthritis occurs more commonly in patients with an impaired immune system and in those with preexisting joint abnormalities such as in rheumatoid arthritis, gout, osteoarthritis, or prosthetic joint.[4] It is important to consider infection as a cause of an acute monoarticular or pauciarticular flare, even in those with an established diagnosis of a chronic rheumatologic condition. The fever and arthritis are less striking in gonococcal arthritis, which is characterized by a migrating polyarticular course.

PHYSICAL EXAMINATION

The manifestations of inflammation were vividly described by Celsus in the first century AD as rubor, tumor, calor, and dolor (redness, swelling, heat, and pain).[11] The inflamed joint is erythematous, warm to the touch, swollen, and painful with passive and active range of motion. Synovial effusion is usually present, though less obvious in certain joints such as the hip or shoulder. A large effusion creates an asymmetry in size with loss of anatomic landmarks; a smaller effusion in the knee may be detected by a "bulge sign" (the examiner presses on the medial aspect of the knee to displace fluid toward the suprapatellar region and then looks for a small bulge in this area after applying pressure on the opposite side of the knee) or patellar ballottement (the examiner taps on the patella while applying pressure to the suprapatellar area to try to elicit a "click" signifying synovial fluid beneath the patella).

Decreased range of motion, muscle spasm, and apprehension of joint examination are prominent features of the examination. The proximal lymph node may be enlarged and tender, indicative of lymphangitic spread. An original source of infection, such as an abscess, cellulitis, gonococcal urethritis, pneumonia, urinary tract infection, or endocarditis, should be sought. Distinct clinical presentations are seen in special situations, which are discussed in the following sections.

Gonococcal Arthritis

Disseminated gonococcal infection is the most common cause of septic arthritis in sexually active adolescents and young adults.[12] There appear to be two distinct clinical presentations. One has been called the *arthritis-dermatitis syndrome* and reflects a bacteremic stage; the other is a localized septic arthritis.[12] The classic triad of clinical findings in disseminated infection is dermatitis, tenosynovitis, and a migratory polyarthritis. The first group is distinguished by tenosynovitis and dermatitis. Skin lesions are present in countable numbers and multiple stages; these lesions are most often maculopapular but are sometimes necrotic, pustular, or vesicular. The lesions are painless and nonpruritic and typically spare the face and scalp. The lesions resolve in several days without scarring.[7] An asymmetric migratory polyarthralgia that affects knees, elbows, wrists, ankles, metacarpophalangeal joints, and associated tendon sheaths is the more common presentation than actual polyarthritis. Synovial fluid cell counts are lower than those commonly seen in bacterial arthritis, and the synovial fluid culture is often negative. The blood culture may be positive. Only 25% of patients have genitourinary symptoms of gonorrhea.[10]

The more focal septic arthritis seen in the second group may occur after a migratory polyarthritis, tenosynovitis, or dermatitis, with the arthritis now settled in one or two joints. The synovial fluid is more purulent, and the culture is more likely to be positive. Blood cultures are typically negative. Taken as a group, cultures of the pharynx, cervix, urethra, and rectum are positive in up to 80% of patients if obtained early on selective media (e.g., Thayer-Martin).[7] Synovial fluid cultures should be plated directly onto chocolate agar. DNA amplification tests may be used to detect *N. gonorrhoeae* in synovial fluid.[13]

Whether these groups represent sequential stages of disease or distinct presentations in different hosts is still debated.[14] This may result in clinical uncertainty about the diagnosis, especially in the context of a wide range of synovial fluid leukocyte counts and negative blood cultures. In this situation, ceftriaxone 1 g/day IV over 48 hours can be a valid diagnostic strategy.

Prosthetic Joint Infection

Millions of people have prosthetic joints. Although the rates of infection after hip or knee arthroplasty have declined significantly to approximately 1%, the large number of prosthetic joints makes this a relatively common problem.[10] It is a serious, potentially devastating problem and is associated with major disability and cost. In most cases the prosthetic joint needs to be removed, and the patient will require up to 6 weeks of IV antibiotics (with or without an antibiotic-impregnated cement spacer), followed by reimplantation of a new prosthetic joint once infection has been eradicated. Biofilms, complex microbial communities formed by bacteria causing prosthetic joint infections, contribute to antibiotic resistance.[15] Coagulase-negative staphylococci are common in this clinical setting and produce an indolent course. Hematogenous seeding at the bone-cement interface with *S. aureus* or group A streptococci may manifest more acutely with sepsis or toxic shock, which is characteristic of these more virulent organisms. Infections in older patients with underlying disease may include gram-negative bacilli (20%) and anaerobes (7%).[16]

One way to classify prosthetic joint infections is by the amount of time elapsed since joint surgery: early (within 3 months), delayed (3 to 24 months), and late (>24 months).[15] Early and delayed infections have their origin at the time of prosthetic placement, whereas late infections are due to hematogenous seeding of bacteria.[15] Infection in a prosthetic joint is often difficult to diagnose, and clinical manifestations may vary depending on the timing of the infection in relation to the surgery. As a rule, the great majority of patients have joint pain with or without radiographic evidence of loosening of the prosthesis. A minority of patients have fever, joint swelling, or sinus tract drainage. It may be difficult to differentiate a delayed-onset infection of a prosthetic joint from a noninfectious inflammation, such as a reaction to components of the prosthetic joint or a mechanical problem with the hardware (e.g., loosening, dislocation, hemarthrosis, and malposition). A helpful observation is that mechanical problems are painful during motion, weight bearing, and pivoting but are comfortable while at rest. Constant joint pain suggests an infection.

Laboratory tests such as acute phase reactants (erythrocyte sedimentation rate [ESR], C-reactive protein [CRP]) or leukocyte count are not helpful because a number of inflammatory conditions can cause elevated levels in any of these tests, and normal values do not rule out infection. Plain radiographs may be helpful, especially if serial studies are available for comparison. Classic findings include lucencies along the bone-cement interface, migration of the prosthesis, and periosteal reactions. These findings are not present in acute or early infections and are difficult to differentiate from mechanical complications in those with delayed-onset infections. A technetium bone scan may take up to 1 year to become negative after surgery[17]; the negative bone scan provides strong evidence against an infectious prosthetic joint. However, positive bone scans or indium leukocyte scans are nonspecific and may be positive because of noninfectious or mechanical problems.[18] Other radiologic techniques such as sequential bone and gallium scanning or combined leukocyte-marrow scintigraphy have shown greater accuracy in the diagnosis of a prosthetic joint infection yet are costly, time-consuming, and not widely available.[19] Ultimately, the diagnosis of a prosthetic joint infection relies on aggressive attempts to isolate an organism by obtaining joint fluid or tissue.

Lyme Disease

The clinical manifestations of Lyme disease can be separated into early localized disease (1 to 30 days), early disseminated disease (days to 10 months), and late disease (months to years) based on elapsed time from tick exposure to symptoms[20] (see Chapter 250). Only 30% of patients with Lyme disease recall a tick bite, but in the setting of known tick exposure, 80% of patients with early, localized Lyme disease suffer arthralgias or migratory arthritis.[20] During this stage the characteristic rash (erythema chronicum migrans) appears with an expanding red border and central clearing, occasionally creating the classic "bull's eye" appearance. Fever, headache, myalgias, arthralgias, and lymphadenopathy may be more noticeable than the skin lesions, which are usually painless.

The manifestations of early, disseminated Lyme disease include multiple systemic features: cardiac problems (pericarditis, atrioventricular nodal heart block, myopathy) in 10% of patients, neurologic problems (facial nerve or Bell's palsy, meningitis, encephalitis, radiculitis with neuropathy) in 10% to 12%, and musculoskeletal problems (migratory polyarthralgias or polyarthritis) in 50%.[20] More prolonged attacks of true arthritis develop in a few joints. In late Lyme disease arthritis, about 60% of patients have a migratory polyarthritis and 10% of patients develop a chronic arthritis that settles in one or two large joints, usually the knees.[21]

In Lyme disease the causative spirochete, *Borrelia burgdorferi*, is difficult to culture from synovial fluid, but sensitive methods of antigen detection (enzyme-linked immunosorbent assay [ELISA]) or polymerase chain reaction (PCR) reveal its presence. Having a high index of suspicion in the right clinical setting makes the diagnosis. In the wrong clinical setting (without sufficiently high pretest probability), serologic tests for Lyme disease are misleading because of the high false-positive rate; therefore such tests should not be ordered indiscriminantly.[22] All patients with true arthritis attributed to early, disseminated, or late Lyme disease should be positive on the Lyme ELISA and confirmed by Western blot.

The outcome is better if diagnosis and treatment are rendered early in this form of infectious arthritis. Medical therapy fails in approximately 50% of patients with late Lyme disease arthritis; progressive joint destruction may then merit synovectomy or total joint arthroplasty.[23]

Injection Drug Use

Infectious arthritis in unusual or axial locations (e.g., sacroiliac joint, sternoclavicular joint, symphysis pubis) should raise suspicion of injection drug use. Similarly, the presence of unusual organisms—*Pseudomonas aeruginosa*, *Serratia marcescens*, and *Candida* species—in joint fluid should lead to open-ended and nonjudgmental queries regarding recreational drug use.[24] Still, most of the joint infections in these joints are due to *S. aureus* with or without injection drug use.[25] Hips and shoulders are other common sites of infection in heroin addicts. In patients who use injection recreational drugs, disseminated gonococcal disease and syphilis should also be considered in the differential diagnosis. The response to antibiotic therapy alone is good (90%), and few patients require surgical drainage despite usually aggressive organisms (e.g., *P. aeruginosa* and *S. aureus*).

Septic Sacroiliitis

Septic sacroiliitis can be an elusive diagnosis for health care providers because of the nonspecific nature of presenting symptoms. Patients may be seen with fever and low back pain or gluteal region pain that is intensified by ambulation.[26] The physical examination alone is inadequate in distinguishing sacroiliitis from muscle pain, disc disease, femoral nerve entrapment in the buttocks (piriformis muscle syndrome), or bursitis. Certain physical examination maneuvers have been devised to try to isolate and stress the sacroiliac joints. Plain radiographs are not helpful in early diagnosis. Focal pain that occurs when shear forces are applied to the sacroiliac joint may indicate septic sacroiliitis, in which case the patient should be referred immediately for a CT scan or MRI. An MRI is uniquely suited to this difficult diagnosis because it alone has the potential to define fluid in the sacroiliac joint, adjacent bone marrow inflammation, and soft tissue abscesses that may extend into the abdominal cavity and the psoas, iliac, and piriform muscles. Because of the complexity of the involved joints and difficult access, these collections need pigtail catheter drainage or surgical debridement.[27]

DIAGNOSTICS

In patients with infectious arthritis, increases in the peripheral WBC count, ESR, and CRP level are frequent but nonspecific findings. Peripheral blood cultures are positive in 40% of cases and are the only sources of microorganisms in 10% of cases.[28] Younger patients suspected of having gonococcal arthritis should have pharyngeal, rectal, and cervical or urethral cultures on specialized gonococcal media. The most important examination for the diagnosis of infectious arthritis is synovial fluid, not only for culture but also for cellular and chemical analysis. Aspiration of inflamed joints provides three important pieces of information: diagnosis of crystal-induced arthritis, degree of inflammation (cell count), and specimen for Gram's stain and culture. Any joint suspected of infection should be aspirated without delay, since the outcome of infectious arthritis depends on early diagnosis and treatment. Sterile technique should be used, and the provider should avoid entering the joint through an area of skin that may be infected. It is important to send blood and synovial fluid cultures for analysis before starting antibiotics.

The most useful components of synovial fluid analysis consists of evaluation for crystals, cell count and differential, protein, Gram's stain, and cultures (aerobic and anaerobic). Synovial fluid protein and glucose are less useful diagnostic tests. Synovial fluid protein is significantly elevated in both infectious arthritis and other forms of inflammatory arthritis. Synovial fluid glucose less than 40 mg/dl or less than 50% of a simultaneous blood glucose is supportive evidence for bacterial arthritis. Synovial fluid lactic acid has high negative predictive value for bacterial arthritis yet is not widely used.[3] With chronic synovitis, fungal and mycobacterial cultures are also sent for analysis, and special stains for acid-fast bacteria and fungi are performed. Synovial fluid WBC counts may be very high (Table 190-1); cell counts in the 100,000/mm^3 range are considered infectious until proven otherwise.[29] There is a considerable overlap in synovial WBC counts among infectious and noninfectious causes of arthritis. Gout, Reiter's syndrome, and rheumatoid arthritis may cause high cell counts normally associated with sepsis, whereas early infectious arthritis or established gonococcal arthritis may cause relatively low cell counts. The predominance of polymorphonuclear leukocytes in synovial fluid is a clue, but is specific only if it exceeds 85%. Intracellular crystals and the profusion of polymorphonuclear cells suggest gout or pseudogout, but free-floating crystals are sometimes seen in infectious arthritis.[30] Synovial fluid PCR may be used to diagnose gonococcal arthritis and Lyme disease arthritis.

Radiographs are not useful in the initial diagnosis of a septic joint. It may take 2 weeks to demonstrate joint space narrowing and marginal erosions—too late to salvage a functional joint. Radiographs are useful in identifying underlying arthritis or osteomyelitis. Gas formation in or around a joint is an important clue to anaerobic organisms or *Escherichia coli*.[31] Such a finding requires early surgical intervention and the removal of any prosthetic material. A three-phase technetium bone scan is helpful in differentiating cellulitis, infectious arthritis, and osteomyelitis.[32] However, arthrocentesis is better. Thus a bone scan, gallium scan, and indium leukocyte scan are of little practical value. A CT scan or MRI is advantageous in difficult diagnostic situations (e.g., sternoclavicular or sacroiliac joint involvement) and as a guide to joint aspiration and anatomic definition of an infected hip.[33]

DIAGNOSTICS

Infectious Arthritis

LABORATORY
CBC and differential
ESR
C-reactive protein
Blood cultures
Rectal, cervical, urethral, or pharyngeal cultures*
Lyme ELISA, Western blot test*

IMAGING
X-ray
CT scan, MRI*

OTHER
Joint aspiration of synovial fluid for crystals, culture, cell count, protein, glucose, and Gram's stain

*If indicated.

TABLE 190-1 Synovial Fluid Analysis

Characteristic	Normal	Noninflammatory (Osteoarthritis)	Inflammatory (Rheumatoid)	Septic (Infection)
Volume	<3.5 ml	>3.5 ml	Large	Large
Clarity	Clear	Transparent	Translucent	Opaque
WBC/mm^3	<200	200-2000	2000-75,000	50,000-100,000
Polymorphonuclear leukocytes	<25%	<25%	>50%	>75%
Culture	Negative	Negative	Negative	Positive
Glucose	Equal to blood	Equal to blood	>50% blood glucose	<50% blood glucose
Protein	1.7 g/dl	<3 g/dl	>3 g/dl	>3 g/dl

WBC, White blood cells.

DIFFERENTIAL DIAGNOSIS

A synovial fluid leukocyte count of more than 2000/mm^3 is considered inflammatory, and a cell count of more than 50,000/mm^3 is considered septic until proven otherwise by Gram's stain and cultures. There is a significant overlap in synovial fluid leukocyte counts in inflammatory conditions from infectious and noninfectious causes. Other types of inflammatory arthritis are distinguished from infectious arthritis by culture and Gram's stain; however, gout, Reiter's syndrome, and rheumatoid arthritis may accrue cell counts in the infectious arthritis range. In such situations, antibiotics should be initiated until cultures are finalized.

DIFFERENTIAL DIAGNOSIS

Rheumatic Disorders

- Bursitis
- Gout
- Pseudogout
- Rheumatoid arthritis
- Reiter's syndrome
- Angioedema
- Rheumatic fever
- Osteoarthritis
- Osteomyelitis
- Cellulitis

Cellulitis, bursitis, acute osteomyelitis, and angioedema should be distinguished by their greater range of motion and less-than-circumferential swelling. Polyarticular infectious arthritis is sometimes seen with staphylococci and streptococci, but also suggests metastatic foci resulting from subacute bacterial endocarditis.[34] Polyarticular noninfectious arthritis is seen with rheumatic fever or poststreptococcal reactive arthritis. In either case, the joint is not the focus of the streptococcal infection. The arthritis of rheumatic fever is migratory and resolves spontaneously in 1 month. Another form of acute reactive arthritis, Reiter's syndrome, is accompanied by urethritis, conjunctivitis, and enthesopathy (i.e., inflamed tendon insertions).

DIFFERENTIAL DIAGNOSIS

Infectious Arthritis

- *Staphylococcus aureus* and streptococci
- Gram-negative organisms (IV drug use, neonatal, older adults)
- Gonococcal arthritis
- Prosthetic joint (coagulase-negative staphylococci)
- Lyme disease
- Septic sacroiliitis
- Viral
- Mycobacterial or fungal

MANAGEMENT

Early initiation of antimicrobial therapy and drainage is required treatment for infectious arthritis. If this condition remains undiagnosed or untreated longer than 5 to 7 days, the prognosis for a functional joint is poor. The initial choice of antibiotic should be sufficiently broad to cover likely sources of infection for an individual, and then the antibiotic may be changed based on the results of the Gram's stain and culture (Table 190-2). Older children and adults do well with nafcillin, oxacillin, or cefazolin, especially if the Gram's stain suggests *S. aureus* and the risk of methicillin-resistant *S. aureus* (MRSA) is low. For patients at high risk for gram-negative septic arthritis (elderly, immunocompromised), cefepime should be considered as an initial broad-spectrum antibiotic.[35] To cover gonococcal arthritis, sexually active young adults should receive ceftriaxone, 1 g IV daily for 7 to 10 days.[36] Pending culture results, infectious arthritis in a prosthetic joint after recent surgery, or in other individuals at risk for MRSA (hemodialysis, diabetes mellitus, nursing home), may require empiric vancomycin to cover the possibility of coagulase-negative staphylococci or MRSA. Aminoglycosides and antipseudomonal β-lactams are sometimes added for synergism in patients who are infected with *S. aureus* or IV drug users in whom *P. aeruginosa* is suspected. Linezolid, daptomycin, and pristinamycin have shown some promise in the treatment of MRSA septic arthritis.[35] It is important to note that aminoglycosides do not work well in abscesses or joints in which the pH is low.[37]

TABLE 190-2 Therapy for Bacterial Arthritis

Infectious Organisms	Therapy*
SEEN ON GRAM'S STAIN	
Gram-positive cocci	
Staphylococcus aureus, Staphylococcus epidermidis, streptococci	Nafcillin or oxacillin
If MRSA or MRSE are likely	Vancomycin
Gram-negative cocci: *Neisseria gonorrhoeae*	Ceftriaxone
Gram-negative bacilli: Enterobacteriaceae, *Haemophilus influenzae*	Piperacillin and aminoglycoside *or* Third-generation cephalosporin
NEGATIVE GRAM STAIN (PENDING CULTURE AND SENSITIVITIES)	
Patient older than 5 years	
S. aureus, group A streptococci	Nafcillin or oxacillin
If MRSA or MRSE likely	Vancomycin
Compromised hosts, older adults	
S. aureus, streptococcal species, gram-negative bacilli	Third-generation cephalosporin *or* Piperacillin-tazobactam
If MRSA or MRSE likely	Add vancomycin
IV drug users: *S. aureus, Pseudomonas* and *Serratia* organisms	Ceftazidime *or* Piperacillin-tazobactam
Sexually active young adult with dermatitis-arthritis syndrome: *N. gonorrhoeae, Neisseria meningitidis*	Ceftriaxone

MRSA, Methicillin-resistant *S. aureus; MRSE,* methicillin-resistant *S. epidermidis.*
*Cefazolin or vancomycin may be substituted for nafcillin in patients who are allergic to penicillin.

Duration of therapy is 2 weeks for *Haemophilus influenzae* and streptococci and 3 weeks for staphylococci or gram-negative bacilli. Shorter courses and oral regimens are often effective in children. Gonococcal arthritis responds quickly and may be treated entirely on an outpatient basis with 2 or 3 days of IV ceftriaxone, followed by early conversion to oral cefixime 400 mg b.i.d. or ciprofloxacin 500 mg b.i.d. to complete a 10- to 14-day course. Patients with underlying rheumatoid arthritis and virulent organisms should be treated for 4 weeks.[38] Newer fluoroquinolones such as gatifloxacin, moxifloxacin, levofloxacin, and trovafloxacin have improved gram-positive coverage. These oral agents may have a possible use in infectious arthritis of adults but are not approved for use in children.[39] Antibiotics have ready access to inflamed joints and should not be given by intraarticular injection or added to solutions for irrigating joints. Antibiotics injected directly into joints may initiate chemical synovitis and prolong postinfectious arthritis.[6]

An infected joint is similar to an abscess that needs daily drainage until the inflammation has resolved. Reactive oxygen species and proteolytic enzymes, which destroy cartilage, are produced by activated leukocytes. Therefore it is important that purulent material and bacterial toxins be removed to preserve cartilage. This is accomplished equally well with either daily arthrocentesis or arthroscopic lavage with placement of drains. Daily arthrocentesis is less expensive and is not complicated by instrumentation morbidity; it also offers the possibility of serial culture and cell counts of synovial fluid to gauge response to therapy. Arthroscopic lavage with debridement and placement of drains or open arthrotomy are appropriate if there is persistence of recurrent effusion and elevation of cell counts after several days of daily arthrocentesis or if loculated fluid is suspected. Hips should be surgically drained at the outset because of their anatomic complexity.[40]

An infected prosthetic joint usually requires drainage, debridement, and removal of all prosthetic components and cement. Even with sensitive organisms, retention of the prosthesis and antibiotic therapy with limited surgical debridement is successful in only about 20% of cases. If revision arthroplasty is attempted at the primary surgery, the success rate is less than 70%. The best approach is a two-step procedure, with removal of prosthesis and cement and 6 weeks of antibiotics followed by revision arthroplasty. An antibiotic-impregnated spacer may be used to maintain the joint space and prevent contracture pending reimplantation of a permanent prosthesis. Six weeks of IV antibiotics are crucial to achieve the 90% success rate.[41]

LIFE SPAN CONSIDERATIONS

Mortality is low when infectious arthritis is diagnosed and treated appropriately. The associated infection carries a significant mortality in older or immunocompromised patients. Toxic shock or a continuing infectious syndrome despite a sterile blood culture is attributable to toxin production by small residual foci of staphylococci or streptococci around dead cartilage or prosthetic joints. There should be no delay in prosthetic joint removal and surgical debridement in the setting of toxic shock or sepsis syndrome, since death may result. Surgery should not be delayed because the problem is typically an abscess, which is unlikely to respond to a continued course of antibiotics.

COMPLICATIONS

Progressive loss of joint function develops in 25% to 50% of patients.[6] A relapse of infectious arthritis may occur if the selection or duration of the antibiotic therapy is inappropriate. Recurrent aseptic joint effusion is common and is referred to as *postinfectious synovitis*. Minor trauma may exacerbate such synovitis. More immediate complications include an associated abscess or bursa infection, which must be drained, and associated osteomyelitis. Ankylosis (fusion), ligamentous instability, and joint contracture are consequences of delayed diagnosis. A total joint arthroplasty can restore mobility in such joints but cannot reverse ligamentous instability or joint contracture. Secondary osteoarthritis is a delayed complication that may require eventual arthroplasty. Some factors that determine outcome are listed in Box 190-1.[42,43]

BOX 190-1

FACTORS AFFECTING OUTCOME IN INFECTIOUS ARTHRITIS

- Delay in diagnosis and treatment beyond 7 days
- Persistently positive culture and effusion after 5 days of treatment
- Prior arthritis, especially rheumatoid arthritis
- Compromised host and older patients
- Virulence of organism: *Staphylococcus aureus* vs. coagulase-negative staphylococci
- Specific joint involved: hips worse than knees
- IV drug use: good prognosis with aggressive organisms
- Appropriate antibiotics
- Effective drainage and debridement
- Physical therapy: initially non–weight bearing, early mobilization, splint contractures

INDICATIONS FOR REFERRAL OR HOSPITALIZATION

A joint infection is a medical emergency. All patients with infectious arthritis should be hospitalized initially because they need to adhere to strict non-weight-bearing activities to preserve cartilage, they require daily aspiration, or they need initial surgical drainage. For patients who have been prescribed bed rest, early mobilization with a passive mobilization device helps prevent adhesions and contractures. Infectious disease, rheumatology, and orthopedic consultations are facilitated when the patient is hospitalized. A physical therapist should be part of the care team, since early mobilization and eventual weight bearing are important. Cartilage has no blood supply and is in part dependent on intermittent compression for nutritional requirements and integrity of structure. It is thus important to try to achieve early mobilization. When the effusion has subsided, early discharge with home IV therapy or oral antibiotics is feasible.

Gonococcal arthritis may, in some cases, be managed as an outpatient. However, gonococcal arthritis may be confused with Reiter's syndrome—a triad of urethritis, conjunctivitis, and arthritis. In the appropriate clinical setting (adequate pretest probability), and if cultures are negative, a rapid response to IV ceftriaxone may be considered diagnostic of gonococcal arthritis. Therefore close observation in a hospital could be essential.[44]

PATIENT AND FAMILY EDUCATION

To remove potential sources of bacteremia, patients should be instructed to be certain that any necessary dental work is done and wounds or ulcers healed before undergoing a total joint arthroplasty. Antibiotic prophylaxis before surgery for total joint arthroplasty is advised to prevent postsurgical infectious arthritis, but prophylaxis before dental work is not advised unless otherwise indicated by the patient's status.[45] Patients with rheumatoid arthritis should be aware that superimposed infectious arthritis is possible. They should disclose any monoarticular flare to their physician for early diagnostic arthrocentesis. Cellulitis, wounds, and ulcers should receive prompt medical attention to prevent bacteremia. Patients recovering from infectious arthritis must be instructed in home physical therapy to prevent contracture and to advance weight bearing after inflammation has subsided. The potential side effects of antibiotics need to be explained, antibiotic-associated diarrhea should be anticipated, and patients with indwelling central lines must be instructed in line care and signs of line infection.

REFERENCES

1. Gillespie WJ: Epidemiology in bone and joint infection, *Infect Dis Clin North Am* 4(3):361-376, 1990.
2. Nade S: Septic arthritis, *Best Pract Res Clin Rheum* 17(2):183-200, 2003.
3. Pioro MH, Mandell BF: Septic arthritis, *Rheum Dis Clin North Am* 23(2):239-258, 1997.
4. Garcia-De La Torre I: Advances in the management of septic arthritis, *Rheum Dis Clin North Am* 29:61-75, 2003.
5. Lowy FD: *Staphylococcus aureus* infections, *N Engl J Med* 339(8):520-532, 1998.
6. Goldenberg DL: Septic arthritis, *Lancet* 351:197-202, 1998.
7. Rice PA: Gonococcal arthritis (disseminated gonococcal infection), *Infect Dis Clin North Am* 19:853-861, 2005.
8. Blackburn WD: Gram-negative septic arthritis. In Espinoza L, editor: *Infections in the rheumatic diseases: a comprehensive review of microbial relations to rheumatic disorders,* Orlando, Fla, 1988, Grune & Stratton.
9. Collo MC, Johnson JL, Finch WR, and others: Evaluating arthritic complaints, *Nurse Pract* 16(2):9-14, 17-18, 20, 1991.
10. Gilliland WR: *Bacterial septic arthritis.* In West SG, editor: *Rheumatology secrets*, ed 2, Philadelphia, 2002, Hanley & Belfus.
11. Inflammation and repair. In Cotran RS, Kumar V, Robbins SL, editors: *Robbins pathologic basis of disease,* ed 4, Philadelphia, 1989, Saunders.
12. Cucurull E, Espinoza LR: Gonococcal arthritis, *Rheum Dis Clin North Am* 24(2):305-322, 1998.
13. Liebling MR, Arkfeld DG, Michelini GA, and others: Identification of *Neisseria gonorrhoeae* in synovial fluid using the polymerase chain reaction, *Arthritis Rheum* 37(5):702-709, 1994.
14. Goldenberg DL: Gonococcal arthritis. In Espinoza L, editor: *Infections in the rheumatic diseases: a comprehensive review of microbial relations to rheumatic disorders,* Orlando, Fla, 1988, Grune & Stratton.
15. Zimmerli W: Prosthetic-joint infections, *N Engl J Med* 351(16):1645-1654, 2004.
16. Gillespie WJ: Infection in total joint replacement, *Infect Dis Clin North Am* 4:465-484, 1990.
17. Smith SL, Wastie ML, Forster I: Radionuclide bone scintigraphy in the detection of significant complications after total knee joint replacement, *Clin Radiol* 56:221, 2001.
18. Brause BD: Infections with prostheses in bones and joints. In Nundell GL, Bennett JE, Dolin J, editors: *Principles and practice of infectious diseases*, ed 4, New York, 1995, Churchill Livingstone.
19. Sia IG, Berbari EF, Karchmer AW: Prosthetic joint infections, *Infect Dis Clin North Am* 19(4):885-914, 2005.
20. Sigal LH: Musculoskeletal manifestations of Lyme arthritis, *Rheum Dis Clin North Am* 24(2):323-351, 1998.
21. Steere AC: Lyme disease, *N Engl J Med* 345(2):115-123, 2001.
22. Steere AC, Taylor E, McHugh GL, and others: The overdiagnosis of Lyme disease, *JAMA* 269(14):1812-1816, 1993.
23. Steere AC: Musculoskeletal manifestations of Lyme disease, *Am J Med* 98(4A):44S-51S, 1995.
24. Brancos MA, Peris P, Miro JM, and others: Septic arthritis in heroin addicts, *Semin Arthritis Rheum* 21(2):81-87, 1991.
25. Gordon RJ, Lowy FD: Bacterial infections in drug users, *N Engl J Med* 353(18):1945-1954, 2005.
26. Ferraro K, Cohen MA: Acute septic sacroiliitis in an injection drug user, *Am J Emerg Med* 22(1):60-61, 2004.
27. Zimmerman B, Mikolich DJ, Lally EV: Septic sacroiliitis, *Semin Arthritis Rheum* 26:592-604, 1996.
28. Smith JW: Infectious arthritis, *Infect Dis Clin North Am* 4(3):523-537, 1990.
29. Goldenberg DL: The evaluation of patients with bacterial arthritis nongonococcal. In Espinoza L, editor: *Infections in the rheumatic diseases: a comprehensive review of microbial relations to rheumatic disorders*, Orlando, Fla, 1988, Grune & Stratton.
30. Baer PA, Tenenbaum J, Fam AG, and others: Coexistent septic and crystal arthritis. Report of four cases and literature review, *J Rheumatol* 13(3):604-607, 1986.
31. Ranjan R, Matei D, Kaufman L: Emphysematous septic arthritis: case report and review of the literature, *J Rheumatol* 22:1776-1778, 1995.
32. Sutter CW, Shelton DK: Three-phase bone scan in osteomyelitis and other musculoskeletal disorders, *Am Fam Phys* 54:1639-1647, 1996.
33. Greenspan A, Tehranzadeh J: Imaging of infectious arthritis, *Radiol Clin North Am* 39(2):267-276, 2001.
34. Dubost JJ, Fis I, Denis P, and others: Polyarticular septic arthritis, *Medicine* 72(5):296-310, 1993.
35. Ross JJ: Septic arthritis, *Infect Dis Clin North Am* 19(4):799-817, 2005.
36. Wise CM, Morris CR, Wasilauskas BL, and others: Gonococcal arthritis in an era of increasing penicillin resistance. Presentations and outcomes in 41 recent cases (1985-1991), *Arch Intern Med* 154(23):2690-2695, 1994.
37. Hamed KA, Tami Y, Proloer CG: Pharmacokinetic optimization of the treatment of septic arthritis, *Clin Pharmacokinet* 31:156-163, 1996.
38. Nolla JM, Gomez-Vaquero C, Fiter J, and others: Pyarthrosis in patients with rheumatoid arthritis: a detailed analysis of 10 cases and literature review, *Semin Arthritis Rheum* 30(2):121-126, 2000.
39. Wuldvogel FN: Use of quinolones for the treatment of osteomyelitis and septic arthritis, *Rev Infect Dis* 11(Suppl 5):S1259-S1263, 1989.
40. Redfield D, Hayes T: Orthopedic infections, *Crit Care Nurs Q* 21(2):24-35, 1998.
41. Harris JM: Orthopedic aspects of septic arthritis. In Espinoza L, editor: *Infections in the rheumatic diseases: a comprehensive review of microbial relations to rheumatic disorders,* Orlando, Fla, 1988, Grune & Stratton.
42. Esterhal JL, Gello I: Adult septic arthritis, *Orthop Clin North Am* 22:503-514, 1991.
43. Kaandorp CJ, Krijnen P, Moens HJ, and others: The outcome of bacterial arthritis: a prospective community-based study, *Arthritis Rheum* 40(5):884-892, 1997.
44. Keat H: Sexually transmitted arthritis syndromes, *Med Clin North Am* 74:1617-1631, 1990.
45. Wahl MJ: Myths of dental-induced prosthetic joint infections, *Clin Infect Dis* 20:1420-1425, 1995.

CHAPTER 191

Knee Pain

Marie-Eileen Onieal

DEFINITION AND EPIDEMIOLOGY

About 10.8 million visits are made to health care provider offices because of a knee problem. It is the most often treated anatomic site by orthopedic surgeons.[1] The multiple structures within the knee make it vulnerable to various types of injuries and degenerative change. Many injuries can be treated conservatively; others require surgery. There also are many extra-articular structures that can become inflamed or injured, causing knee pain.

Musculoskeletal injuries are usually sport specific rather than gender specific; however, anatomic differences can contribute to susceptibility to injury. Injuries to the anterior cruciate ligament (ACL), for example, often occur in soccer, basketball, and volleyball participants. Data collected since 1995 demonstrate that men and women who participate in the same sport have different ACL injury patterns. The incidence of ACL injuries among women basketball players is twice that for men, and female soccer players are four times more likely to experience an ACL tear than their male counterparts. Both women and men incur ACL injuries in noncontact situations. Nearly 60% of ACL injuries in female basketball players occur when landing from a jump.[1]

Knee Pain

The knee is a modified hinge joint that has some rotational mobility when flexed. The knee joint contains three bones, three articulations, five major tendons, four major ligaments, and two menisci. The lateral and medial articulations are between the femoral and tibial condyles. The intermediate articulation is between the patella and the femur. A relatively weak joint, the knee gains its strength from the strong ligaments that attach the femur to the tibia. Five intrinsic ligaments assist in strengthening the articular capsule. The cruciate ligaments connect the femur and tibia within the articular capsule, crossing each other in the form of an X.

As a major weight-bearing joint, the knee is susceptible to many injuries. Torsion is limited in the joint, and any motion that extends beyond the defined range results in a ligamentous injury. Because the knee depends on the integrity of the ligaments to provide its stability, a knee injury can be a calamitous event.

Collateral Ligament Sprains

There are two collateral ligaments: the medial collateral ligament (MCL) and the lateral collateral ligament (LCL). The MCL attaches to the medial condyle of the femur and the tibia. The LCL attaches to the lateral femoral condyle and extends to the lateral tibial plateau. The MCL and the LCL are injured when valgus (MCL) or varus (LCL) stress to the joint extends beyond the normal range of motion. MCL injuries are more common and often include an injury to the medial meniscus. Football players and skiers are more prone to ligamentous injuries, but they can occur just as easily on the dance floor or in the bathroom.

PATHOPHYSIOLOGY

A wrenching motion of the knee while the foot stays firmly planted causes injury to the MCL. In these injuries the knee is in flexion and in slight internal rotation. LCL injuries occur when the varus stress applied to the knee causes a "bend" toward the outside.[2,3] The injuries are graded as first-, second-, or third-degree sprains (Table 191-1).

CLINICAL PRESENTATION

The knee is painful and often swollen and may or may not be ecchymotic over the body of the ligament. Some patients report a feeling that the knee "bent the wrong way" and that the knee became edematous within 20 to 30 minutes. More rapid swelling is an ominous sign.[2]

PHYSICAL EXAMINATION

An examination immediately after the injury is easier and helps to ascertain the severity of the injury. Examination of the knee is more difficult once the joint swells. Both knees should be observed for edema, deformity, muscle atrophy, and patella placement. Fluctuance should be determined with patient first standing and then supine. Tenderness and bony landmarks should be ascertained as well. In the suspected collateral

TABLE 191-1 Collateral Ligament Sprains

First Degree	Second Degree	Third Degree
PATHOLOGY		
Ligament fibers attached	Partial avulsion of fibers from femoral condyle	Complete rupture of ligament (often associated with anterior or posterior cruciate ligament tears or tibial plateau fractures)
FINDINGS		
Tenderness along body of ligament Minimum to no swelling	Pain at joint line of ligament insertion Swelling with tenderness localized to attachment point	Significant pain at ligament insertion and joint line Significant swelling with ecchymosis
No joint widening with ligament stress	Slight to moderate increase in joint widening with stress	Increased joint widening with minimum stress

ligament sprain, there is tenderness along the body of the ligament, and point tenderness at the attachment site is commonly present. In the MCL injury, there may be tenderness at the medial joint line because the MCL attaches to the medial meniscus. Pain at the lateral joint line is equivalent to a joint injury.

Varus or valgus stress on the knee joint determines joint laxity (Figure 191-1). Active range of motion in extension and flexion should be assessed. If active range of motion is not possible, passive extension and flexion should be determined. The unaffected knee should always be examined first to establish the baseline and to allay any anxiety about the evaluation.

DIAGNOSTICS

Plain radiographs exclude fractures and dislocations. More extensive radiologic examinations, such as stress films, CT scans, and MRIs, should be considered in consultation with an orthopedist. It is important to note that in the acutely swollen joint, MRIs are often inconclusive.

A

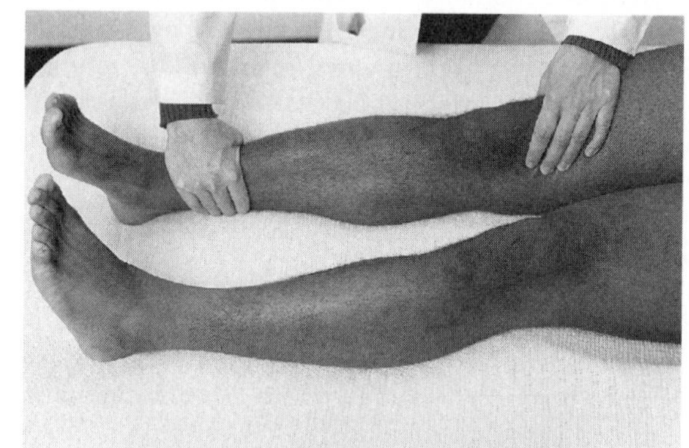

B

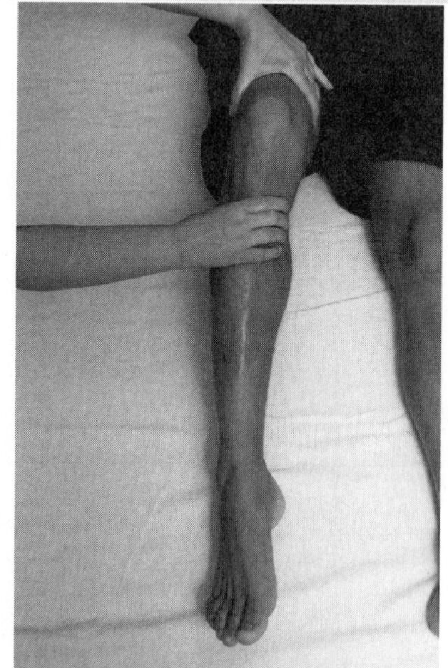

FIGURE 191-1

Varus and valgus stress test of the knee. A, Knee extended. B, Knee flexed. (From Seidel HM: *Mosby's guide to physical examination*, ed 4, St Louis, 1999, Mosby.)

DIAGNOSTICS

Knee Pain

IMAGING	OTHER
X-rays (anteroposterior, lateral, sunrise)	Joint aspiration (e.g., for cell count) if other cause is suspected*
CT scan, MRI*	

*If indicated.

DIFFERENTIAL DIAGNOSIS

As with any joint injury, a fracture or dislocation must be considered. In the knee, consider an ACL or a posterior cruciate ligament (PCL) injury as well.

MANAGEMENT

Isolated first- and second-degree sprains can be managed with RICE (rest, ice, compression [or immobilization], and elevation). If the knee is unstable, an external knee immobilizer is worn at all times. The patient should avoid weight bearing on a swollen or acutely painful knee. Simple straight leg raises and quadriceps-tightening exercises, as well as adductor-strengthening exercises, can be done, even in the immobilizer. Once the swelling and pain subside, a more progressive rehabilitation program should begin.

COMPLICATIONS

Without accurate diagnosis and treatment, the injury can extend, jeopardizing the joint's stability and other structures. The incompletely rehabilitated knee will be weak and potentially unstable. Traumatic arthritis can be a sequela in any joint injury.

INDICATIONS FOR REFERRAL OR HOSPITALIZATION

All severe sprains and fractures should be referred to an orthopedist. Referral to a physical therapist should be considered to assist in complete rehabilitation.

PATIENT AND FAMILY EDUCATION

Explanation of the importance of adherence to the rehabilitative process is imperative. In some instances a knee support for sports is necessary. Pain and swelling are indicators that the knee is being overstressed or has been reinjured.

DIFFERENTIAL DIAGNOSIS

Knee Pain

- Collateral ligament sprains
- Cruciate ligament injury
- Meniscus injuries
- Fracture
- Dislocation
- Effusion
- Hemarthrosis
- Arthritis
- Bursitis
- Synovitis
- Abscess
- Ruptured muscle
- Chondromalacia patellae

CRUCIATE LIGAMENT INJURIES

DEFINITION AND EPIDEMIOLOGY

There are two cruciate ligaments: the ACL and the PCL. The ACL attaches to the anterior part of the intercondylar area of the tibia, posterior to the medial meniscus, and rises superiorly, posteriorly, and laterally to attach to the posterior section of the medial side of the lateral condyle of the femur. The ACL restrains the anterior-to-posterior alignment of the knee, keeping the proper relationship of the femur to the tibia. It is loose with the knee in flexion and tight when the knee is fully extended. It is the weaker of the two cruciate ligaments.

The PCL originates at the posterior part of the intercondylar area of the tibia. It crosses superiorly and anteriorly on the medial side of the ACL and attaches to the anterior part of the lateral surface of the medial femoral condyle. The PCL is tight with the knee in flexion.

A cruciate ligament injury can be a sprain, a partial tear, or a complete disruption of the ligament. Physical examination and radiologic tests as indicated are used to determine the degree of the injury. The ACL is the most commonly involved structure in severe knee injuries. In 70% of patients seen with acute, traumatic hemarthrosis, it is the injured structure.[4] The PCL is less often injured.[2]

PATHOPHYSIOLOGY

The PCL is the stronger ligament and is usually injured through trauma to the anterior surface of the proximal tibia (as in hitting the dashboard).[4] The ACL injury often occurs in combination with ruptures of the MCL and the medial meniscus (O'Donaghue's triad). Once the ligament is torn, the knee is unstable. Swelling occurs rapidly in an ACL or PCL injury because of bleeding from the ligament tear.[5]

CLINICAL PRESENTATION

The patient often recalls hearing a "pop" or feeling the knee "snap" and has an instantaneous sensation of something being "terribly wrong." Pain from the injury prevents a return to the activity. Patients report a distrust of the knee during activities and that the knee "gives out," especially during exertion.

PHYSICAL EXAMINATION

The knee is swollen, and the patient is unable to fully flex or extend the knee. Four standard tests ascertain the integrity of the ligaments. Hamstring spasms and the posterior horn of the meniscus can stabilize the knee, falsely indicating a stable joint; thus it is important for the patient to relax. The normal knee should be examined first to allay anxiety and to establish a baseline, since most people have some degree of laxity in the ligaments.

Lachman's test is used to assess the ACL. The knee should be flexed to about 15 to 30 degrees. One hand is placed just below the knee joint on the posterior aspect of the tibia-fibula. The other hand is placed on the anterior aspect of the femur just above the joint. The examiner lifts up the lower leg while pushing down on the upper leg. If the ACL is intact, the examiner should feel a "knock" or a firm "stop" as the ACL prevents the tibia from sliding forward. In the absence of a firm end point, a ligament tear should be suspected.

The anterior drawer test also is used to assess the ACL (Figure 191-2). The knee should be flexed to about 90 degrees, with the foot kept flat on the examination surface. The examiner sits on the patient's foot and firmly grasps the lower leg, placing the fingers below the popliteal space and the thumbs on the tibial tuberosity. The examiner pulls gently but firmly on the tibia, attempting to slide the tibia forward. A "soft" or absent end point indicates a tear.[3,6]

The posterior drawer test also is used to assess the PCL (see Figure 191-2). With the patient positioned the same as in the anterior drawer test, the examiner pushes posteriorly on the tibia. A torn PCL allows the tibia to slide backward.[6]

The pivot shift test also is used to assess the ACL. It is a more difficult test to master. The examiner grabs the lower leg, flexes the knee, and pushes down on the tibia while flexing and extending the knee. If the ACL is torn, the bones shift erratically with this maneuver.

DIAGNOSTICS

X-ray studies of the knee are indicated. Plain films demonstrate effusions, loose bodies, and avulsion fractures. Segond's fracture, an avulsion of the lateral aspect of the tibial plateau, is pathognomonic of an ACL tear. MRI provides a definitive evaluation of the ligaments.

DIFFERENTIAL DIAGNOSIS

As with any knee injury, damage to other intraarticular structures must be considered. Fracture-dislocations are included in the differential diagnosis.

MANAGEMENT

The degree of the tear with or without instability guides the treatment plan. Partial tears and tears without a concurrent fracture or meniscus tear can often be managed conservatively.[7] An acutely injured knee requires immobilization to decrease swelling and pain. Weight bearing on the affected knee should be avoided. The quadriceps muscle begins to

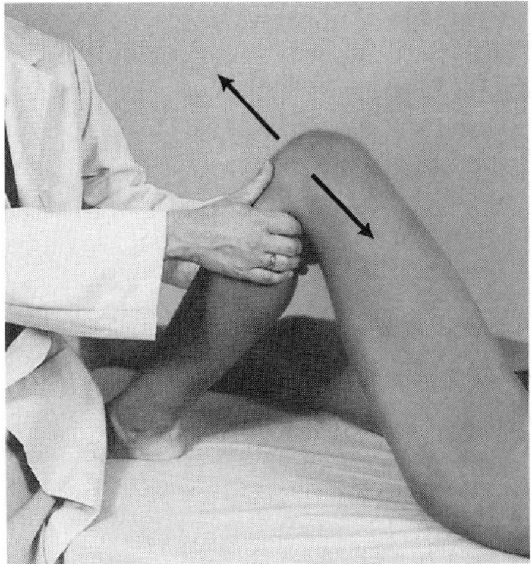

FIGURE 191-2

Drawer test for anterior and posterior stability of the knee. (From Barkauskas VH, Baumann L, Darling-Fisher C: *Health and physical assessment*, ed 2, St Louis, 1998, Mosby.)

atrophy quickly with inactivity; therefore strengthening exercises should begin as tolerated, starting with the simple straight leg raise. The quadriceps muscles are adjunct stabilizers to the ACL, and rehabilitation should stress regaining full range of motion and strength.[2,3]

COMPLICATIONS

The patient with an unstable knee is in jeopardy of fracture; aggravation of the initial injury; or falls as a result of the instability, resulting in other injuries. A knee that has sustained severe trauma is susceptible to the development of arthritis.

INDICATIONS FOR REFERRAL OR HOSPITALIZATION

All persons who have sustained an injury to the cruciate ligaments require an evaluation by an orthopedic surgeon. The timing of surgical repair is controversial, and many patients function normally without surgery.

PATIENT AND FAMILY EDUCATION

It is important for the patient to understand that, despite reconstruction and rehabilitation, the knee is never perfectly normal. The knee can be functional but in some cases will require the use of a custom-made brace.[5]

MENISCUS INJURIES

DEFINITION AND EPIDEMIOLOGY

The menisci are crescent-shaped fibrocartilaginous structures on the articular surface of the tibia. They act as shock absorbers for the knee and help control normal knee motion. Meniscus tears are the third most common of all knee injuries. The medial meniscus is injured or torn more often than the lateral meniscus because of its structure, mobility, and attachment.

PATHOPHYSIOLOGY

The menisci maintain the space between the bones in the knee joint. They are injured when the knee is twisted while in the flexed position. The femur compresses against the tibia and grinds against the meniscus. This grinding motion tears the meniscus as the force exceeds the strength of the fibrocartilage. Once torn, the menisci cannot heal. Menisci tear as a direct result of injury or indirectly as a result of the normal wear and tear on the knee.

CLINICAL PRESENTATION

In an acute injury, joint effusion is always present. There is tenderness along the joint line, and often the person has a sense of instability. Those with a degenerative tear will complain of joint line discomfort and a sense of locking or giving way, especially on descending stairs or walking on uneven surfaces.

PHYSICAL EXAMINATION

Along with effusion in the acute state, quadriceps atrophy is often evident. The joint is stable, but palpating the joint line produces tenderness. McMurray's test helps to ascertain a tear in the cartilage. To perform McMurray's test, the examiner has the patient lie supine with the legs straight. The examiner firmly grasps the heel or ankle with one hand and places the other hand on the knee joint, with the fingers on the medial side and the thumb at the lateral side. The examiner flexes the knee while rotating the tibia internally and externally on the femur. This maneuver will loosen the joint. Then, while flexing and externally rotating the leg, the examiner applies valgus stress to the lateral side of the knee. The examiner holds the valgus stress on the joint while extending the leg and palpating the medial joint line. If a "click" or "pop" is heard or felt, the medial meniscus is torn.

McMurray's test can also be performed with the patient in a sitting position and the knee flexed to 90 degrees (Figure 191-3). The patient should internally rotate the affected leg while the practitioner slowly extends the leg. While performing the maneuver, the practitioner should apply resistance to the knee medially to test the medial meniscus. The practitioner should repeat the maneuver, applying resistance to the knee laterally to test the lateral meniscus. The test is positive if the knee cannot be extended.

In addition to McMurray's test, a simpler test is Apley's compression test (Figure 191-4). This test should be done with the patient prone and the affected leg flexed to 90 degrees. The examiner places his or her knee on the patient's posterior thigh to stabilize it, grabs the foot firmly, leans on the heel to squeeze the menisci between the femur and the tibia, and rotates the tibia. If pain is elicited, there is a tear in the meniscus. The patient should be asked to describe the location of the pain to distinguish a medial meniscus tear from a lateral meniscus tear.

DIAGNOSTICS

The definitive diagnostic test is MRI. Plain films should be obtained to exclude any bony abnormalities.

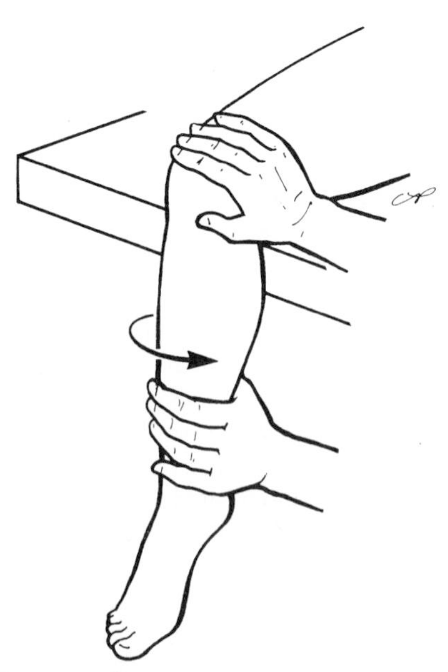

FIGURE 191-3

McMurray's test of the knee. (From Barkauskas VH, Baumann L, Darling-Fisher C: *Health and physical assessment,* ed 2, St Louis, 1998, Mosby.)

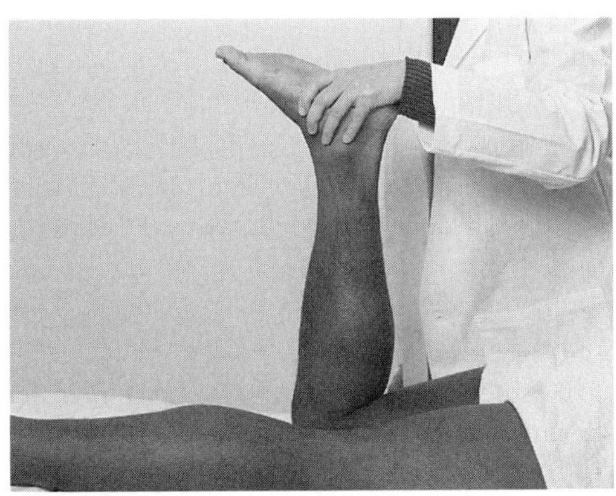

FIGURE 191-4

Apley's assessment of the knee. (From Seidel HM: *Mosby's guide to physical examination,* ed 4, St Louis, 1999, Mosby.)

DIFFERENTIAL DIAGNOSIS

Many times the patient has a sense of joint instability in addition to joint line tenderness; thus the potential for fracture or other structural injury must be considered.

MANAGEMENT

With a minor tear in the meniscus, the treatment is usually conservative. RICE and the use of crutches help quiet the acute phase. Rehabilitation to improve the strength of the quadriceps muscle is imperative. Straight leg raises with the knee in extension, but not locked, can be started immediately and weight bearing gradually increased. Non-weight-bearing activities such as swimming and riding a stationary bicycle are excellent for increasing range of motion and strength.

COMPLICATIONS

Articular damage from the meniscus tear may result in arthritis (see Chapter 194). Because the menisci are stabilizers for the knee, loss of their integrity can lead to more extensive injuries.

INDICATIONS FOR REFERRAL OR HOSPITALIZATION

Orthopedic referral is necessary for patients with persistent locking or swelling in the knee. An orthopedic surgeon or sports medicine specialist should be consulted when persistent effusions do not resolve or respond to conservative measures.

PATIENT AND FAMILY EDUCATION

Maintaining quadriceps strength is essential to minimize the disabilities associated with this injury. Although the knee may not be 100% normal, participation in sports with proper warm-up and equipment can be enjoyed. Achiness and swelling after a particularly strenuous workout or game can be normal. Ice and NSAIDs can help control the symptoms. A patient with persistent swelling, pain, or episodes of instability should be reevaluated.

INFLAMMATORY AND DEGENERATIVE DISORDERS

As people age or become deconditioned as a result of chronic injury or disease, knee pain can be caused by a variety of inflammatory, extraarticular conditions and by age-related degeneration. Anserine bursitis is commonly seen in middle-aged women with osteoarthritis of the knee and a valgus deformity. This disorder produces pain and tenderness over the medial aspect of the knee about 5 cm (2 inches) below the joint line. Obvious swelling is not uncommon. Anserine bursitis is treated conservatively with ice and NSAIDs, but steroid injections may be necessary to alleviate pain in particularly severe cases.

Prepatellar bursitis ("housemaid's knee") manifests as a swelling superficial to the patella. This condition results from trauma such as that which occurs with frequent kneeling and is seen commonly in persons who work on their knees, such as floor or carpet layers. Pain is mild unless direct pressure is applied over the bursa, and there is no pain with weight bearing or range of motion of the knee. The condition is treated with rest, ice, and NSAIDs and is prevented by protecting the knee from repeated trauma.

Popliteal cysts (Baker's cysts) are commonly seen in conjunction with rheumatoid arthritis, osteoarthritis, or internal derangements of the knee. Initially a cystic swelling in the popliteal space may be the only finding. As the cyst increases in size, the possibility of rupture increases. A ruptured cyst will drain into the calf, causing pain, erythema, and swelling, mimicking phlebitis. An ultrasound examination will provide a definitive diagnosis of this condition.

Osteoarthritis is probably the most common cause of knee pain in the older population (see Chapter 194). Pain, stiffness, and decreased function are all cardinal signs. Pain is generally insidious in onset and characterized as mild to moderate. Resting the knee usually alleviates the pain. Osteoarthritis is progressive, and the cartilage damage is permanent. However, conservative treatment, including muscle strengthening, weight loss, analgesics, and NSAIDs, is often effective. Injections of steroids or hyaluronan may provide temporary relief. Severe disease, manifested by resting or night pain and increasing difficulty with ambulation, may require joint replacement surgery.

REFERENCES

1. American Academy of Orthopaedic Surgeons: *Your orthopedic connection,* retrieved Oct 12, 2005, from http://orthoinfo.aaos.org/fact/thr_report.cfm?Thread_ID=88&topcategory=.
2. Schenck R, editor: *Athletic training and sports medicine,* ed 2, Park Ridge, Ill, 1991, American Academy of Orthopaedic Surgeons.
3. American Academy of Orthopaedic Surgeons, American Academy of Pediatrics, Griffin LY, editor: *Essentials of musculoskeletal care,* ed 3, Rosemont, Ill, 2005, American Academy of Orthopaedic Surgeons.
4. Gough JE, Rodriguez LE: Knee injuries. In Wolfson AB, Hendy GW, Hendry PL, and others, editors: *Harwood-Nuss' clinical practice of emergency medicine,* ed 4, Philadelphia, 2005, Lippincott Williams & Wilkins.
5. Levin S: ACL reconstruction: the best treatment option? *Phys Sportsmed* 20:141-161, 1992.
6. Mooar PA: The thigh, knee and patella. In Gates SJ, Mooar PA, editors: *Orthopaedics and sports medicine for nurses: common problems in management,* Baltimore, 1989, Williams & Wilkins.
7. Klippel JH: *Primer on the rheumatic diseases,* ed 12, Atlanta, 2001, Arthritis Foundation.

CHAPTER 192

Low Back Pain

Michele DuBois Finnell

DEFINITION AND EPIDEMIOLOGY

Low back pain (LBP) is one of the most common complaints of patients seen in ambulatory care settings. Between 65% and 80% of the world's population develop back pain at some point during their lives.[1] The risk is increased when the individual is involved in an occupation that requires either prolonged sitting or excessive, repetitive lifting, bending, twisting, or reaching. The most common causes of LBP are ligamentous-muscular injury, degeneration of the spine (osteoarthritis or spondylolysis), and disc herniation. Older individuals may develop spinal stenosis (narrowing of the spinal canal often caused by bone spurs) or spondylolisthesis (slipping of one vertebra over another).

LBP is commonly associated with overuse or an incompetence of the soft tissue structures. Acute LBP is pain that persists for less than 3 weeks, and chronic LBP is defined as that lasting longer than 7 weeks.[2]

LBP is a problem of great magnitude, second only to headache as the most common complaint of pain. Chronic impairment of the back and spine is the most common cause of physical disability in adults younger than 45 years in the United States.[3] At any given time, 31 million Americans will be experiencing some sort of LBP. It is one of the most common causes of disability and lost work time. Although men reportedly have a higher incidence of back pain over their lifetime, women now represent more than 60% of the workforce, and their incidence of back pain will eventually equal that of the men. In addition, a woman's likelihood of experiencing LBP is increased after two or more pregnancies.[4] Back pain in nurses younger than 45 years represents the number one cause of disability in this professional group.[5]

Physician consultation is indicated if back pain is associated with a neurologic deficit, decreased or absent pulses, or bowel or bladder dysfunction.

PATHOPHYSIOLOGY

Structurally, the posterior longitudinal ligaments and opposing anterior longitudinal ligaments, in addition to the supraspinous and interspinous ligaments, provide spinal support at the surface of the vertebral column. In fact, the integrity of the spinous processes is maintained by the interlocking of the facet joints in the vertebral column. The spinal column houses the spinal nerves and is cushioned by the intravertebral discs.[6]

Discerning the source of the back pain may be a challenge to the health care provider because the source is often masked by the reaction of the varied tissues. Degenerative changes in the disc are responsible for most of the pathophysiologic changes of LBP. The impact of stress at the lumbosacral area varies with positioning. The exact amount of pressure being delivered to the area with varied loads shows the vulnerability of this area. The difference in pressure in L3 and L4 discs varies with positioning. There is an increase in pressure of more than 43% between sitting upright or standing compared with being in the supine position.

With repetitive stress, disruption of the muscle fibers or attachments of the ligaments may occur. Injuries such as these will result in bleeding or spasm, causing tenderness and swelling of the affected areas.

As the disc weakens, it may bulge, causing irritation of a nerve root, generally at or below the level of herniation. This results in radicular (sciatic) pain, described as a burning, sharp, intense, or stabbing pain evolving from either the lumbar or sacral area. Radicular pain is worsened by activities that increase intraabdominal pressure, such as coughing, sneezing, or straining at stool. Pain radiating down one or both legs is suggestive of nerve root irritation and is highly sensitive for disc herniation. With radiation to the buttocks, it can also be suggestive of spinal stenosis. The pain may be due to the direct compression of either the dural sac or the nerve root exiting from the involved area. Stenosis will impede flow of cerebrospinal fluid; standing does not provide relief, but sitting or bending forward will because the spinal canal size is increased with this maneuver. Incidental findings of stenosis on x-ray studies or CT scans must be correlated with clinical findings because older patients may have claudication resulting from either peripheral vascular disease or spinal stenosis. Surgery may be indicated after conservative measures fail and disabling pain escalates.[7]

Neurogenic claudication may be present and described as numbness and weakness with activity. This must be differentiated from vascular claudication, which is associated with decreases in peripheral pulses. If bowel or bladder incontinence is reported, immediate evaluation is essential to exclude cauda equina syndrome, which suggests involvement of the S2-4 nerve roots.

CLINICAL PRESENTATION

A complete medical history, including the chief complaint, history of the present illness, past medical history, family history, occupational and social history, and a review of systems, is essential if an injury has precipitated the LBP. It is important to understand the mechanism of injury, which can be achieved with a complete symptom analysis (Box 192-1).

The symptom analysis (e.g., fever, bowel or bladder dysfunction, saddle anesthesia, persistent pain unresponsive to bed rest), when used properly, will provide a wealth of information about the patient's condition. A history of recent trauma, cancer, recent lumbar puncture, concurrent infection, or chronic use of high-dose corticosteroids will help establish an accurate diagnosis.

PHYSICAL EXAMINATION

It is important to evaluate the patient during activity and in several positions. Gait should be observed as the patient walks into the examination room. The examiner should watch for an antalgic gait, foot drop, a widened base of support, joint instability, and posture.

Symmetry of musculature, obvious curvature, and loss of lordosis are assessed with the patient standing. Curvature of the spine does not usually cause back pain, and loss of lordosis

BOX 192-1

SYMPTOM ANALYSIS

Onset: When did the back pain start? What precipitated the pain? Was there an injury? Sudden onset or chronic? Prior history? What treatment has been tried in the past? Does it help? Is it better now, or when it started?
Quality: What is the pain like? Describe it.
Quantity, severity: Rate the pain on a 0 to 10 scale now and when it first started.
Consistency: When does the pain occur? Does it awaken you from sleep? Does it get better with rest?
Location: Point to where the pain is. Does it move? Does it get better with sitting? With standing?
Timing: Is the pain constant? Cyclic? Intermittent? How long does each episode of back pain last?
Aggravating or alleviating symptoms: What makes the pain worse? What makes it better?
Associated symptoms: Any bowel or bladder problems? Any numbness or tingling in extremities?
Present status: Current symptoms? Currently working? What type of work? What other activities are you involved with in your personal life (e.g., taking care of children, elders, house work, weight lifting)?

Nerve root	L4	L5	S1
Pain			
Numbness			
Motor weakness	Extension of quadriceps	Dorsiflexion of great toe and foot	Plantar flexion of great toe and foot
Screening examination	Squat and rise	Heel walking	Walking on toes
Reflexes	Knee jerk diminished	None reliable	Ankle jerk diminished

FIGURE 192-1

Reflex testing. (From Nordin M, Andersson GBJ, Pope MH: *Musculoskeletal disorders in the workplace: principles and practice,* St Louis, 1997, Mosby.)

is often caused by muscle spasm. The spinous processes, sacroiliac joint, sciatic notch, and paraspinal musculature should be palpated to assess for focal tenderness and spasm.

Range of motion and flexibility, including the ability to perform lateral bends, back extension, and toe touches, are examined. Partial assessment of lower extremity strength can be accomplished by asking the patient to walk on his or her heels (anterior tibialis, L4) and toes (gastrocnemius, S1), in addition to tandem walking to assess hip girdle stability.

Motor strength is assessed by testing hip flexor strength (T12-L3), quadriceps strength (L2-4), and hamstring strength (L5-S1), as well as hip abductor (L5) and adductor (L2-4) muscle groups. Comparison of strength from one side to the other is important; the two sides should be equal. Sensation to light touch and pinprick and deep tendon reflexes (DTRs) should also be assessed[8] (Figure 192-1). DTRs are almost always symmetric; however, asymmetric reflexes may be normal for that patient based on a history of previous trauma. It is also helpful to use augmentation (distraction) techniques when testing reflexes to truly assess their presence or absence. Documentation of DTRs with augmentation is essential.[9]

Before examining the patient in a supine position, the examiner should perform a straight leg raise (SLR) with the patient in the sitting position. If the sciatic nerve is irritated, the SLR test will be positive in both the sitting and lying positions (Figure 192-2). The SLR test by itself does not indicate significant nerve root tension or irritation. Pain below the knee at less than 70 degrees of SLR that is aggravated by ankle dorsiflexion or extension and rotation of the limb is suggestive of L5-S1 nerve root tension related to disc herniation. Crossover pain is a stronger indicator of nerve root compression than SLR pain on the affected side. Ninety percent of radiculopathy caused by lumbosacral disc herniation involves nerve roots L4, L5, or S1 at the L4, L5, or S1 disc level.[2,10]

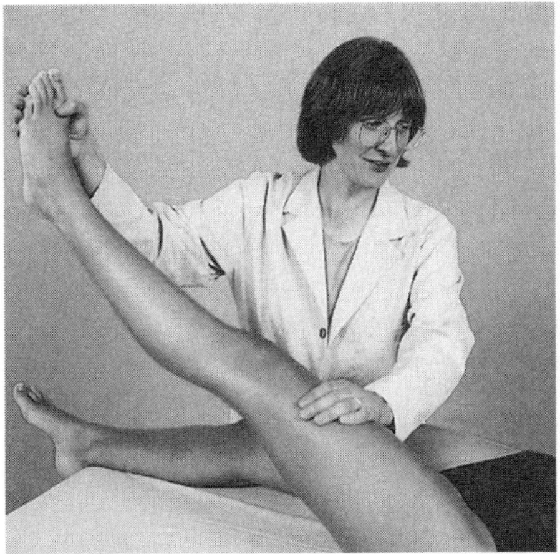

FIGURE 192-2

Straight leg raising test (supine position). (From Barkauskas VH, Baumann L, Darling-Fisher C: *Health and physical assessment,* ed 2, St Louis, 1998, Mosby.)

With the patient in the supine position, the examiner should inspect the lower extremity for passive range of motion. If range of motion is painful without stretching the sciatic nerve, osteoarthritis should be considered in the differential diagnosis. A positive SLR test in both the sitting and lying positions suggests nerve root tension or irritation, which may be caused by a herniated disc. If bladder or bowel dysfunction is present, examination of rectal sphincter tone should also be done to exclude cauda equina syndrome (S2, S3, or S4 injury).

DIAGNOSTICS

With a complete symptom analysis and the physical examination, a diagnosis can usually be made without further diagnostic tests. Routine radiographs of the lumbosacral spine are neither cost-effective nor useful in decision making in patients ages 20 to 50 years. Finding normal disc spaces does not exclude a herniated disc, and encountering a narrowed disc space cannot distinguish between disc rupture and asymmetric degeneration. Osteophytes extending from the vertebral bodies indicate little more than long-existing disc degeneration and attempts of the body to heal itself.

However, certain situations do require x-ray studies to aid in the differential diagnosis (Box 192-2). MRI may be indicated to pinpoint the source of the radiculopathy or if back pain without radiculopathy continues for longer than 6 weeks without improvement despite physical therapy or use of NSAIDs. However, many individuals without back pain have disc bulges or protrusions that may be discovered coincidentally on MRI.[11] Therefore, without the accompanying findings of radiculopathy, neurologic deficits, sexual function deficits, or abnormalities on physical examination, the MRI findings may prove to be nondiagnostic and expensive.[11]

DIAGNOSTICS

Low Back Pain

IMAGING
X-ray*
MRI*

*If indicated.

DIFFERENTIAL DIAGNOSIS

Because back pain is one of the more common primary care complaints, it is important to exclude the possibility of other sources of LBP, particularly osteoporotic compression fracture, infection, trauma, inflammatory disease, myositis, fibromyalgia, neoplasm, malignancy, spinal stenosis, and acute abdominal aneurysm in patients older than 50 years.

The majority of patients with back pain have musculoligamentous injury or degenerative changes, resulting in pain.

BOX 192-2

INDICATIONS FOR IMAGING STUDIES

MAJOR TRAUMA

Suspicion of malignancy: Over age 50, focal persistent bone pain unrelieved by rest, or a history of malignancy

Suspected compression fracture: Prolonged steroid use, postmenopausal woman, or severe trauma

Suspected ankylosing spondylitis: Young male patient, limited spinal range of motion, sacroiliac joint pain

Worsening chronic osteomyelitis: Low-grade fever, high sedimentation rate, focal tenderness, especially after a spinal tap

MAJOR NEUROLOGIC DEFICIT

Localized back pain to the higher lumbar and thoracic regions: Compression fractures and metastatic tumors common in these areas

DIFFERENTIAL DIAGNOSIS

Low Back Pain

- Osteoporotic compression fracture
- Infection
- Trauma
- Inflammatory disease
- Myositis
- Fibromyalgia
- Neoplasm
- Malignancy
- Acute abdominal aneurysm
- Referred pain
- Peripheral neuropathy
- Spinal stenosis

Other sources of LBP include referred pain from other systems (e.g., genitourinary system or reproductive organs). Metabolic diseases, such as diabetes, may cause peripheral neuropathies that result in leg pain, and psychologic stressors cannot be overlooked.

MANAGEMENT

In the acute stage of back pain the initial treatment should attempt to decrease the inflammatory response to the injury, trauma, and stress in the area. Analgesia and control of inflammation will provide comfort (see Table 194-1). Regularly scheduled acetaminophen (Tylenol) is appropriate and beneficial for many patients. Many patients self-treat, having access to NSAIDs over the counter. They may wait to see their health care provider until they no longer can attain relief from pain or they are frustrated with limitations to their mobility. The benefit of the nonsteroidal medications is that they do provide some analgesia along with their antiinflammatory effects. If relief is not adequate with NSAIDs, a muscle relaxant may be added. The addition of a muscle relaxant precludes operating machinery and driving; therefore the patient may be restricted in work assignments. For patients who experience gastrointestinal effects with NSAIDs, a proton pump inhibitor or H_2-blocking drug may be prescribed concomitantly. Patients need to be advised that analgesia is only short term; the key to improvement is mobilization and activity.

Conservative treatment, including antiinflammatory agents and possibly muscle relaxants and analgesics, is the hallmark of management for musculoskeletal LBP. With the initial onset of acute LBP, bed rest is indicated, but only for 2 or 3 days, followed by a return to normal activities of daily living. The use of intermittent heat and/or ice, massage, an aerobic exercise program, abdominal strengthening exercises, and, in some cases, reconditioning exercises with physical therapy is essential to successful recovery. Some patients find wearing an elastic lumbar support helpful. A walking program can be initiated early in the rehabilitation for generalized conditioning and toning. Exercise has been shown to be an effective adjunct to analgesia and is necessary to facilitate recovery.[12] It is helpful to address the patient's fears of reinjury or further exacerbation. Newer modalities for treating back pain, such as acupuncture, may be an appropriate complementary treatment in some patients and require exploration with the provider to determine appropriate timing and to evaluate response to the therapy.[5]

LIFE SPAN CONSIDERATIONS

In the developing spine, contortions associated with spinal malformations are first seen when the child assumes the erect position and begins weight bearing. Numerous structural deficits will be readily visible, and examination of the patient from early childhood into adolescence includes good assessment of the musculoskeletal system. Early identification of structural deficits may well permit correction.

In the young adult, changes in spinal structures may indicate spondylolisthesis. Spinal changes such as spondylolisthesis, caused by excessive extension and flexion as occurs in gymnasts and some other athletes, present challenges to the examiner in determining the source of the pain and the long-term possibility of improvement. Congenital spinal stenosis may be seen, as occurs in achondroplastic dwarfs.[7]

Degenerative changes of the spine occur with the aging process but may not be wholly responsible for back pain. Older individuals may develop degenerative disease that will manifest with lumbago (LBP), leg pain (sciatica), or both. Spinal stenosis (acquired) in the older adult is not uncommon and may affect mobility and lifestyle. The pain associated with spinal stenosis is often claudicating and may be alleviated by stooping forward into an abnormal posture (much like when pushing a grocery cart).[13]

Many treatment modalities are tried with these patients. Local anesthetic blocks may relieve symptoms, although epidural steroids seem to offer to additional benefit. Patients with moderate to severe symptoms may benefit more from surgical decompression than from conservative treatment.[13]

Mechanical-structural changes in the individual may also be responsible for back pain. These involve weight changes, pregnancy, sudden growth spurts in the child or adolescent, and osteoporotic deformities in the aging adult.

COMPLICATIONS

The management of mechanical LBP is uncomplicated and can be accomplished by the health care provider. If a patient has asymmetric reflexes but no other symptoms of a herniated disc other than back pain, no referral is necessary unless symptoms persist for longer than 6 weeks. However, if neurologic symptoms occur or seem to be progressing (e.g., a new onset of sciatica, which may cause a loss of reflexes, muscle weakness, or atrophy) (see Figure 192-1), then treatment options are altered. At that time, further diagnostic testing and referral to an orthopedist or a neurologist are appropriate.

INDICATIONS FOR REFERRAL OR HOSPITALIZATION

In general, mechanical LBP is not an indication for hospitalization. However, cauda equina syndrome or incapacitating back pain that prohibits management at home requires emergent evaluation and possible hospitalization. The onset of neurologic symptoms requires an urgent evaluation but not necessarily admission.

If a patient has a motor or sensory loss, as well as asymmetric reflexes, then referral to a neurologist or an orthopedist is appropriate. Surgery is considered when there is a neurologic deficit or when chronic LBP does not resolve and there is a clear pathologic finding that correlates directly with the clinical examination. If surgery is the recommended treatment option, the surgeon will also make physical therapy recommendations. Physical therapy will assist the patient in learning proper body mechanics and in physical reconditioning. A second referral to the specialist should be considered if symptoms return or persist. In many major medical centers, specialized, multidisciplinary spine centers are available to evaluate and treat patients with chronic back pain.

PATIENT AND FAMILY EDUCATION

Patients should be informed that 85% of those with LBP will recover in 3 to 5 days and will be completely back to normal within 6 to 8 weeks. Problems with bowel or bladder control, leg weakness or persistent leg pain below the knee, symptoms of a urinary tract infection, or an inability to stand on toes should be reported immediately.

Enhanced patient understanding plays a crucial role in reducing and improving back pain and reducing emergency department use. Patients are encouraged to take control of their pain by using the treatment modalities outlined for them, following their medication regimen, and reporting changes in symptoms.

Aerobic activity and physical reconditioning are recommended for all individuals with LBP without radicular symptoms because inactivity and immobilization have not been shown to improve outcomes. Continuation of usual activity maintains conditioning and reduces lost work time. Proper body mechanics for work and home cannot be ignored. Physical therapists will help teach proper body mechanics and provide physical reconditioning exercises. Patients should be encouraged to maintain stretching exercises, abdominal strengthening, and physical activity to reduce the recurrence rate of LBP.[3]

REFERENCES

1. Hochberg MC: *Practical rheumatology*, ed 3, St Louis, 2004, Mosby.
2. Schnare S: Evaluating and managing low back pain, *Contemp Nurse Pract* 10:10-15, 1995.
3. Schoen DC: *Adult orthopaedic nursing*, Philadelphia, 2000, Lippincott.
4. Finnell M: *Primary care seminar: back pain in the primary care setting* (lecture), Boston, Nov 22, 1994, Beth Israel Hospital.
5. Smith-Fassler ME, Lopez-Bushnell K: Acupuncture as complementary therapy for back pain, *Holist Nurs Pract* 15:35-44, 2000.
6. McDonough KA, Wipf JE, Deyo RA: Low back pain. In Branch WT, editor: *Office practice of medicine*, ed 4, Philadelphia, 2003, Elsevier.
7. Esses SI: *Textbook of spinal disorders*, Philadelphia, 1995, Lippincott.
8. Nordin M, Andersson GBJ, Pope MH: *Musculoskeletal disorders in the workplace: principles and practice*, St Louis, 1997, Mosby.
9. Barkauskas VH, Baumann L, Darling-Fisher C: *Health and physical assessment*, ed 2, St Louis, 1998, Mosby.
10. McCance KL, Heuther SE: *Pathophysiology: the biologic basis of disease in adults and children*, ed 3, St Louis, 1998, Mosby.
11. Jarvik JG, Deyo RA: Diagnostic evaluation of low back pain with emphasis on imaging, *Ann Intern Med* 137(7):586-597, 2002.
12. McLain K, Powers C, Thayer P, Seymour RJ: Effectiveness of exercise versus normal activity on acute low back pain: an integrative synthesis and meta-analysis, *Online J Knowl Synth Nurs* 6:7, 1999.
13. Snyder DL: Treatment of degenerative lumbar spinal stenosis, *Am Fam Phys* 70(3):517-520, 2004.

CHAPTER 193

Neck Pain

Joanne N. Casaletto, Rita Beckman-Williams, and Robert J. Riggen

DEFINITION AND EPIDEMIOLOGY

Neck pain is one of the most common patient complaints in primary care. The origins of neck pain are numerous and include the bone, fascia, ligaments, tendons, muscles, and nerves.[1] Recently the facet joints, or zygapophyseal joints, have received increased attention as a source of neck pain, especially after whiplash injury.[2] Neck pain can also be referred from the heart, thyroid, stomach, gallbladder,[1] and vascular system.[3] Injuries from motor vehicle accidents, falls, repetitive motions, or lifting can precipitate symptoms.[1] However, cervical disc injury and radicular pain can often occur without a history of trauma.[1]

Rare conditions that can cause neck pain include meningitis, tumors, fractures, and ankylosing spondylitis.[3] Rheumatoid arthritis can cause neck pain if there is involvement of the C1-2 joint. Other problems encountered include degenerative disc disease, spondylosis, osteoarthritis, cervical strains, and neurologic disorders such as radiculopathy and myelopathy.[3] Cervical spondylotic myelopathy is the most common cause of acquired spastic paraparesis in adults.[4] Common neurologic terminology encountered with cervical problems is listed in Table 193-1.

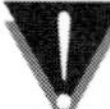

Immediate emergency department referral or physician consultation is indicated for patients with a suspected cervical fracture, new-onset neurologic findings, or signs of meningeal irritation.

Neck pain often manifests with arm pain or radiculopathy (loss of sensory or motor function).[3] The most common cause of radiculopathy is cervical disc herniation.[1] Neck pain is considered chronic if it lasts longer than 3 months. Often the combination of neck pain and radiculopathy can more seriously affect a patient's overall health and mental status than

TABLE 193-1 Physical Examination of Cervical Spine

Physical Examination	Possible Diagnosis
INSPECTION	
Note rash, papules, prominent superior vertebrae, scars, swelling, hematomas, symmetry.	Asymmetry, prominent vertebrae, or swelling related to fracture, subluxation; scars from surgery, old trauma; ecchymosis after trauma
Lordotic cervical spine should be aligned and rest over relaxed shoulders; there should be smooth range of motion and movement when disrobing.	Inability to rotate; fracture of odontoid process
Normal range of motion: Forward flexion: 45 degrees—chin to chest Extension: 55 degrees—eyes parallel to ceiling Lateral band: 45 degrees—ears toward shoulder Rotation: 70 degrees—chin almost touching shoulder	Rotated head: may be spasm, torticollis, or, rarely, subluxation of atlantoaxial joint; limited range because of whiplash pain after motor vehicle accident, fused vertebrae, lymph node enlargement, fracture, and referred pain
POSTERIOR PALPATION	
(Supine patient relaxes muscles.) C2 through large T1 should be aligned; patient should be pain free; spine should be immobile.	Spinous process pain caused by disc herniation or fracture, lateral mobility of spinous process, and crepitus caused by fracture
Note lateral facet joint tenderness or swelling.	Subluxation
Palpate occipital nerves and nuchal ligament from base of skull to C7; head forward flexed.	Ruptured ligament if tenderness; presence of nodules possible indication of trigger points
Trapezius (large muscle) should be bilaterally equal from T12 and laterally to acromion (palpate with hand; turn head away from tested side).	Hard muscle caused by spasm; tenderness from muscle strain; point tenderness caused by fibromyalgia; presence of nodules possible indication of trigger points
Palpate splenius cervicis (small muscle), located superiorly in triangular space between trapezius and sternocleidomastoid.	Spasm; presence of nodules possible indication of trigger points
Palpate levator scapulae, scalene posterior, and scalene medial inferior to splenius cervicis (difficult to palpate).	Strain or spasm, point tenderness fibromyalgia; presence of nodules possible indication of trigger points
ANTERIOR PALPATION	
Examination aids in identifying location of posterior landmarks.	May be thyroid, lymph node, and parotid enlargement
Superior midline hyoid bone corresponds to C3 posteriorly; smooth thyroid cartilage corresponds to C4-5.	
Sternocleidomastoid reaches from sternoclavicular joint to mastoid process.	Injury after motor vehicle accident; swelling possibly indicating hematoma, and may produce torticollis
AUSCULTATION	
Auscultate spinous processes for crepitus.	Cervical spondylosis, rheumatoid arthritis

each problem individually.[5] Shoulder pathologic conditions are often confused with disorders of the cervical spine, since arm pain often occurs concomitantly with neck pain.[6] Headaches emanating from the neck to the frontal region of the head can be caused by disorders of the cervical spine.[7] Also, carpal tunnel syndrome and ulnar nerve entrapments can cause symptoms similar to cervical radiculopathy.[8]

PATHOPHYSIOLOGY

The cervical spine consists of seven cervical vertebrae: the atlas, the axis, and C3-7.[9] The cervical vertebrae are connected to a fairly immobile thoracic spine.[9] The intervertebral discs allow for shock absorption and, together with the vertebrae, allow for flexibility of the spine.[8] The neck muscles surround the trachea and esophagus anteriorly and the seven cervical vertebrae posteriorly. The sternocleidomastoid and trapezius muscles form a triangle laterally, thereby supporting the head and allowing movement. The facet joints extend laterally from the spinous processes of the vertebrae and allow rotational movement. Ligaments also provide support for the spine and allow for flexibility. Sensory nerves permit the perception of pain, temperature, position, and touch, whereas motor nerves control muscle movement.[8]

Pathophysiologic changes in cervical radiculopathy are thought to be a combination of mechanical problems and inflammatory responses.[4] Age-related changes in the cervical disc result in a loss of the disc's height, causing the vertebral bodies to drift toward each other and bulge into the spinal canal.[4] Osteoarthritis causes breakdown of the articular cartilage of the facet joints, as well as microfractures and subsequent cyst and bony spur formation, leading to joint space narrowing. Osteophytes, present in half of people over age 50, are produced from calcium deposits on the vertebral bodies that then can compress nerve roots.[8] Along with these mechanical nerve root changes, it is also believed that an inflammatory response occurs via chemical mediators.[4] These pathologic processes may cause impingement of nerve roots as they emerge from the spinal cord through the neuroforamina, resulting in radicular pain.

Cervical disc herniations occur secondary to posterolateral annular stress and rarely result from trauma.[10] Herniations at the C6-7 level are the most frequent.[10] Disc herniations can be part of the aging process as the discs degenerate and dry and osteophytes form.[11] Herniated cervical discs can resolve, since the increased blood supply brought on from the inflammatory response causes subsequent resorption.[11]

Cervical spondylotic myelopathy is believed to result from a decrease in space available for the spinal cord.[4] Narrowing or stenosis of the anterior-to-posterior diameter of the spinal canal to less than 13 mm (0.5 inch) (normal diameter is 17 to 18 mm [about 0.7 inch]), along with flattening of the cord and vascular changes, contributes to myelopathy.[4]

The facet joints are implicated in whiplash injuries.[2] It is believed that the vertebrae actually rotate backward from C6 upward and are stopped when their articular processes (facet joints) collide.[2]

Cervical headaches are thought to be caused by convergence of trigeminal afferents and cervical afferents.[7] Therefore pain from the cervical spine can be perceived in the frontal regions of the head, the parietal regions, and the orbit.[7]

CLINICAL PRESENTATION

The mechanism of injury should be assessed. Is the pain connected to a particular trauma, awkward posture, repetitive or heavy lifting, or occupational injury? Did the pain start spontaneously without a precipitating cause, as is common with cervical radiculopathy?[1] Sharp neck pain, at times radiating to the head, shoulder, arm, or hand, occurs within hours to days after an acute injury. After a motor vehicle accident, pain may be accompanied by mild amnesia and transient mental dullness. Sudden movement of the head during a sports injury or accident may be the causative factor for a strain or hematoma and may aggravate an existing injury. Sharp, typically burning or achy pain, with or without radiation to shoulder, arm, and hand, occurs with chronic pain.

Cervical strains usually are seen with anterior neck pain along the sternocleidomastoid muscle that is aggravated by rotation to the opposite side.[4] Pain in the posterior neck muscles aggravated by neck flexion implicates a myofascial cause.[4] Pain in the posterior part of the neck aggravated by extension and rotation of the head suggests a disc problem.[4] Symptoms of neck pain, headache, arm pain, shoulder pain, and reduced neck mobility are seen with whiplash-type injuries.[12] However, neck mobility can completely improve in these patients, whereas pain can persist chronically.[12]

A complete history includes location and onset of pain, aggravating and alleviating factors, radiation of pain, and severity of pain on a scale of 0 to 10 (0 is no pain, and 10 is the maximum pain experience). For example, patients with radicular pain often have some relief of symptoms when they raise their hand to the top of their head, relieving tension on the nerve root.[12] A thorough past medical history should include the presence of diseases such as osteoporosis, ankylosing spondylitis, rheumatoid arthritis, or osteoarthritis. A history of hypertension, ulcer disease, or other gastrointestinal disorders may preclude the use of NSAIDs[1] and cyclooxygenase-2 (COX-2) inhibitors. Pregnancy status for women, along with family history of chronic neck or back pain, should be determined. A complete review of symptoms and past medical history ensure appropriate diagnostic studies, education, referral, and care plan. Neurologic history should include the presence and distribution of pain, functional limitations, weakness, paresthesias, numbness, and bladder or bowel dysfunction. It is also important to ask patients whether the pain disrupts their sleep. The presence of fever, unexplained weight loss, previous malignancy, prolonged use of steroids, IV drug use, immunosuppression, and psychologic problems should also be noted.

PHYSICAL EXAMINATION

The examiner should observe the patient initially for signs of pain on introduction and during removal of garments. The provider should also observe the gait for spasticity, which is a possible indicator of myelopathy[1]; inspect the head and neck for loss of cervical lordosis, spinal asymmetry, and muscle atrophy[13]; and inspect the shoulder, scapula, and upper trapezius for winging or drooping, which may indicate C6 or C7 radiculopathy.[1]

Palpation may reveal tenderness, swelling, abnormal masses, and facet alignment. The examiner begins at C2 and palpates each of two lateral facet joints for each spinous process. C7 is the most prominent spinous process, C4 aligns with the top of the thyroid, and C6 is parallel to the cricoid cartilage (see Table 193-1).[13] Cervical lymph node examination may be done while palpating the trapezius muscle, and examination of the thyroid may be done when finding cervical landmarks. Range of motion can then be assessed (see Table 193-1).

Several special maneuvers assist with assessing the integrity of the spine and locating the point of injury (Box 193-1). Spurling's maneuver is useful in differentiating a radicular cause from a muscle or shoulder one.[4] In addition, screening tests for peripheral nerve entrapments, like carpal tunnel syndrome (Chapter 188) and shoulder impingement (Chapter 198), should be performed. Included in the special tests is Adson's maneuver for thoracic outlet syndrome. This syndrome can cause aching pain in the neck and paresthesias to the shoulder, forearm, and hand.[13] This is due to compression of the brachial plexus or subclavian veins or can also be caused by congenital anomalies such as an abnormally long transverse process of C7.[13]

Neurologic examination includes testing of the strength of the intrinsic muscles of the neck. Strength testing is done as the examiner provides resistance with one hand on the patient's head and the other hand on the patient's sternum for forward flexion. Resistance can then be provided on the patient's shoulder for all other motions. Absent or diminished sensation, reflexes, and strength may occur with disc injury. The sensory, motor, and reflex testing of these nerves aids in evaluating the integrity of the spine (Table 193-2). Evaluation of the cranial nerves, as well as the upper and lower extremities, is indicated. The presence of hyperreflexia in the lower extremities, muscle spasticity, or a gait disturbance suggests upper motor neuron dysfunction. One possible cause is cervical myelopathy because of cord compression by a tumor or bony spur.

TABLE 193-2 Neurologic Testing of Cervical Spine

Neurologic Level	Motor	Reflex
C5	Biceps Deltoid	Biceps
C6	Biceps Wrist extensors	Radial
C7	Triceps Wrist flexors Finger extensors	Triceps
C8	Finger flexors interossei muscles (abduct, adduct fingers)	None
T1	Interossei muscles	None

BOX 193-1

SPECIAL MANEUVERS—CERVICAL SPINE

Spurling's test: Extend the neck and laterally rotate the head to the side of the pain. A positive test induces paresthesias to the scapula or upper arm.

Abduction sign: Abducting the arm on the same side of the pain may improve symptoms in patients with cervical radiculopathy.

Axial loading: Press down on top of head to increase cervical pressure. Note pain in dermatone to determine location of cervical injury.

Valsalva's test: Attempt to forcibly exhale with the glottis, nose, and mouth closed. Increases cervical pressure. Pain caused by disc herniation or mass. Note location of neck pain and dermatone pain.

Swallow test: Pain with swallow results from anterior spine mass or infection.

Adson's test (test for thoracic outlet): Abduct and externally rotate shoulder while rotating head toward arm tested. Radicular symptoms indicate that origin of pain is at subclavian artery where C5-T1 nerves travel. Diminished pulse indicates compression of radial artery.

DIAGNOSTICS

X-rays remain the initial diagnostic test in almost every musculoskeletal disorder and can easily detect fractures and tumors.[11] However, disc herniations, cord tumors, and even more advanced degenerative changes can go undetected on x-rays.[11] Flexion-extension views are useful to detect subluxations, instability, and abnormal motion of the cervical spine.[10]

Several x-ray projections show different views of the spine and are used to determine the area that is injured. The anteroposterior view details spinal alignment, uniformity of the disc spaces and vertebrae, and facet dislocation. The open-mouth odontoid view reveals C1 and C2. The cross-table lateral view allows inspection for C1 to T1 spine malalignment or fracture and narrowing of the disc space. Widening of the disc space may indicate a posterior ligament tear. Oblique views permit inspection of the neuroforamina and facets and reveal degenerative disc disease.[10] If x-rays reveal positive findings, then additional studies such as MRI or CT may be indicated. However, even if x-ray results are normal, other diagnostic tests may be indicted if the patient's symptoms worsen, persist, or are accompanied by neurologic signs.

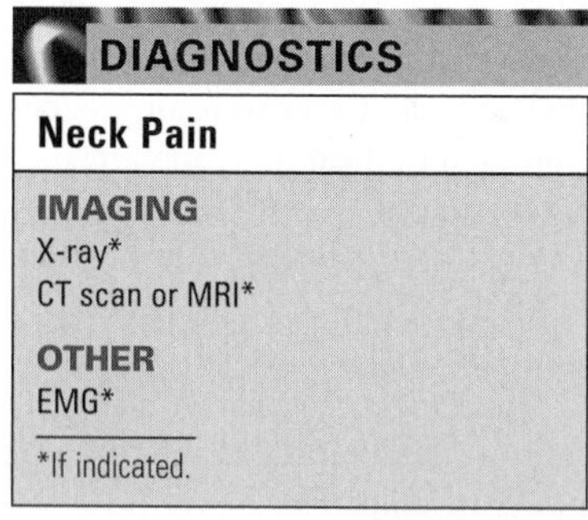
DIAGNOSTICS

Neck Pain

IMAGING
X-ray*
CT scan or MRI*

OTHER
EMG*

*If indicated.

MRI is useful because it can detect disc problems such as degenerative disc disease and disc herniations.[11] MRI can also detect bone tumors or fractures and provides good soft tissue definition.[10,11] CT scan can delineate spinal fractures and is often used in trauma patients.[10] Another advanced diagnostic is discography, a test where contrast material is injected into the disc.[11] This test is often used before surgery or when annular tears are suspected.[11] However, this test can cause pain because of its invasiveness.[10] Electrophysiologic studies may be needed to assess patients with suspected radiculopathy (nerve root irritation) or myelopathy (spinal cord compromise).

DIFFERENTIAL DIAGNOSIS

Acute neck pain may become a chronic problem. Evaluation for fracture or subluxation after trauma may reveal degenerative changes, particularly in older adults. Infection of the bones from septic arthritis, syphilis, or tuberculosis is an uncommon cause of cervical pain. Infection of the meninges will likely be accompanied by headache, fever, and cognitive deficits. A review of systems, past medical history, and physical examination may indicate that pain is referred.

MANAGEMENT

The goals of management are modifying pain, maintaining or restoring strength and flexibility, and assisting with return-to-work issues. Initial treatment consists of ice application for 20 minutes every 2 hours while awake, strategies for relaxation, and gentle range-of-motion exercises performed while showering or after medication. Ice decreases blood flow and hemorrhage into the tissues, along with reducing pain and muscle spasm.[9] NSAIDs are the mainstay of medication treatment. Commonly used initial treatments include ibuprofen or naproxen. Muscle relaxants, such as cyclobenzaprine (Flexeril) 5 to 10 mg, can be used at bedtime, or the 5-mg dose can be taken three times per day.

Narcotic pain medications may be necessary initially in some cases of acute pain, but their use should be time limited. Tramadol (Ultram), a nonnarcotic pain reliever, is another option.[8] Tricyclic antidepressants such as amitriptyline (Elavil) are also being used in low doses and are given at bedtime to assist with sleep and pain control.[8] However, they can have some muscle relaxant properties and should not be taken with muscle relaxers.[14] COX-2 inhibitors such as celecoxib (Celebrex) can also be used instead of NSAIDs in patients with more advanced or chronic symptoms. These drugs should be avoided in patients with a cardiac history or history of hypertension.

DIFFERENTIAL DIAGNOSIS

Neck Pain

- Dislocation, fracture, subluxation
- Disc herniation or radiculopathy
- Cervical stenosis
- Cervical spondylosis (degenerative disc disease)
- Cervical strain, sprain, torticollis
- Infection
- Cervical tumor, metastatic disease
- Spondylolisthesis
- Thoracic outlet syndrome
- Peripheral nerve entrapment
- Osteoporosis, osteomalacia
- Cervicogenic headache
- Whiplash, trauma
- Ankylosing spondylosis
- Rheumatoid arthritis
- Fibromyalgia
- Myofascial pain syndrome
- Rotator cuff disease, shoulder impingement
- Autoimmune disorders

REFERRED PAIN FROM

- Aortic aneurysm
- Heart, lung
- Gallbladder
- Meningitis
- Subarachnoid hemorrhage
- Cancer of the esophagus

RARE DIFFERENTIALS

- Paget's disease
- Polio
- Tetanus
- Tuberculosis
- Syphilis (can cause osteitis and osteophytes)
- Infection of mandible teeth and temporomandibular joint pain

Two or three days after injury, cervical resistance exercises and back strengthening exercises should begin. If pain does not improve within 3 days of an acute injury, or if a patient complains of recurring pain, referral to a physical therapist for soft tissue mobilization, traction, muscle energy techniques, ultrasound treatment, electrical stimulation, and review of cervical exercises is indicated. Traction, provided by the physical therapist, is useful for chronic degenerative disease. Chiropractic manipulation may also be efficacious in the reduction of pain.

Trauma patients must be observed for deteriorating neurologic status; therefore muscle relaxants are contraindicated. Although soft collars are often used, their effectiveness in reducing persistent pain or the length of rehabilitation has not been proved.[15]

If patients were injured at work, all effort should be made to return patients to a modified duty assignment if possible. Sometimes, with acute neck pain, a few days of rest at home and prompt follow-up afterward are indicated. Restrictions for cervical injuries include no lifting, pushing, or pulling greater than 4.5 kg (10 pounds); no repetitive squatting, kneeling, stooping, or twisting; no repetitive upper extremity motions; avoidance of exaggerated neck motions; and no work at or above the shoulder. Also, if skeletal muscle relaxants or narcotic pain relievers are prescribed, the patient should avoid driving or operating machinery.

Co-Management with Specialists

Consultation with orthopedic specialists or neurologists is often indicated in more chronic or severe cases. In workers' compensation cases, a specialist consult or an independent medical examination (IME) is often needed. More advanced treatments such as epidural blocks or anesthetic discograms may be done.[11] Sometimes, surgery may be indicated.

COMPLICATIONS

Complications of cervical disc disease include myelopathy with associated weakness, hyperreflexia, and neurogenic bowel and bladder.[10] Radiculopathy with associated upper extremity weakness and numbness is also a complication.[10]

Whiplash injuries can cause chronic pain because of zygapophyseal joint damage.[2] Third occipital headaches, which originate in the C2-3 zygapophyseal joint, are also complications of whiplash injuries. Altered proprioception or dizziness accompanies chronic neck pain.

Chronic neck pain also affects the patient's psychologic state.[5] Disability and loss of work and wages are long-term problems for persons with work-related neck injuries.

INDICATIONS FOR REFERRAL OR HOSPITALIZATION

Supportive care in an emergency department and orthopedic or neurosurgical consultation are mandatory for all patients with a cervical fracture. C1 vertebral fracture is a life-threatening emergency. Immediate immobilization, stabilization, and transfer to an emergency department are indicated. Shallow dive injuries may cause C5 fractures, resulting in quadriplegia and possibly death. Although rare, C7 fracture and ipsilateral pupil dilation may occur with rear-end whiplash. Trauma patients with neurologic deficits require immediate neurologic consultation. Chronic pain syndrome, characterized by prolonged disability or prescription drug use, may require referral to a chronic pain clinic. A small percentage of patients with neurologic symptoms may benefit from surgery. Consultation with a physiatrist is indicated for persistent point tenderness to evaluate the need for trigger point injections with lidocaine or steroids.

PATIENT AND FAMILY EDUCATION

Maintaining the neck in a neutral posture, demonstrating proper body mechanics, and performing daily back and neck exercises are important practices for patients with a history of neck pain and are essential for patients with a herniated disc. The use of a mirror enables the patient to correct his or her posture with visual feedback. The cervical spine is in correct position when the neck is in alignment with the thoracic spine rather than jutting forward. The shoulders should be relaxed, with the chest held forward and the mandible relaxed. If the patient can visualize a string on the top of the scalp, gently pulling the head superiorly, pressure may be alleviated.

New onset of arm or shoulder paresthesias or severe headache after an injury should be viewed as a warning to return for follow-up. Family members should be given a list of warning signs for decreased level of consciousness and instructed to seek emergency department care without hesitation. A medication education sheet and exercise sheet provide needed sources for reference. Finally, reassurance that discomfort is a normal part of recovery is helpful to patients and families.

HEALTH PROMOTION

Counseling concerning the avoidance of alcohol while swimming and diving, the use of properly adjusted seat belts and headrests, and the use of helmets while riding bicycles or motorcycles or skiing is an important strategy for the prevention of neck injuries. Proper workplace ergonomics, sleeping posture, and reaching and lifting techniques also minimize stress on cervical structures.

REFERENCES

1. Honet JC, Ellenberg MR: What you always wanted to know about the history and physical examination of neck pain but were afraid to ask, *Phys Med Rehabil Clin North Am* 14:473-491, 2003.
2. Ketroser DB: Whiplash, chronic neck pain, and zygapophyseal joint disorders: a selective review, *Minn Med* 83:51-54, 2000.
3. Bogduk N: The anatomy and pathophysiology of neck pain, *Phys Med Rehabil Clin North Am* 14:455-472, 2003.
4. Rao R: Neck pain, cervical radiculopathy, and cervical myelopathy: pathophysiology, natural history, and clinical evaluation, *J Bone Joint Surg* 84-A:1872-1881, 2002.
5. Daffner SD, Hilibrand AS, Hanscom BS, and others: Impact of neck and arm pain on overall health status, *Spine* 28(17):2030-2035, 2003.
6. Wilson C: Rotator cuff versus cervical spine: making the diagnosis, *Nurse Pract* 30(5):45-50, 2005.
7. Bogduk N: The neck and headaches, *Neurol Clin North Am* 22:151-171, 2004.
8. Schmidt Luggen A: A pain in the neck: evaluation and management of cervical problems in older adults, *Adv Nurse Pract* 12(11):28-33, 59, 2004.
9. Windsor RE: *Cervical facet syndrome,* retrieved Nov 2005 from http://www.emedicine.com/sports/topic20.htm.
10. Furman MB, Simon J: *Cervical disc disease,* retrieved Oct 2005 from http://www.emedicine.com/pmr/topic25.htm.
11. Mink JH, Gordon RE, Deutsch AL: The cervical spine: a radiologist's perspective, *Phys Med Rehabil Clin North Am* 14:493-548, 2003.
12. Kasch H, Stengaard-Pedersen K, Arendt-Nielsen L, and others: Headache, neck pain, and neck mobility after acute whiplash injury: a prospective study, *Spine* 26(11):1246-1251, 2001.
13. Greene WB, editor: *Essentials of musculoskeletal care,* ed 2, Rosemont, Ill, 2001, American Academy of Orthopaedic Surgeons.
14. Borg-Stein J: *Oh my aching back: What's new? What works?* (lecture), Boston, Nov 11-13, 2005, Primary Medicine Today.
15. Gennis P, Miller L, Gallagher EJ, and others: The effect of soft cervical collars on persistent neck pain in patients with whiplash injury, *Acad Emerg Med* 3(6):568-573, 1996.

CHAPTER 194

Osteoarthritis

Ann S. Bruner-Welch

DEFINITION AND EPIDEMIOLOGY

Osteoarthritis (OA) is a progressive degenerative joint process. It involves degeneration of the articular (hyaline) cartilage layer on the ends of bones at the joints. OA manifests as a monoarticular or polyarticular phenomenon and is often asymmetric. Occasionally it can appear as a more generalized disease.[1] OA is the most common type of arthritis, and it usually begins asymptomatically in the second or third decade of life. By the fourth decade, most people have some degree of pathologic change on articular weight-bearing surfaces. Symptoms typically begin to appear in the fourth through sixth decades of life. Some degree of symptomatic arthritis is extremely common by the seventh decade. Men and women are equally affected. Risk factors include obesity; prior trauma; genetics; repetitive activities; and metabolic, neurologic, or hematologic conditions.[1]

The carpometacarpal joints of the thumbs, distal interphalangeal joints of the fingers, first metatarsophalangeal joints of the feet, cervical and lumbar spine, and weight-bearing joints such as the hips and knees are most commonly affected. OA can also affect previously injured joints. Pain, stiffness, and limited range of motion are the most common reasons for seeking medical care. The degenerative effects of OA result in physical disability and can have a profound impact on the quality of life.[1,2]

PATHOPHYSIOLOGY

Initially, the cartilage softens and becomes overhydrated and boggy, with decreased quantity and size of proteoglycans within the matrix. Collagen also loses its stiffness with fewer cells and loss of crosslinks as degradation continues.[3] The surface layers fibrillate, and the cartilage loses its thickness, develops surface crevices, and then loses integrity. Loose cartilaginous fragments (known as *loose bodies*) can flake off, blocking range of motion and contributing to pain and disability.[3]

Chondrocytes proliferate with increased metabolic activity as the subchondral bone scleroses under the damaged areas. The bone thickens, stiffens, and then produces cysts, microfractures, and osteophytes at the joint margins.[4] These later findings are often seen on radiographs. The associated increased metabolic activity can be picked up on a bone scan.

The cartilage surface is completely aneural, making the pathogenesis of pain from OA speculative. It is thought to be secondary to increased venous pressure within the bony capillaries and irritation of surrounding supportive tissue. As a result of the joint degradation, the joint capsule may also tighten, resulting in a reactive synovitis and pain. This synovitis is usually sparse in cellular infiltrate and fibrotic in nature. However, it causes an effusion that can stretch and further destabilize the joint capsule.[4]

CLINICAL PRESENTATION AND PHYSICAL EXAMINATION

Insidious, progressive pain or stiffness of one or more joints may be the initial presenting complaint. Symptoms are most prevalent on arising and after a prolonged activity and are relieved by rest.[3] Weight-bearing activities, such as going up or down stairs, getting up from a sitting position, walking, prolonged standing, or changing activity level, can be particularly troublesome. The patient may also complain of crepitus (grinding), swelling, and gradual loss of motion as the disease progresses.[3]

When OA involves the cervical or lumbar spine, neuropathy and radiculopathy may develop as nerves are compressed. OA involving the hip manifests with groin or buttock pain that can radiate to the knee. The pain can cause the patient to "favor" the hip, which in turn can contribute to specific muscle weakness. The resultant gait is known as a Trendelenburg's gait. OA of the knee involves the medial joint compartment 70% of the time, leading to a varus deformity of the extremity. It can then progress to include the lateral joint compartment and patellofemoral articulations as well. Pain on palpation of the medial and lateral joint lines and joint effusions are often seen. Quadriceps muscle atrophy is common on the affected side.[4]

OA of the hands manifests as Heberden's nodes (deformity of the distal interphalangeal joints) and Bouchard's nodes (deformity of the proximal interphalangeal joints). A compression test, as well as pain with palpation of the joint, can detect OA of the carpometacarpal joint. Contracture, deformity, and even joint fusion are common as the disease progresses.[4] Fortunately, OA of the hands is seldom completely disabling.

DIAGNOSTICS

In the early stages of OA, radiographic findings may not be evident.[4] As the disease progresses and joint space is lost, radiographic changes become more prominent. A bone scan may show increased metabolic activity within an arthritic joint.[4]

OA is a nonsystemic disease. There are no serologic markers for OA as yet, but serologic tests are commonly performed to rule out other disorders. See the Diagnostics box for optional testing.

DIAGNOSTICS

Osteoarthritis

LABORATORY
Rheumatoid factor*
Cyclic citrullinated peptide*
Antinuclear antibodies*
CBC and differential*
ESR*
Uric acid*
Joint aspirate for crystals, white blood cells*
C-reactive protein*

IMAGING
X-ray
MRI*
CT scan*

*If indicated.

DIFFERENTIAL DIAGNOSIS

The Differential Diagnosis box lists other diseases that should also be considered and excluded when appropriate. Other arthritic conditions such as rheumatoid arthritis, gout, psoriatic arthritis, and pseudogout are commonly seen with OA.[4]

DIFFERENTIAL DIAGNOSIS

Osteoarthritis

- Lupus erythematosus
- Lyme disease
- Malignancy
- Fracture or dislocation
- Neuropathy
- Osteomyelitis
- Osteonecrosis
- Avascular necrosis
- Bursitis
- Tendinitis
- Gout
- Paget's disease
- Fibromyalgia
- Soft tissue disease

MANAGEMENT

Pharmacologic Management

Acetaminophen. Acetaminophen remains the mainstay of initial treatment for early OA. This is well supported in the literature. The analgesic properties can reduce discomfort without the additional risks of antiinflammatory medications.[5] One gram 4 times daily has been suggested. The maximum daily dose is 4 g (1000 mg PO q 6 hr) for adults. Hepatotoxicity is a concern, particularly if acetaminophen is used in conjunction with alcohol. The maximum daily dose of acetaminophen in patients receiving warfarin therapy should not exceed 2500 mg PO.[6] Patients should be advised to read labels to avoid acetaminophen overdose. Acetaminophen is found in a wide variety of over-the-counter and prescription products such as sleep aids, cold remedies, and prescription pain medications, in addition to being sold by itself.

Tramadol Hydrochloride (Ultram). Tramadol is another nonopioid pain reliever that is indicated for moderate to moderately severe pain; tramadol is not a nonsteroidal antiinflammatory drug (NSAID). The packaging insert should be followed for dosing and precautions. It is also available as a combination drug with acetaminophen. The combination is synergistic and can be given in addition to NSAIDs. It is a centrally acting pain medication taken in place of narcotics such as acetaminophen with hydrocodone (Vicodin), with propoxyphene (Darvocet), or with codeine (Tylenol #3).[2,4]

Nonsteroidal Antiinflammatory Drugs. NSAIDs have long been part of the treatment regimen for OA. NSAIDs are believed to be most beneficial for their analgesic rather than their antiinflammatory properties.[4,7,8]

Cyclooxygenase-2 (COX-2) selective NSAIDs were designed to reduce the gastrointestinal toxicity side effects of traditional NSAIDs. However, two of the three early COX-2 medications, rofecoxib (Vioxx) and valdecoxib (Bextra), were found to have potentially lethal side effects, including cardiac toxicity and an increased incidence of Stevens-Johnson syndrome.[9-17] They have both been removed from the U.S. market.

Celecoxib (Celebrex) remains on the market as of this writing. It remains a good alternative for some patients, especially those on warfarin, those on chronic steroids, or those who have gastrointestinal intolerance for traditional NSAIDs. Most insurance companies still require other medications be tried before approving a prescription of Celebrex. Because of concern that patients taking COX-2 inhibitors may have a higher incidence of vascular events, patients at risk of stroke or myocardial infarction should continue to receive prophylactic aspirin.

Other COX-2 selective medications are currently being studied. Because of the problems linked to Vioxx and Bextra, more stringent studies are being required before their release.

Of the traditional NSAIDs, ibuprofen and naproxen (Naprosyn) were also found to have increased cardiac toxicity.[13] The overall message seems to be that one should be cautious with any NSAID used and carefully consider the patient's overall health and pain symptoms. Patients treated with an NSAID for extended periods should be monitored closely for changes in renal function, liver function, and blood pressure.

Meloxicam (Mobic) is a preferential inhibitor of COX-2, but it is not a true COX-2 inhibitor according to the criteria of the U.S. Food and Drug Administration (FDA). Nonetheless, it seems to be well tolerated, with few side effects or drug-drug interactions.

Of the traditional antiinflammatory drugs, choline salicylate–magnesium salicylate (Trilisate), etodolac (Lodine), salsalate (Disalcid), diclofenac-misoprostol (Arthrotec), and nabumetone (Relafen) are touted as having better gastrointestinal tolerance than other NSAIDs.[8-10] Health care providers should also consider prescribing gastrointestinal protective agents such as H_2 blockers, prostaglandin E_2 inhibitors, or proton pump inhibitors to reduce gastrointestinal intolerance.[7,8] See Table 194-1 for NSAID dosing.

Glucosamine With or Without Chondroitin. Several studies have supported the use of glucosamine with or without chondroitin for OA of the knees.[17-21] Recent multicenter double-blind studies have failed to demonstrate significant pain relief when compared with placebo.[22] If patients want to try this approach, the recommended dosage is 500 mg of glucosamine sulfate t.i.d. Once-daily dosing with 1500 mg has also been shown to be effective.[23] There are few side effects or known drug-drug interactions. Because glucosamine is a dietary supplement and is not regulated by the FDA, the potency and quality may not be consistent between different brands. If one brand is not helpful, the patient may be advised to try another with better results.

Intraarticular Approaches to Treatment

Hyaluronans. Intraarticular injections of exogenous hyaluran can also help reduce the pain of OA of the knees.[24] It seems to be most effective in mild to moderate OA and acts as a lubricant as it improves viscosity within the joint. It has been compared favorably with naproxen in efficacy in double-blind, placebo-controlled studies and has fewer adverse reactions. It is injected once a week for 3 to 5 weeks, depending on the preparation, and it may provide benefit for 6 months or longer.

Intraarticular Corticosteroid Injections. Intraarticular corticosteroid injections can also provide significant pain relief for mild to severe disease. The duration of benefit varies widely. Even in severe disease, injections are not recommended more

TABLE 194-1 Nonsteroidal Antiinflammatory Cost Analysis and Dosing Chart

Medication	OA Dosing	RA Dosing	
COX-2 INHIBITOR			
Celebrex (celecoxib)	100 mg q day–b.i.d. $2.13/pill; $2.13-$4.26/day	200 mg q day $3.16/pill/day	
INDOLEACETIC ACID AND RELATED COMPOUNDS			
Clinoril (sulindac)	150 mg b.i.d. $1/pill; $2/day	200 mg b.i.d. $1.35/pill; $2.70/day	
Indocin* (indomethacin)	25 mg b.i.d.-t.i.d. $0.63/pill; $1.26-$1.89/day	50 mg b.i.d.-t.i.d. $1.04/pill; $2.08-$3.12/day	
Indocin SR (indomethacin)	75 mg q day $2.15/pill/day		
Lodine* (etodolac)	300 mg b.i.d. $1.68/pill; $3.36/day	500 mg b.i.d. $1.86/pill; $3.72/day	
Lodine XL* (etodolac ER)	400 mg q day $1.36/pill/day		
NAPHTHYLALKANONE			
Relafen (nabumetone)	500 mg b.i.d. $2.34/pill; $4.68/day	750 mg b.i.d. $3.06/pill; $6.12/day	
NSAID/GI MUCOSAL PROTECTIVE COMBINATION			
Arthrotec (diclofenac-misoprostol)	50 mg q day $2.21/pill/day	75 mg q day $2.13/pill/day	
OXICAMS			
Feldene* (piroxicam)	10 mg b.i.d. $2.46/pill; $4.92/day	20 mg q day $2.87/pill/day	
Mobic (meloxicam)	7.5 mg q day–b.i.d. $3.53/pill; $3.53-$7.06/day		
PHENYLACETIC ACIDS			
Cataflam (diclofenac potassium)	50 mg b.i.d.-t.i.d. $1.36/pill; $2.72-$4.08/day		
Voltaren* (diclofenac sodium)	50 mg b.i.d.-t.i.d. $2.40/pill; $2.40-$3.60/day	75 mg b.i.d. $1.45/pill; $2.90/day	
Voltaren XR (diclofenac XR)	100 mg q day $5.53/pill/day		
PROPIONIC ACIDS			
Anaprox (naproxen sodium) Aleve (naproxen)	275 mg t.i.d.-q.i.d. $0.12/pill; $0.36-$0.48/day		
Anaprox DS (naproxen sodium)	550 mg q day–b.i.d. $1.33/pill; $1.33-$2.66/day		
Ansaid (flurbiprofen)	50 mg b.i.d.-t.i.d. $1.53/pill; $3.06-$4.59/day	100 mg b.i.d.-t.i.d. $2.73/pill; $5.46-$8.19/day	
Daypro (oxaprozin)	2 600-mg caplets q day $2.44/pill/day		
Motrin* (ibuprofen)	400 mg t.i.d.-q.i.d. $0.07/pill; $0.56-$0.84	600 mg t.i.d.-q.i.d.	800 mg t.i.d.-q.i.d.
Naprelan* (naproxen sodium)	2-375 mg q day $1.33/pill; $2.66/day	2-500 mg q day $1.66/pill; $3.22/day	
Naprosyn (naproxen)	250 mg b.i.d. $0.84/pill; $1.68/day	500 mg b.i.d. $1.20/pill; $2.40/day	
Orudis* (ketoprofen)	75 mg t.i.d. $1.29/pill; $3.87/day		

Data retrieved Feb 28, 2006, from http://www.walgreens.com/library/finddrug/druginfosearch.jsp. All prices quoted are for brand name products; generic formulations are available for some products.
COX-2, Cyclooxygenase-2; *GI*, gastrointestinal; *IM*, intramuscular.
*Generic available.

Continued

TABLE 194-1 Nonsteroidal Antiinflammatory Cost Analysis and Dosing Chart—cont'd

Medication	OA Dosing	RA Dosing
PROPIONIC ACIDS—CONT'D		
Oruvail (ketoprofen)	200 q day $3.66/pill/day	
Toradol (ketorolac) (also available IM or IV)	10 mg q.i.d. $2/pill; $8/day	
PYRROLEACETIC ACIDS		
Tolectin* (tolmetin)	600 mg b.i.d.-t.i.d. $1.96/pill; $3.92-$5.88/day	
SALICYLIC ACIDS		
Disalcid* (salsalate)	500 mg 2 tablets t.i.d. $0.30/pill; $1.80/day	750 mg q.i.d. $0.30/pill; $1.20/day
Dolobid* (diflunisal)	250 mg b.i.d. $1.15/pill; $1.30/day	500 mg b.i.d. $1.63/pill; $3.26/day
Trilisate* (choline–magnesium salicylate) (also available as liquid)	500 mg 3 tablets b.i.d. $0.28/pill; $1.68/day	750 mg t.i.d. $0.36/pill; $1.08/day

often than every 3 to 4 months. Caution should be used with patients who are taking oral prednisone preparations or who have diabetes. All patients should be warned about transient increased pain, warmth, or redness of the joint after an injection. If these symptoms persist, the patient should seek follow-up care.[4,8]

Triamcinolone acetonide (Kenalog) and methylprednisolone acetate (Depo-Medrol) are the preferred corticosteroid preparations because they remain in solution within the joint and do not leave behind crystalline particulate debris. Diabetic patients should be warned to expect a transient elevation in blood glucose levels for about 3 to 4 days.

Nonpharmacologic Management

Exercise has a number of potential benefits for OA management. Aerobic exercise can help with cardiovascular conditioning and weight reduction (if indicated). Physical and occupational therapy can improve muscle strength and functional capacity.[25,26] Stretching programs can help rebalance joints and reduce contractures that lead to excess joint wear. Supportive, well-cushioned shoe wear with lifts or wedges can help adjust for angular deformities. Assistive devices such as canes or walkers can help reduce the load of lower extremity joints. Heat and/or ice may also provide symptomatic relief and improve exercise tolerance. The benefits of weight control are well supported in the literature. If a patient is overweight, losing weight will help reduce symptoms as it helps unload the joint. A good exercise program will help augment a weight control program.[27]

A growing body of evidence suggests that acupuncture may be beneficial, at least short term, as adjunctive treatment for OA and a number of other ailments.[28] It is important, however, to use sterile needles to avoid the risks of HIV, hepatitis, and other communicable diseases that are transmitted by dirty needles.

Other Medications Helpful for Chronic Pain

Other medications, such as gabapentin (Neurontin), selective serotonin reuptake inhibitors, and tricyclic antidepressants, have also been used successfully in the management of chronic pain associated with OA.[9] Topical medications, including rubs and lidocaine patches, may also be of some benefit.[9]

Herbs and Dietary Supplements. Herbal preparations and dietary supplements are often tried by patients with OA. Health care providers should be aware of any supplements being taken by their patients. The Arthritis Foundation has published a guide to many of the most commonly used supplements, along with any associated study results.[29]

Therapeutic magnets and copper bracelets have been used by patients for years to help reduce the chronic pain of OA. Although there is limited scientific evidence to support their efficacy, they seem to cause no harm other than to the pocketbook.

LIFE SPAN CONSIDERATIONS

OA is a disease of older adults. It is not a terminal disease, but it can cause significant disability. The primary goal of management, both conservative and surgical, is to improve the quality of life and reduce pain.

COMPLICATIONS

Pain and immobility that affect the patient's functional capacity and quality of life are the main complications associated with OA. When patients hurt, they find it hard to exercise or to control weight. This can have a detrimental effect globally on the patient's well-being. The risk of falling is higher as a direct effect of a painful or immobile arthritic joint and weakened muscles. This can lead to fractures or other injuries.

Other complications are directly related to the treatment of the disease, including medication side effects, infection or microfractures of damaged joints, or failure involving prosthetic components.

INDICATIONS FOR REFERRAL OR HOSPITALIZATION

Orthopedic consultation is considered when conservative measures fail and/or the patient's quality of life is significantly diminished. Frequent or constant disabling pain, especially pain at rest, and functionally limiting symptoms are the most important criteria for orthopedic consultation.

A number of pain-relieving procedures can be done in a specialty office, including conservative measures such as intraarticular corticosteroid injections or bracing.[30] Arthroscopic surgical procedures can include joint lavage, partial medial or lateral meniscectomy or chondroplasty as indicated, lateral patellar retinacular release, fracture drilling of full-thickness defects, or chondral grafts. Larger or open surgical procedures including osteotomy and partial or total joint arthroplasty are performed commonly. Advanced techniques and technologies have revolutionized joint replacement surgeries, making this an option for younger patients with painful arthritis.

Once a patient has undergone total joint replacement, long-term management may include prophylactic antibiotics for dental work or endoscopy. Annual x-ray examinations to evaluate the position and fixation of prosthetic components may also be recommended.

FUTURE DIRECTIONS

Current research is moving in the direction of disease-modifying agents that are designed to alter the course of OA rather than cover its symptoms. Cartilage cell replacement, stem cell transplantation, gene therapy, and implantable gene chips are proving to be exciting new directions for researchers.[31] The cycline antibiotics, including doxycycline, minocycline, and tetracycline, also seem to have disease-modifying characteristics.[32] Using growth factors to alter disease progression is also being researched.[33,34] Newer medications and advances in prosthetic components to help manage symptoms continue to be explored as well.[35]

PATIENT AND FAMILY EDUCATION

The treatment of OA should begin with a clear explanation of the disease process and likely progression of the disease. Instruction on methods to protect the painful joint should include job or lifestyle modifications. The use of assistive devices, such as a cane, crutches, or a walker, can be helpful. Patients are encouraged to be realistic about their limitations to avoid exacerbations of symptoms.

A number of good websites on the Internet can help further educate the patient on the disease process and newer treatment options.

HEALTH PROMOTION

Obesity and repetitive stress or trauma are specific modifiable risk factors for the development of OA; reduction in one or both may substantially reduce symptoms and disease progression. Maintaining an active lifestyle and weight control can significantly improve the quality of life for these individuals.

REFERENCES

1. National Institute of Arthritis and Musculoskeletal and Skin Diseases: *Handout on health: osteoarthritis*, July 2002, Pub No 02-4617, retrieved Feb 27, 2006, from http://www.niams.nih.gov/hi/topics/arthritis/oahandout.htm.
2. Mayo Clinic: *Osteoarthritis: treatment*, Oct 2005, retrieved Feb 27, 2006, from http://www.mayoclinic.com/health/osteoarthritis/DS00019/DSECTION=8.
3. National Arthritis Foundation: *Osteoarthritis*, 2003, retrieved Feb 27, 2006, from http://www.arthritis.org.sg/101/med/osteo.html.
4. Hinton R, Moody R, Davis A, and others: Osteoarthritis: diagnosis and therapeutic considerations, *Am Fam Phys* 65:5, 2002.
5. Merck Medicus: *Osteoarthritis*, March 2001, retrieved Feb 10, 2007, from http://www.merckmedicus.com/pp/us/hcp/templates/tier2/professionalDev.jsp.
6. Towheed TE: *Acetaminophen for osteoarthritis*, retrieved Feb 27, 2006, from http://www.cochrane.org/reviews/en/aboo4257.html.
7. Michigan Quality Improvement Consortium: *Medical management of adults with osteoarthritis*, 2005, retrieved Feb 27, 2006, from http://www.mqic.org./pdf/osteo05.pdf.
8. American College of Rheumatology Subcommittee on Osteoarthritis Guidelines: Recommendations for the medical management of osteoarthritis of the hip and knee, *Arthritis Rheum* 43(9):1905-1915, 2000.
9. Fredrick M: Life after Vioxx. In Arthritis Foundation: *Arthritis drug guide 2005*, retrieved Feb 27, 2006, from http://www.arthritis.org/conditions/drugguide/life-after-Vioxx.asp.
10. About Arthritis: *Arthritis drugs: what are my options?*, retrieved Feb 10, 2007, from http://arthritis.about.com/cs/druggen/a/arthdrugoptions.htm.
11. Vega C, Barclay L: *Long-term NSAIDs may not be useful for osteoarthritis*, retrieved Nov 1, 2004, from http://www.medscape.com/viewarticle/494858.
12. Graham D, Campen D, Hui R, and others: Risk of acute myocardial infarction and sudden cardiac death in patients treated with cyclooxygenase 2 selective and non-selective non-steroidal anti-inflammatory drugs: nested case control, *Lancet* 365(9458):475-481, 2005.
13. Bell GM, Schnitzer TJ: Cox-2 inhibitors and other nonsteroidal anti-inflammatory drugs in the treatment of pain in the elderly, *Clin Geriatr Med* 17:489-502, 2001.
14. Noble S, King D, Olutade J: Cyclooxygenase-2 enzyme inhibitors: place in therapy, *Am Fam Phys* 61(12):3669-3679, 2000.
15. Zhao SZ, Reynolds MW, Lejkowith J, and others: A comparison of the renal-related adverse drug reactions between rofecoxib and celecoxib, based on the World Health Organization/Uppsala Monitoring Center safety database, *Clin Ther* 23:1478-1491, 2001.
16. Cannon GW, Caldwell JR, Holt P, and others: Rofecoxib, a specific inhibitor of cyclooxygenase 2, with clinical efficacy comparable with that of diclofenac sodium: results of a 1-year randomized, clinical trial in patients with osteoarthritis of the knee and hip, *Arthritis Rheum* 43:978-987, 2000.
17. Clegg DO, Raab L, DiNubile N: *The differential effects of chondroitin sulfate on osteoarthritis symptoms related to degree of radiographic involvement*, poster presentation at Tenth World Conference on Osteoarthritis, Boston, Dec 8-11, 2005.
18. Jacks S: *Osteoarthritis and the ideal treatment*, retrieved Feb 27, 2006, from http://www.vanderbilt.edu/AnS/psychology/health_psychology/glucocond.htm.
19. Hart J: Complementary health: besides pain medication, what else can I do to help ease the pain I have from osteoarthritis? *Health Plus, Health and Wellness*, Nashville, June 19, 2005, Vanderbilt University.
20. Leffler CT, Phillippi AF, Leffler SG: Glucosamine, chondroitin, and manganese ascorbate for degenerative joint disease of the knee or low back: a randomized, double-blind, placebo-controlled pilot study, *Mil Med* 164:85-91, 1999.
21. Morelli V, Naquin C, Weaver V: Alternative therapies for traditional disease states: osteoarthritis, *Am Fam Phys* 67:2, 2003.

22. Clegg D, Reda D, Harris C, and others: Glucosamine, chondroitin sulfate, and the two in combination for painful knee osteoarthritis, *N Engl J Med* 354(8):795-808, 2006.
23. Mayo Clinic: *Osteoarthritis: complementary and alternative medicine,* Oct 2005, retrieved Feb 27, 2006, from http://www.mayoclinic.com/health/osteoarthritis/DS00019/DSECTION=11.
24. Bellamy N, Campbell J, Robinson V, and others: Viscosupplementation for the treatment of osteoarthritis of the knee, *Cochrane Database of Systematic Reviews,* 2, April 19, 2006
25. Felson D: Knee osteoarthritis: does physiotherapy help? *Nature Clin Pract Rheum* 1:16-17, 2005.
26. Petrella RJ: Is exercise effective treatment for osteoarthritis of the knee? *Br J Sports Med* 34:326-331, 2000.
27. Miller G, Nichlas B, Dacis C: Intensive weight loss program improves physical function in older obese adults with knee osteoarthritis, *Obesity* 14(7):1219-1230, 2006.
28. Moore A, McQuay H: Acupuncture: not just needles? *Lancet* 366(9480):100-101, 2005.
29. Welland D: *Arthritis Today's supplement guide,* retrieved Feb 9, 2007, from http://www.arthritis.org/conditions/supplementguide/herbs_d_f.asp.
30. West R: Bracing in the treatment of knee osteoarthritis: O & P options, *Orthop Technol Rev* 5:6, 2003.
31. University of Bristol: *Breakthrough in treatment for osteoarthritis sufferers,* retrieved Dec 19, 2005, from http://www.bris.ac.uk/news/2005/871.html.
32. Brandt K, Mazzuca S, Katz B, and others: Effects of doxycycline on progression of osteoarthritis: results of a randomized, placebo-controlled, double-blind trial, *Arthritis Rheum* 52(7):2015-2025, 2005.
33. Reddi AH: Aging, osteoarthritis and transforming growth factor-b signaling in cartilage, *Arthritis Res Therapy* 8(101):1858, 2006.
34. Schnitzer T: *Advances in osteoarthritis research: investigating subchondral bone as etiologic agent and therapeutic target: an on-line CME activity,* retrieved Feb 10, 2007, from http://doctor.medscape.com/viewprogram/2892.
35. Simon LS: *Future therapeutics for osteoarthritis* (presentation), American College of Rheumatology 2002 Annual Meeting, New Orleans, Oct 26-29, 2002.

CHAPTER 195

Osteomyelitis

Alexander J. Kallen and Thomas H. Taylor

DEFINITION AND EPIDEMIOLOGY

Infection of bone has been classically divided into three groups: (1) hematogenous osteomyelitis, seeded from bacteremia; (2) osteomyelitis associated with a contiguous focus, such as a puncture wound, foreign body, or adjoining soft tissue infection; and (3) osteomyelitis associated with peripheral vascular disease, such as diabetic foot infections or other vascular insufficiency.[1]

These groups may be further divided into acute and chronic varieties. Acute disease is defined by the sudden onset of inflammation, warmth, redness, and edema. Hematogenous osteomyelitis in the young is most likely to be seen acutely, usually with a single organism seeding the medullary cavity, and a good prognosis can be predicted. This entity is most commonly seen in children (50% of cases occur in children less than 5 years old) with a second peak occurring in the elderly.[2]

In contrast to acute disease, chronic osteomyelitis develops over long periods, often months or longer.[3] Osteomyelitis with vascular insufficiency in older adults is an example of these more indolent infections. In this situation an external focus erodes into the superficial periosteum. The flora are usually mixed, and the prognosis varies greatly with factors such as the extent of bone involvement, the presence of sequestra, areas of denuded dead bone, the type of organism, and host conditions. Acute osteomyelitis not diagnosed or inadequately treated may advance to chronic osteomyelitis, resulting in a more complicated clinical picture. Some evidence suggests that the incidence of acute hematogenous osteomyelitis is decreasing (at least in children), whereas the incidence of more chronic osteomyelitis from a contiguous focus may be increasing.[4,5]

A more recent classification scheme by Cierny, Mader, and Pemnick takes into consideration the extent of anatomic involvement (anatomic stage) and host factors (physiologic class), providing a guide to determining the prognosis, extent of surgical intervention, and antibiotic treatment required.[6] Various anatomic stages *may* require further surgical resection, revascularization, muscle flaps, skin grafts, management of dead space, and bone grafts (Table 195-1). Physiologic class is divided into A, B, or C hosts[7] (Box 195-1). A favorable prognosis accompanies A hosts, who have normal vasculature and metabolic factors and a normal immune system. B hosts carry a worse prognosis by virtue of local or systemic compromise. Systemic factors, such as diabetes, smoking, malnutrition, hypoxia, immunosuppression, or immunodeficiency, and local factors, such as lymphedema, venous stasis, arterial insufficiency, or sensory deficits, may require attention during treatment. C hosts represent a group for which treatment of the osteomyelitis may be worse than the disease itself. The Cierny-Mader staging system is important to medical and surgical management but also guides prognosis and education.

TABLE 195-1 Anatomic Classification of Adult Long Bone Osteomyelitis (Cierny-Mader Syndrome)

Stage and Description	Etiologies	Treatment
I. Medullary: Necrosis limited to medullary contents and endosteal surfaces	Hematogenous infection	**Pediatric:** Antibiotics; host alteration (e.g., nutritional support) **Adult:** Unroofing; intramedullary reaming
II. Superficial: Bone necrosis limited to exposed surface	Contiguous soft tissue infection	**Pediatric:** Antibiotics; host alteration **Adult:** Superficial debridement; local or microvasuclar flap coverage; possible ablation
III. Localized: Full-thickness cortical sequestration; infection well marginated, and bone stable before and after debridement	Trauma; evolution of stage I or II; iatrogenic	Antibiotics; host alteration; debridement; dead-space management; temporary stabilization; bone graft optional
IV. Diffuse: Circumferential and/or permeative infection; bone unstable before or after debridement	Trauma; evolution of stage I or II; iatrogenic	Antibiotics; host alteration; debridement; dead-space management; stabilization (internal or external fixation); possible ablation

Modified from Mader JT, Calhoun J: Long-bone osteomyelitis, diagnoses, and management, *Hosp Pract* 29(10):71-76, 1994.

BOX 195-1

PHYSIOLOGIC CLASSIFICATION OF HOSTS WITH OSTEOMYELITIS (CIERNY-MADER SYSTEM)

A. Normal hosts with osteomyelitis
B_{S} Systemic compromise
- Diabetes mellitus
- Extremes of age
- Hypoxia (chronic)
- Immunosuppression
- Immunodeficiency
- Malignancy
- Malnutrition
- Renal failure
- Hepatic failure

B_{L} Local compromise
- Arteritis
- Extensive scarring
- Sensory loss
- Lymphedema
- Major-vessel compromise
- Small-vessel disease
- Venous stasis
- Tissue irradiation
- Tobacco abuse

C. Fragile host; treatment worse than osteomyelitis

PATHOPHYSIOLOGY

Metaphyseal bone, just beneath the epiphysis (or growth plate), is where growing beds of terminal arterioles are prone to deposition of bacteria. Thus the ends of long bones are the most common location of hematogenous osteomyelitis in young patients, whereas the vertebral bodies are a more typical site in adults.[3] Acute inflammation develops at the site, contributing to destruction of bone. This inflammation compromises blood flow and leads to further bone destruction and the formation of sequestra. Antibiotics penetrate these areas poorly, often leading to an inadequate response to treatment with antibiotics alone.[3] The periosteum can thicken and surround this area of dead bone, forming an enclosed capsule (involucrum). In children, Brodie's abscess is an example of this type of enclosed infection commonly found in the metaphysis.[2]

Infecting organisms also differ according to the patient's age and condition and whether the focus is contiguous or hematogenous. A single organism is the norm for hematogenous osteomyelitis. Infants most often harbor *Staphylococcus aureus*, group A and B streptococci, and gram-negative enteric organisms. Children over the age of 1 have most often been infected with *S. aureus* and *Streptococcus pyogenes*. With the advent of Hib conjugate vaccine, *Haemophilus influenzae* is now uncommon in children over the age of 1 year. *S. aureus* is dominant in both hematogenous and contiguous osteomyelitis, but vascular insufficiency with chronic ulcer causes mixed infection with *S. aureus*, streptococci, anaerobes, and gram-negative bacilli.[8] The prevalence of methicillin-resistant *S. aureus* (MRSA), including community-acquired strains, appears to be increasing. This pathogen must therefore be considered in patients with osteomyelitis, especially in those with risk factors for this organism, including dialysis, medical comorbidities, and, most important, a history of previous contact with the health care setting.[9-11]

CLINICAL PRESENTATION

Acute hematogenous osteomyelitis in children or young adults may be associated with fever, leukocytosis, local edema, erythema, and tenderness, although some studies have shown that up to 50% of patients may have milder, vague symptoms.[12] A soft tissue abscess and sinus tract, sometimes exiting many centimeters from the infected bone, may cause practitioners to not consider deeper infection of bone. The fever may be indolent and mild, or high and spiking. On the other hand, chronic osteomyelitis is seldom associated with fever or leukocytosis. Adjacent ulcer and soft tissue cellulitis may mask bone tenderness. In such a situation making the diagnosis of chronic osteomyelitis is difficult. Subacute presentation of osteomyelitis may challenge health care providers caring for patients with fever of unknown origin.

PHYSICAL EXAMINATION

Physical findings are indistinguishable from the clinical presentation. Deep palpation may be necessary to elicit bone tenderness. Ulcers with visible bone or sinus tracts that probe to bone are usually diagnostic of osteomyelitis.[13] Special situations and clinical syndromes are important to recognize and are briefly discussed.

Vertebral Osteomyelitis

Low back pain is a common problem for which a precise source may not be discovered in 80% of patients. Health care providers should be content with uncertainty, but warning signs should lead to further investigation[14] (Box 195-2). Osteomyelitis may be recognized by a radiologic process that involves both sides of the vertebral disc and adjacent vertebrae symmetrically. Malignancy does not cross the disc to involve adjacent vertebrae.[15] Early recognition is important because posterior extension causes epidural abscess and cord compression. Collapsed vertebrae may also threaten the spinal cord. The course may be complicated by paravertebral, retropharyngeal, mediastinal, and subphrenic abscesses, which must be drained.[16]

Pyogenic vertebral osteomyelitis is primarily a disease of adults and is usually hematogenous and insidious in onset. Pain evolves gradually over weeks to months. Fever and leukocytosis are absent in 50% of cases. Although *S. aureus* is the predominant organism, a unique feature of vertebral osteomyelitis is a relatively high rate (30%) of gram-negative infection from a urinary source in older patients.[3,17] In young patients with *Pseudomonas aeruginosa,* vertebral osteomyelitis may be attributed to IV drug use. Unusual pathogens, such as *Candida* species, other fungi, mycobacteria, and gram-negative organisms, emphasize the need to make an etiologic diagnosis whenever possible if treatment is to be successful.

Diabetic Foot

A diabetic foot ulcer is the classic example of contiguous focus osteomyelitis in an area of vascular insufficiency. Although the pulses may be palpable and arterial Doppler studies show good waveforms, 60% of these lesions are associated with relatively high-grade large-vessel obstruction on arteriography.[18] Thus recognition of arterial insufficiency and revascularization are important considerations. In the age of diagnosis-related categories for reimbursement and short hospital stays, the role of amputation in diabetes has, unfortunately, increased. Health care providers must promote prevention, early recognition, and adequate care of diabetic foot ulcers.[19]

Recognition of osteomyelitis in a diabetic foot may be difficult; however, it should be suspected in those with persistent skin ulcerations, particularly those over bony prominences and those in which bone can be directly visualized or easily palpated with a metal probe.[3,20] Additionally, stubborn cellulitis, neuropathic ulcer, and simple edema can be associated signs. Concurrent peripheral neuropathy *can* mask focal tenderness. Fever, leukocytosis, increasing hyperglycemia, and systemic toxicity may all be absent. Because of reactive bone formation in neuropathic feet (Charcot's joint), both plain films and bone scans are problematic.[21] Biopsy of bone is the definitive diagnostic study and supplies good microbiologic evidence to direct antibiotic treatment.[22] However, poor healing at the biopsy site may further compromise the foot. Thus empiric therapy is often undertaken unless debridement is indicated by anatomic criteria. Failure of therapy in later stages is greater than 50%. In those cases, suppression with oral antibiotics or amputation may be a reasonable alternative.[23]

BOX 195-2

THORACIC AND LOW BACK PAIN: WARNING SIGNS SUGGESTING MALIGNANCY OR OSTEOMYELITIS

- Previous cancer
- Weight loss
- Elevated ESR
- Fever, other constitutional symptoms
- Localized tenderness over vertebral body
- Lack of positional relief
- Lack of improvement over time
- Distant foci of infection (endocarditis)
- Indwelling IV catheters
- IV drug abuse
- Neurologic signs (weakness, sensory loss, asymmetric reflexes, loss of bowel or bladder function)
- Thoracic pain

Pseudomonas Infection

Pseudomonas osteomyelitis of the foot is a unique form of infection following a puncture wound such as a nail through the shoe. Sneakers provide a wet, fertile environment for *P. aeruginosa.*[9] *Pseudomonas* organisms also may be associated with IV drug abuse and may involve unusual sites, such as sacroiliac, sternoclavicular, pubic joints, and contiguous bone.[24]

Sickle Cell Disease

Patients with sickle cell disease are at high risk for osteomyelitis, especially in areas where decreased blood flow has led to infarcted bone.[24] Bowel ischemia, a result of intravascular sickling, encourages enteric flora to enter the circulation. *S. aureus* is most common, but enteric gram-negative organisms, especially *Salmonella* organisms, are often encountered.[25] Osteomyelitis may be difficult to distinguish from bone infarction, since they can have similar signs and symptoms. Sequential bone marrow and bone scans may help differentiate between the two entities.[26]

DIAGNOSTICS

Given the spectrum of disease and varied microbiologic characteristics of osteomyelitis, cultures of bone and blood are essential to diagnosis and management. Cultures from sinus tracts or ulcers may not be indicative of organisms in underlying bone. The exception to this is *S. aureus;* cultures of this organism from sinus tracts frequently predict deeper infection.[27,28] Blood cultures are positive in 40% of cases of acute osteomyelitis but are rarely positive in chronic osteomyelitis. In adults with contiguous focus chronic osteomyelitis, culture specimens can be obtained with surgical debridement from bone and soft tissue. Leukocyte counts and erythrocyte sedimentation rates (ESRs) are elevated in acute disease and should be monitored for improvement. C-reactive protein may be more valuable in monitoring the response to therapy because it changes more rapidly than the ESR.[3] Visible bone or sinus tracts that probe to bone are usually diagnostic of chronic osteomyelitis.[13]

Radiologic tests are frequently used to diagnose osteomyelitis. Plain films usually begin to demonstrate destructive processes within 2 weeks of onset in acute osteomyelitis. They are inexpensive and may be helpful in determining extent and activity in chronic osteomyelitis but may be difficult to interpret in the diabetic foot, where neuropathic osteoarthritis is common.

In cases where conventional radiography is ambiguous (i.e., at less than 2 weeks in acute osteomyelitis or with confounding bone disease in chronic osteomyelitis), radiographs may be followed by other radiologic tests. Three- or four-phase bone scans become abnormal in as little as 48 to 72 hours and can differentiate between bone and soft tissue involvement.[29] These tests have a relatively high sensitivity, although their specificity is generally lower because of their inability to distinguish fracture, osteoarthritis, tumor, gouty tophi, and neuropathic bone formation from infection.[30] The sensitivity of bone scans may be diminished in patients with poor vascular flow to the affected area.[9] Gallium scans may overcome this limitation, since they are less dependent on blood flow; however, they are not specific for infection. The disadvantages of gallium scans are poor imaging detail, including problems differentiating cellulitis from osteomyelitis and the need to wait 48 to 72 hours after injection before imaging.[29] Indium-labeled white blood cell scans may add specificity to bone scans when done together, especially in diabetic patients, in whom these tests can differentiate between osteomyelitis and a neuropathic joint. The disadvantages of indium scans are the expense of white blood cell labeling and the limited resolution.[15,31]

Radionucleotide scans (technetium, gallium, indium) do not show anatomic detail. If surgery is contemplated in an adult with chronic or acute osteomyelitis, then CT or MRI will best define sequestra, the anatomic stage, and associated abscess. Both are capable of identifying an abscess and allow for guided needle aspiration of bone. A CT scan is the modality of choice to define bone sequestra and cortical erosion.[30] MRI has among the highest sensitivity and specificity reported for any radiologic test used for the diagnosis of osteomyelitis.[32] It is the preferred imaging modality in cases of vertebral osteomyelitis or diabetic foot (when plain films are not diagnostic) because of its excellent soft tissue resolution.[20,33] Among the disadvantages of MRI are its expense and the fact that young children may require sedation to undergo an examination.[9]

DIAGNOSTICS

Osteomyelitis

LABORATORY
CBC and differential
Blood cultures
ESR
C-reactive protein

IMAGING
X-ray
Bone scan*
Gallium or indium scan*
CT scan, MRI*

OTHER
Open bone biopsy or needle aspiration of bone with culture and sensitivity*

*If indicated.

DIFFERENTIAL DIAGNOSIS

Osteomyelitis at the metaphysis of long bones approximates the joint and must be distinguished from septic arthritis. Examination for joint effusion and arthrocentesis will diagnose a septic joint, and radiologically the bone will be normal. Gout may cause cystic erosion in bone associated with a draining tophus. Although cultures are often positive for skin flora, the drainage is laden with crystals rather than neutrophils. Tophaceous gout is antibacterial and unlikely to be infected. Bone infarcts in hemoglobinopathy are multiple and recurrent, unlike in cases with unifocal osteomyelitis. Posttraumatic periosteal reaction may mimic early osteomyelitis radiologically or may serve as a site for osteomyelitis secondary to recent trauma. Nonspecific periosteal or cortical change caused by adjacent bursitis, abscess, or ulcer is difficult to distinguish from contiguous focus osteomyelitis. Tumor may or may not have distinguishing features on plain films. Old, inactive osteomyelitis may be indistinguishable from active infection radiologically. Finally, a focus of osteomyelitis secondary to subacute bacterial endocarditis must be considered if blood cultures are positive and a new cardiac murmur is appreciated.

DIFFERENTIAL DIAGNOSIS

Osteomyelitis

- Septic arthritis
- Gout
- Posttraumatic periosteal reaction
- Bursitis
- Abscess
- Ulcer
- Tumor
- Subacute bacterial endocarditis
- Hemoglobinopathy (bone infarction)

MANAGEMENT

Anatomic considerations define surgical management. Antibiotics alone often manage acute hematogenous medullary infection in children. Later stages with involucrum need to be surgically unroofed. All more destructive stages require surgical intervention as defined in Table 195-1, as well as prolonged antibiotic therapy based on the sensitivity of organisms obtained by culture of bone at surgery. In stage IV disease, extensive removal of infected bone may require orthopedic rod internal fixation, external fixation, bone graft, and dead space management with antibiotic-impregnated beads and two-phase joint replacement. Plastic surgery may be required to bring skin grafts or tissue flaps over bone to fill defects and revascularize. Vascular surgery may be required to revascularize with bypass grafts or to reroute major vessels away from infected areas.

For the most part, osteomyelitis is treated with 4 to 6 weeks of IV antibiotic therapy and will require placement of a central line.[34] Two recent meta-analyses concluded, however, that no definitive recommendation can be made about the best mode of administration, drugs, or length of treatment for osteomyelitis.[34,35] Sensitive organisms may respond to oral antibiotics that are highly bioavailable. The quinolones, trimethoprim-sulfamethoxazole, clindamycin, linezolid, and rifampin have been used orally to treat osteomyelitis, although rifampin should not be used as a single agent because of rapidly emerging resistance to this agent when it is used alone.[4] Children with acute osteomyelitis may be successfully treated with 2 to 5 weeks of oral antibiotics, after responding to 7 days of parenteral antibiotics.[9,36] The doses of oral penicillins and cephalosporins are higher than doses used for common infections.

Vertebral osteomyelitis is usually treated with IV antibiotics that are appropriate for the isolated organism(s) for a minimum of 6 weeks, although longer courses (12 weeks) are frequently used. Surgery is now infrequently required and is usually reserved for cases with cord compression or spinal instability or cases in which the disease progresses despite adequate therapy.[3] As opposed to vertebral osteomyelitis, in which hematogenous focus yields a single organism, diabetic contiguous focus osteomyelitis yields mixed flora. Counterintuitively, the organisms and antibiotic coverage are easier to predict. Coagulase-positive and coagulase-negative staphylococci, streptococci, anaerobes, and gram-negative bacilli are predictably present in necrotic tissue. An accompanying cellulitis is usually due to streptococci or staphylococci and may be treated with nafcillin or cefazolin alone. However, to treat the ulcer or underlying osteomyelitis, coverage of all organisms is necessary (e.g., ampicillin-sulbactam, piperacillin-tazobactam, or imipenem-cilastatin). Oral therapy with ciprofloxacin-clindamycin combination therapy, or one of the newer oral fluoroquinolones (gatifloxacin, moxifloxacin), may be used in some situations.[37] Presence or suspicion of *Pseudomonas* organisms will necessitate the addition of an antipseudomonal antibiotic, such as piperacillin, ceftazidime, or ciprofloxacin (Table 195-2). Aminoglycosides have poor penetration into bone and do not work well in abscesses, where pH is low.

With the increase in incidence of MRSA infections, questions have arisen about the best agents for treating osteomyelitis caused by this organism. IV vancomycin is frequently used as empiric therapy when this organism is suspected, although failure rates for this antibiotic in *S. aureus* osteomyelitis are considerably higher than failure rates for other commonly used antibiotics.[38] Higher levels of vancomycin are usually needed to optimize penetration of this agent into the infected bone.[39] Trimethoprim-sulfamethoxazole or clindamycin has been used in conjunction with vancomycin to treat susceptible species. There is also now some evidence supporting the use of linezolid to treat MRSA osteomyelitis.[40,41]

The health care provider must monitor the patient for allergic reaction and toxicity of antibiotics, diarrhea caused by *Clostridium difficile*, thrombosis and infection of central lines, and response to therapy. Central lines should be removed soon after completion of antibiotics to avoid providing a focus for further infection. Health care providers should also address nutrition, control of diabetes, reduction of immunosuppressive drugs, rehabilitation for alcohol and substance abuse, smoking cessation for those with vascular insufficiency, treatment of ulcers, and monitoring for patients who are at high risk for developing foot infection. Regular visits to a podiatrist may provide nail care, attention to footwear, wound care, and prophylactic surgery.[42]

LIFE SPAN CONSIDERATIONS

Osteomyelitis is usually not a fatal infection, but associated sepsis may be life threatening. Amputation is a consequence that may require physical therapy, prosthetics, and psychiatric counseling. Chronic use of a suppressive antibiotic is an option if surgery is too life threatening or amputation is being contemplated with understandable reluctance. The patient's quality of life is certainly altered by amputation. However, health care providers may need to provide information regarding below-the-knee amputation and a prosthesis, which may be more functional than a chronically draining site of osteomyelitis in a foot with marginal blood flow.

COMPLICATIONS

Failure of aggressive therapy and relapse are common in patients with diabetes or vascular insufficiency or in compromised hosts. *S. aureus* is noted for associated cellulitis, sepsis, and metastatic foci of infection that may be distant from the site of the osteomyelitis. Fracture through advanced anatomic disease should be preventable by orthopedic evaluation. Sinus tracts, abscesses, and hematomas need to be diagnosed and drained. Infection may threaten adjacent vessels, tendons, and nerves. Chronic osteomyelitis can cause squamous cell carcinoma at the site of chronic drainage.

TABLE 195-2 Empiric Therapy for Osteomyelitis in Adults

Classification	Organism	Empiric Antibiotic
Acute hematogenous osteomyelitis	Staphylococcus aureus, streptococci	Nafcillin, cefazolin*
Contiguous focus vascular insufficiency, diabetic foot, neuropathic ulcer	*S. aureus,* streptococci, gram-negative bacilli, anaerobes	Ampicillin-sulbactam, piperacillin-tazobactam, imipenem-cilastatin, clindamycin-levofloxacin
ADDITIONAL CONSIDERATIONS IN SPECIAL HOSTS		
IV drug abuse	S. aureus; Pseudomonas, Serratia, Enterobacter organisms	Depends on pathogen
Hemoglobinopathies	*Salmonella* organisms	Depends on sensitivity
Immunosuppression	*Enterobacter* organisms, mycobacteria, fungi	Other

*Vancomycin may be substituted or added if patient is at risk for methicillin-resistant *Staphylococcus aureus.*

Amyloidosis has been caused by the systemic response to chronic osteomyelitis. Long-term antibiotic use may be associated with a number of complications, including line infections or thrombosis and adverse drug reactions.

INDICATIONS FOR REFERRAL OR HOSPITALIZATION

Patients with acute osteomyelitis are sick, are often septic, and require IV antibiotics and evaluation by specialists, which often includes an infectious disease specialist and an orthopedic surgeon. There is no question about the need for initial hospitalization, although prolonged antibiotic therapy may be continued at home. Curative therapy for chronic osteomyelitis involves elective admission with surgical debridement, culture of bone, and consultation as defined by individual needs. Same-day surgery programs sometimes accomplish this without hospitalization. Suppressive antibiotic therapy for chronic osteomyelitis may be administered on an outpatient basis.

PATIENT AND FAMILY EDUCATION

In addition to receiving an explanation of the various diagnostic and therapeutic options, patients should understand that "cure" is an elusive concept in this disease. Acute osteomyelitis may relapse years after treatment, and chronic osteomyelitis may smolder indefinitely in a subacute fashion with intermittent drainage. Saying that osteomyelitis is arrested rather than cured is usually appropriate. Patients with extensive bony defects must take precautions against fracture. Patients need to be educated regarding prolonged therapy, central venous lines, relapses, antibiotic complications, amputation, and suppression. Preventive measures include teaching daily foot inspection to patients with diabetes, arthritis, vascular insufficiency, or neuropathy, since these patients are particularly prone to infections in the feet. Diabetic and neuropathic ulcers require prompt medical attention. Insensate feet must be protected from heat, cold, and trauma. Control of diabetes, management of edema, good nutrition, and smoking cessation are all important.

REFERENCES

1. Lew DP, Waldvogel FA: Osteomyelitis, *N Engl J Med* 336:999-1007, 1997.
2. Steer AC, Carapetis JR: Acute hematogenous osteomyelitis in children: recognition and management, *Pediatr Drugs* 6:333-346, 2004.
3. Lew DP, Waldvogel FA: Osteomyelitis, *Lancet* 364:369-379, 2004.
4. Luzzarini L, Mader JT, Calhoun JH: Osteomyelitis in long bones, *J Bone Joint Surg* 86A:2305-2318, 2004.
5. Blyth MJ, Kincaid R, Craigen MA, and others: The changing epidemiology of acute and subacute haematogenous osteomyelitis in children, *J Bone Joint Surg Br* 83:99-102, 2001.
6. Cierny C, Mader JT, Pemnick H: A clinical staging system of adult osteomyelitis, *Contemp Orthop* 10:17-37, 1985.
7. Mader JT, Shirtliff M, Calhoun JH: Staging and staging application in osteomyelitis, *Clin Infect Dis* 25:1303-1309, 1997.
8. O'Hanley P, Swartz MN: Osteomyelitis, *Sci Am Med,* 1995.
9. Gutierrez K: Bone and joint infections in children, *Pediatr Clin North Am* 52:779-794, 2005.
10. Martinez-Aguilar G, Avalos-Mishaan A, Huleton K, and others: Community-acquired, methicillin resistant and methicillin susceptible *Staphylococcus aureus* musculoskeletal infections in children, *Pediatr Infect Dis J* 23:701-706, 2004.
11. Rybak MJ, LaPlante KL: Community-associated methicillin-resistant *Staphylococcus aureus*: a review, *Pharmacotherapy* 25:74-85, 2005.
12. Dahl LB, Hoyland AL, Dramsdahl H, and others: Acute osteomyelitis in children: a population-based retrospective study 1965-1994, *Scand J Infect Dis* 30:573-577, 1998.
13. Grayson ML, Gibbons G, Balogh K: Probing to bone in infected pedal ulcers: a clinical sign of underlying osteomyelitis in diabetic patients, *JAMA* 273:721-723, 1995.
14. Mazanec D: Low back pain: living with ambiguity, *Cleve Clin J Med* 64:407-410, 1997.
15. Haas DW, McAndrew MP: Bacterial osteomyelitis in adults: evolving considerations in diagnosis and treatment, *Am J Med* 101:550-561, 1996.
16. Stravebaugh LJ: Vertebral osteomyelitis, *Postgrad Med* 97:147-154, 1995.
17. Sapico Fl, Montgomerie JZ: Vertebral osteomyelitis, *Infect Dis Clin North Am* 4:539-550, 1990.
18. Caputo GM, Cavanagh PR, Ulbrecht JS, and others: Assessment and management of foot disease in patients with diabetes, *N Engl J Med* 331(13):854-860, 1994.
19. Culleton JL: Preventing diabetic foot complications, *Postgrad Med* 106:74-83, 1999.
20. Lipsky BA, Berendt AR, Deery HG, and others: Diagnosis and treatment of diabetic foot infections, *Clin Infect Dis* 39:885-910, 2004.
21. Longmaid HE, Kruskal JB: Imaging infections in diabetes patients, *Infect Dis Clin North Am* 9:163-182, 1995.
22. Khatri G, Wagner DK, Sohnle PG: Effect of bone biopsy in guiding antimicrobial therapy for osteomyelitis complicating open wounds, *Am J Med Sci* 321(6):367-371, 2001.
23. Karchmer AW, Gibbons GW: Foot infections in diabetes: evaluation and management, *Curr Clin Top Infect Dis* 14:1-22, 1994.
24. Berbari EF, Steckelberg JM, Osmon DR: Osteomyelitis. In Mandell G, Bennett J, Dolen R, editors: *Principles and practice of infectious diseases,* ed 6, Philadelphia, 2005, Churchill Livingstone.
25. Anand AJ, Glatt AE: Salmonella osteomyelitis and arthritis in sickle cell disease, *Semin Arthritis Rheum* 24:211-221, 1994.
26. Skaggs DL, Kim SK, Greene NW, and others: Differentiating between bone infarction and acute osteomyelitis in children with sickle-cell disease with use of sequential radionuclide bone-marrow and bone scans, *J Bone Joint Surg* 83A(12):1810-1813, 2001.
27. Mackowiak PA, Jones SR, Smith JW: Diagnostic value of sinus-tract cultures in chronic osteomyelitis, *JAMA* 239:2772-2775, 1978.
28. Perry CR, Pearson RL, Miller GH: Accuracy of cultures of material from swabbing of the superficial aspect of the wound and needle biopsy in the preoperative assessment of osteomyelitis, *J Bone Joint Surg* 73:745-749, 1991.
29. Siagal G, Azouz EM, Abdenour G: Imaging of osteomyelitis with special reference to children, *Semin Musculoskel Radiol* 8(3):255-265, 2004.
30. Buhne KH, Bohndorf K: Imaging of posttraumatic osteomyelitis, *Semin Musculoskel Rev* 8:199-204, 2004.
31. Schinabeck MK, Johnson JL: Osteomyelitis in diabetic foot ulcers, *Postgrad Med J* 118:11-15, 2005.
32. Berendt AR, Lipsky B: Is this bone infected or not? Differentiating neuro-osteoarthropathy from osteomyelitis in the diabetic foot, *Curr Diabetes Rep* 4:424-429, 2004.
33. Berendt T, Byren I: Bone and joint infection, *Clin Med* 4:510-518, 2004.
34. Lazzarini L, Lipsky BA, Mader JT: Antibiotic treatment of osteomyelitis: what have we learned from 30 years of clinical trials? *Int J Infect Dis* 9:127-138, 2005.
35. Stengel D, Bauwens K, Sehouli J, and others: Systematic review and meta-analysis of antibiotic therapy for bone and joint infections, *Lancet* 1:175-188, 2001.
36. Le Saux N, Howard A, Barrowman NJ, and others: Shorter courses of parenteral antibiotic therapy do not appear to influence response rates for children with acute hematogenous osteomyelitis: a systematic review, *BMC Infect Dis* 2:16-24, 2002.

37. Rissing JP: Antimicrobial therapy for chronic osteomyelitis in adults: role of the quinolones, *Clin Infect Dis* 25:1327-1333, 1997.
38. Tice AD, Hoaglund PA, Shoultz DA: Outcomes of osteomyelitis among patients treated with outpatient parenteral antimicrobial therapy, *Am J Med* 114:723-728, 2003.
39. Boffe El Amari E, Vaugnat A, and others: High versus standard dose vancomycin for osteomyelitis, *Scand J Infect Dis* 36:712-717, 2004.
40. Rao N, Ziran BH, Hall RA, and others: Successful treatment of chronic bone and joint infections with oral linezolid, *Clin Orthop Relat Res* 427:67-71, 2004.
41. Harwood PJ, Giannoudis PV: The safety and efficacy of linezolid in orthopedic practice for the treatment of infections due to antibiotic-resistant organisms, *Expert Opin Drug Safety* 3:405-414, 2004.
42. Muha J: Local wound care in diabetic foot complications, *Postgrad Med* 106:97-102, 1999.

CHAPTER 196

Osteoporosis

Alan Ona Malabanan

DEFINITION AND EPIDEMIOLOGY

Osteoporosis is characterized by increased bone fragility and increased susceptibility to fracture. This increased bone fragility results from decreases in bone mass and deterioration of bone microarchitecture that occur as the result of estrogen deficiency and aging. Osteoporosis is the most common metabolic bone disease, with more than 44 million Americans either having the condition or being at risk for it.[1] It is the leading cause of fractures, accounting for approximately 1.5 million fractures yearly.[2] Osteoporotic fractures are more common than heart attack, stroke, or cancer.[3,4]

Osteoporosis is also defined, by the World Health Organization, as a bone mineral density (BMD) of 2.5 SD or less below the young normal mean (i.e., *T*-score ≤ -2.5).[5] In the absence of osteoporotic fracture, this densitometric definition is the most clinically relevant, but it should not be used as the sole criterion for treatment decision. Much as elevated cholesterol is one risk factor for heart attack, osteoporosis is but one risk factor for osteoporotic fracture. There is no definitive BMD threshold at which osteoporotic fractures occur—only an increasing likelihood of fracture with decreasing BMD. Other risk factors, such as increasing age, family history of hip fracture, current cigarette smoking, or prior fracture, have an impact on this fracture likelihood independent of the BMD.[6]

PATHOPHYSIOLOGY

In addition to providing a supportive and protective framework for the body, bone serves as a large calcium reservoir. Calcium is necessary for proper neural, musculoskeletal, and cardiac function. Normal bone remodeling allows both access to the calcium reservoir and replacement and repair of old and damaged bone. Bone remodeling has two main phases: bone resorption and bone formation.

Bone resorption, which releases calcium into the circulation, is the removal of damaged or old bone by osteoclasts, cells derived from macrophages and monocytes. This process is rapid and occurs in a matter of days to weeks. Osteoblasts, in response to parathyroid hormone (PTH) and other cytokines, secrete RANK ligand (receptor activator of nuclear factor kappa beta) and mCSF (monocyte-colony stimulating factor), which cause monocytes and macrophages to differentiate into osteoclasts and proliferate. Osteoclasts produce powerful degradative enzymes, such as cathepsin K, to break down bone, releasing calcium, phosphorus, and type I collagen crosslinked products into the circulation.[7]

Bone formation occurs when osteoblasts lay down osteoid, an organic matrix composed of type I collagen and other proteins. Bone formation, occurring over months, is a slow process. It is estimated that the skeleton is completely replaced over approximately 4 years. Osteoblasts are also responsible for mineralizing the bone, depositing calcium and phosphorus into the osteoid. This process depends on the presence of adequate amounts of calcium and phosphorus and alkaline phosphatase activity. Poor bone mineralization leads to osteomalacia, a painful softening of the bone.

Normally, bone resorption and bone formation proceed at equal rates. In osteoporosis, however, the rate of bone resorption exceeds that of bone formation, producing a net loss of bone. This uncoupling of bone resorption and bone formation is a consequence of estrogen deficiency and is most pronounced in the first 5 to 10 years after menopause.

Glucocorticoid use is the most common cause of secondary osteoporosis. It causes osteoblast death, decreases levels of estrogen and testosterone, increases the metabolism of vitamin D, and decreases the intestinal absorption of calcium.[8] This increased bone resorption and decreased bone formation lead to a rapid loss of bone, the majority of which occurs in the first 6 months of glucocorticoid use. Other drugs, such as chronic opiates, anticonvulsants, heparin, excessive thyroid hormone, leuprolide, cancer chemotherapeutics, and cigarettes, lead to similar changes in bone metabolism.[9]

Risk Factors

Risk factors, both unmodifiable and modifiable, increase the risk of bone loss or osteoporotic fracture (Box 196-1). These risk factors should be considered when deciding on osteoporosis screening or therapy. Unmodifiable risk factors for osteoporosis include increasing age, personal history of fracture as an adult, Caucasian or Asian race, female gender, and history of fracture in a first-degree relative. Potentially modifiable risk factors for osteoporosis include estrogen deficiency, associated with menopause at younger than age 45 or bilateral ovariectomy and premenopausal amenorrhea; cigarette smoking; low calcium intake; low body weight (<58 kg [127 pounds]); excessive alcohol intake; inadequate physical activity; visual impairment; poor health or frailty; and falls.[2] Minor risk factors for hip fracture in older women include tall height at age 26, fair to poor self-reported health, previous hyperthyroidism, use of long-acting benzodiazepines, excessive caffeine intake, not walking for exercise, weight loss since age 25, being on feet for less than 4 hours per day, inability to rise from a chair without using arms, poor depth perception, poor contrast sensitivity, and tachycardia at rest.[6,10]

BOX 196-1

RISK FACTORS FOR BONE LOSS OR OSTEOPOROTIC FRACTURE

UNMODIFIABLE
- Advanced age
- Female gender
- Caucasian or Asian race
- Personal history of fracture
- History of fracture in a first-degree relative
- Dementia

MODIFIABLE
- Hypogonadism
- Current cigarette smoking
- Excessive alcohol or caffeine use
- Low calcium intake
- Low body weight (<58 kg [127 pounds])
- Inadequate physical activity
- Visual impairment
- Glucocorticoid or anticonvulsant use
- Thyrotoxicosis
- Recurrent falls
- Poor health or frailty

CLINICAL PRESENTATION

Unless an osteoporotic fracture is present, osteoporosis is clinically silent. Low BMD, in the absence of osteoporotic fracture, *does not* cause pain. If pain is present, the presence of fracture should be confirmed or a secondary cause of the low BMD, such as osteomalacia, ruled out.

The sine qua non of osteoporosis is an osteoporotic fracture, a fracture occurring with no or minimum trauma. The presence of a typical osteoporotic fracture in a postmenopausal woman is usually sufficient to diagnose osteoporosis. The typical sites of fractures include the vertebrae, the distal wrist, the proximal femur, and the ribs. Unfortunately, even in the presence of a typical osteoporotic fracture, the diagnosis of osteoporosis is often missed and treatment is never initiated.[11-13] Osteoporosis occurring in men, premenopausal women, or perimenopausal women should lead to a consideration of secondary causes of osteoporosis.[9,14]

PHYSICAL EXAMINATION

Severe or established osteoporosis, that is, osteoporosis with fractures, is readily identifiable. The "dowager's hump" is a thoracic spine kyphotic deformity that occurs with multiple vertebral compression fractures. Vertebral compression fractures may also lead to scoliosis and height loss. A height loss of more than 5 cm (2 inches) or more than 4 cm (1.6 inches) (depending on the research standard used) over 10 years has been associated with low bone density and an increased incidence of vertebral compression fractures.[15-17]

The physical examination in osteoporosis should be directed toward finding signs of secondary osteoporosis. Band keratopathy may suggest a diagnosis of primary hyperparathyroidism. Exophthalmos or lid lag, goiter, tremor, warm moist skin, weight loss, or pretibial myxedema may indicate a diagnosis of hyperthyroidism. Dorsal fat, facial plethora, supraclavicular fat, hypertension, centripetal obesity, proximal muscle weakness, edema, or violaceous abdominal striae may suggest a diagnosis of Cushing's syndrome. Gynecomastia, or decreased facial or axillary hair, and testicular atrophy may suggest hypogonadism. Blue sclera may suggest a diagnosis of osteogenesis imperfecta.

Fall risk should be assessed in each patient seen with osteoporosis. Lower extremity strength, balance, gait, and postural reflexes should be carefully assessed. Poor visual acuity, weak grip strength, difficulty arising from a chair, Romberg's sign, excessive body sway, and an unsteady gait may all be signs of increased fall risk that may benefit from evaluation by a physical therapist or in a specialty fall clinic.

DIAGNOSTICS

Routine chemistry profiles (serum electrolytes, fasting serum calcium and phosphorus, serum glucose, BUN, and creatinine) are usually normal in idiopathic osteoporosis. However, screening laboratory tests may be indicated to exclude underlying pathologic processes suggested by physical examination or presenting symptoms. A serum calcium, PTH, thyroid-stimulating hormone, and 24-hour urine calcium may be the most cost-effective workup for identifying secondary causes of osteoporosis among postmenopausal women.[18] Low vitamin D levels and vitamin D deficiency are a co-existing condition in many patients with osteoporosis, as well as in general medical inpatients.[19,20] A 25-hydroxyvitamin D (*not* 1,25-dihydroxyvitamin D) assessment should be part of the initial evaluation of osteoporosis. The normal range for 25-hydroxyvitamin D in New England is 9 to 52 ng/ml; however, a normal 25-hydroxyvitamin D may still be consistent with vitamin D insufficiency.[20] Many experts believe a 25-hydroxyvitamin D level greater than 32 ng/ml is optimum.[21] A safe and effective method of repleting vitamin D stores in those with normocalcemia and normal renal function is to give 50,000 units of vitamin D weekly for 8 weeks.[22]

Biochemical markers are urine and blood tests that measure breakdown products of bone and collagen. A *biochemical marker* is an indirect measurement of bone turnover (i.e., bone resorption and formation). Bone resorption markers (*N*-telopeptides and *C*-telopeptides) are used to evaluate osteoclast activity, and bone formation markers (bone-specific alkaline phosphatase, osteocalcin, procollagen I extension peptides) are used to evaluate osteoblast activity. High levels imply increased bone turnover. At this time the role of bone markers in primary care is unclear, although specialists may use them. Bone resorption markers help identify response to antiresorptive drug treatment. Six-month intervals are the usual frequency for testing bone markers.

DIAGNOSTICS

Osteoporosis

LABORATORY
CBC and differential
Serum electrolytes
BUN and creatinine
LFTs
Serum calcium with albumin
Serum phosphorus
25-Hydroxyvitamin D
Intact parathyroid hormone*
TSH
Serum and urine protein electrophoresis*
24-Hour urine calcium
24-Hour urine free cortisol*
Urinary *N*-telopeptides*
Serum testosterone*
Tissue transglutaminase antibody*

IMAGING
Bone densitometry
Bone scan*
X-ray*
CT*
MRI*

INVASIVE TESTING
Bone biopsy*

*If indicated.

Plain radiographs are useful primarily in confirming the presence of fracture. They are insensitive to decreases in bone mass. In the absence of fracture the definitive method for diagnosing osteoporosis is bone densitometry, by dual energy x-ray absorptiometry, of the hip and posteroanterior lumbar spine. The wrist may be used in very obese patients, uninterpretable hip and spine scans, and primary hyperparathyroidism. Indications for bone densitometry are listed in Box 196-2. Bone density assessment of other sites such as the finger, wrist, and ankle and the use of other technologies, such as ultrasound, are useful in diagnosing osteoporosis and predicting fracture risk (particularly in woman over 65 years of age) but may not be as useful in ruling out osteoporosis.[23,24]

Bone densitometry provides three pertinent numbers. The first is the actual area density in grams per centimeters squared. This density is then compared with the manufacturer's database for young normal adults and age-matched adults. This comparison results in a *T*-score and a *Z*-score, respectively. The *T*-score is used in diagnosing osteopenia (*T* score <-1.0 and >-2.5) and osteoporosis (≤-2.5). The *Z*-score is ignored, unless it is less than -2.0.

Only bone densitometry of the posteroanterior lumbar spine and hip is recommended for monitoring osteoporosis treatment efficacy, and it is generally performed at 1- to 2-year intervals, depending on the precision of the scan. In general, a 5% density change is considered significant and not caused by measurement statistical variation.[25] Some disease states such as chronic glucocorticoid therapy or paraplegia may lead to more rapid bone density changes. In these cases, assessing bone density every 6 months to 1 year may be indicated.

BOX 196-2

INDICATIONS FOR BONE DENSITOMETRY

WOMEN
- Age of 65 years or more
- Postmenopausal age of less than 65 years with risk factors
- Postmenopausal status with a fracture
- Considering osteoporosis therapy
- Receiving long-term hormone replacement therapy

MEN
- Age of 70 years or more
- Low trauma fractures
- Hypogonadism
- Prevalent vertebral deformities
- Radiographic osteopenia

BOTH
- Hyperparathyroidism
- Chronic glucocorticoid therapy

Data from National Osteoporosis Foundation: *Physician's guide to prevention and treatment of osteoporosis,* Belle Mead, NJ, 1999, Exerpta Medica; Orwoll ES: Osteoporosis in men, *Endocrinol Metab Clin North Am* 272:349-367, 1998; and Bennell K, and others: The role of physiotherapy in the prevention and treatment of osteoporosis, *Manage Ther* 54:198-213, 2000.

DIFFERENTIAL DIAGNOSIS

Osteoporosis is classified as either primary or secondary. Primary osteoporosis includes bone loss arising from menopausal estrogen deficiency or aging. Secondary osteoporosis results from an acquired or inherited disease that interferes with bone remodeling or increases bone turnover.

Postmenopausal osteoporosis should be distinguished from secondary causes of osteoporosis (Box 196-3). Secondary causes of osteoporosis may be potentially reversible. Suspicion of secondary causes of osteoporosis should be high in premenopausal and perimenopausal women, men, those with bone density *Z*-scores of less than -2.0, and those with bone pain in the absence of fracture.

BOX 196-3

SECONDARY CAUSES OF LOW BONE MASS

ENDOCRINE CAUSES
- Hypogonadism
- Cushing's syndrome
- Hyperparathyroidism
- Hyperthyroidism
- Hyperprolactinemia
- Diabetes mellitus type 1
- Acromegaly

GASTROINTESTINAL CAUSES
- Gastrectomy
- Celiac disease
- Malabsorption
- Inflammatory bowel diseases
- Primary biliary cirrhosis
- Hemochromatosis
- Anorexia nervosa

NEUROLOGIC CAUSES
- Multiple sclerosis
- Parkinson's disease
- Spinal cord injury

OSTEOMALACIAS
- Vitamin D deficiency
- Chronic renal failure
- Hypophosphatasia
- Fanconi's syndrome
- Oncogenic osteomalacia
- X-linked hypophosphatemic rickets

MALIGNANCY (MARROW ASSOCIATED)
- Multiple myeloma
- Leukemias and lymphomas
- Systemic mastocytosis
- Tumoral hypercalcemia

CONNECTIVE TISSUE DISEASES
- Rheumatoid arthritis
- Ankylosing spondylitis
- Osteogenesis imperfecta
- Ehlers-Danlos syndrome
- Sarcoidosis
- Homocystinuria

DRUGS
- Glucocorticoids
- Heparin
- Cyclosporin A
- Anticonvulsants
- Gonadotropin-releasing hormone analogs
- Lithium
- Methotrexate
- Cigarette smoking
- Excessive alcohol
- Excessive thyroxine
- Chronic opiates
- Tamoxifen premenopausal use

Data from National Osteoporosis Foundation: *Physician's guide to prevention and treatment of osteoporosis,* Belle Mead, NJ, Exerpta Medica; Harper KD, Weber TJ: Secondary osteoporosis: diagnostic considerations, *Endocrinol Metab Clin North Am* 272:349-367, 1998.

DIFFERENTIAL DIAGNOSIS

Osteoporosis
- Aging
- Estrogen or testosterone deficiency
- Diabetes mellitus
- Cushing's syndrome
- Hyperthyroidism
- Hyperparathyroidism
- Hyperprolactinemia
- Acromegaly
- Hypercalcinuria
- Chronic renal disease
- Renal transplantation
- Liver disease
- Malabsorption
- Eating disorders, malnutrition
- Malignancy, including metastatic diseases, multiple myeloma, lymphoma, leukemia
- Medications
- Osteopetrosis
- Paget's disease
- Rheumatoid arthritis
- Osteogenesis imperfecta
- Marfan's syndrome
- Turner's syndrome
- Klinefelter's syndrome

The presence of a fragility fracture in the absence of low bone density should raise the concern of localized bone destruction, as with metastatic disease or plasmacytoma. Thoracic spine fractures caused by metastasis are more likely when they involve vertebrae above T7.[26] Less common metabolic bone diseases such as Paget's disease and osteopetrosis also may lead to pathologic fractures, despite normal or even high bone density. Further testing, which can include CT scanning, MRI, nuclear medicine bone scanning, or even bone biopsy, may be indicated.

MANAGEMENT

Much of the bone loss of osteoporosis is irreversible, and prevention should be the major focus of health care providers. Ideally, efforts at preventing osteoporosis should begin before puberty and should consist of adequate calcium and vitamin D intake, adequate weight-bearing exercise, and avoidance of cigarette smoking and excessive alcohol. These preventive efforts are also recommended in adults and in those in whom osteoporosis has already developed.

The National Academy of Sciences recommends between 1000 and 1300 mg of elemental calcium (between 3 and 5 cups of milk) daily and between 200 and 600 units of vitamin D daily for adults (Table 196-1).[27] Those who are unable to tolerate dairy may have to use calcium supplements, such as calcium carbonate and calcium citrate. A recent study found that several preparations of calcium carbonate, both oyster shell– and non-oyster shell–based preparations, have trace amounts of lead, the long-term implications of which are unclear.[28,29] Some recommend taking two multivitamins daily (approximately 800 IU of vitamin D/day) to provide adequate vitamin D. This practice may lead to excessive vitamin A intake, which has been associated in retrospective studies with osteoporosis and hip fracture.[30,31] A combination of confirmed

TABLE 196-1 Recommended Calcium and Vitamin D Daily Intake

Age (years)	Calcium (mg/day)	Vitamin D (IU/day)
1-3	500	200
4-8	800	200
9-13	1300	200
14-18	1300	200
19-30	1000	200
31-50	1000	200
51-70	1200	400*
>70	1200	600*

Data from Institute of Medicine: *Dietary reference intakes: calcium, phosphorus, magnesium, vitamin D and fluoride,* Washington, DC, 1997, National Academy Press.
*Evidence exists to recommend a vitamin D daily dosage of 400 to 900 IU/day for these age-groups.

lead-free calcium–vitamin D preparation and one multivitamin daily is probably the best therapeutic alternative.

The major source of vitamin D is sunlight exposure, with cutaneous synthesis of vitamin D from exposure to ultraviolet B radiation. Sunlight exposure (without sun block) to hands, arms, and face for 10 to 15 minutes two or three times a week is recommended by many experts, although the adequacy of this regimen depends on season, latitude, and skin pigmentation.[32] Those at risk for skin cancer may also wish to forgo this source of vitamin D. Studies of calcium and vitamin D intake have shown a modest increase in bone density, with a significant decrease in fracture, in both older men and women, although recent large prospective studies from the United Kingdom have failed to confirm this in ambulatory patients.[18,21,33-36]

Bone is a dynamic tissue that adapts to loading (i.e., weight-bearing exercise) with hypertrophy and increased strength. Exercise is an important part of any osteoporosis therapy.[37,38] Unloading of the skeleton, as occurs with bed rest, space flight, and spinal cord injury, results in dramatic decrements in bone mass.[39,40] Conversely, weight-bearing exercise and weight training may increase bone density, and their effects are dependent on estrogen status. Exercise alone has not been shown to prevent menopausal bone loss, and there is no evidence of a decrease in fracture risk with exercise alone. Some exercise regimens such as Tai Chi, lower limb strengthening, and balance training may decrease risk of fall.[41,42] Exercises to be avoided include high-impact loading, abrupt or explosive movements, resistive trunk flexion, twisting movements, and dynamic abdominal exercises.[41] Referral to a physical therapist for guided exercise may be helpful.

Hip protector pads have been proven to prevent hip fractures. They are indicated for patients with a high risk of falling, those with decreased fat and muscle stores, and those with previous fractures. A study by Cameron and others showed that the use of hip protectors decreased the number of hip fractures from 46.0 to 21.3 fractures per 1000 person-years.[43] Noncompliance with hip protector pads may limit their efficacy, however.[18,44]

In those with osteoporosis, preventive measures of calcium, vitamin D, and exercise alone are not sufficient to prevent osteoporotic fracture. For those with densitometric osteoporosis (*T*-score <-2.5), those with densitometric osteopenia (*T*-score <-1.0 and >-2.5) with multiple risk factors, and particularly those who already have osteoporotic fracture, pharmacologic therapy is imperative. The National Osteoporosis Foundation issued guidelines in 1998, which apply to Caucasian postmenopausal women, suggesting treatment for those with *T*-scores less than -2.0 regardless of risk factors, and those with *T*-scores less than -1.5 in the presence of risk factors.[2] U.S. Food and Drug Administration (FDA)–approved therapies at the time of this writing are listed in Box 196-4.

The only classes of FDA-approved agents at this time that have been proved to prevent both vertebral and nonvertebral fractures in prospective studies are the bisphosphonates and teriparatide. Bisphosphonates, which are synthetic analogs of pyrophosphate, reduce bone resorption and bone loss by binding to bone and poisoning active osteoclasts. Three bisphosphonates are currently FDA approved for the prevention and treatment of postmenopausal osteoporosis: alendronate, risedronate, and ibandronate. Alendronate and risedronate are also approved for use in glucocorticoid-induced osteoporosis. Only alendronate is approved for male osteoporosis, although both alendronate and risedronate are approved for treatment of males with glucocorticoid-induced osteoporosis.

Studies with these agents have shown yearly bone density increases of 2% to 3% at the lumbar spine, which is the skeletal site most responsive to these agents.[45-48] Contraindications include disorders of esophageal motility or active gastroesophageal bleeding, hypocalcemia, and renal disease. The recommended dosage of alendronate for prevention is 5 mg/day (or 35 mg/wk). For the treatment of osteoporosis, the dosage is 10 mg/day or (70 mg/wk). With risedronate, the prevention and treatment dosages are the same: 5 mg/day or 35 mg once a week. Ibandronate is dosed at either 2.5 mg/day or 150 mg once a month. Bisphosphonates should be taken on an empty stomach; with 6 to 8 ounces of water; and 30 minutes before eating (60 minutes for ibandronate), taking other medications, or lying down. To decrease gastrointestinal effects, it is important that patients be given explicit instruc-

BOX 196-4

FOOD AND DRUG ADMINISTRATION–APPROVED THERAPIES FOR OSTEOPOROSIS*

PREVENTION
- Estrogen with or without progesterone
- Raloxifene
- Alendronate
- Risedronate
- Ibandronate

TREATMENT
- Raloxifene
- Alendronate
- Risedronate
- Ibandronate
- Teriparatide
- Calcitonin

*At the time of this writing.

tions on proper administration; esophagitis can be problematic. The weekly dose of a bisphosphonate may be better tolerated than the daily dose,[49] and there is some evidence of decreased gastrointestinal toxicity with daily doses of risedronate 5 mg compared with alendronate 10 mg.[50]

At higher daily doses—risedronate 30 mg and alendronate 40 mg—the effects on the gastric and duodenal mucosa were similar for the two bisphosphonates, and much less than for aspirin 650 mg q.i.d.[51] A recent study comparing weekly doses of 70 mg of alendronate and 35 mg of risedronate found similar tolerability between the two medications, although bone density increase was greater with alendronate.[52]

Bisphosphonates are potent antiresorptive agents and may potentially oversuppress bone turnover. There have been several case reports of osteonecrosis of the jaw, typically associated with cancer patients, high dosages of IV pamidronate or zoledronic acid, and dental work.[53] Cases of unusual fractures occurring with alendronate therapy and associated with low bone turnover have also been described.[54] Suppression of bone turnover has also been found in renal transplant patients treated with modest doses of pamidronate.[55] Caution is recommended in using bisphosphonates in patients at risk for developing complications from low bone turnover. Oral health guidelines are available from the American Dental Association.[56]

Raloxifene is FDA approved for postmenopausal osteoporosis prevention and treatment at a dosage of 60 mg/day. Raloxifene is a selective estrogen receptor modulator (SERM), which acts as an estrogen receptor agonist on the skeleton but as an antagonist on breast and uterine tissue. Raloxifene has been shown to produce roughly a 1.5% to 3% increase in spine and femoral neck density after 3 years, with a 30% reduction in new vertebral fractures.[57] No reduction in nonvertebral fractures has yet been shown. There is an increased risk of venous thromboembolic disease, hot flashes, and leg cramps with raloxifene. Notably, there is also an 84% reduction in the risk of estrogen receptor–positive invasive breast cancers over 4 years,[58] and there are ongoing studies to see if this risk reduction is present in women with a high risk for breast cancer.

Hormone replacement is currently FDA approved only for the prevention of osteoporosis, not for its treatment. Estrogen inhibits bone resorption, decreases bone remodeling, and enhances absorption of calcium. Despite substantial data showing BMD increases with estrogen use, there are insufficient prospective data showing a decreased fracture risk with estrogen use.[59,60] Those women with an intact uterus will require a regimen with progesterone, either daily or cycled (0.625 mg of conjugated equine estrogen daily with 2.5 mg of medroxyprogesterone acetate daily or 5 mg of medroxyprogesterone acetate for 10 to 15 days of a 30-day cycle).

Contraindications to the use of estrogen include undiagnosed vaginal bleeding, pregnancy, active thrombosis or thrombophlebitis, active liver disease, endometrial adenocarcinoma, breast cancer, and other estrogen-dependent tumors. Caution should be taken with a medical diagnosis of endometriosis, uterine leiomyoma, gallbladder disease, or migraine headaches; a family history of breast cancer; or a history of thrombophlebitis. Once estrogen therapy is stopped, bone loss resumes at the same rate as in untreated women.[61,62] With long-term use of estrogen, those at risk for breast cancer and those with a history of uncomfortable side effects should be monitored closely. Most endocrinologists believe that any increase in bone mass is beneficial in preventing further bone loss, regardless of age. Therefore the older woman not previously treated with hormone replacement may benefit from the initiation of hormones to prevent further bone fractures.[63] Concerns about the increased risk of breast cancer and cardiovascular disease associated with long-term (more than 5 years) hormone replacement therapy (estrogen plus progesterone) should be discussed with the patient if hormone replacement therapy is considered.

Subcutaneous PTH is an anabolic bone agent. Anabolic agents stimulate bone formation and increase bone-remodeling rates. Intermittent PTH administration shows an anabolic effect, increasing bone mass, whereas continuous PTH administration leads to bone loss as in primary hyperparathyroidism. A PTH analog (PTH 1-34), administered subcutaneously, has been shown to increase bone density at the hip and spine in postmenopausal women and in both men and women on glucocorticoid therapy.[63-65] An international multicenter study showed that 20 mcg of PTH daily administered to postmenopausal women with established osteoporosis increased bone density by approximately 8% in the spine and approximately 2% at the femoral neck at the end of 1 year. It was shown to decrease vertebral fractures by approximately 65% and nonvertebral fractures by 35%.[66] Adverse effects included nausea, headache, and temporary hypercalcemia.

Etidronate, a first-generation bisphosphonate, is also used for osteoporosis, although it does not have FDA approval for this indication. It increases bone density and decreases the risk of vertebral fractures in postmenopausal women.[67,68] It also has been shown to decrease bone loss in individuals treated with corticosteroids.[69] The recommended daily dose is 5 to 10 mg/kg for 2 weeks (usually 400 mg q.h.s.), followed by 11 to 13 weeks of 1000 to 1500 mg calcium supplementation.

IV pamidronate has also been used for osteoporosis because of its effects on increasing bone density. It has been shown in uncontrolled studies to be useful in children with osteogenesis imperfecta, decreasing the risk of fracture and improving the quality of life.[70] It has been studied in heart transplant recipients and in men with prostate cancer.[71,72] It is FDA approved for the treatment of bone disease associated with multiple myeloma and breast cancer.[73,74] Regimens for breast cancer and myeloma generally involve doses of 90 mg IV administered over 2 to 4 hours monthly. It should not be used in patients with hypocalcemia, uncorrected vitamin D insufficiency, renal failure, or allergy to bisphosphonates. It should be used with caution in those with mild renal insufficiency. It has been associated with myalgias, fevers, leukopenia, and bone pain after the first dose ("Aredia flu") in younger patients.

Zoledronic acid, a potent IV bisphosphonate, has recently been approved for treatment of hypercalcemia of malignancy, bone disease associated with multiple myeloma and breast cancer, and Paget's disease. It is currently being investigated for once-yearly use in postmenopausal osteoporosis.[75] It has adverse effects and precautions similar to those of IV pamidronate.

Calcitonin is a peptide hormone that appears to slow bone loss and temporarily increase vertebral bone mass by decreasing osteoclastic activity. The drug's effect on bone is more pronounced with trabecular bone. The nasal spray produces a 3% increase in vertebral bone only and is not as effective as estrogen and alendronate in forming new bone.[76] Drug delivery is via injection or nasal spray, with the recommended dosage being 50 to 100 units/day three times per week for the injection and 200 units/day, alternating nostrils, for the nasal spray. It is FDA approved for use in postmenopausal women (>5 years postmenopause) with osteoporosis. Supplementation with calcium and vitamin D enhances therapy. Most osteoporosis experts do not advise the use of calcitonin therapy alone in treating established osteoporosis.

Calcitriol therapy has been shown to decrease vertebral fractures after 3 years (from 31.5 per 1000 person-years to 9.9 per 1000 person-years) in postmenopausal women, but adverse effects such as hypercalciuria and hypercalcemia limit its use.[77] Testosterone therapy in hypogonadal older men is useful in increasing bone density.[78] Its efficacy in preventing fractures is not yet established.

Combinations of therapies (e.g., bisphosphonates and estrogen, PTH and estrogen, and PTH and bisphosphonates) may have additive effects on bone density increases.[79-81] It is not clear whether these bone density increases are associated with decreased fracture risk. Recent studies of combination PTH and alendronate have shown no advantage over PTH alone. Sequential use of PTH first, followed by alendronate, appears to produce the best bone density increases.[82-85]

Sodium fluoride is an anabolic agent that causes marked increases in bone formation. However, excessive fluoride use may lead to increased fracture risk, despite bone density increases (fluorosis). Data regarding its efficacy in preventing fracture with slow-release preparations are conflicting, and its use is not recommended.[86]

Co-Management with Specialists

Co-management depends on each patient's particular needs. Fracture management and pain control are the primary reasons for referral. Referrals may also be made to the following specialists:

Endocrinologists or *rheumatologists* specializing in metabolic bone disease for persistent fractures, patients with secondary osteoporosis, premenopausal women or children with osteoporosis, or those with osteoporosis intolerant of FDA-approved therapies

Pain specialist to manage escalating chronic pain associated with debilitating bone and muscle changes associated with fractures

Physical therapist for management of exercise for osteoporosis, spinal and posture strengthening, pain management, and fall and fracture prevention

Nutritionist for balanced diet guidelines regarding calcium and vitamin D intake appropriate for the individual's age and activity level

Orthopedic surgeon for surgical correction of bone fractures

Interventional radiologist for vertebroplasty or kyphoplasty for painful vertebral fractures

LIFE SPAN CONSIDERATIONS

Osteoporotic fractures, especially those of the hip, are associated with increased morbidity and increased mortality. In the first year after hip fracture, one third of patients are discharged to nursing homes, 50% are unable to walk without assistance, and 24% die.[87-89] Mortality rates in men with hip fracture are higher because of co-morbid conditions.[14] In women with vertebral fractures, those with one or more fractures had a 1.23-fold greater age-adjusted mortality rate, with mortality increasing with greater numbers of vertebral fractures.[90]

COMPLICATIONS

Eighty-four percent of those with clinically diagnosed vertebral compression fractures complain of pain. The acute pain of vertebral fracture usually lasts between 2 weeks and 3 months. Chronic back pain from spinal changes, microfractures, and muscle spasms can develop. Patients may develop reduced exercise tolerance and pulmonary reserve. Abdominal protuberance because of loss of height at the lumbar spine may lead to early satiety and resultant weight loss. There is loss of self-esteem and a distortion of body image.[91]

Altered activity or inability to participate in activities of daily living because of pain may persist for a much longer period. In these cases, bed rest and decreased activity for a few days are warranted. The individual should be instructed in proper positioning—either lying supine or side lying with pillows positioned under the knees or between the knees. Medications for pain, such as muscle relaxants for spasms, nonsteroidals (cyclooxygenase-1 [COX-1] and COX-2 inhibitors), and acetaminophen for pain and inflammation, should be prescribed as needed. Narcotics should be used sparingly because of the potential for addiction and associated fall risk. Moist heat or ice may help with pain relief. Moist heat is generally recommended for muscle spasms, and ice is recommended for bone inflammation or pain. The individual in acute pain may need to use a cane or walker to walk safely. Short-term use of a spinal support may be beneficial (Table 196-2). Also available is a posture training support designed to pull the shoulders back with weights as the muscles become stronger.

Chronic pain management may be enhanced with physical therapy. Modalities include transcutaneous electrical nerve stimulation (TENS), electrical muscle stimulation, ultrasound with healed fractures, iontophoresis, and heat or ice. Manual therapy, including joint mobilization, muscle energy techniques, myofascial release, and strain-counterstrain on trigger points in muscle, is beneficial in mobilizing soft tissue and improving muscle imbalance of the spine.

TABLE 196-2 Physical Therapy: Spinal Support

Area	Support
Thoracolumbar area	Body jacket clamshell brace Jewett three-point brace Boston brace
Lumbosacral area	Lumbosacral corset

Vertebroplasty and kyphoplasty are minimally invasive techniques in which polymethylmethacrylate (PMMA) cement is injected into the fractured vertebrae, thereby stabilizing it. The two techniques differ in that vertebroplasty uses a high-pressure injection system and kyphoplasty uses a balloon to expand the collapsed vertebrae and produce a space for the PMMA. Vertebroplasty has a reported rate of success in pain relief of 70% to 90%; the rate for kyphoplasty is 90%. Kyphoplasty has the added benefit of significantly increasing vertebral height. Complication rates are low and include radiculopathy and cord compression. Cement leakage is common, however, particularly in vertebroplasty.[92] This appears an effective therapy for pain relief of vertebral fractures, although the biomechanical effects on the adjacent nonfractured vertebrae are not yet clear.

INDICATIONS FOR REFERRAL OR HOSPITALIZATION

The treatment for fractures is primarily supportive and requires physician consultation. Hospitalization for severe pain or setting of fractures (e.g., hip fractures) requires consultation with a specialist. Monitoring for potential complications after hip fractures or for pain management is indicated.

PATIENT AND FAMILY EDUCATION

Patient education is essential for the prevention and treatment of fractures. Education encompasses nutrition, psychosocial issues, risk factor modification, proper body mechanics and positioning, safety, and fall prevention. Most accidents occur in the home and are related to poor vision, decreased hearing, slowed reflexes, impaired mental status, limited spinal flexibility, decreased lower extremity strength, and unsteady gait. These factors, coupled with decreased muscle and fat mass to cushion the fall, place the individual at jeopardy for injury.[93] Education of individuals prepares them to take an active role in their care (Box 196-5). Family members should be informed of their risk of osteoporosis and encouraged to take preventive measures.

Resources available include the following:

National Osteoporosis Foundation (1232 22nd Street, Washington, DC 20037; http://www.nof.org) has information for both patient and provider.

Boning Up: A Guide to Osteoporosis Prevention has illustrations of good posture and helpful hints. It is available from the National Osteoporosis Foundation.

BOX 196-5

FALL PREVENTION MEASURES

- Regular eye examinations and correction for inadequacies
- Hearing evaluation for sound detection
- Use of assistive devices (cane or walker) as needed
- Use of rubber-soled, flat-soled, fully enclosed shoes
- Use of handrails and steady pieces of furniture
- Use of grab bars, tub seats, and elevated toilets in the bathroom
- Walkways clear of objects and throw rugs
- Proper lighting in hallways and stairways

Living It Safe, an informational guide for patients on fall prevention, is available from the American Academy of Orthopaedic Surgeons, 6300 North River Road, Rosemont, IL 60018; http://www.aaos.org.

REFERENCES

1. National Osteoporosis Foundation: *America's bone health: the state of osteoporosis and low bone mass in our nation,* Washington, DC, 2002, The Foundation.
2. National Osteoporosis Foundation: *Physician's guide to prevention and treatment of osteoporosis,* Belle Mead, NJ, 1999, Exerpta Medica.
3. American Heart Association: *2002 Heart and stroke statistical update,* Dallas, 2001, The Association.
4. American Cancer Society: *Cancer facts and figures 2002,* Atlanta, 2002, The Society.
5. Kanis JA, Melton 3rd LJ, Christiansen C, and others: The diagnosis of osteoporosis, *J Bone Miner Res* 9:1137-1141, 1994.
6. Cummings SR, Fox KM, Ensrud KE, and others: Risk factors for hip fracture in white women: the study of osteoporotic fractures research group, *N Engl J Med* 332:767-773, 1995.
7. Teitelbaum SL: Bone resorption by osteoclasts, *Science* 289:1504-1508, 2000.
8. Lane NA, Lukert B: The science and therapy of glucocorticoid induced bone loss, *Endocrinol Metab Clin North Am* 27:465-483, 1998.
9. Harper KD, Weber TJ: Secondary osteoporosis: diagnostic considerations, *Endocrinol Metab Clin North Am* 27:349-367, 1998.
10. Garnero P, Hausherr E, Chapuy MC, and others: Markers of bone resorption predict hip fracture in elderly women: the EPIDOS Prospective Study, *J Bone Miner Res* 11:1531-1538, 1996.
11. Hajcsar EE, Hawker G, Bogoch ER: Investigation and treatment of osteoporosis in patients with fragility fractures, *CMAJ* 163:819-822, 2000.
12. Freedman KB, Kaplan FS, Bilker WB, and others: Treatment of osteoporosis: are physicians missing an opportunity? *J Bone Joint Surg* 82A:1063-1070, 2000.
13. Mallmin H, Ljunghall S, Persson I, and others: Fracture of the distal forearm as a forecaster of subsequent hip fracture: a population-based cohort study with 24 years of follow-up, *Calcif Tissue Int* 52:269-272, 1993.
14. Orwoll ES: Osteoporosis in men, *Endocrinol Metab Clin North Am* 27:349-367, 1998.
15. Pluijm SM, Tromp AM, Smit JH, and others: Consequences of vertebral deformities in older men and women, *J Bone Miner Res* 15:1564-1572, 2000.
16. Lunt M, Felsenberg D, Reeve J, and others: Bone density variation and its effects on risk of vertebral deformity in men and women studied in 13 European centers: the EVOS study, *J Bone Miner Res* 12:1883-1894, 1997.
17. Sanila M, Kotaniemi A, Viikari J, and others: Height loss rate as a marker of osteoporosis in postmenopausal women with rheumatoid arthritis, *Clin Rheumatol* 13:256-260, 1994.
18. Tannenbaum C, and others: Yield of laboratory testing to identify secondary contributors to osteoporosis in otherwise healthy women, *J Clin Endocrinol Metab* 87:4431, 2002.
19. Leboff MS, and others: Occult vitamin D deficiency in postmenopausal US women with acute hip fracture, *JAMA* 281:1505-1511, 1999.
20. Thomas MK, and others: Hypovitaminosis D in medical inpatients, *N Engl J Med* 338:777-783, 1998.
21. Dawson-Hughes B, and others: Estimates of optimal vitamin D status, *Osteoporosis Intern* 16:713, 2005.
22. Malabanan A, and others: Redefining vitamin D insufficiency, *Lancet* 351:805-806, 1998.
23. Siris ES, and others: Identification and fracture outcomes of undiagnosed low bone mineral density in postmenopausal women: results from the National Osteoporosis Risk Assessment, *JAMA* 286:2815-2822, 2001.

24. Malabanan AO, and others: The utility of portable dual energy x-ray absorptiometry of the wrist in patients referred to a bone health clinic: a pilot study, *J Clin Densitom* 1:245-250, 1998.
25. Health Care Financing Administration: Medicare coverage of and payment for bone mass measurements, *Fed Reg* 63:34320-34328, 1998.
26. Biyani A, Ebraheim NA, Lu J: Thoracic spine fractures in patients older than 50 years, *Clin Orthop* 328:190-193, 1996.
27. Institute of Medicine: *Dietary reference intakes: calcium, phosphorus, magnesium, vitamin D and fluoride,* Washington, DC, 1997, National Academy Press.
28. Ross EA, and others: Lead content of calcium supplements, *JAMA* 284:1425-1429, 2000.
29. Heaney R: Lead in calcium supplements: cause for alarm or celebration? *JAMA* 284:1432-1433, 2000.
30. Melhus H, and others: Excessive dietary intake of vitamin A is associated with reduced bone mineral density and increased risk for hip fracture, *Ann Intern Med* 129:770-778, 1998.
31. Feskanich D, and others: Vitamin A intake and hip fractures among postmenopausal women, *JAMA* 287:47-54, 2002.
32. Holick MF: Vitamin D: photobiology, metabolism, mechanism of actions, and clinical applications. In Favus MJ, editor: *Primer on the metabolic bone diseases and disorders of mineral metabolism,* Philadelphia, 1999, Lippincott Williams & Wilkins.
33. Chapuy MC, and others: Vitamin D_3 and calcium to prevent hip fractures in elderly women, *N Engl J Med* 327:1637-1642, 1992.
34. Dawson-Hughes B, and others: Effect of calcium and vitamin D supplementation on bone density in men and women 65 years of age or older, *N Engl J Med* 337:670-676, 1997.
35. Porterhouse J, and others: Randomised controlled trial of calcium and supplementation with cholecalciferol (vitamin D_3) for prevention of fractures in primary care, *BMJ* 1003, 2005.
36. Grant AM, Cooper C, Torgerson D, and others (RECORD Trial Group): Oral vitamin D_3 and calcium for secondary prevention of low trauma fractures in elderly people (Randomised Evaluation of Calcium or Vitamin D, RECORD): a randomized placebo-controlled trial, *Lancet* 365(9471):1621-1628, 2005.
37. Bennell K, and others: The role of physiotherapy in the prevention and treatment of osteoporosis, *Manage Ther* 5:198-213, 2000.
38. Marcus R: Role of exercise in preventing and treating osteoporosis, *Rheum Dis Clin North Am* 27:131-141, 2001.
39. Arnaud SB, and others: Effects of 1-week head-down tilt bed rest on bone formation and the calcium endocrine system, *Aviat Space Environ Med* 63:14-20, 1992.
40. Biering-SF, and others: Longitudinal study of bone mineral content in the lumbar spine, the forearm and the lower extremities after spinal cord injury, *Eur J Clin Invest* 20:330-335, 1990.
41. Wolf SL, and others: Reducing frailty and falls in older persons: an investigation of Tai Chi and computerized balance training, *J Am Geriatr Soc* 44:489-497, 1996.
42. Campbell AJ, and others: Falls prevention over 2 years: a randomized controlled trial in women 80 years and older, *Age Ageing* 28:513-518, 1999.
43. Cameron ID, and others: Prevention of hip fracture with use of a hip protector, *N Engl J Med* 344:855-857, 2001.
44. Van Schoor NM, Smit JH, Twisk JW, and others: Prevention of hip fractures by external hip protectors: a randomized controlled trial, *JAMA* 289(15):1957-1962, 2003.
45. Liberman UA, and others: Effect of oral alendronate on bone mineral density and the incidence of fractures in postmenopausal osteoporosis: the Alendronate Phase III Osteoporosis Treatment Study Group, *N Engl J Med* 333:1437-1443, 1995.
46. Black DM, and others: Randomised trial of effect of alendronate on risk of fracture in women with existing vertebral fractures, *Lancet* 348:1535-1541, 1996.
47. Orwoll E, and others: Alendronate for the treatment of osteoporosis in men, *N Engl J Med* 343:604-610, 2000.
48. Harris ST, and others: Effects of risedronate treatment on vertebral and nonvertebral fractures in women with postmenopausal osteoporosis: a randomized controlled trial, *JAMA* 282:1344-1352, 1999.
49. Schnitzer T, and others: Therapeutic equivalence of alendronate 70 mg once-weekly and alendronate 10 mg daily in the treatment of osteoporosis: Alendronate Once-Weekly Study Group, *Aging* 12:1-12, 2000.
50. Lanza FL, and others: Endoscopic comparison of esophageal and gastroduodenal effects of risedronate and alendronate in postmenopausal women, *Gastroenterology* 119:866-869, 2000.
51. Lanza F, and others: An endoscopic comparison of the effects of alendronate and risedronate on upper gastrointestinal mucosae, *Am J Gastroenterol* 95:3112-3117, 2000.
52. Rosen CJ, and others (FACT trial investigators): Treatment with once-weekly alendronate 70 mg compared with once weekly risedronate 35 mg in women with postmenopausal osteoporosis: a randomized double-blind study, *J Bone Miner Res* 20(1):141-151, 2005.
53. Marx RE: Pamidronate (Aredia) and zoledronate (Zometa) induced avascular necrosis of the jaw: a growing epidemic, *J Oral Maxillofac Surg* 61(9):1115-1117, 2003.
54. Odvina CV, Zerwekh JE, Rao DS, and others: Severely suppressed bone turnover: a potential complication of alendronate therapy, *J Clin Endocrinol Metab* 90(3):1294-1301, 2005.
55. Coco M, and others: Prevention of bone loss in renal transplant recipients: a progressive, randomised trial of intravenous pamidronate, *J Am Soc Nephrol* 14(10):2669-2676, 2003.
56. Migliorati CA, and others: Managing the care of patients with bisphosphonate-associated osteonecrosis: an American Academy of Oral Medicine position paper, *J Am Dent Assoc* 136(12):1658-1668, 2005.
57. Ettinger B, and others: Reduction of vertebral fracture risk in postmenopausal women with osteoporosis treated with raloxifene: results from a 3-year randomized clinical trial: multiple outcomes of raloxifene evaluation (MORE) investigators, *JAMA* 282:637-645, 1999.
58. Cauley JA, and others: Continued breast cancer risk reduction in postmenopausal women treated with raloxifene: 4-year results from the MORE trial: multiple outcomes of raloxifene evaluation, *Breast Cancer Res Treat* 65:125-134, 2001.
59. PEPI investigators: Effects of hormone therapy on bone mineral density: results from the Postmenopausal Estrogen/Progestin Interventions PEPI Trial, *JAMA* 276:1389-1396, 1996.
60. Villareal DT, and others: Bone mineral density response to estrogen replacement in frail elderly women: a randomized controlled trial, *JAMA* 286:815-820, 2001.
61. Felson DT, and others: The effect of postmenopausal estrogen therapy on bone density in elderly women, *N Engl J Med* 329:1141-1146, 1993.
62. Belchetz PE: Hormonal treatment of postmenopausal women, *N Engl J Med* 330:1062-1071, 1994.
63. Grey AB, Cundy TF, Reid IR: Continuous combined oestrogen/progestin therapy is well tolerated and increases bone density at the hip and spine in post-menopausal osteoporosis, *Clin Endocrinol* 40:671-677, 1994.
64. Neer RM, and others: Effect of parathyroid hormone (1-34) on fractures and bone mineral density in postmenopausal women with osteoporosis, *N Engl J Med* 344:1434-1441, 2001.
65. Bilezikian JP, Kurland ES: Therapy of male osteoporosis with parathyroid hormone, *Calcif Tissue Int* 69:248-251, 2001.
66. Lane NE, and others: Bone mass continues to increase at the hip after parathyroid hormone treatment is discontinued in glucocorticoid induced osteoporosis: results of a randomized controlled clinical trial, *J Bone Miner Res* 15:944-951, 2000.
67. Storm T, and others: Effect of intermittent cyclical etidronate therapy on bone mass and fracture rate in women with post menopausal osteoporosis, *N Engl J Med* 322:1265-1271, 1990.
68. Watts NB, and others: Intermittent cyclical etidronate treatment of postmenopausal osteoporosis, *N Engl J Med* 323:73-79, 1990.
69. Adachi JD, and others: Intermittent etidronate therapy to prevent corticosteroid-induced osteoporosis, *N Engl J Med* 337:382-387, 1997.

70. Glorieux FH, and others: Cyclic administration of pamidronate in children with severe osteogenesis imperfecta, *N Engl J Med* 339:986-987, 1998.
71. Shane ES, and others: Prevention of bone loss after heart transplantation with antiresorptive therapy: a pilot study, *J Heart Lung Transplant* 17:1089-1096, 1998.
72. Smith MR, and others: Pamidronate to prevent bone loss during androgen-deprivation therapy for prostate cancer, *N Engl J Med* 345:948-955, 2001.
73. Berenson JR, and others: Efficacy of pamidronate in reducing skeletal events in patients with advanced multiple myeloma, *N Engl J Med* 334:488-493, 1996.
74. Hortobagyi GN, and others: Efficacy of pamidronate in reducing skeletal complications in patients with breast cancer and lytic bone metastases, *N Engl J Med* 335:1785-1792, 1996.
75. Reid IR, and others: Intravenous zoledronic acid in postmenopausal women with low bone mineral density, *N Engl J Med* 346:1216-1226, 2003.
76. Overgaard K, Hansen MA, Jensen SB, and others: Effect of salcatonin given intranasally on bone mass and fracture rates in established osteoporosis: a dose-response study, *BMJ* 305(6853):556-561, 1992.
77. Tilyard MW, and others: Treatment of postmenopausal osteoporosis with calcitriol or calcium, *N Engl J Med* 326:357-362, 1992.
78. Snyder PJ, and others: Effect of testosterone treatment on bone mineral density in men over 65 years of age, *J Clin Endocrinol Metab* 84:1966-1972, 1999.
79. Wimalawansa SJ: Prevention and treatment of osteoporosis: efficacy of combination of hormone replacement therapy with other antiresorptive agents, *J Clin Densitom* 3:187-201, 2000.
80. Lindsay R, and others: Randomised controlled study of effect of parathyroid hormone on vertebral-bone mass and fracture incidence among postmenopausal women on oestrogen with osteoporosis, *Lancet* 350:550-555, 1997.
81. Rittmaster RS, and others: Enhancement of bone mass in osteoporotic women with parathyroid hormone followed by alendronate, *J Clin Endocrinol Metab* 85:2129-2134, 2000.
82. Finkel JS, and others: The effects of parathyroid hormone, alendronate, or both in men with osteoporosis, *N Engl J Med* 349:1216-1226, 2003.
83. Black DM, and others (PaTH study investigators): One year of alendronate after one year of parathyroid hormone (1-84) for osteoporosis, *N Engl J Med* 353:555-565, 2005.
84. Black DM, and others (PaTH study investigators): The effects of parathyroid hormone and alendronate alone or in combination in postmenopausal osteoporosis, *N Engl J Med* 349:1207-1215, 2003.
85. Cosman F, and others: Daily and cyclic parathyroid hormone in women receiving alendronate, *N Engl J Med* 352:566-575, 2005.
86. Haguenauer D, and others: Fluoride for treating postmenopausal osteoporosis, *Cochrane Database Syst Rev* 4:CD002825, 2000.
87. Kannus P, and others: Epidemiology of hip fractures, *Bone* 18(1 Suppl):57S-63S, 1996.
88. Riggs BL, Melton LJ: The worldwide problem of osteoporosis: insights afforded by epidemiology, *Bone* 17(5 Suppl):505S-511S, 1995.
89. Ray NF, and others: Medical expenditures for the treatment of osteoporotic fractures in the United States in 1995: report from the National Osteoporosis Foundation, *J Bone Miner Res* 12:24-35, 1997.
90. Kado DM, and others: Vertebral fractures and mortality in older women: a prospective study, *Arch Intern Med* 159:1215-1220, 1999.
91. Silverman SL: The clinical consequences of vertebral compression fracture, *Bone* 13:S27-S31, 1992.
92. Garfin SR, and others: New technologies in spine: kyphoplasty and vertebroplasty for the treatment of painful osteoporotic compression fractures, *Spine* 26:1511-1515, 2001.
93. Swezey RL: Site-specific isometric exercises can be done safely at home: preventing osteoporotic fractures: the role of exercise, posture, and safety, *J Musculoskel Med* 14:9-23, 1997.

CHAPTER 197

Paget's Disease of the Bone

Julie P. Fago

DEFINITION AND EPIDEMIOLOGY

Paget's disease is the second most common metabolic bone disease in older adults. Traditionally, medical and surgical specialists have managed the various manifestations of the disease, but now, with more effective treatments available, the primary care team can provide complete management in most cases.

Paget's disease is uncommon before the age of 40 years; however, by the age of 80 years, 1 out of 10 persons is affected by the disease. Between 18% and 25% of the U.S. population have at least one family member with Paget's disease, leading to speculation of a genetic (or environmental) component. Paget's disease is common in England, Western Europe, New Zealand, Australia, and the United States; it is uncommon in Asia, Africa, India, and Scandinavia.

PATHOPHYSIOLOGY

Paget's disease is characterized by a localized increase in bone turnover and blood flow. It can affect one or more sites (monostotic vs. polyostotic). Once the disease is fully established, previously unaffected bones are usually spared. For reasons that are still not well understood, osteoclasts in the affected area are increased in number, size, and activity and cause breakdown of focal areas of bone at great speed. The osteoblasts, which are unaffected by the disease process, try to keep up with the bone degradation by laying down new osteoid as fast as they can. However, the newly formed bone is disorganized and lacks the architectural integrity of normal bone. This results in mechanically weak, highly vascular bone that is prone to deformity and fractures, especially if weight-bearing parts of the skeleton are affected.[1]

CLINICAL PRESENTATION

Although Paget's disease is usually asymptomatic, bone pain is the most common presenting symptom. The pain can be misinterpreted as part of the aging process or as part of another disease process. In one study, one third of patients who came to see their providers with complaints of bone pain were misdiagnosed as having osteoarthritis.[2] Failure to diagnose and initiate early treatment can result in irreversible consequences and significant morbidity.

The degree and character of the bone pain vary with the location and activity of Paget's disease. The most commonly involved sites are the pelvis, femur, tibia, spine, and skull. The hands and feet are only rarely involved. Generally, the affected bone is moderately painful both at rest and during motion. Most patients describe the pain as a deep ache (like a toothache) that can become severe and sharp with weight bearing and when the area is warmed. Hot baths and even warm bedclothes can intensify the pain.[3]

PHYSICAL EXAMINATION

On examination, the affected area is often tender to the touch and may be warm as a result of increased new blood vessel growth within the bone itself. The pagetic bone can be noticeably enlarged. Affected bones may be deformed in a bow shape either from the effects of gravity or from the tension of the attached musculature on the architecturally incompetent pagetic bone. When bones in the lower extremity become deformed, the patient will have an abnormal gait and, often, arthritic changes within the surrounding joints as a result of the mechanical stress.[4] The head size may increase with skull involvement, and frontal bossing may be evident.

Nerve entrapments can occur as a result of bony overgrowth, resulting in a variety of neuropathies, including cranial nerve palsies. Hearing loss may occur as a result of sensory neuropathy and/or conduction impairment resulting from pagetic involvement of the ossicles of the inner ear. When the spine is involved, bony overgrowth can result in spinal stenosis with attendant radiculopathies or motor impairments.[5]

DIAGNOSTICS

Diagnosis is confirmed by checking the serum alkaline phosphatase (SAP) and/or urinary *N*-telopeptide crosslinks (NTx) level, both of which will be elevated in active disease. Their levels correlate with the extent and activity of the disease. Radiographic studies of the affected area(s) usually show a classic mixed sclerotic-sclerolytic ("cotton-wool") pattern, cortical thickening, and bony enlargement. Bone scans show increased uptake in affected areas, but this pattern can be difficult to differentiate from other processes such as cancer and arthritis.

DIAGNOSTICS

Paget's Disease

LABORATORY

Serum alkaline phosphatase
Urinary *N*-telopeptide

IMAGING

Plain x-ray of affected areas
Bone scan
MRI (if neurologic symptoms)

DIFFERENTIAL DIAGNOSIS

The symptoms and signs of Paget's disease must be distinguished from those of several other conditions. When the joints are involved, the differential diagnosis includes osteoarthritis, gout, and pseudogout. Ironically, these three diagnoses can coexist with Paget's disease, can be a complication of Paget's disease, or can mimic the symptoms of Paget's disease when the latter affects the bone adjacent to a joint.

Bone pain that occurs with an elevated SAP level and positive bone scan must be distinguished from malignancy, most commonly a metastasis from a distant site. In early, active Paget's disease the initial wave of osteoclastic resorption can appear as lytic lesions on plain radiographs and thus may mimic such malignancies as multiple myeloma. However, in the great majority of cases, the radiograph will show changes pathognomonic of Paget's disease.

DIFFERENTIAL DIAGNOSIS

Paget's Disease

- Osteoarthritis
- Gout
- Pseudogout
- Malignancy

MANAGEMENT

The goals of treatment are to suppress osteoclastic activity, allowing the osteoblasts to catch up and lay down architecturally normal bone, which in turn reduces symptoms and prevents disease progression. All patients with bone pain or neurologic impingements, or patients who are at risk for complications based on the site of disease (femoral head, tibia, skull), should receive pharmacologic therapy (Box 197-1 and Table 197-1). Although some controversy remains about whether to treat patients solely on the basis of an elevated SAP level, most agree that values three to four times the normal range merit treatment.[6] Bone pain usually responds within 2 to 3 weeks of active drug treatment. Neuropathies, if detected

TABLE 197-1 Pharmacologic Treatment for Paget's Disease

Drug	Dose	Side Effects
Bisphosphonates		
Alendronate	40 mg PO q day for 6 months	Nausea, esophageal ulcers
Risedronate	30 mg PO q day for 2 months	Nausea
Etidronate	400 mg PO q day for 6 months*	Nausea, osteomalacia
Pamidronate	30-60 mg IV q day for 3 days or 60 mg IV once for mild disease (maximum 480 mg)	Mild fever, hypocalcemia, flulike symptoms, transient leukopenia
Tiludronate (Skelid)	800 mg PO q day for 3 months	Back pain, diarrhea, nausea
Calcitonin		
Salmon	50-100 IU SQ q day for 3-6 months, then 3 times per week†	Flushing, nausea, loss of efficacy
Human	0.5-1 mg SQ as above	Flushing, nausea, loss of efficacy
Nasal	200-400 IU q day as above	Nasal irritation, loss of efficacy
Plicamycin‡	15-25 mcg/kg IV q day for 10 days	Bone marrow, kidney, liver toxicity

*Etidronate should be given cyclically with at least 6 months of no treatment between courses.
†Patients with mild disease may need <1 year of treatment; those with moderate to severe disease may need to be treated indefinitely.
‡No longer available in the United States.

BOX 197-1

INDICATIONS FOR DRUG THERAPY IN PAGET'S DISEASE

- Bone or joint pain
- Pagetic lesions in weight-bearing sites
- Involvement of the skull
- Nerve entrapments
- Preparation for elective joint replacement
- Serum alkaline phosphatase levels more than three to four times normal

early, may also respond, but arthropathy will not because it represents fixed-joint degradation. Efficacy of treatment is determined by the amount and duration of the reduction in SAP or NTx.

Bisphosphonates

Bisphosphonates are the most widely used agents for the treatment of Paget's disease. They reduce bone turnover by inhibiting key cellular functions that govern osteoclastic bone resorption. Etidronate (Didronel) was the first bisphosphonate available, although it is not used as commonly now. Alendronate (Fosamax) and risedronate (Actonel) are the oral bisphosphonates of choice for treating Paget's disease in the United States. Clear evidence from randomized controlled trials has shown that both achieve quick normalization of biochemical markers and reduction of pain. In addition, both have prolonged posttreatment effects and low relapse rates.[7,8] However, all bisphosphonates are poorly absorbed from the gut, and absorption is further diminished when taken with 6 to 8 ounces of food. Thus oral bisphosphonates must be taken with plain water on an empty stomach at least ½ hour before a meal. The main side effects are stomach upset and, rarely, esophageal ulceration.

IV bisphosphonates such as pamidronate (Aredia) and zoledronic acid (Zometa) are potent treatment options for those unable to tolerate oral agents. Studies of both agents have shown dramatic and long-lasting improvement in both markers and symptoms.[9,10] Because of its rapid onset of action, intravenous administration is the route of choice for patients with impending fracture, neurologic impingements, hydrocephalus, or severe refractory disease.[3] The side effects are generally minor, but transient hypocalcemia, leukopenia, and flulike symptoms can be seen.

Calcitonin

Calcitonin, although not as potent or long lasting as the bisphosphonates, remains a well-tolerated treatment option.[3] Pain generally remits after 2 to 3 weeks, and as treatment continues, lytic lesions fill in with new normal bone, vascularity decreases, and neurologic deficits (if any) improve.[11] However, the effect of calcitonin wears off with time because of the development of antibodies (in the case of salmon or porcine calcitonin) and/or downregulation of calcitonin receptors.[12] The effective dose of salmon calcitonin is 50 to 100 IU SQ q day for 1 month, followed by injections three times a week for 3 to 6 months as dictated by clinical symptoms and biochemical markers. Nasal salmon calcitonin (200 IU) and human calcitonin (0.5 mg SQ) can be used in a similar schedule. The main side effects of injectable calcitonin are transient flushing and nausea. Vomiting, diarrhea, and abdominal pain can also occur. Nasal calcitonin is generally better tolerated but can cause nasal irritation.

Adjuvant Therapy

NSAIDs can be useful adjuncts for patients with joint or bone pain. When pain is severe, opioids may need to be used until the Paget's disease is controlled. Assistive devices, including shoe lifts, walkers, and canes for equalizing leg length discrepancies, as well as physical therapy for joint symptoms, are often quite helpful. Calcium and/or vitamin D supplements should be considered for those with low dietary intake to ensure adequate bone mineralization.

Ongoing Monitoring

Patients with Paget's disease need to be evaluated periodically. Those with asymptomatic disease in areas of the skeleton where there is little or no risk (e.g., the iliac crest) can be monitored less closely. Conversely, those with active disease in weight-bearing bones or the skull require aggressive follow-up care. Disease activity is monitored using biochemical markers (SAP or NTx), which are usually measured at 3- to 6-month intervals in active disease or yearly in inactive disease. In addition, pain, joint symptoms, neurologic function, and medication side effects need to be assessed at every visit.

LIFE SPAN CONSIDERATIONS

Although untreated Paget's disease can cause pain and deformity, the life span is unaffected unless the patient develops osteosarcoma or severe flattening of the base of the skull with spinal cord compression. Indications for the use of bisphosphonates have been extended to include younger patients to prevent bone deformity of the limbs and the secondary osteoarthritis that is seen with these deformities. The use of bisphosphonates is also recommended to older patients to prevent bone fragility and fracture.[13]

COMPLICATIONS

Bone pain typical of Paget's disease must be distinguished from other long-term consequences of untreated Paget's disease, including neural compromise, fractures, joint deterioration, and sarcomatous transformation. Nerve compression is most common when the spine or skull is involved. Enlarging bone in the vertebrae can compress spinal nerve roots or even the spinal cord itself, resulting in neuropathic pain or myelopathies. Cranial nerves, which exit the skull through tiny foramina, can also be compressed, resulting in facial pain, paralysis, or deafness. Involvement of the base of the skull can result in hydrocephalus (often manifesting as dementia) or brainstem compression.

Pagetic fractures appear with sudden, severe knifelike pain. They may be traumatic or, if the pagetic bone is weakened by extensive lytic disease, can occur spontaneously. Until Paget's disease is controlled, healing is difficult and slow. Pagetic arthropathy occurs when bone adjacent to joint surfaces (e.g., the femoral head or the acetabulum) is affected, resulting in abnormal joint architecture and subsequent degenerative arthritis.

The most dreaded consequence of long-term Paget's disease is osteosarcoma. This is heralded by a sudden increase in pain intensity at a pagetic site. Although it is rare, osteosarcoma has an extremely poor prognosis. The majority of patients die within 1 to 3 years.

INDICATIONS FOR REFERRAL OR HOSPITALIZATION

Medical management of straightforward cases can be easily handled by the health care provider. However, physical therapists are invaluable members of the management team because of their expertise in maximizing physical function and knowledge of assistive devices. Referral to a rheumatologist is indicated if the patient's disease is unresponsive to usual treatment. Orthopedic referral is indicated when an associated arthropathy or spinal stenosis causes unremitting pain or loss of function.

Severe neurologic complications such as hydrocephalus require aggressive inpatient antipagetic therapy combined with neurosurgical intervention. Other causes of hospitalization include fracture, elective joint replacement, or spinal decompression.

PATIENT AND FAMILY EDUCATION

Patients and their families must understand the disease process and medical management to manage Paget's disease optimally. First, they need to be informed about how to take their medications and what side effects could occur. Second, patients need to promptly report any worsening of their symptoms, which could herald disease progression, fracture, or sarcomatous transformation. Those with skull involvement need to understand what neuropathic symptoms to look for and the importance of prompt reporting. For example, progressive hearing loss should not be blamed on age.

In addition, family members should inform their own primary care team of their family history of Paget's disease and should be cautioned to report bone pain or symptoms of nerve compression.

HEALTH PROMOTION

Patients should be encouraged to remain as physically active as possible. If the tibia or proximal femur is affected, heavy weight-bearing exercise should be avoided until the disease is in remission. Swimming, bicycling, and Tai Chi are excellent alternatives for patients with painful arthropathy. Adequate dietary (or supplemental) calcium and vitamin D are important to help maintain bone density.

REFERENCES

1. Sirus ES: Extensive personal experience: Paget's disease of the bone, *J Clin Epidemiol Metab* 80(2):335-339, 1995.
2. Hamdy RC, Moore S, LeRoy J: Clinical presentation of Paget's disease of the bone in older patients, *South Med J* 86(10):1097-1100, 1993.
3. Sirus ES: Paget's disease of the bone. In Favus MJ, editor: *Primer on the metabolic bone diseases and disorders of mineral metabolism*, ed 4, Philadelphia, 2000, Lippincott-Raven.
4. Altman RD: Arthritis in Paget's disease of the bone, *J Bone Metab Res* 14(Suppl 2):85-87, 1999.
5. Poncelet A: The neurologic complications of Paget's disease, *J Bone Metab Res* 14(Suppl 2):88-91, 1999.
6. Selby P, Davie M, Ralston S: Guidelines on the management of Paget's disease of bone, *Bone* 31(3):366-373, 2002.
7. Siris ES, Weinstein RS, Altman R, and others: Comparative study of alendronate versus etidronate for the treatment of Paget's disease of the bone, *J Clin Endocrinol Metab* 81(3):961-967, 1996.
8. Miller PD, Brown JP, Siris ES, and others: A randomized, double-blind comparison of risedronate and etidronate in the treatment of Paget's disease of the bone, *Am J Med* 106(5):513-520, 1999.
9. Grauer A, Klar B, Scharla SH, and others: Long-term efficacy of intravenous pamidronate in Paget's disease of the bone, *Semin Arthritis Rheum* 23(4):283-284, 1994.
10. Reid IR, Miller P, Lyles K, and others: Comparison of a single infusion of zoledronic acid with risedronate for Paget's disease, *N Engl J Med* 353(9):898-908, 2005.
11. Wallach S: Calcitonin: history and prospects: a personal view, *Semin Arthritis Rheum* 23(4):256-260, 1994.
12. Singer FR, Fredericks RS, Minkin C: Salmon calcitonin therapy for Paget's disease of the bone: the problem of acquired clinical resistance, *Arthritis Rheum* 23:1148-1154, 1980.
13. Langston AL, Ralston SH: Management of Paget's disease of bone, *Rheumatology* 43(8):955-959, 2004.

CHAPTER 198

Shoulder Pain

Kathy J. Fabiszewski

DEFINITION AND EPIDEMIOLOGY

Shoulder pain and dysfunction are among the most common musculoskeletal complaints encountered in primary and acute care settings, accounting for approximately 5% of visits to primary care offices, and they are second only to knee pain as a source of impairment in sports and recreational activities.[1-3] The prevalence of shoulder pain ranges from 8% to 20% in those 30 years and older; it is most prevalent in middle-aged and older age-groups.[1] About 4 million people in the United States seek medical care each year for shoulder problems, including 1.5 million visits to orthopedic surgeons annually.[4] Trauma or disease may cause shoulder pain. Injury, coupled with pain, predisposes the individual to functional impairment or disability. The health care provider can, in most cases, diagnose and treat shoulder pain without specialty consultation.

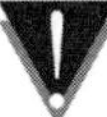
Immediate emergency department referral or orthopedic consultation is indicated for patients with suspected shoulder dislocation or fracture.

Physician consultation is indicated for patients with acromioclavicular separation and functionally significant rotator cuff tears.

PATHOPHYSIOLOGY

The shoulder is the most movable joint in the body and is composed of four separate joints or articulations that are made up of only three bones: the scapula, clavicle, and humerus. The shoulder, or glenohumeral joint (the articulation of the humerus and the glenoid fossa of the scapula), is a closely fitted, complex ball-and-socket joint that is capable of a wide, almost global, range of motion. Adjacent to the glenohumeral joint are the acromioclavicular joint (the articulation between the acromion process and the clavicle) and the sternoclavicular joint (the articulation between the manubrium of the sternum and the clavicle), which form the shoulder girdle. At the scapulothoracic articulation, the scapula is suspended from the posterior thoracic wall by muscular attachments to the ribs and spine.[5] Normal shoulder motion depends on the smooth, integrated movement of these four articulations.

The primary movers of the glenohumeral joint are the pectoralis major and minor (adducts the shoulder), deltoid (abducts the shoulder), teres major, and latissimus dorsi.[5] The trapezius muscles elevate and rotate the scapula. The shoulder joints are stabilized by the soft tissues of the shoulder girdle, including the joint capsule, glenoid labrum, muscles of the rotator cuff, long head of the biceps, and scapular stabilizers.[5] The shoulder socket (glenoid) is shallow and subsequently has little inherent bony stability. This anatomic arrangement provides for greater mobility but is accomplished by compromising some stability, making the shoulder one of the most commonly dislocated joints in the body.

The rotator cuff consists of the musculotendinous attachments of the supraspinatus, infraspinatus, teres minor, and subscapularis muscles, which come together and attach on the greater and lesser tuberosities.[6] Although each muscle and its tendon play a critical role in the stability and movement of the shoulder joint, the primary functions of the rotator cuff are rotation of the humeral head and dynamic stabilization of the glenohumeral joint.[6]

The greater tuberosity of the humerus, tendons of the rotator cuff muscles that elevate the arm, and the subacromial bursa move back and forth through a tight archway of bone and ligament known as the coracoacromial arch. When the arm is raised, the archway becomes smaller, impinging these structures and making them prone to inflammation and degeneration.

CLINICAL PRESENTATION

Shoulder pain symptoms can range from specific to vague.[7] Persistent and recurrent symptoms are common.[1] The patient with a shoulder problem typically complains of shoulder pain, which is aggravated by movement and is often accompanied by limitation of movement. There may or may not be a history of trauma or overuse. Surprisingly, many individuals fail to recollect trauma unless specifically asked. Patients often report difficulty with activities of daily living such as bathing, combing their hair, or dressing, as well as driving, carrying groceries, or exercising. Other symptoms may include stiffness, crepitation, and aching discomfort related to vigorous or sustained use.

Inquiring about hand dominance, employment (e.g., lifting, chronic stress on joints, safety precautions), exercise and recreational activities (extent, type, and frequency), and self-care capacity facilitates identification of contributing factors, potential causes, and the functional impact of the symptomatology. Identifying any history of recent or remote trauma, including the details of injury, is vital. Determining previous diagnostic studies, hospitalizations, surgeries, or therapies guides diagnostic evaluation.

It is also critical to ascertain the exact location and distribution of the pain. It is unusual for pain originating in the shoulder, for example, to radiate below the elbow.[5] Pain involving other joints is suggestive of a generalized arthritic process. Radicular pain arising from C5 and C6 is difficult to differentiate from shoulder pathologic conditions because the sensory distribution runs from the base of the neck to the outer margin of the shoulder.[7] Characterization of the type, intensity, timing, and duration of pain, as well as identification of ameliorating and exacerbating factors, is also essential. The American Shoulder and Elbow Surgeons standardized form for assessment of the shoulder incorporates a synopsis of both patient self-evaluation data and physical examination parameters and is useful in organizing a primary care approach to shoulder pain (Figure 198-1).

PHYSICAL EXAMINATION

Physical examination begins with visual inspection of the shoulder. Anterior and posterior examination for surgical scars, displacement of bony prominences, warmth, swelling, changes in skin color or texture, muscular atrophy, and

SHOULDER ASSESSMENT FORM
AMERICAN SHOULDER AND ELBOW SURGEONS

Examiner:

Name:	Date:
Age: Hand dominance: R L Ambi	Gender: M F
Diagnosis:	Initial Assessment? Y N
Procedure/data:	Follow-up: Y N

PATIENT SELF-EVALUATION

Are you having pain in your shoulder? (Circle the correct answer)	Y	N

Mark where your pain is

Front Back

Do you have pain in your shoulder at night?	Y	N
Do you take pain medication (aspirin, Advil, Tylenol, etc.)?	Y	N
Do you take narcotic pain medication (codeine or stronger)?	Y	N
How many pills do you take each day (average)?	______ pills	

How bad is your pain today (mark line)?

0 ├─┼─┼─┼─┼─┼─┼─┼─┼─┼─┤ 10

No pain at all — Pain as bad as it can be

Does your shoulder feel unstable (as if it is going to dislocate)?	Y	N

How unstable is your shoulder (mark line)?

0 ├─┼─┼─┼─┼─┼─┼─┼─┼─┼─┤ 10

Very stable — Very unstable

Circle the number in the box that indicates your ability to do the following activities: 0 = unable to do; 1 = very difficult to do; 2 = somewhat difficult; 3 = not difficult

Activity	Right Arm	Left Arm
1. Put on a coat	0 1 2 3	0 1 2 3
2. Sleep on your painful or affected side	0 1 2 3	0 1 2 3
3. Wash back/do up bra in back	0 1 2 3	0 1 2 3
4. Manage toileting	0 1 2 3	0 1 2 3
5. Comb hair	0 1 2 3	0 1 2 3
6. Reach a high shelf	0 1 2 3	0 1 2 3
7. Lift 10 lb above the shoulder	0 1 2 3	0 1 2 3
8. Throw a ball overhand	0 1 2 3	0 1 2 3
9. Do usual work–List:	0 1 2 3	0 1 2 3
10. Do usual sport–List:	0 1 2 3	0 1 2 3

FIGURE 198-1

The American Shoulder and Elbow Surgeon's standardized form for assessment of the shoulder. (Reprinted with permission from the American Shoulder and Elbow Surgeons.)

winging of the scapula is necessary. Asymmetry with the uninvolved shoulder should be noted. Classically, there is focal tenderness. Before any shoulder movement is initiated, the examiner should palpate for tenderness in the sternoclavicular joint, the acromioclavicular joint, and the shoulder itself. Both shoulders can be palpated simultaneously to compare the affected side with the unaffected side.[5] Palpating bony landmarks is especially valuable in excluding a joint disorder; palpating the muscular structures is useful in excluding spasm. A simple shoulder examination checklist is provided in Box 198-1.

Active motion should be performed first to determine the integrity of the rotator cuff and to ascertain the location of the pain. Active range of motion of each shoulder should be measured, including forward flexion (normal is 180 degrees), extension (normal is 70 degrees), external rotation (normal is 45 degrees), internal rotation (normal is 60 degrees), abduction (normal is 180 degrees), and adduction (normal is 180 degrees). Any clicks or crepitation suggestive of impingement should be noted. Passive range of motion should be compared with active range of motion and is particularly useful in determining whether adhesive capsulitis (frozen shoulder) is present. A person with adhesive capsulitis can generally still abduct the arm 60 degrees.

Strength testing of the individual rotator cuff muscles is then performed using resisted movements. Table 198-1 summarizes special tests of shoulder function and their associated disorders. Complete neurovascular assessment of the associated shoulder structures should also be performed, documenting sensory, motor, or circulatory impairment. The spine and peripheral joints are examined for evidence of co-existing joint disease.

Evaluation of a painful shoulder is challenging because the problem is often dynamic, with pain occurring only with specific activity. It is necessary to determine whether the discomfort and immobility are articular (bone) or periarticular (soft tissue structure). With bursitis or adhesive capsulitis, for example, both active and passive range of motion will be limited. Weakness on resisted movements suggests a muscle or tendon tear or neurologic compromise.[1]

BOX 198-1

SHOULDER EXAMINATION

INSPECTION

1. Visual inspection comparing affected shoulder with the uninvolved shoulder
2. Range of motion of the cervical spine
3. Active range of motion of the shoulder
   - Wall push (look for winging)
   - Forward elevation, flexion
   - Extension
   - External rotation
   - Internal rotation
   - Abduction
   - Adduction
4. Passive range of motion of the shoulder
   - Impingement test
5. Strength testing of all major muscle groups
   - Flexor-extensor of the wrist
   - Biceps
   - Triceps
   - Supraspinatus isolation
   - Internal rotators
   - External rotators
   - Deltoid
6. Deep tendon reflexes
7. Peripheral pulses (check for bruits)

PALPATION

1. Supraclavicular fissure
2. Sternoclavicular joint
3. Acromioclavicular joint
4. Glenohumeral joint
5. Biceps tendon insertion
6. Muscular structures

DIAGNOSTICS

Diagnostic tests should be used judiciously to confirm or refine suspected clinical diagnoses. It is unwise to base a diagnosis on a radiologic test, since x-ray studies can be misleading or unrevealing. Radiographs and even MRIs are often negative in soft tissue problems in the young athlete; this underscores the importance of a good history and physical examination.[8]

TABLE 198-1 Tests of Shoulder Function

Test	Technique	Interpretation
Apprehension test	Abduct and externally rotate patient's arm to a position where it might easily dislocate.	Impending dislocation is signaled by noticeable look of apprehension on patient's face, with patient resisting further motion.
Drop arm test	Have patient hold affected extremity in a fully abducted position, then ask patient to slowly lower arm to side.	Rotator cuff tearing is suggested if patient's arm drops to side from a position of 90 degrees abduction.
Empty can test	Have patient hold out affected arm as if offering examiner a can of soda, then have patient turn arm to empty the contents.	Rotator cuff tendinitis is suggested if pain is produced by maneuver of "emptying the can."
Impingement test	Have patient elevate arm slowly into overhead position.	Rotator cuff tendinitis is suggested if patient experiences sharp "catches" of pain or impingement with this maneuver.
Yergason's test	Have patient fully flex elbow. Grasp the patient's flexed elbow in one hand while holding patient's wrist in other hand; to test stability of biceps tendon, externally rotate the patient's arm as patient resists and, at same time, pull downward on patient's elbow.	Pain with this maneuver suggests that biceps tendon is unstable in biceps groove; no pain is experienced with a stable tendon.

Plain x-ray films are recommended if there is a history of trauma, if there is reduced range of motion, or if arthritis or neoplastic disease is a consideration. With all significant trauma it is imperative to obtain the appropriate x-ray studies, including standard anteroposterior views of the glenohumeral joint with the arm at 30 degrees external rotation, axillary lateral views, and scapula Y views that detect dislocation not seen on standard views. Occasionally, in atraumatic presentations, calcifications from previous or chronic injuries can be seen. Spurring of the acromial process or calcium deposits in the soft tissues (seen in the tendon in calcific tendinitis) are common findings.[9] A detailed explanation of the reason for the x-ray study enables the radiologist to obtain the appropriate views.[1] X-ray findings of the cervical spine are indicated if cervical radiculopathy is suspected.

MRI has become the imaging technique of choice in detecting soft tissue lesions and in the diagnosis of rotator cuff lesions and impingement.[7] In older patients, however, MRI almost always reveals some "abnormality" that may have nothing to do with the presenting symptoms. Therefore diagnostic imaging studies, which also include ultrasonography and CT scans, as well as invasive studies such as arthrography, are best ordered in consultation with a specialist, particularly when there may be a need for surgical intervention.

DIAGNOSTICS

Shoulder Pain

LABORATORY
CBC and differential*
ESR*
Serologic tests for rheumatologic disease*

IMAGING
X-ray*
- Anteroposterior views
- Axillary lateral views
- Scapula Y view

MRI*
CT scan*
Ultrasound*
Arthrography*
Arthrocentesis*

*If indicated.

Laboratory studies are seldom indicated. However, CBC, erythrocyte sedimentation rate, and serologic tests for rheumatologic diseases should be performed in accordance with the history and examination findings.

DIFFERENTIAL DIAGNOSIS

The ability to correlate the history and physical examination with a functional knowledge of anatomy, an understanding of the mechanism of injury, and an ability to reproduce the symptoms clinically will often diagnose the problem.[8] Shoulder disorders can be categorized as acute or chronic and as either traumatic or atraumatic. The diagnosis of shoulder pain is simplified when there is a history of trauma. If the duration of pain is less than 2 weeks, the patient may recall an injury or fall. The difficulty comes with subacute, smoldering conditions that have an onset 6 weeks to 3 months after the incident or injury.[3]

Although instability is most common in teenagers, gradual onset of shoulder pain on the nondominant side of a middle-aged woman is more likely adhesive capsulitis. Severe acute shoulder pain with restricted movement in a laborer or athlete is likely acute calcific tendinitis.[10] Shoulder pain aggravated by reaching and direct pressure is likely caused by impingement. Pain in the shoulder at night is rotator cuff disease until proven otherwise. Pain in the shoulder with repetitive overhead activity also suggests rotator cuff disease. Pain at rest should suggest that the problem is extrinsic to the shoulder girdle, although acute inflammatory conditions often cause night pain. Pain associated with a throwing motion may be secondary to instability. Pain in the supraclavicular area and toward the vertebral border of the scapula is often referred pain from the neck. Pain radiating down the arm, especially below the elbow, suggests a neurogenic cause.

Tendinitis

Tendinitis occurs when the tendons or surrounding tissue become inflamed, swollen, and tender. Supraspinatus tendinitis is the most common cause of shoulder pain and is usually caused by degenerative changes in that tendon with advancing age.[11] Other common causes of tendinitis include overhead or repetitive activity, a weakened rotator cuff (usually in combination with overhead activity), heavy lifting activities, and muscle strain. In rotator cuff tendinitis, abnormal repetitive stresses cause a mechanical irritation of the structures below the acromial bursa.[9] With calcific tendinitis, calcific deposits form in the rotator cuff tendon, causing local mechanical irritation. Biceps tendinitis, which can result from overuse activities above the head, can lead to subacromial impingement, particularly in internal rotation. Elbow flexion against resistance usually reproduces pain located over the anterior aspect of the shoulder and upper arm.

Tendinitis often has no isolated precipitating event. Most patients complain of a deep ache in the shoulder, with increasing pain on abduction and internal rotation. Determining what position or posture causes pain is diagnostic. Pain with arm elevation, for example, is suggestive of rotator cuff tendinitis or subacromial bursitis. Point tenderness is often localized to the vicinity of the greater tuberosity below the acromion and along the lateral aspect of the humeral head. The reflexive shrug will be noted as the patient tries to abduct the arm. The shrug helps reduce the pain caused by impingement on the acromion.

Generalized muscle weakness on manual muscle testing, especially with internal and external rotation, is characteristic of rotator cuff tendinitis.[9] Also, the empty can test and the impingement test are useful in validating the clinical diagnosis (see Table 198-1).

Bursitis

Bursitis occurs when the bursa becomes inflamed and painful as surrounding muscles move over it. The bursa's primary function is to maintain a gliding surface between muscles and ligaments (see Chapter 184). The most common cause of bursitis is overuse syndromes. Pitching, tennis, swimming, or repetitive use of the arm at or above shoulder level can all cause subacromial bursitis.

Occasionally the calcific deposits in tendinitis may extend the inflammatory process into the subacromial bursa, producing inflammation in the wall of the bursa.

Symptom onset in bursitis is usually abrupt, with pain often felt at the tip of the shoulder or along the upper third of the humerus. The pain is referred down the deltoid muscle into the upper arm. It occurs when the arm is lifted overhead or twisted. In extreme cases pain will be present continuously and may disrupt sleep.

Rotator Cuff Tear or Rupture

In rotator cuff diseases the supraspinatus tendon is the most commonly injured tendon because the tracking of the tendon is directly under the anterior edge of the acromion.[7] Tears in the rotator cuff are more common in older adults because of degenerative changes that take place over time in tendons and lead to structural weakening that predisposes the tendon to tears, particularly after the fifth decade of life.[11] Rotator cuff disease is classified or graded to reflect progressively worsening symptomatology and functional impairment. Grade I disease of the rotator cuff, which is most common in young adults, involves acute inflammation and edema resulting from either acute trauma or repetitive overhead activity. Grade II disease, which is seen in middle-aged adults, is characterized by chronic degenerative changes without actual tear. Grade III disease, commonly observed in older adult populations, represents disruption of tendon integrity (a tear).

Excessive use of the shoulder involving repetitive, stressful movement and injury or repeated injuries will produce this partial or complete rupture or disintegration of the rotator cuff. A weakened rotator cuff at the supraspinatus tendon may tear spontaneously as a result of minimum trauma, such as a fall. Tears tend not to be painful. Muscle atrophy often accompanies rotator cuff tears. Although the rotator cuff is not easily palpable, point tenderness to manual palpation is maximum just below the greater tuberosity of the humerus. Incomplete ruptures produce chronic thickening of the subacromial bursa and impingement syndrome. There is little chance for spontaneous healing of a torn rotator cuff.

The patient with rotator cuff tear typically is seen with complaints of shoulder pain aggravated by activity and radiating to the anterior aspect of the arm. Abduction is painful and weak, and tenderness may be elicited over the insertion of the greater tuberosity.[11] On examination, the patient will be unable to abduct the arm, instead producing a characteristic shoulder shrug. The drop arm test assesses the integrity of the rotator cuff and is positive with significant tears (see Table 198-1).

Subacromial Impingement Syndrome

The tendons comprising the rotator cuff can be worn down by repetitive excursion between the greater tuberosity of the humerus and the acromion and the acromioclavicular ligament.[1] This repetitive trauma can lead to compression of both the tendons and the subacromial bursa, resulting in edema, hemorrhage, inflammation, and ultimately fibrosis. Impingement occurs as a result of acute trauma, repetitive overhead activities, pushing and pulling activities, subtle or overt instability of the glenohumeral joint, and degenerative and inflammatory disorders of the tendons and bursa.[12]

Shoulder Instability, Dislocation, and Subluxation

Shoulder dislocation predisposes the patient to recurrent instability. Instability results from posttraumatic capsular tear or stretch. Athletes are subject to numerous repetitive loads that can lead to symptoms of instability.[13] There are two primary types of shoulder instability: (1) traumatic, unidirectional instability; and (2) atraumatic, multidirectional, bilateral, rehabilitation, inferior capsule shift. Dislocation is much more common in young adults, with the likelihood of redislocation decreasing with advancing age. In older adults rotator cuff tears commonly occur with dislocation. A history of traumatic dislocation and medical or surgical reduction is a powerful risk factor for instability. The patient will simply complain of the shoulder "giving out." Dislocation results from trauma to the shoulder while it is hyperextended. Dislocations are often anterior and are characterized by loss of the shoulder's rounded appearance. The patient typically is seen with the hands held to the side. There is prominence of the acromion, painful limitation of movement, and displacement of the humerus away from the trunk.

The apprehension test detects chronic shoulder dislocation (see Table 198-1). Yergason's test for long head of the biceps tendon stability determines whether the biceps tendon is stable in the occipital groove[14] (see Table 198-1). A palm-up hand position is used to rule out posterior dislocation.

Arthritis

Arthritis of the glenohumeral joint may be secondary to inflammatory arthritis or osteoarthritis. The distinguishing feature of shoulder arthritis is pain at rest, aggravated by movement. The patient reports a grinding or clicking sound with motion. Examination may reveal muscle wasting, crepitation, effusion, and decreased range of motion.

Although the shoulder may undergo arthritic changes from a number of causes, these changes are much better tolerated than arthritic changes occurring in the weight-bearing joints. A hot, red, swollen, and painful shoulder accompanied by fever and chills is suggestive of septic arthritis.

Shoulder Trauma

With severe shoulder trauma the differential diagnosis includes acromioclavicular separation (crepitus and elevation at the acromioclavicular joint), fractures of the clavicle or humerus, strains, sprains, and dislocation. Severe shoulder trauma not promptly responsive to conservative treatment warrants orthopedic referral.

Extrinsic Shoulder Disorders

Shoulder pain may be specific to the shoulder girdle area or may be referred from another location. Referred pain should be suspected when shoulder motion shows a painless complete arc, no specific periarticular shoulder tender point is identified, muscle strength is within normal limits, or pain cannot be reproduced with various tests of the shoulder muscles.

Referred pain from cervical radiculopathies is common.[8] Because it is located in the thoracic dermatome area, shoulder pain can be referred from several interthoracic or abdominal organs innervated by the same nerves.

Myocardial ischemia or infarction may cause pain radiation to the left shoulder. Shoulder symptoms may also be related to diaphragmatic irritation, which shares the same root innervation (C5, C6) as the dermatome covering the shoulder's summit.

Cervical spondylosis, a herniated cervical disc, cervical trauma, or other neck problems may also cause pain radiating to the shoulder, scapula, or upper back. This pain is often felt at the superomedial angle of the scapula and may be verified by Spurling's test in which radicular pain is reproduced with head compression.[10] Spurling's test is a useful tool in differentiating shoulder pathologic conditions from cervical radiculopathy.[7] To test for the Spurling's sign, the patient should extend the neck and laterally tilt the head to the affected side. The examiner should apply downward force to the top of the head. If the test is positive, recreation of the radicular pain or paresthesia will be evident. This occurs due to narrowing of the foramina against the inflamed nerve root or spinal cord from a ruptured disc. Sometimes a spinal fracture, in addition to causing local pain, may radiate pain to the shoulder along the course of any muscle affected by the fracture.

The shoulder may also be affected by a problem of the elbow and the distal end of the humerus, where a fracture can radiate pain proximally to the shoulder; however, this is an uncommon finding.[14]

DIFFERENTIAL DIAGNOSIS

Shoulder Pain

- Dislocation, instability, and subluxation
- Adhesive capsulitis
- Acute calcific tendinitis
- Rotator cuff disease
- Neurogenic cause
- Referred pain
- Malignancy
- Bursitis
- Tendinitis
- Arthritis
- Acromioclavicular joint separation
- Fractures
- Referred shoulder pain
  - Reflex sympathetic dystrophy
  - Thoracic outlet syndrome
  - Cardiovascular causes (pericarditis, ischemia or angina, dissecting aortic aneurysm)
  - Gastrointestinal causes (hepatic inflammation or congestion, cholecystitis, pancreatitis)
  - Pulmonary causes (pleurisy, Pancoast's tumor)
  - Postlaparoscopic surgery
  - Nerve compression or irritation

Reflex sympathetic dystrophy after myocardial infarction, a cerebrovascular accident, and trauma can also cause shoulder pain. The characteristic features are persistent burning pain, diffuse tenderness, immobilization of the shoulder, and vasomotor changes in the hands. Gallbladder disease can cause scapular pain as well as right upper abdominal pain and tenderness. Pain caused by bony malignancy is usually gnawing, constant, and unrelated to movement.

MANAGEMENT

Although neither national specialty guidelines nor evidence-based practice guidelines are available as templates for approaching the management of shoulder pain, certain general principles of management apply to most presentations. Treatment includes both pharmacologic and a variety of non-pharmacologic approaches, including the triad of rest and avoidance of aggravating activities, ice packs or cold for the first few days followed by heat, and graded exercise. Other appropriate therapeutic modalities include physical therapy, NSAIDs, and intraarticular corticosteroid injections. Goals of treatment center on maximizing physical comfort and preserving shoulder joint mobility and function.

When rest is prescribed for the treatment of acute shoulder pain, the patient avoids any activity that precipitates symptoms and especially the offending or "abusive" activity. Although in some situations a sling is useful, immobilization is recommended only in clinical situations where instability is apparent and never for more than 3 or 4 days. Sports and job modifications may be beneficial.[10]

Applications of ice or heat may provide relief. Ice reduces edema and bleeding and is most often recommended after trauma. Both heat and cold have been demonstrated to reduce muscle spasm and pain.[15] Ice applied topically to the affected joint for 30 minutes three or four times a day, particularly after any activity that involves use of the affected extremity, may reduce inflammation and swelling and promote comfort. Ice massage may also be of therapeutic benefit.

Restoration of normal shoulder function should begin as soon as acute pain has subsided. The overall goals of any therapeutic exercise program include maintaining or restoring full range of motion, decreasing inflammation (with ice, NSAIDs, and deep friction massage), and strengthening the rotator cuff musculature. Range-of-motion exercises, including the "pendulum swing" and the "wall climb" (in which the patient "walks" his or her fingers up a wall), can be performed two or three times daily for 5 to 10 minutes and are helpful in maintaining mobility. Strengthening exercises with weight or resistance and stretching-strengthening exercises with Thera-Band are indicated only after the pain has subsided.

Referral to a physical therapist is recommended for a supervised exercise program. Physical rehabilitation programs should focus on restoration of functional ability and resolution of symptoms.[16] Adjunctive physical therapy modalities such as local heat application, electrogalvanic stimulation, ultrasound, and transverse friction massage may promote tissue extensibility and joint function in chronic situations. Acupuncture, when combined with mobilization, may confer short-term analgesic effects in chronic shoulder conditions, including adhesive capsulitis, rotator cuff disease, and osteoarthritis.[17]

Pain-relieving medications may be indicated. The drugs of choice include NSAIDs and acetaminophen (see Table 194-1). Acetaminophen may be recommended for milder analgesia or in patients for whom NSAIDs are contraindicated. Although acetaminophen has no antiinflammatory activity, its analgesic effect is comparable to that of ibuprofen and naproxen with fewer side effects.[18]

Patients should be instructed to use antiinflammatory medication as prescribed, not just when pain is severe. In addition, they should be counseled about the medication's action, dosage, potential adverse effects, and drug-drug interactions. Certain NSAIDs are available over the counter, and these should be discontinued if a prescription-strength product is recommended.[18]

Alternative pharmacotherapeutic options for the treatment of shoulder pain include low-potency opioids such as acetaminophen with codeine or nonopioids such as tramadol (Ultram).

Corticosteroid injections may reduce pain and expedite functional recovery in patients with inflammatory conditions such as bursitis and tendinitis, as well as in rotator cuff impingement that does not improve with conservative therapy (see Chapter 184).

Health-promoting behaviors such as protecting joints, balancing rest and exercise, and maintaining an optimistic attitude can improve outcomes, as can attention to athletic and occupational considerations (e.g., workplace design, worker training, conditioning).[16]

LIFE SPAN CONSIDERATIONS

Children rarely have rotator cuff tears but commonly have shoulder joint instability (subluxations or dislocations of the glenohumeral joint) because of overuse or sports injuries. In young adults tendinitis is the most common cause of shoulder pain, but tears in the rotator cuff are rare. Older patients rarely have problems with instability, but because the rotator cuff apparatus undergoes significant age-related changes, older patients commonly are seen with rotator cuff lesions (tendinitis and tears) and glenohumeral joint problems (adhesive capsulitis and osteoarthritis). These result from the unique anatomy of the shoulder coupled with age-related degenerative changes.[6] Rotator cuff tears often go unrecognized or are clinically confused with degenerative tendinitis or other forms of shoulder disease in older adults.[6] Musculoskeletal disease is the leading cause of functional disability in the older population.[6]

COMPLICATIONS

The most common and worrisome complication of chronic shoulder pain is adhesive capsulitis. Adhesive capsulitis is characterized by a gradual, progressive decline in shoulder mobility, often resulting from prolonged joint immobilization after a painful episode. Diffuse aching pain and limited mobility are common. Pain is related to the stretching of the restricted joint capsule. Both active and passive range of motion of the glenohumeral joint and scapula are limited. Patients may have difficulty with activities of daily living, including dressing, toileting, and even feeding themselves.

INDICATIONS FOR REFERRAL OR HOSPITALIZATION

A referral to an orthopedist may be indicated for more aggressive diagnostic testing, including radiographs to assess for calcifications, spurs, or arthritic changes; MRI; arthrography; ultrasonography; or electromyography for continued muscle weakness. Arthroscopic acromioplasty may be required for debridement of bursa, subacromial decompression, repair of ligaments, and repair of tendons if a tear is present. Total shoulder replacement may be necessary for end-stage arthritic conditions of the glenohumeral joint.

Failure to respond to conservative therapy or escalating symptoms despite conservative therapy, shoulder dislocation or instability, a rotator cuff tear or rupture, severe disabling arthritis, and infection are among the definitive indications for referral. In cases where arthrocentesis or arthroscopy is indicated, referral to a rheumatologist or an orthopedist may be indicated.

PATIENT AND FAMILY EDUCATION

Patient education concerning health promotion and injury prevention is important.[19] Recovery takes time and requires a multidisciplinary approach, including patient participation. If exercise programs are not taken seriously, chronic or recurrent pain and loss of function may result. Recovery from shoulder injury and pain can be an excruciatingly slow process, requiring 6 weeks to 6 months. Education regarding the healing process and the factors that affect healing, including patient motivation, adherence to interventions, social support, nutrition, lifestyle behaviors, exercise, age, occupation, mental status, depression, and co-morbidities, is necessary.

In addition, the importance of exercise and warm-up and stretching before activities should be stressed. Avoidance of repetitive movements and overuse should be carefully explained. For chronic conditions patients should understand that, although the pain may resolve, the condition can recur. Reinforcement of the need for modification of activities, adherence to exercise regimens, ice packs, medications, and gradual resumption of activities is also necessary.

REFERENCES

1. Kern DE: Shoulder pain. In Barker LR, Burton JR, Zieve PD, editors: *Principles of ambulatory medicine*, ed 5, Baltimore, 2003, Williams & Wilkins.
2. Stevenson H, Trojian T: Evaluation of shoulder pain, *J Fam Pract* 51(7):605-611, 2002.
3. Brunet ME, Norwood LA, Sykes TF: What to do for the painful shoulder, *Patient Care* 15:56-83, 1997.
4. National Institutes of Health: *Shoulder problems*, Pub No 01-4865, Washington, DC, 2001, The Institutes.
5. Onieal ME: Problems of the shoulder, *J Am Acad Nurse Pract* 6(6):283-285, 1994.
6. Rousseau P: Rotator cuff tears in the elderly: a brief review of two cases, *J Am Geriatr Soc* 40(6):614-617, 1992.
7. Wilson C: Rotator cuff versus cervical spine: making the diagnosis, *Nurse Pract* 30(5):44-50, 2005.
8. Owens S, Itamura JM: Differential diagnosis of shoulder injuries in sports, *Orthop Clin North Am* 32(3):393-398, 2001.
9. Onieal ME: Rotator cuff tendinitis, *J Am Acad Nurse Pract* 6(7):339-340, 1994.
10. Fongemie AE, Buss DD, Rolnick SJ: Management of shoulder impingement syndrome and rotator cuff tears, *Am Fam Phys* 57(4):667-674, 1998.
11. Simon RR, Koenigsknecht SJ: Fractures and rheumatology. In Simon RR, Koenigsknecht SJ, editors: *Emergency orthopedics: the extremities*, ed 4, New York, 1999, McGraw-Hill.
12. Trojian T, Stevenson JH, Agrawal N: What can we expect from nonoperative treatment options for shoulder pain? *J Fam Pract* 54(3):216-223, 2005.
13. Doukas WC, Speer KP: Anatomy, pathophysiology, and biomechanics of shoulder instability, *Orthop Clin North Am* 32(3):381-389, 2001.
14. Hoppenfeld S: *Examination of the spine and extremities*, London, 1976, Prentice-Hall.
15. Simon RR, Koenigsknecht SJ,: Soft tissue injuries, dislocations, and disorders of the shoulder and upper arm. In Simon RR, Koenigsknecht SJ, editors: *Emergency orthopedics: the extremities*, ed 4, New York, 1999, McGraw-Hill.
16. Kibler WB, McMullen J, Uhl T: Shoulder rehabilitation strategies, guidelines, and practice, *Orthop Clin North Am* 32(3):527-538, 2001.
17. Green S, Buchbinder R, Hetrick S: Acupuncture for shoulder pain, *Cochrane Database of Systematic Reviews* 2:CD005319, 2005.
18. McCarberg BH, Herr KA: Osteoarthritis: how to manage pain and improve patient function, *Geriatrics* 56(10):14-24, 2001.
19. Boyd MD, Gleit CJ, Graham BA, and others: *Health teaching in nursing practice: a professional model*, ed 3, Stamford, Conn, 1998, Appleton & Lange.

CHAPTER 199

Sprains, Strains, and Fractures

Christine Wilson and Mary E. Farrell

DEFINITION AND EPIDEMIOLOGY

Common musculoskeletal injuries include sprains, strains, dislocations, and fractures. Sprains result from a tearing of the ligaments that bind the joint as the joint is forced beyond its normal range of motion. Strains result from the overstretching or overuse of muscles. Dislocations occur when a bone is displaced at the joint so that the articulating surfaces of the bones detach. Partial displacements are called subluxations. A fracture is a break in the cortex of bone. Fractures may be classified as closed or open. A closed (simple) fracture has no associated disruption in the continuity of the overlying skin. An open (compound) fracture has an associated disruption through the skin to the environment.

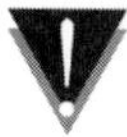

Immediate emergency department referral or physician consultation is indicated for compound fractures or any patient with neurovascular compromise of an extremity.

Strains and sprains are often cared for in private physician offices, clinics, athletic training centers, or simply at home. This makes statistical tracking of these types of injuries an impossibility.[1]

PATHOPHYSIOLOGY

Strains, sprains, and fractures are common musculoskeletal injuries. Strains are minor injuries that result when a muscle is overstretched. No actual muscle damage occurs with a muscle strain, but a sprain involves actual injury to the supporting structures of the affected joint. The degree of damage to these structures depends on the amount of tissue and fiber shearing and tearing that occurs. A grade I sprain usually involves injury with a partial tear of a ligament, grade II also includes a moderate functional impairment, and grade III is a full tear with loss of ligament integrity.

Bone injuries can result in fractures, avulsion fractures, and dislocations. The pulling or pushing of a bone out of its normal position in the joint results in dislocation, which can be complete or incomplete. Avulsion fractures result when a small piece of bone is chipped away, usually after a forceful injury. Stress fractures are small cracks in bone that initially may not be seen on x-ray examination. Repeat x-ray studies after 2 weeks or more may show new bone formation at the fracture site.

CLINICAL PRESENTATION

Sprains may demonstrate swelling, discoloration, and pain with movement. Strains also cause local pain and, if severe, palpable swelling or muscle spasm. Fractures usually manifest with an area of pinpoint pain. There may or may not be associated swelling, discoloration, and decreased range of motion. Dislocations involve the joint and often produce visible deformity. Patients often experience more pain with dislocations than with fractures, as the nerves, tendons, and vessels crossing the joint are disrupted. Injuries that occur as a result of crushing or compression should be evaluated immediately, since they can lead to neurovascular compromise and permanent tissue damage. It is difficult, if not impossible, to exclude a fracture without x-ray studies.

PHYSICAL EXAMINATION

In any trauma, it is essential to exclude or stabilize any life-threatening injuries. A good musculoskeletal examination includes an in-depth history, which should explore the mechanism of injury with a focus on the physical forces incurred by the patient. Often, this assessment is simplified by requesting the patient to use the opposite extremity to reconstruct the exact motion of the affected side during the injury.

A good history of the mechanism of injury will also provide vital information regarding the presence of a compression injury. This will permit accurate diagnosis of these injuries and allow for correct treatment and ongoing monitoring. A past medical history of arthritis, past injuries or surgery that resulted in deformity, or birth defects must be elicited.

Physical examination includes observations of the patient favoring the affected area. Pain, swelling, discoloration, deformity, or open wounds should be noted. The joint above and below the injury should also be examined for injury. Circulatory, motor, and sensory function must be assessed. Palpation for joint laxity can be deferred until a fracture is ruled out.

In an elbow injury the arm is usually flexed at the elbow with the palm toward the chest. From this position, the patient should be asked to move only the lower arm away from the body so that the hand is pointing straight ahead. If elbow pain is elicited, this is indicative of a radial head fracture.

When evaluating fractures, especially in adolescents or children, it is important to recall the classification method developed by Salter-Harris. A type I Salter-Harris fracture occurs when trauma causes complete epiphysis separation only, without any bone fracture.[2] At any age the diagnosis of Salter-Harris type I navicular fracture is made if the clinical examination demonstrates tenderness on palpation at the "snuffbox" (Figure 199-1).

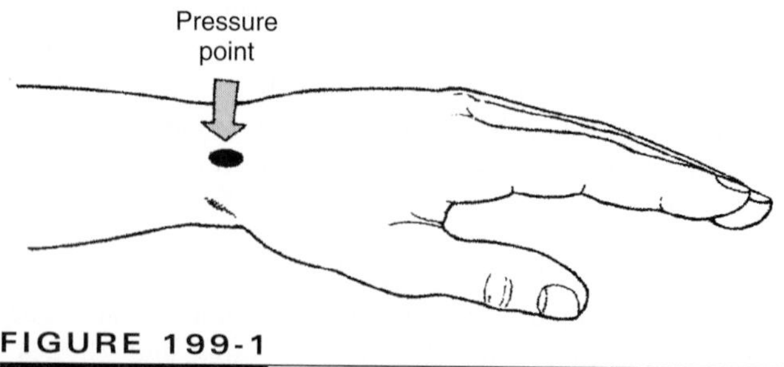

FIGURE 199-1

Palpation for Salter-Harris type I fracture at the "snuffbox" site on the wrist.

Ankle fractures with tenderness through the mortise of the ankle can indicate an associated knee fracture. This indirect fracture of the knee is easily missed on the initial examination; therefore care should be taken to palpate the areas of the upper tibia and fibula and the knee.

Foot fractures of the talus and calcaneus have been misdiagnosed as ankle sprains. A foot fracture must be carefully considered in the differential diagnoses if the patient reports a twisting injury or fall and is walking with an antalgic gait (manner of walking so as to minimize pain in a limb).[3] Talar dome fractures at any age may not be visible on x-ray films for 2 to 4 weeks after injury.[4]

DIAGNOSTICS

Because of the difficulty in determining the type of musculoskeletal injury based on presenting symptoms alone, radiologic examinations are often ordered. Radiologic examinations help diagnosis fractures vs. soft tissue injury only. A history of trauma followed by immediate signs or symptoms of pain, swelling, discoloration, limited range of motion, or decreased strength is an indication for x-ray studies. The ability to bear weight or the absence of swelling, however, may still require x-ray evaluation to rule out fracture.

Fractures are diagnosed when a break in the bone cortex is visible on two radiographic views. *Angulated* fractures refer to either open or closed fractures, usually with more than 30 degrees of angulation. A *transverse* fracture is straight across the bone. *Oblique* fractures are seen diagonally on x-ray films. *Spiral* fractures are seen as wrapping around the bone. A *greenstick* fracture is diagnosed when the bone tears as if a fresh twig were being bent in two. This is commonly seen in children, since they have a more porous cortex, which makes the bone more flexible. An *impacted* fracture occurs when both pieces of the broken bone are crushed into each other. A *comminuted* fracture is observed when the bone ends shatter with multiple fragments. *Stress* fractures are often seen in metatarsals of athletes who run on hard surfaces. The stress from overuse and continued pounding to the bone causes it to fracture, with impaired healing resulting from repeated injury. In the athlete less than 15 years of age the growth plate is still open, and overuse alone may cause a stress fracture in the elbows, knees, tibias, fibulas, heels, and foot.[5] *Jones* fracture involves a fifth metatarsal stress fracture. The fracture itself is distal to the proximal tuberosity and tends not to heal without prolonged immobilization or internal fixation. An *avulsion* or *osteochondral* fracture occurs when the ligament pulls away from the bone, bringing bone fragment(s) with it.

Three common clinical presentations require consideration of additional radiographic views. These are injuries to the navicula, patella, and acromioclavicular joint. Although it is possible to miss a navicular fracture with only a wrist series, the addition of an ulnar deviation view allows more complete assessment of this injury. This view is especially important in the presence of snuffbox tenderness. An injured patella may be better assessed with the sunrise view, which will clearly identify joint effusion and patella fracture. X-ray views taken of a tender acromioclavicular joint while the patient is weight bearing will confirm acromioclavicular separation and allow for grading.

DIAGNOSTICS

Sprains, Strains, and Fractures

IMAGING
X-ray*

*If indicated.

DIFFERENTIAL DIAGNOSIS

Presentation of any musculoskeletal injury requires exclusion of sprains, strains, fractures, dislocations, subluxations, and ligamentous or muscle tears. A large muscle rupture may initially be seen as a convex or concave area with decreased range of motion and pain. Once traumatic injury is excluded, local and systemic causes, such as various forms of arthritis, autoimmune diseases, infection, phlebitis, or tumor, must be considered.

MANAGEMENT

Care of a fracture, strain, or sprain follows these initial guidelines. If appropriate, blood and body fluid precautions should be observed. All jewelry must be removed from the affected limb. Irrigation with normal saline should be considered for any open wounds; then the area should be dressed and bandaged. Impaled objects must be stabilized. If a compartmental or crush injury is suspected, any restrictive dressing or clothing should be removed. Although all orthopedic injuries require assessment of neurovascular function distal to the injury, it is imperative that this function be closely monitored with a compartmental or crush injury.

Any acute orthopedic injury will respond to rest, ice, compression, elevation (RICE), and immobilization. In minor injuries, acetaminophen is often used during the first 24 hours followed by an antiinflammatory nonsteroidal medication. Extremity injuries require constant monitoring of the neurovasculature to prevent complications. If there is no joint involvement and pulses are palpable distal to the injury, the area should be splinted, immobilized, or supported as needed. If there is no palpable pulse and no joint involvement, gentle traction should be applied distally along the long axis until the pulse is palpable. The extremity should then be immobilized.

Extremity injuries involving joints should be immobilized in the presenting position. A sling and swathe can easily splint shoulder injuries. The exception to this is an anterior dislocation of the shoulder, which places the arm in abduction

DIFFERENTIAL DIAGNOSIS

Sprains, Strains, and Fractures

Sprain	Fracture
Strain	• Angulated
Dislocation	• Transverse
Muscle or ligament tear	• Oblique
Arthritis	• Spiral
Infection	• Greenstick
Phlebitis	• Impacted
Tumor	• Comminuted
Autoimmune disorder	• Stress
	• Avulsion

and requires splinting in this position. Wrapping a pillow around the joint and securing it with tape until x-ray films are obtained may comfortably splint severe ankle injuries.

Finger fractures not involving the fingertip should be splinted in the "safe" position, with the metacarpophalangeal joint in 70 degrees of flexion and the proximal interphalangeal joint in 20 degrees of flexion. This position minimizes shortening of the collateral ligaments and subsequent loss of hand function.

If radiographic findings are negative for fracture or dislocation, rest, ice, immobilization, and elevation are recommended. Minor sprains or strains may be immobilized with a simple Ace wrap. An air splint is an appropriate choice for an ankle with an inversion or eversion injury. However, a grade III ankle sprain may need casting and or surgery.[6] With a knee injury, a knee immobilizer should be used to prevent compression on the plexus located in the popliteal space. If an immobilizer is unavailable, a 6-inch Ace bandage may be substituted. An NSAID is usually prescribed if it is not contraindicated. Severe injuries mandate consideration of narcotic analgesic agents. If discomfort persists for more than 10 days, an orthopedic consultation should be considered.

If the back is strained, bed rest is recommended only for the first 24 hours. This should be followed by a slow return to normal activities of daily living. Long-term bracing of back muscles will cause them to remain weak, whereas gentle reconditioning will strengthen them (see Chapter 192).

Clavicular fractures with displacement rarely result in injury to the brachial plexus and adjacent vessels. Clavicular fractures heal well, usually within 2 months. If the fracture does not involve injury to surrounding structures, it is easily managed by making the patient comfortable in a clavicular splint. Although this figure-8 bandage will not reduce a clavicular fracture, it affords great comfort for the patient.

Using RICE has been the standard of care for most sprains and strains for decades and is cited in the patient education information of many national governmental and private organizations.[7-10] Since it is such a well-accepted practice, the need for randomized clinical trials to provide the evidence needed for practice has not been recognized. A few studies have compared compression in ankle injuries using Ace wrap versus other mechanical compression. The studies that have been completed are often not well powered, showed no statistically significant differences in edema or pain, or else have not demonstrated enough improvement in functional outcome to justify the increased cost of an alternative method of compression.[11,12]

Lamb, Nakash, Withers, and colleagues found a paucity of trials addressing mechanical support, so they have designed an emergency department randomized trial, which is ongoing.[11] Wilson and Cooke studied the use of compression for treating ankle sprain and found only 12 trials that addressed this issue.[12] The authors concluded that there was little difference in functional outcome between the type of compression devices used (Ace wrap vs. Tubigrip vs. Aircast) and that early mobility rather than immobilization may lead to the best functional outcome.[12] They found methodologic flaws in all trials, including poor rates of follow up and a concern that subjects in the nonintervention group were those with less severe injuries.

The use of the economical Ace wrap is clinically supported, since the ankle does not have the exposed plexus of nerves and arteries so easily compressed with Ace application to the knee, nor does the ankle Ace wrap tend to roll onto itself, causing uneven compression. The knee is still best supported by a knee immobilizer. Although intuitively the 90-degree angle of the ankle does not allow a cylindric Ace wrap to contour to the anatomy, it is still the standard of care for ankles despite the concerns it may act as an anterior compression band and is unable to prevent inversion or eversion.[12] A stronger mechanical support may actually increase the risk to other joints by transference of the load to the second joint.

Using cyrotherapy instead of heat has been reported in the sports medicine literature as more beneficial. However, in 2004 Bleakly, McDonough, and MacAuley found no statistically significant improvements and called for more trials.[13] NSAIDs have demonstrated some efficacy without adverse side effects.[14,15] One study has now found that, in addition to RICE, low-level laser may decrease edema in grade II ankle sprains.[16]

What is clear is that, in the age of evidence-based practice, this treatment regime (RICE) needs to be examined in randomized trials until a statistically significant advantage can be demonstrated.

LIFE SPAN CONSIDERATIONS

Before full maturation of the skeletal system, patients may sustain fractures as classified by Salter-Harris. Whereas a type I fracture is diagnosed by clinical examination with radiologic confirmation, types II through V are diagnosed by radiography. The most common Salter-Harris fracture is type II.

A type II fracture runs along the epiphysis with an associated triangular break in the metaphysis of the bone. Types III and IV fractures are intraarticular. Type III fractures are uncommon and involve the joint surface as well as the epiphyseal plate and its periphery. Type IV fractures involve the joint surface, epiphysis, epiphyseal plate, and metaphysis. The prognosis for growth is poor in type IV fracture unless reduction and maintenance are flawless.[2] Type V fractures occur when a crushing trauma causes the epiphysis to compress the physis, leading to growth retardation.[2] The physis is the epiphyseal growth plate that connects the epiphysis to the rest of the bone. Trauma to this plate can cause not only a fracture, but also growth changes. If one side of the plate sustains trauma, it may stop producing cells on that side while the rest of the plate continues the growth process. The result is that the growing side enlarges while the injured side stops growing, causing the extremity to become angulated toward the stunted side. Children with angulation-physeal changes should be referred to an orthopedist. The potential for growth stoppage with physeal fractures requires 1 to 2 years of follow-up monitoring. Fractures of the tibia or femur that result in a growth stimulation of up to 1 cm (0.4 inch) are unusual beyond the age ot 12. If this abnormal growth stimulation occurs, it could potentially lead to unequal leg length.[17]

The risk of falling and therefore fractures increases in patients over 65 years. Osteoporosis, poor physical conditioning, co-morbidities, and general frailty exacerbate this risk. Osteoporosis fractures are more common than heart disease or stroke and are a leading cause of disability and nursing home placement (see Chapter 196).

COMPLICATIONS

Complications may occur as a direct result of the injury or as a consequence of treatment provided, and they may be seen within the first hours of injury or weeks after trauma. Critical neurovascular structures lie close to the skeleton; thus disruption of the bone may lacerate, entrap, impale, or compress nerves and vessels at the fracture site. Finger fractures through the volar plate require splinting in extension for 6 weeks. Otherwise the injury to the extensor tendon will cause a mallet finger.

Long bone fractures of the lower extremities at any age require close monitoring. These fractures may have associated blood loss of up to 2 L and may induce hypovolemic shock. The term *compartment* refers to an area where fascia wraps around a muscle group and its supplying arteries, veins, and nerves. Compartment syndrome may occur with any musculoskeletal injury that results in decreased vascular flow to the compartment, thereby causing muscle ischemia and necrosis. Because the fascia is inelastic, anything that increases compression, such as Ace bandages, casts, constrictive jewelry or clothing, or bleeding into an area, can potentiate this risk. The initial compression results in histamine release, which causes increased swelling and capillary dilation. This secondary swelling and dilation increase compression, which leads to further histamine release and more compression. The cyclic process continues, and in 2 to 4 hours irreversible muscle and nerve damage occurs. In 24 to 48 hours complete limb function is lost, and permanent deformity results. The presenting symptoms of this syndrome may include pain, paresthesias, pallor, pulselessness, or paralysis. Nonsurgical treatment includes stopping or decreasing activity to an asymptomatic level.[18] Cooling and elevation may slow or prevent this process. However, surgical intervention may be required to relieve pressure.

Volkmann's contracture is an example of compartment syndrome usually associated with a supracondylar fracture of the elbow. Many different names and descriptions are used to label compartment syndrome. It is essential that presenting signs and symptoms be identified quickly to enable successful intervention.

Acute infection resulting from an open fracture generally occurs within the first 24 to 48 hours. Gas gangrene, a rare occurrence, manifests in a contaminated open fracture approximately 72 hours after injury. Osteomyelitis, a chronic infection, is seen weeks later (see Chapter 195).

After long bone, pelvic, or multiple fractures, fat embolism syndrome may occur within the first 48 to 72 hours. This is manifested by the sudden onset of respiratory distress and extreme arterial hypoxia. Pulmonary emboli are a later complication, generally occurring approximately 2 weeks after the fracture.

Delayed union refers to a fracture that is able to heal but in which the process takes longer than expected. Nonunion occurs if the fracture does not heal sufficiently to support normal limb function and pain continues. Malunion is defined as healing with a poor functional or cosmetic outcome; this generally requires surgical intervention. To protect the fracture site, a cast or brace may be used if complete union fails to occur.

Additional complications include joint stiffness, posttraumatic arthritis, implant failure, and osteochondrosis (avascular necrosis). Reflex sympathetic dystrophy, or reflex sympathetic dystrophy syndrome (also known as complex regional pain syndrome),[19] is a neurologic syndrome that should be suspected if a patient is seen with prolonged, increasing pain extending beyond the anticipated period for healing, along with discoloration and temperature changes of the limb.

Fracture blisters, histologically comparable to second-degree burn blisters, result from a separation of the dermis from the stratified squamous epithelium because of edema; they are most commonly seen with fractures caused by severe twisting, but may appear with other joint or limb trauma. Fracture blisters generally emerge on parts of the body with minimum soft tissue between the skin and bone (e.g., elbow, ankle, foot, shin).[20]

INDICATIONS FOR REFERRAL OR HOSPITALIZATION

Compartment syndrome requires immediate orthopedic referral. If fracture or dislocation is confirmed on x-ray examination, an orthopedist must be consulted.[21] The orthopedist will provide instructions regarding management and hospitalization.

If radiographic findings are positive for fracture or dislocation, an orthopedist is usually consulted. Some primary care practices have guidelines for finger dislocation reductions. The orthopedist is consulted only if the reduction fails. Other types of dislocations, such as a shoulder, require premedication and are usually referred to emergency department physicians or orthopedists.

Physical therapy or occupational therapy referral should be considered in any injury not expected to resolve spontaneously in 10 days. Physical therapy may also be consulted to evaluate ambulation and teach the patient proper use of ambulatory assistive devices. Occupational therapy can be helpful with the appropriate splinting of hand and finger injuries and subsequent rehabilitation.

PATIENT AND FAMILY EDUCATION

In uncomplicated soft tissue injuries, the extremity should be elevated above the level of the heart for the first 24 hours. This implies that the more distal joint should be higher than each preceding proximal joint. Ice should be applied in 20-minute intervals as often as tolerated. Instructions should include placement of a cloth between the ice and skin to prevent cold injury to the skin. Ice therapy can be continued unless muscle spasm occurs, at which time a switch to moist heat is recommended.

The patient should be instructed in how to check for paresthesias, pallor, pulselessness, decreasing circulation, and paralysis in the extremity. Education should address the fact that pain is expected to gradually decrease and that any pain that continues, increases, or is not relieved by medication must be reported to the practitioner.

Ace bandages need to be removed every 2 to 3 hours for 15 minutes and then reapplied snugly. Ace bandages should be removed at night. If a splint or immobilizer is used, specific idiosyncrasies of that particular apparatus should be explained. If no improvement is noted in 4 or 5 days or symptoms persist beyond 10 days, reevaluation and possibly orthopedic referral are indicated.

Patients with casts should be diligent regarding elevation and neurovascular assessment. Patients should also be encouraged to wiggle their fingers or toes to prevent swelling. A cast will conduct cold. Ice contained in a plastic bag and wrapped in a thin cloth will absorb condensation and protect the cast from moisture. The cold will be conducted to the injury, which reduces swelling. Casts should be kept clean and dry. To prevent skin breakdown under or around the edges of the cast, foreign objects such as cast fragments, liquids, lotions, powders, or any device intended to relieve itching should be avoided. Instructions also need to include recommendations for weight bearing, bathing, and follow-up care.

HEALTH PROMOTION

Home and yard safety checks, especially with the older population, should be performed on a regular basis. Poor lighting or outdoor activities at night also account for many injuries. Seasonal issues, including ice or wet surfaces, should be addressed before accidents occur. Warm-up stretches and exercises for any sport are essential. Patients should have yearly physical examinations and ask specifically if their health and physical stature are compatible for the desired sport. Providers should then instruct the parents and children about specific risks. Coaches should be instructed in safe play and pediatric risks involved with their sport and then ensure that children understand and follow the rules. Training programs and instructional programs for both coaches and sports enthusiasts are essential. No sports activity should begin before warm up and stretching exercising, and no sport should be undertaken if the individual is not conditioned for the physical component involved. Safety gear should be checked for fit and worn at all times, and spotters should be used. Properly fitting shoes or protective footwear should be considered in activities that could cause stress injuries to ankles and other joints. First aid equipment and personnel should be available during any organized sport to provide immediate care of injuries. Pain needs to be acknowledged as a warning sign, and activity should be stopped. The health care provider caring for an injured patient should determine when it is safe to return to previous activity levels.

REFERENCES

1. National Center for Injury Prevention and Control, Centers for Disease Control and Prevention: *Unintentional injury prevention,* retrieved Aug 31, 2006, from http://www.cdc.gov/ncipc/duip/ duip.htm.
2. Salter RB: *Textbook of disorders and injuries of the musculoskeletal system,* ed 2, Baltimore, 1983, Williams & Wilkins.
3. Judd DB, Kim DH: Foot fractures frequently misdiagnosed as ankle sprains, *Am Fam Phys* 66(5):785-794, 2002.
4. Wolfe MW, Uhl TL, McCluskey LC: Management of ankle sprains, *Am Fam Phys* 63(1):93-104, 2001.
5. American Academy of Orthopaedic Surgeons: *The young athlete,* retrieved Aug 31, 2006, from http://orthoinfo.aaos.org/brochure/thr_report.cfm?Thread_ID=19&topcategory=Sports%20.
6. Wexler RK: The injured ankle, *Am Fam Phys* 57(3):474-480, 1998.
7. American Academy of Orthopaedic Surgeons: *Sprains and strains,* retrieved Jan 10, 2006, from http://orthoinfo.aaos.org/fact/thr_report.cfm?Thread_ID=45&topcategory=General%20.
8. Medline Plus: *Sprains,* retrieved Jan 10, 2006, from http://www.nlm.nih.gov/medlineplus/ency/article/000041.htm.
9. National Institute of Arthritis and Musculoskeletal and Skin Diseases: *Questions and answers about sprains and strains,* retrieved Feb 10, 2006, from http://www.niams.nih.gov/hi/topics/strain_sprain/strain_sprain.htm#strain_l.
10. American Academy of Family Physicians: *Ankle sprains: healing and preventing injury,* retrieved Aug 31, 2006, from http://familydoctor.org/010.xml.
11. Lamb SE, Nakash RA, Withers EJ, and others (Collaborative Ankle Support Trial research team): Clinical and cost effectiveness of mechanical support for severe ankle sprains: design of a randomised controlled trial in the emergency department, *BMC Musculoskel Dis* 6:1, 2005.
12. Wilson S, Cooke M: Double bandaging of sprained ankles, *Br Med J* 317:722-723, 1998.
13. Bleakly C, McDonough S, MacAuley D: The use of ice in the treatment of acute soft-tissue injury: a systematic review of randomized controlled trails, *Am J Sports Med* 32(1):251-261, 2004.
14. Mazieres B, Rouanet S, Velicy J, and others: Topical ketoprofen patch (100 mg) for the treatment of ankle sprain: a randomized, double-blind, placebo-controlled study, *Am J Sports Med* 33:515-523, 2005.
15. Petrella R, Ekman EF, Schuller R, and others: Efficacy of celecoxib, a COX-2-specific inhibitor, and naproxen in the management of acute ankle sprain: results of a double-blind, randomized controlled trial, *Clin J Sports Med* 14(4):225-231, 2004.
16. Stergiourslas A: Low-level laser treatment can reduce edema in second degree ankle sprains, *J Clin Laser Med Surg* 22(2):125-128, 2004.
17. American Academy of Orthopaedic Surgeons: *Growth plate fractures,* retrieved Aug 31, 2006, from http://orthoinfo.aaos.org/fact/thr_report.cfm?Thread_ID=244&topcategory=Children.
18. Greene WB, editor: *Essentials of musculoskeletal care,* ed 2, Rosemont, Ill, 2000, American Academy of Orthopaedic Surgeons.
19. Reflex Sympathetic Dystrophy Syndrome Association: *Complex regional pain syndrome: treatment guidelines,* retrieved Aug 31, 2006, from http://www.rsds.org/3/clinical_guidelines/index.html#treatment.
20. Strauss E, Petrucelli G, Bong M, and others: Blisters associated with lower extremity fracture: results of a prospective treatment protocol, *Orthop Trauma* 20(9):618-622, 2006.
21. Harvey C: Compartment syndrome: when it is least expected, *Orthop Nurs* 20(3):15-23, 2001.

CHAPTER 200

Stretch Exercises

Anne LeMaitre, Nancy Evans, and
Joanne Sandberg-Cook

GENERAL GUIDELINES

Stretching before and after exercise or athletic activity is widely recommended and practiced. It is generally performed to prevent postexercise pain, improve muscle function, and prevent injury. However, studies proving that stretching actually does prevent postexercise pain or injury are scarce, and some evidence suggests that stretching may not actually be all that effective at preventing pain or injury.[1] Until proven otherwise, health care providers should continue to recommend stretching before exercise. A small body of literature suggests that stretching can help improve range of motion, especially at the hip joint, and can be especially beneficial in an elderly population.[2]

Stretches should not be painful. They are most effective when muscle is maintained in a gently stretched position. Patients should be encouraged to maintain the stretch in a comfortable position, where they feel a mild stretch or tension, but no pain. Muscles respond to pain by contracting and shortening; thus stretching to the point of pain is not beneficial. Patients should be advised that if any stretch causes pain, they should back off and attempt to do the stretch in a more comfortable range. Often it is not the stretch that causes pain, but the technique. If a patient feels pain after stretching but cannot identify a particular stretch as an aggravator, the patient should try doing the stretches at different times during the day.

There is controversy regarding how long a stretch should be held, but it appears that holding a stretch for 15 to 30 seconds is effective. A longer (20- to 30-second) stretch allows muscles to achieve increased lengthening and flexibility, whereas a shorter duration (1 to 15 seconds) is effective in maintaining current muscle flexibility.

Stretches should be done in a relaxed position. An exercise mat should be used on a firm surface if possible. The floor generally provides a better surface than a bed or couch. Any stretching routine should begin with a few moments of deep breathing and relaxation. This is best done while lying supine with bent knees. The patient should focus on taking a few slow, deep, diaphragmatic breaths, then continue breathing slowly while noting any areas of increased tension and trying to release that tension. People often hold tension in their upper trapezius, facial muscles, and low back muscles.

It is common to find that one leg or one side of the body is more flexible than the other side. Each side should be stretched to its comfortable tolerance, and over time the sides should become more equal.

STRETCHES

Low Back Stretch (Figure 200-1)

Lie with your knees bent, feet on the mat. Bring one knee toward your chest until you feel a stretch in your low back or buttock. Use your hands to hold in a comfortably stretched position for 15 to 30 seconds. Return your foot to the mat, then repeat with the opposite leg. Perform alternately, three times on each side.

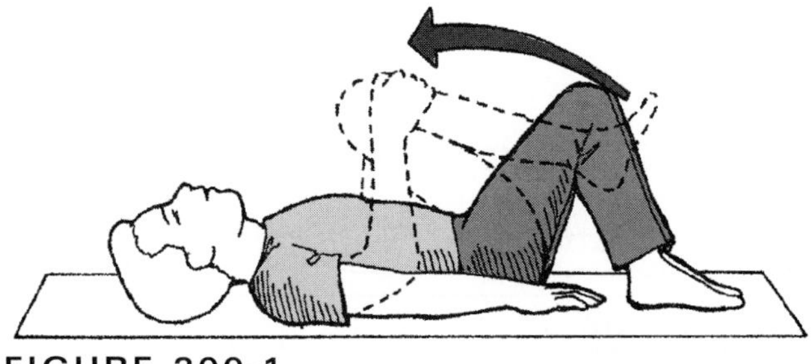

FIGURE 200-1

Low back stretch.

As a progression, bring one knee to your chest and keep it there while bringing the second knee to your chest, again using your hands to assist. Hold, and then lower one knee at a time. Perform three times total.

Hip Flexor Stretch (Figure 200-2)

Begin as in the preceding exercise, but after bringing one knee to your chest, gently lower the opposite knee to the mat, straightening your leg. The stretch should be felt in the front of the hip of the straight leg. Hold 15 to 30 seconds. One leg at a time, return both legs to the starting position. Perform three times for each side.

Alternate Method. If you do not feel a stretch with the above method, lie at the edge of the bed and bring the knee of the leg in the middle of the bed up to your chest. Lower the opposite leg off the edge of the bed, bringing your foot toward the floor until you feel a stretch. Hold as above. Perform three times on one side, then switch to the opposite side.

Lower Trunk Rotation (Figure 200-3)

Lie with your knees bent, feet on the mat. Gently rock your knees from side to side, gradually increasing how far you rock, but never forcing it. You can hold in a stretched position three times for 15 to 20 seconds, but if this is uncomfortable, just continue rocking your knees for 10 to 15 repetitions in a comfortable range.

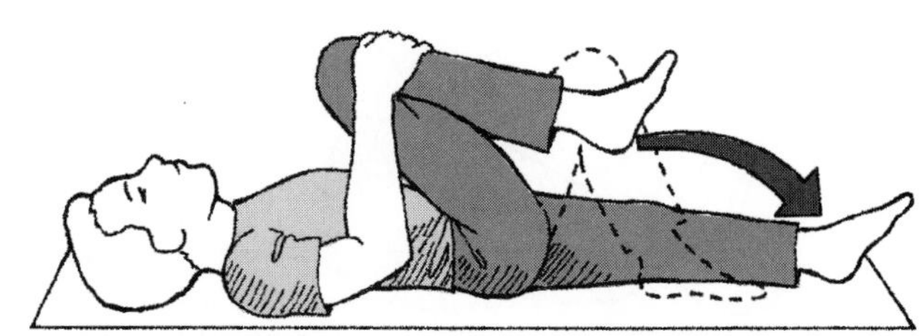

FIGURE 200-2

Hip flexor stretch.

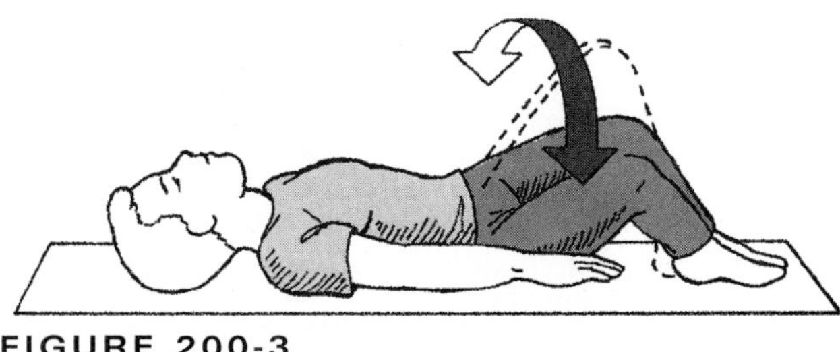

FIGURE 200-3

Lower trunk rotation.

Alternate Method. Bring both knees to your chest as in the first exercise, and rock them from side to side in this position.

Hamstring Stretch (Figure 200-4)

Lie with your knees bent, feet on the mat. Hook both hands behind one knee to support your thigh and straighten this leg. Keep your knee perfectly straight and raise your leg toward the ceiling until you feel a stretch in the back of your leg—it may pull from behind the knee all the way to the ischial tuberosity. Remember to hold in a gently stretched position. Perform three times on each leg. Commonly one leg will be more flexible than the other. Stretch each as tolerated.

Mad Cat Stretch (Figure 200-5)

Gently arch your back up and down—up like an angry cat, then sagging down like a swaybacked horse. Try to move each segment of your spine. You may notice that some parts move freely, whereas other areas are stiff. Focus on increasing movement of the stiff areas.

Rocking Stretch (Figure 200-6)

Begin rocking forward and back slowly and go a bit further each time, until you are able to sit back on your heels, with your arms outstretched in front of you, head down. Hold this position for 15 to 30 seconds. Perform three times.

Extension Stretch (Prone) (Figure 200-7)

Lie on your stomach. While keeping your stomach flat on the mat, rest on your elbows with your arms out in front of you.

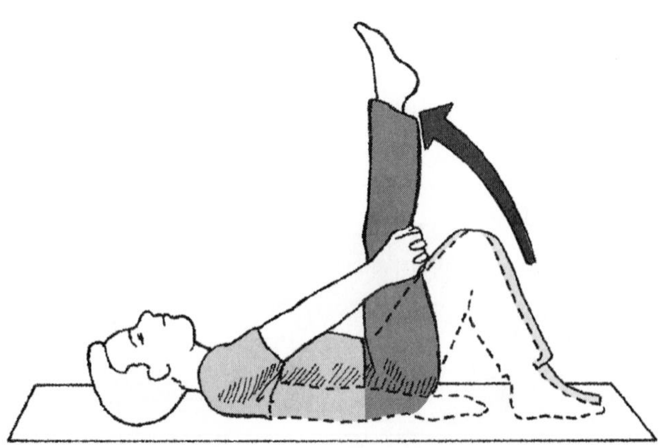

FIGURE 200-4

Hamstring stretch.

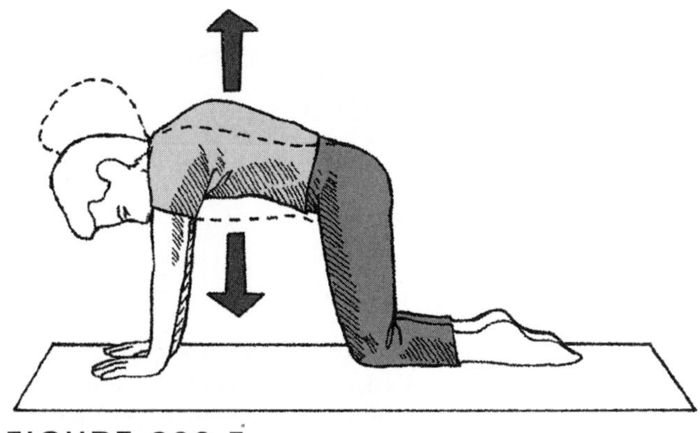

FIGURE 200-5

Mad cat stretch.

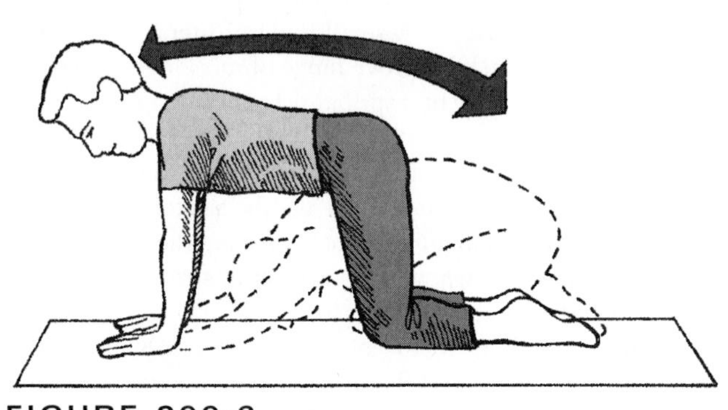

FIGURE 200-6

Rocking stretch.

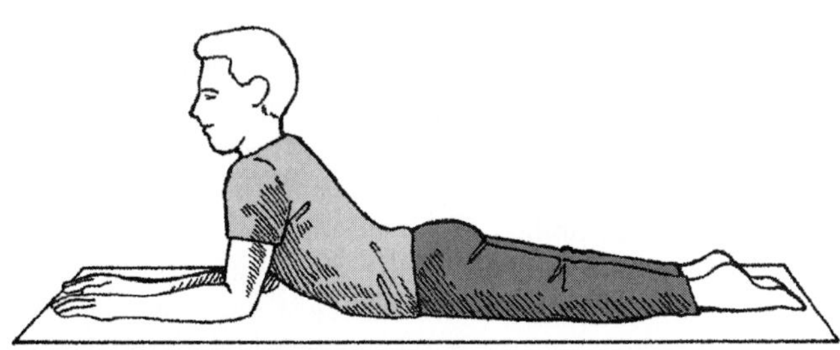

FIGURE 200-7

Extension stretch (prone).

(Your head and shoulders should be up.) Hold 15 to 30 seconds if you feel a stretch. If not, press your hands into the mat and raise yourself so that your stomach, but not your hips, is off the mat, and hold as able (this may not be comfortable for a longer stretch).

Side Stretch (Figure 200-8)

Standing with your feet apart, raise one arm overhead, reaching for the ceiling. Hold if a stretch is felt in the side of your trunk. If not, reach your arm overhead toward the opposite side, then gently slide the opposite hand down

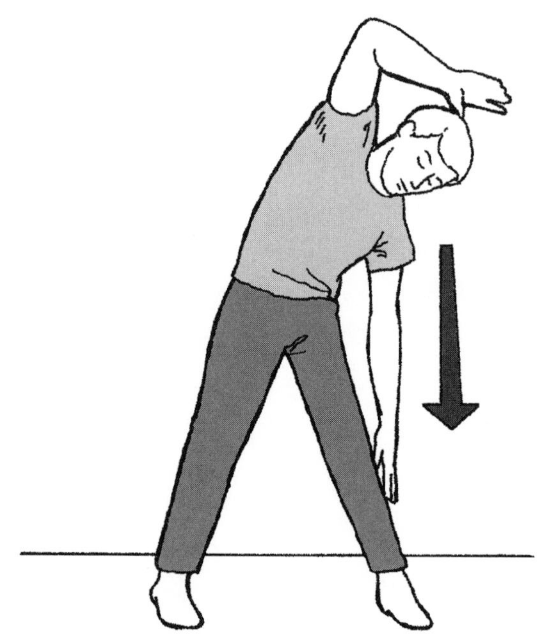

FIGURE 200-8

Side stretch.

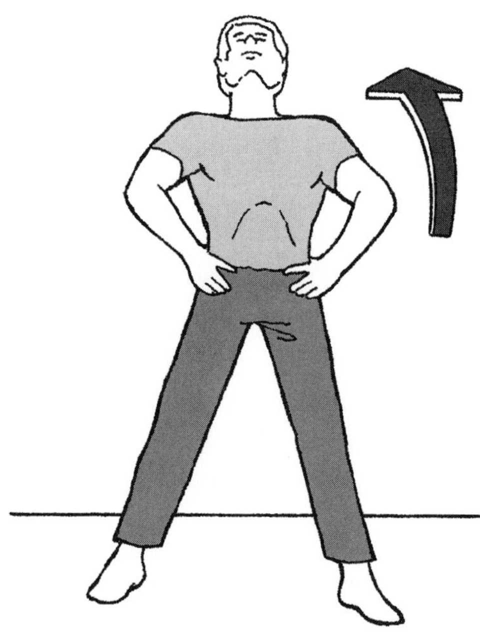

FIGURE 200-9

Extension stretch (standing).

your leg toward the knee. Stop and hold when a stretch is felt, for 15 to 30 seconds. Perform three times on each side, alternating sides.

Extension Stretch (Figure 200-9)

Stand with your feet apart, hands on hips. Slowly arch your back, raising your face to the ceiling. Gently release.

REFERENCES

1. Herbert RD, Gabriel M: Effects of stretching before and after exercise on muscle soreness and risk of injury: systematic review, *BMJ* 325:468, 2002.
2. Zakas A, Balaska P, Grammatikopoulou MG, and others: Acute effects of stretching duration on the range of motion of elderly women, *J Bodywork Movement Ther* 9(4):270-276, 2005.

PART 16

Evaluation and Management of Neurologic Disorders

JOANNE SANDBERG-COOK, *Section Editor*

CHAPTER 201

Amyotrophic Lateral Sclerosis

Noreen M. Leahy

DEFINITION AND EPIDEMIOLOGY

Amyotrophic lateral sclerosis (ALS) is the most common of the progressive motor neuron diseases. New insights into the pathogenesis of ALS have led to exciting advancements in treatment regimens, making this devastating neurodegenerative disease more manageable.[1,2]

ALS is a progressive motor neuron disease that affects both upper motor neurons (UMNs) and lower motor neurons (LMNs) in the corticospinal and corticobulbar tracts, anterior motor horn cells, and bulbar motor nuclei. There are different forms of ALS, including sporadic, familial, and Western Pacific forms. There are also a variety of clinical variants, including progressive muscular atrophy and progressive bulbar palsy, affecting LMNs in limb and bulbar muscles, respectively. Primary lateral sclerosis and progressive pseudobulbar palsy affect UMNs in limb and bulbar muscles. Although these clinical variants may manifest differently early on, they all eventually affect both LMNs and UMNs.[3]

The worldwide incidence rate of ALS is 1 to 3 per 100,000 population, and the prevalence rate is between 3 and 5 per 100,000 population.[3] There appears to be a several-fold higher incidence and prevalence in the Western-specific forms (Guam, Papua New Guinea). The average age of onset is about 55 years, with a slightly increased incidence in men in the United States.[3]

Neurology consultation is indicated for all patients with suspected ALS.

PATHOPHYSIOLOGY

The etiology of ALS remains unknown, although recent literature suggests four major hypotheses as the pathogenesis of the disease. The first describes excitotoxic stimulation as a result of accumulation of glutamate in the central nervous system. It appears that the excess glutamate is toxic to motor neurons. The second hypothesis suggests an autoimmune process with autoantibodies to the calcium channels in motor neurons. The third is a familial hypothesis that neuronal injury is secondary to altered function of superoxide dismutase and subsequent accumulation of free oxygen radicals. There is growing evidence that this oxidative stress, mediated by free radicals, is important in the initiation of the disease. Finally, there is a theory that deficiency in neuronal growth factors leads to degeneration of motor neurons.[3]

The four proposed etiologic mechanisms all lead to neuronal damage of both UMNs and LMNs. The UMNs are initially altered in the motor cortex, thereby affecting the corticospinal and corticobulbar tracts. The LMNs are affected at the anterior motor horn cells in the spinal cord and at the respective motor nuclei in the brainstem. Death of the motor neurons in the brainstem and spinal cord leads to denervation and atrophy of muscle fibers. Selectivity of the neuronal cell death completely spares sensory systems, neuronal systems controlling coordination, and components of the brain controlling cognition. ALS is also selective within the motor system, sparing ocular motility and bowel and bladder function.

CLINICAL PRESENTATION AND PHYSICAL EXAMINATION

A precise documentation of the history of symptoms and a complete neurologic examination are essential. Early LMN cell death leads to an insidious onset of asymmetric weakness that is evident initially in the limbs. The initial presenting symptoms occur in the upper extremities in 40% to 60% of cases and in the lower extremities in 20% of cases. These symptoms include weakness and difficulty performing fine motor tasks. The remaining 20% to 25% of patients with ALS have bulbar symptoms as the initial complaint.[3] These may include dysarthria, dysphagia, and drooling. LMN symptoms include muscle atrophy, hyporeflexia, fasciculations, and muscle cramps. Patients often give a history of early morning cramping while stretching in bed. One of the hallmark physical findings of this disease is fasciculations (spontaneous twitching) that tend to be of low amplitude and high frequency. If the bulbar muscles are initially involved, early symptoms include problems with chewing and swallowing and difficulty with movements of the face and tongue. UMN deterioration of the corticospinal tract leads to spasticity, hyperreflexia, and loss of dexterity. UMN involvement of the corticobulbar tract will cause dysarthria and a pseudobulbar effect. As the disease progresses, both UMN and LMN involvement becomes evident with a more symmetric distribution of the disease. Yet, even in the late stages of disease, sensation, bowel and bladder function, cognition, and ocular motility are spared, although approximately 5% of patients may manifest dementia.[3]

DIAGNOSTICS

The diagnosis of ALS is usually made when there are widespread UMN and LMN signs in the absence of any sensory findings. In 1994 the World Federation of Neurology presented diagnostic criteria for ALS.[4] These include signs of LMN degeneration by clinical, electrophysiologic, or neuropathologic examination and signs of UMN degeneration by clinical examination. The diagnosis also requires a progressive spread of signs within a region or to other regions. The four regions are bulbar, cervical, thoracic, and lumbosacral.

The second part of the diagnosis consists of an absence of electrophysiologic or neuroimaging evidence of other disease processes that might explain the observed clinical or electrophysiologic signs. Based on the World Federation of Neurology diagnostic criteria, the number of regions involved, and the presence and distribution of UMN and LMN signs, a degree of diagnostic certainty can be achieved, although it may not be practical for clinical practice.[1,4]

At this point ALS has are no specific biochemical or laboratory markers. Laboratory and other diagnostic studies may be necessary to exclude other disorders considered in the

DIAGNOSTICS

Amyotrophic Lateral Sclerosis

LABORATORY
CBC and differential
ESR
Serum electrolytes
BUN
Creatinine
Serum glucose
TSH
Lead levels
Calcium
Lyme titer
Vitamin B_{12}
Folate
Cerebrospinal fluid culture
Screening for hereditary disorders*

IMAGING
MRI (head, foramen magnum, and cervical spine)

OTHER
EMG, nerve conduction studies
Lumbar puncture

*If indicated.

differential diagnosis. Electrodiagnostic evaluation with electromyography (EMG) and nerve conduction studies should be performed on every patient with suspected ALS. MRI may reveal changes consistent with UMN dysfunction. Routine laboratory studies, lumbar puncture, Lym titer, and additional serologic studies may be ordered to exclude other disease processes.[1]

DIFFERENTIAL DIAGNOSIS

Differentiating ALS from treatable neurologic disorders was always important in the past because ALS was considered an untreatable disease. Now that ALS has specific treatments, it becomes even more important to diagnose ALS early and initiate the appropriate medical therapy. Atypical features that should alert the practitioner that the patient may have a disease other than ALS include restriction of the disease to just UMNs or LMNs, involvement of neurons other than motor neurons, and EMG findings not consistent with ALS. Compression of the cervical spine, syringobulbia, multifocal motor neuropathy with conduction block, LMN axonal neuropathy, chronic lead poisoning, thyrotoxicosis, inherited enzyme disorders, benign fasciculations, poliomyelitis, and other motor neuron disorders must all be considered when evaluating a patient for possible ALS.[3]

DIFFERENTIAL DIAGNOSIS

Amyotrophic Lateral Sclerosis

Benign fasciculations
Cervical spine compression
Chronic aluminum or lead poisoning
Drug intoxication (phenytoin or strychnine)
Familial amyotrophic lateral sclerosis
Infection
- Herpes zoster
- Poliomyelitis
- Lyme disease
- Tetanus

Adult Tay-Sachs disease
Kennedy's syndrome
Lower motor neuron axonal neuropathy
Multifocal motor neuropathy with conduction block
Syringobulbia
Thyrotoxicosis
Tumor
- Foramen magnum
- Parasagittal tumor

Vitamin deficiency or malabsorption syndrome

MANAGEMENT

Symptom management continues to be the cornerstone of treatment. As more is discovered regarding the mechanisms of this disease, more treatment options become available. Riluzole is an antiglutamate that appears to slow progression of ALS and may improve survival in patients with early bulbar involvement.[5] The efficacy of riluzole has been evaluated in two stratified, randomized, placebo-controlled clinical studies.[6,7] Riluzole significantly reduced mortality over a 21-month period in the first trial and over an 18-month period in the second trial. Early survival improved in both studies, although there was no statistical difference in mortality. The most common side effects described with riluzole are asthenia and nausea. As the dosage is increased, dizziness, diarrhea, and anorexia become more common. The current recommendation for dosing is 50 mg q 12 hr. In addition to the aforementioned side effects, riluzole has been associated with elevations in the serum alanine aminotransferase level in a small proportion of patients. Therefore it has been recommended that liver function tests be obtained at the onset of treatment, monthly during the first 3 months of therapy, and every 3 months thereafter.[5]

The neurotrophic growth factor, insulin-like growth factor-I (IGF-I) has demonstrated conflicting results in clinical trials, and continues to be researched.[8,9] IGF-I is a naturally occurring polypeptide that mediates the activity of growth hormone and has actions similar to those of insulin. Many other treatments are currently under investigation, including antioxidants, heat shock proteins, antibiotics, and gene therapy. It is hoped these agents will work independently or in combination with others to alter the disease course of ALS and establish a new standard of care.[5]

LIFE SPAN CONSIDERATIONS

The median duration of survival for ALS is 23 to 52 months. Most patients die from respiratory failure or infection. The two most important factors in determining survival are the patient's age and the presence or absence of bulbar symptoms at the time of diagnosis. The older the patient, the shorter the duration of survival. Similarly, patients who have bulbar symptoms at the onset of disease have a poorer prognosis and shorter duration of survival.[3]

COMPLICATIONS

Optimum care of these patients can best be provided in collaboration with a specialist. As with any chronic, terminal disease, it is important to maintain a holistic approach toward the patient and family. Providing clear and adequate information in a compassionate fashion, over several visits, early in the disease course contributes to establishment of trust and prevents the patient from becoming overwhelmed.[10] Denial and depression are common early in the disease process and are important to identify and treat to ensure the best quality of life for the patient. The patient should be evaluated for depression at every office visit. Depression is a component of the ALS disease process, and should be explained to the patient. Use of a selective serotonin reuptake inhibitor is a reasonable choice for treatment of depression in patients with ALS, although tricyclic agents can be used effectively if tolerated. The pseudobulbar effect of laughing and crying inappropriately needs to be differentiated from depression.[11] It is also important to involve a multidisciplinary team early, including a social worker; dietitian; and physical, speech, occupational, and respiratory therapists.

Nutritional support can be maximized with early intervention for dysphagia, including referral to a speech therapist and changes in the consistency of foods and fluids. Placement of a gastrostomy tube serves to meet caloric needs and minimize the aspiration of foods and fluids. Tube feedings in these patients can be controversial, and the possible benefits and risks associated with this procedure should be carefully discussed with patients.

Management of respiratory dysfunction in ALS consists of pulmonary function monitoring and the use of respiratory therapy, incentive spirometry, and noninvasive positive pressure ventilation (NIPPV) as needed. Initiation of NIPPV when the patient first demonstrates difficulty with ventilation can provide significant relief of sleep disturbance, which leads to daytime sleepiness, morning headaches, dyspnea, and orthopnea. Serial pulmonary function tests will provide objective evidence of respiratory decline. NIPPV should be initiated when the forced vital capacity is less than 50% of predicted.[2,12] Weakness of respiratory musculature can easily lead to aspiration and pneumonia. Only 4% to 6% of patients with ALS elect to have a tracheostomy and invasive ventilation.[13] Patients' fear of "choking to death" should be addressed with discussions of hypercapneic coma and a peaceful death.

It is important to keep these patients as functional as possible, to anticipate problems, and to ensure patient awareness before problems occur. Cramping, spasticity, and pain are common complaints and should be treated with appropriate pharmacologic agents. The patient should also be vaccinated against pneumococcal infection and influenza.

INDICATIONS FOR REFERRAL OR HOSPITALIZATION

The establishment of advance directives early in the disease course may dictate whether a patient wishes hospitalization for respiratory or other complications. The role of the health care provider is paramount in the organization of the multidisciplinary care required, as well as in identifying and treating any psychosocial issues as they appear.

Impairment of respiratory function in ALS is gradual. During the year preceding death, however, the decline of respiratory function is accelerated. As previously mentioned, it is imperative to promptly treat any sign of respiratory dysfunction or any disorders that will contribute to a rapid respiratory decline. Pneumonia and heart failure should be treated in a hospital setting, especially in the later stages of disease. Most of the hospitalizations will occur in the last year of the patient's life as respiratory function declines.

PATIENT AND FAMILY EDUCATION

ALS is a physically, mentally, and financially debilitating disease. It is important to educate patients and families about its natural history. Discussion topics must include the use of antidepressants, assistive devices, home modifications, gastrostomy tube placement, ventilatory assistance, and hospice care.

In addition, it is important that patients have the necessary physical, mental, and financial support. Forthright discussion with patients and families regarding end-of-life wishes as early as possible will benefit all involved. Patients should be encouraged to appoint a health care proxy and openly discuss end-of-life directives with him or her. Many patients will elect not to have a gastrostomy tube placed and will refuse ventilatory support. Palliative care and hospice services should be introduced early as options that will allow them to maintain independence as long and reasonably as possible, in a manner that respects their rights and provides symptom relief. Patients and caretakers should be referred to local ALS foundations and the Internet for support and educational information.

REFERENCES

1. Elman LB, McCluskey L, Khan T: *Clinical features of amyotrophic lateral sclerosis*, retrieved Feb 13, 2007, from http://www.uptodateonline.com/utd/content/topic.do?topicKey=muscle/13969.
2. Galvez-Jimenez N, Khan T: *Symptom-based management of amyotrophic lateral sclerosis*, retrieved Feb 13, 2007, from http://www.uptodateonline.com/utd/content/topic.do?topicKey=muscle/11391&selectedTitle=6~112.
3. Mitsumoto H: Disorders of upper and lower motor neurons. In Bradley WG, Daroff RB, Fenichel GM, and others, editors: *Neurology in clinical practice: the neurological disorders*, ed 3, Boston, 2000, Butterworth-Heinemann.
4. World Federation of Neurology Research Group on Neuromuscular Diseases Subcommittee on Motor Neuron Disease: El Escorial World Federation of Neurology criteria for the diagnosis of amyotrophic lateral sclerosis, *J Neurol Sci* 124(Suppl):96-107, 1994.
5. Choudry RB, Galvez-Jimenez N, Cudkowicz ME: *Pharmacologic treatment of amyotrophic lateral sclerosis*, retrieved Feb 13, 2007, from http://www.uptodateonline.com/utd/content/topic.do?topicKey=muscle/10778&selectedTitle=5~112.
6. Bengimon G, Lacomblez L, Meininger V: The ALS/riluzole study group: a controlled trial of riluzole in amyotrophic lateral sclerosis, *N Engl J Med* 330:585-591, 1994.
7. Lacomblez L, Bensimon G, Leigh P, and others: Dose ranging study of riluzole in amyotrophic lateral sclerosis, *Lancet* 347:1425, 1996.
8. Lai EC, Felice KJ, Festoff BW, and others: Effect of recombinant human insulin–like growth factor-I on progression of ALS: a placebo-controlled study: the North American ALS/IGF-I Study Group, *Neurology* 49(6):1621-1630, 1997.
9. Borasio GD, Robberecht W, Leigh PN, and others: A placebo-controlled trial of insulin-like growth factor-I in amyotrophic lateral sclerosis: European ALS/IGF-I Study Group, *Neurology* 51:583, 1998.
10. Borasio GD, Sloan R, Pongratz DE: Breaking the news in amyotrophic lateral sclerosis, *J Neurol Sci* 160(Suppl 1):S127-S133, 1998.
11. Borasio GD, Miller RG: Clinical characteristics and management of ALS, *Semin Neurol* 21(2):155-166, 2001.
12. Oppenheimer EA: Treating respiratory failure in ALS: the details are becoming clearer, *J Neurol Sci* 209:1-4, 2003.
13. Gelinas D: Amyotrophic lateral sclerosis and invasive ventilation. In Oliver D, Borasio GD, and Walsh D, editors: *Palliative care in amyotrophic lateral sclerosis*, New York, 2000, Oxford University Press.

CHAPTER 202

Bell's Palsy

Noreen M. Leahy

DEFINITION AND EPIDEMIOLOGY

Bell's palsy is a term used to describe an acute, unilateral, peripheral facial palsy of unknown etiology, which accounts for 60% to 75% of all cases of lower facial motor neuron paralysis.[1] Genetic, autoimmune, infectious, vascular, entrapment, and metabolic causes have been proposed as etiologic factors; viral causation is the most popular theory. With the use of the polymerase chain reaction technique, the herpes simplex virus (HSV) genome has been isolated from the endoneurial fluid of the facial nerve.[2] HSV is believed to be the cause in most cases; thus Bell's palsy may no longer be considered synonymous with *idiopathic facial paralysis*.[3]

Bell's palsy is the most common cause of facial paralysis worldwide, with an incidence of up to 34 per 100,000.[1] Men and women are equally affected. It is more common in young and middle-aged adults. Either side of the face may be affected, and the majority of patients report a recent respiratory tract infection.[4] The incidence is higher during pregnancy, particularly the last trimester or first week postpartum.[1,5,6] It is possibly more common in persons with diabetes and hypertension than in the general population.[1]

Physician consultation is indicated for patients with corneal abrasions or an eyelid that cannot close.

PATHOPHYSIOLOGY

The typical unilateral facial paralysis of Bell's palsy is assumed to be initiated by a triggering event that places physiologic stress on the body (e.g., an upper respiratory tract infection). This stressor promotes the body's protective inflammatory response with its release of acute-phase reactants. The intraneural inflammatory response results in edema of the facial nerve. If the edema is not alleviated, there is ischemia of the nerve, with resulting axonal demyelination and inevitable nerve degeneration. Varying degrees of motor control loss become obvious about 3 days after nerve demyelination. Knowledge of the topographic anatomy of the facial nerve can provide clinical clues to sites of injury; sparing of the forehead muscles typically suggests an upper motor neuron lesion.

CLINICAL PRESENTATION

The typical onset is acute and progressive, with maximum paralysis attained in about half of the cases within 48 to 72 hours and in nearly all cases by day 5. Individuals may report pain behind the ipsilateral ear preceding the facial paralysis by 1 to 2 days. Typically, a smooth forehead, widened palpebral fissure, flattened nasolabial fold, and asymmetric smile are characteristic. Tearing, drooling, postauricular pain, tinnitus, and a mild hearing deficit may occur. Complaints of altered taste (dysgeusia) and an increased sensitivity to sound (hyperacusis) may also be present, as well as a hypoesthesia in one or more branches of the trigeminal nerve.[1,4] A complete and detailed history is essential for diagnosis, since Bell's palsy is a diagnosis of exclusion. Timing of onset is key in the diagnosis; slowly progressive or relapsing courses suggest other entities.

Other associated symptoms include a history of recent infections, especially viral illnesses such as chickenpox, mumps, mononucleosis, coxsackievirus, cytomegalovirus, HIV, and influenza. The presence of chronic illnesses such as diabetes mellitus, hypertension, or hypothyroidism should be ascertained, and the patient should be queried about pregnancy, skin rashes or lesions, and insect (tick) bites, since Bell's palsy is a common neuropathy in Lyme disease.[1] Any history of facial trauma should be carefully noted.

PHYSICAL EXAMINATION

A careful examination of the head and neck with assessment of all cranial nerves is essential, in addition to a general physical examination. Vesicles or eschars in the external ear canal indicate geniculate herpes (Ramsay Hunt syndrome). Special attention to the sensory and motor functions of the branches of the facial nerve is also necessary. Minor asymmetry of the lower face may be a normal deviation. The degree of facial weakness should be documented. A number of grading systems have been developed to objectively define the severity of the palsy.[7,8] Clinicians may find these tools helpful in gauging the severity of neural degeneration and in establishing objective measures of recovery. A photographic record is also helpful in establishing the extent of facial muscle weakness and documenting progressive neural regeneration.

DIAGNOSTICS

Although routine laboratory tests are of little value in the diagnosis of Bell's palsy, diagnostic studies may be useful to exclude varied conditions in the differential diagnosis. If infection is suspected, a CBC and differential are indicated. Lyme titers are useful to exclude Lyme disease. Other serologic tests to consider include thyroid-stimulating hormone, blood glucose, and serum angiotensin-converting enzyme to exclude thyroid dysfunction, diabetes, and sarcoidosis. If indicated, a pregnancy test should also be obtained.

DIAGNOSTICS

Bell's Palsy

LABORATORY
CBC and differential
TSH
Angiotensin-converting enzyme
Serum glucose
Pregnancy test (serum human chorionic gonadotropin)
Lyme titer

IMAGING
MRI*

OTHER
Schirmer's test*
Acoustic reflex*
Electrogustometry*
EMG*
Audiometry*
Electronystagmography*

*If indicated.

Tests usually performed by an otolaryngologist or other specialist include topognostic studies (tests for tactile sensation) such as Schirmer's test (checks for tear production), acoustic reflex, and electrogustometry (salivation test), although these tests have little practical applicability.[1] Electrophysiologic studies involve nerve excitability testing, electromyography, and electroneurography. The percentage of nerve degeneration is useful in predicting recovery. Audiologic studies encompass pure tone audiometry and impedance tests, along with electronystagmography. Neuroimaging studies may be indicated if symptoms are atypical, the course of progression is slow, or recovery extends beyond 6 months.[1] The facial nerve can be visualized on a gadolinium-enhanced MRI, which is the diagnostic choice for cranial nerve pathologic conditions.

DIFFERENTIAL DIAGNOSIS

The list of conditions to be included in the differential diagnosis for unilateral facial paralysis is lengthy. Infectious, traumatic, neoplastic, immunologic, and metabolic conditions (e.g., otitis media, cholesteatoma, tumors, tuberculosis mastoiditis, meningitis, Lyme disease, leukemia, pregnancy, sarcoidosis, diabetes mellitus, and hypothyroidism) should be considered.

MANAGEMENT

Protection of the eye is the single most important goal of care for the patient with Bell's palsy. Exposure keratitis can result in blindness. The cornea should be protected with eyedrops such as methylcellulose twice a day and with an ocular lubricant at bedtime. Protective eyeglasses, moisture chambers, and upper eyelid weights are other options. Eyelids should be closed and patched at night to protect the cornea.[9,10]

Massage of weakened facial muscles may help preserve muscle tone and provide some comfort. A favorable prognostic sign is the lack of complete facial paralysis.[4]

Drug therapy for Bell's palsy remains somewhat controversial. The use of prednisone, beginning with 60 to 80 mg/day during the first 48 hours and then tapering over the next week, and valacyclovir 1 g t.i.d. is standard practice for patients seen within the first week of Bell's palsy onset.[1,11] Associated pain should be managed with nonsteroidal agents if not contraindicated.

Surgical decompression of the facial nerve is not routinely performed.[11,12] Eighty percent to 85% of patients with Bell's palsy recover full function spontaneously with a "watchful waiting" approach; approximately 10% fail to have a return of normal facial function.[4,6,7]

DIFFERENTIAL DIAGNOSIS

Bell's Palsy

Infectious conditions	Metabolic conditions
• Otitis media	• Pregnancy
• Tuberculous mastoiditis	• Diabetes
• Meningitis	• Hypothyroidism
• Lyme disease	Trauma
• Herpes virus	Immunologic
Neoplastic conditions	• Sarcoidosis
• Leukemia	
• Cholesteatoma	
• Parotid or other tumors	

LIFE SPAN CONSIDERATIONS

Bell's palsy occurs three times more often during pregnancy.[5,11] An increase in vascular volume and pregnancy-induced hypertension may contribute to palsy of the facial nerve as a result of edema and entrapment. A viral cause cannot be excluded. For the health care provider giving prenatal care, it is recommended that the advice of an obstetrician be solicited and referral considered. As a rule, a prednisone taper has been shown to be helpful in resolving the inflammation if it is given early in the course of the disease. Valacyclovir may be added to the regimen at 1 g t.i.d. for 1 week. Valacyclovir is category B in pregnancy and should be used in consultation with an obstetrician.

COMPLICATIONS

Evidence of poor functional recovery can be seen in facial asymmetry as a result of muscle weakness and synkinesis. Loss of vision in the affected eye from corneal ulceration is among the worst possible outcomes. Hearing loss and permanent tinnitus are sequelae indicating damage to the auditory nerve. Physician consultation is indicated for patients with corneal abrasions or an eyelid that cannot close.

INDICATIONS FOR REFERRAL OR HOSPITALIZATION

All patients with corneal abrasions or ulcerations should be referred to an ophthalmologist. Any concern for compromise of the eyesight of a patient with poor or no lid closure is also reason for referral to an ophthalmologist. Injection of botulism toxin may be of benefit for those left with facial spasm.[9] For those who fail to recover an acceptable level of motor function, referral to a neurosurgeon or otolaryngologist for autografting or facial reanimation surgery may be of benefit.[9,13] Generally, Bell's palsy does not require hospitalization unless co-existing medical or surgical problems warrant inpatient care.

PATIENT AND FAMILY EDUCATION

Providing a full explanation of Bell's palsy and its usual benign clinical course can allay the fright patients experience from the onset of facial paralysis. The health care provider should caution the patient about corneal abrasion and instruct the patient in using eyedrops during the day and ocular lubricant at night. The provider should teach the patient about patching the eyelid closed at night, taking care to close the eyelid to protect the cornea. Patients should be encouraged to report any ocular pain, discharge, or drainage. Providing information about medications, including the name, therapeutic effects, common side effects, dosing, and any other special considerations, will help engender compliance. The provider also teaches the patient to perform facial muscle exercises in front of a mirror two or three times a day, and encourages follow-up care for evaluation of treatment, provision of emotional support, and documentation of recovery of facial muscle function.

REFERENCES

1. Ronthal M: *Bell's palsy,* retrieved Feb 13, 2007, from http://www.uptodateonline.com/utd/content/topic.do?topicKey=neuropat/6815&selectedTitle=1~33.
2. Murakami S, Mizobuchi M, Nakashiro Y, and others: Bell palsy and herpes simplex virus: identification of viral DNA in endoneurial fluid and muscle, *Ann Intern Med* 124(1 Pt 1):27-30, 1996.

3. Peitersen E: Bell's palsy: the spontaneous course of 2,500 peripheral facial nerve palsies of different etiologies, *Acta Otolaryngol Suppl* (549):4-30, 2002.
4. Macken MP, Sweeney PJ, Hanson MR: Cranial neuropathies. In Bradley WG, Daroff RB, Fenichel GM, and others, editors: *Neurology in clinical practice,* Boston, 2000, Butterworth Heinemann.
5. Billue JB: Bell's palsy: an update on idiopathic facial paralysis, *Nurse Pract* 22(8):88-105, 1997.
6. Shehata HA, Okosun H: Neurological disorders in pregnancy, *Curr Opin Obstet Gynecol* 16:117-122, 2004.
7. Ross BG, Fradet G, Nedzelski JM: Development of a sensitive clinical facial grading system, *Otolaryngol Head Neck Surg* 114(3):380-386, 1996.
8. Chee GH, Nedzelski JM: Facial nerve grading systems, *Facial Plast Surg* 16:315, 2000.
9. Holland NJ, Weiner GM: Recent developments in Bell's palsy, *BMJ* 329:553, 2004.
10. Frock TL, McCaffrey R: Postauricular pain with Bell's palsy, *Nurse Pract* 30(4):58-61, 2005.
11. Grogan PM, Gronseth GS: Practice parameter: steroids, acyclovir, and surgery for Bell's Palsy (an evidence-based review): report of the Quality Standards Subcommittee of the American Academy of Neurology, *Neurology* 56(7):830-836, 2001.
12. Yanagihara N, Hato N, Murakami S, and others: Transmastoid decompression as a treatment of Bell palsy, *Otolaryngol Head Neck Surg* 16:347, 2001.
13. Gilden DH: Clinical practice: Bell's palsy, *N Engl J Med* 351:1323, 2004.

CHAPTER 203

Cerebrovascular Events

John Joseph Graykoski

DEFINITION AND EPIDEMIOLOGY

A stroke is an interruption of blood circulation to the brain causing a neurologic deficit reflecting the area of the brain affected. Stroke can be ischemic or hemorrhagic.[1] Ischemic stroke is most prevalent. It is occlusive in nature. This is the result of atherosclerotic disease and progresses slowly as the affected artery becomes more occluded with plaque. Clotting in the narrowed vessel can bring about full occlusion and resultant symptoms. Another type of ischemic stroke is the result of embolism, or the rupture of atherosclerotic plaque, which travels to the brain and blocks blood flow. Atrial fibrillation can result in clot formation in the heart, which then seeds small embolic particles that travel to the brain. Lacunar strokes are seen more in elderly and diabetic patients. They affect smaller areas of the brain by closing off arterioles.

Hemorrhagic stroke has a lower incidence than ischemic stroke but is more deadly. Subarachnoid stroke can be the result of a congenital (berry) aneurysm rupture, arteriovenous malformation, or trauma.[2] Subarachnoid stroke is a rupture of a large vessel within the protective lining of the brain. Intracerebral stroke is the rupture of a vessel within the brain itself.

Transient ischemic attacks (TIAs) are small ischemic events. Neurologic deficits resolve completely within a few hours but no more than 24 hours. A small study conducted by the University of California and Kaiser Permanente evaluated about 1700 patients who came into the emergency department with TIA. Of those patients, 10% went on to have a stroke within 90 days after the event.[3] Other authorities believe that up to 25% of TIAs signal impending stroke. The American Heart Association has calculated that people with TIAs have nine times the risk of a stroke compared with those who have never had a TIA.[4] These numbers reflect the growing practice of aggressive assessment and early treatment of persons with TIA symptoms.

Stroke is the third leading cause of death in the United States, after coronary heart disease and cancer.[5] There are approximately 700,000 cases of stroke each year, of which 200,000 are recurrences. Of all strokes, 83% are ischemic, 10% are intracerebral hemorrhage, and 7% are subarachnoid hemorrhage. More than 7.5% of ischemic strokes and nearly 38% of hemorrhagic strokes result in death within 30 days. From 1993 to 2003, the stroke death rate fell 18.5%, and the actual number of stroke deaths declined 0.7% (CDC/NCHS).

The rate of stroke death is 56.4 per 100,000 people when all ages, sexes, and races are considered. However, it is a disease of age, with the prevalence being 404.5 per 100,000 in the over-65-year-old population. Women experience stroke at a rate 1.75 times that of men. Hispanics are twice as likely as Caucasians to suffer a stroke. African Americans are four times more likely to have a stroke than Caucasians.[6]

Ischemic strokes tend to occur in older patients with other disease processes, whereas hemorrhagic strokes generally occur in healthy individuals between the ages of 40 and 60. Risk factors for ischemic stroke include hypertension, age, cigarette smoking, male gender, family history, race, previous stroke, carotid stenosis of more than 80%, atrial fibrillation, congestive heart failure, mitral stenosis, prosthetic cardiac valves, myocardial infarction, and drug abuse (e.g., cocaine).[7] Other factors that may contribute to stroke are diabetes, obesity, a sedentary lifestyle, and an elevated serum cholesterol level.

Risk factors for hemorrhagic stroke include intracranial vascular anomalies, hypertension, family history, polycystic kidney disease, Ehlers-Danlos syndrome, systemic lupus erythematosus, neurofibromatosis, and tuberous sclerosis. Pregnancy, cigarette smoking, atherosclerosis, acute alcohol intoxication, and recreational drug use (e.g., cocaine) also increase the risk of hemorrhagic stroke.[8]

Stroke represents a significant burden for long-term care. Fifty percent to 70% of stroke survivors regain functional independence, but 15% to 30% are permanently disabled. Institutional care is required by 20% at 3 months after onset. Approximately 25% of stroke victims die within 1 year of their first stroke.[5]

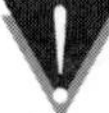

Immediate emergency department referral or physician consultation is indicated for all patients with a suspected cerebrovascular accident.

PATHOPHYSIOLOGY

Ischemic Stroke

In a thrombotic event a critical degree of atherosclerosis causes complete or relatively complete blockage of blood flow through a local area. In an embolic event a clot forms elsewhere (e.g., a fibrillating atrium), breaks off, and travels through the arterial circulation until it lodges in a vessel and blocks the flow of blood distally. The effects of arterial occlusion on brain tissue vary, depending on the location of the occlusion in relation to available collateral and anastomotic channels, and on the degree and duration of the ischemia. The specific neurologic deficit relates to the location and size of the infarction or focus of ischemia. At the time of arterial occlusion, the viscosity of the blood and resistance to flow both increase, and there is sludging within the vessels. The tissue becomes pale. If the ischemia is prolonged, sludging and endothelial damage prevent normal reflow. There is cellular breakdown and swelling.[1]

Hemorrhagic Stroke

Trauma is the most common cause of subarachnoid hemorrhage.[9] Spontaneous subarachnoid hemorrhage is usually the result of rupture of an intracranial saccular aneurysm or arteriovenous malformation on the surface of the brain. A less common type of spontaneous subarachnoid hemorrhage occurs when there is bleeding within the brain tissue itself (intraparenchymal), with subsequent dissection of the hematoma through the brain and into the cerebrospinal fluid. Most of these hemorrhages are caused by hypertension, amyloid angiopathy, intraparenchymal vascular malformations, or tumors.[8]

In either embolic or hemorrhagic stroke, an area immediately surrounding the injury dies within a few minutes from lack of oxygen and the failure of the oxygen-dependent adenosine triphosphate (ATP) metabolic pathway. In a broader area of injury, referred to as the *penumbra,* the damage is more dynamic, extending over 12 to 24 hours. It is believed the release of intracellular calcium initiates the sequence of programmed cell death, or apoptosis.[10]

CLINICAL PRESENTATION

Patients with TIAs and strokes have a similar presentation, although time is a major differentiating factor. The symptoms of cerebral ischemia are widely variable and depend on the vascular territory involved. When the carotid artery circulation is involved, the symptoms reflect ischemia to the ipsilateral eye or brain. The classic visual disturbance (amaurosis fugax) is a transient, painless loss of vision, often described as a "shade" descending over the visual field.[1] Hemispheric brain ischemia usually causes weakness or numbness of the contralateral face or limbs. Language difficulties and cognitive and behavioral changes may also occur.[2] Vertebrobasilar TIAs and strokes may manifest with vertigo, nystagmus, diplopia, dysconjugate gaze, or deficits of cranial nerves III to XII.[2,11]

Many signs and symptoms are common to strokes affecting both anterior (carotid) and posterior (vertebrobasilar) circulation. These include hemiparesis, hemisensory loss, visual field defects, ataxia (difficulty with balance and coordination), dysarthria (difficulty speaking), reflex asymmetry, and Babinski's sign.[11] Headache does not usually occur in ischemic stroke but may in some cases. When present, headache is not nearly as severe as in intracerebral or subarachnoid hemorrhage, and the neck is not stiff. TIAs more commonly precede ischemic stroke than hemorrhagic stroke.

In ischemic stroke the patient usually has a single attack, and the entire illness evolves within a few hours. However, the stroke may occur in a "stuttering" fashion, with intermittent progression of neurologic deficits that extends over several hours or a day or longer. A partial stroke may occur and even recede temporarily for several hours, after which there may be rapid progression to the full-blown stroke. The stroke may involve several parts of the body at once or only one part (e.g., a limb or one side of the face), with the other parts becoming involved in a stepwise fashion until the stroke is fully developed. The stroke may occur during sleep, with the patient remaining unaware until he or she tries to get up and discovers the paralysis.[1]

In subarachnoid hemorrhage the clinical presentation is usually heralded by the abrupt onset of a severe headache ("the worst headache of my life"), nausea and vomiting, signs of meningeal irritation, and varying degrees of neurologic dysfunction. Loss of consciousness at the time of the initial event is common but is usually short lived. Nearly 50% of patients who are seen with aneurysmal subarachnoid hemorrhage give a history of atypical headaches occurring days to weeks before the definitive event.[9] These *sentinel* headaches are characteristically sudden in onset and are often associated with nausea, vomiting, and dizziness, with or without neurologic dysfunction. Some hemorrhagic events may manifest with seizures.

Patients with hypertensive intracerebral hemorrhage may have no consistent warning or prodromal symptoms. In the majority of cases the hemorrhage has its onset while the patient is up and active; onset during sleep is rare. The blood pressure is elevated in almost all cases. The neurologic signs and symptoms vary with the site and size of the extravasation of blood. The patient may lapse almost immediately into stupor and coma, with hemiplegia and steady deterioration to death over the next several hours. More often, the patient complains of a headache, followed within a few minutes by unilateral facial sag, slurred speech, weakness in an arm and leg, and eye deviation away from the paretic limbs. These events, occurring over a period of 5 to 30 minutes, strongly suggest intracerebral bleeding. More advanced cases are characterized by paralysis; aphasia; stupor; coma; deep, irregular respiration; dilated, fixed pupils; and, occasionally, decerebrate rigidity.[1]

PHYSICAL EXAMINATION

Findings on physical examination correspond to the location of the vascular event and associated neurologic deficit. Since TIAs are, by definition, events that last no longer than 24 hours, by the time the patient seeks medical attention all signs and symptoms may have completely resolved, leaving a normal physical examination.

DIAGNOSTICS

Diagnostic studies are necessary to determine the type of stroke and the probable cause, as well as to detect complications. Since management is vastly different, it is important to be able to quickly differentiate ischemic stroke from hemorrhagic stroke and to exclude disorders that may occasionally appear like stroke.

In the initial evaluation the most common imaging procedure performed is a head CT scan.[9] A noncontrast CT scan is better than MRI in discriminating between hemorrhagic and ischemic stroke. Patients who have atypical presentations or who have unusual findings on noncontrast CT scans ought to have a CT scan with contrast or MRI to exclude tumor. CT can miss small subcortical or cortical infarctions or lesions in the posterior fossa. Among patients with ischemic stroke, the CT scan may be normal in the first few hours but will usually show abnormalities after 12 or more hours. In hemorrhagic stroke the head CT scan will usually be abnormal at presentation to the emergency department. If the initial CT scan shows hemorrhage, other studies (e.g., arteriogram) may be necessary to determine whether an underlying vascular malformation is present.[8]

Other diagnostic studies include an ECG, chest radiograph, pulse oximetry or arterial blood gas assessment, CBC with platelets, prothrombin time, partial thromboplastin time, serum glucose, creatinine, BUN, and electrolytes. Depending on the clinical presentation, other tests may be necessary, including examination of the cerebrospinal fluid if central nervous system infection is suspected or when the clinical picture suggests subarachnoid hemorrhage but the head CT scan is negative. An electroencephalogram is indicated when the clinical picture suggests seizure. Carotid ultrasound will assess patency of the carotid arteries. Carotid arteriography or magnetic resonance angiography should be done in patients with severe carotid stenosis on ultrasound evaluation who are considered candidates for endarterectomy. A transesophageal echocardiogram[9] and Holter monitor study may be performed if the presentation is suspicious for an embolic event originating from the heart. Other laboratory tests that may be indicated include a serum cholesterol level, toxicology screening, erythrocyte sedimentation rate, hemoglobin electrophoresis, fibrinogen, serum protein electrophoresis, antiphospholipid antibody level, serologic test for syphilis, protein C level, protein S level, antithrombin III level, lupus anticoagulant, anticardiolipin antibody level, and connective tissue disease screen.

DIAGNOSTICS

Cerebrovascular Events

INITIAL
ECG
Pulse oximetry

LABORATORY
CBC and differential
PT, PTT, International Normalized Ratio
Serum electrolytes
BUN
Creatinine
Serum glucose
Toxic screen*
Lipid profile
ESR
Hemoglobin electrophoresis*
Fibrinogen
Serum protein electrophoresis*
Antiphospholipid antibody*
Fluorescent treponemal antibody absorption test or rapid plasma reagin*
Protein C, protein S*
Antithrombin III*
Lupus anticoagulant*
Anticardiolipin antibody*
Connective tissue disease screening*

IMAGING
CT scan of head (noncontrast)
Transesophageal echocardiogram
Chest x-ray*

OTHER
Carotid ultrasound
EEG*
Arteriography*
ABGs*
Lumbar puncture*
Holter or event monitoring

*If indicated.

DIFFERENTIAL DIAGNOSIS

A number of conditions may be mistaken for TIAs and stroke: migraine and migraine equivalents, simple partial or complex partial seizures, subdural hematoma, brain tumor (primary or

DIFFERENTIAL DIAGNOSIS

Cerebrovascular Events

- Migraine
- Seizures
- Subdural or epidural hematoma
- Tumor (primary, metastatic)
- Syncope
- Hypoglycemia
- Cardiac arrhythmia
- Transient global amnesia
- Encephalopathy
- Conversion disorder
- Carpal tunnel syndrome
- Hyperventilation
- Panic attack
- Infection (meningitis, encephalitis) or systemic infection
- Drug overdose
- Demyelinating disease
- Nonketotic hyperosmolar coma
- Postcardiac arrest ischemia

metastatic), syncope, cardiac arrhythmia, hyperventilation, panic attack, hypoglycemia, demyelinating disease, encephalitis, suicide gestures, conversion disorders, recent cocaine or amphetamine use, transient global amnesia, systemic infection, toxic or metabolic encephalopathy, and carpal tunnel syndrome, among others.[11-13]

MANAGEMENT

Initial management depends on the acuity of presentation. The patient who is seen days after a probable TIA but has no current signs or symptoms of neurologic dysfunction can generally be evaluated and treated in the outpatient setting. Identification of the most likely cause of the TIA is vital to proper management. For example, management of the patient with severe carotid stenosis will be different from that of the patient with atrial fibrillation. Treatment for all patients with a TIA or stroke should include risk factor management.

The patient who is seen acutely with neurologic signs and symptoms compatible with a TIA or stroke should be managed as a medical emergency.[12]

Initial management of suspected stroke includes assessment of the ABCs (airway, breathing, and circulation) and vital signs. The airway should be secured; oxygen administered by nasal cannula; a cardiac monitor, pulse oximeter, and sphygmomanometer attached; an IV access established; a physical examination performed; a 12-lead ECG and portable chest radiograph obtained; laboratory tests (as described previously) ordered; and an urgent, noncontrast head CT scan obtained. If hemorrhage has occurred, a neurosurgeon should be contacted. If ischemic stroke has occurred, thrombolytic therapy should be considered if the patient meets the criteria.

Careful blood pressure management is necessary in the acute ischemic stroke setting. Patients who have a stroke commonly have elevated blood pressure after the acute event. The conscious stroke patient is usually anxious. Often the blood pressure will fall when the patient is moved to a quieter room and allowed to rest after completion of the initial evaluation.[7] There is evidence that an acute hypertensive response may represent a beneficial compensatory response to maintain cerebral perfusion.[14] If the brain is already ischemic, lowering the blood pressure may only exacerbate hypoperfusion and injury. Therefore, except when the blood pressure is extremely high, it is best not to lower it during the first few days after an ischemic infarction. After that time, the blood pressure usually returns to the previous baseline value without additional treatment.[15] Patients with a systolic blood pressure of more than 220 mm Hg or a diastolic blood pressure of more than 120 mm Hg and medical conditions requiring blood pressure control may require medical intervention.

If an antihypertensive drug is necessary, labetalol is currently the drug of choice.[16] The drug is given intravenously, 10 mg, over 1 to 2 minutes. The dose may be repeated or doubled every 10 to 20 minutes, with a maximum dose of 150 mg. If no satisfactory response is obtained with labetalol, a nitroprusside infusion may be started.[16] Use of sublingual calcium antagonists should be avoided because of their rapid absorption and sometimes precipitous decline in blood pressure.[7] If antihypertensive therapy is necessary, blood pressure reduction should be gradual and gentle, and the patient should be carefully monitored. The therapy should be discontinued if there is any neurologic deterioration. In patients with subarachnoid hemorrhage, the blood pressure should be reduced to prestroke levels.

Thrombolytic Therapy

In June 1996 the U.S. Food and Drug Administration approved the use of IV recombinant tissue plasminogen activator (t-PA) for treatment of appropriately selected patients with ischemic stroke if it is administered within 3 hours from the onset of symptoms. Despite an increased incidence of bleeding complications, studies show a significant reduction in neurologic disability in patients treated with t-PA as compared with patients treated in the conventional manner.[7,17] There is no evidence that t-PA is effective after 3 hours of symptoms, and the drug has not been approved for use beyond that point. The time to treatment is the most important determinant of success in treating ischemic stroke (the sooner thrombolytic therapy is started, the better the outcome). Inclusion criteria for use of t-PA include age 18 or older, clinical diagnosis of ischemic stroke, and time of onset less than 180 minutes before t-PA administration. The exclusion criteria list is much longer, focusing primarily on evidence of current bleeding or a risk of bleeding that is sufficient to outweigh potential benefits of t-PA treatment. Because t-PA is the only approved specific treatment for acute ischemic stroke and many patients do not fulfill the criteria for its use, the major goals of stroke management are to limit the size of the infarction, prevent and treat complications, and prevent recurrences.[17]

Surgery

Certain types of stroke may require urgent neurosurgical intervention. Neurosurgical consultation is indicated in cases of subarachnoid hemorrhage, intracerebral hemorrhage, and increased intracranial pressure causing neurologic compromise.

Carotid endarterectomy has been demonstrated to have a beneficial effect (as compared with medical therapy alone) in patients with carotid stenosis greater than 70% to 80%, but the role of endarterectomy for patients with lesser degrees of stenosis has not been clearly established.[7,18] The benefit of surgery must be weighed against potential perioperative morbidity and mortality. Carotid endarterectomy is strongly indicated in patients with a hemispheric TIA and in 70% to 99% of patients with ipsilateral carotid stenosis; it should be undertaken as soon as possible in these patients because of the high risk of a full stroke.[18] Surgery for intracranial or vertebrobasilar disease has not been shown to be of any benefit.

Antiplatelet Agents

Numerous studies have demonstrated a benefit of antiplatelet agents in reducing stroke risk in patients who have had a TIA or minor stroke.[18] The relative benefit of antiplatelet therapy is remarkably constant regardless of age, gender, blood pressure, and the presence or absence of diabetes. Aspirin is the standard medical therapy used for TIAs and ischemic stroke prevention. The optimum dose remains somewhat controversial, but there is increasing evidence that lower doses are as effective as higher doses and have fewer gastrointestinal side effects. Currently prescribed regimens range from 85 to 325 mg q day. A meta-analysis of six major studies involving more than 94,000 people show that the benefits of aspirin in preventing stroke is greater than any risk.[19]

Warfarin (Coumadin) is indicated for TIAs and stroke prevention in patients at risk for cardiac embolism. This includes patients with chronic or paroxysmal atrial fibrillation, left ventricular dysfunction with congestive heart failure, or artificial cardiac valves.

A class of antiplatelet drugs, the thienopyridines, is modestly more effective than aspirin, but the degree of additional benefit is unclear. Two representative drugs from this class are clopidogrel (Plavix) and ticlopidine (Ticlid). Ticlopidine, however, has potential side effects, which can include diarrhea, thrombotic thrombocytopenic purpura, and neutropenia. These risks require hematologic monitoring. Cost is also significantly higher than that for either aspirin or Plavix.[20,21]

LIFE SPAN CONSIDERATIONS

Pregnancy

Stroke during pregnancy is a major tragedy, but fortunately rare. In a retrospective study of hospital admissions for delivery by Jaigobin and Silver, 34 strokes occurred in 50,700 patients.[22] There were 21 infarctions and 23 hemorrhages. The health care provider can best address this through pregnancy preparation counseling for all fertile women, stressing the need for early and complete prenatal care. Extreme weight change, proteinuria, or elevated blood pressure in the gravid patient require early intervention.

Geriatric Patients

Stroke will disproportionately affect older persons. In the elderly, especially those with co-morbid conditions, therapeutic interventions such as surgery or thrombolysis can be contraindicated. In these situations, comprehensive assessment of need will help determine where appropriate care can be provided. Some will retain sufficient capacities that they can return home with supportive services. Others will require skilled nursing care. It is critical that the health care provider come to know a patient's intentions regarding end-of-life care. It is not sufficient to know whether a patient desires intubation or defibrillation in case of respiratory or cardiac arrest. A clear statement regarding the use of feeding tubes or IV hydration can be extremely helpful in directing care. A surrogate decision maker must be identified and his or her role defined through advance directives. But more important, health care providers should learn what a patient values in life in order to help guide decisions when impairments may significantly affect those aspects which bring meaning. In this way care can be tailored to the patient's desires.

COMPLICATIONS

The main complication of a TIA is a subsequent full-blown stroke. A TIA is clearly a warning indicating the necessity for a thorough cardiovascular evaluation and appropriate management.

The complications of stroke affect virtually every organ system. Early complications of stroke include cerebral edema, increased intracranial pressure, pulmonary and urinary tract infections, sepsis, seizures, hypertension, hypotension, cardiac arrhythmias, myocardial ischemia and infarction, deep vein thrombosis, pulmonary embolism, pressure sores, depression, and extension or progression of the stroke. Later complications include permanent residual problems with mobility, activities of daily living, communication, nutrition, swallowing, behavior, continence, sexual function, limb contractures, and dementia.

A patient with an acute stroke should be admitted to the hospital, with management directed toward limiting, if possible, the amount of brain injury and preventing or ameliorating the constellation of potential complications. Complications in the hospitalized stroke patient include pneumonia, seizures, myocardial infarction, deep vein thrombosis, pressure ulcers, hyperglycemia, hypoglycemia, depression, limb contractures, and constipation. Awareness of these potential complications and specific therapies directed toward their prevention will dramatically reduce the stroke patient's morbidity and mortality. Of particular importance is physical, occupational, and speech therapy, which should be initiated as soon as the patient is medically stable and able to participate.

INDICATIONS FOR REFERRAL OR HOSPITALIZATION

All patients with a suspected acute TIA or stroke should be evaluated and managed as an emergency. Time is critical. Any patient seen in an outpatient setting within 3 hours of symptom onset should be transported immediately to the nearest emergency department having CT and the ability to implement a thrombolytic (t-PA) protocol. Clear survival benefits exist in those hospitals having dedicated stroke units.[23] A patient with a suspected TIA with a more remote history and a normal current examination may be evaluated as an outpatient. Physician consultation is warranted, since the specific situation may dictate a sense of urgency similar to that of an acute TIA or stroke and warrant hospitalization for evaluation and treatment.

Even with a remote history and a current normal physical examination, hospitalization may be justified to expedite evaluation and reduce the possibility of a stroke. In certain subgroups of patients with TIAs, including those with multiple frequent and recent (crescendo) TIAs and those with ventricular thrombi, the early risk of stroke is particularly high.[18] The diagnostic evaluation of patients seen within 1 week of a TIA should be completed within 1 week or less. All acute strokes require hospitalization.

PATIENT EDUCATION

Two elements of patient education are paramount: (1) risk factor reduction and (2) stroke symptom recognition and emergency treatment. Hypertension is the most important independent and modifiable risk factor. It is imperative that patients with hypertension be educated about their disease and the importance of medical therapy and lifestyle changes for prevention of complications such as stroke. Cigarette smoking, obesity, diabetes, a sedentary lifestyle, and hypercholesterolemia are other modifiable factors that require patient education. Despite the rapid evolution of stroke care and exciting possibilities being investigated, the most important function for the health care provider is aggressive early identification of at-risk individuals; education for all patients; and appropriate early intervention for those with elevated blood pressure, glucose intolerance, obesity, smoking, and sedentary lifestyles.

The public, particularly those individuals with risk factors, must be educated about the signs and symptoms of TIAs and strokes. The term *brain attack* should be used to convey the same sense of urgency that *heart attack* carries. Factors that have been shown to be associated with delay in treatment include lack of recognition of stroke signs and symptoms, calls made to the health care provider instead of the emergency medical number, living alone, onset while asleep, onset at home rather than at work, and a milder severity of stroke.[17] A study by the American Heart Association revealed that nearly two thirds of the persons surveyed could not identify even one warning sign of a stroke.[12] Patients at risk should be taught to recognize the signs and symptoms of a stroke and to call 911 as soon as symptoms occur.

Those patients who do survive suffer a wide range of physical and psychologic impairments, including impairments of motor, sensory, perceptual, cognitive, and communication skills that may seriously interfere with adequate social interactions and ability to engage in normal activities of daily living. The direct and indirect costs for the patient, family, and society are incalculable.

Rehabilitation services are essential to optimize stroke recovery. Intensive rehabilitation should commence within 48 hours of stabilization. The recovery stage of stroke requires significant adaptive training for the patient, family, and caregivers. The family itself will be stressed by the recovery process and will need access to counseling, peer support, and other community resources.[24]

REFERENCES

1. Adams RD, Victor M: *Principles of neurology*, ed 7, New York, 2001, McGraw-Hill.
2. Stroke, *Dynamed*, retrieved Nov 26, 2001, from http://www.dynamicmedical.com/dynamed.nsf?OpenDatabase.
3. Wilner AN: *Advances in outcomes research* (presentation), 125th Annual Meeting of the American Neurological Association, Boston, Oct 15, 2000, retrieved Nov 27, 2001, from http://www.medscape.com/medscape/cno/2000/ANA/Story.cfm?story_id=1726.
4. American Heart Association: *Stroke*, retrieved Nov 27, 2001, from http://216.185.112.5/presenter.jhtml?identifier=1498.
5. American Heart Association Statistics Committee and Stroke Statistics Subcommittee: Heart disease and stroke statistics—2006 update, *Circulation* 113:e85-e151, 2006, retrieved Feb 10, 2007, from http://circ.ahajournals.org/cgi/content/short/113/6/e85#TBL5.
6. National Center for Health Statistics: *Stroke/cerebrovascular disease*, retrieved Jan 28, 2006, from http://www.cdc.gov/nchs/fastats/stroke.htm.
7. Gasecki AP: *Stroke recurrence and prevention*, paper presented at Neurology for Primary Care Providers Conference, San Diego, May 1997.
8. Sawin PD, Loftus CM: Diagnosis of spontaneous subarachnoid hemorrhage, *Am Fam Phys* 55(1):145-156, 1997.
9. Evans R: *Technology advances our understanding of cerebrovascular events* (presentation), 125th Annual Meeting of the American Neurological Association, Boston, Oct 15, 2000, retrieved Nov 28, 2001, from http://www.medscape.com/medscape/cno/2000/ANA/Story.cfm?story_id=1725.
10. Maeder-Ingvar M, Bogousslavsky J: *Recent advances in cerebrovascular disease*, XVII World Congress of Neurology, June 17, 2001, retrieved Nov 27, 2001, from http://www.medscape.com/medscape/cno/2001/WCNCME/Story.cfm?story_id=2316.
11. Nadeua SE: Transient ischemic attacks: diagnosis and medical and surgical management, *J Fam Pract* 38(5):495-504, 1994.
12. Selman WR, Tarr R, Landis DMD: Brain attack: emergency treatment of ischemic stroke, *Am Fam Phys* 55(8):2655-2662, 1997.
13. Edmeads JG: Transient ischemic attacks: rethinking concepts in management, *Postgrad Med* 96(5):42-54, 1994.
14. Smucker WD, Disabato JA, Krishen AE: Systematic approach to diagnosis and initial management of stroke, *Am Fam Phys* 52(1):225-234, 1995.
15. Biller J, Love BB: Medical management of acute cerebral ischemia in the elderly, *Clin Geriatr Med* 7(3):455-473, 1991.
16. Koller RL, Anderson DC: Intravenous thrombolytic therapy for acute ischemic stroke: weighing the risks and benefits of tissue plasminogen activator, *Postgrad Med* 103(4):221-231, 1998.
17. Broderick JP: Practical considerations in the early treatment of ischemic stroke, *Am Fam Phys* 57(1):73-80, 1998.
18. Feinberg WM: Guidelines for the management of transient ischemic attacks: Ad Hoc Committee on Guidelines for the Management of Transient Ischemic Attacks of the Stroke Council, American Heart Association, *Heart Dis Stroke* 3(5):275-283, 1994.
19. Gorelick PB: Stroke concerns should not limit aspirin use, *Phys Week* 23(1), 2006, retrieved Jan 28, 2006, from http://www.physiciansweekly.com/pc.asp?issueid=304&questionid=298.
20. Hankey GJ, Sudlow CLM, Dunbabin DW: Thienopyridine derivatives (ticlopidine, clopidogrel) versus aspirin for preventing stroke and other serious vascular events in high vascular risk patients, *Cochrane Rev* (2), Oxford, England, 2001, Update Software.
21. Mohr JP, Thompson JL, Lazar RM, and others: A comparison of warfarin and aspirin for the prevention of recurrent ischemic stroke, *N Engl J Med* 345:1444-1451, 1493-1495, 2001.
22. Jaigobin C, Silver FL: Stroke and pregnancy, *Stroke* 31:2948, 2000, retrieved Dec 10, 2001, from http://stroke.ahajournals.org/cgi/content/abstract/31/12/2948.
23. Stroke Unit Trialists' Collaboration: *Organized inpatient (stroke unit) care for stroke*, retrieved Feb 10, 2007, from http://www.cochrane.org/reviews/en/ab000197.html.
24. National Stroke Association: *Recovery and rehabilitation*: retrieved Feb 10, 2007, from http://www.stroke.org/site/PageServer?pagename=REHABT.

CHAPTER 204

Delirium

Karen Dick

DEFINITION AND EPIDEMIOLOGY

Delirium is a serious and significant health problem for older adults and one that requires prompt recognition and treatment. Also known as *acute confusional state*, delirium is often the first and only indicator of underlying physical illness, such as infection, myocardial infarction, or drug toxicity in older adults. According to the *Diagnostic and Statistical Manual of Mental Disorders* (fourth edition, text revision [DSM-IV-TR]), delirium can develop from a general medical condition, substance intoxication or withdrawal, or multiple causes (Box 204-1).[1] It is characterized by a disturbance in attention, consciousness, and cognition. The hallmark of delirium is a clouding of consciousness, with an inability to focus, sustain, or shift attention, as well as a change in cognition, including impairment in short-term memory, disorientation, and perceptual disturbances.[1]

The incidence estimates for delirium in hospitalized medical patients range from 10% to 30% and are as high as 70% in some postoperative (orthopedic or cardiac surgery) patients.[2,3] Delirium is also a common problem in long-term and subacute settings.[4] It has been suggested that many patients who become delirious are never recognized as such and may be incorrectly labeled as having dementia, a psychiatric disorder, or unmanageable behavior.[5] Patients with an underlying dementia are at even greater risk for developing delirium, and the link between dementia and delirium remains poorly understood.[6]

Physician consultation is indicated for patients with delirium.

BOX 204-1

DIAGNOSTIC CRITERIA FOR DELIRIUM

A. Disturbance of consciousness (i.e., reduced clarity of awareness of the environment) with reduced ability to focus, sustain, or shift attention.
B. A change in cognition (such as memory deficit, disorientation, language disturbance) or the development of a perceptual disturbance that is not better accounted for by a preexisting, established, or evolving dementia.
C. The disturbance develops over a short period of time (usually hours to days) and tends to fluctuate during the course of the day.
D. There is evidence from the history, physical examination, or laboratory findings that the disturbance is caused by the direct physiologic consequences of a general medical condition.

From American Psychiatric Association: *Diagnostic and statistical manual of mental disorders,* ed 4, text rev, Washington, DC, 2000, The Association.

PATHOPHYSIOLOGY

The exact cause of delirium remains a topic of disagreement. Several mechanisms have been proposed that might explain the physiologic precipitant underlying the development of delirium[6,7]: (1) an insufficiency of cerebral metabolism as demonstrated by diffuse slowing on an electroencephalogram (EEG) in a patient with delirium; (2) a central abnormality caused by an imbalance of central cholinergic and adrenergic metabolism; (3) activation of cytokines; and (4) a stress reaction as evidenced by abnormally high circulating corticosteroids.

Despite the continuing disagreement as to the exact mechanism, the acetylcholine theory has drawn more attention of late. Patients with Alzheimer's dementia have decreased acetylcholine because of loss of cholinergic neurons and are at high risk of delirium. Anticholinergic drugs are known to precipitate delirium, and certain metabolic abnormalities may decrease acetylcholine synthesis in the central nervous system and contribute to the development of delirium. There is also some evidence that even drugs used commonly in the elderly such as digoxin, furosemide, prednisone, and theophylline may have anticholinergic activity.[8] And finally, increased levels of anticholinergic activity have been shown to correlate with the severity of delirium in some hospitalized elderly patients.[9]

It is likely that a combination of several physiologic, psychologic, and environmental variables, combined with the known effects of the normal aging process, contributes to the development of delirium.

CLINICAL PRESENTATION

Delirium occurs acutely over hours to days and is characterized by fluctuations in mental status over the course of the day. This fluctuating presentation is problematic, since patients may have periods of lucidity interspersed with inattention and high distractibility, motor restlessness, speech that is difficult to follow, and perceptual disturbances that range from misinterpretations of the environment to frank visual hallucinations. Memory, particularly in relation to recent events, is often impaired, and disorientation, most commonly to time (day of the week or time of the year) or place, is usually present. Patients may also exhibit affective signs of fear, anxiety, or anger. They may have a history of a fragmented and disordered sleep-wake cycle. Symptoms may be worse in the late afternoon or evening, which is labeled *sundowning*; however, it is not clear whether sundowning is a component of delirium or a separate clinical condition.[10] Patients with a history of dementia are at greatest risk for sundowning.

Clinical subtypes of delirium that have been identified include hyperactive, hypoactive, and mixed variants.[11] The hyperactive subtype, manifested by agitation and restlessness, is often thought of as the typical presentation of delirium. Surprisingly, these cases account for less than 25% of all cases but have the worst outcomes, including nursing home placement or death in 1 month.[12] The hypoactive subtype includes patients who have decreased alertness, sparse or slow speech, lethargy, slowed movements, and apathy. These patients may be somnolent or stuporous. Because these patients are quiet and do not present increased demands for care or surveillance from family or nursing staff, the chance that these patients will *not* be identified as delirious is high. But in one study of hip fracture patients that looked at both delirium severity and psychomotor types, patients with pure hypoactive delirium had better outcomes than patients with hyperactive delirium, even after adjusting for severity.[12] The mixed variant subtype includes symptoms of both hyperactive and hypoactive delirium, with patients cycling between the two; this accounts for more than 50% of cases. These patients often are not identified as being delirious until they become agitated and confused with more symptoms of the hyperactive state.

Because the diagnosis of delirium is based on history, physical examination, or laboratory evidence of an underlying medical condition, careful attention to other symptomatology and conditions is necessary. For community-dwelling older adults, a detailed history from family members is critical. In long-term care the nursing staff can provide invaluable information as to subtle changes in behavior, appetite, or functional status that may be the warning signs of an underlying problem. Urinary tract infection and pneumonia in the frail nursing home patient often manifest with an altered mental status as the only indicator of an underlying problem.

Polypharmacy and biologic vulnerability for adverse effects make the older person more prone to medication-induced delirium, and a thorough review of all medications, including prescription and over-the-counter preparations, is an essential part of the assessment process.[13] Anticholinergic medications have long been implicated as a risk factor for delirium and, although research results have been mixed as to the strength of the association and the relationship to severity of symptoms, these medications need to be discontinued whenever possible.[14] The patient's use of alcohol and other substances also needs to be evaluated.

It is also important to assess psychosocial and sociocultural factors to better understand the patient's baseline personality and psychologic functioning. For patients admitted to the hospital, information from family members or long-term care facilities can be critical in understanding premorbid behavior and function.

PHYSICAL EXAMINATION

In an attempt to identify the precipitating medical condition, a thorough review of systems and a comprehensive physical examination should be undertaken. This may be difficult, however, if the patient is unable to answer questions or follow even simple commands. A detailed history from family members or other caregivers becomes critical in identifying the onset and development of symptoms and in establishing a sudden change in affect, cognition, or behavior. A neurologic examination is necessary to exclude trauma and focal signs suggestive of a central nervous system disturbance (e.g., tumor, stroke, seizure).

Careful observation of the patient's gait, level of consciousness, speech, appearance, and interactions with others can be most helpful in establishing a diagnosis. Mental status testing is important to establish the degree of cognitive impairment but may have to be modified if the patient is unable to cooperate with the examination. Although it is not specific to delirium, the Folstein Mini-Mental State Examination (MMSE) is the most commonly used evaluation tool.[15] The MMSE measures orientation, memory, attention, calculation, and language functions. Patients with delirium often are unable to pay attention well enough to answer questions on the MMSE. Assessment tools that were developed specifically for purposes of diagnosing delirium include the Delirium Rating Scale[16] and the Confusion Assessment Method.[17] Both are capable of assessing the complex features of delirium and of distinguishing delirium from dementia, and both are feasible for use in delirious patients.[18]

DIAGNOSTICS

More than one medical condition may be contributing to the development of delirium, and multiple causes, including substance intoxication or withdrawal, should be considered. The choice of specific diagnostic studies is guided by the history and physical examination and may include a head CT or MRI, lumbar puncture, an electroencephalogram (EEG), and laboratory studies. A CBC, basic metabolic profile, thyroid function test, drug levels, and urinalysis culture and sensitivity should be checked. Although it is rarely done, the EEG can be helpful in confirming the diagnosis and will show a characteristic slowing of brain wave activity.[19]

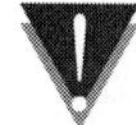

A diagnosis of delirium is considered a medical emergency.

DIFFERENTIAL DIAGNOSIS

DSM-IV-TR diagnostic criteria for delirium mandate that the etiology be specified. Specific causes include systemic diseases, primary cerebral disease, metabolic disturbances, intoxication with exogenous substances (drugs or poisons), and withdrawal from drugs or alcohol.[7]

Delirium must be distinguished from other organic and psychiatric syndromes, including dementia and depression. All three of these conditions have manifestations in common and can occur in the same patient at the same time; the interrelationships between them are complex. It is critical to establish the onset of symptoms, since unlike depression and dementia, the onset of delirium is acute. A psychiatric referral may be necessary to establish a diagnosis.

DIAGNOSTICS

Delirium

LABORATORY
- CBC and differential
- ESR
- Platelet count
- Serum electrolytes
- Serum glucose
- Calcium
- Magnesium
- Phosphorus
- BUN
- Creatinine
- LFTs
- Vitamin B_{12}
- Folate
- Thiamine
- Ammonia
- Thyroid function tests
- Blood and urine toxic screens
- Medication levels
- Urinalysis and culture

IMAGING
- Chest x-ray

OTHER
- ECG
- CT/MRI*
- Lumbar puncture*

*If indicated.

DIFFERENTIAL DIAGNOSIS

Delirium

SYSTEMIC DISEASES
- Infections: urinary tract infection, pneumonia, subacute bacterial endocarditis, meningitis
- Myocardial infarction, congestive heart failure, arrhythmias, pulmonary embolus
- Anemia

PRIMARY CEREBRAL DISEASE
- Cerebrovascular accident
- Transient ischemic attack
- Subdural hematoma
- Temporal arteritis
- Seizure

METABOLIC DISTURBANCES
- Dehydration
- Elevation or decrease in sodium, calcium, magnesium, potassium
- Acid-base imbalance
- Hypoxia
- Hypoglycemia
- Hepatic insufficiency
- Renal insufficiency
- Thyroid dysfunction
- Vitamin deficiencies

INTOXICATION
- Alcohol
- Anticholinergics
- Narcotics
- Sedative-hypnotics
- Antidepressants
- Nonsteroidals
- Heavy metal poisons

WITHDRAWAL
- Alcohol
- Benzodiazepines
- Sedatives and hypnotics
- Narcotics

MANAGEMENT

Treatment of delirium is both definitive and palliative. Current practice remains empirically based without consensus for evidence-based guidelines for diagnosis and management.[20] Definitive care is aimed at identifying and treating the precipitating causes, and palliative care is directed toward the management of symptoms such as agitation, restlessness, and hallucinations.[13] Recent studies have suggested that an interdisciplinary approach may be effective.[20-23] Generally, nonessential medications need to be tapered or discontinued. The sleep-wake cycle needs to be regulated and sensory deficits corrected. The patient should be in a setting that provides necessary medical interventions and close behavioral monitoring and that maintains patient safety. Interventions such as frequent reorientation, reduced stimulation, and a calm and comforting approach can be helpful. Families can often provide a stabilizing presence and can assist with establishing a reassuring and familiar routine. Physical and chemical restraints should be avoided wherever possible.

Haloperidol and droperidol may be useful in controlling agitation and psychosis, and dosing should be guided by the patient's initial response and by frequent reassessment. Newer antipsychotics such as risperidone, quetiapine, and olanzapine may be used in small doses for behavior management in the short term when patient or staff safety is compromised. Benzodiazepines are useful in the treatment of alcohol and sedative withdrawal. The goal of treatment is to promote recovery, prevent additional complications, maintain the patient's safety, and maximize function.

COMPLICATIONS

Delirium contributes to increased morbidity and mortality, longer hospital stays, functional impairment, and more permanent forms of cognitive impairment if it is not recognized and treated in a timely fashion.[24-26] It has been suggested that an episode of delirium may represent the unmasking of an unrecognized dementia in the setting of an acute illness. Patients who become delirious during a hospitalization have longer lengths of stay and higher rates of referral to skilled nursing facilities on discharge. Although it was once thought that delirium was transient, there is now evidence that functional impairment may persist for up to 6 months after treatment.[25] In a prospective study of patients diagnosed with delirium during hospitalization, the 3-year mortality rate was 75% vs. 51% for control patients even when prehospital cognitive, functional, and social measures were taken into account.[27]

INDICATIONS FOR REFERRAL OR HOSPITALIZATION

The need to identify, remove, or treat the underlying condition is critical to modifying the delirious state and preventing subsequent morbidities and complications. Hospitalization is an additional stressor that contributes to delirium, and decisions for treatment should be based on an evaluation of the patient's overall functional status, the caregivers' ability to provide supportive care, and, most important, the patient's safety. Patients are often admitted to the hospital with a diagnosis of mental status change as the search for the underlying cause is actively pursued.

PATIENT AND FAMILY EDUCATION

Patients who have experienced episodes of delirium report feelings of fear and anxiety and often describe vivid hallucinations. Patients and families need reassurance that the delirium is related to a medical condition and is not a sign that the patient is "crazy," is "losing his or her mind," or is becoming "senile." Patients also need an opportunity to reflect on the experience and to express their feelings.

Patients with advanced age, preexisting cognitive impairment, or severe, chronic illnesses, as well as those taking psychoactive medication, are most at risk for delirium.[13,24,25] Although many of these risk factors are not modifiable, it is important that all caregivers be able to recognize the risks and presenting signs and symptoms of delirium.

REFERENCES

1. American Psychiatric Association: *Diagnostic and statistical manual of mental disorders*, ed, 4, text revision, Washington, DC, 2000, The Association.
2. Inouye SK: Delirium in older persons, *N Engl J Med* 354(11):1157-1165, 2006.
3. Sockalingam S, Parekh N, Bogoch II, and others: Delirium in the postoperative cardiac patient: a review, *J Card Surg* 20(6):560-567, 2005.
4. Kiely D, Bergmann MA, Jones RN, and others: Characteristics associated with delirium persistence among newly admitted post acute facility patients, *J Gerontol A Bio Sci Med Sci* 59:344-349, 2004.
5. Foreman MD: Delirium in elderly patients: an overview of the state of the science, *J Gerontol Nurs* 27:12-20, 2001.
6. Inouye SK: Delirium in older persons, *N Engl J Med* 354:1157-1165, 2006.

7. Johnson J: Delirium in the elderly, *Emerg Clin North Am* 8:255-264, 1990.
8. Cole M, McCusker J: Treatment of delirium in older medical inpatients: a challenge for geriatric specialists, *J Am Geriatr Soc* 50:2101-2103, 2002.
9. Mach J, Dysken MW, Kuskowski M, and others: Serum anticholinergic activity in hospitalized older persons with delirium: a preliminary study, *J Am Geriatr Soc* 43:491-495, 1995.
10. Kim P, Louis C, Muralee S, and others: Sundowning syndrome in the older patient, *Clin Geriatr* 13:32-36, 2005.
11. Lipzin B, Levkoff S: An empirical study of delirium subtypes, *Br J Psychiatry* 161:843-845, 1992.
12. Marcantonio E, Ta T, Duthie E, and others: Delirium severity and psychomotor types: their relationship with outcomes after hip fracture repair, *J Am Geriatr Soc* 50(5):850-857, 2002.
13. Jacobsen S: Delirium in the elderly, *Psychiatr Clin North Am* 20:91-109, 1997.
14. Tune L: Anticholinergic effects of medication in elderly patients, *J Clin Psychiatry* 62(Suppl 21):11-14, 2001.
15. Folstein MF, Folstein SE, McHugh PR: "Mini-mental state." A practical method for grading the cognitive state of patients for the clinician, *J Psychiatr Res* 12(3):189-198, 1975.
16. Trzepac P, Dew M: Further analysis of the Delirium Rating Scale, *Gen Hosp Psychiatry* 17:75-79, 1995.
17. Inouye S, van Dyck CH, Alessi CA, and others: Clarifying confusion: the confusion assessment method, *Ann Intern Med* 113:941-948, 1990.
18. Inouye S: The dilemma of delirium, *Am J Med* 97:278-288, 1994.
19. Romano J, Engel G: Delirium, part I, Electroencephalographic data, *Arch Neurol Psychiatry* 51:356-377, 1944.
20. Britton A, Russel R: Multidisciplinary team interventions for delirium in patients with chronic impairment, *Cochrane Database Syst Rev* 1(1):CD000395, 2001.
21. Rizzo JA, Bogardus ST Jr, Leo-Summers L, and others: Multicomponent targeted intervention to prevent delirium in hospitalized elderly patients: what is the economic value? *Med Care* 39(7):740-752, 2001.
22. Milisen K, Foreman MD, Abraham IL, and others: A nurse-led interdisciplinary intervention program for delirium in elderly hip-fracture patients, *J Am Geriatr Soc* 49:5, 2001.
23. Inouye S: Prevention of delirium in hospitalized older patients: risk factors and targeted intervention strategies, *Ann Med* 32:257-263, 2000.
24. Levkoff S, Besdine R, Wetle T: Acute confusional states in the hospitalized elderly, *Ann Rev Gerontol Geriatr* 6:1-26, 1986.
25. Rahkonen T, Makela H, Paanila S, and others: Delirium in elderly people without severe predisposing disorders: etiology and 1-year prognosis after discharge, *Int Psychogeriatr* 12(4):473-481, 2000.
26. Murray A, Levkoff SE, Wetle TT, and others: Acute delirium and functional decline in the hospitalized elderly patient, *J Gerontol* 48:M181-M186, 1993.
27. Curyto K, Johnson J, TenHave T, and others: Survival of hospitalized elderly patients with delirium: a prospective study, *Am J Geriatr Psychiatry* 9:141-147, 2001.

CHAPTER 205

Dementia

Karen Dick

DEFINITION AND EPIDEMIOLOGY

Most people enjoy a fruitful and productive period during their later years. However, for 5% to 10% of the population over age 65, and 45% to 50% of the population over age 85, these years are associated with a serious form of cognitive impairment known as dementia. It is estimated that at least 4.5 million people in the United States—regardless of race, gender, or socioeconomic status—are afflicted with the most common type of dementia, Alzheimer's. The Alzheimer's Association estimates that between 11.3 and 16 million Americans will have dementia of the Alzheimer's type by 2050 unless a cure is found.[1] Dementia is often the reason for institutionalization; the prevalence in nursing home residents is estimated to be between 60% and 80%.[2] It has long been a common belief that memory loss is an inevitable and incurable part of the aging process, making any clinical evaluation useless. However, with the recent advances in research, as evidenced by numerous clinical trials and new drug therapies, early detection, treatment, education, and support for families are even more critical.

The fourth edition of the *Diagnostic and Statistical Manual of Mental Disorders* (DSM-IV-TR) defines dementia as the development of multiple cognitive deficits (including memory impairment) as a result of the direct physiologic effects of a general medical condition, the persisting effects of a substance, or multiple etiologies (e.g., the combined effects of cerebrovascular disease and Alzheimer's disease) (Boxes 205-1 to 205-3).[3] The two most common types of dementia, Alzheimer's disease and vascular dementia, account for about 80% to 90% of all dementias in older adults.[4] Other less common dementias include frontotemporal, Lewy body, Creutzfeldt-Jakob disease, and Parkinson's.

PATHOPHYSIOLOGY

Alzheimer's disease is characterized by amyloid plaques and neurofibrillary tangles. Examinations of the brains of patients with Alzheimer's disease show atrophy of the cerebral cortex that is usually diffuse but may be more pronounced in the frontal, temporal, and parietal lobes.[5] The degree of atrophy may not correlate with the degree of cognitive impairment. The amyloid hypothesis presumes a central role to abnormal amyloid processing, and remains the most widely embraced causative theory.[1] Biochemically, there is disruption to the cortical pathways involved in catecholaminergic, seritonergic, and cholinergic transmission. There is a reduction of choline acetyltransferase, an enzyme found only in cholinergic neurons. Advances in genetic research have included the identification of apolipoprotein E (*ApoE*), a protein involved in cholesterol transport linked to Alzheimer's disease, and the identification of the β-amyloid gene on chromosome 21. Researchers continue to explore the role of inflammation and

BOX 205-1

DIAGNOSTIC CRITERIA FOR DEMENTIA OF THE ALZHEIMER'S TYPE

A. The development of multiple cognitive deficits manifested by both
   (1) memory impairment (impaired ability to learn new information or to recall previously learned information)
   (2) one (or more) of the following cognitive disturbances:
      (a) aphasia (language disturbance)
      (b) apraxia (impaired ability to carry out motor activities despite intact motor function)
      (c) agnosia (failure to recognize or identify objects despite intact sensory function)
      (d) disturbance in executive functioning (i.e., planning, organizing, sequencing, abstracting)

B. The cognitive deficits in Criteria A1 and A2 each cause significant impairment in social or occupational functioning and represent a significant decline from a previous level of functioning.

C. The course is characterized by gradual onset and continuing cognitive decline.

D. The cognitive deficits in Criteria A1 and A2 are not due to any of the following:
   (1) other central nervous system conditions that cause progressive deficits in memory and cognition (e.g., cerebrovascular disease, Parkinson's disease, Huntington's disease, subdural hematoma, normal-pressure hydrocephalus, brain tumor)
   (2) systemic conditions that are known to cause dementia (e.g., hypothyroidism, vitamin B_{12} or folic acid deficiency, niacin deficiency, hypercalcemia, neurosyphilis, HIV infection)
   (3) substance-induced conditions

E. The deficits do not occur exclusively during the course of a delirium.

F. The disturbance is not better accounted for by another Axis I disorder (e.g., Major Depressive Disorder, Schizophrenia).

From American Psychiatric Association: *Diagnostic and statistical manual of mental disorders,* ed 4, text rev, Washington, DC, 2000, The Association.

BOX 205-2

DIAGNOSTIC CRITERIA FOR VASCULAR DEMENTIA

A. The development of multiple cognitive deficits manifested by both
   (1) memory impairment (impaired ability to learn new information or to recall previously learned information)
   (2) one (or more) of the following cognitive disturbances:
      (a) aphasia (language disturbance)
      (b) apraxia (impaired ability to carry out motor activities despite intact motor function)
      (c) agnosia (failure to recognize or identify objects despite intact sensory function)
      (d) disturbance in executive functioning (i.e., planning, organizing, sequencing, abstracting)

B. The cognitive deficits in Criteria A1 and A2 each cause significant impairment in social or occupational functioning and represent a significant decline from a previous level of functioning.

C. Focal neurologic signs and symptoms (e.g., exaggeration of deep tendon reflexes, extensor plantar response, pseudobulbar palsy, gait abnormalities, weakness of an extremity) or laboratory evidence indicative of cerebrovascular disease (e.g., multiple infarctions involving cortex and underlying white matter) that are judged to be etiologically related to the disturbance.

D. The deficits do not occur exclusively during the course of a delirium.

From American Psychiatric Association: *Diagnostic and statistical manual of mental disorders,* ed 4, text rev, Washington, DC, 2000, The Association.

BOX 205-3

DIAGNOSTIC CRITERIA FOR DEMENTIA DUE TO MULTIPLE ETIOLOGIES

A. The development of multiple cognitive deficits manifested by both
   (1) memory impairment (impaired ability to learn new information or to recall previously learned information)
   (2) one (or more) of the following cognitive disturbances:
      (a) aphasia (language disturbance)
      (b) apraxia (impaired ability to carry out motor activities despite intact motor function)
      (c) agnosia (failure to recognize or identify objects despite intact sensory function)
      (d) disturbance in executive functioning (i.e., planning, organizing, sequencing, abstracting)

B. The cognitive deficits in Criteria A1 and A2 each cause significant impairment in social or occupational functioning and represent a significant decline from a previous level of functioning.

C. There is evidence from the history, physical examination, or laboratory findings that the disturbance has more than one etiology (e.g., head trauma plus chronic alcohol use, Dementia of the Alzheimer's type with the subsequent development of Vascular Dementia).

D. The deficits do not occur exclusively during the course of a delirium.

From American Psychiatric Association: *Diagnostic and statistical manual of mental disorders,* ed 4, text rev, Washington, DC, 2000, The Association.

oxidative stress and their effects on neuronal health. Clinical trials are under way investigating the effects of antiamyloid therapies, vitamin E, and nonsteroidal agents on the development of Alzheimer's disease.[2]

Multiple areas of focal ischemic change characterize vascular dementia, formerly known as multiinfarct dementia. The defining lesion is the lacunar infarct. Lacunae are defined as gaps, missing areas, or holes.[6] The infarctions occur in tiny arteries deep in the brain. Patients with hypertension, diabetes, hyperlipidemia, or peripheral vascular occlusive disease are at particular risk.[2]

CLINICAL PRESENTATION

Memory loss, personality changes, language disturbances, and problems with independent activities of daily living (ADLs) are common presenting symptoms of dementia. A concerned family member or friend typically makes the initial presentation to a health care provider. It may take months to years for family members to seek medical attention, since subtle changes in cognition may be overlooked or attributed to old age. Patients with dementia do not typically worry about what is wrong with them. These patients often have little understanding of the seriousness of their symptoms or of safety concerns (e.g., driving, cooking). On the other hand, patients with depression or benign forgetfulness often appear to the health care provider to be overly concerned about minor symptoms (e.g., forgetting a name, misplacing keys). An anecdotal finding in primary care is that those patients worried about memory problems often have only minor problems, whereas the patients who seem unconcerned pose a major worry to providers.

Mild cognitive impairment (MCI) is thought to be a transitional state between normal aging and Alzheimer's disease.

Patients primarily have memory impairment *without* significant deficits in other cognitive domains, have intact ADLs, and do not meet the criteria for dementia. Since it is believed that these patients may progress to Alzheimer's dementia at a rate of 10% to 15% a year, MCI is considered a risk factor for Alzheimer's disease, and these patients need close follow-up monitoring.[7]

Alzheimer's disease is commonly divided into three stages: early, middle, and late (Box 205-4). The initial symptom is typically short-term memory loss. The earliest stage is often accompanied by symptoms of anxiety and depression. Word finding and naming problems may emerge as symptoms progress. The second stage is characterized by a worsening of memory and language as well as judgment. Disorientation to time and place is common. There may be neuropsychiatric symptoms, including paranoia, hallucinations, and delusional thinking. Urinary incontinence may be a problem. The final stage is characterized by motor rigidity; prominent neurologic abnormalities, including apraxia and agnosia; severe cognitive and language impairment; and death. The average duration of the disease from diagnosis until death is 9 years.[5] Staging a patient's disease based on clinical presentation and examination can be helpful to patients and families in planning subsequent care and treatment.

PHYSICAL EXAMINATION

The basic components of an evaluation for dementia include a careful and detailed history from family members or caregivers and a complete physical examination. A thorough review of all medications, including any over-the-counter medications (sleeping medications, anticholinergic cold remedies, and laxatives), should also be addressed. The use of alcohol or other substances should be documented. The physical examination should focus on neurologic signs; blood pressure; carotid bruits; and the assessment of cognition, mood, and function. Many screening tools are available. The Katz Index of Activities of Daily Living, or the get up and go test, can be used to evaluate function.[8,9] The Folstein Mini-Mental State Examination (MMSE) and the Mini-Cog are useful tools for evaluating cognition.[10,11] The Mini-Cog combines the clock drawing test with three-item recall, and performance in diverse populations is comparable to that found with the MMSE.[11] The Geriatric Depression Scale (short form) has been shown to be both valid and reliable in clinical practice.[12] One of the benefits of these tools is the ability to compare scores year to year to provide families with an objective description of disease progression.

BOX 205-4

STAGES OF ALZHEIMER'S DISEASE

EARLY-STAGE DEMENTIA

- Memory loss
- Time and spatial disorientation
- Poor judgment
- Personality changes
- Withdrawal or depression
- Perceptual disturbances

MIDSTAGE DEMENTIA

- Recent and remote memory worsens
- Increased aphasia (slowed speech and understanding)
- Apraxia
- Hyperorality
- Disorientation to place and time
- Restlessness or pacing
- Perseveration
- Irritability
- Loss of impulse control

LATE-STAGE DEMENTIA

- Incontinence of urine and feces
- Loss of motor skills, rigidity
- Decreased appetite and dysphagia
- Agnosia
- Apraxia
- Severely impaired communication
- Possible inability to recognize family members or self in mirror
- Loss of most or all self-care abilities
- Severely impaired cognition
- Depressed immune system

DIAGNOSTICS

Because dementia has no single standard test and Alzheimer's is a disease of exclusion, the diagnostic evaluation should determine whether the patient has a reversible condition that may be contributing to or causing cognitive decline. The most important tests include a CBC, thyroid-stimulating hormone, vitamin B_{12}, folate, rapid plasma reagin, and a metabolic screen. Medications that have measurable levels, such as digoxin, carbamazepine (Tegretol), theophylline, or divalproex sodium (Depakote), should be measured.

Imaging studies are useful in identifying mass lesions, vascular lesions, or infections but do not confirm a diagnosis of Alzheimer's disease. Despite a lack of agreement as to the role of imaging in the workup of dementia, most geriatric specialists recommend a baseline brain imaging study (a noncontrast CT scan is adequate). Referral for neuropsychologic testing can also be useful for differentiating between MCI and dementia, and dementia and depression.

DIFFERENTIAL DIAGNOSIS

Dementia has innumerable causes, which cannot always be determined by diagnostic evaluation. Some dementia syndromes (e.g., Pick's disease, Alzheimer's disease) are characterized by a lack of neurologic signs, whereas others

DIAGNOSTICS

Dementia

LABORATORY

CBC
LFTs
TSH
Vitamin B_{12}
Folate
Rapid plasma reagin
Serum electrolytes
BUN
Creatinine
Serum glucose
Drug and alcohol levels*

IMAGING

CT scan, MRI

*If indicated.

DIFFERENTIAL DIAGNOSIS

Dementia

Alcoholic dementia	Trauma, subdural hematoma, hydrocephalus
Medication, organic toxin, heavy metal intoxication	Depression
Medical illness	Vasculitis
• Liver disease	Alzheimer's dementia
• Hypothyroidism	Vascular dementia
• Chronic hypoglycemia	Pick's disease
• Adrenal insufficiency	Diffuse Lewy body dementia
• Cushing's disease	Huntington's disease
Vitamin deficiency	Creutzfeldt-Jakob disease
• Thiamine	Shy-Drager syndrome
• Vitamin B_{12}	Progressive supranuclear palsy
• Folic acid	Parkinson's disease and other movement disorders
Neoplasm	

are associated with a definitive neurologic disease such as Huntington's disease, diffuse Lewy body disease, or HIV. Delirium and depression are treatable conditions that may manifest with the same symptoms as dementia; however, errors on the MMSE will differ. Patients with dementia have a normal level of consciousness without inattention. Patients with depression often answer questions with "I don't know," whereas those with dementia may confabulate an answer.

Medical illnesses, drug overdoses, adverse effects of medication (especially anticholinergics or anxiolytics), sensory impairments, and nutritional deficits are all part of the differential diagnosis.

MANAGEMENT

Management of dementia depends on the stage of the disease. The family and community supports required are often the same for vascular dementia and Alzheimer's disease. The goal of management includes treatment of all correctable factors that may impair cognition in order to improve daily functioning and delay disability. Activities that promote physical and mental exercise should be encouraged.

It is important to address safety concerns, including driving competency, soon after the diagnosis is made. Laws regarding mandatory reporting of unsafe drivers vary from state to state and can be confirmed by calling the state department of motor vehicles. A kitchen safety evaluation alerts caregivers to possible problems with cooking. A health care proxy and durable power of attorney for health care can help prevent conflicts later in the course of the disease. A discussion of the patient's preference for resuscitation and technology should take place while the patient is still able. Encouraging families to contact the local chapter of the Alzheimer's Association is an important step; through this association caregivers can gain support, obtain reading material to promote understanding of the disease and behavior management, and determine the availability of respite care. Many websites and online support groups can help family members access and share information.

Because management may differ, determining which form of dementia is present is important. In addition, behavior management needs to be individualized. Certain behavioral problems are amenable to medication or to family education regarding the avoidance and management of difficult situations.

Two classes of drugs are currently approved by the U.S. Food and Drug Administration to treat the cognitive symptoms of dementia: the cholinesterase inhibitors and NMDA (*N*-methyl-D-aspartate) receptor antagonists. The cholinesterase inhibitors include donepezil (Aricept), rivastigmine (Exelon), and galantamine (Razadyne). These drugs can be used for the treatment of mild to moderate dementia. Memantine (Namenda) is an NMDA receptor antagonist that can be used in combination with a cholinesterase inhibitor for those with moderate to severe disease. Although these medications do not alter the progression of dementia, they can delay or slow worsening of symptoms.[1] For patients with vascular dementia, optimized treatment of risk factors (e.g., hypertension, hyperglycemia, smoking, hyperlipidemia, diet) may delay further progression.

In general, depressive symptoms are treated with antidepressants even if the patient does not meet the criteria for major depression.[13]

COMPLICATIONS

Dementia has many complications that vary with the stages of illness. In the early stages, getting lost or having a motor vehicle accident puts patients (and others) at risk. In the middle stage, falls, incontinence, and sleep disturbances may cause further problems. Contractures, pressure ulcers, urinary tract infections, and pneumonia, all a result of immobility, are common in late and final stages of the disease. Deconditioning and nutritional deficits are also commonly seen. Patients may develop apraxia and forget how to chew and swallow. Weight loss becomes inevitable. An inability to communicate as a result of aphasia and an inability to tell caretakers about symptoms lead to further frustration and difficulty in diagnosing complications. Death is often the result of infectious complications.

INDICATIONS FOR REFERRAL OR HOSPITALIZATION

Many patients with dementia are frail, older adults with multiple medical, nursing, and social service needs. Involvement of other disciplines is helpful for patients, families, and providers. Physical therapists can optimize function by evaluating and recommending exercises or the appropriate adaptive equipment. Driving evaluations and kitchen and home safety evaluations can be performed by occupational therapists. These therapists can also recommend equipment to help with feeding. Speech therapy is necessary for swallowing or dysphagia assessments in the later stages of dementia. A neurology consultation is often helpful for patients with an unclear clinical picture. A neuropsychologist or geropsychiatrist may be able to differentiate unusual presentations of dementia, especially if depression is present.

Patients with end-stage dementia are eligible for referral to hospice under the Medicare Hospice benefit but must meet criteria related to bed-bound status and stage of disease. These hospice services can be provided in the home or in long-term care facilities.

PATIENT AND FAMILY EDUCATION

The focus of patient education is to maintain independence by emphasizing patients' strengths and allowing them to continue normal activities. A woman who is no longer able to follow a recipe may still be able to knead dough and make a loaf of her special bread with help. A grandmother unable to be left alone with her grandchild is still able to rock an infant to sleep and sing a lullaby she once heard as a child. A carpenter may no longer be able to operate electrical shop tools but may still be able to hammer and glue pieces of furniture that have been precut. Feeling robbed of self-esteem is a major detriment to function; education for families is essential. Behavioral guidance, social supports, and recognition of the difficult caregiver role will benefit both patient and caregiver and may prevent illness or injury.

Families need guidance and suggestions regarding the appropriate settings and activities for their loved ones. The decision about nursing home placement is always difficult and usually comes after community services and family support have been maximized. An acute illness or injury often precedes nursing home placement. Adult day care and group homes are appropriate in the early to middle stages of the disease; special care units are used during the middle stages of dementia. These units represent a wide variation in the philosophies, goals, and design. Although many families are reluctant to enroll their relative in a program or living arrangement specifically for people with dementia, the focus of activities is at an appropriate level so that patients can participate and enjoy. The frustration of not being able to participate in activities that are too difficult is minimized. Staff members are specifically trained to handle behavioral problems in nonpharmacologic ways. Persons with late-stage dementia who are unable to participate in activities are often cared for on the general units of a nursing home.

Families also need to be able to recognize the symptoms of medical illness in a person with dementia; families should understand patients' increased susceptibility to delirium. Pneumonia without a fever or cough, a myocardial infarction without chest pain, and a urinary tract infection with no urinary symptoms are typical. A change in behavior that is noticeable only to those who know the patient well may be the only sign of illness. Families need to be given resource information about support groups, financial and legal matters, and how to tell family and friends about the diagnosis.

If caregivers are unfamiliar with resources, the Alzheimer's Disease Education and Referral Center ([800] 438-4380; http://www.nia.nih.gov/Alzheimers) provides information. The Alzheimer's Association (http://www.alz.org) has state and local chapters and maintains a 24-hour help line at (800) 272-3900. Providers can find guidelines for the evaluation of dementia developed by the American Academy of Neurology, the American Psychiatric Society, and the U.S. Preventive Services Task Force at http://www.guidelines.gov.

REFERENCES

1. Alzheimer's Association: *Alzheimer's disease: causes and risk factors,* retrieved May 29, 2006, from http://www.alz.org/alzheimers_disease_causes_risk_factors.asp.
2. Beers M, Berkow R, editors: *The Merck manual of geriatrics,* ed 3, Whitehouse Station, NJ, 2000, Merck.
3. American Psychiatric Association: *Diagnostic and statistical manual of mental disorders,* ed 4, text rev, Washington, DC, 2000, The Association.
4. Plassman B, Breitner J: The genetics of dementia in late life, *Psychol Clin North Am* 20:59-75, 1997.
5. Kovach C: *Late-state dementia care: a basic guide,* Milwaukee, 1997, Taylor & Francis.
6. Venes D, Thomas C, editors: *Taber's cyclopedic medical dictionary,* ed 19, Philadelphia, 2001, Davis.
7. Grundman M, Petersen RC, Ferris SH, and others: Mild cognitive impairment can be distinguished from Alzheimer disease and normal aging for clinical trials, *Arch Neurol* 6:59-66, 2004.
8. Katz S, Ford AB, Moskowitz RW, and others: Studies of illness in the aged: the index of ADL, *JAMA* 185:914-919, 1963.
9. Mathias S, Nayak US, Issacs B: Balance in elderly patients: the "get up and go" test, *Arch Phys Med Rehabil* 67:387-389, 1986.
10. Folstein M, Folstein S, McHugh P: Mini-mental state: a practical method for grading cognitive state of patients for the clinician, *J Psychiatr Res* 12:189-198, 1975.
11. Scanlan J, Borson S: The mini-cog: receiver operating characteristics with expert and naïve raters, *Int J Geriatr Psychiatry* 16:216-222, 2001.
12. Yesavage J, Brink TL, Rose TL, and others: Development and validation of a geriatric depression screening scale: a preliminary report, *J Psychiatr Res* 17(1):37-49, 1982.
13. Katz I: Diagnosis and treatment of depression in patients with Alzheimer's disease and other dementias, *J Clin Psychiatry* 59(Suppl 9):38-44, 1998.

CHAPTER 206

Dizziness and Vertigo

Nancy McQueen Le

DIZZINESS

DEFINITION AND EPIDEMIOLOGY

Dizziness is a common, nonspecific term used to describe a variety of subjective states with varied etiologies. Clinically it is helpful to classify dizziness into the categories of vertigo, disequilibrium, and presyncope or syncope. Differentiation of the type of dizziness experienced will dictate the direction of evaluation and treatment.

Vertigo is the illusion of movement of either one's self or the environment—spinning, tilting, or moving back and forth. Disequilibrium is a sense of insecurity or imbalance, an unsteadiness in walking. Although this feeling is often described as dizziness, it often occurs in the absence of abnormal head sensations.

Vertigo can be related to a peripheral or central disorder. Peripheral causes may include benign paroxysmal positional vertigo, vestibular neuronitis, acute labyrinthitis, Meniere's disease, ototoxicity, or head trauma. Central disorders include brainstem ischemia, tumors, multiple sclerosis, or a migrainous syndrome. A sense of wooziness or impending faint is often referred to as presyncopal lightheadedness. However, lightheadedness is not exclusive to a presyncopal episode and can be a feeling manifested in some states of disequilibrium or vertiginous conditions. Cardiac conditions associated with lightheadedness or syncope include arrhythmias, sick sinus syndrome, mitral valve prolapse, aortic stenosis, and heart block. Dehydration, hypotension, and cough or Valsalva-related syncope are common causes of vascular-related syncope or presyncope.

It has been noted that less than half of patients complaining of dizziness actually have vertigo.[1] Hain stated that, even after evaluation, the largest diagnostic group is represented by dizziness of uncertain cause.[2]

PATHOPHYSIOLOGY

Vertigo is caused by an imbalance in the vestibular system that may result from lesions in the inner ear, vestibular nerve, brainstem, or cerebellum. Less commonly, vertigo may result from lesions in the subjective sensory pathways of the thalamus or cortex, or stretch receptors in the neck.[1] Disequilibrium may result from visual impairment, bilateral or unilateral vestibular loss, proprioceptive loss, impaired cerebellar function, or involvement of motor (frontal and basal ganglia) centers. Multisensory disequilibrium describes a syndrome of impaired balance caused by some degree of combined dysfunction in the areas of vestibular, visual, and proprioceptive sensation.[3] Lightheadedness or presyncope/syncope is most commonly a result of a cardiovascular problem. Causes include orthostatic hypotension, vasovagal episodes, hyperventilation, and decreased cardiac output. Less common causes of lightheadedness include hypoglycemia and seizure activity. It is rarely a manifestation of impending stroke.

CLINICAL PRESENTATION

Dizziness is an intensely subjective sensation that may be difficult to describe. However, a thorough history will often differentiate the type of dizziness being experienced. It is helpful to start by eliciting a description of the dizziness in the patient's own words, making note of how precise or vague the details are. This description can be further guided through specific questioning and the suggestion of some varied descriptors, especially if the individual is having difficulty articulating his or her sensory experience. Further history is then directed toward defining the characteristics of the dizziness, the time course of individual episodes, the pattern of recurrences, precipitating and relieving factors, and any associated symptoms. A general medical history must be included, with special focus on neurologic and cardiovascular systems, medication history, and functional history.[1,3,4]

True vertigo is such a striking phenomenon that it is usually readily and precisely described as a clear sensation of spinning, tilting, rotating, or swaying. Associated symptoms can include nausea, vomiting, diaphoresis, disequilibrium, nystagmus, or blurry vision. Ear symptoms, including pain or pressure, tinnitus, or altered hearing, may be present. Disequilibrium is described as a sense of imbalance or insecurity on arising or when walking. Patients often say they are dizzy when they are not in fact vertiginous or presyncopal, but rather "off-kilter." They may have begun using a cane or "furniture walking" for unclear reasons. The sense of imbalance may be worse in the dark or may be accompanied by changes in gait characterized by a shortened step length and widened base of support.[3,4] Lightheadedness is classically described as a sense of wooziness or impending faint. It is often accompanied by diaphoresis, apprehension, nausea, and, in the extreme, an actual transient "blackout" with diminished vision but with persisting vague awareness of one's surroundings.

When the description elicited is vague or ill defined, it may reflect multifactorial issues. A specific sensory experience in multisensory disequilibrium may be difficult to describe. Dizziness can also be related to psychogenic causes, such as anxiety states or agoraphobia. However, anxiety and apprehension often accompany dizziness, and these complaints should not be automatically attributed to a psychogenic etiology.

PHYSICAL EXAMINATION

The physical examination in any complaint of dizziness should always include a general medical review. This information will guide a more focused examination.

The neurologic examination should include a cognitive screen. Cranial nerves are assessed with particular emphasis on visual acuity, eye movements, and nystagmus. Motor examination should include evaluation of power, muscle tone, coordination, and deep tendon reflexes. Sensory examination emphasizes basic vision and hearing assessments, as well as testing of primary sensory modalities. Gait and balance evaluation includes observation of stride; arm swing; tandem gait with eyes opened, then closed; and Romberg's sign. A more detailed otologic evaluation includes pneumatic otoscopic examination and hearing assessment with Weber's test and Rinne's test.

Cardiovascular evaluation includes cardiac rate and rhythm, auscultation of heart sounds, carotid bruits, and blood pressure measurement. Orthostatic vital signs, both blood pressure and heart rate, should also be determined.

A neuro-otologic examination refers to a number of special examination procedures considered when problems related to vertigo or disequilibrium are suspected. These procedures specifically assess the vestibulo-ocular and vestibulospinal systems and help distinguish between peripheral disorders and central disorders. They include evaluation for nystagmus using Frenzel's glasses (special gogglelike glasses that remove visual fixation and magnify the eyes), position testing (Hallpike-Dix maneuver) (Box 206-1), head-fixed/body-turn maneuvers, postural sway on a foam surface, and the stepping test (marching in place with the eyes closed).[3]

DIAGNOSTICS

If a vestibular lesion is suspected, the history and examination may be augmented by vestibular laboratory testing, an audiogram, or neuroimaging. Vestibular laboratory testing can help differentiate peripheral from central lesions, confirm lateralization of a documented abnormality, and allow serial evaluation for monitoring purposes.[1,3] Further, it can give valuable functional information and help guide physical therapy interventions. Vestibular laboratory studies include electronystagmography (ENG), rotational testing, and posturography.

Audiology evaluation, including Weber's test and Rinne's test, may have an important adjunctive role in helping establish or confirm a suspected diagnosis. Many disorders resulting in vertigo have associated hearing involvement. The presence or absence of specific hearing findings can help confirm or exclude some conditions. Hearing loss is defined as conductive or sensorineural, based on the etiology.

Neuroimaging may be considered when central (brain) or structural (bony labyrinthine, internal auditory canal) lesions are amenable to visualization. Either a CT scan or MRI is appropriate, depending on what is suspected. Magnetic resonance angiography is used when vertebrobasilar insufficiency is a concern.

BOX 206-1

POSITIONAL NYSTAGMUS TESTING (HALLPIKE-DIX MANEUVER)

1. First check the patient for spontaneous nystagmus while he or she is seated on the examining table.
2. Next, bring the patient quickly back to the recumbent or supine position with the head extended back 30 to 45 degrees over the end of the bed or table, and the head tilted 30 to 45 degrees to one side (i.e., one ear down toward the floor).
3. Repeat the above step two times, once with the head tilted to the left, then again with the head tilted to the right.
4. Observe the patient for latency, duration, direction, and fatigability of nystagmus, both while positioned down and as helped to upright position.

DIAGNOSTICS

Dizziness and Vertigo

VESTIBULAR DISORDERS
Audiogram
CT scan, MRI, magnetic resonance angiography (with gadolinium)*
Vestibular laboratory testing*
Electronystagmography
Posturography

CARDIAC DISORDERS
ECG
Holter or event monitor

LABORATORY
Basic metabolic screen
Electrolytes
CBC and differential
BUN, creatinine
Serum glucose
TSH
Vitamin B_{12}
Fluorescent treponemal antibody absorption test

*If indicated.

When multisystem disequilibrium is suspected or must be excluded, formal ophthalmologic evaluation is necessary. Assessment of peripheral nerve function via electromyography and nerve conduction velocity in these instances can be definitive.

If cardiac issues are suspected, evaluation routinely begins with an ECG. Holter monitoring or telemetry may also be indicated if an arrhythmia is suspected. Serial orthostatic vital signs in conjunction with these studies can provide important data. An echocardiogram may be indicated to further evaluate cardiac status.

An electroencephalogram may be considered if seizure activity should be excluded. Vertigo, disequilibrium, and lightheadedness are not common manifestations of seizures, and thus such testing is commonly under the guidance of a neurologist.

The choice of laboratory diagnostic studies should be guided by presentation and examination. A basic metabolic review usually includes thyroid-stimulating hormone, CBC, electrolytes, serum glucose, BUN, creatinine, vitamin B_{12}, and fluorescent treponemal antibody absorption, as indicated.

DIFFERENTIAL DIAGNOSIS

Clarifying the diagnosis of dizziness begins with differentiating vertigo, disequilibrium, and lightheadedness. Vertigo is a phenomenon resulting from a vast array of causes. Anatomically and neurologically it is helpful to start by determining whether the vertigo is caused by a peripheral or central lesion. Peripheral problems refer to problems of the inner ear or cranial nerve VIII. Peripheral lesions include vestibular neuronitis, labyrinthitis, benign positional vertigo, Meniere's disease, posttraumatic vertigo, acoustic neuroma, and ototoxic drug-induced conditions.[5] The general hallmarks of these conditions include a higher likelihood of associated nausea, a negative neurologic examination, and symptoms that are position related. Central or brain disorders usually involve the brainstem or cerebellum and include vertebrobasilar insufficiency or infarction, multiple sclerosis, posterior fossa tumor, basilar migraine, or central nervous system infection (syphilis).[5] Hallmarks of a central cause include associated neurologic findings and vertigo and nausea that are not position related.

Disequilibrium is sometimes clear from the history. In many cases the descriptions elicited are imprecise or vague yet seem to suggest balance problems rather than actual dizziness. When a description of a balance impairment in the absence of

DIFFERENTIAL DIAGNOSIS

Dizziness and Vertigo

VESTIBULAR DISORDERS
Peripheral
Benign paroxysmal positional vertigo
Vestibular neuronitis
Bacterial labyrinthitis
Meniere's disease
Nerve damage
- Ototoxic drugs
- Head trauma

Acoustic neuroma
Perilymphatic fistula
Physiologic
- Motion sickness
- Height vertigo

Central
Vertebrobasilar insufficiency
- Transitory ischemic attack, cerebrovascular accident

Multiple sclerosis
Tumor in posterior fossa
- Cerebellar pontine angle
- Brainstem
- Cerebellar

Migraine syndrome
CNS infection
Cervical dizziness
- Drop attacks

SYNCOPE
Cardiac arrhythmias
Critical aortic stenosis
Medication effects
Systemic illness
- Infection
- Vasculitis
- Endocrine (in diabetes)

Volume depletion
Valsalva-related syncope
Hypotension
Hypoxia
Severe anemia
Hyperventilation
Hypoglycemia
Psychogenic (anxiety, depression)

DISEQUILIBRIUM (WITHOUT VERTIGO)
Bilateral vestibular loss
Sensory ataxias
- Vitamin B_{12} deficiency
- Tabes dorsalis
- Peripheral neuropathy
- Myelopathy
- Multisystem disequilibrium

Cerebellar degeneration syndromes
Apractic syndromes (frontal lobe syndromes, hydrocephalus, multiinfarct state)
Extrapyramidal syndromes (Parkinson's, progressive supranuclear palsy)

dizziness is clear, the focus turns to evaluation of multisystem impairment, particularly vision and peripheral sensory function. Disequilibrium should be distinguished from complaints that may be based on visual problems or related to psychogenic conditions. Diabetes mellitus is a common cause of a multisystem disequilibrium state. However, a number of other conditions should be considered, including cerebellar disorders, extrapyramidal system disorders, drug toxicity, and posterior fossa tumors.[5]

Lightheadedness is most commonly related to cardiovascular issues. Diagnostic evaluation should exclude cardiac arrhythmias, critical aortic stenosis, vasovagal response, and orthostatic hypotension (autonomic insufficiency, volume depletion with anemia, drug-induced condition). When a psychogenic cause is suspected, it must be considered only in the context of excluding atypical manifestations of other causes. Possible causes to be considered in the evaluation process include anxiety reactions, agoraphobia, hyperventilation, and depression.

MANAGEMENT

Many vestibular disorders are amenable to vestibular rehabilitation and other physical therapy interventions, with a generally limited or symptomatic role for pharmacologic agents. Some conditions respond particularly well to vestibular rehabilitation, and most patients derive some benefit.[3] Treatments are aimed at facilitating vestibular compensation through a specific program of movements and exercises. The goal is to improve functional balance limitations, decrease dizziness, increase activity level, and improve general functional abilities.[3,6-8]

Medications used in treating vestibular disorders target vertigo and the associated nausea, vomiting, and anxiety.[2,7] Indications for use of these medications are dictated by the specific diagnosis. The commonly accepted vestibular suppressants are from the classes of anticholinergics (scopolamine), antihistamines (meclizine, dimenhydrinate [Dramamine], both with anticholinergic effects as well), and benzodiazepines (lorazepam [Ativan], clonazepam [Klonopin], diazepam [Valium]).[2,7]

Antiemetic medications used for the nausea associated with vestibular lesions are phenothiazines (promethazine [Phenergan], prochlorperazine [Compazine]) and antihistamines with anticholinergic properties (meclizine). Meclizine is often the drug of choice because of the vestibular suppressant and antiemetic effects, as well as the low side effect profile.[2,7]

COMPLICATIONS

The risk of falling is greatly increased in the patient with dizziness. This is especially problematic in older patients, in whom the risk of fracture is the highest. Intractable nausea or vomiting associated with dizziness, although rare, can be disabling. Side effects with medications, especially anticholinergics or antihistamines, can include drowsiness, urinary retention, and confusion (especially in older patients). Benzodiazepines should be used cautiously because of the side effect profile and the potential for dependence. Other complications are related to the specific cause of the dizziness and may include visual disturbances, tinnitus, decreased hearing, and balance and gait disorders.

INDICATIONS FOR REFERRAL OR HOSPITALIZATION

Identification of any positive neurologic signs or symptoms or the suspicion of an underlying cardiac disorder warrants prompt referral. Depending on the findings or suspicions, immediate hospitalization or emergency department evaluation by a neurologist or cardiologist may be necessary. Acute labyrinthitis accompanied by a fever always requires urgent referral and treatment.[5] When a diagnosis remains uncertain or the response to standard treatments is suboptimum, further specialty evaluation should be pursued. If these cases involve vertigo or disequilibrium, referral to an otoneurologist or otolaryngologist is indicated for further testing, such as vestibular laboratory evaluation, or recommendations for alternate physical therapy or medication regimens. In most cases of vestibular dysfunction or disequilibrium, referral to physical therapy is recommended for a general functional evaluation or for vestibular rehabilitation. When a change is noted in a previously stable cardiac condition, prompt referral is indicated.

PATIENT AND FAMILY EDUCATION

Patient education should always include information about the diagnostic evaluation and, once a diagnosis is determined, specific information regarding the prognosis, treatment options, and complications. If an exercise program for vestibular compensation is initiated, patients should be told they may initially feel worse, but as they continue the program, symptoms subside. Specific aspects of their program should be reinforced. Other teaching emphasizes how medications can be used to relieve symptoms and the potential side effects of these agents.

The Vestibular Disorders Association is a national organization dedicated to providing information and support to people with dizziness and balance disorders. Patients can be encouraged to contact them at (503) 229-7705 or online at http://www.vestibular.org/find-medical-help.php.

BENIGN PAROXYSMAL POSITIONAL VERTIGO

DEFINITION AND EPIDEMIOLOGY

Benign paroxysmal positional vertigo (BPPV) is a syndrome that may be a manifestation of several varied inner ear conditions. In more than half the cases no certain cause is determined. When a cause can be identified, the two most common are head trauma or a prior viral inner ear infection.[9] However, in the elderly it is estimated that 50% of dizziness is related to BPPV. It is characterized by a sensation of spinning, whirling, or tilting with movement or position change. It is estimated that about half of patients with BPPV will have at least one recurrent episode after a remission, and recurrence can be after a period of years.

PATHOPHYSIOLOGY

Otoconia refers to debris in the inner ear made up of small crystals of calcium carbonate. With certain position changes these crystals shift and disperse within the semicircular canal, sending false signals to the brain.

CLINICAL PRESENTATION

Symptoms of BPPV are precipitated by a change in head position. The most characteristic description is vertigo, which may be spinning or whirling of one's self or the environment. Common movements that precipitate this vertigo are rolling over in bed, arising or turning abruptly, or first lying back on the bed. The symptoms are generally intermittent.

The nystagmus associated with BPPV is characteristic, and any deviation from the typical profiles should raise suspicion of a central lesion. The nystagmus is observed using the Hallpike-Dix maneuver (see Box 206-1). If it is vertical or torsional in nature and lasts less than 30 seconds, it is consistent with a posterior semicircular canal variant. If the nystagmus is direction changing and horizontal (beating toward the ground) and lasts about 1 minute, it is consistent with a horizontal canal variant. Both types should show fatiguing with repeated positioning.

Vertigo that is spontaneous (not position related) and the presence of focal neurologic findings suggest a central etiology. Significant nausea or imbalance is not typical.

PHYSICAL EXAMINATION

With any new complaint of dizziness, a careful history and physical examination as outlined previously is always recommended.

The Hallpike-Dix maneuver can be diagnostic of BPPV if the nystagmus is of the characteristic profile described above. The dizziness and vertigo will be elicited with the affected ear down. In some cases the history is compelling for BPPV but at the time of the examination position testing does not produce the dizziness or nystagmus (likely because of the intermittent nature of BPPV).

The remainder of the neurologic examination should be normal.

DIAGNOSTICS

The diagnosis may be confirmed by history and a positive Hallpike-Dix test. Further testing is warranted if there are positive neurologic findings, any associated features beyond the vertigo and a mild imbalance, or any symptoms or findings that are not movement or position related. If the history is compelling but position testing is not confirmatory, ENG may be helpful.

DIFFERENTIAL DIAGNOSIS

The symptom of vertigo is differentiated from syncope or disequilibrium through a careful history. Vertigo can be a manifestation of peripheral or central disorders of the vestibular system. If there are more symptoms or findings than the vertigo, a mild associated imbalance, and a positive Hallpike-Dix, further diagnoses should be pursed.

MANAGEMENT

BPPV may remit in a few days or weeks without any treatment. In many cases referral for specific vestibular physical therapy will facilitate a quicker and often more prolonged remission. Such therapy consists of habituation exercises designed to train the brain to react less to the confused signals sent from the inner ear. This occurs most effectively if the patient continues with normal head movements despite their causing vertigo. Some exercises can facilitate compensation, such as lying or rolling in a position that will precipitate the vertigo and staying in that position until the vertigo subsides or for 30 seconds. These exercises should be repeated twice a day until the vertigo is gone.

Liberatory maneuvers are specific positioning exercises that are designed to move ear crystal particles from the semicircular canal. Epley's maneuver involves moving the patient from one head-hanging position to another. This presumably rotates the particle(s) out of the semicircular canal and into the utricle of the inner ear, where it is cleared through the endolymphatic duct and no longer affects the dynamics of the semicircular canals. The patient must then not lie flat for 48 to 72 hours to prevent the particles from reentering the posterior canal. The vertigo may recur in a week or two in 10% to 20% of patients, in which case the maneuver should be repeated. Approximately 50% of patients will have a future recurrence. They can be taught to do the maneuver at home.

Medications such as meclizine may be used as a vestibular suppressant if vertigo is severe. However, in BPPV the acute attacks are not suppressed by medications, and the canalith-repositioning maneuvers are more effective in controlling the condition.[8,9] Medications that do cause vestibular suppression slow recovery as they slow compensatory mechanisms.

In rare refractory cases canal plugging surgery may be considered.[8,9]

COMPLICATIONS

As its name implies, BPPV is a benign condition. Associated or indirect complications could include risk of falling or the risks inherent in self-imposed decreased mobility (common because of fear of precipitating the vertigo). Safety issues should be addressed related to driving, if head turning precipitates the vertigo. The condition may interfere with work.

INDICATIONS FOR REFERRAL OR HOSPITALIZATION

If BPPV is the likely diagnosis yet the symptoms are refractory to liberatory maneuvers and physical therapy interventions, referral to a specialist (otoneurologist) may be warranted. Referral to physical therapy for vestibular evaluation and treatment should be considered first line, rather than medication treatment. The Vestibular Disorders Association provides extensive specialty referral sources throughout the United States.[8]

PATIENT AND FAMILY EDUCATION

The experience of acute vertigo can be frightening. Information about the evaluation, prognosis, and treatment options will help alleviate fears of a more serious condition. It is important to emphasize that the most effective treatment (vestibular therapy and exercises) may initially cause increased symptoms, but the treatment must continue for the symptoms to subside. The Vestibular Disorders website has helpful information for patients as well as providers (http://www.vestibular.org).

REFERENCES

1. Baloh RW, Honrubia V: *Clinical neurophysiology of the vestibular system*, ed 2, Philadelphia, 1990, Davis.
2. Hain TC: Treatment of vertigo, *Neurologist* 1(3):125-133, 1995.
3. Furman JM, Cass SP: *Balance disorders: a case study approach*, Philadelphia, 1996, Davis.
4. Burke M: Dizziness in the elderly, *Nurse Pract* 20(12):28-35, 1995.
5. Weiss HD: Dizziness. In Samuels M, editor: *Manual of neurologic therapeutics*, ed 5, Boston, 1991, Little, Brown.
6. Norre ME: Rehabilitation treatments for vertigo and related syndromes, *Crit Rev Phys Rehabil Med* 2(2):101-120, 1990.
7. Rascol O, Hain TC, Brefel C, and others: Antivertigo medications and drug-induced vertigo, *Drugs* 50(5):777-791, 1995.
8. Vestibular Disorders Association: *Treatment for vertigo, imbalance, and dizziness due to vestibular dysfunction*, retrieved Jan 14, 2006, from http://www.vestibular.org/vestibular-disorders/treatment.php.
9. Chang AK, Schoeman G, Hill M: A randomized clinical trial to assess the efficacy of the Epley maneuver in the treatment of acute benign positional vertigo, *Acad Emerg Med* 11(9):918-924, 2004.

CHAPTER 207

Guillain-Barré

Joanne Sandberg-Cook

DEFINITION AND EPIDEMIOLOGY

Guillain-Barré (pronounced *ghee-yan bah-ray*) is an acute clinical syndrome caused by an autoimmune inflammatory destruction of the myelin sheath that covers the peripheral nerves. This destruction causes varying degrees of rapid, progressive, and symmetric loss of motor function and impaired respiratory function. Subtypes of Guillain-Barré syndrome (GBS) include acute inflammatory demyelinating polyradiculoneuropathy, acute motor axonal neuropathy, acute motor sensory axonal neuropathy, Miller Fisher syndrome, and acute panautonomic neuropathy.[1]

The incidence of GBS is 1 or 2 per 100,000 persons, without regard to gender, age, or race.[2] GBS can strike at any age but is at its highest rate in individuals 50 to 74 years of age.[2] The course is more benign in children. The mortality rate is 5% to 10%.[1] Twenty percent to 40% of patients with GBS have weakness after 1 year, 5% have a permanent disability, and 3% may suffer a relapse of muscle weakness and tingling sensations after the initial episode.[2]

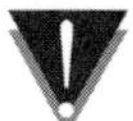

Immediate emergency department referral and hospitalization are indicated for all patients with GBS and impending respiratory failure.

PATHOPHYSIOLOGY

The cause of GBS is unclear, but it is thought to be an autoimmune response triggered by an antecedent illness, often infectious, or a medical condition.[2] The macrophages and T cells attack the myelin sheath of the peripheral and cranial nerves, causing a block in the conduction of nerve impulses. The central nervous system is unaffected. GBS is occasionally triggered by surgery, pregnancy, malignancies (particularly Hodgkin's disease), or vaccinations.[1] The disease may develop in hours, in days, or over 3 to 4 weeks. GBS often occurs 1 to 4 weeks after a respiratory or gastrointestinal infection.[1] *Campylobacter jejuni*, an organism that causes diarrhea, is recognized as the most common organism to precede the syndrome. Other infections that are known to precipitate GBS include hepatitis B, *Mycoplasma pneumoniae*, cytomegalovirus, and Epstein-Barr virus. After infection there may be a severe form of the disease, with increased risk of nerve deterioration, slow recovery, and longer disability.[3]

The 1976 to 1977 swine flu vaccines triggered an increased incidence of GBS in some groups of recipients.[2] The reason for this association has not been determined. During the 1992 to 1993 and the 1993 to 1994 flu seasons, an increased incidence of approximately 1 in 1 million doses was noted when both seasons were combined. However, morbidity and mortality from influenza are greater than the risk of GBS from the vaccine. Other vaccines that are rarely associated with GBS include rabies and vaccinations against group A streptococci.[3]

Certain drugs have been associated with GBS, including gold salts, penicillamine, captopril, danazol, cyclosporine,[4] and heroin.

CLINICAL PRESENTATION

It may be difficult to diagnose GBS in its earliest stages because the signs and symptoms can vary. The initial presentation of GBS is commonly weakness and/or numbness in the lower limbs, which may ascend to the upper extremities, and paresthesia in a "glove and stocking" distribution. Paresthesia occurs first, followed by an ascending muscle weakness and flaccid paralysis. Severe pain in the back, buttocks, thighs, and shoulders is common. Cranial nerve involvement may cause double vision and difficulty swallowing, talking, and chewing.[1] In 25% of patients, weakness of the respiratory muscles necessitates artificial ventilation.[5] Cognitive function and level of consciousness are not affected.

The history should include a review of the symptom duration; medications; diet; and other medical illnesses, particularly any viral respiratory or gastric illness within the past 1 to 4 weeks. The time frame from onset of symptoms to peak disability varies from hours to weeks. Most people reach the stage of greatest weakness within the first 2 weeks after symptoms appear and are at their weakest by the third week of the illness.[1] Symptoms then stabilize at this level for days, weeks, or sometimes months. The recovery period may be a few weeks to 2 years. Residual neurologic disability can be observed in 10% to 40% of cases.[3]

PHYSICAL EXAMINATION

The first physical signs of GBS include varying degrees of progressive weakness and tingling in the legs, which eventually spread to the arms and upper body. Flaccid quadriplegia and bulbar paralysis that ascends from the extremities to the head may occur and is considered a medical emergency. Autonomic dysfunction, including overreactivity or underreactivity of the sympathetic or parasympathetic nervous systems, may occur, leading to disturbances of heart rate and rhythm, blood pressure, and other vasomotor disturbances. Other signs include inappropriate secretion of antidiuretic hormone; depressed or absent deep tendon reflexes; paralysis of extraocular muscles, causing ptosis; and urinary retention.[5] Symptoms can increase in intensity until the muscles cannot be used, leaving the patient almost totally paralyzed and unable to breathe without ventilatory assistance.

The physical examination should include vital signs; assessment of respiratory and urinary function; and a complete neurologic examination that includes the cranial nerves, deep tendon reflexes, and sensory and motor function. Sphincter disturbances are rare; therefore other diagnoses should be considered if these are present. The patellar reflexes are usually lost, with most patients being unable to walk at the peak of illness. Respiratory function can be impaired in many patients, requiring mechanical ventilation.

DIAGNOSTICS

No specific tests exist for GBS, so diagnosis is based mainly on the history and physical examination. Diagnostic tests include CBC (there may be early leukocytosis with a shift to the left that resolves during the course of illness); erythrocyte sedimentation rate; biochemistry with electrolytes; and the following tests depending on which diagnoses are suspected: thyroid-stimulating hormone, chest x-ray study, liver function tests, serologic tests for HIV and Lyme disease, urinary porphyrin screen, and stool for *Clostridium difficile* toxin. A variety of rhythm disturbances can be seen on ECG. Pulmonary function studies, especially forced vital capacity, should be monitored carefully and the patient placed on a ventilator at the first sign of deterioration. A referral is indicated for assessment of nerve conduction velocity (which shows marked slowing of the signals traveling along the nerve) and a lumbar puncture with spinal fluid analysis, which often shows an elevated level of cerebrospinal fluid protein (>400 mg/L).[3]

DIAGNOSTICS

Guillain-Barré

INITIAL
Peak flow meter
Pulse oximetry

LABORATORY
CBC and differential
ESR
Serum electrolytes
BUN
Creatinine
Serum glucose
LFTs
TSH*
HIV*
Lyme titer*
Urinary porphyrin screen*
Stool for *Clostridium difficile**
ABGs*

OTHER
Pulmonary function tests
Electromyogram
Nerve conduction velocity
Lumbar puncture
Chest x-ray*

*If indicated.

DIFFERENTIAL DIAGNOSIS

Because of the lack of objective signs, diagnosis of GBS is difficult in the early stages but is crucial to prevent death from respiratory paralysis. Patients are sometimes misdiagnosed with anxiety or hysteria. Differential diagnoses include spinal cord lesions; myasthenia gravis; poliomyelitis; acquired hypokalemia; periodic paralysis; polymyositis; botulism; acute intermittent porphyria; heavy metals; toxins; lymphoma; lung carcinoma; alcohol abuse; history of hexacarbon abuse; renal failure; hypothyroidism; AIDS; vasculitis; diphtheria; Lyme

DIFFERENTIAL DIAGNOSIS

Guillain-Barré

- Spinal cord lesions
- Myasthenia gravis
- Polio
- Periodic paralysis
- Polymyositis
- Botulism
- Acute, intermittent porphyria
- Heavy metal poisoning
- Alcohol abuse
- Renal failure
- Vitamin B_{12} deficiency
- AIDS
- Vasculitis
- Lyme disease (or other tick-related paralysis)
- Polyneuropathy (hereditary, drug induced)
- Severe hypophosphatemia
- Severe hypokalemia
- Diphtheritic neuropathy
- Brickthorn berry intoxication
- History of hexacarbon abuse
- Lymphoma
- Lung cancer
- Hypothyroidism
- Diabetes

disease; diabetes; vitamin B_{12} deficiency; hereditary causes of polyneuropathy; or conditions secondary to drugs such as gold, disulfiram, phenytoin, or dapsone. Symptoms that have been noted for years suggest a hereditary cause; weeks to months, a toxin or metabolic cause; days, a toxin or GBS.

MANAGEMENT

GBS has no known cure. The goal of management is to expedite recovery, reduce disability, and prevent complications. If the clinical presentation suggests GBS, immediate hospitalization and available ventilator support are essential. Management during hospitalization includes IV fluids, cardiac monitoring, nutritional support, nursing care, prevention of complications, physical and occupational therapy, pain control, improved communication, relief of fear and anxiety, comfort measures, preventive skin care, and home care teaching.

Current medical treatment includes plasma exchange and IV immunoglobulin therapy. Both therapies have been shown to shorten recovery time by as much as 50%. Plasma exchange reduces the severity and duration of the disease by producing a temporary reduction in circulating antibodies.[6] High-dose IV immunoglobulin therapy can mitigate the immune system attack on the nerves. Corticosteroids are no longer used as treatment for GBS, since clinical trials have found no evidence of benefit in these patients.[7]

Most patients recover from even the most severe cases of GBS, although some continue to have a certain degree of weakness. Some patients have a residual disability that requires long-term management and supervision at home. Psychologic counseling and support groups may be needed to help patients and their families adapt to the sudden paralysis and dependence on others.

LIFE SPAN CONSIDERATIONS

GBS occurs in all age-groups, peaking in late adolescence and again in the elderly. Outcomes are worse in those over age 65. The incidence may be lower during pregnancy.[1] Pain in the lower limbs is commonly the early symptom in children under 6.[8] IV immunoglobulin is the treatment of choice in children.[9]

COMPLICATIONS

Ventilator support plus continued monitoring for problems such as arrhythmias, infections, pneumonia, thrombus formation, autonomic dysfunction, bladder atony, gastrointestinal dysfunction, contractures, and pressure ulcers are necessary. Between 4% and 15% of patients die, often of complications related to artificial ventilation.[1]

INDICATIONS FOR REFERRAL OR HOSPITALIZATION

Because GBS is an acute inflammatory disease that can result in respiratory paralysis, it is essential that patients suspected of having this condition be evaluated by a physician. Lumbar puncture is necessary, and the majority of patients require hospitalization. A small number of patients with mild GBS can be managed as outpatients, but they require careful and frequent monitoring.

PATIENT EDUCATION

At diagnosis, the patient and family should be informed of the expected course of the disease and treatment and referred to a support group. The GBS/CIDP Foundation International can be contacted at the Holly Building, 104½ Forrest Avenue, Narberth, PA 19072; (610) 667-0131; http://www.gbsfi.com. Services include arranging visits to patients by recovered persons, providing supplies and literature, fostering research, developing local support groups, and holding an international educational symposium for the medical community and the general public.[9]

Patient education websites include http://www.mayoclinic.com/health/guillain-barre-syndrome/DS00413.

REFERENCES

1. Newswanger DL, Warren CR: Guillain-Barré syndrome, *Am Fam Phys* 69(10):2405-2410, 2004.
2. Safranek T, Lawrence D, Kuriand C, and others: Reassessment of the association between Guillain-Barré syndrome and receipt of swine influenza vaccine in 1976-1977: results of a two state study, *Am J Epidemiol* 133(9):940-951, 1991.
3. Davids H, Oleszek J: *Guillain-Barré syndrome,* retrieved Feb 12, 2007, from http://www.emedicine.com/pmr/topic48.htm.
4. Falk JA, Cordova FC, Popescu A, and others: Treatment of Guillaine-Barré syndrome induced by cyclosporine in a lung transplant patient, *J Heart Lung Transplant* 25(1):140-143, 2006.
5. Hughes RAC, Cornblath D: Guillain-Barré syndrome, *Lancet* 366(9497):1653-1666, 2005.
6. Hughes RA, Wijdicks EF, Barohn R, and others: Practice parameter: immunotherapy for Guillain-Barré syndrome: report of the Quality Standards Subcommittee of the American Academy of Neurology, *Neurology* 61(6):736-740, 2003.
7. Hughes RA, van Der Meche FG: Corticosteroids for treating Guillain-Barré syndrome, *Cochrane Database of Systematic Reviews* 2:CD001446, 2000.
8. Tang T, Noble-Jamieson C: A painful hip as a presentation of Guillain-Barré syndrome in children, *Br Med J* 322(7279):149-150, 2001.
9. Korinthenberg R, Schessl J: Intravenously administered immunoglobulin in the treatment of childhood Guillain-Barré syndrome: a randomized trial, *Pediatrics* 116(1):8-14, 2005.

CHAPTER 208

Headache

Gretchen Van Buren

DEFINITION AND EPIDEMIOLOGY

Headache is experienced by 90% to 95% of the population and is one of the 10 most common complaints in the outpatient setting.[1,2] Many people with headache are never diagnosed by a physician. Some individuals treat headaches at home, with over-the-counter (OTC) medications and home remedies such as ice packs and rest. Research has shown that, even with the development of newer medications, up to 57% of patients with headaches use OTC medications, and many do not seek care for their headaches because they do not believe that satisfactory treatment is available.[3]

Physician consultation is indicated for patients with suspected temporal arteritis, change in mental status, nuchal rigidity, neurologic deficit, or new onset of headache.

It is essential to differentiate secondary from primary headaches because secondary headaches can be harbingers of a potentially more serious medical problem than the benign, primary headaches usually seen in the office setting.[1] Secondary headaches are less common and are usually the result of an underlying disease or condition such as sinusitis, tumor, hemorrhage, temporal arteritis, or meningitis.[1,2] Once identified and treated, secondary headaches may dissipate.

Primary headaches are more common and are not symptomatic of another medical condition. These are distinct disorders that result from pathophysiologic mechanisms. Types of primary headaches include migraine with and without aura, chronic or episodic tension-type headaches, and chronic or episodic cluster headaches.[1,2]

In 1999 the estimated number of migraineurs in the United States was approximately 27 million, and the average annual indirect cost was between $5 billion and $17 billion.[4] These headaches may range in intensity from mild to severe but cause considerable distress. In general, migraine varies by age and sex, increasing in frequency to about age 40 years and declining thereafter in both men and women. Women experience migraine three times more often than men. Similarly, tension-type headache is seen more in women than in men, with a male-female ratio of 4:5.[5] Cluster headache, on the other hand, is more common in men than in women, with a ratio of about 7:1. Cluster attacks usually begin between the ages of 20 and 40.[6]

Clinical and research evidence has demonstrated a relationship between migraine and other disease processes, including epilepsy, major depression, and panic disorder. The neurotransmitter serotonin has been suggested as a basis for both migraine and major depression. Knowing that a co-occurrence exists helps in the treatment of each disease and provides clues to the pathophysiology of migraine.[7]

PATHOPHYSIOLOGY

Headache types have some similarities. Migraine and tension-type headaches have similar features, sparking considerable debate over the existence of a headache continuum. Often the headache is not a "pure" form of one or the other.[2]

The exact mechanism of a headache is still debated. Previously, headaches were thought to be caused by increased blood flow to the head, resulting in distended vessels and pressure on the nerve fibers of the brain.[1] This "vascular theory" was popular for many years, until the 1930s, when Harold Wolfe determined that migraine, specifically, was due to both vascular and chemical changes within the brain.[1,8]

Many theories have since identified several neurochemicals as key elements in migraine development. Serotonin (5-hydroxytryptamine [5-HT]), a powerful vasoconstrictor, sensitizes the blood vessel walls to painful dilation. Other neurochemicals, such as dopamine and the catecholamines, may alter the excitability of the brain and mediate the vasoconstriction or vasodilation of blood vessels.[1] A polypeptide, substance P, may be responsible for propagation of pain impulses from the periphery to the central nervous system. When substance P is released, it interacts with blood vessel walls, resulting in dilation, plasma extravasation, inflammation, and pain.[8]

A similar theory postulates that central brain pathways, which may include the hypothalamus or the brainstem, are involved. Here certain chemicals are released that affect the vasodilation, vasoconstriction, and pain associated with a migraine.[1]

In reviewing the various theories, it is clear that during a headache changes occur in the vasculature of the brain and in the neurochemicals found within the body. These changes are a result of a brain response to a stimulus, or *trigger*. Vasodilation and vasoconstriction subsequently cause the release of neurochemicals, which may be responsible for the headache and for the feelings of impending doom or fatigue that can occur before and after an attack.

CLINICAL PRESENTATION

The International Headache Society has developed criteria for various types of headache disorders. Using the criteria can be tedious and not applicable in many primary care settings, but the information may allow the provider to quickly differentiate the various types of primary headache conditions[9,10] (Boxes 208-1 to 208-4).

Migraine

The two major types of migraine are migraine with aura and migraine without aura. Migraine without aura, also known as *common migraine,* is the more common of the two. In general, the patient complains of an ipsilateral headache. The pain is described as pounding or throbbing, is moderate to severe in intensity, and is aggravated by physical activity. This headache, which is episodic, lasts from 4 to 72 hours and may be associated with nausea, vomiting, photophobia, and phonophobia. These patients usually retreat to a dark, quiet room until the attack is over. They often can identify a trigger that will precipitate the attacks. Triggers are an individual char-

BOX 208-1

INTERNATIONAL HEADACHE SOCIETY CRITERIA FOR MIGRAINE WITHOUT AURA

A. At least five attacks fulfilling criteria B through D
B. Headaches lasting 4 to 72 hours (untreated or unsuccessfully treated)
C. Headache has at least two of the following characteristics:
   1. Unilateral location
   2. Pulsating quality
   3. Moderate or severe intensity (inhibits or prohibits daily activities)
   4. Aggravation by walking stairs or similar routine physical activity
D. During headache, at least one of the following symptoms:
   1. Nausea or vomiting, or both
   2. Photophobia and/or phonophobia
E. No evidence of related organic disease

Modified from Headache Classification Committee of the International Headache Society: Classification and diagnostic criteria for headache disorders, cranial neuralgias, and facial pain, *Cephalalgia* 8(Suppl 7):1-96, 1988.

BOX 208-2

INTERNATIONAL HEADACHE SOCIETY CRITERIA FOR MIGRAINE WITH AURA

A. At least two attacks fulfilling criterion B
B. At least three of the following characteristics:
   1. One or more fully reversible aura symptoms indicating brain dysfunction
   2. At least one aura symptom developing gradually over more than 4 minutes, or two or more symptoms occurring in succession
   3. No single aura symptom lasting more than 60 minutes
   4. Headache following aura with a free interval of less than 60 minutes (may also begin before or simultaneously with the aura)
C. No evidence of a secondary cause

Modified from Headache Classification Committee of the International Headache Society: Classification and diagnostic criteria for headache disorders, cranial neuralgias, and facial pain, *Cephalalgia* 8(Suppl 7):1-96, 1988.

BOX 208-3

INTERNATIONAL HEADACHE SOCIETY CRITERIA FOR EPISODIC TENSION-TYPE HEADACHE

A. At least 10 previous headache episodes fulfilling criteria B through D; number of days with such headache less than 180 per year (<15/mo)*
B. Headache lasting from 30 minutes to 7 days
C. At least two of the following pain characteristics:
   1. Pressing or tightening (nonpulsating) quality
   2. Mild or moderate intensity (may inhibit but does not prohibit activities)
   3. Bilateral location
   4. No aggravation by walking stairs or similar routine physical activity
D. Both of the following:
   1. Absence of nausea and vomiting (anorexia may occur)
   2. Absence of photophobia or phonophobia, or both

Modified from Headache Classification Committee of the International Headache Society: Classification and diagnostic criteria for headache disorders, cranial neuralgias, and facial pain, *Cephalalgia* 8(Suppl 7):1-96, 1988.
*Chronic tension-type headache has similar criteria but occurs >15 days/mo (>180 days/yr) for >6 months. Either condition may be associated with disorder of pericranial vessels.

BOX 208-4

INTERNATIONAL HEADACHE SOCIETY CRITERIA FOR CLUSTER HEADACHE

A. At least five attacks fulfilling criteria B through D
B. Severe unilateral orbital, supraorbital, and/or temporal pain lasting 15 to 180 minutes untreated
C. Headache associated with at least one of the following signs on the side of the pain:
   1. Conjunctival injection
   2. Lacrimation
   3. Nasal congestion
   4. Rhinorrhea
   5. Forehead and facial sweating
   6. Miosis
   7. Ptosis
   8. Eyelid edema
D. Frequency of attacks: from one every other day to eight per day

Modified from Headache Classification Committee of the International Headache Society: Classification and diagnostic criteria for headache disorders, cranial neuralgias, and facial pain, *Cephalalgia* 8(Suppl 7):1-96, 1988.

acteristic and may be difficult to identify because they may not always stimulate a headache. Common triggers include weather changes, foods, alcohol, altitude, delaying or skipping a meal, and hormonal changes.[1,11]

In migraine with aura, or *classic migraine,* the aura usually occurs before the onset of head pain, although sometimes it can extend into the period of headache. The classic aura, or "fortification spectrum," occurs in about 10% of patients and is described as jagged lines similar to the stone fortifications found around a fort.[1,12] Visual auras can also be characterized by spots, shimmering bright lights, or areas of visual loss (scotomas). Somatosensory-type auras can also occur, with tingling or numbness of the fingers, motor disturbances such as hemiparesis or monoparesis, and cognitive disorders.[13] These visual and somatosensory disturbances usually last seconds but can last as long as 20 minutes.[1] The patient then experiences head pain and features similar to those of migraine without aura.

A prodrome can be part of a migraine.[13] Several days before the aura or start of the head pain, the person may have feelings of doom or fatigue. During this period, increased irritability, decreased energy, and food cravings are common complaints. Often this can be an early signal that a severe headache is coming and may enable the patient to use both pharmacologic and nonpharmacologic modalities in the hope of aborting the attack (Table 208-1).

Tension-Type Headache

Acute tension-type headaches are described as feeling like there is a tight band around the head. Nausea and vomiting are not present, and the pain can be mild to moderate in intensity. This headache can last minutes to hours. It usually is not exacerbated by physical activity, but a common trigger is stress. Overall, the acute tension-type headache is a nagging headache that occurs fewer than 15 days per month, is present most of the day, and may start after the person wakes up. It

TABLE 208-1 Abortive Therapies for Headache

Medications	Route	Dosage	Considerations
NSAIDs			
Ibuprofen (Advil, Motrin)	PO	1200 mg ×1, repeat 600 mg ×2 p.r.n.	As with all NSAIDs, side effects include dyspepsia, heartburn, bleeding, and nausea or vomiting; contraindicated in patients with history of ulcer; will have better effect if taken on an empty stomach but might not be well tolerated by patient.
Naproxen sodium (Anaprox DS)	PO	550 mg b.i.d. p.r.n.	
Indomethacin (Indocin)	PO or PR	25-50 mg t.i.d. p.r.n.	Indomethacin suppositories are effective but no longer available in the U.S. and need to be compounded by pharmacist.
Ketorolac (Toradol)	IM	30-60 mg IM p.r.n.	Can be used as an alternative to one of the acute abortives or narcotics; should be used on a limited basis only—5-day course.
GLUCOCORTICOIDS			
Dexamethasone	PO	10-12 mg q day ×1-2 days	Should be limited to <1 treatment per month; hold NSAIDs while administering glucocorticoids; use when usual treatments have not aborted headache and it continues for several days.
Prednisone	PO	Steroid taper over 7 days	
MUSCLE RELAXANTS			
Carisoprodol (Soma)	PO	350 mg ½-1 tablet PO up to q.i.d. p.r.n.	Encourage patient to start with lowest dose and increase as needed to take away tightness; this may often abort a migraine from beginning; used on headaches described as "tight" or "pressure"; used frequently with tension-type headaches; caution patient about sedation.
Metaxalone (Skelaxin)	PO	400 mg 1-2 tablets t.i.d.-q.i.d. p.r.n.	
NARCOTIC ANALGESICS			
Butorphanol tartrate (Stadol)	Nasal	1 mg (1 spray in 1 nostril) followed by 1 mg in 60-90 minutes	Use only occasionally; may be diluted with equal part N/S to decrease side effects; can cause sedation and dysphoria; limit number of bottles per month; frequently used to abort cluster attacks.
Meperidine (Demerol)	PO, IM	75-150 mg stat at headache onset; may repeat q 4-6 hr p.r.n.	Limited use only when other treatments are ineffective; overuse may contribute to rebound headaches; an antinauseant may also be needed. Avoid use in the elderly.
COMBINATION ANALGESICS			
Butalbital combination (Fioricet, Fiorinal)	PO	1-2 PO stat at headache onset; may repeat q 4 hr p.r.n.	Important to tell patient to take sufficient amount of these medications right at start of headache; adding metoclopramide to these may facilitate absorption; because of risk of rebound headache, limit to 2 days per week.
ASA plus caffeine (Excedrin)	PO	1-2 PO stat at headache onset; may repeat q 4 hr p.r.n.	
OTHER			
Isometheptene mucate, dichloralphenazone, and acetaminophen (Midrin)	PO	2 caplets stat, then repeat 1 caplet q 1 hr up to 5 capsules in 24 hours	May cause sedation; maximum dose: 5 caplets/24 hr.
Metoclopramide (Reglan)	PO	10 mg b.i.d. p.r.n.	May facilitate absorption of many abortives; watch for akathisia.
Hydroxyzine	PO	25-mg caplets, 1-2 caplets t.i.d.-q.i.d. p.r.n. for nausea, mild pain, or sleeplessness	Very effective antinauseant; may potentiate some NSAIDs; can be used alone or in combination for mild pain.
ACUTE ABORTIVES			
Triptans			
Sumatriptan (Imitrex)	PO	25-100 mg, up to 200 mg/day p.r.n.	With all triptans, **separate all doses by at least 2 hours;** common side effects are triptan sensations of flushing, tingling, chest tightness, and throat tightness that will subside after 10-20 minutes; contraindicated in presence of hypertension, coronary artery disease, myocardial infarction history, hepatic or renal dysfunction, or pregnancy; first dose of a triptan should be administered under medical supervision.
	Nasal	20 mg for adults, 1 spray in 1 nostril b.i.d. p.r.n.	
	SQ	6 mg SQ b.i.d. p.r.n.	
Zolmitriptan (Zomig)	PO Nasal Fast-melt pill	2.5-5.0 mg b.i.d. p.r.n.; limited to 3 "attacks" per month; maximum dose: 10 mg/day	

Data from Solomon GD, Cady RK, Klapper JA, and others: Standards of care for treating headache in primary care practice, *Cleve Clin J Med* 6(7):373-383, 1996; and Schulman EA, Silberstein SD: Symptomatic and prophylactic treatment of migraine and tension-type headache, *Neurology* 42(2 Suppl):S16-S21, 1992.
ASA, Acetylsalicylic acid; *N/S*, normal saline.

TABLE 208-1 Abortive Therapies for Headache—cont'd

Medications	Route	Dosage	Considerations
ACUTE ABORTIVES—CONT'D			
Triptans—cont'd			
Naratriptan (Amerge)	PO	2.5 mg b.i.d. p.r.n.; limited to 4 "attacks" per month	
Rizatriptan (Maxalt, Maxalt MLT)	PO	5-10 mg; may be repeated in 2 hr; maximum dose: 30 mg/day	Fast-melt preparation may be no faster than PO, but useful when nausea and vomiting are present.
Dihydroergotamine mesylate			
D.H.E. 45	SQ	1 mg b.i.d. p.r.n.	Effective therapy that can last all day but can cause nausea and vomiting; should premedicate with antinauseant, such as promethazine, before administration; leg cramping is common and usually responds to dose reduction.
Migranal 0.5 mg/spray	Nasal	1 spray in each nostril, may repeat in 15 min ×1	
Ergotamine and caffeine (Cafergot)	PO	1-2 tablets at headache onset; may repeat at 30-minute intervals; maximum dose: 6 mg/day	May be more effective if metoclopramide is added; can lead to ergotamine-dependency headaches; its use should be limited to 2 days per week.
	PR	2-mg suppository cut into fourths; repeat ¼ suppository q 30 min until headache abates; limit to 2 suppositories per attack	Causes severe nausea, and dose must be titrated to a subnauseating dose; premedication with an antinauseant is key to success; may not be tolerated by many patients because of severe nausea and vomiting.

rarely awakens the person. Chronic tension-type headache is similar in presentation to the acute type but occurs more often than 15 days per month.

Cluster Headache

The patient with cluster headache, acute or chronic, is usually awakened during the night with severe unilateral, retroorbital pain. A cluster headache reaches maximum intensity in about 15 minutes and usually lasts about 90 minutes, although some can last 3 hours.[6,14] These attacks can occur several times per day. The pain is described as boring, and unlike migraineurs, these patients often cannot sit still. The severe intensity of cluster pain causes restlessness and often pacing. Patients may have thoughts of suicide.[15] Other features of cluster headache include ipsilateral injection of the conjunctiva, lacrimation, rhinorrhea, and a partial Horner's sign. For the patient with acute cluster headache, attacks occur in groups (or clusters) lasting days to weeks and then subside until the next attack. Years can pass between attacks, and often the event occurs at the same time each year. The patient with chronic cluster headache has the same presentation as the patient with the acute type but does not experience any remission longer than 14 days during a 12-month period. These headaches are also relatively resistant to therapy. Although it is well tolerated between attacks, alcohol often will precipitate an attack in patients with acute or chronic cluster headache.[6,14,15]

PHYSICAL EXAMINATION

The history is the most important part of the evaluation. With most primary headache disorders, the diagnosis can be made on the basis of the history alone.[16] It is important that the patient characterize the headache by describing the duration, quality, and location of the pain. The presence or absence of any precipitating factors, or triggers, and the age of onset should be established. Associated symptoms such as nausea, vomiting, or photophobia should be explored. Can the patient be active during these headaches, or does the patient need to lie still in a dark room? How does the patient describe his or her sleep and energy? Sleep is usually labile in the person with headache, and energy may be poor. A medication profile is essential and should include medications that have been tried in the past for headache control. If OTC medications are taken, the number used per month should be identified because patients may not view OTC drugs as medications. Migraine is known to be familial; therefore it is important to determine whether any family member has had headaches, which might have been called "sinus headaches," "sick headaches," or headaches that were disabling. Asking about the presence of any physical abuse is important because it has been shown that a history of abuse contributes to refractory headaches.

A targeted physical examination confirms any information given in the history.[16] The examination in primary headache disorders is usually within normal limits. Key aspects of the physical examination include:

- Funduscopic examination
- Mental status examination
- Palpation of the head, neck, and sinuses
- Evaluation of vital signs
- Palpation of the temporomandibular joint
- Examination of the cranial nerves
- Evaluation of motor and balance

Many patients with tension-type headaches or migraines have tight cervical musculature. Painful biceps insertions, along with general aches and pains along the back, hips, and knees, may herald the beginning of fibromyalgia (see Chapter 186), a condition commonly seen in migraineurs. Pain and pressure on palpation of the sinuses accompanied by purulent nasal discharge may be indicative of sinusitis. The temporomandibular joints may click and pop when the mouth is opened and closed, but rarely is this the cause of a headache. Tension often is exhibited in the musculature surrounding this joint, and the subsequent bruxism may potentiate pain in this area.

Serious symptoms and findings include a headache accompanied by a stiff neck; fever; malaise; nausea or vomiting; and the presence of any aphasia, weakness, or poor coordination. Other danger signs include[1,16]:

- Onset of headache after age 50
- Asymmetry of pupillary responses
- Decreased deep tendon reflexes
- Headache described as "the worst ever experienced"
- Personality change
- Onset of a new or different headache
- Onset of a headache that progressively worsens
- Papilledema
- Painful temporal arteries

Further investigation and referral to a specialist or hospital would be warranted with any of these signs.

DIAGNOSTICS

The use of diagnostic studies depends on the results of the history and physical examination. Most diagnostic studies in the patient with primary headache are unrevealing.[16] If the diagnosis is not clear or the history or physical findings are cause for concern, diagnostic studies should be used to distinguish primary headache from a secondary condition.

Blood tests are generally not indicated, although exceptions include the use of a CBC to exclude anemia or an infectious process, erythrocyte sedimentation rate to help exclude temporal arteritis, and thyroid function tests to identify thyroid dysfunction. Lyme titer or rheumatoid factors may also be indicated in some situations.

Practice guidelines recently developed by the U.S. Headache Consortium advocate three principles for diagnostic testing: (1) testing should be avoided if it will not change the management of the patient, (2) testing is not indicated if the patient is not significantly more likely than the general public to have an abnormality, and (3) testing may make sense in a patient who is excessively concerned that he or she has a serious problem that is causing the headaches. Neuroimaging should be considered when any serious signs or symptoms are present during the physical examination, but it is not indicated if the patient has had these headaches for years, if there are no focal neurologic signs, and if the headache improves without the use of analgesics.

DIAGNOSTICS

Headache

LABORATORY
CBC and differential*
ESR*
Thyroid function tests*
Lyme titer*
Rheumatoid factor*

IMAGING
CT scan, MRI*

*If indicated.

DIFFERENTIAL DIAGNOSIS

The history and physical examination will aid in excluding potential diagnoses. The differential diagnosis includes fever, meningitis, pseudotumor cerebri, hemorrhage, rheumatologic disorders (e.g., lupus erythematosus, rheumatoid arthritis), Lyme disease, temporal arteritis, trigeminal neuralgia, thyroid dysfunction, sleep apnea, tumor, aneurysm, and pheochromocytoma, among many others. Headache is a feature of many disease processes (see the Differential Diagnosis box).

MANAGEMENT

The U.S. Headache Consortium has developed evidence-based practice guidelines for migraine that cover both nonpharmacologic and pharmacologic modalities, with the goals of: reducing the frequency of attacks, improving the response to therapy, and restoring the patient to normal functioning. Control can be achieved after a proper diagnosis is made and proper treatment is prescribed. Currently no cure exists for primary headaches, although control is possible for most patients.[1,13,16-18]

Nonpharmacologic Management

Nonpharmacologic measures attempt to control the headache without medication. These methods include behavior modification, biofeedback, acupressure, and a wellness program. Behavior modification uses several methods, such as relaxation via tapes and stress management, as well as modification of daily activities. Biofeedback involves the use of instrumentation to bring under voluntary control physiologic processes of which the individual is normally unaware. For example, during a migraine attack, vasoconstriction of the periphery causes cold hands. Biofeedback training teaches migraineurs to raise hand temperature and thereby prevent an attack. The

DIFFERENTIAL DIAGNOSIS

Headache

PRIMARY HEADACHE
Migraine
Cluster headache
Tension-type headache

INFECTIOUS OR INFLAMMATORY CAUSES
Fever
Meningitis
Temporal arteritis
Systemic lupus erythematosus
Lyme disease
Trigeminal neuralgia
Rheumatoid arthritis
Systemic lupus erythematosus
Sinusitis
Eye disorder
Abscess
Earache

STRUCTURAL CAUSES
Tumor
Hemorrhage
Aneurysm
Subdural hematoma

METABOLIC CAUSES
Thyroid dysfunction
Pheochromocytoma
Sleep apnea

OTHER CAUSES
Pseudotumor cerebri
Trauma

area between the thumb and the first finger (or other acupressure areas) can be depressed during a headache to offer some relief. It is thought that this pressure causes the release of endogenous endorphins and adrenocorticotropic hormones, which aborts the headache in some people.[1] A wellness program, consisting of balanced meals, regular exercise, and adequate sleep, can also be helpful in controlling headache bouts. Overall, nonpharmacologic approaches may help patients avoid triggers that might be initiating the headache.

Another important nonpharmacologic measure is having the patient keep a headache diary. The diary documents the number of headaches, triggers, and treatment successes and failures.[18] The patient should keep this record daily because attempting to fill it in before a follow-up appointment may be less accurate. It is important for the patient to bring the diary to office visits so information can be shared and the treatment plan adjusted if necessary.

Pharmacologic Management

Pharmacologic treatment can be divided into two areas: abortive and preventive. Some clinicians use a "stepped or staged care" approach when selecting treatment regimens. Here therapy starts with the least potent medication, with increasing potency (and often increasing expense) until headache relief is obtained. Another approach is "stratified care," which matches the level of therapy to the intensity of the headache, regardless of potency or cost. With the stratified approach, providers need to supply education and a range of treatment modalities, allowing the patient to select the most effective treatment. If the attack is severe, early intervention with an appropriate therapy, such as a triptan, is in the patient's best interest.[3,9,17]

Preventive Therapy. Preventive therapy is appropriate for patients if they are unable to deal with their attacks, they experience more than four headaches a month, or the attacks are prolonged and refractory to medicine. Preventive therapy is given daily and, if successful, will decrease headache intensity and frequency. When choosing preventive treatment, the provider must consider the patient's history, including any co-morbid conditions. For example, a connection has been shown between epilepsy and migraine; therefore anticonvulsants, such as divalproex sodium (Depakote), gabapentin (Neurontin), or topiramate (Topamax), can be used to control migraine. A patient with cold hands, Raynaud's phenomenon, or hypertension may do well on calcium channel blockers such as diltiazem (Cardizem) or amlodipine (Norvasc), which vasodilate and decrease blood pressure. A beta blocker, such as propranolol (Inderal) or atenolol, may be chosen for the patient with palpitations caused by mitral valve prolapse or panic disorders. If sleep is a problem or if chronic pain persists in the shoulders, a tricyclic antidepressant, such as amitriptyline (Elavil), may facilitate sleep and also decrease the sensation of pain.[13,19]

The mechanism of action for both beta blockers and calcium channel blockers is not fully understood. Calcium channel blockers prevent calcium from entering the cells and therefore decrease their excitability. This may in turn prevent vascular spasm and headache. Beta blockers affect the β_1-adrenergic receptors and inhibit the usual adrenergic responses.[19] Beyond these mechanisms, it has been theorized that either may have an effect on the serotonergic system within the brain and the vascular system.

Both migraine and tension-type headache may result from an imbalance of neurochemicals. Adjusting these neurochemicals to a more "normal" level may decrease the number and frequency of headaches. The tricyclic antidepressants and the selective serotonin reuptake inhibitors (SSRIs), such as sertraline (Zoloft), modulate the levels of serotonin in the brain. Both the tricyclic antidepressants and the SSRIs have an extensive side effect profile. Weight gain and sexual dysfunction may not be acceptable to patients, although the starting dose for many of the medications can be low. The SSRIs are better tolerated, but they might not be as effective for headaches as the tricyclic antidepressants.[13,19]

Abortive Therapy. Abortive therapy is used to treat the intensity and duration of pain during an attack and to manage associated symptoms such as nausea and vomiting. It is important to prescribe an adequate amount of medication initially. The appropriate medicine depends on the prior response to treatment, the presence of nausea or vomiting, and the interval between headache onset and peak intensity. A patient with a severe migraine or cluster attack that peaks to full intensity within 15 minutes will most likely benefit from parenteral or nasal therapy rather than oral medication.[13] For many patients the pain of the headache is severe, but the associated nausea and vomiting are incapacitating. During a migraine attack, gastric emptying is slowed, causing gastric stasis. Medications that "turn the stomach back on," such as metoclopramide (Reglan), will augment the availability of the abortive therapy, enhance gastric motility, and decrease the nausea.[20] Rectal formulations can also be used when prescribing abortive therapies.

Many of the abortive medications are powerful analgesics. When these medications, including acetaminophen (Tylenol), aspirin, and ibuprofen (Advil), are taken frequently, a condition called *analgesic rebound* can develop in a headache-prone individual.[20] The medications prescribed to abort a headache will essentially potentiate the headache and make it a daily condition.[1] Strict guidelines on the use of abortive medicine, as well as limitations on medication refills, need to be reviewed with the patient to prevent analgesic rebound.[1] Patients should be instructed to limit analgesic use to 2 days per week or less.

Simple analgesics, such as acetaminophen and aspirin, can represent first-line treatment in the management of mild to moderate headaches. Caffeine combinations (Excedrin, Anacin) can potentiate their absorption and analgesia. These medications are available without a prescription.

When simple analgesics are ineffective, combining them with a short-acting barbiturate, such as butalbital (Fioricet, Fiorinal, Esgic), may be effective. These medications should be used with caution because they can cause dependency and rebound headaches if used more than 2 or 3 days per week.[1,20]

Nonsteroidal antiinflammatory drugs (NSAIDs) are helpful in treating an acute attack. Naproxen sodium (Anaprox DS, Aleve) has a longer half life and a better safety profile than some of the other NSAIDs. The addition of metoclopramide to many of the NSAIDs when nausea is present will facilitate their absorption and potentiate their effect.[20]

Ergot derivatives are effective in the treatment of moderate to severe attacks that might not have responded to simple or combination analgesics. Two forms are currently in use: ergotamine tartrate (Cafergot) and dihydroergotamine. Ergotamine tartrate is available in both rectal and oral forms, but the rectal dose is more potent than the oral preparation.[1,13] Dosing regimens need to be reviewed with the patient and adjusted to obtain pain relief without vomiting. Dihydroergotamine is available in both an injectable form and a nasal spray. The injectable form (D.H.E. 45) can be given via the subcutaneous or intramuscular route. The nasal form (Migranal) is easily administered and much more convenient. Because all forms of the ergots can cause nausea and vomiting, premedication with an antiemetic, such as promethazine (Phenergan) or prochlorperazine (Compazine), is necessary. Ergot derivatives may have a high potential for overuse and subsequent rebound headaches; patients need to be made aware of the risk for rebound headaches when this medication is prescribed. With the advent of the 5-HT receptor agonists, the triptans, the use of ergot derivatives is not necessarily first line, although they are effective and less expensive.

Corticosteroids (dexamethasone [Decadron], prednisone) are often used when the patient is unable to abort an attack and the attack continues for several days. They may be given as a one-time dose (dexamethasone 10 mg) or as a tapering dosage (prednisone over 7 days). The side effects with the extended use of corticosteroids are serious and include aseptic necrosis of the hip and gastrointestinal bleeding; therefore frequent use is not recommended.[20]

Newer agents such as the triptans or transnasal butorphanol (TNB [Stadol NS]) have given many migraine and cluster patients relief within a short period. TNB is a powerful agonist-antagonist with a rapid analgesic effect.[20] Sedation is a common side effect, as is dysphoria. It should be used with caution and often is diluted before administration. Recent reports of addiction have caused TNB to be closely scrutinized; now TNB is a scheduled drug and should be prescribed with care and used with close supervision.[19,20]

The triptans target specific receptors, 5-HT, in the brain that are believed to generate headache. Relief can be almost complete, allowing a return to normal daily activities with few side effects. The triptans are arterial constrictors and should be used with caution in the presence of known cardiac disease. Many forms of triptans are available: oral, "quick melt," transnasal, and injectable. The dosing parameters are similar for all the triptans in that a dose may be repeated in 2 hours if the initial dose is ineffective at aborting the headache. As with most abortive medications, the goal is to take the dose of medication required to kill the headache before it becomes severe. The brands of each medication have slight differences; if one triptan is ineffective, another may prove to be effective for that patient.

Patients with cluster headache use many of the same medications and treatment regimens as do patients with migraine or tension-type headache. The cluster attack has such a rapid onset that preventing the attacks may be the key to successful treatment. Preventive therapy includes verapamil and lithium as first-line options. Verapamil is usually well tolerated and does not require the close monitoring necessary with lithium. Calcium channel blockers may prevent the vasospasm that occurs during a cluster attack by blocking the flow of calcium. Lithium, long used for bipolar disorder, also controls cluster headaches. Levels should be monitored, and patient education about the signs and symptoms of lithium toxicity is important. Therapy should be slowly titrated upward. With both regimens, therapy is continued until the patient is free of any attacks for several weeks. Patients are then slowly weaned from the medication.

Because of the rapid onset of the cluster headache, abortive therapy needs to be in either a parenteral or a nasal form. Oxygen can be effective in as many as 75% of patients and should be delivered at a rate of 7 L/min via a nonrebreather face mask. The oxygen should be inhaled at the start of an attack. If this is effective, an oxygen tank should be readily available at all times. Both sumatriptan and butorphanol are effective treatment options for the patient with cluster headache, although overuse may be a concern in patients with chronic cluster headache.

The abortive management of tension-type headaches involves many of the same medications as used for migraine, and the same principles should be used when choosing treatments for these patients. For mild attacks NSAIDs may be helpful. Because there usually is no nausea, antiemetics may not be necessary. Muscle relaxants such as metaxalone (Skelaxin) and carisoprodol (Soma), used cautiously, have been helpful with mild to moderate attacks. Triptan drugs may abort a severe tension attack as well. As with migraine, the use of these medications should be limited to 2 days a week or less to prevent rebound headaches. For many of these patients, stress may be triggering the attack, so nonpharmacologic measures are often helpful.[9]

LIFE SPAN CONSIDERATIONS

As patients age, headaches usually seem to decrease. It is uncommon for headaches to appear after age 50. When an older patient is seen with a history of daily headache, analgesic rebound is often the cause; however, secondary processes need to be excluded.

During pregnancy the headache pattern can change. Many women experience a decrease in headaches during the second and third trimesters, although some see no change in the pattern. For the pregnant woman, headache control is usually limited to abortive medications only, and preventive therapy should be tapered immediately. Acetaminophen and meperidine (Demerol), at dosages within normal parameters, can be safely used during pregnancy.

COMPLICATIONS

Misdiagnosis is the most serious complication. For this reason, all patients who complain of headache pain require a careful history and physical examination. Patients with positive physical findings require appropriate and timely referral. Other complications of headache include status migrainosus; dependency on narcotics, barbiturates, tranquilizers, or other agents; side effects of medication; inadequate treatment; and interruption of the activities of daily living.

INDICATIONS FOR REFERRAL OR HOSPITALIZATION

Most patients with headache can be managed within the primary care setting. Indications for referral to a specialist, a headache clinic, or a neurologist include[1,11,16]:

- The headache is not easily controlled by routine headache medicines, such as dihydroergotamine or sumatriptan.
- Rebound headaches or habituation limits outpatient therapy.
- Headache is new and progressively worsening.
- Headache is described as the "worse headache of my life."
- Headache is affecting the patient's quality of life.
- Headache is accompanied by neurologic symptoms that last longer than 30 minutes or is accompanied by numbness or hemiparesis.

Hospitalization of the patient with headache may be appropriate in some situations. Headaches that are resistant to treatment may be rebound headaches and require IV medication to help abort the headache. Referral to a headache specialist or neurologist for consultation may be advantageous. Consultation may be ongoing to provide frequent monitoring and adjustments. Treatment plans should include a step-by-step algorithm for patients to use when they are in the middle of an attack.

PATIENT AND FAMILY EDUCATION

Knowledge and education are important aspects of patient care. Education allows patients and their family to make choices and may enable them to regain control. During the initial examination and subsequent treatment, open communication and reassurance are necessary because many patients believe that they have a life-threatening condition. It is important they realize that their physical examination findings are normal and that the information received during the history indicates a primary headache disorder. Family members should be included in the treatment plan because headache affects both the patient and the family members.

Educational materials on headaches are widely available. Pharmaceutical companies and national groups such as the American Council for Headache Education (http://www.achenet.org) and the National Headache Foundation (http://www.headaches.org) have developed written information about headaches and their history, pathophysiology, treatment, and prevention. The brochures and videos are available to the public, either free of charge or at a nominal cost. Both national groups encourage headache patients and their families to join for support and information. Websites from both national groups also provide information and support.

HEALTH PROMOTION

As reviewed in the section on management, the nonpharmacologic measures are an important part of headache treatment. This can include the modalities reviewed there but also involve encouraging patients to lead a "regular lifestyle" of going to bed at the same time, getting up at the same time, eating three meals a day, limiting alcohol and caffeine intake, and including exercise as part of the daily routine. This wellness program may abort an attack or prevent triggers from initiating an attack. Being able to identify one's triggers through a daily diary can encourage the headache patient to modify behavior, eating habits, or lifestyle.

REFERENCES

1. Rapoport A, Sheftell F: *Headache disorders: a management guide for practitioners*, Philadelphia, 1996, Saunders.
2. Weiss J: Assessment and management of the client with headaches, *Nurse Pract* 18:44-57, 1993.
3. Matchar DB, McCrory DC, Gray RN: Toward evidence-based management of migraine, *JAMA* 284:2640-2641, 2000.
4. Mannix LK: Epidemiology and impact of primary headache disorders, *Med Clin North Am* 85:887-895, 2001.
5. Lipton RB, Stewart WF, Diamond S, and others: Prevalence and burden of migraine in the United States: data from the American Migraine Study II, *Headache* 41(7):646-657, 2001.
6. Mathew NT: Cluster headache, *Semin Neurol* 17(4):313-323, 1997.
7. Merikangas KR, Stevens DE: Comorbidity of migraine and psychiatric disorders, *Neurol Clin* 15(1):115-123, 1997.
8. Silberstein SD: Advances in understanding the pathophysiology of headache, *Neurology* 42(Suppl 2):S6-S10, 1992.
9. Ward TN: Providing relief from headache pain: current options for acute and prophylactic therapy, *Postgrad Med* 108:121-128, 2000.
10. Headache Classification Committee of the International Headache Society: Classification and diagnostic criteria for headache disorders, cranial neuralgias, and facial pain, *Cephalalgia* 8(Suppl 7):1-96, 1988.
11. Kumar KL, Mathew NT, Silbertstein SD: Migraine: finding the road to relief, *Patient Care* 29(14):90-94, 97-102, 105-110, 1995.
12. Lance JW: Current concepts of migraine pathogenesis, *Neurology* 43(Suppl 3):S11-S15, 1993.
13. Capobianco DJ, Cheshire WP, Campbell JK: An overview of the diagnosis and pharmacologic treatment of migraine, *Mayo Clin Proc* 71:1055-1066, 1996.
14. Walling AD: Cluster headache, *Am Fam Phys* 47:1457-1463, 1993.
15. Campbell JK: Diagnosis and treatment of cluster headache, *J Pain Symptom Manage* 8:155-164, 1993.
16. Solomon GD, Cady RK, Klapper JA, and others: Standards of care for treating headache in primary care practice, *Cleve Clin J Med* 64:373-383, 1996.
17. Morey SS: Guidelines on migraine, part 2, General principles of drug therapy, *Am Fam Phys* 62:1915-1917, 2000.
18. Morey SS: Guidelines on migraine, part 4, General principles of preventive therapy, *Am Fam Phys* 62:2359-2360, 2000.
19. Baumel B: Migraine: a pharmacologic review with newer options and delivery modalities, *Neurology* 44:S13-S17, 1994.
20. Ward TN: Management of an acute primary headache, *Clin Neurosci* 5:50-54, 1998.

CHAPTER 209

Infections of the Central Nervous System

Daniel W. O'Neill and Katherine E. Beben

DEFINITION AND EPIDEMIOLOGY

Infections of the central nervous system (CNS) consist primarily of meningitis (inflammation of the meninges) and encephalitis (inflammation of the brain) and are caused by a variety of pathologic microorganisms. The high morbidity and mortality rates of bacterial meningitis make diagnosis and early treatment a high priority in the primary care setting. Bacterial meningitis is most common in children younger than 2 years, with a peak incidence at 3 to 8 months of age; however, it does occur throughout the life span, with a second peak incidence after 60 years of age. In the United States the annual overall incidence rate is 2 to 5 per 100,000 persons.[1] Despite the use of effective antimicrobial therapy, annual mortality rates remain at 10% to 30%, with up to 50% of survivors having some long-term neurologic sequelae.[1-3]

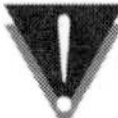

Immediate emergency department referral or physician consultation is indicated for all suspected CNS infections because early treatment reduces morbidity and mortality.

PATHOPHYSIOLOGY

Encephalitis is caused primarily by herpes viruses (40% of cases), arboviruses (transmitted via insects), and enteroviruses, with a peak incidence in the late summer months.[4] Meningitis is defined as either aseptic or septic, depending on the identification of bacteria on the Gram's stain or culture. Aseptic meningitis is caused mostly by enteroviruses, for which there is a good prognosis and no specific therapy. Bacterial meningitis is usually spread hematogenously from another primary source (predominantly the respiratory tract) or via contiguous spread from sinusitis, mastoiditis, or otitis media. The pathogens in meningitis are age specific: group B streptococci and *Escherichia coli* are most common in children under 1 month; *Listeria monocytogenes* is more common in the very young (less than 1 month) and adults over 50 years old; and *Streptococcus pneumoniae* and *Neisseria meningitidis* are the most common causes in children and adults.[2,3] *Haemophilus influenzae* used to be the leading cause of meningitis in young children until the advent of universal vaccination.[1] Because of the widespread overuse of oral antibiotics, there has been a dramatic rise in multidrug-resistant *S. pneumoniae:* nearly one third of isolates show penicillin resistance.[2,3] *N. meningitidis* can occur in epidemic outbreaks in young adults. Elderly adults have a notably higher percentage of infections with gram-negative bacilli and *L. monocytogenes.*

Staphylococci and gram-negative bacilli are the most common causes of postoperative meningitis; staphylococci are common in patients with a cerebrospinal fluid (CSF) shunt. Risk factors for bacterial meningitis are male gender, malignancy and chemotherapy, previous basilar skull fracture or neurosurgery, sickle cell disease, complement deficiency, asplenia, alcoholism, Navajo or Eskimo descent, immunodeficiency (HIV infection or organ transplant recipient), and exposure to a community outbreak.[1] Once the pathogen gains access to the CSF, where there is little natural host defense, it replicates and releases bacterial cell wall proteins, which stimulate cytokine release and capillary leak. This leads to the accumulation of protein and leukocytes, cerebral edema, microvascular thrombosis, and, ultimately, cerebral ischemia and hypoxia.

CLINICAL PRESENTATION

The onset of symptoms of CNS infection can be either acute or subacute, with progression over several days. The classic adult presentation of meningitis is fever, headache, and stiff neck (meningismus). Altered levels of consciousness, seizures, and hypotension predict a poor prognosis.[1] Nausea, vomiting, and photophobia are more common, but can also be seen with migraine. Older adult patients can be seen without fever or meningismus; they are commonly confused or even obtunded, often following an antecedent infection such as bronchitis, pneumonia, sinusitis, or urinary tract infection.[5] Encephalitis manifests with signs and symptoms similar to those of meningitis but with more prevalent alterations in consciousness, focal neurologic signs, seizures, and autonomic and hypothalamic disturbances.[6]

PHYSICAL EXAMINATION

Nuchal rigidity with Kernig's and Brudzinski's signs is detectable in only 50% of cases and thus cannot be used to exclude meningitis. In older adults, nuchal rigidity has an even lower sensitivity and specificity. Kernig's sign is positive if a patient in the supine position resists passive knee extension when the hip is fully flexed on the abdomen. Brudzinski's sign is positive if a patient in the supine position actively flexes the hips when the neck is passively flexed. Purpura or petechiae are often associated with rapidly progressing meningococcemia but can be seen with other infections or can be a sign of disseminated intravascular coagulopathy. In 15% of patients with meningitis, a careful neurologic examination may reveal focal deficits suggestive of brain abscess, cranial nerve inflammation, or cerebral edema. Papilledema is rarely seen; if present, it suggests venous sinus thrombosis, subdural effusion, or brain abscess.[1] Meningitis can lead to signs of increased intracranial pressure (ICP), which include depressed consciousness, sluggishly reactive or dilated pupils, ophthalmoplegia, respiratory depression, bradycardia, hypertension, posturing, hyperreflexia, and spasticity. With clinical presentation alone, it is difficult to distinguish aseptic meningitis from bacterial meningitis or encephalitis.

DIAGNOSTICS

Blood cultures (positive in 80% of patients with bacterial meningitis), CBC, and serum glucose should be obtained immediately. A lumbar puncture (LP) must be obtained in all patients with suspected meningitis or encephalitis, with the following contraindications: cardiorespiratory compromise, evidence of increased ICP, or cellulitis over the LP site.

DIAGNOSTICS

Infections of the Central Nervous System

LABORATORY
CBC and differential
Platelet count
Blood cultures
Serum glucose

IMAGING
CT scan*

OTHER
Lumbar puncture (for cerebrospinal fluid, protein glucose, cell count and differential, Gram's stain and culture; hold extra tubes for special studies)

*If indicated.

Thrombocytopenia is a relative contraindication. If there is evidence of increased ICP or focal neurologic deficits, then an immediate CT scan must be obtained before the LP. The first dose of antimicrobials should be administered *before* the CT scan to avoid critical delays in treatment. The CSF culture can still yield bacteria 1 to 2 hours after the first dose of antibiotics.

Opening CSF pressures should be measured, and a sample of the CSF should be sent for protein, glucose, Gram's stain, culture, and cell count with differential; extra tubes of CSF should be held for special studies, if indicated. Rapid testing of the CSF for antigens of several common pathogens is widely available but not routinely used except in cases of prior antibiotic therapy. Interpretation of CSF values is helpful in distinguishing viral from bacterial infections (Table 209-1), but it has some limitations. Further testing of the CSF with viral cultures, polymerase chain reaction, specialized stains, and cultures may be indicated.

DIFFERENTIAL DIAGNOSIS

Other important viral causes of encephalitis include West Nile virus (epidemic in the United States since an outbreak in New York in 1999 [see Chapter 251]), herpes virus (herpes simplex virus [HSV]-1 and -2 and varicella zoster), mumps virus, influenza virus, lymphocytic choriomeningitis virus, and HIV.[6] Nonviral causes of encephalitis and meningitis include tuberculosis (usually a more indolent course with CSF lymphocytosis and hypoglycemia), spirochetes (e.g., syphilis, Lyme disease), rickettsiae (e.g., Rocky Mountain spotted fever, typhus), protozoa (e.g., malaria), and fungal organisms, each with its own specific therapy.[4] In patients with AIDS, unusual organisms such as *Toxoplasma, Cryptococcus, Histoplasma,* and *Nocardia* organisms; cytomegalovirus; and papovavirus can infect the CNS.[4] Noninfectious causes of encephalitis and meningitis are carcinoma, vasculitis, multiple sclerosis, IV immunoglobulin therapy, drug reactions (e.g., NSAIDs), CNS hemorrhage, and postvaccination aseptic meningitis.[4]

DIFFERENTIAL DIAGNOSIS

Infections of the Central Nervous System

INFECTIOUS
- Herpesvirus
- Mumps virus
- Lymphocytic choriomeningitis virus
- HIV
- Tuberculosis
- Spirochetes
- Rickettsiae
- Protozoa
- Fungal
- Bacteria
- West Nile virus
- Lyme disease

NONINFECTIOUS
- Carcinoma
- Vasculitis
- Multiple sclerosis
- IV immunoglobulin therapy
- Drug reactions
- CNS hemorrhage
- Postvaccination aseptic meningitis

IN PATIENTS WITH AIDS
- *Toxoplasma* organisms
- *Cryptococcus* organisms
- *Histoplasma* organisms
- Cytomegalovirus
- *Nocardia* organisms
- Papovavirus

MANAGEMENT

If bacterial meningitis is suspected, immediate empiric antimicrobial therapy is directed against presumptive pathogens on the basis of age and underlying health status. In most patients, a third-generation cephalosporin such as ceftriaxone (2 g q 12 hr) or cefotaxime (2 g q 6 hr) is recommended.[1,7] This is supplemented with ampicillin (2 g q 4 hr) in adults older than 50 years and in those who are immunocompromised.[1,7] Posttraumatic, neurosurgical, or CSF shunt patients should be started empirically on ceftazidime (2 g q 8 hr) plus vancomycin (1 to 2 g q 12 hr). If gram-positive diplococci are seen on Gram's stain or if a high incidence of penicillin-resistant *S. pneumoniae* (>20%) is known to be present in the community, the addition of vancomycin (1 to 2 g q 12 hr) is currently recommended.[3,7] Other clinical factors and findings on Gram's stain and culture will direct the choice of specific antimicrobial therapy. Adjunctive dexamethasone therapy (10 mg IV q 6 hr for 4 days) *started before or with the first dose of antibiotics* should be used routinely in cases of suspected bacterial meningitis.[1-3,7,8] This is safe and most effective for *H. influenzae* and pneumococcal meningitis in all ages without

TABLE 209-1 Cerebrospinal Fluid Findings in Acute Meningitis

Findings	Normal	Bacterial Meningitis	Viral Meningitis
Opening pressure (mm CSF)	50-195	>180	NL or mildly increased
Cell count (cells/mm^3)	<5 (15% neutrophils)	1000-10,000 (>80% neutrophils)	10-1000 (34% neutrophils)
Protein (mg/dl)	15-50	100-500	50-100
Glucose (mg/dl)	45-80	<40	NL *or* 20-40
CSF:serum glucose	>0.5	<0.4	NL

CSF, Cerebrospinal fluid; *NL,* normal limits.

underlying co-morbidities. If HSV encephalitis is suspected, IV acyclovir (10 mg/kg q 8 hr) should be initiated.[4,6]

COMPLICATIONS

Complications of bacterial meningitis include dehydration, septic shock, hemodynamic compromise, cerebral edema, disseminated intravascular coagulopathy, myocarditis, hyponatremia, seizures, and death (still 20% in some series). Long-term sequelae are seen in 30% of survivors and consist of learning disability, hearing impairment, seizure disorder, visual and motor impairment, ataxia, hydrocephalus, or diabetes insipidus.[1] Permanent neurologic damage is seen in many cases of HSV-1, HSV-2, and eastern equine encephalitis.

INDICATIONS FOR REFERRAL OR HOSPITALIZATION

All cases of suspected meningitis or encephalitis should be immediately referred to a physician experienced in the treatment of CNS infections. All patients with suspected bacterial meningitis should be admitted to the hospital without delay for IV dexamethasone and antimicrobial therapy; 24 hours of respiratory isolation; and close monitoring, possibly in an ICU. IV fluids should be administered cautiously in the absence of hypovolemia to prevent increasing cerebral edema and hyponatremia. If edema is present, mannitol infusions can be used to try to reduce ICP.[4] Consultation with specialists in infectious disease, critical care, neurology, or neurosurgery should be obtained if indicated. Neuropsychiatric testing, rehabilitation specialists, audiologists, psychiatrists, and other counselors may be needed in follow-up care.

PATIENT AND FAMILY EDUCATION

Prevention is a valuable strategy for reducing the morbidity and mortality of bacterial meningitis. The *H. influenzae* type b vaccine has proved to be effective in lowering the attack rate in all ages; it should be strongly encouraged for infants. The 23-valent polysaccharide pneumococcal vaccine should be administered to eligible candidates, including all patients older than 65 years, patients who are immunocompromised, patients with chronic disease, patients without a spleen, or patients in long-term-care facilities.[5] The quadrivalent meningococcal vaccine (MCV4) is available for high-risk patients or travelers to endemic areas and is now recommended as routine vaccination for young adolescents (11- to 12-year-olds).[9,10] To control community outbreaks, chemoprophylaxis with rifampin (600 mg b.i.d. for 2 days) or ciprofloxacin (a single dose of 500 mg) is indicated for close contacts of patients with *N. meningitidis* or *H. influenzae* infection.

HEALTH PROMOTION

The broader implications for public health infrastructure are obvious. Effective surveillance, prevention, and control of vector-borne diseases, including West Nile virus and eastern equine encephalitis, require designated resources in local and state public health departments.[11] This includes public education regarding mosquito control and the prevention of mosquito and tick bites.

REFERENCES

1. Chaudhuri A: Adjunctive dexamethasone treatment in acute bacterial meningitis, *Lancet Neurol* 3:54-62, 2004.
2. Van de Beek D, deGans J, McIntyre P, and others: Steroids in adults with acute bacterial meningitis: a systemic review, *Lancet Infect Dis* 4:139-143, 2004.
3. Pile JC, Longworth DL: Should adults with suspected acute bacterial meningitis get adjunctive corticosteroids? *Cleve Clin J Med* 72(1):67-70, 2005.
4. Kennedy PGE: Viral encephalitis, *J Neurol* 252:268-272, 2005.
5. Miller LG, Choi C: Meningitis in older patients: how to diagnose and treat a deadly infection, *Geriatrics* 52:43-55, 1997.
6. Menaker J, Martin IB, Hirshon JM: Marked elevation of cerebrospinal fluid white blood cell count: an unusual case of *Streptococcus pneumoniae* meningitis, differential diagnosis, and a brief review of current epidemiology and treatment recommendations, *J Emerg Med* 29(1):37-41, 2005.
7. Steiner I, Budka H, Chaudhuri A, and others: Viral encephalitis: a review of diagnostic methods and guidelines for management, *Eur J Neurol* 12:331-343, 2005.
8. Correia JB, Hart CA: Meningococcal disease, *Clin Evid* 12:1164-1181, 2004.
9. Harrison LH: Preventing meningococcal infection in college students, *Clin Infect Dis* 30:648-651, 2000.
10. Centers for Disease Control and Prevention: *Meningococcal diseases and meningococcal vaccine: fact sheet,* April 2005, retrieved Feb 12, 2007, from http://www.cdc.gov/nip/vaccine/mening/mening_fs.htm.
11. Centers for Disease Control and Prevention: Guidelines for surveillance, prevention, and control of West Nile virus infection—United States, *MMWR* 49:25-28, 2000.

CHAPTER 210

Movement Disorders and Essential Tremor

Nancy McQueen Le

MOVEMENT DISORDERS

DEFINITION AND EPIDEMIOLOGY

A number of neurologic disorders cause difficulty with movement, leading to hypokinesis or hyperkinesis. Some manifest as uncontrolled, strikingly awkward muscle contractions of various parts of the body. Others are seen as an awkward, wide-stance gait, and still others involve exceedingly low muscle tone and inability to move various parts of the body.

These movement disorders are caused by dysfunction of the extrapyramidal system of the brain, which extends through the cerebellar and basal ganglia regions.[1,2] Movement disorders may be physical only or may include other manifestations, such as dementia. The disorders are typically divided into categories based on one of the two affected brain regions. They may be inherited, infectious, a result of substance misuse or abuse, a result of trauma, or idiopathic.[1] They may be self-limiting and resolve spontaneously, or chronic and progressive.

PATHOPHYSIOLOGY

The cerebellum is responsible for smooth, coordinated movement of the body. It influences both voluntary and involuntary motion.[1] Cerebellar dysfunction is broken down into three categories: vestibulocerebellar dysfunction (loss of flow from one movement to the next), cerebellar ataxia disorders (steadiness and gait), and cerebellar tremor (rhythmic oscillations with motion).[1] Extremity abnormalities are on the same side as the brain dysfunction. They occur whether the eyes are open or closed.[1] There is no tremor seen with the patient at rest.

The basal ganglia affect posture, muscle tone, and gracefulness. They acquire input from several parts of the body, including the cerebellum, the special sense organs, sensation, and the motor cortex. Dysfunctions of the basal ganglia affect the opposite side of the body and will be found at rest.[1] Symptoms diminish with voluntary movement.

CLINICAL PRESENTATION

The patient may complain of involuntary, awkward body movements. Symptoms can be minor to severe and include tremors, difficulty starting or stopping voluntary motion, and loss of facial muscle tone and expression. Symptoms will be worse in the presence of stress or fatigue.[1,2] A careful medication and drug history is therefore important and should include prescription, over-the-counter, and illicit drug use. Inquiry about alcohol or drug intake is necessary because alcohol intoxication can cause severe ataxia and in other cases improve a tremor, whereas LSD (lysergic acid diethylamide) can produce a parkinsonian picture. Some medications can cause tardive dyskinesia, a permanent change in cell receptor sites that causes slow and awkward movements.

It is important to ascertain the age of onset, progression, factors that make symptoms better or worse, the quality of movements and dysfunction, the region(s) of the body affected, the severity of disability, and timing. A family history of movement disorder should be noted.

PHYSICAL EXAMINATION

A complete neurologic examination, as well as examination of any other pertinent systems, is indicated. Subtle findings in involuntary movement may differentiate between some of the disorders. A good description of the movements, including the side of the body affected and whether the movements occur when the person is at rest or in motion, is crucial.[2-4] Depending on the disorder, deep tendon reflexes (DTRs), muscle tone, gait, Romberg's sign, or Babinski's reflex may be altered.[2] A Mini-Mental State Examination is also important to demonstrate any cognitive dysfunction and to monitor disease progression.[2]

Nystagmus is common with cerebellar disorders.[1] With ataxia, Romberg's test will be difficult, if not impossible, to perform; the gait is often staggering and unsteady. Rapid, alternating movement testing reveals slow, purposeful, jerky, and uncoordinated movement. Performance of the finger-to-nose test may also be jerky and overcorrected. Cerebellar (intention) tremor, like essential tremor, is a rhythmic oscillation of the finger or toe that increases as a target is approached.[1] It begins with intentional movement and is not found at rest. Cerebellar dysfunction can also affect speech, usually causing slurred, slow speech with varying amplitude. There may be a loss of the automatic movements of the body, such as the arm swing.[1,5]

With disorders of the basal ganglia, abnormal movement may be either hyperkinetic or bradykinetic, depending on which part of the basal ganglia is involved. These disorders include tremor; hemiballismus (jumping around of body parts); chorea (facial contortions and flexion-extension movements of the extremities); athetosis (twisting, wormlike movements of the face, arms, and legs, like a screwdriver); or difficult movement of the head, trunk, and extremities.[1,2] Oral motor tone can be impaired, which can affect speech and ability to swallow.

DIAGNOSTICS

Diagnostic studies to consider include a head CT scan or MRI to exclude tumors or cerebellar defects. A positron emission tomography (PET) scan can help exclude parkinsonism and is being evaluated for use in the diagnosis of essential tremor.[5,6] A thyroid panel, including thyroid-stimulating hormone, is recommended to eliminate thyrotoxicosis or hyperthyroidism. An adrenal x-ray study or CT scan, or urine or blood catecholamine levels, can help exclude pheochromocytoma. This analysis should be done when the patient is symptomatic to avoid false-negative test results. Liver function tests will help eliminate hepatic causes for the tremor or ataxia. A CBC and antistreptolysin O titer can help identify infectious causes.[2,3] Serum amino acid levels and urine organic acid analysis can be used to further evaluate metabolic conditions.

DIAGNOSTICS

Movement Disorders

LABORATORY	IMAGING
TSH	MRI, CT scan
LFTs	Consider PET scan
CBC and differential	
Antistreptolysin O titer	
Organic acid screen (urine)	
Amino acid screen (serum)	

DIFFERENTIAL DIAGNOSIS

The cause of movement disorders may be idiopathic or related to a number of degenerative, metabolic, or vascular disorders. Medications should always be reviewed and considered possible precipitants. Neoplasms, infection, anoxia, head trauma, brain surgery, colloid cysts, syringomyelia, and Munchausen's syndrome are also potential causes.

MANAGEMENT

Once the presence of a movement disorder has been determined, a thorough neurologic evaluation is indicated for diagnosis and treatment recommendations. Referral to a neurologist or neurosubspecialist may be indicated. In many cases treatment is directed at controlling or relieving the symptoms; there usually is no cure. For the remaining movement disorders, it is important to treat the underlying condition, such as infection, hormone imbalance, or drug withdrawal.

Disease progression and functional ability should be continually monitored.[3] Haloperidol (Haldol) and phenothiazines may be helpful for chorea and tic syndromes; clonazepam (Klonopin) may be used for myoclonus; and reserpine or haloperidol may be recommended for hemiballismus and tardive dyskinesia.[2,3]

DIFFERENTIAL DIAGNOSIS

Movement Disorders

DEGENERATIVE DISORDERS
- Parkinson's disease
- Huntington's chorea
- Supranuclear palsy
- Hallervorden-Spatz disease
- Olivopontocerebellar atrophies

METABOLIC DISORDERS
- Leigh's disease
- Wilson's disease
- Hormone deficiencies
- Metabolic acidemias
- Organic acidemias

VASCULAR DISORDERS
- Cerebellar or basal ganglia
- Bleed, infarction

MEDICATIONS OR DRUGS
- LSD, methyl-4-phenyl-1,2,3,6-tetrahydropyridine (MPTP)
- Dopamine antagonists
- Dopamine agonists
- Tardive dyskinesia
- CNS stimulants

NEOPLASMS
- Cerebellar or basal ganglia

OTHER CONDITIONS
- Idiopathic infections
- Anoxia
- Head trauma
- Syringomyelia
- Munchausen's syndrome
- Brain surgery
- Colloid cyst

LIFE SPAN CONSIDERATIONS

If the symptoms are severe, activities of daily living, including the ability to feed oneself, may be compromised, and a wheelchair may be necessary. Even with milder symptoms, patients may be self-conscious and experience increased anxiety, which accentuates the disorder.[2] Some patients may be able to learn compensatory strategies to alter or limit unwanted movement.[3] A physical therapist is a valuable resource for this purpose. Unfortunately, the ability to compensate may decrease as the disease progresses.[3] With some of these conditions, such as metabolic or organic acidemias, the life span can be significantly limited; some people die in childhood.

COMPLICATIONS

Some medications may cause undesired side effects. Impotence, exacerbations of asthma or emphysema, or problems with diabetic hypoglycemic control are potential concerns that should be addressed at each office visit. Neuroleptics used to treat these disorders can cause movement disorders, complicating the clinical picture.

The loss of facial expression is also possible.[2] Although this seems benign, facial immobility can affect nonverbal communication. Conscientious patient and family education can promote understanding of the disease process, and alternative ways of communication can be explored.

If the disease process is infectious, confinement is a consideration.

INDICATIONS FOR REFERRAL OR HOSPITALIZATION

Consultation with a physician, often with a neurologist or subspecialist, is indicated for evaluation and management of the various movement disorders. Physical, occupational, and speech therapy, as well as psychiatric consultation, may be beneficial. Hospitalization is generally reserved for complications of disease rather than for the specific disease process itself.

PATIENT AND FAMILY EDUCATION

Understanding the diagnosis and prognosis is beneficial for patients and families. Facilitating the identification of resources to promote awareness of the disease process and treatment options is important. Support and informational groups are available on the Internet, and good information can be found in public and medical libraries.

The following are good resources for patients with movement disorders:

- **We Move (Worldwide Education and Awareness for Movement Disorders)**: http://www.wemove.org
- **Awakenings** (Parkinson's disease): http://www.parkinsonsdisease.com
- **Neurosupport**: http://www.neurosupport.org.uk (supports people with neurologic disorders and their families)

HEALTH PROMOTION

Understanding the specific disease process can be the foundation to better health for these individuals and their families. Appropriate diet, exercise, social support, physical or occupational therapy as indicated, and assistive devices can significantly enhance quality of life.

ESSENTIAL TREMOR

DEFINITION AND EPIDEMIOLOGY

Essential tremor is a benign, chronic neurologic condition that involves symmetric, rhythmic trembling of the upper extremities, head, and/or voice. The legs are less commonly involved. The only clinical finding is the tremor, which may be present at rest and usually progresses over time.[4-6]

The oscillations of 4 to 12 Hz are present throughout voluntary movement and are accentuated as the hand approaches a given target.[2,5] Emotional stress will also increase the symptoms, whereas alcohol or rest will diminish them.[2,4] Known as *benign, familial, hereditary,* or *senile tremor,*[4] this is the most common of the movement disorders. Men and women are affected equally, with a mean age of onset of 45 years. The condition can begin as early as adolescence but most often begins in the sixth or seventh decade of life. An estimated 10 million people in the United States are afflicted with this condition. If more than one person in a family group has the condition, the tremor is termed *familial* or *hereditary tremor.* An autosomal dominant inheritance pattern can be identified in more than 50% of cases. If the tremor begins in old age, it is commonly termed *senile tremor*.[4-6]

PATHOPHYSIOLOGY

Although it is a neurologic disorder, little is known about the etiology of essential tremor.[4] To date, no structural defects have been identified on autopsy, and diagnostic studies are typically normal. It is believed to be caused by focal oscillatory activity within the central nervous system.[6] PET scan studies have found changes in regional blood flow in the cerebellum and inferior olivary nuclei of patients with essential tremor compared with matched control subjects.[6] It is unclear at this time if that finding is specific to essential tremor alone or is also found in other tremors. Because of the autosomal dominant inheritance, a thorough family history may prove helpful in establishing the diagnosis.[4-6] There is high variability in the rate of development of this disease.

CLINICAL PRESENTATION

For essential tremor, the patient's only complaint is that of tremor; any additional neurologic deficits should prompt consideration of an alternative diagnosis.[5,6] The patient typically complains of a tremor at rest. The tremor becomes worse when the patient tries to move his or her hand or fingers in a purposeful manner. Furthermore, the amplitude of the tremor increases as the patient approaches his or her desired target.[2]

The patient may have difficulty writing, eating, or performing other fine motor tasks. The head may nod ("yes" movements) or shake ("no" movements). Eyelid and facial tremor is also common.[3] The voice may quaver or shake. The tremor may be continual; however, it may also be episodic, sporadic, or intermittent.[4] Generally, the tremor disappears during sleep. A careful history of food, coffee or caffeine, antihistamine, medication, or illicit drug intake, as well as other symptoms, is helpful in excluding other causes for the tremor.[2]

Patients often complain that the tremor is worse during periods of increased emotional stress or when they are trying to hurry. The tremor decreases with rest and alcohol; for this reason, a careful inquiry about alcohol consumption should be performed.[2]

The patient will not have problems with weakness or changes in muscle tone, nor will there be problems with coordination despite the tremor. The tremor generally does not affect the lower extremities.[2]

The patient may have had the tremor for several years. A disabling disease progression may be what has brought the patient to the health care provider's attention. A careful history, including the age of onset, rate of progression and symmetry of the tremor, and exacerbating or alleviating factors, should be taken.

PHYSICAL EXAMINATION

An upper extremity tremor that cycles 6 to 10 times per second is obvious. The amplitude of this tremor increases with voluntary movement, particularly as the patient approaches a specific target.[2] The rate of cycles per second should remain unchanged. The fingertip-to-nose test is particularly helpful in eliciting this phenomenon.[3] The patient may have difficulty writing or grasping small objects. Examination should include having the patient draw a circle; this is a useful marker for disease progression, as well as for monitoring treatment efficacy. The drawing should be included in the medical record. The patient's voice may quiver, and the head may shake or nod rhythmically. The eyelids and facial muscles may also twitch. All findings should be documented and updated at subsequent visits.[2,4]

Muscle tone, gait, and posture should all be normal. The lower extremities should be tremor free. The arm swing with walking should be relatively normal. DTRs should also be normal; there should be no clonus.[2] Other findings suggest an alternative diagnosis.

DIAGNOSTICS

The diagnosis is generally based on the history and examination findings. Laboratory or diagnostic testing should be considered when findings other than an isolated, generally symmetric upper extremity tremor is noted.[2]

DIFFERENTIAL DIAGNOSIS

Tremors may originate in the central nervous system, arise from metabolic abnormalities, or be induced by medication or alcohol. Central nervous system tremors may be caused by Parkinson's disease, Huntington's chorea, or Sydenham's chorea (secondary to streptococcal infections), or they may be cerebellar in nature. Metabolic tremors may be related to a thyroid abnormality, pheochromocytoma, or liver disease.

MANAGEMENT

Initially, reassurance may be all that is necessary.[2] If the tremor becomes problematic, a number of medication regimens can help. Finding the medicine that is most effective but has

DIFFERENTIAL DIAGNOSIS

Essential Tremor

CNS TREMORS
- Cerebellar tremor
- Sydenham's chorea secondary to streptococcal infections
- Parkinsonism
- Huntington's chorea

METABOLIC TREMORS
- Hyperthyroidism
- Hypothyroidism
- Pheochromocytoma
- Liver disease

MEDICATIONS OR DRUGS
- Antihistamines
- Stimulants
- Caffeine
- Alcohol withdrawal
- Illicit drugs

TUMORS
- Primary or metastatic neoplasm
- Cervical spine tumor

minimum side effects may require persistent trials and evaluations. Some of the commonly prescribed medications pose a risk for dependence.

The most commonly prescribed medication for this condition is propranolol (Inderal) 80 mg h.s. Symptoms should be reevaluated after 1 to 2 weeks. A number of placebo-controlled studies evaluating a number of beta blockers clearly demonstrate their efficacy, with 40% to 50% of patients experiencing relief.[6,7]

Primidone, at 50 to 350 mg at bedtime, in double-blind, placebo-controlled studies appears to be effective in reducing or eliminating tremor, especially hand tremor.[6] The dosage begins at 25 mg/night and is increased by 50 mg each week until the tremor is controlled. Like propranolol, primidone reduces the amplitude, but not the frequency, of the tremor.

Botulinum toxin (BTX-A) has been used to effectively treat limb, vocal, palatal, and other tremors, in addition to head and hand tremors. One double-blind, placebo-controlled study demonstrated that 75% of BTX-A–treated patients vs. 27% of placebo patients reported mild to moderate benefit at 4 weeks after treatment.[6]

Other medications to consider include nadolol (Corgard) 40 mg/day, clonazepam (Klonopin) 0.5 mg t.i.d., gabapentin (Neurontin) 100 to 2400 mg/day, alprazolam (Xanax) 0.25 to 0.5 mg t.i.d., diazepam (Valium) 2 to 10 mg b.i.d. to t.i.d. increased gradually, topiramate (Topamax) 25 to 300 mg/day, nicardipine hydrochloride (Cardene) 10 to 60 mg/day, nimodipine (Nimotop) 30 to 180 mg/day, and methazolamide (Neptazane) 50 to 100 mg b.i.d. to t.i.d.[3,6,7] These drugs have been used for many years, but limited information is available on their efficacy.

Thalamic stimulation, the implantation of an electrode deep into the thalamus, has been shown to reduce tremor by up to 80%. This deep brain stimulation has proven to be effective with fewer complications than thalamotomy.[8] A real benefit is that this procedure is reversible should other treatments be available in the future. This procedure is expensive and requires close patient follow-up.

Alcohol is often listed as beneficial for tremor sufferers; however, few formal studies have been completed to demonstrate its efficacy.[4-6]

LIFE SPAN CONSIDERATIONS

Although essential tremor is considered a benign condition, it may have a profound effect on the patient's quality of life. The tremor may be embarrassing, particularly in younger patients. The condition may cause the patient to withdrawal socially to avoid the social ramifications.[2,6,7] Careful observation for depression, alcoholism, and suicidal ideation in younger patients is important. Antidepressants and counseling may be required to help patients cope with the disorder.

Severe tremors can significantly interfere with activities of daily living. Basic fine motor activities can be impossible for some patients. Treatment is aimed at controlling the severity of the tremor to facilitate independence.[2,4-7]

COMPLICATIONS

Alcohol dependency is a potential complication. The patient should be advised to avoid overuse. The patient who consumes more than one glass of wine or other alcoholic beverage per day needs to be monitored closely.[3]

All the medications used to treat essential tremor have side effects, and drug-drug interactions are a concern if the patient is taking other medications. It is important to inquire about the tolerability of the medicine at all subsequent patient visits. Inquiry about impaired sexual function and impotence is necessary because the patient generally will not discuss these side effects unless asked directly. Their effects on the patient's life, however, can be significant.

INDICATIONS FOR REFERRAL OR HOSPITALIZATION

Consultation with a physician, possibly a neurologist, is warranted if the cause is unclear. Speech therapy may be helpful if the voice tremor is severe. If conservative management fails to control severe tremors, surgical intervention is available.[4-8] Although studies have evaluated the effectiveness of surgery in reducing tremor in these patients, the numbers are small.[6]

Management questions or difficulty controlling the tremor with prescribed medication also warrants physician consultation.

PATIENT AND FAMILY EDUCATION

The patient should be advised to avoid stimulants such as caffeine, soda, or coffee. Many over-the-counter allergy and cold preparations have stimulants in them that can also accentuate the tremors.

Careful education about the chronicity, progression, and prognosis of the disease is necessary. Although it is medically considered a benign condition, this disorder may have significant psychosocial implications, requiring frequent reevaluation and patient support. Patients also should understand that if the condition is hereditary, their children have a 50% chance of inheriting the same condition.[2,4]

Support groups such as the International Tremor Foundation can be helpful (PO Box 14005, Lenexa, KS 66285-4005; [913] 341-3880 or [888] 387-3667; fax [913] 341-1296; http://www.essentialtremor.org).

HEALTH PROMOTION

Understanding the disease process and receiving support as necessary can help improve the patient's health and quality of life. An appropriate diet and a good exercise program can also be beneficial. Alcohol abuse should always be a concern because consumption can limit the tremor.

REFERENCES

1. Porth CM: *Pathophysiology: concepts of altered health states,* ed 4, Philadelphia, 1994, Lippincott.
2. Olson WH, Brumback RA: *Symptom-oriented neurology: handbook for primary care,* ed 2, St Louis, 1994, Mosby.
3. Weiner W, Goetz C: *Neurology for the non-neurologist,* ed 3, Philadelphia, 1994, Lippincott.
4. Tierney L, McPhee S, Papadakis M: *Current medical diagnosis and treatment,* Norwalk, Conn, 1999, Lange.
5. Louis ED: Clinical practice: essential tremor, *N Engl J Med* 345:887-891, 2001.
6. Koller WC, Deuschl G: Essential tremor, *Neurology* 54(11 Suppl 4):S7, 2000.
7. Evidente VGH: Understanding essential tremor, differential diagnosis and options for treatment, *Postgrad Med* 108:138-140, 143-146, 149, 2000.
8. Schuurman PR, Bosch DA, Bossuyt PMM, and others: A comparison of continuous thalamic stimulation and thalamotomy for suppression of severe tremor, *N Engl J Med* 342:461-468, 2000.

CHAPTER 211

Multiple Sclerosis

Nancy McQueen Le

DEFINITION AND EPIDEMIOLOGY

Multiple sclerosis (MS) is a chronic disease affecting the brain and spinal cord. It is believed to be an autoimmune disease in which the immune system attacks myelin, a fatty tissue that surrounds and protects nerve fibers. The hallmark lesion in MS is called a *plaque* and was first described 2 centuries ago.[1] When viewed microscopically, these plaques are characterized by inflammation, destruction of myelin sheath, and eventual replacement by scar tissue. Lesions are described as demyelinating because of the loss of myelin; however, not all demyelinating lesions are caused by MS. Multiple lesions are seen in multiple locations in the central nervous system (CNS)—hence the name *multiple sclerosis.* Clues to the etiology of MS come from the worldwide and nonrandom pattern of this disease; from the studies of structural and functional changes within the CNS; from neuroimmunologic studies; and from genetic studies, particularly studies of families and twins.[2-6] To date, no single etiologic factor has been identified. Box 211-1 describes the many manifestations of MS.

The onset of MS is likely to occur between 20 and 50 years of age, affecting three times as many females as males. MS affects up to 500,000 Americans and approximately 2.5 million persons worldwide. The worldwide pattern of MS shows that it is rare near the equator, and the highest incidence is across northern Europe, North America, and Australia. It occurs predominantly in Caucasians.[7]

Physician consultation is indicated for all suspected cases of MS.

BOX 211-1

MANIFESTATIONS OF MULTIPLE SCLEROSIS

Relapsing-remitting: Course punctuated by relapses (exacerbations) followed by periods of remission

Primary-progressive: Accumulating disability from initial presentation onward

Secondary-progressive: Accumulating disability after a period of relapsing-remitting disease

Progressive-relapsing: Steadily progressive from onset, but also with acute attacks

Benign: Mild form; patient is fully functional in all neurologic systems

Malignant: Rapidly progressive course with severe disability and death

Transverse myelitis: Inflammation of spinal cord; may be single episode or harbinger of multiple sclerosis (MS)

Optic neuritis: Inflammation of optic nerve, often only symptom; may be first sign of MS

Devic's disease: Neuromyelitis optica, transverse myelopathy, and optic neuritis; considered unfinished form of MS

PATHOPHYSIOLOGY

It is theorized that MS is accompanied by, if not caused by, a disturbance in the function of the immune system. On the basis of animal models and immunopathologic studies of MS lesions, there is increasing evidence that MS results from an unknown trigger that stimulates a cell-mediated perivascular inflammatory response in genetically predisposed persons.

The sequence of these events has become better clarified. CNS-activated T lymphocytes trigger inflammatory processes, which create leaks in the blood-brain barrier. This then causes further damaging effects, resulting in destruction of myelin. This response is an attack on an individual's own cells (autoimmunity). Remyelination is a repair process whereby the brain is able to use brain stem cells that differentiate to rebuild myelin. This is why, particularly early in the disease, symptoms improve or resolve. However, repeated demyelination leads to less effective remyelination, leaving scarred demyelinated areas called plaques. Progressive MS symptoms occur because of cumulative, multiple lesions in the brain and spinal cord.

CLINICAL PRESENTATION

The initial presentation of MS is variable. Often initial symptoms are transient or mild and may not prompt a medical visit. Common initial symptoms include sensory symptoms (paresthesias), optic neuritis, limb weakness, diplopia (intranuclear ophthalmoplegia), nystagmus, unsteady gait, myelopathy (transverse myelitis), and trigeminal neuralgia. Associated findings that increase the likelihood of MS include unexplained excessive fatigue, temperature or heat sensitivity, a history of bandlike sensations around the waist, dysarthria, muscle spasms, and altered bowel or bladder function.

MS has four clinical subtypes standardized by the National Multiple Sclerosis Society.[7] These are relapsing-remitting, primary-progressive, secondary-progressive, and progressive-relapsing (see Box 211-1). This differentiation may not be clear in a particular patient early in the course. However, it becomes important as the disease progresses in terms of recommended treatment options and anticipated prognosis.

As the disease progresses, a variety of typical symptoms and findings will require ongoing medical and rehabilitation management (see Table 211-2).

PHYSICAL EXAMINATION

The initial diagnosis of MS relies heavily on a careful physical and neurologic examination and a focused review of systems. Some patients can be diagnosed clinically on the first visit, but many situations are more difficult, especially when a patient has only transient symptoms or one symptomatic episode. Examination should include a thorough review of systems, with detailed focus on neurologic symptoms. Common initial symptoms or findings include sensory changes, optic neuritis, weakness, double vision, and unsteady gait. Other findings may include nystagmus, speech difficulty, tremor, clumsiness, muscle spasms, bowel or bladder changes, cognitive difficulties, sexual dysfunction, and excessive fatigue.

In a patient with known MS, having a documented neurologic and functional baseline is imperative for evaluating response to treatment or possible exacerbation of the disease. New neurologic findings can be mild or subtle, yet result in significant functional deficits. Functional areas to review or examine might include balance, transfers, and activities of daily living.

DIAGNOSTICS

A health care provider may determine that the patient has a working diagnosis of clinically definite MS, clinically probable MS, laboratory-supported definite MS, or laboratory-probable MS.[8] Diagnostic criteria include:

- At least two distinct episodes of neurologic significance lasting at least 24 hours and occurring at least 1 month apart
- More than one lesion at more than a single site in the CNS on neurologic examination
- Signs and symptoms that cannot be explained by another medical condition

Neuroimaging may reveal areas of demyelination from chronic plaques and active disease. The sensitivity of the test is very high, whereas the specificity is not. The MRI does not always correlate with the patient's clinical picture. Periods of increased MRI activity (enhanced by the use of the contrast agent gadolinium) may be associated with deterioration of the patient's functional abilities. Less often, patients have significant clinical disease with little MRI activity. Clinically, patients who look the same (e.g., have similar disability measures) may have completely different histopathologic results and MRI activity levels. Through the use of serial MRI monitoring, it is now known that gadolinium enhancements may reveal MS before clinical expression of disease activity and that the disease may be active biologically before it becomes clinically apparent.[9]

Evoked potential/evoked response (EP/ER) studies measure the electrical potential in the brain in response to stimulation of a sensory system. These tests are abnormal in the majority of patients with clinically definite MS. These tests also provide a measure of brain and cord *function* that complements the MRI, which provides information about brain *structure*.[10] In patients with only a single spinal cord or brain lesion, EPs may be helpful in establishing a diagnosis of MS. Visual EPs (VEPs) assess nerve conduction through the optic nerve. Brainstem auditory EPs and somatosensory EPs work similarly to assess the integrity of brain and cord pathways. VEPs are the most helpful in providing objective evidence of optic neuritis or an optic nerve lesion, even when the clinical examination is normal. VEPs tend to worsen over time.[10]

Changes in cerebrospinal fluid (CSF) have long been used to support a clinical diagnosis

DIAGNOSTICS

Multiple Sclerosis

LABORATORY
Cerebrospinal fluid IgG
Lyme titer*
ESR*
Antinuclear antibodies*
Vitamin B_{12} levels
Fluorescent treponemal antibody absorption test*

IMAGING
MRI with gadolinium

OTHER
Evoked potential/evoked response studies
Lumbar puncture*

*If indicated.

of MS. A lumbar puncture may be performed if the MRI is not helpful but the clinical picture suggests MS. The most common abnormality is a selective increase in immunoglobulin G. In MS, discrete bands called *single oligoclonal bands* may be seen with electrophoretic separation of CSF proteins. Patients must have two or more of these bands for diagnostic significance.

Further diagnostics should be guided by clinical presentation, physical examination, and consideration of the differential diagnosis.

DIFFERENTIAL DIAGNOSIS

Because many neurologic conditions must be considered, the differential diagnosis is extensive. CNS infections; syphilis; tumors; Lyme disease; vitamin B_{12} deficiency; and autoimmune processes such as systemic lupus erythematosus, sarcoidosis, or vasculitis should be included in the differential diagnosis.

MANAGEMENT

Management of MS is accomplished through a partnership with the patient, family members, and a core team of professionals. In general, the health care provider is the primary patient advocate and coordinates the care plan, educates patients and families in all aspects of the treatment plan, initiates referrals to specialists, triages problems, identifies candidates for research protocols, monitors regular preventive services, and surveys the medication profile. This role may be shared with a neurologist or a center specializing in MS.

The National Multiple Sclerosis Society offers a vast array of resources for care providers, including current research, treatment and care guidelines, and educational programs.[7] Four areas of management for patients with MS include modifying the disease course, treating exacerbations, managing symptoms, and improving function and safety.

Early management of MS begins with initiation of disease-modifying agents as indicated, and as soon as possible. Table 211-1 lists the five current immunomodulating drug therapies approved by the U.S. Food and Drug Administration (FDA) for the treatment of MS. Three are naturally occurring interferons (Betaseron, Avonex, and Rebif), and one is a synthetic protein (glatiramer [Copaxone]). These agents are approved for the treatment of relapsing-remitting MS. An antineoplastic agent (mitoxantrone [Novantrone]) was approved in October 2000 for the treatment of secondary-progressive and progressive-relapsing MS. It is *not* approved for the treatment of relapsing-remitting disease. The interferons, which should not be taken during pregnancy, have a similar biologic activity and an adverse event profile. Patients should be monitored for depression while on treatment. The administration of mitoxantrone requires careful cardiac evaluation and monitoring. It also carries a lifetime accumulated dose limit because of the risk of cardiac toxicity. Of all of these agents, it carries the highest pregnancy risk warning.[11]

Natalizumab (Tysabri) is a monoclonal antibody with immunosuppressant effect that appeared promising in active clinical trials. It was taken off the market in February 2005 after three reported cases (two fatal) of progressive multifocal leukoencephalopathy. After much study the FDA in March 2006 approved resumption of the studies, only for those patients previously enrolled and under strict monitoring guidelines.

Treating an exacerbation typically involves giving high-dose IV steroids over a short period. The goal is to minimize the duration of inflammation and so incur fewer lasting deficits. After an exacerbation most patients benefit greatly from a course of rehabilitation to address any specific new deficits or loss of function, as well as to improve overall physical fitness to maintain function.

Other agents that exert immunosuppressant effects include azathioprine (Imuran), methotrexate (Rheumatrex), cyclophosphamide (Cytoxan), and cladribine (Leustatin). All have been studied, with varying degrees of reported efficacy.[12]

Studies of other experimental therapies, including monoclonal antibodies, vaccines, bee venom therapy, plasmapheresis, and total lymphoid irradiation, have been inconclusive.

Table 211-2 shows symptomatic and rehabilitative therapies that are the biggest challenge in the co-management partnership described above.

DIFFERENTIAL DIAGNOSIS

Multiple Sclerosis

Tumors, especially lymphoma or glioma of brain or spinal cord	Collagen vascular disease
Spinal cord compression	• Systemic lupus erythematosus
• Spondylosis	• Polyarteritis
• Herniated disc	Neurosarcoidosis
• Epidural tumor	Encephalitis
Degenerative disorder	Neurosyphilis
• Motor neuron disease (amyotrophic lateral sclerosis)	HIV encephalopathy
	Lyme disease
	Vitamin B_{12} deficiency
• Spinocerebellar degeneration	Vasculitis

LIFE SPAN CONSIDERATIONS

In some situations, a diagnosis of MS is actually followed by relief, especially for patients who have spent years experiencing strange symptoms and have met with an indeterminable diagnosis. For others the diagnosis is difficult—the variable clinical course of MS leads to an uncertain and unpredictable future. Many persons with MS are still capable of ambulation and regular employment 20 years after diagnosis. The life span is shortened only slightly compared with that of the general population. Several factors are associated with a favorable prognosis: (1) female gender, (2) age of disease onset less than 40 years, (3) sensory symptoms without impairment in ambulation, (4) optic neuritis as an isolated first symptom, and (5) minor abnormalities of the brain MRI at the time of diagnosis.[13]

COMPLICATIONS AND INDICATIONS FOR REFERRAL OR HOSPITALIZATION

If MS is suspected or diagnosed, referral to a neurologist is recommended. The management of care over the long term may have the neurologist take the role of primary manager, with medical issues deferred to the health care provider. In

TABLE 211-1 Disease-Modifying Therapies for Multiple Sclerosis

	Betaseron (Interferon Beta-1b)	Avonex (Interferon Beta-1a)	Copaxone (Glatiramer Acetate)	Novantrone (Mitoxantrone)	Rebif (Interferon Beta-1a)
Description	rDNA technology	rDNA technology	Synthetic mixture of 4 amino acids	Antineoplastic agent	rDNA technology
Action	Antiviral, immunomodulatory	Antiviral, immunomodulatory	Immune system modifier	Immune system modifier	Antiviral, immunomodulatory
Efficacy	Reduces exacerbation rate Tends to slow disease progression	Reduces exacerbation rate Reduces rate of disability progression	Reduces exacerbation rate Trend in slowing disability progression	Reduces exacerbation rate Delays disability progression Reduces number of treated relapses	Reduces exacerbation rate Delays progression of disability
MRI	Decreases lesion load	Changes in lesion load not statistically significant	Data unavailable	Reduces number of *new* lesions detected	Decreases lesion load
Dosing	8 mIU SQ q.o.d.	6 mIU IM weekly	20 mg/day SQ	12 mg/m^2 IV q 3 mo Lifetime cumulative dose limit of 140 mg/m^2 because of cardiac toxicity	44 mcg SQ 3 × per week
Adverse events	Flulike symptoms Injection site reaction Depression Laboratory abnormalities	Flulike symptoms Depression Laboratory abnormalities Asthenia	Immediate postinjection reaction Injection site reaction Chest pain Vasodilation	Myelosuppression Infection Sepsis Cardiac toxicity Heart failure Arrhythmias Renal failure Hyperuricemia Side effects: nausea, hair loss, menstrual disorders	Flulike symptoms Depression Laboratory abnormalities Injection site reactions

other cases the health care provider may remain the primary manager with the neurologist more strictly consultative. Regardless, over the long term a key piece of management should include a rehabilitation approach, with referrals to physical, occupational, and speech therapists or vocational specialists as indicated.

Referral to an ophthalmologist should be considered early on to establish a baseline and for regular monitoring, given the frequency of visual issues with MS. Tone and spasticity may warrant referral to specialized clinic for advanced management, such as botulinum toxin (Botox) or baclofen pump. Skin issues, especially those related to pressure ulcers or bowel and bladder incontinence, must be addressed. Urology consult may be sought for refractory bladder problems, which may affect up to 80% of MS patients,[14] or for evaluation of erectile dysfunction. Psychiatric issues, particularly depression and difficulty coping, are common. Referrals for medication evaluation or counseling may be indicated. If cognitive deficits are suspected or have become evident, a neuropsychologist can help define the deficits and give recommendations regarding safety, behavior, or functional issues such as working, parenting, or managing finances.

Hospitalization may be used short term for administration of IV steroids during an exacerbation. Also, if an infection is more than routine or precipitates an exacerbation, hospitalization may be necessary for medical management. If an exacerbation is significant, or if the patient has suffered progressive, chronic declines in function, admission to a rehabilitation hospital may be warranted for more aggressive and complex rehabilitation management.

Long-term steroid therapy contributes to bone demineralization. Bone densitometry is a useful way to monitor a patient's risk for fractures or further disability. Alendronate (Fosamax) or similar agents may be given for the prevention of osteoporosis, especially in postmenopausal women.

Patients with MS are at higher risk of developing other autoimmune diseases such as thyroid disease, diabetes, or rheumatoid arthritis. These diseases should be screened for and treated as indicated.[15]

PATIENT AND FAMILY EDUCATION

The diagnosis of MS can be devastating for patients and families. Considerable support and education about the disease process, its variability, and available therapies are essential. The health care provider may emphasize interventions that a patient can control rather than what is uncontrollable or unpredictable. Controllable interventions include exercise, rest, nutrition, stress reduction, skin care, and scrutiny of the

TABLE 211-2 Symptomatic and Rehabilitative Therapies for Multiple Sclerosis*

Symptom	Description	Treatment Modalities
Spasticity	Very common Stiff, slow movements; spasms	PT and assistive devices Baclofen intrathecal pump implantation or, rarely, botulinum toxin (Botox) **Drug therapy:** baclofen (Lioresal), tizanidine (Zanaflex), or benzodiazepine
Fatigue	Very frequent Highly debilitating and depressing Often the reason for disability Cause unknown Aggravated by elevated temperature, reversed by cooling	OT for energy conservation techniques Cooling vest or cap Avoidance of heat **Drug therapy:** amantadine (Symmetrel), pemoline (Cylert),† modafinil (Provigil), fluoxetine (Prozac), bupropion (Wellbutrin)
Pain	Fairly common symptom Various disagreeable sensations	Trigeminal neuralgia common Pain from spasms relieved with antispasmodics **Drug therapy:** carbamazepine (Tegretol), gabapentin (Neurontin), pregabalin (Lyrica), duloxetine (Cymbalta), tricyclic antidepressants
Tremor	May involve hand, arm, head, eyes, or voice and may be incapacitating Very difficult symptom to manage	OT help with weighted equipment and environmental strategies **Drug therapy:** propranolol (Inderal), clonazepam (Klonopin), primidone (Mysoline), ondansetron (Zofran)
Weakness		No response to medication, but often compensated for by use of adaptive equipment; weakness possibly worse with baclofen OT/PT evaluation for tailored exercise program
Ataxia	Incoordination and disturbance of balance and gait Worsened by spasticity, weakness, and fatigue Falls common	Home evaluation necessary to assess safety risks
Paresthesias	Numbness, tingling, burning, coldness, revulsion when touched	No specific medical therapy; however, gabapentin, pregabalin, duloxetine, or tricyclic antidepressants may be helpful
Loss of vision	Optic neuritis possibly first sign of MS Disc pallor on ophthalmoscopic examination	Generally treated with corticosteroids Regular eye examinations a must
Dysarthria and dysphagia		Evaluation and interventions of speech and language therapist
Paroxysms	Seizures, tonic spasms	**Drug therapy:** anticonvulsants
Depression	Very common	Antidepressants plus counseling usually helpful Watch for adverse effect of medications
Bowel and bladder	Bladder fails to store or empty as evidenced by postvoid residual Bowel problem generally constipation Fecal incontinence very distressful	Intermittent catheterization sometimes helpful Avoidance of urinary infections Surgery indicated for bladder or bowel when appropriate **Drug therapy:** medications with anticholinergic or muscle relaxant properties, such as oxybutynin (Ditropan), propantheline (Pro-Banthine)
Sexuality	Lack of interest or arousal Changes in self-esteem Problems with intimacy Impotence	None
Cognition	Common complaint Most common deficits: memory (recall of recent events), abstract reasoning, problem solving, verbal fluency, and speed of information processing	Safety assessment Consider neuropsychologic evaluation to aid in recommendations regarding work, parenting, financial management, safety

PT, Physical therapy; *OT,* occupational therapy.
*NOTE: Many medications used for MS worsen weakness and mobility.
†No longer available in the United States.

various unscientifically proven therapies that are available. Family issues should include parenting with disabilities, coping skills, caregiving issues, and relationship issues. Concerns about confidentiality, insurance, employment, and disability issues should also be addressed. Careful explanation about the avoidance of precipitating triggers, including the need for rest, exercise, and a well-balanced diet, may prevent exacerbations. Community support groups may also be helpful.

Research is continuous, and therefore ongoing education about new medications is particularly important. Exciting advances in the understanding and treatment of MS have been made in the past decade, and the future is promising. Resources for patients, family members, and health care professionals include National Multiple Sclerosis Society ([800] 334-4867, http://www.nmss.org), Multiple Sclerosis Association of America (http://www.msaa.com), and Multiple Sclerosis Foundation (http://www.msfocus.org).

REFERENCES

1. Holland N, Murray TJ, Reingold SC: *Multiple sclerosis: a guide for the newly diagnosed,* New York, 1996, Demos Vermande.
2. Trapp BD, Peterson J, Ransohoff RM: Axonal transection in the lesions of multiple sclerosis, *N Engl J Med* 338:278-285, 1998.
3. Cook SD: *Multiple sclerosis and viruses,* excerpts from 4th annual meeting of America's Committee for Treatment and Research in Multiple Sclerosis, Basel, Switzerland, Sept 1997.
4. Sadovnick AD, Ebers GC: Epidemiology of multiple sclerosis: a critical overview, *Can J Neurol Sci* 20:17-29, 1993.
5. Riise T: Cluster studies in multiple sclerosis, *Neurology* 49(2 Suppl 2):S27-S32, 1997.
6. Cook SD, Rohowsky-Kochan C, Banshil S, and others: Evidence for multiple sclerosis as an infectious disease, *Acta Neurol Scand Suppl* 161:34-42, 1995.
7. National Multiple Sclerosis Society: *About MS,* retrieved Jan 29, 2006, from http://www.nmss.org.
8. Tintore M, Rovira A, Riio J, and others: New diagnostic criteria for multiple sclerosis, *Neurology* 60:27-30, 2003.
9. McFarland HF, Frank JA, Albert PS, and others: Using gadolinium-enhancing magnetic resonance imaging lesions to monitor activity in multiple sclerosis, *Ann Neurol* 32:758-766, 1992.
10. The National MS Society: *The MS Information sourcebook,* retrieved Feb 11, 2007, from http://www.nationalmssociety.org/Sourcebook-Evoked.
11. Cook SD: A clinician's approach to modulate disease activity in MS, *Rev Neurol Dis* 2(3):117-123, 2005.
12. Weinstock-Guttman B, Cohen JA: Emerging therapies for multiple sclerosis, *Neurologist* 2:342-355, 1996.
13. Goodkin DE, Neilley LK: *Multiple sclerosis handbook: a primer,* San Francisco, 1996, University of California Regents.
14. Carr LK: Lower urinary tract dysfunction due to multiple sclerosis, *Can J Urol Suppl* 1:2-4, 2006.
15. Bishop B: Diagnostic challenges for patients with multiple sclerosis, *J Nurse Pract* 2(3):200-210, 2006.

CHAPTER 212

Parkinson's Disease

Brenda L. Jordan

DEFINITION AND EPIDEMIOLOGY

Parkinson's disease (PD) is a slowly progressing neurodegenerative disorder with an insidious onset of asymmetric resting tremor, bradykinesia, hypokinesia, and rigidity, sometimes with postural changes. PD is the fourth most common neurodegenerative disease; the age-adjusted prevalence is 1% of the population worldwide, 1.6% in Europe, rising from 0.6% at ages 60 to 64 years to 3.5% at ages 85 to 89 years. In 5% to 10% of those in whom PD develops, symptoms appear before age 40 years, with mean age of onset being 65 years. The incidence worldwide is equal in the two sexes.[1] The risk of developing PD appears to double if a first-degree relative had PD compared with people in the general population.[2,3]

Although the cause of PD is unknown, research has concentrated on genetics, exogenous toxins, and endogenous toxins from cellular oxidative reactions. Those who develop PD may be affected by a combination of genetic and environmental factors, viruses, toxins, drugs containing 1-methyl-4-phenyl-1,2,3,6-tetrahydropyridine (MPTP), well water, vitamin E, and smoking.[4-6] Purely genetic Parkinson's varieties probably affect a small minority of people with the *parkin* gene on chromosome 6, which is possibly associated with Parkinson's. PD may represent different conditions with a final common pathway.

Physician consultation is recommended for patients with treatment failure or disease progression.

PATHOPHYSIOLOGY

PD develops after widespread destruction of pigmented neural cells in the zona compacta of the substantia nigra, causing the nigrostriatal tract to degenerate.[7] Consequently, the dopamine normally secreted in the caudate nucleus and putamen is no longer available. Loss of approximately 80% of the pigmented neurons in the substantia nigra, leading to a 70% to 80% depletion of striatal dopamine, is required for the appearance of clinical parkinsonism.[8] However, the large number of acetylcholine-secreting neurons that transmit excitatory signals remains active. The decreased dopaminergic activity in the striatum leads to an imbalance between dopamine and acetylcholine, and the loss of dopamine receptor sites affects the refinement of voluntary movement.[7] Thus the seven cardinal features of PD are produced: (1) tremor at rest, (2) rigidity, (3) bradykinesia, (4) hypokinesia, (5) flexed posture, (6) loss of postural reflexes with gait disturbance, and (7) freezing phenomenon.

CLINICAL PRESENTATION

The clinical features most suggestive of Parkinson's are asymmetric or unilateral tremor, rigidity and flexed posture, bradykinesia, loss of postural reflexes, and freezing, which clearly respond to treatment with levodopa. Tremor at rest is recognized as the first symptom in 70% of patients with this disease.[7,9] Rest tremor, most common in the distal extremities, characteristically disappears with action but reemerges as the limbs maintain a posture. Rest tremor of the hands increases with walking and may be an early sign when others are not yet present. Tremor misdiagnosis is the most common problem for practitioners without neurology training. In general, tremors may be coarse, medium, or fine in amplitude. Most often, patients with PD exhibit a slow, coarse tremor with a rate varying from two to five oscillations per second, usually averaging four or five oscillations per second when the hand is motionless, and decreasing with postural changes. There is a clear distinction from essential, or intention tremors, which appear only, or primarily, with deliberate, willed movement.[7,9]

Another classic sign is rigidity, which is an increase in muscle tone that can be elicited when one of the patient's limbs, neck, or trunk is passively moved.[7] The increased resistance to passive movement is equal in all directions and usually is manifested by a ratcheting, or cogwheeling, "give" during the movement. Rigidity of the passive limb increases when another limb is engaged in voluntary active movement.[9]

The patient with PD often has a uniquely flexed posture involving the entire body. The head is bowed, the trunk is bent forward, the back is kyphotic, the hands are held in front of the body, and the elbows, hips, and knees are flexed. Deformities of the hands and feet may also be apparent. Lateral tilting of the trunk is common.[9]

The most common features of PD are slowness of movement (hypokinesia), loss of automatic movement (bradykinesia), and difficulty initiating movement (freezing).[7] A tendency to shuffle and a decrease in arm swing may be evident. Masked facies (a reduction in spontaneous facial expression) and decreased frequency of blinking are prevalent. The patient may tend to sit motionless or may be characterized by loss of gesturing. Speech becomes soft (hypophonia), and the voice often has a monotonous tone with lack of inflection (aprosody of speech). Some patients are not able to enunciate clearly (dysarthria) or may experience repetition of syllables (palilalia).[9]

PHYSICAL EXAMINATION

Postural reflexes can be tested by giving a sudden, firm pull on the shoulders from behind, but the health care provider should be prepared to catch the patient. Rigidity, demonstrated by cogwheeling, may be tested by grasping the patient's elbow at antecubital region and slowly flexing and extending the elbow or pronating-supinating the forearm. Walking can also be marked by festination, whereby the patient walks faster and faster with short steps, trying to move the feet forward under the flexed body's center of gravity.[7,9]

The freezing phenomenon, a motor block, is a transient inability to perform active movements. It most often affects the legs but can involve eyelid opening, speaking, and writing.[7,8] The feet may appear to be glued to the ground. Because patients with PD exhibit an increased ability to perform intentional or conscious movement as opposed to automatic movement, freezing can be overcome by having patients intentionally raise their legs as if stepping over objects. Despite severe bradykinesia with marked immobility, patients with PD may rise suddenly and move normally for a short burst of motor activity (kinesia paradoxica).

DIAGNOSTICS

Diagnostic studies are usually not indicated. The earliest pathologic abnormality may be incidental Lewy bodies in the brain (a postmortem finding).[10] Diagnosis is based on the clinical presentation and physical examination. Clinical diagnostic criteria have a sensitivity of 80% and specificity of 30%, compared with the definitive diagnosis at autopsy.[10] A resting tremor almost always suggests PD because it rarely is seen in other syndromes. Perhaps the most important diagnostic aid, although not an absolute confirmation, is a satisfactory response to levodopa. CT or MRI may be considered for identifying patients with lacunae in the basal ganglia because this group may respond poorly to medications.

DIFFERENTIAL DIAGNOSIS

As previously noted, the diagnosis of PD and other forms of parkinsonism is based on the response to levodopa. Bradykinesia and rigidity respond best, but lack of improvement does not exclude the diagnosis of PD. Tremor may never respond satisfactorily.

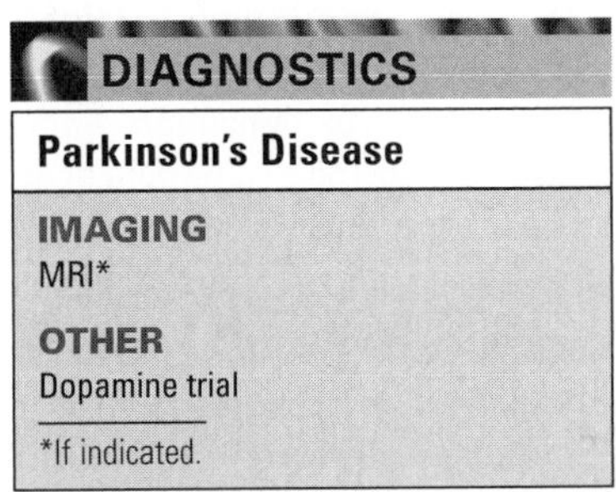
DIAGNOSTICS

Parkinson's Disease

IMAGING
MRI*

OTHER
Dopamine trial

*If indicated.

Diagnosis may be problematic in mild cases, especially if tremor is minimum or absent. For example, mild hypokinesia, or slight tremor, is commonly attributed to old age. The family history, the character of the

DIFFERENTIAL DIAGNOSIS

Parkinson's Disease

IDIOPATHIC PARKINSONISM
- Parkinson's disease

SYMPTOMATIC PARKINSONISM
- Drug-induced condition: dopamine antagonists and depletors
- Hemiatrophy-hemiparkinsonism
- Hydrocephalus
- Hypoxia
- Postencephalitic infection
- Parathyroid dysfunction
- Manganese, carbon dioxide, 1-methyl-4-phenyl-1,2,3,6-tetrahydropyridine (MPTP) cyanide toxicity
- Trauma
- Tumor
- Multiinfarctions
- Parkinson-plus syndromes
- Cortical–basal ganglionic degeneration
- Dementia syndromes
- Lytico-Bodig (Guamanian parkinsonism–dementia–amyotrophic lateral sclerosis)
- Multiple-system atrophy syndromes

HEREDODEGENERATIVE DISEASES
- Hallervorden-Spatz disease
- Huntington's disease
- Mitochondrial cytopathies with striatal necrosis
- Neuroacanthocytosis
- Wilson's disease

OTHER CONDITIONS
- Normal aging
- Essential tremor
- Depression

tremor, and the lack of other neurologic signs should distinguish essential tremor from parkinsonism (see Chapter 210).

Depression, with its associated expressionless face, poorly modulated voice, and reduction in voluntary activity, can be difficult to distinguish from mild parkinsonism, especially because the two disorders may co-exist. In some cases a trial of antidepressant drug therapy may be necessary.

MANAGEMENT

Judicious selection of treatment options can maximize functional gains by symptomatic treatment, but none appears to slow the progress of the disease. Treatment is individualized because each patient has a unique set of signs and symptoms; response to medications; and host of social, occupational, and emotional needs that must be considered. The goal is to maintain independence and functional ability as long as possible. Drug treatment acts in one of two ways: (1) to increase the functional ability of the underactive dopaminergic system or (2) to reduce the excessive influence of the excitatory cholinergic neurons.

Pharmacotherapy

Selegiline. Selegiline (Eldepryl) may be used in early PD but has very mild symptomatic benefit, and its value as a neuroprotector is unclear. Selegiline is a monoamine oxidase B inhibitor that delays the destruction of the nigral neurons and inhibits the metabolic breakdown of dopamine. Some randomly controlled trials have demonstrated the benefit of selegiline in delaying the need for levodopa an average of 9 months if used for patients with early PD.[11-13] Adverse side effects and contraindications in administering and monitoring selegiline should be noted. When given concurrently with levodopa, selegiline can increase the dopaminergic effect and contribute to dopaminergic toxicity. A maximum dosage is currently considered 5 mg b.i.d.

Levodopa. Either levodopa or dopamine agonists can be used initially for symptomatic therapy.[14-16] Levodopa treatment is aimed at restoring the amount of dopamine reaching the basal ganglia. Unfortunately, dopamine does not cross the blood-brain barrier; thus its precursor, levodopa, must be given. Levodopa is metabolized both peripherally and centrally. The peripheral metabolism is responsible for the majority of side effects. Sinemet combines levodopa with carbidopa, which blocks peripheral metabolism, allowing much more of the levodopa to enter the brain than if it were given alone. Sinemet 25/100 contains 25 mg of carbidopa and 100 mg of levodopa. The optimum dosage of carbidopa is 100 to 150 mg/day, which should completely block peripheral metabolism of levodopa. Levodopa is associated with higher risk of dyskinesia than dopamine agonists.

The addition of Carbidopa to Levodopa (Sinemet) increases therapeutic potency and avoids gastrointestinal adverse effects. Therapy should be initiated with immediate-release preparations so initial response can be better evaluated. Slow-release forms of carbidopa-levodopa provide a longer half life and a lower peak plasma level of levodopa, reducing clinical fluctuations.[17,18] Once stable, the patient may be reassessed every 3 to 6 months.

After 2 to 5 years of treatment, more than 50% of patients begin to experience fluctuations in their response to levodopa. This "on-off" effect refers to the shortened duration of improvement after each drug dose, with resultant swings from intense akinesia to uncontrollable hyperactivity. Unfortunately, 75% of patients may have serious complications after 5 years of levodopa therapy. Two randomly controlled trials found no evidence that modified-release levodopa reduced motor complications or improved disease control at 5 years compared with immediate-release levodopa monotherapy in people with early PD.[17,18]

Dopamine Agonists. Evidence exists that dopamine agonist monotherapy and combination therapy reduce the incidence of irreversible motor complications of dyskinesia and fluctuations in motor response related to long-term levodopa treatment. The same systematic review and six long-term randomly controlled trials, however, found that levodopa monotherapy is slightly more effective in treating the disabling motor impairments of PD.[19] Bromocriptine (Parlodel), ropinirole (Requip), and pramipexole (Mirapex) are dopamine agonists that can be effective adjuncts to levodopa in antiparkinsonian therapy to reduce the dosage needed for levodopa alone and to overcome some of the side effects of long-term use of levodopa.[19-21] Therefore dopamine agonists, instead of levodopa, are likely to be beneficial in younger people with early disease.

The agonists tend to induce orthostatic hypotension when first introduced. The best starting regimen is a small dose at bedtime for the first 3 days and then a switch to daytime dosing, with a gradual increase. Bromocriptine and ropinirole may induce psychosis and confusion, whereas pramipexole induces somnolence.[21,22] Overall, however, all are less likely than levodopa to induce dyskinesias, which makes them useful to reduce the severity of "off" states. All dopamine agonists should be used cautiously in patients with cardiac disease.

Catechol *O*-methyltransferase Inhibitors. Catechol *O*-methyltransferase (COMT) inhibitors such as entacapone (Comtan) are ineffective if given alone, but they prolong and potentiate levodopa effect when given in conjunction with levodopa. COMT inhibitors are used to treat motor fluctuations in patient who are experiencing end-of-dose "wearing off" periods.[8]

Anticholinergics. Amantadine (Symmetrel, Symadine), an anticholinergic, may be more useful in controlling tremor and rigidity than bradykinesia but may also cause typical side effects. Anticholinergics should be used in younger patients in whom tremor is the predominant problem. In older patients amantadine may cause mental changes such as depression, anxiety, or psychosis; it probably should not be used in patients over the age of 70.[10] Benztropine (Cogentin) and trihexyphenidyl (Artane) also are useful anticholinergics. The potency of anticholinergics seems to decrease over time, and side effects such as blurred vision, dry mouth, bowel and bladder problems, and cognition changes limit their usefulness. Evidence of benefit of anticholinergics is unclear.

Surgery and Stereotactic Procedures

Limited evidence exists for the benefit of pallidotomy in reducing contralateral tremor and rigidity during "off " time (periods when treatment is not working) and dyskinesia during "on" time (period when treatment is working).[23,24] There is no evidence that pallidotomy reduces the need for medical treatment.[24] Stereotactic procedures may be effective in relieving rigidity, bradykinesia, and tremor for patients responding poorly to pharmacologic management, but evidence of benefit is unclear.[25,26] There is a high incidence of adverse effects with pallidotomy.

Unilateral pallidotomy may greatly improve walking speed and precision of manual performances, but left-sided pallidotomy reduces verbal fluency.[27] Pallidal deep brain stimulation has less frequent adverse effects than pallidotomy.

No randomly controlled trials have been done to compare subthalamic or thalamic surgery and deep brain stimulation with medical treatment.

COMPLICATIONS

Especially significant is depression, which occurs in more than 50% of patients with PD and may precede motor symptoms.[9] There is debate as to whether depression is a reaction to or part of the illness. Most patients with PD exhibit behavioral changes.[28] The patient's attention span is reduced. Passivity and lack of motivation are common. Confusion, agitation, hallucinations, and mania are probably related to activation of dopamine receptors in cortical and limbic structures.[9]

The prevalence of cognitive dysfunction is estimated to be as high as 81%. However, only 15% to 20% exhibit the severe type of dementia seen in Alzheimer's disease.[29] Memory impairment is not a primary feature; rather, the patient is slow in responding to questions. Subtle signs, such as the inability to change mental set rapidly, may be present early in the disease. Concurrent task demand deficiency indicates an attentional control conflict.[9] Onset of true memory impairment soon after diagnosis of PD would suggest a dementia such as Lewy body rather than idiopathic PD.

Sensory symptoms such as pain, burning, and tingling are fairly common in the region of motor involvement.[9] However, uncomfortable sensations tend to disappear with movement. Autonomic disturbances may produce cooler skin, constipation, inadequate bladder emptying, difficulty with erection, and low blood pressure.

The freezing phenomenon may put patients at greater risk of falling. Other concerns include small and slow handwriting (micrographia) and difficulty in shaving, brushing teeth, combing hair, and buttoning.[9] Bradykinesia makes rising from a deep chair, getting out of automobiles, and turning in bed difficult. Drooling saliva results from failure to swallow spontaneously. Choking and aspiration are concerns.

General side effects of overmedication with all dopamine agonists include nervousness, restlessness, and vivid nightmares, which predate hallucinations or delusions. Selegiline's adverse side effects include dizziness, confusion, hallucinations, nausea and vomiting, abdominal pain, and possible fatal reaction with concurrent meperidine or narcotic analgesic. Selegiline also is expensive.

Anticholinergics typically produce dry mouth, blurred vision, constipation, and urinary retention. Delirium is not uncommon, especially in frail older adults. Dopamine agonists tend to induce orthostatic hypotension when first introduced. Patients and their caregivers should be taught the signs and symptoms of confusion and psychosis that are to be reported to their health care provider, as well as any changes in their overall health (e.g., cardiac changes).[9]

INDICATIONS FOR REFERRAL OR HOSPITALIZATION

Collaboration with other health providers is common in the treatment of patients with PD. It is important to consult a neurologist before committing patients to medications. Physician consultation is indicated when patients are not responding to treatment or disease is progressing. Also, if there are signs and symptoms of depression, referral to a psychiatrist should be considered. Neuropsychologic documentation of the precise nature and prevalence of the cognitive deficit has important implications in medical and psychosocial management of patients with PD.[29] Hospitalization may be considered for complications such as pneumonia, deep vein thrombosis, or pulmonary embolus. Physical therapy can improve mobility and strength, which may help maintain independence and prevent injury. Occupational therapy can be useful; adaptive equipment can be provided to the patient or caregivers, and assistance can be provided to adapt the home or workplace as disability progresses.

PATIENT AND FAMILY EDUCATION

Patients should be told that levodopa is more effective when taken on an empty stomach, but this may result in nausea, particularly for the first 3 days. Some patients may report that high-protein meals tend to produce "off" states.[9] The provider should explain that foods containing phenylalanine, leucine, and isoleucine, such as milk and meat, can block the absorption of levodopa from the intestine and its passage into the brain. This effect may be responsible for later diurnal response fluctuations. Side effects of dopamine agonists, including dizziness, confusion, hallucinations, or delusional thinking, should be reviewed with the patient.

Answering questions and addressing concerns honestly are part of establishing a successful provider-patient relationship. Reassurance and encouragement complement medication. The patient should be encouraged to contact a PD support group and a local PD information and referral center. Internet resources are also available for patients with PD. The patient may find the following resources helpful:

American Parkinson Disease Association
135 Parkinson Avenue
Staten Island, NY 10305
(800) 223-2732; California: (800) 908-2732
http://www.apdaparkinson.org

National Parkinson Foundation, Inc.
Bob Hope Parkinson Research Center
1501 NW 9th Avenue
Miami, FL 33136-1494
(800) 327-4545
http://www.parkinson.org

Parkinson's Disease Foundation
1359 Broadway, Suite 1509
New York, NY 10018
(800) 457-6676
http://www.pdf.org

Parkinson Support Groups of America
11376 Cherry Hill Road, #204
Beltsville, MD 20705
(301) 937-1545

National Institute of Neurological Disorders and Stroke
http://www.ninds.nih.gov

REFERENCES

1. de Rijk MC, Tzourio C, Breteler MM, and others: Prevalence of parkinsonism and Parkinson's disease in Europe: the EUROPARKINSON Collaborative Study. European Community Concerted Action on the Epidemiology of Parkinson's disease, *J Neurol Neurosurg Psychiatry* 62(1):10-15, 1997.
2. Marder K, Tang MX, Mejia H, and others: Risk of Parkinson's disease among first-degree relatives: a community-based study, *Neurology* 47(1):155-160, 1996.
3. Jarman P, Wood N: Parkinson's disease genetics comes of age, *BMJ* 318(7199):1641-1642, 1999.
4. Ben-Shlomo Y: How far are we in understanding the cause of Parkinson's disease? *J Neurol Neurosurg Psychiatry* 61:4-16, 1996.
5. de Rijk M, Breteler MM, den Breeijen JH, and others: Dietary antioxidants and Parkinson's disease: the Rotterdam study, *Arch Neurol* 54(6):762-765, 1997.
6. Tzourio C, Rocca WA, Breteler MM, and others: Smoking and Parkinson's disease. An age dependent risk effect? The EUROPARKINSON Study Group, *Neurology* 49(5):1267-1272, 1997.
7. Tierney LM, McPhee SJ, Papadakis MA, editors: *Current medical diagnosis and treatment,* ed 35, Stamford, Conn, 1996, Appleton & Lange.
8. Olanow CW, Kieburtz K, Stern M, and others: Double-blind, placebo-controlled study of entacapone in levodopa-treated patients with stable Parkinson disease, *Arch Neurol* 61:1563, 2004.
9. Tapper VJ: Pathophysiology, assessment, and treatment of Parkinson's disease, *Nurse Pract* 22:76-95, 1997.
10. Hughes AJ, Daniel SE, Blankson S, and others: A clinicopathologic study of 100 cases of Parkinson's disease, *Arch Neurol* 50(2):140-148, 1993.
11. Lees AJ, for Parkinson's Disease Research Group of the United Kingdom: Comparison of therapeutic effects and mortality data of levodopa and levodopa combined with selegiline in people with early, mild Parkinson's disease, *Br Med J* 311:1602-1607, 1995.
12. Przuntek H, Conrad B, Dichgans J, and others: SELEDO: a 5-year long-term trial on the effect of selegiline in early Parkinsonian patients treated with levodopa, *Eur J Neurol* 61(2):141-150, 1995.
13. Larsen JP, Boas J, Erdal JE: Does selegiline modify the progression of early Parkinson's disease? Results from a 5-year study. The Norwegian-Danish Study Group, *Eur J Neurol* 6(5):539-547, 1999.
14. Ahlskog JE: Slowing Parkinson's disease progression, *Neurology* 60:381, 2003.
15. Albin RL, Frey KA: Initial agonist treatment of Parkinson disease: a critique, *Neurology* 60:390, 2003.
16. Miyasaki JM, Martin W, Suchowsky O, and others: Practice parameter: initiation of treatment for Parkinson's disease: an evidence-based review: report of the Quality Standards Subcommittee of the American Academy of Neurology, *Neurology* 58:11, 2002.
17. Dupont E, Andersen A, Boas J, and others: Sustained-release Madopar HBS compared with standard release Madopar in the long-term treatment of de novo parkinsonian patients, *Acta Neurol Scand* 93(1):14-20, 1996.
18. Block G, Liss C, Reines S, and others: Comparison of immediate-release and controlled release carbidopa/levodopa in Parkinson's disease. A multicenter 5-year study. The CR First Study Group, *Eur Neurol* 37(1):23-47, 1997.
19. Ramaker C, van Hilton J: Bromocriptine/levodopa versus levodopa in early Parkinson's disease, *Parkinson Relat Disord* 5(Suppl):82, 1999.
20. Rascol O, Brooks DJ, Korczyn AD, and others: A five-year study of the incidence of dyskinesia in people with early Parkinson's disease who were treated with ropinirole or levodopa, *N Engl J Med* 342(20):1484-1491, 2000.
21. Parkinson's Study Group: Pramipexole versus levodopa as initial treatment for Parkinson's disease, *JAMA* 284:1931-1938, 2000.
22. Rinne U: A 5-year double-blind study with cabergoline versus levodopa in the treatment of Parkinson's disease, *Parkinson Relat Disord* 5(Suppl):84, 1999.
23. Alkhani A, Lozano A: Pallidotomy for Parkinson's disease: a review of contemporary literature, *J Neurosurg* 94:43-49, 2001.
24. de Bie R, de Haan RJ, Nijssen PC, and others: Unilateral pallidotomy in Parkinson's disease: a randomized, single-blind, multicentre trial, *Lancet* 354(9191):1665-1669, 1999.
25. Merello M, Nouzeilles MI, Kuzis G, and others: Unilateral radiofrequency lesion versus electrostimulation of posteroventral pallidum: a prospective randomized comparison, *Mov Disord* 14(1):50-56, 1999.
26. Katayama Y, Kasai M, Oshima H, and others: Double blinded evaluation of the effects of pallidal and subthalamic nucleus stimulation on daytime activity in advanced Parkinson's disease, *Parkinson Relat Disord* 7(1):35-40, 2000.
27. Schmand B, de Bie RM, Koning-Haanstra M, and others: Unilateral pallidotomy in PD: a controlled study of cognitive and behavioural effects, *Neurology* 54(5):1058-1064, 2000.
28. Taylor AE, Saint-Cyr JA: The neuro psychology of Parkinson's disease, *Brain Cogn* 28:281-296, 1997.
29. Braak H, Braak E, Yilmazer D, and others: New aspects of pathology in Parkinson's disease with concomitant incipient Alzheimer's disease, *J Neural Transm Suppl* 48:1-6, 1996.

CHAPTER 213

Seizure Disorder

Karen Gilbert

DEFINITION AND EPIDEMIOLOGY

Epilepsy, a syndrome of recurrent seizures, is a common neurologic condition that currently affects more than 2 million people in the United States, with more than 50,000 to 100,000 new cases reported annually. Although the onset of seizures can occur at any age, incidence rates peak in neonates and young children, plateau, and then rise again in the older adult population. In the United States the prevalence of seizures is approximately 5 to 10 cases per 1000 persons in the general population; the lifetime risk of developing epilepsy in one's lifetime is between 3% and 5%.[1]

A single seizure may result from discrete, temporary abnormalities such as a high fever in small children, hyperventilation, or alcohol withdrawal. A first seizure may manifest in the form of status epilepticus (SE). SE is defined as more than 30 minutes of continuous seizure activity, or two or more seizures without recovery of baseline consciousness between attacks.

Causes of seizures include genetic factors, vascular abnormalities (e.g., strokes, hemorrhages, arteriovenous malformations), significant head trauma, brain tumors, metabolic factors, and infections such as encephalitis and meningitis. Strokes are a common cause of epilepsy, particularly in the elderly. Approximately 10% of patients with cortical infarctions will develop epilepsy. Changes in levels of various electrolytes, in particular hyponatremia and hypercalcemia, may cause isolated seizures. Also, hyperglycemia and hypoglycemia can be responsible for seizure activity, especially in patients with underlying brain injuries.

Genetic predisposition is strongest in forms of epilepsy in which the entire brain is electrically unstable; however, the genetic and biochemical defects have not been well characterized. Childhood absence (petit mal) epilepsy, juvenile myoclonic epilepsy, and generalized convulsive epilepsy are syndromes with a genetic predisposition. These types account for approximately one third of all epilepsy cases, with seizures and electroencephalogram (EEG) abnormalities affecting the entire brain. The remaining types of epilepsy are related to localization, with focal electrical abnormalities usually being the result of a structural lesion. The occurrence of prolonged or complicated febrile seizures in infancy is strongly correlated with the subsequent development of temporal lobe epilepsy.[2]

Physician consultation is indicated for suspected central nervous system (CNS) lesions, SE, initiation of antiepileptic medications, treatment failures, and women with epilepsy who are contemplating pregnancy.

PATHOPHYSIOLOGY

Although the terms *epilepsy* and *seizure disorder* are often used interchangeably, they have two distinct definitions. A seizure can be defined as an isolated event in which a group of neurons produces excessive electrical discharges in the brain. Seizures occur when the balance between excitation and inhibition of the brain's electrical activity becomes abnormally altered in favor of excitation. Seizures can be caused by the excess production or release of an excitatory neurotransmitter, which stimulates neurons to discharge abnormally, or by a loss of inhibitory neuronal activity, which permits abnormal excitation and discharges of neurons to occur. Single seizures can be triggered by hypoxia or metabolic factors, but they do not constitute epilepsy unless they recur in a habitual and unprovoked manner. Epilepsy is characterized by recurrent seizures and is divided into syndromes on the basis of various etiologies, seizure types, associated neurologic symptoms, anatomic correlates, age, and family history. For diagnosis and treatment it is valuable to be able to identify both the type of seizure and the epileptic syndrome.

CLASSIFICATION OF SEIZURES, EPILEPSY, AND EPILEPTIC SYNDROMES

In 1981, a commission for the International League Against Epilepsy (ILAE) developed, revised, and adopted the international classification of epileptic seizures (Box 213-1).[3] Although efforts are being made to revise the classification, the ILEA 1981 version is still widely accepted. The classification includes two broad categories of seizure types: partial, or localization related, and generalized. Partial seizures begin in a limited region of one cerebral hemisphere and show focal EEG abnormalities. Depending on the spread of electrical

BOX 213-1

INTERNATIONAL CLASSIFICATION OF EPILEPTIC SEIZURES

I. **Partial seizures.** Epileptic focus is in one hemisphere of the brain. Also called focal or local seizures.
   A. **Simple partial seizures.** Usually the aura of a complex seizure. Patient has no loss of consciousness.
      1. Motor: tonic or clonic activity of one arm or leg
      2. Sensory: such as an auditory, olfactory, visual hallucination
      3. Autonomic: such as the epigastric rising sensation
      4. Psychic: déjà vu, fear, indescribable feeling
   B. **Complex partial seizure.** Consciousness is altered. Patient may exhibit complex behaviors.
      1. Can begin with a simple partial onset
      2. Can begin with immediate alteration of consciousness
   C. **Partial seizure evolving to generalized.** Patient starts with a simple or complex partial seizure that evolves into a generalized tonic-clonic seizure.

II. **Generalized.** Epileptic focus is not lateralized to one hemisphere. Begins in both hemispheres of the brain simultaneously.
   A. **Nonconvulsive**
      1. Absence (petit mal)
      2. Atonic: loss of muscle tone (drop attacks)
   B. **Convulsive.** Involves motor activity.
      1. Myoclonic: abrupt muscle twitches or jerks
      2. Tonic-clonic (grand mal): tonic, then clonic activity
      3. Tonic: involving increased muscle tone, rigidity
      4. Clonic: muscle contraction and relaxation movements

Modified from Commission on Classification and Terminology of the International League Against Epilepsy: Proposal for revised clinical and electroencephalographic classification of epileptic seizures, *Epilepsia* 22(4):489-501, 1981.

activity, the patient may have varying levels of consciousness. By definition, simple partial seizures are not associated with any alteration of consciousness and are usually the aura, or warning, that the patient experiences before a larger seizure. Occasionally, patients may have simple partial sensory seizures, which are purely subjective. If the seizure activity spreads and involves the brainstem or both hemispheres, consciousness becomes altered and the seizure is classified as complex partial. Altered consciousness and aberrations of behavior, such as automatisms or automatic, repetitive movements, are usually associated with complex partial seizures. If such seizures spread bilaterally and involve the motor cortex, the patient may have a secondarily generalized tonic-clonic seizure.[4]

In contrast, primary generalized seizures occur when the initial electrical activity begins in both cerebral hemispheres. These seizures are usually seen with idiopathic or hereditary types of epilepsy. Consciousness is almost always impaired, and the seizure may be convulsive or nonconvulsive. Motor activity and EEG changes are bilateral. Nonconvulsive seizures, such as absence seizures, may be brief, and the patient may initially be diagnosed as a "daydreamer." The EEG characteristics of generalized spike and wave patterns are crucial for the proper diagnosis of these types of seizures. Convulsive seizures, such as tonic-clonic (grand mal) types, are rarely missed but can be confused with secondarily generalized tonic-clonic seizures. Being able to differentiate between these two types is helpful in prescribing the appropriate treatment, since each type may respond differently to certain antiepileptic medications. In the case of secondarily generalized seizures, it is important to exclude an underlying structural lesion, such as a brain tumor.

To tailor treatment to the individual, it is essential that consideration be given to the seizure type as well as the epileptic syndrome to which it belongs. The International Classification of Epilepsy and Epileptic Syndromes (Box 213-2) was adopted by the ILEA in 1989 and allows the practitioner to categorize cases by seizure type, etiology, precipitating factors, age of onset, and prognosis.[5] This classification separates epilepsy into syndromes that are idiopathic, in which no underlying cause is identified, or symptomatic, which are believed to be secondary to an underlying brain disease.

Although epilepsy can develop at any age, certain syndromes are more age related than others. A variety of epileptic syndromes develop in early childhood. Approximately 70% of childhood epilepsies, particularly the benign partial epilepsies, remit at the time of puberty. Idiopathic, generalized epilepsy usually manifests by 18 years of age. After age 18, focal brain processes should be suspected. Brain tumors are a prominent cause of seizures in adults, whereas strokes are often the cause of seizures that begin late in life.[6] Symptomatic focal epilepsy syndromes account for 30% to 35% of all cases of epilepsy.[1] Seizure manifestations can be helpful in identifying which lobe of the brain is involved.[2,6,7] Table 213-1 outlines the general characteristics of partial seizures in relation to the region of seizure origin. However, not all seizures fit neatly into a particular syndrome. Surgical treatment is often possible if the epileptic focus is in a surgically accessible region of the brain.

BOX 213-2

INTERNATIONAL CLASSIFICATION OF EPILEPSY AND EPILEPTIC SYNDROMES

1. Localization related (focal, partial)
   - 1.1. Idiopathic (benign childhood epilepsy with centerotemporal spikes)
   - 1.2. Symptomatic (e.g., temporal lobe epilepsy, frontal lobe epilepsy)
   - 1.3. Cryptogenic (etiology unknown)
2. Generalized epilepsies
   - 2.1. Idiopathic (juvenile myoclonic, juvenile absence, grand mal on awakening)
   - 2.2. Cryptogenic (Lennox-Gastaut syndrome, West's syndrome)
   - 2.3. Symptomatic
3. Undetermined (neonatal types, Landau-Kleffner syndrome)
4. Special situation related (febrile seizures, metabolic seizures)

Modified from Commission on Classification and Terminology of the International League Against Epilepsy: Proposal for revised clinical and electroencephalographic classification of epileptic seizures, *Epilepsia* 22(4):489-501, 1981.

CLINICAL PRESENTATION

An accurate and detailed history is important. It is essential to obtain history not only from the patient but also from parents, relatives, or friends who have witnessed the seizures. Complicated pregnancy or childbirth, delayed childhood development, childhood diseases such as meningitis and encephalitis, significant head trauma with loss of consciousness, and a family history of epilepsy are among the significant risk factors for the development of epilepsy. New-onset seizures require the determination of any recent history of headache, illness, trauma, focal neurologic deficit, or lightheadedness.

An accurate description is important when attempting to decide whether an event was a seizure. The patient should be questioned to determine if there was a warning before the event. A gastric sensation or a feeling of déjà vu is characteristic of temporal lobe epilepsy. A history of incontinence, injury, tongue biting, postictal confusion, lateralized weakness, or severe headache should raise suspicion of a true epileptic event. A detailed seizure history can also suggest where the seizures are originating, define seizure characteristics and frequency, and determine how the seizures are interfering with the patient's life.

A first seizure may appear in the form of SE. Immediate emergency department referral and physician consultation is indicated for SE or new-onset seizures.

PHYSICAL EXAMINATION

A general physical examination should be performed on all patients with epilepsy and should be directed toward specific disease processes and focal neurologic deficits. Skin and mucous membranes should be assessed to identify areas of injury that may be related to events that occurred while consciousness was altered. Tongue biting and cheek biting are common during tonic-clonic seizures; usually the tongue is bitten on just one side. Cardiovascular assessment is important because syncope and arrhythmias are included in the differential diagnosis of epilepsy. Postural vital signs will determine whether orthostatic hypotension is a consideration.

TABLE 213-1 Clinical Manifestations of Complex Partial Seizures

Site	Aura	Clinical Characteristics	Percentage of Partial Cases
Temporal	Epigastric sensation Déjà vu	Altered consciousness Oral, hand automatisms Moderate postictal confusion	75-85
Frontal	Dizziness or fear	Abrupt onset, rapid clearing Frenetic behavior Sexual automatisms Most occur during sleep	10-15
Parietal	Sensory	With or without altered consciousness Often begins with numbness, tingling, or pain	Rare
Occipital	Visual	May begin with eye twitching May include visual hallucinations May include ictal blindness	5-15

Neurologic signs such as lateralized weakness, papilledema, memory problems, or changes in reflexes can signify a structural lesion in the brain.[4,6] Generally, a patient with epilepsy will have an unremarkable physical examination.

DIAGNOSTICS

Clinical presentation, physical examination, and differential consideration guides diagnostic testing. A new seizure may signify a serious pathologic condition. If infection of the CNS is suspected, a CBC and differential and a lumbar puncture are indicated. A chemistry profile, including calcium, is necessary to exclude hypoglycemia, electrolyte abnormalities, or renal failure. Liver function tests (LFTs) should be obtained to exclude hepatic failure. Alcohol and drug levels may be indicated. An MRI or CT scan is indicated if a tumor, trauma, or a cerebrovascular accident is suspected. An ECG should be obtained to ascertain the presence of arrhythmias or heart block.

Diagnosing and classifying epilepsy and seizure types requires confirmation that the patient does indeed have epileptic seizures. To treat the disorder appropriately, the practitioner must attempt to determine the cause of the epilepsy and classify it according to syndrome. A few diagnostic tests should be part of the initial evaluation.

An EEG is useful because a baseline recording of background brain waves may reveal epileptic abnormalities. The positive predictive value of EEG in most clinics is over 80%, although sensitivity is only 30%.[8] Because the chance of a patient having a seizure during a routine EEG is small, ictal information may not be obtained; however, interictal epileptiform abnormalities may give localizing information and suggest epilepsy. Many patients with focal epilepsy show no focal or generalized EEG abnormalities on routine EEG. Therefore a normal EEG does not exclude a diagnosis of epilepsy. In contrast to focal epilepsy, generalized types of epilepsy often produce abnormalities of spike and wave activity or generalized slowing on routine EEG recordings. Interictal EEG abnormalities—either focal or generalized—are not synonymous with seizure activity, and therefore EEG abnormalities should not be the only basis for treatment.

DIAGNOSTICS

New-Onset Seizure

LABORATORY
Alcohol, drug levels*
Serum electrolytes*
BUN*
Creatinine*
Serum glucose*
Calcium*
CBC and differential*
LFTs*

IMAGING
MRI, CT scan*

OTHER
ECG*
Lumbar puncture*
EEG*

*If indicated.

Although neuroimaging studies can be of great value in diagnosis, the absence of structural abnormalities does not exclude a diagnosis of epilepsy. CT scans are useful for identifying large mass lesions, bleeding, subdural fluid collections, and cerebral infarcts, but they often miss more subtle changes in brain structure. MRIs provide great anatomic detail and are useful in distinguishing small low-grade tumors, scars, and neural migration disorders from each other and from normal variants in brain structure. Except in an emergency, when the immediate availability of a CT scan is an advantage, MRIs should be the primary imaging study in patients with epilepsy.

If a diagnosis of epilepsy cannot be confirmed or excluded after an accurate history, EEG, or imaging study, patients should be referred to a comprehensive epilepsy center in which long-term video and EEG monitoring can be done. This type of monitoring is intended to capture an event on video with simultaneous EEG recording, and it is almost always successful in distinguishing epilepsy from nonepileptic events.

For patients in SE, a battery of laboratory tests is usually performed: CBC, electrolytes, glucose, magnesium, calcium, BUN, creatinine, LFTs, coagulation studies (PT/PTT), alcohol level, toxicology screen, anticonvulsant drug levels, urinalysis, and a pregnancy test. These should be done concurrently with stabilization of the patient. Examination of the cerebrospinal fluid is required if meningitis or encephalitis is suspected. Viral encephalitis should be treated empirically with acyclovir until the results of diagnostic studies for herpes virus are available. Similarly, suspected bacterial meningitis should be treated with appropriate antibiotics until culture results are available.

DIFFERENTIAL DIAGNOSIS

A variety of nonepileptic paroxysmal events can be confused with epileptic seizures. Psychogenic seizures, also called nonepileptic seizures or pseudoseizures, are often mistaken for epileptic seizures; if patients are treated with antiepileptic drugs, this usually increases the seizure frequency. A careful history can help raise the suspicion of psychogenic seizures. In such cases, seizures may be symptoms of conversion disorder and the stress of physical or sexual abuse, a part of post-traumatic stress disorder, attention-seeking behavior, or a means of achieving secondary gain. Treatment involves patient acceptance of the diagnosis of psychogenic seizures and the beginning of a comprehensive psychotherapy program.

The second most common disorder to be confused with epilepsy is syncope. Syncope manifests with loss of consciousness, and convulsive syncope secondary to cerebral ischemia may mimic epileptic seizures. Syncope is often vasovagal, but cardiac causes include heart block or cardiac arrhythmia, and it can be induced by stimuli such as carotid massage, paroxysmal coughing, and voiding. Orthostatic hypotension is a frequent cause of syncope in the elderly. Presyncopal symptoms such as vertigo, sensory disturbances, and tinnitus are sometimes mistaken for epileptic auras or minor seizures.

Other disorders in the differential diagnosis include tumors, cerebrovascular disease, arteriovenous malformation, trauma, CNS infection, migraines, hyperventilation syndrome, movement disorders, transient ischemic attacks, transient global amnesia, and toxic metabolic disturbances such as alcohol withdrawal seizures.[9] Occasionally sleep deprivation may cause generalized tonic-clonic seizures. This phenomenon is not associated with a pathologic disorder.

INITIAL STABILIZATION AND MANAGEMENT OF ACUTE SEIZURES

DIFFERENTIAL DIAGNOSIS

Seizure Disorder

- Psychogenic seizures
- Syncope
- Cardiac arrhythmias
- Migraine
- Hyperventilation
- Movement disorders
- Transient global amnesia
- Transient ischemic attacks
- Cerebrovascular disease
- Toxic metabolic disturbances
- Brain tumor
- Infection
- Alcoholism, drug withdrawal
- Idiopathic
- Trauma
- Sleep deprivation
- Arteriovenous malformation

In the acute setting, most seizures resolve spontaneously within a few minutes and require no specific treatment apart from close observation to ensure that patients do not harm themselves. However, SE is a medical emergency that requires simultaneous medical stabilization (airway, breathing, circulation, and medications to control the seizures) and a search for the underlying cause. The Epilepsy Foundation of America's Working Group on Status Epilepticus defines SE as a continuous seizure lasting 30 minutes or more, or two consecutive seizures in a row without mental clearing.[10] Recently efforts have been made to change the definition from 30 minutes of continuous seizure activity to 10 minutes. This is based on the duration of seizure activity that may produce permanent injury. Generalized convulsive SE (GCSE) is a medical emergency that can lead to transient or permanent brain damage. Early treatment is a key factor in the outcome and prognosis. Initial management should include maintaining homeostasis and providing respiratory support. If seizures persist beyond 30 minutes, a vicious cycle of maladaptive physiologic responses occurs.[11] SE may be complicated by hypotension, hypertension, hyperthermia, hypoglycemia, hypoxemia, acidosis, arrhythmias, rhabdomyolysis, pulmonary edema, fractures, and dislocations.

Mortality and morbidity rates have been related to the cause of SE and the time from the onset until treatment has been initiated. In patients with known epilepsy, one half of the hospital-reported cases of GCSE have been associated with subtherapeutic antiepileptic drug (AED) levels.[12] This is usually due to patients not taking their medication as prescribed. Other common causes of SE are meningitis, head trauma, eclampsia, and progressive neurologic and neurodegenerative disorders.[10] In a study by the Veterans Affairs Status Epilepticus Cooperative Study Group comparing four treatments (lorazepam, phenytoin, phenobarbital, and diazepam) for GCSE, lorazepam was more likely than phenytoin to be successful when used as the initial treatment.[13] Recommendations for treating acute episodes of SE are listed in Table 213-2. The following conditions warrant consideration for admission: SE, incomplete recovery or prolonged postictal state, suspected illness that requires treatment, drug or alcohol withdrawal, febrile illness (adult), expanding mass lesion, history of recent head trauma, or focal signs on examination.[14]

MANAGEMENT

The goal of management in epilepsy is to control seizures with minimum adverse effects. In more than 50% of patients with epilepsy, seizures are completely controlled with medication. Another 20% to 30% of patients have improvement of their symptoms with medications, but they are not seizure free or may suffer significant side effects. The remaining 25% of seizures are medically intractable. Determination of the appropriate medical or surgical treatment is based on a variety of factors. These include patients' perception of how the seizures are interfering with their life goals, economic considerations, personal support from family and friends, and the severity and complexity of the epilepsy in that patient.

Conservative Management

Depending on a number of variables, including the potential for seizure recurrence, first seizures are generally not treated with AEDs. Only about 30% of persons who have a single, unprovoked, generalized tonic-clonic seizure have a second one, whether they are treated with medications or not.[15] Medication may delay recurrence or somewhat reduce its

TABLE 213-2 Recommended Emergency Treatment and Timetable for Status Epilepticus

Time (minutes)	Action
0-5	Diagnose status epilepticus (SE). Give oxygen by nasal cannula or mask; consider intubation if indicated. Establish an IV; obtain blood samples for glucose, serum chemistry, hematology screen, toxicology, and antiepileptic drug levels.
6-9	If hypoglycemia is established or blood glucose is unknown, administer glucose: Adults: Give thiamine 100 mg followed by 50 ml of 50% glucose IV. Children: Give 2 ml/kg of 25% of glucose.
10-20	Administer either 0.1 g/kg of lorazepam at 2 mg/min or 0.2 mg/kg of diazepam at 5 mg/min by IV (if diazepam used, also give phenytoin in follow up).
21-60	IF SE persists, administer 15-20 mg/kg of phenytoin IV no faster than 50 mg/min in adults and 1 mg/kg/min in children. Monitor ECG and blood pressure.*
>60	If SE does not stop after 20 mg/kg of phenytoin, give 20 mg/kg of phenobarbital IV at 100 mg/min. If SE persists, consult anesthesiologist for pentobarbital coma.

Modified from Treatment of Convulsive Status Epilepticus: Recommendations of the Epilepsy Foundation of America's Working Group on Status Epilepticus, *JAMA* 270(7):856, 1993.

*In most centers, fosphenytoin is replacing phenytoin. It is dosed in phenytoin equivalents and can be dosed twice as fast. It also causes less damage if it infiltrates.

likelihood. Factors that should be considered in the decision to treat or not to treat a first seizure include:

- The type of seizure that occurred (Complex partial seizures are more likely to be recurrent than generalized tonic-clonic ones.)
- Environment and occupation (e.g., dangerous work environment such as construction)
- Results of imaging studies and EEG (Treatment is prudent if either is abnormal, since recurrence is likely.)

The decision of whether to treat a patient who has had a single seizure has provoked controversy because of the lack of randomized, unbiased studies. Most studies have combined multiple seizure types, which clouds interpretation of the data. In one randomized multicenter trial of 397 patients seen within 7 days of their first seizure, 36 of 204 treated patients (18%) and 75 of 193 untreated patients (38%) had a recurrent seizure within 2 years.[16] Although these results demonstrate the effectiveness of antiepileptic medication, the recurrence rate even in untreated patients is low enough that most patients with first seizures are not treated.

In a review of the literature by Beghi, Berg, and Hauser,[15] the two most consistent predictors of seizure recurrence are the presence of an abnormal EEG and an underlying cause. In patients with an unprovoked seizure for which there was an underlying antecedent cause (e.g., a previous head injury, mental retardation, or cerebral palsy), the risk of recurrent seizures was double that of patients with an unprovoked seizure for which there was no antecedent cause. After a second seizure, the risk of recurrence increases to more than 80%.[15]

Most epilepsy specialists advocate making treatment decisions after considering the risks and benefits of the treatment for a particular patient. Elements of decision making include the risk to the patient according to the severity, timing, and frequency of seizures; age of seizure onset; and cognitive considerations.[17] In determining risk, it is obvious that patients with generalized tonic-clonic seizures are more at risk for injury than those with simple partial seizures. The timing of seizures is also important. Seizures that occur primarily while the patient is awake pose less risk. Seizures that occur only in relation to special circumstances such as alcohol consumption, sleep deprivation, or pregnancy are sometimes better treated by avoiding those factors than by taking antiepileptic medication. Age and cognition can be factors in decision making. An adolescent who has just learned to drive may be more tolerant of the side effects related to seizure control than a young adult who has just entered college.

Pharmacologic Management

Treatment choices vary with individual differences in etiology, seizure type, age, and psychosocial factors. Controlling seizures with a single drug should be the goal. Each drug should be titrated slowly to determine how it is tolerated, and each drug should be given a fair trial. If seizures are frequent, efficacy can be determined quickly. When medications are changed, the new medication should be added to the existing regimen. When the new medication is well tolerated and an effective dosage has been achieved, the first medication can be slowly reduced. If the patient's seizures remain intractable after trying several single drugs, rational combinations of medications should be tried. Drugs with different mechanisms of action and different side effect profiles usually combine well. To maintain a steady level of the drug in circulation, dosage frequency should be determined by the half life of the drug. Table 213-3 compares the most common AEDs in terms of dosage, peak, half life, side effects, indications, and special considerations.

Side effects occur in approximately 30% to 40% of patients taking AEDs.[18] The side effects should be carefully monitored and the dosages adjusted to minimize the adverse effects of the medication. Rarely, an idiosyncratic reaction can occur, which can be life threatening.

Measurements of blood levels of AEDs are helpful in determining whether a therapeutic dose has been achieved. However, it is most important to follow the patient's response to treatment in relation to efficacy and side effects. With many patients, seizures are controlled with low doses and levels of medications, whereas other patients require and tolerate high levels. Some patients experience significant side effects, even when drug levels are in a normal range. In this case, it may be best to order "free" AED levels, especially if the drug is highly protein bound. Protein binding, absorption, and elimination pharmacokinetics are extremely important factors to consider in predicting side effects and drug-drug interactions. The

TABLE 213-3 Antiepileptic Drug Chart

Drug	Dosage Range	Side Effect Profile	Half Life/Peak Effect	Therapeutic Drug Levels (mcg/ml)	Considerations
Phenobarbital (Luminal)	60-250 mg/day PO in divided or single dose *or* 100-300 mg IV (up to 600 mg to load)	Drowsiness, but tolerance usually develops May cause difficulties with memory and cognition May exacerbate depression in adults	*HL:* 96 hours ±12 *Peak:* Oral: 20-60 minutes IV: 15 minutes	15-40 (levels may not stabilize for 3-4 weeks)	Do not stop abruptly May cause hyperactivity in children Used in partial and generalized seizures Effective for motor seizures
Phenytoin (Dilantin)	300-600 mg/day Loading dose: 1 g IV in divided doses	Gingival hypertrophy Mild sedation Rash, nausea, vomiting Lethargy, nystagmus, ataxia with high doses Difficulty with concentration and memory	*HL:* Oral: 22 hours IV: 10-15 hours *Peak:* 4-12 hours 7-10 days to reach optimum levels	10-20 (levels may stay therapeutic for 7-10 days after stopping) Order free level if patient also taking valproic acid	Used in partial and generalized seizures IV phenytoin and fosphenytoin effective for treating status epilepticus
Carbamazepine (Tegretol)	600-1200 mg in divided doses	Drowsiness, dizziness, nausea, vomiting, which decrease with time Start titration slowly to avoid side effects Diplopia when toxic	*HL:* 12-17 hours *Peak:* 4-5 hours after regular and 3-12 hours after XR or Carbatrol (ER) preparation	4-12 or 8-12 depending on laboratory Takes about 2 days to achieve therapeutic level	Used in partial seizures Not for absence types Should be taken with food Avoid generics in patients with intractable seizures
Primidone (Mysoline)	Slowly titrate up by 125 mg until 250 mg t.i.d.	Drowsiness, ataxia, and vertigo possible; usually decrease with time or dose reduction	*HL:* 12 hours ±6	Levels reported as primidone and phenobarbital Primidone: 5-12 Phenobarbital: 15-40	Used in partial and generalized seizures Effective for motor seizures If patient allergic to phenobarbital, there is cross sensitivity
Divalproex (Depakote)	15-60 mg/kg/day Rarely exceeds 3500-4000 mg/day	Tremor and possible weight gain	*HL:* 6-16 hours *Peak:* 1-4 hours after dose	Normal range 50-100 Levels >100 tolerated by some if well controlled	Effective in generalized seizures May increase free dilantin epoxide—obtain "free" phenytoin levels if needed
Lamotrigine (Lamictal)	Without VPA: 300-500 mg With VPA: 100-150 mg Children: 0.15-1.0 mg/kg/dose b.i.d.	Rash, headache, dizziness, blurred vision Blurred vision more common in patients taking carbamazepine	*HL:* 12-27 hours (with VPA: 70 hours) *Peak:* 1.4-4.8 hour	2.0-4.5 or 3-18 depending on laboratory Lamictal elimination more rapid in patients taking hepatic-enzyme inducing AEDs	Used in partial and generalized seizures Risk of rash higher in patients also taking VPA Titrated to effect, not a certain blood level
Gabapentin (Neurontin)	900-3600 mg/day Titrate to 300 mg t.i.d., then increase by 300-mg increments	Somnolence, dizziness, ataxia, and fatigue Side effects usually short lived Reduced interactions with other AEDs	*HL:* 5-9 hours *Peak:* 2-3 hours	Normal range 2-20 (Neurontin not appreciably metabolized; significance of levels uncertain)	Used in partial seizures Should be taken 2 hours apart from aluminum–magnesium hydroxide (Maalox) to avoid changes in bioavailability

AEDs, Antiepileptic drugs; *HL,* half life; *LFTs,* liver function tests; *VPA,* valproic acid.

TABLE 213-3 Antiepileptic Drug Chart—cont'd

Drug	Dosage Range	Side Effect Profile	Half Life/Peak Effect	Therapeutic Drug Levels (mcg/ml)	Considerations
Topiramate (Topamax)	200-400 mg/day b.i.d. Start low at 25 mg b.i.d., increasing in 25-mg-b.i.d. increments weekly until maximum dosage is reached	Somnolence, dizziness, psychomotor slowing, speech hesitancy, and mood disturbances Also may cause weight loss Increased risk of kidney stones in males	*HL:* 21 hours *Peak:* Within 2 hours after dose	Not completely metabolized, and need for levels is uncertain	Used as an adjunct in partial seizure disorders May decrease estrogen levels in those on oral contraceptives Recommend increased fluid intake
Tiagabine (Gabitril)	12-32 mg Titrate by 4 mg/wk	Somnolence, dizziness, headache, mild memory impairment, abdominal pain	*HL:* 5-13 hours *Peak:* 0.5-1 hour	Not currently established	Used in partial seizures as an adjunctive therapy Adjust dosage if hepatic disease present
Felbamate (Felbatol)	600-3600 mg/day	Insomnia, weight loss, headache Refer to boxed warning re aplastic anemia and hepatic failure	*HL:* 20-23 hours	Monitor concomitant drug levels Monitor frequent CBC and LFTs	Multiple drug interactions with other AEDs; consult a drug text for details Used in partial and generalized seizures
Zonisamide (Zonegran)	100-400 mg/day q.h.s. or b.i.d.	Somnolence, dizziness, anorexia, irritability Rash, renal calculi	*HL:* 63 hours HL decreased with the addition of other AEDs	10-40	Weak carbonic anhydrase inhibitor If patient allergic to sulfa, cross sensitivity may occur
Levetiracetam (Keppra)	1000-3000 mg/day b.i.d.	Somnolence, asthenia, infection, incoordination, behavioral abnormalities	*HL:* 7 hours ±1	3-37	Occasionally associated with increased upper respiratory tract infections
Oxcarbazepine (Trileptal)	600-2400 mg/day 8-10 mg/kg	Dizziness, somnolence, headache, ataxia, diplopia	*HL:* 8-10 hours	Not currently established	Increases phenytoin, phenobarbital, and VPA levels Observe for hyponatremia
Pregabalin (Lyrica)	150-600 mg/day	Dizziness, somnolence, ataxia, weight gain, peripheral edema, blurred vision	*HL:* 6 hours	Not currently established	May lower platelet counts Not metabolized in liver, excreted through kidney

provider should obtain a complete list of medications, including over-the-counter preparations, from the patient. Blood levels should be obtained at least yearly and more often if the patient is having breakthrough seizures, increased side effects, or signs of drug toxicity. In addition, CBC, electrolytes, and LFTs should be performed within a month of beginning a new AED and periodically thereafter.

In making a decision to discontinue AED therapy, the provider and patient should consider the risk/benefit ratio. The risk for relapse is 20% to 40% in the first year of drug withdrawal.[19] Patients with the highest risk for relapse are those with seizure disorder onset during adolescence, an abnormal EEG, an underlying neurologic condition, a definite diagnosis of primary generalized epilepsy, or a history of previous failures at discontinuing AEDs. There is insufficient evidence to establish when to withdraw AEDs in patients who are seizure free.

Surgical Management

Of all patients with epilepsy, 25% are refractory to medical management. Of this 25%, approximately half have focal lesions that are responsible for their seizures; these patients are good candidates for epilepsy surgery. The most common form of epilepsy surgery is a temporal lobectomy. Almost 80% of partial seizures in adults begin in the temporal lobes; a portion of one of the temporal lobes can be removed if tests consistently indicate that the seizures originate in that area. After temporal lobe surgery, success rates (complete seizure control) range from 65% to 95%.[20]

The removal of tumors, abnormal collections of blood vessels, and congenital lesions are other surgical resection options. These conditions can be found anywhere in the brain, and the best results are obtained when both the lesion and the surrounding epileptogenic brain are removed. It is often necessary to perform intracranial EEG mapping to delineate the epileptic zone and to identify cortically important areas such as the language and motor cortex, which must be avoided during surgery.

Another major type of epilepsy surgery involves dividing the corpus callosum. With this type of surgery, the nerve fibers that connect one side of the brain to the other are severed; no tissue is removed. This surgery is most helpful for secondarily generalized tonic-clonic seizures and atonic seizures. Although seizures are not completely stopped by this procedure, they are confined to one hemisphere. Impairment of consciousness, convulsive seizure activity, and falls are often eliminated or greatly reduced.

After surgery, patients remain on antiepileptic medication for several years. Patients who are seizure free for several years can consider a medication taper; however, there is not sufficient evidence to determine whether seizures will recur.

LIFE SPAN CONSIDERATIONS

Although stigma, social isolation, and depression can affect all persons with epilepsy, special concerns are recognized in specific age-groups. Many patients develop epilepsy in early adolescence. This diagnosis can have a profound effect on self-esteem and instill a sense of lacking control because of the unpredictability of seizures. Parental overprotection and preoccupation with the child can lead to problems within the entire family unit. Adolescents should be encouraged to take responsibility for their own care. Providing education and the forum for a trusting relationship is the initial goal for this group of patients. Factual information should be presented in a straightforward, individualized manner, and the young adult should be encouraged to be honest and open about seizure frequency and compliance issues. Collaboration between patient and provider ideally results in a better understanding of the importance of medication, which makes adherence to the treatment plan more likely.

In women with epilepsy there are additional concerns about contraception, fertility, and sexuality. Pregnancy has unpredictable effects on seizure control. Female adolescents should be counseled about family planning and birth control options. Patients taking hepatic enzyme–inducing AEDs should be given a higher-dose oral contraceptive—one with an estrogen content greater than 50 mcg.[21] Women with epilepsy should be encouraged to plan their pregnancies. They should also be given at least 1 mg/day of folic acid supplementation in advance; some AEDs have been shown to inhibit folate action, and folate deficiency is associated with an increased risk of neural tube defects. Overall, AEDs probably double the baseline rate of birth defects. Decisions to continue or to stop taking medication during pregnancy are difficult and should be discussed with a neurologist on an individual basis. Women who continue to take AEDs during pregnancy should be enrolled in the AED pregnancy registry, which can be located through the Epilepsy Foundation of America. Antiepileptic drug levels may fluctuate unpredictably, and dosage modifications may be necessary. AED levels should be checked monthly and free levels obtained whenever possible.

Hormonal changes also have an effect on seizure control. Many women note that seizures tend to occur just before or during their menstrual cycle. This is most likely related to low progesterone levels. Progesterone has been shown to decrease neuronal excitability in animal models.[22] Little is known about the relationship between epilepsy and menopause; however, one preliminary study by Harden, Pulver, Ravdin, and others suggests that hormonal changes that occur during menopause may exacerbate seizures in some women, especially those using estrogen supplementation.[23]

The onset of epilepsy in elders has increased over the past decade. This increase is related to an increase in cerebrovascular disease and brain tumors. Special concerns for older adults include an increased risk of injury or falls during seizures, the effects of AEDs on cognition and physical abilities, and interactions between various medications. Monotherapy is most important for this population to reduce side effects and drug interactions. Dosage changes should be made slowly, since older adults are more sensitive than young patients to even minor changes.

COMPLICATIONS

Medication complications in patients with epilepsy are usually related to seizure events. Injuries that occur during seizures include falls, burns, motor vehicle accidents, and aspiration pneumonia. Risks can be reduced by making lifestyle changes at work and during recreation. Patient advocacy helps ensure safe environments at work and school and can discourage discrimination.

Recent evidence suggests that women and also men taking enzyme-inducing antiepileptic medications are at increased risk for osteoporosis and osteomalacia. This is related to bone metabolism and inadequate absorption of vitamin D.[24]

Convulsive or generalized tonic-clonic SE is a medical emergency that can lead to brain damage or even death.[10] Mortality and morbidity rates are related to the cause of SE and the time from the onset of SE until seizures are controlled. In patients with known epilepsy, one half of the hospital-reported cases of GCSE have been associated with subtherapeutic AED levels.[11] Other causes of SE include brain infection, trauma, and stroke. Most cases of SE can be treated successfully with parenteral drug therapy, including lorazepam, phenytoin, or phenobarbital.[13]

INDICATIONS FOR REFERRAL OR HOSPITALIZATION

Patients with frequent seizures or patients who meet the criteria for SE should be hospitalized for further evaluation and medication adjustment. Patients with seizures that are refractory to conventional therapy should be referred to a neurologist or epileptologist for further evaluation. If adequate seizure control is not achieved, patients should undergo presurgical and diagnostic evaluation with video EEG monitoring at a comprehensive epilepsy center. Patients who are having difficulty tolerating medications should also be referred for a neurology consultation. Patients with structural lesions should be referred promptly to a neurosurgeon for further evaluation.

PATIENT AND FAMILY EDUCATION

Epilepsy provides unique teaching opportunities because it is a chronic condition that affects all aspects of a patient's life. Patient and family education regarding safety is vital. It is imperative that patients avoid high places such as rooftops or ladders, not operate dangerous equipment that could cause cuts or crush injuries, and not swim alone. Family members should be taught simple first aid measures such as turning the patient onto his or her side and not putting objects into the mouth during a tonic-clonic seizure.

Other key areas for patient instruction include:

- The diagnosis
- Diagnostic studies
- Treatment plan
- Medication information
- Alternative or adjunctive therapies
- Safety issues and first aid for seizures
- Support services available (e.g., support groups, centers for independent living) and how to access them

HEALTH PROMOTION

Issues related to driving and other behaviors that impose a great safety risk should be discussed. Each state has varied restrictions for individuals with epilepsy who wish to obtain a driver's license. Information regarding the laws of a particular state can be found by calling the department of motor vehicles. Issues surrounding employment and psychosocial functioning should also be addressed. Resources such as vocational rehabilitation programs, clinical social workers, centers for independent living, and epilepsy support groups should be used.

Overall, moderation should be encouraged. Adequate rest, stress reduction, proper nutrition, and the avoidance of known seizure precipitants can improve seizure control.

Epilepsy is a challenging condition and requires a comprehensive approach to treatment. The goal is to treat the patient but not make the treatment worse than the disease. Efforts to understand the impact of epilepsy on patients will improve the health care provider's ability to treat appropriately and compassionately.

REFERENCES

1. Shorvon S: *Handbook of epilepsy treatment,* Oxford, 2000, Blackwell.
2. French J, Williamson PD, Thadani VM, and others: Characteristics of medial temporal lobe epilepsy, part I, Results of history and physical examination, *Ann Neurol* 34(6):774-780, 1993.
3. Commission on Classification and Terminology of the International League Against Epilepsy: Proposal for revised clinical and electroencephalographic classification of epileptic seizures, *Epilepsia* 22(4):489-501, 1981.
4. Driefuss F: Classification of the epilepsies: influence on management. In Santilli N, editor: *Managing seizure disorders: a handbook for health care practitioners,* Philadelphia, 1996, Lippincott-Raven.
5. Commission on Classification and Terminology of the International League Against Epilepsy: Proposal for revised classification of epilepsy and epileptic syndromes, *Epilepsia* 30(4):389-399, 1989.
6. Annegers J: The epidemiology of epilepsy. In Wylie E, editor: *The treatment of epilepsy: principles and practice,* Baltimore, 2001, Lippincott Williams & Wilkins.
7. Williamson P: Frontal lobe seizures: problems of diagnosis and classification. In Chauvel P, Delgado-Escueta AV, editors: *Advances in neurology,* New York, 1992, Raven Press.
8. Ebersole R, Pedley T, editors: *Current practice of clinical encephalography,* ed 3, Baltimore, 2003, Lippincott Williams & Wilkins.
9. So N, Andermann F: Differential diagnosis. In Engel J, Pedley T, editors: *Epilepsy: a comprehensive textbook,* Philadelphia, 1997, Lippincott-Raven.
10. Working Group on Status Epilepticus: Treatment of status epilepticus, *JAMA* 270:854-859, 1992.
11. Gilbert K: An algorithm for diagnosis and treatment of status epilepticus in adults, *J Neurosci Nurs* 31(1):27-29, 34-36, 1999.
12. Ramsay E: Treatment of status epilepticus, *Epilepsia* 34(Suppl 1):71-81, 1993.
13. Treiman D, Meyers PD, Walton NY, and others: A comparison of four treatments for generalized convulsive status epileptics, *N Engl J Med* 339(12):792-798, 1998.
14. Moore-Sledge CM: Evaluation and management of first seizures in adults, *Am Fam Phys* 56(4):1113-1120, 1997.
15. Beghi E, Berg A, Hauser W: Treatment of single seizures. In Engel J, Pedley T, editors: *Epilepsy: a comprehensive textbook,* Philadelphia, 1997, Lippincott-Raven.
16. First Seizure Trial Group: Randomized clinical trial on the efficacy of antiepileptic drugs in reducing the risk of relapse after a first unprovoked tonic clonic seizure, *Neurology* 43:478-483, 1993.
17. Freeman J, Pedley T: Indications for treatment. In Engel J, Pedley T, editors: *Epilepsy: a comprehensive textbook,* Philadelphia, 1997, Lippincott-Raven.
18. Santilli N: Selection and discontinuation of antiepileptic drugs. In Santilli N, editor: *Managing seizure disorders: a handbook for health care practitioners,* Philadelphia, 1996, Lippincott-Raven.
19. Berg A, Shinnar S, Chadwick D: Discontinuing antiepileptic drugs. In Engel J, Pedley T, editors: *Epilepsy: a comprehensive textbook,* Philadelphia, 1997, Lippincott-Raven.
20. Santilli N, Sierzant T: Surgical management of seizures. In Santilli N, editor: *Managing seizure disorders: a handbook for health care practitioners,* Philadelphia, 1996, Lippincott-Raven.
21. Crawford P: Best practice guidelines for the management of women with epilepsy, *Epilepsia* 46(Suppl 9):117-124, 2005.
22. Morrell M: Hormones and epilepsy through the lifetime, *Epilepsia* 33(Suppl 4):49-57, 1992.
23. Harden CL, Pulver MC, Ravdin L, and others: The effect of menopause and perimenopause on the course of epilepsy, *Epilepsia* 40:1402-1407, 1999.
24. Elliot JO, Darby JM, Jacobson MP: Bone loss in epilepsy; barriers to prevention, diagnosis and treatment, *Epilepsia* 45(Suppl 7):258, 2004.

CHAPTER 214

Trigeminal Neuralgia

Noreen M. Leahy

DEFINITION AND EPIDEMIOLOGY

Trigeminal neuralgia is a common and elusive disorder affecting the sensory branches of the trigeminal nerve. It was first described by John Fothergill in 1773 and is also known as tic douloureux, from the French for *painful spasm*.[1] Women are affected more often than men (3:2), and older adults more often than younger persons. The mean age of onset is 54 years for the idiopathic form and 33 years for the symptomatic form, in which an organic reason is evident.[2]

PATHOPHYSIOLOGY

The fifth cranial nerve, the trigeminal nerve, is a large, mixed sensory and motor nerve that originates in the brainstem and travels in the cervical cord, with the sensory ganglion found in Meckel's cave in the middle cranial fossa. The peripheral branches form three sensory divisions—ophthalmic (V1), maxillary (V2), and mandibular (V3)—which conduct sensory impulses from the greater part of the face and head, from the cornea and conjunctiva, and from the nose and mouth. These impulses eventually terminate in the thalamus, where they are relayed to the appropriate cortical area for interpretation. The motor portion of the nerve supplies the muscles of the jaw and sphenoid areas.

Most cases of trigeminal neuralgia are idiopathic, although some can be attributed to an underlying event such as trauma, multiple sclerosis, or herpes zoster.[1,3] The location of one of the cerebral arteries and its branches is thought to be a factor by creating compression on the nerve as it exits the brainstem. Demyelination, vascular changes, and degenerative changes in the sensory (gasserian) ganglion are postulated to generate altered impulse transmission, allowing ephaptic transmission between nerve fibers mediating light touch and pain.[3,4]

CLINICAL PRESENTATION

The primary feature of this disorder is recurrent paroxysms of pain in the distribution of any branch of the trigeminal nerve. The pain is usually described as burning, stabbing, sharp, penetrating, or electric shock–like and usually is on one side of the face. Males may have unshaven faces or portions thereof. The index of suspicion for multiple sclerosis rises if the patient exhibits bilateral facial pain. The duration of each paroxysm varies from seconds to more than 15 minutes and involves V2 and V3 more often than V1; V1 is more frequently affected by postherpetic neuralgia.[4] Pain may recur once a month or several times per day. If the pain occurs frequently during the day, the patient may complain of unremitting facial discomfort between discrete episodes. Usually, a patient does not awaken from sleep during a paroxysm. Cold weather may dramatically increase the frequency of pain episodes.[1]

During an attack, the patient may cease talking, stop chewing, become very still, rub or pinch the face, avoid making facial expressions during conversation, grimace, or make movements of the face and jaw. Between attacks, the patient is free of symptoms except for fear of an impending attack.

PHYSICAL EXAMINATION

A characteristic feature of trigeminal neuralgia is the trigger zone: a small area of the skin or orobuccal mucosa that the patient can identify as the point that sets off an attack. Trigger points are generally in the distribution of the nerve branch experiencing the pain. Chewing, talking, facial movement, or touch may elicit a paroxysm. Drafts or cool breezes may also precipitate symptoms.[5]

The patient may be reluctant to allow examination of the face for fear of triggering an attack. All cranial nerves should be examined in detail. The remainder of the physical examination, including the neurologic component, is normal.

DIAGNOSTICS AND DIFFERENTIAL DIAGNOSIS

The diagnosis of trigeminal neuralgia is usually made without difficulty from the history and the characteristic manner in which the patient relates the history (the patient is careful not to touch any trigger points or painful areas). However, the classic case presentation of trigeminal neuralgia may not always be encountered. Because there are innumerable causes of facial pain, prudence dictates that alternative diagnoses be investigated and that the patient be reexamined at regular intervals. The differential diagnosis should include headache, particularly migraine; acoustic neuroma; trigeminal neuroma; meningioma; aneurysms; acute polyneuropathy; chronic meningitis; multiple sclerosis; other neuralgias; and dental abnormalities.

Results of laboratory tests are either normal or noncontributory. If alternative diagnoses are suspected, an autoimmune laboratory panel may be indicated. Magnetic resonance angiography of the posterior fossa may be undertaken to differentiate vascular abnormalities. MRI can corroborate multiple sclerosis or mass lesions.

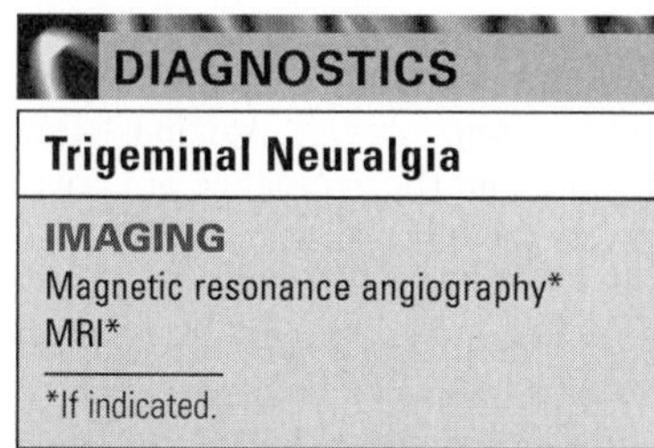

DIAGNOSTICS

Trigeminal Neuralgia

IMAGING
Magnetic resonance angiography*
MRI*

*If indicated.

DIFFERENTIAL DIAGNOSIS

Trigeminal Neuralgia

- Headache
- Acoustic neuroma
- Trigeminal neuroma
- Meningioma
- Aneurysms
- Acute polyneuropathy
- Chronic meningitis
- Multiple sclerosis
- Tumor
- Dental disorders
- Abscess
- Temporomandibular joint syndrome
- Sinusitis
- Migrainous neuralgia

MANAGEMENT

The treatment of trigeminal neuralgia has not changed much over the past decade. Regardless of the intervention adopted, symptoms may remit spontaneously and permanently. The mainstay of pharmacologic treatment centers on the use of anticonvulsants. When using anticonvulsant therapy, the provider should titrate to the maximum

TABLE 214-1 Pharmacotherapy of Trigeminal Neuralgia

Drug	Starting Dose	Maximum Dose	Complications
Carbamazepine (Tegretol)	100-200 mg q day	200-400 mg t.i.d.	Aplastic anemia, agranulocytosis, CNS effects
Phenytoin (Dilantin)	100-300 mg q day	300-500 mg q day	CNS effects, rash
Baclofen (Lioresal)	5-10 mg t.i.d.	30 mg t.i.d	Sedation, dizziness, dyspepsia
Divalproex (Depakote)	250 mg t.i.d.	1000-2500 mg t.i.d.	CNS effects, rash, elevated liver enzymes
Gabapentin (Neurontin)	100-300 mg q day	300-600 mg t.i.d.	CNS effects
Clonazepam (Klonopin)	0.5 mg t.i.d.	1-2 mg t.i.d.	CNS effects
Lamotrigine (Lamictal)	25-50 mg q day	150-200 mg b.i.d.	Rash, Stevens-Johnson syndrome

therapeutic dose necessary to provide pain relief, then titrate down to the lowest effective dose. Abrupt withdrawal of these agents should be avoided. A partial listing of more commonly used agents can be found in Table 214-1. Approximately two thirds of patients will respond to carbamazepine.[1]

If the patient does not respond satisfactorily to the treatments listed in Table 214-1 or has relief only at a dose that causes intolerable adverse effects, combination drug therapy may be started with clonazepam (Klonopin) or a tricyclic antidepressant, such as amitriptyline (Elavil). On occasion, corticosteroids, such as methylprednisolone (Solu-Medrol), may be used. The long-acting prostaglandin E analog misoprostol (Cytotec) has been useful in patients with trigeminal neuralgia associated with multiple sclerosis.[6]

COMPLICATIONS

Complications are usually related to pharmacologic management. Carbamazepine therapy may result in aplastic anemia, drowsiness, dizziness, or ataxia. Other medications also may have untoward effects. Surgical complications include facial numbness and infection, as well as the risk of any surgical procedure. Pain control may also be a significant factor, particularly if patients cannot tolerate the usually prescribed medications. In such an instance, additional management concerns may arise, with weight loss, dehydration, and poor dental hygiene if chewing, liquids, and oral care are triggers, as well as social isolation and depression.

INDICATIONS FOR REFERRAL OR HOSPITALIZATION

The primary care health care provider is often the initial practitioner to evaluate the patient with facial pain. After a thorough history and neurologic examination, a patient presumed to have trigeminal neuralgia should be referred to a neurologist for a more comprehensive physical and imaging examination. Medical treatment may be initiated by the specialist and managed by the health care provider. Care consists of medication initiation, observations for adverse effects, and consultation with the neurologist regarding dose adjustments and response to therapy. Consultation with a specialist is beneficial to the patient and provider in identifying the most efficacious regimen when combination drug therapy is necessary.

Referral to a neurosurgeon is indicated after medical therapies have been exhausted. Surgery is considered when medical regimens do not provide pain relief. Among the surgical interventions that may be appropriate are glycerol block, radiofrequency ablation, microvascular decompression, and stereotactic radiosurgery.[1] Major disadvantages of glycerol blocks, radiofrequency ablation, and decompression surgery include loss of facial sensation, keratitis, facial muscle weakness, spontaneous pain (anesthesia dolorosa), dysesthesias, and recurrent neuralgia.[7,8]

Consultation with a psychologist or psychiatrist may also be indicated, depending on the patient's adaptation skills. Multidisciplinary team meetings may be valuable in planning an approach to care. Referral to a pain center may also be an option for individuals with chronic pain.

PATIENT AND FAMILY EDUCATION

Significant education is necessary to explain the varied medication therapies, all of which are sedating. Caution about use of these medications in conjunction with use of alcohol and other medications is essential. Frequent monitoring of applicable laboratory tests is necessary to prevent commonly known complications of drug therapy. For patients in severe pain or those who are fearful of the next attack, it is important to consider the patient's activities of daily living, including eating, sleeping, and socializing with others. Severe pain may restrict adequate caloric intake; advising the patient to use a straw for liquids may allow intake of nutritional supplements. Maintaining dental hygiene may be challenging, since brushing may elicit pain; use of a Waterpik to clean the teeth may be of benefit to some. A collaborative relationship with the patient enhances a tailored, well-informed approach toward quality care.

REFERENCES

1. Swanson JW, Dodick DW, Capobianco DJ: Headache and other craniofacial pain. In Bradley WG, Daroff RB, Fenichel GM, and others, editors: *Neurology in clinical practice*, Boston, 2000, Butterworth Heinemann.
2. Bowsher D: Trigeminal neuralgia: an anatomically oriented review, *Clin Anat* 10:409-415, 1997.
3. Love S, Coakham HB: Trigeminal neuralgia: pathology and pathogenesis, *Brain* 124:2347, 2001.
4. Bajwa ZH, Ho CC, Khan SA: *Trigeminal neuralgia*, retrieved Sept 2005 from http://www.uptodateonline.com.
5. Adams AC: Facial pain. In Adams AC, editor: *Neurology in primary care*, Philadelphia, 2000, Davis.
6. Reder AT, Arnason BGW: Trigeminal neuralgia in multiple sclerosis relieved by prostaglandin-E analogue, *Neurology* 45:1097-1100, 1995.
7. Liao JJ, Cheng WC, Chang CN, and others: Reoperation for recurrent trigeminal neuralgia after microvascular decompression, *Surg Neurol* 47:562-568, 1997.
8. Barker FG, Janetta PJ, Bissonette DJ, and others: The long-term outcome of microvascular decompression for trigeminal neuralgia, *N Engl J Med* 334(17):1077-1083, 1996.

CHAPTER 215

Tumors of the Brain

Joanne Sandberg-Cook

DEFINITION AND EPIDEMIOLOGY

A tumor is defined as excess tissue that develops when cells duplicate out of control somewhere in the body. A tumor in the brain can be characterized as a benign or malignant expanding lesion and is either a primary tumor originating in the brain or adjacent tissues or a secondary, metastatic tumor that originates elsewhere and spreads to the brain via the blood or lymph systems. All brain tumors cause symptoms by infiltrating, expanding, and displacing healthy brain tissue.

Primary malignant brain tumors represent 1.35% of all primary malignant tumors. There were an estimated 18,820 new brain tumors in the United States in 2006.[1] Metastasis from tumors located in other parts of the body, especially lung or breast, is considerably more common, with an annual incidence of 170,000 cases in the United States.[1] Of all deaths from cancer, 2.4% result from tumors of the brain, with 50% of these patients dying within 1 to 3 years.[1]

Glial tumor is a general term for any tumor of the central nervous system (CNS) and is commonly subdivided into two main categories: astrocytic and oligodendroglial. Glial tumors include astrocytomas, ependymal tumors, glioblastoma multiforme, and primitive neuroectodermal tumors. Many specific tumor types are identified and named for the cell of origin in the CNS. A meningioma originates from the meninges, an adenoma from glandular tissue, a sarcoma from CNS connective tissue, and a neuroma from neurons.[2] Tumor grading is based on the presence or absence of standard pathologic features and how quickly the tumor is likely to grow. Grades range from I to IV, with grade IV being the most aggressive and most difficult to treat. The most commonly used grading system is one developed by the World Health Organization in 1979 and revised in 1999.[3] Currently there is no tumor (TNM) staging system for primary brain tumors. Primary brain tumors can spread within the CNS but rarely to other parts of the body.

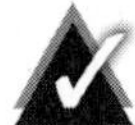

Physician consultation is indicated for all suspected brain tumors.

PATHOPHYSIOLOGY

The nervous system consists of two basic types of cells: neurons and neuroglia. Neurons carry and transmit electric impulses throughout the CNS and peripheral nervous system (PNS). They are responsible for sensation, movement, the senses, and cognitive ability. New neurons are not produced after approximately 2 years of age. Therefore the incidence of tumor formation in neurons is very low.[4]

The neuroglia (nerve glue) cells are the connective tissue cells within the nervous system. There are several types of neuroglia cells, which outnumber neurons 5 to 10:1. Because these cells duplicate and divide throughout life, they are often the origin of primary tumors.[4]

Astrocytes are found in the gray or white matter of the brain. They twist around neurons to help form a supportive transport network, to connect neurons to blood vessels, and to help form the blood-brain barrier. Tumors in these cells are the most common and invasive of all primary brain tumors and have the poorest prognosis.[4]

Oligodendrocytes also construct the semirigid support network between neurons and produce a conductive sheath around the neuronal axons and dendrites. Tumors in the oligodendrocytes are the next most common type of malignant brain tumor.[4]

Microglia are small macrophages within the CNS. Ependymal cells are ciliated CNS epithelial cells that help circulate the cerebrospinal fluid. Neurolemmocytes (Schwann cells) are the oligodendrocytes of the PNS. Satellite cells support ganglia in the PNS.[4]

CLINICAL PRESENTATION

Clinical signs and symptoms tend to be subtle and insidious in onset, often vague and nonfocal at first. Generalized symptoms such as headache or, in more advanced cases, nausea and vomiting reflect increased intracranial pressure. Focal signs, including hemiparesis and aphasia, reflect the location of the tumor.[5]

The most common initial symptom is headache, typically an early morning headache, sometimes rousing the patient from sleep, which comes and goes, does not throb, and gradually improves during the day. The headache worsens with exercise, coughing, or a change in body position.[5]

Seizures are common, especially in patients with low-grade gliomas.[1] Typically the seizures are focal, but they may become generalized and cause loss of consciousness. Mental changes, including problems with memory, speech, communication, reasoning, or concentration, can be seen, as can subtle or dramatic changes in interests, temperament, and affect.[6]

Neurologic changes are often more pronounced and may include loss of balance or coordination, unsteady gait, paralysis, or altered sensation. Blurred or double vision, narrowed fields of vision, crossed eyes, or eye pain can be seen. Hearing problems such as tinnitus, decreased hearing, and earache can occur.

A tumor should be considered in the following specific circumstances: a stroke or seizure in a healthy gravid or postpartum patient, or patients more than 20 years of age who have new seizures or new multiple endocrinopathies.[7]

PHYSICAL EXAMINATION

The health care provider should carefully examine areas that relate to the patient's symptoms. Focus in these areas can sometimes help determine the location and extent of the tumor. Other significant findings are elicited by careful examination of the following:

Eyes: Extraocular movements; pupils equal, round, react to light, and accommodation (PERRLA); visual fields; funduscopic examination; acuity; color discrimination

Ears: Gross hearing, Weber's and Rinne's tests, audiogram as needed

Neck: Range of motion, thyroid nodularity, palpation, nodes, suppleness

Neurologic system: Cranial nerves, deep tendon reflexes, gait, Romberg's sign, Babinski's reflex, cerebellar testing, mental status, stereotactics, extremity sensation, motion and strength, and a full evaluation of focal neurologic deficits

DIAGNOSTICS

The most common diagnostic tests for brain tumors include an MRI with gadolinium enhancement or a CT scan if MRI is contraindicated.[8] If an abnormality is found, a neuro-oncologist may recommend a number of other studies to help define the extent of the tumor before biopsy. Positron emission tomography (PET) scans show chemical functioning of organs and tissues as opposed to structure. A PET scan can detect not only a tumor in the initial stages of growth, but also its type, malignancy, and spread without the need for a risky brain biopsy.[8]

Blood tests may also be indicated, particularly if a prior tumor is being monitored and metastasis is suspected. The tests look at specific hormones produced by cancers (tumor markers) and can help evaluate tumor progression or recurrence.

DIFFERENTIAL DIAGNOSIS

Brain tumor is a distinct pathologic entity that needs to be differentiated from cerebrovascular, demyelinating, inflammatory, and infectious diseases that can cause brain lesions. This is generally possible from clinical and radiologic features. Some exceptions may require additional imaging methods.[9]

Headaches have a variety of causes, the most common being migraine, cluster or tension headaches, and neck strain (see Chapter 208). An inquiry about trauma to exclude various bleeds, whiplash, or a postconcussive headache is important. In addition, infectious causes, including sinusitis, otitis, herpes, meningitis, encephalitis, or abscesses, should be considered in the differential diagnosis. Other dangerous headaches include those associated with spontaneous intracranial hemorrhage, stroke, temporal arteritis, iritis, acute glaucoma, or poisoning (e.g., carbon monoxide exposure).[10]

DIAGNOSTICS

Tumors of the Brain

LABORATORY
Tumor markers*

IMAGING
CT scan, MRI*
PET* (consult with radiologist to determine if contrast is indicated)

*If indicated.

DIFFERENTIAL DIAGNOSIS

Tumors of the Brain

- Migraine
- Cluster headache
- Temporal arteritis
- Vasculitis, Wegener's granulomatosis
- Tension headache
- Sarcoidosis
- Postconcussive headache
- CNS herpes
- Sinusitis
- Pseudotumor
- Otitis
- Cerebrovascular accident
- Meningitis, encephalitis, abscess
- Aneurysm

MANAGEMENT

Primary brain tumors are treated surgically whenever feasible.[5] The tumor must be in a relatively accessible area to spare normal brain or spinal cord tissue as much as possible. Radiation and, finally, chemotherapy are used as adjunctive therapies. Radiotherapy can significantly prolong survival, especially in glial tumors. Tumor treatment is specific to tumor type and grade. Metastatic brain tumors are typically treated with whole brain radiotherapy.[1] Surgical resection may be helpful to patients with a single brain metastasis. Stereotactic radiosurgery may be an alternative to surgery.[1] Primary CNS lymphoma is always treated first with chemotherapy. Resection does not have a role in this disease.[5]

Increased intracranial pressure can be treated with dexamethasone IV or PO. If the patient is having seizures, anticonvulsants are usually prescribed. Prophylactic prescription of anticonvulsants in patients who are not having seizures is not recommended.[11] If brain edema is present, a fluid shunt may be placed.

Clinical trials should be considered when possible. Many newer treatment approaches are currently in clinical trial, including hyperthermia therapy and biologic therapy.[12] Palliative care is essential if the patient is not a candidate for or has failed the previously mentioned therapies (see Chapter 15). Prognosis and advance directives should be discussed openly. Hospice can be helpful in preparing and caring for the patient and family during the terminal phase of the illness.

The emotional implications of a brain or spinal cord tumor diagnosis can be overwhelming for the patient and family. Tremendous support is necessary. Questions should be answered openly and honestly, and resources offered for questions that the health care provider is unable to answer. When developing a treatment plan, the provider should recognize not only the diagnosis but also the individuality of the patient. His or her age, life potential, desires, and physical abilities should be considered. The patient and family should be assisted in developing the treatment plan and advance directives.

LIFE SPAN CONSIDERATIONS

Although the majority of primary CNS tumors occur in patients over the age of 45 years, they are also the most prevalent solid neoplasms of childhood, the second (after leukemia) leading cancer-related cause of death in children, and the third leading cancer-related cause of death in adolescents and adults between the ages of 15 and 34 years.[13] The reported incidence of brain tumor is increasing in persons over the age of 65. This may be related to widespread use of MRI and CT scanning, which identify tumors that otherwise might not come to the attention of health care providers.

COMPLICATIONS

Tumor growth may compress vital brain tissue; block the flow of various fluids; and cause endocrinopathies, weakness or paralysis, and the loss of senses. Vascular compromise, including coagulopathies, disseminated intravascular coagulopathy, cerebrovascular accidents, thrombocytopenia, intracranial hemorrhage or pressure, and thromboses, can also be problematic.[1,4,7] The mass effect from fluid accumulation or tumor growth can further damage delicate brain tissue.

Tumor therapies can also cause difficulties, including immunosuppression, hair loss, weakness, fatigue, cognitive impairment, and gastrointestinal upset or bleeding. Any of the previously discussed therapies can cause neurologic or psychologic problems. Cancer metastasis or recurrence requires continual monitoring.

INDICATIONS FOR REFERRAL OR HOSPITALIZATION

Neurosurgical and oncologic referral for specific diagnosis of tumor type, grading, and definitive treatment is imperative, and early consultation is indicated. The development of new symptoms requires a referral to the specialist for evaluation of specific treatments, tumor progression, or new tumor formation. Specialty care, especially for children and adolescents, may also offer easier access to therapeutic trials. In general, hospitalization is reserved for patients with severe symptoms or unstable clinical findings that cannot be safely or efficiently managed in the outpatient setting. Tumor removal may be performed in a surgical center or limited-stay hospital setting. Postoperative patients may need or benefit from rehabilitation.

PATIENT AND FAMILY EDUCATION

A thorough understanding of the disease process is usually helpful for patients and families. It is important that patients be safe. If the clinical picture includes seizures or loss of consciousness, patients should avoid driving or operating dangerous machinery. Unfortunately, this may affect the patients' mobility and capacity for independent living. Offering alternatives is helpful.

Many useful books are available in public and medical center libraries, and the Internet contains an enormous amount of information and a large number of support groups.

HEALTH PROMOTION

Dietary considerations depend on tumor type, specific medications and treatments, and co-morbid illness.[14] Pharmacists and nutritionists may be helpful resources.

In general, patients should be encouraged to follow a diet and lifestyle that is as normal and healthy as possible. Depression is common in patients with brain tumor and should be addressed when appropriate. Quality of life should be emphasized and support offered when needed. Because prognosis is grim with most malignant brain tumors, advance directives need to be discussed and the patient encouraged to appointment of a health care proxy.

REFERENCES

1. Tam TM: Current role of radiation therapy in the management of malignant brain tumors, *Hematol Oncol Clin North Am* 20:431-453, 2006.
2. Schiff D, Batchelder T: *Classification of brain tumors*, retrieved June 20, 2006, from http://www.uptodate.com.
3. Tatter MD: *The new WHO classification of tumors affecting the central nervous system*, 1998, retrieved June 20, 2006, from http://neurosurgery.mgh.harvard.edu/newwhobt.htm.
4. William J, Weiner G: *Neurology for the nonneurologist*, ed 3, Baltimore, 1994, Lippincott.
5. DeAngelis L: Brain tumors, *N Engl J Med* 344(2):114-123, 2001.
6. Fox SW, Mitchell SA, Booth-Jones M: Cognitive impairment in patients with brain tumors: assessment and intervention in the clinic setting, *Clin J Oncol Nurs* 10(2):169-176, 2006.
7. Cantu RC: *Neurology in primary care*, New York, 1985, Macmillan.
8. *What is PET*, retrieved June 24, 2006, from http://interactive.snm.org/index.cfm?pageID=972.
9. Okamoto K, Furusawa T, Ishikawa K, and others: Mimics of brain tumor on neuroimaging, part II, *Radiat Med* 22(3):135-142, 2004.
10. Remmel K, Bunyan R, Brumback R, and others: *Handbook of symptom-oriented neurology*, ed 3, St Louis, 2002, Mosby.
11. Sperling MR, Ko J: Seizures and brain tumors, *Semin Oncol* 33(3):333-341, 2006.
12. National Cancer Institute: *Adult brain tumors: treatment statement for patients*, retrieved June 19, 2006, from http://www.meb.uni-bonn.de/cancer.gov/CDR0000062697.html.
13. American Cancer Society: *Detailed guide: brain/CNS tumors in children: what are brain and spinal cord tumors in children?*, retrieved June 25, 2006, from http://www.cancer.org/docroot/CRI/content/CRI_2_4_1X_What_are_childrens_brain_and_spinal_cord_tumors_4.asp.
14. American Brain Tumor Association: *A primer of brain tumors*, retrieved June 25, 2006, from http://www.abta.org/buildingknowledge5.htm.

PART 17

Evaluation and Management of Endocrine and Metabolic Disorders

JOANNE SANDBERG-COOK, *Section Editor*

CHAPTER 216

Acromegaly

Alan Ona Malabanan

DEFINITION AND EPIDEMIOLOGY

Acromegaly is an insidious, chronic, debilitating disease arising from the prolonged excessive secretion of growth hormone (GH). This excess GH manifests as excessive bone and soft tissue growth. Untreated or partially treated patients with acromegaly have double the expected mortality rate of age-matched healthy subjects. The increased prevalence of hypertension and diabetes mellitus associated with acromegaly increases cardiovascular morbidity and mortality. Sleep apnea associated with acromegaly may also lead to cardiopulmonary decline. Motor vehicle accidents from daytime somnolence and sleep deprivation contribute to the overall mortality risk. Patients with acromegaly may also have an increased risk for malignancy, particularly of the colon.

Acromegaly is rare, but the diagnosis is commonly delayed or missed. Studies have suggested a prevalence of 40 to 60 cases per 1 million persons and an annual incidence of 3 cases per 1 million persons per year.[1] It is usually diagnosed in middle age, with a mean age at diagnosis of 40 years in men and 45 years in women. When GH excess occurs in children (before the closure of the epiphyseal plates), gigantism results.

Physician consultation is indicated for all patients with suspected acromegaly.

PATHOPHYSIOLOGY

GH is secreted by cells in the anterior pituitary gland. Its secretion is regulated by the two hypothalamic hormones: growth hormone–releasing hormone (GHRH) and somatostatin (SS). GHRH stimulates both GH secretion and production, whereas SS inhibits GH secretion. GH secretion is pulsatile, with brief surges followed by long periods of inactivity. Many physiologic stimuli affect GH secretion, including stress (increased), sleep (increased), meals (increased or decreased), and aging (decreased). The variable nature of a random serum GH level limits its usefulness in diagnosing acromegaly.

Insulin-like growth factor I (IGF-I, or somatomedin C) is a GH-dependent protein produced by the liver. Its serum level is directly proportional to the 24-hour integrated serum GH level, and it is a much better indicator of GH excess than a random serum GH level. The bone and soft tissue growth in acromegaly is a direct result of the effects of GH and IGF-I. In addition, GH has several other metabolic effects, including insulin antagonism, lipolysis, and protein anabolism, resulting in glucose intolerance, decreased fat stores, and increased muscle mass.

The most common cause of GH excess is a GH-secreting pituitary adenoma. Rare (<1%) causes include GHRH-producing tumors such as hypothalamic (hamartomas), bronchial carcinoid, and pancreatic islet cell tumors. Ectopic production of GH has been described in pancreatic islet cell tumors. Acromegaly may be associated with multiple endocrine neoplasia type 1; a triad of pituitary tumor, hyperparathyroidism, and pancreatic tumor; and McCune-Albright syndrome, a genetic disease associated with polyostotic fibrous dysplasia, café au lait spots, and endocrine hyperfunction.

CLINICAL PRESENTATION

Acromegaly in younger patients tends to result from more aggressive tumors and may develop relatively rapidly.[2] In older patients it develops insidiously over many years. As mentioned previously, the diagnosis is often delayed, with most patients having symptoms for 10 to 20 years. Symptoms result from the effects of GH excess or from the pituitary mass's effect on surrounding brain structures. An evaluation of 500 patients with acromegaly revealed the following most common clinical features (in order of frequency): excessive acral growth, enlargement of facial features, soft tissue swelling, excessive sweating, headache, peripheral neuropathy, decreased energy, paresthesia, osteoarthritis, impotence, daytime somnolence, carpal tunnel syndrome, muscular weakness, depression, decreased libido, hypertrichosis, dyspnea, and galactorrhea. About half these patients had hypertension, and 66% had abnormal glucose metabolism (either glucose intolerance or frank diabetes mellitus).[3] Visual field disturbance and amenorrhea may also be presenting complaints.

PHYSICAL EXAMINATION

The earliest and most common physical changes occur in the skin and extremities. The growth of the soft tissues produces facial puffiness; broadening of the nose; furrowing of the brow; skin thickening (bogginess) of the hands and feet; and enlargement of the tongue, uvula, and soft palate, leading to sleep apnea. Vocal cord thickening results in a deeper and coarser voice. Skin tags (acrochordon) are more common in patients with acromegaly, as are colonic polyps.

Facial bone growth leads to coarsened facial features, which are usually recognizable only when they are very severe or after review of the patient's old photographs. These changes include growth of the calvaria and mandible, producing a prominent brow, an enlarged jaw, and dental malocclusion. With growth of the jaw, there is also widening of the spaces between the teeth. Excessive rib growth produces a barrel-shaped chest. Glove and shoe size changes result from bone growth in the hands and feet. Loss of lateral visual fields (bitemporal hemianopsia), papilledema, extraocular palsy, or even rhinorrhea may result from the pituitary tumor's impingement on surrounding structures.

DIAGNOSTICS

Random serum GH levels are not useful in the diagnosis of acromegaly. IGF-I, IGF-binding protein-3, and 24-hour urine study for GH are all GH dependent and are useful as screening tests for acromegaly.[4,5] It is important that these tests be done at laboratories with age-adjusted reference ranges because GH secretion normally decreases with age. Unfortunately, normal and abnormal values for these tests may overlap.

For more than 40 years the definitive test for acromegaly was the oral glucose tolerance test (OGTT),[5] which most

DIAGNOSTICS

Acromegaly

LABORATORY
Serum insulin-like growth factor-I (IGF-I) level
IGF binding protein-3
24-Hour urine study for growth hormone
Plasma growth hormone–releasing hormone*
Oral glucose tolerance test

IMAGING
MRI

OTHER
Oral glucose tolerance test for growth hormone suppression

*If indicated.

clearly demonstrates pathologic GH secretion. In a normal individual, GH secretion is suppressed by an oral glucose load. This test is contraindicated in a patient with poorly controlled diabetes mellitus.

The test is conducted as follows: after an overnight fast, blood is drawn for a baseline serum glucose and GH level. Glucose 75 g is given orally. Samples for serum glucose and GH are then taken every 30 minutes for a total of 120 minutes after the oral glucose challenge. In a normal individual, GH should be suppressed to less than 2 ng/ml by radioimmunoassay and to less than 1 ng/ml by the newer immunoradiometric assay.[6] In a patient with acromegaly there is failure of suppression of GH after a glucose load. As newer assays become more sensitive, it is likely that these criteria will change. Results of the OGTT should always be evaluated together with the IGF-I measurement. Recent research has suggested that a normal OGTT may occur in acromegalic patients with elevated IGF-I levels, so a normal OGTT result does not necessarily rule out acromegaly.[7]

After the biochemical diagnosis of acromegaly, imaging of the pituitary gland should be performed, preferably with MRI. If no pituitary tumor is seen or if generalized pituitary hyperplasia is seen, the possibility of ectopic GHRH production should be considered. A plasma GHRH determination may be helpful in this instance.

DIFFERENTIAL DIAGNOSIS

The primary differential diagnostic consideration in acromegaly is an etiologic one: What is the cause of the GH excess? A few other situations, however, should be examined. Pseudoacromegaly is a syndrome characterized by acromegaloid features and severe insulin resistance without elevated GH or IGF-I levels. Benign familial prognathism may prompt evaluation for acromegaly, but GH and IGF-I levels are normal. Paget's disease of the bone can cause bony deformities, particularly in the skull, but, again, GH and IGF-I levels should be normal. Although the OGTT is the standard test for the diagnosis of acromegaly, in some conditions GH secretion fails to suppress after a glucose load. Among these are severe liver or renal disease, uncontrolled diabetes mellitus, malnutrition, anorexia nervosa, heroin addiction, and levodopa ingestion.[8]

DIFFERENTIAL DIAGNOSIS

Acromegaly

- Pseudoacromegaly
- Benign familial prognathism
- Paget's disease of the bone
- Severe liver disease
- Severe renal disease
- Uncontrolled diabetes
- Malnutrition
- Anorexia nervosa
- Heroin addiction
- Levodopa ingestion

MANAGEMENT AND CO-MANAGEMENT WITH SPECIALISTS

Acromegaly should be co-managed with an endocrinologist experienced in managing acromegaly and hypopituitarism. Early diagnosis is crucial in curing this disease because the success of surgical therapy, the therapy of choice, depends on tumor size. Cure is defined as a reduction in IGF-I to the age-adjusted normal range and a suppressed GH after OGTT to less than 1 ng/ml.[6] For those with small (<10 mm [0.4 inch]), well-localized pituitary tumors, the cure rate is approximately 70% to 80% at major neurosurgical centers.[6,9] The cure rate decreases to less than 50% for tumors larger than 10 mm.

For patients who are not surgical candidates and for patients with postsurgery recurrence, two alternatives exist: pituitary irradiation and medical therapy. Pituitary irradiation effects are delayed. Ten years after irradiation, 50% of patients have adequate GH suppression by old criteria (<5 ng/ml).[10] There is a high risk of hypopituitarism complicating this procedure. Various modalities of radiotherapy are available: stereotactic (proton beam, linac, Gamma Knife), and conventional. Stereotactic, focused radiotherapy may be contraindicated if the tumor is within 5 mm (0.2 inch) of the optic nerve and chiasm. Medical treatment is required for patients in whom radiotherapy is ineffective or contraindicated.

Somatostatin analogs (octreotide) and dopamine agonists (bromocriptine and cabergoline) are the two most commonly used medical therapies. Octreotide is given as three daily subcutaneous injections (100 to 250 mcg/dose) and has produced normalization of IGF-I in 60% and GH of less than 2 ng/ml in 40% of 103 patients studied recently.[11] New long-acting formulations of SS analogs (octreotide-LAR) are now available and have similar efficacy, with the benefit of less frequent administration (intramuscular injection every 2 to 4 weeks).[12,13] Bromocriptine is titrated to a maximum of 20 mg/day and is given orally. It is, however, less effective than octreotide; fewer than 10% treated with bromocriptine have normalization of IGF-I, and fewer than 20% have GH of less than 5 ng/ml.[10] Cabergoline, used in dosages between 1 and 4 mg/wk, has shown more promise, particularly in tumors co-secreting prolactin.[14] The most common side effects are gastrointestinal for bromocriptine (nausea and vomiting), cabergoline (nausea, gastrointestinal cramping), and octreotide (diarrhea, abdominal discomfort, and gallstones). A GH receptor antagonist, pegvisomant, has also been approved for medical therapy of acromegaly and appears to have less impact on glucose homeostasis than somatostatin analogs.[15,16]

LIFE SPAN CONSIDERATIONS

When GH excess occurs in children (before the closure of the epiphyseal plates), gigantism results. Acromegaly in younger patients tends to result from more aggressive tumors and may develop relatively rapidly.[2] In older patients it develops insidiously over many years. Untreated or partially treated patients with acromegaly have double the expected mortality rate of age-matched healthy subjects. The diagnosis is often delayed, with most patients having symptoms for 10 to 20 years.

COMPLICATIONS

The complications associated with advanced acromegaly are numerous and include diabetes, cardiovascular disease, hypertension, sleep apnea, osteoarthritis, peripheral neuropathies, and increased incidence of malignancy. These conditions affect quality of life and increase mortality rates. All cases need to be managed in collaboration with a physician because many of the complications may not remit after treatment of the excess GH. Complications of surgical or radiation therapy include hypopituitarism and may require consultation with an endocrinologist.

INDICATIONS FOR REFERRAL OR HOSPITALIZATION

All patients suspected of having acromegaly should be referred to an endocrinologist experienced in the evaluation and treatment of acromegaly, if possible. The rarity of this condition, its increased mortality rate, and the complexity of its manifestations make this critical. Patients with evidence of pituitary tumor mass effect or hemorrhage need urgent neurosurgical referral.

Advanced acromegaly may lead to neurologic or cardiovascular complications requiring hospitalization. Any patient with new symptoms of headache, visual disturbance, dyspnea, or chest pain should be promptly evaluated.

PATIENT EDUCATION AND HEALTH PROMOTION

The normalization of GH and IGF-I levels is essential in the successful management of acromegaly and requires patient adherence to the prescribed medical therapy. Patients should realize that acromegaly is a chronic and progressive disease, resulting in a multitude of complications that may be avoided or delayed with prompt and appropriate therapy. Patients should be aware that the changes in physical appearance will likely not remit even with successful therapy, but will likely worsen if the condition is not treated. The provider should alert patients to the symptoms of sleep apnea, diabetes mellitus, heart disease, and hypopituitarism so that appropriate evaluation and therapy may be undertaken.

REFERENCES

1. Etxabe J, Gaztambide S, Latorre P, and others: Acromegaly: an epidemiologic study, *J Endocrinol Invest* 16:181-187, 1993.
2. Melmed S, Ho K, Klibanski A, and others: Recent advances in pathogenesis, diagnosis, and management of acromegaly, *J Clin Endocrinol Metab* 80:3395-3402, 1995.
3. Ezzat S, Forster MJ, Berchtold P, and others: Acromegaly: clinical and biochemical features in 500 patients, *Medicine* 73:233-240, 1994.
4. Grinspoon S, Clemmons D, Swearingen B, and others: Serum insulin-like growth factor–binding protein-3 levels in the diagnosis of acromegaly, *J Clin Endocrinol Metab* 80:927-932, 1995.
5. Stoffel-Wagner B, Springer W, Bidlingmaier F, and others: A comparison of different methods for diagnosing acromegaly, *Clin Endocrinol* 46:531-537, 1997.
6. Giustina A, Barkan A, Casanueva FF, and others: Criteria for cure of acromegaly: a consensus statement, *J Clin Endocrinol Metab* 85:526-529, 2000.
7. Dimaraki EV, Jaffe CA, DeMott-Friberg R, and others: Acromegaly with apparently normal GH secretion: implications for diagnosis and follow-up, *J Clin Endocrinol Metab* 87:3537-3542, 2002.
8. Wass JAH, Besser M: Tests of pituitary function. In DeGroot LJ, editor: *Endocrinology*, ed 3, Philadelphia, 1995, Saunders.
9. Kreutzer J, Vance ML, Lopes MBS, and others: Surgical management of GH-secreting pituitary adenomas: an outcome study using modern remission criteria, *J Clin Endocrinol Metab* 86:4072-4077, 2001.
10. Melmed S, Jackson I, Kleinberg D, and others: Current treatment guidelines for acromegaly, *J Clin Endocrinol Metab* 83:2646-2652, 1998.
11. Newman CB, Melmed S, Snyder PJ, and others: Safety and efficacy of long term octreotide therapy of acromegaly: results of a multicenter trial in 103 patients: a clinical research study, *J Clin Endocrinol Metab* 80:2768-2775, 1995.
12. Colao AM, Ferone D, Marzullo P, and others: Long-term effects of depot long-acting somatostatin analog octreotide on hormone levels and tumor mass in acromegaly, *J Clin Endocrinol Metab* 86:2779-2786, 2001.
13. Baldelli R, Colao A, Razzore P, and others: Two-year follow-up of acromegalic patients treated with slow release lantreotide (30 mg), *J Clin Endocrinol Metab* 85(11):4099-4103, 2000.
14. Abs R, Verhelst J, Maiter D, and others: Cabergoline in the treatment of acromegaly: a study in 64 patients, *J Clin Endocrinol Metab* 83:374-378, 1998.
15. Trainer PJ, Drake WM, Katznelson L, and others: Treatment of acromegaly with the growth hormone–receptor antagonist pegvisomant, *N Engl J Med* 342:1171-1177, 2000.
16. Barkan AL, Burman P, Clemmons DR, and others: Glucose homeostasis and safety in patients with acromegaly converted from long-acting octreotide to pegvisomant, *J Clin Endocrinol Metab* 90(10):5684-5691, 2005.

CHAPTER 217

Adrenal Gland Disorders

Dennis M. McCullough

DEFINITION AND EPIDEMIOLOGY

Adrenal gland disorders are conditions marked by inadequate or excessive amounts of glucocorticoid and mineralocorticoid hormones. These conditions can result from overproduction as a consequence of changes in the adrenal gland itself, from hypothalamic or pituitary gland dysfunction, or from the exogenous administration of corticosteroid medications. A second major hormone, aldosterone, a mineralocorticoid, is independently produced in the adrenal cortex and regulates renal and electrolyte (mineral) metabolism. Small amounts of androgens produced by the adrenal cortex also are linked to certain clinical syndromes. Three common types of adrenal gland disorders are discussed: Addison's disease, Cushing's syndrome, and pheochromocytoma.[1]

Addison's Disease

Historically, Addison's disease most commonly occurred as a result of bilateral destruction of the adrenal glands by tuberculosis. More recently, Addison's disease has been associated with autoimmune disturbances.[2] Recent increases in tuberculosis worldwide may alter these patterns. Data suggest that the prevalence of Addison's disease in western countries is 120 per 1 million individuals.[3]

Cushing's Syndrome

Determining the prevalence of Cushing's syndrome is complicated by pseudo-Cushing's syndrome, which is associated with both depression and obesity. Eighty percent of patients with major depression also have abnormal cortisol secretion. Thus a spectrum of disorders is clearly associated with the overproduction of cortisol.[4] Incidental adrenal adenoma found on CT and MRI imaging suggests possible early hypercortisolism and may occur at the rate of 20 to 30 per 1 million individuals.[5]

Pheochromocytoma

A pheochromocytoma is a tumor of chromaffin cells. Ninety percent of these tumors are found in the adrenal medulla. A small percentage may arise intraabdominally along the sympathetic ganglion chain, which also is made up of chromaffin tissue. A malignant process occurs when the tumor spreads beyond chromaffin tissue. Pheochromocytomas are typically unilateral; however, type II bilateral involvement is common in the setting of polyglandular multiple endocrine neoplasia (MEN).

Physician consultation is indicated for patients with adrenal gland disorders.

PATHOPHYSIOLOGY

Hypothalamus-synthesized corticotropin-releasing hormone regulates the secretion of corticotropin, or adrenocorticotropic hormone (ACTH), which in turn regulates the production of glucocorticoids. The glucocorticoids (cortisol) regulate the metabolic processes in the body's response to normal and abnormal physical and psychologic stimuli. This is accomplished by altering physiologic responses that range from hepatic glucose production to inflammatory and vascular reactions.

Underproduction disorders relate to the destruction or dysfunction of some portion of the hypothalamic-pituitary-adrenal axis or to the sudden consequences of withdrawing exogenous corticosteroids after high-dose use. Autoimmune disorders currently account for most cases of Addison's disease. Because more than 90% of both adrenal glands must be destroyed or malfunctioning before clinically recognized adrenal insufficiency is present, destruction by tuberculosis, bilateral hemorrhage or vein thrombosis, medications (rifampin, ketoconazole), and rare infections (meningococcemia, AIDS, histoplasmosis) are among the very rare remaining causes. Inadequate production of cortisol in the context of severe sudden illness or trauma, particularly in chronic users of corticosteroids, is a more common manifestation.

Cushing's syndrome results from ACTH-secreting tumors of the pituitary and occasionally from other conditions, including ectopic secretion of small cell lung carcinomas. Cortisol and ACTH levels are elevated. In rare instances, Cushing's syndrome results from primary overproduction of cortisol by the adrenal gland (low levels of serum ACTH and high levels of serum cortisol). Steroid medications systematically suppress pituitary production of ACTH, particularly when steroids are administered in high doses over long periods. Both short- and long-term regimens (>10 to 14 days) of corticosteroids are a common and appropriate part of the management of asthma, difficult dermatitis problems, various malignancies, rheumatic diseases, and a number of other acute and chronic disorders. Careful monitoring is mandatory to avoid, or to detect early, the impact on endogenous corticosteroid production.

Abnormal production of epinephrine and norepinephrine by a pheochromocytoma has multisystem effects. Renal effects include sodium retention, increased renin secretion, and reduction of hydrostatic pressure. Cardiovascular effects involve peripheral vasoconstrictors and increased cardiac contraction. Tissue oxygen consumption and gluconeogenesis are increased.

CLINICAL PRESENTATION

Addison's disease rarely appears suddenly, although a patient with known Addison's disease who is inadequately supplemented with corticosteroids can exhibit an abrupt onset of nausea, vomiting, hypotension, and acute shock, especially during a period of severe trauma or illness. Most presentations are chronic, with dizziness, nausea, vomiting, chronic abdominal pain, muscle cramps, hyperpigmentation, decreased libido, lethargy, weakness, weight loss, and a progressive decline of health.

Cushing's syndrome almost always manifests with chronic changes; the exception is a patient who has been taking high-dose steroids over a prolonged period. Sudden weight gain, loss of menses, decreased libido, weakness, depression, insomnia, and bruising are all possible presenting symptoms.[6]

With pheochromocytoma, patients may have a family history of the disease, MEN, neurofibromatosis, or multiple neuroma syndrome. Presenting symptoms are episodic and include headache, facial flushing, diaphoresis, and palpitations.[7] The symptomatic episodes last 15 to 30 minutes and may be precipitated by specific activities.

PHYSICAL EXAMINATION

Patients with Addison's disease appear chronically ill. They exhibit weight loss, dehydration, and increased skin pigmentation—a result of melanocyte stimulation by pituitary hormones attempting to drive the adrenal glands. Darkened creases of the palms, elbows, knees, and lips commonly occur. Occasionally, vitiligo is reported.

Patients with Cushing's syndrome have a characteristic habitus similar to, but subtly and importantly different from, that of many patients with exogenous obesity. Central obesity, a moon face appearance caused by thickening of facial fat, the classically described "buffalo hump" dorsocervical fat pad (common with all obesity), increased supraclavicular fat pads, hypertension, thigh muscle weakness and wasting, hirsutism, abdominal skin striae, and acne can be associated signs. Emotional lability or depression may occur as well.

With pheochromocytoma the physical examination is marked by a new onset of moderate to severe hypertension, with systolic pressures above 170 mm Hg. Arrhythmias or sinus tachycardia or bradycardia may be present. The course is characterized by substantial variations in blood pressure measurements.

DIAGNOSTICS

Patients with Addison's disease have an elevated serum ACTH level and suppressed levels of cortisol. Hyponatremia and hyperkalemia related to lost aldosterone production might be a serendipitous finding that suggests Addison's disease. Eosinophilia, azotemia, and hypoglycemia may be present. Adrenal antibody studies to identify autoimmune disorders should be ordered in concert with an endocrinology consultation. Chest x-ray studies and tuberculin testing are essential to exclude underlying tuberculosis.

Metabolic acidosis or decreased potassium or chloride may be present. Cushing's syndrome is most accurately diagnosed by measurement of the 24-hour excretion of cortisol in the urine. This excretion study is thought to be more dependable than serum ACTH and serum cortisol testing. Confirmation of the 24-hour urine cortisol elevation by two or three repeat tests is important because cortisol production can vary markedly from day to day, even in Cushing's syndrome. Pursuit of this elusive diagnosis is an appropriate aspect of a primary care practice. Suppression testing with ACTH is another laborious diagnostic process and may require careful pursuit to separate the physiology of the obese and depressed patients from that of those with true Cushing's syndrome.[8] Consultation is required for testing to separate disorders primary to the pituitary from those primary to the adrenal glands.

Elevated levels of catecholamines in a 24-hour urine collection confirm the diagnosis of pheochromocytoma. To increase accuracy, the collection must occur during a period of hypertension in association with episodes of facial flushing, diaphoresis, or palpitations. Many medications alter the accuracy of the test. Alcohol, amphetamines, quinidine, theophylline, tetracycline, and disulfiram can either raise or lower catecholamine levels. Therefore a careful medication review and consultation of current test guidelines must occur. Specialist consultation concerning test results may be indicated. With abnormal test results, the search for a tumor is undertaken with adrenal CT scan or MRI.[9]

DIAGNOSTICS

Adrenal Gland Disorders

ADDISON'S DISEASE

Laboratory
Serum electrolytes
BUN
Creatinine
Serum glucose
Serum cortisol and serum ACTH
ACTH stimulation test

Imaging
Chest x-ray*

Other
Purified protein derivative

CUSHING'S DISEASE

Laboratory
Creatinine
24-Hour urine for cortisol
ACTH suppression test

PHEOCHROMOCYTOMA

Laboratory
24-Hour urine for catecholamines, metanephrines* and vanillylmandelic acid*

Imaging
CT scan, MRI*

*If indicated.

DIFFERENTIAL DIAGNOSIS

Both Addison's disease and Cushing's syndrome can be difficult to distinguish from normal physiology, particularly because both chronic and acute stresses have such an impact on adrenal hormone production.[10] Addisonian symptoms, when mild, can be produced by eating disorders, alcoholism, malnutrition, hyperthyroidism, diabetes, and the wasting effects of a chronic illness such as AIDS or metastatic cancer. Psychiatric symptoms, including apathy, confusion, and depression, are common with adrenal insufficiency presentations and often confound the clinical assessment. By far the most commonly seen conditions are those associated with exogenous steroid use or with withdrawal or inadequate steroid use in circumstances of stress. Cushing's syndrome can be confused with depression or obesity. Pheochromocytoma is most commonly confused with anxiety or labile "white coat" hypertension.

DIFFERENTIAL DIAGNOSIS

Adrenal Gland Disorders

ADDISON'S DISEASE
- Eating disorders
- Alcoholism
- Malnutrition
- Hyperthyroidism
- Diabetes
- Chronic illness
- Psychogenic illness

CUSHING'S SYNDROME
- Obesity
- Depression

PHEOCHROMOCYTOMA
- Essential hypertension
- Anxiety
- Intracranial neoplasm
- Subarachnoid or intracranial hemorrhage
- Medication withdrawal (clonidine or monoamine oxidase inhibitor)
- Diencephalia epilepsy

MANAGEMENT

An acute adrenal crisis is best managed in the hospital, although treatment for shock with corticosteroids should begin immediately. Chronic adrenal insufficiency is generally a nonemergency and can be treated in an outpatient context with oral hydrocortisone in divided daily doses (total 20 to 30 mg) to allow for restoration of a diurnal pattern. Careful individualized dosing, guided by patients' symptomatic responses, constitutes the core of good management. Mineralocorticoid replacement in Addison's disease with fludrocortisone (0.05 to 0.2 mg/day PO) corrects the renal disturbance and hypotension. The need for replacement doses is monitored by frequent measurement of electrolytes, serum renin, serum ACTH, and judiciously timed serum cortisol levels. Careful dose adjustments can enhance a patient's sense of well-being and quality of life.

Management of Cushing's syndrome depends on the source of the hypercortisolism. Current imaging techniques have enhanced the approach to pituitary surgery and greatly aid in the search for nonadrenal sources of ACTH and adrenal sources of cortisol. Pituitary tumor resection, when indicated, remains the first choice for therapy. Chemotherapy treatments may be used adjunctively. Radiotherapy has a lesser role and is occasionally used for long-term management where surgery fails or is inappropriate. Medical therapies for Cushing's syndrome require consultation with an endocrinologist.

The management issues for pheochromocytoma depend on localization of the tumor. Treatment is surgical removal, if possible.

COMPLICATIONS

Immediate life-threatening complications are generally confined to acute adrenal crisis. With chronic Addison's disease and Cushing's syndrome, complications are prevented by giving careful attention to the side effects of exogenous steroids and to the patient's symptoms, physiologic and emotional functioning, and metabolic status. With chronic adrenal insufficiency, complications from co-morbid conditions that result in periods of sudden adrenal inadequacy can be reduced by the availability of injectable hydrocortisone for home use. With Cushing's syndrome, osteoporosis is a common complication. In addition to monitoring for osteoporosis, providers should observe patients for hypertension and diabetes. Acute hypertensive crisis is a potential complication of pheochromocytoma.

INDICATIONS FOR REFERRAL OR HOSPITALIZATION

If acute adrenal insufficiency is suspected, immediate referral and hospitalization are required. Consultation with an endocrinologist is warranted if the diagnostic evaluation suggests either Addison's disease or Cushing's syndrome. With pheochromocytoma, referral and hospitalization are necessary for hypertensive crisis management. Endocrine and surgical evaluations before resection of the pheochromocytoma are indicated.

Management of an acute adrenal crisis (corticosteroid insufficiency) requires IV administration of hydrocortisone 100 mg q 6 hr for an initial 24 hours, followed by careful dose tapering. Management of hypotension, hypovolemia, and hypoglycemia is accomplished with IV administration of normal saline with 5% dextrose with careful monitoring in the hospital, often in an ICU; consultation is recommended.

Patients who have been taking exogenous steroids at any time during the preceding year are at some risk for inadequate cortisol response when faced with the stress of any surgical procedure. These patients should be considered candidates for perioperative stress doses of hydrocortisone.[11] Consultation with a physician comfortable with prescribing stress steroid doses is advised. In general, for patients with known adrenal insufficiency, hydrocortisone is added to intraoperative IV fluids and infused at a rate of 5 mg/hr. During the first 24 hours after surgery, a total of 150 to 200 mg is administered. The dose is then tapered by 50% per day if the postoperative period is without complications.

PATIENT EDUCATION AND HEALTH PROMOTION

Careful explanation of Addison's disease and Cushing's syndrome and the complications of chronic exogenous steroid dependency is an important component of patient and family education. Patients with adrenal insufficiency require early assessment and medication adjustments with fever and common illnesses. In many of these situations, it is essential that hydrocortisone maintenance doses be doubled quickly. Patients and families must understand the risks of suddenly withdrawing corticosteroid medications.

Medical alert bracelets are vital to improve the recognition of emergency presentations of adrenal insufficiency. Carrying extra oral and emergency parenteral steroids is mandatory when traveling and when in remote places. The impact these diseases may have on lifestyle and reproduction should be explored with patient and family.

Quick access to the health care provider should be an important goal of the provider-patient partnership. A partnership approach and attention to medication use and psychologic and emotional adaptation enables patients and families to have a reasonably full life experience.

REFERENCES

1. Vaughan ED: Diseases of the adrenal gland, *Med Clin North Am* 88(2):443-466, 2004.
2. Karlsson FA: Autoimmune endocrine disease, *Horm Metab Res* 28(7):351-352, 1996.
3. Ten S, New M, Maclaren N: Addison's disease 2001, *J Clin Endocrinol Metab* 84(7):2909-2922, 2001.
4. Peeke PM, Chrousos GP: Hypercortisolism and obesity, *Ann NY Acad Sci* 771:665-676, 1995.
5. Ross NS: Epidemiology of Cushing's syndrome and subclinical disease, *Endocrinol Metab Clin North Am* 23:539-546, 1994.
6. Schuff KG: Issues in the diagnosis of Cushing's syndrome for the primary care physician, *Prim Care* 30(4):791-799, 2003.
7. Manger WM, Eisenhofer G: Pheochromocytoma: diagnosis and management update, *Curr Hypertens Rep* 6(6):477-484, 2004.
8. Orth D: Cushing's syndrome, *N Engl J Med* 332:791-803, 1995.
9. Bornstein SR, Stratakis CA, Chrousos GP: Adrenocortical tumors: recent advances in basic concepts and clinical management, *Ann Intern Med* 130(9):759-771, 1999.
10. Tsigos C, Chrousos GP: Differential diagnosis and management of Cushing's syndrome, *Ann Rev Med* 47:443-461, 1996.
11. Werbel SS, Ober KP: Acute adrenal insufficiency (review), *Endocrinol Metab Clin North Am* 22(2):303-328, 1993.

CHAPTER 218

Diabetes Mellitus

Rosemary Bill-Fleury

DEFINITION AND EPIDEMIOLOGY

Diabetes mellitus (DM) is the most common metabolic disorder seen in primary care and the leading cause of cardiovascular disease, renal failure, blindness, and nontraumatic lower limb amputation. The World Health Organization defines diabetes as a progressive disorder of glucose metabolism with ranges from normal glycemia, impaired glucose tolerance, or impaired fasting glycemia to hyperglycemia.[1] Total prevalence of diabetes in the United States has increased to 18.2 million (6.3% of the population)—13 million diagnosed and 5.2 million undiagnosed. An estimated 90% to 95% of patients with diabetes have adult-onset, or type 2, diabetes; less than 10% have type 1 diabetes[2] (Box 218-1).

The prevalence of diabetes in the United States is twice as high in females as in males. Diabetes in males is more prevalent in individuals of African American, Native American, and Hispanic descent than in Caucasians. Another growing population is young people and children who are overweight or obese. The chance of developing diabetes doubles with every 20% of increased body weight and decade of life.[3]

The long-term sequelae of diabetes are the microvascular and macrovascular complications to target end organs: the eyes, kidneys, heart, blood vessels, and nerves. Diabetes costs in 2002 were an estimated $92 billion a year as a result of long-term complications.[4] This does not include costs associated with medications or disability. To reverse this devastating disease, it is imperative that prevention and aggressive treatment be used to minimize the long-term complications.

BOX 218-1

RECENT CHANGES AND CURRENT CLASSIFICATIONS OF DIABETES FROM THE INTERNATIONAL EXPERT COMMITTEE

- In type 1 diabetes mellitus (DM), insulin deficiency is caused by beta cell destruction and requires exogenous insulin. Ketosis prone and autoimmune in nature, DM may occur in children, young adults, or fragile older adults. Some cases have a genetic or viral basis of development.
- Type 2 diabetes is caused by beta cell dysfunction and/or insulin defect. It is nonketonic in nature. Development occurs later in life secondary to obesity, sedentary lifestyle, medications, or other factors that make the individual glucose intolerant and insulin resistant.
- Secondary diabetes occurs as a result of an underlying medical condition that renders the patient glucose intolerant.
- Gestational diabetes refers to glucose intolerance during pregnancy. These women are at high risk for developing type 2 (non-insulin-dependent) diabetes at a later time.
- Prediabetes, an intermediate stage of glucose imbalance between normal physiology and DM, encompasses impaired fasting glucose (between 110 and 126 mg/dl) and impaired glucose tolerance (between 140 and 200 mg/dl). Persons in this intermediate stage (<200 mg/dl) could go onto develop diabetes and cardiovascular disease.

From the Expert Committee on the Diagnosis and Classification of Diabetes Mellitus: Report of the expert committee on the diagnosis and classification of diabetes mellitus, *Diabetes Care* 26(Suppl 1):S106-S108, 2003.

PATHOPHYSIOLOGY

Diabetes is characterized by glucose intolerance and hyperglycemia. The pathology of diabetes ranges from autoimmune destruction of the beta cells and insulin deficiency (type 1) to defects in insulin secretion, insulin action, insulin resistance, and/or basement membrane thickening (type 2). The morbidity and mortality of the disease are influenced by the patient's glycemic control. Results from the Diabetes Control and Complications Trial (DCCT) (now called Epidemiology of Diabetes Interventions and Complications Study [EDIC]) and the United Kingdom Prospective Diabetes Study (UKPDS) revealed a significant reduction in the complications of retinopathy, nephropathy, and neuropathy with glycemic control within the glycohemoglobin ranges of 6% to 7%.[5]

Type 1 diabetes results from the destruction of the beta cells in the pancreatic islets, causing insulin deficiency. Surgery (e.g., Whipple's procedure or pancreatectomy) or autoimmune damage (e.g., various genetic or environmental insults) can also cause destruction of beta cells. Insulin deficiency impairs the uptake of glucose from intravascular to intercellular spaces, slows lipid synthesis, retards protein synthesis, and stimulates glycolysis.[6]

In type 2 diabetes the pathology is more obscure. Hallmarks of this type are insulin resistance and impaired beta cell function. Hyperglycemia results from increased hepatic glucose production, impaired insulin secretion, and decreased glycogen uptake. Fasting hyperglycemia results from increased hepatic glucose production in the impaired early phase of insulin secretion. Postprandial hyperglycemia is caused by the decreased uptake of glucose from the skeletal muscles. In response to the elevated blood glucose level, the insulin pathways become resistant to hormonal impulses, resulting in hyperinsulinemia. Insulin resistance by definition is the decreased sensitivity of tissue to glucose uptake with normal concentrations of insulin.[6] As hyperglycemia increases, so does insulin resistance. The body is able to adapt and maintain homeostasis for a while, but as hyperglycemia progresses, diabetes occurs. As the degree of glucose intolerance progresses, hyperglycemia results from the insufficient insulin produced by the beta cells.

Primary insulin resistance, a defect in the target cells of insulin receptors and postreceptors, results in altered insulin action and sensitivity. The onset of insulin resistance can occur with hyperinsulinemia, in the fasting or fed state of the individual. The fed state is the time associated with insulin secretion from food intake to carbohydrate metabolism and synthesis of fat and protein.[3] As insulin resistance proceeds to the peripheral levels, glucose transportation or utilization of glucose in the cell is altered. Secondary resistance is caused by hormones or abnormal physiologic states (e.g., puberty, pregnancy, advanced age). Other factors associated with the development of insulin resistance include a high-fat diet, sedentary lifestyle, smoking, and weight gain. Metabolic stress, such as illness and obesity, increases the incidence of insulin resistance. An individual is considered insulin resistant when a daily intake of insulin greater than 1.5 to 2 units/kg body weight is required.

The metabolic syndrome is a group of metabolic components, synergistic in nature, that can lead to cardiovascular disease. These components include abdominal obesity, insulin resistance and hyperglycemia, elevated triglycerides and low high-density lipoproteins (HDLs), hypertension, and proinflammatory state (see Chapter 223).

Researchers are concerned with the increased morbidity associated with metabolic syndrome, endothelial dysfunction, platelet adhesion in a prothrombic state, and their impact on cardiovascular disease.[7] Weight loss, improved glucose tolerance, lipid management, and improved blood pressure may decrease the significance of this syndrome.

CLINICAL PRESENTATION

Polyuria, polydipsia, polyphagia, weight loss, and blurred vision are overt signs of diabetes. However, unexplained fatigue, paresthesia (especially in the feet), recurrent infections, and candidiasis may also signal the onset of the disorder. In type 1 diabetes the individual will be symptomatic for a short time. Then, as the glucosuria increases, nausea, vomiting, shallow breathing, hypotension, and dehydration will lead to ketosis and possibly death. Medical care is essential.

The patient with type 2 diabetes has subtle symptoms that may persist for weeks, months, or even years before detection. Unfortunately, during this time the vascular and neurologic complications begin to develop and progress before the diagnosis is made. Medical conditions that imply underlying diabetes include cranial nerve palsies (cranial nerve III with spared pupillary light reflex), symmetric distal polyneuropathy (stocking and glove), acanthosis nigricans, vitiligo, Dupuytren's contracture, autonomic neuropathy (characterized by tachycardia and orthostatic hypotension), increased incidence of candidal vaginitis, skin infections (furuncles and carbuncles), increased number of urinary tract infections (UTIs), and atrophic changes (hair loss, thinned skin, and decreased body temperature).

PHYSICAL EXAMINATION

The importance of the examination in the patient with diabetes is threefold: (1) to evaluate blood glucose control, since poor control leads to end-organ complications; (2) to assess for the presence or progression of end-organ damage; and (3) to assess for other autoimmune disorders, such as thyroid disorders, or secondary causes of the diabetes.

Annual examinations are comprehensive. Periodic visits, every 3 months for patients with type 1 diabetes and those with type 2 diabetes with one or more complications, should be scheduled to assess end-organ involvement and glucose control. Visits can be stretched to every 6 months if the individual is stable and in control. Each examination should include height, weight, and blood pressure measurements; review of glucose logs; and evaluation of target end-organ involvement[6] (Box 218-2).

BOX 218-2

PHYSICAL EXAMINATION OF PATIENTS WITH DIABETES

Vital signs: Check blood pressure for orthostasis or inappropriate heart rate response (irregular, tachycardia, or bradycardia, especially with activity or position changes).
Eye: Perform funduscopic examination for bleeding, nicking, vascular changes, or retinopathy.
Oral cavity: Check for gum disease, fungal infections, or lesions.
Thyroid: Palpate for enlargement or nodules.
Neck: Auscultate for carotid bruits and evaluate for neck vein distention.
Cardiac: Auscultate heart rate for rhythm, murmurs, clicks, or extra heart sounds.
Abdomen: Assess for hepatomegaly and auscultate for abdominal bruits or aortic pulsations.
Vascular: Palpate pulses for presence and quality. Evaluate hands, fingers, and feet for vibration, sensation, two-point discrimination, and proprioception.
Skin: Examine for signs of irritation, infection, redness, ulcers, lipodystrophy, and hypertrophy; give special attention to feet.
Reproductive system: Evaluate prepubertal individuals for sexual maturation staging.

DIAGNOSTICS

Diagnostic criteria for diabetes, supported by the American Diabetes Association (ADA), no longer require a glucose tolerance test for definitive diagnosis. Initial diagnostic studies should include electrolytes, BUN, creatinine, serum glucose (random or fasting), lipid profile, urinalysis, and, if indicated, a thyroid-stimulating hormone study. A glycosylated hemoglobin assay indicates a percentage of glucose saturation to the hemoglobin and can be expressed with any of the A_1 fractions of the molecule: A_{1a}, A_{1b}, or A_{1c} (the largest). This test evaluates glucose control for the previous 12 weeks and is recommended every 3 months. A urine study for microalbumin evaluates kidney function and should be done yearly after 5 years of diagnosis in the patient with type 1 diabetes and at the onset, and then yearly, in the patient with type 2 diabetes. Twenty-four-hour urine for creatinine clearance is still the definitive test for true evaluation of kidney function. Urine microalbumin spot sample, however, is being used more frequently because of convenience, but treatment should not be based on only one reading. There are variations associated with exercise and posture and day-to-day variability. Insulin levels and C-peptides are helpful in cases that raise concerns about the true diagnosis of type 1 vs. type 2 or glucose intolerance. This is especially helpful when a case of type 1 diabetes has gone into a honeymoon phase. Other markers include islet cell antibodies, glutamic acid decarboxylase islet cell antibody-512, and insulin autoantibody (Box 218-3).

DIAGNOSTICS

Diabetes

LABORATORY
Serum electrolytes
BUN
Creatinine
Serum glucose (random or fasting)
Lipid profile
Urinalysis
TSH*
Glycosylated hemoglobin*

*If indicated.

BOX 218-3

DIAGNOSTIC CRITERIA FOR GLUCOSE CONTROL

- Fasting plasma glucose >126 mg/dl confirmed by a repeat test
- Casual plasma glucose > 200 mg/dl plus classic symptoms of diabetes
- Fasting plasma glucose >110 and <126 mg/dl = impaired glucose tolerance
- Two-hour postprandial plasma glucose >200 mg/dl after 75 g glucose load
- Two-hour postprandial glucose >140 and <200 mg/dl = impaired glucose tolerance

From American Diabetes Association (Committee Report): Nutrition recommendations and principles for people with diabetes mellitus, *Diabetes Care* 28(Suppl 1):S55-S57, 2005.

DIFFERENTIAL DIAGNOSIS

The diagnosis of diabetes has been facilitated by the recent changes in the diagnostic criteria (see Box 218-1). However, secondary causes of diabetes should always be considered. These include excess of counterregulatory hormones (Cushing's syndrome, pheochromocytoma, and acromegaly); significant hypokalemia caused by glucose intolerance; hyperaldosteronism or diuretic use; and destruction in the pancreatic islet from pancreatitis (caused by alcoholism or gallbladder disease), hemochromatosis, or drug-induced islet cell injury. In addition, infection or medication may cause glucose intolerance, whereas the presence of polyuria and polydipsia may indicate DM, diabetes insipidus, or primary polydipsia.

DIFFERENTIAL DIAGNOSIS

Diabetes

- Cushing's syndrome
- Pheochromocytoma
- Acromegaly
- Diabetes insipidus
- Pancreatic disease
- Alcoholism
- Gallbladder disease
- Hemochromatosis
- Drug-induced condition
- Infection

INITIAL STABILIZATION AND MANAGEMENT

Insulin, an anabolic hormone produced by the beta cells of the pancreas, has a vital role in metabolism. Insulin therapy is the primary treatment for type 1 diabetes and is used in patients with type 2 diabetes with persistent hyperglycemia despite oral diabetic agents. Secretion of insulin is biphasic: prandial and basal. The prandial phase controls the initial glucose load and reuptake. The basal phase inhibits glycolysis and gluconeogenesis and maintains insulin in a steady state. Early morning hyperglycemia caused by counterregulatory hormones is controlled by basal insulin, and meal coverage is controlled by prandial insulin. Insulin therapy should pantomime this response. In today's market, insulin therapy is diverse and can cover a multitude of individualized regimens for a more flexible lifestyle. The two types of insulin and three mixtures are derived synthetically from recombinant DNA (human, Humulin) (Table 218-1). Pork-derived regular and NPH insulins, as well as Lente and Ultralente insulins, are no longer produced and soon will be unavailable.

Five insulin analogs made of recombinant human insulin are available. Three are quick acting (lispro, aspart, glulisine), and two are long acting or peakless (glargine and detemir). The three short-acting insulins are better interventions when treating postprandial blood glucose, and the peakless insulins provide true basal coverage of insulin without insulin peaks. The older analogs (lispro, aspart, and glargine) have demonstrated a decrease in the frequency of hypoglycemic episodes and improved glycemic control. Episodes of allergic reactions and lipoatrophy are decreased when synthetic insulin is used instead of animal insulin. The disadvantage of synthetic insulin is its shorter duration. The peakless long-acting insulin analog is being used as a single injection at bedtime to control fasting hyperglycemia and give a basal rate throughout the day. However, it does not cover postprandial hyperglycemia. Mixing of insulin allows a more personalized regimen for better adherence and safety. The four prepared insulin mixtures—lispro 75/25; Novolog 70/30; and mixtures of NPH and regular, 70/30 (human and Humulin) and 50/50—offer ease and safety to the individual. Recent U.S. Food and Drug Administration (FDA) approval of inhaled short-acting insulin (e.g., Exubera) will add yet another option for improved glycemic control.

A new addition to the treatment plan for individuals on insulin (both type 1 and type 2) is pramlintide (Symlin),[8] a synthetic analog of human amylin. Amylin is a hormone produced in the pancreas and becomes deficient as beta cells are destroyed. Its role in diabetes is reducing the amount of glucose in the bloodstream by reducing the amount of food consumed. The release of amylin leads to a decrease in hepatic glycolysis and a slowing of gastric emptying into the small intestine, thereby increasing satiety. The results are decreased glucagon secretion and decreased postprandial glucose spikes. It is used for both type 1 and type 2 patients who have not attained glucose control. Symlin is a subcutaneous injection given 10 to 15 minutes before meals, starting at a low dose of 15 to 60 mcg (type 1) and 30 to 120 mcg (type 2) and titrating slowly. When given with a rapid analog, pramlintide should be decreased by 30% to 50% and taken toward the end of the meal. Side effects include severe hypoglycemia, nausea, anorexia, and gastrointestinal distress. Therefore it is important to titrate slowly and not to increase if side effects are experienced. Severe hypoglycemia can occur from the combination of insulin timing with glucose peaking postprandially. Because of the delay in gastric emptying, Symlin alters the glucose postprandial peak. If insulin is given before the peak in glucose, postprandial hypoglycemia will occur, usually within 3 hours of pramlintide injection.

Diabetes management requires a homeostatic relationship of diet, exercise and activity, illness or disease state, emotional well-being, and insulin or oral diabetic medication. The care for both type 1 and type 2 patients encompasses the same issues and treatment. However, the role of circulating insulin and the progression of complications differ between the two types of diabetes. Insulin therapy is used for type 1 diabetes because of insulin deficiency, whereas diet, weight loss, and exercise are appropriate initial interventions for patients with type 2 diabetes. Individuals with type 2 diabetes with persistent hyperglycemia, ketosis, pregnancy, co-existing factors (e.g., metabolic syndrome), or complications require aggressive therapy to improve glycemic control.

TABLE 218-1 Insulin Types

Type	Onset	Peak	Duration	Comments
SHORT ACTING				
Aspart (Novolog)	5-10 minutes	1-3 hours	3-5 hours	Effective postprandial control—given preprandially Give SQ, mix with NPH
Glulisine (Apidra)	15 minutes	30-90 minutes	3-5 hours	Postprandial control; can mix with NPH
Lispro (Humalog)	15 minutes	30-90 minutes	3-5 hours	Postprandial control; can mix with NPH
Regular (Humulin, Novolin)	0.5-1 hour	2-4 hours	4-8 hours	Prandial glucose control; can mix with NPH
INTERMEDIATE ACTING				
NPH (Humulin, Novolin)	1-1.5 hours	4-12 hours	24 hours	
MIXTURES				
Humalog 75/25	15-30 minutes	30-150 minutes	14-24 hours	75% lispro protamine suspension, 25% lispro
Novolog 70/30	10-20 minutes	1-3 hours	24 hours	70% aspart protamine suspension, 30% aspart
Humulin/ Novolin 70/30	30-60 minutes	2-6 hours	14-24 hours	Mixture of 70% NPH and 30% regular
Humulin 50/50	30-60 minutes	2-5.5 hours	14-24 hours	50% lispro protamine suspension, 50% lispro
LONG ACTING				
Detemir (Levemir)	90 minutes	Peakless	24 hours	Give SQ; do not mix with any insulin Give at supper or bedtime; if b.i.d., give 12 hours apart
Glargine (Lantus)	90 minutes	Peakless	24 hours	Give SQ; do not mix with any insulins Give at bedtime; if b.i.d., give 12 hours apart
Exubera (inhaled)	0-10 minutes	10-20 minutes	30-90 minutes	Take before meals; dose dependent on weight |(kg/body weight × 0.05 mg/dl) Rapid onset like analog; duration similar to that of regular insulin Preliminary pancreas function tests and q 6 months
AMYLIN ANALOG				
Pramlintide (Symlin) (human amylin)				Synthetic analog Give SQ, titrate slowly to 15-60 mcg Use with insulin (but not mixed with insulin); slows gastric emptying Take pramlintide with meal; decrease meal insulin and take it at end of meal Can cause nausea, hypoglycemia, and weight loss

The DCCT (type 1) and UKPDS (type 2)[5] revealed the importance of glycemic control in delaying or preventing vascular and neurologic ravages of the disease. Achievement of near-normal glucose levels (70 to 120 mg/dl) before meals and below 140 mg/dl 2 hours postprandially is the goal for optimum glycemic control. The Diabetes Epidemiology: Collaborative Analysis of Diagnostic Criteria in Europe (DECODE)[9] revealed that postprandial glucose poses a greater risk for cardiovascular disease than fasting blood glucose.

Type 1 Diabetes

When starting an individual on insulin, the health care provider should consider body weight, morphologic development (obese vs. muscular), age (adolescence vs. elderly), and activity (sedentary vs. athletic). Physiologic insulin secretion for adults is approximately 20 to 40 units/day.[10] The recommended starting dose for an adult is approximately 10 to 20 units of insulin in the morning before breakfast. If an individual has fasting blood glucose levels above 250 mg/dl, an additional nighttime dose of five units before bedtime snack (preferably) or before supper should be started, along with a rapid-acting insulin to cover elevated postprandial glucose, especially if the patient is spilling ketones. The type of insulin used depends on the patient's needs and provider's preference (Table 218-2).

Glargine, a true long-acting insulin, given around 8 to 10 PM and lasting for 24 hours, mimics the basal rate of insulin.[11] Therefore this can be an alternative choice when starting individuals on insulin. The insulin dose should be adjusted every 3 or 4 days until the fasting blood glucose level is below 110 mg/dl. The insulin should be increased by increments of 2 to 8 units in an obese individual or by 1 to 4 units in a patient with a thin body frame such as a frail elder, or in patients with frequent episodes of hypoglycemia.[12] Use of standard insulin NPH also could be used to mimic both prandial and basal insulin. The dose when starting is the same but may be increased every 2 or 3 days by 2 to 4 units.

If after a few weeks the individual's glucose range is greater than 150 to 200 mg/dl, at bedtime or before lunch, or if the morning insulin dose exceeds 45 units, the addition of

TABLE 218-2 Management for Type 1 Diabetes

	Breakfast	Lunch	Dinner	Bedtime
Ages 15-18 years	⅔-½ of calculated dose	Sliding scale—¼ of calculated dose	⅓-¼ of calculated dose	¼ of calculated dose
Option 1	NPH + rapid analog	Rapid analog	NPH + rapid analog	
Option 2	Rapid analog	Rapid analog	Rapid analog	Long-acting analog
Option 3	NPH + rapid analog		Rapid analog	NPH or long-acting analog
Option 4	Rapid + long-acting analog	Rapid analog	Rapid analog	Long-acting analog
Option 5	Pump therapy			
Option 6	Exubera	Exubera	Exubera	Long-acting analog

Start with b.i.d. insulin and then titrate upward depending on control. Adolescents may require more insulin per day (1-1.5 units/kg or greater). Add lunchtime insulin if not able to control by AM insulin. If patient very active, may be able to cover with sliding scale of lispro or aspart and bedtime detemir or glargine. Decrease insulin dose with onset of honeymoon phase from 0.1 to 0.5 units/kg body weight.

	Breakfast	Lunch	Dinner	Bedtime
Ages 19-40 years	⅔ of calculated dose		⅓ of calculated dose	
Option 1	NPH + rapid analog		NPH + rapid analog	
Option 2	Long-acting and rapid analog		Rapid analog	Long-acting analog
Option 3	Rapid analog	Rapid analog	Rapid analog	Long-acting analog
Option 4	Pump therapy			

Modified from American Diabetes Association: *Insulin therapy of type 1 diabetic: medical management,* ed 3, Alexandria, Va, 1994, The Association.

rapid-acting lispro or aspart should be initiated. Regular insulin may be used as an alternative but does not offer the immediate mealtime coverage and can mimic a longer-acting insulin. This action increases hyperglycemia postprandially and hypoglycemia before the next meal if mealtime is delayed. Mixing of insulins, including NPH and regular, with the AM or supper doses may help; however, none can be mixed with glargine or detemir. The analogs, if given immediately, may be mixed with NPH; however, some chemical conversions may occur if they are not given instantaneously.[13,14] To achieve tighter control, a second or third injection of lispro or aspart could be added at lunch, and/or the evening dose of insulin could be separated into lispro or aspart insulin given before supper and glargine insulin given before the bedtime snack. Using lispro or aspart insulin before meals allows for more flexibility, better coverage of hyperglycemia, and decreased episodes of hypoglycemia.[15]

Hard-to-control blood glucose levels with wide fluctuations or frequent episodes of hypoglycemia or hyperglycemia may be better managed with carbohydrate-to-insulin ratios (Box 218-4). Adolescent doses are calculated by weight, activity level, and needed insulin requirements to maintain optimum glycemic control (Table 218-3). Requirements for insulin increase during illness, surgery, and growth spurts and in patients with ketoacidosis. Insulin absorption from subcutaneous tissues varies about 25% among patients. The practitioner should be aware of a possible "honeymoon" phase in the patient with newly diagnosed type 1 diabetes with recovering beta cell function. Insulin requirements may decrease to 0.2 to 0.5 unit/kg body weight/day during this short-term phase.[16] The goal of the diabetes plan is to attain glycemic control with appropriate insulin doses but without symptoms of hypoglycemia or hyperglycemia.

BOX 218-4

INSULIN CALCULATIONS

INSULIN-TO-CARBOHYDRATE RATIO FOR FOOD PLANNING

- Add total units of insulin per day; this equals total daily insulin (TDI).
- Divide 450 by TDI. This is the number of carbohydrate grams covered by 1 unit of fast-acting insulin.
  15 g = 1 serving of carbohydrates
- Diabetic patients may have variable insulin-to-carbohydrate ratios during the day. Use several days to determine correct ratio. Adjust by using sensitivity factor.

SENSITIVITY FACTOR FOR INSULIN CORRECTION

- Take the TDI and divide into 1500 to obtain the sensitivity factor.
- Result equals the amount of glucose lowered by 1 unit of rapid-acting insulin.
- Subtract 105 or 110 (baseline sugar [BS]) from the high sugar. This result is what needs to be corrected by the above sensitivity factor.
- Divide the sugar to be corrected by the sensitivity factor.
  Example:
  BS = 220, TDI = 30; 1500/30 = 50 (sensitivity factor); 220 − 105 = 115
  115 divided by sensitivity factor (50) = 2.3 units of insulin extra needed to cover that blood sugar

Data from Beaser RS: *Intensifying insulin treatment programs: Joslin's diabetes deskbook,* Boston, 2001, Joslin Diabetes Center.

Intensified insulin therapy, defined as 4 or more insulin injections in a day, encompasses multiple-dose insulin or infusion pumps to achieve tighter glucose control. This comprehensive plan involves a close partnership with the diabetic individual, the health care provider or diabetic specialist, and the diabetic education team of nurses and nutritionists. To prevent both hypoglycemia and hyperglycemia, factors such as exercise and activity, meals, mealtimes, sleep patterns,

TABLE 218-3 Insulin Dosage over the Life Span

Life Stage	Dosage
Before adolescence	0.7-0.8 units/kg body weight/day Honeymoon phase 0.2-0.6 unit/kg body weight/day
Adolescence	1.2-1.4 units/kg body weight/day
Adult	0.5-1 units/kg body weight/day
Older adult	0.5 units/kg body weight/day
Pregnancy*	
Gestational and type 2 diabetes	0.5-1 units/kg body weight/day 30 units (2:1) NPH plus regular insulin in morning plus 5-10 units regular insulin before evening meal*
Type 1 diabetes:	
First trimester	Decrease preconception dose by 10%-20%
Second and third trimesters	0.9-1.2 units/kg body weight/24 hr
Postpartum and breastfeeding	0.6 units/kg body weight

Modified from White SR, Campbell RK: Pharmacologic therapies for glucose management. In Franz MJ, editor: *Diabetes management therapies—core curriculum for diabetes educators*, Chicago, 2003, American Diabetes Association.
*If insulin is started before the twenty-eighth week in gestational diabetes, decrease the dose by 20%. Some may start with the nighttime injection only, then add the daytime injection.

illness, and psychologic well-being must be considered when calculating insulin doses. Hypoglycemia is a serious side effect of this therapy and prevents some individuals from accepting insulin. One way of controlling day-to-day variations and preventing hypoglycemia is through home blood glucose testing. There are many different brands of glucose monitors. The "best" one is the one the patient uses. To evaluate the range of glucose disparity between plasma and whole blood, a patient should have his or her blood tested using the glucose monitor and the laboratory at the same time. If the range is greater than 20 to 30 points, another glucose monitor should be used.

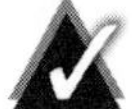

When the patient is using an insulin pump, co-management with an endocrinologist is strongly recommended.

Individuals not appropriate for intensified insulin include (1) those with glycemic control of 70 to 120 mg/dl without complications, (2) those with hypoglycemia unawareness, (3) those who are poorly motivated and unwilling to test their blood glucose frequently, and (4) those who have had diabetes for less than 6 months to 1 year.[10]

Insulin adjustments are made using one type of insulin at a time. One unit of lispro insulin can decrease the blood glucose level by 50 mg/dl. Regular insulin is more variable and can sometimes act like an intermediate insulin. A guideline for initiating intensive insulin therapy is to take the total daily insulin dose and divide it into percentages to be taken before meals and at bedtime. For example, 35% of the total insulin dose should be taken before breakfast, 20% before lunch, 30% before supper, and 15% before bedtime. This needs to be fine tuned if patients work night shifts or eat their larger meal at noon with a smaller meal at nighttime.[10] (See Box 218-4.)

LIFESTYLE CHANGES

Nutritional therapy is essential in management for both type 1 and type 2 diabetes. The goal of nutritional therapy for both types is the development of the meal plan, balancing insulin with food intake and activity to achieve glycemic control. A nutritionist is essential in helping to balance medications and food intake in type 1 diabetes and for weight control and lipid management in type 2. Type 2 individuals must also balance food intake (meals and snacks) with activity and the use of medications.[17] A certified nutritionist can individualize the nutrition guidelines for each individual with diabetes to attain optimum glycemic control and prevent hypoglycemia in short-term illness (Box 218-5). Lifestyle changes such as growth and development, pregnancy, lactation, or recovery from a severe illness need special dietary adjustments with the help of a nutritionist.

Exercise or physical therapy has been shown to improve glycemic control. Exercise suppresses insulin, with increased glucose uptake in skeletal muscle. In the individual without diabetes, counterregulatory hormones increase glucose secretion to balance glucose uptake into skeletal muscle. However, this function is lost in the individual with diabetes. Therefore, to prevent hypoglycemia, the individual with diabetes (especially one on insulin) must balance activity with adequate food and appropriate medication. Postexercise hyperglycemia occurs in an individual with poorly controlled diabetes as a result of decreased circulating insulin and glucose uptake, and increased hormonally regulated hepatic glucose. Ketosis is increased as fatty acids are broken down for energy, resulting in higher blood glucose levels and possible ketosis during exercise.[18]

In the individual with type 2 diabetes, exercise decreases insulin resistance and increases glucose uptake into the cell. Insulin sensitivity caused by the lag effect can last up to

BOX 218-5

NUTRITION GUIDELINES FOR PATIENTS WITH DIABETES

Calories: Adequate amounts for weight control, growth and development, pregnancy, and lactation.
Protein: 10% to 20% of calories; with nephropathy, 0.8 g/kg body weight/day.
Fat: 30% or less from calories with less than 10% of calories from saturated fat; if obese or hyperlipidemic, less than 30% may be needed.
Carbohydrate: Remainder of calories after protein and fat adjustments; percentage varies with individual lifestyle, activity level, and insulin level.
Carbohydrate counting: Calculating dose of fast-acting insulin to correspond with amount of carbohydrate per meal; 15 g of carbohydrate equals 1 unit of lispro or aspart insulin.
Cholesterol: 300 mg/day; if hyperlipidemic, 200 mg/day.
Fiber: 20-35 g/day.
Sodium: 3000 mg/day; for individuals with mild to moderate hypertension, 2400 mg/day; with hypertension and nephropathy, 2000 mg/day.
Alcohol: Limit to two alcoholic beverages per day (12 oz beer, 5 oz wine, or 1½ oz distilled spirits = 1 drink); ingest at meals and substitute for two fat exchanges.

Data from American Diabetes Association (Committee Report): Nutrition recommendations and principles for people with diabetes mellitus, *Diabetes Care* 28(Suppl 1):S55-S57, 2005.

BOX 218-6

EXERCISE RECOMMENDATIONS FOR PATIENTS WITH DIABETES

TYPE 1 DIABETES

1. Eat a carbohydrate snack, 15 to 30 g (glass milk, 1 fruit, ½ banana) for every 30 to 60 minutes of low to moderate exercise.
2. Eat 25 to 50 g of a carbohydrate and protein snack (½ to whole sandwich of meat with glass of milk) for every hour of moderate to high-intensity exercise.
3. Do not exercise when blood glucose level is above 300 mg/dl or if spilling ketones.
4. Be aware of symptoms of hypoglycemia and carry readily absorbable carbohydrate.
5. Diabetics with insensitive feet should avoid running. Those with proliferative retinopathy should avoid Valsalva-like maneuvers, isometric exercises, and high-intensity strenuous exercises.
6. Individuals with hypertension should avoid heavy lifting, Valsalva-like maneuvers, and straining-type exercises.

TYPE 2 DIABETES

1. Exercise when blood glucose level is above 120 mg/dl, 1 to 3 hours after a meal.
2. Decrease insulin that is peaking at time of exercise.
3. Same as recommendations 1, 2, 4, 5, and 6 for type 1 diabetes.

48 hours. Thus medication, especially insulin, needs to be adjusted for the activity or exercise done. Adjustment involves decreasing the insulin that is peaking at the time of exercise. In the patient with type 2 diabetes it would be optimum to decrease medication instead of increasing food consumption for the exercise regimen. Guidelines for exercise in diabetes are reviewed in Box 218-6.[18,19]

Type 2 Diabetes

The mainstay of therapy for the patient with type 2 diabetes is education, diet, and exercise. However, persistent hyperglycemia and end-organ compromise require pharmacologic intervention. Patients with symptomatic hyperglycemia and vascular complications require medication for immediate improvement of glycemic control. Using diet, weight loss, and exercise as treatment options entails a time frame of at least 3 to 6 months to monitor progress. A certified diabetes educator can optimize the time frame efficiently while organizing information for the individual and relaying it as he or she is ready to take on more changes. If time is not an option, then medications must be added to the regimen of diet and exercise.

The variety of oral hypoglycemics, insulin sensitizers, and slowed gastric absorption agents enables treatment individualization for improved glycemic control (Table 218-4). The sulfonylureas are the most widely used first-line oral medications for type 2 diabetes. Their mechanism of action affects both pancreatic and extrapancreatic tissue. Insulin production by indirect stimulation of beta cells is their primary role. Associated benefits are inhibition of glucagon release, increased insulin sensitivity and affinity to postreceptor sites by decreasing insulin resistance, and decreased hepatic insulin release. However, hypoglycemia may be problematic, particularly in older patients.

Meglitinides (repaglinide [Prandin], nateglinide [Starlix]) are nonsulfonylurea insulin stimulators. Repaglinide and nateglinide are used for short and rapid bursts of insulin to control postprandial hyperglycemia and have shorter action times. They do not act on fasting glucose, must be taken before meals, and should be withheld if not eating. These agents are also used in combination with an insulin sensitizer, especially for individuals eating a high-carbohydrate meal who need a higher boost of insulin for shorter period. Nateglinide seems to work slightly faster with fewer episodes of hypoglycemia than repaglinide. Both repaglinide and nateglinide pose risks for drug interactions, causing either hypoglycemia or hyperglycemia (Box 218-7).[20,21]

The two insulin sensitizers have now become first-line agents acting to spare further beta cell destruction and decrease hyperinsulinemia. Biguanides (such as metformin) sensitize liver, small intestine, and peripheral muscle tissue to decrease hepatic glucose production and intestinal glucose absorption. Additional benefits include enhanced glucose uptake into skeletal muscle and tissue, and improved insulin sensitivity. Studies support the effectiveness of monotherapy with the advantage of decreasing endogenous insulin, weight loss, and reduction in low-density lipoprotein (LDL) cholesterol, especially in the obese, insulin-resistant type 2 diabetics. Lactic acidosis is a potential lethal problem. Specific situations prohibiting metformin are given in Box 218-8.[20,21]

Thiazolidinediones (TZDs), pioglitazone and rosiglitazone, act on peripheral and adipose tissues and skeletal muscle to enhance insulin sensitivity and increase glucose uptake and mobilization. Ultimately, this works to decrease insulin resistance, thereby increasing insulin sensitivity and decreasing insulin levels. Improvement of both fasting and postprandial blood glucose levels occurs over time and without stimulating insulin secretion. Both pioglitazone and rosiglitazone are indicated for use as monotherapy or in combination with insulin and exenatide (Byetta). However, they should not be used as first-line therapy if the patient is glucose toxic, since it takes 4 to 8 weeks to fully see the results. Advantages of using TZDs include the delay of beta cell exhaustion, a decrease in insulin resistance, no hypoglycemia (if used alone), and lipid improvement with triglycerides and HDL. Some studies have revealed a slight increase in LDL with rosiglitazone. Disadvantages of this class are weight gain, edema, and a possible increase in liver function enzymes. However, the recommendation is to monitor liver function (LFTs) and stop the drug if serum transaminase exceeds 2.5 times the upper limit. LFTs should then be monitored until they return to normal. Caution is to be used when using TZDs with insulin, since they may cause more peripheral edema (Box 218-9), and in cardiac patients, who may suffer congestive heart failure.[22] Recent and ongoing research on the PPAR family (peroxisome proliferator-activated receptors) has shown a integral relationship with TZDs and their role in fat and carbohydrate metabolism.[21,22]

α-Glucosidase inhibitors (acarbose, miglitol) are antihyperglycemic agents that act in the small intestine, delaying the absorption of glucose. The inhibition of starch and the sucrose enzyme causes lowered postprandial glucose levels. Both

TABLE 218-4 Oral Hypoglycemic Agents

Medication	Dose Range	Actions	Comments
COMBINATIONS			
Rosiglitazone and metformin (Avandamet)	1-4/500	Decreases insulin resistance	Monitor LFTs
Glyburide and metformin (Glucovance)	1.25/250-5/500	Extended release	Titrate slowly, take during meal. Side effects: hypoglycemia, GI distress Same precautions as with metformin
Glipizide and metformin (Metaglip)	5/500 dose Max: 20/2000 mg		Same as above
Pioglitazone and metformin (Actoplus Met)			Same as above
MEGLITINIDES			
Repaglinide (Prandin)	0.5-4 mg b.i.d.-q.i.d.	Increases endogenous insulin postprandially Excreted in bile—short acting	Side effects: hypoglycemia, GI distress Use caution with renal, hepatic insufficiency Take 30 minutes before meals
Nateglinide (Starlix)	60-120 mg		Same precautions as above Take 30 minutes before meals
BIGUANIDES			
Metformin	500-2000 mg; 850 mg-dose available	Decreases hepatic glucose production and increases insulin sensitivity	Take with food Side effects: GI distress and weight loss Do not use if renal or hepatic insufficiency
Metformin extended-release	500-2000 mg		Do not use if renal or hepatic insufficiency
THIAZOLIDINEDIONES			
Rosiglitazone (Avandia)	2-8 mg	Decreases insulin resistance and increases glucose uptake	Side effects: edema May cause anovulatory women to resume ovulation; monitor with use of oral contraceptive pills
Pioglitazone (Actos)	15-45 mg		Contraindicated with renal or hepatic function Side effects: anemia, headache, dizziness, nausea, vomiting Monitor LFTs every 2 months for first year and regularly thereafter
α-GLUCOSIDASE INHIBITORS			
Acarbose (Precose)	25-300 mg	Delays carbohydrate absorption	Side effects: flatulence, diarrhea, abdominal pain
Miglitol (Glyset)	25-300 mg	Treats hypoglycemia with sucrose only	Take during meals, start slowly, and titrate slowly Contraindicated with DKA, inflammatory bowel disease, ulcerative colitis, or bowel obstruction
Exenatide (Byetta)	5, 10 mcg SQ	Lowers postmeal and fasting glucose	Take before breakfast and supper Use with sulfonylurea or metformin Side effects: weight loss, nausea
Glipizide (Glucotrol, Glucotrol XL)	5-40 mg, 5-20 mg	Stimulates insulin secretion, increases absorption of insulin, and improves glucogenesis	Side effects: hypoglycemia, weight gain Take before main meals—better for thinner patients Do not use when nursing or pregnant
Glyburide (Diabeta, Glynase, Micronase)	0.75-12 mg 1.25-20 mg		
Glimepiride (Amaryl)	1-8 mg		Great for use with bedtime insulin
DIPEPTIDYL PEPTIDASE-4 INHIBITORS			
Sitagliptin (Januvia)	100 mg	Enhances incretin system to regulate glucose by affecting alpha and beta cells—increases insulin, decreases glucagons	Decrease dose with renal insufficiency Side effects: headaches, respiratory infection

DKA, Diabetic ketoacidosis; *GI,* gastrointestinal; *LFTs,* liver function tests.

BOX 218-7

HYPOGLYCEMIA AND HYPERGLYCEMIA INDUCED BY PHARMACOKINETICS AFFECTING SULFONYLUREAS

HYPOGLYCEMIA

Displacement from albumin binding site
- Halofenate
- Salicylates
- Some sulfonamides
- Phenylbutazone, oxyphenylbutazone, and sulfinpyrazone

Prolongs half life of sulfonylurea by interfering with metabolism
- Warfarin
- Chloramphenicol
- Monoamine oxidase inhibitors
- Sulfaphenazole
- Pyrazolone derivatives

Decreases urinary excretion of sulfonylurea
- Allopurinol
- Probenecid
- Salicylates
- Pyrazolone derivatives
- Some sulfonamides

HYPERGLYCEMIA

Shortens half life by increasing metabolism of sulfonylurea
- Chronic alcohol use
- Rifampin

Data from American Diabetes Association (Committee Report): Nutrition recommendations and principles for people with diabetes mellitus, *Diabetes Care* 28(Suppl 1):S55-S57, 2005.

BOX 218-8

METFORMIN CONTRAINDICATIONS

CONTRAINDICATIONS TO THE USE OF METFORMIN
- Creatinine levels >1.5 mg/dl in men and 1.4 mg/dl in women
- Hepatic dysfunction
- History of alcoholism
- History of lactic acidosis
- Binge drinking

SITUATIONS REQUIRING WITHHOLDING OF METFORMIN
- Acute myocardial infarction
- Congestive heart failure
- Use of iodine contrast
- Major surgical procedures

BOX 218-9

CONTRAINDICATIONS TO THIAZOLIDINEDIONES

Do not use thiazolidinediones for patients with:
- New York Heart Association Class III or IV heart disease
- Edema or rapid weight gain
- Alanine aminotransferase >2.5 times upper limits of normal
- Symptoms of liver failure: anorexia, jaundice, abdominal pain
- Dark urine with nausea
- Pregnancy

drugs are sufficient as monotherapy, especially in obese individuals eating a high-starch diet. However, they are more effective when used in combination with other hypoglycemic agents or an insulin sensitizer. Contraindications to using acarbose and miglitol include inflammatory bowel disease, colonic ulceration, obstructive bowel disease, gastroparesis, hypoglycemia unawareness when the drug is used with sulfonylureas, type 1 diabetes, and creatinine levels over 2 mg/dl. Close monitoring of individuals with diabetes is needed for medical disorders of digestion or absorption.

Sitagliptin phosphate (Januvia) is a dipeptidyl peptidase 4 (DPP-4) inhibitor recently approved for monotherapy or for combination therapy with an insulin sensitizer (e.g., a biguanide [metformin] or thiazolidinedione) in the treatment of type 2 diabetes.[23] DPP-4s are incretin mimetics. This new class helps to regulate insulin by affecting both alpha and beta cells in response to elevated glucose. Januvia and soon to be released vildagliptin (Galvus) work to release insulin and decrease glucagon levels by slowing the inactivation of incretin hormones. This process then helps to decrease preprandial and postprandial glucose. Januvia is contraindicated in pregnancy and end-stage renal failure and should be used cautiously in patients with renal insufficiency.

Exenatide (Byetta) is also an incretin mimetic.[24] It is given as a subcutaneous injection 15 to 30 minutes before breakfast and evening meals, starting with 5 mcg and titrating to 10 mcg in a month if needed (see Table 218-4). It is not to be used with individuals with gastroparesis or severe kidney disease or in children. There is an increased risk of hypoglycemia when exanatide is combined with oral agents, especially the sulfonylureas. Thus it may be beneficial in some patients to lower the dose of the oral medication. All patients should be advised to monitor their blood glucose levels carefully and discuss the results with the health care provider on a regular basis. In recent studies an advantage of exanatide was found to be the associated weight loss for persons with type 2 diabetes.[24]

Exubera, the first inhaled insulin, recently approved by the FDA, is a rapid-acting insulin used around mealtimes. It can be used for both type 1 and type 2 diabetes; however, it does not replace the longer-acting insulins NPH, glargine, or detemir used in AM or bedtime. This is a new way of giving insulin without needles for better insulin control. Diabetics with asthma, poorly controlled or unstable lung disease, or patients who smoke or have smoked within the past 6 months should not use Exubera. Lung checks (e.g., pulmonary function tests) should be performed before use and every 6 to 12 months thereafter. The device is about the size of an eyeglass case and delivers a dry powder package in 1- to 3-mg inhalable capsules to the lungs.

Insulin may be used as first-line treatment for the patient with type 2 diabetes in the following situations: glycosylated hemoglobin greater than 10% or glucose range over 250 mg/dl, severe illness with associated complications, gestational diabetes, or fragile older adults.[25] However, the most common reason for use of insulin in type 2 diabetes management is failure to respond to the oral antihyperglycemic agents (Box 218-10). A typical scenario with type 2 diabetes is an

BOX 218-10

MANAGEMENT OF TYPE 2 DIABETES

STEP 1

Fasting blood glucose >110 mg/dl or postprandial glucose >200 mg/dl and above ideal body weight—diet and exercise

If within ideal weight or no response within 3 months, go to Step 2

STEP 2

Fasting blood glucose <140 mg/dl, Hgb A1C >6.0

or

Postprandial glucose >160 mg/dl—initiate medical treatment plus Step 1

If inadequate after 3 months, go to Step 3

Fasting blood glucose <140 mg/dl, HgbA1C >6.0	**Fasting blood glucose <150 mg/dl**
Patient obese, dyslipidemic	Patient not obese or dyslipidemic
Choices: metformin b.i.d. or thiazolidinediones (TZDs) q day at low doses	Choices: longer for diet and exercise or metformin b.i.d.

STEP 3

Combination of oral therapy

Choices: Acarbose 25 mg b.i.d., metformin 500 b.i.d.
Pioglitazone (Actos) (15-30 mg), rosiglitazone (Avandia) (2-4 mg) q day, or combination medications

If not responding, add sulfonylureas or meglitinides or exenatide (Byetta) (5-10 mg SQ)

If inadequate after 3 months, go to Step 4

STEP 4

Combination oral therapy and nighttime insulin. Increase oral therapies to maximum.	If fasting blood glucose still high, add 10 units NPH or glargine (Lantus) at nighttime.
If bedtime glucose high, add 2-6 units aspart (Novolog) or lispro (Humalog) at supper. If inadequate after 2-3 months, go to step 5.	

STEP 5

Insulin therapy b.i.d. and TZDs and metformin to decrease insulin resistance

FAILED ORAL THERAPY—INSULIN THERAPY B.I.D., T.I.D., OR Q.I.D.

Stop acarbose and sulfonylureas.

1. Start with glargine, detemir (Levemir), or NPH 10 units and increase to 25% of total daily formula (obese, 0.5 unit/kg/day; nonobese, 0.5-0.7 unit/kg/day).
2. Give four injections of lispro or aspart before meals with glargine or detemir at bedtime.
3. When using glargine, start with 20% of total insulin at bedtime with 30% at breakfast, 20% at lunch, and 30% at supper.
4. Add metformin or insulin sensitizer to keep insulin doses lower.
5. Give two injections of NPH: increase by 50% above formula (½ to ⅔ in AM and ⅓ to ½ in evening).
6. In obese patients with high glucose ranges, follow #2 or use 75/25 or 70/30 (½ to ⅔ in AM and ⅓ to ½ at supper).
7. Give two injections of NPH plus lispro, aspart, or glulisine (Apidra) before breakfast and supper—⅔ in AM and ⅓ at supper.
8. Give three injections: NPH + lispro, aspart, or glulisine in AM; lispro, aspart, or glulisine before supper; and NPH, detemir, or glargine at bedtime.

Data from American Diabetes Association (Committee Report): Nutrition recommendations and principles for people with diabetes mellitus, *Diabetes Care* 28(Suppl 1):S55-S57, 2005.

elevated fasting glucose. This can be treated with a nighttime dose of 5 to 10 units of an intermediate-acting insulin (NPH) or 10 units of a long-acting insulin (glargine or detemir), taken at 8 to 9 PM along with oral agents during the day. If control is still subtherapeutic, then a daytime injection of NPH or Lente or a 75/25 or 70/30 aspart mix should be initiated at a dosage of 10 to 25 units/day.[26]

If a diabetic individual has insulin resistance and/or early morning hyperglycemia, combination with a TZD and metformin or the addition of a long-acting bedtime insulin should be considered. When mixtures of insulin or two injections daily are not maintaining glucose control and/or lifestyle is erratic for standard therapy, an intensive insulin regimen should be initiated using a rapid- and long-acting insulin. Note that, when intensive insulin therapy is initiated, the total daily dose of insulin is reduced by 20% to use as starting nighttime dose of glargine or detemir, and the remainder is divided for meal coverage with rapid-acting insulin. For instance, if total insulin dosage were 40 units/day, a starting dose of 8 units of glargine would be started at 8 to 11 PM and titrated slowly every 4 days.[27]

Combination therapy using the above-mentioned medications along with insulin therapy allows for a more individualized regimen for better glycemic control without side effects and episodes of hypoglycemia. However, diet, exercise, and glucose monitoring are imperative in the ongoing treatment of diabetes. The timing of glucose testing helps with adjusting medications. Fasting and premeal testing gives an overall view of basal control, which should be between 70 and 100 mg/dl. Testing 1 to 2 hours after a meal addresses the impact of insulin secretion and beta cell function; results should be below 130 to 140 mg/dl.[28]

Follow-up care is an integral part of diabetes management. During visits the health care provider evaluates glycemic control, the initiation or progression of vascular complications, and the frequency and severity of hypoglycemic reactions. The patient's ability to understand and manage his or her diabetes improves compliance and prevents problems. The frequency of visits, every 3 to 6 months, depends on diabetic control and complications. Each visit should involve evaluation of blood pressure, weight, height (check against growth chart for age), feet, and blood glucose log. Laboratory tests include a glycohemoglobin test every 3 months. A lipid profile is indicated yearly unless findings are abnormal or are being medically treated; then it is obtained every 4 to 6 months. Yearly screening should include urinary microalbumin and urinalysis, BUN, creatinine, ophthalmologic examinations, and, if indicated cardiovascular, evaluation. A baseline ECG is recommended after age 40. Exercise electrocardiography or peripheral vascular testing should be obtained when indicated.

Pregnancy

Women with diabetes before pregnancy and pregnancy-induced diabetes (gestational diabetes) have special considerations for treatment. If diabetes is untreated or poorly treated, there is an increase in morbidity and mortality for the woman and her infant (Box 218-11). For the woman with type 1 or type 2 diabetes, ideal glycemic control is

BOX 218-11

MATERNAL COMPLICATIONS OF DIABETES

- Hyperglycemia, ketoacidosis
- Pregnancy-induced hypertension
- Pyelonephritis, other infections
- Polyhydramnios
- Preterm labor
- Worsening of chronic complications
- Nephropathy, neuropathy, cardiac disease

Modified from American Diabetes Association: *Medical management of pregnancy complicated by diabetes*, ed 2, Alexandria, Va, 1995, The Association.

strongly recommended both before and during pregnancy to improve the maternal and fetal outcome. The patient with gestational diabetes requires glycemic control during pregnancy. One in every 20 to 30 healthy pregnant women will develop gestational diabetes, carbohydrate intolerance, and insulin resistance. Fetal complications in untreated and poorly treated women include birth injury, macrosomia, hypoglycemia, respiratory distress syndrome, and hyperbilirubinemia (Box 218-12). Maternal complications include an increased incidence of cesarean delivery, preeclampsia, postpartum hemorrhage, development of diabetes later in life.

BOX 218-12

FETAL COMPLICATIONS WITH DIABETIC MOTHERS

- Asphyxia
- Birth injury
- Cardiac hypertrophy
- Congenital anomalies
- Polycythemia and hyperviscosity
- Heart failure
- Hyperbilirubinemia
- Hypocalcemia
- Hypoglycemia
- Hypomagnesemia
- Increased blood volume
- Intrauterine growth retardation
- Macrosomia
- Neurologic instability, irritation
- Organomegaly
- Respiratory distress
- Small left colon syndrome
- Stillbirth
- Transient hematuria

From American Diabetes Association: *Medical management of pregnancy complicated by diabetes*, Alexandria, Va, 1995, The Association.

Glucose intolerance is the cause of increasing insulin resistance during the latter half of pregnancy. Placenta and counterregulatory hormones, along with the stress of the growing fetus, increase insulin resistance, thereby causing hyperglycemia.

Screening for gestational diabetes with a glucose tolerance test is not needed in women under 25 years of age, in women of normal body weight, or in women with no first-degree relative with diabetes.[29] Women who require testing should have a 2- or 3-hour glucose tolerance test performed at 24 to 28 weeks' gestation. Earlier screening at 16 to 20 weeks' gestation is recommended if there is a prior history of gestational diabetes or delivery of a large-for-gestational-age infant. If the glucose tolerance test is negative, it should be repeated at the suggested time of screening (Table 218-5). The screening method is a 50-g glucose load with a 1-hour plasma glucose measurement. If the blood glucose value is 40 mg/dl or greater, then the test should be repeated using either a 75- or 100-g glucose load. Glucose ranges should be as close to 80 to 120 mg/dl as possible.[30] Table 218-6 compares laboratory values.

Management for the patient with gestational diabetes is a priority, and time is of the essence. Treatment for the patient with type 2 diabetes is the same as gestational diabetes. Ideally, glycemic control should be attained preconception to improve both fetal and maternal outcomes. Careful monitoring of blood pressure, renal and retinal status, glycemic control, and fetal well-being by a team of specialists can be necessary throughout the pregnancy. If the woman is taking oral agents, these need to be discontinued and insulin started (see Table 218-3 for insulin dosing during pregnancy). Metformin (pregnancy category B) and the TZDs (pregnancy category C) can be used right up to conception. Postconception dietary management, including an 1800- to 2200-calorie diet, is the

TABLE 218-5 Screening and Diagnosis for Gestational Diabetes*

	Glucose Load		
Plasma Glucose	**50 g**	**75 g**	**100 g**
Fasting		>95	>95 mg/dl
1 hour	<140 mg/dl	>175 mg/dl	>180 mg/dl
2 hour	<120 mg/dl	150 mg/dl	>155 mg/dl
3 hour			>140 mg/dl

Data from American Diabetes Association (Committee Report): Gestational diabetes mellitus, *Diabetes Care* 28(Suppl 1):541, 2005.

*Two or more values exceeding the normal range on the 3-hour glucose tolerance test must be met for diagnosis of gestational diabetes to be made.

TABLE 218-6 Gestational Diabetes Glucose Ranges

	Premeal		2-Hour Postprandial	
	Laboratory	**SMGM**	**Laboratory**	**SMGM**
First trimester	≤105 mg/dl	≤100 mg/dl	≤140 mg/dl	≤120 mg/dl
Second and third trimesters	≤100 mg/dl	≤90 mg/dl	≤120 mg/dl	≤110 mg/dl

SMGM, Self-monitoring glucose monitor.

priority. Monitoring glucose values using a self-monitoring glucose monitor four or more times per day, including fasting and a 2-hour postprandial blood glucose reading, is recommended. Alterations in caloric requirements are needed if the woman is obese and sedentary, or if she is very active. The key to glycemic control is calculating, per meal, appropriate carbohydrates in combination with protein and/or fat to slow glucose release. Exercise is also used to improve glycemic control. Walking or some form of nonstrenuous, aerobic exercise, three or four times per week for 15 to 30 minutes per day, will improve glycemic control. Patients are advised to start slowly and increase gradually to avoid increasing body core temperature. Exercise should be stopped if there are signs of overexertion, hyperthermia, fetal distress, or bleeding or if uterine contractions occur. The obstetrician should be notified if symptoms of fetal distress, bleeding, or contractions develop.[31]

Insulin therapy should be added to improve glucose control when two or more glucose readings exceed the recommended goal range (see Table 218-3). As pregnancy progresses, insulin resistance from hormonal effects can supersede even strict dietary compliance, and insulin therapy is recommended. The starting dosage is approximately 20 to 30 units/day (two thirds in the morning and one third before supper) of a mixture of 75/25 or 70/30 or of NPH and lispro or premeal analogs.[30] However, the exact amount depends on the insulin type and the amount needed for glycemic control. Higher doses of insulin may be necessary in the third trimester, when insulin resistance is the greatest. Adjustments in insulin doses are made in increments of 2 to 4 units every 3 days for minor elevations (120 to 140 mg/dl) or in increments of 5 to 6 units when glucose ranges are higher. Studies have also showed safety and efficacy with using premeal aspart to decrease postprandial blood glucose levels.[32]

The insulin pump is another avenue for controlling preprandial and postprandial glucose. As postprandial hyperglycemia is controlled, it improves outcomes for both fetus and mother. Some endocrinologists are using metformin during pregnancy without ill effects.[33] The hypothesis is that this approach alters the infant's insulin sensitivity. It also has the added benefit of improving the mother's insulin resistance and decreasing weight gain. Gestational diabetes increases the risk of developing diabetes later in life and increases the risk of cardiovascular disease.

Pregnancy in the Patient with Type 1 Diabetes. Pregnancy in the patient with type 1 diabetes is considered a high-risk pregnancy that may result in life-threatening complications for both the mother (see Box 218-11) and fetus (see Box 218-12). Therefore it is imperative that the woman with diabetes attain ideal glycemic control, including a plasma glucose level of 80 to 120 mg/dl and a glycohemoglobin A_{1c} value of 6% to 7%, before pregnancy. However, if pregnancy happens first, glycemic control should be the utmost priority. There is a 1 in 10 chance of congenital anomaly in the growing fetus with poor glycemic control. For the pregnant woman with diabetes the metabolic changes that occur with the growing fetus can accelerate retinal and renal complications. Vascular complications of retinopathy, nephropathy, pregnancy-induced hypertension, and poorly controlled glycemia are strong risk factors for perinatal compromise.[34] These individuals are at high risk and need to be monitored closely by a team of specialists, including an obstetrician, endocrinologist, nephrologist, ophthalmologist, health care provider, nutritionist, and diabetes educator.

Adjustments in insulin doses are needed for glucose control as pregnancy progresses. In the first trimester, insulin doses may be decreased because of hypoglycemia from the increase in fetal glucose transport and a loss of maternal amino acids. During the latter half of the second trimester, there is a rapid diversion to fat metabolism, resulting in higher concentrations of circulating glucose. The longer the postprandial hyperglycemia, the more glucose is transported to the fetus, thus promoting fetal growth. During this time there is also a degree of insulin resistance that occurs from the placental hormone (human placental lactogen), prolactin, and cortisol. Insulin requirements are increased during this stage and into the third trimester, then plateau around the 36th week of gestation.

Everything changes with pregnancy. Dietary requirements, activity and exercise, glucose monitoring, and insulin requirements are adjusted for the pregnant state. Caloric requirements are increased, and snacks are added, particularly during the first trimester, to prevent hypoglycemia. Multiple injections with changes in insulin type (NPH, lispro, aspart, or insulin pump) may be needed for better glycemic control. The advantage of the pump is that it allows for frequent, small dose adjustments in basal and bolus rates using a rapid insulin analog. To achieve safer and improved glycemic control, home monitoring may be increased to eight times per day (fasting, before each meal, 2-hour postprandial, at bedtime, and at 2 or 3 AM). Also, reassessment for signs of retinopathy, nephropathy, and hypertension is necessary because of the metabolic changes of pregnancy.

For both type 1 and 2 pregnant diabetics, certain oral medications are not safe during pregnancy or breastfeeding and will have to be changed (e.g., angiotensin-converting enzyme [ACE] inhibitors, sulfonylureas, and hyperlipidemic agents). Biguanide and TZDs can be used for type 2 diabetics. For about 6 months postpartum, diabetic women may need a change in pharmacologic treatment. After that time, depending on weight, exercise and activity, and food intake, they may return to their prior regimen.

Interestingly, research is currently looking into mothers with type 1 diabetes who begin to produce insulin again during pregnancy. There is a rise in C-peptide levels and drop in insulin requirements. This may be from an increase in mild immunosuppressive hormones (cortisol and progesterone) and growth hormones (prolactin and placental lactogen) that may stop or revive beta cell destruction.

Co-Management with Specialists

Diabetes is a progressive vascular disease requiring collaborative treatment from many specialties to prevent or slow the progression of end-organ complications. Specialists included in the co-management of diabetic individuals throughout the life span include endocrinologists, ophthalmologists, podiatrists, cardiologists, nephrologists, obstetricians, and vascular surgeons. Consultation with an endocrinologist is required for diabetic individuals receiving insulin pump therapy, those with inadequate control (either with hyperglycemia or frequent hypoglycemia), pregnancy, motivational issues, or complications. Referrals include routine yearly visits to an ophthalmologist for evaluation and treatment of retinopathy, cataracts, and retinal hemorrhaging and to a podiatrist for treatment of ulcers, foot deformities, foot infections, callus removal, and nail care. Once renal involvement occurs, nephrology referral is indicated to prevent further renal disease. A vascular surgeon or specialist is needed for treatment of peripheral vascular disease, nonhealing ulcers, or amputation.

Other referrals include consultation with a nutritionist for meal management, caloric requirements, and weight loss; a diabetes educator to improve knowledge and plan of caring for diabetes; an exercise physiologist or physical therapist for exercise guidelines; and a social worker to help with the many fluctuations of emotions that may come throughout their lifetime.[35]

LIFE SPAN CONSIDERATIONS

Diabetes is a progressive disease with acute and chronic phases. It encompasses all ages from newborn to elders. With each stage of development there are issues regarding diabetes management, physical and emotional development, education and understanding, physical disabilities, nutrition, and behavioral and medical problems that will affect the diabetic treatment plan. Adolescents and elders are at greatest risk for failure. Predictors that impede diabetic adherence to therapy include lack of practical knowledge, lack of control, vulnerability, social unacceptance, little or no family support, and fear of hypoglycemia. Other barriers include financial or occupational restraints. Consideration of all these issues is essential for optimum care.

Adolescents pose a particular challenge, since metabolic and biologic changes affect good blood glucose control. Preadolescence or early adolescence (age 12), middle adolescence (13 to 15 years), and late adolescence (16 to 18 years) impose hormonal changes that often cause relative insulin resistance because of changing counterregulatory hormonal responses and declining peripheral insulin action.

During adolescence, emotional and developmental issues are critical. The emotional stages of shock, denial, negotiation, anger, and acceptance can recur as the person ages. Developmental issues of individual identity, sexual identity and exploration, the drive for independence and struggles with parents and authority, and peer acceptance can affect adolescents' ability to manage their diabetes. Other concerns affecting diabetes management include athletic participation, recurrent ketoacidosis, inadequate nutrition and dieting, alcohol, drugs, and sexual activity. The health care provider's ability to communicate and compromise without risking safety will foster the development of a trusting relationship. Education must be factual, specific, consultative vs. directive, and relevant to the adolescent's stage of development and emotional behavior. The treatment plan must be a realistic and workable one agreed on by the patient and the provider. Written instructions are helpful.

During young adulthood, developmental issues of career development, interpersonal relationships, self-image, health perception, and understanding of diabetes can influence glycemic control. As emotional ties to family decline, concerns related to marriage, pregnancy and children, employment, finances, and anticipation of complications can influence diabetes management. Health care providers must provide emotional support, educational review or expansion on previous information, and nutritional and pharmacologic reevaluation. Emphasis should be on blood glucose monitoring, appropriate physical activity, nutrition, and medical intervention to prevent hypoglycemia and maintain glycemic control.

In middle-aged and older persons, concerns about loneliness, economics, and disease progression or failing health can affect diabetic management. Financial concerns can interfere with proper food, prescribed medications, blood testing or insulin equipment, and medical care. Issues of weight loss, physical inactivity, failing vision or blindness, poor dexterity or amputation, memory impairment, hearing loss, gait disturbance or muscle weakness, sexual dysfunction, dialysis, and physical and emotional isolation can affect glycemic control. As complications develop and health begins to falter, denial, anger, hostility, and depression can threaten the emotional well-being of the older patient with diabetes and influence diabetic management. Health care providers must provide emotional support. The maintenance of function, independence, and general well-being, as well as prevention of severe hypoglycemia and vascular compromise, should take precedence over attaining optimum glycemic control. Insulin doses at this time may need to be decreased to prevent hypoglycemia and prevent falls. It is essential that the older patient with diabetes understand and can accomplish the treatment plan. Frequent medical visits, as well as written and simplified instructions, are helpful for older adults with diabetes.

COMPLICATIONS

Psychologic Complications

The diagnosis of DM, like any chronic illness, can be unexpected and potentially devastating. Grief is the most common reaction of an individual diagnosed with DM, and resolution depends on variables such as education, economics, geography, religion, and culture. The integral support of family members and friends affects the long-term acceptance of the disease progression.

Whereas 5% to 8% of the general population will experience a major depressive disorder sometime in their lifetime, there is a threefold to fourfold increase in the prevalence of depression in patients with type 1 or type 2 diabetes.[35] Without treatment, depression in the patient with diabetes can affect glycemic control. This occurs because of poor self-management, either by not testing, not giving correct insulin doses, overeating or undereating, sleep disturbances, or under-exercising or overexercising.[36] Careful coordination of medical therapy and psychotherapy are needed. The newer selective serotonin reuptake inhibitors (SSRIs) are better choices for treatment than most other antidepressant agents, since they do not have hyperglycemic side effects.

Other mental health issues are anxiety, eating disorders, schizophrenia, and subclinical emotional distress that can impede diabetes management, leading to poor glycemic control, poor self-image, confusion of treatment options, and progression of complications leading to poorer quality of life. Treatment options include relaxation, education, better support systems, psychotherapy, and pharmacotherapy.[37]

Macrovascular Complications

Macrovascular disease in the patient with diabetes is characterized by arteriosclerosis and atherosclerosis of moderate- to large-sized arterial and venous vessel walls. Also included is nonatherosclerotic disease leading to vascular insufficiency, claudication, and gangrene. The vascular pathologic condition encompasses cerebral, coronary, and peripheral circulation and is exacerbated by an "atherosclerotic environment" of hypertension, hyperlipidemia, hyperglycemia, obesity, and inflammation. These diffuse atherosclerotic plaques can contribute to tissue ischemia, thrombosis, infarction, and atheroembolism, leading to tissue and organ damage. Also seen is small vessel disease and endothelial dysfunction with inappropriate vasodilatory responses.[38]

The patient with type 2 diabetes presents a particular challenge, since many of the symptoms associated with macrovascular disease are overlooked before the onset or diagnosis of diabetes itself and may be present long before the development of hyperglycemia. Cerebrovascular disease, correlated with the length of time diabetes is present in the patient with type 1 diabetes and the level of glycemic control, carries a five to seven times greater mortality rate than in the nondiabetic population.[39] Slurred speech, intermittent dizziness, transient loss of vision, paresthesia, or weakness of an arm or leg suggests a transient ischemic attack consistent with cerebral disease. In patients with type 1 diabetes these symptoms are usually discernible and easily distinguished from episodes of hypoglycemia, but in patients with type 2 diabetes the diagnosis is often less clear. Auscultation of vascular bruits over the carotid arteries and noninvasive Doppler ultrasound studies can help identify the presence and extent of cerebrovascular disease.[40] Anticoagulant and antiplatelet medications and/or the use of daily aspirin may help prevent a recurrence of symptoms.[7]

Coronary artery disease (CAD) in the patient with diabetes occurs earlier and more extensively than in patients without diabetes, and infarction may occur without typical symptoms. Atypical symptoms of CAD include dyspnea; fatigue; gastrointestinal complaints with exertion; periods of poor glycemic control, particularly if associated with diabetic ketoacidosis; and unexplained congestive heart failure.[41] Typical symptoms of exertional chest pain, chest tightness, and arm pain associated with activity or rest need to be evaluated promptly in these patients. An initial or subsequent myocardial infarction is more likely to precipitate long-term complications (e.g., heart failure or arrhythmia) or death in the patient with diabetes compared with the patient without diabetes. Silent myocardial infarctions are two to three times more common in patients with diabetes. Recent research has revealed a twofold to fivefold fold increase in episodes of congestive heart failure with patients with insulin resistance.[41] Therefore treatment options for decreasing cardiovascular events begin with disease prevention, early detection, and treatment of cardiovascular disease. Early identification, either by screening or diagnostic testing, of those patients needing revascularization is essential (Boxes 218-13 and 218-14). Diabetic patients with cardiovascular disease should be treated with aspirin, ACE inhibitors, target blood pressure control, and lipid therapy. Their medical care should be managed in conjunction with a cardiologist.

BOX 218-13

INDICATIONS FOR CARDIOVASCULAR TESTING

ECG consistent with ischemia
Age >65 years with duration of type 2 diabetes >10 years
Plans to begin vigorous exercise program
Evaluation before renal transplantation
Preoperative clearance for major vascular or noncardiac surgery
Atypical cardiac symptoms
Peripheral or carotid obstructive vascular disease
Two or more of following risk factors in addition to diabetes:

- Total cholesterol ≥240 mg/dl, low-density lipoprotein ≥160 mg/dl, or high-density lipoprotein <35 mg/dl
- Blood pressure >140/90 mm Hg
- Cigarette smoking
- Positive family history of premature coronary artery disease
- Positive microalbuminuria or macroalbuminuria

From Sander GE: Diagnostic evaluation for coronary artery disease in patients with diabetes mellitus. In *Cardiovascular primer*, New Orleans, 2001, Louisiana State University School of Medicine.

Dyslipidemia in patients with predominantly type 2 diabetes is characterized by hypertriglyceridemia, low HDL, and high LDL. There is a twofold to fourfold increase in risk for coronary heart disease. In women with diabetes, there is a five times greater risk for cardiovascular disease as compared to the nondiabetic population.[40] Evaluation for cardiovascular disease includes a fasting lipid profile, C-reactive protein (cardio CRP), blood pressure monitoring, and glycemic control. Cardio CRP is an inflammatory marker and has shown to be a better predictor of cardiovascular events than just LDL.[42,43] TZDs, especially pioglitazone, have been shown to increase HDL and lower LDL. A low-fat, low-cholesterol diet and aerobic exercise are first-line treatment and should be maintained in conjunction with pharmacologic intervention.[40]

Improvement of glycemic control to reach the goals of glycosylated hemoglobin of less than 7%, blood pressure less than 120/80 mm Hg, and LDL of 70 mg/dl will decrease and possibly reverse the ravages of cardiovascular disease.[44] Long-term follow-up on the DCCT/EDIC revealed a 42% reduction in cardiovascular disease with intensive therapy.[5,9] The diabetic individual without cardiovascular disease may be able to use nutritional therapy for 3 to 6 months and drug therapy for LDLs greater than 130 mg/dl. Table 218-7 shows the recommendations for treating high levels of LDL.[45]

BOX 218-14

SCREENING AND DIAGNOSTIC TESTS

- ECG
- Persantine or thallium exercise testing
- Stress echocardiogram
- SPECT sestamibi imaging
- Coronary angiography

TABLE 218-7 Risk Stratification of Lipids

Risk Factor	Lipid Goal
CAD + multiple risk factors	LDL <70 mg/dl
Diabetes (DM), insulin resistance (IR), metabolic syndrome (MS)	
No risk factors	LDL to goal
CAD + risk equivalent	LDL <100 mg/dl
Vascular disease (cerebral, peripheral) and abdominal aortic aneurysm	
Multiple risk factors	LDL <130 mg/dl
0-1 Risk factor	LDL <160 mg/dl
Triglycerides >200 mg/dl	Triglycerides 150 mg/dl
Triglycerides 200-500 mg/dl	Triglycerides, LDL, HDL to goal

Data from Expert panel on detection, evaluation, and treatment of high blood cholesterol in adults. Executive summary of the third report of the national cholesterol education program, *JAMA* 285(19):2486-2497, 2001; and Berra K, Hughes S: Pharmacologic agents to reduce cardiovascular disease risk for the patient with insulin resistance. In Lamendola C, Mason C, editors: *Reducing cardiovascular risk in the insulin resistant patient,* New York, 2001, Preventive Cardiovascular Nurses.

CAD, Coronary artery disease; *HDL,* high-density lipoprotein; *LDL,* low-density lipoprotein.

Major risk factors for coronary vascular disease (CVD) include hypertension, diabetes, smoking, low HDL (44 mg/dl), and family history of premature CVD (at less than 55 years in men and 65 years in women). Treatment starts with lifestyle changes: diet modification of lowered saturated fat and higher polyunsaturated fat, weight loss, increased brisk aerobic exercise for 30 minutes, smoking cessation, reduction of high glycemic carbohydrates, and alcohol consumption of no more than two drinks per day. Drug therapy using statins, fibrates, nicotinic acid, and cholesterol absorptive inhibitors, as monotherapy or in combinations, must be evaluated every 3 to 6 months initially, along with alanine aminotransferase/aspartate aminotransferase ratio, until the goals are achieved. Then monitoring can decrease to yearly.

Occlusive peripheral arterial disease affects about one third of diabetic individuals over 50.[46] The pattern of lower extremity ischemia in these individuals differs from that in the population without diabetes. There is a predilection for macrovascular disease, primarily in the tibial and peroneal arteries. The dorsalis pedis artery and other foot vessels are usually spared. As a direct consequence of poor peripheral circulation, infections, limb ischemia, lower extremity ulceration, and amputations are not uncommon.[47] Early warning signs include claudication (cramping, early fatigue, or leg pain in calves, thighs, and buttocks) relieved by rest; numbness, tingling, and coldness of lower extremities; and slowly healing wounds. Diagnosis by Doppler of lower extremities or by ankle-brachial index confirms the diagnosis. Contrast angiography and arteriography are invasive procedures for evaluating the need for endovascular or revascularization procedures.[46]

CT is used for the evaluation of the aorta and surrounding area. MRI and magnetic resonance angiography allow for measurements of aortic, renal, and carotid arteries as well as the arteries of the lower extremities. Treatment options include walking; exercise programs; aggressive lipid and hypertension management; smoking cessation; relaxation and biofeedback; antiplatelet medications (clopidogrel [Plavix]); cilostazol (Pletal); and vascular interventions, including angioplasty and bypass.[46-49]

Neuropathic Complications

Diabetic neuropathy affects up to 60% of individuals with DM and is one of the most complex and potentially catastrophic of all the diabetic complications. Although the degree and duration of hyperglycemia appear to increase the risk of nerve damage, these two factors do not reliably predict the development of neuropathy. However, recent data from EDIC reveal that intensive therapy improved glycemic control and reduced rates of nerve damage years later.[9] Multiple mechanisms contribute to the pathogenesis of this diabetic complication. There are three major classes of diabetic neuropathies: peripheral or distal polyneuropathy, mononeuropathy, and diabetic autonomic neuropathy.

Peripheral polyneuropathy is the most commonly occurring neuropathic complication. Distal numbness or impaired sensation is typically symmetric and bilateral, and it can occur acutely as a complication of poor glycemic control. Initially, pain sensation and the ability to discriminate sharp stimuli are impaired, along with bilaterally absent knee or ankle jerk reflexes. Progression of sensory deficits can cause destruction of cartilage in foot joints. This destruction results in loss of normal foot architecture, leaving the foot susceptible to an arthropathy known as Charcot's joint. Charcot's joint may be difficult to distinguish from active infection with cellulitis, since both manifest with erythema and swelling.[50] The presence of altered foot sensation suggests that an individual requires daily foot inspection and routine podiatry visits to minimize the risk for complications.

Pain is present in about 25% of all diabetic patients with peripheral neuropathy. Nonpharmacologic treatment for painful peripheral neuropathy is aimed at avoidance of alcohol; improvement of glycemic control; use of relaxation, hypnotic, acupuncture, or biofeedback techniques; use of transcutaneous electrical nerve stimulation (TENS); use of infrared energy (Anodyne); or referral to a pain control clinic. Pharmacologic options include topical capsaicin, which is variably effective; lidocaine patches (Lidoderm); and, in limited situations, narcotics. Sharp pain may respond to anticonvulsants (gabapentin dosed three times daily and slowly titrated upward to maximum of 1200 mg/day; lamotrigine dosed twice daily to maximum of 400 mg/day; and pregabalin 50 to 100 mg b.i.d., which is showing promising results with fewer side effects). Tricyclic antidepressants (amitriptyline, imipramine, nortriptyline, doxepin) alone, given in low doses at bedtime or in combination with SSRIs (paroxetine, citalopram), and/or selective norepinephrine inhibitors (venlafaxine, duloxetine) in small doses during the day may all provide relief of symptoms. Nutraceuticals that have been found to be helpful include evening primrose oil and lipoic acid.[50-52]

The mononeuropathies occur in large nerves or nerve roots and produce radicular symptoms. Large nerve roots in the spinal cord, chest, or abdomen or even cranial nerves can be affected. Mononeuropathy involves both the sensory and motor neurons, producing increased or decreased sensation, weakness, and pain. The pain produced by mononeuropathies can be severe and mimic degenerative disc disease, herpes zoster, carpal tunnel syndrome, Bell's palsy, or intraabdominal conditions. Oculomotor palsy, characterized by ptosis, pain, and sparing of the pupillary reflex, occurs in patients over 50 years of age. Pain and oculomotor function improve gradually over several weeks, and full recovery usually occurs within 3 to 5 months.[51-53]

Autonomic neuropathy affects both sympathetic and parasympathetic fibers. Although any organ system may be affected, the more common effects are found in the gastrointestinal tract, genitourinary tract, and cardiovascular system. Symptoms of gastrointestinal dysfunction include esophageal motility problems and gastroparesis with impaired gastric emptying. The gastroparesis affects food absorption, impairing glycemic control. The erratic nature of gastric emptying also produces nausea and vomiting. Bowel peristaltic dysfunction is evidenced by explosive diarrhea and altered small bowel motility. These symptoms may improve with control of hyperglycemia. Gastroparesis can be addressed through dietary modifications and the use of metoclopramide or cisapride. Various modalities have been tried for controlling diarrhea, including biofeedback, diphenoxylate and atropine (Lomotil), clonidine, bile acid sequestrants (cholestyramine and colestipol), and antibiotics.[53]

Genitourinary symptoms usually consist of neurogenic bladder and sexual dysfunction. Bladder atony, characterized by a residual urine volume greater than 150 ml, may lead to recurrent UTIs and eventual obstructive uropathy. The occurrence of more than two UTIs in 1 year indicates the need for further evaluation. Bethanechol may be helpful as a conservative measure, but surgical intervention with recommended diagnosis by ultrasound (not IV pyelography) may be necessary. Sexual dysfunction in women is characterized by decreased vaginal lubrication and decreased frequency of orgasm. Impotence can affect more than 50% of diabetic men who have had the disease for more than 10 years. Retrograde ejaculations are also common. Psychologic, endocrine-related, medication, or alcohol-induced impotence needs to be excluded before considering vasodilatory substances (sildenafil [Viagra], vardenafil [Levitra], tadalafil [Cialis]), alprostadil injection (Caverject), implantations, or vacuum devices.[50,53]

Cardiovascular autonomic neuropathy has two major associated syndromes: orthostatic hypotension and cardiac denervation. Orthostatic hypotension may be pronounced, with an inability to tolerate rising from a supine to an upright posture unless this is achieved gradually over more than 10 minutes. Cardiac denervation, characterized in later stages by a fixed heart rate in the range of 80 to 100 beats per minute, is unresponsive to stress, exercise, or tilting. These patients may suffer myocardial ischemia or infarction without pain and are at risk for cardiac arrhythmias and sudden death. They should avoid heavy exercise, aerobic exercise, and straining, and are generally not candidates for intensive insulin therapy because of the risk for hypoglycemia and potential cardiac arrhythmias.[50,53]

Nephropathic Complications

Nephropathy results in end-stage renal disease (ESRD), requiring dialysis, in 30% to 40% of patients with type 1 diabetes and represents the second leading cause of death for individuals with diabetes. Sixty percent of all patients with diabetes who ultimately require renal dialysis have type 2 diabetes.[2,54]

Diabetic nephropathy is characterized by proteinuria, hypertension, edema, and renal insufficiency. Once established and without adequate medical intervention, nephropathy progresses through five stages: (1) hypertrophy and hyperfunction, (2) renal lesions, (3) incipient nephropathy, (4) clinical diabetic nephropathy, and (5) ESRD. Histologically there are three classes of renal changes: (1) glomerulosclerosis, (2) structural vascular changes, and (3) tubulointerstitial disease.[54]

The glomerular filtration rate (GFR), which is usually elevated when a person is first diagnosed with diabetes, is directly related to the degree of hyperglycemia but is a poor measure of renal function, since its elevation may ensue over a long "silent" period (about 15 years' duration) as histologic changes in the kidney continue. Serum creatinine, also an unreliable marker for renal disease, might not be elevated until more than 50% of function is lost and may be normal in older patients with renal damage because of decreased muscle mass.[55]

All patients with diabetes should have a urinalysis performed and renal function assessed at least annually. Individuals with proteinuria need close monitoring of renal function, initiation of ACE inhibition, and screening for microalbuminuria. Microalbuminuria analysis can be performed by random spot collection, a 24-hour collection, or a timed (e.g., 4-hour or overnight) collection. Microalbuminuria is diagnostic at greater than 30 mg/24 hr excretion. Two or three positive collections in a 3- to 6-month period should exist before the designation of microalbuminuria is applied. Consultation with a diabetologist or nephrologist should occur when microalbuminuria (30 to 300 mg/24 hr), overt albuminuria (>2 mg/dl), or decreased GFR (<50 ml/min) is present.

Controlling blood pressure is the single most important factor in the prevention and treatment of renal disease in the patient with diabetes. The ADA cites 120/80 mm Hg as the normalized blood pressure goal to prevent complications of cerebral, cardiac, or other organ system functions. In patients with evidence of microvascular or macrovascular complications, a blood pressure greater than 130/80 mm Hg should be considered abnormal.[56,57] Currently, a reasonable blood pressure goal is less than 130/80 mm Hg in individuals with type 2 diabetes and 120/80 mm Hg or lower in those with type 1 diabetes. As with all treatment regimens, diet, exercise, weight loss, and smoking cessation are included. Pharmacologic intervention for blood pressure includes, in order of preference, ACE inhibitors, angiotensin II inhibitors, alpha blockers, beta blockers, calcium channel blockers, and low-dose diuretics.[57,58] Consultation with a cardiologist or nephrologist is recommended with hard-to-control patients.

Microvascular Complications

Retinopathy. All type 1 and type 2 patients will have some form of retinopathy after 20 years of diabetes, and 21% of type 2 patients have retinopathy at the time of diagnosis.[2] Therefore annual screening for retinopathy with a dilated examination by an ophthalmologist is recommended for all individuals with diabetes, beginning at the time of diagnosis for those with type 2. In the 20- to 74-year age-group, diabetic retinopathy is now the leading cause of new-onset blindness in the United States. Poor glucose control, proteinuria, hyperlipidemia, and hypertension are all risk factors associated with the incidence and progression of diabetic retinopathy.

Hypertension increases the blood flow to the retina, which causes a disturbance in the flow of blood to retina and optic nerves. This turbulence also increases the potential for clot formation.[59]

The three stages of diabetic retinopathy are characterized by individual findings and changes:

- Nonproliferative (or background) diabetic retinopathy (NPDR) is the earliest stage, and intraretinal "dot and blot" microaneurysms can be detected. Macular edema, visual changes, eye pain, and hard ring-shaped exudates seen on examination are all reasons to promptly refer the patient to a retinal specialist.
- Preproliferative diabetic retinopathy (PPDR) can be made when the "dot and blot" microaneurysms become clustered, indicating a nonfunctional capacity of the capillary circulation. Cotton-wool spots (soft exudates); "beading" of the retinal veins; and dilated, tortuous retinal capillaries secondary to hypoxia are all seen in this stage.
- Proliferative diabetic retinopathy (PDR), the final and most vision-threatening advancement, is characterized by increased retinal ischemia producing continued abnormal retinal vessel growth and creating neovascularization on the surface of the retina and sometimes extending into the posterior vitreous. As these new vessels bleed, a condition exacerbated by macular edema, the individual will report a new sensation of "floaters" or "cobwebs" in the eye and may experience a sudden, painless loss of vision. Retinal detachment, resulting from the tractional forces of fibrous tissue, blocks the outflow of aqueous humor and increases intraocular pressure. This will manifest as severe pain, loss of vision, and glaucoma.[60]

NPDR and PPDR are treated by strict adherence to blood pressure and blood glucose control and follow-up care by an eye specialist.

Hypoglycemia. Hypoglycemia is a complication of insulin excess and results in various symptoms (Table 218-8). Neuroglycopenia occurs when the brain and central nervous system are not able to maintain normal function because of lowered glucose levels. The lowered serum glucose is classified as mild, moderate, or severe and is dependent on the symptoms of neuroglycopenia and the individual's ability to self-treat.[61] When blood glucose levels are below 70 mg/dl (or higher in a diabetic patient with poor control), the hypothalamus senses the decreased blood glucose and triggers the sensation of hunger. This action stimulates the nervous system to increase gastric juices and stomach contraction. The adrenal medulla secretes epinephrine and cortisol, which stimulate glycogenolysis. This slows glycogenesis (the uptake of glucose) and promotes gluconeogenesis (glucose formation from fatty and amino acids). As the blood glucose level decreases, cerebral function is altered.

Patients with diabetes have different blood glucose ranges for mild to severe hypoglycemia. A previously normal glucose range of 70 mg/dl for one individual may mean hypoglycemia for another. Therefore the individual must monitor episodes of hypoglycemia, symptoms encountered (especially unconscious episodes), and blood glucose ranges. Treatment complications can include an inadequate rise in glucose and an inability to recognize warning signals. *Hypoglycemia unawareness* is the loss of autonomic symptoms that warn the individual of the impending lowered blood glucose level. Uncontrolled diabetes or large swings of hypoglycemia and hyperglycemia are risk factors for this reversible condition.

Intensive insulin therapy and ideal blood glucose control can cause more vulnerability to hypoglycemia. Health care providers must be aware of the influence of medications (Box 218-15) and food on glucose control and be wary of nighttime moderate to severe hypoglycemia. Older adults, type 1 patients, and those with neurologic impairment are at greatest risk for hypoglycemia and should have close watch over insulin adjustments, meals and snacking, and blood glucose monitoring. Severe hypoglycemia left untreated can

TABLE 218-8 Hypoglycemia

Condition	Signs and Symptoms	Treatment
Mild neuroglycopenia	Hungry, weak, shaky, diaphoresis, pallor, tachycardia, paresthesia, difficulty concentrating, irritability but no changes in mental status; individual able to self-treat Plasma glucose <50 mg/dl	10-15 g of simple-acting carbohydrate increases blood glucose level 30-45 mg/dl after 15 minutes. Stop activity and retest in 10-15 minutes; if <60 mg/dl, take additional 10-15 g of carbohydrate; ½ hour later, eat snack or meal consisting of 1 protein and 1 carbohydrate. 20-30 g of carbohydrate may be needed.
Moderate neuroglycopenia	Impaired function of CNS: decreased thinking, increased emotions (anger, irritability), inability to complete tasks, some changes in mental status; individual may be able to self-treat	Take 15-30 g of simple-acting carbohydrate and then follow above instructions.
Severe neuroglycopenia	When glucose levels fall <45 mg/dl, confusion, drowsiness, and progression to unconsciousness; impaired neurologic function; individual not able to self-treat	Take 30-45 g of simple-acting carbohydrate—if able to swallow—or glucagon subcutaneously if not (1 mg for adults; 0.5 mg for children <5 years; 0.25 mg for infants). Cognitive recovery can take up to 2 hours.

Data from Gonder-Frederick L, Cox DJ, Clarke WL: Helping patients understand and recognize hypoglycemia, *Clin Diabetes* 14:86-90, 1996; and Gonder-Frederick LA, Zrebiec J: Hypoglycemia. In Franz MJ, editor: *Diabetes management therapies: core curriculum for diabetes educators,* Chicago, 2003, American Diabetes Association.

BOX 218-15

DRUGS INTERFERING WITH GLYCEMIC CONTROL

INTRINSIC HYPOGLYCEMIC EFFECT

- Alcohol
- Salicylates
- Monoamine oxidase inhibitors
- Beta blockers

INTRINSIC HYPERGLYCEMIC EFFECT

- Acetazolamide
- Beta blockers
- Diazoxide
- Diuretics (thiazides, furosemide)
- Epinephrine
- Estrogens
- Glucagons
- Glucocorticoids
- Indomethacin
- Interferon
- Isoniazid
- Levothyroxine
- Nicotinic acid
- Pentamidine
- Phenytoin

lead to death. Another situation affecting glycemic control is the individual who has encountered a severe hypoglycemic episode and purposefully stays out of control because of fear of a repeat hypoglycemic event. Therefore it is important that providers and diabetic patients collaborate on a treatment plan that is safe and comfortable. Nocturnal noninvasive monitoring devices, GlucoWatch (a wrist watch that sounds an alarm when blood glucose drops below a preset level), and Continuous Glucose Monitoring System (which profiles previous blood glucose levels for a time through interstitial fluids) are ways providers can help decrease episodes of hypoglycemia and recommend safer treatment plans for their patients.

Hyperglycemia. Diabetic ketoacidosis (DKA) and hyperosmolar nonketotic acidosis are two medical emergencies of hyperglycemia that require immediate treatment and possible hospitalization.

DKA involves profound hyperglycemia, osmotic diuresis, dehydration, and acidosis causing an increased anion gap from insulin deficiency. Symptoms associated with this process include a 12- to 24-hour history of polyuria, polydipsia, hyperventilation, and dehydration. A fruity breath, abdominal pain, nausea and vomiting, and changes in consciousness can also be present. Hospitalization can sometimes be avoided if the hyperglycemia, even with positive ketones, is immediately treated with increased levels of insulin[62,63] and dehydration is prevented (Figure 218-1). Once the patient is stable, the cause for DKA should be explored to prevent recurrence. The most common causes include new-onset diabetes, infection, illness or major surgery, and depression (not taking insulin).

Prevention of DKA requires prompt dialogue between the patient and the health care provider to treat increasing hyperglycemia. Sick day management guidelines (Box 218-16) can enable the diabetic patient to actively participate in preventing ketoacidosis.

Hyperosmolar nonketotic syndrome is another emergency and involves the patient with type 2 diabetes. Presenting symptoms include altered consciousness, shallow respiration, polydipsia, hyperglycemia, and profound dehydration. Seizures, coma, or even hemiplegia may be present. This is most common in older adults with type 2 diabetes or in newly diagnosed individuals. Other abnormalities include blood glucose ranges over 600 mg/dl, without ketosis or with slight ketosis; serum osmolarity over 340 mosm/kg water; increased BUN and creatinine; and mild metabolic acidosis. Precipitating causes include medications (see Box 218-15), infection, surgery or severe dialysis, excessive burns, and certain medical conditions (cerebrovascular accident, myocardial infarction, pancreatitis, gastrointestinal hemorrhage, and diabetic gangrene). Treatment includes reversing dehydration and hyperglycemia and correcting any electrolyte abnormalities (Figure 218-2).[62,63]

Insulin Allergy. Local reactions at the injection site are the most common form of allergic reaction to insulin. Delayed hypersensitivity may also occur but remains in the area of injection. The use of synthetic or purified insulin has decreased both local and systemic reactions. Occurrence of reactions may be secondary to improper injection technique, injection of cold insulin, or preservatives. If systemic reactions do occur, the individual may require desensitization (the process of slowly reintroducing the allergy-inducing insulin at minute doses until the body no longer has an allergic response). This procedure requires a series of injections of the insulin.

INDICATIONS FOR REFERRAL OR HOSPITALIZATION

Based on the ADA recommendations, guidelines for hospitalization include:

- Acute metabolic complications: DKA (with ketonuria, blood glucose >250 mg/dl, arterial pH <7.35, and nausea and vomiting), hyperosmolar nonketotic state (with impaired mental status, dehydration, elevated plasma osmolarity, and blood glucose >400 mg/dl), and hypoglycemia with neuroglycopenia
- Newly diagnosed diabetes in children and adolescents
- Poor metabolic control that requires close monitoring
- Uncontrolled or newly diagnosed gestational diabetes requiring insulin
- Institution of insulin pump or other intensive insulin therapy requiring close observation
- Chronic vascular complications of diabetes that progress, requiring intensive treatment

Other situations requiring physician consultation include an inability to attain glucose control (either consistent hyperglycemia or hypoglycemia), pregnancy, and the development of complications.

PATIENT AND FAMILY EDUCATION

Patient education enhances the diabetic individual's ability to attain glycemic control. Education is lifelong as the individual enters different life and emotional stages, resulting in changes,

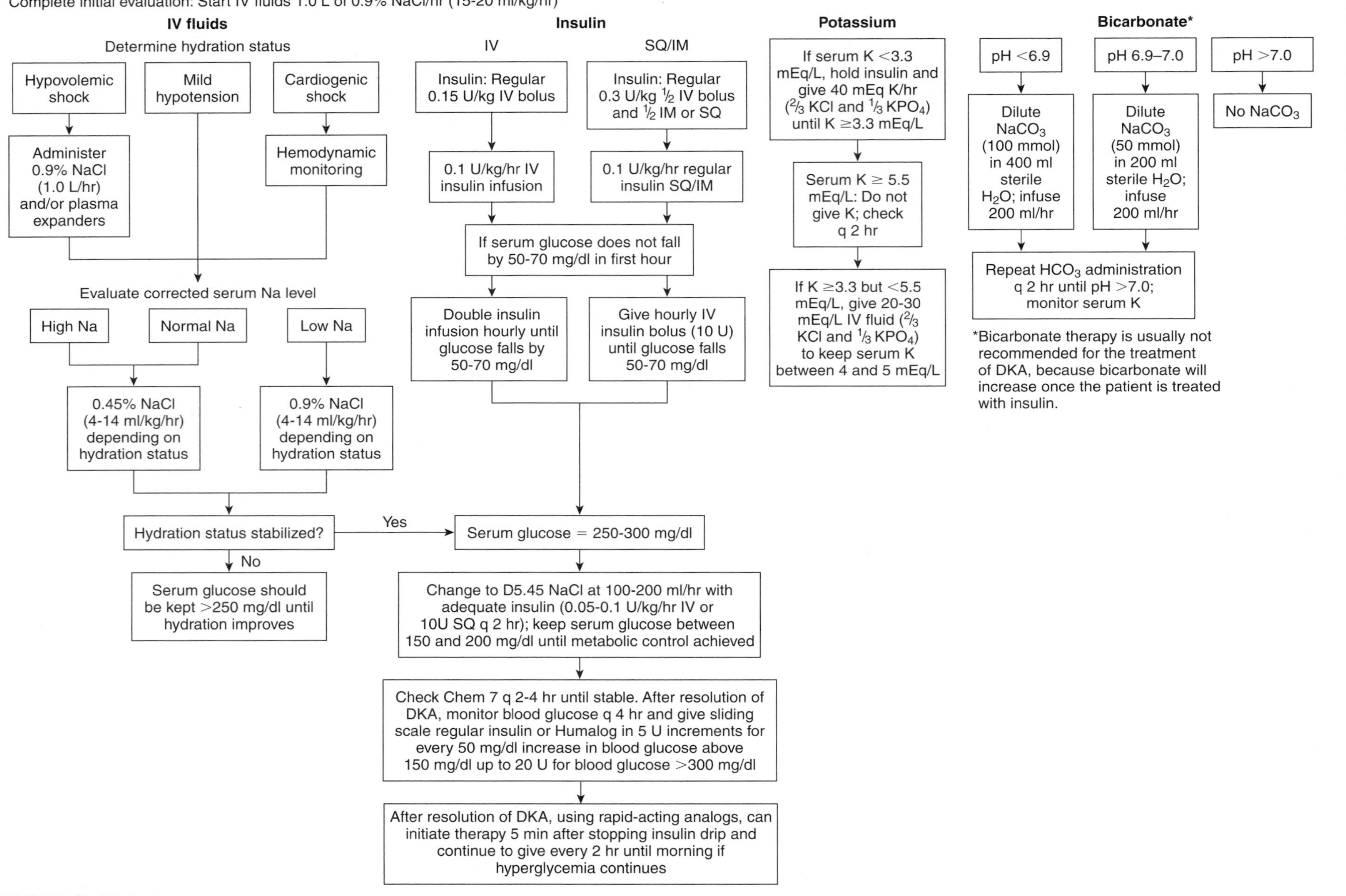

FIGURE 218-1

Management of diabetic ketoacidosis (*DKA*). *D5.45 NaCl*, 5% dextrose in 0.45% NaCl; *K*, potassium; *KCl*, potassium chloride; *KPO_4*, potassium phosphate; *Na*, sodium; *NaCl*, sodium chloride; *$NaCO_3$*, bicarbonate. (Data from American Diabetes Association: Position statement: hyperglycemic crises in patients with diabetes mellitus, *Diabetes Care* 24:585, 2001.)

BOX 218-16

SICK DAY MANAGEMENT OF PATIENTS WITH DIABETES

At time of impending illness when glucose levels are higher, ketones may be present. Some general rules:

1. Monitor blood glucose every 4 hours with symptoms of nausea, anorexia, and rising glucose levels.
2. If blood glucose level is above 275 mg/dl, test for ketones.
3. With elevated blood glucose levels, supplemental lispro or aspart insulin can be given every 1 to 4 hours. Give 10% of total daily dose as supplement if blood glucose level is under 300 mg/dl. If it is above 300 mg/dl, give 20% of total daily dose as supplement. Another method is to use a sliding scale of lispro or aspart insulin while sick until blood glucose levels return to previous control.
4. Maintain adequate hydration by drinking 8 ounces of calorie-free fluid hourly while awake. This can be alternated with a sodium-rich fluid, such as bouillon, consommé, or clear canned soups.
5. Continue to take diabetic medicine, even if anorexic or nauseous. If unable to eat, follow these guidelines using liquids or soft solids: if blood glucose level is 250 mg/dl or higher, drink calorie-free foods; if between 180 and 250 mg/dl, drink equivalent of 15 to 30 g of carbohydrates at meal; if 180 mg/dl or less, drink 45 to 50 g every 3 to 4 hours.
6. Antiemetics should be prescribed for those unable to tolerate fluids by mouth; monitor closely for dehydration—may need IV fluid.
7. Contact health care provider if:
   - Difficulty breathing
   - Vomiting and diarrhea persisting greater than 6 hours
   - Elevated blood glucose of 300 mg/dl or higher unresponsive to increased insulin on two occasions
   - Moderate or large urinary ketones and plasma ketones above 0.6 mmol/L

Modified from King EB, Lipps J: Illness and surgery. In Franz MJ, editor: *Diabetes management therapies: core curriculum for diabetes educators,* Chicago, 2003, American Diabetes Association.

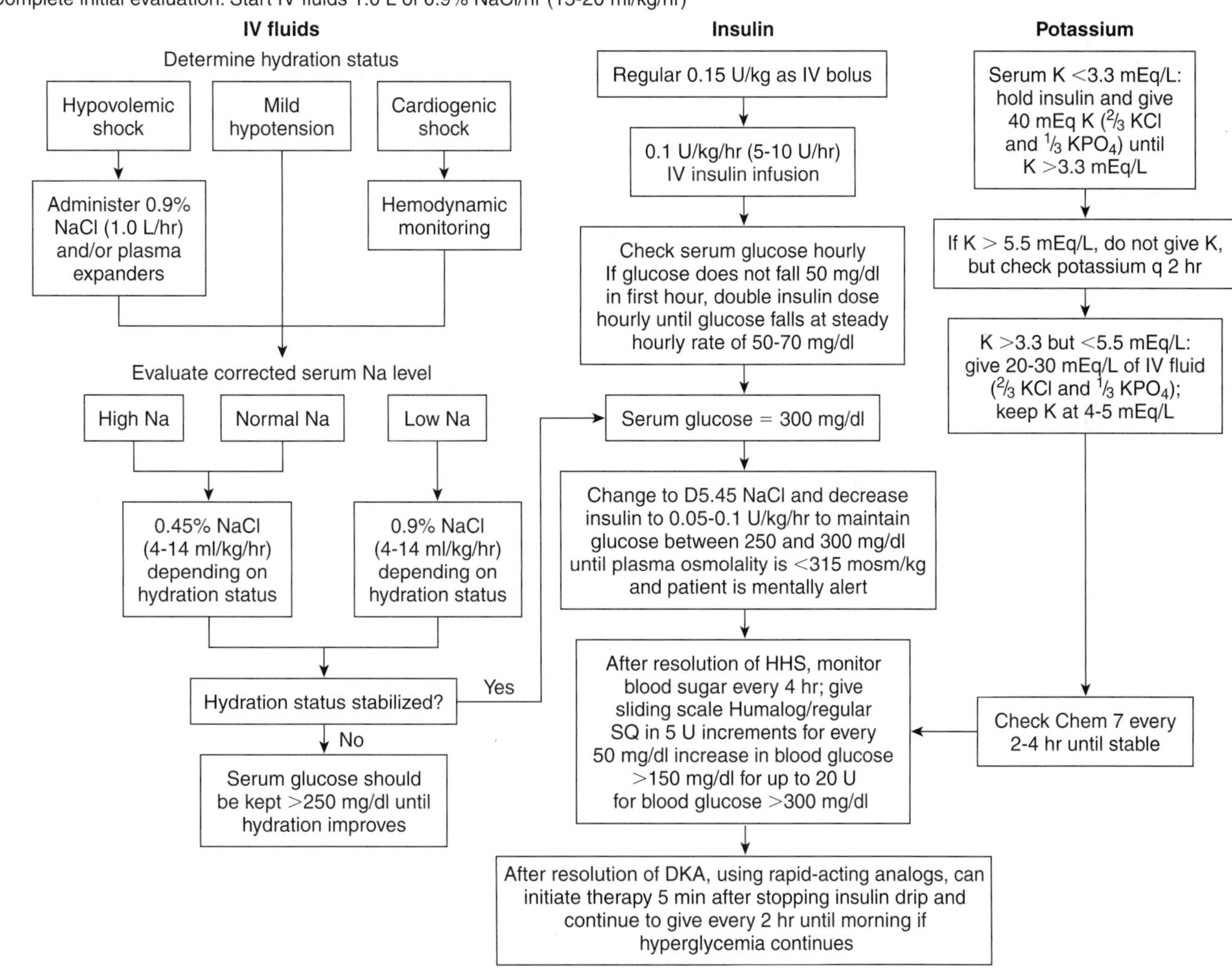

FIGURE 218-2

Hyperosmolar nonketotic syndrome. *D5.45 NaCl,* 5% dextrose in 0.45% NaCl; *HHS,* hyperglycemic hyperosmolar syndrome; *K,* potassium; *KCl,* potassium chloride; *KPO_4,* potassium phosphate; *Na,* sodium; *NaCl,* sodium chloride; *U,* units. (Data from American Diabetes Association: Position statement: hyperglycemic crises in patients with diabetes mellitus, *Diabetes Care* 24:585, 2001.)

reevaluations, and new treatment options. The length of time with the disease alters the amount of knowledge the patient may receive at a particular time. Initially, the patient with diabetes cannot process all that is needed to manage the disease. Therefore survival skills for the patient and the family are devised to maintain a safe environment for managing the disease process. Survival skills encompass the basic pathology of the disease, pharmacologic understanding, and recognition and treatment of hypoglycemia and hyperglycemia. Diabetes educators, support groups, and diabetes classes assist the patient and family in understanding diabetes management. In addition, education includes injection technique, home glucose monitoring, foot care, basic meal planning, and when to notify the health care provider.

As the individual becomes accustomed to the disease, further education is needed. Areas to be reviewed are sick day management, acidosis or situations of impending emergency, the pathology of the disease and complications, carbohydrate counting, adjustment of insulin guidelines, an exercise program with appropriate snacking, management during traveling, preventive care, treatment options for preventing complications of diabetes, nutrition and weight loss, use of glucagon, and diabetic supplies.

Diabetic education reinforced with written material and instruction improves understanding and compliance. The ADA, department of public health, pharmacists, drug representatives and companies, diabetes educators, and diabetic supply companies are great sources for free written materials.

Diabetic Websites

http://www.diabetesmonitor.com
http://www.nutrition.gov (nutrition site)
http://www.kraftdiabeticchoices.com (diabetic meals)
http://www.diabetesatwork.org (work-related issues)
http://www.diabetes.org (materials and information for new diabetics)
http://www.afb.org (visually impaired and blind services)
http://www.aace.com (guidelines for management)

REFERENCES

1. Diabetes Control Program: *Massachusetts guidelines for adult diabetes care*, Boston, June 2005, Massachusetts Department of Public Health.
2. Centers for Disease Control and Prevention: *National diabetes fact sheet: general information and national estimates on diabetes in the United States,* Atlanta, 2005, U.S. Department of Health and Human Services, retrieved Feb 12, 2006, from http://www.cdc.gov/diabetes/pubs/factsheet05.htm.
3. American Diabetes Association: Clinical practice recommendations 2005, *Diabetes Care* 28(Suppl 1):S1-S79, 2005.
4. Centers for Disease Control and Prevention: *CDC national diabetes fact sheet*, Atlanta, 2002, retrieved Feb 12, 2006, from http://www.cdc.gov/diabetes/pubs/factsheet05.htm.
5. Epidemiology of Diabetes Interventions and Complications (EDIC). Design, implementation, preliminary results of a long-term follow-up of the Diabetes Control and Complications Trial cohort, *Diabetes Care* 22(1):99-111, 1999.
6. American Diabetes Association: Diagnosis and classification of diabetes mellitus, *Diabetes Care* 28(Suppl 1):S37-S42, 2005.
7. Berra K: Treatment options for patients with the metabolic syndrome, *J Am Acad Nurse Pract* 15(8):361-370, 2003.
8. Waknine Y: *FDA approvals: Symlin, Mycamine, Fluzone,* retrieved Feb 12, 2007, from http://www.medscape.com/viewarticle/501918?.
9. Nathan D: *Effects of intensive diabetes management on cardiovascular events in the DCCT/EDIC*, presented at American Diabetes Association, San Diego, June 10-14, 2005.
10. Beaser RS: *Joslin's diabetes deskbook*, Boston, 2001, Joslin Diabetes Center.
11. Rosenstock J, Schwartz SL, Clark CM, and others: Basal insulin therapy, *Diabetes Care* 24(4):631-636, 2001.
12. Yki-Jarvinen H, Dressler A, Ziemen M: Less nocturnal hypoglycemia and better post dinner glucose control with bedtime glargine, *Diabetes Care* 23(8):1130-1136, 2000.
13. Lepore M, Pampanelli S, Fanelli C, and others: Pharmacokinetics and pharmacodynamics of subcutaneous injection of long acting human insulin glargine, NPH, and Ultralente and continuous lispro, *Diabetes* 49:2142-2147, 2000.
14. Danne T, Aman J, Schober E, and others: A comparison of postprandial and preprandial administration of insulin aspart in type 1, *Diabetes Care* 26(8):2359-2364, 2003.
15. Novo Nordisk Pharmaceuticals: *Introducing Novolog, insulin aspart* (drug insert), Bagsvaerd, 2001, The Company.
16. King EB, Lipps J: Illness and surgery. In Franz MJ, editor: *A core curriculum for diabetes education: diabetes management therapies,* ed 4, Chicago, 2001, American Association of Diabetes Educators.
17. American Diabetes Association (Committee Report): Nutrition recommendations and principles for people with diabetes mellitus, *Diabetes Care* 28(Suppl 1):S55-S57, 2005.
18. American Diabetes Association: Physical activity/exercise and diabetes, *Diabetes Care* 27(1):S58-S62, 2004.
19. Zinman B, Ruderman N, Campaigne BN, and others: Physical activity/exercise and diabetes mellitus, *Diabetes Care* 26(Suppl 1):S73-S77, 2003.
20. Edelman SV: The role of the thiazolidinediones in the practical management of patients with type 2 diabetes and cardiovascular risk factors, *Rev Cardiovasc Med* 4(Suppl 6):S29-S37, 2003.
21. Beaser RS, Cooppan R, Fonseca V: *Type 2 diabetes*, Boston, 2004, Joslin Diabetes Center.
22. Nesto RW, Bell D, Bonow RO, and others: Thiazolidinedione use, fluid retention, and congestive heart failure: a consensus statement from the American Heart Association and American Diabetes Association, *Diabetes Care* 27(1):256-263, 2004.
23. Osterweil N: *ADA: investigational Januvia put through its paces for diabetes,* June 11, 2006, retrieved Feb 23, 2007, from http://www.medpagetoday.com/2005MeetingCoverage/2005ADAMeeting/tb/3522.
24. Medline Plus, Drugs and Supplements: *Exenatide injection,* retrieved Feb 12, 2007, from http://www.nlm.nih.gov/medlineplus/druginfo/medmaster/a605034.
25. Palumbo PJ: The case for insulin treatment early in type 2, *Cleve Clin J Med* 71(5):385-401, 2004.
26. Mayfield JA, White RD: Insulin therapy for type 2, *Am Fam Phys* 70(3):489-498, 2004.
27. Palumbo PJ: Glycemic control, mealtime glucose excursions, and diabetic complications in type 2 diabetes, *Mayo Clin Proc* 76:609-618, 2001.
28. Bastyr EJ 3rd, Stuart CA, Brodows RG, and others: Therapy focused on lowering postprandial glucose, not fasting glucose, may be superior for lowering HbA1c. IOEZ Study Group, *Diabetes Care* 23(9):1236-1241, 2000.
29. US Preventive Services Task Force: Screening for gestational diabetes, *Am J Nurse Pract* 7(5):22-23, 2003.
30. American Diabetes Association: *Medical management of pregnancy complicated by diabetes,* ed 2, Alexandria, Va, 1995, The Association.
31. Biastre SA, Slocum J: Gestational diabetes. In Franz MJ, editor: *Diabetes in the life cycle and research,* Chicago, 2003, American Diabetes Association.
32. Pettitt DJ, Ospina P, Kolaczynski JW, and others: Comparison of an insulin analog, insulin aspart, and regular human insulin with no insulin in gestational diabetes mellitus, *Diabetes Care* 26(1):183-186, 2003.
33. Rowan J: *Metformin: a logical treatment for type 2 during pregnancy*, Scientific Sessions of American Diabetes Association, San Diego, June 10-14, 2005.

34. Homko CJ, Sargrad KR: Pregnancy with preexisting diabetes. In Franz MJ, editor: *Diabetes in the life cycle and research,* Chicago, 2003, American Diabetes Association.
35. Dixon LB, Wohlheiter K: Diabetes and mental illness: factors to keep in mind, *Consultant* 43(3):337-340, 343-344, 2003.
36. Katon W, Rutter C, Simon G, and others: The association of comorbid depression with mortality in type 2 patients, *Diabetes Care* 28(11):2668-2672, 2005.
37. Rubin RA, Napora JP: Psychosocial assessment. In Franz MJ, editor: *Diabetes education*, Chicago, 2003, American Diabetes Association.
38. Update on the management of diabetes and hypertension, *J Clin Hypertens (Greenwich)* 4(6 Suppl 2):3-10, 2002.
39. McLaughlin T, Reaven G, Abbau F, and others: Is there a simple way to identify insulin resistant individuals at increased risk of cardiovascular disease? *Am J Cardiol* 96(3):399-404, 2005.
40. Gaede P, Vedel P, Larsen N, and others: Multifactorial intervention and cardiovascular disease in patients with type 2 diabetes, *N Engl J Med* 348(5):383-393, 2003.
41. Ingelsson E, Sundstrom J, Arnlov J, and others: Insulin resistance and risk of congestive heart failure, *JAMA* 294(3):334-341, 2005.
42. Ridker PM, Rifai N, Rose L, and others: Comparison of C-reactive protein and low-density lipoprotein cholesterol levels in the prediction of first cardiovascular events, *N Engl J Med* 347(20):1557-1565, 2002.
43. LaRosa JC: *Effect of lowering LDL below currently recommended levels in patients with CAD,* presented American College of Cardiology, Orlando, Fla, March 6-9, 2005.
44. Ashen MD, Blumenthal RR: Low HDL cholesterol levels, *N Engl J Med* 353:1252-1260, 2005.
45. Expert Panel on Detection, Evaluation, and Treatment of High Blood Cholesterol in Adults: Executive summary of the third report of the National Cholesterol Education Program, *JAMA* 285:2486-2497, 2001.
46. Winters S, Jernigan V: Vascular disease risk markers in diabetes: monitoring and intervention, *Nurse Pract* 25(6):40-65, 2000.
47. Caputo GM, Cavanagh PR, Ulbrecht JS: Assessment and management of foot disease in patients with diabetes, *N Engl J Med* 331(13):854-860, 1994.
48. Ahroni JH: Diabetic foot care. In Franz MJ, editor: *Diabetes and complications*, Chicago, 2003, American Diabetes Association.
49. Levin ME: The diabetic foot, *Curr Ther Endocrinol Metab* 6:486-490, 1997.
50. Funnell MM, Feldman EL: Diabetic neuropathy. In Franz MJ, editor: *Diabetes and complications*, Chicago, 2003, American Diabetes Association.
51. Brunton S, McCarber B: Neuropathic pain, *Pri-Med* 9:12-28, 2005.
52. Corbett CF: Practical management of patients with painful diabetic neuropathy, *Diabetes Educ* 31(4):526-532, 2005.
53. Vinik AI, Freeman R, Erbas T: Diabetic autonomic neuropathy, *Semin Neurol* 23(4):365-372, 2003.
54. American Diabetes Association: Diabetic nephropathy, *Diabetes Care* 25(1):S85-S87, 2002.
55. Remuzzi G, Schieppati A, Ruggenenti P: Nephropathy in patients with type 2 diabetes, *N Engl J Med* 346:1145-1151, 2002.
56. Kidney Disease Outcomes Quality Initiative (K/DOQI): K/DOQI clinical practice guidelines on hypertension and antihypertensive agents in chronic kidney disease, *Am J Kidney Dis* 43(5 Suppl 1):S1-S290, 2004.
57. Bakris GL, Williams M, Dworkin L: Preserving renal function in adults with hypertension and diabetes: a consensus approach. National Kidney Foundation Hypertension and Diabetes Executive Committees Working Group, *Am J Kidney Dis* 36(3):646-661, 2000.
58. Schulte M, Mehler PS: Slowing the progression of diabetic nephropathy, *Women's Health* 4(6):437-442, 2001.
59. Kotoula MG, Koukoulis GN, Zintzaras E: Metabolic control of diabetes is associated with an improved response of diabetic retinopathy to panretinal photocoagulation, *Diabetes Care* 28(10):2454-2457, 2005.
60. American Diabetes Association: Screening for diabetic retinopathy, *Diabetes Care* 25(1):S73, 2002.
61. Gabriely I, Shamoon H: Hypoglycemia in diabetes, *Cleve Clin J Med* 17(4):335-341, 2004.
62. American Diabetes Association: Hyperglycemic crisis in patients with diabetes mellitus, *Diabetes Care* 24(1):S85-S86, 2001.
63. Kitabchi A, Wall B: Management of diabetic ketoacidosis, *Am Fam Phys* 60(2):455-464, 1999, retrieved Feb 14, 2007 from: http://www.aafp.org/afp/990800ap/455.

CHAPTER 219

Hirsutism

Michelle Freshman

DEFINITION AND EPIDEMIOLOGY

Hirsutism refers to excessive male pattern hair growth in women resulting from increased levels of circulating androgens. Although areas of coarse, pigmented body hair are not unusual in women, concerns regarding abundance and distribution commonly arise. Thoughtful evaluation of the regions indicative of androgen excess helps discern physiologic from pathologic causes. In each individual, regardless of gender or race, the number of hair follicles is predetermined; what differs is the pigmentation, thickness, and pattern of hair as mediated by localized androgen sensitivity.[1-3] New-onset hirsutism relates to androgen hormone excess. When signs of virilism such as temporal balding or voice deepening accompany hirsutism, an ovarian, adrenal, or exogenous hormone source should be suspected.

Millions of women worldwide are affected by hirsutism. Mild cases are distinguished from clinically significant and progressive ones. Anywhere from 5% to 10% of reproductive-age women are considered hirsute,[4,5] as distinguished from the 75% of women who report unwanted hair but would not qualify as clinically hirsute.[6] At least 25% of normal young women have terminal hair on either their upper lip, areola, or lower abdomen.[7] In fact, coarse, pigmented hair growth on the face, breast, or lower abdomen has also been identified in 17% to 35% of women who have neither androgen excess nor polycystic ovary syndrome (PCOS) and are clinically nonhirsute.[7] Admittedly these definitions are evolving. The sensitivity of subjective scales of abnormal hair growth and the threshold for androgen testing in mild cases have been challenged.[3,8,9] Furthermore, standard charts may suffer from low intra-rater reliability.[10] In one large cohort of subjects who identified themselves as having a minimum of unwanted hair, androgen excess was detected in 50% of cases and correlated with anovulatory or oligomenorrheic status.[6] This correlation was not attributable to differences in race, degree of hair growth, body mass, or family history.[6]

By contrast, among those known to have androgen excess, 70% to 90% are hirsute.[3,6,11] The most common underlying pathologic condition is PCOS, which affects 4% to 8% of premenopausal women.[3,12,13] In fact, 95% of women who are seen with progressive hirsutism have PCOS.[7] PCOS is considered a heterogeneous syndrome. In its mildest form, women have neither gonadotropin nor ovulatory abnormalities but still have higher insulin levels and lower sex hormone–binding globulin (SHBG).[14] In more severe cases, insulin resistance and menstrual cycle irregularities may drive up androgen levels because free testosterone cannot bind to as many sites as a result of reduced levels of circulating SHBG. SHBG levels decrease due to suppressed liver production in response to one of several conditions: hyperinsulinemia, obesity, excess growth hormone, or glucocorticoids.[10] Thus the amount of free testosterone secreted by those with polycystic ovaries is higher than in normally ovulating women and has been correlated with hyperandrogenism.[6,8] A calculated free testosterone from SHBG and total testosterone, rather than by direct assay, is preferred.[8] As has been discovered through research, 40% to 60% of hirsute women without PCOS have elevated levels of androgens, and just as many women with PCOS do not.[11,15] Ultimately 20% of cases are idiopathic, so-called simple or peripheral hirsutism, which is thought to reflect a skin and follicle-level (pilosebaceous unit) abnormality.[11,16]

An important consideration for health care providers is deciding who is at risk for rare but potentially life-threatening conditions. It has been shown that 38% of women with scattered areas of alopecia, especially in the setting of ovulatory dysfunction, as well as 50% of patients with acne, have underlying hyperandrogenism.[8,17] Although many have PCOS, a minority, 1.5% to 5%, have late-onset, nonclassic congenital adrenal hyperplasia (NCAH). Whereas NCAH, hyperandrogenic insulin-resistant acanthosis nigricans (HAIRAN) syndrome, prolactinemia, thyroid disorders, and androgen-secreting neoplasms (ASNs) can be established by a combination of diagnostic testing and imaging, PCOS and idiopathic hirsutism are considered diagnoses of exclusion.[8] Generally fewer than 1% of patients with hyperandrogenism have ovarian or adrenal tumors, half of which are malignant.[18,19]

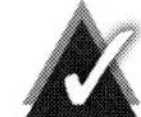

Physician consultation is indicated for all patients with suspected hirsutism.

PATHOPHYSIOLOGY

Hirsutism and virilism result from greater testosterone activity. Testosterone activates the skin and hair follicles via enzyme 5α-reductase, which converts testosterone to its potent metabolite, dihydrotestosterone (DHT). DHT converts short, thin, soft, vellus-type body hair to terminal-type hair. This enzyme makes the difference, given similar androgen profiles, between a woman who is hirsute and one who is not. It is a process mediated by genetic variations between the enzyme and its receptor.[3] Terminal hair expression is ultimately controlled by follicular sensitivity to 5α-reductase.[19] The region of skin involved also influences the likelihood of terminal hair developing from vellus-type hair.[3] Testosterone and its precursors are ultimately excreted via urine as 17-ketosteroids (17-KS). Dehydroepiandrosterone-sulfate (DHEA-S), the largest component of a 17-KS screen, is a useful proxy for the adrenal androgen activity.[15]

As early as 6 years of age, children begin producing androgens. In women these levels peak around age 30.[19] Adrenarche is heralded by hair growth in the axillae, in the lower pubic triangle, and on the arms and lower legs. Normally, boys have more testosterone than girls, which differentiates their distribution of terminal hair.[20] Most centrally located terminal body hair responds to sex hormone production, especially the amount, duration of exposure, and "intrinsic potential of the hair," which together determine the resultant density and diameter.[1,7] The number of hair follicles is said to decline after age 40.[3]

Women with PCOS have abnormal adrenocortical secretion, although only 25% have absolute adrenal excess.[21] A

PCOS individual can suffer from hyperinsulinemia, which stimulates testosterone synthesis through ovarian thecal cell (hyperthecosis) acted on by luteinizing hormone (LH). Hyperinsulinemia is also related to obesity and obesity-related disorders. PCOS is usually identified as an elevated LH-to–follicle-stimulating hormone (LH/FSH) ratio. Gonadotropin-releasing hormone (GnRH) antagonizes LH and FSH by suppressing ovulation and estrogen production through the hypothalamus-pituitary-ovarian axis.

Clinical conditions of androgen excess can relate to the adrenal 19-carbon steroids, androgenic compounds derived from cholesterol. Five products arise from cholesterol conversion: DHEA-S, estradiol, DHT, cortisol, and aldosterone. These result from four pathways, emphasized here to delineate the roles of key intermediate compounds[10,22-24]:

1(a) cholesterol → pregnenolone → 17-hydroxypregnenolone (17-OHPg) → **DHEA** → **DHEA-S**; 1(b) cholesterol → pregnenolone → 17-OHPg → **DHEA** → **androstenedione (AD)** → estrone → estradiol; 1(c) cholesterol → pregnenolone → 17-OHPg → **DHEA** → **AD** → **testosterone** (negative feedback with AD) → estradiol; 1(d) cholesterol → pregnenolone → 17-OHPg → **AD** → **testosterone** (negative feedback with AD) → **DHT**

2(a) through 2(d): The same pathways as above substituting **progesterone** and **17-hydroxypregesterone (17-OHP)** for pregnenolone and 17-OHPg

3 and 4: Two other pathways resulting in cortisol and aldosterone (via **21-hydroxylase**, or 21-OH) starting from (3): cholesterol → pregnenolone → **progesterone** → deoxycorticosterone (by **21-OH enzyme** or ***CYP21A* gene**) → corticosterone (by ***CYP11B1* gene**) → **aldosterone**; and (4) cholesterol → pregnenolone → **pregesterone** → **17-OHP** → **11-deoxycortisol** (by **21-OH** or ***CYP21A* gene**) → **cortisol** (by ***CYP11B1* gene**) *or* pregnenolone → 17-OHPg → **17-OHP** → **11-deoxycortisol** (by **21-OH** or ***CYP21A* gene**) → **cortisol** (by ***CYP11B1* gene**)

Of note, 11-deoxycortisol has a negative feedback loop with AD, which can, in turn, increase testosterone levels.[25]

To varying degrees, ovary and adrenal glands, muscle, fat, and liver tissue contribute to testosterone production.[2] Where ovaries and adrenals overlap in the production of AD and DHEA, their contributions vary; only the adrenals secrete DHEA-S.[10] The liver produces SBHG. Nearly all of testosterone circulates in bound form to SHBG; 1% to 2% is free. When SHBG is suppressed, it can lead to an oversupply of androgen hormones because of decreased binding site availability.[10] Nearly half of testosterone is produced by glandular activity of DHEA and DHEA-S, and the other half is made from AD and DHT precursors, found in the other tissues and converted peripherally. Adrenocorticotropic hormone (ACTH) stimulates DHEA but not DHEA-S.[10]

Androgen excess manifests in abnormal laboratory values. Even patients with normal or slightly elevated levels may suffer from disorders involving peripheral production and clearance abnormality or target organ sensitivity, which leads to hirsutism.[17] Reducing SHBG in turn raises the free testosterone level.[2] SHBG is also diminished in hypothyroidism.[18]

Androgen abnormalities causing hirsutism and occasionally virilism include those found in NCAH, acromegaly (a rare nonandrogenic cause related to growth hormone excess), and Cushing's syndrome with or without virilization caused by tumor (see Chapter 217). Serum DHEA and DHEA-S are highest in an adrenal carcinoma, lowest in adrenal adenoma.[24] Serum DHEA varies directly with ACTH excretion, so a decrease in ACTH corresponds with a decrease in DHEA. Cases where the ACTH is high, but the DHEA and DHEA-S are low, are attributed to Cushing's syndrome or ectopic ACTH syndrome, seen without adrenal growths.[24,25]

In NCAH there is an enzyme deficiency of 21-OH, which causes an accumulation of 17-OHP, which can be captured in a 24-hour urine 17-KS study. In several congenital enzyme deficiency syndromes, including congenital adrenal hyperplasia, prepubertal girls lack the 21-OH enzyme, or *CYP21A* gene. Since insulin and ovarian irregularities have been seen to have a role in the expression of SHBG, multiple interactions are possible.

A study of Chilean adolescent girls with type 1 diabetes mellitus (DM1), compared with normal, nonhirsute controls, demonstrated increasing levels of 17-OHP after GnRH stimulation by leuprolide acetate during late puberty (Tanner stage 5) associated with lower SHBG and a significantly higher free androgen index; this was not the case for controls.[26] Although DM1 status was uniformly associated with hirsutism in these adolescent girls, total testosterone levels did not differ between the two groups; in fact, some evidence suggests that adult Chilean DM1 women may not be as severely hirsute as those hyperandrogenic women without DM1, despite the fact that insulin is key to hair follicle growth.[26] The authors point to the possible interplay of insulin-influenced fat mass (not captured by otherwise matched body mass index) and abnormal ovarian steroid production in late puberty, as precursors to PCOS in this population.[26]

CLINICAL PRESENTATION

Inquiry into familial hair growth, a prior diagnosis of hirsutism, or previous treatment is an important initial screen. Constitutional or familial hirsutism is common in individuals of Mediterranean or Middle Eastern descent, but less common in Asians. Ovarian, adrenal, and menstrual function is normal in 80% of these cases, whereas peripheral androgen marker 3α-diol G correlates with an excess of 17-KS in the urine and increased 5α-reductase activity.[15] Seasonal observations regarding hair growth resulting from neurovascular changes should be considered, since hair growth is more rapid in the summer months.[17]

Use of contraceptives; use by competitive female athletes of anabolic steroids such as nandrolone decanoate, methyltestosterone, or 19-nortestosterone; or use of other progestins such as danazol to treat endometriosis can cause hirsutism, but usually hypertrichosis, or excess vellus-type hair growth.[27] Chronic skin irritation might lead to hair coarsening because of local changes at the pilosebaceous unit.

Gonadal abnormalities are indicative of elevated androgen levels and can be ascertained by a history of abnormal sexual development. Prepubertal androgenism or hermaphroditism might relate to congenital or classic adrenal hyperplasia seen in early adrenarche or with adrenal tumor(s). Genetic testing is helpful in those cases. A menstrual history and menopausal status should be assessed. Any irregular or intermenstrual bleeding may indicate the presence of endometrial neoplasm. Moreover, a pregnancy history significant for hair growth may be useful in diagnosing rare malignant conditions of the ovary or adrenal gland, cancer metastasis, PCOS, or placental aromatase deficiency.[28] Exogenous hormone use may also play a role.

A subset of women is seen with virilization, often accompanied by amenorrhea.[15] Ovarian and adrenal tumors, though rare, are primary considerations.

Patients with PCOS or Cushing's syndrome likely have lipid and insulin abnormalities to differing degrees; the latter syndrome is evidenced by excess ACTH from unsuppressed androgen. Galactorrhea accompanies hyperprolactinemia and is present in 20% of patients with PCOS, stemming from pituitary disorders wherein prolactin stimulates DHEA.[15] Dyslipidemia and hypertension are common in these populations and should be investigated further.

PHYSICAL EXAMINATION

Weight, height, and vital signs are especially pertinent given the profile of a significant proportion of patients with PCOS. Rotterdam criteria established hirsutism, regular ovulatory function, and ultrasonic evidence of multifollicular ovaries as consistent with PCOS; idiopathic hirsutism includes females with normal ovarian anatomy and function.[6] Obesity is seen in patients with PCOS or Cushing's syndrome, although Cushing's syndrome shows up as a mixture of the following, depending on the severity: central obesity, extremity or muscle wasting, red striae, supraclavicular fat pads, moon facies, thin skin or bruising, and sometimes a buffalo hump.

Research in PCOS has determined that body fat varies continuously with gonadotropin abnormalities; obese and nonobese patients with PCOS do not comprise distinct groups.[29] In fact, only 50% of PCOS patients are obese.[17] A rise in blood pressure and concomitant hirsutism could raise the suspicion of excess ACTH.

Typically androgen excess is thought to include hirsutism, acne, and male-pattern alopecia. An essential component of the physical examination must include an objective measurement of hair growth pattern and quantity. Regions of androgen-sensitive growth include the lip, chin, sideburns, chest, upper pubic triangle, and intergluteal area, which, when present in women, may be accompanied by seborrhea, acne, and alopecia.[30] The Ferriman-Gallwey scale is often used as an index (Table 219-1). A score of 8 or more out of 36 is interpreted as evidence of an androgenic excess; a score greater than 15, along with other supporting evidence, is more likely correlated with a neoplasm.[7] Others have modified this classic scale to account for ethnic variation and location-specificity of coarse hair.[3,8,9]

Terminal hair on the upper back, shoulders, or upper abdomen delineates virilism, as does clitoromegaly in excess of 35 mm (1.4 inches).[2,19] The health care provider should look for features of virilism, including those associated with defeminization (antiestrogenic), such as body contour changes, breast size reduction, oligomenorrhea, and vaginal dryness; or

TABLE 219-1 Ferriman-Gallwey Scale: Definition of Hair Grading at 11 Sites*

Site	Grade	Definition
Upper lip	1	Few hairs at outer margin
	2	Small moustache at outer margin
	3	Moustache extending halfway from outer margin
	4	Moustache extending to midline
Chin	1	Few scattered hairs
	2	Scattered hairs with small concentrations
	3, 4	Complete cover, light and heavy
Chest	1	Circumareolar hairs
	2	With midline hair in addition
	3, 4	Fusion of these areas, with three-quarters cover
		Complete cover
Upper back	1	Few scattered hairs
	2	Rather more, still scattered
	3, 4	Complete cover, light and heavy
Lower back	1	Sacral tuft of hair
	2	Rather more, still scattered
	3	Three-quarters cover
	4	Complete cover
Upper abdomen	1	Few midline hairs
	2	Rather more, still scattered
	3, 4	Half and full cover
Lower abdomen	1	Few midline hairs
	2	Midline streak of hair
	3	Midline band of hair
	4	Inverted V-shaped growth
Arm	1	Sparse growth affecting not more than one fourth of limb cover
	2	More than this, cover still incomplete
	3, 4	Complete cover, light and heavy
Forearm	1, 2, 3, 4	Complete cover of dorsal surface, two grades of light and two grades of heavy
Thigh	1, 2, 3, 4	As for forearm
Leg	1, 2, 3, 4	As for forearm

From Mishell DR, Davajan V, Lobo RA: *Infertility, contraception, and reproductive endocrinology,* ed 3, Cambridge, Mass, 1991, Blackwell Scientific.
*Grade 0 at all sites indicates absence of terminal hair.

masculinization (androgenic), such as acne, temporal balding, voice deepening, increased shoulder girth and muscle mass, and clitoromegaly that progresses with increasing androgen levels.[17] Thyroid enlargement and pelvic or abdominal masses should be noted.

Acanthosis nigricans, a pigmented patch on the back of the neck, elbows, knuckles, knees, or intertriginous regions, is seen commonly in obese women and is indicative of insulin resistance. Although this is not a reliable sign of hyperandrogenism, it is found in 30% of hyperandrogenic women.[7,15] A pelvic examination is performed to assess the presence of ovarian cysts. Cysts are palpable 85% of the time.[31] Pregnant women may need careful monitoring in the face of gestational hirsutism, although there is limited intrapregnancy testing available. Typically postpartum patients and their newborns are observed for regression of signs, once malignant causes are excluded.

DIAGNOSTICS

A hormonal evaluation in slow-onset, peripubertally hirsute, nonvirilized, normally menstruating patients is deferred. Diagnosis in this population relies heavily on the physical examination and evidence of virilism. Newly developed hirsutism in postpubertal women and cases of hirsutism and virilization together call for a preliminary investigation, including a serum testosterone level. Normal total testosterone levels range from 0.2 to 2.8 nmol/L, or 70 to 90 ng/dl by other assays.[6,18] Values greater than 3.5 to 6 nmol/L or 150 to 200 ng/dl[18] prompt further investigation for tumors using transvaginal or adrenal ultrasound or adrenal CT studies,[1,30] as would an abnormal free testosterone level greater than or equal to 10.34 pmol/L[11] or 0.75 ng/dl.[6]

Ovarian Source

An LH/FSH ratio can be helpful, but is not an absolute index. This ratio is elevated to 2:1 or 3:1 in approximately three fourths of PCOS cases.[7,12] Testosterone levels show diurnal and menstrual phase–related fluctuation and may not truly indicate circulating levels; thus they are reserved for indeterminate physical findings in the setting of oligoovulation of unknown cause.[3] Therefore the ratio of the total testosterone to SHBG levels may be the preferred diagnostic test in some cases.[8,15] The presence of a pelvic mass warrants a pelvic CT scan.

Adrenal Source

DHEA-S is seen as a screen for adrenal gland production to help distinguish tumors of adrenal origin in the face of virilization and is suspicious if greater than 700 mcg/dl (13.6 μmol/L). 21-OH–deficient NCAH, which affects 1% to 8% of hyperandrogenic women, can be determined by high basal 17-OHP (>200 ng/dl or 6 nmol/L) in the early follicular phase.[3] Since levels are known to vary by age, clinical evidence is still preferred.[8] An elevated DHEA-S level should be followed by an adrenal ultrasound or CT scan. Tumor resection and histopathology determine ASNs, which occur in 1 in 300 to 1 in 1000 hirsute woman.[3] Serum testosterone would be high in patients with Cushing's syndrome caused by an adrenal adenoma or carcinoma. In cases of adrenal carcinoma without Cushing's syndrome, testosterone, DHEA, and DHEA-S are markedly high.[25]

Cortisol Excess

If Cushing's syndrome is suspected, an initial 24-hour urine collection for 17-KS and free cortisol, or overnight dexamethasone suppression test, is advised in the setting of rapid hirsutism or virilization. A 24-hour 17-KS ranges from 5 to 15 mg (17 to 52 μmol) in women under 30 (when it peaks). The relative quantities of these metabolites distinguish among (1) adrenal carcinoma with or without Cushing's syndrome, (2) congenital *CYP11B1* and *CYP21A* gene deficiency syndromes, and (3) ACTH-dependent Cushing's syndrome diagnosis.[25] However, many medications can affect the values.[25]

Insulin Excess

HAIRAN is diagnosed with a fasting basal insulin of 80 μIU/ml, and/or insulin tolerance test of more than 300 μIU/ml.[8] A glucose tolerance test and lipid profile would be valuable if dyslipidemia, insulin resistance, hyperinsulinemia, or diabetes were suspected, since up to 50% of PCOS patients have insulin abnormalities.[3] High circulating insulin levels affects the thecal cells of the ovaries.[3,26]

Prolactin Excess

Galactorrhea warrants measurement of a prolactin level; increased levels are indicative of hyperprolactinemia and possible thyroid dysfunction, although this is rare. In these cases thyroid-stimulating hormone and FSH are also measured. The pituitary is imaged by MRI to search for a prolactinoma.

Thyroid-Stimulating Hormone Excess

Hypothyroidism may result in hypertrichosis.

5α-Reductase Excess

There is no specific test for this enzyme, the effects of which are appreciated clinically. It may be that an otherwise idiopathic presentation of hirsutism relates to local mechanisms at the level of the pilosebaceous unit. Typically there are no adverse sequelae, if all other testing is normal.

DIFFERENTIAL DIAGNOSIS

The onset of hirsutism may correspond to a variety of conditions: recent weight gain, discontinuation of oral contraceptives, initiation of progestins or steroids, insulin disorders, and the onset of menopause or puberty. For patients with PCOS, the constellation of oligomenorrhea, amenorrhea, acne, alopecia, obesity, and ovarian cysts is often seen in conjunction with hirsutism.[15] In menopause, weight gain may stimulate altered sex steroid metabolism, which may influence cancer development.[32] If intermenstrual or irregular bleeding occurs

DIAGNOSTICS

Hirsutism

LABORATORY	IMAGING
Total testosterone	Pelvic ultrasound, pelvic CT scan*
Free testosterone*	Abdominal ultrasound, CT scan*
DHEA*	Adrenal CT scan*
DHEA-S*	Abdominal MRI*
24-Hour urine for 17-hydroxyprogesterone*	**OTHER**
LH/FSH ratio*	ACTH stimulation test*
Prolactin*	Dexamethasone suppression test*
TSH*	24-Hour urinary excretion test for cortisol*
Glucose tolerance test*	Genotyping*
Fasting basal insulin*	
Free cortisol*	
Lipid profile*	

*If indicated.

DIFFERENTIAL DIAGNOSIS

Hirsutism

- Hypertrichosis
- Severe insulin resistance
- Ovarian tumors (androgen secreting)
- Polycystic ovary syndrome
- Idiopathic hirsutism
- Anabolic steroid use
- Androgen therapy (progestin)
- Congenital hyperplasia, nonclassic or late-onset adrenal hyperplasia
- Cushing's syndrome with and without adrenal tumors
- Adrenal tumors (androgen-secreting tumors)
- Gestational androgen excess
- Hyperprolactinemia
- Hypothyroidism
- Severe obesity

in perimenopausal or premenopausal patients more than 35 years old, endometrial cancer needs to be excluded by endometrial biopsy.[1] Finally, a subcategory of normoandrogenic hirsutism is known as idiopathic hirsutism, when the ovulation and androgen levels are normal and ovaries are not polycystic; a 40% subset may prove to be anovulatory with careful testing (luteal phase progesterone of <3 to 5 ng/ml) and actually have PCOS.[16]

A separate condition is hirsutism with concomitant virilism. Adrenal tumors (benign or malignant), enzyme deficiencies, or endocrinopathies are a consideration if virilization accompanies hirsutism. Nonmalignant hyperthecosis of the ovary usually occurs in premenopausal women. Sertoli-Leydig cell tumors of the luteinized thecal cells of the ovary can be present in patients ages 20 to 40, sometimes in conjunction with HAIRAN. In these cases removal of the often unilaterally affected ovary returns testosterone levels to normal and reverses signs of virilism.[33,34] Other ovarian tumors include arrhenoblastomas and hilar cell tumors, which can lead to excess testosterone levels.

Further considerations include congenital adrenal hyperplasia detected either in vivo or early in life, and its milder form indicated by excess cortisol precursors after an ACTH hormone challenge. The milder case is said to affect 1 in 100 to 1000 in the United States and can lead to serious sinus and pulmonary illness and orthostatic syncope.[35] In the presence of elevated ACTH levels, the differential diagnosis should include Cushing's syndrome glucocorticoid resistance, or anabolic steroid use.

The investigation into insulin-resistance conditions is warranted with hirsute patients, since hyperinsulinemia correlates inversely with SHBG concentrations; SHBG is recognized as being inversely proportional to Ferriman-Gallwey scale scores.[30] Finally, a panel of androgen hormones—testosterone, androstenedione, DHEA and DHEA-S—guides pituitary, adrenal or ovarian tumor diagnosis.

Hypertrichosis may be mistaken for hirsutism. Yet, despite an abundance of typically fine, short (<2 cm [0.8 inch]), unpigmented hair, androgens are generally not involved.[36] This type of hair growth results from conditions such as anorexia nervosa, hypothyroidism, porphyria, or dermatomyositis or from drug therapy such as occurs with penicillamine, diazoxide, minoxidil, phenytoin, or cyclosporine.[3,10,19,30] Body hair is often diffusely distributed about the midline, including the face and even the forehead in a nonsexual pattern.[37] In familial, or constitutional, hypertrichosis, genetic factors, rather than disease status, dictate the growth pattern. Unlike hirsutism, abundant familial hair growth patterns cannot be easily treated.[30] A diagnosis of hypertrichosis can be assessed by the hair type and some laboratory testing.

MANAGEMENT

Most often the causes of central hair growth are benign and can be managed effectively with a combination of medical therapy and mechanical hair removal. Because a woman's appraisal of her appearance is influenced by cosmetic and cultural standards, in cases of normal hair growth, reassurance is essential.[38]

A commonly accepted nonpharmacologic strategy is weight reduction.[1,7] Decreasing weight has been proven to lower insulin resistance and reduce hyperandrogenism; in fact, weight gain can worsen hirsutism.[11,30] Weight loss of 10% to 15% may diminish unwanted hair growth and return menses to normal.[1]

Cosmetic measures are advisable in all patients who desire temporary or permanent removal of unwanted hair. Temporary methods include depilatory cream, which dissolves hair but may lead to skin irritation, allergic dermatitis, or permanent skin damage. Although shaving (which may cause stubble to appear coarser and thicker) and plucking (which is uncomfortable and can stimulate hair growth, folliculitis, and scarring) can be used on small areas, waxing removes hair at the base of the pilosebaceous unit and is more effective as a short-term solution, although it may produce superficial burns and infection. Bleaching involves using a diluted cream preparation of hydrogen peroxide and can be effective in temporarily depigmenting hair, although in a matter of weeks, pigmented hair will return as a new growth cycle ensues.[30]

Electrolysis requires the insertion of a fine needle into the base of a hair follicle and the administration of electric current to permanently destroy the follicle. It is a popular, although costly, procedure; moreover, results vary. Caution is advised if acne, skin infection, diabetes mellitus, epilepsy, ischemic heart disease, an in situ pacemaker, or artificial joints are present. Antibiotic prophylaxis is recommended if a patient is at risk for endocardial infection or reactivation of herpes simplex.[38] Patients who choose waxing or electrolysis should be instructed to observe for possible signs of infection. Eflornithine hydrochloride 13.9% topical cream has been shown to slow hair growth by inhibiting ornithine decarboxylase at the follicle, although this is a temporary treatment, requiring 8 to 24 weeks for maximum effect and indefinite use thereafter.[18,39] Laser hair removal via ruby, Alexandrite, diode, or Nd:YAG laser, as well as broad-band intense pulsed light therapy, has been shown to produce long-lasting effects.[40,41] Finally, acupuncture therapy has reduced testosterone levels and body hair.[38]

Since the pattern of hair growth is hormonally mediated, the goal of management is to interrupt the untoward effect of excessive testosterone on the hair follicle. Testosterone excess control depends on ovarian, adrenal, or peripheral tissue production (Table 219-2). Medications are used to suppress androgen secretion in the ovaries and adrenal glands or block testosterone and DHT.

Of the varied pharmacologic options, a first-line approach includes oral estrogen-progesterone agents (oral contracep-

TABLE 219-2 Androgen Production Inhibitors

Agent	Source of Androgen Production
Oral contraceptives	Ovarian, adrenal, peripheral
Corticosteroids	Ovarian, adrenal
Spironolactone	Ovarian, adrenal, peripheral
Cyproterone acetate	Ovarian, peripheral
Ketoconazole	Ovarian, adrenal
Progestins	Ovarian
Gonadotropin-releasing hormone agonist	Ovarian
Topical progesterone	Peripheral
5α-Reductase inhibitors	Peripheral

Modified from Mishell DR, Davajan V, Lobo RA: *Infertility, contraception, and reproductive endocrinology*, ed 3, Cambridge, Mass, 1991, Blackwell Scientific.

tives), which have the added benefit of treating acne and oligomenorrhea. Also, many oral medications slated for acne use diminish hirsutism.[42] Oral contraceptives inhibit LH secretion from the pituitary gland through progestin, reducing bioavailable testosterone, which in turn decreases the stimulation of the ovarian thecal cells and increases SHBG. Contraceptives also decrease adrenal DHEA-S through negative feedback on the glucocorticoid receptor. It is also thought that the progestin might quell production of 5α-reductase and activity at the androgen receptor.[3] The 19-nortestosterone derivatives, such as levonorgestrel, should be avoided, since they block the estrogen-mediated increase in SHBG concentration and are mildly androgenic.[30] Ultimately, the practitioner may want to stop medications after 1 to 2 years to see if any regression has been achieved and observe for return of ovulatory function in premenopausal women.

A second option is spironolactone, which, although better known as a potassium-sparing diuretic, serves as an antiandrogen product. It inhibits pituitary gonadotropin secretion and in turn the binding of testosterone and DHT to the androgen receptor and improves the metabolic clearance of testosterone. It further limits androgen production by inhibiting cytochrome p-450 and is a popular choice for combined therapy with oral contraceptives. Side effects rarely compel patients to discontinue drug therapy; however, nausea, vomiting, abdominal discomfort, diarrhea, fatigue, mental confusion, headache, dizziness, decreased libido, and sun hypersensitivity may follow. Its mild progesterone activity has caused 80% of a sample of women taking it as sole therapy to report menstrual disturbance, especially polymenorrhea, if it is taken cyclically or continuously.[30] A group of researchers claimed the rate of success in treating hirsutism in one series approached 86% when enhanced by electrolysis.[8] Of course, this method should not be used if women are already using a potassium-sparing diuretic (because of the risk of hyperkalemia) or angiotensin II–converting enzyme inhibitors, have renal dysfunction, or are anticipating pregnancy.[15]

Popular therapy combines oral contraceptives and antiandrogens.[43] Patients who do not respond to oral contraceptives or spironolactone treatments may try one of several antiandrogen compounds, such as cyproterone acetate (CPA) or leuprolide, finasteride (which works on 5α-reductase), and GnRH agonists. GnRH does not have an effect on adrenally mediated hyperandrogenism; it is used for ovarian suppression and is best used in tandem with estrogen-progestin therapy.[34] NCAH patients can use glucocorticoids plus oral contraceptives and/or spironolactone,[10] or the antifungal ketoconazole, which opposes testosterone. Of note, various CPA therapies have led to improvement in at least 70% of severely hirsute women.[38] In one study of 40 hirsute women, the efficacies spironolactone, flutamide, and finasteride at a given dose were comparable after 6 months.[44] By contrast, a randomized trial of 70 women showed that finasteride was superior to flutamide in reducing hair, with effects on SHBG and DHEA-S indexes.[45] Patients with accompanying insulin resistance have been started on metformin or troglitazone with improvement.[4,5,46]

Co-Management with Specialists

When an endocrinologist prescribes finasteride, flutamide, or ketoconazole for a patient, liver enzymes should be assessed regularly. Patients must not become pregnant while receiving corrective hormonal therapy. The use of glucocorticoids to reduce hirsutism and induce ovulation in NCAH risks suppression of the hypothalamus pituitary axis (HPA) and induction of Cushingoid features.[3,10] PCOS can also accompany endometrial hyperplasia or other fertility concerns, which is likely to require other specialty collaboration. Finally, an outcome evaluation, such as reevaluating the patient with the Ferriman-Gallwey scale or reviewing the success of mechanical hair removal, is useful.

LIFE SPAN CONSIDERATIONS

Hirsutism is a sensitive issue for adolescent girls, whose desire for peer acceptance may heavily influence body image and resulting health behaviors. In fact, eating disorders related to PCOS are common.[30] Any menstrual cycle irregularities are of concern if they are accompanied by acne, alopecia, and hirsutism, as well as insulin resistance, since this might be a presentation of PCOS. Medication and mechanical hair removal options should be explored. Excessive hair growth can accompany pregnancy but usually disappears within 6 to 15 months postpartum,[35] often without long-term effects to mother or baby, if sinister causes are ruled out.

COMPLICATIONS

Failure to diagnose an adrenal or ovarian tumor that may be malignant is a serious complication of hirsutism. Surgical removal of ovarian or adrenal tumors is recommended, although postsurgical complications, such as adhesions, are possible. Diabetes, hypertension, and the possibility of estrogen-related cancers are often associated with PCOS,[47] necessitating careful follow-up monitoring. In addition, hirsute women may be at increased risk for endometrial cancer.[1] Gestational hyperandrogenism has potential complications for mother and baby.

INDICATIONS FOR REFERRAL OR HOSPITALIZATION

The evaluation of a hirsute patient is performed in consultation with a physician. Patients may be referred to an endocrinologist for androgen studies, or preliminary studies may be performed in primary care. Referral to an endocrinologist is appropriate if hirsutism is accompanied by virilism, which suggests the need for further imaging, androgen, insulin, or dexamethasone studies. Research supports dexamethasone and triptorelin testing to differentiate between adrenal and ovarian sources of androgen excess.[48] An endocrinologist is also consulted for treatment failure or persistent infertility. A nephrologist should evaluate patients with insulin resistance and nephropathy or renal failure. A surgical consultation is indicated for the evaluation of patients with adrenal gland or ovarian tumors.

The psychosocial effects of increasing body hair may warrant a psychiatric consultation if the hair has become a consuming concern. A mental health referral will be useful if there is reason to suspect underlying gonadal abnormality such as chromosomal mosaicism or, in rare cases, hermaphroditism. Genetic counseling, or even fetal testing, may be appropriate in some cases.

PATIENT AND FAMILY EDUCATION

Hirsute patients should be advised to avoid second-generation androgenic oral contraceptives, including norgestrel, levonorgestrel, and norethindrone, in favor of third-generation oral contraceptives.[7,30] Ethinyl estradiol 35 mcg singly, or in combination with CPA 2 mg, offers good effect but must be taken for several years and is often followed by relapse of symptoms after several months of drug hiatus.[49] However, patients using third-generation oral contraceptives should be advised of the possibility of thromboembolic events. All patients taking oral contraceptives should be strictly advised to stop smoking. Use of anabolic steroids for muscle building is strongly discouraged.

Education regarding realistic expectations of cosmetic hair removal, hair loss, and hair growth suppression, as well as a reminder that even a temporary drug holiday will likely return the patient to her previous hirsute status, is essential. It will take anywhere from 6 to 18 months to see a new "set point" in hair growth.[19]

Finally, the provider needs to address increased levels of anxiety and depression in women with PCOS and to provide reassurance about fears of masculinization, ridicule or social rejection, and sexual or gender identity.[30] Because pregnancy is contraindicated during therapy, pregnancy plans should be discussed in advance. Often the discontinuation of therapy will herald a return of hair growth.

HEALTH PROMOTION

Women should be adequately counseled regarding their concerns and realistic expectations regarding future fertility and body image. For patients with PCOS, a diet high in fiber and low in refined carbohydrates is encouraged, as is weight loss. Individual or group psychologic counseling can help with weight management.

REFERENCES

1. Marshburn PB, Carr BR: Hirsutism and virilization: a systematic approach to benign and potentially serious causes, *Postgrad Med* 97(1):99-106, 1995.
2. Agarwal SK, Judd HL: What we see most, we understand least, *Western J Med* 165(6):392-393, 1996.
3. Azziz R: The evaluation and management of hirsutism, *Obstet Gynecol* 101(5):995-1007, 2003.
4. Hock DL, Seifer DB: New treatments of hyperandrogenism and hirsutism, *Obstet Gynecol Clin North Am* 27(3):567-581, vi-vii, 2000.
5. Azziz R, Ehrmann D, Legro RS, and others: Troglitazone improves ovulation and hirsutism in the polycystic ovary syndrome: a multicenter, double blind, placebo-controlled trial, *J Clin Endocrinol Metab* 86(4):1626-1632, 2001.
6. Souter I, Sanchez LA, Perez M, and others: The prevalence of androgen excess among patients with minimal unwanted hair growth, *Am J Obstet Gynecol* 191(6):1914-1920, 2004.
7. Kalve E, Klein JF: Evaluation of women with hirsutism, *Am Fam Phys* 54(1):117-124, 1996.
8. Azziz R, Sanchez LA, Knochenhauer ES, and others: Androgen excess in women: experience with over 1,000 consecutive patients, *J Clin Endocrinol Metab* 89(2):453-462, 2004.
9. Hatch R, Rosenfield RL, Kim MH, and others: Hirsutism, implications, etiology, and management, *Am J Obstet Gynecol* 140(7):815-830, 1981.
10. Neithardt AB, Barnes RB: The diagnosis and management of hirsutism, *Semin Reprod Med* 21(3):285-293, 2003.
11. Carmina E, Rosato F, Janni A, and others: Extensive clinical experience: relative prevalence of different androgen excess disorders in 950 women referred because of clinical hyperandrogenism, *J Clin Endocrinol Metab* 91(1):2-6, 2006.
12. Marshall JC, Eagleston CA: Polycystic ovary syndrome: neuroendocrine aspects of polycystic ovary syndrome, *Endocrinol Metab Clin* 28(2):295-324, 1999.
13. Fraser IS, Kovacs G: Current recommendations for the diagnostic evaluation and follow-up of patients presenting with symptomatic polycystic ovary syndrome, *Best Pract Res Clin Obstet Gynaecol* 18(5):813-823, 2004.
14. Adams JM, Taylor AE, Crowley WF Jr, and others: Polycystic ovarian morphology with regular ovulatory cycles: insights into the pathophysiology of polycystic ovary syndrome, *J Clin Endocrinol Metab* 89(9):4343-4350, 2004.
15. Mishell DR, Stenchever MA, Droegemuller W, and others: *Comprehensive gynecology*, ed 3, St Louis, 1997, Mosby.
16. Azziz R, Carmina E, Sawaya ME: Idiopathic hirsutism, *Endocrine Reviews* 21:347-362, 2000.
17. Taylor AE: Hirsutism and androgen excess. In Carlson KJ, Eisenstat SA, editors: *Primary care of women*, St Louis, 1995, Mosby.
18. Rosenfield RL: Clinical practice. Hirsutism, *N Engl J Med* 353(24):2578-2588, 2005.
19. Rittmaster RS: Hirsutism, *Lancet* 349:191-195, 1997.
20. Bates GW, Cornwell CE: Iatrogenic causes of hirsutism, *Clin Obstet Gynecol* 34(4):849-851, 1991.
21. Yildiz BO, Woods KS, Stanczyk F, and others: Stability of adrenocortical steroidogenesis over time in healthy women and women with polycystic ovary syndrome, *J Clin Endocrinol Metab* 89(11):5558-5562, 2004.
22. Kessel B, Liu J: Clinical and laboratory evaluation of hirsutism, *Clin Obstet Gynecol* 34(4):805-816, 1991.
23. McKenna TJ: Screening for sinister causes of hirsutism, *N Engl J Med* 331(15):1015-1016, 1994.
24. Neiman LK: *Measurement of adrenal androgens*, 2005, retrieved Feb 17, 2007, from http://patients.uptodate.com/topic.asp?file=adrenal/7849.
25. Neiman LK: *Overview of congenital adrenal hyperplasia due to CYP21A2 (21-hydroxylase) deficiency*, 2005, retrieved Feb 17, 2007, from http://patients.uptodate.com/topic.asp?file=adrenal/11964.
26. Codner E, Mook-Kanamori D, Bazaes RA, and others: Ovarian function during puberty in girls with type I diabetes mellitus: response to leuprolide, *J Clin Endocrinol Metab* 90(7):3939-3945, 2005.
27. Gerritsma EJ, Brocaar MP, Hakkesteegt MM, and others: Virilization of the voice in postmenopausal women due to the anabolic steroid nandrolone decanoate (Deca-Durabolin): the effects of medication for 1 year, *Clin Otolaryngol Allied Sci* 19(1):79-84, 1994.
28. McClamrock HD: *Diagnosis and management of gestational hyper-*

androgenism, 2005, retrieved Feb 17, 2007, from http://patients.uptodate.com/topic.asp?file=r_endo_f/9376.
29. Taylor AE, McCourt B, Martin KA, and others: Determinants of abnormal gonadotropin secretion in clinically defined women with polycystic ovary syndrome, *J Clin Endocrinol Metab* 82(7):2248-2256, 1997.
30. Conn JJ, Jacobs HS: The clinical management of hirsutism, *Eur J Endocrinol* 136:339-348, 1997.
31. Ferriman D, Gallwey JD: Clinical assessment of body hair growth in women, *J Endocrinol Metab* 21:144-147, 1961.
32. Lukanova A, Lundin E, Zeleniuch-Jacquotte A, and others: Body mass index, circulating levels of sex-steroid hormones, IGF-I and IGF-binding protein-3: a cross sectional study of healthy women, *Eur J Endocrinol* 150(2):161-171, 2004.
33. Agorastos T, Argyriadis N, Fraggidis G, and others: Postmenopausal virilization due to ovarian hyperthecosis, *Arch Gynecol Obstet* 256(4):209-211, 1995.
34. Chang J: *Use of GnRH agonists in the treatment of hyperandrogenism and hirsutism*, 2005, retrieved Feb 17, 2007, from http://patients.uptodate.com/topic.asp?file=r_endo_f/12136.
35. Kroumpouzos G, Cohen LM: Dermatoses of pregnancy, *J Am Acad Dermatol* 45(1):1-19, 2001.
36. Garcia-Cruz D, Figuera LE, Cantu JM: Inherited hypertrichoses, *Clin Genetics* 61(5):321-329, 2002.
37. Rittmaster RS: Medical treatment of androgen-dependent hirsutism, *J Clin Endocrinol Metab* 80(9):2559-2563, 1995.
38. Schriock EA, Schriock ED: Treatment of hirsutism, *Clin Obstet Gynecol* 34(4):853-863, 1991.
39. Barman-Balfour JA, McClellan K: Topical eflornithine, *Am J Clin Dermatol* 2/3:197-201, 2001.
40. Lask G, Eckhouse S, Slatkine M, and others: The role of laser and intense light sources in photo-epilation: a comparative evaluation, *J Cutan Laser Ther* 1(1):3-13, 1999.
41. Schroeter CA, Groenewegen JS, Reineke T, and others: Hair reduction using intense pulsed light therapy source, *Dermatol Surg* 30(2):168-173, 2004.
42. Shaw JC: Antiandrogen and hormonal treatment of acne, *Dermatol Clin* 14(4):803-811, 1996.
43. Bergfeld WF: Hirsutism in women: effective therapy that is safe for long-term use: symposium: third of four articles on troublesome skin problems, *Postgrad Med* 107(7):93-94, 99-104, 2000.
44. Moghetti P, Tosi F, Tosti A, and others: Comparison of spironolactone, flutamide, and finasteride efficacy in the treatment of hirsutism: a randomized, double blind, placebo-controlled trial, *J Clin Endocrinol Metab* 85(1):89-94, 2000.
45. Muderris II, Bayram F, Guven M: A prospective, randomized trial comparing flutamide (250 mg/d) and finasteride (5 mg/d) in the treatment of hirsutism, *Fertil Steril* 73(5):984-987, 2000.
46. Carmina E: A risk benefit assessment of pharmacological therapies for hirsutism, *Drug Safety* 24(4):267-276, 2001.
47. Marshall K: Polycystic ovary syndrome: clinical considerations, *Altern Med Rev* 6(3):272-292, 2001.
48. Bidzinska B, Tworowska U, Demissie M, and others: Modified dexamethasone and gonadotropin-releasing hormone agonist (Dx-GnRHa) test in the evaluation of androgen source(s) in hirsute women, *Przegl Lek* 57(7-8):393-396, 2000.
49. Kokaly W, McKenna TJ: Relapse of hirsutism following long-term successful treatment with estrogen-progestogen combination, *Clin Endocrinol* 52(3):379-382, 2000.

CHAPTER 220

Hypercalcemia and Hypocalcemia

Kathryn Blum and Kathlyn Nowak
Updated by Alan Ona Malabanan

DEFINITION AND EPIDEMIOLOGY

A stable extracellular calcium concentration is vitally important to a number of physiologic and cellular functions. Aberrations in calcium homeostasis may lead to neuromuscular, cardiac, nephrologic, and gastrointestinal dysfunction.

Hypercalcemia, a high serum ionized calcium, is a disorder in which the calcium level exceeds the upper limit of the normal range (i.e., total calcium >10.5 mg/dl). Conversely, hypocalcemia is a low serum ionized calcium, with a total calcium level below 8.5 mg/dl. Both disorders can be a manifestation of a serious illness such as malignancy or can be detected coincidentally by laboratory testing in a patient with no obvious illness.[1] The imbalance may have varied causes, may be chronic or acute, and may exhibit variable effects.

Ninety-nine percent (1 to 2 kg) of body calcium is used to provide structural support of the bones and teeth. The remaining 1% is found in the extracellular fluid and soft tissues. Approximately 50% of plasma calcium is in the ionized, biologically active form; 10% is complexed in nonionic form; and 40% is protein bound, predominantly to albumin.[2,3] Alterations in albumin level may cause changes in total calcium concentrations, without altering ionized calcium levels. Calcium is a catalyst for muscle contraction (including cardiac), normal neuromuscular excitability, blood coagulation, exocrine and endocrine gland function, cell membrane integrity and permeability, vision, enzyme activity, and cell growth.[4]

The mechanisms regulating extracellular calcium homeostasis are complex and intimately involved with those of phosphorus, both of which are regulated by parathyroid hormone (PTH), and 1,25-dihydroxyvitamin D_3 (calcitriol). These hormones exert their effects through feedback mechanisms on three major organ systems: the skeleton, intestinal tract, and kidneys.

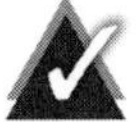

Physician consultation is indicated for patients with serum calcium levels less than 8.5 mg/dl or greater than 10.5 mg/dl.

A decrease in serum ionized calcium stimulates the production of PTH. PTH has a direct effect on calcium and phosphorus through increased osteoclast activity, which is responsible for bone resorption. PTH also directly stimulates the kidney tubules to reabsorb calcium and excrete phosphorus, leading to a rise in serum calcium and a fall in serum phosphorus. PTH also increases renal activation of 25-hydroxyvitamin D, the major circulating vitamin D metabolite, into 1,25-dihydroxyvitamin D, which increases intestinal absorption of calcium.[3,5] Increases in serum calcium and 1,25-dihydroxyvitamin D levels inhibit release of PTH, reversing the process.[3-6]

HYPERCALCEMIA

PATHOPHYSIOLOGY

Hypercalcemia can be categorized as either PTH dependent or PTH independent, depending on whether PTH is nonsuppressed or suppressed, respectively. PTH-dependent hypercalcemia is typically due to primary hyperparathyroidism, and PTH-independent hypercalcemia is typically due to hypercalcemia of malignancy. Primary hyperparathyroidism usually results when an autonomous parathyroid cell line develops. Hypercalcemia of malignancy may develop when bone resorption exceeds bone formation as a result of bony metastases. Solid tumors without metastasis and hematologic malignancies may operate via an alternative mechanism, humoral hypercalcemia of malignancy.[7,8] These tumor cells secrete PTH-related protein, which binds to PTH receptors, initiating bone resorption and renal reabsorption of calcium.[8,9] Milk-alkali syndrome, a combination of hypercalcemia, metabolic alkalosis, and renal insufficiency, develops in response to the simultaneous ingestion of large amounts of calcium and absorbable alkali such as calcium carbonate.[10] Disorders involving vitamin D excess or increased vitamin D activation lead to increased bone resorption and intestinal absorption of calcium.

CLINICAL PRESENTATION

The severity of symptoms in hypercalcemia is influenced by the magnitude of hypercalcemia, rate of rise of calcium, acid-base balance, and presence of hypoalbuminemia. An abnormally high level of calcium may be tolerated chronically, whereas a less elevated but abrupt increase may cause significant symptoms. Clinical manifestations are associated with the depressant effect of calcium on nerve tissue excitability and on the contractility of cardiac, skeletal, and smooth muscle.[9]

Initial symptoms of anorexia, fatigue, malaise, lethargy, nausea, dehydration, vague abdominal pain, and constipation can be easily missed. Central nervous system symptoms include depression, impaired concentration, disorientation and confusion, memory loss, shortened attention span, inappropriate behavior, irritability, and ataxia. If they are allowed to progress, these symptoms may lead to psychosis, stupor, coma, or death. Musculoskeletal effects include muscle fatigue, hypotonia, and weakness. Decreased smooth muscle contractility of the gastrointestinal system causes anorexia, nausea, vomiting, weight loss, abdominal pain, and constipation. Decreased contractility and decreased nerve conduction of the cardiac system produce arrhythmias and increased potential for digitalis toxicity. Renal system effects include polyuria, polydipsia, and nocturia.[11,12]

PHYSICAL EXAMINATION

The physical examination is often unremarkable. Cardiovascular examination may reveal irregularity of rate and rhythm. Band keratopathy, calcium deposition in the cornea, may be present regardless of the cause of hypercalcemia. The presence of a neck mass or breast mass may suggest the cause of the hypercalcemia. Depression of the central nervous system is reflected in hyporeflexia, changes in sensorium, muscle weakness, tremor, lethargy, and ataxia. With severe hypercalcemia, stupor and coma may be result. Occasionally, pseudogout (calcium pyrophosphate dehydrate crystal deposition disease) may cause joint swelling or inflammation.

DIAGNOSTICS

The diagnosis of either hypercalcemia or hypocalcemia is usually made by measuring the serum total calcium level along with a serum albumin level. Hypercalcemia is indicated if the total calcium level is greater than 10.5 mg/dl; a level less than 8.5 mg/dl is diagnostic of hypocalcemia. The level of serum calcium must be correlated with the simultaneous concentration of serum albumin. Serum calcium concentration falls by 0.8 mg/dl for each 1 g/dl decrease of serum albumin. For example, with a serum calcium of 8 mg/dl and an albumin of 2 g/dl (2 g/dl below normal), the corrected serum calcium would be 9.6 mg/dl (2 g/dl × 0.8 = 1.6) and therefore normal.[1,4] The serum pH can be a significant factor in determining true calcium concentration; alkalosis increases the amount of calcium bound to albumin, thereby decreasing the free ionized calcium available for biologic use; the opposite occurs with an acidotic state.[2,4]

When a true calcium imbalance is confirmed, further testing should be pursued to determine the etiology. Initial testing should include measurement of biointact PTH by immunoradiometric assay (IRMA) and vitamin D metabolite, creatinine, amylase, magnesium, and phosphorus levels.[12,13] Measurement of biointact PTH by IRMA is most useful in distinguishing hyperparathyroidism from malignancy and in differentiating hypoparathyroidism from nonparathyroid causes.[12,13] Serum alkaline phosphatase, radiographs, and bone scans can indicate a bony origin of hypercalcemia or hypocalcemia as seen in malignancy, vitamin D excess or deficiency, osteomalacia, or Paget's disease.[12]

DIFFERENTIAL DIAGNOSIS

Hyperparathyroidism and malignancy account for 90% of all cases of hypercalcemia, with 60% attributed to primary hyperparathyroidism.[7,12] Milk-alkali syndrome has recently become the third leading cause of hypercalcemia, possibly because of increased calcium carbonate consumption to prevent osteoporosis.[10] The remaining causes of hypercalcemia include sarcoidosis and other granulomatous disorders, thyrotoxicosis, vitamin A and D intoxication, thiazide diuretics,

DIAGNOSTICS

Hypercalcemia and Hypocalcemia

LABORATORY
Serum calcium
Ionized calcium*
Serum albumin
Serum pH
Parathyroid hormone levels*
Vitamin D metabolites*
Alkaline phosphatase*
Creatinine
Magnesium*
Phosphorus*

IMAGING
X-rays*
Bone scan*

OTHER
ECG*

*If indicated.

DIFFERENTIAL DIAGNOSIS

Hypercalcemia

- Hyperparathyroidism
- Malignancy
- Milk-alkali syndrome
- Sarcoidosis
- Granulomatous disease
- Thyrotoxicosis
- Vitamin A or D toxicity
- Thiazide diuretic use
- Addison's disease
- Renal failure
- Immobilization
- Drug toxicity (lithium, theophylline)

Addison's disease, prolonged immobilization, theophylline or lithium toxicity, and renal failure.[5,12]

MANAGEMENT

With early recognition and rapid intervention, hypercalcemia is a reversible condition. Conversely, the mortality rate of hypercalcemia is 50% without timely intervention.[7] Treatment of hypercalcemia consists of supportive or preventive measures, emergency therapies, and treatment of the underlying disorder. Severe, symptomatic hypercalcemia requires aggressive therapy aimed at decreasing the serum calcium level by increasing renal excretion. Excretion of sodium is accompanied by excretion of calcium; thus inducing natriuresis with saline and furosemide is the emergency treatment of choice.[7,11]

Further medical therapy is specific to treatment of the underlying cause. Parathyroid-induced hypercalcemia often remains silent until the onset of an acute illness or until it is detected by laboratory testing. Surgery is the treatment of choice for symptomatic patients. The asymptomatic patient risks progressive skeletal disease. Medical therapy is directed at both control of hypercalcemia (cinacalcet)[13] and osteoporosis (calcium, bisphosphonates, estrogen, raloxifene). Despite appropriate medical management, surgery is often necessary.

Asymptomatic milk-alkali syndrome is managed primarily through withdrawal of the causative agents. This generally results in rapid correction of both hypercalcemia and metabolic alkalosis.[10] Symptomatic patients are treated with saline (and furosemide, if needed) to induce natriuresis and excretion of calcium.[7,11]

The primary and most effective long-term treatment of malignancy-induced hypercalcemia is antineoplastic therapy aimed at tumor eradication. Medication therapy is directed at inhibiting osteoclast activity.[12] The choice of agent depends on the urgency of treatment, renal status, bone marrow status, and hospitalized vs. nonhospitalized status of patients.[14] Four agents are available that inhibit osteoclastic activity: plicamycin (discontinued in the United States), bisphosphonates, calcitonin, and gallium nitrate.[15] Bisphosphonates are the drugs of choice; they are relatively nontoxic, with maximum effect occurring in 2 to 4 days. Pamidronate is currently the most widely used bisphosphonate; however, zoledronic acid (Zometa), a newer agent, is proving extremely effective and longer lasting.[15,16] Calcitonin works rapidly when effective, although many patients develop tachyphylaxis within 2 to 3 days. Calcitonin in conjunction with a bisphosphonate has good efficacy.[15] Cytotoxic agents such as plicamycin and gallium nitrate should be considered as a last resort, since there is considerably greater toxicity.[12] Hydration and diuresis are a critical concurrent therapy. Medical treatment of hypercalcemia in the face of renal failure is difficult and often requires hemodialysis. Cinacalcet, a calcium mimetic, has recently been approved for the treatment of hypercalcemia of parathyroid carcinoma.[13]

Preventive measures include moderate dietary calcium (1 g/day), adequate hydration (2 L/day), and medication scrutiny. Because immobilization leads to bone resorption, weight-bearing activity is critical.[17] Thiazide diuretics, lithium, vitamins A and D, and theophylline, all of which further contribute to hypercalcemia, should be discontinued. Hypercalcemia decreases cardiac responsiveness to digitalis, necessitating close regulation of this medication.

LIFE SPAN CONSIDERATIONS

The cure rate of hypercalcemia with parathyroidectomy is 90% to 98%, although subsequent therapy for hypocalcemia may be necessary. Primary hyperparathyroidism is common in older women. Confusion may occur with only a slight elevation in serum calcium and is often mistaken as a sign of aging. Fortunately, it is completely reversible with appropriate treatment.[12] Malignancy-induced hypercalcemia usually occurs late in the disease, by which time the survival rate is only 2 to 6 months. If the disease is very advanced and/or the side effects of treatment overshadow the benefits, the decision not to treat may be appropriate.[14]

COMPLICATIONS

Complications of severe hypercalcemia include atonic ileus and obstipation, coma, profound muscular weakness, ataxia, pathologic fractures, renal failure, cardiac arrest, and death.

HYPOCALCEMIA

PATHOPHYSIOLOGY

Hypocalcemia occurs with either an increased loss of calcium from the circulation (deposition in tissue, increased urinary excretion, increased binding within the circulation) or with decreased entry of calcium into the circulation (malabsorption, decreased bone resorption).[18] Hypoparathyroidism causes impaired synthesis and secretion of PTH; lack of PTH is a direct cause of hypocalcemia.[16] Pseudohypoparathyroidism is a genetic deficiency in which the PTH is adequate but there is a peripheral resistance to its effect. Malabsorption syndromes, renal failure, and liver disease interfere with the absorption of both vitamin D and calcium despite elevated levels of PTH.[16] Hypomagnesemia may lead to decreased PTH release and action. Hyperphosphatemia deposits calcium in bone, hypermagnesemia increases peripheral resistance to PTH, and certain substances chelate calcium in the circulation, all effectively leading to hypocalcemia.[19]

CLINICAL PRESENTATION

Clinical manifestations of hypocalcemia are associated with increased excitation of nerve and muscle cells, primarily affecting the neuromuscular and cardiovascular systems.[11,19] Patients often complain of a generalized feeling of hyperirritability with restlessness, jumpiness, and sleeplessness.[6] Early symptoms of hypocalcemia include numbness and tingling, especially around the nose, lips, earlobes, and extremities. As neurologic excitability increases, irritability, depression, memory loss, psychosis, and seizure may occur. Musculoskeletal symptoms manifest as muscle spasm; carpopedal spasm; tetany; and laryngospasm with stridor, which can obstruct the airway, causing asphyxia.[6] Basal ganglia calcification may lead to a Parkinson's-like motor disorder.[18] Gastrointestinal symptoms include intestinal cramps and chronic malabsorption related to increased gastrointestinal motility and spasm.[19]

PHYSICAL EXAMINATION

The physical examination may reveal features of spontaneous neuromuscular irritability with hyperreflexia of deep tendons.[6,16] Chvostek's sign (contraction of the facial muscle in response to tapping the facial nerve against the bone anterior to the ear) and Trousseau's sign (carpal spasm occurring after occlusion of the brachial artery with a blood pressure cuff for 3 minutes) are usually readily elicited.[6,11] A Parkinson's-like tremor may be present.[18] Cardiovascular examination may reveal hypotension, impaired cardiac contractility, and bradyarrhythmias.[1,4,5] Adults suffering from chronic hypocalcemia may display coarse hair, dry and brittle nails, and scaly skin. Subcapsular cataracts can be seen with slit-lamp examination.[6,11]

DIAGNOSTICS

See Diagnostics under Hypercalcemia, p. 1128.

DIFFERENTIAL DIAGNOSIS

Chronic hypocalcemia can be ascribed to several disorders associated with an absence of PTH or with its ineffectiveness. Possible causes include surgery that involves the parathyroid or thyroid, idiopathic hypoparathyroidism, pseudohypoparathyroidism, vitamin D deficiency, malabsorption syndromes, severe renal or liver disease, alcoholism and poor nutritional intake, osteoblastic malignancy, pancreatitis, and hypomagnesemia or hyperphosphatemia. Distinguishing the etiology depends on clinical criteria, including the duration of illness, symptoms of associated disorders, detection of hereditary features, and a history of malnutrition and alcoholism. Acute transient hypocalcemia can be associated with severe sepsis, burns, acute renal failure, extensive blood transfusions with citrated blood, medications, and pancreatitis.[1]

DIFFERENTIAL DIAGNOSIS

Hypocalcemia

- Parathyroid hormone deficiency (surgery, idiopathic hypoparathyroidism, pseudohypoparathyroidism, radiation)
- Vitamin D deficiency
- Malabsorption syndromes
- Renal disease
- Liver disease
- Alcoholism
- Poor nutrition
- Malignancy
- Pancreatitis
- Hypomagnesemia
- Hypermagnesemia
- Hyperphosphatemia
- Severe sepsis
- Burns
- Medications
- Extensive transfusion with citrated blood

MANAGEMENT

All patients with symptomatic hypocalcemia must be treated. Severe, symptomatic hypocalcemia in the presence of tetany, arrhythmias, or seizures should be treated emergently with IV calcium. The treatment of hypocalcemia is guided by the acuity and severity of the hypocalcemia and the associated signs and symptoms. In acute, life-threatening situations, 1 or 2 ampules of calcium gluconate are diluted in 50 to 100 ml of 5% dextrose, infused over 10 to 20 minutes, and followed by a maintenance infusion of 10 ampules of calcium gluconate in 1 L of 5% dextrose at 50 ml/hr, titrated to symptoms and serum calcium level.[20] With less severe symptoms, a more dilute calcium solution is infused over a longer period. Serum calcium should be monitored frequently and the infusion adjusted accordingly.[3,6] Until calcium has been repleted, life-threatening symptoms such as hypotension and arrhythmias are refractory to medical management.[19]

Vitamin D is the cornerstone therapy for chronic hypocalcemia. Calcitriol is recommended (0.25 to 0.5 mcg/day) with calcium supplementation as needed (1 to 1.5 g/day).[6] Vitamin D and calcium can be varied independently. Higher doses of vitamin D allow for more effective absorption of calcium from the intestinal tract. If intestinal absorption is inefficient, higher intakes of oral calcium permit adequate calcium assimilation. Dietary phosphate intake likely should be limited, since excessive phosphate may lower serum calcium. The use of thiazide diuretics with sodium restriction in hypoparathyroidism lowers urinary calcium excretion, thus allowing a lower dose of vitamin D and calcium supplementation.[1] A low serum calcium level associated with a low serum albumin level does not require replacement. Serum pH, potassium, magnesium, and phosphorus levels should be monitored and corrected if necessary. This will usually correct hypocalcemia without further intervention.

LIFE SPAN CONSIDERATIONS

Hypocalcemia can be easily managed throughout the life span with calcium and vitamin D supplementation and monitoring of serum and urinary calcium levels to prevent crisis.

COMPLICATIONS

Complications of hypocalcemia are related to increased neuromuscular irritability and may precipitate laryngospasm, airway obstruction, tetany, seizures, cardiac arrhythmias, coma, or death.

INDICATIONS FOR REFERRAL OR HOSPITALIZATION

Treatment for both hypocalcemic crisis and hypercalcemic crisis always requires hospitalization. Immediate IV correction of the imbalance, either through replacement of calcium in hypocalcemia or through fluid replacement and diuresis in hypercalcemia, with concurrent cardiac monitoring, possible intubation, laboratory analysis, and diligent observation, is required until stabilization occurs. Referral to an endocrinologist or surgeon may be necessary if hyperparathyroidism is diagnosed. Malignancy-induced hypercalcemia should be managed by an oncologist.

PATIENT AND FAMILY EDUCATION AND HEALTH PROMOTION

Patient and family education should emphasize lifestyle changes, including diet, hydration, and mobility. Patients should learn to identify foods that are high in calcium and adjust their diets according to their imbalance. Maintaining mobility to promote uptake of calcium into bone should be stressed, as should the importance of adequate hydration for patients with either hypocalcemia or hypercalcemia. Patients and families should also be taught to recognize signs and symptoms of calcium imbalance. Early manifestations may be treated without hospitalization; however, if neglected, a calcium imbalance can be a truly life-threatening disorder.

REFERENCES

1. Potts JT: Diseases of the parathyroid gland and other hyper- and hypocalcemic disorders. In Isselbacher KJ, Braunwald E, Wilson JD, editors: *Harrison's principles of internal medicine,* ed 13, New York, 1994, McGraw-Hill.
2. Genuth SM: Endocrine regulation of calcium and phosphate metabolism. In Berne RM, Levy M, editors: *Physiology,* ed 4, St Louis, 1998, Mosby.
3. Terry J: The other electrolytes: magnesium, calcium, and phosphorus, *J Intraven Nurs* 14(3):167-176, 1991.
4. Hoppe B: Taking the confusion out of calcium levels, *Nursing* 25(7):32KK-32MM, 1995.
5. Yucha CB, Toto KH: Calcium and phosphorous derangements, *Crit Care Nurs Clin North Am* 6(4):747-766, 1994.
6. Tohme JF, Bilezikian JP: Hypocalcemic emergencies, *Endocrinol Metab Clin North Am* 22(2):363-367, 1993.
7. Clayton K: Cancer-related hypercalcemia: how to spot it, how to manage it, *Am J Nurs* 97(5):42-49, 1997.
8. Rizzoli R, Ferrari SL, Pizurki L, and others: Actions of parathyroid hormone and parathyroid hormone–related protein, *J Endocrinol Invest* 15(9 Suppl 6):51-56, 1992.
9. Kaplan M: Hypercalcemia of malignancy: a review of advances in pathophysiology, *Oncol Nurs Forum* 21(6):1039-1048, 1994.
10. Beall DP, Scofield RH: Milk-alkali syndrome associated with calcium carbonate consumption, *Medicine* 74:89, 1995.
11. Papadakis MA: Fluid and electrolyte disorders. In Tierney LM Jr, McPhee SJ, Papadakis MA, editors: *Current medical diagnosis and treatment,* ed 34, Norwalk, Conn, 1995, Appleton & Lange.
12. Mundy GR: Evaluation and treatment of hypercalcemia, *Hosp Pract* 29(6):79-84, 1994.
13. Silverberg SJ, Faiman C, Bilezikian JP, and others: Cinacalcet HCl effectively treats hypercalcemia in patients with parathyroid carcinoma [abstract], *J Bone Mineral Res* 19:S186, 2004.
14. Schmitt R: Quality of life issues in lung cancer, *Chest* 103(1):515-555, 1993.
15. Pecherstorfer M, Brenner K, Zojer N: Current management strategies for hypercalcemia, *Treat Endocrinol* 2(4):273-292, 2003.
16. Major P, Lortholary A, Hon J, and others: Zolendroic acid is superior to pamidronate in treatment of hypercalcemia of malignancy: a pooled analysis of two randomized, controlled clinical trials, *J Clin Oncol* 19(2):558-567, 2001.
17. Guise TA, Mundy GR: Evaluation of hypocalcemia in children and adults, *J Clin Endocrinol Metab* 80(5):1463-1478, 1995.
18. Rastogi R, Beauchamp NJ, Ladenson PW: Calcification of the basal ganglia in chronic hypoparathyroidism, *J Clin Endocrinol Metab* 88(4):1476-1477, 2003.
19. Ariyan CE, Sosa JA: Assessment and management of patients with abnormal calcium, *Crit Care Med* 32(4 Suppl):S146-S154, 2004.
20. Thakker RV: Hypocalcemia: pathogenesis, differential diagnosis, and management. In Favus M, editor: *Primer on the metabolic bone diseases and disorders of mineral metabolism,* ed 5, Washington, DC, 2003, American Society of Bone and Mineral Research.

CHAPTER 221

Hypernatremia and Hyponatremia

Terry Mahan Buttaro

Physician consultation is indicated for serum sodium levels less than 125 mEq/L or greater than 155 mEq/L.

HYPERNATREMIA

DEFINITION AND EPIDEMIOLOGY

Hypernatremia is one of the more common electrolyte disorders in older adults.[1] Characterized by an increase in the concentration of extracellular serum sodium and defined as a serum sodium level greater than 145 mEq/L, hypernatremia is most commonly associated with a fluid volume deficit. However, it can develop as a result of excessive sodium intake or be related to chronic renal disease or another disorder.[1-3]

PATHOPHYSIOLOGY

Hypernatremia indicates a disruption in water homeostasis. Under normal conditions, water intake and water loss are balanced. When water loss exceeds water intake, serum osmolality rises, and thirst is stimulated. Water balance is achieved as water intake increases. Thirst receptors are stimulated when serum osmolality rises above the normal range of 290 to 295 mosm/kg. Destruction of the thirst centers in the hypothalamus as a result of neoplasm, trauma, or vascular abnormalities leads to an inadequate thirst response and hypernatremia. Patients who are unable to adequately express thirst, such as infants or those with a decreased sensorium, are also at risk for developing hypernatremia. Older adults are at risk because the thirst mechanism decreases with age. Frail, debilitated older adults who live alone are also at greater risk because impaired mobility may limit adequate fluid intake.[1-5]

An excess in water loss in relation to intake leads to increased serum osmolality. In response to this rise in serum osmolality, antidiuretic hormone (ADH), or vasopressin, is secreted from the posterior pituitary gland. ADH increases the permeability of the renal collecting ducts to water. As a result, water is reabsorbed in the collecting ducts, and the urine becomes more concentrated. Patients with a deficit in the production of ADH or a diminished renal response to ADH will develop hypernatremia if water losses are not corrected. Older adults are especially at risk because of the diminished renal concentrating ability that occurs with aging. Patients with diabetes insipidus develop hypernatremia when water intake is not enough to compensate for fluid loss. Also at risk for the development of hypernatremia as a result of losing large amounts of free water are patients who have osmotic diuresis because of hyperglycemia or the administration of osmotic diuretics such as mannitol.[1-6]

Hypernatremia also develops with an increase in insensible water losses. Normally, small amounts of fluids are lost from the skin, respiratory tract, and gastrointestinal tract. Conditions such as fever, tachypnea, diarrhea, vomiting, and burns increase the volume of insensible water loss. Hypernatremia results if these losses are not replaced. Patients who exercise vigorously and drink an insufficient amount of liquid and those with insufficient fluid intake in the setting of fever, vomiting, or diarrhea are at great risk for developing hypernatremia.[1-6]

Hypernatremia occurs less often as a result of excess sodium intake, including rapid administration of IV normal saline or high-solute tube feedings. The sodium excess can cause an increase in serum osmolality and expansion of extracellular volume.[1,2]

CLINICAL PRESENTATION AND PHYSICAL EXAMINATION

The major clinical feature of hypernatremia is a central nervous system disturbance that results from dehydration and shrinkage of brain cells. The purpose of the history is to determine the cause of the increased serum sodium. A recent history of fever, vomiting, diarrhea, or polyuria is significant. Current medications, fluid intake and output over the past 24 hours, and any IV therapy or tube feedings should be reviewed with the past medical history.

Patients may complain of thirst or lightheadedness or, if the hypernatremia is related to a hypothalamic lesion, be completely asymptomatic. The signs and symptoms of hypernatremia are nonspecific and in general do not develop until the serum sodium level becomes greater than 150 mEq/L. Agitation, irritability, confusion, and changes in personality are early signs. Muscle twitching, spasticity, hyperreflexia, and lethargy may also be seen. Coma, seizures, and muscle weakness are later signs. Thirst is always present unless the thirst receptors are nonfunctioning. Other signs of volume depletion include hypotension, tachycardia, and abnormal postural changes in vital signs. Weight loss, flat neck veins, and diminished skin turgor may also be seen, depending on the severity of the volume loss.[1-3,6,7]

Diminished urinary output is also a possible finding, except in patients with diabetes insipidus or osmotic diuresis as the underlying cause of the hypernatremia. Fever, flushing, and dry mucous membranes may also be present.[1-3,6,7]

Classification of the patient's fluid volume status is facilitated by evaluation of the patient's appearance, weight, and postural vital signs and careful examination of the pulmonary, cardiac, and gastrointestinal systems. Neurologic screening, including motor tone, strength, coordination, and cognitive and functional ability, is necessary to determine subtle neurologic changes.

DIAGNOSTICS

Hypernatremia is confirmed by a serum sodium level above 145 mEq/L. Serum glucose, serum electrolytes, BUN, and creatinine are necessary to determine serum osmolality (2(Na) + Serum glucose/18 + BUN/2.8), which will likely be greater than 300 mosm/kg. Other diagnostics to consider depend on the patient history and physical findings and include a CBC and differential if an infection is suspected and a urine sample for

DIAGNOSTICS

Hypernatremia

LABORATORY
Serum glucose
Serum electrolytes
BUN
Creatinine
CBC and differential
Serum protein
Serum osmolality
Urine osmolality
Urine specific gravity

urinalysis and urine osmolality. The urine osmolality is increased to more than 600 mosm/kg, except in patients taking diuretics or in those with diabetes insipidus or osmotic diuresis. Urine specific gravity is not as precise as urine osmolality but is a quick test to determine urine concentration. The urine specific gravity of patients with hypernatremia is elevated, except in the cases noted previously. Urine sodium levels can be elevated, normal, or decreased. Serum protein, hematocrit, and red blood cells will be elevated.[1-3,6,7]

DIFFERENTIAL DIAGNOSIS

It is important that the provider determine the underlying cause of the sodium imbalance because treatment options vary with the etiology. The patient with hypernatremia resulting from diabetes insipidus is treated differently than the patient whose imbalance is a result of excessive diarrhea caused by the use of lactulose.

MANAGEMENT

The primary goal of treatment is the replacement of water loss and restoration of extracellular fluid volume. Oral water replacement is the safest, but replacement can be by nasogastric-gastric infusion or by IV infusion in the hospital. For patients who are hypovolemic as well as hypernatremic, fluid resuscitation with IV normal saline (0.9%) is necessary. Once the vital signs are normalized, the serum sodium can be slowly corrected (0.5 mEq/L/hr) with free water via a nasogastric tube or with hypotonic IV fluid. The IV replacement fluid should be a hypotonic saline solution (0.45% NaCl) or 5% dextrose in water.[1,7] The rate of fluid administration can be calculated by dividing the water deficit by the number of hours over which the fluid is to be replaced.[1,2] Water deficit is calculated as follows:

Adult patient free water deficit = 0.6 × Body weight (kg) × ([Plasma Na/140] − 1)

Elderly patient free water deficit = 0.45 × Body weight (kg) × ([Plasma Na/140] − 1)

After the fluid deficit is calculated, the treatment plan should include replacing the water deficit and maintenance losses (insensible losses, urine, and gastrointestinal losses) over the next 48 to 72 hours (or longer if indicated). Reductions of serum sodium by no more than 1 mEq/L/hr are recommended to avoid cerebral consequences.[8] Elderly patients and patients with chronic hypernatremia should have the water deficit corrected more slowly to prevent cerebral edema. Frequent monitoring of the fluid status and serum electrolytes is necessary while the patient is receiving IV therapy and electrolytes replaced as indicated. Diuretics and laxatives should be held until the deficit is corrected. The need for these medications should then be reevaluated.

The patient with hypernatremia caused by central diabetes insipidus is given vasopressin to decrease renal water losses.[9] If the degree of hypernatremia is moderate (<155 mEq/L), 0.1 to 0.4 ml of desmopressin acetate (DDAVP) may be given intranasally b.i.d. With more severe hypernatremia, aqueous vasopressin is given subcutaneously q 12-24 hr. Nephrogenic diabetes insipidus is treated with a thiazide diuretic (usually hydrochlorothiazide 50 mg q day) and a sodium-restricted diet (2 g/day). Serum sodium levels should be monitored closely.[1-4,7]

DIFFERENTIAL DIAGNOSIS

Hypernatremia

- Water depletion with insufficient water intake
- Excessive sweating and increased insensible water loss
- Diarrheal conditions
- Viral illnesses
- Hepatic encephalopathy with use of lactulose
- Abnormal thirst mechanism
- Increased renal water loss with inadequate fluid intake
- Diabetes insipidus
- Central (pituitary) diabetes insipidus
- Osmotic diuresis
- Glycosuria
- Mannitol use for diuresis
- Chronic renal failure
- Use of loop diuretics
- Water loss from peritoneal dialysis
- Excessive sodium intake with inadequate water intake
- High-solute tube feedings
- Rapid IV normal saline
- Hyperactivity of the adrenal cortex

LIFE SPAN CONSIDERATIONS

Age is a strong risk factor for developing dysnatremia, especially hypernatremia. Aging is associated with a decreased ability to cope with environmental, disease-related, and drug-related stressors in sodium and water balance.[10] Hypernatremia is commonly associated with fever and dehydration and is more common in warm environments. Older patients receiving high-solute tube feedings and diuretic or laxative therapy can also be at increased risk.

COMPLICATIONS

If hypernatremia is not corrected, cerebrovascular damage occurs as a result of brain dehydration and shrinkage. Shock results when a severe volume depletion is not corrected. Patients with cardiac disease should be monitored closely for signs and symptoms of congestive heart failure, which may occur if fluid is replaced too rapidly.[1,2]

INDICATIONS FOR REFERRAL OR HOSPITALIZATION

Hypernatremia may be managed on an outpatient basis if the degree of sodium imbalance is moderate and the patient is alert and able to drink sufficient amounts of fluids. Older adults living alone or those at risk for developing congestive heart failure may best be managed in an inpatient setting. Patients with severe hypernatremia (serum sodium >155 mEq/L) or severe volume depletion should be hospitalized.[1,2,7]

PATIENT AND FAMILY EDUCATION

Patients and families should understand that normally 1500 to 2000 ml of fluid should be consumed each day. Patients at risk for hypernatremia should understand the importance of maintaining proper fluid balance. Older patients in particular need to be aware of the dangers of dehydration, especially in hot weather or if fever is present. Patients who are taking diuretics or medications such as lithium and carbamazepine (Tegretol), which cause hypernatremia, need to be aware of this side effect. Patients who exercise regularly should be educated about the need for adequate fluid intake when exercising. Patients with underlying conditions that put them at risk for hypernatremia need to be educated accordingly.[1,4,6]

HYPONATREMIA

DEFINITION AND EPIDEMIOLOGY

Hyponatremia is a common electrolyte disorder that has been identified as a significant cause of morbidity and mortality in older persons, in hospitalized patients, and more recently in marathon runners.[11,12] It is associated with varied disorders, including infections, traumatic brain injuries, malignancy, untoward medication effects, endocrine disorders, psychogenic polydipsia, the syndrome of inappropriate ADH (SIADH), AIDS, and other illnesses. These conditions seem to be related to a dysfunction in the release of ADH or renal insensitivity to the hormone. However, hyponatremia also results from hyperglycemia or any condition that leads to excess water in relation to body sodium or causes salt loss in excess of water loss.[13]

Defined as a serum sodium concentration of less than 135 mEq/L, hyponatremia can manifest as an acute or a chronic condition. Acute hyponatremia customarily develops in hospitalized patients after surgery and is often associated with fluid overload. Chronic hyponatremia usually occurs outside the hospital, is acquired over a longer period, and is typically associated with less serious neurologic sequelae. It is one of the more common electrolyte disorders in older adults, but premenopausal women and children are also at risk, particularly after surgery.[14-17] In marathon runners the cause can be related to drinking a disproportionate amount of hypotonic fluid or even to NSAID use.[18] Serious morbidity may occur with sodium levels less than 110 mEq/L, with mortality approaching 50% in acute hyponatremia.[13]

Hyponatremia may be classified into one of four categories by the determination of extracellular fluid volume (ECFV).[13] These include hyponatremia with hypervolemia (increased ECFV), hyponatremia with hypovolemia (decreased ECFV), hyponatremia with euvolia (normal ECFV), and pseudohyponatremia.[13,14] The first three hyponatremias are associated with decreased plasma osmolality and are considered hypotonic hyponatremias. Pseudohyponatremia has been identified with both increased and normal osmolality and may be either a hypertonic or isotonic hyponatremia.

PATHOPHYSIOLOGY

As the major extracellular cation, sodium regulates intracellular and extracellular body water and is a determinant of serum osmolality. If serum sodium levels are allowed to fall below normal limits, serum osmolality is decreased and extracellular water is permitted to seep into cells. This results in a hypotonic hyponatremia and the subsequent swelling of cerebral brain cells that causes the neurologic features associated with hyponatremia.

Normally the body responds to an excess amount of water by diuresis. Renal mechanisms and ADH control body fluid volume and the composition of body fluids. An increase in serum osmolality over the normal 275 to 295 mosm/kg stimulates the posterior pituitary to release ADH, which influences the distal tubules and collecting ducts in the kidneys to conserve water. As body fluid accumulates and serum osmolality becomes hypotonic, ADH is inhibited.

Hyponatremia with Increased Extracellular Volume

Hyponatremia with increased ECFV may occur with cirrhosis, congestive heart failure, nephrotic syndrome, or advanced renal failure. In patients with cirrhosis and heart failure, diuretic therapy can actually induce hyponatremia, although heart failure–related hyponatremia is also associated with an increase in arginine vasopressin, causing the renal collecting ducts to increase free water absorption.[19] In cirrhosis the lowered serum sodium can be related to either fluid retention, solute depletion, or both.[20] The hypervolemic hyponatremias are considered edematous conditions and are characterized by urine sodium less than 20 mEq/L and high urine osmolality. In renal failure, however, urine sodium may be more than 20 mEq/L. Unfortunately, in patients on diuretic medications, urine sodium results can be inaccurate, since diuretics can cause elevated urine sodium levels.

Hyponatremia with Decreased Extracellular Volume

Hypovolemic hyponatremia consists of a sodium deficit that occurs in isolation or in addition to a water deficit. This condition can be associated with either nonrenal or renal precipitants; this is distinguished by the evaluation of the urine sodium. With renal-associated disorders (chronic renal disease, osmotic diabetic diuresis, mineralocorticoid deficiency, angiotensin-converting enzyme [ACE] inhibitors, and diuretics), urine sodium is usually greater than 20 mEq/L. In nonrenal disorders (dehydration, diarrhea, vomiting, burns, extreme exercise, diaphoresis, and third-space fluid loss), urine sodium is less than 20 mEq/L and is combined with a high urine osmolality.

Hyponatremia with Normal Extracellular Volume

SIADH is often the cause of hyponatremia associated with normal ECFV and has been identified with many conditions.[18] With SIADH, a stimulus causes an excess production of ADH, which precipitates an increase in water reabsorption, an increase in glomerular filtration rate, and a decrease in sodium reabsorption. SIADH is characterized by hypotonic hyponatremia; euvolemia; increased urinary sodium (usually >20 mEq/L and often >40 mEq/L); a urine osmolality (usually >100 mosm/kg) greater than serum osmolality; and normal renal, cardiac, hepatic, adrenal, and thyroid function. Typically, plasma urea and uric acid are below normal or within normal limits.[21]

Psychogenic polydipsia, beer potamia (the association of severe hyponatremia with ingestion of large quantities of beer), and a reset osmostat have also been identified as precipitants of hypotonic hyponatremia with euvolia. Psychogenic polydipsia can be related to ACE inhibitor or lithium therapy or to a biologic or psychiatric disorder; it may also be a compensatory mechanism for medications that cause dry mouth.[16,21] Individuals with beer potamia derive the vast amount of their caloric intake from large quantities of beer, which contains relatively few solutes.[22] The reduced solute delivery to the distal tubule restricts urine production and results in hyponatremia. The reset osmostat phenomenon, or sick cell syndrome, is found in patients with malnutrition, cancer, or other debilitating conditions. Changes in cellular metabolism cause hypothalamic osmoreceptors to reset to maintain a lowered serum osmolality.[16] The diagnosis of reset osmostat is complex. Usually BUN and creatinine are normal, but urine sodium and osmolality are variable.[16]

Euvolemic hyponatremia has also been identified in varied postoperative situations. Pain and the stress of surgery can stimulate the release of excess ADH, which may cause hyponatremia in the presence of IV hypotonic fluid replacement.[13]

Pseudohyponatremia

Pseudohyponatremia without plasma hypoosmolality has been associated with hyperproteinemia and hyperlipidemia. In these disorders, partial displacement of the sodium-containing plasma by increased numbers of lipids or proteins causes falsely lowered sodium levels. Both conditions are isotonic hyponatremias associated with normal plasma osmolality and are treated with correction of the hyperproteinemia or hyperlipidemia.[1]

Hyperosmolar pseudohyponatremia may be seen with conditions that elevate plasma osmolality, such as hyperglycemia, mannitol excess, and glycerol therapy. The increased serum glucose causes increased plasma osmolality, which shifts body water into the intravascular space and lowers serum sodium. Correction of plasma glucose corrects the hyponatremia.

Pseudohyponatremia may also be caused by the absorption of isotonic irrigant solutions containing glycine or sorbitol after endometrial resection or a urologic procedure.[23] The absorption of the irrigant lowers plasma sodium, but not usually plasma osmolality. Elevated serum osmolality with lowered serum sodium may occur in some cases.[21]

CLINICAL PRESENTATION

The present and past medical history aids in identifying the cause of the lowered serum sodium and helps determine if the onset is acute or chronic. A thorough medication review, including allergies, recent corticosteroid therapy, or over-the-counter medications (e.g., NSAIDs) is essential, since numerous medications will precipitate this disorder. Other history should include any recent illness or surgery, previous illnesses, and any previous psychiatric history. Often the patient's symptoms are quite subtle and the history inconclusive. Nonetheless, hyponatremia should be considered in the differential diagnosis of all individuals who are seen with irritability, restlessness, impaired central nervous system function, history of falls, nonspecific gastrointestinal complaints, flulike symptoms, dysgeusia, unusual water-drinking behavior, or weight changes.[24] Unfortunately, the symptoms commonly associated with hyponatremia may not be apparent until the patient's sodium level has fallen below 120 mEq/L. Still, patients with even mild hyponatremia can experience headache, blurred vision, dizziness, lethargy, weakness, combativeness, extrapyramidal signs, muscle cramps, and fatigue. Stupor, seizures, psychosis, and coma are associated with sodium levels below 110 mEq/L.

PHYSICAL EXAMINATION

The physical signs of hyponatremia can be limited. However, a complete examination, including weight and postural vital signs, can suggest the cause of the disorder, particularly if edema or ascites is present or if the patient appears dehydrated. The evaluation should include determining any neurologic changes (e.g., level of consciousness, change in mental status, seizures) or signs of heart failure, cirrhosis, or hypothyroidism.

DIAGNOSTICS

The history, physical examination, and diagnostic evaluation are critical in discerning the cause and subsequent management of the hyponatremia.[25] Determination of serum glucose, serum electrolytes, BUN, and creatinine is essential to calculate the serum osmolality. This will aid assessment for hyperglycemia and allow mathematical categorization of the hyponatremia into a hypertonic (elevated plasma osmolality), hypotonic (decreased plasma osmolality), or isotonic (normal plasma osmolality) state:

$$2(\text{Na [in mEq/L]}) + \text{K (in mEq/L)} + (\text{BUN [in mg/dl]}/2.8) + (\text{Glucose [in mg/dl]}/18)$$

A lipid profile excludes hyperlipidemia as a cause of isotonic hyponatremia, and a urine sample for sodium, osmolality, specific gravity, and uric acid will classify the hyponatremia appropriately.[25] Other diagnostics that may be necessary include a CBC and differential, liver function studies, calcium,

DIAGNOSTICS

Hyponatremia

LABORATORY
Serum electrolytes
BUN
Creatinine
Serum glucose
Urine for sodium, specific gravity, osmolality
Calcium, magnesium, phosphorus*
LFTs*
CBC and differential*
TSH (if signs of hypothyroidism)*
Fasting lipid profile
Uric acid*
ACTH stimulation test (if recent steroid therapy)*

IMAGING
Chest x-ray (if suspected congestive heart failure)*
CT scan, MRI*

*If indicated.

magnesium, phosphorus, thyroid-stimulating hormone, chest x-ray studies, malignancy evaluations, and definitive neurologic studies.

DIFFERENTIAL DIAGNOSIS

Endurance exercise, metabolic disturbances, severe illness, infection, medications, depression, endocrine abnormalities, nutritional deficiencies, trauma, and cardiovascular and cerebrovascular accidents should be considered in the differential diagnosis. Additionally, the differential diagnosis should include appropriately classifying the fluid volume state.

MANAGEMENT

If the hyponatremia is related to a medication, the medication should be discontinued if at all possible. If the cause is hyperglycemia, correcting the elevated blood glucose should return the serum sodium to normal levels. For hyponatremia not related to a medication or hyperglycemia, the severity of the hyponatremia and volume status guides specific management decisions. Correction of the body water and sodium imbalance is the primary goal, but correction or control of the underlying pathologic condition is also critical.

Hyponatremia with increased extracellular volume (hypervolemia) is associated with lowered serum osmolality (<280 mosm/kg), serum sodium less than 135 mEq/L, and increased urine osmolality. If the cause of the hypervolemic hyponatremia is related to renal failure, the urine sodium will be greater than 20 mEq/L, but otherwise the urine sodium will be less than 20 mEq/L. For asymptomatic patients with serum sodium greater than 125 mEq/L, management consists of fluid restriction (1000 to 1500 ml/day) and dietary sodium restriction (2 to 5 g/day). If the serum sodium is less than 125 mEq/L, the physician should be consulted and the cautious use of loop diuretics considered. In the future for patients with hyponatremia associated with congestive heart failure, a new class of medications, arginine vasopressin receptor agonists, are currently being investigated. It is thought that these medications will allow the excretion of free water, but exclude the excretion of electrolytes.[26]

In hyponatremia with decreased extracellular volume (hypovolemia) associated with a renal disorder, serum osmolality will be less than 275 mosm/kg urine sodium greater than 20 mEq/L, and the BUN and creatinine increased. If diarrhea, vomiting, or dehydration is the cause of the hypovolemic hyponatremia, the serum osmolality will be less than 275 mosm/kg urine sodium less than 20 mEq/L, and the BUN and creatinine increased. Management consists of treating the underlying disorder, eliminating medications associated with the hyponatremia (particularly NSAIDs, thiazide diuretics, and, if necessary ACE inhibitors). Patients with fluid volume deficit may need isotonic fluid replacement. If the serum sodium is less than 125 mEq/L, consultation with the primary care physician is necessary to discuss hospitalization for IV saline.

Hyponatremia associated with euvolemia (normal extracellular volume) requires careful consideration, since the underlying pathologic conditions are considerable. In SIADH, the urine osmolality is usually greater than 100 mosm/kg and urine sodium greater than 20 mEq/L. BUN (<10 mg/dl) and uric acid (<4 mg/dl) are low, and thyroid, renal, adrenal, and hepatic function are normal. Management consists of correcting the underlying pathologic condition and fluid restriction. Consultation with the physician is indicated for a serum sodium less than 125 mEq/L to discuss hospitalization for hypertonic saline infusion or initiation of demeclocycline.

The urine osmolality is less than 100 mosm/kg in polydipsia, beer potamia, and reset osmostat. Treatment of patients with psychogenic polydipsia and beer potamia consists of fluid restriction and behavioral counseling. Management of pseudohyponatremia associated with hyperglycemia consists of correcting the hyperglycemia. If an isotonic genitourinary irrigant is the cause of the hyponatremia, the irrigant should be discontinued. Patients with suspected endurance exercise–induced hyponatremia require hospitalization for judicious IV therapy with hypertonic (3%) or normal (0.9%) saline. No treatment is necessary for hyponatremia related to reset osmostat, hyperlipidemia, or hyperproteinemia.

Co-Management with Specialists

In consultation with a physician, loop diuretics may be used with caution. Furosemide and increased oral sodium may be indicated for patients who are unable to adhere to water restriction. Furosemide is also prescribed in combination with ACE inhibitors to manage hyponatremia in severe congestive heart failure.

Demeclocycline in dosages greater than 600 mg/day (usual daily dosage is 300 to 600 mg PO b.i.d.) inhibits the effect of ADH on the renal tubule and has been used in the long-term management of SIADH and carbamazepine-induced hyponatremia.[23,27] Demeclocycline can increase BUN, precipitate renal toxicity, and induce fluid loss; therefore caution is advised, particularly with congestive heart failure, renal disease, or liver disease.[23,27] Lithium, another ADH inhibitor, has been used

DIFFERENTIAL DIAGNOSIS

Hyponatremia

- Metabolic illness
- Severe illness or infection: AIDS
- Medications: angiotensin-converting enzyme inhibitors, thiazide diuretics, NSAIDs, selective serotonin reuptake inhibitors, oxcarbazepine, carbamazepine, Ecstasy (3,4-methylenedioxymethylamphetamine), neuroleptics, tricyclics, antineoplastics, somatostatin, chlorpropamide
- Depression
- Endocrine abnormalities: hypothyroidism, ACTH deficiency, mineralocorticoid deficiency
- Endurance exercise induced
- Trauma
- Cardiovascular event
- Cerebrovascular accident
- Malignancy
- Pulmonary infections or disorders
- CNS trauma or infections
- Pseudohyponatremia
- Psychogenic polydipsia
- Beer potamia

in the past for the treatment of SIADH despite its potential for precipitating psychogenic polydipsia and thyroid dysfunction.[16,28]

Urea, both oral and IV, has been successfully used to treat varied types of hyponatremia but is contraindicated in patients with gastric ulcers, renal failure, and liver disease.[27,28] Oral nonpeptide vasopressin antagonists may also soon be available and offer added benefit in the treatment of hyponatremia.[29]

COMPLICATIONS

Brain damage or death is the most serious complication of hyponatremia and seems to occur most often in children and premenopausal women.[21] These sequelae are associated with encephalopathy resulting from untreated hyponatremia or central pontine myelinolysis, the untoward consequence of correcting the serum sodium too quickly with IV hypertonic saline.[23]

INDICATIONS FOR REFERRAL OR HOSPITALIZATION

Symptoms of hyponatremia with decreased ECFV are typically those associated with hypovolemia. Treatment of the underlying disorder and isotonic fluid volume replacement in the hospital setting are indicated.[28]

Patients with acute SIADH and serum sodium less than 115 mEq/L should be hospitalized for intensive correction of both the underlying disorder and the SIADH disorder with hypertonic saline (3% NaCl), diuretics, and replacement electrolytes. To prevent central pontine myelinosis and brain damage, care must be taken to prevent hypoxia and to slowly, rather than quickly, repair the hyponatremia with hypertonic IV saline.[22,26] Hypertonic saline should not be administered more rapidly than 10 to 15 mEq/L/24 hr; urinary output and serum electrolytes should be monitored hourly, and the infusion should be discontinued before the serum sodium reaches 130 mEq/L.[30]

PATIENT AND FAMILY EDUCATION

Prevention of hyponatremia is the primary goal. For runners or other patients at risk for exercise-induced hyponatremia, NSAIDs and other medications that induce hyponatremia should be avoided and fluid consumption based on patient thirst.[18] When training for endurance events, participants should be encouraged to weigh in both before and after exercise in an attempt to avoid weight gain and help gauge appropriate amounts of fluid.[18] In addition, participants in endurance events should understand the importance of drinking electrolyte-enhanced fluids rather than ingesting only free water.[30] Education for runners and other athletes competing in endurance events should also include careful explanation of the early symptoms of hyponatremia and its potentially serious sequelae.

Since hyponatremia and its treatment may be anxiety provoking for both patients and families, patients and caregivers (both family and professional) need to understand the nature of the hyponatremic disorder and recognize its associated neurologic symptoms. Instructions regarding the importance of frequent weight measurements, dietary or fluid restriction, intake and output measurement, and medications (and their side effects) should be explicit and understandable. Patients and families also need to understand the importance of calling the health care provider if the fluid restriction causes constipation or other problems. Because fluid restriction can dry oral membranes, good oral hygiene is important. Patients who are bedridden or immobile need good skin care, constant turning, and proper positioning. Frequent follow-up care with continuous evaluation of the treatment plan is imperative.

REFERENCES

1. Kugler JP, Hustead T: Hyponatremia and hypernatremia in the elderly, *Am Fam Phys* 61:3623-3630, 2000.
2. Androgue HJ, Madias NE: Hypernatremia, *N Engl J Med* 342(20):1493-1499, 2000.
3. Fried LF, Palevsky PM: Hyponatremia and hypernatremia, *Med Clin North Am* 81(3):585-609, 1997.
4. Oh MS, Carroll HJ: Disorders of sodium metabolism: hypernatremia and hyponatremia, *Crit Care Med* 20(1):94-103, 1992.
5. Brown RG: Disorders of water and sodium balance, *Postgrad Med* 93(4):227-246, 1993.
6. Bove LA: Restoring electrolyte balance: sodium and chloride, *RN* 59(11):25-29, 1996.
7. Winger JM, Hurnic T: Age-associated changes in the endocrine system, *Nurs Clin North Am* 31(4):827-844, 1996.
8. Stephanides SL: *Hypernatremia*, 2005, retrieved Feb 24, 2007, from http://www.emedicine.com/emerg/topic263.htm.
9. Cooperman M: *Diabetes insipidus*, 2006, retrieved Feb 24, 2007, from http://www.emedicine.com/med/topic543.htm.
10. Hawkins R: Age and gender as risk factors for hyponatremia and hypernatremia, *Clin Chim Acta* 337(1-2):169-172, 2003, retrieved Feb 28, 2007, from http://www.sciencedirect.com/science?_ob=articleURL&_udi+B6T57-49S5X2X-8&_user.
11. Almond CS, Shin AY, Fortescue EB, and others: Hyponatremia among runners in the Boston Marathon, *N Engl J Med* 352(15):1550-1556, 2005.
12. Speedy DBN, Oakes TD, Schneider C: Exercise-associated hyponatremia: a review, *Emerg Med* 13(1):17-27, 2001.
13. Rutecki GW, Whittier FC: Physiologic clues to a state of disordered tonicity, *Consultant* (5):688-690, 700-702, 1994.
14. Tareen N, Martins D, Nagami G, and others: Sodium disorders in the elderly, *J Natl Med Assoc* 97(2):217-224, 2005.
15. Brown OA: Understanding postoperative hyponatremia, *Urol Nurs* 24(3):197-201, 2004.
16. Rousseau P: Hyponatremia among older individuals, *South Med J* 84(9):1114-1118, 1991.
17. Miller M, Hecker MS, Friedlander DA, and others: Apparent idiopathic hyponatremia in an ambulatory geriatric population, *J Am Geriatr Soc* 44(4):404-408, 1996.
18. Rose BD: *Causes of hyponatremia*, retrieved Jan 2, 2006, from http://patients.uptodate.com/topic.asp?file=fldlytes/7034.
19. Oren RM: Hyponatremia in congestive heart failure, *Am J Cardiol* 95(9A):2B-7B, 2005.
20. Castello L, Pirisi M, Sainaghi PP, and others: Quantitative treatment of the hyponatremia of cirrhosis, *Dig Liver Dis* 37(3):176-180, 2005.
21. Mulloy AL, Caruana RJ: Hyponatremic emergencies, *Med Clin North Am* 79(1):155-167, 1995.
22. Reeves WB, Andreoli TE: The posterior pituitary and water metabolism. In Wilson JD, Foster DF, editors: *William's textbook of endocrinology*, ed 8, Philadelphia, 1992, Saunders.
23. Fraser CL, Arieff AI: Epidemiology, pathophysiology, and management of hyponatremic encephalopathy, *Am J Med* 102(1):67-77, 1997.
24. Panayioutou H, Small SC, Hunter JH, and others: Sweet taste (dysgeusia): the first symptom of hyponatremia in small cell carcinoma of the lung, *Arch Intern Med* 155(12):1325-1328, 1995.
25. Saeed BO, Beaumont D, Handley GH: Severe hyponatraemia: investigation and management in a district general hospital, *J Clin Pathol* 55(12):893-896, 2002.

26. Goldsmith SR: Current treatments and novel pharmacologic treatments for hyponatremia in congestive heart failure, *Am J Cardiol* 95(9A):14B-23B, 2005.
27. Soupart A, Decaux G: Therapeutic recommendations for management of severe hyponatremia: current concepts on pathogenesis and prevention of neurologic complications, *Clin Nephrol* 46(3):149-169, 1996.
28. Narins RG, Krishna GG: Disorders of water balance. In Stein JH, Eisenberg JM, Hutton JJ, and others, editors: *Internal medicine,* ed 5, St Louis, 1998, Mosby.
29. Gross P, Wehrle R, Bussemaker E: Hyponatremia: pathophysiology, differential diagnosis, and new aspects of treatment, *Clin Nephrol* 46(4):273-276, 1996.
30. Flynn SD, Sherer RJ: Seizure after exercise in the heat: recognizing life-threatening hyponatremia, *Phys Sports Med* 28:9, 2000, retrieved Jan 2, 2006, from http://www.physsportsmed.com/issues/2000/09_00/flinn.htm.

CHAPTER 222

Lipid Disorders

Mary Young

DEFINITION AND EPIDEMIOLOGY

Despite new knowledge and progress in treatment, lipid disorders remain a significant risk factor in the development of cardiovascular disease (CVD). More than 100 million people in the United States have high cholesterol levels (total cholesterol >200 mg/dl), yet only 40% are being treated. The National Cholesterol Education Program's Adult Treatment Panel III Guidelines (NCEP-ATP III), first published in 2001, have been enhanced by five large recent trials that support and improve current guidelines. Therapeutic lifestyle changes (TLC) remain an important first step, along with aggressive lipid-lowering drugs, to achieve new levels of low-density lipoprotein (LDL): less than 100 mg/dl in high-risk patients, and less than 70 mg/dl in very high–risk patients, which includes patients with diabetes, CVD, or acute coronary syndrome (ACS).[1]

Lipid disorders, or dyslipidemias, are generally the result of a combination of genetic and dietary factors. A serum total cholesterol level of less than 200 mg/dl is considered desirable, but about half of all American adults have a total cholesterol level of 200 mg/dl or greater. More than 40 million, almost 20%, have total cholesterol levels of 240 mg/dl or more and are clearly at increased risk for CVD.

Numerous epidemiologic, clinical, genetic, and laboratory studies support the relationship between elevated cholesterol levels and increased risk of CVD. Several landmark clinical trials have demonstrated dramatic benefits from lipid-lowering medication in reducing morbidity and mortality from CVD, both in patients with established CVD (secondary prevention) and those without known CVD but with risk factors (primary prevention).[2] These benefits affect both men and women, in all age ranges, including the elderly. A 10% reduction in the average cholesterol could produce a 30% reduction in the incidence of CVD.

PATHOPHYSIOLOGY

Cholesterol and other lipids are normal and essential components of human cells. The liver synthesizes much of the body's cholesterol. Additional cholesterol, and a variety of other lipids, is absorbed from the gastrointestinal tract. They are transported via the bloodstream to the liver, where they are processed, and to the rest of the body, where they are used or stored. Since cholesterol and other lipids are insoluble in water, they must be combined with specialized phospholipids and proteins called *apoproteins* to form microscopic packages called *lipoproteins*, which are soluble in the plasma. Lipoproteins take the form of a lipid core containing triglycerides and cholesterol and an outer layer containing the phospholipids and the apoproteins. The apoproteins serve as ligands for the enzymes and receptors that mediate lipid metabolism.

Atherosclerosis is a pathologic process whereby cholesterol is deposited into the walls of arteries. This is influenced by a number of factors, including toxins and inflammatory mediators within the bloodstream and at the level of the vessel wall, and by the characteristics and concentrations of the various lipoproteins. These are characterized by their density and include chylomicrons, very low–density lipoprotein (VLDL), intermediate-density lipoprotein (IDL), LDL, and high-density lipoprotein (HDL).

Low-Density Lipoprotein

LDL carries most of the cholesterol in the plasma and is the cause of atherogenic changes associated with the development of CVD. The principal function of LDL is to transport cholesterol to hepatic and extrahepatic cells. Although LDL particles are small, they carry approximately 70% of the circulating cholesterol in plasma. LDL is removed from the plasma by a single type of receptor located on the surface of many cells throughout the body: the LDL receptor. LDL's primary apoprotein is apoprotein B (apo B), which binds to the LDL receptor during the process by which LDL is brought into the cells. One molecule of apo B is present for each LDL particle, but the quantity of cholesterol per particle can vary considerably. The ratio of LDL cholesterol to apo B correlates with the size of the LDL particles. Low LDL cholesterol/apo B ratios reflect small LDL particles. It has been postulated that these smaller, denser LDL particles are more atherogenic than normal-sized LDL particles. Two theories exist on why this may be true. First, their size allows these particles to filter more easily through the arterial wall, and, second, these particles are especially vulnerable to oxidation. Small, dense LDL particles have been associated with conditions such as insulin resistance, diabetes, hypertriglyceridemia, and low HDL, all of which are independent risk factors for CVD.[3]

It may be that measurements of apo B in the blood correlate even more closely than LDL cholesterol with the risk for CVD, but this test is not available in most laboratories. Elevation of a distinct form of LDL, lipoprotein (a) [Lp(a)], has been identified as an independent risk factor for the development of premature CVD in men. Because there is no scientific proof that lowering Lp(a) will lower cardiovascular risk, assessment of this lipid determination at this time should be limited to research and specialized lipid clinics.

High-Density Lipoprotein

HDL has emerged as a powerful independent predictor of CVD risk. For every 1 mg/dl decrease in HDL, there is a 2% to 3% increase in CVD risk. The role of HDL is twofold. First, when free cholesterol is released from cells into the plasma, it binds to HDL particles, resulting in a reverse cholesterol transport system. Cholesterol is returned to the liver, where it is excreted into bile, converted to bile acids, or reprocessed. Both the liver and intestines synthesize and secrete HDL particles. Second, HDL prevents oxidation of LDL within the arterial wall. There is an inverse relationship between VLDL remnants and small, dense LDL particles—known atherogenic factors—and HDL. Because of the inverse relationship between levels of HDL and CVD risk, low levels of HDL (<40 mg/dl) have been identified as an independent risk factor for CVD regardless of the total cholesterol. Higher HDL cholesterol has a protective effect, and levels over 60 mg/dl are considered to be a negative risk factor, lowering the overall risk.[4]

The ratio of total cholesterol to HDL cholesterol has been correlated to cardiac risk. A total cholesterol/HDL cholesterol ratio of greater than 4.5 is associated with increased cardiac risk. Use of this ratio, however, appears less useful than previously thought. Apoprotein AI (apo AI) is the predominant lipoprotein in HDL, and measurement of apo AI in addition to the apo B found in LDL may, in the future, allow for more accurate assessment of cardiac risk.

Increased levels of physical activity can increase HDL cholesterol levels, and this should be a target for intervention. Also, it appears that modest alcohol consumption increases HDL cholesterol and appears to reduce cardiac risk. Alcohol, however, can also increase triglycerides and have other adverse effects. The intake of one or two alcoholic beverages per day may be beneficial in terms of overall mortality, but consumption of more alcohol than this is clearly detrimental, and in many patients alcohol use can escalate. Recommending alcohol consumption to patients must be done with caution.

Triglycerides

Levels of LDL and HDL cholesterol actually represent a measurement of the amount of cholesterol contained in each kind of lipoprotein particle in the blood. Triglycerides are found in all types of lipoprotein particles. Elevations in triglycerides therefore could represent a number of different abnormalities in lipid metabolism. Nonetheless, elevated triglycerides have been identified as an independent cardiac risk factor and, when extremely elevated, may cause pancreatitis.

Role of Genetics

A person's genetic makeup plays a profound role in his or lipid metabolism and resulting risk for complications. In the well-characterized but relatively rare familial dyslipidemias, single-gene mutations result in a faulty apoprotein, receptor, or enzyme and a particular pattern of dyslipidemia. The most common of these is familial hypercholesterolemia, which is caused by a defect in the gene for the LDL receptor and results in very high levels of serum cholesterol, sometimes over 500 mg/dl. Familial hypertriglyceridemia, familial combined hyperlipidemia, and the other familial hyperlipidemia syndromes are even rarer.

Most individuals with hyperlipidemia do not fit into one of these classic genetic syndromes. Nonetheless, more subtle genetic factors influence their lipid metabolism and predispose them to unfavorable lipid profiles, particularly when exposed to an unhealthy diet and physical inactivity.

Role of Diet and Exercise

Diet and exercise play a significant role in the cause and treatment of lipid disorders. Dietary cholesterol and fats, especially saturated fats, have been identified as factors that contribute to hyperlipidemia. These dietary factors work by down-regulating LDL receptors, resulting in a slowing of the breakdown of LDL particles and increased concentrations in the blood. Obesity is associated with elevated triglycerides, and physical inactivity with low HDL.

Dietary cholesterol is derived only from animal products. Of that which is consumed, 40% is absorbed, contributing to an increase in the endogenous cholesterol and raising total and LDL cholesterol levels in the plasma. It is estimated that for every 100 mg of dietary cholesterol per 1000 calories consumed per day, the serum cholesterol will increase 6 to 10 mg/dl.

There are three major types of dietary fats: saturated, monounsaturated, and polyunsaturated. Each subtype exerts different influences on lipid metabolism, with saturated fats being the most harmful. Saturated fats increase blood cholesterol levels significantly more than dietary cholesterol. Reducing saturated fats in the diet from 14% to 7% of total calories can decrease total blood cholesterol levels by close to 20 mg/dl. Within this category are a number of subtypes (based on the number of carbon bonds), not all of which adversely affect the lipid profile. Unfortunately, the major source of saturated fats in the American diet is from palmitic acid, which does increase lipid levels and is found in meats, eggs, and dairy products. Certain vegetable oils, namely tropical oils such as palm and coconut oil, are highly saturated; raise serum cholesterol significantly; and are typically found in commercially prepared cakes, muffins, cookies, and other baked goods.

Monounsaturated fats are derived from animal and plant oils. The most frequent sources of monounsaturated fats in the American diet are peanuts, olives, avocados, and almonds. Monounsaturated fats do not by themselves raise or lower cholesterol levels but have been shown to help preserve baseline HDL levels when substituted for other fats. Their inclusion is a major feature of the popular Mediterranean diet.

Polyunsaturated fats are considered essential fatty acids because they cannot be synthesized by the body, unlike the saturated and monounsaturated fatty acids. Polyunsaturated fats are derived from vegetable oils consisting of ω-3 fatty acids or ω-6 fatty acids found in fish products. Dietary fish oils have been shown to lower total cholesterol and LDL levels while also lowering HDL levels.

There has been recent evidence for the negative effect of a particular form of unsaturated fats called *trans*–fatty acids.[5] These arise from vegetable oils that are undergoing extensive chemical processing or exposure to excess heat. The most common sources in the American diet are margarine spreads, with the stick form being more concentrated than the tub form. They are also found in commercially produced baked goods and deep fried foods.

The sedentary lifestyle assumed by many Americans has increased the incidence of obesity and hyperlipidemia, and both weight reduction and exercise have shown to decrease LDL and raise HDL. Despite apparent increased awareness of healthy lifestyle choices in the United States, obesity has been on the rise since 1960 and is now considered an epidemic. More than 60% of American adults are overweight or obese, which is more than double the incidence in 1980. Obesity causes an increase in total and LDL cholesterol by decreasing LDL receptor activity. Obesity also decreases HDL cholesterol by increasing triglyceride levels through a mechanism considered more atherogenic than the triglyceride-raising effect of a high-carbohydrate diet or high alcohol intake. Weighing just 9 kg (20 pounds) over one's ideal body weight can increase LDL cholesterol by 10 mg/dl and decrease HDL cholesterol by 3 mg/dl, resulting in a 16% increased risk for the development of CVD.[6,7]

Insulin Resistance, Diabetes, and Metabolic Syndrome

Adult-onset or type 2 diabetes appears to stem from a combination of factors, including progressive insulin resistance and inadequate insulin supply. Insulin resistance may or may not be associated with frank diabetes or even detectable high blood glucose levels. It is strongly influenced by genetic factors and is associated with abdominal obesity. Physical inactivity and a diet high in carbohydrates are major contributing factors. Insulin resistance, together with physical inactivity and obesity, often appears as part of a larger constellation of abnormalities, including hypertension; high triglycerides; low HDL cholesterol; and small, dense LDL particles, which are thought to be particularly atherogenic. Patients with this constellation of abnormalities, labeled *the metabolic syndrome*, have a significantly increased risk for CVD (see Chapter 223).

CLINICAL EVALUATION

The NCEP is an expert panel sponsored by the National Heart, Lung, and Blood Institute that periodically reviews the available evidence and publishes guidelines on the evaluation and treatment of lipid disorders. The panel's most recent report, NCEP-ATP III, reinforces earlier guidelines in the treatment of dyslipidemias, but goes further in recommending tailoring treatment goals to patients according to their overall risk for CVD.[1] Clinical evaluation should thus include a complete medical history, with documentation of any known CVD, symptoms of exertional angina or claudication, hypertension, diet and exercise norms, smoking and alcohol use, obesity, and diabetes. Hypothyroidism and liver and renal disease affect lipid metabolism and should also be evaluated. All cardiac risk factors, including a family history of early CVD, should be reviewed with the patient.

PHYSICAL EXAMINATION

The physical examination should include accurate measurement of blood pressure and height and weight, with determination of body mass index. The waist-hip ratio should be measured, since it has been shown to be more specifically related to the development of CVD than weight alone. As the ratio increases from 1, so does the risk. A good general examination should pay specific attention to any signs of occult cardiac or vascular disease. In the occasional patient with very high cholesterol from a familial hyperlipidemia, the health care provider might find fatty deposits called xanthomas on tendons such as the Achilles and on elbows, knees, and metacarpal joints, or deposits of cholesterol called xanthelasmas on the eyelids. The presence of corneal arcus, an opaque white ring about the corneal periphery, is less predictive of a lipid disorder but should trigger further evaluation if it is seen in the young adult.

DIAGNOSTICS

The NCEP-ATP III guidelines recommend lipid screening every 5 years for all adults over 20 years of age (Figure 222-1).[1]

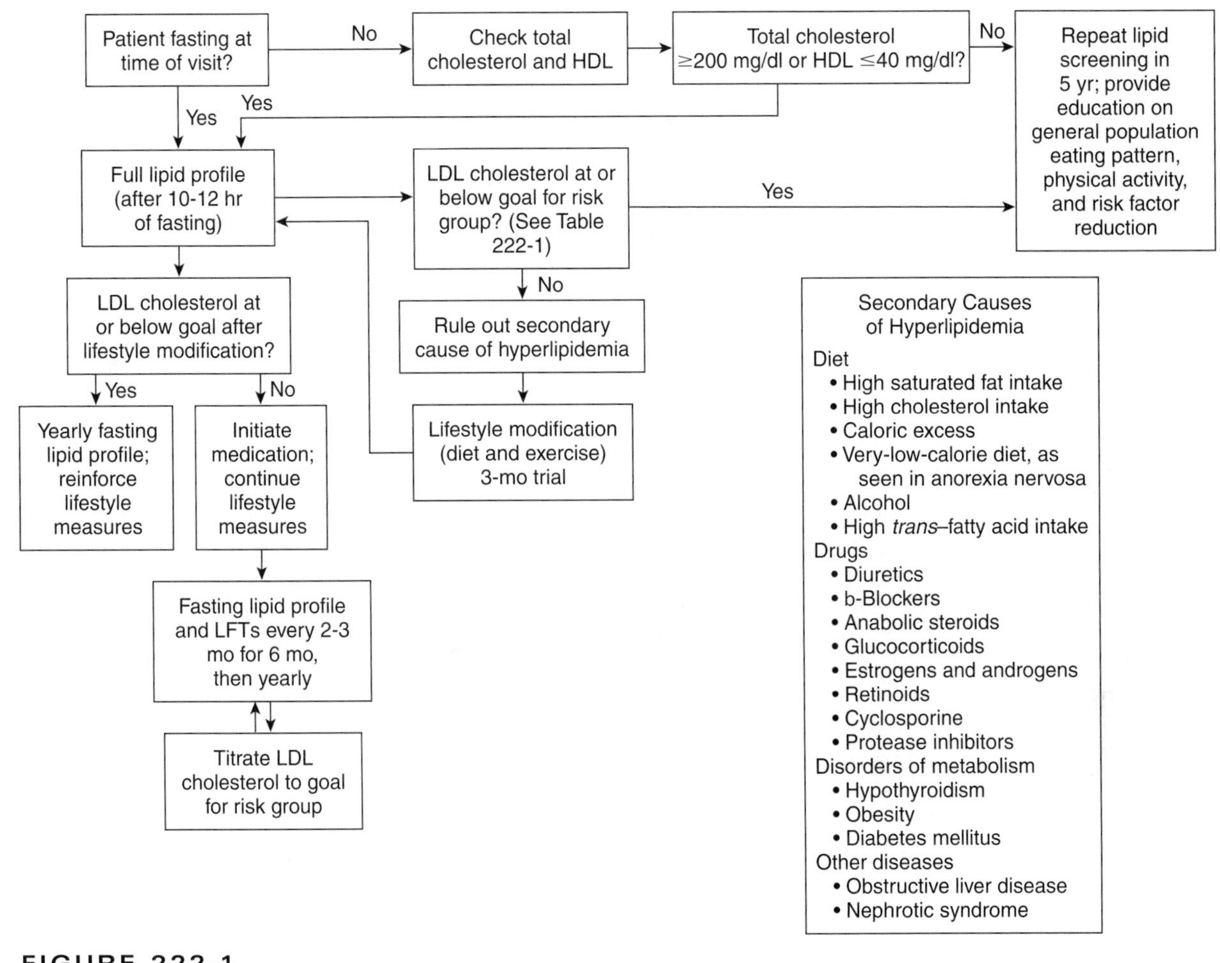

FIGURE 222-1

Screening and treatment of hyperlipidemia should be done for all adults over 20 years of age. *HDL*, High-density lipoprotein; *LDL*, low-density lipoprotein.

If possible, this should be done with a full lipid profile obtained after 10 to 12 hours of fasting. If circumstances do not allow a fasting lipid profile, then total and HDL cholesterol only can be measured with a follow-up fasting profile for those with a total cholesterol of 200 mg/dl or more or with a low HDL cholesterol (<40 mg/dl).[1]

The values in a lipid profile that are actually measured by most laboratories are total cholesterol, HDL cholesterol, and triglycerides. LDL cholesterol is then calculated from these three values according to the following equation:

LDL cholesterol = Total cholesterol − (HDL cholesterol + Triglycerides/5)

Of the three measured values, only triglycerides are significantly affected by dietary intake in the 12 hours preceding the test. This in turn affects the calculated value for LDL cholesterol. If, for whatever reason, the triglyceride level is greater than 400 mg/dl, the LDL cholesterol level cannot be accurately calculated.

Total cholesterol of 240 mg/dl or more is considered high, and 200 to 239 mg/dl is considered borderline high. HDL cholesterol of 40 mg/dl or less is considered low and is an independent risk factor for CVD. Triglyceride levels less than 150 mg/dl are considered desirable, 150 to 199 mg/dl are considered borderline high, 200 to 499 mg/dl are considered high, and 500 mg/dl or greater are considered very high. High triglycerides are also emerging as a risk factor for CVD, particularly when associated with low HDL.

> **DIAGNOSTICS**
>
> **Lipid Disorders**
>
> **LABORATORY**
>
> Cholesterol (random total and high-density lipoprotein [HDL]) every 5 years for all adults >20 years
>
> Lipid profile (10- to 12-hour fasting if total cholesterol is high, if borderline and two or more cardiovascular disease [CVD] risk factors are present, or if HDL cholesterol is <35 mg/dl or overt CVD is present)

Elevated LDL cholesterol is the lipid abnormality most closely associated with the development of CVD, and reduction in LDL cholesterol has been clearly demonstrated to have a dramatic impact on morbidity and mortality. LDL cholesterol remains the primary target of therapy. Decisions to treat elevated LDL cholesterol should prompt a comprehensive assessment of the individual patient's risk for CVD, the initiation of TLCs, and appropriate drug therapy. The desired LDL cholesterol level for a patient depends on an individual risk assessment and is discussed further in the management section.

DIFFERENTIAL DIAGNOSIS

Lipid Disorders

PRIMARY DISORDERS
Familial disorders

SECONDARY DISORDERS
Diet
- High saturated fat intake
- High cholesterol intake
- Caloric excess
- Very low–calorie diet, as seen in anorexia nervosa
- Alcohol
- High *trans*-fatty acid intake

Drugs
- Diuretics
- Beta blockers
- Anabolic steroids
- Glucosteroids
- Estrogens and androgens
- Retinoids
- Cyclosporine
- Protease inhibitors

Disorders of metabolism
- Hypothyroidism
- Obesity
- Diabetes mellitus

Other diseases
- Obstructive liver disease
- Nephrotic syndrome

DIFFERENTIAL DIAGNOSIS

Before embarking on therapy for a dyslipidemia, the health care provider should consider other factors that may influence lipid metabolism. Diet, particularly excesses in overall caloric intake, saturated fat, and dietary cholesterol, can have a profound effect on the lipid profile. In addition, starvation states such as anorexia nervosa can cause an elevation in total serum cholesterol. Overuse of alcohol is associated with hypertriglyceridemia.

The other major causes of secondary dyslipidemia are drugs, disorders of metabolism, and certain disease states. Drugs can affect lipid metabolism in a variety of ways. Glucocorticoids and estrogens have been shown to elevate triglyceride and HDL levels, although anabolic steroids can markedly reduce HDL levels. Thiazide diuretics have been shown to raise total cholesterol, triglyceride, and LDL levels. Alpha blockers may cause increases in HDL, whereas beta blockers can decrease HDL levels and increase triglyceride levels. Angiotensin-converting enzyme inhibitors and calcium channel blockers are thought to be lipid neutral. Elevation of total cholesterol and triglyceride levels is now being reported with the use of protease inhibitors in the treatment of HIV infection. Whether the use of these drugs over time will increase the risk for the development of CVD remains to be seen.

By far the most common metabolic disorders associated with lipid abnormalities are hypothyroidism and diabetes. Therefore a screening test for thyroid-stimulating hormone (TSH) and fasting glucose should be obtained when abnormalities in the lipid profile are discovered. Stabilization to a euthyroid state should be achieved before initiation of lipid treatment. In diabetics, achieving adequate glycemic control will improve the lipid profile and is an integral component of therapy. Other disease states such as the nephrotic syndrome and obstructive liver disease can also cause lipid abnormalities and can be excluded by a thorough medical history; physical examination; and, if appropriate, laboratory tests, including a urinalysis, BUN, creatinine, and liver function tests (LFTs).

MANAGEMENT

There is clear evidence that lowering elevated LDL cholesterol will reduce the risk for new CVD events both in patients without known CVD (primary prevention) and in those with known, preexisting CVD (secondary prevention). Treatment recommendations emphasize grouping patients into more specific categories of risk for cardiac events and tailoring their management accordingly.[1]

Risk Assessment

The NCEP-ATP III recommendations group patients into three categories of risk for CVD and assign each group specific goals for LDL cholesterol. Those with the highest risk for CVD are treated most aggressively.[1]

Patients in the category of highest risk generally have more than a 20% risk for an acute cardiac event in the next 10 years. This category consists of those patients with known CVD and those with a CVD "risk equivalent," or a condition that may yield an equally high risk for a new cardiac event (Figure 222-2). These conditions include other known atherosclerotic diseases such as peripheral vascular disease, aortic aneurysm, or cerebrovascular disease, as well as diabetes. The LDL cholesterol goal for patients in this highest risk category is 70 mg/dl or less. Patients in this group who have LDL cholesterol greater than 100 mg/dl are almost certain to require drug therapy. Those with LDL cholesterol levels between 70 and 100 mg/dl may be initially treated with lifestyle modification, but many advocate early initiation of drug therapy for all patients in this group with LDL cholesterol over 70 mg/dl (Table 222-1).

The intermediate risk category consists of patients with two or more major risk factors for CVD other than diabetes (see Figure 222-2). Patients in this category generally have a 10-year risk for a CVD event of 20% or less. Their goal for LDL cholesterol is less than 130 mg/dl, but decisions about when to initiate drug therapy and when to use lifestyle modification alone may require a more detailed risk assessment. Table 222-2, which is derived from data from the Framingham Heart Study, quantifies patients' 10-year risk for a new CVD event according to a point scoring system based on multiple risk factors. For patients with two or more risk factors and a 10-year risk for a cardiac event between 10% and 20%, lifestyle modification and drug therapy should be considered for all patients with LDL cholesterol of 70 mg/dl or more. The goal for therapy is less than 70 mg/dl. For those with two or more risk factors but a 10-year cardiac risk of less than 10%, the goal remains for LDL cholesterol less than 100 mg/dl. Lifestyle modification should be instituted for LDL cholesterol levels above this. It is reasonable to avoid the use of cholesterol-lowering medication unless the LDL cholesterol level is 160 mg/dl or more.

The category of lowest risk for CVD consists of patients with zero or one major risk factors. They generally have a 10-year risk for a CVD event of 10% or less. Their LDL cholesterol goal is less than 160 mg/dl, but it is reasonable to avoid medication unless their LDL cholesterol level is 190 mg/dl or greater. Although patients in this group have a relatively low 10-year risk for cardiac events, attention must also be paid to their risk for CVD beyond 10 years. This is more difficult to quantify and more difficult to balance against the risks and costs of long-term drug therapy. It is reasonable, though, to initiate lifestyle modification in these patients even with modest elevation of LDL cholesterol (≥130 mg/dl) to reduce their long-term risk of CVD.

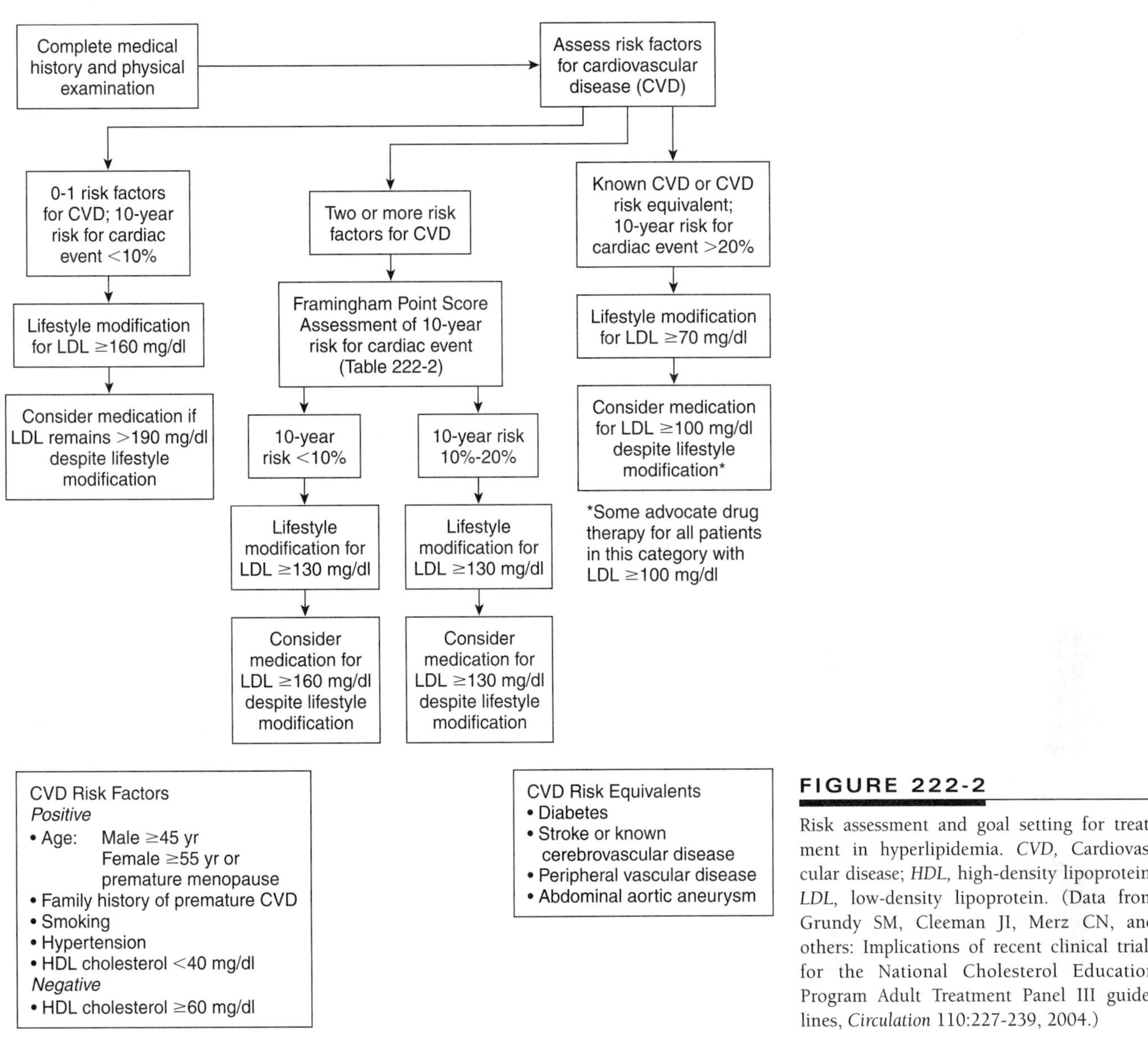

FIGURE 222-2

Risk assessment and goal setting for treatment in hyperlipidemia. *CVD,* Cardiovascular disease; *HDL,* high-density lipoprotein; *LDL,* low-density lipoprotein. (Data from Grundy SM, Cleeman JI, Merz CN, and others: Implications of recent clinical trials for the National Cholesterol Education Program Adult Treatment Panel III guidelines, *Circulation* 110:227-239, 2004.)

Lifestyle Modification

Despite increasing awareness of the importance of diet, exercise, and weight control, obesity in the United States is at an all time high. Many patients, even without hyperlipidemia, would benefit from dietary modification and increased activity. Patients with hyperlipidemia can clearly benefit from such changes.

Diet. Maximum dietary therapy will typically achieve a reduction in LDL cholesterol by 15 to 25 mg/dl, but a healthy balanced diet, exercise, and maintenance of an ideal body weight have benefits well beyond this reduction. Such benefits include a decreased tendency toward other cardiac risk factors, including hypertension, insulin resistance, and diabetes.

Our understanding of the impact of diet on blood lipid levels and cardiac risk is constantly evolving. There has been some evidence that a very low–fat diet (i.e., <10% of calories coming from fat) in conjunction with other lifestyle changes such as exercise, yoga, and meditation can reverse CVD. This degree of restriction, however, is impractical for most patients. Until recently, standard dietary recommendations were to limit total dietary fat to 30% of total calories and saturated fat to 10%. Newer dietary recommendations include a slightly more liberal limit on total fat of 25% to 35% of total calories, with increased restriction of saturated fat to 7%. Saturated fats are primarily found in animal products such as meat and dairy, but also are found in certain vegetable oils such as palm and coconut.

Dietary fat should, whenever possible, be the unsaturated fat found in most vegetable oils and, in particular, the monounsaturated fat found in olive oil and nuts. Evidence for this dietary strategy comes partly from study of the Mediterranean diet. Long known for their lower CVD rates, the populations of countries bordering this sea, such as Italy and Greece, typically have dietary fat intakes equal to or even higher than those of the populations of countries with high rates of CVD. Their consumption of saturated fats, however, is lower, and a higher intake of monounsaturated fats, from olives and olive oil,

TABLE 222-1 NCEP-ATP III LDL Cholesterol Goals and Cutpoints

Risk Category	LDL Cholesterol Goal	Initiate TLC	Consider Drug Therapy[a]
High risk: CVD[b] or CVD risk equivalents[c] (10-year risk >20%)	<100 mg/dl (optional goal: <70 mg/dl)[d]	≥100 mg/dl[e]	≥100 mg/dl[f] (<100 mg/dl: consider drug options)[a]
Moderately high risk: 2+ risk factors[g] (10-year risk 10%-20%)[h]	<130 mg/dl[i]	≥130 mg/dl[e]	≥130 mg/dl (100-129 mg/dl: consider drug options)[j]
Moderate risk: 2+ risk factors[g] (10-year risk <10%)[h]	<130 mg/dl	≥130 mg/dl	≥160 mg/dl
Lower risk: 0-1 risk factor[k]	<160 mg/dl	≥160 mg/dl	≥190 mg/dl (160-189 mg/dl: LDL-lowering drug optional)

From Grundy SM, Cleeman JI, Merz CN, and others: Implications of recent clinical trials for the National Cholesterol Education Program Adult Treatment Panel III guidelines, *Circulation* 110:227-239, 2004.

CVD, Cardiovascular disease; *LDL,* low-density lipoprotein; *TLC,* therapeutic lifestyle changes;

[a]When LDL-lowering drug therapy is employed, it is advised that intensity of therapy be sufficient to achieve at least a 30%-40% reduction in LDL cholesterol levels.

[b]CVD includes history of myocardial infarction, unstable angina, stable angina, or coronary artery procedures (angioplasty or bypass surgery) or evidence of clinically significant myocardial ischemia.

[c]CVD risk equivalents include clinical manifestations of noncoronary forms of atherosclerotic disease (peripheral arterial disease, abdominal aortic aneurysm, and carotid artery disease [transient ischemic attacks or stroke of carotid origin or >50% obstruction of a carotid artery]), diabetes, and 2+ risk factors with 10-year risk for hard CVD >20%.

[d]Very high risk favors the optional LDL cholesterol goal of <70 mg/dl and, in patients with high triglycerides, non-HDL <100 mg/dl.

[e]Any person at high risk or moderately high risk who has lifestyle-related risk factors (e.g., obesity, physical inactivity, elevated triglyceride, low HDL cholesterol, or metabolic syndrome) is a candidate for TLCs to modify these risk factors regardless of LDL cholesterol level.

[f]If baseline LDL cholesterol is <100 mg/dl, institution of an LDL-lowering drug is a therapeutic option on the basis of available clinical trial results. If a high-risk person has high triglycerides or low HDL cholesterol, combining a fibrate or nicotinic acid with an LDL-lowering drug can be considered.

[g]Risk factors include cigarette smoking, hypertension (blood pressure ≥140/90 mm Hg or on antihypertensive medication), low HDL cholesterol (<40 mg/dl), family history of premature CVD (CVD in male first-degree relative <55 years of age; CVD in female first-degree relative <65 years of age), and age (men ≥45 years; women ≥55 years).

[h]Electronic 10-year risk calculators are available at http://www.nhlbi.nih.gov/guidelines/cholesterol.

[i]Optional LDL goal <100 mg/dl.

[j]For moderately high-risk persons, when LDL is 100-129 mg/dl, at baseline or on lifestyle therapy, initiation of an LDL-lowering drug to achieve an LDL <100 mg/dl is a therapeutic option on the basis of available clinical trial results.

[k]Almost all people with 0 or 1 risk factor have a 10-year risk <10%, and thus a 10-year risk assessment is not necessary.

contributes to their increased intake of fat. It is postulated that this diet helps increase HDL and lower LDL cholesterol, thus decreasing the risk for CVD.

There is recent evidence that *trans*–fatty acids, which arise from excessive processing, are also atherogenic.[5] *Trans*–fatty acids are found in margarine spreads, commercially produced baked goods, and deep-fried foods. They should be avoided when possible. Some data support the use of new "cholesterol-lowering" margarine products enriched with plant sterols and stanols, which inhibit the absorption of dietary cholesterol. The long-term safety of these products is currently being studied.

Actual cholesterol in the diet tends to be less detrimental to the lipid profile than saturated fats, and products labeled "low in cholesterol" often mislead patients. Nonetheless, dietary cholesterol does affect serum cholesterol and should be limited to 200 mg/day.

Replacement for fats should come from complex carbohydrates with added emphasis on increasing fiber in the diet to 20 to 30 g/day through the consumption of whole-grain breads and cereals, along with fresh fruits and vegetables. Increased dietary fiber appears to have a direct effect on lowering serum cholesterol.

Food products in the United States are labeled with nutritional information, including the amount of total fat, saturated fat, cholesterol, and dietary fiber. This labeling and the increased awareness of nutrition in our society allow for monitoring of dietary intake and foster adherence to dietary guidelines. For many patients, however, difficulties arise not only with food selection, but also with portion control. Referral to a qualified nutritionist can help patients understand nutrition and meet and maintain their dietary goals.

Exercise. The importance of physical activity cannot be overemphasized. Multiple studies have demonstrated that regular aerobic exercise increases HDL cholesterol and decreases total and LDL cholesterol and triglyceride levels.[6] Regular aerobic exercise can also modulate and improve control of frequent co-existing risk factors such as obesity, hypertension, and insulin resistance. With exercise there is up-regulation of insulin receptors on the cell membrane, thus decreasing the risk for the development of diabetes. Therefore exercise, whenever possible, should be included in the treatment of high blood cholesterol.

All patients with known CVD embarking on a new exercise regimen should have a recent exercise tolerance test and, based on the results, an appropriate, prescribed exercise program. Consideration for exercise testing in individuals with two or more cardiovascular risk factors should be based on the clinical evaluation and the level of exercise intensity to be performed. Low to moderate expenditure, such as moderate walking, can be safely recommended to most asymptomatic individuals without the need for or expense of an exercise test. Even low level activity can have a dramatic impact on health

TABLE 222-2 Point Scoring System for Cardiovascular Disease Risk

ESTIMATE OF 10-YEAR RISK FOR MEN (FRAMINGHAM POINT SCORES)

Age (years)	Points	Age (years)	Points
20-34	−9	55-59	8
35-39	−4	60-64	10
40-44	0	65-69	11
45-49	3	70-74	12
50-54	5	75-79	13

	Points				
Total Cholesterol (mg/dl)	**Age 20-39 Years**	**Age 40-49 Years**	**Age 50-59 Years**	**Age 60-69 Years**	**Age 70-79 Years**
<160	0	0	0	0	0
160-199	4	3	2	1	0
200-239	7	5	3	1	0
240-279	9	6	4	2	1
≥280	11	8	5	3	1

	Points				
Total Cholesterol (mg/dl)	**Age 20-39 Years**	**Age 40-49 Years**	**Age 50-59 Years**	**Age 60-69 Years**	**Age 70-79 Years**
Nonsmoker	0	0	0	0	0
Smoker	8	5	3	1	1

HDL (mg/dl)	Points
≥60	−1
50-59	0
40-49	1
<40	2

Systolic Blood Pressure (mm Hg)	If Untreated	If Treated
<120	0	0
120-129	0	1
130-139	1	2
140-159	1	2
≥160	2	3

Point Total	10-Year Risk (%)	Point Total	10-Year Risk (%)
<0	<1	9	5
0	1	10	6
1	1	11	8
2	1	12	10
3	1	13	12
4	1	14	16
5	2	15	20
6	2	16	25
7	3	≥17	30
8	4		

ESTIMATE OF 10-YEAR RISK FOR WOMEN (FRAMINGHAM POINT SCORES)

Age (years)	Points	Age (years)	Points
20-34	−7	55-59	8
35-39	−3	60-64	10
40-44	0	65-69	12
45-49	3	70-74	14
50-54	6	75-79	16

	Points				
Total Cholesterol (mg/dl)	**Age 20-39 Years**	**Age 40-49 Years**	**Age 50-59 Years**	**Age 60-69 Years**	**Age 70-79 Years**
<160	0	0	0	0	0
160-199	4	3	2	1	1
200-239	8	6	4	2	1
240-279	11	8	5	3	2
≥280	13	10	7	4	2

	Points				
Total Cholesterol (mg/dl)	**Age 20-39 Years**	**Age 40-49 Years**	**Age 50-59 Years**	**Age 60-69 Years**	**Age 70-79 Years**
Nonsmoker	0	0	0	0	0
Smoker	9	7	4	2	1

HDL (mg/dl)	Points
≥60	−1
50-59	0
40-49	1
<40	2

Systolic Blood Pressure (mm Hg)	If Untreated	If Treated
<120	0	0
120-129	1	3
130-139	2	4
140-159	3	5
≥160	4	8

Point Total	10-Year Risk (%)	Point Total	10-Year Risk (%)
<9	<1	17	5
9	1	18	6
10	1	19	8
11	1	20	11
12	1	21	14
13	2	22	17
14	2	23	22
15	3	24	27
16	4	≥25	≥30

From Expert Panel on Detection, Evaluation, and Treatment of High Blood Cholesterol in Adults: Executive summary of the Third Report of the National Cholesterol Education (NCEP) Expert Panel on Detection, Evaluation, and Treatment of High Blood cholesterol in Adults (Adult Treatment Panel III), *JAMA* 265:2486-2497, 2001.
HDL, High-density lipoprotein.

when performed regularly. When a more intensive exercise program is being considered, an exercise test should be obtained, especially for those with multiple risk factors or individuals who have been sedentary. Patients should be encouraged to start slowly and increase their intensity and duration of exercise gradually over several weeks, with the goal of doing moderate exercise for at least 30 minutes 4 or 5 days per week.

Other Risk Factors. The presence of hyperlipidemia can be used as an opportunity to stress the importance of cessation of tobacco use. Tobacco, when combined with other risk factors, dramatically increases the overall risk for CVD. Hypertension and diabetes should also be well controlled to improve overall health outcomes.

Pharmacotherapy

Despite adherence to a prudent diet and exercise program, many will not achieve adequate LDL lowering without the addition of lipid-lowering medications. As described above and outlined in Table 222-1, the recommendation for instituting lipid-lowering drugs, and the goals of therapy, should be based on the presence or absence of other risk factors.

A number of medications are available for the treatment of lipid disorders. These are listed in Table 222-3, along with their expected lipid-lowering potential and side effect profiles. The general drug categories are 5-hydroxy-3-methylglutaryl–coenzyme A (HMG-CoA) reductase inhibitors, or statins; bile acid sequestrants, or resins; nicotinic acid (niacin); fibrates; cholesterol absorption inhibitors; and liposoluble antioxidants.

The most effective and best tolerated drugs for lowering LDL cholesterol are the statins. They also increase HDL cholesterol and decrease triglyceride levels. These are generally the first-line agents for lipid lowering. Several large scale randomized controlled trials have demonstrated dramatic reductions in morbidity and mortality from cardiac events with the use of these agents.[8-12] There is a 1% incidence of hepatic inflammation, and for this reason the liver transaminases, aspartate transaminase and alanine transaminase, should be checked before initiating treatment and monitored every 2 to 3 months for the first 6 months and then every 6 to 12 months thereafter. For elevations in the transaminases of two to two and a half times normal during therapy, treatment should be changed and sources of co-morbid liver toxicity such as alcohol excluded. A rare but serious adverse reaction to the statins is drug-induced myopathy, which can range from mild myalgias to severe muscle breakdown or rhabdomyolysis with the potential for subsequent acute renal failure. Patients taking statins who complain of new muscle pain should have a creatine phosphokinase (CPK) level checked to rule out muscle breakdown. If the CPK is elevated, the drug should be discontinued and the patient monitored for potential renal dysfunction. In the absence of symptoms it is not necessary to routinely monitor CPK.

Recent landmark studies have shown that higher doses of statins are most effective in achieving goal LDL.[7,8] The PROVE IT trial demonstrated the efficacy of early intensive statin therapy in patents with acute myocardial infarction (MI) or unstable angina. Aggressive lipid-lowering therapy initiated at discharge for patients with ACS reduced the risk of long-term cardiovascular outcomes, compared with lower dosage therapy. This trial randomized patients to 80 mg atorvastatin vs. 40 mg pravastatin daily and found that the primary endpoint—all-cause mortality, MI, unstable angina requiring hospitalization, revascularization, or stroke—was reduced in patients receiving 80 mg atorvastatin. Recommendations from this study included using high-dose statins on all patients with ACS and lowering LDL to 70 mg/dl or less.[8]

The ALLHAT study was designed to evaluate treatment of hypertension. A subset of the trial evaluated whether pravastatin therapy reduced all-cause mortality in older patients with moderate hyperlipidemia and hypertension, with one additional risk factor. Total cholesterol results were reduced by 17% for the pravastatin group, vs. 8% for the usual care group. Cardiovascular event rates were not significantly different, except in the African-American subgroup.[10]

The ASCOT-LLA study evaluated more than 19,000 patients and treated them with atorvastatin 10 mg or placebo, randomly. The primary endpoint was nonfatal MI and fatal CVD. At 3.3 years the atorvastatin group had significantly lower primary events than the placebo group. The study was terminated prematurely and indicated that LDL lowering with atorvastatin has great potential to reduce risk for CVD in primary prevention in patients with multiple CVD risk factors.[11]

The Heart Protection Study evaluated more than 20,000 patients at high risk for a CVD event. Simvastatin 40 mg or placebo was randomly assigned. Primary outcomes were total mortality. In the group receiving simvastatin, all-cause mortality was reduced by 13%, and major vascular events were reduced by 24%, coronary death rate by 18%, nonfatal MI and coronary death by 27%, stroke by 25%, and cardiovascular revascularization by 24%. No significant adverse events were recorded, again strongly suggesting the importance of statin therapy.[12]

Bile acid sequestrants (resins) such as cholestyramine have been demonstrated to be safe and effective in lowering LDL modestly when used singularly and can further lower LDL when combined with HMG-CoA reductase inhibitors. They represent a safe alternative to statins in patients with liver disease or those who have had an adverse reaction.

Nicotinic acid (niacin) has good LDL- and triglyceride-lowering and HDL-raising effects. It has been shown to reduce overall mortality rates in secondary prevention trials.[13] It is widely available at reasonable cost in sustained- and immediate-release formulations. Unfortunately, its use is limited by unpleasant side effects, including flushing, itching, rash, and gastrointestinal upset. In rare cases liver toxicity, hyperuricemia, and glucose intolerance have occurred. The frequency and intensity of side effects are usually dose related and can be blunted by the use of sustained-release formulations. With anticipatory guidance, gradual escalation to the mid-range doses of 2 to 3 g/day in divided doses, and pretreatment with aspirin, niacin represents an effective and inexpensive option.

The fibric acids, such as gemfibrozil, are effective in lowering triglycerides and can raise HDL cholesterol. Because

TABLE 222-3 Expected Lipid-Lowering Effects and Side Effects of Available Agents

Drug	Dose/Day	Total Cholesterol	LDL Cholesterol	HDL Cholesterol	Triglycerides	Side Effects	Patient Education
Statins							
Lovastatin (Mevacor)	20-80 mg	↓15%-30%	↓20%-40%	↑5%-10%	↓10%-19%	Well tolerated as a class	Take with evening meal, since most cholesterol is made in evening hours.
Pravastatin (Pravachol)	10-40 mg	↓15%-30%	↓20%-30%	↑5%-10%	↓10%-15%	Increase in transaminases in 1% of patients	Have regular laboratory measurement for efficacy and safety.
Simvastatin (Zocor)	5-80 mg	↓20%-30%	↓23%-40%	↑6%-12%	↓10%-20%	Rare episode of myopathy with or without associated rhabdomyolysis	Call and report any unexplained muscle pains, tenderness, or weakness.
Fluvastatin (Lescol)	20-80 mg	↓20%-30%	↓20%-32%	—	—	Infrequent GI upset, constipation, rash, headaches	Avoid grapefruit juice.
Atorvastatin (Lipitor)	10-80 mg	↓27%-40%	↓36%-60%	↑7%-12%	↓17%-30%		
Rosuvastatin (Crestor)	5-40 mg	—	↓45%-63%	↑8%-12%	↓10%-35%	Asian population may experience a twofold elevation in median exposure to rosuvastatin; consider lower starting dose.	
Cholesterol absorption inhibitors							
Ezetimibe (Zetia)	10 mg	↓13%	↓18%	↑1%	↓8%		
Combination drug (statin with ezetimibe): ezetimibe-simvastatin (Vytorin)	10-10 mg 10-20 mg 10-40 mg 10-80 mg		↓39%-56%				Avoid in patients with moderate to severe hepatic impairment.
Fibric acids							
Gemfibrozil (Lopid)	600-1200 mg	↓6%	↓10%	↑10% (if HDL <35%, ↑25%)	↓35%	LFT abnormality Muscle aches Abdominal pain	Take 30 minutes before breakfast and dinner. Have regular laboratory measurements of efficacy and safety.
Fenofibrite (Tricor)	48 or 145 mg				↑30%		Avoid in patients with renal failure.
Resins	4-24 g	↓10%	↓25%	None	10% of patients will have ↑	Indigestion, bloating, gas, constipation	Mix with uncarbonated liquid. Add high-fiber foods to diet. Drink plenty of fluids. Start with lowest dose and advance as tolerated. Need to take resins 1 hour before or 4 hours after other medication.
Cholestyramine	4-16 g						
Colestipol	5-20 g						
Colesevelam	1.5-3.75 g						
Niacin	2-3 g	↓10%-25%	↓20%-40%	↑15%-30%	↓45%-50%	Flushing, itching, rash, GI upset Increases in glucose, uric acid, and transaminases	Take with aspirin. Avoid taking with hot fluids and ETOH. Start with low dose and increase gradually over several weeks. Call if prolonged nausea occurs. Monitor with laboratory tests.

GI, Gastrointestinal.

their effects at lowering LDL cholesterol are modest, they should be reserved for individuals with very high triglyceride levels. They may be beneficial in patients with metabolic syndrome. Fibrates can also occasionally cause liver toxicity and require monitoring of LFTs.

The newest drugs, cholesterol absorption inhibitors, are especially useful for patients who cannot tolerate statins or who would benefit from combination therapy in an effort to reach goal LDL.

Combining therapy is useful when single drug use and TLC do not achieve LDL goals. The addition of a bile acid sequestrant to a statin can reduce LDL cholesterol by an additional 10%. The combination of two systemic lipid-lowering drugs (e.g., niacin with a statin,[13] or gemfibrozil with a statin) can lead to increased frequency of side effects. LDL cholesterol should be monitored every 6 months when therapy is initiated or doses are changed. Once goal LDL is achieved, monitoring every 6 to 12 months is reasonable.

Pharmacotherapy for Specific Populations

Younger Adults. Premenopausal women and men less than 35 years of age have a relatively low short-term risk of CVD events. As a result, there has been no clear evidence that they will benefit from pharmacologic treatment for high cholesterol. It is, however, known that atherosclerosis begins early in life and that young adults with high cholesterol are predisposed to CVD later in life. It is recommended that younger adults be screened for high cholesterol. This can be used as an opportunity for counseling regarding diet, exercise, weight control, and other risk factors such as tobacco use. Drug therapy in women under 45 and men under 35 years of age should be reserved for those with LDL cholesterol levels of 190 mg/dl or more despite maximum lifestyle modification, or those with other risk factors. Committing a young adult to lifelong drug therapy is a major decision, and consultation with a physician is reasonable.

Middle-Aged Men. The benefits of lowering cholesterol in terms of lowering the risk for CVD had been most clearly demonstrated in men between the ages of 35 and 65. Men in this age-group also have particularly high prevalence of obesity, hypertension, and tobacco use. They should be targeted for aggressive lifestyle modification, lipid screening, and drug therapy when appropriate.

Middle-Aged Women. CVD is often perceived as a disease more prevalent in men, but half of all CVD deaths are in women, and CVD is the leading cause of death in women over the age of 50. The main difference between the sexes is that the onset of CVD in women occurs on average 10 to 15 years later than in men, and rarely before menopause. Women between the ages of 45 and 75 years should be screened and treated, if necessary, for high cholesterol.[14]

For many years it was believed that the presence of estrogen in women's premenopausal years had a protective effect against the development of CVD. For this reason it was widely assumed that estrogen replacement therapy (ERT) in postmenopausal women reduced morbidity and mortality from CVD, and this appeared to be borne out in early clinical trials. In fact, ERT does appear to confer a modest reduction in LDL cholesterol and an increase in HDL cholesterol, but it also appears to increase triglycerides, which, particularly in women, have been shown to be an independent risk factor for CVD. In addition, ERT is associated with an increased risk of the development of blood clots and gallbladder disease and perhaps also a small increased risk of breast cancer. A recent, more comprehensive clinical trial has not shown a benefit in CVD mortality for women taking ERT, and in fact there is a possible trend towards increased mortality early in the course of treatment. The benefits of ERT include protection against osteoporosis and decrease in the symptoms of menopause. Decisions about initiating ERT should include a careful assessment of these factors, but it should not be advocated to reduce CVD risk or overall mortality.[15]

The management of hyperlipidemia in middle-aged women should focus on lifestyle modification and pharmacologic therapy with lipid-lowering medication when indicated according to the standards outlined above. Use of Table 222-2 to quantify the actual risk for the development of CVD will be helpful in directing therapy.

Older Adults. The risk reduction associated with lowering LDL cholesterol appears to persist regardless of age.[16] Decisions regarding treatment in this group should be made on an individual basis, taking the patient's entire clinical situation into account, but lowering cholesterol whether by lifestyle modification or medication is an important aspect of complete medical care.

Metabolic Syndrome. Patients with insulin resistance with or without frank diabetes, and the syndrome of abdominal obesity, physical inactivity, high triglycerides, and low HDL cholesterol, are clearly at increased risk for CVD. It is essential in these patients to work aggressively toward increased physical activity, improvement in diet, and weight loss. Achieving good glycemic control, as always, should be a priority and may lead to improvement in the lipid profile. These patients should be targeted for aggressive treatment of LDL cholesterol even though this may not be the most prominent abnormality in their lipid profile (see Chapter 223).

INDICATIONS FOR REFERRAL

The treatment of lipid disorders for most individuals will not necessitate referral to a specialist. In cases where a primary genetic lipid disorder is suspected, when recommended treatment plans are not successful in achieving treatment goals, when co-morbid conditions such as liver disease limit therapy, or when combination therapy is not successful, referral to a physician or lipid specialty clinic is recommended.

PATIENT EDUCATION

A patient's clear understanding of the essential role of positive lifestyle choices involving diet and exercise is the foundation for the treatment of lipid disorders. Even when drug therapy is prescribed, these lifestyle behaviors should be encouraged. Lifestyle changes can involve multiple behaviors, and thus attainment should be considered a process that occurs over time with support and encouragement. Some patients fail to make behavior changes not from lack of motivation but from real or perceived barriers. Education should focus on the identification of these barriers and the development of interventions and problem-solving techniques that are meaningful and achievable for that individual. Focusing on any achievement, no matter how small, can lead to continued progress toward a healthier lifestyle. Finally, anticipatory education about the potential side effects of medication will increase the likelihood that patients will adhere to treatment plans.

REFERENCES

1. *Third report of the Expert Panel on Detection, Evaluation, and Treatment of High Blood Cholesterol in Adults (Adult Treatment Panel III)*, NIH Pub No 02-5215, Sept 2002, National Institutes of Health, retrieved June 10, 2006, from http://www.nhlbi.nih.gov/guidelines/cholesterol.
2. Grundy SM, Cleeman JI, Merz CN, and others, Coordinating Committee of the National Cholesterol Education Program: Implications of recent clinical trials for the National Cholesterol Education Program Adult Treatment Panel III, *Cardiology* 44(3):720-732, 2004.
3. Cromwell WC, Otvos JD: Low-density lipoprotein particle number and the risk for cardiovascular disease, *Curr Atheroscler Rep* 6(5):381-387, 2004.
4. Drexel H: Reducing risk by raising HDL cholesterol: the evidence. *Oxford Journals, European Heart Journal Supplements* 8(Suppl F):F23-F29, 2006, retrieved Feb 17, 2007, from http://eurheartjsupp.oxfordjournals.org/cgi/content/abstract/8/suppl_F/F23.
5. Mozaffarian D, Katan M, Ascherio A, and others: Trans fatty acids and cardiovascular disease, *N Engl J Med* 354(15):1601-1613, 2006.
6. Stefanick M, Mackey S, Sheehan M, and others: Effects of diet and exercise in men and postmenopausal women with low levels of HDL cholesterol and high levels of LDL cholesterol, *N Engl J Med* 339(1):12-20, 1998.
7. Fogoros RN: *Raising your HDL levels*, retrieved Feb 17, 2007, from http://heartdisease.about.com/cs/cholesterol/a/raiseHDL_2.htm.
8. Cannon CP, Braunwald E, McCabe CH, and others: Intensive versus moderate lipid lowering with statins after acute coronary syndromes: Pravastatin or Atorvastatin Evaluation and Infection–Thrombolysis in Myocardial Infarction 22 (PROVE IT-TIMI 22), *N Engl J Med* 350:1495-1504, 2004.
9. Nissen SE, Tuzcu EM, Schoenhagen P: Effect of intensive compared with moderate lipid-lowering therapy on progression of coronary atherosclerosis, *JAMA* 291(9):1071-1080, 2004.
10. ALLHAT officers and coordinators for the ALLHAT Collaborative Research Group: Major outcomes in moderately hypercholesterolemic, hypertensive patients randomized to pravastatin vs usual care: the Antihypertensive and Lipid-Lowering Treatment to Prevent Heart Attack Trial–Lipid-Lowering Trial (ALLHAT-LLT), *JAMA* 288:2998-3007, 2002.
11. Sever PS, Dahlof B, Poulter NR, and others: Prevention of coronary and stroke events with atorvastatin in hypertensive patients who have average or lower-than-average cholesterol concentrations: the Anglo-Scandinavian Cardiac Outcomes Trial–Lipid-Lowering Arm (ASCOT-LLA): a multicenter randomized controlled trial, *Lancet* 361:1149-1158, 2003.
12. Collins R, Armitage J, Parish S, and others, Heart Protection Study Collaborative group: MRC/BHF Heart Protection Study of cholesterol-lowering with simvastatin in 5963 people with diabetes: a randomised placebo-controlled trial, *Lancet* 361:2005-2016, 2003.
13. Brown BG, Zhao X-Q, Chait A, and others: Simvastatin and niacin, antioxidant vitamins, or the combination for the prevention of coronary disease, *N Engl J Med* 345(22):1583-1592, 2001.
14. Hardesty P, Trupp RJ: Prevention: the key to reducing cardiovascular disease risk in women, *J Cardiovasc Nurs* 20(6):433-442, 2005.
15. Martin KA, Rosen H, Rosenson R, and others: *Postmenopausal hormone therapy and cardiovascular risk*, retrieved March 25, 2006, from http://patients.uptodate.com/topic.asp?file=r_endo_f/18838&title=Hypertension+High+blood+pressure.
16. Shepherd J, Blauw GJ, Murphy MB, and others: Prospective study of pravastatin in the elderly at risk (PROSPER), *Lancet* 360:1623-1630, 2003.

CHAPTER 223

Metabolic Syndrome

Donna Jenell Pease

DEFINITION AND EPIDEMIOLOGY

Metabolic syndrome is a cluster of disorders that was first introduced by Reaven[1] in 1988 and is characterized by insulin resistance with hyperinsulinemia; hypertension; abdominal (central or visceral) obesity; and dyslipidemia consisting of hypertriglyceridemia, low high-density lipoprotein (HDL) cholesterol, and increased small, dense low-density lipoprotein (LDL) particles. More recent characteristics that have been added include elevated C-reactive protein (CRP) levels, increased plasminogen activator inhibitor-1 (PAI-1) levels, microalbuminuria, hyperuricemia, and microvascular angina.[2,3]

In 1998 the World Health Organization defined metabolic syndrome as insulin resistance and/or impaired fasting glucose or glucose intolerance or diabetes mellitus together with two or more of the following components[4]:

- Raised arterial pressure ≥160/90 mm Hg
- Raised plasma triglyceride (≥150 mg/dl or 1.7 mmol/L) and/or low HDL cholesterol (<35 mg/dl or 0.9 mmol/L for men; <39 mg/dl or 1.0 mmol/L for women) levels
- Central obesity (waist-to-hip ratio males >0.90, females 0.85; or body mass index [BMI] >30 kg/m^2)
- Microalbuminuria (urinary albumin excretion rate ≥20 mcg/min or albumin/creatinine ratio ≥20 mg/g)

The third report of the National Cholesterol Education Program's Expert Panel on Detection, Evaluation, and Treatment of High Blood Cholesterol in Adults (NCEP-ATP III) clinical identification of the metabolic syndrome includes three or more of the following components[5]:

- Abdominal obesity, given in waist circumference (men ≥102 cm [≥40 inches]; women ≥88 cm [≥35 inches])
- Triglycerides ≥150 mg/dl
- HDL cholesterol (men <40 mg/dl, women <50 mg/dl)
- Blood pressure ≥130/85 mm Hg
- Fasting glucose ≥110 mg/dl (The American Diabetes Association has recently established a cutpoint of ≥100 mg/dl, above which persons have prediabetes, impaired fasting glucose, or diabetes.)

The International Diabetes Federation consensus worldwide definition of the metabolic syndrome includes[6]:

Central obesity (defined as waist circumference ≥94 cm [37 inches] for Europid men and ≥80 cm [31 inches] for Europid women, with ethnicity-specific values for other groups) plus any two of the following four factors:

- Raised triglyceride levels: ≥150 mg/dl (1.7 mmol/L) or specific treatment for this lipid abnormality
- Reduced HDL cholesterol: <40 mg/dl (1.03 mmol/L) in males and <50 mg/dl (1.29 mmol/L) in females, or specific treatment for this lipid abnormality
- Raised blood pressure: systolic ≥130 mm Hg or diastolic ≥85 mm Hg, or treatment of previously diagnosed hypertension
- Raised fasting plasma glucose ≥100 mg/dl (5.6 mmol/L) or previously diagnosed type 2 diabetes

Not all hyperinsulinemic individuals develop all of the multiple components of this syndrome, but studies have found that the greater the number of associated characteristics an individual exhibits, the greater his or her risk of developing cardiovascular disease (CVD) or dying.[7,8] This syndrome has also been called the *insulin resistant syndrome, Reaven's syndrome, syndrome X, cardiovascular dysmetabolic syndrome,* and *deadly quartet.*[3]

Metabolic syndrome often occurs in the general population, mostly in older individuals and in certain ethnicities. It is estimated that metabolic syndrome is present in more than 20% of the U.S. adult population. The Third National Health and Nutrition Examination Survey found the highest prevalence of metabolic syndrome in Mexican Americans and the lowest in African Americans.[9] Using the Framingham Offspring Study and the San Antonio Heart Study, researchers found that the prevalence of metabolic syndrome among non-Hispanic Caucasians was over 20% and among Mexican Americans over 30%. Rates were highest among Mexican-American women and lowest among Caucasian women.[10] African Americans and Hispanics were found to be more insulin resistant than non-Hispanic Caucasians in the Insulin Resistance Atherosclerosis Study (IRAS).[11] In the United States, approximately one third of overweight or obese persons manifest the metabolic syndrome, and 25% to 35% of nonobese, normal glucose-tolerant U.S. adults have insulin resistance.[1,5]

Both genetic factors and environmental factors have been found to play a role in the incidence of metabolic syndrome. Studies have found a genetic predisposition to the syndrome and the associated cardiovascular risk factors in first-degree relatives of individuals diagnosed with type 2 diabetes.[12,13] Researchers have also found that nonobese individuals with a family history of diabetes, hypertension, or obesity are genetically predisposed to the development of metabolic syndrome.[14]

Various authors have speculated that numerous genes may be involved in this syndrome. One such theory is the "thrifty genes" theory. These thrifty genes ensure optimum storage of surplus energy as abdominal fat during periods of fasting, but when these genes are exposed to the abundance of food in the Western diet, insulin resistance develops. Genes coding for β_2- and β_3-adrenergic receptors, hormone-sensitive lipase, lipoprotein lipase (LPL), skeletal muscle glycogen synthase, and regulation of insulin signaling have also been associated with features of this syndrome.[15]

An environmental factor involved with insulin resistance and obesity is the lifestyle typical of Western civilization, consisting of a high-fat diet and low levels of physical activity. High-energy intake and low-energy output have led to the increased prevalence of obesity seen today. Some studies have shown that tissue sensitivity to insulin declines by about 30% to 40% when an individual becomes more than 35% to 40% over ideal body weight.[16] The fat cells found in abdominal obesity are larger and are more insulin resistant. Abdominal fat is also more metabolically active, and fat lipolysis occurs more often, releasing excess free fatty acids (FFAs) that interfere with hepatic insulin clearance, thus resulting in higher levels of circulating insulin. It has been found that visceral or abdominal obesity may be one of the leading causes of insulin resistance.[17] Visceral adipose tissue also releases cytokines, PAI-1, adiponectin, leptin, and resistin, which are potentially pathogenic and associated with higher CVD risk.[18]

Recently, metabolic syndrome has been recognized as a side effect of several commonly used drugs, such as corticosteroids, antidepressants, antipsychotics, and antihistamines, that can predispose an individual to obesity and glucose intolerance. Protease inhibitors used in the treatment of HIV often induce metabolic syndrome secondary to lipodystrophy and insulin resistance.[18-20]

PATHOPHYSIOLOGY

Visceral or abdominal obesity leads to insulin resistance. Insulin resistance is defined as the impaired insulin-stimulated glucose uptake by skeletal muscle, adipose tissue, or liver. The mechanisms involved in insulin resistance may consist of abnormal insulin molecules, decreased number of insulin receptors, decreased glucose transporters, and defective postreceptor activity.[3] Impairment at the receptor level is usually associated with decreased sensitivity to insulin, whereas postreceptor or cellular defects are associated with decreased responsiveness to insulin.[21] When the cells become resistant to the insulin, the body compensates by producing more insulin to overcome the resistance and to maintain normal glucose levels. Fasting hyperinsulinemia occurs in response to elevated fasting plasma glucose. This hyperinsulinemia leads to the various other abnormalities associated with metabolic syndrome; they include hypertension, dyslipidemia, atherosclerosis, microalbuminuria, proinflammatory state, prothrombotic state, and hyperuricemia.[2,3]

Hypertension

Arterial blood pressure has been found to be inversely related to insulin sensitivity and directly related to fasting plasma insulin concentration. In a retrospective analysis, the European Group for the Study of Insulin Resistance found that for each 10-unit increase in insulin resistance, systolic blood pressure was 1.7 mm Hg higher and diastolic blood pressure was 2.3 mm Hg higher.[22] This small increase is significant considering that prospective studies have found that a 2 mm Hg increase in blood pressure will produce a 17% increase in cerebrovascular disease and a 10% increase in ischemic heart disease.[22]

The hyperinsulinemia associated with insulin resistance may mediate elevated blood pressure in a number of different ways. Increases in plasma insulin concentration cause urinary sodium excretion to decline. This antinatriuretic effect of insulin has been shown to be exerted on both the proximal and distal tubules of the nephron. This renal sodium retention causes expansion of the extracellular fluid volume and leads to the hypertension associated with metabolic syndrome.[16,23] Hyperinsulinemia can also activate the sympathetic nervous system, which leads to an increase in the plasma norepinephrine level. This may cause increased cardiac contractibility, increased heart rate, increased cardiopulmonary blood volume, and direct vasoconstriction of resistant vessels.[16,24] Because insulin is a stimulus for growth of vascular endothelial and smooth muscle cells, hyperinsulinemia may result in a thickening in arterial blood vessel walls.[17] This may lead to hypertension and may also contribute to the CVD associated with metabolic syndrome.

Resnick speculated that there may be an ionic basis to the hypertension and altered insulin metabolism associated with metabolic syndrome and termed this the *ionic hypothesis*.[25] He found that hypertension was caused by increased calcium and decreased magnesium levels and lowered arterial pH in individuals with insulin resistance.

Dyslipidemia

The lipid abnormalities found in metabolic syndrome are elevated triglycerides, low HDL cholesterol, and increased small, dense LDL particles (referred to as *pattern B*, or *atherogenic dyslipidemia*). Insulin impairs the normal suppression of FFA release from the adipose tissue. Increased FFAs released from the adipose tissue and delivered to the liver offer an efficient substrate for enhanced synthesis of triglycerides and very low–density lipoprotein (VLDL). Hyperinsulinemia results in high plasma triglyceride levels by simultaneously increasing production of VLDL and decreasing metabolism of VLDL. Furthermore, when the liver content of lipids is high, gluconeogenesis is increased, resulting in a higher production of glucose by the liver.[3] Finally, HDL cholesterol particles are directly synthesized by the liver but are also derived from liver metabolism of VLDL remnants; therefore reduced VLDL metabolism contributes to a decrease in HDL cholesterol.[26]

Two steps are involved in the formation of small, dense LDL particles and involve lipid transfer protein exchange. When triglyceride from VLDL is exchanged for a cholesterol ester in LDL, the VLDL becomes enriched in cholesterol ester and the LDL becomes enriched in triglyceride. If the triglyceride in LDL is hydrolyzed by LPL or hepatic lipase, a smaller, denser LDL particle will be produced. These small, dense LDL particles lead to atherosclerosis because they are able to bind to and penetrate the arterial wall and more readily undergo oxidative modification.[27] Small, dense LDLs have also been linked to thicker intima media and plaque occurrence in the femoral and carotid arteries.[28,29] These adverse effects in lipoprotein levels increase the risk of atherosclerosis, ischemic heart disease, CVD, and overall cardiovascular mortality.

Prothrombotic State

Studies have found that levels of PAI-1 correlate significantly with insulin resistance. Elevated levels of PAI-1 reflect impaired fibrinolysis, impaired endothelial function, and increased tendency toward acute arterial thrombosis.[30] Insulin resistance also affects other coagulation factors, including platelet aggregability, platelet adhesion, levels of factor VII and factor VIII, tissue plasminogen activator, and fibrinogen.[31]

Proinflammatory State

Inflammation plays a major role in atherogenesis. CRP is a marker of inflammation that has been found to be an independent CVD risk factor and an independent marker of insulin resistance. It has been found that CRP levels and cytokines (tumor necrosis factor-α and interleukin-6) are increased in patients with metabolic syndrome.[2,18]

Microalbuminuria

An association between microalbuminuria and metabolic syndrome has been found secondary to the effects of insulin on renal hemodynamics. The IRAS found that acute hyperinsulinemia causes renal vasodilation, resulting in increased plasma flow, increased glomerular hydrostatic pressure and gradient, and increased glomerular filtration rate. The localized elevated pressure in the glomerular vessels is involved in increased microalbumin secretion.[32,33] Microalbuminuria is a strong predictor of cardiovascular morbidity and mortality.[7,34,35]

Hyperuricemia

Increases in uric acid concentration are commonly seen in association with insulin resistance, hypertension, and dyslipidemia. Studies have found that uric acid concentration is increased in individuals with higher insulin levels, higher insulin response to glucose challenges, higher triglyceride levels, lower HDL cholesterol levels, and higher blood pressure. Researchers have speculated that insulin resistance is correlated with a decreased urinary clearance of uric acid, suggesting a link between insulin metabolism and hyperuricemia[36,37] (Figure 223-1).

Microvascular Angina

Originally H.G. Kemp used the nomenclature *syndrome X* in 1973 to describe microvascular angina as impaired infusion of the microvasculature of the heart occurring in the absence of macrovascular atherosclerosis.[38] The patient with microvascular angina experiences typical anginal chest pain with a positive treadmill test but a completely normal coronary angiogram. Additional studies are ongoing to find a relationship between microvascular angina and metabolic syndrome.[39,40]

Other Pathophysiologic Effects

Several ongoing studies are currently investigating the association between metabolic syndrome, cognitive decline, and sleep apnea.[41-43]

CLINICAL PRESENTATION

Because it is difficult to accurately measure insulin resistance, the diagnosis is usually clinical based on a constellation of physical findings and laboratory characteristics. Insulin resistance can be suspected in the individual who is seen with abdominal obesity, increased triglycerides, low HDL cholesterol, and hypertension.[17]

A physical sign that is suggestive of moderate to severe insulin resistance is the hyperkeratotic condition acanthosis nigricans. This is a diffuse, hyperpigmented, velvety thickening of the cutaneous skin that is found in the neck and axillae. The onset is usually insidious, with the first visible change being darkening of the skin pigmentation so as to appear dirty. As the skin thickens, it becomes velvety, and the skin line is accentuated. Eventually the skin becomes rugose and mammillated.[44,45]

PHYSICAL EXAMINATION

The physical examination consists of accurate measurement of the blood pressure, height and weight, and BMI, or waist-to-hip ratio using the techniques described in the Diagnostics section. A patient with the clinical features of metabolic syndrome should be screened annually for hyperglycemia, glucose intolerance, and type 2 diabetes mellitus. Those who have a diagnosis of metabolic syndrome should also be screened for the cardiovascular complications that accompany the syndrome and managed appropriately. A thorough history

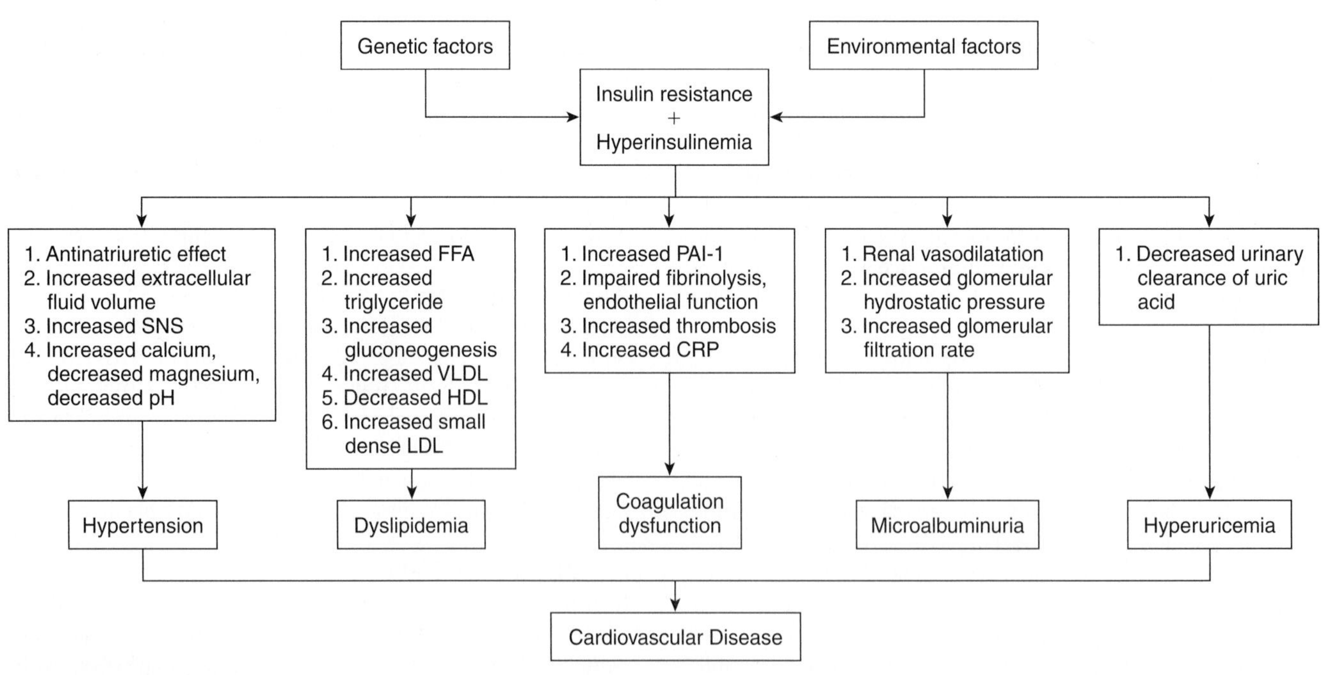

FIGURE 223-1

Role of insulin resistance and cardiovascular disease *(CVD)*. *CRP*, C-reactive protein; *FFA*, free fatty acids; *HDL*, high-density lipoprotein; *LDL*, low-density lipoprotein; *PAI-1*, plasminogen activator inhibitor-1; *SNS*, sympathetic nervous system; *VLDL*, very low–density lipoprotein.

is also important to obtain during the assessment to determine whether the patient is at risk of developing insulin resistance secondary to genetic factors or family history.[46]

DIAGNOSTICS

Several techniques are available for measuring insulin resistance and sensitivity; they include the euglycemic insulin clamp technique, the insulin tolerance test, the insulin suppression test, the frequently sampled IV glucose tolerance test, and the regional arteriovenous balance test.[47] The definitive test for determining insulin resistance is the euglycemic insulin clamp technique. This technique is usually performed in the laboratory setting. It involves infusion of exogenous insulin to maintain a constant plasma insulin level above fasting while glucose is fixed at a basal level through the infusion of glucose at varying rates. Plasma glucose levels are measured every 5 minutes, and if the glucose level falls below basal, the glucose infusion rate is increased to return plasma glucose to basal levels. The total amount of glucose infused over time is a determinant of insulin action on glucose metabolism. Insulin sensitivity is determined by the amount of glucose that has to be infused. If more glucose is infused, the individual is more sensitive to insulin. The insulin-resistant individual requires less glucose to maintain basal plasma glucose levels. This technique is complex and costly and cannot be adapted easily to the clinical setting.[48]

A more practical way of assessing insulin resistance in the clinical setting is through the measurement of the fasting plasma insulin concentration. A significant correlation has been found between fasting insulin levels and insulin action measured by the euglycemic clamp technique. A fasting serum insulin value of 10 mcg/ml indicates insulin resistance.[45] High plasma insulin values with normal glucose levels are suggestive of insulin resistance. The limitation of using the fasting insulin concentration as a diagnostic tool for insulin resistance is the technique's lack of a reliable standardization of the insulin assay procedure.[48]

A variety of measures of body mass and body fat exist that express different aspects of general obesity, fat distribution, patterns, and fat percentage. BMI is calculated as weight divided by height squared and measures percentage of body fat or total adipose tissue. The ratio of waist and hip circumference is highly correlated with visceral adipose tissue. BMI and waist-to-hip ratio are the most routinely used anthropometric indexes because they are easy to use and have a high reliability.[49]

Common laboratory tests can be used to screen for the various other features associated with metabolic syndrome. Impaired fasting glucose (IFG) is measured after an 8- to 12-hour fast; levels between 100 and 126 mg/dl are diagnostic of IFG. Impaired glucose tolerance (IGT) is measured by administering a 75-g load of oral glucose and waiting 2 hours; plasma glucose values between 140 and 200 mg/dl are diagnostic of IGT. HDL and triglyceride blood levels are measured after an 8- to 12-hour fast. Small, dense LDL can be calculated using gradient gel electrophoresis.[29] Microalbumin is measured using a random urine test. A plasma CRP level of more than 3 mg/L indicates an emerging risk factor for CVD.[50] Hyperuricemia can be measured with a serum uric acid test.

DIAGNOSTICS

Metabolic Syndrome

LABORATORY

Euglycemic insulin clamp technique
Glucose tolerance test, fasting blood glucose
Fasting plasma insulin concentration
Fasting lipid profile
Urinalysis (for protein)

DIFFERENTIAL DIAGNOSIS

Metabolic Syndrome

- Type 2 diabetes mellitus
- Impaired glucose tolerance, impaired fasting glucose
- Polycystic ovary syndrome
- Lipodystrophy and lipoatrophic diabetes
- Type A insulin resistance (insulin receptor mutations)
- Type B insulin resistance (anti–insulin receptor antibodies)
- Genetic syndromes

DIFFERENTIAL DIAGNOSIS

Metabolic syndrome is diagnosed based on clinical presentation, so it is important to rule out hypertension, dyslipidemia, or obesity without manifestations of insulin resistance. The differential diagnoses also include type 2 diabetes mellitus or IGT, which can be excluded with laboratory testing. Other diseases characterized by insulin resistance are polycystic ovary syndrome, lipodystrophy and lipoatrophic diabetes, type A insulin resistance (insulin receptor mutations), and type B insulin resistance (anti–insulin receptor antibodies). Genetic syndromes (Down's, Turner's, or muscular dystrophies); neurodegenerative disorders (Werner's syndrome and Friedreich's ataxia); and excess hormonal antagonists such as glucocorticoids, growth hormone, and catecholamines are also characterized by insulin resistance.[45,51]

MANAGEMENT

Recently, the American Diabetes Association and the European Association for the Study of Diabetes released a joint statement regarding the definition and pathogenesis of metabolic syndrome.[52] The concern of these two organizations is that a *syndrome* is an aggregate of specific signs and symptoms usually caused by a unifying pathologic condition and their combination confers a risk that is different from the sum of the parts. Because metabolic syndrome does not meet these criteria, these organizations' recommendation is that providers avoid labeling patients with the term *metabolic syndrome*. Until randomized controlled trials have been completed, there is no appropriate pharmacologic treatment for metabolic syndrome and therefore all cardiovascular risk factors should be treated individually and aggressively. The organizations also recommend that ongoing research of metabolic syndrome continue.

It is imperative to treat the different components of metabolic syndrome appropriately to prevent or lessen the risk of cardiovascular morbidity and mortality. Studies have found that the prevalence of coronary heart disease, myocardial infarction, and stroke are approximately twofold to threefold higher in subjects with metabolic syndrome.[7,53] Methods to treat metabolic syndrome include both nonpharmacologic and pharmacologic measures. These management methods are divided into a three-tiered arrangement: (1) evidence exists for benefit, (2) limited evidence exists for benefit, and (3) evidence of benefit unclear.

Nonpharmacologic treatments for insulin resistance include healthy lifestyle changes in diet and exercise. Because many individuals with metabolic syndrome are overweight, dietary treatment should primarily focus on weight reduction. Weight loss lowers serum cholesterol and triglycerides, raises HDL cholesterol, lowers blood pressure and glucose, reduces insulin resistance, and may decrease serum levels of CRP and PAI-1.

General dietary recommendations include a low intake of saturated fats, *trans*–fatty acids, and cholesterol; reduced consumption of simple sugars; and increased intakes of fruits, vegetables, and whole grains. Dietary carbohydrates with a high glycemic index increase blood glucose levels more rapidly, whereas fiber-rich low-glycemic index foods are digested and absorbed more slowly and can lower triglyceride and raise HDL cholesterol levels. Intake of soluble fiber has been shown to decrease postprandial glucose levels and concentrations of insulin levels. The benefits of a high-fiber diet on decreased levels of fasting plasma insulin were found in both the Coronary Artery Risk Development in Young Adults Study and the Framingham Offspring Study.[54,55] Plant-based foods such as whole grains, fruits, and vegetables have also been found to decrease systolic and diastolic blood pressures and reduce the incidence of coronary heart disease.[54] A monounsaturated fatty acid diet significantly improves insulin sensitivity and the dyslipidemia associated with metabolic syndrome compared with a high–unsaturated fatty acid diet.[56] Dietary trials suggest that treatment of the thrombogenic disorders (elevated plasma fibrinogen and factor VIII coagulant activity levels, raised PAI-1) can be improved with a low-fat diet and a high content of foods rich in complex carbohydrates and dietary fiber.[57,58] "Crash diets" and "extreme diets," consisting of very low calories, high fat, and low carbohydrates, are seldom effective in producing long-term weight loss.

NCEP-ATP III has identified individuals with the metabolic syndrome as candidates for intensified therapeutic lifestyle changes and recommends that they be given the same intensive treatment as people with established heart disease. NCEP-ATP III suggests a therapeutic lifestyle change diet consisting of less than 7% of total calories from saturated fats per day and less than 200 mg of cholesterol per day. NCEP-ATP III also recommends consumption of foods that contain plant stanols and sterols to lower LDL cholesterol and soluble fibers such as cereal grains, beans, peas, legumes, fruits, and vegetables.[59]

Exercise and physical training have been found to be beneficial in the treatment of metabolic syndrome. Exercise improves insulin resistance by increasing glucose utilization by the muscle. Glycogen synthase activity and the number of glucose transporters translocated to the cell surface increase after exercise. Glucose disposal by the skeletal muscle and insulin sensitivity continue for many hours after completion of the exercise. This improvement in insulin sensitivity may prevent the progression of the metabolic abnormalities. The Da Qing IGT and Diabetes study found that diet or exercise led to significant decreases in the incidence of the development of diabetes in individuals with IGT over a 6-year period.[60] Regular aerobic training has also been shown to significantly decrease systolic and diastolic blood pressures. Physical training has been shown to decrease plasma levels of triglyceride by 15% to 30%. Exercise increases LPL activity and improves the removal of VLDL and intermediate-density lipoprotein particles and decreases the levels of small, dense LDL associated with metabolic syndrome. An increase in HDL cholesterol may occur if exercise training is intense and prolonged. Exercise is a potent stimulus for fibrinolysis. Regular physical exercise improves fibrinolytic activity and lowers levels of PAI-1. Exercise and caloric restriction can cause weight loss and a loss of intraabdominal fat, which will decrease the insulin resistance associated with metabolic syndrome.[61]

Recommendations for exercise in individuals with metabolic syndrome are similar to those recommended for individuals with type 2 diabetes (see Box 218-7). The American College of Sports Medicine recommends at least 20 to 30 minutes of continuous aerobic exercise performed at a minimum of 50% of VO_{2max} (maximal oxygen uptake) for at least 5 days a week, and preferably all 7 days, for several weeks to improve cardiovascular fitness. The College recommends that the aerobic exercise be of moderate intensity and involve the legs such as brisk walking, bicycling, and swimming. The exercise session should begin with a 10 minute warm-up consisting of light aerobic activity and stretching and end with a 5- to 10-minute cool down period to lower the heart rate. If the individual is sedentary, a careful cardiovascular assessment may be needed before initiation of an exercise program.[62,63]

Pharmacologic methods involve the treatment of the associated characteristics that are seen with metabolic syndrome. Included would be antihypertensives, 5-hydroxy-3-methylglutaryl–coenzyme A (HMG-CoA) reductase inhibitors (statins), fibric acid derivatives, aspirin therapy, possibly thiazolidinediones, the biguanide metformin, and weight loss medications.

The seventh report of the Joint National Committee on Prevention, Detection, Evaluation, and Treatment of High Blood Pressure recommends that drug therapies be required in persons with categorical hypertension (blood pressure ≥140/90 mm Hg).[64] The classes of antihypertensives that have been found to be effective in reducing blood pressure and increasing insulin sensitivity are α-adrenergic antagonist and the angiotensin-converting enzyme (ACE) inhibitors. Prazosin and doxazosin have been found to increase sensitivity to insulin. α-Adrenergic antagonists play a beneficial role in the dyslipidemia found in metabolic syndrome. They improve lipoprotein metabolism by decreasing triglyceride and VLDL concentrations and increasing HDL cholesterol. ACE inhibitors and angiotensin II receptor blockers (ARBs) do not worsen the insulin resistance or the lipid profile and can actually prevent or retard progression of renal disease. They can also improve the microalbuminuria found in metabolic syndrome. Calcium channel blockers are effective in lowering blood pressure and have no profound adverse effects on lipid or glucose metabolism. Beta blockers are cardioprotective in patients with established CVD and are no longer contraindicated in patients with type 2 diabetes. Beta blockers and diuretics in high doses worsened insulin resistance and decreased glucose uptake by 25% to 32% in studies using the euglycemic clamp technique. Beta blockers may also increase plasma triglyceride levels.[16,17,23,45]

NCEP-ATP III recommends triglyceride levels less than 150 mg/dl, LDL cholesterol levels less than 100 mg/dl, and HDL cholesterol levels more than 40 mg/dl in men or more than 50 mg/dl in women with metabolic syndrome. Statins may lower LDL cholesterol by 18% to 55%, raise HDL cholesterol by 5% to 15%, and lower triglycerides by 7% to 30%. If the triglyceride level is very high (>500 mg/dl), it is recommended that a fibrate (such as gemfibrozil) or nicotinic acid (niacin) be used, which may decrease triglyceride levels by 20% to 50%.[65] Gemfibrozil has been shown to improve insulin action and flow-mediated vasodilation as well as decreases triglyceride levels. Nicotinic acid in high doses can raise plasma glucose levels. Severe myopathy may occur with the combination of a statin plus gemfibrozil.[66]

The Hypertensive Optimal Treatment Trial found that the daily use of aspirin is beneficial in the reduction of myocardial infarction in diabetic and nondiabetic individuals. Aspirin significantly reduced cardiovascular events by 15% and myocardial infarction by 36%.[67] Low-dose aspirin can modify the prothrombotic-proinflammatory state found in metabolic syndrome. The American Heart Association currently recommends use of aspirin prophylaxis in patients whose 10-year risk for coronary heart disease is 10% or greater as determined by the Framingham risk scoring.[68]

The Diabetes Prevention Program was a randomized clinical trial that was conducted to evaluate the safety and efficacy of interventions that may delay or prevent development of diabetes in individuals at increased risk for type 2 diabetes. The study found that intensive lifestyle interventions, including at least 150 minutes of moderate-intensity exercise per week together with a healthy diet, to achieve and maintain a 7% loss of body weight, reduced the incidence of diabetes by 58%, and the use of metformin 850 mg b.i.d. reduced the incidence of diabetes by 31%.[69]

Since obesity has been found to be strongly associated with the metabolic syndrome, weight loss is important in its treatment.[70] Pharmacologic agents available to treat excess adiposity include appetite suppressants and inhibitors of nutrient absorption. The appetite suppressants include phentermine derivatives and sibutramine. These agents are usually taken in the morning and lead to decreased appetite later in the afternoon and evening. Orlistat is an inhibitor of gastrointestinal lipase and prevents the absorption of approximately 30% of the fat that is consumed, so it must be taken at meals. The expected weight loss is typically 5% to 10% of initial weight.[71,72]

Successful surgical procedures to treat obesity include laparoscopic gastric bypass and laparoscopic vertical banded gastroplasty. Weight typically declines about 40% at 1 year and 62% at 5 years. There is usually less weight lost with the laparoscopic vertical banding procedure. Follow-up after these procedures includes monitoring of vitamin and hematologic status, adherence to specific postoperative dietary guidelines, and psychologic issues.[72,73]

Recent research has demonstrated reduction in the cardiovascular risk factors with the use of the thiazolidinediones, which include rosiglitazone and pioglitazone. These drugs improve insulin resistance by sensitizing the muscle and subcutaneous cells to the effects of insulin, thus lowering plasma insulin levels. The use of thiazolidinediones results in decreased blood pressure, improved dyslipidemia by lowering triglyceride levels, decreased lipid oxidation and increased HDL cholesterol levels, improved fibrinolysis and endothelial function, decreased carotid artery intima thickness, and decreased CRP levels. The adverse effects include edema and weight gain. Hepatic aminotransferase levels must be monitored during the use of these drugs.[74-78]

Metformin has been shown to reduce hyperinsulinemia and insulin resistance, lower blood triglyceride levels, assist in weight reduction, and lower plasma PAI-1 levels. Metformin improves the sensitivity of cells to insulin, reduces hepatic glucose production, and increases glucose uptake in muscle and other peripheral tissues. Through these mechanisms of action, metformin has been found to reduce or prevent macrovascular complications. Serum creatinine must be monitored while using metformin.[17,79,80]

Recently, several large trials have shown a reduction in the risk of cardiovascular conditions and the development of type 2 diabetes among patients treated with ACE inhibitors or ARBs. The mechanisms by which ACE inhibitors and ARBs reduce the risk of type 2 diabetes are not clear, but researchers have speculated that the preventive effects might involve increases in bradykinin levels, improved skeletal muscle blood flow, promotion of adipocyte differentiation, or preservation of pancreatic beta cell function.[81]

New studies show that the I_1-imidazoline agonists, moxonidine and rilmenidine, improve glucose metabolism and reduce blood pressure and microalbuminuria associated with the metabolic syndrome. Further research is currently being conducted on these new medications and their beneficial effects on the metabolic syndrome[82-84] (Figure 223-2).

LIFE SPAN CONSIDERATIONS

Insulin resistance may occur at any age. Studies have shown that insulin resistance has been found in overweight African-American children as young as 5 years old. These children also showed elevations in blood pressure and lipid levels.[85] Studies have also shown that childhood obesity increases the risk for metabolic syndrome in adulthood. This risk can be reduced if an obese child reduces his or her relative weight to become a nonobese adult. The baseline assessment of and identification of obese children can possibly lead to the prevention of adult obesity, metabolic syndrome, and cardiovascular risk.[86]

Parents require education on ways to promote healthy lifestyle, proper nutrition, weight loss, and increased physical activity in young obese children. These healthy lifestyle modifications must continue through out the entire life span. The older adult may be at increased risk of developing insulin resistance secondary to increased obesity, decreases in physical activity, and changes in body mass because of muscle loss and increased adipose tissue. Older adults may need to be educated on exercise programs tailored to their needs or modified for the chronic illnesses they have. Dietary recommendations may also need to be modified to provide for the older adult's nutritional needs.[21,87]

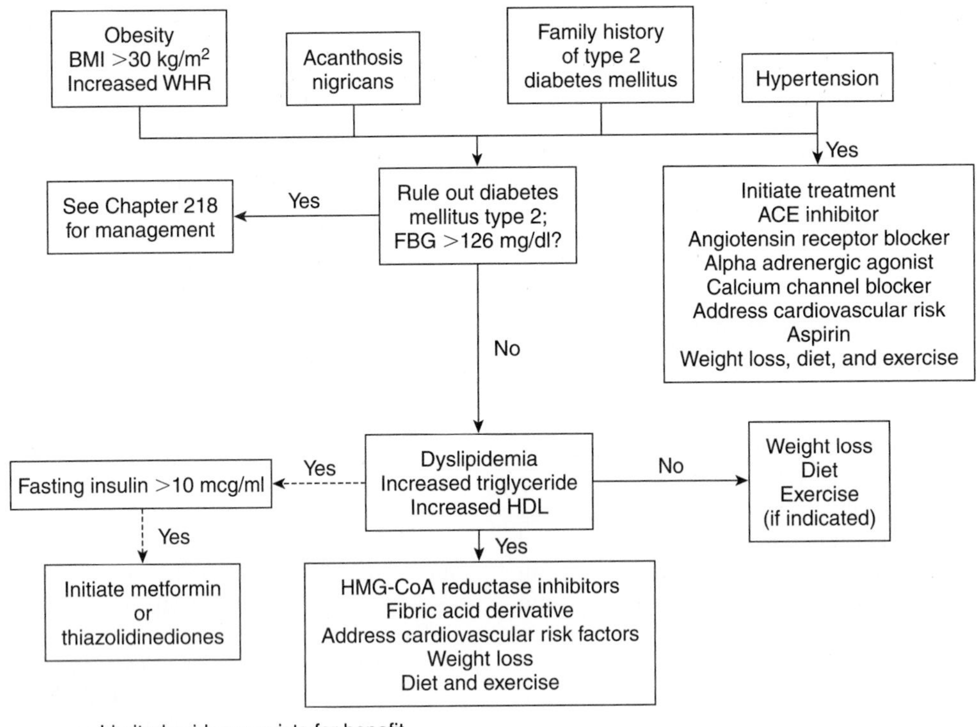

FIGURE 223-2

Algorithm for treatment of metabolic syndrome. *ACE,* Angiotensin-converting enzyme; *BMI,* body mass index; *DM,* diabetes mellitus; *FBG,* fasting blood glucose; *HDL,* high-density lipoprotein; *HMG-CoA,* 5-hydroxy-3-methylglutaryl–coenzyme A; *WHR,* waist-to-hip ratio.

COMPLICATIONS

As discussed earlier, the complications associated with the features of metabolic syndrome include CVD, atherosclerotic vascular disease, ischemic heart disease, coronary artery disease, myocardial infarction, and stroke.[88,89] The Hoorn study recently found that metabolic syndrome was associated with a twofold increase in age-adjusted risk of fatal CVD in men and nonfatal CVD in women.[53]

Insulin resistance is the pathophysiologic hallmark of IGT and type 2 diabetes and may occur decades before the clinical presentation of these diseases. As the beta cell function deteriorates and is no longer able to compensate for the insulin resistance and glucose levels rise, a transition from insulin resistance to IGT with mild increases in postprandial glucose levels occurs and eventually results in type 2 diabetes mellitus.[26]

Very high levels of triglyceride can provoke an acute episode of pancreatitis. Elevated uric acid levels may induce gout or uric acid nephrolithiasis. Elevated PAI-1 may lead to clotting dysfunction and coagulation abnormalities, resulting in an acute cardiovascular event such as stroke or myocardial infarction.[45]

INDICATIONS FOR REFERRAL OR HOSPITALIZATION

A physician consultation is necessary when the hypertension or dyslipidemia (associated with metabolic syndrome) is resistant to therapy. Referral to a dietitian may be beneficial to assist the individual with meal planning and weight loss. A health psychologist can provide psychologic support, as well as support with realistic goal setting, stress management, and behavior modification methods. An exercise physiologist or physical therapist can assist in the development of a safe and effective exercise regimen.[90]

PATIENT AND FAMILY EDUCATION

Education should focus on the pathology of the metabolic syndrome and associated characteristics along with the complications and cardiovascular risks that accompany the syndrome. This instruction should address medication use, mechanism of action, and adverse effects. Education must be provided to the patient and the family members, since meal planning and participation in a physical fitness program will benefit the patient and family members involved. Family support is necessary to assist the patient with the lifestyle changes needed to decrease the risks of complications involved in the syndrome. Explaining the benefits of healthy eating and exercise can empower and motivate the patient. The discussion should involve exploring the patient's feelings towards metabolic syndrome and the treatment regimen. The patient should be instructed on mode, frequency, and intensity of exercise. Preferably, an exercise program of the patient's choice will better ensure adherence. Smoking cessation and limited use of alcohol, including the effects on insulin resistance, triglyceride levels, and cardiovascular risks, should be discussed.[17] Mutual goal setting before the initiation of treatment is necessary for the patient's success. Both written and verbal instructions must be given to the patient and reinforced at each visit.

HEALTH PROMOTION

Health care providers are in a unique position to intervene, motivate, and influence the patient's outcome and the family members through teaching, counseling, and health promotion. As discussed previously, insulin resistance has been found in children as young as 5 years of age; therefore it is imperative to start promoting healthy lifestyles at a very young age. Promotion of weight loss in the individual who is moderately obese can prevent the development of insulin resistance and the complications associated with the syndrome. Practitioners can assist the patient in changing harmful health behaviors through counseling on nutrition and facilitating increases in physical activity. Disease prevention and health promotion before the occurrence of complications associated with metabolic syndrome is more cost-effective in terms of health care dollars and promotes savings in human suffering. Through health promotion and early intervention, the occurrence of and ramifications of metabolic syndrome can surely be decreased or possibly eliminated.

REFERENCES

1. Reaven GM: Role of insulin resistance in human disease, *Diabetes* 37:1595-1607, 1988.
2. Rutter M, and others: C-reactive protein, the metabolic syndrome, and prediction of cardiovascular events in the Framingham Offspring Study, *Circulation* 110(4):380-385, 2004.
3. Timar O, Sestier F, Levy E: Metabolic syndrome X: a review, *Can J Cardiol* 16(6):779-789, 2000.
4. Alberti KGMM, Zimmet PZ: Definition, diagnosis and classification of diabetes mellitus and its complications, part 1, Diagnosis and classification of diabetes mellitus provisional report of a WHO consultation, *Diabet Med* 15(7):539-553, 1998.
5. Third report of the National Cholesterol Education Program (NCEP) Expert Panel on Detection, Evaluation, and Treatment of High Blood Cholesterol in Adults (Adult Treatment Panel III): final report, *Circulation* 106(25):3143-3421, 2002.
6. International Diabetes Federation: *The IDF consensus worldwide definition of the metabolic syndrome,* retrieved Nov 10, 2005, from http://www.idf.org/home/index.cfm?node=1429.
7. Isomaa B, Almgren P, Tuomi T, and others: Cardiovascular morbidity and mortality associated with the metabolic syndrome, *Diabetes Care* 24(4):683-689, 2001.
8. Trevisan M, and others: Syndrome X and mortality: a population-based study: risk factor and life expectancy research group, *Am J Epidemiol* 148(10):958-966, 1998.
9. Park Y, and others: The metabolic syndrome: prevalence and associated risk factors findings in the US population from the Third National Health and Nutrition Examination Survey, 1988-1994, *Arch Intern Med* 163(4):427-436, 2003.
10. Meigs JB, and others: Prevalence and characteristics of the metabolic syndrome in the San Antonio Heart and Framingham Offspring studies, *Diabetes* 52(8):2160-2167, 2003.
11. Haffner SM, and others: Increased insulin resistance and insulin secretion in nondiabetic African-Americans and Hispanics compared with non-Hispanic whites: the Insulin Resistance Atherosclerosis Study, *Diabetes* 45(6):742-748, 1996.
12. Stewart MW, Humphriss DB, Berrish TS, and others: Features of syndrome X in first-degree relatives of NIDDM patients, *Diabetes Care* 18(7):1020-1022, 1995.
13. Gaillard TR, Schuster DP, Bossetti BM, and others: The impact of socioeconomic status on cardiovascular risk factors in African-Americans at high risk for type 2 diabetes: implications for syndrome X, *Diabetes Care* 20(5):745-752, 1997.
14. Hunt KJ, and others: Familial history of metabolic disorders and the multiple metabolic syndrome: the NHLBI family heart study, *Genet Epidemiol* 19(4):395-409, 2000.
15. Groop LC: Pathogenesis of insulin resistance in type 2 diabetes: a collision between thrifty genes and an affluent environment, *Drugs* 58(S1):11-12, 1999.
16. DeFronzo RA, Ferrannini E: Insulin resistance: a multifaceted syndrome responsible for NIDDM, obesity, hypertension, dyslipidemia and atherosclerotic cardiovascular disease, *Diabetes Care* 14(3):173-194, 1991.
17. Baillie GM and others: Insulin and coronary artery disease: is syndrome X the unifying hypothesis? *Ann Pharmacother* 32:233-247, 1998.
18. Grundy SM, and others: Clinical management of metabolic syndrome: report of the American Heart Association/National Heart, Lung, and Blood Institute/American Diabetes Association conference on scientific issues related to management, *Arterioscler Thromb Vasc Biol* 24(2):e19-e24, 2004.
19. Lee GA, Rao MN: The effects of HIV protease inhibitors on carbohydrate and lipid metabolism, *Curr HIV/AIDS Rep* 2(1):39-50, 2005.
20. Sax PE, Kumar P: Tolerability and safety of HIC protease inhibitors in adults, *J AIDS* 37(1):1111-1124, 2004.
21. Muller DC, and others: The effect of age on insulin resistance and secretion: a review, *Semin Nephrol* 16(4):289-298, 1996.
22. Ferrannini E, and others: Insulin resistance, hyperinsulinemia, and blood pressure: role of age and obesity: European Group for the Study of Insulin Resistance (EGIR), *Hypertension* 30(5):1144-1149, 1997.
23. Reaven GM, and others: Hypertension and associated metabolic abnormalities: the role of insulin resistance and sympathoadrenal system, *N Engl J Med* 334(6):374-381, 1996.
24. Reaven GM: Pathophysiology of insulin resistance in human disease, *Physiol Rev* 75(3):473-486, 1995.
25. Resnick LM: Ionic basis of hypertension, insulin resistance, vascular disease, and related disorders: the mechanism of "syndrome X," *Am J Hypertens* 6(4):123S-134S, 1993.
26. Granberry MC, Fonseca VA: Insulin resistance syndrome: options for treatment, *South Med J* 92(1):2-14, 1999.
27. Sniderman AD, and others: Hypertriglyceridemic hyperapoB: the unappreciated atherogenic dyslipoproteinemia in type 2 diabetes mellitus, *Ann Intern Med* 135(6):447-459, 2001.
28. Hulthe J, and others: The metabolic syndrome, LDL particle size, and atherosclerosis: the Atherosclerosis and Insulin Resistance (AIR) study, *Arterioscler Thromb Vasc Biol* 20(9):2140-2147, 2000.
29. Reaven GM, and others: Insulin resistance and hyperinsulinemia in individuals with small, dense, low density lipoprotein particles, *J Clin Invest* 92(1):141-146, 1993.
30. Sakkinen PA, and others: Clustering of procoagulation, inflammation, and fibrinolysis variables with metabolic factors in insulin resistance syndrome, *Am J Epidemiol* 152(10):897-907, 2000.
31. Vinik AI, Erbas T, Park TS, and others: Platelet dysfunction in type 2 diabetes, *Diabetes Care* 24(8):1476-1485, 2001.
32. Mykkanen L, and others: Microalbuminuria is associated with insulin resistance in nondiabetic subjects: the insulin resistance atherosclerosis study, *Diabetes* 47(5):793-800, 1998.
33. Meigs JB, Jacques PF, Selhub J, and others: Fasting plasma homocysteine levels in the insulin resistance syndrome: the Framingham Offspring Study, *Diabetes Care* 24(8):1403-1410, 2001.
34. Palaniappan L, and others: Association between microalbuminuria and the metabolic syndrome: NHANES III, *Am J Hypertens* 16(11Pt 1):952-958, 2003.
35. Liese AD, and others: Microalbuminuria, central adiposity and hypertension in the non-diabetic population of the MONICA Augsburg survey 1994/95, *J Hum Hypertens* 15(11):799-804, 2001.

36. Zavaroni I, and others: Changes in insulin and lipid metabolism in males with asymptomatic hyperuricemia, *J Int Med* 234:24-30, 1993.
37. Reaven GM: Syndrome X: 6 years later, *J Int Med* 736:S13-S22, 1994.
38. Kemp HG: Left ventricular function in patients with the anginal syndrome and normal coronary arteriograms, *Am J Cardiol* 32(3):375-376, 1973.
39. Botker HE, and others: Myocardial insulin resistance in patients with syndrome X, *J Clin Invest* 100(8):1919-1927, 1997.
40. Botker HE, and others: Insulin resistance in microvascular angina (syndrome X), *Lancet* 342(8864):136-140, 1993.
41. Geroldi C, and others: Insulin resistance in cognitive impairment: the InCHIANTI study, *Arch Neurol* 62(7):1067-1072, 2005.
42. Yaffe K, and others: The metabolic syndrome, inflammation, and the risk of cognitive decline, *JAMA* 292(18):2237-2242, 2004.
43. Vgontzas AN, and others: Sleep apnea is a manifestation of the metabolic syndrome, *Sleep Med Rev* 9(3):211-224, 2005.
44. Fitzpatrick TB: *Color atlas and synopsis of clinical dermatology*, ed 3, New York, 1997, McGraw-Hill.
45. Garvey WT, Hermayer KL: Clinical implications of the insulin resistance syndrome, *Clin Cornerstone* 1(3):13-28, 1998.
46. Minchoff LE, Grandin JA: Syndrome X: recognition and management of this metabolic disorder in primary care, *Nurse Pract* 21(6):74-86, 1996.
47. Del Prato S: Measurement of insulin resistance in vivo, *Drugs* 58(Suppl 1):3-6, 1999.
48. American Diabetes Association: Consensus development conference on insulin resistance: 5-6 November 1997, *Diabetes Care* 21(2):310-314, 1998.
49. Liese AD, and others: Development of the multiple metabolic syndrome: an epidemiologic perspective, *Epidemiol Rev* 20(2):157-172, 1998.
50. Pearson TA, Mensah GA, Alexander RW, and others: Markers of inflammation and cardiovascular disease: application to clinical and public health practice: a statement for healthcare professionals from the Centers for Disease Control and Prevention and the American Heart Association, *Circulation* 107(3):499-511, 2003.
51. Moller DE, Flier JS: Insulin resistance: mechanisms, syndromes and implications, *N Engl J Med* 325(13):938-948, 1991.
52. Kahn R, and others: The metabolic syndrome: time for a critical appraisal: joint statement from the American Diabetes Association and the European Association for the Study of Diabetes, *Diabetes Care* 28(9):2289-2304, 2005.
53. Dekker JM, Girman C, Rhodes T, and others: Metabolic syndrome and 10-year cardiovascular disease risk in the Hoorn study, *Circulation* 112(5):666-673, 2005.
54. Liu S, Manson JE: Dietary carbohydrates, physical inactivity, obesity, and the "metabolic syndrome" as predictors of coronary heart disease, *Curr Opin Lipidol* 12(4):395-404, 2001.
55. Ludwig DS, and others: Dietary fiber, weight gain, and cardiovascular disease risk factors in young adults, *JAMA* 282(16):1539-1546, 1999.
56. Riccardi G, Rivellese AA: Dietary treatment of the metabolic syndrome—the optimal diet, *Br J Nutr* 83(Suppl 1):S143-S148, 2000.
57. Jenkins DJ, and others: Dietary fiber, lente carbohydrates and the insulin-resistant diseases, *Br J Nutr* 83(Suppl 1):S157-S163, 2000.
58. Marckmann P: Dietary treatment of thrombogenic disorders related to the metabolic syndrome, *Br J Nutr* 83(Suppl 1):S121-S126, 2000.
59. Expert Panel on Detection, Evaluation, and Treatment of High Blood Cholesterol in Adults: Executive summary of the third report of the National Cholesterol Education Program (NCEP) Expert Panel on Detection, Evaluation, and Treatment of High Blood Cholesterol in Adults (Adult Treatment Panel III), *JAMA* 285(19):2486-2497, 2001.
60. Pan XR, Li GW, Hu YH, and others: Effects of diet and exercise in preventing NIDDM in people with impaired glucose tolerance: the Da Qing IGT and diabetes study, *Diabetes Care* 20(4):537-544, 1997.
61. Shahid SK, Schneider SH: Effects of exercise on insulin resistance syndrome, *Coron Artery Dis* 11(2):103-109, 2000.
62. Thompson PD, and others: Exercise and physical activity in the prevention and treatment of atherosclerotic cardiovascular disease: a statement from the Council on Clinical Cardiology (Subcommittee on Exercise, Rehabilitation, and Prevention) and the Council on Nutrition, Physical Activity, and Metabolism (Subcommittee on Physical Activity), *Circulation* 107(24):3109-3116, 2003.
63. American College of Sports Medicine: Position stand on the recommended quantity and quality of exercise for developing and maintaining cardiorespiratory and muscular fitness in healthy adults, *Med Sci Sports Exerc* 30:975-991, 1998.
64. Chobanian AV, Bakris GL, Black HR, National Heart, Lung, and Blood Institute Joint National Committee on Prevention, Detection, Evaluation, and Treatment of High Blood Pressure. National High Blood Pressure Education Program Coordinating Committee: The Seventh Report of the Joint National Committee on Prevention, Detection, Evaluation, and Treatment of High Blood Pressure: the JNC 7 report, *JAMA* 289(19):2560-2572, 2003.
65. Roberts CK, and others: Reversibility of chronic experimental syndrome X by diet modification, *Hypertension* 37(5):1323-1328, 2001.
66. Avogaro A, and others: Gemfibrozil improves insulin sensitivity and flow-mediated vasodilatation in type 2 diabetic patients, *Eur J Clin Invest* 31(7):603-609, 2001.
67. Hansson L, and others: Effects of intensive blood-pressure lowering and low dose aspirin on patients with hypertension: principal results of the Hypertension Optimal Treatment (HOT) randomized trial, *Lancet* 351(9118):1755-1762, 1998.
68. Pearson TA, and others: American Heart Association guidelines for primary prevention of cardiovascular disease and stroke: 2002 update: consensus panel guide to comprehensive risk reduction for adult patients without coronary or other atherosclerotic vascular diseases, *Circulation* 106(3):388-391, 2002.
69. Diabetes Prevention Program Research Group: Reduction in the incidence of type 2 diabetes with lifestyle intervention or metformin, *N Engl J Med* 346(6):393-403, 2002.
70. Carr DB, and others: Intra-abdominal fat is a major determinant of the National Cholesterol Education Program Adult Treatment Panel III criteria for the metabolic syndrome, *Diabetes* 53(8):2087-2094, 2004.
71. Haddock CK, and others: Pharmacotherapy for obesity: a quantitative analysis of 4 decades of published randomized clinical trials, *Int J Obes Relat Metab Disord* 26:262-273, 2002.
72. Wilson PWF, Grundy SM: The metabolic syndrome: practical guide to origins and treatment, part I, *Circulation* 108(12):1422-1424, 2003.
73. Lee WJ, and others: Effects of obesity surgery on the metabolic syndrome, *Arch Surg* 139(10):1088-1092, 2004.
74. Parulkar AA, and others: Nonhypoglycemic effects of thiazolidinediones, *Ann Intern Med* 134(1):61-71, 2001.
75. Sunayama S, and others: Thiazolidinediones, dyslipidemia and insulin resistance syndrome, *Curr Opin Lipidol* 11(4):397-402, 2000.
76. Rajagopalan R, and others: Effect of pioglitazone on metabolic syndrome risk factors: results of double-blind, multicenter, randomized clinical trials, *Curr Med Res Opin* 21(1):163-172, 2005.
77. Dormandy JA, and others: Secondary prevention of macrovascular events in patients with type 2 diabetes in the PROactive Study (PROspective pioglitazone clinical trial in macrovascular events): a randomized controlled trial, *Lancet* 366(9493):1279-1289, 2005.
78. Satoh N, and others: Antiatherogenic effect of pioglitazone in type 2 diabetic patients irrespective of the responsiveness to its antidiabetic effect, *Diabetes Care* 26(9):2493-2499, 2003.
79. Zimmet P, Collier G: Clinical efficacy of metformin against insulin resistance parameters: sinking the iceberg, *Drugs* 58(Suppl 1):21-28, 1999.
80. Vitale C, and others: Metformin improves endothelial function in patients with metabolic syndrome, *J Intern Med* 258(3):250-256, 2005.
81. Abuissa H, and others: Angiotensin-converting enzyme inhibitors or angiotensin receptor blockers for prevention of type 2 diabetes: a meta-analysis of randomized clinical trials, *J Am Coll Cardiol* 46(5):821-826, 2005.
82. Reid JL: Rilmenidine: a clinical overview, *Am J Hypertens* 13(6 Pt 2):106S-111S, 2000.

83. Prichard BN, Graham BR: I1 imidazoline agonists: general clinical pharmacology of imidazoline receptors: implications for the treatment of the elderly, *Drugs Aging* 17(2):133-159, 2000.
84. Velliquette RA, Ernsberger P: The role of I_1-imidazoline and α_2-adrenergic receptors in the modulation of glucose metabolism in the spontaneously hypertensive obese rat model of metabolic syndrome X, *J Pharmacol Exp Ther* 306(2):646-657, 2003.
85. Young-Hyman D, and others: Evaluation of the insulin resistance syndrome in 5- to 10-year-old overweight/obese African American children, *Diabetes Care* 24(8):1359-1364, 2001.
86. Vanhala M, and others: Relation between obesity from childhood to adulthood and the metabolic syndrome: population based study, *Br Med J* 317(7154):319, 1998.
87. Ferrannini E, and others: Insulin action and age: European Group for the Study of Insulin Resistance (EGIR), *Diabetes* 45(7):947-953, 1996.
88. Bressler P, and others: Insulin resistance and coronary artery disease, *Diabetologia* 39(11):1345-1350, 1996.
89. Stout RW: Insulin and atheroma: 20-yr perspective, *Diabetes Care* 13(6):631-654, 1990.
90. Grundy SM: Hypertriglyceridemia, insulin resistance, and the metabolic syndrome, *Am J Cardiol* 83(9B):25F-29F, 1999.

CHAPTER 224

Parathyroid Gland Disorders

Tara Jayne Hamilton and
Alan Ona Malabanan

DEFINITION AND EPIDEMIOLOGY

The four parathyroid glands, located in the neck, tightly regulate serum levels of ionized calcium through the actions of parathyroid hormone (PTH). PTH is an 84–amino acid peptide that raises serum calcium in three ways: (1) by acting directly on bone to release calcium into the extracellular fluid; (2) by acting directly on the kidney to decrease renal loss of calcium; (3) by acting indirectly on the intestinal tract, via the activation of vitamin D, to increase dietary calcium absorption. Parathyroid disorders cause dysfunction through their effects on bone, kidney, serum calcium, and phosphorus.

The two major categories of parathyroid dysfunction are hyperparathyroidism (the oversecretion of PTH) and hypoparathyroidism (the undersecretion of PTH). PTH levels must be interpreted in the context of the serum calcium level. When considered in this manner, primary hyperparathyroidism can be defined as the inappropriate secretion of PTH in the setting of hypercalcemia. Secondary hyperparathyroidism is an appropriately increased secretion of PTH in the setting of low or normal serum calcium, and can be caused by vitamin D deficiency and renal failure. Tertiary hyperparathyroidism is prolonged secondary hyperparathyroidism in which hypercalcemia develops; it is an initially appropriate secretion that later becomes inappropriate. Hypoparathyroidism is the inappropriately low secretion of PTH in the setting of hypocalcemia.

Automated chemistry measurements have allowed the routine detection of asymptomatic hypercalcemia, increasing the recognition of early primary hyperparathyroidism. The estimated incidence of primary hyperparathyroidism is approximately 1 in 1000, with the peak incidence between the fourth and fifth decades of life. The incidence in women is higher than that in men, approximately 3:1.[1] Exposure to external beam radiotherapy to the head and neck increases the risk of primary hyperparathyroidism in a dose-response relationship.[2] More cases of hyperparathyroidism are discovered in the course of routine measurement of serum calcium. Because of early discovery, these patients are often minimally symptomatic.[3] Secondary hyperparathyroidism is found mainly in patients with renal insufficiency. It is usually present when the glomerular filtration rate falls below 50 ml/min.[4] Vitamin D deficiency is another important cause of secondary hyperparathyroidism, particularly in older adults and institutionalized patients.[5] Secondary hyperparathyroidism may also occur in patients being treated with glucocorticoids, which cause decreased intestinal calcium absorption.

Hypoparathyroidism is primarily a consequence of thyroid and parathyroid surgery. The incidence, which can range between 0.6% and 17%, depends on the skill of the surgeon and the type of operation.[6]

Physician consultation is indicated for all suspected cases of parathyroid disorders.

PATHOPHYSIOLOGY

In 80% to 85% of cases of primary hyperparathyroidism, excess PTH is produced by a single parathyroid adenoma. In 15% to 20% of cases, it is produced by hyperplasia of all four glands. Primary hyperparathyroidism is produced by a parathyroid carcinoma in less than 0.5% of cases.[1]

Excess PTH stimulates osteoclast-mediated bone degradation, releasing calcium and phosphorus into the extracellular space. As a result, prolonged exposure to excess PTH will erode bone, particularly cortical (dense) bone. Trabecular bone is relatively spared. Skeletal sites with primarily cortical bone, such as the wrist and proximal radius, are particularly at increased risk for fracture.

PTH acts on the kidney to increase calcium reabsorption and increase phosphorus losses. The rising serum calcium gradually exceeds the kidney's ability to reabsorb the filtered calcium, thus increasing urinary calcium. Nephrocalcinosis, nephrolithiasis, and renal dysfunction may result. PTH receptors also exist on a variety of tissues, including brain, skin, and heart. The effects of PTH on these tissues are not yet well characterized.

Secondary hyperparathyroidism represents a compensation for decreased serum levels of ionized calcium. The kidney is important in calcium and phosphorus homeostasis, and renal insufficiency disturbs calcium metabolism in three ways. First, decreased phosphorus clearance and hyperphosphatemia cause a decrease in serum ionized calcium levels. Second, a decrease in renal activation of vitamin D decreases intestinal calcium absorption. Third, uremia produces PTH resistance, thus necessitating higher levels of PTH. Finally, uremia decreases the inhibitory effect of calcium on PTH release.[7] As with primary hyperparathyroidism, excess PTH will erode bone.

Prolonged stimulation of the parathyroid glands by hypocalcemia results in hyperplasia of the glands. Occasionally this leads to autonomous parathyroid function and hypercalcemia (tertiary hyperparathyroidism).

Vitamin D deficiency results in a decrease in intestinal calcium absorption. This, coupled with the daily loss of calcium in the urine and the feces, leads to a net loss of calcium. To prevent overt hypocalcemia, the parathyroid glands secrete more PTH, thus releasing calcium from the bone and preserving normal serum calcium levels. Longstanding vitamin D deficiency may lead to overt hypocalcemia if calcium stores in the bone are depleted.

Hypoparathyroidism results from the destruction of the parathyroid glands, whether the result of surgery, radiation, infiltration (hemochromatosis, amyloidosis, hemosiderosis), malignancy, or autoimmune disease. As may be expected, decreased PTH affects the renal conservation of calcium, the intestinal absorption of calcium, and the degradative release of calcium from bone. Hypocalcemia results from these effects. Of note, hypomagnesemia or hypermagnesemia may decrease PTH secretion or diminish PTH action on the bone and should be considered as a potential cause of hypoparathyroidism.

CLINICAL PRESENTATION

Asymptomatic elevation of serum calcium is the most common presentation of primary hyperparathyroidism. The hypercalcemia may be masked by hypoalbuminemia. To correct for hypoalbuminemia, 0.8 mg/dl calcium should be added for every 1 g/dl below 4 g/dl albumin. Usually this hypercalcemia is accompanied by a fasting hypophosphatemia. Kidney stones are another initial presenting complaint. Kidney stones occur more commonly in males and in younger patients.[8] Some cases of primary hyperparathyroidism are found after an evaluation for osteoporosis.

Osteitis fibrosa cystica (OFC) is associated with multiple lytic bone lesions and subperiosteal bone resorption. OFC may be found in conjunction with an acute hyperparathyroid crisis in which the hypercalcemia develops quickly, causing obtundation, volume depletion, and cardiac arrhythmias. Patients with primary hyperparathyroidism may also have slightly worsened hypertension, gastrointestinal complaints, and vague symptoms of fatigue and weakness.

Hyperparathyroidism may occur as part of a familial disorder such as multiple endocrine neoplasia syndrome (MEN). MEN type 1 includes hyperparathyroidism, pituitary tumors, and pancreatic tumors (insulinoma, gastrinoma). MEN type 2A includes hyperparathyroidism, pheochromocytoma, and medullary thyroid carcinoma. In these disorders the hyperparathyroidism is caused by parathyroid hyperplasia.

Secondary hyperparathyroidism is usually found with renal insufficiency and vitamin D deficiency. Patients may be initially seen with bone pain or a pathologic fracture. Risk factors for vitamin D deficiency include minimum sun exposure, minimum vitamin D dietary intake, malabsorption, prior gastric surgery, and medications that may increase the metabolism of vitamin D (e.g., rifampin and anticonvulsants). Other factors, such as aging, sunscreen use, and heavily pigmented skin, decrease sunlight-mediated vitamin D synthesis in the skin. Secondary hyperparathyroidism in chronic kidney disease (CKD) occurs with a host of metabolic derangements, including hypocalcemia, hyperphosphatemia, and low vitamin D. Steps can be taken to minimize the metabolic derangements that occur in CKD, to reduce the morbidity and mortality that can ensue. The most recent National Kidney Foundation Guidelines suggest that PTH be measured in all patients with CKD with a glomerular filtration rate less than 60 ml/min/1.73 m^2. These patients should have their 25-hydroxyvitamin D levels repleted to above 30 ng/ml. If the PTH is over 70 pg/ml in a patient with stage 3 CKD, or over 110 pg/ml in stage 4 CKD, and the patient does not have hypercalcemia then an active vitamin D sterol, such as calcitriol, should be started. For patients on dialysis (stage 5 CKD), an active form of vitamin D should be given if the PTH is over 300 pg/ml.[9]

Hypoparathyroidism manifests as hypocalcemia accompanied by hyperphosphatemia. The presentation can range from symptoms of perioral and digital paresthesias to life-threatening cardiac arrhythmias, seizures, and laryngospasm. The severity of presentation depends on the rapidity of the development of hypocalcemia. It may also depend on the presence of acidemia, which increases ionized calcium, or alkalemia, which decreases ionized calcium. Chronic hypocalcemia can produce premature cataract formation or basal ganglia calcifications, at times with a reversible Parkinson's syndrome.[10]

PHYSICAL EXAMINATION

Physical clues to primary hyperparathyroidism include band keratopathy, a white cloudiness at the border of the cornea. It may be mistaken for arcus senilis and is not specific for hypercalcemia caused by hyperparathyroidism. Occasionally, there may be bony tenderness, particularly of the sternum and tibia. Rarely, there may be a palpable neck mass that is indicative of parathyroid carcinoma.

The physical clues to hypoparathyroidism include the signs indicative of hypocalcemia. Chvostek's sign may be positive in cases of hypocalcemia. This test is performed by tapping (the point of a triangular reflex hammer or a fingertip may be used) over the facial nerve (cranial nerve VII). Contraction of the facial muscles (seen at the corner of the lip and cheek) is a positive test. Trousseau's sign may also be present in hypocalcemia. This test is performed by placing a blood pressure cuff around the biceps and inflating the cuff approximately 10 to 20 mm Hg above the systolic blood pressure. The cuff is left inflated for 3 minutes, or until a positive result is elicited. The test is positive if carpal spasm occurs (flexion at the wrist and extension of the fingers). The presence of Chvostek's and Trousseau's signs can be affected by abnormalities in acid-base balance, potassium level, and magnesium level.

DIAGNOSTICS

Laboratory testing is necessary for the diagnosis of parathyroid disease. The most useful PTH assay is the PTH immunoradiometric assay, which allows measurement of the intact PTH molecule.

Primary hyperparathyroidism requires the assessment of PTH, serum calcium, albumin, 25-hydroxyvitamin D, and fasting phosphorus. Assessing levels of serum 1,25-dihydroxyvitamin D may be useful if medical therapy is planned. A bone mineral density assessment of a cortical bone site (e.g., radius) and a 24-hour urine collection for calcium are useful for assessing the risk for osteoporosis; renal imaging (plain film abdominal radiographs or renal ultrasound) is useful in assessing the presence of nephrolithiasis. An ECG may be useful in assessing hypercalcemic cardiotoxicity (QT shortening). Parathyroid imaging is often not required if an experienced parathyroid surgeon is available and no prior neck surgery has been performed. However, more recently, preoperative imaging has been used to localize the offending adenoma before surgery, allowing a minimally invasive surgical approach. This minimally invasive approach has high success rates and may result in shorter hospital stays postoperatively.[11,12]

Secondary hyperparathyroidism and hypoparathyroidism require assessment of PTH, serum calcium, albumin, and fasting phosphorus. A serum 25-hydroxyvitamin D level, if less than 20 ng/ml, is useful in establishing vitamin D deficiency as the cause of the hyperparathyroidism. A serum magnesium level may also be useful in evaluating hypoparathyroidism. An ECG can reveal hypocalcemic cardiotoxicity (QT lengthening).

DIAGNOSTICS

Parathyroid Gland Disorders

HYPERPARATHYROIDISM

Laboratory
- PTH (PTH immunoradiometric assay)
- Serum calcium
- Albumin
- Fasting phosphorus
- 24-Hour urine calcium
- Serum 1,25-dihydroxyvitamin D*
- Serum 25-hydroxyvitamin D

Imaging
- X-rays of abdomen*
- Renal ultrasound
- Bone mineral densitometry (distal radius)

Other
- ECG*

HYPOPARATHYROIDISM

Laboratory
- PTH
- Serum calcium
- Albumin
- Fasting phosphorus
- Serum 1,25-dihydroxyvitamin D
- Magnesium
- Serum 25-hydroxyvitamin D

Other
- ECG*

*If indicated.

DIFFERENTIAL DIAGNOSIS

By definition, the differential diagnoses for the parathyroid diseases overlap with those of hypercalcemia and hypocalcemia (see Chapter 220). With primary hyperparathyroidism, the most important diagnosis to exclude is familial hypocalciuric hypercalcemia (FHH), an autosomal dominant trait characterized by hypercalcemia and hyperparathyroidism. With FHH, a mutation in the calcium-sensing receptor gene causes a defective calcium-sensing receptor that requires higher levels of calcium to suppress PTH secretion.[13] Patients with FHH do not have the usual sequelae of primary hyperparathyroidism and generally have a benign course. In FHH the fractional excretion of calcium (FE_{Ca}) is generally less than 0.01%. For patients with primary hyperparathyroidism, the FE_{Ca} is more than 0.013%. The formula is as follows:

$$FE_{Ca} = (U_{Ca} \times P_{Cr})/(U_{Cr} \times P_{Ca})$$

DIFFERENTIAL DIAGNOSIS

Parathyroid Gland Disorders

HYPERPARATHYROIDISM
- Primary hyperparathyroidism
- Familial hyperparathyroidism
- Familial hypocalciuric hypercalcemia
- Lithium-related parathyroid disease
- Adenoma
- Radiation-induced hyperparathyroidism
- Multiple endocrine neoplasia syndrome
- Parathyroid carcinoma
- Secondary hyperparathyroidism
- Chronic renal disease
- Vitamin D deficiency
- Thiazide-induced hypercalcemia

HYPOPARATHYROIDISM
- Idiopathic
- Iatrogenic
- Congenital
- Polyglandular autoimmune syndrome
- Metastatic cancer
- Hemochromatosis
- Amyloidosis
- Hypermagnesemia or hypomagnesemia
- Parkinson's syndrome

where U = Urine concentration (mg/dl) of a 24-hour specimen, and P = Plasma concentration (mg/dl) for calcium (Ca) and creatinine (Cr).

An FE_{Ca} should be calculated to rule out FHH before parathyroidectomy for hyperparathyroidism. An FE_{Ca} of less than 0.01% suggests FHH. If needed, genetic analysis for a mutation in the calcium-sensing receptor can be done to confirm the diagnosis. Of note, autoantibodies directed at the calcium-sensing receptor can cause an acquired, immune-mediated disease that resembles FHH.[14]

Another clinical situation that produces a similar picture is lithium-related parathyroid disease. Lithium appears to raise the calcium set point through unclear mechanisms.

For hypoparathyroidism, the most important diagnostic consideration is hypomagnesemia or hypermagnesemia.

MANAGEMENT

The only cure for primary hyperparathyroidism is surgery, and referral to an experienced parathyroid surgeon is important. In most instances, resection of the parathyroid adenoma or 3¾ of the four hyperplastic parathyroid glands corrects the hyperparathyroidism. However, the changing character of primary hyperparathyroidism, with early diagnosis and primarily asymptomatic patients, has led to an increasing role for medical therapy.

There is a conspicuous absence of data regarding the prediction of complications in a patient with asymptomatic primary hyperparathyroidism. In 2002 the National Institutes of Health (NIH) and the National Institute of Diabetes and Digestive and Kidney Diseases issued the following guidelines favoring the choice of surgical over medical management[15]:

- Age <50 years
- Patients who cannot participate in appropriate follow-up
- Serum calcium level 1 mg/dl above the upper limit of normal
- Urine calcium >400 mg/24 hr
- Patients with 30% decrease in renal function
- Patients with complications, including kidney stones, osteoporosis (*T*- score <−2.5), severe psychoneurologic disorders

Longitudinal measurements of bone mineral density in 66 patients with asymptomatic hyperparathyroidism who were managed medically show that their bone disease did not progress at the radius and lumbar spine over 6 years of observation.[16] However, surgery in 34 patients who met the NIH criteria resulted in marked increases in bone mineral density (12.8% at the spine, 12.7% at the femoral neck, and 4% at the distal radius).[17]

Medical management of asymptomatic primary hyperparathyroidism involves maintaining adequate hydration, avoiding medications that may raise calcium (e.g., thiazide diuretics), and maintaining activity (inactivity can increase bone resorption). Dietary calcium excess and deficiency should be avoided—the former for obvious reasons and the latter because of potential increases in PTH as a result of a calcium-deficient diet. A study has suggested that patients with normal levels of 1,25-dihydroxyvitamin D can liberalize their calcium intake (i.e., 1000 mg of elemental calcium daily), whereas patients with elevated levels are advised to ingest less calcium daily to prevent hypercalciuria.[18]

Oral phosphorus supplementation decreases serum calcium but is limited by the risk of ectopic calcification and the potential for further raising PTH. In postmenopausal women, estrogen may decrease serum calcium but does not affect PTH levels. Bisphosphonates have not yet been shown to produce sustained decreases in serum calcium. Preliminary studies of 13 postmenopausal women with mild primary hyperparathyroidism ages 67 to 81 who were treated with alendronate for 2 years demonstrated a decrease in bone turnover markers during treatment and a statistically significant increase in body mass density at the spine (+8.6 ±3.0%), hip (+4.8 ±3.9%), and total body (+1.2 ±1.4%) compared with the nontreatment group. However, there was a transient decrease in serum calcium levels and statistically significant increase in serum PTH levels.[19] Calcimimetic agents that activate the calcium receptor on parathyroid cells show promise for the medical management of primary hyperparathyroidism. Their action seems to inhibit PTH release and decrease serum calcium levels.[20]

Monitoring bone mineral density and 24-hour urinary calcium annually and serum calcium semiannually is prudent. Imaging studies for occult nephrolithiasis and the assessment of creatinine clearance may be helpful.

When vitamin D deficiency and primary hyperparathyroidism co-exist, repletion of vitamin D stores may be linked to increases in bone mineral density. A study of 229 individuals with osteoporosis found five subjects to have both primary hyperparathyroidism and vitamin D deficiency. After replacement of their vitamin D deficiency (50,000 IU twice a week for 5 weeks), increases in bone mineral density of 6.3% and 8.2% in the spine and hip, respectively, were seen despite persistent elevation of PTH.[21] Serum calcium levels were monitored during vitamin D therapy. Another study of 25 patients with primary hyperparathyroidism, mild hypercalcemia, and vitamin D deficiency who underwent vitamin D repletion suggested that vitamin D repletion decreases levels of PTH and alkaline phosphatase without exacerbating hypercalcemia.[22] Bone mineral densities were unchanged in this study.

The management of secondary hyperparathyroidism depends on the cause. For renal failure, renal transplantation usually corrects the hyperparathyroidism, but it may be refractory if longstanding. Specific guidelines, issued by the National Kidney Foundation, are available for management of secondary hyperparathyroidism in chronic kidney disease; readers are referred to the Kidney Disease Outcomes Quality Initiative website (http://www.kidney.org/professionals/KDOQI/index.cfm). For vitamin D deficiency, mild secondary hyperparathyroidism can be corrected with 400 to 800 IU vitamin D daily. More aggressive therapy can be undertaken with 50,000 IU vitamin D weekly for 8 weeks.

Calcitriol (1,25-dihydroxycholecalciferol) and calcium therapy (to raise serum calcium and decrease serum phosphorus) are also useful in lowering PTH levels, but are plagued by problems with hypercalcemia. There are now a number of alternative U.S. Food and Drug Administration–approved therapies for secondary hyperparathyroidism, including two vitamin D analogs, doxercalciferol (Hectorol) and paricalcitol (Zemplar), and a calcium-sensing receptor agonist, cinacalcet (Sensipar).[23-25]

Hypoparathyroidism is difficult to treat. PTH must be given parenterally and therefore is not easily replaced. Therapy usually consists of vitamin D analogs and calcium supplements. Dairy products, which are high in phosphorus, should be avoided. Perhaps the safest medication is calcitriol, but it is also the most expensive. It is preferable to ergocalciferol (vitamin D) because it acts more quickly (days versus weeks) and has a shorter duration of action, which allows rapid titration. Hypercalciuria is the main limitation of calcitriol therapy. The absence of the PTH effect on renal conservation of calcium results in hypercalciuria as intestinal absorption of calcium increases. Calcitriol should be started at 0.25 mcg PO q day and increased as necessary every 2 to 4 weeks to bring serum calcium into the low-normal range without producing hypercalciuria. The judicious use of thiazides may decrease urinary calcium loss and allow the normalization of serum calcium.

COMPLICATIONS

Complications may result from the parathyroid disease process or its treatment. In addition to osteoporosis and nephrolithiasis, surgery for primary hyperparathyroidism may cause hypocalcemia as a result of temporary hypoparathyroidism, vitamin D deficiency, or hungry bone syndrome. With hungry bone syndrome, calcium and phosphorus are rapidly incorporated into bone. This cause of hypocalcemia is more common in patients with higher preoperative serum calcium, alkaline phosphatase, or more severe bone disease.

INDICATIONS FOR REFERRAL OR HOSPITALIZATION

All parathyroid disorders should be referred to a physician or an endocrinologist experienced in the treatment of parathyroid disease. If surgical therapy is indicated, a referral to an experienced parathyroid surgeon is essential.

PATIENT EDUCATION AND HEALTH PROMOTION

For patients with primary hyperparathyroidism, understanding the importance of adequate calcium and fluid intake, as well as continued monitoring of bone and calcium status, is important. Potential complications of parathyroid bone disease, such as wrist and hip fractures, should be carefully explained. For patients with secondary hyperparathyroidism, the importance of calcium and vitamin D supplementation should be stressed. For patients who undergo surgical therapy or who have hypoparathyroidism, it is essential that they recognize the symptoms of hypocalcemia and the consequences of nonadherence to therapy, including tetany, laryngospasm, cardiac arrhythmias, and seizures.

REFERENCES

1. Silverberg SJ, Bilezikian JP: Primary hyperparathyroidism: still evolving? *J Bone Miner Res* 12:856-862, 1997.
2. Schneider AB, Gierlowski TC, Shore-Freedman E, and others: Dose-response relationship for radiation-induced hyperparathyroidism, *J Clin Endocrinol Metab* 80(1):254-257, 1995.
3. Boonen S, Vanderschueren D, Pelemans W, and others: Primary hyperthyroidism: diagnosis and management in the older individual, *Eur J Endocrinol* 151(3):297-304, 2004, retrieved Feb 17, 2007, from http://www.medscape.com/medline/abstract/15362957?src=emed_ckb_ref_.
4. Bushinsky DA: Bone disease in moderate renal failure: cause, nature, and prevention, *Ann Rev Med* 48:167-176, 1997.
5. McKenna MJ: Differences in vitamin D status between countries in young adults and the elderly, *Am J Med* 93:69-77, 1992.
6. Kahky MP, Weber RS: Complications of surgery of the thyroid and parathyroid glands, *Surg Clin North Am* 73:307-321, 1993.
7. Goodman WG, Veldhuis JD, Belin TR, and others: Calcium-sensing by parathyroid glands in secondary hyperparathyroidism, *J Clin Endocrinol Metab* 83(8):2765-2772, 1998.
8. Mollerup CL, Vestergaard P, Frokjaer VG: Risk of renal stone events in primary hyperparathyroidism before and after parathyroid surgery: controlled retrospective follow up study, *BMJ* 325(7368):807, 2002.
9. National Kidney Foundation: K/DOQI clinical practice guidelines for chronic kidney disease: evaluation, classification, and stratification, *Am J Kidney Dis* 39(2 Suppl 1):S1-S266, 2002.
10. Tambyah PA, Ong BKC, Lee KO: Reversible Parkinsonism and asymptomatic hypocalcemia with basal ganglia calcification from hypoparathyroidism 26 years after thyroid surgery, *Am J Med* 94:444-445, 1993.
11. Shabtai M, Ben-Haim M, Muntz Y, and others: 140 consecutive cases of minimally invasive, radio-guided parathyroidectomy: lessons learned and long-term results, *Surg Endosc* 17(5):688-691, 2003.
12. Dillavou ED, Cohn HE: Minimally invasive parathyroidectomy: 101 consecutive cases from a single surgeon, *J Am Coll Surg* 197(1):1-7, 2003.
13. Pollak MR, Brown EM, Chou YH, and others: Mutations in the human Ca(2^+)-sensing receptor gene cause familial hypocalciuric hypercalcemia and neonatal severe hyperparathyroidism, *Cell* 75(7):1297-1303, 1993.
14. Kifor O, Moore FD Jr, Delaney M, and others: A syndrome of hypocalciuric hypercalcemia caused by autoantibodies directed at the calcium sensing receptor, *J Clin Endocrinol Metab* 88(1):60-72, 2003.
15. Bilezikian JP, Potts JT Jr, Fuleihan G-H, and others: Summary statement from a workshop on asymptomatic primary hyperparathyroidism: a prospective for the 21st century, *J Bone Miner Res* 17(Suppl 2):N2-N11, 2002.
16. Silverberg SJ, Gartenberg F, Jacobs TP, and others: Longitudinal measurements of bone density and biochemical indices in untreated primary hyperparathyroidism, *J Clin Endocrinol Metab* 80(3):723-728, 1995.
17. Silverberg SJ, Gartenberg F, Jacobs TP, and others: Increased bone mineral density after parathyroidectomy in primary hyperparathyroidism, *J Clin Endocrinol Metab* 80(3):720-722, 1995.
18. Locker FG, Silverberg SJ, Bilezikian JP: Optimal dietary calcium intake in primary hyperparathyroidism, *Am J Med* 102:543-550, 1997.
19. Rossini M, Gatti D, Isaia G, and others: Effects of oral alendronate in elderly patients with osteoporosis and mild primary hyperparathyroidism, *J Bone Miner Res* 16(1):113-119, 2001.
20. Silverberg SJ, Bone HG 3rd, Marriott TB, and others: Short-term inhibition of parathyroid hormone secretion by a calcium-receptor agonist in patients with primary hyperparathyroidism, *N Engl J Med* 337(21):1506-1510, 1997.
21. Kantorovich V, Gacad MA, Seeger LL, and others: Bone mineral density increases with vitamin D repletion in patients with coexistent vitamin D insufficiency and primary hyperparathyroidism, *J Clin Endocrinol Metab* 85(10):3541-3543, 2000.
22. Grey A, Lucas J, Home A, and others: Vitamin D repletion in patients with primary hyperparathyroidism and coexistent vitamin D insufficiency, *J Clin Endocrinol Metab* 90(4):2122-2126, 2005.
23. Coburn JW, Maung HM, Elangovan L, and others: Doxercalciferol safely suppresses PTH levels in patients with secondary hyperparathyroidism associated with chronic kidney disease stages 3 and 4, *Am J Kidney Dis* 43(5):877-890, 2004.
24. Sprague SM, Llach F, Amdahl M, and others: Paricalcitol versus calcitriol in the treatment of secondary hyperparathyroidism, *Kidney Intern* 63(9):1483-1490, 2003.
25. Block GA, Martin KJ, de Francisco AL, and others: Cinacalcet for secondary hyperparathyroidism in patients receiving hemodialysis, *N Engl J Med* 350(15):1516-1525, 2004.

CHAPTER 225

Thyroid Disorders

Jennifer C. Braimon and Heather Elias

Thyroid disease in its various forms is widely prevalent in the general population. Perhaps 50% of the population has microscopic nodules, 3.5% have occult papillary carcinoma, 15% have palpable goiters, 10% have abnormal thyroid-stimulating hormone (TSH) levels, and 5% of women have overt hypothyroidism or hyperthyroidism.[1]

Hormones secreted by the thyroid gland influence a variety of metabolic processes in the body. Thyroid function is regulated by TSH, which is secreted by basophilic cells in the anterior pituitary gland in response to the secretion of thyrotropin-releasing hormone (TRH) from the hypothalamus. Control of TRH secretion is regulated in a negative-feedback fashion by the thyroid hormones. Low serum levels of thyroid hormones trigger TRH release from the hypothalamus, which in turn causes TSH release from the pituitary. TSH causes increased release of thyroid hormones until a normal serum level is reached. Within the thyroid gland, thyroid function is affected by glandular organic iodine content.

The synthesis of T_4 (thyroxine) and T_3 (triiodothyronine) requires that adequate quantities of iodine enter the thyroid gland. Iodine enters from the bloodstream and is a constituent of both T_4 and T_3. These hormones are transported in the bloodstream bound to plasma proteins. The majority of T_4 is bound; only a small portion is free. However, it is free T_4 concentration in the serum that indicates thyroidal activity. Approximately 80% of serum T_3 is formed in the liver, kidney, and muscle from the deiodination of T_4; the remaining 20% is secreted directly by the thyroid.[2] Alterations in the regulation of hormone secretion can have varied effects on the body (Box 225-1).

Alterations in the function of the thyroid gland may result in hypersecretion and increased metabolism (hyperthyroidism) or hyposecretion and decreased metabolism (hypothyroidism). Enlargement of the gland may also occur and take the form of localized nodules or generalized goiter. Localized nodules may be benign or malignant, and solitary or multiple; goiters may be mild or extensive.

BOX 225-1

PHYSIOLOGIC EFFECTS OF THYROID HORMONES

- Affect fetal development; secreted from 11 weeks in fetus and facilitates normal fetal growth
- Promote basal metabolic function; regulates oxygen consumption and heat production
- Affect cardiovascular muscle contraction
- Stimulate bone resorption and, to some extent, bone formation
- Permit normal glucose metabolism, absorption, and storage
- Function in the synthesis and breakdown of lipids
- Affect the rate of metabolism of many hormones and drugs (depends on amount of thyroid hormones)

THYROID FUNCTION TESTING

Thyroid function can be evaluated in the laboratory through the use of thyroid function tests (TFTs). Thyroid structure and function can be assessed through a variety of imaging techniques and through biopsy.

TSH is the most sensitive indicator of overall thyroid function. Current techniques allow measurement of serum TSH concentrations as low as 0.01 μU/L (third-generation assay, immunometric dual-antibody assay). This generally is the best screening test for thyroid dysfunction. Exceptions include patients with pituitary or hypothalamic (secondary or tertiary) disease and patients immediately after treatment of hypothyroidism or hyperthyroidism (when the TSH response to therapy may lag behind). In addition, various medications and nonthyroidal conditions may affect TSH levels.

TSH measurements are usually sufficient to categorize patients into one of three groups: hyperthyroid (TSH <0.3 μU/L), hypothyroid (TSH >4 μU/L), and euthyroid (TSH = 0.3 to 4 μU/L). Approximately 99% of circulating T_4 and T_3 is bound to serum proteins. It is the free, unbound T_4 that is maintained at a constant level and correlates most with the thyroid state. Free T_4 traverses cell membranes to exert its effects on body tissues. Direct measurements of free T_4 and T_3 are available but are cumbersome and technically demanding. It is usually sufficient to correct the total T_4 (TT_4) level for the concentration of thyroxine-binding globulin (TBG).

TBG determinations are inaccurate in patients with congenital absence of TBG or familial dysalbuminemic hyperthyroxinemia (FDH). Patients with FDH have aberrant albumin that binds T_4 (not T_3) with increased affinity. In FDH, laboratory tests reveal increased TT_4, normal total T_3 (TT_3), normal TSH, and normal free T_4 by equilibrium dialysis. Circumstances that increase TBG include pregnancy; acute hepatitis; inherited abnormalities; and the use of estrogen, oral contraceptives, methadone, or heroin. Decreased TBG results from acromegaly; nephrotic syndrome; cirrhosis; chronic debilitating disease; and treatment with glucocorticoids, androgens, aspirin, NSAIDs, and some penicillins.

If the TSH level is abnormal, T_4 and a marker for binding proteins should be obtained. The T_3U test is the resin or charcoal T_3 (radioactive T_3) uptake test; it estimates the unoccupied binding sites on TBG. The T_3U parallels the concentration of free T_4. The thyroid hormone–binding ratio (THBR) is a standard way of correcting for TBG:

$$\text{THBR} = \text{Patient's } T_3U : \text{Mean laboratory } T_3U$$

Thus the corrected T_4 (T_4 index, or T_7) is calculated as follows:

$$T_4 \text{ index} = TT_4 \times \text{THBR}$$

T_3 determination is useful in diagnosis of T_3 toxicosis (normal TT_4, decreased TSH, and increased TT_3) and in the diagnosis of euthyroid sick patients. With euthyroid sick syndrome, acute nonthyroidal illness, chronic disease, or caloric deprivation causes decreased peripheral conversion of T_4 to T_3 (inhibition of the type 1 deiodinase). Reverse T_3 (rT_3) is a product of T_4 degradation in the peripheral tissues. It is also secreted in insignificant amounts by the thyroid gland. Levels are elevated in states in which T_3 is decreased (e.g., patients who are euthyroid sick).

Autoantibodies to thyroglobulin or thyroid microsomes may be found in patients with autoimmune thyroid disease. Thyroid peroxidase (TPO) is the major microsomal antigen. Anti-TPO antibodies are found in patients with Hashimoto's thyroiditis and in fewer than 85% of patients with Graves' disease (autoimmune hyperthyroidism). Antithyroglobulin antibodies are found in 20% of patients with Hashimoto's thyroiditis and fewer than 20% of patients with Graves' disease. Up to 15% of the general population have antibodies to either of these antigens. Quantifying the antibody titers is not clinically useful, although some studies suggest that the severity of thyroid destruction in Hashimoto's thyroiditis is proportional to the anti-TPO titer. These tests are particularly useful in the evaluation of patients with atypical manifestations of autoimmune thyroid disease (i.e., isolated ophthalmopathy without signs of hyperthyroidism). They are also predictive of postpartum thyroiditis.[3]

Radionuclide imaging cannot be performed for at least 4 weeks in patients who have recently received iodine-containing compounds (i.e., IV contrast). They may also be inaccurate (falsely low uptake) in patients who are following a high-iodine diet.

The pertechnetate scan is often used for imaging the thyroid. Pertechnetate (technetium 99m, $TcO4^-$) has the same size and charge as iodide. It is concentrated but not bound by thyroid tissues. Scans are performed 20 minutes after the administration of $TcO4^-$. Its advantages include low radiation exposure to the patient, availability, and its power of resolution (approximately 5 mm). Rarely there will be a false-positive result (i.e., "hot" or false uptake) in malignant tissues. Iodine isotopes (^{123}I, ^{125}I, and ^{131}I) are concentrated and bound by thyroid tissues. Scans are performed 4 or 24 hours after the administration of ^{123}I or ^{125}I and 48, 72, or 96 hours after the administration of ^{131}I when used to search for metastatic thyroid cancer.

Normally, the isotopes are distributed evenly throughout the thyroid gland. Each thyroid lobe is approximately 3 to 4 cm (1.2 to 1.6 inches) long, 1 to 1.5 cm (0.4 to 0.6 inch) wide, and 1 cm in depth. The isthmus measures about 0.5 cm (0.2 inch) in height and 2 to 3 mm (0.08 to 0.12 inch) in depth. A mottled appearance is seen in Hashimoto's thyroiditis or in recently treated Graves' disease. An inhomogeneous uptake is also seen in multinodular goiters.

Nodules are classified as hot, warm, or cold according to the concentration of isotope in the nodule in comparison with the rest of the thyroid gland. Hot nodules are usually, but not always, benign. Many cold nodules (solid or cystic) are benign; however, most malignancies also appear as cold nodules. The normal radioactive iodine uptake (RAIU) is approximately 30%. Exuberant iodine supplementation is becoming more prevalent and may cause a falsely low RAIU. When ordering isotope scans, the health care provider can order an RAIU alone or with a scan.

Ultrasonography is used to evaluate the anatomy of the thyroid gland and to differentiate solid from cystic nodules. It is useful in detecting abnormalities larger than 0.5 cm (0.2 inch) in diameter. It localizes the position and depth of lesions and can be used to guide fine-needle aspiration (FNA). In a study by Papini, Guglielmi, Bianchini, and colleagues, ultrasound features of thyroid nodules predictive of malignancy included irregular margins (RR 16.83), intranodular vascular spots (RR 14.29), and microcalcifications (RR 4.97). Eighty-seven percent of cancers manifested as a hypoechoic solid nodule on ultrasound.[4] Ultrasound cannot be used to visualize substernal goiters because of interference from bone. CT and MRI are better suited to assess substernal goiters. Cervical lymph nodes are also well visualized on ultrasound. Benign lymph nodes tend to be thin and oval with an echogenic hilus, whereas malignant nodes tend to be round with an undefined hilus and may be vascular.[5] In a retrospective study of the ultrasound appearance of 63 patients with increased cervical lymphadenopathy, a cystic appearance of cervical lymph nodes was characteristic of metastatic papillary thyroid carcinoma: 70% sensitivity, 100% specificity, 100% positive predictive value, 88% negative predictive value, and 90% accuracy.[6]

^{18}F-Fluorodeoxyglucose positron emission tomography (^{18}F-FDG PET) has the highest resolution for detecting aggressive metastatic thyroid cancer lesions. Radiolabeled glucose is injected intravenously, and the scanner produces images that visualize where glucose is utilized. It identifies differences in how quickly cells metabolize glucose. Cancer cells metabolize glucose more quickly than normal cells. PET thyroid incidentalomas have a high risk of malignancy. In a study by Cohen, Arslan, Dehdashti, and colleagues, about 47% of PET thyroid incidentalomas were confirmed thyroid malignancies.[7] In this retrospective study of all patients at their institution who underwent FDG PET scanning between June 1, 1996, and March 15, 2001, the authors identified thyroid incidentalomas in 102 of 4525 patients (2.3%). Eighty-seven of the 102 patients had other malignancies, and therefore no histologic studies were available. The remaining 15 patients underwent FNA biopsy: seven (47%) were diagnosed with thyroid cancer, six (40%) were diagnosed with benign nodular hyperplasia, one had thyroiditis, and one had benign thyroid nodule.

FDG PET scanning is especially useful in patients with elevated thyroglobulin levels and negative ^{131}I whole body scans. The ability of metastatic thyroid lesions to concentrate ^{131}I is usually indicative of a well-differentiated phenotype. Metastases that do not concentrate ^{131}I are typically more aggressive. Most rapidly growing thyroid neoplasms have high metabolic rates. In a study by Wang, Larson, Fazzari, and colleagues,[8] benign and well-differentiated thyroid tumors were found to retain FDG poorly. FDG volume of greater than 125 ml or standard uptake of FDG of more than 10 g/ml suggested a significantly reduced survival. Focal uptake of 18-FDG can also be seen, however, in inflamed lymph nodes, thyroiditis, and benign thyroid nodules.

A core biopsy is used for histologic examination of thyroid tissue (i.e., the architecture is preserved) via closed-needle or open surgery. FNA biopsy obtains material for cytologic examination only. It is simple and safe but should be performed only by experienced practitioners. Initially there had been concern regarding an increased risk of cancer spreading along the needle tract from FNA, but this has not been observed. In experienced hands, FNA biopsy is approximately 95% accurate in excluding cancer.

GOITER (SIMPLE, NONTOXIC)

DEFINITION AND EPIDEMIOLOGY

Enlargement of the thyroid gland is referred to as *goiter*. It may be caused by hormonal or immunologic stimulation or may result from inflammatory, infiltrative, or metabolic conditions, including iodine deficiency or excess, neoplasia, Graves' disease, and thyroiditis.

Nontoxic (simple) goiter occurs when the thyroid gland enlarges in response to inadequate thyroid hormone production. Iodine deficiency remains the most common cause in large areas of Africa, Asia, and South America. The scarcity of iodine in the diet results in the production of TRH, which causes TSH to be secreted in large amounts. The increased TSH has two effects: (1) the retention of all available iodine by the thyroid and (2) the growth of thyroid cells. It is this latter effect that results in thyroid enlargement.

In developed countries, iodine is available in supplemented products such as table salt, fertilizers, animal feeds, and food preservatives. Therefore the most common cause of nontoxic goiter in developed countries is chronic autoimmune thyroiditis.

PATHOPHYSIOLOGY

Initially, the pathology of simple goiters demonstrates a uniformly hypertrophic, hyperplastic, and hypervascular gland. Later, fibrosis may lead to formation of multiple nodules to create a multinodular goiter. These nodules may be "hot" and concentrate iodine or "cold" and not concentrate iodine. When the nodules become autonomous, hyperthyroidism may occur, a condition known as *toxic multinodular goiter.*

Individuals with a nontoxic goiter may or may not have increased levels of TSH. When levels are normal, it is believed the gland enlarges as a response to impaired hormone synthesis by increasing thyroid mass and cellular activity. In individuals with elevated levels of TSH, the thyroid gland increases mass and activity in response to this stimulation.

CLINICAL PRESENTATION

Patients with simple goiter usually are seen with either diffuse or multinodular thyroid enlargement. Symptoms such as difficulty swallowing and neck pressure may be present. Undetected and continued growth may result in the thyroid gland extending downward to a substernal location in the chest. Presentation may include symptoms that result from compression of the trachea, esophagus, and vasculature.

PHYSICAL EXAMINATION

Examination of the thyroid should begin with observation under a good examining light. The normal gland is rarely visible. It is useful to have the patient extend the neck fully to permit inspection of the gland over the trachea. It is also helpful to observe from the side to identify any enlargement between the cricoid cartilage and the suprasternal notch. Any prominence in this area should be measured with a ruler and recorded; a high likelihood of goiter exists if the prominence is larger than 2 mm (0.08 inch). Having the patient swallow a sip of water may enhance visualization of an enlarged gland.

Palpation may be performed either in front of or behind the patient (depending on practitioner's comfort), and the texture is noted. The texture of the thyroid can range from extremely soft to relatively firm; it may be smooth or may contain palpable nodules. Prominent glands should be measured and recorded. Thyroid size should be categorized as normal or goiter.[9] A small goiter is considered to be one to two times the normal size, and a large goiter is greater than twice normal size.

Pemberton's sign is used for examination when substernal goiter is suspected. The patient is asked to elevate both arms until they touch the sides of the head. Flushing of the face, cyanosis, and respiratory distress may occur as a result of impingement of structures within the thoracic inlet.[10] Distention of neck veins may also be apparent in these patients.

DIAGNOSTICS

Laboratory studies may show low or normal free T_4 and, most often, normal levels of TSH. Radioiodine uptake may be high, normal, or low depending on the amount of iodine in the diet and the level of TSH. Isotope scanning results depend on whether nodules are hot or cold. Thyroid ultrasound allows identification of gland size and the number and size of any nodules. If necessary for diagnosis, FNA may be performed.

DIAGNOSTICS

Goiter

LABORATORY
TSH
Free T_4
Antimicrosomal antibodies*

IMAGING
Radionuclide scanning
Thyroid ultrasound

OTHER
Fine-needle aspiration*

*If indicated.

DIFFERENTIAL DIAGNOSIS

Simple goiter must also be differentiated from chronic autoimmune thyroiditis and toxic multinodular goiter. A careful history of symptoms is important. Also, with chronic autoimmune thyroiditis, circulating antimicrosomal antibody levels will be elevated.

DIFFERENTIAL DIAGNOSIS

Goiter

Iodine deficiency or excess
Neoplasia (multinodular, malignant)
Graves' disease
Simple goiter
Thyroiditis
- Chronic autoimmune thyroiditis
- Hashimoto's thyroiditis
- Subacute thyroiditis
- Postpartum thyroiditis

Genetic goiter

MANAGEMENT

The majority of nontoxic goiters grow slowly over many years. The presence of a goiter, with no accompanying symptoms or cosmetic concerns, is not an indication for treatment. Treatment indications include venous flow obstruction, compression of the trachea or esophagus, progressive enlargement of the entire goiter or individual nodules, neck discomfort, or cosmetic concerns.[11] The treatment of nontoxic goiter may involve the use of levothyroxine to suppress glandular function, thyroidectomy, or radioiodine.

Surgical treatment, usually bilateral subtotal thyroidectomy, is the preferred treatment in otherwise healthy, young patients, especially in presence of goiters that grow substernally or continue to enlarge, causing compressive symptoms. There is little evidence that postoperative suppressive T_4 treatment prevents goiter recurrence; therefore it should not be routinely used.[12]

Levothyroxine treatment will suppress TSH, correct any hypothyroidism, and slowly reduce the size of the goiter. However, this therapy may have significant adverse effects, such as decreased bone mineral density, atrial fibrillation, and biochemical hyperthyroidism, if not monitored closely. The best candidates for this form of treatment are young patients with small diffuse goiters and a high normal TSH. T_4 therapy is not recommended for patients with any type of goiter or nodule and a low TSH because this therapy may cause hyperthyroidism, especially in older adults.[12,13] Some sources recommend a trial of suppressive therapy for patients with a solitary and nonfunctioning nodule, negative fine-needle aspirates, and normal or elevated TSH levels with the goal of keeping TSH at low-normal levels. Such therapy may continue for 6 months to 1 year before reevaluation.

Nontoxic multinodular goiter may also be treated with radioiodine to reduce thyroid volume. Therapy with ^{131}I has been found to be an effective alternative with a few side effects.[14,15] This therapy is especially useful in older patients or those with cardiopulmonary disease.

COMPLICATIONS

Nontoxic goiter, even if multinodular, has few complications. Of particular concern is the potential for a multinodular goiter to develop autonomous function with ensuing hyperthyroidism. Close monitoring of TSH enables identification of this potential problem. Surgical patients with a nontoxic goiter may require special observation for airway maintenance and hormone supplementation if indicated.

INDICATIONS FOR REFERRAL OR HOSPITALIZATION

Patients who have any indication for treatment of their goiter may require an endocrinology referral for discussion of an appropriate treatment and a surgical referral if thyroidectomy is selected as the treatment of choice.

PATIENT AND FAMILY EDUCATION AND HEALTH PROMOTION

It is important that patients understand the definition and cause of the nontoxic goiter. Patients need to participate in developing the care plan and understand its rationale. Those who live in inland areas or have seafood allergies should use iodized salt. Patients should understand that nontoxic goiter is a manageable, highly livable condition that will not affect their lives in a negative way if well controlled.

THYROID NODULES AND THYROID CANCER

DEFINITION AND EPIDEMIOLOGY

A thyroid nodule is a palpable abnormality within an apparently normal thyroid gland. By this definition, thyroid nodules include cysts, lobules of normal thyroid tissue, and benign and malignant solid lesions. The term *nodular thyroid disease* is preferred.

With ultrasonography, approximately 50% of all single, palpable nodules are found to be in a multinodular gland. In general, nodules larger than 0.5 to 1 cm (0.2 to 0.4 inch) are palpable. Thyroid adenomas are benign neoplastic nodules within a capsule.

The prevalence of thyroid nodules depends on the method of evaluation. Palpable thyroid nodules are found in 4% to 7% of the general adult population. In a Framingham, Massachusetts, cohort, there was a 4.2% overall incidence (6.4% in women and 1.6% in men).[16] Autopsy and ultrasound studies have quoted a prevalence as high as 50%. The lifetime risk of developing a thyroid nodule is estimated to be between 5% and 10%.[17] Thyroid nodules are common, and most of them are benign. Only 3% to 5% of all thyroid nodules are malignant.

PATHOPHYSIOLOGY

Thyroid nodules may be due to adenomas, cysts, carcinomas, multinodular goiters, Hashimoto's thyroiditis, and subacute thyroiditis. Less common causes of neck lumps include the effects of prior surgery or ^{131}I, parathyroid cysts or adenomas, thyroglossal cysts, nonthyroidal lesions, and lymphomas.

Thyroid adenomas are benign, monoclonal growths. Benign thyroid tumors include embryonal, fetal, follicular, Hürthle cell, and papillary adenomas. They are distinguished by their characteristic histologic appearance.[18] Malignant thyroid tumors include papillary, follicular, medullary, and anaplastic carcinomas.

CLINICAL PRESENTATION AND PHYSICAL EXAMINATION

Thyroid nodules are usually asymptomatic and are identified as a lump by patients or by providers during routine thyroid examinations. Recently, an increasing number of thyroid nodules have been identified incidentally during carotid Doppler ultrasound or other neck imaging studies. Clinical features that increase the likelihood of cancer include a history of head and neck irradiation, a family history of thyroid cancer, an age of less than 20 years or more than 60 years, male gender, and a history of multiple endocrine neoplasia type 2 or medullary thyroid cancer.[19-21] Familial thyroid tumors also occur in Cowden's disease (multiple hamartoma syndrome), Gardner's syndrome (development of multiple tumors with autosomal dominant inheritance), and familial polyposis.

An anaplastic tumor may manifest as an enlarging, painful mass associated with hoarseness, dysphonia, dysphagia, or dyspnea. However, patients with benign goiters may also be seen with compressive symptoms. Patients with anaplastic thyroid cancer may have pathologic fractures of the spine or hip or thoracic outlet syndrome. Patients with toxic nodules may show symptoms of hyperthyroidism. Signs and symptoms of hyperthyroidism or hypothyroidism are usually suggestive of a benign process. However, lymphoma may develop within the thyroid gland of patients with Hashimoto's thyroiditis.

Important features noted during the physical examination include nodule size, consistency, and mobility and the presence and consistency of associated lymphadenopathy. Supraclavicular, anterior cervical, and axillary lymph nodes should be examined. Although most thyroid cancers feel firm or hard, they can be soft and fluctuant on examination. The presence of a new nodule or enlarging nodule while a patient is on T_4 therapy is a cause for concern.

DIAGNOSTICS AND DIFFERENTIAL DIAGNOSIS

TFTs (e.g., TSH) are necessary to exclude hyperthyroidism or hypothyroidism. The routine measurement of serum calcitonin (to exclude medullary thyroid cancer) is not useful or cost-effective.[22]

Historically, radionuclide imaging was the first diagnostic test used in the evaluation of solitary thyroid nodules. Although it is true that most thyroid malignancies appear as cold nodules, most cold nodules are benign. Radionuclide scanning is now used as an initial test if a hyperfunctioning nodule is suspected. It may also be useful if the results of FNA are inconclusive.

High-resolution sonography can clearly distinguish between solid and cystic components. However, ultrasonic findings correlate poorly with disease and are not believed to be useful in the routine evaluation of thyroid nodules. The major indications for use of ultrasound are to aid FNA biopsy, to detect nodules too small to palpate in high-risk patients, and to map the extent of thyroid malignancy.[23]

FNA biopsy is an essential diagnostic procedure for the evaluation of thyroid nodules. It is safe and technically simple but requires an experienced operator and cytopathologist. False-negative and false-positive rates are less than 5% with experienced users. Cytologic results are sufficient in 85% of biopsies for diagnosis.

DIAGNOSTICS

Thyroid Nodules and Thyroid Cancer

LABORATORY
TSH

IMAGING
Thyroid ultrasound*
Radionuclide scan*

OTHER
Fine-needle aspiration

*If indicated.

DIFFERENTIAL DIAGNOSIS

Thyroid Nodules and Thyroid Cancer

NODULES
Adenomas
- Follicular
- Papillary
- Teratoma
- Parathyroid

Cysts
Carcinomas
Multinodular goiters
Hashimoto's thyroiditis
Subacute thyroiditis
Surgery or radiation effects
Parathyroid cysts or adenomas
Thyroglossal cysts
Nonthyroidal lesions
Lymphomas

BENIGN TUMORS
Embryonal
Fetal
Follicular
Hürthle cell adenomas
Papillary adenomas

MALIGNANT CARCINOMAS
Papillary
Follicular
Medullary
Anaplastic

MANAGEMENT

The initial management of a thyroid nodule includes a complete history and physical examination. TSH levels are measured. If there is evidence of a solitary nodule on examination, with normal TSH level, the patient should be referred to a practitioner (usually an endocrinologist) who is experienced in performing FNA biopsies.

If the results of the cytologic tests are benign, no further evaluation is necessary. A repeat FNA biopsy should be reserved for enlarging nodules.[24] Thyroid examinations should be performed every 6 to 12 months. T_4 suppression therapy has been shown to be somewhat effective in patients with multinodular goiters and in patients with diffuse nontoxic goiters (30% reduction in nodule size); it is less effective in the treatment of solitary nodule.[25] Because of the uncertainty of the efficacy of T_4 suppression (evidence of benefit is unclear), therapy should be individualized. T_4 suppression is avoided in postmenopausal women unless they are taking hormone replacement therapy, because of the untoward effects of suppression therapy on bone density. A reasonable strategy is to consider the use of T_4 suppression therapy (TSH = 0.1 to 0.5 μU/ml) in men and premenopausal women. If there is shrinkage, the same dose is continued for approximately 1 year and then decreased to keep the TSH levels between 0.4 and 0.9 μU/ml. A repeat FNA biopsy is performed if the nodules increase in size while the patient is on suppressive therapy.

If the TSH level is elevated on initial evaluation, the patient has two conditions requiring medical attention. In addition to the workup and management of hypothyroidism, the presence of a single dominant nodule necessitates further evaluation by FNA biopsy.

If serum TSH is suppressed, free T_4 and TT_3 values should be obtained and a radionuclide (^{123}I) scan performed. If the nodule is hyperfunctioning, the patient has an autonomously functioning thyroid adenoma. Patients with an adenoma who have thyrotoxicosis should be treated with radioiodine or surgery. Patients with subclinical thyrotoxicosis can be monitored or treated (radioiodine or surgery) depending on adenoma size. There are advantages to both therapies. If the nodule is hypofunctioning on ^{123}I scan, the next step is the FNA biopsy evaluation.

If the cytologic test results are suspicious or positive, referral to an experienced surgeon for resection is necessary. The extent of surgical resection remains controversial. For solitary lesions less than 1 cm (0.4 inch), a lobectomy may be performed. Total thyroidectomy is indicated if there is a history of head or neck irradiation, the tumor extends beyond the thyroid capsule, or the lesion is larger than 1 cm.[22] The thyroid remnant is usually ablated with ^{131}I after surgery. This eases the diagnosis and treatment of metastases (evidence exists for benefit).[26] Prophylactic lymph node dissection is not generally indicated. At the time of surgery, regional lymph nodes are evaluated and removed if abnormal.

Medullary thyroid cancer and anaplastic thyroid cancers are more aggressive than well-differentiated thyroid cancers and therefore are treated differently.[27] If the cytologic results are indeterminate, aspiration should be performed again. If results are still inconclusive, radionuclide imaging may be useful.

Patients with differentiated thyroid carcinoma are followed at 3- to 6-month intervals for 5 years after diagnosis and surgery and then at 6- to 12-month intervals if disease free. Thyroglobulin levels and whole-body scans are followed postoperatively. Serum antithyroglobulin antibodies should be checked; if present, these invalidate serum thyroglobulin measurement. Patients are maintained on suppressive doses of T_4 (the goal is TSH levels of 0.2 to 0.4 μU/ml).[28] Biannual chest x-ray examinations are necessary to exclude pulmonary metastasis in papillary carcinomas.

LIFE SPAN CONSIDERATIONS

The net mortality rate of papillary thyroid cancer is 10% to 20% over 20 to 30 years. Several factors increase the risk of death from cancer: extrathyroidal invasion (six times the risk), metastasis (47 times), age over 45 years (32 times), and tumor larger than 3 cm (1.2 inches) (six times).[3]

Various scoring systems are used to stratify the prognosis of patients with well-differentiated and medullary thyroid cancer. In the *MACIS* scoring system for papillary carcinoma, *M*etastasis, *A*ge, *C*ompleteness of surgery, *I*nvasion, and *S*ize are used to predict survival. The following scores are given:

- .0 for distant metastasis
- 3.1 for age <39 years
- 0.08 × age if >40 years
- 1.0 if surgical removal was incomplete
- 1.0 for extrathyroidal invasion
- 0.3 × size of tumor

A total score of less than 6.0 predicts a 99% chance for 20-year survival; 6.0 to 6.99, 89% chance; 7.0 to 7.99, 56% chance; and over 8.0, 24% chance.

The Mayo Clinic scoring system for follicular carcinoma assigns 1 point to each of the following:

- Age >50 years
- Vascular invasion
- Metastatic disease at diagnosis

A total score of 0 or 1 predicts a 99% chance of 5-year survival and an 86% chance of 20-year survival. A total score of 2 or 3 predicts a 47% chance of 5-year survival and an 8% chance of 20-year survival.

The Mayo Clinic scoring system for medullary thyroid cancer predicts prognosis based on:

- Completeness of resection
- Amyloid staining
- Local invasiveness
- Metastasis

One point is given for each of these items. A total score of 0 predicts a 100% 10-year survival rate; a score of 1 predicts a 78% survival rate; a score of 2 predicts a 26% survival rate; and a score of 3 predicts a 0% 10-year survival rate.

COMPLICATIONS

Complications of thyroid surgery include hypoparathyroidism and hoarseness from recurrent laryngeal nerve damage. Side effects of radioiodine include thyroid tenderness, dry mouth, altered taste, and nausea. Cumulative doses of more than 300 mCi may increase the risk of leukemia. Bone marrow suppression is seen with cumulative doses of more than 500 mCi. Other potential complications of radioiodine include pulmonary fibrosis and ovarian or testicular failure. Treatment doses range from 30 to 150 mCi.

INDICATIONS FOR REFERRAL OR HOSPITALIZATION

Once the initial evaluation has been performed (physical examination and TSH levels), the patient is referred to a practitioner experienced in FNA biopsies. If the cytologic test results are positive or suspicious, the patient should be referred to an experienced thyroid surgeon. After surgery the patient should be referred to thyroid specialist, who can coordinate and administer therapeutic radioiodine. Patients are maintained on suppressive doses of T_4.

Indications for hospitalization include respiratory compromise because of invasive tumors, as well as the administration of radioiodine doses above 30 mCi (requires specialized rooms).

PATIENT AND FAMILY EDUCATION AND HEALTH PROMOTION

Patients should be given instructions regarding precautions after radioiodine treatment or scanning. These instructions include (1) no kissing, exchanging saliva, or sharing food or eating utensils for 5 days; dishes should be washed in a dishwasher; (2) no close contact with infants, young children (<8 years of age), or pregnant women for 5 days; it is permissible to be in the same room; (3) no breastfeeding; (4) flushing toilets twice after urinating and washing hands thoroughly; (5) what to do if a sore throat or neck pain develops (may take acetaminophen or aspirin); and (6) notifying physician if nervousness, tremulousness, or palpitations increase.[29] Patients should be taught how to perform a self-thyroid examination. An informative website for patients with thyroid cancer is http://www.thyca.org/.

HYPERTHYROIDISM

DEFINITION AND EPIDEMIOLOGY

Hyperthyroidism is defined as a clinical syndrome caused by the excess production or release of thyroid hormone and its clinical manifestations. Whereas the term *hyperthyroidism* implies that the thyroid is the source of excess thyroid hormone, *thyrotoxicosis* refers to the syndrome produced by excess thyroid hormone regardless of its source (e.g., overingestion of iodine). Primary hyperthyroidism is independent of TSH. TSH-dependent hyperthyroidism is called *secondary hyperthyroidism*. TRH-dependent hyperthyroidism is referred to as *tertiary hyperthyroidism*.

Graves' disease (autoimmune hyperthyroidism) is the most common cause of hyperthyroidism. There is a female-to-male predominance of 7:1, and it is most common in women ages

TABLE 225-1 Signs and Symptoms of Hyperthyroidism

	Symptoms	Signs
Eyes	Dry eyes, blurry vision	See NO SPECS mnemonic (below)
Neck	Diffuse goiter in patients with Graves' disease	Goiter with thyroid bruit in Graves' disease
Respiratory system	Shortness of breath	Labored respiration
Cardiac system	Palpitation, tachycardia, angina	Systolic hypertension, congestive heart failure, tachycardia, atrial fibrillation
Gastrointestinal system	Hyperphagia, hyperdefecation, weight loss, weight gain (rare), anorexia in older adults	Weight loss, weight gain (rare)
Reproductive system	Amenorrhea, menstrual irregularities, infertility	
Neuromuscular system	Proximal muscle weakness, heat intolerance, tremor	Proximal muscle weakness, hyperreflexia
Skin	Pruritus; hyperhidrosis; warm, moist palms; onycholysis (brittle nails, Plummer's nails)	Smooth, velvety skin; warm, moist palms; onycholysis; pretibial myxedema (Graves' disease)
Skeletal system	Osteoporosis	Thyroid acropachy (Graves' disease)
Psychiatric problems	Anxiety, irritability, nervousness, sleeplessness	Visually manifest
Older adults	Anorexia, constipation, normal pulse, weight loss	

20 to 40 years. Transient hyperthyroidism (thyroiditis) needs to be excluded. Toxic multinodular goiters are usually seen in women over 55 years old who have a long history of goiter. Multinodular goiters with autonomy are more susceptible to iodine-induced hyperthyroidism. Iodine sources include topical povidone-iodine (Betadine), IV contrast medium, and iodine-containing drugs. Postpartum thyroiditis (painless) occurs in approximately 5% to 9% of all pregnant women, 25% of pregnant women with type 1 diabetes, and 75% of women with high microsomal antibody titers before pregnancy.[30,31]

PATHOPHYSIOLOGY

Graves' disease is an autoimmune disorder in which thyroid-stimulating antibodies or immunoglobulins (TSIs) compete with TSH for TSH receptors on the thyroid and activate the production of cyclic adenosine monophosphate; this increases the synthesis and release of thyroid hormones. In Caucasians, there is an increased prevalence of certain human leukocyte antigens (HLA-B8 and HLA-DR3).

Subacute thyroiditis is a postviral illness. The thyroid gland is tender, and there is evidence of multinucleated giant cells on microscopic evaluation. Silent thyroiditis (painless) is believed to be an autoimmune disorder. On microscopic examination, there is evidence of lymphocytic infiltration that may mimic Hashimoto's thyroiditis.

CLINICAL PRESENTATION AND PHYSICAL EXAMINATION

Because thyroid hormone acts on all organs, the clinical presentation is variable. The symptoms of hyperthyroidism are secondary to increased sympathetic activity and increased catabolism. *Apathetic hyperthyroidism* refers to patients who lack these symptoms. It is useful to describe the symptoms by organ system as shown in Table 225-1.

Lid lag may be seen with thyrotoxicosis, regardless of the origin of thyroid hormone. This symptom is caused by increased sympathetic activity. The other eye changes associated with Graves' disease are due to the action of TSIs on the connective tissue behind the eye. The *NO SPECS* mnemonic is used to describe the eye changes in association with Graves' disease, as follows[6]:

- *N*o signs or symptoms
- *O*nly signs, no symptoms
- *S*oft tissue swelling
- *P*roptosis
- *E*xtraocular muscle paresis
- *C*orneal involvement
- *S*ight loss (optic nerve involvement)

With subacute thyroiditis, the thyroid gland is tender, and patients often note a recent viral illness.

DIAGNOSTICS

TSH is the best screening test for primary hyperthyroidism. With primary hyperthyroidism, TSH levels will be low or undetectable. If the TSH is suppressed, a T_3U test (or any test of binding proteins) and T_4 levels should be obtained to determine the degree of hyperthyroidism. Alternatively, a free T_4 level can be obtained. TSH levels will remain suppressed for up to 3 months after treatment, and therefore the free T_4 or free T_4 index must be followed. See Table 225-2 for laboratory results in different types of hyperthyroidism.

Abnormal liver function tests are common in patients with hyperthyroidism. Elevations in alkaline phosphatase, alanine aminotransferase, aspartate aminotransferase, γ-glutamyltransferase, and total bilirubin levels were found in a recent study in 33%, 17%, 26%, 24%, and 8% of patients, respectively.[32]

TABLE 225-2 Thyroid Function Tests in Hyperthyroidism

	T_3	T_4/Free T_4 Index	TSH
Graves' disease	Increase	Increase	Decrease
T_3 toxicosis	Increase	Normal	Decrease
T_4 toxicosis	Normal	Increase	Decrease
Subclinical hyperthyroidism	Normal	Normal	Decrease

BOX 225-2

RADIOIODINE UPTAKE IN DIFFERENT FORMS OF HYPERTHYROIDISM

DECREASED OR ZERO RADIOIODINE UPTAKE
- Thyroiditis (subacute, painless)
- Iodine-induced hyperthyroidism
- Exogenous cause of hyperthyroidism
- Struma ovarii
- Metastatic thyroid cancer postthyroidectomy

NORMAL OR HIGH RADIOIODINE UPTAKE
- Graves' disease
- Toxic nodule
- Toxic multinodular goiter
- TSH-induced hyperthyroidism
- Human chorionic gonadotropin–induced hyperthyroidism

DIAGNOSTICS

Hyperthyroidism

LABORATORY
TSH
T_4, free T_4
Total T_3

IMAGING
Radioiodine uptake scan*
MRI*

*If indicated.

As shown in Box 225-2, a radioiodine uptake is useful in distinguishing Graves' disease from thyroiditis.

A scan is useful in identifying a toxic multinodular goiter or solitary nodular goiter. In patients with a diffusely enlarged gland and obvious signs of eye disease, this test is not necessary for diagnosis of Graves' disease but is needed for calculation of the radioiodine dose necessary if iodine ablation therapy is chosen. The erythrocyte sedimentation rate will be increased in subacute thyroiditis. A careful review of iodine-containing medications is necessary in the evaluation of hyperthyroidism. With TSH-induced (secondary) hyperthyroidism, the TSH is inappropriately elevated in the setting of increased T_4 index. Pituitary adenomas are best visualized on MRI. With TSH adenomas, there is an increased ratio of TSH alpha subunit/TSH.

DIFFERENTIAL DIAGNOSIS

Differential diagnoses are described in the box. Another consideration, "hamburger thyrotoxicosis," refers to an epidemic of thyrotoxicosis in the Midwest that was eventually traced to the ingestion of hamburger meat that included the strap muscles of slaughtered cattle (including thyroid tissue). The U.S. Department of Agriculture now prohibits the use of this material.[33]

DIFFERENTIAL DIAGNOSIS

Hyperthyroidism

THYROID DISORDERS
Graves' disease
Transient hyperthyroidism
- Subacute thyroiditis
- Hashimoto's thyroiditis
- Silent (lymphocytic) thyroiditis (postpartum)

Toxic multinodular goiter
Toxic adenoma (toxic nodular goiter)
Exogenous (factious) hyperthyroidism
Iodine-induced hyperthyroidism (Jod Basedow phenomenon; amiodarone)
Hydatidiform mole, human chorionic gonadotropin–induced hyperthyroidism
TSH-secreting pituitary adenoma
Ectopic thyroxine production
- Struma ovarii
- Metastatic follicular thyroid carcinoma postthyroidectomy

Hereditary familial hyperthyroidism (activating mutation for TSH receptor)

NONTHYROIDAL DISORDERS
Anxiety
Pheochromocytoma
Menopause
Pregnancy
Metastatic carcinoma
Cirrhosis
Hyperparathyroidism
Sprue
Myasthenia gravis
Muscular dystrophy

MANAGEMENT AND LIFE SPAN CONSIDERATIONS

The treatment of hyperthyroidism or thyrotoxicosis depends on the etiology of the disease and the patient's age. To simplify the discussion, the therapeutics are discussed by disease entity.

Graves' Disease

With Graves' disease, symptomatic treatment with beta blockers should be initiated to alleviate the β-adrenergic symptoms of hyperthyroidism (tremor, tachycardia). Propranolol (Inderal) can be used at dosages between 10 and 40 mg PO q 6 hr. The dose is titrated to symptoms. Alternatively, longer-acting preparations can be used. They must be used with caution in patients with congestive heart failure and bronchospasm, and they should be avoided in pregnant women because of untoward effects on the fetus.

Medical therapy is the treatment of choice for patients younger than 20 years of age and for pregnant women. The thioamides (antithyroid drugs) include methimazole (Tapazole) and propylthiouracil (PTU). They inhibit thyroid hormone synthesis by blocking organification. In addition, PTU inhibits the peripheral conversion of T_4 to T_3. PTU is the drug of choice for pregnant women because it crosses the placenta less avidly. Thioamide therapy is described in Table 225-3 and Box 225-3.

Thioamides are generally believed to be the most effective in patients with Graves' disease and small glands. In general, they are used for 6 to 12 months and then discontinued; at that time, 30% of patients are in remission. Radioiodine ablation is generally recommended if relapse occurs. The initial clinical response may lag for 2 weeks given the increased stored thyroid hormone. TFTs are monitored every 4 to 6 weeks until the results are stable. TSH levels may remain suppressed for months, and therefore the T_4 index (or free T_4) should be monitored. In pregnant women, this index should be kept at the high-normal range because of the effect of thioamides in inhibiting the fetal thyroid gland.

TABLE 225-3 Thioamide Therapy

	Prophylthiouracil	Methimazole
Dosage	50-100 mg PO q 6-8 hr	5-20 mg PO q 8 hr, or 15-60 mg/day PO
Tablets	50 mg	5 mg, 10 mg
Protein binding	75%	0%
Half life	75 minutes	4-6 hours
Placental passage	1:1	High
Breast milk concentration	Low	High
Advantages	Inhibits conversion of T_4 to T_3; safer in pregnancy	Long half life

BOX 225-3

SIDE EFFECTS OF THIOAMIDES

- Agranulocytosis occurs in 0.2% to 0.5% of patients, usually reversible with discontinuation of medication.
- Baseline CBC and differential should be obtained before initiation of treatment. Patients should be instructed to discontinue medications and call if there are symptoms of infection (e.g., fever, pharyngitis); a CBC and differential should be obtained.
- Rash, arthralgias, myalgias (lupuslike reaction), and fever (3% to 5% of patients) may occur.
- Transient, propylthiouracil-induced subclinical liver injury is possible; need for baseline LFTs should be questioned.
- Nephrotic syndrome (methimazole) is rare.
- Aplastic anemia and thrombocytopenia are rare.

Radioiodine therapy is the treatment of choice in the United States for patients over 20 years old and for those for whom thioamide therapy has failed (through noncompliance or a relapse after treatment). It is contraindicated during pregnancy and should be avoided in patients with Graves' ophthalmopathy because of the increased risk of exacerbation of eye symptoms after treatment. There is no evidence of increased incidence of long-term malignancies. Because of the high incidence of posttreatment hypothyroidism, TFTs should be monitored closely. Approximately 4 to 6 weeks after treatment, the T_4 index should be checked, and the patient should be reevaluated. If there is no evidence of hypothyroidism at that time, TSH and T_4 index should be monitored monthly for 3 to 4 months and then periodically.

Surgery is recommended for pregnant women who cannot be managed with PTU or who develop side effects from it, for patients who refuse radioiodine and cannot tolerate thioamides, and for patients with an obstructive goiter. Complications include hypothyroidism, hypoparathyroidism, and hoarseness (recurrent laryngeal nerve damage).

No studies to date have demonstrated any of the above treatment options to be superior to the others.

Other much less commonly used medications include cholestyramine (which decreases enterohepatic circulation of thyroid hormone), organic iodides (amiodarone and ipodate, which block T_4 to T_3 conversion), lithium and iodides (which block hormone release), and glucocorticoids (which block T_4 to T_3 conversion).

Subclinical Hyperthyroidism

Subclinical hyperthyroidism is defined as a suppressed TSH with normal serum T_4 and T_3 levels. The etiology of subclinical hyperthyroidism is the same as for overt hyperthyroidism. The majority of cases are due to autonomously functioning thyroid nodules and multinodular goiters. Most elderly patients with subclinical hyperthyroidism have a multinodular goiter.[34] Indications for therapy are based on the known skeletal and cardiovascular consequences of untreated hyperthyroidism. In a meta-analysis by Faber and Galloe, exogenous subclinical hyperthyroidism led to osteoporosis in postmenopausal, but not premenopausal, women.[35] In a community-based study by Sawin, Geller, Wolf, and colleagues, the risk of atrial fibrillation was related to the degree of TSH suppression. The cumulative incidence was 28% in patients with TSH levels less than 0.1 μU/L, 16% when TSH levels were between 0.1 and 01.4 μU/L, and 11% in those with normal TSH levels.[36]

Recommendations for treatment of subclinical hyperthyroidism are based on the recent summary from a clinical consensus group made up of representatives from the American Association of Clinical Endocrinologists, the Endocrine Society, and the American Thyroid Association.[37] Treatment should be considered for endogenous subclinical hyperthyroidism with TSH less than 0.1 μU/L as a result of Graves' or nodular thyroid disease, especially in patients older than 60 years old and for those at increased risk for heart disease, osteopenia, or osteoporosis. In those with TSH levels between 0.1 and 0.5 μU/L, follow-up monitoring alone is appropriate.

Thyroiditis

Thyroiditis may be subacute or painless or may be a result of a toxic nodule or toxic multinodular goiter. Hyperthyroid findings may result.

Subacute Thyroiditis. With subacute thyroiditis, symptomatic treatment with beta blockers can be used during the hyperthyroid phase. Different studies have shown relief of pain with the use of NSAIDs, aspirin, and glucocorticoids. Hyperthyroidism lasts for weeks to months and is followed by hypothyroidism (which lasts for months). Most patients become euthyroid, although 30% may remain hypothyroid. Recurrences are rare.

Painless Postpartum Thyroiditis. With painless postpartum thyroiditis, symptomatic treatment with beta blockers can be used during the hyperthyroid phase. Beta blockers are concentrated in breast milk and must be used with caution. Thyroid hormone therapy can be initiated if hypothyroid phase is severe. TFTs should be monitored closely. Although most patients become clinically euthyroid, up to 30% remain hypothyroid. This condition tends to recur with subsequent pregnancies.

Toxic Nodule. With toxic nodules, radioiodine ablation is the treatment of choice after beta blocker therapy. Some studies demonstrate effective therapy with alcohol ablation through repetitive percutaneous injections under ultrasound guidance. Surgical excision is another option, especially in patients with a large adenoma.

Toxic Multinodular Goiter. With toxic multinodular goiter, radioiodine ablation is the treatment of choice after beta blocker therapy. Other nodules may become toxic in the future and may require repeat doses of ^{131}I. Other treatment options include antithyroid drugs followed by subtotal thyroidectomy.

COMPLICATIONS

Untreated Graves' disease can lead to atrial fibrillation, congestive heart failure, angina, and osteoporosis. Thyroid storm is a rare, life-threatening form of hyperthyroidism that leads to systemic decompensation. The incidence has declined during the past few decades because of advances in medical management, but thyrotoxic crises account for approximately 1% of all hospitalizations for hyperthyroidism. Although it more commonly occurs with Graves' disease, it can be found in conjunction with other causes of hyperthyroidism.

INDICATIONS FOR REFERRAL OR HOSPITALIZATION

Health care providers can perform the initial evaluation for hyperthyroidism. Laboratory confirmation of hyperthyroidism and radioiodine scans should be obtained. Thioamides can be administered by practitioners who are experienced with their use. Treatment options can be discussed with patients; if radioiodine therapy is selected, a consultation with an endocrinologist should be obtained. An endocrinologist and an ophthalmologist should see patients with Graves' ophthalmopathy.

Patients with thyroid storm require hospitalization and should be evaluated by an endocrinologist or by a physician familiar with its treatment. Thyroid storm, or thyrotoxic crisis, requires aggressive inpatient management. The diagnosis is based on clinical findings: temperature of 38.8° to 40.5° C (102° to 105° F), profuse sweating, pulse over 120 to 140 beats per minute, atrial fibrillation, restlessness, confusion, agitation, and coma. Gastrointestinal symptoms may include severe vomiting, diarrhea, and hepatomegaly with jaundice. The goals of therapy are to inhibit thyroid hormone formation and release, provide β-adrenergic blockade, provide supportive therapy, identify and treat any precipitating illness, and initiate long-term therapy to prevent further episodes of thyroid storm.

PATIENT AND FAMILY EDUCATION

Patients should understand the symptoms and treatment of hyperthyroidism and should be instructed in the "danger signs" of thyroid storm. If receiving beta blockers, they are instructed to monitor their pulse and contact their health care provider if their pulse is less than 50 (or 40 if baseline heart rate is low) or greater than 120 beats per minute.

Patients receiving thioamides should be cautioned about the rare but serious effects of agranulocytosis. They should discontinue thioamide therapy if they have signs of infection and a temperature higher than 38.3° C (101° F). Patients should be advised to call their health care provider and have a CBC and differential performed to exclude agranulocytosis. TFTs should be monitored closely during pregnancy. Women with Graves' disease who have received radioiodine ablation in the past should be advised that TSIs could still cross the placenta. They should inform their obstetricians that they have Graves' disease so that the fetal thyroid and heart rate can be closely monitored.

HYPOTHYROIDISM

DEFINITION AND EPIDEMIOLOGY

Hypothyroidism is a condition resulting from the synthesis of thyroid hormone that is insufficient to meet bodily needs. It is the most common disorder of the thyroid gland. This condition usually occurs in the setting of primary hypothyroidism whereby diseases or treatments destroy thyroid tissue or prevalent conditions interfere with thyroid hormone biosynthesis. Rarely, it is caused by inadequate thyroidal stimulation by TSH, which is referred to as *central* or *secondary hypothyroidism*.

If hypothyroidism is congenital or occurs during infancy or childhood, growth and development are slowed and may result in mental retardation, a condition known as *cretinism*. In adulthood, untreated hypothyroidism results in decreased metabolic function and in the deposition of hydrophilic mucopolysaccharides in the skin and other tissues, which results in fluid and sodium retention and impairment of blood circulation and lymphatic drainage. Progressive and severe hypothyroidism with skin thickening and cardiovascular and renal manifestations is known as *myxedema*.[38]

Hypothyroidism is found in 2% of women and 0.2% of men. The prevalence increases with age, with 6% of women and 2.5% of men over 60 years old having this condition. Subclinical hypothyroidism may occur in as many as 15% of persons 60 years of age or older. It has been found that, in 20% to 40% of patients, subclinical hypothyroidism progresses to overt hypothyroidism within 4 years.[39-41]

Appropriate thyroid hormone biosynthesis depends on dietary intake of iodides and on various geographic and environmental factors that may affect a population's ability to obtain the recommended daily allowance of iodine. In the United States, adequate dietary sources of iodine have been established to prevent iodine deficiency disorders, which may manifest as hypothyroidism or goiter. Mountainous areas such as the Himalayas and Andes or lowlands far from the ocean such as central Africa and parts of Europe are important goitrous areas in the world today.[11]

Previous irradiation for head and neck cancers may put a patient at increased risk of developing hypothyroidism. Radioactive treatment with ^{131}I therapy for hyperthyroid disorders results in hypothyroidism in most cases. Subtotal or total thyroidectomy will render a patient hypothyroid.

The most common cause of primary hypothyroidism is chronic autoimmune thyroiditis. This may take atrophic or goitrous forms. When autoimmune thyroiditis co-exists with a goiter, the condition is called *Hashimoto's thyroiditis*. It is believed to be a familial autoimmune condition in which the lymphocytes become sensitized to an individual's own thyroid antigens, resulting in the formation of autoantibodies. The autoantibodies react with the thyroid antigens and destroy functional tissue. This manifests as an increase in TSH and the presence of antithyroid antibodies, including antimicrosomal, anti-TPO, and antithyroglobulin antibodies. Eventually there is a drop in serum T_4 and then T_3. Younger patients most often are seen with goiter, whereas older patients may have more severe disease and a small (atrophic) gland.

Transient primary hypothyroidism may be encountered during the postpartum period, 2 to 6 months after delivery. This condition may be preceded by a brief period of hyperthyroidism and can result in permanent thyroid failure. Post-infectious thyroiditis may follow a similar course. A sentinel viral upper respiratory tract infection followed by an inflamed, large tender thyroid gland, and transient hyperthyroidism followed by transient or permanent hypothyroidism, is the usual observed sequence of events.

Drugs with antithyroid action such as lithium, amiodarone, iodine, and radiographic contrast may cause hypothyroidism. The drug effect may be transient during the period of use or may result in permanent thyroid failure. Patients with underlying chronic autoimmune thyroiditis living in iodine-sufficient geographic areas are more susceptible to hypothyroidism when taking iodine or iodine-containing drugs.

Pituitary (or secondary) causes of hypothyroidism are not common and are usually associated with other signs of pituitary hormone insufficiency. Patients with a history of pituitary disease or tumor may be at risk for thyroid hyposecretion.

PATHOPHYSIOLOGY

Thyroid hormone deficiency has many effects. Cardiac and metabolic consequences include impaired myocardial contractility, cardiomegaly, impaired lipid metabolism with accelerated atherosclerosis, hypertension, depressed ventilatory drive and fatigue, impaired energy utilization, and weight gain. Altered kidney and gastrointestinal performance includes a reduction in glomerular filtration rate and hyponatremia, hypomotility, and constipation, respectively. Musculoskeletal effects include an increased volume of muscle and slowness of contraction leading to myopathic disorders and connective tissue thickening. This can lead to entrapment neuropathies such as carpal tunnel syndrome. In children, delayed skeletal maturation may cause growth retardation. Impaired cellular function in the brain may cause depression or psychiatric disability, and diminished erythropoiesis results in anemia.[11]

Characteristic myxedematous changes seen in untreated advanced disease are largely a result of deposition of hydrophilic mucopolysaccharides, especially hyaluronic acid, in the interstitial tissues. The hydrophilic nature of the mucopolysaccharides and increased capillary permeability to albumin create interstitial edema of heart muscle, striated muscle, and skin.

CLINICAL PRESENTATION

Presentation may range from subclinical hypothyroidism (with an asymptomatic TSH elevation) to overt myxedema (with slowed mentation and visible symptoms). The most common presenting symptom is fatigue. There may also be increased sensitivity to cold, weight gain, hoarseness, puffiness of the face and hands, heavy and irregular menstrual periods, dry skin, dry and brittle hair, depression, paresthesias, muscle aches, and constipation. A careful history will elicit the severity and duration of these symptoms. Goiter may or may not be present. Women are five to seven times more likely to be affected than men, and more women are seen with goiter. Symptoms may be more vague and subtle in older adults and include deafness, confusion, dementia, and ataxia.

PHYSICAL EXAMINATION

The physical examination should focus on the patient's general appearance and degree of energy and animation. Any lethargy or slowness of mentation should be noted. Assessment of physical appearance includes texture, color, and general appearance of the skin. Facial expression and the texture and thickness of the hair should be noted; the patient's voice, which may be deepened, and pulse, which may be slowed, should also be assessed.

The thyroid gland may be large or small on examination and should be evaluated carefully for the presence or absence of nodules. Tenderness of the gland is suggestive of a subacute thyroiditis, whereas a nontender gland is more suggestive of chronic autoimmune thyroiditis. A rubbery, firm, symmetric goiter is characteristic of Hashimoto's thyroiditis. Deep tendon reflexes should be evaluated. Any delay in the relaxation phase, which may be most noticeable in the Achilles tendon, should be noted. The patient's weight should be documented and compared with previous weights to determine if there has been any weight gain. Heart rate and respiratory rate should also be noted and documented.

The presence of headache or visual impairment may suggest secondary hypothyroidism, as may any other features of pituitary hormone excess or deficiencies. Postural hypotension may indicate co-existent endocrine deficiencies such as autoimmune adrenal insufficiency, as seen in Schmidt's syndrome.

DIAGNOSTICS

An ECG examination may reveal low-voltage QRS complexes and P and T waves, as well as cardiac enlargement. This may result from both dilation and pericardial effusion. Bradycardia is usually present, and diastolic blood pressure may be elevated. Respirations may be slow and shallow with advanced disease. Bowel sounds may be diminished and deep tendon reflexes slowed in the relaxation phase. Mentation may also be slowed, and the patient may appear lethargic and expressionless. Occasionally, severe depression or agitation results.

Laboratory tests reveal an elevated TSH level, which may precede symptoms or alterations in thyroid hormones. This condition is referred to as *subclinical hypothyroidism*. More advanced hypothyroidism shows low serum levels of free T_4 and a low free T_4 index. TRH testing to evaluate TSH response and therefore hypothalamic function is rarely used since the introduction of the third-generation TSH. Anti-TPO antibody levels will be elevated in patients with chronic autoimmune thyroiditis. Patients often demonstrate a mild normocytic, normochromic anemia. If menstrual periods are heavy, the anemia may be microcytic. If vitamin B_{12} deficiency is present, the anemia may be macrocytic. Hypercholesterolemia may also be present.

DIAGNOSTICS

Hypothyroidism

LABORATORY
TSH
Antimicrosomal antibodies*
Serum free T_4
Free T_4*
Thyrotropin-releasing hormone*

IMAGING
Thyroid ultrasound*

OTHER
Fine-needle aspiration*

*If indicated.

DIFFERENTIAL DIAGNOSIS

Hypothyroidism

- Chronic autoimmune thyroiditis
- Postpartum thyroiditis
- Radiation-induced thyroid damage
- Postinfectious thyroiditis
- Medication-induced hypothyroidism (amiodarone, lithium, iodide)
- Postsurgical causation
- Idiopathic hypothyroidism
- Pituitary tumor
- Hypothalamic dysfunction
- Nephrotic syndrome
- Chronic nephritis
- Depression

Imaging studies are unnecessary for chronic autoimmune thyroiditis. If imaging is used, the findings may be misleading. The pattern of uptake with goitrous autoimmune thyroiditis may be variable, whereas uptake may be low with atrophic thyroiditis. An ultrasound examination may be indicated to verify the presence of a suspected nodule. FNA biopsy may be necessary to evaluate a suspicious nodule or rapidly enlarging goiter.

DIFFERENTIAL DIAGNOSIS

Chronic autoimmune thyroiditis is differentiated from other causes of hypothyroidism by the presence of thyroid antibodies. TSH levels will distinguish primary hypothyroidism from secondary causes.

Serum TBG concentrations affect serum T_4 concentrations and may mask the diagnosis of hypothyroidism. Certain drugs, such as estrogen, 5-fluorouracil, methadone, clofibrate, heroin, and tamoxifen, may increase TT_4 through increased TBG binding. Other drugs, including androgens, phenytoin, furosemide, salicylates, and corticosteroids, may decrease TT_4 by decreasing TBG binding. A normal TSH level in the presence of these findings would confirm drug effect as long as there are no symptoms of pituitary involvement.

MANAGEMENT

Hypothyroidism is treated with levothyroxine orally in amounts that return the TSH to normal levels. The desired amount is determined by the measurements of TSH and by subjective clinical criteria. The dosage necessary to achieve metabolic homeostasis is usually 1.6 mcg/kg/day. In the United States, 12 different color-coded tablet strengths are available. Supplementation may begin with an initial dosage of 50 mcg/day, with the dosage increased at 4- to 6-week intervals to 100 mcg/day. In patients less than 30 or 40 years old with no history of other medical problems, the initial dosage of T_4 can be 100 mcg/day. Patients with ischemic heart disease or atrial fibrillation (and older patients in whom these conditions may become apparent with treatment) should start at 12.5 to 25 mcg/day and increase by 25 mcg/day every 8 weeks. An euthyroid effect is usually achieved 4 to 6 weeks after the onset of full-dose therapy, which can be adjusted, if necessary, according to TSH determinations. This daily dosage is then monitored once or twice a year to maintain a midnormal TSH. Estrogen administration leads to an increase in TBG levels and thus may increase T_4 requirements in patients with hypothyroidism.[42] If estrogen therapy is initiated in patients with hypothyroidism treated with T_4, TFTs should be rechecked in 12 weeks.

The long half life of levothyroxine (approximately 7 days) allows for daily dosing. Steady state levels are achieved in approximately 5 to 6 weeks. There are wide fluctuations in serum levotriiodothyronine (L-T3) because of its short half life (approximately 1 day).[43] Slow-release formulations of levotriiodothyronine are not currently commercially available. The role of levotriiodothyronine replacement in hypothyroidism remains controversial. Desiccated bovine thyroid is available, which contains a mixture of T_3 and T_4. One grain (60 mg) Armour thyroid contains about 44 mcg T_4 and 9 mcg T_3 and is bioequivalent to 75 to 88 mcg levothyroxine. Despite almost a dozen randomized studies, combination therapy does not appear to be superior to levothyroxine monotherapy for treatment of hypothyroidism.[44-50]

A study by Hennemann, Docter, Visser, and colleagues showed that treatment of hypothyroid rats with a combination of T_4 plus slow-release T_3 led to an improvement in both T_3 and T_4 levels, T_4/T_3 ratios, and serum TSH compared with treatment with levothyroxine alone.[51] Human studies of slow-release T_3 preparations in combination with T_4 are necessary for clinical validation.

Subclinical Hypothyroidism

Subclinical hypothyroidism is defined as an elevated TSH level in the presence of normal thyroid hormone levels. The major causes of subclinical hypothyroidism are the same as for overt hypothyroidism: about 50% are caused by autoimmune thyroiditis, 40% are found in patients with a history of ablative therapy for Graves' disease, and it is also commonly seen with inadequate T_4 replacement for overt hypothyroidism.[52] Two population-based studies concluded the prevalence of subclinical hypothyroidism to be approximately 8% in women and 3% in men. However, in women over 60 years old, the prevalence is 15%, whereas in elderly men, the prevalence is 8%.[53,54]

Patients with type 1 diabetes mellitus or other autoimmune diseases have a higher rate of subclinical hypothyroidism. The development of overt hypothyroidism depends on the value of TSH and the presence of high thyroid antibody titers. In a British study of elderly patients, all patients with an initial TSH level over 20 μU/L and 80% of those with serum antithyroid microsomal antibody titers of 1:1600 or higher developed overt hypothyroidism. Other patients likely to progress to overt hypothyroidism are those with autoimmune thyroid disease and patients who have received radioiodine therapy or radiotherapy.[54] Normalization of serum TSH is more likely to occur in patients with TSH levels less than 10 μU/L and negative antithyroid antibodies.

Several reports suggest subclinical hypothyroidism is associated with neuropsychiatric disease. Patients with depression and subclinical hypothyroidism have a higher prevalence of associated panic disorder and poorer response to antidepressant therapy than euthyroid patients.[55] A cross-sectional study of randomly selected subjects over 65 years old reported an increase in the prevalence of coronary heart disease in patients with serum TSH values greater than 10 μU/L, but not in patients with lower serum TSH concentrations.[56]

The recommendations regarding treatment are that there is not one level of TSH at which clinical action is indicated or contraindicated. However, for those individuals with TSH over 10 μU/L, treatment is more compelling, since it improves cardiac contractility and serum lipid concentrations and secondarily reduces the risk of atherosclerosis. Treatment will also prevent growth of goiter and improve symptoms related to hypothyroidism. In patients with TSH between 4.5 and 10 μU/L, treatment can be considered if patients have typical hypothyroid symptoms that could benefit from T_4. The potential risk of treatment is the development of subclinical hyperthyroidism. If patients are not treated, regular follow-up is indicated. Patients with subtle symptoms such as infertility, menstrual cycle irregularities, depression, and fatigue may also benefit from replacement therapy. Patients without any of these symptoms and with a TSH of less than 10 μU/L may be monitored at yearly intervals with TSH measurement for progression of thyroid failure.[37,57]

LIFE SPAN CONSIDERATIONS

Older adults and those with known heart disease should be started at 25 mcg/day of levothyroxine and increased gradually. This careful administration prevents arrhythmias, angina, and the other cardiac symptoms that may be precipitated by starting at a full daily dose. After the dose has been stabilized, annual TSH measurements are desirable. Patients should understand that supplementation is lifelong, not short term. Given the high prevalence of hypothyroidism in women over 60 years of age and the presence of subtle symptoms, TSH screening is recommended in this age-group.

Patients with known hypothyroidism require close monitoring during pregnancy. TSH should be measured during the prenatal evaluation and in every trimester thereafter. Most often thyroid hormone requirements increase during pregnancy, and close monitoring will ensure appropriate levothyroxine replacement doses. Evidence has emerged that intrauterine fetal development can be adversely affected by untreated hypothyroidism.[58]

Smoking has been found to impair both thyroid hormone secretion and thyroid hormone action. It may contribute to the incidence of subclinical hypothyroidism and may aggravate the clinical manifestations of overt hypothyroidism; therefore smoking cessation is advised.[59]

The consequences of untreated subclinical hypothyroidism include cardiac dysfunction, including atherosclerotic heart disease; elevations in total and low-density lipoprotein cholesterol levels; systemic hypothyroid symptoms; neuropsychiatric dysfunction; and progression to overt hypothyroidism. A large study demonstrated that subjects with modest elevations of TSH (5 to 10 μU/L) had significantly higher mean total cholesterol concentrations than those who were euthyroid (223 vs. 206 mg/dl).[60]

COMPLICATIONS

Myxedema coma, a hypothermic stuporous state that may be characterized by respiratory depression and eventually death, results from untreated hypothyroidism. It may be triggered by environmental stressors such as cold exposure or trauma and by internal stressors such as infection or medications that depress the central nervous system. These patients may require IV levothyroxine and glucocorticoid therapy for any co-existent adrenal insufficiency. Warming for the hypothermia, ventilatory support for the respiratory depression, and treatment of any renal and electrolyte imbalances are necessary.

In patients with underlying coronary disease, angina and arrhythmias may be a complication of therapy and a cause for concern. Some patients also experience palpitations after starting levothyroxine, especially if other medications are added. This is particularly true of stimulants such as caffeine and pseudoephedrine.

Long-term, marked overtreatment with T_4 can result in symptoms of hyperthyroidism. It can also result in bone resorption with significant decreases in bone mineral density.

INDICATIONS FOR REFERRAL OR HOSPITALIZATION

Referral to a surgeon may be necessary for a large goiter that is obstructive. Referral to an endocrinologist may be necessary if there is a solitary nodule requiring biopsy or if regulation of medication is difficult. Persistent symptoms and a normal TSH level or suspicion of secondary hypothyroidism should also prompt an endocrine referral. Hospitalization may be warranted if any of the previously mentioned conditions is severe. Usually, clinical or subclinical hypothyroidism can be managed on an outpatient basis.

PATIENT AND FAMILY EDUCATION AND HEALTH PROMOTION

The most important aspect of education is communicating to the patient and the family that levothyroxine replacement is a permanent and necessary treatment that cannot be discontinued. Patients should be encouraged not to increase their daily dosage without medical supervision, informed not to double the next dose if one is skipped, and advised that osteoporosis is a possible consequence of high doses. They should also understand that annual or biannual monitoring of TSH helps ensure that the medication dosage remains accurate.

EUTHYROID SICK SYNDROME

The *euthyroid sick syndrome* (sick euthyroidism) refers to thyroid function abnormalities in a critically ill euthyroid individual. It is characterized by hypothalamic suppression of TSH release, acute inhibition of peripheral conversion of T_4 to T_3, and increased conversion of T_4 to rT_3. This results in low TSH levels, decreased levels of T_3 (low T_3 syndrome), and increased levels of rT_3. Euthyroid sick syndrome is seen during carbohydrate restriction, liver disease, or severe acute or chronic illness. Patients with the low free T_4 levels in addition to low T_3 levels are severely ill and have an increased mortality

TABLE 225-4 Euthyroid Sick Syndrome

	T_3	T_4	Free T_4	rT_3	TSH
Low T_3 syndrome	Decrease	Normal or increase	Normal or increase	Increase	Low
Low T_4, T_3 syndrome	Decrease	Decrease	Normal	Increase	Low

rate. TT_4 levels can be decreased even initially because of the liberation of fatty acids from ischemic or injured cells, which inhibits the binding of T_4 to TBG. A summary of laboratory tests during acute illness is provided in Table 225-4. These abnormalities resolve when the patient recovers. The TSH level rises to normal or higher than normal levels during the recovery phase; the changes are thought to be a protective adaptation to severe illness. Therapy with T_4 or T_3 has not been shown to improve outcomes and may actually worsen the situation. Given this syndrome, TFTs should not be checked in critically ill patients unless thyroid dysfunction is strongly suspected. If TFTs are checked, TSH alone does not suffice. TFTs should be interpreted in context of the current clinical scenario and time frame of illness.

DRUGS AND THE THYROID GLAND

Pharmacologic agents may cause thyroid dysfunction or abnormalities in TFTs. The most important examples are discussed in this section.

Amiodarone is an iodine-rich pharmacologic agent used in the management of refractory ventricular arrhythmias. It is highly lipophilic and concentrates in the thyroid gland, heart muscles, and adipose tissue. It has a very long half life, and therefore its effects on the thyroid gland can be seen up to 2 to 3 years after discontinuation of the drug. Like iodine or radiographic contrast, its effects on the thyroid gland can be variable depending on the presence of underlying autoimmune disease and the geographic iodine availability. Individuals who have chronic autoimmune thyroiditis or are living in iodine-sufficient areas are more likely to develop hypothyroidism when exposed to iodinated agents, whereas patients with a multinodular goiter or those residing in iodine-deficient areas may be more likely to develop hyperthyroidism.[61] The risk of either thyroid dysfunction is less likely when lower doses are used. In a meta-analysis of four randomized trials, the incidence of thyroid disease was 3.7% after a minimum of 1 year of low-dose therapy.[62,63]

Hypothyroidism is the more common thyroid disorder in patients taking amiodarone in the United States. Symptoms can develop as soon as 2 weeks and as late as 39 months after the initiation of amiodarone therapy.[64] Clinical manifestations and diagnosis of amiodarone-associated hypothyroidism are similar to those of hypothyroidism of any cause. This condition is effectively treated with levothyroxine replacement therapy. It does not necessitate the discontinuation of amiodarone unless this therapy fails to correct the underlying arrhythmia. Goals of therapy include the establishment of a high-normal TSH level and a mid- to low-normal free T_4 level. A larger than normal dose may be required because of amiodarone's effect on T_4 and T_3 production and action.

About 3% of patients treated with amiodarone in the United States become hyperthyroid.[65] This usually occurs between 4 months and 3 years after the start of therapy. It is more common in iodine-deficient areas of the world. The clinical manifestations of amiodarone-induced hyperthyroidism are often masked because its beta-blocking activity minimizes many of the adrenergic effects of thyroid hormone excess. Common symptoms include redevelopment of atrial arrhythmias, exacerbation of ischemic heart disease or congestive heart failure, restlessness, or low-grade fever. When thyrotoxicosis develops in the setting of amiodarone, it could be caused by overactivity of the thyroid gland (type 1) or destructive thyroiditis (type 2), in which there is inflammation of the thyroid gland.[64,65] (See Table 225-5.)

TABLE 225-5 Comparison of Type 1 and 2 Amiodarone-Associated Hyperthyroidism

	Type 1	Type 2
Etiology	Overproduction of thyroid hormone because of Jod Basedow effect (iodine load) in patients with underlying thyroid disease (nodular goiter, Graves' disease)	Destructive thyroiditis from amiodarone, causing release of T_3 and T_4, but not increased production
Physical examination	Diffuse or nodular goiter often present	Normal thyroid
Thyroid antibodies	Present	Absent
24-Hour radioiodide uptake	Normal or increased	Low or absent
Color flow Doppler	Normal or increased	Low
Interleukin-6	Normal	May be up to elevated twofold
Treatment	Thionamides (~40 mg/day) Perchlorate Thyroidectomy if refractory to medical treatment	Prednisone (~40 mg/day) Thyroidectomy if refractory to medical treatment

Amiodarone does not necessarily need to be discontinued immediately.[66] Treatment ultimately depends on the nature of the disease; such cases can be diagnostically challenging and difficult to manage. The differentiation of these two types can be attempted with the evaluation of cytokines, thyroid antibodies, 24-hour radioiodine uptake, and thyroid ultrasound.[66-69] Type 1 hyperthyroidism is treated with antithyroid drugs, and type 2 thyroiditis is treated with oral steroids. If the mechanism of hyperthyroidism is uncertain, a combination of oral steroids and antithyroid drug is a prudent initial approach.[70,71] Ultimately, thyroidectomy may be necessary if hyperthyroidism is refractory to medical intervention.

Ideally, before recommending amiodarone therapy, the health care provider should obtain baseline TFTs and determine the presence of thyroid antibodies. Underlying thyroid disease and family history of thyroid disorders should be noted; this would place the patient at an increased risk of thyroid dysfunction on this drug and would alert clinicians to this possibility. TFTs should be checked at 3-month intervals after start of the medication and for at least 1 year after it is discontinued.

Interferon-α is used in the treatment of hepatitis viruses B and C or malignant disease. Use of this agent can induce the production of thyroid antibodies, resulting in hypothyroidism or thyrotoxicosis or a biphasic thyroiditis. With discontinuation of this agent, these antibodies often disappear.[11]

Lithium, as used in the treatment of psychiatric conditions such as bipolar depression, can induce thyroid dysfunction. It blocks the uptake of iodine and the release of thyroid hormone and can induce chronic autoimmune thyroiditis. Clinical or subclinical hypothyroidism or a goiter in an euthyroid patient is within the spectrum of lithium-induced thyroid disease.[11] TFT abnormalities, including a low TSH, low TT_3, and an elevated rT_3 level, are noted in patients on steroids and pressor agents. Similar abnormalities in T_3 and rT_3 are noted with amiodarone. Much like in sick euthyroid syndrome, these agents block the formation of T_3 from T_4, and most of T_4 is shunted into the formation of rT_3.

THYROID DISEASE IN PREGNANCY

The evaluation and treatment of women with thyroid disease during pregnancy is similar to that of nonpregnant women, but presents some obstacles. Human chorionic gonadotropin (HCG), which is a weak thyroid stimulator, may cause hyperthyroidism during pregnancy. Subclinical hyperthyroidism occurs in 10% to 20% of normal pregnant women during the period of highest HCG concentrations, lasting from fertilization to about 11 weeks.[72] Hyperemesis gravidarum is another cause of HCG-mediated hyperthyroidism. Women usually become euthyroid when the hyperemesis resolves and usually do not require antithyroid treatment. Another cause is trophoblastic hyperthyroidism, which occurs in approximately 60% of women with a hydatidiform mole or choriocarcinoma. The hyperthyroidism can be severe and is treated by removal of the mole or therapy against the choriocarcinoma. Graves' hyperthyroidism is the most frequent cause. It usually becomes less severe during later stages of pregnancy. This is likely mediated by a change in the activity of the TSH receptor antibodies from stimulatory to blocking. Consequences of poorly controlled hyperthyroidism include increased risk of spontaneous pregnancy loss, premature labor, low birth weight, stillbirth, and preeclampsia.[73]

Diagnosis of hyperthyroidism may be challenging. A TSH value of less than 0.01 μU/L and also a high serum free T_4 value are indicative of hyperthyroidism.[74] Because radioiodine is contraindicated during pregnancy, it is often impossible to decipher the cause of the hyperthyroidism. Treatment of pregnant women who are hyperthyroid is difficult, since treatment can be harmful to the fetus. The goal is to maintain maternal T_4 in the high-normal range using the lowest dose of drug possible to prevent fetal hypothyroidism.

Hypothyroidism during pregnancy is less frequent, since many women with hypothyroidism are anovulatory or have high rates of first-trimester miscarriages. Hypothyroidism during pregnancy has been associated with early pregnancy loss, preeclampsia, placental abruption, low birth weight, perinatal mortality, and neuropsychologic dysfunction.[75-77] Thyroid hormone requirements increase in pregnant women with preexisting hypothyroidism because of estrogen-induced elevations in TBG, increased volume of distribution of thyroid hormone, and increased placental transport and degradation of thyroid hormone. For this reason and the significance of maternal euthyroidism for normal fetal growth, serum TSH should be measured 4 to 6 weeks after conception, 4 to 6 weeks after making any change in the dose of T_4, and at least once each trimester. A different approach recommends increasing the dose by 30% as soon as pregnancy is confirmed. A pregnant woman found to have a thyroid nodule should be evaluated in the same way as other patients, except that radioiodine scanning is contraindicated.

REFERENCES

1. Wang C, Crapo LM: Epidemiology of thyroid disease and implications for screening, *Endocrinol Metab Clin North Am* 26(1):189-219, 1997.
2. Surks MI, Ocampo E: Subclinical thyroid disease, *Am J Med* 100(2):217-223, 1996.
3. DeGroot LJ, Larsen PR, Hennemann G: *The thyroid and its diseases*, New York, 1996, Churchill Livingstone.
4. Papini E, Guglielmi R, Bianchini A, and others: Risk of malignancy in nonpalpable thyroid nodules: predictive value of ultrasound and color Doppler features, *J Clin Endocrinol Metab* 87(5):1941-1946, 2002.
5. Choi M, Lee JW, Jang KJ: Distinction between benign and malignant causes of cervical, axillary, and inguinal lymphadenopathy: value of Doppler spectral waveform analysis, *Am J Roentgenol* 165(4):981-984, 1995.
6. Kessler A, Rappaport Y, Blank A, and others: Cystic appearance of cervical LN is characteristic of metastatic papillary thyroid carcinoma, *J Clin Ultrasound* 31(1):21-25, 2003.
7. Cohen MS, Arslan N, Dehdashti F, and others: Risk of malignancy in thyroid incidentalomas identified by fluorodeoxyglucose positron emission tomography, *Surgery* 130(6):941-946, 2001.
8. Wang W, Larson SM, Fazzari M, and others: Prognostic value of [18F]fluorodeoxyglucose positron emission tomographic scanning in patients with thyroid cancer, *J Clin Endocrinol Metab* 85(3):1107-1113, 2000.
9. Siminoski K: Does this patient have a goiter? *JAMA* 273:813-817, 1995.
10. Wallace C, Siminoski K: The Pemberton sign, *Ann Intern Med* 125:568-569, 1996.

11. Braverman LE, Utiger RD: *Werner and Ingbar's the thyroid: a fundamental and clinical text*, ed 8, New York, 2000, Lippincott-Raven.
12. Toft A: Drug therapy: thyroxine therapy, *N Engl J Med* 331:174-180, 1994.
13. Mandel S, Brent GA, Larsen PR: Levothyroxine therapy in patients with thyroid disease, *Ann Intern Med* 119(6):492-502, 1993.
14. Huysmans DA, Hermus AR, Corstens FH, and others: Large, compressive goiters treated with radioiodine, *Ann Intern Med* 121(10):757-762, 1994.
15. Nygaard B, Hegedus L, Gervil M, and others: Radioiodine treatment of multinodular nontoxic goiter, *Br Med J* 307(6908):828-832, 1993.
16. Vander JB, Gaston EA, Dawber TR: Significance of solitary non-toxic thyroid nodules, *N Engl J Med* 251:970, 1954.
17. Mortensen D, Woolner LB, Bennett WA: Gross and microscopic findings in clinically normal thyroid glands, *J Clin Endocrinol Metab* 15:1270, 1955.
18. Hedinger C, Williams ED, Sabin LH: The WHO histological classification of thyroid tumors: a commentary on the second edition, *Cancer* 63:908-911, 1989.
19. Belfiore A, Giuffrida D, La Rosa GL, and others: High frequency of cancer in cold thyroid nodules occurring at young age, *Acta Endocrinol (Copenh)* 121(2):197-202, 1989.
20. Belfiore A, La Rosa GL, La Porta GA, and others: Cancer risk in patients with cold thyroid nodules: relevance of iodine intake, sex, age, and multinodularity, *Am J Med* 93(4):363-369, 1992.
21. Schneider AB, Shore-Freedman E, Ryo UY, and others: Radiation-induced tumors of the head and neck following childhood irradiation, *Medicine (Baltimore)* 64(1):1-15, 1985.
22. Singer PA, Cooper DS, Daniel GH, and others: Treatment guidelines for patients with thyroid nodules and well-differentiated thyroid cancer, *Arch Intern Med* 156(19):2165-2172, 1996.
23. Blum M, Yee J: Advances in thyroid imaging: thyroid sonography; when and how should it be used? *Thyroid Today* 3:1-13, 1977.
24. Lucas A, Llatjos M, Salinas I, and others: Fine-needle aspiration cytology of benign thyroid disease: value of re-aspiration, *Eur J Endocrinol* 132(6):677-680, 1995.
25. Ross DS: Thyroid hormone suppressive therapy of sporadic nontoxic goiter, *Thyroid* 2:263-269, 1992.
26. Mazzaferri EL: Thyroid remnant ^{131}I ablation for papillary and follicular thyroid carcinoma, *Thyroid* 7:265-271, 1997.
27. Heshmati H, Gharib H, van Heerden JA, and others: Advances and controversies in the diagnosis and management of medullary thyroid carcinoma, *Am J Med* 103(1):60-69, 1997.
28. Cooper DS, Specker B, Ho M, and others: Thyrotropin suppression and disease progression in patients with differentiated thyroid cancer: results from the National Thyroid Cancer Treatment Cooperative Registry, *Thyroid* 8(9):737-744, 1998.
29. Grigsby PW, Siegel BA, Baker S, and others: Radiation exposure from outpatient radioactive iodine (^{131}I) therapy for thyroid carcinoma, *JAMA* 283(17):2272-2274, 2000.
30. Singer PA, Cooper DS, Levy EG, and others: Treatment guidelines for patients with hyperthyroidism and hypothyroidism. Standards of Care Committee, American Thyroid Association, *JAMA* 273(1):808-812, 1995.
31. Gerstein H: Incidence of postpartum thyroid dysfunction in patients with type I diabetes mellitus, *Ann Intern Med* 118:419-423, 1993.
32. Biscoveanu M, Hasinski S: Abnormal results of liver function tests in patients with Graves' disease, *Endocrine Pract* 6:367-369, 2000.
33. Hedberg CW, Fishbein DB, Janssen RS, and others: An outbreak of thyrotoxicosis caused by the consumption of bovine thyroid gland in ground beef, *N Engl J Med* 316(16):993-998, 1987.
34. Diez JJ: Hyperthyroidism in patients older than 55 years; an analysis of the etiology and management, *Gerontology* 49:316-323, 2003.
35. Faber J, Galloe AM: Changes in bone mass during prolonged subclinical hyperthyroidism due to L-thyroxine treatment: a meta-analysis, *Eur J Endocrinol* 130:350-356, 1994.
36. Sawin CT, Geller A, Wolf PA, and others: Low serum thyrotropin concentrations as a risk factor for atrial fibrillation in older persons, *N Engl J Med* 331:1249-1252, 1994.
37. Surks MI, Ortiz E, Daniels GH, and others: Subclinical thyroid disease: scientific review and guidelines for diagnosis and management, *JAMA* 291(2):228-238, 2004.
38. Hierholzer K, Finke R: Myxedema, *Kidney Int Suppl* 59:582-589, 1997.
39. Lindsay R, Toft A: Hypothyroidism, *Lancet* 349:413-417, 1997.
40. Dayan C, Daniels G: Medical progress: chronic autoimmune thyroiditis, *N Engl J Med* 335:99-107, 1996.
41. Vanderpump MP, Tunbridge WM, French JM, and others: The incidence of thyroid disorders in the community: a twenty-year follow-up of the Whickham Survey, *Clin Endocrinol* (Oxf) 43(1):55-68, 1995.
42. Arafah BM: Increased need for thyroxine in women with hypothyroidism during estrogen therapy, *N Engl J Med* 344:1743-1749, 2001.
43. LeBoff MS, Kaplan MM, Silva JE, and others: Bioavailability of thyroid hormones from oral replacement preparations, *Metabolism* 31(9):900-905, 1982.
44. Walsh JP, Shiels L, Lim EM, and others: Combined thyroxine/liothyronine treatment does not improve well-being, quality of life, or cognitive function compared to thyroxine alone: a randomized controlled trial in patients with primary hypothyroidism, *J Clin Endocrinol Metab* 88(10):4543-4550, 2003.
45. Sawka AM, Gerstein HC, Marriott MJ, and others: Does a combination regimen of thyroxine (T4) and 3, 5,3'-triiodothyronine improve depressive symptoms better than T4 alone in patients with hypothyroidism? Results of a double-blind, randomized, controlled trial, *J Clin Endocrinol Metab* 88(10):4551-4555, 2003.
46. Saravanan P, Chau WF, Roberts N, and others: Psychological well-being in patients on "adequate" doses of L-thyroxine: results of a large, controlled community-based questionnaire study, *Clin Endocrinol (Oxf)* 57(5):577-585, 2002.
47. Escobar-Morreale HF, Botello-Carretero JI, Gomez-Bueno M, and others: Thyroid hormone replacement therapy in primary hypothyroidism: a randomized trial comparing L-thyroxine plus liothyronine with L-thyroxine alone, *Ann Intern Med* 142(6):412-424, 2005.
48. Saravanan P, Simmons DJ, Greenwood R, and others: Partial substitution of thyroxine (T4) with tri-iodothyronine in patients on T4 replacement therapy: results of a large community-based randomized controlled trial, *J Clin Endocrinol Metab* 90(2):805-812, 2005.
49. Appelhof BC, Fliers E, Wekking EM, and others: Combined therapy with levothyroxine and liothyronine in two ratios, compared with levothyroxine monotherapy in primary hypothyroidism: a double-blind, randomized, controlled clinical trial, *J Clin Endocrinol Metab* 90(5):2666-2674, 2005.
50. Rodriguez T, Lavis VR, Meininger JC, and others: Substitution of liothyronine at a 1:5 ratio for a portion of levothyroxine: effect on fatigue, symptoms of depression, and working memory versus treatment with levothyroxine alone, *Endocr Pract* 11(4):223-233, 2005.
51. Hennemann G, Docter R, Visser TJ, and others: Thyroxine plus low-dose, slow-release triiodothyronine replacement in hypothyroidism: proof of principle, *Thyroid* 14(4):271-275, 2004.
52. Tunbridge WM, Evered DC, Hall R, and others: The spectrum of thyroid disease in a community: the Whickham survey, *Clin Endocrinol (Oxf)* 7(6):481-493, 1977.
53. Parle JV, Franklyn JA, Cross KW, and others: Prevalence and follow-up of abnormal thyrotrophin (TSH) concentrations in the elderly in the United Kingdom, *Clin Endocrinol (Oxf)* 34(1):77-83, 1991.
54. Kabadi UD: Subclinical hypothyroidism. Natural course of the syndrome during a prolonged follow-up study, *Arch Intern Med* 153(8):957-961, 1993.
55. Joffe RT, Levitt AJ: Major depression and subclinical (grade 2) hypothyroidism, *Psychoneuroendocrinology* 17(2-3):215-221, 1992.
56. Lindeman RD, Romero LJ, Schade DS, and others: Impact of subclinical hypothyroidism on serum total homocysteine concentrations, the prevalence of coronary heart disease (CHD), and CHD risk factors in the New Mexico Elder Health Survey, *Thyroid* 13(6):595-600, 2003.
57. Cooper DS: Subclinical hypothyroidism, *N Engl J Med* 345:260-265, 2001.

58. Haddow JE, Palomaki GE, Allan WC, and others: Maternal thyroid deficiency during pregnancy and subsequent neuropsychological development of the child, *N Engl J Med* 341(8):549-555, 1999.
59. Muller B, Zulewski H, Huber P, and others: Impaired action of thyroid hormone associated with smoking in women with hypothyroidism, *N Engl J Med* 333(15):964-969, 1995.
60. Canaris GJ, Manowitz NR, Mayor G, and others: The Colorado thyroid disease prevalence study, *Arch Intern Med* 160(4):526-534, 2000.
61. Martino E, Bartalena L, Bogazzi F, and others: The effects of amiodarone on the thyroid, *Endocr Rev* 22(2):240-254, 2001.
62. Trip MD, Wiersinga W, Plomp TA: Incidence, predictability, and pathogenesis of amiodarone-induced thyrotoxicosis and hypothyroidism, *Am J Med* 91(5):507-511, 1991.
63. Vorperian VR, Havighurst TC, Miller S, and others: Adverse effects of low dose amiodarone: a meta-analysis, *J Am Coll Cardiol* 30(3):791-798, 1997.
64. Bartalena L, Brogioni S, Grasso L, and others: Treatment of amiodarone-induced thyrotoxicosis, a difficult challenge: results of a prospective study, *J Clin Endocrinol Metab* 81(8):2930-2933, 1996.
65. Lambert M, Unger J, De Nayer P, and others: Amiodarone-induced thyrotoxicosis suggestive of thyroid damage, *J Endocrinol Invest* 13(6):527-530, 1990.
66. Osman F, Franklyn JA, Sheppard MC, and others: Successful treatment of amiodarone-induced thyrotoxicosis, *Circulation* 105(11):1275-1277, 2002.
67. Bartalena L, Grasso L, Brogioni S, and others: Serum interleukin-6 in amiodarone-induced thyrotoxicosis, *J Clin Endocrinol Metab* 7(2)8:423-427, 1994.
68. Brennan MD, Erickson DZ, Carney JA, and others: Nongoitrous (type I) amiodarone-associated thyrotoxicosis: evidence of follicular disruption in vitro and in vivo, *Thyroid* 5(3):177-183, 1995.
69. Martino E, Bartalena L, Mariotti S, and others: Radioactive iodine thyroid uptake in patients with amiodarone-iodine-induced thyroid dysfunction, *Acta Endocrinol (Copenh)* 119(2):167-173, 1988.
70. Broussolle C, Ducottet X, Martin C, and others: Rapid effectiveness of prednisone and thionamides combined therapy in severe amiodarone iodine–induced thyrotoxicosis: comparison of two groups of patients with apparently normal thyroid glands, *J Endocrinol Invest* 12(1):37-42, 1989.
71. Cardenas GA, Cabral JM, Leslie CA: Amiodarone induced thyrotoxicosis: diagnostic and therapeutic strategies, *Cleveland Clin J Med* 70(7):624-626, 628-631, 2003.
72. Glinoer D, De Nayer P, Robyn C, and others: Serum levels of intact human chorionic gonadotropin (HCG) and its free alpha and beta subunits in relation to maternal thyroid stimulation during normal pregnancy, *J Endocrinol Invest* 16(11):881-888, 1993.
73. Davis LE, Lucas MJ, Hankins GD, and others: Thyrotoxicosis complicating pregnancy, *Am J Obstet Gynecol* 160:63-70, 1989.
74. Thyroid disease in pregnancy: ACOG practice bulletin: clinical management guidelines for obstetrician-gynecologists, No 37, *Obstet Gynecol* 100:387-396, 2002.
75. Abalovich M, Guttierez S, Alcaraz G, and others: Overt and subclinical hypothyroidism complicating pregnancy, *Thyroid* 12(1):63-68, 2002.
76. Krassas GE, Pontikides N, Kaltsas T, and others: Disturbances of menstruation in hypothyroidism, *Clin Endocrinol (Oxf)* 50(5):655-659, 1999.
77. Casey BM, Dashe JS, Wells CE, and others: Subclinical hypothyroidism and pregnancy outcomes, *Obstet Gynecol* 105(2):239-245, 2005.

PART 18

Evaluation and Management of Hematologic Disorders

JOANNE SANDBERG-COOK, *Section Editor*

CHAPTER 226

Anemia

Katherine Griffis Low

DEFINITION AND EPIDEMIOLOGY

Anemia is not a disease but rather a sign or symptom of an underlying disorder. Anemia is defined as a reduction in the number of red blood cells (erythrocytes [RBCs]), hemoglobin, or hematocrit concentration. Most important, anemia is a condition in which too little oxygen is being transported to the tissues. Inadequate supplies of oxygen in the tissues produce the symptoms of anemia. In general, hemoglobin concentration less than 14 g/dl for men and or less than 12 g/dl for women suggests anemia.[1] Although certain signs and symptoms are sometimes associated with anemia, the diagnosis is often based on laboratory data alone.

PATHOPHYSIOLOGY

Erythropoiesis, the production of erythrocytes, originates in the yolk sac of the embryo, occurs in the liver and spleen during fetal development, and is limited to the axial skeleton and proximal ends of the long bones in the adult.[2] The marrow is a special environment for hematopoietic development; new cells are held within a matrix of reticular cells and fibers. The earliest erythroid progenitor cells are the burst-forming units-erythroid (BFU-E), which divide to become colony-forming units-erythroid (CFU-E) and progress to committed myeloid cells and to proerythroblasts in the bone marrow. This sequence is completed when the nucleus is expelled from the cell, forming a reticulocyte, the immediate precursor of the circulating adult erythrocyte. Under normal conditions the reticulocyte stays in the marrow while hemaglobinization and cell shrinkage continue. When the cell gains mature status, it moves through the sinusoidal wall of the marrow and enters the circulation. Messenger RNA (mRNA) remains within the cell for approximately 24 hours after entering circulation to allow for its identification as an erythrocyte.[3]

The normal proliferation processes of the normoblast (mature proerythroblast) involve four or five cellular divisions to produce the pronormoblast, each of which produces 16 to 32 adult erythrocytes. The normoblast spends approximately 4 days maturing and proliferating in the marrow and an additional 3 days as a marrow reticulocyte before moving into the peripheral circulation. Under the influence of hypoxia or anemia, the normoblast maturation can be shortened with optimum conditions.[2]

At death, normally in the spleen, the erythrocyte contents are released back into circulation and transported to the liver (and spleen) for further breakdown. Globulin, the protein base portion of the molecule, is reduced to amino acids for use throughout the body. Iron is stored in the liver and spleen until needed; the remaining heme is converted to bilirubin and excreted from the body via urine and stool.[4]

Iron is critical for both erythrocyte proliferation and maturation and for hemoglobin synthesis.[5-7] Under normal conditions the turnover rate for erythrocytes is approximately 1% per day; erythrocytes survive 120 ±20 days. Although in response to hypoxia and anemia, marrow precursors may be seen in 2 to 3 days, an increase in the reticulocyte (retic) count will take several more days. The rate of response is affected by the degree of erythropoietin stimulation, which is related to the hypoxia. The most important factor is iron. In persons with no iron stores, the marrow cannot increase erythropoiesis. In contrast, a near optimum response for those persons with a readily abundant supply may increase the production rate three to six times the base.[1,2]

The control of erythropoiesis is dominated by the decreased concentration of hemoglobin in the blood, which leads to changes in tissue hypoxia and in turn triggers receptors within the kidney. The kidney secretes a glycoprotein hormone, erythropoietin (EPO), which is the major humoral regulator for RBC production. EPO induces erythroid precursor cells to differentiate, thereby increasing production.

Anemia can be classified by the deficit in proliferation (hypoproliferative anemia), maturation (ineffective erythropoiesis), or survival (hemolysis). However, it is most commonly associated with the size of the RBC: microcytic, macrocytic, or normocytic. (The reader is referred to any comprehensive hematology textbook for a more detailed discussion of erythropoiesis and the pathophysiology of anemia.) Conditions or diseases that can cause anemia include blood loss (either acute or chronic), malignancies, genetic disorders, immunologic defects, infection, malabsorption problems, dietary deficiencies, drug toxicities, and metabolic disorders.[3]

CLINICAL PRESENTATION

The presentation of anemia can be variable, depending on the rapidity of onset and the ability of the cardiopulmonary system to compensate. If the patient is healthy and the onset of anemia is gradual, there are few signs or symptoms until the hemoglobin value falls below 6 g/dl. However, for the patient with iron deficiency, hemoglobin of less than 11 g/dl may produce significant symptoms. Initially patients may experience fatigue, malaise, dyspnea, and a mild decrease in exercise tolerance. Further declines in hemoglobin may be associated with a markedly reduced exercise capacity, resting tachycardia, and dyspnea requiring supplemental oxygen. Other nonspecific complaints that can accompany a long-term, moderate to severe anemia include wide pulse pressure, a midsystolic or pansystolic murmur, confusion, lethargy, brittle nails, glossitis, angular cheilitis, papillary atrophy of the tongue, and spoon-shaped nails (rare in the United States).[8] Pallor of the mucous membranes, lips, conjunctivae, nail beds, and palmar creases is a common sign of anemia but is of little help in judging its severity.[3]

DIAGNOSTICS

Diagnostic evaluation of anemia includes a CBC with platelet, white cell differential and red cell morphology, reticulocyte (retic) count, peripheral blood smear, and a variety of standard tests. The retic count is the most easily accessible method of evaluating bone marrow production of RBCs (a direct bone marrow examination requires an invasive procedure). The retic count provides an assessment of whether the causative factor of anemia is related to decreased production or increased loss. A normal retic count is 0.5% to 1.5% of the total RBCs. Normal absolute retic count is 25 to 75 × 10^9/L. Any value higher than 100 × 10^9 is considered a normally responding marrow to anemic conditions. Values less than 75 × 10^9 are considered consistent with impaired (decreased) RBC production. However, if reticulocytosis is associated with anemia, then hemolysis needs to be ruled out by observing for hyperbilirubinemia (marker of hemoglobin catabolism), direct cellular injury by increased serum lactate dehydrogenase (LDH), or increased excretion of hemoglobin by low serum haptoglobin. Hemolytic anemias are complex to evaluate and diagnose; if suspected, they should be referred to a hematologist. A low retic count with anemia points to impaired erythropoiesis, and the red cell indexes need review. Impaired erythropoiesis may be due to a reduction in red cell precursors or ineffective production. Ineffective production is reported as erythroid hyperplasia on the bone marrow biopsy and aspiration report, which means the red cells that are being produced are not viable and usually do not leave the marrow. Mean corpuscular volume (MCV) is the single most useful index.[1] Box 226-1 identifies conditions associated with either reticulocytosis or a decreased retic count.

A peripheral blood smear is critical in evaluating anemias. Direct visualization of the RBC size and shape variations, as well as abnormal cell populations too small to change the indexes, can be seen. For example, as iron deficiency progresses, microcytic cells are noted on the smear long before the indexes change.

A hemoglobin electrophoresis allows hemoglobin chains to be separated according to differences in the charges of their subunits. It is essential for accurate diagnosis of thalassemias and hemoglobinopathies.

BOX 226-1

CONDITIONS THAT CAN INFLUENCE RETICULOCYTE COUNTS

INCREASED RETICULOCYTE COUNTS

Hemolytic anemia
- Autoimmune hemolysis
- RBC enzyme deficiencies
- Traumatic or microangiopathic hemolysis
- RBC membrane problems (hereditary spherocytosis and elliptocytosis)

Three to 4 days after acute blood loss
Hemoglobinopathies
Toxin exposures
Hypersplenism
After treatment of anemias
- After adequate doses of iron to treat iron deficiency anemia
- After adequate doses of folate or vitamin B_{12} to correct a megaloblastic anemia

DECREASED RETICULOCYTE COUNTS

Iron deficiency anemia
Aplastic anemia
Untreated megaloblastic anemia
Radiotherapy
Marrow tumors
Myelodysplastic syndromes

DIAGNOSTICS

Anemias

LABORATORY

CBC and differential
Peripheral smear
Reticulocyte count
Ferritin
Total iron-binding capacity*
Transferrin*
Serum iron*
Stool for occult blood × 3*
Hemoglobin electrophoresis*
Folate*
Vitamin B_{12}*
LFTs*
Thyroid function tests*
BUN*
Creatinine*
Glucose-6-phosphate dehydrogenase assay*
Erythropoietin level*
Serum homocysteine*
Methylmalonic acid*
Coombs' direct and indirect tests*

OTHER

Bone marrow biopsy*

*If indicated.

Evaluation of the body's iron stores includes serum ferritin, serum iron, total iron-binding capacity (TIBC), and transferrin saturation percentage. These tests are essential for differentiating the etiology of a microcytic anemia caused by impaired hemoglobin synthesis.

The serum ferritin level reflects total body iron stores. It is the first laboratory value to become abnormal when iron stores are becoming depleted, even before iron deficiency anemia (IDA) is reflected in RBC morphology. The serum ferritin is directly proportional to iron stores: each nanogram per milliliter of serum ferritin reflects 8 to 10 mg of stored iron.[4] Normal value is 12 to 150 mcg/L for women and 10 to 345 mcg/L for men.[1] Serum ferritin levels are low in IDA and normal or elevated in anemia of chronic disease (ACD). Serum ferritin is also elevated in conditions unrelated to anemia such as iron overload (either transfusion-dependent or hereditary hemochromatosis), inflammatory disorders, and alcoholism.

The serum iron reflects the amount of iron bound to transferrin, a plasma carrier protein that regulates iron transport in the blood. Normal values for serum iron are 40 to 150 mcg/dl for women and 40 to 160 mcg/dl for men. The transferrin level is measured indirectly as the TIBC. The TIBC indicates the availability of binding sites on the protein for iron transport. Normal values for TIBC are 250 to 450 mcg/dl (for both women and men).

The percentage of transferrin saturation can be calculated from the TIBC and the serum iron values:

$$\frac{\text{Serum iron}}{\text{TIBC}} \times 100$$

Normal values for percentage of transferrin saturation are 20% to 50%.

Most mild to moderate anemias are usually asymptomatic and are found incidentally on a routine CBC. If data from the patient's history and physical examination suggest an anemia, however, the initial laboratory tests should include a CBC with differential, retic count, and peripheral smear examination of RBC morphology. These results indicate the need for further tests.

Physician consultation is recommended for hemoglobin values less than 10 g/dl in patients with known coronary artery disease, and for any patient with postural vital sign

changes or active bleeding. Physician consultation is also recommended for sickle cell crises, suspected aplastic anemia, or hemolytic anemia.

DIFFERENTIAL DIAGNOSIS

Anemias are generally divided into three categories based on the size of the RBCs produced by the underlying condition or disease. RBCs are normally uniform in size and shape, and alterations in their appearance can suggest a specific cause for the anemia. The degree of anisocytosis (variation in RBC size) is determined by looking at the RBC indexes on the CBC and at cell morphology on the peripheral smear. The most useful RBC index is the MCV. The MCV is a direct measurement averaging the RBC sizes in the sample. The red cell distribution width (RDW) is an indirect measurement that indicates the degree of homogeneity of the sample. For example, uniformly small RBCs will have a low MCV and a normal RDW, whereas a sample with mostly small RBCs but some normal RBCs can have a low MCV with an increased RDW, reflecting the heterogeneity of the sample. Based on the MCV, anemias are classified as microcytic (MCV <80 fl), normocytic (MCV of 80 to 99 fl), or macrocytic (MCV >100 fl).[9] Variations in RBC shape (poikilocytosis) provide important diagnostic clues and in fact are often pathognomonic of underlying disease. Box 226-2 classifies commonly seen hematologic disorders according to RBC morphology.

BOX 226-2

CLASSIFICATION OF ANEMIAS BASED ON RED BLOOD CELL MORPHOLOGY

SIZE

Microcytic (mean corpuscular volume [MCV] <80 fl)
- Iron deficiency
- Thalassemia
- Anemia of chronic disease (occasionally)
- Sideroblastic anemia
- Hemoglobin E disease

Macrocytic (MCV >100 fl)
- Megaloblastic anemia (vitamin B_{12} or folate deficiency)

Normocytic (MCV of 80 to 99 fl)
- Sickle cell disease
- Anemia of chronic disease
- Aplastic anemia
- Hemolytic anemias

SHAPE

Sickle
- Sickle cell disease

Targets
- Thalassemias
- Hemoglobin C
- Hemoglobin E

Spherocytes
- Hereditary spherocytosis
- Immune hemolysis

Elliptocytes
- Hereditary elliptocytosis

MICROCYTIC ANEMIA

IRON DEFICIENCY ANEMIA

IDA is the most common type of anemia in the world and the most common nutrient deficiency. IDA predominantly affects women of reproductive age and older adults. The most common cause is chronic blood loss, especially gastrointestinal blood loss or menorrhagia.[10] Chronic gastrointestinal blood loss should be suspected as a cause of IDA in adult men and postmenopausal women. Box 226-3 lists additional causes of iron deficiency.

Inadequate nutrition and increased requirements for iron are the principal causes for IDA in children and pregnant women. The prevalence of IDA during pregnancy is 3.5% to 7.4% in the first trimester and can increase to 15% to 55% in the third trimester.[11] Nutritional deficiency is more prevalent among poor women. During the past several decades, however, the frequency of nutritional IDA has decreased in women and children in the United States as a result of iron-fortified foods, iron supplementation during pregnancy, better access to health care, and support programs such as WIC (Women, Infants, and Children).[11]

Pathophysiology

Iron is an essential nutrient present in all living cells. In humans more than 70% of the total body iron content is in hemoglobin, with another 5% in myoglobin and other heme-containing enzymes.[12] The remaining 25% of iron is bound to the protein transferrin. The normal man has a total body iron content of about 4000 mg. Women have about 200 mg of total

BOX 226-3

CAUSES OF IRON DEFICIENCY

CONDITIONS LEADING TO MILD IRON DEFICIENCY*

Inadequate diet
Normal or heavy menses
Blood donation
Malabsorption
- Partial gastrectomy
- Malabsorption syndromes

Increased requirements
- Infancy and adolescence (periods of rapid growth)
- Pregnancy

Polycythemia vera treated with phlebotomy

CONDITIONS ASSOCIATED WITH MODERATE TO SEVERE IRON DEFICIENCY

Chronic blood loss
- Gastrointestinal
  - Peptic ulcer disease
  - Varices
  - Malignancy
  - Diverticulitis
- Severe menorrhagia

Severe malabsorption
- Gastrectomy
- Sprue and other malabsorption syndromes

*Usually no associated symptoms.

body iron, a significantly lower amount because of menstrual blood loss and lower dietary intake. The average adult normally loses approximately 1 mg of iron each day through the natural process of desquamation of cells from the skin, gastrointestinal tract, and urinary tract. The adult woman loses an additional 1 mg through normal menstruation.

The recommended daily allowance of iron is 15 mg/day in the diet of nonpregnant women and 30 mg/day for pregnant women. Most American diets consist of approximately 15 mg of elemental iron a day.[13] Dietary iron is absorbed in the duodenum of the small intestine. The amount of iron absorbed from the intestine is determined by several factors, including the iron content of the meal, the form of iron being ingested, the individual's iron status, and the presence or absence of other substances that can enhance or inhibit iron absorption (Box 226-4).[11]

When iron requirements increase or intake declines, the small intestine increases absorption of iron to meet the increased demand. If there is no additional supply of iron to meet this increased demand, the body's iron stores begin to be depleted. At this point several hematologic parameters are affected. The ferritin levels decline as body iron stores decrease. As body iron stores are depleted, the transferrin saturation decreases, leading to a reduced supply of iron to the RBC precursors, resulting in impaired (iron-deficient) erythropoiesis. At this stage, however, an overt microcytic anemia may not yet be present. Once the iron stores are truly depleted and no iron is available for erythropoiesis, an overt microcytic, hypochromic anemia is present, which is manifested in the CBC by a low hemoglobin concentration; the last to change is RBC indexes (decreased MCV, mean corpuscular hemoglobin [MCH], and mean corpuscular hemoglobin concentration [MCHC]). The peripheral smear will show hypochromia, microcytosis, mild anisocytosis, and poikilocytosis. Iron studies will show a low ferritin and high TIBC.

Clinical Presentation

Mild to moderate iron-deficient states are not associated with any clinical symptoms. Severe IDA may be asymptomatic or may be associated with signs and symptoms that are primarily those of severe anemia (i.e., nonspecific to IDA). Patients may complain of fatigue, decreased exercise tolerance, weakness, palpitations, irritability, and headaches. Complaints that are specifically related to iron store depletion include paresthesias; sore tongue; brittle nails; spoon-shaped nails (koilonychia); and pica for starch, ice, or clay.[10] In fact, a craving for ice (pagophagia) is a common symptom of women with IDA.

BOX 226-4

FACTORS THAT INFLUENCE IRON ABSORPTION

SUBSTANCES THAT INHIBIT ABSORPTION
Soy protein
Bran
Dairy products
Tea and coffee
Calcium-rich antacids
Vegetable sources

SUBSTANCES THAT ENHANCE ABSORPTION
Ascorbic acid (vitamin C)
Citric acid
Meat, poultry, and fish sources
Other factors:
- Low iron stores of individual
- Low iron content of meal

Physical Examination

As the severity of the anemia increases, several physical changes may become evident. The patient may demonstrate a more forceful apical pulse, tachycardia with exertion, and a systolic flow murmur. Patients may also demonstrate pallor of the conjunctiva, mucous membranes, nail beds, and palmar creases. The characteristic spooning of the nails may also be present.

Diagnostics

IDA is commonly discovered incidentally during a routine CBC. Once IDA is diagnosed, the history may reveal factors that would cause iron deficiency, such as a recent hemorrhage, gastrointestinal bleeding, menorrhagia, multiple pregnancies, or inadequate nutrition. Iron studies reveal a low serum iron level, decreased serum ferritin, increased TIBC, and decreased percent of transferrin saturation (Box 226-5). Laboratory changes occur gradually as the iron stores are depleted. The earliest laboratory change is a fall in serum ferritin, reflecting depletion of iron stores. This change is followed by a decrease in serum iron and an increase in transferrin, producing a reduction in the percentage of transferrin saturation to less than 15% (this will drop below 10% as the severity progresses) and an associated increase in TIBC. The first change in the CBC is a drop in hemoglobin. Only with increasing severity and duration do the RBCs become microcytic and hypochromic.

The underlying cause of the iron deficiency must be identified. Blood loss by gastrointestinal bleeding or repeated voluntary blood donation should be suspected until proven otherwise. Older adults with suspected IDA should be thoroughly evaluated for gastrointestinal cancers, polypharmacy, and alcohol abuse.

Differential Diagnosis

Only a few diseases need to be considered in the differential diagnosis of a microcytic, hypochromic anemia. The thalassemias typically have a moderate to severe microcytosis with varying degrees of anemia but normal iron studies. ACD presents a more common diagnostic dilemma. With longstanding chronic inflammatory illnesses such as rheumatoid arthritis,

BOX 226-5

LABORATORY STUDIES IN IRON DEFICIENCY ANEMIA

- Hemoglobin: slight decrease to marked decrease
- Serum iron: decreased
- Total iron-binding capacity: increased
- Percent of transferrin saturation: decreased (<10% in severe iron deficiency anemia)
- Serum ferritin: decreased

DIFFERENTIAL DIAGNOSIS

Microcytic Anemia

- Iron deficiency anemia
- Thalassemia
- Anemia of chronic disease
- Sideroblastic anemia
- Lead poisoning, aluminum toxicity

the defective iron supply can result in severe microcytic, hypochromic anemia. Iron studies, especially the serum ferritin level, usually differentiate between a true IDA, ACD, and thalassemia (Table 226-1). Both IDA and ACD have low serum iron levels. The ferritin level is normal or increased in ACD and decreased in IDA. The TIBC is normal or low in ACD and increased in IDA.

Microcytosis can occur in patients with inherited sideroblastic anemias; however, these anemias are rare and are related to X-linked genes. Acquired sideroblastic anemias (idiopathic, secondary to drug or toxin exposure, myeloproliferative, or myelodysplastic disease) can be microcytic but generally are macrocytic. These conditions are characterized by ringed sideroblasts (erythroblasts with one third or more of the nucleus surrounded by ferritin deposits) in the bone marrow and an associated inefficient erythropoiesis.[3] A bone marrow examination is necessary for diagnosis. The anemia tends to be severe (hemoglobin concentration of 6 g/dl) to moderate (hemoglobin concentration of 8 to 10 g/dl) in both forms. Treatment of sideroblastic anemia consists of chronic transfusions and iron chelation therapy (to prevent or treat the transfusion-dependent iron overload). Pyridoxine (vitamin B_6) therapy may sometimes partially correct the anemia in patients with hereditary sideroblastic anemia, leaving them with a milder anemia that does not require as many chronic transfusions.

Management

Treatment of IDA usually begins with an oral iron preparation. The usual therapeutic dosage is 150 to 200 mg of elemental iron per day in divided doses until anemia is corrected. This should be continued empirically for 4 to 6 months or until serum ferritin exceeds 50 mcg/L, then stopped. Common side effects of iron preparations are nausea, constipation, heartburn, upper gastrointestinal discomfort, black stools, and diarrhea. Iron absorption is optimum when iron is taken 30 minutes before meals with ascorbic acid. Absorption can be reduced by as much as 40% to 50% if taken with meals; however, iron on an empty stomach can cause more side effects, leading to noncompliance with medication. Gastrointestinal upset, the most common side effect, may be avoided by starting with a single pill per day and slowly increasing to the recommended dosage.

Once an adequate dosage of iron is reached, changes in the hematologic markers should be seen in just a few weeks. The hemoglobin level should begin to rise within 1 to 2 weeks. The MCV should correct within 1 to 2 months, reflecting the normalization of the erythrocyte size. Supplementation with oral iron should continue until the anemia is corrected, until the underlying cause of the deficiency is corrected, or indefinitely if the cause of the deficiency is chronic.

If the anemia is severe, the patient has an iron malabsorption problem, or oral iron is not tolerated, replacement should be by parenteral iron. Patients should be referred to a hematologist for IV iron administration. Parenteral iron is not without risk. Possible adverse reactions to IV iron include anaphylactic shock, headache, malaise, fever, generalized lymphadenopathy, phlebitis, arthralgias, and urticaria. Therefore administration of IV iron should start with a physician-supervised test dose. The patient should be carefully monitored during the test dose. If the patient tolerates this initial test dose, then the full dose can be administered.

Life Span Considerations

Iron supplementation during pregnancy is almost always required. Pregnancy places a greater demand on iron stores, especially during the last two trimesters. The daily requirement for iron can increase to 5 to 6 mg (the nonpregnant woman requires approximately 1 to 4 mg of iron per day).[11] The additional iron is needed to cover the needs of the developing fetus and placenta and to accommodate the increase in erythrocyte mass that normally occurs during the later stages of pregnancy. Diagnosing IDA during pregnancy can be difficult because of a number of phenomena that normally occur: (1) maternal serum iron is low because of increased

TABLE 226-1 Laboratory Values in Microcytic Anemias

Anemia	Hemoglobin*	MCV	MCHC	Serum Iron†	Serum Ferritin‡	TIBC§	Transferrin Saturation¶
Iron deficiency							
Early	N	N	N	N	N	N	N
Intermediate	N	N	N	↓/N	↓	High N	↓
Late	↓	↓	↓	↓	↓	↑	↓
Thalassemia minor	Low N/↓	↓	N/↓	N	N/≠	N	N
Chronic disease	Low N	N/↓	N/↓	↓	↑	↓	↑
Sideroblastic anemia	↓	↓	↓	↑	↑	N	↑

MCHC, Mean corpuscular hemoglobin concentration; *MCV,* mean corpuscular volume; *TIBC,* total iron-binding capacity.
*N = 12-16 g/dl for women; 13.5-17.5 g/dl for men.
†N = 65-165 mcg/dl for women; 75-175 mcg/dl for men.
‡N = 12-150 mcg/dl for women; 15-300 mcg/dl for men.
§N = 240-450 mcg/dl.
¶N = 20%-50%.

placental uptake, (2) TIBC increases even in pregnant women with sufficient iron stores, and (3) transferrin saturation declines even in nonanemic pregnant women.[11] These factors can make the serum iron, TIBC, and transferrin saturation levels inaccurate. The best indicator of IDA during pregnancy is the serum ferritin level.

Older adults with suspected IDA should be thoroughly evaluated for gastrointestinal cancers, even when their stools are negative for occult blood. Next to ACD, IDA is the most common cause of a microcytic anemia in older adults.[14]

Complications

Untreated IDA is especially worrisome during pregnancy. IDA may be associated with preterm delivery, low birth weight, and learning deficits. Untreated iron deficiency can lead to severe anemia and may be associated with fatigue, falls, and cardiovascular compromise.

Indications for Referral or Hospitalization

Most patients with IDA are diagnosed and treated by their health care providers. Patients who are referred to a hematologist for any of the aforementioned reasons are generally referred back to the health care provider once the anemia has been corrected, or at least once an accurate diagnosis has been made and the patient is receiving stable iron replacement therapy.

Referral to a hematologist should be considered for the following reasons: (1) nonadherence or intolerance to oral iron replacement and persistent IDA, which will require parenteral iron therapy; and (2) persistent microcytic anemia despite iron replacement and the exclusion of other conditions.

Other referrals may be required as evaluation for the cause of the iron deficiency progresses, such as referral to an internist or gastroenterologist to exclude gastrointestinal blood loss or referral to an oncologist to treat any malignancies (either gastrointestinal or gynecologic). Women of reproductive age may require referral to a gynecologist or a hematologist to evaluate severe menorrhagia (the hematology referral may be helpful to rule out von Willebrand's disease as a cause of the menorrhagia).

Healthy patients with IDA do not require hospitalization. Patients who are unable to adequately compensate for a severe anemia may require hospitalization for cardiac or respiratory compromise that may occur.

Patient and Family Education

Patients should receive education about the use of iron supplements to ensure adequate treatment and an understanding of the prescribed regimen. Maximum absorption of iron occurs if it is ingested 30 minutes before meals. Substances that can enhance or inhibit iron absorption are listed in Box 226-4. Calcium can significantly inhibit iron absorption. Multivitamins with calcium or dairy products should be taken 1 to 2 hours after an iron supplement. Ascorbic acid may enhance absorption of iron; therefore concurrent ingestion of foods rich in vitamin C, such as orange juice, should be encouraged.[15]

Numerous iron supplementation preparations are on the market (Table 226-2), some with combinations of iron plus stool softeners, slow-release iron, or iron plus vitamin C. Patients who are intolerant of one preparation may find another that produces fewer or no side effects. Therefore the health care provider should encourage patients to try various preparations before recommending parenteral iron.

TABLE 226-2 Common Iron Supplement Preparations

Preparation	Usual Dosage	Amount of Elemental Iron in Dose (mg)
Ferrous sulfate		
Feosol	200 mg 1-2 q day	65
Slow Fe	160 mg 1-2 q day	50
Ferrous gluconate	324 mg t.i.d.	36
Polysaccharide-iron complex (Niferex)	150 mg 1-2 tablets q day	150
Ferrous fumarate	150 mg 1-2 tablets q day	50

Health Promotion

Nutritional counseling is an important strategy to prevent further episodes of IDA and should include assessment of the patient's dietary intake. Assessment should also include the quantity and timing of iron ingestion and other substances that can interfere with iron absorption, such as tea, coffee, chocolate, dairy products, alcohol, and high-fiber foods. Strict vegetarians who rely on vegetable sources of iron instead of animal sources should be encouraged to supplement their diets with iron-fortified vitamins or to add iron-fortified foods to their diet. Patients whose IDA is secondary to other conditions should be encouraged to seek appropriate medical care.

THALASSEMIA

Definition and Epidemiology

Thalassemia is not a single disorder but rather a group of inherited blood disorders caused by variant or missing genes that affect how the body makes hemoglobin. The resulting anemia depends on the type of thalassemia inherited and varies from asymptomatic to severe hemolytic anemia. All of the thalassemias, except α-thalassemia of a silent carrier, produce some degree of microcytosis and hypochromia.

α-Thalassemia is most commonly found in people with ancestry from Southeast Asia, India, China, or Philippines. β-Thalassemia is more frequent in those of Mediterranean, Middle Eastern, African, or Asian descent. It can be inherited concurrently with genes for the hemoglobinopathies, resulting in conditions such as sickle β-thalassemia (Sβ-thalassemia). Sβ-thalassemia varies according to the amount of β-globin. When no β-globin is produced, the condition is almost identical to sickle cell disease. Severity of the condition is inversely proportional to the amount of β-globin produced. Thalassemia affects males and females equally.

Pathophysiology

The manifestations and severity of clinical symptoms depend on the number of chain deletions in the hemoglobin molecule.[16] Normally, adult RBCs contain predominantly hemoglobin A_1 (96% to 97% of the cell's hemoglobin) and only small amounts of hemoglobin A_2 (2.5%) and hemoglobin F (<1%). The thalassemia abnormalities produce changes in the normal amounts of adult hemoglobin. These quantitative changes are important in the diagnosis of thalassemia.

Inheritance of thalassemia follows an autosomal dominant pattern (Figure 226-1). The two main types of thalassemia are α (alpha) and β (beta), the two protein chains required to make normal hemoglobin. Four genes (two from each parent on chromosome 16) are involved in making α-globin. If one gene is affected, the person is called a *silent carrier* and usually has no symptoms. If two genes are affected, individuals are considered carriers and have mild anemia (α-thalassemia trait or α-thalassemia minor). People with hemoglobin H disease have three genes affected and are moderately to severely anemic.[17] When all four genes are affected, it is called α-thalassemia major (hydrops fetalis), and most affected fetuses are born prematurely and are either stillborn or die shortly after birth.[3] The patients who survive will require life-long transfusions and extensive medical care.

β-Thalassemia genes are located on chromosome 11; each parent provides one to an offspring. An individual is considered a carrier if one gene is affected; this is known as β-thalassemia trait or minor. When both genes are affected, the condition is either β-thalassemia intermedia, causing a moderate anemia, or β-thalassemia major (Cooley's anemia) with severe anemia. Differentiation between β-thalassemia intermedia and major depends on the amount and frequency of transfusions (see below).

Clinical Presentation

Patients with thalassemias are classified as having thalassemia minor (mild), thalassemia intermedia (moderate), or thalassemia major (severe), depending on the severity of their anemia. Throughout the world the majority of patients have thalassemia minor. Patients with α- or β-thalassemia minor generally have either little or no hematologic effects or a mild microcytic hypochromic anemia that is often mistaken for IDA.

Patients with thalassemia intermedia have a moderate microcytic and hypochromic anemia that is not transfusion dependent. Patients with thalassemia intermedia may require occasional transfusions during pregnancy or preoperatively. If patients with thalassemia intermedia begin to develop persistent clinical problems such as abnormal facies, growth

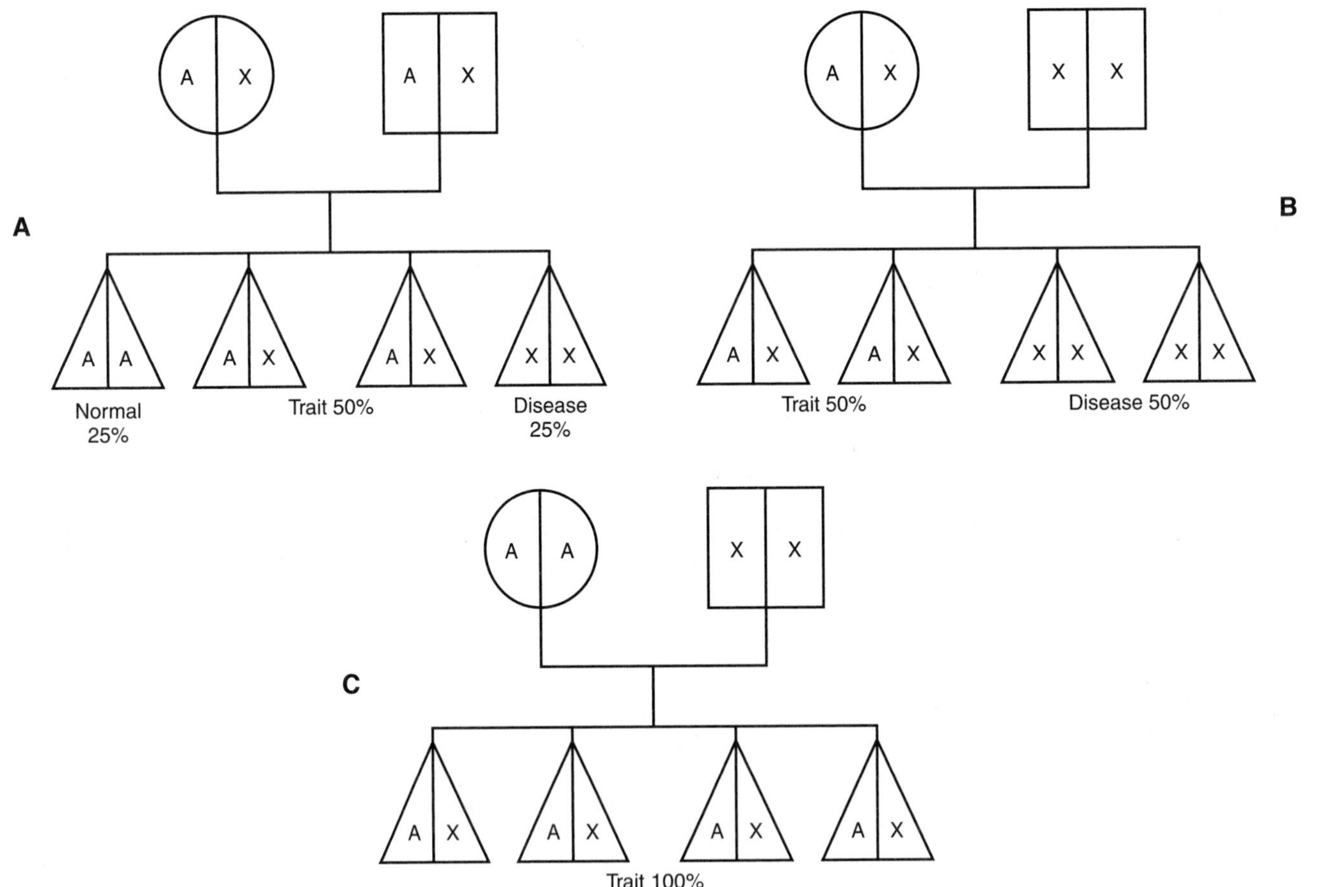

FIGURE 226-1

Inheritance patterns for autosomal genes. **A**, When both parents have a trait, offspring have a 25% chance of being normal, a 25% chance of having the disease, and a 50% chance of having the trait. **B**, When one parent has the disease and the other parent has the trait, offspring have a 50% chance of having the trait and a 50% chance of having the disease. **C**, When one parent has the disease and the other parent is normal, all offspring will have the trait. *A*, Gene for normal hemoglobin; *X*, gene for abnormal hemoglobin (S, C, E) or thalassemia.

retardation, or pathologic fractures, they will require regular transfusions. At this point, these patients are given the diagnosis of thalassemia major.[18]

Patients with β-thalassemia major develop a severe, life-threatening anemia during their first year of life. This profound anemia is associated with developmental problems and decreased life expectancy. These patients require lifelong chronic RBC transfusions to maintain adequate hemoglobin levels and iron chelation.

Physical Examination

The physical examination is remarkable only in patients with thalassemia intermedia and β-thalassemia major. Patients can exhibit the characteristic physical changes of short stature and abnormal facies associated with cranial marrow expansion. In the United States, however, the facial abnormalities are seen primarily in patients with thalassemia intermedia, since most patients with β-thalassemia major are hypertransfused to normal hemoglobin levels, thus preventing the marrow expansion.[18] Children can be diagnosed as early as 3 months of age, with findings of severe anemia; pallor; jaundice; and an enlarged spleen, liver, or heart.

Diagnostics

Patients with thalassemia intermedia or major are diagnosed during the first few years of life. The diagnosis of β-thalassemia minor is based on a mildly decreased hemoglobin concentration, low MCV (<75 fl), normal iron studies, and a normal hemoglobin electrophoresis with high levels of hemoglobin A_2. α-Thalassemia is more difficult to diagnose, since a special test, α-globin DNA mutation analysis, is required; only the largest of medical centers perform this test.

Patients with thalassemia intermedia who maintain adequate hemoglobin levels without requiring transfusions exhibit signs of a mild microcytic anemia with slightly low hemoglobin and a low MCV. Patients with β-thalassemia major who are hypertransfused have either a low or low-normal hemoglobin level and a relatively normal MCV (because they are receiving normal blood during transfusions). Peripheral smears of both patients with thalassemia intermedia and patients with β-thalassemia major have typical target cells present. Patients with β-thalassemia major who do not receive adequate iron chelation therapy reflect their state of overload with very high ferritin, very low TIBC, and percent of transferrin saturation approaching 100%. Patients with thalassemia intermedia may have similar iron studies because they can develop iron overload as a result of iron hyperabsorption rather than from transfusions.

Differential Diagnosis

In most cases the health care provider needs to distinguish thalassemia minor from IDA. Both conditions are microcytic anemias, but results of iron studies are normal in patients with thalassemia minor. In immigrants from Southeast Asia, the differential diagnosis of a mild microcytic anemia must differentiate between β-thalassemia minor and hemoglobin E disease.

Hemoglobin E is the second most common hemoglobinopathy in the world (next to sickle cell disease). It is not a true thalassemia but rather a mild hemolytic anemia. It is characterized by a mild microcytic anemia with many target cells on the peripheral smear. It closely resembles the microcytic anemia of β-thalassemia minor, but hemoglobin E is found only in people of Southeast Asian ancestry. Patients who are homozygous for hemoglobin E (EE) are clinically normal, as are patients with β-thalassemia minor. Patients can also be double heterozygotes for hemoglobin E and sickle cell disease (ES), resulting clinically in a mild sickle cell disease or combined hemoglobin E and β-thalassemia, which results in a moderate to severe transfusion-dependent anemia that will be similar to β-thalassemia major.[19] Hemoglobin E is diagnosed by hemoglobin electrophoresis.

Often, patients with β-thalassemia minor or hemoglobin E are given a diagnosis of IDA because of their mild microcytic anemia and are prescribed a regimen of iron replacement. Failure to correct the anemia with iron supplementation should then lead the provider to suspect thalassemia minor (or hemoglobin E disease if the patient is of Southeast Asian ancestry).

Management

Patients with β-thalassemia minor do not require medical management but should be referred for genetic counseling if family planning is an issue. Patients with thalassemia intermedia can be adequately cared for in a primary care setting, with regular attention to any changes in their anemia. Patients with thalassemia intermedia who begin to develop persistent clinical problems such as abnormal facies, growth retardation, or pathologic fractures should be referred to a hematologist to begin chronic transfusion therapy. Patients with thalassemia intermedia who hyperabsorb iron and develop iron overload require chelation therapy.

In the United States, hematologists who are familiar with the disease manage most patients with β-thalassemia major and intermedia. Management consists of two equally important functions: (1) regular transfusions to maintain an adequate hemoglobin level to allow for normal growth and development and (2) iron chelation therapy to prevent the complications of transfusion-dependent iron overload.

Regular transfusions of packed RBCs are the mainstay of therapy for β-thalassemia major. Transfusions are begun early in childhood to maintain an adequate hemoglobin level to allow for normal growth and development. Transfusions are usually necessary every 3 to 6 weeks to maintain hemoglobin levels at 9 to 10 g/dl.[20]

Chelation therapy is the standard treatment for prevention of complications from iron overload. Complications of iron overload can be profound, since deposition is concentrated in the liver and heart, and are the major cause of death in patients with β-thalassemia major. Deferoxamine is a chelating agent that removes iron from tissues and allows excretion of iron in urine and stools. Deferoxamine must be administered parenterally, generally via a subcutaneous needle, and delivered by slow infusion over at least 8 hours to effectively remove iron. The longer the infusion time, the more effectively the iron is removed. Parenteral therapy is administered 5 to 7 days a week for life. Chelation therapy given as only a single injection with blood transfusions is not effective in any setting.

The normal subcutaneous dose is 50 to 100 mg/kg/day administered by continuous infusion over a 10- to 16-hour period. If subcutaneous administration is not tolerated, IV therapy can be attempted but requires the use of an indwelling venous catheter. The goal of chelation therapy is to reduce body iron stores and maintain a ferritin level of less than 1000 mcg/L, which will significantly reduce the risks associated with iron overload.[21]

Deferasirox is the first oral iron chelator on the U.S. market. It is excreted primarily via the fecal route, with only 8% excreted by the kidneys. Mild increases in serum creatinine during clinical trials were noted in one third of the patients; however, most remained within normal limits. Recommended beginning daily doses start at 20 mg/kg and increase every 3 months based on the monthly serum ferritin trend. Deferasirox is a tablet dissolved in water or juice and consumed on an empty stomach 30 minutes before meals.[22] This provides a much needed alternative to the long infusions otherwise required for iron removal.

Bone marrow transplantation (BMT) is currently the only potential cure for β-thalassemia. Rund and Rachmilewitz reported that more than 1000 transplantations have been done since 1982.[20] BMT is not without serious risks. Transplant success is highest in children and those who are well chelated, have a normal liver, and have no cardiac complications.

Other therapies (including erythropoietin, hydroxyurea, and butyrate derivatives) are currently being investigated for their potential to induce fetal hemoglobin production.[20] Increasing fetal hemoglobin production may prove especially beneficial for patients with thalassemia intermedia as a way to avoid transfusions.

Life Span Considerations

Reproductive issues are a major concern. Well-chelated and well-transfused women may be fertile. Contraception counseling should be offered to all women with thalassemia who are sexually active with male partners. There are no restrictions as to the types of contraception available to women with β-thalassemia.

Complications

Many possible complications are associated with both the regular transfusion regimen and the chelation therapy. However, most of the severe complications are transmittable diseases via the blood pool followed by iron overload.

Transfusions are usually well tolerated, but complications can occur. The development of alloantibodies can make it difficult to find suitable blood donors on a regular basis, requiring lengthy waiting periods of up to 48 hours depending on proximity to regional blood centers. Viral infections such as HIV and hepatitis B and C have become less of an issue because of blood product screening; however, screening is not 100% accurate. Patients should receive hepatitis B vaccine and be screened for hepatitis B antibodies, since immunity is not lifelong and may require boosters. Iron overload is the primary complication of chronic transfusions. Accumulation of excess iron leads to cirrhosis; heart failure; and endocrine problems such as diabetes mellitus, hypothyroidism, growth failure, and delayed sexual development.[20,23]

Chelation therapy can also be problematic. Chronic subcutaneous administration of deferoxamine can cause localized reactions such as scar tissue formation, itching, rash, and local irritation at the site of injection. There are also possible complications if a high dose of deferoxamine is given in the presence of low serum ferritin. These complications include toxic effects on the eye, such as cataracts, night blindness, and reduction of visual fields and acuity (these effects usually regress when deferoxamine therapy is stopped); hearing loss (high-tone deafness is irreversible despite cessation of therapy); and skeletal lesions such as pseudorickets, metaphyseal changes, and short stature (these are also irreversible complications of deferoxamine therapy).[23]

Despite the availability of iron chelation therapy, complications of iron overload are common in patients with thalassemia who are more than 10 years of age. This may be due to inadequate iron chelation early in life with resulting irreversible damage, insufficient chelation therapy, or poor compliance. Iron overload complications include endocrine, cardiac, and hepatic problems (Box 226-6). The presence of cardiac complications is an indication for continuous (24 hours a day, 7 days a week) iron chelation therapy.

Well-chelated patients with thalassemia who maintain a ferritin level of less than 1000 mcg/L do not develop the major complications of iron overload. However, many of them have growth retardation and delayed puberty. Most people with β-thalassemia major are unusually short and may appear younger than their age. Young women are often amenorrheic. An endocrinology consult may be indicated when the patient is nearing the age of puberty. Hormone replacement therapy (estrogen for girls or testosterone for boys) can be initiated to hasten maturation and sexual development.

Indications for Referral or Hospitalization

β-Thalassemia major is a chronic lifelong disease that requires constant attention by health care providers. Ideally, hematologists or health care providers familiar with the disease should manage these patients. Attention to issues of growth and development, compliance with transfusion and chelation therapy, reproductive issues, and assessment for the development of complications require frequent follow-up visits.

BOX 226-6

COMPLICATIONS OF IRON OVERLOAD

ENDOCRINE PROBLEMS

- Growth retardation
- Diabetes mellitus
- Hypothyroidism
- Hypoparathyroidism
- Disturbed pubertal development

CARDIAC PROBLEMS

- Arrhythmias
- Pericarditis
- Cardiac failure

HEPATIC COMPLICATIONS

- Cirrhosis

Even patients with β-thalassemia major who are well transfused and well chelated may experience considerable delays in puberty. These patients should be referred to a reproductive endocrinologist for possible hormone therapy.

Patients with thalassemia who receive chronic transfusion therapy and chelation therapy can lead relatively healthy lives. If they are not compliant, however, the complications of iron overload will eventually lead to increasing morbidity from liver disease and, especially, cardiac disease. When patients with β-thalassemia major are hospitalized for any reason, they should be transfused to maintain an adequate hemoglobin concentration and be maintained on chelation therapy. Now with oral chelation therapy available, compliance should be a lesser problem, and death from iron overload and its complications should also be decreased.

Patient and Family Education

Patients with β-thalassemia major and their families assume a great deal of responsibility for their own health. Chelation therapy occurs at home, and patients must learn how to perform aseptic subcutaneous injections and use the infusion pump. Adhering to the chelation therapy schedule is essential. There are no signs and symptoms of iron overload until a fairly advanced stage; therefore it is hard for young children and especially adolescents to understand the importance of a treatment for which they see no immediate need. Adolescents will have self-image issues. Delayed puberty, the need for daily medication infusions, and frequent trips to the hospital for transfusions will constantly remind them of being different from their peers. The daily (or usually nightly) requirement for infusions can interfere with social life and complicate intimate relationships. The transfusion schedule can interfere with work or school, and most patients with β-thalassemia find that they require a flexible work or school schedule to accommodate their transfusion schedule. The availability of evening and weekend transfusions greatly enhance the patient's well-being and adherence to the treatment schedule.

Although new to the market, deferasirox should prove to increase compliance and therefore decrease side effects from iron overload. Proper preparation of oral chelator and adherence to medication guidelines are important teaching instructions.

Health Promotion

Collaborating with patients and their families is important to promote patients' self-esteem and self-reliance. Patients who believe in the value of their own lives will be more likely to comply with the regular transfusion schedule and their daily chelation therapy.

MACROCYTIC ANEMIA: MEGALOBLASTIC ANEMIA

VITAMIN B_{12} AND FOLATE DEFICIENCY

Definition and Epidemiology

Vitamin B_{12} and folate deficiency are the primary causes of macrocytic anemia. Both vitamins are essential for normal DNA synthesis, and tissues such as bone marrow are highly sensitive to any deficiency. Marrow precursors for all cell lines (erythroid, myeloid, and platelets) become larger than normal and are unable to complete normal growth and maturation, a condition referred to as a megaloblastic bone marrow.[12,24] The resulting ineffective erythropoiesis causes the release of macrocytic RBCs into the circulation and worsening anemia.

Folate deficiency is found in the presence of decreased dietary intake, diseases associated with malabsorption, or increased requirements such as pregnancy. Alcoholism is a common cause of folate deficiency because of alcohol's interference with folate metabolism and the usually poor dietary habits related to alcoholism. In developing countries, malabsorption syndromes such as tropical and nontropical sprue are more common causes.[12] Folate deficiency is also associated with neural tube defects in the fetus.

Pernicious anemia (lack of intrinsic factor [IF]) is the most prevalent cause of vitamin B_{12} deficiency (malabsorption). It is a disease in which atrophy of the parietal cells of the stomach leads to a complete loss of IF.[25] It often co-exists with other autoimmune disorders, gastrointestinal disorders, type 1 diabetes, and thyroid disease. Chronic gastritis can damage parietal cells, and partial or complete gastric resection results in loss of parietal cells and therefore IF. The onset of pernicious anemia usually occurs after age 50 years.

Pathophysiology

Dietary sources of vitamin B_{12} are found only in meat and meat by-products. When vitamin B_{12} from food reaches the small bowel, it is bound to IF, a glycoprotein secreted by parietal cells of the stomach. The vitamin B_{12}–IF (cobalamin-IF) complex is then transported through the terminal ileum into the circulation. Vitamin B_{12} absorption cannot occur in the absence of IF.

Once in the circulation, vitamin B_{12} is bound to the transport protein transcobalamin II, which carries it to the liver, bone marrow, and other proliferating cells. A healthy adult receiving an adequate diet can accumulate from 1 to 10 mg of vitamin B_{12} in the liver, the major storage site.[12] Because the daily requirement of vitamin B_{12} is only 3 to 5 mcg/day, most omnivorous individuals have no difficulty obtaining the necessary amounts from their diets as long as absorption is normal. Only strict vegetarians are at risk for a dietary deficiency, and it would take several years of a strict vegan diet for megaloblastosis to occur.

Dietary folate is readily available in most foods, especially green leafy vegetables; however, folate is heat labile and rapidly destroyed by prolonged cooking or food processing.[26] Body stores are limited to approximately a 3-month reserve. It is possible that a prolonged inadequate diet may not provide sufficient amounts of folate for normal DNA production, especially for patients who are pregnant or have hemolytic anemias (high rates of cell turnover). Dietary folate deficiency is relatively uncommon, since many foods, such as orange juice, are now supplemented. Folate deficiency is commonly associated with chronic alcoholism and can also be caused by the same malabsorption syndromes that lead to vitamin B_{12} deficiency (Box 226-7).

BOX 226-7

COMMON CAUSES OF MEGALOBLASTIC ANEMIA

INADEQUATE INTAKE
- Vegetarian diet devoid of animal proteins (vitamin B_{12})
- Chronic alcoholism (folate)

MALABSORPTION (VITAMIN B_{12} AND FOLATE)
- Lack of intrinsic factor
- Gastric surgery
- Inflammatory bowel disease
- Sprue (tropical and nontropical)
- Celiac disease
- Intestinal tapeworm
- Hyperthyroidism

INCREASED REQUIREMENTS (FOLATE)
- Pregnancy
- Hemolytic anemias

Clinical Presentation

A mild megaloblastic anemia produces few symptoms, and the CBC usually makes the diagnosis incidentally. A severe vitamin B_{12} deficiency includes signs and symptoms of marked anemia and neurologic deficits. Early neurologic symptoms include decreased vibratory sensation, loss of proprioception, peripheral neuropathy, and ataxia. Later involvement results in spasticity, hyperactive reflexes, and a positive Romberg's sign. These neurologic symptoms result from the formation of a demyelinating lesion of the neurons of the spinal cord and cerebral cortex.[12] Neurologic symptoms may be evident in the absence of anemia and may not resolve with correction of the deficiency. Other classic symptoms of B_{12} deficiency include a sore mouth and loss of taste.

Folate deficiency is rarely associated with any symptoms, even in the severe state. Folate deficiency is not associated with neurologic or psychiatric disorders except those caused by neural tube defects.

Physical Examination

The physical examination of a patient with severe megaloblastic anemia may reveal the classic changes associated with any severe anemia. Patients with severe vitamin B_{12} deficiency may have characteristic findings such as a smooth, red, shiny tongue and the aforementioned neurologic changes.

Diagnostics

Findings on the CBC that suggest macrocytic anemia include low hemoglobin levels and an MCV over 100 fl. Severe anemia may also be associated with leukopenia or thrombocytopenia. In addition, the retic count will be low. The peripheral smear is also helpful in diagnosing megaloblastic anemia. Hypersegmented neutrophils and oval macrocytes are the earliest and most specific signs of megaloblastic anemia. Serum cobalamin (vitamin B_{12}) and folate levels may help distinguish the cause of the macrocytosis. Measuring certain metabolites of vitamin B_{12}, methylmalonic acid and homocysteine, provides additional information to help identify the cause of the anemia. The normal range of serum methylmalonic acid is 70 to 270 nm/L, and the normal serum homocysteine level ranges from 5 to 16 nm/L. Homocysteine is elevated in both vitamin B_{12} and folate deficiency. Methylmalonic acid is elevated in vitamin B_{12} deficiency and normal in folate deficiency.

It is important to distinguish vitamin B_{12} deficiency caused by malabsorption from that caused by lack of IF. Many of the medications now used to treat gastroesophageal reflux disease affect absorption. Long-term use of H_2 blockers inhibits release of IF; proton pump inhibitors can reduce absorption of protein-bound cobalamin and can eventually lead to malabsorption. Schilling's test has been the classic method used to verify the diagnosis of pernicious anemia but is now rarely used. An assay for antiintrinsic factor or antiparietal cell antibodies is the currently accepted method for verifying the diagnosis of pernicious anemia. The presence of antiintrinsic factor antibodies is highly specific for pernicious anemia.

Differential Diagnosis

The differential diagnosis involves identifying the cause of the vitamin deficiency itself. It is important to accurately determine the cause of the macrocytic anemia because misdiagnosis can have extremely negative consequences. A vitamin B_{12} deficiency that is inappropriately treated with folic acid may result in permanent neurologic or psychiatric abnormalities.

It may also be necessary to distinguish the macrocytic anemia associated with vitamin B_{12} or folate deficiency from the macrocytosis caused by other conditions such as drug or alcohol abuse, liver disease, hypothyroidism, myelodysplastic syndrome, exposure to chemotherapeutic agents, or hemolysis.[27] It is also essential to consider vitamin B_{12} deficiency in the differential diagnosis of any peripheral neuropathy, dementia, or other psychiatric disorder, especially in older adults.

Management

Initial management of a macrocytic anemia depends on the severity of the anemia. Patients with life-threatening anemia require transfusions of packed RBCs to correct the anemia. Treatment with both B_{12} and folate can be started until a definitive diagnosis is made. If the patient's cardiovascular system is unable to compensate for the degree of anemia, hospitalization is required until the patient is stable.

Patients with asymptomatic anemia should not be treated until an accurate diagnosis is made. Treatment should then be targeted to replacement of the deficient vitamin and correction of the underlying disease, if possible. The usual treatment for vitamin B_{12} deficiency related to IF is 1000 mcg of cyanocobalamin or hydroxocobalamin intramuscular injections every week for 8 weeks and then monthly for life. Reticulocytosis begins in approximately 3 days and peaks in 7 to 10 days after the initiation of vitamin replacement. The anemia should resolve over 3 to 4 weeks.

DIFFERENTIAL DIAGNOSIS

Macrocytic Anemia
- Vitamin B_{12} deficiency
- Folic acid deficiency
- Myelodysplastic syndromes
- Liver disease
- Hypothyroidism
- Hemolysis
- Chemotherapeutic agents
- Hereditary disorder
- Alcoholism
- Drug reaction

The recommended treatment of a macrocytic anemia resulting from folate deficiency is 1 mg of folic acid daily and correction of the underlying cause of the deficiency. Treatment should continue until at least a normal hemoglobin level is reached (usually in about 4 to 6 weeks) and should be continued indefinitely if the patient has an inadequate diet or if the underlying disease persists. Patients with a chronic hemolytic process, such as sickle cell disease, and pregnant patients should receive prophylactic daily supplementation of the same dose.

Patients who have had partial or total gastrectomy, ileal resection, or any other evidence of gastric atrophy or intestinal malabsorption should receive prophylactic treatment of monthly parenteral vitamin B_{12} therapy and daily folic acid supplements.

Life Span Considerations

Studies in the early 1990s by the MRC Vitamin Research Group confirmed preliminary reports of an association between folate deficiency and neural tube defects.[28] Data showed that the risk of neural tube defects is 1 to 5 per 1000 live births for the general population and approximately 10 times this amount among women with previous pregnancies involving neural tube defects. When women received supplements of folic acid before they became pregnant, the incidence of neural tube defects decreased by 72%. In 1992 the Centers for Disease Control and Prevention recommended routine supplementation before pregnancy for all women who wish to become pregnant.[29] The recommended intake is 0.4 mg/day either as a supplement or in the diet.

Annual screening for vitamin B_{12} deficiency is recommended for all older adults.[30] Screening is also recommended for patients with hematologic, neurologic, or psychiatric abnormalities suggestive of vitamin B_{12} deficiency.

Complications

The complication of undiagnosed or mistreated vitamin B_{12} deficiency is irreversible neurologic damage. Manifestations of weakness, ataxia, and poor coordination may not completely resolve with therapy, depending on the duration of the deficiency and the extent of neurologic damage. Mental status changes can range from mild forgetfulness to severe dementia and psychosis. Patients with neurologic damage can have an almost normal blood count with normal indexes, which underscores the need to test for vitamin B_{12} levels in patients with unexplained neurologic deficits.

Indications for Referral or Hospitalization

A health care provider can easily manage patients who are receiving maintenance therapy of either vitamin B_{12} or folate replacement. These patients require regular visits for evaluation of therapy and monthly visits for vitamin B_{12} injections. Periodic evaluations should include a complete history and physical examination to look for the appearance or progression of any neurologic or psychiatric complications, as well as continued assessment of the underlying disease causing the vitamin deficiency. Laboratory evaluations include CBC and serum cobalamin and folate levels. A hematologist should manage patients with refractory anemia.

Patients with a severe macrocytic anemia should be referred to a hematologist for consultation and recommended therapy. Asymptomatic patients can be treated and monitored in an outpatient setting, either by a hematologist or by the patient's health care provider.

As previously stated, patients with a severe, life-threatening anemia may require hospitalization for correction of the anemia. This is especially true for patients with a severe vitamin B_{12} deficiency, who require daily administration of parenteral vitamin B_{12} therapy to begin to correct the vitamin deficiency.

Patient and Family Education

Patients with folate deficiency secondary to an inadequate diet require nutritional counseling to learn how to properly cook and prepare foods without losing their nutritional value. Daily folic acid supplementation may be required for patients on certain drug regimens such as sulfasalazine and patients with other hematologic diseases.

Patients with megaloblastic anemia secondary to vitamin B_{12} deficiency require monthly vitamin B_{12} injections. Patients or caregivers can easily be taught this injection technique so that injections can be administered at home. Parenteral vitamin B_{12} in the absence of pernicious anemia is not effective in increasing energy in older adults. Patients with conditions that require partial or total gastrectomy, ileal resections, and other small bowel removal need counseling on life-long parenteral vitamin B_{12} and folic acid replacement.

Health Promotion

Early recognition and treatment of alcohol abuse is one preventive measure that health care providers can take to reduce the incidence of folate deficiency anemia. Lifestyle modifications include improving dietary sources of folic acid and vitamin B_{12} and taking vitamin supplements if necessary. Health care providers who see older patients should screen for cobalamin deficiency in cases of unexplained mental status changes and should begin therapy with vitamin B_{12} before the onset of symptoms.

NORMOCYTIC ANEMIA

SICKLE CELL DISEASE

Definition and Epidemiology

Sickle cell syndromes are the most common inherited hemoglobinopathies and include homozygous disease (hemoglobin SS), hemoglobin SC (also known as SC disease), Sβ-thalassemia, and a variety of other rare, abnormal hemoglobins. Patients with sickle cell disease have mild to moderate hemolytic anemia that is generally well compensated. The anemia, however, is the least serious manifestation of the disease. The hallmark of sickle cell disease is the acute vaso-occlusive crisis that causes unpredictable, severe pain and organ damage.

One in 10 African Americans carries the gene for sickle cell trait (AS), and about 1 in 400 is affected by the disease (SS). Other types of sickle cell syndromes are found in Mediterranean, Middle Eastern, and Southeast Asian populations. People with only one gene for hemoglobin S are phenotypically normal (sickle cell trait). People who inherit one gene for hemoglobin S from each parent will have SS disease. People with either hemoglobin SC or Sβ-thalassemia have inherited one gene for hemoglobin S and the other gene for either hemoglobin C or β-thalassemia, respectively. The life span of patients with SS disease is approximately 45 years; the life span is 50 to 60 years for patients with other types of sickle cell syndromes, including hemoglobin SC or Sβ-thalassemia.[31]

Pathophysiology

The hemoglobin defect occurs when valine replaces glutamic acid in the beta chain of hemoglobin, resulting in hemoglobin S.[32] Deoxygenated hemoglobin S tends to undergo irreversible polymerization, deforming the erythrocytes and giving them the pathognomonic sickle shape. The sickled cells are rigid and can be easily trapped in the microcirculation, causing obstruction, ischemia, and sometimes infarction. This process leads to the clinical consequences of severe pain and organ damage. These vaso-occlusive episodes, usually referred to as *crises* or *pain crises*, can occur anywhere in the body but commonly affect the joints, extremities, back, chest, abdomen, and lungs.

Clinical Presentation

Sickle cell trait has no clinical manifestations. Manifestations of sickle cell disease vary widely; some affected individuals have few painful crises and rare complications, whereas others are often hospitalized with painful crises or other complications. A study of the natural history of sickle cell disease indicated that about 5% of patients account for almost one third of hospital admissions.[33] Patients with other types of sickle cell syndromes (hemoglobin SC or Sβ-thalassemia) are reported to have milder forms of disease, although this is not always true. For example, patients with hemoglobin SC can exhibit the same range of severity as patients with SS disease.

Physical Examination

Objective manifestations of a moderate to severe hemolytic anemia include jaundice and a physiologic systolic flow murmur. Scleral icterus can range from mild to severe, but often has no association with the severity of disease. The physiologic flow murmur secondary to anemia is often a grade I or II pansystolic murmur, which is heard best along the left sternal border. Cardiomegaly is routinely noted on the radiographs of adults with sickle cell disease and is also a compensatory manifestation of lifelong anemia.

Diagnostics

Accurate diagnosis of any sickle cell syndrome requires a hemoglobin electrophoresis. Patients with sickle cell disease have evidence of a hemolytic anemia: low hemoglobin, chronic reticulocytosis, chronic hyperbilirubinemia, and chronically elevated LDH levels. The peripheral blood smear shows mild to moderate anisocytosis and poikilocytosis with numerous sickle cells and Howell-Jolly bodies (evidence of the patient's functional asplenia). Patients with SC disease have target cells in addition to the sickle cells on their peripheral blood smears.

DIFFERENTIAL DIAGNOSIS

Normocytic Anemia

Sickle cell disorders
- Sickle cell trait
- Sickle cell anemia
- Sβ-Thalassemia
- Sickle cell disease

Hereditary spherocytosis
Hypersplenism
Autoimmune hemolysis
Delayed hemolytic transfusion reaction
Aplastic anemia

Unfortunately, no laboratory tests are diagnostic of an acute painful crisis. Serial determinations of CBC during the crisis may reveal a slight increase in the anemia but give no information about the severity of the crisis.[34]

Differential Diagnosis

Most patients with sickle cell disease are diagnosed at birth. In fact, currently most states have mandatory newborn screening for sickle hemoglobin. However, it is possible for persons with very mild disease to go undiagnosed until they are in their adult years. These patients may be seen with a mild hemolytic anemia (low hemoglobin concentration, slight hyperbilirubinemia with elevated LDH levels, and mild reticulocytosis). A history of occasional, spontaneous painful events, usually abdominal or joint pains, should suggest a hemoglobinopathy. Accurate diagnosis requires hemoglobin electrophoresis to differentiate among the various forms of sickle cell disease. Other possible causes of hemolytic anemia include hereditary spherocytosis, hypersplenism, autoimmune hemolysis, or a delayed hemolytic transfusion reaction.

Management

The frequency and severity of pain crises vary tremendously among patients and even in the same patient over time. Infection and physical or emotional stress may precipitate a crisis, but the majority of crises occur spontaneously with no obvious precipitating events.[34] The sites affected in an acute crisis vary among individuals, but crises tend to recur at the same site(s) for a particular person. The quality of the pain is usually similar as well. Most patients are able to distinguish a "typical" sickle cell pain crisis from other events, such as pyelonephritis or abdominal pain resulting from cholecystitis.

Most crises are mild to moderate in severity and can be managed at home with oral analgesics (either NSAIDs or oral narcotics), adequate hydration, rest, and local measures such as heat or gentle massage. Moderate to severe crises require treatment in an emergency department or a hospital-based outpatient treatment center with parenteral narcotic analgesics and hydration, as well as the same local measures described previously. Often, aggressive and early management of a crisis can prevent hospital admission. Hospitalizations for crises can last from a few days to several weeks. Patients describe a severe crisis as the most intense pain that they have ever experienced. Pain control often requires large quantities of narcotic analgesics. For many patients it is not unusual to administer 4 to 8 mg of hydromorphone as an IV bolus over 10 to 15 minutes every 30 minutes for four to six doses before achieving adequate pain relief. Many adults with sickle cell disease have learned how to manage their pain without the behavioral signs that one would expect from someone experiencing severe pain. Therefore it becomes important when evaluating a sickle cell patient in crisis to believe the patient's report and to treat the pain quickly and appropriately.

Hydroxyurea is becoming standard therapy for patients who experience three or more crises per year. Hydroxyurea induces hemoglobin F formation, which forms soluble hybrid polymers with hemoglobin S, thus reducing hemoglobin S polymer concentration and ameliorating the cellular and tissue damage related to vaso-occlusion.[34] In a randomized, double-blind, placebo-controlled study of 299 patients with SS disease, hydroxyurea reduced the incidence of painful crises.[35] Patient responses have varied; some respond well with a reduction in painful crises, whereas others may see no effect or no obvious reduction in crises. Hydroxyurea is started at a dosage of 15 to 20 mg/kg/day. Patients must be monitored every 2 weeks for signs of toxicity (neutrophil count <2000/mm^3, platelet count <80,000/mm^3, or hemoglobin drop of 2 g/dl) or favorable response. The dose of hydroxyurea can be increased over several months to a maximum dosage of 35 mg/kg/day. Once stable, patients should be monitored monthly.

By definition, patients with sickle cell disease are anemic. The degree of anemia varies, but most have hematocrit concentrations that range from the high teens to the mid-twenties. Patients with hemoglobin SC tend to have hematocrit values in the high twenties to mid-thirties. The baseline hematocrit value tends to remain relatively stable in a given patient. Most patients are able to compensate for their level of anemia and do not require routine transfusions. In fact, transfusing patients to achieve hematocrit concentrations in the mid-thirties or higher can be dangerous, since blood viscosity increases substantially at higher hematocrit levels and the increased viscosity can worsen the tendency to sickle by slowing the RBCs' transit time through low-oxygen regions of the circulation.[36]

Like other people with hemolytic anemias, patients with sickle cell disease require daily folic acid replacement. Folate is necessary for normal erythropoiesis, and in hemolytic anemias it is rapidly consumed by the proliferating erythroid precursors. Supplemental folic acid in the amount of 1 mg/day is enough to maintain the higher rate of erythropoiesis that occurs in chronic hemolysis.

Life Span Considerations

Women with sickle cell disease can carry pregnancies to term but should be considered high risk because of the potential for obstetric complications such as spontaneous abortion, thrombophlebitis, toxemia, and pulmonary embolism after delivery. The frequency of painful crises sometimes increases during pregnancy, but the crises are treated no differently from other crises, with narcotic analgesics and hydration. Pregnancy prevention and family planning options are the same for women with sickle cell disease as they are for other women. In fact, many women experience relief from menses-related crises with the use of oral contraceptives or other hormone contraception methods.

Sickle cell disease is a chronic condition that often leads to psychosocial difficulties, as well as medical problems. Some patients experience frequent complications of their disease, making it almost impossible to participate in normal daily activities, hold a regular job, or attend school on a regular schedule. Many of these patients can benefit from rehabilitation counseling and vocational training. Often, however, adults with sickle cell disease find that they are unable to work because of chronic pain or other multiorgan damage. These individuals are clearly disabled.

Complications

Chronic pain is a substantial problem for most adults with sickle cell disease. The severity of the pain varies greatly among patients and can change over time. Some patients can manage their chronic pain with intermittent use of mild analgesics such as NSAIDs. Most patients, however, require frequent doses of oral narcotic analgesics. Often, these patients become tolerant to narcotics, and the quantity of medication needed to control the pain can escalate over time. This physical tolerance should not be confused with psychologic addiction and drug-seeking behaviors, which are uncommon in this population.

Acute pulmonary disease has become the most common cause of death and the second most common reason for hospitalizations.[37] The term *acute chest syndrome* (ACS) is used to describe an acute pulmonary event that can be either infectious or noninfectious in its etiology. Fever, dyspnea, cough, pulmonary infiltrates, and severe chest pain usually characterize the condition. Clinically, ACS is often more severe than pneumonia in the general population, with severe hypoxia and progressive multilobar involvement despite treatment with antibiotics. Typically the patient is hospitalized for a vaso-occlusive crisis and 1 to 3 days later develops respiratory distress.

The most important step in the treatment of ACS is early recognition. Potential bacterial infections should be treated with appropriate antibiotics. Single-volume exchange transfusions are the treatment of choice for ACS in patients with severe hypoxemia (Pa_{O_2} <60 mm Hg) and can have a dramatic effect on reversing the clinical course, with rapid correction of hypoxia.[38] Simple transfusions raising the hemoglobin concentration to 10 g/dl can also be beneficial in patients with mild to moderate hypoxemia.[37]

Strokes in patients with sickle cell disease are much more common in children than in adults but can occur in the adult population.[39] Stroke in sickle cell disease is a medical emergency. The treatment of choice is an exchange transfusion followed by maintenance hypertransfusion and iron chelation therapy.[40] In 1997 the Stroke Prevention Trial showed that chronic transfusion is highly effective in reducing the risk of first stroke in children with sickle cell disease and an abnormal transcranial Doppler ultrasonogram.[41] It is now recommended that children with sickle cell disease be screened by transcranial Doppler ultrasonography and started on chronic transfusion therapy if results indicate a high risk of stroke. Young patients on chronic transfusion have fewer pain episodes and a reduced risk of ACS.[42] These same patients must be compliant with iron chelation therapy to prevent future complications from iron overload.

Priapism is defined as a persistent, painful erection of the penis that can last from several hours to several days. Priapism lasting more than 3 or 4 hours is a medical emergency, since it can cause impotence. Treatment includes hydration, analgesia, and possible transfusion (either simple or exchange). Other controversial interventions include the use of conjugated estrogens and vasodilators for nonacute cases, and surgical interventions such as aspiration and shunt placement.

There is a high risk of renal dysfunction or failure in adults with sickle cell disease. Renal failure results from sickle cell–induced damage to renal microvasculature.[43] Renal dysfunction is generally diagnosed in the third or fourth decade and eventually progresses to renal failure. Subcutaneous erythropoietin or darbepoetin alfa to maintain appropriate hemoglobin levels is often helpful to try, either to prevent or reduce the need for transfusions in patients with renal insufficiency. Adults with renal failure usually require chronic transfusions and should be offered chelation therapy as necessary. Treatment of end-stage renal disease requires hemodialysis or kidney transplantation.

Skin ulcerations of the lower legs are the most common cutaneous complication of sickle cell disease, causing pain and physical disfigurement. The medial or lateral malleoli are more frequently involved, and ulcerations occur less commonly over the dorsum of the foot, near the Achilles tendon. The size of the ulcers varies from a few millimeters to large, circumferential ulcers that involve the entire ankle or foot. Lesions can extend into the dermis, the underlying subcutaneous tissue, and the underlying muscle fascia. These lesions are highly susceptible to infections and other complications. They are resistant to therapy and often exist for years (some patients report persistent ulcers for more than 10 years). Pain is the major problem and is often severe and unremitting, causing significant disability. In the United States, approximately 25% of patients with sickle cell disease have a history of leg ulcers.[44]

The etiology and pathogenesis of leg ulcers are not well understood. Clinical experience and epidemiology studies suggest a role for three factors: marginal blood supply to the skin of the lower extremities, local edema, and minor trauma.[44] The greatest risk factor for the development of leg ulcers is a history of previous ulcers.

Treatment of existing ulcers can be difficult and frustrating, since there is no effective cure and healing is often only temporary. Zinc is important in wound healing. It is found in RBCs and is lost during hemolysis; therefore zinc deficiency is common in patients with sickle cell disease.[45] The evidence that zinc supplementation benefits the healing of ankle ulcers is controversial; however, zinc supplementation is relatively benign and therefore a reasonable addition to therapy. Other controversial treatments include chronic transfusions and skin grafting for ulcers that are resistant to more conservative therapy, but failure rates for both methods are high.

Prevention includes educating patients about the importance of preventing local trauma by wearing shoes that fit properly, using insect repellents to prevent bites, and promptly treating any minor cuts on the feet and ankles. Patients with a history of ulcers and leg edema are encouraged to wear compression stockings and to perform routine care of the skin with emollients, good local hygiene, and daily inspection for any minor trauma.

The bony skeleton is a common target of the consequences of sickling. Bone marrow necrosis, bone infarcts, avascular necrosis (AVN), and osteomyelitis are common complications. The heads of the femur and humerus are common sites for marrow infarction and necrosis. Infarcts can also occur in the spine, ribs, and sternum. Bone infarcts constitute a painful crisis generally resolving in 1 to 2 weeks. Treatment does not differ from that of any other painful crisis and includes analgesia, hydration, and rest.

AVN commonly affects the hip and shoulder joints and is a more chronic condition than an acute bony infarct. Patients complain of severe chronic pain, limited range of motion, and pain with joint movement. Late stages are evident on plain radiographs, but MRI is much more sensitive in identifying AVN in the early stages. Initially, NSAIDs and narcotic analgesics are the mainstay of treatment. Later stages are usually surgically corrected with core decompression and/or joint replacement.

Retinopathy is a significant problem for patients with sickle cell disease. It is more common in patients with SC disease than in those with homozygous SS disease.[46] The retinopathy resembles that seen in diabetes and is believed to be caused by ischemia to the retina. Annual ophthalmoscopy with pupillary dilation is recommended. Treatment is with laser photocoagulation.

Indications for Referral or Hospitalization

Patients with sickle cell disease can be cared for in a primary care setting. However, the chronic nature of the disease, the frequent need for acute treatment of painful crises, and the high risk for complications generally require care by specialists familiar with the disease. Many of the large urban hospitals in the United States have sickle cell centers where patients receive comprehensive care by multidisciplinary teams of physicians, nurse practitioners, physician assistants, nurses, psychologists, and social workers. These hospital-based centers allow for prompt referral to other specialists such as neurologists, cardiologists, high-risk obstetricians, and ophthalmologists.

Most of the aforementioned complications require hospitalization for treatment. Patients with moderate to severe disease also have many admissions for intractable vaso-occlusive crises. These hospitalizations can last from a couple of days to several weeks.

Consultation with a social worker is recommended for issues related to school, employment, housing, transportation, and medical billing issues.

Patient and Family Education

Patient education begins early in childhood and continues throughout life. Initially, parents are taught how to manage pain crises, to recognize signs of infection, and to administer daily medications.[47] Coping with acute and chronic pain is a lifelong issue and involves learning both pharmacologic and nonpharmacologic interventions. Educating patients on the proper use of oral analgesics and management of painful crises is important and should occur at every opportunity. Patients need to be taught to seek prompt medical attention for any complication and not wait until they can speak to their health care provider.

The importance of preventive care must also be stressed. Routine care should include annual ophthalmologic, gynecologic, and dental examinations; periodic sickle cell clinic visits; and immunizations, including hepatitis A and B, annual influenza vaccine, pneumococcal vaccine, meningococcal vaccine, and *Haemophilus influenzae* vaccine. Patients must also be educated about the importance of maintaining folic acid replacement therapy, even if their disease is mild.

The single most common cause of death in children with SS is *Streptococcus pneumoniae* sepsis. This susceptibility is due to splenic malfunction and failure to make immunoglobulin G (IgG) antibodies to antigens. Prevention is vaccination and prophylactic penicillin. At age 24 months children are given 23-valent pneumococcal polysaccharide vaccine (PPV23). Although most children with sickle cell disease do not respond as well to the vaccine as non-SS children, a rise in IgG antibodies is noted. Prophylactic penicillin begins as a newborn with oral penicillin V 125 mg b.i.d. Dosage is unchanged until age 3, at which time it is increased to 250 mg b.i.d.; it continues until age 5 and then is stopped.[48]

Health Promotion

Adequate hydration, regular exercise, and sufficient sleep play a role in helping patients manage their disease. Teaching children and young adults coping skills can be beneficial and can help them manage both the acute and chronic pain associated with their disease. Annual health screenings, ophthalmologic examinations, and vaccines are recommended but easily overlooked.

ANEMIA OF CHRONIC DISEASE

Definition and Epidemiology

ACD is an anemia of underproduction, usually normocytic, normochromic, with a hemoglobin level above 10 g/L. However, it can be severe, with the MCV reduced in approximately 30% of patients. ACD is one of the most common causes of anemia; over a 2-month period of observation, 52% of hospitalized patients with anemia who were not iron deficient, undergoing hemolysis, or suffering from a hematologic malignancy met the laboratory criteria for ACD.[3] Although anemia is extremely common in cancer patients undergoing chemotherapy, up to 30% of patients with a variety of nonhematologic cancers have anemia before treatment. The presence of anemia may correlate with survival. ACD has also been diagnosed in up to 27% of outpatients with rheumatoid arthritis. Although most hospitalized patients with ACD have active infection, inflammatory conditions, or malignancy, others may have alcoholic liver disease, congestive heart failure, thrombosis, chronic pulmonary disease, diabetes, trauma, or a variety of medical problems. ACD is often confused with IDA when the anemia is microcytic; however, both serum iron and TIBC are low in ACD.

ACD is the most common type of anemia among hospitalized patients.[49] It can mimic or co-exist with other common anemias and cancers.

Pathophysiology

ACD is marked by low serum iron levels, but total iron stores are normal or elevated. Hepcidin is a liver-derived peptide that is a regulator of iron transport. Hepcidin is increased in inflammatory conditions and can lead to many of the iron abnormalities seen in ACD. Hepcidin may play an important role in the pathophysiology of ACD. Additionally there is a relative deficiency of erythropoietin.[3] Although serum erythropoietin levels may be increased, they are not elevated for the degree of anemia. The exact pathogenesis of ACD is unclear but may include several factors, one of which may be a blunted erythropoietin response to anemia. The anemia can be associated with chronic renal failure and therefore erythropoietin deficiency. Erythropoietin is a renal hormone whose normal plasma levels increase logarithmically in response to hemoglobin levels below 12 g/dl.[12] Other possible mechanisms for ACD that have been suggested include a decreased RBC survival time, decreased utilization of reticuloendothelial iron for hemoglobin synthesis, and inflammatory cytokine inhibition of erythropoietin production.[49,50]

Clinical Presentation

ACD is often mild and asymptomatic. Patients generally develop symptoms that are associated with the underlying disease(s) rather than the anemia itself. Progression of anemia results in the usual symptoms of advanced anemia such as fatigue and poor activity tolerance.

Physical Examination

There are usually no changes in the physical examination associated with ACD. Any changes in the physical examination are a result of the patient's underlying disease.

Diagnostics

The CBC will usually reveal a normocytic anemia, but the anemia can occasionally be microcytic. Hemoglobin levels are generally 10 to 11 g/dl. There are no distinctive changes in RBC size or shape, but if microcytosis does occur, the RDW is slightly elevated. Iron studies reveal a low serum iron level, a normal or increased ferritin level, and a normal or elevated TIBC. Bone marrow examination, if done, reveals normal to increased bone marrow iron stores with decreased amounts of bone marrow sideroblasts. The retic count is normal.

Basically, no precise diagnostic criteria exist for ACD. ACD often co-exists with IDA, but laboratory tests can be difficult to distinguish, since frequent overlaps occur. The only true way to distinguish ACD from IDA is by assessment of iron stores (which are absent in IDA and normal or increased in ACD) either by bone marrow aspiration and biopsy or by evaluation of the serum ferritin levels. Although bone marrow aspiration and biopsy are generally completed by hematologist to exclude myelodysplastic syndromes and other diseases, they usually add nothing to an already negative serologic evaluation and physical examination that the less invasive procedure generates.

Differential Diagnosis

If the clinical picture is one of a mild microcytic anemia, the differential diagnosis is between ACD and IDA. Iron studies are the most useful test to differentiate the two (see Differential Diagnosis under Iron Deficiency Anemia, pp. 1185-1186). ACD is a diagnosis of exclusion.

Management

After IDA has been excluded, a mild anemia need not be treated unless symptomatic. The standard treatment for anemia of chronic disease or renal insufficiency is recombinant human erythropoietin (rHuEPO) or darbepoetin alfa (novel erythropoiesis-stimulating protein [NESP]).[51] Intermittent transfusions may be required with more severe anemias. As always, the underlying condition should be treated or optimally controlled. Treatment of the underlying disease(s) will correct the anemia.

Complications

As long as the anemia is mild, the patient should have no complications associated with the anemia itself. Complications of the underlying disease should be managed appropriately.

Indications for Referral or Hospitalization

Once acute reasons for the anemia have been excluded and the diagnosis of ACD confirmed, patients should be monitored by the clinician who is managing the underlying medical condition. The anemia should be monitored with periodic CBCs and iron studies. Referral to a hematologist may be necessary to initiate therapy with rHuEPO or NESP or if the anemia worsens and requires other interventions.

Given that ACD is associated with chronic medical conditions, it is possible that the patient may have an acute reason for anemia, such as a drug or transfusion reaction. If the cause of the anemia is uncertain, referral to, or consultation with, a hematologist is appropriate.

Rarely, ACD requires hospitalization for management. Patients are sometimes hospitalized when the diagnosis is made.

Patient and Family Education

Regular visits with the health care provider should include laboratory studies to monitor for anemia. Patients should be encouraged to contact their provider if they experience any increase in symptoms such as fatigue, decreased exercise tolerance, or shortness of breath.

APLASTIC ANEMIA

Definition and Epidemiology

Aplastic anemia is a life-threatening condition resulting from bone marrow stem cell failure. It is characterized by a marked decrease in all hematopoietic precursors, resulting in pancytopenia. Aplastic anemia can affect all ages and both genders. It is a rare disorder with an estimated incidence of approximately 2 to 6 cases per million people per year.[52]

Pathophysiology

Aplastic anemia is usually related to exposure to specific toxins or medications that can cause bone marrow damage. Box 226-8 includes a few of the more than 500 medications that are associated with aplastic anemia. Aplastic anemia may also be immunologic, resulting from infections or severe disease such as liver failure; however, almost half of all cases of aplastic anemia have an unclear etiology.

Clinical Presentation

Patients may be seen with abnormal bleeding, infection, and anemia (from the pancytopenia). Onset is usually sudden without any other apparent illness. The history may reveal information about a recent viral infection, chronic disease, or exposure to an offending medication or toxin.

BOX 226-8

AGENTS ASSOCIATED WITH APLASTIC ANEMIA

TOXINS

- Radiation
- Alkylating agents
- Insecticides
- Benzene and its derivatives
- Chemotherapeutic agents

MEDICATIONS

- Antibiotics (penicillin, chloramphenicol, cephalosporins, sulfonamides)
- Antidepressants (lithium, tricyclics)
- Antiinflammatory drugs (gold salts, nonsteroidals, salicylates)
- Antimalarials
- Anticonvulsants

OTHER POSSIBLE CAUSES

- Viral: non-A, non-B hepatitis, HIV, Epstein-Barr virus
- Graft-vs.-host disease
- Malignancy
- Pregnancy

Physical Examination

The physical examination may reveal petechiae, ecchymoses, purpura, pallor of the skin and mucous membranes, and mild lymphadenopathy in the late stages. Early stages of aplastic anemia may show no significant changes on physical examination.

Diagnostics

A CBC will show pancytopenia with normocytic and normochromic RBC indexes and morphology. The retic count is also below normal, reflecting the lack of bone marrow activity. A bone marrow biopsy is essential for diagnosis and reveals a severe hypoplasia (<25% cellularity with <30% hematopoietic cells).[17]

Differential Diagnosis

Aplastic anemia is readily detected and easily distinguished from other forms of normocytic, normochromic anemias. Involvement of other cell types (myeloid, platelets) confirms the diagnosis.

Management

Any patient with symptoms suggestive of aplastic anemia should be referred to a hematologist for management. Definitive treatment is either BMT or immunosuppressive therapy.[52,53] Use of blood products to correct the anemia should be minimized to prevent alloimmunization and to reduce the risk of graft failure after BMT. The decision to transfuse a patient with aplastic anemia should be made in consultation with the hematologist who will be treating the patient.

Life Span Considerations

The treatment of choice for aplastic anemia is based on the severity of the anemia and the age of the patient. BMT is more successful in younger patients and is the treatment of choice for children and adolescents. Patients who are more than 40 years of age have a higher risk of transplant-related morbidity and mortality. Immunosuppression therapy is the treatment of choice for adults over 40 years of age.[53]

Complications

Complications of untreated aplastic anemia include sepsis and death resulting from pancytopenia. Complications of BMT include graft failure, graft-vs.-host disease, and a risk of secondary malignancies. Complications of immunosuppressive therapy include relapse and death resulting from pancytopenia or evolution of aplastic anemia to myelodysplasia or leukemia.[53]

Indications for Referral or Hospitalization

All patients who are suspected of having aplastic anemia should be immediately referred to a hematologist for treatment. Patients with severe aplastic anemia require hospitalization for management of the pancytopenia and to begin treatment. Most patients who undergo BMT or immunosuppressive therapy should continue to be monitored by a hematologist or oncologist as necessary.

Patient and Family Education and Health Promotion

Aplastic anemia can be caused by exposure to toxins such as benzene and insecticides. Patients should be taught that proper handling of products such as paints and insecticides includes adequately ventilating the work area and wearing protective clothing such as masks and gloves.

HEMOLYTIC ANEMIA

Definition and Epidemiology

All the hemolytic anemias are associated with an increased rate of RBC destruction. The clinical presentation varies according to the disease. Some patients are seen with chronic hemolytic states that are well compensated, and others have acute, self-limiting hemolytic episodes. The most common chronic hemolytic anemia is sickle cell disease (discussed previously). Most of the other hemolytic anemias (Box 226-9) are rare and are mentioned only briefly here.

BOX 226-9

EXAMPLES OF HEMOLYTIC ANEMIAS

Hemoglobinopathies
Glucose-6-phosphate dehydrogenase deficiency
Membrane structural defects
- Hereditary spherocytosis
- Hereditary elliptocytosis

Autoimmune hemolysis
- Warm-reacting autoimmune hemolytic anemia
- Cold-reacting autoimmune hemolytic anemia

Glucose-6-phosphate dehydrogenase (G6PD) deficiency is an inherited erythrocyte enzyme deficiency that can result in an acute hemolytic anemia. G6PD-induced hemolysis is usually precipitated either by infection or by ingestion of an oxidant drug.

The most common form of G6PD deficiency in the United States is a mild variant of the disorder that typically affects approximately 10% of African-American males.[1] In all, 20% of African-American females carry the X-linked recessive gene for G6PD deficiency. G6PD deficiency is prevalent throughout tropical and subtropical regions of the world because it provides protection against malaria infection.[54] G6PD deficiency can also be inherited along with other hematologic disorders such as sickle cell disease.

A mild chronic hemolytic anemia can also be caused by abnormalities in erythrocyte membrane protein composition. Hereditary spherocytosis and hereditary elliptocytosis are the best examples of this abnormality.[55] The prevalence of hereditary spherocytosis is approximately 1 in 5000 (mostly northern Europeans).[53] Hereditary elliptocytosis is also relatively common, with a prevalence of 1 in 2500 to 1 in 5000, and is observed in all racial and ethnic groups. One form of hereditary elliptocytosis is commonly seen in African Americans. Another form is common in Southeast Asia, especially Papua, New Guinea.[56]

Conditions such as viral or bacterial infections, collagen vascular diseases, or lymphoproliferative disorders are associated with autoimmune hemolytic anemias.

The frequency of an autoimmune hemolytic anemia depends on the prevalence of the associated disease state in the population. Warm-reacting autoantibodies are seen in 80% to 90% of all cases of autoimmune hemolytic anemia. Idiopathic autoimmune hemolytic anemia is most commonly seen in patients older than age 50 years.[57,58]

Pathophysiology

Drugs associated with acute hemolysis in G6PD-deficient patients include aspirin and phenacetin, sulfonamides, nitrofurantoin, and primaquine. Ingestion of an offending drug can result in the denaturation of hemoglobin,[12] leading to an acute hemolytic event. Other precipitants of hemolysis include the ingestion of fava beans or mothballs or a severe bacterial or viral infection.

The functional abnormality in hereditary spherocytosis and hereditary elliptocytosis results from defects in the structural proteins of the erythrocyte cytoskeleton, specifically, a deficiency of the protein spectrin.[55]

In the autoimmune hemolytic anemias, the patient produces autoantibodies that react with the RBCs, causing premature erythrocyte destruction. Two types of autoantibodies are produced: warm-reacting autoantibodies and cold-reacting autoantibodies. Warm-reacting antibodies are reactive with cells at 37° C (98.6° F), and cold-reacting antibodies are reactive at temperatures below 37° C.[59]

Clinical Presentation

Most hemolytic anemias are mild, well compensated, and associated with few signs or symptoms. If the anemia is severe, the patient displays the usual symptoms of severe anemia such as fatigue and exercise intolerance. Patients with G6PD deficiency may have minimum or no clinical signs. Often the first clue that a patient has the deficiency is the onset of an acute hemolytic anemia after ingestion of an oxidant drug. The hemolytic event is self-limiting and usually mild. Patients with the Mediterranean form of G6PD deficiency are at risk for more severe hemolysis.[59]

Both hereditary spherocytosis and hereditary elliptocytosis are usually characterized by a mild hemolytic anemia that is well compensated. Patients with hereditary spherocytosis, however, can have a severe hemolytic anemia, whereas patients with hereditary elliptocytosis rarely have a clinically significant hemolytic anemia. Splenomegaly, aplastic crises, pigment gallstones, and chronic leg ulcers can complicate severe hereditary spherocytosis.[55]

Most commonly, the anemia caused by autoimmune hemolysis is also mild and self-limiting. Patients with a warm-reacting autoimmune hemolytic anemia can have splenomegaly and other symptoms of anemia if the hemolysis is moderate or severe. Patients also show signs and symptoms of the underlying disease. Box 226-10 gives examples of conditions associated with warm and cold antibody autoimmune hemolysis.

Physical Examination

Patients with hemolytic anemias have an essentially normal physical examination. The only remarkable evidence of hemolysis may be scleral icterus, especially in patients with chronic hemolytic anemias such as sickle cell disease.

Diagnostics

During a mild acute hemolytic event, serologic tests show a slight decrease in hemoglobin and the RBC count, an elevated LDH level, and slight hyperbilirubinemia. Patients with chronic hemolytic anemias, even when they are well compensated, have persistent reticulocytosis.

Assays for G6PD are useful and detect most deficient patients. In some milder variants of the disease, however, the screening test may be negative for several weeks after an acute hemolytic event.

A positive family history and the presence of pathognomonic findings on the peripheral blood smear easily diagnose both hereditary spherocytosis and hereditary elliptocytosis. Patients with hereditary spherocytosis have a large number of microspherocytes on the peripheral blood smear and an elevated MCHC on the CBC. The RBCs of patients with hereditary elliptocytosis have a uniform elliptic (oval) shape.

The diagnosis of an autoimmune hemolytic anemia depends on laboratory findings of abnormal autoantibodies. Coombs' test (both direct and indirect) is used to screen for these antibodies. The direct Coombs' test is positive in most cases of autoimmune hemolytic anemia or transfusion reactions and in some cases of drug-induced hemolysis. The indirect Coombs' test is positive in cases of antibody formation from previous transfusions or pregnancy and in drug-induced hemolytic anemia.

BOX 226-10

CONDITIONS ASSOCIATED WITH AUTOIMMUNE HEMOLYSIS

CONDITIONS ASSOCIATED WITH WARM AUTOANTIBODIES

Infections

Collagen vascular diseases
- Systemic lupus erythematosus
- Rheumatoid arthritis

Lymphoproliferative disorders
- Leukemia
- Lymphoma

Drugs
- Quinidine or quinine
- Penicillin
- α-Methyldopa

Chronic renal disease

Idiopathic

CONDITIONS ASSOCIATED WITH COLD AUTOANTIBODIES

Malignancy

Mycoplasma pneumoniae

Viral pneumonia

Idiopathic

Differential Diagnosis

It is important to match the clinical presentation with the possible diagnosis of a hemolytic anemia. Differential diagnoses that should be considered include whether the anemia is acute or chronic and whether the hemolysis is intravascular (as in disseminated intravascular coagulation) or extravascular (as in the hemolytic anemias previously discussed). The presence of any underlying disease will also direct the approach to the diagnosis, since many of the autoimmune disorders have predictable and expected patterns of hemolytic anemia.

Management

Management of a patient with a hemolytic anemia varies according to the individual disease state. Therefore proper management begins with an accurate diagnosis. Patients who are able to compensate for their degree of anemia generally require little intervention. If the hemoglobin level begins to fall well below the patient's baseline, an occasional transfusion of packed RBCs may be necessary. All patients, especially if they have a chronic hemolytic anemia, require folic acid supplementation (1 mg/day) to maintain adequate erythropoiesis.

The acute, self-limiting hemolysis in patients with mild G6PD deficiency rarely requires treatment. The resulting anemia is mild and resolves without intervention. Any patient who sees a health care provider because of an acute hemolytic event resulting from exposure to an oxidant drug should have serial CBCs measured to determine resolution of the ane-

DIFFERENTIAL DIAGNOSIS

Hemolytic Anemia

- Sickle cell disease
- Glucose-6-phosphate dehydrogenase deficiency
- Hereditary disorders (hereditary spherocytosis, hereditary elliptocytosis)
- Autoimmune hemolytic anemia

mia. The most important aspect of management of G6PD deficiency is ensuring the patient's awareness of the condition. All high-risk individuals should be screened, and information about what drugs and foods to avoid should be provided to all patients with the deficiency.

Patients with mild forms of hereditary spherocytosis or hereditary elliptocytosis maintain adequate hemoglobin levels and are in generally good health. Patients with severe hereditary spherocytosis may require a splenectomy to decrease the severity of the anemia.[60] These patients are also candidates for prophylactic cholecystectomy because of the high incidence of pigment gallstones (elective cholecystectomy should definitely be done if gallstones occur).

Patients with autoimmune hemolytic anemia are generally treated with some combination of corticosteroid therapy or immunosuppressive therapy, splenectomy, and transfusion with packed RBCs. The specific therapy varies according to the type and severity of the hemolytic anemia.

Life Span Considerations

Patients with G6PD deficiency, hemoglobinopathy, or a hereditary RBC membrane defect should be aware of the hereditary potential. Professional genetic counseling and screening should be offered to all patients who are considering pregnancy.

Complications

Most of the hemolytic anemias discussed here rarely cause complications, especially if the hemolysis is mild and self-limiting or chronic but well compensated. Patients with more severe forms of hemolytic anemia, especially autoimmune hemolytic anemia, are at risk for acute episodes of severe hemolysis, with the associated morbidity and mortality of a severe anemia.

Indications for Referral or Hospitalization

A referral to a hematologist is prudent when an acute hemolysis does not appear to be resolving or when the anemia is severe or does not respond to treatment. Acute hemolysis that occurs as a result of a mild form of hemolytic anemia does not require hospitalization for management. If the patient also has some other underlying condition or the anemia is severe, however, hospitalization may be required for management. As with any other type of anemia, the need for hospitalization depends on the patient's ability to compensate for the degree of anemia.

Patient and Family Education

Patients should understand the nature of their disorder well enough to be able to explain it to other health care providers. Patients with G6PD deficiency should be given a list of drugs and foods to avoid, including over-the-counter products that contain aspirin or phenacetin. Patients with drug-induced hemolysis should be made aware of the types of drugs to avoid. Those with autoimmune hemolytic anemias should be made aware of the types of situations and conditions that can aggravate their anemia. All patients should be instructed to contact their health care provider if there are any signs of increased anemia.

REFERENCES

1. Greer JP, Foerster J, Lukens JN, and others: *Wintrobe's clinical hematology*, ed 11, Philadelphia, 2004, Lippincott Williams & Wilkins.
2. Hillman RS, Finch CA: *Red cell manual*, ed 7, Philadelphia, 1996, Davis.
3. Hoffman R, Benz EJ Jr, Shattil SJ, and others: *Hematology basic principles and practice*, ed 4, Philadelphia, 2005, Elsevier.
4. Walters GO, Miller FM, Worwood M: Serum ferritin concentration and iron stores in normal subjects, *J Clin Pathol* 26(10):770-772, 1973.
5. Ponka P, Beaumont C, Richardson DR: Function and regulation of transferrin and ferritin, *Semin Hematol* 35(1):35-54, 1998.
6. Conrad ME, Umbreit JN, Moore EG: Iron absorption and transport, *Am J Med Sci* 318(4):213-229, 1999.
7. Ponka P: Cell biology of heme, *Am J Med Sci* 318(4):241-256, 1999.
8. Mazza JJ: *Manual of clinical hematology*, ed 3, Philadelphia, 2002, Lippincott Williams & Wilkins.
9. Abramson SD: Common uncommon anemias, *Am Fam Phys* 54(4):851-858, 1999.
10. Massey AC: Microcytic anemia: differential diagnosis and management of iron deficiency anemia, *Med Clin North Am* 76(3):549-566, 1992.
11. Schwartz WJ 3rd, Thurnau GR: Iron deficiency anemia in pregnancy, *Clin Obstet Gynecol* 38(3):443-454, 1995.
12. Hillman RS, Ault KA: *Hematology in clinical practice: a guide to diagnosis and management*, New York, 1995, McGraw-Hill.
13. Wada L, King JC: Trace element nutrition during pregnancy, *Clin Obstet Gynecol* 37(3):574-586, 1994.
14. Guyatt GH, Patterson C, Ali M, and others: Diagnosis of iron-deficiency anemia in the elderly, *Am J Med* 88(3):205-209, 1990.
15. Hallberg L, Brune M, Rossander L: Iron absorption in man: ascorbic acid and dose-dependent inhibition of phytate, *Am J Clin Nutr* 49(1):140-144, 1989.
16. Lops VR, Hunter LP, Dixon LR: Anemia in pregnancy, *Am Fam Physician* 51(5):1189-1197, 1995.
17. Farhi DC, Chai CC, Edelman AS, and others: *Pathology of bone marrow and blood cells*, Philadelphia, 2004, Lippincott Williams & Wilkins.
18. Pearson HA: Thalassemia intermedia: a Region I conference: proceedings from a conference on thalassemia intermedia, *Genet Res* 11(2):5-10, 1997.
19. Katsanis E, Luke KH, Hsu E, and others: Hemoglobin E: a common hemoglobinopathy among children of Southeast Asian origin, *Can Med Assoc J* 137(1):39-42, 1987.
20. Rund D, Rachmilewitz E: New trends in the treatment of beta-thalassemia, *Crit Rev Oncol Hematol* 33(2):105-118, 2000.
21. Telfer P, Prestcott E, Holden S, and others: Hepatic iron concentration combined with long-term monitoring of serum ferritin to predict complications of iron overload in thalassemia major, *Br J Haematol* 110(4-II):971-977, 2000.
22. Tefferi A: Iron chelation therapy for myelodysplastic syndrome if and when, *Mayo Clin Proc* 81(2):197-198, 2006.
23. Cao A, Gabutti V, Masera G, and others: *1992 Management protocol for the treatment of thalassemia patients*, Flushing, New York, 1992, Cooley's Anemia Foundation.
24. Campbell BA: Megaloblastic anemia in pregnancy, *Clin Obstet Gynecol* 38(3):455-462, 1995.
25. Goldman L, Ausielo D: *Cecil textbook of medicine*, ed 22, Philadelphia, 2004, Saunders.
26. Campbell NR: How safe are folic acid supplements? *Arch Intern Med* 156(15):1638-1644, 1996.
27. Savage DG, Ogundipe A, Allen RH, and others: Etiology and diagnostic evaluation of macrocytosis, *Am J Med Sci* 319(6):343-352, 2000.
28. MRC Vitamin Research Group: Prevention of neural tube defects: results of the Medical Research Council Vitamin Study, *Lancet* 338(8760):131-137, 1991.

29. Centers for Disease Control and Prevention: Recommendations for the use of folic acid to reduce the number of cases of spina bifida and other neural tube defects, *MMWR* 41(RR-14):1-7, 1992.
30. Stabler S: Screening the older population for cobalamin (vitamin B_{12} deficiency), *J Am Geriatr Soc* 43(11):1290-1297, 1995.
31. Koshy M, Dorn L: Continuing care for adult patients with sickle cell disease, *Hematol Oncol Clin North Am* 10(6):1265-1274, 1996.
32. Vichinsky EP, Lubin BH: Sickle cell anemia and related hemoglobinopathies, *Pediatr Clin North Am* 27(2):429-447, 1980.
33. Platt OS, Thorington BD, Brambilla DJ, and others: Pain in sickle cell disease: rates and risk factors, *N Engl J Med* 325(1):11-16, 1991.
34. Ballas SK, Mohandas N: Pathophysiology of vaso-occlusion, *Hematol Oncol Clin North Am* 10(6):1221-1240, 1996.
35. Charache S, Terrin LM, Moore RD, and others: Effect of hydroxyurea on the frequency of painful crisis in sickle cell anemia: investigations of the Multicenter Study of Hydroxyurea in Sickle Cell Anemia, *N Engl J Med* 332(20):1317-1322, 1995.
36. Kaul DK, Fabry ME, Windisch P, and others: Erythrocytes in sickle cell anemia are heterogeneous in their rheological and hemodynamic characteristics, *J Clin Invest* 72(1):22-31, 1983.
37. Vichinsky E, Styles L: Pulmonary complications, *Hematol Oncol Clin North Am* 10(6):1275-1288, 1996.
38. Emre U, Miller ST, Gutierez M, and others: Effect of transfusion in acute chest syndrome of sickle cell disease, *J Pediatr* 127(6):901-904, 1995.
39. Ohene-Frempong K: Stroke in sickle cell disease: demographic, clinical, and therapeutic considerations, *Semin Hematol* 28(3):213-219, 1991.
40. Pegelow CH, Adams RJ, McKie V, and others: Risk of recurrent stroke in patients with sickle cell disease treated with erythrocyte transfusion, *J Pediatr* 126(6):896-899, 1995.
41. Adams RJ: Lessons from the Stroke Prevention Trial in Sickle Cell Anemia (STOP) study, *J Child Neurol* 15(5):344-349, 2000.
42. Miller ST, Wright E, Abboud M, and others: Impact of chronic transfusion on incidence of pain and acute chest syndrome during the Stroke Prevention Trial (STOP) in sickle-cell anemia, *J Pediatr* 139(6):785-789, 2001.
43. Wong WY, Elliott-Mills D, Powars D: Renal failure in sickle cell anemia, *Hematol Oncol Clin North Am* 10(6):1321-1331, 1996.
44. Eckman JR: Leg ulcers in sickle cell disease, *Hematol Oncol Clin North Am* 10(6):1333-1344, 1996.
45. Frost P, Chen JC, Rabbani I, and others: Zinc deficiency in man: studies in sickle cell disease, *Prog Clin Biol Res* 14:211-239, 1977.
46. Clarkson JG: The ocular manifestations of sickle-cell disease: a prevalence and natural history study, *Trans Am Ophthalmol Soc* 90:481-504, 1992.
47. Gil KM, Anthony KK, Carson JW, and others: Daily coping practice predicts treatment effects in children with sickle cell disease, *J Pediatr Psychol* 26(3):163-173, 2001.
48. Gaston MH, Verter JI, Woods G, and others: Prophylaxis with oral penicillin in children with sickle cell anemia: a randomization trial, *N Engl J Med* 314(24):1593-1599, 1986.
49. Sears DA: Anemia of chronic disease, *Med Clin North Am* 76(3):567-579, 1992.
50. Spivak JL: The blood in systemic disorders, *Lancet* 355(9216):1707-1712, 2000.
51. Nissenson AR: Novel erythropoiesis stimulating protein for managing the anemia of chronic kidney disease, *Am J Kid Dis* 38(6):1390-1397, 2001.
52. Fonseca R, Tefferi A: Practical aspects in the diagnosis and management of aplastic anemia, *Am J Med Sci* 313(3):159-169, 1997.
53. Young NS, Barrett AJ: The treatment of severe acquired aplastic anemia, *Blood* 85(12):3367-3377, 1995.
54. Mehta A, Mason PJ, Vulliamy TJ, and others: Glucose-6-phosphate dehydrogenase deficiency, *Baillieres Best Pract Res Clin Haematol* 13(1):21-38, 2000.
55. Smedley JC, Bellingham AJ: Current problems in hematology, part II, Hereditary spherocytosis, *J Clin Pathol* 44(6):441-444, 1991.
56. Davies KA, Lux SE: Hereditary disorders of the red cell membrane skeleton, *Trends Genet* 5:221-227, 1989.
57. Sokol RJ, Booker DJ, Stamps R: The pathology of autoimmune hemolytic anaemia, *J Clin Pathol* 45(12):1047-1052, 1992.
58. Rosenwasser LJ, and others: Immunohematologic diseases, *JAMA* 268(20):2940-2945, 1992.
59. Luzzatto L: Inherited haemolytic states: glucose-6-phosphate dehydrogenase deficiency, *Clin Haematol* 4(1):83-108, 1975.
60. Bolton-Maggs PH: The diagnosis and management of hereditary spherocytosis, *Baillieres Best Pract Clin Haematol* 13(3):327-342, 2000.

CHAPTER 227

Blood Coagulation Disorders

Maura Malone, Laurel McKernan, and Leo Zacharski

DEFINITION AND EPIDEMIOLOGY

Coagulation is the process by which blood changes from a fluid phase needed for tissue perfusion to a cohesive gel that prevents blood loss. This transition is achieved through a complex process involving many different initiatory and inhibitory proteins, as well as certain cells, particularly platelets. The benefits of this mechanism are obvious and are taken for granted except in individuals who have an excess or deficiency in a coagulant or anticoagulant protein, since they may bleed excessively or form pathologic clots (thrombophilia). The normal coagulation mechanism may fail for a wide variety of reasons. A quantitative deficiency or a qualitative abnormality in counterbalancing coagulant or anticoagulant participants may tip the balance toward either bleeding (coagulopathy) or thrombosis. Similarly, a defect at one point in the system can often be compensated for by therapy that targets a different point in the system. Disorders of coagulation factors may be inherited or acquired (e.g., from illness or medications). Three common bleeding disorders are von Willebrand's disease (vWD), hemophilia A, and hemophilia B. The gene for vWD is present in approximately 1% of the general population, and both males and females may be affected. Together, hemophilia A and hemophilia B occur in about 2 per 50,000 males.[1]

Determining the diagnosis required for appropriate management can be challenging, particularly with mild bleeding disorders. Patients are often referred for medical evaluation because of one of the following: a bleeding or thrombotic episode, a positive family history, or an abnormal laboratory test result found, for example, during preoperative screening. The health care provider needs to determine, through clinical and laboratory assessment, whether these referral indicators reflect the presence of a coagulation disorder. Clinical and laboratory assessment go hand in hand, but it is all too common for patients with a clinical disorder to have no abnormality on routine laboratory testing. There are many different coagulation disorders, and this chapter covers the most common, particularly congenital disorders, and discusses practical guidelines for evaluating thrombosing and bleeding disorders.

Extensive studies have shown that an elaborate balance exists between substances in the blood that promote clotting (called coagulation factors) and other substances that preserve blood in fluid form (called anticoagulant factors). This balance is maintained until a blood vessel is injured. The blood coagulation mechanism is designed to interpret such injuries and respond by developing a protective clot at the injury site that stops the flow of blood. Prevention of blood loss from the vasculature with injury is vital, and this process is referred to as *hemostasis*. The clotting mechanism is called a *self-referencing system* because of its ability to turn itself on and off locally to achieve a beneficial effect. It is correctly viewed as an irreducibly complex system because a defect in any one of its many components can lead to malfunction of the entire system.

The normal hemostatic response may be considered to proceed in three phases. In phase 1, blood vessels constrict, reducing blood flow from the site. In phase 2, platelets are activated by tissues, and chemicals are released almost instantaneously, resulting in the formation of a platelet plug. Phase 3 begins within seconds after platelet activation. In this phase a complex cascade, involving more than a dozen protein-clotting factors, is triggered.[2] The end result of this cascade is the production of a powerful enzyme (thrombin) that converts fibrinogen, which is present in solution in the blood, to fibrin. Fibrin is a durable, visible mesh that seals the injured vessel (the scab). Traditionally, this cascade is thought to consist of intrinsic (entirely plasma derived) and extrinsic (tissue factor initiated) pathways.[2] Abnormalities of protein-clotting factors within their pathways can often be detected by common laboratory tests such as the activated partial thromboplastin time (aPTT) and prothrombin time (PT). These tests are contrived in the laboratory to serve different purposes. For example, the PT is preferred for monitoring the therapeutic effect of the common anticoagulant, warfarin. Tissue factor is the substance present on cells and tissues that triggers clot formation both in response to injury and inappropriately in thrombosing disorders. The precise mechanism by which tissue factor initiates clot formation is currently under intense investigation. Such studies hold promise for improving prevention and treatment of bleeding and thrombosing disorders.

Physician consultation should be considered for patients with an elevated or erratic International Normalized Ratio (INR).

Physician consultation is recommended for patients with a falling or unexplained low platelet count.

COAGULOPATHIES

PATHOPHYSIOLOGY AND CLINICAL PRESENTATION

The manifestations of coagulopathies are determined by the type and severity of the defect. Is it a vascular disorder, platelet abnormality, or clotting factor deficiency? Is it acquired or congenital? These questions are answered through clinical and laboratory assessment.

Patients with congenital bleeding disorders usually have a lifelong history of symptoms such as easy bruising and prolonged bleeding with cuts, surgery, or other trauma. Severe deficiencies generally become evident when the affected individual becomes a toddler and is more likely to sustain minor trauma. Bleeding may also occur spontaneously. Mild hereditary deficiencies may go undiagnosed for years or until significant trauma occurs or the individual undergoes surgery. In contrast, acquired disorders may become evident later in life in the absence of a history of bleeding manifestations. Clinical presentation may include a recent onset of increased bruising, bleeding with trauma, or nosebleeds or a recent change in clotting test findings. These changes may be due to effects of medications or other disorders such as liver or renal disease. The type of bleeding reported may indicate which pathway is involved. Excessive bruising, mucosal bleeding, and postsurgical hemorrhage are typical of platelet disorders, whereas a history of frank bleeding after surgery and hemorrhage into the joints and muscles are typical of a marked factor deficiency such as hemophilia A or B. However, there are no rigid distinctions between the types of defects and their clinical manifestations. Clinical symptoms are discussed further in the section on diagnosis.

PHYSICAL EXAMINATION

Bleeding disorders are generally diagnosed by the history and laboratory findings. The physical examination may be negative, especially with mild defects. However, a variety of findings, including bruises, petechiae, gingival bleeding, epistaxis, and hematomas, may be evident, especially in individuals with more severe defects. Some degree of bruising is common in the general population, especially in those with fair complexion, in whom bruises are seen more easily. However, numerous bruises that occur on the trunk in addition to the extremities are more significant.

DIAGNOSTICS AND DIFFERENTIAL DIAGNOSIS

The most valuable diagnostic test for a bleeding disorder is a careful, comprehensive bleeding history. The history should provide clues to the type of bleeding disorder that may be present and to laboratory tests that are indicated for further evaluation. The hemostatic response to trauma determined in the bleeding history is generally a more sensitive test of hemostatic competence than are screening laboratory tests (e.g., when evaluating a patient before surgery).[3] There is no substitute for clinical experience in deciding whether a patient has a coagulation disorder.

The bleeding history has two major elements: the patient's history and the family history. The patient should be asked to describe each event in life that presented a hemostatic challenge. Descriptions should include the duration and intensity of bleeding with minor cuts and scratches, surgery, dental extractions, and menstrual periods. Spontaneous bleeding may occur in the form of joint or soft tissue bleeding, epistaxis, and bruising. Bruising without obvious of trauma is more significant than bruising in response to trauma. It is particularly important to encourage the patient to quantitate the degree of bleeding. This may be done by estimating average bruise counts and location, duration of posttraumatic bleeding, duration and number of pads soaked during menstruation, and so on. Menstrual blood is normally unclotted, and the passage of clots (e.g., with urination, defecation, or pad changes) may be significant. With practice, interviewers will refine their assessment skills and assist their patients in proper interpretations because what is "normal" bleeding to one person may be "heavy" to another. Box 227-1 gives examples of interview questions for use when evaluating a patient for a bleeding disorder.

BOX 227-1

INTERVIEW QUESTIONS FOR EVALUATING A PATIENT WITH A BLEEDING DISORDER

PATIENT HISTORY

- Does the patient have ecchymoses, easy and frequent bruising? How many bruises are present at a given time—one or two, a half dozen or dozen, more? Are they raised or flat? Are they on the chest and trunk or only on the limbs? Are there hematomas with injections?
- Is epistaxis spontaneous, or does it occur with trauma? Is the bleeding one sided or bilateral? Is it seasonal, or does it occur year-round? How many episodes occur in a month? How long do they last, and what measures do you use to stop them? Do large clots form?
- Are there any hemostatic challenges such as injuries or lacerations? How long did the bleeding last—a brief moment or more prolonged duration (minutes, longer)? Did the laceration require sutures? Did the bleeding continue afterward? For how long? Have there been any fractures?
- Have there been any dental extractions? Was there any excessive bleeding? For how long—an hour, half a day, a day, a week?
- Has there been any prior surgery? What kind? Was there any reported excessive bleeding? Were any transfusions required?
- Has there been any significant injury or other trauma that might challenge the coagulation mechanism?
- Is the bleeding immediate, platelet-type bleeding or delayed, with deep hematomas?
- Obtain a detailed menstruation history when appropriate. How long does menstruation last? How heavy is it? What is heavy? Generally, how many pads per day? Is there formation of large clots?
- Has there been any recent illness? Any current medications, including over-the-counter medications (e.g., aspirin)?
- Obtain an obstetric history when appropriate. Was there any bleeding during pregnancy or delivery? Was a transfusion required?

FAMILY HISTORY

- Inquire about immediate family members—brothers, sisters, parents, children. Request documentation when appropriate.
- Inquire about extended family on the maternal and paternal sides—grandparents, aunts and uncles, cousins.
- Review a similar line of questioning as for the patient history for clinical features, surgery, trauma, transfusions, and menstrual history.
- When questioning parents about their children, inquire about cephalhematomas, buccal mucosal bleeding, bleeding from the tongue or tooth extractions, bleeding with separation of the umbilical cord, bruising or hematomas with immunizations, and bruising with the onset of crawling and ambulation.

NOTE: A negative bleeding history in a young child may not rule out a bleeding disorder; rather a hemostatic challenge has not yet been encountered.

The family history is critical in assessing coagulation disorders. The genetic defect in hemophilia A and B (factor VIII and IX deficiency) is X-linked recessive and affects only males. However, the defect in families is carried by females, who are usually asymptomatic. Thus a male patient's maternal grandfather, uncles, and cousins may have bleeding that provides a clue to the diagnosis of hemophilia A or B.

Although the bleeding history is of paramount importance in the evaluation for coagulation disorders, it is not without limitations. The accuracy of information reported largely depends on the interviewer's ability to elicit a description of previous hemostatic challenges. It is easy to miss events or obtain an incomplete history. Mild bleeding disorders are difficult to identify, especially in the absence of a hemostatic challenge, as is often the case in young children. Spontaneous mutations commonly account for cases of hemophilia A and B, and consequently the family history may be negative.

In anticipation of the decision of whether to refer the patient for specialized tests in the face of clinical suspicion, the health care provider should perform certain screening studies. The typical laboratory screen, available in most clinical laboratories, includes the PT, aPTT, platelet count, bleeding time, thrombin time, and fibrinogen level.[3] These studies provide basic information on the integrity of coagulation factor pathways and platelet function.

The platelet count is usually done by automated counters. Low values can be confirmed by estimating the number of platelets present on the peripheral blood smear. Common causes of a low platelet count include immune destruction, drugs, vasculitis, disseminated intravascular coagulation, and chemotherapy.

The bleeding time is a useful screen for platelet disorders if performed by an experienced technologist. It is best done by the same individual using a standardized template method. Prolonged bleeding time generally is defined as more than 8 minutes. Causes of a prolonged bleeding time include thrombocytopenia (platelet count <100,000/mm^3), qualitative platelet defects, vWD, and poor (overly aggressive) technique.

The PT measures the function of the extrinsic system and the common pathway. It is sensitive to abnormalities of factors VII, X, V, II, and fibrinogen. The PTT measures the function of the intrinsic system and the common pathway. It detects abnormalities of prekallikrein; high-molecular-weight kininogen; factors XII, XI, X, IX, VIII, V, II; and fibrinogen.

A prolonged PT or aPTT may be evaluated further by performing mixing studies, which incorporate different ratios of normal (control) and abnormal (patient) plasma. "Correction" of the abnormality on addition of normal plasma suggests the presence of a factor deficiency, whereas failure to correct the abnormality suggests the presence of an inhibitor, such as the lupus anticoagulant. The inhibitor acts to neutralize the added normal plasma, which then fails to correct the abnormal coagulation test. Misinterpretation of the results of mixing studies is a common cause for a request for a coagulation consultation.

If the patient has a negative personal and family bleeding history in spite of challenges to hemostasis, such as surgery or significant trauma, he or she is not likely to have a bleeding disorder, and laboratory evaluation is usually not helpful. If the patient has a negative bleeding history without hemostatic challenges and a positive family history for bleeding, screening tests may be advisable. Diagnosis may be important in planning future care, such as with trauma or elective surgery. Patients may be able to avoid unnecessary blood transfusions if a bleeding disorder is diagnosed and prophylactic treatment provided.

If the patient has a negative bleeding history but abnormal blood tests, other factors need to be considered, such as effects of medications (e.g., aspirin), over-the-counter cold preparations with guaifenesin, allergies (rhinitis), or illness. Circulating anticoagulants are commonly found in patients with an unexplained prolonged aPTT. These may be diagnosed using mixing studies and rarely result in clinical bleeding.

DIAGNOSTICS

Coagulopathies

LABORATORY
PT/PTT
Platelet count
Bleeding time
Thrombin time
Fibrinogen levels
Peripheral smear

DIFFERENTIAL DIAGNOSIS

Coagulopathies

- Hemophilia
- Von Willebrand's disease
- Idiopathic thrombocytopenic purpura
- Vitamin K deficiency
- Liver disease
- Disseminated intravascular coagulation
- Drug-induced condition
- Connective tissue disorder
- Hypersplenism
- Uremia
- Factor XI deficiency
- Hypermobility syndrome

If the patient has a positive bleeding history, it is essential to exclude an anatomic explanation for the bleeding. Unfortunately, routine screening tests are relatively insensitive except in the presence of severe coagulation factor deficiencies. Bleeding disorders that may be associated with normal screening tests include mild hemophilia, vWD, abnormal fibrinogens, factor XIII deficiency, and qualitative platelet disorders. A positive bleeding history in a patient with normal laboratory tests suggests the need for referral to a hematologist with specialty expertise in coagulopathies. A positive history and abnormal laboratory screening tests suggest strongly that a bleeding disorder exists, and referral to a hematologist for further evaluation is needed to determine a specific diagnosis.

It is important to keep in mind that the quality of coagulation test results is highly dependent on the conditions under which the samples are obtained and on the experience and professional quality of the coagulation laboratory. Prompt specimen processing and proper plasma storage are mandatory. Certain tests, such as platelet aggregation studies, require immediate laboratory testing using specialized equipment by highly trained and experienced technicians. Ideally, patients should be medication free for at least 2 weeks and sampled, preferably in the morning, after fasting overnight. It may be inadvisable to make a critical diagnosis on the basis of results obtained on plasma samples after prolonged storage or shipment to a distant laboratory. Travel by the patient to the testing laboratory for blood sampling is optimum.

MANAGEMENT AND INDICATIONS FOR REFERRAL OR HOSPITALIZATION

Since 1975, hemophilia treatment centers (HTCs) have been federally funded to provide comprehensive, specialized care to persons with bleeding disorders. There is evidence that persons who receive care at HTCs have a 40% lower mortality rate associated with bleeding episodes.[4] Therefore management of a patient with a known congenital bleeding disorder by a health care provider should be in conjunction with a hematologist with expertise in blood coagulation and the

TABLE 227-1 Dosing Guidelines for Factor Replacement Therapy for Patients with Hemophilia A (Factor VIII Deficiency) and Hemophilia B (Factor IX Deficiency)*

	Factor VIII	Factor IX†
Type of bleeding episode		
Minor	15-20 units/kg	20-40 units/kg
Major	20-50 units/kg	40-80 units/kg
Life threatening	40-50 units/kg	80-100 units/kg
Factor recovery	**Concentration (plasma derived or recombinant):** 1 IU/kg raises factor level 2% % Correction × Weight (kg) × 0.5 = Dose (IU)	**Plasma derived:** 1 IU/kg raises factor level 1% % Correction × Weight (kg) = Dose (IU) **Recombinant:** 1.2-1.4 IU/kg raises factor level 1% (adults, children) % Correction × Weight (kg) × 1.2-1.4 = Dose (IU)

*Factor dosing depends on type, location, and severity of bleeding episode. Single or multiple doses may be needed based on severity of bleeding episode.
†Recombinant factor IX may require increased dosing to achieve the desired circulating factor IX levels.

guidelines put forth by the Medical and Scientific Advisory Council (MASAC) and adopted by the National Hemophilia Foundation.[5] Once the patient is evaluated by a hematologist, a detailed care plan should be developed that includes the MASAC guidelines for managing the patient if trauma occurs or an invasive procedure is required. Patients with a factor deficiency, such as moderate or severe hemophilia A or B, require replacement with the missing clotting protein. A variety of plasma-derived and recombinant factor concentrates are available, and the hematologist will assist in identifying the appropriate product and dose for the patient (Table 227-1).

It is better to overestimate than to underestimate the risk of bleeding and to treat prophylactically or as soon as possible after bleeding begins, since hemostasis is more difficult to achieve once excessive bleeding has commenced. To ensure rapid and appropriate treatment, a local supply of the appropriate replacement product should be maintained. Most patients with congenital bleeding disorders learn to recognize bleeding episodes soon after they occur and may be trained in self-administration of the clotting factor by IV administration. Generally, any significant trauma will require replacement. Any invasive procedure, even a tooth extraction, may require pretreatment with factor concentrate. Surgery in the patient with a bleeding disorder should be undertaken at a facility equipped with an on-site coagulation laboratory, a full range of treatment products, and expert hematology consultation. Box 227-2 illustrates important issues to consider when assessing the type, degree, and treatment of a bleeding disorder.

BOX 227-2

ASSESSMENT OF BLEEDING EPISODES

- Type of coagulation disorder
- Degree or severity of the disorder
- Presence of co-morbidity as associated with transfusion, such as hepatitis B, hepatitis C, HIV
- Site and extent of bleeding and number of treatments
- History of response to replacement product; history of circulating inhibitors
- Replacement product: choice, dose, half life, risks, benefits
- Any adjunct therapies (e.g., oral antifibrinolytics) required

Trauma or surgery often requires many days of factor replacement accompanied by close monitoring using coagulation factor assays to ensure that hemostatic levels of the deficient clotting protein are present. Mild forms of bleeding disorders such as hemophilia A and vWD may be corrected temporarily by administration of desmopressin acetate (DDAVP), a synthetic analog of vasopressin. This drug is effective, when given either IV or by high-concentrate nasal spray, in increasing levels of factor VIII and von Willebrand's factor (vWF), which is released from vascular endothelial cells. However, not all patients respond to desmopressin, and its use requires demonstration of a rise in clotting factor levels in a trial of this drug performed previously in a controlled setting.

VON WILLEBRAND'S DISEASE

Von Willebrand's disease (vWD) is the most common congenital bleeding disorder and occurs in approximately 1% of the general population.[6] vWD affects both males and females and results from a quantitative or qualitative abnormality in vWF. vWF functions as a bridging molecule that binds to receptors exposed on the platelet surface to link them both to each other and to the area of damage on the blood vessel wall. vWF also serves as the carrier protein for blood coagulation factor VIII and is therefore involved in both platelet and fibrin thrombus formation. Significant deficiencies of vWF are manifested by prolongation of both the bleeding time and the aPTT. vWD can be a challenging disease to diagnose because various conditions (e.g., medications, inflammation, stress, pregnancy) can elevate vWF from abnormally low levels into the normal range, thus masking a true deficient state. vWD bleeding often consists of epistaxis, menorrhagia, excessive bruising, and prolonged bleeding with cuts or dental extractions and in the intraoperative or immediate postoperative period.

There are three major types of vWD. Type I vWD, the most common type representing 70% to 80% of cases, is a quantitative deficiency of vWF.[7] Type IIA and type IIB are characterized by qualitative defects in vWF and represent about 20% to 30% of vWD cases.[7] Type III vWD is a rare and severe homozygous form of type I vWD.[7] It is important to identify the type of vWD so that appropriate treatment can be prescribed. Desmopressin, which is the treatment of choice for a patient with mild to moderate type I vWD, is contraindicated in type IIB vWD.[8,9] The explanation for this is beyond the scope of this text. Because of inherent variability in plasma levels of vWF, a single assay for this protein may not be sufficient for diagnosis. Furthermore, overlap exists between levels present in normal subjects and in those with mild disease. Blood type is also correlated with vWF levels. Relative ranking from higher to lower vWF levels according to blood type is as follows: AB > B > A > O. Typical screening tests for vWD include:

Bleeding time: Normal or prolonged.

PTT: Normal to prolonged.

vWF antigen: Quantitative immunoassay for the amount of vWF protein present. This is typically decreased in type I disease but may be low to normal in type II disease.

vWF activity (ristocetin cofactor C activity): Quantitative measure of the ability of vWF to clump platelets in the presence of the antibiotic ristocetin. vWF activity is decreased in type I disease and disproportionately decreased in type IIA disease.

Factor VIII activity (FVIII:C)—Because vWF functions as a carrier protein for factor VIII, this test generally parallels levels of antigen unless the binding site for factor VIII on vWF is abnormal.

Ristocetin-induced platelet aggregation: Special test used to distinguish between type IIA and type IIB vWD.

vWF multimers: Test that confirms the type of vWD. vWF occurs in the plasma in multimers of various sizes. vWF multimers are clusters consisting of variable numbers of individual vWF molecules. The very large vWF multimers are biologically most active. Type II vWD is characterized by a relatively selective decrease in the larger multimers. This test is therefore helpful in distinguishing between type I and type II vWD.

Once the diagnosis is confirmed, treatment options include desmopressin and plasma-derived factor VIII concentrates that are rich in vWF.[9]

HEMOPHILIA

DEFINITION AND EPIDEMIOLOGY

Hemophilia is an X-linked recessive bleeding disorder characterized by low levels of factor VIII (hemophilia A) or factor IX (hemophilia B).[1] Such deficiencies result in defective fibrin clot formation. Minor injuries are sometimes associated with little bleeding because platelet thrombus formation is normal. However, on later breakdown of the platelet plug, bleeding may occur because of the lack of a stabilizing fibrin clot. Joint and muscle hemorrhages are common in moderate and severe hemophilia. Recurrent hemarthrosis results in hypertrophy and inflammation of the joint synovial tissue, leading to release of proteolytic enzymes that damage the articular cartilage, causing loss of joint function and long-term disability. Limb contractures are common, often requiring physical therapy to regain range of motion. Psoas muscle bleeding may cause vague hip pain or abdominal pain that is often confused with appendicitis or renal colic. Intracranial hemorrhage is a leading cause of death in hemophilia. Most head trauma requires immediate factor replacement.

MANAGEMENT

Treatment of bleeding in the hemophilia patient involves prompt replacement of clotting factors or, in mild hemophilia A, stimulating release of clotting factor from intracellular stores via administration of desmopressin.[10] Even mild hemophilia A patients will require clotting factor replacement for significant injuries or surgery. Symptomatic head trauma must be evaluated by a practitioner with expertise in neurologic injuries, including imaging studies to exclude intracranial bleeding. Soft tissue hematomas may resolve with factor replacement if treated promptly; however, continued bleeding may result in compression of vital structures. Although most patients receive treatment after bleeding is identified, preventive therapy is given before surgery or an invasive procedure. It has been shown that prophylactic infusions of clotting factor for severe hemophilia, especially when begun at an early age, reduce the risk of hemorrhage and prevent associated long-term joint damage.[11]

COMPLICATIONS

Bleeding resulting from disorders of hemostasis may produce a variety of complications. For example, the chronic, recurrent joint bleeding commonly experienced by patients with hemophilia may lead to joint immobility and limb contractures. Chronic bleeding can cause anemia as a result of iron deficiency. Bleeding into various organs can result in dysfunction of that organ. Such bleeding may be fatal if it occurs, for example, in the cranial cavity. Antibodies or inhibitors to infused clotting factor concentrates may develop, making it difficult to control bleeding even with minor injuries.

PATIENT EDUCATION AND LIFE SPAN CONSIDERATIONS

Education is an important and ongoing process. Patients should know the specific name of their bleeding disorder and be able to communicate this diagnosis to future health care providers. They should recognize the signs and symptoms of their disease and know how to respond appropriately to ensure early and effective treatment. Each patient should have an emergency care plan that includes access to a dose of factor, since many hospitals do not maintain a supply of factor products. Work and leisure activities should be reviewed for practices such as contact sports that present a risk for precipitating bleeding episodes. Alcohol and medications such as aspirin and other NSAIDs that aggravate bleeding tendencies should be avoided. Patients are advised to use medications that do not compromise hemostasis, such as acetaminophen for mild discomfort. Medications must be reviewed periodically and new medications evaluated for their potential to increase bleeding. Wearing a medical alert bracelet or necklace is emphasized. The patient's coagulation status must be evaluated before visits to the dentist or for surgical or other invasive procedures. Genetic counseling is recommended as a component of family planning counseling.

THROMBOPHILIA

DEFINITION AND EPIDEMIOLOGY

Thrombosis is the process by which a thrombus (blood clot) forms in the living heart or vasculature. Thrombosis may occur in either the arterial or venous circulation. Sometimes thrombi occur in the patient's veins and arteries, but usually they do not. Thrombi in arteries are commonly associated with atherosclerosis (hardening of the arteries), a condition that does not affect veins. Thrombophilia is a tendency to develop venous thrombosis and is usually a chronic systemic condition.

Thrombosis may occur in any vein (or artery) in the body, but the majority of clots form in the veins of the lower extremity, causing pain, tenderness, and swelling in the distal tissues. Estimates are that more than half a million individuals in the United States experience venous thrombosis each year. Pulmonary embolism resulting in death complicates roughly 200,000 cases per year.[12] The following information focuses on issues surrounding the medical management of inherited venous thrombophilias and thrombosis events.

In the normal state, procoagulant enzymes trigger clot formation to ensure hemostasis after injury. These factors are balanced by inhibitory factors that maintain blood as a liquid. When this equilibrium is disturbed, hypercoagulability results. Fortunately, medical science has produced a steady flow of new findings that have, in many cases, clarified why such clots occur and have provided effective treatment. Clots can occur in superficial veins or deep veins. Thrombi in deep veins, deep vein thrombosis (DVT; see Chapter 133), may be caused by defects in the blood coagulation mechanism that usually do not contribute to clotting in arteries.

Knowledge of components of the normal coagulation mechanism that protect against excessive clot formation prompted investigators to examine substances in the blood for clues to why thrombi develop inappropriately in veins, leading to obstruction of flow and inflammation. This search uncovered many different abnormalities that may either accelerate clot formation beyond control or block reactions needed to keep the blood fluid.[13]

The precise explanation for the occurrence of venous thrombosis in a given location at a specific time may not be apparent in the absence of some obvious predisposing condition. Individuals with various diseases such as cancer or an inflammatory condition, or those who have been immobilized because of surgery, childbirth, injury, or even after a long trip, are more likely to develop venous thrombosis. Other risk factors include advancing age, liver disease, smoking, oral contraceptive use, pregnancy, the presence of the lupus anticoagulant, elevated homocysteine levels, and prior history of DVT. Thrombosis can also occur in otherwise healthy individuals with no obvious explanation.

PATHOPHYSIOLOGY

Virchow's triad continues to define the pathogenesis of DVT, with changes in vessel walls, blood flow, and coagulability of the blood itself contributing to risk. Abnormalities in coagulation proteins may contribute to venous thrombosis. An example is activated protein C-resistance (APC-R). APC-R is commonly due to the presence of an abnormal, or mutated, factor V molecule called factor V Leiden (named for the city in the Netherlands where the mutation was identified).[13] Factor V Leiden occurs in 6% of Caucasians but is rare in individuals of African or Asian decent. The mutated factor V resists breakdown by activated protein C (one of the proteins that helps to keep blood liquid). A person with this defect has about a sevenfold increase in risk for DVT. If this person also takes oral contraceptives, the risk increases to 35-fold, indicating a synergistic interaction between the factor V Leiden mutation and other risk factors.

Other abnormalities that predispose patients to thrombosis include deficiencies of clot inhibitory proteins, including protein C, protein S, and antithrombin III, as well as a mutant form of prothrombin. However, the most prevalent hereditary defect predisposing the patient to DVT is APC-R secondary to the factor V Leiden mutation. An individual with such an abnormality is said to have hereditary thrombophilia. An abnormality in only one of the pair of genes (heterozygote) responsible for the protein is enough to increase the risk of thrombosis. When both members of the gene pair are abnormal (homozygote), a more severe tendency toward thrombosis exists.

CLINICAL PRESENTATION AND PHYSICAL EXAMINATION

Thrombi can form in both superficial and deep veins. Thrombi in the superficial veins manifest with localized tenderness at the site, redness and a feeling of warmth, and possible swelling of the affected limb. Because the vein is close to the surface, it may feel hard or ropelike when examined. The clinical features of DVT include pain, swelling, and erythema of the affected extremity. A positive Homan's sign may also be seen (pain with dorsiflexion of the foot). Physical examination is often neither sensitive nor specific for DVT, and further testing must be done when the condition is suspected (see Chapter133).

DIAGNOSTICS

Doppler ultrasound is generally the first test performed to diagnose a thrombosis event. Ascending venography, a radiologic procedure involving injection of contrast dye into the superficial and deep veins of the leg, permits diagnosis of DVT but is not commonly used.

DIFFERENTIAL DIAGNOSIS

Thrombophilia

- Hereditary
- Acquired
- Disseminated intravascular coagulation
- Malignancy
- Medications (oral contraceptives)
- Autoimmune disease
- Cardiac abnormalities
  - Prosthetic valve
  - Dilated cardiomyopathy
  - Ventricular aneurysm
- Pregnancy
- Nephrotic syndrome

DIFFERENTIAL DIAGNOSIS

Abnormalities that predispose the patient to thrombosis may be acquired (e.g., in association with some other disease such as malignancy or lupus erythematosus) or hereditary (Box 227-3). Thrombophilic disorders are distinguished from one another primarily on the basis of the laboratory

BOX 227-3

SOME CAUSES OF HEREDITARY THROMBOPHILIA

- Activated protein C resistance (factor V Leiden mutation)
- Antithrombin III
- Dysfibrinogenemia
- Factor V Leiden
- Factor XII deficiency
- Homocysteinuria (homocysteinemia)
- Plasminogen deficiency
- Plasminogen activator inhibitor excess
- Protein C deficiency
- Protein S deficiency
- Tissue plasminogen activator deficiency
- Mutant prothrombin
- Factor VIII coagulant activity

evaluation. The decision about which laboratory tests are indicated is determined by the medical history and clinical presentation. The goal of testing is to determine whether a defect is present that may be important for planning future treatment and that may be sought in other family members who may or may not yet have had an episode of venous thrombosis.

MANAGEMENT

Management of venous thrombosis should follow the American College of Chest Physicians guidelines for antithrombotic therapy for prevention and treatment of thrombosis.[14] The diagnosis of hereditary thrombophilia in itself is not necessarily an indication for treatment, especially if thrombosis has not occurred. However, when venous thrombosis does occur in a patient with thrombophilia, treatment is begun immediately with anticoagulants to prevent thrombus growth and possible subsequent pulmonary embolism.

Heparin is the initial treatment because its anticoagulant effect begins immediately. Heparin may be given subcutaneously but is usually given intravenously. Heparin acts together with antithrombin III (ATIII) to block coagulation factor enzymes, especially thrombin. The dose of IV heparin is adjusted according to the aPTT and should be aimed at 1.5 to 2.5 times the normal range for the hospital laboratory; doses causing greater aPTT prolongation place the patient at risk of bleeding.[15]

Initial heparin therapy is typically followed by treatment with warfarin (Coumadin), which may be started immediately or within a few days of beginning heparin. Warfarin is given orally and is absorbed from the intestine along with other nutrients, including vitamin K. Vitamin K is required for the production of certain coagulation factors in their complete, fully active form by the liver. Warfarin competes with vitamin K so that incomplete, less active coagulation factors are produced. This takes time, usually 2 to 3 days. During this period, heparin and warfarin are given together for full protection. When the warfarin becomes effective, as measured by laboratory testing, heparin is discontinued. The patient is then maintained on warfarin as an outpatient usually for a minimum of 3 months after a first episode of thrombosis. In recent years a number of studies have shown that risk of recurrence and prevention of long-term complications of DVT can be minimized by a more prolonged course of therapy. This 3-month treatment is usually reserved for uncomplicated cases of distal thrombosis associated with some precipitating event, such as surgery or trauma, that can be eliminated. A more typical course of warfarin anticoagulation would last 6 months and even up to 1 year in some cases.

Because warfarin and vitamin K are in competition, the effect of warfarin may be exaggerated when dietary vitamin K is inadequate. The effect of warfarin is also exaggerated with liver disease, and many different drugs increase or decrease warfarin's effects. Therefore it is important to identify any medications being used during anticoagulation therapy. When warfarin is stopped, the production of fully active coagulation factors gradually returns over several days. The amount of warfarin required to achieve an optimum degree of therapeutic anticoagulation varies among individuals and is determined by the PT. Guidance on adjusting warfarin dosage according to the PT is provided in Figure 227-1. The degree of anticoagulation reflected by prolongation of the PT is standardized on the INR scale. Expression of the result as the INR is preferred because it eliminates variability between laboratories and reagents used to perform the PT. The degree of warfarin anticoagulation required for maximum protection with minimum risk of bleeding depends on clinical conditions present at that time. The recommended INR range for prophylaxis to reduce the risk of recurrent thrombosis is generally between 2 and 3.[16]

In the past decade, low-molecular-weight forms of heparin (LMW-H) have become available for the treatment of DVT.[17] These also work with ATIII but inhibit activated factor X to a much greater extent than it does thrombin. This ability of LMW-H to block the clotting mechanism "upstream" accounts for many of the advantages of this drug. LMW-H has been shown in large, randomized clinical trials to be at least as effective and safe as either warfarin or standard heparin.[17] Compared with heparin, LMW-H has a longer half life, more consistent and complete absorption when injected subcutaneously, and fewer side effects. LMW-H is as effective when given subcutaneously as when given intravenously and usually does not require laboratory monitoring for dose determination.[18] These advantages may permit management of DVT without hospitalization and also safe, outpatient control of thrombosis with self-administration should warfarin fail.

A pentasaccharide, fondaparinux, is a synthetic inhibitor of activated factor X that has recently been approved by the U.S. Food and Drug Administration for prevention and treatment of DVT. Its mechanism of action is like that of heparin except that it has a longer half life, permitting once daily subcutaneous dosing. It is administered in a fixed dose without laboratory monitoring. A number of other synthetic clotting factor inhibitors are also in development. These advances and others on the horizon offer the prospect of improved care for patients with thrombophilia. They have the advantages of being active orally in a fixed dose, not interacting with food or other medications, and not requiring laboratory monitoring for dosage adjustment.

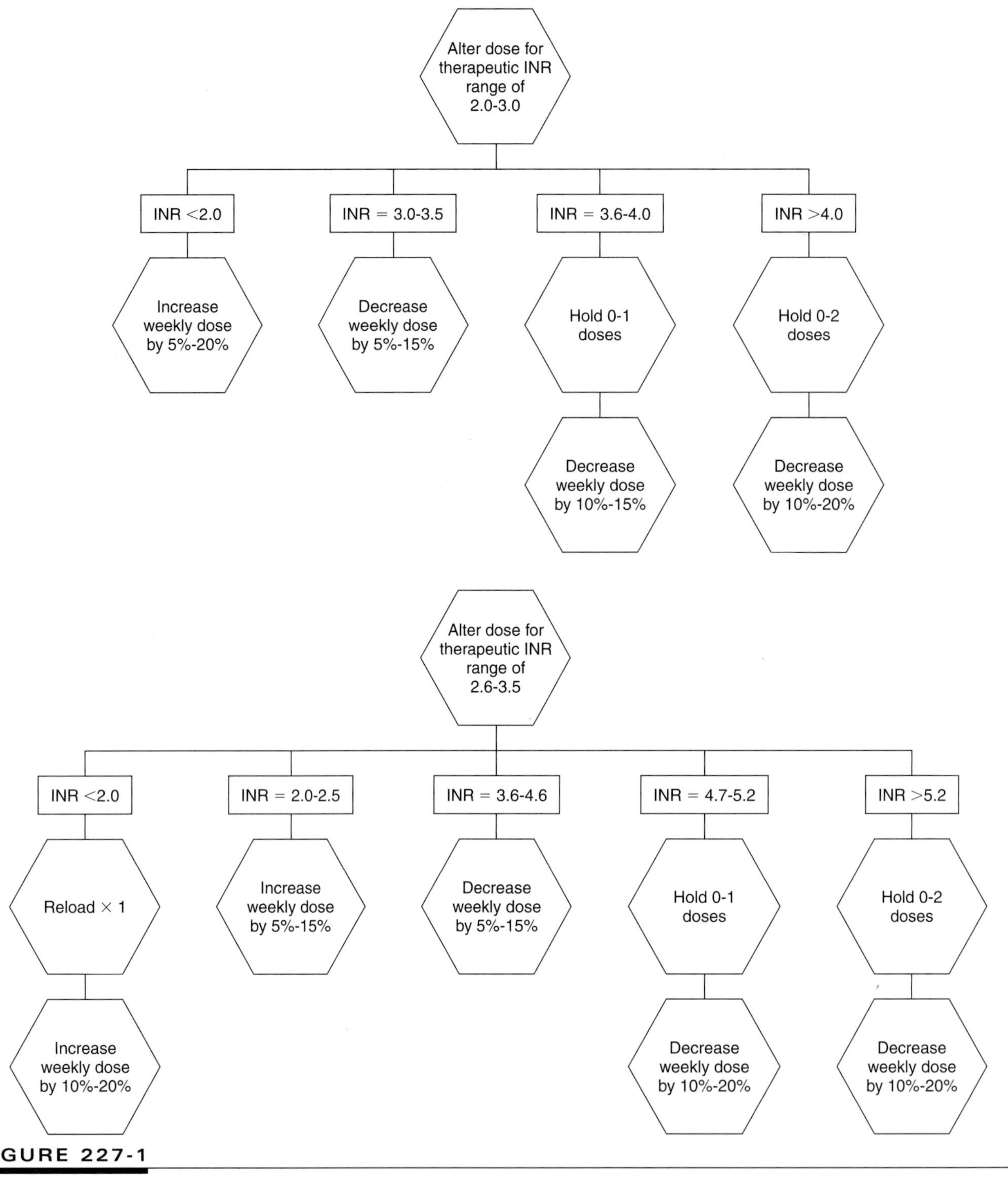

FIGURE 227-1

Warfarin dosage adjustment protocol. *INR,* International Normalized Ratio.(From Establishing an outpatient anticoagulation clinic in a community hospital, *Am J Health Syst Pharm* 53:1154, 1996.)

COMPLICATIONS

Clot formation within intact vessels compromises the vascular supply to the affected areas. With venous thrombosis, the reduced flow of blood from the affected area of the body results in swelling and pain in that part. For example, a thrombus in the veins of the leg can result in swelling and discoloration of the foot and lower leg. When the obstruction is not relieved promptly, the swelling may become chronic and noticeable, especially after patients have been on their feet for a time. A venous clot may extend and break off, producing an embolus that may become lodged in the vessels of the lung (a pulmonary embolus). When such emboli are large or multiple, they can be life threatening. For example, a coronary thrombosis that results in myocardial infarction can result in an arrhythmia (Chapter 124) or congestive heart failure (Chapter 128) secondary to failure of the pumping mechanism of the heart. Thrombosis of a cerebral artery can result in injury to the nervous tissue in the brain, producing changes in sensory or motor function anywhere in the body (Chapter 203). Other examples of complications of arterial thrombosis include infarction of the kidney (renal artery thrombosis) or bowel (mesenteric artery thrombosis).

INDICATIONS FOR REFERRAL OR HOSPITALIZATION

Referral to a hematologist with experience in thrombophilia should be considered for patients with a history of unexplained or recurrent DVT, a family history of thrombosis, or thrombosis at an early age. Prompt investigation for a hereditary cause may result in therapeutic or preventive measures for the patient or family member.

PATIENT AND FAMILY EDUCATION AND LIFE SPAN CONSIDERATIONS

Patient education is an important component of safe and effective outpatient anticoagulation therapy. Patients need to be aware of their diagnosis and factors influencing anticoagulation treatment. Education focuses on the importance of keeping regular follow-up visits; monitoring anticoagulation doses; identifying signs of bleeding; maintaining a consistent diet; noting changes in health, diet, or medications; and avoiding hazardous activities. In addition, a regularly updated pharmacology resource should be consulted for medications that interact with warfarin, and information should be provided to patients, with periodic updates.

Prolonged immobility is discouraged. When the patient is immobilized, such as while driving or flying, he or she should take frequent rest breaks for leg stretching or walking. Patients at risk for thrombus formation need information about the signs and symptoms of clot formation and how to access appropriate care. Genetic counseling and risk management are essential for individuals with inherited disorders.

REFERENCES

1. Venkateswaran L, Williams JA, Jones DJ, and others: Mild hemophilia in children: prevalence, complications, and treatment, *J Pediatr Hematol Oncol* 20(1):32-35, 1998.
2. White GC: Approach to the bleeding patient. In Colman R, editor: *Hemostasis and thrombosis: basic principles and clinical practice,* ed 3, Philadelphia, 1994, Lippincott.
3. Lusher J: Approach to the bleeding patient. In Nathan DG, editor: *Nathan and Oski's hematology of infancy and childhood,* ed 5, Philadelphia, 1998, Saunders.
4. Soucie JM, Nuss R, Evatt B, and others: Mortality among males with hemophilia: relations with source of medical care, *Blood* 96(2):437-442, 2000.
5. National Hemophilia Foundation Medical and Scientific Advisory Council: *Recommendations on the treatment of hemophilia and related bleeding disorders,* New York, 2001, The Foundation.
6. Sham R, Francis C: Evaluation of mild bleeding disorders and easy bruising, *Blood Rev* 8:98-104, 1994.
7. Sadler JE: A revised classification of von Willebrand disease, *Haemophilia* 3(2):11-18, 1997.
8. Mannuccio PM: Desmopressin (DDAVP) in the treatment of bleeding disorders: the first 20 years, *Blood* 9(7):2515-2521, 1997.
9. Blackwell Science: Treatment and management of Von Willebrand disease, *Haemophilia* 3(Suppl 2):4-8, 1997.
10. Coyne MA, Lusher J: Guidelines for emergency care of patients with hemophilia, *Emerg Med* 4(69):69-77, 2000.
11. Nilsson IM, Berntorp E, Ljung R, and others: Prophylactic treatment of severe hemophilia A and B can prevent joint disability, *Semin Hematol* 31(S2):5-9, 1994.
12. Mann KG: Thrombosis: theoretical considerations, *Am J Clin Nutr* 65(5 Suppl):1657S-1664S, 1997.
13. De Stefano V, Finazzi G, Mannucci PM: Inherited thrombophilia: pathogenesis, clinical syndromes, and management, *Blood* 87(9): 3531-3544, 1996.
14. Hirsh J, Raschke R: The Seventh ACCP Conference on Antithrombotic and Thrombolytic Therapy: evidence-based guidelines, *Am Coll Chest Phys* 172S-688S, 2004.
15. Litin SC, Gastineau DA: Concise review for primary-care physicians: current concepts in anticoagulation therapy, *Mayo Clin Proc* 70:266-272, 1995.
16. Ansell JE, Holden A, Nozzolillo E: Oral anticoagulant therapy: practical considerations, *Nurse Pract Forum* 3(2):105-113, 1992.
17. Low molecular weight heparin in the treatment of patients with venous thrombosis. The Columbus Investigators, *N Engl J Med* 337(10):657-662, 1997.
18. Weitz JI: Low-molecular-weight heparins, *N Engl J Med* 337(10):688-698, 1997.

CHAPTER 228

Leukemias

Sara Tinsley

DEFINITION AND EPIDEMIOLOGY

Some of the most challenging and complex cancers to manage in the community setting are the leukemias, hematologic malignancies that affect the bone marrow and lymphatic tissue. There are two types of leukemia: acute and chronic. Acute leukemias are distinguished by an abnormal production of immature white blood cells and a rapid disease progression over approximately 6 months. Chronic leukemias display an overabundance of more mature-appearing but ineffective cells. Disease progression is usually slow, over 2 to 5 years. The overproduction of leukemia cells displaces normal cells in the bone marrow and thus destroys hematopoietic performance. Depending on cell type, treatment of leukemia may be as conservative as observation or as aggressive as bone marrow transplantation. Consequences of the disease state and side effects of treatment options represent a true challenge to the health care provider.[1]

In 2005 there were approximately 34,810 new cases of leukemia in the United States, with chronic and acute leukemia of equal incidence. There were approximately 22,570 deaths from leukemia.[2] The exact etiology of leukemia is unknown. Causes and risk factors for consideration are genetic factors and disorders, exposure to radiation, chemicals, drugs, viruses, and other bone marrow disorders and environmental factors.

Children with genetic disorders such as Down's syndrome have an increased risk of developing acute leukemia. Other conditions that are associated with a high incidence of leukemia include Ellis–van Creveld syndrome, Fanconi's anemia, Kleinfelter's syndrome, Bloom's syndrome, and ataxia-telangiectasia.

Exposure to ionizing radiation is the most conclusive predisposing factor associated with humans and leukemia. This became evident after World War II when a large number of Japanese survivors of the atom bomb explosion displayed an increased incidence of acute myeloid leukemia (AML) and chronic myelogenous leukemia (CML). Pioneer radiologists who were exposed to massive radiation also exhibited a high incidence of leukemia.[3]

Occupational exposure to certain chemicals increases the risk of developing leukemia. Workers exposed to benzene (a hydrocarbon used in industry and in unleaded gasoline), rubber cement, and cleaning solvents are at risk for developing leukemia. Other occupations in which workers are at risk of contracting leukemia are those which expose workers to explosives, dyes, or paints; distilleries; and leather tanning industries. Although the relationship between leukemia and viruses remains unclear, there does appear to be a correlation between retroviruses and T-cell leukemia and hairy cell leukemia.[4]

Polycythemia vera, aplastic anemia, myelodysplastic syndromes, and other diseases of the bone marrow also appear to predispose individuals to leukemia. Environmental factors such as hair dye, cigarette smoking, and sunbathing may also increase the risk of developing leukemia.[5]

Intensive combination chemotherapy for patients with cancer has led to increased survival rates. However, these survivors must be continually evaluated for complications of the long-term cytotoxic treatment. One serious consequence is the development of a second cancer, especially myeloid leukemia. Therapy-related leukemia is generally a fatal disease. The terms *t-MDS* (treatment-related myelodysplastic syndrome) and *t-AML* (treatment-related acute myeloid leukemia) are used to describe a clinical syndrome that may imply a causal relationship, but this relationship remains to be proven.[6]

Physician consultation is indicated for all suspected cases of leukemia.

PATHOPHYSIOLOGY

Leukemia is a malignant disorder of the blood and blood-forming organs—the spleen, lymphatic system, and bone marrow. It is identified as acute or chronic depending on the onset of symptoms and the maturity of the blood cell. With acute leukemia, there is marked abnormality and uncontrolled production of the immature leukocytes. The chronic form of the disease shows an accumulation of mature-appearing cells that have lost the ability to function efficiently. The proliferation of abnormal blood cells infiltrates the bone marrow, the peripheral blood, and other organs, which causes swelling, interferes with normal organ function, and destroys normal hematopoiesis. All blood cell types are formed within the marrow; as leukocyte crowding persists, there is a decrease in the circulating erythrocytes and thrombocytes. This compromise leads to anemia, dyspnea, bruising, the potential for hemorrhage, and further tissue destruction.[7]

The maturation process of various blood cell lines originates from the stem cell. The stem cell line is responsible for the generation of new cells necessary to meet the body's requirements throughout a lifetime.[8] Leukemic cells are designated as either myeloid or lymphoid, according to the type of cell that predominates.

CLINICAL PRESENTATION AND PHYSICAL EXAMINATION

Acute Leukemias

The signs and symptoms of acute lymphocytic leukemia (ALL) and AML may include a viral infection with a low-grade fever, anemia with fatigue, and pallor. Initial manifestations include bleeding gums, epistaxis, ecchymosis, petechiae, and excessive bleeding after minor dental procedures, all caused by thrombocytopenia. Chloromas, the collection of blast cells in the subcutaneous tissues, may imitate a primary or metastatic carcinoma.

In general, the presenting symptoms are nonspecific. Often the health care provider evaluates and treats a sinus, respiratory, perirectal, or urinary tract infection with poor response and may eventually discover leukemia. Since leukemia involves the lymph, spleen, and liver, diffuse lymphadenopathy and hepatosplenomegaly may be present on examination. Patients may complain of bone pain. Younger patients may experience joint pain and swelling that resembles rheumatoid arthritis. Fifty percent of all leukemia patients have some type of ocular involvement. A funduscopic examination may reveal flame-shaped hemorrhages, which are caused by retinal leukemic infiltration; these hemorrhages are a classic sign of leukemia.[9] In AML the skin and gums are often infiltrated with leukemic cells, and therefore an oral examination may be helpful.

Although only 2% of patients have central nervous system (CNS) involvement at the time of initial diagnosis, many may have CNS involvement at some time during the course of their leukemia. The most common signs and symptoms of leukemia that has invaded the CNS are headache, papilledema, vomiting, nuchal rigidity, and cranial nerve palsy. In AML, leukostasis occurs when the blast count exceeds 100,000 cells/mm^3, and the patient is at risk for a fatal cerebral hemorrhage.[10]

Chronic Leukemias

Patients with CML and chronic lymphocytic leukemia (CLL) are usually asymptomatic. There may be subtle changes in the WBC count and differential early in the disease. A cardinal finding on physical examinations of patients with chronic leukemia is splenomegaly. The patient may complain of a mild sensation of fullness in the left upper quadrant or may have an obvious mass. Severe splenomegaly can compress surrounding organs, causing early satiety, weight loss, and peripheral leg edema related to compression of the splenic vein. As the disease progresses, other symptoms occur, such as bone pain, bleeding problems, infection, fatigue, pallor, adenopathy, fevers, and night sweats.[11]

DIAGNOSTICS AND DIFFERENTIAL DIAGNOSIS

Acute Leukemias

To confirm the diagnosis of acute leukemia, a CBC is necessary. Many patients are seen with anemia and thrombocytopenia, but striking abnormalities are noted in the WBC count and differential. The WBC parameters vary within a wide range—from 1000 to 100,000 cells/mm^3. Most patients have counts between 5000 and 30,000 cells/mm^3.[11]

Careful examination of the blood smear is essential. The significant finding on the blood smear is an increased population of blast cells and a decrease of neutrophils and platelets. It is important to realize that as many as 10% of all patients have normal blood counts even when the marrow has been replaced by leukemic cells; therefore a bone marrow aspiration and biopsy are definitive for diagnosis. The bone marrow contents will be hypercellular, with a crowding of blast cells (60% to 90%) and a decrease in normal cellular elements. Auer rods (reddish filaments) incorporated within the blast cells confirm the diagnosis of AML.[10]

Biochemical studies may reveal hyperuricemia. Hyperuricemia occurs because of the high turnover rate of proliferating leukemia cells and the end product of purine catabolism. Electrolyte disorders are common, and in acute leukemia elevated lactate dehydrogenase may occur. Therefore serum chemistries and liver function tests (LFTs) should be ordered initially. Any patient with an increased myeloblast count may be at risk for leukostasis; this condition primarily affects the lungs and brain, but any organ can be involved. Lowering the blast count in a rapid fashion is necessary, usually by chemotherapy and/or leukapheresis. Therefore patients who have acute leukemia should be admitted to a tertiary center for comprehensive and aggressive management.

The differential diagnosis for ALL and AML is lymphoma, although other infiltrative processes such as solid tumors (e.g., breast cancer) must be excluded. Some patients with fever and cytopenia who have a small amount of circulating blast cells must be differentiated from those with reactions occurring in tuberculosis, systemic lupus erythematosus, megaloblastic anemia, and aplastic anemia. Surface antigen and serologic studies can exclude viral infections such as infectious mononucleosis. Cytogenic studies are currently being used as a diagnostic tool in determining the subtype of leukemia.[3]

Chronic Leukemias

At diagnosis, the WBC count may range from fewer than 10,000 to more than 200,000 cells/mm^3, with mature and predominantly myelocytic cells. In general, the red blood cell count is normal, but a slight degree of anemia may occur. Hypereosinophilia and hyperbasophilia are common. Increased levels of uric acid in the blood and urine are also found in patients with CML. Bone marrow biopsy reveals hyperplastic myeloid cells and storage cells similar to Gaucher's cells scattered throughout the marrow. The striking biochemical abnormality in CML is the reduction or absence of leukocyte alkaline phosphatase. This, along with the positive test for Philadelphia chromosome (Ph^1), the hallmark of CML, confirms the diagnosis. CML is the first cancer shown to be associated with a chromosomal abnormality.[11]

CLL is often discovered on a routine office visit when a CBC is ordered. The physical examination may be negative, but some patients have nontender adenopathy or splenomegaly. Patients may report fatigue, night sweats, occasional fever, or malaise. The majority of patients consult their health care provider because of a painless cervical lymph node that waxes and wanes but does not disappear completely.[11]

CLL is suspected whenever an absolute lymphocytosis in the peripheral blood occurs in an adult and is sustained over time. Lymphocytosis also occurs in infectious mononucleosis, pertussis, and toxoplasmosis, but in these conditions the lymphocyte count returns to normal after a few weeks.

A peripheral smear may be adequate for the diagnosis of CLL; a bone marrow biopsy will *always* reveal lymphocytosis in cases of CLL. The lymphocyte count ranges from 10,000 to

DIAGNOSTICS

Leukemia

LABORATORY
CBC and differential
Peripheral blood smear evaluation
Serum electrolytes
Uric acid
LFTs
Urinalysis
Serum protein electrophoresis

OTHER
Bone marrow biopsy

DIFFERENTIAL DIAGNOSIS

Leukemia

- Lymphomas
- Solid tumors
- Systemic lupus erythematosus
- Megaloblastic anemia
- Aplastic anemia
- Lymphoproliferative disorders

150,000/mm³. Because there may be a decrease in immunoglobulin (Ig) levels, a serum protein electrophoresis should be performed; this test may reveal a marked decrease in levels of IgG and slight decreases in IgA and IgM levels. A chest x-ray study may be helpful in detecting hilar and mediastinal adenopathy.[12]

The differential diagnoses for CLL include non-Hodgkin's lymphoma, hairy cell leukemia, and a variety of other lymphoproliferative disorders.

MANAGEMENT

Acute Leukemias

Patients diagnosed with ALL and AML require aggressive chemotherapy. Treatment of AML and ALL involves induction therapy for remission and postremission consolidation or maintenance therapy. The oncologist should be consulted before any medicine is prescribed for a patient who is undergoing chemotherapy for acute leukemia.

Patients with AML may also undergo a hematopoietic stem cell transplant (HSCT). The increasing use of both autologous and allogeneic HSCTs will have a profound effect on the outcome of AML. The impact of these approaches is under research. Management of these patients requires a multidisciplinary approach. Expertise in transfusion management, infectious disease, care of indwelling catheters, nutrition, chemotherapy and side effects, and psychosocial counseling is required.[13]

Approximately 50% of patients with ALL who are less than 15 years of age achieve a long-term, leukemia-free survival. Approximately 70% of all patients with AML who are less than 60 years of age achieve a complete, but short-lived, remission; only 15% remain disease free for 5 years or more. The major cause of failure to achieve remission during induction therapy is death from hemorrhage and infection.[1]

Chronic Leukemias

CML has three phases: chronic phase, accelerated phase, and terminal blast crisis phase. The chronic phase has a duration of approximately 3 to 5 years; the durations of the other phases vary. In contrast, CLL is usually a long-term disease, with reported cases lasting from 1 to 15 years.

Chronic leukemias are managed differently than acute leukemias. CML is treated initially with imatinib mesylate (Gleevec). The U.S. Food and Drug Administration approved Gleevec for CML treatment in May 2001. The translocation between chromosomes 9 and 22, or the Ph[1], disappears in 75% of patients on Gleevec by 18 months of therapy. Alternative treatments include allogeneic HSCT and clinical trials.

CLL and small lymphocytic lymphoma are the same disease, manifested differently. They are treated identically, and the terms are commonly used interchangeably. Initiation of treatment should be individualized and based on prognostic information, including cytogenetic aberrations and stage of disease. Various treatment options exist, including enrollment in a clinical trial, alkylating agent with or without rituximab, purine analog, or alkylating agent–based combination chemotherapy.

In chronic leukemia there may be drug interactions, including an increased effect of anticoagulants, a decreased digoxin level, and an increased drug action of barbiturates. When in doubt, the provider should contact the pharmacist to discuss any potential drug interactions. Any leukemia patient with previously diagnosed diabetes may have episodes of hyperglycemia related to corticosteroid therapy.

Patients diagnosed with leukemia who have undergone chemotherapy or perhaps HSCT are at risk for infection (bacterial, fungal, viral) and other long-term side effects of aggressive treatment. Patients with CLL are predisposed to several infectious complications that are related to the humoral immunocompromise associated with the disease process, as well as to further immunosuppression from steroid therapy and cytotoxic therapy.[14] Periodic visits to the health care provider and the hematologist or oncologist are essential for close monitoring and support.

Patients who have undergone HSCT need close follow-up monitoring, which usually occurs in collaboration with the tertiary center that performed the HSCT. These patients are immunocompromised, and intervening in a timely fashion with antibiotics and antifungal agents when indicated will improve survival and quality of life.

Chemotherapy

Chemotherapy is the cornerstone of treatment for both acute and chronic leukemias. However, chemotherapy management for the leukemias varies (Box 228-1). The goal of chemotherapy is to eradicate leukemic stem cells in acute leukemia and decrease mature leukemia cells in chronic leukemia.

BOX 228-1

MOST COMMONLY USED DRUGS TO TREAT LEUKEMIAS

ACUTE MYELOID LEUKEMIA

- Cytosine arabinoside IV
- Daunorubicin IV

CHRONIC MYELOGENOUS LEUKEMIA

- Busulfan PO
- Hydroxyurea PO
- Imatinib (Gleevec) PO

Advanced Stage

- Cytosine arabinoside IV

ACUTE LYMPHOCYTIC LEUKEMIA

- Vincristine
- L-Asparaginase IV
- Daunorubicin IV
- Prednisone PO

CHRONIC LYMPHOCYTIC LEUKEMIA

- Chlorambucil PO
- Corticosteroids PO

Advanced Stage

- Cyclophosphamide IV
- Doxorubicin IV
- Fludarabine IV

LIFE SPAN CONSIDERATIONS

Leukemia was once thought to be a childhood disease, but 90% of the newly diagnosed cases occur in adults. AML and CLL are the most common adult forms of the disease. ALL accounts for 80% of the childhood forms.[2]

COMPLICATIONS

Chemotherapeutic agents have many side effects, including bone marrow depression, gastrointestinal distress, nausea, vomiting, anorexia, stomatitis, diarrhea, constipation, skin rashes, alopecia, and fatigue. Specific agents have particular side effects. Daunorubicin may cause cardiotoxicity, vincristine may cause peripheral neuropathy, and asparaginase may cause elevated LFTs.

Complications of leukemia include possible sequelae from chemotherapy and HSCT (e.g., secondary malignancies, infection, fertility problems). Neuropathies and cardiopathies may develop and are usually related to the aggressive treatment regimen experienced by the leukemia patient. Despite the development of more effective antibiotics, granulocyte colony-stimulating factor, and granulocyte-macrophage colony-stimulating factor, bacterial and fungal infections continue to be a source of morbidity and mortality in patients with prolonged neutropenia.[13] Other syndromes that are potential complications are discussed next.

Tumor Lysis Syndrome

Acute tumor lysis syndrome (ATLS) is most commonly seen in patients with AML and CML who are undergoing active treatment. ATLS occurs when a great many rapidly proliferating tumor cells are destroyed. Patients with a high WBC count, a heavy tumor burden, lymphadenopathy, and splenomegaly receive cytotoxic chemotherapy that ruptures tumor cell membranes and releases intracellular contents into the bloodstream.[15] ATLS is characterized by the development of acute hyperuricemia, hyperkalemia, hyperphosphatemia, and hypercalcemia, with or without acute renal failure.[15] Prevention and management of these metabolic complications require close monitoring. Renal function and chemistry values should be monitored daily. Fluid balance and electrolyte disturbances should be corrected with vigorous IV hydration and diuretics as indicated. The addition of sodium bicarbonate to maintain urinary alkalinization is recommended, as is the use of allopurinol to decrease serum uric acid levels. Monitoring of daily weights, meticulous assessment of intake and output, and observation for signs and symptoms of fluid overload are also indicated. ATLS ordinarily resolves within 4 to 7 days if adequate renal function is maintained.

Disseminated Intravascular Coagulation

Disseminated intravascular coagulation (DIC) is a hematologic disorder that occurs when there is an alteration in the blood-clotting mechanism. It may be acute or chronic and can be related to either the disease process or the treatment regimen. DIC is the most common serious hypercoagulable state that occurs in patients with cancer.[16] It is an event in which both clotting and hemorrhage exist simultaneously.

Acute leukemia, antineoplastic agents, infection, trauma, and hemolytic transfusion reactions interrupt normal body hemostasis and may initiate an episode of DIC. Spontaneous hemorrhage or the slow occult damage of multiple small clot formation within the lungs, organs of the CNS, or gastrointestinal tract may herald the presentation of DIC. Organ dysfunction from circulatory impairment leads to mental status changes, severe muscle pain, oliguria, and slowed gastrointestinal motility.[15] Symptoms may range from mild chronic episodes to acute and life-threatening incidents.

Abnormal laboratory findings suggest a diagnosis of DIC. A decreased platelet count, a prolonged prothrombin and partial thromboplastin time, and a decreased fibrinogen level with an elevation of fibrin degradation products confirm the diagnosis of DIC.[17]

Treatment of the underlying cause of DIC is vital. Hemorrhage is treated with replacement of fluids and blood component therapy; infection is treated with antibiotics; and cancer is treated with radiotherapy, chemotherapy, or surgery as indicated. Heparin therapy is more commonly used for the chronic DIC of malignancy associated with thrombotic, thromboembolic, or necrotizing complications. Thorough, multiple system assessments in combination with patient and family education and involvement are necessary to prevent further injury and complications associated with DIC.

Leukostasis

The predominant cell in acute leukemia is undifferentiated or immature, usually a blast cell. In leukostasis, blood sludging or stasis occurs when the blood vessels become overcrowded with these blast cells. Individuals with high WBC counts and a large tumor burden are at risk for developing leukostasis. The small, delicate pulmonary and cranial vessels are the most susceptible. If leukostasis is left untreated, rupture and hemorrhage result in ischemia and infarct. Emergent treatment includes high-dose chemotherapy or cranial radiotherapy to decrease the number of circulating blast cells. Leukapheresis (removal of white blood cells from the plasma) may also be indicated.[1]

Pancytopenia

Regardless of the treatment regimen chosen, infection, bleeding, and symptomatic anemia are the most common side effects of leukemia and its therapy. The desired effect of treatment produces severe myelosuppression. Prolonged periods of neutropenia leave the immunocompromised patient especially susceptible to infection. Until normal bone marrow function is restored, the leukemic patient lacks the normal host responses. Treatment with empiric antibiotics to prevent systemic or disseminated infection is indicated once infection is suspected. Prevention of infection must focus on providing meticulous care with any invasive treatment option and limiting unnecessary invasive procedures. Education empowers patients and their families to participate in their own health practices.

Fatigue is one of the most common symptoms associated with cancer and cancer therapies. Chronic low-grade anemia, stress, and alterations in sleeping, eating, and working are known to deplete energy levels. Fatigue can be one of the most disabling complications of cancer and chemotherapy treatments, which allows feelings of hopelessness and power-

BOX 228-2

PATIENT EDUCATION

SEPSIS AND INFECTION

White blood cells are the body's defense against infection. If your WBC count is low, you are at risk for infection and should do the following:

1. Avoid crowds, malls, churches, and movie theaters.
2. Instruct sick friends and relatives to call, not visit.
3. Practice exceptionally careful personal hygiene with multiple handwashings.

Signs and symptoms of infection to report to the health care team: elevated temperature (report a fever of 37.7° C [100° F] or higher); productive cough; wound redness, swelling, or drainage; mouth sores

THROMBOCYTOPENIA

Platelets are the components of blood that play a major part in the clotting mechanism. If your platelets are low, you are at risk for increased bleeding and should do the following:

1. Use electric shavers for shaving (this includes women).
2. Apply extra caution when using any sharp objects.
3. Avoid bumps, bruises, and falls (this is not the time to rearrange furniture).
4. Avoid aspirin and aspirin-containing products.

Signs and symptoms of thrombocytopenia to report to the health care team: increased bruising, nosebleeds, bleeding gums, blood in urine or stool, increased menstrual flow

ANEMIA

You should do the following:

1. Take frequent rest periods.
2. When moving from one position to another, do so slowly.
3. Keep warm.
4. Eat a well-balanced diet and drink plenty of fluids.

Signs and symptoms of anemia to report to the health care team: shortness of breath, ringing in the ears, fainting, pounding heart, increased heart rate, or palpitations

MANAGEMENT OF SIDE EFFECTS OF DISEASE OR TREATMENT

There is the potential for numerous side effects from your disease and the treatment you are receiving. The following are options for managing various side effects. If you are unable to manage these problems effectively, contact your health care team:

Fever: Take acetaminophen (Tylenol) for a temperature over 37.7° C (100° F) and call your health care provider.

Headache: Take acetaminophen; if headache persists or other symptoms (e.g., visual disturbances or seizures) arise, call your health care team immediately.

Mucositis: Ask your health care team to prescribe a medication for sore mouth, and take as directed. Keep mouth clean and moist, rinsing it every 2 hours with ½ teaspoon of salt in 8 ounces of water or with a 1:3 ratio of hydrogen peroxide solution. Brush teeth gently with a soft toothbrush or an oral swab. Use only alcohol-free mouthwash. Drink plenty of liquids. Wear dentures only for meals. Use a lip moisturizer to keep lips from becoming dry and cracked. Avoid highly spiced food, high-acid food, and very hot foods or liquids. Avoid alcohol and tobacco. See your dentist routinely.

Nausea, vomiting, and anorexia: These symptoms affect your ability to maintain a good nutritional state, which is imperative for body repair and healing. Take antinausea medications at the first sign of queasiness; do not wait until vomiting occurs. If the medication does not work, call your health care team for another type of medication; numerous antinausea medications are available. Eat small, frequent, well-balanced meals that are high in protein and calories. Have snacks. If there is a bad taste in your mouth, try chewing gum or sucking on hard candy.

Diarrhea: If you are taking laxatives, *stop*. Take an antidiarrheal preparation such as loperamide (Imodium A-D) after each *watery* stool; follow package instructions. Use the BRAT diet—bananas, rice, applesauce, and dry toast. When free of diarrhea for 24 hours, resume regular diet slowly. Avoid foods that cause diarrhea. If diarrhea persists for 24 hours despite treatment, call your health care team.

Constipation: Many pain medications cause constipation, and prevention is the best treatment. Take a natural laxative with a stool softener at bedtime. Drink at least eight 8-ounce glasses of water each day (if you have had a bone marrow transplant, you may be instructed to drink distilled water). Avoid foods that contribute to constipation. If constipation occurs, increase natural laxative with a stool softener to two or three times a day. Suppositories, enemas, and the more aggressive laxatives (e.g., milk of magnesia or magnesium citrate) may need to be added. When constipation is resolved, remove medications in reverse order, but continue the natural laxative with stool softener. If constipation persists despite treatment, contact your health care team because a more serious problem may exist.

Pain: Take pain medications as prescribed. If you are taking timed-release pain medications, take them regularly to prevent pain. If you are taking pain medications only as needed, take them when the pain begins. Do not wait until pain becomes severe, since the medication will not be as effective. If you are taking narcotics, do not drive, operate dangerous machinery, or drink alcohol. Avoid situations that cause pain to increase. Call your health care team if the pain medication becomes ineffective or if pain changes in intensity or location.

Alopecia: Keep the head warm because a great deal of body heat can be lost through a bare scalp. Wigs, turbans, and caps not only keep the head warm but may also help improve body image. In most cases hair will start to grow back when treatment ends. If eyelashes and eyebrows are gone, wear eye protection, especially when outdoors, to avoid injury to the eyes. Nose hair may also be lost, which may cause discomfort in cold weather; a mask may be helpful.

Fatigue: Maintain good nutrition and take a vitamin supplement. Space exercise and rest periods throughout the day. Use a time log to determine the optimum routine.

Insomnia: Avoid sleeping excessively during the day. Get some exercise daily (this may mean just walking around the house). Do not drink caffeinated beverages before bedtime. Over-the-counter diphenhydramine (Benadryl) may be effective. As a last resort, ask your health care team to consider a sleeping medication.

Depression: Review your medications; many medications and their side effects can affect emotional state. Avoid alcohol because it can have a depressive effect. Discuss your feelings with your health care team. Join a cancer support group; if unable to do this, ask for a referral to a therapist. Eat well, exercise, and get plenty of rest.

Data from Groenwald S, Goodman M, Yarbro CH, and others: *Cancer symptom management*, Boston, 1997, Jones & Bartlett.

lessness to occur. Supportive transfusion or erythropoietin therapies may be used. Many patients find support groups beneficial.[1]

INDICATIONS FOR REFERRAL OR HOSPITALIZATION

All patients with suspected leukemia should be referred to a hematologist or oncologist for bone marrow aspiration and biopsy. Definitive diagnosis and treatment plans vary. In general, patients with acute leukemias are referred to a tertiary care center. Chronic leukemias are often managed in the community by a hematologist or oncologist. However, the health care provider plays a major role in the co-management of the leukemias. A hematology consult is suggested before any invasive procedure such as colonoscopy, cystoscopy, or surgery, whether minor or major.

PATIENT EDUCATION AND HEALTH PROMOTION

The educational goal for leukemia patients and their families is prevention of complications of the disease process and treatment, management of side effects, and access to community resources.

The major life-threatening complication of leukemia is bone marrow suppression. This may be a result of either the disease process itself or the chemotherapy instituted to treat the leukemia. The result of bone marrow suppression is a subnormal functioning of the immune system, which puts the patient at risk for sepsis, thrombocytopenia, and anemia. The health care team will notify the patient and family of laboratory results indicating that the patient is at risk.

It is the health care team's responsibility to educate the patient and family regarding the numerous other side effects of leukemia and its treatment, such as fever; headache; mucositis; nausea, vomiting, and anorexia; diarrhea; constipation; pain; fatigue; insomnia; and depression. Patient instructions are given in Box 228-2. After diagnosis, patients still require cancer screening tests specific for age, including mammograms, Papanicolaou's smears, prostate-specific antigen, and fecal occult blood testing. Other health-promoting activities include stopping smoking, maintaining normal weight, and getting adequate exercise.

REFERENCES

1. Wujcik D: Leukemia. In Groenwald S, and others, editors: *Cancer nursing: principles and practice,* ed 4, Boston, 1997, Jones & Bartlett.
2. American Cancer Society: *Cancer facts and figures,* Atlanta, 2005, The Society.
3. Scheinberg D, Maslak P, Weiss M: Acute leukemias. In DaVita VT Jr, Hellman S, Rosenberg SA, editors: *Cancer: principles and practice of oncology,* ed 6, Philadelphia, 2001, Lippincott Williams & Wilkins.
4. Linet M: Leukemias. In Harras A, editor: *Cancer rates and risks,* ed 4, Bethesda, Md, 1996, National Institutes of Health.
5. Miaskowski E: *Oncology nursing: an essential guide for patient care,* Philadelphia, 1997, Saunders.
6. Thirman M, Larson R: Therapy-related myeloid leukemia, *Hematol Oncol Clin North Am* 2:293-320, 1996.
7. Cotran R, Kumar V, Collins T: *Robbins pathologic basis of disease,* ed 6, Philadelphia, 1999, Saunders.
8. Ososki R: Leukemia. In Otto S, editor: *Oncology nursing,* St Louis, 1997, Mosby.
9. Lien-Gieschen T, McMurtry C: Orbital leukemia, *Nurse Pract* 20(1):75-77, 1996.
10. Miller K, and others: Leukemia. In Osteen R, editor: *Cancer manual,* ed 9, Boston, 1996, American Cancer Society.
11. Kantarjian H, Faderl Stalpaz M: Chronic leukemia. In DaVita VT Jr, Hellman S, Rosenberg SA, editors: *Cancer: principles and practice of oncology,* ed 6, Philadelphia, 2001, Lippincott Williams & Wilkins.
12. Rai K, Keating M: Chronic lymphocytic leukemia. In Holland J, and others, editors: *Cancer medicine,* ed 5, Hamilton, Ontario, Canada, 2000, Decker.
13. Wuest D: Transfusion and stem cell support in cancer treatment, *Hematol Oncol Clin North Am* 2:397-429, 1996.
14. Morrison V: The infectious complications of chronic lymphocytic leukemia, *Semin Oncol* 25(1):98-106, 1998.
15. Shelton BK: Oncology emergencies. In Varriechio C, editor: *A cancer sourcebook for nurses,* London, 1997, Jones & Bartlett.
16. Morris J, Holland J: Oncologic emergencies. In Holland J, and others, editors: *Cancer medicine,* ed 5, Hamilton, Ontario, Canada, 2000, Decker.
17. Arnold SM, Patchell R, Lowy AM, and others: Paraneoplastic syndromes. In DaVita VT Jr, Hellman S, Rosenberg SA, editors: *Cancer: principles and practice of oncology,* ed 6, Philadelphia, 2001, Lippincott Williams & Wilkins.

CHAPTER 229

Lymphomas

John Joseph Graykoski

The lymphomas are a diverse group of neoplasms with varied clinical features and biologic patterns. Clonal expansion of the immune system leads to uncontrolled growth of components of the immune system composed of B, T, and/or null cells. More than 30 neoplasms of the lymphoid system are included in this group of malignancies. They can originate in any site bearing lymphoid tissue such as lymph nodes; spleen; bone marrow; and extranodal sites, including the liver, gut, and rarely other viscera. This chapter addresses the malignant lymphomas, which are typically classified as either Hodgkin's disease (HD) or non-Hodgkin's lymphomas (NHL). The two diseases are differentiated based on pathology and are managed differently. Therefore this chapter addresses each disease separately.

HODGKIN'S DISEASE

DEFINITION AND EPIDEMIOLOGY

The 2006 estimate for new cases of HD in the United States was 7800 (4190 men and 3610 women. It was also estimated that there would be 1490 deaths caused by HD, again evenly divided between males and females.[1] In the United States and some industrialized European nations, there is a bimodal age incidence occurrence. The first incidence peak is seen in people during their twenties and the second peak after age 50 years.[2]

The etiology of the disease is unclear. It has no clear relationship with environmental exposures. Although no specific pathogen has been identified, it is suspected that the Epstein-Barr virus (EBV) is involved, given that patients with a history of infectious mononucleosis have a threefold chance of developing HD and approximately half of all HD nodes have evidence of EBV DNA. However, there appears to be another mechanism because many patients with HD have no evidence of EBV or history of mononucleosis. Also, HD appears with increased frequency in patients with AIDS and in patients after bone marrow transplantation.[3]

CLASSIFICATION

The classification of HD has evolved over time. The older classification is the Rye classification, which associates the histopathologic subtypes to clinical behavior and prognosis. These subtypes are lymphocyte predominance, nodular sclerosis (NS), mixed cellularity (MC), and the uncommon lymphocyte depletion (LD).[2] The World Health Organization (WHO) classification proposed the categories of nodular lymphocyte predominant Hodgkin's lymphoma and classical Hodgkin's lymphoma. Classical Hodgkin's lymphoma is subdivided into NS, lymphocyte-rich classical, MC, and LD. The most common form of HD is NS, which accounts for approximately 60% of cases. The second most common histopathologic finding is MC, which occurs in 20% to 40% of presentations.[3]

PATHOPHYSIOLOGY

The primary neoplastic cell in HD is the polynuclear Reed-Sternberg cell. The majority of the lymphatic tissue of HD is composed of normal-appearing lymphocytes, plasma cells, eosinophils, neutrophils, and histiocytes existing in the varied proportion as reflected in the histologic subtypes. In HD a progressive loss of cell-mediated immunity is associated with the development of cutaneous anergy, lymphocytopenia, and increased susceptibility to organisms associated with depressed cell-mediated immunity and herpes zoster.[2]

CLINICAL PRESENTATION

HD generally manifests as painless lymphadenopathy. Constitutional symptoms that may accompany HD include fevers, night sweats, and weight loss. The patient may also experience pruritus and pain in a lymph node region with alcohol intake. Laboratory evaluation may have nonspecific findings, including a mild lymphocytosis, eosinophilia, and an elevated erythrocyte sedimentation rate (ESR).[3]

PHYSICAL EXAMINATION

Important information in the patient's history includes any constitutional symptoms of weight loss, fever, and night sweats. The history should also include information about functional status, pruritus, and alcohol tolerance.[4] The physical examination includes evaluation of the lymph node regions, size of the liver and spleen, and Waldeyer's ring (tonsils) inspection. Pertinent laboratory values are the CBC, including differential and platelets; ESR; liver function tests; and renal function tests.[4,5]

DIAGNOSTICS

Staging

For more than 25 years, the four-stage clinical and pathologic Ann Arbor system has been the most widely used staging system. It yields important prognostic and treatment information (Table 229-1). In predicting survival, the staging system has two groups. The favorable group includes stages I, II, and IIIA, with disease-specific survival at 15 years being 96%. The less favorable group consists of stages IIIB and IV, with the disease-specific survival being 80%. Overall survival rates are 80% and 60%, respectively, for the two groups.[3]

Diagnosis

Generally, a pathologic diagnosis of HD requires an excisional biopsy of the enlarged lymph node. A needle aspiration or core biopsy may help document recurrent disease, but may give false-negative information because of sampling error for the initial diagnosis and is thus insufficient. A needle or surgical biopsy may be required of any extranodal sites that are suspicious for disease. Other important information can be derived from cytologic examination of effusions.[5] A staging laparotomy is performed in rare circumstances in early stage disease when supradiaphragmatic radiotherapy alone is being considered as the only method of treatment.[4] Polyvalent

TABLE 229-1 Ann Arbor Staging System for Lymphoma

Stage*	Substage†	Definition
I	I	Single node region
	IE	Single extralymphatic site or involvement by direct extension
II	II	Two or more node regions on same side of diaphragm
	IIE	Single node region plus single localized extranodal site
	IIS	Spleen
	IIE+S	Extralymphatic site plus spleen
III	III	Involvement on both sides of diaphragm
IV	IV	Diffuse extralymphatic involvement

From Cheson BJ: Hodgkin's disease and the non-Hodgkin's lymphomas. In Lenhard RE, Osteen RT, Gansler T, editors: *Clinical oncology,* Atlanta, 2001, American Cancer Society.
*Stages can be further classified as A (B symptoms absent) or B (B symptoms [fever, chills, night sweats, weight loss] present) (can be designated at any stage).
†Localized extralymphatic lesions with or without associated lymph node involvement are termed *E* (extranodal) lesions, and those involving the spleen are termed *S*.

DIAGNOSTICS

Lymphomas

LABORATORY
CBC and differential
Serum electrolytes
LFTs
BUN
Creatinine
Serologic evaluation for Epstein-Barr virus
HIV test
Toxoplasmosis titer

IMAGING
Chest x-ray
CT scan of chest, abdomen, pelvis, head
Lumbar puncture
Gallium or thallium scan*

OTHER
Lymph node biopsy
Bone marrow biopsy

*If indicated.

pneumococcal vaccine should be given approximately 2 weeks before staging laparotomy to prevent the possibility of overwhelming sepsis from encapsulated organisms.[6] Other staging diagnostics should include a chest radiograph, chest and abdominal or pelvic CT scans, and a single-photon emission gallium scan. Positron emission tomography (PET) scans are being widely studied and compared with MRI and CT scans for their ability to evaluate abnormal lymph nodes.[3] A bone marrow biopsy is typically performed in patients with HD as part of initial staging.

DIFFERENTIAL DIAGNOSIS

Lymphadenopathy may be a primary or secondary sign of numerous disorders, including infectious diseases, immunologic disorders, and malignant diseases[7] (see Chapter 241). Although malignant lymphadenopathy is rare in the primary care setting, malignant lymphomas should be considered when infection or an inflammatory process has been excluded.[6] A patient with unexplained lymphadenopathy not related to infection or inflammation may need a biopsy to rule out malignancy.[7]

DIFFERENTIAL DIAGNOSIS

Lymphomas

- Infectious process
- Viral syndromes
- Mononucleosis
- HIV
- Bacteremia
- Toxoplasmosis
- Autoimmune disease
- Other malignancy

MANAGEMENT

There may be more than one treatment approach in the management of the patient with HD. The goal is to determine a course of therapy that is potentially curative while minimizing long-term complications.

The course of treatment is based on the stage and prognostic factors. The adverse prognostic factors are advanced age, male gender, histologic subtype, constitutional symptoms, mediastinal mass, number of involved nodal regions, elevated ESR, anemia, and low serum albumin.[5] The treatment for patients with early stage and favorable prognostic factor profile is generally radiation. Patients with early stage disease and an unfavorable risk profile are generally treated with both chemotherapy (typically four cycles) and radiotherapy. Patients in advanced stages receive an extensive course of chemotherapy (eight cycles) with or without consolidating radiotherapy.[5] Eighty percent of patients with bulky mediastinal or retroperitoneal disease who respond to therapy have a persistent radiographic abnormality, which may remain longer than 1 year in half of those cases, without evidence of disease progression. Many of these patients are given additional radiation to sites of bulky disease. They should be observed closely with chest radiographs. Confirmation biopsy and therapy may be needed if the mass continues to enlarge or if disease appears outside of the radiated field. A positive PET scan may also provide evidence to differentiate residual tumor from fibrosis.[3]

Relapsing or Refractory Disease

Although HD is a relatively curable disease, 20% to 30% of patients never achieve a complete remission (CR) or partial remission (PR). Another 20% to 30% relapse after an initial CR. Treatment decisions with patients who have experienced relapse include review of initial therapy and duration of initial response. Patients who experience late relapses from CR or durable PR (>12 months) have a more favorable prognosis and may be treated with combination chemotherapy, with about 15% remaining in remission at 5 years. The prognosis for patients with an early relapse from CR is poor.[3] High-dose therapy with autologous bone marrow or peripheral blood stem cell support may be considered in relapsed patients.[8]

NON-HODGKIN'S LYMPHOMA

DEFINITION AND EPIDEMIOLOGY

The American Cancer Society estimates that 58,870 people (30,689 men and 29,190 women) will be diagnosed with NHL in 2006 and 18,840 people will die.[9] There was a 3.1% decrease in deaths from NHL in all races and in both males and females from 1997 to 2002.[9] During the past 2 decades, the incidence of NHL rose at almost 7% per year, but recently the incidence has leveled, if not decreased. The rise in occurrence was seen most strikingly in older adults and primarily in the diffuse, large B-cell histologic group.[3]

The explanation for the rise in NHL incidence and the cause of NHL are unknown. There is a noted increase in the frequency of aggressive NHL in patients who are on long-term immunosuppressive medicines after allogeneic bone marrow transplant and in patients with inherited immune defects, rheumatoid arthritis, or HIV/AIDS. There is also an association between a variety of infectious agents and lymphomas, including EBV with Burkitt's lymphoma in immunodeficient patients, human herpesvirus 8 with body cavity–based lymphoma, and human T-cell lymphotropic virus 1 with adult T-cell leukemia/lymphoma. *Helicobacter pylori* has been linked to gastric mucosa–associated lymphoid tissue (MALT) lymphomas (or MALTomas).[5] There have also been reports of an association with environmental factors such as pesticides and agricultural chemicals, exercise, smoking, and hair dyes.[3]

Classification

Multiple attempts have been made to classify lymphomas using morphologic characteristics, immunophenotype, and genetic and clinical features to distinguish between the multiple entities that compose the NHLs. The earlier classifications systems, including the Working Formulation (WF) and the Revised European–American Lymphoma (REAL), were recently modified by the WHO. The WF is the most commonly used classification of NHL (Box 229-1). It describes the most common lymphomas. However, it does not recognize a large variety of newly described clinicopathologic entities within the lymphomas. The REAL-WHO classification correlates the lymphoma classification with the normal lymphocyte counterpart. Therefore it is particularly applicable to uncommon lymphomas.[2]

BOX 229-1

CLASSIFICATION OF NON-HODGKIN'S LYMPHOMA: THE WORKING FORMULATION

LOW GRADE

Small lymphocytic
- Chronic lymphocytic leukemia-type
- Plasmacytoid

Follicular, small cleaved cell
Follicular, mixed (small cleaved and large cell)

INTERMEDIATE GRADE

Follicular, large cell
Diffuse, small cleaved cell
Diffuse, mixed cell (small and large cell)
Diffuse, large cell

HIGH GRADE

Immunoblastic (large cell)
Lymphoblastic
Small, noncleaved
- Burkitt's
- Non-Burkitt's

From Emmanouilides C, Casciato DA, Rosen PJ: Hodgkin and non-Hodgkin lymphoma. In Casciato DA, Lowitz BB, editors: *Manual of clinical oncology*, ed 4, Philadelphia, 2000, Lippincott.

PATHOPHYSIOLOGY

The molecular biology research of NHL has identified clues to the pathogenesis of some of these disorders. The translocation of t(14;18) is detectable at 80% to 90% of patient with follicular NHL, and the *BCL2* gene has been cloned at that breakpoint. This gene overexpression prevents apoptosis, or programmed cell death. In mantle cell lymphoma, the *BCL1* gene and cyclin D1 are overexpressed.[3]

CLINICAL PRESENTATION

Patients often are seen with signs or symptoms related to the lymphadenopathy.[3] They may also have constitutional symptoms of fevers, night sweats, and weight loss.[5]

PHYSICAL EXAMINATION

The history and physical examination can yield important information. The presence of constitutional symptoms, as described previously, can have adverse prognostic implications. Other pertinent information includes pain that can be related to sites of disease and co-morbidities such as diabetes or heart disease that may limit treatment options.[5] On physical examination the health care provider should carefully evaluate lymph node areas and the size of the liver and spleen. Other important physical examination findings may include pharyngeal involvement, thyroid mass, pleural effusion, abdominal mass, testicular mass, cutaneous lesions, and Waldeyer's ring. All these findings may direct further investigations and therapies.

DIAGNOSTICS

Laboratory studies should include CBC and screening chemistries, including glucose, calcium, albumin, lactate dehydrogenase, and beta$_2$-microglobulin.[5]

Staging

The initial staging evaluation provides treatment, prognostic, and clinical trial data. The Ann Arbor staging classification is also used in NHL. The International Prognostic Index is widely used to predict outcome. It was initially developed for patients with diffuse aggressive lymphoma, but experience has shown that it applies to patients with almost all subtypes of NHL.[10]

Diagnostic Tests

An initial excisional lymph node biopsy is recommended for precise diagnosis and clarification of the histopathology. Needle biopsies may not provide enough information to distinguish between histologic traits of the different NHLs. An aspirate or core needle biopsy may provide enough information to confirm a suspected recurrence in patients who have previously been diagnosed. The increased use of flow cytometry, cytogenetics, and molecular genetic studies can provide information for analysis from a core needle biopsy and in some instances fine-needle biopsy when dealing with a lymphoma in the mediastinal, retroperitoneal, or other inaccessible locations.[3]

The staging workup should include CT scan of the chest, abdomen, and pelvis and a gallium scan. PET scans are used more frequently than CT, and at least one study has shown that the combination of CT and PET changed the staging of disease by nearly a third when compared with CT alone. This also resulted in a 25% change in choice of treatment.[11]

DIFFERENTIAL DIAGNOSIS

See Hodgkin's Disease, Differential Diagnosis, p. 1219.

MANAGEMENT

The current approach to the treatment of NHL depends on the stage and histologic subtype.

Low-Grade Non-Hodgkin's Lymphoma

Low-grade histologic subtypes include small lymphocytic leukemia, follicular grades I and II. Only about 10% to 15% of patients with grade I or II follicular NHL are initially seen with stages I or II disease. These patients may be treated with local radiotherapy. Advanced stage low-grade NHL is incurable, and there is no evidence that early treatment prolongs survival.[12] Because the therapies have toxicity, treatment is usually given only to patients who are symptomatic. Numerous standard chemotherapies are used, including single agents or combination chemotherapy involving the alkylating agents or purine analogs. Treatment is generally continued until a maximum response in the disease is seen. There is no clear evidence of a survival advantage in maintenance therapy.[2]

Relapsed or Refractory Disease. Patients with low-grade NHL usually relapse. Response with chemotherapy can be achieved with similar regimens, but the response is usually of shorter duration with each treatment. Patients who experience relapse can convert to a high-grade NHL, which has a poor prognosis. Early treatment of these patients may result in the possibility of disease-free survival.[3]

New Approaches. During the past few years, two new classes of drugs have influenced therapy in NHL. These drugs are the purine nucleoside analogs and monoclonal antibodies. Purine nucleoside analogs in combination with other chemotherapy drugs have resulted in impressive response rates for patients with low-grade lymphomas.[13] The first monoclonal antibody to be approved by the U.S. Food and Drug Administration (FDA) for treatment of a human malignancy is rituximab. It is directed against the cells containing the CD20 receptor, which are expressed on more than 90% of B-cell lymphomas. Rituximab is generally well tolerated with the major side effects of fevers and chills. After the first infusion, most patients have no toxicity for the remainder of the treatment.[12,14]

Monoclonal antibodies to other lymphoma antigens and monoclonal antibodies conjugated to radioisotopes have received FDA approval. These include ibritumomab tiuxetan (Zevalin), tositumomab (Bexxar), and Alemtuzumab (Campath). Denileukin diftitox (Ontak) is a form of interleukin-2 and the diphtheria toxin, which is being used for T-cell skin lymphomas.[15] Promising new therapy includes the use of vaccines, prepared from the patient's own tumor cells, that stimulate an antibody reaction to the cancerous cells.[16]

Intermediate or High-Grade Lymphomas

Generally, patients who are seen with local, nonbulky disease may be treated with combination chemotherapy containing doxorubicin and radiotherapy to the site of disease. Patients with bulky disease are generally treated with cyclophosphamide, doxorubicin, vincristine, and prednisone chemotherapy (CHOP). Patients may benefit from radiotherapy if the bulky disease can be encompassed in a radiation port.[2] Recent data show that the addition of rituximab to CHOP chemotherapy resulted in a significantly increased rate of complete response and 2-year event-free survival in older patients with diffuse large B-cell lymphoma compared with CHOP chemotherapy alone.[17]

Within the classification of intermediate or high-grade NHL, there is a subset of less common NHL disease that may have a unique natural history and therapies. These include mantle cell lymphoma, Burkitt's or Burkitt's-like lymphoma, and lymphoblastic lymphoma. Mantle cell lymphoma exhibits the worst features of lymphoma in that it is not curable and has an aggressive clinical course. CR can be achieved, but the disease generally recurs with a median survival of 2½ to 3 years.[3] Patients with mantle cell lymphoma should be considered for clinical trials. Burkitt's or Burkitt's-like lymphoma and lymphoblastic lymphoma are highly aggressive, have exponential growth rate, and disseminate to the bone marrow and meninges. There has been some success in treatment of Burkitt's or Burkitt's-like lymphoma with intensive short-course chemotherapy. Lymphoblastic lymphoma may be treated similarly to lymphoblastic leukemia with dose-intensive cyclophosphamide and anthracycline and standard dose vincristine and asparaginase chemotherapy.[18]

Relapsed or Refractory Disease. Only 40% of patients treated with CHOP chemotherapy are cured. The majority of recurrences happen within 2 years. Late recurrences can demonstrate a low-grade histology, so biopsies of recurrences are necessary. The therapy of patients with relapsed or refractory disease has been investigated with some success.[19,20] Data have supported the use of high-dose chemotherapy with stem cell support in patients who are in the first or subsequent relapse and are still chemosensitive, those with primary induction failure, and those in first remission who were International Prognostic Index (IPI) high-intermediate–risk or high-risk categories. Patients with primary refractory disease and relapsed disease may be considered for allogeneic stem cell therapy. Clinical trials may also be offered to these patients.[17] The biologic therapies of rituximab and ^{131}I -conjugated anti-CD20 antibody (tositumomab) have shown some clinical response.

Marginal Zone Lymphomas

Marginal zone lymphomas consist of MALT NHL, monocytoid B-cell NHL, primary (nodal counterparts to MALTomas), and primary splenic lymphoma with villous lymphocytes. The MALTomas account for about 80% of the indolent NHLs of the stomach. The majority are associated with *H. pylori* and are highly responsive to double or triple antibiotic therapy. Splenic lymphoma is generally disseminated with peripheral blood and bone marrow involvement at diagnosis. A splenectomy can provide a prolonged clinical remission.[3]

Peripheral T-Cell Lymphoma

Peripheral T-cell lymphoma (PTCL) consists of a diverse group of post-thymic T-cell tumors that have a mature T-cell phenotype. They make up fewer than 10% of NHLs in the United States, but they generally first appear with advanced stage disease, constitutional symptoms, and a poorer prognosis in comparison with B-cell lymphoma. Classifications in this lymphoma include PTCL otherwise unspecified (generally 50% of cases), anaplastic large cell lymphoma, angioimmunoblastic T-cell lymphoma, angiocentric lymphoma, adult T-cell leukemia/lymphoma, and a few less common lymphomas. In general, patients with PTCL are treated with aggressive combination chemotherapy such as CHOP. However, often they have a poor response to treatment and a high rate of relapse, with no long-term remissions.[3]

LIFE SPAN CONSIDERATIONS

Patients should be monitored carefully after treatment, and this can be coordinated with the patient's hematology or oncology physician. The necessary radiologic and laboratory studies are usually done by or can be coordinated with the patient's hematologist or oncologist to ensure adequate follow-up evaluation.[21]

Under some circumstances, gonadal dysfunction can affect quality of life after treatment. Transient and sometimes permanent male sterility may occur.[6] Infertility may occur in at least 80% of women over 25 years of age who receive nitrogen mustard, vincristine, procarbazine, or prednisone chemotherapy. This may be reversible after up to three courses of therapy. The newer, nonalkylating agent–containing regimens have a lower risk of infertility. However, sperm banking should be considered before initiating treatment. Pregnancies occurring in patients or their partners do not appear to be associated with complications, congenital abnormalities, or spontaneous abortions.[3]

Improved treatment regimens and survival mean that many patients will return to health care providers for care and monitoring. Advance directives should be discussed with the patient, but with the understanding that some lymphomas can be treated successfully or have an indolent course. Patients are encouraged to prepare a living will and appoint a health care proxy so that both the health care proxy and the health care provider understand their preferences for terminal care.

COMPLICATIONS

Complications from lymphoma can occur during treatment, as a result of treatment, or from the disease itself.

During Therapy

Patients with cancer who undergo chemotherapy and radiotherapy are at risk of infection because of the immunosuppression from the cancer, myelosuppression from chemotherapy, the break in skin barriers from the placement of Port-a-caths and central lines, or shifts in microbial flora. The myelosuppressive effect of chemotherapy can cause neutropenia. Absolute neutropenia is defined as less than 1000/mm^3 neutrophils and bands in the bloodstream and is calculated by multiplying the total number of white cells from the CBC by the total percentage of neutrophils plus bands. The period of neutropenia after chemotherapy is relatively predictable, with the lowest count of neutrophils occurring approximately 10 to 14 days after chemotherapy and recovering in about 3 to 4 weeks after chemotherapy. Although fever can be a presenting sign in a patient with lymphoma, fever in a patient after chemotherapy, especially in a neutropenic patient, may be a sign of life-threatening sepsis. In addition, patients who have undergone splenectomy have a lifelong risk of overwhelming sepsis by encapsulated organisms.[21] Research shows that colony-stimulating factors (CSFs) can reduce the incidence of febrile neutropenia; however, these medications can be inconvenient and expensive and have toxicities, including bone pain. Guidelines for CSF administration have been issued by the American Society of Clinical Oncology, and these medications should be administered based on the recommendation of the treating hematologist or oncologist.[22]

Fatigue is a poorly understood phenomenon that affects the patient's quality of life. It can occur as a result of the treatment or the disease. It may be associated with anxiety or depression or with physiologic processes related to tumor necrosis factor and interleukin-1 and other cytokines. Physiologic conditions such as anemia resulting from the chemotherapy and radiotherapy may also contribute to fatigue. A careful review of symptoms and CBC with differential is important. Current recommendations include education to relieve anxiety, activities that provide distraction, and participation in low-intensity exercise.[18] Packed red blood cell transfusion should be given to patients with severe anemia. Patients with mild anemia may benefit from erythropoietin.[23,24]

Pain is a common complaint in cancer patients. It is experienced by one third of persons receiving treatment and two thirds who have advanced disease. A broad assessment of the symptom is important and should include location, duration, quality, and impact on the patient's life.[25] The range of strategies to relieve pain may target the cause of the pain itself (chemotherapy and radiotherapy), or pharmacologic therapy may rely on the analgesic ladder from the WHO.[26] Nonopioid and adjuvant analgesics such as acetaminophen and NSAIDs may be used. Potential side effects and concerns about gastrointestinal and renal toxicity may limit NSAID use. Other adjuvant analgesics may include steroids as a multipurpose therapy. Antidepressants and anticonvulsants are often used for neuropathic pain. When drug therapy does not resolve pain, consideration can be given for anesthetic, surgical, neurostimulatory, physiatric, or psychologic interventions.[25]

Posttreatment Toxicities

A serious consequence of treatment is the increased risk of a second cancer, including acute myeloid leukemia (AML). The risk of secondary AML extends up to approximately 11 years posttreatment. Radiotherapy with and without chemotherapy may contribute to increased risk of solid tumors in the radiation field. Solid tumors tend to occur in the second decade posttreatment. Breast cancers in this population are often bilateral. Regular breast examination and mammography starting at an early age are recommended as part of routine posttreatment.[3]

More than two thirds of patients who undergo mantle irradiation develop thyroid disease, including hypothyroidism, Graves' disease, silent thyrotoxicosis, and nodules, with a 2% risk of cancer. Mantle field irradiation also adds to the risk of cardiac toxicity.[3]

Other serious treatment complications are cardiotoxicity, which can be fatal, and pulmonary toxicity. High doses of doxorubicin can cause cardiomyopathy. Mantle-field radiotherapy can cause pericarditis, but the incidence of this complication has declined as a result of recent improvements in the delivery of radiotherapy. Mantle field radiotherapy can also cause radiation pneumonitis and chronic restrictive fibrosis. It is unclear whether radiotherapy results in the acceleration of coronary artery disease.[27] Pulmonary fibrosis or restrictive disease has also been associated with bleomycin chemotherapy.

INDICATIONS FOR REFERRAL OR HOSPITALIZATION

A patient should be referred to a hematologist or oncologist after confirming the diagnosis of malignant lymphoma. Patients with high-risk disease should be referred to a comprehensive cancer center whenever possible. These centers can often provide oncology care with access to the latest research treatments.

Patients with a diagnosis of lymphoma in remission should request that the hematologist or oncologist forward treatment records to the health care provider. Follow-up examinations should focus on both the presenting signs and symptoms of the disease and new symptoms or lymphadenopathy. The patient should be referred back to the hematologist or oncologist if constitutional symptoms continue or recur or if suspicious nodes are found.

There is a high prevalence of depression among cancer patients. Patients who are depressed may find help through psychotherapy that involves social support, coping skills, emotional expression, and cognitive restructuring.[28]

The majority of treatments for lymphoma can be administered in an outpatient setting. The patient might be hospitalized for high-dose chemotherapy requiring careful monitoring of laboratory values and blood product support, as well as for episodes of febrile neutropenia.

PATIENT AND FAMILY EDUCATION

One of the most common reactions to the stress of cancer diagnosis and treatment is anxiety and depression. Education about the disease, treatment, and prognosis can help relieve anxiety. Educational and social support resources for patients include American Cancer Society programs such as "I Can Cope" (http://www.cancer.org/docroot/ESN/content/ESN_3_1X_I_Can_Cope.asp), the National Cancer Institute website (http://www.cancer.gov/cancertopics/coping), and Oncolink (http://oncolink.upenn.edu/coping/article.cfm?c=6&s=28&ss=62&id=54).

Nutrition education should begin at diagnosis to prevent complications caused by malnutrition and weight loss often associated with treatment. Dietary counseling should address the need for calorie-, protein-rich foods.[22] Alcoholic beverages should be avoided. Given the treatment-related pulmonary and cardiac toxicity, smoking cessation should be encouraged.

REFERENCES

1. National Cancer Institute: *Cancer stat fact sheet: Hodgkin lymphoma,* retrieved Feb 21, 2007, from http://seer.cancer.gov/statfacts/html/hodg.html?statfacts_page=hodg.html&x=14&y=17.
2. Casciato DA, Lowitz BB: *Manual of clinical oncology,* ed 4, Philadelphia, 2000, Lippincott.
3. Lenhard RE, Osteen RT, Gansler T: *Clinical oncology,* Atlanta, 2001, American Cancer Society.
4. Hoppe RT, and others: *NCCN practice guidelines for Hodgkin's disease,* Rockledge, Penn, 2000, National Comprehensive Cancer Network.
5. DaVita VT Jr, Hellman S, Rosenberg SA, and others, editors: *Cancer: principles and practice of oncology,* ed 6, Philadelphia, 2001, Lippincott.
6. Yarbro CH, Frogge MH, Goodman M, and others, editors: *Cancer nursing,* ed 5, Boston, 2001, Jones & Bartlett.
7. Ferrer R: Lymphadenopathy: differential diagnosis and evaluation, *Am Fam Phys* 58(6):1313-1320, 1998.
8. Moskowitz CH, Nimer SD, Zelenetz AD, and others: A two-step comprehensive high-dose chemoradiotherapy second-line program for relapsed and refractory Hodgkin disease: analysis by intent to treat and development of a prognostic model, *Blood* 97(3):616-623, 2001.
9. National Cancer Institute: *Cancer stat fact sheet: non-Hodgkin lymphoma,* retrieved Feb 21, 2007, from http://seer.cancer.gov/statfacts/html/nhl.html.
10. A predictive model for aggressive non-Hodgkin's lymphoma. The International Non-Hodgkin's Lymphoma Prognostic Factors Project, *N Engl J Med* 329(14):987-994, 1993.
11. Raanani P, Shasha Y, Perry C, and others: Is CT scan still necessary for staging in Hodgkin and non-Hodgkin lymphoma patients in the PET/CT era? *Ann Oncol* 17:117-122, 2006.
12. Horning SJ: Follicular lymphoma: have we made any progress? *Ann Oncol* 11(Suppl 1):S23-S27, 2000.
13. McLaughlin P, Hagemeister FB, Romaguera JE, and others: Fludarabine, mitoxantrone, and dexamethasone: an effective new regimen for indolent lymphoma, *J Clin Oncol* 14(4):1262-1268, 1996.
14. McLaughlin P, Grillo-Lopez AJ, Link BK, and others: Rituximab chimeric anti-CD20 monoclonal antibody therapy for relapsed indolent lymphoma: half of patients respond to a four-dose treatment program, *J Clin Oncol* 16(8):2825-2833, 1998.
15. American Cancer Society: *Detailed guide: lymphoma, non-Hodgkin's type: biological therapy (immunotherapy),* revised Aug 2005, retrieved Jan 22, 2006, from http://www.cancer.org/docroot/CRI/content/CRI_2_4_4X_Biological_Therapy_32.asp?rnav=cri.
16. Santos C, Stern L, Katz L, and others: BiovaxID™ vaccine therapy of follicular lymphoma in first remission: long-term follow-up of a phase II trial and status of a controlled, randomized phase III trial, presented at the 47th annual meeting of the American Hematology Society (ASH), abstract No 2441, Dec 11, 2005, Atlanta.
17. Coiffier B, Lepage E, Briere J, and others: CHOP chemotherapy plus rituximab compared with CHOP alone in elderly patients with diffuse large-B-cell lymphoma, *N Engl J Med* 346(4):235-242, 2002.
18. Zelenetz A, and others: *NCCN practice guidelines for non-Hodgkin's lymphomas,* Rockledge, Penn, 2000, National Comprehensive Cancer Network.
19. Wilson WH, Bryant G, Bates S, and others: EPOCH chemotherapy: toxicity and efficacy in relapsed and refractory non-Hodgkin's lymphoma, *J Clin Oncol* 11(8):1573-1582, 1993.
20. Rodriguez MA, Cabanillas FC, Velasquez W, and others: Results of a salvage treatment program for relapsing lymphoma: MINE consolidated with ESHAP, *J Clin Oncol* 13(7):1734-1741, 1995.
21. Boyer K, Ford M, Judkins A, and others: *Primary care oncology,* Philadelphia, 1999, Saunders.
22. Yarbro CH, Frogge MH, Goodman M, editors: *Cancer symptom management,* ed 2, Boston, 1999, Jones & Bartlett.
23. Ozer H, Armitage JO, Bennett CL, and others: 2000 update of recommendations for the use of hematopoietic colony-stimulating factors: evidence-based, clinical practice guidelines, *J Clin Oncol* 18(20):3558-3585, 2000.

24. Groopman JE, Itri LM: Chemotherapy-induced anemia in adults: incidence and treatment, *J Natl Cancer Inst* 91(19):1616-1634, 1999.
25. Portenoy RK, Lesage P: Management of cancer pain, *Lancet* 353:1695-1700, 1999.
26. World Health Organization: *WHO's pain ladder*, retrieved Feb 28, 2007, from http://www.who.int/cancer/palliative/painladder/en/.
27. Urba WJ, Longo DL: Medical progress: Hodgkin's disease, *N Engl J Med* 326(10):678-687, 1992.
28. Spiegel D: Cancer and depression, *Br J Psychiatry* 168(Suppl 30):109-116, 1996.

CHAPTER 230

Myelodysplastic Syndromes

Anna D. Schaal

DEFINITION AND EPIDEMIOLOGY

The myelodysplastic syndromes (MDSs) are a heterogeneous group of bone marrow disorders characterized by ineffective dysplastic growth of the hematopoietic precursors. Dominant features of this group of diseases include impaired maturation of hematopoietic stem cells and increased cell death, or apoptosis. MDS is not one disease, but a diverse family of malignancies that have variable clinical presentation, biologic activity, and prognosis.

MDS is a relatively rare disease. It is primarily a disease of the elderly with the annual incidence rate rising to 15 to 50 per 100,000 persons per year in those 70 years old and older.[1] Approximately 15,000 new cases of MDS are diagnosed each year in the United States. Males are affected about 1.5 to 2 times as often as females.

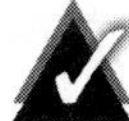

Physician consultation is indicated for all suspected cases of MDS.

PATHOPHYSIOLOGY

The knowledge of pathophysiologic abnormalities that contribute to MDS is advancing at a remarkable pace. Defects in cellular differentiation, responsiveness to cytokines and growth factors, an altered hematopoietic microenvironment, increased apoptosis, and abnormal DNA methylation are all pathways that lead to the ineffective hematopoiesis that is the trademark of MDS (Box 230-1). This ineffective hematopoiesis results in peripheral cytopenias despite a packed, hypercellular bone marrow. In essence, the bone marrow produces cells that are not able to mature into functional red blood cells, white blood cells, and platelets.

BOX 230-1

MYELODYSPLASTIC SYNDROME AT A GLANCE

PATHOGENESIS

- Altered hematopoietic microenvironment
- Increased apoptosis
- Defective cellular differentiation
- Abnormal DNA methylation

CLINICAL FINDINGS

- Usually the end result of underlying cytopenia
- Fatigue, symptoms of anemia, bleeding, and recurrent infections possibly the first sign
- Often diagnosed incidentally by routine CBC

DIAGNOSIS

- Peripheral blood smear review
- Bone marrow biopsy with cytogenetics definitive test for diagnosis
- Hypercellular marrow with peripheral cytopenias is hallmark

TABLE 230-1 International Prognostic Scoring System for Myelodysplastic Syndromes: Survival and Acute Myeloid Leukemia Evolution

	Score				
Prognostic Variables	**0**	**0.5**	**1.0**	**1.5**	**2.0**
Bone marrow blasts (%)	<5	5-10	—	11-20	21-30
Karyotype*	Good	Intermediate	Poor		
Cytopenias	0/1	2/3			

From Greenberg P, Cox C, LeBeau MM, and others: International scoring system for evaluating prognosis in myelodysplastic syndromes [see comment], *Blood* 89(6):2079-2088, 1997 [erratum appears in *Blood* 91(3):1100, 1998].

Scores for risk groups are as follows: Low, 0; intermediate 1, 0.5-1.0; intermediate 2, 1.5-2.0; and high, >2.5.

*Good, normal, –Y, del (5q–), del (20q); poor, complex (>3 abnormalities or chromosome 7 anomalies); intermediate, other abnormalities.

The diagnostic classification of MDS has been a controversial topic for years. Most recently the World Health Organization (WHO) has proposed a new classification system. The acceptable categories include refractory anemia, refractory anemia with ringed sideroblasts, refractory cytopenia with mulitlineage dysplasia, 5q-syndrome, and myelodysplasia unclassifiable.[1] Each category of MDS behaves in a different manner and has different treatment implications.

The International Prognostic Scoring System (IPSS) is another useful classification system that is used to score the number of different variants of MDS (Table 230-1). The scoring is based on three factors: the percentage of blasts in the bone marrow, the specific karyotype or genetic abnormality, and the number of cytopenias. Corresponding scores that range from 0 to 2 help predict both survival and the risk of evolution to acute myeloid leukemia.[2] The IPSS is used to help with projecting prognosis and making treatment decisions.

CLINICAL PRESENTATION AND PHYSICAL EXAMINATION

The clinical presentation of MDS is generally related to symptoms of bone marrow failure, or of the specific cytopenias that each patient is experiencing. If the red blood cells are the prominent lineage that is not maturing, then symptoms of anemia will be present. These may include fatigue, pallor, headaches, shortness of breath (or dyspnea) on exertion, and chest pains or palpitations. If the platelet count is low, symptoms of easy bruising or bleeding will be the dominant presenting symptom. Frequent nose bleeds, petechiae, hematochezia, heavy menstrual bleeding, or large hematomas may encourage a patient to seek medical attention. Finally, if the white blood cells are not maturing, then symptoms of neutropenia—namely, frequent or severe infections—will be the main presenting symptom. Splenomegaly is uncommon in MDS. Increasingly, more and more patients are being diagnosed incidentally from an abnormal CBC done routinely in the primary care setting. In this case, patients feel well and have no subjective or physical examination findings that would make one suspect a myelodysplastic disorder.

DIAGNOSTICS

Myelodysplastic Disorders

LABORATORY
CBC and differential
Peripheral blood smear evaluation

OTHER
Bone marrow biopsy with cytogenetics, flow cytometry, and immunohistochemical staining

DIAGNOSTICS

A number of specific diagnostic tests are required to make the diagnosis of MDS. These include a peripheral blood smear review, a bone marrow biopsy and aspirate with cytogenetic analysis, flow cytometry, and immunohistochemical staining.

The peripheral blood smear will often reveal erythrocytes with anisocytosis, poikilocytosis, or basophilic stippling. The granulocytes may be larger than normal and may lack normal granulation. Platelets may also be larger than normal.

The bone marrow biopsy almost always shows a hypercellular, packed marrow, which is in sharp contrast to the peripheral cytopenia. The hypercellular marrow often demonstrates defects in cellular maturation in all cell lines. For erythroid precursors this includes megaloblastic cells, which are predominantly younger forms and mature cells with distorted nuclei. Ringed sideroblasts will often be identified. These red blood cells are characterized by the presence of excessive cytoplasmic iron granules in a perinuclear distribution.[3] Megakaryocytes are the polynuclear cells responsible for platelet production. In MDS the megakaryocytes are often smaller than normal and hypolobulated. The precursors for white blood cells may also have abnormal granulation and deformed nuclei.

Cytogenetic abnormalities play a role in prognosis. It is estimated that more than 80% of cases of MDS have an altered number or form of chromosomes.[4] Common abnormalities include 5q-, which is a good prognostic indicator, and monosomy 7, which is associated with a poor prognosis and an increased risk of transformation to acute leukemia.

DIFFERENTIAL DIAGNOSIS

Several disorders may mimic the morphologic changes of MDS and should be considered in the differential diagnosis. If macrocytic anemia is the only presenting cytopenia, common types of anemias must first be excluded, including folate and vitamin B_{12} deficiency, iron deficiency, anemia of chronic disease, renal failure, alcohol abuse, hereditary sphereocytosis, and hemolysis. Infection such as HIV, parvovirus, and Epstein-Barr virus should also be ruled out. Drug toxicity or adverse reactions often imitate the cytopenias of MDS. Primary acute

DIFFERENTIAL DIAGNOSIS

Myelodysplastic Disorders

- Vitamin B_{12}, folic acid, or iron deficiency
- Drug toxicity
- Alcohol toxicity
- HIV
- Irradiation
- Parvovirus
- Epstein-Barr virus
- Anemia of chronic disease
- Hemolysis
- Renal failure
- Leukemia

or chronic leukemia or a metastatic solid tumor with bone marrow metastasis should also be considered in the differential diagnosis. Once these disorders have been ruled out, one must consider the diagnosis of myelodysplasia.

MANAGEMENT

The clinical pathway of MDS and response to therapy vary significantly among individuals. The therapy for MDS ranges from supportive care to aggressive treatments. A variety of agents are known to produce a response in MDS. Treatment decisions need to be tailored to the individual patient and should consider age, functional status, and IPSS score. For those who are not good candidates for aggressive treatment strategies or who have failed such treatment attempts, supportive care becomes the foundation of therapy. This approach includes cytokine treatments and transfusion support. There is no evidence of any survival benefit from these treatments; however, they may improve quality of life as they improve symptoms and decrease transfusion requirements. Cytokine treatment consists of erythropoietin (EPO), granulocyte colony-stimulating factor (G-CSF), and granulocyte-macrophage colony-stimulating factor (GM-CSF).

EPO is a hormone that stimulates red blood cell production. Approximately 20% of patients will respond to EPO with an increase in their hemoglobin. The patients who respond are usually those with low or no transfusion requirements.[5] Interestingly, the addition of G-CSF to EPO creates a synergy that improves the erythroid response in up to 50% of patients.[6] G-CSF and GM-CSF both stimulate white blood cell production. The absolute granulocyte count often increases with the use of these cytokines; however, the actual number of infections does not decrease.[7] Because of this, this therapy is generally not used routinely but more often when there is an active infection or an increased risk of infection.

Most patients eventually become red cell transfusion dependent. Transfusions benefit patients in that their symptoms of anemia improve; however, this is only a temporary improvement. The complications of chronic red blood cell transfusions include risk of infection, transfusion reactions, iron overload, and thus accompanying chelation therapy. Quality-of-life issues emerge in the transfusion-dependent patient because of the time, resources, and support burden for patients who are required to go to a clinic for transfusions on a frequent basis.

Fortunately a number of novel agents are now available or in clinical trial for MDS to prolong time to transfusion dependence. 5-Azacitidine, the first agent approved for the treatment of MDS, was approved by the U.S. Food and Drug Administration (FDA) in 2004. 5-Azacitidine inhibits DNA methylation. Hypomethylation restores normal function of silenced growth genes that are responsible for differentiation and proliferation. A clinical trial supported its use, showing improvement in 24% of patients, with 66% of these responders becoming transfusion independent.[8] 5-Azacitidine is delivered in a subcutaneous injection for 7 days every 4 weeks. Its prominent side effects include myelosuppression, pain or skin reaction at injection sites, and nausea.

Thalidomide is an agent that has gained popularity in the treatment of MDS. It is not FDA approved for this use; however, the National Comprehensive Cancer Network (NCCN) recommends its use as a low-intensity therapy.[9] The bone marrow failure characteristic of MDS is in part mediated by angiogenic and proapoptotic cytokines such as tumor necrosis factor-alpha (TNF-alpha) and interleukin-1. Thalidomide acts to down-regulate these cytokines and thus decrease apoptosis and angiogenesis.[10] Approximately 20% of patients will have an improvement in peripheral counts when taking thalidomide.[11] Patients with a low IPSS are better able to maintain a durable duration of response.[12] Thalidomide's major side effect profile includes peripheral neuropathy, sedation, fatigue, constipation, teratogenicity, and thomboembolic events. It is recommended that patients taking thalidomide consider prophylactic anticoagulation.[13]

Lenalidomide (Revlimid) is a 4-aminoglutarimide analog of thalidomide currently being studied in MDS. It also is recommended by the NCCN as a low-intensity agent. It appears to be more potent but lacks the neurotoxicity and teratogenic affects that are problematic with thalidomide. A phase 2 study supports it use in MDS, with 56% of patients responding. The responses ranged from sustained transfusion independence to cytogenetic remissions. The major side effect in early studies was myelosuppression, which is dose dependent. Other adverse reactions were uncommon and generally mild.[14] Lenalidomide is approved and available for use in MDS.

Arsenic trioxide is an agent that has generated interest in the treatment of MDS. Arsenic trioxide can induce differentiation and apoptosis and inhibit cell proliferation or angiogenesis. It is currently under study, with preliminary analysis supporting a 25% response rate with arsenic trioxide alone.[15] Combination therapy of thalidomide and arsenic trioxide has been studied. In a clinical trial using this combination, 28 patients were treated and 25% produced a variety of hematologic responses. Interestingly, some responders were known to have poor prognostic cytogenetics, which suggests a unique sensitivity to this combination program.[16] The major toxicities observed were myelosuppression and fluid retention. Limited evidence from phase 1 and 2 clinical trials exists for benefit of other agents such as antithymocyte globulin, cyclosporine, anti-TNF receptor fusion proteins, and vitamin D analog.[17-19]

Bone marrow transplantation remains the only potential curative treatment for MDS. An allogeneic transplant, either HLA identical related or unrelated, is indicated if the patient meets the rigorous transplant requirements. Unfortunately, with the aged population of MDS patients, few meet this prerequisite. Bone marrow transplant should optimally be performed before disease progression. In patients with less advanced disease, 3-year survival rates of 65% to 75% are achieved. Among patients with advanced disease, the 3-year survival rate drops to 25% to 45%. The incidence of posttransplant relapse is 5% to 35%, worsening with advanced disease.[20]

INDICATIONS FOR REFERRAL OR HOSPITALIZATION

Whenever MDS is suspected, patients are referred to a hematologist for both a review of the peripheral blood smear and a bone marrow biopsy. Hematologists will often chronically follow patients with the help of local health care providers to monitor disease progression and complications. In patients with an absolute neutropenia of less than 1000/mm^3, hospitalization for any febrile illness is warranted. Without prompt initiation of IV antibiotics, patients may quickly become septic and require critical care. Any trend of increasing blast population or worsening transfusion requirements is an indication for hematology follow-up.

COMPLICATIONS

The clinical course of MDS is inevitably progressive. The complications of MDS revolve around the offending cytopenias. Major bleeding episodes and infection are the most common reasons for hospital admissions. Transformation to acute leukemia ranges from 5% to 15% in low-risk groups to 40% to 50% in high-risk groups. This requires prompt intervention with induction chemotherapy if the patient is a candidate. Other less intense treatment regimens such as melphalan are also available.

Fatigue is another major complication of the disease itself. It is extremely common and can often become unrelenting. Patients often describe it as exhaustion. The fatigue can interfere with the patient's functional ability and can result in depression.

MDS is a heterogeneous group of bone marrow disorders that require definitive diagnosis. Each patient must be evaluated and treated on his or her disease specific symptom trajectory. Quality-of-life issues are paramount, since both the disease and its treatments have the potential to disrupt normalcy. Caring support and social intervention can positively modify patients' experience with this disease as they encounter the different management strategies.

PATIENT AND FAMILY EDUCATION

The quality of life of those patients living with myelodysplasia is directly affected by both the disease and its accompanying treatments. The majority of patients who have this disease are elderly, many with other co-morbid conditions. This aging population will often have low physiologic reserves and a prolonged recovery from complications. Quality-of-life issues must be explored, and patients and families should be offered education regarding treatment choices, side effects, inconveniences, and cost to make informed decisions about their care. Patient progress and response to therapies should be reevaluated and discussed with patients and family on a frequent basis.

It is also vital that neutropenic precautions be reviewed when necessary and that patients are aware of who and when to call if they develop fevers, chills, rigors, or persistent bleeding. Patients should also be educated on any clinical trials that may be available for their particular situation.

REFERENCES

1. Steensma DP, Tefferi A: The myelodysplastic syndrome(s): a perspective and review highlighting current controversies (review), *Leuk Res* 27(2):95-120, 2003 [erratum appears in *Leuk Res* 29(1):117, 2005].
2. Greenberg P, Cox C, LeBeau MM, and others: International scoring system for evaluating prognosis in myelodysplastic syndromes [see comment], *Blood* 89(6):2079-2088, 1997 [erratum appears in *Blood* 91(3):1100, 1998].
3. Hillman RS, Ault KA, editors: *Hematology in clinical practice*, ed 3, New York, 2002, McGraw-Hill.
4. Beutler E, Lichtman M, Coller B, and others, editors: *Hematology*, ed 6, New York, 2001, McGraw-Hill.
5. Seipelt G, Ottmann OG, Hoelzer D: Cytokine therapy for myelodysplastic syndrome (review), *Curr Opin Hematol* 7(3):156-160, 2000.
6. Economopoulos T, Mellou S, Papageorgiou E, and others: Treatment of anemia in low risk myelodysplastic syndromes with granulocyte-macrophage colony-stimulating factor plus recombinant human erythropoietin, *Leukemia* 13(7):1009-1012, 1999.
7. Faderl S, Harris D, Van Q, and others: Granulocyte-macrophage colony-stimulating factor (GM-CSF) induces antiapoptotic and proapoptotic signals in acute myeloid leukemia, *Blood* 102(2):630-637, 2003.
8. Kaminskas E, Farrell AT, Wang YC, and others: FDA drug approval summary: azacitidine (5-azacytidine, Vidaza) for injectable suspension (review), *Oncologist* 10(3):176-182, 2005.
9. Greenberg PL, Baer MR, Bennett JM, and others: *Myelodysplastic syndromes*, Jenkintown, Pa, 2005, National Comprehensive Cancer Network.
10. Musto P: Thalidomide therapy for myelodysplastic syndromes: current status and future perspectives (review), *Leuk Res* 28(4):325-332, 2004.
11. Strupp C, Germing U, Aivado M, and others: Thalidomide for the treatment of patients with myelodysplastic syndromes, *Leukemia* 16(1):1-6, 2002.
12. Candoni A, Raza A, Silvestri F, and others: Response rate and survival after thalidomide-based therapy in 248 patients with myelodysplastic syndromes, *Ann Hematol* 84(7):479-481, 2005.
13. Steurer M, Sudmeier I, Stauder R, and others: Thromboembolic events in patients with myelodysplastic syndrome receiving thalidomide in combination with darbepoietin-alpha, *Br J Haematol* 121(1):101-103, 2003.
14. List A, Kurtin S, Roe DJ, and others: Efficacy of lenalidomide in myelodysplastic syndromes [see comment], *N Engl J Med* 352(6):549-557, 2005.
15. Vey N: Arsenic trioxide for the treatment of myelodysplastic syndromes (review), *Expert Opin Pharmacother* 5(3):613-621, 2004.
16. Raza A, Buonamici S, Lisak L, and others: Arsenic trioxide and thalidomide combination produces multi-lineage hematological responses in myelodysplastic syndromes patients, particularly in those with high pre-therapy EVI1 expression, *Leuk Res* 28(8):791-803, 2004.
17. Jonasova A, Neuwirtova R, Cermak J: Promising cyclosporin A therapy for myelodysplastic syndrome, *Leuk Res* 21:842, 1997.
18. Molldrem J, Caples M, Marvroudis D: Antithymocyte globulin for patients with myelodysplastic syndromes, *Br J Haematol* 99:699, 1997.
19. Deeg HJ, Gotlib J, Beckham C: Soluble TNF receptor fusion protein (etanercept) for the treatment of myelodysplastic syndrome, *Leukemia* 16:162, 2002.
20. Benesch M, Deeg HJ: Hematopoietic cell transplantation for adult patients with myelodysplastic syndromes and myeloproliferative disorders (review) [see comment], *Mayo Clin Proc* 78(8):981-990, 2003.

PART 19

Evaluation and Management of Rheumatic and Multisystem Disorders

JOANNE SANDBERG-COOK, *Section Editor*

CHAPTER 231

Common Diagnostics in Rheumatologic Disorders

Robert H. Shmerling

Diagnostic testing in patients with possible or established autoimmune disease may not be helpful or may be misleading because most of these tests have significant limitations in accuracy. Both false-positive results (abnormal findings when the patient is fine) and false-negative results (normal findings when the patient is ill) are common in autoimmune disease. Some are sensitive (usually abnormal findings when disease is present), and others are specific (usually normal findings when disease is absent), but, unfortunately, most are not both. In fact, the symptoms, findings on examination, and, often, the passage of time are the most useful "tests" in patients with possible autoimmune disease.

In clinical practice the most important consideration is predictive value: what does a positive or negative test result mean? Positive predictive value is the likelihood that a positive result is an indication of disease; negative predictive value is the likelihood that a disease is absent if the test result is normal. Predictive value is determined not only by the test's sensitivity and specificity, but also by the likelihood of disease, as clinically assessed, before the test is ordered. If a test is ordered when the chances of disease are low (e.g., rheumatoid factor for a patient with low back pain), an abnormal result will often represent a clinical false-positive finding. Thus how the provider orders a test has a direct effect on its usefulness.

These principles are crucial to interpreting test results in all fields of medicine but particularly in the rheumatic diseases, for which there is often no single result that confirms or excludes a particular illness. It is more common that these disorders are diagnosed by "the big picture," an integration of symptoms and signs, as well as test results. Often routine tests are the most helpful; occasionally more specific (and often more expensive) testing is warranted, especially when the suspicion of rheumatic disease is moderate or high. Selective testing is recommended to avoid unnecessary expense and unhelpful, or even misleading, results. This applies also to combinations of tests, or panels, in which more false-positive results are inevitable as the number of tests increases. It should be noted that for most tests there is no clear consensus regarding when they should be ordered.

ERYTHROCYTE SEDIMENTATION RATE

The erythrocyte sedimentation rate (ESR) is an inexpensive, widely available, and easily measured acute-phase reactant, a family of proteins that appear in the bloodstream in elevated levels during acute inflammation. As such, they are nonspecific, meaning that any cause of inflammation, including infection, tumor, or rheumatic disease, may be associated with an elevated ESR.[1]

Among the rheumatic diseases, the ESR is almost always elevated in giant cell (temporal) arteritis and in most patients with polymyalgia rheumatica (see Chapter 233); in both of these disorders the test is monitored over time, along with symptoms and signs, to help assess disease. Among other rheumatic diseases, including systemic lupus erythematosus (SLE) (see Chapter 236) and rheumatoid arthritis (RA) (see Chapter 235), the test may be suggestive of active illness when the ESR is elevated or of improvement when the ESR is normal, but exceptions to this are common. Among nonrheumatic diseases, patients with subacute bacterial endocarditis (SBE) almost always have an elevation in ESR, but in other infectious, neoplastic, and inflammatory states the ESR may be high or normal.

The test has limited clinical use unless it has previously been proved to correlate well with clinical status, as might be true in a patient with osteomyelitis: the ESR will usually fall with treatment and may rise again if the infection recurs. Other acute-phase reactants (including ferritin, C-reactive protein, transferrin, and haptoglobin) may change in the face of inflammation as well, but these offer no clear advantage compared with ESR.

RHEUMATOID FACTOR AND ANTI–CYCLIC CITRULLINATED PROTEIN

The rheumatoid factor (RF) is an immunoglobulin (Ig) M antibody directed against IgG and is found in most patients with RA, as well as in several other rheumatic and nonrheumatic disorders (Box 231-1). Its usefulness is limited to patients whose chances of having RA, as estimated by the history and physical examination, are neither very low nor very high.[2] Prognostic information provided by RF testing may be more useful than its diagnostic utility because, on average, RF-positive patients with established RA will have more severe joint disease, more frequent disability, and more extraarticular disease (including nodules) compared with RF-negative patients. The higher the titer of a positive RF, the more likely it

BOX 231-1

DISEASES ASSOCIATED WITH POSITIVE RHEUMATOID FACTOR

SYSTEMIC RHEUMATIC DISEASE
- Rheumatoid arthritis
- Sjögren's syndrome

INFECTION
- Subacute bacterial endocarditis
- Hepatitis virus B and C (especially with cryoglobulinemia)
- Viral infection

LUNG DISEASE
- Sarcoidosis
- Interstitial pulmonary fibrosis

MALIGNANCY
- Leukemia (case reports)
- Colon cancer (case reports)

OTHER CHRONIC INFLAMMATORY DISEASE
- Autoimmune hepatitis
- Primary biliary cirrhosis

is that the patient has RA or another RF-associated illness; however, exceptions to this general rule are often encountered. High-titer RF in a patient without other findings of RA should raise the possibility of Sjögren's syndrome, SBE, or cryoglobulinemia. Because many of the non-RA causes of a positive RF finding (see Box 231-1) are associated with arthralgia or even arthritis, there is significant potential for misdiagnosis.[3]

In recent years, researchers have identified a new autoantibody associated with RA, the anti–cyclic citrullinated protein (anti-CCP). This antibody targets citrulline, a modified amino acid. The usefulness of this antibody lies primarily in its specificity, reportedly in the range of 95% to 98%; its sensitivity is less impressive at 40% to 60% in early series.[4,5] It may also identify some RF-negative patients with RA. It could be most helpful in the evaluation of patients with suspected RA for whom uncertainty persists after full evaluation. For example, a patient with hepatitis C, cryoglobulinemia, and arthralgia may be RF positive, raising the possibility of concomitant RA. If anti-CCP is positive, the case for RA becomes much stronger; false-positive anti-CCP results are uncommon in this situation.[4] Similarly, a patient with possible RA who is RF negative but has a positive anti-CCP probably has RA. Anti-CCP antibodies may be present years before the development of RA, a finding reminiscent of the RF in RA and the antinuclear antibodies (ANAs) in SLE.

ANTINUCLEAR ANTIBODIES

ANAs are a heterogeneous family of possibly pathogenic autoantibodies directed against several components of cell nuclei. Almost all patients (95% to 99%) with SLE will have a positive test result; therefore a negative result is a strong argument against that diagnosis. However, up to 20% to 30% of healthy patients will have a positive test result (suggesting low specificity); a positive ANA finding certainly does not establish a diagnosis of SLE.[6] Other ANA-associated diseases include drug-induced lupus, Sjögren's syndrome, mixed connective tissue disease, scleroderma, and RA, but for some of these, sensitivity is not high (Box 231-2). As with RF, the higher the titer of the ANA, the more likely it is that a positive result is truly related to an ANA-associated illness such as SLE, but, again, exceptions are common. The specific antigen responsible for the positive ANA, when identifiable (the specific autoantibody profile), may suggest one disease over another (see Box 231-2), but only anti-Smith (anti-Sm) and anti–double-stranded DNA (anti-dsDNA) have high positive predictive value for SLE. However, they are not highly sensitive, since many lupus patients are negative for anti-dsDNA and anti-Sm. Routine testing for the entire autoantibody profile (antibodies to Sm, dsDNA, Ro, La, ribonucleoprotein) for all patients being tested for ANA has low clinical usefulness.[7]

The ANA and the more specific autoantibody subtypes (including anti-Sm and anti-dsDNA antibodies) may appear before clinical disease; the clinical significance of this observation remains uncertain.[8]

In pregnant women with or without systemic rheumatic disease, anti-Ro (also called SSA) antibodies cross the placenta and are associated with neonatal lupus, a disease in which the newborn may develop rash, thrombocytopenia, and heart block.[9] Consequences may be serious; therefore detection of this antibody before or during pregnancy warrants close monitoring by an obstetrician experienced in managing high-risk pregnancies.

BOX 231-2

RHEUMATIC DISEASES ASSOCIATED WITH A POSITIVE ANA TEST

Systemic lupus erythematosus: 95% to 99% of patients are ANA positive in any pattern; anti-ds-DNA and anti-Sm are highly specific but not sensitive.

Drug-induced lupus: 100% of patients are ANA positive; diffuse pattern is most common; 95% have antihistone antibody specificity.

Sjögren's syndrome: 75% of patients are ANA positive, often in a speckled pattern as a result of anti-Ro (with or without anti-La) specificity.

Scleroderma: 50% to 90% of patients are ANA positive, often in a high-titer speckled or nucleolar pattern.

Mixed connective tissue disease: 95% to 99% of patients are ANA positive; 95% of these cases are due to anti-RNP specificity.

Rheumatoid arthritis: 15% to 30% of patients are ANA positive, usually in a diffuse pattern without presence of specific autoantibodies.

ANA, Antinuclear antibody; *ds-DNA,* double-stranded deoxyribonucleic acid; *RNP,* ribonucleoprotein.

URIC ACID

Serum uric acid (urate) is a by-product of purine metabolism, a pathway crucial to DNA synthesis. Patients develop hyperuricemia because too little is renally excreted, too much is produced, or a combination of the two conditions. Other than obvious contributors (e.g., renal insufficiency), the underlying reason why a person underexcretes or overproduces uric acid is often unclear. Other conditions associated with elevated uric acid include diuretic use, obesity, hypertension, alcohol consumption, and myeloproliferative disorders. Although hyperuricemia generally causes no clinically evident disease, some patients, particularly men and older women (e.g., 5 to 10 years postmenopausal), develop gout or nephrolithiasis (see Chapter 187). Gout is rare when the serum uric acid level is less than 5 to 6 mg/dl, but a sizable subset of gout patients will have a high-normal level of uric acid.

Testing serum for the uric acid level in patients with definite gout is unnecessary unless treatment is planned to lower the uric acid. In addition, testing when gout is suspected but not documented generally yields little useful information because high-normal or high levels are so common in the general population.[10] Conversely, the finding of a low serum uric acid (e.g., <5 mg/dl) is a compelling argument against the diagnosis of suspected gout. For patients treated with allopurinol or probenecid to lower the uric acid level, the dosage of medications is dictated by the serum uric acid level, with a target of 6 mg/dl or less.

HLA-B27

The HLA-B27 immunogenetic marker is associated with spondyloarthropathies (see Chapter 232), which are present in 95% of patients with ankylosing spondylitis and in 50% to 80% of patients with the spondyloarthropathy of inflammatory bowel disease, Reiter's syndrome, or psoriasis. The HLA-B27 molecule may be involved in the pathogenesis of an autoimmune inflammatory response by allowing more efficient or persistent microbial tissue invasion (e.g., in Reiter's syndrome) through molecular mimicry between HLA-B27 and microbial antigens or by other, as-yet-unknown mechanisms. Determining a patient's HLA-B27 status has limited use, except in the case of patients with a moderate pretest probability of ankylosing spondylitis (e.g., patients with morning stiffness in the lower back that improves with exercise, especially if the stiffness is associated with oligoarthralgia, inflammatory eye disease, or radiographic changes of sacroiliitis).[11]

RADIOGRAPHY

Radiographic imaging has a high level of usefulness in evaluating suspected fracture or established, erosive RA and in documenting the presence and severity of osteoarthritis (especially if management would be altered by the radiographic findings, as in the consideration of surgical intervention). However, the level of usefulness is low for the vast majority of patients with low back pain; suspected bursitis; tendinitis; cartilage or ligament injuries; or nonspecific joint pain and early in the course of rheumatic disease, including RA. It takes 3 to 4 months for erosions characteristic of RA to be radiographically detectable. Certain circumstances warrant immediate x-ray studies; these include significant trauma, suspected bone or joint infection (although x-ray findings may be normal if disease has been present less than 10 days), and neck pain in the setting of neurologic findings or erosive RA. Normal or nonspecific radiographic findings are the rule in early RA, SLE, acute gout, and pseudogout.

MISCELLANEOUS

Other diagnostic tests are indicated in select clinical circumstances (Box 231-3).

BOX 231-3

MISCELLANEOUS DIAGNOSTIC TESTS AND THEIR INDICATIONS

Complement: Suspected systemic lupus erythematosus nephritis or cryoglobulinemic vasculitis or glomerulonephritis; may correlate with disease activity[12]

Anti-Scl-70 (topoisomerase): Suspected diffuse scleroderma; less than 50% sensitive

Anticentromere: Suspected CREST syndrome; less than 50% sensitive

Creatine phosphokinase: Suspected myopathy; sensitive measure of muscle injury

Electromyogram and nerve conduction studies: Suspected myopathy or neuropathy, especially if results would alter management (e.g., muscle or nerve biopsy)

Synovial fluid analysis: Suspected infection or crystal disease; less compelling: to determine degree of inflammation or possible hemarthrosis[13]

Antineutrophilic cytoplasmic antibodies: Suspected Wegener's granulomatosis, related renal vasculitides; specific types: anti-PR3 and anti-MPO[14]

Myositis-specific antibodies: Suspected dermatomyositis or polymyositis; 50% sensitivity; effect on diagnosis and management unclear[15]

Tissue biopsy: Suspected vasculitis, sarcoidosis, myositis

CREST, Calcinosis, Raynaud's phenomenon, esophageal dysfunction, sclerodactyly, and telangiectasia; *PR3,* proteinase 3; *MPO,* myeloperoxidase.

REFERENCES

1. Sox HC, Liang MH: The erythrocyte sedimentation rate: guidelines for rational use, *Ann Intern Med* 104:515-523, 1986.
2. Shmerling RH, Delbanco TL: How useful is the rheumatoid factor? An analysis of sensitivity, specificity and predictive value, *Arch Intern Med* 152:2417-2420, 1992.
3. Shmerling RH, Delbanco TL: The rheumatoid factor: an analysis of clinical utility, *Am J Med* 91:528-534, 1991.
4. Kessel A, Rosner I, Zukerman E, and others: Use of antikeratin antibodies to distinguish between rheumatoid arthritis and polyarthritis associated with hepatitis C infection, *J Rheumatol* 27:610-612, 2000.
5. Lee DM, Schur PH: Clinical utility of the anti-CCP assay in patients with rheumatic diseases, *Ann Rheum Dis* 62:870-874, 2003.
6. Slater CA, Davis RB, Shmerling R: Antinuclear antibody testing: a study of clinical utility, *Arch Intern Med* 156:1421-1425, 1996.
7. Homburger HA: Cascade testing for autoantibodies in connective tissue diseases, *Mayo Clin Proc* 70:183-184, 1995.
8. Arbuckle MR, McClain MT, Rubertone MV, and others: Development of autoantibodies before the clinical onset of systemic lupus erythematosus, *N Engl J Med* 349:1526-1533, 2003.
9. Buyon JP, Winchester RJ, Slade SG, and others: Identification of mothers at risk for congenital heart block and other neonatal lupus syndromes in their children: comparison of enzyme-linked immunosorbent assay and immunoblot for measurement of anti-SS-A/Ro and anti-SS-B/La antibodies, *Arthritis Rheum* 36:1263-1273, 1993.
10. Liang MH, Fries JF: Asymptomatic hyperuricemia: the case for conservative management, *Ann Intern Med* 88:666-670, 1978.
11. Olajos A, Suranyi P: The value of HLA-B27 typing in the diagnosis of early, oligosymptomatic spondyloarthropathies, *Br J Rheumatol* 35:192, 1996.
12. Hebert LA, Cosio FG, Neff JC: Diagnostic significance of hypocomplementemia, *Kidney Int* 39:811-821, 1991.
13. Shmerling RH, Delbanco TL, Tosteson AN, and others: Synovial fluid tests: what should be ordered? *JAMA* 264:1009-1014, 1990.
14. Savige J, Gillis D, Benson E, and others: International consensus statement on testing and reporting of antineutrophil cytoplasmic antibodies (ANCA), *Am J Clin Pathol* 111:507-513, 1999.
15. Love LA, Leff RL, Fraser DD, and others: A new approach to the classification of idiopathic inflammatory myopathy: myositis-specific autoantibodies define useful homogeneous patient groups, *Medicine (Baltimore)* 70(6):360-374, 1991.

CHAPTER 232

Ankylosing Spondylitis and Related Disorders

Susan Hoch

ANKYLOSING SPONDYLITIS

DEFINITION AND EPIDEMIOLOGY

The seronegative spondyloarthropathies are a group of inflammatory arthritides, sharing many clinical, radiographic, and genetic features. The seronegative spondyloarthropathies include (1) ankylosing spondylitis, (2) reactive arthritis and Reiter's syndrome, (3) psoriatic arthritis, and (4) arthritis associated with inflammatory bowel disease (IBD). These illnesses are characterized by the presence of sacroiliitis, peripheral joint inflammation, and eye inflammation. Ankylosing spondylitis is the prototype of the seronegative spondyloarthropathies.

Ankylosing spondylitis has an estimated hospital prevalence of 0.1% to 0.2% in North America.[1] It tends to be familial and follows the population frequency of HLA-B27. The male-female ratio, according to most studies, is between 2.5:1 and 5:1. It may be more severe in men. The disease usually begins in the third or fourth decade of life.

PATHOPHYSIOLOGY

A strong association exists with the genetically determined histocompatibility antigen, HLA-B27. Of note, however, is the fact that HLA-B27 by itself is neither necessary nor sufficient for development of these diseases.[2] The association with HLA-B27 is the highest in ankylosing spondylitis, where it is 95%, but only 2% to 10% of HLA-B27-positive individuals develop ankylosing spondylitis. The explanation for the link between HLA-B27 and the spondyloarthropathies remains unknown.

The pathognomonic features of ankylosing spondylitis are (1) inflammation of the bony insertions of ligaments and tendons (entheses), known as enthesitis or enthesopathy; and (2) new bone formation. The pathophysiology of this disease begins with ligamentous inflammatory granulation tissue that is gradually replaced by fibrocartilage and then ossifies.

CLINICAL PRESENTATION

Low back pain caused by sacroiliitis is the initial complaint of approximately 60% of patients. The back pain of sacroiliitis is inflammatory and can be distinguished clinically from back pain of other etiologies. It is usually insidious in onset; it is chronic, lasting for more than 3 months, with periods of exacerbation and remission. It is diffuse, poorly localized, and described as a deep ache or nagging discomfort in the lower back below the waist, in the buttocks, or in the hips. As in other types of inflammatory joint pain, the inflammatory back pain of ankylosing spondylitis worsens with bed rest and improves with exercise. Sleep disturbance is common, and patients may describe having to get up in the middle of the night to "walk the pain off." The back pain is worse in the morning and is associated with morning stiffness that is inflammatory in nature (i.e., lasts longer than 30 minutes). Patients can have intermittent sciatica occurring on alternating sides, which is pathognomonic for ankylosing spondylitis.

Spondylitis occurs in approximately 50% of patients with ankylosing spondylitis and begins in the lumbosacral spine. As the disease progresses, the upper portions of the spine are involved.

Patients may have peripheral joint involvement, and the diagnosis of ankylosing spondylitis can be made with only minimum sacroiliitis. Peripheral joint involvement is usually asymmetric, often involving large joints, and is most frequently found in the lower limbs. More than 30% of patients develop chronic peripheral joint arthritis. Involvement of the hip joint can be an early manifestation in ankylosing spondylitis. Other inflammatory enthesopathic (at ligament and tendon insertions) areas of involvement peculiar to ankylosing spondylitis are the sternoclavicular joint, the costochondral joint, the Achilles tendon, and the plantar fascia. Small joints of the hands and feet are infrequently involved, unlike in rheumatoid arthritis.

Extraarticular manifestations of the disease include low-grade fever, fatigue, and weight loss. Inflammatory eye disease, usually acute anterior uveitis, manifests as a painful and often red eye and occurs in up to 30% of patients during the course of their disease. The inflammation is acute in onset 90% of the time, and in approximately 95% of patients the uveitis is unilateral or unilateral-alternating.[3] Cardiac involvement, most commonly aortic valve insufficiency, can be clinically silent or can dominate the picture.

PHYSICAL EXAMINATION

Examination of the spine will show loss of the normal lumbar lordosis. Palpable muscle spasm of the paraspinal muscles is frequently present. Measurement of spine mobility is decreased in most patients and can be documented by (1) Schober's flexion test of the lumbosacral spine, (2) Moll's lateral flexion test of the thoracic spine, or (3) measurement of chest expansion.[4] Schober's flexion test measures lumbosacral flexion by having the patient stand erect and marking two points 15 cm apart in the midline—5 cm below and 10 cm above the level of the dimples of Venus. The patient is then asked to bend forward, reaching for the floor as far as possible. Normal flexion is defined as an increase in the distance between the two points of 5 cm or more in a patient under the age of 50. Moll's lateral flexion test measures lateral thoracic spine flexion by having the patient stand erect with the hands behind the head. One mark is placed in the midaxillary line at the iliac crest, and another mark is placed 20 cm above the iliac crest. The patient is asked to tilt, bending the trunk to the opposite side as far as possible, and the distance between the two marks is measured. Normal thoracic spine tilt or lateral flexion is 3 cm. Chest expansion is measured with the patient standing erect with the hands on the head. With a centimeter tape at the nipple line, the patient is asked to first maximally expire and then maximally inspire. The chest circumference should normally increase by at least 5 cm with full inspiration.

Extraarticular manifestations can produce physical findings such as the heart murmur of aortic valve insufficiency or the red, inflamed eye associated with acute iritis.

DIAGNOSTICS

The rheumatology community has developed three clinical criteria for the diagnosis of ankylosing spondylitis[5]: (1) low back pain and stiffness of greater than 3 months' duration, improving with exercise, not relieved by rest; (2) limited range of motion of the lumbar spine; and (3) limited chest expansion. The presence of sacroiliitis on radiologic examination associated with one clinical criterion is considered to be diagnostic of definite ankylosing spondylitis.[6] Many patients will have negative findings on plain radiographs because their disease has not been severe enough or of long enough duration to produce radiographic changes. MRI is able to identify sacroiliitis earlier than standard plain x-ray studies.[7] As visualized on MRI, early sacroiliitis includes irregularity of the sacroiliac joints, with subchondral bone resorption giving a rosary-bead effect, and pseudowidening. More advanced sacroiliitis produces sclerosis, with the joint becoming indistinct and narrow over time. Complete bony fusion is seen late in the disease. Characteristic spine x-ray findings in ankylosing spondylitis include syndesmophyte formation, which leads to bony bridging from one vertebral body to the next, producing a "bamboo" spine appearance. MRI studies of the spine in ankylosing spondylitis are useful for evaluating the presence of inflammation as measured by enhancement after injection of gadolinium.[8] Often these inflammatory changes can be early in disease before significant radiographic changes. X-ray changes in the hip occur in up to 50% of patients and are often bilateral and symmetric with uniform joint space narrowing in ankylosing spondylitis as compared with osteoarthritis.

Laboratory findings can include a normochromic, normocytic anemia of chronic disease and an elevated erythrocyte sedimentation rate (ESR) or C-reactive protein (CRP); however, anemia and elevated inflammatory markers are not necessary for the diagnosis. Rheumatoid factor and antinuclear antibodies are typically negative. HLA-B27 testing is inappropriate for screening an asymptomatic population. In the clinical setting, it should not be thought of as a routine diagnostic test; since the test result does not absolutely confirm or exclude ankylosing spondylitis, in general it is not useful enough diagnostically to warrant its expense.[9]

DIAGNOSTICS

Ankylosing Spondylitis and Related Disorders

LABORATORY
CBC and differential
ESR
HLA-B27*
Antinuclear antibody
C-reactive protein*
Uric acid*
ELISA for *Borrelia burgdorferi* (Lyme disease)*
Rheumatoid factor*

IMAGING
X-ray of spine, including sacroiliac joints
X-ray of small joints of hands and feet
MRI of sacroiliac joints

OTHER
Joint fluid analysis

*If indicated.

DIFFERENTIAL DIAGNOSIS

For patients with sacroiliitis or spinal disease, the principal diseases to consider are Reiter's syndrome, psoriatic spondylitis, and spondylitis of IBD, all of which are discussed later in this chapter. In the absence of axial involvement, the most common chronic inflammatory arthritides that can be confused with ankylosing spondylitis in the 20- to 40-year age-group are (1) seronegative rheumatoid arthritis and (2) Lyme arthritis. Rheumatoid arthritis is more likely to involve the upper extremity (especially small) joints, characteristically has hand involvement, and is symmetric. Distinguishing rheumatoid arthritis from the seronegative spondyloarthropathies often requires prolonged observation of the patient. The presence of anti–cyclic citrullinated peptide antibodies may be helpful in distinguishing early rheumatoid arthritis from ankylosing spondylitis.[10] Lyme arthritis, which most commonly involves the knee, is suggested by a history of tick exposure and of erythema migrans and is established by enzyme-linked immunosorbent assay (ELISA) for *Borrelia burgdorferi* antibody, which can be confirmed by Western blot analysis.[11]

Anatomic causes of noninflammatory back pain, such as a herniated intervertebral disc, and noninflammatory arthritis of the spine, such as degenerative joint disease or disseminated idiopathic skeletal hyperostosis, produce different pain, noninflammatory in nature, which is relieved by rest and aggravated by motion.

MANAGEMENT

Ankylosing spondylitis and the other seronegative spondyloarthropathies respond symptomatically to NSAIDs. The hip arthritis, sacroiliitis, and spondylitis of ankylosing spondylitis respond particularly well to the indole-derivative class of NSAIDs, including indomethacin, tolmetin, and sulindac. High-dose aspirin (4 to 8 g/day) is usually not effective. Other nonsteroidal agents, particularly the ketoprofens such as ibuprofen and naproxen, are variably effective if used at high doses. The cyclooxygenase-2 (COX-2)–specific inhibitor celecoxib appeared to be equivalent to ketoprofen in a short-term study and may potentially have less gastrointestinal toxicity.[12] Biologic anti–tumor necrosis factor (TNF) agents have been proven effective in the treatment of patients with ankylosing spondylitis.[13] Because of their cost and potential side effects, criteria for the use of these agents have been devel-

DIFFERENTIAL DIAGNOSIS

Ankylosing Spondylitis and Related Disorders

- Amyloidosis
- Behçet's syndrome
- Degenerative joint disease
- Disseminated idiopathic skeletal hyperostosis
- Familial Mediterranean fever
- Herniated intervertebral disc
- Lyme arthritis
- Polyarticular symmetric disease
- Psoriatic spondylitis
- Reiter's syndrome
- Seronegative rheumatoid arthritis
- Spondylitis of inflammatory bowel disease
- Systemic sclerosis
- Vasculitis with abdominal involvement

oped.[14] These criteria include meeting the diagnostic criteria for definite ankylosing spondylitis, as discussed previously, and the presence of active disease for at least 1 month. Failure of previous treatment with at least two NSAIDs or intolerability is suggested. Sulfasalazine and methotrexate, both considered disease-modifying antirheumatic drugs, have efficacy for those patients with peripheral arthritis,[15] and failure with one of these is recommended as a criterion for anti-TNF therapy. However, since neither sulfasalazine nor methotrexate has been shown to be effective for axial disease, those patients are candidates for anti-TNF therapy.

Studies with both etanercept and infliximab in ankylosing spondylitis show sustained reduction of spinal inflammation as assessed on MRI, and sustained improvement in clinical measurements and in health-related quality-of-life indexes in patients treated over several years.[16-19] The optimum dosage and dosing intervals have not been determined, nor is there available long-term data regarding progression of disease. There is a suggestion that patients treated with etanercept or infliximab for ankylosing spondylitis have a decreased incidence of uveitis.[20] Etanercept and infliximab are currently approved for ankylosing spondylitis; preliminary studies show efficacy of adalimumab as well.[21]

Contraindications to the use of anti-TNF agents are similar to those for patients with rheumatoid arthritis and include active infection, untreated tuberculosis, heart failure, pregnancy, and demyelinating disease. Side effects are rare but include infection and reactivation of latent tuberculosis as in rheumatoid arthritis. In ankylosing spondylitis, as opposed to rheumatoid arthritis, these drugs can be used as single agents without methotrexate or other immunosuppressive medication.

Pain management is important to minimize spinal deformity and allow patients to exercise. Patients stoop with pain, thereby increasing the likelihood of the spine fusing in a kyphotic position. Analgesics such as acetaminophen, muscle relaxants, and low-dose corticosteroids (5 to 7.5 mg/day) can be beneficial adjunct therapy. Patients often find the use of heat and massage helpful. Using small doses of narcotic pain relievers intermittently for short periods may be appropriate in selected situations. Local injections of corticosteroids can treat pain from enthesopathy. Sacroiliac joint pain may benefit from corticosteroid injection under fluoroscopic or CT guidance.

LIFE SPAN CONSIDERATIONS

The prognosis with ankylosing spondylitis is variable. Death from the disease itself is very unusual. Some patients have minimum aggravating symptoms that are limited to the low back and pelvis. Less commonly, patients may have progressive widespread disease with skeletal deformity and functional loss, requiring chronic medication and physical therapy. Chronic medical therapy can shorten the patient's life span as a result of medication side effects. Pregnancy in patients with ankylosing spondylitis does not improve symptoms, unlike what is observed in rheumatoid arthritis. The majority of women with ankylosing spondylitis have unchanged or temporarily aggravated disease activity during pregnancy. The disease has no effect on fertility, course of pregnancy, or delivery. However, the offspring of patients with ankylosing spondylitis have an increased risk of developing ankylosing spondylitis themselves.

COMPLICATIONS

Visual loss secondary to inflammatory eye disease is a major cause of disability in this disease. A variety of neurologic complications of ankylosing spondylitis can be seen in long-standing disease. These include cord compression secondary to spinal fracture of a fused spine; atlantoaxial subluxation resulting from chronic cervical involvement; cauda equina syndrome with slowly progressive sensory loss in the lumbosacral dermatomes with less frequent weakness, pain, and sphincter disturbance; and tarsal tunnel syndrome caused by ankle arthritis. Cardiovascular involvement, while rare, can include ascending aortitis, aortic valve insufficiency, and conduction abnormalities. Pulmonary involvement can be seen in ankylosing spondylitis with upper lobe fibrocystic changes and chest wall restriction with restrictive lung disease. Ankylosing spondylitis is associated with bone loss and osteoporosis, particularly in the lumbar spine, placing these patients at risk for spinal fracture. Amyloid deposition is a rare complication after years of inflammatory disease and can produce nephrotic syndrome or renal failure.

INDICATIONS FOR REFERRAL OR HOSPITALIZATION

Referral to a physical therapist is appropriate to promote pain relief, minimize deformity, and maintain independent function.[22] Referral to an orthopedic surgeon is indicated in the 20% to 30% of patients who develop hip arthritis that is severe enough to produce night pain, rest pain, and pain on weight bearing, impairing the ability to walk.[23] Immediate referral to an ophthalmologist is warranted for acute eye pain. Periodic ophthalmic monitoring is recommended when iritis has been a manifestation. Evaluation by a cardiologist is indicated in the presence of an aortic valve murmur. Hospitalization is rarely indicated in patients with ankylosing spondylitis. Acute catastrophic neurologic complications, congestive heart failure secondary to progressive aortic valve insufficiency, and significant gastrointestinal bleeding resulting from NSAIDs are the most likely reasons for hospitalization.

PATIENT EDUCATION

Optimum management is enhanced when patients understand the chronic nature of the disease and their role in preventing disability and deformity. Patients need to learn to rest when tired and to discontinue any activity that causes joint pain to avoid disease flares. Extension exercises and regular physical activity are beneficial. Walking (shallow water) or running (deep water) in a pool are excellent exercises for increasing and maintaining trunk and neck muscle strength. Swimming is recommended because it avoids excessive stressful weight bearing. The backstroke is particularly good for stretching anterior chest muscles and strengthening posterior chest and neck extensor muscles, thereby decreasing the tendency toward kyphosis. Ongoing attention to daytime and nighttime posture minimizes deformity, and sleeping without a pillow under the head or knees is important to avoid flexion deformity.

REACTIVE ARTHRITIS AND REITER'S SYNDROME

DEFINITION AND EPIDEMIOLOGY

Reactive arthritis refers to an acute sterile inflammatory arthropathy following an infection where there is no microbial invasion of the synovium or joint space and where the prior infection is remote from the joint. Reiter's syndrome, as first described by Hans Reiter in 1916, is an example of a reactive arthritis defined by the classic triad of conjunctivitis, urethritis, and arthritis. Because as many as two thirds of patients are initially seen with an incomplete syndrome and do not fulfill all three criteria, *reactive arthritis* is a preferred and more general term. Reactive arthritis has been observed after both sexually transmitted and dysenteric infection and can be initiated by a number of infectious organisms. The most common infectious agents associated with reactive arthritis and Reiter's syndrome are *Salmonella, Shigella, Yersinia, Campylobacter,* and *Chlamydia* organisms.

The exact prevalence of reactive arthritis and Reiter's syndrome in the general population has not been determined, but it is not rare. In one study, of 260 individuals infected with *Salmonella typhimurium* during an outbreak of gastroenteritis, 19 patients (7%) developed reactive arthritis.[24] The common infection *Chlamydia trachomatis* can lead to the sexually transmitted form of Reiter's syndrome. The peak incidence of reactive arthritis and Reiter's syndrome is during the third decade of life. Postvenereal Reiter's syndrome affects men more commonly, with male/female ratios ranging from 9:1 to 5:1. The dysenteric form of Reiter's syndrome and reactive arthropathy affects males and females equally.

PATHOPHYSIOLOGY

Like ankylosing spondylitis, Reiter's syndrome has a strong association with the histocompatibility antigen HLA-B27. HLA-B27 is observed in 60% to 80% of patients with Reiter's syndrome and appears to be associated with increased disease susceptibility and severity of disease expression. As in rheumatoid arthritis, there is inflammatory synovitis with infiltration of polymorphonuclear leukocytes, lymphocytes, and plasma cells. However, unlike rheumatoid arthritis, production of synovial pannus is rare. As in ankylosing spondylitis, there is inflammation at the insertions of ligaments and tendons (enthesopathy). Erosions, bony proliferation, and periosteal new bone formation may occur.

The relationship between the antecedent infection and the development of reactive arthritis or Reiter's syndrome is not completely understood. The HLA-B27 molecule participates in binding antigenic peptides and presenting them to CD8 T cells. That the disease does occur in patients with AIDS, who presumably lack a full complement of functional CD4 T cells, suggests a role for CD8 cells in reactive arthritis. It is of interest that most of the infectious agents associated with reactive arthritis survive and multiply within cells. Antigenic bacterial peptides derived from these intracellular organisms may then trigger reactive arthritis. The exact mechanism by which this happens is not known. One possible hypothesis is that sharing of an amino acid sequence between bacterially derived peptides and self-antigens may induce autoreactivity.

CLINICAL PRESENTATION AND PHYSICAL EXAMINATION

Reactive arthritis or Reiter's syndrome can occur without documented prior infection. When there has been an antecedent infection, arthritic symptoms tend to occur 10 to 20 days later. Less than 40% of patients are seen with the classic triad. The eye and genitourinary tract features of the triad may take as long as 5 years to appear. Urethritis in men may be transient, and the genitourinary symptoms (cervicitis, cystitis, or mild urethritis) in women are often missed, occult, or not reported.[25] The eye inflammation manifests classically as conjunctivitis, but blepharitis, keratitis, iritis, or uveitis can also be seen. The arthropathy of Reiter's syndrome is distinctive and characterized by lower extremity, asymmetric joint involvement; "sausage digits"; heel pain; Achilles tendinitis; plantar fasciitis; and sacroiliitis.[26] Hip involvement is common. Approximately 50% of patients develop sacroiliitis, and some progress to spondylitis. Like patients with ankylosing spondylitis, they have inflammatory back pain (see Ankylosing Spondylitis, p. 1233).

A classic enthesopathic feature is dactylitis, which produces a sausage digit as a result of inflammation of the bony insertions of ligaments and tendons throughout the entire length of a digit. These sausage digits are characteristic of Reiter's syndrome and psoriatic arthritis. Enthesopathic involvement of the anterolateral ribs, pubic symphysis, and iliac crest may manifest with pain and/or swelling in these areas.

Dermatologic manifestations include painless, shallow lingual or palatal ulcerations; keratoderma blenorrhagica; and circinate balanitis. These tend to correlate with severity of disease. Keratoderma blenorrhagica is the most common dermatologic manifestation of Reiter's syndrome, appearing as painless papulosquamous lesions on the palms or soles. The histopathology of keratoderma blenorrhagica is indistinguishable from that of pustular psoriasis. Circinate balanitis occurs in males and is seen as painless, shallow ulcerative lesions on the glans of the penis, which may go unnoticed.

The course of the disease is highly variable with the initial episode often lasting 2 to 3 months. Some patients have recurrent acute attacks, often with disease-free intervals. About a third of patients have sustained disease activity with a chronic course.[27] Less than 20% of patients develop chronic, destructive, and potentially debilitating disease.

DIAGNOSTICS

For the most part, laboratory test results are nonspecific, consistent with an inflammatory process, and similar to those in ankylosing spondylitis. The ESR and C-reactive protein are elevated. There is often peripheral leukocytosis with thrombocytosis and often a mild anemia. There is usually a synovial fluid leukocytosis, often with a polymorphonuclear leukocyte predominance that is suggestive of a septic arthritis. The x-ray studies of sausage digits, Achilles tendinitis, and plantar fasciitis reveal the fluffy periosteal reaction of new bone formation. Periarticular demineralization or osteopenia is notably absent in Reiter's syndrome as compared with rheumatoid arthritis. The syndesmophytes in the vertebral spine are not as fine as in ankylosing spondylitis, are nonmarginal and denser, and may be asymmetric and skip portions of the spine.

DIFFERENTIAL DIAGNOSIS

Distinguishing between psoriatic arthritis and Reiter's syndrome can be difficult because the arthritis is similar and the skin histology is identical. Only the finding of nail pitting, characteristic of psoriatic arthritis, differentiates the two. More important, Reiter's syndrome or reactive arthritis may be misdiagnosed as seronegative rheumatoid arthritis. Reiter's syndrome can have symmetric peripheral joint involvement, but sacroiliitis is uncommon in rheumatoid arthritis. In rheumatoid arthritis, hip disease is a late sequela, and sausage digits, Achilles tendinitis, plantar fasciitis, and other presentations of enthesopathy do not occur. Dactylitis is not a feature of rheumatoid arthritis. Lyme disease manifests with chronic knee arthritis and can be differentiated from Reiter's syndrome by a positive *B. burgdorferi* antibody assay.[9]

MANAGEMENT

Reiter's syndrome responds to the same drugs as ankylosing spondylitis.[28] Sulfasalazine at a dosage of 2 g/day is more effective than placebo and well tolerated in patients with chronically active reactive arthritis not responding NSAID therapy.[28] Methotrexate, 15 to 25 mg q week, has been used with some success.[29]

The utility of antibiotics in the treatment of patients with reactive arthritis is unclear. In one study, patients with chlamydial infection and reactive arthritis responded to long-term (3-month) tetracycline therapy with decreased duration of illness.[30] A more recent study suggests that a 3-month course of ciprofloxacin in patients with reactive arthritis may affect the long-term prognosis, with fewer patients developing chronic arthritis.[31] Reactive arthritis associated with HIV infection has been reported to improve after antiretroviral treatment, with a rise in CD4 T cell count.[32]

There is increasing interest in the possibility that anti-TNF therapy may be effective in patients with reactive arthritis and spondyloarthropathy. One study showed clinical efficacy in a limited number of patients with reactive and undifferentiated arthritis treated with etanercept.[33] In this study, synovial pathologic condition improved in a majority of the patients.

COMPLICATIONS

The course of Reiter's syndrome is highly variable. Some patients develop chronic, disabling arthritis and are forced to consider alternative employment options.[27]

INDICATIONS FOR REFERRAL

Most patients with Reiter's syndrome can be managed by the primary care provider with initial diagnostic studies and management suggestions from a rheumatologist. In cases where the skin disease is prominent or painful, referral to a dermatologist may be helpful. A physical therapist or occupational therapist should be consulted for suggestions regarding exercise regimens or teaching on joint protection and energy conservation. As noted above, patients with chronic, disabling arthritis may benefit from vocational counseling.

PATIENT EDUCATION

Patient education should be directed toward managing the disease chronically and developing thorough familiarity with drugs and side effects. Patients receiving NSAIDs are advised to take these medications with food and be warned of the risk of gastrointestinal bleeding associated with these medications. In cases where gastrointestinal symptoms occur, consideration should be given to ulcer prevention with H_2 blockers and antacids. Patients who receive second-line agents such as sulfasalazine or methotrexate should be managed according to guidelines for patients with rheumatoid arthritis on these medications, with regular laboratory screening.

PSORIATIC ARTHRITIS

DEFINITION AND EPIDEMIOLOGY

Psoriatic arthritis is an inflammatory arthritis associated with the dermatologic condition of psoriasis. Approximately 6% of patients with mild to moderate psoriasis will develop inflammatory arthritis. Patients with severe psoriasis have a 30% to 40% incidence of joint disease, with men and women being affected equally.[27] The most common age at onset is 30 to 40 years. More extensive spinal involvement occurs in men who are positive for HLA-B27.

PATHOPHYSIOLOGY

Immune, genetic, and environmental factors influence disease expression. Some patients have elevated serum immunoglobulin (Ig) A and IgG, the presence of IgG rheumatoid factor, and even elevated immune complexes. Peripheral joint disease has been linked to HLA-B38, and axial disease to HLA-B27. Patients have been known to have flares after trauma to a joint or infection with group A streptococci. Immune mechanisms are suggested by a possible molecular similarity between streptococcal and epidermal components, which could allow T-cell clones directed against streptococcus to initiate the skin disease.

CLINICAL PRESENTATION AND PHYSICAL EXAMINATION

Psoriatic arthritis may occur before the onset, concomitantly with, or after the onset of the skin disease.[34] Arthritis precedes the rash in 15% to 20% of patients. In these patients, nail pitting is often present before rash as an early clue to the diagnosis. The arthritis is heterogeneous, with five different clinical presentations being recognized: oligoarticular asymmetric, 48%; spondyloarthropathy, 24%; polyarticular symmetric, 18%; distal phalangeal, 8%; and arthritis mutilans, 2%. Only the distal interphalangeal (DIP) joint and arthritis mutilans types are clinically unique to psoriatic arthritis, thus excluding them from other inflammatory arthritides. Typically, patients, over time, develop overlapping forms of the disease, and most patients eventually develop DIP involvement. As in Reiter's syndrome, sausage digits occur (see p. 1236). Arthritis mutilans is a destructive form of arthritis in which there is significant bone erosion with decreased bone length, producing redundant skin and "opera glass" deformity. The spondylitis, when seen, is similar to that of Reiter's syndrome and can occur without sacroiliitis, be asymmetric, and skip portions of the spine.[6] Sacroiliitis in psoriatic arthritis is often asymmetric, as opposed to in ankylosing spondylitis where bilateral sacroiliac involvement is more common. Systemic involvement is limited to eye inflammation, which occurs in approximately 30% of patients. HIV infection in patients with psoriatic arthritis causes increased proliferation of the skin disease and is associated with rapidly progressive polyarticular joint involvement.

DIAGNOSTICS

Laboratory tests are mostly nonspecific, as they are in the other seronegative spondyloarthropathies. Tests for rheumatoid factor and antinuclear antibodies are negative. The ESR and C-reactive protein may be elevated. Hyperuricemia may result from the high-purine turnover in psoriatic skin lesions. Psoriatic synovial histology is similar to rheumatoid synovial histology, with lymphocyte and plasma cell infiltration and microvascular changes.

The radiographic changes in hands and feet are distinctive.[6] Subchondral erosions and erosions with new bone formation, called proliferative erosions, are seen. In late disease, radiographs of the DIP joints may show whittling and a "pencil in cup" appearance, which is believed to be pathognomonic of psoriatic arthritis. Osteoporosis is notably absent, and periosteal reaction can be seen along the bone shafts of sausage digits.

DIFFERENTIAL DIAGNOSIS

It is often difficult to distinguish between Reiter's syndrome and psoriatic arthritis. The skin lesions of both diseases are histologically similar. Both can manifest with eye disease. Nail pitting suggests psoriatic arthritis, whereas nail onycholysis can be seen in both diseases.

Polyarticular symmetric disease can appear exactly like seronegative rheumatoid arthritis, and it may be impossible to differentiate the two. Antibodies against cyclic citrullinated peptide can be found in a small but significant proportion of patients with psoriatic arthritis and appear to be associated with polyarthritic disease and possibly erosive disease.[35] The monarticular arthritis of Lyme disease involving the knee can be differentiated from oligoarticular asymmetric psoriatic arthritis by *B. burgdorferi* antibody assay.[11] Degenerative joint disease of the DIP joints looks similar to that of psoriatic DIP joints, but patients with psoriatic arthritis have morning stiffness for longer than 30 minutes, whereas those with degenerative joint disease do not.

MANAGEMENT

NSAIDs may be helpful in controlling the arthritis; however, many patients have continued active disease despite these agents and require second-line therapy. Sulfasalazine in doses of 2 to 3 g/day may provide control of joint symptoms.[36] Methotrexate, 15 to 25 mg PO once a week, has been the standard drug used in patients with erosive joint disease and aggressive skin disease.[37] In the past, azathioprine, gold, hydroxychloroquine (Plaquenil), retinoids, and cyclosporine were used in patients with psoriatic arthritis who were unresponsive to methotrexate. Over the past few years, all three anti-TNF agents (etanercept, infliximab, and adalimumab) have shown great promise in controlling both joint and skin disease in psoriatic arthritis and are now all approved for treatment of this disease.[38] The anti-TNF agents show sustained benefits in psoriatic arthritis with inhibition of radiologic progression and improvement in disability and quality-of-life indexes.[39-41] Oral steroids are not recommended for the treatment of psoriatic arthritis because of the flare of skin disease that may occur with withdrawal of steroid medication.

Patients with a history of alcohol ingestion who are receiving methotrexate need to be monitored with percutaneous liver biopsies, since the incidence of methotrexate-induced cirrhosis in patients with psoriasis who consume alcohol is significant. Patients treated with methotrexate should not drink alcohol. Patients with severe, erosive joint disease may become permanently disabled, requiring work disability or assistance with activities of daily living. The risks and benefits of anti-TNF agents in psoriatic arthritis are the same as those described for patients with ankylosing spondylitis (see p. 1235).

Suppression of the psoriatic skin disease is essential for the patient's comfort and appearance. It may also be important in the management of the associated arthritis, since flares in the skin disease may correlate with flares in the joint disease.

COMPLICATIONS

Acute iritis can lead to loss of vision. Cirrhosis of the liver can occur in patients treated with methotrexate who consume alcohol. Infection has been reported in psoriatic patients undergoing intraarticular injection, aspiration, or surgery. Therefore careful preparation of the skin before surgery or arthrocentesis is necessary.

INDICATIONS FOR REFERRAL

Most patients with psoriatic arthritis can be managed by the primary care provider. In cases where the joint or skin disease is disabling, referral to a rheumatologist or dermatologist for consultation may be helpful. As in other cases of inflammatory arthritis, referral to a physical therapist or occupational therapist for joint-protective exercise regimens, as well as teaching in joint protection and energy conservation, is very helpful. Patients disabled by joint disease may need vocational counseling.

PATIENT EDUCATION

Patients should be counseled about the chronic nature of this disease. Medication regimens can be complicated and need to be reviewed periodically. Patients taking methotrexate should understand that permanent sterility is possible and should be urged to use reliable birth control because of the possibility of birth defects. These patients should not drink alcohol. Appropriate forms of exercise may include range-of-motion and stretching exercises, as well as swimming.

ARTHRITIS OF INFLAMMATORY BOWEL DISEASE

DEFINITION AND EPIDEMIOLOGY

The arthritis of inflammatory bowel disease (IBD) is an inflammatory arthritis associated with ulcerative colitis and with Crohn's disease. Peripheral arthritis occurs in 15% to 20% of patients with IBD. Spondylitis and sacroiliitis are less common and are associated with HLA-B27 approximately 50%

of the time. Approximately 16% of patients with Crohn's disease or regional enteritis will have radiographic evidence of sacroiliitis.[42] Sex distribution of ankylosing spondylitis in Crohn's disease is equal. Sacroiliac joint involvement is strongly associated with acute uveitis and occurs in 17% of patients with ulcerative colitis. In ulcerative colitis the presence of ankylosing spondylitis has an equal sex distribution.

PATHOPHYSIOLOGY

Arthritis is one of several extraintestinal manifestations associated with ulcerative colitis and Crohn's disease. The mechanism of this association is not clearly understood; the arthritic manifestations of the disorder may be an immunologic phenomenon.

CLINICAL PRESENTATION AND PHYSICAL EXAMINATION

Two forms of arthritis occur in IBD: peripheral joint disease (a systemic manifestation of the IBD varying with bowel disease activity) and ankylosing spondylitis, which is unrelated to IBD activity. The peripheral arthritis is acute or subacute and is more common in the lower extremities than in the upper extremities. It tends to be associated with active IBD and flares when the bowel disease flares.[43]

The spondylitis seen in association with IBD is insidious and chronic and does not correlate with bowel disease activity. The joint involvement is identical to that of ankylosing spondylitis. Patients may develop inflammatory eye disease, usually uveitis, which manifests as an acute, red, painful eye. This presentation is more commonly unilaterally but can be bilateral.

The clinical presentation may include complaints of joint pain, back pain, or morning stiffness. Mild abdominal pain with reports of bloody or mucous stools may antedate or occur with the joint disease, indicating a direct causal relationship between the two, but joint disease may be seen as the first symptom.

DIAGNOSTICS

Indicators of inflammation, including ESR and C-reactive proteins, are often elevated. A mild hypochromic anemia is common. Joint fluid findings are consistent with inflammatory arthritis, showing cell counts of 1500 to 50,000 cells/mm^3.

DIFFERENTIAL DIAGNOSIS

Inflammatory arthritis is seen in conjunction with gastrointestinal manifestations in a number of diseases, including vasculitis with abdominal involvement, systemic sclerosis complicated by motility dysfunction, amyloidosis, Behçet's syndrome, and familial Mediterranean fever.[43] This involvement is differentiated from the arthritis of IBD by the fact that the abdominal disease occurs as a complication of the disease and is not related to the cause of the arthritis.

MANAGEMENT

Sulfasalazine 2 to 3 g/day, which often controls the bowel disease, can be helpful in controlling the joint disease. Corticosteroids usually control both bowel and joint disease but are not indicated for long-term use because of drug toxicity. Azathioprine has been beneficial in patients whose disease is not controlled with sulfasalazine. NSAIDs, when tolerated, are useful for the control of joint pain. Infliximab appears to be effective and well tolerated in patients with Crohn's disease and ulcerative colitis and is being used increasingly to treat disease resistant to standard therapy. Infliximab appears to be steroid sparing and is being used increasingly as a maintenance therapy. Extraintestinal manifestations of Crohn's disease, including arthritis, appear to respond well to infliximab.[44] The response of arthritis associated with ulcerative colitis has not been studied.

COMPLICATIONS

Complications primarily arise with uncontrolled bowel disease. Abdominal pain and bloody diarrhea with weight loss can be severely disabling and may require hospitalization. Corticosteroid-treated patients with IBD are at risk for steroid-induced osteoporosis and should be given appropriate calcium and vitamin D supplementation, as well as prophylactic treatment with a bisphosphonate, to prevent steroid-driven bone loss.

INDICATIONS FOR REFERRAL

Referral to a rheumatologist or a gastroenterologist may be indicated for confirmation of the diagnosis or treatment suggestions. Referral to a physical or occupational therapist can be beneficial for patients dealing with severe joint disease. Dietary modifications may be helpful in controlling bowel disease, and referral to a dietitian may be useful.

PATIENT EDUCATION

Patients need to understand the chronicity of this disease and the relationship between their bowel disease and their arthritis. Unlike psoriatic arthritis, there does not seem to be a correlation between the activity of the bowel and joint disease. Total colectomy may provide a cure for patients with ulcerative colitis and effect remission in the associated arthritis. This is not necessarily true for patients with Crohn's disease, since the bowel inflammation can affect the remaining gastrointestinal tract even if the colon is removed. Patients need to understand their medication regimens and potential toxicities. Patients taking prednisone should be cautioned not to discontinue this medication abruptly. Dietary modifications may be crucial, and patients are often advised to adhere to a low-residue diet.

REFERENCES

1. Gran JT, Husby G: The epidemiology of ankylosing spondylitis, *Semin Arthritis Rheum* 22(5):319-334, 1993.
2. Schumacher TM, Genant HK, Kellet MJ, and others: HLA-B27 associated arthropathies, *Radiology* 126:289-297, 1978.
3. Tay-Kearney M, Schwam BL, Lowder C, and others: Clinical features and associated diseases of HLA-B27 uveitis, *Am J Ophthalmol* 121:47-56, 1996.
4. Merritt JL, McClean TJ, Erickson RP, and others: Measurement of trunk flexibility in normal subjects: reproducibility of three clinical methods, *Mayo Clin Proc* 61(3):192-197, 1986.
5. Van der Linden S, Valkenburg HA, Cats A: Evaluation of diagnostic criteria for ankylosing spondylitis: spondyloarthropathies, *Arthritis Rheum* 27:361-368, 1984.
6. El-Khoury GY, Kathol MH, Brandser EA: Seronegative spondyloarthropathies, *Radiol Clin North Am* 34(2):343-357, 1996.

7. Oostveen J, Prevo R, den Boer J, and others: Early detection of sacroiliitis on magnetic resonance imaging and subsequent development of sacroiliitis on plain radiography: a prospective longitudinal study, *J Rheum* 26(9):1953-1958, 1999.
8. Baraliakos X, Landewe R, Hermann KG, and others: Inflammation in ankylosing spondylitis: a systematic description of the extent and frequency of acute spinal changes using magnetic resonance imaging, *Ann Rheum Dis* 64:730-734, 2005.
9. Khan MA, Khan MK: Diagnostic value of HLA-B27 testing in ankylosing spondylitis and Reiter's syndrome, *Ann Intern Med* 96(1):70-76, 1982.
10. Correa PA, Tobon GJ, Citera G, and others: Anti-cyclic citrullinated peptide antibodies in rheumatoid arthritis: relation with clinical features, cytokines and HLA DRB1, *Biomedica* 24(2):140-152, 2004.
11. Centers for Disease Control and Prevention: Recommendations for test performance and interpretation from the Second National Conference on Serologic Diagnosis of Lyme Disease, *MMWR* 44(31):590-591, 1995.
12. Dougados M, Behier JM, Jolchine I, and others: Efficacy of celecoxib, a cyclooxygenase 2-specific inhibitor, in the treatment of ankylosing spondylitis: a 6 week controlled study with comparison against placebo and against a conventional nonsteroidal anti-inflammatory drug, *Arthritis Rheum* 44(1):180-185, 2001.
13. Braun J, Baraliakos X, Brandt J, and others: Therapy of ankylosing spondylitis, part II, Biological therapies in the spondyloarthritides, *Scand J Rheumatol* 34(3):178-190, 2005.
14. Braun J, Pham T, Sieper J, and others: International ASAS consensus statement for the use of anti-tumor necrosis factor agents in patients with ankylosing spondylitis, *Ann Rheum Dis* 62(9):817-824, 2003.
15. Creemers MC, van Riel PL, Franssen MJ, and others: Second-line treatment in seronegative spondyloarthropathies, *Curr Opinion Rheum* 13(4):245-249, 2001.
16. Baraliakos X, Davis J, Tsuji W, and others: Magnetic resonance imaging examinations of the spine in patients with ankylosing spondylitis before and after therapy with the tumor necrosis factor alpha receptor fusion protein etanercept, *Arthritis Rheum* 52(4):1216-1223, 2005.
17. Baraliakos X, Brandt J, Listing J, and others: Outcome of patients with active ankylosing spondylitis after 2 years of therapy with etanercept: clinical and magnetic resonance imaging data, *Arthritis Rheum* 53(6):856-863, 2005.
18. Heiberg MS, Nordvag BY, Mikkelsen K, and others: The comparative effectiveness of tumor necrosis factor blocking agents in patients with rheumatoid arthritis and patients with ankylosing spondylitis: a 6 month, longitudinal, observational, multicenter study, *Arthritis Rheum* 52(8):2506-2512, 2005.
19. Davis JC, van der Heijde D, Dougados M, and others: Reductions in health-related quality of life in patients with ankylosing spondylitis and improvements with etanercept therapy, *Arthritis Rheum* 53(4):494-501, 2005.
20. Braun J, Baraliakos X, Listing J, and others: Decreased incidence of anterior uveitis in patients with ankylosing spondylitis treated with the anti-tumor necrosis factor agents infliximab and etanercept, *Arthritis Rheum* 52(8):2447-2451, 2005.
21. Haibel H, Rudwaleit M, Brandt HC, and others: Adalimumab reduces spinal symptoms in active ankylosing spondylitis: clinical and magnetic resonance imaging results of a 52-week open-label trial, *Arthritis Rheum* 54(2):678-681, 2006.
22. Oh TH, Brander VA, Hinderer SR, and others: Rehabilitation in joint and connective tissue diseases, part II, Inflammatory and degenerative spine diseases, *Arch Phys Med Rehabil* 76(5):S41-S46, 1995.
23. Sorokin R: Management of the patient with rheumatic disease going to surgery, *Med Clin North Am* 77(2):453-464, 1993.
24. Inman RD, Johnston ME, Hodge M, and others: Postdysenteric reactive arthritis: a clinical and immunogenetic study following an outbreak of salmonellosis, *Arthritis Rheum* 31(11):1377-1383, 1988.
25. Smith DL, Bennett RM, Regan MG: Reiter's disease in women, *Arthritis Rheum* 23(3):335-340, 1980.
26. Arnett FC, McLusky E, Schacter BZ: Incomplete Reiter's syndrome: discriminating features and HLA-W27 in diagnosis, *Ann Intern* Med 84:8-12, 1975.
27. Fox R, Calin A, Gerber RC, and others: The chronicity of symptoms and disability in Reiter's syndrome: an analysis of 131 consecutive patients, *Ann Intern Med* 91(2):190-193, 1979.
28. Clegg DO, Reda DJ, Weisman MH, and others: Comparison of sulfasalazine and placebo in the treatment of reactive arthritis (Reiter's syndrome): a Department of Veterans Affairs Cooperative Study, *Arthritis Rheum* 39(12):2021-2027, 1996.
29. Lally EV, Ho G: A review of methotrexate therapy in Reiter syndrome, *Semin Arthritis Rheum* 15(2):139-145, 1985.
30. Lauhio A, Leirisalo-Repo M, Lahdevirta J, and others: Double-blind, placebo-controlled study of 3-month treatment with lymecycline in reactive arthritis, with special reference to chlamydia arthritis, *Arthritis Rheum* 34(1):6-14, 1991.
31. Flagg SD, Meador R, Hsia E, and others: Decreased pain and synovial inflammation after etanercept therapy in patients with reactive and undifferentiated arthritis: an open-label trial, *Arthritis Rheum* 53(4):613-617, 2005.
32. McGonagle D, Reade S, Marzo-Ortega H, and others: Human immunodeficiency virus associated spondyloarthropathy: pathogenic insights based on imaging findings and response to highly active antiretroviral treatment, *Ann Rheum Dis* 60(7):696-698, 2001.
33. Ruzicka T: Psoriatic arthritis: new types, new treatments, *Arch Dermatol* 132(2):215-219, 1996.
34. Smiley JD: Psoriatic arthritis, *Bull Rheum Dis* 44(4):1-2, 1996.
35. Bobliolo L, Alpini C, Caporali R, and others: Antibodies to cyclic citrullinated peptides in psoriatic arthritis, *Arthritis Rheum* 39(12):2012-2020, 1996.
36. Clegg DO, and others: Comparison of sulfasalazine and placebo in the treatment of psoriatic arthritis: a Department of Veterans Affairs Cooperative Study, *J Rheum* 32(3):511-515, 2005.
37. Cuellar ML, Espinoze LR: Methotrexate use in psoriasis and psoriatic arthritis, *Rheum Dis North Am* 23(4):797-809, 1997.
38. Brandt J, Braun J: Anti-TNF-alpha agents in the treatment of psoriatic arthritis, *Expert Opin Biol Ther* 6(2):99-107, 2006.
39. Mease PJ, Kivitz CE, Burch FX, and others: Etanercept treatment of psoriatic arthritis: safety, efficacy, and effect on disease progression, *Arthritis Rheum* 50(7):2264-2272, 2004.
40. Antoni CE, Kavanaugh A, Kirkham B, and others: Sustained benefits of infliximab therapy for dermatologic and articular manifestations of psoriatic arthritis: results from the infliximab multinational psoriatic arthritis controlled trial (IMPACT), *Arthritis Rheum* 52(4):1227-1236, 2005.
41. Mease PJ, Gladman DD, Ritchlin CT, and others: Adalimumab for the treatment of patients with moderately to severely active psoriatic arthritis: results of a double-blind randomized, placebo-controlled trial: spondylitis and regional enteritis, *Arthritis Rheum* 52:3279-3289, 2005.
42. Mueller CE, Seeger JF, Martel W: Ankylosing spondylitis and regional enteritis, *Radiology* 112(3):579-581, 1974.
43. Mielants H, Veys EM: Enteropathic arthritis. In Schumacher HR, editor: *Primer on the rheumatic diseases*, ed 10, Atlanta, 1993, Arthritis Foundation.
44. Rispo A, Scarpa R, Di Girolamo E, and others: Infliximab in the treatment of extra-intestinal manifestations of Crohn's disease, *Scand J Rheum* 34(5):387-391, 2005.

CHAPTER 233

Polymyalgia Rheumatica and Temporal Arteritis

Susan Hoch

DEFINITION AND EPIDEMIOLOGY

Polymyalgia rheumatica (PMR) is a musculoskeletal syndrome seen in persons over 50 years of age. This disorder is characterized by pain and stiffness in the neck, shoulder girdle, and pelvic girdle; an elevated erythrocyte sedimentation rate (ESR) and an elevated C-reactive protein (CRP); and a dramatic, rapid response to corticosteroids. It can occur alone or in association with giant cell (temporal) arteritis (GCA). GCA is a systemic inflammatory vasculitis of large and medium-sized arteries, commonly affecting the branches of the proximal aorta that supply the neck and the extracranial structures of the head. Approximately 40% to 50% of patients with GCA have symptoms of PMR, and, conversely, 15% to 20% of patients with PMR have GCA.

The average annual incidence of PMR is 52.5 per 100,000 persons 50 years of age and older.[1] It is more common in Caucasians than in other groups, and the highest recorded incidence is in Northern Europe and northern United States. Typically, patients are older than 50 years of age, and 90% are over 60 years of age. The male/female ratio is 1:2.

GCA has a prevalence of 133 per 100,000 population in people 50 years of age. The disease is rare before age 50, and the mean age at onset is 71 years. The incidence increases with age. It has a striking predilection for Caucasians and is more common in females. The male/female ratio is 1:2 to 1:5.

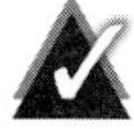

Physician consultation is indicated for patients with suspected PMR. Physician consultation is indicated for patients with tender temporal arteries or with suspected temporal arteritis.

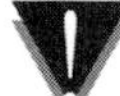

New-onset headache or visual symptoms in an elderly patient with or without musculoskeletal symptoms should prompt consideration of GCA. GCA is a medical emergency with the potential for the occurrence of sudden and irreversible blindness.

PATHOPHYSIOLOGY

PMR and GCA are related disorders that seem to represent a continuum of disease. The current hypothesis is that an infectious cause (or causes) appears to precipitate a cellular immune response directed at the walls of specific arteries. Why these diseases specifically target individuals above the age of 50 is not known. This initial arterial insult appears to initiate a series of cellular and immunologic events with influx of interferon-γ (IFN-γ), producing T cells, macrophages, and giant cells.[2] The artery itself responds with proliferation of smooth muscle cells and the eventual production of a lumen-obstructing neointima. Molecular studies have shown differing tissue cytokine profiles in PMR and GCA that may be related to disease expression.[3] Patients with PMR symptoms seem to have higher production of interleukin-2, whereas higher levels of synthesis of IFN-γ, interleukin-1β, and platelet-derived growth factor seem to correlate with ischemic symptoms.[3,4] There appears to be an association between the histocompatibility antigen HLA-DR4 in both patients with PMR and GCA. In patients with large-vessel (nontemporal artery) GCA, there appears to be overrepresentation of the *HLA-DRB1*0404* allele, suggesting that GCA itself is a heterogeneous entity.[5] Similarly, a small proportion of patients with PMR without vascular symptoms are discovered to have arteritis on blind biopsies.

These studies suggest that heterogeneity either in the triggering agent or in the host's immunologic and vascular response may correlate with the variations in the clinical presentation of these syndromes.[5] GCA most commonly affects the arteries originating from the arch of the aorta. Large-vessel GCA generally involves the subclavian, axillary, and brachial arteries and may or may not be associated with cranial GCA. Autopsies on patients who died of GCA show severe involvement most commonly in the superficial temporal, vertebral, ophthalmic, and posterior ciliary arteries. The central retinal, carotid, subclavian, brachial, and abdominal arteries and the aorta may also be affected. Intracranial arteries are infrequently involved. The arterial lesion may be segmental or patchy with skip areas. Blindness is usually a result of occlusion of the posterior ciliary artery and less commonly of the central retinal artery.

CLINICAL PRESENTATION

The onset of PMR symptoms may be abrupt or subacute. Several weeks to months may elapse before the diagnosis is made. Symmetric pain and stiffness in the neck, shoulders, and hips are present, and patients report feeling as though they have aged several decades. Difficulty in rising from a chair is reported, and gelling occurs after immobility. Morning stiffness, the time it takes for patients to reach their baseline agility and limberness, is inflammatory in nature and lasts more than 60 minutes—often as long as 2 to 3 hours. Range of motion of the hips and shoulders is usually normal, but adhesive capsulitis of the shoulder with significant loss of motion (a frozen shoulder) is sometimes present. Constitutional symptoms, including fever, weight loss, lassitude, fatigue, and anorexia, are common. Muscle pain without significant muscle weakness is common. The pain is characterized by the patient as diffuse and often limits mobility. Patients will report difficulty getting in and out of a car or difficulty combing their hair. However, true muscle weakness is not usually present, although pain may limit effort in strength testing. Synovial swelling in joints such as wrists and knees has been reported but is uncommon.

GCA has varied presentations.[6] Patients may be initially seen with PMR with or without symptoms of arteritis. Headache, found in two thirds of patients, may be continuous or intermittent; can be located temporally or occipitally; and can be throbbing, aching, or sharp. A new headache in a patient over 60 years of age must raise the suspicion of GCA. A history of scalp tenderness at any time but particularly in association with headache suggests GCA. Jaw claudication (jaw pain on chewing) is pathognomonic of GCA. In addition, 20% of patients may have fever (as high as 39° C [102.2° F]), and 40% experience weight loss. Fatigue and anorexia occur. Approximately 15% of patients have fever of unknown origin. Visual symptoms, including diplopia, ptosis, amaurosis fugax, and blindness, occur in 30% of patients. Fifteen percent of patients have permanent visual loss. Eye involvement is often initially unilateral and may become bilateral without treatment within 1 to 10 days. Neurologic complications occur in 31% of patients, with neuropathies occurring in 14% and strokes in 7%. Respiratory symptoms such as cough, sore throat, and hoarseness occur in 10% of patients. Tongue claudication or dysphagia secondary to ischemia of the muscles of deglutition can occur. In addition, tongue numbness, tinnitus, vertigo, and hearing loss have been reported. The presence of an abnormal temporal artery on physical examination and anemia appear to be the best predictors of severe ischemic manifestations of GCA.[7]

PHYSICAL EXAMINATION

Most patients with PMR have normal findings on joint examination, although joint and muscle tenderness may be present. The knee and wrist may show mild swelling, usually without loss of motion. There is no muscle atrophy or true muscle weakness. When muscle strength is being tested in the upper arms, the patient is asked to abduct his or her arms to 90 degrees and resist the examiner's arms pressing downward. These patients may be unable to maintain their arms in the horizontal position because of pain elicited by the examiner's maneuver rather than because of weakness. Trigger point tenderness and pain on mild squeezing of the extremities, so characteristic of fibromyalgia, is unusual. Often it is helpful to watch patients get up out of a chair and walk, since the stiffness and gelling can be striking.

All patients seen with symptoms of PMR should be examined for GCA. In normal individuals the temporal artery pulsations are easily palpable. With GCA there may be a decrease in pulsation or lack of pulsation in an involved temporal artery. The temporal, occipital, or other scalp or cervical arteries may be enlarged, erythematous, and tender. Bruits or pulse deficits may be present over the carotid, subclavian, or brachial arteries. Carotidynia may be present. Patients with visual symptoms may have funduscopic findings of disc pallor and edema, cotton-wool spots, and retinal hemorrhage progressing to optic atrophy.

DIAGNOSTICS

Most patients with PMR have an elevated ESR above 40 to 50 mm/hr, and many have ESRs above 80 mm/hr. However, 7% of patients are seen with ESRs below 40 mm/hr.[8] Patients with PMR and low ESRs appear to differ from patients with PMR and high ESRs only by the increased frequency of systemic symptoms in the high ESR group.[8] Elevated serum concentrations of CRP may be more sensitive than a high ESR for diagnosing PMR or monitoring a relapse.[9] Normochromic, normocytic anemia may be present, and liver function tests (LFTs), particularly for alkaline phosphatase, may show mild elevations. Muscle enzymes, muscle biopsy, and nerve conduction studies are normal. Rheumatoid factor (RF) and antinuclear antibody tests are negative.

DIAGNOSTICS

Polymyalgia Rheumatica

LABORATORY
CBC and differential
ESR
C-reactive protein (CRP)
LFTs
Creatine phosphokinase
Rheumatoid factor*
Antinuclear antibodies*
TSH*
Serum protein electrophoresis*

OTHER
Muscle biopsy
Nerve conduction studies

*If indicated.

DIAGNOSTICS

Temporal Arteritis

LABORATORY
ESR
CBC and differential
LFTs

OTHER
Temporal artery biopsy
Prednisone trial

Recent studies of MRI and shoulder ultrasonography in patients with PMR have confirmed the presence of subacromial-subdeltoid bursitis in the majority of cases of PMR.[10,11] Inflammation of these bursae, as well as iliopectineal bursitis and co-existent hip synovitis, may explain the symptoms of diffuse shoulder and hip girdle pain and stiffness in these patients.[11]

It has been suggested that a dramatic and rapid response to low-dose corticosteroids (≤15 mg/day) after 2 or 3 days of treatment may be an additional criterion for the diagnosis of PMR.[12] No other disease will have 100% improvement within 48 hours with steroid therapy.[13]

Like PMR, laboratory studies in GCA show evidence of inflammation. Characteristically the ESR and CRP are elevated. A normochromic, normocytic anemia is commonly observed. There is often a thrombocytosis. Patients may have mildly elevated findings on LFTs, usually for alkaline phosphatase. When liver biopsies have been performed on these patients, granulomatous changes have been found, but this is not part of the usual diagnostic evaluation in this disease.

The major clinical question in establishing a diagnosis of GCA is whether to perform a temporal artery biopsy or not. A positive temporal artery biopsy assuredly documents the diagnosis of GCA, yet a negative biopsy in a setting of high clinical suspicion does not exclude this condition. This remains an area of some controversy. Biopsies may be falsely negative because of the high incidence of skip lesions. Performing bilateral temporal artery biopsy has been found to increase the diagnostic yield by only 3% compared with unilateral biopsy.[14] Some rheumatologists believe that, because of this low positive biopsy rate, biopsies should not be done unless patients have other system involvement not explainable by GCA. In lieu of biopsy, a diagnostic trial of 40 to 60 mg of prednisone for 10 days to 2 weeks may be considered with monitoring of clinical symptoms and ESR. Others believe that the long-term commitment to high-dose corticosteroids in this elderly patient population is associated with significant toxicity, and therefore it is useful to try to confirm by biopsy who indeed has temporal arteritis.

Regardless of the decision to biopsy or not, providers should not hesitate to begin high-dose prednisone if there is clinical suspicion of GCA. The biopsy can be arranged in a couple of days, and the pathologic condition will not change. The consequences of delay in the institution of corticosteroids in a patient with GCA symptoms can be blindness or stroke. Based on the patient's initial clinical response, the decision to biopsy can be made at a less emergent moment.

DIFFERENTIAL DIAGNOSIS

Rheumatoid arthritis is difficult to differentiate from PMR in elders, particularly in the early stages, when there is little detectable synovitis and the RF is negative.[15] Measurement of the level of anti–cyclic citrullinated peptide antibodies may be useful because these antibodies are highly suggestive of rheumatoid arthritis.[16] Continued observation or a diagnostic trial of steroids can help resolve the dilemma. Patients with little or no observable joint findings after several weeks are unlikely to have rheumatoid arthritis. Patients with symmetric synovitis of their proximal interphalangeal, metacarpophalangeal, or metatarsophalangeal joints are not likely to have PMR. Polymyositis can manifest much like PMR, but patients with polymyositis have muscle weakness and may have muscle atrophy. They also have abnormal findings on muscle enzyme studies, muscle biopsies, and nerve conduction studies. Myeloma and hypothyroidism may appear similar to PMR, but serum protein electrophoresis in myeloma and thyroid function tests in hypothyroidism will be abnormal. Fibromyalgia manifests with muscle pain and tenderness, but patients have characteristic pain on palpation of trigger points and have a normal ESR. Degenerative joint disease can manifest with neck, shoulder, and hip pain but will not have inflammatory morning stiffness, as in PMR. Patients with DJD have noninflammatory morning stiffness that lasts less than 30 minutes. Parkinsonism can manifest with muscle aching and severe stiffness but will not have an elevated ESR. In addition, patients with parkinsonism may have cogwheel rigidity and tremor on examination.

Other forms of systemic vasculitis, such as Wegener's granulomatosis, hypersensitivity vasculitis, and polyarteritis nodosa, can involve the temporal arteries (see Chapter 237). Therefore all patients with symptoms of GCA who have signs or symptoms of other organ involvement require a biopsy to establish the cause of their arteritis.

Finally, the presence of any systemic inflammatory disease other than GCA is believed to exclude a diagnosis of primary PMR.

DIFFERENTIAL DIAGNOSIS

Polymyalgia Rheumatica

- Rheumatoid arthritis
- Polymyositis
- Myeloma
- Hypothyroidism
- Fibromyalgia
- Degenerative joint disease
- Parkinson's disease

DIFFERENTIAL DIAGNOSIS

Temporal Arteritis

- Wegener's granulomatosis
- Hypersensitivity vasculitis
- Polyarteritis nodosa

MANAGEMENT

PMR is usually curable, although relapses do occur. The duration of the disease can be as short as 6 weeks or as long as several years. It is important to keep in mind that PMR is a heterogeneous disorder with significant variation between patients in treatment duration and required dose of corticosteroids for control of symptoms and disease process.[17] Nonetheless, many physicians treat patients with an initial dosage of 10 to 15 mg/day of prednisone for 2 to 4 weeks. The patient is monitored for control of musculoskeletal symptoms, and the ESR and CRP are followed closely. With control of symptoms and normalization of ESR and CRP, tapering can then begin. The goal is to taper the dose of prednisone as quickly as possible while maintaining a normal ESR and CRP and the patient in an asymptomatic state. Again, there is no single widely accepted steroid-tapering protocol for PMR, but many physicians will taper by no more than 1 mg every week or two above 10 mg prednisone and by 1 mg monthly below 10 mg. With this schedule, many patients will discontinue prednisone after slightly more than 1 year of treatment.[18]

GCA is considered a medical emergency. Treatment is begun immediately. As previously noted, in a patient with new-onset headache, temporal artery symptoms, and a suspicion of GCA, there is no reason to wait to start steroids. Corticosteroids should be initiated at a dosage of 40 to 60 mg/day, the higher dosage where there is a stronger clinical suspicion. This high-dose steroid therapy should then be continued for 4 to 6 weeks with frequent monitoring of the patient's clinical condition and sedimentation rate. In general, there is little risk of eye complications and blindness occurring in patients with normal ESRs and CRPs. The steroid dosage is tapered rapidly to 20 mg/day by decrements of 2.5 to 5 mg every other week. A good rule of thumb for GCA and other forms of vasculitis, including systemic lupus erythematosus, is to taper steroids no faster than 10% of the dose per week. Steroids are then tapered slowly as recommended for PMR.

Methotrexate has shown efficacy in some studies as a steroid-sparing agent in combination with prednisone.[19] Recent case studies have suggested that infliximab, a tumor necrosis factor–blocking agent, may be effective in the treatment of GCA.[20] Alternate-day use of steroids is not advised. Treatment for 1 to 2 years is typical. Treatment may be necessary for as long as 5 years. Recurrences usually appear during the first 18 months after diagnosis and within 12 months of discontinuation of therapy.

Patients with both PMR and GCA should be managed to minimize the risks associated with long-term corticosteroid usage in this elderly population. Serum potassium should be checked regularly and potassium supplements prescribed if hypokalemia occurs. Serum glucose should be monitored. A baseline bone densitometry study should be performed to check for pre-existing osteoporosis. Because of the risk of steroid-induced osteopenia and osteoporosis, all patients with PMR and GCA should be supplemented with 1200 mg/day of elemental calcium and 400 mg/day vitamin D. Treatment with either raloxiphene or a bisphosphonate should be initiated either to prevent the development of corticosteroid-induced osteoporosis or to treat pre-existing osteoporosis in a patient who is now receiving corticosteroids. Daily weight bearing exercise should be encouraged. Patients receiving corticosteroids for either PMR or GCA should be considered immunocompromised and should receive immunization with both pneumococcal and influenza vaccines.

LIFE SPAN CONSIDERATIONS

Studies of the natural history of PRM and GCA have not shown a reduction in survival in comparison with the general population.

COMPLICATIONS

The most significant and most common complication of PMR is GCA. Other complications frequently seen in patients with PMR are secondary to long-term corticosteroid therapy, including osteoporosis, infection, cataract formation, hypertension, hypokalemia, and glucose intolerance.

Blindness, which occurs in 15% of patients with GCA, is the most common complication of GCA. Several studies have tried to predict which patients with GCA may be at increased risk of blindness. In one recent study of 161 patients, the best predictors of irreversible blindness were the presence of amaurosis fugax and cerebrovascular accidents, suggesting that patients with other ischemic manifestations are at higher risk for ischemic visual loss.[21] Another study of a similar number of patients has suggested that thrombocytosis with a platelet count greater than 400,000/mm^3 may be a risk factor for permanent visual loss.[22] This study raises the issue of whether there is a role for antiplatelet therapy in the treatment of GCA. Further suggestive evidence of the potential role for antiplatelet therapy in preventing cranial ischemic complications in GCA comes from a retrospective study of 166 patients with biopsy-confirmed GCA.[23] This study found that, of the 36 patients who received aspirin before being diagnosed with GCA, only three (8%) developed cranial ischemia as compared to 40 (29%) of the non-aspirin-treated group.[23]

There is an increased risk of aortic aneurysm and dissection in patients with GCA, which is often a late complication and may be fatal.[24] In one series, patients with GCA were 17 times more like to develop thoracic aortic aneurysms and 2.4 times more like to develop abdominal aortic aneurysms than controls.[24] Yearly chest x-ray examinations have been recommended to identify patients at risk. CT may be of use in monitoring patients with identified aneurysms. Myocardial infarction is another potential complication of GCA. Neurologic complications of GCA include optic neuropathies, ocular motility disorders, acute auditory nerve infarction, mononeuritis multiplex, transient ischemic attack, and stroke.[25] Complications of long-term, high-dose steroid use in GCA are similar to those observed in PMR but may occur more frequently and be more severe given the higher doses of corticosteroids and longer duration of treatment for GCA.

CONSIDERATIONS FOR REFERRAL OR HOSPITALIZATION

Physician consultation is indicated in suspected cases of PMR to assist with the differential diagnosis and determination for steroid therapy. A rheumatologist should be consulted for (1) patients who do not respond to standard steroid therapy; (2) patients with other rheumatic or neurologic disorders, making management difficult; and (3) patients with other system involvement. All patients suspected of having GCA should have physician consultation. Temporal artery biopsy is performed by an ophthalmologist, general surgeon, or plastic surgeon. A rheumatologist is consulted for patients with biopsy-proven GCA who do not respond to steroids.

PMR rarely warrants hospitalization unless there are life-threatening side effects of treatment, such as diabetes that is out of control or gastrointestinal bleeding. With GCA, symptoms of stroke, aortic aneurysm, or myocardial infarction would warrant hospitalization.

PATIENT EDUCATION

Patients with PMR should be educated about its association with GCA. Patients should be aware of the necessity to report immediately any new headache, change in vision, scalp tenderness, difficulty chewing, or other new symptom.

Education about the dangers of corticosteroid therapy is important. The patient should be informed of the potential life-threatening risk of sudden withdrawal of corticosteroids secondary to hypoadrenalism. Obtaining a medical alert bracelet indicating the use corticosteroids should be recommended. Patients need to be aware of common steroid side effects and the importance of contacting their health care provider should they develop such symptoms as increased thirst, polyuria, and weight loss. Medications should be taken with food. If symptoms of heartburn or nausea occur, ulcer prophylaxis with proton pump inhibitors or H_2 blockers is indicated. The patient should understand the risks of the development of corticosteroid-induced bone loss and the importance of behaviors such as daily weight bearing exercise and adequate (1200 mg) calcium and (400 mg) vitamin D intake, as well as the use of antiresorptive medication.

REFERENCES

1. Hunder GG: Giant cell arteritis and polymyalgia rheumatica, *Med Clin North Am* 81(1):195-219, 1997.
2. Weyand CM, Goronzy JJ: Pathogenic principles in giant cell arteritis, *Intern J Cardiol* 75(Suppl 1):S9-S15, 2000.
3. Weyand CM, Tetzlaff N, Bjornsson J, and others: Disease patterns and tissue cytokine profiles in giant cell arteritis, *Arthritis Rheum* 40(1):19-26, 1997.
4. Weyand CM, Hafner V, Kaiser M, and others: Giant cell arteritis—a molecular approach to the multiple facets of the syndrome, *Annales Med Int* 149(7):420-424, 1998.
5. Brack A, Martinez-Taboada V, Stanson A, and others: Disease pattern in cranial and large-vessel giant cell arteritis, *Arthritis Rheum* 42(2):311-317, 1999.
6. Hunder GG: Giant cell (temporal) arteritis, *Rheumatol Clin North Am* 16:399-409, 1990.
7. Gonzalez-Gay MA, Barros S, Lopez-Diaz MJ, and others: Giant cell arteritis: disease patterns of clinical presentation in a series of 240 patients, *Medicine* 84(5):269-276, 2005.
8. Proven A, Gabriel SE, O'Fallon WM, and others: Polymyalgia rheumatica with low erythrocyte sedimentation rate at diagnosis, *J Rheum* 26(6):1333-1337, 1999.
9. Hoffman GS, Cid MC, Hellmann DB, and others: A multicenter, randomized, double-blind, placebo-controlled trial of adjuvant methotrexate treatment for giant cell arteritis, *Arthritis Rheum* 46:1309-1318, 2002.
10. Pavlica P, Barozzi L, Salvarani C, and others: Magnetic resonance imaging in the diagnosis of PMR, *Clin Exp Rheum* 18(4 Suppl 20):S38-S39, 2000.
11. Cantini F, Salvarani C, Olivieri I, and others: Shoulder ultra-

sonography in the diagnosis of polymyalgia rheumatica: a case-control study, *J Rheum* 28(5):1049-1055, 2001.
12. Cohen MD, Ginsburg WW: Polymyalgia rheumatica, *Rheum Dis North Am* 16:325-339, 1990.
13. Michet CJ, Evans JM, Fleming KC, and others: Common rheumatologic diseases in elderly patients, *Mayo Clin Proc* 70:1205-1214, 1995.
14. Boyev LR, Miller, NR, Green WR: Efficacy of unilateral versus bilateral temporal artery biopsies for the diagnosis of giant cell arteritis, *Am J Ophthalmol* 128(2):211-215, 1999.
15. Hunder GG, Goronzy J, Weyand C: Is seronegative RA in the elderly the same as polymyalgia rheumatica? *Bull Rheum Dis* 43(1):1-3, 1994.
16. Lopez-Hoyos M, Ruiz de Alegria C, Blanco R, and others: Clinical utility of anti-CCP antibodies in the differential diagnosis of elderly-onset rheumatoid arthritis and polymyalgia rheumatica, *Rheumatology* 43(5):655-657, 2004.
17. Weyand CM, Fulbright JW, Evans JM, and others: Corticosteroid requirements in polymyalgia rheumatica, *Arch Intern Med* 159(6):577-584, 1999.
18. Cohen MD, Abril A: Polymyalgia rheumatica revisited, *Bull Rheum Dis* 50(8):1-4, 2001.
19. Jover JA, Hernandez-Garcia C, Morado IC, and others: Combined treatment of giant-cell arteritis with methotrexate and prednisone: a randomized, double-blind, placebo-controlled trial, *Ann Intern Med* 134(2):106-114, 2001.
20. Cantini F, Niccoli L, Salvarani C, and others: Treatment of longstanding active giant cell arteritis with infliximab: report of four cases, *Arthritis Rheum* 44(12):2933-2935, 2001.
21. Gonzalez-Gay MA, Garcia-Porrua C, Llorca J, and others: Visual manifestations of giant cell arteritis: trends and clinical spectrum in 161 patients, *Medicine* 79(5):283-292, 2000.
22. Liozon E, Herrman F, Ly K, and others: Risk factors for visual loss in giant cell (temporal) arteritis: a prospective study of 174 patient, *Am J Med* 111(3):211-217, 2001.
23. Nesher G, Berkun Y, Mates M, and others: Low-dose aspirin and prevention of cranial ischemic complications in giant cell arteritis, *Arthritis Rheum* 50(4):1332-1337, 2004.
24. Evans JM, O'Fallon WM, Hunder GG: Increased incidence of aortic aneurysm and dissection in giant cell (temporal) arteritis, *Ann Intern Med* 122:502-507, 1995.
25. Caselli RJ, Hunder GG: Neurologic complications of giant cell (temporal) arteritis, *Semin Neurol* 14(4):349-353, 1994.

CHAPTER 234

Raynaud's Phenomenon

Lin A. Brown

DEFINITION AND EPIDEMIOLOGY

Raynaud's phenomenon is a vasospastic disorder that affects the blood flow to the digits. When these changes occur in isolation with a normal physical examination, the disorder is known as *primary Raynaud's phenomenon*. There are no associated autoimmune diseases, and rarely are autoantibodies present. Primary Raynaud's phenomenon characteristically occurs in women in their second to third decade of life. It is not uncommon and is thought to affect 5% to 20% of women and 4% to 14% of men.[1]

Secondary Raynaud's phenomenon is seen in patients who also have an autoimmune disorder such as progressive systemic sclerosis (scleroderma), systemic lupus erythematosus, dermatomyositis, polymyositis, or mixed connective tissue disease. In addition to autoimmune diseases, Raynaud's phenomenon has been seen in association with migraine headaches and chest pain.[2] Secondary Raynaud's phenomenon can also be seen as part of the *CREST* constellation (*C*alcinosis, *R*aynaud's phenomenon, *E*sophageal dysmotility, *S*clerodactyly, and *T*elangiectasia). Patients with systemic lupus erythematosus who have Raynaud's phenomenon often have antiphospholipid antibodies.

Secondary Raynaud's phenomenon is more severe than primary disease with a greater likelihood of ulcerations and severe ischemic changes.

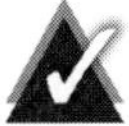

Physician consultation is recommended for patients with persistent pallor, coldness or tissue breakdown in the digits, or reduced pulses in the extremities.

PATHOPHYSIOLOGY

The vascular endothelium, smooth muscle cells, and nerve terminals form an integrated unit that works in response to elements in the microenvironment to determine the final balance between vasodilation and vasoconstriction. These elements are influenced by a variety of factors, including temperature, physical activity, emotional state, and direct trauma.[3]

In Raynaud's phenomenon the blood vessels constrict in response to cold or stress. This may be related to increased activation of the sympathetic nerves. In addition, there appears to be an alteration in vascular function on the cellular level, particularly in vascular smooth muscle. The resultant disturbance in circulation causes a series of color changes in the skin: white, blanched, or pale as the blood flow is reduced (Color Plate 41); blue as the affected digit loses oxygen from the decreased blood flow; and red or flushed as blood flow returns. Finally, as the attack subsides and the circulation returns to normal, usual skin color is restored. In the white or blue stages, numbness, tingling, and coldness can be felt. In the red stage a feeling of warmth, burning, or swelling may be reported. Not infrequently, pain is experienced.

CLINICAL PRESENTATION

The vasospasm of Raynaud's phenomenon causes classic tricolor changes of first white (pallor), then blue (cyanosis), and then red (reperfusion hyperemia) after the vasospasm ends.[1] Episodes can be triggered by cold exposure, rapid changes in ambient temperature, or emotional stress. Attacks can occur in single or multiple digits and can spread to other digits, the other hand, or the feet. Cutaneous vasospasm can be seen at other sites, including ears, nose, face, knees, and nipples.[4] Patients can experience pain, numbness, and burning. Patients with a history of digital frostbite can subsequently experience Raynaud's in the affected digits.

PHYSICAL EXAMINATION

On examination, the aforementioned classic tricolor changes can often be observed with sharp demarcation of where the spasm occurs. Submerging the patient's hand in ice water can occasionally precipitate attacks. Physical examination of the digits can reveal dilated capillary loops at the base of the nail beds. Tissue breakdown and ulcerations, or pitted scars of former attacks, can also be present.

DIFFERENTIAL DIAGNOSIS

Raynaud's Phenomenon

PRIMARY DISORDER
Raynaud's phenomenon

SECONDARY DISORDER
Drug-induced condition
Trauma (electric shock or repetitive injury)
Occupational injury or exposure
Connective tissue disease
- Rheumatoid arthritis
- Scleroderma
- Systemic lupus erythematosus
- Polymyositis
- Dermatomyositis

Hematologic disorders
- Polycythemia
- Cryoglobulinemia
- Waldenström's macroglobulinemia
- Cold agglutinins
- Cryofibrinogemia
- Myeloproliferative disorder

Occlusive disease or disorder
- Atherosclerosis
- Thromboembolism
- Thoracic outlet syndrome
- Buerger's disease (thromboangiitis obliterans)
- Takayasu's arteritis

Neurologic disorder
- Cervical disc disease
- Tumor
- Cerebrovascular accident
- Poliomyelitis

Pulmonary hypertension
Reflux sympathetic dystrophy
Chilblain

DIAGNOSTICS

The diagnosis of Raynaud's phenomenon is based on a clinical history of the classic tricolor changes. Capillaroscopy of the nail fold allows direct visualization of the capillaries, helping to distinguish primary from secondary Raynaud's.[5] Antinuclear antibody positivity is a predictor of progression to, or association with, a connective tissue disease. In particular, the presence of an anticentromere antibody is associated with the development of CREST, whereas the anti-Scl-70 antibody is more often seen in scleroderma.[6]

DIFFERENTIAL DIAGNOSIS

The differential diagnosis of Raynaud's phenomenon is extensive and can be divided into several categories. These include occupational exposures, drug exposures, occlusive vascular disease, connective tissue disease, hematologic disorders, and others.[7] Primary Raynaud's phenomenon can be difficult to distinguish from other causes of vasospasm in the differential diagnosis. Observation of the tricolor changes is helpful.

Patients with primary Raynaud's phenomenon without the presence of autoantibodies tend to do well without medical intervention. The absence of nail fold capillary abnormalities in patients with autoantibodies improves the prognosis. Patients with CREST are usually spared the life-threatening organ involvement seen in scleroderma. They are still subject to the pulmonary hypertension.

DIAGNOSTICS

Raynaud's Phenomenon

INITIAL
Nail fold capillaroscopy

LABORATORY
Antinuclear antibody
Anti-Scl-70
Anticentromere antibody

MANAGEMENT

In its most benign form, Raynaud's phenomenon can be a mild inconvenience. Most patients suffer from discomfort when Raynaud's phenomenon is triggered but have no permanent damage. Nifedipine, a calcium channel blocker, may help prevent vasospasm.[8] If vasospasms are not controlled, other vasodilators such as hydralazine and prazosin can be added, provided that the blood pressure is not adversely affected. Losartan or pentoxifylline can also be used. Many other drugs are being studied, including selective serotonin reuptake inhibitors and sildenafil. So far, limited evidence exists for benefit of any one treatment. The herbal ginkgo biloba was studied in a double blind placebo-controlled trial and was found to reduce the number of attacks by 56% when compared with placebo.[9] Antiplatelet therapy with aspirin should be considered for all patients with secondary Raynaud's with a history of ischemic ulcers.[10]

In patients for whom standard medical therapy has failed and who are at risk for permanent ischemic damage, chemical ganglion sympathectomies can be tried. Sympathectomy has been used to treat patients with Raynaud's for decades. This can be achieved chemically with lidocaine blocks delivered locally or cervically. A vascular or hand surgeon can perform permanent digital sympathectomy if medical therapies fail. It is unclear whether the benefits of this procedure persist over time, and newer medical strategies may be more appropriate.

Alternatively, patients are hospitalized for IV administration of prostaglandin, such as prostaglandin E_1.[11] This therapy is reserved for those with secondary Raynaud's and severe digital ischemia. Oral and inhaled prostaglandin preparations are being studied in Japan, Europe, and the United States. So far their usefulness is limited to patients with pulmonary hypertension. There have been mixed results with the treatment of Raynaud's phenomenon.[3]

COMPLICATIONS

In some patients the protracted ischemia results in ulcerations that can become superinfected. Treatment of the infection can be challenging, since local delivery of antibiotics is difficult given the impaired blood flow. Rarely, ischemia can be so profound that loss of tissue and bone stock can occur, resulting in autoamputation of digits.

INDICATIONS FOR REFERRAL OR HOSPITALIZATION

Referral to a rheumatologist is necessary to exclude the presence of associated autoimmune disease. In severe cases consultation with a vascular surgeon or anesthesiologist may be indicated. Patients who are in intractable pain or at risk for autoamputation of a digit or severe infection should be hospitalized under the care of a rheumatologist. A vascular surgeon should be consulted early if possible digit loss is suspected. Anesthesia can also be helpful in providing chemical ganglion sympathectomies for the relief of pain. Referral to an occupational therapist for evaluation and education can be helpful. Some patients have found biofeedback useful for management and reduction of Raynaud's attacks.

PATIENT EDUCATION

Patient education is crucial, and the potentially serious nature of this disorder should be emphasized. Patients should avoid exposing their hands to the cold if at all possible. Mittens, which are preferable to gloves, should be worn as soon as the weather begins to get cool. For some patients, mittens need to be worn when grocery shopping, since reaching for food items in refrigerator or freezer sections can often trigger attacks. Keeping core temperature higher by wearing hats and layering clothing may also be of benefit. Sudden temperature changes should be avoided. For many patients, emotional stress can trigger episodes; relaxation techniques, behavioral modification, and biofeedback may play a role in limiting attacks. Most critically, patients should discontinue cigarette smoking if they are smokers. Medications to be avoided include decongestants, amphetamines, estrogen, and beta blockers.

If Raynaud's occurs with the use of vibrating machinery such as jack hammers or chain saws, patients may need vocational counseling.

REFERENCES

1. Wigley FM: Clinical practice: Raynaud's phenomenon, *N Engl J Med* 347:1001, 2002.
2. O'Keeffe ST, Tsapatsaris NP, Beetham WP: Increased prevalence of migraine and chest pain in patients with primary Raynaud's disease, *Ann Intern Med* 116(12):985-989, 1992.
3. Boin F, Wigley F: Understanding, assessing and treating Raynaud's phenomenon, *Curr Opin Rheumatol* 17(6):752-760, 2005.
4. Cooke JP, Marshall JM: Mechanisms of Raynaud's disease, *Vasc Med* 10(4):293-307, 2005.
5. Maurizio C, Pizzorni C, Sulli A: Capillaroscopy, *Best Pract Res Clin Rheumatol* 19(3):437-452, 2005.
6. Sarkozi J, Bookman AA, Lee P, and others: Significance of anticentromere antibody in idiopathic Raynaud's syndrome, *Am J Med* 83:893-898, 1987.
7. Silver R: Raynaud's phenomenon. In Stein J, Eisenberg JM, Hutton JJ, and others, editors: *Internal medicine*, ed 5, St Louis, 1998, Mosby.
8. Rodeheffer RJ, Rommer JA, Wigley F, and others: Controlled double-blind trial of nifedipine in the treatment of Raynaud's phenomenon, *N Engl J Med* 308:880-883, 1983.
9. Muir AH, Robb R, McLaren M, and others: The use of ginkgo biloba in Raynaud's disease: a double-blind placebo-controlled trial, *Vasc Med* 7(4):265-267, 2002.
10. Wigley F: *Clinical manifestations and diagnosis of the Raynaud phenomenon*, retrieved Feb 2, 2006, from http://www.uptodate.com.
11. Simms RW, Farber H, Kissen E, and others: Intravenous epoprostenol for severe digital ischemia in scleroderma, *Arthritis Rheum* 9:1704, 2004.

CHAPTER 235

Rheumatoid Arthritis

Dorothy Johnson and
Francisco P. Quismorio, Jr.

DEFINITION AND EPIDEMIOLOGY

Rheumatoid arthritis (RA) is an autoimmune disorder characterized by symmetric inflammatory polyarthritis and varying degrees of extraarticular involvement. Most patients experience a chronic fluctuating course of the disease that may result in joint destruction, deformity, disability, and premature death.[1-4] Major economic and emotional disabilities can result from RA and can have a significant impact on patients' families and loved ones. More than 9 million physician visits and more than 250,000 hospitalizations occur in the United States each year because of RA.[1-6]

RA affects 1% of the adult population in the United States, with women affected two or three times more often than men. The prevalence increases with age. Despite extensive research, the etiology of RA remains unknown; however, most investigators believe that a combination of genetic, environmental, hormonal, and reproductive factors is important. RA probably occurs in a genetically susceptible person with an abnormal immune response to an undetermined antigen(s). Genetic studies have shown that RA is strongly linked to *HLA-DRB 1* alleles, which encode similar sequences (*shared epitope*).[7] Other susceptibility genes, including T-cell receptor signaling, have recently been identified. Smoking, an environmental factor, has also been shown to increase risk for the disease.[7]

PATHOPHYSIOLOGY

The main target of inflammation is the synovial lining of diarthrodial joints. The earliest changes in the synovial membrane are seen in the capillaries and small blood vessels. There is proliferation of the lining cells and early infiltration by T lymphocytes. Later, there is diffuse infiltration with B and T lymphocytes, macrophages, and plasma cells. The synovial membrane undergoes hyperplastic thickening with the proliferation of lining cells and fibroblasts and formation of new blood vessels. This granulation tissue, called *pannus*, invades the cartilage and subchondral bone and is primarily responsible for the destruction of joint structures in RA.[1-4]

Immune complexes in the synovial tissue activate the complement system, which then participates in the inflammatory process. Kinins, prostaglandins, cytokines, and other mediators increase the permeability of blood vessels and attract leukocytes and lymphocytes into the joint. Neutrophils and macrophages ingest immune complexes and release enzymes that degrade articular cartilage and joint structures. Rheumatoid factor (RF), antibodies to citrullinated proteins, and possibly other autoantibodies produced locally in the synovium participate in the formation of pathogenic immune complexes.[1-4,8-10]

T cells are the major infiltrating lymphocytes in the rheumatoid synovium. Many autoantigens are targeted by the immune system in RA, and some autoantigens are T-cell targets. Activated T cells proliferate, expand, and stimulate monocytes, macrophages, and synovial fibroblasts to secrete cytokines, including interleukin-1 (IL-1) and tumor necrosis factor-α (TNF-α). Both cytokines stimulate mesenchymal cells to secrete matrix metalloproteinases that destroy cartilage and bone. Activated T cells stimulate B cells to produce immunoglobulins, including RF.[1-4,10]

Venules and small blood vessels become occluded by hypertrophied endothelial cells: fibrin, platelets, and inflammatory cells. The decreased circulation along with the increased metabolic demands of hypertrophy and hyperplasia results in hypoxia and metabolic acidosis. Acidosis stimulates the release of hydrolytic enzymes from synovial cells into the surrounding tissue, causing erosion of articular cartilage and inflammation of ligaments and tendons.[1-4,10]

CLINICAL PRESENTATION

The onset of RA is usually insidious, occurring over a period of several weeks or months, but in 10% to 15% of patients the onset is acute. The initial symptoms include general systemic manifestations of inflammation, weakness, weight loss, malaise, fatigue, anorexia, aching, and stiffness. Localized symptoms include painful, tender, swollen joints. Morning stiffness lasts for as long as 1 to 2 hours.[1-4,11]

The small joints of the hands, metacarpophalangeal and proximal interphalangeal joints, wrists and small joints of the feet, and metatarsophalangeal joints are commonly affected initially. Joint involvement is bilateral and symmetric. The hips, knees, ankles, shoulders, and cervical spine may also be involved.[1-4,11]

PHYSICAL EXAMINATION

A complete medical history should be obtained in a comfortable setting. Particular attention should be paid to the location, quality, quantity, course, and alleviating factors of the patient's pain. Functional activities, activities of daily living, instrumental activities of daily living, and social support should be assessed. The patient should be evaluated for comorbid medical conditions such as hypertension, diabetes, or heart disease.[2]

Physical examination of the peripheral joints and the axial skeleton is central to the evaluation of a patient with RA. The joints should be examined in an organized manner, and report of joint pain, tenderness, degree of swelling, range of motion, and deformity should be recorded. On palpation, the inflamed joint feels warm and tender and the synovial membrane feels thickened and boggy. The skin over the affected joint may look thin and shiny and have a ruddy color. During the joint examination the examiner should support painful or weak joints.[11,12]

The physical examination should include evaluation for the presence of extraarticular manifestations. Subcutaneous nodules, which are present in 20% of patients with RA, are found over pressure areas, such as the extensor surface of the elbow and other areas of trauma. Rheumatoid nodules may occasionally be found on the cardiac valves, pericardium, pleura, lung parenchyma, and spleen. Other extraarticular manifestations of RA can include signs of vasculitis (mononeuritis multiplex, skin infarcts, and ulceration), ocular signs

(Sjögren's syndrome, episcleritis, and scleritis), respiratory symptoms (interstitial lung disease or pleurisy), cardiac involvement (pericarditis or valvular heart disease), and peripheral nerve entrapments.[1,2,12]

Sjögren's syndrome, seen in up to 30% of patients with RA, is characterized by dry eyes (keratoconjunctivitis sicca) and dry mouth (xerostomia) and is caused by immune-mediated destruction of the salivary and lacrimal glands. Felty's syndrome, an uncommon feature seen in longstanding RA, is characterized by skin ulcers, leukopenia, splenomegaly, and increased risk for bacterial infections.[1-4,11,12]

DIAGNOSTICS

The diagnosis of RA is primarily based on the clinical history and physical findings. Laboratory tests, including radiographs, are used to confirm the diagnosis, to exclude other conditions, and, more important, to predict the prognosis and develop a treatment plan for the individual patient.

Because RA can affect many organs, it is important to obtain laboratory tests as a baseline evaluation and periodically during the course of treatment. Baseline evaluation should include a CBC; acute-phase reactants, including erythrocyte sedimentation rate (ESR) and C-reactive protein (CRP); serum creatinine; hepatic panel; urinalysis; RF; and anti–cyclic citrullinated peptide (anti-CCP) antibodies. Normocytic, normochromic anemia is very common in RA. Evaluation of renal and hepatic functions is necessary because many antirheumatic agents have renal and hepatic toxicity and may be contraindicated if these organs are severely impaired.[2,3,8,9]

RF in RA is an immunoglobulin (Ig) M autoantibody that is directed against antigenic determinants in the IgG molecule. Not all RA patients have a positive RF at the time of diagnosis, but 70% to 80% of patients will become positive during the course of disease. RA patients with high titer of RF tend to have more severe joint and extraarticular disease and worse prognosis than RF-negative patients. The titer of RF does not change rapidly with treatment, so frequent monitoring is not recommended.[1-4,11]

DIAGNOSTICS

Rheumatoid Arthritis

LABORATORY

- ESR
- C-reactive protein
- Rheumatoid factor
- CBC and differential count
- BUN, creatinine
- Hepatic panel (alanine aminotransferase, aspartate aminotransferase, albumin and alkaline phosphatase)
- Urinalysis
- Synovial fluid analysis
- Imaging
- Hepatitis B and C panel
- Anti–cyclic citrullinated peptide antibody

IMAGING

- Radiography of selected involved joints

Acute-phase reactants are proteins that are synthesized rapidly by the liver in the presence of inflammation or tissue necrosis and include CRP, fibrinogen, complement proteins, and several other proteins. Measurement of serum concentration of CRP and ESR is widely used to assess the activity of the inflammatory process and aid in monitoring response to therapy.[1-4,11]

Radiographs

Because the hands and feet are often involved in RA, x-ray studies of these and other affected joints help with the diagnosis and establish a baseline for future evaluation of the effectiveness of treatment. The radiographs of the joints and bones are often normal at the onset of the disease, but bone erosions can develop within the first 2 years. The American College of Rheumatology established criteria for the classification of RA that can be used as guidelines for patient diagnosis and for research classification.[1-4,11]

Synovial Fluid Analysis

Aspiration of an inflamed joint and examination of the synovial fluid are important to the diagnosis of RA. Normal synovial fluid is clear, viscous, and low in volume with a WBC count of 2000 cells/mm^3. In RA the joint fluid is inflammatory with poor viscosity and a high WBC count of more than 10,000 cells/mm^3 with a predominance of neutrophils.[1-4,11]

DIFFERENTIAL DIAGNOSIS

The differential diagnosis must consider other causes of inflammatory arthritis. Initially, systemic lupus erythematosus, psoriatic arthritis, and seronegative spondyloarthropathies (ankylosing spondylitis, reactive arthritis, enteropathic arthritis, Reiter's syndrome) may be indistinguishable from RA. Usually the presence of extraarticular manifestations of these disorders helps establish the correct diagnosis. Although antinuclear antibodies (ANAs) may be present in RA patients' anti–double stranded DNA (anti-dsDNA) and anti-Smith (anti-Sm) antibodies, the specific types of ANA associated with systemic lupus erythematosus are negative.[1-4]

Soft tissue disorders such as fibromyalgia, a generalized pain disorder, tendinitis, bursitis, and, in older adults, polymyalgia rheumatica may confound the diagnosis of RA early in the course of the disease. Viral infections such as human parvovirus, hepatitis viruses B and C, and HIV infection can cause symmetric polyarthritis and chronic arthralgia and should be considered in the differential diagnosis.[1-4]

MANAGEMENT

An assessment of the patient's prognosis should be made before selecting the treatment regimen. Poor prognosis is suggested by early age of onset, high serum titer of RF and anti-CCP antibodies, elevated ESR, and swelling of more than two joints. Poor prognostic extraarticular signs are rheumatoid nodules, Sjögren's syndrome, episcleritis, scleritis, interstitial lung disease, pericardial involvement, systemic vasculitis, and Felty's syndrome.[1,2]

DIFFERENTIAL DIAGNOSIS

Rheumatoid Arthritis

- Fibromyalgia
- Osteoarthritis
- Viral syndrome
- Soft tissue syndromes
- Spondyloarthropathies
- Systemic lupus erythematosus
- Scleroderma
- Dermatomyositis polymyositis
- Polymyalgia rheumatica
- Systemic vasculitis

Nonpharmacologic Treatment

Instruction in joint protection, conservation of energy, strengthening exercises, and a range-of-motion program is beneficial for all RA patients. Regular participation in dynamic and aerobic conditioning exercise program improves joint symptoms, muscle strength, functional abilities, and psychologic well-being. Consultation with occupational and physical therapists for assistive and adaptive devices and education about care of joints are recommended.

Complementary and alternative therapy is of growing interest and use to RA patients. Many patients receiving conventional medical therapy are also using acupuncture, acupressure, herbs, and other complementary modalities.[12]

Pharmacologic Therapy

Choosing a pharmacologic agent for an individual patient is based on consideration of cost, efficacy, safety, and convenience. Pharmacologic therapy often consists of a combination of NSAIDs, disease-modifying antirheumatic drugs (DMARDs), anti-TNF-α agents, and glucocorticoids[12-14] (Table 235-1).

Nonsteroidal Antiinflammatory Drugs. Salicylates, NSAIDs, or selective cyclooxygenase-2 (COX-2) inhibitors to reduce joint pain and swelling and to improve joint function are usually the initial drug treatment. These drugs have analgesic and antiinflammatory effects but do not alter the course of disease or prevent joint destruction. They should not be used alone as the treatment of RA.

Adverse cardiovascular effects of selective COX-2 agents have been identified and include hypertension, myocardial infarction, stroke, and exacerbation of congestive heart failure. These agents should be avoided or used with caution in those patients with cardiovascular risk factors.[12,15-18]

Disease-Modifying Antirheumatic Drugs. All patients with RA are candidates for DMARD therapy. DMARDs have the potential to reduce or prevent joint damage and preserve joint integrity and function and alter the course of the disease. Any RA patient taking NSAIDs with ongoing signs or symptoms of active RA such as fatigue, morning stiffness, elevated ESR, synovitis, extraarticular features, or radiographic changes should have DMARD therapy started promptly.

Many factors influence the choice of a DMARD. Patients and their providers must select the initial DMARD based on the efficacy, ease of administration, requirements for monitoring, cost, adverse reactions, co-morbid diseases, and the prognosis of the disease. Commonly used DMARDs include methotrexate, leflunomide, hydroxychloroquine, sulfasalazine, etanercept, infliximab, and anakinra. Less commonly used DMARDs are gold salts, D-penicillamine, azathioprine, minocycline, and cyclosporine.[19-22] Intramuscular gold has not been available commercially for the past several years, and its use has been supplanted by the newer DMARDs (see Table 235-1).

TABLE 235-1 Disease-Modifying Antirheumatic Drugs

Medication	Usual Maintenance Dose
Infliximab	3-5 mg/kg IV q 8 wk
Etanercept	25 mg SQ 2 times a week
Anakinra subcutane	100 mg SQ q day
Methotrexate	7.5-20 mg PO q wk 7.5-20 mg SQ q wk
Hydroxychloroquine	200 mg b.i.d.
Sulfasalazine	500-1000 mg b.i.d.-t.i.d.
Auranofin gold	3 mg PO b.i.d.

Anti–Tumor Necrosis Factor-α Therapy. Biologic agents that selectively block cytokines are now widely used in the treatment of RA. The most clinically effective anticytokine agent is an antagonist to TNF-α; the three available preparations in the United States are etanercept, infliximab, and adalimumab.[22-24]

Interleukin-1 Receptor Antagonist. IL-1 is a cytokine that has been shown to play a major role in RA synovial inflammation and joint destruction. IL-1 receptor antagonist (IL-1Ra) acts to block the binding of IL-1a and IL-1b to the IL-1 receptors, preventing the activation of target cells. Anakinra subcutane, a recombinant form of IL-1Ra, is being used in the treatment of RA.[25]

Glucocorticoids. Low-dose oral glucocorticoids (<10 mg/day of prednisone) are highly effective in relieving symptoms in active RA. The benefits should be weighed against adverse effects such as osteoporosis, hypertension, weight gain, possible hyperglycemia, cataracts, and increased skin fragility. Effectiveness of treatment should be assessed at each follow-up visit. Symptoms of inflammation indicate active disease and may necessitate changing treatment regimens. Intaarticular injection of glucocorticoids is efficacious and widely used if one or two joints are actively inflamed.[1,2,22]

Co-Management with Specialists

The rheumatologist should provide support and consultation to the patient and his or her health care provider. Because the level, training, and experience in the diagnosis and treatment of RA vary among health care providers, the responsibility for diagnosis, development of a treatment plan, and monitoring of therapy should be assigned to the rheumatologist. A general maintenance plan should be developed for the patient with all health care providers participating.

LIFE SPAN CONSIDERATIONS

RA has considerable impact on quality of life. Significant work disability has been identified in patients with RA, with about half of patients who are working at the onset of disease becoming work disabled within 10 years. Direct and indirect monetary costs of RA are enormous. Pregnancy should be avoided in those RA patients taking immune-modulating medications. Approximately half of the RA patients who choose to become pregnant will experience a temporary remission in disease activity for the duration of the pregnancy. Early death has been identified in RA patients, with the life span decreased by about 10 years.[26]

COMPLICATIONS

Joint deformity, with the resulting sequelae of muscle, tendon, and ligament weakening or deconditioning and joint immobilization, is the most important complication. Small-vessel vasculitis can cause neuropathy and skin ulcers. Cervical spine involvement can cause neck pain or abnormal neurologic findings because of myelopathy.

Complications related to adverse reactions to medications include osteoporosis, osteonecrosis (avascular necrosis), retinal toxicity, gastrointestinal irritation and bleeding, and hepatic toxicity. Opportunistic infections may develop with the anti-TNF-α agents, systemic corticosteroids, and other immunosuppressive agents. The development of tuberculosis is a major concern among patients on anti-TNF agents.[1-4,23]

INDICATIONS FOR REFERRAL OR HOSPITALIZATION

Referral to a rheumatologist for diagnosis and treatment of RA is strongly recommended. A rheumatologist should manage medication regimens and monitor for adverse drug reactions. Referral to an orthopedic surgeon specializing in joint replacement should be considered for end-stage joint disease. Quality of life is improved and pain relieved in most patients after joint replacement surgery. Physical and occupational therapists should be consulted for exercise programs and adaptive devices.[27,28] A rheumatology nurse specialist can provide information about lifestyle changes and community programs such as those sponsored by the Arthritis Foundation. Because most patients experience a period of grief after diagnosis, referral to a clinical psychologist or social worker should be considered. Life role adjustments will be made because of the disease, and many patients will benefit from psychologic counseling through this transition.[26-28]

PATIENT AND FAMILY EDUCATION

Patients should be educated about lifestyle modifications such as increased bed rest for disease flare-ups, use of adaptive aids to facilitate function, prioritizing and planning activities to accommodate fatigue, and use of splints for painful and swollen wrists and hands. Podiatric care for foot pain should be provided, along with special shoe wear and flexible orthotic devices. Education about the need for a regular aerobic and muscle-strengthening exercise program is essential to help reduce stiffness, avoid joint contractures, and prevent osteoporosis.

The health care provider should advise the patient about the benefit of warm showers in the morning and frequent position changes to alleviate stiffness. The use of pillows to position joints at night is contraindicated, since this may predispose the patient to flexion deformities.

The health care provider should also educate the patient and family regarding medication use; restrictions; and side or adverse effects, including pregnancy and fetal effects. Warnings against stopping certain medications without notifying the health care provider should be stressed. Instructions should be given about dietary restrictions or recommendations as they relate to medications.[26-28]

Self-management programs, educational information, and exercise programs from the Arthritis Foundation are available to the patients in print form and online. Most material is available in Spanish and English.

REFERENCES

1. Harris ED: Rheumatoid arthritis: pathophysiology and implications for therapy, *N Engl J Med* 322:1277-1289, 1990.
2. Klippel JH, editor: *Primer on the rheumatic diseases,* ed 11, Atlanta, 1997, Arthritis Foundation.
3. Albani S, Carson D: Rheumatoid arthritis. In Koopman WJ, editor: *Arthritis and allied conditions,* ed 13, Baltimore, 1996, Williams & Wilkins.
4. Newman S, Fitzpatrick R, Revenson T, and others: *Understanding rheumatoid arthritis,* London, 1996, Routledge.
5. Silman AJ, Hochberg MC: *Epidemiology of the rheumatic diseases,* New York, 1993, Oxford University Press.
6. Allaire SL, Prashker M, Meenan R: The costs of rheumatoid arthritis, *Pharmoeconomics* 6:513-522, 1994.
7. Van der Helm-van Mil AH, Wesoly JZ, Huizinga TW: Understanding the genetic contribution to rheumatoid arthritis, *Curr Opin Rheumatol* 17:299-304, 2005.
8. Vander Cruyssen B, Peene I, Cantaert IEA, and others: Anti-citrullinated protein/peptide in rheumatoid arthritis: specificity and relation with rheumatoid factor, *Auto Rev* 4:468-474, 2005.
9. Hitchon CA, Alex P, Eridile LB, and others: A distinct multicytokine profile is associated with anti-cyclical citrullinated peptide antibodies in patients with early untreated inflammatory arthritis, *J Rheumatol* 12:2336-2346, 2004.
10. Choy EHS, Panayi GS: Mechanisms of disease: cytokine pathways and joint inflammation in rheumatoid arthritis, *N Engl J Med* 344:907-916, 2001.
11. Arnett FC, Edworthy SM, Bloch DA, and others: The American Rheumatism Association 1987 revised criteria for the classification of rheumatoid arthritis, *Arthritis Rheum* 31:315-324, 1988.
12. Affleck G, Tennen H, Pfeiffer C, and others: Appraisals of control and predictability in adapting to chronic disease, *J Pers Soc Psychol* 53(2):273-279, 1987.
13. Polley HF, Hunder GG: *Physical examination of the joints,* ed 2, Philadelphia, 1978, Saunders.
14. American College of Rheumatology: Guidelines for the management of rheumatoid arthritis, *Arthritis Rheum* 46:328-346, 2002.
15. Hudson M, Richard H, Pilote L: Differences in outcomes of patients with congestive heart failure prescribed celecoxib, rofecoxib, or non-steroidal anti-inflammatory drugs: population based study, *BMJ* 330:1370(7504), 2005.
16. Shaya FT, Blume SW, Blanchette CM, and others: Selective cyclooxygenase-2 inhibition and cardiovascular effects: an observational study in a Medicaid population, *Arch Intern Med* 165:181, 2005.
17. Kimmel SE, Berlin JA, Reilly M, and others: Patients exposed to rofecoxib, celecoxib have different odds of nonfatal myocardial infarction, *Ann Intern Med* 142:157, 2005.
18. Johnsen SP, Larsson H, Tarone RE, and others: Risk of hospitalization for myocardial infarcation among users of rofecoxib, celecoxib and other NSAIDs: a population-based case-control study, *Arch Intern Med* 165(9):198-984, 2005.
19. Solomon SD, McMurray JJ, Pfeiffer MA, and others: Cardiovascular risk associated with celecoxib in a clinical trial for colorectal adenoma prevention, *N Engl J Med* 352:1071, 2005.
20. Van der Heijde DW, Johannes WG, Jacobs MD, and others: The effectiveness of early treatment with "second-line" antirheumatic drugs: a randomized, controlled trial, *Ann Intern Med* 124:699-707, 1996.
21. Tsakonas E, Fitzgerald AA, Fitzcharles MA, and others: Consequences of delayed therapy with second-line agents in rheumatoid arthritis: a 3-year follow-up on the Hydroxychloroquine in Early Rheumatoid Arthritis (HERA) study, *J Rheumatol* 27:623-629, 2000.
22. Albers JM, Paimela L, Kurki P, and others: Treatment strategy, disease

activity, and outcome in four cohorts of patients with early rheumatoid arthritis, *Ann Rheum Dis* 60:453-458, 2001.

23. Weinblatt ME, Kremer JM, Bankhurst AD, and others: A trial of etanercept, a recombinant tumor necrosis factor receptor: Fc fusion protein, in patients with rheumatoid arthritis receiving methotrexate, *N Engl J Med* 340:253-259, 1999.
24. Heiberg MS, Nordvag BY, Mikkelsen K, and others: The comparative effectiveness of tumor necrosis factor–blocking agents in patients with rheumatoid arthritis and patients with ankylosing spondylitis: a 6 month, longitudinal, observational, multicenter study, *Arthritis Rheum* 8:2506-2512, 2005.
25. Jiang Y, Genant HK, Watt I, and others: A multicenter, double-blind, dose-ranging, randomized, placebo-controlled study of recombinant human interleukin-1 receptor antagonist in patients with rheumatoid arthritis, *Arthritis Rheum* 43(5):1001-1009, 2000.
26. Schiaffino KM, Revenson TA, Gibofsky A: Assessing the impact of self-efficacy beliefs of adaptation to rheumatoid arthritis, *Arthritis Care Res* 4:150-157, 1991.
27. Komatireddy GR, Leitch RW, Cella K, and others: Efficacy of low resistance muscle training in patients with rheumatoid arthritis functional class II and III, *J Rheumatol* 24:1531-1539, 1997.
28. Neuberger GB, Press AN, Lindsley HB, and others: Effects of exercise on fatigue, aerobic fitness, and disease activity measures with rheumatoid arthritis, *Res Nurs Health* 20:195-204, 1997.

CHAPTER 236

Systemic Lupus Erythematosus

Francisco P. Quismorio, Jr., and
Dorothy Johnson

DEFINITION AND EPIDEMIOLOGY

Systemic lupus erythematosus (SLE) is a chronic multisystem inflammatory rheumatic disease that may cause diverse symptoms such as fatigue, joint pain, skin rashes, seizures, edema, and chest pain.[1,2] SLE has a predilection for women, particularly during the prime childbearing years of 15 to 35. The most characteristic laboratory finding in SLE is the presence of a wide variety of autoantibodies, including antinuclear antibodies (ANAs). SLE can damage many organ systems, notably the kidneys, lungs, heart, and brain, and may result in severe disability and even death.

SLE is not an uncommon rheumatic disease, with the incidence and prevalence rates that are difficult to measure with great precision. These rates vary by geographic distribution and by demographic characteristics. Data from European and American surveys suggest that the prevalence of SLE among Caucasians ranges from 12 to 39 per 100,000 persons.[3] The reported incidence rates of SLE in the United States also vary from 1.8 to 7.6 cases per 100,000 persons per year. SLE is up to 10 times more common in women than in men.[3] The disease is more common in African-American women, among whom the prevalence may be as high as 1 in 250. In addition, African-American patients with SLE are more likely to experience severe organ damage.[4] Epidemiologic data have suggested that the incidence of the disease may be increasing.[5]

The cause of SLE is unknown.[1,2] Its association with certain genotypes such as the *C4* null allele and various HLA haplotypes, as well as the 25% rate of concordance in identical twins, suggests that the disease is likely a result of an interaction between genetic makeup and one or more environmental triggers. Genetic studies have identified chromosomal regions that exhibit significant linkage with SLE.[6] Because certain drugs can induce lupus-like syndromes, it is speculated that certain environmental agents may promote the development of SLE. An amino acid, L-canavanine, which is found in alfalfa sprouts, has been associated with the development of an SLE-like disease in macaque monkeys; this, together with reports of disease exacerbation in SLE patients after ingestion of alfalfa tablets, suggests a role for dietary factors. Other potential environmental triggers include a wide range of viruses, including the Epstein-Barr virus,[7] physical trauma, and emotional stress. Differences in the level and metabolism of estrogen, androgen, and other sex hormones may partly account for the female predilection for the disease.

PATHOPHYSIOLOGY

The pathophysiologic hallmark of SLE is the development of antibodies directed against components of "self" tissues, particularly structures found within cell nuclei. The LE cell test, the first laboratory diagnostic test for the disease, described in 1948 by Hargraves, is predicated on the presence of ANA specific for deoxyribonucleoprotein.[1] Since then, a wide variety of autoantibodies have been reported in SLE, including antibodies directed against DNA and other nuclear constituents, red blood cells, platelets, white blood cells, and phospholipids. Autoantibodies form immune complexes in the circulation or in situ and become deposited in kidneys, skin, lungs, and other target organs. Circulating immune complexes are normally solubilized and cleared from the circulation by the reticuloendothelial system. In SLE, there is an aberrant clearance of immune complexes that may be related to defective solubilization of antigen-antibody complexes and abnormalities of complement and cell receptor functions. Individuals with genetic deficiencies of the early complement components C1q, C2, and C4 are at an increased risk for lupus-like autoimmune disease. Defective apoptosis (programmed cell death) with phagocytosis of cell debris allowing nuclear antigens to become antigenic, abnormalities in T and B cell functions, cytokines, innate immunity, and other immune mechanisms that promote self-tolerance all contribute to the development of autoimmunity in SLE.[8]

The deposition of immune complexes in tissues generates a local inflammatory response that may have organ-specific effects. Inflammation in blood vessels can cause vasculitis, which may result in vessel occlusion, ischemia, or infarction of the affected organ. Inflammation of serosal surfaces (visceral membrane linings) may result in pleurisy or pericarditis. The deposition of pathogenic immune complexes in the renal glomeruli can result in the development of lupus nephritis.

CLINICAL PRESENTATION AND PHYSICAL EXAMINATION

SLE is a systemic inflammatory disorder characterized by varied presentation, disease relapses, and remissions. The disease can develop acutely, with obvious severe manifestations that include arthritis, nephritis, serositis, or vasculitis, or it may become apparent in an individual who has had mild symptoms and subtle physical findings (e.g., fatigue, arthralgia, skin rashes) sporadically for many years. The disorder is often misdiagnosed, since many of the early symptoms of SLE are nonspecific (e.g., fatigue, oral ulcers, joint pain) and the ANA test is positive in approximately 5% of healthy persons. The American College of Rheumatology has developed and validated a set of criteria for the classification of SLE[9] (Box 236-1).

Malaise and fatigue, often profound, are common but nonspecific complaints. Anorexia and weight loss may be seen in those patients with active disease, as can fevers, lymphadenopathy, tachycardia, and anemia.

The malar (or butterfly) skin rash, one of the most recognizable features of SLE, is observed in only 35% of patients. This is a photosensitive erythematous rash on the cheeks and over the bridge of the nose that tends to spare the nasolabial folds. Discoid lupus rash is seen in 20% of patients with SLE. In a more benign clinical form of lupus, termed *discoid lupus*

BOX 236-1

REVISED CRITERIA FOR CLASSIFICATION OF SYSTEMIC LUPUS ERYTHEMATOSUS*

1. Malar rash: Fixed erythema, flat or raised, over the malar eminences, tending to spare the nasolabial folds
2. Discoid rash: Erythematous raised patches with adherent keratotic scaling and follicular plugging; atrophic scarring may occur in older lesions
3. Photosensitivity: Skin rash as a result of unusual reaction to sunlight, by patient or physician observation
4. Oral ulcers: Oral or nasopharyngeal ulceration, usually painless, observed by a physician
5. Arthritis: Nonerosive arthritis involving two or more peripheral joints, characterized by tenderness, swelling, or effusion
6. Serositis
   a. Pleuritis—convincing history of pleuritic pain or rub heard by a physician or evidence of pleural effusion *or*
   b. Pericarditis—documented by ECG or rub or evidence of pericardial effusion
7. Renal disorder
   a. Persistent proteinuria—greater than 0.5 g/day or greater than 3+ if quantitation not performed *or*
   b. Cellular casts—may be red cell, hemoglobin, granular, tubular, or mixed
8. Neurologic disorder
   a. Seizures—in the absence of offending drugs or known metabolic derangements (e.g., uremia, ketoacidosis, or electrolyte imbalance) *or*
   b. Psychosis—in the absence of offending drugs or known metabolic derangements (e.g., uremia, ketoacidosis, or electrolyte imbalance)
9. Hematologic disorder
   a. Hemolytic anemia—with reticulocytosis *or*
   b. Leukopenia—less than 4000/mm^3 total on two or more occasions *or*
   c. Lymphopenia—less than 1500/mm^3 on two or more occasions *or*
   d. Thrombocytopenia—less than 100,000/mm^3 in the absence of offending drugs
10. Immunologic disorder
   a. Anti-DNA—antibody to native DNA in abnormal titer *or*
   b. Anti-Sm—presence of antibody to Sm nuclear antigen *or*
   c. Positive antiphospholipid antibodies based on abnormal serum level IgG or IgM anticardiolipin, positive test for lupus anticoagulant *or*
   d. False-positive serologic test for syphilis known to be positive for at least 6 months and confirmed by *Treponema pallidum* immobilization or fluorescent treponemal antibody absorption test
11. Antinuclear antibody: An abnormal titer of antinuclear antibody by immunofluorescence or an equivalent assay at any point in time and in the absence of drugs known to be associated with "drug-induced lupus" syndrome

Tan EM, Cohen AS, Fries JF, and others: The 1982 revised criteria for the classification of systemic lupus erythematosus, *Arthritis Rheum* 25(11):1271-1277, 1982; and Hochberg MC: Updating the American College of Rheumatology revised criteria for the classification of systemic lupus erythematosus, *Arthritis Rheum* 40:1725, 1997.

*The proposed classification is based on 11 criteria. For the purpose of identifying patients in clinical studies, a person shall be said to have systemic lupus erythematosus if any 4 or more of the 11 criteria are present, serially or simultaneously, during any interval of observation.

erythematosus, the disease is predominantly cutaneous with no or mild visceral involvement. Discoid lupus skin lesions are thick, round, erythematous plaques on the face, scalp, and extremities that heal with scarring, atrophy, depigmentation, and loss of hair. Mucous membrane ulcers are also common, occurring in the oral and nasal cavities.

Approximately one third of SLE patients experience Raynaud's phenomenon, a vasospastic syndrome characterized by episodic changes in blood flow to the extremities, accompanied by sequential color change and often unpleasant tingling or painful sensations (see Chapter 234). Livedo reticularis is a purplish mottling or lacelike appearance of the skin, especially in the extremities, and is associated with antiphospholipid syndrome (see below). Cutaneous vasculitis may manifest as tender skin nodules, splinter hemorrhages, palpable purpura or skin infarcts, and ulcerations. Bruising or petechiae caused by immune thrombocytopenia may also occur.

Joint pain (arthralgia) occurs in 80% to 90% of patients with SLE, and inflammatory arthritis can be objectively documented in about 50% of patients. The arthritis of SLE is generally milder than rheumatoid arthritis. It is nonerosive, and fewer than 10% of the patients will develop joint deformities, called Jaccoud's arthropathy. Osteoporosis is common and is multifactorial in etiology, including corticosteroid therapy, chronic inflammation, and physical inactivity. In those patients with renal insufficiency, metabolic bone disease related to vitamin D deficiency and secondary hyperparathyroidism may be a contributing factor. Inflammatory myositis manifesting as proximal muscle weakness with elevated creatine phosphokinase can be seen in SLE.

Chest pain is a common complaint and is often musculoskeletal in origin. More significantly, SLE can cause serious cardiopulmonary disease, including pleurisy, pericarditis, pneumonitis, interstitial lung disease, pulmonary hemorrhage, myocarditis, and valvular heart disease.

A subset of SLE patients develop antiphospholipid syndrome, characterized by hypercoagulability, recurrent venous or arterial thrombosis, repeated abortions and fetal loss, and the presence of antiphospholipid antibodies as measured by anticardiolipin antibodies or lupus anticoagulant. These patients have an increased risk for pulmonary embolism that can result in pulmonary hypertension, strokes, abortion and fetal loss, Libman-Sacks endocarditis, and valvular heart disease.

Lupus patients are at a greatly increased risk of developing ischemic heart disease.[10] It has been reported that SLE patients in the age range of 35 to 44 years have a 50-fold increased risk for myocardial infarction.[11] The prevalence of symptomatic coronary artery disease (CAD) in large longitudinal studies is at least 10%, and, depending on the diagnostic technique used, subclinical CAD is detected in 35% of patients.[12] The full reasons for the increased risk are unclear but may relate in part to hypertension, alterations in lipid metabolism associated with nephrotic syndrome and the long-term use of corticosteroids, and endothelial damage due to chronic inflammatory process. Hypertension is common and may be associated with underlying lupus nephritis, the use of corticosteroids, and possibly NSAIDs as contributing factors.

Mood changes, depression, and migraine headaches are common. SLE can cause wide-ranging neuropsychiatric abnormalities, the most common being cognitive dysfunction with confusion and impaired memory and concentration. Psychosis, seizures, altered consciousness, stroke, and neuropathies may develop. The pathogenesis of neuropsychiatric manifestations probably involves different mechanisms, including small vessel vasculopathy, thrombosis associated with antiphospholipid syndrome, effects of complement split products, cytokines, and antineuronal antibodies.

Lupus nephritis will develop along the course of the disease in 25% to 50% of patients. Persistent proteinuria greater than 500 mg/day, cellular casts, and red blood cells in the urine sediment are observed. There is a spectrum of renal involvement ranging from mesangial lupus nephritis with increased cellularity and deposition of immune complexes limited to the mesangium to severe diffuse proliferative glomerulonephritis with involvement of all glomeruli. Evaluation and staging of renal disease in SLE require a kidney biopsy, and the histopathologic findings are useful in assessing prognosis and determining a therapeutic regimen. Hemodialysis or kidney transplantation becomes necessary in those who develop end-stage renal disease. Most patients who undergo kidney transplantation do relatively well because of the immunosuppression required for preventing graft rejection. Lupus nephritis recurs at a rate of approximately 6% in the transplanted kidney.

DIAGNOSTICS

During a disease exacerbation of SLE, laboratory tests reveal nonspecific evidence of systemic inflammation with an elevated erythrocyte sedimentation rate, C-reactive protein, and serum gamma globulins.[1,2] Anemia is common and may result from one or a combination of several mechanisms, including iron deficiency; chronic systemic inflammation causing an anemia of chronic disease; autoimmune hemolysis with a positive Coombs' test; bone marrow damage; and, in patients with renal insufficiency, inadequate erythropoietin response. Leukopenia, lymphopenia, and thrombocytopenia are characteristic hematologic features of the disease and appear to be mediated by organ-specific autoantibodies. Immune thrombocytopenic purpura may be the presenting manifestation of SLE. Thrombocytopenia is associated with antiplatelet and antiphospholipid antibodies.

DIAGNOSTICS

Systemic Lupus Erythematosus

LABORATORY	
Urinalysis	Total antinuclear antibodies
CBC and differential	Serum gamma globulins
BUN	Anti-dsDNA, anti-Sm, anti-Ro, anti-La, antiribonucleoprotein
Creatinine	CH_{50}, C3, C4*
ESR	PT/PTT*
Rheumatoid factor	Lupus anticoagulant*
C-reactive protein	Anticardiolipin antibodies

*If indicated.

A urinalysis should always be obtained during a flare and to monitor the disease because patients without previous kidney involvement can develop lupus nephritis de novo. BUN, creatinine, 24-hour urine protein excretion, and creatinine clearance should be monitored for changes indicating new renal involvement or worsening renal function.

Although the "total" ANA test is the most sensitive diagnostic test, a positive test result is not specific for SLE. In contrast, anti-Smith (anti-Sm) and anti–double-stranded DNA (anti-dsDNA) autoantibodies are more specific for the diagnosis of lupus.[9] Both types of autoantibodies are present in 30% to 40% of patients; thus a negative test for either anti-Sm or anti-dsDNA does not necessarily exclude a diagnosis of SLE.[9] The presence of anti-Ro/SSA and anti-La/SSB in 30% and 15% of patients, respectively, is associated with subacute cutaneous lupus, secondary Sjögren's syndrome, and neonatal lupus syndrome.[1,2]

Antiphospholipid antibodies (aPLs) are a heterogeneous group of autoantibodies in SLE and are commonly tested by immunoglobulin (Ig) G and IgM anticardiolipin antibodies and by lupus anticoagulant. A prolonged activated partial thromboplastin time (aPTT) may suggest the presence of a lupus anticoagulant; however, the most commonly used assay for lupus anticoagulant is the dilute Russell's viper venom test (DRVVT). Antiphospholipid antibodies may sometimes cause a biologic false-positive test for syphilis (Venereal Disease Research Laboratory [VDRL] or rapid plasma reagin); however, a syphilitic infection is excluded by negative specific antitreponemal tests.[13] Other autoantibodies, including rheumatoid factor and antiribonucleoprotein, can be seen in SLE patients. Anti–cyclic citrullinated peptide antibody, a characteristic finding in rheumatoid arthritis, has been reported in a few SLE patients.

In contrast to other systemic rheumatic disorders, serum complement levels may decrease in SLE, indicating the deposition of immune complexes in tissues. In many patients, a fall in the serum concentration of C3 is associated with flares of nephritis. Complement can be activated in inflammation of other tissues, including the skin. Direct immunofluorescent test on a biopsy specimen of normal-appearing skin in SLE shows the presence of IgG, IgM, IgA, C3, and/or C1q deposits at the dermal-epidermal junction (lupus band test).

DIFFERENTIAL DIAGNOSIS

SLE can be mistaken for a number of diseases, particularly other systemic rheumatic conditions, including rheumatoid arthritis, mixed connective tissue disease, dermatomyositis, systemic vasculitis, as well as fibromyalgia, multiple sclerosis, and other nonrheumatic disorders. Individuals with fibromyalgia who have a low titer of ANA may be misdiagnosed as having SLE. Acute parvovirus infection with arthritis can mimic SLE, and serologic tests may be positive.[14] Drug-induced lupus may develop in patients taking procainamide, hydralazine, quinidine, anticonvulsants, antithyroid medications, or other medications.

DIFFERENTIAL DIAGNOSIS

Systemic Lupus Erythematosus

- Fibromyalgia
- Mixed connective tissue disease
- Rheumatoid arthritis
- Dermatomyositis, polymyositis
- Primary Sjögren's syndrome
- Systemic sclerosis (scleroderma)
- Systemic vasculitides (e.g., Wegener's granulomatosis, polyarteritis)
- Drug-induced lupus
- Multiple sclerosis
- Lymphoma and other malignancies
- Psychiatric disorders

MANAGEMENT

Individuals diagnosed with SLE require guidance and education about the disease.[1] Avoidance of strong sunlight is emphasized because many patients are photosensitive such that sun exposure may precipitate lupus skin rash and exacerbation of disease activity. Patients are advised to use sunscreen with a sun protection factor (SPF) of at least 15 and sun protective clothing to avoid excessive exposure. In a few documented cases, exposure to unshielded fluorescent lighting has exacerbated disease activity. Modest physical exercise is considered helpful in maintaining cardiopulmonary fitness, avoiding obesity, and improving mood. Diet is important and often overlooked. Studies in mice with lupus-like syndromes show that diets enriched with fish oil–derived fatty acids protect mice from the development of glomerulonephritis, whereas mice fed diets enriched with lipids derived from beef tallow have an accelerated disease process.[15] Although this has not been confirmed in SLE patients, the frequent occurrence of lipid abnormalities and the accelerated atherosclerosis in the lupus population suggest that avoidance of diets high in saturated fats is reasonable. When indicated, statins can be safely prescribed to treat hypercholesterolemia in SLE patients. Because of the frequent occurrence of osteoporosis in these patients, attention should be paid to ensuring adequate calcium and vitamin D in the patient's diet.

Regular health checkups with other specialties are important in the patient with lupus. Regular gynecologic care is important, considering recent studies showing an increased incidence of cervical dysplasia and human papillomavirus infection among SLE patients.[16] Obviously the issues regarding pregnancy and hormone replacement are complex in these patients and require communication among obstetrician/gynecologist, rheumatologist, and health care provider. The patient with SLE will need dental consultation with attention to antibiotic prophylaxis, given the risk for infective endocarditis, especially in those with valvular heart abnormalities.[17] When secondary Sjögren's syndrome is present, accelerated problems with caries and gingivitis are often seen. Ophthalmologic monitoring is important to detect the onset of dry eyes (Sjögren's syndrome) and to check for ocular side effects of hydroxychloroquine, chloroquine, and corticosteroids.

NSAIDs are generally employed for the treatment of pain, particularly joint pain, fever, and serositis. Careful monitoring for NSAID toxicity is advised. Salicylate hepatitis can be seen occasionally in SLE patients. An unusual syndrome of aseptic meningitis can occur with the use of ibuprofen and other NSAIDs in SLE. All NSAIDs, including the cyclooxygenase-2 (COX-2) selective NSAIDs, have effects on renal functions that can exacerbate hypertension, edema, and renal insufficiency in patients with lupus nephritis. COX-2 selective NSAIDs should be avoided in patients with cardiovascular risk factors. Hydroxychloroquine is widely prescribed and is effective in managing the musculoskeletal, cutaneous, and serosal manifestations of the disease (Table 236-1). It has been shown to be effective in allowing tapering of steroids and reducing flares of disease.[18]

Corticosteroids remain the mainstay of drug therapy for SLE, and the dosage depends on the severity and extent of the disease. For discoid and other lupus skin lesions, treatment with local corticosteroid cream, ointment, or injection is often helpful. For patients with joint pain, fatigue, and milder disease who have failed to respond to hydroxychloroquine, low-dose corticosteroids (<10 mg/day) may improve the quality of life. For patients with major organ involvement (pericarditis, thrombocytopenia, autoimmune hemolytic anemia, nephritis, neuropsychiatric lupus) or multiorgan life-threatening disease, corticosteroids are given in higher dosages, ranging from 40 to 100 mg/day to "pulse" therapy of 1 g methylprednisolone IV q day for 3 days.

After the initial active disease begins to come under control, a variety of immunosuppressive agents are added to control disease and allow tapering of corticosteroids (steroid-sparing effect). The choice of immunosuppressive agent depends in part on the organ involvement. For diffuse lupus nephritis (Class IV), studies have shown that the combination of IV cyclophosphamide and prednisone is associated with better renal outcome than prednisone alone.[19] Mycophenolate mofetil has also been shown in recent controlled trials to be effective in lupus nephritis and with a better safety profile than cyclophosphamide.[20] For patients with severe persistent arthritis, methotrexate has been used. Azathioprine has shown efficacy in both renal and nonrenal lupus. Intravenous gamma globulin is efficacious in severe immune thrombocytopenic purpura and in other organ-threatening lupus.

The treatment of antiphospholipid syndrome in SLE involves anticoagulation for thrombosis or pregnancy prophylaxis; however, certain aspects of therapy remain controversial.[13] Clearly the patient who has experienced recurrent thrombosis or a major thrombotic event such as a pulmonary embolism or stroke should be treated with anticoagulation. These patients need to maintain anticoagulation at medium to high therapeutic range. Whether lifetime anticoagulation should be recommended for all the patients remains unresolved. For pregnant SLE patients with aPL and prior fetal loss, subcutaneous low-molecular-weight heparin and low-dose aspirin are recommended. Pregnant SLE patients with prior history of both obstetric and thrombotic complications are given a therapeutic dose of heparin and low-dose aspirin. A pregnant SLE patient with moderate to high titer of aPL antibodies but without prior thrombotic or obstetric complications is given low-dose aspirin alone. Many rheumatologists also recommend low-dose aspirin daily for SLE patients with moderate or high titers of aPL antibodies but without a previous history of thrombotic event or pregnancy loss; however, the value of the regimen remains to be validated.

Patients with SLE who are at risk for osteoporosis require attention to bone health. Osteoporosis prophylaxis with calcium supplementation and vitamin D is appropriate. Measurement of bone density and implementation of osteoporosis therapy such as bisphosphonates may be required. Avoidance of prolonged high doses of corticosteroids and use of steroid-sparing immunosuppressives may help limit steroid-induced bone loss. Estrogens, on the other hand, should be used with caution because they may exacerbate disease activity and thrombotic tendencies in some patients.

Optimum control of blood pressure is important because SLE patients are at increased risk for cardiovascular disease. High blood pressure increases the risk of kidney involvement or may result from kidney involvement. Systemic corticosteroids contribute to hypertension. Patients with Raynaud's phenomenon may benefit from the use of calcium channel blockers such as nifedipine or angiotensin receptor blockers such as losartan.[21]

Many persons with SLE have difficulty maintaining employment and household work roles.[22] The Americans with Disabilities Act may be able to support patients in efforts to obtain flexible work hours, placement of filters on fluorescent lights, or other accommodations to preserve employment or enhance productivity. Methods of reducing the amount of energy expended in commuting, in doing household work, and in maintaining social activities should be explored. Women can be encouraged to adopt a manager rather than "doer" homemaker role; family counseling may help members manage family role changes necessitated by the disease.[22] The level of social support has been linked to health status, and studies have shown that persons with rheumatic diseases with higher levels of social support have better function.[22] Telephone counseling programs have been effective in reducing feelings of depression and anxiety, as well as in improving

TABLE 236-1 Drugs Used in Treatment of Systemic Lupus Erythematosus

Drug	Dosage	Length of Treatment
Hydroxychloroquine	200 mg q day to b.i.d.	Long term
Chloroquine	250 mg q day	Long term
Prednisone (mild disease)	5-10 mg q day	Intermittent courses
Prednisone (organ-threatening disease)	30-100 mg q day	Intermittent courses
Azathioprine	75-200 mg q day	6 months or longer
Mycophenolate (PO)	Up to 2000 mg/day	6 months or longer
Cyclophosphamide (IV)	0.5-1 g/m2 monthly for 6 months	6 months or longer
Methotrexate (with folic acid, 1 mg q day)	7.5-15 mg q wk	

function and providing support.[23,24] Some patients benefit from treatment with antidepressant medications.

Influenza vaccine should be administered yearly. Administration of pneumococcal vaccine should be considered for all patients with lupus, given evidence of splenic dysfunction in these patients. As mentioned previously, patients with lupus are at increased risk for infective endocarditis and therefore should receive antibiotic prophylaxis while undergoing dental, genitourinary, and other invasive procedures.[1,2]

LIFE SPAN CONSIDERATIONS

The prognosis for patients with SLE has improved dramatically since its first description, when the disease was universally fatal. At present, more than 90% of patients with SLE live 10 years after the onset of symptoms, although the survival rate for those with organ-threatening disease is somewhat lower.[1,2] Certain subsets of the population appear to experience worse disease. African-Americans generally have more severe disease and a poorer prognosis.[4] The reasons for this are unclear but may relate, in part, to socioeconomic factors and reduced access to health care.

Pregnancy may be problematic for both mother and fetus, especially for women with antiphospholipid syndrome. Patients with SLE have increased fetal losses and are at increased risk for preeclampsia and premature rupture of membranes, resulting in prematurity, intrauterine growth retardation, and pregnancy loss. Maternal risks include disease flares during pregnancy, exacerbation of pre-existing hypertension, worsening of renal status, and pulmonary embolism. Both prednisone and methylprednisolone can be safely used in pregnancy because they are inactivated by placental enzymes and do not affect the fetus. However, pregnancy-induced diabetes or hypertension can have effects on fetal well-being. The presence of maternal anti-Ro/SSA during pregnancy is associated with an increased risk for neonatal lupus syndrome in the baby. a condition characterized by congenital heart block and transient lupus skin rash. A high-risk obstetric service, when available, should follow pregnant SLE patients to monitor the progress of the pregnancy, including fetal heart rhythm.

Women who wish to avoid pregnancy should use birth control methods, at least during disease exacerbations, especially in those with nephritis and in those taking methotrexate, leflunomide, or cyclophosphamide. Both injectable medroxyprogesterone (Depo-Provera) and progesterone-only minipills can be safely used by patients with lupus, as can barrier methods. Anecdotal experience suggests that estrogen-containing oral contraceptives, especially in high doses, may exacerbate the disease in some patients.

As young women with lupus live longer, the issue of hormone replacement at menopause becomes one of increasing concern. Though studies are ongoing to determine whether hormone replacement at menopause exacerbates lupus, concerns about the adverse effects of hormone therapy in all menopausal women continue. Certainly in a patient with high to moderate aPL antibodies, both estrogen and the selective estrogen receptor–modulating drug raloxifene should be avoided because of their association with hypercoagulability and venous thrombosis.

COMPLICATIONS

Fever in the patient with SLE should always raise the question of whether it represents a flare of the underlying illness or an infectious process. In particular, fever in the absence of other signs of active SLE or fever associated with leukocytosis should prompt search for an infection and appropriate culture. In patients taking corticosteroids or immunosuppressive agents, opportunistic organisms such as *Listeria monocytogenes, Pneumocystis jiroveci, Cryptococcus neoformans,* and others should be considered. Tuberculosis remains a significant infection in these patients. Fever with digital infarcts and joint pain could represent a flare of lupus but could also be caused by infective endocarditis. In evaluating these patients, the health care provider should promptly perform microbiologic cultures of blood, urine, cerebrospinal fluid, sputum, joint fluid, and other specimens, if available.

Previous sections have discussed some of the complications of lupus, including renal disease and renal failure, deep vein thrombosis and pulmonary embolism, stroke, coronary artery disease, and osteoporosis. Many of these complications are accelerated or worsened by corticosteroids. In particular, aseptic necrosis of bone (osteonecrosis), especially the femur, is an unfortunate complication. It can be seen in lupus patients who have received corticosteroids, but is much more prevalent among the steroid-treated patients.

Many rheumatologists use immunosuppressive agents to limit corticosteroid-induced side effects (steroid sparing). However, these agents have toxicities of their own. Of note, cyclophosphamide is associated with sustained amenorrhea and premature ovarian failure, particularly in the patient who is older than 30 years. There is also an increased risk for cancer.[25]

Common causes of death from SLE are complications of infections, renal disease and its sequelae, premature atherosclerotic heart disease, thromboembolic events, neuropsychiatric lupus, and suicide. Early death results from complications of active disease, whereas later deaths are associated with accelerated atherosclerosis and other complications related to therapy.

INDICATIONS FOR REFERRAL OR HOSPITALIZATION

Patients with SLE should be referred to a specialist at diagnosis for several reasons. Confirmation of the diagnosis of this serious illness is important because it is a life-altering chronic disease. Even patients with relatively mild or even asymptomatic lupus require periodic assessment of disease severity and activity, an evaluation best performed by a physician familiar with lupus. Given the myriad choices for management in this disease, the rheumatologist's involvement in patient care is important, even in mild cases. In uncontrolled disease with life-threatening organ involvement and in special complications such as pregnancy and antiphospholipid antibody syndrome, management by a rheumatologist is in the patient's best interest. Obviously other specialists, such as a dermatologist, an ophthalmologist, a high-risk obstetrician, a nephrologist, a cardiologist, an orthopedic surgeon, and a hematologist, are often consulted to manage specific problems related to SLE. Psychiatric or psychologic consultation may assist the patient in dealing with the lifestyle changes wrought by this illness and in managing depression. An occupational therapist should design and teach methods of conserving energy and prescribe appropriate assistive technology.[26] A physical therapist should be consulted to design an appropriate exercise regimen. Nutrition counseling is indicated for those patients with obesity, diabetes, hyperlipidemia, or renal insufficiency.

PATIENT AND FAMILY EDUCATION

As with any chronic illness, education is essential to enable the patient with SLE to skillfully self-manage the disease on a day-to-day basis. Medication management; appropriate, disease-relevant health habits; and self-monitoring activities should be encouraged. Lower socioeconomic status is associated with poorer outcome in SLE, in part because of less adherence to complex treatment regimens and self-monitoring actions, as well as a greater sense of learned helplessness.[4] These conditions can be influenced by educational programs.

The SLE self-help course, a group education and support program, has been developed to assist persons with disease-related self-management activities. Course evaluation has indicated improved feelings of self-worth and self-efficacy, increased enabling skills, and lowered uncertainty and depression, in addition to increased knowledge about the disease.[27] Recent changes have made the course more relevant to persons of Hispanic origin.[28] The course is available through local chapters of the Arthritis Foundation ([800] 283-7800) or the Lupus Foundation of America ([301] 670-9292; [800] 558-0121; Spanish: [800] 558-0231).

REFERENCES

1. Klippel JH, editor: *Primer on the rheumatic diseases,* ed 12, Atlanta, 2001, Arthritis Foundation.
2. Wallace DJ, Hahn BH, editors: *Dubois' lupus erythematosus,* ed 6, Baltimore, 2002, Lippincott Williams & Wilkins.
3. Petri M: Epidemiology of systemic lupus erythematosus, *Best Pract Res Clin Rheumatol* 6:847-858, 2002.
4. Liang MH, Partridge AJ, Daltroy LH, and others: Strategies for reducing excess morbidity and mortality in blacks with systemic lupus erythematosus, *Arthritis Rheum* 34(9):1187-1196, 1991.
5. Uramoto KM, Michet CJ Jr, Thumboo J, and others: Trends in the incidence and mortality of systemic lupus erythematosus 1950-1992, *Arthritis Rheum* 42(9):46-50, 1999.
6. Wakeland EK, Liu K, Graham RR, and others: Delineating the genetic basis of systemic lupus erythematosus, *Immunity* 15(3):397-408, 2001.
7. James JA, Neas BR, Moser KL, and others: Systemic lupus erythematosus in adults is associated with previous Epstein-Barr virus exposure, *Arthritis Rheum* 44(5):1122-1126, 2001.
8. Criscione LG, Pisetsky DS: The pathogenesis of systemic lupus erythematosus, *Bull Rheum Dis* 52:1-4, 2003.
9. Tan EM, Cohen AS, Fries JF, and others: The 1982 revised criteria for the classification of systemic lupus erythematosus, *Arthritis Rheum* 25(11):1271-1277, 1982.
10. Ward MM: Premature morbidity from cardiovascular and cerebrovascular diseases in women with systemic lupus erythematosus, *Arthritis Rheum* 42:338-346, 1999.
11. Manzi S, Meilahn EN, Rairie JE, and others: Age-specific incidence rates of myocardial infarction and angina in women with systemic lupus erythematosus: comparison with the Framingham study, *Am J Epidemiol* 145(5):408-415, 1997.
12. Nikpour M, Urowitz MB, Gladman DD: Premature atherosclerosis in systemic lupus erythematosus, *Rheum Dis Clin North Am* 31:329-354, 2005.
13. Sammaritano LR: Antiphospholipid syndrome (review), *South Med J* 98:617-625, 2005.
14. Trapani S, Ermini M, Falcini F: Human parvovirus B19 infection: its relationship with systemic lupus erythematosus, *Semin Arthritis Rheum* 28:319-325, 1999.
15. Prickett JD, Robinson DR, Steinberg AD: Dietary enrichment with the polyunsaturated fatty acid eicosapentaenoic acid prevents proteinuria and prolongs survival in NZB x NZW F1 mice, *J Clin Invest* 68:556-559, 1981.
16. Dhar JP, Kmak D, Bhan R, and others: Abnormal cervicovaginal cytology in women with lupus: a retrospective cohort study, *Gynecol Oncol* 82(1):4-6, 2001.
17. Miller CS, Egan RM, Falace DA, and others: Prevalence of infective endocarditis in patients with systemic lupus erythematosus, *J Am Dental Assoc* 130(3):387-392, 1999.
18. A randomized study of the effect of withdrawing hydroxychloroquine sulfate in systemic lupus erythematosus: the Canadian Hydroxychloroquine Study Group, *N Engl J Med* 324:150-154, 1991.
19. Austin HA 3rd, Klippel JH, Balow JE, and others: Therapy of lupus nephritis: controlled trial of prednisone and cytotoxic drugs, *N Engl J Med* 314(10):614-619, 1986.
20. Ginzler EM, Dooley MA, Aranow C, and others: Mycophenolate mofetil or intravenous cyclophosphamide for lupus nephritis, *N Engl J Med* 353:2219-2229, 2005.
21. Dziadzio M, Denton CP, Smith R, and others: Losartan therapy for Raynaud's phenomenon and scleroderma: clinical and biochemical findings in a 15-week, randomized, parallel-group, controlled trial. *Arthritis Rheum* 42(12):2646-2655, 1999.
22. Allaire S: Employment and household work disability in women with rheumatoid arthritis, *J Appl Rehabil Couns* 23:44-51, 1992.
23. Horton R, Peterson MG, Powell S, and others: Users evaluate Lupusline, a telephone peer counseling service, *Arthritis Care Res* 10(4):257-263, 1997.
24. Austin JS, Maisiak RS, Macrina DM, and others: Health outcome improvements in patients with systemic lupus erythematosus using two telephone counseling interventions, *Arthritis Care Res* 9(5):391-399, 1996.
25. Boumpas DT, Austin AH 3rd, Vaughan EM, and others: Risk for sustained amenorrhea in patients with systemic lupus erythematosus receiving intermittent pulse cyclophosphamide therapy, *Ann Intern Med* 119(5):366-369, 1993.
26. Wegener ST, editor: *Clinical care in the rheumatic diseases,* Atlanta, 1996, American College of Rheumatology.
27. Braden CJ: Patterns of change over time in learned response to chronic illness among participants in a Systemic Lupus Erythematosus Self-Help Course, *Arthritis Care Res* 4:158-167, 1991.
28. Robbins L, Allegrante JP, Paget SA: Adapting the Systemic Lupus Erythematosus Self-Help (SLESH) course for Latino SLE patients, *Arthritis Care Res* 6:97-103, 1993.

CHAPTER 237

Vasculitis

Derrick J. Todd and Simon M. Helfgott

DEFINITION AND EPIDEMIOLOGY

The vasculitides include a diverse group of uncommon disorders characterized by immune system–mediated inflammation resulting in destruction of blood vessel walls. Clinical signs and symptoms result from the subsequent impairment of blood flow through these damaged blood vessels to the distal tissues and organs. Patients with a vasculitic syndrome often suffer from multiorgan dysfunction. Accordingly, these conditions are serious and often fatal if not recognized early and treated aggressively, usually with long-term immunosuppressive therapy. Although the specific vasculitides typically affect only certain organs, virtually any may be involved.

Since the vasculitic syndromes are uncommon and data on disease incidence are imprecise, conclusions about the epidemiology of these conditions are difficult to make. For most conditions, age of onset is variable, ranging from infancy to old age. Some vasculitides, however, affect only certain age-groups; for example, giant cell arteritis (GCA, or temporal arteritis) does not occur in individuals younger than 50 years of age, Takayasu's arteritis is virtually never seen in patients older than 40 years of age, and Kawasaki's disease is a vasculitis of childhood. Ethnic differences among vasculitides are less distinct; GCA tends to afflict individuals of Northern European ancestry, whereas there appears to be a higher incidence of Takayasu's arteritis in women of East-Asian descent.

Classification of Vasculitic Syndromes

Ideally, classification of the vasculitides would be based on the underlying disease mechanisms of the various disorders. However, our understanding of the immunopathogenesis of the vasculitides remains far from complete. For this reason, vasculitides are often classified according to the size of the involved blood vessels (Box 237-1). This classification scheme does not necessarily account for disease mechanisms, but it is practical in that the clinical features of vasculitic syndromes that involve similar-sized vessels tend to affect common organ systems.

Large-vessel vasculitides include GCA, the most common of all systemic vasculitides, and Takayasu's arteritis. These diseases typically involve the aorta or its major branches, including the carotid, subclavian, mesenteric, renal, and iliac arteries. Clinically, these syndromes manifest as large-territory claudication or infarction of the involved vascular tree. The medium-vessel vasculitides include polyarteritis nodosa (PAN) and Kawasaki's disease. These conditions can cause aneurysms of the involved arteries, which may supply the heart, kidney, gastrointestinal tract, and gonads. The many types of small-vessel vasculitides cause ischemia at the level of the arterioles or capillaries and typically affect the skin, kidneys, lung, gastrointestinal tract, and peripheral nervous system, as well as other sites that tend to be more disease specific.

BOX 237-1

THE VASCULITIDES

LARGE VESSELS

- Giant cell arteritis
- Takayasu's arteritis

MEDIUM VESSELS

- Polyarteritis nodosa
- Kawasaki's disease
- Primary angiitis of the central nervous system

SMALL TO MEDIUM VESSELS*

- Wegener's granulomatosis
- Microscopic polyangiitis
- Churg-Strauss syndrome

SMALL VESSELS

- Leukocytoclastic angiitis
- Goodpasture's syndrome
- Henoch-Schönlein purpura
- Cryoglobulinemic vasculitis
- Drug-induced vasculitis
- Behçet's syndrome
- Relapsing polychondritis
- Lupus vasculitis
- Rheumatoid vasculitis
- Sjögren's syndrome vasculitis

*Antineutrophil cytoplasmic antibody–associated vasculitides.

PATHOPHYSIOLOGY

The pathophysiology of the vasculitides is varied. Multinucleated giant cells may be observed in biopsies of the temporal artery in patients with GCA and are the hallmark of this diagnosis. Hepatitis B virus surface antigen has been found in the serum of some patients with PAN, suggesting a role for this virus in the pathogenesis of PAN. Infection with hepatitis C virus can lead to the formation of cryoglobulins, which are immune complexes that deposit in blood vessel walls and result in vascular inflammation and destruction. Three small to medium-sized vessel vasculitides, Wegener's granulomatosis (WG), Churg-Strauss syndrome (CSS), and microscopic polyangiitis (MPA), are associated with an autoantibody, the antineutrophil cytoplasmic antibody (ANCA). The role of ANCA, if any, in the pathogenesis of these conditions has not been fully elucidated. Necrotizing granulomas are a histologic feature of WG and CSS. Unique to CSS are large numbers of circulating and tissue-based eosinophils.

Patients with a drug-induced vasculitis may have immune complex formation consisting of the foreign protein (offending drug) and its binding antibody.[1] In some instances, this may represent a true serum-sickness reaction in which the patient's immune system generates antibodies against foreign protein (historically antisera). Alternatively, some medications (e.g., propylthiouracil, hydralazine, minocycline) cause a vasculitis that is associated with strongly positive ANCA serology. The contribution of ANCA in the pathogenesis of drug-induced vasculitis is also unclear. Rarely, patients with connective tissue diseases such as rheumatoid arthritis, systemic lupus erythematosus, or Sjögren's syndrome may develop a small-vessel vasculitis, although it is not clear how the underlying disease process in these cases contributes to the systemic vasculitis.

CLINICAL PRESENTATION AND PHYSICAL EXAMINATION

Clinical manifestations of systemic vasculitis are protean, and therefore diagnosis (and treatment) is often delayed. In general, most vasculitic syndromes have characteristic clinical, laboratory, or pathologic features that allow for their identification and classification. A systematic approach to the vasculitides, based chiefly on clinical presentation and physical examination findings, can expedite the process.

Constitutional symptoms, including fever, malaise, fatigue, anorexia, weight loss, arthralgias, and myalgias, are almost uniformly present and therefore do not distinguish among the vasculitides. The absence of any of these should call into question the diagnosis of vasculitis. Fever, when present, rarely exceeds 38.9° C (102° F) and is not typically associated with rigors or chills.

GCA is the prototypical large-vessel vasculitis. GCA is the most common of all vasculitides, although it is found almost exclusively in patients over 50 years of age (see Chapter 233).[2] The presentation of GCA is varied and includes the new onset of headache, scalp tenderness, cranial pain, visual disturbances, or jaw claudication in an elderly patient with constitutional symptoms. Arm claudication from subclavian artery stenosis can occur. Patients might complain of arm pain when using a hairdryer, and a subclavian bruit may be present. Fever of unknown origin is a less common presentation. Blindness from ophthalmic artery occlusion is a dreaded complication of unrecognized GCA and, if not treated immediately, is often irreversible. Aortic aneurysms occur, usually in the ascending thoracic aorta. Involvement of large vessels below the diaphragm (e.g., celiac, mesenteric, renal, and iliac arteries) is rare. Approximately half of patients with known GCA also complain of diffuse shoulder and pelvic girdle achiness and carry the diagnosis of polymyalgia rheumatica (PMR). On the other hand, GCA occurs in only about 20% of patients with known PMR.[3]

Takayasu's arteritis is another large-vessel vasculitis, which primarily affects women younger than 40 years of age. Patients with this vasculitis classically are seen without palpable pulses, and there may be signs of unequal blood pressures, arm claudication, or bruits in the neck or arms. Other presentations include cerebrovascular accident, heart failure, or ruptured aortic aneurysm. Since these are all extremely unusual events in young persons, Takayasu's arteritis should be considered in the appropriate clinical setting.[4]

PAN is defined as a necrotizing arteritis that predominantly affects medium but also small arteries. Destruction of the blood vessel wall leads to the development of microaneurysms, which interfere with blood flow to affected organs. In addition to constitutional symptoms, common features of PAN include palpable purpura from skin involvement, hypertension from renal involvement, postprandial abdominal pain from mesenteric artery involvement, testicular or ovarian pain from gonadal artery involvement, and peripheral neuropathy (see below).[5] Some patients with PAN may have chronic infection with hepatitis B virus.

Kawasaki's disease is a medium-vessel vasculitis of infancy and childhood classically seen with high fever, bilateral conjunctivitis, tender cervical lymphadenopathy, desquamating rash, peripheral edema, and "strawberry tongue." Affected children are at risk for coronary aneurysms, the major cause of death. Aspirin and IV immunoglobulin constitute the definitive therapy.

Primary angiitis of the central nervous system (PACNS) is a very rare vasculitic condition that exclusively affects the brain and/or spinal cord, usually of older adults. Patients typically are seen with subacute dementia and personality changes. PACNS is often not recognized until late into the disease course when stroke and coma occur. Brain biopsy is often required to confirm the diagnosis.[6] Understandably, this condition is associated with significant morbidity and mortality.

WG is a small- to medium-vessel ANCA-associated vasculitis. Although varied in presentation, the classic triad of involvement is that of the upper airway, lower airway, and kidneys.[7] Disease of the ears, nose, and throat is common and can manifest as recurrent sinusitis, mucosal ulcerations, hearing loss, and epistaxis. Hemoptysis from pulmonary hemorrhage and stridor from subglottic stenosis often herald lower airway involvement, and both can be life threatening. Renal involvement usually requires laboratory analysis to identify (see below). Additional manifestations of WG can include palpable purpura; mononeuritis multiplex; central nervous system disease; and, less commonly, ocular, gastrointestinal, skeletal muscle, joint, or cardiac involvement. Overt joint swelling (i.e., arthritis) is uncommon. More often, patients complain of nonspecific arthralgias and myalgias.

CSS is an ANCA-associated small- to medium-vessel vasculitis characterized by asthma and eosinophilia. One should suspect the condition when a middle-aged or elderly patient develops new-onset asthma, which often precedes vasculitis by up to 3 years. CSS vasculitis frequently affects the upper and lower respiratory tracts, the peripheral nervous system as mononeuritis multiplex, and the heart as myocarditis or coronary arteritis. Other common involvement includes that of the central nervous system, the gastrointestinal tract, skeletal muscle, joints, palpable purpura, and glomerulonephritis.

MPA is a third ANCA-associated small- to medium-vessel vasculitis, which has only recently been established as an entity distinct from PAN. Unlike WG and CSS, which cause granulomatous vasculitis, MPA is characterized by a necrotizing inflammation of involved vessels. Features of MPA include palpable purpura, glomerulonephritis, necrotizing alveolitis, mononeuritis multiplex, and gastrointestinal disease.

In the evaluation of most small-vessel vasculitides, the presence of palpable purpura is perhaps the most helpful physical examination finding (Color Plate 24). These lesions are usually multiple, more often seen in distal lower extremities. They occur as a result of extravasation of red blood cells and white blood cells outside the destroyed blood vessel wall of the small arterioles. They vary in size from a few millimeters to 1 to 2 cm (0.4 to 0.8 inch) in diameter. Occasionally, they are itchy. Other skin lesions, including livedo reticularis, nonpalpable purpura, and cutaneous ulcers, can also be seen.

The small- and medium-vessel vasculitides can involve a peripheral nerve, and a careful neurologic examination may detect these findings (e.g., sensory dysesthesia, motor weakness, optic neuritis). Classic findings include wrist drop, foot drop, or a facial droop. Vasculitic involvement of a single peripheral nerve is termed *mononeuritis*. Mononeuritis multiplex describes the cumulative involvement of multiple peripheral nerves over time and is highly suspicious for the presence of a vasculitis in the proper clinical setting.

Henoch-Schönlein purpura (HSP) is a small-vessel vasculitis that may affect people of all ages, usually from early childhood to middle age. Typically, there is involvement of the joints (with pain and/or swelling), skin (palpable purpura), gastrointestinal tract (abdominal pain, bleeding), and kidneys (microscopic hematuria, rising serum creatinine). Although this is usually a benign disorder in children, it may be a more serious condition in adults in whom renal involvement is more likely to lead to end-stage renal disease.[5]

Cryoglobulinemic vasculitis occurs in the setting of patients with serum cryoglobulins. Patients typically have chronic infection with hepatitis C virus, although cryoglobulins can occur in other settings (i.e., malignancy, chronic infection, and systemic rheumatologic disease). Cryoglobulinemic vasculitis classically causes glomerulonephritis, arthralgias, palpable purpura, and peripheral neuropathy. Gastrointestinal involvement also occurs, although rarely.

Leukocytoclastic angiitis typically involves the smallest blood vessels in the skin. In most cases, the skin is the only organ involved, although more widespread involvement may be observed in more severe cases. Patients are seen with palpable purpura that may be slightly itchy; purpura may develop over the trunk and chest as well. The most common predisposing factor is the ingestion about 7 to 10 days earlier of a drug known to predispose patients to cutaneous vasculitis. The most common inciting drugs include antibiotics such as penicillins and sulfonamides, hydralazine, and propylthiouracil.[5]

DIAGNOSTICS

Establishing the diagnosis of vasculitis requires a high degree of clinical suspicion, since the multiorgan involvement can mimic many other conditions. Common diagnostic studies for all vasculitides should include a CBC with differential, serum electrolytes, BUN, creatinine, liver studies, erythrocyte sedimentation rate (ESR), C-reactive protein (CRP), urinalysis with sediment, and chest x-ray examination. The CBC often shows anemia of chronic disease and reactive thrombocytosis. Eosinophilia supports CSS in the correct clinical setting. Elevated BUN and creatinine can occur in many of the vasculitides. Liver studies (albumin, transaminases, bilirubin, and alkaline phosphatase) can be elevated in some of the vasculitides, in particular GCA. ESR and CRP are markers of inflammation and are usually elevated. A freshly spun urine sediment should be carefully examined for the presence of red cell casts and dysmorphic red blood cells, which would suggest glomerulonephritis. Chest radiograph can show a variety of abnormalities, depending on the underlying vasculitic process. A widened mediastinum in a patient with large-vessel vasculitis raises the concern of a proximal (thoracic) aortic aneurysm. Pulmonary nodules, hemorrhage, or infiltrates can be seen in many of the small-vessel vasculitides. Of course, chest x-ray studies can also show an infectious pulmonary process in patients with known vasculitis on immunosuppressive therapy. Patients should also have additional diagnostic testing for occult infectious and neoplastic processes as appropriate for their presentation.

In the specific evaluation of patients with suspected large-vessel vasculitis, a thorough history, physical examination, and basic studies as listed above are often enough to make the diagnosis. ESR and CRP are likely to be elevated and appear to correlate with disease activity in GCA. ESR is notoriously unreliable in patients with Takayasu's arteritis, however. Additional laboratory testing is unlikely to be of diagnostic benefit. Magnetic resonance arteriography (MRA) of the great vessels of the thorax can confirm suspected disease and reveal subclinical arterial stenoses as well. MRA is increasingly replacing traditional angiography, a procedure that carries a higher morbidity. Temporal artery biopsy showing granulomatous inflammation confirms the diagnosis of GCA.

In patients with suspected medium-vessel vasculitis, few additional laboratory studies are of value. In PAN, hepatitis B viral serology can demonstrate hepatitis B–positive core antigen, indicating chronic infection. ANCA is occasionally positive, with a pANCA pattern (described in next paragraph) and antimyeloperoxidase specificity. MRA is rarely helpful in any of the medium-vessel vasculitides because involved vessels are smaller than the limits of resolution of the study. Angiography can show characteristic aneurysms of involved arteries, confirming the diagnosis. Occasionally, PAN can be described fortuitously in a pathologic specimen following cholecystectomy or orchiectomy.

In contrast to large- and medium-vessel vasculitides, where few diagnostic tests have been developed, an armamentarium of blood tests exists to work up suspected small-vessel vasculitis. These include ANCA, complements, anti–glomerular basement membrane (anti-GBM) antibodies, cryoglobulins, hepatitis C viral serology, HIV serology, rheumatoid factor, and antinuclear antibodies (ANA). ANCA can show two patterns of staining, perinuclear (pANCA) and cytoplasmic (cANCA). In general, pANCA is associated with antimyeloperoxidase antibodies and is seen in MPA and CSS, whereas cANCA is associated with antiproteinase 3 antibodies and is seen with WG. Serum complements are low in some of the small-vessel vasculitides (e.g., HSP, cryoglobulinemic vasculitis, lupus vasculitis), but not in others such as ANCA-associated vasculitides. Although not truly a vasculitic processes, anti-GBM disease and Goodpasture's disease are on the differential diagnosis of pulmonary-renal syndromes. Thus anti-GBM antibodies should be measured if considering the diagnosis of small-vessel vasculitis. Cryoglobulins, hepatitis C–specific antibody, or rheumatoid factor can each be seen in patients with cryoglobulinemic vasculitis. Serum cryoglobulins must be obtained with great care because of the manner in which the specimen needs to be processed. If allowed to cool below body temperature, cryoglobulins can precipitate prematurely, resulting in a false-negative test. Thus it is recommended that cryoglobulins be collected in a separate specimen tube. The tube should be maintained at body temperature (e.g., held in a warm hand or water bath) while being transported to the laboratory and then immediately centrifuged. Measurement of an ANA can occasionally be of benefit in patients with newly diagnosed lupus vasculitis or Sjögren's vasculitis. Often these patients have significant involvement of their underlying connective tissue disease process.

Further imaging studies beyond a baseline chest radiograph should be tailored to disease involvement. Sinusitis or other upper airway involvement necessitates a CT scan of the head and neck and or sinuses. Chest CT should be performed in patients with significant pulmonary symptoms. MRI of the brain with contrast may rarely show a pattern consistent with central nervous system vasculitis. Electromyogram can confirm the presence of peripheral nerve involvement by vasculitis.

Biopsy of involved organs is often necessary to confirm the presence of a small-vessel vasculitis. Histologic evidence of blood vessel wall necrosis and inflammation establishes the diagnosis. Almost any organ can be biopsied, but the simplest tissue to obtain is clearly the skin. Thus any patient with suspected vasculitis should be examined carefully for skin lesions that can be biopsied. Another useful biopsy site is the sural nerve, a pure sensory nerve near the ankle that is easily accessible for biopsy. When this procedure is performed, the adjacent gastrocnemius muscle should also be sampled to increase the diagnostic yield. To establish the diagnosis, it may be necessary to biopsy other organs such as the lung, kidney, or even brain, depending on disease involvement. Successful lung biopsy generally requires that the procedure be done via an open lung approach or videoscopic-assisted thoracoscopy. Needle aspiration or biopsy via bronchoscopy is rarely helpful, and the same is true for biopsy of the bowel during endoscopic procedures. Neither is diagnostic because specimens do not contain arterioles, the vessels involved in the vasculitic process.

DIAGNOSTICS

Vasculitis

GENERAL ASSESSMENT

CBC with differential
Serum electrolytes
BUN
Creatinine
LFTs
ESR
C-reactive protein
Urinalysis
Chest x-ray

FURTHER EVALUATION OF LARGE-VESSEL VASCULITIS

MRA of affected area
Temporal artery biopsy
Catheterization with angiography

FURTHER EVALUATION OF MEDIUM-VESSEL VASCULITIS

Hepatitis B viral serology
HIV serology
Consider antineutrophil cytoplasmic antibody (ANCA)
Catheterization with angiography
Biopsy of affected tissue, if feasible

FURTHER EVALUATION OF SMALL-VESSEL VASCULITIS

ANCA
Complements (C3, C4, CH_{50})
Anti–glomerular basement membrane antibodies
Cryoglobulins
Hepatitis C viral serology
HIV serology
Rheumatoid factor
Antinuclear antibodies
CT scan of involved area (head, neck, chest)
MRI brain with contrast if CNS involved
EMG affected extremities
Biopsy of affected tissue

DIFFERENTIAL DIAGNOSIS

In general, the differential diagnosis of vasculitis includes infectious diseases, such as subacute bacterial endocarditis, or bacteremia, such as meningococcemia. Other multisystem disorders, including syphilis and antiphospholipid syndrome, can mimic vasculitis. Similarly, cholesterol emboli syndrome may mimic vasculitis. Affected patients are older and may be using an anticoagulant medication or have undergone some vascular manipulation, such as angiography, or sustained aortic trauma days to weeks earlier. The presentation is characterized by fever, bilateral palpable purpura over the legs and feet, renal insufficiency, and eosinophilia.

MANAGEMENT

The choice of therapy in systemic vasculitis depends on the severity of the involvement. For example, drug-induced vasculitis may be treated successfully simply by withholding the offending agent. Patients with systemic disease of a more serious nature generally require high-dose corticosteroids either orally or intravenously. Oral dosages are generally 0.5 to 1 mg/kg/day of prednisone or its equivalent. For more serious disease, IV corticosteroid preparations (e.g., methylprednisolone) can be given for a faster mode of onset. Steroids are the mainstay of treatment for the large-vessel vasculitides, and few of the other agents discussed below show any benefit in treating GCA.

Certain vasculitides, such as WG and MPA, warrant additional immunosuppressive therapy. Such is also the case for other vasculitides like PAN, lupus vasculitis, or rheumatoid vasculitis when they affect the central nervous system, kidneys, heart, lungs, or other vital organs. Cyclophosphamide is traditionally the agent of choice to induce remission of vasculitis in any of these conditions. It has also been used to maintain remission. However, less toxic agents such as methotrexate and azathioprine may also show benefit in maintaining remission. Methotrexate and azathioprine can also act as steroid-sparing agents in patients with disease refractory to corticosteroid therapy or in those who have developed serious corticosteroid-induced side effects (e.g., avascular necrosis). Less clear is the role for other drugs, such

DIFFERENTIAL DIAGNOSIS

Vasculitis

- Allergic angiitis
- Atheroembolic vasculitis
- Serum sickness
- Infectious endocarditis
- Viral myocarditis
- Viral infections
- Medications (antibiotics, sulfa drugs, NSAIDs)
- Lymphoproliferative disorders
- Inflammatory bowel disease
- Buerger's disease
- Fibromuscular dysplasia
- Antiphospholipid antibody syndrome
- Thrombotic thrombocytopenic purpura
- Chilblain
- Atrial myxoma
- Ergotamine abuse
- Pseudoxanthoma elasticum

as mycophenolate mofetil and tumor necrosis factor-α antagonists.

Since patients diagnosed with vasculitis generally require steroids for longer than 1 month, they should also be maintained on supplemental calcium, vitamin D, and if necessary a bisphosphonate to protect against bone loss. Blood pressure and blood glucose should be monitored carefully. In addition, patients on high-dose steroids (>20 mg/day of prednisone) generally require prophylaxis against pneumocystis pneumonia. Trimethoprim-sulfamethoxazole is the agent of choice, although oral atovaquone, oral dapsone, or inhaled pentamidine can also be used in patients with sulfa allergies.

COMPLICATIONS

Serious complications from systemic vasculitis may often be life threatening and include stroke, seizure, renal failure, pulmonary hemorrhage, myocardial infarction, thoracic aortic aneurysm, mesenteric infarct, or gangrene of distal extremities. The use of high-dose corticosteroids may predispose patients to the development of obesity, osteoporosis, hyperglycemia, hypertension, infections, and osteonecrosis. The use of other immunosuppressive agents can cause bone marrow suppression, may predispose to infections, and in the long term may also increase the risk for the development of malignancies.

INDICATIONS FOR REFERRAL OR HOSPITALIZATION

All patients suspected of having a vasculitis should be referred to a rheumatologist for diagnosis and management because these conditions can be severe and life threatening.

PATIENT AND FAMILY EDUCATION

Patients diagnosed with vasculitis must understand the potentially serious nature of their condition. Although some forms of vasculitis (e.g., drug induced or HSP) are a limited, one-time event, most are chronic. Mortality resulting from vasculitis has been greatly reduced thanks to earlier diagnosis and intervention with immunosuppressant therapies. Long-term survivors, however, are susceptible to complications of treatment or the disease process itself, including accelerated atherosclerosis and a higher incidence of infections resulting from immunosuppression.

Signs of worsening disease may include new rash, sensory loss, hemoptysis, hematuria, or proteinuria. A sudden headache or loss of vision should be reported immediately. Side effects of high-dose steroids, including hypertension, obesity, cataracts, skin thinning, and osteoporosis, should be reviewed with both the patient and family.

Given the potentially life-threatening complications of both the diseases and treatment regimen, an open and accessible patient-provider relationship is essential.

REFERENCES

1. Choi HK, Merkel PA, Walker AM, and others: Drug-associated neutrophil cytoplasmic antibody-positive vasculitis: prevalence among patients with high titers of antimyeloperoxidase antibodies, *Arthritis Rheum* 43:405-413, 2000.
2. Hunder GG: Epidemiology of giant-cell arteritis, *Cleve Clin J Med* 69:SII79-82, 2002.
3. Chuang TY, Hunder GG, Ilstrup DM, and others: Polymyalgia rheumatica: a 10 year epidemiologic and clinical study, *Ann Intern Med* 97:672-680, 1982.
4. Dillon MJ, Ansell BM: Vasculitis in children and adolescents, *Rheum Dis Clin North Am* 21:1115-1136, 1995.
5. Jeanette JC, Falk RJ: Medical progress: small-vessel vasculitis, *N Engl J Med* 337:1512-1523, 1997.
6. Calabrese LH, Duna GF, Lie JT: Vasculitis in the central nervous system, *Arthritis Rheum* 40(7):1189-1201, 1997.
7. Hoffman GS, Kerr GS, Leavitt RY, and others: Wegener's granulomatosis: an analysis of 158 patients, *Ann Intern Med* 116:488-498, 1992.

CHAPTER 238

Barotrauma and Other Diving Injuries

Joanne Sandberg-Cook

The popularity of scuba diving has increased over the past several decades, along with the number of patients who are at risk for injuries sustained while diving. These injuries are diverse and vary in severity from the benign to the life threatening. Many diving injuries require sophisticated medical attention emergently. These include near drowning, hypothermia, arterial gas embolism (AGE), severe decompression sickness (DCS), and poisonous bites or stings. Other diving injuries are not as serious, enabling patients to be seen by their own health care provider or at a nearby facility.

DECOMPRESSION SICKNESS AND BAROTRAUMA

PREDIVE PHYSICAL EXAMINATION AND DIAGNOSTICS

Because few health care providers are trained in sports or diving medicine, it may be necessary for the diver to assess injuries on site and educate health care providers. The prediving physical examination is an opportunity for both the diver and the health care provider to be aware of potential problems. A careful history is imperative.

Diving is relatively contraindicated in any patient with a history of frequent ear infections, serous otitis, chronic sinus infections, or asthma. Tubes in the ears or chronic or intermittent aspiration suggesting an incompetent larynx are absolute contraindications, as is chronic lung disease, emphysema, and a history of spontaneous pneumothorax.[1] Known coronary artery disease, heart failure, certain dysrhythmias, and valvular disease are also contraindications. A patent foramen ovale increases the odds for developing DCS twofold to fivefold.[2] Epilepsy and unstable diabetes are both contraindications to diving because of the possibility of loss of consciousness. Obesity is a hazard in that it may reflect poor physical conditioning and may predispose a diver to DCS on the basis of nitrogen's lipid solubility.

The physical examination should reveal a normal eye, ear, nose, and throat. The tympanic membrane should be intact, and each ear should be autoinflated, using a modified Valsalva's maneuver. Normal neurologic examination findings with intact reflexes and strength are essential. The range of motion for all joints should be within normal limits. Lung and heart examination findings should be completely benign without rales, wheezes, murmurs, or extra sounds. Cardiac stress testing may be recommended for divers ages 45 and older, as for any other activity requiring physical exertion. Older divers are at higher risk for chronic disease and should consider annual physical evaluation for diving fitness.[3]

Recommended studies before diving include a chest x-ray examination, ECG, and visual acuity testing. Pulmonary function tests, bone and joint x-rays studies, and periodic audiograms are recommended for commercial divers.[1]

PATHOPHYSIOLOGY

Most of the injuries sustained while diving stem directly from the differences in physical properties between liquids and gases.[4] A basic understanding of the laws of physics, particularly those laws which deal with the pressure and density relative to liquids and gases, is important. Barotrauma, the most common diving-related injury, develops when an air-filled body space fails to equilibrate its pressure with the environment when the pressures in that environment change. Barotrauma can occur during either descent or ascent.[2] The trauma during ascent is typically more severe, since expanding gas volumes in a confined space can cause serious damage to tissues.

DCS is the result of bubble formation from tissue inert gas supersaturation during decompression. During a dive the body absorbs nitrogen from the breathing gas in proportion to the surrounding pressure. Nitrogen at higher pressures can alter the electrical properties of brain function (nitrogen narcosis). Every 50 feet of depth is the equivalent of one alcoholic drink, causing many of the same impairments in judgment and coordination as alcohol intoxication.[5] If the pressure is removed too quickly, the nitrogen comes out of solution and forms bubbles in the tissue and in the bloodstream. These bubbles can cause different problems depending on where they form.

Risk factors for DCS include rapid ascent, deeper and longer dives, repeated dives, and failure to follow appropriate decompression procedures. Dive tables or decompression computers are used to calculate the rate of ascent based on the depth of the dive and are essential to safe diving. Following appropriate decompression procedures can reduce but not eliminate the risk of DCS.[6]

Air embolism (AGE) occurs when a diver surfaces without exhaling or when the rate of ascent exceeds the rate at which expanding gas can exit through the tracheobronchial tree. Trapped air in the lungs expands and may rupture lung tissue, releasing gas bubbles into the circulation. These bubbles are then carried to vital organs, causing life-threatening conditions or sudden death.[1] The term *dysbarism* has been used to describe these pressure-related injuries that result in permanent tissue damage. *Barotrauma* refers to injury of the lung, middle or inner ear, sinus, or gastrointestinal tract caused by differences in pressure. *Decompression illness* is now the preferred term when describing an injured diver who is suffering from either AGE or DCS.

CLINICAL PRESENTATION

DCS can manifest acutely, even while the diver is still in the water, but delayed presentation is more frequent. The vast majority of symptoms start within 24 hours of surfacing, although altitude exposure, including commercial air travel, can precipitate DCS after a longer time. Individual differences in physical fitness, body weight, gender, fatigue, hydration, and age may make some divers more prone to DCS in spite of the use of appropriate decompression procedures.

Type I DCS can manifest with dull pain in limbs or joints, especially in the upper extremities.[5] Skin itching, rash, and localized swelling (lymphedema) are also common manifestations of type I DCS. Type II DCS is more severe and characterized by neurologic or pulmonary symptoms, including chest pain and cough. Nervous system involvement most often manifests as patchy numbness or paresthesias, but paralysis can also occur. Headache, dizziness (including vertigo), urinary or anal sphincter disorders (usually urinary retention), or mental status changes can also be seen. Hypovolemic shock can occur as a result of fluid shifts from intravascular to extravascular spaces.[5]

PHYSICAL EXAMINATION

A careful history of the dive is essential. Knowing where the dive took place, how deep it was, and how much time was spent at specific depths is crucial. Questions about the diver's predive condition, including drug or alcohol intake, should be asked. Knowledge of first aid administered at the site is helpful. Multiple systems can be affected, but the neurologic and respiratory systems in particular must be carefully assessed. Disorientation, dizziness, fatigue, and joint pain with limited ability to move are common complaints. The joint pain of limb DCS can sometimes be relieved by inflating a blood pressure cuff around the affected joint, although this is not a reliable sign. Physical findings may also include skin blotching, weakness, ataxia, paresthesias, or paralysis. Hypotension, tachycardia, chest pain, and cough are common symptoms. Collapse with loss of consciousness may indicate hypovolemic shock.[5]

DIFFERENTIAL DIAGNOSIS

Many of the signs of DCS are identical to those of more common syndromes, including dehydration, electrolyte imbalance, viral syndromes, and exhaustion. The differential diagnosis for a patient with symptoms within 48 hours of a dive should always include decompression injury.[6] A central nervous system lesion could certainly cause many of the neurologic symptoms discussed above. Sprains, strains, fracture, arthritis, and herniated disc can all cause musculoskeletal pain. Congestive heart failure and pulmonary edema can cause symptoms similar to those of AGE. Dermatitis, allergic reactions, abrasions, contusions, or envenomations can all lead to dermatologic symptoms, including cellulitis, rash, itching, or burning. Heat exhaustion or heat stroke can lead to muscle cramping or mental status changes. Deep vein thrombosis and thrombophlebitis can certainly be a cause of limb pain but not usually joint pain.

Pulmonary barotrauma with AGE is second only to drowning as a cause of death in divers.[4] Trapped air in the lung expands and ruptures alveolar tissue, releasing air bubbles into the circulation. If a bubble lodges in the brain, stroke, seizures, paralysis, and unconsciousness can occur. Air bubbles traveling to the heart can lead to myocardial infarction or cardiac arrest. AGE can also cause minor symptoms such as numbness, tingling, or weakness of a limb. Vision and hearing losses have also been seen, all without loss of consciousness.

DIFFERENTIAL DIAGNOSIS

Barotrauma

SYSTEMIC SYMPTOMS
- Dehydration
- Electrolyte imbalance
- Viral syndromes
- Exhaustion

NEUROLOGIC SYMPTOMS
- CNS lesions, cerebrovascular accident
- Heat exhaustion, heat stroke

MUSCULOSKELETAL SYMPTOMS (LIMB PAIN)
- Sprains, strains, fractures
- Arthritis
- Herniated disc
- Deep vein thrombosis, phlebitis

CARDIAC OR PULMONARY SYMPTOMS
- Congestive heart failure
- Pulmonary edema
- Angina

DERMATOLOGIC SYMPTOMS
- Allergic reactions
- Abrasions
- Contusions
- Envenomations
- Cellulitis

The pathognomonic features of air embolism (AGE) include marbling of the skin of the upper body, gas emboli in the retina, and areas of pallor on the tongue, although this is rarely seen.[1] Pneumothorax can occur in conjunction with AGE or may occur in isolation and become evident at a later time. The patient may be in respiratory distress with mild to moderate pain. Tachypnea, pallor, decreased or absent oxygen saturation, and diminished breath sounds may be noted. Mediastinal air can track cephalad into the soft tissues of the neck and cause changes in the voice.[7] A chest x-ray examination will usually confirm the diagnosis, although CT scans may be required.

MANAGEMENT

Medical stabilization at the nearest facility with rapid transport to the nearest recompression (hyperbaric) chamber is essential. This could include emergency care at the scene, including CPR and intubation if indicated. Injured divers are often hypovolemic, requiring aggressive IV hydration, but placing the patient in Trendelenburg position is contraindicated.[5] Unless contraindicated, an aspirin is indicated.[5] Immediate treatment with inhaled 100% oxygen is highly effective in reducing symptoms while awaiting transport. The breathing of 100% oxygen reduces bubble size and enhances oxygen delivery to ischemic tissues. However, even if the symptoms improve with 100% oxygen, the patient will still require decompression. Divers often are seen by health care providers several days after the onset of symptoms, but recompression may still be beneficial.[6]

Emergency management of AGE is the same as for DCS and includes on-site use of 100% inhaled oxygen therapy, medical stabilization, and transport to a recompression chamber. However, patients with mild presenting symptoms may relapse while undergoing recompression. This relapse may be on the basis of bubble interaction with blood vessel wall causing an inflammatory response.[7] This response leads to blood vessel occlusion and cell damage, which can result in clinical deterioration or even death in spite of recompression treatments.[5] These patients are often observed in hospital and discharged with careful instructions to return if symptoms increase. Persistent problems maintaining adequate oxygen saturation may require hospitalization for chest tube placement and ongoing assessment of respiratory status.

LIFE SPAN CONSIDERATIONS

Children under the age of 12 are usually not certified to dive, since they may lack the maturity to appreciate the inherent dangers and need for absolute adherence to the rules. Diving in pregnancy is not recommended because of risk to the fetus from the unknown effects of nitrogen diffusion across the placenta. Older adults, who are more likely to have medical problems that could affect diving, should seek medical clearance before diving and thereafter annually or as health status changes.

COMPLICATIONS

Complications of decompression illness include cardiac arrest, drowning or near drowning, hypoxia, and permanent neurologic damage.[5] Initial symptoms that appear minimum can worsen over the first few hours; thus it is recommended that patients with even mild symptoms be referred to a facility with a recompression chamber and medical personnel with knowledge of diving injuries.[7]

Ear Barotrauma

Ear barotrauma was first described in 1897 and remains an important problem for both occupational and recreational divers. Again, the pathophysiology is related to an inability to equalize pressures during descent or ascent. The injuries can range from injury to the tympanic membrane (including rupture), to severe middle ear damage, to inner ear labyrinthine window rupture. Symptoms associated with these problems include dizziness, tinnitus, nausea, ear pain, jaw or neck pain, and hearing difficulty.[5]

Examination of the ear canal may reveal bloody drainage and acute damage to the tympanic membrane. Inflammation of the eardrum or collection of fluid behind the eardrum may be seen. Nystagmus, hearing loss, and loss of balance may also be noted. The Weber's and Rinne's tests may be helpful in distinguishing conductive hearing loss (caused by middle ear barotrauma) from sensorineural hearing loss (implicating either inner ear barotrauma or inner ear DCS).[1]

Management. All patients must refrain from diving until symptoms have cleared. If symptoms are limited to the ear, referral to recompression centers is indicated only for treatment of inner ear DCS.[1] Systemic decongestants may provide symptomatic relief. Antibiotics may be necessary if purulent secretions are present. Topical antiinflammatory, antibiotic drops may be helpful in alleviating the pain of otitis externa. Occasionally, mild systemic analgesics may be needed. Most tympanic membrane ruptures heal within 4 or 5 days.

Inner ear barotrauma with vertigo and tinnitus will require a period of bed rest, usually in hospital, with medication to control vertigo and possibly sedatives to help the patient rest comfortably.[8] Surgical exploration to repair a round window rupture may be required. Referral to an audiologist for hearing evaluation may be necessary if hearing loss is severe or persistent.

Varying degrees of hearing loss, vestibular dysfunction resulting in chronic vertigo, balance disorders, and gait disorders are the most serious complications of ear barotrauma.[7] Permanent inner ear damage can be a contraindication to further diving.[8]

Sinus Barotrauma

Sinus barotrauma is associated with severe pain during descent. The frontal sinus is most commonly involved. Epistaxis occurs in about half of cases.[1] This can be a problem for divers who have experienced it before and those with a history of chronic sinus problems.

Management. Topical and systemic nasal decongestants may provide both relief and prophylaxis for divers who are predisposed to this complication. Antibiotics may be indicated when infection is suspected. Patients who do not respond to conservative therapy should be referred to an otolaryngologist for ongoing management.[1]

MARINE ANIMAL BITES AND STINGS

A common source of injuries to divers is inadvertent contact with marine life. Bites and stings from sea creatures are common and range from the annoying to life threatening. These injuries usually require immediate treatment, but patients who sustain multiple or deep wounds or serious systemic illness will require follow-up by health care providers. This discussion is limited to some of the more common or toxic species found in the Western Hemisphere.

CLINICAL PRESENTATION

Often it is not possible to identify the marine animal that caused the injury. The envenomations of the lionfish and the stingray are notable for severe reactions. Symptoms, including hypotension, heart failure, respiratory distress, and death, can occur, although the number of confirmed human deaths from these encounters is much less than commonly believed.[9] Milder and delayed reactions can include regional lymphadenopathy, fever, malaise, nausea, vomiting, and delirium. The wounds inflicted are most commonly mild (erythema only) but often extremely painful. More severe encounters can result in vesicle formation, cellulitis, and necrotic breakdown. Recovery can take months, especially if the wounds are complicated by secondary infection.[4]

Coral scrapes are the most commonly seen injuries. The soft living material on the surface of rough coral is easily deposited into a cut or scrape. This can cause inflammation, infection, and delayed wound healing. Treatment consists of initially scrubbing the wound with soap and water then flushing with copious amounts of water. Flushing the wound with half strength hydrogen peroxide and covering with an antibiotic ointment and dry sterile dressing further ensures a clean wound.[10]

The sting of the sculpin, a common member of the scorpion fish family found off the coast of Southern California, produces severe pain and occasionally nausea and vomiting. The venom produces protein that is rapidly broken down in the presence of heat. Treatment is immersion in as hot water as can be tolerated for 60 to 90 minutes. Once the pain is relieved, the wound should be flushed of debris and monitored for infection.

The stingray can also be found in large numbers off the coast of Southern California, Florida, and other warmer waters. Typically a swimmer will step on the stingray lying on the bottom in shallow water. Pain can be excruciating and can be accompanied by systemic symptoms such as vomiting, headache, fainting, shortness of breath, paralysis, and collapse. Treatment should include immersion in hot water to tolerance for up to 90 minutes and transport to the nearest medical facility as soon as possible.[10]

The jellyfish envenomation is of low toxicity but quite painful, and in susceptible people an allergic reaction can occur. First aid consists of removal of any adherent tentacles followed by a vinegar rinse. The wound is then washed with soap and water and treated with a topical hydrocortisone cream. Pain can be controlled with acetaminophen or ibuprofen.

The Portuguese man-of-war, found in tropical and subtropical regions of the Pacific, in the northern Atlantic Gulf Stream, and in the Caribbean, is infamous for its painful sting and systemic manifestations. This animal has a "sail" that floats with the wind and often one or more tentacles that can extend 10 m (33 feet) or more and can be separated from the sail and drift invisibly toward the surface. Exposure to the tentacle and its powerful venom is what causes the injury.[11] Symptoms include severe pain, vomiting, and difficulty breathing. Anaphylactic shock is treated with epinephrine and other supportive measures. First aid generally consists of copious flushing with either sea or fresh water, removal of visible tentacles with tweezers or a gloved hand, and applications of ice to control pain. Rubbing should be avoided and the application of vinegar, often helpful for other marine animal stings, is controversial.[12]

MANAGEMENT

Good and immediate first aid is essential to uncomplicated healing. This should include immediate assessment of the patient's general status, especially if there is airway, breathing, or circulatory compromise requiring stabilization or resuscitation.[2] Gentle removal of visible spines, control of bleeding, analgesia, and transport to the nearest emergency department are recommended initial treatments.

In the emergency department, stings are managed immediately by removing tentacles and spines (if not done at the dive site) and irrigating the area. Local anesthesia should be used. Open wounds require careful and thorough irrigation and debridement of foreign bodies. Heat treatment using immersion of the affected limb into water no hotter than 45.4° C (114° F) can be effective with specific envenomations (see above).[10]

Wound care is then directed toward healing without secondary infection. Skin irritations and itching can be treated with warm or cool compresses and mild steroid creams. The patient's tetanus status should be ascertained and vaccine administered if more than 10 years have elapsed since the last immunization.

INDICATIONS FOR REFERRAL

All patients with DCS and pulmonary barotrauma (dysbarism) must be stabilized on site and referred to the nearest recompression chamber facility. This referral can be made more than 24 hours after a dive with treatment success. Evaluation by a sports medicine physician with specialized knowledge of diving injuries is preferred whenever possible. Patients with ear barotrauma may need to be seen and managed by an otolaryngologist, especially if they are not responding to conservative therapy. The health care provider can manage bites and stings as long as wound healing is uncomplicated. Referral for surgical debridement may be necessary for nonhealing wounds.

PATIENT EDUCATION

All divers are required to complete a standard course in diving principles and first aid. Diving certification agencies have uniform standards established by the Recreational Scuba Training Council.[5] A basic life support certification is highly recommended. Extra training in the use of oxygen in an emergency is also recommended. Divers should make every effort to avoid contact with marine life and wear protective clothing while diving. Venomous species are widespread throughout tropical, subtropical, and temperate waters, and the ability to visually identify these fish is advised. Appropriate gear in cold water will help to prevent hypothermia. Recreational divers are encouraged to use dive tables and computers conservatively.[1] Immunizations, especially tetanus, should be current.

The Divers Alert Network (DAN) is a nonprofit organization that provides expert medical information to the diving public and to medical providers treating diving-related injuries, promotes and supports diving research, and maintains a 24-hour emergency telephone line for diving accidents. DAN can provide medical providers with the location of the nearest recompression chamber. Health care providers who encounter patients with possible diving-related injuries can use DAN for both emergent and nonemergent consultations and questions, especially for cases in which decompression injuries are suspected.

DAN can be contacted at Peter B. Bennett Center, 6 W. Colony Place, Durham, NC 27705; http://www.diversalertnetwork.org. Emergency medical numbers are as follows:

- Diving emergencies (Remember: Call local EMS first, then DAN!)
  (919) 684-8111
  (919) 684-4DAN (collect)
  (800) 446-2671 (toll-free)
  (919) 684-9111 (Latin America Hotline)
- Travel assistance for nondiving emergencies
  (800) DAN-EVAC (326-3822)

If outside the United States, Canada, Puerto Rico, Bahamas, and British or U.S. Virgin Islands, call (919) 684-3483 (collect).

- Nonemergency medical questions
  (800) 446-2671 or (919) 684-2948, Mon-Fri, 9 AM–5 PM (ET)
- All other inquiries
  (800) 446-2671 or (919) 684-2948

REFERENCES

1. Bove A, Davis JC: *Diving medicine,* Philadelphia, 1997, Saunders.
2. Chandy D, Weinhouse G: *Complications of diving,* retrieved Feb 2, 2005, from http://www.uptodate.com.
3. Bove AA, editor: *Medical examination of sports scuba divers,* ed 3, San Antonio, Tex, 1998, Medical Seminars.
4. Mebane GV, editor: *DAN dive and travel medical guide,* Durham, NC, 1995, Diver Alert Network.
5. Pulley SA: Decompression sickness, *eMedicine J* 2(9), 2005, retrieved March 4, 2007, from http://www.emedicine.com/emerg/topic121.htm.
6. Emerson GM: What you need to know about diving medicine but won't find in a textbook, *Emerg Med* 14:371-376, 2002.
7. Moon RE: Treatment of diving emergencies, *Crit Care Clin* 15:429-456, 1999.
8. DAN Divers Alert Network: *Diving medicine FAQs: diving with existing ear injuries,* retrieved Jan 16, 2006, from http://www.diversalertnetwork.org.
9. Gallagher SA: Lionfish and stonefish, *eMedicine J* 2(7), 2001.
10. Auerbach PS: Marine life trauma, *Alert Diver,* Jan-Feb 1998, retrieved Jan 15, 2006, from http://www.diversalertnetwork.org.
11. DAN Divers Alert Network: *Diving medicine FAQs:* Physalia physalis *(Portuguese man-of-war),* retrieved Jan 16, 2006, from http://www.diversalertnetwork.org/medical/faq/index.asp.
12. *The Portuguese man of war: a dangerous ocean organism of Hawaii,* retrieved Jan 16, 2006, from http://www.aloha.com/~lifeguards/portugue.html.

CHAPTER 239

Fatigue

Michelle Freshman

DEFINITION AND EPIDEMIOLOGY

Fatigue is common, often seen as an attendant rather than a primary complaint. The subjective nature of this problem compels a practitioner to rely almost entirely on the patient's perception of diminished performance. Fatigue has been cited as a chief complaint in 5% of primary care visits, accounting for more than 10 million visits a year, representing 25% of ambulatory care visits, and totaling $1 billion.[1] In fact, there is some concern that it may be underreported.[2] Attempts to catalog the source have determined that 20% to 45% of cases are related to physical causes, and 40% to 80% are due to emotional ones.[1] Although it is recognized that both physical and emotional components are involved, research has not yet delineated the relationship between these domains. Some researchers define fatigue as a marked decrease in a patient's ability to exert himself or herself physically or mentally during usual activities. Others incorporate depressed affect in their definition, as well as interactions with psychologic and somatic pain.[3]

Fatigue may accompany infections or parallel a precipitous decline in health status and persist over months. In contrast to illness-related fatigue, physiologic fatigue is said to result from poor sleep hygiene, pregnancy, postpartum status, or stress.[4] Health-destructive practices such as intentional sleep deprivation; a diet of nutritionally deficient foods; a sedentary lifestyle; and excessive intake of alcohol, caffeine, or stimulant drugs also result in protracted fatigue. Physiologic fatigue is easily managed if the offending habits, medications, sleep disturbances, or exertional demands can be rectified.

Many medications cause fatigue. A sampling includes antipsychotics, cancer chemotherapy drugs (interferon-alfa, high-dose corticosteroids, vincristine, cisplatin), cardiac drugs (calcium channel blockers, beta blockers, diuretics), phenobarbital, carbamazepine, H_1- and H_2-receptor blockers, benzodiazepines, and sedative tricyclic antidepressants. A common source of pharmacologically induced fatigue is the chronic use of hypnotics, hypnotic withdrawal, or minor tranquilizers. Antihistamines that have anticholinergic effects can produce fatigue as a side effect.

A large population at risk for debilitating fatigue is postpartum women. Blood loss at the time of delivery coupled with sleep deprivation and the demands of caring for a newborn can contribute to profound fatigue. Postpartum "blues" occur in 50% to 85% of pregnancies.[5] One in 1000 manifest psychosis, with a 4% mortality.[5] Although serious postpartum sequelae affect less than 10% of delivered patients, the discerning practitioner can help avert serious illness in those patients who do complain of fatigue. It is important to remember that concerned family members may be the first ones to approach the practitioner with concerns about a postpartum patient.

Finally, perimenopausal women may also complain of fatigue. Vasomotor symptoms can impact sleep and, in some cases, metrorrhagia can cause significant anemia with resultant fatigue.

PATHOPHYSIOLOGY AND CLINICAL PRESENTATION

The pathophysiology of fatigue is entirely dependent on its etiology. Given the subjective nature of this complaint, a careful review of symptoms and a physical examination are required. Inquiry is first directed to sleep habits, noise, privacy, temperature discomfort, snoring, safety, difficulties with partner, and bedtime irregularity (see Chapter 19). Irregular sleeping patterns, generalized apathy, loneliness, vegetative symptoms, a change in circumstances (e.g., recent loss, a new job), anorexia, crying, hopelessness, and suicidal ideation must also be gleaned.

A symptom profile is constructed by assessing the effects of rest periods, such as bedtime sleep, naps, weekends, and vacation, on the perceived state of fatigue. The Fatigue Scale is a popular inventory; a score of 8 or greater out of 11 is positive.[6] A medication inventory of prescribed, over-the-counter, and self-prescribed remedies, including alcohol, should be elicited. Of particular concern is the use of caffeine, nicotine, amphetamines, cocaine, or central nervous system (CNS) depressants. Screening for contacts with infectious agents or vectors, including pets and other animals, may be informative if viral or bacterial symptoms are present. Pertinent family history, including a history of malignancies or recent family illnesses, should also be gathered. One pernicious environmental toxin resulting from a workplace or residential heating unit malfunction is carbon monoxide, which can manifest as fatigue or, after substantial poisoning, coma and death.

Concurrent CNS illness or chronic pain produces fatigue. It is useful to know whether the patient has accompanying neurologic deficits such as dysphasia, tremor, gait disturbance, or dysgraphia. Fatigue often accompanies deconditioning after a prolonged illness or hospitalization. If fatigue increases during the day but is relieved by rest, rheumatologic or other organic causes are considered. Fatigue that has increased over months suggests potentially insidious disease. Recurrent, irresistible attacks of daytime sleepiness—often in conjunction with a triad of cataplexy, sleep paralysis, and hypnagogic hallucinations—suggests narcolepsy.

PHYSICAL EXAMINATION

For patients with fatigue, the physical examination is an adjunct to a thorough history of the complaint. Initially, habitus, including neck girth (a measure correlated with sleep apnea); speech; cognition; balance; and gait are assessed. Measurements of postural blood pressure and pulse, with attention to pulse character, may indicate postural hypotension or cardiac arrhythmia, which can precipitate fatigue. Skin should be examined for dryness, jaundice, pallor, or lesions. Thinning hair, glossy tongue, poor skin turgor or wound healing, easy bruising, and body wasting can be signs of poor nutritional status. Thyromegaly and lymphadenopathy should be noted.

A complete examination of the cardiorespiratory system should be performed with attention to the presence of respiratory rales or consolidation determined by tactile fremitus and adventitious, irregular, or rapid breath sounds. Jugular venous distention, cardiac murmurs, or peripheral edema should be noted. The abdominal examination should carefully exclude ascites, bruits, organomegaly, and gastrointestinal bleeding. Neuromuscular coordination and movement, exertional strain, and joint function are included to determine whether chronic disease or acute infection exists. All age- and history-appropriate cancer screenings, including breast, cervical, prostate, and colon examinations, are recommended.

DIAGNOSTICS

Diagnostic investigation requires persistence, since fatigue may be a manifestation of any number of organic diseases. Generally, an initial screen in cases of fatigue with a suspected physical cause should include a CBC with differential; chemistry profile, including serum electrolytes, serum glucose, calcium, albumin, creatinine, BUN, and liver enzymes; erythrocyte sedimentation rate; thyroid-stimulating hormone; urinalysis; and occult blood in stool. A secondary adrenal insufficiency would be implicated if peak cortisol and growth hormone responses after insulin tolerance testing are abnormal in the setting of autoimmune disorders, a gastrointestinal hemorrhage, or postpartum history.[7] Immunoglobulin levels, Lyme titer, rheumatoid factor, cortisol, adrenocorticotropic hormone (ACTH), and serum creatine kinase-MB might be added depending on leading signs. Any abnormal results require follow-up evaluation.

In addition, clinical information can be obtained from a pharyngeal culture; monospot test; syphilis titer; and testing for hepatitis, HIV, or tuberculosis if the history and physical examination support this investigation. A chest x-ray film is ordered for suspected lung, cardiac, or disseminated disease. A

DIAGNOSTICS

Fatigue

LABORATORY
- CBC and differential
- ESR
- Rheumatoid factor*
- Immunoglobulins*
- Serum electrolytes
- Serum glucose
- BUN
- Creatinine
- Iron studies*
- Vitamin B_{12}
- Folate
- Urinalysis
- Throat culture
- Monospot*
- Rapid plasma reagin*
- PPD*
- HIV*
- Lyme titer*
- TSH
- Calcium, albumin
- LFTs
- Hepatitis panel*
- Stool for occult blood
- ACTH*
- Peak cortisol*
- Creatine kinase-MB, if time frame appropriate*

IMAGING
- Chest x-ray*
- Abdominal or pelvic ultrasound, CT*
- Brain MRI with gadolinium*

OTHER
- ECG*
- Echocardiogram *
- EMG*
- Nerve conduction study*
- Toxicology screen*
- 24-Hour urine collection*
- Sleep study*

*If indicated.

patient with primary sleep disorder should be referred to a sleep disorder clinic. For patients in whom postpolio syndrome (PPS) is suspected, a nerve conduction study and an electromyogram can differentiate such cases from myasthenia gravis or other neuropathies, which are central as opposed to peripheral.[8] Although myasthenia gravis may be considered a disease of older age, it can be seen in women ages 20 to 40 years of age, often triggered by an infection.[9]

DIFFERENTIAL DIAGNOSIS

The differential diagnosis for fatigue is divided into four categories: physiologic, physical, psychiatric, and situational. Physiologic fatigue results from adverse external influences such as poor sleep hygiene, substance abuse, or medication side effects. Physical disorders include acute and chronic illnesses resulting from a host of systemic conditions such as chronic anemia. Some patients suffer from restless leg syndrome or periodic limb movement, which causes undetectable sleep interruption but nonrefreshing sleep as a result.[10] Any cardiac, pulmonary, hematologic, endocrine, rheumatoid, neuromuscular, skin, renal, immune, or CNS disorders may individually or collectively contribute to fatigue.[6] Systemic disorders result from inflammation, malignancy, infection, noxious fumes, or ingested poisons.

Fatigue accompanies cardiac, pulmonary, hematologic, and metabolic disturbances. The mechanisms in most of these cases involve reduced oxygen intake, pulmonary congestion or inelasticity, or severe iron deficiency. A calorie-consuming malignancy such as pancreatic cancer is known to manifest with marked fatigue and few other symptoms. Morbid obesity can be a cause of fatigue, particularly in cases of sleep apnea, which may cause hemoglobin desaturation, leading to pulmonary hypertension. The decreased metabolic activity associated with hypothyroidism commonly produces sluggishness and depression, whereas hyperthyroidism in older patients can manifest as fatigue, weight loss, and apathy. Uncontrolled diabetes mellitus causes fatigue because of significant calorie and fluid depletion. In cases of acute or chronic infection, fever and lymphadenopathy often accompany fatigue because of the long-term assault on immunologic resources. Fatigue is also associated with rheumatologic diseases but is not usually the only symptom. Patients with multiple sclerosis commonly experience profound fatigue.

Another source of chronic fatigue is the relatively prevalent phenomenon of PPS, which affects 25% to 40% of victims of poliomyelitis 30 years after the initial illness.[8] Approximately 1.6 million people have had acute poliomyelitis in the United States.[8] It is projected that between 66% and 80% of these patients will experience some later degree of disability, usually in the form of weakness, heat or cold intolerance, or easy fatigability.[8]

Fatigue persisting for at least 6 months and accompanied by a 50% decrease in activity level and exclusion of all other medical and psychiatric explanations warrants consideration of chronic fatigue syndrome (CFS).[4] Muscle or joint pain, headaches, sore throat, enlarged and painful nodes, and mental dullness or confusion severe enough to affect routine activity are common symptoms. Nonrestorative sleep and an extreme reaction to exertion are also reported. The reported ratio of women to men is 3:1, and the syndrome is seen more commonly among those in their early thirties.[3] Some sources claim that more than two thirds of patients with CFS have psychiatric disorders, most often mood, somatoform, and anxiety disorders.[4]

CFS is a diagnosis of exclusion. No definitive test exists for the syndrome. Between 20% and 60% of patients improve in 1 to 2 years, whereas others have conditions that wax and wane for years.[11] Therapies that have been helpful, in addition to lifestyle adjustment, include use of antidepressants and cognitive reframing strategies.[11] Myofascial conditions or fibromyalgia may be difficult to distinguish from CFS. Myofascial pain syndrome involves painful, tender areas in muscles that twitch on palpation or produce an area of referred pain. This localized, short-term condition lacks systemic manifestations other than fatigue. Fibromyalgia, in contrast, has uniform trigger point associations, with fatigue and other systemic features (see Chapter 186).

Slow-onset fatigue is commonly related to psychologic distress.[12] Fatigue is often observed in depression. Research on clinically diagnosed depression has established the contribution of neurotransmitter chemistry. In addition, chronic anxiety or stress can produce neck and shoulder muscle fatigue, irregular sleeping patterns, or irritable bowel symptoms. Among the mental illnesses that tax energy reserves are anxiety, eating, or depressive disorders. Generalized anxiety produces autonomic hyperactivity, sleep disturbances, dry mouth, and bowel distress.[12]

Of note, situational factors such as increased work, school or relationship stress, unemployment, delayed effects of trauma, or bereavement provoke fatigue. CFS patients can also have depressive illness, although premorbid depression is not necessarily a precursor.

DIFFERENTIAL DIAGNOSIS

Fatigue

PHYSIOLOGIC CAUSES
- Poor sleep hygiene
- Substance abuse
- Medication side effects
- Postpartum
- Health-destructive behaviors

PHYSICAL CAUSES
- Anemias
- Malignancy
- Chronic obstructive pulmonary disease
- Congestive heart failure
- HIV
- Thyroid dysfunction
- Diabetes mellitus
- Acute or chronic infection
- Rheumatic disorders
- Renal insufficiency
- Postpolio syndrome
- Chronic fatigue syndrome
- Sleep apnea
- Restless leg syndrome

PSYCHOLOGIC CAUSES
- Depression
- Chronic anxiety
- Mania, psychosis
- Eating disorders

SITUATIONAL CAUSES
- Role stress
- Unemployment
- Posttraumatic stress disorder
- Grief

MANAGEMENT

The patient with fatigue requires support. The provider must acknowledge the fatigue as a valid complaint, worthy of further exploration. Behavioral, situational, and environmental contributions to sleep disturbance should be identified for optimum improvement (see Chapter 19). Treatment of primary, secondary, and chronic insomnia focuses on the sleep cycle and behavioral maladaptation. One interesting study found evidence to support the theory that primary insomniacs experience a state of hyperarousal, as defined by increased glucose metabolism in the brain on positron emission tomography and elevated ACTH and cortisol levels.[13] Depression should be confirmed before medication for short-term sleep management is prescribed. When generalized anxiety disorder is identified, use of benzodiazepines other than on a short-term basis is discouraged in favor of buspirone and other antidepressants such as venlafaxine.[14]

Chronic muscle fatigue and joint pain sufferers can influence the onset and toll of their illness by maintaining normal weight; avoiding exercising to the point of muscle pain; keeping body temperature warmer than air temperature (to avoid the muscle tension associated with cold); and using stress reduction, energy conservation, and time management techniques. The provider can empower the patient to have a sense of control over the situation by encouraging him or her to network, obtain relevant publications, and attend support groups. Cognitive behavioral therapies have also been used. If endurance can be improved, a regimen of increased exercise ameliorates fatigue by improving cardiovascular functioning,[15] depth of sleep, and sense of well-being.

If the diagnosis is elusive, the patient is asked to keep a fatigue diary. Recording the time of onset, duration, severity, accompanying symptoms, relief measures, exercise, mood, diet, medications, and stressors not only helps the health care provider, but will be helpful if future consultation is necessary.

For the subset of patients who are physically disabled by fatigue, employment considerations and alternative compensation might require a practitioner's involvement. A patient may wish to file for temporary disability, workers' compensation, job reassignment, long-term disability, or government disability funds.

LIFE SPAN CONSIDERATIONS

A patient's age and life span stressors influence the evaluation. Teenagers and newly independent young adults should be screened for deleterious health habits, given a natural tendency toward experimentation with alcohol, drugs, and irregular sleep and nutrition. Transitions and losses resulting from changes such as marriage or the death of a parent can be destabilizing. Situational depression or anxiety accompanies these developmental transitions and can cause fatigue. Hormonal fluctuations causing "hot flashes" frequently interrupt sleep in perimenopausal women; serotonin receptor blockers have helped. Older patients who have nightmares or who sleepwalk may have precipitant underlying disease or may be using medications or alcohol, which can contribute to this phenomenon.[16]

COMPLICATIONS

Complications of fatigue include daytime sleepiness, risk of injury or accident, poor performance, and cognitive and functional impairment in managing independent activities of daily living.

INDICATIONS FOR REFERRAL OR HOSPITALIZATION

The collaborating physician is consulted in the evaluation of the patient with fatigue when symptoms elude treatment or explanation. Specialist involvement is dictated by the suspected cause of the fatigue. When fatigue is longstanding, mental health referral is helpful for support. Referral is also indicated for progressive symptoms, a lack of response to therapy, or indications of life-threatening illness. It is important to consider services available to the patient with a chronic fatigue condition such as CFS or PPS, which greatly affects the quality of life and work. Cognitive behavioral therapy has been effective with adult outpatients with CFS.[17]

Postpartum patients with fatigue are screened for anemia, thyroid and endocrine disorders, and urinary tract infections. When fatigue is associated with acute depression, psychosis, cardiomyopathy, congestive heart failure or chronic obstructive pulmonary disease exacerbation, or obstructive sleep apnea resulting from morbid obesity or anatomic abnormality, patients should be referred to the appropriate specialist or acute care setting.

PATIENT AND FAMILY EDUCATION

It is important to acknowledge fatigue as a legitimate symptom of various underlying illnesses. The importance of proper nutrition, sleep, and exercise should be stressed to patients in concrete terms. This approach optimizes their health, assists them in maintaining an optimum quality of life, and protects against debilitating stressors and communicable illnesses. Consultation with a nutritionist, review of sleep hygiene, and an exercise tolerance test are recommended when indicated.

Alcohol, drug, tobacco, and caffeine consumption has an adverse effect on restful sleep. Patients are advised to discontinue caffeine 4 to 6 hours before bed and to avoid late-night snacks and stimulants such as tobacco and alcohol. Regular sleep and wake times, minimum environmental stimuli such as noise or light, regulated ambient temperature, and early afternoon or morning exertion or exercise encourage good sleep hygiene.

REFERENCES

1. Libbus MK: Women's beliefs regarding persistent fatigue, *Issues Ment Health Nurs* 17:589-600, 1996.
2. Passik SD, Kirsh KL, Donaghy K, and others: Patient-related barriers to fatigue communication: initial validation of the fatigue management barriers questionnaire, *J Pain Symptom Manage* 24(5):481-493, 2002.
3. Gorensek MJ: Definition of fatigue and the problem of chronic fatigue, *Prim Care* 18(2):397-407, 1991.
4. Portwood MF: Chronic fatigue syndrome: a diagnosis for consideration, *Nurs Pract* 13(2):11-23, 1988.
5. Atkinson LS, Baxley EG: Postpartum fatigue, *Am Fam Phys* 50(1):113-118, 1994.
6. Aggarwal VR, McBeth J, Zakrzewska JM, and others: The epidemiology of chronic syndromes that are frequently unexplained: do they have common associated factors? Int J Epidemiol 35(2):468-476, 2006.
7. Greenfield JR, Samaras K: Evaluation of pituitary function in the fatigued patient: a review of 59 cases, *Eur J Endocrinol* 154(1):147-157, 2006.
8. LeCompte CM: Post polio syndrome: an update for the primary health care provider, *Nurs Pract* 22(5):133-154, 1997.
9. Suarez GA: Myasthenia gravis: diagnosis and treatment, *Rev Neurol* 29(2):162-165, 1999.

10. Insomnia: assessment and management in primary care: National Heart, Lung, and Blood Institute Working Group on Insomnia, *Am Fam Phys* 59(11):3029-3038, 1999.
11. Buchwald D, Gantz NM, Katon WJ, and others: Tips on chronic fatigue syndrome, *Patient Care* 25:45-58, 1991.
12. Epstein KR: The chronically fatigued patient, *Med Clin North Am* 79(2):315-327, 1995.
13. Silber MH: Chronic insomnia, *N Engl J Med* 353(8):803-810, 2005.
14. Lydiaer RB: An overview of generalized anxiety disorder: disease state—appropriate therapy, *Clin Ther* 22(Suppl A):A3-A24, 2000.
15. Potempa K, Lopez M, Reid C, and others: Chronic fatigue, *Image J Nurs Sch* 18(4):165-169, 1986.
16. Vgontzas AN: Sleep and its disorders, *Ann Rev Med* 50:387-400, 1999.
17. Price JR, Couper J: Cognitive behaviour therapy for chronic fatigue syndrome in adults: Cochrane Depression, Anxiety, and Neurosis Group, *Cochrane Database Syst Rev* (2):CD001027, 2000.

CHAPTER 240

Immunodeficiency

Matthew Stiles McDonald

DEFINITION AND EPIDEMIOLOGY

Our immune system is the result of millions of years of evolution all leading to one over-arching goal: to protect us from our environment. When working properly, immunity enables us to conduct all the normal affairs of running the human body, such as taking in nutrients, breathing air potentially contaminated with microorganisms or pollution, and eliminating organisms that could potentially do us harm. When immunity develops abnormally (primary or inherited immunodeficiency) or later becomes compromised by any mechanism (secondary or acquired immunodeficiency), the result could prove catastrophic for the affected individual.

One need only recall the images of young David Vetter, aka the "Bubble Boy," who lived almost all of his 12 years in a sealed enclosure, to understand the precarious situation caused by the lack of a functional immune system (Figure 240-1). Fortunately, conditions such as David Vetter's are uncommon, probably affecting less than 1 in 100,000 live births, although the exact incidence is unknown.[1] But more common primary immunodeficiencies, such as isolated immunoglobulin (Ig) A deficiency, can affect as many as 1 in 500 individuals; all told, immunodeficiency is seen in around 1 in 2000 live births.[2,3] Furthermore, there have been more than 100 primary immunodeficiencies described since Colonel Ogden Bruton first discovered agammaglobulinemia in 1952.[4]

Acquired immunodeficiencies tend to be more common than inherited forms, and even the newest health care provider understands the toll that human immunodeficiency virus/acquired immunodeficiency syndrome (HIV/AIDS), the most

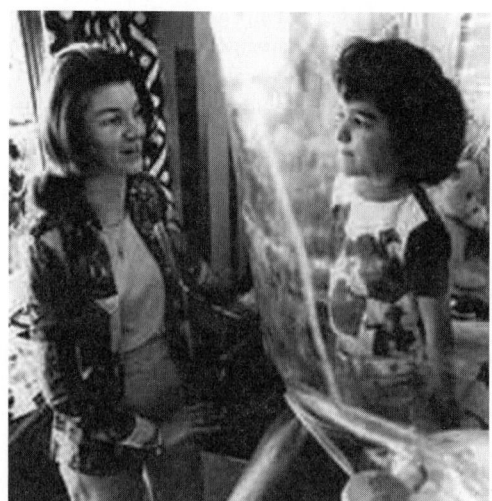

FIGURE 240-1

Carol Ann Vetter and her son David, aka the "Bubble Boy." (Courtesy NASA.)

common secondary immunodeficiency in the United States, can take on patients, families, and the health care system. Acquired immunodeficiency is discussed in Chapter 246 and is not covered thoroughly here.

Generally, whether inherited or acquired, most immunodeficiencies manifest as an unusual susceptibility to infection. The type of infection can often provide a clue to the underlying mechanism of disease and to its potential treatment.[2,5-7] Although recurrent infections can often be masked with antibiotics, other allergic or autoimmune symptoms can also be clues that the patient may have an underlying immunodeficiency.

Consultation with an allergist or clinical immunologist is indicated for all patients with suspected immunodeficiency disorders.[3]

PATHOPHYSIOLOGY

Primary immunodeficiencies are by definition congenital, and most arise from single-gene defects, although others come under the influence of multiple genes.[8] They can be caused by mutations in somatic genes, where they are usually recessive, or linked to sex chromosomes. Most appear by the age of 6 years, but milder forms may never cause enough morbidity to facilitate diagnosis. One concrete rule is that the earlier a patient shows signs of an immunodeficiency, the more severe the underlying disease.[6] The causes of secondary immunodeficiencies can be influenced by genetics, but more often outside or environmental factors cause these diseases. For example, with AIDS, the patient's T-helper cells are destroyed by HIV, thus leading to a cell-mediated deficiency.

Understanding how the immune system is structured can provide clues as to the underlying mechanisms of a suspected immunodeficiency, as well as allow for classification of immunodeficiencies. The immune system is composed of two main divisions. The innate immune system is that section which provides nonspecific defense. Examples of innate immunity include physical barriers such as intact skin or mucus in the lungs, which blocks entry of harmful bacteria or viruses; immune cells (macrophages, neutrophils, etc.), which recognize and target primitive protein sequences common to most nonself organisms; and finally protein components (such as complement or cytokines), which circulate throughout the blood ready to latch on to foreign proteins. Whether a lowly snail or sprinting cheetah, all living organisms, including humans, possess some of these same innate tactics for fighting off the environment.

The adaptive immune system, on the other hand, is an evolutionary advance that we share only with fellow vertebrates. Here, foreign proteins (antigens) are recognized and processed by immune effector cells. This process, called immune priming, induces changes in the development and maturation of other cells (B and T cells), which then specifically target the new invader for destruction. These respective cell lines produce antigen-specific antibodies (via B cells, or humoral immunity) or target the antigen for cell-mediated destruction (via T cells, or cell-mediated immunity).

Both these divisions are complex and are further regulated by added levels of intricacy. Failure of just one protein in one pathway can subsequently lead to partial or total deficiency of immune function. This is the pathophysiologic underpinning of immunodeficiency. Deficiencies in the innate immune system include barrier disorders (such as cystic fibrosis), neutrophil or phagocyte defects, and complement deficiencies. Disorders of the adaptive immune system usually manifest as B- or T-cell defects, antibody deficiencies, or severe combined immunodeficiencies (SCIDs).

Relative frequencies of various immune disorders can also help guide diagnosis. The most common disorders are antibody deficiencies (50%), followed by combined B- and T-cell deficiencies (20%), phagocytic defects (18%), cellular defects (10%), and complement deficiencies (2%).[6,9]

CLINICAL PRESENTATION

Immunodeficient patients are unusually vulnerable to repeated or chronic infections. According to the American Academy of Allergy, Asthma and Immunology, findings suggestive of immune dysfunction include eight or more new infections in 1 year, two or more serious sinus infections in 1 year, 2 or more months on antibiotics with little or no effect, two or more pneumonias within 1 year, failure to thrive, recurrent deep skin or organ abscesses, persistent oral or skin candidiasis after 1 year of age, need for IV antibiotics to clear infections, and a family history of immune disorders.[1-7] In addition, serious or repeated infections with normally nonpathogenic organisms are a potential clue that immune dysfunction is a consideration.

Knowing how the immune system is organized and how deficiencies in its various components will manifest themselves clinically can often provide clues to the health care provider of an immunodeficiency (Table 240-1). For example, recurrent sinopulmonary infections with encapsulated bacteria such as *Streptococcus*, *Staphylococcus*, or *Haemophilus* organisms can be suggestive of an antibody deficiency or B-cell disturbance, since humoral immunity is generally responsible for dispatching these types of pathogens. However, wide use of antibiotics can mask or cloud the diagnosis of a specific immunodeficiency. Thus it is sometimes important to watch for common associations seen in these diseases. Common related conditions include chronic diarrhea, eczema, hepatosplenomegaly, hematologic disorders, autoimmune diseases, and failure to thrive in infants and children.

An example here would be Wiskott-Aldrich syndrome (WAS), which like other humoral deficiencies is characterized by recurrent infections with pneumococci. But WAS is also associated with platelet maturation anomalies through the underlying genetic defect and thus could manifest with prolonged bleeding, easy bruising, eczema, etc. There is also a tendency in WAS to later develop T-cell anomalies.

Primary T-cell disorders manifest as unusual susceptibility to viruses, fungi, some parasites, and other bacteria that are the targets of this class of cell. Common T-cell mutations affect the manner in which the T cells mature or become activated, but some will also be confined to how these cells communicate with others (i.e., defects in their receptors and/or production of cytokines).

Even more severe are combined immunodeficiency disorders (CID or SCID), which may knock out multiple immune cell pathways, usually as a result of an enzyme or early

TABLE 240-1 Medical History in Patients with Recurrent Infection

Parameter	Association with Infection
AGE AT ONSET	
4-5 months	Combined T- and B-cell deficiency
7-9 months	B-cell deficiency
SITE OF INFECTION	
Otitis media	B-cell deficiency
Sinusitis	B-cell deficiency
Pneumonia	B-cell deficiency
Meningitis	B-cell deficiency
Gingivitis	Neutrophil and phagocytic defects
Skin infections	Neutrophil and phagocytic defects
Organ abscesses	Neutrophil and phagocytic defects
MICROBIOLOGY OF INFECTION	
Viruses (herpes, varicella, cytomegalovirus)	T-cell deficiency
Fungi	
Candida organisms	T-cell deficiency
Aspergillus organisms	T-cell deficiency or phagocytic defect
PARASITES	
Giardia lamblia	B-cell deficiency
Pneumocystis carinii	T-cell deficiency
Toxoplasma gondii	T-cell deficiency
BACTERIA	
Mycobacteria	T-cell deficiency
Encapsulated organisms	B-cell or complement deficiency
Low-virulence organisms	Neutrophil or phagocytic defects
GASTROINTESTINAL DISTURBANCES	
Malabsorption, diarrhea	B- or T-cell deficiency
Lactose intolerance	B-cell deficiency
Celiac disease	B-cell deficiency
FAMILY HISTORY	
X linked	B- or T-cell deficiency
Autosomal recessive	B- or T-cell deficiency
ADVERSE VACCINE OR TRANSFUSION REACTION	
Paralytic polio from OPV	B-cell or combined T- and B-cell deficiency
Transfusion reaction	B-cell (IgA) or phagocytic (chronic granulomatous disease) deficiency

Reprinted with permission from Adkinson NF, Yunginger JW, Busse WW, editors: *Middleton's allergy: principles and practice*, ed 6, St Louis, 2003, Mosby.

maturation defect. Both B and T cell lines can be affected, leading to early and devastating infections. This is the type of disease that affected David Vetter. Without prompt treatment with bone marrow transplant or more recently, gene therapy, these children's lives are usually measured in days to months rather than years.

Secondary immunodeficiencies are acquired or associated with some underlying disorder and are not caused by intrinsic abnormalities in the development and function of the immune system. HIV infection and malnutrition are the most common causes of secondary immunodeficiency.[10] Other causes include malignancy, immunosuppressive agents, and systemic inflammatory diseases such as rheumatoid arthritis and systemic lupus erythematosus.[11] Secondary immunodeficiencies must be considered in the differential diagnosis of patients with multiple or recurrent infections.

PHYSICAL EXAMINATION

A careful history usually provides evidence that identifies the nature of the immune system defect. The history should include a detailed description of infections, including age of onset, site(s), patterns of recurrence, response to treatment, and pathogens if known. More severe immunodeficiency disorders such as SCID, characterized by defects in both B and T cells, can manifest with life-threatening infections in the first few months of life.[11] The patient's immunization history and response to immunizations should be assessed. A history of normal response to smallpox vaccination or contact dermatitis from poison ivy suggests an intact cellular immunity.[2] Associated symptoms such as eczema, diarrhea, or arthritis should be noted. Risk factors for HIV infection should be assessed. A history of weight loss, enlarged lymph nodes, night sweats, fever, ecchymosis, pruritus, or epistaxis should be obtained. The past medical history should determine childhood illnesses, including developmental delay or failure to thrive, recurrent infections, autoimmune diseases, cancer, and a history of splenectomy. A family history of unexplained death from infection may be significant.[11]

A complete physical examination should be performed with the goal of identifying the site and source of infection and any chronic indictors of immune dysfunction. It is important to review the growth parameters such as height and weight, since failure to thrive is one of the more common features of adaptive immunodeficiency. Findings of ocular telangiectasia, tympanic membrane scarring, tonsillar absence, lymphadenopathy, periodontitis, dental erosions, gingivostomatitis, mucocutaneous candidiasis, eczema, vitiligo, oculocutaneous albinism, hepatosplenomegaly, clubbing or fungal infections of the nails, petechiae, and pallor can all be associated with various immunodeficient states.[6,7] Also, the tendency for immunodeficiency to be part of other congenital syndromes should cause the provider to look for body dysmorphisms. Examples of these include micrognathia, short philtrum, and ear abnormalities seen with DiGeorge's syndrome; short-limbed dwarfism associated with some T-cell disorders; or prominent forehead, deep-set eyes, broad nasal bridge, and prognathism associated with hyperimmunoglobulinemia E syndrome.[8] A full neurologic examination should also be performed. Broad-based gait in a young child could be the first sign of ataxia-telangiectasia before immunodeficiency becomes apparent.[12]

DIAGNOSTICS

When an immunodeficiency disorder is suspected, initial laboratory work should include studies that are broadly informative, readily available, and cost-effective. A CBC with differential is important for detecting neutropenia and relative levels of various leukocytes. A peripheral smear should be done concurrently to look for abnormal white cell morphology. These can help to exclude neutropenia, lymphopenia, etc. Thrombocytopenia can be consistent with WAS. Metabolic profiles can be helpful for excluding potential immune-

DIAGNOSTICS

Immunodeficiency

LABORATORY	
CBC and differential	C-reactive protein
ESR	Immunoglobulins
Serology and cultures*	**OTHER**
HIV	Nitroblue tetrazolium test*
Qualitative immunoglobulin panel	Skin testing (PPD, mumps)
CH_{50}	PFTs*
Fasting glucose	

*If indicated.

DIFFERENTIAL DIAGNOSIS

Immunodeficiency

Primary
- Congenital

Secondary
- Infectious diseases
- Malignancies
- Immunosuppressive agents
- Malnutrition
- Hereditary metabolic defects
- Chromosomal abnormalities

modulating diseases such a diabetes mellitus. HIV testing should be performed. When possible, it is important to identify all organisms infecting the patient. To this end, blood, urine, sputum, and wound cultures, as well as consultation with a serologist, can be helpful. An erythrocyte sedimentation rate and C-reactive protein should be performed for evidence of inflammation. Pulmonary function testing should be considered when the patient's symptoms have a chronic respiratory component, since immunodeficiencies can alter lung function over time.

Immune testing should also begin broadly, but clinical symptoms can help guide which tests are ordered. Health care providers may also obtain quantitative serum immunoglobulin as part of the initial screening, since antibody disorders are the most common immunodeficiencies.

Other specialized immune testing can be ordered and performed by the clinical immunologist. Delayed-type hypersensitivity (DTH) skin testing is a common test of T-cell function, and positive reactions to common antigens such as *Candida* organisms, tetanus, and mumps can help rule out T-cell disorders in up to 85% of adults.[7] There is more controversy in using DTH testing in infants and young children who have not yet developed an exposure history adequate enough to turn a skin test positive. Although some providers perform skin testing in children, there seems to be no utility of testing children less than 1 year of age.[3,6]

Other specialized tests examine antibody production (e.g., IgE levels, antibody responses to protein or polysaccharide antigens, isohemagglutinins, IgG subclasses), T cells (functional assessment, quantification of T-cell subtypes), phagocytic function (nitroblue tetrazolium test, flow cytometry for diseased cell markers such as CD18), and complement deficiencies (complement levels C3, C4, CH_{50}).[3,5-8,13] Checking sweat chloride and cystic fibrosis transmembrane regulator gene assays can help to rule out cystic fibrosis. Further evaluations, including enzyme measurements, genetic and chromosomal studies, chemotaxic assays, and surgical biopsies (e.g., lymph nodes, colon), may also be considered by the clinical immunologist.[7]

DIFFERENTIAL DIAGNOSIS

The differential diagnosis should include primary and secondary causes of immune dysfunction. Both B- and T-cell deficiencies can occur in association with secondary immunodeficiencies. Categories of secondary immunodeficiencies include infectious diseases, specifically HIV/AIDS; malignancies; immunosuppressive agents; malnutrition; hereditary metabolic defects; and chromosomal abnormalities. For newborns, providers should also consider congenital *TORCH* (*T*oxoplasmosis, *O*ther infections, *R*ubella, *C*ytomegalovirus, or *H*erpes simplex) infections.

MANAGEMENT

There are two goals of treatment when providing care for a patient with a primary immunodeficiency: (1) minimize the occurrence and impact of infections on the overall health of the individual, and (2) replace the defective component of the immune system by passive transfer or transplantation when possible.[13]

All providers should have a low threshold for treating immunodeficient patients with antibiotics after appropriate cultures are obtained. The health care provider should keep in mind that these patients may require more aggressive and prolonged therapy and that there should always be attempts to narrow the antibiotic spectrum based on culture and sensitivity results. Providers should also have a low threshold for further evaluation of opportunistic infections, such as when viruses, parasites, or fungi are suspected. Like all of those on repeated or chronic antibiotics, immunodeficient patients should be monitored for complications of antibiotic use, including renal and liver impairment, *Clostridium difficile* overgrowth, and fungal infections. Some groups of patients, such as those with chronic lung disease, should also be considered candidates for prophylactic antimicrobials. These antibiotic regimens usually involve a 1- to 2-month course of sequential antibiotics of different functional classes to minimize resistance.[14,15] The recommendations for these prophylactic regimens are constantly changing for each condition, and therefore the clinical immunologist should have updated reference material on appropriate selections.[3]

Replacement of defective immune components can be achieved by a variety of means depending on the component in question. These include administration of exogenous immunoglobulins, cytokine therapy, enzyme replacement, plasma infusion, growth factors, or reconstitution of stem cells via transplantation or gene therapy (Table 240-2).

IV immunoglobulin (IVIg) is used in a variety of humoral and cellular immunodeficiencies, including X-linked agammaglobulinemia, common variable immunodeficiency (CVID), hyper-IgM syndrome, WAS, and SCID.[2,3,6,10,15] The rationale for this treatment is to replace absent or dysfunctional antibodies with normal components. And there is longstanding evidence to show that this treatment can be helpful in the aforementioned conditions.[16,17] The use of IVIg in patients with IgA deficiency and some forms of CVID (those without

TABLE 240-2 Selected Primary Immunodeficiency Disorders

Disorder	Functional Immunodeficiency	Inheritance Pattern	Therapy
B-CELL DISORDERS			
X-linked agammaglobulinemia	Antibody Pre–B-cell maturation	XL	Antibiotics Immunoglobulin
Common variable hypogammaglobulinemia	Antibody Cell-mediated immunity B-cell maturation	AR	Antibiotics Immunoglobulin
Transient hypogammaglobulinemia of infancy	None: immunoglobulins low, but antibodies present Usually resolves by 16-30 months	Unknown	Antibiotics Immunoglobulins
Selective IgA deficiency	IgA B-cell maturation	XL AR?	Antibiotics Immunoglobulins in rare cases
IgG subclass deficiency	IgG and IgA Chromosomal deletion	AR	
T-CELL DEFICIENCIES			
DiGeorge's syndrome	T-cell deficiency Faulty embryonic development of third and fourth pharyngeal pouches: hypoplasia or aplasia of thymus gland		Transplantation of fetal thymic tissue Calcium and vitamin D Bone marrow transplantation
Chronic mucocutaneous candidiasis	T-cell deficiency No T-cell receptor for *Candida* antigens		Antifungal agents
COMBINED B- AND T-CELL DISORDERS			
Severe combined immunodeficiency syndrome	Antibody B- and T-cell maturation Adenosine deaminase deficiency (ADA)	XL AR	Bone marrow transplantation Irradiated erythrocytes to replace ADA Gene therapy
Wiskott-Aldrich syndrome	IgM T-cell function decreasing as disease progresses	XL	Antibiotics Bone marrow transplantation
Ataxia-telangiectasia	IgA Variable T-cell deficiency	AR	Antibiotics Bone marrow transplantation
PHAGOCYTE DISORDERS			
Chronic granulomatous disease	Neutrophil function	XL	Antibiotics Interferon-γ

AR, Autosomal recessive; *IgA,* immunoglobulin A; *IgG,* immunoglobulin G; *IgM,* immunoglobulin M; *XL,* X linked.

detectable IgA) is complicated by the fact that some of these patients' IgA deficits are due to the presence of anti-IgA antibodies. Since IVIg can contain trace amounts of both IgA and IgM, giving a patient with these autoantibodies a large infusion of IVIg could cause anaphylaxis. Accordingly, testing to identify the presence of anti-IgA antibodies can be done and special preparations of IVIg without IgA obtained.[7]

Administration of IVIg is usually initiated at 300 to 400 mg/kg/month and then subsequently titrated monthly based on trough levels. Trough levels are drawn after 4 weeks of treatment, and the recommended goal is to keep trough levels above 500 mg/dl.[6,7] There is some evidence to suggest that keeping trough levels above 600 mg/dl can be beneficial.[6] Adverse reactions to IVIg often occur on or near the infusion day and may be lessened by slowing infusion rate, attempting to control any concurrent infections, or switching manufacturers.[6,7] Common reactions include fever, chills, nausea, emesis, and myalgias. Uncommon and more severe adverse effects consist of anaphylactic symptoms of hypotension, respiratory distress, and flushing. These constitute a medical emergency and require immediate evaluation and resuscitation. If anaphylaxis occurs and the patient absolutely needs this replacement, the clinical immunologist may consider slow infusions with the subcutaneous form of the drug and pretreatment with diphenhydramine and/or corticosteroids.

The definitive treatment for SCID or CID is reconstitution of functional cells via stem cell transplantation (SCT) or gene therapy.[3] Pluripotent stem cells have the ability to become any leukocyte within the white blood cell milieu. So by infusing these healthy predecessor cells after native cells have been destroyed via chemotherapeutic means, the provider should be able to completely replace diseased cells with healthy ones. SCT has been successful in cellular deficiencies; almost all SCIDs; and a variety of other conditions such as DiGeorge's syndrome, leukocyte adhesion deficiency, and WAS.[13,18-21] SCT is most successful when using HLA-identical sibling bone marrow donors.[3] The adverse effects of the SCT process are numerous.[22]

Gene therapy has been shown to reconstitute functionality to native immune cells in two SCIDs, common gamma-chain deficiency and adenosine deaminase (ADA) deficiency.[3,22-24] Briefly, copies of healthy genes are added to delivery vectors that insert the healthy gene into diseased cells, thereby using the cell's own machinery to then produce normal gene products. Although gene therapy holds promise, these techniques are still experimental. Given that several of the patients with ADA deficiency treated with gene therapy have later developed lymphoma, some further modifications are probably needed before this could become widely available.[25]

Other modalities of immune function replacement are tailored to the specific pathophysiology of each disease. Apart from SCT, patients with DiGeorge's syndrome can also be treated with the thymic hormone thymosin or with transplantation of fetal thymic tissue with the goal of restoring T-cell function.[26,27] ADA deficiency has also been treated with replacement of the ADA enzyme using a polyethylene glycol formulation.[7] Complement deficiencies can be treatment with blood factor–rich fresh-frozen plasma. Replacement with the cytokine interferon-γ is used to treat patients with chronic granulomatous disease.[7] Progenitor cell growth factors like granulocyte-macrophage colony-stimulating factor are used to stimulate white blood cell proliferation in the presence of neutropenia.[2]

LIFE SPAN CONSIDERATIONS

Some immunodeficiencies are mild and may even go unnoticed throughout a person's life. Such can be the case with isolated IgA deficiency, which affects 1 in 500 of Americans and at one spectrum can be asymptomatic. Approximately two thirds of immunodeficient patients will live to adulthood.[2] However, many will have a shortened life span because of their disease. Death can result from overwhelming infections, chronic stigmata, or complications of the disease and some of the treatment modalities themselves. Frank discussions with patients and their families are important to help them anticipate potential deterioration of health, and the use of community or mental health resources can be helpful for patients and their families.

COMPLICATIONS

Complications associated with immunodeficiency or its management depend on the specific disease entity. In general, the complications of poorly controlled chronic or recurrent infections are common (e.g., bronchiectasis with recurrent pulmonary infections). Some patients' diseases have a tendency to worsen over time. Some patients may even be at greater risk for malignancy or autoimmune diseases. For example, patients with CVID are at a greater risk of developing lymphoma. Complications can also occur secondary to treatment.

INDICATIONS FOR REFERRAL

All patients should be referred to a clinical immunologist when the diagnosis of an immunodeficiency disorder is suspected, unless that disorder is already known to be secondary and thus other specialists may be better suited to caring for the patient. For example, HIV/AIDS patients are now often cared for by infectious disease consultants or specialists in HIV medicine.

Once a definitive diagnosis of primary immunodeficiency is made and the care plan is developed by the clinical immunologist, the patient can be monitored in a collaborative fashion. Infections can be diagnosed and managed by the health care provider. Patients should be closely monitored for the development of autoimmune diseases and malignancy. The majority of malignancies are seen in patients with ataxia-telangiectasia, WAS, and CVID.[26] Those requiring specialized therapy such as immunoglobulin replacement therapy or bone marrow or stem cell transplant should receive this care under the supervision of a clinical immunologist. Relatives of affected individuals should be referred for genetic testing and counseling as appropriate. It is especially important to screen for carrier status all female relatives of patients with X-linked disorders and both parents of a patient with a suspected disorder known to have an autosomal recessive inheritance pattern.[3] Intrauterine diagnosis of some primary immunodeficiencies is possible for those with known familial disorders.[27]

PATIENT EDUCATION AND HEALTH PROMOTION

Patients with primary immunodeficiency disorders should understand the importance of avoiding contact with individuals with known contagious diseases, and they should be able to identify and report signs and symptoms of infection. It is essential that these patients seek care at the first sign of infection. Good personal hygiene and adaptation of health behaviors such as regular exercise and stress management should be recommended to promote good health and support immune function. Social service providers can help with affordability issues, and national organizations such as the Immune Deficiency Foundation (40 W. Chesapeake Ave., Suite 308, Towson, MD 21204; [800] 296-4433; http://www.primaryimmune.org) or the Jeffrey Modell Foundation (747 Third Ave., New York, NY 10017; [212] 819-0200; http://www.jmfworld.org) can provide specific educational and support materials to patients, families, and providers.

Although there are no special dietary restrictions for immunodeficient patients, special consideration should be given to those with malabsorption or chronic diarrhea as part of their clinical picture to ensure adequate nutrition delivery.

Patients with congenital immunodeficiencies should have current childhood, adolescent, and adult vaccinations as recommended by the National Immunization Program of the Centers for Disease Control and Prevention.[28] Recommendations in the 2006 guidelines were as follows: Infants and children should be vaccinated for tetanus (DT), polio (IPV), *Haemophilus influenzae* (Hib), pneumococcus (PCV7), pneumococcus (PPV23), and hepatitis A (if indicated). The recommendations for adults are similar with the addition of hepatitis B if indicated. Anthrax, polio (IPV), rabies, and inactivated typhoid can be used if indicated. In general, live attenuated vaccines (BCG, influenza LAIV, typhoid Ty21a, vaccinia, MMR, and yellow fever) are contraindicated because of the risk of vaccine-induced infection. There are two exceptions to this recommendation. First, the live attenuated form of the influenza vaccine (LAIV) cannot be used, but the inactivated form can be given to children and adults with primary immunodeficiency. Second, varicella vaccine is contraindicated in patients with T-cell involvement, but humoral deficient patients may be given the vaccine. For current guidelines, providers should check with their local or national health agency in charge of vaccine recommendations.

Transfusions of whole blood are contraindicated in immunodeficient patients, since the donor blood could contain lymphocytes that could induce a graft-vs.-host rejection. Appropriate preparation of blood products before transfusion should include means such as irradiation to minimize the risk of infection, especially with viruses like cytomegalovirus or the hepatitides.

The use of surgical treatments for immunodeficient patients is by and large controversial and untested. Generally there are no indications for tonsillectomy, adenoidectomy, or splenectomy in these patients. In fact, these procedures should be limited to certain circumstances, such as to control bleeding secondary to WAS-induced thrombocytopenia. Some proponents have recommended tympanostomy tube placement for those with recurrent otitis, but evidence is lacking on whether this provides significant advantage for this population. Further studies with regards to surgical interventions are needed.

REFERENCES

1. McGhee SA, Stiemh ER, McCabe ER: Potential costs and benefits of newborn screening for severe combined immunodeficiency, *J Pediatr* 147(5):603-608, 2005.
2. Kasper DL, Braunwald E, Jameson JL, and others: *Harrison's principles of internal medicine*, ed 16, New York, 2005, McGraw-Hill.
3. Bonilla FA, Bernstein L, Khan DA, and others: Practice parameters for the diagnosis and management of primary immunodeficiencies, *AAAAI Pract Parameters* 95:S20, 2005.
4. Bruton OC: Agammaglobulinemia, *J Pediatr* 9:722, 1952.
5. Bonilla FA, Geha RS: Primary immunodeficiency diseases, *J Allergy Clin Immunol* 111(2):S571, 2003.
6. Ballow M, O'Neill KM: Approach to patient with recurrent infections. In Adkinson NF, Yunginger JW, Busse WW, editors: *Middleton's allergy: principles and practice*, ed 6, Philadelphia, 2003, Mosby.
7. Cunningham-Rundles C: Primary immunodeficiency diseases. In Adelman DC, Corren J, Casale TB, editors: *Manual of allergy and immunology*, ed 4, Philadelphia, 2002, Lippincott Williams & Wilkins.
8. Buckley RH: Primary immunodeficiency diseases. In Adkinson NF, Yunginger JW, Busse WW, editors: *Middleton's allergy: principles and practice*, ed 6, Philadelphia, 2003, Mosby.
9. Ballow M: Primary immunodeficiency disorders: antibody deficiency, *J Allergy Clin Immunol* 109:581-591, 2002.
10. Beers MH, Berkow R: *The Merck manual of diagnosis and therapy*, ed 17, Whitehouse Station, NJ, 1999, Merck Research Laboratories.
11. Woroniecka M, Ballow M: Office evaluation of children with recurrent infection, *Pediatr Clin North Am* 47(6):1211-1224, 2000.
12. Regueiro JR, Porras O, Lavin M, and others: Ataxia telangiectasia: a primary immunodeficiency revisited, *Immunol Allergy Clin North Am* 20:177-206, 2000.
13. Hyde RM: *Immunology*, ed 3, Philadelphia, 1995, Williams & Wilkins.
14. International Union of Immunological Societies: Primary immunodeficiency diseases, *Clin Exp Immunol* 118(Suppl 1):1-28, 1999.
15. Lilic D, Sewel WA: IgA deficiency: what we should or should not be doing, *J Clin Pathol* 54:337-338, 2001.
16. Oates JA, Wood AJJ: The use of intravenous immune globulin in immunodeficiency diseases, *N Engl J Med* 325(2):110-117, 1991.
17. Schwartz SA: Intravenous immunoglobulin treatment of immunodeficiency disorders, *Pediatr Clin North Am* 47(6):1355-1369, 2000.
18. Amrolia P, Gaspar HB, Hassan A, and others: Nonmyeloablative stem cell transplantation for congenital immunodeficiencies, *Blood* 96:1239-1246, 2000.
19. Bensoussan P, Le Deist F, Latger-Cannard V, and others: T-cell immune constitution after peripheral blood mononuclear cell transplantation in complete DiGeorge's syndrome, *Br J Haematol* 117:899-907, 2002.
20. Bordigoni P, Auburtin B, Carret AS, and others: Bone marrow transplantation as treatment for X-linked immunodeficiency with hyper-IgM, *Bone Marrow Transplant* 22:1111-1114, 1998.
21. Buckley RH: A historical review of bone marrow transplantation for immunodeficiencies, *J Allergy Clin Immunol* 113:793-800, 2004.
22. Buckley RH: Molecular defects in human severe combined immunodeficiency and approaches to immune reconstitution, *Ann Rev Immunol* 22:625-655, 2004.
23. Cavazzana-Calvo M, Hacein-Bey S, De Saint Basile G, and others: Gene therapy of human severe combined immunodeficiency (SCID)-X1 disease, *Science* 288:669-672, 2000.
24. Hacein-Bey-Albine S, Le Deist F, Carlier F, and others: Sustained correction of X-linked severe combine immunodeficiency by ex-vivo gene therapy, *N Engl J Med* 346:1185-1193, 2002.
25. Hacein-Bey-Abina S, Von Kalle C, Schmidt M, and others: LMO2-associated clonal T-cell proliferation in two patients after gene therapy for SCID-X1, *Science* 302(5644):415-419, 2003.
26. Filipovich AH, Heinitz KJ, Robison LL, and others: The immunodeficiency cancer registry: a research resource, *Am J Pediatr Hematol Oncol* 9(2):183-184, 1987.
27. Buckley RH: Immunodeficiency diseases, *JAMA* 268(20):2797-2806, 1992.
28. Advisory Committee on Immunization Practices: Recommended childhood and adolescent immunization schedule—United States 2006, *MMWR* 54(52):Q1-Q4, 2006.

CHAPTER 241

Lymphadenopathy

Michelle Freshman

DEFINITION AND EPIDEMIOLOGY

Lymphadenopathy refers to lymph nodes that have enlarged or changed in consistency. Lymphadenitis is defined as tender, warm, erythematous nodes, and suppurative lymphadenitis includes fluctuance. In 56% of physical examinations, there are incidental but palpable nodes.[1] Lymph nodes typically vary between 0.5 and 2.5 cm (0.2 and 1 inch) in diameter.[2] These enlargements are often related to inflammation or infection in younger patients but become more suspicious in older patients. Neck masses in patients between 15 and 35 years of age are most often associated with an infection such as mononucleosis, but congenital disorders and neoplasms may also cause neck masses in this age-group. With the exception of thyroid disease, 90% of neck masses in patients over 50 years of age are malignant.[3] The "rule of 80s" refers to patients over 40 years of age who regularly smoke cigarettes or drink alcohol and who are seen with a neck mass: 80% of all nonthyroid neck masses are neoplastic, 80% of those are malignant, 80% of those are metastatic, and 80% of those arise from primary sites above the clavicle.[4] Three or more disparate node enlargements constitute generalized lymphadenopathy.

PATHOPHYSIOLOGY

The lymph nodes are integral to the lymphatic drainage system and provide filtration of foreign substances through the action of lymphocytes, monocytes, and macrophages. They are located in clusters around the lymphatic veins, where excess interstitial fluid is accumulated, processed, and later returned to hematologic circulation. More than 1000 lymph nodes exist in the body, with one third of these located in the head and neck. Only a small number of lymph nodes are normally palpable.[3] The lymphatic system is made up of head and neck (internal and external drainage), supraclavicular, deltopectoral, axillary, epitrochlear, inguinal, and popliteal regions.

Because development of the lymphatic system is linked to venous development, the lymphatic ducts run along venous tracks.[3] Lymph fluid ultimately reaches one of two large ducts in the thorax: the right lymphatic duct or the thoracic duct. The right lymphatic duct drains lymph from the right upper body—mediastinum, lungs, and esophagus—into the right supraclavicular vein; the thoracic duct drains lymph from the rest of the body, including the abdominal cavity and reproductive organs, into the left supraclavicular vein.

Lymph nodes filter foreign substances and protein byproducts from the bloodstream and swell in response to viral or bacterial antigens. This swelling is caused by the proliferation of monocytes (the precursors to macrophages) or B and T lymphocytes. Along with the lymph nodes, other lymphoid organ tissues—including the tonsils, spleen, and sometimes the liver—may enlarge. Splenomegaly associated with lymphadenopathy may reflect lymphocytosis generated by infection, various types of immune hyperplasia, macrophage proliferation, or a tumor. Generalized lymphadenopathy may indicate systemic disease or malignancy, since the lymph system can be infiltrated by malignant cells and other cells not normally present in the nodes.

CLINICAL PRESENTATION

Because lymphadenopathy is often related to infection or inflammation in patients less than 50 years old, a thorough symptom analysis, including infectious contacts or exposures (e.g., deer ticks, bird droppings, cat feces), may suggest a nonmalignant condition.[5] Foreign travel or travel to endemic infectious areas of the United States requires investigation. Questions regarding occupational exposure to livestock, asbestos, or silicone are also useful. Patients should be asked about any previous abdominal, thoracic, breast, head and neck, pelvic, reproductive organ, or lower extremity surgery or injury; silicon implant products or prostheses; cancer diagnosis or family history; irradiation; and chemotherapy.

A review of systems should include all areas of the skin for irregular or nonhealing lesions. A history of scalp pruritus (e.g., seborrheic dermatitis, scabies infection), conjunctivitis, eye pain, photophobia, visual complaints, unilateral ear pain, difficulty hearing, nose or throat pain or discharge, odynophagia, impaired swallowing, acidic food intolerance, voice changes or persistent hoarseness, mastoid swelling or pain, dental maladies, dental malocclusion, facial paralysis, and muscular strain of the head or neck should be obtained from the patient.

A woman's breastfeeding history may indicate mastitis. Gastrointestinal symptoms suggestive of malabsorption, complaints of diarrhea or constipation, or back pain with relief in the fetal position can be associated with abdominal or inguinal lymphadenopathy.[6] Any signs of external or internal bleeding, such as hemoptysis, hematuria, melena, or menorrhagia, should be pursued to exclude malignancy. New medications and long-term prescriptions are worth reviewing for potential drug hypersensitivities. Phenytoin use and typhoid vaccination can result in generalized lymphadenopathy.[2] Inquiry into the incidence and frequency of blood transfusions, sexually transmitted diseases, cigarette smoking and chewing tobacco, and illegal drug or alcohol abuse is also necessary. Tobacco and alcohol used together increase the risk of head and neck cancer greatly.[4] Iodine deficiency is a risk factor for thyroid cancer.[4]

Essential to the diagnosis is the duration and extent of the lymph node enlargement. It is also important to establish unilateral or bilateral involvement, pain, and other subjective symptoms.

PHYSICAL EXAMINATION

The history and location of the lymphadenopathy guide the physical examination. Patient age and likely etiology may warrant measurement of vital signs.

Differentiating between normally palpable cervical, axillary, and inguinal lymph nodes and enlarged nodes can be subtle. Smaller nodes greater than 1.5 cm (0.6 inch) and larger nodes in excess of 3 cm (1.2 inch) are considered abnormal.[2] The node should be characterized by degree of fluctuance,

BOX 241-1

LYMPHADENOPATHY: IMPORTANT FINDINGS ON PHYSICAL EXAMINATION

Nonneoplastic: Enlarged, flat, relatively soft
Neoplastic: Enlarged, irregular, and rubbery hard
Infectious: Enlarged, with a variable degree of hardness (may be fluctuant), tenderness, erythema, heat, and pain
Other factors: Presence or absence or hepatosplenomegaly

From Hess CE: Approach to patients with lymphadenopathy and splenomegaly. In Thorup OA, editor: *Leavell and Thorup's fundamentals of clinical hematology,* Philadelphia, 1987, Saunders.

firmness, matted or shoddy quality, mobility or immobility, and tenderness or nontenderness. Unilateral or bilateral involvement, hard and fixed position, and symmetry or asymmetry may indicate or exclude malignancy (Box 241-1). Skin quality, accompanying or overlying vessels, and visible pulsations or bruits should be assessed.[3]

A swollen node that is warm, tender, and rapidly enlarging may represent lymphadenitis and is suggestive of an infection at the drainage terminal. Lymphedema is an interruption and blockage in drainage and may result from a variety of causes. Primary lymphedema refers to congenital malformations; secondary refers to traumatic injury resulting from cancer obstruction, radiation, recurrent infection, or surgery.

Evaluation of the cervical nodes requires full muscle relaxation and midline positioning. Both anterior and posterior cervical node enlargement can indicate carcinomas of the head or neck. The presence of posterior cervical adenopathy more often suggests an infectious etiology.[6] A supraclavicular node can be elicited by Valsalva's maneuver in thin individuals.[6] Axillary nodes are terminal lymph drains for the upper extremities and can become enlarged as a result of cellulitis of the arm or hand or breast malignancies. Observed in both abducted and adducted positions, most axillary adenopathy is benign.[6] However, a woman of any age with a positive axillary node requires a mammography to exclude breast cancer. Liver and spleen examinations are essential.

Inguinal or retroperitoneal nodes may be difficult to palpate unless they are grossly enlarged; however, pain or a feeling of fullness may be present.[7] Unilateral or bilateral presentation is an important consideration, since the former is more often malignant. Bilateral presentation is also less common, except in syphilis.[6] Men can be seen with unilateral malignant lymphedema of the leg in cases of disseminated prostate cancer; it is termed *lymphoma* in women, who are usually over 40 years of age with a characteristic postsurgical, radiation, or infection history.[8]

DIAGNOSTICS

A peripheral blood smear may be one of the most beneficial initial screens for lymphadenopathy.[1,6] Routine diagnostics to exclude infectious diseases may be indicated and include CBC with differential; a throat culture; a heterophil antibody test or monospot; an enzyme-linked immunosorbent assay/Western blot; and rapid plasma reagin (RPR), a Venereal Disease Research Laboratory test, or a fluorescent treponemal antibody absorption test for secondary stage syphilis, especially if the presentation includes palmar rash. If indicated, Lyme disease titers should be obtained.

Other cultures and screening tests should not be ordered unless the history or physical examination suggests specific conditions such as systemic lupus erythematosus (see Chapter 236) or other autoimmune disease, for which an erythrocyte sedimentation rate, antinuclear antibodies, anti-DNA antibodies, and rheumatoid factor might follow. Liver function tests are important in the presence of hepatomegaly; splenomegaly is an unusual and more ominous finding; renal disease or metastasis would be suggested by abnormal urinalysis, BUN, and creatinine. Thyroid studies are warranted in suspected cases of thyroiditis, goiter, or carcinoma, for which a serum calcitonin might provide further confirmatory evidence. Serum or urine monoclonal proteins could inform diagnoses of chronic leukocytic leukemia, multiple myeloma, non-Hodgkin's lymphoma, or amyloidosis.[9] Hypogammaglobulinemia implicates common variable immunodeficiency and Whipple's disease among the differential diagnoses.[9] A chest radiograph with hilar adenopathy is more likely to indicate tuberculosis, sarcoidosis, or infection than a local or disseminated malignancy. In fact, a study of 35 hospitalized pneumococcal pneumonia cases without lymphoma demonstrated that 54% had intrathoracic lymphadenopathy on CT scan and 100% had ipsilateral pneumonia, which meant that it was not necessary to suspect other sources.[10] Malignancy is said to occur in 1.1%

DIAGNOSTICS

Lymphadenopathy

LABORATORY

CBC and differential
Peripheral blood smear
Heterophil antibody (monospot)*
HIV polymerase chain reaction (PCR)*
Rapid plasma reagin or VDRL*
Throat culture*
PPD*
Sputum culture*
LFTs*
Hepatitis panel*
Epstein-Barr serology*
Rubella serology*
Cytomegalovirus PCR*
Toxoplasma serology*
Histoplasma serology*
Coccidioidomycosis serology*
Brucella serology*
Tularemia serology*
Typhoid fever blood culture*
Lyme titer*
Urinalysis*
BUN, creatinine*
TSH*
ESR*
Antinuclear antibodies*
Rheumatoid factor*
Serum creatine kinase*
Monoclonal proteins in serum and/or urine*
Serum angiotensin-converting enzyme*
Serum complement level*

IMAGING

Chest x-ray*
CT*
Ultrasound*
Bone scan*
Positive emission tomography with ^{18}F fluorodeoxyglucose*

OTHER

Cat-scratch disease and Sjögren's syndrome: skin and lip biopsies*
Fine-needle aspiration cytology*
Lymph node biopsy*
Lesion biopsy*
Bone marrow biopsy*
Dematomyositis: muscle biopsy*
EMG*

*If indicated.

of primary care cases of lymphadenopathy.[11] Ultrasound (to avoid administering iodine contrast to thyroid lesions), CT,[12] and positive technetium scans are reserved for soft tissue masses. A bone scan is ordered to confirm metastasis.

Firm, immobile, nontender nodes greater than 1 cm (0.4 inch) are an indication for biopsy, whether by fine-needle aspiration or open excision, as is slowly progressive lymphadenopathy in a patient who lacks other symptoms.[6] Inguinal nodes have the least yield on biopsy; typically supraclavicular, cervical, axillary, and epitrochlear nodes are preferred.[9] Parotid gland and neck biopsy risks damage to the facial nerves and spinal accessory nerve.[9] Typing and clinical staging of lymphomas require a specialist (see Chapter 229).

DIFFERENTIAL DIAGNOSIS

Lymphadenopathy may be related to an acute infectious process, a longstanding illness, malignancy, endocrine disorders, drug sensitivity, or other conditions. The mnemonic *CHICAGO* stands for *C*ancers, *H*ypersensitivities, *I*nfections, *C*onnective tissue disease, *A*typical lymphoproliferative disorders, *G*ranulomatous lesions, and *O*ther unusual causes.[9] Drugs specifically known to produce lymphadenopathy include diphenylhydantoin, hydralazine, para-aminosalicylic acid, and allopurinol. Illnesses associated with lymphadenopathy include HIV/AIDS; syphilis; chancroid; Hodgkin's disease; leukemia; and perhaps systemic lupus erythematosus, rheumatoid arthritis, and chronic fatigue syndrome.

Most infectious processes that coincide with lymphadenopathy last fewer than 2 weeks. More troublesome is lymphadenopathy lasting longer than 2 weeks; however, enlarged lymph nodes lasting more than 1 year without a change in size are more likely to be benign.[11] Mononucleosis classically manifests with lymphadenopathy, pharyngitis, and fever, although gonococcal pharyngitis is possible, as is adenovirus. Parasitic toxoplasmosis can arise from contact with cat feces. Varicella, brucellosis, histoplasmosis, fungal coccidioidomycosis, and cytomegalovirus are other infectious considerations. Hyperthyroidism, sarcoidosis, amyloidosis, and lipid storage diseases should also be included in the differential.

Head and neck area lymphadenopathy coupled with a history of smoking or alcohol use should raise a high index of suspicion for cancer if accompanied by hoarseness, hemoptysis, otalgia or hearing loss, facial nerve deficits, nasal obstruction or bleeding, throat pain or difficulty swallowing, or nonhealing ulcers.[4] Cervical mycobacterial lymphadenitis, or scrofula, an extrapulmonary form of tuberculosis, accounts for 5% of head and neck lymphadenopathy cases and should be of particular concern in immunocompromised or AIDS patients.[13] Parotid swelling, or less commonly salivary gland enlargement, might signal the onset of mumps, known to be more severe in adults and teens. In fact, a mumps epidemic recently surfaced in Great Britain, which is of special concern, since up to 20% of adult men have unilateral orchitis as a complication.[14]

A supraclavicular node enlargement or an asymptomatic, generalized lymphadenopathy pose the greatest risk for malignancy.[3,6] Virchow's node, a pathologic left anterior supraclavicular node, portends an abdominal or thoracic neoplasm; the Delphian node, at the midline prelaryngeal level, is considered a sinister sign in thyroid or laryngeal cancer.[9]

Axillary node enlargement suggests infection but may represent breast neoplasm, melanoma, Hodgkin's disease, or non-Hodgkin's lymphoma. The epitrochlear node may signal an infection such as secondary syphilis, lepromatous leprosy, leishmaniasis, connective tissue disorder, lymphoma, or leukemia.[9]

A Sister Mary Joseph's nodule in the periumbilical region may be a metastatic deposit or enlarged anterior abdominal node.[9] Inguinal lymphadenopathy may be confused with a

DIFFERENTIAL DIAGNOSIS

Lymphadenopathy

Disorder	Associated Findings
Mononucleosis-type syndromes	Fatigue, malaise, fever, atypical lymphocytosis
Epstein-Barr virus*	Splenomegaly in 50% of patients
Toxoplasmosis*	80%-90% of patients asymptomatic
Cytomegalovirus*	Often mild symptoms; possibly hepatitis
Initial stages of HIV infection*	Flulike illness, rash
Cat-scratch disease	Fever in one third of patients; cervical or axillary nodes
Pharyngitis caused by group A streptococcus, gonococcus	Fever, pharyngeal exudates, cervical nodes
Tuberculosis lymphadenitis*	Painless, matted cervical nodes
Secondary syphilis*	Rash
Hepatitis B*	Fever, nausea, vomiting, icterus
Lymphogranuloma venereum	Tender, matted inguinal nodes
Chancroid	Painful ulcer, painful inguinal nodes
Lupus erythematosus*	Arthritis, rash, serositis; renal, neurologic, hematologic disorders
Rheumatoid arthritis	Arthritis
Lymphoma*	Fever, night sweats, weight loss in 20%-30% of patients
Leukemia*	Blood dyscrasias
Serum sickness*	Fever, malaise, arthralgia, urticaria, exposure to antisera or medications
Sarcoidosis	Hilar nodes, skin lesions, dyspnea
Kawasaki's disease*	Fever, conjunctivitis, rash, mucous membrane lesions
LESS COMMON CAUSES OF LYMPHADENOPATHY	
Lyme disease*	Rash, arthritis
Measles*	Fever, conjunctivitis, rash, cough
Rubella*	Rash
Tularemia	Fever, ulcer at inoculation site
Brucellosis*	Fever, sweats, malaise
Plague	Fever, acute illness with cluster of tender nodes
Typhoid fever*	Fever, chills, headache, abdominal complaints
Still's disease*	Fever, rash, arthritis
Dermatomyositis*	Proximal weakness, skin changes
Amyloidosis*	Fatigue, weight loss

Modified from Ferrer R: Lymphadenopathy: differential diagnosis and evaluation, *Am Fam Phys* 58(6):1318, 1998.
*Causes of generalized lymphadenopathy.

hernia; vessel malformations; lipomas; or ectopic endometrial, testicular, or splenic tissue.[6] Cat-scratch disease, lymphogranuloma venereum, or herpesvirus can manifest with a unilateral, tender, and enlarged inguinal node. An asymptomatic unilateral enlargement suggests a malignant neoplasm or lymphoma.[6]

Whether symptomatic or not, node characteristics, including pain, may not reveal the diagnosis, even in cases of cancer, although they are suggestive. Although pain is often associated with infection or rapidly growing nodes within their capsule, hemorrhage resulting from tissue death in a cancerous node also causes pain.[1] Splenomegaly may corroborate infectious mononucleosis or one of the lymphomas or leukemias. Fever, weight loss (10% in 6 months), night sweats, and pruritus—known as the "B" symptoms—occur in approximately 30% of cases of Hodgkin's disease and 10% of cases of non-Hodgkin's lymphoma.[1,15] These symptoms are found in 8% of patients with stage I Hodgkin's disease and 68% in stage IV disease.[11] Hodgkin's disease is particularly prevalent in young adults but, if treated early, has excellent long-term survival rates.[16] Immunohistochemical studies will identify Reed-Sternberg cells of Hodgkin's disease[9] (see Chapter 229).

MANAGEMENT

Symptomatic relief of viral infections and appropriate antibiotic therapy for bacterial, mycobacterial, fungal, rickettsial, and chlamydial infections are indicated if the pathogen is known. Abscesses and other deep structure infections are treated in the hospital and may require surgery for drainage. Congenital or benign growths, such as lipomas or pilar cysts, can be surgically removed. Evidence of malignancy requires referral to the appropriate specialist. Patients with lymphadenopathy of unclear etiology also require physician consultation. Corticosteroid or indiscriminate antibiotic use is not recommended.[9]

Co-Management with Specialists

It is imperative that patients with malignancies have continued primary care surveillance to monitor for physical and psychosocial complications. It is also important that patients receive drug level monitoring, counseling, and weight management during chemotherapy. Monoclonal antibodies coupled with radiation have significantly improved head and neck cancer survival rates.[17] Patients and family should receive support for psychologic distress that may result from functional loss, hair loss, and other cosmetic change. Advance directives are often most comfortably discussed with health care providers and communicated to the consultant. End-of-life care may be best managed at home with the help of the family, community volunteers, and hospice services.

LIFE SPAN CONSIDERATIONS

With lymphadenopathy, an age greater than 50 years is correlated with an increased likelihood of malignancy.[3] As patients age, some lose muscular mass in the neck. As a result, some structures, including the hyoid bone, carotid bulbs, and thyroid, may become more pronounced or appear asymmetric and be mistaken for abnormalities.[4] Older adults can develop immunoblastic lymphadenopathy with a host of symptoms, including combined autoimmune hemolytic anemia, polyclonal gammopathy, hepatosplenomegaly, and rash.[7] Older patients diagnosed with life-threatening infections or malignancies may decline treatment, especially if they suffer from other chronic diseases. Patients and their families will certainly need guidance and support through these difficult decisions.

COMPLICATIONS

Given the variety of structures in the head and neck, a single enlarged node or a group of nodes might be mistaken for benign or congenital growths. Unfortunately, if an oropharyngeal or laryngeal cancer is missed, local metastasis may result. Untreated or inadequately treated group A β-hemolytic streptococci may lead to rheumatic heart disease and glomerulonephritis and therefore warrant sufficient testing. A negative rapid strep test should be followed by a throat culture and possibly the antistreptolysin-O titer to identify chronic carriers.[18] Tonsillar capsule abscesses can follow chronic or recurrent infections.[18] Infection can travel along the carotid sheath to the chest; therefore a CT scan might be required to determine surgical strategy.[18] Complications related to prescribed drugs, especially antibiotics and chemotherapeutic agents, are common.

INDICATIONS FOR REFERRAL OR HOSPITALIZATION

Patients with unusual infectious diseases (e.g., those resulting from foreign travel or communicable illnesses), cases of rare animal or environmental exposure, chronic inflammatory diseases such as systemic lupus erythematosus, or a diagnosis of malignancy should be referred to the appropriate specialist. The crucial decision point for health care providers is *when* to biopsy a node for a definitive diagnosis. A referral to an otolaryngologist or general surgeon might precede a visit to the oncologist. Immunosuppressed patients with AIDS, malignancy, or other illnesses may require hospitalization for intensive nutritional, antiinfective, and chemotherapeutic support. Positron emission tomography using ^{18}F fluorodeoxyglucose is considered the "best noninvasive imaging technique" to determine response to treatment or relapse, with a sensitivity of 76% and a specificity of 94%.[19] The algorithms for fine-needle aspiration and high-tech imaging have become increasingly complex.[20,21]

PATIENT AND FAMILY EDUCATION

Patients with lymphadenopathy need reassurance that many cases are benign and require only watchful waiting. Nodes that persist for more than 4 weeks require further investigation. Ongoing cancer screening for early cancer detection significantly increases the odds for survival.

HEALTH PROMOTION

Because many diseases involving lymph node enlargement in otherwise healthy adults are sexually transmitted, patients should be well informed of their health risks for genital and oral contagion. Frank discussion with patients, as well as support of communication and condom use between partners, is critical. Cancer prevention strategies include eliminating all forms of tobacco, reducing alcohol consumption, and protecting skin from ultraviolet radiation and occupational hazards. Health behaviors that fortify the immune system such as proper nutrition, sleep, exercise, emotional support, and stress management promote health and assist recovery. Patients are often able to find educational and social support in local or state chapters of national disease foundations.

REFERENCES

1. Pangalis GA, Vassilakopoulos TP, Boussiotis VA, and others: Clinical approach to lymphadenopathy, *Semin Oncol* 20(6):570-582, 1993.
2. *Lymphadenopathy: professional guide to signs and symptoms,* ed 3, Springhouse, Penn, 2001, Springhouse.
3. Olsen KD: Evaluation of masses in the neck, *Prim Care* 17(2):415-435, 1990.
4. Prisco MK: Evaluating neck masses, *Nurs Pract* 25(4):30-32, 35-36, 38, 2000.
5. Shaffer S: Benign lymphoproliferative disorders, *Semin Oncol Nurs* 12(1):29-37, 1996.
6. Segal GH, Clough JD, Tubbs RR: Autoimmune and iatrogenic causes of lymphadenopathy, *Semin Oncol* 20(6):611-626, 1993.
7. Dowd TR, Stewart FM: Primary care approach to lymphadenopathy, *Nurs Pract* 19(12):36-44, 1994.
8. McGee S: *Evidence-based physical diagnosis,* Philadelphia, 2001, Saunders.
9. Habermann TM, Steensma DP: Lymphadenopathy: subspecialty clinics: hematology, *Mayo Clin Proc* 75(7):723-732, 2000.
10. Stein DL, Haramati LB, Spindola-Franco H, and others: Intrathoracic lymphadenopathy in hospitalized patients with pneumococcal pneumonia, *Chest* 127(4):1271-1275, 2005.
11. Bazemore AW, Smucker DR: Lymphadenopathy and malignancy, *Am Fam Phys* 66(11):2103-2110, 2003.
12. Magarelli N, Guglielmi G, Savastano M, and others: Superficial inflammatory and primary neoplastic lymphadenopathy: diagnostic accuracy of power-Doppler sonography, *Eur J Radiol* 52(3):253-263, 2004.
13. Weber AL, Siciliano A: CT and MR imaging evaluation of neck infections with clinical correlations, *Radiol Clin North Am* 38(5):941-968, 2000.
14. Gupta RK, Best J, MacMahon E: Mumps and the UK epidemic 2005, *BMJ* 330:1132-1135, 2005.
15. Erikson JM: Update on Hodgkin's disease, *Nurs Pract* 19(11):63-68, 1994.
16. Morrison C, Gordon S, Yeo TP: Hodgkin's disease in primary care, *Nurs Pract* 25(7):44, 47-50, 2000.
17. Bonner JA, Harari PM, Giralt J, and others: Radiotherapy plus cetuximab for squamous-cell carcinoma of the head and neck, *N Engl J Med* 354(6):567-578, 2006.
18. Richardson MA: Otolaryngology for the internist, *Med Clin North Am* 83(1):75-83, 1999.
19. Jerusalem G, Hustinx R, Beguin Y, and others: Evaluation of therapy for lymphoma, *Semin Nucl Med* 35(3):186-196, 2005.
20. Gupta RK, Naran S, Lallu S, and others: The diagnostic value of fine needle aspiration cytology (FNAC) in the assessment of palpable supraclavicular lymph nodes: a study of 218 cases, *Cytopathology* 14(4):201-207, 2003.
21. Divgi C: Imaging: staging and evaluation of lymphoma using nuclear medicine, *Semin Oncol* 32(1 Suppl 1):511-518, 2005.

CHAPTER 242

Weight Loss

Michelle Freshman

DEFINITION AND EPIDEMIOLOGY

The average American is able to maintain his or her body weight within a range of 0.5 to 1 kg (1.1 to 2.2 pounds) annually.[1] Although not all weight loss is ominous, an unintentional loss in excess of 5% of body weight in 6 months or 10% within 1 year typically warrants further investigation.[1-4] Even intentional weight loss in elders, whether medically advised or self-directed, has been associated with increased mortality and hip fracture.[5,6] Among older adults in particular, involuntary weight loss may result from a broad spectrum of physiologic or psychosocial factors.

Within the nursing home population, the Omnibus Budget Reconciliation Act of 1987 established strict criteria for unintentional weight loss: 5% decrease in body weight in 30 days or 10% in 6 months.[7] Such a threshold has been shown to be highly predictive of mortality and has been associated with increased morbidity.[3,4,7] One study indicated that 50% to 65% of nursing home residents were unexpectedly thinner over time.[8] Hospitalized older adults are also at increased risk. Although annual prevalence and incidence within this subgroup have not been well established, the 2-year mortality rate among a group of 91 older adults was reported to be 25% among those initially hospitalized with an unexplained weight loss,[3] a trend borne out in other investigations.[3-5,9,10] Moreover, 20% of 850 patients treated in England from a pool of 1611 surveyed demonstrated malnutrition on admission.[11] Despite a thorough workup and the progression of time, weight loss may remain unexplained in up to one fourth of patients.[5]

PATHOPHYSIOLOGY

Protein-energy malnutrition occurs when the supply of proteins or calories is inadequate to maintain weight. In most industrial societies a combination of the conditions marasmus (insufficient calories) and kwashiorkor (protein deficiency) occurs, as evidenced by changes in body composition, systemic weakness, and laboratory abnormalities.[12] Muscle wasting follows fat losses and may disproportionately affect skeletal and cardiac muscle if cachexia has developed.

Unintentional weight loss can be categorized by one of the following: decreased caloric intake, decreased caloric absorption, and increased metabolic demands that are not met by sufficient caloric intake. Decreased caloric intake may result from behavioral adaptation to what is an unsatisfactory eating experience. Referred to as *functional anorexia*, it may be due to apathy, mechanical obstacles to mastication, a depressed sense of taste and smell, delayed gastric emptying time, or pain with elimination. Decreased caloric absorption results from malabsorption, vomiting, diarrhea, and urinary frequency, which may in turn lead to decreased caloric intake. Increased metabolism occurs with infection, hyperactivity, hyperthyroidism, and tumor growth through neurohormonal mechanisms.

There is a pathophysiologic connection between weight loss and infection through the diminished capacity of cell-mediated and humoral immune systems to mount an adequate response; other humoral system secretions in the setting of illness produce anorexia.[3] Cytokines such as cachectin (tumor necrosis factor) and interleukins, humoral substances, hypersensitivity to cholecystokinins, and corticotrophin-releasing factor are biochemical drivers currently under study.[10,13] Regardless of the cause, the pathway by which weight loss occurs has not yet been fully explained.[3]

CLINICAL PRESENTATION

Patients may be unaware of weight changes. In the absence of consistent health records, they may only recall the observations of others or demonstrate unconsciously cinched-in clothing as evidence of weight loss. A record of the quantity, quality, and regularity of intake is of utmost importance. Situational stress or anxiety can explain unintentional weight loss. Changes in mood, affect, or coping can point to a psychogenic origin.[14]

An inquiry into food affordability, availability, preparation, and safety and social isolation is essential. An older patient with early dementia may have trouble sequencing the steps necessary to procure and prepare food. Recent adoption of proscribed food practices, such as veganism or religious fasting, coupled with inadequate education can lead to unintentional weight loss. Exotic travel, environmental, residential, or work exposures to infection or toxins may be a factor.

For those who report polyphagia or polydipsia and appear to have lost weight, a set of endocrine disorders should be included in the differential diagnosis, including hypothyroidism, hyperthyroidism, diabetes mellitus, diabetes insipidus, hyperparathyroidism, pheochromocytoma, and adrenal insufficiency. Symptoms associated with decreased intake such as fever, night sweats, dyspnea, and mental status changes suggest underlying infection, malignancy, or possible neurologic impairment. In those who suffer from Parkinson's disease or advanced Alzheimer's dementia, mental confusion and apathy may inadvertently lead to meal skipping.

Swallowing difficulties may cause a patient to adjust the types or amounts of food eaten. Common reasons for decreased appetite include dysgeusia, sticking or choking sensation, pain with chewing, dry mouth, unpleasant smell of food, heartburn, and gastric pain before or after eating or associated with eating fatty or acidic foods. Disturbances such as severe reflux, nausea, vomiting, abdominal bloating, flatulence, constipation, and diarrhea affect intake. Individuals may also try to prevent diarrhea by avoiding food.[9] Milk products associated with these latter complaints might signal lactose intolerance. Bloody, painful, or urgent stool can indicate hemorrhoids, inflammatory bowel disease, or malignancy. Fatty, odorous stool can point to gallbladder disease or malabsorption syndromes. Paroxysmal, sustained midabdominal pain can mark pancreatic insufficiency and lead to malabsorption.[11] A history of chronic diarrhea, whether secondary to bacterial or parasitic exposure or a result of underlying illness or recent hospitalization, should be elicited, as should erratic, severe abdominal pain associated with pseudo-obstruction.

Premorbid health conditions can tax a patient's reserves to a degree that interferes with adequate nutrition and hydration. Fatigue, shortness of breath, or impaired mobility may make the duration of a meal exhausting, resulting in decreased intake. Older adults experience diminished senses of taste, smell, and thirst.[15] It is critical to obtain a smoking, alcohol, and drug history. Patients who abuse alcohol may substitute it for food, leading to vitamin deficiencies, which cause anorexia. A history of behaviors that put people at risk for disease, including HIV, should be elicited along with a history of eating disorders. Immunocompromised states can exist along with wasting syndrome.

Surgery can take a toll on health status. In a study of older adults, where the majority had normal prealbumin, transferrin, and body mass index (BMI) values before undergoing elective coronary artery bypass graft repair, 95% had a reduced BMI 4 to 6 weeks after surgery.[16] The lower the posthospitalization weight, the higher the likelihood of rehospitalization.[16] Surgical repair or resection of the intestine may risk bowel torsion or obstruction. This could lead to constipation and subsequent anorexia. In these cases, bacterial overgrowth is of potential concern.

A review of medications, especially if there is evidence of polypharmacy, is necessary. Drugs that affect taste and smell include digoxin, theophylline, and angiotensin-converting enzyme inhibitors. Many other medications, including antiviral agents, macrolide antibiotics, and antineoplastic medications, can cause anorexia.[14] Anticholinergics produce dry mouth and, along with narcotics, potassium, iron, NSAIDs, and calcium channel agonists, slow bowel transit.[4,7] Psychotropic drugs can disturb eating behaviors.[7] Excessive use of diuretics or laxatives should also be explored. Amphetamine use, digitalis, and thyroid medication can all cause anorexia.

PHYSICAL EXAMINATION

General appearance, habitus, affect, speech, cognition, and recall provide basic information. Weight loss can be determined if a previsit weight is available and should be calculated as a percentage change from baseline. Weight charts are not as useful in patients over 75 years of age. Serial skin fold measurement may be helpful to determine the percentage of body fat. Muscle wasting at the temples and intercostal spaces, which is more commonly seen in older adults, should be assessed in context. Vital signs may indicate orthostasis or arrhythmias, suggestive of underlying cardiac disease and disability. Dyspnea, arrhythmias, diminished breath sounds, jugular venous distention, wheezing, and ankle edema suggest cardiopulmonary problems that may interfere with appetite or energy demands. Functional limitations are usually evident with minimum exertion.[9]

Pallor, jaundice, rash, skin texture and turgor, hair consistency and distribution, and poor wound healing should be noted. Hyperpigmentation of the joints, waist, mouth, and palmar creases is associated with adrenal insufficiency.[17] Exophthalmos typifies hyperthyroidism. An oropharyngeal examination is essential for glossitis, ulcers, exudates, masses, ill-fitting or odorous dentures, tooth or gum decay, and missing teeth. The temporomandibular joint should be palpated and gently extended to assess pain or crepitation. Lymphadenopathy, neck masses, and a diminished swallow reflex may warrant further studies. Thyroid enlargement requires further testing for thyroid dysfunction.

Breast examination is important given the increasing incidence of cancers associated with aging. An abdominal examination that is positive for acute rigidity, masses, hepatomegaly, midepigastric tenderness, or ascites may indicate problems of digestion, absorption, or liver disease. A pelvic examination with cervical screening should be included, if indicated. Rectal ulcers, lesions or fissures, hemorrhoids, swollen prostate or nodule, and painful defecation resulting from underlying disease processes may be seen on examination or follow-up studies.

Finally, a subset of unexplained weight loss is frailty. Frailty is associated with slow, ataxic gait; strength loss; fear of falling; poor appetite; cognitive decline; and depressed affect and is correlated with sarcopenia, osteopenia, and immunologic markers such as catabolic cytokines and coagulopathy.[18]

DIAGNOSTICS

Ultrasensitive thyroid chemistries to exclude hyperthyroidism are especially warranted in women over 40 years of age and generally in those over 70 years of age who have signs of tachycardia and fatigue[19] (see Chapter 225). An abnormal CBC with differential is helpful in determining the presence of infection or malignancy. A positive screen for anemia should be followed by evaluation of serum iron, ferritin, thiamine, vitamin B_{12}, and folate levels. A chemistry profile, including calcium, potassium, alkaline phosphatase, liver function studies, serum electrolytes, serum glucose, serum albumin (which is sensitive to hydration status), BUN, and creatinine, would suggest nutritional deficiencies or other underlying diseases. The combination of low serum albumin and high alkaline phosphatase, in a retrospective inpatient analysis, was 17% sensitive but 87% specific for neoplasia.[1] One study found measurements of transferrin, prealbumin, and retinol-binding protein, in the inpatient setting, particularly useful (despite their expense) in determining frailty, since these markers have relatively short half lives.[16] A urinalysis can reveal infection or unmask diabetes or uremia associated with early anorexia.[3] Glucose tolerance testing is appropriate for suspected diabetes. A chest x-ray study is helpful if pulmonary pathologic condition is suspected. Age- and history-appropriate cancer screenings should be incorporated.

Although a stool evaluation for occult blood is indicated if a rectosigmoid source is suspected, testing for ova and parasites, culture, or fat content is based on clinical presentation and physical signs. If the patient's history suggests a possible esophageal stricture or gastric or duodenal ulcer, several tests are available. An upper gastrointestinal series with or without small bowel follow through, endoscopy, and/or barium swallow may help clarify symptoms in the setting of food-sticking sensation, low hematocrit, positive *Helicobacter pylori* status, or chronic diarrhea. Pelvic, renal, and abdominal ultrasounds; echocardiography; and lung studies should be reserved for confirming suspected abdominal, renal, gynecologic, cardiac, or pulmonary causes of weight loss. Sigmoidoscopy or colonoscopy, Doppler-flow ultrasonography, or magnetic resonance angiography are appropriate for a high suspicion of intestinal or mesenteric arterial disease.

DIAGNOSTICS

Weight Loss

LABORATORY
TSH
CBC and differential
Calcium
Serum electrolytes
Alkaline phosphatase
Serum glucose
LFTs
Cholesterol
BUN
Creatinine
Serum albumin
Iron, vitamin B_{12}, folate, ferritin*
Thiamine
Urinalysis
Stool for occult blood
Stool for ova and parasites*
Stool for fecal fat*
Stool for culture*

IMAGING
Ultrasound (abdominal, pelvic, renal)*
CT scan or MRI*
Chest x-ray
Upper GI

OTHER
Endoscopy*
Barium swallow*
Echocardiogram
Colonoscopy

*If indicated.

Finally, a low score on the Mini-Mental State Examination for cognitive functioning (<24) should raise the question of dementia. A positive depression inventory should lead a provider to further explore situational or psychologic diagnoses. Because judicious testing has been shown to reveal about 75% of the cases of weight loss among older adults, a straightforward approach is best guided by physical examination and history.[5,9]

DIFFERENTIAL DIAGNOSIS

From a summary of seven studies, it can be concluded that the three most common diagnoses associated with weight loss are cancer, gastrointestinal disorders, and psychiatric problems.[4] Weight loss can result from a multitude of other organ system illnesses: cardiac, respiratory, endocrine, rheumatologic, immunologic, and neurologic.

As noted above, the psychiatric component is said to be significant: 25% of older adults seen in outpatient settings have been found to have any of a constellation of depressive symptoms; 10% of those surveyed had major depressive disorders.[9] Furthermore, 25% of patients diagnosed with Alzheimer's disease are thought to be both depressed and demented; all eventually suffer from decreased thirst and appetite.[9] Schizophrenia and mania can be recognized in later life.

A fair number of cases of weight loss may defy diagnosis; follow-up evaluation and support are useful in this population, even though most weight loss proves not to be deleterious over time.[1,3,5] One interesting rubric is worth noting. The difference between a patient's actual loss and perceived loss has been used to predict the nature of the cause: an underestimation of greater than 0.5 kg (1.1 pound) is correlated with organic disease with a sensitivity of 40% and a specificity of 92%; and overestimation of greater than 0.5 kg is predictive of inorganic disease with a sensitivity of 70% and a specificity of 81%.[12]

MANAGEMENT

The primary goals are to provide adequate energy, protein, and micronutrients and to treat the underlying disease.

DIFFERENTIAL DIAGNOSIS

Weight Loss

DECREASED CALORIC INTAKE
- Malignancies
- Gastrointestinal or bowel distress
- Depression, anxiety, stress, hypomania
- Anorexia nervosa, bulimia
- Poor nutrition
- Alcoholism
- Congestive heart failure
- Chronic respiratory disease
- HIV/AIDS or infectious diseases
- Poor dentition
- Decreased smell or taste
- Functional obstacles to eating
- Decreased access to food
- Dementia
- Social isolation
- Drug side effects

DECREASED CALORIC ABSORPTION
- Uncontrolled diabetes mellitus
- Renal disease
- Small bowel disease
- AIDS wasting syndrome
- Post–gastrectomy surgery
- Alcoholism or liver disease
- Repeated vomiting or diarrhea from illness or chemotherapy
- Gallbladder disease
- Open skin wounds

INCREASED METABOLIC DEMANDS
- Hyperthyroidism
- Malignancies
- Fever
- Mania
- Chronic respiratory disease
- Cocaine abuse

Medications can reverse nausea, increase appetite, or both and include the progestins, megestrol acetate, and the cannabanoid dronabinol. Other agents include cyproheptadine (an antihistamine and serotonergic), olanzapine (an antipsychotic), mirtazapine (an antidepressant), thalidomide, melatonin, ω3-fatty acids (antiinflammatories), and prednisone (corticosteroid).[5] Megestrol acetate has been shown to improve appetite, enjoyment of life, and well-being; in a geriatric population, its use led to weight gain after 3 months.[20] Some research suggests that appetite-stimulation may be of limited utility.[5] Young patients with anorexia from AIDS wasting syndrome can be given cyproheptadine, but this medication should be avoided in older patients.[4] Anabolic steroids, like testosterone, might be used with cancer cachexia syndrome.[21] Antidepressants should be chosen carefully because some selective serotonin reuptake inhibitors are known to decrease appetite.

Smaller food portions and a calorie-rich breakfast for those with advanced cirrhosis may enhance nutritional intake. With severe wasting or when oral feeding is not safe or desirable, enteral tube feedings or parenteral feedings can supplement or supplant oral feedings. Finally, weight-bearing exercise may have dual benefits for appetite and bone and muscle preservation.

LIFE SPAN CONSIDERATIONS

As older adults experience the physiologic changes that uniquely predispose them to weight loss, it is important to monitor weight and nutrition before weight loss occurs. Body mass peaks in men during their forties and in women during their fifties, although the peak may be a decade later.[3,11] This results from shifts in muscle and fat stores and fat atrophy, causing a 1- to 2-kg (2.2- to 4.4-pound) decrease per decade.[11] Smell and taste sensations also change, which diminishes the pleasurable experience of eating. Because older age brings limitations in abilities and the potential for social isolation, a thorough evaluation of functional independence and safety may clarify meal-related problems. Weight loss that is related to a disease process, acute illness, or depression may be difficult to recover, particularly in older adults, so optimum management requires a team effort.[4] This is particularly true in institutional settings, where contributing factors such as dependency or illness can be assessed more globally. Anticipating malnutrition and weight loss during acute episodes is likely to be crucial to the care of the vulnerable patient, since catching up on depleted stores is difficult.[22]

INDICATIONS FOR REFERRAL OR HOSPITALIZATION

If available, the services of a dietitian or nutritionist are invaluable. Occupational, physical, and speech therapists can help patients with functional or swallowing problems. Medical specialists, including oncologists, neurologists, and psychologists, should be consulted when necessary.

Any patient with severe anorexia, weight loss in excess of 35% of ideal body weight, hypokalemia, hypotension, or prerenal azotemia related to dehydration requires immediate hospitalization to prevent sudden death.[19] Patients with wasting syndromes, including cancer, HIV/AIDS, or failure to thrive, may require hospitalization for nasal or gastric tube placement and feedings or parenteral nutrition. An unchecked decline in weight and functional status can result in a spiraling decline in health with potentially dire consequences.

COMPLICATIONS

Complications include severe malnutrition, weakness, loss of muscle mass, orthostatic hypotension, falls, immobility, and skin breakdown and mortality due to infection. Immunocompromised patients and older adults are at special risk for weight loss. Because the course of a debilitative process and recovery is compounded by weight loss,[16] patients who are at risk require nutritional evaluation and support whether in hospital or home settings.

PATIENT AND FAMILY EDUCATION

Teaching patients simple nutritional concepts and encouraging them to keep a food diary may be helpful. Suggestions for increasing meal attractiveness include flavor enhancement through polyunsaturated butters, oils, dressings, jellies, and creamers. Increased fiber and increased fluid content should be encouraged. Zinc deficiency can lead to dysgeusia, so adding a multivitamin along with protein-rich snacks and nutritional supplements may significantly improve appetite and intake.[3,9] Facilitating food procurement with prepackaged meals or home-delivered foods can make a difference. Increasing activity, social engagement, and a sense of functional capability in the face of dysfunction or physical limitation also improve quality of life. Appetite may also be improved with a simplified regimen that reduces the number of medications taken, eliminating those which might be contributing to the problem. Because weight loss can be a late sign of renal or cardiac disease, it is important to encourage patients or their advocates to look for medical guidance to optimize their quality of life.[17]

HEALTH PROMOTION

Primary prevention of weight loss includes promoting activities that support safe access to food, medical and dental services, and socialization for those at social or financial risk of decreased intake. Preventing communicable diseases, receiving scheduled Pneumovax and flu vaccines, managing sleep requirements, and making adjustments in diet for tastes and preferences all help safeguard nutritional status. Managing side effects such as constipation, nausea and vomiting, and gas; focusing on the favorite meal of the day; and choosing easy-to-prepare foods with adequate flavorings are important strategies to optimize the experience.

REFERENCES

1. Wise GR, Craig D: Evaluation of involuntary weight loss: where do you start? *Postgrad Med* 95(4):143-150, 1994.
2. Gregg EW, Gerzoff RB, Thompson TJ, and others: Intentional weight loss and death in overweight and obese adults 35 years of age and older, *Ann Intern Med* 138:383-389, 2003.
3. Reife CM: Significance of involuntary weight loss, *Med Clin North Am* 79(2):299-313, 1995.
4. Wallace JI, Schwartz RS: Involuntary weight loss in elderly outpatients: recognition, etiologies, and treatment, *Clin Geriatr Med* 13(4):717-735, 1997.
5. Alibhai SMH, Greenwood C, Payette H: An approach to the management of unintentional weight loss in elderly people: review synthese, *Can Med Assoc J* 172(6):773-780, 2005.
6. Wannamethee SG, Sharper AG, Lennon L: Reasons for intentional weight loss, unintentional weight loss, and mortality in older men, *Arch Intern Med* 165(9):1035-1040, 2005.
7. Fabiny AR, Kiel DP: Assessing and treating weight loss in nursing home residents, *Clin Geriatr Med* 13(4):737-751, 1997.
8. Bouras EP, Lange SM, and Scolapio JS: Rational approach to patients with unintentional weight loss (review), *Mayo Clin Proc* 76(9):923-929, 2001.
9. Robbins LJ: Evaluation of weight loss in the elderly, *Geriatrics* 44(4):31-37, 1989.
10. Huffman GB: Evaluating and treating unintentional weight loss in the elderly, *Am Fam Phys* 65(4):640-650, 2002.
11. Edington J, Boorman J, Durrant ER, and others: Prevalence of malnutrition on admission to four hospitals in England: the malnutrition prevalence group, *Clin Nutr* 19(3):191-195, 2000.
12. McGee S: *Evidence-based physical diagnosis,* Philadelphia, 2001, Saunders.
13. Mattox TW: Treatment of unintentional weight loss in patients with cancer, *Nutr Clin Pract* 20(4):400-410, 2005.
14. Williams B, Waters D, Parker K: Evaluation and treatment of weight loss in adults with HIV disease, *Am Fam Phys* 60(3):843-854, 1999.
15. Lipschitz DA: Screening for nutritional status in the elderly, *Prim Care* 21(1):55-67, 1994.
16. DiMaria-Ghalili RA, Amella E: Nutrition in older adults, *Am J Nurs* 105(3):40-50, 2005.
17. Holmes HN, editor: *Professional guide to signs and symptoms,* ed 3, Springhouse, Penn, 2001, Springhouse.
18. Vanitallie TB: Frailty in the elderly: contributions of sarcopenia and visceral protein depletion, *Metabolism* 52(10 Suppl 2):22-26, 2003.
19. Kennedy JW, Caro JF: The ABCs of managing hyperthyroidism in the older patient, *Geriatrics* 51(5):22-32, 1996.
20. Yeh SS, Wu SY, Lee TP, and others: Improvement in quality of life measures and stimulation of weight gain after treatment with megestrol acetate oral suspension in geriatric cachexia: results of a double-blind, placebo-controlled study, *J Am Geriatr Soc* 48(5):485-492, 2000.
21. Puccio M, Nathanson L: The cancer cachexia syndrome, *Semin Oncol* 24(3):277-287, 1997.
22. Moriguti JC, Ferriolli E, de Castilho Cacao J, and others: Involuntary weight loss in elderly individuals: assessment and treatment, *Sao Paulo Med J* 119(2):72-77, 2001.

PART 20

Evaluation and Management of Infectious Diseases

JOANNE SANDBERG-COOK, *Section Editor*

CHAPTER 243

Emerging and Reemerging Infectious Diseases

Thomas H. Taylor

DEFINITIONS

Emerging infectious diseases cause public health problems and are defined as diseases resulting from newly discovered and previously unknown infections. Increased international travel and trade, deforestation and changing ecosystems, and rapid adaptation of microorganisms have all contributed to this problem.[1] The 2002 to 2003 epidemic of severe acute respiratory syndrome (SARS), caused by a newly emergent and variant *Coronavirus* organism (SARS-CoV), is an example and also illustrates the globalization of health care, as this pathogen spread rapidly in Asia to Hong Kong, Singapore, China, Taiwan, and eventually Canada and other countries via modern-day travelers. Global health care initiatives, organized by the WHO, were able to miraculously contain and identify the definitive pathogen in record time, with international cooperation, laboratory collaboration, education, and use of routine health care measures: case definition for rapid recognition, isolation of cases, quarantine of contacts, and personal protective measures.

Reemerging infectious diseases are those previously known and recently reactivated diseases that had formerly caused so few infections that they were no longer considered a public health problem.[1] Dengue fever (DF) is an example of a reemerging infectious disease, whose vector, *Aedes aegypti* mosquito, has distributed it from Africa throughout the Americas via expanding world commerce. The disease was held in check by after World War II mosquito control programs, designed to eradicate yellow fever. With the gradual discontinuation of those programs, the *A. aegypti* mosquito has expanded its geographic distribution in South America, the Caribbean, and now southern United States, where cases of DF are more prevalent and more severe than in the past.

EPIDEMIOLOGY

The Bible recounts the plagues of Egypt. During the Age of Exploration, Spanish *conquistadores* delivered smallpox to the New World, and returned to the Old World with syphilis. In some sense, all infectious diseases emerged and reemerged, to make up our present array of diversified pathogens. With the advent of the antibiotic era in the 1940s, some predicted infectious diseases would become obsolete, and infectious disease physicians dwindled in numbers. Thanks to vaccines, the rashes of measles, rubella, and chickenpox are unknown to recently trained health care providers. The global effort to successfully eradicate smallpox is commendable, and international vaccination efforts promise to eradicate polio. Simple education initiatives, globally enacted by the WHO, may soon eradicate guinea worm. But how does one explain the rapid succession of newly identified pathogens: reemergent and now resistant bacteria, reemergent diarrheal illnesses in developing nations, new respiratory pathogens, and vector-borne illnesses (Table 243-1)? Why has life expectancy of Africans actually decreased, and why should developed nations be concerned?

New to the epidemiology of emerging and reemerging pathogens is the concept of globalization of health care. AIDS may have emerged by jumping from African green monkeys to malnourished African populations, and resistance to antiretroviral therapy arose in first-world nations, unable to fully comprehend rapid mutation mechanisms in retroviruses and complex antiretroviral regimens. We are each our brother's keeper. Whether or not we devote resources to control multidrug-resistant (MDR) tuberculosis in Haiti, Peru, and the jails of former U.S.S.R. has consequences for us all. Widespread and geographically diverse outbreaks of *Salmonella*, *Cyclospora*, and *Escherichia coli* O157:H7 diarrheal illnesses are directly related to the globalization of our food supply. International travelers returned to many destinations with leptospirosis after engaging in extreme sports in Malaysian Borneo.[2,3] Trends toward urbanization and overcrowding have been linked to outbreaks of MDR tuberculosis. Civil wars and ethnic cleansing have spawned outbreaks of cholera in camps for displaced populations. Deforestation and irrigation have contributed to more resistant species of malaria in sub-Saharan Africa and the Amazon River basin. Reforestation of farmlands, reemergence of deer herds, and our desire to live in ecozones (edge areas) contributed to the reemergence of Lyme disease in the United States. Animal contact exposes bird farmers and open market tourists to avian influenza A (H5N1). Exotic tourism in rainforests exposes travelers to reemergent DF.

Natural disasters and infrastructure deterioration have an impact on plague in India and resistant *Salmonella* and *Campylobacter* organisms in tsunami- or monsoon-stricken Southeast Asia. International poverty and malnutrition explain why rotavirus, which infects children under age 5 equally throughout the world, is eminently survivable in Western nations, but increasingly causes high infant mortality in third-world nations. Bioterrorism expressed itself with anthrax in the United States and has alerted us to the possibility of plague, tularemia, and Q fever. Epidemics of IV drug abuse and sexual tourism have contributed to resurgence of HIV and hepatitis C in specific populations. Prescribing practices and antibiotic use in animal feed have contributed to emergence of MDR enteric pathogens, vancomycin-resistant enterococci (VRE), methicillin-resistant *Staphylococcus aureus* (MRSA), and penicillin-resistant *Streptococcus pneumoniae* (PRSP). Resistant gram-negative bacterial pathogens are now widely distributed in underdeveloped nations. Emerging resistance to trimethoprim-sulfamethoxazole and fluoroquinolones has prompted agencies drafting travelers' diarrhea guidelines to stop recommending prophylactic antibiotic use. And so the rubric of globalization is multifaceted when applied to emerging pathogens and health care.

PATHOGENS

Our interconnected world enhances factors mentioned above by allowing pathogens rapid access to new immunologically naive populations and by facilitating spread of new agents and antimicrobial resistance. Major emerging pathogens are

TABLE 243-1 Recent Evolution of Emerging Pathogens

Year	Organism	Diseases
1973	Rotavirus	Diarrhea, with high infant mortality
1975	Parvovirus B19	Erythema infectiosum
1976	*Cryptosporidium parvum*	Outbreaks of watery diarrhea
1977	Ebola virus	Ebola hemorrhagic fever
1977	Hantaan virus	Hemorrhagic fever renal syndrome
1977	*Legionella pneumophila*	Legionnaires' disease
1977	*Campylobacter jejuni*	Diarrhea; already a global pathogen
1980	Human T-lymphotropic virus type 1 (HTLV-1)	T-cell lymphoma/leukemia
1981	Toxic shock syndrome toxin 1 (TSST-1)	Toxic shock syndrome
1982	*Escherichia coli* O157:H7	Enterohemorrhagic colitis Hemolytic uremic syndrome
1982	Human T-lymphotropic virus type 2 (HTLV-2)	Hairy cell leukemia
1982	*Borrelia burgdorferi*	Lyme disease
1983	Human immunodeficiency virus	Acquired immunodeficiency syndrome (AIDS)
1985	*Helicobacter pylori*	Peptic ulcer disease Gastric cancer
1986	Vancomycin-resistant enterococcus (VRE)	Antibiotic resistance
1986	*Cyclospora cayetanensis*	Diarrhea outbreaks
1988	Human herpesvirus 6 (HHV-6)	Roseola infantum (exanthema subitum)
1988	Hepatitis E	Non-A, non-B hepatitis, enteric transmission
1989	*Ehrlichia chaffeensis*	Human monocytic ehrlichiosis
1989	Hepatitis C	Non-A, non-B hepatitis, parenteral transmission
1992	*Bartonella henselae*	Cat-scratch disease Bacillary angiomatosis
1993	Sin Nombre virus	Hantavirus pulmonary syndrome
1994	*Anaplasma phagocytophilum*	Human granulocytotropic anaplasmosis
1994	Hendra virus	Encephalitis transmitted from horses to humans
1995	Human herpesvirus 8 (HHV-8)	Kaposi's sarcoma in AIDS patients
1996	New variant Creutzfeldt-Jakob disease agent	Progressive spongiform encephalopathy
1997	Avian influenza A (H5N1)	Bird influenza transmitted to humans
1999	Nipah virus	Encephalitis transmitted from pigs to humans
2001	Human metapneumovirus	Acute respiratory syncytial virus–like pneumonia; primarily in infants and elderly
2002	Vancomycin-resistant *Staphylococcus aureus* (VRSA)	Antibiotic resistance
2003	SARS coronavirus	Severe influenza-like pneumonia
2006	Human bocavirus	Mild respiratory disease in children

concentrated in the following niches: respiratory pathogens, diarrheal illness, vector-borne and zoonotic disease, and antibiotic resistance. Brief review of some emerging infections will be helpful to differential diagnosis and future practices.

Acute Respiratory Diseases

Human Metapneumovirus. Human metapneumovirus (hMPV) is a newly recognized cause of respiratory tract illness, discovered in 2001 by researchers applying molecular polymerase chain reaction (PCR) techniques to children with previously unexplained pneumonia. The illness ranges from upper respiratory tract illness (URI) or common cold symptoms to lower respiratory tract illness (LRI), such as exacerbations of asthma (14% of LRI illnesses), croup (18%), bronchiolitis (59%), and pneumonia (8%). The clinical illness is indistinguishable from respiratory syncytial virus (RSV), but is often milder and affects a slightly older group of children (6 to 12 months of age), as opposed to RSV, which affects many infants before 2 months of age. At least 5% to 7% of children hospitalized with LRI have hMPV as the cause. Serologic studies demonstrate antibodies to hMPV in virtually all children by age 5 years. Although recognized as pediatric diseases, both RSV and hMPV have recently emerged as major causes of severe LRI in immunocompromised hosts and the elderly. Like RSV and influenza, hMPV circulates in winter months. Since influenza, RSV, and hMPV share common seasonality and common hosts, co-infection with these pathogens is well documented and may contribute to more severe illness. The virus is difficult to grow, and serologic tests are yet to be standardized. Diagnosis is best made with real-time PCR on bronchial secretions. No vaccine or antiviral therapy is available, but studies show ribavirin and IV immunoglobulin (Ig) inhibit hMPV in vitro. Repeated encounters with asymptomatic infection or common cold symptoms maintains immunity in adults.[4-6]

Severe Acute Respiratory Syndrome Coronavirus. Coronaviruses are pathogens in animals and humans, well known as a cause of common colds. The winter of 2002 to 2003 saw emergence of a new coronavirus in Guangdong Province,

China, which caused a severe and often fatal (10%) pneumonia, with prominent systemic symptoms. An incubation period of 4 to 7 days, sometimes as long as 2 weeks, was followed by fever; a flulike illness; and, a few days later, symptoms of pneumonia, diarrhea, leukopenia, thrombocytopenia, and characteristically lymphopenia. About 25% of patients developed severe pneumonia complicated by acute respiratory distress syndrome (ARDS). Mortality ran as high as 50% in elderly patients and hosts with underlying respiratory disease, diabetes, cardiac disease, and chronic hepatitis. Ironically, common cold symptoms were absent, and rash was unusual. Chest x-ray studies showed peripheral interstitial diffuse infiltrates characteristic of atypical pneumonia. Early consolidation and other common complications of bacterial pneumonia, such as hilar adenopathy, pleural effusions, cavitations, and nodular infiltrates, were unlikely.[7] Long-term morbidity has not yet been described. Laboratory diagnosis was best made by antibody detection, which appears about 10 days into the illness, or reverse transcription PCR (RT-PCR) on bronchial secretions, but RT-PCR was used on blood, urine, stool, and upper and lower respiratory samples as well.[8]

The intrigue of SARS lay in its abrupt emergence as a new viral pathogen from a presumed animal coronavirus that jumped species, spread rapidly from human to human locally and then internationally, had high morbidity and mortality rates associated with spread in naive populations, was rapidly isolated followed by availability of a diagnostic test, and thus represented remarkable containment of an international epidemic. Although the United States had only eight laboratory-confirmed cases, more than 8000 cases and 780 deaths were reported from 29 countries before the outbreak ended in June 2003. An exposure-based case definition facilitated early isolation of possible cases, pathogen precautions (contact, droplet, and airborne), quarantine of contacts, and travel advisories. We have not seen another case to date, but concern lingers, since some patients secreted virus for prolonged periods in stool, and persons with subclinical infection may still harbor the organism. Isolation of SARS-CoV from open-market animals included the palm civet and a ferret badger, and the virus could still be circulating in animals, only to reemerge as a human pathogen.[9-11]

Avian Influenza A (H5N1). Avian influenza circulates widely in birds, but does not usually infect mammalian cells. However, human influenza pandemics have been caused by viruses closely related to avian strains, and it is thought that major antigenic shift, or rearrangement of avian influenza genes into human influenza virus, has spawned such events. The pandemics of 1957 and 1968 were attributed to such genetic reassortment, the intracellular mixing and genetic recombination of bird and human influenza viruses. This is in contrast to annual antigenic drift, or minor antigenic changes on surface glycoproteins, hemagglutinin, and neuraminidase that are caused by common point mutations and give rise to new strains of influenza, for which we must be immunized each year but that do not cause major pandemics. Our thoughts about the origins of pandemics and annual outbreaks of influenza have been shaken by the recent sequencing of the influenza virus that caused the 1918 pandemic, which killed 20 million to 30 million worldwide.[12,13] This pandemic was caused by an avian influenza virus that arose not by major gene rearrangements, but by antigenic drift, which made the avian influenza virus recognizable to receptors on mammalian cells and contained enhanced virulence factors.[14] Avian influenza is a more direct threat, as a source of the next influenza pandemic, than we once thought.

In 1997 a small outbreak of avian influenza A (H5N1) occurred within the live poultry markets of Hong Kong. This outbreak was unique in that the virus jumped species and caused severe illness in 18 previously healthy adults, six of whom died. There was no human-to-human transmission, and the outbreak was contained by culling the entire poultry population of Hong Kong.[15]

In 2003 the same virus reemerged as an unprecedented poultry outbreak in many Asian countries: China, Cambodia, Laos, Vietnam, Thailand, Indonesia, South Korea, and Japan. Human cases of avian influenza A (H5N1) have followed in three waves, from December 2003 through 2005, and parallel the geographic spread of the poultry epidemic. As of March 2007, there have been 277 laboratory-confirmed human cases, with 167 (44%) fatalities.[16] Although there have been family clusters, human-to-human transmission remains limited and unsustained. Most human cases had direct exposure to diseased birds. Of great concern is the expanding geographic distribution of the poultry epidemic, along migration routes of geese and ducks, to Siberia, Kazakhstan, Mongolia, Eastern Europe, and more recently Africa. As of this writing, there has been no avian or human H5N1 influenza in North America, but the West Coast can be reached via Arctic flyways.[17]

The influenza vaccine will not protect us from avian influenza (H5N1), but 30,000 to 50,000 die each year in the United States from current endemic influenza strains, and immunization will prevent other influenza illnesses from being confused with avian influenza, should human-to-human transmission become more facile. Refrigeration does not kill influenza viruses, and it is important to separate raw meat from ready-to-eat foods, to use different chopping boards or knives, to avoid eating raw or soft-boiled eggs, to wash hands and surfaces after handling frozen or fresh poultry, and to cook food thoroughly. Poultry meat needs to reach 70° C (158° F) internally. It is wise to avoid live poultry markets in areas touched by the avian influenza epidemic. The H5N1 avian influenza virus is resistant to amantadine and rimantadine, antivirals effective against human influenza A. Oseltamivir (Tamiflu) and zanamivir (Relenza) remain effective against avian influenza, but inappropriate use may promote drug resistance, and self-treatment may prevent etiologic diagnosis. It is important to document any cases of suspected influenza H5N1 and report them to public health departments.[18]

Diagnosis of influenza H5N1 is by viral culture and RT-PCR detection of H5N1-specific PCR. Rapid antigen tests have been insensitive. Clinically, influenza H5N1 may be distinguished from common colds and influenza A and B by a paucity of upper respiratory tract symptoms, such as nasal congestion and conjunctivitis. A noninflammatory, watery diarrhea is more common with influenza H5N1 and may precede respiratory symptoms by several days.[18] In contrast to influenza A and B, where rapid antigen tests are best performed on posterior nasal secretions, avian influenza H5N1 RT-PCR is best detected on pharyngeal or bronchial lavage specimens. Cases of H5N1 influenza may be suspected after travel to endemic countries and after contact with domestic fowl, wild birds, or suspected human cases; patients should undergo rapid antigen testing for influenza A and B to help determine whether they should be isolated and further tested for influenza H5N1. There is a bird vaccine active against influenza H5N1, but large doses are required for humans, and adjuvant human vaccines are still under development. However, there is no guarantee that present avian influenza H5N1 vaccines will be effective against next generation H5N1 virus, after further antigenic drift or antigenic shift produces the next pandemic influenza virus.[18,19]

Acute Diarrheal Illnesses

Vibrio cholerae. Cholera is a classic example of reemerging epidemics through the ages, brought on by natural disasters, civil war, and displaced populations. We are now in the seventh pandemic. The first six pandemics, caused by the classic biotype *Vibrio cholerae* O1, occurred before 1926, originated in Asia and India, and were eventually exported to Europe and the Americas. The seventh pandemic is caused by a new classic biotype, El Tor, first isolated in Egypt. It causes milder disease, which remained sporadic and endemic throughout Africa, Europe, and Asia for many years. Recent extension of the pandemic to naive populations in Latin America began in 1991,[20] and emergence of a new subtype, *Vibrio cholerae* O139, began in India and Bangladesh in 1992. Past exposure to *V. cholerae* O1 offers no immunity to *V. cholerae* O139, and the new strain is resistant to trimethoprim-sulfamethoxazole.[21] Infants and young children bear the brunt of epidemics in third-world nations, where 80% of all diarrheal deaths occur in children under the age of 5.[22]

Cholera is a natural aquatic inhabitant, which lives attached to algae, crustaceans, and plankton. Cholera periodically emerges from its dormant state, inspired by warm waters (e.g., El Niño), and its growth is facilitated by changes in nutrients and salinity (e.g., from monsoons, tsunamis, and typhoons).[23] In its activated state it grows and, once humans are infected, spreads rapidly as a water-borne or food-borne pathogen. Person-to-person spread is unlikely because of the large inoculum required for infection. Disasters provide ready availability of contaminated water and food. Under such circumstances there are also outbreaks of bacillary dysentery caused by *Shigella* species, which requires a small inoculum and is spread person to person. *Cryptosporidium parvum* causes large outbreaks of watery diarrhea via contamination of water supplies. Nontyphoidal *Salmonella* species require a large inoculum and cause small outbreaks of diarrhea through ingestion of contaminated food. *Cyclospora cayetanensis* is a parasite that caused thousands of cases of diarrhea in Canada and the United States when contaminated raspberries were imported from Guatemala in 1996.[24]

Severe dehydration, electrolyte imbalance, renal failure, and metabolic acidosis can all be fatal complications of cholera, and oral or IV rehydration is paramount. Mortality is as high as 10% in epidemic settings without adequate health care support, but only 3% in centers versed in simple hydration techniques. Antibiotics are secondary in importance to hydration in the treatment of cholera. One 300-mg dose of doxycycline, 1 g of ciprofloxacin, or one tablet of trimethoprim-sulfamethoxazole b.i.d. for 3 days is effective treatment, if the organism is sensitive. But emerging antibiotic resistance is a problem for developing nations. Vaccines have not produced effective or long-lasting immunity, and none is currently recommended.[25] Fortunately, cholera is a predictably reemergent disease, less likely to be encountered during routine travel, but most likely to be encountered after natural disasters, in refugee camps, and in urban slums where it is endemic. Simple measures to dispose of human waste, avoid contaminated water, and provide a potable water supply all work well in developing nations.[26]

***Escherichia coli* O157:H7.** *E. coli* O157:H7 was first recognized as a food-borne pathogen in the United States in 1982. Outbreaks occurred via distribution of contaminated hamburger meat, and enterohemorrhagic *E. coli* (EHEC) soon became the most common cause of bloody diarrhea. The CDC estimates 73,000 illnesses annually in the United States, resulting in more than 2000 hospitalizations and 60 deaths.[27] *E. coli* O157:H7 is a zoonotic emerging pathogen, which normally resides in the gut of healthy cattle. Evolution of cattle feeding in the United States from hay to grain has lowered colonic pH, thus giving *E. coli* O157:H7 a competitive advantage over other *E. coli* strains in the cattle colon. Early outbreaks of *E. coli* O157:H7–mediated disease were traced to unpasteurized apple cider, which was made from fallen apples in orchards where cattle grazed, thus contaminating it with feces.[28] Discovery of this relationship has resulted in recognition of the need to pasteurize apple cider. Improved cooking standards in fast-food restaurants have decreased the incidence of *E. coli* O157:H7 in ground beef foods, but the problem has shifted to water-borne and vegetable-associated disease. Our preference for organic foods, rejection of chemical fertilizer for cow manure, and concomitant contamination of water and vegetables with *E. coli* O157:H7 have introduced new sources of what use to be the "hamburger disease."[29]

Another unique aspect of *E. coli* O157:H7 is the spectrum of disease this organism may confer, from mild diarrhea to severe hemorrhagic colitis. Further, association of *E. coli* O157:H7 diarrhea with childhood hemolytic uremic syndrome (HUS) has come to exemplify how a pathogen at one site can explain a disease at another uninfected site. HUS was previously an unexplained illness, defined by hemolysis, thrombocytopenia, and acute renal failure, often in children. EHEC has evolved by acquiring a symbiotic relationship with a bacteriophage that encodes a shiga-like toxin (SLT), a toxin also present in *Shigella dysenteriae*. SLT attaches to a receptor, globotriaosylceramide (GB), on enterocytes in the gut. GB receptors also exist on endothelial cells of glomerular capillaries and other small capillary beds. Damage to these capillary beds, by circulating SLT, explains the occurrence of acute renal failure, microangiopathic hemolytic anemia, and thrombocytopenia, which define HUS.[30] Further investigation demonstrates that HUS is the most common cause of acute renal failure in children. Neutralizing antibodies to SLT develop in most children before the age of 10 and decline as they age. Thus persons most severely affected by *E. coli* O157:H7 are the young and the elderly. *E. coli* O157:H7 has emerged as a common cause of HUS, a disease not previously recognized as infectious.[31] Other examples of emergent infectious causes of disease of uncertain etiology are *Campylobacter jejuni* as one of the many causes of Guillain-Barré syndrome,[32] and the link between *Helicobacter pylori* and peptic ulcer disease.

Treatment of EHEC diarrhea requires hydration and correction of electrolyte imbalance. Antibiotic treatment causes release of SLT, and had been thought to worsen the risk of HUS,[33] although a recent meta-analysis did not show an increased risk of HUS associated with antibiotic administration.[34] By the time HUS appears, the acute diarrhea has already subsided, so antibiotics are not likely to help.

Clostridium difficile. Antibiotic-associated diarrhea (AAD) has been with us since the advent of broad-spectrum antibiotics, which alter anaerobic and enteric bowel flora, allowing antibiotic-resistant *Clostridium difficile* to grow and produce diarrhea and more severe pseudomembranous colitis. There has been a gradual increase in *C. difficile*–associated disease over the past 10 to 15 years, but more urgent concern is raised by several recent studies showing both increasing rates and increasing severity of *C. difficile* colitis.[35] The new epidemic is occurring in widespread geographic areas; causes disease in previously healthy patients[36]; and is dominated by a previously uncommon strain of *C. difficile*, which produces a new binary toxin, similar to the more virulent binary toxin in *Clostridium perfringens*. The new strain also contains a mutation in the tcdC regulatory gene, and consequently produces greater amounts of toxins A and B responsible for diarrhea. Interestingly, this new strain is more resistant to the extended-spectrum fluoroquinolones: levofloxacin, gatifloxacin, and moxifloxacin. Recent overuse of these fluoroquinolones may have selected out this particular strain of *C. difficile*, much as clindamycin selected out past strains of *C. difficile* and was more closely associated with AAD than other antibiotics. The new epidemic strain of *C. difficile* is not resistant to either metronidazole or vancomycin.[37-39]

Treatment of the new strain of *C. difficile* remains essentially the same as for past strains, but we need to be more alert to the increasing possibility of AAD and its increasing severity to prevent complications of toxic megacolon, colonic perforation, transverse volvulus, and protein-losing enteropathy. Broad-spectrum antibiotics should be stopped, if at all possible. Hydration and electrolyte replacement are of foremost importance. Although 10-day regimens of metronidazole 500 mg PO t.i.d. or vancomycin 125 to 250 mg PO q.i.d. are equally effective, metronidazole is preferred due to the greater cost of oral vancomycin and the possible selection of VRE or, more recently, vancomycin-resistant *S. aureus* (VRSA).[40]

Recurrent *C. difficile* diarrhea follows a course of treatment in up to 20% of cases, and multiple relapses occur in at least 6%. Repeat testing for *C. difficile* toxin should not be done if diarrhea is improving, since toxin and culture may remain positive in many improving patients. True relapses should be treated with another course of metronidazole, with the dosage gradually tapered each week (i.e., 500 mg t.i.d., then the same dose b.i.d., q day, every other day, and every third day). Patients with multiple recurrences are placed on long-term metronidazole, the lowest dose that controls symptoms, for 2 to 4 months. When bowel health has improved, another attempt at weaning may be tried. Long-term vancomycin use is expensive and encourages colonization with VRE. IV vancomycin should not be considered because it does not get into the bowel lumen in significant concentrations, and vancomycin neither is absorbed orally nor progresses to the colon if there is an ileus. Severely ill patients should be treated with IV metronidazole, which is excreted lower down in the bile and to some extent directly into the colon. In severely ill patients, liquid vancomycin may be placed into nasogastric tubes, high rectal tubes, and ostomies, in addition to IV metronidazole. A surgeon should be consulted, since complications of toxic megacolon and colon perforation may require colectomy or diverting colostomy.

Epidemic *C. difficile* places new emphasis on preventive measures. Antibiotic use should be limited to the shortest effective course and the narrowest spectrum antibiotic for each pathogen. Broad-spectrum empiric regimens should be narrowed as culture results return, and more specific diagnosis may allow for early discontinuation. Isolation and cohorting of cases should be accompanied by gowns, gloves, and handwashing. Alcohol scrubs do not inactivate *C. difficile* spores, so soap and water are required to remove them from hands. Electronic thermometers should be replaced by disposable thermometers. Broad-spectrum antimicrobial use should be subject to approval by an infectious disease expert, and use of clindamycin, gatifloxacin, moxifloxacin, and levofloxacin should be limited.[41,42]

Vector-Borne Diseases

West Nile Virus. West Nile virus is the best example of an arthropod-borne virus, with recent evolution to more aggressive disease and wide geographic spread. It is discussed in Chapter 251, and mentioned here only to be complete. Similarly, Rift Valley fever (caused by flood water–breeding *Aedes* mosquitoes) and Japanese encephalitis (caused by ground pool–breeding *Culex* mosquitoes) have reemerged, with spread to wider geographic areas over the past decade.

Dengue Fever. DF is spread by the *A. aegypti* mosquito, which originated in Africa. The reemergence of dengue is the story of spread of this mosquito by international commerce throughout Africa, the Middle East, Asia, the West Pacific, and Latin America and more recently to the Caribbean and southern United States.[43] Elimination of mosquito control programs fostered the success of *A. aegypti* and facilitated spread of DF. The global distribution and impact of DF is now similar to that of malaria.

An interesting aspect of DF is the spectrum of disease, from mild viral illness to dengue septic shock (DSS) and dengue hemorrhagic fever (DHF). Dengue virus has four serotypes. Immunity to one virus is not cross protective to the other three, and it is the second infection, with a second serotype, that leads to extensive immunologic reaction, damage to small capillary beds, and more severe disease. When epidemics were small and isolated, patients would be less likely to sustain the second devastating infection. Now several serotypes may circulate in one sustained outbreak, affording greater opportunity for a second infection. Most deaths now occur in children under the age of 15. There is no effective treatment, other than supportive measures and fluid resuscitation for DSS, and vaccine development is problematic, given the immunologic nature of DSS and DHF.[44,45]

An incubation period of 4 to 7 days is followed by chills, fever, headache with characteristic retro-orbital pain, severe musculoskeletal pain, abdominal tenderness, back pain, and hyperesthesia of skin. As fever resolves, a maculopapular rash appears, which may be scarlatiniform or petechial. The illness may be biphasic, with acute illness followed by prolonged weakness, fatigue, and depression.

Leukopenia, neutropenia, thrombocytopenia, transaminitis, and severe musculoskeletal symptoms may help distinguish DF from other viral illness or typhoid fever in a returning traveler. Viremia reaches high levels, and viral blood culture, PCR, and serum IgM may all be used to make the diagnosis. Second exposures to dengue virus may be complicated by DHF, DSS, ARDS, hepatitis, myositis, rhabdomyolysis, or acute renal failure, which is more likely to be found in infants and elderly patients.

Zoonosis

Hendra and Nipah Viruses. Hendra and Nipah are similar viruses, and both have caused recent outbreaks of flulike illness followed by encephalitis. Hendra virus infects horses, with secondary transmission to human trainers, only by close contact with the horse. Both equine and human infections have been fatal and confined to small outbreaks in Australia.[46] Nipah virus caused an outbreak in pigs in Malaysia that spread to Singapore. In contrast to Hendra virus, this infection was highly contagious and spread rapidly among pigs and their handlers. Of 265 humans infected, 40% died of encephalitis, and others suffered marked sequelae.[47] Search for a reservoir host has led to bats, where both viruses are maintained. These potentially devastating viruses are currently limited to Australia, Malay Peninsula, Bangladesh, Thailand, and Cambodia, but the range of their reservoir host, the pteropid fruit bat, is much wider, and it is likely we will see more outbreaks.

Monkeypox and Herpes B Virus. Traffic in exotic animals or exposure to pets or even laboratory animals can be harmful to your health. Monkeys are hosts for both monkeypox and herpes B virus. Monkeypox is a disease similar to smallpox and has previously circulated in central Africa. Monkeys, like humans, are incidental hosts, and the reservoir is likely to be found in many species of rodents and squirrels in the region. The smallpox vaccine is also effective against monkeypox, and so monkeypox in humans was markedly decreased by smallpox vaccination programs. Now that smallpox vaccination is no longer required in any country and civil wars have increased dependence on hunting, human monkeypox has reemerged in central Africa. In 2003 there was an outbreak of monkeypox in the United States, with 72 cases reported from six Midwestern states. Investigation revealed most cases followed the acquisition of a new prairie dog, also infected with monkeypox. A shipment of infected Gambian giant rats had been cohorted with prairie dogs, and the disease was transmitted to human exotic pet owners. In contrast to smallpox, monkeypox produces noteworthy adenopathy, demonstrates lower person-to-person transmission, and has a lower mortality rate of 1% to 10%. Real-time PCR, IgG and IgM enzyme-linked immunosorbent assay, indirect fluorescent antibody assay, and viral culture are all helpful in diagnosis. Treatment is supportive, and smallpox vaccination is recommended during the 10- to 14-day incubation period for persons with known exposure.[48,49]

Cercopithecine herpesvirus 1 (B virus) infects rhesus macaques, frequently used in research laboratories. It causes asymptomatic infection, but remains latent in up to 70% of animals in macaque colonies. Like other herpes viruses, B virus can reactivate and spread to other monkey species or humans, often with devastating consequences. Bites, scratches, mucosal inoculation, and needle sticks may all lead to local vesicle formation. Nondescript fever and malaise progress to myelitis, ascending paralysis, and diffuse hemorrhagic encephalitis. Wounds should be washed extensively with soap, iodine, or bleach. Mucosal splashes should be heavily irrigated. Oral valacyclovir, 1 g PO q 8 hr for 14 days, is recommended for postexposure prophylaxis. Early treatment with IV acyclovir or ganciclovir has arrested disease in some cases, but oral valacyclovir may need to be continued for months to years to prevent reactivation.[50,51]

Antibiotic Resistance

MRSA has emerged as a major pathogen in hospitals nationwide, and vancomycin-intermediate *S. aureus* (VISA) and VRSA have emerged in small numbers.[52] *S. aureus* is an important cause of community-associated disease, especially in colonized patients. The United States prevalence of *S. aureus* nasal carriage in 2001 to 2002 was 32.4%, but only 0.8% of the population was colonization with MRSA.[53] Over the past 10 years, an increasing number of patients from the community have been admitted to hospitals with MRSA, but have been known carriers or were associated with known links to hospital-associated MRSA (HA-MRSA) through recent hospitalization, infusion centers, dialysis units, or nursing homes.[54] I suspect that the proportion of the U.S. population colonized with MRSA is growing, since we have witnessed an emergence of community-associated MRSA (CA-MRSA) infections in patients without recent exposure to antibiotics or hospitalization.[55-58] The current epidemic began in 1999, when a series of fatal cases of CA-MRSA infections occurred in Native American children in the Midwest, with no link to health care settings.[59,60] Now 60% to 75% of all community-acquired isolates of *S. aureus* are methicillin resistant, and thus resistant to all β-lactam and cephalosporin antibiotics.[61]

CA-MRSA infections are distinct from HA-MRSA infections because they are associated with a gene encoding the Panton-Valentine leukocidin (PVL) toxin. PVL is a cytotoxin that causes destruction of leukocytes and tissue necrosis and is associated with a predilection to skin and soft tissue infections, as well as abscesses, necrotizing fasciitis, necrotizing pneumonia, and sepsis.[62] CA-MRSA is also more likely to carry genetic factors (*agr*1 and *agr*3) that cause aggressive expression of toxins and other virulence factors.[63] A clue to the presence of a toxin-producing strain of CA-MRSA is the early presence of a necrotic center, which sometimes leads to the misdiagnosis of recluse spider bite. We are thus faced with the paradox that CA-MRSA is more likely to affect young, healthy outpatients, without the usual exposure to antibiotics and hospitals, and with higher morbidity and mortality than HA-MRSA.

Compared with HA-MRSA, CA-MRSA isolates are more likely to carry a distinct resistance gene, staphylococcal chromosomal cassette *mec* type IV (SCC*mecA* type IV), and are more sensitive to clindamycin, trimethoprim-sulfamethoxazole, doxycycline, and fluoroquinolones.[64] HA-MRSA is unlikely to be sensitive to these antibiotics. A sensitivity pattern suggesting CA-MRSA in young, healthy outpatients, with MRSA soft-tissue infection, should raise concern for more serious infection and complications such as necrotizing fasciitis, metastatic abscess, pneumonia, empyema, or endocarditis. Unfortunately, resistance to macrolides, tetracyclines, and fluoroquinolones may emerge under therapy, and treatment with trimethoprim-sulfamethoxazole and clindamycin has not been widely studied in serious CA-MRSA infections. Clindamycin is problematic, because it is exported from the bacteria by the same inducible efflux pump (MLS_B) that renders the MRSA resistant to macrolides, and it should not be used if there is resistance to erythromycin or azithromycin. Vancomycin, linezolid, or daptomycin should be the initial drug in all serious community-acquired *S. aureus* infections, pending sensitivities, with the caveat that vancomycin and daptomycin are not good antibiotics for MRSA lung infections because of poor concentrations in lung tissue and high failure rates. Linezolid is thus an important option for CA-MRSA pneumonias.[65]

Other important topics—such as Sin Nombre virus, the cause of hantavirus pulmonary syndrome, and other categories of emerging antibiotic resistance, such as VRE and PRSP—are covered in other chapters. Overuse of antibiotics, steroids, immunosuppressant therapy, transplantation services, evolution of trauma centers, and the extensive use of plastic lines and drainage tubes all set patients up for reemergence of resistant gram-positive infections, gram-negative infections with extended-spectrum β-lactamases, and a plethora of emerging fungal infections. On the bright side, international cooperation has eliminated smallpox, polio eradication is possible, and the world has shown it can work as one when faced with emerging infectious diseases.

BOX 243-1

PATHOGENESIS OF EMERGING AND REEMERGING INFECTIOUS DISEASES: GLOBAL PROBLEM

- Global travel allows for rapid dissemination of new pathogens.
- Urbanization as rural populations move to cities creates overcrowding and poverty.
- Civil wars and ethnic cleansing create displaced populations without health care.
- Irrigation, deforestation, and reforestation all upset ecosystems of vectors and animals.
- Living in ecozones and population migration increase contact with insects and animals.
- Infrastructure deterioration caused by poverty or natural disasters deters health care delivery.
- IV drug abuse, sexual mores, and sexual tourism facilitate pathogen spread.
- Inappropriate use of antibiotics or antibiotic use in animal feed spawn resistance.
- Contagion spreads via bioterrorism.

REFERENCES

1. WHO: *Global infectious disease surveillance,* June 1998, retrieved March 7, 2006, from http://www.who.int/mediacentre/factsheets/fs200/en/print.html.
2. Centers for Disease Control and Prevention: Outbreak of acute febrile illness among participants in Eco-Challenge-Sabah 2000—Malaysia, 2000, *MMWR* 49:816-817, 2000.
3. Centers for Disease Control and Prevention: Update: outbreak of acute febrile illness among athletes participating in Eco-Challenge-Sabah 2000—Borneo, Malaysia, 2000, *MMWR* 50:21-24, 2000.
4. Williams JV, Harris PA, Tollefson SJ, and others: Human metapneumovirus and lower respiratory tract disease in otherwise healthy infants and children, *N Engl J Med* 350:443-450, 2004.
5. Mejias A, Chavez-Bueno S, Ramilo O: Human metapneumovirus: a not so new virus, *Pediatr Infect Dis J* 23:1-10, 2004.
6. Van Den Hoogan BG, Osterhaus ME, Fouchier RA: Clinical impact and diagnosis of human metapneumovirus infection, *Pediatr Infect Dis J* 23:S25-S32, 2004.
7. Peiris JSM, Phil D, Yuen KY, and others: Current concepts: the severe acute respiratory distress syndrome, *N Engl J Med* 349:2431-2440, 2003.
8. Cockerill FR, Smith FR: Response of the clinical microbiology laboratory to emerging (new) and reemerging infectious diseases, *J Clin Microbiol* 42:2359-2365, 2004.
9. Low DE, McGeer A: Perspective: SARS—1 year later, *N Engl J Med* 349:2381-2382, 2003.
10. Centers for Disease Control and Prevention: *In the absence of SARS-CoV transmission worldwide: guidance for surveillance, clinical and laboratory evaluation, and reporting,* 2003, retrieved March 8, 2007, from http://www.cdc.gov/ncidod/sars/absenceofsars.htm.
11. Guan Y, Zheng BJ, He YQ, and others: Isolation and characterization of viruses related to the SARS coronavirus from animals in southern China, *Science* 302:276-278, 2003.
12. Tumpey TM, Basler CF, Aguilar PV, and others: Characterization of the reconstructed 1918 Spanish influenza pandemic virus, *Science* 310:77-80, 2005.
13. Taubenberger JK, Reid AH, Lourens RM, and others: Characterization of the 1918 influenza virus polymerase genes, *Nature* 437:889-893, 2005.
14. Sampathkumar P, Maki DG: Avian H5N1 influenza: are we inching closer to a global pandemic? *Mayo Clin Proc* 80:1552-1555, 2005.
15. Yuen KY, Chan PKS, Peiris M, and others: Clinical features and rapid viral diagnosis of human disease associated with avian influenza A H5N1 virus, *Lancet* 351:467-471, 1998.
16. World Health Organization: *Cumulative number of confirmed human cases of avian influenza A/(H5N1) reported to WHO,* March 1, 2007, retrieved March 15, 2007, from http://www.who.int/csr/disease/avian_influenza/country/cases_table_2007_03_01/en/index.html.
17. Tiensin T, Chaitawesub P, Songserm T, and others: Highly pathogenic avian influenza H5N1, Thailand, 2004, *Emerg Infect Dis* 11:1664-1672, 2005.
18. Writing committee, World Health Organization consultation on human influenza A/H5: Current concepts: avian influenza A (H5N1) infections in humans, *N Engl J Med* 353:1374-1385, 2005.
19. Bartlett J, Hayden FG: Influenza A (H5N1): Will it be the next pandemic influenza? Are we ready? *Ann Intern Med* 143:460-462, 2005.
20. Centers for Disease Control and Prevention: Update: cholera—Western Hemisphere, 1992, *MMWR* 42:89-91, 1993.
21. Centers for Disease Control and Prevention: Imported cholera associated with a newly described toxigenic *Vibrio cholerae* O139 strain—California, 1993, *MMWR* 42:501-503, 1993.

22. World Health Organization: *World health report 2003: shaping the future*, Geneva, 2003, The Organization.
23. Lipp EK, Huq A, Colwell RR: Effects of global climate on infectious disease: the cholera model, *Clin Microbiol Rev* 15:757-770, 2002.
24. Centers for Disease Control and Prevention: Outbreaks of *Cyclospora cayetanensis* infection—United States, 1996, *MMWR* 45:549-551, 1996.
25. Centers for Disease Control and Prevention: Update: *Vibrio cholerae* O1—Western Hemisphere, 1991-1994, and *V. cholerae* O139—Asia, 1994, *MMWR* 44:215-219, 1995.
26. Seas C, Gotuzzo E: Cholera: overview of epidemiologic, therapeutic, and preventive issues learned from recent epidemics, *Int J Infect Dis* 1:37, 1996.
27. Frenzen PD, Drake A, Angulo FJ: Emerging Infections Program FoodNet Working Group: economic cost of illness due to *Escherichia coli* O157 infections in the United States, *J Food Protection* 68(12):2623-2630, 2005.
28. Cody SH, Glynn MK, Farrar JA, and others: An outbreak of *Escherichia coli* O157:H7 infection from unpasteurized apple juice, *Ann Intern Med* 130:202-209, 1999.
29. Blaser MJ: Bacteria and diseases of unknown cause: hemolytic-uremic syndrome, *J Infect Dis* 189:552-555, 2004.
30. Moake JL: Mechanisms of disease: thrombotic microangiopathies, *N Engl J Med* 347:589-600, 2002.
31. Griffin PM, Mead PS, Sivapalasingam S: *Escherichia coli* O157:H7 and other enterohemorrhagic *E. coli*. In Blaser MJ, Smith PD, Ravdin JI, and others, editors: *Infections of the gastrointestinal track*, ed 2, Philadelphia, 2002, Lippincott Williams & Wilkins.
32. Rees JH, Soudain SE, Gregory NA, and others: *Campylobacter jejuni* infection and Guillain-Barré syndrome, *N Engl J Med* 333:1374-1379, 1995.
33. Wong CS, Jelacic S, Habeeb RL, and others: The risk of hemolytic-uremic syndrome after antibiotic treatment of *Escherichia coli* O157:H7 infections, *N Engl J Med* 342:1930-1991, 2000.
34. Safdar N, Said A, Gangnon RE, and others: Risk of hemolytic-uremic syndrome after antibiotic treatment of *Escherichia coli* O157:H7 enteritis: a meta-analysis, *JAMA* 288:996-1001, 2002.
35. Archibald LK, Banerjee SN, Jarvis WR: Secular trends in hospital-acquired *Clostridium difficile*–associated disease in the United States, 1987-2001, *J Infect Dis* 189:1585-1589, 2004.
36. Centers for Disease Control and Prevention: Severe *Clostridium difficile*–associated disease in populations previously at low risk—four states, 2005, *MMWR* 54:1201-1205, 2005.
37. Muto CA, Pokrywka M, Shutt K, and others: A large outbreak of *Clostridium difficile*–associated disease with an unexpected proportion of deaths and colectomies at a teaching hospital following increased fluoroquinolone use, *Infect Control Hosp Epidemiol* 26:273-280, 2005.
38. McDonald LC, Killgore GE, Thompson A, and others: An epidemic, toxin gene–variant strain of *Clostridium difficile*, *N Engl J Med* 353:2433-2441, 2005.
39. Loo VG, Poirier L, Miller MA, and others: A predominantly clonal multi-institutional outbreak of *Clostridium difficile*–associated diarrhea with high morbidity and mortality, *N Engl J Med* 353:2442-2449, 2005.
40. Teasley DG, Olson MM, Gebhard RL, and others: Prospective randomized trial of metronidazole versus vancomycin for *Clostridium difficile*–associated diarrhea and colitis, *Lancet* 2:1043-1046, 1983.
41. Bartlet JG, Perl TM: The new *Clostridium difficile*: what does it mean? *N Engl J Med* 353:2503-2505, 2005.
42. Centers for Disease Control and Prevention: *Information about a new strain of* Clostridium difficile, 2005, March 8, 2007 from http://www.cdc.gov/ncidod/dhqp/id_CdiffFAQ_newstrain.html.
43. Centers for Disease Control and Prevention: Underdiagnosis of dengue—Lorado, Texas, 1999, *MMWR* 50:57-59, 2001.
44. Gubler DJ: Epidemic dengue/dengue hemorrhagic fever as a public health, social, and economic problem in the 21st century, *Trends Microbiol* 10:100-103, 2002.
45. Willis BA, Nguyen MD, Ha TL, and others: Comparison of three fluid solutions for resuscitation in dengue shock syndrome, *N Engl J Med* 353:877-889, 2005.
46. Murray K, Selleck P, Hooper P, and others: A morbillivirus that caused fatal disease in horses and humans, *Science* 268:94-97, 1995.
47. Chua KB: Nipah virus outbreak in Malaysia, *J Clin Virol* 26:265-275, 2003.
48. Nalca A, Rimoin AW, Bavari S, and others: Reemergence of monkeypox: prevalence, diagnosis, and countermeasures, *Clin Infect Dis* 41:1765-1771, 2005.
49. Huhn GD, Bauer AM, Yorita K, and others: Clinical characteristics of human monkeypox and risk factors for severe disease, *Clin Infect Dis* 41:1742-1751, 2005.
50. Holmes GP, Hilliard JK, Klontz KC, and others: B virus (*Herpesvirus simiae*) infection in humans: epidemiologic investigation of a cluster, *Ann Intern Med* 112:833-839, 1990.
51. Cohen JI, Davenport DS, Stewart JA, and others: Recommendations for prevention of and therapy for exposure to B virus (cercopithecine herpesvirus 1), *Clin Infect Dis* 35:1191-1203, 2002.
52. Whitener CJ, Park SY, Browne FA, and others: Vancomycin-resistant *Staphylococcus aureus* in the absence of vancomycin exposure, *Clin Infect Dis* 38:1049-1055, 2004.
53. Kuehnert MJ, Kruszon-Moran D, Hill HA, and others: Prevalence of *Staphylococcus aureus* nasal colonization in the United States, 2001-2002, *J Infect Dis* 193:172-179, 2006.
54. Salgado CD, Farr BM, Calfee DP: Community-acquired methicillin-resistant *Staphylococcus aureus*: a meta-analysis of prevalence and risk factors, *Clin Infect Dis* 36:131-139, 2003.
55. Centers for Disease Control and Prevention: Methicillin-resistant *Staphylococcus aureus* infections in correctional facilities—Georgia, California, and Texas, 2001-2003, *MMWR* 52:992-996, 2003.
56. Centers for Disease Control and Prevention: Methicillin-resistant *Staphylococcus aureus* infections among competitive sports participants—Colorado, Indiana, Pennsylvania, and Los Angeles County, 2000-2003, *MMWR* 52:793-795, 2003.
57. Centers for Disease Control and Prevention: Outbreaks of community-associated methicillin-resistant *Staphylococcus aureus* skin infections—Los Angeles County, California, 2002-2003, *MMWR* 52:88, 2003.
58. Bergier EM, Frenette K, Barrett NL, and others: A high morbidity outbreak of methicillin-resistant *Staphylococcus aureus* among players of a college football team, facilitated by body shaving and turfburns, *Clin Infect Dis* 39:1446-1453, 2004.
59. Herold BC, Immergluck LC, Maranan MC, and others: Community-acquired methicillin-resistant *Staphylococcus aureus* in children with no identified predisposing risk, *JAMA* 279:593-598, 1998.
60. Centers for Disease Control and Prevention: Four pediatric deaths from community-acquired methicillin-resistant *Staphylococcus aureus*—Minnesota and North Dakota, 1997-1999, *MMWR* 48:707-710, 1999.
61. Kaplan SL, Hulten KG, Gonzalez BE, and others: Three year surveillance of community-acquired methicillin-resistant *Staphylococcus aureus* infections in children, *Clin Infect Dis* 40:1785-1791, 2005.
62. Francis JS, Doherty MC, Lopatin U, and others: Severe community-onset pneumonia in healthy adults caused by methicillin-resistant *Staphylococcus aureus* carrying the Panton-Valentine leukocidin genes, *Clin Infect Dis* 40:100-107, 2005.
63. Miller LG, Perdreau-Remington F, Rieg G, and others: Necrotizing fasciitis caused by community-associated methicillin-resistant *Staphylococcus aureus* in Los Angeles, *N Engl J Med* 352:1445-1453, 2005.
64. King MD, Humphrey BJ, Wang YF, and others: Emergence of community-acquired methicillin-resistant *Staphylococcus aureus* USA 300 clone as the predominant cause of skin and soft-tissue infections, *Ann Intern Med* 144:309-317, 2006.
65. Moellering RC: The growing menace of community-acquired methicillin-resistant *Staphylococcus aureus* (editorial), *Ann Intern Med* 309:368-370, 2006.

CHAPTER 244

Fever

Elizabeth A. Talbot

A clinical encounter with a febrile patient can be challenging. This chapter defines fever and clarifies the types and patterns of fever, provides an approach to evaluating the febrile patient, reviews special circumstances such as fever of unknown origin (FUO) and fever in young children, and provides principles for empiric management.

DEFINITION AND EPIDEMIOLOGY

Fever is a state of elevated core temperature, which is often, but not necessarily, part of the host's defensive responses to the invasion of microorganisms or inanimate matter recognized as pathogenic or alien by the host.[1] Fever is a rise in body temperature above normal, which raises several important considerations, including definition of normal body temperature, appreciation of inherent host variability, and limitations to accurate temperature measurement.

Although most patients and providers believe that a core temperature of 37° C (98.6° F) is normal, research shows that 36.8° C (98.2° F) ±1° C (1.8° F) is closer to normal for a healthy population.[2] In addition, a healthy person's body temperature varies during the day. Diurnal variation may be as much as 1° C (highest in the early evening and lowest in the early morning).[2,3] "Normal" body temperature also varies by population. For example, compared with men, women have on average higher temperatures: 0.2° C on average and 0.5° C while ovulating.[4] The elderly[5] and those with certain illnesses such as chronic renal insufficiency may have lower "normal" body temperature.[2]

Ability to detect a fever is affected by the accuracy of the device used, correct positioning of the device probe, choice of anatomic site for measurement, and the patient's condition. The anatomic sites for measuring core body temperature include axilla, rectum, mouth, tympanic membrane, and skin; the latter is accomplished by applying to the forehead a plastic strip embedded with temperature-sensitive crystals. There are excellent reviews describing which site is optimum for which population,[2] but oral is generally preferred for an ambulatory adult population, and axillary may be best for neonates.

CLINICAL PRESENTATION

Hyperpyrexia is a fever in excess of 41.5° C (106.7° F), which can result from various causes, including high environmental temperatures, strenuous physical exercise, or illness.[3] A temperature of 41° C (105.8° F) may lead to brain damage, whereas a temperature in excess of 43° C (109.4° F) is invariably fatal. Hyperthermia is extremely elevated body temperature, which occurs when thermoregulatory systems of heat production or heat dissipation fail. Heat stroke, severe burns, and thyroid storm may be associated with hyperthermia. Malignant hyperthermia is an autosomal dominant hereditary condition of fever over 40° C (104° F), muscular rigidity, and hemodynamic instability that occurs after general anesthesia. Neuroleptic malignant syndrome is also a condition of high fever and muscular rigidity, but it includes mental status changes and dysautonomias. It is caused by withdrawal of central nervous system (CNS) dopaminergic agents or by use of CNS antidopaminergic agents, such as haloperidol.[3]

Central fever is fever attributed to CNS disorders, including CNS malignancy, trauma, and hemorrhage. A febrile patient with a CNS disorder can, of course, have an alternate cause for fever (such as an infection); therefore central fever is a diagnosis of exclusion. Occasionally patients may lie about or fabricate the presence of fever for a variety of reasons; this is known as *factitious fever*. Factitious fever is more common among women and those who have worked in a medical profession. In contrast, patients with Munchausen's syndrome may create infection that is reflected by physiologic fever. Care of such patients requires specialty referral, once it has been identified by the astute health care provider.

Fever patterns include sustained fever (temperature is constantly elevated within a degree on a daily basis), intermittent fever (temperature returns to normal at least once a day), remittent fever (temperature decreases but not to normal), relapsing fever (elevated temperature is interspersed with sustained periods of normal temperatures), and hectic fever (temperatures fluctuate widely).[6,7] *Relative bradycardia* refers to the occurrence of fever without expected elevation of pulse (~10 beats per minute per degree elevation).

Hypothermia is temperature of 36° C (97° F) or less, which can result from exposure to cold environment, hypothyroidism, uremia, and overwhelming infection. The latter scenario usually signifies that a patient is unable to mount an appropriate fever, a poor prognostic sign.

HISTORY, PHYSICAL EXAMINATION, AND DIFFERENTIAL DIAGNOSIS

Evaluation of Fever Without Clear Etiology

Often a febrile episode is mild and self-limiting. If the patient comes for medical attention, the history and associated signs and symptoms often make the cause obvious. Occasionally, however, a febrile illness may be more severe or prolonged and not have an apparent cause. There are many causes of fever, including infection, malignancy, medication, blood products, connective tissue disease, and thrombi. The differential diagnosis of fever must be generated with additional patient context, such as epidemiologic information, a thorough history, and the clinical presentation.

Epidemiologic information about locally circulating illnesses may greatly inform the differential diagnosis of fever even before the patient is interviewed. Obviously, in the absence of travel, only locally and seasonally prevalent diseases should be considered. For example, a community-acquired acute febrile cough illness in a normal host occurring in the winter in New England should prompt testing for pertussis before testing for tuberculosis (TB). The state, county, city, or local health department can serve as a resource for providers to find out more about the local epidemiology of certain illnesses. This is especially true of reportable diseases, but public health officials often are aware of outbreaks or the circulation of nonreportable diseases as well, such as the arrival of seasonal influenza, a school varicella outbreak, or the occurrence of summer enteroviral meningoencephalitis.

A complete history of the febrile illness should be obtained, including exposures to ill persons or animals, recent travel, and associated symptoms, which are helpful in focusing the diagnostic evaluation. The fever pattern, several of which are defined above, may provide a diagnostic clue but is rarely conclusive.[7] For example, relative bradycardia may suggest typhoid fever, leptospirosis, or drug fever in the right clinical context; a relapsing fever pattern may suggest an infection caused by *Borrelia* or *Streptobacillus* organisms; a hectic fever may raise consideration of TB or lymphoma.

Eliciting a history of exposures to animals, animal products, or insects may help elucidate the cause of a fever. For example, rabies, cat-scratch disease, pasteurellosis, toxoplasmosis, leptospirosis, anthrax, brucellosis, psittacosis, and rat-bite fever are associated with animal or animal product exposure, whereas Rocky Mountain spotted fever, babesiosis, ehrlichiosis, and Lyme disease can all follow an insect (tick) bite.

Discovery that a febrile patient has recently traveled to the tropics raises an important differential diagnosis. Many infections acquired during travel are actually not classic tropical diseases. Routine respiratory viruses can be acquired during or after travel and should be considered in the right clinical context. It is noteworthy that influenza, although exceedingly rare in the United States in the summer, circulates year round in most of the tropics. Many of the classic tropical diseases, including Japanese encephalitis, Rift Valley fever, ebola, and yellow fever, are extremely rare in ill returning travelers.[8] But several tropical diseases must be considered, most importantly malaria, since it is relatively common in ill returning travelers and can be life threatening. Dengue virus is probably more common than malaria and usually self-limiting.[8] Typhoid fever, tularemia, extraintestinal amebiasis, plague, and TB should also be considered for the patient with a clinically compatible illness.

The value of obtaining a complete medical history to elucidate the cause and significance of fever cannot be overemphasized. The most important example is that of the immunocompromised state. Clearly the differential diagnosis of any fever shifts dramatically for patients with a medical history that includes bone marrow transplant; HIV infection; malignancy; or drug-induced immune dysfunction, such as chemotherapy or corticosteroid use. In addition, eliciting a history of a recent surgical procedure or implantation of a foreign body, including prostheses and urinary or intravascular catheters, should direct the initial diagnostic investigation. A review of the patient's immunization and tuberculin skin test status and past infections can be helpful. For example, a recent history of otitis media, urinary tract infection, or pneumonia may signify progressive infection, such as mastoiditis, renal abscess, or empyema, respectively.

Detailed medication use history is vital in the evaluation of fever because many medications can cause fever ("drug fever"). Commonly implicated classes of medications include antihypertensives, antiarrhythmic medications, antibiotics, thyroid medication, and antiepileptics. Drug fever may occur anytime from shortly after initiation to years after starting an implicated medication. Occasionally, there are clues to the diagnosis of drug fever, such as eosinophilia, rash, mild transaminitis, or elevated erythrocyte sedimentation rate (ESR), but often drug fever is a diagnosis of exclusion. Stopping the suspected drug usually results in defervescence within 72 hours, and the fever resumes when the drug is restarted.

Signs of infection should be diligently sought by thorough physical examination. Skin, sinus, nasal, ear, dental, and throat examinations are essential. Regional lymph node enlargement suggests a localized infectious process, whereas generalized lymphadenopathy may suggest systemic infection such as HIV or malignancy such as lymphoma. Detection of a new or changed heart murmur, especially in the setting of cutaneous stigmata, is a valuable clue to endocarditis. Adventitious or asymmetric breath sounds may indicate pneumonia or pulmonary emboli or effusions. An abdominal mass, hepatosplenomegaly, or tenderness should prompt further investigation for an abdominal fever source. Calf tenderness with a palpable vascular cord is evidence of thrombophlebitis. An abnormal joint examination can suggest osteomyelitis or infectious or rheumatologic arthritis. Breast, pelvic, penile, and rectal examinations are indicated when infections or neoplasms are suspected.

Diagnostics. The cause of the fever is often apparent once the history is taken and the physical examination is completed. Appropriate diagnostic and therapeutic maneuvers are then obvious. For a febrile patient who remains without a suspected or confirmed etiology, reasonable diagnostic maneuvers may include CBC with differential, liver function tests, urinalysis, blood (and other potential source) cultures, and C-reactive protein or ESR to confirm a systemic process. The ESR is a sensitive but nonspecific test, but if the ESR is greater than 100 mm/hr, temporal arteritis, osteomyelitis, and endocarditis should be considered. Serologic testing is reserved when the history and physical examination suggest a particular diagnosis. CT and MRI may be useful for detecting abscesses or mass lesions. Echocardiogram is mandatory if there are cardiac findings, persistent bacteremia, or stigmata of endocarditis.

Evaluation of Fever of Unknown Origin

In contrast to fever without clear etiology, there are strictly defined syndromes of FUO, including classic FUO, nosocomial FUO, neutropenic FUO, and FUO associated with HIV.[9] The most common FUO in most primary care settings is classic FUO, defined as fever in excess of 38.3° C (101° F) after 3 days of hospitalization or three outpatient visits or 1 week of intensive outpatient investigations persisting beyond 3 weeks, for which intensive investigation fails to yield a diagnosis.[9] Studies show that the leading causes of classic FUO in adults are infectious (such as TB, occult abscesses, and bacterial endocarditis) and malignant (especially lymphoma, leukemia, and renal cell carcinoma). Rheumatologic diseases, such as rheumatoid arthritis and temporal arteritis, occasionally also cause FUO. In children, FUO is less likely to be from malignant causes than from infectious causes, including viral illnesses and cat-scratch disease (*Bartonella* organisms). Important noninfectious causes of FUO in the pediatric population are systemic onset juvenile rheumatoid arthritis and Takayasu's arteritis. Hereditary periodic fever syndromes such as familial Mediterranean fever or hyperimmunoglobulin D syndrome can also cause fever in children and adults.[2]

Diagnostics. During evaluation of a patient with FUO, hospitalization may be warranted to allow detailed history, physical examination, and diagnostic maneuvers. By the time a patient is diagnosed with FUO, many standard laboratory evaluations and imaging studies have already been completed. Additional, more invasive evaluation such as bone marrow, temporal artery, or liver biopsy or lumbar puncture should be done when clinical and laboratory findings indicate these systems as potential sources.

LIFE SPAN CONSIDERATIONS

Fever is a common presenting complaint of children and infants seen in emergency departments (EDs). In 2003 the American College of Emergency Physicians updated its clinical policy for children coming to the ED with fever.[10] The policy applies to healthy term infants and children between the ages of 1 day and 36 months. Guidance that may be useful in primary care includes that febrile infants between the ages of 1 and 28 days old should be presumed to have a serious bacterial infection. The policy also clearly discourages a trial of antipyresis in clinical decision making, since a number of research trials have not demonstrated that response to antipyretic therapy indicates lower likelihood of serious bacterial infection.[11] A chest radiograph should be done for febrile children younger than 3 months and for older children with high temperatures (>39° C [102.2° F]) and a WBC count over 20,000/mm^3. Empiric antibiotics may be appropriate for previously healthy, well-appearing children ages 3 to 36 months with fever 39° C or higher and a WBC count of 15,000/mm^3 or more.[10]

Older adults are less likely to develop the high fevers of childhood; some seniors, even those with severe infections, may not be able to mount a febrile response at all. Hypothermia is very common in this age-group because of failing hypothalamic thermoregulatory systems.

MANAGEMENT

Treatment of the cause is the best treatment for fever. Surprisingly, though, there is no clear consensus whether fever itself should be treated, that is, suppressed with antipyretics. Fever is an adaptive response that has widely evolved among most members of the animal kingdom, strongly suggesting an adaptive role for fever.[2,3] Much experimental data suggest that fever is associated with improved outcome in infection, and, conversely, some data suggest that suppressing fever may delay recovery from infection.[2]

In spite of some controversy, there are circumstances when fever should be treated. For example, any patient whose fever exceeds 41° C (105.8° F) should be treated as soon as possible with antipyretics and cooling measures to avoid brain damage.[3] Children are more susceptible to harmful effects of elevated temperatures, manifesting seizures particularly at younger ages (3 months to 5 years). Patients with underlying cardiovascular disease may not tolerate increased metabolic demands of prolonged high fever, since a 1° C (1.8° F) increase in temperature increases the basal metabolic rate by more than 10%.[3] In many settings of fever and identified infection, antipyretics can be given at regular intervals for symptomatic relief.

Antipyretic drugs include steroids, aspirin and other NSAIDs, and acetaminophen. Acetaminophen is usually the first line of treatment for fever. The risk of Reye's syndrome makes aspirin contraindicated in children. Physical methods such as sponging with cool water or alcohol and applying cold packs or cooling blankets may be effective, but are generally not considered first-line interventions.

In the absence of increased water intake, fever produces dehydration; can cause confusion, delirium, and seizures; and increases myocardial oxygen consumption by inducing tachycardia. Therefore treatment for fever should include close attention to maintaining hydration and nutrition.

INDICATIONS FOR REFERRAL OR HOSPITALIZATION

Hospitalization may be indicated if the patient is unable to maintain hydration; is hemodynamically unstable; or has a suspected infection that can lead to rapid deterioration such as endocarditis, necrotizing fasciitis, or bacterial meningitis.

PATIENT AND FAMILY EDUCATION

Patients should be advised to call the health care provider for fever that is higher than 38.6° C (101.5° F) for more than 24 hours. Immunosuppressed patients, including those with AIDS and those taking chemotherapeutic drugs, are advised to seek immediate care if they have a temperature above 37.8° C (100° F). Parents should be especially cautioned against the use of aspirin in their febrile children because of risk of Reye's syndrome.[3]

REFERENCES

1. IUPS Commission for Thermal Physiology: Glossary of terms for thermal physiology, third edition, *Jap J Physiol* 51:245-280, 2001.
2. Mackowiak PA: Temperature regulation and pathogenesis of fever. In Mandell G, Douglas J, Bennett R, editors: *Principles and practice of infectious diseases*, ed 6, Philadelphia, 2006, Churchill Livingstone.
3. Dinarello CA, Gelfand JA: Fever and hyperthermia. In Fauci AS, editor: *Harrison's principles of internal medicine*, ed 16, New York, 2005, McGraw-Hill.
4. McCance KL, Huether SE: *Pathophysiology: the biological basis for disease in adults and children*, ed 3, St Louis, 1998, Mosby.
5. Norman DC, Yoshikawa TT: Fever in the elderly, *Infect Dis Clin North Am* 10(1):93-99, 1996.
6. McGee S: Temperature. In *Evidence-based physical diagnosis*, Philadelphia, 2001, Saunders.
7. Cunha BA: The clinical significance of fever patterns, *Infect Dis Clin North Am* 10(1):33-44, 1996.
8. Freedman DO, Weld LH, Kozarsky PE, and others: Spectrum of disease and relation to place of exposure among ill returned travelers, *N Engl J Med* 354:119-130, 2006.
9. Durack DT, Street AC: Fever of unknown origin—reexamined and redefined. In Remington JS, Swartz MN, editors: *Current clinical topics in infectious diseases* 11:35-51, 1991.
10. American College of Emergency Physicians Clinical Policies Committee, American College of Emergency Physicians Clinical Policies Subcommittee on Pediatric Fever: Clinical policy for children younger than 3 years presenting to the emergency department with fever, *Ann Emerg Med* 42(4):530-545, 2003.
11. Prinzhorn J: Fever management in children who are febrile is questionable, *Pediatr Nurs* 30(4):322, 2004.

CHAPTER 245

Tuberculosis

Patricia Polgar Bailey

DEFINITION AND EPIDEMIOLOGY

Tuberculosis (TB) is an airborne infectious disease caused by *Mycobacterium tuberculosis*, an acid-fast aerobic bacterium that is capable of remaining alive outside the host for a relatively long time. In the United States the vast majority of TB cases are caused by *M. tuberculosis*, also referred to as the *tubercle bacillus*. However, several closely related mycobacteria can cause disease in humans, including *M. bovis*, the cause of TB in cattle; *M. avium*, one of the causes of TB in birds; and *M. africanum*. TB caused by these organisms was relatively rare in the United States until they were identified as the cause of opportunistic infections in patients infected with HIV. *M. microti*, another mycobacterium, does not cause TB in humans.[1]

TB has reemerged as one of the most pressing public health problems in the United States and throughout the world. In 1993 the World Health Organization (WHO) declared TB to be a "global health emergency," and a 1995 report identified it as the leading single-infection killer of adults. *M. tuberculosis* infects a third of the world's population, more than 8 million people develop active TB annually, and approximately 2 million people die from the disease every year.[2,3] Southeast Asia currently has the highest prevalence of TB, with one third of new cases occurring in this area every year, but the incidence per capita is highest in sub-Saharan Africa, where it parallels the HIV/AIDS epidemic.[3,4] In 2004, 1.7 million people died of TB, 15% of whom were co-infected with HIV. Persons with active TB who receive no treatment can infect an average of 10 to 15 people annually.[3,5]

During the mid-twentieth century the United States benefited from relatively successful control of TB. From 1953 to 1985, the reported cases of TB in the United States dropped from 84,000 to 22,000.[2] From 1985 to 1992, there was an unprecedented resurgence of TB in the United States. From 1993 to 2005, the annual TB rate decreased steadily, although this decline has recently decelerated, raising the concern that the progress toward eliminating TB is slowing. In 2005 there were a total of 14,093 TB cases (4.8 cases per 100,000 population), which represented a 3.8% decline in the rate from 2004. Although the TB rates were the lowest recorded since national reporting began in 1953, the decline has slowed from an average of 7.1% per year (1993 to 2000) to an average of 3.8% per year (2001 to 2005). In addition, the number of multidrug-resistant (MDR) TB cases in the United States has increased 13.3% with 128 cases reported in 2004, up from 113 in 2003.[2] MDR TB is defined as resistance to at least isoniazid and rifampin, and during the 1990s MDR TB emerged as a significant threat to TB control, both in the United States and worldwide. MDR TB treatment requires the use of second-line drugs that are less effective, more toxic, and costlier than first-line isoniazid- and rifampin-based regimens. The 13.3% increase in MDR TB cases represents the largest increase since 1993.[6]

Historically, TB in the United States was a disease that affected primarily older adults; increasingly, younger adults and children are being affected.[1] Minority populations are disproportionately affected by TB; Hispanics, African Americans, and Asians have TB rates 7.3, 8.3, 19.6 times higher than Caucasians, respectively. For 2005 and for the second consecutive year, more TB cases were reported among Hispanics than any other racial and ethnic groups. In 2005 the TB rate of foreign-born persons in the United States was 8.7 times that of U.S.-born persons.[2] TB is largely a social disease, and homeless and incarcerated individuals are at increased risk of infection with TB.[7,8] TB control can be particularly problematic in correctional and detention facilities, in which persons from diverse backgrounds and communities live together for varying and sometimes extended periods. In July 2006 the Centers for Disease Control and Prevention (CDC) published guidelines for the prevention and control of TB in jails, prisons, and other correctional and detention facilities.[9] Providers working in these settings should familiarize themselves with the recommendations, which can be found in *MMWR* or on the Internet at http://www.cdc.gov/mmwr.

Transmission of *M. tuberculosis* in health care institutions was a contributing factor to the resurgence of TB during the period from 1985 to 1992, and recommendations were developed to prevent transmission in these settings. In 2003, persons who had worked in health care during the 2 years prior to their TB diagnosis accounted for 3.1% of TB cases nationwide. However, the elevated risk among health care workers may be attributable to other factors (e.g., birth in a country with a high incidence of TB). A recent large multistate occupational survey indicted that health care workers, with the exception of respiratory therapists, do not have a higher risk for TB than the general population.[3]

Many factors have contributed to the increased incidence of TB, including the HIV epidemic and higher rates of poverty, homelessness, incarceration, and drug use. An increasing number of immigrants, many of whom live in crowded housing and have inadequate health care, and an increasing number of residents in long-term care facilities have also contributed to this public health problem. Deterioration in the health care infrastructure and reductions in TB outreach programs, which historically improved compliance with treatment regimens, have also contributed to the resurgence of TB.

The decelerating decline of the overall national TB rate, the persistent disparities in TB rates between U.S.-born and foreign-born persons and between Caucasians and ethnic minorities, and the increase in MDR TB cases all threaten progress toward the goal of eliminating TB in the United States.[2] Major challenges to successful control of TB in the United States include detecting and treating TB in the non-U.S.-born population, eliminating delays in detecting and reporting cases of pulmonary TB and protecting contacts of TB-infected persons, and preventing and responding to TB outbreaks. In addition, there is a large reservoir of persons living in the United States with latent TB infection (LTBI) who are at risk for progression to TB disease. Finally, the successful control of TB depends on maintaining clinical and public health expertise in TB management in an era of declining TB incidence.[3]

Treatment of TB benefits both the individual patient and the community as a whole. Therefore any public health program or health care provider undertaking to treat a patient with TB is assuming a public health function that includes not only prescribing an appropriate medication regimen but also ensuring adherence to the regimen until treatment is completed.[10]

Physician consultation is recommended for any patient suspected of having pulmonary or extrapulmonary TB.

PATHOPHYSIOLOGY

TB is spread primarily through direct infection (person to person), but it can also be spread indirectly via the airborne transmission of the tubercle bacilli, which can remain suspended in the air for several hours. Transmission, which may occur if these bacilli-laden sputum droplets (each containing one to three organisms) are inhaled, depends on three factors: the infectiousness of the person with TB, the environment in which the exposure occurred, and the duration of exposure.[1] Although theoretically one organism implanted in the alveolus can initiate this process, five to 200 organisms are usually required.[11] Most of the larger inhaled particles become lodged in the upper respiratory tract, where infection is unlikely to take place. Infection begins if the droplet nuclei reach the alveolar macrophage and multiplication of the tubercle bacilli is initiated. A small number of mycobacteria spread through the lymph system to regional lymph nodes and via the bloodstream to more distant tissues and organs, including areas in which TB is more likely to develop, such as the apices of the lung, the kidneys, the brain, and the bone. Eighty-five percent of all TB cases involve the lungs; other common sites include the pleura, central nervous system (CNS), lymphatic system, genitourinary system, and bones and joints. TB can also become disseminated and then is referred to as *miliary TB*.

TB disease has two distinct epidemiologic patterns. Reactivation, or postprimary, disease is the most common clinical form of TB. Most symptomatic cases of TB arise in persons with a history of TB infection who were inadequately treated or not treated. The second epidemiologic profile, primary infection, does not usually appear as a symptomatic infection except in persons infected with HIV. More than 90% of persons with primary infection are entirely asymptomatic, and infection with TB is identified only by a positive reaction to a tuberculin skin test.

Certain medical conditions increase the risk that TB infection will progress to active disease. The risk may be three times greater (as with co-existent diabetes mellitus) to 100 times greater (as with HIV infection) for persons who have these conditions compared with those who do not.[1] Medical conditions that increase the risk of active TB are listed in Box 245-1.

BOX 245-1

CONDITIONS THAT INCREASE THE RISK OF ACTIVE TUBERCULOSIS

- HIV infection
- Recent infection with *Mycobacterium tuberculosis* (within the past 2 years)
- Chest radiographic findings suggestive of previous tuberculosis (in a person who receives inadequate or no treatment)
- Diabetes mellitus
- Silicosis
- Substance abuse (notably drug injection)
- Prolonged corticosteroid therapy
- Other immunosuppressive therapy
- Cancer of the head and neck
- Hematologic and reticuloendothelial diseases (e.g., leukemia and Hodgkin's disease)
- End-stage renal disease
- Intestinal bypass or gastrectomy surgery
- Chronic malabsorption syndrome
- Low body weight (≥10% below the ideal)

CLINICAL PRESENTATION

Persons who have been infected with *M. tuberculosis* but do not have active disease are completely asymptomatic. For the majority of persons, the only evidence of LTBI is an immune response against mycobacterial antigens, which is demonstrated by a positive skin test, or in certain circumstances, a whole blood antigen–stimulated assay result (e.g., the QuantiFERON-TB Gold [QFT-G] test).[3] There is no radiographic evidence of TB in persons with LTBI.

Symptoms of pulmonary TB (the most common site) include fatigue, anorexia, weight loss, night sweats, cough, chest pain, hemoptysis, irregular menses, and a low-grade fever. Symptoms in adults are often subtle and may appear in conjunction with or simulate other illnesses and therefore are often not associated with TB. However, one third of persons with pulmonary TB are asymptomatic on initial presentation.[1,12]

Approximately 15% of cases of TB are extrapulmonary, with common sites including the bones and joints, genitourinary system, lymphatic system, and the CNS. The symptoms of extrapulmonary TB depend on the site affected. TB of the spine often causes back pain, whereas TB of the genitourinary system may result in hematuria or persistent dysuria.

PHYSICAL EXAMINATION

A complete physical examination is an essential part of the evaluation but cannot be used alone to confirm or exclude TB. Even if the physical examination is entirely negative, it can provide useful information about the patient's overall condition. Certain findings, although not diagnostic of TB, may be suggestive of the diagnosis. Rales in the upper posterior portion of the chest, evidence of pleural effusion, lymphadenopathy, weight loss, and fever may increase the suspicion for TB. Confirmation of TB is based on the diagnostic evaluation presented in the next section.

DIAGNOSTICS

Screening is the first step in the diagnostic evaluation of TB and is performed to identify infected patients at high risk for TB who would benefit from preventive therapy, as well as patients with TB who need treatment. Because the vast majority of patients infected with TB are asymptomatic, health care providers should administer the tuberculin skin test to all high-risk persons as part of their routine evaluation. Persons with any of the medical conditions listed in Box 245-1 should be screened annually unless there is prior documentation of a positive tuberculin skin test.[13] Other high-risk groups include close contacts of a person with infectious disease; foreign-born persons from areas in which TB is common (e.g., Asia, Africa, and Latin America); the medically underserved and low-income populations, including high-risk racial and ethnic groups (e.g., Asians and Pacific Islanders, African Americans, Hispanics, and Native Americans), migrant farm workers, and homeless persons; residents of long-term care facilities (e.g., correctional facilities and nursing homes); and other groups identified as having a disproportionate prevalence of TB. Routine institutional screening is also recommended for health care workers and the staff of long-term institutional facilities who may have occupational exposure to TB or who would pose a risk to large numbers of susceptible persons if they developed active disease (e.g., staff member of an AIDS hospice).[1]

The standard and preferred method of screening for TB infection is the Mantoux tuberculin skin test, which is administered by injecting 5 tuberculin units (0.1 ml) of purified protein derivative (PPD) intradermally into either the volar or dorsal surface of the forearm. The injection should be made with a disposable tuberculin syringe with the needle bevel pointing upward. The injection should produce a discrete, pale elevation of the skin (a wheal) that is 6 to 10 mm (0.2 to 0.4 inch) in diameter and disappears within several hours. If a wheal is not produced, the injection was probably too deep and will likely result in a false-negative reading. In the absence of a wheal, the skin test should be repeated. The amount of induration, rather than the erythema, is measured. All reactions, even those classified as negative, should be recorded in millimeters of induration. If no induration is found, "0 mm" should be recorded.

The skin test is read within 48 to 72 hours. If the patient fails to show up for a scheduled reading within 72 hours, a positive reaction may still be measurable up to 1 week later. However, all negative responses not documented within 72 hours should be repeated.[1] The criteria for determining whether a skin test is significant depend on a patient's risk for developing disease or ability to mount a reaction to the PPD. The criteria for a positive PPD test are listed in Box 245-2. Once a patient has had a positive tuberculin skin test, no subsequent tuberculin skin testing should be performed.

A variety of factors can cause a false-negative tuberculin skin test, including the recipient's age, the simultaneous administration of a live vaccine, concomitant infections, metabolic deficiencies, underlying disease, and improper placement or storage of the PPD. Live vaccinations such as the measles, mumps, rubella (MMR) vaccine and the oral poliovirus vaccine may cause a false-negative response of the tuberculin skin text for up to 2 months after immunization. However, results of the PPD skin test performed simultaneously with inoculation of these vaccines are unaffected.[13] Other potential causes of false-negative test results are listed in Box 245-3.

BOX 245-2

CRITERIA FOR A POSITIVE TUBERCULIN SKIN TEST

INDURATION ≥5 MM

Persons with HIV infection
Household or close contacts of persons with tuberculosis (TB) infection
Persons with fibrotic lesions or evidence of old, healed TB on chest x-ray studies
Patients who are immunosuppressed

INDURATION ≥10 MM

Foreign-born persons from countries with high TB prevalence
Medically underserved, low-income populations, including high-risk minority populations
Homeless persons
Prisoners
Alcoholics
IV drug users
Persons with other medical factors known to increase the risk of TB, including:

- Silicosis
- Diabetes
- Immunosuppressive or steroid therapy
- Chronic obstructive pulmonary disease
- Hematologic and reticuloendothelial disease
- End-stage renal disease
- Intestinal bypass
- Postgastrectomy
- Carcinomas of the oropharynx and upper gastrointestinal tract
- Persons ≥10% below ideal body weight

Health care workers
Persons with prior bacille Calmette-Guérin vaccination

INDURATION ≥15 MM

Persons at low risk for TB

BOX 245-3

POTENTIAL CAUSES OF FALSE-NEGATIVE TUBERCULIN TEST REACTIONS

- Age (>45 years, newborns)
- Immunosuppression (e.g., corticosteroids, chemotherapy, or other agents)
- Systemic viral, fungal, and bacterial infections
- Live virus vaccinations (e.g., measles, mumps, rubella; trivalent oral poliovirus vaccine)
- Malnutrition, cachexia, or nutritional derangement (e.g., severe protein deficiency, zinc deficiency)
- Chronic renal failure
- Hematologic or lymphoreticular disorders (e.g., Hodgkin's disease)
- Sarcoidosis
- Stress (e.g., burns, postoperative status, mental illness)
- Jejunoileal bypass surgery
- Alcoholism
- Mechanical (injection too deep, inexperienced reader)
- Improper storage (exposure to light or heat)

Modified from American Thoracic Society: Diagnostic standards and classification of tuberculosis, *Am Rev Respir Dis* 142(3):725-735, 1990; and Bass JB: *Tuberculin skin testing and other tests for latent tuberculosis infections,* retrieved Aug 1, 2006, from http://63.240.11.74/topic.asp?file=tubercul/7414.

Because there are many potential causes of a false-negative tuberculin test, the absence of a positive reaction does not exclude TB disease or infection. Anergy, which is a decreased or absent, delayed-type hypersensitivity response, can be caused by severe or febrile illness, miliary or pulmonary disease, and most of the factors listed in Box 245-3. Of all patients with TB, 10% to 25% have negative reactions to the tuberculin skin test. Approximately one third of patients with HIV infection and more than 60% of patients with AIDS have skin test reactions of less than 5 mm, even though they have been infected with *M. tuberculosis.*[1]

Differentiating between a negative skin test reaction that results from noninfection and one that results from anergy is made possible by the simultaneous administration of the Mantoux test and at least one other delayed-type hypersensitivity antigen. One of several antigens to which most adult patients have been exposed, such as tetanus toxoid, mumps, or the *Candida* species, is administered in the same way as the Mantoux test. A reaction of 3 mm or greater to any of the antigens, including PPD, excludes anergy. Persons who have a positive reaction to the tuberculin should be regarded as having been infected with *M. tuberculosis,* regardless of their reaction to the antigen testing. The results of the anergy test should be recorded in millimeters of induration, similar to the PPD reading. If the person is determined to be anergic, the probability of disease or infection should be assessed on the basis of risk factors and presentation. In the absence of findings consistent with active disease, anergic individuals with a high risk of exposure should be considered for preventive therapy. Low CD4 T-lymphocyte counts ($\leq$200/mm^3) have been closely correlated with anergy, but anergy can also occur in persons with relatively high CD4 counts. Similarly, reactivity to the tuberculin skin test and control antigens may be present at very low CD4 levels; therefore TB screening should be performed unless anergy has been previously documented.[1]

False-negative reactions can result from a decreased or waning delayed-type hypersensitivity reaction over time, especially among older adults who may have been infected years before being screened for TB. Although previously infected with TB, their hypersensitivity to the PPD antigen has been blunted over time. Although they may not respond to the initial skin test, the skin test may stimulate or "boost" their ability to react to the tuberculin on a subsequent test. Therefore skin testing is repeated in 1 to 3 weeks. A positive reaction to the second test probably represents a boosted reaction rather than a reaction to new infection. On the basis of this two-step testing, the patient should be classified as previously infected, and management should proceed accordingly.[1] Guidelines for interpreting the results of a two-step tuberculin skin testing are included in Box 245-4.

Many foreign countries vaccinate against TB using the bacille Calmette-Guérin (BCG) vaccine. Sensitivity to tuberculin varies significantly among persons who have received the BCG vaccination; this variance depends in part on the strain of BCG used and the person vaccinated. A history of BCG vaccination often confuses the diagnostic picture because there is no reliable way to determine whether a reaction to the tuberculin skin test is due to the BCG vaccine or to infection with *M. tuberculosis.* Nevertheless, a prior history of BCG vaccination is not considered a contraindication to PPD tuberculin skin testing. A reaction to the tuberculin skin test is probably a result of infection with *M. tuberculosis* rather than the BCG vaccine if the induration is large, if significant time has elapsed since BCG vaccination, if the person has had recent exposure to someone with infectious TB, if there is a family history of TB, if the person comes from an area in which TB is endemic, or if the chest x-ray study shows evidence of previous TB infection. Patients who have received the BCG vaccine should be screened, evaluated, and managed in a manner similar to those who have not been vaccinated with BCG.[1,13]

BOX 245-4

CRITERIA FOR INTERPRETATION OF TWO-STEP TUBERCULIN SKIN TESTING

- If the first test is positive, consider the person infected.
- If the first test is negative, give second test 1 to 3 weeks later.
- If the second test is positive, consider the person infected. If the second test is negative, consider the person uninfected.

Modified from Centers for Disease Control and Prevention: *Core curriculum on tuberculosis: what the clinician should know,* ed 3, Atlanta, 1994, US Department of Health and Human Services.

The QFT-G test is a new blood assay, approved by the U.S. Food and Drug Administration (FDA) to aid in the diagnosis of LTBI and active TB.[14] QFT-G can be used in all situations in which a tuberculin skin test is used. The QFT-G is an enzyme-linked immunosorbent assay that detects the release of interferon-γ from sensitized white blood cells in fresh, heparinized whole blood. Blood is collected no more than 12 hours before testing and then incubated for 16 to 24 hours with a mixture of synthetic peptides that simulate two antigenic proteins secreted by all *M. tuberculosis* strains, as well as by pathogenic strains of *M. bovis*. The synthetic peptides make the QFT-G a more specific test for *M. tuberculosis* than either the PPD or the older QuantiFERON-TB (QFT) test, which was approved by the FDA in 2001 but has been replaced by QFT-G. The QFT-G has greater specificity than either the tuberculin skin test or earlier QFT because the latter two tests both measured response to PPD, which is made from a polyvalent pool of antigens.[14] These antigens are part of many nontuberculosis bacteria and of the BCG vaccine, and as a result, false-positive tuberculin skin tests were common. Another advantage of the QFT-G test is that results are available 24 hours after blood collection, in contrast to the 2- or 3-day wait with tuberculin skin testing. In addition, two-step skin testing is recommended in certain situations, but with the QFT-G, two-step testing is neither necessary nor recommended. In addition, the QFT-G eliminates the need for proper intradermal injection technique, whereas with PPD lack of proper technique can result in the PPD solution being "washed out," resulting in a possible false-negative result. The QFT-G is cost-effective and efficient in that it eliminates the need for a second visit for test reading and, in populations that include many BCG-vaccinated people (i.e., many non-U.S.-born persons), should lead to fewer false-positive results.

DIAGNOSTICS

Tuberculosis

INITIAL
PPD (NOTE: Patients with a previous history of a positive PPD should not undergo this test again.)

LABORATORY
Sputum culture for acid-fact bacilli × 3*

IMAGING
Chest x-ray*

*If indicated.

However, although the QFT-G seems to have greater specificity, its sensitivity in detecting *M. tuberculosis* in young children and immunocompromised persons has not yet been determined.[14] In addition, although QFT-G testing may save time for clinic staff, the labor and cost burden is shifted to microbiology staff. Also, the cost of the test kit, the need for rapid specimen transport, and associated laboratory costs all need to be factored into the cost of the test. Finally, the difficulty of processing nonurgent blood specimens within 12 hours will be a barrier to using the QFT-G in many settings.

Both the tuberculin skin test and the QFT-G require sound clinical judgment in the interpretation of the results. Immunocompromised patients can have a diminished response to both the tuberculin skin test and QFT-G; therefore a negative test on either is not sufficient to exclude either latent or active TB in these patients.[14] Although the QFT-G is now approved, more research is needed to learn about the test's specificity and sensitivity and clarify its indications for use. Consensus guidelines on the use of the QFT-G are available from the Centers for Disease Control and Prevention.[15]

Persons with a positive tuberculin skin test or QFT-G should have an anteroposterior chest x-ray study to exclude active pulmonary TB and to detect fibrotic lesions, which may suggest an old TB infection or silicosis. Once these conditions have been excluded, no subsequent chest radiographs are indicated unless the person is symptomatic. In addition, anergic persons who have symptoms consistent with TB or have risk factors for TB should have a chest x-ray examination. Abnormalities in the apical and posterior segments of the upper lobe or in the superior segments of the lower lobe are those most often seen with pulmonary TB. Infiltrates without cavities and mediastinal or hilar lymphadenopathy may also be seen. HIV infection and other immunocompromising illnesses may result in unusual chest x-ray findings. Chest x-ray findings may be suggestive of TB but are never diagnostic. Nevertheless, they may be used to exclude the possibility of pulmonary TB.[1]

Persons suspected of having pulmonary or laryngeal TB should have at least three sputum cultures performed to detect the presence of acid-fast bacilli (AFB). A positive smear is strongly suggestive but not diagnostic of TB because the AFB on a smear may be due to mycobacteria other than *M. tuberculosis*. It is also possible for those with TB to have negative AFB smears. Species of mycobacteria are identified using a variety of methods, including nucleic acid probes, liquid chromatography, and polymerase chain reactions. The diagnosis is confirmed by a positive culture of *M. tuberculosis* complex, *M. avium*, or *M. intracellulare*. The mycobacterium isolates are then tested for drug susceptibility. Drug susceptibility is important to ensure appropriate treatment and should be repeated within 2 months if there has not been an adequate response to treatment.

DIFFERENTIAL DIAGNOSIS

The differential diagnosis of TB varies depending on the type of TB and the site of involvement. The signs and symptoms associated with pulmonary TB are consistent with those of other respiratory illnesses such as pneumonia, acute bronchitis, or carcinoma. Extrapulmonary TB can occur in any organ; therefore persistent signs and symptoms in any organ should lead to consideration of TB.

MANAGEMENT

The management of TB depends entirely on the current clinical classification system of disease, which is based on the pathogenesis of the disease and the diagnostic results. The classification system is described in Table 245-1, and the CDC and American Thoracic Society's (ATS's) complete recommendations for the treatment of TB can be found in *MMWR*[10] or on the Internet at http://www.cdc.gov/ mmwr. Currently, 10 drugs are approved by the FDA for treatment of TB. In addition, the fluoroquinolones, although not approved by the FDA for treatment of TB, are used relatively often for TB caused by drug-resistant organisms or for patients who are intolerant of some of the first-line drugs.[10]

Class 0 and class 1 TB require no treatment. Patients with class 1 TB should have another tuberculin skin test performed within several months given the history of known exposure to TB.

Patients with class 2 TB have been infected with TB but do not have any evidence of disease. The main purpose of preventive therapy is to decrease the risk that LTBI will progress to clinically active TB disease. Isoniazid (INH) is most commonly used for preventive therapy and is highly effective when taken as prescribed. Isoniazid is bactericidal, relatively nontoxic, inexpensive, and easily administered. The degree of protection conferred by isoniazid varies depending on the percentage of mycobacteria eradicated. Isoniazid has been shown to reduce the incidence of disease by 54% to 90%; the primary reason for this variation in efficacy appears to be the actual amount of isoniazid taken during the year it was prescribed.

Isoniazid remains less widely prescribed in the United States than it should be. Some studies have shown that fewer than one third of patients at risk for TB are screened with the tuberculin skin test; of those with class 2 TB, only 5% of those eligible for preventive therapy were offered it by their health care provider.[16] Preventive therapy should be considered for persons younger than 35 who have tuberculin skin tests of 10 mm or greater and who have any risk factors for TB. Patients younger than 35 with no known risk factors should be evaluated for preventive therapy if their reaction to the tuberculin skin test was 15 mm or

DIFFERENTIAL DIAGNOSIS

Tuberculosis

- Pneumonia
- Acute bronchitis
- Carcinoma
- Sarcoidosis
- Wegener's granulomatosis
- Lymphoma

TABLE 245-1 Clinical Classification System for Tuberculosis (TB)

Class	Type	Description
0	No TB exposure Not infected	No history of exposure Negative reaction to tuberculin skin test
1	TB exposure No evidence of infection	History of exposure Negative reaction to tuberculin skin test
2	TB infection No disease	Positive reaction to tuberculin skin test Negative bacteriologic studies (if done) No clinical or radiographic evidence of TB
3	Current TB disease	*Mycobacterium tuberculosis* cultured (if done) *or* Positive reaction to tuberculin skin test *and* Clinical or radiographic evidence of current disease
4	Previous TB disease	History of episode(s) of TB *or* Abnormal but stable radiographic findings Positive reaction to the tuberculin skin test Negative bacteriologic studies (if done) *and* No clinical or radiographic evidence of current disease
5	TB suspected	Diagnosis pending

From Centers for Disease Control and Prevention: *Core curriculum on tuberculosis: what the clinician should know,* ed 3, Atlanta, 1994, US Department of Health and Human Services.

greater. Unless otherwise indicated, isoniazid preventive therapy should be offered to individuals with class 2 TB (tuberculin positive), regardless of their history of BCG vaccination.

The major side effect of isoniazid is hepatitis. Other problems associated with isoniazid include peripheral neuropathy, gastrointestinal upset, and mild CNS effects. From 10% to 20% of patients started on isoniazid develop mild abnormalities of liver function, which often resolve even if isoniazid therapy is continued. Isoniazid should be discontinued if any of the liver function tests (LFTs) reach three to five times the upper limit of normal.[17] The risk for isoniazid-induced hepatitis increases directly with increasing age; therefore isoniazid is recommended for patients older than 35 only if they are at high risk for developing TB. Baseline and monthly LFTs and a monthly clinical evaluation should be performed for all persons undergoing isoniazid therapy.[13] High-priority candidates for TB preventive therapy, regardless of age, are listed in Box 245-5. Alcohol consumption has also been identified

BOX 245-5

HIGH-PRIORITY CANDIDATES FOR TUBERCULOSIS-PREVENTIVE THERAPY

Preventive therapy should be recommended for the following persons with a positive skin test, regardless of age (criterion for a positive reaction in millimeters of induration is listed in parentheses):

- Persons with known or suspected HIV infection, including persons who inject drugs whose HIV status is unknown (≥5 mm)
- Close contacts of persons with infectious clinically active TB (≥5 mm)
- Persons who have chest x-ray findings suggestive of previous TB and who have received inadequate or no treatment (≥5 mm)
- Persons who inject drugs and are known to be HIV negative (≥10 mm)
- Recent tuberculin skin test converters (≥10-mm increase within a <2-year period for those <35 years of age; ≥15-mm increase for those ≥35 years of age)
- Persons with medical conditions that increase the risk of TB, such as diabetes mellitus, prolonged corticosteroid therapy, immunosuppressive therapy, some hematologic and reticuloendothelial diseases, IV drug use, end-stage renal disease, and clinical situations associated with rapid weight loss (≥10 mm)

as a contributing risk factor in the development of isoniazid-induced hepatitis. Other drugs that increase the risk of isoniazid-induced hepatitis include acetaminophen, phenytoin (Dilantin), steroids, methimazole (Tapazole), estropipate (Ogen, Ortho-Est), and metoclopramide (Reglan, Maxolon). Isoniazid administration increases the serum levels of certain drugs, including phenytoin, theophylline, carbamazepine (Tegretol), benzodiazepines, and anticoagulants. During isoniazid administration the serum levels of these drugs should be monitored more closely. Drugs that decrease the serum concentration of isoniazid include antacids, corticosteroids, and laxatives.

Peripheral neuropathy is associated with the administration of isoniazid and most likely results from interference with pyridoxine absorption. It is recommended that pyridoxine (10 to 50 mg/day) be administered in conjunction with isoniazid to patients who have medical problems where neuropathy is already common, such as diabetes, uremia, alcoholism, and malnutrition. In addition, pyridoxine should be administered to pregnant women and to patients with a seizure disorder who are undergoing isoniazid therapy.

The usual preventive therapy regimen is isoniazid 300 mg/day for 6 to 12 months; the duration of therapy depends on the risk factors for TB and the associated co-morbidity. Six months of therapy has been shown to confer a high degree of protection (approximately 69%) if the medication is taken as prescribed. Twelve months of therapy reduces the risk by more than 90% if the entire course of therapy is completed. Patients infected with HIV should receive 12 months of therapy.[1]

For persons with a positive tuberculin skin test and evidence of silicosis or old fibrotic lesions without evidence of clinically active disease, alternative regimens include 4 months of isoniazid and rifampin or 12 months of isoniazid. For persons who have had close contact with individuals with isoniazid-resistant TB, preventive therapy with rifampin for 6 months or more should be considered. Rifampin preventive therapy can also be considered for patients who are isoniazid intolerant.[1]

Rifampin is bactericidal and easily administered. The most common side effect is gastrointestinal upset. Other adverse reactions include rashes, hepatitis, and, rarely, thrombocytopenia and cholestatic jaundice. Rifampin is a cytochrome P450 (hepatic microsomal enzyme) inducer that may increase the clearance of drugs metabolized by the liver, including oral hypoglycemic agents, glucocorticoids, estrogens, warfarin (Coumadin) derivatives, methadone, theophylline, antiarrhythmic agents (quinidine, verapamil, mexiletine), anticonvulsants, ketoconazole, and cyclosporin. By interfering with estrogen metabolism, rifampin may also interfere with the effectiveness of oral contraceptives.[17]

Based on adverse event data, the CDC and ATS revised their guidelines and, in 2003, recommended against the use of rifampin and pyrazinamide (PZA) for treatment of LTBI. A CDC cohort analysis in 2003 found the rates of severe liver injury and death related to the use of rifampin and PZA to be significantly higher than the rates for isoniazid-associated liver injury in the treatment of LTBI.[17] On the basis of these findings, the ATS and CDC now recommend that this regimen generally not be offered to persons with LBTI, unless the potential benefits of this regimen outweigh the risk for severe liver injury and death associated with rifampin-PZA. The CDC recommends that a TB and LTBI expert be consulted before rifampin-PZA is offered. In addition, patients should be asked about whether they have a history of liver disease or adverse effects from isoniazid or other drugs; be informed of potential hepatotoxicity of the rifampin-PZA regimen; and be advised against the concurrent use of potentially hepatotoxic drugs, including over-the-counter drugs such as acetaminophen.[18]

Treatment of class 3, or clinically active, TB requires multidrug therapy. The specific drug regimen should be developed in consultation with a specialist familiar with the management of TB. Four drugs are included in the initial regimen: isoniazid, rifampin, pyrazinamide (PZA), and ethambutol or streptomycin; the purpose is to prevent the development of MDR TB. Once the drug susceptibility results are known, the regimen is adjusted. If susceptibility to isoniazid and rifampin is demonstrated, administration of these two drugs is continued after the initial 2 months of multidrug therapy. Three-drug therapy (isoniazid, rifampin, PZA) is sometimes used as initial therapy if drug resistance is unlikely.[1]

The most important side effect of PZA is hepatotoxicity. However, the risk for liver injury does not seem to increase when this drug is co-administered with isoniazid and rifampin. Other adverse effects include hyperuricemia (acute gout is uncommon), arthralgias, skin rashes, and gastrointestinal side effects. Salicylates are often effective in relieving PZA-related arthralgias.[17] Baseline and monthly LFTs and monthly uric acid levels should be obtained for patients taking PZA.

The most common adverse reactions to ethambutol are optic neuritis, decreased visual acuity, and the loss of red-green perception. These side effects appear to be dose related and are more common in patients with renal failure, probably as a result of decreased clearance of the drug. All patients taking this drug should receive monthly red-green discrimination and visual acuity testing. Ototoxicity is the most common serious side effect of streptomycin, often resulting in vertigo or hearing loss. Nephrotoxicity occurs less commonly, but both of these adverse effects are more common in patients who are older than 60 or who have renal damage.

Second-line antitubercular drugs, such as para-aminosalicylic acid, ethionamide, and cycloserine, tend to be less effective and more toxic than the first-line drugs previously discussed. They are generally used only in cases of drug-resistant TB or atypical mycobacterial infections. Research on newer antitubercular drugs continues to be of importance, especially in this era of emerging drug resistance.

The antitubercular drug regimens used to treat extrapulmonary TB are similar to those used to treat pulmonary TB. Additional therapies such as corticosteroid therapy or surgery may be required depending on the site of TB infection. The type of follow-up and bacteriologic evaluation required is determined by the site of infection.

The diagnosis of nonclinically active TB (class 4) is defined by a history of previous episodes of TB or stable radiographic findings in a patient with a positive tuberculin skin test. Sputum cultures, if obtained, are negative, and there is no radiographic evidence of clinically active disease. Patients with class 4 TB may be treated in several ways depending on TB risk factors and the co-existing medical conditions. Some patients may have completed a course of preventive therapy, and some may be receiving preventive therapy; for others, preventive therapy may not be indicated. Current, clinically active TB must be excluded before a patient can be classified as class 4.

Patients are categorized as having class 5 TB while the evaluation for TB is still being done and the diagnosis of TB is pending. Patients remain in this class until all diagnostic studies have been performed but should not remain in this class for more than 3 months. If clinically active TB is strongly suspected, patients are started on multidrug therapy while the evaluation is still pending. If a diagnosis of clinically active TB (class 3) is confirmed, multidrug therapy is continued. If TB disease is excluded, the drug regimen is altered accordingly. For example, if a diagnosis is changed to infectious (class 2) TB, preventive therapy is continued if indicated. If active TB is highly possible, it is imperative to start multidrug therapy initially and alter the regimen accordingly, because progressing from single-drug therapy (e.g., isoniazid) to multidrug therapy once a diagnosis of active disease is confirmed increases the risk of spreading the disease and of developing drug-resistant TB.

One of the most significant problems associated with TB control is adherence to antitubercular regimens. Approximately 25% of patients receiving TB treatment do not complete their prescribed regimen within 12 months.[1] Inconsistent or partial treatment has resulted in TB that is resistant to isoniazid and rifampin (MDR TB). MDR TB accounts for about 1% of new TB cases and is a particular problem in certain areas of the world, such as the former Soviet Union, because of the breakdown in health system infrastructure and subsequent incomplete or inadequate treatments.[4] Although MDR TB is generally treatable, the drug regimens required to treat it take longer and are considerably more expensive and toxic.

Directly observed therapy (DOT) is one way to ensure medication compliance. WHO introduced the DOTS (directly observed therapy short course) program in 1991, which includes five essential components: case detection by sputum-smear microscopy, government commitment to TB control, regular supply of TB drugs, supervised treatment, and reports on the progress of the health system. WHO has helped more than 180 countries implement DOTS, which is also used in the United States.[4] Cases of TB are subject to mandatory reporting in all 50 states, the District of Columbia, U.S. dependencies and possessions, and independent nations within the United States (e.g., Native American lands). TB in the United States is closely monitored by local, federal, and state health departments.[8] As part of DOT, a health care provider or other designated person directly observes the patient taking each dose of TB medication. DOT is routinely implemented in many areas, such as homeless shelters and institutional settings. Trained personnel can provide DOT daily or intermittently in the office, clinic, or field (patient's home, workplace, corner bar, or any site that is mutually agreeable).[10] Antitubercular regimens can often be prescribed to be taken two or three times weekly, making DOT less burdensome. DOT has been shown to be cost-effective when such intermittent regimens are used and is now the core management strategy for all patients with TB.[1,10]

The law in every state requires that a diagnosis of TB be reported to the local health department. All drug susceptibility test results should be forwarded to the health department. Reporting TB is important for source and contact identification, epidemiologic surveillance, and the provision of resources for case management.

Co-Management with Specialists

Consultation with a specialist is required for the management of all patients requiring multidrug therapy, those with active clinical disease (class 3), and those for whom the evaluation is pending (class 5). In addition, consultation is indicated for patients with evidence of TB infection (class 2) and co-existent medical conditions, especially those which alter immune responsiveness, which may increase the risk of developing clinically active disease.

LIFE SPAN CONSIDERATIONS

One approach to improving TB detection and control has been to integrate TB skin testing and LTBI treatment with services routinely accessed by clients, such as methadone maintenance clinics. Prenatal care offers another opportunity to see patients on a regular basis. Pregnant women should receive tuberculin skin testing unless otherwise indicated. Women with evidence of LTBI (class 2) should be considered for isoniazid preventive therapy using the standard criteria. Although isoniazid is not contraindicated in pregnancy, the treatment of LTBI during pregnancy is controversial because of the risk of isoniazid-associated hepatitis. Both the American College of Obstetricians and Gynecologists and the CDC recommend deferring LTBI treatment until after birth, except for women with conditions such as HIV or recent infection with TB that would promote transmission of the organism to the placenta.[19] Pregnant women with clinically active TB (class 3) must receive adequate therapy as soon as TB is suspected, since risk of transmission to the fetus is high. Untreated TB presents a much greater danger to a woman and her fetus than does treatment of the disease. The preferred initial drug regimen includes isoniazid, rifampin, and ethambutol. These drugs do cross the placenta but have no demonstrated teratogenic side effects. A woman on antitubercular therapy should not be discouraged from breastfeeding; although small concentrations of the drug are found in breast milk, they do not cause toxicity in newborns. Streptomycin is contraindicated during pregnancy, and PZA is not routinely used because its effects on the fetus are still unknown.[1,10,16]

Older adults receiving antitubercular therapy must be monitored closely for drug side effects. Many of the adverse reactions increase with advancing age and decreased renal function.

COMPLICATIONS

Complications of TB can result from the disease process itself or can be secondary to drug therapy. The death rate of untreated pulmonary TB is approximately 60%, with a median time until death of 2½ years. Patients with miliary or disseminated TB often become ill before radiographic changes are apparent or a diagnosis of TB has been made. Without treatment, the prognosis for miliary TB is poor. However, miliary TB responds to the same drug regimens used to treat other forms of TB.

Persons taking antitubercular drugs need to be monitored closely for side effects and drug toxicities. Baseline laboratory evaluations and monthly examinations are indicated for most of the drugs used to treat TB.

TB and HIV/AIDS form a lethal combination, since each disease speeds the progress of the other. Because HIV weakens the immune system, someone who is infected with HIV and TB is many times more likely to develop active TB than someone infected with TB who is HIV negative. TB is the leading cause of death among people who are HIV positive and accounts for approximately 13% of AIDS-related deaths worldwide.[5]

INDICATIONS FOR REFERRAL OR HOSPITALIZATION

Most patients with clinically active pulmonary TB should be considered for hospitalization during the first couple of weeks of therapy. After 2 weeks of multidrug therapy, the infectiousness of these patients is reduced significantly and they are no longer a threat to public health. Patients with extrapulmonary TB generally are much less infectious and can be managed as outpatients.

Persons with MDR TB should be referred to an infectious disease specialist or a pulmonologist with expertise in the treatment of TB. Immunocompromised patients with active TB or any patients with disseminated disease should also be referred.

PATIENT AND FAMILY EDUCATION

Patient education is critical to controlling the resurgence of TB. The public must be educated about the role of TB screening and the need to identify persons infected with TB before active disease develops so they can benefit from preventive therapy. Bilingual and bicultural outreach staff workers are needed to work with immigrant individuals and communities to counter opposition to LBTI therapy based on cultural misunderstandings about its purpose and fears of stigmatization based on adherence to a long-term medication regimen. The importance of medication adherence must be carefully explained to patients receiving isoniazid or multidrug therapy. Untreated TB can lead to reactivation of the disease in the future, progression of the disease, continued spread of the disease, and the development of drug resistance. In addition, the potential drug side effects must be carefully discussed, and patients should be instructed to contact their health care provider as soon as any signs or symptoms associated with drug toxicity develop.

REFERENCES

1. Centers for Disease Control and Prevention: *Core curriculum on tuberculosis: what the clinician should know*, ed 3, Atlanta, 1994, US Department of Health and Human Services.
2. Centers for Disease Control and Prevention: Trends in tuberculosis—United States, 2005, *MMWR* 55(11):305-308, 2006.
3. American Thoracic Society, Centers for Disease Control and Prevention, Infectious Disease Society of America: Controlling tuberculosis in the United States, *Am J Respir Med* 172:1169-1227, 2005.
4. Murray S: Challenges of tuberculosis, *CMAJ* 174(1):33-34, 2006.
5. Global Health Reporting: *Tuberculosis: overview*, retrieved July 24, 2006, from http://www.globalhealthreporting.org/tb.asp.
6. Centers for Disease Control and Prevention: Emergence of *Mycobacterium tuberculosis* with extensive resistance to second-line drugs—worldwide, 2000-2004, *MMWR* 55(11):301-306, 2006.
7. Miller T, Hilsenrath P, Lykens K, and others: Using cost and health impacts to prioritize the targeted testing of tuberculosis in the United States, *Ann Epidemiol* 16:305-312, 2006.
8. Myers W, Westenhouse J, Flood J, and others: An ecological study of tuberculosis transmission in California, *Am J Pub Health* 96(4):685-690, 2006.
9. Centers for Disease Control and Prevention: Prevention and control of tuberculosis in correctional and detention facilities: recommendations from CDC, *MMWR* 55(RR-9):1-54, 2006.
10. Centers for Disease Control and Prevention: Treatment of tuberculosis, *MMWR* 52(RR11):1-77, 2003.
11. Danneburg AM: Immune mechanisms in the pathogenesis of pulmonary tuberculosis, *Rev Infect Dis* 11(Suppl 2):S369-S378, 1989.
12. Comstock GW, Reichman LB, Starke JR: Can we control TB this time? *Patient Care* 1995.
13. McColloster P, Neff NE: Outpatient management of tuberculosis, *Am Fam Phys* 53(5):1579-1594, 1996.
14. Todd B: The QuantiFERON-TB Gold test, *Am J Nurs* 106(6):33-34, 37, 2006.
15. Mazurek G, Villarino M: Guidelines for using the QuantiFERON-TB test for diagnosing latent *Mycobacterium tuberculosis* infection, *MMWR* 52(RR02):15-18, 2003, retrieved March 8, 2007, from: http://www.cdc.gov/mmwr/preview/mmwrhtml/rr5202a2.htm.
16. American Thoracic Society: Control of tuberculosis in the United States, *Am Rev Respir Dis* 146(6):1623-1633, 1992.
17. American Thoracic Society: Treatment of tuberculosis and tuberculosis infection in adults and children, *Am J Respir Crit Care Med* 149(5):1359-1374, 1994.
18. Centers for Disease Control and Prevention: Update: adverse event data and revised American Thoracic Society/CDC recommendations against the use of rifampin and pyrazinamide for treatment of latent tuberculosis infection—United States, 2003, *MMWR* 52(31):735-739, 2003.
19. Sackoff J, Pfeiffer M, Driver D, and others: Tuberculosis prevention for non-U.S.-born pregnant women, *Am J Obstet Gynecol* 194:451-456, 2006.

CHAPTER 246

HIV Infection

Bryan J. Marsh

DEFINITION AND EPIDEMIOLOGY

Human immunodeficiency virus type 1 (HIV-1) is a member of the family of viruses known as retroviruses. HIV-1 was first isolated in 1985, at which time it was identified as the etiologic agent underlying the recently identified epidemic of acquired immunodeficiency syndrome (AIDS). HIV-1 is a zoonosis that was transmitted from chimpanzees to humans three or more times early in the twentieth century. HIV-2 is a genetically distinct retrovirus that was transmitted from monkeys to humans and also causes AIDS (though possibly more slowly than does HIV-1), but which is much less prevalent, both globally and in the United States, than is HIV-1.

HIV infection presents a number of challenges for the health care provider, including when to consider the diagnosis and test for infection, when to initiate antiretroviral therapy (ART) and with which antiretrovirals (ARVs), how to monitor disease progression and treatment efficacy, the need for close attention to avoid dangerous drug-drug interactions when patients are being treated with ART, how to incorporate risk reduction counseling into clinical care to further reduce HIV transmission, and when to recommend postexposure prophylaxis after a possible exposure to HIV.

The first AIDS case definition was developed by the Centers for Disease Control and Prevention (CDC) in 1987 as a tool to aid in the study of the epidemiology of the AIDS epidemic. This definition encompassed a mixture of syndromes, primarily opportunistic infections and malignancies, associated with advanced immune dysfunction.[1] The AIDS case definition has subsequently been expanded several times and now requires that an individual have laboratory documentation of HIV infection and either (1) one of a broad spectrum of opportunistic infections, malignancies, and nonspecific syndromes; or (2) a CD4 cell count of less than 200/mm^3.[2] Because AIDS is a clinical case definition used primarily for epidemiologic monitoring, once an individual is diagnosed with AIDS, that individual will always carry the diagnosis of AIDS, even after immune restoration such that the CD4 cell count is greater than 200/mm^3 and all complications of AIDS have resolved.

In addition to the AIDS case definition, several systems classify HIV-infected patients by degree of immune dysfunction, usually based on a combination of laboratory and clinical criteria. The most widely used classification system in the United States, established by the CDC in 1993, combines three clinical classes (A if asymptomatic, B if symptomatic but not included in category C, and C if symptomatic with an AIDS-defining condition) and three immunologic classes (1 if CD4 is >500/mm^3, 2 if CD4 is 200-500/mm^3, and 3 if CD4 is <200/mm^3).[2] Insurance and other agencies occasionally require that patients be defined by the CDC classification system, but these classification systems were developed before the dynamic nature of HIV infection became clear and before effective treatment became available, and they have little utility to the clinician caring for HIV-infected patients.

Transmission of HIV can occur sexually, parenterally through either injection drug use or blood product transmission, and vertically from mother to child during pregnancy or subsequently through breastfeeding. The risk of sexual transmission varies depending on the nature of the sexual encounter, but is generally in the range of 0.1% to 1% per episode of vaginal or rectal sex when no barrier protection is used. The risk of transmission through oral sex is markedly lower. Factors that increase the risk of transmission include other active sexually transmitted diseases (STDs) and a high HIV viral load. Transmission from blood products was virtually eliminated in the United States in 1985 when it became possible to screen blood donations for HIV infection. The risk of transmission from an untreated HIV-infected mother to child is between 20% and 30% during pregnancy, with a subsequent risk of transmission through breastfeeding that is cumulative and depends on duration and consistency of breastfeeding.

The CDC estimates that approximately 1 million people were living with HIV infection in the United States at the end of 2004.[3] At that time, the cumulative number of AIDS cases reported to the CDC was 902,223, of which 81% were males, 19% females; this number also included 9348 children less than 13 years old. Since 1997, the number of non-Hispanic African Americans living with AIDS has outnumbered the number of non-Hispanic Caucasians. The three states reporting the highest number of cumulative AIDS cases were New York, California, and Florida. Total deaths were 505,801, including 5168 children under age 15 years.

AIDS has been a reportable condition since 1987, but HIV has never been a nationally reportable disease, and consequently the understanding of U.S. epidemiology has been based primarily on AIDS cases. This has provided a picture of trends in the epidemic that is a number of years out of date and has become even less accurate more recently, with the introduction of therapy that can prevent progression of HIV infection to AIDS. Based on results from states in which HIV is a reportable condition, it is estimated that men who have sex with men (MSM) now account for approximately half of all new HIV infections in the United States, followed by heterosexual transmission (34%) and injecting drug use (15%). Among women with newly diagnosed HIV infection, however, almost 80% of cases are secondary to heterosexual transmission.[3] Important trends include a growing disproportion of cases in minorities, a growing proportion of cases in the southern states, and a resurgence in cases among MSM in at least some areas in the United States.

HIV has had a relatively minor impact on U.S. health care and economy, but this is not the case in many economically disadvantaged countries around the world. The Joint United Nations Programme on HIV/AIDS estimates that more than 40 million people worldwide were living with HIV/AIDS as of the end of 2005; of these, 38.0 million were adults, 17.5 million were women, and 2.3 million were children less 15 years old.[4] Approximately 95% of people living with HIV now live in the developing world, and the vast majority of them do not have access to any form of effective treatment for HIV and thus will likely die from AIDS. During 2005 alone, 4.9 million people became infected and AIDS caused the deaths of an estimated 3.1 million people, including 1.1 million women and 570,000 children less than 15 years old.

PATHOPHYSIOLOGY

Although some aspects of the HIV life cycle and HIV/AIDS pathophysiology still require further study, the general outline is well established. To infect a cell, HIV must attach to two cell surface proteins: first, CD4 and, second, one of the two chemokine receptors, CCR5 or CXCR4, which are often referred to as co-receptors. The virus then fuses with the cell surface, followed by release of viral RNA and proteins into the infected cell. The viral RNA is then reverse transcribed to DNA (hence the name *retrovirus*), and this DNA is transported into the cell nucleus and incorporated into the cellular genome. Various cells, including monocytes-macrophages and dendritic cells, are susceptible to HIV infection, but the CD4 T lymphocyte is the primary target. A CD4 T lymphocyte that is infected by HIV can remain metabolically inactive with latent HIV infection, or it can be activated with resultant active HIV replication. Through mechanisms that are not entirely understood, with the replication of HIV in activated CD4 T cells, and the resultant high-level viremia with the subsequent infection of more CD4 T cells, there is an inexorable decline in the total pool of CD4 T cells in the infected person. As the total number of CD4 T cells declines, as measured by the number of circulating CD4 T cells in peripheral blood (often referred to as the "CD4 count" or "T-cell count"), there is a steady decline in the functional capacity of the immune system. After sufficient damage, the infected person starts to suffer from complications of this immune dysfunction, and eventually will develop one or more of the many complications of AIDS and succumb to the disease. These AIDS-defining conditions seldom occur until the CD4 T-cell count drops below 200 cells/mm^3.

The rate of progression of immune dysfunction, monitored by the decline of the CD4 T-cell count in peripheral blood, varies significantly between individuals. Without ART, the average time from initial HIV infection until the development of a first complication of AIDS is about 8 years, and the average time from this first complication to death is another year; however, some individuals progress to AIDS in a few years (occasionally as short as 1 year), and some rare individuals (known as long-term nonprogressors) maintain a normal CD4 T-cell count indefinitely and never develop AIDS.

CLINICAL PRESENTATION

The clinical presentation of a person with HIV infection varies tremendously, but the spectrum of presentations is determined by the stage of disease, and most important by whether the person is experiencing primary HIV infection (PHI), is in the period of clinical latency, or has progressed to AIDS.

PHI refers to the time after infection but before the infected person has established a comprehensive immunologic response to infection; in other words, the period when HIV can be identified in the person's blood but before standard serologic tests for HIV have become positive. This period before seroconversion typically lasts several weeks, but may be as long as 3 months. During this time the infected person may experience a seroconversion illness, which is often described as flulike but is highly variable and most often consists of fever, myalgia, headache, and a pleomorphic rash.

During the years between PHI and AIDS, a person infected with HIV is typically asymptomatic; however, assorted clinical syndromes may occur during this period. These are important to be aware of, both for management of a known HIV-infected patient and as indications to consider underlying HIV in as yet undiagnosed patients. Occasionally opportunistic infections occur at a CD4 range of more than 200 cells/mm^3, but in the United States the more frequent, though still rare, severe complications at these higher CD4 counts are malignancies, the most important of which are lymphomas of various types (excluding the primary CNS lymphoma of advanced AIDS) and cervical and anal carcinoma. The one severe infection that does occur at a higher rate in this CD4 range is tuberculosis (TB). Less severe complications in this range include shingles, severe psoriasis, severe (particularly bacteremic) pneumococcal disease, recurrent oral and vaginal candidiasis, oral hairy leukoplakia (OHL), and idiopathic thrombocytopenia. The occurrence of any of these conditions in a patient without known HIV infection should result in assessment of risk of HIV infection and frequently in HIV serologic testing.

When a person infected with HIV has progressed to the severe immune dysfunction present in AIDS, he or she becomes at risk for all the potential complications thereof, and development of any one of these mandates testing for HIV infection. The risk of developing an HIV-associated complication increases steadily as the CD4 count drops below 200/mm^3. A few of the more common of the earlier complications include *Pneumocystis jiroveci* pneumonia (PCP), Kaposi's sarcoma (KS, a primarily cutaneous malignancy that manifests as raised violaceous macules), cryptococcal meningitis, and esophageal candidiasis. At lower CD4 counts, especially at less than 50 cells/mm^3, additional complications may develop, including *Toxoplasma* encephalitis, disseminated *Mycobacterium avium intracellulare* complex infection, cytomegalovirus (CMV) retinitis, progressive multifocal leukoencephalopathy, AIDS dementia, primary CNS lymphoma, and AIDS wasting syndrome.

The evaluation of a person newly diagnosed with HIV is extensive. If the patient has an acute illness, whether from acute or chronic HIV infection, evaluation and management of that illness takes priority, but whether the patient is ill or asymptomatic, the assessment needs to include a comprehensive history and physical examination and extensive laboratory evaluation and other testing. Aspects of the history that require particular attention include:

- Assessment of patients' understanding of the new diagnosis and of the implications for their future, both short and long term. In particular, it is important to define patients' emotional state and ensure their safety, both from potential self-harm and from abuse by a partner, family, or others secondary to the depression and stigmatization often associated with a new diagnosis of HIV infection.
- The development of a trusting and therapeutic relationship with patients. A first medical appointment after a new diagnosis of HIV infection provides a unique opportunity for the health care provider to establish rapport with patients that is crucial for future health care. This requires the provider to balance the need to inquire about deeply personal, always emotionally intense, and sometimes shaming history and the importance of ensuring that patients understand that the primary purpose in collecting this information is to ensure comprehensive care. Successful negotiation of this encounter will facilitate future care, whereas an encounter that leaves the patient uncomfortable with or untrusting of the provider will affect the patient's willingness to return, to provide sensitive information, and to work productively with the provider. Depending on the patient's health and potential risk to others, it may be appropriate to defer some of this history and discussion for subsequent meetings. Should this be the case, it is often helpful to frame the subjects for future discussion so it is easier to return to them at the appropriate time.
- Medical history. This should be comprehensive, but should also address in detail aspects of history that may give clues to possible exposures that increase the risk of certain opportunistic infections, including a detailed travel and exposure history. A history of prior STDs and exposure to TB is particularly important.
- Sexual history. This should include an attempt to define patients' sexual orientation; history of sexual behavior; prior use of condoms; ability to negotiate sexual activity and condom use (especially in a current relationship); and circumstances in which patients may be less able to constrain their sexual behavior, whether due to peer pressure, concerns about safety, or loss of inhibition secondary to substance abuse.
- Substance abuse history. Details of the history and current use of illicit drugs, the use of alcohol, and the abuse of prescription medications aids in individual patient care, informs the choice of ART, and defines the need for risk reduction interventions.
- Alternative therapies. Since some alternative, herbal, or vitamin therapies are contraindicated for use in combination with some ARVs, the use of any of these therapies needs to be carefully defined and then researched for safety.

The physical examination needs to be comprehensive, both for general health assessment and for detection of complications of HIV infection. Particular attention should be paid to the neurologic examination (for both focal and cognitive deficits), the skin (for KS and assorted dermatitides), oropharynx (for thrush, OHL, periodontitis, KS, etc.), liver, and genitals (for STDs). If the patient has a CD4 count under 100/mm^3, the routine examination should always include a retinal examination (for CMV and other causes of retinitis).

DIAGNOSTICS

Diagnosis of HIV Infection

The diagnosis of chronic HIV-1 infection is established by the laboratory confirmation of the presence of antibodies to HIV-1, often referred to as serologic testing. When HIV serologic tests are ordered, two different diagnostic assays are performed. First, an enzyme-linked immunosorbent assay

(ELISA) is performed as a screening test. The sensitivity of the HIV ELISA is so high that almost no false-negative test results occur, but as a consequence the rate of false-positive results, especially in a low-risk patient, is significant. A negative ELISA thus excludes chronic HIV infection, and there is no role for subsequent Western blot testing. A positive ELISA, however, must be confirmed by Western blot testing, which is performed automatically in the United States when a specimen is ELISA positive. Western blot testing identifies the presence of a number of discrete antibodies against HIV, and the results of the test are defined by the number of these antibodies (referred to as *bands*) which are present. No positive bands is defined as a negative test, one band as indeterminate, and more than one band as positive. A negative Western blot excludes chronic HIV infection (and thus establishes that the ELISA was false positive secondary to nonsignificant cross-reacting antibodies), and a positive Western blot definitively diagnoses chronic HIV infection.

An indeterminate Western blot can be due to one of three causes: a cross-reacting antibody to one of the HIV-specific antibodies that are assayed for by the HIV Western blot (i.e., a false positive); PHI, so soon after infection that the patient has made significant antibody against one HIV antigen but not yet against others; and HIV-2 infection, assuming the original Western blot was HIV-1 specific and not a combination HIV-1/HIV-2 Western blot. HIV-2 is very rare in the United States, so the important differential diagnosis is usually to distinguish between a false-positive test and PHI. The likelihood of these two possibilities is influenced by the pretest probability that the patient being tested could have PHI. If the patient has a low risk of recent HIV infection and is without a syndrome suggestive of PHI, then the likelihood that the indeterminate Western blot is false positive is very high; but if the individual has recently participated in activities associated with a high risk of HIV acquisition, or if the individual has been tested because of a syndrome highly suggestive of PHI, then the possibility that the Western blot is indeterminate due to HIV seroconversion and indicative of PHI is more significant. Depending on the estimate of likelihood of PHI, an individual who tests indeterminate can be further worked up in one of two ways:

- If there is a low likelihood of PHI, the approach to exclude recent HIV infection involves repeating the serologic test after allowing sufficient time for seroconversion to occur. If the serologic testing is repeated 1 month after the initial indeterminate test was obtained, the majority of patients undergoing seroconversion will test positive; if it is repeated at 3 months, close to 100% will have converted and no further testing is indicated. Viral load testing usually should not be obtained in this setting, since the risk of a false-positive result, and the added emotional distress and medical workup that this entails, outweighs the low likelihood of obtaining a true positive result.
- If there is a significant likelihood of PHI, such as a recent potential high-risk exposure to HIV or any recent risk and a syndrome suggestive of PHI, an alternative approach to confirming the diagnosis can be considered. In the setting of PHI the degree of HIV viremia is exceptionally high, and a standard quantitative HIV assay (most commonly polymerase chain reaction [PCR] and branched chain DNA [bDNA]) will invariably be positive at very high titer. The advantages of the earlier diagnosis obtained with this approach, rather than waiting 1 to 3 months to obtain a repeat serologic test, include less opportunity for loss to follow up; referral to a research center or HIV specialist for consideration of treatment of PHI; and early intervention to reduce risky behavior for further transmission. This last advantage is of particular importance, since the very high viremia associated with PHI results in a period of markedly increased transmissibility.

It is important to be certain that a patient entering care who reports a prior diagnosis of HIV infection truly is infected, so an HIV serology should be repeated if an actual report of HIV serologic testing is not available. It is reasonable to make an exception to this if there is documentation of repeated positive viral load testing.

New patients whose serostatus is unknown or questionable should be counseled about the distinctions of anonymous vs. confidential testing. Concerns about inadvertent disclosures or the reactions of insurance companies may result in a desire for anonymous testing.

Laboratory and Other Testing of Patient with Newly Diagnosed HIV

When an individual is diagnosed with HIV, extensive additional testing should be performed. This is to determine the degree of immunosuppression and thus the need for ART and other therapy, the presence of significant co-morbid conditions, the need for appropriate immunizations, and aspects of physiologic function that may affect the choice of ART.

The most important assay to establish current immunologic status is the determination of the CD4 count, which is reported as both an absolute and a percent. In addition, quantifying the amount of HIV in the patient's plasma, known as the *HIV viral load* or *viral burden*, provides additional information about immune function (the higher the viral load, the more immunologically compromised the patient), but more important provides an estimate of the expected rate of immunologic decline (as measured by falling CD4) and is important to establish at baseline, since decline in viral load after starting ART is the most important initial marker of efficacy of ART.

The plasma viral load can be measured by two technologies, reverse transcriptase PCR (RT-PCR) and bDNA. The results of these tests are reported as the number of copies of viral RNA per milliliter of plasma. During the chronic phase of HIV infection, the viral load is typically between 10,000 and 100,000 copies/ml, with lower values predictive of a slower than average rate of progression and a higher viral load predictive of more rapid progression. Finally, most patients with newly diagnosed HIV should undergo viral resistance testing, usually with an HIV genotype assay, to exclude the presence of infection with a virus resistant to one or more of the available ARVs.

Routine baseline testing should usually include CBC and a comprehensive metabolic profile, including liver function tests, amylase and lipase, a fasting lipid profile, and serologic tests for syphilis, *Toxoplasma gondii*, and CMV.

Some of the more important additional testing at baseline is to exclude co-infection with hepatitis B and C virus (HBV and HBC) and TB. Testing for the hepatitis viruses is performed through the same algorithm as for patients without HIV. Testing for TB, however, is more complex. The diagnosis of latent TB in a patient with HIV is complicated by the steady decline in the reliability of the purified protein derivative (PPD) test as the CD4 count declines, to the point where it is highly compromised if the CD4 count is less than 200/mm^3 and essentially worthless if less than 50/mm^3. Therefore, although it is always appropriate to perform PPD testing on patients with HIV, this testing should usually be repeated if patients have a low enough CD4 that they are started on ART and always should be repeated after patients with a nadir CD4 of less than 200/mm^3 have been on ART long enough to suppress the HIV viral load and raise the CD4 over 200/mm^3. The definition of a positive PPD in patients with HIV infection is an induration 5 mm or more. Because the risk for a patient with HIV and latent TB of developing active TB is exceptionally high (an annual risk of approximately 10%), treatment of latent TB is always indicated once active TB is excluded.

DIFFERENTIAL DIAGNOSIS

The differential diagnosis for a patient with a clinical syndrome consistent with a diagnosis of AIDS is fairly narrow. In the rare instances in which patients appear with such an illness, test negative for HIV on routine testing, and have no other evident cause for immunosuppression (such as an underlying malignancy or treatment with a known immunosuppressing mediation therapy), they should be immediately referred for expert consultation. There are many congenital immunodeficiency states, but the vast majority become evident in childhood (see Chapter 240). One interesting but exceptionally rare condition of unknown etiology that mimics HIV and does first appear in adults is idiopathic CD4 lymphocytopenia (ICL). ICL is diagnosed in the presence of persistently low CD4 counts (<300/mm^3, or <20% of total lymphocytes) without laboratory evidence of HIV infection or other cause.[5]

Measurement of the CD4 count should never be used as a surrogate for serologic diagnosis of HIV infection or as sufficient for diagnosis of ICL, especially in the setting of an acute illness. During an acute infectious illness of sufficient severity, it is not unusual for patients to develop transient lymphopenia with absolute CD4 lymphopenia that can even enter the AIDS range. In addition, the HIV viral load should not be used to diagnose HIV infection, save for the rare times when it is used to diagnose PHI.

MANAGEMENT

The management of HIV includes highly active antiretroviral therapy (HAART) when indicated, close attention to medication adherence, prevention of opportunistic infections with chemoprophylaxis, appropriate immunization, close monitoring for complications of HIV and of the therapy for HIV, management of co-morbid conditions, and attempts to minimize behavior that can result in HIV transmission. In addition, because HIV is now a treatable disease with a long life expectancy, all usual aspects of primary health care must also be provided. An excellent set of up-to-date guidelines for many aspects of HIV care is maintained at the U.S. Department of Health and Human Services AIDSinfo website, http://www.aidsinfo.nih.gov.

Treatment with HAART is one of the more complex areas of modern medicine; when done correctly, it can convert HIV from a progressive and inevitably fatal disease to a chronic disease with potentially normal life expectancy, but when done poorly, it can result in viral resistance to all antivirals and consequently untreatable progressive disease. HAART should thus only be prescribed by clinicians with significant training and experience in its use.

Current guidelines that address the initiation of HAART attempt to balance the obvious benefits of HAART with the disadvantages of treatment, which include the risk of development of resistance precluding future therapy, drug toxicities, and the medicalization of life in someone who may be clinically entirely well.[6,7] The consensus in the United States is that treatment should always be initiated in a patient with clinical AIDS or a CD4 less than 200/mm^3, and that treatment should usually be offered to patients whose CD4 is somewhere in the range of 200 to 350/mm^3, but seldom at higher CD4 counts. This recommendation is based on the efficacy, tolerability, and toxicity of current agents and on the results of retrospective cohort analyses, which demonstrate that mortality does not significantly increase until treatment is deferred to CD4 counts below 200/mm^3.[8,9] The viral load, which in the past has been incorporated into treatment decisions, is currently deemphasized. An important implication of the range of CD4 at which treatment can appropriately be initiated is that initiation of HAART in an asymptomatic patient is never urgent, and there is usually time to educate the patient and to address other active problems that might adversely affect therapy, including depression related to the new diagnosis.

Whether patients diagnosed with PHI should be treated with HAART is an area of debate. A theoretic benefit of treatment of PHI is that this might minimize early immunologic damage and allow development of a more robust immunologic response to HIV, resulting in better immunologic control of HIV when HAART is withdrawn and a longer period before treatment of chronic infection would become necessary. Unfortunately, studies of treatment of PHI with currently available agents have not shown a convincing benefit and so treatment is not generally recommended. Nevertheless, this remains an active and important area of research, and referral to a research center should be strongly considered.[10,11]

One other absolute indication for HAART is the treatment of a pregnant woman to prevent mother-to-child transmission. Optimum HAART in a pregnant woman can reduce the risk of vertical transmission from approximately 25% to less than 2%, and recommended regimens have no known significant fetal toxicity.[12] This benefit is so significant that elective cesarean section is no longer indicated in the optimally treated pregnant woman.

There are now 20 ARVs (and four formulations containing either two or three of these agents) approved for treatment of HIV in the United States, representing four different classes of agents: nucleoside analog reverse transcriptase inhibitors (NRTIs), nonnucleoside reverse transcriptase inhibitors (NNRTIs), protease inhibitors (PIs), and fusion inhibitors.

Despite the innumerable possible combinations of three agents, clinical trials and extensive experience have defined a few preferred regimens for first-line therapy, the easiest of which involves two or three pills once daily (Table 246-1), although many alternatives are used based on patient-specific factors. First-line treatment usually consists of a combination of two NRTIs and either a PI or an NNRTI. The specific choice of agents is driven by a preferred schedule (once vs. twice a day; with or without food; in the morning or before bed), drug interactions with other medications the patient is on or may need to start, co-morbid conditions, pregnancy or desire for pregnancy, and patient concerns about specific possible adverse drug reactions.

The short-term goal of HAART is to suppress viral replication to such a degree that there is no detectable HIV in peripheral blood, whether measured by RT-PCR or bDNA. When that is the case, the result of viral load testing is reported as below the lower limit of detection for the assay, which is less than 50 copies/ml for RT-PCR and less than 75 copies/ml for bDNA; this is often referred to as an *undetectable viral load*. The amount of time it takes to obtain an undetectable viral load after initiating HAART depends on the baseline viral load, so the goal is to reduce tenfold to 100-fold the first viral load obtained 4 to 6 weeks after initiation of therapy. If that is not attained, then the patient should be assessed for viral resistance, medication adherence, and appropriateness of HAART. CD4 counts need not be measured soon after initiation of HAART, but with successful suppression of viral replication, the CD4 count should start to increase; typically it increases 100 to 200/mm^3/yr on HAART.

When a patient is on stable HAART and has attained an undetectable viral load, it is crucial to monitor the patient carefully for ongoing efficacy (with viral load and CD4 testing, usually every 3 months), safety (with the specific laboratory testing determined by the given regimen), and adherence. If patients are less than 95% adherent, they run an unacceptably high risk of developing resistance to the agents in the regimen, demonstrated by virologic rebound after initial suppression to undetectable levels, with consequent need to change ARVs, and—if repeated more than a few times—eventual loss of all effective therapy.

The reason to check viral loads every 3 months when someone is on HAART is to detect virologic rebound. When this occurs, it is crucial to address medication adherence and then to consider defining the degree of viral resistance to the HAART regimen. Resistance can be determined by either a genotypic or phenotypic assay, but in either case the interpretation of these and the choice of subsequent regimens if resistance is present should be handled by an HIV specialist.

An often overlooked aspect of the care of patients on HAART is the danger of drug-drug interactions with many of the ARVs. These interactions can affect both the non-ARV, most often by decreasing metabolism (potentially to a life-threatening degree), and the ARV, most concerningly by decreasing ARV concentrations to subtherapeutic levels and thus increasing the likelihood of resistance and failure. It is thus imperative that drug interactions be researched before starting any new medication, whether prescription or over the counter.

When ART is not indicated, the patient should be evaluated in the clinic and by laboratory testing, primarily CD4 and viral load, every 3 to 4 months. If other treatable co-morbid conditions have been identified, such as HBC or latent TB, this may be an appropriate time to address them.

Although HAART has the most profound impact on survival of all aspects of treatment of HIV, other components of care should not be forgotten. Chemoprophylaxis and immunizations should be provided when indicated, and routine health care should be provided. For a patient with AIDS who is starting HAART, primary chemoprophylaxis (the administration of a medication to prevent a first episode of an opportunistic infection) can reduce the risk of developing an opportunistic infection before adequate immune restoration; whereas for patients with AIDS for whom immune restoration will not occur (either because of untreatable HIV secondary to the development of antiviral resistance, or to patient choice to defer ART), appropriate prophylaxis can provide a moderate prolongation of life expectancy. Decisions about when to start and stop prophylactic medications will usually be made by the HIV specialist, but excellent guidelines for chemoprophylaxis and immunizations are readily available, some of which are summarized in Tables 246-2 and 246-3.[13]

In addition, a number of conditions require particularly careful monitoring and evaluation for people with HIV, no matter what the CD4:

- Latent TB. Given the high risk of developing active TB in a patient co-infected with HIV and TB, annual PPD screening is mandatory.
- Screening for human papillomavirus (HPV)–associated disease. Cervical carcinoma develops more frequently in HIV-infected women and requires close screening and aggressive management. As a result of similar pathophysiology, HPV-associated anal carcinoma occurs much more frequently in MSM with HIV; annual rectal examinations should be performed, as should workup of any consistent symptoms. Anal Papanicolaou's smears are performed at some centers, but are not currently standard of care.
- Screening for STDs. This is important both because many patients with HIV remain at risk for infection with STDs, and because the presence of an STD increases the risk of HIV transmission.
- Management of chronic HBV and HCV. The leading cause of death for people co-infected with HIV and HCV is liver

TABLE 246-1 Preferred Antiretroviral Regimen for Antiretroviral Therapy–Naive Patients

Basis for Therapy	Regimens	Pills/Day
Nonnucleoside reverse transcriptase inhibitors	Efavirenz + (lamivudine *or* emtricitabine) + (zidovudine *or* tenofovir DF)	2-3
Protease inhibitors	Lopinavir-ritonavir (coformulation) + (lamivudine *or* emtricitabine) + zidovudine	6-7

Adapted from U.S. Department of Health and Human Services: *AIDSinfo drug database,* retrieved March 13, 2007 from http://aidsinfo.nih.gov/DrugsNew/Default.aspx?MenuItem=Drugs&ClassID=8&TypeID=1

TABLE 246-2 Primary Prophylaxis of AIDS-Indicator Disease

Pathogen	Indication	First Choice	Alternatives
STRONGLY RECOMMENDED AS STANDARD OF CARE			
Pneumocystis carinii (Pneumocystis jiroveci)	CD4 count <200/mm^3 or oropharyngeal candidiasis or unexplained fever ≥2 weeks	TMP-SMZ	Dapsone, or dapsone plus pyrimethamine plus leucovorin, or aerosolized pentamidine, via Respirgard II nebulizer
Mycobacterium tuberculosis			
Isoniazid sensitive	PPD or tuberculin skin test reaction ≥5 mm *or* prior positive PPD result without treatment or contact with case of tuberculosis	Isoniazid plus pyridoxine for 9 months	Rifampin
Isoniazid resistant	Same; high probability of exposure to isoniazid-resistant tuberculosis	Rifampin for 4-6 months	Uncertain
Multidrug (isoniazid and rifampin) resistant	Same; high probability of exposure to multidrug-resistant tuberculosis	Choice of drugs requires consultation with public health authorities	None
Toxoplasma gondii	IgG antibody to *Toxoplasma* and CD4 count <100/mm^3	TMP-SMZ	Dapsone *plus* pyrimethamine *plus* leucovorin
Mycobacterium avium-intracellulare complex	CD4 count <50/mm^3	Clarithromycin or azithromycin	Rifabutin; azithromycin plus rifabutin
Streptococcus pneumoniae	All patients	Pneumococcal vaccine (CD4 ≥200/mm^3)	None
Varicella zoster virus (VZV)	Significant exposure to chickenpox or shingles for patients who have no history of either condition or, if available, negative antibody to VZV	Varicella zoster immune globulin (VZIG), ideally within 48 hours	Acyclovir
GENERALLY RECOMMENDED			
S. pneumoniae	All patients	Pneumovax	None
Hepatitis B virus	All susceptible (anti-HB_c-negative) patients	Routine immunization	None
Influenza virus	All patients (annually, before influenza season)	Whole or split virus	Influenza antiviral
NOT RECOMMENDED FOR MOST PATIENTS; INDICATED ONLY IN UNUSUAL CIRCUMSTANCES			
Candida species	CD4 count <50/mm^3	Fluconazole	
Bacteria	Neutropenia	Granulocyte colony-stimulating factor (GCSF) or granulocyte-macrophage colony-stimulating factor (GM-CSF)	
Cryptococcus neoformans	CD4 count <50/mm^3	Fluconazole	Itraconazole
Histoplasma capsulatum	CD4 count <100/mm^3 and endemic geographic area	Itraconazole	None
Cytomegalovirus (CMV)	CD4 count <50/mm^3 and CMV antibody positivity	Oral ganciclovir	None
Coccidioidomycosis	CD4 count <200/mm^3	Fluconazole	None

IgG, Immunoglobulin G; *PPD,* purified protein derivative; *TMP-SMX,* trimethoprim-sulfamethoxazole.

disease, so management of chronic hepatitis is an integral aspect of patient care. Unfortunately, though, therapy for HCV remains poorly effective and poorly tolerated, and criteria for whom to treat and when to treat have not been established, so management of HCV in a patient co-infected with HIV should be addressed by an HIV expert. The health care provider can play an important role by reinforcing the importance of alcohol abstinence and providing immunization for HBV and hepatitis A virus for all nonimmune patients. There are fewer data on co-infection with HBV, but the issues are similar.

- Cardiovascular disease risk. Several ARVs, primarily PIs, increase the risk of cardiovascular disease, mediated primarily but not entirely by dyslipidemia and insulin resistance. It is thus important to address modifiable risk factors, to monitor lipids and glucose, and to treat metabolic abnormalities when they develop.

LIFE SPAN CONSIDERATIONS

The life expectancy of a patient newly diagnosed with HIV has steadily increased since the onset of the epidemic, and continues to do so. The largest impact on life expectancy occurred

TABLE 246-3 Immunizations for HIV-Infected Adults

Immunization	Comments
Haemophilus influenzae B (Hib) vaccine	Should be considered.
Hepatitis A vaccine	Should be screened first for past infection. Although not specifically recommended for HIV-infected individuals, hepatitis A vaccine is recommended for sexually active men who have sex with men, injecting and noninjecting drug users, and persons with clotting factor disorders.
Hepatitis B vaccine	Should be screened first for past infection. Should be offered to sexually active men who have sex with men, commercial sex workers, injecting drug users, heterosexual men and women with STDs or different sex partners, and household or sexual contacts of HbsAg carriers.
Immune globulin	Recommended to prevent measles or hepatitis A after exposure.
Influenza vaccine	Recommended annually. Usually produces protective antibodies in HIV-infected persons with minimum manifestations of HIV disease and high CD4 T-cell counts. Alternatives for influenza prophylaxis include rimantadine or amantadine.
Measles-mumps-rubella (MMR) vaccine	Although live-virus or live-bacteria vaccines should not be administered to HIV-infected individuals, MMR is considered safe and is recommended when indicated.
Pneumococcal vaccine	Recommended at 6-year intervals.
Varicella-zoster immune globulin (VZIG)	Indicated for severely immunocompromised persons after significant exposure to chickenpox or herpes zoster. An alternative to VZIG is a 3-week course of oral acyclovir.
Other vaccines	Vaccines containing killed or inactivated antigens such as diphtheria-tetanus-pertussis vaccine, enhanced inactivated polio vaccine, meningococcal vaccine, rabies vaccine, cholera vaccine, plague vaccine, and anthrax vaccine may be used for the same indications as for persons with a healthy immune system. Yellow fever vaccine, oral polio vaccine, and bacillus Calmette-Guérin (BCG) are contraindicated. Inactivated (parenteral) typhoid vaccine or typhoid (Vi) polysaccharide vaccine should be used in place of live oral typhoid (Ty21a) vaccine.

STDs, Sexually transmitted diseases.

in the mid-1990s with the introduction of HAART, but improvements in the safety and efficacy of available ARVs, the growing number of agents, and growing sophistication in the management of people living with HIV have resulted in constant incremental improvements in life expectancy. The most important predictor of life expectancy is thus no longer the CD4 and viral load at baseline, but the patients' ability to tolerate and maintain a high level of adherence to ARVs. Population statistics are thus not helpful in defining the prognosis for an individual patient, and the emphasis needs to be on the patient's idiosyncratic circumstances. Under ideal circumstances, though, it is reasonable to hope for a dramatic extension of, and possibly even unaffected, life expectancy.

Because life expectancy is long, it has become important to address long-term life plans and family planning with all patients infected with HIV. Discussions about desires and plans for children are particularly important. For an HIV-infected woman, the decision to become pregnant is usually complicated. If she has an uninfected male partner, the logistics of insemination are fairly straightforward, but the management of the pregnancy is intensive.

COMPLICATIONS

The most important complications that a person with HIV is at risk for are those which are secondary to immune dysfunction, as reflected in the CD4 count. These are discussed in the section on clinical presentation.

In addition to complications of immune dysfunction, it is important to monitor HIV-infected patients closely for complications of HAART. Antiviral therapy has a dramatic impact on life expectancy when prescribed appropriately, but these medications have a number of significant toxicities that must be actively monitored to reduce the risk of a spectrum of problems, ranging from cosmetic to life threatening. The potential toxicities vary depending on the specific regimen, so appropriate monitoring is defined uniquely for every patient. A few general recommendations are warranted:

- Metabolic toxicities. The PI and, to a lesser degree, the NNRTI and NRTI classes of ARVs all carry a risk of metabolic side effects that require monitoring. The most significant of these is dyslipidemia, which should be assessed by measuring a fasting lipid profile at baseline and then 1 to 3 months after any change in a pertinent medication. When ARV-induced dyslipidemia does develop, options for management include usual lipid-lowering therapy (diet, exercise, and medications) and change in ART if an equally effective alternative is available. A second complication is insulin resistance, which should be monitored at a minimum by appropriate interview at regular clinic appointments.
- Lipodystrophy. Lipodystrophy refers to a change from baseline in the relative proportion of fat, whether centrally with intraabdominal, breast, or dorsocervical fat accumulation, or peripherally with limb and buttock subcutaneous fat atrophy. These toxicities have no clearly attributable risk of increased mortality, but can be profoundly disfiguring. Since these changes are not readily reversible, they need to be watched for carefully and an appropriate medication change considered as needed.
- Liver disease. All but two of the currently available ARVs are associated with one or more liver toxicities, ranging from otherwise asymptomatic hyperbilirubinemia, to

fulminant and potentially fatal drug-induced hepatitis, to slowly progressive but also potentially fatal hepatic steatosis–lactic acidosis. It is thus important to define the nature of hepatotoxicity that is associated with a given regimen and monitor appropriately, whether by interview or laboratory testing.

- Drug interactions. It cannot be overemphasized that there are innumerable potential drug interactions with essentially all ART regimens, so any unusual symptom should always raise the concern of an adverse drug reaction to a new medication, whether prescribed, over the counter, herbal, or illicit, and a detailed history of the use of all medications and nutraceuticals should be obtained.

INDICATIONS FOR REFERRAL OR HOSPITALIZATION

All HIV-infected patients should be under the care of a primary health care provider and a clinician with HIV expertise, so referral to an HIV specialist should be recommended to all HIV-infected patients who enter care, whether newly diagnosed or changing health care providers. Depending on the providers' expertise, the complexity and nature of the active medical issues, challenges of travel and other constraints on accessing care, and patient preferences, the division of responsibilities between the health care provider and the specialist can vary, so it is important to explicitly define their respective roles. Patients often wonder why they need to see a health care provider when they are seen by an HIV specialist four or more times per year, and so may need to be reminded that, given the long life expectancy that can now be anticipated for HIV-infected patients, health maintenance and other aspects of primary care are as important to them as to the general population.

For HIV-infected patients who are in care, it is as important not to overreact to nonsevere acute illness as it is to be attentive to potential complications of HIV. In particular, most nonopportunistic infections can be managed just as they would be in an immunocompetent host, especially if the CD4 count is more than 200/mm^3. On the other hand, any more serious illness, any syndrome consistent with an opportunistic infection, or any potentially infectious disease that cannot be readily diagnosed as a community-acquired infection should prompt rapid consultation with an HIV specialist.

PATIENT AND FAMILY EDUCATION

Patient education for an HIV-infected patient needs to be extensive and ongoing. The initial diagnosis is often overwhelming, and basic education about HIV will often need to be repeated several times. The education needs to start by ensuring that the patient understands both the natural history of HIV and the potential immense benefit of current therapy, although it is a challenge to convey both the severity of the disease and the optimism that HAART can provide. This discussion often transitions into family planning and the need to discuss the nature of the risks associated with pregnancy. Initial discussions also need to define the nature of medical care for someone living with HIV, including the frequency of appointments, the significance of the CD4 count and viral load, the nature of medical therapy, the importance of strict adherence to ART when started, and any other pertinent aspects of care. In addition, initial education often needs to address misconceptions that the patient might have about HIV.

Further education needs to address both HIV-specific and usual aspects of general health maintenance. The patient should be informed about how to avoid exposure to infectious diseases, which includes discussion of food and water safety, pet hygiene, and international travel. The importance of patient-specific health maintenance issues should be addressed, including cigarette, alcohol, and other substance abuse. Nutritional counseling should be routinely provided.

The provider should also explicitly discuss the public health issues of HIV infection. This usually starts with a discussion of the mechanisms of transmission of HIV and how to prevent transmission. It might thus be necessary to instruct the patient on male or female condom use or on how to ensure that needles and other paraphernalia used for illicit drugs are sterile. This conversation also needs to address notification and testing of current and past partners, both sexual and needle-sharing, and of children born to an infected woman. It is thus important that the provider understand what resources are available for anonymous or confidential testing and for contact notification, which includes programs run by the department of health in every state.

REFERENCES

1. Council of State and Territorial Epidemiologists; AIDS Program, Center for Infectious Diseases: Revision of the CDC surveillance case definition for acquired immunodeficiency syndrome, *MMWR* 36(Suppl 1):1S-15S, 1987.
2. Centers for Disease Control and Prevention: *HIV/AIDS surveillance report* 9(2):18, 1997.
3. Center for Disease Control and Prevention: *The cumulative estimated number of diagnoses of AIDS through 2004 in the United States*, retrieved Feb 20, 2006, from the http://www.cdc.gov/hiv/topics/surveillance/basic.htm#aidscases.
4. UNAIDS and World Health Organization: *AIDS epidemic update: December 2005*, Geneva, 2005, UNAIDS.
5. Fauci AS: CD4+ T-lymphocytopenia without HIV infection: no lights, no camera, just facts, *N Engl J Med* 328(6):429-431, 1993.
6. Yeni PG, Hammer SM, Hirsch MS, and others: Treatment for adult HIV infection, *JAMA* 292:251-265, 2004.
7. US Department of Health and Human Services: *Guidelines for the use of antiretroviral agents in HIV-1-infected adults and adolescents*, retrieved Feb 20, 2006, from http://aidsinfo.nih.gov/ContentFiles/AdultandAdolescentGL.pdf.
8. Yeni P, Hammer S, Carpenter C, and others: Antiretroviral treatment for adult HIV infection in 2002, *JAMA* 288:222-235, 2002.
9. Lane HC, Neaton J: When to start therapy for HIV infection: a swinging pendulum in search of data, *Ann Intern Med* 138(8):680-681, 2003.
10. Pao D, Fisher M, Hue S, and others: Transmission of HIV-1 during primary infection: relationship to sexual risk and sexually transmitted infections, *AIDS* 19(1):85-90, 2005.
11. Martinez LJ: Treatment during PHI as a method of altering the epidemic spread of HIV, *Res Initiat Treat Action* 7(2):20-25, 2002.
12. US Department of Health and Human Services: *Recommendations for use of antiretroviral drugs in pregnant HIV-1–infected women for maternal health and interventions to reduce perinatal HIV-1 transmission in the United States*, October 12, 2006, retrieved March 8, 2006, from http://aidsinfo.nih.gov/ContentFiles/PerinatalGL.pdf.
13. Centers for Disease Control and Prevention: *Guidelines for the prevention of opportunistic infections in persons infected with human immunodeficiency virus*, July 14, 2002, retrieved March 8, 2007, from http://aidsinfo.nih.gov/ContentFiles/OIpreventionGL.pdf.

CHAPTER 247

Influenza

Judy Ptak

DEFINITION AND EPIDEMIOLOGY

Influenza is an acute infection of the respiratory tract caused by influenza virus type A or B. It is usually a self-limiting disease that occurs in outbreaks, primarily during the winter months in temperate climates, and may occur year round in the tropics. Influenza is highly contagious and occurs in all age-groups. It tends to occur in outbreaks that can rapidly affect 10% to 40% of the population.[1]

PATHOPHYSIOLOGY

Influenza is transmitted from person to person via respiratory secretions that contain virus. These respiratory secretions are spread in the form of droplets that are produced when a person talks, coughs, or sneezes. Virus is detectable and may be shed in respiratory secretions up to 24 hours before the onset of symptoms.

Once virus reaches the epithelium cells of the respiratory tract, it penetrates the cells and begins replication. This viral replication leads to cell death and release of large amounts of virus that can infect adjacent cells. This quickly causes desquamation of the ciliated epithelium. Onset of the acute symptoms coincides with this desquamation.[1]

CLINICAL PRESENTATION

After an incubation period of 1 or 2 days there is an abrupt onset of symptoms. These symptoms include fever, chills, headache, malaise, myalgia, and loss of appetite. Respiratory symptoms are also present but are usually overshadowed by the severity of the systemic symptoms. Respiratory symptoms include dry cough, nasal congestion and clear discharge, and sore throat. The cough is usually the most prominent of these respiratory symptoms.

The patient's temperature rises rapidly after onset, peaking at 37.7° to 40° C (100° to 104° F) in about 12 hours. The fever typically begins to decline on the second or third day and may last as long as 4 to 8 days. Systemic symptoms become less prominent as the fever decreases. A convalescent phase of 1 to 2 weeks follows the acute febrile stage. Cough, malaise, and fatigue, often extreme, are often seen during the convalescent phase.

Some patients have mild illness that resembles the common cold. Older adults, people with underlying chronic diseases, and women in the third trimester of pregnancy may experience a rapidly worsening course of influenza.

PHYSICAL EXAMINATION

Uncomplicated cases of influenza have minimum physical findings. At the onset of symptoms the patient's face is often flushed, and the eyes may be watery and red. There may be fever. The skin may be hot and moist. Cervical lymph nodes may be enlarged and tender. The pharynx is usually unremarkable, and the chest examination is usually normal.[2]

DIAGNOSTICS

Virus can be isolated from nose and throat specimens such as nasal swabs or washings, sputum, and throat swabs. Virus can be detected in cell cultures in 2 to 7 days. There are several techniques to detect the presence of viral antigens in nose and throat specimens that yield results rapidly, ranging from 1 hour to 24 to 48 hours. These rapid tests may not be as sensitive as cell culture, however, and they may be most useful in the management of individual patients at high risk for serious complications from influenza, who may benefit most from appropriate antiviral treatment. These rapid diagnostic tests for influenza may also be helpful in institutional settings where prophylaxis for other residents is indicated.[3]

Infection with influenza virus can also be confirmed by showing at least a fourfold rise in antibody titer in convalescent serum taken 10 to 20 days after an acute serum sample.

Clinical diagnosis in the setting of a confirmed influenza outbreak is very accurate.

DIFFERENTIAL DIAGNOSIS

On an individual basis in the absence of a known outbreak of influenza, it may be difficult to distinguish a case of the flu from many of the other respiratory viruses such as the common cold and respiratory syncytial virus. Other conditions to consider are *Mycoplasma pneumoniae,* bacterial pneumonia, and severe streptococcal pharyngitis.

MANAGEMENT

Treatment of influenza is primarily symptomatic. Patients should rest as much as possible. They should maintain an adequate fluid intake. Antipyretics and analgesics can be used to control fever and relieve headache and myalgia.

In the United States four antiviral medications are currently approved for treatment of influenza: amantadine (Symmetrel), rimantadine (Flumadine), zanamivir (Relenza), and oseltamivir (Tamiflu). Amantadine and rimantadine are no longer generally recommended for chemoprophylaxis and treatment of influenza A. Resistance develops quickly during treatment, and these agents are not recommended until susceptibility to these antivirals has been reestablished among circulating influenza A viruses.[4] Oseltamivir may be used for chemoprophylaxis and treatment of uncomplicated influenza A and B. Zanamivir may be used for treatment only of influenza A and B. When used as treatment for influenza, these drugs must be started within 48 hours of the onset of symptoms and can reduce the severity of the symptoms and the duration of symptoms by about 1 day.[4] Recommendations for the prophylaxis of influenza with antiviral drugs are listed in Box 247-1.

LIFE SPAN CONSIDERATIONS

Influenza can cause death in any age-group; however, mortality is highest in older people. In the United States, about 30,000 people die each year from influenza or its complications. People 65 years old or older account for more than 90% of these deaths. In a large retrospective study of women between 15 and 64 years old, Neuzil, Reed, and Mitchell found

BOX 247-1

RECOMMENDATIONS FOR PROPHYLAXIS OF INFLUENZA WITH ANTIVIRAL DRUGS

- Persons at high risk who have not been vaccinated
- Persons at high risk who are vaccinated after influenza activity has begun
- Unvaccinated household members of persons at high risk
- Unvaccinated persons who provide care to those at high risk
- Persons who have immunodeficiency

From Smith N, Bresee J, Shay D, and others, Advisory Committee on Immunization Practices: Prevention and control of influenza, *MMWR* 55(RR19):1-42, 2006.

a significant increase in acute cardiopulmonary hospitalizations and deaths during influenza season.[5]

COMPLICATIONS

The primary complications of influenza are pulmonary. The most notable pulmonary complications are primary influenza pneumonia, which is rare, or secondary bacterial pneumonia. Other pulmonary complications include croup in children and exacerbation of chronic pulmonary disease. Central nervous system complications such as Guillain-Barré syndrome and encephalitis occur rarely after influenza infection. The association with influenza infection and Reye's syndrome in children prompted the recommendation that aspirin be avoided when treating children with influenza. Other complications that have been associated with influenza infection are myositis, which is seen primarily in children, and toxic shock syndrome.

INDICATIONS FOR REFERRAL OR HOSPITALIZATION

Patients who do not begin to gradually improve a few days after the onset of symptoms should be reevaluated and referred as appropriate. Hospitalization may be indicated for patients with underlying chronic conditions that are complicated by the added stress of influenza infection. Anyone who is rapidly getting worse should be considered for hospitalization.

PATIENT AND FAMILY EDUCATION

Patients and their families should be educated about the need to get the influenza vaccine on a yearly basis. Basic personnel hygiene measures such as good handwashing and covering coughs and sneezes may help reduce the risk of acquiring and spreading influenza.

HEALTH PROMOTION

The influenza vaccine is the primary method of preventing influenza infection. People at risk for complications from influenza infection, as well as people who are likely to transmit influenza to those at high risk for complications, should be encouraged to receive the influenza vaccine. The vaccine should be given each year at least 2 weeks before the expected start of the influenza season. In the temperate climates mid-October to the start of the flu season is the preferred time to vaccinate people.

Two types of vaccine are currently available in the United States. The "flu shot" contains three inactivated strains of influenza virus: two influenza A subtypes and one influenza B type. It is approved for all people 6 months of age or older who do not have an egg allergy. The second type of influenza vaccine is the nasal spray. This vaccine contains live attenuated strains of the influenza virus. It is currently approved only for healthy nonpregnant people between the ages of 5 and 49 years old. On an annual basis the U.S. Food and Drug Administration determines the three influenza strains to be included in the next year's vaccine based on which viruses are most likely to cause epidemics in the coming winter.[6] Recommendations for the use of influenza vaccines are listed in Box 247-2.

BOX 247-2

RECOMMENDATIONS FOR USE OF INFLUENZA VACCINE

People 50 years or older
Residents of long-term-care facilities
Adults and children with chronic pulmonary or cardiovascular disease (including asthma)
Adults and children requiring care for chronic metabolic disease, renal dysfunction, hemoglobinopathy, or immunosuppression (including HIV)
Adults and children with any condition that can compromise respiratory function or the handling of respiratory secretions or that can increase the risk for aspiration
Children ages 6 to 23 months
Children ages 24 to 59 months and their household contacts and out-of-home caregivers
Children and adolescents (ages 6 months to 18 years) who are receiving long-term aspirin therapy
Women who will be pregnant during the influenza season (usually December through March)
People who can transmit influenza to those at high risk:
- Health care personnel
- Employees of long-term-care facilities
- Employees of residences for people at high risk

Providers of home care to people at high risk:
- Household members (including children) of people at high risk

Groups to consider for vaccination:
- People at high risk traveling to locations where influenza may be circulating
- People providing essential community services
- Students and others in institutional settings
- Any person who wishes to reduce the risk of infection with influenza

From Smith N, Bresee J, Shay D, and others, Advisory Committee on Immunization Practices: Prevention and control of influenza, *MMWR* 55(RR19):1-42, 2006.

REFERENCES

1. Mandell GL, Bennett JE, Dolin R: *Mandell, Douglas, and Bennett's principles and practice of infectious diseases,* ed 5, New York, 2000, Churchill Livingstone.
2. Fauci A, Braumwald E, Isselbacher K, and others: *Harrison's principles of internal medicine,* ed 14, New York, 1998, McGraw-Hill.
3. Coonrad JD: Influenza: will new diagnostic tests and antiviral drugs make a difference? *Chest* 119(6):1630-1632, 2001.
4. Smith N, Bresee J, Shay D, and others, Advisory Committee on Immunization Practices: Prevention and control of influenza, *MMWR* 55(RR10):1-42, 2006.
5. Neuzil KM, Reed GW, Mitchell EF Jr, and others: Influenza-associated morbidity and mortality in young and middle-aged women, *JAMA* 281(10):901-907, 1999.
6. Couch RB: Prevention and treatment of influenza, *N Engl J Med* 343(24):1778-1787, 2000.

CHAPTER 248

Infectious Mononucleosis

Patricia Polgar Bailey

DEFINITION AND EPIDEMIOLOGY

Infectious mononucleosis (IM) is an acute, self-limiting, generally benign illness that occurs in both children and adults after primary infection with Epstein-Barr virus (EBV), cytomegalovirus (CMV), and other infectious agents. The classic manifestation of this syndrome includes fever, malaise, pharyngitis, lymphadenopathy, and atypical lymphocytosis, although atypical presentations, including symptomatic pulmonary involvement, also occur.[1] This syndrome was first described in the 1880s; however, the term *infectious mononucleosis* was not used until the 1920s. The link between EBV and IM was not discovered until the late 1960s.[2]

In this chapter, the term *Epstein-Barr virus–associated infectious mononucleosis* (EBV-IM) is used to refer to IM caused by acute EBV infection. The term *non–Epstein-Barr virus–associated IM* (non-EBV-IM) is used to refer to the clinical syndrome of IM that is caused by an agent other than EBV. The term *IM* is used to refer to the triad of fever, pharyngitis, and lymphadenopathy regardless of the infectious agent. This chapter deals primarily with the presentation, evaluation, and management of EBV-IM, the most common type of acute IM, which is seen in 20% to 70% of adolescents and young adults.[3]

The peak rate of EBV-IM occurs between the ages of 15 and 19 years in industrialized countries, and the annual incidence in this age-group is 345 to 671 cases per 100,000.[3] In persons younger than 10 and older than 30 years, the annual incidence of EBV-IM decreases dramatically to less than 1 case per 1000 persons, but mild infection in young adults may be underdiagnosed. It is most common in populations with many young adults, such as active-duty military personnel and college students, in whom the annual incidence ranges from 11 to 48 cases per 1000.[1] The incidence of EBV-IM is 30 times higher in Caucasians than in African Americans. No gender differences have been noted. Interestingly, more than 90% of adults worldwide have serologic evidence of prior EBV infection, which indicates that a significant number of EBV infections are atypical or without clinical manifestations.[2] The chance of developing IM after EBV infection appears to increase from childhood to young adulthood; it is estimated that less than 10% of children develop IM after EBV exposure, but up to 20% to 70% of adolescents have a chance of developing EBV-IM after acute EBV infection.[2] IM is relatively uncommon in adults, accounting for less than 2% of adults who see their health care provider with a sore throat.[1]

PATHOPHYSIOLOGY

IM can be caused by a variety of infectious agents other than EBV, including CMV, herpesvirus 6, HIV, adenovirus, hepatitis A virus, influenza A and B viruses, and rubella virus. In addition, IM is also associated with some neoplasms. Transmission of IM varies, depending on the specific causative infectious agent. Transmission of EBV-IM occurs through exposure to oropharyngeal secretions, although blood products have also been reported as a source of transmission. EBV is a relatively fragile DNA herpesvirus that cannot survive for long outside the host. The virus initially infects the oral epithelial cells and then spreads to the B lymphocytes, which then circulate through the reticuloendothelial system, causing a significant but time-limited immunologic response. Many of the signs and symptoms associated with the clinical presentation of EBV-IM are the result of this immunologic response. The incubation time of EBV-IM is usually between 4 and 8 weeks. Acute EBV infection stimulates the production of antibodies against EBV antigens, which remain present lifelong.[1,2]

CLINICAL PRESENTATION

The classic triad of symptoms of acute IM includes fever, pharyngitis, and lymphadenopathy. The typical adolescent with EBV-IM is seen with sore throat, fever, and lymph node and tonsillar enlargement. Additional common presenting symptoms include pharyngeal inflammation and transient palatal petechiae. Older adults are less likely to have sore throat and adenopathy but more likely to have hepatomegaly and jaundice.[1] However, IM often manifests atypically, making diagnosis difficult. Pharyngitis is usually diffuse, with exudates present in approximately 30% of cases. Lymphadenopathy usually affects the anterior and posterior cervical chain and may also be diffuse. Temperatures may be as high as 40° C (104° F) and may last as long as 2 weeks. Symptoms that may precede, as well as persist throughout, the acute phase of illness include malaise, anorexia, and fatigue. Symptoms of EBV-IM usually peak approximately 7 days after onset and become less pronounced during the next 1 to 3 weeks. Based on reports, splenic enlargement occurs in 40% to 100% of cases, although studies that have included ultrasonography as part of the evaluation suggest that splenomegaly may be more common than not.[2]

Less common signs and symptoms of EBV-IM include upper airway compromise, abdominal pain, rash, hepatomegaly, jaundice, and eyelid edema. The rash, which occurs in approximately 5% to 10% of individuals, may be macular, urticarial, petechial, or erythema multiforme.[2,4]

PHYSICAL EXAMINATION

On physical examination the patient may appear ill or may not, depending on degree of fever, associated signs and symptoms, and length of time since onset of symptoms. The classic clinical manifestation of fever, pharyngitis, and lymphadenopathy raises suspicion for EBV-IM. The anterior and posterior cervical chains should be assessed for lymphadenopathy, which may be diffuse. An abdominal examination identifies splenomegaly and hepatomegaly, which are complications of EBV-IM, especially in older adults. Rash and jaundice should be noted, since they are associated with EBV-IM in some cases.

DIAGNOSTICS

The most useful laboratory test is the serologic test for heterophil antibodies. These may be demonstrable at the onset of illness or may appear later in the course of the illness. The

DIAGNOSTICS

Infectious Mononucleosis

LABORATORY
Heterophil antibody
Viral capsid antigen IgG and IgM*
Epstein-Barr virus nuclear antigen*
CBC and differential*
LFTs*

IMAGING
Abdominal ultrasonography*

*If indicated.

accuracy of the test varies depending on the specific kit and reagent used, with sensitivity ranging from 63% to 84% and specificity ranging from 84% to 100%. The likelihood of positive heterophil antibodies in response to acute infection increases in direct response to the length of time since onset of symptoms. In addition, individuals more than 4 years of age are more likely to have positive antibodies in response to acute illness.[2]

False-positive heterophil antibody results, albeit rare, have also been associated with lymphoma, viral hepatitis, and autoimmune disease. In addition, 10% to 43% of individuals with acute IM may have titers that are lower than the range associated with positive infection.[2,4,5]

If the heterophil antibody test is negative but EBV-IM is still highly suspect, then further testing may be helpful. More sensitive tests have been developed that detect viral capsid antigen (VCA) immunoglobulin (Ig) G and IgM. When the results are negative, these tests are better than heterophil antibody tests in ruling out EBV-IM, since they are better able to detect acute infection, but when the results are positive, the tests are similar in their ability to rule in disease.[1] VCA IgG and IgM generally become positive within 1 to 2 weeks of infection, but VCA IgM becomes undetectable after 6 months. Antibody to Epstein-Barr nuclear antigen (EBNA) is not usually detectable until 6 to 8 weeks after the onset of symptoms, but can help distinguish between acute and previous infections. If EBNA is positive in the presence of acute symptoms and suspected IM, then previous infection is suggested. Liver enzymes are elevated in approximately 50% of persons with IM.[1]

Hoagland's criteria for the diagnosis of IM are the most widely cited and include at least 50% lymphocytes and at least 10% atypical lymphocytes in the presence of fever, pharyngitis, and adenopathy and confirmed by a positive serologic test. These criteria are quite specific but not highly sensitive, since only 50% of patients with symptoms consistent with IM and a positive heterophil antibody test meet all of Hoagland's criteria. Therefore these criteria, although frequently cited, are most useful for research purposes.[1]

DIFFERENTIAL DIAGNOSIS

The triad of fever, pharyngitis, and lymphadenopathy are associated with a number of diagnoses in addition to acute IM, including streptococcal pharyngitis and one of several viral pharyngitides, acute CMV infection, and acute HIV infection.[1] The reported incidence of IM in patients with peritonsillar abscess ranges from 2% to 20%; therefore it is recommended that all patients with peritonsillar abscess be fully clinically assessed and screened for IM.[6] If symptoms have been present for only a few days, group A β-hemolytic streptococcal pharyngitis or a viral upper respiratory tract infection should be considered. It is important to remember, however, that individuals with a positive streptococcal culture may also have acute IM. Individuals with a negative throat culture for group A β-hemolytic streptococcus and symptoms that persist for more than a week are highly suspect for acute IM.

DIFFERENTIAL DIAGNOSIS

Infectious Mononucleosis

INFECTIOUS CAUSES
- Bartonellosis (cat-scratch disease)
- *Corynebacterium diphtheriae*
- Cytomegalovirus
- Epstein-Barr virus
- Hepatitis A and B viruses
- HIV
- Human herpesvirus 6
- Lyme disease
- Malaria
- Meningococcemia
- Rubella
- *Salmonella* bacteremia
- *Streptococcus* pharyngitis
- Syphilis
- Toxoplasmosis
- Trichinosis
- Tuberculosis
- Viral pharyngitis

NONINFECTIOUS CAUSES
- Juvenile rheumatoid arthritis
- Kawasaki's disease
- Lymphoma
- Sarcoidosis
- Systemic lupus erythematosus

DRUGS
- Dapsone
- Phenytoin
- Sulfonamides

It may not be possible to distinguish clinically between IM caused by EBV infection and an IM-like syndrome caused by toxoplasmosis or CMV, and in fact the management of these syndromes is essentially the same. However, diagnostic testing to determine the etiology is important in pregnant women, since toxoplasmosis and acute HIV and CMV infections are associated with significant pregnancy complications. If acute HIV infection is suspected, a quantitative polymerase chain reaction test should be done.[1]

MANAGEMENT

Treatment of uncomplicated EBV-IM is primarily supportive, including adequate hydration, NSAIDs or acetaminophen for fever reduction and myalgias, throat lozenges or sprays, and gargling with a 2% lidocaine solution to relieve pharyngeal discomfort.[1] Aspirin should be avoided, since it has been associated with Reye's syndrome in a few cases of acute EBV.[7] Bed rest may be helpful during the acute phase of the illness depending on the degree of fatigue. Individuals with splenomegaly should be encouraged to refrain from strenuous physical activity for 3 to 4 weeks to avoid the risk of splenic rupture before resolution of the splenomegaly. Studies have shown that neither corticosteroids nor acyclovir reduced the severity or duration of symptoms. Therefore current management guidelines do not include the use of either of these agents in the treatment of acute uncomplicated EBV-IM,[1,2] although corticosteroids may be useful in the treatment of several complications associated with EBV-IM such as airway obstruction.[8] Most patients with EBV-IM recover spontaneously in approximately 2 to 4 weeks.[2]

LIFE SPAN CONSIDERATIONS

Older individuals are at risk for misdiagnosis of EBV-IM because the disease is relatively uncommon in older adults, occurring in only 3% to 10% of those 40 years of age or older. In addition, older adults with acute IM often manifest the disease differently; fever is present in more than 90% of individuals, but pharyngitis and lymphadenopathy are seen in less than 50% of patients.[3] The risk of EBV-associated liver disease is more common in older adults, however, and hepatitis, cholestasis, and hepatomegaly are seen in substantial numbers of older adults with EBV-IM as well. Jaundice is seen in more than 20% of older individuals.[3] Similarly, the risk of EBV-IM-associated hepatic failure and other complications increases with age. Nonetheless, the prognosis for EBV-IM is good even in older individuals.

COMPLICATIONS

The most common complications of EBV-IM, albeit rare, include upper airway obstruction, hepatomegaly, splenomegaly, and splenic rupture. Patients with IM are likely to have splenomegaly, even if it is not detected on physical examination. Ultrasonography done on patients hospitalized with IM revealed that only 17% of the enlarged spleens and 8% of the enlarged livers were palpable on physical examination.[1] Because splenomegaly increases the risk of splenic rupture, athletes should not compete in contact or collision sports for 3 to 4 weeks after onset of symptoms. Splenic rupture is estimated at 0.1% based on retrospective studies.[1]

In 1% to 2% of cases, EBV-IM has been associated with neurologic complications, including cranial nerve palsies, Guillain-Barré syndrome, encephalitis, and peripheral neuropathies. In rare cases EBV-IM has been associated with fatal conduction abnormalities and myocarditis. In addition, there is increasing evidence that EBV infection may be implicated in the development of multiple sclerosis, in particular contributing to the initiation of this disease.[9] Various ophthalmologic problems have been associated with EBV-IM, including keratitis, uveitis, retinopathy, and periorbital cellulitis. Complications of EBV-IM can also result in a variety of renal pathologic conditions, including nephritic syndrome, hemolytic uremic syndrome, and renal failure. Hematologic complications include aplastic anemia, thrombocytopenia, and acute monoarthritis.[2,7]

The association between EBV-IM and chronic fatigue has been controversial for some time. Transient fatigue is part of acute IM; however, the evidence for EBV-associated chronic fatigue is questionable. In fact, the Centers for Disease Control and Prevention do not consider workup for EBV infection to be useful in the evaluation of individuals suffering from chronic fatigue. Several studies have found that psychiatric morbidity and distress are associated with delayed recovery or development of chronic fatigue syndrome, although it has been difficult to confirm these findings.[10]

INDICATIONS FOR REFERRAL OR HOSPITALIZATION

IM caused by EBV is generally a self-limiting disease of young adults. However, mild liver enzyme abnormalities are not uncommon, and hepatitis is a rare but well-recognized complication of EBV infection that generally resolves spontaneously. IM is rarely seen in older adults; however, the potential for complications appears to increase in the older population, and several cases of severe cholestatic jaundice associated with IM have been reported in this age-group. Abdominal imaging should be obtained in such cases to rule out a malignant extrahepatic biliary obstruction, and acute EBV infection should be considered in patients with cholestasis. Because this complication is rare, it is generally not established until more common causes have been eliminated and serology consistent with EBV infection has been obtained.[11] The rate of peritonsillar abscess has been estimated as high as 23%.[6] Peritonsillar abscess can be a medical emergency, requiring surgical drainage and antibiotic therapy. Because of associated dysphagia and possible respiratory compromise, hospitalization may be indicated while treatment is initiated.

PATIENT AND FAMILY EDUCATION

Education about the nature of the illness and prognosis is important. Acute IM has been referred to colloquially as the "kissing disease," and it is important to communicate that transmission through oropharyngeal secretions occurs in a variety of ways other than kissing. Changes in routines and schedules during the first few of weeks should be encouraged to allow for sufficient rest. The fact that acute IM is usually an uncomplicated, self-limiting illness is reassuring, especially during the first few weeks when the manifestations are most pronounced. However, education about the possible complications is important so that proper treatment can be initiated should any complications occur.

REFERENCES

1. Ebell M: Epstein-Barr virus infectious mononucleosis, *Am Fam Phys* 70(7):1279-1287, 1289-1290, 2004.
2. Godshall SE, Kirschner JT: Infectious mononucleosis: complexities of a common syndrome, *Postgrad Med* 107(7):175-186, 2000.
3. Auwaerter PG: Infectious mononucleosis, *JAMA* 281(5):454-459, 1999.
4. Schooley RT: Epstein-Barr virus (infectious mononucleosis). In Mandell GL, Bennett JE, Dolin R, editors: *Mandell, Douglas, and Bennett's principles and practice of infectious diseases,* ed 4, New York, 1995, Churchill Livingstone.
5. White PD, Thomas JM, Amess J, and others: Incidence, risk and prognosis of acute and chronic fatigue syndromes and psychiatric disorders after glandular fever, *Br J Psychiatry* 173:475-481, 1998.
6. Ryan C, Dutta C, Simo R: Role of screening for infectious mononucleosis in patients admitted with isolated unilateral peritonsillar abscess, *J Laryngol Otol* 118:362-365, 2004.
7. Bailey RE: Diagnosis and treatment of infectious mononucleosis, *Am Fam Phys* 49(4):879-888, 1994.
8. Thompson S, Doerr T, Hengerer A: Infectious mononucleosis and corticosteroids, *Arch Otolaryngol Head Neck Surg* 131:900-904, 2005.
9. Goldacre J, Wotton C, Seagroatt V, and others: Multiple sclerosis after infectious mononucleosis: record linkage study, *J Epidemiol Commun Health* 58:1032-1035, 2004.
10. Buchwald DS, Rea TD, Katon WJ, and others: Acute infectious mononucleosis: characteristic of patients who report failure to recover, *Am J Med* 109(7):531-537, 2000.
11. Tahan V, Ozaras R, Uzunismail H, and others: Infectious mononucleosis presenting with severe cholestatic liver disease in the elderly, *J Clin Gastroenterol* 33(1):88-89, 2001.

CHAPTER 249

Infectious Diarrhea

Terry Davies, Thomas H. Taylor, and
Joanne Sandberg-Cook

DEFINITION AND EPIDEMIOLOGY

Diarrhea is an alteration in a normal bowel movement characterized by an increase in volume or frequency of stools. Infectious diarrhea is diarrhea with an infectious etiology, often accompanied by symptoms of nausea, vomiting, or abdominal cramping. Infectious diarrhea can be further defined as inflammatory or noninflammatory. Acute diarrhea is an episode of diarrhea lasting less than 14 days.[1] Infectious diarrheal diseases are the second leading cause of morbidity and mortality worldwide. In the United States some 211 million to 375 million episodes of diarrheal illness occur each year, resulting in 3100 deaths.[2]

PATHOPHYSIOLOGY

The small intestine absorbs approximately 8.5 L of fluid daily, while the colon absorbs another 1.5 L. An estimated 200 ml of fluid is lost in stool. Pathogens such as viruses, bacteria, or parasites can cause diarrhea. Viruses usually occur on a year-round basis but peak in the winter months. Bacterial illnesses are more common in the summer or early fall. Causes of acute infectious diarrhea are categorized as noninflammatory or inflammatory (see Differential Diagnosis box, p. 1324). Infectious diarrhea, the most common type of diarrhea, is spread by food or water contamination, person-to-person contact, the fecal-oral route, or animals.[3,4]

Risk factors include travel, ingestion of certain foods (chicken, meat, fried rice, mayonnaise or cream, eggs, seafood), and an immunocompromised state. Daycare employees, institutionalized persons, and patients with certain medical conditions (Reiter's syndrome, thyroiditis, pericarditis, and glomerulonephritis) may also be at increased risk for contracting infectious diarrhea.[5]

CLINICAL PRESENTATION

The medical history is most helpful in determining the cause of infectious diarrhea. The patient's normal bowel pattern should be ascertained. Questions about when the diarrhea began, whether the onset was abrupt or gradual, and the characteristic of the stool are all necessary. The provider should also ask about bowel symptoms such as abdominal pain, rectal discomfort, blood or mucus in the stool, weight loss, and nocturnal diarrhea. The presence of associated nausea, vomiting, and fever is ascertained. Signs of dehydration include increased thirst, oliguria, dizziness, and dark or concentrated urine.

Recent travel (<6 months) and consumption of raw meat, eggs, shellfish, or unpasteurized milk should be noted. Episodes of swimming in or drinking untreated water, including mountain streams, ponds, or wells, are documented. An occupational history as a caregiver, food handler, or animal handler is noted. A family history of recent diarrheal illness, especially if meals have been shared, raises the suspicion of food poisoning.

Acute diarrhea accounts for 90% of cases and is typically self-limiting. Symptoms range from mild abdominal cramping with three or fewer loose stools per day to profuse diarrhea with fever, bloody stools, severe abdominal pain, and dehydration.

PHYSICAL EXAMINATION

The physical examination includes weight and temperature and orthostatic vital signs (blood pressure and heart rate lying, sitting, and standing) to assess volume depletion (dry mucous membranes, decreased skin turgor, absent jugular venous pulsation). The patient's mental status should be noted along with a close assessment for skin color, temperature, rashes, or joint inflammation (Reiter's syndrome). The head and neck should be assessed for evidence of conjunctivitis (suggesting Reiter's syndrome), infection, thyromegaly, or lymphadenopathy.

Particular emphasis during the abdominal examination is necessary to detect abdominal distention, peristalsis, masses, organomegaly, tenderness, rigidity, rebound, guarding, fecal impaction, or bleeding. In the female patient with lower abdominal symptoms, a pelvic examination is imperative. In the geriatric patient, fecal impaction must be ruled out.[1]

DIAGNOSTICS

For the patient who has mild, afebrile, acute diarrhea, diagnostic evaluation is typically not indicated. This diarrhea is usually viral and considered benign. Symptoms usually resolve within 1 week, often within 1 to 3 days, and a diagnosis is rarely documented.

A stool sample for fecal leukocytes should be taken for patients with a fever over 38.8° C (102° F), bloody diarrhea, abdominal pain, more than six unformed stools in a 24-hour period, profuse watery diarrhea, and dehydration, or for patients who are frail and elderly or immunocompromised.

A CBC, serum electrolytes, BUN, and creatinine are necessary. Stool evaluation for occult blood and fecal leukocytes may be indicated in certain circumstances (see above). Normally no fecal leukocytes or polymorphonuclear cells are found in the stool. These are associated with *Campylobacter, Shigella*, or *Salmonella* organisms; *Clostridium difficile;* and enterohemorrhagic *Escherichia coli*. If fecal leukocytes are present, typically in inflammatory diarrhea, the stool should be further evaluated for ova and parasites and a stool culture. If *C. difficile* is suspected, a stool sample for both culture and *C. difficile* toxin is necessary.

DIAGNOSTICS

Infectious Diarrhea

LABORATORY

- CBC and differential*
- Serum electrolytes
- Serum glucose
- BUN
- Creatinine*
- Stool for occult blood and fecal leukocytes*
- Stool for ova and parasites, cultures for *Clostridium difficile**

*If indicated.

DIFFERENTIAL DIAGNOSIS

Differential diagnoses to consider with acute diarrhea are classified as noninflammatory and inflammatory. The inflammatory pathogens usually affect the integrity of the lower intestinal mucosa. They can manifest with fever and bloody stools. The noninflammatory pathogens usually affect the upper gastrointestinal tract. There may or may not be fever, but bloody diarrhea is an uncommon presenting symptom.

Physician consultation is indicated if diarrhea is accompanied by high fever, abdominal pain, dehydration, or bloody stools.

Travelers' Diarrhea

Travelers' diarrhea is a clinical syndrome resulting from the ingestion of microbe-contaminated food or water. The diarrhea can occur during or up to 10 days after travel.[6] It affects 20% to 50% of travelers to developing countries, including parts of the Caribbean, southern Asia, and Africa. Travelers' diarrhea generally lasts approximately 3 to 5 days. It is usually a self-limiting illness, and the patient rarely develops complications. Postinfection sequelae have been described,[7] including reactive arthritis, Guillain-Barré syndrome, and irritable bowel syndrome. The causative bacterial agents include enterotoxigenic *E. coli* (ETEC), enteroaggregative *E. coli* (EAEC), *Campylobacter jejuni*, *Salmonella* organisms, and *Shigella* organisms.[7]

A variety of other organisms, including viruses (rotavirus, norovirus [previously Norwalk-like virus]) and parasites (*Entamoeba histolytica*, *Cryptosporidium parvum*, *Giardia* organisms), can cause 10% to 20% of cases of travelers' diarrhea.

ETEC is the cause of most travelers' diarrhea. The diarrhea occurs within 24 to 72 hours with mild watery diarrhea and occasionally fever or vomiting. The diarrhea is self-limiting. Treatment includes oral fluid replacement (commercial or homemade solutions [Box 249-1]). Travelers must remember to use only sealed or carbonated beverages. Loperamide (Imodium), 4 mg PO at onset and 2 mg after each loose stool up to 16 mg/day, can be helpful. Antibiotics may shorten the duration of illness to 24 to 36 hours. A 3-day course of ciprofloxacin 50 mg PO b.i.d. or azithromycin as a single 1000-mg dose may be prescribed. Bismuth subsalicylate (Pepto-Bismol) has both antimicrobial and antiinflammatory effects and may be taken as 2 tablets every 30 to 60 minutes up to eight doses per day.[6]

Prevention is the cornerstone of treatment. Travelers' diarrhea can be avoided by not drinking untreated water or ice cubes or unpasteurized milk, and not eating raw fruits and vegetables and undercooked meat. Chemoprophylactic agents, including bismuth subsalicylate and *Lactobacillus acidophilus*, are recommended, but the benefit is uncertain. Antibiotics are typically not prescribed as a preventive measure for most travelers. Widespread antibiotic resistance to ampicillin, to trimethoprim-sulfamethoxazole (Bactrim DS), and, increasingly, to quinolones have made these agents less useful for the treatment of travelers' diarrhea.[7] In addition, they are not effective against viral or parasitic infections and may provide a false sense of security.

Noninflammatory Diarrhea

Noninflammatory diarrhea does not invade the tissue but colonizes the small bowel mucosa. This causes the small bowel to secrete excess fluid and electrolytes. Therefore there is little

DIFFERENTIAL DIAGNOSIS

Diarrhea

INFECTIOUS DIARRHEA	NONINFECTIOUS DIARRHEA
Noninflammatory Type	Drugs
Viruses	• Laxatives
• Rotavirus	• Antibiotics
• Norovirus	• Antiarrhythmic agents
Bacteria	• Diuretics
• Enterotoxigenic *Escherichia coli*	Lactose intolerance
• *Clostridium perfringens*	Toxins
• *Staphylococcus aureus*	• Heavy metals
• *Bacillus cereus*	• Insecticides
• *Vibrio cholerae*	Endocrine disorders
Parasites	Thyroid disease
• *Giardia lamblia*	Diabetes
• *Cryptosporidium* organisms	Irritable bowel syndrome
Inflammatory Type	Inflammatory bowel disease
Bacteria	Crohn's disease
• *Campylobacter jejuni*	Malignancies
• *Shigella* organisms	HIV disease
• Enterohemorrhagic *E. coli*	Tropical sprue
• *Clostridium difficile*	Celiac sprue
• *Vibrio parahaemolyticus*	Scleroderma
• *Salmonella* organisms	Short bowel syndrome
Parasites	Whipple's disease
• *Entamoeba histolytica*	

BOX 249-1

HOMEMADE ORAL REHYDRATING SOLUTIONS

One serving
8 oz of apple juice or juice diluted with water 1:1
½ tsp honey (do not use in children younger than 1 year) or corn syrup
Pinch of salt
Followed by
8 oz clear water
¼ tsp baking soda
Or
One liter
4½ cups water
¼ tsp salt substitute (with potassium)
½ tsp baking soda
½ tsp salt
2 to 3 Tbsp sugar, honey (do not use in children younger than 1 year), or corn syrup
Or
Rehydration with active diarrhea
¼ cup baby rice cereal
8 oz water
Pinch of salt
Flavoring or ½ to 1 tsp of sugar may make this more palatable
Drink one serving after each loose stool

Adapted from Kelly D, Nadeau J: Oral rehydration solution: a "low-tech" oft neglected therapy, retrieved March 12, 2006, from http://www.healthsystem.virginia.edu/internet/digestive-health/nutritionarticles/KellyArticle.pdf.

damage to the tissue.[7] Symptoms include massive volumes of diarrhea that is watery but not bloody. It is associated with cramping in the periumbilical region, bloating, nausea, or vomiting. This large amount of volume loss may quickly lead to dehydration associated with hypokalemia and metabolic acidosis. Noninflammatory diarrhea is usually caused by either a toxin-producing bacterium such as ETEC, *Staphylococcus aureus, Bacillus cereus, Clostridium perfringens, Vibrio cholerae,* rotavirus, and norovirus or parasites such as *Giardia lamblia* or cryptosporidia (see Differential Diagnosis box, p. 1324). If the diarrhea is caused by viral enteritis or *S. aureus*, food poisoning should be suspected.[1,5]

C. perfringens causes illness 8 to 4 hours after consumption of contaminated meat, poultry, or legumes. Symptoms include diarrhea and crampy abdominal pain that usually lasts 24 hours. Treatment includes fluid replacement. Antibiotics are not indicated.[5]

S. aureus food poisoning has a rapid onset within 2 to 6 hours and resolves within 10 hours. Symptoms include vomiting and diarrhea. Treatment includes fluid replacement. *S. aureus* has been associated with institutional outbreaks.[5]

V. cholerae is a classic example of reemerging epidemics through the ages, brought on by natural disasters, civil war, and displaced populations. Infants and young children bear the brunt of epidemics in third-world nations, where 80% of all diarrheal deaths occur in children under the age of 5.[8]

Cholera is a natural aquatic inhabitant, which lives attached to algae, crustaceans, and plankton. Cholera periodically emerges from its dormant state, inspired by warm waters (e.g., El Niño), and its growth is facilitated by changes in nutrients and salinity (e.g., from monsoons, tsunamis, and typhoons).[9] In its activated state it grows and, once humans are infected, spreads rapidly as a water-borne or food-borne pathogen. Person-to-person spread is unlikely because of the large inoculum required for infection. Disasters provide ready availability of contaminated water and food.

Severe dehydration, electrolyte imbalance, renal failure, and metabolic acidosis can all be fatal complications of cholera, and oral or IV rehydration is paramount. Mortality is as high as 10% in epidemic settings without adequate health care support, but only 3% in centers versed in simple hydration techniques. Antibiotics are secondary in importance to hydration in the treatment of cholera. One 300-mg dose of doxycycline, 1 g of ciprofloxacin, or one tablet trimethoprim-sulfamethoxazole b.i.d. for 3 days is effective treatment, if the organism is sensitive. But emerging antibiotic resistance is a problem for developing nations. Vaccines have not produced effective or long-lasting immunity, and none is currently recommended.[10] Fortunately, cholera is a predictably reemergent disease, less likely to be encountered during routine travel, but most likely to be encountered after natural disasters, in refugee camps, and in urban slums where it is endemic. Simple measures to dispose of human waste, avoid contaminated water, and provide a potable water supply all work well in developing nations.[11]

Rotavirus is a viral agent associated with viral gastroenteritis that is transmitted via the fecal-oral route. It occurs predominantly in children under 5 years of age during the colder months. Worldwide, rotavirus kills an estimated 610,000 children each year. In the United States the virus accounts for 70,000 hospitalizations annually.[12] Infection can occur in adults. The virus manifests with vomiting lasting from less than 24 hours up to 4 to 8 days, accompanied by diarrhea and a low-grade fever. The stools are watery and yellow and may contain mucus and blood. The diarrhea is often so severe that, if untreated, it can lead to dehydration and shock very quickly. Rotavirus is found in stool cultures; polymerase chain reaction (PCR) will also detect the virus. Treatment includes oral fluid replacement, antiemetics, or bismuth subsalicylate. Recently, a vaccine has been approved for general use in more than 20 countries, including the European Union, and is under review in the United States. The vaccine confers 85% to 98% protection from severe rotavirus diarrhea.[12]

Norovirus (previously Norwalk-like virus) is a food-borne and water-borne agent that affects older children and adults. More than 90% of viral gastroenteritis in the United States is caused by noroviruses. It is transmitted via the fecal-oral route. The onset of symptoms occurs from 1 to 3 days after infection and is associated with a gradual or abrupt onset of abdominal cramping and nausea that progress to vomiting and diarrhea. The patient may experience from four to eight watery stools without mucus or bleeding along with general malaise, myalgia, and a low-grade fever (38.3° to 38.8° C [101° to 102° F]). Stool leukocytes are typically not present. No diagnostic tests are available to detect the virus in stool samples. It can be detected using the PCR test. Treatment is oral fluid replacement, antiemetics, or bismuth subsalicylate.[13]

Giardiasis (caused by *G. lamblia*) is a protozoal infection that is transmitted by fecal contamination of water or food, person-to-person contact, or anal-oral intercourse. The parasite is found in untreated rivers, streams, ponds, and well water. Common in daycare centers, dormitories, and institutions, giardiasis can be acute or chronic with an incubation period of 1 to 3 weeks; the onset can be gradual or sudden. The diarrhea ranges from mild to severe and is greasy with a foul odor, but the stools are not bloody or purulent. Nausea, vomiting, and abdominal cramping are less common. Stool samples should be tested for ova and parasites 1 week after the onset of diarrhea (number of organisms varies day to day). Three stool specimens are collected every 2 days.[14] Treatment varies, although it is recommended that treatment be initiated for patients in high-risk areas. The drug of choice is tinidazole 2 g PO as a single dose. Although it is expensive, a short course is well tolerated. Another choice is metronidazole 250 to 750 mg PO t.i.d. for 5 to 7 days. Children should be treated with furazolidone 100 mg q.i.d. for 7 to 10 days and nitazoxanide 500 mg b.i.d. orally for 3 days.[14]

Cryptosporidiosis is another protozoal infection that is transmitted fecal-orally person-to-person or by contaminated food or water (drinking, swimming pool, hot tubs, lakes, rivers, and ponds) that may be contaminated with sewage or feces. Once a person is infected, the parasite lives in the intestinal tract and is shed in the stool. Once outside the body, it can live on surfaces for an extended period and is difficult to eradicate even with bleach-based cleaners. Outbreaks may occur in households, daycare centers, and sexual partners. Immunosuppressed patients, especially patients with AIDS, are at higher risk. Clinically, the illness may be mild and self-limiting or be severe with explosive, frequent, watery diarrhea. Mucus may be present in the stool, but usually no blood or leukocytes are present. Other symptoms include low-grade fever, anorexia, myalgia, malaise, abdominal cramping, vomiting, and dehydration. These symptoms can last from a few days to a few weeks. The diagnosis is confirmed by three fresh stool samples over 5 to 7 days. Other diagnostics include the PCR test and serum antibody tests. Also available are commercial antigen detection kits. Most cases are self-limiting and just require oral rehydration. Antibiotic medications have not been particularly helpful. Nitazoxanide (Alina) has recently been approved for use in children and adults with healthy immune systems. The usual adult dosage is 500 mg PO b.i.d. for 3 days. For AIDS patients, antiretroviral medications that will strengthen the immune system seem to be most helpful. Other medications that have been used with some success include paromomycin (Humatin), azithromycin, and octreotide. Hyperimmune bovine colostrums and lactobacillus have also been tried without consistent success.[15,16]

Inflammatory Diarrhea

Inflammatory diarrhea occurs when the cells of the intestinal mucosa are destroyed by the offending pathogen. These pathogens affect the large intestine, so the amount of diarrhea is minimal.[7] Symptoms include fever and bloody diarrhea (dysentery) along with left lower quadrant cramping, an urgent need to defecate, and tenesmus. Fecal leukocytes may be present. Inflammatory diarrhea is usually caused by shigellosis, salmonellosis, *Campylobacter* or *Yersinia* infection, amebiasis, or a toxin such as *C. difficile* or *E. coli* O157:H7 (see Differential Diagnosis box, p. 1324). Cytomegalovirus can cause intestinal ulceration with watery or blood diarrhea in the immunocompromised or HIV patient.[1]

C. jejuni is common and the leading cause of food-borne diarrhea in the United States. Transmission occurs when contaminated raw or undercooked food is ingested or with direct contact with infected animals. The illness is self-limiting and manifests with a prodrome of fever, headache, and myalgia. Diarrhea occurs in 12 to 48 hours and may be associated with fever and crampy abdominal pain. It may continue for 3 to 4 weeks. Diagnosis is confirmed by a stool specimen for culture. Treatment consists of erythromycin 250 mg PO q.i.d. for 5 to 7 days. An alternative choice is a fluoroquinolone such as ciprofloxacin 500 mg PO b.i.d. Caution should be exercised due to increasing resistance to fluoroquinolones. Gentamicin, imipenem, or chloramphenicol intravenously is indicated for systemic infections.[17]

Shigellosis is caused by *Shigella sonnei* in the United States and by *Shigella flexneri* and *Shigella dysenteriae* in developing countries. It is transmitted person to person. Clinical symptoms include mild watery diarrhea to severe dysentery, along with fever, after 1 to 7 days. Diagnosis is confirmed with fecal leukocytes and a stool culture. If it is untreated, diarrhea and fever will persist. Treatment includes fluid replacement and antibiotic therapy.[18] Trimethoprim-sulfamethoxazole (160/800 mg) PO b.i.d. or ampicillin 500 mg PO q.i.d. for 5 to 7 days is the drug of choice. However, there are now resistant strains. Ciprofloxacin 500 mg PO b.i.d. or azithromycin or IV ceftriaxone 50 mg/kg/day are alternative choices. Single doses of ciprofloxacin or azithromycin have also shown success. A serious complication is hemolytic uremic syndrome.[18]

Antibiotic-associated diarrhea (AAD), primarily *C. difficile*, has been a problem since the advent of broad-spectrum antibiotics, which alter anaerobic and enteric bowel flora, allowing antibiotic-resistant *C. difficile* to grow and produce diarrhea and more severe pseudomembranous colitis. There has been a gradual increase in *C. difficile*–associated disease over the past 10 to 15 years, but more urgent concern is raised by several recent studies showing both increasing rates and increasing severity of *C. difficile* colitis.[19] The new epidemic is occurring in widespread geographic areas; causes disease in previously healthy patients[20]; and is dominated by a previously uncommon strain of *C. difficile*, which produces a new binary toxin, similar to the more virulent binary toxin in *C. perfringens*. Recent overuse of fluoroquinolones may have selected out this particular strain of *C. difficile*, much as clindamycin selected out past strains of *C. difficile* and was more closely associated with AAD than other antibiotics. The new epidemic strain of *C. difficile* is not resistant to either metronidazole or vancomycin.[21-23]

Although any antibiotic can cause *C. difficile* colitis, the most common offending antibiotics are third-generation cephalosporins and clindamycin. The illness may completely resolve after discontinuation of the offending medication, but also can appear up to 3 months after the medication has been taken. Clinically, the patient develops a fever; elevated WBC count; and profuse, foul-smelling diarrhea. The diagnosis is confirmed by stool culture for *C. difficile* toxin. The goals of treatment include preventing spread of infection to other patients and improving the patient's condition. Management includes stopping the offending antibiotic and, if indicated, administering metronidazole 500 mg PO t.i.d. or vancomycin 125 to 250 mg PO q.i.d. for 7 to 10 days.[24,25]

Recurrent *C. difficile* diarrhea follows a course of treatment in up to 20% of cases, and multiple relapses occur in at least 6%. Repeat testing for *C. difficile* toxin should not be done if diarrhea is improving, since toxin and culture may remain positive in many improving patients. True relapses should be treated with another course of metronidazole, with the dosage gradually tapered each week (i.e., 500 mg t.i.d., then the same dose b.i.d., q day, every other day, and every third day). IV vancomycin should not be considered because it does not penetrate the gastric mucosa. If diarrhea persists despite treatment, cholestyramine 4 g/day with or without lactobacilli 1 to 2 g PO q.i.d. is added to the treatment regimen. Antimotility agents should be avoided. There is new evidence that resistant strains of *C. difficile* are emerging.[21-23]

Epidemic *C. difficile* places new emphasis on preventive measures. Antibiotic use should be limited to the shortest effective course and the narrowest spectrum antibiotic for each pathogen. Broad-spectrum empiric regimens should be narrowed as culture results return, and more specific diagnosis may allow for early discontinuation. Isolation and cohorting of cases should be accompanied by gowns, gloves, and hand-washing. Alcohol scrubs do not inactivate *C. difficile* spores, so soap and water are required to remove them from hands. Electronic thermometers should be replaced by disposable thermometers. Broad-spectrum antimicrobial use should be subject to approval by an infectious disease expert, and use of clindamycin, gatifloxacin, moxifloxacin, and levofloxacin should be limited.[21-23]

Vibrio parahaemolyticus is associated with uncooked seafood. Symptoms occur within 4 hours to 4 days after ingestion. Watery diarrhea is accompanied by abdominal cramps, nausea, vomiting, fever, and chills. Diagnosis is confirmed with a stool culture. Treatment recommendations include oral hydration and, if the illness is severe, tetracycline 500 mg PO q.i.d. for 5 to 7 days.[26]

Salmonella is transmitted through the ingestion of contaminated food, especially eggs and poultry, improperly washed fruits and vegetables, or water. Pet turtles have been implicated in the transmission. Clinical symptoms can last up to 2 weeks, but appear 2 to 4 hours after exposure and are associated with diarrhea, cramps, nausea, vomiting, and fever. Diagnosis is confirmed with stool culture. Fecal leukocytes may be present. Patients at risk include those using antacids, antibiotics, antimotility drugs, or immunosuppressive agents and those with HIV infection or sickle cell disease.[27]

E. histolytica infection, or amebiasis, is a parasitic illness that causes death worldwide. It commonly occurs in the tropics, Mexico, Central and South America, India, Asia, and Africa. Individuals at risk include travelers, immigrants, sexual contacts, and institutionalized patients. Illness occurs 2 to 6 weeks after the ingestion of cysts from contaminated water and food or from person-to-person contact. The illness may initially be mild with gradually increasing severity of symptoms. The patient may have 10 to 12 liquid stools per day with blood and mucus in the stool, plus malaise, weight loss, and diffuse abdominal pain. Hepatomegaly is rarely seen. However, close observation is indicated if this occurs because hepatic abscess can occur. Hospitalization is common for affected individuals. Medication treatment includes metronidazole 750 mg PO t.i.d. for 7 to 10 days followed by iodoquinol 650 mg PO t.i.d. for 20 days, diloxanide furoate 500 PO t.i.d. for 10 days (not commercially available; obtained from the Centers for Disease Control and Prevention), or paromomycin 500 mg PO t.i.d. for 10 days.[1]

Escherichia coli O157:H7

E. coli O157:H7 was first recognized as a food-borne pathogen in the United States in 1982. Outbreaks occurred via distribution of contaminated hamburger meat, and EHEC soon became the most common cause of bloody diarrhea; The CDC estimates 73,000 illnesses annually in the United States, resulting in more than 2000 hospitalizations and 60 deaths.[28] *E. coli* O157:H7 is a zoonotic emerging pathogen, which normally resides in the gut of healthy cattle. Early outbreaks of *E. coli* O157:H7–mediated disease were traced to unpasteurized apple cider, which was made from fallen apples in orchards where cattle grazed, thus contaminating it with feces.[29] Discovery of this relationship has resulted in recognition of the need to pasteurize apple cider. Improved cooking standards in fast-food restaurants have decreased the incidence of *E. coli* O157:H7 in ground beef foods, but the problem has shifted to water-borne and vegetable-associated disease. Our preference for organic foods, rejection of chemical fertilizer for cow manure, and contamination of water and vegetables with *E. coli* O157:H7 have introduced new sources of what use to be the "hamburger disease."[29]

Another unique aspect of *E. coli* O157:H7 is the spectrum of disease this organism may confer, from mild diarrhea to severe hemorrhagic colitis. Treatment of EHEC diarrhea requires hydration and correction of electrolyte imbalance. Antibiotic treatment causes release of shiga-like toxin, a toxin also present in *S. dysenteriae,* and had been thought to worsen the risk of hemolytic uremic syndrome (HUS),[30] although a recent meta-analysis did not show an increased risk of HUS associated with antibiotic administration.[31] By the time HUS appears, the acute diarrhea has already subsided, so antibiotics are not likely to help.

MANAGEMENT

Medications can be used for symptomatic relief of nausea and vomiting, abdominal cramping, and diarrhea. These are generally used in older children and healthy adults. Absorbents and antisecretory agents such as bismuth subsalicylate (Kaopectate, Pepto Bismol) and antispasmodic-anticholinergic sedatives such as atropine sulfate, scopolamine hydrobromide, hyoscyamine sulfate, and phenobarbital are used to decrease abdominal cramping. Antisecretory agents such as bismuth subsalicylate also have an antiinflammatory effect and are commonly used if there is vomiting and abdominal cramping. These products may cause salicylate toxicity and should be used cautiously. Patients taking warfarin should be warned as well because anticoagulation will be affected. Concomitant use of bismuth subsalicylate with antibiotics may decrease the effectiveness of the antibiotics.[32]

Antimotility agents that are used in noninflammatory diarrhea include loperamide, diphenoxylate hydrochloride–atropine sulfate (Lomotil), or tincture of opium. Loperamide is preferred in children, pregnant women, and immunocompromised patients. If nausea is the main complaint, treatment with promethazine (Phenergan), prochlorperazine (Compazine), or another antiemetic is recommended.[1] Antimotility agents should not be used in patients with bloody diarrhea or fecal leukocytosis.

Empiric treatment with antibiotics should be considered in the presence of fecal leukocytes without a confirmed positive stool culture; with occult blood; if the patient has fever with profuse, watery diarrhea (>8 stools/day), appears dehydrated, has had symptoms for more than 1 week, and is immunocompromised; or if hospitalization is considered. *Salmonella, Shigella,* or *Campylobacter* pathogens are the most likely cause of the infection in these cases. Ciprofloxacin or norfloxacin can be initiated until the stool culture results are verified but should not be used in children or pregnant or lactating women. If the diarrhea persists for longer than 2 weeks, *Giardia* organisms may be suspected and metronidazole can be initiated. Specific therapy is initiated once the pathogen is identified.[32]

COMPLICATIONS

Complications from diarrhea are usually the result of dehydration. Regardless of the cause, attention should be directed toward fluid and electrolyte replacement. Electrolyte disorders, particularly hypocalcemia, hypomagnesemia, and hypokalemia, are common in persistent diarrhea. Continuous diarrhea can require hospitalization for fluid and electrolyte replacement if the patient is unable to maintain hydration with oral fluid replacement. Sepsis and cardiovascular collapse are potential complications, and infants, older adults, and immunosuppressed patients are more susceptible to these complications. Refractory diarrhea is usually a symptom of a more serious illness and requires diagnostic evaluation and immediate physician consultation.[32]

Further, association of *E. coli* O157:H7 diarrhea with childhood HUS has come to exemplify how a pathogen at one site can explain a disease at another uninfected site. HUS was previously an unexplained illness, defined by hemolysis, thrombocytopenia, and acute renal failure, often in children. EHEC have evolved by acquiring a symbiotic relationship with a bacteriophage that encodes SLT, a toxin also present in *Shigella dysenteriae*. SLT attaches to a receptor, globotriaosylceramide (GB), on enterocytes in the gut. GB receptors also exist on endothelial cells of glomerular capillaries and other small capillary beds. Damage to these capillary beds, by circulating SLT, explains the occurrence of acute renal failure, microangiopathic hemolytic anemia, and thrombocytopenia, which define HUS.[31,33] Further investigation demonstrates that HUS is the most common cause of acute renal failure in children. Neutralizing antibodies to SLT develop in most children before the age of 10 and decline as they age. Thus persons most severely affected by *E. coli* O157:H7 are the young and the elderly. *E. coli* O157:H7 has emerged as a common cause of HUS, a disease not previously recognized as infectious.[34]

INDICATIONS FOR REFERRAL OR HOSPITALIZATION

If dehydration is severe or vomiting is protracted, IV fluids should be initiated. If symptoms of the illness persist beyond 3 weeks despite treatment measures, the provider should consider chronic lactose intolerance; giardiasis; malignancies; and disease states such as diabetes, thyrotoxicosis, lupus, HIV infection, or irritable bowel syndrome. Physician consultation is imperative in these cases.

PATIENT AND FAMILY EDUCATION

The following are some general recommendations that should be discussed with the patient and family:

- Practice good handwashing after each bowel movement to reduce the possibility of spreading disease to other family members.
- Immunocompromised patients are at greater risk of severe infection and should be diligent about proper safe food handling and preparation.
- Drink frequent, small sips of fluids (water, tea, bouillon, flat cola, flat ginger ale, or sports drink) to avoid dehydration.
- Avoid foods and let your stomach rest until bowel movements begin to return to normal or until you begin to feel better. Gradually add small amounts of food (e.g., crackers, toast, rice, bananas), avoiding those that may aggravate symptoms (e.g., dairy products, caffeine, high-fat or high-fiber foods, carbonated beverages, sugar-free products, and alcohol).
- It is better to avoid antidiarrheal products because most cases of diarrhea are self-limiting.
- Rest.
- If symptoms persist or are accompanied by mental confusion, fever with temperature higher than 38.3° C (101° F), chills, vomiting, weakness (especially muscle weakness), dizziness, dry mouth, extreme thirst, little or no urinary output, severe abdominal discomfort, blurred vision, or black or bloody stools, immediately notify the health care provider.
- Some medications, particularly bismuth subsalicylate, will cause stools to appear black
- Children, daycare workers, or food handlers should remain at home until the diarrhea resolves.

HEALTH PROMOTION OR ILLNESS PREVENTION

Prevention of diarrhea should be the primary goal. Important information to convey to patients includes:

- Handwashing remains the best preventive measure. Always wash hands after handling chicken or other raw meats. Wash cutting boards frequently (plastic cutting boards that can be washed in a dishwasher are preferable). Change sponges and wash kitchen countertops frequently. Sponges should be washed and disinfected daily (by microwaving on high or placing in boiling water for 2 minutes).
- Use a meat thermometer to check temperature of roasts, chicken, and hamburger. When traveling, especially out of the country, drink and brush teeth with bottled water and eat only washed then peeled fruits and vegetables. Avoid iced drinks, and never drink untreated water.
- Avoid high-risk foods, such as raw seafood, raw eggs, unpasteurized dairy products, and undercooked poultry and beef.
- Avoid foods that have sat out at room temperature for more than 2 hours.
- Defrost meats in the microwave (as directed) or refrigerator.
- Cook foods to the proper temperature.

REFERENCES

1. Dupont HL, Practice Parameters Committee of American College of Gastroenterology: Guidelines in acute infectious diarrhea in adults, *Am J Gastroenterol* 92(11):1962-1975, 1997.
2. Herikstad H, Yang S, Van Gilder TJ: A population-based estimate of the burden of diarrhoeal illness in the United States: FoodNet, 1996-7, *Epidemiol Infect* 129(1):9-17, 2002.
3. Ahlquest DA, Camilleri M: Diarrhea and constipation. In Kasper DL, Fauci AS, Longo DL, and others, editors: *Harrison's principles of internal medicine*, ed 16, New York, 2005, McGraw-Hill.
4. Thielman NM, Guerrant RL: Acute infectious diarrhea, *N Engl J Med* 350(1):38-47, 2004.
5. Fauci A, Braunwald E, Isselbacher K, and others, editors: *Harrison's principles of internal medicine*, ed 14, New York, 1998, McGraw-Hill.
6. Connor BA, Landsberg BR: Persistent traveler's diarrhea, *Infect Med* 20:5, retrieved Dec 19, 2005, from http://www.medscape.com/viewarticle/455532.
7. Wanke CA: *Epidemiology and causes of acute diarrhea in the United States and other developed countries*, retrieved March 31, 2006, from http://www.utdol.com/utd/content/topic.do?topicKey=gi_infec/13221&view=text.

8. World Health Organization: *World health report 2003: shaping the future,* Geneva, 2003, The Organization.
9. Lipp EK, Huq A, Colwell RR: Effects of global climate on infectious disease: the cholera model, *Clin Microbiol Rev* 15:757-770, 1993.
10. Centers for Disease Control and Prevention: *Update: Vibrio cholerae* O1—Western hemisphere, 1991-1994, and *V cholerae* O139—Asia, 1994, *MMWR* 44:215-219, 1995.
11. Seas C, Gotuzzo E: Cholera: an overview of epidemiologic, therapeutic and preventive issues learned from recent epidemics, *Int J Infect Dis* 1:37, 1996.
12. Glass RI: New hope for defeating rotavirus, *Sci Am* 294(4):47-55, 2006.
13. Blacklow NR: Epidemiology of viral gastroenteritis in adults, retrieved March 27, 2006, from http://www.utdol.com/utd/content/topic.do?topicKey=gi_infec/11294&view=print.
14. Leder K, Weller PF: *Giardiasis in adults,* retrieved Dec 19, 2005, from http://patients.uptodate.com/topic.asp?file=parasite/7013.
15. Centers for Disease Control and Prevention: *Fact sheet for the general public: Cryptosporidium infection,* retrieved April 1, 2006, from http://www.cdc.gov/ncidod/dpd/parasites/cryptosporidiosis/factsht_cryptosporidiosis.htm.
16. Kourtis A: *Cryptosporidiosis,* retrieved March 12, 2007, from http://www.emedicine.com/ped/topic516.htm.
17. Blaser MJ: Infections due to *Campylobacter* and related species. In Kasper DL, Fauci AS, Longo DL, and others, editors: *Harrison's principles of internal medicine,* ed 16, New York, 2005, McGraw-Hill.
18. Keusch GT, Kopecko DJ: Shigellosis. In Kasper DL, Fauci AS, Longo DL, and others, editors: *Harrison's principles of internal medicine,* ed 16, New York, 2005, McGraw-Hill.
19. Archibald LK, Banerjee SN, Jarvis WR: Secular trends in hospital-acquired *Clostridium difficile*–associated disease in the United States, 1987-2001, *J Infect Dis* 189:1585-1589, 2004.
20. Centers for Disease Control and Prevention: Severe *Clostridium difficile*–associated disease in populations previously at low risk—four states, *MMWR* 54:1201-1205, 2005.
21. Muto CA, Pokrywka M, Shutt K, and others: A large outbreak of *Clostridium difficile*–associated disease with an unexpected proportion of deaths and colectomies at a teaching hospital following fluoroquinolone use, *Infect Control Hosp Epidemiol* 26:273-280, 2005.
22. McDonald LC, Killgore GE, Thompson A, and others: An epidemic, toxin gene-variant strain of *Clostridium difficile, N Engl J Med* 353:2433-2441, 2005.
23. Loo VG, Poirer L, Miller MA, and others: A predominantly clonal multi-institutional outbreak of *Clostridium difficile*–associated diarrhea with high morbidity and mortality, *N Engl J Med* 353:2442-2449, 2005.
24. Bricker E: *Antibiotic treatment for* Clostridium difficile*–associated diarrhea in adults,* retrieved Dec 19, 2005, from http://www.medscape.com/viewarticle/502155?src=search.
25. Centers for Disease Control and Prevention: *Information about a new strain of* Clostridium difficile, retrieved Dec 1, 2005, from http://www.cdc.gov/ncidod/dhqp/id_CdiffFAQ_newstrain.html.
26. Waldor MK, Keusch GT: Cholera and other vibrioses. In Kasper DL, Fauci AS, Longo DL, and others, editors: *Harrison's principles of internal medicine,* ed 16, New York, 2005, McGraw-Hill.
27. Lesser CF, Miller SI: Salmonellosis. In Kasper DL, Fauci AS, Longo DL, and others, editors: *Harrison's principles of internal medicine,* ed 16, New York, 2005, McGraw-Hill.
28. Frenzen PD, Drake A, Angulo FJ: Emerging infections program, FoodNet Working Group. Economic cost of illness due to *Escherichia coli* O157 infections in the United States, *J Food Protection* 68(12):2623-2630, 2005.
29. Cody SH, Glynn MK, Farrar JA, and others: An outbreak of *Escherichia coli* O157:H7 infection from unpasteurized apple juice, *Ann Intern Med* 130:202-209, 1999.
30. Blaser MJ: Bacteria and diseases of unknown cause: hemolytic-uremic syndrome, *J Infect Dis* 189:552-555, 2004.
31. Safdar N, Said A, Gangnon RE, and others: Risk of hemolytic-uremic syndrome after antibiotic treatment of *Escherichia coli* O157:H7 enteritis: a meta-analysis, *JAMA* 288:996-1001, 2002.
32. Guerrant RL, Van Gilder T, Steiner TS, and others: Practice guidelines for the management of infectious diarrhea, *Clin Infect Dis* 32:331-350, 2001.
33. Moake JL: Mechanisms of disease: thrombotic microangiopathies, *N Engl J Med* 347:589-600, 2002.
34. Griffen PM, Mead PS, Sivapalasingam S: *Escherichia coli* O157:H7 and other enterohemorrhagic *E coli.* In Blaser MJ, Smith PD, Ravdin JI, and others, editors: *Infections of the gastrointestinal tract,* ed 2, Philadelphia, 2002, Lippincott Williams & Wilkins.

CHAPTER 250

Lyme Disease

Martin Jan Bergman

DEFINITION AND EPIDEMIOLOGY

Lyme disease is an infectious disease caused by the spirochete *Borrelia burgdorferi,* which is transmitted to humans by the bite of the deer tick *Ixodes scapularis* or *Ixodes pacificus.* It is often accompanied by a classic rash and may involve the central nervous system (CNS), cardiac system, and musculoskeletal system. When diagnosed in a timely fashion, it is curable with conventional antibiotics, but both underdiagnosis and overdiagnosis have been a problem.

Since its first description in 1977, Lyme disease has captured the attention of the medical community and the public.[1] The investigative process involved in recognizing the disease and determining the vector and the causative agent represents a classic study in epidemiologic research. In the fall of 1975, two mothers, concerned about an unusual cluster of juvenile rheumatoid arthritis (JRA) in their communities and not satisfied with the explanations given to them by their health care providers, notified the Connecticut Health Department and the Rheumatology Clinic at Yale University. An initial survey done by Steere, Malawista, Sydman, and colleagues revealed a cluster of 51 cases of JRA in three communities along the eastern shore of the Connecticut River.[1] Peculiar to these cases, in addition to the "clustering" of a relatively uncommon entity, was the involvement of 12 adults with the disease, the marked seasonality of the initial presentation, and the association of the illness with an unusual rash, similar to erythema chronicum migrans. This rash was first described by a Swedish physician, Afzelius, in 1910 and was known to be associated with the bite of the sheep tick *Ixodes ricinus.* A few years later, a new member of the genus *Ixodes, I. dammini* (also called *I. scapularis),* was identified in the region where the new entity, Lyme disease (named for one of the towns, Lyme, Connecticut), was prevalent. This was followed by Burgdorfer's isolation of a spirochete, later characterized as a member of the genus *Borrelia,* from the gut of *I. dammini;* it is now recognized as the causative agent, *B. burgdorferi.*[2]

Much has been learned about the disease, including other manifestations, diagnostic modalities and treatments, the life cycle of the vector, and the life cycle of the organism. With this knowledge has also come much misinformation, hysteria, and exploitative behavior by the general public and less scrupulous health professionals.

Although it was best described in the late 1970s, it is obvious from studies that this disease has been around for many years. The spirochete has been isolated from the gut of a 50-year-old museum specimen, and the Europeans have known of a similar disease, Bannwarth's syndrome, since the early twentieth century.[3] Cases have been increasing at nearly an exponential rate since Steere's first description. The Centers for Disease Control and Prevention show 19,804 cases being reported in 2004 in all of the United States except Montana. The majority of the cases have been found in the Northeast, Mid-Atlantic, Great Lakes, and West Coast regions, and of these a disproportionate number have been reported in New York, Connecticut, Pennsylvania, and New Jersey.[4] There is no racial or sexual predominance in this disease, but the incidence of the disease does seem to have an association with encroachment of the woodlands by community development.

To understand the disease and its epidemiology, it is necessary to understand the life cycle of its primary vector, *I. scapularis.*[2] New eggs hatch in the early spring, and the as-yet-uninfected larvae seek their first blood meal. The host of choice is the white-footed mouse, which is also the reservoir for the *B. burgdorferi* organism. After this meal, the now-infected ticks molt over the winter and emerge the next spring in the nymph stage. These ticks, which prefer to live in tall grasses or woods, are aggressive feeders, seeking their next blood meal from any warm-blooded, carbon dioxide–exhaling creature, including humans. It is this stage that is responsible for the vast majority of infections. After this blood meal, the tick again molts, to the adult stage, and may again seek a blood meal in the early fall and then mate, generally on the white-tailed deer, starting the cycle again. There does not appear to be any transovarial transmission of the disease; thus the newborn tick will again emerge infection free.

Physician consultation is recommended for patients with a positive Lyme titer or suspected Lyme disease.

PATHOPHYSIOLOGY

Because Lyme disease is a classic arthropod-borne infection, the risk of infection in hosts, such as humans, depends on a number of factors. The infection rates of the tick vary from location to location, so that tick infection density plays a role. High-prevalence areas may have infection rates of 20% to 30% of nymphs to 50% to 65% of adult ticks, but, obviously, the host must come into contact with the tick to be bitten. The tick must then be embedded and feed long enough to transmit the disease. This is generally thought to require at least 24 hours and probably closer to 48 hours. This, then, affords some time for application of simple preventive measures, such as avoidance of grassy areas, long clothing, and tick removal. Even when embedded and feeding, for reasons not entirely clear and probably relating to host defenses and differences in infecting organisms, only 1% to 3% of reported tick bites ultimately cause Lyme disease.[5]

CLINICAL PRESENTATION AND PHYSICAL EXAMINATION

Once infected by *B. burgdorferi,* a patient may have any number of presentations. This is described as three, potentially overlapping stages: localized disease, early disseminated disease, and chronic disease. Any individual may manifest symptoms in any of these levels of disease; patients may first be seen with signs and symptoms of disseminated or late disease or may progress in a stepwise fashion from localized to early disseminated to chronic disease.

Localized Disease

Usually within 1 week to 1 month of the tick bite, the classic rash of erythema migrans (EM) appears.[2,5] This generally occurs in the late spring and early summer and is reported in 60% to 80% of patients with Lyme disease. Usually appearing at the site of the initial bite, or the groin, axilla, or scalp, the rash is classically described as a large circular rash, at least 5 cm (2 inches) in diameter with central clearing (bull's eye), that expands rapidly, at a rate of about 20 cm^2/day (7.8 $inches^2$) and lasts approximately 1 to 2 weeks (Color Plates 42 and 43). This means that, if there is a question as to the proper diagnosis, the rash can be measured and outlined with a marker. The patient can return to the office or clinic the next day, and at that time the rash can be remeasured and should have enlarged noticeably. This also helps distinguish the rash from a tick bite reaction, which is an indurated erythematous lesion generally less than 3 cm (1.2 inches) in diameter (about the size of a quarter) that does not expand.[6]

Most patients with EM have some associated constitutional signs; these may include fatigue, myalgias, arthralgias, headache, conjunctivitis, lymphadenopathy, fevers, and a stiff neck. These are the symptoms which are generally described by the media as a flulike illness. Absent, however, are the sore throat, rhinorrhea, and cough that are often seen with common seasonal viral illnesses. These constitutional symptoms suggest dissemination and tend to blur the distinction between localized and disseminated disease.[6]

Not all rashes appear in the classic fashion. The rash may be irregular in shape, and the central clearing may not be present. Central necrosis or vesicles may be noted. The rash is usually asymptomatic, but there may be warmth, tenderness, and occasional pruritus. Often these rashes are believed to be spider bites. In the Northeast United States the brown recluse spider, which is known for its bite, is essentially absent, yet the diagnosis of a brown recluse bite is often made in patients subsequently shown to have Lyme disease.[6]

Early Disseminated Disease

Early in the course, multiple skin lesions may appear, suggesting dissemination. These lesions are generally smaller than the original lesion and are not at the site of the original bite. In addition, they are more evanescent than the primary lesion and are less likely to have prominent local symptoms.

As the disease disseminates, more constitutional symptoms may be seen along with more evidence of other organ system involvement. These symptoms may occur anywhere from 1 week to 7 months from the original bite; typically they occur 1 to 2 months later. Nervous system dissemination occurs early in the course of the disease.[7] This may manifest in a peripheral form such as Bell's palsy, as any cranial neuropathy, or as a peripheral sensorimotor radiculoneuritis. Even cases of neurogenic bladder have been described. There may be subtle signs of encephalitis manifested by changes in mood or emotional lability, or the disease may appear as frank meningitis. The severity of the headache and neck stiffness, however, is less than that of bacterial meningitis. At this time, dissemination to the heart may also occur, with the conduction system being the most commonly affected. The most common abnormality noted is a nonspecific ST-T wave change, but any conduction abnormality, including complete heart block, can occur. Fortunately, these conditions respond well to antibiotic therapy, so that, when necessary, the use of a pacemaker is usually temporary. On rare occasions the patient may have true myocarditis with global dysfunction, but, fortunately, this is exceedingly uncommon and usually responds to antibiotics.

The musculoskeletal system is another system that is often involved.[7] Initially, patients may notice a migratory polyarthralgia, which generally settles into a monoarticular or an oligoarticular presentation. Most commonly, the joints involved are large weight-bearing joints, with the knee being the most common site. Polyarticular involvement, although described, is unusual and should steer the provider toward another diagnosis, such as rheumatoid arthritis (RA) or systemic lupus erythematosus (SLE), rather than Lyme disease. The involved joint, although markedly inflamed, is surprisingly asymptomatic, with patients complaining more of swelling than of pain. Examination of the fluid reveals significant inflammation, and studies of the fluid for Lyme disease are uniformly positive. Untreated, the arthropathy of Lyme disease remits and recurs, with attacks occurring approximately once or twice a year but lasting for months at a time. However, most patients respond to antibiotic therapy. Occasionally, even with adequate therapy, a patient may develop a chronic, noninfectious arthritis that requires treatment other than antibiotics.

Chronic Disease

Left untreated or unrecognized, the *Borrelia* infection becomes chronic. The primary sites of chronicity are the joints, as previously discussed, and the CNS. An atrophic lesion of the skin, acrodermatitis atrophicans, has also been described, but this lesion is more common in Europe than in the United States and probably reflects differences in the infecting organisms seen in different locations.

Neuroborreliosis can manifest in many different ways, ranging from subtle changes of cognition to frank neuropathies. The nervous system seems to be infected relatively early in the course of the infection, often within the first month after exposure. Symptoms may start as mood changes and cognitive deficits. Abnormalities on MRI may be noted. Whether these lesions represent actual infection or "microinfarcts" is not clear. A confusional state, suggesting encephalitis, may develop as well. Bandlike neuropathies are not uncommon and are believed to be caused by direct invasion of the nerve by the organism, although molecular mimicry with autoimmune reactions and lymphokines has also been implicated in this presentation, as well as in the encephalopathies. In addition, the damage to the nervous system caused by the infection (or the host's immune response) can delay healing and result in some degree of residual damage and dysfunction.[8,9]

Another of the chronic manifestations of Lyme disease is fibromyalgia.[10] This chronic pain syndrome, which is associated with fatigue, malaise, sleep disturbance, and tender trigger points on examination, can be extremely disconcerting to the patient, especially given the public's widespread concern about Lyme disease. Noninfectious in nature, it responds to pain control, sleep correction, and aerobic exercise but not to repeated courses of antibiotics (see Chapter 186).

DIAGNOSTICS

The diagnosis is generally straightforward but requires a high degree of clinical suspicion and appropriate use of laboratory studies. If a patient is seen with an expanding, bull's-eye rash, the diagnosis is established. No further testing is necessary or indicated.[10] Testing too early in the course of the infection, before the body can produce an antibody response, can result in a false-negative finding and the impression that the rash is not caused by Lyme disease. The testing for Lyme disease, when indicated clinically and not used as a screening test, generally consists of measuring antibodies directed against the organism (an enzyme-linked immunosorbent assay [ELISA] is used) and then confirming the specificity of the testing with Western blot (WB) testing.[10] After an initial infection, the body will start to make antibodies of the immunoglobulin (Ig) M class. This usually begins 1 to 2 weeks after exposure and is then followed, in an additional 4 weeks, by the production of antibodies of the IgG class. Both of these antibodies may persist after treatment and do not indicate persistence of infection. Antibiotics given early in the course of the disease can abort this antibody production and make laboratory interpretation difficult. This is one of the arguments against empiric use of antibiotics in all but established cases of Lyme disease. The initial study should always be confirmed by WB analysis because cross-reactivity with normal host flora and other disease states can lead to false-positive results and erroneous treatment regimens. In the presence of the appropriate clinical presentation and positive laboratory testing and confirmation, the diagnosis is established and therapy should be begun.

The stage of the disease must be considered when interpreting the results. For patients with a chronic manifestation, an isolated positive IgM titer without a concurrent rise in the IgG titer should raise suspicion about the validity of the study. Similarly, in a previously untreated patient with a chronic manifestation of the disease, the absence of an IgG antibody response should be considered before initiation of a treatment regimen.

In general, the antibody production is "locally produced"; that is, the antibody will be produced in excess in the affected site. Therefore patients with CNS involvement would be expected to have antibodies not only in their blood but also in their cerebrospinal fluid (CSF). Measuring this antibody production through lumbar puncture is an essential part of the diagnosis of neuroborreliosis. In the more acute forms, pleocytosis with lymphocytic predominance, elevated protein levels (including low levels of oligoclonal banding), and positive Lyme titers by ELISA and WB are expected. If meningitis is part of the early disseminated syndrome, these antibodies may be absent because the body has not yet had a chance to respond with antibody production. In the later stages of CNS disease, positive antibodies in either the blood or CSF are nearly universal and should always be sought. Polymerase chain reaction (PCR) studies, which measure DNA from the organism, are even more specific and are currently recommended in CSF testing as well. In patients with a chronic polyneuropathy, the CSF may be negative, but results of peripheral blood testing are nearly always positive.

DIAGNOSTICS

Lyme Disease

LABORATORY
ELISA*
Western blot*
IgM, IgG*
Polymerase chain reaction*

IMAGING
MRI*

OTHER
Lumbar puncture*
Synovial fluid analysis*

*If indicated.

A similar antibody response and testing regimen is recommended for Lyme arthritis; however, this time the synovial fluid should be studied. The joint fluid is highly inflammatory, and Lyme titers of both the blood and the fluid are nearly universally positive. PCR can be done to confirm the presence of the organism as well.

The role of MRI testing, which is generally nonspecific in its findings for Lyme disease, and the role of neuropsychiatric studies remain unclear. The latter may be very sensitive and specific for Lyme disease but requires a skilled evaluator and is generally not covered by most insurance plans, nor is it commonly available outside of academic centers.

New laboratory studies are being investigated that will detect the organism at an earlier stage and will be more specific for infection rather than exposure. Their availability and utility are not yet established. PCR, although very specific, is technically demanding and requires that the living organism be found in the studied fluid. Unfortunately, if the small sample studied does not contain the living organism, the test will be negative, even in an established disease. The Lyme urine antigen test has given unreliable results and should not be used in the diagnosis of Lyme disease.[10,11]

DIFFERENTIAL DIAGNOSIS

Depending on the stage of infection, Lyme disease may be confused with a number of other diseases. Some of this confusion may be related to the myth of Lyme disease being the "great imitator," akin to syphilis. As can be seen from the previous sections, the more common presentations of Lyme disease are stereotypical.

During the summer months the differential diagnosis of Lyme disease always includes the far more common and benign "summer flu." Coryza, cough, and congestion will help differentiate the viral illness from *Borrelia* infection. The EM rash may be confused with a simple cellulitis or a spider bite. As previously noted, the local arachnid population should be considered. On the East Coast of the United States, where brown recluse spiders are unusual, that diagnosis should be made reluctantly. Other arthropod-borne infections such as Rocky Mountain spotted fever, babesiosis, and chronic granulocytic ehrlichiosis can cause rashes and constitutional symptoms similar to those of Lyme disease and are in fact transmitted by the *I. scapularis* tick.[9] Proper laboratory testing and recognition of other related symptoms and signs will help differentiate these from Lyme disease.

In its disseminated stages, Lyme disease can be easily confused for other conditions. When a patient with any nervous system involvement is being treated, the caveat "common things happen commonly" should be kept in mind. Thus, although Lyme disease should be included in the differential

DIFFERENTIAL DIAGNOSIS

Lyme Disease

- Influenza
- Cellulitis
- Bell's palsy
- Bacterial meningitis
- Reiter's syndrome
- Gonorrheal arthropathy
- Crystalline-induced arthritis
- Rheumatoid arthritis
- Infection
- Tumor
- Multiple sclerosis
- Vasculitides
- Depression
- Fibromyalgia
- Collagen vascular disease

diagnosis of a facial nerve palsy, even in endemic regions, the more common cause of this abnormality is still idiopathic Bell's palsy. In addition, although Lyme meningitis may be present, failure to diagnose and treat pyogenic meningitis could have lethal complications. A lumbar puncture done at this time should show a lymphocytic or monocytic predominance if Lyme disease is the cause, distinguishing it from the polymorphonuclear reaction of pyogenic meningitis. An elevation of the CSF protein level may be seen in both. Testing of either blood or CSF at this stage is almost uniformly positive for Lyme disease.

The arthropathy of Lyme disease is generally pauciarticular and thus can be confused with any of the other causes of oligoarthritis, such as reactive arthritis, gonorrheal infection, crystalline-induced arthritis, or even early RA. In some patients this arthropathy has been erroneously diagnosed as a sprain or internal derangement, leading to unnecessary arthroscopic procedures. Any patient with an inflammatory arthritis, particularly of the knee, should be evaluated for Lyme disease. If the arthropathy becomes more generalized, it is less likely to be Lyme disease and more likely to be a rheumatologic illness such as RA or SLE. In the latter, rashes and neurologic involvement may confuse the presentation. Unlike Lyme disease, these conditions will not respond to antibiotics, although patients have received multiple courses of IV antibiotics after the misdiagnosis of Lyme disease.

New-onset heart block, especially in an unusual setting, such as a younger patient without a cardiac history, requires evaluation for the infection. The cardiac manifestations are otherwise relatively limited and should not be confused with other cardiac disease. Rarely, a cardiomyopathy can occur that should be excluded from the more common forms such as atherosclerotic and hypertensive cardiomyopathies.

The later manifestations of CNS involvement generally cause the most diagnostic confusion. Radicular pain may be caused by trauma or by nerve encroachment from disc disease, infections such as syphilis or herpes zoster, or tumors. Multiple levels, a seasonal onset, and bilaterality tend to favor the diagnosis of Lyme disease but are not specific findings. Headaches and memory deficits can be caused by Lyme disease, tumor, multiple sclerosis, vasculitides, collagen vascular diseases, fibromyalgia, or depression. Only a careful history, physical examination, and appropriate laboratory testing will help differentiate these problems.

MANAGEMENT

The treatment of Lyme disease depends on the clinical manifestations. Currently, no human vaccinations are available for prevention of the disease. As with most infections, it is generally easier to eradicate the infection, with less toxic or aggressive techniques, the earlier the diagnosis is made.

For most of the symptoms, except the true CNS manifestations, the treatment of choice is oral antibiotics.[3,6,12-14] In general, doxycycline 100 mg b.i.d. for 10 to 12 days is sufficient to treat EM rashes, myalgias and arthralgia, and mild heart block. Alternate therapies include amoxicillin 500 mg t.i.d. for 2 to 3 weeks and cefuroxime axetil (Ceftin) 500 mg b.i.d. for 2 to 3 weeks. The arthritis is generally treated for 28 days via the oral route or, now less commonly, for 14 to 28 days with IV ceftriaxone 2 g/day. The longer courses of antibiotics are generally reserved for later or for more severe manifestations. In children younger than 9 years old, in whom tetracyclines are to be avoided, the drugs of choice are amoxicillin 250 mg t.i.d. or 25 to 50 mg/kg/day in three divided doses or cefuroxime axetil 125 mg or 30 mg/kg b.i.d., both for 2 to 4 weeks, depending on the presentation.[12-14] What appears to be Bell's palsy, if there are absolutely no other CNS symptoms, can also be treated with the above oral regimens. However, if there is any possibility of more extensive CNS involvement, a lumbar puncture should be performed and treatment decisions based on the results.

For all other CNS involvement or serious cardiac manifestations, or in the case of true treatment failures, the treatment of choice is a third-generation cephalosporin given intravenously.[14-16] The most common regimen is ceftriaxone 2 g/day for 2 to 4 weeks, although cefotaxime 2 g q 8 hr may also be used. In children the dosage is 75 to 100 mg/kg/day (maximum of 2 g) for ceftriaxone and 150 mg/kg/day (maximum of 6 g) in three or four[15,16] divided doses for cefotaxime. If a true cephalosporin allergy is found, treatment with chloramphenicol 50 mg/kg/day in four divided doses has been recommended, although strong consideration of a rapid desensitization regimen to a cephalosporin and treatment with that drug is preferred.

It is not uncommon for patients to develop fevers, chills, myalgias, and rashes early in the course of the antibiotic regimen. Called the Jarisch-Herxheimer reaction and also seen in treatment for syphilis, it is the body's response to the rapid lysis of the infecting organism and should not lead to premature abortion of the therapy.

Treatment failures occur in approximately 10% of cases and can generally be treated intravenously. If the treatment still fails, reconsideration of the original diagnosis is necessary.[8] If the cause is fibromyalgia, treatment is rest, exercise, aerobic conditioning, and low doses of antidepressant medications to correct the sleep disturbance—not repeated courses of antibiotics or new combinations of antibiotics.[15,16]

A few scenarios that are often encountered need special mention. Even in endemic areas, only 1% to 3% of tick bites cause infection. Thus there currently is no indication for empiric treatment of a tick bite, unless the patient manifests symptoms of Lyme disease.[13] However, a study has shown that a single dose of 200 mg doxycycline given within 72 hours of a known tick bite (after removal of the embedded tick) can have some efficacy in preventing disease.[17] Treatment too early in the course of the disease can abrogate the initial antibody response, making later diagnosis difficult, and may subject the patient to a greater risk of side effects from the treatment than from the disease.

Seronegative Lyme disease (where test results are negative for Lyme disease, but the patient has Lyme disease) is a rare but well-recognized entity. Generally, it occurs in a patient who took an inadequate amount or duration of antibiotics early in the course of the disease. In this situation all other possible explanations for the symptomatology must be excluded, and fixed end points of treatment must be established before therapy is begun. Open-ended therapies of long duration have not been shown to have any efficacy and subject patients to potentially serious toxicities. In addition, a previous response to an antibiotic should never be used as a criterion for making the diagnosis and continuing treatment.[16,17]

The patient who tests positive for Lyme disease on a screening test presents a different problem. In this situation the patient has clearly been exposed to the organism, but more often than not, the symptom that resulted in the positive test is not caused by Lyme disease. A thorough history and physical examination should determine whether there are any obvious signs of Lyme disease. If any are present, they should be treated with the appropriate regimen. If such signs are absent, a frank discussion with the patient about the risks of treatment (e.g., photosensitivity to tetracyclines, allergic reactions) vs. the potential benefits of treatment is necessary to develop an appropriate treatment plan. If treatment is chosen, it should be via the oral route and for 2 to 4 weeks' duration (e.g., doxycycline 100 mg b.i.d. for 2 to 4 weeks).[9]

COMPLICATIONS

Although there are few complications when Lyme disease is diagnosed and treated properly, pregnancy requires special consideration.[3] Obviously, having an infection during pregnancy can be cause for great concern for any expectant parent. The spirochete has been shown to cross the placenta and infect the fetus, but, fortunately, this is a rare occurrence. In fact, studies concerned with the risk of miscarriage and congenital defects in patients with Lyme disease have not shown any increase in either compared with other pregnancies in the same region.[18] The best approach is to treat the infected mother with amoxicillin 500 mg PO t.i.d. for 3 to 4 weeks for early localized disease and with ceftriaxone 2 g/day IV for 3 to 4 weeks for disseminated disease (tetracyclines are contraindicated in pregnancy).[19] Although no guarantees can be made, the expectant parents can in general be reassured of a normal outcome of the pregnancy.

INDICATIONS FOR REFERRAL OR HOSPITALIZATION

In general, the management of early localized disease and the more common disseminated features does not require consultation with a specialist. Uncommon rashes may confound the practitioner and require consultation. Patients may require consultation with a specialist when the disease is more advanced and procedures such as a lumbar puncture or arthrocentesis are being contemplated. Because patients do not always welcome these procedures, it is often best to refer the patient for a definitive procedure and evaluation, rather than potentially subjecting the patient to a procedure that may need to be repeated in the near future. In patients who have unusual manifestations such as polyarticular involvement, persistent synovitis, multiple neurologic deficits, or seronegative Lyme disease or in those for whom therapy has failed in the past, a referral to a rheumatologist, a neurologist, or an infectious disease specialist will help secure a proper diagnosis and ensure proper therapy. It is worth repeating that even in endemic regions, other diseases such as RA, SLE, idiopathic Bell's palsy, and fibromyalgia are common entities that need to be considered, independent of Lyme disease.

Lyme disease, for the most part, is treated on an outpatient basis, requiring admission to a hospital only when the presenting feature would otherwise warrant it, independent of the cause. Thus a patient with acute meningitis or heart failure as a result of a high-degree heart block should be admitted to a hospital, but this admission would have been made regardless of the ultimate cause of the symptom. As a rule, in patients who have not taken a cephalosporin in the past for other reasons, home IV therapy companies will require that the first dose be given in a controlled environment (e.g., a short procedure unit or a physician's office). Antibiotic desensitization should always be done in a controlled setting, where emergency measures to treat anaphylaxis are readily available. With these exceptions, Lyme disease is easily managed in the outpatient setting.

PATIENT AND FAMILY EDUCATION

Although diagnosis and treatment are necessary in the management of this disease, the best approach to Lyme disease is avoidance of the tick bite. Patients should be instructed to wear light-colored, long-legged, and long-sleeved clothing, with socks tucked in, whenever walking through potentially endemic areas. This will make it harder for the tick to find skin to burrow into and will allow easy identification of the tick on the outside of the clothing. Insect repellents, such as deet (diethyltoluamide), should also be considered, since these will also decrease the chance of tick bites. On returning from a wooded or grassy area, patients should make a thorough search of all body areas. Any nonembedded tick can be removed and destroyed. If an embedded tick is found, it should be grasped firmly at the base of the head with a pair of tweezers and gently removed. Care should be taken to avoid crushing the embedded tick while it is still attached or removing the body of the tick while leaving the mouth parts attached. Measures such as applying petroleum jelly, oils, or lighted cigarettes to the tick to aid in removal are not effective and are potentially dangerous. The bite site should be observed for the next week for signs of induration, with any expanding rash or viral-type symptoms reported to the practitioner.

Lyme disease continues to spread as humans encroach on the wilderness, increasing the likelihood of an encounter with an infected tick. Although Lyme disease causes unwarranted anxiety and fear, with understanding of the disease process and recognition of its manifestations, the practitioner should be able to treat and cure this condition.

REFERENCES

1. Steere AC, Malawista SE, Sydman DR, and others: Lyme arthritis: an epidemic of oligoarticular arthritis in children and adults in three Connecticut communities, *Arthritis Rheum* 20(1):7-17, 1977.

2. Nocton JJ, Steere AC: Lyme disease, *Adv Intern Med* 40:69-117, 1995.
3. Zemel LS: Lyme disease: a pediatric perspective, *J Rheumatol* 19(Suppl 34):1-13, 1992.
4. Centers for Disease Control and Prevention: *Lyme disease statistics*, retrieved Nov 11, 2004, from http://www.cdc.gov/ncidod/dvbid/lyme/ld_statistics.htm.
5. Centers for Disease Control and Prevention: Lyme disease—United States, 1999, *MMWR* 50:181-185, 2001,
6. Nadelman RB, Wormser GP: Erythema migrans and early Lyme disease, *Am J Med* 98(Suppl 4A):15S-24S, 1995.
7. Steere AC, Taylor E, McHugh GL, and others: The overdiagnosis of Lyme disease, *JAMA* 269(14):1812-1816, 1993.
8. Sigal LH: Anxiety and persistence of Lyme disease, *Am J Med* 98(Suppl 4A):74S-83S, 1995.
9. Krause PJ, Telford SR 3rd, Spielman A, and others: Concurrent Lyme disease and babesiosis. Evidence for increased severity and duration of illness, *JAMA* 275(21):1657-1660, 1996.
10. Steere AC: Lyme disease, *N Engl J Med* 345(2):115-125, 2001.
11. Centers for Disease Control and Prevention: Notice to readers: caution regarding testing for Lyme disease, *MMWR* 54(05):125, 2005.
12. Shapiro ED: Lyme disease in children, *Am J Med* 98(Suppl 4A):69S-73S, 1995.
13. Dattwyler RJ, Left BJ, Kunkel MJ, and others: Ceftriaxone compared with doxycycline for the treatment of acute disseminated Lyme disease, *N Engl J Med* 337(5):289-294, 1997.
14. Treatment of Lyme disease, *Med Lett* 47(1209):41-43, 2005.
15. Treatment of Lyme disease, *Med Lett* 42(1077):37-39, 2000.
16. Klempner MS, Hu LT, Evans J, and others: Two controlled trials of antibiotic treatment in patients with persistent symptoms and a history of Lyme disease, *N Engl J Med* 345(2):85-92, 2001.
17. Nadelman RB, Nowakowski J, Fish D, and others: Prophylaxis with single-dose doxycycline for the prevention of Lyme disease after an *Ixodes scapularis* tick bite, *N Engl J Med* 345(2):79-84, 2001.
18. Elliott D, Eppe S, Klein J: Teratogen update: Lyme disease, *Teratology* 64(5):276-281, 2001, retrieved March 13, 2007, from http://www3.interscience.wiley.com/cgi-bin/abstract/85515844/ABSTRACT.
19. Shapiro ED: Doxycycline for tick bites—not for everyone, *N Engl J Med* 345:133-134, 2001.

CHAPTER 251

West Nile Virus

Thomas H. Taylor

DEFINITIONS

West Nile virus (WNV) is an arboviral infection of the family *Flaviviridae*, from *flavus*, Latin for yellow, which includes the prototype, yellow fever, as well as dengue fever, Japanese encephalitis (JE), St. Louis encephalitis (SLE), and tick-borne encephalitis. These viruses have a common predisposition to cause acute febrile illness (West Nile fever [WNF]) and central nervous system (CNS) infection (West Nile encephalitis [WNE] or aseptic meningitis). They may invade muscle, joints, and liver and thus give rise to complications of myositis, arthritis, and hepatitis and cause considerable morbidity. The terms *encephalitis, meningitis, myelitis*, and *neuritis* refer to inflammation of brain, leptomeninges, spinal cord, and nerve roots, respectively. *Radiculitis* refers to involvement primarily of the sensory nerve root, and *acute flaccid paralysis* (AFP) refers to a myelitis involving the anterior horn cells, or motor cells, of the spinal cord. Both conditions may complicate WNV infection. Meningoencephalitis—inflammation of both meninges and brain—is common in WNV infection.

Transmission of arboviral infection (*ar* for arthropod and *bo* for borne, or arthropod-borne viral infection) is predominantly by mosquitoes, but also ticks. Birds are the WNV reservoir (amplifying host). Horses and humans are susceptible but dead end hosts. Many other vertebrates are susceptible to infection, but like humans, most do not sustain high-level viremias for long enough periods to become a reservoir.[1]

EPIDEMIOLOGY

The evolution of WNV represents a true emerging infectious disease, with rapid spread throughout North America and now progressing to the Caribbean,[2] suggestive of what we might expect from the next influenza pandemic or acts of bioterrorism. WNV was first isolated from a febrile female patient in the West Nile district of Uganda in 1937, but was not associated with neurologic disease at that time. WNV did have close serologic identity with JE virus and SLE virus, two closely related and highly neurotropic viruses. For 3 decades WNF, associated with fever, arthritis, and rash, circulated in Africa and the Middle East, with little neuroinvasive disease. In the 1960s outbreaks of equine and human WNE occurred in the Middle East and the Mediterranean Basin. A subtype of WNV, Kunjin virus, appeared in Australasia in 1973, causing a large epidemic, but also with little neuroinvasive disease. From 1975 to 1993 there were no major epidemics of WNV, but the 1990s brought increasingly frequent and severe outbreaks of West Nile neuroinvasive disease (WNND) to Europe, Russia, and the Middle East, along avian migration routes; these outbreaks were associated with parallel events in many vertebrate species.[3] In 1999 WNV crossed the Atlantic and produced an outbreak of WNND in boroughs of New York City, epidemiologically associated with mosquito exposure.[4] The New World strain was closely related to a newly emergent clade 1a strain circulating in the Middle East, and may have arrived via a febrile traveler, a transported mosquito, or a storm-blown avian host.[5,6] Like its Middle East counterpart, this virus was neuroinvasive and rapidly spread from New York via bird migration routes along the entire East Coast and subsequently westward to involve all states in 2005, except Alaska and Hawaii (see Figure 251-1).

The virus is maintained in a bird-mosquito-bird cycle, since wild birds develop high levels of viremia over long but relatively asymptomatic intervals, which facilitates transmission to many mosquitoes (amplification) (see Figure 251-2). *Corvidae* birds (crows and jays) and certain passerine species (songbirds) are susceptible to neuroinvasive disease and have a high mortality, leading to bird die-offs, such as occurred in New York, in parallel with the human epidemic in 1999.[7] Avian and mosquito active surveillance is now recommended by the Centers for Disease Control and Prevention (CDC) to facilitate early warning of impending community outbreaks. Mosquitoes of the *Culex* family transmit the WNV to humans and horses, which are incidental hosts with low-level viremia of short duration (i.e., dead end hosts). There has been no incidental human-to-human or other vertebrate–to-human transmission. However, transmission via transfusion, trans-

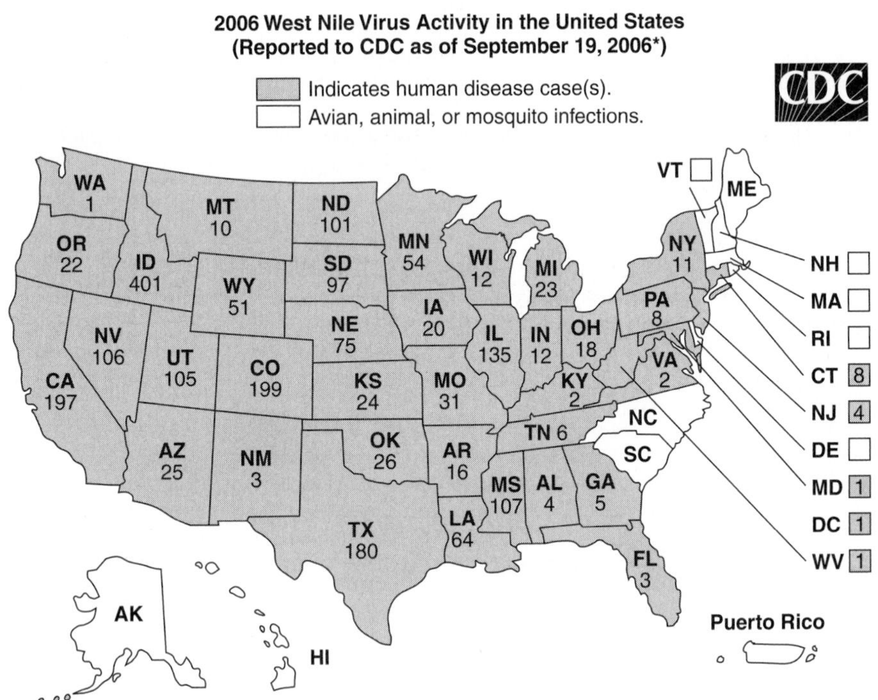

*Map shows the distribution of avian, animal, or mosquito infection occurring during 2006 with number of human cases, if any, by state. If West Nile virus (WNV) infection is reported to CDC from any area of a state, that entire state is shaded.

Data table:
As of September 19, 2006, avian, animal, or mosquito WNV infections have been reported to CDC ArboNET from Alabama, Arizona, Arkansas, California, Colorado, Connecticut, Delaware, District of Columbia, Florida, Georgia, Idaho, Illinois, Indiana, Iowa, Kansas, Kentucky, Louisiana, Maine, Maryland, Massachusetts, Michigan, Minnesota, Mississippi, Missouri, Montana, Nebraska, Nevada, New Hampshire, New Jersey, New Mexico, New York, North Carolina, North Dakota, Ohio, Oklahoma, Oregon, Pennsylvania, Rhode Island, South Carolina, South Dakota, Tennessee, Texas, Utah, Vermont, Virginia, Washington, West Virginia, Wisconsin, and Wyoming.

Human cases have been reported in Alabama, Arizona, Arkansas, California, Colorado, Connecticut, District of Columbia, Florida, Georgia, Idaho, Illinois, Indiana, Iowa, Kansas, Kentucky, Louisiana, Maryland, Michigan, Minnesota, Mississippi, Missouri, Montana, Nebraska, Nevada, New Jersey, New Mexico, New York, North Dakota, Ohio, Oklahoma, Oregon, Pennsylvania, South Dakota, Tennessee, Texas, Utah, Virginia, Washington, West Virginia, Wisconsin, and Wyoming.

Maps detailing county-level human, mosquito, veterinary, avian, and sentinel data are published each week on the collaborative USGS/CDC WNV website: http://westnilemaps.usgs.gov/.

For information on WNV activity in Canada please see:
http://www.phac-aspc.gc.ca/wnv-vwn/index.html
http://www.cnphi-wnv.ca/healthnet/Welcome.do

FIGURE 251-1

West Nile virus map, 2006. (From Centers for Disease Control and Prevention: 2006 West Nile virus activity in the United States [reported to CDC as of March 6, 2007], retrieved March 13, 2007, from http://www.cdc.gov/ncidod/dvbid/westnile/Mapsactivity/ surv&control06Maps.htm.)

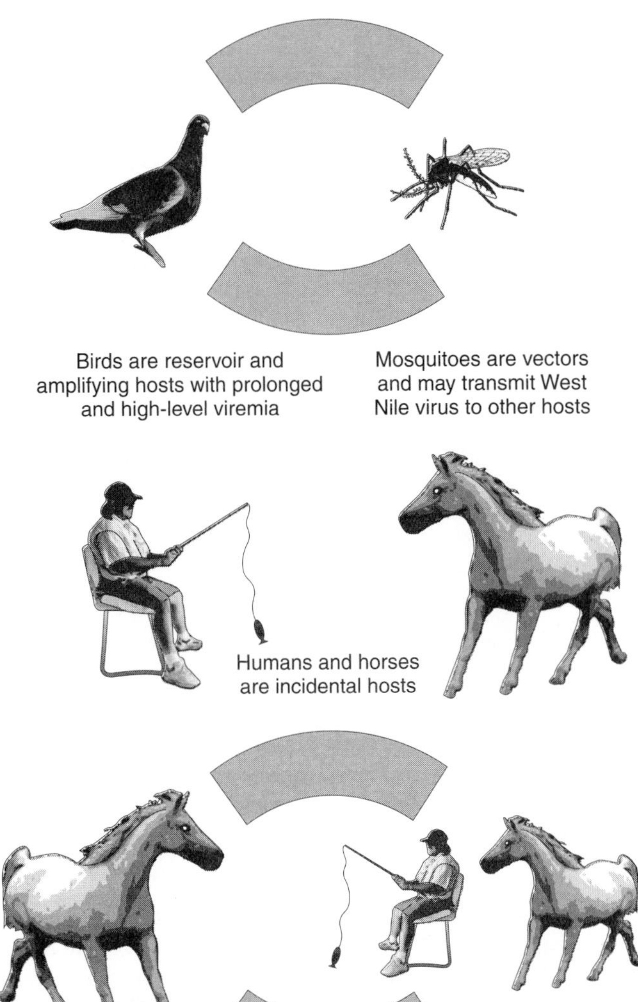
Birds are reservoir and amplifying hosts with prolonged and high-level viremia
Mosquitoes are vectors and may transmit West Nile virus to other hosts
Humans and horses are incidental hosts
Brief and low-level viremia makes them dead-end hosts

FIGURE 251-2

West Nile virus (*WNV*) cycle.

plantation, laboratory inoculation, breast milk, hemodialysis, and in utero infection has occurred.[8-14] Most cases in North America have occurred in the late summer and early fall, in conjunction with high rates of mosquito WNV carriage. Children have high rates of infection, but low rates of neuroinvasive disease.[15] Adults over 65 have higher mortality and 110 times the incidence of WNND compared with children.[16]

CLINICAL PRESENTATION

As with SLE and JE, most infection with WNV is asymptomatic. Following outbreaks in Ohio, seroprevalence remained low at 3%, but estimations of 1 WNF to 5 asymptomatic infections and 1 WNND to 150 asymptomatic infections can be calculated from recent outbreaks.[4,16] After an incubation period of 2 to 14 days (14 days or longer in immunocompromised hosts), WNF is characterized by a flulike illness, fever, arthralgia, myalgia, rash, malaise, and headache. Gastrointestinal symptoms have included nausea, vomiting, and diarrhea. Generalized lymphadenopathy, splenomegaly, and hepatomegaly are common.[17] Rash appears early in 50% to 60% of cases and is a nonspecific maculopapular rash that most often begins on the trunk. Although WNV was confirmed serologically, the acute-phase serum tested negative at the time of rash in 57% of patients.[18] Convalescent serum is often needed to confirm the diagnosis in this early and nonspecific stage of illness.

Weakness is a prominent feature of more severe disease, and myelitis, caused by infection of motor anterior horn cells, may lead to AFP reminiscent of poliomyelitis.[19,20] As in poliovirus, and more closely related JE and SLE, a biphasic illness eventuates in aseptic meningitis (30%) and encephalitis (60%), as the second phase of illness following WNF.[17] Prominent findings in patients with encephalitis are movement disorders: tremor, parkinsonism, gait disturbances, myoclonus, and rarely seizure disorder. These motor disturbances appear early, have a pathophysiologic correlation with lesions seen on MRI in the basal ganglia and thalamus, and may resolve over ensuing months.[21] AFP can be recognized as progressive weakness and loss of deep tendon reflexes. There have been reports of Guillain-Barré syndrome (GBS) following WNV infection, also associated with gradual, ascending loss of muscle weakness and loss of deep tendon reflexes.[22] GBS is an autoimmune acute inflammatory demyelinating polyradiculopathy distinguished by preceding sensory paresthesias, symmetric ascending weakness, and autonomic dysfunction (see Chapter 207). Sensory and autonomic nerve involvement is not seen with AFP, precipitated by acute viral infection of the motor anterior horn cells. It is important to distinguish between AFP and GBS, since AFP is associated with little long-term improvement and GBS is largely reversible over a few months.[23]

Aseptic (nonbacterial) meningitis and encephalitis commonly follow the symptoms of WNF by 4 to 7 days, but may appear without recognized prodrome as stiff neck (meningismus), headache, and sensitivity to light (photophobia). These symptoms may further proceed to encephalitis characterized by alterations in consciousness: lethargy, confusion, stupor, and coma. More focal encephalopathic findings include difficulty with word finding, speech, and memory; seizures; cranial neuropathy; upper motor neuron paralysis with hyperreflexia; and extensor plantar responses. The hypothalamic-pituitary axis may become involved and is associated with CNS-mediated fever, hyponatremia resulting from syndrome of inappropriate antidiuretic hormone (SIADH), or diabetes insipidus (urinary water loss) caused by insufficient antidiuretic hormone.

PHYSICAL EXAMINATION

The general examination should include awareness of rash, arthritis, adenopathy, and splenomegaly. Photophobia is recognized by excessive reaction to bright light. Nuchal rigidity is recognized by passive flexing of the neck, which induces involuntary hip flexion (Brudzinski's sign). More diffuse meningeal irritation is elicited by Kernig's sign: with hip flexed, attempts to extend the knee produce resistance and pain in the hamstring and back. Meningeal irritation in children may be recognized by tripoding, or sitting on the examination table supported by buttocks and both hands placed posteriorly, so as to maintain a rigid spine. Encephalitis is recognized by testing multiple areas of cognitive function, degree of alertness, speech, motor and sensory function, and cranial nerves. AFP may be recognized by abrupt onset of weakness and decreased deep tendon reflexes and may be distinguished from GBS by lack of autonomic or sensory nerve involvement.[23] Disease may progress rapidly, and frequently repeated examinations are required to assess the need for increasing levels of supportive care.

DIAGNOSTICS

Patients older than 50 years, with febrile illness, meningitis, or encephalitis who are seen during the summer or fall, should be considered for WNV laboratory confirmation. Serologic testing is the most effective method to confirm clinical suspicion of WNV infection. Enzyme-linked immunosorbent assay (ELISA) of immunoglobulin M (IgM) in serum or cerebrospinal fluid (CSF) is indicative of recent infection and 90% sensitive after 8 days of illness.[24] Individuals recently infected with or vaccinated against related viruses such as yellow fever, dengue fever, and JE may have false-positive serologic results for WNV.[17] The problem of cross-reactivity with flaviviruses, including SLE virus circulating in the Northern Hemisphere, can be corrected by confirmatory testing with a plaque-reduction neutralization assay.[25] IgM antibody to WNV may persist for as long as 16 months postinfection, which lessens the specificity of this test in serum.[26] However, IgM does not cross the blood-brain barrier, and the presence of IgM in the CSF is strong evidence of local production and thus acute WNND infection. Molecular amplification assays (e.g., polymerase chain reaction [PCR]) in serum are low yield (14%) because of the usually low levels and transient nature of viremia in humans. PCR has moderate sensitivity (57%), detecting WNV in CSF, but is most useful in blood supply screening and active surveillance of bird and mosquito populations.[27] Tissue samples from postmortem examinations may be tested by immunofluorescent antibody and viral culture.[28]

CBCs may be normal or moderately increased with a relative lymphocytosis, but 15% may demonstrate lymphopenia. Hyponatremia may be indicative of SIADH, which is often seen with any encephalitis. The patient may have transaminitis consistent with a usually mild hepatitis. In such cases, serum amylase and lipase should be checked for concomitant pancreatitis. Muscle enzymes such as creatine phosphokinase and myoglobin may be elevated to mild or severe degrees. Lumbar puncture should be performed and reveals a CSF pleocytosis in the range of cell counts often seen in aseptic meningitis (10 to 1000 cells/mm^3), with predominance of lymphocytes, mildly increased protein, and normal glucose. There may be a predominance of neutrophils in early stages of encephalitis. This is in contradistinction to GBS, in which there is a paucity of cells, usually less than 10/mm^3, and a dramatic increase in CSF protein, referred to as *albuminocytologic dissociation*.[29] Thus lumbar puncture can be helpful in distinguishing between AFP and GBS, for which the prognosis is quite different.

TABLE 251-1 Diagnostic Tests for West Nile Virus

Diagnostic Test	Result
INITIAL DIAGNOSTICS	
CBC/differential	Normal or moderately increased
Serum electrolytes, blood urea nitrogen, and creatinine	Fluid and electrolyte imbalance (e.g., hyponatremia [SIADH])
Liver function tests	Elevated transaminases
Amylase,* lipase*	Pancreatitis
Cerebrospinal fluid (CSF)	Pleocytosis <1000 cells/mm^3, lymphocyte predominance Protein increased, but usually <100 mg/dl Glucose normal
Serum or CSF IgM antibody	Positive: 50% on admission, 95% by day 10 of illness
Nucleic acid amplification (PCR)	Positive: 50% in CSF, but less in serum
IMAGING	
CT	Normal
MRI (preferred imaging technique)	Meningeal, periventricular, basal ganglia enhancement May be normal with clinical degrees of encephalitis

IgM, Immunoglobulin M; *PCR,* polymerase chain reaction; *SIADH,* syndrome of inappropriate antidiuretic hormone.
*If indicated.

Cerebral CT is often normal. Cerebral MRI is more likely to reveal abnormalities (30%), such as enhancement of the leptomeninges or the periventricular areas, but is only diagnostic of meningitis or encephalitis in general. MRI is the imaging procedure of choice, but it is possible to have clinical degrees of encephalitis without MRI abnormalities. T2-weighted images showing high-intensity signals in the thalamus and basal ganglia may be early indications of encephalitis.[4,21,30]

Diagnostic tests for WNV are listed in Table 251-1.

DIFFERENTIAL DIAGNOSIS

Bacterial meningitis must quickly be distinguished from aseptic meningitis by a lumbar puncture, which identifies acute bacterial meningitis by cell count greater than 1000 cells/mm^3, neutrophil predominance, and growth of common bacterial offenders. It is helpful clinically to distinguish between aseptic meningitis and encephalitis, but diagnostically the same agents may affect both meninges and brain in varying degrees. Most causes of encephalitis are viral. Although the list is long, many viral causes of meningoencephalitis seen in North America are listed in the Differential Diagnosis box, p. 1339. Nonviral causes that should be considered include drug reactions, carcinomatous meningitis, vasculitis, Behçet's syndrome, endocarditis, demyelinating diseases, postinfectious encephalitis, Lyme disease, leptospirosis, *Listeria* organisms, cat-scratch disease, *Mycoplasma* organisms, and various species of *Rickettsia* and *Ehrlichia*. Patients with AIDS have well-known opportunistic causes of encephalitis: toxoplasmosis, cyto-

DIFFERENTIAL DIAGNOSIS

Viral Causes of Acute Encephalomyelitis

Alphavirus
- Eastern equine
- Western equine
- Venezuelan equine

Flavivirus
- St. Louis
- West Nile
- Japanese
- Dengue
- Tick borne
- Yellow fever

Bunyavirus
- Hepatitis A

Arenavirus
- Lymphocytic choriomeningitis
- Machupo
- Lassa

Reovirus
- Colorado tick fever

Rhabdovirus
- Rabies
- *Lyssavirus* species

Filovirus
- Ebola
- Marburg

Retrovirus
- HIV

Herpesvirus
- Herpes simplex virus types 1 and 2
- Varicella-zoster
- Herpes B
- Cytomegalovirus
- Human herpesvirus 6
- Human herpesvirus 7
- Epstein-Barr

megalovirus, mycobacteria, lymphoma, and progressive multifocal leukoencephalopathy (JC virus). Hypogammaglobulinemic patients may suffer from encephalitis and myositis caused by chronic enterovirus infection. Patients with T-cell depletion, often from chemotherapy, exhibit unusual forms of encephalitis from various herpesviruses, inclusion body encephalitis from measles, and adenovirus.

Seasonal variation is helpful in identifying the arboviruses. Alphavirus, flavivirus, and bunyavirus groups are prevalent when mosquito vectors are active in late summer and early fall in North America. Tick vectors—tick-borne encephalitis in Europe, analogous tick-borne Powassan viral encephalitis in North America, Lyme disease, and *Rickettsia* and *Ehrlichia* organisms—are active in late spring and early summer. Enteroviruses are the most common cause of encephalitis in warm months, when fecal/oral-water spread is common, but enterovirus circulates at lower levels throughout the year. Herpesvirus and mumps occur more uniformly throughout the year. Lymphocytic choriomeningitis is most prevalent in late fall and winter, when rodents come into homes. Leptospirosis is most likely in summer, when rodents are about and urinating in bodies of water frequented by humans.

Geographic distribution and travel histories are important. The *Flaviviridae* viruses have distinct distribution patterns. WNV is now common in the Middle East, Eastern Europe, and North America. Eastern equine encephalitis occurs in small outbreaks along the Atlantic and Gulf Coasts and Great Lakes. SLE and LaCrosse encephalitis occur in larger outbreaks, and they are now widely distributed in North America. The original names no longer reflect their present geographic distribution. Tick-borne encephalitis is found in the distribution of *I. ricinus* and *Ixodes persulcatus* ticks in Eastern Europe and the adjoining Asian continent. JE manifests in large epidemics and is widespread over a third of the globe from Pakistan, India, Australia, and Asia to the eastern border of what once was the United Soviet Socialist Republic (USSR). Lyme disease encephalitis is concentrated in the Northeast and north central Midwest United States and in Europe.

Age can be helpful. WNV causes encephalitis much more commonly in elderly patients, whereas LaCrosse virus causes encephalitis in children. The ratio of asymptomatic infection or febrile illness to encephalitis is small (1:100) in the arboviral diseases, except for eastern equine encephalitis, where infection produces encephalitis with high frequency (1:10) at all ages. AFP has a more limited differential etiology. This includes the prototype poliovirus, which is close to extinction worldwide, and, more likely, circulating vaccine poliovirus strains that have reverted toward wild type. Some enteroviruses and other arboviruses may mimic WNV in their ability to cause AFP.

MANAGEMENT

There is no specific antiviral drug for WNV infection, and treatment is supportive. All patients should be hospitalized and lumbar puncture performed to discern treatable bacterial meningitis, to rule out other treatable causes of encephalitis such as herpesvirus encephalitis, and to observe for progression of encephalitis and AFP. Prolonged periods of unconsciousness may be followed by remarkable periods of recovery, and the health care provider must ensure management of ventilators, bladder catheters, nutrition, IV lines, decubitus ulcers, aspiration pneumonia, urinary tract infection, line sepsis, venous thromboembolism, and seizures. Although steroids and osmotic agents have not been studied as adjunctive therapy, they may be used to manage acute cerebral edema. Ribavirin and interferon-α showed limited effect against WNV in animal models,[31,32] but a retrospective review of their use in Israel showed no effect on mortality.[33] Passive immunization with pooled human IV immunoglobulin (IVIG) may offer some cross-reacting antibodies from circulating antibody to SLE, and now from antibody to WNV in North America. Studies in mice have shown pooled IVIG to have prophylactic and therapeutic efficacy.[34] In one anecdotal report from Israel, IVIG given to a compromised host produced a dramatic response.[35] Results of a large controlled trial completed in December of 2006 (evidence-based category III) remain pending as of this writing.

LIFE SPAN CONSIDERATIONS

Hospitalized patients with WNND, mostly encephalitis, have an upfront mortality of 10% to 15%. Weakness and fatigue in hospitalized patients was predictive of higher mortality (30%). This figure does not tell the whole story, since 50% of patients leave the hospital with significant residua, and an additional 12% die in the next year. Chronic sequelae persist at 1 year in 35%, and include headache, chronic fatigue, weakness, cognitive dysfunction, depression, ataxia, seizures, and chronic aspiration.[16,36-38]

COMPLICATIONS

In addition to the chronic sequelae of severe encephalitis mentioned above, WNV may infect certain organ systems in a selective manner. Arthritis and myalgias are common, but frank myositis, with high serum myoglobin levels, may eventuate in rhabdomyolysis, and acute renal failure may ensue.[39] Cardiomyopathy may be a further consequence of WNV predilection for muscle.[32] As in other flavivirus-induced conditions, infection of the liver manifests as transaminitis, and progression to fulminant hepatitis has occurred.[40] Pancreatitis may reflect infection of pancreas and pancreatic duct.[41]

Chorioretinitis is the most common ophthalmologic manifestation of WNV infection, but anterior uveitis, occlusive retinal vasculitis, and optic neuritis have all been reported. In one survey all patients with ophthalmic manifestations of WNV also had systemic symptoms of WNF or meningoencephalitis.[42] Acute pathologic conditions in the hypothalamic-pituitary axis may result in central hyperthermia, SIADH with hyponatremia, and diabetes insipidus. Acute myelitis causes AFP, which is often asymmetric and irreversible.[20,23] Basal ganglia pathologic conditions are reflected in chronic tremor, myoclonus, parkinsonism, and gait disturbances.[21]

In one study, one in utero infection resulted in birth at 38 weeks' gestation of an infant with bilateral chorioretinitis and marked destruction of cerebral white matter. Four other cases of WNV infection in pregnancy were discovered and apparently did not result in damage to the fetus. Three of these infants tested negative for WNV, and one was not tested for WNV.[15]

INDICATIONS FOR REFERRAL OR HOSPITALIZATION

Patients with diagnosed WNF may be monitored in the primary care setting, but all patients with suspected WNND should be admitted to a hospital, where a lumbar puncture and MRI can be performed. Meningitis and encephalitis have nonspecific presentations, and an infectious disease expert should be consulted immediately to aid in differential diagnosis and consider empiric treatment for bacterial meningitis or herpesvirus encephalitis pending confirmation of a specific diagnosis.

Patients need close monitoring for progression of encephalitis to stages of stupor and coma, at which point they should be in an ICU, where a team from nursing, critical care, and pulmonary medicine will watch for aspiration, airway protection, ventilator support, IV fluids, deep venous thrombosis, pulmonary embolism, and skin breakdown. A nutrition team may need to manage a long course of hyperalimentation. AFP may result in paralysis of respiratory muscles and need for various degrees of long-term respiratory support. Even without AFP, intensive physical and occupational therapy may be required because of chronic weakness from encephalopathy, tremor, parkinsonism, and gait disturbances from basal ganglia pathologic condition. Speech therapy may be needed to manage aspiration and speech issues. Depression is common and may have a physiologic origin in encephalitis, which will require psychiatric consultation and antidepressants, before postencephalitis rehabilitation strategies can progress. A psychologist may be required to perform more formal testing of cognitive function. Chaplain services and alternative spiritual leaders should be welcome.

Recovery from encephalitis and sequelae takes months to years, but higher levels of function may eventually ensue, and remarkable recoveries over time have occurred. Long-term rehabilitation care may be rewarding. Severely compromised patients, especially those with severe cognitive dysfunction, inability to eat, or inadequate airway protection, may not make a meaningful recovery, and withdrawal of support is indicated, with help from family, nursing, physicians, chaplain services, and other spiritual leaders.

HEALTH PROMOTION

WNV is a disease for which an ounce of prevention is worth a ton of cure. Mosquito control and bite reduction can be accomplished individually and outside regional vector-control programs, which may use insecticide spray campaigns, when an outbreak is eminent. Each of us should eliminate mosquito larva breeding sites such as standing water in birdbaths, flowerpots, construction sites, and swimming pool covers. Insect repellents containing deet (diethytoluamide) in high concentrations (20%) are applied to skin. The insecticide permethrin is applied to clothing, mosquito nets, and tents. The combination of deet on skin and permethrin on clothes is better than either agent used alone. Watch for allergic skin reactions to deet. Toxic encephalopathy may occur in young children, and deet should not be used for children under 2 months of age. Older children, under 10 years of age, may use concentrations of deet up to 10%. Avon Skin-So-Soft and citronella products are much less effective, so long-sleeved shirts, long pants, clothing insecticides, and mosquito nets should be the mainstay in young children. Avoid dusk and dawn exposure to mosquitoes, since this is their preferred feeding time.[17]

Screening of the U.S. blood supply has been in effect since June 2003. This has greatly reduced, but not eliminated, the risk of blood product transmission, and it is estimated that screening for WNV is more cost-effective than screening for hepatitis C virus or HIV.[43]

Although there is a vaccine for horses, human vaccine is still in early stages of development. A live chimeric vaccine contains genetic material from WNV in a dengue virus vector. A live attenuated subtype of WNV (Kunjin virus), with little neurotropic potential, is in stage I trials. However, U.S. private industry vaccine development programs require financial incentive, which is lacking in WNV infection. Given that most infections are asymptomatic, that only 1 in 150 patients with infection develop WNND, that seroconversion is only 3% in communities that have faced outbreaks,[44] that 42 states reported fewer than 3000 cases of WNV in 2005, that live vaccines may have complications, and that we live in a litigious society, there may be little incentive for development of a human vaccine. There is some evidence that presently available JE vaccine produces cross-reacting antibodies to WNV and has moderate efficacy.[45]

Health care providers all need to be aware of the clinical signs of WNF and WNND, including meningitis, encephalitis, and AFP, and patient guides do exist.[46] The Kansas Department of Health implemented an extensive WNV education campaign, but follow-up evaluation demonstrated that media messages were not reaching targeted populations, and risk perception remained low.[47] Awareness of the dangers of mosquito and tick exposure, the diseases they transmit, protective measures, and early signs of specific disease is an educational goal that is yet to be achieved.

REFERENCES

1. Van der Meulen KM, Pensaert MB, Nauwynck HJ: West Nile virus in the vertebrate world, *Arch Virol* 150:637-657, 2005.
2. Quirin R, Salas M, Zientara S, and others: West Nile virus, Guadeloupe, *Emerg Infect Dis* 10(4):706-708, 2003.
3. Zeller HG, Schuffenecker I: West Nile virus: an overview of its spread in Europe and the Mediterranean Basin in contrast to its spread in the Americas, *Eur J Clin Microbiol Infect Dis* 23:147-156, 2004.
4. Nash D, Mostashari F, Fine A, and others: The outbreak of West Nile virus infection in the New York City area in 1999, *N Engl J Med* 344(24):1807-1814, 2001.
5. Giladi M, Metzkor-Cotter E, Martin DA, and others: West Nile encephalitis in Israel, 1999: the New York connection, *Emerg Infect Dis* 7(4):659-661, 2001.
6. Ceccaldi PE, Lucas M, Despres P: New insights on the neuro-pathogenicity of West Nile virus, *FEMS Microbiol Lett* 233:1-6, 2004.
7. Yaremych SA, Warner RE, Mankin PC, and others: West Nile virus and high death rate in American crows, *Emerg Infect Dis* 10(4):709-711, 2004.
8. Pealer LN, Marfin AA, Petersen LR, and others: Transmission of West Nile virus through blood transfusion in the United States in 2002, *N Engl J Med* 349(13):1236-1245, 2003.
9. Kleinschmidt-DeMasters BK, Marder BA, Levi ME, and others: Naturally acquired West Nile virus encephalomyelitis in transplant recipients, *Arch Neurol* 61:1210-1220, 2004.
10. Centers for Disease Control and Prevention: West Nile virus infections in organ transplants—New York and Pennsylvania, August-September, 2005, *MMWR* 54(40):1021-1023, 2005.
11. Centers for Disease Control and Prevention: Possible West Nile virus transmission to an infant through breast-feeding—Michigan, 2002, *MMWR* 51:877-878, 2002.
12. Centers for Disease Control and Prevention: Laboratory-acquired West Nile virus infections—United States, 2002, *MMWR* 51:1133-1135, 2002.
13. Centers for Disease Control and Prevention: Intrauterine West Nile virus infection—New York, 2002, *MMWR* 51:1135-1136, 2002.
14. Centers for Disease Control and Prevention: Possible dialysis-related West Nile virus transmission—Georgia, 2003, *MMWR* 53:738-739, 2004.
15. Hayes EB, O'Leary DR: West Nile virus infection: a pediatric perspective, *Pediatrics* 113:1375-1381, 2004.
16. Mandalakas AM, Kippes C, Sedransk J, and others: West Nile virus epidemic, northeast Ohio, 2002, *Emerg Infect Dis* 11(11):1774-1777, 2005.
17. Peterson LR, Marfin AA: West Nile virus: a primer for the clinician, *Ann Intern Med* 137:173-179, 2002.
18. Ferguson DD, Gershman K, LeBailly A, and others: Characteristics of the rash associated with West Nile fever, *Clin Infect Dis* 41:1204-1207, 2005.
19. Centers for Disease Control and Prevention: Acute flaccid paralysis syndrome associated with West Nile virus infection—Mississippi and Louisiana, July-August 2002, *MMWR* 51(37):825-827, 2002.
20. Jeha LE, Sila CA, Lederman RJ, and others: West Nile virus infection: a new paralytic illness, *Neurology* 61:55-59, 2003.
21. Sejvar JJ, Haddad MB, Tierney BC, and others: Neurologic manifestations of West Nile virus infection, *JAMA* 290(4):511-515, 2003.
22. Ahmed F, Libman R, Wesson K, and others: Guillain-Barré syndrome: an unusual presentation of West Nile virus infection, *Neurology* 55:144-146, 2000.
23. Sejvar JJ, Leis AA, Stokic DS, and others: Acute flaccid paralysis and West Nile virus infection, *Emerg Infect Dis* 9(7):788-793, 2003.
24. New York City Department of Health: *West Nile virus surveillance and control: an update for health-care providers in New York City*, New York, 2001, City Health Information.
25. Martin DA, Biggerstaff BJ, Johnson AJ, and others: Use of IgM cross-reactions in differential diagnosis of human flaviviral encephalitis infections in the United States, *Clin Diagn Lab Immunol* 9:544-549, 2002.
26. Roehrig JT, Nash D, Maldin B, and others: Persistence of virus-reactive serum IgM antibody in confirmed West Nile virus encephalitis cases, *Emerg Infect Dis* 9(3):376-379, 2003.
27. Sampathkumar P: West Nile Virus: epidemiology, clinical presentation, diagnosis, and prevention, *Mayo Clin Proc* 78:1137-1144, 2003.
28. Huang C, Slater B, Rudd R, and others: First isolation of West Nile virus from a patient with encephalitis in the United States, *Emerg Infect Dis* 8:1367-1371, 2002.
29. Ropper AH: The Guillain-Barré syndrome, *N Engl J Med* 326(17):1130-1136, 1992.
30. Tyler KL: West Nile virus infection in the United States, *Arch Neurol* 61:1190-1195, 2004.
31. Jordan I, Briese T, Fischer N, and others: Ribavirin inhibits West Nile virus replication and cytopathic effect in neural cells, *J Infect Dis* 182(4):1214-1217, 2000.
32. Campbell GL, Marfin AA, Lanciotti RS, and others: West Nile virus, *Lancet Infect Dis* 2(9):519-529, 2002.
33. Chowers MY, Marfin AA, Lanciotti RS, and others: Clinical characteristics of the West Nile fever outbreak, Israel 2000, *Emerg Infect Dis* 7:675-678, 2001.
34. Ben-Nathan D, Shlomo N, Tam G, and others: Prophylactic and therapeutic efficacy of human intravenous immunoglobulin in treating West Nile virus infection in mice, *J Infect Dis* 188:5-12, 2003.
35. Shimoni Z, Niven MJ, Pitlick S, and others: Treatment of West Nile encephalitis with intravenous immunoglobulin (letter), *Emerg Infect Dis* 7(4):759, 2001.
36. Green MS, Weinberger M, Ben-Ezer J, and others: Long-term death rates, West Nile virus epidemic, Israel 2000, *Emerg Infect Dis* 11(11):1754-1757, 2005.
37. Weiss D, Carr D, Kellachan J, and others: Clinical findings of West Nile virus infection in hospitalized patients, New York and New Jersey 2000, *Emerg Infect Dis* 7(4):654-658, 2001.
38. Pepperell C, Rau N, Krajden S, and others: West Nile virus infection in 2002: morbidity and mortality among patients admitted to hospital in southcentral Ontario, *CMAJ* 168(11):1399-1405, 2003.
39. Smith RD, Konoplev S, DeCourten-Myers G, and others: West Nile virus encephalitis with myositis and orchitis, *Hum Pathol* 35:254-258, 2004.
40. Georges AJ, Lesbordes JL, Georges-Courbot MC, and others: Fatal hepatitis from West Nile virus, *Ann Inst Pasteur Virol* 138:237-244, 1987.
41. Perelman A, Stern J: Acute pancreatitis in West Nile fever, *Am J Trop Med Hyg* 23:1150-1152, 1974.
42. Garg S, Jampol LM: Systemic and intraocular manifestations of West Nile virus infection, *Surv Ophthalmol* 50:3-13, 2005.
43. Custer B, Busch MP, Marfin AA, and others: The cost-effectiveness of screening the U.S. blood supply for West Nile virus, *Ann Intern Med* 143:486-492, 2005.
44. Mostashari F, Bunning ML, Kitsutani PT, and others: Epidemic West Nile encephalitis, New York 1999: results of a household-based seroepidemiological survey, *Lancet* 358:261-264, 2001.
45. Yamshchikov G, Borisevich V, Kwok CW, and others: The suitability of yellow fever and Japanese encephalitis vaccines for immunization against West Nile virus, *Vaccine* 23:4785-4792, 2005.
46. Mackenzie DL: Combat West Nile virus, *Nurs Manage* 34(8):24-26, 2003.
47. Averett E, Neuberger JS, Hansen G, and others: Evaluation of West Nile virus education campaign, *Emerg Infect Dis* 11(11):1751-1753, 2005.

PART 21

Evaluation and Management of Oncologic Disorders

JOANN TRYBULSKI, *Section Editor*

CHAPTER 252

Collaborative Management of the Oncology Patient

Jane Williams

Optimum cancer care depends on careful planning across multidisciplinary care settings to reduce the risk of fragmentation and ensure a continuum of care. Many patients belong to managed care insurance plans that require the primary health care provider to maintain the gatekeeper role. Also, many oncology patients live hundreds of miles away from the cancer center and need qualified care close to home. It is important that the health care provider be viewed as a valuable member of the cancer care team, not as a resented formality. Therefore it is necessary that all providers have a basic understanding of cancer-specific risk factors, presenting signs and symptoms, diagnostic tools, treatment options, prognosis, psychosocial issues, and available support systems.

CANCER RISKS

Approximately three fourths of all cancer risks are elements that individuals can control themselves. These include dietary habits, the use of tobacco products or alcohol, sun exposure, lack of physical activity, and risky sexual behaviors. Emphasizing healthy lifestyle practices is a principal component of primary care, not only for cancer prevention but also for overall disease prevention.

SCREENING FOR CANCER

The American Cancer Society offers cancer-specific guidelines for screening asymptomatic patients, and evidence-based screening guidelines can also be obtained from the National Cancer Institute.[1,2] The health care provider needs to be involved in high-quality screening activities, which include the following comprehensive examinations: breast, gynecologic (women), genitourinary (men), colorectal, skin, and oral head and neck. Screening tests should be performed according to age-appropriate recommended guidelines and need to include mammography, cervical smears, colorectal screening, and prostate screening. The health care provider will most likely be the one to detect cancer and will be the first source of information regarding diagnosis and possible treatment options before referring the patient to the oncologist or cancer center.

New information about genetic testing is widely available. Although only 5% to 10% of cancers are hereditary, providers must be diligent in obtaining accurate family histories to establish the possibility of a hereditary cancer syndrome. If this possibility does exist, the patient should be informed about the potential personal risk for cancer and about available surveillance and management strategies, including self-examinations, screening examinations, diagnostic tests, and cancer prevention strategies. Patients at high risk for certain cancers may need additional screening. For example, women suspected of being at risk for hereditary breast and ovarian syndromes need to increase clinical breast examinations to annually if between ages 20 and 40 years (some authorities even recommend every 6 months) and have annual mammograms or other imaging studies beginning at least 10 years earlier than the youngest age of diagnosis in a relative. In addition, an annual CA_{125} and transvaginal ultrasound screening for ovarian cancer is advised. Other high-risk guidelines can be obtained from the American Cancer Society.[2] If indicated, a referral to a National Cancer Institute–designated comprehensive cancer center that offers genetic testing and counseling is appropriate.

PATIENT MANAGEMENT ISSUES

After a diagnosis of cancer, a timely referral for treatment increases the opportunity for optimum outcomes. In many cases these outcomes include improved rates of cure, longer survival rates, and improved quality of life.

With shortened hospital stays, the management of cancer patients has moved from the hospital to the home. In such cases, collaboration with the oncology team in managing symptoms and monitoring for complications becomes essential. There needs to be clear communication with the oncology team regarding current treatment, including side effects and expected outcome, current condition and prognosis, patient understanding, frequency of reports to and from the oncology team, and future treatment plans. Communication must clearly define areas of responsibility between the primary health care provider and oncology and should be task oriented. For example, if the health care provider agrees to monitor laboratory values for neutropenia, anemia, thrombocytopenia, kidney function, and liver function, he or she must be aware of critical laboratory parameters that require management by the oncology team or referral to a specialist. Additionally, the primary health care provider can reinforce to the patient the signs and symptoms that indicate need for urgent evaluation, such as fever, mental status change, increasing pain, or persistent vomiting. The health care provider should recognize how treatment may affect blood glucose, blood pressure, thyroid function, kidney function, or liver enzymes and should be able to determine whether symptoms are related to cancer or cancer treatment or other known or new conditions. Referral back to the oncology team is required for symptoms that are difficult to manage; critical laboratory studies; new suspicious findings; or oncologic emergencies such as spinal cord compression, hypercalcemia, tumor lysis syndrome, syndrome of inappropriate antidiuretic hormone, or superior vena cava syndrome (see Chapter 257).

Febrile neutropenia—temperature over 38° C (100.4° F) and absolute neutrophil count less than 500/mm^3—is a common complication of patients on chemotherapy and needs immediate attention. Standard procedures include hospitalization with chest x-ray examination, urine culture and sensitivity, blood cultures, and, if a central line is in place, culture of the line.

Long-term surveillance is important, especially for young survivors but also for the older population as we develop more effective cancer treatments. Complications may affect the cardiovascular system, including increased risk of hypertension and hyperlipidemia from vascular endothelial injury and increased plasma renin and aldosterone levels.[3] Serious cardiovascular complications have been reported after cisplatin-based therapy. Peripheral neuropathy may occur with cisplatin or taxane therapies. Tinnitus and high-frequency hearing loss are related to peripheral neuropathy. Bleomycin-related acute pulmonary toxicity is increased in cigarette smokers.[3] Young survivors may have problems with reproduction after radiotherapy or chemotherapy, and radiotherapy and chemotherapy may also increase the risk of additional primary malignancies in long-term survivors.

Caring for the cancer patient can place inordinate burdens on family and friends. Assessing the caregivers' readiness and availability to care for the patient is imperative. The primary caregiver must be aware of the established support systems and the availability of additional community resources such as breast cancer support groups, the United Ostomy Associations of America, I Can Cope, Candlelighters, Us TOO, and CanCare. The local American Cancer Society chapter is another excellent resource, and many communities have faith-based support services. Successful home care also depends on such factors as cultural beliefs, role delineation, and resolution of any existing interpersonal conflicts. Additionally, personal values surrounding narcotic analgesic use and beliefs about death and dying should be explored.

ROLE OF THE PRIMARY HEALTH CARE PROVIDER

The primary health care provider is an essential resource between appointments with the oncologist, especially if the oncologist is in another city or if the health care provider is seeing the patient for management of other chronic conditions. If the provider is not receiving reports and updates from the oncologist, he or she should contact the oncologist and request to receive all vital information that will affect patient outcomes. This allows the primary health care provider to adequately monitor various symptoms, accurately answer patient questions regarding treatment side effects, and reinforce information given by the oncologist. Establishment of a collaborative relationship between the oncology team and the health care provider ensures safe and continuous care, minimizes potential complications, and promotes patient and provider confidence.

Health care reform has redirected patient care. Both patients with cancer and cancer survivors are especially vulnerable to the risk of fragmentation of care when migrating from specialist to generalist or from hospital to home care. Consistent personnel who know the patient's situation are the key components for successful delivery of health care. It is the responsibility of the patient and all members of the multidisciplinary health care team to identify needs and form a collaborative plan so that outcomes of care can be optimized.

REFERENCES

1. American Cancer Society: *Cancer-specific prevention and early detection,* 2006, retrieved March 4, 2007, from http://www.cancer.org/docroot/PED/content/PED_2_3X_ACS_Cancer_Detection_Guidelines_36.asp?sitearea=PED.
2. National Cancer Institute: *Cancer-specific early detection,* 2006, retrieved March 4, 2007, from http://www.nci.nih.gov./cancertopics/screening.
3. Vaughn DJ, Gretchen AG, Meadows AT: Long-term medical care of testicular cancer survivors, *Ann Intern Med* 136(6):463-470, 2002.

CHAPTER 253

Basic Principles of Oncology Treatment

Karen Borden and Debra Connolly

Treatment of any cancer is multifaceted and involves a multidisciplinary team that includes physician specialists, nurse practitioners, physician assistants, nurses, pharmacists, social workers, and other health care professionals. Primary health care providers act as patient advocates and play a central role in coordinating the effort among all involved disciplines.

The oldest treatment for cancer is surgery. The early 1800s marked the modern era of elective surgery for visceral tumors in frontier America.[1] Surgery is effectively used for cancer prevention, diagnosis, definitive treatment, rehabilitation, and palliation. Using combinations of surgery, chemotherapy, radiotherapy, biotherapy, and hormonal and genetic therapy, the health care team has significantly lengthened disease-free intervals and achieved recognizable survival benefits. Radiotherapy and chemotherapy, historically relegated to palliative roles, have become adjunctive treatments for local disease and are even curative for some early-stage cancers.[2]

The first approach to any cancer treatment is determined by tumor type. One major role of surgery is to obtain tissue for an accurate histologic diagnosis.[1] Once a histologic diagnosis has been established, the patient's disease is staged, which is an essential component of cancer management. Staging is performed to assess the extent of disease and determine prognosis and choice of therapy. There are various cancer staging systems. Some are used for multiple cancers, whereas others are specific for individual cancers.[3] Common parameters in most staging systems include cell type, location of primary tumor, tumor grade, tumor size and number, lymph node involvement, and presence of metastases.[3]

In the earliest stages of the disease, the tumor is localized and a cure is possible through local or regional therapy. If the tumor stage is higher, the cancer is no longer localized and the chance of curing the patient diminishes. Once the tumor type and stage are determined, the treatment plan is created. This plan considers the risk/benefit ratio of various options, the patient's overall physical condition, the patient's consent, the availability of treatment facilities, and any financial restrictions.

RADIOTHERAPY (RADIATION THERAPY)

Radiotherapy may be the sole treatment for cancer but is often combined with surgery or chemotherapy and biologic therapy to eliminate or shrink tumors. Although treatment techniques and equipment may vary, the important principles of radiotherapy form a basis on which a course of treatment is chosen and designed for each patient.[2]

There are three delivery modes of radiotherapy. The first and most commonly used are teletherapy or external beam. Second, brachytherapy delivers radiation from a source placed within the body or body cavity. Lastly, radionuclides deliver systemic radiation.

Teletherapy produces x rays of varying energies (orthovoltage or megavoltage). The higher the voltage, the greater the depth of penetration of the x-ray beam. Disadvantages of teletherapy include poor depth of penetration, severe skin reactions resulting from high doses at the skin level, and bone necrosis (bone absorbs more radiation than soft tissue). Megavoltage equipment has distinct advantages over an orthovoltage beam. Megavoltage equipment provides deeper penetration, more uniform absorption of radiation, and greater skin sparing.[4]

The dose of radiation is determined by the radiosensitivity of the tumor. The gray (abbreviated Gy) system international unit is the accepted term for radiation dosages: 1 Gy equals 100 rad (radiation absorbed dose); 1 cGy equals 1 rad.[5] In some cases a sterotactic external beam radiation (SEBR) is used. SEBR is used to deliver high-intensity external radiation to a small target lesion with minimum damage to the surrounding tissue. Often this is used to treat primary brain tumors or isolated metastatic brain lesions.[6] Brachytherapy involves placement of these sources of radioactive material within or near a tumor and is the treatment of choice for a variety of malignancies. It is often combined with teletherapy and may be used preoperatively or postoperatively. Radioactive isotopes for brachytherapy application are contained in a variety of forms such as wires, ribbons, tubes, needles, grains, seeds, or capsules. The source is selected by the radiotherapist according to the site to be treated, size of the lesion, and whether the implant is temporary or permanent. Brachytherapy is given at either a low-dose rate or a high-dose rate, which produces the same effect in a shorter period.[4]

It is usually assumed that DNA is the critical target for the effects of radiotherapy. A cell damaged by radiation loses its reproductive integrity but may divide at least once before its offspring are reproductively sterile. Some delay in division is usually produced, even in cells that are not damaged lethally.[2] Other factors that affect the biologic response to radiotherapy include oxygen effect (well-oxygenated tumors have a greater response), linear energy transfer (the rate at which energy is lost from different types of radiations while traveling through matter), relative biologic effectiveness, and fractionation.[2]

After the patient has been evaluated and a decision to use external beam therapy has been made, a simulation is performed. Simulation localizes the tumor and defines the volume to be treated. The field of treatment is delineated by tattooing the area to be irradiated. Special immobilization devices, such as custom casts or molds, may be used.[4]

For patients not receiving whole-body irradiation, certain treatment-related side effects may develop. Predictable side effects of radiation therapy for a particular tumor type often occur. Factors that predict side effects include the exact body tissue treated, the daily dose and total dosage given, the particular method of radiation delivery, and individual factors (e.g., the patient's age and genetic makeup). Many symptoms do not develop until 10 to 14 days into treatment, and some do not subside until 2 or more weeks after treatments have ended.[2] Common side effects include fatigue, anorexia, mucositis, xerostomia, radiation caries, esophagitis, dysphagia, nausea, vomiting, diarrhea, tenesmus, cystitis, urethritis, alopecia, skin reactions, and bone marrow depression.[5]

In the future, radiation oncology will be characterized by continuous improvement of treatment techniques and increased application of multimodal therapy. Radiotherapy has come a long way since its beginning in the 1800s. The future holds promise for advances in cancer treatment, with radiotherapy playing a major role in primary treatment and in combined modality approaches.

The primary health care provider's responsibility is to monitor for common gastrointestinal and dermatologic complications and collaborate with oncologists or radiotherapists in implementing a management strategy.

CHEMOTHERAPY

The word *chemotherapy* was introduced by Paul Ehrlich in the early 1900s.[7] Chemotherapeutic agents have traditionally been classified by their mechanism of action, chemical structure, or biologic source. Alkylating agents were the first modern chemotherapeutic agents and were a product of the secret weapons programs in the two world wars. After an explosion in Italy, physicians noticed that many of the soldiers exposed to the resultant gases died from atrophy of the lymph glands and bone marrow suppression.[5] After this discovery, a similar chemical called nitrogen mustard was given to patients with metastatic lymphomas; this resulted in transient but promising antitumor responses (Table 253-1).[8]

In the last decade, molecular analysis of the DNA of both normal and neoplastic cells has defined the mechanisms by which chemotherapy causes cell death. Understanding how chemotherapy works and how genetic change can result in resistance to therapy has enabled new types of treatment. These therapies combine molecular, genetic, and biologic strategies to increase the sensitivity of abnormal cells to treatment and to protect the normal tissues of the body from therapy-induced side effects.[7] Discovery of these new strategies could change the way therapy is delivered over the next few years and improve treatment outcomes, especially in patients with cancers that are resistant to standard therapy.

TABLE 253-1 Common Oncology Medications

Drugs	Uses
PLATINUM COMPLEXES	
Carboplatin, cisplatin	Ovarian cancer; endometrial, head and neck, lung, testicular, breast cancers; relapsed acute leukemia; non-Hodgkin's lymphoma; testicular, ovarian, bladder, uterine, cervical, lung, head, and neck sarcoma
NITROGEN MUSTARDS	
Chlorambucil, cyclophosphamide, estramustine, ifosfamide, mechlorethamine, melphalan	CLL; HD; NHL; ovarian cancer; choriocarcinoma; lymphosarcoma
AZIRIDINE	
Thiotepa	Ovarian, breast, superficial bladder cancer; HD; CML; CLL; bronchogenic carcinoma; malignant effusions (intracavitary); BMT for refractory leukemia, lymphoma
ALKYL SULFONATE	
Busulfan	CML; BMT
NITROSOUREAS	
Carmustine, lomustine, streptozocin	Brain and refractory brain cancer; multiple myeloma; HD; NHL; melanoma; BMT; GI carcinomas; NSCLC; pancreatic islet cell carcinoma; carcinoid colon; hepatoma
NONCLASSIC ALKYLATORS	
Dacarbazine, procarbazine, altretamine	Malignant melanoma; HD; sarcoma; neuroblastoma; NHL; brain, lung, ovarian, breast, cervical cancer
ANTIMETABOLITES	
Methotrexate, fludarabine, mercaptopurine, thioguanine, cladribine, pentostatin, cytarabine, floxuridine, fluorouracil, gemcitabine	Breast, head, neck, GI, lung cancer; ALL; CNS leukemia; Burkitt's lymphoma; CLL; CML; AML; multiple myeloma; hairy-cell leukemia; NHL; lymphoma; pancreatic, renal cell, prostate, ovarian cancer
Hydroxyurea (Hydrea, substituted urea)	CML; ALL; ovarian, head and neck cancer; melanoma; essential thrombosis; polycythemia
NATURAL PRODUCTS	
Bleomycin, dactinomycin, daunorubicin, doxorubicin, idarubicin, mitoxantrone, mitomycin, etoposide, teniposide, docetaxel, paclitaxel, vinblastine, vincristine, vinorelbine, irinotecan, topotecan	Skin, bladder, breast, ovarian, testicular, vulvar, penile, thyroid, gastric, colorectal, uterine, cervical, pancreatic, and renal cancers; reticulum cell sarcoma; HD; squamous cell cancer of head and neck; Wilm's tumor; Ewing's sarcoma; AML; ALL; NHL; SCLC; CML; NSCLC; melanoma; rhabdomyosarcoma
Asparaginase (enzyme)	ALL; CML; AML

ALL, Acute lymphocytic leukemia; *AML,* acute myelogenous leukemia; *BMT,* bone marrow transplant; *CLL,* chronic lymphocytic leukemia; *CML,* chronic myelogenous leukemia; *GI,* gastrointestinal; *HD,* Hodgkin's disease; *NHL,* non-Hodgkin's lymphoma; *NSCLC,* non-small cell lung cancer.

Administering and monitoring chemotherapy requires an understanding of the principles of carcinogenesis and cellular kinetics.[8] Carcinogenesis is the process by which one or more normal cells undergo genetic changes, leading to malignant transformation. The direct exposure of DNA to a carcinogen may lead to irreversible genetic damage that allows this malignant transformation. The cell cycle is a sequence of steps through which both normal and abnormal cells grow and reproduce.[9] This process involves five phases: M, the period of cell division, or mitosis; G_1, the postmitotic period (in the proliferative cycle); G_0, the postmitotic period (temporarily out of the proliferative cycle); S, the period of DNA synthesis; and G_2, the premitotic period (RNA and protein synthesis). These cell-cycle kinetics are altered when a cell becomes malignant. Chemotherapeutic agents can be classified according to the phase of the cell cycle in which they are active (Box 253-1).

Chemotherapy is used as an induction treatment for advanced disease, as an addition to local methods of treatment, or as the primary treatment for patients with localized cancer. Chemotherapeutic agents may also be directly instilled into tumor sanctuaries (e.g., the brain or meninges) or perfused into specific regions of the body most affected by the cancer (e.g., intraperitoneal).[7]

BOX 253-1

CELL-CYCLE ACTIVITY

S-PHASE AGENTS

Antimetabolites
- Cytarabine
- Doxorubicin
- Fludarabine
- Gemcitabine
- Hydroxyurea
- Mercaptopurine
- Methotrexate
- Prednisone
- Procarbazine
- Thioguanine

CELL-CYCLE PHASE–NONSPECIFIC AGENTS

Alkylating agents
Antibiotics
Nitrosoureas
Miscellaneous

M-PHASE AGENTS

Vinca alkaloids
- Vinblastine
- Vincristine
- Vinorelbine

Podophyllotoxins
- Etoposide
- Teniposide

Taxanes
- Docetaxel
- Paclitaxel

G_2-PHASE AGENT

Bleomycin

G_1-PHASE AGENTS

Asparaginase
Corticosteroids

Among patients receiving chemotherapy, there is a wide diversity in both therapeutic response and toxicity observed. This variability can be attributed to differences in patient characteristics, the chemotherapeutic agents given, and the type of tumor being treated.[9] Patient factors include toxicity response, organ dysfunction, previous treatments, and age. The occurrence and severity of toxicity are widely variable among patients and may require a dose reduction or a treatment delay.

Chemotherapy may be given as neoadjuvant (preoperative) therapy, as adjuvant (postoperative) therapy, or as palliative therapy for advanced disease. Administering a combination of clinically effective antitumor drugs is the standard chemotherapeutic approach for most malignancies. This technique provides maximum cell kill for resistant cells, reduces the development of resistant cell lines, and minimizes toxicity.[7]

The oncologist and primary health care provider often work collaboratively in managing common side effects of chemotherapy. These common adverse effects of cancer and its therapy include fatigue, anorexia, diarrhea, constipation, nausea and vomiting, cardiotoxicity, neurotoxicity, pulmonary toxicity, hepatotoxicity, hemorrhagic cystitis, nephrotoxicity, and gonadal toxicity.[7]

BIOLOGIC THERAPIES

Progress in molecular biology and biotechnology has had a major impact on the way patients with cancer are treated today. With a greater understanding of the molecular nature of cancer and the immune system, newer agents have been developed for a variety of purposes. For example, growth-stimulating factors are currently being used to support the immune system so patients can receive optimum doses of chemotherapeutic agents. Alternatively, biologic therapies such as interferon and interleukin-2 are also being used for their ability to control tumor growth and generation and to restore, augment, or modulate patients' ability to fight cancer. Antibody-based immunotherapies, otherwise known as monoclonal antibodies, have been found to be effective both alone and in combination with other therapies for the treatment of cancer. Although many of the monoclonal antibodies are still under clinical investigation, they offer a safe and specific new approach to treating cancer cells and sparing normal tissue.[10,11] Gene therapy is an attempt to alter patients' genetic material to fight or prevent disease. Current and future research endeavors include combining chemotherapy, biologic therapy, and gene therapy to achieve optimum patient outcomes.

Primary health care providers have multiple responsibilities to patients receiving therapy for cancer. Understanding the implications of different tumor types and monitoring for treatment side effects are essential when caring for these patients. Direct communication and collaboration between the oncologist and health care provider are necessary for the recognition of subtle but potentially life-threatening changes in the patient's condition.

REFERENCES

1. Rosenberg S: Principles of cancer management in surgical oncology. In DeVita VT, Hellman S, Rosenberg SA, editors: *Cancer: principles and practice of oncology*, ed 5, Philadelphia, 1997, Lippincott.

2. Hellman S: Principles of cancer management in radiation therapy. In DeVita VT, Hellman S, Rosenberg SA, editors: *Cancer: principles and practice of oncology*, ed 5, Philadelphia, 1997, Lippincott.
3. National Cancer Institute: *Staging: questions and answers*, retrieved March 12, 2007, from http://www.cancer.gov/cancertopics/factsheet/Detection/Staging.
4. Iwamato RR: Radiation therapy. In Varricchio C, Pierce M, Walker CL, and others, editors: *A cancer sourcebook for nurses*, ed 7, Atlanta, 1997, American Cancer Society.
5. Bucholtz JD: Radiation. In Gross J, Johnson BJ, editors: *Handbook for oncology nursing*, ed 3, Boston, 1998, Jones & Bartlett.
6. Chao C: *Radiation oncology: management decisions*, ed 2, Philadelphia, 2002, Lippincott Williams & Wilkins.
7. Hubbard SM, Gakassi A: Chemotherapy. In Gross J, Johnson BL, editors: *Handbook of oncology nursing*, ed 3, Boston, 1998, Jones & Bartlett.
8. DeVita V: Principles of cancer management in chemotherapy. In DeVita VT, Hellman S, Rosenberg SA, editors: *Cancer: principles and practice of oncology*, ed 5, Philadelphia, 1997, Lippincott.
9. Page R, Rhodes V, Pazdur R: Cancer chemotherapy. In Pazdur R, Coia L, Haskins WJ, and others, editors: *Cancer management: a multidisciplinary approach*, ed 5, New York, 2001, PRR.
10. Chabner B, Longo D: *Cancer chemotherapy and biotherapy: principles and practice*, ed 3, Philadelphia, 2001, Lippincott Williams & Wilkins.
11. Yarbro C, Frogge MH, Goodman M, and others: *Cancer nursing: principles and practice*, ed 5, Boston, 2000, Jones & Bartlett.

CHAPTER 254

Unknown Primary Carcinoma

Renato Lenzi

DEFINITION AND EPIDEMIOLOGY

Unknown primary carcinoma (UPC) is defined as the presence of documented metastatic cancer in the absence of an identifiable primary tumor site. Because identification of the primary site forms the basis for formulating prognosis and assigning the appropriate therapy of malignant diseases, the absence of a primary site poses a major challenge. In patients with UPC, the reason the primary site cannot be diagnosed remains unknown. Investigators have speculated that the tumor either remains below the limits of clinical or radiographic detection or regresses spontaneously.

Of the large population of patients referred to a cancer center, approximately 1% have metastases from an unknown primary site.[1] Higher prevalence rates of 3% to 15% have been reported, probably reflecting differences in referral patterns, demographics, and the type and extent of the evaluation performed. Patients with UPC are heterogeneous in their clinical presentation and have widely varying clinical courses. As a group, these patients have a poor median survival of 11 months. Except for a slight preponderance of male patients, the demographics (age and ethnicity) generally mirror those of the general cancer patient population.[1]

PATHOPHYSIOLOGY

Findings of chromosome 1 deletion, translocations, and gene amplification in UPC suggest that these tumors may rapidly progress to reach the ability to metastasize. It has been speculated that specific genetic changes of UPC may support metastatic but not local growth. Although UPCs would be expected to have a high rate of *p53* mutations because of their metastatic nature and clinical aggressiveness, the measured frequency of *p53* mutations is low (26%).[2] Furthermore, there appear to be no differences in microvessel density between metastases from unknown primary sites and those from primary tumors originating in the colon or breast.[3]

CLINICAL PRESENTATION

The clinical presentations of patients with UPC vary widely, probably reflecting the heterogeneous nature of the underlying malignancies. Subgroups of patients with similar clinical presentations have been identified as having disease that is responsive to therapy and/or longer survival times. These "favorable" subsets include (1) women with peritoneal carcinomatosis, (2) women with metastatic adenocarcinoma or carcinoma confined to the axillary nodes, (3) patients with inguinal node metastases with histologic features of squamous cell carcinoma, (4) patients with squamous cell carcinoma confined to lymph nodes in the high or middle neck, and (5) patients with neuroendocrine tumors. Moreover, it has been

TABLE 254-1 Tumor Histology of 1109 Patients with Unknown Primary Carcinoma

Histology	Patients	% of Total
Adenocarcinoma	646	58.3
Well differentiated	14	
Moderately differentiated	45	
Poorly differentiated	220	
Mucinous	46	
No descriptor/other	321	
Carcinoma	317	28.6
Poorly differentiated	161	
Undifferentiated	21	
Large cell	9	
Small cell	14	
No descriptor/other	112	
Squamous	68	6.1
Neuroendocrine	48	4.3
Adenosquamous	7	0.6
Pathology not available for review/other	23	2.1

Data from Abbruzzese JL, Abbruzzese MC, Lenzi R: Unpublished data, Houston, 2005, M.D. Anderson Cancer Center.

shown that patients initially seen with lymph node involvement have longer median survival times than patients with lung, liver, or bone metastasis.[1]

The tumor histology of 1109 consecutive UPC patients is summarized in Table 254-1. Glandular differentiation sufficient to permit a diagnosis of adenocarcinoma was identified in approximately 60% of patients with UPC. Nearly 30% patients were diagnosed with carcinoma, and more than half of these had evidence of poorly differentiated or undifferentiated carcinoma. Squamous cell carcinoma and neuroendocrine carcinoma together accounted for 10% of patients and were associated with more favorable median survival times. Patients with carcinoma also had a longer median survival time (12 months) than patients with two adenocarcinomas (9 months), but their survival advantage was not as pronounced as that of patients with squamous cell carcinoma (24 months) and neuroendocrine carcinoma (33 months).

PHYSICAL EXAMINATION

The initial evaluation should focus on signs and symptoms that could identify the primary site (e.g., blood in stool, persistent cough) and should include an inquiry regarding the family history of cancer. The physical examination should include a search for skin lesions; a careful breast and pelvic examination (for women); and a testicular, rectal, and prostate examination (for men). Areas with lymph nodes should be examined for adenopathy.

DIAGNOSTICS

A limited and focused evaluation that includes a pathologic review; careful physical examination; CBC; chemistry survey (SMA-20); chest radiography; a CT scan of the chest, abdomen, and pelvis in all patients; prostate-specific antigen levels in men; and a mammography in women has been shown to be effective in identifying the more treatable primary malignancies.[4] Additional studies are performed as needed to pursue abnormalities that are revealed during the initial evaluation. This strategy identified a primary malignancy in 20% (179 patients) of a consecutive group of 879 patients referred with suspected UPC.[4] Positron emission tomography (PET) scan should also be considered in patients with cervical metastasis for the diagnosis of a primary and of additional unrecognized regional and distant metastatic lesions.[5] Breast MRI should be done if a breast primary malignancy is suspected and mammography is negative. Careful review of biopsy material is the most important single step in determining the primary site or identifying a unique histologic subset that is amenable to therapy.[4]

DIAGNOSTICS

Unknown Primary Carcinoma

PATHOLOGY

Review of biopsy material
- Morphology
- Immunohistochemistry*
- Molecular and chromosomal studies*

Repeat biopsy*

LABORATORY

CBC and differential
Complete chemistry profile
Prostate-specific antigen (for men)
β-Human chorionic gonadotropin and alpha-fetoprotein (if extragonadal germ cell syndrome is suspected)

IMAGING

Chest x-ray
CT scan of chest, abdomen, pelvis
Mammogram, breast MRI

*If indicated to perform additional studies such as immunohistochemistry.

Good communication between the primary health care provider and pathologist is needed to plan the optimum use of immunohistochemical staining, electron microscopy, or molecular studies for the evaluation of each patient. Carefully selected special studies can be extremely useful in diagnosing the primary type in patients with morphologically undifferentiated or poorly differentiated neoplasms and in patients with well-differentiated carcinomas that cannot be further classified solely on morphologic criteria.[6]

DIFFERENTIAL DIAGNOSIS

At the beginning of the diagnostic evaluation, it is important to establish unequivocally whether the patient indeed has a neoplastic process. A small but significant percentage of the patients referred with a diagnosis of metastatic carcinoma of unknown primary are found on further evaluation not to have cancer.[1] In the majority of these cases the diagnosis of neoplastic disease was made on the basis of radiographic studies only, and the initial evaluation did not include a biopsy. For example, a patient with osteoporosis and compression fractures of single or multiple vertebral bodies may be initially diagnosed with metastatic bone lesions.

Clarification of the diagnosis is usually accomplished with a biopsy of the suspected metastatic site. Appropriate caution needs to be used in planning invasive diagnostic modalities because complications can result from the diagnostic procedure itself. For example, a liver biopsy may result in excessive bleeding if the liver lesion suspected of being neoplastic is actually a hemangioma. Additional imaging studies may need to be performed to better define the lesion for biopsy (in this case, MRI or a tagged red cell scan). In some cases, lesions that appear to be metastatic may indeed represent the primary

DIFFERENTIAL DIAGNOSIS

Unknown Primary Carcinoma Conditions Responsive to Therapy

- Women with peritoneal carcinomatosis
- Women with isolated axillary node involvement
- Squamous cell carcinoma in high or middle neck nodes
- Squamous cell carcinoma in inguinal nodes
- Neuroendocrine carcinoma
- Extragonadal germ cell syndrome

cancer. For example, multiple liver lesions thought to be metastatic from an unknown site may represent a primary multifocal hepatocellular carcinoma. Sometimes the primary tumor displays an unusual pattern of tumor growth, and more specialized imaging studies may be necessary.[7]

MANAGEMENT

The treatment of patients in whom the primary site or a unique histologic subtype (e.g., melanoma, lymphoma, sarcoma) has been identified should follow disease-specific guidelines. The treatment of patients with features matching one of the subsets is as follows.

Male gender, an age less than 50 years, and rapidly growing and poorly differentiated carcinomas involving predominantly midline structures (mediastinum, retroperitoneum) are typical features of the extragonadal germ cell syndrome. A careful pathologic review will identify the true germ cell histologic types; molecular studies of chromosome 12 may be needed to establish the diagnosis.[8] These patients should be treated aggressively with chemotherapy regimens used for germ-cell cancer. Patients with poorly differentiated carcinomas without histologic evidence of germ cell features are much less responsive to therapy but should be given a trial of platinum-based chemotherapy.[9]

In women the most common cause of carcinomas confined to the axillary nodes is occult breast cancer. MRI should be performed if mammogram and breast ultrasound are not diagnostic. When a breast primary carcinoma is in the diagnostic differential, biopsy material should be analyzed for estrogen, progesterone receptors, and gross cystic disease fluid protein.[10,11] If the pathologic findings are consistent with primary breast cancer, these patients should be treated similarly to patients with a breast primary tumor of a corresponding stage.[12] Overall, the survival rate appears to be similar to that of patients with breast cancer. Inguinal node metastases of unknown origin with histologic features of squamous cell carcinoma (a rare clinical presentation) require careful inspection of the skin, anus, and distal genitourinary tract and a gynecologic examination in women. Patients in whom the primary tumor cannot be identified and who do not have additional sites of disease should undergo lymph node dissection of the affected area. Local radiotherapy is often administered after surgery.

Squamous cell carcinoma is found in more than 70% of patients with involved nodes high in the neck or in the middle neck. The most common occult primary sites include the nasopharynx, tonsil, base of the tongue, and hypopharynx. These patients should undergo CT or MRI studies of the head and neck and a thorough ear, nose, and throat evaluation, including endoscopic evaluation with biopsy (random and abnormal appearing areas). Tonsillectomy increases the diagnostic yield of the head and neck evaluation and may improve patient outcome.[13] If no primary tumor is found, the patient should undergo neck dissection followed by radiotherapy. Patients with extensive adenopathy are often treated with platinum-based chemotherapy.

Poorly differentiated neuroendocrine carcinoma is a clinicopathologic entity that has been recognized for its responsiveness to therapy. Immunohistochemical stains are usually positive for chromogranin and/or synaptophysin. These patients often are seen with diffuse hepatic or bone metastases. Poorly differentiated neuroendocrine carcinomas do not have the indolent histologic or clinical features of typical carcinoid tumors, islet cell tumors, or paragangliomas, for which observation is often appropriate; they are often responsive to cisplatin-based chemotherapy.[14]

Well-differentiated neuroendocrine tumors, although often not responsive to chemotherapy, usually follow an indolent course resulting in longer than average survival for patients with UPC. The majority of patients with UPC do not fit into one of the previously described subsets.

Chemotherapy, with either investigational or standard agents, should be offered to patients with adequate performance status. The chemotherapeutic agents studied for the treatment of these patients have included 5-fluorouracil, platinum compounds, taxanes, etoposide, gemcitabine, and irinotecan.[15-17] A combination of carboplatin and paclitaxel is a commonly used regimen for these patients, resulting in overall response rates of approximately 30% to 40%. Best results have been observed in patients with nodal or pleural disease and in women with peritoneal carcinomatosis. Patients with multiorgan involvement or bone or liver metastases have a lower rate of response of approximately 15% and a shorter median survival.[18] In a study of patients treated with carboplatin, paclitaxel, and etoposide, a 3-year survival rate of 14% was observed.[19] Regimens including gemcitabine and sequential multiple drug combinations have shown similar rates of response and survival.[20,21]

Co-Management with Specialists

The delivery of care to patients with UPC often requires a multidisciplinary team to provide adequate integration and planning of multimodality care. This care involves specialists in medical oncology, radiotherapy, surgery, and pain and symptom management.

LIFE SPAN CONSIDERATIONS

The median survival for patients with UPC is relatively short (11 months). Consideration should be given to prompt identification of patients belonging in the more treatable subsets. This can usually be accomplished if the limited and focused evaluation previously described is used; the goal is timely administration of therapy without the undue delay of prolonged and unproductive testing. Relevant prognostic factors that have been described include number of metastatic sites, axillary node involvement (in women), sex, performance status, and lactate dehydrogenase levels.[1,22]

COMPLICATIONS

As with other patients with metastatic cancer, patients with UPC are at risk for a broad spectrum of complications. Complications directly related to the disease process include spinal cord compression from metastatic disease, hypercalcemia of malignancy, urethral and biliary obstruction, pleural and pericardial effusions, and ascites. Complications related to treatment include chemotherapy-induced alopecia, nausea, vomiting, diarrhea, and mucositis, as well as febrile neutropenia, anemia, and thrombocytopenia, which often require the transfusion of blood products. Narcotic analgesics are often necessary for pain control and may cause respiratory depression, hallucinations, somnolence, nausea, vomiting, and severe constipation.

Radiation treatment may cause fatigue and, depending on the anatomic area being treated, hair loss, esophagitis with dysphagia, gastritis, diarrhea, rectal pain or burning, and cystitis or dysuria.

Clinically significant anxiety and depression are often observed in these patients.

INDICATIONS FOR REFERRAL OR HOSPITALIZATION

Diagnostic evaluation and therapeutic decisions for patients with UPC are complex and require referral to a physician who specializes in the treatment of cancer patients. Hospitalization may be required for adequate management of symptoms and complications related to either the disease process (e.g., spinal cord compression, bleeding, hypercalcemia, intractable pain) or treatment side effects (e.g., intractable nausea and vomiting, febrile neutropenia, thrombocytopenia with bleeding). Hospitalization may also be required for the administration of chemotherapy or for procedures such as surgical stabilization of metastatic bone lesions or excision of limited metastatic disease.

PATIENT AND FAMILY EDUCATION

A diagnosis of UPC is a major challenge for patients and families. The lack of knowledge of the primary tumor results in diagnostic and therapeutic uncertainties and can generate anxiety in the health care provider and patient.[4] It is important to emphasize that, although the primary site is not known, there are guidelines to help choose the most effective treatment for each patient. Patients need education regarding the side effects of chemotherapy and radiotherapy and need to be taught to recognize the complications that require immediate medical attention. It is also important to educate patients in the appropriate use of pain medications. Finally, it is often necessary to educate and communicate with these patients on emotionally charged topics such as do-not-resuscitate status and the shift from chemotherapy to supportive care only. Training staff in these difficult aspects of patient communication will increase their confidence in dealing with these issues.[23]

REFERENCES

1. Abbruzzese JL, Abbruzzese MC, Hess KR, and others: Unknown primary carcinoma: natural history and prognostic factors in 657 consecutive patients, *J Clin Oncol* 12:1272-1280, 1994.
2. Bar-Eli M, Abbruzzese JL, Lee-Jackson D, and others: p53 gene mutation spectrum in human unknown primary tumors, *Anticancer Res* 13:1619-1623, 1993.
3. Hillen HF, Hak LE, Joosten-Achjanie SR, and others: Microvessel density in unknown primary tumors, *Int J Cancer* 74:81-85, 1997.
4. Abbruzzese JL, Abbruzzese MC, Lenzi R, and others: Analysis of a diagnostic strategy for patients with suspected tumors of unknown origin, *J Clin Oncol* 13:2094-2103, 1995.
5. Rusthoven KE, Koshy M, Paulino AC: The role of fluorodeoxyglucose positron emission tomography in cervical lymph node metastases from an unknown primary tumor, *Cancer* 101:2641-2649, 2004.
6. Dennis JL, Hvidsten TR, Wit EC, and others: Markers of adenocarcinoma characteristic of the site of origin: development of a diagnostic algorithm, *Clin Cancer Res* 11:3766-3772, 2005.
7. Lenzi R, Kim EE, Raber MN, and others: Detection of primary breast cancer presenting as metastatic carcinoma of unknown primary origin by 111 In-pentetreotide scan, *Ann Oncol* 9:213-216, 1998.
8. Motzer RJ, Rodriguez E, Reuter VE, and others: Molecular and cytogenetic studies in the diagnosis of patients with poorly differentiated carcinomas of unknown primary site, *J Clin Oncol* 13:274-282, 1995.
9. Lenzi R, Hess KR, Abbruzzese MC, and others: Poorly differentiated carcinoma and poorly differentiated adenocarcinoma of unknown origin: favorable subsets of patients with unknown-primary carcinoma? *J Clin Oncol* 15:2056-2066, 1997.
10. O'Connell FP, Wang HH, Odze RD: Utility of immunohistochemistry in distinguishing primary adenocarcinomas from metastatic breast carcinomas in the gastrointestinal tract, *Arch Pathol Lab Med* 129:338-347, 2005.
11. Tomos C, Soslow R, Chen S, and others: Expression of WTl, CA 125, and GCDFP-15 as useful markers in the differential diagnosis of primary ovarian carcinomas versus metastatic breast cancer to the ovary, *Am J Surg Pathol* 29:1482-1489, 2005.
12. Ellerbroek N, Holmes F, Singletary E, and others: Treatment of patients with isolated axillary nodal metastases from an occult primary carcinoma consistent with breast origin, *Cancer* 66:1461-1467, 1990.
13. Issing WJ, Taleban B, Tauber S: Diagnosis and management of carcinoma of unknown primary in the head and neck, *Eur Arch Otorhinolaryngol* 260:436-443, 2003.
14. Hainsworth JD, Johnson DH, Greco FA: Poorly differentiated neuroendocrine carcinoma of unknown primary site: a newly recognized clinicopathologic entity, *Ann Intern Med* 109:364-371, 1988.
15. Lenzi R, Raber MN, Frost P, and others: Phase II study of cisplatin, 5-fluorouracil and folinic acid in patients with carcinoma of unknown primary origin, *Eur J Cancer* 29A:1634, 1993.
16. Hainsworth JD, Erland JB, Kalman LA, and others: Carcinoma of unknown primary site: treatment with 1-hour paclitaxel, carboplatin, and extended-schedule etoposide, *J Clin Oncol* 15:2385-2393, 1997.
17. Culine S, Lortholary A, Voigt JJ, and others: Cisplatin in combination with either gemcitabine or irinotecan in carcinomas of unknown primary site: results of a randomized phase II study—trial for the French Study Group on Carcinomas of Unknown Primary (GEFCAPI 01), *J Clin Oncol* 21:3479-3482, 2003.
18. Briasoulis E, Kalofonos H, Bafaloukos D, and others: Carboplatin plus paclitaxel in unknown primary carcinoma: a phase II Hellenic Cooperative Oncology Group Study, *J Clin Oncol* 18:3101-3107, 2000.
19. Greco FA, Burris HA 3rd, Erland JB, and others: Carcinoma of unknown primary site, *Cancer* 89:2655-2660, 2000.
20. Pouessel D, Culine S, Becht C, and others: Gemcitabine and docetaxel as front-line chemotherapy in patients with carcinoma of an unknown primary site, *Cancer* 100:1257-1261, 2004.
21. Greco FA, Rodriguez GI, Shaffer DW, and others: Carcinoma of unknown primary site: sequential treatment with paclitaxel/carboplatin/etoposide and gemcitabine/irinotecan: a Minnie Pearl Cancer Research Network phase II trial, *Oncologist* 9:644-652, 2004.
22. Culine S, Kramar A, Saghatchian M, and others: Development and validation of a prognostic model to predict the length of survival in patients with carcinomas of an unknown primary site, *J Clin Oncol* 20:4679-4683, 2002.
23. Baile WF, Lenzi R, Kudelka AP, and others: Improving physician-patient communication in cancer care: outcome of a workshop for oncologists, *J Cancer Educ* 12:166-173, 1997.

CHAPTER 255

Gastrointestinal Symptoms in the Oncology Patient

Jane Williams and Marcia L. Patterson

Cancer patients can experience numerous disorders of the digestive system. These disorders can be treatment related (chemotherapy, radiation, surgery) or disease related (neoplasm, infection, function, obstruction, motility alterations, or malabsorption). The prevention of complications and early detection of lower grade toxicities lead to fewer and more easily managed sequelae and improved quality of life. This chapter focuses on the most common problematic symptoms, which include nausea and vomiting, constipation and diarrhea, anorexia, and the oral manifestations of mucositis and xerostomia.

PATHOPHYSIOLOGY

Chemotherapy-Induced Nausea and Vomiting

Nausea and vomiting (N&V) are mediated centrally and occur when the vomiting center (VC) receives specific information (mediated by neurotransmitters such as serotonin, acetylcholine, histamine, dopamine, and substance P) from the gastrointestinal (GI) tract, the chemoreceptor trigger zone (CTZ), the vestibular apparatus, or the cerebral cortex and limbic system.[1,2]

Chemotherapy-induced N&V (CINV) is particularly common in the oncology patient, and its control is critical in treatment compliance; preservation of quality of life; and prevention of such complications as weight loss, dehydration, and electrolyte imbalances. The three types of CINV are acute, delayed, and anticipatory.[1,2]

Acute N&V occurs within the first 24 hours of chemotherapy administration, whereas delayed emesis occurs more than 24 hours after chemotherapy. Anticipatory N&V is a conditioned response resulting from memory of emesis with previous chemotherapy administration. Delayed and anticipatory N&V can be more difficult to control, and the risk of both increases if the acute phase is poorly controlled. Hence optimum antiemetic control is essential from the beginning of chemotherapy.[2-4]

Several patient-related factors affect the severity of CINV, including gender, age, and alcohol intake. N&V are not as well controlled in females as in males, particularly if the females are young (<30 years of age) or menstruating. Individuals with a high alcohol intake (>5 drinks/day) have better control of vomiting than those with low or no alcohol intake. Patients with a history of motion sickness or a propensity for N&V (pregnancy, migraine headaches) may be more prone to delayed or anticipatory N&V.[2,4]

In addition to CINV, N&V can result from radiotherapy to the abdomen, pelvis, or brain; medications such as analgesics, antimicrobials, and iron; intestinal obstruction; fluid and electrolyte imbalances; metabolic alterations; constipation; tumor invasion of the GI tract; cytokine release from tumor; and brain metastasis.[1,2,5]

Constipation

Constipation may be described as stool that is infrequent, dry, hard, and difficult to pass, or a feeling of incomplete evacuation.[6] It is important to consider the patient's perception of well-being and usual pattern of evacuation rather than a standard norm. The most common constipating chemotherapeutic agents are the vinca alkaloids, which result in autonomic nerve dysfunction and can lead to decreased peristalsis and paralytic ileus. CINV may also contribute to constipation through decreased oral intake and administration of 5-HT_3 antagonists. Cancer patients may also be prone to constipation from the use of narcotic agents, aluminum antacids, calcium, anticonvulsants, anticholinergic drugs, antispasmodics, diuretics, tricyclic antidepressants, antiinflammatory drugs, and muscle relaxants. Primary or metastatic tumors of the bowel may result in extraluminal compression on the intestine itself, which blocks the passage of stool, or in interference with the colon's neural innervation. This can also be seen with pelvic cancer, malignant ascites, paraneoplastic syndromes, spinal cord compression, hypercalcemia, organ failure, or debility with advanced disease. Fatigue and immobility may also be contributing factors.[6,7]

Diarrhea

Diarrhea is, by definition, present when stool volume amounts to more than 200 g/day.[8] However, in the clinical setting, it is typically diagnosed when stools are frequent, loose, and watery.[1] The most common causes of cancer-related diarrhea are abdominal irradiation; GI surgery; bone marrow transplant; and chemotherapeutic agents such as 5-fluorouracil, irinotecan, and docetaxel. Additionally, diarrhea can be a manifestation of certain types of tumor such as carcinoid, or it may be a side effect of certain medications or tube feedings.[1,9] Patients who are immunosuppressed are more susceptible to infectious organisms, such as *Clostridium difficile*, which causes excessive mucosal secretion of fluid and electrolytes by the bowel mucosa. Pseudodiarrhea may occur with intestinal ileus or obstruction.

Anorexia

Anorexia is characterized by a decrease in appetite and food intake. The resulting weight loss may lead to cachexia, a syndrome of progressive wasting that may be irreversible and fatal. Interferences of physiologic, psychologic, and social stimuli can decrease food intake and nutritional status. Appetite suppression results from the secretion of cytokines that act as anorexigenic agents. Physiologic factors include nausea and vomiting, dysgeusia or taste alterations, constipation, dysphagia, odynophagia, fatigue, infection, and stomatitis. Psychologic factors include anxiety and depression. Social factors include personal or cultural preferences, or the loss of the patient's usual eating companions when hospitalized. Medical causes can be related to tumors, bowel obstruction, fever, metabolic disorders (hepatic and renal dysfunction), and ectopic hormone production by tumors. Head and neck surgery may affect the ability to eat normally because of altered facial architecture. Radiotherapy can lead to glossitis, stomatitis, esophagitis, and altered taste. In addition to chemotherapeutic agents, antibiotics, antifungal agents, and pain medications may produce a loss of appetite.[1]

Mucositis

All mucous membranes are at risk for the effects of systemic chemotherapy, but the most common sites for mucositis are the oral cavity and the esophagus. The most common mucosatoxic agents are 5-fluorouricil, methotrexate, bleomycin, actinomycin D (dactinomycin), etoposide, cytarabine, cyclophosphamide, floxuridine, docetaxel, paclitaxel, vinblastine, doxorubicin, daunorubicin, mitoxantrone, chlorambucil, vindesine (not commercially available in the United States), thioguanine, amsacrine, and plicamycin.[5,10] With radiation, tissues that are in the treatment field will be predisposed to mucositis. The risk of developing mucositis is not the same for all patients and is not the same for each drug regimen. The mucosa may become dry, inflamed, ulcerated, and painful. Pain is the major clinical problem and may render the patient unable to practice adequate oral hygiene, eat properly, or communicate.

Xerostomia

Xerostomia is a decrease in the quantity and quality of saliva, resulting in thick, ropy saliva that interferes with nutrition, taste, and speech. It may be of long duration, lasting months to years. Common causes include surgery or radiotherapy to the head and neck region, anticholinergic and opioid medications, oral infections, and dehydration.[5]

CLINICAL PRESENTATION

The presenting symptoms vary based on which GI disturbance the patient is experiencing. In general, patients with any significant GI disturbance demonstrate signs and symptoms related to reduced oral intake and altered bowel function and are at risk for dehydration and electrolyte imbalance. Constitutional symptoms such as fatigue, malaise, and weight loss are common. Dry mouth, dizziness, reduced urinary output, and hypotension may indicate dehydration. A general overview of all organ systems provides the necessary information to narrow down the differential diagnoses. A thorough assessment of GI symptoms is essential, including quantification of the daily fluid and food intake, the number and characteristics of bowel movements per day, the number and characteristics of recent emetic episodes, and a description of any abdominal pain. Any significant symptoms should be further assessed by asking about factors that exacerbate or relieve symptoms; the quality, severity, timing, and duration of symptoms; and relationship to intake of food or medications.

PHYSICAL EXAMINATION

The health care provider should assess for significant weight loss (>1% to 2% per week). The oral cavity should be inspected for integrity of mucosa, ulcerations, thrush or exudate, erythema, and gingivitis. Using a gloved finger and tongue depressor helps ensure thorough examination of the oral mucosa and oropharynx. The abdomen should be inspected, auscultated, and palpated. Inspection is done first and may reveal striae, distention, and contour abnormalities. Jaundice can be detected by inspecting the skin and sclerae. Auscultation of bowel sounds in all quadrants is done next, with palpation and percussion performed last. Rebound tenderness, visible peristalsis, distention, or altered bowel sounds may indicate obstruction. Paralytic obstruction is characterized by absent bowel sounds, whereas hyperactive high-pitched bowel sounds can indicate mechanical obstruction. Palpation can detect presence of stool, masses, hepatosplenomegaly, inguinal lymphadenopathy, and asymmetry of contour. Ascites can be detected by testing for fluid wave or shifting dullness of the abdomen. Digital rectal examinations are avoided if the patient is neutropenic or thrombocytopenic or has received radiotherapy to the rectum. A guideline for grading the severity of N&V can be found in Box 255-1.

DIAGNOSTICS

Laboratory data serve to confirm or rule out a diagnosis and warn of potential complications in a cancer patient suffering from altered GI function. For example, a chemistry profile consisting of electrolytes, BUN, and creatinine aids in the diagnosis of fluid and electrolyte imbalances that can result from prolonged vomiting, diarrhea, and anorexia. Kidney function can deteriorate rapidly in a dehydrated patient who has received nephrotoxic chemotherapy. Additional chemistries that are helpful include magnesium and phosphorus. These can drop precipitously in a patient with altered GI function, especially after receiving chemotherapy that affects excretion, such as cisplatin and ifosfamide. Ileus can be caused by hypomagnesemia, hypophosphatemia, hypokalemia, or hypercalcemia. A CBC can detect neutropenia, thrombocytopenia, and anemia, all of which can be related to GI symptomatology. A urinalysis is indicated if urinary tract infection is a suspected cause of the N&V. Serum albumin, particularly prealbumin, can be useful in assessing nutritional status. A liver panel, amylase, lipase, prothrombin time, and albumin may be ordered if hepatic dysfunction is suspected.

BOX 255-1

SEVERITY GRADING FOR NAUSEA AND VOMITING

GRADE 1

- Loss of appetite without alteration in eating habits
- One episode of vomiting in 24 hours

GRADE 2

- Oral intake decreased without significant weight loss, dehydration, or malnutrition
- IV fluids indicated for less than 24 hours
- Two to five episodes of vomiting in 24 hours

GRADE 3

- Inadequate oral caloric or fluid intake; IV fluids, tube feedings, or total parenteral nutrition indicated for 24 hours or more
- Six or more episodes of vomiting in 24 hours

GRADE 4

- Life-threatening consequences

Modified from National Cancer Institute: *Nausea and vomiting PDQ*, retrieved March 5, 2007, from http://cancernet.nci.nih.gov/cancertopics/pdq/supportivecare/nausea/healthprofessional.

DIAGNOSTICS

Gastrointestinal Symptoms in the Oncology Patient

LABORATORY
CBC and differential
Serum electrolytes
BUN
Creatinine
Serum glucose
Serum calcium*
Serum magnesium*
Serum phosphorus*
Serum human chorionic gonadotropin*
LFTs*
Serum albumin and total protein*
Stool for occult blood and *Clostridium difficile**
Urinalysis*

IMAGING
KUB*

*If indicated.

The tests mentioned are basic panels that are generally ordered in cancer patients with GI symptoms. Additional tests are indicated based on the differential diagnoses for that particular patient. For example, stool testing for occult blood (three sequential specimens) should be ordered if GI bleeding is suspected, and stool testing for *C. difficile* is indicated for relentless diarrhea, particularly in a patient who has received broad-spectrum antibiotics. Additional stool studies such as Gram stain, leukocytosis, and vancomycin-resistant enterococci may be indicated. An abdominal series is helpful in diagnosing intestinal obstruction and ileus. If the GI symptoms raise suspicions of obstruction, perforation, or disease progression, a CT scan of the abdomen and pelvis is generally performed.

DIFFERENTIAL DIAGNOSIS

It is important to recognize other conditions with presentations similar to those of cancer-related GI symptoms. Gastroenteritis, hepatitis, pancreatitis, cholecystitis, peptic ulcer disease, ileus, obstruction, uremia, urinary tract infection, hypercalcemia, and psychogenic or anticipatory vomiting should be considered when evaluating the patient with GI complaints. Other possibilities include anorexia nervosa, irritable bowel syndrome, increased intracranial pressure, spinal cord compression, vestibular disorders, and acute myocardial infarction. Pregnancy is a possibility that must be considered in sexually active women of childbearing age. Knowing the details of the symptom's onset, along with the patient's past medical history, risk factors for other diseases, and side effects of current treatment, is essential in identifying the most likely cause of the GI symptoms.

DIFFERENTIAL DIAGNOSIS

Gastrointestinal Symptoms in the Oncology Patient

- Irritable bowel
- Gastroenteritis
- Hepatitis
- Pancreatitis
- Peptic ulcer disease
- Ileus
- Uremia
- Urinary tract infection
- Constipation
- Pregnancy
- Increased intracranial pressure
- Vestibular disorder
- Acute myocardial infarction
- Anorexia nervosa
- Psychogenic vomiting

MANAGEMENT

Nausea and Vomiting

N&V are amongst the most uncomfortable and dreaded symptoms experienced by oncology patients. In recent years, significant progress has been made in understanding, preventing, and controlling N&V in cancer patients. An effective antiemetic regimen interrupts the stimulation of the VC. U.S. Food and Drug Administration approval of the 5-HT_3 antagonists in the early 1990s revolutionized antiemetic control with CINV. More recently a new class of antiemetics called neurokinin-1 (NK1) antagonists has resulted in further advances, particularly with delayed emesis. A combination of antiemetic agents is generally used to maximize prevention and control of both acute and delayed emesis.[3,11,12]

The major predictor of CINV is the emetic potential of the chemotherapeutic agent. Chemotherapy may be classified as having low, moderate, or severe emetic potential. Agents that are considered highly emetogenic include cisplatin, actinomycin D, mechlorethamine, streptozocin, cyclophosphamide, carmustine, doxorubicin, epirubicin, idarubicin, oxaliplatin, cytarabine, and ifosfamide. Intermediate-risk agents include irinotecan, mitoxantrone, paclitaxel, docetaxel, mitomycin, topotecan, gemcitabine, etoposide, and teniposide. Low-risk agents include vinorelbine, fluorouracil, methotrexate, bleomycin, L-asparaginase, vinblastine, vincristine, busulfan, and tamoxifen.[1,12]

Evidence-based studies continue to support the efficacy of 5-HT_3 antagonists and dexamethasome in both acute and delayed emesis when given with chemotherapeutic agents with moderate or high emetic potential.[12] Until recently, efficacy among all of the 5-HT_3 antagonists was similar. However, palonosetron, a very long–acting second-generation 5-HT_3 antagonist, provides superior control of delayed emesis, particularly with moderately emetogenic chemotherapy. The recent introduction of aprepitant, the first NK1 antagonist, has resulted in superior prevention of both acute and delayed emesis when given with highly emetogenic chemotherapy.[3,5,11,12]

Studies are ongoing, and new pharmaceutical agents are being developed, resulting in constantly evolving antiemetic guidelines. Guidelines reflecting current standard of care are published by various national and professional organization, such as National Comprehensive Cancer Network and American Society of Clinical Oncology.[3,4,11,12] These guidelines can be referenced if specific information is desired.

In general, the 5-HT_3 antagonists are well tolerated with minimum side effects. The major side effects reported are constipation and headache and, less commonly, bradycardia.[2] Occasionally, a patient cannot tolerate 5-HT_3 antagonists, or the N&V are not related to chemotherapy administration, and another antiemetic agent is indicated. Metoclopramide is a dopamine receptor antagonist and, when combined with dexamethasone, is particularly beneficial for delayed emesis after chemotherapy. Phenothiazines (prochlorperazine) and butyrophenones (haloperidol, droperidol) are somewhat effective, but less so than metoclopramide, and they induce more extrapyramidal symptoms, especially in patients under 30 years of age. Benzodiazepines such as lorazepam and antihistamines such as diphenhydramine are useful adjuncts for their antianxiety effect and prevention of the extrapyramidal reactions associated with some antiemetics, although they are not recommended for single-agent use. Cannabinoids, both inhaled (marijuana) and oral (dronabinol [Marinol]), have been found to have some antiemetic activity, but significantly less than other agents and with undesirable side effects.[1,2,5,12]

Some patients can learn to interrupt the association of N&V with chemotherapy through the use of behavioral interventions. Progressive muscle relaxation, hypnosis, imagery, biofeedback, or distraction may be valuable. Any adverse sounds or smells that stimulate the VC should be minimized in the environment. Patients who experience sustained episodes of N&V may be encouraged to avoid eating their "favorite foods" to possibly avoid food aversions after treatment subsides.

Constipation

The management of constipation should first include the prevention and elimination of precipitating factors. Once constipation occurs, bowel management includes increasing fluid intake to 2 quarts of fluid per day. Regular exercise should be encouraged for all patients. A physical therapist can be consulted for coordination of an exercise regimen for bedbound patients and those with physical limitations. Fiber intake should be increased by consuming more fruits (including figs, dates, prunes), vegetables, and whole grains. Two to four ounces of prune juice or a hot liquid before a large meal may be helpful.[7,9] The patient should be given privacy for defecation; the use of a bedpan should be avoided if at all possible. Patients receiving narcotics should also receive a senna derivative and a stool softener.[7,9] If the constipation continues, use of osmotic laxatives is encouraged. Polyethylene glycol is an example of an osmotic laxative that is well tolerated and effective.[9] Rectal agents should be avoided in cancer patients who are at risk for thrombocytopenia or leukopenia. If a patient is immunocompromised, there should be no manipulation of the anus because this can lead to fissures or abscesses, which are portals of entry for infection.[1]

Diarrhea

The management of diarrhea may begin with dietary interventions such as low-fiber, high-calorie, and high-protein meals. Identification and avoidance of aggravating foods, such as milk products or high-fat foods, is helpful. Pharmacologic measures may also be used. Anticholinergic drugs such as diphenoxylate plus atropine, or loperamide, reduce gastric secretions and decrease intestinal peristalsis. Opiate drugs bind to receptors on the smooth muscle of the bowel, slowing intestinal motility and increasing fluid absorption. Octreotide acetate, which is reserved for patients with excessive diarrhea, inhibits the release of intestinal hormones (including serotonin and gastrin), prolongs intestinal transit time, and increases intestinal water and electrolyte transport. Psyllium may be effective in controlling high-output diarrhea. Topical agents containing hydrocortisone or dibucaine are useful for perianal irritation. Glucocorticoid retention enemas are often used for radiation-induced proctitis. Antidiarrheal medications should be avoided in patients with GI infections and in those with the pseudodiarrhea that occurs with an ileus or partial small bowel obstruction.[1,6,13]

Anorexia

Anorexia can be managed through education, behavioral changes, and pharmacologic methods. Consultation with a nutritionist can be valuable for exploring high-calorie options, food supplements, appetizing recipes, and visually appealing presentations. Simple measures such as avoiding metal utensils and eating a few slices of pickle may decrease the sense of metallic taste. Increased physical activity and smaller, more frequent meals may also be helpful. Simple maneuvers such as having a family member share a meal, serving a favorite wine or beer, or using special table settings may be helpful.

Several pharmacologic agents have been helpful in managing anorexia. The most common is megestrol acetate, which may inhibit tumor necrosis factor and increase weight gain. Other agents include metoclopramide, which increases gastric emptying and is useful for patients with early satiety or delayed gastric emptying; cannabinoids, which appear to increase appetite and control N&V; and dexamethasone, which stimulates appetite and induces a sense of well-being. Patients who continue to have significant anorexia or weight loss may require formal nutritional support, such as enteral or parenteral feeding.[1,13]

Mucositis and Stomatitis

The systematic performance of oral hygiene may be of greater value in preventing or reducing stomatitis than the actual agents used. Therefore it is important to develop with the patient a plan for oral care that includes daily plaque removal and mouth rinses at least after meals and at bedtime. Soft toothbrushes and dental floss should be used regularly unless there is danger of mucosal injury or evidence of thrombocytopenia. In that instance, foam brushes can be used. Mouth rinses should be nonirritating and nondrying and include normal saline and sodium bicarbonate peroxide. Hydrogen peroxide has an antifibroblastic effect and should be avoided because of the possible impairment of wound healing.[13] Cryotherapy, or sucking on ice chips or popsicles, may reduce the severity of mucositis.[14,15] The lips should be lubricated often to keep them moist and comfortable.

Topical formulations that are available to relieve the pain and inflammation of stomatitis are numerous and should be individualized for each patient. Camp-Sorrell has several excellent tables for oral care and the prevention of complications.[6] An example of a good universal solution is a combination of aluminum and magnesium hydroxide (Maalox) or bismuth subsalicylate (Kaopectate), viscous lidocaine, and diphenhydramine. Palifermin, currently the only agent approved for treatment of oral mucositis, is approved for use in patients with hematologic malignancies undergoing stem cell transplant.[13] In general, patients should avoid all tobacco products; alcohol; and foods that cause irritation such as hot, spicy, or rough foods.[10]

Xerostomia

The thick, ropy saliva of xerostomia makes eating difficult and unpleasant. Oral care before meals may help freshen the mouth. Increasing fluids during meals will help moisten food and aids in swallowing. Patients should be encouraged to eat soft foods that are moistened with milk or gravy and to avoid dry, spicy, and acidic foods. The use of humidified air may help prevent mucous membranes from drying and cracking. Lubricating agents such as saliva substitutes are expensive and may or may not be useful. Some authorities have suggested swishing liquid corn oil or vegetable oil in the mouth. Papain and amylase will dissolve and break up thick saliva in some patients. Papain is found naturally in papaya and meat tenderizers. Amylase is found in papaya but can sting the mouth. Prolonged xerostomia can result in dental caries, and therefore regular dental check-ups are important.[13]

COMPLICATIONS

Complications of GI symptoms are varied and depend on the severity or grade of toxicity. For example, significant mucositis in the presence of neutropenia can be life threatening and requires aggressive antibiotic management. Severe GI toxicities can create friable, edematous, and ulcerative mucosal insults, resulting in anorexia, malabsorption, malnutrition, dehydration, and intractable pain. Mechanical or paralytic obstruction of the bowel is serious and difficult to diagnose early in its presentation; any suspicion of this complication should be promptly referred to a GI specialist and surgeon.

INDICATIONS FOR REFERRAL OR HOSPITALIZATION

Persistent or worsening GI symptoms may indicate a treatment complication or disease progression, and referral to a specialist or hospitalization may be necessary. A detailed history and physical examination will determine the differential diagnosis and the need for referral or hospitalization. Common causes of hospitalizations for treatment-related GI complications include acute or refractory N&V, acute or refractory pain, GI bleed, dysphagia, dehydration, orthostatic hypotension, intractable diarrhea, and constipation.

PATIENT AND FAMILY EDUCATION

Patients and families need to understand the importance of notifying the health care provider if GI symptoms occur. Written instructions, as well as verbal discussion of treatments for N&V, diarrhea, constipation, and oral hygiene, will assist patients in controlling problematic symptoms. A list of symptoms that indicate a need to call the health care provider should also be available to the patient and family. Prompt recognition and reporting of GI symptoms, particularly when accompanied by fever, chills, or signs of dehydration, may help avoid serious sequelae.

REFERENCES

1. National Cancer Institute: *PDQ supportive care/screening*, retrieved March 5, 2007, from http://www.cancer.gov/cancertopics/factsheet/Information/PDQ.
2. Grunberg SM, Gralla RJ: Management of nausea and vomiting. In Pazdur R, Coia LR, Hoskins WJ, and others, editors: *Cancer management: a multidisciplinary approach*, ed 8, New York, 2004, CMP Healthcare Media.
3. Viale PH: Integrating aprepitant and palonesetron into clinical practice: a role for the new antiemetics, *Clin J Oncol Nurs* 9(1):77-84, 2005.
4. Roscoe JA, Bushunow P, Morrow GR, and others: Patient expectation is a strong predictor of severe nausea after chemotherapy, *Cancer* 101(11):2701-2708, 2004.
5. Crawley MM, Benson LM: Current trends in managing oral mucositis, *Clin J Oncol Nurs* 9(5):584-592, 2005.
6. Camp-Sorrell D: Chemotherapy: toxicity management. In Groenwald SL, Frogge MH, Goodman M, and others, editors: *Cancer nursing: principles and practice*, ed 5, Boston, 2000, Jones & Bartlett.
7. Bisanz A: Managing bowel elimination problems in patients with cancer, *Oncol Nurs Forum* 24(4):679-686, 1997.
8. Soffer EE: Diarrhea. In Andreoli TE, Bennett JC, Carpenter CJ, and others, editors: *Cecil essentials of medicine*, ed 5, Philadelphia, 2001, Saunders.
9. Cherny NI: Taking care of the terminally ill cancer patient: management of gastrointestinal symptoms in patients with advanced cancer, *Ann Oncol* 15(Suppl 4):iv205-iv213, 2004.
10. Kostler WJ, Hejna M, Wenzel C, and others: Oral mucositis complicating chemotherapy and/or radiotherapy: options for prevention and treatment, *CA J Clin* 51(5):290-315, 2001.
11. Hesketh PJ: New treatment options for chemotherapy-induced nausea and vomiting, *Support Care Cancer* 12:550-554, 2004.
12. Kris MG, Hesketh PJ, Herrstedt J, and others: Consensus proposals for the prevention of acute and delayed vomiting and nausea following high-emetic-risk chemotherapy, *Support Care Cancer* 13(2):85-96, 2005.
13. Wadler S, Benson AB, Englegking C, and others: Recommended guidelines for the treatment of chemotherapy-induced diarrhea, *J Clin Oncol* 16(9):3169-3178, 1998.
14. Rubenstein EB, Peterson DE, Schubert M, and others: Clinical practice guidelines for the prevention and treatment of cancer therapy–induced oral and gastrointestinal mucositis, *Cancer* 100:2026-2046, 2004.
15. Edelman MJ, Gandara DR, Perez EA, and others: Phase I trial of edatrexate plus carboplatin in advanced solid tumors: amelioration of dose-limiting mucositis by ice chip cryotherapy, *Invest New Drugs* 16(1):69-75, 1998.

CHAPTER 256

Management of Cancer Pain

Updated by Kelli Gershon

DEFINITION AND EPIDEMIOLOGY

Fear of pain and suffering is a common experience for most patients who are diagnosed with cancer. Dealing with the pain caused by cancer is an additional issue for cancer patients and their families. Health care providers are faced with several barriers in their efforts to effectively manage pain.[1] Knowledge deficits exist because of a lack of academic attention to pain mechanisms and treatment in most medical, nursing, and pharmacy curricula. Attitudes about pain and misconceptions about related issues—particularly treatment with opioids—and difficulties in dealing with the subjective nature of pain contribute to the reluctance to aggressively use the necessary tools to manage pain. Fears of addiction and dependence are major factors in undertreatment despite considerable evidence that the development of these problems is rare even with the prolonged use of opioids. Impediments also include the monitoring and regulatory controls applied to opioid use, particularly in states that require triplicate prescriptions.[2]

The International Association for the Study of Pain defines pain as "an unpleasant sensory and emotional experience associated with actual or potential tissue damage, or described in terms of such damage." The association goes on to say that pain is always subjective. This means that the patient's self-report of pain is the only true indicator of its presence and severity. However, because pain is subjective, it may be difficult to assess and treat if a patient's cognition is affected by either disease or medication. The impact of pain is unique to the individual and may be affected by a multitude of other symptoms that cancer patients experience.[3]

PATHOPHYSIOLOGY

The key to treating pain effectively is to identify the underlying cause(s) wherever possible. Pain can be nociceptive or neuropathic or a combination of both. A "chronic cancer pain" complaint can be aggravated by factors such as infection, trauma, or progression; therefore careful assessment is essential. Factors such as inflammation and myofascial pain may contribute to the overall pain problem.[4]

Nociceptive pain is the most common mechanism and is a function of the normal nervous system. Nociceptors are the receptors that respond to noxious stimuli and transmit a message through the peripheral nerves, to the spinal cord, and then up to the cerebral cortex, where the message is interpreted. Some motor responses (e.g., withdrawal of an extremity from a heat source) are initiated from the spinal cord, whereas others are initiated by higher brain centers. Nociceptive pain may also be classified as somatic (i.e., arising from soft tissue and musculoskeletal structures) or visceral (i.e., arising from the internal organs). Nociceptive pain is characteristically described as dull, sharp, aching, or heavy, although other adjectives might be used. There are fewer pain fibers in the viscera and a convergence of visceral and cutaneous afferent fibers at the dorsal horn of the spinal cord, which accounts for the fact that visceral pain may be referred to other areas. Many cancer pain syndromes demonstrate classic referral patterns. For example, pain associated with cancer of the pancreas is often experienced as pain in the middle or upper back.

Neuropathic pain does not rely on the activation of the nociceptors. It develops as a result of injury to the peripheral nerves, spinal cord, or brain tissue. Nerves are injured or damaged by being cut, crushed, compressed, stretched, burned, frozen, or exposed to toxic agents such as chemotherapeutic drugs or viruses. The result of the injury is a cascade of events that creates both anatomic and neurochemical changes in the neurons. A severed peripheral nerve may send out tendrils as it tries to regrow, but the tendrils may tangle together to form a neuroma, which can be painful under light pressure. An imbalance in the number of sodium channels along the axon may occur as the nerve tries to repair itself, allowing for generation of ectopic impulses. Common examples of neuropathic pain syndromes include postherpetic neuralgia, phantom pain, postthoracotomy, and peripheral neuropathy. Neuropathic pain is characteristically described as burning, tingling, shocking, or jolting. Neuropathic pain often has a delayed onset from the time of the precipitating injury. For example, postherpetic neuralgia can occur more than 3 months after the skin lesions of herpes have healed. Over that time the perception of normally mild and nonpainful stimuli (e.g., touch) can change to being exquisitely sensitive or painful (allodynia). Neuropathic pain may also be accompanied by sympathetic dysfunction. An injured nerve may develop an electrical or a chemical interaction with sympathetic nerve fibers, providing continuous stimuli to peripheral nerves.[5]

Many pain syndromes are accompanied by inflammation that either contributes to or is the primary underlying mechanism of the pain. The inflammatory response includes the release of prostaglandins and leukotrienes that sensitize peripheral nerves to painful stimuli. Associated swelling causes pressure on the nerves or other sensitive structures. With bone metastases, inflammation may account for much of the pain.

CLINICAL PRESENTATION

Pain associated with cancer has many presentations. It may evolve slowly from an awareness of discomfort with increasing intensity, or it may be acute and severe in onset. Many times patients' chronic cancer pain will be well managed, but then they experience a sudden worsening in their pain or different type of pain. Because it is possible for pain to be experienced before a tumor is clinically detectable, caution should be exercised even in patients for whom no evidence of disease can be found—and especially in patients who have a history of cancer and have been free of disease for some time. It is important to be aware that patients who experience a sudden worsening of pain or a new pain might fear relapse or disease progression.

A thorough history includes identification of the pattern, characteristics, severity, and impact of the pain. Many instruments can be used to conduct a comprehensive pain assessment. The severity of pain cannot be measured by any direct or physiologic means; patient report is the only valid means of establishing the degree or intensity of the pain. The most convenient method, and one that most patients can use, is to ask for a rating on a 0-to-10 scale, where 0 indicates no pain and 10 indicates the worst pain imaginable. Other scales can be used if preferred by the patient. Several versions of a "faces scale" show a range of happy to sad or hurting faces accompanied by a numerical scale. These scales are useful for children (ages 3 and up) or for patients with communication difficulties (e.g., a language barrier or an inability to speak). It is important to use one scale consistently with the individual so that you have a sense of the change in status or impact of your interventions over time. While doing the pain assessment, it is important to review other symptoms, which may have an impact on a patient's pain level and treatment plan. Tools used to assess multiple symptoms include the Edmonton Symptom Assessment Scale (ESAS) and the M.D. Anderson Symptom Inventory (MDASI).

To interpret the ratings given by patients, providers must remember that these are *subjective* measures and therefore have no "normal values." In general, ratings of 1 to 3 are considered to be mild pain, 4 to 6 are described as moderate, and 7 or greater as severe.[6] Because there is considerable individual variation in the way patients use these scales, comparison among patients should be avoided except for aggregate analysis for research and quality assurance purposes.

Since pain is a subjective complaint, it can be influenced or distorted by delirium, somatization, and chemical coping. It is imperative to assess not only the pain complaint but also the patient's cognitive status and coping techniques. Cognition can be assessed using standardized tools such as the Memorial Delirium Assessment Scale or Mini-Mental State Examination. Somatization and chemical coping can be difficult to detect, but a careful medical history and patient interview may clue a practitioner to these types of coping strategies. Red flags that a pain complaint may be influenced by one of these include rapid opioid escalation, continued complaints of severe pain despite aggressive titration, and history of substance abuse.

PHYSICAL EXAMINATION

Patients can experience significant pain without appearing to be suffering. Coping abilities vary widely among individuals. With persistent pain, physiologic and psychosocial adaptations usually occur; signs, including elevated pulse and blood pressure, and even behaviors such as grimacing may not be seen. The physical examination should focus initially on the painful area(s) to identify any lesions, inflammation, vascular changes, edema, or pain on palpation. Sensory changes in the affected part or new areas should also be carefully assessed because such changes often herald new disease or injury from other sources, such as chemotherapy. Changes in motor capacity, joint range of motion, and muscle strength should also be observed. The patient needs to be observed during ambulation, wherever possible, to determine the impact of pain on movement and functional ability. If the patient complains of back pain, there should be a high suspicion that impending cord compression is possible. Assessment questions for possible cord compression include a history of sensory changes (leg weakness), autonomic dysfunction (loss of bladder or bowel function), and pain (usually sudden onset). One test is to apply firm compression over the spinous processes to determine if vertebral pain is elicited; if it is, further workup is indicated.

DIAGNOSTICS

No specific imaging or laboratory technique exists with which to directly study pain. The diagnostic evaluation should be guided by the location and nature of the pain and by an understanding of the natural history of the underlying disease. Relevant x-ray studies and scans should be reviewed and repeated periodically. CT scans may be indicated to identify masses that involve the vital organs or lymphadenopathy. Plain films and a bone scan should be obtained if bone metastases are suspected. The bone scan is a sensitive test that can show disease before it is visible on x-ray films; however, it is not as specific and may be positive for other inflammatory processes. Plain films may be negative until 30% to 50% of the cortical bone has been destroyed. An MRI is usually necessary to evaluate for nerve root or epidural cord compression. Epidural cord compression is an oncologic emergency, and the patient may complain of back pain without any signs of neurologic impairment. Patients with a history of tumors that tend to metastasize to the bone (especially breast, lung, lymphoma, and prostate) should undergo an MRI promptly to exclude cord impingement. With cord compression, the earliest possible intervention (e.g., steroids, surgery, radiotherapy) is critical to preserve neurologic function.[7,8] If neuropathic pain is being assessed, an electromyography (EMG) might be beneficial to show nerve compression or injury or nerve root injury.

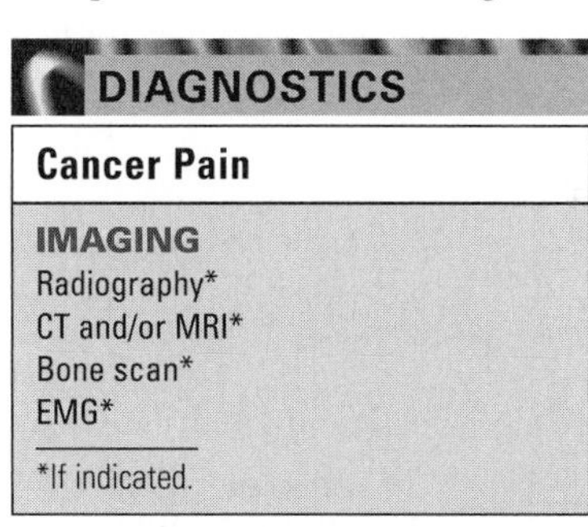
DIAGNOSTICS

Cancer Pain

IMAGING
Radiography*
CT and/or MRI*
Bone scan*
EMG*

*If indicated.

DIFFERENTIAL DIAGNOSIS

Cancer Pain

Tumor-related pain
- Peripheral neuropathies
- Cervical, brachial, and lumbosacral
- Bone metastasis
- Epidural cord compression

Treatment-related pain
- Chemotherapy
- Radiotherapy
- Biologic therapy
- Postsurgical
- Acute and postherpetic neuralgia
- Mucositis

Preexisting chronic pain
Abdominal obstruction
Nonmalignant pain
Infection

DIFFERENTIAL DIAGNOSIS

Pain is a significant problem for a majority of cancer patients at some point during the course of their disease. Although pain can occur at any time and can be related to tumor involvement or tumor treatment, the incidence and severity of pain may increase as the disease progresses. Common treatment-related cancer pain syndromes include those associated with surgery, chemotherapy, radiotherapy, and biologic therapy.[9,10] Surgical patients may, for example, experience postmastectomy, post-thoracotomy, or phantom pain. Some chemotherapeutic agents, such as the vinca alkaloids and cisplatin, can cause peripheral neuropathies; extravasational agents can cause significant tissue and nerve damage. Radiation effects can be early (e.g., mucositis) or late (e.g., brachial plexopathy or osteoradionecrosis). Biologic agents such as interferon can cause peripheral neuropathy and joint pain, both of which can be transient or chronic.

Tumor-related pain can result from the compression of pain-sensitive structures by a mass (e.g., epidural cord compression), or it can be related to direct infiltration, especially of the nervous and musculoskeletal systems. Pain resulting from bone metastasis is one of the most severe and disabling types of pain. Patients may also experience pain that is unrelated to the tumor or its treatment. Many patients have preexisting chronic pain problems (e.g., low back pain, migraine, diabetic neuropathy). These syndromes must be assessed and included in the treatment plan.

Other causes of pain must always be considered. Infection of any malignant wounds can cause sudden and severe pain that is easily improved with appropriate antimicrobial medications. Herpes zoster is common in immunocompromised patients. It can be in either the acute or chronic stage and causes sharp, burning, or aching pain and follows a dermatomal distribution. Obstruction, constipation, ileus, peptic ulcer disease, gallbladder disease, pancreatitis, and appendicitis are examples of diseases and conditions that can cause abdominal pain. Mucositis may cause severely painful lesions of the oral mucosa.

BOX 256-1

PAIN MANAGEMENT PEARLS

Pain is a multidimensional experience that requires multidimensional assessment.
Pain and other symptoms can change rapidly. Regular and frequent assessment are necessary.
Reassure the patient and family that most pain can be relieved.
Reassure the patient and family about their concerns and fears regarding opioids.
Explain to the patient the difference between physical dependence, addiction, and tolerance.
Encourage normal activity to the fullest extent possible.
Treat pain promptly and aggressively.
Rational pain management tailors the regimen to the type and intensity of pain.
Regular around the clock administration with adequate breakthrough dosing and adjuvants as required plus proactive antiemetic and laxative regimens are the hallmarks of rational and effective pain management in cancer patients.
Optimize opioids before adding adjuvants.
Opioid conversion tables are inexact; patients should be observed carefully whenever regimen changes are made.
Consider nonpharmacologic options to control pain, such as anesthetic and neurosurgical approaches, in intractable pain syndromes where the risk-to-benefit ratio favors benefit.
Beware of overzealous opioid use in the patient who is experiencing delirium and somatization.
Beware of the pitfalls of polypharmacy.
Treating the patient who suffers from total pain (nociception, psychological distress, and spiritual distress) means treating the whole patient (body, mind, and spirit).

From Reddy S: Pain management. In Elsayem A, Driver L, Bruera E, editors: *The M.D. Anderson symptom control and palliative care handbook,* San Antonio, Tex, 2003, University of Texas Health Science Center Printing Service.

MANAGEMENT

Effective pain management, particularly for the patient with advanced cancer, requires a comprehensive approach that often involves the use of multiple modalities (Box 256-1). A thorough assessment and physical examination are very important in effective pain management. If the type of pain and pathophysiology of pain can be determined, the treatment can then be specific for that type of pain. Providers should remember that cancer patients often have pain in multiple body areas from several sources; pain relief regimens need to accommodate this characteristic.[11]

Opioids (the preferred term for narcotic analgesics) are the mainstay of pain management.[6] However, adjuvant pharmacologic management and surgical, anesthetic, and nonpharmacologic interventions play an important role in care. Initial therapy for minor pain (1 to 3 on a scale of 1 to 10) can include NSAIDs if the patient is not taking any analgesics.[6] Adjuvant drugs to enhance pain control (e.g., the tricyclic antidepressants and anticonvulsant drugs for neuropathic pain or those targeted to manage side effects) are appropriate at any stage, if indicated.

Unfortunately, opioids are among the most underused and misunderstood category of drugs. To use opioids effectively, it is important to distinguish between key terms that are often misapplied in practice: *addiction, dependence,* and *tolerance.* The phenomenon known as *pseudoaddiction* must also be recognized.

Addiction (psychological addiction) is chiefly a psychologic and behavioral problem in which controlled substances are used for reasons other than pain. For someone who is addicted, obtaining and taking drugs become the primary focus of existence, and drug use is continued despite the risks (social and physical) involved. Illegitimate drug use resulting in addiction is destructive. In contrast, legitimate use of opiates for pain relief can improve the body's overall ability to fight off and cope with disease and significantly improve the patient's quality of life and ability to function and carry out normal life activities, limited only by the disease and related disability. If a patient has no history of dependence, it is rare for pain treatment to lead to addiction. If a patient has a history of dependence, aggressive pain management is still possible with good assessment, close observation, and open communication.

Dependence, sometimes known as physical addiction, is not synonymous with or diagnostic of addiction. Dependence is a physiologic process resulting from adaptation to the presence of a drug. Its only clinical significance is the potential for a withdrawal syndrome (e.g., vomiting, diarrhea, cramping, and diaphoresis). The avoidance of withdrawal may promote drug-seeking behaviors, but this has no clinical significance to the patient with pain as long as the dose is properly tapered when no longer needed to relieve the pain.

Patients are often reluctant to take opioids in the early stages of cancer because they believe morphine is for dying patients. They also fear that they may become "immune" to them—that is, the drug will not work when it is "really needed." It may be that patients confuse tolerance with "immunity." Tolerance is a phenomenon whereby a higher dose of a drug is required over time to maintain the same therapeutic effect. The possible development of tolerance is sometimes of great concern to health care providers who worry about the amount of medications that they give to a patient. Fortunately, tolerance is much less of a problem than once thought; to the extent it does occur, it can be overcome by upward dose titration, or an opioid rotation. Experience with cancer patients has shown that patients with stable pain may stay on the same dose for years without decreasing efficacy.[12] When dose escalation (especially a rapid increase) is required, progression of disease is the most common reason for the change.[10,12] Other causes for dose escalation include delirium, somatization, and chemical coping. Opioid medications do not have a ceiling dose and so can be continually titrated based on need.

Pseudoaddiction is a recently recognized phenomenon. Many patients who have been labeled as "difficult" and "drug seeking" are in fact simply being undertreated for their pain.[13] Factors contributing to the development of pseudoaddiction include the administration of opioids at intervals greater than their expected duration of action or doses that are too low or of insufficient potency for the type of pain experienced. Patients who have endured unrelieved pain may become more aggressive in seeking relief and may increase their dose; as a consequence, they may call frequently and earlier than expected for more medication. These patients might be labeled as "clock watchers" and may ask for their pain medications at exactly the prescribed time. Although these actions may serve as warning signs to alert the practitioner to abuse, the adequacy of treatment must be assessed thoroughly before a judgment can be made.

Opioids are classified as pure agonists, mixed agonist-antagonists, or partial agonists. The pure agonists can be relied on to produce effective analgesia and, except for meperidine (Demerol), can be titrated to pain relief without having a ceiling effect (Box 256-2). Meperidine is not recommended for routine use in the cancer population. The metabolite normeperidine often causes central nervous system excitability (delirium, tremors, seizures, and even death), and the potential is enhanced in older persons and in patients with renal insufficiency or hepatic impairment.[14,15]

The mixed agonist-antagonist opioids produce analgesia but can also reverse analgesia. These drugs are also associated with a fairly high incidence of psychotomimetic side effects and, like meperidine, are not recommended for routine use. The most serious consequence arises when agonist-antagonists are given to a patient who has been taking a pure agonist opioid. In this situation, the agonist-antagonist acts as an antagonist by displacing the agonist from the opiate receptors, which precipitates withdrawal and reverses analgesia.

BOX 256-2

OPIOID AGONISTS USED FOR CANCER PAIN

Codeine (Tylenol #3 or #4*)
Fentanyl (Sublimaze, Duragesic)
Hydrocodone (Vicodin,* Lortab*)
Hydromorphone (Dilaudid)
Levorphanol (Levo-Dromoran)
Methadone (Dolophine)
Morphine (MSIR, Roxanol, MS Contin,† Oramorph,† Kadian†)
Oxycodone (Percocet,* Percodan,‡ Roxicodone, OxyContin†)

NOTE: The following medications are not recommended for the relief of cancer pain: propoxyphene, meperidine, mixed agonist-antagonist, partial agonists, and placebos.[6]

*Combination containing acetaminophen.
†Sustained or controlled-release delivery system.
‡Combination containing aspirin.

Withdrawal and exacerbation of pain not only impair quality of life but also pose considerable risk to critically ill and debilitated patients. For this reason, the injudicious use of naloxone, a pure opioid antagonist, is also to be avoided because respiratory depression is rare in the opioid-tolerant patient. In rare cases, the rapid infusion of naloxone can even lead to severe pulmonary edema.[16,17] The action of partial agonists is not well understood, and, in general, they have limited usefulness in the treatment of cancer pain.

The key principle for effective pain control with opioids is to titrate the dose to achieve the desired outcome.[6] Considerable variability in dosage exists from one patient to another. Some opioids (e.g., morphine and hydromorphone) are classified as strong, and others (e.g., codeine and hydrocodone) are classified as weak. However, these opioids are actually capable of producing equally effective analgesia if given in sufficient doses. The "weak" opioids are usually combined with aspirin or acetaminophen, and dosing is limited by the potential for renal and hepatic toxicity associated with the nonopioid drug.

Table 256-1 demonstrates the relative equianalgesic doses for some of the commonly used opioids. Morphine is used for comparison because it is the most widely used opioid and more is known about its pharmacokinetics, but any of the agonist opioids can be used. Using the table, the health care provider can change one drug or route to another. For example, a dose of hydromorphone requires only 1.5 mg to produce approximately the same analgesia as 10 mg of morphine. Opioids administered via the gastrointestinal tract are subject to a first-pass effect, whereby a portion of the drug is metabolized to nonanalgesic substances as it is routed through the hepatic circulation before being circulated systemically. If a patient is receiving adequate analgesia from 10 mg of morphine sulfate given parenterally, it takes 30 mg to achieve the *same* effect if given orally because approximately 20 mg is metabolized before reaching the systemic circulation. The parenteral-to-oral ratio varies from drug to drug. It must be remembered that these equianalgesic comparisons are only guides; the relationship between the drugs is not absolute. In addition, the longer a patient is taking an opioid, the less

TABLE 256-1 Opioid Conversion Table

Drug	Parenteral Dose (mg) Equivalent to 10 mg IV/SQ Morphine	Oral Dose (mg) Equivalent to 30 mg Oral Morphine	Parenteral-to-Oral Ratio	Dosing Interval (hours)
Morphine	10	30	1:3	2-4 for immediate release; 8-24 for sustained release
Codeine	100 (SQ only)	300	1:3	2-4
Hydromorphone	1.3-1.5	7.5	1:5	2-4
Levorphanol	2	4	1:2	4-12
Methadone*	1-10	2-20	1:2 or 3	8-24
Oxycodone	N/A	20-30	N/A	2-4 for immediate release; 8-12 for sustained release
Fentanyl	0.1-0.2 mg	N/A	N/A	1-2

Parenteral Morphine (mg/24 hours)	Duragesic Patch Equivalent (mcg/hour)
8-22	25
23-37	50
38-52	75
53-67	100
68-92	125
83-97	150

Data from *Ripamonti C, Groff L, Brunelli C, and others: Switching from morphine to oral methadone in treating cancer pain: what is the equianalgesic dose ratio? *J Clin Oncol* 16(10):3216-3221, 1998; Reddy S: Pain management. In Elsayem A, Driver L, Bruera E, editors: *The M.D. Anderson symptom control and palliative care handbook,* San Antonio, Tex, 2003, University of Texas Health Science Center Printing Service; McAuley D: *Narcotic analgesic converter,* 2007, retrieved March 16, 2007, from http://www.globalrph.com/narcoticonv.htm; and Derby S: Opioid conversion guidelines for management of adult cancer pain, *Am J Nurs* 99(10):62-65, 1999.

accurate these relationships are because of what is called *cross-tolerance*. In fact, often when a patient who has been using opioids over time changes from one opioid to another, the amount of the new opioid being used might need to be anywhere from 10% to 50% of the amount the chart recommends.

The oral route of administration is the route of choice in most situations because of simplicity and cost-effectiveness.[14,18,19] However, opioids are extremely versatile drugs and can be given via numerous routes. The choice of route and drug depends on a variety of patient factors, including (1) the nature and stability of the pain, (2) the functional status of the gastrointestinal tract, (3) patient and caregiver abilities to manage the regimen (e.g., cognitive function, psychomotor skills), (4) side effects, (5) dosage forms and availability, and (6) cost. More invasive routes of administration, such as parenteral, epidural, and intrathecal, increase the risk for complications (e.g., infection), are usually more costly, and should be reserved for carefully selected patients. The subcutaneous route and rectal route are under utilized and can deliver excellent pain control in patients who cannot tolerate oral medication but who want to be managed at home. Caution should be exercised when using topical pain medications prepared at compounding pharmacies because they have not been standardized and proven in clinical trials.

Opioids should be administered on an around-the-clock schedule that is based on their expected duration of action. As needed (p.r.n.) dosing leads to greater peaks and valleys in analgesic blood levels between doses, especially if patients wait until the pain is severe before requesting medication. The administration of medications on an as-needed basis is most appropriate for isolated moments of incident pain in an otherwise pain-free patient, or in postoperative pain management. Cancer pain is best treated with a long-acting, around-the-clock medication with a short-acting pain medication for breakthrough. The short-acting medication dose should be between 10% and 30% of the total daily dose. If two or three breakthrough doses are required routinely, the long-acting medication can then be titrated.

Rapid dose titration is needed for severe, uncontrolled pain or in response to interventions such as surgery. Short-term use of parenteral administration may be required. In such situations, use of the patient-controlled analgesia pump is ideal. The on-demand patient-administered dose used as needed with or without a continuous (basal) infusion allows for individualized dosing and sustained analgesia. If the patient shows evidence of delirium, somatization, or chemical coping, the on-demand patient-administered dose should be avoided because of the possibility of opioid-induced neurotoxicity.

As a way to better understand the use of long-acting opioids in combination with short-acting opioids, a patient with insulin-dependent diabetes serves as an example of the principle.[17] Typically, a long-acting form of insulin serves as the baseline. However, blood glucose levels are not steady: they respond to a host of influences. Regular insulin is given to treat episodic hyperglycemia. Pain is also a dynamic state influenced by a host of factors. Controlled-release drugs, continuous infusions, and transdermal delivery systems can be used to provide sustained analgesia, much like long-acting insulin.[20,21] Transdermal delivered medication should be used when a patient's pain is stable because of the difficulty in titrating the slow-release medication. Regular, short-acting opioids can be used to treat the breakthrough pain associated with activity, treatments, or other factors. They can also be used as a preventive approach to pain control. When an event or activity (e.g., walking) is known to provoke pain, the as-needed dose should be taken about 30 to 45 minutes in advance of that activity whenever possible.

COMPLICATIONS

Vigilant management is critical to the success of pain therapy and is needed to avoid the complications associated with pain therapy. Side effects are among the most common reasons cited for opioid failure and premature abandonment of therapy.[22] A patient who experiences nausea, sedation, or clouded thinking has often been improperly labeled as being allergic to opioids. Fortunately, a true allergy to opioids is rare. Some side effects, particularly nausea and sedation, are usually transient and improve once tolerance develops. Tolerance to another side effect of opioids, respiratory depression, develops rapidly and is rare after a few days of drug exposure. Most patients develop a tolerance to the emetic and sedating effects over several days. Sedation is most likely to be related to sleep deprivation, which is to be expected in patients who have experienced unrelieved pain. Daytime sedation usually abates within 72 hours on a stable dose of opioids, and sleep is restored. Instead of sacrificing pain control if sedation persists, sedation can be treated by increasing caffeine intake or adding a stimulant such as methylphenidate (Ritalin) or modafinil (Provigil).

Nausea and vomiting can be managed with antiemetics on a scheduled basis initially and then as needed once the opioid dose is stabilized. Metoclopramide is a good antinausea medication because of its peripheral effects (improved gastric motility) and central effects (antidopaminergic effect on the chemoreceptor trigger zone). Often nausea is directly related to decreased bowel function and resolves when the constipation is corrected. Unfortunately, patients do not develop a tolerance to the constipating effects of opioids, and it is a rare patient who does not need an aggressive bowel management program. For patients who have not had a bowel movement in more than 3 to 5 days, it is essential that a serious effort be made to restore bowel function. Proper hydration and a diet with foods rich in fiber are important. However, when patients are on opioids for chronic use, they will need scheduled laxatives. Standard practice is to use senna with stool softeners just to maintain their normal bowel regimen. If this does not work, more aggressive therapies such as polyethylene glycol (Miralax), lactulose, bisacodyl (Dulcolax) suppositories, or magnesium citrate can be used. Caution should be used with polyethylene glycol because, if not enough water is consumed, constipation may result. Prepared enemas can also be purchased. In a refractory situation, laxatives and enemas may need to be repeated every 6 hours.[23] Once a reasonable regimen has been restored, a prophylactic regimen should be initiated using a combination of a senna laxative and stool softener (Senekot-S) titrated to maintain a normal, comfortable bowel movement at least every other day. The bowel regimen is similar to the pain regimen with standard "around the clock" medications (laxative with stool softener) and some type of preparation (suppository, enema, etc.) for breakthrough if no bowel movement occurs within 3 days. If, at any time, there is concern that an ileus or malignant bowel obstruction is present, the patient needs to be medically evaluated, which might mean having appropriate diagnostics (e.g., x-ray study).

All opioids have the potential to cause delirium. Patients who have rapid escalation of opioids, develop renal or hepatic failure, or have other pathophysiologic causes for delirium are at higher risk. The other causes include multiple medications, sepsis, electrolyte imbalances, dehydration, brain tumors, hypoxia, co-morbid medical conditions, and paraneoplastic syndrome. Identifying the cause of the delirium and then reversing it, if possible, are the appropriate treatment for delirium. If opioids are suspected to be the cause, an opioid rotation is required. (See Chapter 204.)

Less common opioid side effects include urinary retention and myoclonus. Urinary retention is often transient and can be temporarily relieved with straight catheterization or a change to another opioid. Myoclonus, the intermittent muscle jerking that occurs especially during sleep, is usually seen at higher opioid doses and with long-term opioid use. It is important to monitor for myoclonus because it can lead to seizures if treatment is not initiated. If myoclonus persists, the opioid may need to be decreased or changed. Other complications of pain management include an increased risk of gastrointestinal bleeding with the use of NSAIDs or corticosteroids.

INDICATIONS FOR REFERRAL OR HOSPITALIZATION

A pain and/or palliative care specialist should be consulted if efforts to titrate the dose to desired effect and manage the related side effects are not successful. If pain specialists are not available, a local hospice organization is an excellent resource. Consultation is essential whenever a more invasive route of administration or other intervention is indicated. Typically pain is not the only symptom experienced by cancer patients; therefore a palliative care consult might be beneficial to manage an array of symptoms. It should be remembered that some pain problems are relatively easily managed through the use of simple procedures performed in a pain center (e.g., epidural steroid injections, trigger point injections, celiac plexus block). Multidisciplinary pain specialty teams are being established to combine the expertise of such diverse fields as neurology, anesthesia, neurosurgery, nursing, psychology, and physical medicine.

PATIENT AND FAMILY EDUCATION

Patient education regarding the management of side effects is essential to ensuring good pain management. Patients should be encouraged to anticipate that side effects will improve with adaptation and that they can be treated without sacrificing pain relief. General education regarding around-the-clock dosing and as-needed dosing needs to be provided to patients and families. Patients should be instructed to contact their health care provider if they require three or more breakthrough doses daily. When starting patients on opioids it is important to educate them on constipation prevention and the symptoms of opioid-induced neurotoxicity. These include sedation, delirium, hallucinations, and myoclonus and require immediate contact with a physician. Patients and families should also be encouraged to discuss with the health care provider their concerns about pain management, including the fear of pain, the fear of addiction, and possible misconceptions about the management of cancer pain. This approach will involve patients in the care plan and promote pain control.

REFERENCES

1. Hill CS, Fields WS, Thorpe DM: A call to action to improve relief of cancer pain. In Hill CS, Fields WS, editors: *Drug treatment of cancer pain in a drug-oriented society: advances in pain research and therapy*, New York, 1989, Raven Press.
2. Hill CS: A review and commentary on the negative influence of licensing and disciplinary boards and drug enforcement agencies on pain treatment with opioid analgesics, *J Pharm Care Pain Symp Control* 1:33, 1993.
3. McCaffery M, Pasero A: *Pain: clinical manual*, ed 2, St Louis, 1999, Mosby.
4. Payne R: Pathophysiology of cancer pain. In Foley KM, Bonica JJ, Ventafridda V, editors: *Advances in pain research and therapy*, vol 16, New York, 1990, Raven Press
5. Fields HL: *Pain*, New York, 1987, McGraw-Hill.
6. Panchal SJ, Angelescu DL, Bendettti C, and others: Adult cancer pain. In *National Comprehensive Cancer Network clinical practice guidelines in oncology v.1.2006*, retrieved Sept 8, 2006, from http://www.nccn.org/professionals/physician_gls/PDF/pain/pdf.
7. Fisher G, Mayer DK, Struthers C: Bone metastases, part I, Pathophysiology, *Clin J Oncol Nurs* 1:29-35, 1997.
8. Weinstein SM: Management of spinal neoplasm and its complications. In Berger A, Portenoy RK, Weissman DE, editors: *Principles and practices of supportive oncology*, Philadelphia, 1998, Lippincott-Raven.
9. Foley KM: The treatment of cancer pain, *N Engl J Med* 313:84-95, 1985.
10. Cherny JI, Portenoy RK: The management of cancer pain, *CA Cancer J Clin* 44:262-303, 1994.
11. Carr D, Goudas L, Lawrence D, and others: *Management of cancer pain*, vol 1, AHRQ Evidence Reports, #35, Pub No 02-E002, Oct 2001, retrieved Sept 7, 2006, from http://www.ahrq.gov/downloads/pub/evidence/pdf/cansymp/cansymp.pdf.
12. Foley KM: Changing concepts of tolerance to opioids: what the cancer patient has taught us. In Chapman CR, Foley KM, editors: *Current and emerging issues in cancer pain: research and practice*, New York, 1993, Raven Press.
13. Weissman DE, Haddox JD: Opioid pseudoaddiction: an iatrogenic syndrome, *Pain* 35:363-366, 1989.
14. Jacox A, Carr DB, Payne R: *Management of cancer pain: clinical practice guideline no 9*, AHCPR Pub No 94-0592, Rockville, Md, 1994, Agency for Health Care Policy and Research, US Department of Health and Human Services, Public Health Service.
15. Kaiko RF, Foley KM, Grabinski PY, and others: Central nervous system excitatory effects of meperidine in cancer patients, *Ann Neurol* 13:180-185, 1983.
16. Schwartz JA, Koenigsberg MD: Naloxone-induced pulmonary edema, *Ann Emerg Med* 16:1294-1296, 1987.
17. Thorpe DM: The insulin-dependent diabetic as a model for pain management, *Dimens Oncol Nurs* 4:36-38, 1990.
18. Burke J, German D, Lee A, and others: *NPPR nurse practitioner's prescribing reference*, New York, 2006, Prescribing Reference, Inc.
19. Hill CS: Oral opioid analgesics. In Patt RB, editor: *Cancer pain*, Philadelphia, 1993, Lippincott.
20. Portenoy RK: Continuous infusion of opioid drugs in the treatment of cancer pain: guidelines for use, *J Pain Symptom Manage* 1:223-228, 1986.
21. Payne R: Transdermal fentanyl: suggested recommendations for clinical use, *J Pain Symptom Manage* 7:40-44, 1992.
22. Texas Cancer Council Workgroup on Pain Control in Cancer Patients, Hill CS, editor: *Guidelines for treatment of cancer pain*, ed 2, Austin, Tex, 1997, The Council.
23. Bisanz A: Managing bowel elimination problems in patients with cancer, *Oncol Nurs Forum* 24:679-686, 1997.

CHAPTER 257

Oncology Complications and Paraneoplastic Syndromes

Jane Williams and Zita Dubauskas

An oncologic emergency is an acute, potentially life-threatening event that is directly or indirectly related to cancer or its treatment. If it is left unrecognized and untreated, significant morbidity or death may result. An oncologic emergency may also occur in an individual not previously diagnosed with cancer. Because cancer manifests itself in various ways, it must be considered part of the differential diagnosis of many complex medical events. In addition, because the nature of these entities is emergent and requires treatment of the underlying cancer, all these syndromes require urgent referral to an oncologist.

Common structural emergencies consist of superior vena cava syndrome (SVCS) and spinal cord compression (SCC). Metabolic emergencies include hypercalcemia, syndrome of inappropriate antidiuretic syndrome (SIADH), and tumor lysis syndrome (TLS). Other oncologic emergencies not discussed in this chapter include sepsis and disseminated intravascular coagulation.

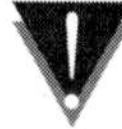

Immediate emergency department referral or physician consultation is indicated for patients with angioedema, dyspnea, stridor, papilledema, seizures, and other signs of SVCS.

Immediate emergency department referral or physician consultation is indicated for back pain accompanied by focal weakness, ataxia, or bowel or bladder dysfunction.

Immediate emergency department referral or physician consultation is indicated for patients with serum calcium levels of greater than 12 mg/dl.

Immediate emergency department referral or physician consultation is indicated for patients with TLS.

Immediate emergency department referral or physician consultation is indicated for patients with serum sodium levels of 125 mEq/L or less.

SUPERIOR VENA CAVA SYNDROME

DEFINITION AND EPIDEMIOLOGY

SVCS occurs when blood flow through the superior vena cava (SVC) is obstructed. Lung cancer is responsible in approximately 70% of SVCS cases.

PATHOPHYSIOLOGY

Any pathologic process that invades the lymphatics or structures of the superior mediastinum can encroach on the thin-walled, compliant SVC and cause obstruction of venous return to the heart. SVCS may result from external compression, direct invasion, or thrombosis of the SVC. The most common cause of SVC obstruction is malignancy, usually lung cancer, lymphoma, or breast cancer.[1] The most common nonmalignant cause of SVCS is thrombosis of the SVC associated with indwelling central venous catheters.[2]

CLINICAL PRESENTATION AND PHYSICAL EXAMINATION

SVCS is usually insidious in onset. The severity of presentation depends on the underlying cause, rapidity of obstruction, concurrent thrombosis, location of obstruction, and adequacy of collateral circulation. Swelling of the face, neck, or chest or orthopnea is the classic presenting complaint.[2] Other symptoms include headache, dizziness, visual disturbances, hoarseness, chest pain, and dysphagia. Physical findings include venous distention in the upper body, facial edema, cyanosis, arm and hand edema, telangiectasias of the chest and upper back, tachypnea, hoarseness, and stridor.[1,2] Neurologic abnormalities resulting from increased intracranial pressure include papilledema, agitation, lethargy, confusion, seizures, and coma.

DIAGNOSTICS

A chest x-ray examination commonly reflects a superior mediastinal mass or widening (64%), pleural effusion (26%), a right hilar mass (12%), or adenopathy; however, 16% of patients may have normal radiographic findings.[1] An MRI or a CT scan of the chest is indicated to localize the level of SVC obstruction and identify the presence of intrinsic or extrinsic obstruction, superimposed thrombosis, collateral circulation, mediastinal adenopathy, masses, and other sites of unrecognized disease in the chest. Because the underlying pathologic condition in many patients with new-onset SVCS is not identified, other diagnostic evaluations (biopsies) are almost always required before the definitive therapy can be administered.

DIFFERENTIAL DIAGNOSIS

With SVCS, idiopathic mediastinal fibrosis, tuberculosis, histoplasmosis, and aneurysm of the aortic arch are among the differential diagnoses.[1] Other diagnoses to consider are constrictive pericarditis and thrombosis from indwelling catheters or pacemakers leads.

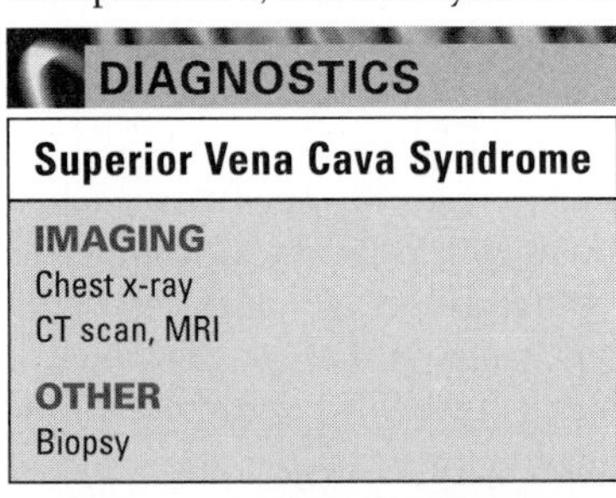
DIAGNOSTICS

Superior Vena Cava Syndrome

IMAGING
Chest x-ray
CT scan, MRI

OTHER
Biopsy

DIFFERENTIAL DIAGNOSIS

Superior Vena Cava Syndrome

- Idiopathic mediastinal fibrosis
- Tuberculosis
- Histoplasmosis
- Goiter
- Aortic aneurysm
- Thrombosis
- Constrictive pericarditis

MANAGEMENT AND COMPLICATIONS

Treatment is directed at the underlying cause. The treatment of SVCS should be guided by the stage and histologic features of the primary process. Chemotherapy alone or in combination with radiotherapy is the treatment of choice for SVCS caused by small cell lung cancer (SCLC) and non-Hodgkin's lymphoma, whereas non-SCLC is best treated with radiotherapy, endovascular stent placement, or both.[1-3] Temporary measures to alleviate discomfort include bed rest with elevation of the upper body, supplemental oxygen, and limited IV fluids. Venipuncture and IV lines should not be placed in the upper extremities. There may be temporary symptomatic improvement with diuretic therapy and reduced sodium diets, but dehydration may increase the risk for thrombosis and exacerbate the SVCS. The use of short-term corticosteroids to reduce the inflammation and edema associated with the tumor is controversial; however, corticosteroids and bronchodilators are indicated if stridor or airway compromise is present. Intubation or an emergency tracheostomy may be necessary. Patients with central nervous system (CNS) signs require high doses of dexamethasone to relieve increased intracranial pressure.[1] If the SVCS is a result of thrombosis, thrombolytic agents (urokinase or streptokinase) are effective if initiated within 7 days of symptom onset. Other less commonly used treatments include balloon angioplasty, caval stenting, and surgical bypass.[2] If left untreated, patients will develop marked venous distention, laryngeal edema, stridor, increased intracranial pressure, sagittal sinus thrombosis, and cerebral edema.

SPINAL CORD COMPRESSION

DEFINITION AND EPIDEMIOLOGY

Neoplastic epidural SCC occurs in approximately 5% to 10%[4] of patients with cancer, with the majority of cord compressions in adults arising from metastatic breast, lung, or prostate cancer. Other cancers that cause spinal cord metastases include non-Hodgkin's lymphoma, melanoma, renal cell carcinoma, sarcoma, multiple myeloma, and unknown primary carcinoma. Approximately 20% of cases of SCC are seen as the initial manifestation of malignancy.[4-6]

PATHOPHYSIOLOGY

SCC usually results when metastasis from a vertebral body extends into the epidural space or when a vertebral body collapses, resulting in a compression fracture. Direct extension of a paraspinous tumor through a vertebral foramen will also compress the spinal cord.[4] Rarely, a tumor may emanate from the epidural space without any bony involvement. The compression of the spinal cord impairs blood flow, resulting in spinal cord edema, ischemia, and infarction.

CLINICAL PRESENTATION AND PHYSICAL EXAMINATION

The signs and symptoms of SCC depend on the area of spinal cord involved. The thoracic spine is involved most often (70%), followed by the lumbosacral (20%) and cervical (10%) vertebrae. In 70% to 95% of patients the presenting symptom is a constant, dull, aching back pain that is often worse when the patient is supine (opposite of the usual finding with a herniated disc).[4] The pain, which antedates the diagnosis of SCC by days to many months, is exacerbated by movement, sneezing, straining, or neck flexion.[4,5] Weakness, especially of the lower extremities, is the second most common symptom.

It may be preceded or accompanied by sensory loss or paresthesia that ascends to the level of compression.[2] The loss of proprioception produces ataxia. Autonomic dysfunctions such as urinary frequency, urgency, urinary retention, constipation, and sexual impotence are late manifestations and are associated with a poor prognosis.[4,5] Physical findings may include tenderness on palpation of the involved vertebrae, hyperactive deep tendon reflexes, an extensor plantar response, a palpable bladder, and diminished rectal tone.[2]

DIAGNOSTICS

After an accurate neurologic history and physical examination, an MRI is the preferred diagnostic test for SCC. A CT scan or myelography is reserved for patients who cannot undergo an MRI (e.g., patients who have cardiac pacemakers or are claustrophobic).[4] Plain films of the spine lack sufficient sensitivity, with false-negative rates of 10% to 17%.[7] Patients with cancer who are seen with a new complaint of back pain should undergo an evaluation for SCC.

DIFFERENTIAL DIAGNOSIS

Other clinical situations may mimic SCC by causing motor or sensory deficits of the neck or upper and lower back or by causing pain. These situations include thoracic outlet syndromes, osteoarthritis of the spine, periarthritis of the shoulder, a herniated disc, sacroiliitis, facet joint degenerative arthritis, spinal stenosis, irritation of the sciatic nerve, compression fracture from osteoporosis, epidural abscess, ankylosing spondylitis, leaking aortic aneurysm, and renal stones.

MANAGEMENT

Clear indications of SCC in the cancer patient (e.g., focal weakness, ataxia, bowel or bladder dysfunction accompanied by back pain) demand an emergent evaluation and a referral. Immediate therapy with steroids (dexamethasone is most commonly used) may reduce vasogenic edema. The optimum loading dose and maintenance dose are controversial. An IV loading dose of 10 to 100 mg is given, followed by 4 to 24 mg q 6 hr. After 2 days, therapy is switched to 4 to 8 mg oral dexamethasone q 6 hr. Steroid doses are tapered every 4 days.[4] If neurologic decline results from dose reduction, the dose is maintained at effective levels during definitive treatment.

The decision to proceed with surgery, radiotherapy, or chemotherapy is based on the type of cancer. Radiotherapy alone is the definitive treatment for most patients.[4] Surgical decompression is indicated in the following situations: the histopathology of the cancer is unknown, neurologic deterioration develops during or after radiotherapy, the cancer is radiation resistant, a pathologic fracture causes compression by bone, or the spine is unstable.[2,4] Chemotherapy can be used for chemosensitive tumors (e.g., lung cancer, lymphoma) and is usually used as an adjunct to radiotherapy.[2,4]

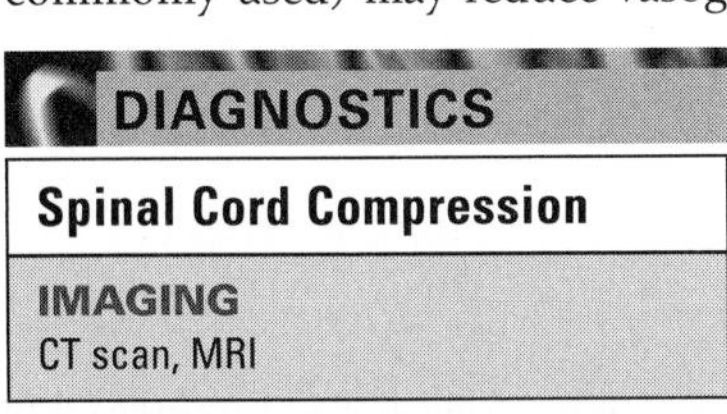

DIAGNOSTICS

Spinal Cord Compression

IMAGING

CT scan, MRI

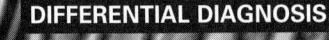

DIFFERENTIAL DIAGNOSIS

Spinal Cord Compression

- Thoracic outlet syndrome
- Osteoarthritis
- Periarthritis of shoulder
- Sacroiliitis
- Herniated disc
- Facet joint degenerative arthritis
- Spinal stenosis
- Sciatic nerve irritation
- Epidural abscess
- Leaking aortic aneurysm
- Renal stones
- Ankylosing spondylitis
- Compression fractures

COMPLICATIONS

If left untreated or undiagnosed, SCC can result in paraplegia, quadriplegia, or loss of bowel or bladder function. In most patients, motor function and sphincter control cannot be regained once they have been lost. Neurologic deficits are more likely to reverse with a gradual rather than a rapid compression.[4,5]

HYPERCALCEMIA

DEFINITION AND EPIDEMIOLOGY

The most common metabolic emergency in patients with cancer is hypercalcemia, developing in 10% to 20% patients with solid tumors.[8] The most common malignancies associated with hypercalcemia are cancers of the breast, lung, kidney, head and neck, esophagus, thyroid, and prostate; lymphomas; and multiple myeloma. Hypercalcemia develops when the rate of calcium mobilization from bone exceeds the renal threshold for calcium excretion. The serum calcium level is greater than 11 mg/dl.[2,9]

PATHOPHYSIOLOGY

In ambulatory patients, 90% of cases of hypercalcemia are caused by either hyperparathyroidism or malignancy; hyperthyroidism is also an important cause in the ambulatory population.[10] The mechanisms involved in hypercalcemia of malignancies were thought to be related primarily to bone resorption resulting from metastatic bone lesions. Although bone metastasis results in hypercalcemia, recent evidence suggests that certain tumors secrete a variety of hormonal factors that stimulate osteoclast activity, resulting in the release of calcium from the bone. Several of these humoral factors are parathyroid hormone–related protein (PTH-rP), osteoclast-activating factors, transforming growth factors, hematopoietic colony-stimulating factors, prostaglandins (E series), and 1,25-dihydroxyvitamin D. Other phenomena that can contribute to and worsen hypercalcemia are immobility, dehydration, and renal insufficiency.[9,11]

CLINICAL PRESENTATION AND PHYSICAL EXAMINATION

Most patients with hypercalcemia see their health care provider with nonspecific symptoms of fatigue (70%), anorexia (60%), nausea, constipation (60%), weight loss (60%), bone pain (60%), polyuria, polydipsia, or dehydration.[8,9,12,13] The neurologic symptoms begin with vague muscle weakness, lethargy, apathy, and hyporeflexia and then progress to stupor and coma.[8,9,12,13] Ventricular extrasystoles and idioventricular rhythms can occur, especially in the presence of digoxin. The most important renal signs are nephrogenic diabetes insipidus

DIAGNOSTICS

Hypercalcemia

LABORATORY
Serum calcium
Serum phosphorus
Serum albumin
Total protein
Ionized serum calcium

OTHER
ECG

and acute and chronic renal failure.[8]

DIAGNOSTICS

With hypercalcemia, serum calcium level is elevated and serum phosphorus level is often low. Because calcium binds to albumin, total calcium measurements can be greatly affected by changes in albumin concentrations. Hypoproteinemia is often seen in cancer patients; therefore the measurement of total serum calcium may understate the severity of the disorder. It is useful to obtain an initial measurement of ionized serum calcium; alternatively, total serum calcium can be adjusted for the level of serum protein using the following equation:

Corrected calcium (mg/dl) = Measured calcium (mg/dl) – [Albumin (g/dl) + 4]

Other changes include a shortened QT interval on ECG.[9]

DIFFERENTIAL DIAGNOSIS

Other than neoplasia, causes of hypercalcemia to consider include primary or secondary hyperparathyroidism, acromegaly, adrenal insufficiency, sarcoidosis or other granulomatous disorders, Paget's disease of bone, hypophosphatasia, familial hypocalciuric hypercalcemia, and renal failure. Other causes are immobilization, complications of renal transplantation, medication-induced hypercalcemia (thiazide diuretics, lithium), excessive intake of vitamin D or A, and milk-alkali syndrome (secondary to calcium ingestion for osteoporosis prevention or in some cases related to overuse of calcium carbonate in patients with peptic ulcer disease or gastroesophageal reflux).[9,11]

MANAGEMENT

Oral or parenteral rehydration is recommended as initial therapy for all patients with hypercalcemia. IV normal saline is generally preferred for hospitalized patients, with infusion rates of 250 to 500 ml/hr in the initial hours.[2] Strict attention to adequate urinary output and fluid balance is critical. Furosemide is primarily used to prevent hypervolemia after euvolemia is achieved with saline infusion. If renal function is normal, 20 to 40 mg furosemide IV may be initiated after volume expansion is achieved, with subsequent doses given if the urinary output is less than 150 to 200 ml/hr.[2]

DIFFERENTIAL DIAGNOSIS

Hypercalcemia

- Primary or secondary hyperparathyroidism
- Acromegaly
- Adrenal insufficiency
- Sarcoidosis
- Granulomatous disease
- Paget's disease of the bone
- Hypophosphatasia
- Familial hypocalciuric hypercalcemia
- Renal failure or transplantation
- Medication-induced hypercalcemia
- Excessive vitamin D or A ingestion
- Immobilization
- Milk-alkali syndrome

Hospitalization is recommended for patients with a serum calcium level of 12 mg/dl or greater (3.0 mmol/L) for patients who have symptoms other than mild fatigue and constipation. For moderate to severe hypercalcemia (total calcium ≥12 mg/dl), saline hydration alone does not generally reduce the serum calcium, and antiresorptive drug therapy should be instituted within 24 hours. Third-generation bisphosphonates (pamidronate or zoledronate) are potent inhibitors of osteoclast activity. When compared with pamidronate, zoledronate showed superior results in terms of complete response rate (88% vs. 70%) and response duration (32 vs. 18 days). Moreover, zoledronate offers the convenience of a 15-minute infusion as opposed to a 2-hour infusion.[14] In patients with osteolysis mediated by PTH-rP (epidermoid carcinomas) in which bisphosphonates may be inferior, treatment with gallium nitrate may be considered.

In addition, salmon calcitonin (4 IU/kg) reduces serum calcium by inhibiting bone resorption and increasing renal calcium excretion. Given its rapid onset of action, serum calcium levels should be remeasured several hours after treatment. If the patient is found to be calcitonin sensitive, treatment may be repeated every 6 to 12 hours (4 to 8 IU/kg). A reduction in serum calcium is achieved in 12 to 48 hours.[2,4,8-10,13]

COMPLICATIONS

Without treatment, symptoms progress to profound alterations in mental status, psychotic behavior, seizures, coma, and ultimately death. Prolonged hypercalcemia eventually causes permanent renal tubular abnormalities with renal tubular acidosis, glucosuria, aminoaciduria, and hyperphosphaturia. Sudden death from cardiac arrhythmias may occur when serum calcium rises acutely.[9,11]

TUMOR LYSIS SYNDROME AND HYPERURICEMIA

DEFINITION AND EPIDEMIOLOGY

TLS is a metabolic imbalance that occurs with the rapid killing and lysis of neoplastic cells and the subsequent release of large quantities of intracellular potassium, phosphorus, and nucleic acids into the bloodstream. Patients with large tumor burdens of malignancies that are highly radiosensitive or chemosensitive such as acute leukemia, high-grade lymphoma, and, to a lesser degree, solid tumors (e.g., breast cancer, SCLC, squamous cell carcinoma of the head and neck, hepatoblastoma, multiple myeloma) and myeloproliferative disorders are at high-risk for the development of this syndrome.[5,9]

PATHOPHYSIOLOGY

The metabolic consequences of cell death include the catabolism of nucleic acid purines by xanthine oxidase to produce uric acid. High levels of uric acid crystallize in the distal tubule of the nephron, with resultant acute obstructive uropathy and renal failure. The massive release of other intracellular products, such as potassium and phosphorus, may lead to life-threatening concentrations. This syndrome is characterized by hyperuricemia, uric acid nephropathy, hyperkalemia, hyperphosphatemia, hypocalcemia, and hyperazotemia. The severity of the syndrome depends on the extent of tumor burden and preexisting renal insufficiency.[5,9]

CLINICAL PRESENTATION AND PHYSICAL EXAMINATION

Although urate nephropathy with TLS is sometimes reported at the time of the initial cancer diagnosis, most cases develop within 1 or 2 days of the initiation of cytotoxic treatment. Patients develop rapidly progressive oliguria with signs of uremia. Edema, fluid overload, hypertension, congestive heart failure, and seizures may result. Acute hyperkalemia and hypocalcemia may result in cardiac arrhythmias, tetany, syncope, and sudden death. Hypocalcemia may cause mild muscle cramps, tetany, and seizures. Hyperphosphatemia may aggravate renal failure. Acidosis and anuria may result. These metabolic changes may occur individually or simultaneously.

DIAGNOSTICS

Serum electrolytes, uric acid, phosphorus, calcium, and creatinine should be checked several times per day for 3 or 4 days after initiation of cytotoxic therapy. Hyperkalemia poses the greatest immediate threat, with the elevation of serum potassium often being the first sign of TLS. If hyperkalemia or hypocalcemia develops, an ECG should be evaluated and possible cardiac arrhythmia monitored. Common ECG changes include peaked T-waves and QRS widening.

DIFFERENTIAL DIAGNOSIS

Gout is the most common cause of hyperuricemia. Other causes of uremia include primary hyperuricemia from specific enzyme defects (Lesch-Nyhan syndrome, glycogen storage disease) and decreased renal clearance of uric acid secondary to intrinsic kidney disease.[5,9]

MANAGEMENT AND COMPLICATIONS

Treatment is aimed at prevention by identifying patients at risk. Prophylactic measures include the initiation of allopurinol, a xanthine oxidase inhibitor, 300 to 900 mg/day starting 1 or 2 days before therapy and continuing until there is evidence of TLS. Dose adjustments should be made for patients with renal insufficiency. More rapid control and lower levels of plasma uric acid have been observed with the administration of rasburicase, a recombinant urate oxidase. Rasburicase is significantly more expensive than allopurinol and is U.S. Food and Drug Administration–approved for use in pediatrics.[8] One should also avoid routinely using drugs that make the urine alkaline. Other prophylactic treatment includes vigorous IV hydration with approximately 3000 ml/ day and diuresis with urinary pH of at least 7.0 before any chemotherapy or cytotoxic therapy is begun. The alkalinization of urine is a controversial topic. Although it is recommended to avoid crystallization of uric acid, it may cause precipitation of calcium-phosphate complexes in the renal tubules.[9] The urine may be alkalinized by adding 100 mEq sodium bicarbonate to each liter of IV fluid. Hyperkalemia can be managed with an oral sodium-potassium exchange resin (sodium polystyrene sulfonate [Kayexalate] 15 g PO q 6 hr) or combined with insulin glucose therapy. Loop diuretics are also useful in the elimination of excess potassium. In the setting of hyperkalemia-induced cardiac arrhythmias, calcium gluconate offers immediate but transient benefits. Generally, calcium replacement is not indicated because of the risk of producing acute nephrocalcinosis and increased renal failure by the precipitation of calcium phosphate in the kidney. Hyperphosphatemia can be controlled with the ingestion of aluminum hydroxide antacid. The hypocalcemia usually responds to the correction of hyperphosphatemia. Any of the previously mentioned imbalances may be severe enough to require temporary hemodialysis.[5,9]

DIAGNOSTICS

Tumor Lysis Syndrome

LABORATORY
Serum electrolytes
Uric acid
Phosphorus
Calcium
Creatinine

OTHER
ECG*

*If indicated.

DIFFERENTIAL DIAGNOSIS

Tumor Lysis Syndrome

- Gout
- Enzyme defects resulting in primary hyperuricemia
- Decreased renal clearance of uric acid

SYNDROME OF INAPPROPRIATE ANTIDIURETIC HORMONE

DEFINITION AND EPIDEMIOLOGY

SIADH is a paraneoplastic syndrome that develops when excessive amounts of antidiuretic hormone (ADH) are present, causing excessive amounts of water retention. Ectopic ADH secretion has been noted in SCLC and in primary tumors with metastatic lesions to the brain and lung.[2,5]

PATHOPHYSIOLOGY

SIADH is characterized by excessive urinary loss of sodium and excessive retention of water by the renal tubules, as well as by the reduced levels of serum sodium and serum osmolality. Because the normal regulation of ADH release occurs from both the CNS and the chest via baroreceptors, any disorders affecting the CNS (structural, metabolic, psychiatric, or pharmacologic) or the lungs may cause SIADH. With excessive ADH secretion, excessive water is reabsorbed in the collecting ducts, and a dilutional hyponatremia occurs.

CLINICAL PRESENTATION AND PHYSICAL EXAMINATION

With mild hyponatremia, early manifestations include thirst, anorexia, mild nausea and vomiting, weight gain without edema, muscle cramps, headache, and mild lethargy.[5,11] Patients become more symptomatic as hyponatremia develops rapidly or as sodium levels fall below 115 mg/dl. Signs and symptoms include hyporeflexia, confusion, oliguria, seizures, and coma.[5,11]

DIAGNOSTICS

With SIADH, the serum sodium level is less than 135 mEq/L, plasma osmolality is less than 280 mosm/kg, urine osmolality is greater than 500 mosm/kg, and urinary sodium is greater than 20 mEq/L.[2] Creatinine should be measured. Thyroid and adrenal dysfunction may also need to be excluded.[11] A chest x-ray and CT scan may be ordered to evaluate pulmonary or neurologic disorders that may cause excessive ADH production.

DIAGNOSTICS

Syndrome of Inappropriate Antidiuretic Hormone

LABORATORY	
Serum electrolytes	Creatinine
Serum osmolality	TSH*
Urine sodium	**IMAGING**
Urine osmolality	Chest x-ray*
BUN	CT scan*

*If indicated.

DIFFERENTIAL DIAGNOSIS

The differential diagnosis of hyponatremia includes liver disease, congestive heart failure, renal failure, hypothyroidism, adrenal insufficiency, psychogenic polydipsia, and idiosyncratic drug reaction (thiazide diuretics, angiotensin-converting enzyme inhibitors). Other causes include CNS infection (meningitis, abscess), CNS trauma (hemorrhage, stroke), and pulmonary infections (tuberculosis).[2,11]

MANAGEMENT AND COMPLICATIONS

Treatment of mild to moderate SIADH (serum sodium level of 120 to 134 mEq/L) with minimum symptoms consists of limiting fluid intake to 500 to 1000 ml/24 hr. If SIADH is refractory or if patients can be managed on an outpatient basis, demeclocycline 600 to 1200 mg/day in divided doses may be used.[2] Patients with significant neurologic impairments (coma, seizures) require hospitalization for treatment with 3% saline by slow infusion at a rate sufficient to increase the serum sodium level by 0.5 to 1.0 mEq/L/hr not to exceed a 20 mEq/L rise in serum sodium concentration during the first 48 hours to avoid development of central pontine myelinolysis.[11] Untreated SIADH or too rapid an increase in serum sodium may result in severe neurologic impairment or death.[2]

INDICATIONS FOR REFERRAL OR HOSPITALIZATION

All the complications discussed in this chapter are considered emergencies. Patients usually require hospitalization and are often sent to an emergency medical center. Because most of these complications are related to progression of the cancer, patients may need to be referred to an oncologist for further management.

DIFFERENTIAL DIAGNOSIS

Syndrome of Inappropriate Antidiuretic Hormone

- Small cell cancer of the lung
- Metastatic cancer to brain or lungs
- Liver disease
- Congestive heart failure
- Renal failure
- Adrenal insufficiency
- Medication-induced hyponatremia
- Pseudohyponatremia
- Hypothyroidism
- Polydipsia
- Reset osmostat
- Beer potamia
- CNS infection
- CNS trauma (stroke, hemorrhage)
- Pulmonary infection (tuberculosis)

PATIENT AND FAMILY EDUCATION

In any emergency, patients and families are frightened, but they also want honest explanations regarding their situation. Patients should be told possible causes for the symptoms being experienced and the possible plan of action, and they should be reassured that the oncologist is being notified immediately. Once treatment is initiated, the patient will benefit from reinforcement from the health care provider regarding instructions for medications, activities, and further warning signs that need to be reported.

REFERENCES

1. Yahalom J: Superior vena cava syndrome. In DeVita VT, Hellman S, Rosenberg SA, editors: *Cancer: principles and practice of oncology*, Philadelphia 2005, Lippincott-Raven.
2. Escalante CP, Gollamudi SV, Bonin SR: Oncologic emergencies and paraneoplastic syndromes. In Pazdur R, Coia LR, Hoskins WJ, and others, editors: *Cancer management: a multidisciplinary approach*, New York, 2005, PRR.
3. Tierney LM, Messina LM: Blood vessels and lymphatics. In Tierney LM, McPhee SJ, Papakis MA, editors: *Current medical diagnosis and treatment*, Norwalk, Conn, 1998, Appleton & Lange.
4. Baehring J: Spinal cord compression. In DeVita VT, Hellman S, Rosenberg SA, editors: *Cancer: principles and practice of oncology*, Philadelphia, 2005, Lippincott-Raven.
5. Rugo HS: Cancer. In Tierney LM, McPhee SJ, Papakis MA, editors: *Current medical diagnosis and treatment*, Norwalk, Conn, 1998, Appleton & Lange.
6. Schiff D, O'Neill BP, Suman VJ: Spinal epidural metastasis as the initial manifestation of malignancy: clinical features and diagnostic approach, *Neurology* 49(2):452-456, 1997.
7. Schiff D: *Clinical features and diagnosis of epidural spinal cord compression, including cauda equine syndrome*, 2006, retrieved March 7, 2007, from http://patients.uptodate.com/topic.asp?file=genl_onc/5033&title=Epidural+spinal+cord+compression.
8. Spinazze S, Schrijvers D: Metabolic emergencies, *Crit Rev Oncol Hematol* 58:79-89, 2006.
9. Tito Fojo A: Metabolic emergencies. In DeVita VT, Hellman S, Rosenberg SA, editors: *Cancer: principles and practice of oncology*, Philadelphia, 2005, Lippincott-Raven.
10. Agus ZS, Berenson JR: *Treatment of hypercalcemia*, 2006, retrieved March 6, 2007, from http://patients.uptodate.com/topic.asp?file=minmetab/4862.
11. Okuda T, Kurokawa K, Papakis MA: Fluid and electrolyte disorders. In Tierney LM, McPhee SJ, Papakis MA, editors: *Current medical diagnosis and treatment*, Norwalk, Conn, 1998, Appleton & Lange.
12. Kaye TB: Hypercalcemia: how to pinpoint the cause and customize treatment, *Postgrad Med* 97:153-160, 1995.
13. Edelson GW, Kleerekoper M: Hypercalcemic crisis, *Med Clin North Am* 79:79-92, 1995.
14. Major P, Lortholary A, Hon J, and others: Zoledronic acid is superior to pamidronate in the treatment of hypercalcemia of malignancy: a pooled analysis of two randomized, controlled clinical trials, *J Clin Oncol* 19:558, 2001.

PART 22

Evaluation and Management of Mental Health Disorders

PATRICIA POLGAR BAILEY, *Section Editor*

CHAPTER 258

Alcohol Abuse

Joseph Rampulla

DEFINITION AND EPIDEMIOLOGY

Alcoholism is a term used to describe recurrent maladaptive drinking that is difficult to control and results in adverse consequences. Alcoholism generally refers to long-term problematic alcohol consumption, whereas more specific terms (e.g., *alcohol intoxication, alcohol withdrawal*) are best used to describe an acute condition. Alcohol abuse, or "problem drinking," refers to a pattern of intermittent maladaptive alcohol consumption that includes continued drinking despite knowledge of specific medical consequences; drinking despite medical recommendations to stop; drinking while driving, working, or operating hazardous equipment; and recurrent problems such as arrests, work impairment, a failure to meet financial obligations, and alcohol-related family problems. Alcohol has a ubiquitous and normative presence in human society; as a result, problems with alcohol use are found among all ethnic, economic, and gender groups.

Alcohol abuse usually includes episodes of binge drinking, which is defined by the Substance Abuse and Mental Health Services Administration as drinking five or more drinks on at least one occasion in a 30-day period.[1] A drink is usually considered to be 12 ounces of beer, 5 ounces of table wine, or 1.5 ounces of distilled spirits. Alcohol abuse is generally considered a less severe condition than dependence, but binge drinkers probably contribute to more highway fatalities than dependent alcoholics.[2] Alcohol dependence develops when repetitive heavy drinking causes cellular adaptive changes; the individual then requires a baseline level of alcohol to maintain homeostasis. The development of alcoholism is multifactorial, and there is little question that the risk for developing alcoholism runs in families.

In 2002 it was estimated that 120 million persons (51% of the U.S. population) 12 years of age or older had used alcohol in the past month, with approximately 54 million engaging in binge drinking.[3] The overall trend in reported alcohol use among teenagers has been slowly declining since a peak in 1997.[4] This unfortunately coincides with an increase in the abuse of prescription medications by teens.

Physician consultation is indicated for delirium tremens (DTs), withdrawal symptoms, and psychotic behavior.

PATHOPHYSIOLOGY

Ethyl alcohol is a low-molecular-weight alcohol that primarily acts as a central nervous system sedative; this effect is thought to be related primarily to its effects on the γ-aminobutyric acid (GABA) system and possibly to alterations in cellular membrane fluidity. The perceived stimulant effect of alcohol may be caused by depressant effects on the cerebral cortex, resulting in disinhibition and excitement. It is likely that alcohol somehow affects all neurotransmitter-receptor complexes, including opiate-mediated dopamine levels in the brain reward center and *N*-methyl-D-aspartate glutaminergic receptors.[5] Serotonin neurotransmission dysfunction appears to contribute to early-onset alcoholism.[6]

Alcohol is absorbed from the stomach and small intestine; the presence of food delays absorption. Infinitely miscible in water, alcohol distributes to all bodily tissues in concentrations roughly proportional to their water content. Alcohol is metabolized in the liver by two principal pathways: (1) alcohol dehydrogenase (ADH) catalyzes degradation of alcohol to acetaldehyde, which is then metabolized by aldehyde dehydrogenase; and (2) the liver's microsomal ethanol oxidizing system increases in activity with chronic exposure to alcohol. Both of these pathways reduce a co-factor, nicotinamide-adenine dinucleotide, to NADH. Excess NADH produces a wide range of metabolic derangements, including fatty liver, hypertriglyceridemia, and hypoglycemia.[7]

In the absence of liver failure, the hepatic metabolism of alcohol and several other drugs is somewhat increased in chronic alcoholics. It takes 1 hour for most individuals to oxidize 7.5 to 10 ml of alcohol, with the excess accumulating and causing toxicity. The effects of alcohol toxicity are roughly related to both the blood alcohol concentration (BAC) and the tolerance of the individual. BAC is influenced by the amount and rate of ingestion and absorption, body weight, and rate of metabolism. Women generally achieve a higher BAC per drink than men, possibly because of their smaller body water compartment and lesser gastric ADH activity.[7] BAC can be estimated by measuring the amount in saliva or expired air. A level of 0.10% (100 mg/dl) is generally considered the BAC that results in clinical intoxication. Taking individual differences into account, a BAC of 50 mg/dl causes mild tranquilization; a BAC of 50 to 150 mg/dl causes impairment in coordination, speech, judgment, and concentration. BACs above 150 mg/dl cause delirium or stupor. Levels of consciousness decline at 300 to 400 mg/dl, leading to unconsciousness and, with increasing BAC levels, respiratory depression, cardiovascular collapse, and death.

Partial tolerance to alcohol develops and is associated with cross-tolerance to other drugs that affect the GABA system, such as benzodiazepines and barbiturates. Tolerance develops in several ways: (1) intracellular adaptation; (2) metabolically, such that the liver metabolizes alcohol more rapidly, and (3) behaviorally, through the person changing his or her lifestyle to accommodate dependence. In patients who are alcohol dependent, an abstinence syndrome develops when alcohol levels decline.

Alcohol Withdrawal (Abstinence)

Withdrawal from alcohol produces a range of manifestations, from mild emotional symptoms to life-threatening autonomic instability. Because withdrawal syndrome develops when the BAC falls below the level to which the individual has adapted, highly tolerant individuals may experience withdrawal even with a substantial level of alcohol in their system. Concomitant misuse of other substances complicates the presentation of patients in withdrawal (see Chapter 267). Within a few hours after the last drink, anxiety, headache, nausea, hypervigilance, tachycardia, and mild tremors develop. Diaphoresis; photophobia; hyperreflexia; a more rapid pulse; elevated blood pressure; more pronounced tremors; and auditory, visual, or tactile hallucinations constitute manifestations of more severe withdrawal. Some form of hallucination is common, and they persist in a small number of patients long after withdrawal. Tonic-clonic seizures, which are usually self-limiting and short lived, may occur during the first week of withdrawal and typically 12 to 48 hours after the last drink. With uncomplicated alcohol withdrawal, temperature does not usually rise to greater than 38.1° C (100.5° F). Major withdrawal can be dangerous because it may herald the development of DTs, may aggravate a serious co-morbid condition such as coronary artery disease and cerebrovascular disease, or may provoke status epilepticus.

DTs are a severe withdrawal syndrome characterized by deterioration of mental status and instability of the autonomic nervous system. DTs usually develop within 24 to 72 hours of the last drink. The development of disorientation, confusion, frank hallucinations, and elevated temperature in the setting of alcohol withdrawal should be considered an urgent situation. The mortality rate for DTs has been declining in recent years with better recognition and more aggressive treatment.

CLINICAL PRESENTATION

The earliest manifestations of alcoholism are psychosocial, including behavioral and emotional instability; family and marital dysfunction; and difficulties with work, school, and the law. Alcoholism affects those around the patient. The first indicator of a problem is often a secondary report from the patient's spouse, child, or employer. A history of arrests for driving while intoxicated, disorderly behavior, or assault is highly suggestive of alcoholism. Patients with alcoholism or other substance use disorders are likely to benefit from early intervention, which makes screening appropriate in the primary care setting.

As a screening tool, the *CAGE* questionnaire—which focuses on Concern about drinking, being Annoyed by criticism about drinking, having Guilt about drinking, and taking an "Eye-opener" drink in the morning—can be woven into standard history taking (Box 258-1).[8] These questions should be asked if the patient reports drinking or drug use when asked about medications or lifestyle. The CAGE questions were derived from the 24-question Michigan Alcoholism Screening Test. Two or more positive answers suggest an alcohol use disorder, but like any structured questionnaire this should be interpreted contextually. A patient who answers "yes" to one question but is grossly tremulous is more likely to have a problem than a patient who scores a 4 but drinks only twice a year. Answers of "yes" to any question should be pursued by follow-up questions. Asking the two questions "Have you, in the past year, drunk or used more drugs than you meant to?" and "Have you felt that you wanted or needed to cut down on your drinking or drug use in the past year?" may be as effective as CAGE with the advantage of screening for both alcohol and drug concerns.[9]

BOX 258-1

CAGE QUESTIONNAIRE

Have you ever felt you ought to . . .	**C**ut down on your drinking?
Have people . . .	**A**nnoyed you by criticizing your drinking?
Have you ever felt bad or . . .	**G**uilty about your drinking?
Have you ever had an . . .	**E**ye-opener drink first thing in the morning?

From Ewing J: Detecting alcoholism: the CAGE questionnaire, *JAMA* 252:1905-1907, 1984.

Health problems that suggest the presence of alcoholism include emotional difficulties, poor nutrition, trauma, seizures, unexplained tachycardia, refractory hypertension, dyspepsia, liver disease, pancreatitis, and peripheral neuropathy (see the Complications section).

PHYSICAL EXAMINATION

There often are no abnormal physical findings unless the patient is intoxicated, is in withdrawal, or indulges in chronic heavy alcohol use. The patient's general mental status and vital signs should be noted. Postural blood pressure and pulse changes may indicate gastrointestinal bleeding. The smell of alcohol strongly suggests alcohol dependence, since even the heaviest drinkers will not drink before a primary care appointment. The head should be observed for signs of recent or old trauma, facial flushing, and rhinophyma. Facial puffiness in the morning often follows a drinking binge. Unusual bruises, abrasions, and burns should raise the suspicion of an alcohol problem. Older drinkers, especially older patients who have recently been prescribed medications that interact with alcohol, are prone to falls. Ataxia characterized by a wide or stepping gait may result from secondary cerebellar deterioration. Early peripheral neuropathy is suggested by diminished lower extremity touch or temperature sensations.

DIAGNOSTICS

Several laboratory values are altered by excessive alcohol use. No laboratory test demonstrates better screening properties than the *CAGE* questionnaire. Mean corpuscular volume is elevated from impaired folate utilization and probably from direct bone marrow toxicity. It may not return to normal for months, even with folate substitution. Affected liver enzymes include γ-glutamyltransferase (GGT), aspartate aminotransferase (AST), alanine aminotransferase (ALT), and alkaline phosphatase. All liver enzyme levels are nonspecific when interpreted in isolation. The GGT returns to normal after approximately 3 weeks of abstinence and is useful for tracking abstinence. In contrast to chronic viral hepatitis, alcohol causes the AST level to rise in excess of the ALT level. Carbohydrate-deficient transferrin levels are elevated in male patients who have been drinking heavily for 1 week or longer and may be a useful indicator of the severity of drinking.[10]

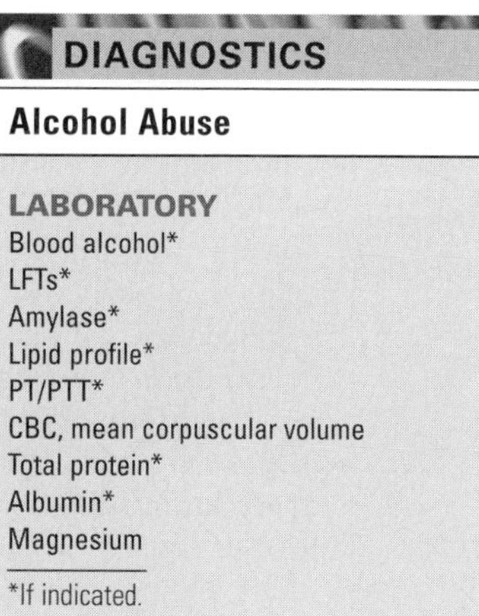
DIAGNOSTICS

Alcohol Abuse

LABORATORY
- Blood alcohol*
- LFTs*
- Amylase*
- Lipid profile*
- PT/PTT*
- CBC, mean corpuscular volume
- Total protein*
- Albumin*
- Magnesium

*If indicated.

DIFFERENTIAL DIAGNOSIS

Because alcoholism affects every body system, the physical symptoms and findings may indicate numerous pathologic conditions. Hypertension, hyperlipidemia, cardiac arrhythmias, cardiac myopathy, liver disease, peptic ulcer disease, pancreatitis, or injury may be the first physical indication of this disorder.

Psychologic disorders that may be associated with alcoholism include anxiety, depression, and social isolation and dysfunction. Other forms of substance abuse should also be considered in the differential diagnosis. Alcohol and nicotine are the earliest and most enduring substances of abuse that persons with major mental illness use for self-medication.

MANAGEMENT

When alcoholism is suspected, a follow-up appointment should be scheduled to further explore the issue. This discussion is usually better accepted when addressed in the context of the patient's overall health and quality of life. Patients may be susceptible to using other substances, and this should be kept in mind. The provider's concerns about drinking and the evidence that supports these concerns should be shared and reinforced. It is helpful if a spouse or significant other is willing to accompany the patient to the appointment, although patients often reject this suggestion in the beginning. A brief intervention by a health care provider and advice to cut down on drinking may ultimately be the most effective interventions for reducing drinking problems. The approach should be empathetic, nonaccusatory, and concerned. In brief, health care providers should (1) provide feedback on their impression of the problem (including historical and physical evidence about alcoholism and its severity), (2) inform the patient about safe consumption limits while offering recommendations about changing and sources of help, (3) assess the patient's readiness to change and to negotiate goals and strategies, and (4) arrange a follow-up visit.[11] Brief interventions for heavy-drinking college students have been associated with reduction in drinking and adverse consequences, although it is not clear how much improvement is due to the intervention and how much to the students' normal maturation.[12]

In a formal intervention the important people in a patient's life (e.g., spouse, work supervisor, and health care provider) meet together to confront the patient, express concern, and help the patient recognize the need for treatment. This type of intervention should be conducted with an experienced consultant; it should be rehearsed, with the logistics of referral worked out in advance.

Alcoholics Anonymous (AA) is the prototype community self-help group and for decades has provided millions of people with a foundation for alcoholism recovery. The focus and tone of individual meetings can differ, and patients may need to attend several before finding a meeting in which they feel comfortable. In brief, the 12 steps of recovery (12-step program) in AA ask that participants begin to acknowledge that they have a problem, that there is a spiritual dimension to life beyond their control, that personal relationships should be healed, and that recovering persons should use experiences and insight to help other alcoholics. These principles are the same at all AA meetings, and the only requirement for attendance is a desire to stop using alcohol or mind-altering drugs. The advantage of the recommendation to attend "90 meetings in 90 days" is that it helps patients get into a routine of AA attendance, begin to understand that their problems are shared by others, and begin to establish a relationship with a member who has achieved successful sobriety. Some patients engage better with cognitive behavior–oriented groups such as Rational Recovery; others benefit from church attendance. In-depth, insight-oriented psychotherapeutic approaches have not been shown to be helpful in assisting with early recovery, but they may be helpful for patients who have established long-term sobriety.

DIFFERENTIAL DIAGNOSIS

Alcohol Abuse

- Hypertension
- Cardiac arrhythmias
- Liver disease
- Pancreatitis
- Endocrine disorder
- Anxiety
- Substance abuse

Family members often experience more distress than the patient. Most counseling centers have services for family members, including Al-Anon meetings. Al-Anon and its affiliate, Alateen, provide group support for family members. The major goals for family members of alcoholics are to understand that they are not to blame for the patient's alcoholism, to recognize the role that the patient's alcoholism plays in family functioning, and to limit enabling behaviors.

Pharmacologic adjuncts include medications to prevent major withdrawal, drugs to reduce craving, antidepressants (usually selective serotonin reuptake inhibitors) for persistent dysthymia or co-existing depression, and disulfiram (Antabuse) as aversive therapy. Patients should also receive thiamine, multivitamin, and folic acid supplementation. Selective serotonin reuptake inhibitors may be helpful for mood stability and reduced alcohol consumption, particularly if there is co-existing depression.[13]

Benzodiazepines have consistently been shown to be the safest and most effective drugs to assist with alcohol detoxification. Outpatient detoxification is labor intensive and requires the patient to have good involved social support and the provider to have ready inpatient backup. If outpatient detoxification is preferred, one sample general guideline for detoxification begins with 50 to 100 mg of chlordiazepoxide and then 25 to 50 mg q 4-6 hr p.r.n. The patient returns the next day and then receives 25 mg once or twice a day p.r.n.[14] The patient should be referred for inpatient detoxification if he or she resumes drinking or has worsening withdrawal symptoms while following this regimen. Higher doses are generally used when patients are admitted for inpatient detoxification. Inpatient detoxification consists of usually brief (approximately 1 week) admission to a facility, during which the patient is monitored and given medication to prevent major withdrawal symptoms. Initially, sufficient medication is given to produce mild sedation, and this is tapered over several days. Patients attend AA meetings and group and individual counseling while plans for aftercare are developed.

Acamprosate is a novel anticraving medication that has recently been approved in the United States after several years of widespread use in Europe. It appears to reduce the activity of hyperactive glutaminergic neurons and to stimulate GABA transmission.[13] Acamprosate is given three times per day, and complete abstinence is not a prerequisite for treatment. Dosage needs to be adjusted in patients with renal impairment. Patients treated with acamprosate have shown a greater rate of treatment completion, abstinence, and reduced drinking days with minimum side effects compared to those receiving a placebo. However, trials that did not provide social support or did not require abstinence before starting the drug did not find any statistical benefit of acamprosate over placebo.[15-17]

Naltrexone is an opioid antagonist that may reduce the desire to drink and support abstinence at a dosage of 50 mg/day.[16] Because it is mildly hepatotoxic, liver function test results should be evaluated before treatment and at 1, 3, and 6 months. A recent study questions the effectiveness of naltrexone. No difference was found between those patients receiving counseling and naltrexone and those receiving counseling and placebo interventions.[18]

Some practitioners begin aversive treatment with disulfiram after the first couple of days of verifiable abstinence. Disulfiram interferes with the metabolism of acetaldehyde, causing headache, flushing, nausea, vomiting, and, sometimes, chest pain. It is used as an adjunct to counseling and may help patients resist temptation in the early stages of recovery.[14] It is generally contraindicated in patients who are not currently engaged in counseling and in patients who have neurologic impairment, cardiovascular disease, and a history of past drinking while taking disulfiram. Patients need to be warned explicitly about the nature of the reaction and warned to avoid any alcohol-containing products. Patients should know to come to the emergency department if a reaction occurs.

COMPLICATIONS

The earliest physical complications are usually related to trauma or poisoning. Drinking is a factor in almost half of all motor vehicle fatalities, half of all violent deaths, and approximately one third of all suicides. Alcohol-related motor vehicle deaths have steadily declined during the past decade from 8.9 to 5.8 per 100,000.[5] Approximately 25% of teens involved in fatal alcohol crashes had been drinking alcohol.[19] Trauma accompanies alcoholism so often that a history of two or more major injuries after 18 years of age is strongly suggestive of alcoholism. Also, alcoholism greatly increases the risk of becoming homeless. Overall quality of life is perceived as very poor by alcoholics and appears to improve with reduction in drinking or abstinence.[20] Older alcohol abusers are more likely to develop long-term impairments in ability to work and in their ability to function independently at home.[21]

Nutritional and Metabolic

Drinking causes nutritional deficiencies in two primary ways. As a source of energy, alcohol may be consumed in preference to food, leading to deficiencies of macronutrients. Alcohol hinders the absorption of any vitamin that is absorbed in the small intestine, most notably thiamine (B_1), folic acid, pyridoxine (B_6), niacin, and vitamin A. Pancreatitis, chronic gastritis, and liver disease are common co-morbid conditions that impair the absorption and use of nutrients. Alcohol ketosis results from starvation after a period of heavy drinking that has caused vomiting and an inability to hold down food or fluids. This condition resolves with the administration of IV glucose solutions, but thiamine must be administered first to prevent toxic cerebral accumulation of glucose. Chronic alcohol ingestion suppresses the production and function of the white blood cells, which results in increased susceptibility to tuberculosis, pneumonia, and skin infections.[22] Hyperuricemia, blood sugar dysregulation, and hypogonadism are caused by excess NADH.

Neurologic

Alcohol and its metabolite acetaldehyde are direct neurotoxins whose effects are compounded by associated nutritional deficiencies. The entire picture of the effects of alcohol on the brain is not clear. Although brain atrophy appears to be more common among older drinkers than among abstainers, the reverse is true for white matter defects.[23] "Moderate" alcohol consumption has even been linked with a lower risk of both Alzheimer's disease and vascular dementia.[24]

Familiar syndromes that are clearly related to excessive alcohol use include Wernicke's encephalopathy, Korsakoff's psychosis, hepatic encephalopathy, convulsive disorders, and neuropathy.[25] Wernicke-Korsakoff syndrome is the frequent co-existence of Wernicke's encephalopathy and Korsakoff's psychosis. Wernicke's encephalopathy is an acute neurologic syndrome that is characterized by confusion, ocular palsies (nystagmus, paralysis of the external ocular muscles), and ataxia. The primary cause is thiamine deficiency, and the acute syndrome can be treated with IV thiamine. Treatment must be initiated quickly, because the damage can become irreversible. Korsakoff's psychosis is an amnestic syndrome that often appears after episodes of Wernicke's encephalopathy or DTs. It is characterized by impaired memory, with the preservation of most other neurologic functions. Impairments in recent memory and the ability to encode new information are the most evident deficits. Confabulation is common but not universal. Wernicke-Korsakoff syndrome can improve over time with alcohol abstinence, vitamin supplementation, and compensatory cognitive strategies. A more generalized dementia from the direct toxic effects of alcohol and its metabolites generally improves after 3 weeks of abstinence.

Hepatic encephalopathy is the deterioration of mental status in patients with cirrhosis and may result from portal-systemic shunting of venous blood and a subsequent failure to detoxify several toxins, most notably ammonia and GABA. Precipitants include drinking binges, central nervous system depressants, and physiologic stressors such as gastrointestinal bleeding and infections. It begins with inattention, reversal of the sleep-wake cycle, and asterixis, and it may progress to delirium and coma. Treatment is abstinence and administration of a cathartic disaccharide.

The most common alcohol-related cause of generalized seizures is alcohol withdrawal. Individuals with alcoholism are also prone to other seizure foci as a result of head trauma and metabolic derangements. Peripheral neuropathy is characterized by limb paresthesias, diminished sensation, and sometimes shooting neuropathic pains. This may progress to permanent motor weakness and chronic pain. Manifestations of peripheral neuropathy are often complicated by co-existing alcoholic cerebellar degeneration.[25]

Cardiovascular

Alcoholism has several cardiovascular consequences, possibly the most serious of which is dilated cardiomyopathy. Acetaldehyde is directly toxic to the myocardium. This is often aggravated by a co-existing thiamine deficiency (beriberi). Orthopnea is usually the first symptom, and an enlarged heart is noted on chest films. The "holiday heart" syndrome, in which the patient experiences runs of tachyarrhythmias, including atrial fibrillation, is probably an antecedent of cardiomyopathy.[7] Excessive alcohol use causes 5% to 20% of hypertension in the United States, which usually improves with abstinence. Drinking three or more standard drinks per day doubles the risk of hypertension that is resistant to therapy.[26] Binge drinking appears to cause wider swings in blood pressure than steady alcohol consumption, and this is thought to contribute to increased susceptibility to "Monday morning heart attacks."[27] On the other hand, numerous studies repeatedly demonstrate the cardioprotective effects of low to moderate alcohol use, possibly because of beneficial effects on lipid profiles and reduced platelet aggregation.[26,28]

Gastrointestinal

Alcoholism contributes to four major esophageal disorders. Alcohol decreases lower esophageal pressure, contributing to reflux esophagitis; frequent vomiting can result in mucosal tears of the lower esophagus (Mallory-Weiss syndrome); portal hypertension causes esophageal varices; and, when used with nicotine, alcohol increases the incidence of esophageal adenocarcinoma.[29] Erosive gastritis is probably a result of the direct toxic effects of alcohol on the mucosa and increased susceptibility to *Helicobacter pylori* infections. Alcoholism is the major cause of chronic pancreatitis, which can result in a chronic pain syndrome and pancreatic insufficiency with diabetes often unresponsive to oral agents. Acute exacerbations of pancreatitis can be life threatening from necrosis and acute respiratory distress syndrome. Heavy prolonged alcohol use is associated with the progression of colon adenomas to high-risk adenomas or colorectal cancer.[30]

Alcoholic liver disease has three major pathologic forms—fatty liver, alcoholic hepatitis, and cirrhosis—all of which may exist simultaneously. Excess NADH contributes to the deposition of hepatic fat and an enlarged liver that usually improves with abstinence. Alcoholic hepatitis results from an acute inflammatory response to alcohol and its metabolites. Patients may be seen with right upper quadrant pain, icterus, and AST increased in comparison to ALT. Cirrhosis and fibrotic derangement of liver acini may be subclinical and insidious or may first be noted with the onset of an acute complication, such as ruptured esophageal varices. Coagulopathies develop as a consequence of impaired clotting factor synthesis. Edema develops as a consequence of depressed albumin synthesis.

Fetal Alcohol Syndrome

Pregnancy is perhaps the most important contraindication to alcohol use; a safe level of drinking during pregnancy has not been defined. The major manifestations of fetal alcohol syndrome (FAS) are intellectual impairment and developmental delays, growth retardation, and characteristically abnormal facial features (short palpebral fissures, flattening of the midface, and a thin upper lip). More subtle behavioral and learning difficulties are termed *fetal alcohol effect*, but these cannot be diagnosed before the child reaches school age.

INDICATIONS FOR REFERRAL OR HOSPITALIZATION

Inpatient treatment should be considered for patients who have a history of severe withdrawal, who are drinking all day long, who are medically ill, or who are abusing other substances. Patients with repeated seizures, severe intoxication, or mental status changes that are not obviously attributable to intoxication, recent head trauma, fevers, postural hypotension or tachycardia, shortness of breath, chest pain, severe abdominal pain, severe vomiting, or diarrhea often need to be seen in the emergency department for stabilization and consideration for hospitalization. Pregnant women who are alcohol dependent should be referred for inpatient detoxification; this needs to be coordinated with the patient's obstetric team and often involves making arrangements for child care, and it should be done in conjunction with a treatment program that has experience with the treatment of pregnant women. If a patient does not yet have prenatal care, such care should be arranged urgently.

PATIENT AND FAMILY EDUCATION

The health care provider should carefully explain the dangers associated with alcohol and explore treatment options with the patient. The importance of safety considerations for patients and others should be stressed. Encouragement and support are essential to enable the patient to make the necessary lifestyle changes to attain sobriety. Patients will often ask about or allude to the idea of resuming alcohol use in a controlled manner. This may be possible for some patients and life threatening for others. Studies on returning to controlled drinking conflict. It is probably best to advise continued abstinence in patients who have had health or repeated social problems related to their drinking.

The following are resources for patients with alcoholism:

Al-Anon Family Group Headquarters, Inc.
1600 Corporate Landing Pkwy.
Virginia Beach, VA 23454
To locate a meeting: (888) 4AL-ANON (425-2666); corporate headquarters: (757) 563-1600
http://www.al-anon.org

Alcoholics Anonymous
PO Box 459
New York, NY 10163
(212) 870-3400
http://www.alcoholics-anonymous.org

Rational Recovery Systems, Inc.
PO Box 800
Lotus, CA 95651
(530) 621-4374 or (530) 621-2667
Fax: (530) 622-4296
http://www.rational.org

REFERENCES

1. Substance Abuse and Mental Health Services Administration: *National household survey on drug abuse: population estimates, 1996,* DHHS Pub No (SMA) 97-3137, Washington, DC, 1997, US Department of Health and Human Services.
2. Duncan DF: Chronic binge drinking and drunk driving, *Psychol Rep* 80:681-682, 1997.
3. Substance Abuse and Mental Health Services Administration Office of Applied Studies: *2002 National household survey on drug abuse and health: national findings,* DHHS Pub No (SMA) 03-3836, NSDUH Series H-22, Rockville, Md, 2005, US Department of Health and Human Services.
4. Johnston LD, O'Malley PM, Bachman JG, and others: *The monitoring the future survey results on drug use: 1975-2004,* NIH Pub No 02-5728, Bethesda, Md, 2005, National Institute of Drug Abuse.
5. Tsai G, Gastfriend DR, Coyle JT: The glutamatergic basis of human alcoholism, *Am J Psychiatry* 152:332-340, 1995.
6. Heinz A, Mann K, Weinberger DR, and others: Serotonergic dysfunction, negative mood states, and response to alcohol, *Alcohol Clin Exp Res* 25:487-495, 2001.
7. Lieber CS: Medical disorders of alcoholism, *N Engl J Med* 333:1058-1065, 1995.
8. Ewing J: Detecting alcoholism: the CAGE questionnaire, *JAMA* 252:1905-1907, 1984.
9. Brown RL, Leonard T, Saunders LA, and others: A two-item conjoint screen for alcohol and other drug problems, *J Am Board Fam Pract* 14(2):95-106, 2001.
10. Gronhoek M, Henriksen JH, Becker U: Carbohydrate-deficient transferrin: a valid marker of alcoholism in population studies: results from the Copenhagen City Heart Study, *Alcohol Clin Exp Res* 19:457-461, 1995.
11. Samet JH, Rollnick S, Barnes H: Beyond CAGE: a brief clinical approach after detection of substance abuse, *Arch Intern Med* 156:2287-2293, 1996.
12. Baer JS, Kivlahan DR, Blume AW, and others: Brief intervention for heavy-drinking college students: 4 year follow-up and natural history, *Am J Pub Health* 91:1310-1316, 2001.
13. Gastfriend DR, Elman I, Solhkha R: Pharmacotherapy of substance abuse and dependence, *Psychiatr Clin North Am* 5:211-229, 1998.
14. Clark WD: Alcohol problems. In Noble J, Greene HL 2nd, Levinson W, and others, editors: *Textbook of primary care medicine,* ed 2, St Louis, 1996, Mosby.
15. Mason BJ: Treatment of alcohol-dependent outpatients with acamprosate: a clinical review, *J Clin Psychiatr* 62(Suppl 20):42-48, 2001.
16. Volpicelli JR, Alterman AI, Havashida M, and others: Naltrexone in the treatment of alcohol dependence, *Arch Gen Psychiatr* 49(11):876-880, 1992.
17. Acamprosate campral for alcoholism, *Med Lett Drugs Ther* 47(1119):1-3, 2005.
18. Krystal JH, Cramer JA, Krol WF, and others: Naltrexone in the treatment of alcohol dependence, *N Engl J Med* 345(24):1734-1739, 2001.
19. National Highway Traffic Safety Administration, National Center for Statistics and Analysis: *Alcohol involvement in fatal motor vehicle traffic crashes, 2003* (DOT HS 809 822), Springfield, Va, March 2005, US Department of Transportation, retrieved March 14, 2007, from http://www-nrd.nhtsa.dot.gov/Pubs/809822.PDF.
20. Foster JH, Powell JE, Marshall EJ, and others: Quality of life in alcohol-dependent subjects—a review, *Qual Life Res* 8(3):255-261, 1999.
21. Osterman J, Sloan FA: Effects of alcohol consumption on disability among the near elderly: a longitudinal analysis, *Milbank Q* 79:487-515, iii, 2001.
22. Schuckit MA: Alcohol and alcoholism. In Wilson JD, Braunwald E, Isselbacher KJ, and others, editors: *Harrison's principles of internal medicine,* ed 12, New York, 1991, McGraw-Hill.
23. Mukamal KK, Longstreth WT Jr, Mittleman MA, and others: Alcohol consumption and subclinical findings on magnetic resonance imaging of the brain in older adults: the cardiovascular health study, *Stroke* 32:1939-1946, 2001.
24. Ruitenberg A, van Swieten JC, Witteman JC, and others: Alcohol consumption and risk of dementia: the Rotterdam Study, *Lancet* 359(9303):281-286, 2002.
25. Levesque CA, Sabin TD: Dementing illnesses. In Noble J, Greene HL 2nd, Levinson W, and others, editors: *Textbook of primary care medicine,* ed 2, St Louis, 1996, Mosby.
26. Cushman WC: Alcohol consumption and hypertension, *J Clin Hypertens* 3:166-172, 2001.
27. Marques-Vidal P, Arveiler D, Evans A, and others: Different alcohol drinking and blood pressure relationships in France and Northern Ireland: the PRIME study, *Hypertension* 38(6):1361-1366, 2001.
28. Smart R, Ogborne A: Beliefs about the cardiovascular benefits of drinking wine in the adult population of Ontario, *Am J Drug Alcohol Abuse* 28(2):371-378, 2002.
29. Burakoff R: Esophagus. In Noble J, Greene HL 2nd, Levinson W, and others, editors: *Textbook of primary care medicine,* ed 2, St Louis, 1996, Mosby.
30. Bardou M, Montembault S, Giraud V, and others: Excessive alcohol consumption favours high risk polyp or colorectal cancer occurrence among patients with adenomas: a case control study, *Gut* 50(1):38-42, 2002.

CHAPTER 259

Anxiety Disorders

Willadene "Billie" Walker Schmucker

DEFINITION AND EPIDEMIOLOGY

Anxiety is normally a helpful emotion that rouses the individual to action and alerts the individual to danger. Everyone has anxiety; it is common to feel anxiety before a first date, when beginning a new job, or before an examination. In general, anxiety is a state of tension that occurs in the body as a warning to keep the body safe and out of danger. An anxiety disorder, on the other hand, often disrupts daily life. Individuals with anxiety disorders feel anxious most of the time and without apparent reason. The anxious feelings can be so uncomfortable that an individual may stop everyday activities to avoid the discomfort or may have immobilizing bouts of anxiety. Because anxiety is an emotion common to everyone, there is also considerable misunderstanding about anxiety disorders. A common misconception is that individuals should be able to overcome their symptoms through sheer willpower.

Anxiety is commonly defined as an unpleasant and overriding mental tension that has no apparent identifiable cause and is accompanied by physical distress and disruption in activities of daily living. Uhde and Nemiah provide a more formal definition of anxiety: a pathologic state characterized by a feeling of dread and accompanied by somatic signs indicative of a hyperactive autonomic nervous system, differentiated from fear, which has a known cause.[1] Anxiety is considered a disorder when it becomes a problem in daily life. There are several anxiety disorders: generalized anxiety disorder (GAD), simple phobias, panic disorder (sometimes accompanied by agoraphobia), posttraumatic stress disorder (PTSD), obsessive-compulsive disorder (OCD), social phobias (general social phobia and performance anxiety), and atypical anxiety.[2]

Anxiety disorders are the most common mental disorders in the United States and throughout the world. In any given year, 19% of the U.S. population suffers from one or another of the six anxiety disorders identified by the fourth edition of the *Diagnostic and Statistical Manual of Mental Disorders* (DSM-IV).[3-6] GAD is common in Western society, and surveys suggest that as many as 4% of the U.S. population suffers from GAD, whereas 3% of Britain's population suffers from this disorder.[7] Other common anxiety disorders in the United States include specific phobias (9.0%), social phobias (8.0%), panic disorder (2.3%), and OCD (2.0%).[6,8] As a group, anxiety disorders afflict nearly 9% of Americans during any 6-month period.[9] In addition, with undiagnosed anxiety disorders, an undetermined amount of the health care dollars is spent on additional medical testing to exclude a medical condition.

Symptoms of anxiety disorders can be so severe that sufferers are almost totally disabled—too terrified to leave their homes, to enter the elevator that takes them to their offices, or to shop for food. National Institute of Mental Health (NIMH) research shows that anxiety disorders (1) have an age of onset from late childhood to adulthood; (2) affect a higher ratio of females to males as a group across several of the individual disorders; and (3) have a family link to prevalence, with an 80% to 90% concordance in monozygotic twins for GAD.[2] Many people have a single anxiety disorder, but it is not unusual for an anxiety disorder to be accompanied by another illness, such as depression, an eating disorder, alcoholism, drug abuse, or another anxiety disorder. In these cases the other illnesses also need to be treated.[10] According to NIMH sources, anxiety disorders are real, identifiable brain diseases, and gradually an understanding is developing regarding the specific circuits in the brain that are malfunctioning in PTSD, OCD, and perhaps panic disorder. It is also possible that anxiety disorders arise from a combination of genetic vulnerability with an environmental "second hit."

Anxiety disorders carry with them a profound burden of disability for patients in primary care settings. A significant amount of the disability and work loss associated with physical illness may in fact be attributable primarily to co-morbid mental disorders. The majority of individuals with anxiety and depression receive most or all of their mental health care from primary care physicians.[11] Anxiety has been shown to be as serious as depression in terms of their association with functional impairment and work loss.[12] Effective anxiety interventions will likely result in large gains in health functioning and decreased health care costs.[13]

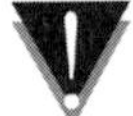

Immediate psychiatric evaluation is required for all patients with suicidal or homicidal ideation.

PATHOPHYSIOLOGY

Since the 1990s, which was designated by Congress as the Decade of the Brain, the NIMH has supported sizable and multifaceted research programs on anxiety disorders and their causes, diagnosis, treatment, and prevention. This research involves studies of anxiety disorders in human subjects and investigations of the biologic basis for anxiety and related phenomena in animals. A large database of information regarding the pathophysiology of anxiety disorders has been derived from these investigations. For example, in positron emission tomography (PET) studies of OCD, a decreased metabolism has been demonstrated in the orbital gyrus, caudate nuclei, and cingulate gyrus; with panic, an increased PET blood flow has been demonstrated in the right parahippocampus; in anxiety, this increase in blood flow is demonstrated in the frontal lobe.[11] Using classification criteria from the DSM-IV, studies have shown that mitral valve prolapse is present in 50% of the subjects identified with panic disorder.[1]

Probably no single situation or condition causes anxiety disorders. Instead, physical and environmental triggers may combine to create a particular anxiety illness. More recent studies have indicated that biochemical imbalances may be the source. Scientists speculate that all thoughts and feelings result from complex electrochemical interactions in the central nervous system. Moreover, some studies indicate that infusions of certain biochemicals can cause a panic attack in some individuals. According to this theory, the treatment of anxiety should correct these biochemical imbalances.[9]

Other theories from the psychologic field of study have been used to define the cause of anxiety disorders. Psychoanalytic theory attributes anxiety to unconscious impulses that threaten to burst into consciousness and produce anxiety. According to this theory, defense mechanisms are used to ward off anxiety. Learning theory attributes the cause of anxiety to frustration or stress. Norepinephrine, serotonin, and dopamine regulate mood, movement, and blood pressure, and they stimulate and initiate postsynaptic impulse conduction. Debate exists as to the exact imbalance that leads to an anxiety disorder. Excess levels of serotonin or norepinephrine characterize anxiety, but there is disagreement regarding whether the problem reflects excess production, blockage, or impaired uptake of these neurotransmitters. Another explanation of anxiety disorders relates to the hypothesis that some individuals have an overly sensitive response system.

The treatment of chemical imbalances underlies the treatment of all anxiety disorders. Because the biologic function of "anxiety" is a useful and protective natural function of the body, the elimination of anxiety is not possible or desired. However, *control* of the noxious symptoms of an anxiety disorder is desired and necessary to prevent the long-term adverse effects on the body of the almost constant hyperproduction of certain neurochemicals. It is hypothesized that noradrenergic, γ-aminobutyric acid (GABA)–ergic, and serotonergic neuronal systems in the frontal lobe and limbic system are the areas from which the pathophysiology of anxiety disorders arises.[1]

CLINICAL PRESENTATION

One of the most striking aspects of anxiety disorders is the similar statements that patients voice during the initial interview (Box 259-1). It is essential that the health care provider pay close attention to the words patients use to describe their feelings. Key words to note include *tense, uptight, on edge, hassled, nervous, dread, jumpy, jittery, edgy, vulnerable, worried,* and *anxious.* Individuals with panic disorder often believe they are going to die during a panic attack and often convince others of this fact; they are in such distress that, to all outward evaluation, it seems they are indeed going to die. A rapidly worsening medical condition, substance-induced anxiety, and a psychologic response to stressors associated with a medical condition should be excluded. Anxiety disorder should be considered a potential diagnosis in the presentation of physical symptoms such as shortness of breath, nervousness, gastrointestinal upset, palpitations, fatigue, muscle aches, tension, and sleep disorders.[14] It is easy to overlook biologic inheritance, but genes influence health and behavior from birth to death. In an initial interview, investigation of family members with similar symptoms is an important consideration.

BOX 259-1

COMMON STATEMENTS VOICED DURING INITIAL INTERVIEW

- I have butterflies in my stomach.
- There is a lump in my throat.
- I think I'm going crazy.
- I don't go out anymore.
- I know something bad is going to happen.
- I feel a black cloud over my head.
- My mind just goes blank.
- I know this isn't rational, but I can't seem to shake this feeling of doom.
- I have been feeling "on edge" a lot lately.
- I know something awful is wrong with me.
- I can feel my heart beating in my chest.
- I can't breathe.
- I'm going to die.
- I'm so easily fatigued/irritable/restless.
- I have had a lot of worries lately.
- I have been under a lot of stress.
- I shake all the time.
- My hands sweat.
- I have to go to the bathroom so much.

PHYSICAL EXAMINATION

Anxiety disorders emerge from a malfunction of neurobiologic substances that alert individuals to danger.[12] A complete physical examination is necessary to exclude any underlying physical condition. The physical complaints related to an anxiety disorder include dizziness, lightheadedness, diarrhea, frequent urination and urgency, tachycardia, shortness of breath, tingling in the extremities, tremors, hyperreflexes, gastrointestinal distress, palpitations, hypertension, syncope, muscle tightness, sweating, nausea, and vomiting. However, individuals may not "fit" the expected profile for the symptoms observed. Young, healthy appearing individuals are seen with shortness of breath, heart palpitations, a fear of dying, and other symptoms. Older patients also experience anxiety symptoms, but because they "fit" the expected profile for many disease processes, the diagnosis of anxiety is often overlooked.

DIAGNOSTICS

Diagnostic tests should be guided by the history and physical examination. ECG and baseline laboratory studies are also indicated. In addition, many tests are available as an initial screen for anxiety disorders. Standardized instruments include the Zung Anxiety Self-Assessment Scale and the Hamilton Anxiety and Depression Scales. Although these tests are easily administered and scored, they do not replace a formal evaluation but rather serve as a database. It is essential to remember that individuals may be physically ill and have an anxiety disorder. Individuals under stress from medical conditions may also experience nonpathologic anxiety.

According to Valente, diagnosing untreated anxiety disorders may be challenging. Patients complain of diverse somatic symptoms during brief primary care visits.[14] The DSM-IV diagnostic criteria have shortcomings; mild symptoms may be overlooked because symptoms of physical illness and anxiety overlap (Box 259-2). Serious

DIAGNOSTICS

Anxiety Disorders

LABORATORY

TSH*
CBC and differential*
Serum electrolytes*
BUN*
Creatinine*
Serum glucose*

*If indicated.

BOX 259-2

DIAGNOSTIC CRITERIA FOR GENERALIZED ANXIETY DISORDER

A. Excessive anxiety and worry (apprehensive expectation) occurring more days than not for at least 6 months about a number of events or activities (such as work or school performance).
B. The person finds it difficult to control the worry.
C. The anxiety and worry are associated with three (or more) of the following six symptoms (with at least some symptoms present for more days than not for the past 6 months). NOTE: Only one item is required in children.
   (1) Restlessness or feeling keyed up or on edge
   (2) Being easily fatigued
   (3) Difficulty concentrating or mind going blank
   (4) Irritability
   (5) Muscle tension
   (6) Sleep disturbance (difficulty falling or staying asleep, or restless, unsatisfying sleep)
D. The focus of anxiety and worry is not confined to features of an Axis I disorder, e.g., the anxiety or worry is not about having a Panic Attack (as in Panic Disorder), being embarrassed in public (as in Social Phobia), being contaminated (as in Obsessive-Compulsive Disorder), being away from home or close relatives (as in Separation Anxiety Disorder), gaining weight (as in Anorexia Nervosa), having multiple physical complaints (as in Somatization Disorder), or having a serious illness (as in Hypochondriasis), and the anxiety and worry do not occur exclusively during Posttraumatic Stress Disorder.
E. The anxiety, worry, or physical symptoms cause clinically significant distress or impairment in social, occupational, or other important areas of functioning.
F. The disturbance is not due to the direct physiologic effects of a substance (e.g., a drug of abuse, a medication) or a general medical condition (e.g., hyperthyroidism) and does not occur exclusively during a Mood Disorder, a Psychotic Disorder, or a Pervasive Developmental Disorder.

From American Psychiatric Association: *Diagnostic and statistical manual of mental disorders,* ed 4 (text rev), Washington DC, 2000, The Association.

sequelae of anxiety disorders include suicide risk, alcohol or chemical dependency, sexual dysfunction, and vulnerability to physical illness.[14] Screening for anxiety disorders is necessary because a large and growing percentage of anxious individuals are now treated in primary care settings.

DIFFERENTIAL DIAGNOSIS

Hyperthyroidism, hypoglycemia, hyperglycemia, pheochromocytoma, cardiac conditions, vestibular dysfunctions, hyperparathyroidism, temporal lobe epilepsy, and other organic conditions should be considered in the differential diagnosis. Alcohol and drug dependencies, factitious disorders, malingering, adjustment reactions, borderline personality disorders, dementia, delirium, psychoses, schizophrenia, depression, somatization disorders, dysthymia, and other psychiatric illnesses must be considered.

Co-morbid conditions and mixed disorders often occur with the anxiety disorders; there is a complicated two-way interaction between anxiety disorders and co-morbid medical disorders. Although anxiety can mimic or exacerbate various medical conditions, it can also be the result or expression of those same disorders. Approximately 25% of medical patients

DIFFERENTIAL DIAGNOSIS

Anxiety Disorders

MEDICAL DISORDERS
- Cardiac conditions
- Central nervous system disorders
- Hyperglycemia or hypoglycemia
- Hyperparathyroidism
- Hyperthyroidism
- Medications
- Nutritional problems
- Pheochromocytoma
- Respiratory disorders
- Stimulants (e.g., caffeine)
- Temporal lobe epilepsy
- Vestibular dysfunctions

PSYCHIATRIC DISORDERS
- Acute situational anxiety
- Adjustment reaction
- Alcohol and drug dependencies
- Borderline personality disorder
- Delirium
- Dementia
- Depression
- Dysthymia
- Factitious disorder
- Generalized anxiety disorder
- Malingering
- Panic disorder
- Phobias
- Posttraumatic stress disorder
- Psychosis
- Schizophrenia
- Somatization disorder

complaining of anxiety have an underlying physical pathologic condition at the root of their complaint.[15] Anxiety may actually be an early reaction to the onset of major medical problems and may be caused by underlying cardiopulmonary, endocrine, gastrointestinal, neurologic, metabolic, and drug-related causes. Factors that increase the likelihood of underlying illness include an onset of anxiety symptoms after 35 years of age, a lack of a personal or family history of anxiety disorders, the absence of significant stressors or emotional traumas, and a poor response to standard antianxiety medications.[16]

MANAGEMENT

Treatment that has shown to be most effective for the anxiety disorders combines education, brief counseling, self-management techniques, and medications.[14] Education includes an explanation of the biologic etiology of anxiety; a provision of written information; an explanation of available treatments; and an emphasis on the effectiveness of treatments, strategies for coping, and relaxation.[17] Anxiety disorders respond most effectively when there is an understanding of individual symptoms and an ability to identify cues and learn self-management techniques. Progressive relaxation, routine noncompetitive exercise, music, and medication help reduce anxiety.[18] Studies demonstrate a synergistic effect of multiple treatment approaches.[19]

Pharmacotherapy has not shown equal efficacy across all the anxiety disorders.[20] Medications have been most effective in treating panic disorder, while showing generally lesser efficacy in the treatment of GAD and social anxiety disorder (SAD). The effectiveness of medications appears to be marginal to good in PTSD and OCD but relatively ineffective in the treatment of specific phobias and therefore is rarely used for the treatment of those.[20]

Nonetheless, the pharmacologic treatment of anxiety has increased with the advent of more specific drug therapies. Nine classes of drugs may be used to treat anxiety. Barbiturates (which are seldom used because of their potential for toxicity, interaction, and abuse), glycerol derivatives, benzodiazepines, antihistamines, tricyclic antidepressants, selective serotonin reuptake inhibitor (SSRI) antidepressants, antipsychotics, azaperone, and beta blockers are commonly used as treatments for primary anxiety disorders. Benzodiazepines used in the treatment of anxiety disorders are often associated with therapeutic dependence. This therapeutic drug dependence is frequently associated with dependence on alcohol and certain illicit drugs and associated with "addiction," although emergence of withdrawal symptoms on cessation of the drug is the only feature that benzodiazepines have in common with these other drugs. Unlike addiction, therapeutic dependence on benzodiazepines is not associated with tolerance (the need to escalate the dosage to produce the same anxiolytic effect or the initial dosage producing a decreased effect), craving for the medication, and adverse health or social consequences, such as an all-encompassing preoccupation with the drug.[20] In addition, there is no evidence that individuals without a history of substance abuse are more likely to abuse benzodiazepines than other drugs.[20] However, the common perception is still that benzodiazepines are "addictive," and practice generally involves the short-term use of benzodiazepines to reduce symptoms until other medications become effective. If used, benzodiazepines should be tapered slowly after a limited period of use. Medication management alone provides some symptom relief, but the prognosis improves if self-management strategies are included.[15]

SSRIs are helpful with virtually all anxiety disorders, with the initial starting doses and final effective dose varying by disorder. Any of the SSRIs—citalopram (Celexa), paroxetine (Paxil), fluoxetine (Prozac), sertraline (Zoloft), or venlafaxine (Effexor)—can be effective; however, patients must understand there is a 3- to 5-week initial period before the medication becomes fully effective. Benzodiazepines should be used sparingly and for short periods until the SSRIs become effective. This strategy has proven to be particularly helpful in the treatment of panic disorder. However, the advantage of the antidepressant-benzodiazepine combination was not reported in studies looking at the treatment of SAD and therefore it is unclear whether this combination is as helpful in anxiety disorders other than panic disorder.[20] Buspirone (BuSpar) is a good choice as an initial medication for patients without depressive symptoms. The recommended beginning dose of buspirone is 5 to 10 mg b.i.d. Patients with anxiety disorders often "overreact" to medications, so medications should be started slowly. Beginning doses of the SSRIs are 10 mg for citalopram, 5 to 10 mg for paroxetine, 10 mg for fluoxetine, 25 mg for sertraline, and 37.5 mg for venlafaxine. Doses are titrated according to the side effect profile and at 1- to 2-week intervals. Side effects for the SSRIs include gastrointestinal distress, dry mouth, and sexual dysfunction. Abrupt cessation of SSRIs may also lead to withdrawal symptoms, although these tend to be milder in comparison with the benzodiazepine withdrawal syndrome. Therefore the dosage of SSRIs should be tapered carefully before their cessation, but can proceed at a faster rate than benzodiazepine tapering.[20]

Drug-drug interactions need to be assessed before medications are prescribed. OCD can be treated effectively with SSRIs, and several medications, including clomipramine (Anafranil) and fluvoxamine (Luvox), are specific to symptoms of OCD. Tricyclic antidepressants are also sometimes useful, but the side effect profile and the potential for lethal overdose make these medications a less likely choice.

If patients continue to experience symptoms after a fair trial on medication, a referral is recommended; this dual-treatment approach has been shown to be most effective. Recent research also demonstrates the importance of ethnicity in psychopharmacologic management of depression and anxiety disorders, with sometimes profound implications for efficacy and safety. Because different ethnic groups respond differently to therapy, health care providers are advised to use ethnically sensitive approaches to assessment and treatment.[19]

Education regarding the adverse effects that caffeine, alcohol, and over-the-counter and prescribed stimulants have on anxiety is useful. Patients often do not wish to reduce their use of these chemicals, but education about the biologic effects may encourage them to do so.

Coordination of health care services with individuals who have anxiety disorders may prove difficult. Clearly, the "health care provider" shopping performed by patients with anxiety disorders leads to frustration of both the provider and the patient. Often heard are the following phrases: "No one can tell me what is wrong," "I have been everywhere but I can't get any relief," and "I am so worried about my health." The coordination between the primary health care provider and mental health care provider is essential to provide successful treatment.[21]

One difficulty reported in several studies is the accurate diagnosis of anxiety disorders.[22] DSM-IV, the standard for mental health care providers, can be cumbersome and difficult to use by health care providers. To simplify the task for health care providers, the American Psychiatric Association published a primary care version of the DSM-IV in 1995. This version, the *DSM-IV-PC* (primary care), groups psychiatric disorders by their presenting symptoms.[22] It is hoped that the use of this manual will increase the accurate diagnosis and treatment of anxiety disorders and thereby substantially improve outcomes.

LIFE SPAN CONSIDERATIONS

Anxiety disorders occur across the life span and are associated with distressing physical symptoms and a tendency to worry about health issues. These symptoms often bring patients to health care providers, who may be frustrated by seemingly unexplained somatic complaints. Extensive studies document that parental anxiety disorders are a potent risk for child psychiatric disorders and behavioral problems. Although some of this risk is attributable to shared genetic vulnerability, it is likely that parenting by an ill mother also contributes substantially to the development of such disorders. In one study of children whose mothers had anxiety disorders, as many as 80% had emotional disturbances.[23]

GAD and panic disorder are common in depressed older adults and often co-exist with other mental health problems, such as depression. Co-morbid GAD and panic disorder appear to significantly affect the severity of late-life major depressive disorder and response to treatment. Individuals with co-morbid anxiety and depression are seen with more severe somatic symptoms and a higher frequency of suicidal ideation. In addition, recent research suggests that older adults with co-morbid GAD have greater memory decline than those without co-morbid anxiety.[24]

The family members of patients with anxiety disorders may also be affected. Different psychosocial factors are likely to have an impact on anxiety disorders at different stages of life. Anxiety impairs quality of life; when the underlying disorder is treated, quality of life improves. Bereavement and loss, childbearing, the postpartum period, life changes (e.g., retirement), and the loss of health and independence in older adults are all times for the potential emergence of anxiety disorders. Health care providers are likely to see these patients and should be aware of this potential. Older patients have a potential risk for falls and are vulnerable to cognitive impairments, memory impairments, and disorientation from the medications used to treat their anxiety.

COMPLICATIONS

Only one in four patients with an anxiety disorder is correctly diagnosed and treated.[25] Undiagnosed anxiety disorders have a negative impact on many aspects of life; they interfere with and diminish a patient's quality of life. Anxiety disorders increase health concerns and the use of medical services, including urgent care costs and visits. Beyond the direct cost of frequent and often unnecessary visits, undiagnosed anxiety disorders adversely affect social and occupational functioning, causing frequent work absences and the loss of untold hours of productivity. Serious complications of untreated anxiety include alcohol and chemical dependency, suicide risk, sexual dysfunction, and an increased vulnerability to physical illness.[25]

INDICATIONS FOR REFERRAL OR HOSPITALIZATION

Meredith, Sherbourne, Jackson, and colleagues demonstrated that health care providers often do not detect anxiety disorders and that the outcome of detection and referral of patients with anxiety disorders significantly increases a positive health outcome.[26] Referral to a mental health practitioner should be considered when an anxiety disorder is diagnosed and the initial treatment has not been successful. Although health care providers can treat anxiety disorders, studies have shown improved outcomes with specialized mental health care.[27]

Individuals with anxiety disorders are often hospitalized to exclude co-morbid medical conditions. Medical causes must be excluded when an individual is seen in acute distress with complaints of cardiovascular symptoms such as palpitations, sweating, and chest pain. Anxiety disorders often accompany stroke and diseases of the cardiovascular, endocrine, neurologic, metabolic, and respiratory systems. The co-morbid medical condition often indicates a need for hospitalization, but treatment of the anxiety disorder often shortens the hospitalization and increases positive outcomes.[19]

Patients with suicidal ideation require careful psychiatric evaluation and potential hospitalization. A mental health evaluation is recommended when a patient's thought processes are significantly impaired or when psychosis is present (see Chapter 265). Evaluation of dementia, delirium, and psychosis also requires referral to a mental health care provider.

PATIENT AND FAMILY EDUCATION

The educational component of the treatment of anxiety disorders is the core to treatment success and positive outcome; this fact cannot be overemphasized. The patient's ability to develop positive coping strategies depends on the education of both the patient and family members.[23]

A variety of techniques can be used to educate patients with anxiety disorders. Some of these techniques include positive self-talk, imagery, a daily mood log, realistic goals, exercise, relaxation exercises, behavioral therapy, family therapy, insight-oriented psychotherapy, hypnosis, supportive therapy, cognitive therapy, brief psychotherapy, and systematic desensitization.

Because of the nature of the disease process, patients with anxiety disorders are particularly difficult to educate at times. The motor and visceral effects of anxiety also have effects on thinking, perception, and learning. This fact needs to be considered in the education of both patients and their families. Anxiety tends to produce confusion and distort perception, not only of time and space but also of people and the meaning of events. These distortions can interfere with learning by lowering concentration, reducing recall, and impairing the ability to relate one item to another (association).[2] The provision of written information is often necessary to overcome the difficulties these patients experience.

Education should include the fact that anxiety disorders can be treated effectively. To reduce anxiety, patients must learn and practice difficult skills. Consistent and reliable support, coaching, and the belief that "you can do it" from significant others are helpful.[14] Investigating a patient's preferred learning style is an important consideration. Patients gradually learn strategies for coping with anxiety if provided with the support and instructional materials necessary to accomplish their goal. Educational audiotapes, videos, books, how-to manuals, relaxation techniques, breathing exercises, self-talk instruction, nonnegative thinking guidance, and distraction techniques are useful teaching methods. Just informing an individual on "how to fix the problem," "get control," or "set your mind to it" is not effective. Short-term psychotherapy is effective in helping individuals understand anxiety, identify cues, and learn self-management techniques. Research shows that individual and family education is an integral part of the treatment package for anxiety disorders and that treatment outcomes are significantly improved with the use of a combined treatment strategy. Studies have also shown a synergistic effect of proven psychosocial treatments and proven drug treatments.[19]

The following brochures, which provide more detailed information on various anxiety disorders and related topics, are available by from the NIMH (http://www.nimh.nih.gov):

- Understanding Panic Disorder (NIH Pub. No. 93-3482)
- *Obsessive-Compulsive Disorder* (NIH Pub. No. 94-3755)
- *Medications* (DHHS Pub. No. [ADM] 92-1509)

HEALTH PROMOTION

Anxiety is a part of our everyday life; all the generally accepted positive lifestyle behaviors promote the management of anxiety: sufficient rest, a healthy and balanced diet, regular exercise, routine medical check-ups, and maintenance of a routine. A family history of relatives with anxiety disorders increases the individual's risk for the development of an anxiety disorder. Education is the key to early intervention.

Anxiety often refers to the feeling or emotion of fear when the cause of the emotion is sometimes obscure; the events of September 11, 2001, have brought to the forefront identifiable fears. People during this time of terrorism are not unclear about the source of their fear. They know exactly what they are afraid of, and it is not an irrational anxiety. The key to limiting the growth of anxiety disorders resulting from a steady state of heightened fear is education.[28] The way to promote health and deal with rational fears is through the use of reason and logic.

REFERENCES

1. Uhde TW, Nemiah JC: Panic and generalized anxiety disorders. In Kaplan HI, Sadock BJ, editors: *Comprehensive textbook of psychiatry*, ed 7, Baltimore, 2000, Williams & Wilkins.
2. National Anxiety Foundation: *What are anxiety disorders?*, retrieved March 14, 2007, from http://www.lexington-on-line.com/naf.whatare.html.
3. Kessler R, Chiu W, Demler O, and others: Prevalence, severity and comorbidity of 12-month DSM-IV disorders in the National Comorbidity Survey Replication, *Arch Gen Psychiatry* 62:617-627, 2005.
4. Demyttenaere K, Bruffaerts R, Posada-Villa J, and others: Prevalence, severity, and unmet need for treatment of mental disorders in the World Health Organization World Mental Health Surveys, *JAMA* 291:2581-2590, 2004.
5. Comer R: *Abnormal psychology*, New York, 2004, Worth.
6. American Psychiatric Association: *Diagnostic and statistical manual of mental disorders*, ed 4 (text rev), Washington, DC, 2000, The Association.
7. Roemer L, Orsillo S, Barlow D: Generalized anxiety disorder. In Barlow DH, editor: *Anxiety and its disorders: the nature and treatment of anxiety and panic*, ed 2, New York, 2002, Guildford.
8. Ingersoll R, Burns L: Prevalence of adult disorders. In Welfel E, Ingersoll R, editors: *The mental health desk reference*, New York, 2001, Wiley.
9. American Psychiatric Association: *Let's talk facts about anxiety disorders*, retrieved Nov 25, 2005, from http://healthyminds.org/factsheets/LTF-Anxiety.pdf.
10. US Department of Health and Human Services, National Institutes of Health: *Anxiety disorders*, retrieved March 14, 2007, from http://www.nimh.nih.gov/publicat/anxiety.cfm#anx1.
11. Lucey JV, Costa DC, Adshead G, and others: Brain blood flow in anxiety disorders, *Br J Psychiatry* 171:346-350, 1997.
12. Young A, Klpa R, Sherbourne C, and others: The quality of care for depressive and anxiety disorders in the United States, *Arch Gen Psychiatry* 58:55-61, 2001.
13. Stein M, Roy-Byrne P, Craske M, and others: Functional impact and health utility of anxiety disorders in primary care outpatients, *Med Care* 43(12):1164-1170, 2005.
14. Valente S: Diagnosis and treatment of panic disorder and generalized anxiety in primary care, *Nurse Pract* 21:26-38, 1996.
15. Sherbourne CD, Wells KB, Meredith LS, and others: Comorbid anxiety disorder and the functioning and well-being of chronically ill patients of general medical providers, *Arch Gen Psychiatry* 53(10):889-895, 1996.
16. Rosenbaum JF, Pollack MH: Anxiety. In Cassem NH, editor: *Massachusetts General Hospital handbook of general hospital psychiatry*, ed 4, St Louis, 1997, Mosby.
17. Wise MG, Griffies WS: A combined treatment approach to anxiety in the medically ill, *J Clin Psychiatry* 56(Suppl 2):14-19, 1995.
18. Leaman TL: Generalized anxiety disorder: an evolving concept, *Anxiety Profil* 1:4-5, 1993.
19. Barlow DH, Lehman CL: Advances in the psychosocial treatment of anxiety disorders, *Arch Gen Psychiatry* 53:727-735, 1996.
20. Starcevic V: Issues in the pharmacological treatment of anxiety disorders, *Aust Psychiatry* 31(4):371-374, 2005.
21. Eisenberg L: Treating depression and anxiety in primary care: closing the gap between knowledge and practice, *N Engl J Med* 326:1080-1085, 1992.
22. American Psychiatric Association: *Diagnostic and statistical manual of mental disorders*, ed 4 (primary care), Washington, DC, 1995, The Association.
23. Shear MK, Mammen O: Anxiety disorders in primary care: a life-span perspective, *Bull Menninger Clin* 612:A37-A53, 1997.
24. DeLuca A, Lenze E, Mulsant B, and others: Comorbid anxiety disorder in late life depression: association with memory decline over 4 years, *Int J Geriatr Psychiatry* 20:848-854, 2005.
25. Gorman JM, Papp LA: Drug treatment strategies for GAD, *Anxiety Profil* 1:6-8, 1993.
26. Meredith LS, Sherbourne CD, Jackson CA, and others: Treatment typically provided for comorbid anxiety disorders, *Arch Fam Med* 6(3):231-237, 1997.
27. Jonas BS, Franks P, Ingram DD: Are symptoms of anxiety and depression risk factors for hypertension? *Arch Fam Med* 6:244-256, 1997.
28. Cox S: *Terrorism fear and what you can do to alleviate it*, Lexington, Ky, 2006, National Anxiety Foundation, retrieved March 14, 2007, from http://lexington-on-line.com/naf.html.

CHAPTER 260

Bipolar Disorder

Claire Barrett

DEFINITION AND EPIDEMIOLOGY

People experience a wide range of moods throughout their lifetimes, and often from one day to the next. This is an expected part of living and usually is not problematic. However, some people experience mood disorders that are more extreme fluctuations of their baseline mood. These fluctuations affect thoughts, feelings, physical health, behavior, and social functioning. Bipolar disorder is a mood disorder characterized by a vacillation between depressed (low) and manic (elevated) mood states.

Symptoms of the disorder may vary over time within the same patient or may remain similar across episodes. These symptoms also vary across a population afflicted with the disease. Because bipolar disorder is characterized by mood cycles, the clinical presentation may vary widely from a manic to a depressed episode. There are medications to treat the symptoms, and therefore early recognition of the disorder can aid in recovery. If left untreated, symptoms may become severe. Because episodes are often recurrent, it is important to have a treatment plan and for the patient and the practitioner to maintain open communication.

Bipolar disorder is most thoroughly explained in the fourth edition of the *Diagnostic and Statistical Manual of Mental Disorders* (DSM-IV).[1] The clinical presentation is characterized by one or more manic or mixed episodes during a patient's lifetime. The patient has often also had a major depressive episode, but such an episode is not necessary for diagnosis.

Approximately 1% of the population experiences a bipolar I disorder over the course of lifetime. The prevalence for bipolar II disorder is probably significantly higher because it is underdiagnosed. The lifetime prevalence for a major depressive disorder is approximately 15%, but this proportion may approach 25% in women.[2] In contrast to major depression, bipolar disorder affects men and women equally. However, gender may play a role in the timing of bipolar episodes.[2] Men are more likely to have a manic episode first, whereas women are more likely to have an initial depressive episode.[1] Women may also experience an onset of symptoms during the postpartum period, and women who have the disorder are at increased risk for experiencing additional episodes postpartum.[1] The premenstrual period may also be associated with the exacerbation of symptoms.[1]

In a study across several countries, bipolar disorder rates are notably consistent, whereas major depression rates vary widely.[3] Although the differential incidence of the disorder by racial or ethnic group has not been reported, mood disorders and schizophrenia have been underdiagnosed and overdiagnosed in patients whose cultures or races differ from that of their health care providers.[2] This may be related both to stereotypes and assumptions about races or ethnic groups and to the way in which people of different cultural, ethnic, or racial groups describe their symptoms.

The age of onset for a bipolar disorder can fall within a wide range but is generally between 15 and 30 years. Newly diagnosed mania rarely occurs in children or in adults over the age of 65 years. The initial episodes may be depressive; approximately 10% to 15% of adolescents with major depressive episodes are diagnosed with bipolar disorder later in life.[2]

There seems to be a genetic link among mood disorders, with the risk increasing with increases in the proportion of genes shared with an afflicted person.[4] This link is supported by a concordance rate for monozygotic twins that is approximately three times that noted in dizygotic twins.[4,5] In a National Institute of Mental Health–Yale University study, affective disorders occurred much more frequently in first-degree relatives of patients with affective disorders than in relatives of patients in a control group.[5] Despite the evidence supporting a genetic link, a specific mode of genetic transmission has not yet been found.[4]

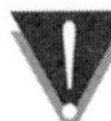
Immediate psychiatric evaluation is required for all patients with suicidal or homicidal ideation. Approximately 25% of individuals with bipolar disorder will attempt suicide.[6]

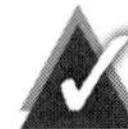
Physician consultation is indicated for patients with psychosis or violent behavior.

PATHOPHYSIOLOGY

Bipolar disorder is a biologic illness; however, its specific cause is still unknown. Reports from neuroimaging studies suggest that the thalamus, hypothalamus, amygdala, caudate, prefrontal cortex, and cerebellum may be involved in pathophysiology.[7] The neurotransmitters serotonin, norepinephrine, dopamine, and acetylcholine and second-messenger pathways have also been implicated.[8] In many patients, dysregulation of the hypothalamic-pituitary-adrenal axis and of circadian rhythms has been identified.[4] The search for gene carriers has been the subject of much study, but no single gene has been identified.[9,10] It is probable that there is a complex interaction between genetic and environmental factors.

CLINICAL PRESENTATION

Observation of the patient's behaviors and attention to the patient's description of symptoms are valuable for diagnosis. The clinical presentation of bipolar disorder varies depending on whether the presenting episode is manic or depressive. Subtypes of bipolar disorder include bipolar I disorder, in which the disorder appears for the first time with a manic episode and almost always has depressions as well. In bipolar II disorder, hypomania rather than mania occurs. Bipolar II disorder is more difficult to diagnose because hypomania may not be seen as problematic; the person is seen as happy or energetic, especially if he or she is able to avoid serious consequences. The person then may see a health care provider only during depressive episodes, thus jeopardizing effective treatment.

A working knowledge of the common symptoms enables appropriate questions to be directed toward the patient during any stage of illness. Manic states involve heightened mood, sexuality, and impulsivity. Increased energy results in a decreased need for sleep, faster speech, and physical activity. Although mania is often thought to be a grouping of exaggerated positive characteristics, certain stages of mania are quite painful to the patient. Increased irritability, paranoia, and suspicion may also be evident.[11]

Mania can begin as hypomania, a state most easily described as a less severe manic phase and one in which the patient's mood might be euphoric and self-confident. Thinking may be affected at times, since thoughts move quickly. However, the patient may enjoy this feeling because it allows for increased productivity, creativity, and energy.[11]

The progression from hypomania to a full-blown manic episode is gradual, but the actual time involved varies from person to person and episode to episode. During acute mania, cognition and perception often become psychotic; delusions or hallucinations may be experienced. Because thinking is so quick and tangential, patients are often highly distractible. When the affected patient is speaking, cognitive symptoms become obvious to others because of loose associations between ideas and, at times, the flight of ideas from one topic to another. Behavior can be bizarre and inappropriate and can seem disorganized.[11]

Patients with bipolar disorder can become violent and destructive or, more specifically, homicidal or suicidal. Although the beginning stage of mania is usually pleasurable, the later stages can be frightening and, finally, painful. By the height of the mania, the patient is in great pain but is usually apathetic.[12] During all stages of mania; it is crucial to assess a patient's risk of harm to self or others.

Depressive episodes are on the opposite end of the mood spectrum and have a very different presentation from that of mania. Although speech, movement, and thoughts are increased and quicker in mania, depression tends to decrease pleasure and to slow speech, thoughts, energy, and sexuality. Mood is negative and pessimistic, and the patient can be irritable, paranoid, and angry.[11]

Depression can be simple or psychotic. Simple depression usually includes morbid preoccupations and, frequently, suicidal thoughts. Sleeping and eating patterns are often altered and are characterized by decreased appetite and difficulty in getting to sleep or staying asleep.[11] Psychotic depression can also include mood-congruent hallucinations and delusions similar to those exhibited in mania. Mixed episodes are those in which symptoms of mania and depression occur at the same time.

The course of an individual's illness may be influenced by high rates of co-morbid alcohol or substance abuse. Almost two thirds of patients with the disorder will meet the diagnostic criteria for an addictive disorder over their lifetime.

PHYSICAL EXAMINATION

The physical examination may reveal symptoms indicative of bipolar disorder, but the time frame and controlled setting limit the range of observable symptoms. The provider's office does not allow for observation of the patients as they function in their own environment, where many of the previously described symptoms could be observed. In addition, patients in an acute state of mania or depression are much less likely than a healthy individual to keep a scheduled appointment. Signs and symptoms of mania or depression likely to be observed during a physical examination are rapid, slowed, or incoherent speech; changes in weight; irritability; grandiosity; distractibility; and overt psychosis.

DIAGNOSTICS

The commonly accepted method of diagnosing bipolar disorder is the use of DSM-IV criteria. Although the criteria for diagnosis are listed in the following paragraphs, the DSM-IV itself should be consulted for the most comprehensive information. An understanding of the criteria for a manic or major depressive episode, as well as the criteria for several disorders important in the differential diagnosis, is imperative for the diagnosis of bipolar I disorder. The essential feature of bipolar I disorder is a clinical course that includes one or more manic or mixed episodes. Often the patient has had one or more episodes of major depression; however, such an episode is not necessary for diagnosis.[1] Mood problems resulting from the use of substances, medical conditions, or other diagnoses are not counted toward the diagnosis.[1]

A major depressive episode is manifested by feeling sad, blue, or "down in the dumps" or by losing interest in normally enjoyable activities and by having at least four of the following:

- Insomnia or hypersomnia
- Significant weight loss or gain
- Impaired concentration, indecisiveness
- Psychomotor agitation or retardation
- Loss of energy, fatigue
- Feelings of worthlessness or guilt
- Thoughts of suicide or death

The feelings must be present daily or almost daily for at least 2 weeks.

In addition to meeting the preceding symptom criteria, the episode must not meet criteria for a mixed episode, and it must cause clinically significant distress or difficulties in important areas of functioning (e.g., social, occupational). In addition, symptoms must not be a result of the direct effects of a substance or medical condition, and they may not be better explained by bereavement[2] (see Chapter 261 for more information on depression).

To meet the criteria for a manic episode, defined as a period of abnormally and persistently elevated, expansive, or irritable mood,[1] the mood must last at least 1 week unless hospitalization is necessary sooner. Three or four of the following must be manifested in a significant and persistent manner:

- Inflated self-esteem or grandiosity
- Decreased need for sleep
- More talkative than usual or pressure to keep talking
- Flight of ideas, racing thoughts
- Distractibility
- Increased goal-directed activity or psychomotor agitation
- Excessive involvement in pleasurable activities, which might result in painful consequences

These symptoms must not be part of a mixed episode. The mood disturbance must also be severe enough to result in impaired occupational, social, or relationship functioning; to necessitate hospitalization to prevent harm; or to include psychotic features. Again, the symptoms may not be better explained by the physiologic effects of a substance or medical condition.[1]

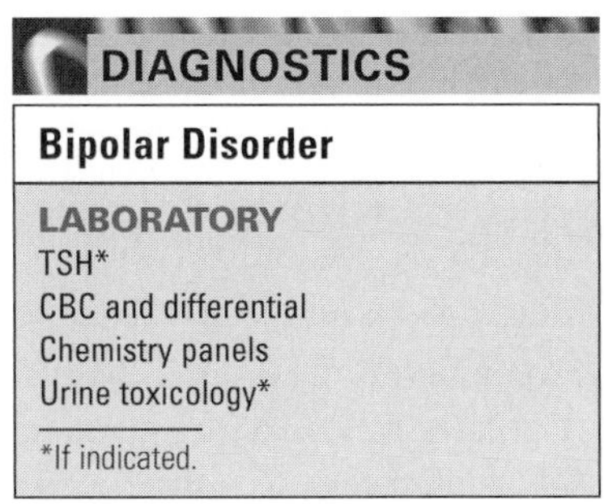
DIAGNOSTICS

Bipolar Disorder

LABORATORY
TSH*
CBC and differential
Chemistry panels
Urine toxicology*

*If indicated.

DIFFERENTIAL DIAGNOSIS

The diagnosis of a psychiatric illness differs from that of a physical illness because there are no laboratory tests from which to draw conclusive diagnoses. Diagnosis and treatment are based on the patient's report of symptoms, observation, and the elimination of other diagnoses. This emphasizes the importance of obtaining a thorough history. When possible, family interviews can be helpful in providing a more objective description of recent events. Schizophrenia; schizoaffective disorder; posttraumatic stress disorder; abuse of alcohol, cocaine, or amphetamines; and personality disorders can mimic or co-exist with bipolar disorder.[13,14] In the primary care setting, providers see patients with medical illnesses with symptoms that resemble manic episodes, including thyrotoxicosis, partial complex seizures, systemic lupus erythematosus, cerebrovascular accident, HIV, tertiary syphilis, and steroid-induced mood symptoms.[13,15] For this reason, evaluation should include physical examination with particular focus on neurologic and endocrine systems; observation for signs of abuse of alcohol or other substances; and laboratory testing that includes thyroid function tests, CBC, chemistry panels, and urine toxicology for possible substance abuse. Patients previously treated for depression with medication or electroconvulsive therapy may exhibit signs of mania; in such cases, a diagnosis should not be based on these symptoms.[1]

Bipolar I disorder is distinguished from other mood disorders by matching the criteria for diagnosis with the patient's symptoms. It is distinguished from major depressive disorder by the presence of only one manic or mixed episode in the patient's lifetime. It is less easily distinguished from bipolar II disorder, in which the only difference is the presence of one or more manic or mixed episodes (bipolar I) as opposed to hypomanic episodes (bipolar II). Cyclothymic disorders also share similar criteria with bipolar I disorder and are differentiated by the duration and nature of symptoms. With cyclothymic disorder, the hypomanic and depressive symptoms are present but do not meet the criteria for manic episodes or major depressive episodes.[1]

DIFFERENTIAL DIAGNOSIS

Bipolar Disorder

- Bipolar I and II
- Depression
- Cyclothymic disorder
- Schizoaffective disorder
- Schizophrenia
- Hyperthyroidism/hypothyroidism
- Pheochromocytoma
- Hypercortisolemia
- Metabolic disorder
- Posttraumatic stress disorder
- Substance abuse

MANAGEMENT

During the acute phase of the illness, the focus should be on management of the presenting symptoms and on ensuring the patient's safety. Patients in this phase may be suicidal, be psychotic, or display such poor judgment that they pose an imminent risk to self. Hospitalization may be necessary until the severity of symptoms abates. The continuation phase can last weeks to months. The goal is to reach full remission of symptoms and to restore the patient to full functioning. The maintenance phase aims to maintain remission and should last at least 1 year after resolutions of symptoms.

The major components of treatment include psychopharmacology, psychotherapy, and education. Psychotherapy is indicated to facilitate the resolution of issues that may contribute to or be exacerbated by the symptoms. Co-morbid substance abuse and personality disorders seem to predict poorer outcomes for patients with bipolar disorder, and therapy can be helpful in managing these conditions.[16] Specific cognitive behavioral strategies should focus on medication compliance, psychoeducation, and good sleep habits. The sleep cycle is very fragile in bipolar patients, and its disturbance is a source of destabilization in the illness.[6] Family therapy can enable the patient and significant others to work through problems resulting from or contributing to the disorder. Support groups, such as the National Alliance on Mental Illness and the Depression and Bipolar Support Alliance, allow individuals and significant others to receive support from peers who understand.

A psychiatrist or health care provider skilled in the use of psychiatric medications should manage all medications used to treat bipolar disorder. Pregnant women or women who may become pregnant pose significant complications in prescribing. Any possibility of pregnancy should be carefully explored during the assessment. A psychiatric evaluation is standard before beginning treatment, and system functions should be monitored throughout the course of treatment. Because toxic and therapeutic levels of lithium are often close, serum levels should be carefully monitored.

Medications commonly used during a manic episode to reduce symptoms include mood stabilizers (e.g., lithium carbonate), anticonvulsants, and atypical antipsychotics (e.g., olanzapine). The choice of a mood stabilizer is often based on previous history, side effect profiles, and any co-existing medical illness. For example, lithium is contraindicated in patients with severe renal disease, and valproate is contraindicated in patients with hepatic impairment.

Hypomania may be a precursor of either a manic or a depressive episode. It is often characterized by a decrease in sleep time. Administration of a mood stabilizer or a low dose of a stabilizing antipsychotic may end the hypomanic state.[17]

The Expert Consensus Guidelines, a series of treatment guidelines based on current research and on the expert opinion of many psychiatric practitioners, suggest the following[6]:

- For nonpsychotic mania, the initial options are a combination of a traditional mood stabilizer and an antipsychotic, or monotherapy with a mood stabilizer. Psychotic mania should be treated with an antipsychotic alone as the first option or with a mood stabilizer for the second line. The treatment of choice for hypomania is a mood stabilizer alone. Mood stabilizers are the main foundation for maintenance therapy.

- Bipolar disorder is a chronic illness; therefore ongoing treatment with medication and psychotherapy is indicated. Good treatment can reduce the frequency and severity of episodes.
- Electroconvulsive therapy remains a reliable and effective treatment for manic episodes nonresponsive to psychopharmacology.
- Treatment of the depressed phase of bipolar disorder has not been extensively studied and is controversial. In many cases, a mood stabilizer alone, usually lithium, may be useful. Unlike treatment of an episode of unipolar depression, antidepressant treatment of the depressed phase of bipolar disorder should be limited to the acute episode. Antidepressants should not be used without the concomitant administration of a mood stabilizer.
- For more information about the Expert Consensus Guidelines, see http://www.psychguides.com.

LIFE SPAN CONSIDERATIONS

As patients with bipolar disorder age, it may be beneficial to consult a geriatric psychiatrist or similarly trained professional. With increasing age and without treatment, the interval between mood episodes decreases and the duration of the episodes increases.[18] The ongoing use of powerful medications may require monitoring of various body systems for adverse effects or decreased tolerance.

COMPLICATIONS

The complications of bipolar disorder are primarily psychosocial. Recurrences of symptoms often result in the stigma associated with inappropriate behavior. Relationships and employment are jeopardized by behaviors that are perceived as harmful to the patient and others. Diminished financial status and credit are often the result of excessive spending and disregard for repayment during manic episodes.

Harm to self or others is the most severe consequence of bipolar disorder. Patients should be regularly monitored for mood changes that may indicate an impending acute episode. Because alcoholism is often a secondary complication associated with the disorder, the risks and consequences of alcoholism must also be considered if present. Careful exploration of suicidal or homicidal ideation is ongoing. It is important that the provider determine the level of impulsivity and impaired judgment, as well as consider whether impairment may result in unreported feelings. Although the provider should view the patient's perceptions as important, these accounts may not be indicative of the actual level of danger because objectivity is obscured during an episode. In these cases, collateral informants, clinical judgment about impulsivity, knowledge of a history of dangerous or violent behavior, and knowledge of the patient's ability to convey risk accurately are infinitely valuable pieces of information.

INDICATIONS FOR REFERRAL OR HOSPITALIZATION

Treatment for bipolar disorder is best administered by a psychiatrist or psychiatric nurse practitioner. Hospitalization on a psychiatric unit may be necessary if the mood disorder presents a danger to the patient or others or gravely impairs the patient's ability to provide for his or her basic needs. Mania may precipitate anger and violence at the threat of intervention. Anger, delusions, and hallucinations can result in homicidality or suicidality. In depressed patients an inability to care for self and a failure to thrive can warrant hospitalization. Certainly, suicide is also a risk during a major depressive episode. To ensure patient safety, it is important that medication management and control of the disorder occur in a secure setting, where patients will not be allowed to harm themselves or others.

PATIENT AND FAMILY EDUCATION

Of all patients with bipolar disorder, 85% to 95% will have a recurrence.[5] Therefore it is important to educate the patient and family about the signs and symptoms of an impending episode of depression or mania. Because the early stages of mania can be pleasant, the health care provider should discuss likely progression of the disorder to more unpleasant stages. Encouraging continuity with medications through education about risks and benefits can prove helpful in the quest to maintain stable mood. As always, efforts to minimize side effects, maximize patient involvement in treatment, and address patient concerns are valuable. It is important to encourage the patient to become as informed about the illness as possible. There are many published biographies, self-help books, and informative sites on the Internet that can serve as valuable resources.

Education of family and friends can increase support for the patient. By teaching significant others about the disorder and risks associated with the refusal of treatment options, the provider can ensure everyone participates in noticing the warning signs and creating plans with the patient to manage symptoms and increase safety.

REFERENCES

1. American Psychiatric Association: *Diagnostic and statistical manual of mental disorders,* ed 4 (text rev), Washington, DC, 2000, The Association.
2. Kaplan HI, Sadock BJ, Grebb JA: *Kaplan and Sadock's synopsis of psychiatry,* ed 7, Baltimore, 1994, Williams & Wilkins.
3. Weissman MM, Bland RC, Canino GJ, and others: Cross-national epidemiology of major depression and bipolar disorder, *JAMA* 276(4):293-299, 1996.
4. Tsuang MT, Faraone SV, Green R: Genetic epidemiology of mood disorders. In Papolos DF, Lachman HM, editors: *Genetic studies in affective disorders,* New York, 1994, John Wiley & Sons.
5. Charney EA, Weissman MM: Epidemiology of depressive and manic syndromes. In Georgotas A, Cancro R, editors: *Depression and mania,* New York, 1988, Elsevier.
6. Keck PE, Perlis RH, Otto MW, and others: *Treatment of bipolar disorder 2004: the expert consensus guideline series,* New York, 2004, McGraw-Hill.
7. Calabrese JR, Bowden CL, Sachs GS, and others: A double-blind placebo-controlled study of lamotrigine monotherapy in outpatients with bipolar I depression, *J Clin Psychiatr* 60(2):79-88, 1999.
8. Potash JB, DePaulo JR: Searching high and low: a review of the genetics of bipolar disorder, *Bipolar Disord* 2:8, 2000.
9. Craddock N, Jones I: Molecular genetics of bipolar disorder, *Br J Psychiatry* 178:S128, 2001.
10. Goodwin F, Jamison KR: *Manic depressive illness,* New York, 1990, Oxford University Press.
11. Schad-Somers SP: *On mood swings,* New York, 1990, Plenum Press.
12. Sachs G: Approach to the patient with elevated, expansive, or irritable

mood. In Stern TA, Herman JB, Slavin PL, editors: *The MGH guide to psychiatry in primary care,* New York, 1998, McGraw-Hill.
13. Blazer D: Mood disorders. In Kaplan HI, Sadock BJ, editors: *Comprehensive textbook of psychiatry,* ed 5, Baltimore, 1995, Williams & Wilkins.
14. Hilty DM, Brady KT, Hales RE: A review of bipolar disorder among adults, *Psychiatr Serv* 50:201-213, 1999.
15. Jefferson JW: Lithium. In Goodnick PA, editor: *Predictors of treatment response in mood disorders,* Washington, DC, 1996, American Psychiatric Press.
16. Freeman MP, Stoll AL: Mood-stabilizer combination: a review of safety and efficacy, *Am J Psychiatry* 155:12-21, 1998.
17. Krauthammer C, Klerman GL: Secondary mania: manic syndromes associated with antecedent physical illness or drugs, *Arch Gen Psychiatry* 30:74-79, 1978.
18. Winokur G, Coryell W, Akiskal HS, and others: Alcoholism in manic-depressive (bipolar) illness, and the primary-secondary distinction, *Am J Psychiatry* 152(3):365-372, 1995.

CHAPTER 261

Depressive Disorders

Debra Fournier

DEFINITION

Normal variations exist in mood and affect (outward display of mood). Factors, including age, personality development, and genetically predisposed temperament, influence how any one person may interpret events, behave, and modulate his or her emotions. Specific criteria exist to separate these normal displays of personality from episodes of diagnosable mood disorders that may benefit from treatment. Mood disorders, according to the fourth edition of the *Diagnostic and Statistical Manual of Mental Disorders* (DSM-IV), are defined by mood *episodes.*[1] Major depressive disorder (referred to as MDD or depression throughout this chapter) is the most common of the depressive disorders and is diagnosed when all criteria are met for at least one major depressive episode, without evidence of manic or hypomanic behavior. Dysthymic disorder involves a vaguer presentation of depressed mood over a longer period. The symptoms must not be better explained by any other medical or psychiatric condition, must cause significant impairment in function, and must be prominent for more days than not in a 2-week period for a diagnosis of MDD, and a 2-year period for dysthymic disorder. The diagnosis Depressive Disorder Not Otherwise Specified (NOS) is used to describe patterns of symptoms that do not fit into the above categories, yet for which depressed mood remains the predominant symptom.

The World Health Organization has developed a method for evaluating cost of care and disease burden outside of mortality statistics alone. Disability adjusted life years (DALYs) reflect the number of healthy years lost, or expected to be lost, because of a specific illness or injury.[2] Using this calculation, depression is the fourth leading cause of global disease burden in the past 2 decades. Worldwide, it is associated with the largest nonfatal burden.[3] Some estimates report that by 2020, MDD will be second only to ischemic heart disease in measures of overall disability.[4] In addition to lost work time and impairment in interpersonal and role functioning, people with MDD have been noted to use medical services at an increased rate. For example, a study of Medicaid recipients found that people with MDD receive the majority of their care in the general (primary care) setting. They cost the system more than twice (2.33) as much as someone without a diagnosable mental health problem in areas of general medical care and drug costs. Specialty care (mental health) was less utilized by those with MDD, and overall costs were surpassed only by those with diagnoses of bipolar disorder and psychotic disorders.[5]

EPIDEMIOLOGY

Information on the epidemiology of MDD comes primarily from four large studies since the publication of the DSM-III in 1980. Initially, estimates of the prevalence of lifetime and current MDD were 5.2% and 3.0%, respectively.[6] As the use of structured surveys and interviews became more reliable, researchers concluded that the prevalence of lifetime MDD in adults ages 18 to 65 was 13% to 16%, with 5.3% to 8.6% of this population currently meeting criteria for the diagnosis.[7-9]

Women are approximately twice as likely as men to experience MDD in their lifetime. Adults ages 30 to 60 have the highest rates of MDD, in samples of people less than 65. In the studies cited above, the first diagnosed depressive episode was noted to be at approximately age 30, yet clinical reports and guidelines suggest that the first episode of MDD most often occurs between the ages of 18 and 22.[1] Of greater concern, treatment is often not sought until approximately 3 years after the onset of symptoms. One study found little difference between ethnic groups[8]; however, another found Native Americans to be 1.5 times more likely than Caucasian Americans and twice as likely as other ethnic groups to have lifetime depression, with no difference in rates of MDD between Hispanic and African Americans.[9] This differed greatly from the original findings of the 1980s, which reported African Americans to be the most at-risk ethnic group.[6] Research consistently suggests no differences in numbers when considering education, urban vs. rural, or geographic region. Income is inversely related to prevalence of lifetime MDD. People who were divorced, widowed, or separated are twice as likely to have MDD as those who were married or never married.[6-10]

Two specific populations have been omitted from these large-scale studies: (1) the elderly and (2) children and adolescents. Prevalence rates for these age-groups vary widely, perhaps because of the complexity of changing roles, developing personalities, cognitive development or deterioration, and medical co-morbidities. Several studies that screened adolescents for *subclinical* depression found rates as high as 30%.[11] Rates of diagnosed MDD are less clear, yet correlates of medical illness and impaired function match those of their adult counterparts. When controlling for medical illness, screening positive for probable depressive disorder was associated with poorer functioning in overall role activity and less educational achievement. Clinically, available interventions are offered when subclinical symptoms have been identified, thereby ideally reducing later complications of adult MDD.

In general, the prevalence of MDD has been noted to be slightly lower in older adults (>65) than in those 30 to 60 years of age. Although prevalence rates in older adults are 4% to 8%, the incidence (number of new cases in 1 year) has been noted to be as high as 15%.[12,13] Estimates of MDD in older adults vary widely by setting. Healthy older adults living in the community have an estimated prevalence of MDD of 3%. Of those who frequently access primary care services, rates increase to 17% to 37%, and 12% to 30% of those living in long-term care facilities meet diagnostic criteria for MDD.[14,15] Depression is thought to be present in 20% of older patients diagnosed with Alzheimer's type dementia, and depression with psychotic features has been estimated to be as high as 45% in hospitalized elders with a history of some depressive symptoms.[13] Subclinical or minor depression is estimated to occur twice as frequently, with similar impact on function.[12] Factors such as physical illness, hospitalization, death of a partner, cognitive decline, and decreased income are more powerful predictors of MDD than age alone. It is expected that, as the retiring generation lives longer (women outliving men), with more medical problems, more hospitalizations, and less income, rates of MDD will continue to trend higher (Box 261-1).

PATHOPHYSIOLOGY

With technologic advances allowing for the evaluation of brain metabolism, neurotransmitter activity, and subtle differences in size of regions of the brain, literature related to the pathophysiology of neurologic disorders is abundant. Several theories have emerged regarding the biologic genesis of depression. Increased blood flow in the amygdala region and dysfunction in the limbic-prefrontal cortex communication systems have been identified in people with MDD.[16-19] Cortisol levels have been evaluated and explored as a potential measure for diagnosing MDD. Studies have found increased basal levels of cortisol in people with depression, as well as a general dysregulation of the stress-response function mediating cortisol. The hypothalamus-pituitary-adrenal (HPA) axis is responsible for regulating the body's response to stress and is mediated by cortisol release. In people with MDD, it is slower to recover from stress-stimuli.[17,19-21]

Postmortem studies have associated decreased hippocampal volume with the presence of depression in those who committed suicide.[17] Decreased hippocampal volume may be linked to damage caused by prolonged exposure to glucocorticoids (cortisol),[22] rather than a preexisting structural factor in the development of MDD. Disruption to sleep patterns has been strongly associated with the occurrence of MDD, yet it remains unclear whether this is a risk factor or sequela of the disorder.[1]

The biologic theory that has the strongest implication for pharmacologic treatment involves the relationship between synaptic levels of neurotransmitters and MDD. Although norepinephrine and dopamine levels are implicated in symptom manifestation, the strongest research associates lower levels of serotonin with the diagnosis of MDD.[17,19] More recent studies suggest that, rather than having a central role in the

BOX 261-1

FAST FACTS ABOUT DEPRESSION AND SUICIDE

- In the United States, the lifetime prevalence for major depressive disorder is 15%.
- Ratio of women/men = 2:1.
- Depression is first diagnosed around age 30, although symptoms often start 10 years earlier and treatment is often not sought until age 33.
- Depression is the leading cause of nonfatal disease burden worldwide.
- Most people with depression seek and receive treatment in the primary care setting.
- Suicide is the third leading cause of death in Americans ages 15 to 24.
- Depression is often underdiagnosed and undertreated, yet it can be diagnosed in less than a few minutes and is treatable.

Data from References 2, 12, 50, 52.

BOX 261-2

NEUROBIOLOGIC CHANGES ASSOCIATED WITH DEPRESSION

- Serotonin, norepinephrine, and dopamine depletion or deficiency
- Hypothalamus-pituitary-adrenal axis dysregulation (leading to increased levels of corticotropin-releasing factor and cortisol)
- Structural and metabolic differences in areas of the brain such as the hippocampus, amygdala, and prefrontal cortex

modulation of mood and sleep, serotonin levels may be more closely linked with the regulation of other neurobiologic systems in the brain, designed to respond to stressful or emotional stimuli.[23] Box 261-2 highlights the neurobiologic changes associated with MDD.

Depression has a strong familial association; MDD is 1.5 to 3 times more common in first-degree biologic relatives of those with the disorder compared with the general population.[1] Environmental factors and personality development are closely linked with coping styles. Psychodynamic theories of the manifestation of mental illness include the need for mastery of developmental tasks, the healthy interpretation of events, and successful interpersonal interactions. Logically, children of parents with depressive symptoms are more inclined to develop difficulties with role functioning, including behavioral problems, substance abuse, and depressed mood.[1,24] Several twin studies, however, connect MDD in part to a genetic predisposition.[25,26] It is still unclear whether this genetic connection is related to an inherited modifier to the HPA axis or serotonin deficiency or a specific chromosomal pattern.

CLINICAL PRESENTATION

The majority of people with depressive disorders are seen by their health care providers for initial treatment, yet may not identify the depressive symptoms as their chief complaint. Many patients may focus on vague somatic concerns rather than identifying or sharing emotions such as sadness or hopelessness. Family members or a provider who has established rapport with the patient may notice increased irritability. Irritability is likely to be the predominant symptom in children, whereas depressed mood and hopelessness are more apparent in adults, and somatic concerns dominate older adults' presentation. Loss of interest or pleasure in previously enjoyable events and social withdrawal are almost always present. Appetite is usually less than normal, and insomnia is prevalent, yet may be missed, since the person with depression may complain of fatigue or anergia without significant physical stimuli. Preoccupations with perceived personal deficits, along with an exaggerated sense of guilt or worthlessness, are also common. Impaired concentration, difficulty with decision making, and mild memory impairment is possible and must not be confused with cognitive changes associated with dementia. Thoughts of death vary from "the world would be better off without me," to engaging in dangerous behaviors without concern for personal safety, to specific plans for suicide.[1]

Depression is often a chronic condition. Depressive episodes may be separated by periods of partial or full recovery of varying lengths of time. Sixty percent of people who experience one depressive episode are likely to have another, 70% of those who have had two depressive episodes are likely to have a third, and 90% of those who have had three episodes will have more. Between 5% and 10% of people who have a depressive episode may later have a manic episode (see Chapter 260). Factors such as incomplete recovery, co-morbid substance use, and personality disorders may have some predictive value in estimating the course of the illness, with these factors associated with more frequent episodes and increased severity of impairment.[27]

The presentation, communication, and interpretation of symptoms related to depressive disorders can be complicated by culture because research shows that the cultural background of the provider interpreting the symptoms affects how those symptoms are interpreted. In the broadest of definitions, culture refers to the context in which one was raised and norms with which one identifies. Family patterns, religious beliefs, societal and generational norms, and past experience all influence how symptoms of mental health problems are disclosed. A strong patient-provider relationship enhances the ability to detect and effectively manage mental health problems, regardless of cultural expectations or differences in subtle presentations of symptoms.

PHYSICAL EXAMINATION

During a clinical visit, the provider can elicit risk factors for depression through careful interview. Psychosocial stressors, sleep patterns, nutritional habits, and physical activity can be important indicators of a depressive disorder, since many of these realms are often impaired when depression is present. As mentioned above, many people may come to the health care provider with vague somatic concerns. Even when depression is suspected, all other medical and psychiatric diagnoses must be explored. Many medical conditions and medications are associated with symptoms of depression, and complications of common medical conditions (including mortality) are greater in people who have also been diagnosed with MDD.[5,12]

DIAGNOSTICS

Currently no laboratory tests or imaging studies can definitively diagnose MDD, in spite of the progress made in the exploration of biologic correlates of mental illness as described above. Blood tests to evaluate nutritional, endocrine, and thyroid function are critical in ruling out medical, reversible causes for presenting symptoms. Imaging of the head and cardiac stress tests may also be helpful in considering ischemic disease, emboli, or traumatic injury as complicating factors.

MDD is diagnosed by interview, when criteria are met for a depressive episode and there is no history of manic or hypomanic behavior (refer to Chapter 260). A depressive episode is present when five of the following symptoms occur, more days than not, in a 2-week period and cause significant impairment in any realm of functioning: depressed mood, loss of interest or pleasure, significant unintended change in weight or appetite, significant change in sleep pattern, change in psychomotor activity (increased restlessness or psychomotor retardation), fatigue or loss of energy, feelings of worthlessness or guilt, impaired concentration or decision-making ability, and recurrent thoughts of death or suicide. At least one of the symptoms must be depressed mood (subjective or observed) or anhedonia (loss of pleasure), and symptoms must not be better explained by another medical or psychiatric disorder.[1] Box 261-3 includes full DSM-IV criteria for MDD.

Several structured interviews are available for the diagnosis of depressive disorders. The Structured Clinical Interview for DSM Diagnoses can be separated into modules for specific disorders. The Hamilton Depression Scale and the Beck Depression Inventory involve self-report of symptoms and do not require interviewer time. The Geriatric Depression Scale includes some modifications to better assess the presence of depression that may be complicated by multiple physical conditions or medication effects common in the older population.[28] The PRIME-MD is a tool designed for the use of health care providers in their daily practice, considering the pressures of time in the outpatient clinical setting.[29] All these scales have significant sensitivity and specificity in identifying depressive disorders, concordant with specialty reviewers.[30]

BOX 261-3

DSM-IV DIAGNOSTIC CRITERIA FOR MAJOR DEPRESSIVE DISORDER

A. Five (or more) of the following symptoms have been present during the same 2-week period and represent a change from previous functioning; at least one of the symptoms is either (1) depressed mood or (2) loss of interest or pleasure.
   NOTE: Do not include symptoms that are clearly due to general medical condition, or mood-incongruent delusions or hallucinations.
   (1) Depressed mood most of the day, nearly every day, as indicated either by subjective report (e.g., feels sad or empty) or observation made by others (e.g., appears tearful). NOTE: In children and in adolescents, can be irritable mood
   (2) Markedly diminished interest or pleasure in all, or almost all, activities most of the day, nearly every day (as indicated by either subjective report or observations made by others)
   (3) Significant weight loss when not dieting or weight gain (e.g., a change of more than 5% of body weight in a month), or decrease or increase in appetite early every day. NOTE: In children, considerable failure to make expected weight gains
   (4) Insomnia or hypersomnia nearly every day
   (5) Psychomotor agitation or retardation nearly every day (observable by others, not merely subjective feelings of restlessness or being slowed down)
   (6) Fatigue or loss of energy nearly every day
   (7) Feelings of worthlessness or excessive or inappropriate guilt (which may be delusional) nearly every day (not merely self-reproach or guilt about being sick)
   (8) Diminished ability to think or concentrate, or indecisiveness, nearly every day (either by subjective account or as observed by others)
   (9) Recurrent thoughts of death (not just fear of dying), recurrent suicidal ideation without a specific plan, or a suicide attempt or a specific plan for committing suicide

B. The symptoms do no meet the criteria for a Mixed Episode.

C. The symptoms cause clinically significant distress or impairment in social, occupational, or other important areas of functioning.

D. The symptoms are not due to the direct physiologic effects of a substance (e.g., a drug of abuse, a medication) or a general medical condition (e.g., hypothyroidism).

E. The symptoms are not better accounted for by Bereavement, i.e., after the loss of a loved one, the symptoms persist longer than 2 months or are characterized by marked functional impairment, morbid preoccupation with worthlessness, suicidal ideation, psychotic symptoms, or psychomotor retardation.

From American Psychiatric Association: *Diagnosis and statistical manual of mental disorders,* ed 4 (text rev), Washington, DC, 2000, The Association.

Specifiers, further describing the characteristics of the disorder, may be included yet are more commonly diagnosed by a mental health provider. These include depression:

- With or without psychotic features
- That is chronic
- With catatonic features
- With melancholic features
- With atypical features
- With postpartum onset
- That is a single episode or recurrent
- With seasonal pattern

The diagnostic criteria for MDD must be initially met, and the specifiers are used only to describe the pattern of onset or predominant symptom presentation.[1]

A diagnosis of dysthymic disorder requires the presence of depressed mood (subjectively or reported by others) for more days than not over a 2-year period accompanied by two of the following: poor appetite or overeating, insomnia or hypersomnia, low energy, low self-esteem, poor concentration, and feelings of hopelessness. The presence of any specific mood episode must be excluded, and the symptoms must not be better accounted for by another medical or psychiatric diagnosis. Dysthymic disorder is less common than MDD and often has an earlier onset. Children are more commonly seen with irritability rather than reporting depressed mood. The prevalence of dysthymic disorder is lower than that of MDD, with a lifetime community prevalence of 6%; however, dysthymic disorder may precede MDD. In these cases the likelihood of full remission between episodes is decreased.[1]

Depressive disorder NOS includes some symptoms of other depressive disorders, although full criteria for another diagnosis are not met due to duration of symptoms or severity of functional impairment. This category is also often used when medical or other psychiatric complications have not yet been fully explored, yet all symptoms for a major depressive episode are met.[1]

DIFFERENTIAL DIAGNOSIS

The following conditions may manifest with symptoms such as sad mood, anhedonia, fatigue, and change in appetite and must be considered before a diagnosis of MDD is made: viral infection, hypothyroidism, hypoparathyroidism, hypoadrenocorticism, leukemia, lymphoma, cancer (pancreatic and others), cerebrovascular disease (transient ischemic attacks, stroke, vascular dementia), myocardial infarction, vitamin B_{12} deficiency, malnutrition, and traumatic brain or spinal cord injury.[12,14] When onset and intensity of depressive symptoms parallel the pattern of the medical illness, yet persist in the context of optimum treatment for the medical condition, mood disorder due to general medical condition, with depressive features, can be diagnosed.[1] Treatment options mirror those of MDD, and optimum treatment of depressive symptoms is associated with better overall prognosis.

DIFFERENTIAL DIAGNOSIS

Depressive Disorders

MEDICAL CONDITIONS
- Viral infection
- Hypothyroidism
- Hypoparathyroidism
- Hypoadrenalcorticism
- Leukemia
- Lymphoma
- Cancer
- Cerebrovascular disease
- Myocardial infarction
- Vitamin B_{12} deficiency
- Malnutrition
- Traumatic brain or spinal cord injury

MEDICATIONS
- Cardiovascular drugs
- Antiparkinsonian drugs
- Antianxiety or sedative agents
- Antiinflammatory medications
- Antiinfectives, antibiotics
- Stimulants
- Hormones
- Antihistamines

Many medications cause side effects that may manifest as depressive symptoms. Cardiovascular drugs such as clonidine or beta blockers may cause sedation and fatigue. Antiparkinsonian drugs such as levodopa and amantadine may be associated with psychomotor retardation. Antianxiety or sedative medications such as benzodiazepines may not be metabolized in the older person as quickly as expected, and accumulated metabolites may lead to general central nervous system depressive effects. Antiinflammatory and antibiotic medications, stimulants, hormones, and antihistamines all may have an additional impact on the older adult.[14] These potential medication effects must be considered and offending medications eliminated, when possible, to evaluate for a new diagnosis of MDD.

MANAGEMENT

Several classes of medications have emerged for the treatment of depression. Monoamine oxidase (MAO) inhibitors and tricyclic antidepressants (TCAs) were the standard of care until the first selective serotonin reuptake inhibitor (SSRI) was approved for use in the late 1980s. Although when comparing efficacy of reducing symptoms of MDD alone, these agents are equal, SSRIs offer a gentler side effect profile, have fewer drug interactions, and are less likely to be lethal in overdose.[31-33] MAO inhibitors increase the level of tyramine, making it necessary for patients taking these drugs to restrict ingestion of tyramine-containing foods to avoid dangerous cardiotoxic effects. TCAs carry a risk of arrhythmia, are highly anticholinergic, and are lethal in overdose.[32,33] Newer, atypical agents alter levels of norepinephrine in addition to serotonin with consistent efficacy in the management of depressive symptoms.

Given equal efficacy between the general classes of medications, specific agents should be chosen based on individual considerations of predominant symptoms, potential side effects, risk for interactions, and co-morbid conditions.[31,34] Tables 261-1 and 261-2 highlight conditions that may be considered when choosing an antidepressant, dosing recommendations, and prevalence of side effects for the most commonly prescribed agents. For example, an elderly woman with insomnia and decreased appetite may benefit from mirtazapine, since it is likely to cause somnolence and stimulate appetite. In this case, the individual or her caregivers must also be aware of the risk for hypotension with mirtazapine, since it may increase her risk for injury related to dizziness or falls. These tables are designed to serve as a quick reference for choosing the most appropriate medication, not to substitute for full review of prescribing information and contraindications. Box 261-4 includes basic tips for prescribing antidepressant medications.

Once an agent has been selected, the initial dose should be maintained for 1 to 2 weeks before increasing to the target dose. Faster titrations are safe within an inpatient or supervised setting, but may be associated with higher incidence of side effects. A trial of 6 to 8 weeks is necessary to determine effectiveness or response.[31,34] Once MDD is diagnosed and treated for the first time and symptoms are managed with an acceptable dosage, medications should continue for 6 to 9 months. The likelihood of recurrent episodes increases if full remission of symptoms is not initially achieved. If medications were stopped after 9 months of adequate treatment with full remission and a second depressive episode occurs, the same agent may be selected with similar strategy, yet should continue for at least 1 year. Once someone has experienced a third depressive episode, lifelong treatment with medications is recommended.[31]

Some evidence suggests that after several years of use, a specific agent may lose its effectiveness. Although the reason for this change is not well understood, there is evidence to suggest that effective treatment can still occur with a different medication from within the same class.[33,35] Frequent and thorough follow-up appointments enhance the adherence to a plan to continue medications once some symptom relief has been achieved. Incomplete and inadequate treatment is associated with more frequent episodes of recurrent depression.

Hypothyroidism, as discussed above, may initially manifest with symptoms of depression. Although some evidence suggests that augmentation of antidepressants with thyroid supplementation in euthyroid patients has some benefit,[34] SSRIs alone have no direct effect on the regulation of the hypothalamic-pituitary-thyroid axis.[35,36] Some literature also suggests that augmentation of an SSRI with lithium may be helpful, yet because of the degree of follow up required, specialty care is recommended for any strategy involving more than one agent.

Psychotherapy is effective at reducing symptoms of depression. If used alone, a longer course of treatment is expected before full remission of initial symptoms. Many studies suggest that a combination of medications and therapy offers the best odds for recovery.[31] Psychotherapy is most likely to play a role in reducing relapse or a recurrence of depression for most people.[31] Several types of therapy have demonstrated this effectiveness in clinical trials, including interpersonal therapy, cognitive therapy, behavioral therapy, combination cognitive behavior therapy, and brief dynamic therapy.[31,37] All psychotherapy requires a referral to a specialty provider.

Nutrition plays a role in mood. Glycemic variability, vitamin deficiencies, and electrolyte imbalances may all be enhanced or stabilized with the benefit of improved mood. It is clear that adequate intake of good nutritional value has a role in the management and perhaps the prevention of mild

TABLE 261-1 Choosing Medications for Treatment of Major Depressive Disorder

Medication	Therapeutic Dose*	Conditions That May Also Benefit	Cautions
Duloxetine	20-60 mg	Neuropathic pain	
Escitalopram	5-20 mg		
Citalopram	10-60 mg		
Sertraline	50-200 mg	Posttraumatic stress disorder	May cause diarrhea May cause sexual dysfunction
Fluoxetine	10-80 mg; also available in once a week dosing	Premenstrual dysphoric disorder	Long half life May cause sexual dysfunction
Paroxetine	20-60 mg	Anxiety	Immediate release has short half life
Paroxetine CR	25-62.5 mg		May cause sexual dysfunction
Fluvoxamine	50-300 mg	Obsessive compulsive disorder	May cause gastrointestinal upset May cause sexual dysfunction
Bupropion	225-450 mg	Nicotine dependence Anergia	Lowers the seizure threshold (contraindicated if eating disorder or seizure disorder present)
Bupropion SR	150-300 mg (give in divided doses)		
Venlafaxine	75-375 mg	Anergia	May cause sexual dysfunction
Venlafaxine XR		Anxiety disorders (higher doses)	May elevate blood pressure
Mirtazapine	15-60 mg	Insomnia Decreased appetite	Sedation Weight gain Hypotension
Trazodone	150-600 mg	Insomnia	Liver dysfunction Sedation
Amitriptyline	75-300 mg	Migraines Insomnia Neuropathic pain	Sedation Anticholinergic Weight gain Possible arrhythmia Confusion
Nortriptyline	40-200 mg	Migraines Neuropathic pain	

Data from References 31-35.
*Starting dose = first lowest in the range of therapeutic dose.

to moderate symptoms of depression. Strategies of supplementation, however, are not validated in the literature for the treatment of MDD.[38]

Bright light therapy has been researched for efficacy in the management of depression with seasonal and nonseasonal patterns. Although large clinical trials are still lacking, there is some evidence to suggest that it produces a modest improvement in symptoms of depressed mood, especially for people who also have sleep disorders, yet hypomania is a potential side effect.[39]

Electroconvulsive therapy (ECT) may be considered after resistance to pharmacologic interventions has been established. ECT requires management by a specialist team and often includes a brief inpatient stay. Based on the current literature, little is clear about factors that may predict an effective response to ECT intervention. Investigations of symptom severity, age, previous pharmacology trials, and presenting symptomatology have been completed without consistent results. Although the number of recommended sessions may vary, evidence now suggests that efficacy can be predicted after the third session.[40]

New research on repetitive transcranial magnetic stimulation offers some promise for additional specialty procedures for the management of MDD that may be resistant to psychotropic medications, yet few trials exist to demonstrate its efficacy.[41]

LIFE SPAN CONSIDERATIONS

An initial symptom of childhood and adolescent depression is often irritability rather than depressed mood and sadness. Randomized controlled trials suggest that combination treatment strategies (employing SSRIs and cognitive behavior therapy) are as effective for children as for adults.[42] Recently, concerns were raised about an association between the use of SSRIs and rates of suicides in adolescents.[43] Thorough reviews have challenged this warning, and national rates of adolescent suicides have decreased with the rising use of SSRI therapy.[44,45] Suicide is a risk for any child, adolescent, adult, or elder with symptoms of depression, at any stage of intervention and recovery.

MDD is rarely first diagnosed over age 65, although mood disorder due to general medical condition, with depressive features, is a diagnosis often made later in life. In the absence of a long-term relationship between older adult and provider, initially distinguishing between dementia and depression may be difficult. Dementia is often slow in onset with a stable or steady decline in function, whereas depression may appear more rapidly with an inconsistent or fluctuating course.

TABLE 261-2 Side Effects of Common Antidepressants

Adverse Reaction	Prevalence			
	High (>30%)	Moderate (10%-30%)	Low (2%-10%)	Very Low (<2%)
Drowsiness or sedation	Mirtazapine Trazodone Amitriptyline	Citalopram Fluoxetine Fluvoxamine Paroxetine Sertraline Venlafaxine	Duloxetine Escitalopram Bupropion Nortriptyline	
Insomnia		Citalopram Fluoxetine Duloxetine Escitalopram Fluvoxamine Paroxetine Sertraline Bupropion Venlafaxine	Mirtazapine Trazodone Amitriptyline	Nortriptyline
Excitement		Fluvoxamine Sertraline Bupropion Venlafaxine	Citalopram Fluoxetine Escitalopram Paroxetine Mirtazapine Nortriptyline	Duloxetine Trazodone Amitriptyline
Confusion		Fluoxetine Amitriptyline Nortriptyline	Fluvoxamine Mirtazapine Bupropion Venlafaxine	Citalopram Duloxetine Escitalopram Paroxetine Sertraline Trazodone
Headache		Citalopram Fluoxetine Escitalopram Fluvoxamine Paroxetine Sertraline Bupropion Venlafaxine	Mirtazapine Trazodone Amitriptyline	Duloxetine Nortriptyline
Dry mouth	Mirtazapine Amitriptyline	Citalopram Fluoxetine Duloxetine Fluvoxamine Paroxetine Sertraline Bupropion Venlafaxine Trazodone Nortriptyline	Escitalopram	
Constipation		Duloxetine Fluvoxamine Paroxetine Mirtazapine Bupropion Venlafaxine Amitriptyline Nortriptyline	Citalopram Fluoxetine Escitalopram Sertraline Trazodone	

Data from References 31-35.

TABLE 261-2 Side Effects of Common Antidepressants—cont'd

	Prevalence			
Adverse Reaction	**High (>30%)**	**Moderate (10%-30%)**	**Low (2%-10%)**	**Very Low (<2%)**
Sweating		Citalopram Fluvoxamine Paroxetine Bupropion Venlafaxine Amitriptyline	Fluoxetine Duloxetine Escitalopram Sertraline Mirtazapine	Trazodone Nortriptyline
Tremor		Fluoxetine Fluvoxamine Paroxetine Sertraline Bupropion Amitriptyline Nortriptyline	Citalopram Duloxetine Escitalopram Mirtazapine Venlafaxine Trazodone	
Orthostatic hypotension or dizziness		Fluoxetine Paroxetine Sertraline Venlafaxine Trazodone Amitriptyline	Citalopram Duloxetine Escitalopram Fluvoxamine Mirtazapine Bupropion Nortriptyline	
ECG changes		Amitriptyline	Trazodone Nortriptyline	Citalopram Fluoxetine Duloxetine Escitalopram Fluvoxamine Paroxetine Sertraline Mirtazapine Bupropion Venlafaxine Nortriptyline
Gastrointestinal distress	Fluvoxamine Sertraline Venlafaxine	Citalopram Fluoxetine Duloxetine Escitalopram Paroxetine Bupropion Trazodone	Mirtazapine Amitriptyline	
Rash			Fluoxetine Fluvoxamine Sertraline Bupropion Venlafaxine Amitriptyline	Citalopram Duloxetine Paroxetine Mirtazapine Escitalopram Trazodone Nortriptyline
Weight gain	Mirtazapine Amitriptyline	Paroxetine	Citalopram Fluoxetine Escitalopram Sertraline Fluvoxamine Trazodone Nortriptyline	Duloxetine Bupropion Venlafaxine
Sexual disturbance	Citalopram Fluoxetine Fluvoxamine Paroxetine Sertraline Venlafaxine	Mirtazapine	Duloxetine Escitalopram Amitriptyline	Bupropion Trazodone Nortriptyline

BOX 261-4

PRESCRIBING TIPS

- Some people will respond to antidepressants at initial doses.
- Higher doses of selective serotonin reuptake inhibitors (SSRIs) may be more effective if there is a co-morbid anxiety disorder.
- Reduce starting doses by 50% in the elderly, people with impaired renal function, or those especially sensitive to side effects.
- Refer to package inserts for contraindications in people with severe renal or hepatic impairment and when switching to a new antidepressant (tapering and wash-out periods are necessary for some agents).
- Serotonin syndrome (confusion, hyperreflexia, myoclonus, fever) may occur when more than one serotonergic agent is prescribed.
- Serotonin withdrawal (flulike symptoms, anxiety) may occur when an SSRI is stopped suddenly.
- The risk for suicide is not reduced by antidepressant medication.

Data from References 31, 32, and 34.

Somatic concerns, sad mood, difficulty concentrating, and disruptions to appetite and sleep patterns are more likely to be prominent in the presentation of MDD and concealed by the patient with dementia. An awareness of deficits and profound sadness and anergia are more associated with MDD, whereas patients with dementia may not seem quite as concerned about their inaccurate responses.[14] Depression and dementia may co-exist, and optimum treatment of both conditions is required to reduce functional impairment.[12,13]

Treatment strategies for any depressive disorder in the elderly, once appropriately diagnosed, mirror those for healthy adults. Consideration of side effect profiles and possible drug interactions, however, becomes more critical. Initial doses should be half that of the adult starting dose, and titration that occurs more slowly will reduce the risk of complicating side effects or drug interactions. Longer courses of treatment are often required for full remission of symptoms, yet prognosis is the same as for younger adults.[13,14] Social support, however, plays a more influential role in reducing functional impairment when depressive symptoms are present in this population.[46]

COMPLICATIONS

Depression has been researched both as a preexisting risk factor for people to develop cardiac disease and diabetes, and as a postevent predictor of poorer outcomes (increased mortality and general decreased function).[47-49] Strong associations have emerged suggesting that the rates of depression are higher when a co-occurring medical condition exists, and the presence of depression is an indicator of increased mortality. The prevalence of suicidal ideation is also increased for people with depression and a serious medical diagnosis.[29]

Suicide

According to the Centers for Disease Control and Prevention, suicide is the third leading cause of death in Americans ages 15 to 24.[50] In 2003, suicide was the eighth leading cause of death in men in the United States.[50] Geographic patterns indicate that suicide is more prevalent in Alaska, Florida, and Midwestern states such as Wyoming, Colorado, Idaho, Arizona, New Mexico, Nevada, North Dakota, and South Dakota, with lowest rates in Ohio, Michigan, Illinois, New York, New Jersey, Massachusetts, Rhode Island, and Connecticut.[51] It is unclear, however, if geography alone is a factor or if these prevalence data are mediated by other risk factors for depression and suicide.

Worldwide, 90% of people who have committed suicide had been diagnosed with a mental illness (including 60% with depression; other diagnoses included substance use disorders and psychotic disorders).[10,52] Risk factors for suicide include unemployment, marital isolation, low socioeconomic status, family history of mental illness, family history of suicide, exposure to the suicidal behavior of others (including via media), family violence, personal history of physical or sexual abuse, alcohol or drug use, incarceration, and previous suicide attempts.[10,52] Although women are more likely to attempt suicide, men are more likely to die by suicide.[52] Given that suicide by firearms is now the most common method for both men and women,[50] it is hypothesized that this ratio of lethality will soon equalize.

The rates of suicide in the elderly are five times higher than in younger adults. The presence of a medical illness increases the probability of death by suicide, yet this outcome has shown to be directly mediated by the presence of depression. Older Caucasian men (age >65) and young African-American men (ages 19 to 29) have the highest relative rates of suicide.[12,52] Studies evaluating differences in suicide rates between ethnic groups suggest that, when controlling for the presence of MDD, Americans of Mexican and Puerto Rican descent are at lower risk for suicide.[10]

Thoughts of death are common in people with depression. Given the risk of suicide in this population, anyone with MDD or subclinical symptoms must be carefully assessed. There are four components to a thorough suicide assessment (Box 261-5). First, it is important to understand the specific thoughts that someone may be having related to death. Hopelessness for the future—thoughts such as "The world would be better off without me" or "I wish I could go to sleep and not wake up"—must be explored further to determine level of risk. For example, the provider can say, "What you're telling me sounds incredibly difficult to manage. Has it been so bad that you've had thoughts of ending your own life?" If patients have not thought of suicide, they are likely to answer quickly and volunteer reasons such as religious belief or family considerations. If they have thought of taking their own life, they are likely to answer more slowly, wary of the potential reaction from the provider. Clinicians with less experience with psychiatry often fear that they will somehow contribute to the risk of suicide by asking the questions. This is a myth.

Once the patient has shared his or her suicidal ideation, the assessment must continue with an evaluation of specific plan, access to means, and intention to implement that plan. Many

BOX 261-5

ASSESSING RISK FOR SUICIDE

- Thoughts of suicide
- Plan to commit suicide
- Means to complete the plan
- Intention to follow through with the plan

people who have thought of suicide, and who have had ideas about a plan, also have strong convictions about the circumstances under which they would or would not follow through with this plan. Others may have thought about ways to die, yet have not developed methods to access the means necessary for completion. Collaboration and consultation are critical in managing people with depression and thoughts of suicide.

"Contracting for safety" is a therapeutic intervention some specialty providers use. It is not a legal agreement and, even if in writing, does not protect a provider from liability. It is a "promise" between the patient with suicidal ideation and the provider, reflective of a spoken or written commitment that the person will not act on his or her thoughts or carry out the plan for suicide. This is only as effective as the relationship between patient and provider and depends on the provider's commitment to the person with depression.

Suicidal ideation requires careful assessment. Emergency psychiatric assessment for hospitalization is indicated for anyone considered at high risk for self-harm.

INDICATIONS FOR REFERRAL OR HOSPITALIZATION

The majority of people with depressive disorders are treated in outpatient primary care settings. Many conditions, however, may require services from a mental health provider. It is advisable for health care providers to know the resources and systems to access mental health care in their area, to facilitate urgent referrals, and to provide accurate information to patients in need of those referrals. Box 261-6 includes referral criteria.

Screening tools and intensive case management services are structural interventions under exploration to enhance the management of MDD in the primary care setting. Many clinics also incorporate behavioral health specialists in the outpatient clinic to increase the ease of referral and reduce the stigma of seeking services.[53,54]

BOX 261-6

WHEN TO REFER TO MENTAL HEALTH SPECIALISTS

Emergent intervention is needed as soon as possible if:
- Patients are experiencing serotonin syndrome or serotonin withdrawal.
- Patients are assessed as being at risk of harming themselves or others.
- Patients are so profoundly impaired by their symptoms that their own health is acutely suffering.
- The provider is unsure of this risk.

Urgent intervention is needed within 1 week when:
- The patient is assessed as being at high risk for suicide, yet is currently safe.
- Other psychiatric co-morbidities are present.
- There is an indication for electroconvulsive therapy.

Follow up with specialty provider is needed within 1 month when:
- Recurrent symptoms are not responding to treatments provided in the primary care setting.
- Complications with medication management require frequent follow up.
- Dementia is also present.
- Patients may benefit from psychotherapy, family education, or group support.

PATIENT AND FAMILY EDUCATION

Loved ones and family members may notice improvement in someone receiving treatment before the patient feels better. Depressed mood and hopelessness are often the last symptoms to respond to medications. During times of remission, the risk for suicide persists. Patients and families require education regarding the recurrent nature of depression and the risk for suicide. Information about the importance of complete remission of symptoms is also needed to improve prognosis and prevent complications related to other medical illnesses. Social support may help identify warning signs of a recurring depressive episode and precipitate earlier treatment, which in turn predicts a better treatment response. Support groups or resources for families are often available through community mental health centers. National resources include the National Institute of Mental Health and the National Alliance on Mental Illness.

HEALTH PROMOTION

Regardless of predisposing factors, healthy lifestyle choices offer some protective value related to the onset of MDD given a particular stressor. Diets low in sugars and carbohydrates and high in ω3-fatty acids and antioxidants have been associated with a generally stable and content mood.[38] Mineral supplementation is not recommended as effective prevention for MDD. Exercise has been associated with acute improvements in mood as well as long-term benefits. As with most diseases and disorders, lifestyle modifications may reduce the risk of onset and deter the course of an illness, yet may not fully mediate the impact of biologic influences.

REFERENCES

1. American Psychiatric Association: *Diagnostic and statistical manual of mental disorders,* ed 4 (text rev), Washington, DC, 2000, The Association.
2. World Health Organization: *Disability adjusted life years (DALY),* retrieved Jan 29, 2006, from http://www.who.int/healthinfo/boddaly/en/print.html.
3. Ustun TB, Ayuso-Mateos JL, Chatterji S, and others: Global burden of depressive disorders in the year 2000, *Br J Psychiatry* 184:386-392, 2004.
4. Lecrubier Y: The burden of depression and anxiety in general medicine, *J Clin Psychiatry* 62(Suppl 8):4-9, 2001.
5. Thomas MR, Waxmonsky JA, Gabow PA, and others: Prevalence of psychiatric disorders and costs of care among adult enrollees in a Medicaid HMO, *Psychiatr Serv* 56(11):1394-1401, 2005.
6. Weissman MM, Leaf PJ, Holzer CE, and others: The epidemiology of depression: an update on sex differences in rates, *J Affect Disorders* 7:179-188, 1984.
7. Kessler RC, Nelson CB, McGonagle KA, and others: Comorbidity of DSM-III-R major depressive disorder in the general population, *Br J Psychiatry* 168:17-30, 1996.
8. Kessler RC, Berglund P, Demler O, and others: The epidemiology of major depressive disorder: results from the national comorbidity survey replication (NCS-R), *JAMA* 289(23):3095-3105, 2003.
9. Hasin DS, Goodwin RD, Stinson FS, and others: Epidemiology of major depressive disorder: results from the national epidemiologic survey on alcoholism and related conditions, *Arch Gen Psychiatry* 62:1097-1106, 2005.
10. Oquendo MA, Ellis SP, Greenwald S, and others: Ethnic and sex differences in suicide rates relative to major depression in the United States, *Am J Psychiatry* 158:1652-1658, 2001.
11. Asarnow JR, Jaycox LH, Duan N, and others: Depression and role impairment among adolescents in primary care clinics, *J Adolesc Health* 37:477-483, 2005.

12. Alexopoulos GS: Depression in the elderly, *Lancet* 365:1961-1970, 2005.
13. Blazer D: Depression in late life: a review and commentary, *J Gerontol* 58A(3):249-265, 2003.
14. Birrer RB, Vemuri SP: Depression in later life: a diagnostic and therapeutic challenge, *Am Fam Phys* 69(10):2375-2382, 2004.
15. Smalbrugge M, Pot AM, Jongenelis K, and others: Prevalence and correlates of anxiety among nursing home patients, *J Affect Disorders* 88(2):145-153, 2005.
16. Herman JP, Ostrander MM, Mueller NK, and others: Limbic system mechanisms of stress regulation: hypothalamo-pituitary-adreno-cortical axis, *Progress Neuro-Psychopharm Biol Psychiatry* 29:1201-1213, 2005.
17. Garlow SJ, Messelman DL, Nemeroff CB: The neurochemistry of mood disorders: clinical studies. In Charney DS, Nestler EJ, Bunney BS, editors: *Neurobiology of mental illness,* New York, 1999, Oxford University Press.
18. Coryell W, Nopoulos P, Drevets W, and others: Subgenual prefrontal cortex volumes in major depressive disorder and schizophrenia: diagnostic specificity and prognostic implications, *Am J Psychiatry* 162:1706-1712, 2005.
19. Duman RS: The neurochemistry of mood disorders: preclinical studies. In Charney DS, Nestler EJ, Bunney BS, editors: *Neurobiology of mental illness,* New York, 1999, Oxford University Press.
20. Posener JA, Debattists C, Veldhuis JD, and others: Process irregularity of cortisol and adrenocorticotropin secretion in men with depressive disorder, *Psychoneuroendocrinology* 29:1129-1137, 2004.
21. Burke HM, Davis MC, Otte C, and others: Depression and cortisol responses to psychological stress: a meta-analysis, *Psychoneuroendo-crinology* 30:846-856, 2005.
22. Campbell S, MacQueen G: The role of the hippocampus in the pathophysiology of major depression, *J Psychiatry Neurosci* 29(6):417-426, 2004.
23. Neumeister A, Young T, Stastny J: Implications of genetic research on the role of the serotonin in depression: emphasis on the serotonin type 1A receptor and the serotonin transporter, *Psychopharmacology* 174:512-524, 2004.
24. Rice F, Harold GT, Thapar A: The link between depression in mothers and offspring: an extended twin analysis, *Behav Genet* 35(5):565-577, 2005.
25. Shih RA, Belmonte PL, Zandi PP: A review of the evidence from family, twin and adoption studies for a genetic contribution to adult psychiatric disorders, *Int Rev Psychiatry* 16(4):260-283, 2004.
26. McGuffin P, Knight J, Breen G, and others: Whole genome linkage scan of recurrent depressive disorder from the depression network study, *Hum Molec Genet* 14(22):3337-3345, 2005.
27. Mulder RT, Joyce PR, Frampton C, and others: Six months of treatment for depression: outcome and predictors of the course of illness, *Am J Psychiatry* 163:95-100, 2006.
28. D'Ath P, Katona P, Mullan E, and others: Screening, detection and management of depression in elderly primary care attenders: the acceptability and performance of the 15 item Geriatric Depression Scale (GDS15) and the development of short versions, *Fam Pract* 11(3):260-266, 1994.
29. Goodwin RD, Kroenke K, Hoven CW, and others: Major depression, physical illness, and suicidal ideation in primary care, *Psychosom Med* 65:501-505, 2003.
30. Watson LC, Pignone MP: Screening accuracy for late-life depression in primary care: a systematic review, *J Fam Pract* 52(12):956-964, 2003.
31. Depression Guideline Panel: *Depression in primary care: treatment of major depression,* Clinical Practice Guideline, 2(5), AHCPR Pub No 93-0551, Washington, DC, 1993, US Department of Health and Human Services, Public Health Service, Agency for Health Care Policy and Research.
32. Arana GW, Rosenbaum JF: *Handbook of psychiatric drug therapy,* ed 4, Philadelphia, 2000, Lippincott.
33. Bezchlibnyk-Butler KZ, Jeffries JJ, editors: *Clinical handbook of psychotropic drugs,* ed 12 (rev), Seattle, 2002, Hogrefe & Huber.
34. Sutherland JE, Sutherland SJ, Hoehns JD: Achieving the best outcome in treatment of depression, *J Fam Pract* 52(3):201-209, 2003.
35. Joffe RT, Levitt AJ, Sokolov ST, and others: Response to an open label trial of a second SSRI in major depression, *J Clin Psychiatry* 57(3):114-115, 1996.
36. Schüle C, Baghi TC, Alajbegovic L, and others: The influence of 4-week treatment with sertraline on the combined T3/TRH test in depressed patients, *Eur Arch Psychiatry Clin Neurosci* 255:334-340, 2005.
37. Westbrook D, Kirk J: The clinical effectiveness of cognitive behaviour therapy: outcome for a large sample of adults treated in routine practice, *Behav Res Ther* 43:1243-1261, 2005.
38. Bodner LM, Wisner KL: Nutrition and depression: implication for improving mental health among childbearing-aged women, *Biol Psychiatry* 58:679-685, 2005.
39. Tuunainen A, Kripke DF, Endo T: Light therapy for non-seasonal depression, *Cochrane Database Syst Rev* (2):CD004050.pub2; DOI: 10.1002/14651858; CD004050.pub.2, 2004.
40. Tsuchiyama K, Nagayama H, Yamada K, and others: Predicting efficacy of electroconvulsive therapy in major depressive disorder, *Psychiatry Clin Neurosci* 59:546-550, 2005.
41. Loo CK, Mitchell PB: A review of the efficacy of transcranial magnetic stimulation (TMS) treatment for depression, and current and future strategies to optimize efficacy, *J Affect Disorders* 88:255-267, 2005.
42. Clarke G, Debar L, Lynch F, and others: A randomized effectiveness trial of brief cognitive-behavioral therapy for depressed adolescents receiving antidepressant medication, *J Am Acad Child Adolesc Psychiatry* 44(9):888-898, 2005.
43. Hamrin V, Scahill L: Selective serotonin reuptake inhibitors for children and adolescents with major depression: current controversies and recommendations, *Issues Mental Health Nurs* 26(45):433-450, 2005.
44. Isacsson G, Holmgren P, Ahlner J: Selective serotonin reuptake inhibitor antidepressants and the risk of suicide: a controlled forensic database study of 14,857 suicides, *Acta Psychiatry Scand* 111(4):286-290, 2005.
45. Weller FB, Tucker S, Weller RA: The selective serotonin reuptake inhibitors controversy in the treatment of depression in children, *Curr Psychiatry Rep* 7(2):87-90, 2005.
46. Hays JC, Saunders WB, Flint EP, and others: Social support and depression as risk factors for loss of physical function in late life, *Aging Mental Health* 1(3):209-220, 1997.
47. Bhogal SK, Teasell R, Foley N, and others: Lesion location and post-stroke depression; systematic review of the methodological limitations in the literature, *Stroke* 35:794-802, 2004.
48. Petersen T, Iosifescu DV, Papakostas GI, and others: Clinical characteristics of depressed patients with diabetes mellitus, *Int Clin Psychopharmacol* 21(1):43-47, 2006.
49. Schins A, Honig A, Crijns H, and others: Increased coronary events in depressed cardiovascular patients: 5-HT_{2a} receptor as missing link, *Psychosom Med* 65:729-737, 2003.
50. Centers for Disease Control and Prevention: *Suicide fact sheet,* retrieved March 14, 2007, from http://www.cdc.gov/ncipc.
51. Centers for Disease Control and Prevention: *Injury mortality maps of the United States: 1989-1998,* Atlanta, 2001, retrieved Jan 22, 2006, from http://webappa.cdc.gove/cdc_mxt3.
52. National Institute of Mental Health: *Depression,* retrieved Jan 22, 2006, from http://www.nimh.nih.gov/healthinformation/depression-menu.cfm.
53. Gask L: Overt and covert barriers to the integration of primary and specialist mental health care, *Soc Sci Med* 61:1785-1794, 2005.
54. Gilbody SM, Whitty PM, Grimshaw JM, and others: Improving the detection and management of depression in primary care, *Qual Safety Health Care* 12:149-155, 2003.

CHAPTER 262

Eating Disorders*

Barbara E. Wolfe, Eran D. Metzger,
Laurie L. Flanagan, and David C. Jimerson

DEFINITION AND EPIDEMIOLOGY

Anorexia nervosa and bulimia nervosa are psychiatric disorders characterized by excessive concern with body shape and weight. Impaired psychosocial functioning often accompanies these disorders, and serious medical consequences may arise as a result of the behavioral manifestations of the illness. Diagnostic criteria and clinical characteristics are reviewed in detail later.

The lifetime prevalence of anorexia nervosa is approximately 0.5% to 1% among young adult women, although the lifetime prevalence has been reported to be as high as 2% in an urban-suburban population.[1,2] Lifetime prevalence of bulimia nervosa is approximately 1% to 3% among female adolescents and young adults,[3,4] with a more recent report as high as 4.6% in urban-suburban–dwelling young women.[2] Typically bulimia nervosa is more common than anorexia, although the reverse may be true in some cultures.[5] Women are 10 times more likely than men to be affected by an eating disorder. Caucasian women tend to report greater disturbances in eating, as well as body dissatisfaction, compared with minority groups, although ethnic differences appear to diminish when formal clinical disorders are examined.[6] Age of onset is typically during adolescence and young adulthood. The course of the illness is variable and is often influenced by medical complications and psychiatric co-morbidity. Anorexia nervosa is associated with an increased mortality rate,[7] with evidence that suicide may be a leading cause of death among patients referred to a tertiary care treatment program.[8]

PATHOPHYSIOLOGY

Psychologic and environmental factors are likely to influence the development of an eating disorder. In addition, research has focused on understanding potential biologic influences, including variations in neurochemicals involved in the modulation of eating behavior. Laboratory studies have shown that stimulation of carbohydrate intake may result from increased activity of norepinephrine and neuropeptide Y in the hypothalamus. Serotonin and cholecystokinin suppress food intake and increase satiety. Dopamine and opiates influence food cravings and the food reward system.[9] Studies in laboratory animals suggest that leptin decreases food intake while also increasing the use of energy.[10]

Studies have demonstrated abnormalities in several of these neurochemical systems in patients with active symptoms of anorexia nervosa and bulimia nervosa.[11] However, little is known regarding which of these alterations may be a consequence of the illness itself. Although some abnormalities return to normal with the remission of symptoms, certain changes (e.g., in the serotonin system) may be more persistent.

CLINICAL PRESENTATION

Patients with anorexia nervosa typically exhibit denial regarding the potential seriousness of their reduced weight state. Despite life-threatening cachexia, these patients maintain a need to lose weight, often reflecting distortions in body image. Many patients with anorexia nervosa have other coexisting psychiatric disorders.[12] Depression is common, with depressive symptoms often remitting after weight restoration. An estimated 25% to 50% of patients with anorexia nervosa have a lifetime history of an anxiety disorder, including obsessive-compulsive disorder, panic disorder, social phobia, or generalized anxiety disorder. Recent data suggest that the anxiety disorders predate the onset of an eating disorder, pointing to a potential vulnerability to the development of an eating disorder.[13] Up to one third of patients with anorexia nervosa, particularly those with the binge-eating/purging type, have a co-morbid alcohol or substance abuse or dependence disorder.

Patients with bulimia nervosa characteristically demonstrate feelings of shame and embarrassment regarding their symptoms. Efforts to maintain the secrecy of the disorder are often accompanied by social withdrawal and a denial of illness. Psychiatric co-morbidity is common.[12] As many as half of the patients with bulimia nervosa have a lifetime history of major depression. Alcohol and substance abuse or dependence disorders are also common, perhaps reflecting increased impulsivity in this patient group. Approximately one third of patients with bulimia nervosa have a lifetime history of an anxiety disorder, which generally includes social phobia, obsessive-compulsive disorder, or generalized anxiety disorder.

Other conditions that may be evident on presentation include personality disorders and trauma history. Dependent, avoidant, obsessive-compulsive, and borderline are the most commonly occurring personality disorders in patients with eating disorders.[12] Borderline personality disorder appears to more frequent in bulimia nervosa than in anorexia nervosa, perhaps contributing to impulse dysregulation and self-destructive behavior at times observed in this patient group. Sexual trauma in patients with eating disorders has been widely reported in the literature, although a causal relationship between an eating disorder and trauma history remains to be elucidated.

PHYSICAL EXAMINATION

A comprehensive psychiatric history, medical history, and physical examination are customarily recommended for the initial assessment of a patient with an eating disorder. The initial appearance of a patient with anorexia nervosa may be deceptive if the health care provider is under the assumption that all such patients appear outwardly cachectic. Loose-fitting or baggy clothes are common attire for patients with this disorder and often disguise weight loss. Body weight for a female adolescent with anorexia nervosa is typically below a body mass index of 17.5 kg/m^2.[14] Vital sign abnormalities include depression of core body temperature and bradycardia

*Supported in part by a USPHS grant (R01 MH057395) from the National Institute of Mental Health.

(e.g., pulse in the range of 40 to 60 beats per minute). However, heart rate may manifest tachycardia in the event of dehydration, or tachyarrhythmia secondary to ipecac-induced cardiomyopathy. Blood pressure is generally low, and postural changes in heart rate and blood pressure typically exceed the normal range.

Dry skin and decreased turgor indicate dehydration, and temporal wasting may be apparent. Thinning hair, a sign of malnutrition, is often noted. Lanugo, a covering of dry, downy hair, may be observed over the neck, cheeks, forearms, and legs. The skin may adopt a yellow hue as a result of hypercarotenemia. Examination of the mouth often reveals poor dentition related to self-induced vomiting. These dental changes are most commonly observed on the interior aspects of the molars, which exhibit a subtle loss of luster and mild discoloration where the gastric acid has eroded the enamel. Skin abrasion or scarring over the carpometacarpal joints (Russell's sign) is additional evidence of a history of self-induced vomiting.

Examination of the chest and abdomen reveals protruding ribs and a dramatically reduced abdominal girth, with protrusion of the iliac crests. Cardiac auscultation often uncovers abnormalities in heart rhythm. A neurologic examination may show motor weakness that accompanies muscle wasting. Hypothyroidism secondary to malnutrition may result in a characteristic latency in deep tendon reflexes.

Unlike patients with anorexia nervosa, patients with bulimia do not typically have the physical signs of severe cachexia, but laboratory studies may reveal evidence of malnutrition related to abnormal dietary patterns. Physical signs of self-induced vomiting (dental erosion, Russell's sign) may be apparent in patients who use this method of purging. Patients who binge and self-induce vomiting may also have enlarged salivary glands, particularly the parotid glands. Preliminary research suggests a correlation between salivary gland enlargement and elevated serum amylase.[15] Rarely, binge eating and self-induced vomiting can result in severe medical complications such as esophagitis, esophageal tears, or gastric perforation.

DIAGNOSTICS

The fourth edition of the *Diagnostic and Statistical Manual of Mental Disorders* (DSM-IV) published specific criteria defining anorexia nervosa and bulimia nervosa (Boxes 262-1 and 262-2).[16] Individuals who do not meet formal criteria for

DIAGNOSTICS

Eating Disorders

LABORATORY	
CBC and differential*	LFTs*
Serum electrolytes	Cholesterol
Calcium*	TSH, T_3
Phosphorus*	FSH, LH*
Magnesium*	Urinalysis
BUN	**OTHER**
Creatinine	ECG

*If indicated.

BOX 262-1

DIAGNOSTIC CRITERIA FOR ANOREXIA NERVOSA

A. Refusal to maintain body weight at or above a minimally normal weight for age and height (e.g., weight loss leading to maintenance of body weight less than 85% of that expected; or failure to make expected weight gain during period of growth, leading to body weight less than 85% of the expected).
B. Intense fear of gaining weight or becoming fat, even though underweight.
C. Disturbance in the way in which one's body weight or shape is experienced, undue influence of body weight or shape on self-evaluation, or denial of the seriousness of the current low body weight.
D. In postmenarcheal females, amenorrhea, i.e., the absence of at least three consecutive menstrual cycles. (A woman is considered to have amenorrhea if her periods occur only following hormone, e.g., estrogen, administration.)

Specify type:

- **Restricting Type:** During the current episode of Anorexia Nervosa, the person has not regularly engaged in binge-eating or purging behavior (i.e., self-induced vomiting or the misuse of laxatives, diuretics, or enemas).
- **Binge-Eating/Purging Type:** During the current episode of Anorexia Nervosa, the person has regularly engaged in binge-eating or purging behavior (i.e., self-induced vomiting or the misuse of laxatives, diuretics, or enemas).

From American Psychiatric Association: *Diagnostic and statistical manual of mental disorders*, ed 4 (text rev), Washington, DC, 2000, The Association.

BOX 262-2

DIAGNOSTIC CRITERIA FOR BULIMIA NERVOSA

A. Recurrent episodes of binge eating. An episode of binge eating is characterized by both of the following:
   (1) Eating in a discrete period of time (e.g., within any 2-hour period) an amount of food that is definitely larger than most people would eat during a similar period of time and under similar circumstances
   (2) A sense of lack of control over eating during the episode (e.g., a feeling that one cannot stop eating or control what or how much one is eating)
B. Recurrent inappropriate compensatory behavior in order to prevent weight gain, such as self-induced vomiting; misuse of laxatives, diuretics, enemas, or other medications; fasting; or excessive exercise.
C. The binge eating and inappropriate compensatory behaviors both occur, on average, at least twice a week for 3 months.
D. Self-evaluation is unduly influenced by body shape and weight.
E. The disturbance does not occur exclusively during episodes of Anorexia Nervosa.

Specify type:

- **Purging Type:** During the current episode of Bulimia Nervosa, the person has regularly engaged in self-induced vomiting or the misuse of laxatives, diuretics, or enemas.
- **Nonpurging Type:** During the current episode of Bulimia Nervosa, the person has used other inappropriate compensatory behaviors, such as fasting or excessive exercise, but has not regularly engaged in self-induced vomiting or the misuse of laxatives, diuretics, or enemas.

From American Psychiatric Association: *Diagnostic and statistical manual of mental disorders*, ed 4 (text rev), Washington, DC, 2000, The Association.

anorexia nervosa or bulimia nervosa may fall under the diagnostic category of Eating Disorder Not Otherwise Specified. This latter diagnostic category currently includes the DSM-IV provisional diagnosis (in need of further study) identified as Binge Eating Disorder, which characterizes individuals who experience regular binge eating but do not engage in routine compensatory behaviors to prevent weight gain.

DIFFERENTIAL DIAGNOSIS

Alternative medical and psychiatric diagnoses should be considered during the initial evaluation, particularly when the clinical presentation is atypical. Such characteristics include an unusual age of onset or an absence of symptoms related to a preoccupation with body weight and shape. Medical illnesses that may mimic some aspects of anorexia nervosa include peptic ulcer disease, hyperthyroidism, primary or secondary adrenocortical insufficiency, AIDS, and cancer. A voracious appetite is associated with the rarely occurring Kleine-Levin syndrome. A change in body weight and eating patterns can accompany psychiatric conditions such as drug abuse (e.g., alcohol, cocaine and other stimulants), major depression, and schizophrenia. A preoccupation with body shape, without the additional eating disorder diagnostic characteristics, raises the possibility of body dysmorphic disorder.

MANAGEMENT

Successful management of patients with eating disorders involves ongoing and thorough assessment, planning, intervention, and evaluation. It depends on proficient communication and collaborative efforts with other health care professionals who are involved in the care or treatment of the patient. Communication with the patient is crucial to establish the critically needed therapeutic alliance.

For patients with anorexia nervosa, medical stability and restoration of body weight to the point of resumption of normal bodily function (e.g., restoration of menses) are primary concerns. Monitoring body weight provides an index of nutritional changes, with frequency of assessment based on the patient's weight status. For the adolescent patient, ongoing monitoring of developmental growth is important and includes regular measurement of body height and weight. Weight gain is achieved based on the patient's ability to increase caloric intake. Caloric intake may initially start in the range of 1000 to 1600 kcal/day, with a progressive increase to allow for body weight restoration and maintenance.[14] Targeted weight gain parameters generally range from 0.2 to 0.4 kg (0.5 to 1 pound) per week for nonhospitalized individuals and 0.9 to 1.4 kg (2 to 3 pounds) per week for hospitalized patients.[14]

DIFFERENTIAL DIAGNOSIS

Eating Disorders

MEDICAL
- AIDS
- Cancer
- Hyperthyroidism
- Kleine-Levin syndrome
- Peptic ulcer disease
- Primary or secondary adrenocortical insufficiency

PSYCHIATRIC
- Body dysmorphic disorder
- Drug abuse
- Major depression
- Schizophrenia

Refeeding during a significantly low-weight malnourished state requires careful assessment of vital signs, electrolytes, and signs and symptoms of fluid overload. Excessive or rapid refeeding has been associated with seizures, cardiac arrhythmias, delirium, and, in rare instances congestive heart failure.[17] Vitamin, mineral, and food supplements may be necessary during the initial weight gain phase.

Periodic monitoring of serum electrolytes should be considered in cases of anorexia nervosa or bulimia nervosa, and particularly for individuals with frequent purging behaviors, who are at increased risk for hypokalemia.[18] A finding of hypokalemia should be followed up with an ECG, with attention given to possible cardiac conduction and rhythm disturbances.

The potential role of psychotropic medications in the initial treatment of an eating disorder is evaluated in the context of presenting symptoms and co-morbid conditions. In general, medications are not a first-line treatment for anorexia nervosa unless co-morbid conditions such as major depression, severe anxiety disorder, or psychosis necessitate such interventions.[14] There is little evidence from well-controlled clinical trials that psychotropic medications contribute to weight gain in anorexia nervosa, although preliminary data suggest that antidepressant medications of the serotonin selective reuptake inhibitor (SSRI) class (e.g., fluoxetine) may help prevent relapse after weight restoration.[19] After treatment of malnutrition, psychosocial interventions are thought to be particularly helpful.

For bulimia nervosa, treatment primarily focuses on reducing the binge and purge behavior. Outpatient psychotherapy is often effective for bulimia nervosa and is advantageous as an initial treatment modality for many patients. Of the various psychotherapeutic modalities, currently cognitive behavior therapy appears to have the most evidence demonstrating efficacy with bulimia nervosa.[14] Medications may be part of an initial treatment plan for patients with bulimia nervosa, particularly since placebo-controlled trials have shown that administration of an antidepressant agent may contribute to a diminished frequency of binge-eating and purging behaviors, even in the absence of current depression. Medications also may be particularly beneficial for patients who show a limited response to an initial period of psychotherapy or manifest a co-morbid condition. The SSRIs have received particular attention, in part because of their relatively favorable side effect profile.[20] Tricyclic antidepressants are an alternative for patients who are refractory to SSRIs, although these medications may require more frequent monitoring of blood pressure and cardiac function. Use of tricyclic antidepressant agents necessitates extreme caution with patients at risk for suicide attempt. Monoamine oxidase inhibitors are generally avoided given that adherence to the required low-tyramine diet may prove difficult for a patient with an eating disorder. Clinical consensus suggests that a combined approach of psychotherapy and medications may be more efficacious than either modality alone.[14]

Management of eating disorders is ideally conducted by a multidisciplinary team, which often includes a health care provider, dietitian, and individual psychotherapist. Consultation with an endocrinologist may be particularly helpful in assessing the cause of amenorrhea during the initial evaluative phase. Referral for a dental examination is indicated for patients engaged in self-induced vomiting. A psychiatric clinician can make important contributions to the assessment and treatment planning phases, as well as provide individual or group psychotherapy and a referral to appropriate support groups. A family therapist may also play an important role in the treatment of children and older patients. The psychiatric clinician or a consultant psychopharmacologist often manages psychotropic medication intervention.

LIFE SPAN CONSIDERATIONS

Although the onset of eating disorders typically occurs during adolescence or young adulthood, the illness can be present and recur during other life phases. Relapse is likely to happen during periods of increased stress. Patients with bulimia nervosa are most vulnerable to relapse during the first 6 months after psychiatric treatment for the disorder.[21] Eating disorders are often chronic conditions; although symptoms of bulimia nervosa are responsive to treatment, complete abstinence from binge eating may be a difficult goal in short-term treatment.[22] Certain metabolic sequelae of an eating disorder, such as decreased bone mineral density, may have residual consequences later in life. Pregnancy, while rare in anovulatory states such as anorexia nervosa, poses significant concerns for patients with an active eating disorder and requires frequent assessment of adequate nutrition, weight gain, and eating disorder symptoms.[23]

COMPLICATIONS

Clinical laboratory abnormalities are often encountered in patients with eating disorders, particularly when malnutrition is marked and purging behaviors are frequent. For non-hospitalized, normal-weight individuals, initial laboratory tests often include a CBC, electrolytes, BUN, creatinine level, thyroid function tests, and urinalysis.[14] In the presence of severe symptoms or poor nutritional states, liver function tests and the measurement of serum calcium, phosphorus, and magnesium may be indicated.[14] An initial ECG may be particularly valuable in the presence of severely low body weight, significant malnutrition, or a history of regular abuse of ipecac. Levels of serum follicle-stimulating hormone (FSH) and luteinizing hormone (LH) are included as part of an evaluation of persistent amenorrhea for individuals at normal weight. Serum estradiol levels and the measurement of bone mineral density (e.g., dual energy x-ray absorptiometry) provide indexes of bone loss and the risk for fracture and may be indicated for individuals with prolonged low-weight states.

The hematologic profile associated with anorexia nervosa reflects nutrition-related anemia and may also reveal leukopenia and thrombocytopenia. Mineral and electrolyte abnormalities can include decreased chloride, calcium, magnesium, and phosphate. BUN levels may be increased as a result of dehydration or decreased in association with muscle wasting. Malnutrition may result in elevated serum levels of hepatic enzymes and cholesterol. Commonly observed endocrine alterations include elevations in serum cortisol and growth hormone levels. A history of secondary amenorrhea is characteristically associated with decreased levels of FSH, LH, estrogen, and progesterone. Although levels of TSH are often normal, a malnutrition-related sick euthyroid syndrome is associated with reduced concentrations of serum tri-iodothyronine (T_3).

Anemia is common, particularly among patients who are strict vegetarians. In patients with frequent self-induced vomiting, electrolyte measurements may reveal increased concentrations of serum bicarbonate, which suggests metabolic alkalosis. Less commonly, laxative abuse may contribute to decreased serum bicarbonate levels. Self-induced vomiting, laxative abuse, and diuretic abuse may result in hypokalemia, hypochloremia, and hypomagnesemia. Severe hypokalemia, with an increased risk for life-threatening arrhythmia, can occur in patients with bulimia nervosa but is a relatively uncommon finding in outpatients. Repeated use of ipecac to induce vomiting may increase the risk for cardiomyopathy resulting from emetine toxicity.

ECG disturbances occur in both anorexia nervosa and bulimia nervosa. In anorexia nervosa, severe malnutrition is commonly associated with bradycardia. Abnormalities in heart rhythm, including prolonged QT intervals, may rarely be associated with sudden death. As previously noted, hypokalemia may be observed in both disorders, contributing to prolonged ventricular repolarization as reflected in QT prolongation or U waves.

INDICATIONS FOR REFERRAL OR HOSPITALIZATION

Weight loss and medical complications may become severe enough to warrant hospitalization. Significant electrolyte disturbances, for example, can require inpatient cardiac monitoring. Severe malnutrition may result in transient cognitive impairment to the extent that the patient is incapable of making a valid decision about care; in such instances, involuntary hospitalization may be necessary to ensure safety. Hospitalization is also indicated in the presence of significant co-morbid psychiatric conditions such as depression with suicidal ideation.

Although uncommon, enteral and parenteral alimentation may be considered during hospitalization when a severely malnourished patient is medically compromised and unable to comply with less invasive measures. These modes of refeeding can be accompanied by serious medical risks and may require intensive medical monitoring for potential problems. A refusal of life-sustaining care may require legal petitioning for a medical guardian.

Hospitalization provides patients with an opportunity to discontinue potentially harmful forms of purging while receiving intensive psychologic, nursing, and medical support. Laxatives, diuretics, and diet pills can usually be discontinued rapidly, with symptomatic treatment of the resultant constipation or edema. Medical-psychiatric inpatient units often have specific, behaviorally oriented protocols for working with patients with eating disorders. Partial hospital programs provide an alternative to inpatient hospitalizations for symptomatic patients who can be treated in a less restrictive setting.

PATIENT AND FAMILY EDUCATION

Education about the disorder, medical consequences, nutritional needs, and treatment options is important for patients and families. Information regarding specific interventions (e.g., medication treatment) is necessary not only for informed consent but also for enhancing adherence to the treatment regimen. For younger patients, it is often important to educate family members about the etiology, course of illness, prognosis, and treatment of the disorder. Attention to these needs helps build the alliance required for treatment adherence and longitudinal medical monitoring.

HEALTH PROMOTION

Risk factors are not fully understood, and it is unlikely that there will prove to be a single cause for eating disorders; however, there are several identifiable at-risk groups for whom primary prevention may be important. Adolescence, for example, is a time of developmental body change, weight gain, challenge to self-esteem, peer pressure, and increased external influences related to body image. Teens may be particularly vulnerable to media messages that portray an unrealistic waiflike figure as the "ideal" body shape. In an era where more than one third of the U.S. adult population is overweight, dieting behavior is rampant. Dieting behavior is thought to be a potential risk factor for an eating disorder because it often precedes the onset of illness. Individuals participating in activities such as ballet, gymnastics, wrestling, or crew may be subject to pressures related to minimizing body weight. Thus they may be vulnerable to the use of compensatory behaviors to prevent weight gain. Although all these groups may be at risk, it is clear that no single stressor provides a comprehensive explanation for the development of an eating disorder. Thus the context in which a set of risk factors operates is likely to be important for expression of the disorder in the person who may, for example, be biologically or genetically vulnerable.

Although in their infancy, primary prevention strategies are currently being tested by the research community. There seems to be little argument about the potential value of primary prevention, but less agreement with regard to the content of such programs. Some critics fear that educational components focused on compensatory behaviors used to prevent weight gain, for example, have the potential for introducing unhealthy behaviors to vulnerable individuals who may have not otherwise known about them. Programs that focus on positive eating habits, nutritional values, positive-self-esteem, and coping strategies seem likely to be beneficial, although the long-term effectiveness in preventing an eating disorder remains unknown.

REFERENCES

1. Walters EE, Kendler KS: Anorexia nervosa and anorexic-like syndromes in a population-based female twin sample, *Am J Psychiatry* 152(1):64-71, 1995.
2. Favaro A, Ferrara S, Santonastaso P: The spectrum of eating disorders in young women: a prevalence study in a general population, *Psychosom Med* 65:701-708, 2003.
3. Garfinkel PE, Lin E, Goering P, and others: Bulimia nervosa in a Canadian community sample: prevalence and comparison of subgroups, *Am J Psychiatry* 152(7):1052-1058, 1995.
4. Kendler KS, MacLean C, Neale M, and others: The genetic epidemiology of bulimia nervosa, *Am J Psychiatry* 148(12):1627-1637, 1991.
5. Nakamura K, Yamamoto M, Yamazaki O, and others: Prevalence of anorexia nervosa and bulimia nervosa in a geographically defined area in Japan, *Int J Eat Disord* 28(2):173-180, 2000.
6. Wildes JE, Emery RE: The roles of ethnicity and culture in the development of eating disturbances and body dissatisfaction: a meta-analytic review, *Clin Psychol Rev* 21(4):521-551, 2001.
7. Sullivan PF: Mortality in anorexia nervosa, *Am J Psychiatry* 152(7):1073-1074, 1995.
8. Birmingham CL, Su J, Hlynsky JA, and others: The mortality rate from anorexia nervosa, *Int J Eat Disord* 38(2):143-146, 2005.
9. Woods SC, Seeley RJ, Porte D, and others: Signals that regulate food intake and energy homeostasis, *Science* 280:1378-1383, 1998.
10. Friedman JM, Halaas JL: Leptin and the regulation of body weight in mammals, *Nature* 395:763-770, 1998.
11. Kuikka JT, Tammela L, Karhunen L: Reduced serotonin transporter binding in binge eating women, *Psychopharmacology* 155:310-314, 2001.
12. Braun DL, Sunday SR, Halmi KA: Psychiatric comorbidity in patients with eating disorders, *Psychol Med* 24(4):859-867, 1994.
13. Kaye WH, Bulik CM, Thornton L, and others: Comorbidity of anxiety disorders with anorexia and bulimia nervosa, *Am J Psychiatry* 161(12):2215-2221, 2004.
14. American Psychiatric Association: *Practice guideline for the treatment of patients with eating disorders*, ed 3, Arlington, Va, 2006, The Association.
15. Metzger ED, Levine JM, McArdle CR, and others: Salivary gland enlargement and elevated serum amylase in bulimia nervosa, *Biol Psychiatry* 45(11):1520-1522, 1999.
16. American Psychiatric Association: *Diagnostic and statistical manual of mental disorders*, ed 4 (text rev), Washington, DC, 2000, The Association.
17. Kohn MR, Golden NH, Shenker IR: Cardiac arrest and delirium: presentations of the refeeding syndrome in severely malnourished adolescents with anorexia nervosa, *J Adolesc Health* 22:239-243, 1998.
18. Wolfe BE, Metzger ED, Levine JM, and others: Laboratory screening for electrolyte abnormalities and anemia in bulimia nervosa: a controlled study, *Int J Eat Disord* 30(3):288-293, 2001.
19. Kaye WH, Nagata T, Weltzin TE, and others: Double-blind placebo-controlled administration of fluoxetine in restricting and restricting-purging type anorexia nervosa, *Biol Psychiatry* 49(7):644-652, 2001.
20. Jimerson DC, Wolfe BE, Brotman AW, and others: Medications in the treatment of eating disorders, *Psychiatr Clin North Am* 19(4):739-754, 1996.
21. Olmsted MP, Kaplan AS, Rockert W: Rate and prediction of relapse in bulimia nervosa, *Am J Psychiatry* 151(5):738-743, 1994.
22. Fairburn CG, and others: The natural course of bulimia nervosa and binge eating disorder in young women, *Arch Gen Psychiatry* 57(7):659-665, 2000.
23. Wolfe BE: Reproductive health in women with eating disorders, *J Obstet Gynecol Neonatal Nurs* 34(2):255-263, 2005.

CHAPTER 263

Grief

Alice Bolton

DEFINITION AND EPIDEMIOLOGY

Grief, also referred to as *bereavement*, is the normal emotional and physical response to the death of a loved one but also occurs in the aftermath of other losses.[1] Grief is associated with a wide range of emotions, including sadness, anger, guilt, and despair, and is the most psychologically distressing event that most people will ever experience.[2] It is dynamic, pervasive, highly individualized, and found in all age-groups.[3]

Approximately 2 million to 2.5 million people die yearly in the United States, and it is estimated that each death leaves an average of five people bereaved, resulting in more than 10 million people in the United States grieving each year. Approximately 10% to 20% of persons develop complicated grief, a more severe and prolonged grief reaction.[4,5]

Grieving usually occurs after a person experiences the death of a family member, spouse, child, close friend, or pet. A grief response can also occur in response to other losses, such as a job or career loss, loss of physical health or abilities, miscarriage, divorce, financial loss, or the diminishing health of a spouse or loved one. The initial painful experience of disbelief, shock, loss, and sadness is often followed by a sense of emptiness, hopelessness, and loss of interest in usual activities, followed by a prolonged phase of restitution and recovery, which for many individuals represents a departure from the state of health and well-being they are used to.[6]

Many health care providers are uncomfortable talking about death with patients, even though it is an issue that every person will eventually have to deal with. As with every important life transition, perspectives on death are influenced and shaped by cultural norms and beliefs. Talking about death and loss can be an emotionally laden experience for both the patient and the provider, and it can be a temptation to respond in clichés. To prevent such responses, providers must be aware of their own feelings about death and loss. Providers can be most helpful during this time by providing support in a way that is consistent with the values, spirituality, and beliefs of each individual.

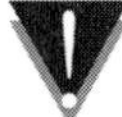

Immediate psychiatric evaluation is required for all patients with suicidal or homicidal ideation.

CLINICAL PRESENTATION

The length of the grief response varies. Estimates of 2 months to 2 years have been given. Individuals experience stages of grief: denial, anger, bargaining, depression, and acceptance.[7] The process is ongoing, does not follow a rigid order or time frame, and may vary or even skip stages. The stages of grief are not necessarily all obvious. They may be repeated many times and are often not completed before moving on to another stage. Kübler-Ross, one of the first observers of these phases, recognized that not everybody progresses through all the phases, or in the same way, but describing bereavement in terms of phases has given us a useful framework for thinking about grief, especially from a Western perspective.[8]

However, many cultures have different ways of coping with grief. Some cultures expect and encourage expressions of grief, whereas in other cultures these expressions are suppressed. For example, grieving among the Navajo is limited to a period of 4 days, and after that one is expected to show no signs of grief. In Samoan culture one is also expected to recover rapidly from the loss of a loved one, and expressions of grief considered normal in the United States are unknown in this Pacific Island culture.[8] In contrast, Orthodox Judaism understands grieving as a discipline, "one in which the mourner is not only allowed, but expected, to be engaged."[9] In Orthodox Jewish culture, the days, then the months, and then all the years after a death are marked with specific practices prescribed for each unit of time. Japanese Buddhists believe in maintaining contact with dead ancestors, and many homes have an altar dedicated to them. In contrast, the Hopi Indians believe that contact with death brings pollution, so they remove all reminders of their deceased relatives.[10]

Gender differences in grief responses have long been noted. Historically, researchers labeled these gender differences in grief "feminine" and "masculine"—the former characterized by openly displaying intense affect, seeking support, and sharing emotions with others. People who did not express their grief in this way, usually men, were considered to be responding in an inappropriate, unhealthy way.[11] More recently, it has been suggested that it might be more useful to characterize grief reactions as a continuum stretching from *instrumental* grief (cognitive, problem-solving ways of dealing with grief), which is generally more characteristic of the way men respond to grief, to *intuitive* grief (emotive, help-seeking ways of dealing with loss), which is generally more descriptive of the way women handle loss.[11] A instrumental griever might respond to his or her grief in honoring the deceased by building a memorial, finding ways to solve the problems arising from the loss, or even finding safe situations to express the loss. In contrast, an intuitive griever might experience the pain of the loss more deeply and be inclined to express emotions more openly and seek support from individuals or groups. Keeping this model in mind can be helpful in encouraging people find outlets for their grief that correspond to their place on the continuum.[11]

PHYSICAL EXAMINATION

Physical complaints, which are often vague, are common during the grieving period. Office visits to the health care provider may become more frequent. Sleep and appetite disturbances are often reported. Women have been reported to have more sickness than men after the death of a family member.[12]

DIAGNOSTICS

Although there are no definitive laboratory tests to diagnose grief, research has demonstrated the neuroanatomy of grief through MRI studies.[13] At this time, research findings are not sufficiently significant to enable a diagnosis of grief by laboratory testing. The physical symptoms of patients must be taken seriously, with disorders such as diabetes, anemia, hypothyroidism, hyperthyroidism, and gastrointestinal or cardiac abnormalities excluded as indicated.

DIFFERENTIAL DIAGNOSIS

Symptoms commonly associated with grief, such as sadness, low energy, and sleep and appetite disturbances, are also typical depression symptoms. However, the current official psychiatric nomenclature, based on the current diagnostic manual of the American Psychiatric Association, the *Diagnostic and Statistical Manual of Mental Disorders* (DSM-IV),[14] distinguishes between normal grief (bereavement) and depressive disorder precipitated by loss of a loved one. According to the DSM-IV, "Periods of sadness are inherent in the human aspects of the human experience" that should not be diagnosed as major depressive disorder (MDD) unless the criteria for severity, duration, and clinically significant distress or impairment are met.[6,14]

A syndrome of persistent symptoms and impairment related to grief has been described and referred to as *complicated grief* or, less commonly, traumatic grief. Complicated grief can sometimes co-occur with MDD or posttraumatic stress disorder (PTSD), but it has a distinct phenomenology, clinical course, and outcomes and thus warrants a separate diagnosis.[6] Characteristic features of complicated grief include persisting preoccupation with thoughts about the loved one along with longing, yearning, and inability to accept the death; distressing intrusive thoughts about the death; and avoidance of reminders about the loss.[6] Diagnostic criteria for complicated grief have been identified by Horowitz, Sonneborn, and Sugahara, and colleagues[15] and validated by Langner and Maercker.[16] These criteria include a loss that occurred at least 14 months ago; severe emotional symptoms related to memories of and yearnings for the lost relationship that interfered with daily functioning during the previous month; isolating behaviors; avoidance of contact with circumstances or situations that remind the person of the deceased; loss of interest in social, recreational, or work activities to a problematic degree; severe disruption in sleep patterns; and feelings of being alone or empty.[15]

Complicated grief and depression should be considered when diagnosing a grief reaction, and although they are related and often co-occur, they do constitute distinct reactions to loss.[17] An MDD is characterized by a change from a previous level of functioning during a 2-week period, with either a depressed mood or a loss of pleasure or interest in almost all activities. Symptoms associated with this disorder are prevalent all or most of the day. These include weight loss or gain not related to dieting; increased or decreased appetite; sleep disturbances; low energy or fatigue daily; psychomotor retardation or agitation; diminished concentration; inability to make decisions; excessive guilt or feelings or worthlessness; or a suicidal ideation, intent, plan, or attempt. To establish the diagnosis, these symptoms cannot result from a substance abuse disorder or medical condition and may significantly interfere with the person's ability to function. According to the DSM-IV, the diagnosis MDD should be considered when the duration of grief lasts more than 2 months and is associated with persistent feelings of guilt (not related to the loved one's death), preoccupation with thoughts about death (other than the loved one's), feelings of worthlessness, psychomotor retardation, and the inability to perform daily activities.

PTSD may be present if the death occurred in a violent or traumatic manner, especially if the patient witnessed it. PTSD is characterized by recurrent and disturbing recollections about the death; avoidance of situations having to do with the death; and increased arousal such as difficulty sleeping, difficulty concentrating, and outbursts of anger.[1]

DIFFERENTIAL DIAGNOSIS

Grief

GRIEF

- May be present up to 2 months after loss
- Guilt related to the deceased
- Thoughts of death related to the deceased
- Intact self-esteem
- Short-lived functional impairment
- No hallucinations; may "hear" voice of deceased or "see" image of deceased

COMPLICATED GRIEF

- Occurs up to 14 months
- Persistent feelings of being alone or empty
- Functional impairment
- Isolation
- Avoidance of situations reminiscent of the deceased

MAJOR DEPRESSIVE DISORDER

- Severe and persistent symptoms after bereavement, lasting 2 weeks or more
- Thoughts of death
- Feelings of worthlessness
- Prolonged and marked functional impairment
- Possible auditory or visual hallucinations unrelated to the deceased

POSTTRAUMATIC STRESS DISORDER

- May be present if the death occurred in a violent or traumatic manner
- Most likely if violent or traumatic death was witnessed
- Recurrent, disturbing recollections of the death
- Avoidance of situations having to do with the death
- Increased arousal (difficulty sleeping and concentrating, angry outbursts)

MANAGEMENT

Grief is a "normal" experience, and social support can often be helpful during the bereavement process. However, people do not always get the response they need from family and friends. People often seek help from health care providers for issues directly or indirectly related to their loss. Health care providers, like the rest of society, often find death and grief difficult to deal with. This is probably particularly true because there are few shared expectations in our societies concerning rituals, expressions of grief, and the provision of comfort. In health care settings, death and grieving may carry associations of failure that are difficult for the provider to accept.[2]

Management for uncomplicated grief includes empathetic responses from health care providers, support groups, books, and provision of symptom relief. Support group information should be available to the patient. The health care provider should be knowledgeable about the group, its affiliations, and its leadership. Understanding the way in which an individual processes and copes with grief is helpful. For example, an instrumental griever may appreciate information rather than counseling in response to his or her distress, whereas an intuitive griever responding to the same type of loss might appreciate counseling and support groups more.

Medication is the final consideration in treatment of the grief response. The primary concern should be to allow the process to unfold and progress toward resolution. However, in some cases short-term symptom relief is indicated. Benzodiazepines (clonazepam, lorazepam, and alprazolam) prescribed in small doses for infrequent use may be helpful for the anxiety and insomnia associated with grief.[18] However, current research is inconclusive regarding the use of benzodiazepines during bereavement.[19] There is a risk for addiction when prescribing such medications, and therefore they should not be prescribed for patients with any type of substance abuse history. In addition, when these medications are prescribed, the patient must be monitored for signs of tolerance as well as substance abuse. Taking more of the drug to achieve the desired affect is a clear indication of trouble. Limiting the number of tablets dispensed is an effective way to monitor use and prevent abuse. Clonazepam or lorazepam 0.5 mg b.i.d. or t.i.d. is usually more than adequate to provide relief of anxiety or insomnia. No more than 15 to 20 tablets need be dispensed weekly. Benzodiazepines should be used with extreme caution in older adults because of the great risk for falls and mental confusion in this age-group.[18] Follow-up office visits at frequent intervals (every 2 weeks) provide an opportunity to offer emotional support, assess the person's progress, and identify any complications.

Antidepressants may be indicated for some persons during the grief process.[20] Those who have not responded to short-term use of antianxiety agents (2 weeks) may benefit from a selective serotonin reuptake inhibitor (SSRI) or tricyclic agent. Although the SSRIs (fluoxetine, sertraline, paroxetine, citalopram, escitalopram) usually produce a maximum antidepressant benefit in 2 to 5 weeks, many patients report a decrease in anxiety within a week or even days of beginning therapy. Although some drug interactions have been reported, SSRIs have proven to be relatively safe. The side effect profile is usually benign when therapy is initiated with a low dose (half the recommended starting dose). Older adults most often respond favorably to one fourth of the recommended starting dose. Sedation and some anxiolytic effect can be achieved using tricyclic antidepressants (nortriptyline, doxepin) and trazodone. Limited evidence exists for use of bupropion sustained release for bereavement.

A bedtime dose of trazodone or mirtazapine (atypical antidepressants) or a tricyclic agent can provide immediate relief of insomnia; the antidepressant effect occurs in approximately 3 to 6 weeks. The tricyclics have a greater potential for adverse interactions yet can be safely prescribed if used with caution. Prescribing tricyclics for older adults is usually not advised because of the anticholinergic effects.[18] Awareness of potential drug-drug interactions is needed before prescribing any agent.

LIFE SPAN CONSIDERATIONS

Grieving occurs in all age-groups. Children may fear abandonment or the loss of others they love, and they may feel guilt or responsibility for the loss.[21] They may begin to have behavioral problems at home or school. Evidence exits that the loss of a parent in childhood is linked to psychosocial problems in adulthood when remaining family relationships are poor.[22,23]

Ten percent to 20% of clinically recognized pregnancies end in miscarriage, with up to 20% of affected women still remaining grief-stricken 6 to 8 weeks after the loss, and again 6 months after loss.[24] There is a growing body of evidence that clinicians tend to be to quick to pathologize such bereavement, perhaps hoping in the process to provide intervention and resolution. One recent study involving both English- and Spanish-speaking women showed preliminary evidence for the benefits of phone-administered interpersonal counseling.[24]

For most parents, the birth of a child is a time of joy and celebration. However, nearly 4% of parents receive distressing news about their child's health at the time of birth and may go through a bereavement process as they adapt to their child's condition.[25]

COMPLICATIONS

Complications of grief include major depression, complicated grief, physical illness, and suicide. A thorough history, including a brief psychosocial assessment, is needed to screen the at-risk population. It is helpful to ask questions related to living arrangements, availability of transportation, friends, socialization, and diet. Inquiries about feelings of sadness or depression, thoughts of suicide, and coping skills are necessary. Illness resulting from accidents is common during the bereavement period. Stress-related illness and substance abuse are common during the first year of grieving.

Complicated grief can occur in the aftermath of loss but needs to be differentiated from depression. Key features of complicated grief include (1) a sense of disbelief regarding the death; (2) anger and bitterness over the death; (3) recurrent pangs of painful emotions, with intense yearnings and longing for the deceased; and (4) preoccupations with thoughts of the loved one, often including distressing intrusive thoughts related to the death.[5,26,27] Complicated grief is a risk especially for older adults, for individuals who lose a spouse or child, for individuals in poor health, and for those with severe co-existing and preexisting stressors.[28] Individuals who have had dependent relationships, have lacked social support, or have had ambivalent relationships with the person who died are also at risk for complicated grief.[29,30] A recent randomized control trial[5] demonstrated that persons with complicated grief responded better to targeted complicated grief treatment than they did to interpersonal psychotherapy, but more work is needed in this area. In other studies, antidepressant medication has been shown to make small changes in complicated grief symptoms.[20]

A major depressive episode is an additional risk. Several screening tools are helpful in diagnosing an MDD (see Chapter 261 for the assessment and management of depression).

Assessment for suicide risk is necessary at each visit. Office appointments should be scheduled at frequent intervals to assess the patient's response to medication and risk factors. Patients are often treated by several health care providers, all of whom may prescribe medications and other interventions. For the patient's safety and to avoid duplication and drug interactions, it is essential that all providers be aware of what medications and other therapies are being prescribed and by whom.

INDICATIONS FOR REFERRAL OR HOSPITALIZATION

Complicated grief and major depression can be difficult and time consuming to treat in the primary care setting. Often patients are seen with somatic symptoms that require frequent clinic visits, assessments, and testing. Patients may not be able to clearly express their concerns, and they may require more time than the routine visit allows. Antidepressant medications may take from 2 to 5 weeks to reach a beneficial effect, and dose titrations or a trial of an alternative antidepressant may delay the treatment progress. Anxiety may be a component of the depression and complicate the person's recovery.

A referral to psychiatric care may be threatening to a patient because of the persisting bias toward mental illness in today's society. Psychiatric care is sometimes associated with incapacitation or insanity. Immediate psychiatric intervention is indicated for suicidal thoughts, intent, and attempts; for individuals who have not responded to one or two trials of antidepressants; for persons who require more time than the provider has available; and for those whom the provider is not comfortable treating. The patient can be prepared for referral if the psychiatric intervention is not an emergency. Approaches that are empathetic and honest are best. Presenting depression as a treatable, biologic disorder similar to other medical conditions is often helpful.

Immediate hospitalization is indicated when patients pose a threat to themselves or others. Health care providers must be aware of the mental health act in their practice locale and take appropriate action. All states have provisions for involuntary placement for evaluation in mental health emergencies.

Some health care providers refer persons with uncomplicated grief reactions for mental health services. Advance practice registered nurse practitioners in mental health, licensed clinical social workers, mental health counselors, and psychologists can assess, diagnose, and treat mental health disorders.

Many people are not covered by prescription plans, and for these people the cost of medications may be prohibitive. Many pharmaceutical companies make medications available through patient assistance drug programs. The patient assistance program can be initiated by calling the specific drug company. In addition, psychotherapy is not covered benefit in many insurance plans, and patients may not be able to pay out of pocket for these expenses. Local mental health clinics and providers offering services on a sliding scale may be an option.

PATIENT AND FAMILY EDUCATION

Grieving is a normal process in response to loss. An awareness of the predisposing factors to complicated grief may aid in its prevention. The maintenance of mental, physical, and spiritual well-being may be a positive indicator of successful grieving.[30]

Emotional support is essential as an individual progresses through the grieving process. It is helpful for a person to know that the feelings associated with grieving are natural and that the intensity of these feelings will wax and wane as the process continues.

Weight loss is not uncommon during this period, since grieving is often accompanied by a loss of appetite. People are often unaware of the importance of nutrition to emotional health. Nutrition education stressing the importance of eating balanced meals may be helpful. A liquid dietary supplement may be indicated if there is the potential for a nutritional deficit. These supplements may be substituted for one or two meals or used as additional supplements.

Some find support and comfort in their faith and spiritual practices. Others may reject their religious ties, blaming God for their loss. Assurance that this is often part of the normal grieving process may be helpful.

Maintaining a routine, in so far as possible, is an important component of maintaining a healthy lifestyle. Patients should be encouraged to maintain regular bed and waking times each day. Scheduling activities outside the home is also important. Maintaining social contacts is essential, but people also need to know that quiet time alone is acceptable and may be helpful. Exercise in some form is beneficial and need not be strenuous.

Medication education is important. People should understand the rationale, side effects, risks, and use of the medication prescribed. A list of concurrent medications should always be reviewed for potential drug interactions or duplications. This approach offers an opportunity to assess an individual's knowledge of the medication and health status and also provides an opportunity for teaching. Education about the use of as-needed medication should also be reviewed, since this concept is often misunderstood. Specific instructions are needed rather than "when," "if," or "as you need it" statements, and assessment and education about medication should be ongoing. Although most patients do not intend to abuse medication, dependence can occur unintentionally.

Most people do think of alcohol as a drug and often minimize their intake. The potential for drug and alcohol interaction should be assessed as medications are reviewed. Education about the antidepressant effects of alcohol is especially needed in this population.

It is often helpful to include the family in grief education to discuss the nature of the grief response, in particular the universality and individuality of the phenomenon and the fact that it is a process. Expectations of family and friends can help or hinder bereavement process. Education is the key to better understanding, and the resolution of grief depends on it. The following resources can provide further assistance and additional information:

Grief Recovery Institute
(800) 907-9600
http://www.grief.net

AARP grief and loss programs
http://www.aarp.org/families/grief_loss

Mental Health America
(800) 969-6642
http://www.nmha.org

National Institute of Mental Health
(866) 615-6464
http://www.nimh.nih.gov

American Psychiatric Association
(703) 907-7300
http://www.psych.org

REFERENCES

1. Reynold S: Grief, *JAMA* 293(21):2616, 2005.
2. Viney A: Bereavement as a health issue, *Healthcare Counsel Psychother J* 5(3):6-9, 2005.
3. Cowles K, Rodgers B: The concept of grief: a foundation for nursing research and practice, *Res Nurs Health* 14(2):119-127, 1991.
4. US Census Bureau: *Vital statistics for the United States*, Washington, DC, 2006, US National Center for Health Statistics.
5. Shear K, Frank E, Houck, P, and others: Treatment of complicated grief, *JAMA* 293:2601-2608, 2005.
6. Glass R: Is grief a disease? Sometimes, *JAMA* 293(21):2058, 2005.
7. Kübler-Ross E, Wessler S, Avioli L: On death and dying, *JAMA* 221(2):174-179, 1972.
8. Dalzell R: Making sense of grieving, *Healthcare Counsel Psychother J* 5(3):20-21, 2005.
9. Winner L: *Mudhouse Sabbath*, Brewster, Mass, 2003, Paraclete.
10. Comer R: *Abnormal psychology*, New York, 2004, Worth.
11. Versalle A, McDowell E: The attitudes of men and women concerning gender differences in grief, *Omega* 50(1):53-67, 2004-2005.
12. Vahtera J, Kivimaki M, Vaananen A, and others: Sex differences in health effects of family death or illness: are women more vulnerable than men? *Psychosom Med* 68(2):283-291, 2006.
13. Gundel H, O'Connor M, Littrell B, and others: Functional neuroanatomy of grief: an FMRI study, *Am J Psychiatry* 10:1946-1953, 2003.
14. American Psychiatric Association: *Diagnostic and statistical manual of mental disorders*, ed 4 (text rev), Washington, DC, 2000, The Association.
15. Horowitz M, Sonneborn D, Sugahara C, and others: Self-regard: a new measure, *Am J Psychiatry* 153(3):382-385, 1996.
16. Langner R, Maercker A: Complicated grief as a stress response disorder: evaluating diagnostic criteria in a German sample, *J Psychosom Res* 58(3):235-242, 2005.
17. Boelen P, van den Bout J: Complicated grief, depression, and anxiety as distinct postloss syndromes: a confirmatory factor analysis, *Am J Psychiatry* 162(11):2175-2177, 2005.
18. Shear MK, Frank E, Foa E, and others: Traumatic grief treatment: a pilot study, *Am J Psychiatry* 158(9):1506-1508, 2001.
19. Warner J, Metcalfe C, King M: Evaluating the use of benzodiazepines following recent bereavement, *Br J Psychiatry* 178(1):36-41, 2001.
20. Zisook S, Shuchter SR, Pedrelli P, and others: Bupropion sustained release for bereavement: results of an open trial, *J Clin Psychiatry* 62(4):227-230, 2001.
21. Stuber M, Merskhai V: What do we tell children? Understanding childhood grief, *Western J Med* 174(3):187-191, 2001.
22. Luecken L: Attachment and loss experiences during childhood are associated with hostility, depression and social support, *J Psychosom Res* 49(1):85-91, 2000.
23. Macias C, Jones D, Harvey J, and others: Bereavement in the context of serious mental illness, *Psychiatry Serv* 55(4):421-426, 2004.
24. Neugebauer R, Ritsher J: Depression and grief following early pregnancy loss, *Int J Childbirth Educ* 20(3):21-24, 2003.
25. Barnett D, Clements M, Kaplan-Estrin M, and others: Building new dreams: supporting parents' adaptation to their child with special needs, *Infants Young Children* 16(5):184-199, 2003.
26. Horowitz M, Siegel B, Holen A, and others: Diagnostic criteria for complicated grief disorder, *Am J Psychiatry* 154:904-910, 1997.
27. Prigerson H, Shear M, Jacobs S, and others: Consensus criteria for traumatic grief: a rational and preliminary empirical test, *Br J Psychiatry* 174:67-73, 1999.
28. Arnold J, Gemma P, Cushman L: Exploring parental grief: combining quantitative and qualitative measures, *Arch Psychiatric Nursing* 19(6):245-255, 2005.
29. Boerner K, Wortman C, Bonanno G: Resilient or at risk? A 4-year study of older adults who initially showed high or low distress following conjugal loss, *J Gerontol B Psychol Sci Soc Sci* 60(2):67-73, 2005.
30. Pearce M, Chen J, Silverman GK, and others: Religious coping, health and health services among bereaved adults, *Int J Psychiatry Med* 32(2):179-199, 2002.

CHAPTER 264

Posttraumatic Stress Disorder

Debra Fournier

DEFINITION

Stress is a universal experience. Personality structure, coping style, and the psychosocial environment mediate how stressful experiences are interpreted and integrated. Mental health is often defined as one's ability to adapt to adversity, integrate new experiences, and continue to love and work. Events of extreme stress, or trauma, are common. Reasons for maladaptive reactions to overwhelming experiences have been explored since the time of Homer, with multiple tales of physical effects (e.g., blindness) resulting from witnessing traumatic events, such as homicide. Academic writings speculating on these reactions, their etiology, and symptom presentation became prolific in the late nineteenth century with Oppenheim's description of "traumatic neurosis" and "cardiac neurosis," associating physical pathologic conditions with psychologic experience. Later, Briquet, Charcot, Janet, Breuer, and Freud all discussed the connection between horrific experiences and complex anxiety reactions.[1] The categorization of these symptoms has evolved from such terms as *hysteria, shell shock,* and *rape trauma,* to *posttraumatic stress disorder* (PTSD), as ultimately defined in the *Diagnostic and Statistical Manual of Mental Disorders* (DSM-IV).[2] PTSD was initially defined by a standardized collection of symptoms in 1980, following undisputable patterns of symptoms in Vietnam veterans. PTSD is now recognized as a seriously impairing potential consequence of having experienced a traumatic event.

Trauma is often subjectively defined, dependent on the individual's reaction to an event, not necessarily the event itself. The distinction between a stressful event and a traumatic event is based on the severity of that event and the impact or the consequences. Clinically, traumatic events are therefore often defined based on the ability to maintain individual functioning and the absence of additional mental health symptoms. Traumatic events are defined by the DSM-IV as events that involve "actual or threatened injury or death or serious injury," witnessing such an event, or learning about such an event affecting a close loved one.[2] Potentially traumatic events can be categorized into natural disasters, accidents, and incidents of interpersonal violence (Box 264-1).

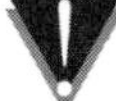

Patients who have suicidal or homicidal ideation, or an inability to maintain their own safety in their environment, require emergency assessment in a local hospital emergency department or by a psychiatric emergency response team. (Refer to section on suicide, Chapter 261.)

A referral should be made to a mental health specialist for anyone with symptoms of PTSD and impairment in daily functioning.

BOX 264-1

TYPES OF POTENTIALLY TRAUMATIC EVENTS

NATURAL DISASTERS
- Hurricane
- Flood
- Tornado
- Blizzard
- Earthquake

ACCIDENTS
- Fire
- Motor vehicle crash
- Airplane crash
- Sudden illness

INTERPERSONAL VIOLENCE
- Physical assault
- Sexual assault
- Homicide
- Terrorism
- Combat

EPIDEMIOLOGY

Potentially traumatic events are not uncommon. In general population samples, the majority of people report having experienced one or more potentially traumatic events. In samples of people seeking general medical care (primary care offices, general internal medicine clinics), the prevalence of potentially traumatic events is slightly higher than in general population estimates.[3,4] In samples of those receiving services from community mental health centers and hospitals, researchers have reported that 98% to 100% have experienced at least one potentially traumatic event (Table 264-1).[5] Life-changing events, such as receiving a terminal diagnosis or having a child with a terminal diagnosis, although less studied, have also been identified as traumas.[6]

PTSD prevalence data vary widely based on variables in existence before the trauma and surrounding and following the trauma. Specific types of traumatic events are also differently associated with the likelihood of PTSD development. Considering all these factors, it is estimated that at any given time, the prevalence of PTSD in the United States is 8%. Women are approximately four times more likely to have PTSD than men, even when controlling for the high asso-

TABLE 264-1 Prevalence of Posttraumatic Stress Disorder (PTSD)

	Prevalence of Exposure to Traumatic Event	Prevalence of (Lifetime) PTSD
General population	50%-75%	5%-10%
Civilian primary care patients	83%	12%-37%
Veterans	90%	18%-49%
Chronically mentally ill	98%	43%

Data from References 2, 5, 16, 19, 24, and 46; and Elliot DM, Brierre J: Posttraumatic stress associated with delayed recall of sexual abuse: a general population study, *J Traum Stress* 8(4):629-648, 1995.

ciation of PTSD and sexual trauma.[2,7] Natural disasters, such as floods, have a 16% association with PTSD development,[8] acutely following the disaster, yet with decreasing rates in community samples after 1 year. Childhood sexual abuse and rape are associated with the highest incidence of PTSD (22% to 50%).[9]

PATHOPHYSIOLOGY

The normal physiologic response to an event that poses a threat is commonly thought of as "fight or flight." The body does not distinguish between an event that is physically threatening and one that is psychologically threatening. Primitively, blood flow is increased to the large muscle groups, in a state of alarm, preparing for a "fight or flight." The digestive system is slowed while the legs and heart are activated to work harder. This is largely regulated through cortisol mediated by the hypothalamus-pituitary-adrenal (HPA) axis. Ideally, this system operates as a negative feedback loop; when enough cortisol is detected in the body to meet the demand of the threat, the HPA axis is triggered to slow down and not release additional cortisol.

Cortisol has been studied in relation to major depressive disorder (MDD), with a strong association between elevated cortisol levels and the diagnosis of MDD. In people with PTSD, lower cortisol levels have been noted. It has been suggested that several aspects of the HPA axis are altered when one is exposed to chronic stress or threat, resulting in an ineffective system for responding to further stressors.[10-14] Stress intolerance is common in people with PTSD and may be explained by this inefficiency.[10,14] There is some evidence to suggest that genetics may play a role in the function of the HPA axis. Personality characteristics, developmental age at the time of the first trauma exposure, and cognitive appraisals of events all have been explored as affecting the cortisol response.[11] Few studies are able to compare the cortisol levels of people *before* a traumatic exposure, yet in one prospective study of new firefighters, salivary cortisol was measured on initial training and 1 year later. Presumably, after 2 years of potentially traumatic experiences, those firefighters with more PTSD symptoms would have lower cortisol levels. Although there was no difference in baseline cortisol levels, the group with lower cortisol did score higher on measures of hostility at baseline, suggesting perception and personality as mediators.[15]

Although the HPA axis and cortisol response have been the most researched biologic association with PTSD, there are other hypotheses and findings. Variations in activity in the limbic system (where the associations of emotion and memory are processed via the hippocampus and the amygdala) have been noted in imaging studies.[14] An endogenous opioid response, stress-induced analgesia, has been noted and validated through studies of naloxone (Narcan) used to reverse the physiologic effect.[10,13,14] The γ-aminobutyric acid (GABA) pathway is involved in the formation of memory. Exposure to extreme stress may down-regulate this system, allowing for a unique encoding of memory. This may explain why substance use and abuse (especially of central nervous system depressants such as alcohol and benzodiazepines) is common in people with PTSD, since it may physiologically repress the traumatic memory.[13]

Other systems of the adrenergic response and neurotransmitter activity are affected in the acute and chronic phases of PTSD, supporting the use of β-adrenergic antagonists and selective serotonin reuptake inhibitors (SSRIs), respectively.[10,14]

CLINICAL PRESENTATION

Not everyone who experiences a traumatic event develops PTSD. Crises and traumatic events have other sequelae. After a potentially traumatic event, people may initially experience somatic concerns, depressed mood, amnesia, feelings of guilt or shame, or no apparent symptoms. Recurrent, troublesome thoughts or memories of the event; avoidance of reminders (or triggers) of the event; and a general hypervigilance are characteristic of PTSD. Emotional numbing and dissociation (extreme separation from reality in response to overwhelming emotion) may also occur. In response to a traumatic event, people may experience intense hopelessness or acute anxiety and may suffer impairment in their ability to form and maintain healthy relationships, regulate emotions, tolerate non-life-threatening stress, and maintain an understanding of reality. These symptoms may be better explained by other DSM diagnoses such as depressive disorders, anxiety disorders (other than PTSD), personality disorders, and thought disorders and require further assessment and possible referral.

Factors affecting risk and resiliency have been investigated and are discussed as pretrauma, peritrauma and posttrauma (Box 264-2). In the prospective study of firefighters mentioned earlier, researchers assessed personality characteristics, depression, anxiety, and PTSD symptoms at the time of entering the profession and up to 2 years after initiation. Presumably the firefighters had comparable levels of exposure, experiencing multiple potentially traumatic events during the 2-year period. Pretrauma personality characteristics of hostility (high) and self-efficacy (low) were associated with more PTSD symptoms, peaking 1 year after initial study; these firefighters sustained a

BOX 264-2

VARIABLES ASSOCIATED WITH INCREASED RISK OF POSTTRAUMATIC STRESS DISORDER

PRETRAUMA
- Youth
- Poor family structure
- Lack of social support
- Lower education
- Major depressive disorder
- Female gender

PERITRAUMA
- Close proximity
- Severity of event
- Dissociation
- Prolonged or repeated exposure
- Perceived life threat

POSTTRAUMA
- Repeated exposures
- Homecoming environment
- Poor emotional support
- Isolation

Data from References 2, 3, 16.

significantly higher level of distress than those without these personality features.[15]

Conversely, advanced age, sense of control during the event, and enhanced social support during the disclosure or aftermath of the event serve as protective factors.[16] Resilience, including features of hardiness, self-esteem, adaptability, humor, and development of strength through stress, is associated with overall better outcomes of less symptom severity and minimum impact on physical health. However, spirituality or strength of spiritual beliefs is associated with more severe PTSD and poor physical health outcomes, perhaps since it emerges as a coping strategy, rather than a preexisting factor.[17]

In general, events that occur in isolation and that challenge preexisting world views lead to more impairment, whereas community disasters explained by chance or "bad luck," with a shared experience of loss, have a lower association with posttrauma complications. For example, rape, which is an individualized event carrying some cultural stigma in disclosure and often perpetrated by a known, previously trusted assailant, is the event most likely to predict PTSD.[18]

As described above, not everyone who experiences a trauma develops PTSD. Symptoms may develop within the first month of trauma exposure and resolve (acute stress disorder), exist for 3 months and then resolve (acute PTSD), or persist for longer than 3 months (chronic PTSD). Symptoms or impairment in functioning may resolve spontaneously with formal treatment. Recurrence of symptoms is common in the face of triggers (reminders of the traumatic event) or subsequent trauma exposure.[2]

PHYSICAL EXAMINATION

Physical injury may occur as a direct result of trauma, leaving a visible, objective reminder of an event such as physical assault or combat. When clinical examination findings suggest maltreatment, providers must follow state reporting laws regarding the disclosure of abuse.

More commonly, the psychologic effects of a past trauma may be observable during a routine examination with attention to behavior. Guarded movements, emotional numbing, or inappropriate affect suggest anxiety about the physical examination that may be connected to a history of trauma. It is generally *not* common for patients seen in a primary or acute care setting to disclose their personal history specific to traumatic exposure, since they may not consider such experience relevant to their overall health status.

Although PTSD cannot be diagnosed by physical examination, the presence of traumatic events can be elicited during a careful history (much the same way as assessing for substance use or sexual history). In the absence of formal screening instruments, specific behavioral or historical questions, including psychoeducation about the prevalence of extreme stress, may be helpful. For example, at the time of a new assessment, a provider may ask the patient, "We know that stress, in our past and current environments, can sometimes influence our physical health. What was the most stressful thing you ever experienced? Do you think that event has any impact on you now?" Disclosure of specific details about a particular trauma is not encouraged in this setting. Should a patient begin to share such details, it is helpful to provide some respectful redirection to focus on current functioning and health status. Information obtained in the history may lead to required adjustments in technique or time allotment for a comprehensive examination. Women who have survived sexual trauma may, for example, feel especially vulnerable during a physical examination. It is imperative to establish a relationship that honors safety. Patients can be empowered to request that the examination be stopped at any time or to have a support person present to minimize distress or reactions to potential triggers.

Providers must be mindful that the majority of people seeking care in the primary care settings have experienced trauma.[19] Respect for this history and awareness of current sequelae are required for a competent physical assessment. Techniques such as carefully explaining each assessment and reason for touch enhance the patient's sense of safety and should be employed during every examination, not only with patients confirmed to have histories of interpersonal trauma.

The relationship between health care provider and patient is critical to maintain. As described in the Complications section below, the course of many medical illnesses is complicated by traumatic exposure and PTSD. Screening for PTSD in the primary care setting; providing a safe, validating environment; and referring patients for trauma-specific treatment will ideally reduce the risk of complications related to medical disease management.

DIAGNOSTICS

Currently, there are no laboratory or imaging tests that diagnose PTSD. As mentioned above, several physiologic changes have been noted in association with symptoms of acute and chronic PTSD; however, researchers are not yet able to confidently use these findings for diagnostic purposes.

Once an event has been defined as a trauma, the diagnosis of PTSD specifically includes a constellation of symptoms from three clusters: reexperiencing, avoidance-numbing, and hypervigilance. Symptoms from each cluster have to be noted at least 1 month after the experience of a traumatic event and must be associated with functional impairment that is not better explained by another disorder. If these symptoms occur within 1 month of the experience, acute stress disorder may be diagnosed. PTSD may be diagnosed at anytime greater than 1 month after the event, even if symptoms were not present immediately (delayed onset), and would be considered chronic if the duration of symptoms is greater than 3 months.[2] (Box 264-3 lists the full DSM-IV criteria for PTSD.)

Mental health professionals commonly use clinician interviews such as the Structured Clinical Interview for DSM-IV[20] and the Clinician Administered PTSD Scale[21] to diagnose PTSD. Self-report screening tools and symptom checklists are more often used in general settings, and recent studies validate the diagnostic reliability of shortened forms including 2 to 6 items.[22,23] PTSD is a risk factor for poor physical health and a potential outcome of a terminal diagnosis. Regardless of the sequence of diagnoses, it is clear that, when serious medical illness and PTSD are noted in the same individual (regardless of age), prognosis is poorer than in the absence of comorbidity. Given this finding, it is imperative to screen for PTSD in primary care to facilitate overall improvement in

BOX 264-3

DSM-IV DIAGNOSTIC CRITERIA FOR POSTTRAUMATIC STRESS DISORDER

A. The person has been exposed to a traumatic event in which both of the following were present:
   (1) The person experienced, witnessed, or was confronted with an event or events that involved actual or threatened death or serious injury, or a threat to the physical integrity of self or others.
   (2) The person's response involved intense fear, helplessness, or horror. NOTE: In children this may be expressed instead by disorganized or agitated behavior.

B. The traumatic event is persistently experienced in one (or more) of the following ways:
   (1) Recurrent and intrusive distressing recollections of the event, including images, thoughts, or perceptions. NOTE: In young children, repetitive play may occur in which themes or aspects of the trauma are expressed.
   (2) Recurring distressing dreams of the event. NOTE: In children, there may be frightening dreams without recognizable content.
   (3) Acting or feeling as if the traumatic event were recurring (includes a sense of reliving the experience, illusions, hallucinations, and dissociative flashback episodes, including those that occur on awakening or when intoxicated). NOTE: In young children, trauma-specific reenactment may occur.
   (4) Intense psychologic distress at exposure to internal or external cues that symbolize or resemble an aspect of the traumatic event.
   (5) Physiologic reactivity on exposure to internal or external cues that symbolize or resemble an aspect of the traumatic event.

C. Persistent avoidance of stimuli associated with the trauma and numbing of general responsiveness (not present before the trauma), as indicated by three (or more) of the following:
   (1) Efforts to avoid thoughts, feelings, or conversations associated with the trauma
   (2) Efforts to avoid activities, places, or people that arouse recollections of the trauma
   (3) Inability to recall an important aspect of the trauma
   (4) Markedly diminished interest or participation in significant activities
   (5) Feeling of detachment or estrangement from others
   (6) Restricted range of affect (e.g., unable to have loving feelings)
   (7) Sense of a foreshortened future (e.g., does not expect to have a career, marriage, children, or a normal life span)

D. Persistent symptoms of increased arousal (not present before the trauma), as indicated by two (or more) of the following:
   (1) Difficulty falling or staying asleep
   (2) Irritability or outbursts of anger
   (3) Difficulty concentrating
   (4) Hypervigilance
   (5) Exaggerated startle response

E. Duration of the disturbance (symptoms in criteria B, C, and D) is more than 1 month.

F. The disturbance causes clinically significant distress or impairment in social, occupational, or other important areas of functioning.

Specify if:
- **Acute:** if duration of symptoms is less than 3 months
- **Chronic:** if duration of symptoms is 3 months or more

Specify if:
- **With delayed onset:** if onset of symptoms is at least 6 months after the stressor

From American Psychiatric Association: *Diagnostic and statistical manual of mental disorders,* ed 4 (text rev), Washington, DC, 2000, The Association.

functioning secondary to physical diagnoses. The broader use of these shorter, self-report tools enhances the likelihood that health care providers will become more aware of their patients' traumatic histories, thereby improving their ability to comprehensively care for other chronic illnesses.

DIFFERENTIAL DIAGNOSIS

Because the symptoms of PTSD are so diverse, and often some symptoms manifest more severely than others, an early, accurate diagnosis is often complicated. PTSD is distinguished from other diagnoses by the presence of a traumatic event, the connection between reexperiencing and avoidance symptoms and that event or reminders of the event, and duration of impairment. Other mental health diagnoses can co-exist as long as each set of criteria is independently met and not better explained by the presence of the other condition. Most commonly, PTSD exists with MDD,[24,25] substance use disorders,[13,25] and borderline personality disorder.[26]

DIFFERENTIAL DIAGNOSIS

Posttraumatic Stress Disorder

- Borderline personality disorder
- Adjustment disorder
- Acute stress disorder
- Schizophrenia
- Major depressive disorder
- Attention deficit disorder
- Dissociative identity disorder
- Generalized anxiety disorder
- Panic disorder

MANAGEMENT

In the primary care setting, the provider's role following a patient's traumatic experience is one of initial assessment and referral. PTSD is not an illness to be managed by general medical practitioners. General clinicians, however, may be involved in prescribing medications for symptoms and, although not providing therapy, need to have an understanding of evidence-based treatments.

Most models of treatment are based on several key principles related to PTSD:

- There has been an experience of overwhelming stress.
- Coping or survival strategies that may have been employed at the time of exposure (e.g., in childhood), although effective then, may not have evolved or been adapted for adult scenarios.
- Physiologic and psychologic interpretation of stressors is altered, usually sensitized.
- Memories are disorganized and have disproportionate meaning.
- Traumatic exposure has an impact on a person's physical and psychologic well-being for years following the event.
- Treatment can be effective in managing reminders, tolerating stress, and enhancing coping strategies to ultimately achieve better integration of the experience.

Because of the diverse symptom presentation of PTSD, medications are chosen based on the most distressing or impairing facet of the disorder, and polypharmacy is common. Medications such as SSRIs are the most common and, to date, the most empirically supported pharmacologic intervention for PTSD.[27,28] Clinical and empiric evidence supports the efficacy of these agents in reducing PTSD symptoms of anxiety, depressed mood, anger, and numbing, and further research is under way to explore an adaptation of these drugs and their effect on serotonin receptors.[10,14,29] Arousal symptoms may be effectively managed with β-adrenergic blockers, benzodiazepines, or anticonvulsants. Dissociation and flashbacks may respond to new generation antipsychotic agents such as quetiapine.[13,14,30]

Several models of psychotherapy have been evaluated in clinical practice across various population samples. Regardless of type of traumatic history, differences in symptoms, and duration of symptoms, the research supports the efficacy of these models. Models of cognitive behavior therapy (CBT) have the most empiric support.[31-34] Generally, treatment includes an exploration of automatic thoughts and beliefs that may be associated with maladaptive behavioral responses to triggers or reminders of the traumatic event. After developing a therapeutic rapport, specifically trained, skilled therapists lead the patient through steps of psychoeducation, relaxation training, challenging of belief systems, and habituation to triggers or memories. As the number of clinical trials continues to expand, information is emerging about how to assess and predict which patients may respond best to CBT or may be better suited for a less-intensive style of therapy—an exploration that grew out of incidental findings of high rates of attrition.[34,35] Other exposure-based therapies include eye movement desensitization retraining and the counting technique.[31] Both of these latter treatments include habituation and stress tolerance skill building. There is also a role for peer support. Symptoms of PTSD are common in women after a diagnosis of breast cancer, for example. These symptoms are dramatically reduced through peer support group participation.[6] However, caution is encouraged in other forums of peer support, since without skilled facilitation, retelling stories of trauma or hearing the traumas of others may be retraumatizing in itself and has the potential to exacerbate symptoms.

LIFE SPAN CONSIDERATIONS

Children may demonstrate symptoms of PTSD differently from adults, depending on language development and emotional maturity. Dreams or nightmares may have characteristic monsters or the absence of a rescuing hero, and characteristics of the traumatic event may be mirrored in play. Common somatic symptoms in children include stomachaches and headaches. Patterns of diminished interest, hypervigilance, and social withdrawal are more accurately assessed by supervising adults (teachers, daycare providers), rather than endorsed by the child. Adolescents with PTSD may exhibit extreme behavior such as anger and overt disobedience or complete withdrawal and social isolation. Differential diagnoses specific to children with the above behaviors include attention deficit hyperactivity disorder, oppositional defiant disorder, MDD, and bipolar affective disorder.[2]

Women are four times more likely to have PTSD than men. During pregnancy, women are at increased risk for domestic violence (see Chapter 24). Women who have histories of traumatic events, especially those which occurred in childhood, may have an increase in distressing symptoms in pregnancy and may require more medical follow-up. Various stages of early parenting may also trigger reminders of past events or vulnerabilities. The prevalence of PTSD in pregnant, low-income women is 8% to 14%, slightly higher than in community samples. One study found, however, that fewer than 15% of these women with PTSD had ever sought treatment.[36] Physical violence during pregnancy poses direct risk to the unborn child. Yet little is known about how the neurobiologic changes associated with PTSD may affect the child of a woman with PTSD. Women who were pregnant in September 2001 and who developed PTSD after the terrorist attacks on the World Trade Center were compared with pregnant women with the same exposure, but no PTSD symptoms. Women with PTSD and their babies were found to have significantly lower levels of cortisol than women and children without PTSD.[37] It remains to be seen if this low cortisol level will predispose these children to a higher risk of PTSD development on further traumatic exposure.

The most common new trauma experienced by older adults is domestic violence.[38,39] Older adults, with any traumatic history, often are seen with somatic concerns,[25,38] seemingly without connection to specific events, and tend to have stronger avoidance symptoms than their younger counterparts,[25] placing them at higher risk for being underdiagnosed. Assessment techniques for traumatic exposure and PTSD symptoms in the older adult do not differ from those discussed for the general population.[40] Cultural or generational differences may exist, however, in regards to beliefs about disclosure or the event itself; if not carefully considered, these beliefs may be a barrier to effective treatment. Prevalence data in older adults depend largely on the World War II population, with rates of PTSD ranging from 18% to 50% in veterans and a rate of almost 70% in prisoners of war.[25]

Modifications to evidence-based treatments for older adults have not been reviewed or recommended. One study explored the potential benefit of adding an educational video to the advocacy interventions for older adults after reporting a violent crime. Although this increased their level of education and understanding related to potential symptoms or sequelae, this intervention had no impact on actual symptoms of depression or anxiety 6 weeks later.[39]

As adults with PTSD age and develop cognitive impairments, exacerbations of PTSD symptoms related to triggers or misinterpretations of the sensory environment may result in an increase in challenging or aggressive behaviors.[41] Although this is supported in clinical experience, no trials have explored additional interventions or modifications to current treatment recommendations for dementia in people with PTSD.

COMPLICATIONS

PTSD is associated with severe impairments in all areas of functioning: employment, relationships, and self-care. In people with PTSD, the risk of further victimization, self-harm, and suicide is high, especially if symptoms go largely untreated. As mentioned above, PTSD commonly co-occurs with substance use and abuse. In addition to complications consistent with an increase in substance use and unhealthy lifestyle choices, declining physical health has been directly linked in clinical and statistic models to trauma exposure and the diagnosis of PTSD.[42]

The experience of adverse events in childhood has been associated with an increase in obesity, smoking, physical activity, and depressed mood. Yet even when controlling for these traditional risk factors for ischemic heart disease (IHD), one large study found an association between childhood experiences and IHD.[43]

People with PTSD have higher rates of anemia, arthritis, asthma, back pain, cardiovascular disease, diabetes, eczema, kidney disease, lung disease, and gastric ulcers. In most models the diagnosis of PTSD is a stronger predictor of poor health than trauma history, physical injury, lifestyle factors, or depression.[44-46] People with PTSD also have higher rates of service utilization. For example, women with PTSD, participating in an urban area HMO, had a 104% increase in total annual medical cost compared with women without PTSD. Primary care costs were twice as high as for patients with few or no symptoms, when controlling for depression and chronic illness.[47]

Clinicians who provide care to traumatized individuals also face a risk: vicarious traumatization, a syndrome characterized by a change in the provider's belief system because of the cumulative experience of bearing witness to the traumatic stories of many patients. Depression, pessimism, and an altered world view are potential effects of this type of specific care. Strategies for increased awareness of this risk, balance and variety in the work setting, and collaboration and supervision reduce the chances of developing vicarious traumatization.

INDICATIONS FOR REFERRAL OR HOSPITALIZATION

Once a health care provider determines that a patient has a traumatic exposure history and suspects that current symptoms or complications may be related, the patient should be referred to a specialty provider. Knowing the area or facility resources and understanding the specialty care available will facilitate a cohesive collaborative relationship. Not all psychotherapists and psychiatrists have training or experience in evidence-based treatment for PTSD.

PATIENT AND FAMILY EDUCATION

For family members of those having experienced a known trauma, education regarding the possible sequelae is imperative. Initially, loved ones are encouraged to support and validate the survivor's experience of trauma, thereby increasing their potentially protective factors by offering a positive homecoming moment. Understanding symptoms of PTSD and the increased risk for suicide will also facilitate prompt treatment for the survivor of trauma. Information for patients and families is available from the National Center for Posttraumatic Stress Disorder (with special information to help families of soldiers returning from war), Centers for Disease Control and Prevention, the National Institute of Mental Health (with publications also available in Spanish), and the National Alliance on Mental Illness (with information regarding local support groups for families).

HEALTH PROMOTION

Good physical health, including adequate nutrition, healthy weight and exercise routines, appropriate sleep patterns, and stress management techniques, help buffer the effects of trauma. Health care providers are in a privileged role of often being the first to learn of a patient's traumatic experience. Regardless of external pressures of time and schedule, the provider's response during this initial disclosure is critical. A validating, supportive, resourceful encounter enhances the patient's preexisting protective factors and, despite trauma exposure, can help prevent the development of impairing conditions such as PTSD.

REFERENCES

1. Van der Kolk BA, McFarlane AC, Weisaeth L: *Traumatic stress: the effects of overwhelming experience on mind, body, and society,* New York, 1996, Guilford Press.
2. American Psychiatric Association: *Diagnostic and statistical manual of mental disorders*, ed 4 (text rev), Washington, DC, 2000, The Association.
3. Walker JL, Carey PD, Mohr N, and others: Gender differences in the prevalence of childhood sexual abuse in the development of pediatric PTSD, *Arch Womens Mental Health* 7:111-121, 2004.
4. Tagay S, Herpertz S, Langkafel M, and others: Posttraumatic stress disorder in a psychosomatic outpatient clinic: gender effects, psychosocial functioning, sense of coherences, and service utilization, *J Psychosom Res* 58(5):439-446, 2005.
5. Mueser KT, Trumbetta SL, Rosenberg SD, and others: Trauma and posttraumatic stress disorder in severe mental illness, *J Consult Clin Psychol* 66(3):493-499, 1998.
6. Levine EG, Eckhard J, Targ E: Change in post-traumatic stress symptoms following psychosocial treatment for breast cancer, *Psycho-Oncology* 14:618-635, 2005.
7. Stein MB, Walker JR, Forde DR: Gender difference in susceptibility to posttraumatic stress disorder, *Behav Res Therapy* 38:619-628, 2000.
8. North CS, Kuwaski A, Spitznagel EL, and others: The course of PTSD, major depression, substance abuse, and somatization after a natural disaster, *J Nervous Mental Dis* 192(12):823-829, 2004.
9. Grubagh AL, Magruder KM, Waldrop AE, and others: Subthreshold PTSD in primary care: prevalence, psychiatric disorders, healthcare use, and functional status, *J Nervous Mental Dis* 193(10):658-664, 2005.
10. Friedman MJ: What might the psychobiology of posttraumatic stress disorder teach us about future approaches to pharmacotherapy? *J Clin Psychiatry* 61(Suppl 7):44-51, 2000.
11. Olf M, Langeland W, Gersons BPR: The psychobiology of PTSD: coping with trauma, *Psychoendocrinology* 30:974-982, 2005.
12. Fries E, Hesse J, Hellhammer J, and others: A new view on hypocortisolism, *Psychoendocrinology* 30:1010-1016, 2005.
13. Hageman I, Anderson HS, Jergensen MB: Posttraumatic stress disorder: a review of psychobiology and pharmacotherapy, *Acta Psych Scand* 104:411-422, 2001.
14. Van der Kolk BA: The psychobiology and psychopharmacology of PTSD, *Hum Psychopharmacol Clin Exper* 16:S49-S64, 2001.
15. Heinrichs M, Wagner D, Schoch W, and others: Predicting posttraumatic stress symptoms from pretraumatic risk factors: a 2-year prospective follow-up study in firefighters, *Am J Psychiatry* 162:2276-2286, 2005.
16. Schnurr PP, Lunney CA, Sengupta A: Risk factors for the development versus maintenance of posttraumatic stress disorder, *J Traum Stress* 17(2):85-95, 2004.
17. Connor KM, Davidson JRT, Lee LC: Spirituality, resilience, and anger in survivors of violent trauma: a community survey, *J Traum Stress* 16(5):487-494, 2003.
18. Bruce SE, Weisberg RB, Dolan RT, and others: Trauma and posttraumatic stress disorder in primary care patients, *Primary Care J Clin Psychiatry* 3(5):211-217, 2001.

19. Niles BL, Mori DL, Lambert JF, and others: Depression in primary care: comorbid disorders and related problems, *J Clin Psychol Med Settings* 12(1):71-77, 2005.
20. Spitzer RL, Williams JB, Bibbin M, and others: *Structured clinical interview for DSM-IV*, New York, 1994, New York State Psychiatric Institute.
21. Weathers FW, Keane TM, Davidson JRT: Clinician administered PTSD scale: a review of the first 10 years of research, *Depression Anxiety* 13:132-156, 2001.
22. Brewin CR: Systematic review of screening instruments for adults at risk for PTSD, *J Traum Stress* 18(1):53-62, 2005.
23. Lang AJ, Stein MB: An abbreviated PTSD checklist for use as a screening instrument in primary care, *Behav Res Therapy* 43:585-594, 2005.
24. National Center for PTSD: *Returning from the war zone: a guide for families*, Nov 2005, retrieved Feb 20, 2006, from http://www.ncptsd.va.gov/ncmain/ncdocs/manuals/nc_manual_returnwarz_gp.html?opm=1&rr=rr1562&srt=d&echorr=true.
25. Averill PM, Beck JG: Posttraumatic stress disorder in older adults: a conceptual review, *J Anxiety Dis* 14(2):133-156, 2000.
26. Golier JA, Yehuda R, Bierer LM, and others: The relationship of borderline personality disorder to posttraumatic stress disorder and traumatic events, *Am J Psychiatry* 160(11):2018-2024, 2003.
27. Davidson JRT, Connor KM, Hertzberg MA, and others: Maintenance therapy with fluoxetine in posttraumatic stress disorder, *J Clin Psychopharmacol* 25:166-169, 2005.
28. Brady K, Pearlstein T, Asnis GM, and others: Efficacy and safety of sertraline treatment of posttraumatic stress disorder, *JAMA* 283(14):1837-1844, 2000.
29. Cooper J, Carty J, Creamer M: Pharmacotherapy for posttraumatic stress disorder: empirical review and clinical recommendations, *Aust NZ J Psychiatry* 39:674-682, 2005.
30. Ahearn EP, Mussey M, Johnson C, and others: Quetiapine as an adjunctive treatment for posttraumatic stress disorder: an open-label study, *Int Clin Psychopharmacol* 21:29-33, 2006.
31. Shalev AY, Friedman MJ, Foa EB, and others: Integration and summary. In Foa EB, Keane TM, Friedman MJ, editors: *Effective treatments for PTSD: practice guidelines from the International Society for Traumatic Stress Studies*, New York, 2000, Guilford Press.
32. Butler AC, Chapman JE, Forman EM, and others: The empirical status of cognitive-behavioral therapy: a review of meta-analysis, *Clin Psychol Rev* 26:17-31, 2006.
33. Foa EB, Hembree EA, Cahill SP, and others: Randomized trial of prolonged exposure for posttraumatic stress disorder with and without cognitive restructuring: outcome at academic and community clinics, *J Counsel Clin Psychol* 73(5):953-964, 2005.
34. McDonagh A, Friedman MJ, McHugo G, and others: Randomized trial of cognitive-behavioral therapy for chronic posttraumatic stress disorder in adult female survivors of childhood sexual abuse, *J Counsel Clin Psychol* 73(3):515-524, 2005.
35. Bradley R, Greene J, Russ E, and others: A multidimensional meta-analysis of psychotherapy for PTSD, *Am J Psychiatry* 162:214-227, 2005.
36. Cook CAL, Flick LH, Homan SM, and others: Posttraumatic stress disorder in pregnancy: prevalence, risk factors, and treatment, *Obstet Gynecol* 103(4):710-717, 2004.
37. Yehuda R, Engel SM, Brand SR, and others: Transgenerational effects of posttraumatic stress disorder in babies of mothers exposed to the World Trade Center attacks during pregnancy, *J Endocrinol Metab* 90(7):4115-4118, 2005.
38. Grey MJ, Acierno R: Symptom presentations of older adult crime victims: description of a clinical sample, *Anxiety Dis* 16:299-309, 2002.
39. Acierno R, Rheingold AA, Resnick HS, and others: Preliminary evaluation of a video-based intervention for older adult victims of violence, *J Traum Stress* 17(6):535-541, 2004.
40. Acierno R, Resnick H, Kilpatrick D, and others: Assessing elder victimization, *Soc Psychiatry Psychiatr Epidemiol* 38:644-653, 2003.
41. Cook JM, Ruzek JI, Cassidy E: Possible association of posttraumatic stress disorder with cognitive impairment among older adults, *Psychiatric Serv* 54(9):1223-1225, 2003.
42. Alonzo AA: The experience of chronic illness and posttraumatic stress disorder: the consequences of cumulative adversity, *Soc Sci Med* 50:1475-1484, 2000.
43. Dong M, Giles WH, Felitti VJ, and others: Insights into causal pathways for ischemic heart disease: adverse childhood experiences study, *Circulation* 110:1761-1766, 2004.
44. Schnurr PP, Green BL: Understanding relationships among trauma, posttraumatic stress disorder, and health outcomes. In Schnurr PP, Green BL, editors: *Trauma and health: physical health consequences of exposure to extreme stress*, Washington, DC, 2004, American Psychiatric Association.
45. Kean EM, Kelsay K, Wamboldt F, and others: Posttraumatic stress in adolescents with asthma and their parents, *J Am Acad Child Adolesc Psychiatry* 45(1):78-86, 2006.
46. Weisberg RB, Bruce SE, Machan JT, and others: Nonpsychiatric illness among primary care patients with trauma histories and posttraumatic stress disorder, *Psychiatr Serv* 53(7):848-854, 2002.
47. Walker EA, Katon W, Russo J, and others: Health care costs associated with posttraumatic stress disorder symptoms in women, *Arch Gen Psychiatry* 60:369-374, 2003.

CHAPTER 265

Psychotic Disorders

Cindy Campbell

DEFINITION AND EPIDEMIOLOGY

Psychosis in itself is not a diagnosis but rather a presenting set of symptoms.[1] It may be a diagnostic symptom of a number of psychiatric disorders, or it may indicate an underlying metabolic or neurologic illness or a toxic reaction to a medication. The fourth edition of the *Diagnostic and Statistical Manual of Mental Disorders* (DSM-IV) defined psychosis as an impairment in reality testing that can include such symptoms as hallucinations and delusions.[2] Hallucinations may be auditory, visual, tactile, somatic, olfactory, or gustatory.[2] Hallucinations need to be differentiated from illusions, which have as their basis some external stimuli that is then misinterpreted. A delusion is any persistent belief with no factual basis. Types of delusions include paranoid delusions, ideas of reference, thought insertion, and thought broadcasting.

Psychosis can be a symptom of a number of underlying conditions such as schizophrenia and dementia. It is estimated that the lifetime prevalence of schizophrenia is 1%; that is, approximately 1 out of every 100 people in the world suffers from schizophrenia during his or her lifetime.[2] An estimated 2.5 million people with this disorder are currently living in the United States.[3] Schizophrenia often appears between the person's mid-teens and late twenties.[2] Schizophrenia affects equal numbers of men and women; however, in men the disorder often begins earlier and may be more severe.[4] Although schizophrenia appears in all socioeconomic groups, it is found more frequently in the lower socioeconomic groups, which has led some to theorize that the stress of poverty may be a cause of the disorder. However, it could also be that schizophrenia causes people to fall from higher to lower socioeconomic levels or to remain poor because of decreased functioning. This has been referred to as the *downward drift theory*.[5]

It is estimated that between 2% and 4% of individuals over 65 years old have a diagnosis of Alzheimer's-type dementia.[2] In older adults, psychosis often occurs in association with a diagnosis of dementia.

In addition to schizophrenia and Alzheimer's-type dementia, there is an array of mental health disorders in which psychosis is a key feature, including brief psychotic disorder, schizophreniform and schizoaffective disorders, delusional disorder, shared psychotic disorder, and substance-induced psychotic disorders. Psychotic disorders can also be caused by a general health condition, in which hallucinations or delusions are caused by a medical illness or brain damage.[5] Providers in primary care settings need to be aware of the possibility of psychosis developing in response to a medical condition.[5]

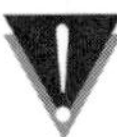

Immediate psychiatric evaluation is required for all patients with suicidal or homicidal ideation.

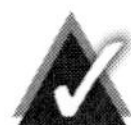

Physician consultation is indicated for increased psychotic behavior or for the development of tardive dyskinesia (TD).

PATHOPHYSIOLOGY

Research to identify the etiology of schizophrenia is ongoing. The most promising theory is the biologically based neurotransmitter and receptor site theory.[6] This theory involves a number of transmitter systems—dopamine, serotonin, and γ-aminobutyric acid—all of which appear to play a role. No single neurotransmitter system is ultimately responsible for schizophrenia. Schizophrenia is likely a complex combination of neurotransmitter availability, receptor sensitivity, and other mediating neural pathways. It is believed that either an alteration in neurotransmitters or a genetic vulnerability is inherited. The combination of genetics and life stressors leads to schizophrenia.[6]

Alzheimer's-type dementia is the most common type of dementia. Some families experience higher rates of Alzheimer's disease than others; therefore there is believed to be some genetic component.[7] Other theories include disorders of the neurotransmitters, an infectious process, or exposure to toxins.[7]

CLINICAL PRESENTATION

Psychosis may manifest in a variety of ways. A patient may be actively psychotic and obviously hallucinating; this is evident if the patient responds to unseen stimuli by talking out loud when nobody else is present. However, often the presentation is not so obvious. Patients experiencing a schizophrenic decompensation are reluctant to discuss their unusual thought processes. The more obvious thought disturbances are paranoid delusions, ideas of reference, thought insertion, and thought broadcasting. A paranoid delusion may include the belief that one is being monitored electronically by unknown persons. An individual who attaches special and personal meaning to the actions of others or to various objects or events, such as a conversation on the radio or a newspaper article, is said to be experiencing delusions of reference.[5] Those with delusions of control believe that their feelings, thoughts, and actions are being controlled by someone else. Thought insertion is the belief that thoughts are being placed inside one's head. Thought broadcasting is the belief that one's thoughts are being broadcast to the world at large.

A psychosis may appear as speech disorganization, behavior disorganization, or catatonia. These conditions are more likely to be found in children.[8] Disorganized speech may be evidenced by an inability to complete a train of thought or to speak words in a comprehensible order. Disorganized behavior is observed as an inability to complete any goal-directed activity such as activities of daily living. Catatonia is an extreme lack of reaction to outside stimuli; the individual may stare into space for hours, completely unresponsive to any verbal or physical stimuli. A less obvious sign of psychosis is thought blocking, which is evidenced by lengthy pauses between words and frequent losses of trains of thought. Thought blocking may be so severe that the individual forgets the question before formulating a response.

The symptoms are often grouped in three categories: positive symptoms, negative symptoms, and psychomotor symptoms. Positive symptoms are pathologic excesses or bizarre additions to a person's behavior such as delusions, disorganized thinking and speech, hallucinations, and inappropriate affect. Negative symptoms are those which appear to be pathologic deficits, or characteristics that are lacking in an individual such as blunted or flat affect, loss of volition, and social withdrawal. Psychomotor symptoms include awkward movements or repeated grimaces and odd gestures, which may have a ritualistic or magical meaning for the individual.[5]

Psychosis related to dementia often manifests as aggressive behavior accompanied by paranoia and delusions. Current estimates project that somewhere between 30% and 73% of individuals with Alzheimer's disease experience psychotic symptoms.[9,10] Individuals with Alzheimer's disease may suddenly fail to recognize their spouse and, believing there is a stranger in the home, may become combative. Such experiences may exacerbate paranoia and delusional thinking.

PHYSICAL EXAMINATION

A comprehensive physical examination is essential to exclude an underlying medical cause of psychosis. It is important that the health care provider not make an immediate psychiatric diagnosis in an individual previously undiagnosed with a psychiatric disorder. A thorough medical evaluation is also indicated, even in patients with a known psychiatric history. Psychosis may hamper communication about serious medical illness.

DIAGNOSTICS

Numerous conditions may cause psychosis. It is necessary to first establish the origin of psychotic symptoms, which will dictate treatment. To determine if a medical or psychiatric diagnosis is appropriate, certain laboratory tests are necessary, including CBC, BUN, glucose, creatinine, electrolytes, liver function tests, and urine toxin screen.[11] Results of these tests help the provider reach an appropriate diagnosis. The DSM-IV also has specific criteria by which to define schizophrenia and brief psychotic disorder (Boxes 265-1 and 265-2).

A mental status examination is also essential to establish the patient's orientation and ability to perform executive functioning and to obtain a general overview of the patient's cognitive impairment. This information aids in determining a differential diagnosis. Neuropsychologic testing is another valuable tool for establishing an accurate psychiatric diagnosis. Testing consists of a battery of written and verbal tests administered and interpreted by a qualified licensed practitioner.

No specific diagnostic tests are indicative of schizophrenia or dementia. Research to determine the role certain structural abnormalities play in the development and treatment of schizophrenia continues. Depending on the situation, a CT scan may be used to determine the presence of structural abnormalities. A CT scan is required if neurologic indicators are present, if the patient is experiencing a psychosis of sudden onset, or if the patient is experiencing a psychosis for the first time.[11] MRI, positron emission tomography, and single proton

BOX 265-1

DIAGNOSTIC CRITERIA FOR SCHIZOPHRENIA

A. *Characteristic symptoms:* Two (or more) of the following, each present for a significant portion of time during a 1-month period (or less if successfully treated):
   (1) Delusions
   (2) Hallucinations
   (3) Disorganized speech (e.g., frequent derailment or incoherence)
   (4) Grossly disorganized or catatonic behavior
   (5) Negative symptoms (i.e., affective flattening, alogia, or avolition)
   NOTE: Only one Criterion A symptom is required if delusions are bizarre or hallucinations consist of a voice keeping up a running commentary on the person's behavior or thoughts, or two or more voices conversing with each other.

B. *Social/occupational dysfunction:* For a significant portion of the time since the onset of the disturbance, one or more major areas of functioning such as work, interpersonal relations, or self-care are markedly below the level achieved prior to the onset (or when the onset is in childhood or adolescence, failure to achieve expected level of interpersonal, academic, or occupational achievement).

C. *Duration:* Continuous signs of the disturbance persist for at least 6 months. This 6-month period must include at least 1 month of symptoms (or less if successfully treated) that meet Criterion A (i.e., active-phase symptoms) and may include periods of prodromal or residual symptoms. During these prodromal or residual periods, the signs of the disturbance may be manifested by only negative symptoms or two or more symptoms listed in Criterion A present in an attenuated form (e.g., odd beliefs, unusual perceptual experiences).

D. *Schizoaffective and Mood Disorder exclusion:* Schizoaffective Disorder and Mood Disorder with Psychotic Features have been ruled out because either (1) no Major Depressive, Manic, or Mixed Episodes have occurred concurrently with the active-phase symptoms; or (2) if mood episodes have occurred during active-phase symptoms, their total duration has been brief relative to the duration of the active and residual periods.

E. *Substance/general medical condition exclusion:* The disturbance is not due to the direct physiologic effects of a substance (e.g., a drug of abuse, a medication) or a general medical condition.

F. *Relationship to a Pervasive Developmental Disorder:* If there is a history of Autistic Disorder or another Pervasive Developmental Disorder, the additional diagnosis of Schizophrenia is made only if prominent delusions or hallucinations are also present for at least a month (or less if successfully treated).

Classification of longitudinal course (can be applied only after at least 1 year has elapsed since the initial onset of active-phase symptoms):

- **Episodic with Interepisode Residual Symptoms** (episodes are defined by the reemergence of prominent psychotic symptoms); *also specify if:* **With Prominent Negative Symptoms**
- **Continuous** (prominent psychotic symptoms are present throughout the period of observation); *also specify if:* **With Prominent Negative Symptoms**
- **Single Episode in Partial Remission;** *also specify if:* **With Prominent Negative Symptoms**
- **Single Episode in Full Remission**
- **Other or Unspecified Pattern**

From American Psychiatric Association: *Diagnostic and statistical manual of mental disorders,* ed 4 (text rev), Washington, DC, 2000, The Association.

BOX 265-2

DIAGNOSTIC CRITERIA FOR BRIEF PSYCHOTIC DISORDER

A. Presence of one (or more) of the following symptoms:
(1) Delusions
(2) Hallucinations
(3) Disorganized speech (e.g., frequent derailment or incoherence)
(4) Grossly disorganized or catatonic behavior
NOTE: Do not include a symptom if it is a culturally sanctioned response pattern.

B. Duration of an episode of the disturbance is at least 1 day but less than 1 month, with eventual full return to premorbid level of functioning.

C. The disturbance is not better accounted for by a Mood Disorder with Psychotic Features, Schizoaffective Disorder, or Schizophrenia and is not due to the direct physiologic effects of a substance (e.g., a drug of abuse, a medication) or a general medical condition.

Specify if:

- **With Marked Stressor(s)** (brief reactive psychosis): if symptoms occur shortly after and apparently in response to events that, singly or together, would be markedly stressful to almost anyone in similar circumstances in the person's culture
- **Without Marked Stressor(s):** if psychotic symptoms *do* not occur shortly after, or are not apparently in response to events that, singly or together, would be markedly stressful to almost anyone in similar circumstances in the person's culture
- **With Postpartum Onset:** if onset within 4 weeks postpartum

From American Psychiatric Association: *Diagnostic and statistical manual of mental disorders*, ed 4 (text rev), Washington, DC, 2000, The Association.

DIAGNOSTICS

Psychotic Disorders

LABORATORY
CBC and differential
BUN
Creatinine
Serum glucose
Serum electrolytes
LFTs
Urine for toxic screen

IMAGING
CT scan*

*If indicated.

emission CT scans indicate that enlarged ventricles, decreased temporal and hippocampus size, increased basal ganglia, and abnormal glucose utilization in the prefrontal cortex are consistently found in patients with schizophrenia when examined as a group.[2] Autopsies have shown that neurofibrillary tangles and protein-based neuritic plaques are present in greater numbers and locations in the brains of individuals with Alzheimer's disease than in the brains of patients with other dementias and forms of aging.[7] However, this is only relevant postmortem and is not useful in the diagnosis and treatment of patients.

DIFFERENTIAL DIAGNOSIS

Numerous conditions may be responsible for psychosis. Medical conditions to consider in the differential diagnosis include metabolic disorders (e.g., hypoglycemia, hypothyroidism, hyperthyroidism, porphyria), nutritional deficiencies, neurologic disorders (e.g., brain lesion, encephalitis, Parkinson's disease, Huntington's chorea, cerebrovascular accident, seizure disorder), exposure to heavy metals, and medication toxicity (e.g., digitalis, theophylline, steroids, antiparkinsonian medications).[11] Psychiatric diagnoses to consider include schizophrenia, major depression with psychotic features, bipolar disorder, substance abuse or withdrawal (alcohol, benzodiazepines, LSD [lysergic acid diethylamide], PCP [phencyclidine hydrochloride], stimulants, cocaine, marijuana), and medication toxicity (anticholinergics). In older adults it is necessary to consider dementia (Alzheimer's dementia; vascular dementia; or dementia resulting from a specific medical condition such as HIV, Parkinson's disease, and others). In children it is necessary to exclude pervasive developmental disorders.[12,13]

DIFFERENTIAL DIAGNOSIS

Psychotic Disorders

Heavy metal exposure
Medication or substance toxicity
- Antiparkinsonian drugs
- Digitalis
- Steroids
- Theophylline
- Anticholinergics
- Substance abuse

Metabolic disorder
- Hypoglycemia
- Hypothyroidism
- Hyperthyroidism
- Porphyria

Neurologic disorder
- Brain lesion
- Cerebrovascular accident
- Encephalitis
- Huntington's chorea
- Parkinson's disease
- Seizure disorder

Nutritional deficiencies
Psychiatric disorders
- Bipolar disorder
- Dementia
- Major depression
- Schizophrenia

MANAGEMENT

The treatment of choice for psychosis is the use of antipsychotic medications, which date back to the 1940s and the development of phenothiazines. Antipsychotic medications can now be differentiated into two groups: (1) the first-generation, or typical, antipsychotic drugs, which were developed throughout the 1960s, 1970s, and 1980s; and (2) the more recent second-generation, or "atypical," antipsychotics. These medications are also referred to as *neuroleptics* because they often produce undesired movement effects similar to the symptoms of neurologic diseases.[5] First-generation antipsychotics are further classified as low-, medium-, or high-potency neuroleptics. The low-potency antipsychotic drugs (chlorpromazine [Thorazine], thioridazine [Mellaril], and mesoridazine [Serentil]) are highly sedating and are associated with increased anticholinergic side effects such as weight gain, constipation, blurred vision, urinary retention, and dry mouth. They have a lower potential for causing extrapyramidal side effects (EPSs). At present, thioridazine is used only when all other attempts at stabilization have been exhausted because of the potential for cardiac QTc prolongation.

The high-potency antipsychotics (haloperidol [Haldol], thiothixene [Navane], fluphenazine [Prolixin], perphenazine [Trilafon], molindone [Moban], pimozide [Orap], trifluoperazine [Stelazine], loxapine [Loxitane]) tend to be less sedating but have an increased tendency to cause EPSs. The atypical antipsychotic drugs (clozapine [Clozaril], risperidone [Risperdal], olanzapine [Zyprexa], quetiapine [Seroquel], ziprasidone [Geodon], aripiprazole [Abilify]) are reported to have decreased tendency to cause EPSs and may have a decreased tendency to cause tardive dyskinesia (TD). However, these medications are too new for this to be established with certainty. All antipsychotic medications have the potential to cause TD. They also have the potential to lower the seizure threshold and therefore should be used with caution in patients with seizure disorder.[13,14] The serious side effects associated with these medications suggest that they be prescribed in consultation with the physician or psychiatric provider.

Antipsychotic drugs, particularly the conventional ones, reduce the positive symptoms of schizophrenia, such as hallucinations and delusions, more completely or at least more quickly, than the negative symptoms such as flat affect, alogia (poverty of speech), and loss of volition.[15] Although antipsychotic drugs are now widely accepted, adherence is a problem, largely because of the drugs' powerful side effects. Discussions with patients regarding medication options need to include clear explanations of all risks and benefits of treatment choices. All atypical antipsychotics now carry a black box warning regarding the potential for increasing glucose levels and risk for development of diabetes mellitus. Before initiation of these medications it is recommended that fasting glucose and lipid profiles and a baseline weight be established.[16]

Supportive psychotherapy for both the patient and family is equally important. It is well known that the impact of schizophrenia can be greatly reduced with early aggressive intervention.[6] Other treatment options necessary at various times during the course of the disease include case management and vocational rehabilitation. As with any major disorder, patient and family education and the use of community resources are essential. Respite care is also a useful intervention for families experiencing caregiver stress.

Co-Management with Specialists

A psychiatric health care provider treats most patients with psychosis. Therefore treatment with the health care provider and any other specialty providers must be closely coordinated. Antipsychotic medications should never be discontinued abruptly and, ideally, dosages should never be decreased without serious consideration by the patient, family, and the psychiatric health care provider. Although a patient may appear to be completely free of psychosis, this is usually a result of the antipsychotic medication. Because each psychotic episode incurs a risk that the patient may not return to the previous level of functioning, lowering or discontinuing antipsychotic medications is a serious decision.

Accurate medication records are necessary because of interactions and potentiation of medications and because many medications can exacerbate psychosis. Although the use of the medication in question may be necessary, collaboration with the psychiatric health care provider can allow for an adjustment in the antipsychotic medications.

LIFE SPAN CONSIDERATIONS

The use of antipsychotic medications in children and adolescents has not yet been approved by the U.S. Food and Drug Administration. Nevertheless, in many cases it is necessary to use these medications for patients less than 18 years of age who are experiencing psychotic symptoms. Consideration should be given to the age and weight of the child, and consent must be obtained from the custodial parents or legal guardian and from the child if possible.[17] As always, the dose should be started low and slowly titrated up to the minimum effective dose. Atypical antipsychotic medications should be selected for use in children. These medications may have a decreased incidence of TD, but the incidence of TD increases with length of time on the medication. When making the initial assessment of children, it is necessary to obtain information from parents, siblings, and teachers.[8,13]

It is always necessary to determine pregnancy before initiating antipsychotic medications in women of childbearing age. In certain extenuating circumstances it may be necessary to use antipsychotic medications during pregnancy. In such cases, the benefits must clearly outweigh the risks. A thorough discussion of the potential side effects must be held, and a referral to a neonatologist is recommended.

Antipsychotic medications should be used with care in older adults. A much lower dose of medication is often required because of the decreased ability to metabolize it.[18] Older adults may be taking a multitude of medications, and drug interactions must be carefully assessed. The risk of lowered blood pressure and orthostatic changes with these medications is a primary concern, since dizziness can result in falls and fractures.[19] The anticholinergic side effects of the antipsychotic medications may increase confusion in this population. All atypical antipsychotics now carry a black box warning regarding the increased risk of death when used to treat dementia in the elderly.

COMPLICATIONS

All antipsychotic medications have the potential to cause uncomfortable side effects, which often cause patients to stop taking their medications. EPSs include dystonia, tremors, akathisia (an intolerable restlessness and need to pace), and a shuffling gait. Medications available to combat these unpleasant side effects include benztropine (Cogentin) and trihexyphenidyl (Artane). However, these medications have their own side effects, which can include increased psychosis and anticholinergic effects. Amantadine (Symmetrel) is also used for gait disturbances and muscle stiffness. Other treatment options for antipsychotic side effects include the beta blocker propranolol (Inderal) for tremors and akathisia and benzodiazepines for akathisia. Propranolol may worsen postural hypotension, and benzodiazepines should be avoided if possible because of their potential for both addiction and increased risk for falls in older adults.

The most frightening side effect of the antipsychotic medications is TD. It is a sometimes irreversible condition characterized by involuntary muscle movements of the mouth, jaw, and tongue. The incidence of TD is estimated to be between 3% and 5% per year.[2] There is no known treatment, but clonazepam (Klonopin) may ease the symptoms. If symptoms of TD develop, the antipsychotic medication must be tapered immediately and then discontinued if possible. Of the patients who are able to be kept off of antipsychotic medications, approximately one third experience resolution of TD within 3 months, and approximately 50% within 18 months.[2]

The decision regarding whether a patient can remain free of antipsychotic medications is best made by the patient and the specialty psychiatric health care provider.

The atypical antipsychotic clozapine has the potential to cause life-threatening agranulocytosis. Consequently, one of the requirements is that all patients taking this medication have their WBC count and absolute neutrophil count (ANC) monitored weekly. This may change to biweekly after 6 months of normal results, and then monthly after an additional 6 months of normal results. The medication is dispensed from the pharmacy after confirmation of an acceptable WBC and ANC count.

Neuroleptic malignant syndrome (NMS) is the most serious complication of antipsychotic administration and is potentially fatal. Although the clinical presentation of NMS may vary, it is usually associated with an elevated temperature and muscle rigidity. In addition, at least two of the following must be present: diaphoresis, dysphagia, tremor, incontinence, mutism, tachycardia, labile blood pressure, leukocytosis, elevated creatine phosphokinase, and a change in level of consciousness.[2] NMS usually occurs within the first 3 months of initiating the medication but can occur at any time, even after the patient has been maintained on a medication for months.[2]

Weight gain, hyperlipidemia, hyperglycemia, and diabetes mellitus are seen as health risks of antipsychotic therapy.[20] Hyperprolactinemia is a less common occurrence. Newer studies complicate the treatment horizon by suggesting there are few advantages to using the newer atypical antipsychotics.[21] What is clear is that we continue to accumulate new information as more research is done and we must remain current as this new information becomes available.

Psychosis has many complications. In patients with schizophrenia, psychosis may progressively worsen over time, resulting in decreased functional ability, particularly if medications are not taken consistently. Each exacerbation of the illness has the potential to last longer and be more severe. It is possible that the patient may never return to the previous level of functioning.

Whether a result of schizophrenia or dementia, treatment-resistant psychosis may result in the need for a series of medication trials, which can be frustrating for both the patient and the caregivers. Care must be taken to provide a safe environment during this process. Patients with psychosis may also have a potential for violence. This potential must be carefully and continually assessed, since patients may feel threatened by the environment as a result of the hallucinations.

INDICATIONS FOR REFERRAL OR HOSPITALIZATION

Psychosis is often only a symptom of a severe brain disorder and therefore needs to be managed by a psychiatric health care provider. Any patient experiencing psychosis needs to have the benefit of a full psychiatric evaluation to ensure proper diagnosis and treatment. Psychosis in children or adolescents should be managed by a psychiatric health care provider, preferably one with a specialty in child and adolescent psychiatry.

Hospitalization is often necessary during an acute exacerbation of a psychotic illness. This determination is best made by a psychiatric health care professional. However, any health care provider who believes a patient to be in imminent danger of harming either himself or herself or someone else should immediately initiate procedures for a psychiatric consultation.

PATIENT AND FAMILY EDUCATION

Patients and their families must be educated about psychosis and the available treatments so that they may make informed health care decisions. The side effects of medications are often frightening to both patients and families. A thorough discussion of the potential side effects and a plan to manage them can greatly alleviate the concerns of patients and families when deciding whether to use an antipsychotic medication. They must also be informed that psychosis is a biochemical illness with extreme psychosocial ramifications that respond to chemical intervention. As with any serious illness, patients must understand that, even if they are feeling better, medications need to be continued.

HEALTH PROMOTION

Hyperglycemia, hyperlipidemia, and weight gain can be managed with a combination of diet and exercise. It must be acknowledged, however, that many of the symptoms of a psychotic disorder include low motivation and indifference to personal appearance and hygiene. Consequently expectations must be kept realistic and achievable and should be highly individualized.

REFERENCES

1. Preston J, Johnson J: *Clinical psychopharmacology made ridiculously simple*, ed 3, Miami, 1997, MedMaster.
2. American Psychiatric Association: *Diagnostic and statistical manual of mental disorders*, ed 4 (text rev), Washington, DC, 2000, The Association.
3. Bichsel S: Schizophrenia and severe mental illness: guidelines for assessment, treatment and referral. In Welfel ER, Ingersoll R, editors: *The mental health desk reference*, New York, 2001, Wiley.
4. Usall J, Haro J, Ochoa S, and others: Influence of gender on social outcome in schizophrenia, *Acta Pysch Scand* 106(5):337-342, 2002.
5. Comer R: *Abnormal psychology*, New York, 2004, Worth.
6. Munich R: Contemporary treatment of schizophrenia, *Bull Menninger Clin* 61:189-220, 1997.
7. Tariot P: Neurobiology and treatment of dementia. In Salzman C, editor: *Clinical geriatric psychopharmacology*, ed 2, Baltimore, 1992, Williams & Wilkins.
8. Volkmar F: Childhood and adolescent psychosis: a review of the past 10 years, *J Am Acad Child Adolesc Psychiatry* 35:843-851, 1996.
9. Lacro J, Jeste D: Geriatric psychosis, *Psychiatr Q* 68:247-259, 1997.
10. Wilson R, Gilley DW, Bennett DA, and others: Hallucinations, delusions, and cognitive decline, *J Neurol Neurosurg Psychiatry* 69(2):172-177, 2000.
11. Hyman S: *Manual of psychiatric emergencies*, ed 2, Boston, 1988, Little, Brown.
12. Gartner J, Weintraub S, Carlson G: Childhood-onset psychosis: evolution and comorbidity, *Am J Psychiatry* 154:256-261, 1997.
13. Dulcan M, Martini D: *Concise guide to child and adolescent psychiatry*, ed 2, Washington, DC, 1999, American Psychiatric Press.
14. Green W: *Child and adolescent psychopharmacology*, ed 2, New York, 1995, Williams & Wilkins.
15. Torrey E: Studies of individuals with schizophrenia never treated with antipsychotic medications: a review, *Schizophrenia Res* 58(2-3):101-115, 2002.
16. Henderson D: Schizophrenia and comorbid metabolic disorders, *J Clin Psychiatry* 66(Suppl 6):11-20, 2005.

17. McClellan J, Werry J: Practice parameters for the assessment and treatment of children and adolescents with schizophrenia, *J Am Acad Child Adolesc Psychiatry* 33(5):616-635, 1994.
18. Salzman C: *Psychiatric medications for older adults: the concise guide*, New York, 2001, Guilford Press.
19. Lamy P, Salzman C, Nevis-Olesen J: Drug prescribing patterns, risks, and compliance guidelines. In Salzman C, editor: *Clinical geriatric psychopharmacology*, ed 2, Baltimore, 1992, Williams & Wilkins.
20. Sussman N: Review of atypical antipsychotics and weight gain, *J Clin Psychiatry* 62(Suppl 23):5-12, 2001.
21. Gardner D, Baldessarini R, Waraich P: Modern antipsychotic drugs: a critical overview, *CMAJ* 172(13):1703-1711, 2005.

CHAPTER 266

Somatization Disorder

Alice Bolton, Cindy Campbell, and
Willadene "Billie" Walker Schmucker

DEFINITION AND EPIDEMIOLOGY

Somatization disorder represents the extreme end of a continuum of somatoform disorders. These disorders are characterized by a history of symptoms that cannot be explained by organic causes or be attributed to anxiety, depression, or hypochondriasis. Somatization disorder is characterized by a history of at least eight unexplained symptoms in four or more bodily systems and represents somatoform disorder in its most extreme form.[1] Such patients describe high levels of distress and functional disability and have excessive resource utilization. Somatization disorder generally develops before 30 years of age and is characterized by frequent, varied, and long-lasting somatic complaints that have no basis in physical dysfunction. People with somatization disorder often describe their symptoms in dramatic or exaggerated terms, do not accept the psychologic basis of their problems, and insist on obtaining medical help for them.[1] Health care providers often find them frustrating or irritating because they do not get better and keep coming back or go from provider to provider in search of relief. As a result, somatization disorder represents a significant cost to the health care system.

There are six types of somatoform disorders: (1) body dysmorphic disorder, (2) conversion disorder, (3) hypochondriasis, (4) somatization disorder, (5) somatoform pain disorder, and (6) undifferentiated somatoform disorder.[2] The essential feature of these disorders is the presence of a physical or somatic complaint in the absence of any demonstrable organic findings or any known physiologic mechanisms that can account for the complaint or explain the findings. There is also the presumption of associated psychologic factors or unconscious conflicts to account for the syndrome.[3]

Somatization disorder was first described by Pierre Briquet in 1859 and was previously known as Briquet's syndrome.[1] In contrast to the other somatoform disorders, a diagnosis of somatization disorder requires that a person have multiple ailments that include several pain symptoms rather than complaints limited to one organ system.[1] To meet the criteria for classification as a somatization disorder, the patient must have experienced symptoms before 30 years of age and must have at least four pain symptoms, two gastrointestinal symptoms, one sexual symptom, and one pseudoneurologic symptom.[2] These unexplained symptoms are not intentionally feigned or produced.[2] The severity of somatization disorder is assessed from a total count of any of the following: complaints, the search for medical treatment, the use of medication, or lifestyle adjustments for different symptoms.[4]

The onset of a somatization disorder usually occurs in adolescence or early adulthood. It occurs predominantly in women: between 0.2% and 2% of all women in the United States experience a somatization disorder in any given year, compared with less than 0.2% of men.[5] This is consistent with research conducted by Faravelli, Guerrini-Degl'Innocenti, Aiazzi, and colleagues, in which all somatoform disorders were much more common in women, with somatization, conversion, and body dysmorphic disorders found only among females in their inquiry.[6] Somatization disorder often runs in families; 10% to 20% of close female relatives of women with the disorder develop it themselves.[1] It also tends to be associated with sociopathy and alcoholism in male relatives.[7] Kroenke, Spitzer, deGruy, and colleagues report that the diagnosis of a somatization disorder involves lifetime symptoms, with more than one fourth of all health care provider visits attributable to somatoform disorders.[8] All somatoform disorders seem to be more common in less educated, lower socioeconomic groups and in persons of low occupational status. Studies have shown a concordance rate of 29% in monozygotic twins and 10% in dizygotic twins.[9] Cultural factors may influence the gender ratio for somatization disorder. This particular somatoform disorder occurs only rarely in men in the United States; a higher frequency is reported in Greek and Puerto Rican men.[2]

PATHOPHYSIOLOGY

Somatization is one of the oldest of all known psychologic diagnoses. The first reference to this type of phenomenon appeared in Egyptian documents in approximately 1900 BC; it was also commented on by the Greeks. In its modern form, it was first defined in 1859 by Briquet, a French physician who identified patients with medical symptoms but no demonstrable medical disease.[10] The cause of somatization disorder is unknown. Rossi and Cheek have suggested that patients with this disorder have no conscious control over their somatization because it is tied to neuropsychophysiologic state–dependent memory, but they do have control over whether they embellish their symptoms and disabilities.[11]

The suspected etiology of somatization disorder lies in the mind-body connection.[12] One body of research reports an interrelated link between psychosocial and genetic factors, including identification with a parent who models the sick role, suppression or repression of anger toward others and turning this anger inward toward self, a punitive personality organization with a strong superego, and low self-esteem. There seems to be a genetic link, with a 10% to 20% incidence of mothers or sisters of patients also being afflicted.[9] Some studies have suggested a neuropsychologic basis for somatization disorder. These investigations propose that patients with this disorder have characteristic attentional and cognitive impairments that result in a faulty perception and assessment of somatosensory input. Impairments include excessive distractibility, an inability to habituate to repetitive stimuli, and partial and circumstantial associations. Cultural and ethnic factors are important to note because they influence the patient's self-report of symptoms.[13]

CLINICAL PRESENTATION

Patients with somatization disorder often have "seen every health care provider in town." The nature of the disorder is chronic and lifelong, generally beginning in adolescence and lasting through the life cycle if left untreated. Individuals often are seen with complex and inconsistent medical histories. Laboratory tests are generally not significantly abnormal, and reported symptoms may be the result of a faulty assessment of somatosensory input by the individual.

It is necessary to review 35 symptoms as part of the assessment for somatization disorder. To receive this diagnosis, the patient must display 13 or more of these 35 symptoms, and these symptoms must lack an acceptable medical explanation. If the physical examination reveals no acceptable medical explanation, the following seven symptoms are recommended as an initial screen for somatization disorder: (1) pain in extremities, (2) shortness of breath, (3) amnesia, (4) burning sensation in sexual organs or rectum (other than during intercourse), (5) difficulty swallowing, (6) vomiting, and (7) painful menstruation.[11] Patients with somatization disorder often report a belief that they have "always been sickly" and that "nobody has been able to help me." Somatization disorder has a fluctuating course, and afflicted individuals are rarely asymptomatic. It is unusual for them to go for more than 1 year without some medical attention. These individuals describe their symptoms in vivid, colorful, exaggerated, emotional, and dramatic terms. Instead of simply saying "I can't swallow," a patient with somatization disorder would likely say, "I can't swallow; it's as if I have someone's hands around my throat, squeezing his fingers deeply into my neck." These individuals often dress in an exhibitionistic manner and are sometimes seductive. They usually describe significant distress and interpersonal problems and often report marital, occupational, and social problems. When describing their histories, they are often vague, imprecise, inconsistent, and disorganized. Suicide threats are common, but actual suicides are rare.[9]

PHYSICAL EXAMINATION

Somatoform disorders are a diagnostic challenge because the symptoms encountered are nonspecific and can overlap with a multitude of medical conditions. Caution is always necessary so that underlying and potentially treatable mental and general medical disorders are not overlooked.[8] A thorough physical examination is necessary, even in patients with a psychiatric history. As is always the case, it is important that the health care provider not be swayed by a suspicion of a psychiatric diagnosis in patients previously undiagnosed with a psychiatric disorder. Although the provider may be tempted to forgo the physical examination in a patient previously diagnosed with a somatoform disorder, these individuals can also develop serious medical illnesses.

DIAGNOSTICS

Given the array of potential symptoms, an appropriate clinical investigation is indicated. The fourth edition of the *Diagnostic and Statistical Manual of Mental Disorders* (DSM-IV) has specific criteria for defining a somatization disorder (Box 266-1). The initial diagnostic tests should be guided by the history and physical examination. However, characteristically there is a lack of findings on diagnostic studies.[2] Health care providers treating this condition often find themselves walking a fine line between an appropriate clinical investigation and an exhaustive but unproductive battery of tests.[14] Neuropsychologic testing is a valuable tool in establishing an accurate psychiatric diagnosis. This procedure consists of a battery of written and

BOX 266-1

DIAGNOSTIC CRITERIA FOR SOMATIZATION DISORDER

A. A history of many physical complaints beginning before age 30 years that occur over a period of several years and result in treatment being sought or significant impairment in social, occupational, or other important areas of functioning.
B. Each of the following criteria must have been met, with individual symptoms occurring at any time during the course of the disturbance:
   (1) *Four pain symptoms:* a history of pain related to at least four different sites or functions (e.g., head, abdomen, back, joints, extremities, chest, rectum, during menstruation, during sexual intercourse, or during urination)
   (2) *Two gastrointestinal symptoms:* a history of at least two gastrointestinal symptoms other than pain (e.g., nausea, bloating, vomiting other than during pregnancy, diarrhea, or intolerance of several different foods)
   (3) *One sexual symptom:* a history of at least one sexual or reproductive symptom other than pain (e.g., sexual indifference, erectile or ejaculatory dysfunction, irregular menses, excessive menstrual bleeding, vomiting throughout pregnancy)
   (4) *One pseudoneurologic symptom:* a history of at least one symptom or deficit suggesting a neurologic condition not limited to pain (conversion symptoms such as impaired coordination or balance, paralysis or localized weakness, difficulty swallowing or lump in throat, aphonia, urinary retention, hallucinations, loss of touch or pain sensation, double vision, blindness, deafness, seizures; dissociative symptoms such as amnesia; or loss of consciousness other than fainting)
C. Either (1) or (2)
   (1) After appropriate investigation, each of the symptoms in Criterion B cannot be fully explained by a known general medical condition or the direct effects of a substance (e.g., a drug of abuse, a medication).
   (2) When there is a related general medical condition, the physical complaints or resulting social or occupational impairment are in excess of what would be expected from the history, physical examination, or laboratory findings.
D. The symptoms are not intentionally produced or feigned (as in factitious disorder or malingering).

From American Psychiatric Association: *Diagnostic and statistical manual of mental disorders,* ed 4 (text rev), Washington, DC, 2000, The Association.

verbal tests given by a licensed individual who is qualified to administer the tests and interpret the results.

DIFFERENTIAL DIAGNOSIS

Symptom presentation may be indicative of numerous medical conditions. Three clues may indicate the presence of somatization disorder: (1) the physical complaints often involve multiple organ systems; (2) the symptoms have appeared early (before age 30), appear to be chronic, and lack physical findings or structural abnormalities; and (3) there is an absence of diagnostic abnormalities that are characteristic of the indicated medical condition.[2] Many medical conditions, including hyperparathyroidism, porphyria, multiple sclerosis, and lupus, also manifest as vague somatic symptoms and must be excluded in the differential diagnosis.[2] It is essential to remember that such presentations in an older patient are most likely indicative of a medical condition.[1]

A number of psychiatric disorders must also be considered; these include schizophrenia, panic disorder, generalized anxiety disorder, mood disorders, posttraumatic stress disorder, factitious disorder, and malingering.[2,14,15]

DIFFERENTIAL DIAGNOSIS

Somatization Disorder

MEDICAL DISORDERS
- Hyperparathyroidism
- Systemic lupus erythematosus
- Multiple sclerosis
- Porphyria

PSYCHIATRIC DISORDERS
- Factitious disorder
- Generalized anxiety disorder
- Malingering
- Mood disorders
- Panic disorder
- Posttraumatic stress disorder
- Schizophrenia

MANAGEMENT

It is helpful to view the development of somatization disorder as an unhealthy coping skill,[16] which often lasts for many years. The symptoms may fluctuate over time but rarely resolve or disappear completely without psychotherapy.[1] Because any number of symptoms may be present, it is important to focus on symptom relief. If the patient is experiencing a high level of anxiety or significant depressive symptoms, a selective serotonin reuptake inhibitor (SSRI) antidepressant may be helpful. It is essential that the patient be involved in some type of therapy, the goal of which is to develop healthier methods of coping. Cognitive behavior therapy is also useful and can assist with the reduction of somatization by not reinforcing this behavior.[15] Group therapy in combination with regular consultation with a health care provider can also be helpful in treating somatoform disorders. The patient may have additional medical or psychiatric illnesses that require appropriate treatment.

Because these patients often seek health care from many providers, it is of utmost importance to obtain a thorough history, including current medications and treatments. Queries about past and current interventions to seek symptom relief may help the provider discover a duplication of treatment interventions or dangerous drug interactions. Communication among all health care providers is necessary. Records from previous and current providers may be required.

When narcotic analgesics or other controlled substances are considered in treatment, precautions must be taken to avoid dependence or addiction.

LIFE SPAN CONSIDERATIONS

By definition, symptoms of somatoform disorder begin before age 30. Women are diagnosed more often with the disorder in the United States; men of Puerto Rican or Greek descent are diagnosed more often. Recent research by Brown, Schrag, and Trimble showed that persons with somatization reported higher levels of family conflict and significantly lower levels of family cohesion than the comparison group.[17] The study found an association between somatization disorder and being raised in an environment with frequent arguments, emotional distance, poor support, and high levels of physical and emotional abuse.

COMPLICATIONS

Complications associated with any somatoform disorder include unnecessary medical treatment and operations, financial distress, impairment in work and social activities, family discord, iatrogenic effects from multiuse and overuse of medical interventions, substance-related disorders, and suicide.[2,18] Treatment is often sought from several providers, which places the patient at risk for dangerous interactions from treatment combinations. Each operation or hospitalization adds health risks. Time is lost from work, which often creates job insecurity. Families suffer from loss of the patient's interaction, loss of parental guidance, or loss of spousal support. The risk for dependence on narcotic analgesics is great. Depression and suicide risk increase as the condition progresses.

INDICATIONS FOR REFERRAL OR HOSPITALIZATION

Somatoform disorders present a challenge in primary care. Because the condition is not readily recognized, considerations for referral are not definitively identified. The primary care provider might consider the following as guidelines for referral: the patient's medical and surgical history, the frequency and nature of primary care and specialist office visits, and response to interventions. A psychosocial assessment may provide clues to the causative nature of the disorder. Childhood abuse has been correlated with the development of somatoform disorders.[19] A mental health referral is made after the provider has excluded any physical reason for the patient's symptoms.

With the advent of managed care, hospitalizations for somatoform disorder have been limited. Outpatient evaluations are more prevalent. Patients with a somatoform disorder and a co-morbid personality disorder may be at risk for suicide. For the patient's safety, any indication of suicide risk requires an immediate referral to a psychiatric health care provider. All states have provisions for emergency inpatient evaluation for patients who pose a danger to themselves or others. Providers should be familiar with the mental health act in their practice locale.

PATIENT EDUCATION

Many patients are prescribed medications for symptom relief. Education about the side effects, risks, purposes, and use of medications is stressed. A review of medications and an assessment of the effectiveness of the intervention are made at each office visit. Patients are advised to write down their questions and concerns before the visit; such communication may provide clues to a diagnosis.

Although often seen in primary care, somatization is not often treated in this setting. Nevertheless, the health care provider in primary care often continues to be the medical provider. The challenge to the provider is to distinguish somatic symptoms from those with an actual biologic origin. The provider has the opportunity to assess and educate the patient about treatment. Educating the patient about the importance of continuing mental health treatment is essential. A decrease in the use of health care has been associated with patients' ability to distinguish between mental health issues and physical symptoms.[18]

HEALTH PROMOTION

Health promotion is difficult to define in this diagnosis. The nature of the disorder is to displace emotional responses with magnified physical symptomatology. Those persons identified as being at risk for developing the disorder should receive psychotherapy and other supportive interventions early in life. Those persons diagnosed would benefit from ongoing treatment focusing on developing and maintaining effective coping skills and on developing and maintaining a healthy lifestyle, including regular exercise, appropriate diet, routine physical examination, adequate rest, and maintenance of a routine.

REFERENCES

1. Comer R: *Abnormal psychology*, ed 5, New York, 2004, Worth.
2. American Psychiatric Association: *Diagnostic and statistical manual of mental disorders*, ed 4 (text rev), Washington, DC, 2000, The Association.
3. Barsky AJ, Borus JF: Somatization and medicalization in the era of managed care, *JAMA* 27:1931-1934, 1995.
4. Servan-Schreiber D, Tabas G, Kolb R: Somatizing patients, part II, Practical management, *Am Fam Phys* 61:1423-1428, 1431-1432, 2000; retrieved Nov 30, 2005, from http://www.aafp.org/afp/20000215/1073.html.
5. Ladwig K, Marten M, Erazo M, and others: Identifying somatization disorder in a population-based health examination survey: psychological burden and gender differences, *Psychosomatics* 42(6):511-518, 2001.
6. Faravelli C, Guerrini-Degl'Innocenti B, Aiazzi L, and others: Epidemiology of somatoform disorders: a community survey in Florence, *J Affect Disord* 20(2):135-141, 1990.
7. Berkow R: Somatoform disorders. In Beers MH, Berkow R, editors: *The Merck manual of diagnosis and therapy*, ed 17, Whitehouse Station, NJ, 2002, Merck, retrieved Nov 30, 2005, from http://www.merck.com/mrkshared/mmanual/section15/chapter186/186a.jsp .
8. Kroenke K, Spitzer RL, deGruy FV 3rd, and others: Multisomatoform disorder, *Arch Gen Psychiatry* 54(4):352-358, 1997.
9. Kaplan H, Sadock B: *Synopsis of psychiatry, behavioral sciences, clinical psychiatry*, ed 6, Baltimore, 1991, Williams & Wilkins.
10. Richardson R, Engel C: Evaluation and management of medically unexplained physical symptoms, *Neurologist* 10(1):18-30, 2004.
11. Rossi E, Cheek D: *Mind-body therapy: methods of ideodynamic healing in hypnosis*, Baltimore, 1988, Norton.
12. McClendon P: *The mind-body connection*, retrieved Nov 30, 2005, from http://www.clinicalsocialwork.com/mind-body.html.
13. Noyes R, Holt CS, Happel RL, and others: A family study of hypochondriasis, *J Nerv Ment Dis* 185(4):223-232, 1997.
14. Peveler R, Kilkenny L, Kinmouth A: Medically unexplained physical symptoms in primary care: a comparison of self-report screening questionnaires and clinical opinion, *J Psychosom Res* 42:245-252, 1997.
15. Gooch J, Wolcott R, Speed J: Behavioral management of conversion disorder in children, *Arch Phys Med Rehabil* 78:264-268, 1997.
16. Badura A, Reiter RC, Altmaier EM, and others: Dissociation, somatization, substance abuse, and coping in women with chronic pelvic pain, *Obstet Gynecol* 90(3):405-410, 1997.
17. Brown R, Schrag A, Trimble M: Dissociation, childhood interpersonal trauma and family functioning in persons with somatization disorder, *Am J Psychiatry* 162:899-905, 2005.
18. Morse D, Suchman A, Frankel R: The meaning of symptoms in 10 women with somatization disorder and a history of childhood abuse, *Arch Fam Med* 6:468-476, 1997.
19. Farley M, Keaney J: Physical symptoms, somatization, and dissociation in women survivors of childhood sexual assault, *Women Health* 25:33-45, 1997.

CHAPTER 267

Substance Abuse

Joseph Rampulla

DEFINITION AND EPIDEMIOLOGY

Patients afflicted with substance abuse and addiction have health, emotional, family, social, legal, and spiritual troubles that are vexing to the patient, the family, and the health care provider. The HIV epidemic, the cocaine surge of the 1980s, the heroin surge of the 1990s, designer drugs, methamphetamine, and the recognition of the morbidity and mortality associated with substance abuse have increasingly brought this problem to the attention of health care providers. Patients with an addiction usually incur higher medical costs than patients with other chronic conditions.[1]

The term *substance abuse* refers to a maladaptive pattern of substance use in which people rely on a drug excessively and regularly, damaging social and interpersonal relationships; failing to fulfill major role obligations at work, school, or home; and putting themselves or others in danger.[2,3] A more advanced pattern, *substance dependence*, also known as *addiction*, refers to a syndrome in which there is overriding concern with the use and acquisition of a drug, despite the negative consequences. Addiction involves drug obsession; self-dose escalation; and health, family, emotional, and economic deterioration as people center their lives on it. Addiction also usually implies a degree of tolerance and physiologic dependence. The term *abuse* usually refers to a problematic pattern of substance use that is not necessarily associated with a defined withdrawal syndrome. Not all patients who develop a physiologic dependence are "addicted." Physiologic dependence inevitably develops with the therapeutic use of several medications, such as opiates that are appropriately prescribed for chronic pain and corticosteroids that are prescribed for refractory inflammatory conditions. Although these patients may experience abstinence syndromes, they usually do not display addictive behaviors and should not be diagnosed with a substance use disorder on this basis alone.

The term *abstinence* can refer to the stereotyped adverse physiologic or psychologic syndromes of drug withdrawal; this term is often used interchangeably with the term *withdrawal*. An individual who is abstinent is drug free, whereas an individual in recovery is in the long-term process of attending to the spiritual, physical, and psychosocial needs that have been affected by addiction. *Withdrawal* refers to the process of removing the drug of dependence from the body, whereas *detoxification* generally refers to the process of administrating tapering doses of the same or cross-tolerant drugs to assist with withdrawal.

Tolerance refers to the need to increase the amount of drug to achieve the same effects. Because individuals who are tolerant have adapted to a certain level of drug use, they can experience both intoxication and abstinence at the same time. *Relapse* is the return to problematic drug use after a significant period of abstinence; it may involve a different drug than the patient's original drug of choice. A common example of this is the abstinent opioid addict who develops alcoholism.

In 2002, 19.5 million U.S. adults, representing 8.3% of the population, were estimated to be current users of illicit drugs.[4] Approximately 50% of American youth are estimated to have tried an illicit drug by grade 12.[5] The misuse and abuse of prescription medications is a growing problem in all segments of the population, beginning in preadolescent children. The National Survey on Drug Use and Health, conducted by the Substance Abuse and Mental Services Administration (SAMHSA), estimates that in 2003, 6.3 million Americans, ages 12 years and older, abused prescriptions drugs (took prescription drugs not prescribed for them or took medication solely for pleasure or entertainment) in the month preceding the survey. Most people abused pain relievers (4.7 million), but a substantial number also abused tranquilizers (1.8 million), stimulants (1.2 million), and sedatives (0.3 million).[6]

Although serious substance abuse disorders are rarely permanently reversed by a single treatment episode, counseling by a health care provider can reduce substance abuse and its hazards over time. Alcohol and nicotine are the most widely abused substances in the United States, resulting in the greatest burden of substance use–related suffering, meriting discussion in separate chapters. Nicotine dependence is discussed in Chapter 24, and Chapter 258 is devoted to alcohol abuse.

Physician consultation is required for buprenorphine and buprenorphine-naloxone (Suboxone) maintenance treatment.

PATHOPHYSIOLOGY

Addictive disorders are chronic relapsing conditions. The cause of addictive disorders is probably the result of interactions among genetic and temperament susceptibility, psychosocial factors, and drug availability. Major hazards include overdose; withdrawal symptoms; violence and unintentional injuries; pregnancy and neonatal complications; social, economic, and family dysfunction; and the complications of injection drug use (IDU). Drugs can be conveniently, although not precisely, classified as central nervous system (CNS) depressants, opioids, stimulants, psychotomimetics and hallucinogens, inhalants, nicotine, and anabolic steroids.

On a neurobiologic level, addiction appears to be driven by activation of the dopaminergic neurons in the ventral tegmental area–nucleus accumbens of the brain in complex interaction with endogenous opioids (endorphins), γ-aminobutyric acid (GABA), serotonin channels, acetylcholine, and adrenergic systems.[7] Drugs act at various sites to stimulate brain reward, thereby reinforcing repeated use. Long-term alterations in brain reward pathways may explain persistent heightened vulnerability to drug effects and continued dependence long after the clinical physical dependence has resolved. Such alterations may in part explain the chronic relapsing nature of addiction.

Major Drugs of Abuse

Drugs from one class can be used to enhance the desired or attenuate the undesired effects of drugs from another class. Understanding the features of these drug classes should be tempered by the knowledge that addicted patients usually take drugs from more than one category at a time.

Central Nervous System Sedatives. The major CNS sedatives are alcohol, barbiturates, benzodiazepines, and other compounds that are similar to either barbiturates or benzodiazepines. GABA is the major inhibitory neurotransmitter that lowers cell excitability, and sedatives generally depress brain activity by augmenting the GABA systems. Mild manifestations of sedative intoxication include tranquilization, fine lateral nystagmus, and slightly decreased alertness. Moderate intoxication is manifested as ataxia, slurred speech, coarse nystagmus, and sedation. An overdose of these substances produces somnolence, staggering, and marked dysarthria; this can progress to coma, respiratory depression, and death. The major hazards of sedative abuse include a dangerous abstinence syndrome, unintentional injuries, and overdose. Alcohol alters CNS membrane fluidity and interacts with GABA receptors, producing sedative effects (see Chapter 258). Although the perinatal effects of maternal alcohol use are well known, such research regarding other sedatives is sparse.

Barbiturates, which are derivatives of barbituric acid, both enhance and mimic the effect of GABA, thus depressing all brain activity. They are classified by their onset and duration of action, although their wide distribution in body fat and muscle compartments makes the relationship between serum concentration and action variable. Their prescribed use for sedation has largely been replaced by benzodiazepines, but phenobarbital is still useful for epilepsy, and butabarbital combinations are effective for headaches. Barbiturates have a much narrower therapeutic index than do benzodiazepines. Chronic use may cause slowed learning, impaired memory, sleep disturbances, and emotional lability. The short-acting (e.g., pentobarbital) and intermediate-acting (e.g., amobarbital) barbiturates are most often abused. Long-acting barbiturates (e.g., phenobarbital) are not considered intoxicating, but individuals with addiction often take them in high doses with alcohol, producing dangerous impairment and toxicity. The chronic metabolism of barbiturates induces hepatic enzymes that can speed the metabolism of other sedatives, phenytoin, and warfarin. Because tolerance to barbiturates is incomplete, chronic users are still vulnerable to overdose. The drugs methaqualone and glutethimide are synthetic compounds that are similar in toxicity and effect to barbiturates.

Benzodiazepines, formerly referred to as minor tranquilizers, facilitate the action of GABA at specific sites. They are often prescribed for relief of anxiety, insomnia, or muscle spasm or tension; for acute management of agitation; and for acute treatment of convulsions. Cross-tolerance and a wide therapeutic index make benzodiazepines good agents to assist with alcohol detoxification. In general, benzodiazepines are effective and have a wide margin of safety; however, their misuse is widespread among addicts. Their abuse potential seems to be associated with speed of onset and potency, with rapidly acting drugs (e.g., diazepam, clonazepam, and alprazolam) having the greatest potential for abuse, and slower-acting compounds (e.g., oxazepam and prazepam [not available in the United States]) having the least. The high potency of clonazepam and alprazolam, with 1 mg roughly equivalent to 10 mg of diazepam, appears to contribute to their abuse potential and street value.[8] All benzodiazepines are metabolized to inactive compounds in the liver. Longer-acting benzodiazepines first require hepatic oxidation, which produces active drug metabolites. Flunitrazepam (Rohypnol) is a high-potency and short-acting benzodiazepine that has been implicated in acquaintance rape. It is prescribed for insomnia in many countries and is smuggled into the United States for illicit use. Zolpidem and zaleplon are newer short-acting synthetic hypnotics that are similar in action to the benzodiazepines.

γ-Hydroxybutyrate (GHB) is an emerging sedative of abuse that is a synthetic formulation of a normally occurring neurotransmitter. It induces anesthesia, absence seizures, and probably dependence. It is often synthesized in home laboratories; several deaths have been attributed to the ingestion of home GHB recipes that include lye. Estimates of overdose and other GHB-related medical emergencies are imprecise because GHB is short acting and difficult to detect with laboratory tests.[9]

The severity of withdrawal from sedatives is generally proportional to the level and duration of use, with barbiturates and rapidly acting, high-potency benzodiazepines producing the most severe syndromes. Restlessness, anxiety, and mild tremors usually develop approximately 12 to 24 hours after discontinuation of a short-acting drug. The onset may be delayed for several days if the primary drug is long acting. Chronic liver dysfunction may increase drug storage and thereby delay the manifestations of withdrawal. Escalating symptoms, increased tremors, dissociative and perceptual symptoms, increased pulse and blood pressure, and hyperreflexia develop. At this point the patient becomes prone to convulsions, even if properly treated. If the patient is left untreated, withdrawal can progress to an acute psychosis that resembles delirium tremens. Patients experiencing high-dose sedative withdrawal need to be treated on an inpatient basis with a long-acting sedative like phenobarbital. Patients may be given a challenge dose of pentobarbital to estimate their habit and to guide dosing.[8]

Low-dose sedative withdrawal is a different phenomenon that is primarily characterized by waxing and waning anxiety, insomnia, irritability, and mild tremors. These individuals may be addicted or may instead be physiologically dependent on therapeutic benzodiazepine regimens. Tapering the benzodiazepine dose may take as long as 6 months. Patients usually benefit from additional psychosocial support and must be cautioned that they may experience a recurrence of the original anxiety symptoms.

Opioids. Opioids produce their effects by interacting with endogenous opioid receptors throughout the CNS and intestines. Morphine is the prototypical opioid, with heroin (diacetylmorphine) the form most often seriously abused. There has been an increasing trend in new heroin use since 1992, although this trend appears to be leveling off. Heroin is illegal in the United States and is sold on the streets as a white or brown powder; it is usually diluted with sugar, talc, baking soda, aspirin, or quinine. It is sometimes mixed with scopolamine, strychnine, or other poisons. Heroin may be insufflated (snorted), smoked, or dissolved and injected. Most heroin users eventually turn to IV use and rarely return to other routes.[10] Synthetic opioids include methadone, propoxyphene, meperidine, and fentanyl. Tramadol is a newer synthetic with both mu and kappa opioid activity. Overuse can provoke convulsions, but so far reports of abuse have been low.[11]

There has been an emerging problem with the illicit use of the sustained-release formulations of the prescription analgesic oxycodone. The sustained-release coating is easily bypassed by crushing the pill, making a high-potency drug available for rapid effects. Tablets are reported to sell on the street for $0.50 to $1 per milligram.[12] Fentanyl transdermal patches and hydrocodone tablets are other commonly diverted and abused prescription opiates.

Opioids are useful for relief of pain and suffering, for cough suppression, and for their antidiarrheal effects. With a few individual differences, most opioids display similar pharmacologic actions and vary mostly in kinetics. Although chronic administration inevitably produces some degree of physiologic dependence, susceptibility to the development of addiction varies among individuals. Addiction, overdose, and premature labor are the most serious complications directly caused by opiates, with most other complications caused by IV drug use and hazardous lifestyles. The long-term mortality rate for heroin addicts may be 50 to 100 times that of the general population.[13] Aloofness, calmness, and mild sedation characterize opioid intoxication. A warm flush and sudden sensation of pleasure accompany injection, sometimes with mild nausea and vomiting. Individuals experience vague itching and characteristically scratch their nose. Opioid intoxication usually produces drowsiness and slowed movement but with less mental slowing than with sedative intoxication. Pupils constrict and respiratory rate and bowel motility decrease, effects that persist even if the individual has a high level of tolerance. Blood pressure and pulse are mildly decreased.

Stupor that progresses to coma, markedly slow and shallow respirations, and pulmonary edema characterize opioid overdose. Meperidine overdose and/or cerebral anoxia may produce dilated pupils; meperidine or propoxyphene overdose may produce seizures. Acute frothy pulmonary edema and eosinophilia are the prominent features of a hypersensitivity type of overdose. Naloxone, an intravenously administered pure opioid antagonist, reverses the stupor, usually precipitating an opioid abstinence syndrome. It is short acting, and the patient should be observed for at least 24 hours, especially if overdose with a long-acting opioid is suspected. A legion of other toxic, neurologic, and metabolic causes should be sought when a patient who is stuporous does not respond to naloxone.

A stereotypic abstinence syndrome develops as blood levels of opiates decline. The timing of this syndrome varies with the duration of the drug's effect; withdrawal from long-acting opiates begins later and lasts longer. Severity is proportional to the size and duration of the habit. The syndrome starts with overwhelming fatigue and is followed by restlessness, pupillary dilation, temperature intolerance, general aches and arthromyalgias, increased respiratory rate and yawning, runny eyes and nose, piloerection, sweating, and hyperactive bowels. Nausea, vomiting, and an elevated blood pressure and pulse may occur. Vital signs may reveal little about withdrawal severity, with respiratory rate being the most affected by opioid withdrawal. The most reliable physical signs are pupillary dilation and constantly hyperactive bowel sounds. The patient is unable to sleep despite the administration of sedatives. Objectively, the syndrome resembles an acute episode of influenza that is accompanied by parasympathetic hyperactivity and intense drug craving. The syndrome can precipitate premature labor but otherwise is not dangerous. Protracted, low-level symptoms may persist for months or years.

Pharmacologic treatment of abstinence is discussed in the section on management.

Central Nervous System Stimulants. CNS stimulants encompass a wide array of drugs that increase alertness, cause excitation, and sometimes cause euphoria. Stimulant drugs include cocaine, amphetamines, and methylphenidate, as well as several amphetamine-like psychotomimetic compounds. Use of stimulants in the United States appeared to have declined in recent years, until the recent surge in methamphetamine or amphetamine abuse. The ingredients needed for conversion of pseudoephedrine to methamphetamine are relatively easy to obtain, leading to an epidemic of methamphetamine abuse and complications in the United States.

Major stimulants are often used in combination with opioids or sedatives. Mild stimulant intoxication is manifest by increased alertness, hyperactivity, anorexia, elevated blood pressure, and pulse elevation. Intoxication is manifest by euphoric excitement, hyperstimulation, and grandiosity. Chronic stimulant users develop nervousness, irritability, insomnia, and often paranoia. Depression, hypersomnia, lethargy, poor concentration, and drug craving characterize stimulant withdrawal.

Cocaine hydrochloride has the properties of a CNS and peripheral nervous system stimulant and local anesthetic. The major methods of cocaine use involve sniffing, injecting, or vaporization (smoking "crack"). Cocaine enhances the effects of dopamine, serotonin, and norepinephrine by elevating synaptic levels. MRI changes have been noted with both cocaine administration and drug-free episodes of cocaine craving.[14]

Restlessness, agitation, paranoia, and panic characterize acute toxicity. Blood pressure and pulse increase, and pupils dilate. Overdose can produce cardiac arrhythmias, including ventricular fibrillation and seizures. Vasospasm can cause myocardial, cerebral, or hepatic infarction, even in users with normal arteries. This also contributes to the premature separation of membranes when used during pregnancy. Cocaine effects vary depending on the route of administration. The onset is within minutes when inhaled nasally and within seconds when injected or smoked. The duration of effect is brief. The withdrawal syndrome appears quickly, reinforcing frequent administration and the accumulation of metabolites. Alcohol and cocaine together form cocaethylene, a compound that appears to intensify cocaine's euphoric effects and possibly increases the risk for sudden death. The need for frequent multiple injections of cocaine probably increases the risk of acquiring HIV infection compared with other IV drugs of abuse. Prostitution often accompanies crack cocaine addiction, making cocaine smoking an independent risk factor for sexually transmitted disease. The prenatal effects of maternal cocaine use have not been as drastic as originally feared. Cocaine-exposed infants and young children display delayed motor development and impaired ability to regulate attention.[15]

Amphetamine and amphetamine-like stimulants have effects that are qualitatively similar to those of cocaine, but their effects are more prolonged. The two most commonly abused forms of these substances are methamphetamine, which is synthesized in home laboratories, and methylphenidate, which is diverted from pharmaceutical supplies. The methods of methamphetamine use involve the oral route, sniffing, smoking, and injection. Tolerance develops rapidly, and users become sensitized and seizure prone. Chronic heavy use causes a paranoid psychosis that is difficult to manage, and it may cause long-term degeneration of dopaminergic neurons. IV amphetamine use is associated with the development of vasculitis.[16] Inadvertent subcutaneous injections of methylphenidate produce deep purulent abscesses. Burns and inhalation are common hazards of home methamphetamine synthesis.

Adolescent use of 3,4-methylenedioxymethamphetamine (MDMA), also known as "ecstasy," has increased in recent years.[17] MDMA has a chemical structure similar to that of both amphetamines and mescaline and produces both stimulant and hallucinogenic effects. MDMA stimulates the release of serotonin, producing a feeling of empathy and closeness and an enhanced sense of pleasure, confidence, and endurance, with effects lasting several minutes to hours. Psychologic effects include confusion, depression, sleep problems, and anxiety that may persist for weeks. Physical effects include muscle tension, involuntary teeth clenching, blurred vision, faintness, elevated blood pressure and pulse, and altered control of body temperature. The drug, which allows users to dance for extended periods, is usually used in hot crowded nightclubs, increasing the risk for hyperthermia, dehydration, and heart or kidney failure. The drug appears to cause long-lasting serotonin neuron loss and memory damage.[17]

Stimulant users who have persistent depression may benefit from antidepressant therapy, but no medication has been demonstrated to effectively treat stimulant withdrawal or drug craving. Sedation is often necessary during acute toxicity, and medications are often needed for detoxification from a co-existing dependence on sedatives or opioids.

Psychotomimetics and Hallucinogens. Psychotomimetics and hallucinogens are an informal category of drugs that alter perceptions and/or mimic psychotic or dissociative states. Included in this category are cannabinoids, lysergic acid diethylamide (LSD) and similarly acting hallucinogens, and phencyclidine (PCP). As with stimulant drugs, no medication has been demonstrated to effectively treat hallucinogen withdrawal or drug craving. Sedation is often needed during episodes of acute toxicity.

Cannabinoids, in the form of marijuana, are the active ingredients in the leaves or resin of the *Cannabis sativa* hemp plant; they are either smoked or taken orally. Marijuana is the most commonly abused illicit substance. Intoxication produces a mildly dissociated and dreamy mental state, an elevated pulse, dilated pupils, an increased appetite, and a characteristic odor. In high doses it may produce hallucinations and, idiosyncratically, paranoia. Marijuana use is greatest in adolescence and young adulthood and possibly hinders emotional development and initiative. Heavy users appear to be prone to a mild abstinence syndrome that consists of nervousness, restlessness, and appetite and sleep disturbance.

PCP and the related compound ketamine are dissociative anesthetics whose action closely mimics schizophrenia. PCP is most commonly smoked but can be absorbed via any route. Toxicity is dose dependent, with individuals varying markedly in their responses. Mild toxicity induces giddiness, elation, expansiveness, and mild dissociative states. Highly toxic individuals display disorientation, a bizarre affect, rotary nystagmus, ataxia, tachycardia, and a dissociative lack of concern with pain or the external world. These individuals are prone to self-mutilation and are difficult to contain despite sedation. Deaths from overdose are caused by hypertensive crisis, respiratory arrest, and status epilepticus.

The true hallucinogenic drugs are ergots (LSD), phenylalkylamines (mescaline), indolealkylamines (psilocybin), and the amphetamine-like drug MDMA (ecstasy). As with cannabis, young people are the main users of hallucinogens. LSD is the prototype and appears to produce its action by serotonin inhibition and dopamine stimulation. It is highly potent, and its effects are noted with oral ingestions of tiny fractions of a gram.

Tolerance to hallucinogens develops rapidly, sometimes after a single dose. Giddiness, visual and other sensory distortions, marked dissociation, widely dilated pupils, and peripheral vasoconstriction characterize intoxication. Patients may develop acute panic or psychosis. The effects last 8 to 12 hours; some patients report recurrent manifestations months to years later.

Inhalants. The term *inhalant* describes an informal grouping of differing substances that are used by inhaling their vapors. Solvents (e.g., acetone, benzene, toluene), nitrous oxide gas, and volatile nitrites (e.g., amyl nitrite, butyl nitrite) are members of this group. Solvent inhalation produces a rapid onset of sedative-like intoxication, including dizziness, drowsiness, slurred speech, and ataxia. Chronic complications include cerebral atrophy, peripheral neuropathy, toxic hepatitis, and bone marrow toxicity, as well as the complications associated with lead poisoning and other impurities. Nitrous oxide is usually obtained from medical or laboratory supplies or from commercial aerosol sprays. It displaces CNS oxygen rapidly after inhalation, causing an acute euphoric state followed by a brief period of sedation; the major hazard is anoxia. The effect of the volatile nitrites is short-lived flushing, dizziness, euphoria, and hypotension. Chronic use can lead to methemoglobinemia, which is evidenced by cyanosis that does not respond to oxygen administration.

Anabolic Steroids. Anabolic steroids are synthetic derivatives of testosterone that are used to enhance athletic performance and build lean muscle mass. They are usually smuggled from outside the United States and sold surreptitiously in gymnasiums. Internet user groups have been a recent supply source. Injection is the most common route of use, which makes the user susceptible to the hazards of unsterile injections. Toxicity is characterized by aggression, irritability, impulsiveness, and elation. Users also have disturbed hormonal cycles, acne, hair loss, excessive muscle growth, testicular atrophy or clitoral hypertrophy, breast enlargement or atrophy, liver toxicity, and elevated low-density lipoprotein. A common pattern of use is "cycling," which involves taking these drugs for weeks and then stopping them for short periods. Lethargy, restlessness, insomnia, and anorexia often occur with abstinence.

Injection Drug Use. IDU violates the first line of defense of the body, leaving the user vulnerable to infection, chemical impurities, and immediate drug toxicity. This method of use is obviously a greater hazard when injection equipment is shared. The Centers for Disease Control and Prevention report that in 2005, 14% of HIV infections in adults were acquired by injecting drugs.[18] HIV-1 has been found to remain viable in used syringes for as long as 6 weeks.[19] Immunologic abnormalities include hypergammaglobulinemia, which may be related to repeated IV introduction of impurities or hepatitis C. Chronic rheumatologic conditions are a consequence, as sometimes are false-positive serologic tests for syphilis. Neurologic complications include brain abscesses from endocarditis, cerebral anoxia, and transverse myelitis. Lung granulomas and abscesses can result from particles and pathogens that filter through the pulmonary circulation. Endocarditis may result from bacteria and fungi that settle in the endocardium. In the United States, IDU is the major means of transmission for hepatitis viruses B and C and has been linked to serious outbreaks of hepatitis D. Most injection drug users have serologic evidence of remote hepatitis virus B exposure. Renal disease may be the result of immune complex deposition, endocarditis, or nephrotoxic impurities. Vertebral osteomyelitis from hematologic seeding of the cancellous bone is the most common serious musculoskeletal condition associated with IDU. Cellulitis, subcutaneous abscesses, and fascial abscesses are a common result of injection infiltration outside of the vein. Phlebitis is common, particularly when irritating drugs are injected.

Poor venous access complicates the care of these patients, particularly when the management of co-morbid conditions calls for frequent laboratory testing. This is a major disincentive for addicts to seek health care. Needle exchange and other "harm reduction" methods have been used with some success and much controversy to reduce the public and individual health hazards of IDU.

CLINICAL PRESENTATION AND PHYSICAL EXAMINATION

Patients may have no history of a recognized addictive disorder, may be actively addicted, may be in early recovery, or may have a history of addiction and be well established in recovery. As a screening tool, the *CAGE* questions regarding *C*oncern about drinking, being *A*nnoyed by others criticizing your drinking, feeling *G*uilt about drinking, and taking an "*E*ye-opener" drink in the morning can be adapted to include other drugs[20] (see Box 258-1). These questions can be woven into a standard history and should be asked if patients report drinking or drug use when asked about medications or lifestyle. Poor compliance and requests for disability testimony by an otherwise healthy patient should raise concerns about the presence of substance abuse. Behavioral problems appear first, and early manifestations of addiction are rarely apparent with routine examination. The time of the last substance use can be asked when reviewing medications, and the temporal relationship between substance use and symptoms should be considered.

Addiction-related causes of fever are endocarditis, acute retroviral syndrome–associated and HIV-associated infections, anticholinergic ingestion, and sedative withdrawal. Withdrawal from opioids will cause chills and sweats that are not accompanied by fever. A simultaneously elevated pulse and blood pressure often result from sedative withdrawal or stimulant toxicity. Weight may fluctuate because of an irregular diet, wasting infections, or chronic liver disease. Generalized edema may be due to liver failure from chronic hepatitis, kidney failure from glomerulopathies, or heart failure from valvular insufficiency or cardiomyopathy. Overwhelming lethargy and fatigue accompany withdrawal from stimulants and very early opioid withdrawal. Varying degrees of lethargy are seen with co-existing vegetative depressions, chronic hepatitis, and kidney failure. Headaches commonly accompany alcohol and cocaine withdrawal. Sudden headaches may be related to cocaine-induced venospasms. Many addicts have a history of head trauma or brain abscess; therefore it is helpful if cranial nerve deficits are noted in initial examinations. Visual changes may be caused by retinal emboli from IDU or from several complications of HIV infection. Sedatives may cause diplopia. The sclerae should be examined for icterus. Opioid withdrawal or cannabis, stimulant, or hallucinogen intoxications dilate the pupils, and the use of opioids causes pupils to constrict. Sedative and alcohol intoxication causes nystagmus. Rotary nystagmus is a unique feature of PCP intoxication. Nasal heroin or cocaine use causes mucosal inflammation. Perforation of the nasal septum is caused by mucosal vasoconstriction and subsequent tissue ischemia with cocaine use. Inhalation of hot crack vapors can cause flaming pharyngitis and tonsillar swelling. In addition to well-known HIV-related adenopathy, IV drug users often have swollen lymph nodes in response to local injections. The cervical spine is a possible focus of osteomyelitis.

Because of hypersensitivity, nasal heroin use causes a bronchitis that resembles severe asthma. The bronchitis tends to get worse with each subsequent exposure and is difficult to control with steroids and bronchodilators if the patient continues to inhale heroin. Cocaine may make the heart hyperdynamic through its adrenergic effects, or it may slow myocardial impulses through its anesthetic effects. Ischemic chest pain can result from vasospasm that damages the intima and predisposes the patient to subsequent coronary artery disease. A variety of cocaine-induced arrhythmias can cause sudden death. Patients with endocarditis are usually febrile, with a new or changed murmur, petechiae, and possible signs of metastatic infections. A wide pulse pressure may represent secondary aortic regurgitation. The strain of acute sedative withdrawal may precipitate a serious cardiac event in a patient with preexisting cardiac disease.

Evidence of ascites should be determined in a patient with increasing abdominal girth. Mild tenderness in the right upper quadrant may be the only clinical manifestation of chronic hepatitis. The visceral pain and hyperactive bowel sounds from opioid withdrawal can be severe enough to mimic an acute abdominal emergency. Bleeding in the stool may be from alcohol-induced gastritis, liver congestion, coagulopathies, or hemorrhoids from opioid-related constipation.

The usual life of a patient with addiction leaves little time and energy for concern regarding regular Papanicolaou's (Pap) tests and breast, testicular, rectal, and prostate examinations. In addition to neglecting these health maintenance examinations, addicts often exchange sex for drugs, adding to the concern about sexually transmitted diseases. Many addicts also have a history of sexual trauma and avoid genital examinations, which they can find frightening. The possibility of pregnancy is a consideration with all fertile female patients.

Vertebral tenderness raises the question of osteomyelitis or epidural abscess. Swollen and tender joints suggest septic arthritis from injected pathogens, gonorrhea, or syphilis. Arthromyalgias may be a prominent feature of opioid withdrawal. Arthromyalgias also commonly accompany polyarteritis syndromes, which are associated with IV amphetamine abuse and with hepatitis C. Localized muscle hypertrophy and calcification from repeated needle manipulation ("drug abuser's elbow") may be seen as a worrisome mass.

Developing relationships with patients over time is the most useful way for the health care provider to understand the neurologic and psychiatric conditions. Intoxication with alcohol or sedatives causes incoordination. Broad-based gaits are associated with alcohol-induced cerebellar degeneration. Intention tremors are the conspicuous physical sign of sedative withdrawal. Compression and trauma are the most common causes of mononeuropathy. Neuropathy of the ulnar or radial nerves sometimes follows prolonged periods of unconsciousness and results from compression of the nerves against the bony prominences. Peripheral manifestations of alcoholism or thiamine deficiency include proximally progressing decreased peripheral sensation and deep tendon reflexes. Symmetric hyperreflexia suggests stimulant drug toxicity or sedative withdrawal, whereas sedative toxicity causes reflexes to be sluggish. Seizure disorders are complicated by multiple drug use, head trauma, and past cerebral anoxia. Stimulant toxicity and withdrawal from sedatives or alcohol are the most common causes of drug-related convulsions. Substance abuse is the most common precipitant of psychiatric symptoms.

Edema of the hands without co-existing ankle or facial edema is usually a result of damaged veins. Needle marks from cocaine injection are usually multiple and recent, whereas those from heroin use are more deliberately tracked along large veins. Venous insufficiency and attendant complications are common, especially in older addicts. Injection of irritating substances causes chemical phlebitis with varying degrees of severity. Palmar erythema suggests chronic liver disease. Patients often have scars from cigarette burns or wrist cutting.

DIAGNOSTICS

The use of laboratory tests should be individualized and based on the clinical presentation. Toxicology testing is essential in evaluating many emergency situations. Drug screening may be useful in monitoring patients in treatment programs or receiving prescriptions for controlled substances, but it may give little information about addiction per se because screening tests reflect use during a fairly narrow period. Commercially prepared urine enzyme immune assays are the most commonly used drug screening tests, giving a positive or negative test for several classes but not all drugs of abuse. Drugs concentrate in the urine, making urine tests generally better for screening purposes than serum tests. Chromatography tests are necessary for specific serum levels of specific substances. Because psychiatric symptoms are so often caused or influenced by substance use, toxicology tests may be most useful in evaluating refractory psychiatric symptoms.

Anemia and thrombocytopenia are often a result of liver disease or HIV infection. Liver function abnormalities are often due to viral hepatitis or alcoholism. Hepatitis and syphilis serologic screening should be conducted at some point. Patients should be counseled and offered HIV testing in the office or given information about anonymous HIV test sites. Urine or blood human chorionic gonadotropin testing for pregnancy may be indicated and, if positive, may be helpful in guiding the pace, intensity, and nature of treatment plans. Baseline renal function tests are useful in detecting glomerulonephropathies associated with IV drug use. Baseline thyroid function tests are useful because sedatives and stimulants can mimic hypothyroidism or hyperthyroidism, respectively, whereas their abstinence syndromes cause the reverse effects. Patients usually need frequently neglected routine health maintenance screening tests such as Pap smears and lipid levels.

MANAGEMENT

Conveying a hopeful attitude is important. There is no way to predict when a single episodic encounter may be the time that the patient makes substantial progress. Because substance use disorders are often chronic conditions that progress slowly over time, health care providers address a patient's substance abuse problems, monitor progress, and provide regular supportive counseling. This provides the patient with a stable relationship during which reducing harm and keeping up with health maintenance can pay off in long-term benefits.

The primary care brief intervention format of (1) providing feedback of relevant data, (2) emphasizing patient responsibility and self-efficacy, (3) advising about recommended change, (4) providing a menu of helpful options, and (5) taking an empathetic approach is helpful whether or not the patient enters a formal treatment program. Patients should be counseled about risk-reduction strategies such as not sharing needles, using condoms, and not driving while using. The provider should be familiar with local treatment, consultation, and case management services and have a handy referral list.

Although several studies suggest that an inpatient detoxification is unlikely to affect the long-term course of addiction, it may be needed to stabilize the patient and facilitate entry into more long-term treatment. Other treatment often is impossible without detoxification first. Individual motivated patients sometimes significantly reduce drug use after a brief detoxification without other services.[21]

Common formal treatment programs include outpatient methadone maintenance, long-term residential treatment programs, outpatient drug-free programs, and short-term inpatient rehabilitation programs. Some patients find regular acupuncture to be an effective treatment for detoxification and craving. Most outpatient substance abuse counseling is based on cognitive behavior therapy or 12-step models (see Chapter 258). Patients in longer-term recovery often benefit from insight-oriented therapy. Intensive outpatient or partial hospitalization programs for less stable patients are designed to provide a daily therapeutic milieu while having the advantage of allowing patients to stay at home or even participating in the evening while working during the day. Long-term residential programs offer a drug-free therapeutic living environment that is staffed by counselors and usually other recovering addicts. The optimum duration of involvement in long-term residential treatment appears to be 6 months. These programs are especially helpful in supporting the recovery of addicts who are homeless and reintegrating them into society. Residential programs for these patients usually require a more lengthy stay. Adolescent programs should include strong peer and family components. The primary care provider may become a collaborative part of the treatment team and/or continue to treat the patient's medical conditions, encourage continuing participation in the program, and schedule follow-up visits after treatment termination to monitor progress and help prevent relapse.

How to judiciously prescribe controlled substances is one of the major difficulties providers face in caring for these patients. Drug-seeking patients may feign symptoms and request medications for longer than their medical conditions dictate. Medications that can be abused may reinitiate craving and addiction in patients who have achieved drug abstinence, whereas inadequately treated pain, depression, or anxiety may also be a trigger for relapse. Recognizing that symptom relief is a legitimate goal of care, the guidelines of the Drug Enforcement Agency (DEA) ask providers to consider the following when controlled substances are indicated: the severity of the patient's symptoms and ability to tolerate them, the patient's reliability in taking medications, and the addiction liability of the medication.[22] The DEA also recognizes that patients have a corresponding obligation to comply with the prescriber's instructions.[23]

Opiates, barbiturates, and stimulants are schedule II drugs and have the highest potential for abuse. In general, prescribing opiates to treat opiate withdrawal is restricted to methadone programs and acute medical situations such as hospital admission. Schedule III and IV medications are considered by the DEA to have a lower potential for abuse. Prescriptions of controlled substances should be written only for recognized indications and for limited amounts, and they are usually recommended for finite periods. The number of doses to be dispensed should be written out both in longhand and numerically to discourage alteration. Recent research suggests that the nonmedical use of opioids is a predictable parallel phenomenon of their prescriptive availability and that the potential for and extent of diversion are directly related to the relative potency of the drug and the amount prescribed. The goal is not to refrain from opioid use for patients when it is indicated or to treat fewer patients. Rather, the goal is to have less abuse and diversion while simultaneously providing therapy to patients.[24] This is one of the reasons why it is good practice to consult with addiction or pain specialists when prescribing controlled substances to patients with addiction or who might be at risk for addiction.

Antidepressant medications (usually selective serotonin reuptake inhibitors) may be useful for dysthymic states that persist after detoxification. The antidepressant trazodone is a useful adjunctive medication for persistent insomnia. It has a low potential for overdose and addiction, but its efficacy varies. When used to assist with sleep, trazodone is taken in a low dose approximately 30 to 40 minutes before going to bed.

Antagonist drugs are designed to block or change the effect of the addictive drug and thereby help people avoid falling back into a pattern of abuse or dependence after stopping a drug. Disulfiram (Antabuse) has been used for years to help people stay away from alcohol once they stop drinking it. Naloxone and naltrexone are narcotic antagonists that are sometimes used to treat people with opioid dependence.[25] These drugs attach to endorphin receptor sites throughout the brain and make it impossible for opioids to exert their usual effects. There is less incentive to continue to use drugs, since no high is experienced. Narcotic antagonists may also be useful in the treatment of cocaine dependence.[26] Although narcotic antagonists are effective, especially in emergencies (e.g., to rescue people from opioid overdoses), some clinicians believe they are too dangerous for regular treatment of opioid dependence. These drugs must be administered carefully because they have the potential to throw a person with an opioid addiction into serious withdrawal. Partial antagonists, which produce less severe withdrawal symptoms, have also been used.

Medical management of opioid dependence includes tapering doses of the long-acting opioid methadone, the α_2-adrenergic antihypertensive clonidine, or the mixed opioid agonist-antagonist drug buprenorphine. Clonidine attenuates some abstinence symptoms and, in combination with other medication for myalgias, abdominal cramps, and insomnia, can help patients withdraw from opioids. Once abstinence is established, patients can begin taking naltrexone, an antagonist that blocks the effect of opioids and assists some highly motivated addicts to maintain drug abstinence. Patients should be cautioned that naltrexone will block the effects of opioid analgesics, and liver function tests (LFTs) should be monitored.

A drug-related lifestyle may be as big of a problem as, or a bigger problem than, the direct effect of drug use. Methadone maintenance programs were developed in the 1960s to give heroin-addicted individuals a laboratory opioid, methadone, as a substitute for heroin. Although drugs users develop methadone addiction, this was considered to be a safe alternative to heroin addiction, since it could be maintained under supervision, it could be administered orally once daily, and it eliminated the dangers of IV needles. Although methadone programs seemed to be effective, they became less popular in the 1980s because of the dangers of methadone. In addition, many clinicians believe that substituting one addiction for another is not an acceptable alternative and that an additional drug problem sometimes complicates the initial one.[3] Methadone can also be harder to withdraw from than heroin, since the withdrawal symptoms last twice as long.[27] However, recently outpatient opioid maintenance programs (including methadone and buprenorphine, a newly developed substitute drug) have received new interest, partly because of new research and partly because of the rapid spread of HIV by IV drug users.[28] IV drug use is also an indirect cause of 60% of HIV cases in childhood, which has renewed interest in outpatient opioid treatment programs.[29] Although patients remain physiologically dependent, these programs have repeatedly demonstrated effectiveness in reducing illicit opioid use and the harm associated with opioid addiction.

Methadone detoxification may be prescribed only through specially licensed drug treatment programs or for patients who are acutely hospitalized for a co-existent medical condition. Methadone maintenance involves the administration of high oral doses of methadone to substitute for and to block the effect of illicit opioids. At this point, methadone maintenance is the treatment of choice for heroin addicts who are pregnant. Their neonates are born physically dependent but can be safely withdrawn in the nursery. Higher dosages (80 to 100 mg/day) appear to be more effective than lower dosages.[30] Remaining on methadone for 1 year or longer is associated with better overall outcomes in terms of alcohol use, illicit drug use, and criminal involvement.[31] Outpatient treatment programs are more effective when they are combined with education (including AIDS education), psychotherapy, family therapy, and employment counseling. The major hazards of opioid maintenance programs may be related to the harsh social milieu and lack of ancillary services in some programs.

Whereas methadone has been the primary pharmacotherapy for the treatment of opioid addiction in the United States, buprenorphine has been used for this purpose in France since 1996. Buprenorphine was approved for the treatment of opioid dependence by the U.S. Food and Drug Administration (FDA) in 2002 under schedule III, which is a less restrictive category than methadone. A sublingual formulation of buprenorphine and naloxone (Suboxone) is the latest medication approved for treatment of opioid addiction. Buprenorphine has combined opioid and antagonist properties, and naloxone is a pure opioid antagonist that is included to discourage IV abuse of the tablets.

Buprenorphine and naloxone are the first opioids available to physicians in the United States to prescribe in the office-based setting for opioid dependence.[32] In a recent comparative trial of buprenorphine and methadone, buprenorphine was found to have comparable efficacy. Based on objective measures of adverse effects and patient self-reports of side effects, buprenorphine appears to be safe and has a mild side effect profile. Based on research thus far, there is little evidence that buprenorphine is associated with elevated LFTs, either producing new liver function elevations or exacerbating previous abnormal values.[32]

The process of Suboxone treatment consists of three phases: (1) induction, (2) stabilization, and (3) maintenance. During induction buprenorphine is introduced and illicit use is discontinued or markedly reduced. Some patients may need to be induced with pure buprenorphine rather than buprenorphine-naloxone combination if the patients are dependent on long-acting opiates such as methadone. The stabilization phase begins after the patient is no longer experiencing withdrawal symptoms. During this period there is more frequent patient contact, monitoring, counseling, and usually dosage adjustments. After stabilization patients move into a long-term maintenance phase to participate in counseling and function without physiologic need for a fix. Major difficulties with buprenorphine and naloxone include subsequent pain management, management of overdose, treatment noncompliance, and drug diversion. Management of pain that requires opioids exceeding the buprenorphine ceiling effect may necessitate discontinuance of Suboxone.[33] Currently only physicians with special certification are permitted by the FDA to prescribe buprenorphine and naloxone

Several behavioral therapies, such as aversion therapy and teaching of alternative behaviors, have been used in the treatment of substance-related disorders. Aversion therapy is an approach based on classical conditioning, in which people are presented with an unpleasant stimulus at the moment they are taking a drug. Aversion therapy has been used more often with alcohol abuse and dependence than with other substance-related disorders. Two other behavioral approaches, alternative behaviors and contingency management, encourage people to substitute other behaviors (relaxation, meditation, biofeedback) when they feel the urge to drink or use other drugs, or patients are offered incentives for continued abstinence. Both these therapies are most effective when individuals are motivated to continue them.[3] With behavioral self-control training and relapse-prevention training, individuals keep track of their substance use and are taught to plan ahead of time regarding how they will handle certain situations. Both these approaches appear to be most effective for people who abuse alcohol and are not dependent on it, but they have been used with some success in the treatment of marijuana and cocaine abuse.[3,34]

Many patients with substance abuse disorders have been helped through the drug self-help movement, which dates back to 1935, when two Ohio men met to discuss alternative treatment possibilities. This first discussion led to others and eventually to the formation of Alcoholics Anonymous. Related self-help programs have developed for other substance-related disorders, including Narcotics Anonymous and Cocaine Anonymous, and for people who live and care for persons with substance abuse disorders, including Al-Anon and Alateen. Many self-help programs have expanded into residential treatment centers or therapeutic communities, where people with a history of substance abuse live, work, and socialize in a drug-free environment.[3]

COMPLICATIONS

Drug abuse has myriad complications, which affect patients and families socially, psychologically, legally, and physically. Every body system can be affected, placing the patient at risk for cardiac arrhythmias; infections; injuries; seizures; coma; and liver, heart, or kidney failure.

INDICATIONS FOR REFERRAL OR HOSPITALIZATION

Referral to an inpatient or outpatient addiction program should always be discussed with actively addicted patients. Referral to the emergency department should be considered for patients with unexplained fevers, delirium, overdose, severe sedative withdrawal, vital sign instability, severe headaches, chest pain, acute shortness of breath, acute abdominal pain and gastrointestinal bleeding, or active suicidality. These patients often need to be stabilized and considered for hospitalization. Hospitalized substance abusers are notoriously difficult patients who are often unwelcome and sometimes undertreated for discomfort. In addition to assisting with the medical aspects of care, the health care provider collaborates with the inpatient team to help humanize the patient and help the hospital staff recognize and work with problematic behaviors. Patients on methadone should be kept on their usual dosage and receive normal or slightly higher doses of pain medication as indicated by their medical conditions.

Medical clearance is often requested of the health care provider before a patient is admitted to a detoxification or rehabilitation program. A brief history and physical examination are necessary to identify and stabilize acute health problems. It is helpful to know what resources are available at the program, since it may or may not have medical support or medication on site. It should be clear, to both the patient and the program, that "medically clear" does not mean the patient does not have outstanding health problems that need future attention; it is simply an assessment that the patient is stable enough to enter a program.

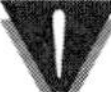

Emergency department consultation should be considered for patients with unexplained fevers, delirium, overdose, severe sedative withdrawal, vital sign instability, severe headaches, chest pain, acute shortness of breath, acute abdominal pain and gastrointestinal bleeding, or active suicidality.

PATIENT AND FAMILY EDUCATION

Both patients and families need to understand that resources are available to help with addiction. As with the patient, it is important to convey a feeling of hopefulness to significant others. The importance of recognizing symptoms of infections and other complications, plus the need to seek treatment when necessary, should be emphasized. The disease, treatment, nutritional counseling, and side effects of prescribed medications should be carefully explained. In many cases patients are not amenable to formal treatment, abstinence, detoxification, or maintenance. Counseling regarding harm-reduction strategies usually focuses on IDU hazards, but can also include seizures, violence, crime, and unintentional injury avoidance. Frequent follow-up is important both to promote health and to help patients and families cope with the devastating effects of substance abuse.

The following are sources of information for patients with substance abuse problems:

Substance Abuse and Mental Health Services Administration (SAMHSA)
1 Choke Cherry Road
Rockville, MD 20857
(240) 276-2000
http://www.samhsa.gov

National Directory of Drug and Alcohol Abuse Treatment Programs, 2006, available from SAMHSA, (800) 729-6686; https://ncadistore.samhsa.gov/whatsnew

Treatment improvement protocols (TIPs), a service of SAMHSA's Center for Substance Abuse Treatment, available through the National Clearinghouse for Alcohol and Drug Information, (800) 729-6686; https://ncadistore.samhsa.gov/whatsnew

SAMHSA Substance Abuse Treatment Facility Locator, http://findtreatment.samhsa.gov/

Hazelden
CO3, PO Box 11
Center City, MN 55012-0011
(800) 257-7810
http://www.hazelden.org

REFERENCES

1. Garnick DW, Hendricks AM, Comstock C, and others: Do individuals with substance abuse diagnoses incur higher charges than individuals with other chronic conditions? *J Subst Abuse Treat* 14(5):457-465, 1997.
2. American Psychiatric Association: *Diagnostic and statistical manual of mental disorders,* ed 4 (text rev), Washington, DC, 2000, The Association.
3. Comer R: *Abnormal psychology*, New York, 2004, Worth.
4. Substance Abuse and Mental Health Services Administration: *Results from the 2002 National Survey on Drug Use and Health: National Findings, Office of Applied Studies*, NHSDA Series H-22, DHHS Pub No SMA 03-3836, Rockville, Md, 2003, The Administration.
5. Johnston LD, O'Malley PM, Bachman JG, and others: *Monitoring the future national survey results on drug use*, 1975-2004, vol II, *College students and adults ages 19-45,* NIH Pub No 05-5728, Bethesda, Md, 2005, National Institute on Drug Abuse.
6. Volkow N: Confronting the rise in abuse of prescription drugs, *NIDA Notes* 19(5):3, 2005.
7. Hyman SE: Why does the brain prefer opium to broccoli? *Harvard Rev Psychiatry* 2:43-46, 1994.
8. Wesson DR, Center for Substance Abuse Treatment: *Detoxification from alcohol and other drugs,* DHHS Pub No (SMA) 95-3046, Treatment Improvement Protocol (TIP) Series, No 19, Rockville, Md, 1995, US Department of Health and Human Services.
9. National Institute of Drug Abuse: Conference highlights increasing GHB abuse, *NIDA Notes* 16(2), 2001, retrieved March 1, 2007, from http://www.nida.nih.gov/NIDA_notes/NNvol16N2/Conference.html.
10. Strang J, Griffiths P, Powis B, and others: How constant is an individual's route of heroin administration? Data from treatment and non-treatment samples, *Drug Alcohol Depend* 46(1-2):115-118, 1997.
11. Cicero TJ, Adams EH, Geller A, and others: A postmarketing surveillance program to monitor Ultram (tramadol hydrochloride) abuse in the United States, *Drug Alcohol Depend* 57(1):7-22, 1999.
12. US Department of Justice: *Drugs and chemicals of concern: oxycodone,* Washington, DC, Aug 2001, The Department, retrieved Aug 12, 2002, from http://www.deadiversion.usdoj.gov/drugs_concern/oxycodone/summary.htm.
13. Hser YI, Hoffman V, Grella CE, and others: A 33-year follow-up of narcotic addicts, *Arch Gen Psychiatry* 58(5):503-508, 2001.
14. Breiter HC, Gollub RL, Weisskoff RM, and others: Acute effects of cocaine on human brain activity and emotion, *Neuron* 19(3):591-611, 1997.
15. Smeriglio VL, Wilcox HC: Prenatal drug exposure and child outcome, *Clin Perinatol* 26:1-16, 1999.
16. Younger DS: Vasculitis of the nervous system, *Curr Opin Neurol* 17(3):317-336, 2004.
17. Bolla KI, McCann UD, Ricaurte GA: Memory impairment in abstinent MDMA ("ecstasy") users, *Neurology* 51:1532-1537, 1998.
18. Centers for Disease Control and Prevention: *HIV/AIDS surveillance report 2005,* retrieved March 14, 2007, from http://www.cdc.gov/hiv/topics/surveillance/resources/reports/2005report/pdf/2005Surveillance Report.pdf.

19. Heimer R, Abdal N: Viability of HIV-1 in syringes: implications for interventions among injection drug users, *AIDS Reader* 10:410-417, 2000.
20. Ewing J: Detecting alcoholism: the CAGE questionnaire, *JAMA* 252:1905-1907, 1984.
21. Chutuape MA, and others: Detoxification beneficial as a stand-alone treatment, *DATA* 20:1-6, 2001.
22. Joranson DE, Carrow GM, Ryan KM, and others: Pain management and prescription monitoring, *J Pain Symptom Manage* 23(3):231-238, 2002.
23. Severinghaus J, Kinney J: Medical management. In Kinney J, editor: *Clinical manual of substance abuse,* ed 2, St Louis, 1996, Mosby.
24. Dasgupta N, Kramer E, Zalman M, and others: Association between non-medical and prescriptive usage of opioids, *Drug Alcohol Depend* 82:135-142, 2006.
25. Kirchmayer U, Davoli M, Verster A, and others: A systematic review on the efficacy of naltrexone maintenance treatment in opioid dependence, *Addiction* 97(10):1241-1249, 2002.
26. O'Brien C, McKay J: Pharmacological treatments for substance abuse disorders. In Nathan P, Gorman J, editors: *A guide to treatments that work,* ed 2, London, 2002, Oxford University Press.
27. Backmund M, Meyer K, Eichenlaub D, and others: Predictors for completing an inpatient detoxification program among intravenous heroin users, methadone substituted and codeine substituted patients, *Drug Alcohol Depend* 64(2):173-180, 2001.
28. Gossup M, Marsden J, Steward D, and others: Outcomes after methadone maintenance and methadone reduction treatments: 2 year follow-up results from the National Treatment Outcome Research Study, *Drug Alcohol Depend* 62(3):255-264, 2001.
29. Brown L: Enrollment of drug abusers in HIV clinical trials: a public health imperative for communities of color, *J Psycho Drugs* 25(1):45-48, 1993.
30. Strain EC, Bigelow GE, Liebson IA, and others: Moderate vs high-dose methadone in the treatment of opioid dependence: a randomized control trial, *JAMA* 281(11):1000-1005, 1999.
31. Simpson DD, Joe GW, Rowan-Szal GA: Drug abuse treatment retention and process effects on follow-up outcomes, *Drug Alcohol Depend* 47(3):227-235, 1997.
32. Lofwall M, Stitzer M, Bigelow G, and others: Comparative safety and side effect profiles of buprenorphine and methadone in the outpatient treatment of opioid dependence, *Addictive Dis Treat* 4(2):49-64, 2005.
33. McNicholas L, SAMHSA Center for Substance Abuse Treatment: *Clinical guidelines for the use of buprenorphine in the treatment of opioid addiction,* DHHS Pub No (SMA) 04-3939, Treatment Improvement Protocol (TIP) Series, No 40, Rockville, Md, 2004, US Department of Health and Human Services.
34. Foxhall K: Preventing relapse: looking at data differently led to today's influential relapse prevention therapy, *APA Monitor* 32(6):46-47, 2001.

INDEX

Page numbers followed by *f* indicate figures; *t*, tables; *b*, boxes